Please send me the following Facts and Comparisons publications:

- ☐ Drug Facts and Comparisons
  - ☐ Loose-leaf edition @ $165.00 (includes book and 11 monthly updates)
  - ☐ Microfiche format @ $165.00 (includes 11 monthly updates)
  - ☐ Annual hardbound edition @ $95.50
- ☐ Patient Drug Facts @ $65.95 (includes book and 3 quarterly updates)
- ☐ Drug Interaction Facts @ $82.50 (includes book and 3 quarterly updates)
- ☐ Drug Newsletter @ $54.00 (for 12 monthly issues)
- ☐ Pharmacy Law Digest @ $65.50
- ☐ 1993 American Drug Index @ $37.95

Method of Payment

☐ Payment enclosed.* Make check payable to Facts and Comparisons.

☐ Bill me (plus handling).

☐ Charge to my credit card number:

☐ MasterCard ☐ VISA ☐ American Express

Card # ____________________

Exp. date ____________________

Signature ____________________

Name ____________________

Company ____________________

Address ____________________

City, State, Zip ____________________

Profession ____________________ P.O.# ____________

* Please include sales tax where applicable. Prices quoted in US funds and subject to change.

BI 93

To order other Facts and Comparisons Publications, mail this handy return card to us today. For even faster service – call toll free, **800/223-0554** now.

facts and comparisons

111 West Port Plaza • Suite 423 • St. Louis, Missouri 63146-3098

Please send me the following Facts and Comparisons publications:

- ☐ Drug Facts and Comparisons
  - ☐ Loose-leaf edition @ $165.00 (includes book and 11 monthly updates)
  - ☐ Microfiche format @ $165.00 (includes 11 monthly updates)
  - ☐ Annual hardbound edition @ $95.50
- ☐ Patient Drug Facts @ $65.95 (includes book and 3 quarterly updates)
- ☐ Drug Interaction Facts @ $82.50 (includes book and 3 quarterly updates)
- ☐ Drug Newsletter @ $54.00 (for 12 monthly issues)
- ☐ Pharmacy Law Digest @ $65.50
- ☐ 1993 American Drug Index @ $37.95

Method of Payment

☐ Payment enclosed.* Make check payable to Facts and Comparisons.

☐ Bill me (plus handling).

☐ Charge to my credit card number:

☐ MasterCard ☐ VISA ☐ American Express

Card # ____________________

Exp. date ____________________

Signature ____________________

Name ____________________

Company ____________________

Address ____________________

City, State, Zip ____________________

Profession ____________________ P.O.# ____________

* Please include sales tax where applicable. Prices quoted in US funds and subject to change.

BI 93

NO POSTAGE
NECESSARY
IF MAILED
IN THE
UNITED STATES

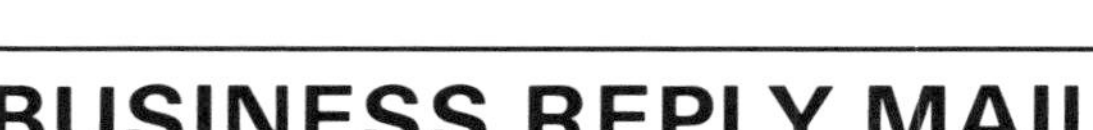

BUSINESS REPLY MAIL
FIRST CLASS MAIL PERMIT NO. 3515 ST. LOUIS, MO

POSTAGE WILL BE PAID BY ADDRESSEE

Facts and Comparisons
111 West Port Plaza, Suite 423
St. Louis, MO 63146-9811

NO POSTAGE
NECESSARY
IF MAILED
IN THE
UNITED STATES

BUSINESS REPLY MAIL
FIRST CLASS MAIL PERMIT NO. 3515 ST. LOUIS, MO

POSTAGE WILL BE PAID BY ADDRESSEE

Facts and Comparisons
111 West Port Plaza, Suite 423
St. Louis, MO 63146-9811

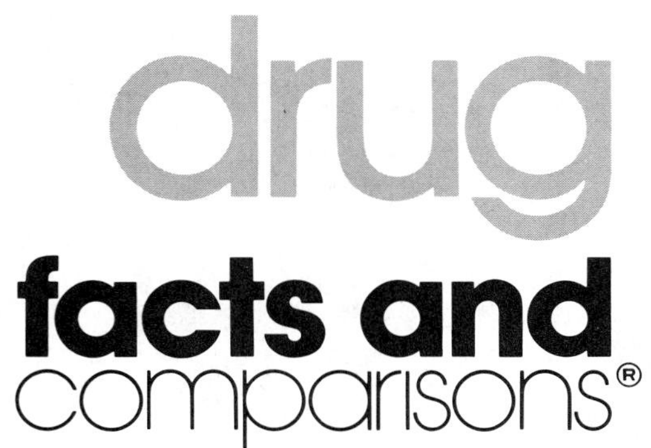

1993 edition

drug facts and comparisons®

1993 edition

Facts and Comparisons
St. Louis
A **Wolters Kluwer** Company

Drug Facts and Comparisons,® 1993 Edition

ISBN 0-932686-93-1
ISSN 0277-9714

Printed in the United States of America

The information contained in this publication is intended to supplement the knowledge of health care professionals regarding drug information. This information is advisory only and is not intended to replace sound clinical judgment or individualized patient care in the delivery of health care services. Facts and Comparisons disclaims all warranties, whether expressed or implied, including any warranty as to the quality, accuracy or suitability of this information for any particular purpose.

Published by
Facts and Comparisons
111 West Port Plaza, Suite 423
St. Louis, Missouri 63146-3098
314/878-2515
Toll free Customer Service 1-800-223-0554

Facts and Comparisons Staff:

C. Sue Sewester
publisher

Bernie R. Olin, PharmD
editor-in-chief

Steven K. Hebel, BS Pharm
associate editor

Charles E. Dombek, BS Pharm, MA, MIM
assistant editor

Erwin K. Kastrup, BS Pharm, DSc
founding editor

Facts and Comparisons Editorial Advisory Panel:

Dennis J. Cada, PharmD
Executive Editor, The Formulary
Director of Pharmacy
South Coast Medical Center

Timothy R. Covington, PharmD, MS
Anthony and Marianne Bruno Professor of Pharmacy
School of Pharmacy, Samford University

Daniel A. Hussar, PhD
Remington Professor of Pharmacy
Philadelphia College of Pharmacy and Science

Louis Lasagna, MD
Dean, Sackler School of Graduate Biomedical Sciences
Academic Dean, School of Medicine
Tufts University

James R. Selevan, BSEE, MD
Executive Director, The Formulary
Chairman, Pharmacy and Therapeutics Committee
South Coast Medical Center

David S. Tatro, PharmD
Drug Information Consultant
Assistant Clinical Professor
College of Pharmacy
University of California, San Francisco

Thomas L. Whitsett, MD
Professor of Medicine and Pharmacology
Director of Clinical Pharmacology Program
University of Oklahoma Health Sciences Center

Contributing Review Panel:

Jonathan Abrams, MD
Professor of Medicine
University of New Mexico
Albuquerque, New Mexico

Ezra A. Amsterdam, MD, FACC
Professor, Internal Medicine
Director, Cardiac Care Unit
University of California at Davis and Sacramento
School of Medicine and Medical Center

Danial E. Baker, PharmD
Associate Professor of Pharmacy Practice
Director, Drug Information Center
Washington State University College of Pharmacy
Spokane, Washington

Jimmy D. Bartlett, OD, DOS
Associate Professor of Optometry
Department of Optometry
School of Optometry
University of Alabama at Birmingham

Dale Berg, MD
Instructor of Medicine
Medical College of Wisconsin
Milwaukee, Wisconsin

R. Keith Campbell, RPh, FAPP
Associate Dean/Professor of Pharmacy
Washington State University
College of Pharmacy
Pullman, Washington

Melvin D. Cheitlin, MD
Professor of Medicine
University of California, San Francisco, Cardiology Division
Associate Chief, Cardiology Division
San Francisco General Hospital
San Francisco, California

Stephen L. Dahl, PharmD
University of Missouri – Kansas City
School of Medicine
Kansas City, Missouri

N. Rex Ghormley, OD, FAAO
Contact Lens Consultants, President
St. Louis, MO
Adjunct Assistant Professor
School of Optometry
University of Missouri – St. Louis

Ellen L. Hamburg, PharmD
Adjunct Assistant Professor of Pharmacy
College of Pharmacy
University of New Mexico
Albuquerque, New Mexico

Siret D. Jaanus, PhD
Professor of Pharmacology
Southern California College of Optometry
Fullerton, California

Susan O'Donoghue, MD
Associate Director, Cardiac Arrhythmia Center
Washington Hospital Center
Washington, DC

Edward V. Platia, MD
Director, Cardiac Arrhythmia Center
Washington Hospital Center
Professor of Medicine
George Washington University, School of Medicine

Michael T. Reed, PharmD
Associate Professor of Pharmacy
College of Pharmacy
University of New Mexico
Albuquerque, New Mexico

J. James Rowsey, MD
Director of Corneal Services
Department of Ophthalmology
Dean A. McGee Eye Institute
University of Oklahoma

Udho Thadani, MD, FACC
Professor of Medicine
Vice Chief of Cardiology and Director of Clinical Research
University of Oklahoma Health Sciences Center
Oklahoma City, Oklahoma

Thom J. Zimmerman, MD, PhD
Chairman of Department of Ophthalmology and Visual Sciences
Professor of Pharmacology & Toxicology
University of Louisville

Preface

Facts and Comparisons® provides a broad range of drug information to fulfill the everyday needs of practicing health-care professionals. Developed in 1945 by pharmacist Erwin K. Kastrup, *Facts and Comparisons* was designed to provide objective information in a format to facilitate comparisons of drug products. Although the basic concepts remain the same, the content of *Facts* continues to evolve to reflect the changing information needs of health-care professionals.

Facts and Comparisons, a loose-leaf text, is kept up-to-date through the issue of monthly updates. In 1977, the Microfiche Edition was introduced to provide the same monthly updated information in a microfilm format. The Annual Bound Edition of *Facts and Comparisons* was first published in 1978. In 1982, the title became *Drug Facts and Comparisons,* which better describes the nature of the reference.

The introduction of new drugs and products emphasizes the need for current information. In the past year, much of the text has been significantly revised. Hundreds of new drug products, dosage forms and formula changes are included. This edition incorporates 27 new drugs: Aldesleukin *(Proleukin),* azithromycin *(Zithromax),* cefprozil *(Cefzil),* clarithromycin *(Biaxin),* didanosine *(Videx),* enoxacin *(Penetrex),* felodipine *(Plendil),* finasteride *(Proscar),* flumazenil *(Mazicon),* foscarnet *(Foscavir),* histrelin *(Supprelin),* isosorbide mononitrate *(Ismo),* lomefloxacin *(Maxaquin),* loracarbef *(Lorabid),* mivacurium *(Mivacron),* nabumetone *(Relafen),* oxandrolone *(Oxandrin),* pamidronate *(Aredia),* pentostatin *(Nipent),* pravastatin *(Pravachol),* quinapril *(Accupril),* sermorelin *(Geref),* sertraline *(Zoloft),* simvastatin *(Zocor),* teniposide *(Vumon),* ticlopidine *(Ticlid)* and zalcitabine *(Hivid).*

Significant new dosage forms added include: Butorphanol, nasal *(Stadol NS),* carteolol, ophthalmic *(Ocupress),* diltiazem, IV *(Cardizem IV),* glyburide, micronized *(Glynase),* ketorolac, oral *(Toradol),* liothyronine, IV *(Triostat),* nicardipine, IV and sustained release *(Cardene IV, Cardene SR),* nicotine, transdermal *(Habitrol, Nicoderm, Nicotrol, ProStep)* and triamcinolone acetonide, nasal *(Nasacort).*

Sections that have undergone major revisions include: Antiarrhythmic Agents, Anticoagulants, Anticonvulsants, Biphosphonates, Digestive Enzymes, Fluoroquinolone Antibiotics, HMG-CoA Reductase Inhibitors, Influenza Virus Vaccines, Iron Salts, IV Nutritionals, Macrolide Antibiotics, NSAIDs, Ophthalmic Beta Blockers, Smoking Deterrents, Sulfonylureas, Sympathomimetic Bronchodilators and Topical Agents. Also, more than 135 tables and diagrams have been added or extensively revised.

New investigational drugs in this edition include: AIDS drugs update, amlodipine, bisoprolol, gepirone, paroxetine, remoxipride, taxol and teicoplanin.

As this edition goes to press, we begin the process of revision for the 1994 edition. As always, *Facts and Comparisons* remains dedicated to fulfilling the drug information needs of health-care professionals. Comments, criticisms and suggestions are always welcome.

B.R.O.

Table of Contents

Note: A detailed table of contents appears on the first page of each chapter.

Introduction

Drug Facts and Comparisons is a comprehensive drug information compendium. Organized by therapeutic drug classes, the unique format is designed to provide a wide scope of drug information in a manner which facilitates comparisons among drugs. A comprehensive index, a detailed table of contents for each chapter and extensive cross referencing enable the reader to quickly locate needed information. All readers are urged to review the following information to assure efficient and effective use of *Drug Facts and Comparisons.*

Editorial Policy:

The principle editorial guidelines are: Accurate, unbiased information; concise, standardized presentation; comparative, objective format; timely delivery. Review of FDA-approved product labeling, thousands of biomedical journal articles and textbooks, and policies and recommendations from many authoritative and official groups (eg, Centers for Disease Control, National Academy of Sciences, Joint National Committee on Detection, Evaluation, and Treatment of High Blood Pressure, National Heart, Lung and Blood Institute, American Thoracic Society, National Cancer Institute, National Information Center for Orphan Drugs and Rare Diseases, Food and Drug Administration) form the base of evaluation of information for *Drug Facts and Comparisons*.

Editorial policy is guided by the distinguished Facts and Comparisons Editorial Advisory Panel. This is an authoritative group of nationally and internationally recognized clinicians, scientists, physicians, pharmacists and pharmacologists. Pages are reviewed by these panel members and in addition, many other prominent health-care professionals provide review in their specific areas of expertise for *Drug Facts and Comparisons*. Indications and dosage recommendations are FDA-approved unless otherwise specified. Legitimate "unlabeled" uses and dosages are included when appropriate and given special emphasis. Input from a special panel of drug interaction experts is also a feature.

This collection of wisdom is then molded and refined into the *Drug Facts and Comparisons* monographs and product listings. Many sources of information are constantly monitored so that *Drug Facts and Comparisons* contains the most comprehensive, current drug product data base available. There is not a more complete text available presenting such clinical prescribing and drug product information.

Most of the products listed are protected by letters of patent, and their names are trademarked and registered by the firm whose name appears with the product. The product distributor is given in parentheses next to the brand name who may or may not be the actual manufacturer or fabricator of the final dosage form. When more than one company distributes a generic product, the generic product name is listed, followed by "Various, eg," in parentheses with a selected list of distributors. Listing of specific products is an indication only of market availability, and is not an endorsement or recommendation.

Products that contain the same active ingredients are listed together for comparison and as an aid in product selection. However, drug product interchange is regulated by state laws; listing of products together does not imply that products are therapeutically equivalent or legally interchangeable. Caution is particularly advised when attempting to compare extended release or delayed release dosage forms.

Organization:

Information in *Drug Facts and Comparisons* is organized by therapeutic use. Each of the twelve chapters is divided into groups and subgroups to facilitate comparisons of drugs and drug products with similar uses. The first page of each chapter provides a detailed outline, including page references, of the information presented in that chapter.

Products most similar in content or use are listed together. This format of presenting the FACTS makes it easy to make COMPARISONS of identical, similar or related products. Because drugs are listed by use, some drugs with multiple uses may be listed in more than one section of the book.

Index:

The alphabetical index includes page references for all drugs by their generic name, brand name, synonyms, common abbreviations, and therapeutic group names. Drug products recently withdrawn from the market that are listed in the book for reference purposes are included in the index with the designation (W). A separate index is included with the COLOR LOCATOR.

Drug Monographs:

Prescribing information is presented in comprehensive drug monographs. General information on a group of closely related drugs (eg, Thiazide Diuretics) may be presented in a group monograph. Specific information relating to a particular drug is presented in an individual monograph under the generic name of the drug. All monographs are divided into sections identified with bold titles for ease in locating the desired information.

Actions: This section gives a brief summary of the known pharmacologic and pharmacokinetic properties.

Indications: All indications or uses listed are FDA approved unless specifically designated as *"Unlabeled Uses"*.

Contraindications: This section specifies those conditions in which the drug should NOT be used.

Warnings and Precautions: These sections list conditions in which use of the drug may be hazardous, precautions to observe and parameters to monitor during therapy.

Drug Interactions: A brief summary of documented, clinically significant drug-drug, drug-food and drug-lab test interactions is provided.

Adverse Reactions: Reported adverse reactions are presented. Incidence data on adverse effects are included when available.

Overdosage: The clinical manifestations of toxicity and treatment of overdosage are given for most agents.

Patient Information: Essential information required by the patient for safe and effective self-administration of the medication is included.

Administration and Dosage: Dosage ranges and methods of administration are presented.

Product Listings:

Individual products are listed following each monograph. The format and components of the product listings are discussed below and illustrated on the opposite page.

1. Cross references to the appropriate drug monograph(s) for complete prescribing information appear at the top of the page.

2. Products are grouped by dosage form or strength.

3. Identical brand name products are listed in alphabetical order.

4. The name of the distributor is given in parentheses next to the product name.

5. Products available by their generic name from multiple sources are indicated as available from (Various) distributors and in selected cases, specific generic manufacturers are listed.

6. Package sizes are given for all dosage forms and strengths of each product.

7. Product identification imprint codes are indicated by the symbol #.

8. Distribution status of products is indicated as *Rx* or *otc*.

9. Controlled substances are designated by their schedule (*c-II, c-III, c-IV*, or *c-V*).

10. Sugar free liquid preparations are designated by *sf*.

11. Combination products are listed in tables to facilitate comparisons. Products most similar in formulation are listed next to each other.

12. Products with identical formulations are listed together.

13. The Cost Index, located on the right side of the product listings, is designed to give an indication of the relative cost of similar or identical products. It's simply a ratio of the average wholesale prices for equivalent quantities of a drug. The Cost Indices for dosage forms of different strengths are adjusted to accurately compare equivalent amounts of products. The basis for the Cost Index calculation is given at the bottom of each table of product listings.

    As an example of the Cost Index, if product A has a Cost Index of 45, and product B has a Cost Index of 15, product A is 3 times as expensive as product B (based on average wholesale cost).

    The Cost Index is only an indication of *relative wholesale costs.* The Cost Index is NOT a rating or recommendation. It is based only on average wholesale price and is presented for informational purposes only, without consideration of potential differences in the quality of similar products.

342f **TETRACYCLINES (Cont.)**

1 Complete prescribing information for these products begins on page 341.

OXYTETRACYCLINE

Administration and Dosage:

Oral: See Tetracycline HCl.

Parenteral:

Adults – The usual daily dose is 250 mg administered once every 24 hours or 300 mg given in divided doses at 8 to 12 hour intervals.

Children (over 8 years of age) – 15 to 25 mg/kg, up to a maximum of 250 mg per single daily injection. Dosage may be divided and given at 8 to 12 hour intervals. **C.I.*** 13

		Product	Form	Packaging	C.I.*
	Rx	**Oxytetracycline HCl** (Various, eg, Balan, Bioline, Dixon-Shane, Geneva, Goldline, Major, Moore, Parmed, Rugby, Schein) 5	**Capsules:** 2 250 mg (as HCl)	In 100s and 1000s.	6+
	Rx	**E.P. Mycin** (Edwards)		6 In 100s.	30
	Rx	**Terramycin** (Pfizer)		7 (#Terramycin Pfizer 073). Yellow. In 100s and 500s.	100
	Rx	**Uri-Tet** (American Urologicals) 4		In 100s.	51
8	*Rx*	**Terramycin IM** (Various, eg, Roerig, Texas Drug)	**Injection:** 50 mg per ml with 2% lidocaine	In 2 ml amps and 10 ml vials.	904
	Rx	**Terramycin IM** (Roerig)	**Injection:** 125 mg per ml with 2% lidocaine	In 2 ml amps.	1294

* Cost Index based on cost per 500 mg oxytetracycline oral or IM.

\# Product identification code.

COUGH PREPARATIONS (Cont.)

Refer to the general discussion of these products beginning on page 199.

Content given per 5 ml.

Antitussive Combinations, Liquids (Con

		Product & Distributor	Decongestant	Antihistamine	Antitussive	
10	*otc sf*	**Colrex Cough Syrup** (Reid-Rowell)	5 mg phenylephrine HCl	2 mg chlorphenir-amine maleate	10 mg dextromethor-phan HBr	4.5
11	*otc sf*	**Codimal DM Syrup** (Central)	5 mg phenylephrine HCl	8.33 mg pyrilamine maleate	10 mg dextromethor-phan HBr	4% Sa
3	*otc*	**Myminicol Liquid** (My-K Labs)	12.5 mg phenylpro-panolamine HCl	2 mg chlorphenir-amine maleate	10 mg dextromethor-phan HBr	
	otc	**Pertussin AM Liquid** (Canaan Labs)				9.5 So
	otc	**Threamine DM Syrup** (Various)				
12	*otc*	**Triaminicol Multi-Symptom Cold Syrup** (Sandoz)				
	otc	**Tricodene Forte Liquid** (Pfeiffer)				
	otc	**Triminol Cough Syrup** (Rugby)				
	otc sf	**Trind DM Liquid** (Mead Johnson Nutritional)	12.5 mg phenylpro-panolamine HCl	2 mg chlorphenir-amine maleate	7.5 mg dextromethor-phan HBr	5% So
	otc	**Cheracol Plus Liquid** (Upjohn)	8.3 mg phenylpro-panolamine HCl	1.3 mg chlorphenir-amine maleate	6.7 mg dextromethor-phan HBr	8% So
	otc	**Halls Mentho-Lyptus Decongestant Liquid** (Warner-Lambert)	18.75 mg phenylpro-panolamine HCl		7.5 mg dextromethor-phan HBr	7 m 6.3 22%
9	*c-v*	**Tricodene Syrup** (Pfeiffer)		4.17 mg pyrilamine maleate	8.1 mg codeine phosphate	Te m

* Cost Index based on cost per 5 ml. *sf* – Sugar free.

(Continued on following page)

Color Locator

The Color Locator is an aid in identifying tablets and capsules by their appearance. The products pictured include commonly used prescription drug products. Because of the similarity in size, shape and color of products with significantly different ingredients, product identification should be confirmed by identifying imprints.

Organization

Products are arranged by dosage form, color, size and shape. Every effort has been made to accurately reproduce the color of each product. However, variations will occur and exact reproductions are sometimes not possible. See the Table of Contents below for dosage form arrangement. The index begins on page CL-41.

Contents

Each product pictured is identified with the product trade name, strength and manufacturer. For products with a product identification code imprint, the ID Code is included following the manufacturer's name. Products are also indicated as prescription (℞) or controlled substance (C-II, C-III, C-IV or C-V).

Slight variations of color and ID code may occur. Drug manufacturers are expanding the use of product imprints to identify products by name or ID code. During this transition, various lots of the same product may have differing imprints. The ID code following the manufacturer name may not appear on all products pictured.

Table of Contents

Light Yellow Tablets

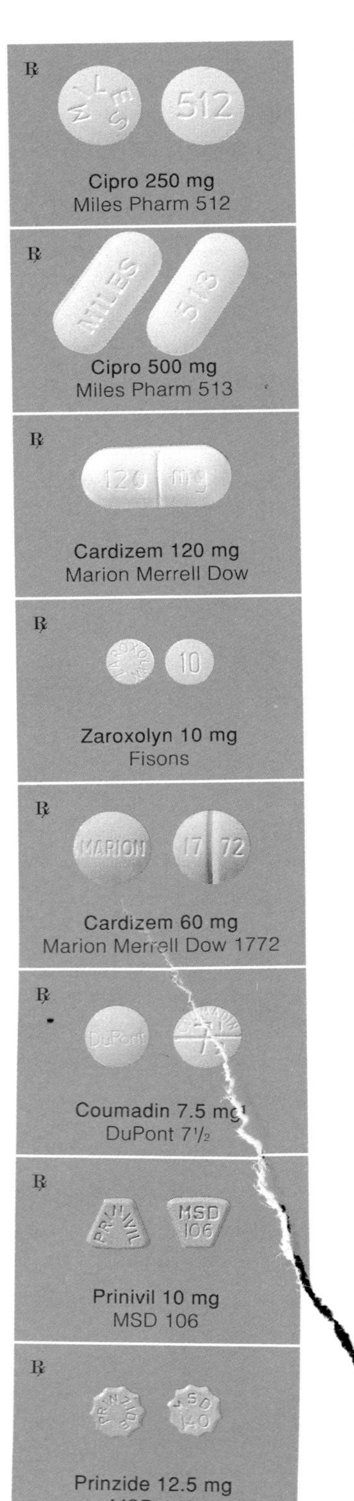

℞ Cipro 250 mg
Miles Pharm 512

℞ Cipro 500 mg
Miles Pharm 513

℞ Cardizem 120 mg
Marion Merrell Dow

℞ Zaroxolyn 10 mg
Fisons

℞ Cardizem 60 mg
Marion Merrell Dow 1772

℞ Coumadin 7.5 mg
DuPont 7½

℞ Prinivil 10 mg
MSD 106

℞ Prinzide 12.5 mg
MSD 140

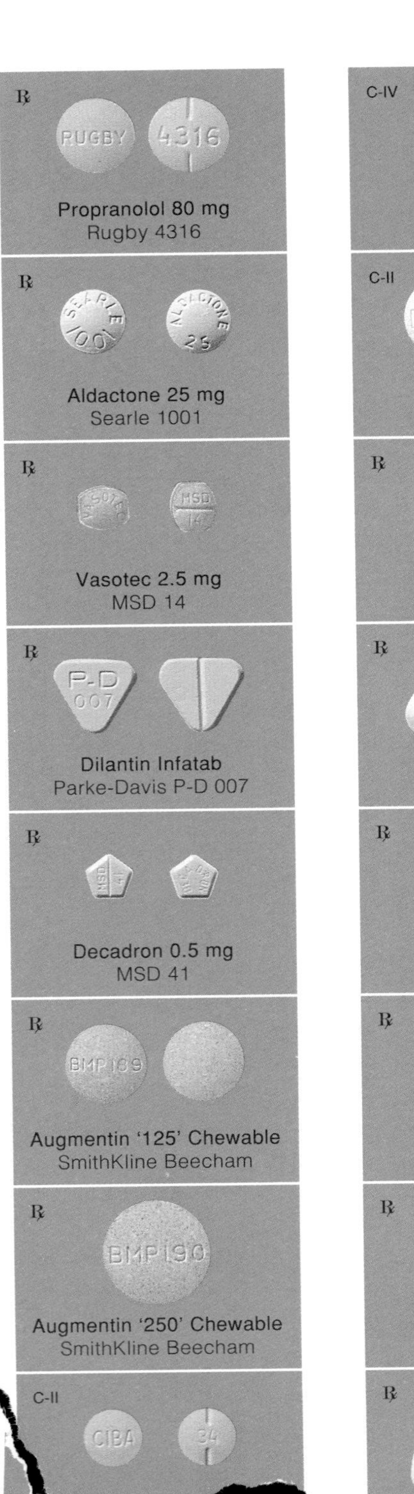

℞ Propranolol 80 mg
Rugby 4316

℞ Aldactone 25 mg
Searle 1001

℞ Vasotec 2.5 mg
MSD 14

℞ Dilantin Infatab
Parke-Davis P-D 007

℞ Decadron 0.5 mg
MSD 41

℞ Augmentin '125' Chewable
SmithKline Beecham

℞ Augmentin '250' Chewable
SmithKline Beecham

C-II Ritalin 20

C-IV Diazepam 5 mg
Rugby 3592

C-II Percodan
DuPont

℞ Naprosyn 250 mg
Syntex

℞ Naprosyn 500 mg
Syntex

℞ Zestril 40 mg
ICI Pharma 134

℞ Floxin 200 mg
Ortho

℞ Floxin 300 mg
Ortho

℞ Floxin 400 mg
Ortho

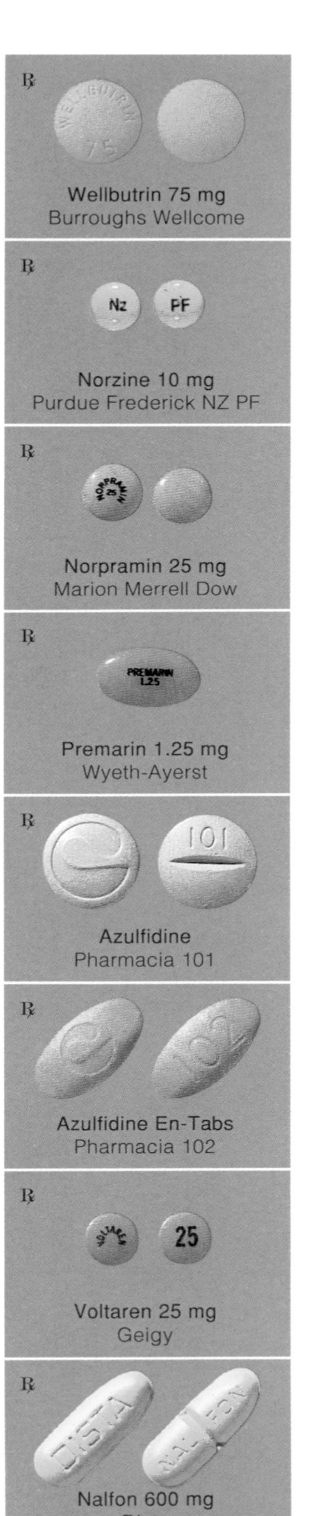

Wellbutrin 75 mg
Burroughs Wellcome

Norzine 10 mg
Purdue Frederick NZ PF

Norpramin 25 mg
Marion Merrell Dow

Premarin 1.25 mg
Wyeth-Ayerst

Azulfidine
Pharmacia 101

Azulfidine En-Tabs
Pharmacia 102

Voltaren 25 mg
Geigy

Nalfon 600 mg
Dista

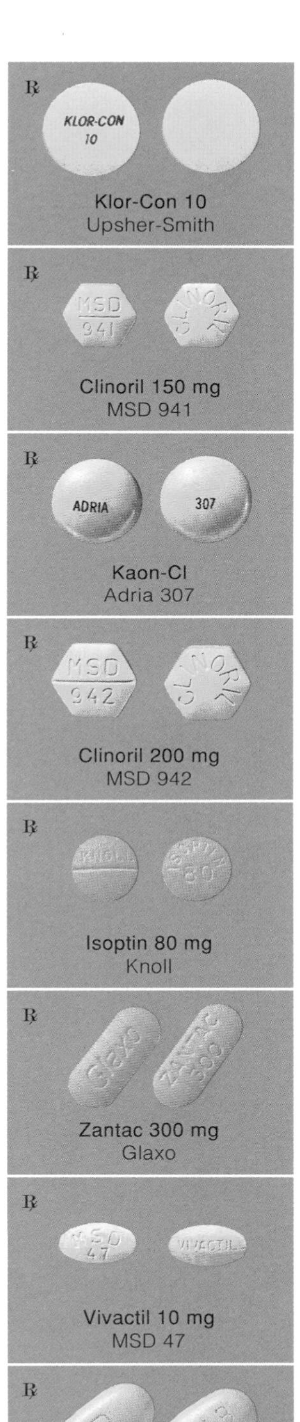

Klor-Con 10
Upsher-Smith

Clinoril 150 mg
MSD 941

Kaon-Cl
Adria 307

Clinoril 200 mg
MSD 942

Isoptin 80 mg
Knoll

Zantac 300 mg
Glaxo

Vivactil 10 mg
MSD 47

K-Tab 10 mEq
Abbott

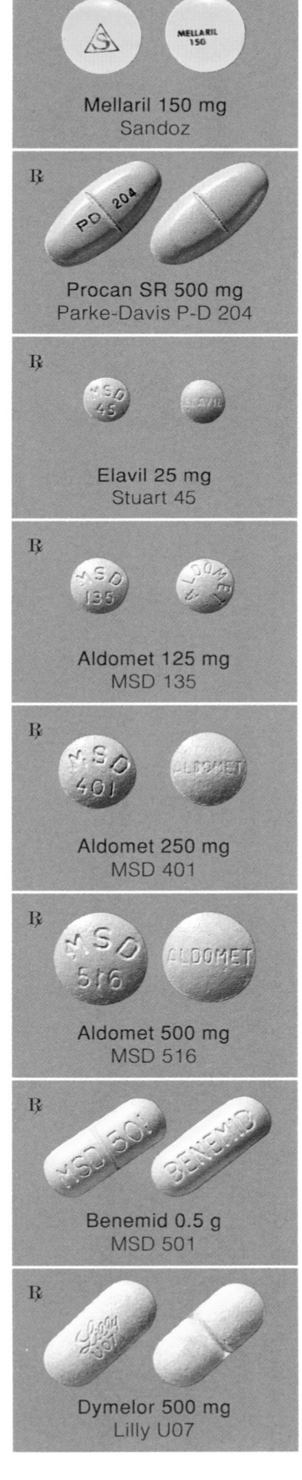

Mellaril 150 mg
Sandoz

Procan SR 500 mg
Parke-Davis P-D 204

Elavil 25 mg
Stuart 45

Aldomet 125 mg
MSD 135

Aldomet 250 mg
MSD 401

Aldomet 500 mg
MSD 516

Benemid 0.5 g
MSD 501

Dymelor 500 mg
Lilly U07

Green Tablets

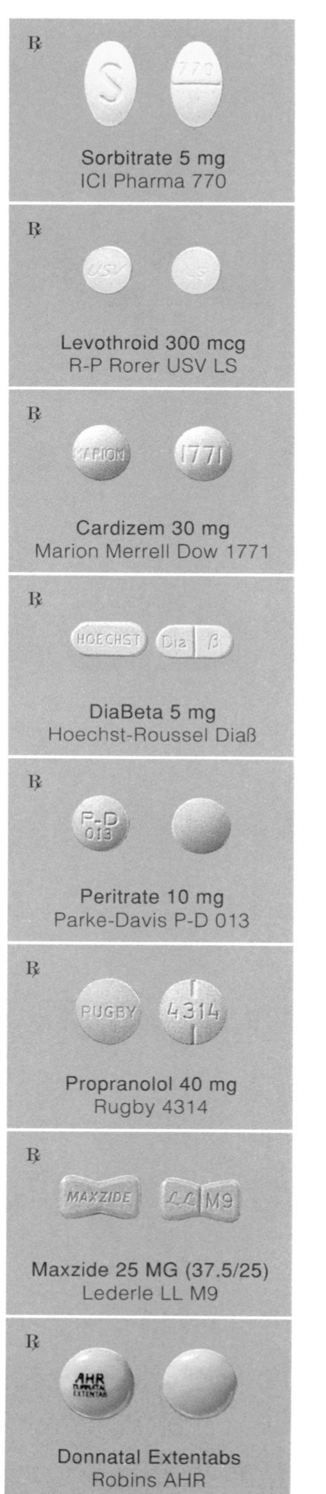

℞ Sorbitrate 5 mg
ICI Pharma 770

℞ Levothroid 300 mcg
R-P Rorer USV LS

℞ Cardizem 30 mg
Marion Merrell Dow 1771

℞ DiaBeta 5 mg
Hoechst-Roussel Diaß

℞ Peritrate 10 mg
Parke-Davis P-D 013

℞ Propranolol 40 mg
Rugby 4314

℞ Maxzide 25 MG (37.5/25)
Lederle LL M9

℞ Donnatal Extentabs
Robins AHR

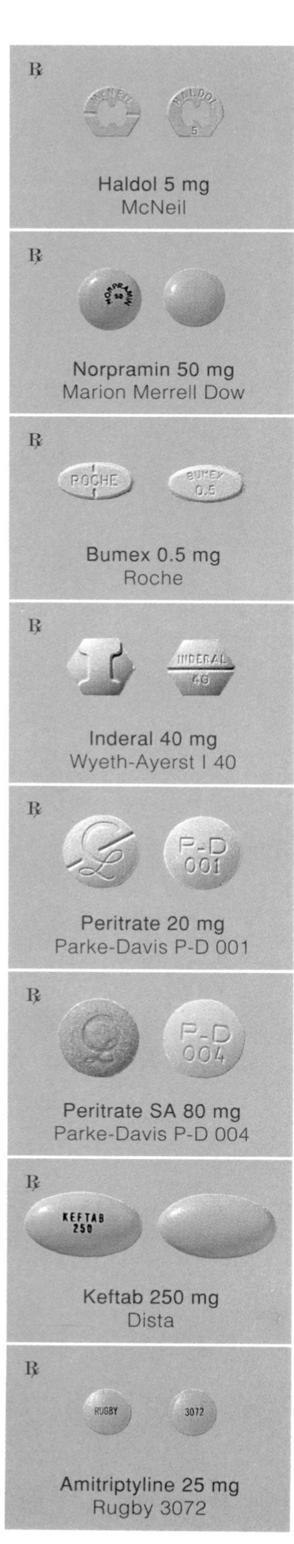

℞ Haldol 5 mg
McNeil

℞ Norpramin 50 mg
Marion Merrell Dow

℞ Bumex 0.5 mg
Roche

℞ Inderal 40 mg
Wyeth-Ayerst I 40

℞ Peritrate 20 mg
Parke-Davis P-D 001

℞ Peritrate SA 80 mg
Parke-Davis P-D 004

℞ Keftab 250 mg
Dista

℞ Amitriptyline 25 mg
Rugby 3072

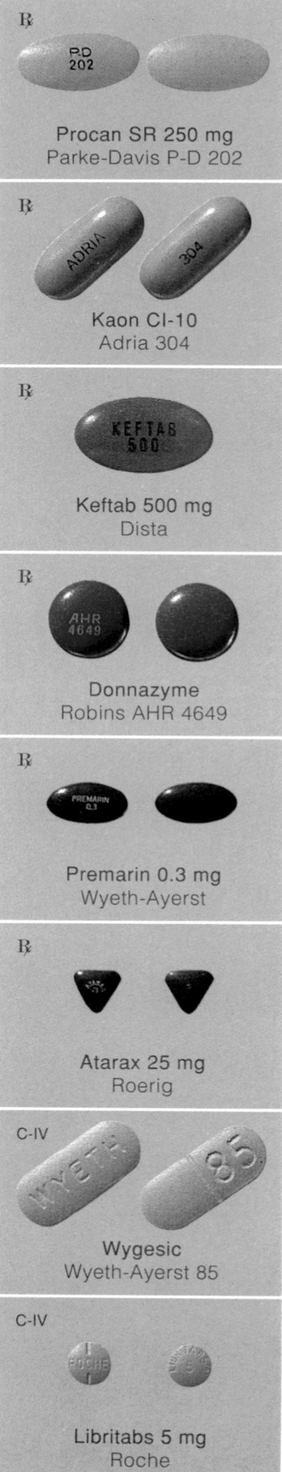

℞ Procan SR 250 mg
Parke-Davis P-D 202

℞ Kaon Cl-10
Adria 304

℞ Keftab 500 mg
Dista

℞ Donnazyme
Robins AHR 4649

℞ Premarin 0.3 mg
Wyeth-Ayerst

℞ Atarax 25 mg
Roerig

C-IV Wygesic
Wyeth-Ayerst 85

C-IV Libritabs 5 mg
Roche

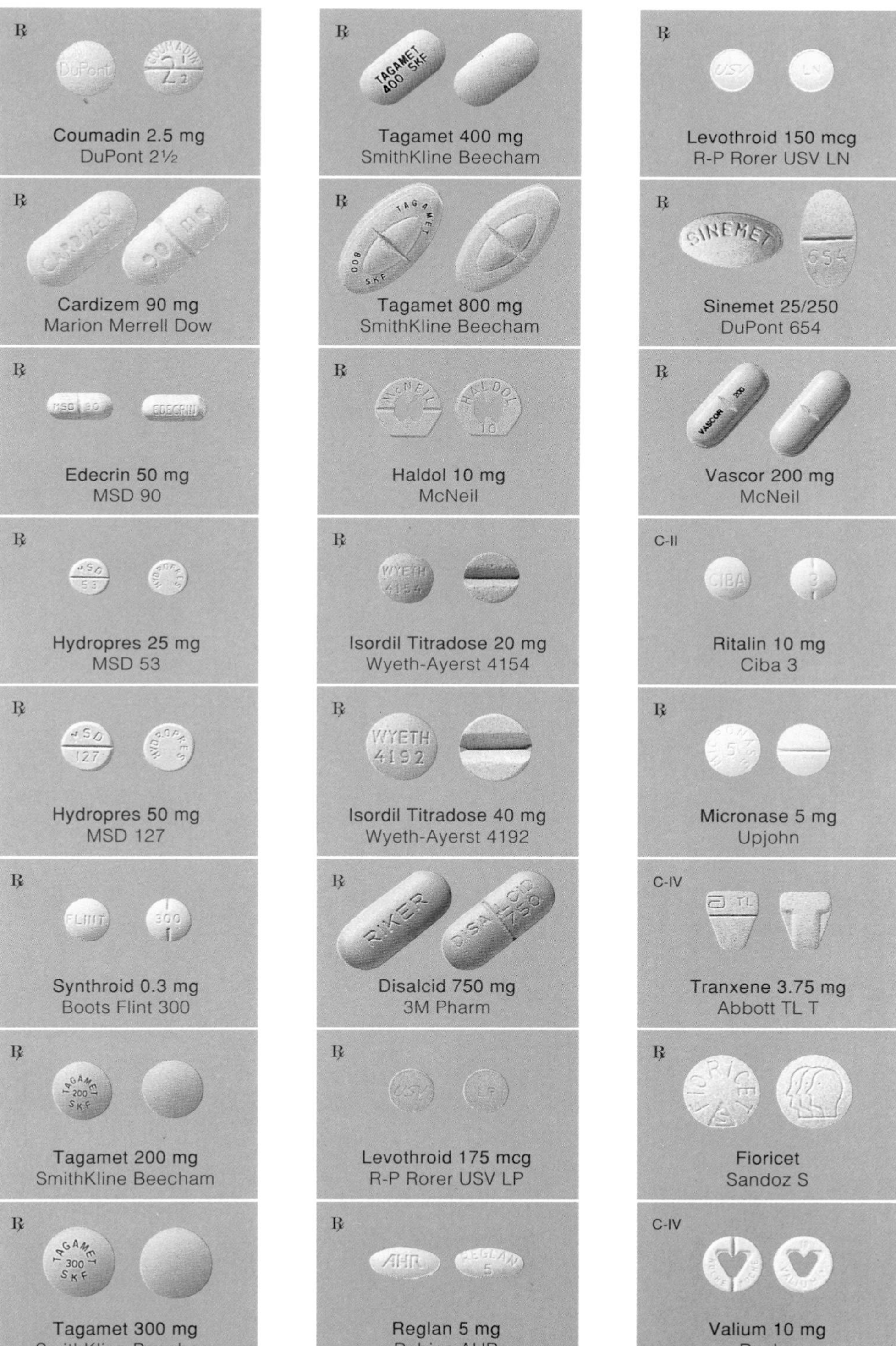

℞ Coumadin 2.5 mg DuPont 2½	℞ Tagamet 400 mg SmithKline Beecham	℞ Levothroid 150 mcg R-P Rorer USV LN
℞ Cardizem 90 mg Marion Merrell Dow	℞ Tagamet 800 mg SmithKline Beecham	℞ Sinemet 25/250 DuPont 654
℞ Edecrin 50 mg MSD 90	℞ Haldol 10 mg McNeil	℞ Vascor 200 mg McNeil
℞ Hydropres 25 mg MSD 53	℞ Isordil Titradose 20 mg Wyeth-Ayerst 4154	C-II Ritalin 10 mg Ciba 3
℞ Hydropres 50 mg MSD 127	℞ Isordil Titradose 40 mg Wyeth-Ayerst 4192	℞ Micronase 5 mg Upjohn
℞ Synthroid 0.3 mg Boots Flint 300	℞ Disalcid 750 mg 3M Pharm	C-IV Tranxene 3.75 mg Abbott TL T
℞ Tagamet 200 mg SmithKline Beecham	℞ Levothroid 175 mcg R-P Rorer USV LP	℞ Fioricet Sandoz S
℞ Tagamet 300 mg SmithKline Beecham	℞ Reglan 5 mg Robins AHR	C-IV Valium 10 mg Roche

Blue Tablets

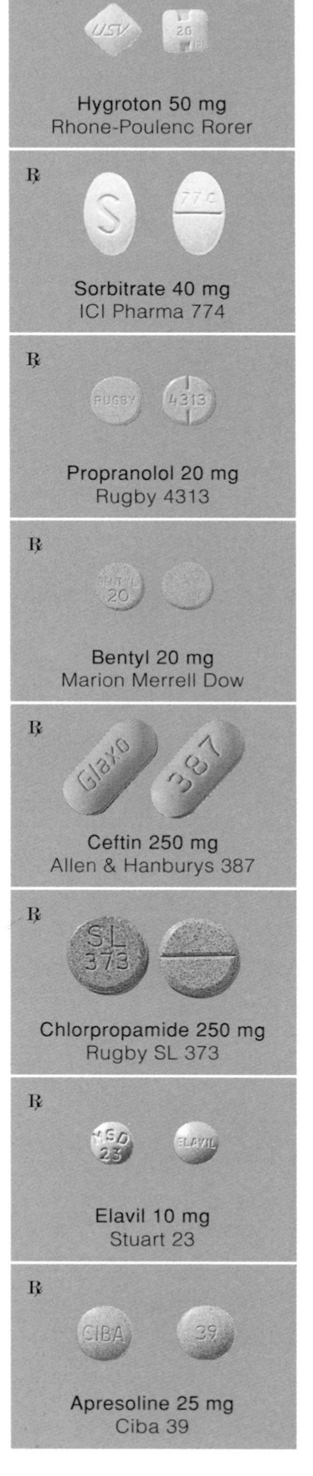
℞
Hygroton 50 mg
Rhone-Poulenc Rorer
℞
Sorbitrate 40 mg
ICI Pharma 774
℞
Propranolol 20 mg
Rugby 4313
℞
Bentyl 20 mg
Marion Merrell Dow
℞
Ceftin 250 mg
Allen & Hanburys 387
℞
Chlorpropamide 250 mg
Rugby SL 373
℞
Elavil 10 mg
Stuart 23
℞
Apresoline 25 mg
Ciba 39

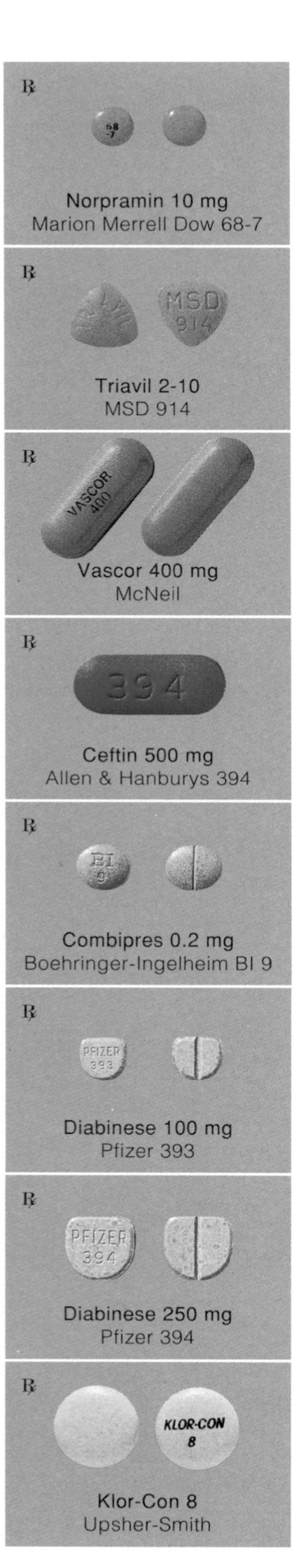
℞
Norpramin 10 mg
Marion Merrell Dow 68-7
℞
Triavil 2-10
MSD 914
℞
Vascor 400 mg
McNeil
℞
Ceftin 500 mg
Allen & Hanburys 394
℞
Combipres 0.2 mg
Boehringer-Ingelheim BI 9
℞
Diabinese 100 mg
Pfizer 393
℞
Diabinese 250 mg
Pfizer 394
℞
KLOR-CON 8
Klor-Con 8
Upsher-Smith

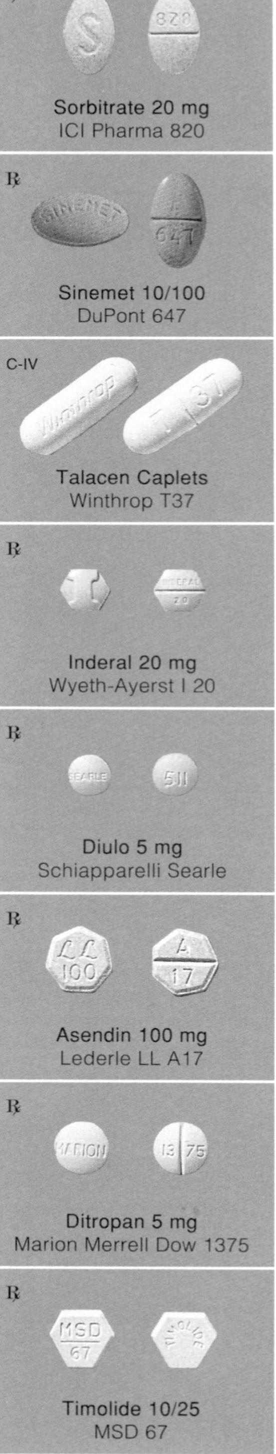
℞
Sorbitrate 20 mg
ICI Pharma 820
℞
Sinemet 10/100
DuPont 647
C-IV
Talacen Caplets
Winthrop T37
℞
Inderal 20 mg
Wyeth-Ayerst I 20
℞
Diulo 5 mg
Schiapparelli Searle
℞
Asendin 100 mg
Lederle LL A17
℞
Ditropan 5 mg
Marion Merrell Dow 1375
℞
Timolide 10/25
MSD 67

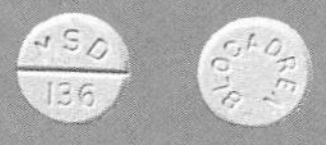

℞
Blocadren 10 mg
MSD 136

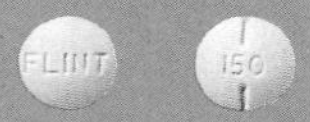

℞
Synthroid 0.15 mg
Boots Flint 150

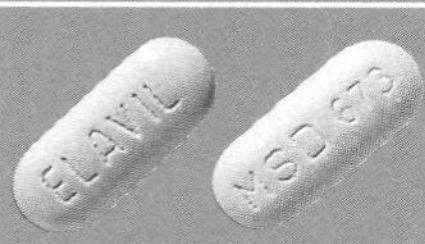

℞
Elavil 150 mg
Stuart 673

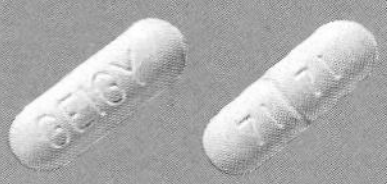

℞
Lopressor 100 mg
Geigy 71 71

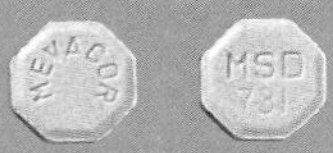

℞
Mevacor 20 mg
MSD 731

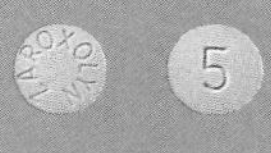

℞
Zaroxolyn 5 mg
Fisons

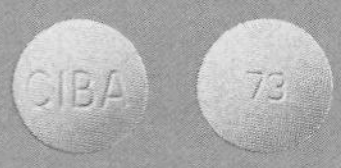

℞
Apresoline 50 mg
Ciba 73

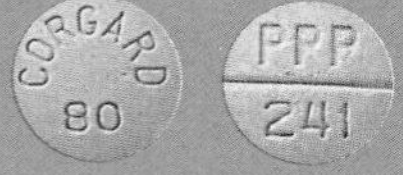

℞
Corgard 80 mg
Bristol PPP 241

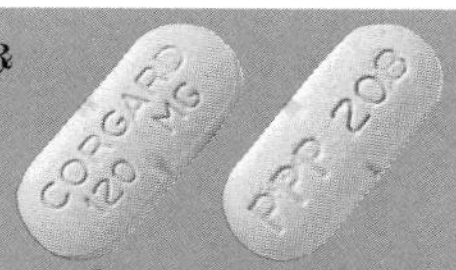

℞
Corgard 120 mg
Bristol PPP 208

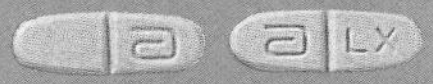

℞
Ogen 2.5 mg
Abbott LX

C-IV 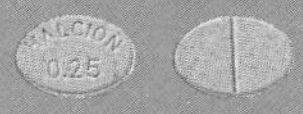
Halcion 0.25 mg
Upjohn

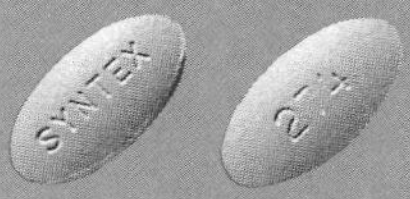

℞
Anaprox 275 mg
Syntex 274

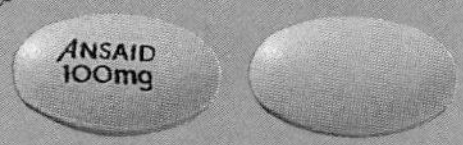

℞
Ansaid 100 mg
Upjohn

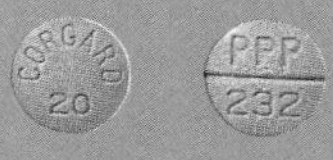

℞
Corgard 20 mg
Bristol PPP 232

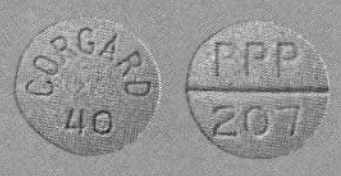

℞
Corgard 40 mg
Bristol PPP 207

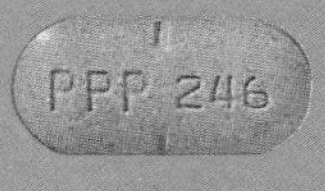

℞
Corgard 160 mg
Bristol PPP 246

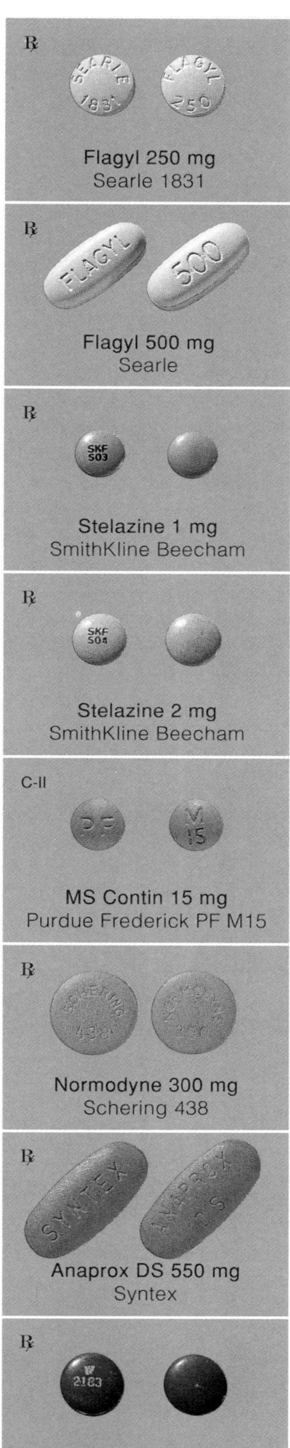

℞
Flagyl 250 mg
Searle 1831

℞
Flagyl 500 mg
Searle

℞
Stelazine 1 mg
SmithKline Beecham

℞
Stelazine 2 mg
SmithKline Beecham

C-II
MS Contin 15 mg
Purdue Frederick PF M15

℞
Normodyne 300 mg
Schering 438

℞
Anaprox DS 550 mg
Syntex

℞
Urised
Webcon W 2183

CL - 10 Dark Blue to Lavender Tablets

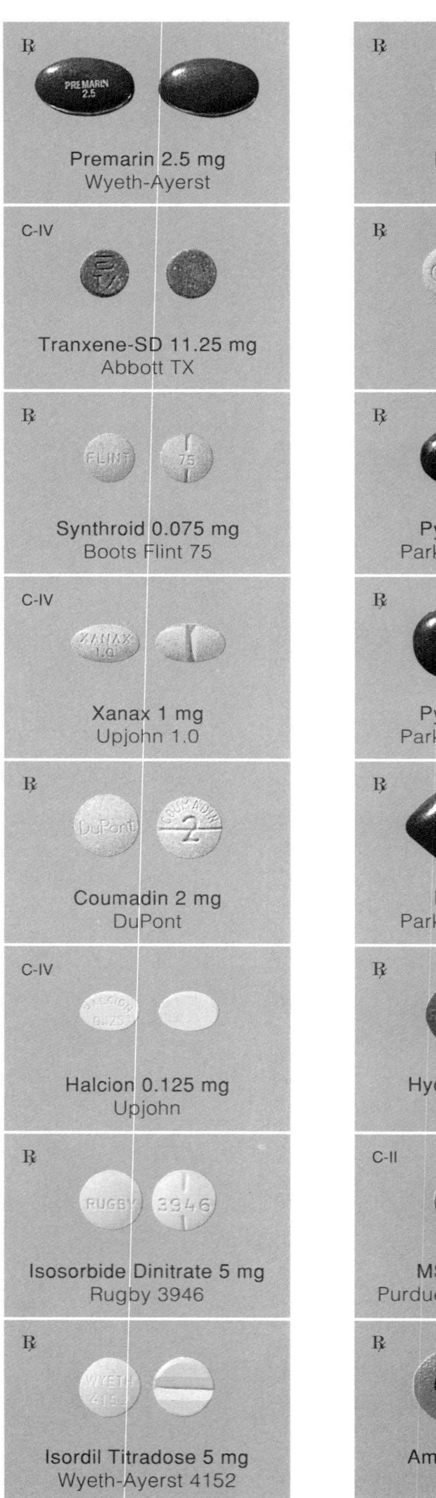

℞
Premarin 2.5 mg
Wyeth-Ayerst

C-IV
Tranxene-SD 11.25 mg
Abbott TX

℞
Synthroid 0.075 mg
Boots Flint 75

C-IV
Xanax 1 mg
Upjohn 1.0

℞
Coumadin 2 mg
DuPont

C-IV
Halcion 0.125 mg
Upjohn

℞
Isosorbide Dinitrate 5 mg
Rugby 3946

℞
Isordil Titradose 5 mg
Wyeth-Ayerst 4152

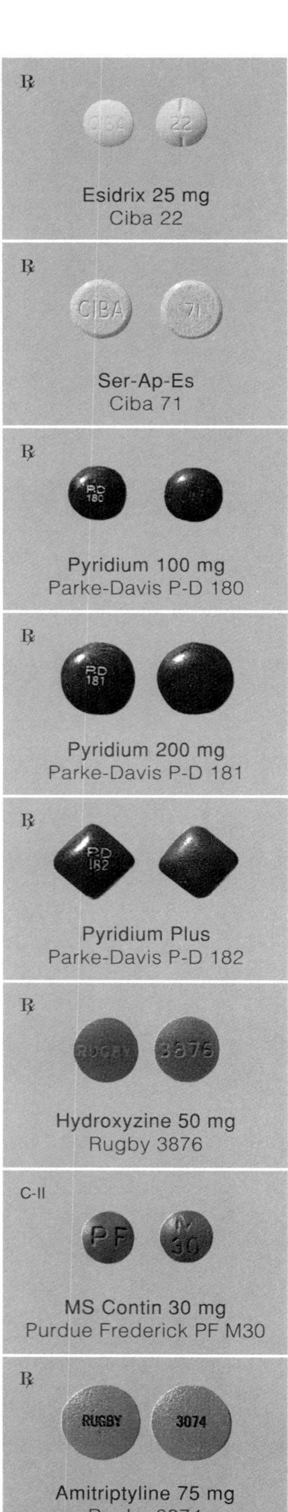

℞
Esidrix 25 mg
Ciba 22

℞
Ser-Ap-Es
Ciba 71

℞
Pyridium 100 mg
Parke-Davis P-D 180

℞
Pyridium 200 mg
Parke-Davis P-D 181

℞
Pyridium Plus
Parke-Davis P-D 182

℞
Hydroxyzine 50 mg
Rugby 3876

C-II
MS Contin 30 mg
Purdue Frederick PF M30

℞
Amitriptyline 75 mg
Rugby 3074

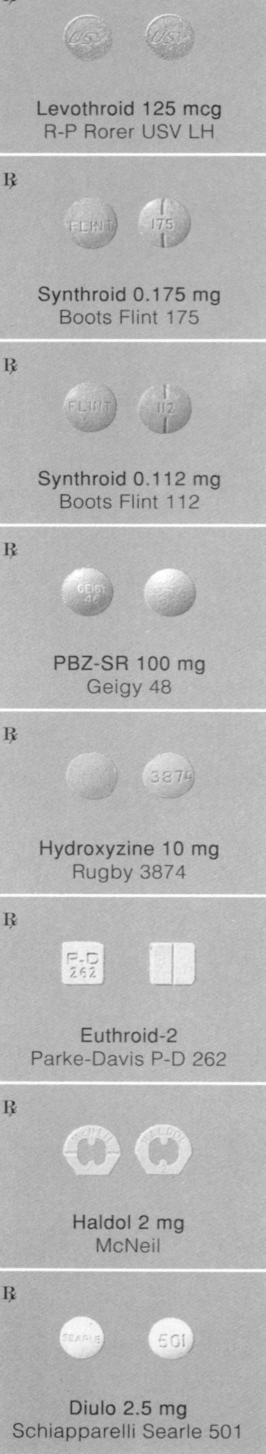

℞
Levothroid 125 mcg
R-P Rorer USV LH

℞
Synthroid 0.175 mg
Boots Flint 175

℞
Synthroid 0.112 mg
Boots Flint 112

℞
PBZ-SR 100 mg
Geigy 48

℞
Hydroxyzine 10 mg
Rugby 3874

℞
Euthroid-2
Parke-Davis P-D 262

℞
Haldol 2 mg
McNeil

℞
Diulo 2.5 mg
Schiapparelli Searle 501

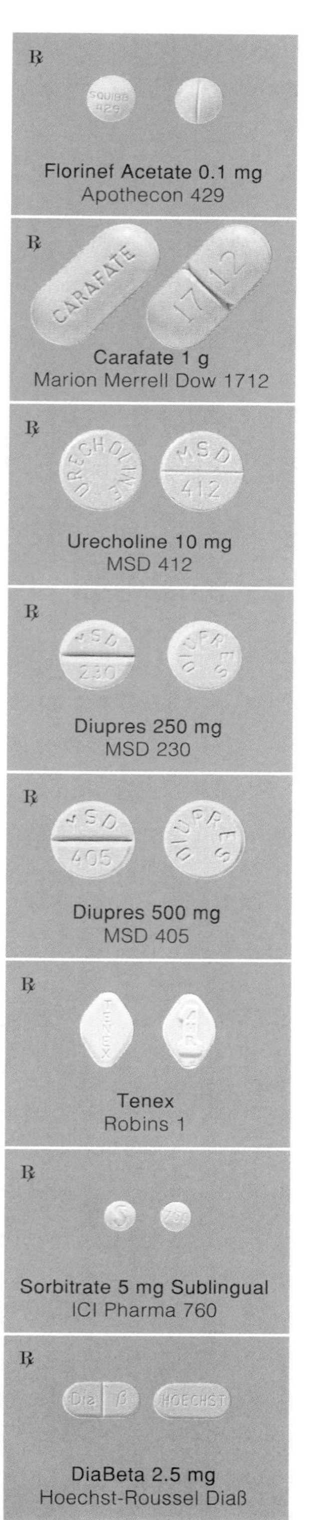

℞ Florinef Acetate 0.1 mg
Apothecon 429

℞ Carafate 1 g
Marion Merrell Dow 1712

℞ Urecholine 10 mg
MSD 412

℞ Diupres 250 mg
MSD 230

℞ Diupres 500 mg
MSD 405

℞ Tenex
Robins 1

℞ Sorbitrate 5 mg Sublingual
ICI Pharma 760

℞ DiaBeta 2.5 mg
Hoechst-Roussel Diaß

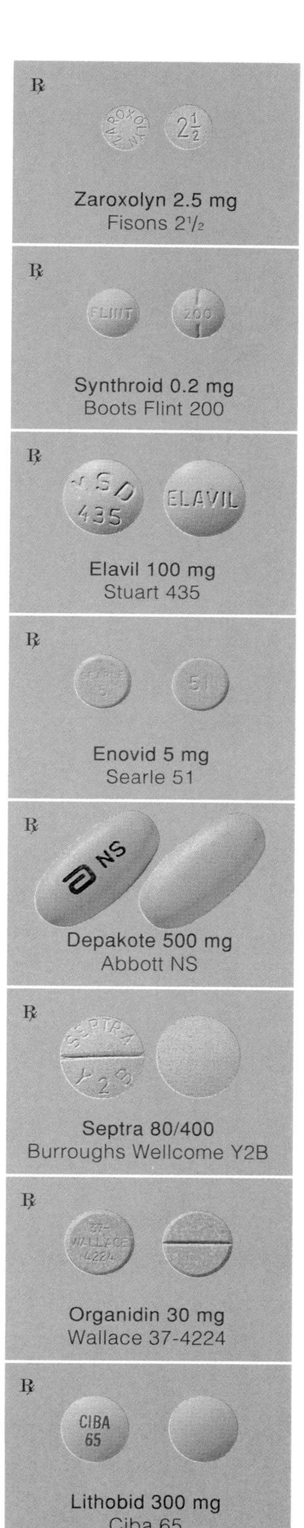

℞ Zaroxolyn 2.5 mg
Fisons 2½

℞ Synthroid 0.2 mg
Boots Flint 200

℞ Elavil 100 mg
Stuart 435

℞ Enovid 5 mg
Searle 51

℞ Depakote 500 mg
Abbott NS

℞ Septra 80/400
Burroughs Wellcome Y2B

℞ Organidin 30 mg
Wallace 37-4224

℞ Lithobid 300 mg
Ciba 65

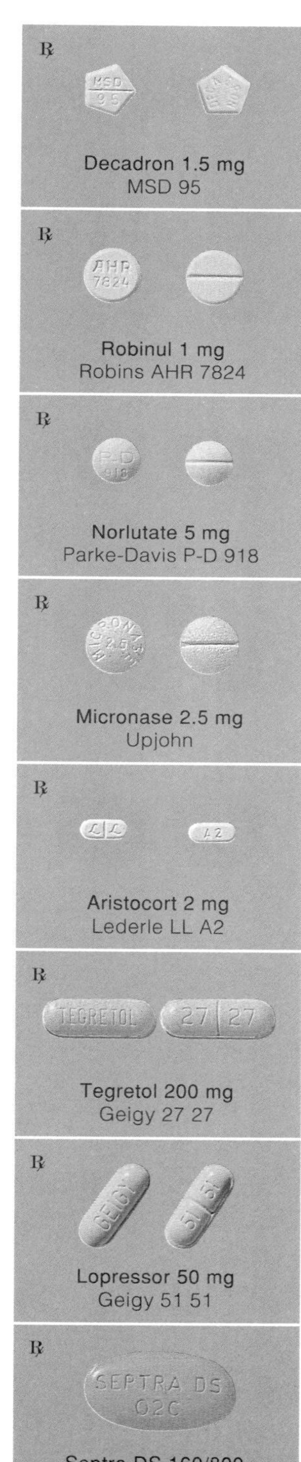

℞ Decadron 1.5 mg
MSD 95

℞ Robinul 1 mg
Robins AHR 7824

℞ Norlutate 5 mg
Parke-Davis P-D 918

℞ Micronase 2.5 mg
Upjohn

℞ Aristocort 2 mg
Lederle LL A2

℞ Tegretol 200 mg
Geigy 27 27

℞ Lopressor 50 mg
Geigy 51 51

℞ Septra DS 160/800
Burroughs Wellcome 02C

Red to Salmon Tablets

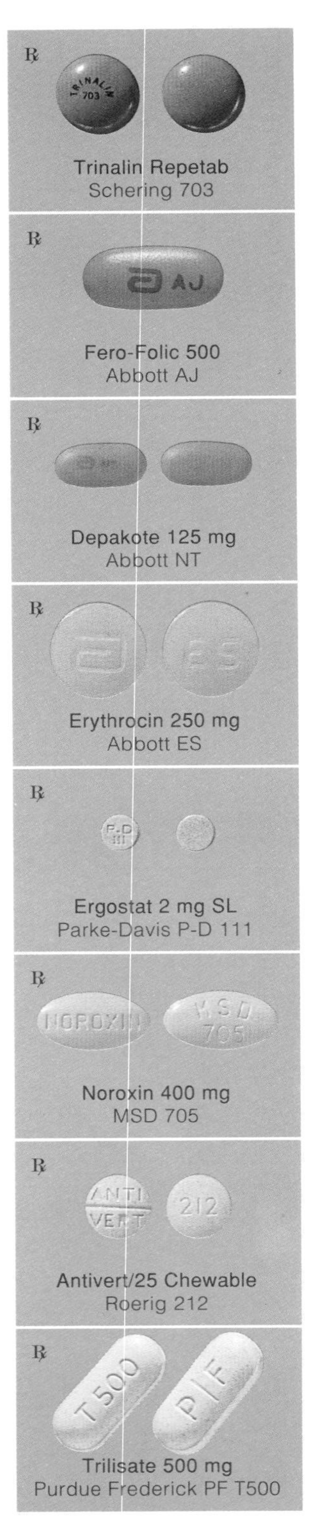

℞ Trinalin Repetab
Schering 703

℞ Fero-Folic 500
Abbott AJ

℞ Depakote 125 mg
Abbott NT

℞ Erythrocin 250 mg
Abbott ES

℞ Ergostat 2 mg SL
Parke-Davis P-D 111

℞ Noroxin 400 mg
MSD 705

℞ Antivert/25 Chewable
Roerig 212

℞ Trilisate 500 mg
Purdue Frederick PF T500

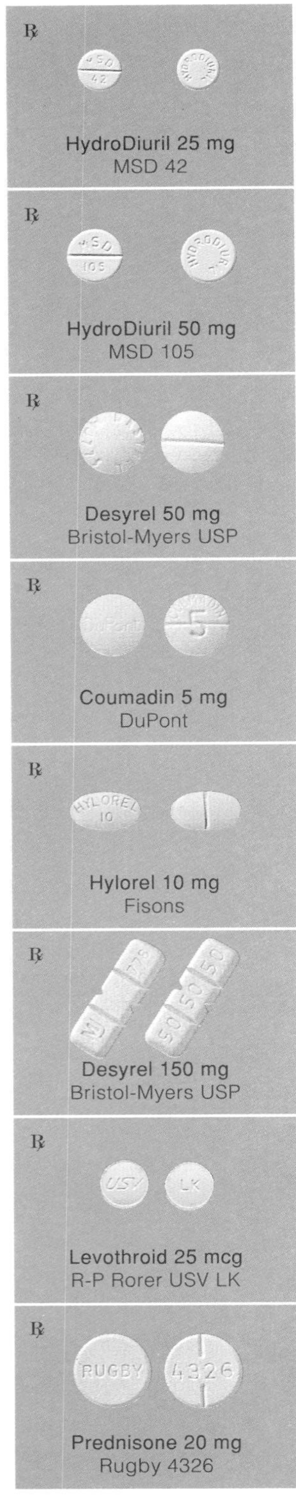

℞ HydroDiuril 25 mg
MSD 42

℞ HydroDiuril 50 mg
MSD 105

℞ Desyrel 50 mg
Bristol-Myers USP

℞ Coumadin 5 mg
DuPont

℞ Hylorel 10 mg
Fisons

℞ Desyrel 150 mg
Bristol-Myers USP

℞ Levothroid 25 mcg
R-P Rorer USV LK

℞ Prednisone 20 mg
Rugby 4326

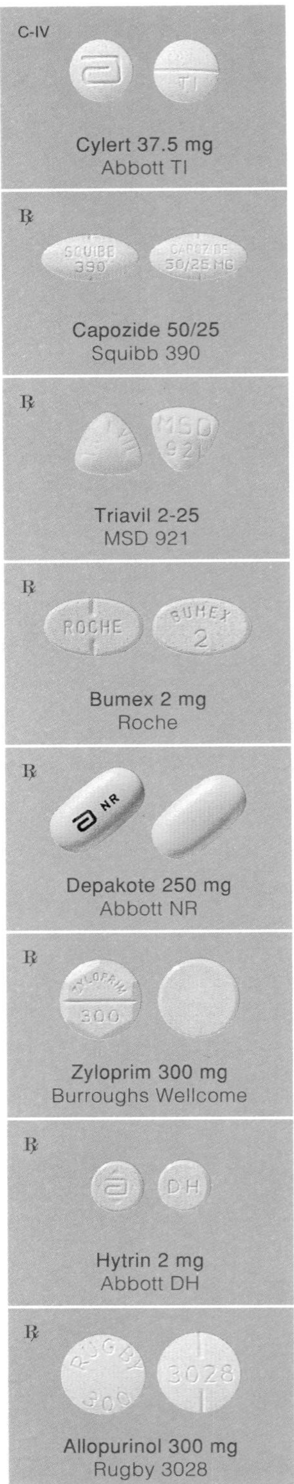

C-IV Cylert 37.5 mg
Abbott TI

℞ Capozide 50/25
Squibb 390

℞ Triavil 2-25
MSD 921

℞ Bumex 2 mg
Roche

℞ Depakote 250 mg
Abbott NR

℞ Zyloprim 300 mg
Burroughs Wellcome

℞ Hytrin 2 mg
Abbott DH

℞ Allopurinol 300 mg
Rugby 3028

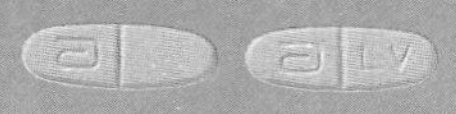

℞
Ogen 1.25 mg
Abbott LV

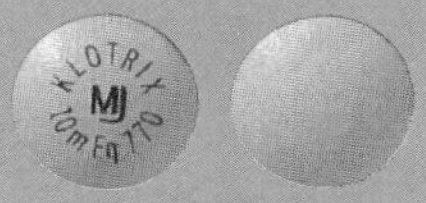

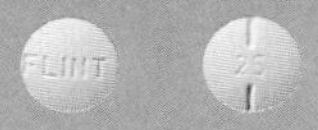

℞
Synthroid 0.025 mg
Boots Flint 25

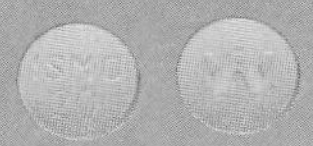

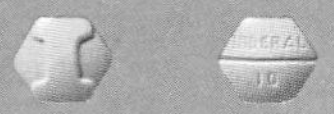

℞
Inderal 10 mg
Wyeth-Ayerst I 10

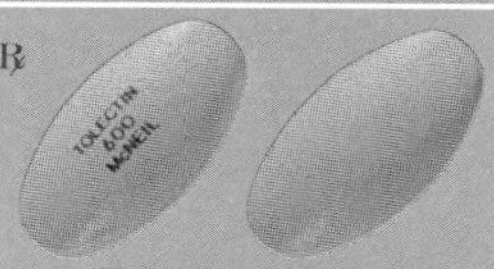

℞
Enduron 2.5 mg
Abbott

℞
Dolobid 250 mg
MSD 675

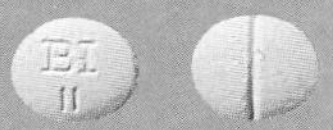

℞
Catapres 0.3 mg
Boehringer-Ingelheim BI 11

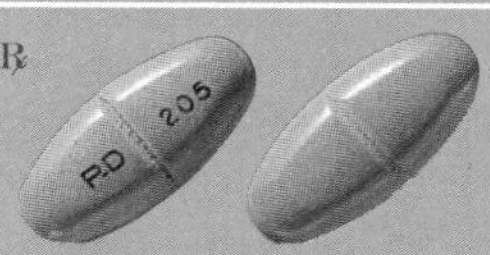

℞
Trandate 100 mg
Glaxo

℞
Trandate 300 mg
Glaxo

℞
Klotrix 10 mEq
Bristol MJ 770

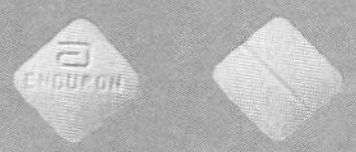

℞
Ismo
Wyeth-Ayerst W 20

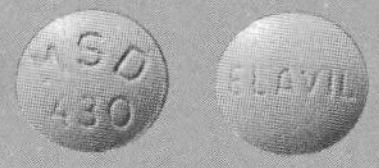

℞
Tolectin 600 mg
McNeil

℞
Elavil 75 mg
Stuart 430

C-IV
Klonopin 0.5 mg
Roche

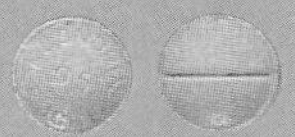

℞
Procan SR 750 mg
Parke-Davis P-D 205

℞
Dolobid 500 mg
MSD 697

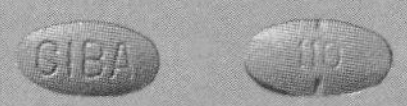

℞
Ludiomil 25 mg
Ciba 110

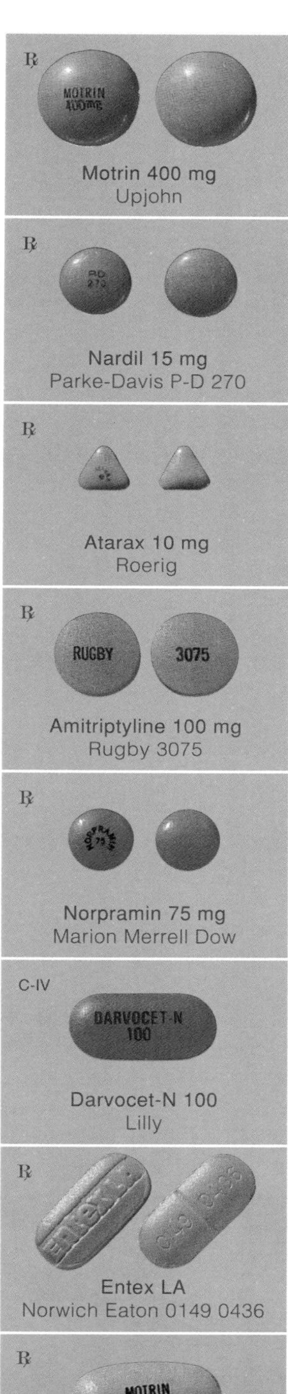

℞
Motrin 400 mg
Upjohn

℞
Nardil 15 mg
Parke-Davis P-D 270

℞
Atarax 10 mg
Roerig

℞
Amitriptyline 100 mg
Rugby 3075

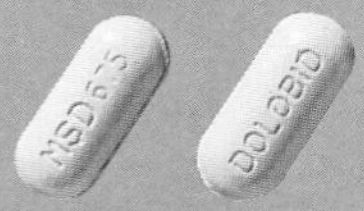

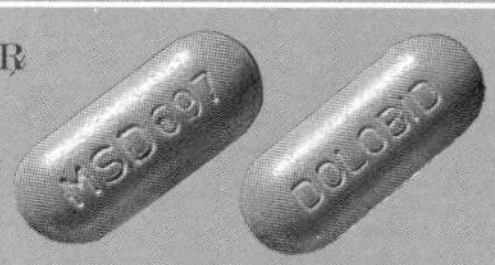

℞
Norpramin 75 mg
Marion Merrell Dow

C-IV
Darvocet-N 100
Lilly

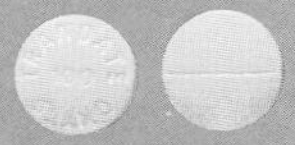

℞
Entex LA
Norwich Eaton 0149 0436

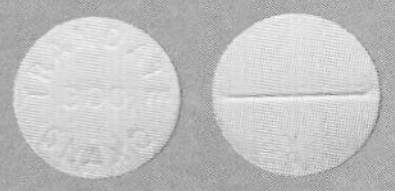

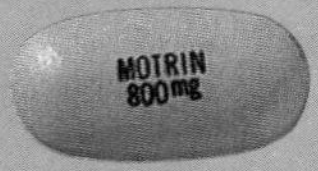

℞
Motrin 800 mg
Upjohn

Orange to Light Orange Tablets

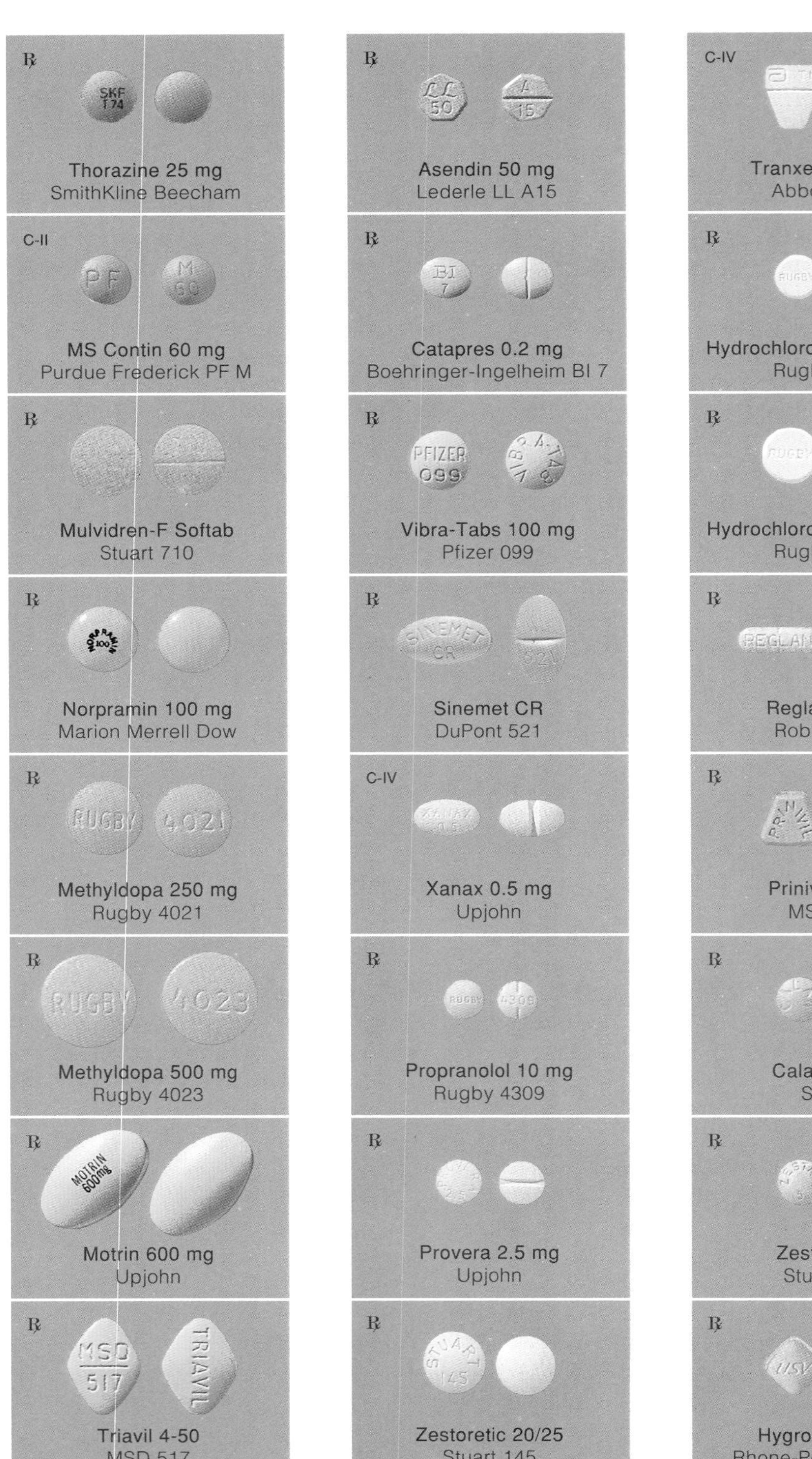

℞ Thorazine 25 mg
SmithKline Beecham

C-II MS Contin 60 mg
Purdue Frederick PF M

℞ Mulvidren-F Softab
Stuart 710

℞ Norpramin 100 mg
Marion Merrell Dow

℞ Methyldopa 250 mg
Rugby 4021

℞ Methyldopa 500 mg
Rugby 4023

℞ Motrin 600 mg
Upjohn

℞ Triavil 4-50
MSD 517

℞ Asendin 50 mg
Lederle LL A15

℞ Catapres 0.2 mg
Boehringer-Ingelheim BI 7

℞ Vibra-Tabs 100 mg
Pfizer 099

℞ Sinemet CR
DuPont 521

C-IV Xanax 0.5 mg
Upjohn

℞ Propranolol 10 mg
Rugby 4309

℞ Provera 2.5 mg
Upjohn

℞ Zestoretic 20/25
Stuart 145

C-IV Tranxene 7.5 mg
Abbott TM T

℞ Hydrochlorothiazide 25 mg
Rugby 3922

℞ Hydrochlorothiazide 50 mg
Rugby 3919

℞ Reglan 10 mg
Robins AHR

℞ Prinivil 40 mg
MSD 237

℞ Calan 40 mg
Searle

℞ Zestril 5 mg
Stuart 130

℞ Hygroton 25 mg
Rhone-Poulenc Rorer

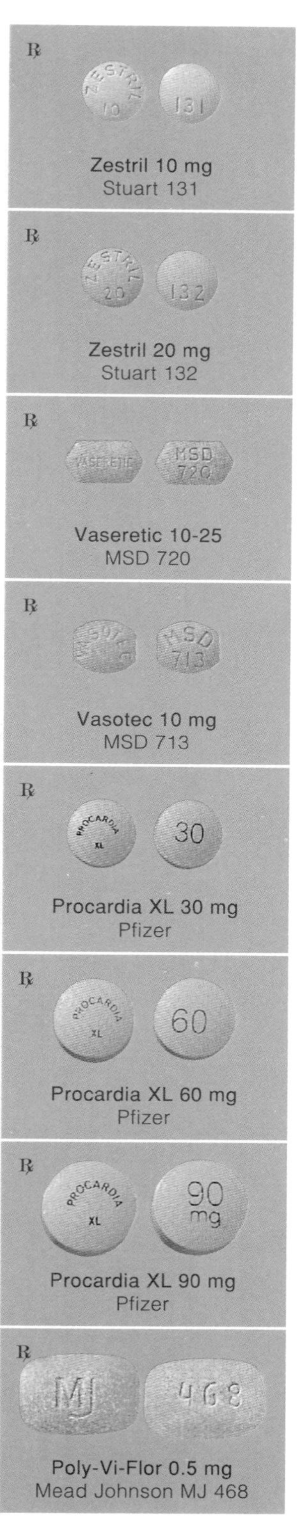

Zestril 10 mg
Stuart 131

Zestril 20 mg
Stuart 132

Vaseretic 10-25
MSD 720

Vasotec 10 mg
MSD 713

Procardia XL 30 mg
Pfizer

Procardia XL 60 mg
Pfizer

Procardia XL 90 mg
Pfizer

Poly-Vi-Flor 0.5 mg
Mead Johnson MJ 468

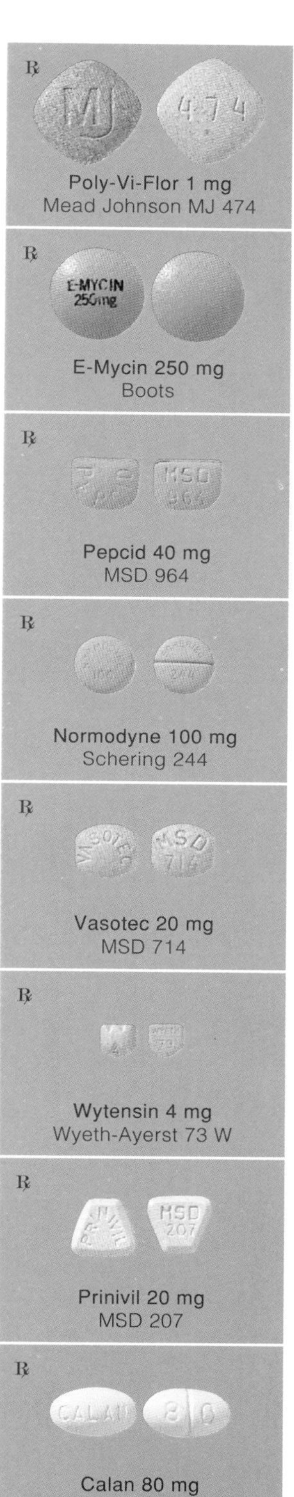

Poly-Vi-Flor 1 mg
Mead Johnson MJ 474

E-Mycin 250 mg
Boots

Pepcid 40 mg
MSD 964

Normodyne 100 mg
Schering 244

Vasotec 20 mg
MSD 714

Wytensin 4 mg
Wyeth-Ayerst 73 W

Prinivil 20 mg
MSD 207

Calan 80 mg
Searle

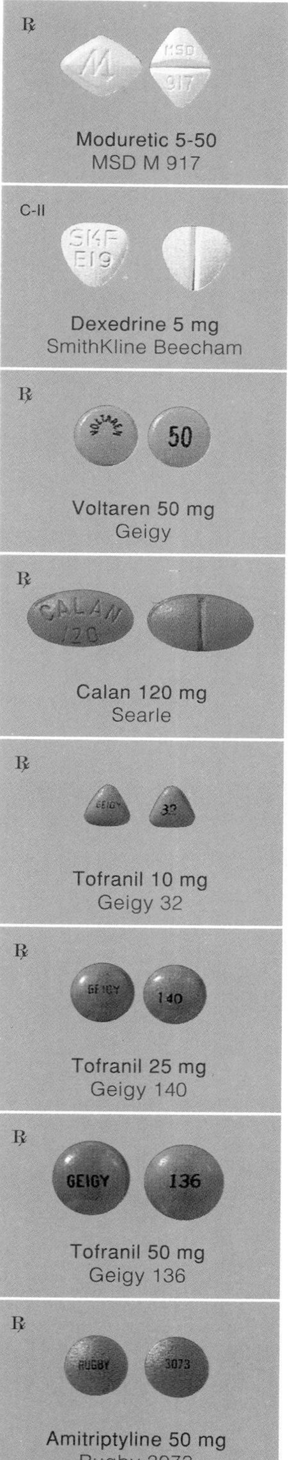

Moduretic 5-50
MSD M 917

C-II
Dexedrine 5 mg
SmithKline Beecham

Voltaren 50 mg
Geigy

Calan 120 mg
Searle

Tofranil 10 mg
Geigy 32

Tofranil 25 mg
Geigy 140

Tofranil 50 mg
Geigy 136

Amitriptyline 50 mg
Rugby 3073

Brown to Multi-Colored Tablets

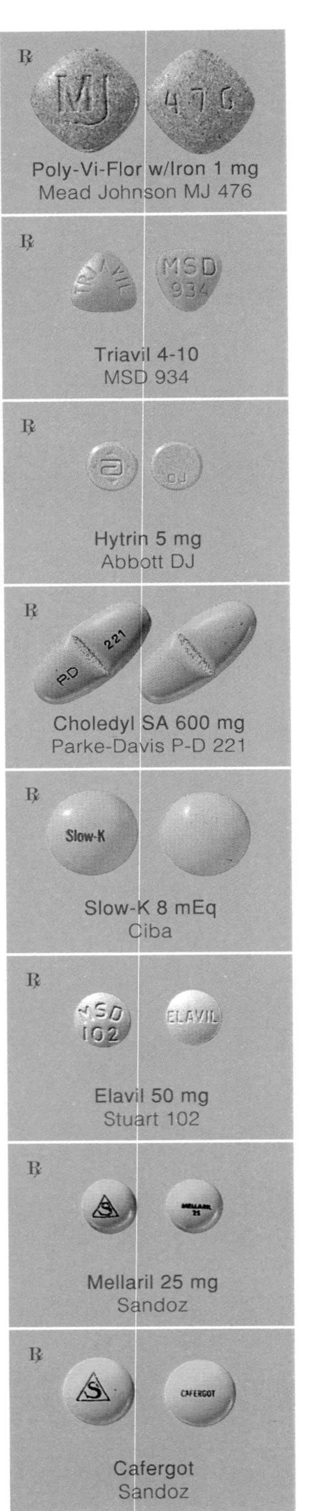

℞ Poly-Vi-Flor w/Iron 1 mg
Mead Johnson MJ 476

℞ Triavil 4-10
MSD 934

℞ Hytrin 5 mg
Abbott DJ

℞ Choledyl SA 600 mg
Parke-Davis P-D 221

℞ Slow-K 8 mEq
Ciba

℞ Elavil 50 mg
Stuart 102

℞ Mellaril 25 mg
Sandoz

℞ Cafergot
Sandoz

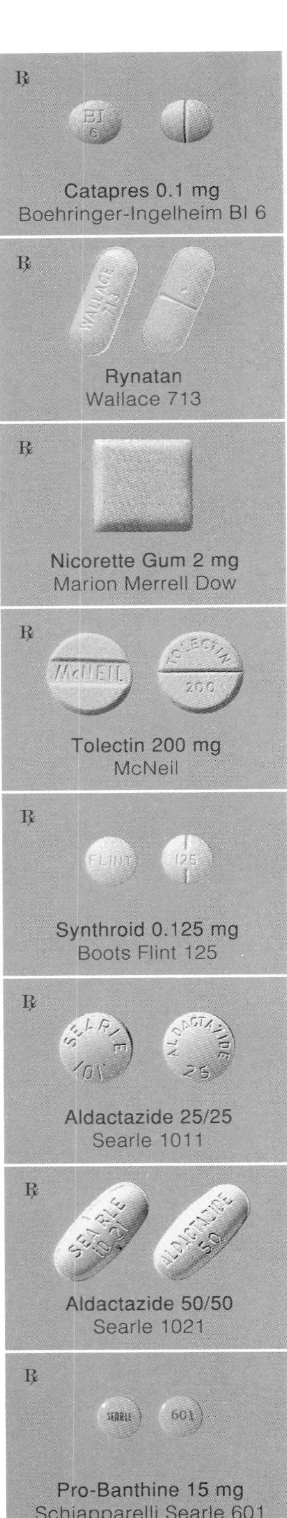

℞ Catapres 0.1 mg
Boehringer-Ingelheim BI 6

℞ Rynatan
Wallace 713

℞ Nicorette Gum 2 mg
Marion Merrell Dow

℞ Tolectin 200 mg
McNeil

℞ Synthroid 0.125 mg
Boots Flint 125

℞ Aldactazide 25/25
Searle 1011

℞ Aldactazide 50/50
Searle 1021

℞ Pro-Banthine 15 mg
Schiapparelli Searle 601

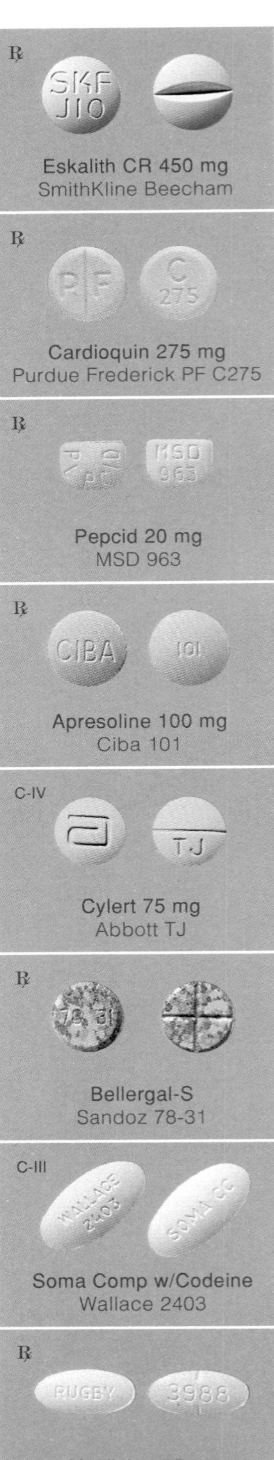

℞ Eskalith CR 450 mg
SmithKline Beecham

℞ Cardioquin 275 mg
Purdue Frederick PF C275

℞ Pepcid 20 mg
MSD 963

℞ Apresoline 100 mg
Ciba 101

C-IV Cylert 75 mg
Abbott TJ

℞ Bellergal-S
Sandoz 78-31

C-III Soma Comp w/Codeine
Wallace 2403

℞ Meclizine 25 mg
Rugby 3988

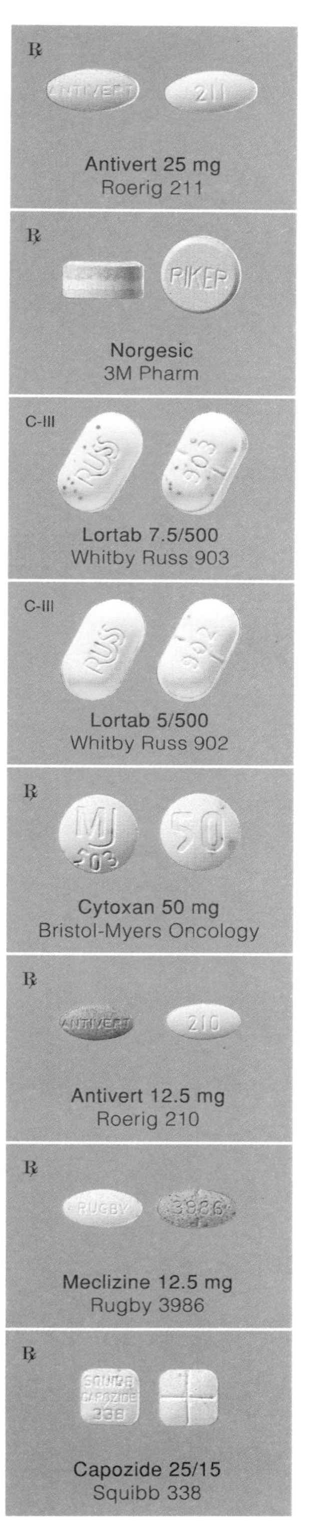

℞ Antivert 25 mg
Roerig 211

℞ Norgesic
3M Pharm

C-III Lortab 7.5/500
Whitby Russ 903

C-III Lortab 5/500
Whitby Russ 902

℞ Cytoxan 50 mg
Bristol-Myers Oncology

℞ Antivert 12.5 mg
Roerig 210

℞ Meclizine 12.5 mg
Rugby 3986

℞ Capozide 25/15
Squibb 338

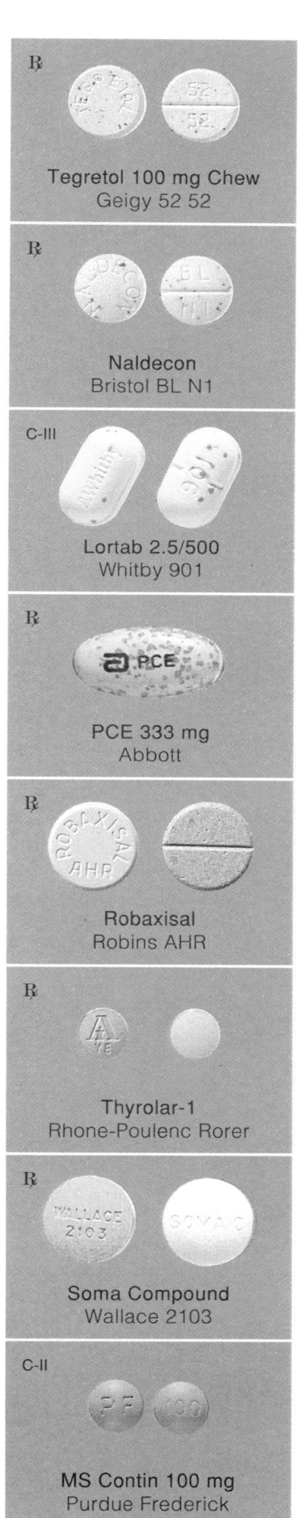

℞ Tegretol 100 mg Chew
Geigy 52 52

℞ Naldecon
Bristol BL N1

C-III Lortab 2.5/500
Whitby 901

℞ PCE 333 mg
Abbott

℞ Robaxisal
Robins AHR

℞ Thyrolar-1
Rhone-Poulenc Rorer

℞ Soma Compound
Wallace 2103

C-II MS Contin 100 mg
Purdue Frederick

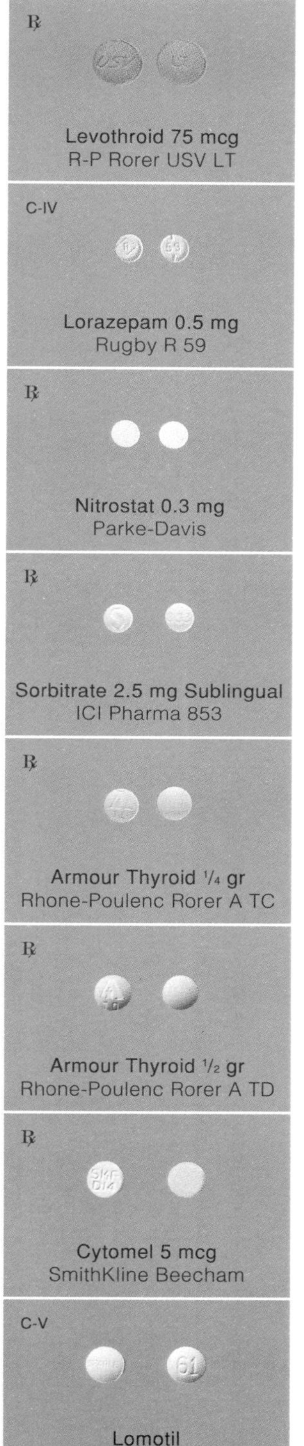

℞ Levothroid 75 mcg
R-P Rorer USV LT

C-IV Lorazepam 0.5 mg
Rugby R 59

℞ Nitrostat 0.3 mg
Parke-Davis

℞ Sorbitrate 2.5 mg Sublingual
ICI Pharma 853

℞ Armour Thyroid 1/4 gr
Rhone-Poulenc Rorer A TC

℞ Armour Thyroid 1/2 gr
Rhone-Poulenc Rorer A TD

℞ Cytomel 5 mcg
SmithKline Beecham

C-V Lomotil
Searle 61

White Round Tablets

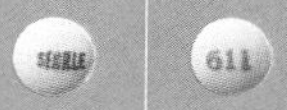

℞
Pro-Banthine 7.5 mg
Schiapparelli Searle 611

℞
Ventolin 2 mg
Glaxo

C-IV
Lorazepam 1 mg
Rugby R 57

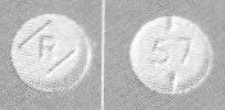

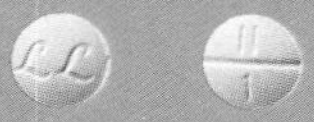

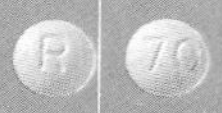

℞
Dipyridamole 25 mg
Rugby R 70

C-II
Demerol HCl 50 mg
Winthrop W D 35

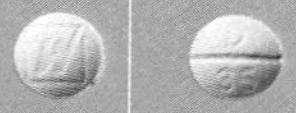

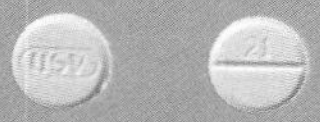

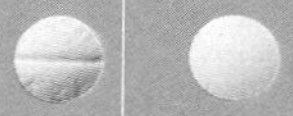

℞
Myleran 2 mg
Burroughs Wellcome K2A

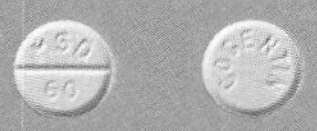

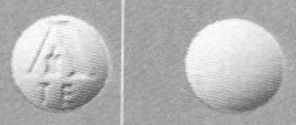

℞
Armour Thyroid 1 gr
Rhone-Poulenc Rorer A TE

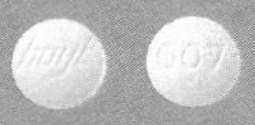

℞
Cogentin 0.5 mg
MSD 21

℞
Proventil 2 mg
Schering 252

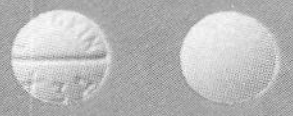

℞
Lanoxin 0.25 mg
Burroughs Wellcome X3A

℞
Neptazane 50 mg
Lederle LL N1

C-IV
Cylert 18.75 mg
Abbott TH

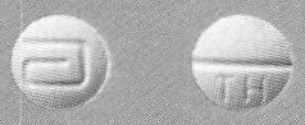

℞
Hygroton 100 mg
Rhone-Poulenc Rorer

℞
Cogentin 2 mg
MSD 60

℞
Luride-SF 1 mg
Colgate-Hoyt 007

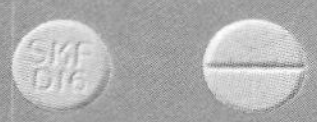

℞
Cytomel 25 mcg
SmithKline Beecham

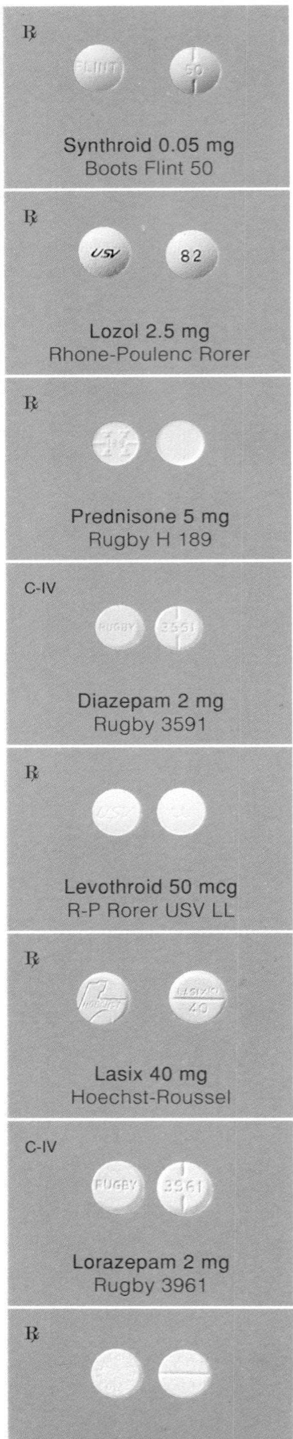

℞
Synthroid 0.05 mg
Boots Flint 50

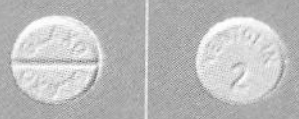

℞
Lozol 2.5 mg
Rhone-Poulenc Rorer

℞
Prednisone 5 mg
Rugby H 189

C-IV
Diazepam 2 mg
Rugby 3591

℞
Levothroid 50 mcg
R-P Rorer USV LL

℞
Lasix 40 mg
Hoechst-Roussel

C-IV
Lorazepam 2 mg
Rugby 3961

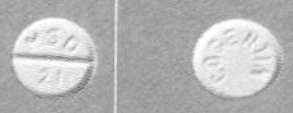

℞
Mysoline 50 mg
Wyeth-Ayerst

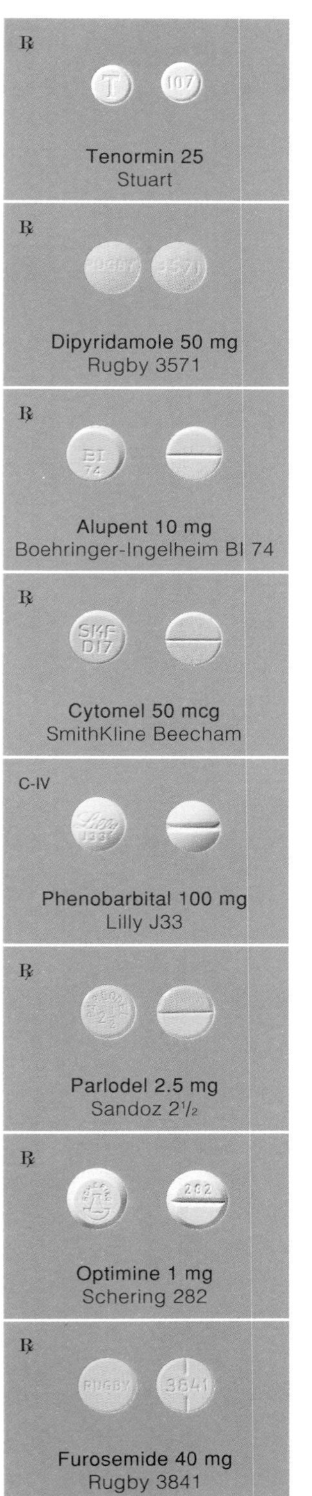

℞
Tenormin 25
Stuart
℞
Dipyridamole 50 mg
Rugby 3571
℞
Alupent 10 mg
Boehringer-Ingelheim BI 74
℞
Cytomel 50 mcg
SmithKline Beecham
C-IV
Phenobarbital 100 mg
Lilly J33
℞
Parlodel 2.5 mg
Sandoz 2½
℞
Optimine 1 mg
Schering 282
℞
Furosemide 40 mg
Rugby 3841

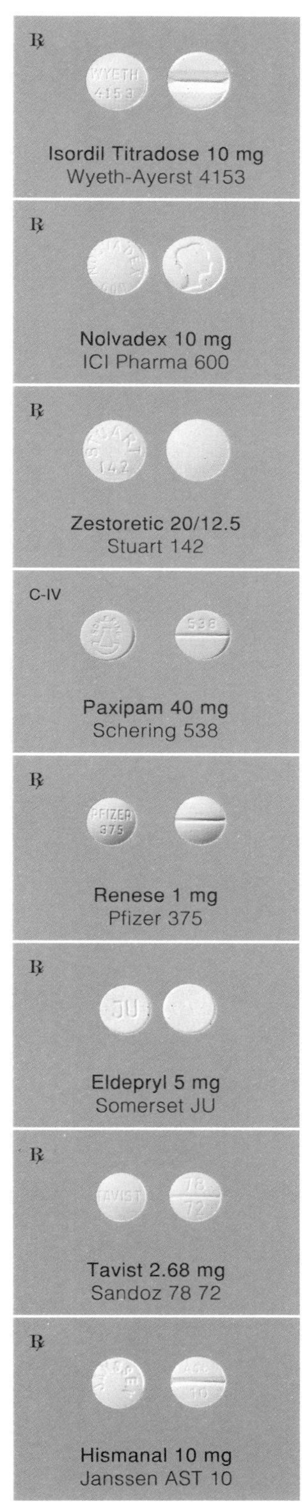

℞
Isordil Titradose 10 mg
Wyeth-Ayerst 4153
℞
Nolvadex 10 mg
ICI Pharma 600
℞
Zestoretic 20/12.5
Stuart 142
C-IV
Paxipam 40 mg
Schering 538
℞
Renese 1 mg
Pfizer 375
℞
Eldepryl 5 mg
Somerset JU
℞
Tavist 2.68 mg
Sandoz 78 72
℞
Hismanal 10 mg
Janssen AST 10

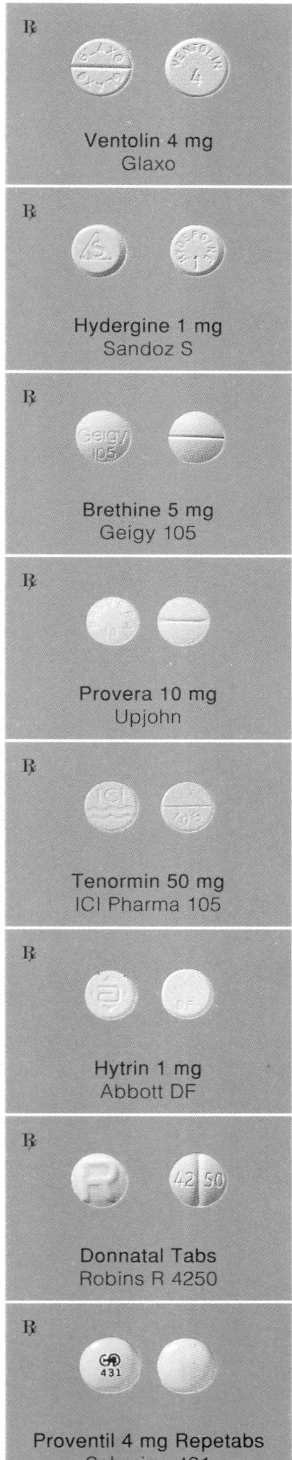

℞
Ventolin 4 mg
Glaxo
℞
Hydergine 1 mg
Sandoz S
℞
Brethine 5 mg
Geigy 105
℞
Provera 10 mg
Upjohn
℞
Tenormin 50 mg
ICI Pharma 105
℞
Hytrin 1 mg
Abbott DF
℞
Donnatal Tabs
Robins R 4250
℞
Proventil 4 mg Repetabs
Schering 431

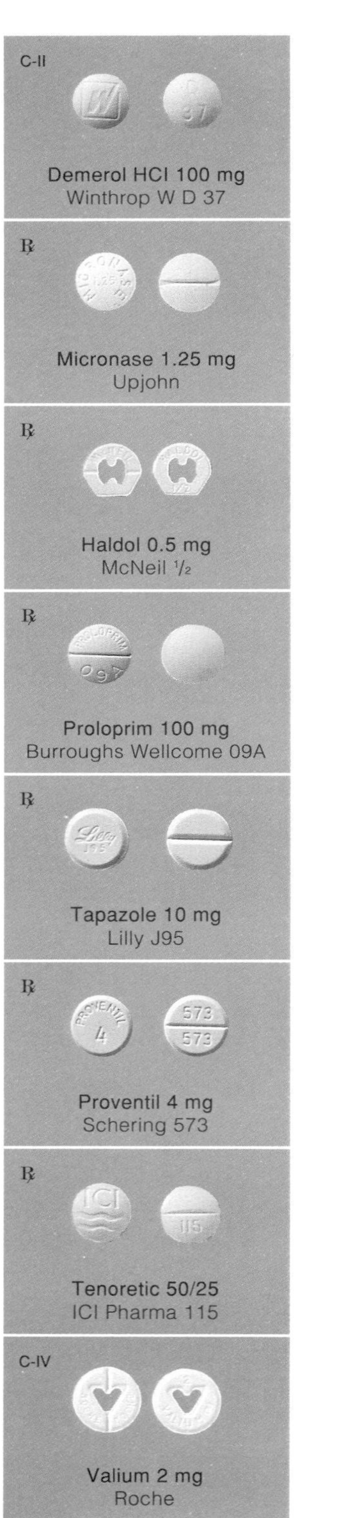

C-II
Demerol HCl 100 mg
Winthrop W D 37

℞
Micronase 1.25 mg
Upjohn

℞
Haldol 0.5 mg
McNeil ½

℞
Proloprim 100 mg
Burroughs Wellcome 09A

℞
Tapazole 10 mg
Lilly J95

℞
Proventil 4 mg
Schering 573

℞
Tenoretic 50/25
ICI Pharma 115

C-IV
Valium 2 mg
Roche

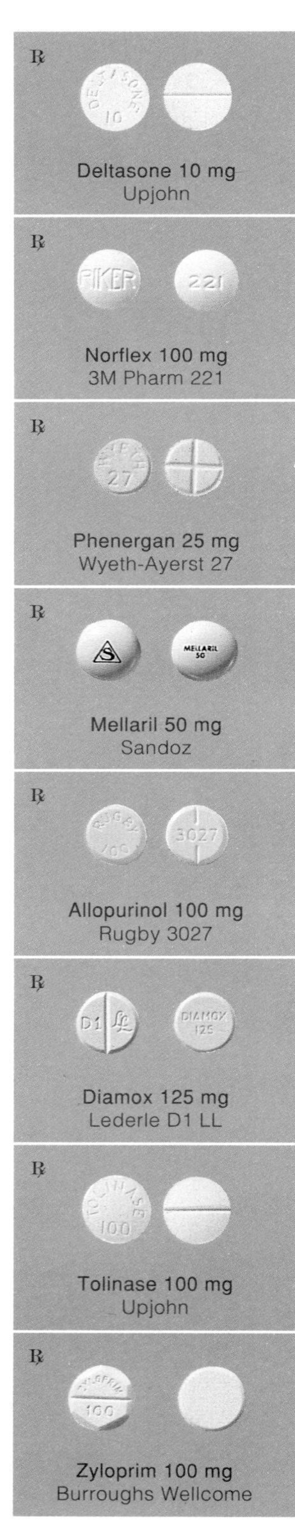

℞
Deltasone 10 mg
Upjohn

℞
Norflex 100 mg
3M Pharm 221

℞
Phenergan 25 mg
Wyeth-Ayerst 27

℞
Mellaril 50 mg
Sandoz

℞
Allopurinol 100 mg
Rugby 3027

℞
Diamox 125 mg
Lederle D1 LL

℞
Tolinase 100 mg
Upjohn

℞
Zyloprim 100 mg
Burroughs Wellcome

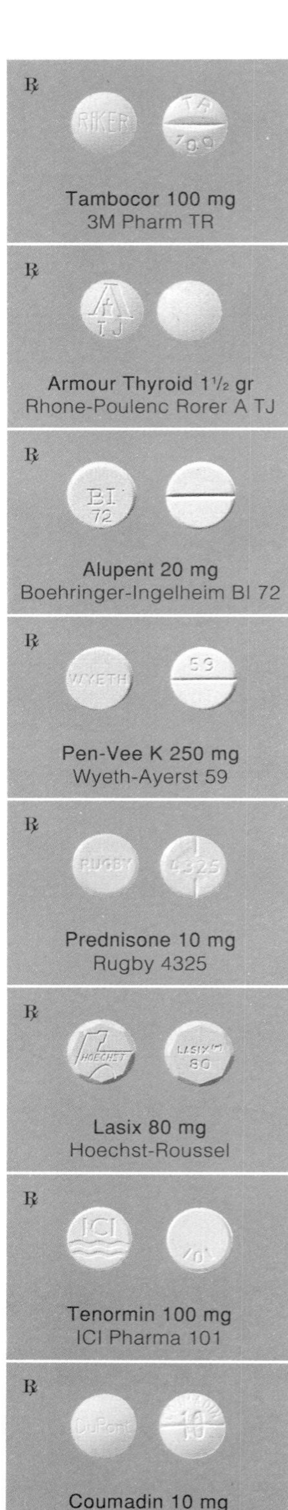

℞
Tambocor 100 mg
3M Pharm TR

℞
Armour Thyroid 1½ gr
Rhone-Poulenc Rorer A TJ

℞
Alupent 20 mg
Boehringer-Ingelheim BI 72

℞
Pen-Vee K 250 mg
Wyeth-Ayerst 59

℞
Prednisone 10 mg
Rugby 4325

℞
Lasix 80 mg
Hoechst-Roussel

℞
Tenormin 100 mg
ICI Pharma 101

℞
Coumadin 10 mg
DuPont

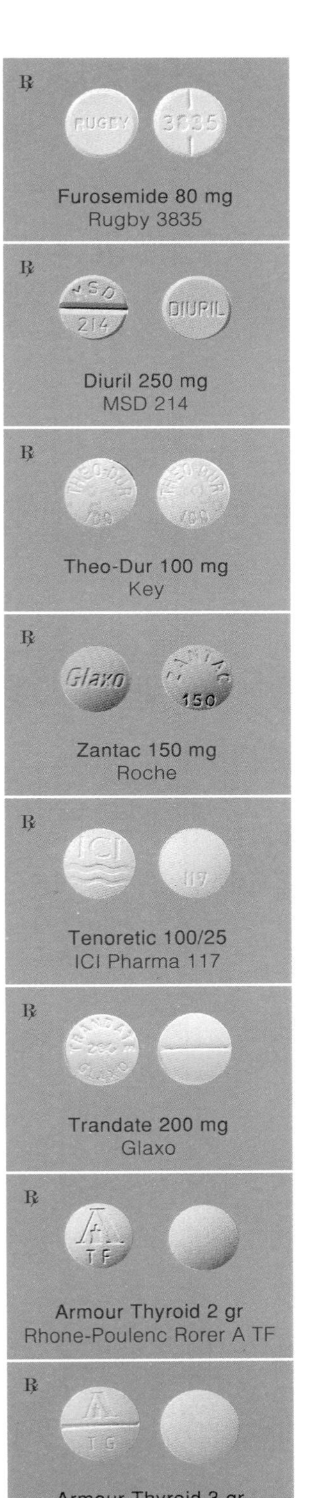

℞ Furosemide 80 mg
Rugby 3835

℞ Diuril 250 mg
MSD 214

℞ Theo-Dur 100 mg
Key

℞ Zantac 150 mg
Roche

℞ Tenoretic 100/25
ICI Pharma 117

℞ Trandate 200 mg
Glaxo

℞ Armour Thyroid 2 gr
Rhone-Poulenc Rorer A TF

℞ Armour Thyroid 3 gr
Rhone-Poulenc Rorer A TG

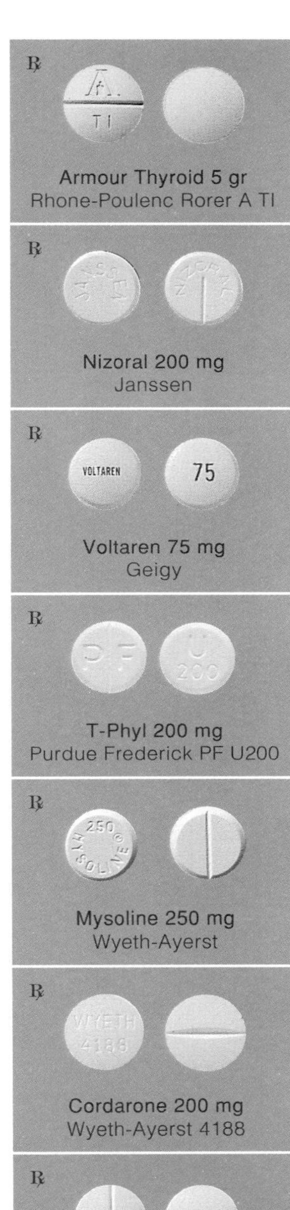

℞ Armour Thyroid 5 gr
Rhone-Poulenc Rorer A TI

℞ Nizoral 200 mg
Janssen

℞ Voltaren 75 mg
Geigy

℞ T-Phyl 200 mg
Purdue Frederick PF U200

℞ Mysoline 250 mg
Wyeth-Ayerst

℞ Cordarone 200 mg
Wyeth-Ayerst 4188

℞ Penicillin V K 250 mg
Mylan M 95

℞ Normodyne 200 mg
Schering 752

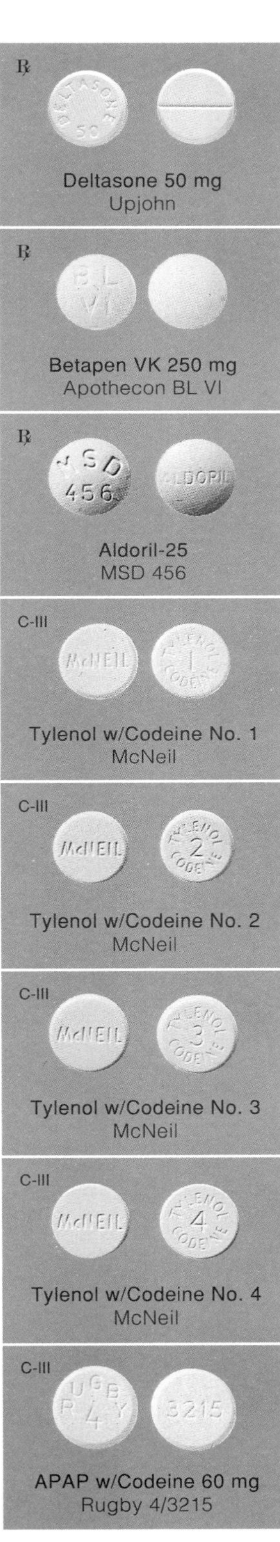

℞ Deltasone 50 mg
Upjohn

℞ Betapen VK 250 mg
Apothecon BL VI

℞ Aldoril-25
MSD 456

C-III Tylenol w/Codeine No. 1
McNeil

C-III Tylenol w/Codeine No. 2
McNeil

C-III Tylenol w/Codeine No. 3
McNeil

C-III Tylenol w/Codeine No. 4
McNeil

C-III APAP w/Codeine 60 mg
Rugby 4/3215

White Round Tablets

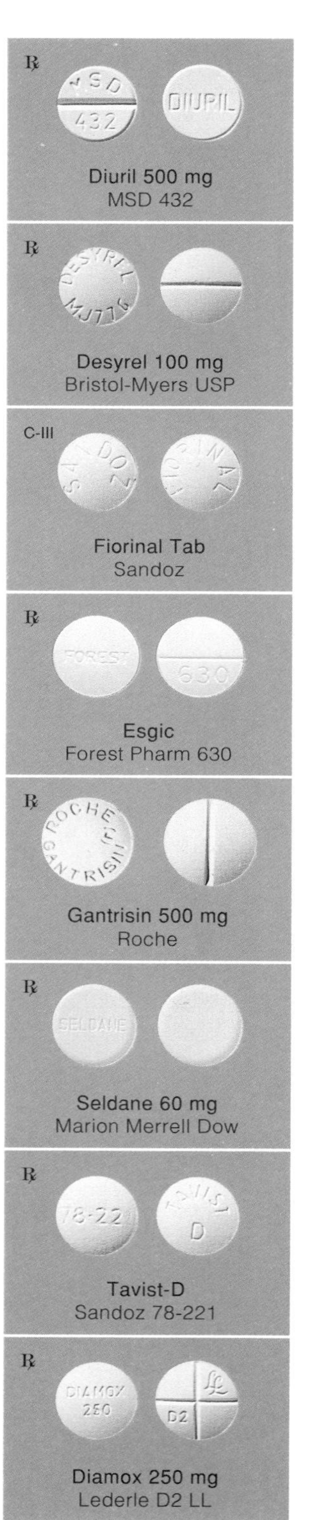

Diuril 500 mg
MSD 432
Desyrel 100 mg
Bristol-Myers USP
C-III
Fiorinal Tab
Sandoz
Esgic
Forest Pharm 630
Gantrisin 500 mg
Roche
Seldane 60 mg
Marion Merrell Dow
Tavist-D
Sandoz 78-221
Diamox 250 mg
Lederle D2 LL

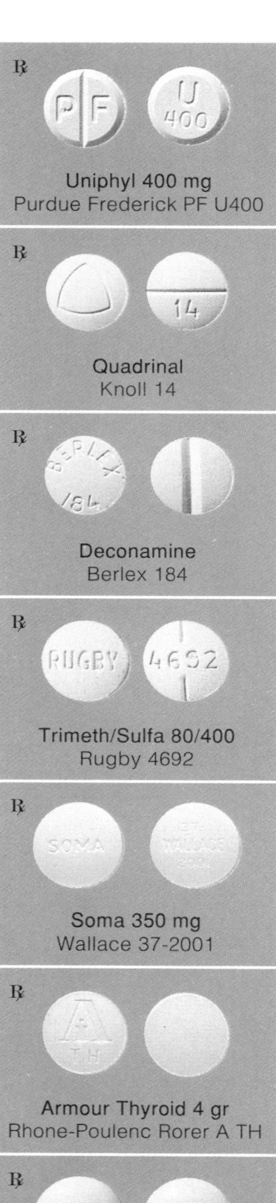

Uniphyl 400 mg
Purdue Frederick PF U400
Quadrinal
Knoll 14
Deconamine
Berlex 184
Trimeth/Sulfa 80/400
Rugby 4692
Soma 350 mg
Wallace 37-2001
Armour Thyroid 4 gr
Rhone-Poulenc Rorer A TH
Motrin 300 mg
Upjohn
C-III
Empirin w/Codeine No. 3
Burroughs Wellcome

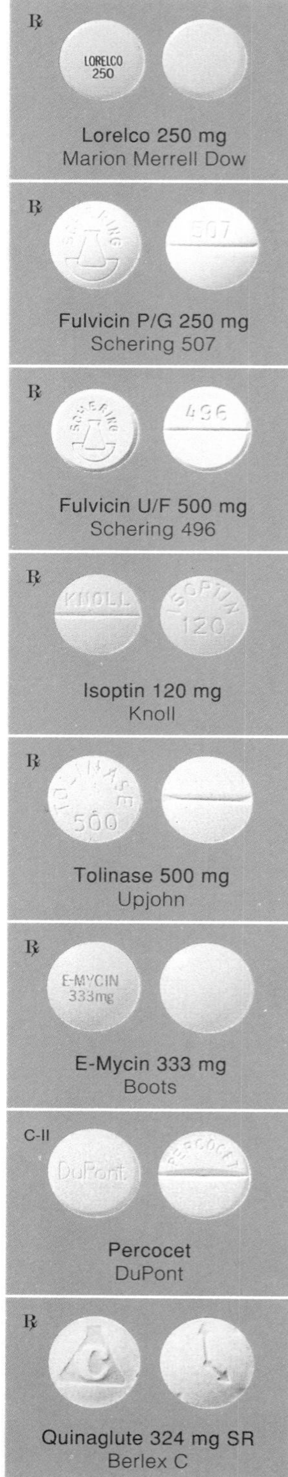

Lorelco 250 mg
Marion Merrell Dow
Fulvicin P/G 250 mg
Schering 507
Fulvicin U/F 500 mg
Schering 496
Isoptin 120 mg
Knoll
Tolinase 500 mg
Upjohn
E-Mycin 333 mg
Boots
C-II
Percocet
DuPont
Quinaglute 324 mg SR
Berlex C

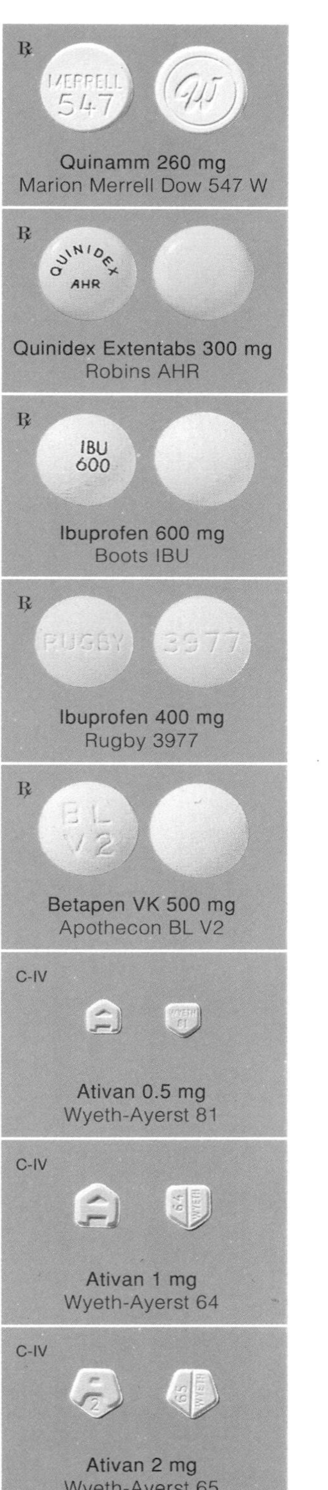

℞
Quinamm 260 mg
Marion Merrell Dow 547 W

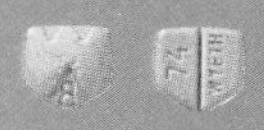

℞
Quinidex Extentabs 300 mg
Robins AHR

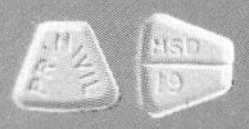

℞
Ibuprofen 600 mg
Boots IBU

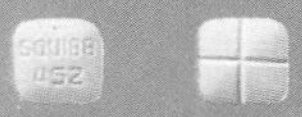

℞
Ibuprofen 400 mg
Rugby 3977

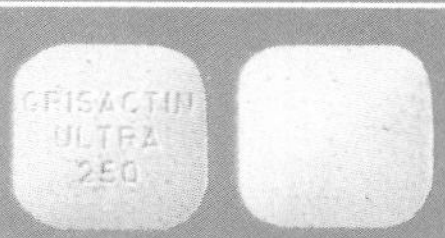

℞
Betapen VK 500 mg
Apothecon BL V2

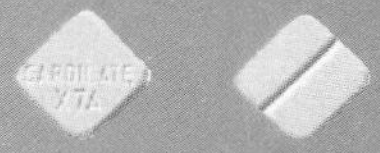

C-IV
Ativan 0.5 mg
Wyeth-Ayerst 81

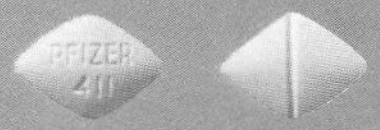

C-IV
Ativan 1 mg
Wyeth-Ayerst 64

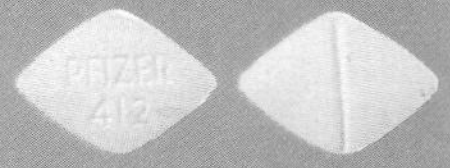

C-IV
Ativan 2 mg
Wyeth-Ayerst 65

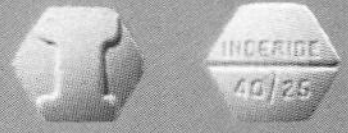

℞
Wytensin 8 mg
Wyeth-Ayerst 74 W

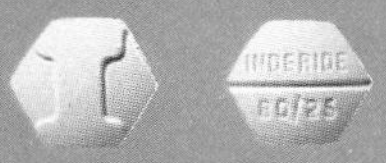

℞
Prinivil 5 mg
MSD 19

℞
Capoten 25 mg
Squibb 452

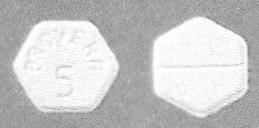

℞
Grisactin Ultra 250 mg
Wyeth-Ayerst

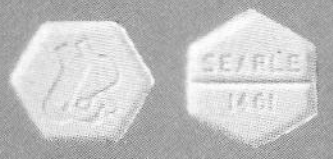

℞
Cardilate 10 mg
Burroughs Wellcome X7A

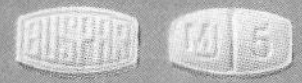

℞
Glucotrol 5 mg
Roerig Pfizer 411

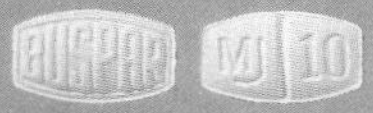

℞
Glucotrol 10 mg
Roerig Pfizer 412

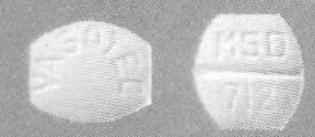

℞
Inderide 40/25
Wyeth-Ayerst

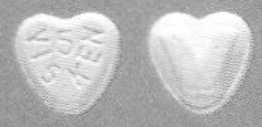

℞
Inderide 80/25
Wyeth-Ayerst

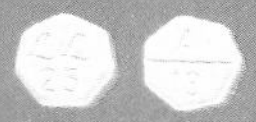

℞
Asendin 25 mg
Lederle LL A13

℞
Provera 5 mg
Upjohn

℞
Cytotec 200 mcg
Searle 1461

℞
BuSpar 5 mg
Bristol-Myers USP

℞
BuSpar 10 mg
Bristol-Myers USP

℞
Vasotec 5 mg
MSD 712

℞
Visken 5 mg
Sandoz

White Odd-Shaped to Oval Tablets

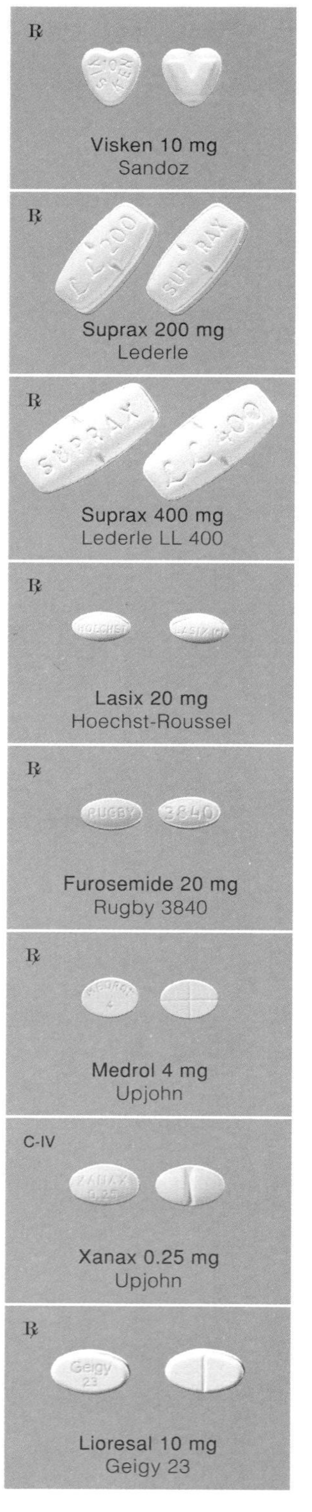

Visken 10 mg
Sandoz

Suprax 200 mg
Lederle

Suprax 400 mg
Lederle LL 400

Lasix 20 mg
Hoechst-Roussel

Furosemide 20 mg
Rugby 3840

Medrol 4 mg
Upjohn

C-IV

Xanax 0.25 mg
Upjohn

Lioresal 10 mg
Geigy 23

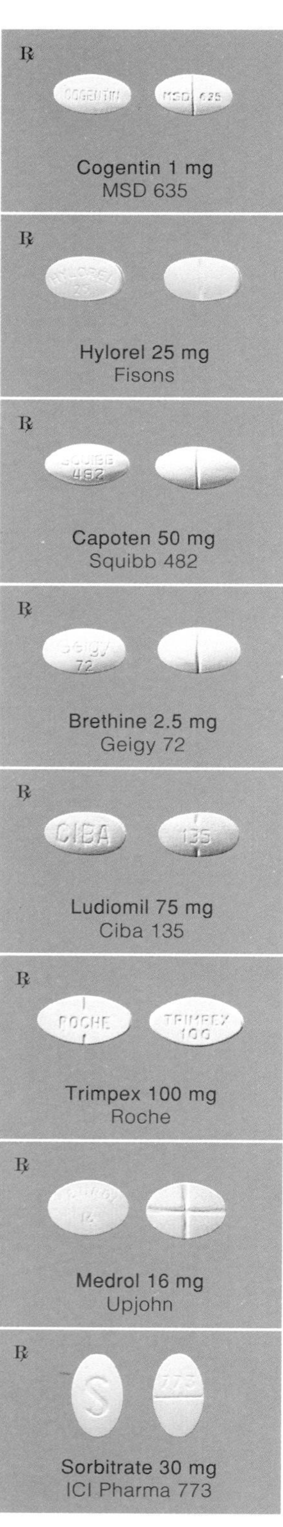

Cogentin 1 mg
MSD 635

Hylorel 25 mg
Fisons

Capoten 50 mg
Squibb 482

Brethine 2.5 mg
Geigy 72

Ludiomil 75 mg
Ciba 135

Trimpex 100 mg
Roche

Medrol 16 mg
Upjohn

Sorbitrate 30 mg
ICI Pharma 773

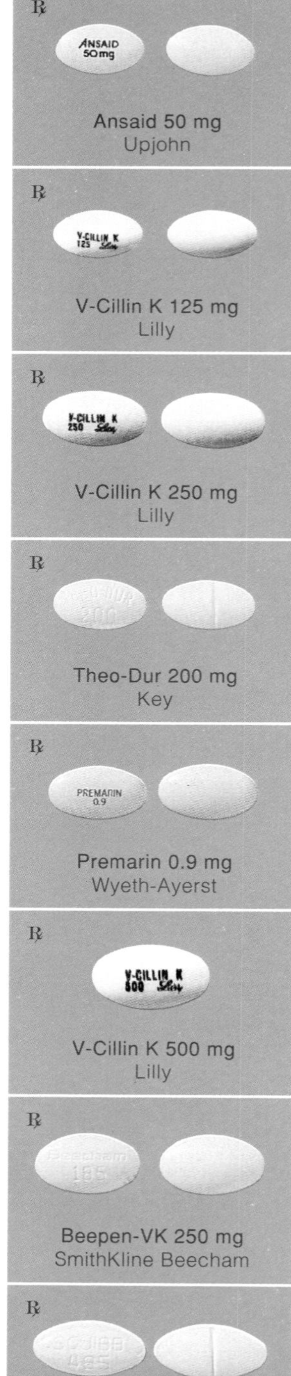

Ansaid 50 mg
Upjohn

V-Cillin K 125 mg
Lilly

V-Cillin K 250 mg
Lilly

Theo-Dur 200 mg
Key

Premarin 0.9 mg
Wyeth-Ayerst

V-Cillin K 500 mg
Lilly

Beepen-VK 250 mg
SmithKline Beecham

Capoten 100 mg
Squibb 485

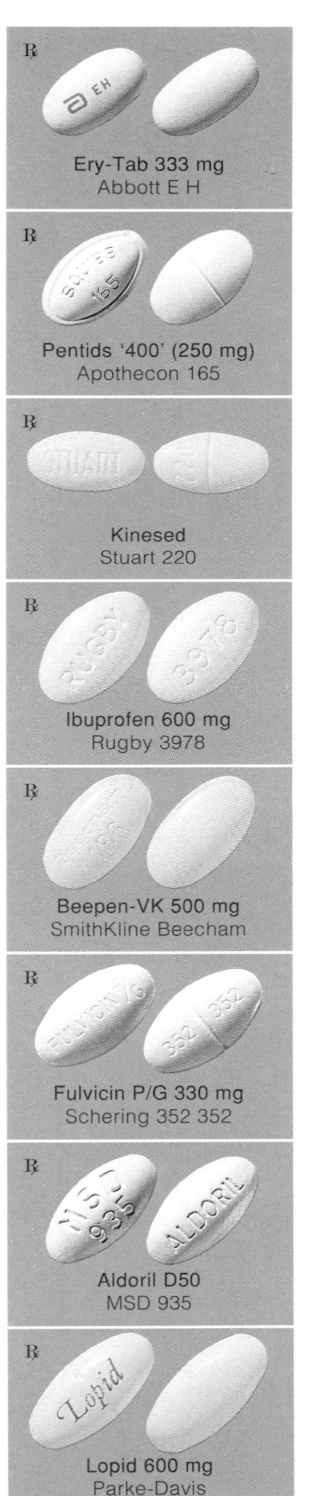

℞ Ery-Tab 333 mg
Abbott E H

℞ Pentids '400' (250 mg)
Apothecon 165

℞ Kinesed
Stuart 220

℞ Ibuprofen 600 mg
Rugby 3978

℞ Beepen-VK 500 mg
SmithKline Beecham

℞ Fulvicin P/G 330 mg
Schering 352 352

℞ Aldoril D50
MSD 935

℞ Lopid 600 mg
Parke-Davis

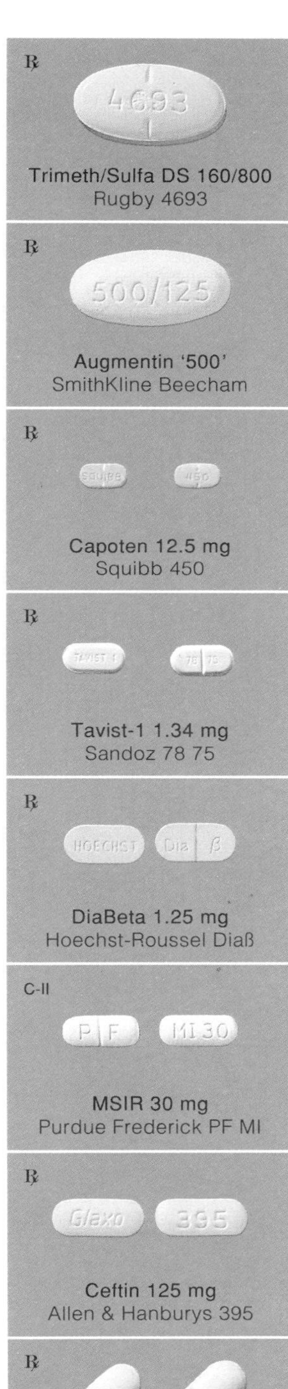

℞ Trimeth/Sulfa DS 160/800
Rugby 4693

℞ Augmentin '500'
SmithKline Beecham

℞ Capoten 12.5 mg
Squibb 450

℞ Tavist-1 1.34 mg
Sandoz 78 75

℞ DiaBeta 1.25 mg
Hoechst-Roussel Diaß

C-II MSIR 30 mg
Purdue Frederick PF MI

℞ Ceftin 125 mg
Allen & Hanburys 395

℞ Dymelor 250 mg
Lilly U03

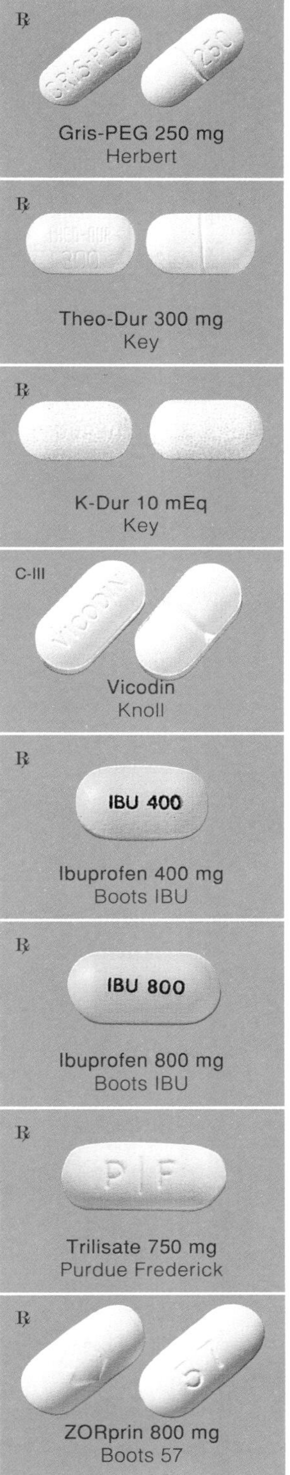

℞ Gris-PEG 250 mg
Herbert

℞ Theo-Dur 300 mg
Key

℞ K-Dur 10 mEq
Key

C-III Vicodin
Knoll

℞ Ibuprofen 400 mg
Boots IBU

℞ Ibuprofen 800 mg
Boots IBU

℞ Trilisate 750 mg
Purdue Frederick

℞ ZORprin 800 mg
Boots 57

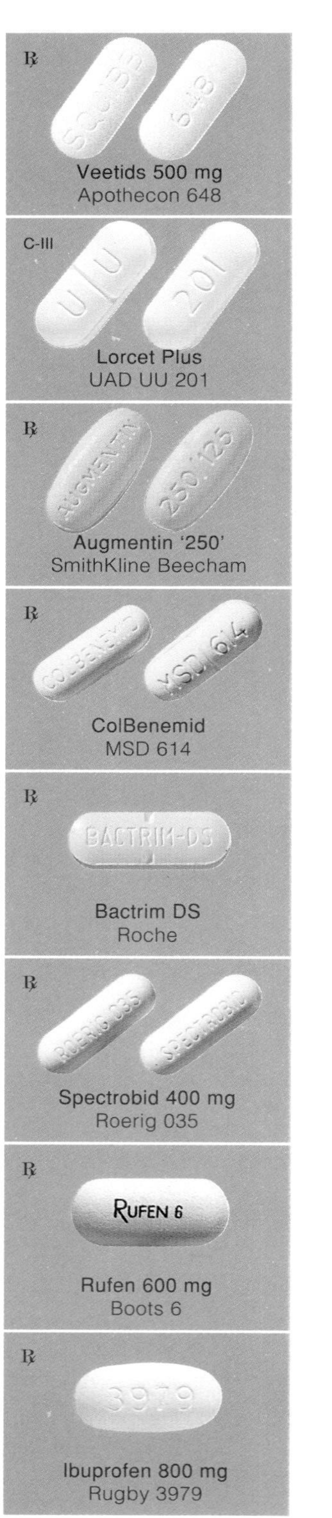

Veetids 500 mg
Apothecon 648

Lorcet Plus
UAD UU 201

Augmentin '250'
SmithKline Beecham

ColBenemid
MSD 614

Bactrim DS
Roche

Spectrobid 400 mg
Roerig 035

Rufen 600 mg
Boots 6

Ibuprofen 800 mg
Rugby 3979

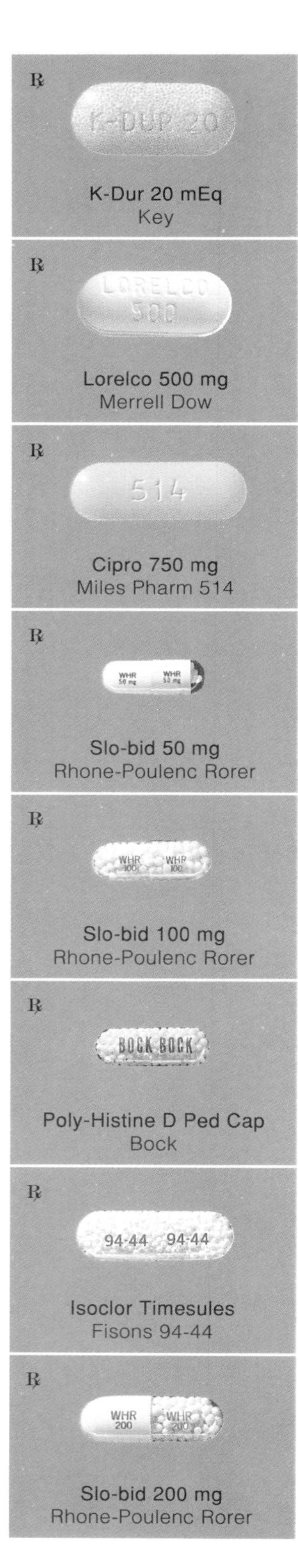

K-Dur 20 mEq
Key

Lorelco 500 mg
Merrell Dow

Cipro 750 mg
Miles Pharm 514

Slo-bid 50 mg
Rhone-Poulenc Rorer

Slo-bid 100 mg
Rhone-Poulenc Rorer

Poly-Histine D Ped Cap
Bock

Isoclor Timesules
Fisons 94-44

Slo-bid 200 mg
Rhone-Poulenc Rorer

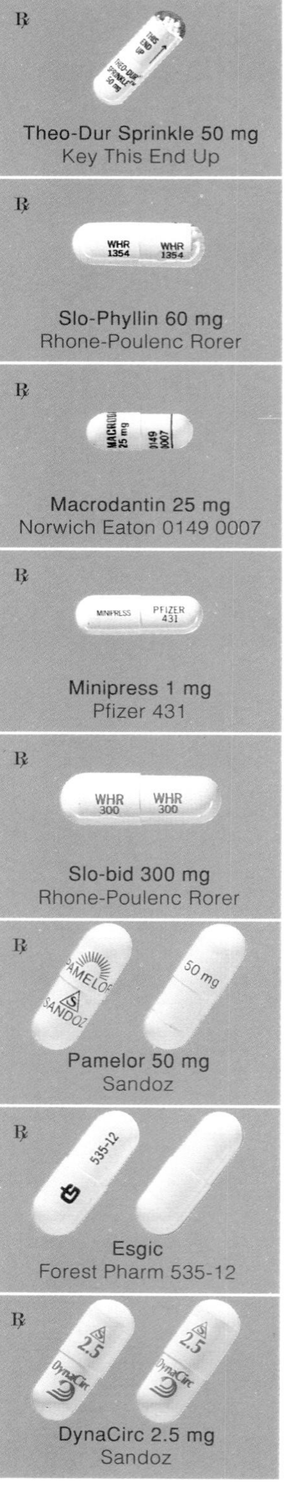

Theo-Dur Sprinkle 50 mg
Key This End Up

Slo-Phyllin 60 mg
Rhone-Poulenc Rorer

Macrodantin 25 mg
Norwich Eaton 0149 0007

Minipress 1 mg
Pfizer 431

Slo-bid 300 mg
Rhone-Poulenc Rorer

Pamelor 50 mg
Sandoz

Esgic
Forest Pharm 535-12

DynaCirc 2.5 mg
Sandoz

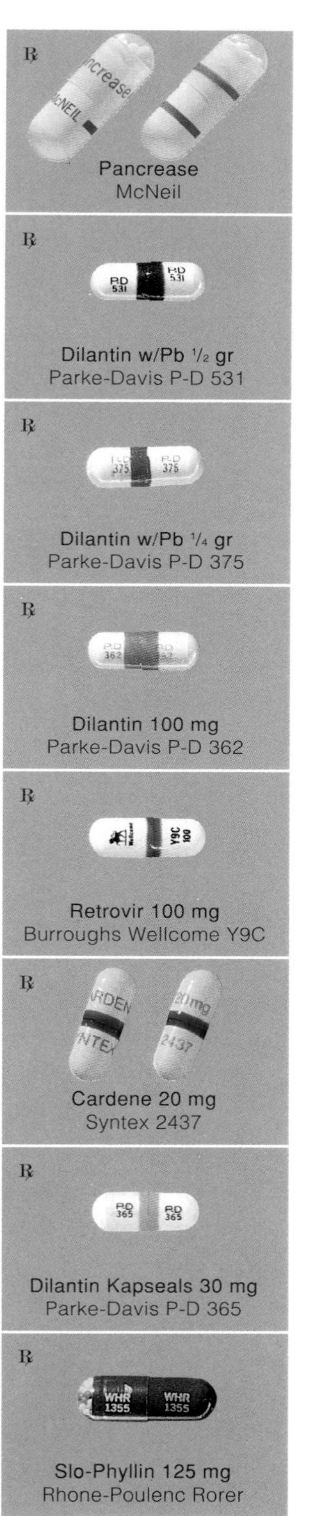

℞ Pancrease
McNeil

℞ Dilantin w/Pb 1/2 gr
Parke-Davis P-D 531

℞ Dilantin w/Pb 1/4 gr
Parke-Davis P-D 375

℞ Dilantin 100 mg
Parke-Davis P-D 362

℞ Retrovir 100 mg
Burroughs Wellcome Y9C

℞ Cardene 20 mg
Syntex 2437

℞ Dilantin Kapseals 30 mg
Parke-Davis P-D 365

℞ Slo-Phyllin 125 mg
Rhone-Poulenc Rorer

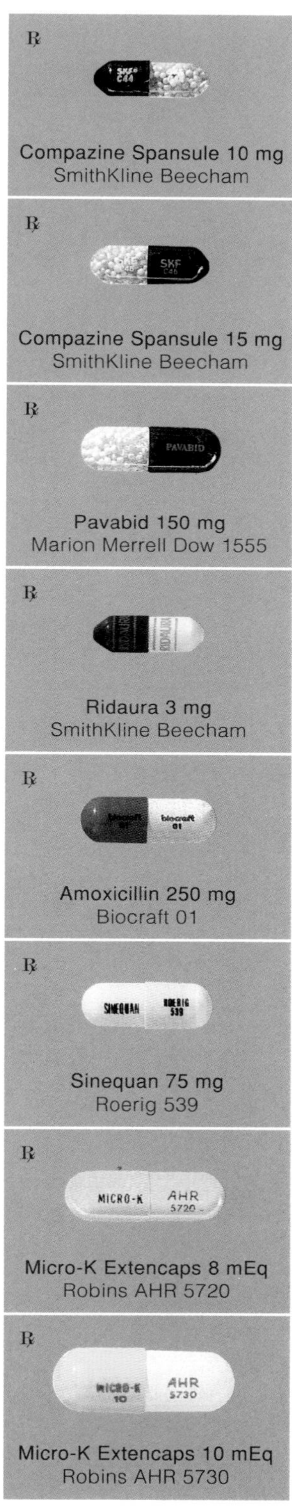

℞ Compazine Spansule 10 mg
SmithKline Beecham

℞ Compazine Spansule 15 mg
SmithKline Beecham

℞ Pavabid 150 mg
Marion Merrell Dow 1555

℞ Ridaura 3 mg
SmithKline Beecham

℞ Amoxicillin 250 mg
Biocraft 01

℞ Sinequan 75 mg
Roerig 539

℞ Micro-K Extencaps 8 mEq
Robins AHR 5720

℞ Micro-K Extencaps 10 mEq
Robins AHR 5730

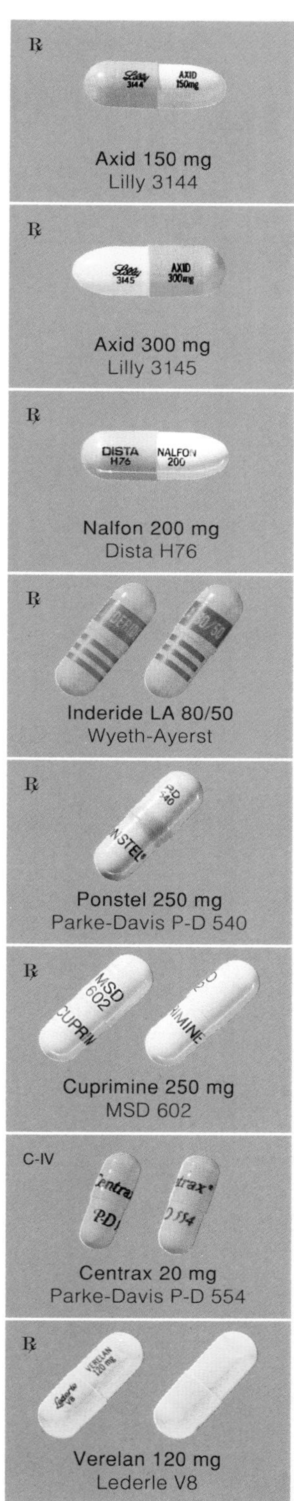

℞ Axid 150 mg
Lilly 3144

℞ Axid 300 mg
Lilly 3145

℞ Nalfon 200 mg
Dista H76

℞ Inderide LA 80/50
Wyeth-Ayerst

℞ Ponstel 250 mg
Parke-Davis P-D 540

℞ Cuprimine 250 mg
MSD 602

C-IV Centrax 20 mg
Parke-Davis P-D 554

℞ Verelan 120 mg
Lederle V8

Yellow to Green Capsules

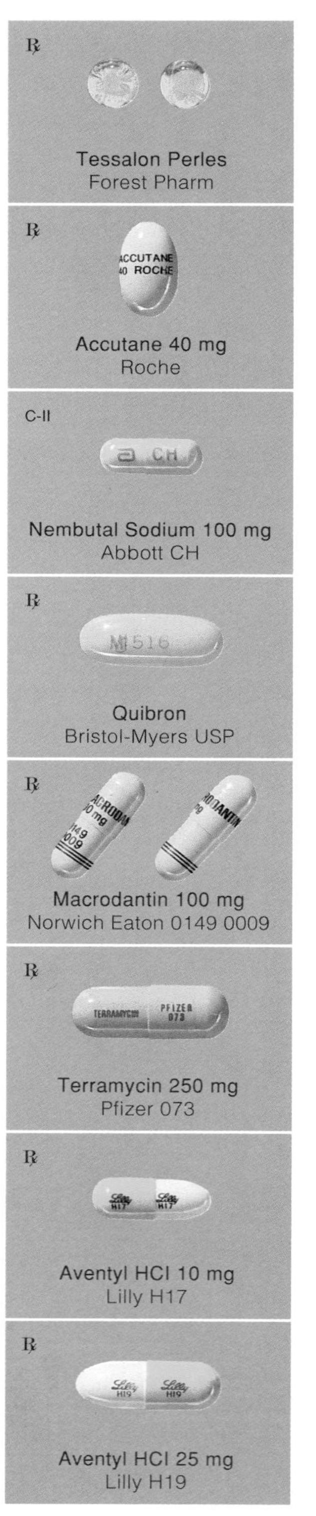

℞
Tessalon Perles
Forest Pharm

℞
Accutane 40 mg
Roche

C-II
Nembutal Sodium 100 mg
Abbott CH

℞
Quibron
Bristol-Myers USP

℞
Macrodantin 100 mg
Norwich Eaton 0149 0009

℞
Terramycin 250 mg
Pfizer 073

℞
Aventyl HCl 10 mg
Lilly H17

℞
Aventyl HCl 25 mg
Lilly H19

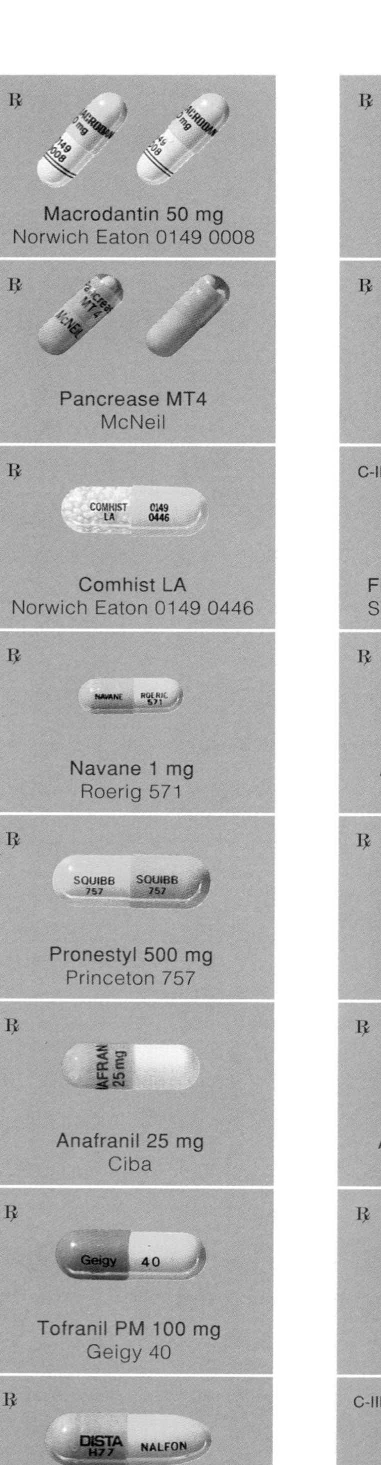

℞
Macrodantin 50 mg
Norwich Eaton 0149 0008

℞
Pancrease MT4
McNeil

℞
Comhist LA
Norwich Eaton 0149 0446

℞
Navane 1 mg
Roerig 571

℞
Pronestyl 500 mg
Princeton 757

℞
Anafranil 25 mg
Ciba

℞
Tofranil PM 100 mg
Geigy 40

℞
Nalfon 300 mg
Dista H77

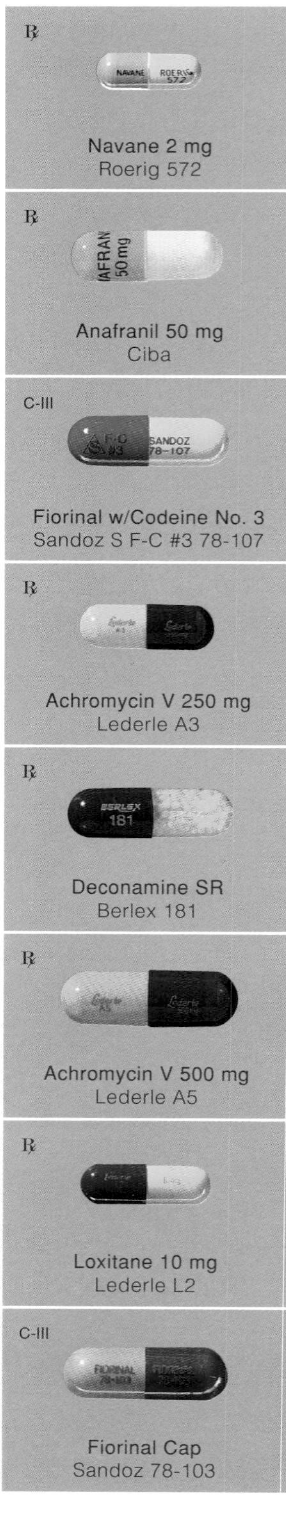

℞
Navane 2 mg
Roerig 572

℞
Anafranil 50 mg
Ciba

C-III
Fiorinal w/Codeine No. 3
Sandoz S F-C #3 78-107

℞
Achromycin V 250 mg
Lederle A3

℞
Deconamine SR
Berlex 181

℞
Achromycin V 500 mg
Lederle A5

℞
Loxitane 10 mg
Lederle L2

C-III
Fiorinal Cap
Sandoz 78-103

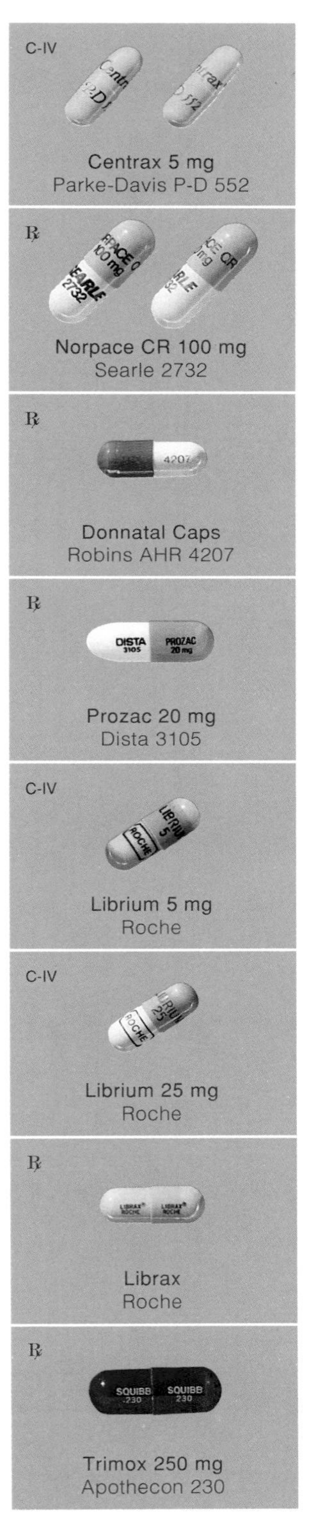

C-IV
Centrax 5 mg
Parke-Davis P-D 552

℞
Norpace CR 100 mg
Searle 2732

℞
Donnatal Caps
Robins AHR 4207

℞
Prozac 20 mg
Dista 3105

C-IV
Librium 5 mg
Roche

C-IV
Librium 25 mg
Roche

℞
Librax
Roche

℞
Trimox 250 mg
Apothecon 230

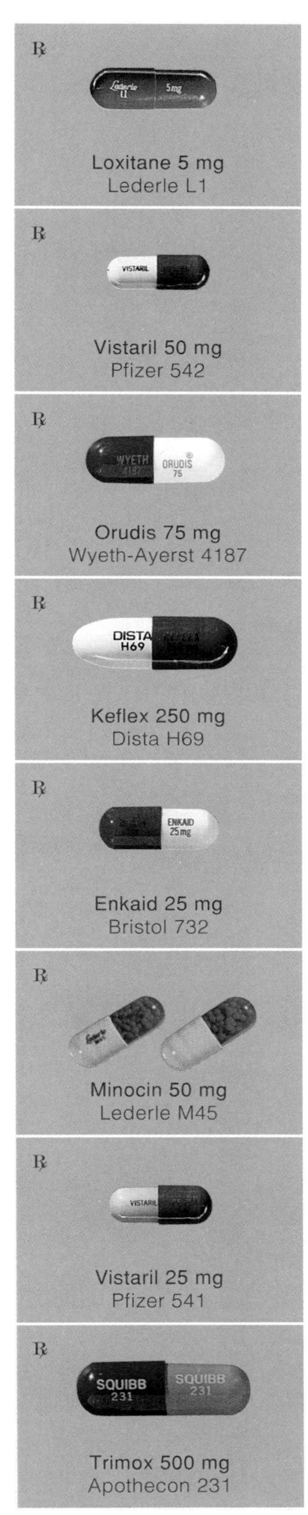

℞
Loxitane 5 mg
Lederle L1

℞
Vistaril 50 mg
Pfizer 542

℞
Orudis 75 mg
Wyeth-Ayerst 4187

℞
Keflex 250 mg
Dista H69

℞
Enkaid 25 mg
Bristol 732

℞
Minocin 50 mg
Lederle M45

℞
Vistaril 25 mg
Pfizer 541

℞
Trimox 500 mg
Apothecon 231

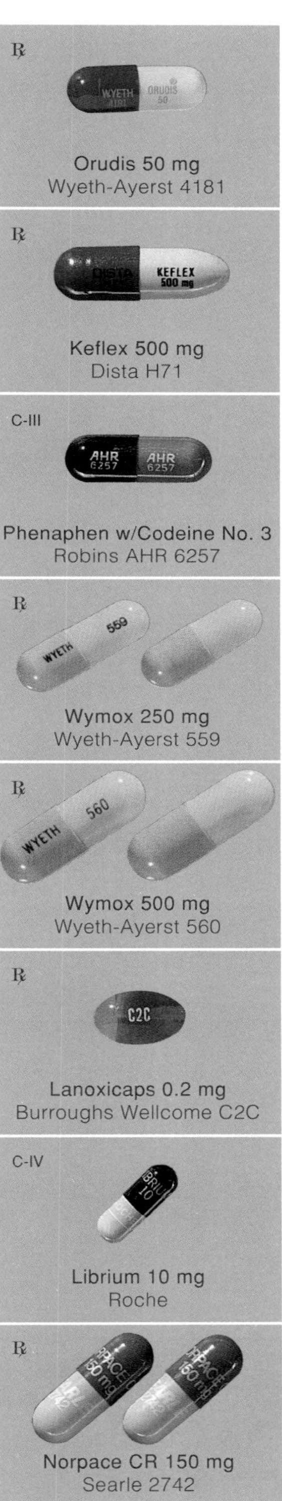

℞
Orudis 50 mg
Wyeth-Ayerst 4181

℞
Keflex 500 mg
Dista H71

C-III
Phenaphen w/Codeine No. 3
Robins AHR 6257

℞
Wymox 250 mg
Wyeth-Ayerst 559

℞
Wymox 500 mg
Wyeth-Ayerst 560

℞
Lanoxicaps 0.2 mg
Burroughs Wellcome C2C

C-IV
Librium 10 mg
Roche

℞
Norpace CR 150 mg
Searle 2742

Green to Blue Capsules

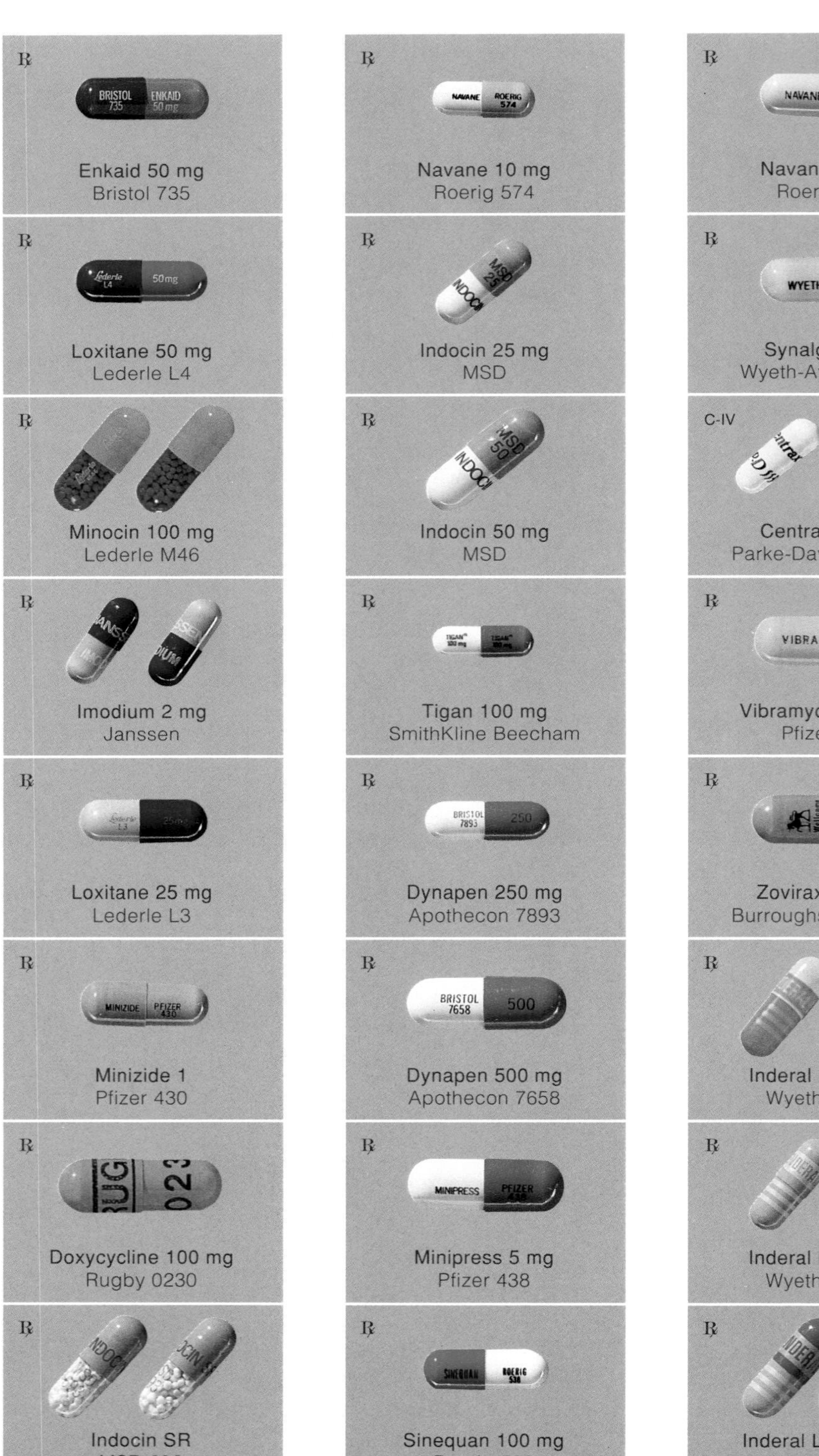

℞ Enkaid 50 mg Bristol 735	℞ Navane 10 mg Roerig 574	℞ Navane 20 mg Roerig 577
℞ Loxitane 50 mg Lederle L4	℞ Indocin 25 mg MSD	℞ Synalgos D-C Wyeth-Ayerst 4191
℞ Minocin 100 mg Lederle M46	℞ Indocin 50 mg MSD	C-IV Centrax 10 mg Parke-Davis P-D 553
℞ Imodium 2 mg Janssen	℞ Tigan 100 mg SmithKline Beecham	℞ Vibramycin 100 mg Pfizer 095
℞ Loxitane 25 mg Lederle L3	℞ Dynapen 250 mg Apothecon 7893	℞ Zovirax 200 mg Burroughs Wellcome
℞ Minizide 1 Pfizer 430	℞ Dynapen 500 mg Apothecon 7658	℞ Inderal LA 60 mg Wyeth-Ayerst
℞ Doxycycline 100 mg Rugby 0230	℞ Minipress 5 mg Pfizer 438	℞ Inderal LA 80 mg Wyeth-Ayerst
℞ Indocin SR MSD 693	℞ Sinequan 100 mg Roerig 538	℞ Inderal LA 120 mg Wyeth-Ayerst

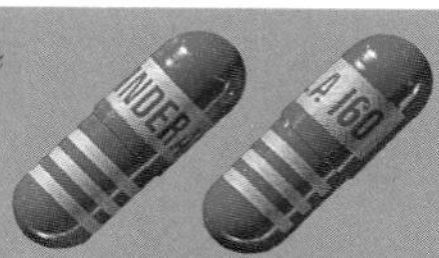

℞
Inderal LA 160 mg
Wyeth-Ayerst

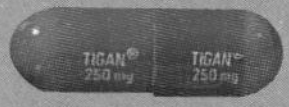

℞
Tigan 250 mg
SmithKline Beecham

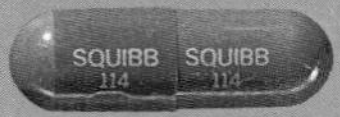

℞
Velosef 500 mg
Apothecon 114

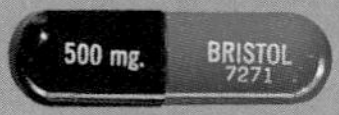

℞
Ultracef 500 mg
Bristol 7271

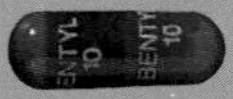

℞
Bentyl 10 mg
Marion Merrell Dow

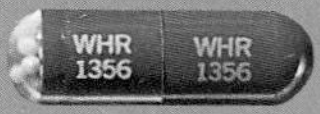

℞
Slo-Phyllin 250 mg
Rhone-Poulenc Rorer

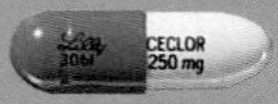

℞
Ceclor 250 mg
Lilly 3061

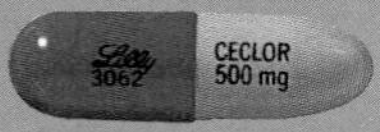

℞
Ceclor 500 mg
Lilly 3062

C-II 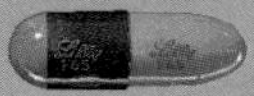
Tuinal 100 mg
Lilly F65

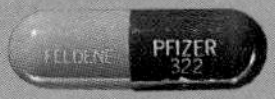

℞
Feldene 10 mg
Pfizer 322

C-IV 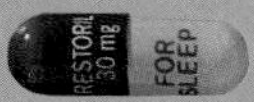
Restoril 30 mg
Sandoz For Sleep

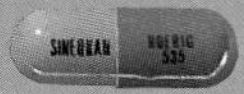

℞
Sinequan 25 mg
Roerig 535

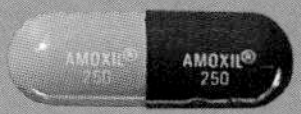

℞
Amoxil 250 mg
SmithKline Beecham

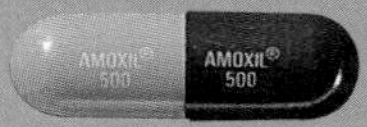

℞
Amoxil 500 mg
SmithKline Beecham

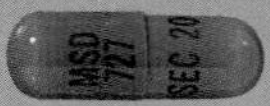

℞
Prilosec 20 mg
MSD 727

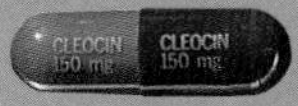

℞
Cleocin HCl 150 mg
Upjohn

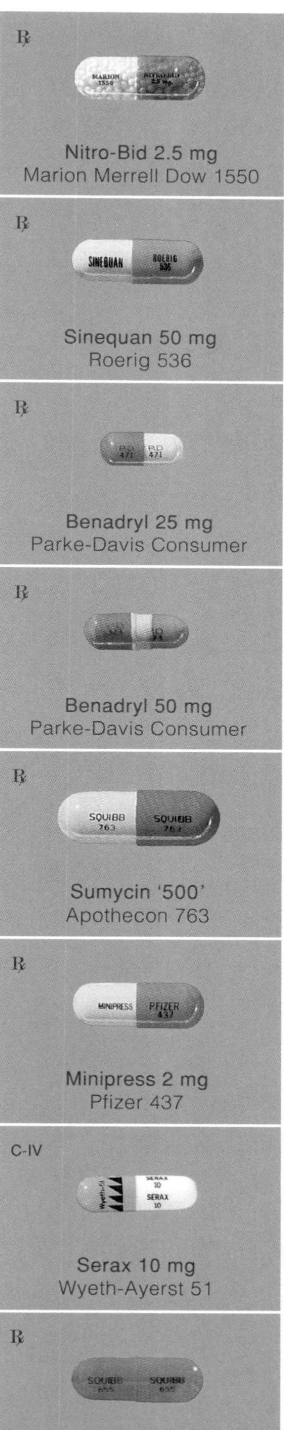

℞
Nitro-Bid 2.5 mg
Marion Merrell Dow 1550

℞
Sinequan 50 mg
Roerig 536

℞
Benadryl 25 mg
Parke-Davis Consumer

℞
Benadryl 50 mg
Parke-Davis Consumer

℞
Sumycin '500'
Apothecon 763

℞
Minipress 2 mg
Pfizer 437

C-IV
Serax 10 mg
Wyeth-Ayerst 51

℞
Sumycin 250 mg
Apothecon 655

Pink to Red Capsules

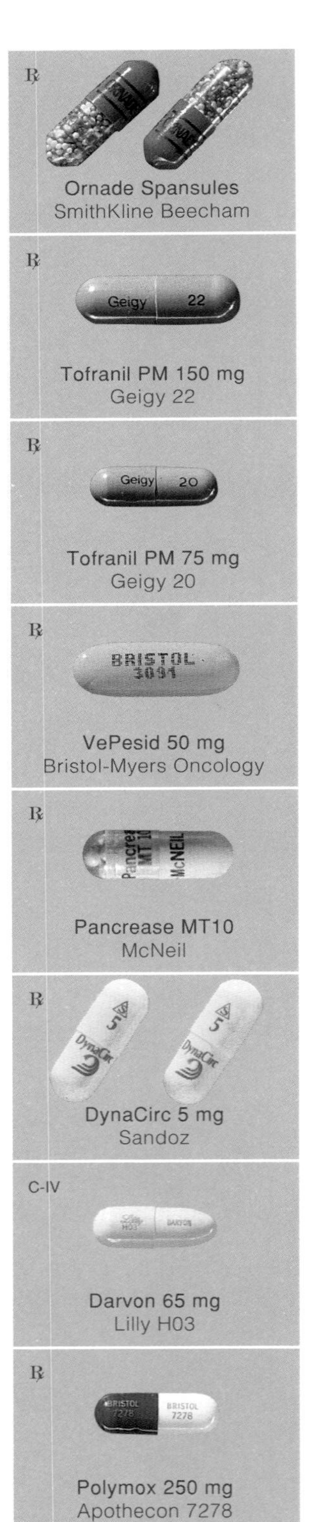

℞
Ornade Spansules
SmithKline Beecham

℞
Tofranil PM 150 mg
Geigy 22

℞
Tofranil PM 75 mg
Geigy 20

℞
VePesid 50 mg
Bristol-Myers Oncology

℞
Pancrease MT10
McNeil

℞
DynaCirc 5 mg
Sandoz

C-IV
Darvon 65 mg
Lilly H03

℞
Polymox 250 mg
Apothecon 7278

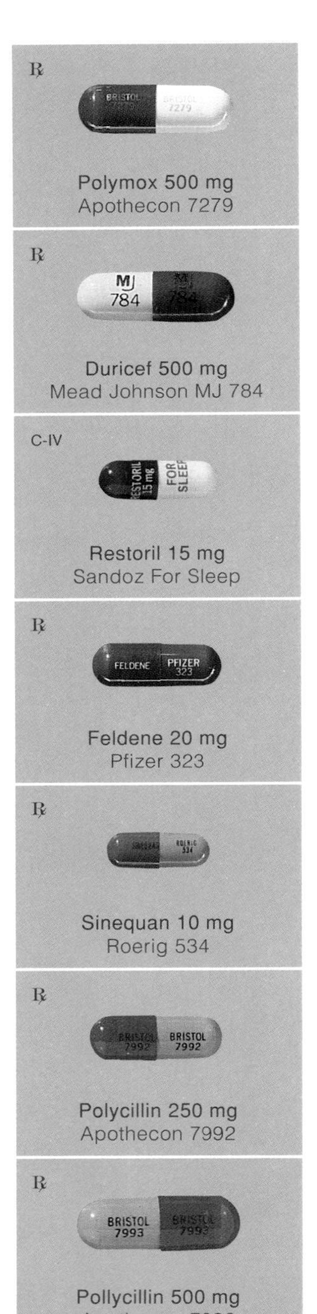

℞
Polymox 500 mg
Apothecon 7279

℞
Duricef 500 mg
Mead Johnson MJ 784

C-IV
Restoril 15 mg
Sandoz For Sleep

℞
Feldene 20 mg
Pfizer 323

℞
Sinequan 10 mg
Roerig 534

℞
Polycillin 250 mg
Apothecon 7992

℞
Pollycillin 500 mg
Apothecon 7993

℞
Lodine 200 mg
Wyeth-Ayerst

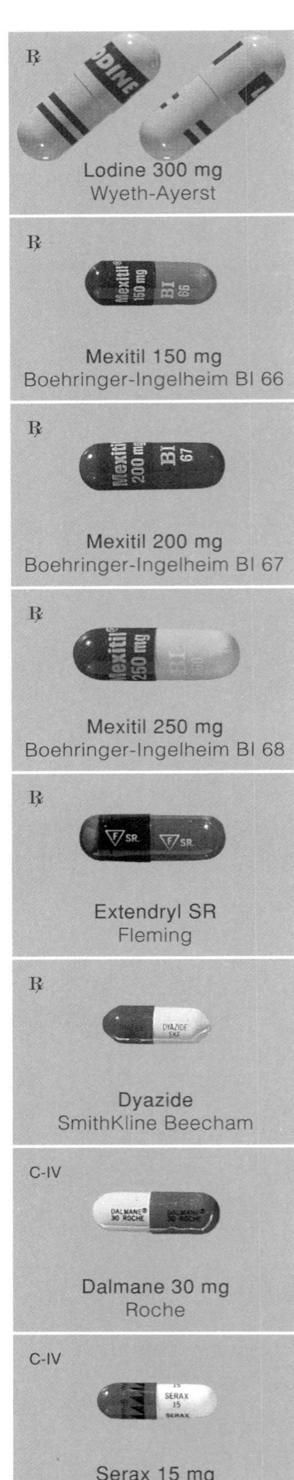

℞
Lodine 300 mg
Wyeth-Ayerst

℞
Mexitil 150 mg
Boehringer-Ingelheim BI 66

℞
Mexitil 200 mg
Boehringer-Ingelheim BI 67

℞
Mexitil 250 mg
Boehringer-Ingelheim BI 68

℞
Extendryl SR
Fleming

℞
Dyazide
SmithKline Beecham

C-IV
Dalmane 30 mg
Roche

C-IV
Serax 15 mg
Wyeth-Ayerst 6

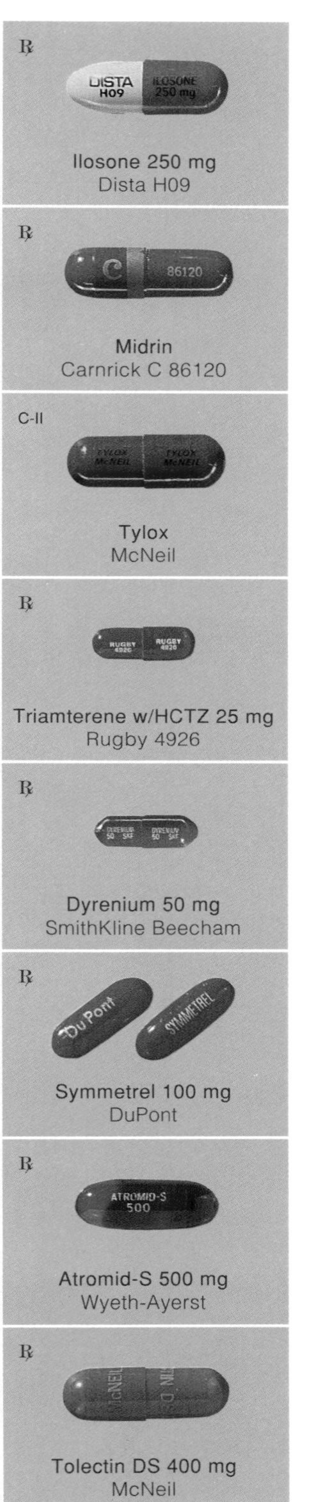

℞ Ilosone 250 mg
Dista H09

℞ Midrin
Carnrick C 86120

C-II Tylox
McNeil

℞ Triamterene w/HCTZ 25 mg
Rugby 4926

℞ Dyrenium 50 mg
SmithKline Beecham

℞ Symmetrel 100 mg
DuPont

℞ Atromid-S 500 mg
Wyeth-Ayerst

℞ Tolectin DS 400 mg
McNeil

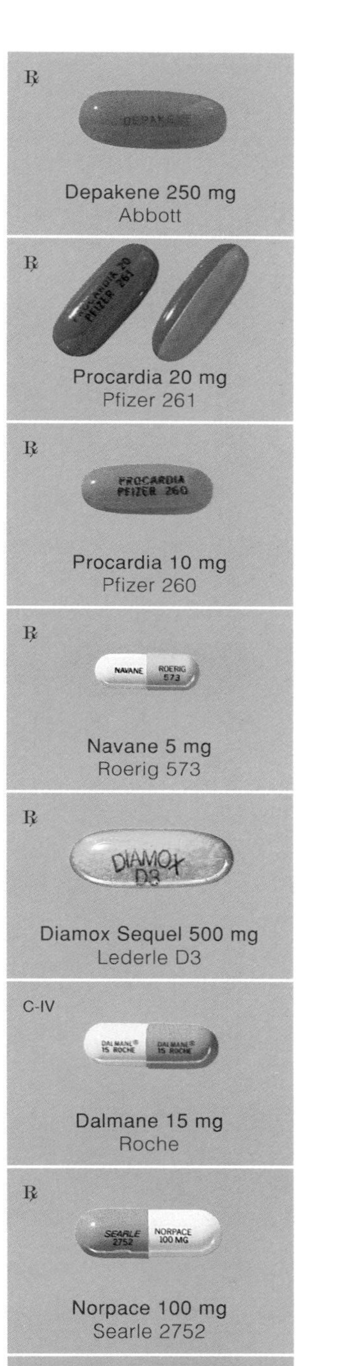

℞ Depakene 250 mg
Abbott

℞ Procardia 20 mg
Pfizer 261

℞ Procardia 10 mg
Pfizer 260

℞ Navane 5 mg
Roerig 573

℞ Diamox Sequel 500 mg
Lederle D3

C-IV Dalmane 15 mg
Roche

℞ Norpace 100 mg
Searle 2752

℞ Entex
Norwich Eaton 0149 0412

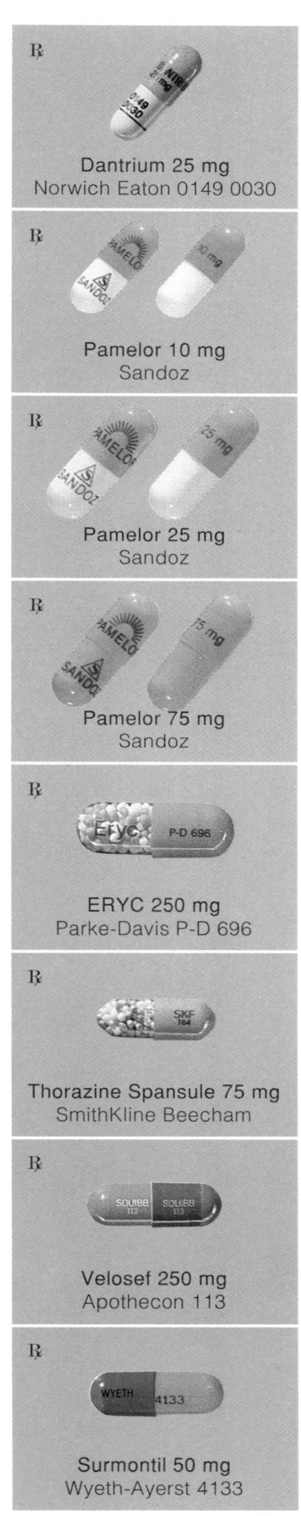

℞ Dantrium 25 mg
Norwich Eaton 0149 0030

℞ Pamelor 10 mg
Sandoz

℞ Pamelor 25 mg
Sandoz

℞ Pamelor 75 mg
Sandoz

℞ ERYC 250 mg
Parke-Davis P-D 696

℞ Thorazine Spansule 75 mg
SmithKline Beecham

℞ Velosef 250 mg
Apothecon 113

℞ Surmontil 50 mg
Wyeth-Ayerst 4133

Orange to Brown Capsules

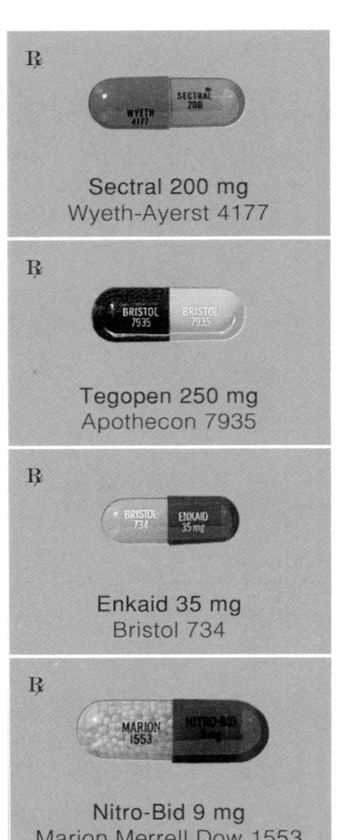

Sectral 200 mg
Wyeth-Ayerst 4177

Tegopen 250 mg
Apothecon 7935

Enkaid 35 mg
Bristol 734

Nitro-Bid 9 mg
Marion Merrell Dow 1553

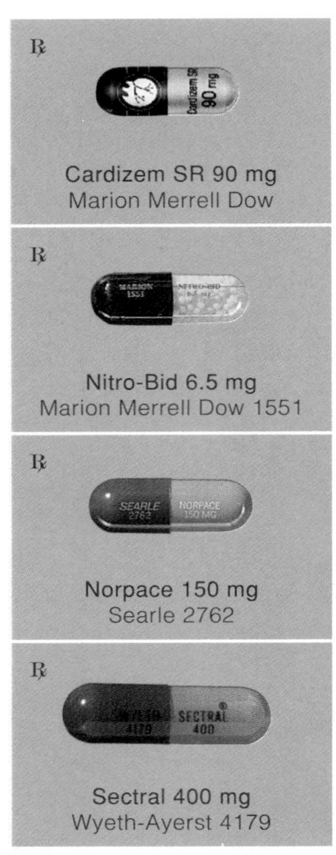

Cardizem SR 90 mg
Marion Merrell Dow

Nitro-Bid 6.5 mg
Marion Merrell Dow 1551

Norpace 150 mg
Searle 2762

Sectral 400 mg
Wyeth-Ayerst 4179

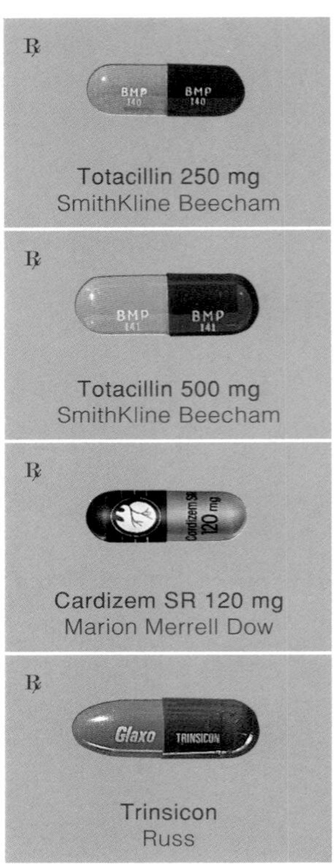

Totacillin 250 mg
SmithKline Beecham

Totacillin 500 mg
SmithKline Beecham

Cardizem SR 120 mg
Marion Merrell Dow

Trinsicon
Russ

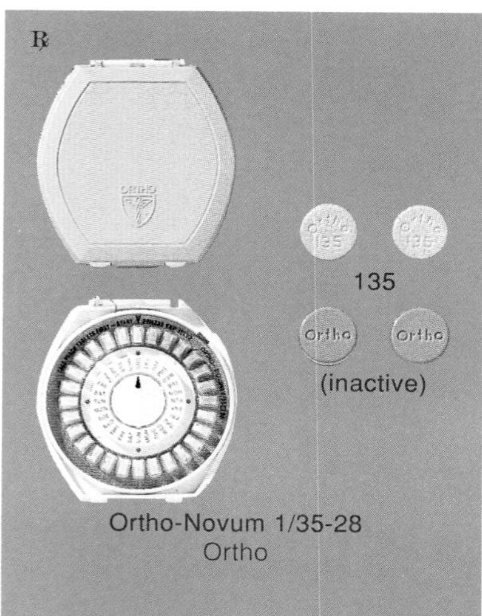

Ortho-Novum 1/35-28
Ortho

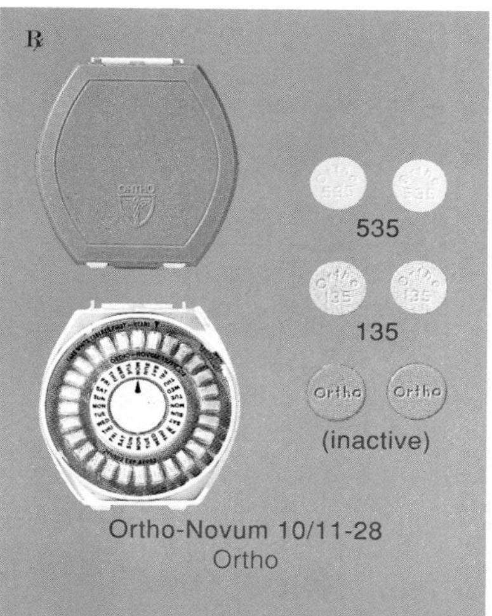

Ortho-Novum 10/11-28
Ortho

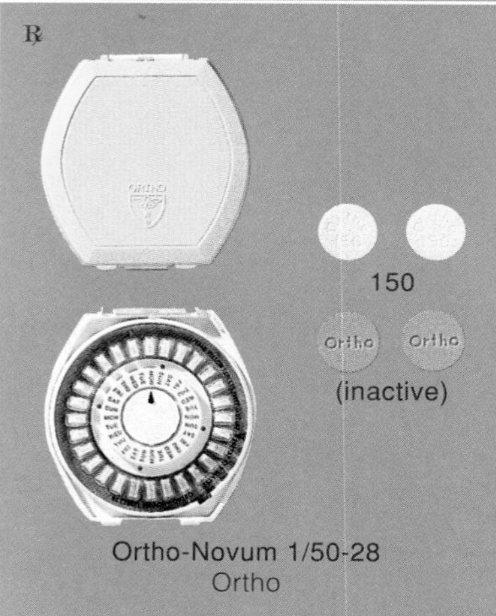

Ortho-Novum 1/50-28
Ortho

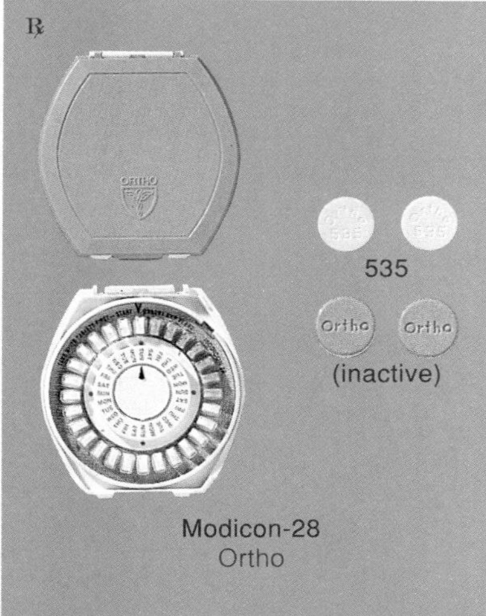

Modicon-28
Ortho

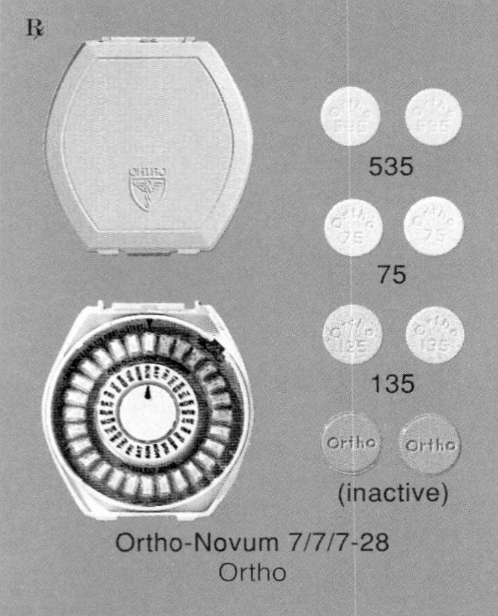

Ortho-Novum 7/7/7-28
Ortho

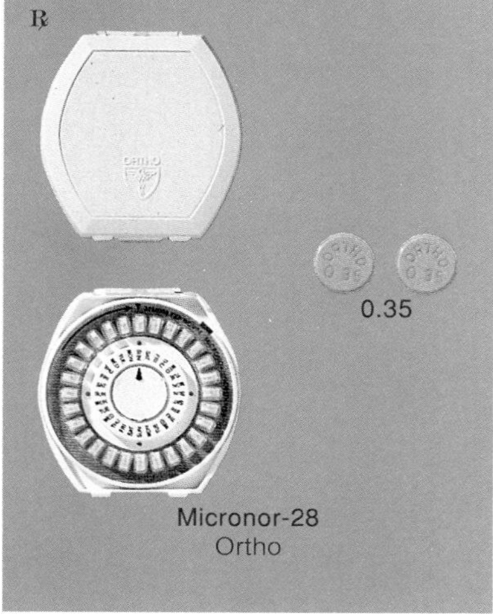

Micronor-28
Ortho

℞

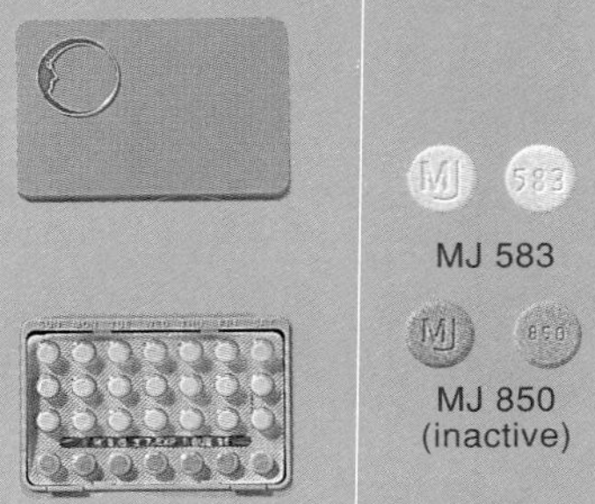

MJ 583
MJ 850
(inactive)

Ovcon 35-28
Mead Johnson

℞

7
(inactive)
NORINYL® 1+35
28-DAY Tablets

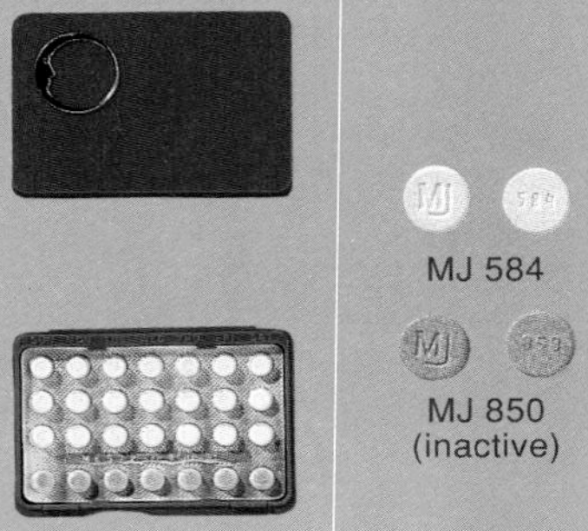

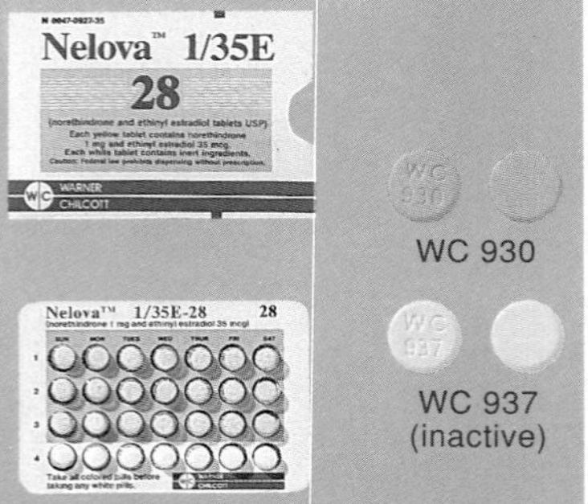

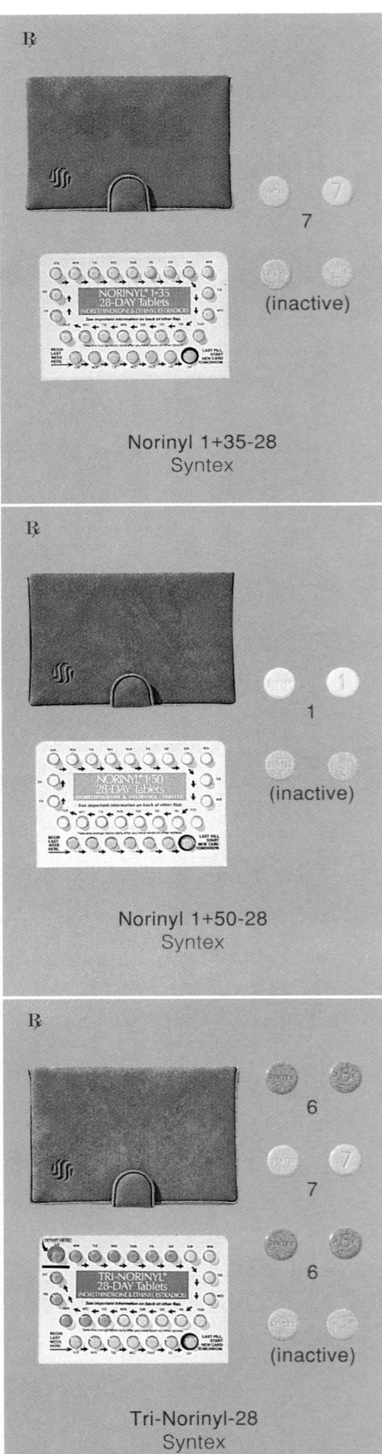

Norinyl 1+35-28
Syntex

℞

MJ 584
MJ 850
(inactive)

Ovcon 50-28
Mead Johnson

℞

1
(inactive)
NORINYL® 1+50
28-DAY Tablets

Norinyl 1+50-28
Syntex

℞

Nelova™ 1/35E
28
WARNER
CHILCOTT
WC 930
WC 937
(inactive)

Nelova 1/35E-28
Warner Chilcott

℞

6
7
6
(inactive)
TRI-NORINYL®
28-DAY Tablets

Tri-Norinyl-28
Syntex

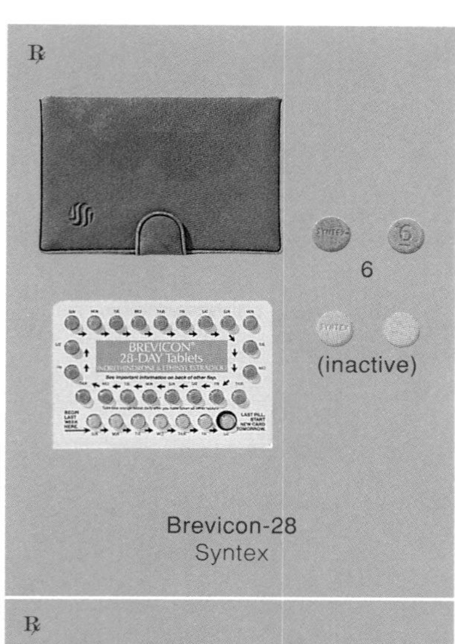

Brevicon-28
Syntex

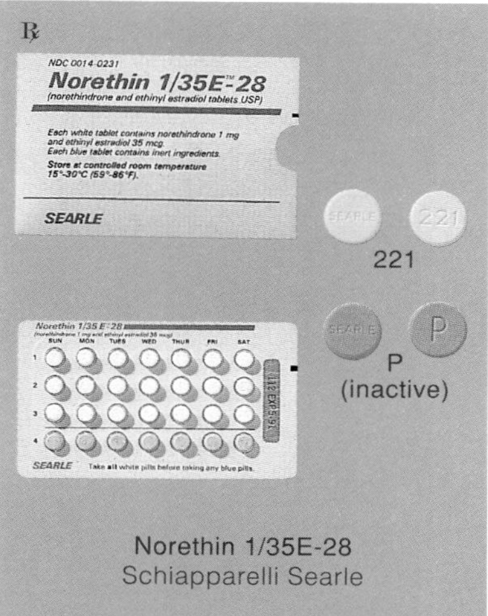

Norethin 1/35E-28
Schiapparelli Searle

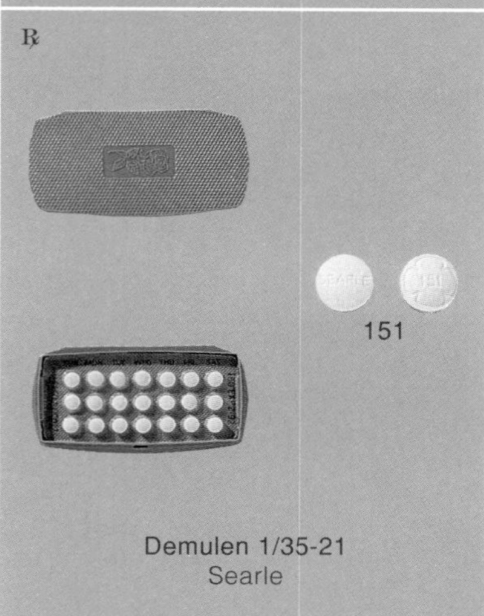

Demulen 1/35-21
Searle

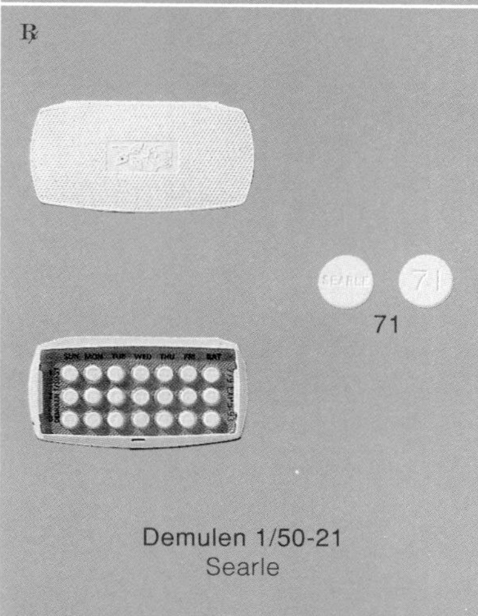

Demulen 1/50-21
Searle

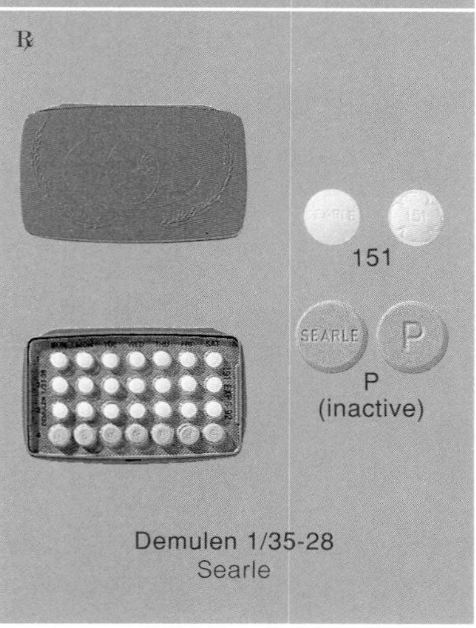

Demulen 1/35-28
Searle

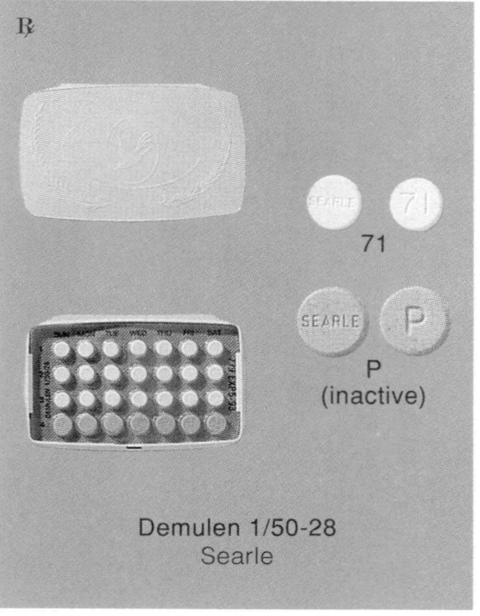

Demulen 1/50-28
Searle

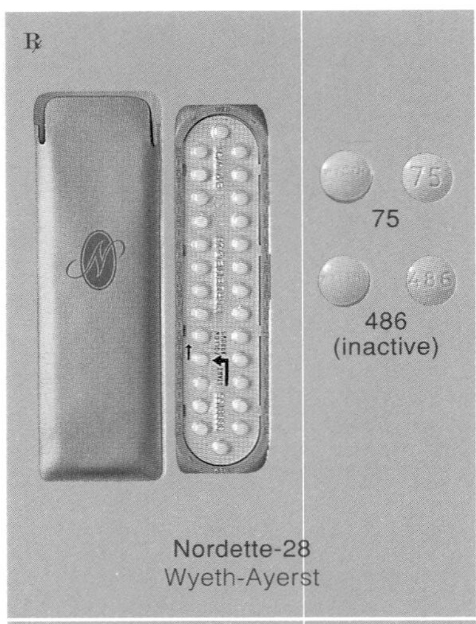

Nordette-28
Wyeth-Ayerst

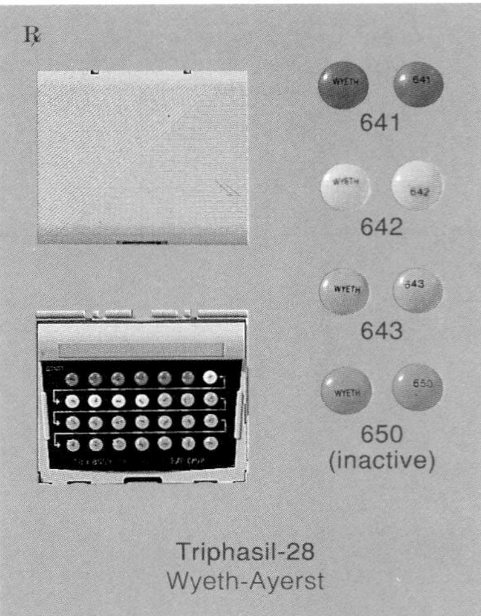

Triphasil-28
Wyeth-Ayerst

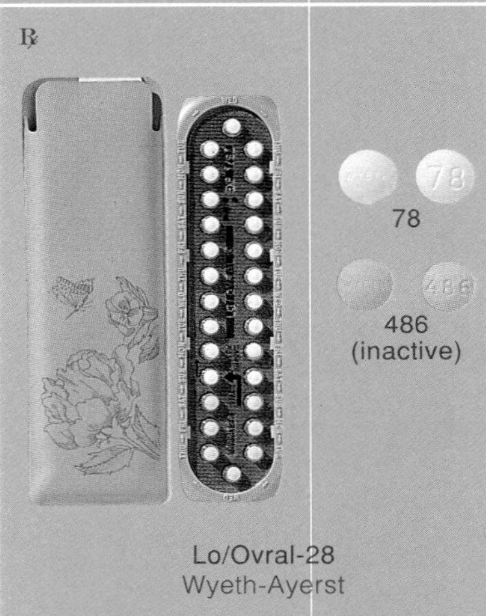

Lo/Ovral-28
Wyeth-Ayerst

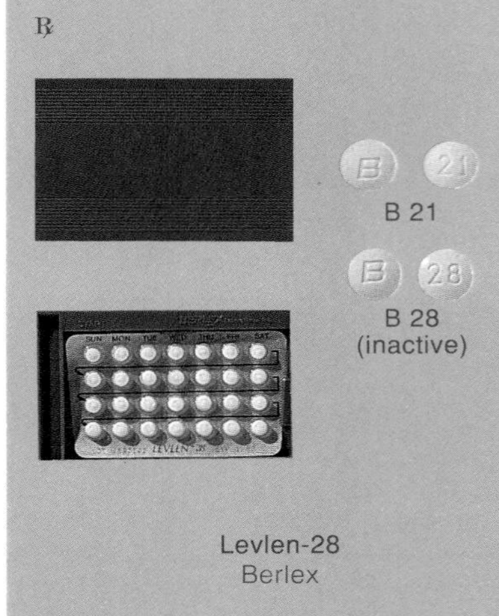

Levlen-28
Berlex

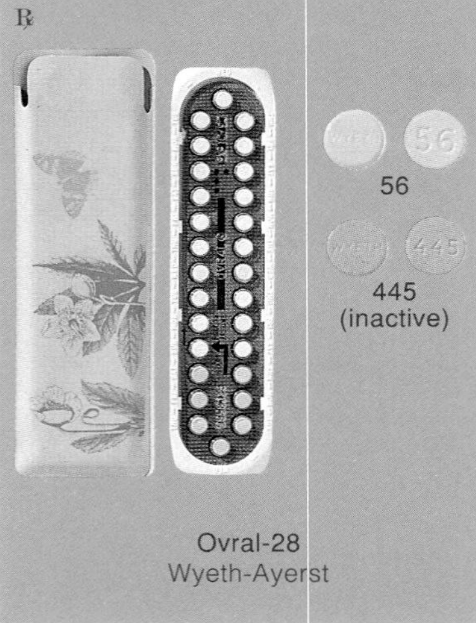

Ovral-28
Wyeth-Ayerst

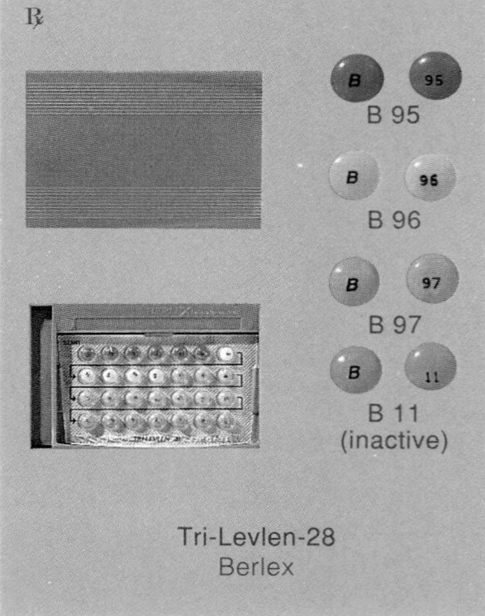

Tri-Levlen-28
Berlex

chapter 1

nutritional products

Recommended Dietary Allowances (RDA) are published by the Food and Nutrition Board, National Research Council-National Academy of Sciences, as a guide for nutritional problems and to provide standards of good nutrition for different age groups. They are revised periodically.

The RDA values are *not requirements;* they are *recommended* daily intakes of certain essential nutrients. Based on available scientific knowledge, they are believed to be adequate for known nutritional needs for most *healthy* persons under usual environmental stresses. The recommended allowances vary for age and sex, with extra allowances for women during pregnancy and lactation. The most commonly used RDA values (the "reference male" and "reference female") are those of adults 23 to 50 years of age. With the exception of energy (kilocalories), the RDA provide for individual requirement variations and prevent symptoms of clinical deficiency of 97% of the population.

RDA have been established for 10 of the 13 known essential nutrients; present knowledge of human nutritional needs of vitamin K, pantothenic acid and biotin is incomplete. Therefore, to ensure adequate nutrient intake, obtain the recommended allowances from as varied a selection of foods as possible. Nutritionists suggest that dietary planning include regular intake of each of the four basic food groups:

1. Milk, cheese, dairy products – Minimum 2 servings/day.
2. Meat, poultry, fish, beans – Minimum 2 servings/day.
3. Vegetables, fruit – Minimum 4 servings/day.
4. Bread, cereal (whole-grain and enriched or fortified) – Minimum 4 servings/day.

Such a balance, in sufficient quantities will provide about 1200 kcal, enough protein, and most of the vitamins and minerals required daily. A person may increase nutrient and energy intake by consuming larger quantities (or more servings/day) of the four basic food groups. Nutrient and energy intake may also be increased by selecting food from the fifth group, fats-sweets-alcohol, which provides mainly energy.

RDA quantities apply only to healthy persons and are not intended to cover therapeutic nutritional requirements in disease or other abnormal states (ie, metabolic disorders, weight reduction, chronic disease, drug therapy). Although certain single nutrients in larger quantities may have pharmacologic actions, these are unrelated to nutritional functions. There is no convincing evidence that consuming excessive quantities of single nutrients will cure or prevent nonnutritional diseases.

The "official" listings of United States Recommended Daily Allowances (US-RDAs) should not be confused with the RDA values. US-RDA are derived from the 1968 RDA and serve as legal standards for nutritional labeling of food and dietary food and dietary supplement products controlled by the Food and Drug Administration. Generally, they represent the higher value of the male or female RDA and are grouped into only three age brackets plus one category for pregnant or lactating women. Prior to 1972, these allowances were erroneously listed as minimum daily requirements (MDR). A second fallacy perpetuated by US-RDA labeling of foods is the implication that a food is defective if it does not contain all the officially êstablished nutrients in their full US-RDA quantities. No individual food is nutritionally complete, but several foods together should complement each other to provide maximal nutrient balance and to minimize naturally occurring toxic principles consumed from any individual foodstuff.

The Recommended Dietary Allowances (RDA) for adult males and adult females are included in each individual vitamin monograph. The table on the following page presents the listing of vitamin and mineral RDA values for all age groups as published in *Recommended Dietary Allowances,* 9th Edition, National Academy of Sciences, Washington, D.C., 1980.

RECOMMENDED DIETARY ALLOWANCES[1]

Patient Parameters						Fat-Soluble Vitamins				Water-Soluble Vitamins							Minerals						
Age (years) or Condition	Weight[2] (kg)	Weight[2] (lb)	Height[2] (cm)	Height[2] (in)	Protein g	Vitamin A μg RE[3]	Vitamin D IU[4]	Vitamin E IU[5]	Vitamin K μg	Ascorbic Acid (C) mg	Thiamine (B_1) mg	Riboflavin (B_2) mg	Niacin (B_3) mg	Pyridoxine (B_6) mg	Folate μg	Cyanoco-balamin (B_{12}) μg	Calcium mg	Phosphorus mg	Magnesium mg	Iron mg	Zinc mg	Iodine μg	Selenium μg
Infants																							
0.0-0.5	6	13	60	24	13	375	300	4	5	30	0.3	0.4	5	0.3	25	0.3	400	300	40	6	5	40	10
0.5-1	9	20	71	28	14	375	400	6	10	35	0.4	0.5	6	0.6	35	0.5	600	500	60	10	5	50	15
Children																							
1-3	13	29	90	35	16	400	400	9	15	40	0.7	0.8	9	1	50	0.7	800	800	80	10	10	70	20
4-6	20	44	112	44	24	500	400	10	20	45	0.9	1.1	12	1.1	75	1	800	800	120	10	10	90	20
7-10	28	62	132	52	28	700	400	10	30	45	1	1.2	13	1.4	100	1.4	800	800	170	10	10	120	30
Males																							
11-14	45	99	157	62	45	1000	400	15	45	50	1.3	1.5	17	1.7	150	2	1200	1200	270	12	15	150	40
15-18	66	145	176	69	59	1000	400	15	65	60	1.5	1.8	20	2	200	2	1200	1200	400	12	15	150	50
19-24	72	160	177	70	58	1000	400	15	70	60	1.5	1.7	19	2	200	2	1200	1200	350	10	15	150	70
25-50	79	174	176	70	63	1000	200	15	80	60	1.5	1.7	19	2	200	2	800	800	350	10	15	150	70
51 +	77	170	173	68	63	1000	200	15	80	60	1.2	1.4	15	2	200	2	800	800	350	10	15	150	70
Females																							
11-14	46	101	157	62	46	800	400	12	45	50	1.1	1.3	15	1.4	150	2	1200	1200	280	15	12	150	45
15-18	55	120	163	64	44	800	400	12	55	60	1.1	1.3	15	1.5	180	2	1200	1200	300	15	12	150	50
19-24	58	128	164	65	46	800	400	12	60	60	1.1	1.3	15	1.6	180	2	1200	1200	280	15	12	150	55
25-50	63	138	163	64	50	800	200	12	65	60	1.1	1.3	15	1.6	180	2	800	800	280	15	12	150	55
51 +	65	143	160	63	50	800	200	12	65	60	1	1.2	13	1.6	180	2	800	800	280	10	12	150	55
Pregnant					60	800	400	15	65	70	1.5	1.6	17	2.2	400	2.2	1200	1200	320	30	15	175	65
Lactating – 1st 6 mo.					65	1300	400	18	65	95	1.6	1.8	20	2.1	280	2.6	1200	1200	355	15	19	200	75
Lactating – 2nd 6 mo.					62	1200	400	16	65	90	1.6	1.7	20	2.1	260	2.6	1200	1200	340	15	16	200	75

Reproduced from: *Recommended Dietary Allowances,* 10th edition, 1989, National Academy of Sciences, National Academy Press, Washington, DC.

[1] The allowances, expressed as average daily intakes over time, are intended to provide for individual variations among most normal persons as they live in the US under usual environmental stresses. Diets should be based on a variety of common foods in order to provide other nutrients for which human requirements have been less well defined.

[2] Weights and heights of Reference Adults are actual medians for the US population of the designated age, as reported by NHANES II. The median weights and heights of those under 19 years of age were taken from Hamill PV et al. *Am J Clin Nutr* 1979;32:607-29. The use of these figures does not imply that the height-to-weight ratios are ideal.

[3] Retinol equivalents. 1 retinol equivalent = 1 μg retinol or 6 μg β-carotene.

[4] As cholecalciferol. 10 μg cholecalciferol = 400 IU of vitamin D.

[5] α-Tocopherol equivalents. 1 mg d-α-tocopherol = α-TE = 1.49 IU.

Fat-Soluble Vitamins

VITAMIN A

Actions:

Pharmacology: Vitamin A is found only in animal sources; it occurs in high concentrations in the liver of the cod, halibut, tuna and shark. It is also prepared synthetically. Absorption from an aqueous vehicle is greater than when given in an oily solution.

One IU vitamin A is equal to 0.3 mcg all-*trans*-retinol. Vitamin A activity is expressed as retinol equivalents (RE). One RE has the activity of 1 mcg all-*trans*-retinol (3.33 IU), 6 mcg (10 IU) β-carotene or 12 mcg carotenoid provitamins. Beta-carotene (provitamin A) is converted to retinol primarily in the intestinal mucosa.

Retinol combines with opsin, the rod pigment in the retina, to form rhodopsin, which is necessary for visual adaptation to darkness. Vitamin A prevents retardation of growth and preserves the integrity of the epithelial cells. Its deficiency is characterized by nyctalopia (night blindness), keratomalacia (necrosis of the cornea), keratinization and drying of the skin, lowered resistance to infection, retardation of growth, thickening of bone, diminished production of cortical steroids and fetal malformations.

Pharmacokinetics: Because vitamin A is fat soluble, absorption requires bile salts, pancreatic lipase and dietary fat. It is transported in the blood to the liver by the chylomicrons of the lymph. Normal serum vitamin A is 80 to 300 IU/ml. The vitamin is stored (primarily as the palmitate) both in parenchymal liver cells and in non-parenchymal fat-storing cells in the liver. The normal adult liver contains approximately 100 to 300 mcg/g, providing 2 years' requirements of vitamin A. Vitamin A is mobilized from liver stores and transported in plasma as retinol, bound to retinol-binding protein (RBP).

The excretion pathways are uncertain; a major portion appears to be excreted in the bile bound to a glucuronide and a small amount is excreted in the urine.

Indications:

Treatment of vitamin A deficiency: Deficiencies occur rarely in well nourished individuals; conditions which may cause vitamin A deficiency include: Biliary tract or pancreatic disease, sprue, colitis, hepatic cirrhosis, celiac disease, regional enteritis, extreme dietary inadequacy and partial gastrectomy and cystic fibrosis.

Parenteral administration is indicated when oral administration is not feasible as in anorexia, nausea, vomiting, preoperative and postoperative conditions, or in the "malabsorption syndrome" with accompanying steatorrhea.

Contraindications:

Hypervitaminosis A; oral use in malabsorption syndrome; hypersensitivity; IV use.

Warnings:

Pregnancy: Category C. Safety of amounts exceeding 5000 IU oral or 6000 IU parenteral daily during pregnancy has not been established. Avoid use of vitamin A in excess of the RDA during normal pregnancy. Animal reproduction studies have shown fetal abnormalities associated with overdosage in several species. One case of an infant with congenital renal anomalies has been reported.

Lactation: The US-RDA of vitamin A is 6000 units for nursing mothers. Human milk supplies sufficient vitamin A for infants unless maternal diet is grossly inadequate.

Renal function impairment: Vitamin A toxicity and elevated plasma calcium and alkaline phosphatase concentrations have been reported in chronic renal failure patients undergoing hemodialysis.

Precautions:

Closely supervise prolonged daily administration over 25,000 IU. Evaluate vitamin A intake from fortified foods, dietary supplements, self-administered drugs and prescription drug sources.

Blood level assays are not a direct measure of liver storage. Liver storage should be adequate before discontinuing therapy.

Single vitamin A deficiency is rare. Multiple vitamin deficiency is expected in any dietary deficiency.

Acne: Efficacy of large systemic doses of vitamin A in the treatment of acne has not been established; in view of the potential for toxicity, avoid this use. However, see topical vitamin A (tretinoin) and isotretinoin (see individual monographs).

Drug Interactions:

Cholestyramine may reduce absorption of vitamin A due to the reduced availability of fat-solubilizing bile salts.

Mineral oil use may interfere with the intestinal absorption of vitamin A.

Oral contraceptives significantly increase plasma vitamin A levels.

Adverse Reactions:

See Overdosage. Anaphylactic shock and death have been reported after IV use.

(Continued on following page)

Fat-Soluble Vitamins (Cont.)

VITAMIN A (Cont.)

Overdosage:

Toxicity manifestations depend on patient's age, dosage, duration of administration, RBP levels and the liver's ability to store or secrete vitamin A.

Acute toxicity: Signs of increased intracranial pressure develop within 8 to 12 hours, and cutaneous desquamation follows in a few days. A single dose of 25,000 IU/kg has caused acute toxicity.

Infants – Doses of > 350,000 IU cause acute intoxication.

Adults – Doses of > 2 million IU cause acute intoxication.

Chronic toxicity: 4000 IU/kg administered for 6 to 15 months.

Infants (3 to 6 months old) – 18,500 IU (water dispersed) daily for 1 to 3 months.

Adults – 1 million IU daily for 3 days, 50,000 IU daily for longer than 18 months or 500,000 IU daily for 2 months.

Hypervitaminosis A syndrome generally manifests as a cirrhotic-like liver syndrome. The following symptoms have been reported as manifestations of chronic overuse:

General – Malaise; lethargy; night sweats; abdominal discomfort; anorexia; vomiting.

Skeletal – Slow growth; hard tender cortical thickening over radius and tibia; migratory arthralgia; premature closure of epiphysis; bone pain.

CNS – Irritability; headache; vertigo; increased intracranial pressure as manifested by bulging fontanelles, papilledema and exophthalmos.

Dermatologic – Lip fissures; drying and cracking skin; alopecia; scaling; massive desquamation; increased pigmentation; generalized pruritus; erythema; inflammation of the tongue, lips and gums.

Miscellaneous – Hypomenorrhea; hepatosplenomegaly; jaundice; edema of lower extremities; leukopenia; vitamin A plasma levels > 1200 IU/dl; polydipsia; polyuria; hypercalcemia.

Treatment – Discontinue vitamin A. If hypercalcemia persists, give IV saline, prednisone and calcitonin, as required. Perform liver function tests; liver damage may be permanent.

Patient Information:

Avoid prolonged use of mineral oil and cholestyramine while taking this drug.

Do not exceed recommended dosage, especially during pregnancy.

Notify physician if signs of overdosage (eg, nausea, vomiting, anorexia, malaise, drying/cracking of skin/lips, irritability, loss of hair) or bulging fontanelle in infants occur.

Administration and Dosage:

Recommended dietary allowances (RDA): Adult males, 1000 mcg RE; adult females, 800 mg RE (RE = retinol equivalents: 1 RE = 1 mcg retinol or 6 mcg β-carotene).

For a complete listing of RDA by age, sex or condition, refer to page 5

Treatment of deficiency states: Adults and children (> 8 years old) –

Severe deficiency with xerophthalmia: 500,000 IU/day for 3 days, followed by 50,000 IU/day for 2 weeks.

Severe deficiency: 100,000 IU/day for 3 days, followed by 50,000 IU/day for 2 weeks.

Follow-up therapy: Adults: 10,000 to 20,000 IU/day for 2 months.

Children (1 to 8 years old): 5,000 to 10,000 IU/day for 2 months.

Parenteral (IM) – Adults: 100,000 IU/day for 3 days, then 50,000 IU/day for 2 weeks.

Children (1 to 8 years old): 17,500 to 35,000 IU/day for 10 days.

Infants: 7,500 to 15,000 IU/day for 10 days.

Storage: Protect IM product from light.

	Product	Form/Strength	Packaging	C.I.*
otc	**Aquasol A** (Astra)	**Drops:** 5,000 IU/0.1 ml	In 30 ml w/dropper.	65
otc	**Vitamin A** (Various, eg, Dixon-Shane, Lilly, Schein)	**Capsules:** 10,000 IU	In 100s, 250s and 1000s.	10+
Rx[1]	**Vitamin A** (Various, eg, Lilly, Rugby, Schein)	**Capsules:** 25,000 IU	In 100s, 250s, 500s & 1000s.	5.8+
Rx	**Aquasol A** (Astra)		Red. In 100s.	35
Rx[1]	**Vitamin A** (Various, eg, Major, Rugby, Schein)	**Capsules:** 50,000 IU	In 100s, 250s, 500s & 1000s.	5+
Rx	**Del-Vi-A** (Del-Ray)		Amber. In 100s.	10
Rx	**Aquasol A** (Astra)		Red. In 100s and 500s.	30
Rx	**Aquasol A** (Astra)	**Injection:** 50,000 IU/ml	In 2 ml vials.[2]	425

* Cost Index based on cost per 10,000 IU.

[1] Some products may be available *otc* according to distributor discretion.

[2] With 0.5% chlorobutanol, polysorbate 80, butylated hydroxyanisole and butylated hydroxytoluene.

VITAMIN D

Actions:

Pharmacology: Vitamin D is a fat-soluble vitamin derived from natural sources such as fish liver oils or from conversion of provitamins (ergosterol and 7-dehydrocholesterol) derived from foodstuffs. One USP unit or one IU of vitamin D activity is equal to 0.025 mcg vitamin D_3 (1 mg = 40,000 units). "Vitamin D" refers to both ergocalciferol (D_2) and cholecalciferol (D_3). Vitamin D_2, essentially a plant vitamin, is used in fortified milk and cereals. Natural supplies of vitamin D depend on ultraviolet light for conversion of 7-dehydrocholesterol to vitamin D_3 or ergosterol to vitamin D_2.

Vitamin D is hydroxylated by the hepatic microsomal enzymes to 25-hydroxy-vitamin D (25-[OH]-D_3 or calcifediol). Calcifediol is hydroxylated primarily in the kidney to 1, 25-dihydroxy-vitamin D (1, 25-$[OH]_2$-D_3 or calcitriol). Calcitriol is believed to be the most active form of vitamin D_3 in stimulating intestinal calcium and phosphate transport.

Dihydrotachysterol is a synthetic reduction product of tachysterol, a close isomer of vitamin D. Dihydrotachysterol is hydroxylated in the liver to 25-hydroxydihydrotachysterol, the major circulating active form of the drug. It does not undergo further hydroxylation by the kidney, and therefore is the analog of 1,25-dihydroxy-vitamin D.

The metabolic pathway of vitamin D activation

Ergosterol (Provitamin D_2)	UV light →	Ergocalciferol (Vitamin D_2)	Liver →	25-hydroxyergocalciferol[1] (25 [OH]-D_2)	Kidney →	1,25-dihydroxyergocalciferol[2] (1,25 $[OH]_2$-D_2)
7-dehydrocholesterol (Provitamin D_3)	Skin via UV light →	Cholecalciferol[1] (Vitamin D_3)	Liver →	Calcifediol[2] (25 [OH]-D_3)	Kidney →	Calcitriol[3] (1,25 $[OH]_2$-D_3)
Dihydrotachysterol	Liver →	25-hydroxy-dihydrotachysterol[2]				

[1] The kidney, in the absence of PTH, converts vitamin D_3 to 24,25$(OH)_2$-D_3, which is much less active than 1,25$(OH)_2$-D_3.

[2] Major transport form of vitamin D; minor intrinsic activity. [3] Physiologically active forms.

Physiological function: Vitamin D is considered a hormone. Although not a natural human hormone, vitamin D_2 apparently can substitute for D_3 in every metabolic step. Vitamin D, in conjunction with PTH and calcitonin, regulates calcium homeostasis. Vitamin D metabolites promote active absorption of calcium and phosphorus by the small intestine, increase rate of accretion and resorption of minerals in bone and promote resorption of phosphate by renal tubules. Vitamin D is also involved in magnesium metabolism.

Vitamin D deficiency leads to progressive hearing loss, rickets in children and osteomalacia in adults. Vitamin D reverses symptoms of nutritional rickets or osteomalacia unless permanent deformities have occurred. Response to vitamin D varies, as seen in idiopathic hypercalcemia at one extreme and vitamin D-resistant rickets at the other.

Pharmacokinetics: Absorption – Vitamin D is readily absorbed from the small intestine. Vitamin D_3 may be absorbed more rapidly and more completely than vitamin D_2. Bile is essential for adequate absorption. Absorption is reduced in liver or biliary disease and steatorrhea.

Distribution – Stored chiefly in the liver, vitamin D is also found in fat, muscle, skin and bones. In plasma, it is bound to alpha globulins and albumin.

Metabolism – There is a lag of 10 to 24 hours between administration of ergocalciferol and initiation of its action in the body. Maximal hypercalcemic effects occur about 4 weeks after daily administration of a fixed dose and the duration of action can be $\geq$ 2 months. The serum half-life of calcifediol is approximately 16 days. The elimination half-life of calcitriol is 3 to 6 hours; pharmacologic activity persists for 3 to 5 days. Dihydrotachysterol has a rapid onset of effect and is less persistent after cessation of treatment.

Excretion – The primary route of excretion of vitamin D is in the bile; only a small percentage is found in the urine.

(Continued on following page)

VITAMIN D (Cont.)

Indications:

Refer to individual product listings.

Contraindications:

Hypercalcemia; evidence of vitamin D toxicity; malabsorption syndrome; hypervitaminosis D; abnormal sensitivity to the effects of vitamin D; decreased renal function.

Warnings:

Hypersensitivity to vitamin D may be one etiological factor in infants with idiopathic hypercalcemia. In these cases, severely restrict vitamin D intake.

Concomitant calcium administration: Adequate dietary calcium is necessary for clinical response to vitamin D therapy.

Monitoring: Dosage adjustment is required as soon as there is clinical improvement. Individualize dosage. Start therapy at the lowest possible dose and do not increase without careful monitoring of the serum calcium. Estimate daily dietary calcium intake and adjust the intake when indicated. Patients with normal renal function taking calcitriol should avoid dehydration. Maintain adequate fluid intake. In vitamin D-resistant rickets, the range between therapeutic and toxic doses is narrow. When high therapeutic doses are used, follow progress with frequent serum and urinary calcium, phosphate and urea nitrogen determinations.

Periodically determine serum calcium, phosphate, magnesium and alkaline phosphatase; monitor 24 hour urinary calcium and phosphate, especially in hypoparathyroid and dialysis patients. During the initial phase, determine serum calcium twice weekly. Maintain serum calcium levels between 9 and 10 mg/dl.

Hypercalcemia: The product of serum calcium multiplied by phosphate (Ca x P) should not exceed 70; exceeding the solubility product may result in precipitation of calcium phosphate. Progressive hypercalcemia due to overdosage may be so severe as to require emergency attention. Chronic hypercalcemia can lead to generalized vascular calcification, nephrocalcinosis and other soft tissue calcification. Radiographic or slit lamp evaluation of suspect anatomical regions may be useful for early detection.

In patients with normal renal function, chronic hypercalcemia may be associated with an increase in serum creatinine. While this is usually reversible, it is important in such patients to pay careful attention to factors which may lead to hypercalcemia.

A fall in serum alkaline phosphatase levels usually precedes hypercalcemia and may indicate impending hypercalcemia. Should hypercalcemia develop, discontinue the drug immediately. After achieving normocalcemia, readminister at a lower dosage.

Renal function impairment: The kidneys of uremic patients cannot adequately synthesize calcitriol, the active hormone formed from precursor vitamin D. Resultant hypocalcemia and secondary hyperparathyroidism are a major cause of the metabolic bone disease of renal failure. However, other bone-toxic substances which accumulate in uremia (eg, aluminum) may also contribute.

The beneficial effect of calcitriol in renal osteodystrophy appears to result from correction of hypocalcemia and secondary hyperparathyroidism. It is uncertain whether calcitriol produces other independent beneficial effects. In patients with renal osteodystrophy accompanied by hyperphosphatemia, maintain a normal serum phosphorus level by dietary phosphate restriction or administration of aluminum gels to prevent metastatic calcification.

Because of the effect on serum calcium, administer to patients with renal stones only when potential benefits outweigh possible hazards.

Pregnancy: Category C. Safety of amounts in excess of 400 IU/day is not established. Avoid doses greater than the RDA during a normal pregnancy. Animal studies have shown fetal abnormalities associated with hypervitaminosis D. Calcifediol and calcitriol are teratogenic in animals when given in doses several times the human dose. The offspring of a woman administered 17 to 36 mcg/day of calcitriol (17 to 144 times the recommended dose) during pregnancy manifested mild hypercalcemia in the first two days of life which returned to normal at day 3. There are no adequate and well controlled studies in pregnant women; use during pregnancy only if the potential benefits outweigh the potential hazards to the fetus.

Lactation: Vitamin D is excreted in breast milk in limited amounts. In a mother given large doses of vitamin D, 25-hydroxycholecalciferol appeared in the milk and caused hypercalcemia in the child. Monitoring of the infant's serum calcium concentration is required in that case. Exercise caution when administering to a nursing mother.

Children: Safety and efficacy in children of doses exceeding the RDA and in children undergoing dialysis have not been established. Pediatric doses must be individualized and monitored under close medical supervision.

(Continued on following page)

VITAMIN D (Cont.)

Precautions:

Use caution in patients with coronary disease, renal function impairment and arteriosclerosis, especially in the elderly.

Concomitant vitamin D intake: Evaluate vitamin D ingested in fortified foods, dietary supplements and other concomitantly administered drugs. It may be necessary to limit dietary vitamin D and its derivatives during treatment.

Hypoparathyroidism: Calcium, parathyroid hormone or dihydrotachysterol may be needed.

Tartrazine sensitivity: Some of these products contain tartrazine, which may cause allergic-type reactions (including bronchial asthma) in susceptible individuals. Although incidence of sensitivity is low, it is frequently seen in patients with aspirin hypersensitivity. Specific products containing tartrazine are identified in the product listings.

Drug Interactions:

Vitamin D Drug Interactions

Precipitant drug	Object drug*		Description
Vitamin D	Antacids, magnesium-containing	↑	Hypermagnesemia may develop in patients on chronic renal dialysis.
Vitamin D	Digitalis glycosides	↑	Hypercalcemia in patients on digitalis may precipitate cardiac arrhythmias.
Vitamin D	Verapamil	↑	Atrial fibrillation has recurred when supplemental calcium and calciferol have induced hypercalcemia.
Cholestyramine	Vitamin D	↓	Intestinal absorption of vitamin D may be reduced.
Mineral oil	Vitamin D	↓	Absorption of vitamin D is reduced with prolonged use of mineral oil.
Phenytoin, Barbiturates	Vitamin D	↓	Half-life of vitamin D may be decreased.
Thiazide diuretics	Vitamin D	↑	Hypoparathyroid patients on vitamin D may develop hypercalcemia due to thiazide diuretics.

* ↑ = Object drug increased ↓ = Object drug decreased

Adverse Reactions:

Early: Weakness; headache; somnolence; nausea; vomiting; dry mouth; constipation; muscle pain; bone pain; metallic taste.

Late: Polyuria; polydipsia; anorexia; irritability; weight loss; nocturia; mild acidosis; reversible azotemia, generalized vascular calcification, nephrocalcinosis; conjunctivitis (calcific); pancreatitis; photophobia; rhinorrhea; pruritus; hyperthermia; decreased libido; elevated BUN; albuminuria; hypercholesterolemia; elevated AST and ALT; ectopic calcification; hypertension; cardiac arrhythmias; overt psychosis (rare).

In clinical studies on hypoparathyroidism and pseudohypoparathyroidism, hypercalcemia was noted on at least one occasion in about 1 in 3 patients and hypercalciuria in about 1 in 7. Elevated serum creatinine levels were observed in about 1 in 6 patients (approximately one half of whom had normal levels at baseline).

Overdosage:

Symptoms: Administration to patients in excess of their daily requirements can cause hypercalcemia, hypercalciuria and hyperphosphatemia. Concomitant high intake of calcium and phosphate may lead to similar abnormalities. Doses of 60,000 IU/day can cause hypercalcemia.

Hypercalcemia leads to anorexia, nausea, weakness, weight loss, vague aches and stiffness, constipation, diarrhea, mental retardation, tinnitus, ataxia, hypotonia, depression, amnesia, disorientation, hallucinations, syncope, coma, anemia and mild acidosis. Impairment of renal function may cause polyuria, nocturia, hypercalciuria, polydipsia, reversible azotemia, hypertension, nephrocalcinosis, generalized vascular calcification, irreversible renal insufficiency or proteinuria. Widespread calcification of soft tissues, including heart, blood vessels, renal tubules and lungs can occur. Bone demineralization (osteoporosis) may occur in adults; decline in average linear growth rate and increased bone mineralization may occur in infants and children (dwarfism). Effects can persist $\geq$ 2 months after ergocalciferol treatment, 1 month after cessation of dihydrotachysterol therapy, 2 to 4 weeks for calcifediol and 2 to 7 days for calcitriol. Death can result from cardiovascular or renal failure.

(Overdosage continued on following page)

Complete prescribing information for these products begins on page 8

Fat-Soluble Vitamins (Cont.)

VITAMIN D (Cont.)

Overdosage (Cont.):

Treatment of hypervitaminosis D with hypercalcemia consists of immediate withdrawal of the vitamin, a low calcium diet, generous fluid intake and urine acidification along with symptomatic and supportive treatment.

Hypercalcemic crisis with dehydration, stupor, coma and azotemia requires more vigorous treatment. The first step is hydration; saline IV may quickly and significantly increase urinary calcium excretion. A loop diuretic (eg, furosemide) may be given with the saline infusion to further increase calcium excretion. Other measures include administration of citrates, sulfates, phosphates, corticosteroids, EDTA and plicamycin. Persistent or markedly elevated serum calcium levels may be corrected by dialysis against a calcium-free dialysate. With appropriate therapy, and when no permanent damage has occurred, recovery is probable.

Treatment of accidental overdosage consists of general supportive measures. Refer to General Management of Acute Overdosage. If ingestion is discovered within a short time, emesis or gastric lavage may be of benefit. Mineral oil may promote fecal elimination. Treat hypercalcemia as outlined above.

Patient Information:

Compliance with dosage instructions, diet and calcium supplementation are essential.

Swallow whole; do not crush or chew.

Eating a balanced diet and periodic exposure to sunlight usually satisfies normal vitamin D requirements. Never use vitamin supplements as a substitute for a balanced diet.

Notify physician if any of the following occurs: Weakness, lethargy, headache, anorexia, weight loss, nausea, vomiting, abdominal cramps, diarrhea, constipation, vertigo, excessive thirst, excessive urine output, dry mouth or muscle or bone pain.

Avoid concurrent prolonged use of mineral oil. If on chronic renal dialysis, avoid magnesium-containing antacids while taking this drug. See Drug Interactions.

Administration:

Individualize dosage. The effectiveness of therapy is predicated on adequate daily intake of calcium either by calcium supplementation or proper dietary measures. Refer to page 5 for a complete listing of RDAs.

DIHYDROTACHYSTEROL (DHT)

Dihydrotachysterol is a synthetic reduction product of tachysterol, a close isomer of vitamin D; 1 mg is approximately equivalent to 3 mg (120,000 IU) vitamin D_2.

Indications:

Treatment of acute, chronic and latent forms of postoperative tetany, idiopathic tetany and hypoparathyroidism.

Dosage:

Initial dose: 0.8 to 2.4 mg daily for several days.

Maintenance dose: 0.2 to 1 mg daily, as required, for normal serum calcium levels. Average dose is 0.6 mg daily. May be supplemented with oral calcium.

	Product	Form	Description	C.I.*
Rx	**DHT** (Roxane)	**Tablets:** 0.125 mg	Lactose, sucrose. (54 280). White. In 50s and UD 100s.	490
		0.2 mg	Lactose, sucrose. (54 903). Pink. In 100s and UD 100s.	310
		0.4 mg	Lactose, sucrose. (54 772). White. In 50s.	275
		Intensol Solution: 0.2 mg/ml	20% alcohol. In 30 ml w/ dropper.	370
Rx	**Hytakerol** (Winthrop Pharm.)	**Capsules:** 0.125 mg	In 50s.	1250
		Oral Solution: 0.25 mg per ml in oil	In 15 ml.	1105

* Cost Index based on cost per 0.2 mg dihydrotachysterol.

Complete prescribing information for these products begins on page 8

Fat-Soluble Vitamins (Cont.)

CALCITRIOL (1,25 dihydroxycholecalciferol; 1,25 $[OH]_2$–D_3)

Indications:

Management of hypocalcemia in patients on chronic renal dialysis.

May reduce elevated parathyroid hormone levels in some patients.

Unlabeled use: Calcitriol, orally (0.5 mcg/day for 6 months) and topically (0.5 mcg/g petrolatum once daily for 8 weeks), decreased the severity of psoriatic lesions in patients with psoriasis vulgaris.

Dosage:

Dialysis patients: 0.25 mcg/day. If a satisfactory response is not observed, increase dosage by 0.25 mcg/day at 4 to 8 week intervals. During this titration period, obtain serum calcium levels at least twice weekly; if hypercalcemia is noted, discontinue use until normocalcemia is attained.

Patients with normal or only slightly reduced serum calcium levels may respond to doses of 0.25 mcg every other day. Most patients undergoing hemodialysis respond to doses between 0.5 and 1 mcg/day.

Oral calcitriol may normalize plasma ionized calcium in some uremic patients, yet fail to suppress parathyroid hyperfunction. In these individuals with autonomous parathyroid hyperfunction, oral calcitriol may be useful to maintain normocalcemia, but has not been shown to be adequate treatment for hyperparathyroidism.

Hypoparathyroidism: Initial dose is 0.25 mcg/day given in the morning. If a satisfactory response in the biochemical parameters and clinical manifestations of the disease is not observed, increase dose at 2 to 4 week intervals. During the dosage titration period, obtain serum calcium levels at least twice weekly and, if hypercalcemia is noted, immediately discontinue use until normocalcemia ensues. Carefully consider lowering dietary calcium intake.

Adults and children ($\geq$ 6 years) – 0.5 to 2 mcg daily. *(1 to 5 years)* – 0.25 to 0.75 mcg daily. The number of treated patients with pseudohypoparathyroidism $<$ 6 years of age is too small to make dosage recommendations.

	Product	Form/Strength	Description	C.I.*
Rx	**Rocaltrol** (Roche)	**Capsules:** 0.25 mcg	Sorbitol. (Rocaltrol 0.25 Roche). Light orange. In 30s and 100s.	790
		0.5 mcg	Sorbitol. (Rocaltrol 0.5 Roche). Dark orange. In 100s.	630
Rx	**Calcijex** (Abbott)	**Injection:** 1 mcg/ml	In 1 ml amps.	2295
		2 mcg/ml	In 1 ml amps.	1935

CALCIFEDIOL (25-hydroxycholecalciferol; 25 $[OH]$–D_3)

Indications:

Management of metabolic bone disease or hypocalcemia in patients on chronic renal dialysis.

Increases serum calcium levels and decreases alkaline phosphatase, parathyroid hormone levels, subperiosteal bone resorption, histological signs of hyperparathyroid bone disease and mineralization defects in some patients.

Dosage:

Initial dose: 300 to 350 mcg/week, administered daily or on alternate days. If a satisfactory response is not obtained, dosage may be increased at 4 week intervals. During this period, obtain serum calcium levels at least weekly; if hypercalcemia is noted, discontinue use until normocalcemia is attained.

Some patients with normal serum calcium levels may respond to doses of 20 mcg every other day. Most patients respond to doses between 50 and 100 mcg/day or between 100 and 200 mcg on alternate days.

	Product	Form/Strength	Description	C.I.*
Rx	**Calderol** (Organon)	**Capsules:** 20 mcg	White. In 60s.	825
		50 mcg	Orange. In 60s.	755

* Cost Index based on cost per 0.5 mcg calcitriol or 50 mcg calcifediol.

Complete prescribing information for these products begins on page 8

Fat-Soluble Vitamins (Cont.)

ERGOCALCIFEROL (D_2)

Ergocalciferol 1.25 mg provides 50,000 IU of vitamin D activity.

Indications:

Treatment of refractory rickets (also known as vitamin D-resistant rickets), familial hypophosphatemia and hypoparathyroidism.

Dosage:

Recommended dietary allowances (RDAs): Adults (< 25 years) 400 IU; (> 25 years) 200 IU. For a complete listing of RDAs by age, sex and condition, refer to page 2a. Daily dosage of 400 IU satisfies requirements for all age groups, unless there has been exposure to ultraviolet irradiation.

Individualize dosage. The range between therapeutic and toxic doses is narrow.

Blood calcium, phosphorus and BUN determinations must be made every 2 weeks or more frequently if necessary. X-ray bones monthly until the condition is corrected and stabilized. Ensure adequate calcium intake. Maintain serum calcium concentration between 9 and 10 mg/dl.

Vitamin D resistant rickets: 12,000 to 500,000 IU daily.

Hypoparathyroidism: 50,000 to 200,000 IU/day plus 500 mg elemental calcium 6 times daily.

Familial hypophosphatemia: 10,000 to 80,000 IU daily plus 1 to 2 g/day elemental phosphorus.

IM therapy: Required in patients with GI, liver or biliary disease associated with malabsorption of vitamin D.

	Product	Form	Packaging	C.I.*
otc	**Calciferol Drops** (Schwarz Pharma Kremers Urban)	**Liquid:** 8,000 IU per ml	In 60 ml[1].	670
otc	**Drisdol Drops** (Winthrop Pharm.)		In 60 ml[1].	1845
Rx	**Vitamin D** (Various, eg, Dixon-Shane, Major, Moore, Rugby, Schein, URL)	**Capsules:** 50,000 IU	In 100s and 1000s.	15+
Rx	**Deltalin Gelseals** (Lilly)		In 100s.	55
Rx	**Drisdol** (Winthrop Pharm.)		Tartrazine. In 50s.	260
Rx	**Calciferol** (Schwarz Pharma Kremers Urban)	**Tablets:** 50,000 IU	Sugar. (KU 1). Yellow. Oval. In 100s.	95
Rx	**Calciferol** (Schwarz Pharma Kremers Urban)	**Injection:** 500,000 IU per ml	In 1 ml amps.[2]	2000

CHOLECALCIFEROL (D_3)

Cholecalciferol 1 mg provides 40,000 IU vitamin D activity.

Indications:

Dietary supplement, treatment of vitamin D deficiency or prophylaxis of deficiency.
Unlabeled uses: Hypocalcemic tetany and hypoparathyroidism.

Dosage: 400 to 1000 IU daily.

	Product	Form	Packaging	C.I.*
otc *sf*	**Delta-D** (Freeda)	**Tablets:** 400 IU D_3	In 250s and 500s.	22
otc *sf*	**Vitamin D_3** (Freeda)	**Tablets:** 1000 IU D_3	In 100s.	21

* Cost Index based on cost per 50,000 IU ergocalciferol or 1000 IU cholecalciferol.

sf – Sugar free.

[1] In propylene glycol.

[2] In sesame oil.

VITAMIN E

Actions:

Although the exact biochemical mechanisms of vitamin E in the body are unclear, it is an essential element of human nutrition. Many of its actions are related to its antioxidant properties. Vitamin E may protect cellular constituents from oxidation and prevent the formation of toxic oxidation products; it preserves red blood cell (RBC) wall integrity and protects them against hemolysis; it may act as a cofactor in enzyme systems. Enhancement of vitamin A utilization and suppression of platelet aggregation have also been attributed to vitamin E.

Clinical deficiency of vitamin E is rare, since adequate amounts are supplied in the normal diet. Sources of vitamin E include vegetable oils, vegetable shortening and margarine. Other food sources include leafy vegetables, milk, eggs and meats. Absorption depends on the ability to digest and absorb fat; bile is essential. There is no single storage organ, but adipose tissue, liver and muscle account for most of the body's tocopherol.

Low tocopherol levels have been noted in: Premature infants; severe protein-calorie malnourished infants with macrocytic megaloblastic anemia; prolonged fat malabsorption (ie, cystic fibrosis, hepatic cirrhosis, sprue); malabsorption syndromes (ie, celiac disease, GI resections); acanthocytosis; patients with abetalipoproteinemia. Low levels of vitamin E make the erythrocyte more susceptible to destruction by oxidants. Vitamin E deficiency may result in hemolysis; also consider the possibility of deficiency in spinocerebellar syndromes.

Vitamin E requirements: The daily vitamin E requirement is related to the dietary intake of polyunsaturated fatty acids (PUFA), primarily linoleic acid. Vitamin E requirements may be increased in patients taking large doses of iron; diets containing selenium, sulfur-amino acids or antioxidants may decrease the daily requirement. Vitamin E supplementation has been effective in preventing the hemolytic anemia and relieving the edema and skin lesions which develop in low birthweight premature infants fed artificial formulas containing iron and high concentrations of PUFA. Commercial infant formulas currently available provide an adequate ratio of vitamin E to PUFA; formulas for premature infants have a lower level of iron to preclude interference with vitamin E use. Thus, there is no longer a need to routinely administer vitamin E supplementation to prevent anemia.

Indications:

Treatment of vitamin E deficiency.

Unlabeled uses: Vitamin E has been used in certain premature infants to reduce the toxic effects of oxygen therapy on the lung parenchyma (bronchopulmonary dysplasia) and the retina (retrolental fibroplasia). It has also been used to prevent hemolytic anemia in infants, and has been investigated for the prevention of periventricular hemorrhage in premature infants.

It has also been used in cancer, skin conditions, nocturnal leg cramps, sexual dysfunction, heart disease, aging, premenstrual syndrome and to increase athletic performance. However, data does not support use of vitamin E in these conditions.

Contraindications:

Vitamin E should not be administered IV, since the role of IV vitamin E in the deaths of 38 infants receiving the drug remains unclear.

Drug Interactions:

Oral anticoagulants: The hypoprothrombinemic effects may be increased, possibly with bleeding.

Adverse Reactions:

Hypervitaminosis E symptoms include fatigue, weakness, nausea, headache, blurred vision, flatulence and diarrhea.

Patient Information:

Swallow capsules whole; do not crush or chew.

(Continued on following page)

Fat-Soluble Vitamins (Cont.)

VITAMIN E (Cont.)

Administration and Dosage:

Recommended dietary allowances (RDAs): Adult males, 15 IU; adult females, 12 IU. For a complete listing of RDAs by age, sex and condition, refer to page 5

The potencies of the several forms of vitamin E vary; therefore, dosage is usually standardized in International Units (IU), based on activity. The following table indicates the relative potency of 1 mg of the various forms of vitamin E available:

Relative Potencies of Vitamin E	
1 mg dl-alpha tocopheryl acetate = 1 IU	1 mg d-alpha tocopherol = 1.49 IU
1 mg dl-alpha tocopherol = 1.1 IU	1 mg d-alpha tocopheryl acid succinate = 1.21 IU
1 mg d-alpha tocopheryl acetate = 1.36 IU	1 mg dl-alpha tocopheryl acid succinate = 0.89 IU

Free tocopherols can be oxidized and destroyed under adverse conditions; the esters available, acetate and succinate, are very stable in light. Keep in dry, airtight container.

	Product	Form/Strength	Package	C.I.*
otc	**Vitamin E** (Various, eg, Schein)	**Tablets:** 200 IU[1]	In 100s.	NA
		400 IU[1]	In 50s and 100s.	NA
otc	**Vitamin E** (Various, eg, Dixon-Shane, Geneva Marsam, Schein)	**Capsules:** 100 IU[1]	In 100s, 250s, 500s and 1000s.	15+
		200 IU[1]	In 100s, 250s, 500s and 1000s.	10+
		400 IU[1]	In 50s, 60s, 90s, 100s, 250s, 500s, 1000s.	5+
		500 IU[1]	In 100s and 1000s.	NA
		600 IU[1]	In 60s, 100s, 250s and 1000s.	NA
		1000 IU[1]	In 30s, 50s, 60s, 100s, 250s, 500s & 1000s.	5+
otc	**Aquasol E** (Astra)	**Capsules:** 73.5 mg[2]	In 100s.	165
otc sf	**E-200 I.U. Softgels** (Nature's Bounty)	**Capsules:** 147 mg[2]	In 100s.	NA
otc	**E-Vitamin Succinate** (Forest)	**Capsules:** 165 mg[3]	In 100s.	20
otc sf	**Amino-Opti-E** (Tyson)		In 100s.	NA
otc	**Aquasol E** (Astra)	**Capsules:** 400 IU[1]	In 30s.	75
otc	**E-400 I.U. in a Water Soluble Base** (Nature's Bounty)		In 100s.	NA
otc	**E-Vitamin Succinate** (Forest)	**Capsules:** 330 mg[3]	In 100s.	25
otc sf	**Vita-Plus E Softgels** (Scot-Tussin)	**Capsules:** 400 IU[1]	In 100s.	4
otc sf	**E-Complex-600** (Nature's Bounty)	**Capsules:** 600 IU[1]	In 50s.	NA
otc sf	**E-1000 I.U. Softgels** (Nature's Bounty)	**Capsules:** 1000 IU[1]	In 50s.	NA
otc	**Aquasol E** (Astra)	**Drops:** 50 mg[4] per ml	In 12 and 30 ml.	570

* Cost Index based on cost per 100 IU.

sf – Sugar free.

[1] Form of vitamin E unknown; content given in IU.

[2] As d-alpha tocopheryl acetate.

[3] As d-alpha tocopheryl acid succinate.

[4] As dl-alpha tocopheryl acetate.

Water-Soluble Vitamins

THIAMINE HCl (B_1)

Actions:

Thiamine combines with adenosine triphosphate (ATP) to form thiamine pyrophosphate, a coenzyme. Its role in carbohydrate metabolism is the decarboxylation of pyruvic and alpha keto acids. An increase in serum pyruvic acid is one sign of the deficiency state. The need for thiamine is greater when the carbohydrate content of the diet is high. Significant B_1 depletion can occur in 3 weeks of total thiamine dietary absence.

Pharmacokinetics: Maximum oral absorption is 8 to 15 mg daily. Oral absorption may be increased by administering in divided doses with food. Tissue stores are saturated when intake exceeds minimal requirement ($\approx$ 1 mg/day); excess thiamine is excreted in urine. With normal renal function, 80% to 96% of an IV dose is excreted in urine.

Clinical pharmacology: Beriberi, a deficiency state, is characterized by GI manifestations, peripheral neurologic changes and cerebral deficits. *Wet beriberi* includes cardiovascular symptoms characterized by dyspnea on exertion, palpitations, ECG abnormalities and high-output cardiac failure.

Wernicke's encephalopathy is characterized by horizontal nystagmus, bilateral sixth nerve palsy, ataxia and confusion. Conditions associated with development are excessive alcohol consumption, prolonged IV feeding, hyperemesis gravidarum, anorexia nervosa, prolonged fasting, refeeding after starvation and gastric plication.

Indications:

Treatment or prophylaxis of thiamine deficiency.

Parenteral: When the oral route is not feasible (eg, anorexia, nausea, vomiting, severe alcoholism, preoperative and postoperative conditions); impaired GI absorption in malabsorption syndromes; beriberi.

Unlabeled use: Oral thiamine has been studied as a mosquito repellant; further verification is needed.

Contraindications:

Hypersensitivity to thiamine.

Warnings:

Sensitivity reactions can occur. Deaths have resulted from IV use. An intradermal test dose is recommended in patients with suspected sensitivity.

Wernicke's encephalopathy: Thiamine deficient patients may experience a sudden onset or worsening of Wernicke's encephalopathy following glucose administration; in suspected thiamine deficiency, administer thiamine before or along with dextrose-containing fluids.

Single vitamin B_1 deficiency is rare. Suspect multiple vitamin deficiencies.

Pregnancy: Category A (parenteral). Studies have not shown an increased risk of fetal abnormalities if administered during pregnancy. The possibility of fetal harm appears remote; however, use during pregnancy only if clearly needed.

Lactation: It is not known whether this drug is excreted in breast milk. Use with caution in nursing women.

Adverse Reactions:

Feeling of warmth; pruritus; urticaria; weakness; sweating; nausea; restlessness; tightness of the throat; angioneurotic edema; cyanosis; pulmonary edema; hemorrhage into the GI tract; cardiovascular collapse; death.

Parenteral: Some tenderness and induration may follow IM use.

(Continued on following page)

Water-Soluble Vitamins (Cont.)

THIAMINE HCl (B_1) (Cont.)

Administration and Dosage:

Recommended dietary allowances (RDAs): Adult males, 1.2 to 1.5 mg; adult females, 1.1 mg. Thiamine is recommended at 0.5 mg/1000 Kcal intake. For a complete listing of RDAs by age, sex and condition, refer to page 5.

Wet beriberi with myocardial failure: Treat as an emergency cardiac condition. Administer 10 to 30 mg IV 3 times daily.

Beriberi: 10 to 20 mg IM 3 times/day for 2 weeks. Give an oral therapeutic multivitamin containing 5 to 10 mg thiamine daily for 1 month to achieve body tissue saturation.

Incompatibility: B_1 is unstable in neutral or alkaline solutions; do not use in combination with alkaline solutions (eg, **carbonates, citrates, barbiturates, erythromycin lactobionate IV**). Solutions containing sulfites are incompatible with thiamine.

				C.I.*
otc	**Thiamine HCl** (Various, eg, Dixon-Shane, Freeda, Geneva Marsam, Genetco, Lilly, Major, Nature's Bounty, Purepac, Rugby, Schein)	**Tablets:** 50 mg	In 100s, 200s, 1000s and UD 100s.	5+
		100 mg	In 100s, 250s, 500s, 1000s and UD 100s.	3.5+
		250 mg	In 100s, 250s, 1000s and UD 100s & 1000s.	1.5+
		500 mg	In 100s and 1000s.	1+
otc	**Thiamilate** (Tyson)	**Tablets, enteric coated:** 20 mg	In 100s.	NA
Rx	**Thiamine HCl** (Various, eg, Dixon-Shane, Elkins-Sinn, Goldline, Lilly, Major)	**Injection:** 100 mg per ml	In 1 ml amps and syringes and 1, 2, 10 and 30 ml vials.	15+
Rx	**Biamine** (Forest)		In 30 ml vials.[1]	15

* Cost Index based on cost per 25 mg.

[1] With 0.5% chlorobutanol.

RIBOFLAVIN (B_2)

Actions:

Riboflavin functions in the body as a coenzyme in the forms of flavin adenine dinucleotide (FAD) and flavin mononucleotide (FMN), which play a vital metabolic role in numerous tissue respiration systems. Symptoms of riboflavin deficiency include corneal vascularization, cheilosis, glossitis and seborrheic dermatitis, especially in skin folds. Corneal vascularization is usually accompanied by itching and burning, blepharospasm and photophobia.

Indications:

Treatment and prevention of riboflavin deficiency.

Precautions:

Riboflavin deficiency seldom occurs alone and is often associated with deficiency of other B vitamins and protein.

Patient Information:

Riboflavin may cause a yellow/orange discoloration of the urine.

Administration and Dosage:

Recommended Dietary Allowances (RDAs): Adult males, 1.4 to 1.8 mg; adult females, 1.2 to 1.3 mg. For a complete listing of RDAs by age, sex or condition, refer to page 5.

Treatment of deficiency states: 5 to 25 mg daily.

				C.I.*
otc	**Riboflavin** (Various, eg, Freeda, IDE, Nature's Bounty, Rugby)	**Tablets:** 25 mg	In 100s and 250s.	6.2+
		50 mg	In 100s, 500s and 2500s.	5.2+
		100 mg	In 100s, 250s and 500s.	3.6+

CALCIUM PANTOTHENATE (B_5; Pantothenic Acid)

Actions:

Pantothenic acid is a precursor of coenzyme A, which is a cofactor for a variety of enzyme-catalyzed reactions involving transfer of acetyl groups. It is associated with oxidative metabolism of carbohydrates; gluconeogenesis; synthesis of fatty acids, sterols, steroid hormones and porphyrins.

Pantothenic acid deficiency has not been recognized in humans with a normal diet, due to the ubiquitous occurrence of this vitamin in ordinary foods. However, a deficiency syndrome was experimentally induced in volunteers. Symptoms included fatigue, headache, sleep disturbances, abdominal cramps, nausea and flatulence. Paresthesias in the extremities, muscle cramps and impaired coordination also occurred.

Indications:

Pantothenic acid deficiency.

Administration and Dosage:

The magnitude of need is not definitely known. From 4 to 7 mg/day has been recommended for adults.

				C.I.*
otc	**Calcium Pantothenate** (Various, eg, Freeda, Rugby, Schein)	**Tablets:** 100 mg	In 100s.	3+
		250 mg	In 100s.	1+
		500 mg	In 100s.	1+
otc *sf*	**Calcium Pantothenate** (Freeda)	**Tablets:** 25 mg	In 250s and 500s.	4
otc *sf*	**Calcium Pantothenate** (Freeda)	**Tablets:** 218 mg	In 100s, 250s and 500s.	1.5
		545 mg	In 100s, 250s and 500s.	1

* Cost Index based on cost per 25 mg riboflavin or 10 mg calcium pantothenate.

sf – Sugar free.

NIACIN (B_3; Nicotinic Acid)

Actions:

Niacin, vitamin B_3, is the common name for nicotinic acid. Nicotinic acid functions in the body as a component of two coenzymes: NAD (nicotinamide adenine dinucleotide, coenzyme I) and NADP (nicotinamide adenine dinucleotide phosphate, coenzyme II), which serve a role in oxidation-reduction reactions essential for tissue respiration. Nicotinic acid is present in NAD and NADP in its active form, nicotinamide (niacinamide). The niacin deficiency state *pellagra* is characterized by mucous membrane, GI and CNS manifestations, a triad often referred to as dermatitis, diarrhea and dementia.

Pharmacology: Although nicotinic acid and nicotinamide function identically as vitamins, their pharmacologic effects differ. In large doses (up to 6 g/day), nicotinic acid is effective in reduction of serum lipids (both LDL cholesterol and triglycerides; see Antihyperlipidemic Agents monograph). The mechanism of this action may involve: Decreased production of VLDL by the liver; inhibition of lipolysis in adipose tissue; decreased esterification of triglycerides by the liver; increased action of lipoprotein lipase. In large doses, peripheral vasodilation is produced, predominantly in the cutaneous vessels of the face, neck and chest. Nicotinic acid causes a release of histamine, which acts directly on peripheral vessels, producing vasodilation and increased blood flow. Nicotinamide does not affect blood lipid levels or the cardiovascular system.

Pharmacokinetics: Niacin is rapidly absorbed from the GI tract; peak serum concentrations usually occur within 45 minutes. The plasma elimination half-life is about 45 minutes. The major metabolites include nicotinuric acid, N-methyl-nicotinamide and 2-pyridone. Approximately ⅓ of an oral dose is excreted unchanged in the urine.

The following prescribing information pertains primarily to therapeutic uses of niacin in doses exceeding basic nutritional intake (RDA levels).

Indications:

Correction of niacin acid deficiency; prevention and treatment of pellagra.

Nicotinic acid: Adjunctive therapy in patients with significant hyperlipidemia who do not respond adequately to diet and weight loss (see Antihyperlipidemic Agents monograph).

Contraindications:

Hepatic dysfunction; active peptic ulcer.

Warnings:

Schizophrenia: There is no convincing evidence to support the use of megadoses of nicotinic acid in the treatment of schizophrenia as part of what is referred to as "orthomolecular psychiatry." Furthermore, high doses are associated with considerable toxicity, including liver damage, hypotension, peptic ulceration, hyperglycemia, hyperuricemia, dermatoses, cardiac arrhythmias, tachycardia, heartburn, nausea, vomiting, diarrhea and other effects commonly seen with lower doses such as flushing and pruritus.

Pregnancy and lactation: (Category C if used in doses above the RDA). Use doses in excess of nutritional requirements during pregnancy or lactation only when clearly needed and when the potential benefits outweigh the potential hazards to the fetus or nursing infant.

Children: Safety and efficacy in children have not been established in doses which exceed nutritional requirements.

Precautions:

Closely observe patients with coronary disease, gallbladder disease, a history of jaundice, liver disease, peptic ulcer or arterial bleeding.

Monitoring: Monitor liver function tests and blood glucose frequently.

Diabetes: Observe diabetic or potential diabetic patients closely for decreased glucose tolerance. Adjustment of diet or hypoglycemic therapy may be necessary.

Gout: Elevated uric acid levels have occurred; use caution in patients predisposed to gout.

Flushing appears frequently with oral therapy and may occur within the first 2 hours of administration. This is transient and will usually subside with continued therapy. The flush response can be attenuated with a dose of a prostaglandin inhibitor, such as aspirin, administered at a dose of approximately 325 mg 30 minutes to 1 hour before the niacin administration.

Tartrazine sensitivity: Some of these products contain tartrazine, which may cause allergic-type reactions (including bronchial asthma) in susceptible individuals. Although the incidence of tartrazine sensitivity in the general population is low, it is frequently seen in patients who also have aspirin hypersensitivity. Specific products containing tartrazine are identified in the product listings.

(Continued on following page)

NIACIN (B_3; Nicotinic Acid) (Cont.)

Drug Interactions:

Lovastatin: Coadministration of niacin may have resulted in rhabdomyolysis in one patient.

Sulfinpyrazone's uricosuric effect may be inhibited by nicotinic acid.

Adverse Reactions:

Flushing (see Precautions), pruritus and GI distress appear frequently with nicotinic acid oral therapy.

GI: Activation of peptic ulcer; nausea; vomiting; abdominal pain; diarrhea.

The hepatotoxicity of nicotinic acid (including cholestatic jaundice) has occurred with as little as 750 mg/day for < 3 months. Hepatitis occurred with sustained release nicotinic acid with as little as 500 mg/day for 2 months. Crystalline (non-sustained release) niacin may be less hepatotoxic.

Dermatologic: Severe generalized flushing; sensation of warmth; keratosis nigricans; pruritus; skin rash; dry skin; itching; tingling.

Miscellaneous: Toxic amblyopia; hypotension; transient headache; atrial fibrillation and other cardiac arrhythmias; decreased glucose tolerance.

Laboratory test abnormalities: Decreased glucose tolerance; abnormalities of hepatic function tests; hyperuricemia.

Patient Information:

Cutaneous flushing and a sensation of warmth, especially in the area of the face, neck and ears, may occur within the first 2 hours. Itching or tingling and headache may also occur. These effects are transient and will usually subside with continued therapy.

May cause GI upset; take with meals.

If dizziness (postural hypotension) occurs, avoid sudden changes in posture.

Extended release products – Take whole; do not break, crush or chew before swallowing.

Administration and Dosage:

Recommended Dietary Allowances (RDAs): Adult males, 15 to 20 mg; adult females, 13 to 15 mg. Niacin is recommended at 6.6 mg/1000 Kcal intake. For a complete listing of RDAs by age, sex and condition, refer to page 5.

Oral: Begin therapy with small doses and increase dose in gradual increments, observing for adverse effects and efficacy.

Niacin deficiency – up to 100 mg/day.

Pellagra – Up to 500 mg/day.

Hyperlipidemia – 1 to 2 g 3 times daily. Do not exceed 6 g/day.

Parenteral: Use only for vitamin deficiencies (not for treatment of hyperlipidemia) and when oral therapy is impossible. The length of parenteral treatment depends upon the patient's response and upon how soon oral medication and a complete and well balanced diet may be taken. Administer by slow IV injection, SC or IM. The IV route is recommended whenever possible.

	Product	Form	Packaging	C.I.*
otc	**Nicotinic Acid (Niacin)** (Various)	**Tablets:** 25 mg	In 100s, 1000s and UD 100s.	NA
otc[1]	**Nicotinic Acid (Niacin)** (Various, eg, Freeda, Nature's Bounty)	**Tablets:** 50 mg	In 100s, 200s, 250s, 300s, 500s, 1000s and UD 100s, 250s and 1000s.	15+
otc[1]	**Nicotinic Acid (Niacin)** (Various, eg, Dixon-Shane, Freeda, Nature's Bounty, Schein)	**Tablets:** 100 mg	In 100s, 250s, 300s, 500s, 1000s and UD 100s, 250s and 1000s.	10+
otc[1]	**Nicotinic Acid (Niacin)** (Various, eg, Nature's Bounty)	**Tablets:** 250 mg	In 100s and 1000s.	35+
otc[1]	**Nicotinic Acid (Niacin)** (Various, eg, Major)	**Tablets:** 500 mg	In 100s, 250s, 500s and 1000s.	2+
Rx	**Niacor** (Upsher-Smith)		(Niacor). White, scored. In 100s.	NA
Rx	**Nicolar** (Rhone-Poulenc Rorer)		Tartrazine. (NE). Yellow, scored. In 100s.	4

* Cost Index based on cost per 100 mg.

[1] Some products may be available *Rx* according to distributor discretion.

(Products continued on following page)

Water-Soluble Vitamins (Cont.)

NIACIN (B_3; Nicotinic Acid) (Cont.)

	Product (Distributor)	Form/Strength	Description/Packaging	C.I.*
otc sf	**Slo-Niacin** (Upsher-Smith)	**Tablets, timed release:** 250 mg	Pink. In 100s and 1000s.	10
otc sf	**Slo-Niacin** (Upsher-Smith)	**Tablets, timed release:** 500 mg	Pink. In 100s and UD 100s.	5
otc sf	**Slo-Niacin** (Upsher-Smith)	**Tablets, timed release:** 750 mg	Pink. In 100s.	5
otc[1]	**Nicotinic Acid (Niacin)** (Various, eg, Dixon-Shane, Geneva Marsam, Goldline, Major, Moore, Schein, Vitarine)	**Capsules, timed release:** 125 mg	In 100s and 1000s.	10+
otc	**Nicobid Tempules** (Rhone-Poulenc Rorer)		(2835/USV). Black/clear. In 100s.	15
otc[1]	**Nicotinic Acid (Niacin)** (Various, eg, Dixon-Shane, Genetco, Geneva Marsam, Major, Nature's Bounty, Parmed, Rugby, Schein, Vitarine)	**Capsules, timed release:** 250 mg	In 100s and 1000s.	6.5+
otc	**Nicobid Tempules** (Rhone-Poulenc Rorer)		(2840/USV). Green/clear. In 100s.	10
otc	**Niac** (Forest)	**Capsules, timed release:** 300 mg	In 100s.	25
otc[1]	**Nicotinic Acid (Niacin)** (Various, eg, Dixon-Shane, Genetco, Major, Moore, Parmed, Rugby, Vitarine)	**Capsules, timed release:** 400 mg	In 100s and 1000s.	5.6+
otc	**Nia-Bid** (Geriatric Pharm.)		In 100s.	NA
otc	**Niacels** (Hauck)		In 100s.	20
otc	**Nico-400** (Jones Medical)		In 100s.	35
Rx	**Nicotinic Acid (Niacin)** (Various, eg, Goldline, Major, Nature's Bounty, Rugby, Schein)	**Capsules, timed release:** 500 mg	In 100s and 250s.	5+
otc	**Nicobid Tempules** (Rhone-Poulenc Rorer)		(2841/USV). Blue/white. In 100s.	5
otc	**Nicotinex** (Fleming)	**Elixir:** 50 mg per 5 ml	14% alcohol. Sherry wine base. In pt and gal.	60
Rx	**Nicotinic Acid (Niacin)** (Various)	**Injection:** 100 mg per ml	In 30 ml vials.	NA

NICOTINAMIDE (Niacinamide)

Actions: Nicotinamide is used by the body as a source of niacin. Lipid metabolism, tissue respiration and glycogenolysis require nicotinamide. Nicotinamide does not have hypolipidemic or vasodilating effects.

Indications: Prophylaxis and treatment of pellagra.

Administration and Dosage: Therapeutic dose is 50 mg 3 to 10 times daily.

	Product (Distributor)	Form/Strength	Description/Packaging	C.I.*
otc[1]	**Nicotinamide (Niacinamide)** (Various, eg, Freeda, Nature's Bounty, Rugby, Schein, Sidmak, UDL, Vangard, Vitarine)	**Tablets:** 50 mg	In 100s, 1000s and UD 100s.	65+
		100 mg	In 100s, 1000s and UD 100s.	6.8+
		125 mg	In 100s, 500s and 1000s.	12+
		250 mg	In 100s, 500s and 1000s.	6.5+
		500 mg	In 100s and 1000s.	4.9+

* Cost Index based on cost per 100 mg.

[1] Some products may be available *Rx*, according to distributor discretion.

PYRIDOXINE HCl (B_6)

Actions:

Natural substances that have vitamin B_6 activity, pyridoxine in plants, and pyridoxal or pyridoxamine in animals, are converted to physiologically active forms of vitamin B_6, pyridoxal phosphate (codecarboxylase) and pyridoxamine phosphate.

Vitamin B_6 acts as a coenzyme in the metabolism of protein, carbohydrates and fat. In protein metabolism, it participates in the decarboxylation of amino acids; conversion of tryptophan to niacin or serotonin (5-hydroxytryptamine); and deamination, transamination and transulfuration of amino acids. In carbohydrate metabolism, it is responsible for the breakdown of glycogen to glucose-1-phosphate.

The total adult body pool consists of 16 to 25 mg pyridoxine. The need for pyridoxine increases with the amount of protein in the diet.

Pharmacokinetics: Pyridoxine is readily absorbed from the GI tract. Its biologic half-life appears to be 15 to 20 days. Vitamin B_6 is degraded to 4-pyridoxic acid in the liver. This metabolite is excreted in the urine.

Indications:

Pyridoxine deficiency, including: Inadequate diet; drug-induced deficiency (eg, isoniazid, hydralazine, oral contraceptives); inborn errors of metabolism (eg, B_6-dependent seizures or B_6-responsive anemia).

The parenteral route is indicated when oral use is not feasible (eg, anorexia, nausea, vomiting, preoperative and postoperative conditions, impaired GI absorption).

Unlabeled uses: Hydrazine poisoning. Although experience is limited, reversal of neurologic symptoms and CNS depression have been reported.

Premenstrual syndrome (PMS) has been treated with pyridoxine 40 to 500 mg/day, but with conflicting results.

Hyperoxaluria type I (and oxalate kidney stones) has been treated with pyridoxine in low doses (25 to 300 mg/day).

Nausea and vomiting in pregnancy is sometimes treated with pyridoxine.

Contraindications:

Sensitivity to pyridoxine.

Warnings:

Pregnancy and lactation: Category A. Pyridoxine requirements are increased during pregnancy and lactation. Pyridoxine varies in concentration in breast milk in response to changes in maternal intake of the vitamin. Use doses in excess of the RDA for lactating females with caution. Pyridoxine may inhibit lactation by prolactin suppression.

Children: Safety and efficacy have not been established for use in children.

Precautions:

Pyridoxine deficiency alone is rare; multiple vitamin deficiencies can be expected in any inadequate diet. Some drugs may result in increased pyridoxine requirements, including: Cycloserine, hydralazine, isoniazid, oral contraceptives and penicillamine.

Abuse and dependence have been noted in adults given 200 mg/day followed by withdrawal.

Drug Interactions:

Pyridoxine Drug Interactions			
Precipitant drug	Object drug*		Description
Pyridoxine	Levodopa	↓	Pyridoxine reduces levodopa's effectiveness by increasing its peripheral metabolism; therefore, lower levels are available for CNS penetration. Avoid supplemental vitamins that contain > 5 mg pyridoxine in the daily dose.
Pyridoxine	Phenobarbital	↓	Phenobarbital serum levels may be decreased.
Pyridoxine	Phenytoin	↓	Phenytoin serum levels may be decreased.

* ↓ = Object drug decreased

Adverse Reactions:

Sensory neuropathic syndromes; unstable gait; numb feet; awkwardness of hands; perioral numbness; decreased sensation to touch, temperature and vibration; paresthesia; somnolence; low serum folic acid levels.

Overdosage:

Ataxia and severe sensory neuropathy have occurred in patients who had consumed pyridoxine (50 mg to 2 g) over a long period of time. When pyridoxine is discontinued, symptoms will lessen. It may take 6 months for sensation to return to normal.

(Continued on following page)

Water-Soluble Vitamins (Cont.)

PYRIDOXINE HCl (B_6) (Cont.)

Administration and Dosage:

Recommended Dietary Allowances (RDAs): Adult males, 1.7 to 2 mg; adult females, 1.4 to 1.6 mg. Requirements are greater in persons having certain genetic defects or those receiving INH or oral contraceptives. For a complete listing of RDAs by age, sex and condition, see page 5.

Dietary deficiency: 10 to 20 mg daily for 3 weeks. Follow-up treatment is recommended daily for several weeks with an oral therapeutic multivitamin containing 2 to 5 mg pyridoxine. Correct poor dietary habits and encourage an adequate, well balanced diet.

Vitamin B_6 dependency syndrome: May require a therapeutic dosage of as much as 600 mg/day and 30 mg/day for life.

Deficiencies due to isoniazid: Some advocate pyridoxine prophylaxis for all isoniazid patients; others advocate prophylaxis only for those predisposed to neuropathy. Recommended prophylactic doses range from 6 to 100 mg daily, but the lower doses appear more common. Treatment of established neuropathy requires 50 to 200 mg daily.

INH poisoning (> 10 g), give an equal amount of pyridoxine: 4 g IV followed by 1 g IM every 30 minutes. Pyridoxine can be toxic, but doses of 70 to 357 mg/kg have been administered without incident.

	Product	Form	Packaging	C.I.*
otc	**Pyridoxine HCl** (Various, eg, Geneva Marsam, Schein)	**Tablets:** 25 mg	In 100s and 1000s.	20+
otc	**Nestrex** (Fielding)		Dextrose. In 100s.	95
otc	**Pyridoxine HCl** (Various, eg, Dixon-Shane, Geneva Marsam, Moore, Schein)	**Tablets:** 50 mg	In 100s and 1000s.	10+
otc	**Pyridoxine HCl** (Various, eg, Dixon-Shane, Moore, Schein)	**Tablets:** 100 mg	In 100s and 1000s.	2.4+
otc	**Vitamin B_6** (Mission)	**Tablets, timed release:** 100 mg	In 100s.	
Rx	**Pyridoxine HCl** (Various, eg, Major, Moore, Schein)	**Injection:** 100 mg per ml	In 10 and 30 ml vials.	30+
Rx	**Beesix** (Forest)		In 30 ml vials.[1]	40

CYANOCOBALAMIN (B_{12})

Actions:

Vitamin B_{12} is essential to growth, cell reproduction, hematopoiesis and nucleic acid and myelin synthesis. For use of vitamin B_{12} in treatment of pernicious anemia, see monograph in Blood Modifiers section.

Indications:

Nutritional vitamin B_{12} deficiency.

These products are NOT indicated for treatment of pernicious anemia.

Contraindications:

Hypersensitivity to cyanocobalamin.

Administration and Dosage:

Recommended Dietary Allowances (RDAs): Adults, 2 mcg. For a complete listing of RDAs by age, sex and condition, refer to page 5.

Nutritional deficiency: 25 to 250 mcg/day.

	Product	Form	Packaging	C.I.*
otc	**Vitamin B_{12}** (Various, eg, Dixon-Shane, Geneva Marsam, Rugby, Schein)	**Tablets:** 25 mcg	In 100s.	11+
		50 mcg	In 100s and 1000s.	4.5+
		100 mcg	In 100s and 1000s.	2.5+
		250 mcg	In 100s.	2.5+
otc	**Ener-B** (Nature's Bounty)	**Nasal gel:** 400 mcg/unit	In 0.1 ml units (12s)	NA

* Cost Index based on cost per 50 mg pyridoxine or 25 mcg cyanocobalamin.

[1] With 1.5% benzyl alcohol.

PARA-AMINOBENZOIC ACID (PABA)

Actions:

Although not considered to have the status of a vitamin, this accessory food factor is found naturally associated with B complex vitamins. Small amounts are present in cereal, eggs, milk and meats. Detectable amounts are normally found in human blood, spinal fluid, urine and sweat.

PABA is a component of several biologically important systems and participates in a number of fundamentally biologic processes. It has been suggested that PABA has an antifibrosis action due to mediation of increased oxygen uptake at the tissue level. Pathological fibrosis is believed to occur from either too much serotonin or too little monoamine oxidase (MAO) activity over a period of time. MAO requires an adequate supply of oxygen to function properly. By increasing oxygen supply at the tissue level, PABA may enhance MAO activity and prevent or bring about regression of fibrosis. These effects are speculative.

Indications:

"Possibly effective" in the treatment of scleroderma, dermatomyositis, morphea, linear scleroderma, pemphigus and Peyronie's disease.

Topical PABA is useful as a sunscreen (see Sunscreens section).

Contraindications:

Concurrent sulfonamide therapy.

Warnings:

Pregnancy and lactation: Safety for use has not been established. Use only when clearly needed and when potential benefits outweigh potential hazards to the fetus or nursing infant.

Precautions:

Anorexia or nausea: Should anorexia or nausea occur, interrupt therapy until the patient is eating normally again. This permits prompt subsidence of symptoms and also avoids the possible development of hypoglycemia.

Renal disease: Use cautiously.

Hypersensitivity: If a hypersensitivity reaction occurs, discontinue the drug. Refer to Management of Acute Hypersensitivity Reactions.

Drug Interactions:

Dapsone's antimalarial effect may be antagonized by PABA due to interference with its primary mechanism of action.

Adverse Reactions:

Anorexia, nausea, fever and rash have occurred infrequently, subsiding with discontinuation of the drug. After desensitization, treatment can be resumed.

Administration and Dosage:

Take with food. Take tablets with an adequate amount of liquid to prevent GI upset.

Adults: 12 g daily in 4 to 6 divided doses.

Children: 1 g/10 lb (4.55 kg) daily in divided doses.

				C.I.*
otc	**Para-Aminobenzoic Acid** (Various)	**Tablets:** 30 mg	In 100s, 250s and 500s.	1233+
		100 mg	In 100s, 250s and 500s.	412+
		500 mg	In 100s.	90+
Rx	**Potaba** (Glenwood)	Potassium Para-Aminobenzoate: **Tablets:** 500 mg	(Potaba 54). In 100s and 1000s.	450
		Capsules: 500 mg	(Potaba 51). In 250s and 1000s.	420
		Envules (Powder for Reconstitution): 2 g	In 50s.	430
		Powder	In 100 g and 1 lb.	393

* Cost Index based on cost per 1 g.

VITAMIN C (Ascorbic Acid)

Actions:

Vitamin C is an essential vitamin in man; however, its exact biological functions are not fully understood. It is essential for the formation and the maintenance of intercellular ground substance and collagen, for catecholamine biosynthesis, for synthesis of carnitine and steroids, for conversion of folic acid to folinic acid and for tyrosine metabolism.

The deficiency state *scurvy* is characterized by degenerative changes in the capillaries, bone and connective tissues. Mild vitamin C deficiency symptoms may include faulty bone and tooth development, gingivitis, bleeding gums and loosened teeth. Febrile states, chronic illness and infection increase the need for ascorbic acid. Premature and immature infants require relatively large amounts of the vitamin. Hemovascular disorders, burns and delayed fracture and wound healing are indications for an increase in daily intake.

Absorption of dietary ascorbate from the intestines is nearly complete. Vitamin C is readily available in citrus fruit, tomatoes, potatoes and leafy vegetables.

Indications:

Prevention and treatment of scurvy. Parenteral administration is desirable in an acute deficiency or when absorption of oral ascorbic acid is uncertain.

Unlabeled uses: Vitamin C in high doses has been advocated for prevention of the common cold, for treatment of asthma, atherosclerosis, wounds, schizophrenia and for treatment of cancer; however, clinical data do not justify these uses.

Vitamin C ($\geq$ 2 g/day) may be used as a urinary acidifier in conjunction with methenamine therapy. Data regarding the efficacy of ascorbic acid for this purpose are conflicting. Failure of vitamin C to significantly lower urine pH may be attributed to inadequate dosage ($<$ 2 g/day).

Vitamin C in doses of at least 150 mg has been used to control idiopathic methemoglobinemia (less effective than methylene blue).

Warnings:

Excessive vitamin C doses: Diabetics, patients prone to recurrent renal calculi, those undergoing stool occult blood tests and those on sodium restricted diets or anticoagulant therapy should not take excessive doses of vitamin C over an extended period of time.

Pregnancy: Category C. It is not known whether ascorbic acid can cause fetal harm or can affect reproduction capacity. Give to pregnant women only if clearly needed.

Do not administer ascorbic acid to pregnant women in excess of the amount needed for treatment. The possibility of the fetus adapting to high levels of the vitamin could result in a scorbutic condition after birth when the intake drops to normal levels. This action is controversial.

Lactation: Administer with caution to a nursing mother. Ascorbic acid is excreted in breast milk, but does not necessarily increase in response to increasing doses.

Precautions:

Tartrazine sensitivity: Some of these products contain tartrazine, which may cause allergic type reactions (including bronchial asthma) in susceptible individuals. Although the incidence of sensitivity is low, it is frequently seen in patients who also have aspirin hypersensitivity. Specific products containing tartrazine are identified in the product listings.

Sulfite sensitivity: Some of these products contain sulfites which may cause allergic-type reactions in certain susceptible people. The overall prevalence of sulfite sensitivity in the general population is unknown and probably low. Sulfite sensitivity is seen more frequently in asthmatic than in nonasthmatic people.

Drug Interactions:

Contraceptives, oral and estrogens: Ascorbic acid increases serum levels of estrogen and estrogen contained in oral contraceptives, possibly resulting in adverse reactions.

Warfarin: The anticoagulant action of warfarin may be reduced.

(Drug Interactions continued on following page)

VITAMIN C (Ascorbic Acid) (Cont.)

Drug Interactions (Cont.):

Drug/Lab test interactions: Large doses (> 500 mg) of vitamin C may cause false-negative urine **glucose determinations.**

No exogenous vitamin C should be ingested for 48 to 72 hours before amine-dependent stool **occult blood** tests are conducted because possible false-negative results may occur.

Adverse Reactions:

Large doses may cause diarrhea and precipitation of cystine, oxalate or urate renal stones if the urine becomes acidic during therapy.

Transient mild soreness may occur at the site of IM or SC injection. Too rapid IV administration may cause temporary faintness or dizziness.

Administration and Dosage:

Recommended Dietary Allowances (RDAs): Adults, 60 mg. For a complete listing of RDAs by age, sex and condition, refer to page 5.

Administer IV, IM or SC. Avoid too rapid IV injection. Absorption and utilization are somewhat more efficient with the IM route, which is usually preferred.

Infants: Average daily protective requirement is 30 mg. The usual curative dose is 100 to 300 mg daily, continued as long as clinical symptoms persist or until saturation, as indicated by excretion tests, has been attained.

Premature infants: May require 75 to 100 mg/day.

Adults: The average protective dose is 70 to 150 mg daily. For scurvy, 300 mg to 1 g daily is recommended. However, up to 6 g/day has been administered parenterally to normal adults without evidence of toxicity.

Enhanced wound healing – Doses of 300 to 500 mg daily for 7 to 10 days both preoperatively and postoperatively are adequate, although considerably larger amounts have been recommended.

Burns – Individualize dosage. For severe burns, daily doses of 1 to 2 g are recommended.

In other conditions in which the need for vitamin C is increased, 3 to 5 times the daily optimum allowances appears adequate.

	ASCORBIC ACID			C.I.*
otc	**Ascorbic Acid** (Various, eg, Lannett)	**Tablets:** 25 mg	In 1000s.	5.6+
otc	**Ascorbic Acid** (Various, eg, Goldline, Lannett)	**Tablets:** 50 mg	In 1000s and UD 100s.	3.9+
otc	**Ascorbic Acid** (Various, eg, Century, Dixon-Shane, Lannett, UDL, West-Ward)	**Tablets:** 100 mg	In 100s, 500s, 1000s and UD 100s.	5.2+
otc	**Ascorbic Acid** (Various, eg, Approved Pharm[1], Dixon-Shane, Geneva Marsam, Lannett, Moore, Roxane, UDL, West-Ward)	**Tablets:** 250 mg	In 30s, 100s, 500s, 1000s and UD 100s.	3.4+
otc	**Ascorbic Acid** (Various, eg, Approved Pharm[1], Century, Dixon-Shane, Geneva Marsam, Lannett, Lederle, Roxane, Rugby, UDL, West-Ward)	**Tablets:** 500 mg	In 100s, 250s, 500s, 1000s and UD 100s.	2.5+
otc	**Ascorbic Acid** (Various, eg, Approved Pharm.[1])	**Tablets:** 1000 mg	In 50s and 100s.	NA

* Cost Index based on cost per 100 mg.

[1] With or without rose hips.

(Continued on following page)

Complete prescribing information for these products begins on page 25.

Water-Soluble Vitamins (Cont.)

ASCORBIC ACID (Cont.)

				C.I.*
otc	**Ascorbic Acid** (Various, eg, Rugby)	**Tablets, chewable:** 100 mg	In 100s, 250s and 1000s.	NA
otc	**Flavorcee** (Hudson)		Orange flavor. In 100s.	38
otc	**Ascorbic Acid** (Various, eg, Dixon-Shane, Geneva Marsam)	**Tablets, chewable:** 250 mg	In 100s and 1000s.	11+
otc	**Flavorcee** (Hudson)		Orange flavor. In 250s.	21
otc	**Ascorbic Acid** (Various, eg, Dixon-Shane, Scientific Nutrition)	**Tablets, chewable:** 500 mg	In 90s, 100s and 1000s.	7.8+
otc	**Flavorcee** (Hudson)		With rose hips. Sodium free. In 90s.	NA
otc	**Ascorbic Acid** (Various, eg, Approved Pharm.[1])	**Tablets, timed release:** 500 mg	In 100s.	NA
otc sf	**Ascorbic Acid Caplets**[1] (Approved Pharm.)	**Tablets, timed release:** 1000 mg	Sodium free. In 50s, 100s and 250s.	NA
otc sf	**Ascorbic Acid Caplets** (Approved Pharm.)	**Tablets, timed release:** 1500 mg	Rose hips. Sodium free. In 50s.	3.3
otc	**Ascorbic Acid** (Various, eg, Geneva Marsam)	**Capsules, timed release:** 500 mg	In 100s	8+
otc	**Ascorbicap** (ICN)		Tartrazine. In 50s and 250s.	22
otc	**Cebid Timecelles** (Hauck)		In 100s.	19
otc	**Cetane** (Forest)		In 100s.	11
otc	**Cevi-Bid** (Geriatric)		In 30s, 100s and 500s.	26
otc sf	**N'ice Vitamin C Drops** (SmithKline Beecham Consumer)	**Lozenges:** 60 mg	Menthol, sorbitol and tartrazine. Orange, lemon and grape flavors. In 16s.	NA
otc sf	**C-Crystals** (Nature's Bounty)	**Crystals:** 5 g per teaspoonful	In 180 g.	NA
otc sf	**Vita-C** (Freeda)	**Crystals:** 4 g per teaspoonful	Sodium free. In 100 and 500 g.	6.4
otc sf	**Dull-C** (Freeda)	**Powder:** 4 g per teaspoonful	Sodium free. In 100 and 500 g.	6.4
otc	**Ce-Vi-Sol** (Mead Johnson Nutritional)	**Liquid:** 35 mg per 0.6 ml	5% alcohol. In 50 ml w/dropper.	226
otc	**Cecon** (Abbott)	**Solution:** 100 mg per ml	In 50 ml w/dropper.	140
otc	**Ascorbic Acid** (Various, eg, Barre, Rugby)	**Syrup:** 500 mg per 5 ml	In 120 and 480 ml.	1+
Rx	**Ascorbic Acid** (Various, eg, Loch, Lyphomed, Pasadena)	**Injection:** 250 mg per ml	In 2 ml amps and 2 and 30 ml vials.	90+
Rx	**Ascorbic Acid** (Various, eg, American Regent, Major, Pasadena, Schein)	**Injection:** 500 mg per ml	In 2 ml amps and 50 ml vials.	13+
Rx	**Cevalin** (Lilly)		In 1 ml amps.[2]	346

* Cost Index based on cost per 100 mg.
sf- Sugar free.

[1] With or without rose hips.
[2] With 0.5% sodium hydrosulfite.

(Continued on following page)

Complete prescribing information for these products begins on page 25.

Water-Soluble Vitamins (Cont.)

	Product	Form	Description	C.I.*
SODIUM ASCORBATE				
otc *sf*	**Sodium Ascorbate** (Freeda)	**Tablets:** 585 mg (equiv. to 500 mg ascorbic acid)	Buffered. In 100s, 250s and 500s.	11
otc *sf*	**Sodium Ascorbate** (Freeda)	**Crystals:** 1020 mg (equiv. to 900 mg ascorbic acid) per ¼ teaspoonful	Buffered. In 120 and 480 g.	6.6
Rx	**Sodium Ascorbate** (Various, eg, Interstate)	**Injection:** 250 mg/ml (equiv. to 222 mg/ml ascorbic acid)	In 30 ml vials.	42+
Rx	**Cenolate** (Abbott)	**Injection:** 562.5 mg per ml (equiv. to 500 mg/ml ascorbic acid)	In 1 and 2 ml amps.[1]	196
CALCIUM ASCORBATE				
otc *sf*	**Calcium Ascorbate** (Freeda)	**Tablets:** 610 mg (equiv. to 500 mg ascorbic acid)	Buffered. Sodium free. In 100s, 250s and 500s.	17
otc *sf*	**Calcium Ascorbate** (Freeda)	**Powder:** 1 g (equiv. to 826 mg ascorbic acid) per ¼ teaspoonful	Buffered. In 120 and 480 g.	71
ASCORBIC ACID COMBINATIONS				
otc	**Chewable C** (Approved Pharm.)	**Tablets, chewable:** 100 mg vitamin C as sodium ascorbate and ascorbic acid	Sugar, fructose. Orange flavor. In 100s.	NA
otc	**Chewable C** (Approved Pharm.)	**Tablets, chewable:** 250 mg vitamin C as sodium ascorbate and ascorbic acid	Orange flavor. In 100s.	NA
otc	**Chewable C** (Approved Pharm.)	**Tablets, chewable:** 300 mg vitamin C as ascorbic acid and sodium ascorbate with rose hips	Lemon flavor. In 100s.	NA
otc	**Chewable C** (Approved Pharm.)	**Tablets, chewable:** 500 mg vitamin C as sodium ascorbate and ascorbic acid	Orange flavor. In 100s.	NA
otc	**C-Max** (Bio-Tech)	**Tablets, gradual release:** 1000 mg vitamin C, 40 mg magnesium, 5 mg zinc, 10 mg potassium, 1 mg manganese and 10 mg pectin in a rose hips base	In 100s.	NA
otc	**Vicks Vitamin C Drops** (Richardson-Vicks)	**Lozenges:** 60 mg vitamin C as sodium ascorbate and ascorbic acid	Orange or lemon flavor. In 14s and 30s.	NA

* Cost Index based on cost per 100 mg ascorbic acid.
sf – Sugar free.
[1] With 0.5% sodium hydrosulfite.

BIOFLAVONOIDS (Vitamin P)

Citrus bioflavonoids, formerly referred to as Vitamin P, are derived from the rind of green citrus fruits, and are also found in rose hips and black currants.

These products were previously used to decrease capillary permeability and fragility and were classified as hemostatic agents. Their mechanism of action is unknown.

Unlabeled uses: This group of compounds has been widely used for many diseases including: Rheumatic fever; decidual bleeding in pregnancy; habitual abortion; poliomyelitis; prevention of hemorrhage in anticoagulated patients; rheumatoid arthritis; periodontal disease; diabetic retinitis; various thrombocytopenic and nonthrombocytopenic hemorrhagic disorders; herpes labialis. Unfortunately, many of these uses have not been tested in controlled clinical trials; hence, *there is little evidence that they are effective for any indication. There is no established need in human nutrition.*

	Product	Composition	Supplied	C.I.*
otc	**Citro-Flav 200** (Goldline)	**Capsules:** 200 mg citrus bioflavonoids complex	In 100s.	1.9
otc *sf*	**Pan C-500** (Freeda)	**Tablets:** 100 mg hesperidin, 100 mg citrus bioflavonoids, and 500 mg vitamin C	Sodium free. In 100s, 250s and 500s.	2.9
otc	**Amino-Opti-C** (Tyson)	**Tablets, sustained release:** 250 mg lemon bioflavonoids, rutin, hesperidin, 1000 mg vitamin C and rose hips powder	In 100s.	2.9
otc *sf*	**C Factors "1000" Plus** (Solgar)	**Tablets:** 1000 mg vitamin C with rose hips, 250 mg citrus bioflavonoids, 50 mg rutin, 25 mg hesperidin complex	Sodium free. Capsule shape. In 50s, 100s and 250s.	NA
otc	**Peridin-C** (Beutlich)	**Tablets:** 150 mg hesperidin complex, 50 mg hesperidin methyl chalcone (bioflavonoids) and 200 mg ascorbic acid	In 100s and 500s.	4.9
otc *sf*	**Span C** (Freeda)	**Tablets:** 300 mg citrus bioflavonoids and 200 mg vitamin C (ascorbic acid; from rose hips)	Sodium free. In 100s, 250s and 500s.	2.7
otc *sf*	**Flavons-500** (Freeda)	**Tablets:** 500 mg citrus bioflavonoids complex and hesperidin complex	Sodium free. In 100s and 250s.	2.8
otc *sf*	**C Speridin** (Marlyn)	**Tablets, sustained release:** 100 mg hesperidin, 100 mg lemon bioflavonoids and 500 mg ascorbic acid	In 100s.	1.3
otc *sf*	**Super Complex C-500 Caplets** (Approved Pharm.)	**Tablets:** 25 mg citrus hesperidin complex; 100 mg citrus bioflavonoid complex; 50 mg rutin; 500 mg ascorbic acid; 100 mg rose hips, acerola, green pepper and black currant concentrate	Sodium free. In 100s.	NA
otc *sf*	**Citrus-flav C 500** (Fibertone)	**Tablets:** 200 mg citrus bioflavonoids complex, 200 mg vitamin C, 40 mg hesperidin complex, 50 mg acerola, 10 mg rutin in a citrus base of orange and lemon powder, grapefruit concentrate powder and citrus pectin	Sodium free. In 100s and 250s.	1

* Cost Index based on cost per capsule or tablet.
sf – Sugar free.

(Continued on following page)

Water-Soluble Vitamins (Cont.)

BIOFLAVONOIDS (Vitamin P) (Cont.)

	Product	Content	Notes	C.I.*
otc	**Bio-Acerola C Complex** (Solgar)	**Wafers:** 500 mg vitamin C, 10 mg citrus bioflavonoids, 5 mg rutin in a natural base of acerola, rose hips, buckwheat, black currant and green pepper concentrate powders	Cane sugar. Cherry flavoring. In 50s and 100s.	NA
otc	**Super Citro Cee** (Marlyn)	**Tablets, sustained release:** 500 mg lemon bioflavonoids, 50 mg rutin, 500 mg ascorbic acid and 500 mg rose hips powder	In 50s, 100s and 200s.	1.5
otc *sf*	**Ester-C Plus** (Solgar)	**Capsules:** 500 mg vitamin C, 25 mg citrus bioflavonoid complex, 10 mg acerola, 10 mg rose hips, 5 mg rutin, 62 mg calcium	Sodium free. In 50s.	NA
otc *sf*	**Extra Potency Ester-C Plus** (Solgar)	**Tablets:** 1000 mg vitamin C, 200 mg citrus bioflavonoid complex, 25 mg acerola, 25 mg rutin, 25 mg rose hips, 125 mg calcium	Sodium free. In 30s.	NA
otc *sf*	**Ester-C Plus Multi-Mineral** (Solgar)	**Capsules:** 425 mg vitamin C, 50 mg citrus bioflavonoid complex, 12.5 mg acerola, 12.5 mg rose hips, 5 mg rutin, 25 mg calcium, 13 mg magnesium, 12.5 mg potassium, 2.5 mg zinc	Sodium free. In 60s.	NA
otc *sf*	**Quercetin** (Freeda)	**Tablets:** 50 mg bioflavonoid (from eucalyptus)	Sodium free. In 100s and 250s.	2.7
		250 mg bioflavonoid (from eucalyptus)	Sodium free. In 100s and 250s.	7.6

* Cost Index based on cost per capsule, tablet or wafer.
sf – Sugar free.

CALCIUM

For information on parenteral calcium products, refer to Intravenous Nutritional Therapy, Electrolytes section.

Actions:

Calcium is the fifth most abundant element in the body; the major fraction is in bone. It is essential for the functional integrity of the nervous and muscular systems, for normal cardiac function, for cell permeability and for blood coagulation. It also functions as an enzyme cofactor and affects the secretory activity of endocrine and exocrine glands.

Adequate calcium intake is particularly important during periods of bone growth in childhood and adolescence, and during pregnancy and lactation. An adequate supply of calcium is necessary in adults, especially those over 40 years of age, to prevent a negative calcium balance which may contribute to the development of osteoporosis.

Patients with advanced renal insufficiency exhibit phosphate retention and some degree of hyperphosphatemia. The retention of phosphate plays a pivotal role in causing secondary hyperparathyroidism associated with osteodystrophy and soft tissue calcification. Calcium acetate, when taken with meals, combines with dietary phosphate to form insoluble calcium phosphate which is excreted in the feces.

Elemental Calcium Content of Calcium Salts		
Calcium salt	% Calcium	mEq Ca^{++}/g
Calcium glubionate	6.5	3.3
Calcium gluconate	9.3	4.6
Calcium lactate	13	9.2
Calcium citrate	21	12
Calcium acetate	25	12.6
Tricalcium phosphate	39	19.3
Calcium carbonate	40	20

Calcium must be in a soluble, ionized form to be absorbed. Solubility (except calcium lactate) is increased by acidic pH. Give with meals to maximize acidity and solubility. Differences in absorption and bioavailability between various calcium salts appear to exist, as well as between different preparations of the same salt.

Indications:

As a dietary supplement when calcium intake may be inadequate (eg, childhood and adolescence, chronic renal failure, pregnancy, lactation, postmenopausal females, the aged).

In the treatment of calcium deficiency states which may occur in diseases such as: Tetany of newborn; end stage renal disease, mild to moderate renal insufficiency; renal osteodystrophy; acute and chronic hypoparathyroidism; pseudohypoparathyroidism; postmenopausal and senile osteoporosis; rickets and osteomalacia. Some studies have suggested that the use of calcium citrate is more effective than calcium carbonate in the treatment of postmenopausal osteoporosis.

Calcium acetate (PhosLo): Control of hyperphosphatemia in end stage renal failure; does not promote aluminum absorption.

Unlabeled uses: Calcium supplementation may lower blood pressure in some hypertensive patients with indices suggesting calcium "deficiency." However, other hypertensives may experience a pressor response.

In one study, calcium administration significantly reduced premenstrual symptoms of fluid retention, pain and negative affect.

Contraindications:

Renal calculi; hypophosphatemia; hypercalcemia.

Warnings:

PhosLo: End stage renal failure patients may develop hypercalcemia when given calcium with meals. Do not give other calcium supplements concurrently with *PhosLo.* Chronic hypercalcemia may lead to vascular and other soft tissue calcification. Monitor serum calcium levels twice weekly during the early dose adjustment period. Do not allow serum calcium times phosphate product to exceed 66.

Pregnancy: Category C (PhosLo): It is not known whether *PhosLo* can cause fetal harm when administered to a pregnant woman or can affect reproduction capacity. Give to a pregnant woman only if clearly needed.

(Continued on following page)

CALCIUM (Cont.)

Precautions:

Hypercalcemia/hypercalciuria may result when therapeutic amounts are given for prolonged periods; it is most likely to occur in hypoparathyroid patients receiving high doses of vitamin D. Avoid by frequent monitoring of plasma and urine calcium levels. For symptoms and treatment refer to the vitamin D monograph.

Calcium citrate: Renal function impairment – Avoid concurrent aluminum-containing antacids.

Drug Interactions:

Calcium Drug Interactions

Precipitant drug	Object drug*		Description
Thiazide diuretics	Calcium salts	↑	Hypercalcemia resulting from renal tubular reabsorption, or bone release of calcium by thiazides may be amplified by exogenous calcium.
Calcium salts	Atenolol	↓	Mean peak plasma levels and bioavailability of atenolol may be decreased, possibly resulting in decreased beta blockade.
Calcium salts	Iron salts	↓	GI absorption of iron may be reduced.
Calcium carbonate	Quinolones	↓	The bioavailability of norfloxacin may be reduced; ciprofloxacin and ofloxacin do not appear to be affected.
Calcium salts	Sodium polystyrene sulfonate	↓	Coadministration in patients with renal impairment may result in an unanticipated metabolic alkalosis and a reduction of the resin's binding of potassium.
Calcium salts	Tetracyclines	↓	The absorption and serum levels of tetracyclines are decreased; a decreased anti-infective response may occur.
Calcium salts	Verapamil	↓	Clinical effects and toxicities of verapamil may be reversed.

* ↑ = Object drug increased ↓ = Object drug decreased

Drug/Food interaction: Diets high in dietary fiber have been shown to decrease absorption of calcium due to decreased transit time in the GI tract and complexing of fiber with the calcium.

Adverse Reactions:

GI disturbances are rare. Mild hypercalcemia ($Ca^{++} > 10.5$ mg/dl) may be asymptomatic or manifest itself as: Anorexia; nausea; vomiting; constipation; abdominal pain; dry mouth; thirst; polyuria. More severe hypercalcemia ($Ca^{++} > 12$ mg/dl) is associated with confusion, delirium, stupor and coma.

The risk of hypercalcemia with calcium acetate may be less than that of calcium carbonate and calcium citrate.

Overdosage:

Administration of *PhosLo* in excess of the appropriate daily dosage can cause severe hypercalcemia (see Adverse Reactions). Severe hypercalcemia can be treated by acute hemodialysis and discontinuing therapy.

Patient Information:

Notify physician if any of the following occurs: Anorexia, nausea, vomiting, constipation, abdominal pain, dry mouth, thirst or polyuria.

Take with or following meals to enhance absorption.

Take with a large glass of water.

Administration and Dosage:

Recommended Dietary Allowances (RDAs): Adults (25 to > 51 years of age), 800 mg. For a complete listing of RDAs by age, sex and condition, refer to page 5.

Dietary supplement: The usual daily dose is 500 mg to 2 g, 2 to 4 times daily.

An NIH Consensus Development conference recommends a calcium intake for adults of 1000 to 1500 mg/day to reduce bone loss associated with aging.

PhosLo: 2 tablets with each meal. The dosage may be increased to bring the serum phosphate value < 6 mg/dl, as long as hypercalcemia does not develop. Most patients require 3 to 4 tablets with each meal.

(Products listed on following pages)

Complete prescribing information for these products begins on page 31.

	Product	Form/Strength	Description/Packaging	C.I.*
CALCIUM GLUBIONATE, 6.5% calcium.				
otc	**Neo-Calglucon** (Sandoz)	**Syrup:** 1.8 g calcium glubionate (115 mg calcium) per 5 ml	Saccharin, sorbitol, sucrose. In 480 ml.	167
CALCIUM GLUCONATE, 9% calcium.				
otc	**Calcium Gluconate** (Various, eg, Dixon-Shane, Genetco, Lannett, Lilly, Major, Roxane, Rugby, Schein, URL, West-Ward)	**Tablets:** 500 mg (45 mg calcium)	In 100s, 1000s and UD 100s.	84+
		650 mg (58.5 mg calcium)	In 100s, 1000s and UD 100s.	41+
		975 mg (87.75 mg calcium)	In 100s, 500s, 1000s and UD 100s.	68+
		1 g (90 mg calcium)	In 1000s.	50+
CALCIUM LACTATE, 13% calcium.				
otc	**Calcium Lactate** (Various, eg, Dixon-Shane, Geneva Marsam, Rugby)	**Tablets:** 325 mg (42.25 mg calcium)	In 1000s.	45+
		650 mg (84.5 mg calcium)	In 100s and 1000s.	30+
CALCIUM CITRATE, 21% calcium.				
otc	**Citracal** (Mission)	**Tablets:** 950 mg (200 mg calcium)	In 100s.	60
otc	**Citracal Liquitab** (Mission)	**Tablets, effervescent:** 2376 mg (500 mg calcium)	Aspartame (12 mg phenylalanine). Citrus flavor. In 30s.	NA
CALCIUM ACETATE, 25% calcium.				
otc	**Phos-Ex 62.5 Mini-Tabs** (Vitaline)	**Tablets:** 250 mg (62.5 mg calcium)	In 250s and 1000s.	NA
otc	**Phos-Ex 167** (Vitaline)	**Tablets:** 668 mg (167 mg calcium)	Mint flavor. Oblong. In 180s and 1000s.	NA
Rx	**PhosLo** (Braintree)	**Tablets:** 667 mg (169 mg calcium)	In 200s.	NA
otc	**Phos-Ex 250** (Vitaline)	**Tablets:** 1000 mg (250 mg calcium)	Lemon meringue flavor. Oblong. In 180s and 1000s.	NA
otc	**Phos-Ex 125** (Vitaline)	**Capsules:** 500 mg (125 mg calcium)	In 180s and 1000s.	NA
TRICALCIUM PHOSPHATE (Calcium Phosphate, Tribasic), 39% calcium.				
otc *sf*	**Posture** (Whitehall)	**Tablets:** 1565.2 mg (600 mg calcium)	In 60s.	28

* Cost Index based on cost per 100 mg calcium.

Complete prescribing information for these products begins on page 32.

CALCIUM CARBONATE. 40% calcium. For calcium carbonate antacids, see the Antacids monograph.

	Product	Formulation	Description / Packaging	C.I.*
otc	**Calcium Carbonate** (Various, eg, Rugby)	**Tablets:** 650 mg (260 mg calcium)	In 1000s.	19+
otc *sf*	**Calciday-667** (Nature's Bounty)	**Tablets:** 667 mg (266.8 mg calcium)	In 60s.	24
otc	**Calcium Carbonate** (Roxane)	**Tablets:** 1.25 g (500 mg calcium)	Film coated. In 100s and UD 100s.	25
otc	**Os-Cal 500** (Marion Merrell Dow)		Corn syrup. (OsCal). In 60s and 120s.	42
otc *sf*	**Oyst-Cal 500** (Goldline)		Tartrazine. Lime green. Film coated. Oblong. In 60s, 120s and 1000s.	16
otc *sf*	**Oystercal 500** (Nature's Bounty)		In 60s.	8
otc	**Oyster Shell Calcium-500** (Vangard)		In 100s, UD 100s and 640s.	NA
otc	**Calcium 600** (Various, eg, Dixon-Shane, Major, Rugby, Schein)	**Tablets:** 1.5 g (600 mg calcium)	In 60s, 120s and 1000s.	34
otc	**Cal-Plus** (Geriatric Pharm.)		In 100s.	NA
otc *sf*	**Caltrate 600** (Lederle)		(LL C 600). Film coated. In 60s.	35
otc	**Gencalc 600** (Goldline)		White. Film coated. Oblong. In 60s.	14
otc	**Nephro-Calci** (R & D)		In 100s and 500s.	9
otc	**Caltrate, Jr.** (Lederle)	**Tablets, chewable:** 750 mg (300 mg calcium)	(LL). Orange flavor. In 60s.	38
otc	**Calci-Chew** (R & D)	**Tablets, chewable:** 1.25 g (500 mg calcium)	Sugar. Assorted flavors. In 100s.	18
otc	**Os-Cal 500** (Marion Merrell Dow)		Dextrose. (OsCal). Bavarian cream/coconut flavor. In 60s.	38
otc	**Oysco 500** (Rugby)		In 60s.	16
otc	**Calci-Mix** (R & D)	**Capsules:** 1250 mg powdered calcium carbonate (500 mg calcium)	To be mixed with food. In 100s.	NA
otc	**Calcium Carbonate** (Roxane)	**Oral Suspension:** 1.25 g (500 mg calcium) per 5 ml	Sorbitol. In 500 ml and UD 5 ml.	24
otc	**Cal Carb-HD** (Konsyl Pharm)	**Powder:** 6.5 g (2400 mg calcium) per packet	Simethicone. In 210 g bottles and 7 g packets.	40
otc	**Florical** (Mericon)	**Capsules and tablets:** 364 mg calcium carbonate (145.6 mg calcium) and 8.3 mg sodium fluoride *Dose:* 1 capsule or tablet daily.	In 100s and 500s.	109

* Cost Index based on cost per 100 mg calcium. *sf* – Sugar free.

[1] Konsyl Pharmaceuticals, 4200 South Hulen St., Suite 513 Fort Worth, TX 76109; (817) 763-8011.

PHOSPHORUS REPLACEMENT PRODUCTS

For information on parenteral phosphate, refer to the monograph in the IV Nutritional Therapy section.

Actions:

Pharmacology: Phosphorus is an important component of all cells in the body; 80% to 85% of body phosphorus is present in the skeletal system. The remainder functions intracellularly for 1) Energy transport and production in the form of ATP and ADP; 2) phospholipids in cell membranes responsible for nutrient transport; 3) part of nucleic acids (RNA, DNA); 4) buffering systems and calcium transport.

Phosphate administration lowers urinary calcium levels and increases urinary phosphate levels and urinary pyrophosphate inhibitor. Orthophosphates appear to decrease the aggregation and number of oxalate crystals in the urine of calculous patients.

Indications:

Dietary supplements of phosphorus, particularly if the diet is restricted or if needs are increased.

Contraindications:

Addison's disease; hyperkalemia; acidification of urine in urinary stone disease; patients with infected urolithiasis or struvite stone formation; severely impaired renal function (< 30% of normal); presence of hyperphosphatemia.

Warnings:

Pregnancy: Category C. It is not known whether this product can cause fetal harm or can affect reproduction capacity when administered to a pregnant woman. Use only when clearly needed.

Lactation: It is not known whether this drug is excreted in breast milk. Exercise caution when administering to a nursing woman.

Precautions:

Sodium/Potassium restriction: Use with caution if patient is on sodium or potassium restricted diet. These products provide significant amounts of sodium or potassium.

Special risk patients: Use with caution when the following medical problems exist: Cardiac disease (particularly in digitalized patients); acute dehydration; renal function impairment or chronic renal disease; extensive tissue breakdown; myotonia congenita; cardiac failure; cirrhosis of the liver or severe hepatic disease; peripheral and pulmonary edema; hypernatremia; hypertension; preeclampsia; hypoparathyroidism; osteomalacia; acute pancreatitis; rickets (rickets may benefit from phosphate therapy; however, use caution).

Kidney stones: Warn patients with kidney stones of the possibility of passing old stones when phosphate therapy is started.

Monitoring: The following determinations are important in patient monitoring (other tests may be warranted in some patients): Renal function; serum calcium; serum phosphorus; serum potassium; serum sodium. Monitor at periodic intervals during therapy.

Drug Interactions:

Phosphate Drug Interactions			
Precipitant drug	Object drug *		Description
Antacids	Phosphates	↓	Antacids containing magnesium, aluminum or calcium may bind the phosphate and prevent its absorption.
Calcium Vitamin D	Phosphates	↓	The effects of phosphates may be antagonized in the treatment of hypercalcemia.
Potassium-containing agents Potassium-sparing diuretics	Phosphates	↑	Hyperkalemia may occur with concurrent use. Periodically monitor patient's serum potassium level.

* ↑ = Object drug increased   ↓ = Object drug decreased

(Continued on following page)

PHOSPHORUS REPLACEMENT PRODUCTS (Cont.)

Adverse Reactions:

Individuals may experience a mild laxative effect for the first few days. If this persists, reduce the daily intake until this effect subsides, or, if necessary, discontinue use.

GI upset (eg, diarrhea, nausea, stomach pain, vomiting) may occur with phosphate therapy. The following side effects have been reported less frequently: Headaches; dizziness; mental confusion; seizures; weakness or heaviness of legs; unusual tiredness or weakness; muscle cramps; numbness, tingling, pain or weakness of hands or feet; numbness or tingling around lips; fast or irregular heartbeat; shortness of breath or troubled breathing; swelling of feet or lower legs; unusual weight gain; low urine output; unusual thirst; bone and joint pain (possible phosphate-induced osteomalacia). High serum phosphate levels may increase the incidence of extra-skeletal calcification.

Administration and Dosage:

Recommended dietary allowances (RDAs): Adults, 800 to 1200 mg. For a complete listing of RDAs by age, sex and condition, refer to page 2a.

In the product table, contents given per capsule, tablet or 75 ml reconstituted liquid.

Capsules must be reconstituted. Do *not* swallow capsules. Refer to manufacturers' labeling for reconstitution of capsules and powder.

	Product and distributor	Phosphorus		Potassium		Sodium		Recommended adult dose	How supplied	C.I.*
		mg	mM	mg	mEq	mg	mEq			
Rx	**Uro-KP-Neutral**[1] **Tablets** (Star)	250	8	49.4	1.27	250.5	10.9	1 or 2 tablets 4 times daily with full glass of water	Peach. Film coated. Capsule shape. In 100s.	1.8
Rx	**K-Phos Neutral**[2] **Tablets** (Beach)	250	8	45	1.1	298	13		(Beach 1125). White, scored. Film coated. Capsule shape. In 100s and 500s.	1
otc	**Neutra-Phos**[3] **Capsules** (Willen)	250	8	278	7	164	7	1 capsule or 1 powder packet reconstituted in 75 ml water 4 times daily. Provides 250 mg phosphorus per dose (1 g daily)	In 100s.	1.3
otc sf	**Neutra-Phos**[3] **Powder** (Willen)								Fruit flavor. In 64 g bottle and 1.25 g packets.	1.1
otc	**Neutra-Phos-K**[4] **Capsules** (Willen)	250	8	556	14.25	0	0		In 100s.	1.6
otc sf	**Neutra-Phos-K**[4] **Powder** (Willen)								In 71 g bottle and 1.45 g packets (100s).	1.3

* Cost Index based on cost per minimum recommended adult dose.

[1] From disodium and dipotassium phosphate anhydrous and monobasic sodium anhydrous.

[2] From dibasic sodium phosphate anhydrous, monobasic sodium phosphate and monobasic potassium phosphate monohydrate.

[3] From monobasic and dibasic sodium and potassium phosphates.

[4] From dibasic and monobasic potassium phosphates.

FLUORIDE

Actions:

Pharmacology: Sodium fluoride acts systemically before tooth eruption, and topically post-eruption, by increasing tooth resistance to acid dissolution, by promoting remineralization and by inhibiting the cariogenic microbial process. Acidulation provides greater topical fluoride uptake by dental enamel than neutral solutions. Phosphate protects enamel from demineralization by the acidulated formulation. Topical application of fluoride works superficially on enamel and plaque, and can reduce dental caries by 30% to 40%. Fluoride supplements may reduce the incidence of caries by up to 60%.

Pharmacokinetics: Fluoride is absorbed in the GI tract, lungs and skin. About 90% of oral fluoride is absorbed in the stomach. Absorption is related to solubility; sodium fluoride is almost completely absorbed. Calcium, iron or magnesium ions may delay absorption. Following ingestion, 50% of fluoride is deposited in bone and teeth. The major route of excretion is the kidneys; it is also excreted by sweat glands, the GI tract and in breast milk.

Indications:

Prevention of dental caries: Both neutral and acidulated phosphate fluoride effectively control dental decay. Use where water supplies are low in fluoride (< 0.7 ppm). Fluoride also controls rampant dental decay which frequently follows xerostomia-producing radiotherapy of head and neck tumors.

In communities without fluoridated water, the American Dental Association's Council on Dental Therapeutics recommends continuing fluoride supplements until the age of 13; the American Academy of Pediatrics recommends supplementation until 16 years of age.

Unlabeled uses: Sodium fluoride may be effective in treating osteoporosis. Doses (as fluoride) up to 60 mg daily or more are used in conjunction with calcium supplements, vitamin D or estrogen. However, large doses may result in a higher frequency of side effects. Some data suggest that doses < 50 mg/day are efficacious with fewer adverse reactions. No commercially available products contain high sodium fluoride doses for this use; therefore a large number of tablets would be required to obtain this dosage. Fluoride supplementation is not recommended for the prophylaxis of osteoporosis due to the potential for increased incidence of fractures (see Precautions).

Contraindications:

When the fluoride content of drinking water exceeds 0.7 ppm; low sodium or sodium free diets; hypersensitivity to fluoride.

Do not use 1 mg tablets in children < 3 years old or when the drinking water fluoride content is ≥ 0.3 ppm. Do not use 1 mg/5 ml rinse (as a supplement) in children < 6 years old.

Warnings:

Pregnancy: Consult physician before using.

Lactation: Consult physician before using.

Children: See Contraindications.

Precautions:

Fractures: Some epidemiological studies suggest that the incidence of certain types of bone fractures (crippling skeletal fluorosis) may be higher in some communities with naturally high or adjusted fluoride levels. However, other studies have not detected increased incidence of bone fractures. Crippling skeletal fluorosis is more common in parts of the world with high natural fluoride (> 10 ppm), but is extremely rare in the US.

Mucositis: Gingival tissues may be hypersensitive to some flavors or alcohol.

Tartrazine sensitivity: Some of these products contain tartrazine, which may cause allergic-type reactions (including bronchial asthma) in susceptible individuals. Although the incidence of tartrazine sensitivity in the general population is low, it is frequently seen in patients who also have aspirin hypersensitivity. Specific products containing tartrazine are identified in the product listings.

Drug Interactions:

Drug/Food interaction: Incompatibility of dairy foods with systemic fluoride has occurred due to formation of calcium fluoride, which is poorly absorbed.

Adverse Reactions:

Dermatologic: Eczema; atopic dermatitis; urticaria; allergic rash and other idiosyncrasies (rare).

Miscellaneous: Gastric distress; headache; weakness. Rinses and gels containing stannous fluoride may produce surface staining of the teeth; this does not occur with non-stannous fluoride topical preparations. Acidulated fluoride may dull porcelain and composite restorations.

(Continued on following page)

FLUORIDE (Cont.)

Overdosage:

Chronic overdosage of fluorides may result in dental fluorosis (a mottling of tooth enamel) and osseous changes.

Acute overdosage: Symptoms – In children, acute ingestion of 10 to 20 mg sodium fluoride may cause excessive salivation and GI disturbances; 500 mg may be fatal. The oral lethal dose is 70 to 140 mg/kg (5 to 10 g in adults).

GI: Salivation, nausea, abdominal pain, vomiting and diarrhea are frequent due to conversion of sodium fluoride to corrosive hydrofluoric acid in the stomach.

CNS: Because of the calcium-binding effect of fluoride, CNS irritability, paresthesias, tetany, convulsions and respiratory and cardiac failure may occur. Fluoride has a direct toxic action on muscle and nerve tissue, and it interferes with many enzyme systems.

Hypocalcemia, hypoglycemia and delayed hyperkalemia are frequent laboratory findings.

Treatment: Usual supportive measures. Refer to General Management of Acute Overdosage. Precipitate the fluoride by using gastric lavage with 0.15% calcium hydroxide. Administer IV glucose in saline for a forced diuresis; IV calcium may be indicated for tetany. Administer calcium IM (10 ml of 10% calcium gluconate, 5 ml in children) every 4 to 6 hours until recovery is complete. Maintain electrolytes, normal blood pH and adequate urine output. Removing fluoride with dialysis and hemoperfusion may also be beneficial.

Patient Information:

Tablets and drops – Milk and other dairy products may decrease absorption of sodium fluoride; avoid simultaneous ingestion.

Tablets – Dissolve in the mouth, chew, swallow whole, add to drinking water or fruit juice or add to water for use in infant formulas or other food.

Drops – Take orally, undiluted, or mix with fluids or food.

Rinses and gels are most effective immediately after brushing or flossing and just prior to sleep. Expectorate any excess. *Do not swallow.* Do not eat, drink or rinse mouth for 30 minutes after application.

Notify dentist if teeth become mottled.

Administration and Dosage:

Use according to directions accompanying the product.

Fluoride Dosage	
Route/Age	Daily dose
Oral:	
Fluoride content of drinking water (< 0.3 ppm):	
< 2 years	0.25
2 to 3 years	0.5 mg
3 to 12 years	1 mg
Fluoride content of drinking water (0.3 - 0.7 ppm):	
< 2 years	0.125 mg
2 to 3 years	0.25 mg
3 to 14 years	0.25 - 0.75 mg
Topical (rinse):	
Children (6 to 12 years)	5 to 10 ml[1]
Adults and children (> 12 years)	10 ml[1]

[1] Use once daily (*Point-Two,* once weekly) after thoroughly brushing teeth and rinsing mouth. Rinse around and between teeth for 1 minute, then spit out.

(Products listed on following page)

FLUORIDE, ORAL

	Product	Form	Description	C.I.*
Rx	**Sodium Fluoride**[1] (Various, eg, Major, Rugby)	**Tablets, chewable:** 0.5 mg (from 1.1 mg sodium fluoride)	In 1000s.	12+
Rx	**Fluoritab** (Fluoritab)		Dye free. Pineapple flavor. In 1000s and 5000s.	NA
Rx *sf*	**Luride Lozi-Tabs** (Colgate-Hoyt)		Grape and assorted fruit flavors. In 120s. Grape also in 1200s.	77
Rx *sf*	**Pharmaflur 1.1** (Pharmics)		Grape flavor. In 120s.	66
Rx	**Sodium Fluoride**[1] (Various, eg, Geneva, Major, Rugby, Schein)	**Tablets, chewable:** 1 mg (from 2.2 mg sodium fluoride)	In 100s, 1000s and UD 1000s.	12+
Rx	**Fluoritab** (Fluoritab)		Dye free. Pineapple and cherry flavors in 100s and 5000s. Cherry also in 1000s.	36
Rx	**Karidium** (Lorvic)		White. In 180s and 1000s.	60
Rx *sf*	**Luride Lozi-Tabs** (Colgate-Hoyt)		Cherry and assorted fruit flavors. In 120s and 1000s. Cherry also in 5000s.	92
Rx *sf*	**Luride-SF Lozi-Tabs** (Colgate-Hoyt)		In 120s.	110
Rx *sf*	**Pharmaflur** (Pharmics)		Cherry flavor. In 1000s.	NA
Rx *sf*	**Pharmaflur df** (Pharmics)		Dye free. Cherry flavor. In 120s.	68
Rx *sf*	**Flura** (Kirkman)	**Tablets:** 1 mg (from 2.2 mg sodium fluoride)	In 100s and 1000s.	NA
Rx	**Karidium** (Lorvic)		White. In 180s and 1000s.	NA
Rx	**Sodium Fluoride** (Rugby)	**Drops:** 0.125 mg per drop (from ≈ 0.275 mg sodium fluoride)	In 30 ml.	NA
Rx	**Karidium** (Lorvic)		In 30 and 60 ml w/dropper.	NA
Rx *sf*	**Luride** (Colgate-Hoyt)		Peach flavor. In 30 ml.	504
Rx *sf*	**Fluoritab** (Fluoritab)	**Drops:** 0.25 mg per drop (from 0.55 mg sodium fluoride)	In 22.8 ml.	130
Rx	**Flura-Drops** (Kirkman)		In 24 ml.	NA
Rx *sf*	**Pediaflor** (Ross)	**Drops:** 0.5 mg per ml (from 1.1 mg sodium fluoride)	< 0.5% alcohol, sorbitol. Cherry flavor. In 50 ml w/ dropper.	364
Rx *sf*	**Flura-Loz** (Kirkman)	**Lozenges:** 1 mg (from 2.2 mg sodium fluoride)	Raspberry flavor. In 100s and 1000s.	NA
Rx *sf*	**Phos-Flur** (Colgate-Hoyt)	**Solution:**[2] 0.2 mg per ml (from 0.44 mg sodium fluoride)	Cherry flavor. In 250, 500 ml & gal. Cinnamon (w/saccharin), grape and wintergreen flavors. In 500 ml.	NA

* Cost Index based on cost per tablet or ml.
[1] May be regular or chewable.
sf – Sugar free.
[2] May be used as a rinse or supplement.

FLUORIDE, TOPICAL

	Product (Manufacturer)	Strength	Description	C.I.*
otc	**Listermint with Fluoride** (Warner-Lambert)	**Rinse:** 0.01% (from 0.02% sodium fluoride)	Saccharin, 6.65% SD alcohol 38-B. In 180, 300, 360, 480, 540, 720, 960 & 1740 ml.	18
otc	**ACT** (Johnson & Johnson)	**Rinse:** 0.02% (from 0.05% sodium fluoride)	7% alcohol. In 90, 360 and 480 ml.	NA
otc	**Fluorigard** (Colgate-Palmolive)		6% alcohol. Tartrazine. In 180, 300 & 480 ml.	NA
Rx	**Fluorinse** (Oral-B)	**Rinse:** 0.09% (from 0.2% sodium fluoride)	Alcohol free. Mint and cinnamon flavors. In 480 ml.	28
Rx	**Point-Two** (Colgate-Hoyt)		6% alcohol. Mint flavor. In 240 ml and gal.	NA
Rx	**Gel Kam** (Scherer)	**Gel:** 0.1% (from 0.4% stannous fluoride)	Cinnamon flavor. In 65 and 122 g and 105 g (Dental Therapy-Pak [2]).	103
otc	**Gel-Tin** (Young Dental)		Lime, grape, cinnamon, raspberry, mint and orange flavors. In 60 g.	66
otc	**Stop** (Oral-B)		Grape, cinnamon, bubblegum, piña colada and mint flavors. In 120 g.	NA
Rx	**Karigel** (Lorvic)	**Gel:** 0.5% (from 1.1% sodium fluoride)	pH 5.6. Orange flavor. In 30, 130 and 250 g.	103
Rx	**Karigel-N** (Lorvic)		Neutral pH. In 24 and 120 g.	128
Rx	**Prevident** (Colgate-Hoyt)		Mint, berry, cherry and fruit sherbet flavors. In 24 and 60 g. Lime flavor in 60 g.	NA
Rx	**Thera-Flur** (Colgate-Hoyt)	**Gel-Drops:** 0.5% (from 1.1% sodium fluoride)	pH 4.5. Lime flavor. In 24 ml.	NA
Rx	**Thera-Flur-N** (Colgate-Hoyt)		Neutral pH. In 24 ml.	NA
Rx	**Minute-Gel** (Oral-B)	**Gel:** 1.23% (as acidulated phosphate fluoride)	Spearmint, strawberry, grape, apple-cinnamon, cherry cola and bubblegum flavors. In 480 ml.	104

* Cost Index based on cost per tablet, g or ml.

ZINC SUPPLEMENTS

For information on parenteral zinc, refer to the monograph in the IV Nutritional Therapy section.

Actions:

Pharmacology: Normal growth and tissue repair depend upon adequate zinc. Zinc acts as an integral part of several enzymes important to protein and carbohydrate metabolism.

Zinc deficiency manifestations include: Anorexia; growth retardation; impaired taste and olfactory sensation; hypogonadism; alopecia; hepatosplenomegaly; dwarfism; rashes; cutaneous lesions; glossitis; stomatitis; blepharitis; paronychia; impaired healing.

Pharmacokinetics: Zinc salts are poorly absorbed from the GI tract; 20% to 30% of dietary zinc is absorbed. The major stores of zinc are in skeletal muscle and bone; zinc is also found in hair, nails, prostate, spermatazoa and the choroid of the eye. The main excretion route is through the intestine. Only minor amounts are lost in the urine (≈ 2%).

Contraindications:

Pregnancy (see Warnings); lactation.

Indications:

As a dietary supplement; use to treat or prevent zinc deficiencies.

Unlabeled uses: For acrodermatitis enteropathica and delayed wound healing associated with zinc deficiency, doses of 220 mg zinc sulfate 3 times daily are used. Zinc sulfate has also been used to treat acne, rheumatoid arthritis and Wilson's disease. However, data conflict and are insufficient to recommend these uses.

In one study, zinc gluconate appeared to significantly shorten the duration of the common cold. Patients (n = 65) dissolved one tablet containing 23 mg zinc (one-half tablet for children) in the mouth every 2 hours until all symptoms were absent for 6 hours; 11% were asymptomatic within 12 hours, 22% within 24 hours. Zinc sulfate should not be used. Further study is needed.

Warnings:

Excessive intake in healthy persons may be deleterious. Eleven healthy men who ingested 150 mg zinc twice daily for 6 weeks showed significant impairment of lymphocyte and polymorphonuclear leukocyte functions and a significant decrease in high-density lipoproteins (HDL). No clinical side effects were seen during the study.

Pregnancy: Although zinc deficiency during pregnancy has been associated with adverse perinatal outcomes, other studies report no such occurrences. Therefore, since zinc deficiency is very rare, the routine use of zinc supplementation during pregnancy is not recommended. However, a *dietary* zinc intake of 15 mg/day is recommended

Lactation: Breast milk concentrations of zinc decrease over time following delivery; extra dietary intake of zinc of 7 mg/day for the first 6 months of lactation and 4 mg/day during the second 6 months are recommended.

Precautions:

Do not exceed prescribed dosage; will cause emesis if administered in single 2 g doses.

Drug Interactions:

Zinc Drug Interactions			
Precipitant drug	Object drug *		Description
Zinc salts	Fluoroquinolones	↓	The GI absorption and serum levels of some fluoroquinolones may be decreased, possibly resulting in a decreased anti-infective response.
Zinc salts	Tetracyclines	↓	The GI absorption and serum levels of tetracyclines may be decreased, possibly resulting in a decreased anti-infective response. Doxycycline does not appear to be affected.

* ↓ = Object drug decreased

Drug/Food Interactions: Bran products (including brown bread) and some foods (eg, protein, phytates, some minerals) may decrease zinc absorption.

Adverse Reactions:

Nausea; vomiting.

Overdosage:

Symptoms: Nausea; severe vomiting; dehydration; restlessness; sideroblastic anemia (secondary to zinc-induced copper deficiency).

Treatment: Reduce dosage or discontinue to control symptoms.

Patient Information:

If GI upset occurs, take with food, but avoid foods high in calcium, phosphorus or phytate.

(Continued on following page)

ZINC SUPPLEMENTS (Cont.)

Administration and Dosage:

Recommended dietary allowances (RDAs): Adults, 12 to 15 mg. For a complete listing of RDAs by age, sex and condition, refer to page 5

Dietary supplement: Average adult dose is 25 to 50 mg zinc daily. Take zinc with food to avoid gastric distress; however, some studies indicate that ingestion with some foods (eg, those that contain bran, phytates, protein, some minerals) may inhibit zinc absorption.

ZINC SULFATE (23% zinc)				C.I.*
otc	**Zinc 15** (Mericon)	**Tablets:** 66 mg (15 mg zinc)	In 100s.	26
otc	**Orazinc** (Mericon)	**Tablets:** 110 mg (25 mg zinc)	In 100s.	44
otc	**Zinc Sulfate** (Various, eg, Rugby)	**Tablets:** 200 mg (45 mg zinc)	In 1000s.	6+
Rx	**Zinc Sulfate** (Various)	**Capsules:** 220 mg (50 mg zinc)	In 100s, 1000s and UD 100s.	NA
otc	**Orazinc** (Mericon)		In 100s and 1000s.	40
otc	**Verazinc** (Forest)		In 100s.	52
otc	**Zinc-220** (Alto)		Pink and blue. In 100s, 1000s and UD 100s.	36
Rx	**Zincate** (Paddock)		In 100s and 1000s.	42

ZINC GLUCONATE (14.3% zinc)				C.I.*
otc	**Zinc Gluconate** (Various, eg, IDE)	**Tablets:** 10 mg (1.4 mg zinc)	In 250s.	38+
otc	**Zinc Gluconate** (Various, eg, IDE)	**Tablets:** 15 mg (2 mg zinc)	In 250s.	29+
otc	**Zinc Gluconate** (Various, eg, IDE, Major, Mission, Moore)	**Tablets:** 50 mg (7 mg zinc)	In 100s and 250s.	12+
otc	**Zinc Gluconate** (Major)	**Tablets:** 78 mg (11 mg zinc)	In 100s and 300s.	1

COMPLEX ZINC CARBONATES				
otc	**Zinc** (Sublingual Products)	**Liquid:** 15 mg/ml	Fructose, corn syrup solids, sorbitol, parabens. Fruit flavor. In 30 ml with dropper.	NA

* Cost Index based on cost per 15 mg zinc.

MAGNESIUM

For information on parenteral magnesium, refer to the monographs in the IV Nutritional Therapy and Anticonvulsant sections.

Actions:

Pharmacology: Magnesium is an electrolyte which is necessary in a number of enzyme systems, phosphate transfer, muscular contraction and nerve conduction. Magnesium deficiency may occur in: Malabsorption syndromes; prolonged diarrhea or steatorrhea; vomiting; pancreatitis; aldosteronism; renal tubular damage; chronic alcoholism; prolonged IV therapy with magnesium-free solutions; diuretic therapy; during hemodialysis; renal tubular damage; disorders associated with hypokalemia and hypocalcemia; in patients on digitalis therapy. While there are large stores of magnesium present intracellularly and in bone in adults, these stores often are not mobilized sufficiently to maintain plasma levels; therefore serum levels may not reflect total magnesium stores.

Indications:

As a dietary supplement.

Unlabeled uses: A pyridoxine/magnesium oxide combination has been used to prevent recurrence of calcium oxalate kidney stones.

Oral magnesium gluconate may be a cost-effective and clinically effective alternative to oral ritodrine as a tocolytic for continued inhibition of contractions following parenteral magnesium sulfate. Further study is needed.

Warnings:

Pregnancy: There is weak evidence that magnesium supplementation reduces the risk of poor perinatal outcome. However, since magnesium deficiency is rare, there appears to be no need for routine supplementation during pregnancy.

Precautions:

Renal disease: Do not use without physician supervision due to potential accumulation.

Excessive dosage may cause diarrhea and GI irritation.

Drug Interactions:

Magnesium Drug Interactions

Precipitant drug	Object drug *		Description
Magnesium salts	Aminoquinolines	⬇	The absorption and therapeutic effect of the aminoquinolines may be decreased.
Magnesium salts	Digoxin	⬇	Magnesium salts may absorb digoxin in the GI tract, decreasing its bioavailability; however, this has only been reported for magnesium-containing antacids.
Magnesium salts	Nitrofurantoin	⬇	Adsorption of nitrofurantoin onto magnesium salts may occur, decreasing the bioavailability and possibly the anti-infective effect of nitrofurantoin.
Magnesium salts	Penicillamine	⬇	The GI absorption of penicillamine may be decreased, possibly decreasing its pharmacologic effects; however this has only been reported for magnesium-containing antacids
Magnesium salts	Tetracyclines	⬇	The GI absorption and serum levels of tetracyclines may be decreased; a decreased antimicrobial response may occur.

* ⬇ = Object drug decreased

Overdosage:

Symptoms: Hypermagnesemia following oral ingestion in the absence of renal disease is unlikely; however, it may occur with overdosage. Symptoms may include: Hypotension, nausea, vomiting, urinary retention, bradycardia, cutaneous vasodilation (3 to 9 mEq/L); ECG changes, hyporeflexia, secondary CNS depression (5 to 10 mEq/L); respiratory changes, coma (> 9 to 10 mEq/L); asystolic arrest (> 14 to 15 mEq/L).

Treatment: Reversal of toxicity with calcium is immediate but transient. Dialysis is the treatment of choice (both peritoneal and hemodialysis).

Administration and Dosage:

1 g Mg = 83.3 mEq (41.1 mmol).

Dietary supplement: 54 to 483 mg/day in divided doses. Refer to product labeling.

Recommended dietary allowances (RDAs): Adult – Males, 350 to 400 mg; females, 280 to 300 mg. For a complete listing of RDAs by age, sex and condition, refer to page 5.

Magnesium-containing antacids may also be used; refer to the Antacids monograph.

(Products listed on following page)

MAGNESIUM (Cont.)

	Product	Formulation	How supplied	C.I.*
otc	**Mag-200** (Optimox)	**Tablets:** 400 mg magnesium (oxide)	In 120s.	NA
otc	**Mag-Ox 400** (Blaine)	**Tablets:** 400 mg magnesium oxide (241.3 mg magnesium)	Scored. In 100s and 1000s.	NA
otc	**Almora** (Forest)	**Tablets:** 500 mg magnesium gluconate (27 mg magnesium)	In 100s.	178
otc	**Magonate** (Fleming)		In 100s and 1000s.	136
otc	**Magtrate** (Mission)	**Tablets:** 500 mg magnesium gluconate (29 mg magnesium	In 100s.	98
otc *sf*	**Chelated Magnesium** (Freeda)	**Tablets:** 500 mg magnesium amino acids chelate (100 mg magnesium)	In 100s, 250s and 500s.	20
otc	**Slow-Mag** (Searle)	**Tablets, sustained release:** 535 mg magnesium chloride hexahydrate (64 mg magnesium)	In 60s.	84
otc	**Uro-Mag** (Blaine)	**Capsules:** 140 mg magnesium oxide (84.5 mg magnesium)	In 100s and 1000s.	NA
otc	**Magonate** (Fleming)	**Liquid:** 54 mg/5 ml magnesium (as gluconate)	Melon flavor. In pt and gal.	NA

MANGANESE

For information on parenteral manganese, refer to the monograph in the IV Nutritional Therapy section.

Actions:

Pharmacology: Manganese is a cofactor in many enzyme systems; it stimulates synthesis of cholesterol and fatty acids in the liver and influences mucopolysaccharide synthesis. It is concentrated in mitochondria, primarily of the pituitary gland, pancreas, liver, kidney and bone.

Indications:

As a dietary supplement.

Administration and Dosage:

20 to 50 mg daily.

The need for manganese in human nutrition has been established, but no RDA has been determined. Manganese deficiency is unlikely because dietary intake usually satisfies the need; therefore, 2 to 5 mg/day via the diet is recommended.

	Product	Formulation	How supplied	C.I.*
otc *sf*	**Chelated Manganese** (Freeda)	**Tablets:** 20 mg	In 100s, 250s and 500s.	18
		50 mg	In 100s, 250s and 500s.	16

* Cost Index based on cost per 27 mg magnesium or 5 mg manganese.
sf – Sugar free.

POTASSIUM REPLACEMENT PRODUCTS

For information on parenteral potassium, refer to the IV Nutritional Therapy section.

Actions:

Pharmacology: Potassium, the principal intracellular cation of most body tissues, participates in a number of essential physiological processes, such as maintenance of intracellular tonicity and a proper relationship with sodium across cell membranes, cellular metabolism, transmission of nerve impulses, contraction of cardiac, skeletal and smooth muscle, acid-base balance and maintenance of normal renal function. Normal potassium serum levels range from 3.5 to 5 mEq/L. The active ion transport system maintains this gradient across the plasma membrane.

mEq/g of Various Potassium Salts	
Potassium salt	mEq/g
Potassium gluconate	4.3
Potassium citrate	9.8
Potassium bicarbonate	10
Potassium acetate	10.2
Potassium chloride	13.4

Potassium homeostasis: The potassium concentration in extracellular fluid is normally 4 to 5 mEq/L; the concentration in intracellular fluid is approximately 150 to 160 mEq/L. Plasma concentration provides a useful clinical guide to disturbances in potassium balance. By producing large differences in the ratio of intracellular to extracellular potassium, relatively small absolute changes in extracellular concentration may have important effects on neuromuscular activity.

Despite wide variations in dietary intake of potassium (eg, 40 to 120 mEq/day), plasma potassium concentration is normally stabilized within the narrow range of 4 to 5 mEq/L by virtue of close renal regulation of potassium balance. Renal potassium excretion is accomplished largely by potassium secretion in the distal portion of the nephron; essentially all filtered potassium is reabsorbed in the proximal tubule. The potassium that appears in the urine is added to the filtrate by a distal process of sodium-cation exchange. Fecal excretion of potassium is normally only a few mEq per day and does not play a significant role in potassium homeostasis.

Natural potassium sources: Foods rich in potassium include: Beef; veal; ham; chicken; turkey; fish; milk; bananas; dates; prunes; raisins; avocado; watermelon; canteloupes; apricots; molasses; beans; yams; broccoli; brussels sprouts; lentils; potatoes; spinach.

Hypokalemia: Gradual potassium depletion may occur whenever the rate of potassium loss through renal excretion or GI loss exceeds the rate of potassium intake. Potassium depletion is usually a consequence of prolonged therapy with oral diuretics, primary or secondary hyperaldosteronism, diabetic ketoacidosis, severe diarrhea (especially if associated with vomiting) or inadequate replacement during prolonged parenteral nutrition. Potassium depletion due to these causes is usually accompanied by a concomitant deficiency of chloride and is manifested by hypokalemia and metabolic alkalosis.

The use of potassium salts in patients receiving diuretics for uncomplicated essential hypertension is often unnecessary when such patients have a normal diet. However, if hypokalemia occurs, dietary supplementation with potassium-containing foods may be adequate. In more severe cases, potassium salt supplementation may be indicated.

Potassium depletion sufficient to cause 1 mEq/L drop in serum potassium requires a loss of about 100 to 200 mEq potassium from the total body store.

Symptoms – Weakness; fatigue; ileus; tetany; polydipsia; flaccid paralysis or impaired ability to concentrate urine (in advanced cases). ECG may reveal atrial and ventricular ectopy, prolongation of QT interval, ST segment depression, conduction defects, broad or flat T waves or appearance of U waves.

Indications:

Treatment of hypokalemia in the following conditions: With or without metabolic alkalosis; digitalis intoxication; familial periodic paralysis; diabetic acidosis; diarrhea and vomiting; surgical conditions accompanied by nitrogen loss, vomiting, suction drainage, diarrhea and increased urinary excretion of potassium; certain cases of uremia; hyperadrenalism; starvation and debilitation; corticosteroid or diuretic therapy.

Prevention of potassium depletion when dietary intake is inadequate in the following conditions: Patients receiving digitalis and diuretics for congestive heart failure; significant cardiac arrhythmias; hepatic cirrhosis with ascites; states of aldosterone excess with normal renal function; potassium-losing nephropathy; certain diarrheal states.

When hypokalemia is associated with alkalosis, use potassium chloride. When acidosis is present, use the bicarbonate, citrate, acetate or gluconate potassium salts.

Unlabeled use: In patients with mild hypertension, the use of potassium supplements (24 to 60 mmol/day) appears to result in a long-term reduction of blood pressure.

(Continued on following page)

POTASSIUM REPLACEMENT PRODUCTS (Cont.)

Contraindications:

Severe renal impairment with oliguria or azotemia; untreated Addison's disease; hyperkalemia from any cause (eg, systemic acidosis, acute dehydration, extensive tissue breakdown); adynamia episodica hereditaria; acute dehydration; heat cramps; patients receiving potassium-sparing diuretics (spironolactone, triamterene or amiloride) or aldosterone-inhibiting agents.

Solid dosage forms of potassium supplements are contraindicated in any patient in whom there is cause for arrest or delay in tablet passage through the GI tract. Wax matrix potassium chloride preparations have produced esophageal ulceration in cardiac patients with esophageal compression due to an enlarged left atrium; give potassium supplementation as a liquid preparation to these patients.

Warnings:

Hyperkalemia: In patients with impaired potassium excretion, potassium salts can produce hyperkalemia or cardiac arrest. This occurs most commonly in patients given IV potassium, but may also occur in patients given oral potassium. Potentially fatal hyperkalemia can develop rapidly and may be asymptomatic.

Hyperkalemia may be manifested only by an increased serum potassium concentration and characteristic ECG changes (eg, peaking of T waves, loss of P wave, depression of ST segment, prolongation of the QT interval, lengthened P-R interval, widened QRS complex). However, the following may also occur: Parasthesias; heaviness; muscle weakness and flaccid paralysis of the extremities; listlessness; mental confusion; decreased blood pressure; shock; cardiac arrhythmias; heart block.

In response to a rise in the concentration of body potassium, renal excretion of the ion is increased. With normal kidney function, it is difficult to produce potassium intoxication by oral administration. However, administer potassium supplements with caution, since the amount of deficiency and corresponding daily dose is unknown. Frequently monitor the clinical status, periodic ECG and serum potassium levels. This is particularly important in patients receiving digitalis and in patients with cardiac disease. There is a hazard in prescribing potassium in digitalis intoxication manifested by atrioventricular (AV) conduction disturbance.

GI lesions: Potassium chloride tablets have produced stenotic or ulcerative lesions of the small bowel and death. These lesions are caused by a concentration of potassium ion in the region of a rapidly dissolving tablet, which injures the bowel wall and produces obstruction, hemorrhage or perforation. The reported frequency of small bowel lesions is much less with wax matrix tablets (< 1 per 100,000 patient-years) and microencapsulated tablets than with enteric coated tablets (40 to 50 per 100,000 patient-years). Upper GI bleeding, esophageal ulceration and stricture, gastric ulceration and lower GI ulceration have occurred with wax matrix preparations. The total number of GI lesions is < 1 per 47,000 patient-years. Discontinue either type of tablet immediately and consider the possibility of bowel obstruction or perforation if severe vomiting, abdominal pain or distention or GI bleeding occurs.

Patients at greatest risk for developing potassium chloride-induced GI lesions include: The elderly, the immobile and those with scleroderma, diabetes mellitus, mitral valve replacement, cardiomegaly or esophageal stricture/compression.

Reserve slow release potassium chloride preparations for patients who cannot tolerate liquids or effervescent potassium preparations, or for patients in whom there is a problem of compliance with these preparations.

Some studies suggest the "microencapsulated" preparations are less likely to cause GI damage; however, evidence conflicts and a specific recommendation of one solid oral product over another (wax matrix or microencapsulated) cannot be made. Avoid enteric coated products.

Metabolic acidosis and hyperchloremia: In some patients (eg, those with renal tubular acidosis), potassium depletion is rarely associated with metabolic acidosis and hyperchloremia. Replace potassium with potassium bicarbonate, citrate, acetate or gluconate.

Renal function impairment requires careful monitoring of the serum potassium concentration and appropriate dosage adjustment.

Pregnancy: Category C. It is not known whether potassium salts can cause fetal harm when administered to a pregnant woman or can affect reproduction capacity. Give to a pregnant woman only if clearly needed.

Lactation: It is not known whether this drug is excreted in breast milk. Exercise caution when administering to a nursing woman. The normal potassium content of breast milk is ≈ 13 mEq/L. As long as body potassium is not excessive, the contribution of potassium salts should have little or no effect on the level of breast milk.

Children: Safety and efficacy for use in children have not been established.

(Continued on following page)

POTASSIUM REPLACEMENT PRODUCTS (Cont.)

Precautions:

Hypokalemia is ordinarily diagnosed by demonstrating potassium depletion in a patient and by a careful clinical history. In interpreting the serum potassium level, consider that acute alkalosis can produce hypokalemia in the absence of a deficit in total body potassium, while acute acidosis can increase the serum potassium concentration to the normal range, even in the presence of a reduced total body potassium. Treatment, particularly in the presence of cardiac disease, renal disease or acidosis, requires careful attention to acid-base balance and monitoring of serum electrolytes, ECG and clinical status of the patient.

The administration of concentrated dextrose or sodium bicarbonate may cause an intracellular potassium shift. This may cause hypokalemia which, in turn, may lead to serious cardiac arrhythmias.

Administering potassium to hypokalemic hypertensives may lower blood pressure.

Monitoring: When blood is drawn for analysis of plasma potassium, it is important to recognize that artificial elevations can occur after improper venipuncture technique or as a result of in vitro hemolysis of the sample.

Tartrazine sensitivity: Some of these products contain tartrazine, which may cause allergic-type reactions (including bronchial asthma) in susceptible individuals. Although the incidence of tartrazine sensitivity in the general population is low, it is frequently seen in patients who also have aspirin hypersensitivity. Specific products containing tartrazine are identified in the product listings.

Drug Interactions:

Potassium Preparation Drug Interactions			
Precipitant drug	Object drug*		Description
ACE inhibitors	Potassium preparations	↑	Concurrent use may result in elevated serum potassium concentrations in certain patients
Potassium-sparing diuretics	Potassium preparations	↑	Potassium-sparing diuretics will increase potassium retention and can produce severe hyperkalemia
Potassium preparations	Digitalis	↑	In patients receiving digoxin, hypokalemia may result in digoxin toxicity. Therefore, use caution if discontinuing a potassium preparation in patients maintained on digoxin

*↑ = Object drug increased

In addition, potassium citrate, a urinary alkalinizer, may affect the renal excretion and pharmacologic effects of various agents (refer to the Citrate and Citric Acid Solutions monograph).

Adverse Reactions:

Most common: Nausea, vomiting, diarrhea, flatulence and abdominal discomfort due to GI irritation are best managed by diluting the preparation further, by taking with meals or by dose reduction.

Rare: Skin rash.

Most severe: Hyperkalemia; GI obstruction, bleeding, ulceration or perforation.

Overdosage:

For symptoms and treatment of potassium overdosage and hyperkalemia, refer to the monograph in the IV Nutritional Therapy section.

Patient Information:

May cause GI upset; take after meals or with food and with a full glass of water.

Do not chew or crush tablets; swallow whole.

Oral liquids, soluble powders and effervescent tablets: Mix or dissolve completely in 3 to 8 ounces of cold water, juice or other suitable beverage and drink slowly.

Following release of potassium chloride, the expended wax matrix, which is not absorbable, can be found in the stool. This is no cause for concern.

Do not use salt substitutes concurrently, except on the advice of a physician.

Notify physician if tingling of the hands and feet, unusual tiredness or weakness, a feeling of heaviness in the legs, severe nausea, vomiting, abdominal pain or black stools (GI bleeding) occurs.

(Continued on following pages)

POTASSIUM REPLACEMENT PRODUCTS (Cont.)

Administration and Dosage:

The usual dietary intake of potassium ranges between 40 to 150 mEq/day.

Individualize dosage. Usual range is 16 to 24 mEq/day for the prevention of hypokalemia to 40 to 100 mEq/day or more for the treatment of potassium depletion.

Potassium intoxication may result from any therapeutic dosage.

	Product	Liquids		C.I.*
Rx	**Potassium Chloride** (Various, eg, Barre-National, Geneva, Major, Parmed, PBI, Rugby, Schein)	20 mEq/15 ml potassium and chloride (10% KCl)	In pt and gal.	252+
Rx *sf*	**Cena-K** (Century)		In pt and gal.	270
Rx	**Kaochlor 10%** (Adria)		5% alcohol, tartrazine, saccharin, sorbitol, sucrose. Citrus flavor. In 480 ml.	1514
Rx *sf*	**Kaochlor S-F** (Adria)		5% alcohol, saccharin. Fruit flavor. In 480 ml.	218
Rx *sf*	**Kay Ciel** (Forest)		4% alcohol. In 118 ml, pt and gal.	3848
Rx	**Klorvess** (Sandoz)		0.75% alcohol. Saccharin, sucrose. Cherry flavor. In 480 ml.	2180
Rx *sf*	**Potasalan** (Lannett)		4% alcohol. Orange flavor. In pt and gal.	270
Rx	**Rum-K** (Fleming)	30 mEq/15 ml potassium and chloride (15% KCl)	Butter-rum flavor. In pt and gal.	550
Rx	**Potassium Chloride** (Various, eg, Barre-National, Geneva, Major, PBI, Rugby, Schein)	40 mEq/15 ml potassium and chloride (20% KCl)	In pt and gal.	178+
Rx *sf*	**Cena-K** (Century)		In pt and gal.	NA
Rx *sf*	**Kaon-Cl 20%** (Adria)		5% alcohol, saccharin. Cherry flavor. In 480 ml.	964
Rx	**Potassium Gluconate** (Various, eg, Major, PBI)	20 mEq/15 ml potassium (as potassium gluconate)	In 118 ml, pt, gal and UD 5 and 15 ml (100s).	NA
Rx *sf*	**Kaon** (Adria)		5% alcohol. Saccharin. Grape flavor. In 480 ml.	325
Rx	**Kaylixir** (Lannett)		5% alcohol. Saccharin. In pt and gal.	70
Rx	**K-G Elixir** (Geneva)		5% alcohol. In 480 ml.	127
Rx	**Tri-K** (Century)	45 mEq/15 ml potassium (from potassium acetate, potassium bicarbonate and potassium citrate)	In pt and gal.	46
Rx	**Twin-K** (Boots)	20 mEq/15 ml potassium (as potassium gluconate & potassium citrate)	Sorbitol, saccharin. In 480 ml.	261
Rx *sf*	**Kolyum** (Fisons)	20 mEq potassium and 3.4 mEq chloride/15 ml (from potassium gluconate and potassium chloride)	Sorbitol, saccharin. Cherry flavor. In pt and gal.	410

* Cost Index based on cost per 40 mEq potassium.
sf – Sugar free.

POTASSIUM REPLACEMENT PRODUCTS (Cont.)

Powders

	Product	Content	Other	Cost Index*
Rx	**K + Care** (Alra)	15 mEq potassium chloride per packet	Saccharin. Fruit or orange flavor. In 30s and 100s.	NA
Rx	**K-Lor** (Abbott)		Saccharin. Fruit flavor. In 100s.	3687
Rx	**Potassium Chloride** (Various, eg, Geneva, Schein)	20 mEq potassium chloride per packet	In 30s and 100s.	662+
Rx *sf*	**Gen-K** (Goldline)		Orange/fruit flavor. In 30s.	700
Rx	**Kato** (ICN)		0.25 mEq sodium/packet. In 30s & 120s.	2127
Rx *sf*	**Kay Ciel** (Forest)		Saccharin. In 30s and 100s.	4464
Rx	**K + Care** (Alta)		Saccharin. Fruit or orange flavor. In 30s and 100s.	NA
Rx	**K-Lor** (Abbott)		Saccharin. Fruit flavor. In 30s and 100s.	2851
Rx *sf*	**Klor-Con** (Upsher-Smith)		Saccharin. Fruit flavor. In 30s and 100s.	573
Rx	**Micro-K LS** (Robins)		Extended-release. Sucrose. In 30s and 100s.	1809
Rx	**K + Care (Alra)**	25 mEq potassium chloride per packet	Saccharin. Orange flavor. In 30s and 100s.	NA
Rx *sf*	**Klor-Con/25** (Upsher-Smith)		Saccharin. Fruit flavor. In 30s, 100s and 250s.	544
Rx	**K • Lyte/Cl** (Mead-J)	25 mEq potassium chloride per dose	Fruit punch flavor. In 225 g (30 doses).	864
Rx *sf*	**Klorvess Effervescent Granules** (Sandoz)	20 mEq each potassium & chloride (potassium chloride, bicarbonate and citrate & lysine hydrochloride)/packet	Sodium free. Saccharin. In 30s.	2173
Rx *sf*	**Kolyum** (Fisons)	20 mEq potassium and 3.4 mEq chloride (from potassium gluconate and potassium chloride) per packet	Sorbitol, saccharin. Cherry flavor. In 30s.	2743

Effervescent Tablets (Dissolve in water)

	Product	Content	Other	Cost Index*
Rx	**K+ Care ET** (Alra)	20 mEq potassium (from potassium bicarbonate)	Saccharin. In 30s and 100s.	NA
Rx *sf*	**Klorvess** (Sandoz)	20 mEq potassium (from potassium chloride and bicarbonate and lysine hydrochloride)	Sodium free. Saccharin. White. In 60s and 1000s.	2680
Rx	**K•Lyte/Cl** (Bristol)	25 mEq potassium (from potassium Cl and bicarbonate, l-lysine monohydrochloride and citric acid)	Saccharin, docusate sodium. Fruit punch or citrus flavor. In 30s, 100s and 250s.	1386
Rx	**K•Lyte/Cl 50** (Bristol)	50 mEq potassium (from potassium Cl and bicarbonate, l-lysine monohydrochloride and citric acid)	Saccharin, docusate sodium. Fruit punch or citrus flavor. In 30s & 100s.	1183
Rx	**K+ Care ET** (Alra)	25 mEq potassium (from potassium bicarbonate)	Saccharin. Orange or lime flavor. In 30s and 100s.	661

* Cost Index based on cost per 40 mEq potassium. *sf* – Sugar free.

(Continued on following page)

POTASSIUM REPLACEMENT PRODUCTS (Cont.)

Effervescent Tablets (Cont.) (Dissolve in water)

Rx	**Effer-K** (Nomax)	25 mEq potassium (as bicarbonate and citrate)	Saccharin. Orange or lime flavor. In 30s, 100s & 250s.	492
Rx	**Effervescent Potassium** (Rugby)		Saccharin. Lime, orange or fruit punch flavors. In 30s.	794
Rx *sf*	**Klor-Con/EF** (Upsher-Smith)		Saccharin. Orange flavor. In 30s and 100s.	518
Rx	**K•Lyte** (Bristol)		Saccharin, docusate sodium, dextrose. Orange or lime flavor. In 30s, 100s and 250s.	1386
Rx	**K•Lyte DS** (Bristol)	50 mEq potassium (from potassium bicarbonate and citrate and citric acid)	Saccharin, docusate sodium, lactose. Orange or lime flavor. In 30s and 100s.	1183

Capsules and Tablets

				C.I.*
Rx	**Kaon-Cl** (Adria)	**Tablets, controlled release:** 6.7 mEq (500 mg) potassium chloride in a wax matrix	Tartrazine, sucrose. (Adria/307). Yellow. Sugar coated. In 100s, 250s & 1000s.	1664
Rx	**Potassium Chloride** (Various, eg, Abbott, Geneva, Goldline, Major, Rugby, Warner Chilcott)	**Tablets, controlled release:** 8 mEq (600 mg) potassium chloride in a wax matrix	In 100s and 1000s.	NA
Rx	**Klor-Con 8** (Upsher-Smith)		Blue. Film coated. In 100s, 500s and UD 100s.	630
Rx	**Slow-K** (Summit)		(Slow-K). Sucrose. Buff. Sugar coated. In 100s, 1000s and UD 100s.	1493
Rx	**K+ 10** (Alra)	**Tablets, controlled release:** 10 mEq (750 mg) potassium chloride in a wax matrix	Film coated. In 100s, 500s, 1000s and UD 100s.	362
Rx	**Kaon Cl-10** (Adria)		Sucrose. (Adria/304). Green. Sugar coated. Capsule shape. In 100s, 500s, 1000s and Stat-Pak 100s.	1162
Rx	**Klor-Con 10** (Upsher-Smith)		Yellow. Film coated. In 100s, 500s and UD 100s.	568
Rx	**Klotrix** (Bristol)		Orange. Film coated. In 100s, 1000s and UD 100s.	972
Rx	**K-Tab** (Abbott)		Yellow. Film coated. Oval. In 100s, 1000s, 5000s and Abbo-Pac 100s.	1464

* Cost Index based on cost per 40 mEq potassium. *sf* – Sugar free.

(Continued on following page)

POTASSIUM REPLACEMENT PRODUCTS (Cont.)

		Capsules and Tablets (Cont.)		C.I.*
Rx	**Potassium Chloride** (Various, eg, Major, Rugby)	**Tablets, extended release:** 750 mg potassium chloride equivalent to 10 mEq potassium in a wax matrix	In 100s and 1000s.	858+
Rx	**K-Dur 10** (Key)	**Tablets, controlled release:** 750 mg microencapsulated potassium chloride equivalent to 10 mEq potassium	(K-Dur 10). White. Oblong. In 100s and UD 100s.	1032
Rx	**Ten-K** (Summit)		White, scored. Capsule shaped. Polymeric coated crystals. In 100s, 500s and UD 100s.	894
Rx	**K-Dur 20** (Key)	**Tablets, controlled release:** 1500 mg microencapsulated potassium chloride equivalent to 20 mEq potassium	(K-Dur 20). White, scored. Oblong. In 100s, 500s, 1000s and UD 100s.	977
Rx	**Micro-K Extencaps** (Robins)	**Capsules, controlled release:** 600 mg potassium chloride equivalent to 8 mEq potassium. Microencapsulated particles	(Micro-K AHR/5720). Orange. In 100s, 500s and UD 100s.	1139
Rx	**Potassium Chloride** (Various, eg, EtheX, Goldline, Major, Moore, Parmed, Rugby, Schein, Warner-Chilcott)	**Capsules, controlled release:** 10 mEq (750 mg) potassium chloride. Microencapsulated particles	In 100s and 500s.	NA
Rx	**K-Lease** (Adria)		(13/308). Green. In 100s, 500s, 1000s and 2500s.	620
Rx	**K-Norm** (Fisons)		Sugar. (K-Norm 10). Clear. In 100s and 500s.	855
Rx	**Micro-K 10 Extencaps** (Robins)		(Micro-K 10 AHR/5730). Orange/white. In 100s, 500s and UD 100s.	1000
otc	**Potassium Gluconate** (Various, eg, Rugby)	**Tablets:** 500 mg potassium gluconate (83.45 mg potassium)	In 100s and 1000s.	948+
otc	**Potassium Gluconate** (Mission)	**Tablets:** 595 mg potassium gluconate (99 mg potassium)	In 100s.	637

* Cost Index based on cost per 40 mEq potassium.

Salt Replacement Products

SODIUM CHLORIDE

For information on parenteral sodium products, refer to the monograph in the IV Nutritional Therapy section.

Indications:

Prevention or treatment of extracellular volume depletion, dehydration or sodium depletion (eg, due to excessive salt restriction); aid in the prevention of heat prostration.

Warnings:

Acclimatization: Inappropriate salt administration in an effort to acclimatize to a hot environment can be dangerous. Balanced electrolytes and adequate hydration are essential.

Salt tablets may pass through the GI tract undigested. Avoid their use in treating heat cramps since they may cause vomiting, pooling of oral fluids and potassium depletion. Use oral salt solutions instead.

Pregnancy: Seek professional advice before using these products.

Lactation: Seek professional advice before using these products.

Precautions:

Supplementation: Individuals with adequate dietary sodium intake and normal renal function should not require sodium chloride supplementation. Balanced electrolyte supplements may be preferred to prevent hypokalemia.

Use with caution in the presence of congestive heart failure, kidney dysfunction, peripheral or pulmonary edema or preeclampsia.

Overdosage:

Symptoms: Overdosage may cause serious electrolyte disturbances. Ingestion of large amounts of sodium chloride irritates the GI mucosa and may result in nausea, vomiting, diarrhea and abdominal cramps. Edema is a sign of excess total body sodium.

Manifestations of hypernatremia may include:

Neurologic – Irritability; restlessness; weakness; obtundation progressing to convulsions and coma.

Cardiovascular – Hypertension; tachycardia; fluid accumulation.

Respiratory – Pulmonary edema; respiratory arrest.

Treatment includes usual supportive measures. Refer to General Management of Acute Overdosage. Use appropriate measures to empty the stomach. Magnesium sulfate may be given as a cathartic. Provide an adequate airway and ventilation. Maintain vascular volume and tissue perfusion.

Administration and Dosage:

Refer to specific product labeling for dosage guidelines.

				C.I.*
otc	**Sodium Chloride** (Purepac)	**Tablets:** 650 mg	In 100s.	35
otc	**Sodium Chloride** (Various)	**Tablets:** 1 g	In 100s and 1000s.	NA
otc	**Sodium Chloride** (Lilly)	**Tablets:** 2.25 g	In 100s and 500s.	99
otc	**Slo-Salt** (Mission)	**Tablets, slow release:** 600 mg	In 100s.	54
otc	**Slo-Salt-K** (Mission)	**Tablets, slow release:** 410 mg sodium chloride and 150 mg potassium chloride in wax matrix	In 1000s.	NA

* Cost Index based on cost per tablet.

Oral Electrolyte Mixtures

Actions:

Pharmacology: Used properly, mixtures with electrolytes, water and glucose prevent dehydration or achieve rehydration, and maintain strength and feeling of well being. They contain sodium, chloride, potassium and bicarbonate to replace depleted electrolytes and restore acid-base balance. Glucose facilitates sodium transport, which aids in sodium and water absorption.

Indications:

For maintenance of water and electrolytes following corrective parenteral therapy for severe diarrhea; for maintenance to replace mild to moderate fluid losses when food and liquid intake are discontinued; to restore fluid and minerals lost in diarrhea and vomiting in infants and children.

Contraindications:

Severe, continuing diarrhea or other critical fluid losses; intractable vomiting; prolonged shock, renal dysfunction (anuria, oliguria). These conditions require parenteral therapy.

Administration and Dosage:

Individualize dosage. Follow the guidelines listed on the product labeling.

Ricelyte: Children $<$ 2 years of age – Consult physician.

Children $\geq$ 2 years of age – Administer every 3 to 4 hours, up to 2 quarts per day.

Resol: Individualize dosage based on extent of weight loss and dehydration as assessed by the physician.

Pedialyte/Rehydralyte: Offer frequently in amounts tolerated. Adjust total daily intake to meet individual needs, based on thirst and response to therapy. In the following table, suggested intakes for replacement are based on fluid losses of 5% or 10% of body weight, including maintenance requirement.

Pedialyte/Rehydralyte Dosage for Infants/Young Children

Age	Weight (approx.) kg	Weight (approx.) lb	*Pedialyte* oz/day	*Rehydralyte* Replacement for 5% dehydration (oz/day)	*Rehydralyte* Replacement for 10% dehydration (oz/day)
2 wks	3.2	7	13-16	18-21	23-26
3 mos	6	13	28-32	38-42	48-52
6 mos	7.8	17	34-40	47-53	60-66
9 mos	9.2	20	38-44	53-59	68-74
1 yr	10.2	23	41-46	58-63	75-80
1.5 yr	11.4	25	45-50	64-69	83-88
2 yr	12.6	28	48-53	69-74	90-95
2.5 yr	13.6	30	51-56	74-79	97-102
3 yr	14.6	32	54-58	78-82	102-106
3.5 yr	16	35	56-60	83-87	110-114
4 yr	17	38	57-62	85-90	113-118

Extemporaneous oral rehydration solution (developed by the World Health Organization): To be added to 1 L of water. Follow physician's instructions for administration.

	Na^+/Cl^-	K^+	Citrate	Glucose
Source	NaCl or table salt	KCl or potassium salt[1]	sodium bicarbonate (baking soda)	Glucose or sucrose (cane sugar)
Weight (g)	3.5	1.5	2.5	20[2]
Household measure	0.5 tsp	0.25 tsp	0.5 tsp	2 tbsp[3]
mmol/L	90/80	20	30	111

[1] See potassium salt substitutes. [2] If sucrose is used, 40 g. [3] If sucrose is used, 4 tbsp.

	Product	Electrolyte content (mEq/L) Na^+	K^+	Cl^-	Citrate	Ca^{++}	Mg^{++}	Phosphate	Other Content	Calories per fl. oz.	How Supplied
otc	**Rehydralyte Solution** (Ross)	75	20	65	30				25 g/L dextrose	3	In 240 ml ready-to-use.
otc	**Ricelyte Oral Solution** (Mead Johnson)	50	25	45	34				30 g/L rice syrup solids	4.2	Fruit flavor. In ≈ 1 L ready-to-use.
otc	**Resol Solution** (Wyeth-Ayerst)	50	20	50	34	4	4	5	20 g/L glucose	2.5	In 240 ml ready-to-use.
otc	**Pedialyte Solution** (Ross)	45	20	35	30				25 g/L dextrose	3	Regular or fruit flavor. In 240 & 960 ml ready-to-use.

Systemic Alkalinizers

CITRATE AND CITRIC ACID SOLUTIONS

Actions:

Pharmacology: Citrate and citric acid solutions are systemic and urinary alkalinizers. Preparations containing potassium citrate are preferred in patients requiring potassium or those who require sodium restriction. Conversely, sodium citrate may be administered when potassium is undesirable or contraindicated. Potassium citrate and sodium citrate are capable of buffering gastric acidity (pH > 2.5). The effects are essentially those of chlorides before absorption, and subsequently, those of bicarbonates.

Pharmacokinetics: Potassium citrate and sodium citrate are absorbed and metabolized to potassium bicarbonate and sodium bicarbonate, thus acting as systemic alkalinizers. The citric acid is metabolized to carbon dioxide and water; therefore, it has only a transient effect on systemic acid-base status. It functions as a temporary buffer component.

Oxidation is virtually complete; < 5% of the citrates are excreted in the urine unchanged.

Indications:

Treatment of chronic metabolic acidosis, particularly when caused by renal tubular acidosis.

Conditions where long-term maintenance of an alkaline urine is desirable, in treatment of patients with uric acid and cystine calculi of the urinary tract and in conjunction with uricosurics in gout therapy to prevent uric acid nephropathy.

Nonparticulate neutralizing buffers.

Contraindications:

Severe renal impairment with oliguria, azotemia or anuria; untreated Addison's disease; adynamia episodica hereditaria; acute dehydration; heat cramps; severe myocardial damage; hyperkalemia.

Sodium citrate: Sodium restricted patients.

Warnings:

Pregnancy: Polycitra-K is not expected to cause fetal harm when administered in dosages that will not result in hyperkalemia.

Lactation: Exercise caution when administered to a nursing woman.

Precautions:

Urolithiasis: Citrate mobilizes calcium from bones and increases its renal excretion; this, along with the elevated urine pH, may predispose to urolithiasis.

Hyperkalemia/Alkalosis: Patients with low urinary output and abnormal renal mechanisms may develop hyperkalemia or alkalosis, especially in the presence of hypocalcemia.

Sodium salts: Use cautiously in patients with cardiac failure, hypertension, impaired renal function, peripheral and pulmonary edema and preeclampsia. Monitor serum electrolytes, particularly the serum bicarbonate level, in patients with renal disease.

GI effects: Dilute with water to minimize GI injury associated with the oral ingestion of concentrated potassium salts. Take after meals to avoid saline laxative effect.

Drug Interactions:

Urinary Alkalinizer Drug Interactions

Precipitant drug	Object drug *		Description
Urinary alkalinizers (eg, potassium citrate, sodium citrate)	Chlorpropamide Lithium Methenamine Methotrexate Salicylates Tetracyclines	⬇	Urinary alkalinizers may increase the excretion and decrease the serum levels of these agents, possibly decreasing their pharmacologic effects.
Urinary alkalinizers (eg, potassium citrate, sodium citrate)	Anorexiants Flecainide Mecamylamine Quinidine Sympathomimetics	⬆	Urinary alkalinizers may decrease the excretion and increase the serum levels of these agents, possibly increasing their pharmacologic effects.

* ⬆ = Object drug increased ⬇ = Object drug decreased

Adverse Reactions:

Hyperkalemia: Listlessness, weakness, mental confusion, tingling of extremities and other symptoms associated with high serum potassium. Hyperkalemia may exhibit the following ECG abnormalities: Disappearance of the P wave; widening or slurring of the QRS complex; changes of the ST segment; tall peaked T waves.

(Continued on following page)

Systemic Alkalinizers (Cont.)

CITRATE AND CITRIC ACID SOLUTIONS (Cont.)

Overdosage:

Symptoms: Overdosage with sodium salts may cause diarrhea, nausea, vomiting, hypernoia (excessive mental activity) and convulsions. Overdosage with potassium salts may cause hyperkalemia and alkalosis, especially in the presence of renal disease. Treat hyperkalemia immediately, because lethal levels can be reached in a few hours.

Treatment: For treatment of hyperkalemia, refer to the Potassium monograph in the IV Nutritional Therapy section; for treatment of sodium overdosage, refer to the Sodium Chloride monograph in the Salt Replacement Products section.

Patient Information:

Dilute with water; follow with additional water, if desired.

Take after meals.

Notify physician if diarrhea, nausea, stomach pain, vomiting or convulsions occur.

Administration and Dosage:

Dilute in water before taking; follow with additional water, if desired. Monitor urinary pH with *Hydrion* paper (pH 6 to 8) or *Nitrazine* paper (pH 4.5 to 7.5).

Dosage: Adults – 15 to 30 ml diluted with water, after meals and before bedtime.
Children – 5 to 10 ml diluted with water, after meals and before bedtime. The solution, not the crystals, is recommended for pediatric administration since dosage can be more easily regulated.

Neutralizing buffer: A single dose of 15 ml diluted with 15 ml water.

Rx	**Polycitra** (Willen)	**Syrup:** 550 mg potassium citrate monohydrate, 500 mg sodium citrate dihydrate and 334 mg citric acid monohydrate per 5 ml. (1 mEq potassium and 1 mEq sodium per ml and is equivalent to 2 mEq bicarbonate)	Sugar. Alcohol free. In 473 ml.
Rx sf	**Polycitra-LC** (Willen)	**Solution:** 550 mg potassium citrate monohydrate, 500 mg sodium citrate dihydrate and 334 mg citric acid monohydrate per 5 ml. (1 mEq potassium and 1 mEq sodium per ml and is equivalent to 2 mEq bicarbonate)	Alcohol free. In 473 ml.
Rx sf	**Polycitra-K** (Willen)	**Solution:** 1100 mg potassium citrate monohydrate and 334 mg citric acid monohydrate per 5 ml. (2 mEq potassium per ml and is equivalent to 2 mEq bicarbonate)	Alcohol free. In 473 ml.
Rx sf	**Polycitra-K** (Willen)	**Crystals:** 1100 mg potassium citrate monohydrate and 334 mg citric acid monohydrate per 5 ml when reconstituted. (2 mEq potassium per ml and is equivalent to 2 mEq bicarbonate)	In UD packets (100) to make 15 ml when reconstituted.
Rx	**Oracit** (Carolina Medical Products)	**Solution:** 490 mg sodium citrate and 640 mg citric acid per 5 ml. (1 mEq sodium per ml and is equivalent to 1 mEq bicarbonate)	Parabens. In 500 ml and UD 15 and 30 ml.
Rx sf	**Bicitra** (Willen)	**Solution:** 500 mg sodium citrate dihydrate and 334 mg citric acid monohydrate per 5 ml. (1 mEq sodium per ml and is equivalent to 1 mEq bicarbonate)	Alcohol free. In 120 and 473 ml, gal and UD 15 and 30 ml.

sf – Sugar free.

Systemic Alkalinizers (Cont.)

SODIUM BICARBONATE

For information on parenteral sodium bicarbonate products, refer to the monograph in the IV Nutritional Therapy section.

One g of sodium bicarbonate provides 11.9 mmol sodium and 11.9 mmol bicarbonate.

Indications:

A gastric, systemic and urinary alkalinizer.

Precautions:

Use cautiously in patients with edematous sodium-retaining states, congestive heart failure or renal impairment. Prolonged therapy may lead to systemic alkalosis.

Administration and Dosage:

Usual dose is 325 mg to 2 g, 1 to 4 times daily. Maximum daily intake is 16 g (200 mEq) in patients < 60 years old and 8 g (100 mEq) in those older than 60 years of age.

otc	**Sodium Bicarbonate** (Various, eg, Rugby)	**Tablets:** 325 mg	In 1000s.
		650 mg	In 1000s.
		Powder	In 120 and 300 g and 1 lb.

	Product & Distributor	A IU	D IU	C mg	Content Given Per	Other Content and How Supplied	**C.I.***
otc	**Ultra Vitamin A & D Tablets** (Nature's Bounty)	25,000	1000		tablet	In 100s.	43
otc	**Cod Liver Oil Concentrate Capsules** (Schering)	10,000	400		capsule	In 40s and 100s.	215
otc	**Super D Perles** (Upjohn)					Tartrazine. In 100s.	132
otc	**Vitamin A & D Tablets** (Nature's Bounty)	10,000	400		tablet	In 100s.	38
otc	**Cod Liver Oil Concentrate w/Vitamin C Tablets** (Schering)	4,000	200	50	chewable tablet	Tartrazine, sugar. In 100s.	97
otc	**Cod Liver Oil Concentrate Tablets** (Schering)	4,000	200		chewable tablet	Tartrazine, sugar. In 100s.	72
otc *sf*	**Triple Vita Drops** (PBI)	1,500	400	35	1 ml	Alcohol free. In 50 ml.	100
otc	**Tri-Vi-Sol Drops** (Mead J Nutritional)					In 30 and 50 ml.	247
otc	**Tri Vit Drops** (Barre)					Cherry flavor. In 50 ml.	NA
otc *sf*	**Vi-Daylin ADC Drops** (Ross)					< 0.5% alcohol. Pineapple-fruit flavor. In 50 ml.	250
otc	**Cod Liver Oil Capsules** (Various, eg, Balan, Bioline, Dixon-Shane, Goldline, Moore, Nature's Bounty, Rugby, Schein, Squibb Mark, URL)	1,250	135		capsule	In 40s, 100s, 250s and 1000s.	24+
otc	**Scott's Emulsion** (Beecham)	1,250	100		5 ml	In 187.5 and 375 ml.	136
otc	**Cod Liver Oil Liquid USP** (Various, eg, Balan, Denison, Halsey, Humco, Lannett, Purepac, Squibb Mark, Whiteworth)	850	85		g	In 120, 240 and 360 ml, pt and gal.	123+

* Cost Index based on cost per content listed.
sf – Sugar free.

Content given per tablet.

	Product & Distributor	Ca[1] mg	D IU	P mg	Other Content and How Supplied	C.I.*
otc	**Calcium 600 Tablets** (Schein)	600	125		In 60s.	65
otc *sf*	**Calcium 600 + D Tablets** (Nature's Bounty)				Sodium free. Film coated. In 60s.	62
otc	**Calcium with Vitamin D Tablets** (Schein)				Green, oval. In 60s.	115
otc *sf*	**Caltrate 600 + Iron Tablets** (Lederle)				18 mg Fe.[2] Sodium free. (Lederle C45). Red, scored. Film coated. Capsule shape. In 60s.	250
otc *sf*	**Caltrate 600 + D Tablets** (Lederle)				Sodium free. (LL C40). Tan, scored. Film coated. Capsule shape. In 60s.	214
otc	**Fergon Iron Plus Calcium Caplets** (Winthrop)				18 mg Fe.[2] Timed release. Coated. In 60s.	212
otc *sf*	**Posture-D Tablets** (Whitehall)				Scored, coated. In 60s.	202
otc	**NeoVadrin Calcium 600 with Vitamin D Tablets** (Mission)	600	100		In 60s.	NA
otc	**NeoVadrin + Iron & Vitamin D Tablets** (Mission)				18 mg Fe.[2] In 60s.	NA
otc *sf*	**Calel D Tablets** (Rorer)	500	200		Sodium free. In 75s.	195
otc	**Os-Cal 500 + D Tablets** (Marion Merrell Dow)	500	125		In 60s.	225
otc *sf*	**Oyster Calcium Tablets** (Nature's Bounty)	375	200		800 IU vitamin A. In 100s.	50
otc	**Citracal 1500 + D Tablets** (Mission)	315	200		In 60s.	213
otc	**Posture-D Tablets** (Whitehall)	300	62.5		(Posture D). In 100s.	NA
otc	**Cal-Bid Tablets** (Geriatric Pharm.)	250	125		100 mg vitamin C. In 100s.	197
otc	**Calcium Oyster Shell Tablets** (Schein)				Tartrazine. Green. In 250s and 1000s.	35
otc	**Caltro Tablets** (Geneva Generics)				Green. In 100s and 1000s.	48
otc	**Os-Cal 250 + D Tablets** (Marion Merrell Dow)				(Marion Os-Cal 1650). Lt green. Film coated. In 100s and 240s.	114
otc	**Oyst-Cal-D Tablets** (Goldline)				Tartrazine. Green. Film coated. In 100s, 240s and 1000s.	63
otc *sf*	**Oystercal-D 250 Tablets** (Nature's Bounty)				In 100s and 250s.	45
otc	**Oysco 'D' Tablets** (Rugby)				Green. In 100s, 250s, 1000s.	50
otc	**NeoVadrin Oystershell Calcium with Vitamin D Tablets** (Mission)	250	120		Tartrazine. In 100s.	NA
otc	**Calcet Tablets** (Mission)	153	100		Yellow, coated. Bolus shaped. In 100s.	137

* Cost Index based on cost per tablet.
sf – Sugar free.
[1] Expressed in mg elemental calcium.
[2] As ferrous fumarate.

(Continued on following page)

Content given per capsule, tablet or wafer.

	Product & Distributor	Ca[1] mg	D IU	P mg	Other Content and How Supplied	C.I.*
otc *sf*	**Super CalciCaps Tablets** (Nion)	400	133	42	In 90s.	106
otc	**Dical-D Wafers** (Abbott)	232	200	180	Chewable. Sucrose and dextrose. Vanilla flavor. In 51s.	238
otc *sf*	**Bone Meal with Vitamin D Tablets** (Nature's Bounty)	220	100	100	0.45 mg Fe, 3.25 mg Cu, 20 mcg Zn, 2.75 mcg Mn, 0.925 mg Mg. In 100s, 250s.	NA
otc	**CalciCaps Tablets** (Nion)	125[2]	67	60	In 100s and 500s.	49
otc	**CalciCaps with Iron Tablets** (Nion)				7 mg Fe.[3] Tartrazine. In 100s and 500s.	58
otc	**Dical-D Tablets** (Abbott)	117	133	90	In 100s and 500s.	112
otc	**Dical Captabs** (Rugby)	116[4]	133	90	Capsule shape. In 1000s.	40
otc	**Dibasic Calcium Phosphate with Vitamin D Pulvules** (Lilly)	116	33	90	In 100s.	122
otc	**Diostate D Tablets** (Upjohn)	114	133	88	Tartrazine. In 100s.	78
otc	**Osteon-D Tablets** (Pasadena)	100	67	67	40 mg Mg. In 180s.	75

VITAMIN COMBINATIONS, MISCELLANEOUS

Content given per capsule or tablet.

	Product and Distributor	A IU	E mg	B_3 mg	C mg	Other Content	How Supplied	C.I.*
otc	**A.C.N. Tablets** (Person & Covey)	25,000		25	250		In 100s.	186
otc *sf*	**Oxi-Freeda Tablets** (Freeda)	5000[8]	150[10]	40	100	20 mg B_1, 20 mg B_2, 20 mg B_5, 20 mg B_6, 10 mcg B_{12}, 15 mg chelated Zn, 50 mcg Se, 40 mg glutathione, 75 mg L-cysteine	In 100s and 250s.	399
otc *sf*	**Anti-Oxidant Capsules** (Murdock)	5000	134[5]		90	15 mg Zn, 100 mcg Se, 30 mg glutathione	Sodium free. In 90s.	219
otc	**Ocuvite Tablets** (Lederle)	5000[8]	30[9]		60	40 mg Zn, Cu, 40 mcg Se	Film coated. Eye shape. In 60s.	NA
otc *sf*	**KLB6 Complete Tablets** (Nature's Bounty)	833.3	5[10]	3.3	10	200 mg soya lecithin, 25 mg kelp, 40 mg cider vinegar, 83.3 mg wheat bran, 66.7 IU, D 0.067 mg FA, 0.25 mg B_1, 0.28 mg B_2, 8.3 mg B_6, 1 mcg B_{12}, 0.05 mg biotin	In 100s.	78
otc *sf*	**C & E Capsules** (Nature's Bounty)		400[7]		500		In 50s and 100s.	186
otc	**Ecee Plus Tablets** (Edwards)		165[6]		100	70 mg Mg sulfate, 80 mg Zn sulfate	Orange. In 100s.	250

* Cost Index based on cost per capsule, tablet or wafer.
sf – Sugar free.
[1] Expressed in mg elemental calcium.
[2] Dibasic calcium phosphate, calcium gluconate and calcium carbonate.
[3] From ferrous gluconate.
[4] Dicalcium phosphate and calcium gluconate.
[5] As d-alpha tocopherol.
[6] As d-alpha tocopheryl acid succinate.
[7] In IU; as mixed tocopherols complex.
[8] As beta carotene.
[9] As dl-alpha tocopheryl acetate.
[10] Form of vitamin E unknown, content given in IU.

Content given per capsule or tablet.

	Product and Distributor	Ca[1] mg	E mg	B_6 mg	C mg	Other Content	How Supplied	C.I.*
otc *sf*	**Ze Caps Capsules** (Everett)		200[2]			9.6 mg Zn (as gluconate)	Sodium free. In 60s.	183
otc *sf*	**Herbal Cellulex Tablets** (Nature's Bounty)				83	33 mg K, 9 mg Fe	In 90s.	133
otc *sf*	**Dolomite Tablets** (Nature's Bounty)	130				78 mg Mg	In 100s and 250s.	24
otc	**Beelith Tablets** (Beach)			20		600 mg Mg oxide	In 100s.	190
otc *sf*	**Chelated Calcium Magnesium Tablets** (Nature's Bounty)	500				250 mg Mg	Protein coated. In 50s.	53
otc *sf*	**Chelated Calcium Magnesium Zinc Tablets** (Nature's Bounty)	333				133 mg Mg, 8.3 mg Zn	In 100s.	44
otc *sf*	**KLB6 Softgels** (Nature's Bounty)			3.5		100 mg soya lecithin, 25 mg kelp, 40 mg cider vinegar	In 100s.	70
otc	**Ultra KLB6 Tablets** (Nature's Bounty)			16.7		400 mg lecithin, 33.3 mg kelp, 80 mg cider vinegar	In 100s.	82
otc *sf*	**Mag-Cal Tablets** (Fibertone)	416.7[3] 166.7[1]				66.7 IU D_3, 83.3 mg Mg, 0.167 mg Cu, 0.83 mg Mn, 1.67 mg K, 0.167 mg Zn	In 90s and 180s.	51
otc *sf*	**Bo-Cal Tablets** (Fibertone)	250				125 mg Mg, 100 IU D_3, 0.75 mg Boron	In 120s.	36
otc	**Calfos-D Tablets** (Pal-Pak)	116				100 IU D, 90 mg P	Tan, scored. In 1000s.	22
otc *sf*	**Multi-Mineral Tablets** (Nature's Bounty)	166.7				75.7 mg P, 25 mcg I, 3 mg Fe, 66.7 mg Mg, 0.33 mg Cu, 2.5 mg Zn, 12.5 mg K, 8.3 mg Mn	In 100s.	51
otc	**Efamol PMS** (Murdock)	20	12[4]	21	100	30 Mg, 3 mg Zn, 45 mg gamma-linolenic acid, 115 mg cis-linoleic acid, 35 mg alpha-linolenic acid, 14 mg eicosapentaenoic acid, 9 mg docosahexaenoic acid	In 30s and 90s.	

* Cost Index based on cost per capsule or tablet.
sf – Sugar free.
[1] Calcium content expressed in mg elemental calcium.
[2] As dl-alpha tocopheryl acetate.
[3] Carbonate.
[4] Form of vitamin E unknown, content given in IU.

B VITAMIN COMBINATIONS, ORAL

Content given per capsule, tablet or 5 ml.

	Product & Distributor	B_1 mg	B_2 mg	B_3 mg	B_5 mg	B_6 mg	B_{12} mcg	FA mg	Other Content	How Supplied	C.I.*
otc sf	**B-150 Tablets** (Nature's Bounty)	150	150	150	150	150	150	0.15	150 mcg d-biotin, 150 mg base of choline, inositol, PABA, lecithin	In 30s.	385
otc sf	**B-125 Tablets** (Nature's Bounty)	125	125	125	125	125	125	0.125	125 mcg d-biotin, 125 mg base of choline, inositol, PABA, lecithin	In 50s.	NA
otc	**B-Complex "100" Tablets** (Vitaline)	100	100	100	100	100	100	0.4	30 mg PABA, 100 mg inositol, 100 mcg biotin, 100 mg choline bitartrate	Regular and controlled release. In 90s and 1000s.	33
otc sf	**NeoVadrin B Complex "100" Tablets** (Mission)								100 mg PABA, 100 mg inositol, 100 mcg biotin and 100 mg choline bitartrate	In 100s.	NA
otc sf	**B-100 Tablets** (Nature's Bounty)	100	100	100	100	100	100	0.1	100 mcg d-biotin, 100 mg base of PABA, choline, inositol and lecithin	In 50s and 100s.	237
otc	**Balanced B-100 Tablets** (Fibertone)								100 mg PABA, 100 mg inositol and 100 mcg d-biotin	Sustained release. In 50s and 90s.	NA
otc	**Mega-B Tablets** (Arco)								100 mg PABA, 100 mg inositol, 100 mcg d-biotin and 100 mg choline bitartrate	In 30s, 100s and 500s.	280
otc sf	**NeoVadrin B Complex "50" Tablets** (Mission)	50	50	50	50	50	50	0.4	50 mg PABA, 50 mg inositol, 50 mcg biotin and 50 mg choline bitartrate	In 100s.	NA
otc sf	**Super Quints-50 Tablets** (Freeda)	50	50	50	50	50	50	0.4	30 mg PABA, 50 mcg d-biotin, 50 mg inositol	In 100s, 250s and 500s.	191
otc	**B-Complex "50" Tablets** (Vitaline)	50	50	50	50	50	50	0.1	30 mg PABA, 50 mg inositol, 50 mcg biotin, 50 mg choline bitartrate	Regular or controlled release. In 90s and 1000s.	26
otc sf	**Ultra B-50 Tablets** (Nature's Bounty)								50 mg PABA, 50 mg inositol, 50 mcg d-biotin, 50 mg choline and lecithin	In 60s and 180s.	NA

* Cost Index based on cost per tablet.
sf – Sugar free.

(Continued on following page)

B VITAMIN COMBINATIONS, ORAL (Cont.)

Content given per capsule, tablet or 5 ml.

	Product & Distributor	B_1 mg	B_2 mg	B_3 mg	B_5 mg	B_6 mg	B_{12} mcg	FA mg	Other Content	How Supplied	C.I.*
otc sf	**B-50 Tablets** (Nature's Bounty)	50	50	50	50	50	50	0.1	50 mcg d-biotin, 50 mg base of choline, inositol, PABA, lecithin	In 50s and 100s.	143
otc sf	**B-50 Time Release Tablets** (Nature's Bounty)								50 mcg d-biotin, 50 mg base of choline, inositol, PABA, lecithin	Timed release. In 60s.	142
otc sf	**Vital B-50 Tablets** (Goldline)								50 mcg d-biotin, 50 mg PABA, 50 mg choline bitartrate, 50 mg inositol and 20 mg bromelain	Timed release. In 60s.	175
otc	**Neurodep-Caps** (Medical Prod.)	125				125	1000			In 50s.	NA
otc	**Apatate Liquid** (Kenwood)	15				0.5	25			Alcohol free. Cherry flavor. In 120 and 240 ml.	554
otc	**Becotin Pulvules** (Dista)	10	10	50	25	4.1	1			In 100s.	252
otc	**Secran Liquid** (Scherer)	10		10			25		17% alcohol	In 480 ml.	204
Rx	**Sorbi-Tinic-F Liquid** (Ortega)	10				5	25	0.333	12 mg Fe, 100 mg l-lysine HCl, sorbitol, sucrose	In pt and gal.	265
otc	**Orexin Softab Tabs** (J & J-Merck)	8.1				4.1	25		Saccharin, mannitol	Chewable. Pink. In 100s.	426
otc	**Trophite Liquid** (SK Consumer)	10					25			In 118 ml.	571
otc sf	**B-Complex and B-12 Tablets** (Nature's Bounty)	7	14	4.5			25		10 mg protease	In 90s.	47
otc	**Surbex Filmtabs** (Abbott)	6	6	30	10	2.5	5			Film coated. In 100s.	220
otc	**Tega-Atric Elixir** (Ortega)	0.83	0.4	8.3	1.67	1.67	16.7		18% alcohol, I, 2.5 mg Fe, 0.33 mg Zn, choline, Mn	Sherry base. In pt.	198
otc	**Vitamin B Complex Elixir** (Lilly)	2.7	1.35	6.8	2.7	0.55	3		500 mg soluble liver fraction, 17% alcohol, saccharin	In 473 ml.	314
otc	**Lederplex Capsules** (Lederle)	2.25	2.6	30	15	3	9			(L6). Brown. In 100s.	144
otc	**Triasyn B Caps and Tabs** (Lannett)	2	3	20						In 500s and 1000s.	20
otc	**Almebex Plus B_{12} Liquid** (Dayton)	1	2	5		0.4	5		33 mg choline, 10% alcohol	In pt with vitamin B_{12} in separate glass container.	15

* Cost Index based on cost per capsule, tablet or 5 ml.
sf – Sugar free.

(Continued on following page)

B VITAMIN COMBINATIONS, ORAL (Cont.)

Content given per capsule, tablet or 5 ml.

	Product & Distributor	B_1 mg	B_2 mg	B_3 mg	B_5 mg	B_6 mg	B_{12} mcg	FA mg	Other Content	How Supplied	C.I.*
otc	**B-Nutron Tablets** (Nion)	2	2	25	2	2	16.7		3000 IU vitamin A, 10 mg vitamin E, 333 mg vitamin C, 16.7 mg Zn and 6.7 mcg Se	In 100s and 500s.	102
otc	**Lederplex Liquid** (Lederle)	1.13	1.3	15	7.5	1.5	4.5		Sucrose, honey	Orange flavor. In 360 ml.	256
otc	**Vitamin B Complex Pulvules** (Lilly)	1	2	10	3.33	0.4	1			In 100s.	209
otc	**Gevrabon Liquid** (Lederle)	0.83	0.42	8.3	1.67	0.17	0.17		2.5 mg Fe, 16.7 mg choline, 16.7 mcg I, Mg, Mn, Zn, 18% alcohol, sucrose	Sherry flavor. In 480 ml.	191
otc	**Vitamin-Mineral-Supplement Liquid** (PBI)								16.67 mcg I, 2.5 mg Fe, 0.33 mg Mg, 0.33 mg Zn, 0.33 mg Mn, 16.67 mg choline, 18% alcohol	In pt and gal.	94
otc	**Lanoplex Elixir** (Lannett)	0.67	1	6.7		0.33			11% alcohol	Sherry flavor. In pt and gal.	60
Rx	**Senilezol Elixir** (Edwards)	0.42	0.42	1.67	0.83	0.17	0.83		3.3 mg ferric pyrophosphate and 15% alcohol	In 480 ml.	238
otc	**Lipovite Capsules** (Rugby)	0.3	0.3	3.3	1.67	0.3	1.67		111 mg choline bitartrate	In 60s.	117
otc	**Geriplex-FS Liquid** (Parke-Davis)	0.2	0.28	2.5		0.17	0.83		2.5 mg Fe, 18% alcohol, sorbitol, saccharin	In 480 ml.	164
otc	**Eldertonic Elixir** (Mayrand)	0.17	0.19	2.22	1.11	0.22	0.67		0.22 mg Mg, 0.22 mg Mn, 1.67 mg Zn, 13.5% alcohol	Sherry base. In 240 ml, pt, qt and gal.	152
otc *sf*	**Brewers Yeast Tablets** (Nature's Bounty)	0.08	0.025	0.22						In 250s and 500s.	21
otc	**Mucoplex Tablets** (ICN)		1.5				5		750 mg liver fraction	In 100s and 250s.	209
Rx	**Megaton Elixir** (Hyrex)			4.4	1.1	0.44	1.33	0.1	4 mg Fe, 0.44 mg Mn, 1.67 mg Zn, 13% alcohol	Sherry base. In 480 ml.	163
Rx	**May-Vita Elixir** (Mayrand)			40	10	4	12	1	36 mg Fe, 15 mg Zn, 4 mg Mn, 13% alcohol	In 45 ml and pt.	NA

* Cost Index based on cost per capsule, tablet or 5 ml.   *sf* – Sugar free.

B VITAMINS, PARENTERAL

Content given per ml.

	Product & Distributor	B_1 mg	B_2 mg	B_3 mg	B_5 mg	B_6 mg	Other Content	Content Given Per	How Supplied	C.I.*
Rx	**B-Ject-100** (Hyrex)	100	2	100	2	2		1 ml	In 10 and 30 ml vials.[1]	1088
Rx	**Becomject-100** (Mayrand)								In 30 ml vials.[1]	1093

B VITAMINS WITH VITAMIN C, PARENTERAL

Content given per ml.

	Product & Distributor	B_1 mg	B_2 mg	B_3 mg	B_5 mg	B_6 mg	B_{12} mcg	C mg	Other Content	Content Given Per	How Supplied	
Rx	**Key-Plex Injection** (Hyrex)	50	5	125	6	5	1000	50		1 ml	In 10 ml vials.[1]	1104
Rx	**Vicam Injection** (Keene)										In 10 ml vials.[1]	1506
Rx	**Neurodep Injection Lyophilized** (Medical Products)	50	5	125	6	5		50	1% benzyl alcohol	1 ml	In 10 ml multidose vials.	NA
Rx	**B Complex with Vitamin C and B12-10,000** (Lyphomed)	20	3	75	5	5	1000	100		1 ml	In 10 ml multiple dose covials.[2]	1400
Rx	**Scorbex/12 Injection** (Pasadena)										In 10 ml vials.[2]	1390

* Cost Index based on cost per ml.
[1] With benzyl alcohol.
[2] With benzyl alcohol, methyl and propyl parabens and sodium bisulfite.

B VITAMINS WITH VITAMIN C, ORAL

Content given per capsule or tablet.

	Product & Distributor	B_1 mg	B_2 mg	B_3 mg	B_5 mg	B_6 mg	B_{12} mcg	C mg	Other Content	How Supplied	C.I.*
otc	**Enviro-Stress Tablets** (Vitaline)	50	50	100	50	50	25	600	0.4 mg FA, 30 mg Zn, 30 IU vitamin E, Mg, Se, PABA	In 90s and 1000s.	139
otc *sf*	**T-Vites Tablets** (Freeda)	25	25	150	25	25		100	30 mcg biotin, 30 mg PABA, 10 mg K, 125 mg Mg, 2 mg Mn and 20 mg Zn	In 100s, 250s and 500s.	208
otc	**Vio-Bec Capsules** (Solvay Pharm.)	25	25	100	40	25		500		In 100s.	230
otc *sf*	**Marbec Tablets** (Marlyn)	25	25	100	23	25	25	300	120 mg brewer's yeast	In 100s.	89
otc	**Thera-Combex H P Kapseals** (Parke-Davis)	25	15	100	20	10	5	500	Bisulfites	In 100s.	232
otc	**Beminal 500 Tablets** (Whitehall)	25	12.5	100	20	10	5	500	Lactose	In 100s.	215
otc	**ThexForte Caplets** (Medtech)	25	15	100	10	5		500		In 75s.	148
otc	**BC-Vite Tablets** (Drug Industries)	25	5	50	10	1	2	150		In 100s and 500s.	NA
otc	**Vicon-C Capsules** (Whitby)	20	10	100	20	5		300	70 mg Mg, 50 mg dried Zn	In 30s, 60s, 500s and UD 100s.	222
otc	**Viogen-C Capsules** (Goldline)								Tartrazine. 50 mg Mg, 50 mg dried Zn	Yellow and orange. In 100s.	135
otc	**Vitazin Capsules** (Misemer)								70 mg Mg, 220 mg Zn	Maroon. In 100s.	288
otc	**Allbee-T Tablets** (Robins)	15.5	10	100	23	8.2	5	500	Lactose, desiccated liver	(AHR). Orange. Film coated. Capsule shape. In 100s.	173

* Cost Index based on cost per capsule or tablet.
sf – Sugar free.

(Continued on following page)

B VITAMINS WITH VITAMIN C, ORAL (Cont.)

Content given per capsule, tablet or 5 ml.

	Product & Distributor	B_1 mg	B_2 mg	B_3 mg	B_5 mg	B_6 mg	B_{12} mcg	C mg	Other Content	How Supplied	C.I.*
Rx	**B-C With Folic Acid Tablets** (Geneva G)	15	15	100	18	4	5	500	0.5 mg folic acid	Orange. Capsule shape. In 100s.	112
Rx	**Berocca Tablets** (Roche)								0.5 mg folic acid, sugar	Light green. Capsule shape. In 100s and 500s.	428
Rx	**B-Plex Tablets** (Goldline)								0.5 mg folic acid	Yellow. Oblong. In 100s.	120
Rx	**Strovite Tablets** (Everett)									In 100s.	250
Rx	**Larobec Tablets** (Roche)	15	15	100	18		5	500	0.5 mg folic acid	(Larobec Roche). Orange. In 100s.	332
otc	**Allbee w/C Caplets** (Robins)	15	10.2	50	10	5		300	Saccharin, lactose	(AHR Allbee C). Yellow. In UD 100s.	158
otc sf	**Arcobee with C Capsules** (Nature's Bounty)									In 100s.	88
otc	**Econo B & C Caplets** (Vangard)								Tartrazine	In 100s, 1000s and UD 100s.	116
otc sf	**Gen-bee with C Caplets** (Goldline)									Yellow, oblong. In 130s and 1000s.	51
otc	**Therapeutic B Complex with Vitamin C Capsules** (Upsher-Smith)									In UD 100s.	119
otc	**Vita-bee w/C Captabs** (Rugby)								Tartrazine	In 100s and 1000s.	56
otc	**Stress Formula 500 Tablets** (Schein)	15	10	100	20	5	12	500	30 IU vitamin E, 0.4 mg folic acid, 45 mcg biotin	In 60s and 250s.	
otc	**Surbex-T Filmtabs** (Abbott)	15	10	100	20	5	10	500		(A). Orange. In 100s, UD 100s.	270
otc sf	**Surbu-Gen-T Tablets** (Goldline)									Orange. Film coated. Oval. In 100s.	75
otc sf	**C-B Time Liquid** (Arco)	15	10	100	20	5	5	300		Alcohol free. In 120 ml.	NA
otc	**Bee-T-Vites Tablets** (Rugby)	15	10	100	20	5	4	300		Film coated. In 100s.	93
otc sf	**Glutofac Tablets** (Kenwood)	15	10	50	20	50		300	133 mg Mg, 25 mcg Se, 18 mg Zn, 25 mcg chromium complex	Green. In 90s.	316

* Cost Index based on cost per capsule, tablet or 5 ml. *sf* – Sugar free.

(Continued on following page)

B VITAMINS WITH VITAMIN C, ORAL (Cont.)

Content given per capsule or tablet.

	Product & Distributor	B_1 mg	B_2 mg	B_3 mg	B_5 mg	B_6 mg	B_{12} mcg	C mg	Other Content	How Supplied	C.I.*
otc	**Probec-T Tablets** (J & J-Merck)	12.2	10	100	18.4	4.1	5	600	Sucrose	In 60s.	423
otc *sf*	**Mega B with C Tablets** (Nature's Bounty)	10	15	25	100	10	25	500	Tartrazine, 400 mcg FA, 100 mcg biotin, 125 mg choline bitartrate, 250 mg inositol, 50 mg PABA	In 60s.	198
otc	**Stresscaps Capsules** (Lederle)	10	10	100	20	2	6	300		(Lederle S5). Brown. In 100s.	235
otc	**C-B Time 500 Tablets** (Arco)	10	10	50	10	5	10	500		Timed release. In 30s, 100s and 500s.	163
otc *sf*	**B-Complex + C Tablets** (Nature's Bounty)	10	10	50	10	5	10	200		Timed release. In 100s.	102
otc	**C-B Time Tablets** (Arco)									Timed release. In 120s.	136
otc	**Surbex with C Filmtabs** (Abbott)	6	6	30	10	2.5	5	250		Film coated. In 100s and 480s.	274
otc	**Mechol Tablets** (Manne)	5	2	20		5		75	100 mg soy protein, debittered brewer's yeast	In 120s and 1000s.	NA
Rx	**Nephrocaps Capsules** (Fleming)	1.5	1.7	20	5	10	6	100	1 mg FA and 150 mcg biotin	In 100s.	150
Rx	**Nephro-Vite Rx** (R & D)	1.5	1.7	20	10	10	6	60	1 mg FA, 300 mcg d-biotin, $<$ 0.3 mg Mg	Lactose. Yellow. Film coated. In 100s.	NA
otc	**Nephro-Vite B & C Tablets** (R & D)	1.5	1.7	20	10	10	6	60	800 mcg FA, 300 mcg biotin	In 100s.	156

* Cost Index based on cost per capsule or tablet.

sf – Sugar free.

MULTIVITAMINS, PARENTERAL

	Product & Distributor	Content[1] given per	A IU	D IU	E mg	B_1 mg	B_2 mg	B_3 mg	B_5 mg	B_6 mg	B_{12} mcg	C mg	biotin mcg	FA mg	Other Content and How Supplied	C.I.*
Rx	**M.V.I.-12 Injection** (Armour)	5 ml	3,300	200	10[2]	3	3.6	40	15	4	5	100	60	0.4	In 2 vial sets: Vial 1[3] (5 ml single dose, 50 ml multiple dose) and vial 2[4] (5 ml single dose, 50 ml multiple dose).	4020
Rx	**M.V.I.-12 Unit Vial** (Armour)	10 ml													In 10 ml two-chambered vials.[5]	4025
Rx	**M.V.C. 9 + 3 Injection** (Lyphomed)	5 ml													In 2 vial sets: Vial 1[6] (5 ml single dose and 50 ml maxi-vials) and vial 2[4] (5 ml single dose and 50 ml maxi-vials).	8760
		10 ml													In 10 ml two-chambered Vita-Gard vials.[6]	5500
Rx	**M.V.I. Pediatric Powder for Injection** (Armour)	5 ml	2,300	400	7[2]	1.2	1.4	17	5	1	1	80	20	0.14	200 mcg vitamin K. In single and multiple dose vials.[5]	8200
Rx	**M.V.C. 9 + 4 Pediatric Powder for Injection** (Lyphomed)														200 mcg vitamin K. With 375 mg mannitol. In 10 ml vials.	NA

* Cost Index based on cost per content given.
[1] After combining vials, if necessary.
[2] As dl-alpha tocopheryl acetate.
[3] With propylene glycol, polysorbate 80 and polysorbate 20.
[4] With propylene glycol.
[5] With polysorbate 20 and polysorbate 80.
[6] With propylene glycol and polysorbate 20.

MULTIVITAMINS, CAPSULES AND TABLETS

Content given per capsule or tablet.
For a comparison of the potencies of various forms of vitamin E, see p14.

	Product & Distributor	A IU	D IU	E mg	B_1 mg	B_2 mg	B_3 mg	B_5 mg	B_6 mg	B_{12} mcg	C mg	FA mg	Other Content and How Supplied	C.I.*
otc *sf*	**Multi 75 Tablets** (Fibertone)	25,000	500	150[3]	75	75	75	75	75	75	250	0.4	Ca, Fe, biotin, I, Mg, Zn, Cu, PABA, K, Mn, Cr, Se, Mo, Ge, B, Si, choline bitartrate, inosol, rutin, lemon bioflavonoid complex, hesperidin, betaine, glutamic acid HCl. Timed release. In 50s, 100s & 250s.	192
otc *sf*	**Quintabs Tablets** (Freeda)	10,000	400	25[2]	25	25	100	25	25	25	300	0.1	50 mg inositol and 30 mg PABA. In 100s, 250s and 500s.	167
otc	**Day-Vite Tablets** (Drug Industries)	10,000	1000	6.7[3]	5	5	25	10	2	2	100		In 100s and 500s.	110
otc	**Optilets-500 Filmtabs** (Abbott)	10,000	400	30[1]	15	10	100	20	5	12	500[4]		Film coated. In 100s and 120s.	278
Rx	**Al-Vite Tablets** (Drug Industries)	10,000	400	18.3[5]	20	10	100	20	6	†	200		Orange. In 100s and 500s.	310
otc *sf*	**Adavite Tablets** (Nature's Bounty)	5,500	400	30[1]	3	3.4	30	10	3	9	120	0.4	15 mcg biotin. In 100s.	135
otc	**Theravee Tablets** (Vangard)												15 mcg biotin. In UD 100s.	101
otc *sf*	**Theragenerix Tablets** (Goldline)	5,500	400	30[1]	3	3.4	30	10	3	9	120	0.4	15 mcg biotin & 2500 IU beta carotene. Red. Oval. In 130s & 1000s.	54
otc	**Therems Tablets** (Rugby)												15 mcg biotin. Red. In 130s and 1000s.	62
otc	**Theragran Tablets** (Apothecon)	5,000	400	30[1]	3	3.4	30	10	3	9	90	0.4	35 mcg biotin and 1250 IU beta carotene. Sucrose. (Theragran 842). In 30s, 100s, 180s, 1000s and UD 100s.	168

* Cost Index based on cost per capsule or tablet.
[1] As dl-alpha tocopheryl acetate.
[2] As d-alpha tocopheryl acid succinate.
sf – Sugar free.
[3] As d-alpha tocopherol acetate.
[4] As sodium ascorbate.
[5] As d-alpha tocopheryl acetate.
† ½ NF unit B_{12} with intrinsic factor concentrate.

(Continued on following page)

MULTIVITAMINS, CAPSULES AND TABLETS (Cont.)

Content given per capsule or tablet.
For a comparison of the potencies of various forms of vitamin E, see p 14.

	Product & Distributor	A IU	D IU	E mg	B_1 mg	B_2 mg	B_3 mg	B_5 mg	B_6 mg	B_{12} mcg	C mg	FA mg	Other Content and How Supplied	C.I.*
otc *sf*	**Theravim Tablets** (Nature's Bounty)	5,000	400	30[3]	3	3.4	30	10	3	9	120	0.5	2500 IU beta carotene, 15 mcg biotin. In 130s.	61
otc *sf*	**One-A-Day Plus Extra C Tablets** (Miles Inc.)	5,000	400	30	1.5	1.7	20	10	2	6	300	0.4	(One-A-Day). Orange. Capsule shape. In 60s.	173
otc *sf*	**One-A-Day Essential Tablets** (Miles Inc.)	5,000	400	30[1]	1.5	1.7	20	10	2	6	60	0.4	(One-A-Day). Brown. In 60s and 100s.	111
otc	**One-Tablet-Daily Tablets** (Various, eg, Goldline, Rexall)												In 30s, 100s, 250s, 365s & 1000s.	28+
otc	**Sesame Street Vitamins Chewable Tablets** (McNeil-CPC)			30[3]									300 mcg biotin. In 60s.	NA
otc	**Dayalets Filmtabs** (Abbott)	5,000	400	30[1]	1.5	1.7	20		2	6	60	0.4	Film coated. In 100s.	205
otc *sf*	**Vita-Bob Capsules** (Scot-Tussin)												In 100s.	98
otc	**Sigtab Tablets** (Upjohn)	5,000	400	15[1]	10.3	10	100	20	6	18	333[4]	0.4	Sucrose. In 90s and 500s.	321
otc	**Zymacap Capsules** (Upjohn)	5,000	400	15[1]	2.25	2.6	30	15	3	9	90	0.4	In 90s.	236

* Cost Index based on cost per capsule or tablet.
sf – Sugar free.
[1] As dl-alpha tocopheryl acetate.
[2] As sodium ascorbate and ascorbic acid.
[3] Form of vitamin E unknown; content given in IU.
[4] As sodium ascorbate.

(Continued on following page)

MULTIVITAMINS, CAPSULES AND TABLETS (Cont.)

Content given per capsule, tablet or wafer.
For a comparison of the potencies of various forms of vitamin E, see p. 14

	Product & Distributor	A IU	D IU	E mg	B_1 mg	B_2 mg	B_3 mg	B_5 mg	B_6 mg	B_{12} mcg	C mg	FA mg	Other Content and How Supplied	C.I.*
otc	**Unicap** (Upjohn)	5,000	400	30[1]	1.5	1.7	20		2	6	60	0.4	Tartrazine. **Capsules:** Yellow. In 90s, 120s and 240s.	133
				15[1]									**Tablets:** Yellow. In 120s.	133
otc *sf*	**Multi-Day Tablets** (Nature's Bounty)	5,000	400	30[5]	1.5	1.7	20	10	2	6	60	0.4	In 100s and 365s.	45
otc	**Unicap Jr. Chewable Tablets** (Upjohn)	5,000	400	15[1]	1.5	1.7	20		2	6	60[2]	0.4	Sucrose, mannitol. Orange flavor. In 120s.	118
otc	**Multa-Gen 12+E Capsules** (Jones Medical)	5,000	400	15[1]	2	2	20		1	3	37.5	0.2	Maroon. In 100s.	39
otc	**Vita-Kid Chewable Wafers** (Solgar)	5,000	400	8.26[3]	2	2	10		2	5	100	0.3	Orange flavor. In 50s.	NA
otc	**Halercol Capsules** (Hauck)	5,000	400	0.74[4]	1.5	2	20	1	0.1	1	37.5		In 100s.	64
otc	**Vita-Kaps Filmtabs** (Abbott)	5,000	400		3	2.5	20		1	3	50[2]		Film coated. In 100s, 480s and 1000s.	141
otc	**Hexavitamin** (Various, eg, Amide, Baxter, Lannett, Raway, Upsher-Smith, West-Ward)	5,000	400		2	3	20				75		**Capsules:** In 100s, 1000s and UD 100s.	70+
													Tablets: In 100s, 500s, 1000s and UD 100s.	40+
otc	**Hepicebrin Tablets** (Lilly)												Sucrose, sodium bisulfite. In 100s.	99
otc	**Therabid Tablets** (Mission)	5,000	200	24.8[3]	15	10	100	20	10	5	500		Green. In 60s and 1000s.	244
otc	**Chew-Vites Chewable Tablets** (Vortech)	2,500	400	15[5]	1.05	1.2	13.5		1.05	4.5	60[2]	0.3	In 100s and 1000s.	51
otc	**NeoVadrin Children's Chewable Tablets** (Mission)	2,500	400	15[1]	1.05	1.2	13.5		1.05	4.5	60[6]	0.3	Dextrose. In 100s.	55

* Cost Index based on cost per capsule, tablet or wafer.
[1] As dl-alpha tocopheryl acetate.
[2] As sodium ascorbate.
[3] As d-alpha tocopheryl acid succinate.
[4] As d-alpha tocopheryl acetate.
[5] Form of vitamin E unknown; content given in IU.
[6] As sodium ascorbate and ascorbic acid.

(Continued on following page)

MULTIVITAMINS, CAPSULES AND TABLETS (Cont.)

Content given per tablet.
For a comparison of the potencies of various forms of vitamin E, see p14.

	Product & Distributor	A IU	D IU	E mg	B_1 mg	B_2 mg	B_3 mg	B_5 mg	B_6 mg	B_{12} mcg	C mg	FA mg	Other Content and How Supplied	C.I.*
otc	**Hulk Hogan Plus Extra C Chewable Tablets** (S.G. Labs)	2,500	400	15[1]	1.05	1.2	13.5		1.05	4.5	300	0.3	Sucrose. In 60s.	NA
otc sf	**Bugs Bunny With Extra C Children's Chewable Tablets** (Miles Inc)	2,500	400	15[1]	1.05	1.2	13.5		1.05	4.5	250[4]	0.3	Sorbitol, aspartame and xylitol. Fruit flavors. In 60s.	149
otc	**Flintstones With Extra C Children's Chewable Tablets** (Miles Inc)												Sucrose, fructose. In 60s and 100s.	149
otc	**Scooby-Doo Children's Chewable Tablets Plus Extra C** (Vita-Fresh)	2,500	400	15[3]	1.05	1.2	13.5		1.05	4.5	250	0.3	In 60s.	NA
otc sf	**Bugs Bunny Children's Chewable Tablets** (Miles Inc)	2,500	400	15[3]	1.05	1.2	13.5		1.05	4.5	60[2]	0.3	Sorbitol, aspartame and xylitol. Fruit flavors. In 60s.	120
otc	**Flintstones Children's Chewable Tablets** (Miles Inc)												Sucrose. In 60s and 100s.	120
otc	**Scooby-Doo Children's Chewable Tablets** (Vita-Fresh)	2,500	400	15[3]	1.05	1.2	13.5		1.05	4.5	60	0.3	In 60s.	NA
otc	**Fruity Chews Tablets** (Goldline)	2,500	400	15[3]	1.05	1.2	13.5		1.05	4.5	60[4]	0.3	Chewable. In 100s.	164
otc	**Bounty Bears Tablets** (Nature's Bounty)	2,500	400	15[1]	1.05	1.2	13.5		1.05	4.5	60	0.3	Chewable. In 100s.	53
otc	**Poly-Vi-Sol Chewable Tablets** (Mead Johnson Nutritional)												Sucrose. Fruit flavor. In 60s and 100s.	140
otc sf	**Spider-Man Children's Chewable Vitamin Tablets** (Nature's Bounty)												Xylitol and sorbitol. In 75s and 130s.	76
otc	**Vi-Daylin Chewable Tablets** (Ross)	2,500	400	15[3]	1.05	1.2	13.5		1.05	4.5	60[4]	0.3	Sucrose. Cherry flavor. In 100s.	164
otc	**Sesame Street Vitamin Chewable Tablets** (McNeil-CPC)	2,500	400	10[1]	0.7	0.8	9	5	0.7	3	40	0.2	150 mg biotin. In 60s.	NA
otc sf	**Stress "1000" Tablets** (Nature's Bounty)			22[5]	15	15	100	20	5	12	1,000		In 60s.	NA
otc	**EPlus Tablets** (Drug Industries)			73.5[5]	5		20		2		50		In 100s and 500s.	160

* Cost Index based on cost per tablet.
sf – Sugar free.
[1] Form of vitamin E unknown; content given in IU.
[2] As sodium ascorbate.
[3] As dl-alpha tocopheryl acetate.
[4] As sodium ascorbate and ascorbic acid.
[5] As d-alpha tocopheryl acetate.

(Continued on following page)

MULTIVITAMINS, CAPSULES AND TABLETS (Cont.)

Content given per capsule or tablet.
For a comparison of the potencies of various forms of vitamin E, see p14.

	Product & Distributor	A IU	D IU	E mg	B_1 mg	B_2 mg	B_3 mg	B_5 mg	B_6 mg	B_{12} mcg	C mg	FA mg	Other Content and How Supplied	C.I.*
otc	**Allbee C-800 Tablets** (Robins)			45[1]	15	17	100	25	25	12	800		(AHR). Orange. Film coated. In 60s.	200
otc	**Vita Bee C-800 Tablets** (Rugby)												In 60s.	116
otc *sf*	**Stress Formula "605" Tablets** (Nature's Bounty)			30[2]	15	15	100	20	5	12	605	0.4	45 mcg biotin. In 60s.	111
otc	**Stress Formula Vitamins** (Various, eg, Approved Pharm, Mission, Moore, Rexall, Schein)			30[1]	15	15	100	20	5	12	600	0.4	45 mcg biotin. **Capsules:** In 100s. **Tablets:** In 60s, 100s, 250s, 300s, 400s and 600s.	99+ 118+
otc	**Stresstabs Advanced Formula Tablets** (Lederle)			30[2]	15	10	100	20	5	12	500	0.4	45 mcg biotin. In 60s.	246
Rx	**Cefol Filmtab Tablets** (Abbott)			30[2]	15	10	100	20	5	6	750	0.5	Green. Film coated. In 100s.	426

* Cost Index based on cost per capsule or tablet.
sf – Sugar free.
[1] Form of vitamin E unknown; content given in IU.
[2] As dl-alpha tocopheryl acetate.

MULTIVITAMINS, DROPS AND LIQUIDS

For a comparison of the potencies of various forms of vitamin E, see p14.

	Product & Distributor	Content Given Per	A IU	D IU	E mg	B_1 mg	B_2 mg	B_3 mg	B_5 mg	B_6 mg	B_{12} mcg	C mg	Other Content	How Supplied	C.I.*
otc sf	**LKV-Drops** (Freeda)	0.6 ml	2,500	200	5[1]	1	1	10	3	1	4	50	75 mcg biotin	In 60 ml powder and liquid.	208
otc	**Multi Vit Drops** (Barre-National)	1 ml	1,500	400	4.13[2]	0.5	0.6	8		0.4	2	35		Alcohol free. Lemon-orange flavor. In 50 ml.	112
otc sf	**Multi-Vita-Drops** (PBI)	1 ml	1,500	400	5[1]	0.5	0.6	8		0.4	2	35		Alcohol free. In 50 ml.	100
otc	**Poly-Vi-Sol Infants' Drops** (Mead Johnson Nutritional)													Fruit-like flavor. In 30 and 50 ml.	341
otc sf	**Vi-Daylin Multivitamin Drops** (Ross)	1 ml	1,500	400	4.13[2]	0.5	0.6	8		0.4	1.5	35	< 0.5% alcohol	Fruit flavor. In 50 ml.	276
otc	**Theragran Liquid** (Apothecon)	5 ml	10,000	400		10	10	100	21.4	4.1	5	200	Sugar	In 120 ml.	302
otc	**Thera Multi-vitamin Liquid** (Major)													In 120 ml.	283
otc	**Syrvite Liquid** (Various, eg, Barre-National, Dixon-Shane, Harber, Major, Moore, Schein)	5 ml	2,500	400	15[3]	1.05	1.2	13.5		1.05	4.5	60		In 240 ml, pt and gal.	80+
otc	**Vi-Daylin Multivitamin Liquid** (Ross)	5 ml	2,500	400	11[4]	1.05	1.2	13.5		1.05	4.5	60	≤ 0.5% alcohol, glucose, sucrose	Lemon/orange flavor. In 240 and 480 ml.	278
otc	**Homicebrin Liquid** (Lilly)	5 ml	2,500	400		1	1.2	10		0.8	3	60	5% alcohol, sorbitol, saccharin, glucose	In 473 ml.	228

* Cost Index based on cost per content given.
sf – Sugar free.
[1] Form of vitamin E unknown; content given in IU.
[2] As d-alpha tocopheryl acid succinate.
[3] As dl-alpha tocopheryl acetate.
[4] As d-alpha tocopheryl acetate.

MULTIVITAMINS WITH IRON

These products contain supplemental iron; hematinic products containing therapeutic amounts of iron (> 25 mg) with vitamins are listed on page 217
For a comparison of the potencies of various forms of vitamin E, see p14.
Content given per tablet.

	Product & Distributor	Fe[1] mg	A IU	D IU	E mg	B_1 mg	B_2 mg	B_3 mg	B_5 mg	B_6 mg	B_{12} mcg	C mg	FA mg	Other Content and How Supplied	C.I.*
otc *sf*	**Stress Formula "605" with Iron Tablets** (Nature's Bounty)	27			30[3]	15	15	100	20	5	12	605	0.4	45 mcg biotin. In 60s.	118
otc	**Stress Formula 500 Plus Iron Tablets** (Schein)	27			30[2]	15	10	100	20	5	12	500	400	45 mcg biotin. In 60s and 250s.	
otc *sf*	**Unicap Plus Iron Tablets** (Upjohn)	22.5	5,000	400	30[2]	1.5	1.7	20	10	2	6	60	0.4	Sucrose, Ca. In 120s.	161
otc	**Femiron Multi-Vitamins and Iron Tablets** (Beecham)	20	5,000	400	15[2]	1.5	1.7	20	10	2	6	60	0.4	In 40s and 120s.	70
otc *sf*	**Multi-Day Plus Iron Tablets** (Nature's Bounty)	18	5,000	400	15[2]	1.5	1.7	20		2	6	60	0.4	Tartrazine. In 100s and 365s.	39
otc *sf*	**Dayalets Plus Iron Filmtabs** (Abbott)	18	5,000	400	30[3]	1.5	1.7	20		2	6	60	0.4	Film coated. In 100s.	227
otc *sf*	**Theragran Jr. With Iron Chewable Tablets** (Squibb Mark)	18	5,000	400	30[3]	1.5	1.7	20		2	6	60[4]	0.4	Sorbitol. In 75s.	103
otc *sf*	**One Tablet Daily With Iron** (Various, eg, Goldline, Rexall)	18	5,000	400	30[3]	1.5	1.7	20	10	2	6	60	0.4	In 100s, 250s and 365s.	29+
otc	**Bioday with Iron Tablets** (Bioline)													Red. In 100s and 1000s.	41
otc	**Scooby-Doo Children's Chewable Plus Iron Tablets** (Vita-Fresh)	15	2,500	400	15[3]	1.05	1.2	13.5		1.05	4.5	60	0.3	Fruit flavors. In 60s.	200

* Cost Index based on cost per tablet.
sf – Sugar free.

[1] Iron content expressed in mg elemental iron.
[2] Form of vitamin E unknown; content given in IU.
[3] As dl-alpha tocopheryl acetate.
[4] As sodium ascorbate and ascorbic acid.

(Continued on following page)

MULTIVITAMINS WITH IRON (Cont.)

Note: These products contain supplemental iron; hematinic products containing therapeutic amounts of iron (> 25 mg) with vitamins are listed on page 217
For a comparison of the potencies of various forms of vitamin E, see p14. Content given per capsule, tablet, 5 ml liquid or 1 ml drops.

	Product & Distributor	Fe[1] mg	A IU	D IU	E mg	B_1 mg	B_2 mg	B_3 mg	B_5 mg	B_6 mg	B_{12} mcg	C mg	FA mg	Other Content and How Supplied	C.I.*
otc	**Bounty Bears Plus Iron Tablets** (Nature's Bounty)	15	2,500	400	15[4]	1.05	1.2	13.5		1.05	4.5	60	0.3	Chewable. In 100s.	48
otc sf	**Bugs Bunny Plus Iron Tablets** (Miles Inc.)													Chewable. Sorbitol. Fruit flavors. In 60s.	133
otc	**Flintstones Plus Iron Tablets** (Miles Inc.)													Chewable. Sucrose. In 60s and 100s.	133
otc	**Hulk Hogan Plus Iron Chewable Tablets** (S.G. Labs)													Sucrose. In 60s.	NA
otc	**PeeWee's Children's Chewable Vitamins** (Mission)													Sugar. In 100s.	NA
Rx	**Vicef Capsules** (Drug Industries)	14.4			100[4]	10		25		10	50	100	1.5	In 60s and 1000s.	260
otc	**Fruity Chews with Iron Chewable Tablets** (Goldline)	12	2,500	400	15[2]	1.05	1.2	13.5		1.05	4.5	60[3]	0.3	8 mg Zn, 0.8 mg Cu. Pink. Animal shapes. In 100s.	53
otc	**Vi-Daylin Plus Iron Tablets** (Ross)													Chewable. Sucrose. Orange flavor. In 100s.	173
otc	**Vi-Daylin Plus Iron Liquid** (Ross)	10	2,500	400	11[5]	1.05	1.2	13.5		1.05	4.5	60		< 0.5% alcohol. Lemon lime flavor. In 240 and 480 ml.	322
otc sf	**Multi-Vita Drops w/Iron** (PBI)	10	1,500	400	5[4]	0.5	0.6	8		0.4		35		In 50 ml.	100
otc	**Poly-Vi-Sol with Iron Drops** (Mead Johnson Nutritional)													In 50 ml.	132

* Cost Index based on cost per capsule, tablet, 5 ml liquid or 1 ml drops.
sf – Sugar free.

[1] Iron content expressed in mg elemental iron.
[2] As dl-alpha tocopheryl acetate.
[3] As sodium ascorbate and ascorbic acid.
[4] Form of vitamin E unknown; content given in IU.
[5] As d-alpha tocopheryl acetate.

(Continued on following page)

MULTIVITAMINS WITH IRON (Cont.)

Note: These products contain supplemental iron; hematinic products containing therapeutic amounts of iron (> 25 mg) with vitamins are listed on page 217
For a comparison of the potencies of various forms of vitamin E, see p.14 Content given per capsule or 1 ml drops.

	Product & Distributor	Fe[1] mg	A IU	D IU	E mg	B_1 mg	B_2 mg	B_3 mg	B_5 mg	B_6 mg	B_{12} mcg	C mg	FA mg	Other Content and How Supplied	C.I.*
otc *sf*	**Polyvitamin Drops with Iron** (Rugby)	10	1,500	400	5[2]	0.5	0.6	8		0.4		35		In 50 ml.	95
otc *sf*	**Vi-Daylin Multivitamin + Iron Drops** (Ross)	10	1,500	400	4.1[3]	0.5	0.6	8		0.4		35		< 0.5% alcohol. Fruit flavor. In 50 ml.	276
otc *sf*	**Tri-Vi-Sol with Iron Drops** (Mead Johnson Nutritional)	10	1,500	400								35		In 50 ml.	248
otc *sf*	**Vi-Daylin ADC Vitamins + Iron Drops** (Ross)													Fruit flavor. In 50 ml.	250
otc	**Simron Plus Capsules** (Merrell Dow)	10								1	3.33	50	0.1	Maroon. In 100s.	787

* Cost Index based on cost per capsule or 1 ml drops.
sf – Sugar free.
[1] Iron content expressed in mg elemental iron.
[2] As dl-alpha tocopheryl acetate.
[3] As d-alpha tocopheryl acid succinate.

MULTIVITAMINS WITH IRON AND OTHER MINERALS

Content given per tablet. For a comparison of the potencies of various forms of vitamin E, see p. 14

	Product & Distributor	Fe[1] mg	A IU	D IU	E mg	B_1 mg	B_2 mg	B_3 mg	B_5 mg	B_6 mg	B_{12} mcg	C mg	FA mg	Other Content	How Supplied	C.I.*
otc	**Decagen Tablets** (Goldline)	30	9,000	400	30[2]	10	10	20	20	5	10	90	0.4	Ca, Cr, Cu, I, K, Mg, Mn, Mo, P, Se, 15 mg Zn, 25 mcg vit K, 45 mcg biotin	Maroon. Film coated. Oval. In 130s.	99
otc	**Myadec Tablets** (Parke-Davis)														In 100s.	146
otc	**NeoVadrin Therapeutic M Tablets** (Mission)	27	7,500	400	30[3]	3	3.4	30	10	3	9	120	0.4	Ca, Cl, Cr, Cu, I, K, Mg, Mn, Mo, P, Se, 15 mg Zn, biotin	In 30s and 100s.	NA
otc	**Theravee-M Tablets** (Vangard)	27	5,500	400	30[3]	3	3.4	30	10	3	9	120	0.4	Ca, Cl, Cr, Cu, K, I, Mg, Mn, Mo, Se, Zn, P, 15 mcg biotin	In 100s, 1000s and UD 100s.	56
otc	**Therems-M Tablets** (Rugby)													Cl, Cr, Cu, I, K, Mg, Mn, Mo, Se, 15 mg Zn, 15 mcg biotin	In 130s and 1000s.	56
otc *sf*	**Adavite-M Tablets** (Hudson)	27	5,000	400	30[3]	3	3.4	30	10	3	9	120	0.4	Ca, Cl, Cr, Cu, I, K, Mg, Mn, Mo, P, Se, 15 mg Zn, 15 mcg biotin, 2500 IU beta carotene	In 130s.	NA
otc	**Theragenerix-M Tablets** (Goldline)	27	5,000	400	30[2]	3	3.4	30	10	3	9	120	0.4	Ca, Cl, Cr, Cu, I, K, 15 mcg biotin, Mg, Mn, Mo, P, Se, 15 mg Zn, 2500 IU beta carotene	Maroon. Film coated. Oval. In 130s and 1000s.	52
otc *sf*	**Theravim-M Tablets** (Nature's Bounty)	27	5,000	400	30[3]	3	3.4	30	10	3	9	120	0.4	Ca, Cl, Cr, Cu, I, K, Mg, Mn, Mo, P, Se, 15 mg Zn, 15 mcg biotin, 2500 IU beta carotene	In 130s.	64

* Cost Index based on cost per tablet.
sf – Sugar free.

[1] Iron content expressed in mg elemental iron.
[2] As dl-alpha tocopheryl acetate.
[3] Form of vitamin E unknown; content given in IU.

(Continued on following page)

MULTIVITAMINS WITH IRON AND OTHER MINERALS (Cont.)

Content given per tablet.
For a comparison of the potencies of various forms of vitamin E, see p14.

	Product & Distributor	Fe[1] mg	A IU	D IU	E mg	B_1 mg	B_2 mg	B_3 mg	B_5 mg	B_6 mg	B_{12} mcg	C mg	FA mg	Other Content	How Supplied	C.I.*
otc *sf*	**ABC to Z Tablets** (Nature's Bounty)	27	5,000	400	30[2]	2.25	2.6	20	10	3	9	90	0.4	Ca, Cl, Cr, Cu, I, K, Mg, Mn, Mo, P, Se, 45 mcg biotin, 25 mcg vitamin K, 15 mg Zn	In 100s.	88
otc *sf*	**Multi-Day with Calcium and Extra Iron Tablets** (Nature's Bounty)	27	5,000	400	30[3]	1.5	1.7	20	10	2	6	60	0.4	Ca	In 100s.	69
otc	**Optilets-M-500 Filmtabs** (Abbott)	20	10,000	400	30[3]	15	10	100	20	5	12	500		Cu, I, Mg, Mn, 1.5 mg Zn	Film coated. In 100s and 120s.	290
otc *sf*	**Nova-Dec Tablets** (Rugby)	20	10,000	400	30[3]	10	10	100	20	5	6	250	0.4	Cu, I, Mg, Mn, 20 mg Zn	In 130s.	63
otc *sf*	**Unicap T Tablets** (Upjohn)	18	5,000	400	30[4]	10	10	100	25	6	18	500	0.4	Tartrazine, Cu, I, K, Mn, Se, 15 mg Zn.	In 60s.	210
otc *sf*	**Unicap M Tablets** (Upjohn)	18	5,000	400	30[4]	1.5	1.7	20	10	2	6	60	0.4	Tartrazine. Ca, Cu, I, K, Mn, P, 15 mg Zn	In 120s and 500s.	133
otc	**Avail Tablets** (Beecham)	18	5,000	400	30[2]	2.25	2.55	20		3	9	90	0.4	Ca, Cr, I, Mg, Se, 22.5 mg Zn	(Avail). Peach. In 60s and 100s.	144
otc	**Centrum Jr. + Iron Tablets** (Lederle)	18	5,000	400	30[3]	1.5	1.7	20	10	2	6	60	0.4	Ca, Cr, Cu, I, Mg, Mn, Mo, P, 15 mg Zn, 45 mcg biotin, 10 mcg vitamin K	(Centrum Jr. Lederle C2). Chewable. In 60s.	192
otc *sf*	**Flintstones Complete Chewable Tablets** (Miles Inc.)													Sorbitol. Ca, Cu, I, Mg, P, 15 mg Zn, 40 mcg biotin	In 60s.	182
otc	**Sesame Street Vitamins and Minerals Chewable Tablets** (McNeil-CPC)													300 mcg biotin, 100 mg Ca, 150 mcg I, 15 mg Zn, 2 mg Cu	In 60s.	NA

* Cost Index based on cost per tablet.
sf – Sugar free.

[1] Iron content expressed in mg elemental iron.
[2] As dl-alpha tocopheryl acetate.
[3] Form of vitamin E unknown; content given in IU.
[4] As dl-alpha tocopherol acetate.

(Continued on following page)

MULTIVITAMINS WITH IRON AND OTHER MINERALS (Cont.)

Content given per tablet.
For a comparison of the potencies of various forms of vitamin E, see p14.

	Product & Distributor	Fe[1] mg	A IU	D IU	E mg	B_1 mg	B_2 mg	B_3 mg	B_5 mg	B_6 mg	B_{12} mcg	C mg	FA mg	Other Content	How Supplied	C.I.*
otc *sf*	**Daily-Vite w/Iron & Minerals Tablets** (Rugby)	18	5,000	400	30[2]	1.5	1.7	20	10	2	6	60	0.4	Ca, Cl, Cr, Cu, I, K, Mg, Mn, Mo, P, Se, 15 mg Zn, biotin, vitamin K	In 100s.	64
otc	**Hulk Hogan Complete Chewable Tablets** (S.G. Labs)													Ca, Mg, Zn, Mn, Cu, I, P, 40 mcg biotin	Sucrose. In 60s.	NA
otc	**Multi-Day Plus Minerals Tablets** (Nature's Bounty)													Ca, Cl, Cr, Cu, I, K, Mg, Mn, Mo, P, Se, Zn, 50 mcg vitamin K, 30 mcg biotin	In 100s.	73
otc	**Centrovite Jr. Tablets** (Rugby)	18	5,000	400	15[2]	1.5	1.7	20	10	2	6	60	0.4	Cu, I, Mg, Zn	In 60s.	71
otc	**Unicomplex-M Tablets** (Rugby)	18	5,000	400	15[3]	1.5	1.7	20	10	2	6	60	0.4	Ca, Cu, I, K, Mn, Zn	In 90s and 1000s.	56
otc	**Stuart Formula Tablets** (J & J-Merck)	18	5,000	400	15[3]	1.2	1.7	20		2	6	60	0.4	Ca, I, Mg, P	In 100s and 250s.	165
otc	**Gevral Tablets** (Lederle)	18	5,000		30[3]	1.5	1.7	20		2	6	60	0.4	Ca, I, Mg, P	Sucrose. (LL G1). Brown. In 100s.	175
otc *sf*	**One-A-Day Stressgard Tablets** (Miles Inc.)	18	2,500	400	30[3]	15	10	100	20	5	12	600	0.4	Cu, 15 mg Zn, 2500 IU beta carotene	(One-A-Day). In 60s.	NA
otc	**One-A-Day Maximum Formula Tablets** (Miles Inc.)	18	1,500	400	30[3]	1.5	1.7	20	10	2	6	60	0.4	Ca, Cl, Cr, Cu, I, K, Mg, Mn, Mo, P, Se, 15 mg Zn, 30 mcg biotin, 5,000 IU beta carotene	In 30s, 60s and 100s.	187
otc *sf*	**Quintabs-M Tablets** (Freeda)	15	10,000	400	50[2]	30	30	150	30	30	30	300	0.4	Ca, Cu, K, Mg, Mn, Se, Zn, PABA	In 100s, 250s and 500s.	153

* Cost Index based on cost per tablet.
sf – Sugar free.
[1] Iron content expressed in mg elemental iron.
[2] Form of vitamin E unknown; content given in IU.
[3] As dl-alpha tocopheryl acetate.

(Continued on following page)

MULTIVITAMINS WITH IRON AND OTHER MINERALS (Cont.)

Content given per capsule or tablet.
For a comparison of the potencies of various forms of vitamin E, see p14.

	Product & Distributor	Fe[1] mg	A IU	D IU	E mg	B_1 mg	B_2 mg	B_3 mg	B_5 mg	B_6 mg	B_{12} mcg	C mg	FA mg	Other Content	How Supplied	C.I.*
otc	**Generix-T Tablets** (Goldline)	15	10,000	400	5.5[2]	15	10	100	10	2	7.5	150		Cu, I, Mg, Mn, 1.5 mg Zn	Orange. Oval. In 100s and 1000s.	102
otc	**Mi-Cebrin T Tablets** (Dista)														Sucrose. (Dista C20). In 30s, 100s, 1000s & UD 100s.	352
otc	**Multilex-T & M Tablets** (Rugby)	15	10,000	400	5.5[3]	15	10	100	10	2	7.5	150		Cu, I, Mg, Mn, Zn	In 100s and 1000s.	70
otc	**Mi-Cebrin Tablets** (Dista)	15	10,000	400	5.5[2]	10	5	30	10	1.7	3	100		Cu, I, Mg, Mn, 1.5 mg Zn	Sucrose. (Dista C19). In 60s, 100s & UD 100s.	245
otc	**Multilex Tablets** (Rugby)														In 100s.	53
otc	**Vitarex Tablets** (Pasadena)	15	10,000	200	15[2]	15	10	100	20	5	5	250		Ca, Cu, I, K, Mg, Mn, P, Zn	In 100s.	136
otc	**Fosfree Tablets** (Mission)	14.5	1,500	150		5	2	10	1	3	2	50		Ca	Pink. In 60s and 120s.	227
otc	**Mevanin-C Capsules** (Beutlich)	14	3,000	300		2	2	5		0.5	1	200	0.1	Ca, Cu, I, K, Mg, Mn, 0.42 mg Zn, hesperidin complex	Red and white. In 90s and 450s.	253
otc	**Vita-Plus H Softgels** (Scot-Tussin)	13.4	5,000	400	3[3]	3	2.5	20	5	1.5	2.5	50		Ca, K, Mg, Mn, P, 1.4 mg Zn	In 50s.	NA
otc	**Thera-M Tablets** (Various, eg, Dixon-Shane, Major, Med-Corp, Raway)	12	10,000	400	15[2]	10.3	10	100	18.4	4.1	5	200		Cu, I, Mg, Mn, 1.5 mg Zn	In 100s, 250s, 1000s and UD 100s.	46+
otc	**Circavite-T Tablets** (Circle)	12	10,000	400	15[3]	10.3	10	100	18.4	4.1	5	200		Cu, I, Mg, Mn, 1.5 mg Zn	Maroon. In 100s.	100

* Cost Index based on cost per capsule or tablet.
[1] Iron content expressed in mg elemental iron.
[2] Form of vitamin E unknown; content given in IU.
[3] As dl-alpha tocopheryl acetate.

(Continued on following page)

MULTIVITAMINS WITH IRON AND OTHER MINERALS (Cont.)

Content given per capsule, tablet or 15 ml liquid. For a comparison of the potencies of various forms of vitamin E, see p14.

	Product & Distributor	Fe[1] mg	A IU	D IU	E mg	B_1 mg	B_2 mg	B_3 mg	B_5 mg	B_6 mg	B_{12} mcg	C mg	FA mg	Other Content	How Supplied	C.I.*
otc	**Poly-Vi-Sol w/Iron Chewable Tablets** (Mead-J)	12	2,500	400	15[3]	1.05	1.2	13.5		1.05	4.5	60	0.3	Cu, 8 mg Zn	In 100s and Circus Shape 60s and 100s.	166
otc	**Vi-Daylin Multivitamins + Iron Chewable Tabs** (Ross)	12	2,500	400	15[2]	1.05	1.2	13.5		1.05	4.5	60	0.3	Sucrose	Orange flavor. In 100s.	187
otc	**Unicomplex T & M Tablets** (Rugby)	10	5,000	400	15[3]	10	10	100	20	2	4	300	0.4	Ca, Cu, I, K, Mg, Mn	In 60s.	98
otc	**VitaKaps-M Tabs** (Abbott)	10	5,000	400		3	2.5	20		1	3	50		Cu, I, Mn, 7.5 mg Zn	Film coated. In 100s.	185
otc sf	**Unicap Senior Tablets** (Upjohn)	10	5,000	200	15[2]	1.2	1.4	16	10	2.2	3	60	0.4	Ca, Cu, I, K, Mg, Mn, P, 15 mg Zn	In 120s.	136
otc	**Sesame Street Vitamins and Minerals Chewable Tablets** (McNeil-CPC)	10	2,500	400	10[5]	0.7	0.8	9	5	0.7	3	40	0.2	150 mcg biotin, 80 mg Ca, 70 mcg I, 8 mg Zn, 1 mg Cu	In 60s.	NA
otc	**Advanced Formula Centrum Liquid** (Lederle)	9	2,500	400	30[5]	1.5	1.7	20	10	2	6	60		300 mcg biotin, I, Zn, Mn, Cr, Mo, 6.6% alcohol	In 236 ml.	NA
otc sf	**Hi-Po-Vites Tablets** (Hudson)	5.8	10,000	400	10.3[3]	25	25	50	12.5	15	50	150	0.4	Ca, Cu, I, Mg, Mn, P, Zn, biotin, PABA, choline bitartrate, betaine, inositol, desiccated liver	In 100s.	198
otc sf	**Ultra Vita Time Tablets** (Nature's Bounty)														With rutin, bioflavonoids, bone meal and lecithin. In 50s and 100s.	167
otc	**Sunshine Chewable Tablets** (Fibertone)	5	5,000	400	67[5]	15	15	25	20	15	15	150	0.1	Ca, Cu, Mn, Zn, K iodide, biotin, betaine, PABA, choline bitartrate, inositol, hesperidin	With rutin, bioflavonoids and lecithin. Citrus flavor. In 60s.	NA
otc sf	**Vitalets Tablets** (Freeda)	3.3	5,000	400	5[5]	2.5	0.9	20	3	2	5	60		25 mcg biotin, Mn, Ca	Chewable. In 100s & 250s.	109
Rx	**Eldec Kapseals** (P-D)	3.3	1,667		10[4]	10	0.9	17	10	0.7	2	67	0.3	Ca, I	(P-D 337). In 100s.	368

* Cost Index based on cost per capsule or tablet.
sf – Sugar free.
[1] Iron content expressed in mg elemental iron.
[2] As dl-alpha tocopherol acetate.
[3] As d-alpha tocopheryl acid succinate.
[4] As dl-alpha tocopheryl acetate.
[5] Form of vitamin E unknown; content given in IU.

MULTIVITAMINS WITH FLUORIDE, CAPSULES AND TABLETS

Used for prophylaxis of vitamin deficiencies and as an aid in the prevention of dental caries in infants and children where the fluoride content of the drinking water does not exceed 0.7 ppm. For complete prescribing information on fluoride-containing products, refer to page 37

Content given per capsule or tablet.

For a comparison of the potencies of various forms of vitamin E, see p. 14

	Product & Distributor	F[1] mg	A IU	D IU	E mg	B_1 mg	B_2 mg	B_3 mg	B_5 mg	B_6 mg	B_{12} mcg	C mg	FA mg	Other Content and How Supplied	C.I.*
Rx	**Adeflor M Tablets** (Upjohn)	1	6,000	400		1.5	2.5	20	10	10	2	100		250 mg Ca, 30 mg Fe. Sorbitol, sucrose. Pink, elliptical. In 100s.	320
Rx	**Natabec with Fluoride Capsules** (Parke-Davis)	1	4,000	400		3	2	10		3	5	50		240 mg Ca, 30 mg Fe. (P-D 534). In 100s.	283
Rx	**Adeflor Chewable Tablets** (Upjohn)	1	4,000	400		2	2	18	5	1	2	75		Saccharin, sorbitol. (Adeflor Chewable 1.0). Light purple. Raspberry flavor. In 100s.	237
Rx	**Mulvidren-F Softab Tablets** (Stuart)	1	4,000	400		1.6	2	10	2.8	1	3	75		Saccharin. Chewable. (Stuart 710). Orange, scored. In 100s.	223
Rx	**Florvite Tablets** (Everett)	1	2,500	400	15[2]	1.05	1.2	13.5		1.05	4.5	60	0.3	Chewable. Sucrose. In 100s and 1000s.	160
Rx	**Florvite + Iron Tablets** (Everett)													Sucrose. 12 mg Fe, Cu, 10 mg Zn. Chewable. Grape flavor. In 100s.	165
Rx	**Poly-Vi-Flor Chewable Tablets 1.0 mg** (Mead Johnson Nutritional)													Sucrose. In 100s and 1000s.	210
Rx	**Poly-Vi-Flor with Iron 1.0 mg Chewable Tablets** (Mead Johnson Nutritional)													Cu, 12 mg Fe, 10 mg Zn. In 100s and 1000s.	219
Rx	**Soluvite C.T. Tablets** (Pharmics)													Chewable. In 100s.	NA
Rx	**Poly Vitamins w/Fluoride Tablets** (Various, eg, Rugby, Schein)	1	2,500	400	15[4]	1.05	1.2	13.5		1.05	4.5	60	0.3	In 100s and 1000s.	66+
Rx	**Polytabs-F Tablets** (Major)	1	2,500	400	15[2]	1.05	1.2	13.5		1.05	4.5	60[3]	0.3	Chewable. In 100s and 1000s.	60
Rx	**Vi-Daylin/F Chewable Tablets** (Ross)													Sucrose. Cherry flavor. In 100s.	204

* Cost Index based on cost per capsule or tablet.
[1] Fluoride content expressed in mg elemental fluoride.
[2] As dl-alpha tocopheryl acetate.
[3] As ascorbic acid and sodium ascorbate.
[4] Form of vitamin E unknown; content given in IU.

(Continued on following page)

MULTIVITAMINS WITH FLUORIDE, CAPSULES AND TABLETS (Cont.)

Content given per tablet.
For a comparison of the potencies of various forms of vitamin E, see p 14

	Product & Distributor	F[1] mg	A IU	D IU	E mg	B_1 mg	B_2 mg	B_3 mg	B_5 mg	B_6 mg	B_{12} mcg	C mg	FA mg	Other Content and How Supplied	C.I.*
Rx	**PolyVitamin w/Iron Fluoride Tablets** (Rugby)	1	2,500	400	15[2]	1.05	1.2	13.5		1.05	4.5	60	0.3	12 mg Fe. In 100s and 1000s.	68
Rx	**Vi-Daylin/F + Iron Chewable Tablets** (Ross)	1	2,500	400	15[3]	1.05	1.2	13.5		1.05	4.5	60	0.3	12 mg Fe. Sucrose. Pink. Cherry flavor. In 100s.	183
Rx	**Tri-Vi-Flor 1.0 mg Tablets** (Mead Johnson Nutritional)	1	2,500	400								60		Sucrose. Chewable. In 100s and 1000s.	190
Rx	**Triple Vitamins with Fluoride Chewable Tablets** (Major)													In 100s.	NA
Rx *sf*	**O-Cal f.a. Tablets** (Pharmics)	0.5	5000	400	30[2]	3	3	20		4	12	90	1	200 mg Ca, 100 mg Mg, 66 mg Fe, 150 mcg I, 2 mg Cu and 15 mg Zn. Dye free. In 500s	
Rx	**Adeflor Chewable Tablets** (Upjohn)	0.5	4,000	400		2	2	18	5	1	2	75		Saccharin, sorbitol. (Adeflor Chewable 0.5). Pink. Cherry flavor. In 100s.	237
Rx	**Florvite Tablets Half Strength** (Everett)	0.5	2,500	400	15[3]	1.05	1.2	13.5		1.05	4.5	60	0.3	Sucrose. Chewable. In 100s.	160
Rx	**Poly-Vi-Flor Chewable Tablets 0.5 mg** (Mead Johnson Nutritional)													Sucrose. In 100s.	210
Rx	**Poly-Vi-Flor w/Iron 0.5 mg Chewable Tablets** (Mead Johnson Nutritional)													Cu, 12 mg Fe, 10 mg Zn. Sucrose. In 100s.	219
Rx	**Poly Vitamins w/Fluoride Tablets** (Various, eg, Goldline, Rugby)	0.5	2,500	400	15[2]	1.05	1.2	13.5		1.05	4.5	60	0.3	In 100s and 1000s.	54+
Rx	**Cari-Tab Tablets** (Jones Medical)	0.5	2,000	200								75		Chewable. (Cari). Red, scored. Raspberry flavor. In 100s.	217
Rx	**Poly-Vi-Flor Chewable Tablets 0.25 mg** (Mead Johnson)	0.25	2,500	400	15[3]	1.05	1.2	13.5		1.05	4.5	60	0.3	In 100s.	210

* Cost Index based on cost per tablet. *sf* – Sugar free.
[1] Fluoride content expressed in mg elemental fluoride.
[2] Form of vitamin E unknown; content given in IU.
[3] As dl-alpha tocopheryl acetate.

MULTIVITAMINS WITH FLUORIDE DROPS

For a comparison of the potencies of various forms of vitamin E, see p14.

	Product & Distributor	Content Given Per	F[1] mg	A IU	D IU	E mg	B_1 mg	B_2 mg	B_3 mg	B_5 mg	B_6 mg	B_{12} mcg	C mg	Other Content and How Supplied	C.I.*
Rx	**Adeflor Drops** (Upjohn)	0.6 ml	0.5	2,000	400						1		50	Saccharin. In 50 ml.	260
Rx	**Florvite Drops** (Everett)	1 ml	0.5	1,500	400	5[3]	0.5	0.6	8		0.4	2	35	In 50 ml.	245
Rx *sf*	**Multi-Vita-Drops w/Fluoride** (PBI)	1 ml	0.5	1,500	400	5[3]	0.5	0.6	8		0.4	2	35	Alcohol free. In 50 ml.	100
Rx	**Polyvitamin w/Fluoride Drops** (Rugby)													In 50 ml.	105
Rx *sf*	**Polyvite with Fluoride Drops** (Geneva)													Alcohol free. Pineapple flavor. In 50 ml.	94
Rx	**Poly-Vi-Flor 0.5 mg Drops** (Mead Johnson Nutritional)	1 ml	0.5	1,500	400	5[2]	0.5	0.6	8		0.4	2	35	In 50 ml.	315
Rx	**Multivitamin with Fluoride Drops** (Major)	1 ml	0.5	1,500	400	4.1[4]	0.5	0.6	8		0.4	2	35	In 50 ml.	106
Rx	**Poly-Vi-Flor with Iron 0.5 mg Drops** (Mead Johnson Nutritional)	1 ml	0.5	1,500	400	4.1[4]	0.5	0.6	8		0.4		35	10 mg Fe.[5] In 50 ml.	315
Rx	**ADC with Fluoride Drops** (Major)	1 ml	0.5	1,500	400								35	In 50 ml.	126
Rx *sf*	**Triple-Vita-Flor Drops** (PBI)													Alcohol free, cherry flavor. In 50 ml.	100
Rx *sf*	**Triplevite with Fluoride Drops** (Geneva)													Alcohol free. Cherry flavor. In 50 ml.	103
Rx	**Tri-Vi-Flor 0.5 mg Drops** (Mead Johnson Nutritional)													In 50 ml.	287
Rx	**Tri-Vitamin w/Fluoride Drops** (Rugby)													In 50 ml.	88
Rx	**Tri Vit w/Fluoride Drops** (Barre)													In 50 ml.	NA

* Cost Index based on cost per content listed.
sf – Sugar free.
[1] Fluoride content expressed in mg elemental fluoride.
[2] Form of vitamin E unknown; content given in IU.
[3] As dl-alpha tocopheryl acetate.
[4] As d-alpha tocopheryl acid succinate.
[5] Iron content expressed in mg elemental iron.

(Continued on following page)

MULTIVITAMINS WITH FLUORIDE DROPS (Cont.)

For a comparison of the potencies of various forms of vitamin E, see p14.

	Product & Distributor	Content Given Per	F[1] mg	A IU	D IU	E mg	B_1 mg	B_2 mg	B_3 mg	B_5 mg	B_6 mg	B_{12} mcg	C mg	Other Content and How Supplied	C.I.*
Rx	**Poly-Vi-Flor 0.25 mg Drops** (Mead Johnson Nutritional)	1 ml	0.25	1,500	400	5[5]	0.5	0.6	8		0.4	2	35	In 50 ml.	314
Rx	**Polyvite with Fluoride Drops** (Geneva)													Pineapple flavor. In 50 ml.	106
Rx	**Multi-Vita-Drops w/Fluoride** (PBI)													Alcohol free. In 50 ml.	116
Rx	**Florvite Drops** (Everett)	1 ml	0.25	1,500	400	5[2]	0.5	0.6	8		0.4	2	35	In 50 ml.	254
Rx	**Multivitamin and Fluoride Drops** (Major)													In 50 ml.	138
Rx	**Florvite + Iron Drops** (Everett)	1 ml	0.25	1,500	400	5[5]	0.5	0.6	8		0.4		35	10 mg Fe.[3] In 50 ml.	254
Rx	**Poly-Vi-Flor with Iron 0.25 mg Drops** (Mead Johnson Nutritional)	1 ml	0.25	1,500	400	3.3[4]	0.5	0.6	8		0.4		35	10 mg Fe.[3] In 50 ml.	314
Rx *sf*	**Vi-Daylin/F Drops** (Ross)	1 ml	0.25	1,500	400	4.1[4]	0.5	0.6	8		0.4		35	< 0.1% alcohol. Fruit flavor. In 50 ml.	310
Rx *sf*	**Vi-Daylin/F + Iron Drops** (Ross)													10 mg Fe.[3] < 0.1% alcohol. Fruit flavor. In 50 ml.	309
Rx	**Triple-Vita-Flor Drops** (PBI)	1 ml	0.25	1,500	400								35	Alcohol free. In 50 ml.	100
Rx	**Triplevite with Fluoride Drops** (Geneva)													Alcohol free. In 50 ml.	160
Rx	**Tri-Vi-Flor 0.25 mg Drops** (Mead Johnson Nutritional)													In 50 ml.	284
Rx *sf*	**Vi-Daylin/F ADC Drops** (Ross)													0.3% alcohol. Fruit flavor. In 50 ml.	283
Rx	**Tri-Vi-Flor 0.25 mg with Iron Drops** (Mead Johnson Nutritional)	1 ml	0.25	1,500	400								35	10 mg Fe.[3] In 50 ml.	286
Rx *sf*	**Vi-Daylin/F ADC + Iron Drops** (Ross)													10 mg Fe.[3] Fruit flavor. In 50 ml.	283
Rx	**Tri Vit w/Fluoride Drops** (Barre)													In 50 ml.	NA

* Cost Index based on cost per content listed.
[1] Fluoride content expressed in mg elemental fluoride.
[2] As dl-alpha tocopheryl acetate.
sf – Sugar free.
[3] Iron content expressed in mg elemental iron.
[4] As d-alpha tocopheryl acid succinate.
[5] Form of vitamin E unknown; content given in IU.

MULTIVITAMINS WITH CALCIUM AND IRON

Content given per tablet.
For a comparison of the potencies of various forms of vitamin E, see p14.

	Product & Distributor	Ca[1] mg	Fe[1] mg	A IU	D IU	E mg	B_1 mg	B_2 mg	B_3 mg	B_5 mg	B_6 mg	B_{12} mcg	C mg	FA mg	Other Content	How Supplied	C.I.*
otc sf	**One-A-Day Within Tablets** (Miles Inc)	450	27	5,000	400	30[3]	1.5	1.7	20	10	2	6	60	0.4	15 mg Zn, tartrazine	In 60s and 100s.	131
Rx	**Natafort Filmseal Tablets** (Parke-Davis)	350	65	6,000	400	30[2]	3	2	20		15	6	120	1	I, Mg, 25 mg Zn	(P-D 282). Film coated. In 100s.	325
otc sf	**K.P.N. Tablets** (Freeda)	333	11	2,666	133	10[3]	2	2	10	3.3	0.83	2	33	0.13	I, Cu, Mn, K, Mg, 0.03 mg Zn	In 100s, 250s and 500s.	99
otc	**Engran-HP Tablets** (Squibb)	325	9	4,000	200	15[2]	0.85	1	10		1.25	4	30	0.4	I, Mg, tartrazine, sugar	In 100s.	290
Rx	**Zenate Prenatal Tablets** (Solvay Pharm.)	300	65	5,000	400	30[2]	3	3	20		10	12	80	1	I, Mg, 20 mg Zn	(RR 1146). Blue. Capsule shape. Film coated. In 100s.	289
Rx	**Filibon Forte Tablets** (Lederle)	300	45	8,000	400	45[2]	2	2.5	30		3	12	90	1	I, Mg, sucrose	(LL F6). Pink, scored. Film coated. Capsule shape. In 100s.	305
Rx	**Par-F Tablets** (Pharmics)	250	60	5,000	400	30	3	3.4	20	10	12	12	120	1	I, Cu, Mg, 15 mg Zn	In 100s.	NA
Rx	**Prenate 90 Tablets** (Bock)	250	90	4,000	400	30[3]	3	3.4	20		20	12	120	1	DSS, Cu, I, 25 mg Zn	(PN/90). White. Film coated. Oval. In 100s.	260
Rx	**Natacomp-FA Tablets** (Trimen)	250	60	8,000	400	30[3]	3	3.4	20	10	12	12	120	1	Cu, I, Mg, 15 mg Zn	(Trimen). Pink. Film coated. Oval. In 100s.	220
Rx	**Materna Tablets** (Lederle)	250	60	5,000	400	30[2]	3	3.4	20	10	10	12	100	1	Cr, Cu, I, Mg, Mn, Mo, 25 mg Zn, 30 mcg biotin, sucrose	(Materna M40). Off-white, scored. Film coated. Capsule shape. In 100s.	284
Rx	**Mynatal Capsules** (ME Pharm)		65	5,000	400	30	3	3.4	20	10	10	12	120	1	30 mcg biotin, Ca, Cr, Cu, I, Mg, Mn, Mo, 25 mg Zn	In 100s and 500s.	NA

* Cost Index based on cost per tablet

sf – Sugar free.

[1] Calcium and iron content expressed in mg elemental calcium and iron.

[2] As dl-alpha tocopheryl acetate.

[3] Form of vitamin E unknown; content given in IU.

(Continued on following page)

MULTIVITAMINS WITH CALCIUM AND IRON (Cont.)

Content given per capsule or tablet.
For a comparison of the potencies of various forms of vitamin E, see p14.

	Product & Distributor	Ca[1] mg	Fe[1] mg	A IU	D IU	E mg	B_1 mg	B_2 mg	B_3 mg	B_5 mg	B_6 mg	B_{12} mcg	C mg	FA mg	Other Content	How Supplied	C.I.*
Rx	**Secran Prenatal Tablets** (Scherer)	250	60	8,000	400	30[2]	1.7	2	20		2.5	8	60	1	Mg, 20 mg Zn	In 100s and 240s.	118
Rx	**Niferex-PN Forte Tablets** (Central)	250	60	5,000	400	30[3]	3	3.4	20		4	12	80	1	Cu, I, Mg, 25 mg Zn	(Central 1/0). White, scored. Film coated. Capsule shape. In 100s.	268
Rx	**Pramet FA Filmtabs** (Ross)	250	60	4,000	400		3	2	10	0.9	5	3	100	1	Cu, I	Controlled release. (147). Blue. Film coated. In 100s.	312
Rx	**Filibon F.A. Tablets** (Lederle)	250	45	8,000	400	30[3]	1.7	2	20		4	8	60	1	I, Mg, Sucrose	(LL F5). Pink, scored. Film coated. Capsule shape. In 100s.	280
Rx	**Pramilet FA Filmtabs** (Ross)	250	40	4,000	400		3	2	10	1	3	3	60	1	Cu, I, Mg, 0.085 mg Zn	(121). Pink. Film coated. In 100s.	278
otc	**En-Cebrin Pulvules (Capsules)** (Lilly)	250	30	4,000	400		3	2	10	5	1.7	5	50		Cu, I, Mg, Mn, 1.5 mg Zn	In 100s.	231
otc	**Os-Cal Plus Tablets** (Marion Merrell Dow)	250	16.6	1,666	125		0.5	0.66	3.3		0.5		33		Mn, 0.75 mg Zn	In 100s.	203
otc	**Os-Cal Fortified Tablets** (Marion Merrell Dow)	250	5	1,668	125	0.7[4]	1.7	1.7	15		2		50		Mg, Mn, 0.5 mg Zn	In 100s.	203
Rx	**Natabec Rx Kapseals** (Parke-Davis)	240	30	4,000	400		3	2	10		3	5	50	1		(P-D 547). Blue with pink band. In 100s.	282
otc	**Natabec FA Kapseals** (Parke-Davis)	240	30	4,000	400		3	2	10		3	5	50	0.1	Mg	(P-D 541). Pink with white band. In 100s.	260
otc	**Natabec Kapseals** (Parke-Davis)	240	30	4,000	400		3	2	10		3	5	50		Mg	(P-D 390). Pink with blue band. In 100s.	260

* Cost Index based on cost per capsule or tablet.
[1] Calcium and iron content expressed in mg elemental calcium and iron.
[2] Form of vitamin E unknown; content given in IU.
[3] As dl-alpha tocopheryl acetate.
[4] As dl-alpha tocopherol acetate.

(Continued on following page)

MULTIVITAMINS WITH CALCIUM AND IRON (Cont.)

Content given per tablet.
For a comparison of the potencies of various forms of vitamin E, see p14.

	Product & Distributor	Ca[1] mg	Fe[1] mg	A IU	D IU	E mg	B_1 mg	B_2 mg	B_3 mg	B_5 mg	B_6 mg	B_{12} mcg	C mg	FA mg	Other Content	How Supplied	C.I.*
Rx *sf*	**o-cal f.a. Tablets** (Pharmics)	200	66	5,000	400	30[2]	3	3	20		4	12	90	1	0.5 mg F, 100 mg Mg, 150 mcg I, 2 mg Cu, 15 mg Zn	Dye free. In 500s.	NA
Rx	**Adequate M Improved Tablets** (Ortega)	200	65	8,000	400	30[3]	2.55	3	20		10	12	90	1	I, Mg, 25 mg Zn	In 100s.	150
Rx	**Par-Natal Plus 1 Improved Tablets** (Parmed)	200	65	4,000	400	11[4]	1.5	3	20		10	12	120	1	Cu, 25 mg Zn	In 100s and 500s.	136
Rx	**Stuartnatal 1 + 1 Tablets** (Stuart)	200	65	4,000	400	11[4]	1.5	3	20		10	12	120	1	Cu, 25 mg Zn	(Stuart 021). Yellow. In 100s & 500s.	290
Rx	**Lactocal-F Tablets** (Laser)	200	65	4,000	400	30[3]	3	3.4	20		5	12	100	1	Cu, I, Mg, 15 mg Zn	White. In 100s.	217
Rx	**Prenatal-1 + Iron Tablets** (Major)	200	65	4,000	400	11[4]	1.5	3	20		10	12	120	1	Cu, 25 mg Zn	In 100s and 500s.	119
Rx	**Natalins Rx Tablets** (Mead Johnson Labs)	200	60	4,000	400	15[3]	1.5	1.6	17	7	4	2.5	80	1	Cu, Mg, 25 mg Zn, 0.03 mg biotin	In 100s and 1000s.	322
Rx	**Norlac Rx Tablets** (Solvay Pharm.)	200	60	8,000	400	30[3]	2	2	20		4	8	90	1	Cu, I, Mg, 15 mg Zn	(Rowell 1611). Peach. In 100s.	306
otc	**Prenatal w/Folic Acid Tablets** (Geneva)	200	60	8,000	400	30[3]	1.7	2	20		4	8	60	0.8	I, Mg	Pink. Oblong. In 100s.	112
otc *sf*	**Prenavite Tablets** (Rugby)	200	60	8,000	400	30[2]	1.7	2	20		4	8	60	0.8	I, Mg	In 100s and 500s.	73
otc	**Prenatal-S Tabs** (Goldline)	200	60	4,000	400	11[5]	1.5	1.7	18		2.6	4	100	0.8	25 mg Zn	Pink. In 100s & 1000s.	65
otc	**Stuart Prenatal Tabs** (Stuart)	200	60	4,000	400	11[5]	1.5	1.7	18		2.6	4	100	0.8	25 mg Zn	(Stuart 071). In 100s.	286
otc	**Natalins Tablets** (Mead Johnson Nutritional)	200	45	5,000	400	30[5]	1.7	2	20		4	8	90	0.8	I, Mg	(MJ). Film coated. In 100s and 1000s.	286

* Cost Index based on cost per tablet.
sf – Sugar free.
[1] Calcium and iron content expressed in mg elemental calcium and iron.
[2] Form of vitamin E unknown; content given in IU.
[3] As dl-alpha tocopheryl acetate; content given in IU.
[4] Form of vitamin E unknown.
[5] As dl-alpha tocopheryl acetate.

(Continued on following page)

MULTIVITAMINS WITH CALCIUM AND IRON (Cont.)

Content given per capsule or tablet. For a comparison of the potencies of various forms of vitamin E, see p. 14

	Product & Distributor	Ca[1] mg	Fe[1] mg	A IU	D IU	E mg	B_1 mg	B_2 mg	B_3 mg	B_5 mg	B_6 mg	B_{12} mcg	C mg	FA mg	Other Content	How Supplied	C.I.*
otc	**Nestabs Tablets** (Fielding)	200	36	8,000	400	30[3]	3	3	20		3	8	120	0.8	I, 15 mg Zn	Pink. In 100s.	150
Rx	**Nestabs FA Tablets** (Fielding)	200	36	5,000	400	30[3]	3	3	20		3	8	120	1	I, 15 mg Zn	In 100s.	225
otc	**Nutricon Tablets** (Pasadena)	200	20	2,500	200	11[4]	1.5	1.5	10	5	2	5	50	0.4	Cu, I, Mg, 3.75 mg Zn, 0.6 mg biotin	In 120s.	91
Rx	**Mission Prenatal Rx Tablets** (Mission)	175	60	8,000	400		4	2	20	10	20	8	240	1	Cu, I, 15 mg Zn	Pink. Film coated. In 100s.	240
otc	**Nutrex Tablets** (Abana)	162	27	5,000	400	30[2]	2.25	2.6	20	10	3	9	90	0.4	Cl, Cr, Cu, I, K, Mg, Mn, Mo, P, Se, 15 mg Zn, 45 mcg biotin, 25 mcg vitamin K	In 100s.	175
otc	**Centrum Jr. + Extra Calcium Chewable Tablets** (Lederle)	160	18	5,000	400	30[3]	1.5	1.7	20	10	2	6	60	0.4	Cr, Cu, I, Mg, Mn, Mo, P, 15 mg Zn, 10 mcg vit K, 45 mcg biotin	(Centrum Jr LL C60). Scored. Cherry flavor. In 60s.	149
otc	**Calcet Plus Tabs** (Mission)	152.8	18	5,000	400	30[3]	2.25	2.55	30	15	3	9	500	0.8	15 mg Zn	In 60s.	262
otc	**Chromagen OB Capsules** (Savage)	125	33	4,000	200	15[3]	1.5	1.7	10		5	6	75	0.4	Cu, DSS, I, Mg, 12.5 mg Zn	Maroon. In 100s.	139
otc	**Filibon Tablets** (Lederle)	125	18	5,000	400	30[3]	1.5	1.7	20		2	6	60	0.4	I, Mg	(LL F4). Pink. Film coated. Capsule shape. In 100s and 120s.	222
otc	**Centrum Jr. + Extra C Chewable Tablets** (Lederle)	108	18	5,000	400	30[4]	1.5	1.7	20	10	2	6	300	0.4	Cr, Cu, I, Mg, Mn, Mo, P, 15 mg Zn, 10 mcg vitamin K and 45 mcg biotin	(Centrum Jr Extra C LL C39). Scored. In 60s.	149

* Cost Index based on cost per capsule or tablet.
[1] Calcium and iron content expressed in mg of elemental calcium and iron.
[2] As dl-alpha tocopheryl acetate.
[3] Form of vitamin E unknown; content given in IU.
[4] As d-alpha tocopheryl acetate.

(Continued on following page)

MULTIVITAMINS WITH CALCIUM AND IRON (Cont.)

Content given per capsule or tablet. For a comparison of the potencies of various forms of vitamin E, see p14.

	Product & Distributor	Ca[1] mg	Fe[1] mg	A IU	D IU	E mg	B_1 mg	B_2 mg	B_3 mg	B_5 mg	B_6 mg	B_{12} mcg	C mg	FA mg	Other Content	How Supplied	C.I.*
otc sf	**Bugs Bunny Vitamins and Minerals Chewable Tablets** (Miles Inc.)	100	18	5,000	400	30[4]	1.5	1.7	20	10	2	6	60	0.4	Cu, I, Mg, P, 15 mg Zn, 40 mcg biotin	Fruit flavor. In 60s.	182
Rx	**Pre-H Cal Tablets** (T.E. Williams)	95	51.5	4,000	400		3	3		3	5	2.5	50	0.5	Cu	(Pre-H-Cal). Pink, scored. Film coated. Oval. In 60s.	328
otc	**Gynovite Plus Tablets** (Optimox)	83	3	833	67	55[2]	1.7	1.7	3.3	1.7	3.3	21	30	0.067	Boron, betaine, biotin, Cr, Cu, hesperidin, I, inositol, Mg, Mn, PABA, pancreatin, rutin, Se, 2.5 mg Zn	In 180s.	200
otc sf	**Nature's Bounty 1 Tablets** (Nature's Bounty)	50	10	10,000	400	30[4]	25	25	50	50	50	50	250	0.4	50 mcg biotin, choline, inositol, PABA, P, I, Cr, Mg, 15 mg Zn, Mn, Se, Cu, K, Cl, Mo	Timed release. In 30s and 60s.	192
otc	**Soft-Stress Capsules** (Marlyn)	50	4.5	6,250	100	50[4]	6.25	6.25	6.25	6.25	6.25	6.25	125	0.05	Choline, Cr, Cu, K, Mg, P, PABA, Se, 6.25 mcg biotin, octacosanol, inositol, lecithin, 3.75 mg Zn	In 30 paks of 4.	433
otc	**Theragran-M Tablets** (Apothecon)	40	27	5,000	400	30[3]	3	3.4	30	10	3	9	90	0.4	Cl, Cr, Cu, I, K, Mg, Mn, Mo, P, Se, 15 mg Zn, 35 mcg biotin, 1,250 IU beta carotene	(Squibb 849). Film coated. In 100s and 180s.	224
otc	**Scooby-Doo Children's Complete Formula Tablets** (Vita-Fresh)	25	18	5,000	400	30[3]	1.5	1.7	20	10	2	6	60	0.4	Cu, I, Mg, P, 15 mg Zn, 45 mcg biotin, aspartame	Chewable. In 60s.	160

* Cost Index based on cost per capsule or tablet.
sf – Sugar free.
[1] Calcium and iron content expressed in mg elemental calcium and iron.
[2] As d-alpha tocopheryl acid succinate.
[3] As dl-alpha tocopheryl acetate.
[4] Form of vitamin E unknown; content given in IU.

MULTIVITAMINS WITH MINERALS (Cont.)

Content given per capsule or tablet.
For a comparison of the potencies of various forms of vitamin E, see p14.

	Product & Distributor	A IU	D IU	E mg	B_1 mg	B_2 mg	B_3 mg	B_5 mg	B_6 mg	B_{12} mcg	C mg	FA mg	Zn mg	Other Content	How Supplied	C.I.*
Rx	**Vademin-Z Capsules** (Hauck)	12,500	50	50[1]	10	5	25	10	2		150		20	Mg, Mn	In 60s and 500s.	367
otc	**Total Formula Tablets** (Vitaline)	10,000	400	24.8[2]	15	15	25	25	25	25	100	0.4	30	Ca, Cr, Cu, 20 mg Fe, I, K, Mg, Mn, Mo, P, Se, Si, vanadium, 70 mcg vitamin K, 300 mcg biotin, choline, bioflavonoids, hesperidin, inositol, PABA, rutin	In 90s and 1000s.	92
Rx	**Vicon Forte Capsules** (Russ)	8,000		50[3]	10	5	25	10	2	10	150	1	18.4	Mg, Mn	(Glaxo). Orange and black. In 60s, 500s and UD 100s.	279
otc	**Multilyte Effervescent Tablets** (Inter-Hermes Pharma)	5,000	400	15[3]	3	3.4	36	14	4.4	6	120	0.4	10.5	100 mcg biotin, Ca, K, Mg, Mn, phenylalanine.	Orange flavor. In 12s.	NA
otc sf	**Formula VM-2000 Tablets** (Solgar)	5,000	200	67.1[4]	50	50	50	50	50	50	150	0.4	15	Boron, Ca, Cr, Cu, 5 mg Fe, I, K, Mg, Mn, Mo, Se, 7500 IU beta carotene, betaine, 50 mcg biotin, choline, bioflavonoids, amino acids, glutamic acid, hesperidin, inositol, l-glutathione, PABA, rutin	In 30s, 60s, 90s and 180s.	NA
otc	**OCuZIN Tablets** (Cynacon-OCuSOFT)	5,000		30							60			Cu, Se, 40 mg Zn	In 60s.	NA
otc	**Vi-Zac Capsules** (Russ)	5,000		50[3]							500		18.4		(Glaxo). Orange. In 60s.	264
otc sf	**Glutofac Tablets** (Kenwood)	5,000		30[3]	15	10	50	20	50		300		5	Cu, Mg, Se, Cr	In 90s.	NA

* Cost Index based on cost per capsule or tablet.
sf – Sugar free.
[1] As dl-alpha tocopheryl acetate.
[2] As d-alpha tocopheryl succinate.
[3] Form of vitamin E unknown; content given in IU.
[4] As d-alpha tocopherol.

(Continued on following page)

MULTIVITAMINS WITH MINERALS (Cont.)

Content given per capsule, tablet or 5 ml.
For a comparison of the potencies of various forms of vitamin E, see p14.

	Product & Distributor	A IU	D IU	E mg	B_1 mg	B_2 mg	B_3 mg	B_5 mg	B_6 mg	B_{12} mcg	C mg	FA mg	Zn mg	Other Content	How Supplied	C.I.*
Rx	**Eldercaps Capsules** (Mayrand)	4,000	400	25[1]	10	5	25	10	2		200	1	25.3	Mg, Mn	In 100s.	270
otc	**Vicon Plus Capsules** (Russ)	4,000		50[1]	10	5	25	10	2		150		18.4	Mg, Mn	(Glaxo). Red and yellow. In 60s.	240
otc *sf*	**Kenwood Therapeutic Liquid** (Kenwood)	3,333	133	1.5[2]	2	1	20	2	0.33		50			Ca, K, Mg, Mn, P	Alcohol free. In 360 ml.	273
otc	**Maximum Red Label Tablets** (Vitaline)	833	66.7	55.1[3]	16.7	8.3	31.7	66.7	16.7	16.7	200	0.1	5	Ca, Cr, Cu, 20 mg Fe, I, K, Mg, Mn, Mo, Se, Si, vanadium, 50 mcg biotin, choline, inositol, bioflavonoids, l-lysine, PABA, SOD	In 180s.	92
otc	**Maximum Green Label Tablets** (Vitaline)		16.7											Ca, Cr, I, K, Mg, Mn, Mo, Se, Si, vanadium, 50 mcg biotin, choline, bioflavonoids, inositol, SOD, l-lysine, PABA	In 180s.	92
otc	**Maximum Blue Label Tablets** (Vitaline)													Ca, Cr, Cu, I, K, Mg, Mn, Mo, Se, Si, vanadium, 50 mcg biotin, choline, bioflavonoids, inositol, SOD, l-lysine, PABA	In 180s.	92
otc	**Clusivol Syrup** (Whitehall)	2,500	400		1	1	5	3	0.6	2	15		0.5	Mg, Mn, sucrose, dextrose	Candy flavor. In 240 and 480 ml.	NA
otc	**Po-Pon-S Tablets** (Shionogi)	2,000	100	5[1]	5	3	35	15	4	6	100			Ca, P	Sugar coated. Oval. In 60s and 240s.	99
otc	**ADEKs Tablets** (Scandipharm)	4,000	400	150[1]	1.2	1.3	10	10	1.5	12	60	0.2		3 mg beta carotene, 50 mcg biotin, 150 mcg K, Zn, fructose, sorbitol	In 60s and 100s.	NA

* Cost Index based on cost per capsule, tablet or 5 ml.
sf – Sugar free.
[1] Form of vitamin E unknown; content given in IU.
[2] As dl-alpha tocopherol acetate.
[3] As d-alpha tocopheryl succinate.

(Continued on following page)

MULTIVITAMINS WITH MINERALS (Cont.)

Content given per capsule, tablet or 5 ml.
For a comparison of the potencies of various forms of vitamin E, see p14.

	Product & Distributor	A IU	D IU	E mg	B_1 mg	B_2 mg	B_3 mg	B_5 mg	B_6 mg	B_{12} mcg	C mg	FA mg	Zn mg	Other Content	How Supplied	C.I.*
otc	**Cezin Capsules** (UAD)				20	10	100	20	5		300		80	70 mg Mg	In 100s.	NA
otc	**Mediplex Tabules (Tablets)** (U.S. Pharmaceutical Corp.)			54.5[3]	25	10	100	25	10	25	300		18.4	Cu, Mg, Mn	Oval. In 100s.	300
otc	**Besta Capsules** (Hauck)			45[2]	20	15	50	5	25	4	300		18.21	Mg	(Besta Hauck 202). Orange. In 100s.	220
otc	**Tega Atric M Elixir** (Ortega)				0.83	0.42	8.3	1.7	0.16	0.16			0.33	18% alcohol, 2.5 mg Fe, I, Mg, Mn, choline	Sherry wine base. In pt.	198
otc *sf*	**Hair Booster Vitamin Tablets** (Nature's Bounty)						35	100		6		0.4	15	Cu, 18 mg Fe, I, Mn, choline, inositol, PABA, protein, tartrazine.	In 60s.	177
otc	**B•C•E & Zinc Tablets** (Schein)			45[1]	15	10.2	100	25	10	6	600		22.5		In 60s and 250s.	130
otc	**Z-gen Tablets** (Goldline)			45[3]	15	10.2	100	25	10	6	600		22.5		Green. Film coated. Oval. In 60s and 1000s.	113
otc	**Bee-Zee Tablets** (Rugby)														In 60s.	102
otc	**Z-Bec Tablets** (Robins)														(Z-BEC AHR). Green. Film coated. Capsule shape. In 60s, 500s and Dis-co pack 100s.	200

* Cost Index based on cost per capsule, tablet or 5 ml.
sf – Sugar free.
[1] As dl-alpha tocopheryl acetate.
[2] Form of vitamin E unknown; content given in IU.
[3] As dl-alpha tocopherol acetate.

(Continued on following page)

MULTIVITAMINS WITH MINERALS (Cont.)

Content given per tablet.
For a comparison of the potencies of various forms of vitamin E, see p14.

	Product & Distributor	A IU	D IU	E mg	B_1 mg	B_2 mg	B_3 mg	B_5 mg	B_6 mg	B_{12} mcg	C mg	FA mg	Zn mg	Other Content	How Supplied	C.I.*
Rx	**Vio-Bec Forte Tablets** (Solvay Pharm.)			30[1]	25	25	100	40	25	5	500	0.5	25	Cu	(RR 1218). Brown. Film coated. Capsule shape. In 100s.	216
otc	**Stress Formula 500 Plus Zinc Tablets** (Schein)			30[2]	15	10	100	20	5	12	500	0.4	23.9	45 mcg biotin, 3 mg copper	In 60s and 250s.	NA
otc	**Stress Formula 600 Plus Zinc Tablets** (Schein)			30[1]	20	10	100	25	5	12	600	0.4	23.9	Cu, Mg, 45 mcg biotin	In 60s and 250s.	130
otc	**Surbex 750 with Zinc Filmtab Tablets** (Abbott)			30[1]	15	15	100	20	20	12	750	0.4	22.5		Film coated. In 50s.	321
otc *sf*	**Stress Formula "605" with Zinc Tablets** (Nature's Bounty)			30[1]	20	10	100	25	5	12	605	0.4	23.9	Cu, 45 mcg biotin	In 60s.	NA
otc	**Stresstabs + Zinc Tablets** (Lederle)			30[1]	15	10	100	20	5	12	500	0.4	23.9	Cu, 45 mcg biotin	In 60s.	232
otc	**Efamol PMS Soft Gel Capsules** (Murdock)			12[2]					21		100		3	20 mg Ca, 30 mg Mg, 45 mg gamma-linolenic acid, 115 mg cis-linoleic acid, 35 mg alpha-linolenic acid, 14 mg eicosapentaenoic acid, 9 mg docosahexaenoic acid	In 30s and 90s.	NA

* Cost Index based on cost per tablet.
sf – Sugar free.
[1] As dl-alpha tocopheryl acetate.
[2] Form of vitamin E unknown; content given in IU.

GERIATRIC SUPPLEMENTS WITH MULTIVITAMINS AND MINERALS

Content given per capsule or tablet. For a comparison of the potencies of various forms of vitamin E, see p14.

	Product & Distributor	A IU	D IU	E mg	B_1 mg	B_2 mg	B_3 mg	B_5 mg	B_6 mg	B_{12} mcg	C mg	Fe[1] mg	FA mg	Ca[1] mg	Zn mg	Other Content	How Supplied	C.I.*
otc *sf*	**Megadose Tablets** (Arco)	25,000	1,000	100[2]	80	80	80	80	80	80	250	1.2	0.4	4.5	3.58	80 mg choline, 80 mg inositol, 80 mcg biotin, 80 mg PABA, rutin, 30 mg bioflavonoids, 30 mg betaine, glutamic acid, 5 mg hesperidin, Cu, I, K, Mg, Mn	In 30s, 100s and 250s.	422
otc *sf*	**Mega VM-80 Tablets** (Nature's Bounty)	10,000	1,000	100[2]	80	80	80	80	80	80	250	1.2	0.4	4.5	3.58	80 mg choline, 80 mg inositol, 80 mcg biotin, 80 mg PABA, rutin, 30 mg bioflavonoids, 30 mg betaine, 30 mg glutamic acid, 5 mg hesperidin, Cu, I, K, Mg, Mn	In 30s, 60s and 100s.	262
otc	**Vita-Plus G Softgels** (Scot-Tussin)	10,000	400	2[3]	5	2.5	40	4	1	2	75	30		75	0.5	K, Mg, Mn, 58 mg P	In 100s.	110
Rx	**Cezin-S Caps** (UAD)	10,000	50	50	10	5	50	10	2		200		0.5		80	70 mg Mg, 4 mg Mn	In 100s.	NA
otc	**Viopan-T Tablets** (Trimen)	8,000	400	30[2]	10	10	100	5	2	6	200	15	0.4	100	15	25 mg choline, 25 mg l-lysine, 10 mcg biotin, Cu, I, K, Mg, Mn, 42 mg P	(Trimen). Red. Film coated. In 100s.	200
otc	**Centrum Silver Gel-Tabs** (Lederle)	6,000	400	45[2]	1.5	1.7	20	10	3	25	60	9	0.025	200		30 mcg biotin, Cu, I, Mg, P, Zn, Cl, Cr, Mn, Mo, Ni, Se, Si, V, 10 mcg K	In 60s.	NA
otc	**Gerimed Tabs** (Fielding)	5,000	400	30[2]	3	3	25		2	6	120			370	15	Mg, 130 mg P	Red. In 60s.	198
Rx	**Strovite Plus Tablets** (Everett)	5,000		30[3]	20	20	100	25	25	50	500	27	0.8		22.5	150 mcg biotin, Cr, Cu, Mg, Mn	In 100s.	310
otc	**Geriplex FS Kapseals** (Parke-Davis)	5,000		5[3]	5	5	15			2	50	6		59	0.5	20 mg choline, sodium bisulfite, Cu, Mn, 100 mg DSS, 150 mg aspergillus oryzae enzymes	(P-D 544). In 100s.	359

* Cost Index based on cost per capsule or tablet.
sf – Sugar free.

[1] Calcium and iron content expressed in mg elemental calcium and iron.
[2] Form of vitamin E unknown; content given in IU.
[3] As dl-alpha tocopheryl acetate.

(Continued on following page)

GERIATRIC SUPPLEMENTS WITH MULTIVITAMINS AND MINERALS (Cont.)

Content given per capsule or tablet.
For a comparison of the potencies of various forms of vitamin E, see p. 5.

	Product & Distributor	A IU	D IU	E mg	B_1 mg	B_2 mg	B_3 mg	B_5 mg	B_6 mg	B_{12} mcg	C mg	Fe[1] mg	FA mg	Ca[1] mg	Zn mg	Other Content	How Supplied	C.I.*
otc sf	**Ultra-Freeda Tablets** (Freeda)	3,333	133	66.7[2]	16.7	16.7	33	33	16.7	33	333	5	0.27	66.7	7.5	33 mg choline, 33 mg inositol, 833 IU beta carotene, 33 mg bioflavonoids, 16.7 mg PABA, 100 mcg biotin, Cr, I, K, Mg, Mn, Mo, Se	In 90s, 180s and 270s.	NA
otc sf	**Ultra-Freeda Iron Free Tablets** (Freeda)																In 90s, 180s and 270s.	NA
otc sf	**Optivite P.M.T. Tablets** (Optimox)	2,083	16.7	16.7[2]	4.2	4.2	4.2	4.2	50	10.4	250	2.5	0.03	†	4.2	52 mg choline bitartrate, Cr, Cu, I, K, Mg, Mn, Se, bioflavonoids, betaine, PABA, rutin, pancreatin, biotin	In 180s.	139
otc	**Hep-Forte Capsules** (Marlyn)	1,200		6.7[3]	1	1	10	2	0.5	1	10		0.06		2	21 mg choline, 10 mg inositol, 3.3 mg biotin, 10 mg dl-methionine, 194.4 mg desiccated liver, 64.8 mg liver concentrate, 64.8 mg liver fraction number 2, lecithin	In 100s, 300s and 500s.	81

* Cost Index based on cost per capsule or tablet.
sf – Sugar free.
† – Amount not supplied by manufacturer.

[1] Calcium and iron content expressed in mg elemental calcium and iron.
[2] Form of vitamin E unknown; content given in IU.
[3] As d-alpha tocopherol.

(Continued on following page)

GERIATRIC SUPPLEMENTS WITH MULTIVITAMINS AND MINERALS (Cont.)

Content given per 15 ml.

	Product & Distributor	A IU	D IU	E mg	B_1 mg	B_2 mg	B_3 mg	B_5 mg	B_6 mg	B_{12} mcg	C mg	Fe[1] mg	FA mg	Ca[1] mg	Zn mg	Other Content	How Supplied	C.I.*
otc	**Vigortol Liquid** (Rugby)				2.5	1.25	25	5	0.5	0.5		10			1	50 mg choline, 50 mg inositol, I, K, Mg, Mn, 18% alcohol, calcium saccharin	Sherry wine base. In pt.	226
otc	**Viminate Elixir** (Various, eg, Barre-National, Bioline, Major, Moore)				2.5	1.25	25	5	0.5	0.5		7.5			1	50 mg choline, I, Mg, Mn, alcohol	In pt and gal.	236+
otc	**Geravite Elixir** (Hauck)				1	1.2	100			10						15% alcohol, 150 mg l-lysine	Wine flavor. In pt and gal.	629

MULTIVITAMINS WITH HORMONES, ORAL

Products in this group are recommended as nutritional supplements for the patient needing mild hormonal effects.
Content given per capsule.

	Product & Distributor	B_1 mg	B_2 mg	B_3 mg	B_5 mg	B_6 mg	B_{12} mcg	C mg	Fe[1] mg	Methyltestos-terone (mg)	Conjugated Estrogens (mg)	Other Content	How Supplied	C.I.*
c-III	**Mediatric Capsules** (Wyeth-Ayerst)	10	5	50	20	3	2.5	100[2]	9[3]	2.5	0.25	1 mg methamphet-amine HCl	(Ayerst 252). In 100s.	836

* Cost Index based on cost per capsule or 15 ml.
[1] Calcium and iron content expressed in mg elemental calcium and iron.
[2] From sodium ascorbate and ascorbic acid.
[3] From dried ferrous sulfate.

LIPOTROPICS WITH VITAMINS

Content given per capsule, tablet or 5 ml.

	Product & Distributor	Choline (mg)	Inositol (mg)	Methionine (mg)	B_1 mg	B_2 mg	B_3 mg	B_5 mg	B_6 mg	B_{12} mcg	C mg	Other Content	How Supplied	C.I.*
otc	**Lipotriad Liquid** (Numark)	334[1]	†		1	1	10	5	1	5		Saccharin, parabens	Alcohol free. In pt.	462
otc	**Lipogen Capsules** (Various, eg, Goldline, Rugby)	111[2]	111		0.33	0.33	3.33	1.7	0.33	1.7	††		In 60s and 100s.	156+
otc	**Lipotriad Capsules** (Numark)	111	†		0.33	0.33	3.33	1.66	0.33	1.66		1667 IU vitamin A (as beta-carotene), 10 IU E, Zn, Cu	(Numark). In 100s and 1000s.	192
otc	**Lipoflavonoid Capsules** (Numark)	111[2]	111		0.33	0.33	3.33	1.66	0.4	1.66	100	100 mg lemon bioflavonoid complex	In 100s and 500s.	422
otc	**Cholinoid Capsules** (Goldline)	111[2]	111		0.33	0.33	3.33	1.7	0.33	1.7	100	100 mg lemon bioflavonoid complex	Red and beige. In 100s.	198
otc	**Akoline C.B. Capsules** (Akorn)	111[2]	111	28	0.33	0.33	3.33	0.39	0.33	1.7	100	100 mg lemon bioflavonoid complex	In 100s.	184
otc	**Akoline C.B. Caplets** (Akorn)											100 mg lemon bioflavonoid complex, 6.7 mg Zn	In 100s.	190
otc	**Liponol Capsules** (Rugby)	115[2]	83	110	3	3	10	2	2	2		56 mg desiccated liver, 30 mg liver concentrate, sorbitol	In 60s.	138
otc	**Methatropic Capsules** (Goldline)											56 mg desiccated liver, & 30 mg liver concentrate	Pink. In 100s and 1000s.	160
otc *sf*	**Cholidase Tablets** (Freeda)	185[3]	150						2.5	5		7.5 mg vitamin E[4]	In 100s, 250s and 500s.	142

* Cost Index based on cost per capsule, tablet or 5 ml.
sf – Sugar free.
† – Amount not supplied by manufacturer.
†† May or may not contain vitamin C.
[1] From tricholine citrate.
[2] From choline bitartrate.
[3] From choline dihydrogen citrate.
[4] As d-alpha tocopherol.

Intravenous nutritional therapy is required when normal enteral feeding is not possible or is inadequate for nutritional requirements. Specific nutritional requirements and administration mode depend on the nutritional status of the patient and the duration of parenteral therapy. To meet IV nutritional requirements, one or more of the following nutrients may be required:

Protein Substrates
- Amino Acids – General Formulations
- Amino Acids – Renal Failure Formulations
- Amino Acids – Hepatic Failure/Encephalopathy Formulations
- Amino Acids – Metabolic Stress Formulations

Energy Substrates
- Dextrose
- IV Fat Emulsion

Electrolytes

Vitamins

Trace Metals

The following general discussion reviews peripheral and central routes of administration, and provides basic guidelines for the use of the various components of IV nutritional therapy.

PERIPHERAL PARENTERAL NUTRITION:

Peripheral protein sparing: Amino acids with maintenance electrolytes (with or without dextrose) prevent protein catabolism in patients with adequate body fat and with no clinically significant protein malnutrition, for short periods of time. Lipolysis provides energy from oxidation of free fatty acids and ketone bodies; minimal nitrogen is lost since proteolysis does not occur. For peripheral IV infusion, 1 to 1.5 g/kg/day of amino acids achieves optimal fat mobilization and spares protein catabolism.

ProcalAmine is a unique product that provides a physiological ratio of biologically utilizable essential and nonessential amino acids, glycerin (glycerol) and maintenance electrolytes. Glycerin preserves body protein and participates as an active energy substrate through its phosphorylation to α-glycerophosphate.

Peripheral total parenteral nutrition (TPN): Peripheral TPN is for patients requiring parenteral nutrition in whom the central venous route is not indicated. Amino acids with electrolytes, combined with 5% or 10% dextrose and used in conjunction with IV fat emulsions (and usually vitamins and trace metals), reduce protein catabolism in patients moderately catabolic or depleted and minimize liver glycogen depletion. Peripheral infusions may provide inadequate maintenance requirements for patients with greatly increased metabolic demands or with severe nutritional deficiencies requiring repletion. Oral calories may also be added as tolerated.

CENTRAL TOTAL PARENTERAL NUTRITION:

Amino acids combined with hypertonic dextrose and IV fat emulsions infused via a central venous catheter promote protein synthesis in hypercatabolic or severely depleted patients or those requiring long-term parenteral nutrition. Appropriate electrolytes, vitamins and trace minerals are added to provide total parenteral nutrition.

Actions:

Amino acids promote the production of proteins (anabolism) needed for synthesis of structural components, reduce the rate of protein breakdown (catabolism), promote wound healing and act as buffers in the extracellular and intracellular fluids.

Dextrose is a source of calories; nonprotein calories are required for efficient utilization of amino acids. It decreases protein and nitrogen losses, promotes glycogen deposition and prevents ketosis (see individual monograph).

IV fat emulsions provide a mixture of fatty acids utilized as a source of energy and to prevent essential fatty acid deficiency (EFAD) (see individual monograph).

Fluid/Electrolytes/Trace metals are provided to compensate for normal sensible and insensible losses, as well as the additional losses often present in patients requiring parenteral nutrition (see individual section).

Indications:

Parenteral nutrition is indicated to prevent nitrogen and weight loss or to treat negative nitrogen balance when: (1) The alimentary tract, by the oral, gastrostomy or jejunostomy route, cannot or should not be used; (2) GI absorption of protein is impaired by obstruction, inflammatory disease or its complications or antineoplastic therapy; (3) bowel rest is needed because of GI surgery or its complications such as ileus, fistulae or anastomotic leaks; (4) metabolic requirements for protein are substantially increased, as with extensive burns, infections, trauma or other hypermetabolic states; (5) morbidity and mortality may be reduced by replacing amino acids lost from tissue breakdown, thereby preserving tissue reserves, as in acute renal failure; (6) tube feeding methods alone cannot provide adequate nutrition.

(Indications continued on following page)

Indications: (Cont.)

After the patient's nutritional deficits, reserves and current status are assessed, set rational and precise nutritional goals. Dosage, route of administration and concomitant infusion of nonprotein calories depend on nutritional and metabolic status, anticipated duration of parenteral nutritional support and vein tolerance.

Peripheral parenteral nutrition: Administration of nutritional solutions through peripheral veins is appropriate if caloric needs are minimal, if they can be partially met by enteral alimentation, if nutritional therapy will only be required for 5 to 14 days, or if central venous access is not feasible.

Central parenteral nutrition: Amino acids, combined with hypertonic dextrose and IV fat emulsions infused via a central venous catheter, promote protein synthesis in hypercatabolic or severely depleted patients or in those requiring long-term parenteral nutrition.

Specific disease states in which total parenteral nutrition requires special considerations are:

Renal failure
Acute metabolic stress
Hepatic failure/Hepatic encephalopathy
See individual sections for specific discussions.

Total nutrient admixtures (TNA): A combination of amino acids, dextrose and lipids in one container has been used. Also known as multicomponent admixtures, all-in-one, 3-in-1 or triple mix, TNA offers the advantage of substituting some dextrose calories with lipids, thereby reducing the incidence of carbohydrate-related complications (eg, impaired glucose control). It also appears to be utilized better by the liver due to the continuous administration of lipids, and is less likely to interfere with immune functions. Refer also to the admixture incompatibilities/compatibilities section under Administration.

Contraindications:

Protein substrates: Hypersensitivity to any component; decreased (subcritical) circulating blood volume; inborn errors of amino acid metabolism (eg, maple syrup urine disease, isovaleric acidemia); anuria.

General amino acid formulations: Severe renal failure; severe liver disease; hepatic coma or encephalopathy; metabolic disorders involving impaired nitrogen utilization.

Renal failure formulations: Severe electrolyte and acid-base imbalance; hyperammonemia.

Hepatic failure/Hepatic encephalopathy formulations: Anuria.

High metabolic stress formulations: Anuria; hyperammonemia; hepatic coma; severe electrolyte or acid-base imbalance.

Warnings:

Prevention of complications: IV nutritional therapy may be associated with complications that can be prevented or minimized by careful attention to solution preparation, administration and patient monitoring. It is essential to follow a carefully prepared protocol based on current medical practices, preferably administered by an experienced team.

Amino acid metabolism: Hyperchloremic metabolic acidosis may result from amino acids provided as hydrochloride salts that release hydrochloride when utilized. To prevent or control this, supply a portion of the cations as acetate or lactate salts. Sodium and potassium phosphates are also available.

Hepatic function impairment may result in serum amino acid imbalances, metabolic alkalosis, prerenal azotemia, hyperammonemia, stupor and coma. Instances of asymptomatic hyperammonemia have occurred in patients without overt liver dysfunction. Amino acid products specifically formulated for patients with hepatic failure are discussed separately in this section. Give conservative doses of amino acids to patients with known or suspected hepatic dysfunction.

Hyperammonemia occurs most often in children and adults with renal or hepatic disease and results from a diminished ability to handle a protein load. It is of special significance in infants as it can result in mental retardation. This reaction is dose-related and more likely to develop during prolonged therapy; treatment involves adjusting the dosage or decreasing amino acids.

Ketosis – Administration of amino acids without carbohydrates may result in the accumulation of ketones; correct ketonemia by administering carbohydrates.

Pregnancy: Category C. It is not known whether IV nutritional therapy can cause fetal harm when administered to a pregnant woman or can affect reproduction capacity. Use only when clearly needed and when the potential benefits outweigh the hazards to the fetus.

Lactation: Exercise caution when administering to a nursing woman.

Children: The effect of amino acid infusions without dextrose on carbohydrate metabolism of children is not known. Use special caution in pediatric patients with acute renal failure, especially low birth weight infants. Laboratory and clinical monitoring must be extensive and frequent.

(Warnings continued on following page)

Warnings (Cont.):

Infection control: Parenteral nutrition is associated with a constant risk of sepsis. Careful, aseptic technique in the preparation of solutions and insertion and maintenance of central venous catheters is imperative. A 0.22 micron filter is often recommended to block particulate matter and bacteria. Presence of *Staphylococcus* or *Candida* suggests catheter sepsis. Early symptoms of infection include fever, chills, glucose intolerance and a change in the level of consciousness.

If other sources are not apparent and if fever persists, change solution, delivery system and catheter site. Culture catheter tip and draw blood cultures.

Precautions:

Monitoring: Laboratory monitoring and clinical evaluation are necessary for proper monitoring before and during administration. Do not withdraw venous blood for blood chemistries through the same peripheral infusion site; interference with estimations of nitrogen containing substances may occur. The following general protocol is suggested:

General Patient Monitoring During IV Nutritional Therapy
Baseline studies: CBC, platelet count, prothrombin time, weight, body length and head circumference (in infants), electrolytes, CO_2, BUN, glucose, creatinine, total protein, cholesterol, triglycerides (if on fat emulsion), uric acid, bilirubin, alkaline phosphatase, LDH, AST, albumin and other appropriate parameters.
Daily studies during stabilization (average 3 to 5 days): Urine glucose, acetone and ketones each shift, intake/output, weight, plasma and urine osmolarity, electrolytes, trace elements, CO_2, BUN, creatinine.
Routine studies after stabilization:
Daily – Intake/output, weight, urine glucose and osmolarity and ketones.
Two to three times weekly – Electrolytes, BUN, blood glucose, plasma transaminases, bilirubin, blood acid-base status, ammonia, creatinine.
Weekly: CBC, prothrombin time, plasma total protein and fractions, hemoglobin, body length and head circumference (in infants), cholesterol, triglycerides, uric acid, albumin, LDH, AST, alkaline phosphatase.
Periodic: Nitrogen balance, trace elements, total lymphocyte count, iron status.

BUN: IV infusion of amino acids may induce a rise in BUN, especially in patients with GI bleeding or impaired hepatic or renal function. Perform appropriate laboratory tests periodically and discontinue infusion if BUN exceeds normal postprandial limits and continues to rise. A modest rise in BUN normally occurs as a result of increased protein intake. Patients with azotemia should not receive amino acids without regard to total nitrogen intake.

Protein sparing: If daily increases in BUN (range, 10 to 15 mg/dl) for > 3 days occur, discontinue protein sparing therapy and institute a regimen with full nonprotein caloric substrates.

Cardiac effects: Avoid circulatory overload, particularly in patients with cardiac insufficiency. In patients with myocardial infarction, infusion of amino acids should always be accompanied by dextrose, since in anoxia, free fatty acids cannot be utilized by the myocardium, and energy must be produced anaerobically from glycogen or glucose.

Hypertonic solutions containing dextrose should not be administered by peripheral vein infusions. Do not use hypertonic solutions in the presence of intracranial or intraspinal hemorrhage or if the patient is already dehydrated.

Glucose imbalances:

Hyperglycemia – Glucose intolerance is the most common metabolic complication; metabolic adaptation to large glucose loads requires up to 72 hours, although severely septic or hypermetabolic patients may not be able to handle the glucose load. A too rapid infusion of amino acid-carbohydrate mixtures may result in hyperglycemia, glycosuria and a hyperosmolar syndrome, characterized by mental confusion and loss of consciousness. Reducing the administration rate, decreasing the dextrose concentration or administering insulin will minimize these reactions.

Hyperglycemia may not be reflected by glycosuria in renal failure. Therefore, determine blood glucose frequently, often every 6 hours, to guide dosage of dextrose and insulin if required. Infusion of hypertonic dextrose carries a greater risk of hyperglycemia in low birth weight or septic infants.

Excess carbohydrate calories may result in fatty infiltration of the liver. Excess carbon dioxide from administration of too much glucose can compromise weaning of hypermetabolic patients from mechanical ventilation or can precipitate acute respiratory failure.

Rebound hypoglycemia may result from sudden cessation of a concentrated dextrose solution due to continued endogenous insulin production. Withdraw parenteral nutrition mixtures slowly. Administer a solution containing 5% or 10% dextrose when hypertonic dextrose infusions are abruptly discontinued.

(Precautions continued on following page)

Precautions (Cont.):

Essential fatty acid deficiency (EFAD) results from long-term fat-free IV feeding; symptoms include dry, scaly skin, eczematous rash, hair loss, poor wound healing and fatty degeneration of the liver. In adults, administer at least 500 ml fat emulsion per week to prevent EFAD (see individual monograph).

Electrolyte abnormalities: Intracellular ion deficits may arise due to two mechanisms. As protein is used for increased energy demands in a catabolic patient, intracellular ions are lost. In addition, as anabolism occurs, ions are employed in building new cells. Focus attention on supplying adequate potassium, phosphate, magnesium and calcium. Observe patients for clinical signs of paresthesias, neuromuscular weakness and changes in level of consciousness; monitor laboratory results.

The presence of impaired renal function, pulmonary disease, or cardiac insufficiency presents danger of retention of fluids.

Sodium: Use solutions containing sodium ions cautiously in patients with CHF, severe renal insufficiency, and edema with sodium retention.

Potassium: Use solutions containing potassium ions cautiously in patients with hyperkalemia or severe renal failure, and in conditions in which potassium retention is present.

Acetate: Use solutions containing acetate ions cautiously in patients with metabolic or respiratory alkalosis and in those conditions in which there is an increased level or impaired utilization of this ion, such as severe hepatic insufficiency.

Cancer chemotherapy patients: The American College of Physicians discourages the routine use of parenteral nutrition in patients undergoing cancer chemotherapy since no benefit has been determined (ie, there was no improvement in overall or short-term survival and no greater improvement in chemotherapy response).

Sulfite sensitivity: Some of these products contain sulfites which may cause allergic-type reactions including anaphylactic symptoms and life-threatening or less severe asthmatic episodes in certain susceptible persons. The overall prevalence of sulfite sensitivity in the general population is unknown and probably low. Sulfite sensitivity is seen more frequently in asthmatic or atopic persons.

Drug Interactions:

Tetracycline, because of its antianabolic activity, may reduce the protein sparing effects of infused amino acids.

Adverse Reactions:

Catheter complications: Phlebitis and venous thrombosis may occur at the site of venipuncture or along the vein. If this occurs, discontinue use or choose another administration site. Use of large peripheral veins, inline filters and slower infusion rates may reduce the incidence of local venous irritation. Infection at the injection site and extravasation may occur.

Nausea, fever and flushing of the skin have occurred.

Metabolic complications include: Metabolic acidosis and alkalosis; hypophosphatemia; hypocalcemia; osteoporosis; glycosuria; hyperglycemia; hypo- or hypermagnesemia; osmotic diuresis; dehydration; hypervolemia; rebound hypoglycemia; hypo- or hypervitaminosis; electrolyte imbalances; hyperammonemia; elevated hepatic enzymes.

Phosphorus deficiency may lead to impaired tissue oxygenation and acute hemolytic anemia. Relative to calcium, excessive phosphorus intake can precipitate hypocalcemia with cramps, tetany and muscular hyperexcitability.

Complications known to occur from the placement of central venous catheters are pneumothorax, hemothorax, hydrothorax, artery puncture and transection, injury to the brachial plexus, malposition of the catheter, formation of arteriovenous fistula, phlebitis, thrombosis and air and catheter embolus.

Reactions reported in clinical studies as a result of infusion of the parenteral fluid were water weight gain, edema, increase in BUN and mild acidosis.

Administration:

Total daily dose depends on daily protein requirements and on the patient's metabolic and clinical responses. The determination of nitrogen balance and accurate daily body weights, corrected for fluid balance, are probably the best means of assessing protein requirements. In addition, guide dosage by the patient's fluid intake limits, glucose and nitrogen tolerances as well as by metabolic and clinical response.

Protein: Recommended dietary allowances of protein are approximately 0.9 g/kg for a healthy adult and 1.4 to 2.2 g/kg for healthy growing infants and children. Protein and caloric requirements in traumatized or malnourished patients may be substantially increased. Daily doses of approximately 1 to 1.5 g/kg for adults and 2 to 3 g/kg for infants are generally sufficient to promote positive nitrogen balance, although higher doses may be required in severely catabolic states. Such higher doses require frequent laboratory evaluation.

(Administration continued on following page)

Administration (Cont.)

Energy requirements: To ensure proper caloric intake, the required calorie and energy needs may be estimated using the basal metabolic rate; energy expenditure and disease states need to be considered as well. The energy required for proper amino acid utilization is derived from glycogenolysis, lipolysis or infusion of dextrose or fat emulsions. After glycogen is depleted, in the absence of exogenous calories, fat becomes the major energy source. Parenterally administered amino acids will not be retained and utilized for anabolic purposes unless adequate nonprotein calories are provided simultaneously.

IV fat emulsion should comprise no more than 60% of the total caloric intake, with carbohydrates and amino acids comprising the remaining 40% or more.

Electrolyte requirements: In adults, ≈ 60 to 180 mEq of potassium, 10 to 30 mEq of magnesium and 10 to 40 mM of phosphate per day appear necessary to achieve optimum metabolic response; individualize each requirement. Give sufficient quantities of the major extracellular electrolytes, sodium, calcium and chloride. (Calcium prevents hypocalcemia that may accompany phosphate administration.) Consider the electrolyte content of the amino acid infusion when calculating daily electrolyte intake.

HepatAmine contains < 3 mEq chloride/L and ≤ 10 mM/L of phosphate. Some patients, especially those with hypophosphatemia, may require additional phosphate.

Fluid balance: Provide sufficient water to compensate for insensible, urinary and other (eg, nasogastric suction, fistula drainage, diarrhea) fluid losses. Average daily adult fluid requirements are between 2500 and 3000 ml, but may be much higher with losses such as fistula drainage or in burn patients.

Vitamin therapy: If a patient's nutritional intake is primarily parenteral, provide vitamins (especially the water soluble vitamins). Iron is added to the solution or given IM in depot form as indicated. Folic acid and vitamin K are required additives.

Pediatric requirements are constrained by the greater relative fluid and caloric requirements per kg of the infant. Amino acids are best administered in a 2.5% concentration. For most pediatric patients, 2.5 g amino acids/kg/day with dextrose alone or with IV fat calories of 100 to 130 kcal/kg/day are recommended for maintenance. Start with nutritional solution of half strength at a rate of about 60 to 70 ml/kg/day. Within 24 to 48 hours, the volume and concentration of the solution can be increased until full strength pediatric solution is given at a rate of 125 to 150 ml/kg/day.

A basic central line solution for pediatric use should contain 25 g of amino acids and 200 to 250 g of glucose per 1000 ml. Such a solution given at a rate of 145 ml/kg/day provides 100 to 130 kcal/kg/day.

Administer supplemental electrolytes and vitamins (including agents such as carnitine) as necessary. Iron is more critical in infants because of increasing red cell mass required for growth. Monitor serum lipids for EFAD in patients maintained on fat-free TPN.

To ensure the precise delivery of the small volumes of fluid necessary, use accurately calibrated and reliable infusion systems.

Preparation/stability of solutions: Aseptically prepare solutions under a laminar flow hood. Use promptly after mixing. Store under refrigeration for a brief period of time only (< 24 hours). Do not exceed 24 hours for administration time of a single bottle.

Admixture incompatibilities/compatibilities: Because of the potential for incompatibility in the complex formulations, keep additives to a minimum. Do not administer simultaneously with **blood** through the same infusion site because of possible pseudoagglutination. **Antibiotics, steroids** and **pressor agents** should not be added to these solutions. **Bleomycin** is incompatible with amino acids.

Vitamins, electrolytes, trace minerals, heparin and **insulin** are compatible with these solutions.

Total nutrient admixture (TNA; all-in-one; 3-in-1; triple mix): The combination of amino acids, dextrose and lipids (also known as total nutrient admixture) in one container is generally compatible. When utilizing this type of admixture, consider the following: (1) The order of mixing is important – add amino acids to the fat emulsion or the dextrose; (2) do not add the electrolytes directly to the fat emulsion – add them to the dextrose or amino acids first; (3) TNAs with electrolytes will eventually aggregate; (4) if not used immediately, refrigerate.

Administration sets: Replace all IV sets every 24 hours. Follow appropriate guidelines for care and maintenance of long-term indwelling catheters (eg, Broviac or Hickman).

(Products listed on following pages)

For a complete discussion of the use of protein substrates as a compound of intravenous nutritional therapy, refer to the general monograph beginning on page 100

Protein Substrates

AMINO ACID INJECTION (General formulations)

Actions: Crystalline amino acid injections are hypertonic solutions of balanced essential and nonessential l-amino acids; d-amino acids are not readily utilized by the body. Depending on the amount of caloric supplementation, these amino acids provide a substrate for protein synthesis (anabolism) or enhance conservation of existing body protein (protein sparing effect).

Dosage:

Peripheral protein sparing: Administer amino acids in a dose of 1 to 1.7 g/kg/day via a peripheral vein. If daily increases in BUN in the range of 10 to 15 mg/dl for > 3 days occur, discontinue and implement a regimen with full nonprotein calorie substrates.

ProcalAmine – Approximately 3 L/day will provide 90 g of amino acids, 390 nonprotein calories and recommended daily intake of principal intra- and extracellular electrolytes for the stable patient. In adults, begin with 3 L on the first day with close monitoring of the patient.

Peripheral vein administration: Mix amino acid injections with low concentrations of dextrose solutions (5% or 10%) and administer by peripheral vein with fat emulsions.

Central vein administration: Typically, 500 ml amino acid injection mixed with 500 ml concentrated dextrose injection, electrolytes and vitamins is administered over an 8 hour period.

Strongly hypertonic mixtures of amino acids and dextrose may be safely administered by continuous infusion only through a central venous catheter with the tip located in the superior vena cava. The initial rate of IV infusion should be 2 ml/min and may be increased gradually to the maximum required dose, as indicated by frequent determinations of urine and blood sugar levels. May be started with infusates containing lower concentrations of dextrose and gradually increased to estimated caloric needs as the patient's glucose tolerance increases. If the administration rate falls behind schedule, do not attempt to "catch up" to planned intake. Do not exceed 24 hours administration time for a single bottle. In addition to meeting protein needs, the administration rate is also governed by the patient's glucose tolerance, especially during the first few days of therapy.

(Products listed on following pages)

Protein Substrates (Cont.)

CRYSTALLINE AMINO ACID INFUSIONS

	Aminosyn 3.5% (Abbott)	Aminosyn II 3.5% (Abbott)	Aminosyn 5% (Abbott)	Aminosyn II 5% (Abbott)	Travasol 5.5% (Clintec)	TrophAmine 6% (McGaw)
Amino Acid Concentration	3.5%	3.5%	5%	5%	5.5%	6%
Nitrogen (g/100 ml)	0.55	0.54	0.79	0.77	0.925	0.93
Amino Acids (Essential) (mg/100 ml)						
Isoleucine	252	231	360	330	263	490
Leucine	329	350	470	500	340	840
Lysine	252	368	360	525	318	490
Methionine	140	60	200	86	318	200
Phenylalanine	154	104	220	149	340	290
Threonine	182	140	260	200	230	250
Tryptophan	56	70	80	100	99	120
Valine	280	175	400	250	252	470
Amino Acids (Nonessential) (mg/100 ml)						
Alanine	448	348	640	497	1140	320
Arginine	343	356	490	509	570	730
Histidine[1]	105	105	150	150	241	290
Proline	300	253	430	361	230	410
Serine	147	186	210	265		230
Taurine						15
Tyrosine	31	95	44	135	22	140
Aminoacetic Acid (Glycine)	448	175	640	250	1140	220
Glutamic Acid		258		369		300
Aspartic Acid		245		350		190
Cysteine						< 14
Electrolytes (mEq/L)						
Sodium	7	16.3		19.3		5
Potassium			5.4			
Chloride					22	< 3
Acetate	46	25.2	86	35.9	48	56
Phosphate (mM/L)						
Osmolarity (mOsm/L)	357	308	500	438	575	525
Supplied in (ml)	1000[2]	1000[3]	500[4] 1000[4]	500[3] 1000[3]	500[5] 1000[5] 2000[5]	500[6]
Labeled Indications						
Peripheral Parenteral Nutrition	Yes	Yes	Yes	Yes	Yes	Yes
Central TPN	No	No	Yes	Yes	Yes	Yes
Protein Sparing	Yes	Yes	Yes	Yes	Yes	No

[1] Histidine is considered an essential amino acid in infants and in renal failure.
[2] With 7 mEq/L sodium from the antioxidant sodium hydrosulfite.
[3] Includes 20 mg/dl sodium hydrosulfite.
[4] Includes 5.4 mEq/L potassium from the antioxidant potassium metabisulfite.
[5] With ≈ 3 mEq/L sodium bisulfite.
[6] With < 50 mg sodium metabisulfite per 100 ml.

(Continued on following page)

Protein Substrates (Cont.)

CRYSTALLINE AMINO ACID INFUSIONS

	Aminosyn 7% (Abbott)	Aminosyn-PF 7% (Abbott)	Aminosyn II 7% (Abbott)	Aminosyn 8.5% (Abbott)
Amino Acid Concentration	7%	7%	7%	8.5%
Nitrogen (g/100 ml)	1.1	1.07	1.07	1.34
Amino Acids (Essential) (mg/100 ml)				
Isoleucine	510	534	462	620
Leucine	660	831	700	810
Lysine	510	475	735	624
Methionine	280	125	120	340
Phenylalanine	310	300	209	380
Threonine	370	360	280	460
Tryptophan	120	125	140	150
Valine	560	452	350	680
Amino Acids (Nonessential) (mg/100 ml)				
Alanine	900	490	695	1100
Arginine	690	861	713	850
Histidine[1]	210	220	210	260
Proline	610	570	505	750
Serine	300	347	371	370
Taurine		50		
Tyrosine	44	44	189	44
Aminoacetic Acid (Glycine)	900	270	350	1100
Glutamic Acid		576	517	
Aspartic Acid		370	490	
Cysteine				
Electrolytes (mEq/L)				
Sodium		3.4	31.3	
Potassium	5.4			5.4
Chloride				35
Acetate	105	32.5	50.3	90
Phosphate (mM/L)				
Osmolarity (mOsm/L)	700	586	612	850
Supplied in (ml)	500[2]	250[3] 500[3]	500[4]	500[2] 1000[2]
Labeled Indications				
Peripheral Parenteral Nutrition	Yes	Yes	Yes	Yes
Central TPN	Yes	Yes	Yes	Yes
Protein Sparing	Yes	No	Yes	Yes

[1] Histidine is considered an essential amino acid in infants and in renal failure.
[2] Includes 5.4 mEq/L potassium from the antioxidant potassium metabisulfite.
[3] From the antioxidant sodium hydrosulfite.
[4] Includes 20 mg/dl sodium hydrosulfite.

(Continued on following page)

Protein Substrates (Cont.)

CRYSTALLINE AMINO ACID INFUSIONS

	Aminosyn II 8.5% (Abbott)	**Travasol 8.5% without electrolytes** (Clintec)	**FreAmine III 8.5%** (McGaw)
Amino Acid Concentration	8.5%	8.5%	8.5%
Nitrogen (g/100 ml)	1.3	1.43	1.3
Amino Acids (Essential) (mg/100 ml)			
Isoleucine	561	406	590
Leucine	850	526	770
Lysine	893	492	620
Methionine	146	492	450
Phenylalanine	253	526	480
Threonine	340	356	340
Tryptophan	170	152	130
Valine	425	390	560
Amino Acids (Nonessential) (mg/100 ml)			
Alanine	844	1760	600
Arginine	865	880	810
Histidine[1]	255	372	240
Proline	614	356	950
Serine	450		500
Taurine			
Tyrosine	230	34	
Aminoacetic Acid (Glycine)	425	1760	1190
Glutamic Acid	627		
Aspartic Acid	595		
Cysteine			< 20
Electrolytes (mEq/L)			
Sodium	33.3		10
Potassium			
Chloride		34	< 3
Acetate	61.1	73	72
Phosphate (mM/L)			10
Osmolarity (mOsm/L)	742	890	810
Supplied in (ml)	500[2] 1000[2]	500[3] 1000[3] 2000[3]	500[4] 1000[4]
Labeled Indications			
Peripheral Parenteral Nutrition	Yes	Yes	Yes
Central TPN	Yes	Yes	Yes
Protein Sparing	Yes	Yes	Yes

[1] Histidine is considered an essential amino acid in infants and in renal failure.
[2] Includes 20 mg/100 ml sodium hydrosulfite.
[3] With 3 mEq/L sodium bisulfite.
[4] With < 0.1 g sodium bisulfite per 100 ml.

(Continued on following page)

Protein Substrates (Cont.)

CRYSTALLINE AMINO ACID INFUSIONS

	TrophAmine 10% (McGaw)	Aminosyn 10% (Abbott)	Aminosyn-PF 10% (Abbott)	Aminosyn II 10% (Abbott)	Aminosyn (pH6) 10% (Abbott)
Amino Acid Concentration	10%	10%	10%	10%	10%
Nitrogen (g/100 ml)	1.55	1.57	1.52	1.53	1.57
Amino Acids (Essential) (mg/100 ml)					
Isoleucine	820	720	760	660	720
Leucine	1400	940	1200	1000	940
Lysine	820	720	677	1050	720
Methionine	340	400	180	172	400
Phenylalanine	480	440	427	298	440
Threonine	420	520	512	400	520
Tryptophan	200	160	180	200	160
Valine	780	800	673	500	800
Amino Acids (Nonessential) (mg/100 ml)					
Alanine	540	1280	698	993	1280
Arginine	1200	980	1227	1018	980
Histidine[1]	480	300	312	300	300
Proline	680	860	812	722	860
Serine	380	420	495	530	420
Taurine	25		70		
Tyrosine	240	44	40	270	44
Aminoacetic Acid (Glycine)	360	1280	385	500	1280
Glutamic Acid	500		620	738	
Aspartic Acid	320		527	700	
Cysteine	< 16				
Electrolytes (mEq/L)					
Sodium	5		3.4	45.3	
Potassium		5.4			2.7
Chloride	< 3				
Acetate	97	148	46.3	71.8	111
Phosphate (mM/L)10					
Osmolarity (mOsm/L)	875	1000	829	873	993
Supplied in (ml)	500[2]	500[3] 1000[3]	1000[4]	500[5] 1000[5]	500[6] 1000[6]
Labeled Indications					
Peripheral Parenteral Nutrition	Yes	Yes	Yes	Yes	Yes
Central TPN	Yes	Yes	Yes	Yes	Yes
Protein Sparing	No	Yes	No	Yes	Yes

[1] Histidine is considered an essential amino acid in infants and in renal failure.
[2] With < 50 mg sodium metabisulfite per ml.
[3] Includes 5.4 mEq/L potassium from the antioxidant potassium metabisulfite.
[4] With 230 mg sodium hydrosulfite per 100 ml.
[5] With 20 mg sodium hydrosulfite per 100 ml.
[6] Potassium derived from the antioxidant potassium metabisulfite.

(Continued on following page)

Protein Substrates (Cont.)

	CRYSTALLINE AMINO ACID INFUSIONS				
	Travasol 10% (Clintec)	**FreAmine III 10%** (McGaw)	**Novamine** (Clintec)	**Novamine 15%** (Clintec)	**Aminosyn II 15%** (Abbott)
Amino Acid Concentration	10%	10%	11.4%	15%	15%
Nitrogen (g/100 ml)	1.65	1.53	1.8	2.37	2.3
Amino Acids (Essential) (mg/100 ml)					
Isoleucine	600	690	570	749	990
Leucine	730	910	790	1040	1500
Lysine	580	730	900	1180	1575
Methionine	400	530	570	749	258
Phenylalanine	560	560	790	1040	447
Threonine	420	400	570	749	600
Tryptophan	180	150	190	250	300
Valine	580	660	730	960	750
Amino Acids (Nonessential) (mg/100 ml)					
Alanine	2070	710	1650	2170	1490
Arginine	1150	950	1120	1470	1527
Histidine[1]	480	280	680	894	450
Proline	680	1120	680	894	1083
Serine	500	590	450	592	795
Taurine					
Tyrosine	40		30	39	405
Aminoacetic Acid (Glycine)	1030	1400	790	1040	750
Glutamic Acid			570	749	1107
Aspartic Acid			330	434	1050
Cysteine		< 24			
Electrolytes (mEq/L)					
Sodium		10			62.7
Potassium					
Chloride	40	< 3			
Acetate	87	≈ 89	114	151	107.6
Phosphate (mM/L)		10			
Osmolarity (mOsm/L)	1000	≈ 950	1057	1388	1300
Supplied in (ml)	250[2,3] 500[2,3] 1000[2,3] 2000[2]	500[4] 1000[4]	500[5] 1000[5]	500[5] 1000[5]	2000[6]
Labeled Indications					
Peripheral Parenteral Nutrition	Yes	Yes	Yes	Yes	Yes
Central TPN	Yes	Yes	Yes	Yes	Yes
Protein Sparing	Yes	Yes	Yes	No	No

[1] Histidine is considered an essential amino acid in infants and in renal failure.
[2] Acetate in Viaflex container = 60 mEq/L; osmolarity is 970 mOsm/L.
[3] Sizes also come in Viaflex containers.
[4] With < 0.1 g sodium bisulfite per 100 ml.
[5] With 30 mg sodium metabisulfite.
[6] With 60 mg sodium hydrosulfite per 100 ml.

(Continued on following page)

Protein Substrates (Cont.)

CRYSTALLINE AMINO ACID INFUSIONS WITH ELECTROLYTES

	ProcalAmine (McGaw)	**FreAmine III 3% w/Electrolytes** (McGaw)	**Aminosyn 3.5% M** (Abbott)	**Aminosyn II 3.5% M** (Abbott)	**3.5% Travasol w/Electrolytes** (Clintec)	**5.5% Travasol w/Electrolytes** (Clintec)
Amino Acid Concentration	3%	3%	3.5%	3.5%	3.5%	5.5%
Nitrogen (g/100 ml)	0.46	0.46	0.55	0.54	0.591	0.925
Amino Acids (Essential) (mg/100 ml)						
Isoleucine	210	210	252	231	168	263
Leucine	270	270	329	350	217	340
Lysine	220	220	252	368	203	318
Methionine	160	160	140	60	203	318
Phenylalanine	170	170	154	104	217	340
Threonine	120	120	182	140	147	230
Tryptophan	46	46	56	70	63	99
Valine	200	200	280	175	161	252
Amino Acids (Nonessential) (mg/100 ml)						
Alanine	210	210	448	348	728	1140
Arginine	290	290	343	356	364	570
Histidine[1]	85	85	105	105	154	241
Proline	340	340	300	253	147	230
Serine	180	180	147	186		
Tyrosine			31	95	14	22
Glycine	420	420	448	175	728	1140
Glutamic Acid				258		
Aspartic Acid				245		
Cysteine	< 20	< 20				
Electrolytes (mEq/L)						
Sodium	35	35	47	36	25	70
Potassium	24	24.5	13	13	15	60
Magnesium	5	5	3	3	5	10
Chloride	41	41	40	37	25	70
Acetate	47	44	58	25	52	102
Phosphate (mM/L)	3.5	3.5	3.5	3.5	7.5	30
Osmolarity (mOsm/L)	735	≈ 405	477	425	450	850
Nonprotein Calories (g/100 ml) (glycerin)	3					
Supplied in (ml)	1000[2]	1000[3]	1000[4]	1000[5]	500[6] 1000[6]	500[6] 1000[6] 2000[6]
Labeled Indications						
Peripheral Parenteral Nutrition	Yes	Yes	Yes	Yes	Yes	Yes
Central TPN	No	No	No	No	No	Yes
Protein Sparing	Yes	Yes	Yes	Yes	Yes	Yes

[1] Histidine is considered an essential amino acid in infants and in renal failure.
[2] With < 50 mg K^+ metabisulfite and 3 mEq Ca/L.
[3] With < 0.05 g of the antioxidant potassium metabisulfite.
[4] Includes 7 mEq/L sodium from the antioxidant sodium hydrosulfite.
[5] With 20 mg sodium hydrosulfite per 100 ml.
[6] With 3 mEq/L sodium bisulfite.

(Continued on following page)

Protein Substrates (Cont.)

CRYSTALLINE AMINO ACID INFUSIONS WITH ELECTROLYTES

	Aminosyn 7% w/Electrolytes (Abbott)	Aminosyn II 7% with Electrolytes (Abbott)	Aminosyn 8.5% w/Electrolytes (Abbott)	Aminosyn II 8.5% with Electrolytes (Abbott)	FreAmine III 8.5% w/Electrolytes (McGaw)	Travasol 8.5% w/Electrolytes (Clintec)	Aminosyn II 10% with Electrolytes (Abbott)
Amino Acid Concentration	7%	7%	8.5%	8.5%	8.5%	8.5%	10%
Nitrogen g/100 ml	1.1	1.07	1.34	1.3	1.3	1.43	1.53
Amino Acids (Essential) (mg/100 ml)							
Isoleucine	510	462	620	561	590	406	660
Leucine	660	700	810	850	770	526	1000
Lysine	510	735	624	893	620	492	1050
Methionine	280	120	340	146	450	492	172
Phenylalanine	310	209	380	253	480	526	298
Threonine	370	280	460	340	340	356	400
Tryptophan	120	140	150	170	130	152	200
Valine	560	350	680	425	560	390	500
Amino Acids (Nonessential) (mg/100 ml)							
Alanine	900	695	1100	844	600	1760	993
Arginine	690	713	850	865	810	880	1018
Histidine[1]	210	210	260	255	240	372	300
Proline	610	505	750	614	950	356	722
Serine	300	371	370	450	500		530
Tyrosine	44	189	44	230		34	270
Glycine	900	350	1100	425	1190	1760	500
Glutamic Acid		517		627			738
Aspartic Acid		490		595			700
Cysteine					< 20		
Electrolytes (mEq/L)							
Sodium	70	76	70	80	60	70	87
Potassium	66	66	66	66	60	60	66
Magnesium	10	10	10	10	10	10	10
Chloride	96	86	98	86	60	70	86
Acetate	124	50	142	61	125	141	72
Phosphate (mM/L)	30	30	30	30	20	30	30
Osmolarity (mOsm/L)	1013	869	1160	999	1045	1160	1130
Supplied in (ml)	500[2]	500[3]	500[2]	500[3]	500[4] 1000[4]	500[5] 1000[5] 2000[5]	1000[3]
Labeled Indications							
Peripheral Parenteral Nutrition	Yes	Yes	Yes	Yes	Yes	Yes	Yes
Central TPN	Yes	Yes	Yes	Yes	Yes	Yes	Yes
Protein Sparing	Yes	Yes	Yes	Yes	Yes	Yes	Yes

[1] Histidine is considered an essential amino acid in infants and in renal failure.
[2] Includes 5.4 mEq/L potassium from the antioxidant potassium metabisulfite.
[3] Includes sodium from the antioxidant sodium hydrosulfite.
[4] With < 0.1 g sodium bisulfite per 100 ml.
[5] With 3 mEq/L sodium bisulfite.

(Continued on following page)

Protein Substrates (Cont.)

CRYSTALLINE AMINO ACID INFUSIONS WITH DEXTROSE

	Travasol 2.75% in 5% Dextrose[1] (Clintec)	Travasol 2.75% in 10% Dextrose[1] (Clintec)	Travasol 2.75% in 25% Dextrose[1] (Clintec)	Aminosyn II 3.5% in 5% Dextrose[1] (Abbott)	Aminosyn II 3.5% in 25% Dextrose[1] (Abbott)
Amino Acid Concentration	2.75%	2.75%	2.75%	3.5%	3.5%
Dextrose Concentration	5%	10%	25%	5%	25%
Nitrogen (g/100 ml)	0.46	0.46	0.46	0.54	0.54
Amino Acids (Essential) (mg/100 ml)					
Isoleucine	132	132	132	231	231
Leucine	170	170	170	350	350
Lysine	159	159	159	368	368
Methionine	159	159	159	60	60
Phenylalanine	170	170	170	104	104
Threonine	115	115	115	140	140
Tryptophan	50	50	50	70	70
Valine	126	126	126	175	175
Amino Acids (Nonessential) (mg/100 ml)					
Alanine	570	570	570	348	348
Arginine	285	285	285	356	356
Histidine[2]	120	120	120	105	105
Proline	115	115	115	252	252
Serine				186	186
Tyrosine	11	11	11	94	94
Aminoacetic Acid (Glycine)	570	570	570	175	175
Glutamic Acid				258	258
Aspartic Acid				245	245
Cysteine					
Electrolytes (mEq/L)					
Sodium				18	18
Potassium					
Magnesium					
Chloride	11	11	11		
Acetate	16	16	16	25.2	25.2
Phosphate (mM/L)					
Osmolarity (mOsm/L)	530	785	1540	585	1515
Supplied in (ml)	500 ml with 500 ml dextrose	500 ml with 500 ml dextrose	500 ml with 500 ml dextrose	1000 ml with 1000 ml dextrose[3]	500 ml with 500 ml dextrose[3]
Labeled Indications					
Peripheral Parenteral Nutrition	Yes	Yes	Yes	Yes	No
Central TPN	Yes	Yes	Yes	No	Yes

[1] Solution composition represents admixture of dual-chamber *Quick Mix* or *Nutrimix* container.
[2] Histidine is considered an essential amino acid in infants and in renal failure.
[3] With 30 mg sodium hydrosulfite per 100 ml.

(Continued on following page)

Protein Substrates (Cont.)

	CRYSTALLINE AMINO ACID INFUSIONS WITH DEXTROSE			
	Travasol 4.25% in 5% Dextrose[1] (Clintec)	**Aminosyn II 4.25% in 10% Dextrose**[1] (Abbott)	**Travasol 4.25% in 10% Dextrose**[1] (Clintec)	**Aminosyn II 4.25% in 20% Dextrose**[1] (Abbott)
Amino Acid Concentration	4.25%	4.25%	4.25%	4.25%
Dextrose Concentration	5%	10%	10%	20%
Nitrogen (g/100 ml)	0.7	0.65	0.7	0.65
Amino Acids (Essential) (mg/100 ml)				
Isoleucine	203	280	203	280
Leucine	263	425	263	425
Lysine	246	446	246	446
Methionine	246	73	246	73
Phenylalanine	263	126	263	126
Threonine	178	170	178	170
Tryptophan	76	85	76	85
Valine	195	212	195	212
Amino Acids (Nonessential) (mg/100 ml)				
Alanine	880	422	880	422
Arginine	440	432	440	432
Histidine[2]	186	128	186	128
Proline	178	307	178	307
Serine		225		225
Tyrosine	17	115	17	115
Aminoacetic Acid (Glycine)	880	212	880	212
Glutamic Acid		314		314
Aspartic Acid		298		298
Cysteine				
Electrolytes (mEq/L)				
Sodium		19		19
Potassium				
Magnesium				
Chloride	17		17	
Acetate	22	30.6	22	30.6
Phosphate (mM/L)				
Osmolarity (mOsm/L)	680	894	935	1295
Supplied in (ml)	500 ml with 500 ml dextrose	1000 ml with 1000 ml dextrose[3]	500 ml with 500 ml dextrose	1000 ml with 1000 ml dextrose[3]
Labeled Indications				
Peripheral Parenteral Nutrition	Yes	Yes	Yes	No
Central TPN	Yes	No	Yes	Yes

[1] Solution composition represents admixture of dual-chamber *Quick Mix* or *Nutrimix* container.
[2] Histidine is considered an essential amino acid in infants and in renal failure.
[3] With 30 mg sodium hydrosulfite per 100 ml.

(Continued on following page)

Protein Substrates (Cont.)

	CRYSTALLINE AMINO ACID INFUSIONS WITH DEXTROSE		
	Aminosyn II 4.25% in 25% Dextrose[1] (Abbott)	**Travasol 4.25% in 25% Dextrose**[1] (Clintec)	**Aminosyn II 5% in 25% Dextrose**[1] (Abbott)
Amino Acid Concentration	4.25%	4.25%	5%
Dextrose Concentration	25%	25%	25%
Nitrogen (g/100 ml)	0.65	0.65	0.77
Amino Acids (Essential) (mg/100 ml)			
Isoleucine	280	203	330
Leucine	425	263	500
Lysine	446	246	525
Methionine	73	246	86
Phenylalanine	126	263	149
Threonine	170	178	200
Tryptophan	85	76	100
Valine	212	195	250
Amino Acids (Nonessential) (mg/100 ml)			
Alanine	422	880	496
Arginine	432	440	509
Histidine[2]	128	186	150
Proline	307	178	361
Serine	225		265
Tyrosine	115	17	135
Aminoacetic Acid (Glycine)	212	880	250
Glutamic Acid	314		369
Aspartic Acid	298		350
Cysteine			
Electrolytes (mEq/L)			
Sodium	19		22.2
Potassium			
Magnesium			
Chloride		17	
Acetate	30.6	22	35.9
Phosphate (mM/L)			
Osmolarity (mOsm/L)	1536	1690	1539
Supplied in (ml)	750 and 1000 ml and 750 and 1000 ml dextrose[3]	500 ml with 500 ml dextrose[3]	500, 750 and 1000 ml and 500, 750 and 1000 ml dextrose[3]
Labeled Indications			
Peripheral Parenteral Nutrition	No	Yes	No
Central TPN	Yes	Yes	Yes

[1] Solution composition represents admixture of dual-chamber *Quick Mix* and *Nutrimix* container.
[2] Histidine is considered an essential amino acid in infants and in renal failure.
[3] With 30 mg sodium hydrosulfite per 100 ml.

(Continued on following page)

Protein Substrates (Cont.)

	CRYSTALLINE AMINO ACID INFUSIONS WITH ELECTROLYTES IN DEXTROSE	
	Aminosyn II 3.5% M[1] **in 5% Dextrose** [2] (Abbott)	**Aminosyn II 4.25% M**[1] **in 10% Dextrose** [2] (Abbott)
Amino Acid Concentration	3.5%	4.25%
Dextrose Concentration	5%	10%
Nitrogen (g/100 ml)	0.535	0.65
Amino Acids (Essential) (mg/100 ml)		
Isoleucine	231	280
Leucine	350	425
Lysine	368	446
Methionine	60	73
Phenylalanine	104	126
Threonine	140	170
Tryptophan	70	85
Valine	175	212
Amino Acids (Nonessential) (mg/100 ml)		
Alanine	348	422
Arginine	356	432
Histidine[3]	105	128
Proline	252	307
Serine	186	225
Tyrosine	94	115
Aminoacetic Acid (Glycine)	175	212
Glutamic Acid	258	314
Aspartic Acid	245	298
Cysteine		
Electrolytes (mEq/L)		
Sodium	41	43.7
Potassium	13	13
Magnesium	3	3
Chloride	36.5	36.5
Acetate	25.1	30.5
Phosphorus (mM/L)	3.5	3.5
Osmolarity (mOsm/L)	616	919
Supplied in (ml)	500 and 1000 ml and 500 and 1000 ml dextrose[4]	500 ml and 500 ml dextrose[4]
Labeled Indications		
Peripheral Parenteral Nutrition	Yes	Yes
Central TPN	No	Yes
Protein Sparing	No	No

[1] With maintenance electrolytes.
[2] Solution composition represents admixture of *Nutrimix* dual-chamber container.
[3] Histidine is considered an essential amino acid in infants and in renal failure.
[4] With 30 mg sodium hydrosulfite per 100 ml.

For a complete discussion of the use of protein substrates for intravenous nutritional therapy, refer to the general monograph beginning on page 100

Protein Substrates (Cont.)

AMINO ACID FORMULATIONS FOR RENAL FAILURE

Actions:

Patients with renal decompensation have different amino acid requirements than those with normal renal function. Use in uremic patients is based on the minimal requirements for each of the 8 essential amino acids. These products contain histidine, an amino acid considered essential for infant growth and for uremic patients.

In renal failure, nonspecific nitrogen-containing compounds are broken down in the intestine. The ammonia formed is absorbed and incorporated by the liver into nonessential amino acids, provided essential amino acid requirements are being met. Exogenously supplying only essential amino acids allows urea nitrogen to be recycled which can serve as a precursor for nonessential amino acid synthesis. Therefore, administration to uremic patients, particularly those who are protein deficient, results in the utilization of retained urea, and may be followed by a drop in BUN and resolution of many azotemic symptoms.

Infusion of essential amino acids and hypertonic dextrose promotes protein synthesis, improves cellular metabolic balance, decreases the rate of rise of BUN and minimizes deterioration of serum potassium, magnesium and phosphorus balance in patients with impaired renal function. This therapy may decrease morbidity associated with acute renal failure and promote earlier return of renal function. Although controversial, these formulations may have no clinically significant advantage over the general formulations containing both essential and nonessential amino acids in most uremic patients.

Indications:

For nutritional support of uremic patients, particularly when oral nutrition is impractical, not feasible or insufficient.

Essential amino acid injection does not replace dialysis and conventional supportive therapy in patients with renal failure. To promote urea reutilization, provide adequate calories with minimal amounts of essential amino acids and restrict the intake of nonessential nitrogen.

Children: Use with caution in pediatric patients, especially low birth weight infants, due to limited clinical experience. Laboratory and clinical monitoring must be extensive and frequent. Use a low initial dose and increase slowly.

The absence of arginine in *NephrAmine* and *Aminess* may accentuate the risk of hyperammonemia in infants. *Aminosyn-RF* and *RenAmin* contain arginine.

Dosage:

Provide adequate calories simultaneously. Administer essential amino acid/dextrose mixtures by continuous infusion through a central venous catheter. Use slow initial infusion rates, generally 20 to 30 ml/hour for the first 6 to 8 hours. Increase by 10 ml/hour each 24 hours, up to a maximum of 60 to 100 ml/hour.

Administration rate is governed by the patient's nitrogen, fluid and glucose tolerance. Uremic patients are frequently glucose intolerant, especially in association with peritoneal dialysis, and may require exogenous insulin to prevent hyperglycemia. To prevent rebound hypoglycemia when hypertonic dextrose infusions are abruptly discontinued, administer a 5% dextrose solution.

Adults:

Aminosyn-RF – 300 to 600 ml. Mix 300 ml with 500 ml of 70% dextrose to provide a solution of 1.96% essential amino acids in 44% dextrose (calorie:nitrogen ratio = 504:1).

Aminess – 400 ml. Mix 400 ml with 500 ml of 70% dextrose to yield a solution of 2.3% essential amino acids in 39% dextrose (calorie:nitrogen ratio = 450:1).

NephrAmine – 250 to 500 ml. Mix 250 ml w/500 ml of 70% dextrose to yield solution of 1.8% essential amino acids in 47% dextrose (calorie:nitrogen ratio = 744:1).

RenAmin – 250 to 500 ml.

Children: Individualize dosage. A dosage of 0.5 to 1 g/kg/day will meet the requirements of the majority of pediatric patients. Use a low initial daily dosageand increase slowly; > 1 g/kg/day is not recommended.

(Products listed on following page)

Protein Substrates (Cont.)

AMINO ACID FORMULATIONS FOR RENAL FAILURE (Cont.)

	Aminosyn-RF 5.2% (Abbott)	**Aminess 5.2%** (Clintec)	**5.4% NephrAmine** (McGaw)	**RenAmin** (Clintec)
Amino Acid Concentration	5.2%	5.2%	5.4%	6.5%
Nitrogen (g/100 ml)	0.79	0.66	0.65	1
Amino Acids (Essential) (mg/100 ml)				
Isoleucine	462	525	560	500
Leucine	726	825	880	600
Lysine	535	600	640	450
Methionine	726	825	880	500
Phenylalanine	726	825	880	490
Threonine	330	375	400	380
Tryptophan	165	188	200	160
Valine	528	600	640	820
Histidine	429	412	250	420
Amino Acids (Nonessential) (mg/100 ml)				
Cysteine			< 20	
Arginine	600			630
Alanine				560
Proline				350
Glycine				300
Serine				300
Tyrosine				40
Electrolytes (mEq/L)				
Sodium			5	
Acetate	≈ 105	50	≈ 44	60
Potassium	5.4			
Chloride			< 3	31
Osmolarity (mOsm/L)	475	416	435	600
Supplied in (ml)	300[1]	400[2]	250[3]	250[4] 500[4]

[1] With 60 mg potassium metabisulfite per 100 ml.
[2] In 500 ml bottle.
[3] With < 0.05 g sodium bisulfite per 100 ml.
[4] With ≈ 3 mEq sodium bisulfite.

For a complete discussion of the use of protein substrates as a compound of intravenous nutritional therapy, refer to the general monograph beginning on page 100.

Protein Substrates (Cont.)

AMINO ACID FORMULATIONS FOR HIGH METABOLIC STRESS

Actions:

These formulations are mixtures of essential and nonessential amino acids with high concentrations of the branched chain amino acids (BCAA), isoleucine, leucine and valine.

Acute metabolic stress is characterized by increased urinary nitrogen excretion and hyperglycemia; glucose utilization and fat store mobilization are impaired. The primary substrates used to meet energy requirements of muscle are BCAAs.

Indications:

To prevent nitrogen loss or treat negative nitrogen balance in adults if: (1) The alimentary tract, by oral, gastrostomy or jejunostomy route, cannot or should not be used, or adequate protein intake is not feasible by these routes; (2) GI protein absorption is impaired; or (3) nitrogen homeostasis is substantially impaired as with severe trauma or sepsis.

Dosage:

Daily amino acid doses of ≈ 1.5 g/kg for adults with adequate calories generally satisfy protein needs and promote positive nitrogen balance. Higher doses may be required in severely catabolic states. Fat emulsion may help meet energy requirements.

For severely catabolic, depleted patients or those requiring long-term TPN, consider central venous nutrition. Start TPN with infusates containing lower concentrations of dextrose; gradually increase dextrose content to estimated caloric needs as glucose tolerance increases. *FreAmine HBC* 750 ml and 250 ml 70% dextrose or 500 ml *Aminosyn-HBC* 7% and 500 ml concentrated dextrose, with added electrolytes, trace metals and vitamins, may be given over 8 hours. *BranchAmin* 4% must be admixed with a complete amino acid injection, with or without a concentrated caloric source.

For moderately catabolic, depleted patients in whom the central venous route is not indicated, diluted *FreAmine HBC* or *Aminosyn-HBC* 7% with minimal caloric supplementation may be infused by peripheral vein, supplemented, if desired, with fat emulsion.

Usual administration of 4% BCAA Injection is used as a supplement to parenteral nutrition solutions to achieve an amino acid solution that is ≈ 50% w/w BCAA. One method for achieving this ratio is the admixture of two volumes of 4% BCAA Injection at 4 g/dl concentration with one volume of an amino acid solution of 8 to 10 g/dl concentration. The supplemental amino acid mixture is given with energy substrates to provide at least 35 kcal/kg ideal body weight as nonprotein calories.

AMINO ACID FORMULATION IN HEPATIC FAILURE/HEPATIC ENCEPHALOPATHY

Actions:

This formulation is a mixture of essential and nonessential amino acids with high concentrations of the BCAAs, isoleucine, leucine and valine.

Hepatic failure/Hepatic encephalopathy: The etiopathology of hepatic encephalopathy is unknown and multifactorial. The rationale for BCAA therapy is based on studies in which BCAA infusions reversed the abnormal plasma amino acid pattern characterized by lower BCAA levels and elevated levels of aromatic amino acids and methionine. Normalization of these amino acids improved mental status and EEG patterns. Nitrogen balance was significantly improved and mortality reduced in these typically protein-intolerant patients who received substantial amounts of protein equivalents.

Indications:

For the treatment of hepatic encephalopathy in patients with cirrhosis or hepatitis. Provides nutritional support for patients with these diseases of the liver who require parenteral nutrition and are intolerant of general purpose amino acid injections, which are contraindicated in patients with hepatic coma.

Dosage:

Give 80 to 120 g amino acids (12 to 18 g nitrogen)/day. Typically, 500 ml *HepatAmine* mixed with ≈ 500 ml of 50% dextrose supplemented with electrolytes and vitamins is given over 8 to 12 hours. This results in a total daily fluid intake of ≈ 2 to 3 L. Patients with fluid restrictions may only tolerate 1 to 2 L. Although nitrogen requirements may be higher in severely hypercatabolic or depleted patients, provision of additional nitrogen may not be possible due to fluid intake limits, nitrogen or glucose intolerance.

Use slow initial infusion rates; gradually increase to 60 to 125 ml/hr.

Peripheral vein administration is indicated with or without parenteral carbohydrate calories for patients in whom the central venous route is not indicated and who can consume adequate calories enterally. Prepare infusates by dilution of *HepatAmine* with Sterile Water for Injection or 5% to 10% Dextrose to prepare isotonic or slightly hypertonic solutions; accompany with adequate caloric supplementation.

(Products listed on following page)

Protein Substrates (Cont.)

AMINO ACID FORMULATIONS FOR HIGH METABOLIC STRESS AND IN HEPATIC FAILURE/HEPATIC ENCEPHALOPATHY (Cont.)

	STRESS FORMULATION			HEPATIC FORMULATION
	4% BranchAmin (Clintec)	**FreAmine HBC 6.9%** (McGaw)	**Aminosyn-HBC 7%** (Abbott)	**HepatAmine** (McGaw)
Amino Acid Concentration	4%	6.9%	7%	8%
Nitrogen (g/100 ml)	0.443	0.97	1.12	1.2
Amino Acids (Essential) (mg/100 ml)				
Isoleucine	1380	760	789	900
Leucine	1380	1370	1576	1100
Lysine		410	265	610
Methionine		250	206	100
Phenylalanine		320	228	100
Threonine		200	272	450
Tryptophan		90	88	66
Valine	1240	880	789	840
Amino Acids (Nonessential) (mg/100 ml)				
Alanine		400	660	770
Arginine		580	507	600
Histidine[1]		160	154	240
Proline		630	448	800
Serine		330	221	500
Tyrosine			33	
Glycine		330	660	900
Cysteine		<20		<20
Electrolytes (mEq/L)				
Sodium		10	7[4]	10
Chloride		<3		<3
Acetate		≈57	72	≈62
Phosphate (mM/L)				10
Osmolarity (mOsm/L)	316	620	665	785
Supplied in (ml)	500	750[2,3]	500[4] 1000[4]	500[2]
Labeled Indications				
Peripheral Parenteral Nutrition	Yes[5]	Yes	Yes	Yes
Central TPN	Yes[5]	Yes	Yes	Yes

[1] Histidine is considered an essential amino acid in infants and in renal failure.
[2] With < 100 mg sodium bisulfite/100 ml.
[3] In 1000 ml bottles.
[4] With 60 mg sodium hydrosulfite.
[5] Must be admixed with a complete amino acid injection.

For a complete discussion of the use of protein substrates as a component of intravenous nutritional therapy, refer to the general monograph beginning on page 100.

Protein Substrates (Cont.)

CYSTEINE HCl

Actions:

Cysteine is a sulfur-containing amino acid. It is synthesized from methionine via the trans-sulfuration pathway in the adult, but newborn infants lack the enzyme necessary to effect this conversion. Therefore, cysteine is generally considered an essential amino acid in infants.

Metabolism of cysteine produces pyruvate and inorganic sulfate as end products. Cysteine is introduced directly into the pathway of carbohydrate metabolism at the pyruvate stage with all three carbons convertible to glucose. The sulfur is primarily transformed to inorganic sulfate, which is introduced into complex polysaccharides among other structural components.

In premixed solutions of crystalline amino acids, cysteine is relatively unstable over time, eventually converting to insoluble cystine. To avoid such precipitation, cysteine is provided as an additive for use with crystalline amino acid solutions immediately prior to administration.

Indications:

Use only after dilution as an additive to *Aminosyn* to meet the IV amino acid nutritional requirements of infants receiving total parenteral nutrition.

Administration and Dosage:

Use only after dilution in *Aminosyn.* Combine each 0.5 g of cysteine with 12.5 g of amino acids, such as that present in 250 ml of *Aminosyn* 5%, then dilute with 250 ml of 50% Dextrose or lesser volume as indicated. Equal volumes of *Aminosyn* 5% and 50% Dextrose produce a final solution containing *Aminosyn* 2.5% and 25% Dextrose, which is suitable for administration by central venous infusion.

Storage: Avoid excessive heat. Do not freeze. Begin administration of the final admixture within 1 hour of mixing; otherwise, immediately refrigerate the mixture and use within 24 hours.

Rx	**Cysteine HCl** (Various, eg, Abbott, Gensia)	**Injection:** 50 mg per ml	In 10 ml additive syringe and single dose vials.

Carbohydrates

DEXTROSE (d-GLUCOSE)

Actions:

Pharmacology: A source of calories and fluids in patients unable to obtain adequate oral intake. Parenterally injected dextrose undergoes oxidation to carbon dioxide and water, and provides 3.4 calories per gram of d-glucose monohydrate (molecular weight 198.17). A 5% solution is isotonic and is administered by IV infusion into peripheral veins. Concentrated dextrose infusions are used to provide increased caloric intake with less fluid volume; they may be irritating if given by peripheral infusions. Therefore, administer highly concentrated solutions only by central venous catheters.

Dextrose injections may induce diuresis. Dextrose is readily metabolized, may decrease body protein and nitrogen losses, promotes glycogen deposition, and decreases or prevents ketosis if sufficient doses are provided.

Caloric Content and Osmolarity of the Various Concentrations of Dextrose

Dextrose concentration		Caloric content (Cal/L)	Osmolarity (mOsm/L)
%	g/L		
2.5	25	85	126
5	50	170	253
10	100	340	505
20	200	680	1010
25	250	850	1330
30	300	1020	1515
40	400	1360	2020
50	500	1700	2525
60	600	2040	3030
70	700	2380	3535

Indications:

2.5%, 5% and 10%: Used for peripheral infusion to provide calories whenever fluid and caloric replacement are required.

25% (hypertonic): Acute symptomatic episodes of hypoglycemia in the neonate or older infant to restore depressed blood glucose levels and control symptoms.

50%: Used in the treatment of insulin hypoglycemia (hyperinsulinemia or insulin shock) to restore blood glucose levels.

10%, 20%, 30%, 40%, 50%, 60%, and 70% (hypertonic): For infusion after admixture with other solutions such as amino acids.

Unlabeled uses: Hypertonic solutions of 25% to 50% have been used as a sclerosing agent for the treatment of varicose veins, as an irritant to produce adhesive pleuritis and to reduce cerebrospinal pressure and cerebral edema caused by delirium tremens or acute alcohol intoxication.

Contraindications:

In diabetic coma while blood sugar is excessively high.

Concentrated solutions: When intracranial or intraspinal hemorrhage is present; in the presence of delirium tremens in dehydrated patients; in patients with severe hydration, anuria, hepatic coma or glucose-galactose malabsorption syndrome.

Warnings:

Fluid/Solute overload: Dextrose solutions IV can cause fluid or solute overload resulting in dilution of serum electrolyte concentrations, overhydration, congested states or pulmonary edema.

Hypertonic dextrose solutions may cause thrombosis if infused via peripheral veins; therefore, administer via a central venous catheter.

Diabetes mellitus: Use dextrose-containing solutions with caution in patients with subclinical or overt diabetes mellitus or carbohydrate intolerance.

Rapid administration of hypertonic solutions may produce significant hyperglycemia or hyperosmolar syndrome, especially in patients with chronic uremia or carbohydrate intolerance.

(Warnings continued on following page)

Carbohydrates (Cont.)

DEXTROSE (d-Glucose) (Cont.)

Warnings (Cont.):

Pregnancy: Category C. It is not known whether dextrose can cause fetal harm when administered to a pregnant woman or can affect reproduction capacity. Use only when clearly needed. Dextrose crosses the placenta; however, insulin does not cross the placenta and the fetus is responsible for its own insulin production in response to the dextrose. Therefore, administer dextrose to a pregnant woman with caution. One report recommends an infusion rate of 3.5 to 7 g/hour since doses > 10 g/hr cause increases in fetal insulin.

Lactation: Exercise caution when administering dextrose to a nursing woman.

Children: Use with caution in infants of diabetic mothers, except as may be indicated in hypoglycemic neonates.

Precautions:

Monitoring: Perform clinical evaluations and laboratory determinations to monitor fluid balance, electrolyte concentrations and acid-base balance.

Hyperglycemia and glycosuria may be functions of rate of administration or metabolic insufficiency. To minimize these conditions, slow the infusion rate, monitor blood and urine glucose; if necessary, administer insulin. When concentrated dextrose infusion is abruptly withdrawn, administer 5% or 10% dextrose to avoid rebound hypoglycemia.

Extravasation: Administer so that extravasation does not occur. If thrombosis occurs during administration, stop injection and correct.

Hypokalemia: Excessive administration of potassium free solutions may result in significant hypokalemia. Add potassium to dextrose solutions and administer to fasting patients with good renal function, especially those on digitalis therapy.

Vitamin B complex deficiency may occur with dextrose administration.

Drug Interactions:

Corticosteroids: Cautiously administer parenteral fluids, especially those containing sodium ions, to patients receiving corticosteroids or corticotropin.

Adverse Reactions:

Febrile response; infection at the injection site; tissue necrosis; venous thrombosis or phlebitis extending from the site of injection; extravasation; hypovolemia; hypervolemia; dehydration; mental confusion or unconsciousness. These may occur because of the solution or administration technique. Use the largest available peripheral vein and a well placed small bore needle.

Hypertonic solutions are more likely to cause irritation; administer into larger central veins. Significant hyperglycemia, hyperosmolar syndrome and glycosuria may occur with too rapid administration of hypertonic solutions.

Overdosage:

In the event of a fluid or solute overload during parenteral therapy, reevaluate the patient's condition and institute appropriate corrective treatment.

Administration and Dosage:

Do not administer concentrated solutions SC or IM.

The concentration and dose depend on the patient's age, weight and clinical condition. Add electrolytes based on fluid and electrolyte status.

The maximum rate at which dextrose can be infused without producing glycosuria is 0.5 g/kg/hour. About 95% is retained when infused at 0.8 g/kg/hour.

Insulin-induced hypoglycemia: Determine blood glucose before injecting dextrose. In emergencies, promptly administer without waiting for pretreatment test results.

Adults - 10 to 25 g. Repeated doses may be required in severe cases.

Neonates - 250 to 500 mg/kg/dose (5 to 10 ml of 25% dextrose in a 5 kg infant) to control acute symptomatic hypoglycemia.

Severe cases or older infants - Larger or repeated single doses up to 10 or 12 ml of 25% dextrose may be required. Subsequent continuous IV infusion of 10% dextrose may be needed to stabilize blood glucose levels.

Admixture incompatibilities: Additives may be incompatible. When introducing additives, use aseptic technique, mix thoroughly and do not store.

Do not administer dextrose simultaneously with **blood** through the same infusion set because pseudoagglutination of red cells may occur.

Storage/Stability: Do not use unless solution is clear. Discard unused portion. Protect from freezing and extreme heat.

(Products listed on following page)

Carbohydrates (Cont.)

DEXTROSE IN WATER INJECTION

Rx	**D-2.5-W** (Various, eg, Abbott, Clintec)	2.5%	In 1000 ml.
Rx	**D-5-W** (Various, eg, Abbott, Clintec, IMS, McGaw)	5%	In 25, 50, 100, 150, 250, 500 and 1000 ml vials and 10 ml syringes, 25 ml fill in 150 ml, 50 ml fill in 250 ml and 100 ml fill in 250 ml vials.
Rx	**D-10-W** (Various, eg, Abbott, Clintec, Elkins-Sinn, McGaw, Solopak, Winthrop)	10%	In 3 ml amps, 250, 500 and 1000 ml vials, 17 ml fill in 20 ml, 500 ml fill in 1000 ml, and 1000 ml fill in 2000 ml vials.
Rx	**D-20-W** (Various, eg, Abbott, Clintec, McGaw)	20%	In 500 ml vials, 500 ml fill in 1000 ml and 1000 ml fill in 2000 ml.
Rx	**D-25-W** (Various, eg, Abbott, IMS)	25%	In 10 ml syringes.
Rx	**D-30-W** (Various, eg, Abbott, Clintec, McGaw)	30%	In 500 and 1000 ml, 500 ml fill in 1000 ml and 1000 ml fill in 2000 ml.
Rx	**D-40-W** (Various, eg, Abbott, Clintec, McGaw)	40%	In 500 and 1000 ml, 500 ml fill in 1000 ml and 1000 ml fill in 2000 ml.
Rx	**D-50-W** (Various, eg, Abbott, Astra, Clintec, IMS, McGaw, Lyphomed, Pasadena, Schein)	50%	In 500, 1000 and 2000 ml and 50 ml amps, vials and syringes and 500 ml fill in 1000 ml and 1000 ml fill in 2000 ml.
Rx	**D-60-W** (Various, eg, Abbott, Clintec, McGaw)	60%	In 500 and 1000 ml, 500 ml fill in 1000 ml and 1000 ml fill in 2000 ml.
Rx	**D-70-W** (Various, eg, Abbott, Clintec, McGaw)	70%	In 70, 1000 and 2000 ml, 500 ml fill in 1000 ml and 1000 ml fill in 2000 ml.

For specific information on dextrose, refer to the individual monograph.

Carbohydrates (Cont.)

ALCOHOL (ETHANOL) IN DEXTROSE INFUSIONS

Actions:

Alcohol in dextrose solutions are an intravenous source of carbohydrate calories that restore blood glucose levels. Each ml of alcohol provides 5.6 calories; each gram of d-glucose monohydrate provides 3.4 calories. Dextrose may aid in minimizing liver glycogen depletion and exerts a protein-sparing action.

Pharmacokinetics: Metabolism – Ethyl alcohol is metabolized at a rate of approximately 10 to 20 ml/hour. Sedative effects of alcohol occur if the rate of infusion exceeds the rate of metabolism. Dextrose (d-glucose) can be infused at a maximum rate of approximately 0.5 to 0.85 g/kg/hour without producing significant glycosuria. Thus, the maximum rate that alcohol can be infused without producing sedative effects is well below the maximum rate of utilization of dextrose. Alcohol is metabolized (mostly in the liver) to acetaldehyde or acetate; the rate of oxidation is linear with time. Starvation lowers the rate of metabolism and insulin increases the rate.

Indications:

Increasing caloric intake and replenishing fluids.

Unlabeled use: Premature labor – Infusion of a 10% solution of ethyl alcohol IV causes a decrease in uterine activity during labor, presumably by inhibiting the release of oxytocin from the posterior pituitary, and has been used to prevent premature delivery. However, this use has largely been replaced by other therapies (eg, β-adrenergic therapy).

Contraindications:

Epilepsy; urinary tract infection; alcoholism; diabetic coma.

Warnings:

Special risk patients: Use alcohol cautiously in shock, following cranial surgery and in actual or anticipated postpartum hemorrhage.

Diabetic patients: Alcohol decreases blood sugar in these patients. In the untreated diabetic, the rate of alcohol metabolism is slowed.

Vitamin deficiencies: As a nutrient, alcohol supplies only calories; given alone it may cause or potentiate vitamin deficiencies and liver function disturbances.

IV administration of this solution can cause fluid or solute overload resulting in dilution of serum electrolyte concentrations, overhydration, congested states or pulmonary edema.

Extravasation: Avoid extravasation during IV administration; do not give SC.

Pseudoagglutination/Hemolysis: Do not administer simultaneously with blood because of possibility of pseudoagglutination or hemolysis.

Hepatic/Renal function impairment: Use alcohol cautiously.

Pregnancy: Category C. It is not known whether alcohol can cause fetal harm when administered to a pregnant woman or can affect reproduction capacity. Use only when clearly needed. Alcohol crosses the placenta rapidly and enters the fetal circulation.

Fetal Alcohol Syndrome (FAS), a pattern of fetal anomalies, is associated with chronic maternal alcohol consumption of 60 to 75 ml absolute alcohol (4 to 5 drinks) per day; mild FAS is associated with ingestion of as little as 30 ml per day. Features of FAS involve craniofacial, limb, growth, and CNS anomalies. Other reported problems involve cardiac and urogenital defects, liver abnormalities and hemangiomas. Behavioral problems may be long-term. Moderate drinking (> 1 ounce absolute alcohol twice/week) is associated with second trimester spontaneous abortions.

Administration of alcohol prior to delivery may cause intoxication and depression of the newborn.

Lactation: Alcohol passes freely into breast milk approximately equivalent to maternal serum levels; however, effects on the infant are generally insignificant until maternal blood levels reach 300 mg/dl. The American Academy of Pediatrics considers alcohol use in the mother compatible with breastfeeding, although adverse effects may occur.

Alcohol may cause potentiation of severe hypoprothrombic bleeding, a pseudo-Cushing syndrome and a reduction in the milk-ejecting response.

Children: Safety and efficacy in children have not been established. See Administration and Dosage.

Precautions:

Administer slowly and observe patient for restlessness or narcosis.

Gout: Alcohol increases serum uric acid and can precipitate acute gout.

Monitoring: Clinical evaluation and periodic laboratory determinations are necessary to monitor changes in fluid balance, electrolyte concentrations and acid-base balance.

(Continued on following page)

ALCOHOL (ETHANOL) IN DEXTROSE INFUSIONS (Cont.)

Drug Interactions:

The following interactions may occur with alcohol administration. Those interactions that may only occur with long-term oral alcohol ingestion have not been included.

Alcohol Drug Interactions			
Precipitant drug	Object drug*		Description
Barbiturates, Benzodiazepines, Chloral hydrate, Glutethimide, Meprobamate, Metoclopramide, Phenothiazines	Alcohol	↑	Increased CNS depressant effects may occur.
Cephalosporins[1], Chlorpropamide, Disulfiram, Furazolidone, Metronidazole, Procarbazine	Alcohol	↑	A disulfiram-like reaction consisting of facial flushing, lightheadedness, weakness, sweating, tachycardia, nausea or vomiting may occur.
Alcohol	Antidiabetic agents (insulin, phenformin, sulfonylureas)	↑	Because of altered glucose metabolism, the pharmacologic effects of these agents may be increased by alcohol resulting in hypoglycemia. In addition, alcohol may contribute to the lactic acidosis that is sometimes observed following phenformin administration. Both hypo- and hyperglycemia have occurred with sulfonylureas and alcohol.
Alcohol	Bromocriptine	↑	Intolerance of bromocriptine due to the severity of side effects has occurred with concurrent alcohol.
Alcohol	Salicylates	↑	Alcohol may potentiate aspirin-induced GI blood loss and bleeding time prolongation.

* ↑ = Object drug increased [1] Those agents with a methyltetrazolethiol moiety.

Adverse Reactions:

Fever; infection at the injection site; venous thrombosis or phlebitis; extravasation; hypervolemia. These may occur because of the solution or administration technique.

Alcoholic intoxication may occur with too rapid infusion. Vertigo, flushing, disorientation (especially in elderly patients), or sedation may also occur. An alcoholic odor may be noted on the breath. Generally, these effects can be avoided by slowing the rate of infusion. Too rapid infusion of hypertonic solutions may cause local pain and, rarely, excessive vein irritation. Use the largest available peripheral vein and a well placed small bore needle.

Overdosage:

In the event of alcoholic intoxication or sedation, slow the infusion or discontinue temporarily. If overhydration or solute overload occurs, reevaluate the patient and institute appropriate corrective measures.

Administration and Dosage:

Administer by slow IV infusion only; do not give SC. Individualize dosage. The average adult can metabolize approximately 10 ml/hour (200 ml of 5% solution or 100 ml of 10% solution). The usual adult dosage is 1 to 2 L and rarely exceeds 3 L of a 5% solution in a 24 hour period. Children may be given 40 ml/kg/24 hours or from 350 to 1000 ml, depending on size and clinical response.

Storage/Stability: Do not use unless solution is clear and seal is intact. Discard unused portion. Protect from freezing and extreme heat.

		Cal/L	mOsm/L	How Supplied
Rx	**5% Alcohol and 5% Dextrose in Water** (Abbott, Clintec)	450	1114	In 1000 ml.
Rx	**5% Alcohol and 5% Dextrose in Water** (McGaw)		1125	In 1000 ml.
Rx	**10% Alcohol and 5% Dextrose in Water** (McGaw)	720	1995	In 1000 ml.

Refer to the general discussion beginning in the IV Nutritional Therapy monograph.

Lipids

INTRAVENOUS FAT EMULSION

Warning:

Deaths in preterm infants after infusion of IV fat emulsions have occurred. Autopsy findings included intravascular fat accumulation in the lungs. Treatment of premature and low birth weight infants with IV fat emulsion must be based on careful benefit-risk assessment. Strict adherence to the recommended total daily dose is mandatory; hourly infusion rate should be as slow as possible and should not exceed 1 g/kg in 4 hours. Premature and small for gestational age infants have poor clearance of IV fat emulsion and increased free fatty acid plasma levels following fat emulsion infusion; therefore, administer less than the maximum recommended doses in these patients to decrease the likelihood of IV fat overload. Monitor the infant's ability to eliminate the infused fat from the circulation (such as triglycerides or plasma free fatty acid levels). The lipemia must clear between daily infusions.

Actions:

Pharmacology: Intravenous fat emulsions are prepared from either soybean or safflower oil and provide a mixture of neutral triglycerides, predominantly unsaturated fatty acids. The major component of fatty acids are linoleic, oleic, palmitic, stearic and linolenic acids; see product listings for content. In addition, these products contain 1.2% egg yolk phospholipids as an emulsifier and glycerol to adjust tonicity. The emulsified fat particles are approximately 0.4 to 0.5 microns in diameter, similar to naturally occurring chylomicrons. IV fat emulsions are isotonic and may be given by central or peripheral venous routes.

These products are metabolized and utilized as a source of energy, causing an increase in heat production, decrease in respiratory quotient and an increase in oxygen consumption following administration. The infused fat particles are cleared from the blood stream in a manner thought to be comparable to the clearing of chylomicrons.

Essential Fatty Acid Deficiency (EFAD): Linoleic, linolenic and arachidonic acids are essential in humans. Linoleic acid, the metabolic precursor to both linolenic and arachidonic acid, cannot be synthesized in vivo. When there is a deficiency of linoleic acid, the enzyme system that converts linoleic acid to arachidonic acid (a tetraene) acts on oleic acid to synthesize eicosatrienoic acid (a triene) which lacks the physiologic functions of arachidonic acid. Biochemically, EFAD is defined as a triene to tetraene ratio > 0.4. Clinical manifestations of EFAD include scaly dermatitis, alopecia, growth retardation, poor wound healing, thrombocytopenia and fatty liver. IV fat emulsion prevents or reverses biochemical and clinical manifestations of EFAD.

Indications:

Source of calories and essential fatty acids for patients requiring parenteral nutrition for extended periods of time (usually for > 5 days).

Source of essential fatty acids when a deficiency occurs.

Contraindications:

Disturbance of normal fat metabolism such as pathologic hyperlipemia, lipoid nephrosis or acute pancreatitis, if accompanied by hyperlipemia. Egg yolk phospholipids are present; do not give to patients with severe egg allergies.

Warnings:

Special risk patients: Exercise caution in administering to patients with severe liver damage, pulmonary disease, anemia, blood coagulation disorders, or when there is danger of fat embolism.

Pregnancy: Category C. It is not known whether IV fat emulsions can cause fetal harm when administered to a pregnant woman or can affect reproduction capacity. Use only when clearly needed.

Precautions:

Jaundiced or premature infants: Use with caution because free fatty acids displace bilirubin bound to albumin.

Too rapid administration can cause fluid or fat overloading. This can result in dilution of serum electrolyte concentrations, overhydration, pulmonary edema, impaired pulmonary diffusion capacity or metabolic acidosis.

Monitoring: When IV fat emulsion is administered, monitor the patient's capacity to eliminate the infused fat from the circulation. The lipemia must clear between daily infusions. Closely monitor the hemogram, blood coagulation, liver function tests, plasma lipid profile and platelet count (especially in neonates). Discontinue use if a significant abnormality in any of these parameters is attributed to therapy.

(Continued on following page)

INTRAVENOUS FAT EMULSION (Cont.)

Adverse Reactions:

Most frequent: Sepsis due to administration equipment and thrombophlebitis due to vein irritation from concurrently administered hypertonic solutions. These adverse reactions are inseparable from the TPN procedure with or without IV fat emulsion.

Less frequent (more directly related to IV fat emulsion):

Immediate (acute) ($<$ 1%) – Dyspnea; cyanosis; hyperlipemia; hypercoagulability; nausea; vomiting; headache; flushing; increase in temperature; sweating; sleepiness; chest and back pain; slight pressure over the eyes; dizziness; irritation at the infusion site; thrombocytopenia in neonates (rare).

Long-term (chronic) – Hepatomegaly; jaundice due to central lobular cholestasis; splenomegaly; thrombocytopenia; leukopenia; transient increases in liver function tests; overloading syndrome (focal seizures, fever, leukocytosis, splenomegaly and shock).

The deposition of brown pigmentation in the reticuloendothelial system (the so-called "IV fat pigment") has occurred. Cause and significance of this phenomenon are unknown.

Overdosage:

Stop the infusion until visual inspection of the plasma, determination of triglyceride concentrations or measurement of plasma light-scattering activity by nephelometry indicates the lipid has cleared. Reevaluate the patient and institute appropriate corrective measures.

Dosage:

Total parenteral nutrition: As part of TPN, administer IV via a peripheral vein or by central venous catheter. Fat emulsion should comprise no more than 60% of the patient's total caloric intake, with carbohydrates and amino acids comprising the remaining 40% or more of caloric intake.

Adults – 10%: Initial infusion rate is 1 ml/min for the first 15 to 30 minutes. If no adverse reactions occur, the infusion rate can be increased to 2 ml/min. Infuse only 500 ml the first day and increase dose the following day. Do not exceed a daily dosage of 2.5 g/kg.

20%: Initial infusion rate is 0.5 ml/min for the first 15 to 30 minutes. Infuse only 250 ml *(Liposyn II)* or 500 ml *(Intralipid)* the first day and increase dose the following day. Do not exceed a daily dosage of 3 g/kg.

Children – 10%: Initial infusion rate is 0.1 ml/min for the first 10 to 15 minutes.

20%: Initial infusion rate is 0.05 ml/min for the first 10 to 15 minutes.

If no untoward reactions occur, increase rate to 1 g/kg in 4 hours. Do not exceed daily dosage of 3 g/kg.

The dosage for premature infants starts at 0.5 g fat/kg/24 hours (5 ml *Intralipid* 10%; 2.5 ml *Intralipid* 20%) and may be increased in relation to the infant's ability to eliminate fat. The maximum dosage recommended by the American Academy of Pediatrics is 3 g fat/kg/24 hours.

Fatty acid deficiency: To correct EFAD, supply 8% to 10% of the caloric intake by IV fat emulsion to provide an adequate amount of linoleic acid (4% of caloric intake as linoleate).

(Continued on following page)

Lipids (Cont.)

INTRAVENOUS FAT EMULSION (Cont.)

Administration:

Fat emulsion is supplied in single dose containers; do not store partially used bottles or resterilize for later use. Do not use filters. Do not use any bottle in which there appears to be separation of the emulsion.

Fat emulsions may be simultaneously infused with amino acid-dextrose mixtures by means of a Y-connector located near the infusion site using separate flow rate controls for each solution. Keep the lipid infusion line higher than the amino acid-dextrose line. Since the lipid emulsion has a lower specific gravity, it may be taken up into the amino acid-dextrose line.

Fat emulsions may also be infused through a separate peripheral site.

Total nutrient admixture (TNA): IV fat emulsions are compatible with dextrose and amino acids, when properly mixed, for use in TPN therapy. This is also referred to as all-in-one, 3-in-1 and triple-mix. The following proper mixing sequence must be followed to minimize pH-related problems by ensuring that typically acidic dextrose injections are not mixed with lipid emulsions alone: (1) Transfer dextrose injection to the TPN admixture container; (2) transfer amino acid injection; (3) transfer the IV fat emulsion.

Amino acid injection, dextrose injection and the IV fat emulsion may be simultaneously transferred to the admixture container. Use gentle agitation to avoid localized concentration effects. Additives must not be added directly to the fat emulsion and in no case should the fat emulsion be added to the TPN container first. Shake bags gently after each addition to minimize localized concentration. If evacuated glass containers are used, add the dextrose and amino acid injections first, followed by the fat emulsion and then additives. Shake bottles gently after each addition.

Use these admixtures promptly; store under refrigeration (2 to 8°C; 36 to 46°F) for ≤ 24 hours and use completely within 24 hours after removal from refrigeration.

The prime destabilizers of emulsions are excessive acidity (low pH) and inappropriate electrolyte content. Give careful consideration to additions of divalent cations (calcium and magnesium) which cause emulsion instability. Amino acid solutions exert a buffering effect protecting the emulsion.

Inspect the admixture carefully for "breaking or oiling out" of the emulsion, which is described as the separation of the emulsion and can be visibly identified by a yellowish streaking or the accumulation of yellowish droplets in the admixed emulsion. Also examine the admixture for particulates. The admixture must be discarded if any of the above is observed.

Heparin may be added to activate lipoprotein lipase at a concentration of 1 or 2 units/ml prior to administration.

Lipid-containing fluids have a propensity to extract phthalates from phthalate-plasticized polyvinyl chloride (PVC). Although the amount is very small and no adverse clinical effects have been reported from administration of such amounts of phthalate, consider administration through a nonphthalate infusion set. Commercially available products may be accompanied by nonphthalate infusion sets.

	Oil (%)		Fatty acid content (%)									
Product & Distributor	Safflower	Soybean	Linoleic	Oleic	Palmitic	Linolenic	Stearic	Egg yolk phospholipids (%)	Glycerin (%)	Calories/ml	Osmolarity (mOsm/L)	How Supplied
Intralipid[1] 10% (Clintec)		10	50	26	10	9	3.5	1.2	2.25	1.1	260	In 50, 100, 250 and 500 ml.
Intralipid[1] 20% (Clintec)		20	50	26	10	9	3.5	1.2	2.25	2	260	In 50, 100, 250 and 500 ml.
Liposyn II[2] 10% (Abbott)	5	5	65.8	17.7	8.8	4.2	3.4	1.2	2.5	1.1	276	In 100, 200 and 500 ml.
Liposyn II[2] 20% (Abbott)	10	10	65.8	17.7	8.8	4.2	3.4	1.2	2.5	2	258	In 200 and 500 ml.
Liposyn III[2] 10% (Abbott)		10	54.5	22.4	10.5	8.3	4.2	1.2	2.5	1.1	284	In 100, 200 and 500 ml.
Liposyn III[2] 20% (Abbott)		20	54.5	22.4	10.5	8.3	4.2	1.2	2.5	2	292	In 200 and 500 ml.

[1] Store at 25°C (77°F) or below; do not freeze.

[2] Store at 30°C (86°F) or below; do not freeze.

For information on oral sodium chloride, refer to the Minerals and Electrolytes, Oral section.

Electrolytes

SODIUM CHLORIDE

Actions:

Pharmacology: Normal osmolarity of the extracellular fluid ranges between 280 to 300 mOsm/L; it is primarily a function of sodium and its accompanying ions, chloride and bicarbonate. Sodium chloride is the principal salt involved in maintenance of plasma tonicity. One g of sodium chloride provides 17.1 mEq sodium and 17.1 mEq chloride.

Hyponatremia (< 135 mEq/L): Symptoms may include weakness, nausea, disorientation, lethargy and headache; severe cases may progress to seizures and coma.

Indications:

For parenteral restoration of sodium ion in patients with restricted oral intake. Sodium replacement is specifically indicated in patients with hyponatremia or low salt syndrome. Sodium Chloride may also be added to compatible carbohydrate solutions such as Dextrose in Water to provide electrolytes.

Sodium Chloride Injections are also indicated as pharmaceutic aids and diluents for the infusion of compatible drug additives.

0.9% Sodium Chloride (Normal Saline), which is isotonic, restores both water and sodium chloride losses. Other indications for parenteral 0.9% saline include: Diluting or dissolving drugs for IV, IM or SC injection; flushing of IV catheters; extracellular fluid replacement; treatment of metabolic alkalosis in the presence of fluid loss and mild sodium depletion; as a priming solution in hemodialysis procedures and to initiate and terminate blood transfusions without hemolyzing red blood cells.

0.45% Sodium Chloride (Hypotonic) is primarily a hydrating solution and may be used to assess the status of the kidneys, since more water is provided than is required for salt excretion. It may also be used in the treatment of hyperosmolar diabetes where the use of dextrose is inadvisable and there is a need for large amounts of fluid without an excess of sodium ions.

3% or 5% Sodium Chloride (Hypertonic) is used in hyponatremia and hypochloremia due to electrolyte and fluid loss replaced with sodium-free fluids; drastic dilution of body water following excessive water intake; emergency treatment of severe salt depletion.

Bacteriostatic Sodium Chloride: Only for diluting or dissolving drugs for IV, IM or SC injection. See Contraindications and Warnings.

Concentrated Sodium Chloride: As an additive in parenteral fluid therapy for use in patients who have special problems of sodium electrolyte intake or excretion. It is intended to meet the specific requirements of the patient with unusual fluid and electrolyte needs. After available clinical and laboratory information is considered and correlated, determine the appropriate number of milliequivalents of Concentrated Sodium Chloride Injection, USP and dilute for use.

Contraindications:

Hypernatremia; fluid retention; when the administration of sodium or chloride could be clinically detrimental.

3% and 5% sodium chloride solutions: Elevated, normal or only slightly decreased plasma sodium and chloride concentrations.

Bacteriostatic sodium chloride: Newborns (see Warnings); for fluid or sodium chloride replacement.

Warnings:

Fluid/solute overload: Excessive amounts of sodium chloride by any route may cause hypokalemia and acidosis. Administration of IV solutions can cause fluid or solute overload resulting in dilution of serum electrolyte concentrations, congestive heart failure (CHF), overhydration, congested states or acute pulmonary edema, especially in patients with cardiovascular disease and in patients receiving corticosteroids or corticotropin or drugs that may give rise to sodium retention. The risk of dilutional states is inversely proportional to the electrolyte concentration. The risk of solute overload causing congested states with peripheral and pulmonary edema is directly proportional to the electrolyte concentration.

Infusion of > 1 L of isotonic (0.9%) sodium chloride may supply more sodium and chloride than normally found in serum, resulting in hypernatremia; this may cause a loss of bicarbonate ions, resulting in an acidifying effect. Infusion during or immediately after surgery may result in excessive sodium retention.

Hypertonic solutions: When administered peripherally, slowly infuse through a small bore needle placed well within the lumen of a large vein to minimize venous irritation. Carefully avoid infiltration.

(Warnings continued on following page)

SODIUM CHLORIDE (Cont.)

Warnings (Cont.):

Bacteriostatic Sodium Chloride: Do not use in newborns. Benzyl alcohol as a preservative in Bacteriostatic Sodium Chloride Injection has been associated with toxicity in newborns. This toxicity may result from both high cumulative amounts (mg/kg) of benzyl alcohol and the limited detoxification capacity of the neonate liver. These solutions have not been reported to cause problems in older infants, children and adults. It is estimated that a 30 ml IV dose may be given to adults without toxic effects. Data are unavailable on the toxicity of other preservatives in newborns. Use preservative-free Sodium Chloride Injection for flushing intravascular catheters. Where a sodium chloride solution is required for preparing or diluting medications for use in newborns, use only preservative-free 0.9% Sodium Chloride.

Concentrated Sodium Chloride Injection is hypertonic and must be diluted before use. Inadvertent direct injection or absorption of concentrated Sodium Chloride Injection may give rise to sudden hypernatremia and such complications as cardiovascular shock, CNS disorders, extensive hemolysis, cortical necrosis of the kidneys and severe local tissue necrosis (if administered extravascularly). Do not use unless solution is clear.

Surgical patients should seldom receive salt-containing solutions immediately following surgery unless factors producing salt depletion are present. Because of renal retention of salt during surgery, additional electrolyte given IV may result in fluid retention, edema and overloading of the circulation.

Renal function impairment: Infusions of sodium ions may result in excessive sodium retention; administer with care.

Pregnancy: Category C. It is not known whether sodium chloride can cause fetal harm when given to a pregnant woman or can affect reproduction capacity. Use only if clearly needed.

Lactation: It is not known whether sodium chloride is excreted in breast milk. Exercise caution when administering sodium chloride to a nursing woman.

Children: Safety and efficacy have not been established.

Precautions:

Monitoring: Clinical evaluation and periodic laboratory determinations are necessary to monitor changes in fluid balance, electrolyte concentrations and acid-base balance during prolonged parenteral therapy or whenever the condition of the patient warrants such evaluation. Significant deviations from normal concentrations may require tailoring of the electrolyte pattern.

Extraordinary electrolyte losses (eg, during protracted nasogastric suction, vomiting, diarrhea, GI fistula drainage) may necessitate additional electrolyte supplementation. Supply additional essential electrolytes, minerals and vitamins as needed.

Hypokalemia may result from excessive administration of potassium-free solutions.

Special risk patients: Administer cautiously to patients with decompensated cardiovascular, cirrhotic and nephrotic disease, circulatory insufficiency, hypoproteinemia, hypervolemia, urinary tract obstruction, CHF and to patients with concurrent edema and sodium retention, those receiving corticosteroids or corticotropin and those retaining salt.

Elderly or postoperative patients: Exercise care in administering sodium-containing solutions in renal or cardiovascular insufficiency, with or without CHF.

3% and 5% sodium chloride solutions: Infuse very slowly and use with caution to avoid pulmonary edema; observe patients constantly.

Adverse Reactions:

Reactions due to solution or technique of administration: Febrile response; local tenderness; abscess; tissue necrosis or infection at injection site; venous thrombosis or phlebitis extending from injection site; extravasation; hypervolemia.

Hypernatremia may be associated with edema and exacerbation of CHF due to retention of water, resulting in expanded extracellular fluid volume.

Ion excess/deficit: Symptoms may result from an excess or deficit of one or more of the ions present in the solution; therefore, frequent monitoring of electrolyte levels is essential. If infused in large amounts, chloride ions may cause a loss of bicarbonate ions, resulting in an acidifying effect.

(Adverse Reactions continued on following page)

SODIUM CHLORIDE (Cont.)

Adverse Reactions (Cont.):

Postoperative salt intolerance: Symptoms include – Cellular dehydration; weakness; disorientation; anorexia; nausea; distention; deep respiration; oliguria; increased BUN.

Too rapid infusion of hypertonic solutions may cause local pain and venous irritation. Adjust rate of administration according to tolerance. Use of the largest peripheral vein and a well-placed small bore needle is recommended. (See Warnings.)

If an adverse reaction occurs, discontinue the infusion, evaluate the patient, institute appropriate countermeasures and save the remainder of the fluid for examination.

Overdosage:

Parenteral preparations are unlikely to pose a threat of sodium chloride or fluid overload except possibly in newborn or very small infants. If these occur, reevaluate the patient and institute appropriate corrective measures.

Administration of too much sodium chloride may result in serious electrolyte disturbances with resulting retention of water, edema, loss of potassium and aggravation of an existing acidosis.

When intake of sodium chloride is excessive, excretion of crystalloids is increased in an attempt to maintain normal osmotic pressure. Thus there is increased excretion of potassium and of bicarbonate and, consequently, a tendency toward acidosis. There is also a rapid elimination of any foreign salt, such as iodide and bromide, being used for therapy.

Administration and Dosage:

Individualize dosage. Frequent laboratory determinations and clinical evaluation are essential to monitor changes in fluid balance, blood glucose and electrolytes.

In the average adult, daily requirements of sodium and chloride are met by the infusion of 1 L of 0.9% sodium chloride (154 mEq each of sodium and chloride). Base fluid administration on calculated maintenance or replacement fluid requirements.

Do not use plastic container in series connection.

If administration is controlled by a pumping device, take care to discontinue pumping action before the container runs dry or air embolism may result.

IV catheters: Prior to and after administration of the medication, entirely flush the catheter with 0.9% Sodium Chloride for Injection. Use in accord with any warnings or precautions appropriate to the medication being administered.

Calculation of sodium deficit: To calculate the amount of sodium that must be administered to raise serum sodium to the desired level, use the following equation (TBW = total body water): Na deficit (mEq) = TBW (desired – observed plasma Na).

Base the repletion rate on the degree of urgency in the patient. Use of hypertonic saline (eg, 3% or 5%) will correct the deficit more rapidly.

Concentrated Sodium Chloride: The dosage as an additive in parenteral fluid therapy is predicated on specific requirements of the patient. The appropriate volume is then withdrawn for proper dilution. Having determined the mEq of sodium chloride to be added, divide by four to calculate the number of ml to be used. Withdraw this volume and transfer into appropriate IV solutions such as 5% Dextrose Injection. The properly diluted solution may be given IV.

Admixture incompatibilities: Some additives may be incompatible. Consult a pharmacist. When Sodium Chloride Injections are used as diluents for infusion of compatible drug additives, refer to dosage and administration information accompanying additive drugs. Check specific references for any possible incompatibility with sodium chloride.

To minimize the risk of possible incompatibilities arising from mixing this solution with other additives that may be prescribed, inspect the final infusate for cloudiness or precipitation immediately after mixing, prior to administration and periodically during administration. Do not store.

Stability and storage: Replace IV apparatus at least once every 24 hours. Use only if solution is clear. Protect from freezing; avoid excessive heat. Store at 15° to 30°C (59° to 86°F). Brief exposure up to 40°C (104°F) does not adversely affect the product.

Electrolytes (Cont.)

SODIUM CHLORIDE INTRAVENOUS INFUSIONS FOR ADMIXTURES

		Sodium (mEq/L)	Chloride (mEq/L)	Osmolarity (mOsm/L)	How Supplied
Rx	**0.45% Sodium Chloride (½ Normal Saline)** (Various, eg, Abbott, Astra, Clintec, McGaw)	77	77	≈ 155	In 25, 50, 150, 250, 500 and 1000 ml.
Rx	**0.9% Sodium Chloride (Normal Saline)** (Various, eg, Abbott, Astra, Clintec, Elkins-Sinn, Gensia, McGaw, Lyphomed, Rugby, Smith & Nephew SoloPak)	154	154	≈ 310	In 2, 3, 5, 10, 20, 25, 30, 50, 100, 150, 250, 500, 1000 ml and 2 ml fill in 3 ml.
Rx	**3% Sodium Chloride** (Various, eg, Clintec, McGaw)	513	513	1030	In 500 ml.
Rx	**5% Sodium Chloride** (Various, eg, Abbott, Clintec, McGaw)	855	855	1710	In 500 ml.

SODIUM CHLORIDE DILUENTS

Rx	**Bacteriostatic Sodium Chloride Injection**[1] (Various, eg, American Regent, Elkins-Sinn, Lyphomed, Major, Rugby)	0.9% sodium chloride	In 2, 10, and 30 ml.

CONCENTRATED SODIUM CHLORIDE INJECTION

Not for direct infusion. *Must* be diluted before use.

Rx	**Sodium Chloride Injection** (Various, eg, Abbott, IMS, Lyphomed)	14.6% sodium chloride	In 20, 40 and 200 ml.
Rx	**Sodium Chloride Injection** (Various, eg, American Regent, Gensia, IMS, Lyphomed, Pasadena)	23.4% sodium chloride	In 30, 50, 100 and 200 ml.

[1] With benzyl alcohol or parabens.

For information on oral potassium, refer to the Mineral and Electrolytes, Oral section. For information on potassium phosphate, refer to specific monograph in this section.

POTASSIUM SALTS

Actions:

Pharmacology: The principal intracellular cation, potassium is essential for maintenance of intracellular tonicity; transmission of nerve impulses; contraction of cardiac, skeletal and smooth muscle; and maintenance of normal renal function. Potassium participates in carbohydrate utilization and protein synthesis and is critical in the regulation of nerve conduction and muscle contraction, particularly in the heart.

Hypokalemia: Gradual potassium depletion occurs via renal excretion, through GI loss or because of inadequate intake (excretion > intake). Depletion usually results from diuretic therapy, primary or secondary hyperaldosteronism, diabetic ketoacidosis, severe diarrhea (especially if associated with vomiting) or inadequate replacement during prolonged parenteral nutrition.

Potassium depletion sufficient to cause 1 mEq/L drop in serum potassium requires a loss of about 100 to 200 mEq of potassium from the total body store.

Symptoms – Weakness; fatigue; ileus; polydipsia; flaccid paralysis or impaired ability to concentrate urine (in advanced cases).

ECG may reveal premature atrial and ventricular contractions, prolongation of QT interval, ST segment depression, broad and flat T waves or appearance of U waves. Severe cases may lead to muscular weakness, paralysis and respiratory failure.

Pharmacokinetics: Normally about 80% to 90% of the potassium intake is excreted in the urine with the remainder voided in the stool and, to a small extent, in perspiration. The kidneys do not conserve potassium well; during fasting or in patients on a potassium-free diet, potassium loss from the body continues, resulting in potassium depletion. A deficiency of either potassium or chloride will lead to a deficit of the other.

Indications:

Prevention and treatment of moderate or severe potassium deficit when oral replacement therapy is not feasible.

Potassium acetate is useful as an additive for preparing specific IV fluid formulas when patient needs cannot be met by standard electrolyte or nutrient solutions.

Potassium acetate is also indicated for marked loss of GI secretions by vomiting, diarrhea, GI intubation or fistulas; prolonged diuresis; prolonged parenteral administration of potassium-free fluids such as normal saline and dextrose solutions; diabetic acidosis, especially during vigorous treatment with insulin and dextrose infusions; metabolic alkalosis; attacks of hereditary or familial periodic paralysis; hyperadrenocorticism; primary aldosteronism; overmedication with adrenocortical steroids, testosterone or corticotropin; the healing phase of scalds or burns; cardiac arrhythmias, especially due to digitalis glycosides.

Contraindications:

Diseases where high potassium levels may be encountered; hyperkalemia; renal failure and conditions in which potassium retention is present; oliguria or azotemia; anuria; crush syndrome; severe hemolytic reactions; adrenocortical insufficiency (untreated Addison's disease); adynamica episodica hereditaria; acute dehydration; heat cramps; hyperkalemia from any cause; early postoperative oliguria except during GI drainage.

Warnings:

Potassium intoxication: Do not infuse rapidly. High plasma concentrations of potassium may cause death through cardiac depression, arrhythmias or arrest. Monitor potassium replacement therapy whenever possible by continuous or serial ECG. In addition to ECG effects, local pain and phlebitis may result when a > 40 mEq/L concentration is infused.

Renal impairment or adrenal insufficiency may cause potassium intoxication. Potassium salts can produce hyperkalemia and cardiac arrest. Potentially fatal hyperkalemia can develop rapidly and be asymptomatic. Use with great caution, if at all.

Concentrated potassium solutions are for IV admixtures only; do not use undiluted. Direct injection may be instantaneously fatal.

Metabolic alkalosis: Potassium depletion is usually accompanied by an obligatory loss of chloride resulting in hypochloremic metabolic alkalosis. Treat the underlying cause of potassium depletion and administer IV potassium chloride.

Use solutions containing acetate ion carefully in patients with metabolic or respiratory alkalosis, and in conditions in which there is an increased level or impairment of utilization of this ion.

Metabolic acidosis: Treat associated hypokalemia with an alkalinizing potassium salt (eg, bicarbonate, citrate, gluconate, acetate).

(Warnings continued on following page)

POTASSIUM SALTS (Cont.)

Warnings (Cont.)

Musculoskeletal/Cardiac effects: When serum sodium or calcium concentration is reduced, moderate elevation of serum potassium may cause toxic effects on the heart and skeletal muscle. Weakness and later paralysis of voluntary muscles, with consequent respiratory distress and dysphagia, are generally late signs, sometimes significantly preceding dangerous or fatal cardiac toxicity.

Renal function impairment: Normal kidney function permits safe potassium therapy. Although temporary elevation of serum potassium level due to renal insufficiency secondary to dehydration or shock may mask an intracellular potassium deficit, do not replenish potassium until renal function is reestablished by overcoming dehydration and shock. Discontinue potassium-containing solutions if signs of renal insufficiency develop during infusions.

Pregnancy: Category C. It is not known whether potassium salts can cause fetal harm when administered to a pregnant woman or can affect reproduction capacity. Give to a pregnant woman only if clearly needed.

Lactation: Exercise caution when administering to a nursing woman.

Precautions:

Monitoring: Base therapy on close medical supervision with frequent ECGs and serum potassium determinations. Plasma levels are not necessarily indicative of tissue levels.

Special risk patients: Use with caution in the presence of cardiac disease, particularly in digitalized patients or in the presence of renal disease, metabolic acidosis, Addison's disease, acute dehydration, prolonged or severe diarrhea, familial periodic paralysis, hypoadrenalism, hyperkalemia, hyponatremia and myotonia congenita.

Fluid/Solute overload: IV administration can cause fluid or solute overloading resulting in dilution of serum electrolyte concentrations, overhydration, congested states or pulmonary edema.

The risk of dilutional states is inversely proportional to the electrolyte concentration of administered parenteral solutions. The risk of solute overload causing congested states with peripheral and pulmonary edema is directly proportional to the electrolyte concentrations of such solutions.

Drug Interactions:

Potassium Preparation Drug Interactions			
Precipitant drug	Object drug*		Description
ACE inhibitors	Potassium preparations	↑	Concurrent use may result in elevated serum potassium concentrations in certain patients.
Potassium-sparing diuretics/potassium-containing salt substitutes	Potassium preparations	↑	Potassium-sparing diuretics and potassium-containing salt substitutes will increase potassium retention and can produce severe hyperkalemia.
Potassium preparations	Digitalis	↑	In patients receiving digoxin, hypokalemia may result in digoxin toxicity. Therefore, use caution if discontinuing a potassium preparation in patients maintained on digoxin.

* ↑ = Object drug increased

Adverse Reactions:

Hyperkalemia: Adverse reactions involve the possibility of potassium intoxication. Signs and symptoms include: Paresthesias of extremities; flaccid paralysis; muscle or respiratory paralysis; areflexia; weakness; listlessness; mental confusion; weakness and heaviness of legs; hypotension; cardiac arrhythmias; heart block; ECG abnormalities such as disappearance of P waves, spreading and slurring of the QRS complex with development of a biphasic curve and cardiac arrest. See Overdosage.

Other: Nausea; vomiting; abdominal pain; diarrhea.

Reactions due to solution or technique of administration: Febrile response; infection at injection site; venous thrombosis; phlebitis extending from injection site; extravasation; hypervolemia; hyperkalemia; venospasm.

(Continued on following page)

POTASSIUM SALTS (Cont.)

Overdosage:

If excretory mechanisms are impaired or if potassium is administered too rapidly IV, potentially fatal hyperkalemia can result (see Contraindications and Warnings). It is important to consider the entire clinical picture and not rely solely on potassium levels since only extracellular potassium can be measured, yet intracellular potassium accounts for 98% of the total body amount.

Symptoms: Mild (> 5.5 to 6.5 mEq/L) to moderate (> 6.5 to 8 mEq/L) hyperkalemia may be asymptomatic and manifested only by increased serum potassium concentration and characteristic ECG changes. Other symptoms include muscular weakness, progressing to flaccid quadriplegia and respiratory paralysis; however, these generally do not develop unless potassium concentrations exceed 8 mEq/L. Dangerous cardiac arrhythmias often occur before onset of complete paralysis. Note that hyperkalemia produces symptoms paradoxically similar to those of hypokalemia.

ECG – Progressive increase in height and peaking of T waves; lowering of the R wave; decreased amplitude and ultimate disappearance of P waves; prolongation of PR interval and QRS complex; shortening of the QT interval; and finally, ventricular fibrillation and death.

Treatment: Terminate potassium administration. Monitor ECG. Infusion of combined dextrose and insulin in a ratio of 3 g dextrose to 1 unit regular insulin may be administered to shift potassium into cells. Administer sodium bicarbonate 50 to 100 mEq IV to reverse acidosis and also produce an intracellular shift. Give 10 to 100 ml calcium gluconate or calcium chloride 10% to reverse ECG changes. To remove potassium from the body use sodium polystyrene sulfonate resin or hemodialysis or peritoneal dialysis.

In digitalized patients, too rapid lowering of serum potassium can cause digitalis toxicity (see Drug Interactions).

Administration and Dosage:

mEq/g of Various Potassium Salts

Potassium salt	mEq/g
Potassium acetate	10.2
Potassium chloride	13.4
Dibasic potassium phosphate[1]	11.5
Monobasic potassium phosphate[1]	7.3

[1] Commercial preparations of potassium phosphate injection contain a mixture of both mono- and dibasic salts (see Potassium Phosphate monograph).

Do not administer undiluted potassium. Potassium preparations must be diluted with suitable large volume parenteral solutions, mixed well and given by slow IV infusion.

Too rapid infusion of hypertonic solutions may cause local pain and, rarely, vein irritation. Adjust rate of administration according to tolerance. Use of the largest peripheral vein and a small bore needle is recommended.

The usual additive dilution of potassium chloride is 40 mEq/L of IV fluid. The maximum desirable concentration is 80 mEq/L, although extreme emergencies may dictate greater concentrations.

In critical states, potassium chloride may be administered in saline (unless saline is contraindicated) since dextrose may lower serum potassium levels by producing an intracellular shift.

Avoid "layering" of potassium by proper agitation of the prepared IV solution. Do not add potassium to an IV bottle in the hanging position.

Individualize dosage. Guide dosage and rate of infusion by ECG and serum electrolyte determinations. The following may be used as a guide:

Potassium Dosage/Rate of Infusion Guidelines

Serum K^+	Maximum infusion rate	Maximum concentration	Maximum 24 hour dose
>2.5 mEq/L	10 mEq/hr	40 mEq/L	200 mEq
<2 mEq/L	40 mEq/hr	80 mEq/L	400 mEq

Add electrolytes to the mixed solutions only after considering electrolytes already present and potential incompatibilities such as calcium and phosphate or sulfate.

Children: IV infusion up to 3 mEq/kg or 40 mEq/m^2/day. Adjust volume of administered fluids to body size.

(Products listed on following page)

Electrolytes (Cont.)

POTASSIUM ACETATE

Must be diluted before use.

Rx	**Potassium Acetate** (Various, eg, Abbott, American Regent, IMS, Lyphomed)	**Injection:** 2 mEq/ml	In 20, 50 and 100 ml vials.
Rx	**Potassium Acetate** (Various, eg, Lyphomed, McGuff)	**Injection:** 4 mEq/ml	In 50 ml vials.

POTASSIUM CHLORIDE FOR INJECTION CONCENTRATE

Concentrate *must* be diluted before use.

Rx	**Potassium Chloride** (McGaw)	**Injection:** 2 mEq/ml	In 250 and 500 ml.
Rx	**Potassium Chloride** (Various, eg, Abbott, Baxter, Lyphomed)	**Injection:** 10 mEq	In 5, 10, 50 and 100 ml vials and 5 ml additive syringes.
Rx	**Potassium Chloride** (Various, eg, Abbott, American Regent, Baxter, Lyphomed)	**Injection:** 20 mEq	In 10 and 20 ml vials, 10 ml additive syringes, 10 ml amps.
Rx	**Potassium Chloride** (Various, eg, Abbott, Baxter, Lyphomed)	**Injection:** 30 mEq	In 15, 20, 30 and 100 ml vials and 20 ml additive syringes.
Rx	**Potassium Chloride** (Various, eg, Abbott, American Regent, Baxter, Lyphomed, McGuff)	**Injection:** 40 mEq	In 20, 30, 50 and 100 ml vials, 20 ml amps, 20 ml additive syringes.
Rx	**Potassium Chloride** (Various, eg, American Regent, McGuff)	**Injection:** 60 mEq	In 30 ml vials.
Rx	**Potassium Chloride** (Various, eg, Lyphomed)	**Injection:** 90 mEq	In 30 ml vials.

For information on oral calcium, refer to the Minerals and Electrolytes, Oral section.

Electrolytes (Cont.)

CALCIUM

Actions:

Pharmacology: Calcium is the fifth most abundant element in the body with > 99.5% of total body stores in skeletal bone. It is essential for the functional integrity of the nervous and muscular systems, for normal cardiac contractility and the coagulation of blood. It also functions as an enzyme cofactor and affects the secretory activity of endocrine and exocrine glands. Normal levels are 8.5 to 10.5 mg/dl.

Hypocalcemia: Symptoms – Tetany; paresthesias; laryngospasm; muscle spasms; seizures (usually grand mal); irritability; depression; psychosis; prolonged QT interval; intestinal cramps and malabsorption; respiratory arrest. Prolonged hypocalcemia may be associated with ectodermal defects including the nails, skin and teeth.

Pharmacokinetics: Approximately 80% of body calcium is excreted in the feces as insoluble salts; urinary excretion accounts for the remaining 20%.

Indications:

Hypocalcemia: For a prompt increase in plasma calcium levels (eg, neonatal tetany and tetany due to parathyroid deficiency, vitamin D deficiency, alkalosis); prevention of hypocalcemia during exchange transfusions; conditions associated with intestinal malabsorption.

Calcium chloride and gluconate: Adjunctive therapy in the treatment of insect bites or stings, such as Black Widow spider bites to relieve muscle cramping; sensitivity reactions, particularly when characterized by urticaria; depression due to overdosage of magnesium sulfate; acute symptoms of lead colic; rickets; osteomalacia.

Calcium chloride: To combat the deleterious effects of severe hyperkalemia as measured by ECG, pending correction of increased potassium in the extracellular fluid.

Cardiac resuscitation – Particularly after open heart surgery, when epinephrine fails to improve weak or ineffective myocardial contractions.

Calcium gluconate: To decrease capillary permeability in allergic conditions, nonthrombocytopenic purpura and exudative dermatoses such as dermatitis herpetiformis; for pruritus of eruptions caused by certain drugs; in hyperkalemia, calcium gluconate may aid in antagonizing the cardiac toxicity, provided the patient is not receiving digitalis therapy.

Unlabeled uses: Calcium salts have been used to treat verapamil overdose, treat acute hypotension from verapamil and prevent initial hypotension in patients requiring verapamil for whom decreases in blood pressure could be detrimental.

Contraindications:

Hypercalcemia; ventricular fibrillation; digitalized patients.

Warnings:

Extravasation: **Calcium chloride** and **gluconate** can cause severe necrosis, sloughing and abscess formation with IM or SC admininstration. Take great care to avoid extravasation or accidental injection into perivascular tissues.

Hypocalcemia of renal insufficiency: **Calcium chloride** is an acidifying salt and is therefore usually undesirable for treating this condition.

Pregnancy: Category C. It is not known whether this drug can cause fetal harm when given to a pregnant woman or can affect reproduction capacity. Use only when clearly needed.

Lactation: It is not known whether **calcium gluconate** is excreted in breast milk. Exercise caution when administering to a pregnant woman.

Precautions:

Cardiovascular effects: It is particularly important to prevent a high concentration of calcium from reaching the heart because of the danger of cardiac syncope.

(Continued on following page)

CALCIUM (Cont.)

Drug Interactions:

Calcium Drug Interactions			
Precipitant	Object drug*		Description
Thiazide diuretics	Calcium salts	↑	Hypercalcemia resulting from renal tubular reabsorption, or bone release of calcium by thiazides may be amplified by exogenous calcium.
Calcium salts	Atenolol	↓	Mean peak plasma levels and bioavailability of atenolol may be decreased, possibly resulting in decreased beta blockade.
Calcium salts	Digitalis glycosides	↑	Inotropic and toxic effects of these agents are synergistic; arrhythmias may occur, especially if calcium is given IV. Avoid IV calcium in patients receiving digitalis glycosides; if necessary, give slowly in small amounts.
Calcium salts	Sodium polystyrene sulfonate	↓	Coadministration in patients with renal impairment may result in an unanticipated metabolic alkalosis and a reduction of the resin's binding of potassium.
Calcium salts	Verapamil	↓	Clinical effects and toxicities of verapamil may be reversed.

* ↑ = Object drug increased. ↓ = Object drug decreased.

Drug/Lab test interaction: Transient elevations of plasma 11-hydroxy-corticosteroid levels (Glenn-Nelson technique) may occur when IV calcium is administered, but levels return to control values after 1 hour. In addition, IV calcium gluconate can produce false-negative values for serum and urinary magnesium.

Adverse Reactions:

IM administration: Mild local reactions may occur **(calcium gluceptate)**. Local necrosis and abscess formation may occur with **calcium gluconate**, and severe necrosis and sloughing may occur with IM or SC administration of **calcium chloride.**

IV administration: Rapid IV administration may cause bradycardia, sense of oppression, tingling, metallic, calcium or chalky taste or "heat waves". Rapid IV administration of **calcium gluconate** may cause vasodilation, decreased blood pressure, cardiac arrhythmias, syncope and cardiac arrest. **Calcium chloride** injections cause peripheral vasodilation and a local burning sensation; blood pressure may fall moderately.

Overdosage:

Symptoms: Inadvertent systemic overloading with calcium ions can produce an acute hypercalcemic syndrome characterized by a markedly elevated plasma calcium level, weakness, lethargy, intractable nausea and vomiting, coma and sudden death.

Treatment: It may be life-saving to rapidly lower blood calcium to safe levels. It is now agreed that the most effective mode of therapy is IV infusion of sodium chloride plus administration of potent natriuretic agents, such as furosemide. Sodium competes with calcium for reabsorption in the distal renal tubule and furosemide potentiates this effect. Together they cause a marked increase in renal clearance of calcium and reduction of hypercalcemia.

Administration and Dosage:

Elemental Calcium Content of Calcium Salts		
Salt	% Calcium	mEq/g
Calcium chloride	27.3	13.6
Calcium gluconate	9.3	4.65
Calcium gluceptate	8.2	4.1

Calcium gluconate is generally preferred over calcium chloride as it is less irritating.

IV administration: Warm solutions to body temperature and administer slowly (0.5 to 2 ml/minute); stop if the patient complains of discomfort. Resume when symptoms disappear. Following injection, the patient should remain recumbent for a short time. Repeated injections may be necessary because of the rapid excretion of calcium. Inject **calcium chloride** and **gluconate** through a small needle into a large vein to minimize venous irritation.

(Administration and Dosage continued on following page)

CALCIUM (Cont.)

Administration and Dosage (Cont.):

IM administration of **calcium gluceptate** and **gluconate** may be tolerated; however, reserve this route for emergencies when technical difficulty makes IV injection impossible. Administer **calcium gluconate** only by the IV route and **calcium chloride** by the IV or intraventricular route.

Admixture incompatibilities: Calcium salts should not generally be mixed with **carbonates, phosphates, sulfates** or **tartrates** in parenteral admixtures; they are conditionally compatible with potassium phosphates, depending on concentration. Calcium ions will chelate **tetracycline.**

CALCIUM GLUCONATE 1 g (10 ml) contains 93 mg (4.65 mEq) calcium.

Administration and Dosage:

For IV use only, either directly or by infusion; SC or IM injection may cause severe necrosis and sloughing. Do not exceed a rate of 0.5 to 2 ml/minute. Calcium gluconate may also be administered by intermittent infusion at a rate not exceeding 200 mg/min, or by continuous infusion. Discontinue injection if the patient complains of discomfort. Do not use IM, as abscess formation and local necrosis may occur.

Adults: 2.3 to 9.3 mEq (5 to 20 ml) as required. Daily dosage range is 4.65 to 70 mEq daily.

Children: 2.3 mEq/kg/day or 56 mEq/m²/day, well diluted and slowly given in divided doses.

Infants: Not more than 0.93 mEq (2 ml).

Emergency elevation of serum calcium: Adults – 7 to 14 mEq (15 to 30.1 ml) IV. *Children* – 1 to 7 mEq (2.2 to 15 ml). *Infants* – $<$ 1 mEq (2.2 ml). Depending on patient response, these doses can be repeated every 1 to 3 days.

Hypocalcemic tetany: Adults – 4.5 to 16 mEq of calcium (9.7 to 34.4 ml) may be given IM until therapeutic response occurs. *Children:* 0.5 to 0.7 mEq/kg (1.1 to 1.5 ml/kg) IV 3 or 4 times daily or until tetany is controlled. *Neonates* – 2.4 mEq/kg/day (5.2 ml/kg/day) in divided doses.

Hyperkalemia with secondary cardiac toxicity: Administer IV to provide 2.25 to 14 mEq (4.8 to 30.1 ml) while monitoring the ECG. If necessary, repeat doses after 1 to 2 minutes.

Magnesium intoxication: Adults – Initial dose is 4.5 to 9 mEq (9.7 to 19.4 ml) IV. Adjust subsequent doses to patient response. If IV administration is not possible, give 2 to 5 mEq (4.3 to 10.8 ml) IM.

Exchange transfusion: Adults – Approximately 1.35 mEq (2.9 ml) IV concurrent with each 100 ml of citrated blood. *Neonates* – Administer IV at a dosage of 0.45 mEq (1 ml)/100 ml of exchanged citrated blood.

Stability: If precipitation has occurred in syringes, do not use. If precipitation is present in vials or amps dissolve by heating to 80°C (146°F) in a dry heat oven for a minimum of 1 hour. Shake vigorously; allow to cool to room temperature. Do not use if precipitate remains.

Rx	**Calcium Gluconate** (Various, eg, American Regent, Astra, Elkins-Sinn, IDE, IMS, Lyphomed, McGuff, Rugby)	**Injection:** 10%	In 10 ml amps and syringes, 10 and 50 ml single dose vials and 100 and 200 ml pharmacy bulk vials.[1]

CALCIUM GLUCEPTATE 1.1 g (5 ml) contains 90 mg (4.5 mEq) calcium.

Administration and Dosage:

IM: 2 to 5 ml (0.44 to 1.1 g). Inject 5 ml (1.1 g) doses in the gluteal region or, in infants, in the lateral thigh.

IV: 5 to 20 ml (1.1 to 4.4 g). Warm solution to body temperature and administer slowly ($\leq$ 2 ml/min).

Exchange transfusions in newborns: 0.5 ml (0.11 g) after every 100 ml of blood exchanged.

Storage/stability: Do not administer unless solution is clear; do not use if crystals are present. Discard unused portion.

Rx	**Calcium Gluceptate** (Abbott)	**Injection:** 1.1 g per 5 ml	In 5 ml amps and 5 ml fill in 10 ml vial.[2]

[1] Not for direct infusion; dilute prior to use.

[2] With 5 mg/ml monothioglycerol.

Electrolytes (Cont.)

CALCIUM CHLORIDE 1 g (10 ml) contains 273 mg (13.6 mEq) calcium.

Administration and Dosage:

For IV use only. Injection is irritating to veins and must not be injected into tissues, since severe necrosis and sloughing may occur. Avoid extravasation. Administer slowly (not to exceed 0.5 to 1 ml/minute).

Intraventricular administration: In cardiac resuscitation, injection may be made into the ventricular cavity; do not inject into the myocardium. Intraventricular injection may be administered by personnel who are well trained in the technique and familiar with possible complications. Break off the IV needle supplied with the syringe and replace with a suitable intracardiac needle by affixing it firmly to the Luer taper provided on the syringe. After the injection has been completed, remove the needle/syringe assembly from the injection site by grasping the needle at the Luer fitting.

The intraventricular dose usually ranges from 200 to 800 mg (2 to 8 ml).

Hypocalcemic disorders: Adults – 500 mg to 1 g at intervals of 1 to 3 days, depending on response of patient or serum calcium determinations. Repeated injections may be required. *Children* – 0.2 ml/kg up to 1 to 10 ml/day.

Magnesium intoxication: Give 500 mg promptly; observe patient for signs of recovery before further doses are given.

Hyperkalemic ECG disturbances of cardiac function: Adjust dosage by constant monitoring of ECG changes during administration.

Cardiac resuscitation: Adults – Dose ranges from 500 mg to 1 g IV or 200 to 800 mg injected into the ventricular cavity. *Children* – 0.2 ml/kg.

Rx	**Calcium Chloride** (Various, eg, Abbott, American Regent, Astra, IMS, Lyphomed, Moore, VHA)	**Injection:** 10%	In 10 ml amps, vials and syringes.

CALCIUM PRODUCTS COMBINED, PARENTERAL

Rx	**Calphosan** (Glenwood)	**Injection:** 50 mg calcium glycerophosphate and 50 mg calcium lactate per 10 ml in sodium chloride solution (0.08 mEq Ca/ml)	In 60 ml vials.[1]

[1] With 0.25% phenol.

For information on oral magnesium, refer to the Minerals and Electrolytes, Oral section. For information on the use of magnesium sulfate as an anticonvulsant, refer to the monograph in the Anticonvulsants section.

MAGNESIUM

Actions:

Pharmacology: Magnesium is a cofactor in a number of enzyme systems, and is involved in neurochemical transmission and muscular excitability. As a nutritional adjunct in hyperalimentation, the precise mechanism of action for magnesium is uncertain.

Magnesium deficiency is rare in well nourished individuals, except in malabsorption syndromes. Magnesium deficiency may occur in malabsorption syndromes, chronic alcoholism, malnutrition, intestinal bypass surgery, diuretic therapy, severe diarrhea, prolonged nasogastric suction, steatorrhea, during hemodialysis, diabetes mellitus, pancreatitis, primary aldosteronism and renal tubular damage. Early symptoms of hypomagnesemia (< 1.5 mEq/L) may develop as early as 3 to 4 days or within weeks. Predominant deficiency effects are neurological (eg, muscle irritability, clonic twitching, tremors). Hypocalcemia and hypokalemia often follow low serum levels of magnesium. While large stores of magnesium are found intracellularly and in bone in adults, they often are not mobilized sufficiently to maintain plasma levels. Parenteral magnesium therapy repairs the plasma deficit and causes deficiency signs and symptoms to cease. The normal adult body contains 20 to 30 g (2000 mEq) magnesium.

Magnesium prevents or controls convulsions by blocking neuromuscular transmission and decreasing the amount of acetylcholine liberated at the end plate by the motor nerve impulse. Magnesium is said to have a depressant effect on the CNS, but it does not adversely affect the mother, fetus or neonate when used as directed in eclampsia or preeclampsia. Normal plasma magnesium levels range from 1.5 to 2.5 mEq.

Magnesium acts peripherally to produce vasodilation. With low doses, only flushing and sweating occur; larger doses cause a lowering of blood pressure and CNS depression. The central and peripheral effects of magnesium poisoning are antagonized by IV administration of calcium.

One g of magnesium sulfate provides 8.12 mEq of magnesium.

Hypermagnesemia: As plasma magnesium rises above 4 mEq/L, the deep tendon reflexes are first decreased and then disappear as the plasma level approaches 10 mEq/L. At this level respiratory paralysis may occur. Heart block also may occur at this or lower plasma levels of magnesium. Serum magnesium concentrations in excess of 12 mEq may be fatal.

Pharmacokinetics: IM injection results in therapeutic plasma levels within 60 minutes and persists for 3 to 4 hours. IV doses provide immediate effects that last for 30 minutes. Effective anticonvulsant serum levels range from 2.5 to 7.5 mEq/L. Magnesium is excreted by the kidneys at a rate proportional to the plasma concentration and glomerular filtration.

Indications:

Hypomagnesemia: Magnesium sulfate is used as replacement therapy in magnesium deficiency especially in acute hypomagnesemia accompanied by signs of tetany similar to those observed in hypocalcemia. In such cases, the serum magnesium (Mg^{++}) level is usually below the lower limit of normal (1.5 to 2.5 or 3 mEq/L) and the serum calcium (Ca^{++}) level is normal (4.3 to 5.3 mEq/L) or elevated.

Total parenteral nutrition patients may develop hypomagnesemia (<1.5 mEq/L) without supplementation. Magnesium is added to correct or prevent hypomagnesemia.

Preeclampsia/eclampsia/nephritis (magnesium sulfate): Prevention and control of convulsions of severe preeclampsia and eclampsia and for control of hypertension, encephalopathy and convulsions associated with acute nephritis in children (see monograph in Anticonvulsants, Miscellaneous section).

Unlabeled uses: Inhibition of premature labor (tocolytic); however, it is not a first-line agent.

Administration to suspected acute myocardial infarction patients immediately after admission to counteract post-infarctional hypomagnesemia and subsequent arrhythmias.

Magnesium IV is effective as a bronchodilator and, therefore, may be useful in some asthmatic patients.

Since magnesium deficiency may play a role in chronic fatigue syndrome, it has been suggested that magnesium administration may be beneficial in this condition; however, there are conflicting reports and further study is needed.

(Continued on following page)

MAGNESIUM (Cont.)

Contraindications:

Magnesium sulfate: Heart block or myocardial damage; IV magnesium to patients with preeclampsia during the 2 hours preceding delivery.

Magnesium chloride: Renal impairment; marked myocardial disease; comatose patients.

Warnings:

Renal function impairment: Because magnesium is excreted by the kidneys, use with caution. Parenteral use in the presence of renal insufficiency may lead to magnesium intoxication.

Elderly: Geriatric patients often require reduced dosage because of impaired renal function. In patients with severe impairment, dosage should not exceed 20 g in 48 hours. Monitor serum magnesium in such patients.

Pregnancy: Category A. Studies in pregnant women have not shown that magnesium sulfate injection increases the risk of fetal abnormalities if administered during all trimesters of pregnancy. If this drug is used during pregnancy, the possibility of fetal harm appears remote. However, because studies cannot rule out the possibility of harm, use during pregnancy only if clearly needed.

When administered by continuous IV infusion (especially for > 24 hours preceding delivery) to control convulsions in toxemic mothers, the newborn may show signs of magnesium toxicity, including neuromuscular or respiratory depression (see Overdosage).

Lactation: Since magnesium is distributed into milk during parenteral magnesium sulfate administration, use with caution in nursing women.

Children: Safety and efficacy in children have not been established.

Precautions:

Flushing/Sweating: Administer with caution if flushing or sweating occurs.

Hypomagnesemia: Do not administer magnesium sulfate injection unless hypomagnesemia is confirmed.

Monitoring: Maintain urine output at a level of ≥ 100 ml every 4 hours. Monitor serum magnesium levels and clinical status to avoid overdosage in preeclampsia. See Overdosage for serum level/toxicity relationships.

Clinical indications of a safe dosage regimen include the presence of the patellar reflex (knee jerk) and absence of respiratory depression (≈ 16 breaths or more per minute). Serum magnesium levels usually sufficient to control convulsions range from 3 to 6 mg/dl (2.5 to 5 mEq/L). Strength of deep tendon reflexes begins to diminish when magnesium levels exceed 4 mEq/L. Reflexes may be absent at 10 mEq/L, where respiratory paralysis is a potential hazard. Keep an injectable calcium salt immediately available to counteract potential hazards of magnesium intoxication in eclampsia.

Drug Interactions:

Neuromuscular blocking agents, nondepolarizing: Neuromuscular blocking effects may be increased by concurrent magnesium sulfate. Prolonged respiratory depression with extended periods of apnea may occur.

Adverse Reactions:

Adverse effects are usually the result of magnesium intoxication and include: Flushing; sweating; hypotension; stupor; depressed reflexes; flaccid paralysis; hypothermia; circulatory collapse; cardiac and CNS depression proceeding to respiratory paralysis (the most life-threatening effect).

Hypocalcemia with signs of tetany secondary to magnesium sulfate therapy for eclampsia has occurred.

Overdosage:

Symptoms: Sharp drop in blood pressure and respiratory paralysis. ECG changes may include increased PR interval, increased QRS complex and prolonged QT interval. Disappearance of the patellar reflex is a useful clinical sign to detect the onset of magnesium intoxication.

Although patients usually tolerate high concentrations of magnesium in plasma, there are occasional instances when cardiac consequences may be seen in the form of complete heart block at concentrations well below 10 mEq/L.

Other signs include muscle weakness, hypotension, sedation and confusion. As plasma concentrations of magnesium begin to exceed 4 mEq/L, deep-tendon reflexes are decreased and may be absent at levels approaching 10 mEq/L.

When magnesium sulfate injection is administered parenterally in doses that are sufficient to induce hypermagnesemia, the drug has a depressant effect on the CNS and, via the peripheral neuromuscular junction, on muscle.

(Overdosage continued on following page)

MAGNESIUM (Cont.)

Overdosage (Cont.):

Symptoms (Cont.):

Approximate Correlation of Magnesium Toxicity vs Serum Level	
Serum level (mEq/L)	Effect
1.5 to 2.5	Normal serum concentration
4 to 7	"Therapeutic" level for preeclampsia/eclampsia/ convulsions
7 to 10	Loss of deep tendon reflexes, hypotension, narcosis
12 to 15	Respiratory paralysis
> 15	Cardiac conduction affected. PR interval lengthening, QRS widening, dysrhythmias
> 25	Cardiac arrest

Treatment: Provide artificial ventilation until a calcium salt (10 to 20 ml of a 5% solution, diluted with isotonic Sodium Chloride for Injection if desired) can be injected IV to antagonize the effects of magnesium. A dose of 5 to 10 mEq calcium will usually reverse the respiratory depression and heart block. Physostigmine 0.5 to 1 mg SC may be helpful. Peritoneal dialysis or hemodialysis are also effective.

Hypermagnesemia in the newborn may require resuscitation and assisted ventilation via endotracheal intubation or intermittent positive pressure ventilation as well as IV calcium.

Administration and Dosage:

IV administration: Do not exceed 1.5 ml/min of a 10% concentration (or its equivalent), except in cases of severe eclampsia with seizures. Dilute IV infusion solutions to a concentration of ≤ 20% prior to IV administration. The most commonly used diluents are 5% Dextrose Injection and 0.9% Sodium Chloride Injection.

IM administration: Deep IM injection of the undiluted (50%) solution is appropriate for adults, but dilute to ≤ 20% concentration prior to IM injection in children.

Admixture incompatibilities: Magnesium sulfate in solution may result in a precipitate formation when mixed with solutions containing: Alcohol (in high concentrations); alkali carbonates and bicarbonates; alkali hydroxides; arsenates; barium; calcium; clindamycin phosphate; heavy metals; hydrocortisone sodium succinate; phosphates; polymyxin B sulfate; procaine HCl; salicylates; strontium; tartrates.

Hyperalimentation: Maintenance requirements are not precisely known. Maintenance dose range: *Adults* – 8 to 24 mEq/day. *Infants* – 2 to 10 mEq/day.

Mild magnesium deficiency: Adults – 1 g (8.12 mEq; 2 ml of 50% solution) IM every 6 hours for 4 doses (total of 32.5 mEq/24 hours).

Severe hypomagnesemia: IM – As much as 2 mEq/kg (0.5 ml of 50% solution) within 4 hours if necessary. *IV* – 5 g (≈ 40 mEq)/L of 5% Dextrose Injection or 0.9% Sodium Chloride solution, infused over 3 hours. In the treatment of deficiency states, observe caution to prevent exceeding the renal excretory capacity.

Seizures associated with preeclampsia/eclampsia/nephritis: Refer to Anticonvulsants, Miscellaneous for complete dosing information.

Rx	**Magnesium Chloride** (Various, eg, American Regent, McGuff)	**Injection:** 20% (1.97 mEq/ml)	In 50 ml multiple dose vials.
Rx	**Magnesium Sulfate** (Various, eg, Astra, Lyphomed, Pasadena)	**Injection:** 10% (0.8 mEq/ml)	In 20 and 50 ml vials and 20 ml amps.
Rx	**Magnesium Sulfate** (Various, eg, Abbott)	**Injection:** 12.5% (1 mEq/ml)	In 20 ml vials.
Rx	**Magnesium Sulfate** (Various, eg, Abbott, American Regent, Astra, IMS, Lyphomed, McGuff, Pasadena, Smith & Nephew Solopak)	**Injection:** 50% (4 mEq/ml)	In 2, 5, 10, 20 and 50 ml vials, 5 and 10 ml syringes, 2 and 10 ml amps.

For information on oral sodium bicarbonate, refer to the Minerals and Electrolytes, Oral section.

SODIUM BICARBONATE

Actions:

Pharmacology: Increases plasma bicarbonate; buffers excess hydrogen ion concentration; raises blood pH; reverses the clinical manifestations of acidosis.

One g of sodium bicarbonate provides 11.9 mEq sodium and 11.9 mEq bicarbonate.

Pharmacokinetics: Sodium bicarbonate in water dissociates to provide sodium (Na^+) and bicarbonate (HCO_3^-) ions. Sodium is the principal cation of the extracellular fluid. Bicarbonate is a normal constituent of body fluids and the normal plasma level ranges from 24 to 31 mEq/L. Plasma concentration is regulated by the kidney. Bicarbonate anion is considered "labile" since, at a proper concentration of hydrogen ion (H^+), it may be converted to carbonic acid (H_2CO_3), then to its volatile form, carbon dioxide (CO_2), excreted by the lungs. Normally, a ratio of 1:20 (carbonic acid:bicarbonate) is present in the extracellular fluid. In a healthy adult with normal kidney function, practically all the glomerular filtered bicarbonate ion is reabsorbed; $<$ 1% is excreted in the urine.

Indications:

Metabolic acidosis: In severe renal disease, uncontrolled diabetes, circulatory insufficiency due to shock, anoxia or severe dehydration, extracorporeal circulation of blood, cardiac arrest and severe primary lactic acidosis where a rapid increase in plasma total CO_2 content is crucial. Treat metabolic acidosis in addition to measures designed to control the cause of the acidosis (eg, insulin in uncomplicated diabetes, blood volume restoration in shock). Since an appreciable time interval may elapse before all ancillary effects occur, bicarbonate therapy is indicated to minimize risks inherent to acidosis itself.

At one time it was suggested to administer bicarbonate during cardiopulmonary resuscitation following cardiac arrest; however, recent evidence suggests that little benefit is provided and its use may be detrimental. For treatment of acidosis in this clinical situation, concentrate efforts on restoring ventilation and blood flow. According to the American Heart Association guidelines, use as a last resort after other standard measures have been utilized.

Urinary alkalinization: In the treatment of certain drug intoxications (eg, salicylates, lithium) and in hemolytic reactions requiring alkalinization of the urine to diminish nephrotoxicity of blood pigments.

Severe diarrhea which is often accompanied by a significant loss of bicarbonate.

Neutralizing additive solution: To reduce the incidence of chemical phlebitis and patient discomfort due to vein irritation at or near the infusion site by raising the pH of IV acid solutions.

Contraindications:

Losing chloride by vomiting or from continuous GI suction; receiving diuretics known to produce a hypochloremic alkalosis; metabolic and respiratory alkalosis; hypocalcemia in which alkalosis may produce tetany, hypertension, convulsions or congestive heart failure (CHF); when the administration of sodium could be clinically detrimental.

Neutralizing additive solution: Do not use as a systemic alkalinizer.

Warnings:

Cardiac effects: Cardiac arrest – The risk of rapid infusion must be weighed against the potential for fatality due to acidosis.

CHF – Since sodium accompanies bicarbonate, use cautiously in patients with CHF or other edematous or sodium-retaining states.

Fluid/Solute overload: IV administration can cause fluid or solute overloading resulting in dilution of serum electrolyte concentrations, overhydration, congested states or pulmonary edema. The risk of dilutional states is inversely proportional to the electrolyte concentrations of administered parenteral solutions. The risk of solute overload causing congested states with peripheral and acute pulmonary edema is directly proportional to the electrolyte concentrations of such solutions. Rapid or excessive administration of Sodium Bicarbonate Injection may produce tetany due to a decrease in ionized calcium and hypokalemia as potassium reenters the cells. Hypertonic solutions may cause vein damage. Avoid extravasation.

Renal function impairment: Administration of solutions containing sodium ions may result in sodium retention. Use with caution. Also use cautiously in patients with oliguria or anuria.

Elderly/Postoperative patients: Exercise particular care when administering sodium-containing solutions to elderly or postoperative patients with renal or cardiovascular insufficiency, with or without CHF.

(Warnings continued on following page)

SODIUM BICARBONATE (Cont.)

Warnings (Cont.):

Pregnancy: Category C. It is not known whether sodium bicarbonate can cause fetal harm when administered to a pregnant woman. Use only if clearly needed.

Lactation: It is not known whether this drug is excreted in breast milk. Exercise caution when administering to a nursing woman.

Neonates and children (< 2 years old): Rapid injection (10 ml/min) of hypertonic sodium bicarbonate solutions may produce hypernatremia, a decrease in cerebrospinal fluid pressure and possible intracranial hemorrhage. Do not administer > 8 mEq/kg/day. A 4.2% solution is preferred for such slow administration.

Precautions:

Monitoring: Adverse reactions may result from an excess or deficit of one or more of the ions in the solution; therefore, frequent monitoring of electrolyte levels is essential.

Avoid overdosage and alkalosis by giving repeated small doses and periodic monitoring by appropriate laboratory tests.

Potassium depletion may predispose to metabolic alkalosis, and coexistent hypocalcemia may be associated with carpopedal spasm as the plasma pH rises. Minimize by treating electrolyte imbalances prior to or concomitantly with bicarbonate.

Chloride loss: Patients losing chloride by vomiting or GI intubation are more susceptible to developing severe alkalosis if given alkalinizing agents.

Neutralizing additive solution: Administer this solution promptly. When introducing additives, mix thoroughly and do not store. Raising the pH of IV fluids with neutralizing additive solution will only reduce the incidence of chemical irritation caused by the infusate; it will not diminish any foreign body effects caused by the needle or catheter.

Extraordinary electrolyte losses such as may occur during protracted nasogastric suction, vomiting, diarrhea or GI fistula drainage may necessitate additional electrolyte supplementation.

Drug Interactions:

Sodium Bicarbonate Drug Interactions			
Precipitant drug	Object drug*		Description
Sodium bicarbonate	Chlorpropamide Lithium Methotrexate Salicylates Tetracyclines	↓	The renal clearance of these agents may be increased due to alkalinization of the urine, possibly resulting in a decreased pharmacologic effect
Sodium bicarbonate	Anorexiants Flecainide Mecamylamine Quinidine Sympathomimetics	↑	The renal clearance of these agents may be decreased due to alkalinizaton of the urine, possibly resulting in increased pharmacologic or toxic effects

* ↑ = Object drug increased ↓ = Object drug decreased

Adverse Reactions:

Symptoms: Extravasation of IV hypertonic solutions of sodium bicarbonate may cause chemical cellulitis (because of their alkalinity), with tissue necrosis, ulceration or sloughing at the site of infiltration. Prompt elevation of the part, warmth and local injection of lidocaine or hyaluronidase are recommended to prevent sloughing.

Too rapid infusion of hypertonic solutions may cause local pain and venous irritation. Adjust the rate of administration according to tolerance. Use of the largest peripheral vein and a well placed small bore needle is recommended.

Too rapid or excessive administration may result in hypernatremia and alkalosis accompanied by hyperirritability or tetany. Hypernatremia may be associated with edema and exacerbation of CHF due to the retention of water, resulting in an expanded extracellular fluid volume.

Reactions that may occur because of the solution or the technique of administration include febrile response, infection at the site of injection, venous thrombosis or phlebitis extending from the injection site, extravasation and hypervolemia.

Treatment: If an adverse reaction does occur, discontinue the infusion, evaluate the patient, institute appropriate therapeutic countermeasures and save the remainder of the fluid for examination if deemed necessary.

(Continued on following page)

SODIUM BICARBONATE (Cont.)

Overdosage:

Symptoms: Excessive or too rapid administration may produce alkalosis. Severe alkalosis may be accompanied by hyperirritability or tetany.

Treatment: Discontinue sodium bicarbonate. Control symptoms of alkalosis by rebreathing expired air from a paper bag or rebreathing mask or, if more severe, by parenteral injections of calcium gluconate (to control tetany and hyperexcitability). Correct severe alkalosis by IV infusion of 2.14% ammonium chloride solution, except in patients with hepatic disease, in whom ammonia use is contraindicated. Sodium chloride (0.9%) IV or potassium chloride may be indicated if there is hypokalemia.

Administration and Dosage:

Administer IV or SC following dilution to isotonicity (1.5%). For IV administration, suitable concentrations range from 1.5% (isotonic) to 8.4% (undiluted), depending on the clinical condition and requirements of the patient. Suitable dilution can be calculated from the following formula:

$$conc_1 \times volume_1 = conc_2 \times volume_2$$

Thus, 8.4% x 50 ml = 1.5% x 280 ml; or 7.5% × 50 ml = 1.5% × 250 ml; or 4.2% × 10 ml = 1.5% × 28 ml.

The diluent may be Sterile Water for Injection, Sodium Chloride Injection, 5% Dextrose or other standard electrolyte solutions. For SC administration, an isotonic solution (1.5%) of sodium bicarbonate can be prepared by diluting 1 ml (84 mg) of 8.4% solution with 4.6 ml Sterile Water for Injection. For 7.5% solution, dilute 1 ml (75 mg) with 4 ml Sterile Water for Injection. For 4.2% solution, dilute 1 ml (42 mg) with 1.8 ml Sterile Water for Injection.

Cardiac arrest: Bicarbonate administration in this situation may be detrimental. See Indications. Administer according to results of arterial blood pH and $PaCO_2$ and calculation of base deficit. Flush IV lines before and after use.

Adults – A rapid IV dose of 200 to 300 mEq of bicarbonate, given as a 7.5% or 8.4% solution. Observe caution where rapid infusion of large quantities of bicarbonate is indicated. Bicarbonate solutions are hypertonic and may produce an undesirable rise in plasma sodium concentration. In cardiac arrest, however, the risks from acidosis exceed those of hypernatremia.

In emergencies, administer 300 to 500 ml of 5% sodium bicarbonate injection as rapidly as possible without overalkalinizing the patient. To avoid overalkalinizing a patient whose own body mechanisms for correcting metabolic acidosis may be maximally stimulated, only one-third to one-half of the calculated dose is administered as rapidly as indicated by the patient's cardiovascular and fluid balance status. Then, redetermine serum pH and bicarbonate concentration.

Infants (≤ 2 years of age) – 4.2% solution for IV administration at a rate not to exceed 8 mEq/kg/day to guard against the possibility of producing hypernatremia, decreasing CSF pressure and inducing intracranial hemorrhage.

Initial dose: 1 to 2 mEq/kg/min given over 1 to 2 minutes followed by 1 mEq/kg every 10 minutes of arrest. If base deficit is known, give calculated dose of 0.3 × kg × base deficit. If only 7.5% or 8.4% sodium bicarbonate is available, dilute 1:1 with 5% Dextrose in Water before administration.

Severe metabolic acidosis: Administer 90 to 180 mEq/L (≈ 7.5 to 15 g) at a rate of 1 to 1.5 L during the first hour. Adjust to the patient's needs for further management.

(Administration and Dosage continued on following page)

Complete prescribing information for these products begins on page 145

Electrolytes (Cont.)

SODIUM BICARBONATE (Cont.)

Administration and Dosage (Cont.):

Less urgent forms of metabolic acidosis: Sodium Bicarbonate Injection may be added to other IV fluids. The amount of bicarbonate to be given to older children and adults over a 4 to 8 hour period is approximately 2 to 5 mEq/kg, depending on the severity of the acidosis as judged by the lowering of total CO_2 content, blood pH and clinical condition. Initially, an infusion of 2 to 5 mEq/kg over 4 to 8 hours will produce improvement in the acid-base status of the blood.

Alternatively, estimates of the initial dose of sodium bicarbonate may be based on the following equation:

$$0.5\ (L/kg) \times \text{body weight (kg)} \times \text{desired increase in serum } HCO_3^-\ (mEq/L) = \text{bicarbonate dose (mEq)}$$

or

$$0.5\ (L/kg) \times \text{body weight (kg)} \times \text{base deficit (mEq/L)} = \text{bicarbonate dose (mEq)}.$$

The next step of therapy is dependent on the clinical response of the patient. If severe symptoms have abated, reduce frequency of administration and dose.

If the CO_2 plasma content is unknown, a safe average dose of sodium bicarbonate is 5 mEq (420 mg)/kg.

It is unwise to attempt full correction of a low total CO_2 content during the first 24 hours, since this may accompany an unrecognized alkalosis due to delayed readjustment of ventilation to normal. Thus, achieving total CO_2 content of about 20 mEq/L at the end of the first day will usually be associated with a normal blood pH. Further modification of the acidosis to completely normal values usually occurs in the presence of normal kidney function when and if the cause of the acidosis can be controlled. Total CO_2 brought to normal or above normal within the first day may be associated with grossly alkaline blood pH.

If administration is controlled by a pumping device, discontinue pumping action before the container runs dry or air embolism may result.

Neutralizing additive solution: One vial of neutralizing additive solution added to 1 L of any of the commonly used parenteral solutions including Dextrose, Sodium Chloride, Ringer's, etc, will increase the pH to a more physiologic range (specific pH may vary slightly).

Note: Some products such as amino acid solutions and multiple electrolyte solutions containing dextrose will not be brought to near physiologic pH by the addition of sodium bicarbonate neutralizing additive solution. This is due to the relatively high buffer capacity of these fluids.

Admixture incompatibilities: Avoid adding sodium bicarbonate to parenteral solutions containing **calcium**, except where compatibility is established; precipitation or haze may result. **Norepinephrine** and **dobutamine** are incompatible.

Storage/Stability: Store at 15° to 30°C (59° to 86°F). Avoid excessive heat. Protect from freezing. Brief exposure up to 40°C does not adversely affect the product. Replace administration apparatus at least once every 24 hours.

(Products listed on following page)

Complete prescribing information for these products begins on page 145

Electrolytes (Cont.)

SODIUM BICARBONATE (Cont.)

Rx	**Sodium Bicarbonate** (Abbott)	**Injection:** 4.2% (0.5 mEq/ml)	In 10 ml (5 mEq) syringes.
Rx	**Sodium Bicarbonate** (Astra)		In 2.5 and 5 ml fill in 5 and 10 ml syringes.
Rx	**Sodium Bicarbonate** (Lyphomed)		In 10 ml (5 mEq) Bristoject syringes.
Rx	**Sodium Bicarbonate** (Abbott)	**Injection:** 5% (0.6 mEq/ml)	In 500 ml[1] (297.5 mEq).
Rx	**Sodium Bicarbonate** (Baxter)		In 500 ml (297.5 mEq).
Rx	**Sodium Bicarbonate** (McGaw)		In 500 ml[1] (297.5 mEq).
Rx	**Sodium Bicarbonate** (Abbott)	**Injection:** 7.5% (0.9 mEq/ml)	In 50 ml (44.6 mEq) amps and 50 ml (44.6 mEq) syringes.
Rx	**Sodium Bicarbonate** (American Regent)		In 50 ml (44.6 mEq) vials.
Rx	**Sodium Bicarbonate** (Astra)		In 44.6 ml fill in 50 ml syringes.
Rx	**Sodium Bicarbonate** (Lyphomed)		In 50 ml (44.6 mEq) single-dose vials, 50 ml (44.6 mEq) Bristoject syringes and 200 ml (179 mEq) *MaxiVials*.
Rx	**Sodium Bicarbonate** (Abbott)	**Injection:** 8.4% (1 mEq/ml)	In 50 ml (50 mEq) fliptop vials and 10 ml (10 mEq) and 50 ml (50 mEq) syringes.
Rx	**Sodium Bicarbonate** (American Regent)		In 50 ml (50 mEq) vials.
Rx	**Sodium Bicarbonate** (Astra)		In 10 and 50 ml syringes.
Rx	**Sodium Bicarbonate** (Lyphomed)		In 50 ml (50 mEq) vials and 10 and 50 mEq Bristoject syringes.
Rx	**Neut** (Abbott)	**Neutralizing Additive Solution**[2]: 4% (0.48 mEq/ml)	In 5 ml (2.4 mEq) fliptop and pintop vials.[1]
Rx	**Sodium Bicarbonate** (Lyphomed)	**Neutralizing Additive Solution**[2]: 4.2% (0.5 mEq/ml)	In 5 ml fill in 6 ml vials (2.5 mEq).

[1] With EDTA.

[2] For use as a neutralizing additive solution to acidic large volume parenterals.

Complete prescribing information for these products begins on page 145

Electrolytes (Cont.)

SODIUM LACTATE

Actions:

Pharmacology: One liter of ⅙ Molar sodium lactate (isotonic) administered IV is potentially equivalent in alkalinizing effect to approximately 280 ml of 5% sodium bicarbonate. One g of sodium lactate provides 8.9 mEq of sodium and of lactate.

Sodium lactate is metabolized to bicarbonate in the liver. The alkalinizing effects of sodium lactate result from simultaneous removal of lactate and hydrogen ions. Lactate is metabolized to glycogen and ultimately converted to carbon dioxide and water in the liver. The conversion of sodium lactate to bicarbonate requires 1 to 2 hours.

Indications:

As an alkalinizing agent for the treatment of metabolic acidosis resulting from starvation, acute infections, diabetic acidosis, diarrhea and vomiting, or renal failure.

Warnings:

Hepatic function impairment/severe illness: Conversion of lactate to bicarbonate may be impaired in the severely ill and in persons with hepatic disease.

Severe acidosis: Not intended nor effective for correcting severe acidotic states that require immediate restoration of plasma bicarbonate levels. Sodium lactate has no advantage over sodium bicarbonate and may be detrimental in the management of lactic acidosis.

Rx	**1/6 Molar Sodium Lactate** (Various, eg, Abbott, Baxter, McGaw)	**Injection:** 167 mEq/L each of sodium and lactate ions	In 500 and 1000 ml.

SODIUM ACETATE

Actions:

Pharmacology: The acetate ion is metabolized to bicarbonate almost on an equimolar basis. Metabolism occurs outside the liver. One g of sodium acetate provides 7.3 mEq of sodium and of acetate.

Indications:

Useful in acidotic states. Used as a source of sodium in large volume IV fluids to prevent or correct hyponatremia in patients with restricted intake. Useful for preparing IV fluid formulas when patient needs cannot be met by standard electrolyte or nutrient solutions.

Rx	**Sodium Acetate** (Various, eg, Abbott, American Regent, Lyphomed)	**Injection:** 2 mEq each of sodium and acetate per ml (16.4%)	In 20, 50 and 100 ml vials.
Rx	**Sodium Acetate** (Various, eg, American Regent, LyphoMed)	**Injection:** 4 mEq each of sodium and acetate per ml (32.8%)	In 50 and 100 ml vials.

TROMETHAMINE

Actions:

Pharmacology: Tromethamine, a highly alkaline, sodium-free organic amine, acts as a proton acceptor to prevent or correct acidosis. When administered IV as a 0.3 M solution, it combines with hydrogen ions from carbonic acid to form bicarbonate and a cationic buffer. It also acts as an osmotic diuretic, increasing urine flow, urinary pH and excretion of fixed acids, carbon dioxide and electrolytes.

Pharmacokinetics: At pH 7.4, 30% of tromethamine is not ionized and therefore is capable of reaching equilibrium in total body water. This portion may penetrate cells and may neutralize acidic ions of the intracellular fluid. The drug is rapidly eliminated by the kidneys; ≥ 75% appears in urine after 8 hours and the remainder within 3 days.

Indications:

Prevention and correction of systemic acidosis in the following conditions: Metabolic acidosis associated with cardiac bypass surgery; correction of acidity of Acid Citrate Dextrose (ACD) blood in cardiac bypass surgery; cardiac arrest.

Contraindications:

Anuria; uremia.

Warnings:

Administer slowly: Correct only the existing acidosis; avoid overdosage and alkalosis.

Duration of therapy: Because clinical experience has been limited generally to short-term use, do not administer for > 1 day except in a life-threatening situation.

Respiratory depression, although infrequent, may be more likely in patients with chronic hypoventilation or those treated with drugs which depress respiration. Large doses may depress ventilation due to increased blood pH and reduced CO_2 concentration. Adjust dosage so that blood pH does not increase above normal. If respiratory acidosis is present concomitantly with metabolic acidosis, the drug may be used with mechanical assistance to ventilation.

Perivascular infiltration of this highly alkaline solution may cause inflammation, vascular spasms and tissue damage (eg, necrosis, sloughing, chemical phlebitis, thrombosis). Place the needle within the largest available vein and infuse slowly (see Adverse Reactions).

Hemorrhagic hepatic necrosis has occurred in newborns when a hypertonic solution of tromethamine was administered via the umbilical vein.

Renal function impairment demands extreme care because of potential hyperkalemia and possible decreased excretion of tromethamine. Monitor ECG and serum potassium.

Pregnancy: Category C. It is not known whether tromethamine can cause fetal harm when administered to a pregnant woman or can affect reproduction capacity. Give to a pregnant woman only if clearly needed.

Children: Severe hemorrhagic liver necrosis has occurred in neonates.

Hypoglycemia may occur when administered to premature or even full term neonates.

Precautions:

Monitoring: Measure blood pH, pCO_2, bicarbonate, glucose and electrolytes before, during and after administration.

Adverse Reactions:

Generally, side effects are infrequent. Transient depression of blood glucose; respiratory depression, hemorrhagic hepatic necrosis (see Warnings).

Local reactions that may occur because of the solution or the technique of administration include: Febrile response; infection at injection site; venous thrombosis or phlebitis extending from the site of extravasation; hypervolemia.

(Continued on following page)

TROMETHAMINE (Cont.)

Overdosage:

Symptoms: Overdosage, in terms of total drug or too rapid administration, may cause alkalosis, overhydration, solute overload and severe prolonged hypoglycemia (several hours).

Treatment: Discontinue infusion and institute appropriate countermeasures.

Administration and Dosage:

Administer by slow IV infusion, by addition to pump oxygenator ACD blood or other priming fluid, or by injection into the ventricular cavity during cardiac arrest.

For peripheral vein infusion, use a large needle in the largest antecubital vein or place an indwelling catheter in a large vein of an elevated limb to minimize chemical irritation by the alkaline solution.

Avoid overtreatment (alkalosis). Measure pretreatment and subsequent blood values (eg, pH, pCO_2, pO_2, glucose, electrolytes) and urinary output to monitor dosage and progress of treatment. Limit dosage to increase blood pH to normal limits (7.35 to 7.45) and to correct acid-base derangements. Drug retention may occur, especially in patients with impaired renal function.

Dosage may be estimated from the buffer base deficit of the extracellular fluid (mEq/L) using the Siggaard-Andersen nomogram. The following formula is a general guide:

Tromethamine solution (ml of 0.3M) =
body weight (kg) X base deficit (mEq/L) X 1.1†

Determine need for additional solution by serial measurements of existing base deficit.

Acidosis during cardiac bypass surgery: Average dose of approximately 9 ml/kg (2.7 mEq/kg or 0.32 g/kg). A total single dose of 500 ml (150 mEq or 18 g) is adequate for most adults. Larger single doses (up to 1000 ml) may be required in severe cases. Do not exceed individual doses of 500 mg/kg over a period of not less than 1 hour.

Acidity of ACD priming blood: Stored blood has a pH range from 6.22 to 6.8. Use from 0.5 to 2.5 g (15 to 77 ml) added to each 500 ml of ACD blood to correct acidity. Usually, 2 g (62 ml) added to 500 ml of ACD blood is adequate.

Acidosis associated with cardiac arrest: Administer at the same time that other standard resuscitative measures are being applied.

If the chest is open, inject 2 to 6 g (62 to 185 ml) directly into the ventricular cavity. Do not inject into the cardiac muscle. If the chest is not open, inject from 3.6 to 10.8 g (111 to 333 ml) into a large peripheral vein. Additional amounts may be required to control systemic acidosis persisting after cardiac arrest is reversed.

Stability/Storage: Highly alkaline solutions may erode glass; discard solutions of tromethamine 24 hours after reconstitution. Protect from freezing and extreme heat.

Rx	**Tham** (Abbott)	**Injection:** 18 g (150 mEq) per 500 ml (0.3M)	In 500 ml single dose container.[1]

† Factor of 1.1 accounts for an approximate reduction of 10% in buffering capacity due to sufficient acetic acid to lower pH of the 0.3M solution without electrolytes to approximately 8.6.

[1] With acetic acid.

PHOSPHATE

Actions:

Pharmacology: A prominent component of all body tissues, phosphorus participates in bone deposition, regulation of calcium metabolism, buffering effects on acid-base equilibrium and various enzyme systems. In the extracellular fluid, phosphate exists as both a monovalent and a divalent form, the ratio of which is pH-dependent.

Normal serum inorganic phosphate levels are as follows: *Adults* – 3 to 4.5 mg/dl. *Children* – 4 to 7 mg/dl.

Hypophosphatemia: Moderate (*serum level* $\leq$ 2.5 mg/dl) – Symptoms include muscle weakness, malaise, paresthesias, CNS irritability, confusion, obtundation.

Severe (serum level $<$ 1 mg/dl) – Seizures, coma, respiratory failure, hemolytic anemia, rhabdomyolysis, tremors, platelet and leukocyte dysfunction.

Pharmacokinetics: Phosphate infused IV is excreted in the urine. Plasma phosphate is filtered by the renal glomeruli, and $>$ 80% is actively reabsorbed by the tubules.

Indications:

A source of phosphate to add to large volume IV fluids, to prevent or correct hypophosphatemia in patients with restricted oral intake.

Additive for preparing specific IV fluid formulas when needs of patient cannot be met by standard electrolyte or nutrient solutions.

Contraindications:

High phosphate or low calcium levels.

Potassium phosphate: Hyperkalemia.

Sodium phosphate: Hypernatremia.

Warnings:

Electrolyte intoxication: To avoid phosphate, sodium or potassium intoxication, infuse solutions slowly.

Hypocalcemic tetany: Infusions of high concentrations of phosphate reduce serum calcium and produce symptoms of hypocalcemic tetany. Monitor calcium levels.

Cardiac effects: Use sodium phosphate with caution in patients with cardiac failure or who are on other edematous or sodium-retaining medications. Use potassium phosphate with caution in the presence of cardiac disease, particularly in digitalized patients. High plasma concentrations of potassium may cause death through cardiac depression or arrhythmias.

Adrenal insufficiency: Administration of phosphate products in patients with adrenal insufficiency may cause sodium or potassium phosphate intoxication.

Renal function impairment: Administration may cause sodium or potassium phosphate intoxication.

Hepatic function impairment: Use sodium phosphate with caution in patients with cirrhosis.

Pregnancy: Category C. It is not known whether sodium phosphate can cause fetal harm when administered to a pregnant woman or can affect reproduction capacity. Give phosphate to a pregnant woman only if clearly needed.

Lactation: It is not known whether this drug is excreted in breast milk. Exercise caution when administering to a nursing woman.

Precautions:

Monitoring: Guide replacement therapy by the serum inorganic phosphate level and the limits imposed by the accompanying sodium or potassium ion.

Drug Interactions:

For information on drug interactions involving potassium, refer to the Potassium Salts monograph in this section.

(Continued on following page)

PHOSPHATE (Cont.)

Adverse Reactions:

Phosphate intoxication results in reciprocal hypocalcemic tetany.

Overdosage:

Potassium phosphate may cause combined potassium and phosphate intoxication.

Symptoms: Paresthesias of the extremities; flaccid paralysis; listlessness; confusion; weakness and heaviness of the legs; hypotension; cardiac arrhythmias; heart block; ECG abnormalities (eg, disappearance of P waves, spreading and slurring of the QRS complex with development of a biphasic curve, cardiac arrest).

Treatment: Immediately discontinue infusions. Restore depressed serum calcium levels; reduce elevated potassium levels.

Administration and Dosage:

Commercial injections are mixtures of the monobasic and dibasic salt forms. To avoid confusion, prescribe and dispense in terms of millimoles (mM) of phosphorus.

For IV use only. Dilute and thoroughly mix in a larger volume of fluid. Individualize dosage. Monitor serum sodium (or potassium), inorganic phosphorus and calcium levels.

Total parenteral nutrition (TPN): Approximately 10 to 15 mM of phosphorus (equivalent to 310 to 465 mg elemental phosphorus) per liter of TPN solution is usually adequate to maintain normal serum phosphate; larger amounts may be required in hypermetabolic states. Consider the amount of sodium (or potassium) which accompanies the addition of phosphate; monitor serum electrolytes and ECG.

Infants receiving TPN: 1.5 to 2 mM/kg/day.

Rx	**Potassium Phosphate** (Various, eg, Abbott, American Regent, Lyphomed)	**Injection:** Provides 3 mM phosphate and 4.4 mEq potassium per ml	In 5, 10, 15, 30, and 50 ml vials.
Rx	**Sodium Phosphate** (Various, eg, Abbott, American Regent, Lyphomed)	**Injection:** Provides 3 mM phosphate and 4 mEq sodium per ml	In 10, 15, 30 and 50 ml vials.

AMMONIUM CHLORIDE

Actions:

Pharmacology: When loss of hydrogen and chloride ions occurs, serum bicarbonate and pH rise and serum potassium falls. The ammonium ion is converted into urea in the liver. The liberated hydrogen and chloride ions in blood and extracellular fluid result in decreased pH and corrected alkalosis. Ammonium chloride also lowers urinary pH which increases the excretion rate of basic drugs (eg, amphetamines, quinidine).

One g ammonium chloride provides 18.7 mEq of chloride.

Indications:

Treatment of hypochloremic states and metabolic alkalosis.

Contraindications:

Renal function impairment; hepatic function impairment (see Warnings); metabolic alkalosis due to vomiting of hydrochloric acid when it is accompanied by loss of sodium (excretion of sodium bicarbonate in the urine).

Warnings:

Hepatic function impairment, severe (as occurs in uremia, cirrhosis or hepatitis): The liver may fail to convert the ammonia to urea. This may result in marked ammonia retention with intoxication and hepatic coma.

Pregnancy: Category C. It is not known whether this drug can cause fetal harm when administered to a pregnant woman or affect reproductive capacity. Use only if clearly needed.

Precautions:

Ammonium toxicity: Observe patients receiving ammonium chloride for symptoms of ammonia toxicity (eg, pallor, sweating, irregular breathing, retching, bradycardia, cardiac arrhythmias, local and general twitching, tonic convulsions, coma).

Use with caution in primary respiratory acidosis, and high total CO_2 and buffer base.

Administer slowly IV to avoid pain, toxic effects and local irritation at the venipuncture site and along the course of the vein.

Adverse Reactions:

Serious metabolic acidosis (see Overdosage).

Rapid IV administration may cause pain or irritation at the injection site or along the vein.

Reactions which may occur because of solution or administration technique include: Febrile response; injection site infection; venous thrombosis or phlebitis extending from injection site; extravasation; hypervolemia (from large volume diluent).

Overdosage:

Symptoms: Serious degree of metabolic acidosis; confusion; disorientation; coma.

Treatment: Acidosis – Administer sodium bicarbonate or sodium lactate.

Administration and Dosage:

Administer by slow IV infusion.

Dosage depends on the patient's condition and tolerance. Add the contents of one to two vials (100 to 200 mEq) to 500 or 1000 ml isotonic (0.9%) Sodium Chloride Injection. Do not exceed a concentration of 1% to 2% ammonium chloride or an administration rate of 5 ml/min in adults ($\approx$ 3 hours for infusion of 1000 ml). Monitor dosage by repeated serum bicarbonate determinations.

Storage/Stability: Avoid excessive heat; protect from freezing. When exposed to low temperatures, concentrated solutions may crystallize. If crystals form, warm the solution to room temperature in a water bath prior to use.

Rx	**Ammonium Chloride** (Abbott)	**Injection:** 26.75% (5 mEq/ml) To be diluted before infusion	In 20 ml (100 mEq) vials.[1]

[1] With 2 mg EDTA.

For information on oral iodine, manganese and zinc, refer to the Minerals and Electrolytes, Oral section. Iodine is also used as a thyroid agent (see monograph in Thyroid Drugs section) and as an expectorant (see monograph in Respiratory Drugs chapter).

Trace Metals

Actions:

Chromium: Trivalent chromium is part of glucose tolerance factor, an essential activator of insulin-mediated reactions. Chromium helps maintain normal glucose metabolism and peripheral nerve function.

Serum chromium is bound to transferrin (siderophilin). Administration of chromium supplements to chromium deficient patients can result in normalization of the glucose tolerance curve from the diabetic-like curve typical of chromium deficiency. This response is viewed as a more meaningful indicator than serum chromium levels.

Copper serves as a cofactor for serum ceruloplasmin, an oxidase necessary for proper formation of the iron carrier protein, transferrin. Copper also helps maintain normal rates of red and white blood cell formation. The daily turnover of copper through ceruloplasmin is approximately 0.5 mg.

Iodine: Absorption from the GI tract is rapid and complete. Skin and lungs can also absorb iodine. On administration, iodide equilibrates in extracellular fluids and although all body cells contain iodide, it is specifically concentrated by the thyroid gland, which is estimated to contain 7 to 8 mg total iodine.

Other important organs to take up iodide are salivary glands, gastric mucosa, choroid plexus, skin, hair, mammary glands and placenta. Iodine in saliva and gastric mucosal secretions is reabsorbed and recycled. The circulating iodine is hormonal thyroxine of which 30 to 70 mcg is protein bound and 0.5 mcg is free thyroxine.

Manganese serves as an activator for several enzymes. During minimal intake, 20 mcg/day is retained. Manganese is bound to a specific transport protein, transmanganin, and is widely distributed, but it concentrates in mitochondria-rich tissues such as brain, kidney, pancreas and liver.

Molybdenum is a constituent of the enzymes xanthine oxidase, sulfite oxidase and aldehyde oxidase. Tissue storage of molybdenum varies with the intake levels and is affected by the amount of copper and sulfate in the diet. Consistent levels are observed in liver, kidney and adrenal cortex.

Selenium is part of glutathione peroxidase which protects cell components from oxidative damage due to peroxides produced in cellular metabolism.

Pediatric conditions, Keshan disease and Kwashiorkor have been associated with low dietary intake of selenium. The conditions are endemic to geographic areas with low selenium soil content. Dietary supplementation with selenium salts reduces the incidence of the conditions among affected children.

Zinc serves as a cofactor for $>$ 70 different enzymes. Zinc facilitates wound healing, helps maintain normal growth rates, normal skin hydration and the senses of taste and smell. Zinc resides in muscle, bone, skin, kidney, liver, pancreas, retina, prostate and particularly in the red and white blood cells. Zinc binds to plasma albumin, α_2-macroglobulin and some plasma amino acids including histidine, cysteine, threonine, glycine and asparagine.

At plasma levels $<$ 20 mcg/dl, dermatitis followed by alopecia has been reported for TPN patients.

(Actions continued on following page)

Trace Metals (Cont.)

Actions (Cont.):

The following table summarizes deficiency symptoms, excretion routes and normal plasma levels for various trace metals. The serum level at which deficiency symptoms appear for many of these elements is not well defined.

Trace Metals: Deficiency/Excretion/Plasma Levels			
Trace metal	Symptoms of deficiency	Excretion	Normal plasma levels
Copper	Leukopenia, neutropenia, anemia, decreased ceruloplasmin levels, impaired transferrin formation of secondary iron deficiency, skeletal abnormalities, defective tissue formation.	Bile (80%), intestinal wall (16%), urine (4%)	80-163 mcg/dl
Chromium	Impaired glucose tolerance, peripheral neuropathy, ataxia, confusional state.	Kidneys (3-50 mcg/day), bile	1-5 mcg/L[1]
Iodine	Impaired thyroid function, goiter, cretinism.	Kidneys, bile	0.5-1.5 mcg/dl
Manganese	Nausea, vomiting, weight loss, dermatitis, changes in growth and hair color.	Bile; if obstruction present, then pancreatic juice or return to intestinal lumen. Urine (negligible)	6-12 mcg/L (whole blood)
Molybdenum	Tachycardia, tachypnea, headache, night blindness, nausea, vomiting, central scotomas, edema, lethargy, disorientation, coma, hypermethioninemia, hypouricemia, hypouricuria, low urinary excretion of inorganic sulfate and elevated urinary excretion of thiosulfate.	Primarily renal, some biliary	nd
Selenium	Muscle pain & tenderness, cardiomyopathy, Kwashiorkor, Keshan disease.	Urine, feces, lungs, skin	nd
Zinc	Diarrhea, apathy, depression, parakeratosis, hypogeusia, anorexia, dysosmia, geophagia, hypogonadism, growth retardation, anemia, hepatosplenomegaly, impaired wound healing.	90% in stools; urine, perspiration	100 $\pm$ 12 mcg/dl

[1] Not considered a meaningful index of tissue stores. nd = No data

Indications:

Supplement to IV solutions given for TPN.

Contraindications:

Do not give undiluted by direct injection into a peripheral vein because of the potential for infusion phlebitis, tissue irritation and potential to increase renal loss of minerals from a bolus injection.

Molybdenum without copper supplementation: Copper-deficient patients. See Warnings.

Warnings:

Renal failure or biliary tract obstruction: Metals may accumulate. Serial determinations of serum trace metal concentrations may be a valuable guideline.

Consider the possibility of **copper** and **manganese** retention in patients with biliary tract obstruction. Ancillary routes of manganese excretion include pancreatic secretions or reabsorption into the lumen of the duodenum, jejunum or ileum.

Adjust, reduce or omit trace metal supplements in renal dysfunction or GI malfunction. Consider contributions from blood transfusions. Frequently determine plasma levels.

Wilson's disease: Avoid administering **copper** supplements to patients with this genetic disorder of copper metabolism.

Decreased serum levels: Administration of **copper** in the absence of **zinc** and of zinc in the absence of copper may cause decreases in plasma levels. Perform periodic determinations of plasma zinc and copper for subsequent administrations.

Copper deficiency: **Molybdenum** promotes the mobilization of tissue **copper** and increases urinary excretion of copper; excessive amounts produce a copper deficiency. Frequently check the metabolism of copper in patients receiving molybdenum.

(Warnings continued on following page)

Trace Metals (Cont.)

Warnings (Cont.):

Multiple trace element solutions present a risk of overdosage when the need for one trace element is appreciably higher than that for the other trace elements present in the formulation. Administration of trace metals as separate entities may be required.

Hypersensitivity: Sensitization to **iodides** and deaths due to anaphylactic shock following administration have been reported. (See Adverse Reactions.) Evaluate the patient for hypersensitivity before initiating TPN supplementation. If a patient develops a reaction, withdraw TPN immediately and institute appropriate measures. Refer to Management of Acute Hypersensitivity.

Pregnancy: Category C. It is not known whether trace metals can cause fetal harm or can affect reproductive capacity. Give to a pregnant woman only if clearly indicated.

Molybdenum crosses the placenta. Presence of **selenium** in placenta and umbilical cord blood has been reported.

Precautions:

Replacement trace metal therapy beyond maintenance requirements may be necessary in protracted vomiting or diarrhea, in patients with fistula drainage or nasogastric suction or in acute catabolic states.

Diabetes mellitus: In assessing the contribution of chromium supplements to maintenance of glucose homeostasis, give consideration to the possibility that the patient may be diabetic.

Iodine is readily absorbed through skin, lungs and mucous membranes. Give consideration to the environment, topical skin disinfection and wound treatment practices with surgical swabs and solutions containing iodine and povidone iodine. Air in the coastal areas is known to contain more iodine than inland areas.

Benzyl alcohol: Some of these products contain benzyl alcohol, which has been associated with a fatal "gasping" syndrome in premature infants.

Adverse Reactions:

Symptoms of toxicity are unlikely to occur at recommended doses.

Hypersensitivity to **iodides** may result in angioneurotic edema, cutaneous and mucosal hemorrhages, fever, arthralgia, lymph node enlargement and eosinophilia. See Warnings.

Overdosage:

Chromium: Nausea, vomiting, GI ulcers, renal and hepatic damage, convulsions and coma.

Copper: Prostration, behavior change, diarrhea, progressive marasmus, hypotonia, photophobia, hepatic damage and peripheral edema have occurred with a serum copper level of 286 mcg/dl. Penicillamine is an effective antidote.

Iodine: Symptoms of chronic poisoning include metallic taste, sore mouth, increased salivation, coryza, sneezing, swelling of the eyelids, severe headache, pulmonary edema, tenderness of salivary glands, acneiform skin lesions and skin eruptions. Abundant fluid and salt intake helps in elimination of iodides.

Manganese: "Manganese madness", irritability, speech disturbances, abnormal gait, headache, anorexia, apathy and impotence.

Molybdenum: Gout-like syndrome with increased blood levels of molybdenum, uric acid and xanthine oxidase.

No data on treatment of molybdenosis in humans is available. Among animals, treatment with copper, sulfate ions and tungsten enhances excretion of molybdenum. The sulfur-containing amino acids, methionine and cysteine, may afford limited protection.

Selenium: Toxicity symptoms include hair loss, weak nails, dermatitis, dental defects, GI disorders, nervousness, mental depression, metallic taste, vomiting and garlic odor of breath and sweat. Acute poisoning due to ingestion has resulted in death with histopathological changes including fulminating peripheral vascular collapse, internal vascular congestion, diffusely hemorrhagic, congested and edematous lungs and brick-red color gastric mucosa. Death was preceded by coma. No effective antidote is known.

Zinc: Single IV doses of 1 to 2 mg/kg have been given to adult leukemic patients without toxic manifestations. However, acute toxicity was reported in an adult when 10 mg zinc was infused over 1 hour on each of 4 consecutive days. Profuse sweating, decreased consciousness, blurred vision, tachycardia (140/min) and marked hypothermia (94.2°F) on the fourth day were accompanied by a serum zinc concentration of 207 mcg/dl. Symptoms abated within 3 hours.

Patients receiving an inadvertent overdose (50 to 70 mg zinc/day) developed hyperamylasemia (557 to 1850 Klein units; normal, 130 to 310).

Death resulted from 1683 mg zinc IV over 60 hours to a 72-year-old patient. Symptoms included hypotension (80/40 mm Hg), pulmonary edema, diarrhea, vomiting, jaundice and oliguria with a serum zinc level of 4184 mcg/dl.

Calcium supplements may confer a protective effect against zinc toxicity.

(Continued on following page)

Complete prescribing information for these products begins on page 157.

Trace Metals (Cont.)

Administration:

Administer IV after dilution. Frequently monitor plasma levels and clinical status.

Preparation: Trace metals are usually physically compatible together, and with the electrolytes usually present in amino acid/dextrose solution used for TPN.

ZINC

Administration and Dosage:

Metabolically stable adults: 2.5 to 4 mg/day. Add 2 mg/day for acute catabolic states.

Stable adults with fluid loss from the small bowel: Give an additional 12.2 mg zinc per L of TPN solution, or an additional 17.1 mg per kg of stool or ileostomy output.

Full-term infants and children (≤ 5 years of age): 100 mcg/kg/day.

Premature infants (birth weight < 1500 g and up to 3 kg): 300 mcg/kg/day.

Rx	**Zinc Sulfate** (Various, eg, American Regent, Loch, Lyphomed, McGuff, Raway)	**Injection:** 1 mg/ml (as sulfate [as 4.39 mg heptahydrate or 2.46 mg anhydrous])	In 10 and 30 ml vials.
Rx	**Zinca-Pak** (Smith & Nephew SoloPak)		In 10 and 30[1] ml vials.
Rx	**Zinc Sulfate** (Various, eg, Loch, Raway)	**Injection:** 5 mg/ml (as 21.95 mg sulfate)	In 5 and 10 ml vials.
Rx	**Zinca-Pak** (Smith & Nephew SoloPak)		In 5 ml vials.
Rx	**Zinc** (Various, eg, Abbott)	**Injection:** 1 mg/ml (as 2.09 mg chloride)	In 10 ml vials.

COPPER

Administration and Dosage:

Adults: 0.5 to 1.5 mg/day.

Children: 20 mcg/kg/day.

Rx	**Copper** (Abbott)	**Injection:** 0.4 mg/ml (as 1.07 mg cupric Cl)	In 10 ml vials.
Rx	**Cupric Sulfate** (Various, eg, American Regent, Loch, Lyphomed)	**Injection:** 0.4 mg/ml (as 1.57 mg sulfate)	In 10 and 30 ml vials.
Rx	**Cupric Sulfate** (Various, eg, Loch, LyphoMed)	**Injection:** 2 mg/ml (as 7.85 mg sulfate)	In 10 ml vials.

MANGANESE

Administration and Dosage:

Adults: 0.15 to 0.8 mg/day.

Children: 2 to 10 mcg/kg/day.

Rx	**Manganese Chloride** (Various, eg, Abbott)	**Injection:** 0.1 mg/ml (as 0.36 mg manganese chloride)	In 10 ml vials.
Rx	**Manganese Sulfate** (Various, eg, American Regent, Lyphomed)	**Injection:** 0.1 mg/ml (as 0.31 mg sulfate)	In 10 and 30 ml vials.

[1] With 0.9% benzyl alcohol.

Complete prescribing information for these products begins on page 157.

Trace Metals (Cont.)

MOLYBDENUM

Administration and Dosage:

Metabolically stable adults: 20 to 120 mcg/day. For pediatric patients, calculate the additive dosage level by extrapolation.

Deficiency state resulting from prolonged TPN support: 163 mcg/day for 21 days reverses deficiency symptoms without toxicity.

	Product	Form	Packaging
Rx	**Ammonium Molybdate** (Various, eg, American Regent)	**Injection:** 25 mcg/ml (as 46 mcg/ml ammonium molybdate tetrahydrate)	In 10 ml vials.
Rx	**Molypen** (Lyphomed)		In 10 ml vials.

CHROMIUM

Administration and Dosage:

Adults: 10 to 15 mcg/day.

Metabolically stable adults with intestinal fluid loss: 20 mcg/day.

Children: 0.14 to 0.2 mcg/kg/day.

	Product	Form	Packaging
Rx	**Chromium** (Various, eg, Abbott, McGuff)	**Injection:** 4 mcg/ml (as 20.5 mcg chromic chloride hexahydrate)	In 10 and 30 ml vials.
Rx	**Chromic Chloride** (Various, eg, Lyphomed)		In 10 and 30[1] ml vials.
Rx	**Chromium Chloride** (Various, eg, American Regent, Raway)		In 10 and 30 ml vials.
Rx	**Chroma-Pak** (Smith & Nephew SoloPak)		In 10 and 30[1] ml vials.
Rx	**Chromic Chloride** (Various)	**Injection:** 20 mcg/ml (as 102.5 mcg chromic chloride hexahydrate)	In 10 ml vials.
Rx	**Chroma-Pak** (Smith & Nephew SoloPak)		In 5 ml vials.

SELENIUM

Administration and Dosage:

Metabolically stable adults: 20 to 40 mcg/day.

Deficiency state resulting from prolonged TPN support: 100 mcg/day for 24 and 31 days, respectively, reverses deficiency symptoms without toxicity.

Children: 3 mcg/kg/day.

	Product	Form	Packaging
Rx	**Selenium** (Various, eg, American Regent, McGuff)	**Injection:** 40 mcg/ml (as 65.4 mcg selenious acid)	In 10 ml vials.
Rx	**Sele-Pak** (Smith & Nephew SoloPak)		In 10 and 30[1] ml vials.
Rx	**Selepen** (Lyphomed)		In 10 and 30[1] ml vials.

IODINE

Administration and Dosage:

Metabolically stable adults: 1 to 2 mcg/kg/day (normal adults, 75 to 150 mcg/day).

Pregnant and lactating women; growing children: 2 to 3 mcg/kg/day.

	Product	Form	Packaging
Rx	**Iodopen** (Lyphomed)	**Injection:** 100 mcg/ml (as 118 mcg sodium iodide)	In 10 ml vials.

[1] With 0.9% benzyl alcohol.

Complete prescribing information for these products begins on page 157.

Trace Metals (Cont.)

TRACE METAL COMBINATIONS

Administration and Dosage:

See manufacturers' product labeling for individual dosing information.

Therapeutic supplements to provide replacement for extraordinary losses of individual trace metals may be added.

Content given per ml solution.

	Product and Distributor	Chromium (as chloride) mcg	Copper (as sulfate) mg	Iodide (as sodium iodide) mcg	Manganese (as sulfate) mg	Selenium (as selenious acid) mcg	Zinc (as sulfate) mg	How Supplied
Rx	**Pedtrace-4** (Lyphomed)	0.85	0.1		0.025		0.5	In 3 and 10 ml vials.
Rx	**Multiple Trace Element Neonatal** (American Regent)	0.85	0.1		0.025		1.5	In 2 ml vials.
Rx	**Neotrace-4** (Lyphomed)							In 2 ml vials.
Rx	**PedTE-PAK-4** (Smith & Nephew SoloPak)	1	0.1		0.025		1	In 3 ml vials.
Rx	**P.T.E.-4** (Lyphomed)							In 3 ml vials.
Rx	**Multiple Trace Element Pediatric** (American Regent)	1	0.1		0.03		0.5	In 10 ml vials.
Rx	**Trace Metals Additive in 0.9% NaCl** (Abbott)	2	0.2[1]		0.16[1]		0.8[1]	In 5 and 10 ml vials, 50 ml vials and 5 ml syringes.
Rx	**M.T.E.-4** (Lyphomed)	4	0.4		0.1		1	In 3, 10 and 30[2] ml vials.
Rx	**MulTE-PAK-4** (Smith & Nephew SoloPak)							In 3, 10 and 30 ml vials.
Rx	**Multiple Trace Element** (American Regent)							In 3 and 10 ml vials.
Rx	**Multiple Trace Element Concentrated** (American Regent)	10	1		0.5		5	In 1 and 10 ml vials.
Rx	**ConTE-PAK-4** (Smith & Nephew SoloPak)							In 1, 10[2] and 30[2] ml vials.
Rx	**M.T.E.-4 Concentrated** (Lyphomed)							In 1 and 10[2] ml vials.
Rx	**PTE-5** (Lyphomed)	1	0.1		0.025	15	1	In 3 and 10 ml vials.
Rx	**M.T.E.-5** (Lyphomed)	4	0.4		0.1	20	1	In 10 ml vials.
Rx	**MulTE-PAK-5** (Smith & Nephew SoloPak)							In 3 and 10 ml vials.
Rx	**Multiple Trace Element with Selenium** (American Regent)							In 3, 10 and 30[2] ml vials.
Rx	**M.T.E.-5 Concentrated** (Lyphomed)	10	1		0.5	60	5	In 1 and 10[2] ml vials.
Rx	**Multiple Trace Element with Selenium Concentrated** (American Regent)							In 1 ml fill in 2 ml vials and 10[2] ml vials.
Rx	**M.T.E.-6** (Lyphomed)	4	0.4	25	0.1	20	1	In 10 ml vials.
Rx	**M.T.E.-7**[3] (Lyphomed)							In 10 ml vials.
Rx	**M.T.E.-6 Concentrated** (Lyphomed)	10	1	75	0.5	60	5	In 1 and 10[2] ml vials.

[1] As chloride. [2] With 0.9% benzyl alcohol. [3] With 25 mcg molybdenum.

Refer to the general discussion of Trace Metals.
Complete prescribing information for Electrolytes begins on page 131

Trace Metals (Cont.)

TRACE METALS AND ELECTROLYTE COMBINATIONS

Administration and Dosage:

Not for direct infusion. These concentrated solutions are for IV admixtures only. Dilute to appropriate strength with suitable IV fluid prior to administration.

Adults: Add 20 ml/L (40 ml of double electrolyte products per 2 L) amino acid/dextrose solution (TPN) or other suitable IV solution.

Trace Elements (mg/ml)	**Tracelyte** (Lyphomed)	**Tracelyte w/ Double Electrolytes** (Lyphomed)	**Tracelyte-II** (Lyphomed)	**Tracelyte-II w/ Double Electrolytes** (Lyphomed)
Chromium (as chloride) (mcg/ml)	0.6	0.3	0.6	0.3
Copper (as sulfate)	0.06	0.03	0.06	0.03
Manganese (as sulfate)	0.015	0.0075	0.015	0.0075
Zinc (as sulfate)	0.15	0.075	0.15	0.075
Electrolytes (mEq/ml)				
Acetate	2.03	2.03	1.475	1.475
Calcium	0.25	0.25	0.225	0.225
Chloride	1.675	1.675	1.75	1.75
Gluconate	0.25	0.25		
Magnesium	0.4	0.4	0.25	0.25
Potassium	2.025	2.025	1	1
Sodium	1.25	1.25	1.75	1.75
Osmolarity (mOsm/L)	7570	7570	6200	6200
How Supplied	20 ml vials[1]	40 ml vials[2]	20 ml vials[1]	40 ml vials[2]

[1] To prepare 1 liter solution.
[2] To prepare 2 liter solution.

Intravenous Replenishment Solutions

COMBINED ELECTROLYTE SOLUTIONS

Electrolyte content given in mEq/L.

	Product & Distributor	Na^+	K^+	Ca^{++}	Mg^{++}	Cl^-	Lactate	Acetate	Gluconate	Citrate	Osmolarity (mOsm/L)	How Supplied
Rx	**Plasma-Lyte 56**[1] (Baxter)	40	13		3	40		16			111	In 1000 ml.
Rx	**Ringer's Injection** (Various, eg, Abbott, Baxter, McGaw)	≈ 147	4	≈ 4		≈ 156					≈ 310	In 250, 500 and 1000 ml.
Rx	**Lactated Ringer's Injection** (Various, eg, Abbott, Baxter, McGaw)	130	4	3		≈ 109	28				≈ 273	In 150, 250, 500 and 1000 ml.
Rx	**Plasma-Lyte R**[1] (Baxter)	140	10	5	3	103	8	47			312	In 1000 ml.
Rx	**Isolyte S**[2] (McGaw)	140	5		3	98		27	23		295	In 1000 ml.
Rx	**Isolyte S pH 7.4**[3,4] (McGaw)	141	5		3	98		27	23		295	In 500 and 1000 ml.
Rx	**Normosol-R**[5] (Abbott)	140	5		3	98		27	23		295	In 500 and 1000 ml.
Rx	**Normosol-R pH 7.4**[6] (Abbott)										295	In 500 and 1000 ml.
Rx	**Plasma-Lyte 148**[1] (Baxter)										294	In 500 and 1000 ml.
Rx	**Plasma-Lyte A pH 7.4**[4] (Baxter)										294	In 500 and 1000 ml.
Rx	**Isolyte E**[7] (McGaw)	140	10	5	3	103		49		8	310	In 1000 ml.
Rx	**0.15% Potassium Chloride in 0.9% Sodium Chloride Injection** (Various, eg, Baxter, McGaw)	154	20			174					≈ 350	In 1000 ml.
Rx	**0.22% Potassium Chloride in 0.9% Sodium Chloride Injection** (McGaw)	154	30			184					365	In 1000 ml.
Rx	**0.3% Potassium Chloride in 0.9% Sodium Chloride Injection** (Various, eg, Baxter, McGaw)	154	40			194					≈ 390	In 1000 ml.

[1] pH ≈ 5.5.
[2] pH ≈ 6.7.
[3] With 1 mEq/L phosphate.
[4] pH ≈ 7.4.
[5] pH ≈ 5.5-7.
[6] pH ≈ 7.2-7.8.
[7] pH ≈ 6.

Intravenous Replenishment Solutions (Cont.)

COMBINED ELECTROLYTE CONCENTRATES

These concentrated solutions are not for direct infusion. They are for prescription compounding of IV admixtures only. Dilute to appropriate strength with suitable IV fluid prior to administration. Electrolyte concentrations listed are based on amount when diluted in one liter. Osmolarity is based on the concentrate.

	Electrolyte content given in mEq/L after dilution. Product & Distributor	Na^+	K^+	Ca^{++}	Mg^{++}	Cl^-	Acetate	Gluconate	Osmolarity (mOsm/L)	How Supplied
Rx	**Hyperlyte** (McGaw)	25	≈40	5	8	≈33	≈41	5	6015	In 25 ml fill in 30 ml vials.
Rx	**Lypholyte** (Lyphomed)								7562	In 20, 40, 100 and 200 ml flip-top vials.
Rx	**Multilyte-40** (Lyphomed)								6015	In 25 ml flip-top vials.
Rx	**Nutrilyte** (American Regent)								7562	In 20 and 100 ml.
Rx	**Lypholyte**-II (Lyphomed)	35	20	4.5	5	35	29.5		6200	In 20 & 40 ml single dose flip-top vials & 100 and 200 ml flip-top vials.
Rx	**TPN Electrolytes** (Abbott)	35	20	4.5	5	35	29.5		6200	In 20 ml flip-top vials.
Rx	**Nutrilyte** II (American Regent)	35	20	4.5	5	35	29.5		6212	In 20 and 100 ml vials.
Rx	**TPN Electrolytes** II (Abbott)	18	18	4.5	5	35	10.5		4320	In 20 ml flip-top and pin-top vials and 20 ml syringes.
Rx	**TPN Electrolytes** III (Abbott)	25	40.6	5	8	33.5	40.6	5	7520	In 20 ml flip-top and pin-top vials and 20 ml syringes.
Rx	**Hyperlyte CR** (McGaw)	25	20	5	5	30	30		5500	In 250 ml Super-Vials.
Rx	**Hyperlyte R** (McGaw)	25	20	5	5	30	25		4205	In 25 ml fill in 30 ml vials.
Rx	**Multilyte-20** (Lyphomed)								4205	In 25 ml flip-top vials.

DEXTROSE-ELECTROLYTE SOLUTIONS

Electrolyte content given in mEq/L.

	Product & Distributor	Dextrose (g/L)	Calories (Cal/L)	Na^+	K^+	Ca^{++}	Mg^{++}	Cl^-	Phosphate	Lactate	Acetate	Osmolarity (mOsm/L)	Other Content & How Supplied
Rx	**Dextrose 2.5% with 0.45% Sodium Chloride** (Various, eg, Abbott, Baxter, McGaw)	25	85	77				77				280	In 250, 500 and 1000 ml.
Rx	**Dextrose 5% with 0.11% Sodium Chloride** (McGaw)	50	170	19				19				290	In 500 ml.
Rx	**Dextrose 5% with 0.2% Sodium Chloride** (Various, eg, Abbott, Baxter, McGaw)	50	170	34-38.5				34-38.5				320-330	In 250, 500 and 1000 ml.
Rx	**Dextrose 5% with 0.33% Sodium Chloride** (Various, eg, Abbott, Baxter, McGaw)	50	170	51-56				51-56				355-365	In 250, 500 and 1000 ml.
Rx	**Dextrose 5% with 0.45% Sodium Chloride** (Various, eg, Abbott, Baxter, McGaw)	50	170	77				77				≈ 405	In 250, 500 and 1000 ml.
Rx	**Dextrose 5% with 0.9% Sodium Chloride** (Various, eg, Baxter, McGaw)	50	170	154				154				≈ 560	In 250, 500 and 1000 ml.
Rx	**Dextrose 10% with 0.2% Sodium Chloride** (Various, eg, Abbott, McGaw)	100	340	34-38.5				34-38.5				575-582	In 250 and 500 ml.
Rx	**Dextrose 10% with 0.3% Sodium Chloride** (Abbott)	100	340	51				51				607	In 250 ml.
Rx	**Dextrose 10% with 0.45% Sodium Chloride** (McGaw)	100	340	77				77				660	In 1000 ml.
Rx	**Dextrose 10% with 0.9% Sodium Chloride** (Various, eg, Abbott, Baxter, McGaw)	100	340	154				154				813	In 500 and 1000 ml.

(Continued on following page)

Intravenous Replenishment Solutions (Cont.)

DEXTROSE-ELECTROLYTE SOLUTIONS (Cont.)

Electrolyte content given in mEq/L.

	Product & Distributor	Dextrose (g/L)	Calories (Cal/L)	Na^+	K^+	Ca^{++}	Mg^{++}	Cl^-	Phosphate	Lactate	Acetate	Osmolarity (mOsm/L)	Other Content & How Supplied
Rx	**0.179% Potassium Chloride in 5% Dextrose and Lactated Ringer's** (Baxter)	50	170	130	24	3		129		28		565	In 1000 ml.
Rx	**0.328% Potassium Chloride in 5% Dextrose and Lactated Ringer's** (Baxter)	50	170	130	44	3		149		28		605	In 1000 ml.
Rx	**Potassium Chloride 0.075% in D-5-W** (Various, eg, Baxter, McGaw)	50	170		10			10				≈ 272	In 1000 ml.
Rx	**Potassium Chloride 0.15% in D-5-W** (Various, eg, Baxter, McGaw)	50	170		20			20				≈ 293	In 1000 ml.
Rx	**Potassium Chloride 0.224% in D-5-W** (Baxter)	50	170		30			30				312	In 1000 ml.
Rx	**Potassium Chloride 0.3% in D-5-W** (Baxter)	50	170		40			40				333	In 500 and 1000 ml.
Rx	**0.075% Potassium Chloride in 5% Dextrose and 0.2% NaCl** (Various, eg, Abbott, Baxter)	50	170	34-38.5	10			44-48.5				340-349	In 1000 ml.
Rx	**0.15% Potassium Chloride in 5% Dextrose and 0.2% Sodium Chloride** (Various, eg, Abbott, Baxter, McGaw)	50	170	34-38.5	20			54-58.5				360-370	In 250, 500 and 1000 ml.
Rx	**0.22% Potassium Chloride in 5% Dextrose & 0.2% NaCl** (Various, eg, Abbott, Baxter, McGaw)	50	170	34-38.5	30			64-68.5				380-389	In 1000 ml.
Rx	**0.3% Potassium Chloride in 5% Dextrose and 0.2% Sodium Chloride** (Various, eg, Abbott, Baxter, McGaw)	50	170	34-38.5	40			74-78.5				400-409	In 1000 ml.
Rx	**0.15% Potassium Chloride in 5% Dextrose and 0.33% Sodium Chloride** (Various, eg, Abbott, Baxter, McGaw)	50	170	51-56	20			71-76				395-405	In 500 and 1000 ml.
Rx	**0.224% Potassium Chloride in 5% Dextrose & 0.33% NaCl** (Various, eg, Abbott, Baxter)	50	170	51-56	30			81-86				415-425	In 1000 ml.

(Continued on following page)

Intravenous Replenishment Solutions (Cont.)

DEXTROSE-ELECTROLYTE SOLUTIONS (Cont.)

	Electrolyte content given in mEq/L. Product & Distributor	Dextrose (g/L)	Calories (Cal/L)	Na^+	K^+	Ca^{++}	Mg^{++}	Cl^-	Phosphate	Lactate	Acetate	Osmolarity (mOsm/L)	Other Content & How Supplied
Rx	**0.3% Potassium Chloride in 5% Dextrose and 0.33% Sodium Chloride** (Various, eg, Abbott, Baxter)	50	170	51-56	40			91-96				434-446	In 1000 ml.
Rx	**0.075% Potassium Chloride in 5% Dextrose and 0.45% Sodium Chloride** (Various, eg, Baxter, McGaw)	50	170	77	10			87				≈ 425	In 1000 ml.
Rx	**0.15% Potassium Chloride in 5% Dextrose and 0.45% Sodium Chloride** (Various, eg, Baxter, McGaw)	50	170	77	20			97				≈ 445	In 500 and 1000 ml.
Rx	**0.22% Potassium Chloride in 5% Dextrose and 0.45% Sodium Chloride** (Various, eg, Baxter, McGaw)	50	170	77	30			107				≈ 465	In 1000 ml.
Rx	**0.3% Potassium Chloride in 5% Dextrose and 0.45% Sodium Chloride** (Various, eg, Baxter, McGaw)	50	170	77	40			117				≈ 490	In 1000 ml.
Rx	**0.15% Potassium Chloride in 5% Dextrose and 0.9% Sodium Chloride** (Various, eg, Baxter, McGaw)	50	170	154	20			174				≈ 600	In 1000 ml.
Rx	**0.22% Potassium Chloride in 5% Dextrose and 0.9% Sodium Chloride** (McGaw)	50	170	154	30			184				620	In 1000 ml.
Rx	**0.15% Potassium Chloride in 10% Dextrose and 0.2% Sodium Chloride** (McGaw)	100	340	34	20			54				615	In 250 ml.
Rx	**0.3% Potassium Chloride in 5% Dextrose and 0.9% Sodium Chloride** (Various, eg, Baxter, McGaw)	50	170	154	40			194				≈ 640	In 1000 ml.

[1] With sodium sulfite.

(Continued on following page)

Intravenous Replenishment Solutions (Cont.)

DEXTROSE-ELECTROLYTE SOLUTIONS (Cont.)

Electrolyte content given in mEq/L.

	Product & Distributor	Dextrose (g/L)	Calories (Cal/L)	Na^+	K^+	Ca^{++}	Mg^{++}	Cl^-	Phosphate	Lactate	Acetate	Osmolarity (mOsm/L)	How Supplied
Rx	**Isolyte G with 5% Dextrose** (McGaw)	50	170	65	17			149				555	70 mEq NH_4^+. In 1000 ml.[1]
Rx	**5% Dextrose and Electrolyte #75** (Baxter)	50	180	40	35			48	15	20		402	In 250, 500 and 1000 ml.
Rx	**Isolyte M with 5% Dextrose** (McGaw)	50	170	38	35			44	15		20	400	In 500 ml.[1]
Rx	**Dextrose 5% in Ringer's** (Various, eg, Abbott, Baxter, McGaw)	50	170	≈ 147	4	≈ 4.5		≈ 156				≈ 560	In 150, 250, 500 and 1000 ml.
Rx	**Dextrose 2.5% in Half-Strength Lactated Ringer's** (Various, eg, Abbott, Baxter, McGaw)	25	≈ 89	≈ 65.5	2	≈ 1.5		≈ 55		14		≈ 264	In 250, 500 and 1000 ml.
Rx	**Dextrose 5% in Lactated Ringer's** (Various, eg, Abbott, Baxter, McGaw)	50	170-180	130	4	3		109-112		28		525-530	In 250, 500 and 1000 ml.
Rx	**5% Dextrose and Electrolyte No. 48** (Baxter)	50	180	25	20		3	24	3	23		348	In 250, 500 and 1000 ml.
Rx	**Isolyte H with 5% Dextrose** (McGaw)	50	170	42	13		3	39			17	370	In 500 and 1000 ml.[1]
Rx	**Normosol-M and 5% Dextrose** (Abbott)	50	170	40	13		3	40			16	363	In 500 & 1000 ml.
Rx	**Plasma-Lyte 56 and 5% Dextrose** (Baxter)												In 500 and 1000 ml.
Rx	**Isolyte P with 5% Dextrose** (McGaw)	50	170	25	20		3	23	3		23	350	In 250 and 500 ml.[1]

[1] With sodium bisulfite.

(Continued on following page)

Intravenous Replenishment Solutions (Cont.)

DEXTROSE-ELECTROLYTE SOLUTIONS (Cont.)

Electrolyte content given in mEq/L.

	Product & Distributor	Dextrose (g/L)	Calories (Cal/L)	Na^+	K^+	Ca^{++}	Mg^{++}	Cl^-	Phosphate	Lactate	Acetate	Gluconate	Osmolarity (mOsm/L)	Other Content & How Supplied
Rx	**Isolyte S with 5% Dextrose** (McGaw)	50	170	142	5		3	98			30	23	555	In 1000 ml.[1]
Rx	**Normosol-R and 5% Dextrose** (Abbott)	50	185	140	5		3	98			27	23	552	In 500 & 1000 ml.[2]
Rx	**Plasma-Lyte 148 and 5% Dextrose** (Baxter)	50	190	140	5		3	98			27	23	547	In 500 and 1000 ml.
Rx	**10% Dextrose with Electrolytes** (Abbott)	100	340	80	20		6	80	7 (mM)			21	730	In 500 ml in 1000 ml partial fill container.[2]
Rx	**10% Dextrose and Electrolyte No. 48** (Baxter)	100	†	25	20		3	24	3	23			600	In 250 ml.[1]
Rx	**Isolyte R with 5% Dextrose** (McGaw)	50	170	41	16	5	3	40			24		380	In 1000 ml.[1]
Rx	**Plasma-Lyte M and 5% Dextrose** (Baxter)	50	180	40	16	5	3	40		12	12		377	In 500 and 1000 ml.
Rx	**Plasma-Lyte R and 5% Dextrose** (Baxter)	50	181	140	10	5	3	103		8	47		564	In 1000 ml.[1]
Rx	**Isolyte E with 5% Dextrose** (McGaw)	50	170	141	10	5	3	103			49		565	8 mEq citrate. In 1000 ml.[1]

[1] With sodium bisulfite. [2] With sodium metabisulfite. † Not indicated by manufacturer.

Intravenous Replenishment Solutions (Cont.)

HYPERTONIC DEXTROSE SOLUTIONS WITH ELECTROLYTES

Electrolyte content given in mEq/L.

	Product & Distributor	Dextrose (g/L)	Calories (Cal/L)	Na^+	K^+	Ca^{++}	Mg^{++}	Cl^-	Phosphate	Lactate	Acetate	Gluconate	Osmolarity (mOsm/L)	Other Content & How Supplied
Rx	**50% Dextrose with Electrolyte Pattern N** (McGaw)	500	1700	90	80		16	150	28				2875	16 mEq sulfate. In 500 ml in 1000 ml partial fill containers.[1]
Rx	**50% Dextrose with Electrolyte Pattern A** (McGaw)	500	1700	84	40	10	16	115				13	2800	16 mEq sulfate. In 500 ml in 1000 ml partial fill containers.[2]
Rx	**50% Dextrose with Electrolyte Pattern B** (McGaw)	500	1700	32		9	16	32				4.2	2615	16 mEq sulfate. In 500 ml in 1000 ml partial fill containers.[2]

[1] With sodium metabisulfite. [2] With sodium bisulfite.

INVERT SUGAR-ELECTROLYTE SOLUTIONS

Invert sugar is composed of equal parts of dextrose (glucose) and fructose (levulose). It has the same caloric value as dextrose but is more rapidly utilized. Fructose augments utilization of dextrose. Used for nonelectrolyte fluid and caloric replacement.

Refer to dextrose monograph for further information.

	Electrolyte content given in mEq/L. Product & Distributor	Invert Sugar (g/L)	Calories (Cal/L)	Na^+	K^+	Ca^{++}	Mg^{++}	Cl^-	Phosphate	Lactate	Osmolarity (mOsm/L)	How Supplied
Rx	**5% Travert and Electrolyte No. 2** (Baxter)	50	196	56	25		6	56	12.5	25	449	In 1000 ml.[1]
Rx	**10% Travert and Electrolyte No. 2** (Baxter)	100	384	56	25		6	56	12.5	25	726	In 1000 ml.[1]

[1] With sodium bisulfite.

Amino Acids

L-TRYPTOPHAN

The FDA has recommended a nationwide recall of all over-the-counter supplements containing L-tryptophan as the sole major component due to a possible link with the eosinophilia myalgia syndrome. Eosinophilia myalgia is a rare blood disorder characterized by "flu-like" symptoms, including muscle pain, weakness, joint pain, swelling of arms and legs, fever and rash. Consult your doctor before using any products containing L-tryptophan.

For oral amino acid therapy. Tryptophan 60 mg provides the equivalent of 1 mg of niacin through metabolic conversion. L-tryptophan also is a precursor of serotonin.

Unlabeled Uses: L-tryptophan has been used as a hypnotic agent. Doses of 4 to 5 g reduce sleep latency, increase sleep time and reduce the number of awakenings. Based on the theory that depression is associated with serotonin deficiency, L-tryptophan has been used as an antidepressant.

Drug Interactions:

Fluoxetine: Coadministration with L-tryptophan may produce symptoms related to both central toxicity (agitation, aggressiveness, worsening of obsessive-compulsive symptoms) and peripheral toxicity (eg, nausea and vomiting).

Monoamine oxidase inhibitors: Concurrent use with L-tryptophan may result in neurologic and behavioral syndromes (eg, confusion, disorientation, myoclonic jerks, hyperreflexia) due to an increase in serotonin activity.

Dosage: 500 mg to 2 g daily.

	Product	Form	Packaging	C.I.*
otc	**L-Tryptophan** (Nature's Bounty)	**Tablets:** 200 mg	In 30s and 100s.	154
otc	**L-Tryptophan** (Various, eg, Approved, Goldline, Moore, Raway, Rexall, Rugby, Schein, Scherer, URL, Vangard)	**Tablets:** 500 mg	In 24s, 30s, 50s, 60s, 100s & UD 100s.	109+
otc	**Trofan** (Upsher-Smith)		In 30s, 100s and UD 100s.	576
otc	**Tryptacin** (Arther)		In 100s, 250s & UD 100s.	455
otc	**L-Tryptophan** (Various, eg, Miller, Tyson & Assoc.)	**Capsules:** 500 mg	In 50s, 60s and 100s.	33+
otc sf	**L-Tryptophan** (Various, eg, Nature's Bounty, Rugby)	**Tablets:** 667 mg	In 30s and 100s.	135
otc sf	**Tryptacin** (Arther)	**Tablets:** 1000 mg	Scored. In 100s, 250s and UD 100s.	455
otc	**Trofan-DS** (Upsher-Smith)	**Tablets:** 1 g	(#Trofan DS 1GM). In 30s, 100s and UD 100s.	925

GLUTAMIC ACID

Indications: Dietary supplement.

Dosage: 500 to 1000 mg daily or as directed. Take with liquids.

	Product	Form	Packaging	C.I.
otc	**Glutamic Acid** (Various, eg, Freeda, Nature's Bounty, West-Ward)	**Tablets:** 500 mg	In 100s, 500s and 1000s.	27
otc	**Glutamic Acid** (J.R. Carlson)	**Capsules:** 500 mg	In 100s and 300s.	49

* Cost Index based on cost per tablet, capsule or 15 ml. Powdered doseforms based on cost per g.
sf – Sugar free.

Amino Acids (Cont.)

L-LYSINE

An essential amino acid which improves utilization of vegetable proteins.

Unlabeled Uses: Oral L-lysine has been promoted as treatment and as a prophylactic agent in herpes simplex infections; however, controlled studies do not support these claims.

Dosage: 334 to 1500 mg daily.

				C.I.*
otc	**L-Lysine** (Various, eg, Moore, Rugby)	**Tablets:** 312 mg	In 100s.	36
otc	**Enisyl** (Person & Covey)	**Tablets:** 334 mg	In 100s.	673
otc	**L-Lysine** (Various, eg, Approved, Balan, Goldline, Moore, Pasadena, Rexall, Rugby, Schein, Scherer, URL)	**Tablets:** 500 mg	In 60s, 100s and 250s.	45+
otc	**Enisyl** (Person & Covey)		In 100s and 250s.	89
otc	**L-Lysine** (Various, eg, Miller,Tyson & Assoc.)	**Capsules:** 500 mg	In 100s.	100+
otc	**L-Lysine** (Approved Pharm.)	**Tablets:** 1000 mg	In 60s.	121

otc **Lycolan** (Lannett)

Indications: Dietary supplement.

Dosage: *Adults* – 15 to 30 ml, 3 times daily before meals.

Children (6 to 12 years) – 15 ml, 3 times daily before meals.

Elixir: 1.8 g glycine and 0.1 g l-lysine/15 ml. 12% alcohol. Wine flavor. In pt. 150

METHIONINE

Indications: Dietary supplement.

Dosage: 500 mg daily. The recommended daily allowance has not been established.

				C.I.*
otc	**Uranap** (Vortech)	**Capsules:** 200 mg	In 100s.	190
Rx	**Methionine** (Various, eg, Lannett, Schein)	**Tablets:** 500 mg	In 100s, 500s and 1000s.	50+
Rx	**Methionine** (Tyson and Assoc.)	**Capsules:** 500 mg	In 30s.	299
otc	**Uranap 500** (Vortech)		In 100s and 1000s.	186

THREONINE

Indications: Dietary supplement.

Dosage: 500 mg daily, preferably on an empty stomach, or as directed.

				C.I.*
otc	**Threonine** (Various, eg, Solgar, Tyson & Assoc.)	**Capsules:** 500 mg	In 60s and 100s.	332+
otc	**Threonine** (Freeda)	**Tablets:** 500 mg	In 100s and 250s.	370

* Cost Index based on cost per capsule, tablet or 15 ml.

Amino Acids Combinations

		Amino Acids with Vitamins and Minerals		C.I.*
otc	**Dequasine** (Miller)	**Tablets:** 20 mg l-lysine, 100 mg l-cysteine, 50 mg dl-methionine, 200 mg vitamin C, 5 mg iron with Cu, I, Mg, Mn and Zn. *Dose:* 1 tablet daily.	In 100s.	140
otc	**Aminoprel** (Pasadena)	**Capsules:** 30 mg aspartic acid, 19 mg serine, 18 mg glycine, 11 mg alanine, 12 mg arginine, 8 mg histadine, 71 mg lysine, 12 mg tyrosine, 5 mg tryptophan, 17 mg phenylalanine, 3 mg cystine, 18 mg methionine, 14 mg threonine, 23 mg leucine, 17 mg isoleucine, 20 mg valine, 38 mg glutamic acid, 542 mg protein hydrolysate complex (45% amino acids), 50 mg l-lysine monohydrochloride, 13 mg dl-methionine, 2 mg Fe, 0.16 mg Cu, 0.025 mg I, 0.33 mg Mn, 3 mg K, 0.33 mg Zn, 3 mg Mg, 17 mg vitamin C, 0.33 mg B_6. *Dose:* 2 capsules 3 times daily with meals.	In 180s.	153
otc *sf*	**Eaase** (NeuroGenesis/ Matrix)	**Capsules:** 375 mg D, L-phenylalanine, 50 mg L-glutamine, 278 IU vitamin A, 0.375 mg B_1, 0.8 mg B_2, 1.25 mg B_5, 1 mg B_6, 1 mcg B_{12}, 0.03 mg FA, 30 mg C, 0.05 mg biotin, 10 mg B_3, 50 mg Ca, 25 mg Mg, 0.01 mg Cr. *Dose:* 2 capsules 3 times daily.	Yeast and preservative free. In 42s and 180s.	NA
otc *sf*	**PhenaCal** (NeuroGenesis/ Matrix)	**Capsules:** 500 mg D, L-phenylalanine, 15 mg L-glutamine, 25 mg L-tyrosine, 10 mg L-carnitine, 10 mg L-arginine pyroglutamate, 10 mg L-ornithine/L-aspartate, 0.033 mg Cr, 0.012 mg Se, 0.33 mg vitamin B_1, 5 mg B_2, 3.3 mg B_3, 0.33 mg B_5, 0.33 mg B_6, 1 mcg B_{12}, 5 IU E, 0.05 mg biotin, 0.066 mg FA, 1 mg Fe, 2.5 mg Zn, 35 mg Ca, 0.25 mg I, 0.33 mg Cu, 25 mg Mg. *Dose:* 6 capsules daily.	Yeast and preservative free. In 42s and 180s.	NA
otc *sf*	**Saave +** (NeuroGenesis/ Matrix)	**Capsules:** 460 mg D, L-phenylalanine, 25 mg L-glutamine, 333.3 IU vitamin A, 2.417 mg B_1, 0.85 mg B_2, 33 mg B_3, 15 mg B_5, 3 mg B_6, 5 mcg B_{12}, 0.067 mg FA, 100 mg C, 5 IU E, 0.05 mg biotin, 25 mg Ca, 0.01 mg Cr, 1.5 mg Fe, 25 mg Mg, 2.5 mg Zn. *Dose:* 3 to 6 capsules daily.	Yeast and preservative free. In 42s and 180s.	NA
otc *sf*	**Tropamine +** (NeuroGenesis/ Matrix)	**Capsules:** 250 mg D, L-phenylalanine, 150 mg L-tyrosine, 50 mg L-glutamine, 1.67 mg vitamin B_1, 2.5 mg B_2, 16.7 mg B_3, 15 mg B_5, 3.3 mg B_6, 5 mcg B_{12}, 0.067 mg FA, 100 mg C, 25 mg Ca, 0.01 mg Cr, 1.5 mg Fe, 25 mg Mg, 5 mg Zn. *Dose:* $\leq$ 6 capsules daily.	Yeast and preservative free. In 42s and 180s.	NA
otc	**Herpetrol** (Alva)	**Tablets:** L-lysine, vitamin A, E, B_2, C and Zn. *Dose:* 4 tablets daily until symptoms subside.	In 42s and 84s.	94
otc	**A/G-Pro** (Miller)	**Tablets:** 542 mg protein hydrolysate (45% amino acids), 50 mg l-lysine, 12.5 mg dl-methionine, 16.7 mg vitamin C, 0.33 mg B_6, 1.66 mg iron with Cu, I, K, Mg, Mn and Zn. *Dose:* 2 tablets 3 times daily before meals.	In 180s.	94
otc	**Jets** (Freeda)	**Tablets, chewable:** 300 mg lysine, 25 mg vitamin C, 25 mcg B_{12}, 5 mg B_6, 10 mg B_1.	In 30s, 250s and 500s.	131
otc	**PDP Liquid Protein** (Wesley Pharm.)	**Liquid:** 15 g protein (from hydrolyzed animal collagen), l-tryptophan and 72 Calories per 30 ml. *Dose:* 30 ml daily.	Sorbitol, saccharin. Cherry flavor. In qt.	150

* Cost Index based on cost per capsule, tablet or 15 ml.

Amino Acid Derivatives

LEVOCARNITINE (L-Carnitine)

Actions:

L-carnitine is a naturally occurring amino acid derivative, synthesized from methionine and lysine, required in energy metabolism. It facilitates long-chain fatty acid entry into cellular mitochondria, delivering substrate and subsequent energy production. Commercial synthesis of carnitine produces a D and L racemic mixture. In the biologic system, only the L isomer is present. The D isomer has pharmacologic effects but does not participate in lipid metabolism. Most carnitine is excreted in urine and feces. In renal failure, carnitine levels may rise.

Primary systemic carnitine deficiency resulting in impairment in fatty acid metabolism manifests itself as elevated triglycerides and free fatty acids, diminished ketogenesis and lipid infiltration of liver and muscle. Severe chronic deficiency may be associated with hypoglycemia, progressive myasthenia, hypotonia, lethargy, hepatomegaly, encephalopathy, hepatic coma, cardiomegaly, congestive heart failure, cardiac arrest, neurologic disturbances and, in infants, impaired growth and development.

Primary carnitine deficiency is a rare inborn error of metabolism in which biosynthesis or use of L-carnitine is impaired and normal dietary sources (eg, meat, milk) are inadequate or ineffectual in compensating for the deficiency.

Indications:

For therapy of patients with primary systemic carnitine deficiency.

Unlabeled uses: L-carnitine may be of benefit in secondary carnitine deficiency (due to defects of intermediary metabolism or other conditions).

L-carnitine appears effective in modifying abnormal plasma lipoprotein patterns. Most studies have dealt with hemodialysis patients. Carnitine apparently normalizes the abnormal lipid profile produced by loss of plasma L-carnitine (53% to 78%) in the hemodialysis procedure.

It has also been used to improve athletic performance, and may be of use in valproate toxicity.

Warnings:

Carnitine deficiency: D, L-carnitine, sold in health food stores as vitamin B_T, competitively inhibits L-carnitine and can cause a deficiency.

Pregnancy: Category B. There are no adequate and well controlled studies in pregnant women. Use during pregnancy only if clearly needed.

Lactation: Carnitine is a normal component of breast milk. L-carnitine supplementation in nursing mothers has not been studied.

Precautions:

Monitoring should include periodic blood chemistries, vital signs, plasma carnitine concentrations and overall clinical condition.

Adverse Reactions:

Most common: Transient GI complaints (41%) including: Nausea, vomiting, abdominal cramps, diarrhea; avoid by slow consumption or greater dilution of liquid. Decreasing dosage may diminish or eliminate drug-related body odor (11%) or GI symptoms.

Mild myasthenia has occurred in uremic patients on D, L-carnitine but not L-carnitine.

Overdosage:

Treatment includes usual supportive measures. Refer to General Management of Acute Overdosage.

Administration:

Solution: Adults – Give 1 to 3 g/day for a 50 kg subject. Use higher doses with caution. Start dosage at 1 g/day, and increase slowly while assessing tolerance and response.

Children – 50 to 100 mg/kg/day. Give higher doses with caution. Start dosage at 50 mg/kg/day, and increase slowly to a maximum of 3 g/day while assessing tolerance and therapeutic response.

Give alone or dissolve in drinks or liquid food. Space doses evenly (every 3 or 4 hours), preferably with or after meals; consume slowly to maximize tolerance.

Tablets: Adults – 990 mg, 2 or 3 times a day, depending on clinical response.

Infants and children – Between 50 and 100 mg/kg/day, in divided doses, with a maximum of 3 g/day. Dosage depends on clinical response.

				C.I.*
Rx	**Carnitor** (Sigma-Tau)	**Tablets:** 330 mg	In 90s.	NA
otc	**L-Carnitine** (Various, eg, R & D Labs, Tyson)	**Capsules:** 250 mg	In 30s and 60s.	5.1+
Rx	**Carnitor** (Sigma-Tau)	**Solution:** 100 mg per ml	Sucrose. Cherry flavor. In 118 ml.	NA
Rx	**VitaCarn** (Kendall McGaw)		Sucrose. Cherry flavor. In 118 ml.	1+

* Cost Index based on cost per 100 mg.

Lipotropic Products

The need for lipotropics in human nutrition has not been established. The lipotropic factors choline, inositol and betaine have not been proven therapeutically valuable, although they have been used for treatment of liver disorders and disturbed fat metabolism.

Choline (trimethylethanolamine), a component of the major phospholipid, lecithin, demonstrates lipotropic action, functions as a methyl group donor and is a precursor of the neurochemical transmitter, acetylcholine. Choline and lecithin (because of its choline content) have been advocated for tardive dyskinesia, Huntington's chorea, Tourette's syndrome, Friedreich's ataxia, presenile dementia, fatty liver and cirrhosis. Intestinal bacteria metabolize choline to trimethylamine, which imparts an unpleasant odor to the breath and body. Lecithin does not produce this odor. Choline also causes clinical depression in some patients.

Inositol, an isomer of glucose, is present in cell membrane phospholipids and plasma lipoproteins. No specific role in human nutrition has been established.

Linoleic and linolenic acid are polyunsaturated fatty acids that serve as precursors of important biochemical compounds, such as arachidonic acid, which gives rise to a wide variety of prostaglandins. Linoleic acid is regarded as an essential fatty acid because it cannot be synthesized in vivo and because it has a defined metabolic significance; it helps to support normal growth and development and helps prevent the clinical appearance of essential fatty acid deficiency (EFAD). The metabolic significance of linolenic acid is unclear. Use of these precursors to alter disease states requires more research.

CHOLINE

Administration and Dosage: 650 mg to 2 g daily or as directed.

otc	**Choline** (Various, eg, Approved, Rugby)	**Tablets:** 250 mg, 300 and 500 mg	In 100s.
		650 mg	In 90s and 100s.
otc	**Choline Bitartrate** (Various, eg, City Chem, Fibertone, Spectrum)	**Tablets:** 250 mg	In 100s, 250s, 500s and 1000s.
		Powder:	In 120 g and 1 lb.
Rx	**Choline Chloride** (Various, eg, Baker, Biochemical, City Chem, Spectrum)	**Powder:**	In 120 and 500 g and 1 and 5 lb.
otc	**Choline Dihydrogen Citrate** (Freeda)	**Tablets:** 650 mg	In 250s.
		Powder:	In 120 g and 1 lb.

INOSITOL

Administration and Dosage: 1 to 3 g daily in divided doses.

otc	**Inositol** (Various, eg, Biochemical, Freeda, Nature's Bounty, Rugby)	**Tablets:** 250 mg	In 100s.
		500 mg	In 100s.
		650 mg	In 90s and 100s.
		Powder:	In 25, 60, 100, 120 and 500 g and 1 lb.

Lipotropic Combinations

otc	**Lecithin** (Various, eg, Approved, Dixon-Shane, Goldline, Moore, Nature's Bounty, Rugby, Schein, West-Ward)	A source of choline, inositol, phosphorus, linoleic & linolenic acids. *Dose:* 1-2 caps/day. **Capsules:** 420 mg	In 60s.
		1.2 g	In 100s, 250s and 1000s.
		Tablets: 1.2 g	In 50s.
		Granules:	In 210, 240, 420 g & 1 lb.
		Liquid:	In 480 ml.
otc	**PhosChol** (Advanced Nutritional Technology)	Phosphatidylcholine (highly purified lecithin) **Softgels:** 200 mg	In 100s and 300s.
		565 mg	In 100s and 300s
		900 mg	In 100s and 300s.
		Liquid conc.: 3000 mg/5 ml	In 240 and 480 ml.
otc	**Pertropin** (Lannett)	**Capsules:** 7 mins. linolenic acid, other essential unsaturated free fatty acids and 5 IU vitamin E. *Dose:* 1 or 2 capsules 3 or 4 times daily.	In 100s.

OMEGA-3 (N-3) POLYUNSATURATED FATTY ACIDS

Cold water fish oils contain large amounts of omega-3 (N-3) polyunsaturated fatty acids, eicosapentaenoic acid (EPA) and docosahexaenoic acid (DHA). Diets high in omega-3 fatty acids may lower very low-density lipoproteins (VLDL), triglyceride and total cholesterol concentrations; increase concentrations of high-density lipoproteins (HDL); prolong bleeding times; decrease platelet aggregation; reduce plasma fibrinogen (data conflict); inhibit leukocyte function.

Studies on the effects of omega-3 fatty acids on the lipoproteins closely associated with atherosclerosis (LDL and HDL) show variable results and require further investigation.

Some studies have actually shown an increase in LDL-cholesterol levels in patients and healthy subjects receiving omega-3 fatty acids at doses currently recommended by the manufacturers (4.6 to 13.3 g/day). Although the optimal dose has not been established, significant effects of the omega-3 fatty acids may only be observed with 20 g or more per day. Some of the available products also contain cholesterol and saturated fat, which may play a role in the increased LDL-cholesterol levels.

Patients on diets with high levels of fish oils have increased EPA levels and decreased arachidonic acid levels in plasma lipids and platelet membranes. Also, increased synthesis of prostaglandin I_3 and decreased platelet synthesis of thromboxane A_2 have been noted. Prostaglandin I_3, an antiaggregation substance, and thromboxane A_2, a potent stimulator of platelet aggregation and secretion, are usually in balance. It is believed EPA is utilized by vessel walls to synthesize prostaglandin I_3, and arachidonic acid is utilized by platelets to synthesize thromboxane A_2. Therefore, the higher EPA levels and lower arachidonic acid levels produced by a diet high in fish oils could cause decreased platelet aggregation. Vitamin E in the product could also contribute to decreased platelet aggregation.

Indications:

Omega-3 fatty acids may be used as nondrug dietary supplements for patients at early risk of coronary artery disease primarily because of the effects on platelets and lipids.

The American Heart Association recommends consumption of fish; however, it does not find justification for fish oil capsule supplementation.

Unlabeled uses: Omega-3 fatty acids have been studied as adjunctive treatment of rheumatoid arthritis (20 g/day have been used). These agents may also be of benefit in the treatment of psoriasis (10 to 15 g/day); however, data is conflicting. Omega-3 fatty acids (18 g/day) may be beneficial in preventing early restenosis after coronary angioplasty in combination with dipyridamole and aspirin in high risk male patients.

Warnings, Precautions and Adverse Reactions:

Diarrhea has occurred in patients taking 4 to 6 capsules per day.

Increased bleeding time and *inhibition of platelet aggregation* have occurred. Use caution in patients receiving **anticoagulants** or **aspirin**.

Diabetes mellitus: In one study the fasting and mean glucose levels increased and insulin secretion was impaired in six patients with non-insulin dependent diabetes mellitus (NIDDM) following 1 month of omega-3 fatty acid administration (5.4 g/day). However, increased insulin sensitivity in NIDDM patients has occurred. Use with caution in NIDDM patients.

Pregnancy: Until further information is available, do not use omega-3 fatty acids in these patients.

Children: Until further information is available, do not use omega-3 fatty acids in these patients.

Administration and Dosage:

Nutritional supplement: 1 to 2 capsules 3 times daily with meals.

(Products listed on following page)

OMEGA-3 (N-3) POLYUNSATURATED FATTY ACIDS (Cont.)

	Product/ Distributor	mg/ capsule	N-3 fat content (mg) EPA	DHA	Other Content	How Supplied	C.I.*
otc *sf*	**Promega Pearls Softgels** (Parke-Davis)	600	168	72	< 2 mg cholesterol, 1 IU vitamin E,[1] < 2% RDA of vitamins A, B_1, B_2, B_3, Fe and Ca	In 60s and 90s.	NA
otc	**Cardi-Omega 3 Capsules** (Thompson Medical)	1000	180	120	< 2% RDA of vitamins A, B_1, B_2, B_3, C, D, Fe and Ca	Sodium free. Peppermint flavor. In 60s.	240
otc	**Marlipids** III **Capsules** (Fibertone)				5 IU vitamin E[1]	In 100s.	88
otc *sf*	**EPA Capsules** (Nature's Bounty)				1 IU vitamin E[1]	In 50s and 100s.	136
otc	**Max EPA Capsules** (Various, eg, Jones Medical, Moore, Rexall, Schein)				5 mg cholesterol, < 2% RDA of vitamins A, B_1, B_2, B_3, C, Ca, Fe	In 60s, 90s & 100s.	45+
otc *sf*	**Promega Softgels** (Parke-Davis)	1000	280	120	< 1 mg cholesterol, 1 IU vitamin E[1] (6% RDA), vitamins A, B_1, B_2, B_3, Ca & Fe (< 2% RDA)	Sodium free. In 30s and 60s.	212
otc *sf*	**Sea-Omega 50 Softgels** (Rugby)	1000	300	200	1 IU vitamin E[1]	Sodium free. In 50s.	297
otc	**Sea-Omega 30 Softgels** (Rugby)	1200	180	140	2 IU vitamin E[1]	In 100s.	95
otc	**Marine Lipid Concentrate Softgels** (Vitaline)	1200	360	240	5 IU vitamin E[1]	Sodium free. In 90s.	NA
otc	**SuperEPA 1200 Softgels** (Advanced Nutritional)	1200	360	240	5 IU vitamin E[1]	In 60s, 90s and 180s.	NA
otc	**SuperEPA 2000 Capsules** (Advanced Nutritional)	1000	563	312	20 IU vitamin E[1]	In 30s, 60s and 90s.	NA

* Cost Index based on cost per capsule.
sf – Sugar free.
[1] As d-alpha tocopherol.

Enteral nutrition products may be administered orally, via nasogastric tube, via feeding gastrostomy or via needle-catheter jejunostomy. The defined formula diets may be monomeric or oligomeric (amino acids or short peptides and simple carbohydrates) or polymeric (more complex protein and carbohydrate sources) in composition. Modular supplements are used for individual supplementation of protein, carbohydrate or fat when formulas do not offer sufficient flexibility.

There are different criteria for evaluating and categorizing these products; no single system of classification is ideal. Caloric density, generally in the range of 1, 1.5 or 2 Cal/ml, influences the density of other nutrients. Protein content is also a major determinant. Osmolality may be important in patients who experience diarrhea and cramping with high osmolality formulas. Consider products with low fat content in patients with significant malabsorption, hyperlipidemia or severe exocrine pancreatic insufficiency. Medium chain triglycerides are a useful energy source in patients with malabsorption, but do not provide essential fatty acids. Lactose, poorly tolerated by patients lacking lactase activity, has been eliminated from many of the nutritionally complete enteral formulas. In general, with the exception of lactose or specific allergies (eg, corn, gluten), the source of the protein or carbohydrate is not critical. Various amounts of vitamins, electrolytes and minerals are included in the formulations. Consider sodium and potassium content in patients with renal or hepatic disease. Also, consider vitamin K content in patients receiving warfarin, since the hypoprothrombinemic effect may be decreased. Although many of the products have been formulated to contain lesser amounts of vitamin K, caution is still warranted.

Some enteral preparations list the osmolality or osmolarity of the formula at standard dilution. However, when the term osmolarity is used, it cannot be determined whether the osmolarity was calculated from osmolality or if the term osmolarity is being used erroneously. Also, when samples of a specific product from the same lot or different lots were reconstituted, or if the powder was reconstituted by using the provided scoop vs reconstitution by weight, there was a wide variation in osmolality. Be aware of these potential discrepancies when utilizing osmolality information.

Cost of products is influenced by composition (oligomeric or polymeric) and form (ready-to-use or powder). In general, polymeric products cost less than oligomeric products. The form of the product indirectly affects its cost due to the amount of labor involved in preparation.

Specialized formulas are indicated for specific disease states and may be nutritionally incomplete.

Hepatic failure/encephalopathy formulas contain high concentrations of branched chain amino acids (BCAA) and low concentrations of aromatic amino acids (AAA) in an attempt to correct the abnormal plasma amino acid profiles.

Renal failure formulas contain only essential amino acids as the source of protein.

Trauma or high stress formulas contain high concentrations of BCAA, but unlike the hepatic products, are not restricted in the amounts of AAA.

Monitoring of patients receiving enteral nutritional therapy includes the following: Weight, fluid balance, serum electrolytes, glucose tolerance, liver and renal function, albumin and general condition. Watch for GI overload or obstruction and abdominal distention; check tube placement for proper position. Initiate therapy with a slow but gradual advancement in administration rate.

Several case reports and single-dose studies suggest that phenytoin administration during enteral nutritional therapy may result in decreased phenytoin concentrations; however, this has not been substantiated. Monitor phenytoin concentrations in these patients. Consider giving phenytoin 2 hours before and after the enteral feeding, or stopping the enteral therapy for 2 hours before and after phenytoin administration.

Enteral Nutritional Product Categories	
Modular Supplements	*Defined Formulas*
Protein	Milk-based formulas
Carbohydrate	Specialized formulas
Fat	Hepatic failure/encephalopathy
	Renal failure
	Trauma/stress
	Pulmonary
	Nutritionally complete, lactose free formulas

Content listed is based on standard dilutions. Refer to manufacturer's literature for mixing directions, other dilutions and storage conditions.

(Continued on following page)

Modular Supplements

PROTEIN PRODUCTS

	Product	Description	How Supplied
otc	**Gevral Protein** (Lederle)	**Powder:** Ca caseinate and sucrose. Each ⅓ cup (≈26 g) contains: 15.6 g protein, 7.05 g carbohydrate, 0.52 g fat, < 50 mg Na, ≥ 13 mg K and 95.3 Calories *Dose:* 26 g in 8 oz liquid.	< 1% alcohol. In 8 oz and 5 lb.
otc	**ProMod** (Ross)	**Powder:** D-whey protein concentrate and soy lecithin. Each 26.4 g provides 20 g protein, 2.4 g fat, 2.68 g carbohydrate, 176 mg Ca, 60 mg Na, 260 mg K, 132 mg P and 112 Calories *Dose:* Add 1 scoop (6.6 g) to liquid, food or enteral formula.	In 275 g cans.
otc	**Propac** (Sherwood)	**Powder:** Each tablespoon (4 g) contains 3 g protein (from whey protein), 0.24 g carbohydrate from lactose, 0.32 g fat, 2 mg Cl, 20 mg K, 9 mg Na, 14 mg Ca, 12 mg P, 2 mg Mg and 16 Calories *Dose:* Add 1 tablespoon to liquid.	In 20 g packets and 350 g cans.

GLUCOSE POLYMERS

Actions:

These glucose polymers are derived from cornstarch by hydrolysis.

Indications:

Supplies calories in persons with increased caloric needs or persons unable to meet their caloric needs with usual food intake. Supplies carbohydrate calories in protein, electrolyte and fat restricted diets. Also used to increase the caloric density of traditional foods, liquid and tube feedings.

Dosage:

Add to foods or beverages or mix in water. Small, frequent feedings are more desirable than large amounts given infrequently. May be used for extended periods with diets containing all other essential nutrients, or as an oral adjunct to IV administration of nutrients. Not a balanced diet; do not use as a sole source of nutrition.

Content given per 100 ml liquid or 100 g powder.

	Product & Distributor	CHO (g)	Calories	Sodium (mg)	Chloride (mg)	Potassium (mg)	Calcium (mg)	Phosphorus (mg)	How Supplied
otc	**Polycose Liquid** (Ross)	50	200	70	140	6	20	3	In 126 ml.
otc	**Polycose Powder** (Ross)	94	380	110	223	10	30	5	In 350 g.
otc	**Moducal Powder** (Mead Johnson Nutritional)	95[1]	380	70	150	< 10	—	—	In 368 g.[2]
otc	**Sumacal Powder** (Sherwood)	95[1]	380	100	210	< 39	< 20	< 31	In 400 g.[2]

[1] Maltodextrin.

[2] Contains 0.4 g/100 g minerals (ash).

Modular Supplements (Cont.)

CORN OIL

Indications:

Increasing caloric intake.

Precautions:

Use in the presence of gallbladder disease or diabetes only on the advice of a physician.

Dosage:

Adults: 45 ml, 2 to 4 times daily, after or between meals.

Children: 30 ml, 1 to 4 times daily, after or between meals.

otc	**Lipomul** (Roberts[1])	**Liquid:** 10 g corn oil per 15 ml in a vehicle containing polysorbate 80, glyceride phosphates and 6.3 mg saccharin (from sodium saccharin) with 0.05% sodium benzoate, 0.05% benzoic acid, 0.07% sorbic acid, BHA and vitamin E. Each serving (45 ml) contains 270 Calories and 30 g fat.	Citrus-vanilla flavor. In 473 ml.

SAFFLOWER OIL

Indications:

Dietary management of patients requiring caloric supplementation (ie, fatty acid deficiencies). Supplies essential fatty acids.

Precautions:

Use in the presence of gallbladder disease or diabetes only on the advice of a physician.

Do not administer to patients with a severe malabsorption syndrome.

Dosage:

Oral: May give by tablespoon. Flavor additives may improve patient acceptance.

Tube feeding: Can be added to a patient's formula depending upon the degree of caloric supplementation needed.

Shake well before using.

otc	**Microlipid** (Sherwood)	**Emulsion:** 50% fat emulsion. Safflower oil, polyglycerol esters of fatty acids, soy lecithin, xanthan gum and ascorbic acid. Contains 4500 Calories and 500 g fat per L. *Osmolality* – 60 mOsm/kg water	In 120 ml.

MEDIUM CHAIN TRIGLYCERIDES (MCT)

Medium chain triglycerides are more rapidly hydrolyzed than conventional food fat, require less bile acid for digestion, are carried by the portal circulation and are not dependent on chylomicron formation or lymphatic transport. Does not provide essential fatty acids.

Indications:

A special dietary supplement for use in the nutritional management of patients who cannot efficiently digest and absorb conventional long chain food fats.

Precautions:

Hepatic cirrhosis: In persons with advanced cirrhosis, large amounts of MCT may elevate blood and spinal fluid levels of medium chain fatty acids (MCFA) due to impaired hepatic clearance of MCFA which are rapidly absorbed via the portal vein. These elevated levels have caused reversible coma and precoma in subjects with advanced cirrhosis, particularly with portacaval shunts. Use with caution in persons with hepatic cirrhosis and complications such as portacaval shunts or tendency to encephalopathy.

Dosage:

15 ml, 3 to 4 times per day. Mix with fruit juices, use on salads and vegetables, incorporate into sauces or use in cooking or baking. Do not use plastic containers or utensils.

otc	**MCT** (Mead Johnson Nutritionals)	**Oil:** Lipid fraction of coconut oil consisting primarily of the triglycerides of C_8 (≈ 67%) and C_{10} (≈ 23%) saturated fatty acids. Contains 115 Calories/15 ml	In qt.

[1] Roberts Pharmaceutical Corp., Meridian Center III, 6 Industrial Way West, Eatontown, NJ 07724

Defined Formula Diets

Milk-based formulas

		Content per Liter											
		Protein		Carbohydrate		Fat							
	Product & Distributor	g	Source	g	Source	g	Source	Na (mg)	K (mg)	mOsm/ kg H_2O	Cal/ ml	Other Content	How Supplied
otc	**Meritene Liquid** (Sandoz Nutrition)	58	concentrated sweet skim milk, Na caseinate	110	lactose, hydrolyzed corn starch, sugar	32	corn oil, mono- and diglycerides	880	1600	510[1]	0.96	Vit A, B_1, B_2, B_3, B_5, B_6, B_{12}, C, D, E, folic acid, biotin, choline, Ca, Cl, Cu, Fe, I, Mg, Mn, P, Zn	*Gluten free.* Chocolate and vanilla flavors. In 250 ml ready-to-use.
otc	**Sustacal Powder**[2] (Mead Johnson Nutritionals)	86.5	nonfat milk	202.6	sugar, corn syrup solids	38.8	unknown	1329.6	3840.2		1.01	Vit A, B_1, B_2, B_3, B_5, B_6, B_{12}, C, D, E, folic acid, biotin, Ca, Cl, Cu, Fe, I, Mg, Mn, P, Zn	Vanilla. In 1.9 oz. packets and 1 lb cans. Chocolate. In 1.9 oz. packets.
otc	**Lonalac Powder** (Mead Johnson Nutritionals)	53.8	casein	74.9	lactose	55.9	coconut oil	40.1	1983	360	1.01	Vit A, B_1, B_2, B_3, Ca, Cl, Mg, P	In 1 lb cans.
otc	**Meritene Powder**[2] (Sandoz Nutrition)	69	nonfat milk, whole milk, Ca caseinate	120	lactose, sugar, hydrolyzed corn starch, fructose	34	milk fat, soy lecithin	1100	2800	690	1.1	Vit A, B_1, B_2, B_3, B_5, B_6, B_{12}, C, D, E, K, folic acid, biotin, choline, Ca, Cl, Cu, Fe, I, Mg, Mn, P, Zn	*Gluten free.* Plain, chocolate, eggnog, vanilla and milk chocolate flavors. In 1 and 4½ lb.

[1] Vanilla.
[2] Content given for powder mixed with whole milk.

(Continued on following page)

Defined Formula Diets (Cont.)

Milk-based formulas (Cont.)

		Content per Liter											
		Protein		Carbohydrate		Fat							
	Product & Distributor	g	Source	g	Source	g	Source	Na (mg)	K (mg)	mOsm/kg H_2O	Cal/ml	Other Content	How Supplied
otc	**Compleat Regular Formula Liquid** (Sandoz Nutrition)	43	beef, nonfat milk	130	nonfat milk, fruits and vegetables, maltodextrin	43	beef, corn oil, mono- and diglycerides	1300	1400	450	1.1	Vit A, B_1, B_2, B_3, B_5, B_6, B_{12}, C, D, E, K, FA, biotin, choline, Ca, Cl, Cr, Cu, Fe, I, Mg, Mn, Mo, P, Se, Zn	In 250 ml ready-to-use bottles and cans and Closed System.
otc	**Forta Shake Powder**[1] (Ross)	9	nonfat dry milk	26	sucrose	< 1	unknown	115	440	NA	140 (per 39.6 g mix)	Vit A, B_1, B_2, B_3, B_5, B_6, B_{12}, C, D, E, folic acid, biotin, Ca, Cu, Fe, I, Mg, Mn, P, Zn	Tartrazine. Vanilla & eggnog. In 1 lb cans, 1.4 oz pkts. Chocolate. In 1 lb 2.7 oz cans, 1.6 oz pkts.
otc	**Travasorb Renal Powder**[2] (Clintec Nutrition)	8	crystalline amino acids	94.7	glucose oligosaccharides, sucrose	6.2	MCT (fractionated coconut oil), sunflower oil, lecithin	0	0	≈ 590	467 per packet	Vit B_1, B_2, B_3, B_5, B_6, C, folic acid, biotin, choline	*For renal failure.* Apricot and strawberry flavors. In 112 g packets.
otc	**Sustacal Pudding**[3] (Mead Johnson Nutritionals)	6.8	nonfat milk	32	sugar, lactose, modified food starch	9.5	partially hydrogenated soy oil	120	320	NA	1.6 (per 141.5 g)	Vit A, B_1, B_2, B_3, B_5, B_6, B_{12}, C, D, E, FA, biotin, Ca, Cl, Cu, Fe, I, Mg, Mn, P, Zn	Vanilla (contains tartrazine), chocolate and butterscotch. In 5 oz.
otc	**Sustagen Powder** (Mead Johnson Nutritionals)	112.9	nonfat milk, dry whole milk, calcium caseinate	316	dextrose, lactose, corn syrup solids, sugar (chocolate)	16.9	milk fat	1044	3375	1100	1.8	Vit A, B_1, B_2, B_3, B_5, B_6, B_{12}, C, D, E, K, folic acid, biotin, choline, Ca, Cl, Cu, Fe, I, Mg, Mn, P, Zn	Vanilla and chocolate flavors. In 1 lb.

NA = Not applicable.
[1] Content given per serving (1.4 oz or 39.6 g mix).
[2] Content given per packet (112 g).
[3] Content given per 5 oz (141.5 g) serving.

(Continued on following page)

Defined Formula Diets (Cont.)

Specialized formulas

		Content per Liter											
		Protein		Carbohydrate		Fat							
	Product & Distributor	g	Source	g	Source	g	Source	Na (mg)	K (mg)	mOsm/kg H_2O	Cal/ml	Other Content	How Supplied
otc	**Amin-Aid Instant Drink Powder** (Kendall McGaw)	19.4	essential amino acids	365.5	maltodextrins, sucrose	44.9	partially hydrogenated soybean oil, lecithin, mono- and diglycerides	< 115	0	700	2		*For acute or chronic renal failure.* Lemon-lime (contains tartrazine), orange, berry and strawberry flavors. In 148 g packets.
otc	**Replena Liquid** (Ross)	30	sodium and calcium caseinates	255.7	hydrolyzed corn starch, sucrose	95.8	hi-oleic safflower oil, soy oil, soy lecithin	784	1118	615	2	Vit A, B_1, B_2, B_3, B_5, B_6, B_{12}, C, D, E, K, folic acid, Ca, Cl, Cu, Fe, I, Mg, Mn, P, Se, Zn[1]	*For acute or chronic renal failure.* Lactose and gluten free, vanilla flavor. In 8 oz ready-to-use cans.
otc	**Travasorb Hepatic Powder** (Clintec Nutrition)	29.4	L-amino acids	215.3	glucose oligosaccharides, sucrose	14.7	MCT (fractionated coconut oil), sunflower oil, lecithin	235	882	600	1.1	Vit A, B_1, B_2, B_3, B_5, B_6, B_{12}, C, D, E, K, folic acid, Ca, Cl, Cu, Fe, I, Mg, Mn, P, Zn[1]	*For liver failure.* Apricot and strawberry flavors. In 96 g packets.
otc	**Hepatic-Aid II Instant Drink Powder** (Kendall McGaw)	44.1	amino acids (high BCAA, low AAA)	168.5	maltodextrins, sucrose	36.2	partially hydrogenated soybean oil, lecithin, mono- and diglycerides	< 115	0	560	1.2		*For chronic liver disease.* Chocolate, eggnog and custard flavors; some contain tartrazine, consult package label. In 88.7 g packets.
otc	**Accupep HPF** (Sherwood)	40	hydrolyzed lactalbumin	188	maltodextrin	10	MCT oil (fractionated coconut oil), corn oil, mono- and diglycerides	680	1150	490	1	Vit A, B_1, B_2, B_3, B_5, B_6, B_{12}, C, D, E, K, folic acid, Ca, Cl, Cu, Fe, I, Mg, Mn, P, Zn[1]	*For GI conditions.* In 128 g packets.

[1] Also contains biotin and choline.

(Continued on following page)

Defined Formula Diets (Cont.)

Specialized formulas (Cont.)

		Content per Liter								mOsm/ kg H_2O	Cal/ ml	Other Content	How Supplied
		Protein		Carbohydrate		Fat		Na (mg)	K (mg)				
	Product & Distributor	g	Source	g	Source	g	Source						
otc	**Glucerna Liquid** (Ross)	41.8	amino acids, Ca and Na caseinate	93.7	hydrolyzed cornstarch, fructose, soy fiber	55.7	hi-oleic safflower oil, soy oil, soy lecithin	928	1561	375	1	Vit A, B_1, B_2, B_3, B_5, B_6, B_{12}, C, D, E, K, folic acid, Cl, Ca, P, Mg, I, Mn, Cu, Zn, Fe, Se, Cr, Mo[1]	*For abnormal glucose tolerance.* Vanilla flavor. In 8 oz ready-to-use cans.
otc	**Traum-Aid HBC Powder** (Kendall McGaw)	56	amino acids	166	maltodextrins	12.4	partially hydrogenated soybean oil, MCT, lecithin	533	1167	760	1	Vit A, B_1, B_2, B_3, B_5, B_6, B_{12}, C, D, E, K, folic acid, Ca, Mg, Mn, Fe, Cu, Zn, Cr, Se, Mo, Cl, P, I[1]	*For trauma and sepsis.* Tartrazine. Lemon creme flavor. In 125.8 g packets.
otc	**Stresstein Powder** (Sandoz Nutrition)	70	amino acids (44% BCAA)	170	hydrolyzed cornstarch	28	MCT, soybean oil, polyglycerol esters of fatty acids.	650	1100	910	1.2	Vit A, B_1, B_2, B_3, B_5, B_6, B_{12}, C, D, E, K, folic acid, Ca, P, I, Fe, Mg, Cu, Zn, Cl, Mn, Se, Cr, Mo[1]	*For severe metabolic stress, trauma and sepsis.* In 102 g packets.
otc	**TraumaCal Liquid** (Mead Johnson Nutritionals)	82.3	Ca and Na caseinate, amino acids	143.5	corn syrup, sugar	68.4	soybean oil, MCT (fractionated coconut oil), lecithin	1182	1393	490	1.5	Vit A, B_1, B_2, B_3, B_5, B_6, B_{12}, C, D, E, K, folic acid, Ca, P, I, Fe, Mg, Mn, Cu, Zn, Cl[1]	*For multiple trauma and major burns.* Lactose free. Vanilla flavor. In 8 oz ready-to-use cans.
otc	**Pulmocare Liquid** (Ross)	62.5	Ca and Na caseinate	105.5	hydrolyzed cornstarch, sucrose	92	corn oil, lecithin	1308	1730	490	1.5	Vit A, B_1, B_2, B_3, B_5, B_6, B_{12}, C, D, E, K, folic acid, Cl, Ca, P, Mg, I, Mn, Cu, Zn, Fe[1]	*For pulmonary patients.* Lactose free. Vanilla and strawberry flavors. In 8 oz ready-to-use cans.

[1] Also contains biotin and choline.

(Continued on following page)

Defined Formula Diets (Cont.)

Lactose Free Products

		Content per Liter											
		Protein		Carbohydrate		Fat		Na	K	mOsm/	Cal/	Other	
	Product & Distributor	g	Source	g	Source	g	Source	(mg)	(mg)	kg H_2O	ml	Content	How Supplied
otc	**Half Strength Entrition Entri-Pak Liquid** (Biosearch)	17.5	Na and Ca caseinates	68	maltodextrin	17.5	corn oil, soy lecithin, mono- and diglycerides	350	600	120	0.5	Vit A, B_1, B_2, B_3, B_5, B_6, B_{12}, C, D, E, K, Ca, P, Mg, I, Fe, Zn, Mn, Cu, Cl[1]	In 1 L pouch.
otc	**Pre-Attain Liquid** (Sherwood)	20	Na caseinate	60	maltodextrin	20	corn oil, soy lecithin	340	575	150	0.5	Vit A, B_1, B_2, B_3, B_5, B_6, B_{12}, C, D, E, K, Ca, Cl, Cu, I, Fe, Mg, Mn, P, Zn[1]	In 250 ml cans and 1000 ml pre-filled closed systems.
otc	**Citrotein Powder** (Sandoz Nutrition)	41	egg white solids	120	sugar, hydrolyzed cornstarch	1.6	mono- and diglycerides, partially hydrogenated soybean oil	670	550	490[2]	0.67	Vit A, B_1, B_2, B_3, B_5, B_6, B_{12}, C, D, E, Ca, P, I, Fe, Mg, Cu, Zn, Cl, Mn[1]	*Cholesterol free.* Orange (tartrazine), grape & punch flavors. In 1.57 oz packets, 14.16 oz cans.
otc	**Precision Isotonic Diet Powder**[3] (Sandoz Nutrition)	7.5	egg white solids, Na caseinate	37.5	maltodextrin, sucrose	7.8	partially hydrogenated soybean oil, mono- and diglycerides	200	250	300	250[3]	Vit A, B_1, B_2, B_3, B_5, B_6, B_{12}, C, D, E, K, Ca, P, I, Fe, Mg, Cu, Zn, Cl, Mn, Se, Cr, Mo[1]	*Cholesterol, purine & gluten free.* Vanilla and orange flavors. In 58.4 g packets.
otc	**Entrition Entri-Pak Liquid** (Biosearch)	35	Ca and Na caseinates	136	maltodextrin	35	corn oil, soy lecithin, mono- and diglycerides	700	1200	300	1	Vit A, B_1, B_2, B_3, B_5, B_6, B_{12}, C, D, E, K, Ca, Cl, Cu, I, Fe, Mg, Mn, P, Zn[1]	In 1 L pouch.
otc	**Entrition RDA Entri-Pak Liquid** (Biosearch)	36	Na and Ca caseinates	135	maltodextrin	35	corn oil, soy lecithin, mono- and diglycerides	800	1333	300	1	Vit A, B_1, B_2, B_3, B_5, B_6, B_{12}, C, D, E, K, Ca, P, Mg, Fe, Zn, Mn, Cu, I, Cl, Se, Cr, Mo[1]	In 1.5 L pouch.

[1] Also contains biotin, choline and folic acid. [2] Orange flavor. [3] Content given per 2.06 oz (58.4 g) packet

(Continued on following page)

Defined Formula Diets (Cont.)

Lactose Free Products (Cont.)

		Content per Liter								mOsm/ kg H_2O	Cal/ ml	Other Content	How Supplied
		Protein		Carbohydrate		Fat		Na (mg)	K (mg)				
	Product & Distributor	g	Source	g	Source	g	Source						
otc	**Travasorb MCT Powder** (Clintec Nutrition)	49.3	lactalbumin, Na and K caseinate	122.8	corn syrup solids	33	sunflower oil, MCT (fractionated coconut oil)	350	1000	312	1	Vit A, B_1, B_2, B_3, B_5, B_6, B_{12}, C, D, E, K, Ca, Cl, Cu, Fe, I, Mg, Mn, P, Zn[1]	*Gluten free.* In 89 g packets.
otc	**PediaSure Liquid** (Ross)	30	Na caseinate, whey protein concentrate	109.8	hydrolyzed cornstarch, sucrose	49.8	hi-oleic safflower oil, soy oil, MCT (fractionated coconut oil), mono- and diglycerides, soy lecithin	380	1308	<310	1	Vit A, B_1, B_2, B_3, B_5, B_6, B_{12}, C, D, E, K, inositol, Cl, Ca, P, Mg, I, Mn, Cu, Zn, Fe[1]	*Gluten free.* Vanilla flavor. In 240 ml ready-to-use cans.
otc	**Vitaneed Liquid** (Sherwood)	40	pureed beef, Ca and Na caseinates, dietary fiber from soy	128	maltodextrin, pureed fruits and vegetables	40	corn oil, soy lecithin	680	1250	300	1	Vit A, B_1, B_2, B_3, B_5, B_6, B_{12}, C, D, E, K, Ca, Cl, Cu, Fe, I, Mg, Mn, P, Zn[1]	In 250 ml ready-to-use cans and 1000 ml prefilled systems.
otc	**Travasorb HN Powder**[2] (Clintec Nutrition)	15	enzymatically hydrolyzed lactalbumin	58.3	glucose oligosaccharides	4.5	MCT (fractionated coconut oil), sunflower oil	307	390	560	333.3 (per packet)	Vit A, B_1, B_2, B_3, B_5, B_6, B_{12}, C, D, E, K, Ca, Cl, Cu, Fe, I, Mg, Mn, P, Zn[1]	*Gluten free.* In 83.3 g packets.
otc	**Travasorb STD Powder**[2] (Clintec Nutrition)	10	enzymatically hydrolyzed lactalbumin	63.3	glucose oligosaccharides	4.5	MCT (fractionated coconut oil), sunflower oil	307	390	560	333.3 (per packet)	Vit A, B_1, B_2, B_3, B_5, B_6, B_{12}, C, D, E, K, Ca, Cl, Cu, Fe, I, Mg, Mn, P, Zn[1]	*Gluten free.* In 83.3 g packets.

[1] Also contains biotin, choline and folic acid.
[2] Content given per 83.3 g packet.

(Continued on following page)

Defined Formula Diets (Cont.)

Lactose Free Products (Cont.)

	Product & Distributor	Content per Liter								mOsm/ kg H_2O	Cal/ ml	Other Content	How Supplied
		Protein		Carbohydrate		Fat		Na (mg)	K (mg)				
		g	Source	g	Source	g	Source						
otc	**Replete Liquid** (Clintec Nutrition)	62.4	K and Ca caseinate	112.8	maltodextrin, sucrose	33.2	corn oil, lecithin	500	1560	350	1	Vit A, B_1, B_2, B_3, B_5, B_6, B_{12}, C, D, E, K, folic acid, Ca, Cl, Cu, Fe, I, Mg, Mn, P, Zn[1]	*Cholesterol free, gluten free.* Vanilla flavor. In 250 ml ready-to-use containers.
otc	**Peptamen Liquid** (Clintec Nutrition)	40	23% of proteins from BCAA, enzymatically hydrolyzed whey proteins	127	maltodextrin, starch	39	MCT (fractionated coconut oil), sunflower oil, lecithin	500	1250	260	1	Vit A, B_1, B_2, B_3, B_5, B_6, B_{12}, C, D, E, K, folic acid, Ca, Cl, Cu, Fe, I, Mg, Mn, P, Zn[1]	*Cholesterol free, gluten free.* In 500 ml ready-to-use cans.
otc	**Attain Liquid** (Sherwood)	40	Na and Ca caseinate	135	maltodextrin	35	MCT (fractionated coconut oil), corn oil, soy lecithin	805	1600	300	1	Vit A, B_1, B_2, B_3, B_5, B_6, B_{12}, C, D, E, K, folic acid, Ca, Cl, Cu, Fe, I, Mg, Mn, P, Zn, Cr, Se, Mo[1]	In 250 ml ready-to-use cans and 1000 ml closed system.
otc	**Profiber Liquid** (Sherwood)	40	Na and Ca caseinate, dietary fiber from soy	132	hydrolyzed cornstarch	40	corn oil, soy lecithin	730	1250	300	1	Vit A, B_1, B_2, B_3, B_5, B_6, B_{12}, C, D, E, K, folic acid, Ca, Cl, Cr, Cu, Fe, I, Mg, Mn, Mo, P, Se, Zn[1]	In 250 ml ready-to-use cans and 1000 ml closed system.
otc	**Impact Liquid** (Sandoz Nutrition)	56	Na and Ca caseinates, L-arginine	132	hydrolyzed cornstarch	28	structured lipids from palm kernel oil and sunflower oil, refined menhaden oil, hydroxylated soy lecithin	1100	1300	375	1	Vit A, B_1, B_2, B_3, B_5, B_6, B_{12}, C, E, D, K, folic acid, Ca, Fe, P, I, Mg, Zn, Cu, Cl, Mn, Se, Cr, Mo[1]	In 250 ml ready-to-use cans.

[1] Also contains biotin and choline.

(Continued on following page)

Defined Formula Diets (Cont.)

Lactose free products (Cont.)

		Content per Liter								mOsm/ kg H_2O	Cal/ ml	Other Content	How Supplied
		Protein		Carbohydrate		Fat		Na	K				
	Product & Distributor	g	Source	g	Source	g	Source	(mg)	(mg)				
otc	**Nutren 1.0 Liquid** (Clintec Nutrition)	40	K and Ca caseinates	127.2	maltodextrin, corn syrup, sucrose[1]	38	MCT (fractionated coconut oil), corn oil, lecithin	500	1252	300-390	1	Vit A, B_1, B_2, B_3, B_5, B_6, B_{12}, C, D, E, K, folic acid, biotin, choline, Ca, Cl, Cu, Fe, I, Mg, Mn, P, Zn	*Cholesterol and gluten free.* Unflavored, vanilla, chocolate and strawberry flavors. In 250 ml.
otc	**Sustacal Liquid** (Mead Johnson Nutritionals)	61.2	Ca and Na caseinates, soy protein isolate	139.3	sucrose, corn syrup	23.2	partially hydrogenated soy oil, lecithin	917	2086	650, 690[2]	1	Vit A, B_1, B_2, B_3, B_5, B_6, B_{12}, C, D, E, K, folic acid, biotin, choline, Ca, P, I, Fe, Mg, Cu, Zn, Mn, Cl	Vanilla, chocolate, strawberry and eggnog flavors. In 240, 360 ml and qt ready-to-use cans.
otc	**Tolerex Powder** (Procter & Gamble Pharm.)	20.6	free amino acids	226.3	predigested carbohydrates	1.45	safflower oil	468	1172	550	1	Vit A, B_1, B_2, B_3, B_5, B_6, B_{12}, C, D, E, K, folic acid, biotin, choline, Ca, P, I, Fe, Mg, Cu, Zn, Mn, Se, Mo, Cr	Assorted flavors. In 80 g packets.
otc	**Vivonex T.E.N. Powder** (Procter & Gamble Pharm.)	38.2	free amino acids	205.6	predigested carbohydrates	2.77	safflower oil	460	782	630	1	Vit A, B_1, B_2, B_3, B_5, B_6, B_{12}, C, D, E, K, folic acid, biotin, choline, Ca, P, I, Fe, Mg, Cu, Zn, Mn, Se, Mo, Cr, Cl	Assorted flavors. In 80.4 g packets.

[1] Sucrose not in unflavored varieties.
[2] Chocolate flavor.

(Continued on following page)

Defined Formula Diets (Cont.)

Lactose free products (Cont.)

	Product & Distributor	Protein g	Protein Source	Carbohydrate g	Carbohydrate Source	Fat g	Fat Source	Na (mg)	K (mg)	mOsm/ kg H_2O	Cal/ ml	Other Content	How Supplied
otc	**Portagen Powder** (Mead Johnson Nutritionals)	35.4	Na caseinate	114.6	corn syrup solids, sucrose	47.9	MCT (fractionated coconut oil), corn oil, soy lecithin	542	1250	320	1	Vit A, B_1, B_2, B_3, B_5, B_6, B_{12}, C, D, E, K, folic acid, biotin, choline, inositol, Ca, P, I, Fe, Mg, Cu, Zn, Mn, Cl	In 1 lb cans.
otc	**Vital High Nitrogen Powder** (Ross)	41.7	essential amino acids, partially hydrolyzed whey, meat and soy	184.7	hydrolyzed cornstarch, sucrose	10.8	safflower oil, MCT (fractionated coconut oil), mono- & diglycerides, soy lecithin	472	1167	500	1	Vit A, B_1, B_2, B_3, B_5, B_6, B_{12}, C, D, E, K, folic acid, biotin, choline, Ca, P, Mg, Fe, Cu, Zn, Mn, I, Cl	Vanilla flavor. In 79 g packets.
otc	**Entrition HN Entri-Pak Liquid** (Biosearch)	44	Na and Ca caseinates, soy protein isolate	114	maltodextrin	41	corn oil, soy lecithin, mono and diglycerides	920	1579	300	1	Vit A, B_1, B_2, B_3, B_5, B_6, B_{12}, C, D, E, K, folic acid, biotin, choline, Ca, Cl, Cu, Fe, I, Mg, Mn, P, Zn	In 1 liter pouch.
otc	**Precision High Nitrogen Diet Powder**[1] (Sandoz Nutrition)	12.5	egg white solids	62	maltodextrin, sucrose	0.36	MCT, partially hydrogenated soybean oil	280	260	525	300	Vit A, B_1, B_2, B_3, B_5, B_6, B_{12}, C, D, E, K, folic acid, biotin, choline, Ca, P, I, Fe, Mg, Cu, Zn, Cl, Mn, Se, Cr, Mo	*Cholesterol and gluten free.* Vanilla and citrus flavors. In 83 g packets.

[1] Content given per 83 g packet.

(Continued on following page)

Defined Formula Diets (Cont.)

Lactose free products (Cont.)

		Content per Liter								mOsm/ kg H_2O	Cal/ ml	Other Content	How Supplied
		Protein		Carbohydrate		Fat		Na (mg)	K (mg)				
	Product & Distributor	g	Source	g	Source	g	Source						
otc	**Criticare HN Liquid** (Mead Johnson Nutritionals)	38	enzymatically hydrolyzed casein	220	maltodextrin, modified cornstarch	5.3	safflower oil, mono- and diglycerides	630	1320	650	1.06	Vit A, B_1, B_2, B_3, B_5, B_6, B_{12}, C, D, E, K, folic acid, Ca, P, I, Fe, Mg, Cu, Zn, Mn, Cl[1]	Cholesterol free. In 240 ml ready-to-use.
otc	**Isocal Liquid** (Mead Johnson Nutritionals)	34	Ca and Na caseinates, soy protein isolate	135	maltodextrin	44	soy oil, MCT (fractionated coconut oil), lecithin	530	1320	270	1.06	Vit A, B_1, B_2, B_3, B_5, B_6, B_{12}, C, D, E, K, folic acid, Ca, P, I, Fe, Mg, Cu, Zn, Mn, Cl, Se, Cr, Mo[1]	In 240, 360 ml and qt ready-to-use.
otc	**Isocal HN Liquid** (Mead Johnson Nutritionals)	43.9	Ca and Na caseinate, soy protein isolate	122.4	maltodextrin	45.2	soy oil, MCT (fractionated coconut oil)	802	1055	NA	1.06	Vit A, B_1, B_2, B_3, B_5, B_6, B_{12}, C, D, E, K, folic acid, Ca, P, I, Fe, Mg, Cu, Zn, Mn, Cl, Se, Cr, Mo[1]	In 237 ml ready-to-use.
otc	**Jevity Liquid** (Ross)	44.3	Ca and Na caseinates, soy fiber	151.4	hydrolyzed cornstarch	36.7	MCT (fractionated coconut oil) soy oil, corn oil, soy lecithin	928	1561	310	1.06	Vit A, B_1, B_2, B_3, B_5, B_6, B_{12}, C, D, E, K, folic acid, Ca, P, Mg, Fe, Mn, Cu, Zn, I, Cl, Se, Cr, Mo[1]	In 240 ml and qt ready-to-use.
otc	**Resource Liquid** (Sandoz Nutrition)	37	Ca and Na caseinates, soy protein isolate	140	sugar, hydrolyzed cornstarch	37	corn oil, soy lecithin	890	1600	430	1.06	Vit A, B_1, B_2, B_3, B_5, B_6, B_{12}, C, D, E, K, folic acid, Ca, P, I, Fe, Mg, Cu, Zn, Mn, Cl[1]	*Gluten free.* Vanilla, chocolate and strawberry flavor. In 237 ml.

[1] Also contains biotin and choline.

(Continued on following page)

Defined Formula Diets (Cont.)

Lactose free products (Cont.)

	Product & Distributor	Content per Liter								mOsm/ kg H_2O	Cal/ ml	Other Content	How Supplied
		Protein		Carbohydrate		Fat		Na	K				
		g	Source	g	Source	g	Source	(mg)	(mg)				
otc	**Osmolite Liquid** (Ross)	37.1	Ca and Na caseinate, soy protein isolate	144.7	hydrolyzed cornstarch	38.4	MCT (fractionated coconut oil), corn oil, soy oil, soy lecithin	633	1013	300	1.06	Vit A, B_1, B_2, B_3, B_5, B_6, B_{12}, C, D, E, K, folic acid, choline, biotin, Cl, Ca, P, Mg, I, Mn, Cu, Zn, Fe	In 8 oz and qt ready-to-use.
otc	**Osmolite HN Liquid** (Ross)	44.4	Ca and Na caseinate, soy protein isolate	138.9	hydrolyzed cornstarch	36.7	MCT (fractionated coconut oil), corn oil, soy oil, lecithin	928	1561	300	1.06	Vit A, B_1, B_2, B_3, B_5, B_6, B_{12}, C, D, E, K, folic acid, choline, biotin, Cl, Ca, P, Mg, I, Mn, Cu, Zn, Fe	In 8 oz and qt ready-to-use.
otc	**Ensure Liquid and Powder** (Ross)	37.1	Ca and Na caseinate, soy protein isolate	144.7	corn syrup, sucrose	37.1	corn oil, soy lecithin	844	1561	470	1.06	Vit A, B_1, B_2, B_3, B_5, B_6, B_{12}, C, D, E, K, folic acid, choline, biotin, Cl, Ca, P, Mn, I, Mg, Cu, Zn, Fe	Assorted flavors. In 8 oz and qt ready-to-use and 400 g powder.
otc	**Ensure HN Liquid** (Ross)	44.3	Ca and Na caseinate, soy protein isolate	140.9	corn syrup, sucrose	35.4	corn oil, soy lecithin	802	1561	470	1.06	Vit A, B_1, B_2, B_3, B_5, B_6, B_{12}, C, D, E, K, folic acid, choline, biotin, Cl, Ca, P, Mg, Fe, Mn, Cu, Zn, I	Vanilla flavor. In 8 oz and qt ready-to-use. Chocolate flavor. In 8 oz ready-to-use.

(Continued on following page)

Defined Formula Diets (Cont.)

Lactose free products (Cont.)

		Content per Liter								mOsm/kg H_2O	Cal/ml	Other Content	How Supplied
		Protein		Carbohydrate		Fat		Na (mg)	K (mg)				
	Product & Distributor	g	Source	g	Source	g	Source						
otc	**Ultracal Liquid** (Mead Johnson Nutritional)	44	Ca and Na caseinate, soy fiber, oat fiber	123	maltodextrin	45	MCT (fractionated coconut oil), soy oil, mono- and diglycerides, soy lecithin	930	1610	310	1.06	Vit A, B_1, B_2, B_3, B_5, B_6, B_{12}, C, D, E, K, folic acid, choline, biotin, Ca, P, I, Fe, Mg, Cu, Zn, Mn, Cl, Se, Cr, Mo	In 8 oz ready-to-use cans.
otc	**Compleat Modified Formula** (Sandoz Nutrition)	43	beef, Ca caseinate	140	maltodextrin, pureed fruits & vegetables	37	corn oil, mono- and diglycerides	1000	1400	300	1.07	Vit A, B_1, B_2, B_3, B_5, B_6, B_{12}, C, D, E, K, folic acid, choline, biotin, Ca, P, I, Fe, Mg, Cu, Zn, Cl, Mn, Se, Cr, Mo	In 250 ml cans and 1000 ml closed systems. Ready-to-use.
otc	**Enrich Liquid with Fiber** (Ross)	39.7	Ca and Na caseinates, soy protein isolate, soy fiber	161.6	hydrolyzed cornstarch, sucrose	37.1	corn oil, soy lecithin	844	1688	480	1.1	Vit A, B_1, B_2, B_3, B_5, B_6, B_{12}, C, D, E, K, folic acid, choline, biotin, Cl, Ca, P, Mg, Fe, Mn, Cu, Zn, I	Assorted flavors. In 8 oz and qt ready-to-use.
otc	**Precision LR Diet Powder**[1] (Sandoz Nutrition)	7.5	egg white solids	71	maltodextrin, sucrose	0.45	MCT, partially hydrogenated soybean oil, mono- and diglycerides	200	250	510	317	Vit A, B_1, B_2, B_3, B_5, B_6, B_{12}, C, D, E, K, folic acid, choline, biotin, Ca, P, I, Fe, Mg, Cu, Zn, Mn, Se, Cr, Mo	*Cholesterol and gluten free.* Tartrazine (orange flavor). Orange and cherry flavors. In 3 oz packets.

[1] Content given per packet.

(Continued on following page)

Defined Formula Diets (Cont.)

Lactose free products (Cont.)

		Content per Liter								mOsm/ kg H_2O	Cal/ ml	Other Content	How Supplied
		Protein		Carbohydrate		Fat		Na	K				
	Product & Distributor	g	Source	g	Source	g	Source	(mg)	(mg)				
otc	**Isosource Liquid** (Sandoz Nutrition)	43.2	Ca and Na caseinate, soy protein isolate	175.5	maltodextrin	43.9	MCT, canola oil, lecithin	760	1182	390	1.2	Vit A, B_1, B_2, B_3, B_5, B_6, B_{12}, C, D, E, K, folic acid, biotin, choline, Ca, Cl, Cu, Fe, I, Mg, Mn, P, Zn, Se, Cr, Mo	*Gluten free.* Vanilla flavor. In 250 and 1000 ml closed systems. Ready-to-use.
otc	**Isotein HN Powder** (Sandoz Nutrition)	68	delactosed lactalbumin, Na caseinate	160	hydrolyzed cornstarch, fructose, mono-saccharides	34	partially hydrogenated soybean oil, MCT, mono- and diglycerides	620	1100	300	1.2	Vit A, B_1, B_2, B_3, B_5, B_6, B_{12}, C, D, E, K, folic acid, choline, biotin, Ca, P, I, Fe, Mg, Cu, Zn, Cl, Mn, Se, Cr, Mo	*Gluten free.* Vanilla flavor. In 2.9 oz packets.
otc	**Isosource HN Liquid** (Sandoz Nutrition)	56.1	Ca and Na caseinate, soy protein isolate	165	maltodextrin	43.9	MCT, canola oil, soy lecithin	760	1772	390	1.2	Vit A, B_1, B_2, B_3, B_5, B_6, B_{12}, C, D, E, K, folic acid, choline, biotin, Ca, P, I, Fe, Mg, Cu, Zn, Cl, Mn, Se, Cr, Mo	*Gluten free.* Vanilla flavor. In 250 ml cans and 1000 ml closed system. Ready-to-use.
otc	**Comply Liquid** (Sherwood)	60	Ca and Na caseinate	180	hydrolyzed cornstarch, sucrose[1]	60	corn oil, soy lecithin	1100	1850	410	1.5	Vit A, B_1, B_2, B_3, B_5, B_6, B_{12}, C, D, E, K, folic acid, biotin, choline, Ca, Cl, Cu, Fe, I, Mg, Mn, P, Zn	Unflavored. In 250 ml cans. Vanilla, orange and banana flavors. In 250 ml cans and 1000 ml prefilled systems.

[1] Sucrose not in unflavored variety.

(Continued on following page)

Defined Formula Diets (Cont.)

Lactose free products (Cont.)

		Content per Liter											
		Protein		Carbohydrate		Fat							
	Product & Distributor	g	Source	g	Source	g	Source	Na (mg)	K (mg)	mOsm/kg H_2O	Cal/ml	Other Content	How Supplied
otc	**Nutren 1.5 Liquid** (Clintec Nutrition)	60	casein	169.6	maltodextrin, corn syrup, sucrose	67.6	MCT (fractionated coconut oil), corn oil	752	1880	410-590	1.5	Vit A, B_1, B_2, B_3, B_5, B_6, B_{12}, C, D, E, K, folic acid, biotin, choline, Ca, Cl, Cu, Fe, I, Mg, Mn, P, Zn	*Cholesterol and gluten free.* Unflavored, vanilla and chocolate flavors. In 250 ml.
otc	**Ensure Plus Liquid** (Ross)	55	Ca and Na caseinate, soy protein isolate	199.6	corn syrup, sucrose	53.2	corn oil, soy lecithin	1055	1941	690	1.5	Vit A, B_1, B_2, B_3, B_5, B_6, B_{12}, C, D, E, K, folic acid, biotin, choline, Cl, Ca, P, Mg, Mn, I, Fe, Cu, Zn	Assorted flavors. In 8 oz and qt ready-to-use.
otc	**Resource Plus Liquid** (Sandoz Nutritional)	54.9	Ca and Na caseinates, soy protein isolate	200	maltodextrin, sucrose	53.3	corn oil, lecithin	899	1740	600	1.5	Vit A, B_1, B_2, B_3, B_5, B_6, B_{12}, C, D, E, K, folic acid, biotin, choline, Ca, P, I, Fe, Mg, Cu, Zn, Cl, Mn	*Gluten free.* Vanilla, chocolate and strawberry flavors. In 8 oz ready-to-use.
otc	**Sustacal HC Liquid** (Mead Johnson Nutritionals)	61	Ca and Na caseinate	190	corn syrup solids, sugar	58	corn oil, lecithin	850	1480	650	1.5	Vit A, B_1, B_2, B_3, B_5, B_6, B_{12}, C, D, E, K, folic acid, biotin, choline, Ca, P, I, Fe, Mg, Cu, Zn, Mn, Cl	Eggnog, chocolate and vanilla flavors. In 8 oz ready-to-use.

(Continued on following page)

Defined Formula Diets (Cont.)

Lactose free products (Cont.)

	Product & Distributor	Content per Liter								mOsm/kg H_2O	Cal/ml	Other Content	How Supplied
		Protein		Carbohydrate		Fat		Na	K				
		g	Source	g	Source	g	Source	(mg)	(mg)				
otc	**Ensure Plus HN Liquid** (Ross)	62.6	Ca and Na caseinate, soy protein isolate	199.7	hydrolyzed cornstarch, sucrose	49.8	corn oil, soy lecithin	1182	1815	650	1.5	Vit A, B_1, B_2, B_3, B_5, B_6, B_{12}, C, D, E, K, choline, Cl, Ca, P, Mg, I, Mn, Cu, Zn, Fe[1]	Vanilla and chocolate. In 8 oz ready-to-use.
otc	**Magnacal Liquid** (Sherwood)	70	Ca and Na caseinate	250	maltodextrin, sucrose	80	partially hydrogenated soy oil, soy lecithin, mono- and diglycerides	1000	1250	590	2	Vit A, B_1, B_2, B_3, B_5, B_6, B_{12}, C, D, E, K, choline, Ca, Cl, Cu, Fe, I, Mg, Mn, P, Zn[1]	Vanilla flavor. In 120 and 250 ml ready-to-use.
otc	**Isocal HCN Liquid** (Mead Johnson Nutritionals)	75	Ca and Na caseinate	200	corn syrup	102	soy oil, MCT (fractionated coconut oil), lecithin	800	1700	640	2	Vit A, B_1, B_2, B_3, B_5, B_6, B_{12}, C, D, E, K, choline, Ca, P, I, Fe, Mg, Cu, Zn, Mn, Cl, Se, Cr, Mo[1]	In 8 oz ready-to-use.
otc	**Nutren 2.0 Liquid** (Clintec Nutrition)	80	casein	196	maltodextrin, corn syrup solids, sucrose	106	MCT, corn oil	1000	2500	710	2	Vit A, B_1, B_2, B_3, B_5, B_6, B_{12}, C, D, E, K, choline, Ca, Cl, Cu, Fe, I, Mg, Mn, P, Zn[1]	*Cholesterol and gluten free.* Vanilla flavor. In 250 ml ready-to-use.
otc	**Forta Drink Powder**[2] (Ross)	5	whey protein concentrate	15	sucrose	< 1	unknown	50	70	NA	85	Vit A, B_1, B_2, B_3, B_5, B_6, B_{12}, C, D, E, Ca, Cu, Fe, I, Mg, Mn, P, Zn[1]	Orange and fruit punch flavors. In 482 g cans.

NA = Not available.

[1] With folic acid and biotin.

[2] Content given per serving (0.8 oz mix).

Infant Foods

Uses: Formula for bottle-fed infants; as a supplement to breast feeding.

Precautions:
In conditions where the infant is losing abnormal quantities of one or more electrolytes, it may be necessary to supply electrolytes from sources other than the formula. With premature infants weighing < 1500 g at birth, it may be necessary to supply an additional source of sodium, calcium and phosphorus during the period of very rapid growth.

	Product & Distributor	Dilution	Content per Dilution									Other Content	How Supplied
			Protein		Carbohydrate		Fat		Na	K			
			g	Source	g	Source	g	Source	(mg)	(mg)	Cal		
otc	**Enfamil Human Milk Fortifier** (Mead Johnson Nutritionals)	4 packets (3.8 g) added to breast milk	0.7	whey protein, casein	2.7	corn syrup solids, lactose	< 0.1	unknown	7	15.6	14	Vit A, B_1, B_2, B_3, B_5, B_6, B_{12}, C, D, E, K, folic acid, biotin, Ca, P, Zn, Mn, Cu, Cl	In 0.96 g packets (100s).
otc	**Enfamil Premature 20 Formula** (Mead Johnson Nutritionals)	120 ml ready-to-use	2.4	nonfat milk, whey protein concentrate	8.9	corn syrup solids, lactose	4.1	coconut and soy oils, medium chain triglycerides	31.2	82.3	80	Vit A, B_1, B_2, B_3, B_5, B_6, B_{12}, C, D, E, K, folic acid, biotin, choline, inositol, Ca, P, Mg, Zn, Fe, Mn, Cu, I, Cl	In 120 ml nursettes.
otc	**Similac PM 60/40 Liquid** (Ross)	120 ml ready-to-use	1.9	whey protein concentrate, Na caseinate	8.2	lactose	4.4	coconut oil, mono- and diglycerides	19.2	68.8	80	Vit A, B_1, B_2, B_3, B_5, B_6, B_{12}, C, D, E, K, folic acid, biotin, choline, inositol, Ca, P, Mg, Zn, Fe, Mn, Cu, I, Cl	In 120 ml bottles.

(Continued on following page)

Infant Foods (Cont.)

	Product & Distributor	Dilution	Content per Dilution									Other Content	How Supplied
			Protein		Carbohydrate		Fat		Na (mg)	K (mg)	Cal		
			g	Source	g	Source	g	Source					
otc	**Similac** (Ross)	1 liter	15	nonfat milk	72.3	lactose	36.3	Powder: Coconut & corn oils. Liquid & concentrate: Coconut & soy oils, mono- & diglycerides, soy lecithin	189	730	676	Vit A, B_1, B_2, B_3, B_5, B_6, B_{12}, C, D, E, K, folic acid, biotin, choline, inositol, Ca, P, Mg, Zn, Fe, Mn, Cu, I, Cl	In 390 ml concentrate, 240 ml and 1 qt ready-to-use, 120 and 240 ml nursettes and 1 lb powder.
otc	**Enfamil** (Mead Johnson Nutritionals)	1 liter	14.7	nonfat milk, reduced minerals whey	68.7	lactose	37.3	soy and coconut oils, soy lecithin, mono- and diglycerides	180	720	667	Vit A, B_1, B_2, B_3, B_5, B_6, B_{12}, C, D, E, K, folic acid, biotin, choline, inositol, Ca, P, Mg, Zn, Fe, Mn, Cu, I, Cl	In 390 ml concentrate, 240 ml & 1 qt ready-to-use, 120, 180 & 240 ml nursettes & 1 lb powder.
otc	**RCF Liquid** (Ross)	390 ml concentrate	12.9	soy protein isolate	†		23.2	soy oil, coconut oil, mono- and diglycerides, soy lecithin	189	468	260	Vit A, B_1, B_2, B_3, B_5, B_6, B_{12}, C, D, E, K, folic acid, biotin, choline, inositol, Ca, Mg, P, Zn, Fe, Mn, Cu, I, Cl	In 390 ml concentrate.

† Contains no carbohydrates; add a carbohydrate before feeding.

ENTERAL NUTRITIONAL THERAPY (Cont.)

Infant Foods with Iron

	Product & Distributor	Dilution	Content per Dilution										Other Content	How Supplied
			Protein		Carbohydrate		Fat		Iron (mg)	Na (mg)	K (mg)	Cal		
			g	Source	g	Source	g	Source						
otc	**Lofenalac Powder** (Mead Johnson Nutritionals)	1 liter	22	casein hydrolysate, amino acids	86.7	corn syrup solids, modified tapioca starch	26	corn oil	12.5	313	680	667	Vit A, B_1, B_2, B_3, B_5, B_6, B_{12}, C, D, E, K, folic acid, biotin, choline, inositol, Ca, P, Mg, Zn, Mn, Cu, I, Cl	*Low phenylalanine.* In 1 lb powder.
otc	**Similac w/Iron** (Ross)	1 liter	15	nonfat milk	72.3	lactose	36.3	Powder: Coconut and corn oils. Liquid and Concentrate: Coconut and soy oils, mono- and diglycerides, soy lecithin	12.2	189	730	676	Vit A, B_1, B_2, B_3, B_5, B_6, B_{12}, C, D, E, K, folic acid, biotin, choline, inositol, Ca, P, Mg, Zn, Mn, Cu, I, Cl	In 390 ml concentrate, 240 ml and 1 qt ready-to-use, 120 and 240 ml nursettes and 1 lb powder.
otc	**SMA Iron Fortified** (Wyeth-Ayerst)	1 liter	15	nonfat milk, reduced minerals whey	72	lactose	36	oleo, coconut, safflower and soybean oils, soy lecithin	12	150	560	667	Vit A, B_1, B_2, B_3, B_5, B_6, B_{12}, C, D, E, K, folic acid, biotin, choline, Ca, P, Mg, Cl, Cu, Zn, Mn, I	In 390 ml concentrate, 240 ml, 1 qt ready-to-use and 1.06 oz unit-of-use packets and 1 lb powder.
otc	**SMA with Whey** (Wyeth-Ayerst)	1 liter	15	skim milk, reduced minerals whey	72	lactose	36	oleo, coconut, safflower and soybean oils, soy lecithin	1.5	150	360	670	Vit A, B_1, B_2, B_3, B_5, B_6, B_{12}, C, D, E, K, folic acid, biotin, choline, Ca, P, Mg, Cl, Cu, Zn, Mn, I	In 120 ml.

(Continued on following page)

Infant Foods with Iron (Cont.)

	Product & Distributor	Dilution	Content per Dilution										Other Content	How Supplied
			Protein		Carbohydrate		Fat		Iron (mg)	Na (mg)	K (mg)	Cal		
			g	Source	g	Source	g	Source						
otc	**SMA Lo-Iron** (Wyeth-Ayerst)	1 liter	15	nonfat milk, reduced minerals whey	72	lactose	36	oleo, coconut, safflower and soybean oils, soy lecithin	1.5	150	560	667	Vit A, B_1, B_2, B_3, B_5, B_6, B_{12}, C, D, E, K, folic acid, biotin, choline, Ca, P, Mg, Cl, Cu, Zn, Mn, I	In 390 ml concentrate, 120 ml and 1 qt ready-to-use, 1.06 oz unit-of-use packets and 1 lb powder.
otc	**Enfamil w/Iron** (Mead Johnson Nutritionals)	1 liter	14.4	nonfat milk, reduced minerals whey	66	lactose	36	soy and coconut oils, soy lecithin, mono- and diglycerides	12	173	691	640	Vit A, B_1, B_2, B_3, B_5, B_6, B_{12}, C, D, E, K, folic acid, biotin, choline, inositol, Ca, P, Mg, Zn, Mn, Cu, I, Cl	In 390 ml concentrate, 240 ml and 1 qt ready-to-use, 180 ml nursettes and 1 lb powder.
otc	**Advance Liquid** (Ross)	1 liter	20	nonfat milk, soy protein isolate	55.1	corn syrup	27	soy oil, corn oil, mono- and diglycerides, soy lecithin	7	189	788	540	Vit A, B_1, B_2, B_3, B_5, B_6, B_{12}, C, D, E, K, folic acid, biotin, choline, inositol, Ca, P, Mg, Zn, Mn, Cu, I, Cl	In 390 ml concentrate and 1 qt ready-to-use.

Hypoallergenic Infant Foods

For infants and children with chronic diarrhea; malabsorption; galactosemia; intestinal resection; cystic fibrosis; short gut syndrome; steatorrhea; severe protein-calorie malnutrition; vegetarianism; colic; sensitivity or allergy to corn or cow's milk; lactase deficiency; lactose intolerance. Also for adults with allergy or sensitivity to cow's milk or in maintenance of nutrition during test or elimination diets.

	Product & Distributor	Dilution	Content per Dilution											Other Content	How Supplied
			Protein		Carbohydrate		Fat		Iron (mg)	Na (mg)	K (mg)	Cal			
			g	Source	g	Source	g	Source							
otc	**Soyalac** (Loma Linda)	1 liter	20.7	soybean solids, amino acids	66.7	corn syrup, sucrose	36.7	soy oil, soy lecithin	12	293	780	667		Vit A, B_1, B_2, B_3, B_5, B_6, B_{12}, C, D, E, K, folic acid, biotin, choline, inositol, Ca, P, Mg, I, Zn, Cu, Mn, Cl	In 384 ml concentrate, 1 qt ready-to-use and 400 g powder.
otc	**I-Soyalac** (Loma Linda)	1 liter	20.7	soy protein isolate, amino acids	66.7	sucrose, tapioca dextrin	36.7	soy oil, soy lecithin	12.7	280	780	667		Vit A, B_1, B_2, B_3, B_5, B_6, B_{12}, C, D, E, K, folic acid, biotin, choline, inositol, Ca, P, Mg, I, Zn, Cu, Mn, Cl	Corn free. In 384 ml concentrate and 1 qt ready-to-use.
otc	**Alimentum** (Ross)	1 liter	18.3	casein hydrolysate, amino acids	68	sucrose, modified tapioca starch	36.9	MCT (fractionated coconut oil), safflower oil, soy oil	12	293	787	676		Vit A, B_1, B_2, B_3, B_5, B_6, B_{12}, C, D, E, K, folic acid, biotin, choline, inositol, Ca, Cl, Cu, I, Mg, Mn, P, Zn	Corn free. In 1 qt ready-to-use.
otc	**Isomil** (Ross)	1 liter	17.7	soy protein isolate	67.3	corn syrup, sucrose; concentrate also contains cornstarch	36.4	Powder: Corn, soy & coconut oils. Concentrate & Liquid: Soy & coconut oils, mono & diglycerides, soy lecithin	12	293	720	676		Vit A, B_1, B_2, B_3, B_5, B_6, B_{12}, C, D, E, K, folic acid, biotin, choline, inositol, Ca, P, Mg, Zn, Mn, Cu, I, Cl	In 390 ml concentrate, 240 ml and 1 qt ready-to-use and 14 oz powder.

(Continued on following page)

Hypoallergenic Infant Foods (Cont.)

	Product & Distributor	Dilution	Content per Dilution										Other Content	How Supplied
			Protein		Carbohydrate		Fat		Iron (mg)	Na (mg)	K (mg)	Cal		
			g	Source	g	Source	g	Source						
otc	**Isomil SF** (Ross)	1 liter	17.7	soy protein isolate, amino acids	67.3	hydrolyzed cornstarch	36.4	soy oil, coconut oil, mono- and diglycerides, soy lecithin	11.5	282	691	676	Vit A, B_1, B_2, B_3, B_5, B_6, B_{12}, C, D, E, K, folic acid, biotin, choline, inositol, Ca, P, Cu, Mg, Zn, Mn, I, Cl	*Sucrose free.* In 390 ml concentrate and 1 qt ready-to-use.
otc	**Nursoy Liquid** (Wyeth-Ayerst)	1 liter	21	soy protein isolate, l-methionine	69	sucrose	36	oleo, coconut, safflower and soybean oils, soy lecithin	11.5	200	700	667	Vit A, B_1, B_2, B_3, B_5, B_6, B_{12}, C, D, E, K, folic acid, choline, inositol, biotin, Ca, P, Cl, Mg, Mn, Cu, Zn, I	In 390 ml concentrate and 1 qt ready-to-use.
otc	**Pregestimil Powder** (Mead Johnson Nutritionals)	1 liter	18.7	enzymatically hydrolyzed casein, amino acids	68.7	corn syrup solids, modified corn starch, dextrose	26	corn oil, MCT (fractionated coconut oil), high oleic safflower oil	12.5	260	727	667	Vit A, B_1, B_2, B_3, B_5, B_6, B_{12}, C, D, E, K, folic acid, biotin, choline, inositol, Ca, P, Cu, Mg, Zn, Mn, I, Cl	In 1 lb.
otc	**Nutramigen** (Mead Johnson Nutritionals)	1 liter	18.7	enzymatically hydrolyzed casein, amino acids	89.3	corn syrup solids, modified cornstarch	26	corn oil	12.5	313	727	667	Vit A, B_1, B_2, B_3, B_5, B_6, B_{12}, C, D, E, K, folic acid, biotin, choline, inositol, Ca, P, Cu, Mg, Zn, Mn, I, Cl	In 1 lb powder, 390 ml concentrate and 1 qt ready-to-use.
otc	**ProSobee** (Mead Johnson Nutritionals)	1 liter	20	soy protein isolate, amino acids	66.7	corn syrup solids	35.3	Powder: Coconut & corn oil. Liquid: Soy & coconut oil, lecithin, mono- and diglycerides	12.5	240	813	667	Vit A, B_1, B_2, B_3, B_5, B_6, B_{12}, C, D, E, K, folic acid, biotin, choline, inositol, Ca, P, Cu, Mg, Zn, Mn, I, Cl	*Sucrose free.* In 390 ml concentrate, 240 ml and 1 qt ready-to-use and 14 oz powder.

Food Modifiers

These products are used as modifiers for infant formulas or as dietary supplements.

LACTOSE

otc	**Lactose** (Various, eg, Humco, Paddock)	**Powder**	In 1 lb.

CALCIUM CASEINATE

otc	**Casec** (Mead Johnson Nutritionals)	**Powder:** Contains 88 g protein, 1.6 g calcium, 120 mg sodium, 2 g fat and 370 calories per 100 g	In 75 g.

LACTASE ENZYME

Use: To digest lactose contained in milk for patients with lactose intolerance.

Administration and Dosage:

Liquid: 5 to 15 drops per quart of milk, depending on level of lactose conversion desired.

Tablets: 1 to 3 tablets with a meal will normally neutralize a lactose challenge equal to 1 glass of milk.

Capsules: 1 or 2 capsules taken with milk or dairy products. If the patient is severely intolerant to lactose, increase dosage until a satisfactory dose is achieved as recognized by resolution of the symptoms.

To pretreat milk, add the contents from 1 or 2 capsules to each quart of milk.

If the patient cannot swallow capsules, sprinkle the contents of the capsules onto dairy products before consuming.

otc	**LactAid** (LactAid Inc.)	**Liquid:** Beta-D-galactosidase derived from Kluyveromyces lactis yeast (≥ 1250 NLU[1] per 5 drop dosage) in carrier of glycerol (50%), water (30%) and inert yeast dry matter (20%)	In units of 12, 30 and 75 one quart dosages at 5 drops per dose.
		Caplets: ≥ 3000 FCC lactase units of beta-D-galactosidase from *Aspergillis oryzae*	In 12s, 100s and UD 50s.
otc	**Lactogest** (Thompson)	**Capsules:** 125 mg lactase enzyme	In 50s.
otc	**Lactrase** (Schwarz Pharma Kremers Urban)	**Capsules:** 250 mg standardized enzyme lactase	(Kremers Urban 505). Orange and white. In 100s and blisterpack 10s and 30s.
otc	**SureLac** (Caraco)	**Tablets:** 3000 FCC lactase units	Sorbitol or mannitol. Chewable. In 60s.
otc	**Dairy Ease** (Winthrop)	**Tablets, chewable:** 3300 FCC lactase units	Mannitol. In 60s.

ALPHA-D-GALACTOSIDASE ENZYME

Actions: Alpha-D-galactosidase enzyme hydrolyzes raffinose, verbascose and stachyose into the digestible sugars sucrose, fructose, glucose and galactose.

Use: Treatment of gassiness or bloat as a result of eating a variety of grains, cereals, nuts, seeds or vegetables containing the sugars raffinose, stachyose or verbascose. This includes all or most legumes and all or most cruciferous vegetables (eg, oats, wheat, beans, peas, lentils, peanuts, soy-content foods, pistachios, broccoli, brussels sprouts, cabbage, carrots, corn, onions, squash).

Precautions:

Galactosemics should not use without physician advice since one of the breakdown sugars is galactose.

Administration and Dosage:

Use 3 to 8 drops per average serving. Approximately 5 drops on the first portion of food consumed will deal with the entire subsequent portion.

Use a higher or lower number of drops depending on the quantity of food eaten, levels of alpha-linked sugars in the food and the gas-producing propensity and tolerance of the person.

otc	**Beano** (LactAid Inc.)	**Liquid:** Alpha-D-galactosidase derived from *Aspergillus niger,* a fungal source (≥ 175 GALU[2] per 5 drop dosage) in carrier of water and glycerol	In 75 serving size at 5 drops per dose.

[1] Neutral lactase units. [2] Galactose units.

chapter 2

blood modifiers

Actions:

Pharmacology: Iron, an essential mineral, is a component of hemoglobin, myoglobin and a number of enzymes. The total body content of iron is approximately 50 mg/kg in men (3.5 g in the average 70 kg man) and 35 mg/kg in women. Iron is primarily stored as hemosiderin or ferritin, found in the reticuloendothelial cells of the liver, spleen and bone marrow. Approximately two-thirds of total body iron is in the circulating red blood cell mass in hemoglobin, the major factor in oxygen transport.

Pharmacokinetics: Absorption/Distribution – The average dietary intake of iron is 18 to 20 mg/day; however, only about 10% of this iron is absorbed (1 to 2 mg/day) in individuals with adequate iron stores. Absorption is enhanced (20% to 30%) when storage iron is depleted or when erythropoiesis occurs at an increased rate. Iron is primarily absorbed from the duodenum and upper jejunum by an active transport mechanism. The ferrous salt form is absorbed three times more readily than the ferric form. The common ferrous salts (sulfate, gluconate, fumarate) are absorbed almost on a milligram-for-milligram basis, but differ in the content of elemental iron. Sustained release or enteric coated preparations reduce the amount of available iron; absorption from these doseforms is reduced because iron is transported beyond the duodenum. Dose also influences the amount of iron absorbed. The amount of iron absorbed increases progressively with larger doses; however, the percentage absorbed decreases. Food can decrease the absorption of iron by 40% to 66%; however, gastric intolerance may often necessitate administering the drug with food.

Excretion – Iron is transported via the blood and bound to transferrin. The daily loss of iron from urine, sweat and sloughing of intestinal mucosal cells amounts to approximately 0.5 to 1 mg in healthy men. In menstruating women, ≈ 1 to 2 mg is the normal daily loss.

Elemental Iron Content of Iron Salts

Iron salt	% Iron
Ferrous sulfate	20
Ferrous sulfate, exsiccated	≈ 30
Ferrous gluconate	≈ 12
Ferrous fumarate	33

Indications:

For the prevention and treatment of iron deficiency anemias.

Unlabeled use: Iron supplementation may be required by most patients receiving epoetin therapy. Failure to administer iron supplements (oral or IV) during epoetin therapy can impair the hematologic response to epoetin.

Contraindications:

Hemochromatosis; hemosiderosis; hemolytic anemias.

Warnings:

Chronic iron intake: Individuals with normal iron balance should not take iron chronically.

Precautions:

Intolerance: Discontinue use if symptoms of intolerance appear.

GI effects: Occasional GI discomfort, such as nausea, may be minimized by taking with meals and by slowly increasing to the recommended dosage.

Tartrazine sensitivity: Some of these products contain tartrazine, which may cause allergic-type reactions (including bronchial asthma) in susceptible individuals. Although the incidence of tartrazine sensitivity in the general population is low, it is frequently seen in patients who also have aspirin hypersensitivity. Specific products containing tartrazine are identified in the product listings.

Sulfite sensitivity: Some of the products contain sulfites, which may cause allergic-type reactions (eg, hives, itching, wheezing, anaphylaxis) in certain susceptible persons. Although the overall prevalence of sulfite sensitivity in the general population is probably low, it is seen more frequently in asthmatics or in atopic nonasthmatic persons. Specific products containing sulfites are identified in the product listings.

(Continued on following page)

Drug Interactions:

Iron Salts Drug Interactions			
Precipitant drug	Object drug *		Description
Antacids	Iron salts	↓	GI absorption of iron may be reduced.
Ascorbic acid	Iron salts	↑	Ascorbic acid may enhance the absorption of iron from the GI tract; however, this increase may not be significant.
Chloramphenicol	Iron salts	↑	Serum iron levels may be increased.
Cimetidine	Iron salts	↓	GI absorption of iron may be reduced.
Iron salts	Levodopa	↓	Levodopa appears to form chelates with iron salts, decreasing levodopa absorption and serum levels.
Iron salts	Methyldopa	↓	Extent of methyldopa absorption may be decreased, possibly resulting in decreased efficacy.
Iron salts	Penicillamine	↓	Marked reduction in GI absorption of penicillamine may occur, possibly due to chelation.
Iron salts	Quinolones	↓	GI absorption of quinolones may be decreased due to formation of a ferric ion-quinolone complex.
Iron salts Tetracyclines	Tetracyclines Iron salts	↓ ↓	Coadministration may decrease absorption and serum levels of tetracyclines. Absorption of iron salts may also be decreased.

* ↑ = Object drug increased ↓ = Object drug decreased

Drug/Food interactions: Eggs and milk inhibit iron absorption. Coffee and tea consumed with a meal or 1 hour after a meal may significantly inhibit the absorption of dietary iron; clinical significance has not been determined. Administration of calcium and iron supplements with food can reduce ferrous sulfate absorption by one-third. If combined iron and calcium supplementation is required, iron absorption is not decreased if calcium carbonate is used and the supplements are taken between meals.

Adverse Reactions:

GI irritation; anorexia; nausea; vomiting; constipation; diarrhea. Stools may appear darker in color.

Iron-containing liquids may cause temporary staining of the teeth. Dilute the liquid to reduce this possibility. When iron-containing drops are given to infants, some darkening of the membrane covering the teeth may occur.

Overdosage:

Symptoms: The oral *lethal* dose of elemental iron is about 200 to 250 mg/kg; however, considerably less has been fatal. Symptoms may present when 30 to 60 mg/kg is ingested. Acute poisoning will produce symptoms in four stages:

1) Within 1 to 6 hours: Lethargy; nausea; vomiting; abdominal pain; tarry stools; weak-rapid pulse; hypotension; dehydration; acidosis; coma.

2) If not immediately fatal, symptoms may subside for about 24 hours.

3) Symptoms return 12 to 48 hours after ingestion and may include: Diffuse vascular congestion; pulmonary edema; shock; acidosis; convulsions; anuria; hyperthermia; death.

4) If patient survives, in 2 to 6 weeks after ingestion, pyloric or antral stenosis, hepatic cirrhosis and CNS damage may be seen.

Treatment: Maintain proper airway, respiration and circulation. If the patient is a candidate for emesis, induce with syrup of ipecac; follow with gastric lavage using tepid water or 1% to 5% sodium bicarbonate to convert the ferrous sulfate to ferrous carbonate, which is poorly absorbed and less irritating. Systemic chelation therapy with deferoxamine is generally recommended for patients with serum iron levels > 300 mg/dl; IM therapy may suffice, but severe poisoning (ie, shock, coma) may require IV administration (see deferoxamine mesylate in the Antidotes section). Oral use of deferoxamine is controversial and generally discouraged. Saline cathartics may be used. Specific treatment for shock, convulsions, acidosis and renal failure may be necessary. Treatment includes usual supportive measures. Refer to General Management of Acute Overdosage.

Patient Information:

Take on an empty stomach; if GI upset occurs, take after meals or with food.

Avoid coadministration with antacids, tetracyclines or fluoroquinolones.

Drink liquid iron preparations in water or juice and through a straw to prevent tooth stains.

Medication may cause black stools, constipation or diarrhea.

Do not chew or crush sustained release preparations.

(Continued on following page)

Administration and Dosage:

Recommended Dietary Allowances (RDAs): Adult males (≥ 19 years old) – 10 mg; adult females (11 to 50 years old) – 15 mg, (≥ 51 years old) – 10 mg; pregnancy – 30 mg; lactation – 15 mg. For a complete listing of RDAs by age, sex or condition, refer to page 2a.

Iron replacement therapy in deficiency states: Adults – 100 to 200 mg (2 to 3 mg/kg) elemental iron daily in three divided doses is the usual therapeutic dose.

Children (2 to 12 years) – 3 mg/kg/day in 3 to 4 divided doses; (6 months to 2 years) – up to 6 mg/kg/day in 3 to 4 divided doses.

Infants – 10 to 25 mg daily in 3 to 4 divided doses.

The length of iron therapy depends upon the cause and severity of the iron deficiency. In general, approximately 4 to 6 months of oral iron therapy is required to reverse uncomplicated iron deficiency anemias.

Iron supplementation: Consider only in individuals with documented risk factors for iron deficiency.

Pregnancy – 30 mg elemental iron daily (not taken with meals) should be adequate to meet the daily requirement of the last 2 trimesters.

FERROUS SULFATE. 20% elemental iron.				**C.I.***
otc	**Mol-Iron** (Schering-Plough)	**Tablets:** 195 mg (39 mg iron)	Sugar. In 100s.	12
otc	**Feratab** (Upsher-Smith)	**Tablets:** 300 mg (60 mg iron)	In 100s.	NA
otc	**Ferrous Sulfate** (Various, eg, Geneva, Major, Parmed, Rugby, Schein)	**Tablets:** 324 mg (65 mg iron)	Plain or enteric coated. In 100s, 1000s, 5000s and UD 100s.	2.4+
otc	**Ferrous Sulfate** (Various, eg, Geneva, Parmed, Rugby)	**Capsules:** 250 mg (50 mg iron)	In 100s and 1000s.	8.2+
otc	**Ferospace** (Hudson)		In 60s.	9.2
otc	**Fero-Gradumet Filmtab** (Abbott)	**Tablets, timed release:** 525 mg (105 mg iron)	Castor oil. Red. Film coated. In 100s.	18
otc	**Fer-In-Sol** (Mead Johnson Nutritionals)	**Syrup:** 90 mg (18 mg iron) per 5 ml	Sugar, sorbitol, sodium bisulfite. 5% alcohol. In pt.	88
otc	**Ferrous Sulfate** (Various, eg, Barre, Goldline, Major, Rugby, Schein)	**Elixir:** 220 mg (44 mg iron) per 5 ml	In pt and gal.	7+
otc	**Feosol** (SmithKline-Beecham)		Saccharin, sucrose, glucose. 5% alcohol. In pt.	21
otc	**Ferrous Sulfate** (Various, eg, Barre, Major, Schein)	**Drops:** 75 mg (15 mg iron) per 0.6 ml	In 50 ml.	25+
otc	**Fer-In-Sol** (Mead Johnson Nutritionals)		Sugar, sorbitol, sodium bisulfite, 0.2% alcohol. In 50 ml w/dropper.	80
otc	**Fer-Iron** (Rugby)	**Drops:** 75 mg (15 mg iron) per 0.6 ml	Sugar, sorbitol, sodium bisulfite, 0.2% alcohol. In 50 ml.	21+

* Cost Index based on cost per 180 mg iron.

Complete prescribing information for these products begins on page 208

FERROUS SULFATE EXSICCATED

Dried ferrous sulfate is prepared by exposing well crushed crystals of ferrous sulfate to 70° to 80°F (21° to 27°C) stirring frequently, and then powdering. This salt is more stable in air than the fully hydrated ferrous sulfate. Contains ≈ 30% elemental iron.

	Product	Form	Description	C.I.*
otc	**Fer-In-Sol** (Mead Johnson Nutritionals)	**Capsules:** 190 mg (60 mg iron)	Lecithin. In 100s.	17
otc	**Feosol** (SmithKline-Beecham)	**Tablets:** 200 mg (65 mg iron)	Glucose. Triangular. In 100s, 1000s and UD 100s.	8.6
otc	**Feosol** (SmithKline-Beecham)	**Capsules, timed release:** 159 mg (50 mg iron)	Sucrose. (Feosol). In 30s, 60s, 500s and UD 100s.	45
otc	**Ferrous Sulfate** (Various, eg, Parmed)	**Capsules, timed release:** 250 mg dried ferrous sulfate equivalent (50 mg iron)	In 100s and 1000s.	NA
otc	**Ferralyn Lanacaps** (Lannett)		Red and clear. In 100s, 500s and 1000s.	49
otc	**Ferra-TD** (Goldline)		Red and clear. In 100s and 1000s.	12
otc	**Slow FE** (Ciba Consumer)	**Tablets, slow release:** 160 mg (50 mg iron)	Lactose. (Ciba). In 30s, 60s and 100s.	33

FERROUS GLUCONATE. 11.6% elemental iron.

	Product	Form	Description	C.I.*
otc	**Ferrous Gluconate** (Various, eg, Major, Parmed, Rugby)	**Tablets:** 300 mg (34 mg iron)	In 100s and 1000s.	7.3+
otc	**Fergon** (Winthrop Consumer)	**Tablets:** 320 mg (37 mg iron)	Sucrose. In 100s and 1000s.	15
otc	**Ferralet** (Mission)		In 100s.	13
otc	**Ferrous Gluconate** (Various, eg, Dixon-Shane, Geneva, Goldline, Schein, URL)	**Tablets:** 325 mg (38 mg iron)	In 100s and 1000s.	4.6+
otc	**Ferralet Slow Release** (Mission)	**Tablets, sustained release:** 320 mg (37 mg iron)	In 30s.	33
otc	**Simron** (Marion Merrell Dow)	**Capsules, soft gelatin:** 86 mg (10 mg iron)	Maroon. In 100s.	292
otc	**Fergon** (Winthrop Consumer)	**Elixir:** 300 mg (34 mg iron) per 5 ml	7% alcohol, glucose, saccharin. In pt.	34

* Cost Index based on cost per 180 mg iron.

Complete prescribing information for these products begins on page 208

FERROUS FUMARATE. 33% elemental iron.

	Product	Dosage form	Description	C.I.*
otc	**Femiron** (Menley & James)	**Tablets:** 63 mg (20 mg iron)	In 40s and 120s.	24
otc	**Fumerin** (Laser)	**Tablets:** 195 mg (64 mg iron)	Sugar coated. In 100s and 1000s.	10
otc	**Fumasorb** (MiLance)	**Tablets:** 200 mg (66 mg iron)	In 30s and 60s.	9.8
otc	**Ircon** (Kenwood)		In 100s.	8.6
otc	**Hemocyte** (U.S. Pharm.)	**Tablets:** 324 mg (106 mg iron)	In 100s.	8
otc	**Ferrous Fumarate** (Various, eg, Major, Rugby, Schein)	**Tablets:** 325 mg (106 mg iron)	In 1000s.	1+
otc	**Ferretts** (Pharmics)		Sugar. In 100s.	NA
otc	**Nephro-Fer** (R & D Labs)	**Tablets:** 350 mg (115 mg iron)	In 100s.	6.3
otc	**Feostat** (Forest)	**Tablets, chewable:** 100 mg (33 mg iron)	Chocolate flavor. In 100s and 1000s.	21
otc	**Span-FF** (Lexis)	**Capsules, controlled release:** 325 mg (106 mg iron)	Sucrose. In 60s, 100s and 500s.	NA
otc	**Feostat** (Forest)	**Suspension:** 100 mg (33 mg iron) per 5 ml	In 240 ml.	50
otc	**Feostat** (Forest)	**Drops:** 45 mg (15 mg iron) per 0.6 ml	In 60 ml.	46

POLYSACCHARIDE-IRON COMPLEX

	Product	Dosage form	Description	C.I.*
otc	**Niferex** (Central)	**Tablets:** 50 mg iron	Brown. Film coated. In 100s.	22
otc	**Hytinic** (Hyrex)	**Capsules:** 150 mg iron	In 50s and 500s.	9.4
otc	**Niferex-150** (Central)		(Central). Orange and brown. In 100s and 1000s.	16
otc	**Nu-Iron 150** (Mayrand)		In 100s.	14
otc *sf*	**Niferex** (Central)	**Elixir:** 100 mg iron per 5 ml	10% alcohol. Dye free. In 240 ml.	25
otc *sf*	**Nu-Iron** (Mayrand)		10% alcohol. In 237 ml.	21

Modified Iron Products

	Product	Dosage form	Description	C.I.*
otc	**Fermalox** (Rhone-Poulenc Rorer)	**Tablets:** 200 mg ferrous sulfate (40 mg iron), 100 mg magnesium hydroxide and 100 mg dried aluminum hydroxide	In 100s.	32
otc	**Ferocyl** (Hudson)	**Tablets, sustained release:** 150 mg ferrous fumarate (50 mg iron) and 100 mg docusate sodium	In 100s.	10
otc	**Ferro-Sequels** (Lederle)		(LL F2). Green. Film coated. Capsule shape. In 30s, 100s and UD 30s and 100s.	NA
otc	**Ferro-Docusate T.R.** (Parmed)	**Capsules, timed release:** 150 mg ferrous fumarate (50 mg iron) and 100 mg docusate sodium	Sucrose. In 100s.	14
otc	**Ferro Dok TR** (Major)		In 100s.	13
otc	**Ferro-DSS S.R.** (Geneva Marsam)		Green. In 100s.	8.6

* Cost Index based on cost per 180 mg iron.
sf – Sugar free.

Complete prescribing information for these products begins on page 208

IRON WITH VITAMIN C

ASCORBIC ACID (Vitamin C) may enhance the absorption of iron.
Content given per capsule or tablet.

	Product and Distributor	Fe (mg)	Vitamin C: Ascorbic Acid (mg)	Vitamin C: Sodium Ascorbate (mg)	Other Content & How Supplied	C.I.*
	Tablets					
otc	**Mol-Iron with Vitamin C Tablets** (Schering-Plough)	39[1]	75		Sugar. In 100s.	443
otc	**Ferancee-HP Tablets** (J & J-Merck)	110[2]	600[4]		Red. Film coated. Oval. In 60s.	356
otc	**Vitron-C-Plus Tablets** (Fisons)	132[2]	250		Lactose. In 100s.	290
	Tablets, Chewable					
otc	**Niferex with Vitamin C Tablets** (Central)	50[3]	100	169	In 50s.	684
otc	**Vitron-C Tablets** (Fisons)	66[2]	125		Saccharin. Fruit flavor. In 100s and 1000s.	290
otc	**Ferancee Tablets** (J & J-Merck)	67[2]	150[4]		Tartrazine, saccharin, sugar. In 100s.	377
	Capsules and Tablets, Timed Release					
Rx	**Cevi-Fer Capsules** (Geriatric Pharm.)	20[2]	300		1 mg folic acid. In 30s and 100s.	4374
otc	**Irospan Tablets** (Fielding)	60[1]	150		In 100s.	480
otc	**Irospan Capsules** (Fielding)				In 60s.	550
otc	**Fe-O.D. Tablets** (Trimen)	100[2]	500		In 100s.	287
otc	**Fero-Grad-500 Filmtabs** (Abbott)	105[1]		500	Red. Film coated. In 100s, 500s and UD 100s.	441
otc	**Hemaspan Tablets** (Bock)	110[2]	200[4]		20 mg DSS. (Bock 330). Tan. In 30s and 100s.	395

* Cost Index based on cost per 180 mg iron.
[1] From ferrous sulfate.
[2] From ferrous fumarate.
[3] From polysaccharide-iron complex.
[4] Form of vitamin C unknown.

IRON DEXTRAN

Warning:

The parenteral use of complexes of iron and carbohydrates has resulted in fatal anaphylactic-type reactions. Deaths associated with such administration have been reported; therefore, use iron dextran injection only in those patients in whom the indications have been clearly established and laboratory investigations confirm an iron deficient state not amenable to oral iron therapy.

Actions:

Pharmacology: Iron dextran, a hematinic agent, is a complex of ferric hydroxide and dextran for IM or IV use. The iron dextran complex is dissociated by the reticuloendothelial system, and the ferric iron is transported by transferrin and incorporated into hemoglobin and storage sites.

Indications:

For treatment of patients with documented iron deficiency in whom oral administration is unsatisfactory or impossible.

Unlabeled use: Iron supplementation may be required by most patients receiving epoetin therapy. Failure to administer iron supplements (oral or IV) during epoetin therapy can impair the hematologic response to epoetin.

Contraindications:

Hypersensitivity to the product; all anemias not associated with iron deficiency.

Warnings:

Maximum dose: 2 ml of undiluted iron dextran is the maximum recommended daily dose.

Delayed adverse reactions: The following pattern of signs/symptoms has been reported as a delayed (1 to 2 days) reaction at recommended doses: Modest-high fever; chills; backache; headache; myalgia; malaise; nausea; vomiting; dizziness. These reactions have been reported in an unexpectedly high incidence with certain batches. Therefore, in estimating the benefit/risk of treatment for an individual patient, assume that such a delayed reaction may occur.

Hypersensitivity reactions: Have epinephrine immediately available in the event of acute hypersensitivity reactions. (Usual adult dose: 0.5 ml of a 1:1000 solution by SC or IM injection.) Refer to Management of Acute Hypersensitivity Reactions.

Hepatic function impairment: Use this preparation with extreme caution in the presence of serious impairment of liver function.

Carcinogenesis: A risk of carcinogenesis may exist for the IM injection of iron-carbohydrate complexes. Such complexes produce sarcoma when large doses are injected in rats, mice, and rabbits and possibly in hamsters.

The long latent period between the injection of a potential carcinogen and the appearance of a tumor makes it impossible to accurately measure the risk in humans. There have been, however, several reports in literature describing tumors at the injection site in humans who had previously received iron-carbohydrate complexes IM.

Pregnancy: In animal studies, iron dextran during pregnancy caused an increase in the number of stillbirths and fetal anomalies, fetal edema and a decrease in neonatal survival. In addition, the fetus can obtain from 80% to 90% of the iron administered to the pregnant dam during the third trimester. Whether this represents a danger to the fetus and whether the drug is effective in treating maternal iron deficiency under these circumstances is not known. Therefore, do not use in pregnancy or in women of childbearing potential unless potential benefits outweigh possible hazards.

Precautions:

Iron overload: Unwarranted therapy with parenteral iron will cause excess storage of iron with the consequent possibility of exogenous hemosiderosis. Such iron overload is particularly apt to occur in patients with hemoglobinopathies and other refractory anemias which might be erroneously diagnosed as iron deficiency anemia.

Allergies/Asthma: Use with caution in patients with history of significant allergies/asthma.

Arthritis: Patients with iron deficiency anemia and rheumatoid arthritis may have an acute exacerbation of joint pain and swelling following IV administration.

Adverse Reactions:

Anaphylactic reactions including fatal anaphylaxis; other hypersensitivity reactions including dyspnea, urticaria, other rashes, itching, arthralgia, myalgia and febrile episodes; variable degree of soreness and inflammation at or near injection site, including sterile abscesses (IM); brown skin discoloration at injection site (IM); lymphadenopathy; local phlebitis at injection site (IV); peripheral vascular flushing with overly rapid IV administration; hypotensive reaction; possible arthritic reactivation in patients with quiescent rheumatoid arthritis; leukocytosis, frequently with fever, headache, backache, dizziness, malaise, transitory paresthesias, nausea and shivering.

(Continued on following page)

IRON DEXTRAN (Cont.)

Administration and Dosage:

Iron deficiency anemia: Dosage – Use periodic hematologic determinations as a guide in therapy. Recognize that iron storage may lag behind the appearance of normal blood morphology. Although there are significant variations in body build and weight distribution among males and females, the following table and formula represent a simple and convenient means for estimating the total iron required. This total iron requirement reflects the amount of iron needed to restore hemoglobin to normal or near normal levels plus an additional 50% allowance to provide adequate replenishment of iron stores in most individuals with moderately or severely reduced levels of hemoglobin.

The formula should not be used for patients weighing ≤ 30 pounds (adjustments have been made in the table values to account for the lower normal hemoglobins for those patients weighing ≤ 30 pounds).

Note: The table and accompanying formula are applicable for dosage determinations only in patients with iron deficiency anemia; they are not to be used for dosage determinations in patients requiring iron replacement for blood loss.

Iron Dextran Dosage Determination for Iron Deficiency Anemia

$$\frac{\text{mg blood iron}}{\text{lb body weight}} = \frac{\text{ml blood}}{\text{lb body weight}} \times \frac{\text{g hemoglobin}}{\text{ml blood}} \times \frac{\text{mg iron}}{\text{g hemoglobin}}$$

a) Blood volume .... 8.5% body weight

b) Normal hemoglobin (males and females)

> 30 pounds .... 14.8 g/dl

≤ 30 pounds .... 12 g/dl

c) Iron content of hemoglobin 0.34%

d) Hemoglobin deficit

e) Weight

Based on the above factors, individuals with normal hemoglobin levels will have approximately 20 mg of blood iron per pound of body weight.

Total Amount of Iron Dextran Required (to the nearest ml) for Restoration of Hemoglobin and Replacement of Depleted Iron Stores, Based on Observed Hemoglobin and Body Weight

Patient weight		Amount required (ml) based on observed hemoglobin			
lb	kg	4 g/dl	6 g/dl	8 g/dl	10 g/dl
10	4.5	3	3	2	2
20	9.1	7	6	4	3
30	13.6	10	8	7	5
40	18.1	18	14	11	8
50	22.7	22	18	14	10
60	27.2	26	21	17	12
70	31.8	31	25	19	14
80	36.3	35	28	22	16
90	40.8	39	32	25	18
100	45.4	44	35	28	20
110	49.9	48	39	30	21
120	54.4	53	42	33	23
130	59	57	46	36	25
140	63.5	61	50	39	27
150	68.1	66	53	41	29
160	72.6	70	57	44	31
170	77.1	74	60	47	33
180	81.7	79	64	50	35

The total amount of iron (in mg) required to restore hemoglobin to normal levels and to replenish iron stores may be approximated from the following formula:

$$0.3 \times \text{body weight in lb} \times \left(100 - \frac{\text{hemoglobin [g/dl]} \times 100}{14.8}\right)$$

To calculate dose in ml, divide this result by 50.

(Administration and Dosage continued on following page)

IRON DEXTRAN (Cont.)

Administration and Dosage (Cont.)

Administration: IV injection – The total amount of iron dextran required for the treatment of iron deficiency anemia is determined from the preceding formula or table (see Dosage section).

Test dose: Prior to administering the first therapeutic dose, give all patients an IV test dose of 0.5 ml. Although anaphylactic reactions known to occur following administration are usually evident within a few minutes or sooner, it is recommended that a period of ≥ 1 hour elapse before the remainder of the initial therapeutic dose is given.

Individual doses of ≤ 2 ml may be given on a daily basis until the calculated total amount required has been reached.

Give undiluted and slowly (≤ 1 ml/min).

IM injection – The total amount required for the treatment of iron deficiency anemia is determined from the preceding formula or table (see Dosage section).

Test dose: Prior to administering the first therapeutic dose, give all patients an IM test dose of 0.5 ml administered in the same recommended test site and by the same technique as described for IV injection. Although anaphylactic reactions known to occur following administration are usually evident within a few minutes or sooner, it is recommended that a period of ≥ 1 hour elapse before the remainder of the initial therapeutic dose is given.

If no adverse reactions are observed, the injection can be given according to the following schedule until the calculated total amount required has been reached. Each day's dose should ordinarily not exceed 0.5 ml (25 mg iron) for infants < 10 lb, 1 ml (50 mg iron) for children < 20 lb and 2 ml (100 mg iron) for other patients.

Inject only into the muscle mass of the upper outer quadrant of the buttock (never into the arm or other exposed areas) and inject deeply with a 2 or 3 inch 19 or 20 gauge needle. If the patient is standing, have them bear their weight on the leg opposite the injection site, or if in bed, have them in a lateral position with injection site uppermost. To avoid injection or leakage into the subcutaneous tissue, a Z-track technique (displacement of the skin laterally prior to injection) is recommended.

Iron replacement for blood loss: Some individuals sustain blood losses on an intermittent or repetitive basis. Such blood losses may occur periodically in patients with hemorrhagic diatheses (eg, familial telangiectasia, hemophilia, GI bleeding) and on a repetitive basis from procedures such as renal hemodialysis. Direct iron therapy in these patients toward replacement of the equivalent amount of iron represented in the blood loss. The table and formula described under *Iron deficiency anemia* are not applicable for simple iron replacement values.

Quantitative estimates of the individual's periodic blood loss and hematocrit during the bleeding episode provide a convenient method for the calculation of the required iron dose.

The following formula is based on the approximation that 1 ml of normocytic, normochromic red cells contains 1 mg elemental iron:

Replacement iron (in mg) = Blood loss (in ml) x hematocrit

Example: Blood loss of 500 ml with 20% hematocrit

Replacement iron = 500 x 0.2 = 100 mg

$$\text{Iron dextran dose} = \frac{100\text{ mg}}{50} = 2\text{ ml}$$

Rx	**InFeD** (Schein)	**Injection:** 50 mg iron per ml (as dextran)[1]	In 2 ml amps and 10 ml vials.

[1] With ≈ 0.9% sodium chloride.

Complete prescribing information for iron begins on page 208

In these products:

IRON in combination with *VITAMIN* B_{12} *or FOLIC ACID* is used to treat iron deficiency anemia in conjunction with certain nutritional deficiencies.

B COMPLEX vitamins function as coenzymes in carbohydrate, protein or amino acid metabolism, synthesis of DNA and other molecules, maturation of red blood cells, nerve cell function or oxidation-reduction reactions.

ASCORBIC ACID (Vitamin C) may enhance the absorption of iron.

Warnings:

Folic acid alone is improper therapy in the treatment of pernicious anemia and other megaloblastic anemias where vitamin B_{12} is deficient. Where anemia exists, establish its nature and determine underlying causes.

Folic acid, especially in doses > 0.1 mg daily, may obscure pernicious anemia, in that hematologic remission may occur while neurological manifestations remain progressive. Concomitant parenteral therapy with vitamin B_{12} may be necessary in patients with deficiency of vitamin B_{12}. Pernicious anemia is rare in women of childbearing age, and the likelihood of its occurrence along with pregnancy is reduced by the impairment of fertility associated with vitamin B_{12} deficiency.

Capsules and Tablets

Content given per capsule or tablet.

	Product & Distributor	Fe (mg)	B_{12} (mcg)	C (mg)	FA (mg)	Other Content and How Supplied	C.I.*
Rx	**Hemocyte-F Tablets** (US Pharm.)	106[1]			1	Maroon. Sugar coated. In 100s.	3.4
otc	**Ircon-FA Tablets** (Kenwood)	82[1]			0.8	In 100s.	1.9
Rx	**Tolfrinic Tablets** (B.F. Ascher)	200[1]	25	100		Lactose. Dark brown. Film coated. In 100s.	3.4
otc	**Vita-Feron Tablets** (Vitaline)	150	6		0.8	In 90s.	NA
Rx	**Niferex-150 Forte Capsules** (Central)	150[2]	25		1	Sucrose. In 100s and 1000s.	5.7
Rx	**Fero-Folic-500 Filmtabs** (Abbott)	105[3]		500	0.8	Controlled release. (AJ). Red. Film coated. In 100s and 500s.	6.2
Rx	**Fumatinic Capsules** (Laser)	90[1]	15	100	1	Sustained release. Red and orange. In 100s and 1000s.	5.5
otc	**Ferralet Plus Tablets** (Mission)	46[4]	25	400	0.8	In 60s.	7.2

* Cost Index based on cost per 180 mg iron.

[1] From ferrous fumarate.

[2] From polysaccharide-iron complex.

[3] From ferrous sulfate.

[4] From ferrous gluconate.

(Continued on following page)

IRON WITH VITAMINS (Cont.)

Capsules and Tablets (Cont.)

Content given per tablet.

	Product & Distributor	Fe mg	A IU	D IU	E IU	B_1 mg	B_2 mg	B_3 mg	B_5 mg	B_6 mg	B_{12} mcg	C mg	FA mg	Other Content and How Supplied	C.I.*
otc	**Generet-500 Tablets** (Goldline)	105[1]				6	6	30	10	5	25	500[2]		Timed release. In 60s.	4.4
otc	**Iberet-500 Filmtabs** (Abbott)													Controlled release. Red. Film coated. In 30s, 60s, 100s, 500s and Abbo-Pac 100s.	9.2
Rx	**Multibret-500 Hematinic Tablets** (Copley)													Timed release. In 60s.	NA
otc	**Iberet Filmtabs** (Abbott)	105[1]				6	6	30	10	5	25	150[2]		Controlled release. Red. Film coated. In 60s.	8.7
otc	**Stuartinic Tablets** (J & J-Merck)	100[3]				4.9	6	20	9.2	0.8	25	500[4]		Yellow. Film coated. Oval. In 60s.	7.4
otc	**Gerivites Tablets** (Rugby)	50[1]				5	5	30	2	0.5	3	75		In 40s, 100s and 1000s.	3
otc	**Livitamin Tablets** (SK-Beecham)	16.4[3]				3	3	10	2	3	5	100		Chewable. Tartrazine, Cu. In 100s.	30
Rx	**Hemocyte Plus Tabules** (US Pharm.)	106[3]				10	6	30	10	5	15	200[2]	1	Cu, Mg, Mn, Zn. In 100s.	6.1
Rx	**Iberet-Folic-500 Filmtabs** (Abbott)	105[1]				6	6	30	10	5	25	500[2]	0.8	Controlled release. (AK). Red. Film coated. In 60s and 100s.	10
Rx	**Multibret-Folic-500 Tablets** (Copley)													Timed release. In 60s.	NA
otc *sf*	**Parvlex Tablets** (Freeda)	100[3]				20	20	20	1	10	50	50	0.1	Cu, Mn. In 100s and 250s.	2.2

* Cost Index based on cost per 180 mg iron.
sf – Sugar free.
[1] From ferrous sulfate.
[2] As sodium ascorbate.
[3] From ferrous fumarate.
[4] From ascorbic acid and sodium ascorbate.

(Continued on following page)

IRON WITH VITAMINS (Cont.)

Capsules and Tablets (Cont.)

Content given per tablet.

	Product & Distributor	Fe mg	A IU	D IU	E IU	B_1 mg	B_2 mg	B_3 mg	B_5 mg	B_6 mg	B_{12} mcg	C mg	FA mg	Other Content and How Supplied	C.I.*
Rx	**Tabron Tablets** (Parke-Davis)	100[1]			30[2]	6	6	30	10	5	25	500	1	50 mg DSS. Film sealed. In 100s.	8.3
otc	**Allbee C-800 plus Iron Tablets** (Robins)	27[1]			45[3]	15	17	100	25	25	12	800	0.4	Lactose. Red. Film coated. Elliptical. In 60s.	11
otc	**Surbex 750 with Iron Filmtabs** (Abbott)	27[4]			30[2]	15	15	100	20	25	12	750[5]	0.4	Film coated. In 50s.	16
otc	**Theragran Stress Formula Tablets** (Apothecon)	27[1]			30[2]	15	15	100	20	25	12	600	0.4	45 mcg biotin. In 75s.	NA
otc	**Stress Formula 500 Plus Iron Tablets** (Schein)	27[1]			30[2]	15	10	100	20	5	12	500	0.4	45 mcg biotin. In 60s.	1
otc	**Stress Formula w/Iron Tablets** (Goldline)													45 mcg biotin. Red. Film coated. Oblong. In 60s.	1.2
otc	**Stresstabs + Iron Tablets** (Lederle)	27[1]			30[2]	10	10	100	20	5	12	500	0.4	45 mcg biotin. (LL S2). Orange-red. Film coated. Capsule shape. In 30s and 60s.	1.9

* Cost Index based on cost per 180 mg iron.
[1] From ferrous fumarate.
[2] As dl-alpha tocopheryl acetate.
[3] Form of vitamin E content unknown.
[4] From ferrous sulfate, exsiccated.
[5] From sodium ascorbate.

(Continued on following page)

IRON WITH VITAMINS (Cont.)

Capsules and Tablets (Cont.)

Content given per tablet.

	Product & Distributor	Fe mg	A IU	D IU	E IU	B_1 mg	B_2 mg	B_3 mg	B_5 mg	B_6 mg	B_{12} mcg	C mg	FA mg	Other Content and How Supplied	C.I.*
Rx	**Niferex-PN Tablets** (Central)	60[1]	4,000	400		3	3	10		2	3	50[2]	1	Ca, Zn, sorbitol. (131/05). Blue. Film coated. Oval. In 30s, 100s & 1000s.	5.9
Rx	**Nu-Iron V Tablets** (Mayrand)													Ca. Maroon. Film coated. In 100s.	5.8
Rx	**B C w/Folic Acid Plus Tablets** (Geneva)	27[3]	5,000		30[4]	20	20	100	25	25	50	500	0.8	0.15 mg biotin, Cr, Cu, Mg, Mn, Zn. In 100s.	11
Rx	**Berocca Plus Tablets** (Roche)													0.15 mg biotin, Cr, Cu, Mg, Mn, Zn. (Berocca Plus Roche). Yellow. Capsule shape. In 100s.	30
Rx	**Berplex Plus Tablets** (Schein)													0.15 mg biotin, Cr, Cu, Mg, Mn, Zn. In 100s.	11
Rx	**Formula B Plus Tablets** (Major)													0.15 mg biotin, Cr, Cu, Mg, Mn, Zn. In 100s and 500s.	8.9
otc	**Mission Prenatal H.P. Tablets** (Mission)	30[5]	4,000	400		5	2	10	1	25	2	100	0.8	Ca. In 100s.	11
otc	**Mission Prenatal F.A. Tablets** (Mission)	30[5]	4,000	400		5	2	10	1	10	2	100	0.8	Ca, Zn. In 100s.	10
otc	**Mission Prenatal Tablets** (Mission)	30[5]	4,000	400		5	2	10	1	3	2	100	0.4	Ca. In 100s.	9.8
otc	**Iromin-G Tablets** (Mission)	30[5]	4,000	400		5	2	10	1	25	2	100	0.8	Ca. In 100s.	8.7
Rx	**Nestabs FA Tablets** (Fielding)	36.3[3]	5,000	400	30[6]	3	3	20		3	8	120	1	Ca, I, Zn. In 100s.	8.4
Rx *sf*	**Vitafōl Caplets** (Everett)	65[3]	6,000	400	30[7]	1.1	1.8	15		2.5	5	60	1	Ca. Pink. Film coated. In 100s and 1000s.	4.7

* Cost Index based on cost per 180 mg iron.
sf– Sugar free.
[1] From polysaccharide-iron complex.
[2] From sodium ascorbate.
[3] From ferrous fumarate.
[4] As dl-alpha-tocopheryl acetate.
[5] From ferrous gluconate.
[6] Form of vitamin E unknown.
[7] As d-alpha tocopherol succinate.

(Continued on following page)

Capsules and Tables (Cont.)

Content given per capsule or tablet.

	Product & Distributor	Fe mg	A IU	D IU	E IU	B_1 mg	B_2 mg	B_3 mg	B_5 mg	B_6 mg	B_{12} mcg	C mg	FA mg	Other Content and How Supplied	C.I.*
otc	**Compete Tablets** (Mission)	27[1]	5,000	400	45[2]	2.25	2.6	30		25	9	90	0.4	Zn. In 100s.	8.1
otc	**Gevral T Tablets** (Lederle)	27[3]	5,000	400	45[4]	2.25	2.6	30		3	9	90	0.4	Ca, Cu, I, Mg, P, Zn. (LL G2). Maroon. Film coated. In 100s.	12
otc *sf*	**Freedavite Tablets** (Freeda)	30[3]	5,000	400	3[5]	5	3	25	5	2	2	60		Choline, inositol, potassium iodide, Ca, Cu, K, Mg, Mn, Se, Zn. In 100s, 250s and 500s.	4.7
otc	**Mission Surgical Supplement Tablets** (Mission)	27[1]	5,000	400	45[2]	2.5	2.6	30	16.3	3.6	9	500		Zn. In 100s.	11
otc	**Theragenerix-H Tablets** (Goldline)	66.7[3]	8,333	133	5[4]	3.3	3.3	33.3	11.7	3.3	50	100[6]	0.33	Cu, Mg. Pink. Sugar coated. Oblong. In 100s.	2.6
otc	**Thera Hematinic Tablets** (Major)													Cu, Mg. In 250s and 1000s.	1.6
Rx	**Theragran Hematinic Tablets** (Apothecon)	66.7[3]	1,400	140	5[4]	3.3	3.3	33.3	11.7	3.3	50	100	0.33	Cu, Mg. Lactose, sucrose, sodium bisulfite. In 90s.	11
otc	**Theravee Hematinic Tablets** (Vangard)	66.7	8,333	133	5[4]	3.3	3.3	33.3	11.7	3.3	50	100	0.33	Cu, Mg. In 100s and UD 100s.	3.1
otc *sf*	**Yelets Tablets** (Freeda)	19.8[3]	10,000	400	10[2]	10	10	25	10	10	10	100	0.1	PABA, lysine, glutamic acid, Ca, I, Mg, Mn. In 100s, 250s and 500s.	10
Rx	**Zodeac-100 Tablets** (Econo Med)	60[3]	8,000	400	30[2]	1.7	2	20	11	4	8	120	1	300 mcg biotin, Ca, Cu, I, Mg, Zn. Orange. In 100s.	3.5
otc *sf*	**Geritol Complete Tablets** (SK-Beecham)	50	6,000	400	30[2]	1.5	1.7	20	10	2	6	60	0.4	45 mcg biotin, Ca, Cl, Cr, Cu, I, K, Mg, Mn, Mo, Ni, P, Se, Si, Sn, V, Zn, vitamin K. In 14s, 40s, 100s and 180s.	5.4
otc *sf*	**Geriot Tablets** (Goldline)	50[3]	6,000	400	30[4]	1.5	1.7	20	10	2	6	60	0.4	45 mcg biotin, Ca, Cl, Cr, Cu, I, K, Mg, Mn, Mo, Ni, P, Se, Si, Zn, vitamin K. Maroon. Film coated. Oval. In 100s.	2.1

* Cost Index based on cost per 180 mg iron.
sf – Sugar free.
[1] From ferrous gluconate.
[2] Form of vitamin E content unknown.
[3] From ferrous fumarate.
[4] As dl-alpha-tocopheryl acetate.
[5] From sodium ascorbate.
[6] As d-alpha tocopherol.

(Continued on following page)

IRON WITH VITAMINS (Cont.)

Capsules and Tablets (Cont.)

Content given per tablet.

	Product & Distributor	Fe mg	A IU	D IU	E IU	B_1 mg	B_2 mg	B_3 mg	B_5 mg	B_6 mg	B_{12} mcg	C mg	FA mg	Other Content and How Supplied	C.I.*
otc	**Arbon Plus Tablets** (Forest)	27[1]	5,000	400	30[2]	2.25	2.6	20	10	3	9	90	0.4	150 mcg biotin, Ca, Cu, I, K, Mg, Mn, P, Zn. In 100s.	6.8
otc	**Alpha Zeta Tablets** (Parmed)				30[3]									45 mcg biotin, Ca, Cl, Cr, Cu, I, K, Mg, Mn, Mo, P, Se, Zn. In 30s.	6.1
otc	**Centurion A-Z Tablets** (Mission)	27[4]			30[2]									0.45 mg biotin, Ca, Cl, Cr, Cu, I, K, Mg, Mn, Mo, P, Se, Zn, vitamin K_1. In 130s.	4.1
otc *sf*	**ABC to Z Tablets** (Nature's Bounty)	18[1]	5,000	400	30[3]	1.5	1.7	20	10	2	6	60	0.4	30 mcg biotin, Ca, Cl, Cr, Cu, I, K, Mg, Mn, Mo, Ni, P, Se, Si, Sn, V, Zn, vitamin K_1. In 100s.	6.5
otc	**Advanced Formula Centrum Tablets** (Lederle)													30 mcg biotin, B, Ca, Cl, Cr, Cu, I, K, Mg, Mn, Mo, Ni, P, Se, Si, Sn, V, Zn, vitamin K_1. In 30s, 60s, 100s and 200s.	10
otc	**Arbon Tablets** (Forest)				30[2]									Ca, Cu, I, Mg, P, Zn. In 100s and 1000s.	7.7
otc	**Certagen Tablets** (Goldline)				30[3]									30 mcg biotin, Ca, Cl, Cr, Cu, I, K, Mg, Mn, Mo, Ni, P, Se, Si, Sn, V, Zn, vitamin K_1. Peach. Film coated. Oblong. In 100s and 1000s.	9.3
otc *sf*	**K-Dec Tablets** (Schein)													30 mcg biotin, Ca, Cl, Cr, Cu, I, K, Mg, Mn, Mo, Ni, P, Se, Si, Sn, V, Zn, vitamin K_1. In 130s.	2.7
otc	**Centrovite Advanced Formula Tablets** (Rugby)													30 mcg biotin, Ca, Cl, Cr, Cu, I, K, Mg, Mn, Mo, Ni, P, Se, Si, Sn, V, Zn, vitamin K_1. Dextrose, lactose, sucrose. In 100s.	4.9

* Cost Index based on cost per 180 mg iron.
sf – Sugar free.

[1] From ferrous fumarate.
[2] Form of vitamin E content unknown.
[3] As dl-alpha-tocopheryl acetate.
[4] Form of iron content unknown.

IRON WITH VITAMINS (Cont.)

Liquids

Content given per 15 ml.

	Product & Distributor	Fe mg	B_1 mg	B_2 mg	B_3 mg	B_5 mg	B_6 mg	B_{12} mcg	C mg	FA mg	Other Content	How Supplied	C.I.*
Rx *sf*	**Niferex Forte Elixir** (Central)	300[1]						75		3	10% alcohol	In 120 ml.	8.7
Rx *sf*	**Nu-Iron Plus Elixir** (Mayrand)										10% alcohol	Dye free. In 237 ml.	5.5
otc	**Troph-Iron Liquid** (Menley & James)	60[2]	30					75			Saccharin, glucose	In 120 ml.	37
otc	**Incremin with Iron Syrup** (Lederle)	90[2]	30				15	75			900 mg l-lysine. 0.75% alcohol, sorbitol	Regular and cherry flavors. In 118 and 473 ml.	25
Rx	**Vitafōl Syrup** (Everett)	90[2]			39.9		6	25.02		0.75		Raspberry-mint flavor. In 473 ml.	19
otc *sf*	**Vitalize SF Liquid** (Scot-Tussin)	66[2]	30				15	75			300 mg l-lysine.	Alcohol and dye free. In 120 and 240 ml, pt and gal.	15
otc *sf*	**Kovitonic Liquid** (Freeda)	42[2]	5				10	30		0.1	10 mg l-lysine. Sorbitol	In 120 & 240 ml and pt.	20
otc	**Geritol Tonic Liquid** (SK-Beecham)	50[3]	2.5	2.5	50	2	0.5	0.75			25 mg methionine, 50 mg choline bitartrate, 12% alcohol	In 120 and 360 ml.	16
otc	**Iberet-Liquid** (Abbott)	78.75[4]	4.5	4.5	22.5	7.5	3.75	18.75	112.5		1% alcohol, sorbitol	Raspberry-mint flavor. In 240 ml.	23
otc	**Iberet-500 Liquid** (Abbott)	78.75[4]	4.5	4.5	22.5	7.5	3.75	18.75	375		1% alcohol, sorbitol	Citrus flavor. In 240 ml.	28

* Cost Index based on cost per 180 mg iron.
sf – Sugar free.
[1] From polysaccharide-iron complex.
[2] From ferric pyrophosphate.
[3] From ferric ammonium citrate.
[4] From ferrous sulfate.

IRON AND LIVER COMBINATIONS

Complete prescribing information for iron begins on page 208

IRON and LIVER combinations are recommended for iron deficiency anemia in conjunction with certain nutritional deficiencies.

Precautions:

The ingredients in these products are not sufficient, nor are they intended, for the treatment of pernicious anemia. The use of folic acid without adequate vitamin B_{12} therapy in patients with pernicious anemia may result in hematologic remission, but neurological progression.

LIVER (concentrate, fraction or desiccated) is used as a source of vitamin B complex.

B COMPLEX VITAMINS function as coenzymes in nutrient metabolism and maturation of red blood cells.

ASCORBIC ACID (Vitamin C) may enhance the absorption of iron.

Capsules and Tablets

Content given per capsule or tablet.

	Product & Distributor	Fe mg	Liver	B_1 mg	B_2 mg	B_3 mg	B_5 mg	B_6 mg	B_{12} mcg	C mg	Other Content	How Supplied	C.I.*
otc	**Arcotinic Tablets** (Arco)	102.5[1]	200 mg (desiccated)							250		In 100s.	NA
otc	**Feocyte Tablets** (Dunhall)	110[2]	†					2	50	100	0.8 mg folic acid, Cu	Prolonged action. In 100s and 1000s.	4.8
otc	**Rogenic Tablets** (Forest)	60[3]	25 mg (desiccated)					6	25	100		Slow release. In 100s and 1000s.	5.6
otc *sf*	**I-L-X B_{12} Tablets** (Kenwood)	37.5[4]	130 mg (desiccated)	2	2	20			12	120		In 100s.	7.2
otc	**Livitamin Capsules** (SK-Beecham)	33[5]	150 mg (desiccated)	3	3	10	2	3	5	100	Cu	In 100s.	16

* Cost Index based on cost per 180 mg iron.

† Content unknown.

sf – Sugar free.

[1] From ferrous fumarate and ferrous sulfate, exsiccated.

[2] From ferrous fumarate, ferrous gluconate and ferrous sulfate, dried.

[3] From ferrous fumarate, ferrous sulfate and ferrous gluconate.

[4] From ferrous gluconate.

[5] From ferrous fumarate.

IRON AND LIVER COMBINATIONS (Cont.)

Refer to the general discussion of these products on page 224

Liquids

Content given per 15 ml.

	Product & Distributor	Fe mg	Liver	B_1 mg	B_2 mg	B_3 mg	B_5 mg	B_6 mg	B_{12} mcg	Other Content	How Supplied	C.I.*
otc	**Liquid Geritonic** (Geriatric Pharm)	105[1]	375 mg liver fraction 1	3	3	30		0.3	9	60 mg inositol, 180 mg glycine, 375 mg yeast concentrate, Ca, I, K, Mg, Mn, P. 20% alcohol	In 240 ml and gal.	22
otc	**I-L-X B_{12} Elixir** (Kenwood)	102[1]	98 mg liver fraction 1	5	2	10			10	8% alcohol	In 360 ml.	12
otc	**I-L-X Elixir** (Kenwood)	70[2]	98 mg liver concentrate 1:20	5	2	10				8% alcohol	In 360 ml.	16
otc	**Arcotinic Liquid** (Arco)	64.8	180 mg liver fraction 1	4.5	4.5	30	4	1.5	6	3% alcohol	In 360 ml.	NA
otc	**Livitamin Liquid** (SK-Beecham)	35.5[3]	500 mg liver fraction 1	3	3	10	2	3	5	Cu	In 240 ml, pt and gal.	41

* Cost Index based on cost per 180 mg iron.
1 From iron ammonium citrate, brown.
2 From ferrous gluconate.
3 From peptonized iron.

IRON AND LIVER COMBINATIONS (Cont.)

Refer to the general discussion of these products on page 224

Parenteral

Dose: 1 to 2 ml IM 1 to 3 times weekly.

Content given per ml.

	Product & Distributor	Fe mg	B_{12} equivalent mcg	B_1 mg	B_2 mg	B_3 mg	B_5 mg	B_6 mg	B_{12} mcg	Other Content	How Supplied	C.I.*
Rx	**Rogenic** (Forest)	20[1]	10					500			In 10 ml vials.[2]	17
Rx	**Hemocyte** (US Pharm)	3[3]	1		0.75	50	1.25		15	2% procaine HCl	In 30 ml vials.[2]	53
Rx	**Hytinic** (Hyrex)										In 30 ml vials.[2]	53
Rx	**Licoplex DS** (Keene)										In 30 ml vials.[2]	40
Rx	**Hemocyte-V** (US Pharm)	3.6[3]	2	10	0.5	10	1	1	15	glucose	In 10 ml vials.[4]	NA
Rx	**Liver-Iron B Complex w/ Vitamin B_{12}** (Akorn)										In 30 ml vials.[4]	NA

* Cost Index based on cost per 50 mg iron.
[1] Peptonized iron.
[2] With 2% benzyl alcohol.
[3] From ferrous gluconate.
[4] With 0.5% chlorobutanol and 2% benzyl alcohol.

IRON WITH VITAMIN B_{12} AND INTRINSIC FACTOR

These products contain Intrinsic Factor derived from stomach extract to promote the absorption of vitamin B_{12}. Although previously used to treat anemias responsive to oral hematinics, parenteral cobalamin therapy is preferred in treating B_{12} deficiencies, including pernicious anemia.

One NF unit of *Vitamin B_{12} with Intrinsic Factor Concentrate* (IFC) contains not more than 15 mcg B_{12} and 300 mg IFC.

Content given per capsule.

	Product & Distributor	Fe mg	B_{12}[1] mcg	IFC[2]	B_1 mg	B_2 mg	B_3 mg	C mg	FA mg	Other Content	How Supplied	C.I.*
Rx	**Pronemia Hematinic Capsules** (Lederle)	115[3]	15	75 mg				150	1	Sucrose	(LL P9). Maroon. In 30s.	14
Rx	**Contrin Capsules** (Geneva)	110[3]	15	240 mg				75	0.5		Red/maroon. In 100s.	2.4
Rx	**Ferotrinsic Capsules** (Rugby)										In 100s and 1000s.	1.3
Rx	**Livitrinsic-f Capsules** (Goldline)										Maroon/red. In 100s.	2.1
Rx	**Trinsicon Capsules** (Whitby)										Pink and red. In 60s, 500s and UD 100s.	NA

* Cost Index based on cost per 180 mg iron.

[1] B_{12} activity derived from cobalamin or liver.

[2] Intrinsic factor as concentrate or from stomach preparations.

[3] From ferrous fumarate.

(Continued on following page)

IRON WITH VITAMIN B_{12} AND INTRINSIC FACTOR (Cont.)

Content given per capsule or tablet.

	Product & Distributor	Fe mg	B_{12}[1]	IFC[2]	B_1 mg	B_2 mg	B_3 mg	C mg	FA mg	Other Content	How Supplied	C.I.*
Rx	**Fergon Plus Caplets** (Sanofi Winthrop)	58[3]	½ NF unit B_{12} with IFC					75			Pink. Sugar coated. In 100s.	12
Rx	**TriHEMIC 600 Tablets** (Lederle)	115[4]	25 mcg B_{12}	75 mg IFC				600	1	50 mg DSS, 30 IU vitamin E[5]. Lactose	(LL T1). Red. Film coated. Capsule shape. In 30s and 500s.	13
Rx	**Heptuna Plus Capsules** (Roerig)	100[6]	5 mcg B_{12}, 50 mg desiccated liver	25 mg IFC	3.1	2	15	150[7]		0.9 mg B_5, 1.6 mg B_6, Ca, Cu, I, K, Mg, Mn, Mo, P	Red and white. In 100s.	4.1
Rx	**Livitamin w/Intrinsic Factor Capsules** (SK-Beecham)	33[4]	5 mcg B_{12}, 150 mg desiccated liver, ⅓ NF unit B_{12} with IFC		3	3	10	100		2 mg B_5, 3 mg B_6, Cu	Green. In 100s.	18
Rx	**Chromagen Capsules** (Savage)	66[4]	10 mcg B_{12}	100 mg desiccated stomach substance				250			Maroon. In 100s and 500s.	8.4

* Cost Index based on cost per 180 mg iron.
[1] B_{12} activity as derived from cobalamin or the various liver preparations.
[2] Intrinsic factor as concentrate or from stomach preparations.
[3] From ferrous gluconate.
[4] From ferrous fumarate.
[5] From dl-alpha-tocopheryl acetate.
[6] From ferrous sulfate, dried.
[7] From sodium ascorbate.

FOLIC ACID (Folacin; Pteroylglutamic Acid; Folate)

Actions:

Exogenous folate is required for nucleoprotein synthesis and maintenance of normal erythropoiesis. Folic acid stimulates production of red and white blood cells and platelets in certain megaloblastic anemias.

Dietary folic acid is present in foods, primarily as reduced folate polyglutamate. It must undergo hydrolysis, reduction and methylation in the GI tract before it is absorbed. Conversion to tetrahydrofolate, the active form, may be B_{12} dependent; supplies are maintained by food and enterohepatic recirculation. Oral synthetic folic acid is a monoglutamate and is completely absorbed following administration, even in the presence of malabsorption syndromes.

Indications:

Treatment of megaloblastic anemias due to a deficiency of folic acid as seen in sprue, anemias of nutritional origin, pregnancy, infancy, or childhood.

Contraindications:

Not effective in the treatment of pernicious, aplastic or normocytic anemias.

Warnings:

Pernicious anemia: Doses above 0.1 mg daily may obscure pernicious anemia. Patients with untreated pernicious anemia may show hematologic improvement with daily folic acid (as low as 0.25 mg/day). In such cases, irreversible neurological damage may progress after 3 months, despite the absence of anemia. Rule out suspected pernicious anemia prior to folic acid therapy by means of a Schilling test and a vitamin B_{12} blood level determination.

Resistance to treatment may be due to depressed hematopoiesis, alcoholism, the presence of antimetabolic drugs, and to deficiencies of vitamins B_6, B_{12}, C, and E.

Usage in Lactation: Folic acid is excreted in breast milk; milk:plasma ratio equals approximately 0.02.

Usage in Pregnancy: Pregnant women are more prone to develop folate deficiency as reflected in larger dosage recommendations. Folate deficient mothers may be more prone to complications of pregnancy and fetal abnormalities.

Drug Interactions:

Oral contraceptives may impair folate metabolism and produce folate depletion, but the effect is mild and unlikely to cause anemia or megaloblastic changes.

Phenytoin: An increase in seizure frequency and a decrease in serum concentration to subtherapeutic levels have been reported in patients receiving folic acid (particularly 15 to 20 mg/day) with phenytoin. The mechanism appears to be increased metabolic clearance of phenytoin and/or a redistribution of phenytoin in the CSF and brain. **Phenytoin** and **primidone** are reported to cause a decrease in serum folate levels, and may produce symptoms of folic acid deficiency in 27% to 91% of patients (but clinically important megaloblastic anemia in $< 1\%$) on long-term therapy. If folic acid is required, a higher dose of phenytoin may be needed. Monitor hydantoin plasma levels and the patient's seizure control. Adjust the dose accordingly. **P-aminosalicylic acid** and **sulfasalazine** may cause a similar deficiency.

Pyrimethamine: Folic acid may interfere with the antimicrobial actions against toxoplasmosis.

Pyrimethamine, trimethoprim, or **triamterene:** A dihydrofolate reductase deficiency caused by administration of folic acid antagonists, may interfere with folic acid utilization.

Adverse Reactions:

Allergic sensitization has been reported.

(Continued on following page)

FOLIC ACID (Folacin; Pteroylglutamic Acid; Folate) (Cont.)

Patient Information:

Take only under medical supervision.

Administration and Dosage:

Give orally, except in severe intestinal malabsorption.

Give IM, IV or SC if disease is very severe or GI absorption is very severely impaired.

Usual therapeutic dosage: Up to 1 mg daily. Resistant cases may require larger doses.

Maintenance dosage level: When clinical symptoms have subsided and the blood picture has normalized, use the dosage below. Never give less than 0.1 mg/day. Keep patients under close supervision and adjust maintenance dose if relapse appears imminent. In the presence of alcoholism, hemolytic anemia, anticonvulsant therapy or chronic infection, the maintenance level may need to be increased.

Infants – 0.1 mg/day.
Children (under 4) – up to 0.3 mg/day.
Adults and children (over 4) – 0.4 mg/day.
Pregnant and lactating women – 0.8 mg/day.

Recommended Dietary Allowances (RDAs): Adult males and females, 0.4 mg. For a complete listing of RDAs by age and sex, refer to page 5.

Stability: At concentrations usually used for parenteral nutrition, folate will remain stable in solution providing the pH of the solution remains above 5.

				C.I.*
otc[1]	**Folic Acid** (Fibertone)	**Tablets:** 0.1 mg	In 100s, 250s, 500s and 1000s.	18
otc[1]	**Folic Acid** (Various)	**Tablets:** 0.4 mg	In 100s.	5+
otc[1]	**Folic Acid** (Various)	**Tablets:** 0.8 mg	In 100s and UD 100s.	2+
Rx	**Folic Acid** (Various)	**Tablets:** 1 mg	In 100s, 1000s and UD 32s & 100s.	2+
Rx	**Folvite** (Lederle)		(#LL F1). Orange. In 100s, 1000s and UD 100s.	20
Rx	**Folic Acid** (LyphoMed)	**Injection:** 5 mg/ml	In 10 ml vials.[2]	29
Rx	**Folvite** (Lederle)		In 10 ml vials.[3]	34
Rx	**Folic Acid** (Various)	**Injection:** 10 mg/ml	In 10 ml vials.	5+

* Cost Index based on cost per mg. # Product identification code.

[1] Although most folic acid products carry the *Rx* legend, products which provide 0.4 mg or less (or 0.8 mg for pregnant or lactating women) may be *otc* items.

[2] With 1.5% benzyl alcohol and EDTA.

[3] With 1.5% benzyl alcohol.

LEUCOVORIN CALCIUM (Folinic Acid; Citrovorum Factor)

Actions:

Pharmacology: Leucovorin is one of several active, chemically reduced derivatives of folic acid. It is useful as an antidote to drugs which act as folic acid antagonists. Leucovorin is a mixture of the diasteroisomers of the 5-formyl derivative of tetrahydrofolic acid (THF). The biologically active compound of the mixture is the l-isomer, known as citrovorum factor or folinic acid. Leucovorin does not require reduction by the enzyme dihydrofolate reductase in order to participate in reactions utilizing folates as a source of "one-carbon" moieties. l-Leucovorin is rapidly metabolized to 1,5-methyltetrahydrofolate, which can in turn be metabolized via other pathways back to 5, 10-methyl-ene-tetrahydrofolate, which is converted to 5-methyltetrahydrofolate by an irreversible, enzyme-catalyzed reduction using the cofactors $FADH_2$ and NADPH.

Administration of leucovorin can counteract the therapeutic and toxic effects of folic acid antagonists such as methotrexate (MTX), which act by inhibiting dihydrofolate reductase.

In contrast, leucovorin can enhance the therapeutic and toxic effects of fluoropyrimidines used in cancer therapy, such as 5-fluorouracil (5-FU). Concurrent administration of leucovorin does not appear to alter the plasma pharmacokinetics of 5-FU. 5-FU is metabolized to fluorodeoxyuridylic acid, which binds to and inhibits the enzyme thymidylate synthase (an enzyme important in DNA repair and replication). The reduced folate, 5,10-methylenetetrahydrofolate, acts to stabilize the binding of fluorodeoxyuridylic acid to thymidylate synthase and thereby enhances the inhibition of this enzyme.

Pharmacokinetics:

Leucovorin Pharmacokinetics[1]

Parameter	IV	IM	Oral
Total reduced folates:			
Mean peak conc. (ng/ml)	1259 (range, 897-1625)	436 (range, 240 to 725)	393 (range, 160 to 550)
Mean time to peak	10 min	52 min	2.3 hrs
Terminal half-life	6.2 hrs	6.2 hrs	5.7 hrs
5-Methyl-THF[2]			
Mean peak conc. (ng/ml)	258	226	367
Mean time to peak	1.3 hrs	2.8 hrs	2.4 hrs
5-Formyl-THF[3]			
Mean peak conc. (ng/ml)	1206	360	51
Mean time to peak	10 min	28 min	1.2 hrs

[1] Following administration of a 25 mg dose.
[2] The major metabolite to which leucovorin is primarily converted in the intestinal mucosa and which becomes the predominant circulating form of the drug.
[3] The parent compound.

The initial rise in total reduced folates is primarily due to the parent compound (5-formyl-THF). A sharp drop in parent compound follows and coincides with the appearance of the active metabolite (5-methyl-THF).

Following IV administration, the area under the plasma concentration vs time curves (AUC) for l-leucovorin, d-leucovorin and 5-methyl-THF were 28.4 ± 3.5, 956 ± 97 and 129 ± 12 mg • min/L. When a higher dose of d,l-leucovorin was used, similar results were obtained. The d-isomer persisted in plasma at concentrations greatly exceeding those of the l-isomer. There was no difference between IM and IV administration in the AUC for total reduced folates, 5-formyl-THF or 5-methyl-THF. The AUC of total reduced folates after oral administration was 92% of the AUC after IV administration.

Following oral administration leucovorin is rapidly absorbed and expands the serum pool of reduced folates. At a dose of 25 mg, almost 100% of the l-isomer but only 20% of the d-isomer is absorbed. Oral absorption of leucovorin is saturable at doses $>$ 25 mg. The apparent bioavailability of leucovorin was 97% for 25 mg, 75% for 50 mg and 37% for 100 mg.

(Actions continued on following page)

LEUCOVORIN CALCIUM (Folinic Acid; Citrovorum Factor) (Cont.)

Actions (Cont.):

Clinical trials: In a randomized clinical study in patients with advanced metastatic colorectal cancer, three treatment regimens were compared. Leucovorin 200 mg/m² and 5-FU 370 mg/m² vs leucovorin 20 mg/m² and 5-FU 425 mg/m² vs 5-FU 500 mg/m². All drugs were given by slow IV infusion daily for 5 days repeated every 28 to 35 days. Response rates were 26%, 43% and 10% for the high-dose leucovorin, low-dose leucovorin and 5-FU alone groups, respectively. Respective median survival times were 12.2 months, 12 months and 7.7 months. The low-dose leucovorin regimen gave a significant improvement in weight gain of > 5%, relief of symptoms and improvement in performance status. The high-dose regimen gave a significant improvement in performance status and trended toward improvement in weight gain and in relief of symptoms.

In a second randomized clinical study, the 5-FU monotherapy was replaced by a regimen of sequentially administered MTX, 5-FU and leucovorin. Response rates with leucovorin 200 mg/m² and 5-FU 370 mg/m² vs leucovorin 20 mg/m² and 5-FU 425 mg/m² vs sequential MTX and 5-FU and leucovorin were, respectively, 33%, 31% and 4%. Respective median survival times were 402 days, 418 days and 223 days. No significant difference in weight gain of > 5% or in improvement in performance status was seen between the treatment arms.

Indications:

Oral and parenteral: Leucovorin "rescue" after high-dose methotrexate therapy in osteosarcoma.

To diminish the toxicity and counteract the effects of impaired methotrexate elimination and of inadvertent overdosages of folic acid antagonists.

Parenteral: Treatment of megaloblastic anemias due to folic acid deficiency when oral therapy is not feasible.

In combination with 5-fluorouracil to prolong survival in the palliative treatment of patients with advanced colorectal cancer.

Contraindications:

Pernicious anemia and other megaloblastic anemias secondary to the lack of vitamin B_{12} (see Warnings).

Warnings:

Anemias: Leucovorin is improper therapy for pernicious anemia and other megaloblastic anemias secondary to the lack of vitamin B_{12}. A hematologic remission may occur while neurologic manifestations continue to progress.

5-Fluorouracil dosage/toxicity: Leucovorin enhances the toxicity of 5-FU. When these drugs are administered concurrently in the palliative therapy of advanced colorectal cancer, the dosage of 5-FU must be lower than usually administered. Although the toxicities observed in patients treated with the combination of leucovorin plus 5-FU are qualitatively similar to those observed in patients treated with 5-FU alone, GI toxicities (particularly stomatitis and diarrhea) are observed more commonly and may be more severe and of prolonged duration in patients treated with the combination.

In a controlled trial, toxicity, primarily GI, resulted in 7% of patients requiring hospitalization when treated with 5-FU alone or 5-FU in combination with 200 mg/m² leucovorin and 20% when treated with 5-FU in combination with 20 mg/m² leucovorin. In another trial, hospitalizations related to treatment toxicity also appeared to occur more often in patients treated with low-dose leucovorin/5-FU combination than in patients treated with the high-dose combination (11% vs 3%). Therapy with leucovorin/5-FU must not be initiated or continued in patients who have symptoms of GI toxicity of any severity, until those symptoms have completely resolved. Patients with diarrhea must be monitored with particular care until the diarrhea has resolved, as rapid clinical deterioration leading to death can occur. In an additional study utilizing higher weekly doses of 5-FU and leucovorin, elderly or debilitated patients were found to be at greater risk for severe GI toxicity.

Since leucovorin enhances the toxicity of 5-FU, administer the combination for advanced colorectal cancer under the supervision of a physician experienced in the use of antimetabolite cancer chemotherapy. Take particular care in the treatment of elderly or debilitated colorectal cancer patients, as these patients may be at increased risk of severe toxicity.

Methotrexate concentrations: Monitoring of the serum MTX concentration is essential in determining the optimal dose and duration of treatment with leucovorin. Delayed MTX excretion may be caused by a third space fluid accumulation (ie, ascites, pleural effusion), renal insufficiency or inadequate hydration. Under such circumstances, higher doses of leucovorin or prolonged administration may be indicated. Doses higher than those recommended for oral use must be given IV.

(Warnings continued on following page:

LEUCOVORIN CALCIUM (Folinic Acid; Citrovorum Factor) (Cont.)

Warnings (Cont.):

Calcium content: Because of the calcium content of the leucovorin solution, inject no more than 160 mg/min IV (16 ml of a 10 mg/ml, or 8 ml of a 20 mg/ml solution per minute).

Folic acid antagonist overdosage: In the treatment of accidental overdosages of folic acid antagonists, administer leucovorin as promptly as possible. As the time interval between antifolate administration (eg, MTX) and leucovorin rescue increases, leucovorin's effectiveness in counteracting toxicity decreases.

Benzyl alcohol: Because of the benzyl alcohol contained in the 1 ml amp and in certain diluents used for leucovorin injection, when doses > 10 mg/m² are administered, reconstitute leucovorin injection with Sterile Water for Injection, USP, and use immediately (see Administration and Dosage). Benzyl alcohol has been associated with a fatal "Gasping Syndrome" in premature infants.

Pregnancy: Category C. It is not known whether leucovorin can cause fetal harm when administered to a pregnant woman or can affect reproduction capacity. Give to a pregnant woman only if clearly needed.

Lactation: It is not known whether this drug is excreted in breast milk. Exercise caution when administering to a nursing woman.

Precautions:

Parenteral administration is preferable to oral dosing if there is a possibility that the patient may vomit or not absorb the leucovorin. Leucovorin has no effect on non-hematologic toxicities of MTX such as the nephrotoxicity resulting from drug or metabolite precipitation in the kidney.

Monitoring: Obtain a CBC with differential and platelets prior to each treatment with the leucovorin/5-FU combination. During the first two courses a CBC with differential and platelets must be repeated weekly and thereafter once each cycle at the time of anticipated WBC nadir. Perform electrolytes and liver function tests prior to each treatment for the first three cycles, then prior to every other cycle. Institute dosage modifications of 5-FU as follows, based on the most severe toxicities:

5-Fluorouracil Dosage Modifications Based on Toxicities			
Diarrhea or stomatitis	WBC/mm³ nadir	Platelets/mm³ nadir	5-FU dose
Moderate	1000-1900	25,000-75,000	decrease 20%
Severe	< 1000	< 25,000	decrease 30%

If no toxicity occurs, the 5-FU dose may increase 10%.

Defer treatment until WBCs are 4000/mm³ and platelets are 130,000/mm³. If blood counts do not reach these levels within 2 weeks, discontinue treatment. Follow up patients with physical examination prior to each treatment course and with appropriate radiological examination as needed. Discontinue treatment when there is clear evidence of tumor progression.

Drug Interactions:

Leucovorin Drug Interactions			
Precipitant drug	Object drug*		Description
Leucovorin	Anticonvulsants	↓	Folic acid in large amounts may counteract the antiepileptic effect of phenobarbital, phenytoin and primidone, and increase the frequency of seizures in susceptible children. Although this interaction has not been reported with leucovorin, consider the possibility when using these drugs concomitantly.
Leucovorin	5-Fluorouracil	↑	Leucovorin may enhance the toxicity of 5-FU (see Warnings).
Leucovorin	Methotrexate	↓	Small quantities of systemically administered leucovorin enter the CSF primarily as 5-methyltetrahydrofolate and remain 1 to 3 orders of magnitude lower than the usual MTX concentrations following intrathecal administration. However, high doses of leucovorin may reduce the efficacy of intrathecally administered MTX.

* ↑ = Object drug increased ↓ = Object drug decreased

(Continued on following page)

LEUCOVORIN CALCIUM (Folinic Acid; Citrovorum Factor) (Cont.)

Adverse Reactions:

Allergic sensitization, including anaphylactoid reactions and urticaria, has been reported following administration of both oral and parenteral leucovorin. No other adverse reactions have been attributed to the use of leucovorin alone.

The following table summarizes significant adverse events occurring in 316 patients treated with the leucovorin/5-FU combinations compared with 70 patients treated with 5-FU alone for advanced colorectal carcinoma.

Adverse Reactions with the Leucovorin/5-Fluorouracil Combination

	High leucovorin[1]/5-FU (n=155)		Low leucovorin[2]/5-FU (n=161)		5-FU alone (n=70)	
Adverse reaction	Any (%)	Grade 3+ (%)	Any (%)	Grade 3+ (%)	Any (%)	Grade 3+ (%)
Leukopenia	69	14	83	23	93	48
Thrombocytopenia	8	2	8	1	18	3
Infection	8	1	3	1	7	2
Nausea	74	10	80	9	60	6
Vomiting	46	8	44	9	40	7
Diarrhea	66	18	67	14	43	11
Stomatitis	75	27	84	29	59	16
Constipation	3	–	4	–	1	–
Lethargy/Malaise/ Fatigue	13	3	12	2	6	3
Alopecia	42	5	43	6	37	7
Dermatitis	21	2	25	1	13	–
Anorexia	14	1	22	4	14	–
Hospitalization for toxicity	5%		15%		7%	

[1] High leucovorin = 200 mg/m².
[2] Low leucovorin = 20 mg/m².
Any = Percentage of patients reporting toxicity of any severity.
Grade 3+ = Percentage of patients reporting toxicity of Grade 3 or higher.

Overdosage:

Excessive amounts of leucovorin may nullify the chemotherapeutic effect of folic acid antagonists.

Administration and Dosage:

Oral administration of doses > 25 mg is not recommended.

Advanced colorectal cancer: Either of the following two regimens is recommended:

1) Leucovorin 200 mg/m² by slow IV injection over a minimum of 3 minutes, followed by 5-FU 370 mg/m² by IV injection.
2) Leucovorin 20 mg/m² by IV injection followed by 5-FU 425 mg/m² by IV injection.

Treatment is repeated daily for 5 days. This 5 day treatment course may be repeated at 4 week (28 day) intervals for 2 courses and then repeated at 4 to 5 week (28 to 35 day) intervals provided that the patient has completely recovered from the toxic effects of the prior treatment course.

In subsequent treatment courses, adjust the dosage of 5-FU based on patient tolerance of the prior treatment course. Reduce the daily dosage of 5-FU by 20% for patients who experienced moderate hematologic or GI toxicity in the prior treatment course, and by 30% for patients who experienced severe toxicity (see Precautions). For patients who experienced no toxicity in the prior treatment course, 5-FU dosage may be increased by 10%. Leucovorin dosages are not adjusted for toxicity.

Several other doses and schedules of leucovorin/5-FU therapy have also been evaluated in patients with advanced colorectal cancer; some of these alternative regimens may also have efficacy in the treatment of this disease. However, further clinical research will be required to confirm the safety and efficacy of these alternative treatment regimens.

(Administration and Dosage continued on following page)

LEUCOVORIN CALCIUM (Folinic Acid; Citrovorum Factor) (Cont.)

Administration and Dosage (Cont.):

Leucovorin rescue after high-dose MTX therapy: The recommendations for leucovorin rescue are based on an MTX dose of 12 to 15 g/m² administered by IV infusion over 4 hours (see Methotrexate monograph). Leucovorin rescue at a dose of 15 mg (≈ 10 mg/m²) every 6 hours for 10 doses starts 24 hours after the beginning of the MTX infusion. In the presence of GI toxicity, nausea or vomiting, administer leucovorin parenterally.

Determine serum creatinine and MTX levels at least once daily. Continue leucovorin administration, hydration and urinary alkalinization (pH of ≥ 7) until the MTX level is < 5 x 10^{-8} M (0.05 micromolar). Adjust the leucovorin dose or extend leucovorin rescue based on the following guidelines:

Guidelines for Leucovorin Rescue Dosage and Administration		
Clinical situation	Laboratory findings	Leucovorin dosage and duration
Normal MTX elimination	Serum MTX level ≈ 10 micromolar at 24 hours after administration, 1 micromolar at 48 hours, and < 0.2 micromolar at 72 hours	15 mg orally, IM or IV every 6 hours for 60 hours (10 doses starting at 24 hours after start of MTX infusion)
Delayed late MTX elimination	Serum MTX level remaining > 0.2 micromolar at 72 hours and > 0.05 micromolar at 96 hours after administration	Continue 15 mg orally, IM or IV every 6 hours, until MTX level is < 0.05 micromolar
Delayed early MTX elimination or evidence of acute renal injury	Serum MTX level of ≥ 50 micromolar at 24 hours, or ≥ 5 micromolar at 48 hours after administration or a ≥ 100% increase in serum creatinine level at 24 hours after MTX administration (eg, an increase from 0.5 mg/dl to a level of ≥ 1 mg/dl)	150 mg IV every 3 hours, until MTX level is < 1 micromolar; then 15 mg IV every 3 hours until MTX level is < 0.05 micromolar

Patients who experience delayed early MTX elimination are likely to develop reversible renal failure. In addition to appropriate leucovorin therapy, these patients require continuing hydration and urinary alkalinization, and close monitoring of fluid and electrolyte status, until the serum MTX level has fallen to < 0.05 micromolar and the renal failure has resolved.

Some patients will have abnormalities in MTX elimination or renal function following administration, which are significant but less severe than the abnormalities described in the table above. These abnormalities may or may not be associated with significant clinical toxicity. If significant clinical toxicity is observed, extend leucovorin rescue for an additional 24 hours (total of 14 doses over 84 hours) in subsequent courses of therapy. Always consider the possibility that the patient is taking other medications which interact with MTX (eg, medications which may interfere with MTX elimination or binding to serum albumin) when laboratory abnormalities or clinical toxicities are observed.

Impaired MTX elimination or inadvertent overdosage: Begin leucovorin rescue as soon as possible after an inadvertent overdosage and within 24 hours of MTX administration when there is delayed excretion (see Warnings). Administer leucovorin 10 mg/m² IV, IM or orally every 6 hours until the serum MTX level is < 10^{-8} M. In the presence of GI toxicity, nausea or vomiting, administer leucovorin parenterally.

Determine serum creatinine and MTX levels at 24 hour intervals. If the 24 hour serum creatinine has increased 50% over baseline or if the 24 or 48 hour MTX level is > 5 x 10^{-6} M or > 9 x 10^{-7} M, respectively, increase the dose of leucovorin to 100 mg/m² IV every 3 hours until the MTX level is < 10^{-8} M.

Use hydration (3 L/day) and urinary alkalinization with sodium bicarbonate solution concomitantly. Adjust the bicarbonate dose to maintain the urine pH at ≥ 7.

Megaloblastic anemia due to folic acid deficiency: Up to 1 mg leucovorin daily. There is no evidence that doses > 1 mg/day have greater efficacy than those of 1 mg; additionally, loss of folate in urine becomes roughly logarithmic as the amount administered exceeds 1 mg.

(Administration and Dosage on followng page)

LEUCOVORIN CALCIUM (Folinic Acid; Citrovorum Factor) (Cont.)

Administration and Dosage (Cont.):

Storage/Stability: Leucovorin powder for injection contains no preservative. Reconstitute with Bacteriostatic Water for Injection, USP, which contains benzyl alcohol, or with Sterile Water for Injection, USP. When reconstituted with Bacteriostatic Water for Injection, USP, the resulting solution must be used within 7 days. If the product is reconstituted with Sterile Water for Injection, USP, it must be used immediately.

Because of the benzyl alcohol contained in the 1 ml amp and in Bacteriostatic Water for Injection, USP, when doses > 10 mg/m² are administered, reconstitute the leucovorin amps with Sterile Water for Injection, USP, and use immediately. Because of the calcium content of the leucovorin solution, inject no more than 160 mg/min IV (16 ml of a 10 mg/ml, or 8 ml of a 20 mg/ml solution per minute).

Protect from light.

	Product	Form	Description	C.I.*
Rx	**Leucovorin Calcium** (Various, eg, Barr, Lederle)	**Tablets:** 5 mg (as calcium)	In 30s, 100s and UD 50s.	1.7+
Rx	**Wellcovorin** (Burroughs Wellcome)		Lactose. (Wellcovorin 5). Off-white, scored. In 20s, 100s and UD 50s.	3.4
Rx	**Leucovorin Calcium** (Lederle)	**Tablets:** 10 mg (as calcium)	Lactose. (LL 10 C 12). Yellowish-white, scored. Square, convex. In 12s, 24s and UD 50s.	1.7
Rx	**Leucovorin Calcium** (Lederle)	**Tablets:** 15 mg (as calcium)	Lactose. (LL 15 C 35). Yellowish-white, scored. Oval, convex. In 12s, 24s and UD 50s.	1.6
Rx	**Leucovorin Calcium** (Barr)	**Tablets:** 25 mg (as calcium)	(485). Light green. In 25s.	2.7
Rx	**Wellcovorin** (Burroughs Wellcome)		Lactose. (Wellcovorin 25). Peach, scored. In 25s and UD 10s.	3.3
Rx	**Leucovorin Calcium** (Lederle)	**Injection:** 3 mg/ml (as calcium)	In 1 ml amps.[1]	2.9
Rx	**Leucovorin Calcium** (Lederle)	**Powder for Injection:** 50 mg/vial (as calcium)[2]	In vials.	2.6
Rx	**Leucovorin Calcium** (Lederle)	**Powder for Injection:** 100 mg/vial (as calcium)[2]	In vials.	2.1
Rx	**Wellcovorin** (Burroughs Wellcome)		In vials.	1
Rx	**Leucovorin Calcium** (Lederle)	**Powder for Injection:** 350 mg/vial (as calcium)[2]	In vials.	1.2

* Cost Index based on cost per mg.

[1] With 0.9% benzyl alcohol.

[2] Preservative free.

Actions:

Pharmacology: Vitamin B_{12} (cyanocobalamin and hydroxocobalamin) is essential to growth, cell reproduction, hematopoiesis and nucleoprotein and myelin synthesis. Its physiologic role is associated with methylation, participating in nucleic acid and protein synthesis. Cyanocobalamin participates in red blood cell formation through activation of folic acid coenzymes. Cyanocobalamin has hematopoietic activity apparently identical to that of the anti-anemia factor in purified liver extract. Hydroxocobalamin (vitamin B_{12_a}), an analogue of cyanocobalamin in which a hydroxyl radical replaces the cyano radical, functions the same as cyanocobalamin.

The normal range of plasma B_{12} is 150 to 750 pg/ml, which represents about 0.1% of the total body content. The total daily loss ranges from 2 to 5 mcg. Because of its slow rate of utilization and considerable body stores, vitamin B_{12} deficiency may take many months to appear.

The average diet supplies about 5 to 15 mcg/day of vitamin B_{12}. Vitamin B_{12} is bound to intrinsic factor during transit through the stomach; separation occurs in the terminal ileum in the presence of calcium, and vitamin B_{12} enters the mucosal cell for absorption. It is then transported by specific B_{12} binding proteins, transcobalamin I and II. Transcobalamin II is the delivery protein for vitamin B_{12}. In addition, approximately 1% to 3% of the total amount ingested is absorbed by simple diffusion, but this mechanism is significant only with large doses.

Pharmacokinetics: Absorption of vitamin B_{12} depends on the presence of sufficient intrinsic factor and calcium. In general, absorption of B_{12} is inadequate in malabsorptive states and in pernicious anemia (unless intrinsic factor is simultaneously administered).

Cyanocobalamin is rapidly absorbed from IM and SC injection sites; the plasma level peaks within 1 hour. Once absorbed, it is bound to plasma proteins, stored mainly in the liver and is slowly released when needed to carry out normal cellular metabolic functions. Within 48 hours after injection of 100 to 1000 mcg of vitamin B_{12}, 50% to 98% of the dose appears in the urine. The major portion is excreted within the first 8 hours. More rapid excretion occurs with IV administration; there is little opportunity for liver storage.

Hydroxocobalamin (vitamin B_{12_a}) is more highly protein bound and is retained in the body longer than cyanocobalamin. However, it has no advantage over cyanocobalamin. Administration of hydroxocobalamin has resulted in antibody formation to the hydroxocobalamin-transcobalamin II complex and thus cyanocobalamin may be preferred.

Indications:

Vitamin B_{12} deficiency due to malabsorption syndrome as seen in pernicious anemia; GI pathology, dysfunction or surgery; fish tapeworm infestation; malignancy of pancreas or bowel; gluten enteropathy, sprue; small bowel bacterial overgrowth; total or partial gastrectomy; accompanying folic acid deficiency.

Increased requirements associated with pregnancy, thyrotoxicosis, hemolytic anemia, hemorrhage, malignancy and hepatic and renal disease.

Vitamin B_{12} absorption test (Schilling test).

Unlabeled Use: Hydroxocobalamin has been used to prevent and to treat cyanide toxicity associated with sodium nitroprusside. It lowers red blood cell and plasma cyanide concentrations by combining with cyanide to form cyanocobalamin, which is nontoxic and excreted in the urine.

Contraindications:

Hypersensitivity to cobalt, vitamin B_{12} or any component of these medications.

Warnings:

Parenteral administration is preferred for pernicious anemia. Avoid the IV route.

An inadequate therapeutic response may be due to infection, uremia, bone marrow suppressant drugs (ie, chloramphenicol), concurrent iron or folic acid deficiency or misdiagnosis.

Vitamin B_{12} deficiency allowed to progress for more than 3 months may produce permanent degenerative lesions of the spinal cord.

Optic nerve atrophy: Patients with early Leber's disease (hereditary optic nerve atrophy) who have been treated with cyanocobalamin suffer severe and swift optic atrophy.

Hypokalemia, possibly fatal, could occur upon conversion of megaloblastic to normal erythropoiesis with B_{12} therapy as a result of increased erythrocyte potassium requirements.

"Gasping syndrome": Some of these products contain benzyl alcohol, which has been associated with a fatal "gasping syndrome" in premature infants.

(Warnings continued on following page)

Warnings (Cont.):

Usage in Pregnancy: (Category C – Parenteral). Adequate and well controlled studies have not been performed in pregnant women. However, B_{12} is an essential vitamin and needs are increased during pregnancy. Amounts of vitamin B_{12} recommended by the Food and Nutrition Board, National Academy of Science-National Research Council (4 mcg daily) should be consumed during pregnancy.

Usage in Lactation: Vitamin B_{12} is excreted in breast milk in concentrations that approximate the mother's vitamin B_{12} blood level. Amounts of B_{12} recommended by the Food and Nutrition Board, National Academy of Science-National Research Council (4 mcg daily) should be consumed during lactation.

Usage in Children: The Food and Nutrition Board, National Academy of Science-National Research Council recommends a daily intake of 0.5 to 3 mcg daily for children.

Precautions:

Test dose: Give an intradermal test dose in patients sensitive to the cobalamines.

Folate: Doses exceeding 10 mcg daily may produce hematologic response in patients with folate deficiency. Indiscriminate use may mask the true diagnosis of pernicious anemia.

Doses of folic acid greater than 0.1 mg/day may result in hematologic remission in patients with vitamin B_{12} deficiency. Neurologic manifestations will not be prevented with folic acid, and if not treated with vitamin B_{12}, irreversible damage will result.

Single deficiency (vitamin B_{12} alone) is rare. Expect multiple vitamin deficiency in any dietary deficiency.

Polycythemia vera: Vitamin B_{12} deficiency may suppress the signs of polycythemia vera. Treatment with vitamin B_{12} may unmask this condition.

Monitoring therapy: During treatment of severe megaloblastic anemia, monitor serum potassium levels closely for the first 48 hours and replace potassium if necessary. Obtain reticulocyte counts, hematocrit and vitamin B_{12}, iron and folic acid plasma levels prior to treatment and between the fifth and seventh days of therapy, and then frequently until the hematocrit is normal. If folate levels are low, also administer folic acid. Continue periodic hematologic evaluations throughout the patient's lifetime.

Vegetarian diets containing no animal products (including milk products or eggs) do not supply any vitamin B_{12}. Vegetarians should take oral vitamin B_{12} regularly.

Pernicious anemia patients have about 3 times the incidence of stomach carcinoma as the general population; perform appropriate tests for this condition when indicated.

Drug Interactions:

Neomycin, colchicine, para-aminosalicylic acid, timed-release potassium, or excessive **alcohol** intake (longer than 2 weeks) may cause malabsorption of vitamin B_{12}.

Chloramphenicol and other bone marrow suppressant drugs may cause a lack of therapeutic response to vitamin B_{12}, due to interference with erythrocyte maturation.

Cimetidine decreases digestion and release of food-bound B_{12} by decreasing gastric acid and pepsin release. The availability of B_{12} for combination with gastric intrinsic factor is reduced, impairing absorption.

Nitrous oxide: Moderately severe neuropathy has been reported in two patients with previously undiagnosed B_{12} deficiency 2 months after being anesthetized with nitrous oxide during abdominal surgery.

Drug/lab tests: **Methotrexate, pyrimethamine** and most **antibiotics** invalidate folic acid and vitamin B_{12} diagnostic microbiological blood assays.

Adverse Reactions:

The following reactions are associated with parenteral vitamin B_{12}:

Hypersensitivity: Anaphylactic shock and death.

Cardiovascular: Pulmonary edema; congestive heart failure early in treatment; peripheral vascular thrombosis.

Dermatological: Itching; transitory exanthema; urticaria.

Local: Pain at injection site.

Ophthalmic: Severe and swift optic nerve atrophy (see Warnings).

Miscellaneous: Feeling of swelling of the entire body; hypokalemia; mild transient diarrhea; polycythemia vera.

Patient Information:

Patients with pernicious anemia will require monthly injections of vitamin B_{12} for the rest of their lives. Failure to do so will result in return of the anemia and in development of incapacitating and irreversible damage to the nerves of the spinal cord.

A well balanced dietary intake is necessary; correct poor dietary habits.

Do not take folic acid instead of vitamin B_{12} because folic acid may prevent anemia, but allow progression of subacute combined degeneration.

(Continued on following page)

Complete prescribing information for these products begins on page 237

CYANOCOBALAMIN CRYSTALLINE

Administration and Dosage:

Addisonian pernicious anemia: Parenteral therapy is required for life; oral therapy is not dependable. Administer 100 mcg daily for 6 or 7 days by IM or deep SC injection. If there is clinical improvement and a reticulocyte response, give the same amount on alternate days for 7 doses, then every 3 to 4 days for another 2 to 3 weeks. By this time, hematologic values should have become normal. Follow this regimen with 100 mcg monthly for life. Administer folic acid concomitantly if needed.

Other patients with vitamin B_{12} deficiency: In seriously ill patients, administer both vitamin B_{12} and folic acid while awaiting laboratory results. It is not necessary to withhold therapy until the precise cause of B_{12} deficiency is established. Children may be given a total dosage of 1 to 5 mg over a period of 2 or more weeks in doses of 100 mcg; maintenance dosage is 30 to 50 mcg every 4 weeks. Closely observe serum potassium for the first 48 hours; administer potassium if necessary.

Oral – Up to 1000 mcg/day. Give patients with normal intestinal absorption a daily oral multivitamin preparation containing 15 mcg vitamin B_{12}. Oral vitamin B_{12} therapy is not usually recommended for vitamin B_{12} deficiency. The maximum amount of vitamin B_{12} that can be absorbed from a single oral dose is 2 to 3 mcg. The percent absorbed decreases with increasing doses.

IM or SC – 30 mcg daily for 5 to 10 days followed by 100 to 200 mcg monthly. If the patient is critically ill, has neurologic or infectious disease or hyperthyroidism, considerably higher doses may be indicated. However, the optimum obtainable neurologic response may be expected with a dosage of vitamin B_{12} sufficient to produce good hematologic response. Coadminister folic acid early in the treatment if necessary.

Schilling test: The flushing dose is 1000 mcg IM.

Storage: Protect parenterals from light. Avoid freezing.

	Product	Form	Package	C.I.*
otc	**Vitamin B_{12}** (Various)	**Tablets:** 500 mcg	In 100s, 250s and 1000s.	1+
otc	**Vitamin B_{12}** (Various)	**Tablets:** 1000 mcg	In 30s, 60s, 100s and 500s.	1+
Rx	**Vitamin B_{12}** (Various)	**Injection:** 30 mcg/ml	In 30 ml vials.	17+
Rx	**Vitamin B_{12}** (Various)	**Injection:** 100 mcg per ml	In 1, 10, 30 ml vials and 1 ml Tubex.	4+
Rx	**Crystamine** (Dunhall)		In 10 and 30 ml vials.[1]	24
Rx	**Rubramin PC** (Apothecon)		In 10 ml vials and 1 ml unimatic.[1]	71
Rx	**Vitamin B_{12}** (Various)	**Injection:** 1000 mcg per ml	In 1, 10 and 30 ml vials and 1 ml amps and 1 ml disp syringe.	1+
Rx	**Cobex** (Pasadena)		In 10 and 30 ml vials.	1
Rx	**Crystamine** (Dunhall)		In 10 and 30 ml vials.[1]	3
Rx	**Crysti-12** (Hauck)		In 10 and 30 ml vials.	2
Rx	**Cyanoject** (Mayrand)		In 10 and 30 ml vials.[1]	3
Rx	**Cyomin** (Forest)		In 30 ml vials.[1]	3
Rx	**Rubesol-1000** (Central)		In 10 and 30 ml vials.[1]	3
Rx	**Rubramin PC** (Apothecon)		In 1 and 10 ml vials and 1 ml unimatic.[1]	20
Rx	**Sytobex** (Parke-Davis)		In 10 ml vials.[2]	5

* Cost Index based on cost per 100 mcg.

[1] With benzyl alcohol.

[2] With methyl and propyl parabens.

Complete prescribing information for these products begins on page 237

HYDROXOCOBALAMIN, CRYSTALLINE (Vitamin B_{12a})

Administration and Dosage:

Administer IM only. The recommended dosage is 30 mcg/day for 5 to 10 days, followed by 100 to 200 mcg monthly. Children may be given a total of 1 to 5 mg over 2 or more weeks in doses of 100 mcg, then 30 to 50 mcg every 4 weeks for maintenance. Institute concurrent folic acid therapy early in the treatment if needed.

	Product		How Supplied	C.I.*
Rx	**Hydroxocobalamin** (Various)	**Injection:** 1000 mcg/ml	In 10 and 30 ml vials.	1+
Rx	**Alphamin** (Vortech)		In 10 ml vials.[1]	7
Rx	**AlphaRedisol** (MSD)		In 10 ml vials.[1]	18
Rx	**Codroxomin** (Forest)		In 10 ml vials.[1]	9
Rx	**Hybalamin** (Mallard)		In 10 ml vials.	7
Rx	**Hydrobexan** (Keene)		In 10 ml vials.[1]	6
Rx	**Hydro-Crysti 12** (Hauck)		In 10 ml vials.	10
Rx	**Hydroxo-12** (Ortega)		In 10 ml vials.[1]	6
Rx	**LA-12** (Hyrex)		In 10 ml vials.[1]	7

LIVER PREPARATIONS

Crude liver extracts are a source of vitamin B_{12} (extrinsic factor). Purified crystalline cyanocobalamin is the preferred source of B_{12} in deficiency states.

Refer to cyanocobalamin monograph (p.237) for complete prescribing information.

ORAL LIVER PREPARATIONS

	Product		How Supplied	C.I.*
Rx	**Biopar Forte** (USV)	**Tablets:** 0.5 oral unit vitamin B_{12} with intrinsic factor concentrate and 25 mcg cobalamin *Dose:* 1 to 3 tablets daily.	In 30s.	231

PARENTERAL LIVER PREPARATIONS

Inject IM only.

	Product		How Supplied	C.I.*
Rx	**Liver, Crude** (Various)	**Injection:** 2 mcg B_{12} per ml	In 10 & 30 ml vials.	8+
Rx	**Liver, Refined** (Various)	**Injection:** 10 mcg B_{12} per ml	In 10 & 30 ml vials.	13+
Rx	**Liver, Refined** (Various)	**Injection:** 20 mcg B_{12} per ml	In 10 & 30 ml vials.	9+

PARENTERAL LIVER COMBINATIONS

Content given per ml.

	Product & Distributor	Liver Inj. B_{12} Equiv. (mcg)	Cryst. B_{12} (mcg)	FA (mg)	How Supplied	C.I.*
Rx	**Crysti-Liver** (Hauck)	10	100	0.4	In 10 ml vials.[2]	95
Rx	**Folabee** (Vortech)				In 10 ml vials.[2]	99
Rx	**Hepfomin-R** (Keene)				In 10 ml vials.[2]	48
Rx	**Hyliver Plus** (Hyrex)				In 10 ml vials.[2]	119
Rx	**Lifoject** (Mayrand)				In 10 ml vials.[2]	106
Rx	**Lifolbex** (Central)				In 10 ml vials.[2]	114
Rx	**Lifomin-R** (Kay Pharm.)				In 10 ml vials.[2]	50
Rx	**Liver Combo No. 5** (Rugby)				In 10 ml vials.[2]	37
Rx	**Livifol** (Dunhall)				In 10 ml vials.[2]	83
Rx	**Livroben** (Forest)				In 10 ml vials.[2]	110
Rx	**Vifex** (Mallard)				In 10 ml vials.[2]	78

* Cost Index based on cost per tablet, ml or 100 mcg.

[1] With methyl and propyl parabens.

[2] With phenol.

Actions:

Pharmacology: Vitamin K promotes the hepatic synthesis of active prothrombin (factor II), proconvertin (factor VII), plasma thromboplastin component (factor IX) and Stuart factor (factor X). The mechanism by which vitamin K promotes formation of these clotting factors is not known.

Phytonadione (vitamin K_1) and menadione (vitamin K_3) are lipid soluble synthetic analogs of vitamin K. Menadiol sodium diphosphate (vitamin K_4) is a water soluble derivative which is converted to menadione in vivo. Phytonadione possesses essentially the same type and degree of activity as the naturally occurring vitamin K. Phytonadione has a more rapid and prolonged effect than menadione and menadiol sodium diphosphate, and is generally more effective, particularly in the treatment of oral anticoagulant-induced hypoprothrombinemia. Vitamin K_4 is approximately one-half as potent as menadione.

In the prophylaxis and treatment of hemorrhagic disease of the newborn, phytonadione has demonstrated a greater margin of safety than menadiol sodium diphosphate.

Pharmacokinetics: Phytonadione is absorbed from the GI tract via intestinal lymphatics only in the presence of bile salts. Menadiol sodium diphosphate enters the bloodstream directly, and is absorbed in the absence of bile. Although initially concentrated in the liver, vitamin K is rapidly metabolized and very little tissue accumulation occurs.

Parenteral phytonadione and menadiol sodium diphosphate are generally detectable within 1-2 hours. Phytonadione usually controls hemorrhage within 3 to 6 hours. A normal prothrombin level may be obtained in 12-14 hours. Oral phytonadione exerts its effect in 6-10 hours. Response to parenteral vitamin K_4 may require 8 to 24 hours.

Minimum daily requirements for vitamin K have not been officially established, but have been estimated to be 10 to 20 mcg for infants, 15 to 100 mcg for children and adolescents and 70 to 140 mcg for adults. Usually, dietary vitamin K will satisfy these requirements, except during the first 5 to 8 days of the neonatal period.

Indications:

Coagulation disorders due to faulty formation of factors II, VII, IX and X when caused by vitamin K deficiency or interference with vitamin K activity.

Oral: Anticoagulant-induced prothrombin deficiency (see Warnings); hypoprothrombinemia secondary to salicylates or antibacterial therapy; hypoprothrombinemia secondary to obstructive jaundice and biliary fistulas, but only if bile salts are administered concomitantly with phytonadione.

Parenteral: Hypoprothrombinemia secondary to conditions limiting absorption or synthesis of vitamin K. Obstructive jaundice, biliary fistula, sprue, ulcerative colitis, celiac disease, intestinal resection, cystic fibrosis of the pancreas, regional enteritis, drug-induced hypoprothrombinemias due to interference with vitamin K metabolism (eg, antibiotics and salicylates).

Phytonadione administered parenterally is also indicated for the prophylaxis and therapy of hemorrhagic disease of the newborn.

Contraindications:

Hypersensitivity to any component.

Do not administer **menadiol sodium diphosphate** to women during the last few weeks of pregnancy or during labor as a prophylactic measure against physiologic hypoprothrombinemia or hemorrhagic disease of the newborn. Do not administer to infants.

Warnings:

Usage in impaired hepatic function: Hypoprothrombinemia due to hepatocellular damage is not corrected by administration of vitamin K. Repeated large doses of vitamin K are not warranted in liver disease if the initial response is unsatisfactory (Koller test). Failure to respond to vitamin K may indicate a coagulation defect or a condition unresponsive to vitamin K. In hepatic disease, large doses may further depress liver function.

Paradoxically, giving excessive doses of Vitamin K or its analogs in an attempt to correct hypoprothrombinemia associated with severe hepatitis or cirrhosis may actually result in further depression of the prothrombin concentration.

Oral anticoagulant-induced hypoprothrombinemia: For the treatment of oral anticoagulant-induced hypoprothrombinemia, phytonadione is preferred. Menadiol sodium diphosphate is ineffective. *Vitamin K will not counteract the anticoagulant action of heparin.*

Phytonadione promotes synthesis of prothrombin by the liver, but does not directly counteract the effects of the oral anticoagulants. Immediate coagulant effect should not be expected. It takes a minimum of 1 to 2 hours for a measurable improvement in the prothrombin time (PT). The prothrombin test is sensitive to the levels of factors II, VII and X. Fresh plasma or blood transfusions may be required for severe blood loss.

With phytonadione use and anticoagulant therapy indicated, the patient is faced with the same clotting hazards prior to starting anticoagulant therapy. Phytonadione is not a clotting agent, but overzealous therapy may restore original thromboembolic phenomena conditions. Keep dosage as low as possible and check PT regularly.

(Warnings continued on following page)

Warnings (Cont.):

Hemorrhagic disease of the newborn: In the prophylaxis and treatment of hemorrhagic disease of the newborn, menadiol sodium diphosphate is not as safe as phytonadione.

In infants (particularly prematures), excessive doses of vitamin K analogs may cause increased bilirubinemia during the first few days of life. Severe hemolytic anemia, hemoglobinuria, kernicterus, brain damage and death in neonates may also occur. Use of these drugs by the mother during the last few weeks of pregnancy may induce these toxic reactions in the neonate; therefore, do not give menadione derivatives to pregnant women or to newborn infants.

Usage in Pregnancy: Category C. Vitamin K crosses the placenta. There is no adequate information on whether this drug may affect fertility in humans or have teratogenic or other adverse effects on the fetus. Give to a pregnant woman only if clearly needed.

Menadione has caused retardation of skeletal ossification and an increase in fetal resorptions in rats.

Usage in Lactation: Vitamin K is excreted in breast milk. Consider this if the drug must be used in a nursing mother.

Precautions:

Benzyl alcohol contained in some products has been associated with toxicity in newborns. Specific products containing benzyl alcohol are identified in the product listings.

Sulfite Sensitivity: Sulfites may cause allergic-type reactions (eg, hives, itching, wheezing, anaphylaxis) in certain susceptible persons. Although the overall prevalence of sulfite sensitivity in the general population is probably low, it is seen more frequently in asthmatics or in atopic nonasthmatic persons. Specific products containing sulfites are identified in the product listings.

Drug Interactions:

Coumarin and **indandione:** Anticoagulant effects are antagonized by vitamin K. Temporary resistance to oral anticoagulants may result, especially when larger doses are used. If relatively large doses have been employed, it may be necessary when reinstituting anticoagulant therapy to use larger doses of the prothrombin-depressing anticoagulant, or to use one with a different mechanism, such as heparin.

Mineral oil or **cholestyramine** may decrease absorption of the oil soluble vitamins, phytonadione and menadione, with concurrent oral administration.

Drug/Lab Tests: In adults, prolongation of PT has been reported after maximum doses of vitamin K. Menadione has interfered with the modified Reedy, Jenkins, Thorn procedure for determining urinary 17-hydroxycorticosteroids, producing falsely elevated levels.

Adverse Reactions:

Allergic reactions: Rash and urticaria; anaphylactoid reactions may also occur.

Parenteral administration: Rarely, pain, swelling and tenderness at the injection site; after repeated injections, reactions resembling erythema perstans. Delayed cutaneous reactions (pruritic erythematous placques) at the site of IM injection.

Transient "flushing sensations" and "peculiar" sensations of taste; rarely, dizziness, rapid and weak pulse, profuse sweating, brief hypotension, dyspnea and cyanosis.

Hyperbilirubinemia has been reported in newborns, particularly premature infants. This may result in kernicterus which can lead to brain damage or death. Immaturity is an important factor in the development of toxic reactions to vitamin K analogs, as full-term and larger premature infants demonstrate greater tolerance. These effects are more frequent with soluble menadione derivatives.

Menadiol sodium diphosphate can induce erythrocyte hemolysis in persons with G-6-PD deficiency.

Phytonadione: Deaths have occurred after IV administration (see Warning Box, p.243).

MENADIOL SODIUM DIPHOSPHATE (K_4)

Administration and Dosage:

Oral: For hypoprothrombinemia secondary to obstructive jaundice and biliary fistulas give 5 mg daily. For hypoprothrombinemia secondary to the administration of antibacterials or salicylates give 5 to 10 mg daily.

Parenteral: Inject SC, IM or IV. The response after IV administration may be more prompt, but more sustained action follows IM or SC use.

Adults: 5 to 15 mg once or twice daily. *Children:* 5 to 10 mg once or twice daily. **C.I.***

Rx	**Synkayvite** (Roche)	**Tablets:** 5 mg	(#Roche 37 Synkayvite 5). White. In 100s.	68
		Injection: 5 mg per ml	In 1 ml amps.[1]	1156
		10 mg per ml	In 1 ml amps.[1]	844
		37.5 mg per ml	In 2 ml amps.[1]	311

* Cost Index based on cost per 5 mg. # Product identification code.

[1] With phenol and sodium metabisulfite.

Complete prescribing information for these products begins on page 241

PHYTONADIONE (K_1, Phylloquinone, Methylphytyl Napthoquinone)

Warning:

IV use: Severe reactions, including fatalities, have occurred during and immediately after IV injection, even with precautions to dilute the injection and to avoid rapid infusion. These severe reactions resemble hypersensitivity or anaphylaxis, including shock and cardiac or respiratory arrest. Some patients exhibit these severe reactions on receiving vitamin K for the first time. Therefore, restrict the IV route to those situations where other routes are not feasible and the serious risk involved is justified.

Administration and Dosage:

If possible, discontinue or reduce the dosage of drugs interfering with coagulation mechanisms (eg, salicylates, antibiotics) as an alternative to phytonadione.

Inject SC or IM when possible. In older children and adults, inject IM in the upper outer quadrant of the buttocks. In infants and young children, the anterolateral aspect of the thigh or the deltoid region is preferred. When IV administration is unavoidable, inject very slowly, not exceeding 1 mg per minute.

Anticoagulant-induced prothrombin deficiency in adults: 2.5 to 10 mg or up to 25 mg (rarely, 50 mg) initially. Determine subsequent doses by prothrombin time (PT) response or clinical condition. If in 6 to 8 hours after parenteral administration (or 12 to 48 hours after oral administration), the PT has not been shortened satisfactorily, repeat dose. If shock or excessive blood loss occurs, use whole blood or component therapy.

Hemorrhagic disease of the newborn:

Prophylaxis – Single IM dose of 0.5 to 1 mg within 1 hour after birth; 1 to 5 mg may be given to the mother 12 to 24 hours before delivery.

Oral doses of 2 mg have been shown to be adequate for prophylaxis.

Treatment – 1 mg SC or IM. Higher doses may be necessary if the mother has been receiving oral anticoagulants. Empiric administration of vitamin K_1 should not replace proper laboratory evaluation. A prompt response (shortening of the PT in 2 to 4 hours) is usually diagnostic of hemorrhagic disease of the newborn; failure to respond indicates another diagnosis or coagulation disorder. Give whole blood or component therapy if bleeding is excessive. This therapy, however, does not correct the underlying disorder; administer phytonadione concurrently.

Hypoprothrombinemia due to other causes in adults: 2.5 to 25 mg (rarely, up to 50 mg); amount and route of administration depends on severity of condition and response obtained. Avoid oral route when clinical disorder would prevent proper absorption. Give bile salts with tablets when endogenous supply of bile to GI tract is deficient.

Storage: Protect from light at all times.

				C.I.*
Rx	**Mephyton** (MSD)	**Tablets:** 5 mg	(MSD 43). Yellow, scored. In 100s.	439
Rx	**AquaMEPHYTON** (MSD)	**Injection (aqueous colloidal solution):**		
		2 mg per ml	In 0.5 ml amps.[1]	4726
		10 mg per ml	In 1 ml amps[1] and 2.5 and 5 ml vials.[1]	1927
Rx	**Konakion** (Roche)	**Injection (aqueous dispersion). FOR IM USE ONLY:**		
		2 mg per ml	In 0.5 ml amps.[2]	5478
		10 mg per ml	In 1 ml amps.[3]	2263

* Cost Index based on cost per 5 mg.

[1] With polyoxyethylated fatty acid derivative, dextrose and benzyl alcohol.

[2] With polysorbate 80, phenol, propylene glycol, sodium acetate and glacial acetic acid.

[3] With polysorbate 80, propylene glycol, sodium acetate and glacial acetic acid.

EPOETIN ALFA (Erythropoietin; EPO)

Actions:

Erythropoietin is a glycoprotein which stimulates red blood cell production. It is produced in the kidney and stimulates the division and differentiation of erythroid progenitors in the bone marrow. Epoetin alfa, a 165 amino acid glycoprotein manufactured by recombinant DNA technology, has the same biological effects as endogenous erythropoietin. It has a molecular weight of 30,400 daltons and is produced by mammalian cells into which the human erythropoietin gene has been introduced. The product contains the identical amino acid sequence of natural erythropoietin.

Pharmacology: Endogenous production of erythropoietin is regulated by the level of tissue oxygenation. Hypoxia and anemia generally increase the production of erythropoietin, which in turn stimulates erythropoiesis. In normal subjects, plasma erythropoietin levels range from 0.01 to 0.03 U/ml and increase up to 100- to 1000-fold during hypoxia or anemia. In patients with chronic renal failure (CRF), erythropoietin production is impaired; this deficiency is the primary cause of their anemia.

Epoetin alfa stimulates erythropoiesis in anemic patients on dialysis and those who do not require regular dialysis. The first evidence of a response to epoetin alfa administration is an increase in the reticulocyte count within 10 days, followed by increases in the red cell count, hemoglobin and hematocrit, usually within 2 to 6 weeks. Once the hematocrit reaches the target range (30% to 33%), that level can be sustained by epoetin alfa therapy in the absence of iron deficiency and concurrent illnesses.

The rate of hematocrit increase varies between patients and is dependent upon the dose of epoetin alfa within a therapeutic range of approximately 50 to 300 U/kg 3 times weekly; a greater biologic response is not observed at doses exceeding 300 U/kg 3 times weekly. Other factors affecting the rate and extent of response include availability of iron stores, baseline hematocrit and concurrent medical problems. Responsiveness in HIV-infected patients is dependent on the endogenous serum erythropoietin level prior to treatment. Patients with levels ≤ 500 mU/ml receiving zidovudine (AZT) ≤ 4200 mg/week may respond; patients with levels > 500 mU/ml do not appear to respond. In four trials, 60% to 80% of patients had levels ≤ 500 mU/ml. Response is manifested by reduced transfusion requirements and increased hematocrit.

Pharmacokinetics: Epoetin alfa IV is eliminated via first-order kinetics with a circulating half-life of 4 to 13 hours in patients with CRF. Within the therapeutic dosage range, detectable levels of plasma erythropoietin are maintained for at least 24 hours. After SC administration of epoetin alfa to patients with CRF, peak serum levels are achieved within 5 to 24 hours after administration and decline slowly thereafter. There is no apparent difference in half-life between patients not on dialysis (serum creatinine > 3) and patients maintained on dialysis. The half-life in healthy volunteers is ≈ 20% shorter than in CRF patients.

Clinical trials: The rate of increase in hematocrit is dependent upon the dose of epoetin alfa administered and individual patient variation.

Hematocrit Increase Based on Epoetin Alfa Dose		
	Hematocrit increase	
Starting dose (3 times weekly, IV)	Hematocrit points/ day	Hematocrit points/ 2 weeks
50 U/kg	0.11	1.5
100 U/kg	0.18	2.5
150 U/kg	0.25	3.5

Over this dosage range, approximately 95% of all patients responded with a clinically significant increase in hematocrit, and by the end of approximately 2 months of therapy, virtually all patients were transfusion-independent. Once the target hematocrit was achieved, the maintenance dose was individualized.

Dialysis patients – Thirteen clinical studies were conducted involving IV administration to a total of 1010 anemic patients on dialysis for 986 patient-years of epoetin alfa therapy. In the three largest trials, the median dose necessary to maintain the hematocrit between 30% to 36% was approximately 75 U/kg 3 times weekly. In the US multicenter Phase III study, approximately 65% of the patients required doses of 100 U/kg 3 times weekly, or less, to maintain their hematocrit at approximately 35%. Almost 10% of patients required ≤ 25 U/kg 3 times weekly, and approximately 10% required a dose of > 200 U/kg 3 times weekly to maintain their hematocrit at this level.

(Actions continued on following page)

EPOETIN ALFA (Erythropoietin; EPO) (Cont.)

Actions (Cont.):

Clinical trials (Cont.):

Patients with CRF not requiring dialysis – Four clinical trials were conducted in 181 epoetin alfa-treated patients for approximately 67 patient-years of experience. These patients responded to therapy in a manner similar to that of patients on dialysis. These patients demonstrated a dose-dependent and sustained increase in hematocrit when epoetin alfa was administered either IV or SC. Doses of 75 to 150 U/kg *per week* maintain hematocrits of 36% to 38% for up to 6 months.

AZT-treated HIV-infected patients – In four placebo controlled trials enrolling 297 anemic (hematocrit < 30%) HIV-infected (AIDS) patients receiving concomitant therapy with AZT, epoetin alfa reduced the mean cumulative number of units of blood transfused per patient by ≈ 40% in patients with endogenous erythropoietin levels ≤ 500 mU/ml (n = 89) vs placebo. Among those patients who required transfusions at baseline, 43% epoetin alfa vs 18% placebo were transfusion-independent during the second and third months of therapy. Epoetin alfa therapy also resulted in significant increases in hematocrit compared to placebo. There was a statistically significant reduction in transfusion requirements in epoetin alfa-treated patients whose mean weekly AZT dose was ≤ 4200 mg/week. In patients whose prestudy endogenous serum erythropoietin levels were > 500 mU/ml, epoetin alfa therapy did not reduce transfusion requirements or increase hematocrit.

Indications:

Treatment of anemia associated with CRF, including patients on dialysis (end-stage renal disease) and patients not on dialysis, to elevate or maintain the red blood cell level (as manifested by the hematocrit or hemoglobin determinations) and to decrease the need for transfusions.

Not intended for patients who require immediate correction of severe anemia. Epoetin alfa may obviate the need for maintenance transfusions but is not a substitute for emergency transfusion.

Treatment of anemia related to therapy with AZT in HIV-infected patients: To elevate or maintain the red blood cell level (as manifested by the hematocrit or hemoglobin determinations) and to decrease the need for transfusions in these patients when the endogenous erythropoietin level is ≤ 500 mU/ml and the dose of AZT is ≤ 4200 mg/week.

Not indicated for the treatment of anemia in HIV-infected patients due to other factors such as iron or folate deficiencies, hemolysis or GI bleeding which should be managed appropriately.

Unlabeled uses: Epoetin alfa in doses of 150 U/kg SC 3 times per week for 12 weeks is effective in reversing anemia in cancer patients receiving chemotherapy. Hematocrits in these patients rose significantly compared to placebo and side effects were minimal. The use of epoetin alfa may be an effective alternative to transfusion in these patients.

Epoetin alfa is effective in increasing the procurement of autologous blood in patients about to undergo elective surgery. In one study, patients received 600 U/kg IV twice a week for 21 days, 25 to 35 days before surgery. The volume of red blood cells donated was 41% higher compared to placebo. Increasing the amount of autologous blood preoperatively decreases the need for homologous blood transfusion.

Contraindications:

Uncontrolled hypertension; hypersensitivity to mammalian cell-derived products or to human albumin.

Warnings:

Hypertension: Up to 80% of patients with CRF have a history of hypertension. Do not treat patients with uncontrolled hypertension; monitor blood pressure adequately before initiation of therapy. Blood pressure may rise during therapy, often during the early phase of treatment when the hematocrit is increasing, whether on dialysis or not.

For patients who respond with a rapid increase in hematocrit (eg, > 4 points in any 2 week period), reduce the dose because of the possible association of excessive rate of rise of hematocrit with an exacerbation of hypertension.

To prevent hypertension and its sequelae, carefully monitor and aggressively control blood pressure. Hypertensive encephalopathy has been observed in CRF patients treated with epoetin alfa. When hematocrit is increasing, approximately 25% of patients on dialysis may require initiation of, or increases in, antihypertensive therapy and dietary restrictions. If blood pressure is difficult to control, reduce the dose. If necessary, epoetin alfa may be withheld until blood pressure control is reestablished.

In contrast to CRF patients, epoetin alfa has not been linked to exacerbation of hypertension, seizures and thrombotic events in HIV-infected patients. However, withhold epoetin alfa in these patients if pre-existing hypertension is uncontrolled and do not start until blood pressure is controlled.

(Warnings continued on following page)

EPOETIN ALFA (Erythropoietin; EPO) (Cont.)

Warnings (Cont.):

Seizures: The relationship to seizures is uncertain. The baseline incidence of seizures in the untreated dialysis population appears to be 5% to 10% per patient-year. There have been 47 seizures in 1010 patients on dialysis treated with epoetin alfa with an exposure of 986 patient-years for a rate of approximately 0.048 events per patient-year. In patients on dialysis, there was a higher incidence of seizures during the first 90 days of therapy (occurring in approximately 2.5% of patients). Decrease the dose of epoetin alfa if the hematocrit increase exceeds 4 points in any 2 week period. Monitor the presence of premonitory neurologic symptoms closely. Patients should avoid potentially hazardous activities such as driving or operating heavy machinery during this period.

Thrombotic events: During hemodialysis, patients treated with epoetin alfa may require increased anticoagulation with heparin to prevent clotting of the artificial kidney. Clotting of the vascular access (A-V shunt) has occurred at an annualized rate of about 0.25 events per patient-year on epoetin alfa therapy.

Overall, for patients with CRF (whether on dialysis or not), other thrombotic events (eg, myocardial infarction, cerebrovascular accident, transient ischemic attack) have occurred at an annualized rate of < 0.04 events per patient-year of epoetin alfa. Monitor patients with pre-existing vascular disease closely.

Allergic reactions: Skin rashes and urticaria are rare, mild and transient. There is no evidence of antibody development to erythropoietin, including those receiving IV epoetin alfa for > 2 years. Nevertheless, if an anaphylactoid reaction occurs, immediately discontinue the drug and initiate appropriate therapy. Refer to Management of Acute Hypersensitivity Reactions.

Pregnancy: Category C. Adverse effects occurred in rats when given in doses 5 times the human dose. There are no adequate and well controlled studies in pregnant women. Use in pregnancy only if the potential benefit justifies the potential risk to the fetus.

In some female patients, menses have resumed following epoetin alfa therapy; discuss the possibility of potential pregnancy and evaluate the need for contraception.

Lactation: It is not known whether epoetin alfa is excreted in breast milk. Exercise caution when administering to a nursing woman.

Children: Safety and efficacy have not been established.

Precautions:

Hematology: The elevated bleeding time characteristic of CRF decreases toward normal after correction of anemia in epoetin alfa-treated patients. Reduction of bleeding time also occurs after correction of anemia by transfusion.

Allow sufficient time to determine a patient's responsiveness before adjusting the dose. Because of the time required for erythropoiesis and the red cell half-life, an interval of 2 to 6 weeks may occur between the time of a dose adjustment (initiation, increase, decrease or discontinuation) and a significant change in hematocrit.

Porphyria exacerbation has been observed rarely in epoetin alfa-treated patients with CRF. However, epoetin alfa has not caused urinary excretion of porphyrin metabolites in healthy volunteers, even in the presence of a rapid erythropoietic response. Nevertheless, use with caution in patients with known porphyria.

Bone marrow fibrosis is a complication of CRF and may be related to secondary hyperparathyroidism or unknown factors. The incidence of bone marrow fibrosis was not increased in a study of patients on dialysis who were treated with epoetin alfa for 12 to 19 months, compared to controls.

Delayed or diminished response: If the patient fails to respond or to maintain a response, consider and evaluate the following etiologies.

1) Functional iron deficiency may develop with normal ferritin levels but low transferrin saturation (< 20%), presumably due to the inability to mobilize iron stores rapidly enough to support increased erythropoiesis. Virtually all patients will eventually require supplemental iron therapy.
2) Underlying infectious, inflammatory or malignant processes.
3) Occult blood loss.
4) Underlying hematologic diseases (eg, thalessemia, refractory anemia or other myelodysplastic disorders).
5) Vitamin deficiencies: Folic acid or vitamin B_{12}.
6) Hemolysis.
7) Aluminum intoxication.
8) Osteitis fibrosa cystica.
9) Increase in AZT dosage.

(Precautions continued on following page)

EPOETIN ALFA (Erythropoietin; EPO) (Cont.)

Precautions (Cont.):

Laboratory monitoring: Patients with CRF not requiring dialysis – Monitor blood pressure and hematocrit no less frequently than for patients maintained on dialysis. Closely monitor renal function and fluid and electrolyte balance, as an improved sense of well-being may obscure the need to initiate dialysis in some patients.

Determine the hematocrit twice a week until it has stabilized in the target range and the maintenance dose has been established. After any dose adjustment, determine the hematocrit twice weekly for at least 2 to 6 weeks until the hematocrit has stabilized; then monitor at regular intervals.

Perform complete blood count with differential and platelet counts regularly. Modest increases have occurred in platelets and white blood cell counts, but values remained within normal ranges.

Monitor serum chemistry values (including blood urea nitrogen [BUN], uric acid, creatinine, phosphorus and potassium) regularly. In patients on dialysis, modest increases occurred in BUN, creatinine, phosphorus and potassium. In some patients, modest increases in serum uric acid and phosphorus were observed. The values remained within the ranges normally seen in patients with CRF.

AZT-treated, HIV-infected patients – Measure hematocrit once a week until hematocrit is stabilized; measure periodically thereafter.

Iron evaluation: Prior to and during therapy, evaluate the patient's iron stores, including transferrin saturation (serum iron divided by iron binding capacity) and serum ferritin. Transferrin saturation should be at least 20%, and ferritin should be at least 100 ng/ml. Supplemental iron may be required to increase and maintain transferrin saturation that will support epoetin alfa-stimulated erythropoiesis.

Diet: As the hematocrit increases and patients experience an improved sense of well-being, reinforce the importance of compliance with dietary guidelines and frequency of dialysis.

Hyperkalemia is not uncommon in patients with CRF. In patients on dialysis, hyperkalemia has occurred at an annualized rate of approximately 0.11 episodes per patient-year of epoetin alfa therapy, often in association with poor compliance to medication, dietary guidelines and frequency of dialysis.

Dialysis management: Therapy with epoetin alfa results in an increase in hematocrit and a decrease in plasma volume that could affect dialysis efficiency. This has not adversely affected dialyzer function or the efficiency of high-flux hemodialysis.

Renal function: In short-term trials (< 1 year) in patients with CRF not on dialysis, changes in creatinine and creatinine clearance were not significantly different in epoetin alfa-treated patients, compared with placebo-treated patients.

Adverse Reactions:

CRF patients: Epoetin alfa is generally well tolerated. The following adverse reactions are frequent sequelae of CRF and are not necessarily due to epoetin alfa therapy:

Epoetin Alfa Adverse Reactions in CRF Patients

Adverse reaction	Epoetin alfa (n = 200)	Placebo (n = 135)
Hypertension	24%	19%
Headache	16%	12%
Arthralgias	11%	6%
Nausea	11%	9%
Edema[1]	9%	10%
Fatigue[1]	9%	14%
Diarrhea	9%	6%
Vomiting	8%	5%
Chest pain[1]	7%	9%
Skin reaction[1] (administration site)	7%	12%
Asthenia[1]	7%	12%
Dizziness[1]	7%	13%
Clotted access	7%	2%
Seizure	1.1%	1.1%
CVA/TIA[1]	0.4%	0.6%
Myocardial infarction[1]	0.4%	1.1%

[1] Incidence of reaction more frequent with placebo.

(Adverse Reactions continued on following page)

EPOETIN ALFA (Erythropoietin; EPO) (Cont.)

Adverse Reactions (Cont.):

CRF patients (Cont.):

Most common – Incidence (number of events per patient-year) in patients on dialysis (> 567 patients): Hypertension (0.75); headache (0.4); tachycardia (0.31); nausea/vomiting (0.26); clotted vascular access (0.25); shortness of breath (0.14); hyperkalemia (0.11); diarrhea (0.11).

Events that occurred within hours of administration of epoetin alfa were rare, mild and transient, and included flu-like symptoms (eg, arthralgias and myalgias).

Allergic reactions – Skin rashes and urticaria are rare, mild and transient. If an anaphylactoid reaction occurs, immediately discontinue the drug and initiate appropriate therapy. See Warnings.

Seizures – There have been 47 seizures in 1010 patients on dialysis treated with epoetin alfa with an exposure of 986 patient-years for a rate of approximately 0.048 events per patient-year. However, there appeared to be a higher rate of seizures during the first 90 days of therapy (occurring in approximately 2.5% of patients). See Warnings.

Hypertension – During the early phase of treatment when hematocrit is increasing, approximately 25% of patients on dialysis may require initiation or increases in antihypertensive therapy. Hypertensive encephalopathy and seizures have been observed. See Warnings.

AZT-treated HIV-infected patients: Adverse experiences were consistent with the progression of HIV infection.

Epoetin Alfa Adverse Reactions in AZT-Treated Patients

Adverse reaction	Epoetin alfa (n = 144)	Placebo (n = 153)
Pyrexia	38%	29%
Fatigue[1]	25%	31%
Headache	19%	14%
Cough	18%	14%
Diarrhea[1]	16%	18%
Rash	16%	8%
Congestion, respiratory	15%	10%
Nausea	15%	12%
Shortness of breath	14%	13%
Asthenia[1]	11%	14%
Skin reaction (injection site)	10%	7%
Dizziness[1]	9%	10%

[1] Incidence of reaction more frequent with placebo.

Allergic reactions – Two AZT-treated, HIV-infected patients had urticarial reactions within 48 hours of their first exposure to medication. One was treated with epoetin alfa and one was treated with placebo. Both patients had positive immediate skin tests against their medication with a negative saline control. The basis for this apparent preexisting hypersensitivity to components of the formulation is unknown, but may be related to HIV-induced immunosuppression or prior exposure to blood products.

Seizures – In double-blind and open label trials, 10 patients experienced seizures. In general, these seizures appear to be related to underlying pathology such as meningitis or cerebral neoplasms, not epoetin alfa therapy.

Overdosage:

The maximum amount that can be safely administered in single or multiple doses has not been determined. Doses of up to 1500 U/kg 3 times weekly for 3 to 4 weeks have been given without any direct toxic effects.

Epoetin alfa can cause polycythemia if the hematocrit is not carefully monitored and the dose appropriately adjusted. If the target range is exceeded, epoetin alfa may be temporarily withheld until the hematocrit returns to the target range; therapy may then be resumed using a lower dose (see Administration and Dosage). If polycythemia is of concern, phlebotomy may be indicated to decrease the hematocrit to within acceptable ranges.

(Continued on following page)

EPOETIN ALFA (Erythropoietin; EPO) (Cont.)

Administration and Dosage:

CRF patients:

Epoetin Alfa: General Therapeutic Guidelines in CRF Patients	
Starting dose	50 to 100 U/kg 3 times weekly IV: Dialysis patients. IV or SC: Non-dialysis CRF patients.
Reduce dose when:	1) Target range is reached, or 2) Hematocrit increases > 4 points in any 2 week period.
Increase dose if:	Hematocrit does not increase by 5 to 6 points after 8 weeks of therapy, and hematocrit is below target range.
Maintenance dose	Individualize. General dosage change: 25 U/kg (3 times weekly)
Target hematocrit range	30% to 33% (maximum, 36%)

In patients on dialysis, epoetin alfa usually has been administered as an IV bolus 3 times weekly. While the administration is independent of the dialysis procedure, it may be administered into the venous line at the end of the dialysis procedure to obviate the need for additional venous access. In patients with CRF not on dialysis, epoetin alfa may be given either as an IV or SC injection.

When the hematocrit reaches 30% to 33%, decrease the dosage by approximately 25 U/kg 3 times weekly to avoid exceeding the target range. Once the hematocrit is within the target range, individualize the maintenance dose.

At any time, if the hematocrit increases by more than 4 points in a 2 week period, immediately decrease the dose. After the dose reduction, monitor the hematocrit twice weekly for 2 to 6 weeks and make further dose adjustments.

As the hematocrit approaches or exceeds 36%, temporarily withhold epoetin alfa until the hematocrit decreases to the target range of 30% to 33%; reduce the dose by approximately 25 U/kg 3 times weekly upon reinitiation of therapy.

If a hematocrit increase of 5 to 6 points is not achieved after an 8 week period and iron stores are adequate (see Precautions, Delayed or diminished response), the dose may be increased in increments of 25 U/kg 3 times weekly. Further increases of 25 U/kg 3 times weekly may be made at 4 to 6 week intervals until the desired response is attained.

Maintenance – Individualize dosage.

Target hematocrit range: 30% to 33%. As the hematocrit approaches or exceeds 36%, temporarily withhold until the hematocrit is ≤ 33%. To reinitiate therapy, reduce the dose by approximately 25 U/kg 3 times weekly or omit doses and allow 2 to 6 weeks for stabilization of response.

Dialysis patients: Median dose is 75 U/kg 3 times weekly (range, 12.5 to 525 U/kg). See Actions for more discussion.

Nondialysis CRF patients: Usual dose is 75 to 150 U/kg *per week*. See Actions for more discussion.

Delayed or diminished response – Over 95% of patients with CRF responded with clinically significant increases in hematocrit, and virtually all patients were transfusion-independent within approximately 2 months of initiation of therapy.

If a patient fails to respond or maintain a response, consider other etiologies and evaluate as clinically indicated. See Precautions section for discussion of delayed or diminished response.

(Administration and Dosage continued on following page)

EPOETIN ALFA (Erythropoietin; EPO) (Cont.)

Administration and Dosage (Cont.):

AZT-treated, HIV-infected patients: Prior to beginning therapy, determine the endogenous serum erythropoietin level prior to transfusion. Available evidence suggests that patients receiving AZT with endogenous serum erythropoietin levels > 500 mU/ml are unlikely to respond to therapy.

Initial dose – For patients with serum erythropoietin levels ≤ 500 mU/ml who are receiving a dose of AZT ≤ 4200 mg/week, the recommended starting dose is 100 U/kg as an IV or SC injection 3 times weekly for 8 weeks.

If the response is not satisfactory in terms of reducing transfusion requirements or increasing hematocrit after 8 weeks of therapy, the dose can be increased by 50 to 100 U/kg 3 times weekly. Evaluate response every 4 to 8 weeks thereafter and adjust the dose accordingly by 50 to 100 U/kg increments 3 times weekly. If patients have not responded satisfactorily to a 300 U/kg dose 3 times weekly, it is unlikely that they will response to higher doses.

Monitor hematocrit weekly during the dose adjustment phase of therapy.

Maintenance dose – When the desired response is attained, titrate the dose to maintain the response based on factors such as variations in AZT dose and the presence of intercurrent infectious or inflammatory episodes. If the hematocrit exceeds 40%, discontinue the dose until the hematocrit drops to 36%. When resuming treatment, reduce the dose by 25%, then titrate to maintain the desired hematocrit.

Pre-therapy iron evaluation: Prior to and during therapy, evaluate the patient's iron stores, including transferrin saturation and serum ferritin. See Precautions.

Preparation: Do not shake. Shaking may denature the glycoprotein, rendering it biologically inactive. Use only one dose per vial; do not re-enter the vial. Discard unused portions. Contains no preservatives. Do not give in conjunction with other drug solutions.

Storage: Procrit – Store at 2° to 8°C (36° to 46°F). Do not freeze.

Rx	**Epogen** (Amgen)	**Preservative Free Injection:**[1] 2,000 units	In 1 ml vials.
		3,000 units	In 1 ml vials.
		4,000 units	In 1 ml vials.
		10,000 units	In 1 ml vials.
Rx	**Procrit** (Ortho Biotech)	**Preservative Free Injection:**[1] 2,000 units	In 1 ml vials.
		3,000 units	In 1 ml vials.
		4,000 units	In 1 ml vials.
		10,000 units	In 1 ml vials.

[1] With 2.5 mg albumin (human) per vial.

FILGRASTIM (Granulocyte Colony Stimulating Factor; G-CSF)

Actions:

Filgrastim was approved by the FDA in February 1991. Filgrastim is a human granulocyte colony stimulating factor (G-CSF), produced by recombinant DNA technology. Filgrastim is produced by *Escherichia coli* bacteria inserted with the human G-CSF gene. G-CSF regulates the production of neutrophils within the bone marrow; endogenous G-CSF is a glycoprotein produced by monocytes, fibroblasts and endothelial cells. It has minimal direct in vivo or in vitro effects on the production of other hematopoietic cell types.

Pharmacology: Colony stimulating factors are glycoproteins which act on hematopoietic cells by binding to specific cell surface receptors and stimulating proliferation, differentiation commitment and some end-cell functional activation.

Endogenous G-CSF is a lineage-specific colony stimulating factor with selectivity for the neutrophil lineage. It is not species-specific and primarily affects neutrophil progenitor proliferation, differentiation, and selected end-cell functional activation (including enhanced phagocytic ability, priming of the cellular metabolism associated with respiratory burst, antibody-dependent killing, and the increased expression of some functions associated with cell surface antigens).

Pharmacokinetics: Absorption and clearance follow first-order pharmacokinetics without apparent concentration dependence. A positive linear correlation occurs between the parenteral dose and both the serum concentration and area under the concentration-time curves. Continuous IV infusion of 20 mcg/kg filgrastim over 24 hours resulted in mean and median serum concentrations of approximately 48 and 56 ng/ml, respectively. SC administration of 3.45 and 11.5 mcg/kg resulted in maximum serum concentrations of 4 and 49 ng/ml, respectively, within 2 to 8 hours. The volume of distribution averaged 150 ml/kg in both healthy subjects and cancer patients. The elimination half-life in both healthy subjects and cancer patients was approximately 3.5 hours. Clearance rates were approximately 0.5 to 0.7 ml/min/kg. Single parenteral doses or daily IV doses, over a 14 day period, resulted in comparable half-lives. The half-lives were similar for IV administration (231 minutes following doses of 34.5 mcg/kg) and for SC administration (210 minutes following doses of 3.45 mcg/kg). Continuous 24 hour IV infusions at 20 mcg/kg over an 11 to 20 day period produced steady-state serum concentrations of filgrastim with no evidence of drug accumulation over the time period investigated.

Clinical trials: In studies involving 96 patients with various non-myeloid malignancies, filgrastim administration resulted in a dose-dependent increase in circulating neutrophil counts over the dose range of 1 to 70 mcg/kg/day. This increase in neutrophil counts was observed whether filgrastim was administered IV (1 to 70 mcg/kg twice daily), SC (1 to 3 mcg/kg once daily), or by continuous SC infusion (3 to 11 mcg/kg/day). With discontinuation of filgrastim therapy, neutrophil counts returned to baseline, in most cases within 4 days. Isolated neutrophils displayed normal phagocytic and chemotactic activity in vitro.

The absolute monocyte count increased in a dose-dependent manner in most patients receiving filgrastim; however, the percentage of monocytes in the differential count remained within the normal range. In all studies to date, absolute counts of both eosinophils and basophils did not change and were within the normal range following administration of filgrastim. Increases in lymphocyte counts following administration have occurred in some healthy subjects and cancer patients.

White blood cell differentials obtained during clinical trials have demonstrated a shift towards granulocyte progenitor cells (left shift), including the appearance of promyelocytes and myeloblasts, usually during neutrophil recovery following the chemotherapy-induced nadir. In addition, Dohle bodies, increased granulocyte granulation and hypersegmented neutrophils have been observed. Such changes were transient and were not associated with clinical sequelae nor were they necessarily associated with infection.

Filgrastim is safe and effective in accelerating the recovery of neutrophil counts following a variety of chemotherapy regimens. Patients with small cell lung cancer received SC administration of filgrastim (4 to 8 mcg/kg/day, days 4 to 17) or placebo. In this study, filgrastim prevented infection as manifested by febrile neutropenia, decreased hospitalization and decreased IV antibiotic usage. No difference in survival or disease progression was demonstrated.

(Actions continued on following page)

FILGRASTIM (Granulocyte Colony Stimulating Factor; G-CSF) (Cont.)

Actions (Cont.):

Clinical trials (Cont.):

In another study in patients with small cell lung cancer, patients were randomized to receive filgrastim (n = 99) or placebo (n = 111) starting on day 4 after receiving standard dose chemotherapy with cyclophosphamide, doxorubicin and etoposide:

Clinical Effects of Filgrastim[1]		
Parameter	Filgrastim	Placebo
Infection (at least one infection, all cycles)	40%	76%
Hospitalization (first cycle)	52%	69%
IV antibiotic usage (first cycle)	38%	60%
Severe neutropenia (ANC <500/mm³)		
First cycle	84%	96%
All cycles	57%	77%
Median duration		
First cycle	2 days	6 days
All cycles	1 day	3 days
Mean severity[2]		
First cycle	496/mm³	204/mm³
All cycles	403/mm³	161/mm³

[1] Incidence obtained during the first cycle of chemotherapy, over all cycles, or both.
[2] Measured by ANC nadir.

Indications:

To decrease the incidence of infection, as manifested by febrile neutropenia, in patients with non-myeloid malignancies receiving myelosuppressive anti-cancer drugs associated with a significant incidence of severe neutropenia with fever.

Obtain a complete blood count and platelet count prior to chemotherapy, and twice per week during therapy to avoid leukocytosis and to monitor the neutrophil count (see Precautions). In clinical studies, therapy was discontinued when the absolute neutrophil count (ANC) was ≥ 10,000/mm³ after the expected chemotherapy-induced nadir.

Contraindications:

Hypersensitivity to *E coli*-derived proteins.

Warnings:

Pregnancy: Category C. There are no adequate and well controlled studies in pregnant women. Use during pregnancy only if the potential benefit justifies the potential risk to the fetus.

In rabbits, increased abortion and embryolethality were observed at doses of 80 mcg/kg/day. Administration to pregnant rabbits (100 mcg/kg/day) during the period of organogenesis was associated with increased fetal resorption, genitourinary bleeding, developmental abnormalities, and decreased body weight, live births and food consumption. In rats, offspring of dams treated at > 20 mcg/kg/day exhibited a delay in external differentiation (detachment of auricles and descent of testes) and slight growth retardation, possibly due to lower body weight of females during rearing and nursing. Offspring of dams treated at 100 mcg/kg/day exhibited decreased body weights at birth, and a slightly reduced 4 day survival rate.

Lactation: It is not known whether filgrastim is excreted in breast milk. Exercise caution if administering to a nursing woman.

Children: Safety data indicate that filgrastim does not exhibit any greater toxicity in children than in adults. Filgrastim has been used to treat 128 pediatric severe chronic neutropenia patients (3 months to 18 years of age); doses used were 0.6 to 120 mcg/kg/day for up to 3 years. Such doses were well tolerated, and the overall pattern of adverse events in children and adults appeared to be similar. While subclinical increases in spleen size detected by imaging studies occurred more often in children than in adults, the clinical significance of these radiographic findings relative to normal growth and development is not known. In addition, 12 pediatric patients with neuroblastoma received up to six cycles of cyclophosphamide, cisplatin, doxorubicin and etoposide chemotherapy concurrently with filgrastim; in this population, filgrastim was well tolerated. There was one report of palpable splenomegaly associated with therapy; however, the only consistently reported adverse event was musculoskeletal pain, which is no different from the experience in the adult population.

(Continued on following page)

SARGRAMOSTIM (Granulocyte Macrophage Colony Stimulating Factor; GM-CSF)

Actions:

Sargramostim was approved by the FDA in March 1991.

Sargramostim is a recombinant human granulocyte-macrophage colony stimulating factor (rhu GM-CSF) produced by recombinant DNA technology in a yeast *(S cerevisiae)* expression system. GM-CSF is a hematopoietic growth factor which stimulates proliferation and differentiation of hematopoietic progenitor cells. Sargramostim is a glycoprotein of 127 amino acids. The amino acid sequence differs from the natural human GM-CSF by substituting leucine at position 23; the carbohydrate moiety may be different from the native protein.

Pharmacology: GM-CSF belongs to a group of growth factors termed colony stimulating factors which support survival, clonal expansion and differentiation of hematopoietic progenitor cells. GM-CSF induces partially committed progenitor cells to divide and differentiate in the granulocyte-macrophage pathways.

GM-CSF can also activate mature granulocytes and macrophages. GM-CSF is a multilineage factor and, in addition to dose-dependent effects on the myelomonocytic lineage, can promote the proliferation of megakaryocytic and erythroid progenitors. However, other factors are required to induce complete maturation in these two lineages. The various cellular responses (division, maturation, activation) are induced through GM-CSF binding to specific receptors expressed on the cell surface of target cells.

The biological activity of GM-CSF is species-specific. Chemotactic, antifungal and antiparasitic activities of granulocytes and monocytes are increased by exposure to sargramostim. Sargramostim increases the cytotoxicity of monocytes toward certain neoplastic cell lines and activates polymorphonuclear neutrophils to inhibit the growth of tumor cells.

Pharmacokinetics: In two patients receiving 250 mcg/m^2 by 2 hour IV infusion, serum sargramostim concentrations ranged from 22,000 to 23,000 pg/ml at the termination of the infusion. The pharmacokinetic profile, based on five patients receiving 500 to 750 mcg/m^2 by 2 hour IV infusion, revealed a rapid initial decline in GM-CSF serum concentration (alpha half-life ≈ 12 to 17 minutes) followed by a slower decrease (beta half-life ≈ 2 hours). In four patients receiving 125 mcg/m^2 SC every 12 hours, sargramostim was detected in the serum within 5 minutes after administration (range, 55 to 450 pg/ml). Peak levels were observed 2 hours after injection (range, 350 to 3,900 pg/ml), and sargramostim remained at detectable levels 6 hours following injection (range, 150 to 2,700 pg/ml).

Antibody formation: Neutralizing antibodies were detected in 5 of 165 patients (3%) after receiving sargramostim by continuous IV infusion (3 patients) or SC injection (2 patients) for 28 to 84 days in multiple courses. All 5 patients had impaired hematopoiesis before administration and consequently the effect of the development of anti-GM-CSF antibodies on normal hematopoiesis could not be assessed. Drug-induced neutropenia, neutralization of endogenous GM-CSF activity, and diminution of the therapeutic effect of sargramostim secondary to formation of neutralizing antibody remain a theoretical possibility.

Clinical trials: Myeloid reconstitution after autologous bone marrow transplantation – Sargramostim is safe and effective in accelerating myeloid engraftment in autologous bone marrow transplantation (BMT). After autologous BMT in patients with non-Hodgkin's lymphoma (NHL), acute lymphoblastic leukemia (ALL) or Hodgkin's disease, sargramostim accelerated myeloid engraftment, decreased median duration of antibiotic administration, reduced the median duration of infectious episodes and shortened the median duration of hospitalization.

Three single-center, randomized, placebo controlled and double-blinded studies (n = 128) were conducted to evaluate the safety and efficacy of sargramostim for promoting hematopoietic reconstitution following autologous BMT. Treatment with 250 mcg/m^2/day given by a 2 hour IV infusion or placebo was initiated within 2 to 4 hours of the marrow infusion and continued for 21 consecutive days post-transplantation. The majority of the patients had lymphoid malignancy (87 NHL, 17 ALL), 23 patients had Hodgkin's disease, and 1 patient had acute myeloblastic leukemia (AML). Preoperative regimens in the three studies included cyclophosphamide (total dose, 120 to 150 mg/kg) and total body irradiation. Various other chemotherapeutic regimens were used in patients with Hodgkin's disease and NHL without radiotherapy. Compared to placebo, administration of sargramostim in two studies significantly improved the following hematologic and clinical endpoints: Time to neutrophil engraftment, duration of hospitalization and infection experience or antibacterial usage. In the third study there was a positive trend toward earlier myeloid engraftment in favor of sargramostim. A subgroup analysis of the data from all three studies revealed that the median time to engraftment for patients with Hodgkin's disease, regardless of treatment, was 6 days longer when compared to patients with NHL and ALL, but that the overall beneficial sargramostim treatment effect was the same.

(Actions continued on following page)

SARGRAMOSTIM (Granulocyte Macrophage Colony Stimulating Factor; GM-CSF) (Cont.)

Actions (Cont.):

Clinical trials (Cont.):

Myeloid reconstitution after autologous bone marrow transplantation (Cont.) – Patients with lymphoid malignancy (NHL and ALL):

Autologous BMT: Combined Analysis from Placebo Controlled Clinical Trials of Responses in Patients with NHL and ALL

Treatment	Median values (days)				
	ANC[1] ≥ 500/mm³	ANC ≥ 1000/mm³	Duration of hospitalization	Duration of infection	Duration of antibacterial therapy
Sargramostim (n = 54)	18	24	25	1	21
Placebo (n = 50)	24	32	31	4	25

[1] Absolute neutrophil count.

Patients with Hodgkin's disease: A trend toward earlier myeloid engraftment (ANC ≥ 500 cells/mm³) was noted. Sargramostim-treated patients (n = 22) engrafted earlier (by 5 days) than the placebo-treated subjects.

Bone marrow transplantation failure or engraftment delay – In one study, 140 patients experiencing graft failure following allogeneic or autologous BMT were evaluated in comparison to 103 historical controls; 163 had lymphoid or myeloid leukemia, 24 had NHL, 19 had Hodgkin's disease and 37 had other diseases (eg, aplastic anemia, myelodysplasia, nonhematologic malignancy). Three categories of patients were eligible: 1) Patients displaying a delay in engraftment; 2) patients displaying a delay in engraftment who had evidence of an active infection and; 3) patients who lost their marrow graft after a transient engraftment.

One hundred day survival was improved in patients treated with sargramostim after graft failure following either autologous or allogeneic BMT. In addition, the median survival was improved by greater than two-fold. Median survival of patients treated with sargramostim after autologous failure was 474 days vs 161 days for the historical patients. After allogeneic failure, median survival was 97 days vs 35 days, respectively. Improvement in survival was better in patients with fewer impaired organs.

Indications:

Myeloid reconstitution after autologous bone marrow transplantation: Acceleration of myeloid recovery in patients with non-Hodgkin's lymphoma (NHL), acute lymphoblastic leukemia (ALL) and Hodgkin's disease undergoing autologous bone marrow transplantation (BMT). Hematologic response to sargramostim can be detected by complete blood count (CBC) with differential performed twice per week.

Insufficient data are presently available to support the efficacy of sargramostim in accelerating myeloid recovery following peripheral blood stem cell transplantation.

Bone marrow transplantation failure or engraftment delay: For patients who have undergone allogeneic or autologous BMT in whom engraftment is delayed or has failed.

Survival benefit may be relatively greater in those patients who demonstrate one or more of the following characteristics: Autologous BMT failure or engraftment delay; no previous total body irradiation; malignancy other than leukemia; or a multiple organ failure score ≤ 2. Hematologic response can be detected by CBC with differential performed twice weekly.

Unlabeled uses: GM-CSF has been used in the following conditions:

To increase WBC counts in patients with myelodysplastic syndromes and in AIDS patients receiving zidovudine.

To decrease nadir of leukopenia secondary to myelosuppressive chemotherapy and decrease myelosuppression in preleukemic patients.

To correct neutropenia in aplastic anemia patients.

To decrease transplantation-associated organ system damage, particularly in the liver and kidney (consistent with the observation that the duration of neutropenia correlates with organ system injury).

Contraindications:

Excessive leukemic myeloid blasts in the bone marrow or peripheral blood (≥ 10%); known hypersensitivity to GM-CSF, yeast-derived products or any component of the product.

(Continued on following page)

SARGRAMOSTIM (Granulocyte Macrophage Colony Stimulating Factor; GM-CSF) (Cont.)

Warnings:

Cardiovascular symptoms: Occasional transient supraventricular arrhythmia has occurred during administration, particularly in patients with a previous history of cardiac arrhythmia. However, these arrhythmias have been reversible after discontinuation of sargramostim. Use with caution in patients with preexisting cardiac disease.

Respiratory symptoms: Sequestration of granulocytes in the pulmonary circulation has occurred following sargramostim infusion, occasionally with dyspnea. Give special attention to respiratory symptoms during or immediately following infusion, especially in patients with preexisting lung disease. In patients displaying dyspnea during administration, reduce the rate of infusion by half. Subsequent IV infusions may be administered following the standard dose schedule with careful monitoring. If respiratory symptoms worsen despite infusion rate reduction, discontinue infusion. Administer with caution in patients with hypoxia.

Fluid retention: Peripheral edema, pleural or pericardial effusion have occurred in patients after administration. In 156 controlled study patients using a dose of 250 mcg/m^2/day by 2 hour IV infusion, the incidence of fluid retention (sargramostim vs placebo) were: Peripheral edema (11% vs 7%); pleural effusion (1% vs 0%); pericardial effusion (4% vs 1%). In patients with preexisting pleural and pericardial effusions, administration of sargramostim may aggravate fluid retention; however, fluid retention associated with or worsened by sargramostim has been reversible after interruption or dose reduction with or without diuretic therapy. Use with caution in patients with preexisting fluid retention, pulmonary infiltrates or congestive heart failure.

Renal and hepatic dysfunction: In some patients with preexisting renal or hepatic dysfunction in uncontrolled clinical trials, sargramostim has induced elevation of serum creatinine or bilirubin and hepatic enzymes. Dose reduction or interruption of administration has resulted in a decrease to pretreatment values. However, in controlled trials the incidences of renal and hepatic dysfunction were comparable between sargramostim 250 mcg/m^2/day by 2 hour IV infusion and placebo patients. Biweekly monitoring of renal and hepatic function in patients displaying renal or hepatic dysfunction prior to initiation of treatment is recommended during administration.

Hypersensitivity reactions: Use appropriate precautions during parenteral administration of recombinant proteins in case an allergic or untoward reaction occurs. Transient rashes and local injection site reactions have occasionally been observed. Serious allergic or anaphylactic reactions have been reported rarely. If any anaphylactoid reaction occurs, immediately discontinue and initiate appropriate therapy. Refer to Management of Acute Hypersensitivity Reactions.

Pregnancy: Category C. It is not known whether sargramostim can cause fetal harm when administered to a pregnant woman or can affect reproduction capacity. Give to a pregnant woman only if clearly needed.

Lactation: It is not known whether sargramostim is excreted in breast milk. Exercise caution when administering to a nursing woman.

Children: Safety and efficacy in children have not been established; however, available data indicate that sargramostim does not exhibit any greater toxicity in children than adults. A total of 113 pediatric subjects between the ages of 4 months and 18 years have been treated with 60 to 1,000 mcg/m^2/day IV and 4 to 1,500 mcg/m^2/day SC. In 53 pediatric patients in controlled studies at a dose of 250 mcg/m^2/day by 2 hour IV infusion, the type and frequency of adverse events were comparable to those in adults.

Precautions:

Growth factor potential: Sargramostim is a growth factor that primarily stimulates normal myeloid precursors. However, the possibility that sargramostim can act as a growth factor for any tumor type, particularly myeloid malignancies, cannot be excluded. Exercise caution when using this drug in any malignancy with myeloid characteristics.

Sargramostim has been administered to patients with AML and myelodysplastic syndromes (MDS) in uncontrolled studies without evidence of increased relapse rates or acceleration of disease progression. Use in patients with AML or MDS is not recommended due to a possibility of proliferative effects on abnormal myeloid cells.

Progression of underlying neoplastic disease (NHL, ALL or Hodgkin's disease) was not observed during sargramostim administration in clinical trials; however, should disease progression be detected, discontinue therapy. In controlled studies, the 12 month relapse rate was comparable in patients treated with sargramostim or placebo.

First dose effects: Hypotension with flushing and syncope has occurred rarely following the first administration. These signs have resolved with symptomatic treatment and have not recurred with subsequent doses in the same cycle of treatment.

(Precautions continued on following page)

SARGRAMOSTIM (Granulocyte Macrophage Colony Stimulating Factor; GM-CSF) (Cont.)

Precautions (Cont.):

Rapid increase in peripheral blood counts: Stimulation of marrow precursors with sargramostim may result in a rapid rise in white blood cell (WBC) count. If the ANC exceeds 20,000 cells/mm^3 or if the platelet count exceeds 500,000/mm^3, interrupt administration or reduce the dose by half. Base the decision to reduce the dose or interrupt treatment on the clinical condition of the patient. Excessive blood counts have returned to normal or baseline levels within 3 to 7 days following cessation of therapy. Perform biweekly monitoring of CBC with differential (including examination for the presence of blast cells) to preclude development of excessive counts.

Patients receiving purged bone marrow: Sargramostim is effective in accelerating myeloid recovery in patients receiving bone marrow purged by monoclonal antibodies. Data obtained from uncontrolled studies suggest that if in vitro marrow purging with chemical agents causes a significant decrease in the number of responsive hematopoietic progenitors the patient may not respond to sargramostim. When the bone marrow purging process preserves a sufficient number of progenitors, a beneficial effect of sargramostim on myeloid engraftment has occurred.

Previous exposure to intensive chemotherapy/radiotherapy: In patients who before autologous BMT have received extensive radiotherapy to hematopoietic sites for the treatment of primary disease in the abdomen or chest, or have been exposed to multiple myelotoxic agents (eg, alkylating agents, anthracycline antibiotics, antimetabolites) the effect of sargramostim on myeloid reconstitution may be limited.

Concomitant use with chemotherapy and radiotherapy: Because of potential sensitivity of rapidly dividing hematopoietic progenitor cells to cytotoxic chemotherapeutic or radiologic therapies, sargramostim should not be administered within 24 hours preceding or following chemotherapy, or within 12 hours preceding or following radiotherapy.

Monitoring: Sargramostim can induce variable increases in WBC or platelet counts. To avoid potential complications of excessive leukocytosis (WBC $>$ 50,000 cells/mm^3; ANC $>$ 20,000 cells/mm^3), perform a CBC twice per week during therapy. Biweekly monitoring of renal and hepatic function in patients with renal or hepatic dysfunction prior to initiation of treatment is recommended during administration.

Drug Interactions:

Drugs which may potentiate the myeloproliferative effects of sargramostim, such as **lithium** and **corticosteroids,** should be used with caution.

Adverse Reactions:

Sargramostim is generally well tolerated. The frequency and type of adverse events were similar between sargramostim and placebo control groups. Diarrhea, asthenia, rash, peripheral edema, malaise and urinary tract disorder were the only adverse reactions observed more often in the sargramostim group than in the placebo group.

Sargramostim Adverse Reactions (%)[1]

Adverse reaction	Sargramostim (n=79)	Placebo (n=77)	Adverse reaction	Sargramostim (n=79)	Placebo (n=77)
General			*Skin & appendages*		
Fever	95	96	Alopecia	73	74
Mucous membrane disorder	75	78	Rash	44	38
Asthenia	66	51	*Respiratory*		
Malaise	57	51	Dyspnea	28	31
Edema	34	35	Lung disorder	20	23
Peripheral edema	11	7			
Sepsis	11	14			
GI			*GU*		
Nausea	90	96	Urinary tract disorder	14	13
Diarrhea	89	82	Kidney function abnormal	8	10
Vomiting	85	90	*Other*		
Anorexia	54	58	Blood dyscrasia	25	27
GI disorder	37	47	Hemorrhage	23	30
GI hemorrhage	27	33	CNS disorder	11	16
Stomatitis	24	29			
Liver damage	13	14			

[1] Following BMT or peripheral stem cell transplantation in three controlled studies.

(Adverse Reactions continued on following page)

SARGRAMOSTIM (Granulocyte Macrophage Colony Stimulating Factor; GM-CSF) (Cont.)

Adverse Reactions (Cont.):

In some patients with preexisting renal or hepatic dysfunction enrolled in uncontrolled clinical trials, administration of sargramostim has induced elevation of serum creatinine or bilirubin and hepatic enzymes (see Warnings).

Headache (26%), pericardial effusion (25%), arthralgia (21%) and myalgia (18%) were also reported in the graft failure study.

In uncontrolled Phase I/II studies with sargramostim in 215 patients, the most frequent adverse events were fever, asthenia, headache, bone pain, chills and myalgia. These systemic events were generally mild or moderate and were usually prevented or reversed by the administration of analgesics and antipyretics such as acetaminophen. In these uncontrolled trials, other infrequent events reported were dyspnea, peripheral edema and rash.

In patients with preexisting peripheral edema, pleural or pericardial effusion, administration of sargramostim may aggravate fluid retention (see Warnings).

In one patient with Hodgkin's disease treated with a 24 hour 250 mcg/m^2 IV infusion after autologous BMT, in whom sargramostim administration was pursued despite massive weight gain and development of significant peripheral edema, a capillary leak syndrome occurred. Carefully monitor body weight and hydration status during administration.

Adverse events observed in pediatric patients in controlled studies were comparable to those observed in adult patients.

Overdosage:

The maximum amount that can be safely administered in single or multiple doses has not been determined. Doses up to 100 mcg/kg/day (4,000 mcg/m^2/day or 16 times the recommended dose) were administered to 4 patients in a Phase I uncontrolled clinical study by continuous IV infusion for 7 to 18 days. Increases in WBC up to 200,000 cells/mm^3 were observed. Adverse events reported were: Dyspnea, malaise, nausea, fever, rash, sinus tachycardia, headache and chills. All these events were reversible after discontinuation of sargramostim.

In case of overdosage discontinue therapy and carefully monitor the patient for WBC increase and respiratory symptoms.

Administration and Dosage:

Myeloid reconstitution after autologous bone marrow transplantation: 250 mcg/m^2/day for 21 days as a 2 hour IV infusion beginning 2 to 4 hours after the autologous bone marrow infusion, and not less than 24 hours after the last dose of chemotherapy and 12 hours after the last dose of radiotherapy. If a severe adverse reaction occurs, reduce or temporarily discontinue the dose until the reaction abates. If blast cells appear or progression of the underlying disease occurs, discontinue the treatment.

In order to avoid potential complications of excessive leukocytosis (WBC $>$ 50,000 cells/mm^3; ANC $>$ 20,000 cells/mm^3), a CBC with differential is recommended twice per week during sargramostim therapy. Discontinue treatment if the ANC exceeds 20,000 cells/mm^3.

Bone marrow transplantation failure or engraftment delay: 250 mcg/m^2/day for 14 days as a 2 hour IV infusion. The dose can be repeated after 7 days off therapy if engraftment has not occurred. If engraftment still has not occurred, a third course of 500 mcg/m^2/day for 14 days may be tried after another 7 days off therapy. If there is still no improvement, it is unlikely that further dose escalation will be beneficial. If a severe adverse reaction occurs, the dose can be reduced or temporarily discontinued until the reaction abates. If blast cells appear or disease progression occurs, discontinue the treatment.

In order to avoid potential complications of excessive leukocytosis (WBC $>$ 50,000 cells/mm^3; ANC $>$ 20,000 cells/mm^3) a CBC with differential is recommended twice per week during therapy. Interrupt or reduce the dose by half if the ANC exceeds 20,000 cells/mm^3.

(Administration and Dosage continued on following page)

SARGRAMOSTIM (Granulocyte Macrophage Colony Stimulating Factor; GM-CSF) (Cont.)

Administration and Dosage (Cont.):

Preparation:

1. Reconstitute with 1 ml Sterile Water for Injection, USP (without preservative). The reconstituted solutions are clear, colorless and isotonic with a pH of 7.4 ± 0.3. Do not re-enter or reuse the single use vial. Discard any unused portion.
2. During reconstitution direct the Sterile Water for Injection, USP at the side of the vial and gently swirl the contents to avoid foaming during dissolution. Avoid excessive or vigorous agitation; do not shake.
3. Perform dilution for IV infusion in 0.9% Sodium Chloride Injection, USP. If the final concentration is < 10 mcg/ml, add albumin (human) at a final concentration of 0.1% to the saline prior to addition of sargramostim to prevent adsorption to the components of the drug delivery system. For a final concentration of 0.1% albumin (human), add 1 mg albumin (human) per 1 ml 0.9% Sodium Chloride Injection, USP.
4. Do not use an in-line membrane filter for IV infusion.
5. Sargramostim contains no antibacterial preservative; therefore, administer as soon as possible, and within 6 hours following reconstitution or dilution for IV infusion. Store solutions under refrigeration at 2° to 8°C (36° to 46°F); do not freeze. Sargramostim vials are intended for single use only; discard any unused solution after 6 hours.
6. In the absence of compatibility and stability information, do not add other medication to infusion solutions containing sargramostim. Use only 0.9% Sodium Chloride Injection, USP to prepare IV infusion solutions.

Storage: Refrigerate the sterile powder, the reconstituted solution and the diluted solution for injection at 2° to 8°C (36° to 46°F). Do not freeze or shake. Do not use beyond the expiration date printed on the vial.

Rx	**Leukine** (Immunex)	**Powder for Injection, lyophilized**[1]: 250 mcg	Preservative free. In single-use vials.
Rx	**Prokine** (Hoechst-Roussel)		Preservative free. In single-use vials.
Rx	**Leukine** (Immunex)	**Powder for Injection, lyophilized**[1]: 500 mcg	Preservative free. In single-use vials.
Rx	**Prokine** (Hoechst-Roussel)		Preservative free. In single-use vials.

[1] With 40 mg mannitol, 10 mg sucrose and 1.2 mg tromethamine, USP.

Venous thrombi consist mainly of fibrin and red blood cells. Arterial thrombi are composed mainly of platelet aggregates. Theoretically then, anticoagulant drugs should be effective for reducing risks involved with venous thrombi formation and antiplatelet drugs should be more effective for reducing risks of arterial thrombi formation.

Many drugs have been shown to interfere with platelet function including clofibrate, tricyclic antidepressants, dextrans and β-blockers. The drugs most commonly used for their antiplatelet effects are aspirin, sulfinpyrazone and dipyridamole.

DIPYRIDAMOLE

Actions:

Pharmacology: It is believed that platelet reactivity and interaction with prosthetic cardiac valve surfaces, resulting in abnormally shortened platelet survival time, is a significant factor in thromboembolic complications occurring in connection with prosthetic heart valve replacement.

Dipyridamole has been found to lengthen abnormally shortened platelet survival time in a dose-dependent manner. In three randomized controlled clinical trials involving 854 patients who had undergone surgical placement of a prosthetic heart valve, dipyridamole with warfarin decreased the incidence of postoperative thromboembolic events by 62% to 91% compared to warfarin alone. In three additional studies involving 392 patients taking dipyridamole and coumarin-like anticoagulants, the incidence of thromboembolic events ranged from 2.3% to 6.9%. Dipyridamole does not influence prothrombin time or activity measurements when administered with warfarin.

Mechanism: Dipyridamole is a platelet adhesion inhibitor, although the mechanism of action has not been fully elucidated. The mechanism may relate to 1) inhibition of red blood cell uptake of adenosine, itself an inhibitor of platelet reactivity, 2) phosphodiesterase inhibition leading to increased cyclic-3', 5'-adenosine monophosphate within platelets, and 3) inhibition of thromboxane A_2 formation which is a potent stimulator of platelet activation.

Hemodynamics – Intraduodenal doses of 0.5 to 4 mg/kg dipyridamole produced dose-related decreases in systemic and coronary vascular resistance leading to decreases in systemic blood pressure and increases in coronary blood flow. Onset of action in animals was about 24 minutes and effects persisted for about 3 hours.

In humans, the same qualitative hemodynamic effects have been observed. However, acute IV administration of dipyridamole may worsen regional myocardial perfusion distal to partial occlusion of coronary arteries.

Pharmacokinetics: Metabolism – Following an oral dose of dipyridamole, the average time to peak concentration is about 75 minutes.

The decline in plasma concentration fits a two-compartment model. The α half-life (the initial decline following peak concentration) is $\approx$ 40 minutes. The β half-life (the terminal decline in plasma concentration) is $\approx$ 10 hours. Dipyridamole is highly bound to plasma proteins. It is metabolized in the liver where it is conjugated as a glucuronide and excreted with the bile.

Indications:

Dipyridamole is indicated as an adjunct to coumarin anticoagulants in the prevention of postoperative thromboembolic complications of cardiac valve replacement.

Unlabeled Uses: The antiplatelet effect of dipyridamole, alone and in combination with aspirin, is being evaluated in the prevention of myocardial reinfarction and reduction of mortality post MI. Preliminary data suggest that such therapy may be beneficial, particularly if initiated early after infarction.

The FDA has proposed to withdraw approval of dipyridamole-containing products for long-term therapy of chronic angina (see page 617).

Contraindications:

None known.

Warnings:

Usage in Pregnancy: Category B. Reproduction studies have been performed in mice, rats and rabbits at doses up to 125 mg/kg (15.6 times the maximum recommended daily human dose) and have revealed no evidence of impaired fertility or harm to the fetus. There are, however, no adequate and well-controlled studies in pregnant women. Use during pregnancy only if clearly needed.

Usage in Lactation: Dipyridamole is excreted in breast milk. Exercise caution when administering to a nursing woman.

Usage in Children: Safety and efficacy in children below the age of 12 years have not been established.

(Continued on following page)

DIPYRIDAMOLE (Cont.)

Precautions:

Hypotension: Use with caution in patients with hypotension since it can produce peripheral vasodilation.

Drug Interactions:

Warfarin: Adminstered concomitantly with warfarin, bleeding was no greater in frequency or severity than that observed when warfarin was administered alone.

Adverse Reactions:

Adverse reactions at therapeutic doses are usually minimal and transient. On long-term use, initial side effects usually disappear. The following reactions were reported in two heart valve replacement trials comparing dipyridamole and warfarin therapy to either warfarin alone or warfarin and placebo:

CNS: Dizziness 13.6%, headache 2.3%.

GI: Abdominal distress 6.1%.

Dermatologic: Rash 2.3%.

Other: Diarrhea, vomiting, flushing and pruritis. Angina pectoris has been reported rarely.

On those uncommon occasions when adverse reactions have been persistent or intolerable, they have ceased on withdrawal of the medication.

Overdosage:

Hypotension, if it occurs, is likely to be of short duration, but a vasopressor may be used if necessary. Since dipyridamole is highly protein bound, dialysis is not likely to be of benefit.

Administration and Dosage:

Adjunctive use in prophylaxis of thromboembolism after cardiac valve replacement: The recommended dose is 75 to 100 mg, 4 times daily as an adjunct to the usual warfarin therapy. Please note that aspirin is not to be administered concomitantly with coumarin anticoagulants.

				C.I.*
Rx	**Persantine** (Boehringer Ingelheim)	**Tablets:** 25 mg	(#BI/17). Orange, sugar coated. In 100s, 1000s and UD 100s.	21
		50 mg	(#BI/18). Orange, sugar coated. In 100s, 1000s and UD 100s.	17
		75 mg	(#BI/19). Orange, sugar coated. In 100s, 500s and UD 100s.	15

* Cost Index based on cost per 300 mg (minimum daily dose).

Product identification code.

TICLOPIDINE HCl

Actions:

Ticlopidine was approved by the FDA in October 1991.

Pharmacology: Ticlopidine is a platelet aggregation inhibitor. When taken orally, ticlopidine causes a time and dose-dependent inhibition of both platelet aggregation and release of platelet granule constituents, as well as a prolongation of bleeding time. Ticlopidine interferes with platelet membrane function by inhibiting ADP-induced platelet-fibrinogen binding and subsequent platelet-platelet interactions. The effect on platelet function is irreversible for the life of the platelet.

In healthy volunteers, substantial inhibition (> 50%) of ADP-induced platelet aggregation is detected within 4 days after administration of ticlopidine 250 mg twice daily, and maximum platelet aggregation inhibition (60% to 70%) is achieved after 8 to 11 days. Lower doses cause less and more delayed platelet aggregation inhibition, while doses > 250 mg twice daily give little additional effect on platelet aggregation, but an increased rate of adverse effects. After discontinuation of ticlopidine, bleeding time and other platelet function tests return to normal within 2 weeks in the majority of patients. At the recommended therapeutic dose (250 mg twice daily), ticlopidine has no known significant pharmacological actions in man other than inhibition of platelet function and prolongation of the bleeding time.

Pharmacokinetics: Ticlopidine is rapidly absorbed (> 80%), with peak plasma levels occurring at approximately 2 hours after dosing, and is extensively metabolized. Administration after meals results in a 20% increase in the area under the plasma concentration-time curve (AUC).

Ticlopidine displays non-linear pharmacokinetics and clearance decreases markedly on repeated dosing. In older volunteers, the apparent half-life after a single 250 mg dose is about 12.6 hours; with repeat dosing at 250 mg twice daily, the terminal elimination half-life rises to 4 to 5 days and steady-state levels of ticlopidine in plasma are obtained after ≈ 14 to 21 days.

Ticlopidine binds reversibly (98%) to plasma proteins, mainly to serum albumin and lipoproteins. The binding to albumin and lipoproteins is nonsaturable over a wide concentration range. Ticlopidine also binds to alpha-1 acid glycoprotein; at concentrations attained with the recommended dose, ≤ 15% in plasma is bound to this protein.

Ticlopidine is metabolized extensively by the liver; only trace amounts of intact drug are detected in the urine. Following an oral dose, 60% is recovered in the urine and 23% in the feces. Approximately, one-third of the dose excreted in the feces is intact ticlopidine, possibly excreted in the bile. Ticlopidine is a minor component in plasma (5%) after a single dose, but at steady state is the major component (15%). Approximately 40% to 50% of the metabolites circulating in plasma are covalently bound to plasma proteins, probably by acylation. Although analysis of urine and plasma indicates at least twenty metabolites, no metabolite which accounts for the activity of ticlopidine has been isolated.

Clearance decreases with age. Steady-state trough values in elderly patients (mean age 70 years) are about twice those in young populations.

Hepatically impaired patients: The average plasma concentration in patients with advanced cirrhosis was slightly higher than that seen in older subjects.

Renally impaired patients: Patients with mildly (creatinine clearance [Ccr] 50 to 80 ml/min) or moderately (Ccr 20 to 50 ml/min) impaired renal function were compared to healthy subjects (Ccr 80 to 150 ml/min). AUC values of ticlopidine increased by 28% and 60% in mild and moderately impaired patients, respectively, and plasma clearance decreased by 37% and 52%, respectively, but there were no statistically significant differences in ADP-induced platelet aggregation. Bleeding times showed significant prolongation only in the moderately impaired patients.

Clinical trials: Patients experiencing stroke precursors – In a trial comparing ticlopidine and aspirin (The Ticlopidine Aspirin Stroke Study; TASS), 3069 patients (1987 men, 1082 women) who had experienced such stroke precursors as transient ischemic attack (TIA), transient monocular blindness (amaurosis fugax), reversible ischemic neurological deficit or minor stroke were randomized to ticlopidine 250 mg twice daily or aspirin 650 mg twice daily. The study was designed to follow patients for at least 2 and up to 5 years. Over the duration of the study, ticlopidine significantly reduced the risk of fatal and nonfatal stroke by 24% from 18.1 to 13.8 per 100 patients followed for 5 years, compared to aspirin. During the first year, when the risk of stroke is greatest, the reduction in risk of stroke (fatal and nonfatal) compared to aspirin was 48%; the reduction was similar in men and women.

(Actions continued on following page)

TICLOPIDINE HCl (Cont.)

Actions (Cont.):

Clinical trials (Cont.):

Patients who had a completed atherothrombotic stroke – In a trial comparing ticlopidine with placebo (The Canadian American Ticlopidine Study; CATS) 1073 patients who had experienced a previous atherothrombotic stroke were treated with ticlopidine 250 mg twice daily or placebo for up to 3 years. Ticlopidine significantly reduced the overall risk of stroke by 24% from 24.6 to 18.6 per 100 patients followed for 3 years, compared to placebo. During the first year, the reduction in risk of fatal and nonfatal stroke over placebo was 33%.

Indications:

To reduce the risk of thrombotic stroke (fatal or nonfatal) in patients who have experienced stroke precursors, and in patients who have had a completed thrombotic stroke.

Because ticlopidine is associated with a risk of neutropenia/agranulocytosis, which may be life-threatening (see Warnings), reserve for patients who are intolerant to aspirin therapy where indicated to prevent stroke.

Unlabeled uses: Ticlopidine has also been utilized in various other conditions; further study is needed:

Ticlopidine Unlabeled Uses

Condition	Result
Intermittent claudication	Improved maximum walking and pain-free distance
Chronic arterial occlusion	Improved lower extremity ulcer healing, vascular improvement
Subarachnoid hemorrhage	Reduced incidence of neurological deficit
Uremic patients with AV shunts or fistulas	Reduced incidence of vascular occlusion
Open heart surgery	Preoperative use reduces degree of platelet count drop during extracorporeal circulation
Coronary artery bypass grafts	Decreased graft occlusion
Primary glomerulonephritis	Reduced degree of proteinuria and hematuria, improved creatinine clearance
Sickle cell disease	Reduced incidence, duration, severity of infarctive crises

Contraindications:

Hypersensitivity to the drug; presence of hematopoietic disorders such as neutropenia and thrombocytopenia; presence of a hemostatic disorder or active pathological bleeding (such as bleeding peptic ulcer or intracranial bleeding); severe liver impairment.

Warnings:

Neutropenia defined as an absolute neutrophil count (ANC) < 1200 neutrophils/mm³ occurred in 50 of 2048 (2.4%) stroke patients who received ticlopidine in clinical trials. Neutropenia is calculated as follows: ANC = WBC x % neutrophils.

Severe neutropenia (< 450 neutrophils/mm³) or agranulocytosis occurred in 17 patients (0.8%) who received ticlopidine. When the drug was discontinued, the neutrophil counts returned to normal (> 1200 neutrophils/mm³) within 1 to 3 weeks.

Mild to moderate neutropenia (451 to 1200 neutrophils/mm³) occurred in 33 patients (1.6%) who received ticlopidine. Eleven of the patients discontinued treatment and recovered within a few days. In the remaining 22 patients, the neutropenia was transient and did not require discontinuation of therapy.

The onset of severe neutropenia occurred 3 weeks to 3 months after the start of therapy with no documented cases of severe neutropenia beyond that time. The bone marrow typically showed a reduction in myeloid precursors. It is therefore essential that CBCs and white cell differentials be performed every 2 weeks starting from the second week to the end of the third month of therapy, but more frequent monitoring is necessary for patients whose absolute neutrophil counts have been consistently declining or are 30% less than the baseline count.

If clinical evaluation and repeat laboratory testing confirm the presence of neutropenia, discontinue the drug. In clinical trials, when therapy was discontinued immediately upon detection of neutropenia, the neutrophil counts returned to normal within 1 to 3 weeks.

After the first 3 months of therapy, CBCs need to be obtained only for patients with signs or symptoms suggestive of infection.

(Warnings continued on following page)

TICLOPIDINE HCl (Cont.)

Warnings (Cont.):

Thrombocytopenia: Rarely, thrombocytopenia may occur in isolation or together with neutropenia. If clinical evaluation and repeat laboratory testing confirm the presence of thrombocytopenia (< 80,000 cells/mm³), discontinue the drug.

Cholesterol elevation: Ticlopidine therapy causes increased serum cholesterol and triglycerides. Serum total cholesterol levels are increased 8% to 10% within 1 month of therapy and persist at that level. The ratios of lipoprotein subfractions are unchanged.

Hematological effects: Rare cases of pancytopenia and thrombotic thrombocytopenia purpura, some of which have been fatal, have occurred.

Anticoagulant drugs: If a patient is switched from an anticoagulant or fibrinolytic drug to ticlopidine, discontinue the former drug prior to ticlopidine administration.

Hepatic function impairment: Because of limited experience in patients with severe hepatic disease, who may have bleeding diatheses, the use of ticlopidine is not recommended.

Renal function impairment: There is limited experience in patients with renal impairment. In controlled clinical trials, no unexpected problems have been encountered in patients having mild renal impairment and there is no experience with dosage adjustment in patients with greater degrees of renal impairment. Nevertheless, for renally impaired patients it may be necessary to reduce ticlopidine dosage or discontinue it altogether if hemorrhagic or hematopoietic problems are encountered (see Pharmacokinetics).

Elderly: Clearance of ticlopidine is somewhat lower in elderly patients and trough levels are increased. No overall differences in safety or efficacy were observed between elderly patients and younger patients, but greater sensitivity of some older individuals cannot be ruled out.

Pregnancy: Category B. Doses of 400 mg/kg in rats, 200 mg/kg/day in mice and 100 mg/kg in rabbits produced maternal toxicity as well as fetal toxicity, but there was no evidence of a teratogenic potential of ticlopidine. There are no adequate and well controlled studies in pregnant women. Use during pregnancy only if clearly needed.

Lactation: Ticlopidine is excreted in the milk of rats. It is not known whether this drug is excreted in human breast milk. Because of the potential for serious adverse reactions in nursing infants from ticlopidine, decide whether to discontinue nursing or to discontinue the drug, taking into account the importance of the drug to the mother.

Children: Safety and efficacy in patients < 18 years of age have not been established.

Precautions:

Increased bleeding risk: Use with caution in patients who may be at risk of increased bleeding from trauma, surgery or pathological conditions. If it is desired to eliminate the antiplatelet effects of ticlopidine prior to elective surgery, discontinue the drug 10 to 14 days prior to surgery. Increased surgical blood loss has occurred in patients undergoing surgery during treatment with ticlopidine. In TASS and CATS it was recommended that patients have ticlopidine discontinued prior to elective surgery. Several hundred patients underwent surgery during the trials, and no excessive surgical bleeding was reported.

Prolonged bleeding time is normalized within 2 hours after administration of 20 mg methylprednisolone IV. Platelet transfusions may also be used to reverse the effect of ticlopidine on bleeding.

GI bleeding: Ticlopidine prolongs template bleeding time. Use with caution in patients who have lesions with a propensity to bleed (such as ulcers). Use drugs that might induce such lesions with caution in patients on ticlopidine.

(Continued on following page)

TICLOPIDINE HCl (Cont.)

Drug Interactions:

The dose of drugs metabolized by hepatic microsomal enzymes with low therapeutic ratios, or being given to patients with hepatic impairment, may require adjustment to maintain optimal therapeutic blood levels when starting or stopping concomitant therapy with ticlopidine.

Ticlopidine Drug Interactions			
Precipitant drug	Object drug*		Description
Antacids	Ticlopidine	↓	Administration of ticlopidine after antacids has resulted in an 18% decrease in ticlopidine plasma levels.
Cimetidine	Ticlopidine	↑	Chronic cimetidine administration has reduced the clearance of a single ticlopidine dose by 50%.
Ticlopidine	Aspirin	↑	Ticlopidine potentiated the effect of aspirin on collagen-induced platelet aggregation. Ticlopidine-mediated inhibition of ADP-induced platelet aggregation is not affected. Coadministration is not recommended.
Ticlopidine	Digoxin	↓	Digoxin plasma levels may be slightly decreased (≈ 15%).
Ticlopidine	Theophylline	↑	Theophylline elimination half-life was significantly increased (from 8.6 to 12.2 hr) with a comparable reduction in total plasma clearance in healthy volunteers.

* ↑ = Object drug increased ↓ = Object drug decreased

Drug/Food interaction: The oral bioavailability of ticlopidine is increased by 20% when taken after a meal. Administration with food is recommended to maximize GI tolerance.

Adverse Reactions:

Adverse reactions were relatively frequent, with > 50% of patients reporting at least one. Most (30% to 40%) involved the GI tract. Most adverse effects are mild, but 21% of patients discontinued therapy because of an adverse event, principally diarrhea, rash, nausea, vomiting, GI pain and neutropenia. Most adverse effects occur early in the course of treatment, but a new onset of adverse effects can occur after several months.

Ticlopidine Adverse Reactions vs Aspirin and Placebo (%)			
Adverse reaction	Ticlopidine (n = 2048)	Aspirin (n = 1527)	Placebo (n = 536)
Any reaction	60	53.2	34.3
Diarrhea	12.5	5.2	4.5
Nausea	7	6.2	1.7
Dyspepsia	7	9	0.9
Rash	5.1	1.5	0.6
GI pain	3.7	5.6	1.3
Neutropenia	2.4	0.8	1.1
Purpura	2.2	1.6	0
Vomiting	1.9	1.4	0.9
Flatulence	1.5	1.4	0
Pruritus	1.3	0.3	0
Dizziness	1.1	0.5	0
Anorexia	1	0.5	0
Abnormal liver function test	1	0.3	0

GI: Ticlopidine therapy has been associated with a variety of GI complaints including diarrhea and nausea. The majority of cases are mild, but about 13% of patients discontinued therapy. They usually occur within 3 months of initiation of therapy and typically are resolved within 1 to 2 weeks without discontinuation of therapy. If the effect is severe or persistent, discontinue therapy.

Hemorrhagic: Ticlopidine has been associated with a number of bleeding complications such as ecchymosis, epistaxis, hematuria, conjunctival hemorrhage, GI bleeding and perioperative bleeding. Intracerebral bleeding was rare with an incidence no greater than that seen with comparable agents (ticlopidine 0.5%, aspirin 0.6%, placebo 0.75%).

(Adverse Reactions continued on following page)

TICLOPIDINE HCl (Cont.)

Adverse Reactions (Cont.):

Rash: Ticlopidine has been associated with a maculopapular or urticarial rash (often with pruritus). Rash usually occurs within 3 months of initiation of therapy, with a mean onset time of 11 days. If drug is discontinued, recovery occurs within several days. Many rashes do not recur on drug rechallenge. There have been rare reports of severe rashes.

Adverse reactions occurring in 0.5% to 1% of patients: GI fullness; urticaria; headache; asthenia; pain; epistaxis; tinnitus.

In addition, rarer, relatively serious events have also been reported: Pancytopenia; hemolytic anemia with reticulocytosis; allergic pneumonitis; systemic lupus (positive ANA); peripheral neuropathy; vasculitis; serum sickness; arthropathy; hepatitis; cholestatic jaundice; nephrotic syndrome; myositis; hyponatremia; immune thrombocytopenia; thrombocytopenic thrombotic purpura.

Lab test abnormalities: Elevations of alkaline phosphatase and transaminases generally occurred within 1 to 4 months of therapy initiation. The incidence of elevated alkaline phosphatase (> 2 times upper limit of normal) was 7.6% in ticlopidine patients, 6% in placebo patients, and 2.5% in aspirin patients. The incidence of elevated AST (> 2 times upper limit of normal) was 3.1% in ticlopidine patients, 4% with placebo and 2.1% with aspirin. Occasionally patients developed minor elevations in bilirubin. Perform liver function testing whenever liver dysfunction is suspected, particularly during the first 4 months of treatment.

Overdosage:

One case of deliberate overdosage has been reported. A 38-year-old male took a single 6000 mg dose (equivalent to 24 standard 250 mg tablets). The only abnormalities reported were increased bleeding time and increased ALT. No special therapy was instituted and the patient recovered without sequelae.

Single oral doses of 1600 and 500 mg/kg were lethal to rats and mice, respectively. Symptoms of acute toxicity were GI hemorrhage, convulsions, hypothermia, dyspnea, loss of equilibrium and abnormal gait.

Patient Information

A decrease in the number of white blood cells (neutropenia) can occur, especially during the first 3 months of treatment. If neutropenia is severe, it could result in an increased risk of infection. It is critically important to obtain the scheduled blood tests to detect neutropenia. Patients should contact their physicians if they experience any indication of infection such as fever, chills or sore throat, all of which may be consequences of neutropenia.

It may take longer than usual to stop bleeding when taking ticlopidine. Patients should report any unusual bleeding to their physician. Patients should tell physicians and dentists that they are taking ticlopidine before any surgery is scheduled and before any new drug is prescribed.

Promptly report side effects such as severe or persistent diarrhea, skin rashes or subcutaneous bleeding, or any signs of cholestasis, such as yellow skin or sclera, dark urine or light colored stools.

Take ticlopidine with food or just after eating in order to minimize GI discomfort.

Administration and Dosage:

Recomended dose: 250 mg twice daily taken with food.

Rx	**Ticlid** (Syntex)	**Tablets:** 250 mg	(Ticlid 250). White. Oval. Film coated. In 30s and 100s.

Blood coagulation resulting in the formation of a stable fibrin clot involves a cascade of proteolytic reactions involving the interaction of clotting factors, platelets and tissue materials. Clotting factors (see table) exist in the blood in inactive form and must be converted to an enzymatic or activated (a) form before the next step in the clotting mechanism can be stimulated. Each factor is stimulated in turn until an insoluble fibrin clot is formed.

Two separate pathways, intrinsic and extrinsic, lead to the formation of a fibrin clot. Both pathways must function for hemostasis.

Intrinsic pathway – All the protein factors necessary for coagulation are present in circulating blood. Clot formation may take several minutes and is initiated by activation of factor XII.

Extrinsic pathway – Coagulation is activated by release of tissue thromboplastin, a factor not found in circulating blood. Clotting occurs in seconds because factor III bypasses the early reactions.

Refer to the next page for the complete coagulation pathway.

Anticoagulants used therapeutically include heparin, warfarin (a coumarin derivative) and anisindione (an indandione derivative).

Blood Clotting Factors

Factor	Synonym	Vitamin K-dependent
I	Fibrinogen	no
II	Prothrombin	yes
III	Tissue thromboplastin, tissue factor	no
IV	Calcium	no
V	Labile factor, proaccelerin	no
VII	Proconvertin	yes
VIII	Antihemophilic factor, AHF	no
IX	Christmas factor, plasma thromboplastin component, PTC	yes
X	Stuart factor, Stuart-Prower factor	yes
XI	Plasma thromboplastin antecedent, PTA	no
XII	Hageman factor	no
XIII	Fibrin stabilizing factor, FSF	no
HMW-K	High molecular weight Kininogen, Fitzgerald factor	no
PL	Platelets or phospholipids	no
PK	Prekallikrein, Fletcher factor	no
Protein C[1]		yes
Protein S[2]		yes

[1] Partially responsible for inhibition of the extrinsic pathway. Inactivates factors V and VIII and promotes fibrinolysis. Activity declines following warfarin administration.

[2] A cofactor to accelerate the anticoagulant activity of protein C. Decreased levels occur following warfarin administration.

(Continued on following page)

COAGULATION PATHWAY

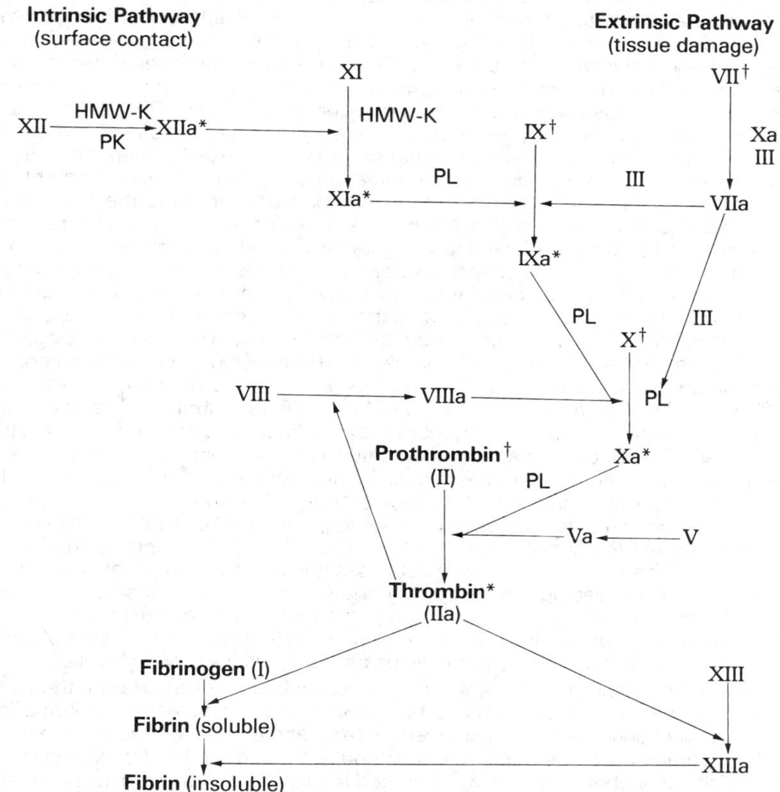

* Site of activity for heparin

† Site of activity for warfarin and anisindione

HEPARIN

Actions:

Pharmacology: Commercial preparations of heparin are derived from bovine lung or porcine intestinal mucosa; although chemical and biological differences exist, there is no clinical difference in the antithrombotic effects. Heparin calcium is reported to cause a lower incidence of local hematoma than heparin sodium; however, differences in side effects or efficacy have not been documented. The anticoagulant potency of heparin is standardized by bioassay and is expressed in "units" of activity. Because the number of USP units per milligram vary, express dosage only in "units". (Heparin sodium, USP and heparin calcium, USP should contain not less than 140 USP heparin units/mg.)

The major rate-limiting step in the coagulation cascade is the activation of factor X, which is involved in both intrinsic and extrinsic pathways (refer to the Anticoagulant introduction). Small amounts of heparin in combination with antithrombin III (heparin cofactor) inhibit thrombosis by inactivating factor Xa and inhibiting the conversion of prothrombin to thrombin. Once active thrombosis has developed, larger amounts of heparin can inhibit further coagulation by inactivating thrombin and preventing the conversion of fibrinogen to fibrin. In combination with antithrombin III, heparin inactivates factors IX, X, Xa, XI, XII and thrombin, inhibiting conversion of fibrinogen to fibrin. The heparin-antithrombin III complex is 100 to 1000 times more potent as an anticoagulant than antithrombin III alone. Heparin also prevents the formation of a stable fibrin clot by inhibiting the activation of factor XIII (the fibrin stabilizing factor). Other effects include the inhibition of thrombin-induced activation of factors V and VIII.

Commercial products contain both low and high molecular weight heparin fractions. Low molecular weight heparin has a greater inhibitory effect on factor Xa, and less antithrombin activity than the high molecular weight fraction.

Heparin inhibits reactions that lead to clotting, but does not significantly alter the concentration of the normal clotting factors of blood. Although clotting time is prolonged by full therapeutic doses, in most cases it is not measurably affected by low doses of heparin. Bleeding time is usually unaffected. The drug has no fibrinolytic activity; it will not lyse existing clots, but it can prevent extension of existing clots.

Heparin also enhances lipoprotein lipase release, (which clears plasma of circulating lipids), increases circulating free fatty acids and reduces lipoprotein levels.

Pharmacokinetics: Absorption/Distribution – Heparin is not absorbed from the GI tract and must be given IV or SC. An IV bolus results in immediate anticoagulant effects. The duration of action is dose-dependent. Peak plasma levels of heparin are achieved 2 to 4 hours following SC administration, although there are considerable individual variations. Once absorbed, heparin is distributed in plasma and is extensively protein bound.

Metabolism/Excretion: Following administration, heparin demonstrates a biphasic elimination curve. The absence of a relationship between plasma half-life and pharmacologic half-life may reflect factors such as protein binding. Heparin is rapidly cleared from plasma with an average half-life of 30 to 180 minutes. The half-life of heparin is dose-dependent and may be significantly prolonged at higher doses (150 minutes at 400 units/kg). Heparin is partially metabolized by liver heparinase and by the reticuloendothelial system. There may be a secondary site of metabolism in the kidneys. Apparent volume of distribution is 40 to 60 ml/kg. In patients with deep venous thrombosis, the plasma clearance is more rapid and the half-life is shorter than in patients with pulmonary embolism. Heparin half-life may be prolonged in liver disease. Heparin is excreted in urine as unchanged drug (up to 50%) particularly after large doses. Some urinary degradation products have anticoagulant activity.

Indications:

Prophylaxis and treatment of venous thrombosis and its extension; pulmonary embolism; peripheral arterial embolism; atrial fibrillation with embolization.

Diagnosis and treatment of acute and chronic consumption coagulopathies (disseminated intravascular coagulation [DIC]).

Low dose regimen for prevention of postoperative deep venous thrombosis (DVT) and pulmonary embolism in patients undergoing major abdominothoracic surgery or patients who are at risk of developing thromboembolic disease.

According to the National Institutes of Health Consensus Development Conference, low-dose heparin is the treatment of choice as prophylaxis for DVT and pulmonary embolism in urology patients $>$ 40 years of age, pregnant patients with prior thromboembolism, stroke patients and patients with heart failure, acute MI or pulmonary infection; it is also recommended as a suggested prophylaxis in high-risk surgery patients, moderate and high-risk gynecologic patients without malignancy, neurology patients with extracranial problems and patients with severe musculoskeletal trauma.

Prevention of clotting in arterial and heart surgery, blood transfusions, extracorporeal circulation, dialysis procedures and blood samples for laboratory purposes.

(Indications continued on following page)

HEPARIN (Cont.)

Indications (Cont.):

Unlabeled uses: Prophylaxis of left ventricular thrombi and cerebrovascular accidents post-MI.

Continuous infusion for treatment of myocardial ischemia in unstable angina refractory to conventional treatment. Heparin decreases the number of anginal attacks and silent ischemic episodes and reduces the daily duration of ischemia. Intermittent heparin is not as effective.

Prevention of cerebral thrombosis in the evolving stroke.

As an adjunct in treatment of coronary occlusion with acute myocardial infarction (MI). Although there is some controversy regarding the efficacy of heparin therapy with concurrent antiplatelet therapy (eg, aspirin) in the prevention of rethrombosis/reocclusion after primary thrombolysis with thrombolytics (eg, alteplase, anistreplase, streptokinase) during acute MI, it is recommended by the American College of Cardiology and the American Heart Association. Generally, administer heparin IV immediately after thrombolytic therapy, usually within 2 to 8 hours (depending on the thrombolytic used), and maintain the infusion for at least 24 hours. Begin aspirin therapy immediately as soon as the patient is admitted, and continue its administration.

Contraindications:

Hypersensitivity to heparin; severe thrombocytopenia; uncontrolled bleeding (except when it is due to DIC); any patient for whom suitable blood coagulation tests cannot be performed at the appropriate intervals (there is usually no need to monitor coagulation parameters in patients receiving low-dose heparin).

Warnings:

IM administration: Avoid IM administration because of the danger of hematoma formation.

Hemorrhage can occur at virtually any site in patients receiving heparin. An unexplained fall in hematocrit, fall in blood pressure or any other unexplained symptom should lead to serious consideration of a hemorrhagic event. An overly prolonged coagulation test or bleeding can usually be controlled by withdrawing the drug. Signs and symptoms will vary according to the location and extent of bleeding and may present as paralysis, headache, chest, abdomen, joint or other pain, shortness of breath, difficulty breathing or swallowing, unexplained swelling or unexplained shock. GI or urinary tract bleeding may indicate an underlying occult lesion. Certain hemorrhagic complications may be difficult to detect.

Adrenal hemorrhage resulting in acute adrenal insufficiency has occurred. Discontinue therapy in patients who develop signs and symptoms of acute adrenal hemorrhage or insufficiency. Initiation of therapy should not depend on laboratory confirmation of diagnosis, since any delay in an acute situation may result in the patient's death.

Ovarian (corpus luteum) hemorrhage developed in a number of women of reproductive age receiving anticoagulants. This complication, if unrecognized, may be fatal.

Retroperitoneal hemorrhage may occur.

Germinal matrix-intraventricular hemorrhage occurs fourfold higher in low-birth-weight infants receiving heparin therapy.

Use heparin with extreme caution in disease states in which there is increased danger of hemorrhage. These include:

Cardiovascular – Subacute bacterial endocarditis; arterial sclerosis; dissecting aneurysm; increased capillary permeability; severe hypertension.

CNS – During and immediately following spinal tap, spinal anesthesia or major surgery, especially of the brain, spinal cord or eye.

Hematologic – Hemophilia; some vascular purpuras; thrombocytopenia.

GI – Ulcerative lesions, diverticulitis or ulcerative colitis; continuous tube drainage of the stomach or small intestine.

Obstetric – Threatened abortion; menstruation.

Other – Liver disease with impaired hemostasis; severe renal disease.

Hyperlipidemia: Heparin may increase free fatty acid serum levels by induction of lipoprotein lipase. The catabolism of serum lipoproteins by this enzyme produces lipid fragments which are rapidly processed by the liver. Patients with dysbetalipoproteinemia (type III) are unable to catabolize the lipid fragments, resulting in hyperlipidemia.

Benzyl alcohol, contained in some of these products as a preservative, has been associated with a fatal "gasping syndrome" in premature infants.

Resistance: Increased resistance to the drug is frequently encountered in fever, thrombosis, thrombophlebitis, infections with thrombosing tendencies, MI, cancer and postoperative states.

(Warnings continued on following page)

HEPARIN (Cont.)

Warnings (Cont.):

Thrombocytopenia has occurred in patients receiving heparin with a reported incidence of up to 30%. The development of thrombocytopenia does not necessarily imply a causal relationship. Often patients have other potential causes for thrombocytopenia; they can be ill, receiving several medications or in a postoperative phase. Exclude these potential causes for thrombocytopenia before implicating heparin. The incidence of heparin-associated thrombocytopenia is higher with bovine than with porcine heparin (15.6% vs 5.8%). The severity also appears to be related to the dose of heparin, with low-dose therapy resulting in fewer complications.

Early thrombocytopenia (Type I) develops 2 to 3 days after starting heparin, tends to be mild and is due to a direct action of heparin on platelets.

Delayed thrombocytopenia (Type II) develops 7 to 12 days after either low-dose or full-dose heparin, can have serious consequences and may reflect the presence of an immunoglobulin that induces platelet aggregation.

Mild thrombocytopenia (platelet count > 100,000/mm³) may remain stable or reverse even if heparin is continued. However, closely monitor thrombocytopenia of any degree. If a count falls below 100,000/mm³ or if recurrent thrombosis develops, discontinue heparin. If continued heparin therapy is essential, administration of heparin from a different organ source can be reinstituted with caution.

White clot syndrome – Rarely, patients may develop new thrombus formation in association with thrombocytopenia resulting from irreversible aggregation of platelets induced by heparin, the so-called "white clot syndrome." The process may lead to severe thromboembolic complications (eg, skin necrosis, gangrene of the extremities possibly leading to amputation, MI, pulmonary embolism, stroke, possibly death). Monitor platelet counts before and during therapy. If significant thrombocytopenia occurs, immediately terminate heparin and institute other therapeutic measures.

Hypersensitivity: Heparin is derived from animal tissue; use with caution in patients with a history of allergy. Before a therapeutic dose is given, a trial dose may be advisable. Have epinephrine 1:1000 immediately available. Refer to Management of Acute Hypersensitivity Reactions.

Vasospastic reactions may develop 6 to 10 days after starting therapy and last 4 to 6 hours. The affected limb is painful, ischemic and cyanotic. An artery to this limb may have been recently catheterized. After repeated injections, the reaction may gradually increase to generalized vasospasm with cyanosis, tachypnea, feeling of oppression and headache. Protamine sulfate has no marked effect. Itching and burning, especially on the plantar side of the feet, is possibly based on a similar allergic vasospastic reaction. Chest pain, elevated blood pressure, arthralgias or headache have also been reported in the absence of definite peripheral vasospasm.

Elderly: A higher incidence of bleeding has occurred in women > 60 years of age.

Pregnancy: Category C. Safety for use during pregnancy has not been established. Heparin does not cross the placenta. However, its use during pregnancy has been associated with 13% to 22% unfavorable outcomes, including stillbirths and prematurity. This contrasts with a 31% incidence with coumarin derivatives. Heparin is probably the preferred anticoagulant during pregnancy, but it is not risk free. Rare heparin-induced osteoporosis has occurred. Use with caution during pregnancy, especially during the last trimester and during the immediate postpartum period, because of the risk of maternal hemorrhage.

Lactation: Heparin is not excreted in breast milk.

Children: See Administration and Dosage. Safety and efficacy have not been determined in newborns; germinal matrix intraventricular hemorrhage occurs more often in low-birth-weight infants receiving heparin.

Use heparin lock flush solution with caution in infants with disease states in which there is an increased danger of hemorrhage. The use of the 100 unit/ml concentration is not advised because of the risk of bleeding, especially in low-birth-weight infants.

Precautions:

Hyperkalemia may develop, probably due to induced hypoaldosteronism. Use with caution in patients with diabetes or renal insufficiency. Monitor patient closely.

Monitoring: The most common test used to monitor heparin's effect is Activated Partial Thromboplastin Time (APTT). The APTT is widely used, quick, easily done and reproducible. Other tests used include Activated Coagulation Time (ACT) and Lee White-Whole Blood Clotting Time (WBCT). The ACT is also rapid and readily available. The WBCT is time consuming and unreliable; it is used as a standard with which to compare newer tests. If the coagulation test is unduly prolonged or if hemorrhage occurs, discontinue the drug promptly (see Overdosage). Perform periodic platelet counts, hematocrit and tests for occult blood in stool during the entire course of therapy, regardless of route of administration.

(Continued on following page)

HEPARIN (Cont.)

Drug Interactions:

Heparin Drug Interactions			
Precipitant drug	Object drug*		Description
Cephalosporins	Heparin	↑	Several parenteral cephalosporins have caused coagulopathies; this might be additive with heparin, possibly increasing the risk of bleeding.
Nitroglycerin	Heparin	↓	The pharmacologic effects of heparin may be decreased, although information on the interaction is conflicting.
Penicillins	Heparin	↑	Parenteral penicillins can produce alterations in platelet aggregation and coagulation tests. These effects might be additive with heparin, possibly increasing the risk of bleeding.
Salicylates	Heparin	↑	An increased risk of bleeding is possible during concurrent administration.

* ↑ = Object drug increased ↓ = Object drug decreased

Drug/Lab test interactions: Significant elevations of **aminotransferase** (AST and ALT) levels have occurred in a high percentage of patients. Cautiously interpret aminotransferase increases that might be caused by heparin.

If heparin comprises ≥ 10% of the total volume of a sample for blood gas analysis, errors in measurements of **carbon dioxide pressure, bicarbonate concentration** and **base excess** may occur.

Adverse Reactions:

Hemorrhage is the chief complication (≤ 10%). See Warnings.

Local: Avoid IM use. Local irritation, erythema, mild pain, hematoma or ulceration may follow deep SC use, but are more common after IM use. Histamine-like reactions and subcutaneous and cutaneous necrosis have been observed.

Hypersensitivity: Most common – Chills; fever; urticaria. *Rare* – Asthma; rhinitis; lacrimation; headache; nausea; vomiting; shock; anaphylactoid reactions. Allergic vasospastic reactions with painful, ischemic, cyanotic limbs may develop 6 to 10 days after starting therapy and last 4 to 6 hours. Whether these are identical to the thrombocytopenia-associated complications is undetermined. See Warnings.

Other: Thrombocytopenia (see Warnings); osteoporosis (after long-term, high doses); cutaneous necrosis, suppressed aldosterone synthesis, delayed transient alopecia, priapism, rebound hyperlipidemia (after discontinuation).

Overdosage:

Symptoms: Bleeding is the chief sign of heparin overdosage. Nosebleeds, hematuria or tarry stools may be the first sign of bleeding. Easy bruising or petechial formations may precede frank bleeding.

Treatment: Protamine sulfate (1% solution) will neutralize heparin (see individual monograph). Each mg of protamine neutralizes ≈ 100 USP heparin units.

Administration and Dosage:

Give by intermittent IV injection, continuous IV infusion or deep SC (ie, above the iliac crest of abdominal fat layer) injection. Avoid IM injection.

Continuous IV infusion is generally preferable due to the higher incidence of bleeding complications with other routes.

Adjust dosage according to coagulation test results prior to each injection. Dosage is adequate when WBCT is approximately 2.5 to 3 times control value, or when APTT is 1.5 to 2 times normal.

When given by continuous IV infusion, perform coagulation tests every 4 hours in the early stages. When administered by intermittent IV infusion, perform coagulation tests before each dose during early stages and at appropriate intervals thereafter. After deep SC injection, perform tests 4 to 6 hours after the injections.

(Administration and Dosage continued on following page)

HEPARIN (Cont.)

Administration and Dosage (Cont.):

General heparin dosage guidelines: Although dosage must be individualized, the following may be used as guidelines:

Heparin Dosage Guidelines		
Method of administration	Frequency	Recommended dose[1]
Subcutaneous[2]	Initial dose	10,000 – 20,000 units[3]
	Every 8 hours	8,000 – 10,000 units
	Every 12 hours	15,000 – 20,000 units
Intermittent IV	Initial dose	10,000 units[4]
	Every 4 to 6 hours	5,000 – 10,000 units[4]
IV Infusion	Continuous	20,000 – 40,000 units/day[3]

[1] Based on a 68 kg (150 lb) patient.
[2] Use a concentrated solution.
[3] Immediately preceded by IV loading dose of 5,000 units.
[4] Administer undiluted or in 50 to 100 ml 0.9% Sodium Chloride.

Children: In general, the following dosage schedule may be used as a guideline:

Initial dose – 50 units/kg IV bolus.

Maintenance dose – 100 units/kg/dose IV drip every 4 hours, or 20,000 units/m²/24 hours continuous IV infusion.

Low-dose prophylaxis of postoperative thromboembolism: Low-dose heparin prophylaxis, prior to and after surgery, will reduce the incidence of postoperative DVT in the legs and clinical pulmonary embolism. Give 5000 units SC 2 hours before surgery and 5000 units every 8 to 12 hours thereafter for 7 days or until the patient is fully ambulatory, whichever is longer. Administer by deep SC injection above the iliac crest or abdominal fat layer, arm or thigh using a concentrated solution. Use a fine guage needle (25 to 26 guage) to minimize tissue trauma. Reserve such prophylaxis for patients > 40 years of age undergoing major surgery. Exclude patients on oral anticoagulants or drugs that affect platelet function (see Drug Interactions) or in patients with bleeding disorders, brain or spinal cord injuries, spinal anesthesia, eye surgery or potentially sanguineous operations.

If bleeding occurs during or after surgery, discontinue heparin and neutralize with protamine sulfate. If clinical evidence of thromboembolism develops despite low-dose prophylaxis, give full therapeutic doses of anticoagulants until contraindicated. Prior to heparinization, rule out bleeding disorders; perform appropriate coagulation tests just prior to surgery. Coagulation test values should be normal or only slightly elevated at these times.

Surgery of the heart and blood vessels: Give an initial dose of not less than 150 units/kg to patients undergoing total body perfusion for open heart surgery. Often, 300 units/kg is used for procedures < 60 minutes and 400 units/kg is used for procedures > 60 minutes.

Extracorporeal dialysis: Follow equipment manufacturers' operating directions.

Blood transfusion: Add 400 to 600 units per 100 ml whole blood to prevent coagulation. Add 7500 units to 100 ml 0.9% Sodium Chloride Injection (or 75,000 units/L of 0.9% Sodium Chloride Injection); from this sterile solution, add 6 to 8 ml per 100 ml whole blood. Perform leukocyte counts on heparinized blood within 2 hours of addition of heparin. Do not use heparinized blood for isoagglutinin, complement, erythrocyte fragility tests or platelet counts.

Laboratory samples: Add 70 to 150 units per 10 to 20 ml sample of whole blood to prevent coagulation of sample. (See *Blood transfusion*.)

Clearing intermittent infusion (heparin lock) sets: To prevent clot formation in a heparin lock set, inject dilute heparin solution (Heparin Lock Flush Solution, USP; or a 10 to 100 units/ml heparin solution) via the injection hub in a quantity sufficient to fill the entire set to the needle tip. Replace this solution each time the heparin lock is used. Aspirate before administering any solution via the lock to confirm patency and location of needle or catheter tip. If the administered drug is incompatible with heparin, flush the entire heparin lock set with sterile water or normal saline before and after the medication is administered; following the second flush, the dilute heparin solution may be reinstilled into the set. Consult the set manufacturer's instructions.

Since repeated injections of small doses of heparin can alter APTT, obtain a baseline APTT prior to insertion of a heparin lock set.

(Administration and Dosage continued on following page)

HEPARIN (Cont.)

Administration and Dosage (Cont.):

Preparation of solution: Slight discoloration does not alter potency.

When heparin is added to infusion solution for continuous IV administration, invert container ≥ 6 times to ensure adequate mixing and to prevent pooling of heparin.

Converting to oral anticoagulant therapy: Perform baseline coagulation tests to determine prothrombin activity when heparin activity is too low to affect the prothrombin time (PT) or the International Normalized Ratio (INR). For immediate anticoagulant effect, give heparin in usual therapeutic doses. When the results of the initial prothrombin determinations are known, initiate the oral anticoagulant in the usual amount. Thereafter, perform coagulation tests and prothrombin activity at appropriate intervals. To ensure continuous anticoagulation, continue full heparin therapy for several days after the PT or INR has reached the therapeutic range. Heparin therapy may then be discontinued. Measure PT or INR at least 5 hours after last IV bolus dose and 24 hours after last SC dose of heparin. If continuous IV heparin infusion is used, PT or INR can usually be measured at any time. When the prothrombin activity reaches the desired therapeutic range, discontinue heparin and continue oral anticoagulants.

HEPARIN SODIUM INJECTION, USP

A sterile solution of heparin sodium in water for injection.

		Multiple Dose Vials		C.I.*
Rx	**Heparin Sodium** (Various, eg, Apothecon, Elkins-Sinn, Geneva, Lyphomed, Moore, Organon, Schein, Upjohn)	**Injection:** 1,000 units per ml	In 5, 10 and 30 ml vials.	3.1+
Rx	**Liquaemin Sodium**[1] (Organon)		In 10 and 30 ml vials.[2]	3.8
Rx	**Heparin Sodium** (Various, eg, Elkins-Sinn, Lyphomed, Organon, Schein, Upjohn, URL)	**Injection:** 5,000 units per ml	In 10 ml vials.	1.3+
Rx	**Liquaemin Sodium**[1] (Organon)		In 10 ml vials.[2]	2.8
Rx	**Heparin Sodium** (Various, eg, Elkins-Sinn, Lilly, Lyphomed, Moore, Organon, Pasadena, Schein, Upjohn)	**Injection:** 10,000 units per ml	In 4, 5 and 10 ml vials.	1.5+
Rx	**Liquaemin Sodium**[1] (Organon)		In 4 ml vials.[2]	2.4
Rx	**Heparin Sodium** (Various, eg, Lilly, Moore, Schein)	**Injection:** 20,000 units per ml	In 2, 5 and 10 ml vials.	1+
Rx	**Liquaemin Sodium**[1] (Organon)		In 2 and 5 ml vials.[2]	2.8
Rx	**Heparin Sodium** (Various, eg, Schein)	**Injection:** 40,000 units per ml	In 2 and 5 ml vials.	5.2+
		Single Dose Ampules and Vials		
Rx	**Heparin Sodium** (Various, eg, Lyphomed)	**Injection:** 1,000 units per ml	In 1 ml amps and vials.	22+
Rx	**Liquaemin Sodium Preservative Free**[1] (Organon)		In 1 ml amps.	NA
Rx	**Heparin Sodium** (Various, eg, Lyphomed, Organon, Upjohn)	**Injection:** 5,000 units per ml	In 1 ml vials.	4.4+
Rx	**Liquaemin Sodium Preservative Free**[1] (Organon)		In 1 ml amps.	NA
Rx	**Heparin Sodium** (Various, eg, Lyphomed, Organon, Pasadena, Upjohn, Winthrop)	**Injection:** 10,000 units per ml	In 1 ml vials.	2.9+
Rx	**Liquaemin Sodium Preservative Free**[1] (Organon)		In 1 ml amps.	NA
Rx	**Heparin Sodium** (Various, eg, Lyphomed, Schein)	**Injection:** 20,000 units per ml	In 1 ml vials.	2.9+
Rx	**Liquaemin Sodium**[1] (Organon)		In 1 ml vials.[2]	2.7
Rx	**Liquaemin Sodium**[1] (Organon)	**Injection:** 40,000 units per ml	In 1 ml vials.[2]	2.9

* Cost Index based on cost per 5,000 units.

[1] From porcine intestinal mucosa.

[2] With 1% benzyl alcohol.

(Continued on following page)

Complete prescribing information for these products begins on page 269

HEPARIN SODIUM INJECTION, USP (Cont.)

		Unit-Dose		C.I.*
Rx	**Heparin Sodium**[1] (Elkins-Sinn)	**Injection:** 1,000 units per dose	In 1 and 2 ml Dosette vials.[2]	13
Rx	**Heparin Sodium**[1] (Wyeth-Ayerst)		In 1 ml Tubex.[2]	21
Rx	**Heparin Sodium**[1] (Wyeth-Ayerst)	**Injection:** 2,500 units per dose	In 1 ml Tubex.[2]	20
Rx	**Heparin Sodium**[1] (Elkins-Sinn)	**Injection:** 5,000 units per dose	In 0.5 and 1 ml Dosette vial.[2]	3.5
Rx	**Heparin Sodium**[1] (Wyeth-Ayerst)		In 0.5 and 1 ml Tubex.[2]	9.3
Rx	**Heparin Sodium**[1] (Winthrop)		In 1 ml fill in 2 ml Carpuject.[2]	7.7
Rx	**Heparin Sodium**[1] (Wyeth-Ayerst)	**Injection:** 7,500 units per dose	In 1 ml Tubex.[2]	7.1
Rx	**Heparin Sodium**[1] (Elkins-Sinn)	**Injection:** 10,000 units per dose	In 0.5 and 1 ml Dosette vials.[2]	2.3
Rx	**Heparin Sodium**[1] (Wyeth-Ayerst)		In 1 ml Tubex.[2]	6.4
Rx	**Heparin Sodium**[1] (Wyeth-Ayerst)	**Injection:** 20,000 units per dose	In 1 ml Tubex.[2]	6

HEPARIN SODIUM AND SODIUM CHLORIDE

Rx	**Heparin Sodium**[1] **and 0.9% Sodium Chloride** (Clintec)	**Injection:** 1000 units 2000 units	In 500 ml Viaflex. In 1000 ml Viaflex.	203 108
Rx	**Heparin Sodium**[1] **and 0.45% Sodium Chloride** (Abbott)	**Injection:** 12,500 units 25,000 units	In 250 ml.[3] In 250 and 500 ml.[3]	21 11

HEPARIN CALCIUM INJECTION

A preservative free, sterile solution of heparin calcium in water.

				C.I.*
Rx	**Calciparine**[1] (DuPont)	**Injection:** 5,000 units per dose	In 0.2 ml disp. syringe.	14

HEPARIN SODIUM LOCK FLUSH SOLUTION

Used as an IV flush to maintain patency of indwelling IV catheters in intermittent IV therapy or blood sampling; not intended for therapeutic use.

				C.I.*
Rx	**Heparin Lock Flush** (Various, eg, Abbott, Lyphomed, Solopak, Winthrop, Wyeth-Ayerst)	**Injection:** 10 units per ml	In 1, 2, 5, 10 and 30 ml vials and 1, 2, 2.5, 3 and 5 ml disp. syringe.	162+
Rx	**Hep-Lock**[1] (Elkins-Sinn)		In 1 and 2 ml Dosette vials, 1 and 2.5 ml Dosette cartridge needle units and 10 and 30 ml vials.[2]	182
Rx	**Hep-Lock U/P**[1] (Elkins-Sinn)		Preservative free. In 1 ml Dosette vials.	NA
Rx	**Heparin Lock Flush** (Various, eg, Abbott, Lyphomed, Solopak, Winthrop, Wyeth-Ayerst)	**Injection:** 100 units per ml	In 1, 2, 5, 10 and 30 ml vials, 1 ml amps and 1, 2, 2.5, 3 and 5 ml disp. syringe.	16+
Rx	**Hep-Lock**[1] (Elkins-Sinn)		In 1 and 2 ml Dosette vials, 1 and 2.5 ml Dosette cartridge needle units and 10 and 30 ml vials.[2]	18
Rx	**Hep-Lock U/P**[1] (Elkins-Sinn)		Preservative free. In 1 ml Dosette vials.	NA

* Cost Index based on cost per 5000 units.
[1] From porcine intestinal mucosa.
[2] With benzyl alcohol.
[3] With EDTA.

Coumarin and Indandione Derivatives

Actions:

Pharmacology: Coumarins (warfarin) and indandiones (anisindione) interfere with the hepatic synthesis of vitamin K-dependent clotting factors (refer to the Anticoagulant introduction) which results in an in vivo depletion of clotting factors VII, IX, X and II (prothrombin). Anticoagulant effects are dependent on the half-lives of these clotting factors, which are 6, 24, 36 and 50 hours, respectively. Hence, the reduction in the rate of synthesis of the clotting factors determines the clinical response. Although factor VII is quickly depleted and an initial prolongation of the prothrombin time (PT) is seen in 8 to 12 hours, maximum anticoagulation (thus, antithrombotic effects) is not approached for 3 to 5 days as the other factors are depleted and the drug achieves steady state.

Oral anticoagulants have no direct effect on an established thrombus, nor do they reverse ischemic tissue damage. However, once thrombosis has occurred, anticoagulant treatment may prevent further extension of the formed clot and prevent secondary thromboembolic complications which may result in serious and possibly fatal sequelae.

Warfarin is available as a racemic mixture containing the R(+) and S(–) enantiomers in equal proportions; however, the S-isomer is 3 to 6 times more potent as an anticoagulant than the R-isomer.

Pharmacokinetics:

Various Pharmacokinetic Parameters of Oral Anticoagulants			
Oral anticoagulant	Half-life (days)	Peak activity (days)	Duration[1] (days)
Coumarin derivative			
Warfarin	1-2.5[2]	1.5-3	2-5
Indandione derivative			
Anisindione	3-5	2-3	1-3

[1]Following drug discontinuation [2]S-isomer ≈ 2 days; R-isomer ≈ 1.33 days

Absorption - The oral anticoagulants are generally rapidly and completely absorbed. Although serum levels are easily attained, therapeutic effect is more dependent on depletion of clotting factors; duration of effect may vary more in relation to their half-lives.

Distribution - Oral anticoagulants are highly bound to plasma proteins (97% to > 99%), primarily albumin. Therefore, potential exists for interaction with other drugs capable of displacing these agents from binding sites. (See Drug Interactions.)

Metabolism/Excretion - These agents are metabolized by hepatic microsomal enzymes and are excreted primarily in the urine and feces as inactive metabolites.

Indications:

Warfarin/Anisindione: Prophylaxis and treatment of venous thrombosis and its extension; treatment of atrial fibrillation with embolization; prophylaxis and treatment of pulmonary embolism.

Warfarin: Prophylaxis of atrial fibrillation with embolism. As an adjunct in the prophylaxis of systemic embolism after myocardial infarction (MI).

Anisindione: As an adjunct in the treatment of coronary occlusion.

Warfarin is generally the drug of choice. Anisindione has greater incidence of severe adverse reactions including cutaneous, hepatic and hematologic effects.

Unlabeled uses: Oral anticoagulants have been used to prevent recurrent transient ischemic attacks and to reduce the risk of recurrent MI, but data conflict. Warfarin has shown potential benefit as an adjunct in the treatment of small cell carcinoma of the lung, given concomitantly with chemotherapy and radiation.

Contraindications:

Pregnancy (see Warnings); hemorrhagic tendencies; hemophilia; thrombocytopenic purpura; leukemia; recent or contemplated surgery of the eye or CNS, major regional lumbar block anesthesia, or surgery resulting in large, open surfaces; patients bleeding from the GI, respiratory or GU tract; threatened abortion; aneurysm (cerebral, dissecting aortic); ascorbic acid deficiency; history of bleeding diathesis; prostatectomy; continuous tube drainage of the small intestine; polyarthritis; diverticulitis; emaciation; malnutrition; cerebrovascular hemorrhage; eclampsia and preeclampsia; blood dyscrasias; severe uncontrolled or malignant hypertension; severe renal or hepatic disease; pericarditis and pericardial effusion; subacute bacterial endocarditis; visceral carcinoma; following spinal puncture and other diagnostic or therapeutic procedures (ie, IUD insertion) with potential for uncontrollable bleeding; history of warfarin-induced necrosis.

(Continued on following page)

Warnings:

Monitoring: Prothrombin time (PT) – Treatment is highly individualized. Control dosage by periodic determination of PT or other suitable coagulation tests (eg, INR; see below). Whole blood clotting and bleeding times are not effective measures. Routine monitoring of the activated partial thromboplastin time (APTT) is not recommended when patients are receiving only oral anticoagulant therapy. Monitor PT daily during the initiation of therapy and whenever any other drug is added to or discontinued from therapy which may alter the patient's response (see Drug Interactions). Concurrent heparin therapy will elevate the PT 10% to 20%; if target PT levels are not increased by the same percentage during concurrent therapy, the patient could be inadequately anticoagulated when the heparin therapy is discontinued. Also, patients subject to factors rendering them more or less sensitive to anticoagulant therapy may require more frequent laboratory monitoring and dosage adjustment (see Precautions). Once stabilized, monitor PT every 4 to 6 weeks.

International Normalized Ratio (INR) – PT, the most common monitoring method for oral anticoagulation, is performed by adding a thromboplastin/calcium mixture to citrated plasma. However, thromboplastins vary greatly in their responsiveness to the anticoagulant effects depending on their source and method of preparation, differing not only between manufacturers but from lot to lot as well. Also, results vary among labs using different thromboplastins. This could result in inappropriate management of therapy.

Therefore, a system of standardizing the PT was introduced by the World Health Organization in 1983. It is based on the determination of an International Normalized Ratio which provides a common basis for PT results and interpretations of therapeutic ranges. The INR is derived from calibrations of commercial thromboplastin reagents against a sensitive human brain thromboplastin, the International Reference Preparation (IRP). It is recommended that laboratories adopt a standard thromboplastin and report PT as INR. For a discussion of the relationship between PT and INR in clinical practice, refer to Administration and Dosage.

Hemorrhage/Necrosis: The most serious risks associated with anticoagulant therapy are hemorrhage in any tissue or organ and, less frequently, necrosis or gangrene of skin and other tissues; this has resulted in death or permanent disability. The risk of hemorrhage is related to the level of intensity and duration of therapy. Necrosis appears to be associated with local thrombosis and usually appears within a few days of the start of therapy. In severe cases, debridement or amputation of the affected tissue, limb, breast or penis has been reported. Careful diagnosis is required to determine whether necrosis is caused by an underlying disease. Discontinue therapy when anticoagulants are the suspected cause of developing necrosis; consider heparin therapy.

Hemorrhagic tendency may be manifested by hematuria, skin petechiae, hemorrhage into or from a wound or ulcerating lesion or petechial and purpuric hemorrhages throughout the body. Caution patients to report any signs of bleeding, bruising, red or dark brown urine or black or red stools. Examine patients daily and test urine to detect hematuria. Bleeding complications in the GU tract may range in severity from microscopic to gross hematuria to extensive uterine hemorrhage. When an ulcerative lesion of the GI tract is suspected or when therapy is administered postoperatively to patients who have had an operative procedure on the GI tract, examine stools frequently for evidence of hemorrhage into the bowel. GI hemorrage may be secondary to peptic ulceration or silent neoplasm and is responsible for 25% of all deaths due to oral anticoagulant therapy.

Bleeding during anticoagulant therapy does not always correlate with prothrombin activity. Bleeding that occurs when the PT or INR is within the therapeutic range warrants investigation since it may unmask a previously unsuspected lesion (eg, tumor, ulcer).

Independent risk factors that may provide a basis for predicting major bleeding with anticoagulants include: $\geq$ 65 years of age; history of stroke; history of GI bleeding; serious comorbid condition (eg, recent MI, renal insufficiency, severe anemia); atrial fibrillation.

"Purple toe syndrome": Anticoagulant therapy may enhance the release of atheromatous plaque emboli thereby increasing the risk of complications from systemic cholesterol microembolization including the "purple toe syndrome." Discontinuation of therapy is recommended when such phenomena are observed. While the "purple toe syndrome" is reported to be reversible, other complications of microembolization may not be reversible.

Excessive uterine bleeding may occur, but menstrual flow is usually normal. Women may be at risk of developing ovarian hemorrhage at the time of ovulation.

Oral anticoagulants should not be used in the treatment of acute completed strokes due to the risk of fatal cerebral hemorrhage.

Adrenal hemorrhage with resultant acute adrenal insufficiency has occurred. Discontinue therapy if patients develop signs and symptoms of acute adrenal hemorrhage or insufficiency. Measure plasma cortisol levels and promptly institute aggressive IV corticosteroid therapy. Do not depend on laboratory confirmation of diagnosis before initiating therapy; any delay in an acute situation may result in death.

(Warnings continued on following page)

Coumarin and Indandione Derivatives (Cont.)

Warnings (Cont.):

Special risk patients: There is an increased risk with use of anticoagulants in the following conditions: Trauma; infection (concomitant antibiotic therapy may alter intestinal flora); renal insufficiency; prolonged dietary insufficiencies (eg, sprue, vitamin K deficiency); severe to moderate hypertension; polycythemia vera; vasculitis; severe allergic disorders; anaphylactic disorders; indwelling catheters; severe diabetes; surgery or trauma resulting in large exposed raw surfaces. Thoroughly evaluate the benefits vs the enhanced risk of hemorrhage, thrombosis or embolization.

Use with caution in patients with active tuberculosis, severe diabetes, history of ulcerative disease of the GI tract and during menstruation and the postpartum period.

Protein C deficiency: Known or suspected hereditary, familial or clinical deficiency in protein C has been associated with necrosis following warfarin therapy. Tissue necrosis may occur in the absence of protein C deficiency. Concurrent anticoagulation therapy with heparin for 5 to 7 days before initiation of warfarin therapy may minimize the incidence of this reaction. Discontinue therapy when warfarin is the suspected cause of developing necrosis. Suspect this condition if there is a history of recurrent episodes of thromboembolic disorders in the patient or in the family.

Agranulocytosis and hepatitis have been associated with anisindione use. Perform liver function and blood studies periodically. Instruct patients to report to the physician symptoms such as marked fatigue, chills, fever or sore throat; discontinue the drug promptly since these symptoms may signal the onset of severe toxicity. If leukopenia or evidence of hypersensitivity occurs, discontinue the drug. Test the urine periodically for albumin whenever anisindione is used because of the possibility of renal damage.

Rebound hypercoagulability was thought to occur upon sudden anticoagulant withdrawal, but has not been reproducible. Also there is no evidence that thrombosis will recur following abrupt withdrawal. Therefore, tapering the dose to discontinuation appears unnecessary, although tapering the dose gradually over 3 to 4 weeks is recommended if possible.

Hypersensitivity reactions (delayed) are rare and occur within 1 to 3 months following the start of anisindione; 10% of cases are fatal. Discontinue the medication at the first sign of hypersensitivity reactions. Symptoms include:

Dermatologic – Erythema to macular or eczematous rash; fatal exfoliative dermatitis; exudative erythema multiforme; alopecia.

Hematologic – Eosinophilia; leukopenia; thrombocytopenia; agranulocytosis; pancytopenia; neutropenia.

Renal – Nephropathy; nephritis; acute tubular necrosis; nephrotic azotemia; oliguria; anuria; albuminuria.

GI – Enanthema with diarrhea; severe stomatitis; ulcerative colitis; paralytic ileus.

Hepatic – Mixed hepatocellular damage; cholestasis; hepatitis; jaundice.

Other – Microadenopathy; fever.

Hepatic/Renal function impairment: Use with caution.

Elderly patients may be more sensitive to these agents.

Pregnancy: Category X. Oral anticoagulants pass the placental barrier. Fetal hemorrhage (possibly fatal), optic atrophy, brain abnormalities, diaphragmatic hernia, hydrocephaly, microcephaly, spontaneous abortion, stillbirth, congenital malformations including nasal hypoplasia and other abnormalities resembling chondrodysplasia punctata and CNS defects and prematurity may occur. Approximately 30% of exposed fetuses may experience a problem related to anticoagulants.

If a patient becomes pregnant during therapy, apprise her of the potential risks to the fetus, and discuss the possibility of terminating the pregnancy. If oral anticoagulants are used in pregnant women, do not administer during the first trimester, and discontinue prior to labor and delivery.

Some clinicians suggest the replacement of oral anticoagulants with heparin therapy before term. Heparin is withheld during early labor and reinstituted 6 hours postpartum. After 5 to 7 days, therapy with oral anticoagulants may be resumed if indicated.

Lactation: Warfarin appears in breast milk in an inactive form. Infants nursed by warfarin-treated mothers had no change in PT. Effects in premature infants have not been evaluated.

Anisindione or its metabolites may be excreted in breast milk in amounts sufficient to cause a prothrombopenic state and bleeding in the newborn.

Children: Safety and efficacy in children < 18 years old have not been established. Oral anticoagulants may be beneficial in children with rare thromboembolic disorder secondary to other disease states such as the nephrotic syndrome or congenital heart lesions. Heparin is probably the initial anticoagulant of choice because of its immediate onset of action.

(Continued on following page)

Coumarin and Indandione Derivatives (Cont.)

Precautions:

Patient selection: Use care in the selection of patients to ensure cooperation, especially from alcoholic, senile or psychotic patients.

Enhanced anticoagulant effects: Several endogenous factors that may result in an increased response to the oral anticoagulants or an increased PT or INR include: Carcinoma; hepatic disorders including hepatitis or obstructive jaundice; biliary fistula; febrile states; preparatory bowel sterilization; recent surgery; x-ray therapy; vitamin K deficiency; steatorrhea; CHF; diarrhea; poor nutritional state or collagen disease; renal insufficiency; hyperthyroidism. Also, female and elderly patients are more sensitive to these agents.

Decreased anticoagulant effects: Endogenous factors that may reduce the response to the oral anticoagulants or decrease the PT or INR include: Edema; hyperlipidemia; diabetes mellitus; hypothyroidism; hereditary resistance to oral anticoagulants. Patients with a genetic resistance to oral anticoagulants also have an increased need for vitamin K.

Tartrazine sensitivity: Some of these products contain tartrazine, which may cause allergic-type reactions (including bronchial asthma) in susceptible individuals. Although the incidence of tartrazine sensitivity in the general population is low, it is frequently seen in patients who also have aspirin hypersensitivity. Specific products containing tartrazine are identified in the product listings.

Drug Interactions:

The oral anticoagulants have a great potential for clinically significant drug interactions. Warn all patients about potential hazards and instruct against taking **any** drug, including nonprescription products, without the advice of a physician or pharmacist. In addition, advise against sudden change in life habits (eg, drastic change in diet or alcohol consumption).

Careful monitoring and appropriate dosage adjustments usually will permit safe administration of combined therapy. Critical times during therapy occur when an interacting drug is added to or discontinued from a patient stabilized on anticoagulants.

Oral Anticoagulant Drug Interactions				
Precipitant drug		Object drug*		Description
Acetaminophen Androgens Beta blockers Clofibrate Corticosteroids Cyclophosphamide Dextrothyroxine Disulfiram Erythromycin Fluconazole Gemfibrozil Glucagon Hydantoins[1]	Influenza virus vaccine Isoniazid Ketoconazole Miconazole Moricizine Propoxyphene Quinolones Sulfonamides Tamoxifen Thioamines Thyroid hormones	Anticoagulants	↑	These agents may increase the anticoagulant effect of warfarin or anisindione. The risk of bleeding may be increased. The mechanism of the interaction is unknown or complicated.
Amiodarone Chloramphenicol Cimetidine Ifosfamide[2] Lovastatin Metronidazole Omeprazole	Phenylbutazones[2] Propafenone Quinidine Quinine SMZ-TMP Sulfinpyrazone	Anticoagulants	↑	These agents may increase the anticoagulant effect of warfarin or anisindione due to inhibition of the anticoagulant's hepatic metabolism. The risk of bleeding may be increased.
Chloral hydrate Loop diuretics Nalidixic acid		Anticoagulants	↑	These agents may increase the anticoagulant effect of warfarin or anisindione due to displacement from binding sites. The risk of bleeding may be increased.
Aminoglycosides Mineral oil Tetracyclines Vitamin E		Anticoagulants	↑	These agents may increase the anticoagulant effect of warfarin or anisindione due to interference with vitamin K. The risk of bleeding may be increased.

* ↑ = Object drug increased

[1] Hydantoin serum levels may also be increased.

[2] May also displace the anticoagulant from protein binding sites.

(Drug Interactions continued on following page)

Coumarin and Indandione Derivatives (Cont.)

Drug Interactions (Cont.):

Oral Anticoagulant Drug Interactions				
Precipitant drug		Object drug*		Description
Cephalosporins[1] Diflunisal NSAIDs Penicillins Salicylates		Anticoagulants	↑	These agents may increase the anticoagulant effect of warfarin and increase the risk of bleeding due to effects on platelet function, and, in the case of NSAIDs, GI irritant effects.
Ascorbic acid Dicloxacillin Ethanol[2] Ethchlorvynol	Griseofulvin Nafcillin Sucralfate Trazodone	Anticoagulants	↓	These agents may decrease the anticoagulant effect of warfarin or anisindione. The mechanism of the interaction is unknown.
Aminoglutethimide Barbiturates Carbamazepine	Etretinate Glutethimide Rifampin	Anticoagulants	↓	These agents may decrease the anticoagulant effect of warfarin or anisindione due to induction of the anticoagulant's hepatic microsomal enzymes.
Cholestyramine[3] Contraceptives, oral[4] Estrogens[4]	Thiopurines[5] Spironolactone[6] Thiazide diuretics[6] Vitamin K[7]	Anticoagulants	↓	These agents may decrease the anticoagulant effect of warfarin or anisindione due to various mechanisms.

* ↑ = Object drug increased ↓ = Object drug decreased

1 Those agents with a methyltetrazolethiol side chain.

2 Chronic consumption may increase the clearance of the anticoagulant; moderate to small doses do not alter the anticoagulant effect.

3 Reduced anticoagulant absorption and possibly increased elimination.

4 Increased risk of thromboembolism in rare instances which is in contrast to the intended effect of the anticoagulant.

5 Thiopurine-induced increase in synthesis or activation of prothrombin.

6 Diuretic-induced hemoconcentration of clotting factors.

7 Vitamin K overcomes interference of vitamin K-dependent clotting factors by anticoagulants.

Drug/Lab test interaction: Oral anticoagulants may cause red-orange discoloration of alkaline urine; this may interfere with some lab tests.

Adverse Reactions:

Hemorrhage is the principal adverse effect of oral anticoagulants; skin necrosis has occurred rarely (see Warnings). Hemorrhage from any tissue or organ is a consequence of the anticoagulant effect. The signs and symptoms will vary according to the location and degree or extent of the bleeding. Hemorrhagic complications may present as: Paralysis; headache; chest, abdomen, joint or other pain; shortness of breath; difficult breathing or swallowing; unexplained swelling; unexplained shock. Therefore, consider the possibility of hemorrhage in evaluating the condition of any anticoagulated patient with complaints that do not indicate an obvious diagnosis.

Other adverse reactions include: Nausea; diarrhea; pyrexia; dermatitis; exfoliative dermatitis; urticaria; alopecia; sore mouth; mouth ulcers; red-orange urine; priapism (causal relationship not established); paralytic ileus and intestinal obstruction from submucosal or intramural hemorrhage.

Warfarin: Other side effects are infrequent and include:

Cutaneous – Necrosis or gangrene of the skin and other tissues (see Warnings).

GI – Vomiting; anorexia; abdominal cramping; diarrhea; hepatotoxicity; cholestatic jaundice.

Miscellaneous – Fever; systemic cholesterol microembolization ("purple toes" syndrome; see Warnings); hypersensitivity reactions (see Warnings); compressive neuropathy secondary to hemorrhage adjacent to a nerve (rare); leukopenia.

(Adverse Reactions continued on following page)

Adverse Reactions (Cont.):

Anisindione: Dermatitis has been the only reported reaction consistently associated with anisindione. The following reactions have been reported with other indandione anticoagulants and therefore might also occur with anisindione: Headache; sore throat; blurred vision; paralysis of accommodation; steatorrhea; hepatitis; liver damage; renal tubular necrosis; albuminuria; anuria; myeloid immaturity; leukocyte agglutinins; red cell aplasia; atypical mononuclear cells; leukopenia; leukocytosis; anemia; thrombocytopenia; eosinophilia; agranulocytosis; jaundice; nephropathy.

Overdosage:

Symptoms: Early – Microscopic hematuria; excessive menstrual bleeding; melena; petechiae; oozing from superficial injuries (eg, nicks made by shaving, bleeding from gums after brushing teeth, excessive bruising).

Treatment: Excessive anticoagulation, with or without bleeding, is readily controlled by discontinuing therapy and, if necessary, by administration of oral or parenteral phytonadione (see individual monograph).

In excessive prothrombinopenia with mild or no bleeding, omission of one or more doses may suffice; if necessary, give small doses of oral phytonadione (2.5 to 10 mg). If minor bleeding persists or progresses to frank bleeding, give 5 to 25 mg parenteral phytonadione. Such use of phytonadione reduces response to subsequent anticoagulant therapy; therefore, use caution in determining the need for this vitamin. A hypercoagulable state may occur following the rapid reversal of a prolonged PT or INR. Smaller doses (5 to 15 mg) of phytonadione may be sufficient, except in cases of severe hemorrhage.

In emergency situations, clotting factors can be returned to normal by administering 200 to 500 ml of fresh frozen plasma or by giving commercial Factor IX complex. Consider fresh whole blood transfusions in cases of severe bleeding or prothrombinopenic states unresponsive to phytonadione. Purified Factor IX preparations should not be used because they cannot increase the levels of prothrombin. Factor VII and Factor X are also depressed along with the levels of Factor IX as a result of warfarin treatment. Packed red blood cells may also be given if significant blood loss has occurred. Carefully monitor infusions of blood or plasma to avoid precipitating pulmonary edema in elderly patients or patients with heart disease.

Resumption of anticoagulant administration reverses the effect of phytonadione and a therapeutic PT or INR can again be obtained by careful dosage adjustment.

Patient Information:

Dosing is highly individual and may have to be adjusted several times based on lab test results. Strict adherence to prescribed dosage schedule is necessary.

Do not take or discontinue any other medication, except on advice of physician or pharmacist. Avoid alcohol, salicylates and drastic changes in dietary habits.

Oral anticoagulants may cause a red-orange discoloration of alkaline urine.

Notify physician if unusual bleeding or bruising, red or dark brown urine (blood), red or tar black stools or diarrhea occurs.

Do not change from one brand to another without consulting a physician or pharmacist.

Consult physician before undergoing dental work or elective surgery.

Administration and Dosage:

Dosage: Individualize dosage. Adjust the dosage based on the results of the one stage PT. Different thromboplastin reagents vary substantially in their responsiveness to warfarin-induced effects on PT. To define the appropriate therapeutic regimen it is important to be familiar with the sensitivity of the thromboplastin reagent used in the laboratory and its relationship to the International Reference Preparation (IRP), a sensitive thromboplastin reagent prepared from human brain.

Early clinical studies of oral anticoagulants, which formed the basis for recommended therapeutic ranges of 1.5 to 2.5 times control PT, used sensitive human brain thromboplastin. When using the less sensitive rabbit brain thromboplastins commonly employed in PT assays today, adjustments must be made to the targeted PT range that reflect this decrease in sensitivity. Available clinical evidence indicates that prolongation of the PT to 1.2 to 1.5 times control, when measuring with the less sensitive thromboplastin reagents, is sufficient for prophylaxis and treatment of venous thromboembolism and minimizes the risk of hemorrhage associated with more prolonged PT values. In cases where the risk of thromboembolism is great, such as in patients with recurrent systemic embolism, maintain a PT of 1.5 to 2 times control. A ratio of > 2 appears to provide no additional therapeutic benefit in most patients and is associated with a higher risk of bleeding.

(Administration and Dosage continued on following page)

Coumarin and Indandione Derivatives (Cont.)

Administration and Dosage (Cont.):

Dosage (Cont.):

For the three commercial rabbit brain thromboplastins currently used in North America, a PT ratio of 1.3 to 2 is equivalent to an INR of 2 to 4. For other thromboplastins, the INR can be calculated as:

$$INR = (\text{observed PT ratio})^{ISI}$$

where the ISI (International Sensitivity Index) is the calibration factor and is available from the manufacturers of the thromboplastin reagent and observed PT ratio is:

$$\frac{\text{PT observed}}{\text{PT control}}$$

Following are the recommended therapeutic ranges for oral anticoagulant therapy from the American College of Chest Physicians (ACCP) and the National Heart, Lung and Blood Institute (NHLBI):

ACCP/NHLBI Recommended Therapeutic Range for Oral Anticoagulant Therapy		
Condition	PT ratio[1]	INR
Acute MI[2]	1.3 to 1.5	2 to 3
Atrial fibrillation[2]	1.3 to 1.5	2 to 3
Mechanical prosthetic valves	1.5 to 2	3 to 4.5
Pulmonary embolism, treatment	1.3 to 1.5	2 to 3
Systemic embolism		
Prevention	1.3 to 1.5	2 to 3
Recurrent	1.5 to 2	3 to 4.5
Tissue heart valves[2]	1.3 to 1.5	2 to 3
Valvular heart disease[2]	1.3 to 1.5	2 to 3
Venous thrombosis		
Prophylaxis (high-risk surgery)	1.3 to 1.5	2 to 3
Treatment	1.3 to 1.5	2 to 3

[1] ISI of 2.4
[2] To prevent systemic embolism

Loading dose: Heparin is preferred if rapid anticoagulation is necessary. Administer oral anticoagulants at anticipated maintenance dosage levels or a slightly higher loading dose (eg, 10 mg/day of warfarin for 2 to 4 days); then adjust the daily dosage based on the results of PT or INR determinations. Use of a large loading dose (eg, 30 mg warfarin) may increase incidence of bleeding complications; it does not offer more rapid protection vs thrombi formation, and is not recommended.

Transfer from heparin therapy: To provide continuous adequate anticoagulation in a patient on heparin, switch to oral anticoagulation. Since there is a delayed onset of oral anticoagulant effects, give heparin and warfarin simultaneously from the first day, or alternatively, start warfarin on the third to sixth day of heparin therapy. Use concurrent therapy until a therapeutic PT or INR is achieved.

Elderly: Lower dosages are recommended.

Duration of therapy: In the determination of the duration of long-term anticoagulant therapy, consider history of recurrent thromboembolism, underlying diseases, reason for anticoagulant therapy (eg, atrial fibrillation) and risks of adverse effects.

Treatment during dentistry and surgery (warfarin): The management of patients who undergo dental and surgical procedures requires close liaison between attending physicians, surgeons and dentists. In patients who must be anticoagulated prior to, during or immediately following dental or surgical procedures, adjusting the dosage to maintain the PT at the low end of the therapeutic range (or maintain the corresponding INR value) may safely allow for continued anticoagulation. Limit the operative site to permit effective use of local measures for hemostasis. Under these conditions, dental and surgical procedures may be performed without undue risk of hemorrhage.

Minidose warfarin may be beneficial as prophylaxis against venous thrombosis after major surgery. In one study, 1 mg daily given before surgery (mean 20 days) significantly lowered the incidence of DVT compared to controls; there was no difference between the 1 mg/day and the full-dose anticoagulation group. APTT and PT were not prolonged beyond normal on the day of surgery using the minidose therapy.

(Products listed on following page)

Complete prescribing information for these products begins on page 277.

Coumarin and Indandione Derivatives (Cont.)

WARFARIN SODIUM

Dosage[1]:

Induction: Initiate with 10 mg/day for 2 to 4 days; adjust daily dosage according to PT or INR determinations. Use of a large loading dose (eg, 30 mg) may increase the incidence of hemorrhagic and other complications, does not offer more rapid protection against thrombi formation and is not recommended.

Elderly/Debilitated patients or patients with increased sensitivity: Use lower dose.

Maintenance: 2 to 10 mg daily, based on PT or INR.

Bioequivalence problems have been documented for warfarin sodium products marketed by different manufacturers. Brand interchange is not recommended. **C.I.***

	Product	Form	Description	C.I.*
Rx	**Coumadin** (DuPont)	**Tablets:** 1 mg	Lactose. (Coumadin 1). Pink, scored. In 100s, 1000s and UD 100s.	17
Rx	**Warfarin Sodium** (Various, eg, Major, PBI)	**Tablets:** 2 mg	In 100s, 250s, 500s, 1000s and UD 100s.	1.8+
Rx	**Coumadin** (DuPont)		Lactose. (Coumadin 2). Lavender, scored. In 100s, 1000s and UD 100s.	8.8
Rx	**Panwarfin** (Abbott)		Lactose. (2). Lavender. In 100s and UD 100s.	6
Rx	**Sofarin** (Lemmon)		Lactose. (832 Warfarin 2). Lavender, scored. In 100s.	10
Rx	**Warfarin Sodium** (Various, eg, Major, Parmed, PBI)	**Tablets:** 2.5 mg	In 100s, 250s, 500s, 1000s and UD 100s.	1.5+
Rx	**Coumadin** (DuPont)		Lactose. (Coumadin 2½). Green, scored. In 100s, 1000s and UD 100s.	7.3
Rx	**Panwarfin** (Abbott)		Lactose. Orange. In 100s and UD 100s.	5
Rx	**Sofarin** (Lemmon)		Lactose. (832 Warfarin 2½). Orange, scored. In 100s.	5
Rx	**Warfarin Sodium** (Various, eg, Major, Parmed, PBI)	**Tablets:** 5 mg	In 100s, 250s, 500s, 1000s and UD 100s.	1+
Rx	**Coumadin** (DuPont)		Lactose. (Coumadin 5). Peach, scored. In 100s, 1000s and UD 100s.	3.8
Rx	**Panwarfin** (Abbott)		Lactose. (5). Peach. In 100s, 500s and UD 100s.	2.5
Rx	**Sofarin** (Lemmon)		Lactose. (93 Sofarin 5). Pink, scored. In 100s and 1000s.	2.8
Rx	**Warfarin Sodium** (Major)	**Tablets:** 7.5 mg	In 100s.	1+
Rx	**Coumadin** (DuPont)		Lactose. (Coumadin 7½). Yellow, scored. In 100s & UD 100s.	3.8
Rx	**Panwarfin** (Abbott)		Lactose, tartrazine. Yellow. In 100s & UD 100s.	2
Rx	**Coumadin** (DuPont)	**Tablets:** 10 mg	Dye free. Lactose. (Coumadin 10). White, scored. In 100s and UD 100s.	2.8
Rx	**Panwarfin** (Abbott)		Lactose. (10). White. In 100s and UD 100s.	1.8

ANISINDIONE

Dosage[1]:

300 mg the first day, 200 mg the second day, 100 mg the third day and 25 to 250 mg daily for maintenance. **C.I.***

	Product	Form	Description	C.I.*
Rx	**Miradon** (Schering)	**Tablets:** 50 mg	Lactose. (ANK or 795). Pink, scored. In 100s.	3.3

* Cost Index based on cost per minimum daily maintenance dose.

[1] Refer to Administration and Dosage section for further information about initial, induction or loading doses.

PROTAMINE SULFATE

Actions:

Pharmacology: Protamines are strongly basic simple proteins of low molecular weight, rich in arginine. They occur in sperm of salmon and certain other fish species. Given alone, protamine sulfate has an anticoagulant effect. However, when given with heparin (strongly acidic), a stable salt forms resulting in loss of anticoagulant activity of both drugs.

Pharmacokinetics: Protamine sulfate has a rapid onset of action which persists approximately 2 hours. Heparin is neutralized within 5 minutes after IV injection. The metabolic fate of the heparin-protamine complex is not known, but one theory is that protamine sulfate in the heparin-protamine complex may be partially metabolized or may be cleaved by fibrinolysin, thus freeing heparin.

Indications:

Treatment of heparin overdosage.

Contraindications:

Hypersensitivity to the drug.

Warnings:

Recurrent bleeding: Hyperheparinemia or bleeding has occurred in some patients 30 minutes to 18 hours after cardiac surgery (under cardiopulmonary bypass) in spite of complete neutralization of heparin by adequate doses of protamine at the end of the operation. Therefore, observe patients closely after cardiac surgery. Administer additional doses of protamine sulfate if indicated by coagulation studies, such as the heparin titration test with protamine activated clotting time (ACT) or activated partial thromboplastin time (APTT) and the plasma thrombin time.

Too rapid administration can cause severe hypotensive and anaphylactoid reactions. Have facilities available to treat shock.

Pulmonary edema: High-protein, noncardiogenic pulmonary edema associated with the use of protamine has occurred in patients on cardiopulmonary bypass who are undergoing cardiovascular surgery. The etiologic role of protamine in the pathogenesis of this condition is uncertain, and multiple factors have been present in most cases. The condition has been reported in association with administration of certain blood products, other drugs, cardiopulmonary bypass alone, and other etiologic factors. It is difficult to treat, and it can be life-threatening.

Circulatory collapse, severe and potentially irreversible, associated with myocardial failure and reduced cardiac output, can also occur. The mechanism(s) of this reaction and the role played by concurrent factors are unclear.

Hypersensitivity: Patients with a history of allergy to fish may develop hypersensitivity reactions, although, to date, no relationship has been established between allergic reactions to protamine and fish allergy.

Previous exposure to protamine through use of protamine-containing insulins or during heparin neutralization may predispose susceptible individuals to the development of untoward reactions from the subsequent use of this drug. Reports of the presence of antiprotamine antibodies in the serums of infertile or vasectomized men suggest that some of these individuals may react to use of protamine sulfate.

Complete activation by the heparin-protamine complexes, release of lysosomal enzymes from neutrophils, and prostaglandin and thromboxane generation have been associated with the development of anaphylactoid reactions. Fatal anaphylaxis has been reported in one patient with no prior history of allergies. Give protamine only when resuscitation techniques and treatment of anaphylactic and anaphylactoid shock are readily available. Have epinephrine 1:1000 immediately available. Refer to Management of Acute Hypersensitivity Reactions.

Pregnancy: Category C. It is not known whether the drug can cause fetal harm when administered to a pregnant woman or can affect reproduction capacity. Administer to a pregnant woman only if clearly needed.

Lactation: It is not known whether this drug is excreted in breast milk. Administer cautiously to a nursing mother.

Children: Safety and efficacy in children have not been established.

Precautions:

Anticoagulant effects: Because of the anticoagulant effect, do not give > 100 mg over a short period unless a larger requirement is necessary.

Heparin rebound: Protamine sulfate can be inactivated by blood; when it is used to neutralize large doses of heparin, a heparin "rebound" may be encountered. This complication is treated by additional protamine sulfate injections as needed.

(Continued on following page)

PROTAMINE SULFATE (Cont.)

Adverse Reactions:

Sudden fall in blood pressure; bradycardia; transitory flushing and feeling of warmth; dyspnea; nausea; vomiting; lassitude; pulmonary edema (see Warnings); back pain in conscious patients undergoing such procedures as cardiac catheterization; anaphylaxis that may result in severe respiratory distress, circulatory collapse, capillary leak and noncardiogenic pulmonary edema (see Warnings); acute pulmonary hypertension; circulatory collapse (see Warnings).

Overdosage:

Symptoms: Overdose of protamine sulfate may cause bleeding. Protamine has a weak anticoagulant effect due to an interaction with platelets and with many proteins including fibrinogen. Distinguish this effect from the rebound anticoagulation that may occur 30 minutes to 18 hours following the reversal of heparin with protamine.

Rapid administration of protamine is more likely to result in bradycardia, dyspnea, a sensation of warmth, flushing and severe hypotension. Hypertension has also occurred.

The median lethal dose of protamine sulfate in mice is 100 mg/kg. Serum concentrations of protamine sulfate are not clinically useful. Information is not available on the amount of drug in a single dose that is associated with overdosage or is likely to be life-threatening.

Treatment: In managing overdosage, consider the possibility of multiple drug overdoses, interaction among drugs and unusual drug kinetics.

Replace blood loss with blood transfusions or fresh frozen plasma. If the patient is hypotensive, consider fluids, epinephrine, dobutamine or dopamine. Refer to Management of Acute Overdosage.

Administration and Dosage:

Protamine sulfate 1 mg neutralizes approximately 90 USP units of heparin activity derived from lung tissue or about 115 USP units derived from intestinal mucosa.

Since heparin disappears rapidly from circulation, the protamine dose required also decreases rapidly with time elapsed since IV heparin injection. For example, if protamine is given 30 minutes after heparin, half the usual dose may be sufficient.

Give very slowly IV over 10 minutes in doses not to exceed 50 mg. Guide dosage by blood coagulation studies.

Incompatibilities: Certain antibiotics, including several cephalosporins and penicillins.

Prepared solution: Protamine sulfate injection is for use without further dilution; if further dilution is desired, use Dextrose 5% in Water or normal saline.

Storage/Stability: Refrigerate at 2° to 8°C (36° to 46°F); Do not store diluted solutions; they contain no preservative. **C.I.***

Rx	**Protamine Sulfate** (Various, eg, Elkins-Sinn, Lilly, Lyphomed)	**Injection:** 10 mg/ml	In 5 and 25 ml amps and 5, 10 and 25 ml vials.	383+

* Cost Index based on cost per 10 mg.

ALTEPLASE, RECOMBINANT

Actions:

Alteplase, a tissue plasminogen activator (tPA) produced by recombinant DNA, is used in the management of acute myocardial infarction (AMI). It is a sterile, purified glycoprotein of 527 amino acids. It is synthesized using the complementary DNA (cDNA) for natural human tissue-type plasminogen activator obtained from a human melanoma cell line.

Biological potency, determined by an in vitro clot lysis assay, is expressed in International Units as tested against the WHO standard. The specific activity is 580,000 IU/mg.

Pharmacology: Mechanism – Alteplase is an enzyme (serine protease) which has the property of fibrin-enhanced conversion of plasminogen to plasmin. It produces limited conversion of plasminogen in the absence of fibrin. When introduced into the systemic circulation at pharmacologic concentration, alteplase binds to fibrin in a thrombus and converts the entrapped plasminogen to plasmin. This initiates local fibrinolysis with limited systemic proteolysis. Following administration of 100 mg, there is a decrease (16% to 36%) in circulating fibrinogen. In a controlled trial, 8 of 73 patients (11%) receiving alteplase (1.25 mg/kg over 3 hours) experienced a decrease in fibrinogen to below 100 mg/dl.

Pharmacokinetics: Alteplase is cleared rapidly from circulating plasma at a rate of 550 to 680 ml/min, primarily by the liver. More than 50% present in plasma is cleared within 5 minutes after the infusion has been terminated, and approximately 80% is cleared within 10 minutes.

Clinical trials: AMI – Coronary occlusion due to a thrombus is present in the infarct-related coronary artery in approximately 80% of patients experiencing a transmural myocardial infarction evaluated within 4 hours of onset of symptoms.

In patients studied in a controlled trial with coronary angiography at 90 and 120 minutes following infusion, infarct artery patency was observed in 71% and 85% of patients (n = 85), respectively. In a second study, patients received coronary angiography prior to and following infusion within 6 hours of symptoms; reperfusion of the obstructed vessel occurred within 90 minutes after the commencement of therapy in 71% of 83 patients.

In a double-blind randomized trial (138 patients), patients infused with alteplase within 4 hours of onset of symptoms experienced improved left ventricular function at day 10, compared to the placebo group, when ejection fraction was measured by gated blood pool scan (53.2% vs 46.4%). Relative to baseline (day 1) values, the net changes in ejection fraction were +3.6% and –4.7% for the treated and placebo group, respectively. Also, there was a reduced incidence of clinical congestive heart failure (CHF) in the treated group (14%) compared to the placebo group (33%).

In a second double-blind randomized trial (136 patients), patients infused with alteplase within 2.5 hours of onset of symptoms experienced improved left ventricular function at a mean of 21 days, compared to the placebo group, when ejection fraction was measured by gated blood pool scan (54% vs 48%) and by contrast ventriculogram (62% vs 54%). Although the contribution of tPA alone is unclear, the incidence of non-ischemic cardiac complications when taken as a group (ie, CHF, pericarditis, atrial fibrillation, conduction disturbance) was reduced when compared to placebo patients.

Pulmonary emboli – In a comparative randomized trial (n = 45), 59% of 22 patients treated with alteplase (100 mg over 2 hours) experienced moderate or marked lysis of pulmonary emboli when assessed by pulmonary angiography 2 hours after treatment initiation. Alteplase patients also experienced a significant reduction in pulmonary embolism-induced pulmonary hypertension within 2 hours of treatment. Pulmonary perfusion at 24 hours was significantly improved.

Indications:

Acute myocardial infarction: Management of AMI in adults for the lysis of thrombi obstructing coronary arteries, the improvement of ventricular function and reduction of the incidence of CHF.

Start treatment as soon as possible after the onset of AMI symptoms.

Pulmonary embolism: Management of acute massive pulmonary embolism (PE) in adults.

For the lysis of acute pulmonary emboli, defined as obstruction of blood flow to a lobe or multiple segments of the lungs, and for the lysis of pulmonary emboli accompanied by unstable hemodynamics, eg, failure to maintain blood pressure without supportive measures.

Confirm the diagnosis by objective means, such as pulmonary angiography or noninvasive procedures such as lung scanning.

Unlabeled uses: Alteplase has been investigated in the treatment of unstable angina pectoris. In patients with unstable angina pectoris, alteplase may result in coronary thrombolysis and reduction of ischemic events.

(Continued on following page)

ALTEPLASE, RECOMBINANT (Cont.)

Contraindications:

Because thrombolytic therapy increases risk of bleeding, alteplase is contraindicated in: Active internal bleeding; history of cerebrovascular accident; recent (within 2 months) intracranial or intraspinal surgery or trauma; intracranial neoplasm, arteriovenous malformation or aneurysm; bleeding diathesis; severe uncontrolled hypertension.

Warnings:

Bleeding is the most common complication. The bleeding associated with thrombolytic therapy can be divided into two broad categories:

1) Internal bleeding involving the GI tract, GU tract, retroperitoneal or intracranial sites.
2) Superficial or surface bleeding, observed mainly at invaded or disturbed sites (eg, venous cutdowns, arterial punctures, sites of recent surgical intervention).

The concomitant use of heparin anticoagulation may contribute to the bleeding. Some of the hemorrhagic episodes occurred one or more days after the effects had dissipated, but while heparin therapy was continuing.

As fibrin is lysed during therapy, bleeding from recent puncture sites may occur. Therefore, thrombolytic therapy requires careful attention to all potential bleeding sites (including catheter insertion sites, arterial and venous puncture sites, cutdown sites and needle puncture sites). Avoid IM injections and nonessential handling of the patient during treatment with alteplase. Perform venipunctures carefully and only as required. Minimize arterial and venous punctures.

Should an arterial puncture be necessary during an infusion, it is preferable to use an upper extremity vessel that is accessible to manual compression. Apply pressure for at least 30 minutes, apply a pressure dressing and check the puncture site frequently for evidence of bleeding. Avoid noncompressible arterial puncture (ie, avoid internal jugular and subclavian punctures to minimize bleeding from noncompressible sites).

If serious bleeding (not controllable by local pressure) occurs, terminate the infusion and any concomitant heparin. Protamine can reverse heparin effects.

In the following conditions, the risks of therapy may be increased and should be weighed against the anticipated benefits:

- Recent (within 10 days) major surgery, eg, coronary artery bypass graft, obstetrical delivery, organ biopsy, previous puncture of noncompressible vessels
- Cerebrovascular disease
- Recent GI or GU bleeding (within 10 days)
- Recent trauma (within 10 days)
- Hypertension: Systolic BP $\geq$ 180 mm Hg or diastolic BP $\geq$ 110 mm Hg
- High likelihood of left heart thrombus, eg, mitral stenosis with atrial fibrillation
- Acute pericarditis
- Subacute bacterial endocarditis
- Hemostatic defects including those secondary to severe hepatic or renal disease
- Significant liver dysfunction
- Pregnancy
- Diabetic hemorrhagic retinopathy, or other hemorrhagic ophthalmic conditions
- Septic thrombophlebitis or occluded AV cannula at seriously infected site
- Advanced age, ie, $>$ 75 years old
- Patients currently receiving oral anticoagulants, eg, warfarin sodium
- Any other condition in which bleeding constitutes a significant hazard or would be particularly difficult to manage because of its location

Arrhythmias may result from coronary thrombolysis associated with reperfusion. These arrhythmias (such as sinus bradycardia, accelerated idioventricular rhythm, ventricular premature depolarizations, ventricular tachycardia) are not different from those often seen in the ordinary course of AMI and may be managed with standard antiarrhythmic measures. Have antiarrhythmic therapy for bradycardia or ventricular irritability available when infusions of alteplase are administered.

Pulmonary embolism: The treatment of pulmonary embolism with alteplase has not been shown to constitute adequate clinical treatment of underlying deep vein thrombosis. Furthermore, consider the possible risk of reembolization due to the lysis of underlying deep venous thrombi.

Pregnancy: Category C. It is not known whether alteplase can cause fetal harm when administered to a pregnant woman or can affect reproduction capacity. Give to a pregnant woman only if clearly needed.

Lactation: It is not known whether alteplase is excreted in breast milk. Exercise caution when administering to nursing women.

Children: Safety and efficacy for use in children have not been established.

(Continued on following page)

ALTEPLASE, RECOMBINANT (Cont.)

Precautions:

Implement standard management of MI or PE concomitantly with treatment.

Hypersensitivity: No serious or life-threatening reactions have occurred, and there is no experience with readministration of tPA. If an anaphylactoid reaction occurs, discontinue the infusion immediately and initiate appropriate therapy. Refer to Management of Acute Hypersensitivity Reactions.

Sustained antibody formation in patients receiving one dose of tPA has not been documented, but readminister with caution. Detectable antibody levels (single point measurement) were reported in one patient but subsequent antibody test results were negative.

Laboratory test abnormalities: During therapy, if coagulation tests or measures of fibrinolytic activity are performed, the results may be unreliable unless specific precautions are taken to prevent in vitro artifacts. Alteplase present in blood in pharmacologic concentrations remains active in vitro. This can lead to degradation of fibrinogen in blood samples removed for analysis. Collection of blood samples in the presence of aprotinin (150 to 200 units/ml) can, to some extent, mitigate this phenomenon.

Drug Interactions:

Aspirin, dipyridamole: In addition to bleeding associated with heparin and vitamin K antagonists, drugs that alter platelet function may increase risk of bleeding if given prior to, during or after alteplase therapy (see Administration and Dosage).

Heparin has been given with and after alteplase infusions to reduce risk of rethrombosis. Either heparin or alteplase may cause bleeding complications; carefully monitor for bleeding, especially at arterial puncture sites (see Administration and Dosage).

Adverse Reactions:

Bleeding (most frequent): Bleeding associated with thrombolytic therapy can be divided into two types:

1) Internal bleeding, involving GI tract, GU tract, retroperitoneal or intracranial sites.

2) Superficial or surface bleeding, observed mainly at invaded or disturbed sites (eg, venous cutdowns, arterial punctures, sites of recent surgical intervention).

The following incidence of significant bleeding (estimated as > 250 ml blood loss) has been reported in studies in over 800 patients treated at all doses:

Incidence of Significant Bleeding

Site of Bleeding	Total Dose	
	≤ 100 mg	> 100 mg
GI	5%	5%
GU	4%	4%
ecchymosis	1%	< 1%
retroperitoneal	< 1%	< 1%
epistaxis	< 1%	< 1%
gingival	< 1%	< 1%

The incidence of intracranial bleeding (ICB) is as follows:

Incidence of Intracranial Bleeding

Dose	Patients	%
1 to 1.4 mg/kg	237	0.4
100 mg	3272	0.4
150 mg	1779	1.3

These data indicate that a dose of 150 mg should not be used because it has been associated with an increase in ICB.

Although fatalities due to ICB have been observed during and after therapy, an analysis of data from three controlled clinical trials in AMI revealed no evidence of increased overall in-hospital mortality. While not statistically significant, in-hospital mortality in patients treated with alteplase was lower (4.7%; 11/232) compared to patients not receiving alteplase (6.8%; 11/162).

If serious bleeding in a critical location (intracranial, GI, retroperitoneal, pericardial) occurs, immediately discontinue alteplase and any concomitant heparin therapy.

Fibrin, which is part of the hemostatic plug formed at needle puncture sites, will be lysed during therapy. Therefore, alteplase therapy requires careful attention to potential bleeding sites, eg, catheter insertion sites, arterial puncture sites.

Other reactions: Occasional mild hypersensitivity reactions (eg, urticaria). Nausea, vomiting, hypotension and fever are frequent sequelae of MI and may or may not be attributable to therapy.

(Continued on following page)

ALTEPLASE, RECOMBINANT (Cont.)

Administration and Dosage:

For IV administration only.

Acute myocardial infarction: Administer as soon as possible after the onset of symptoms. Lysis of coronary artery thrombi has been documented in 71% of patients treated within 6 hours of the onset of symptoms. Improvement of ventricular function and reduction of the incidence of CHF has occurred in patients treated within 4 hours of the onset of symptoms.

Recommended dose – 100 mg given as 60 mg (34.8 million IU) in the first hour (of which 6 to 10 mg is given as a bolus over the first 1 to 2 minutes), 20 mg (11.6 million IU) over the second hour, and 20 mg (11.6 million IU) over the third hour. For smaller patients (< 65 kg), a dose of 1.25 mg/kg given over 3 hours, as described above, may be used.

Concomitant administration – Although the use of anticoagulants and antiplatelet drugs during and following alteplase has not been shown to be of unequivocal benefit, heparin has been given concomitantly for ≥ 48 hours in > 90% of patients. Aspirin or dipyridamole has been given either during or following heparin treatment (see Drug Interactions).

Pulmonary embolism: Recommended dosage – 100 mg administered by IV infusion over 2 hours. Institute or reinstitute heparin therapy near the end of or immediately following the alteplase infusion when the partial thromboplastin time or thrombin time returns to twice normal or less.

Do not use a dose of 150 mg because it has been associated with an increase in intracranial bleeding.

Reconstitution: Do not use if vacuum is not present. Add the appropriate volume of the accompanying Sterile Water for Injection to the vial. Reconstitute only with Sterile Water for Injection without preservatives. Do not use Bacteriostatic Water for Injection. The reconstituted preparation results in a colorless to pale yellow transparent solution containing 1 mg/ml at approximately pH 7.3. The osmolality is approximately 215 mOsm/kg.

Reconstitute with a large bore needle (eg, 18 gauge), directing the stream of Sterile Water for Injection into the lyophilized cake. Slight foaming upon reconstitution is usual; standing undisturbed for several minutes is usually sufficient to allow dissipation of any large bubbles.

Because alteplase contains no antibacterial preservatives, reconstitute immediately before use. The solution may be used for direct IV administration within 8 hours following reconstitution when stored between 2° and 30°C (36° and 86°F). Before further dilution or administration, visually inspect for particulate matter and discoloration whenever solution and container permit.

May be administered as reconstituted at 1 mg/ml. As an alternative, the reconstituted solution may be further diluted immediately before administration with an equal volume of 0.9% Sodium Chloride Injection or 5% Dextrose Injection to yield a concentration of 0.5 mg/ml. Either polyvinyl chloride bags or glass bottles are acceptable. Alteplase is stable for up to 8 hours in these solutions at room temperature. Exposure to light has no effect on stability. Avoid excessive agitation during dilution; mix by gentle swirling or slow inversion. Do not use other infusion solutions. Discard unused solution.

IV incompatibilities: Do not add other medications to infusion solution.

Storage: Store lyophilized alteplase at controlled room temperature not to exceed 30°C (86°F), or under refrigeration (2° to 8°C; 36° to 46°F). During extended storage, protect from excessive exposure to light.

Rx	**Activase** (Genentech)	**Lyophilized powder for injection:** 20 mg (11.6 million IU) per vial[1]	In vials with diluent (20 ml Sterile Water for Injection).
		50 mg (29 million IU) per vial[1]	In vials with diluent (50 ml Sterile Water for Injection).

[1] With l-arginine and polysorbate 80.

ANISTREPLASE (Anisoylated Plasminogen Streptokinase Activator Complex; APSAC)

Actions:

Pharmacology: Anistreplase, the p-anisoylated derivative of the lys-plasminogen-streptokinase activator complex, is an inactive derivative of a fibrinolytic enzyme with the catalytic center of the activator complex temporarily blocked by an anisoyl group. The anisoyl group does not decrease the high fibrin-binding ability of the complex. Anistreplase is made in vitro from lys-plasminogen and streptokinase. Anistreplase differs from the complex initially formed in vivo upon administration of streptokinase; the latter complex contains predominantly glu-plasminogen. Activation of anistreplase occurs with release of the anisoyl group by deacylation, a non-enzymatic first-order process with a half-life in vitro in human blood of about 2 hours. In solution, deacylation of anistreplase starts immediately and the enzymatically active lys-plasminogen-streptokinase activator complex is progressively formed. The production of plasmin from plasminogen by deacylated anistreplase can take place in the bloodstream or within the thrombus; the latter process is catalytically more efficient but both may contribute to thrombolysis. The half-life of fibrinolytic activity of the circulating anistreplase is 70 to 120 minutes (mean 94 minutes).

Clinical trials: Randomized, controlled studies have demonstrated that anistreplase reduces mortality when administered within 6 hours of the onset of the symptoms of acute myocardial infarction (AMI). The benefit of mortality reduction occurs acutely and is maintained for at least 1 year.

In a study of 1258 patients (AIMS trial), mortality at 30 days postinfarction was decreased 47.2% in patients receiving anistreplase as compared with placebo. At 1 year, the reduction in mortality was maintained (38%). The incidence of heart failure was less in patients treated with anistreplase (17.9%) compared with patients who received placebo (23.3%).

In a double-blind, randomized trial of anistreplase compared with heparin bolus, left ventricular function was improved and infarction size reduced. There was significantly higher left ventricular ejection fraction for the anistreplase treatment group (53%) compared with the heparin treatment group (47.5%) when measured 4 days after treatment. This difference was maintained when patients were reexamined by radionuclide ventriculography at day 19, even when patients who experienced successful angioplasty were excluded from the analysis. About 3 weeks after treatment, mean infarct size was 24% lower in the patients treated with anistreplase compared with those treated with heparin. Similarly, if those patients who experienced successful angioplasty were excluded from the analysis, the mean infarct size in patients treated with anistreplase was significantly less than that of heparin-treated patients.

In randomized comparative studies, reperfusion rates of between 50% and 68% have been reported in patients receiving anistreplase within 6 hours of symptom onset. However, for maximum rates of reperfusion, initiate treatment as soon as possible after onset of symptoms.

In two studies, anistreplase and intracoronary streptokinase were compared in patients with angiographically proven coronary artery occlusion. Reperfusion occurred about 45 minutes after the start of therapy for both treatment groups. When therapy was initiated within 4 hours of onset of AMI symptoms, reperfusion rates of 59% (n = 87) and 68% (n = 41) were observed for anistreplase compared with 59% (n = 85) and 70% (n = 43) for streptokinase. Of those patients who had coronary artery reperfusion, angiographically demonstrated reocclusion occurred within 24 hours in 3% to 4% of those treated with anistreplase and in 7% to 12% of those treated with streptokinase.

In a well controlled randomized study, a patency rate of 72% was obtained with anistreplase compared with 53% for IV streptokinase. Patency for the 107 patients was determined by posttreatment angiography.

Anistreplase was also found to have a favorable risk/benefit profile in elderly patients (> 65 years, n = 940) who participated in clinical trials. Use of anistreplase in patients > 75 years old has not been adequately studied.

Indications:

Management of AMI in adults, for the lysis of thrombi obstructing coronary arteries, the reduction of infarct size, the improvement of ventricular function following AMI, and the reduction of mortality associated with AMI. Initiate treatment as soon as possible after the onset of AMI symptoms (see Pharmacology).

Contraindications:

Because thrombolytic therapy increases the risk of bleeding, anistreplase is contraindicated in the following situations: Active internal bleeding; history of cerebrovascular accident; recent (within 2 months) intracranial or intraspinal surgery or trauma (see Warnings); intracranial neoplasm, arteriovenous malformation or aneurysm; known bleeding diathesis; severe, uncontrolled hypertension; severe allergic reactions to either anistreplase or streptokinase.

(Continued on following page)

ANISTREPLASE (Anisoylated Plasminogen Streptokinase Activator Complex; APSAC) (Cont.)

Warnings:

Bleeding: (See Adverse Reactions). The most common complication associated with anistreplase therapy is bleeding. The types of bleeding associated with thrombolytic therapy can be divided into two broad categories:

1. Internal bleeding involving the GI tract, GU tract, retroperitoneal, ocular or intracranial sites
2. Superficial or surface bleeding, observed mainly at invaded or disturbed sites (eg, venous cutdowns, arterial punctures, sites of recent surgical intervention).

The concomitant use of heparin anticoagulation may contribute to the bleeding. Some of the hemorrhagic episodes occurred 1 or more days after the effects of anistreplase had dissipated, but while heparin therapy was continuing.

As fibrin is lysed during anistreplase therapy, bleeding from recent puncture sites may occur. Therefore, thrombolytic therapy requires careful attention to all potential bleeding sites (including catheter insertion sites, arterial and venous puncture sites, cutdown sites and needle puncture sites).

Avoid IM injections and nonessential handling of the patient during treatment with anistreplase. Perform venipunctures carefully and only as required.

Should an arterial puncture be necessary following administration of anistreplase, it is preferable to use an upper-extremity vessel that is accessible to manual compression. Apply a pressure dressing, and check the puncture site frequently for evidence of bleeding.

Carefully evaluate each patient being considered for therapy with anistreplase and weigh anticipated benefits against potential risks associated with therapy.

In the following conditions, the risks of anistreplase therapy may be increased and should be weighed against the anticipated benefits:

- recent (within 10 days) major surgery (eg, coronary artery bypass graft, obstetrical delivery, organ biopsy, previous puncture of noncompressible vessels)
- cerebrovascular disease
- recent GI or GU bleeding (within 10 days)
- recent trauma (within 10 days) including cardiopulmonary resuscitation
- hypertension: systolic BP $\geq$ 180 mmHg or diastolic BP $\geq$ 110 mmHg
- high likelihood of left heart thrombus (eg, mitral stenosis with atrial fibrillation)
- subacute bacterial endocarditis
- acute pericarditis
- hemostatic defects including those secondary to severe hepatic or renal disease
- pregnancy
- age $>$ 75 years
- diabetic hemorrhagic retinopathy or other hemorrhagic ophthalmic conditions
- septic thrombophlebitis or occluded AV cannula at seriously infected site
- patients currently receiving oral anticoagulants (eg, warfarin sodium)
- any other condition in which bleeding constitutes a significant hazard or would be particularly difficult to manage because of its location.

Arrhythmias may result from coronary thrombolysis associated with reperfusion. These arrhythmias (such as sinus bradycardia, accelerated idioventricular rhythm, ventricular premature depolarizations, ventricular tachycardia) are not different from those often seen in the ordinary course of AMI and may be managed with standard antiarrhythmic measures. It is recommended that antiarrhythmic therapy for bradycardia or ventricular irritability be available when injections of anistreplase are administered.

Hypotension, sometimes severe, not secondary to bleeding or anaphylaxis, has occasionally been observed soon after IV administration. Monitor patients closely. Should symptomatic or alarming hypotension occur, administer appropriate symptomatic treatment.

Pregnancy: Category C. It is not known whether anistreplase can cause fetal harm when administered to a pregnant woman or if the drug can affect reproduction capacity. Use in pregnancy only if clearly needed.

Lactation: It is not known whether anistreplase is excreted in breast milk. The physician should decide whether the patient should discontinue nursing or not receive anistreplase.

Children: Safety and efficacy of anistreplase in children have not been established.

(Continued on followinge page)

ANISTREPLASE (Anisoylated Plasminogen Streptokinase Activator Complex; APSAC) (Cont.)

Precautions:

Implement standard management of MI concomitantly with treatment. Minimize invasive procedures (see Warnings).

Hypersensitivity: Anaphylactoid reactions have rarely been reported. Accordingly, adequate treatment provisions such as epinephrine should be available for immediate use. Refer to Management of Acute Hypersensitivity Reactions.

Readministration: Because of the increased likelihood of resistance due to antistreptokinase antibody, anistreplase may not be as effective if administered > 5 days after prior anistreplase or streptokinase therapy or streptococcal infection, particularly between 5 days and 6 months. Increased antistreptokinase antibody levels between 5 days and 6 months after these drugs may also increase the risk of allergic reactions. Repeated administration of anistreplase within 1 week of the initial dose has occurred in a small number of patients treated for AMI and non-AMI conditions. The incidence of hematomas/bruising was somewhat greater with repeat doses, but otherwise the adverse event profile was similar to that of patients who received one dose.

Drug Interactions:

Anticoagulants (eg, **heparin, warfarin**) and **antiplatelet agents** (eg, **aspirin, dipyridamole**): Anistreplase alone or in combination with these agents may cause bleeding complications. Therefore, careful monitoring is advised, especially at arterial puncture sites. In clinical studies, a majority of patients treated received anticoagulant therapy postdosing with anistreplase and a minority received heparin pretreatment with anistreplase. The use of antiplatelet agents increased the incidence of bleeding events similarly in patients treated with anistreplase or non-thrombolytic therapy. There was no evidence of a synergistic effect of combined anistreplase and antiplatelet agents on bleeding events. In addition, there was no difference in the incidence of hemorrhagic CVAs in anistreplase-treated patients who did or did not receive aspirin.

Drug/Laboratory test interactions: IV administration of anistreplase will cause marked decreases in plasminogen and fibrinogen and increases in thrombin time, activated partial thromboplastin time and prothrombin time. Results of coagulation tests or measures of fibrinolytic activity performed during anistreplase therapy may be unreliable unless specific precautions are taken to prevent in vitro artifacts. Anistreplase, when present in blood in pharmacologic concentrations, remains active under in vitro conditions. This can lead to degradation of fibrinogen in blood samples removed for analysis. Collection of blood samples in the presence of aprotinin (2000 to 3000 KIU/ml) can, to some extent, mitigate this phenomenon.

Adverse Reactions:

Bleeding: The incidence of bleeding (major or minor) varied widely from study to study and may depend on the use of arterial catheterization and other invasive procedures, patient population or concomitant therapy. The overall incidence of bleeding in patients treated with anistreplase in clinical trials (n = 5275) was 14.6% (non-puncture-site bleeding 10.2%, puncture-site bleeding 5.7%). Puncture site bleeding occurred more frequently in clinical trials in which the patients underwent immediate coronary catheterization (13.3%, n = 637) compared with those who did not (3%, n = 2023). Incidence of presumed intracranial bleeding within 7 days postdosing with anistreplase was 0.57% (n = 5275; 0.34%, etiology confirmed hemorrhagic; 0.23%, etiology not confirmed) compared to 0.16% (n = 1249) after non-thrombolytic therapy.

In the AIMS trial, the overall incidence of bleeding in patients treated with anistreplase was 14.8% compared with 3.8% for placebo. In this study there was no difference between anistreplase and placebo in the incidence of major bleeding events.

Incidence of Specific Bleeding Events with Anistreplase		
Type of Bleeding	Anistreplase (n = 500)	Placebo (n = 501)
Puncture site	4.6%	< 1%
Non-puncture site hematoma	2.8%	< 1%
Hematuria/genitourinary	2.4%	< 1%
Hemoptysis	2.2%	< 1%
GI hemorrhage	2%	1.4%
Intracranial	1%	< 1%
Gum/mouth hemorrhage	1%	0
Epistaxis	< 1%	< 1%
Anemia	< 1%	< 1%
Eye hemorrhage	< 1%	< 1%
Hemorrhage (unspecified)	< 1%	0

(Adverse Reactions continued on following page)

ANISTREPLASE (Anisoylated Plasminogen Streptokinase Activator Complex; APSAC) (Cont.)

Adverse Reactions (Cont.):

Should serious bleeding (not controlled by local pressure) occur in a critical location (intracranial, gastrointestinal, retroperitoneal, pericardial), immediately terminate any concomitant heparin and consider protamine to reverse heparinization. If necessary, the bleeding tendency can be reversed with appropriate replacement therapy.

Minor bleeding can be anticipated mainly at invaded or disturbed sites. If such bleeding occurs, take local measures to control the bleeding (see Warnings).

Cardiovascular: The most frequently reported adverse experiences in anistreplase clinical trials (n = 5275) were arrhythmia/conduction disorders which occurred in 38% of patients treated with anistreplase and 46% of non-thrombolytic control patients. Hypotension occurred in 10.4% of patients treated with anistreplase compared to 7.9% for patients who received non-thrombolytic treatment (see Warnings).

Allergic-type reactions: Anaphylactic and anaphylactoid reactions have been observed rarely (0.2%) in patients treated with anistreplase and are similar in incidence to streptokinase (0.1% anaphylactic shock in one study). These include symptoms such as bronchospasm or angioedema.

Other milder or delayed effects such as urticaria, itching, flushing, rashes and eosinophilia have been occasionally observed. A delayed purpuric rash appearing 1 to 2 weeks after treatment has occurred in 0.3% of patients. The rash may also be associated with arthralgia, ankle edema, GI symptoms, mild hematuria and mild proteinuria. The syndrome was self-limiting and without long-term sequelae. See Precautions.

Risk of viral transmission: Six batches of anistreplase (five different batches of lys-plasminogen) were used in clinical trials designed specifically to monitor possible hepatitis non-A, non-B transmission. No case of hepatitis was diagnosed in patients receiving anistreplase.

Causal relationship unknown (may also be associated with AMI or other therapy) reported in clinical trials (< 10%): Chills; fever; headache; shock; cardiac rupture; chest pain; emboli; purpura; sweating; nausea or vomiting; thrombocytopenia; elevated transaminase levels; arthralgia; agitation; dizziness; paresthesia; tremor; vertigo; dyspnea; lung edema.

Administration and Dosage:

Administer as soon as possible after the onset of symptoms. The recommended dose is 30 units of anistreplase administered only by IV injection over 2 to 5 minutes into an IV line or vein.

Reconstitution: Slowly add 5 ml of Sterile Water for Injection, USP by directing the stream of fluid against the side of the vial. Gently roll the vial, mixing the dry powder and fluid. *Do not shake.* Try to minimize foaming. The reconstituted preparation is a colorless to pale yellow transparent solution. Withdraw the entire contents of the vial.

Admixture incompatibility: The reconstituted solution should not be further diluted before administration or added to any infusion fluids. No other medications should be added to the vial or syringe containing anistreplase.

Storage/Stability: Store lyophilized anistreplase between 2° to 8°C (36° to 46°F). If not administered within 30 minutes of reconstitution, discard.

Rx	**Eminase** (Beecham)	**Powder, lyophilized:** 30 units[1]	In vials.

[1] Potency is expressed in units of anistreplase by using a reference standard which is specific for anistreplase and is not comparable with units used for other fibrinolytics.

Warnings:

Use in hospitals where the recommended diagnostic and monitoring techniques are available. Consider thrombolytic therapy in all situations where the potential benefits outweigh the risk of potentially serious hemorrhage. When internal bleeding occurs, it may be more difficult to manage than that which occurs with conventional anticoagulant therapy.

Institute treatment as soon as possible after onset of pulmonary embolism, preferably within 7 days. Any delay in instituting lytic therapy to evaluate the effect of heparin decreases the potential for optimal efficacy.

When urokinase is used to treat coronary artery thrombosis associated with evolving transmural myocardial infarction, institute therapy within 6 hours of onset of symptoms.

Actions:

Pharmacology: Urokinase acts on the endogenous fibrinolytic system. It directly converts plasminogen to the enzyme plasmin. Plasmin degrades fibrin clots and fibrinogen. Intravenous infusion for lysis of pulmonary embolism is followed by increased fibrinolytic activity. This effect disappears within a few hours after discontinuation, but a decrease in plasma levels of fibrinogen and plasminogen and an increased amount of circulating fibrin(ogen) degradation products (FDP/fdp) may persist for 12 to 24 hours. There is a lack of correlation between embolus resolution and changes in coagulation and fibrinolytic assay results. Because FDP/fdp has an anticoagulant effect, bleeding may be difficult to control.

Streptokinase acts with plasminogen to produce an "activator complex" that converts plasminogen to the proteolytic enzyme plasmin. Plasmin degrades fibrin clots as well as fibrinogen and other plasma proteins. Plasmin is inactivated by circulating inhibitors, such as α-2-macroglobulin. These inhibitors are rapidly consumed at high doses of streptokinase.

Intravenous infusion of streptokinase is followed by increased fibrinolytic activity, which decreases plasma fibrinogen levels for 24 to 36 hours. The decrease in plasma fibrinogen is associated with decreases in plasma and blood viscosity and red blood cell aggregation. The hyperfibrinolytic effect disappears within a few hours after discontinuation, but a prolonged thrombin time may persist for up to 24 hours due to the decrease in plasma levels of fibrinogen and an increase in the amount of circulating FDP. Depending upon the dosage and duration of infusion of streptokinase, the thrombin time will decrease to less than two times the normal control value within 4 hours, and return to normal by 24 hours.

Intravenous administration reduces blood pressure and total peripheral resistance with a corresponding reduction in cardiac afterload.

Variable amounts of circulating antistreptokinase antibody are present in individuals as a result of recent streptococcal infections. The recommended dosage schedule usually obviates the need for antibody titration.

(Actions continued on following page)

Actions (Cont.):

Pharmacokinetics: These agents are administered by IV or intracoronary infusion. Intravenous infusion of urokinase is cleared rapidly by the liver; serum half-life is 20 minutes or less. Expect patients with impaired liver function (eg, cirrhosis) to show a prolongation in half-life. Small fractions of urokinase are excreted in bile and urine. The $t_{1/2}$ of the streptokinase activator complex is about 23 minutes; the complex is inactivated, in part, by antistreptococcal antibodies. The mechanism of elimination is unknown; no metabolites of streptokinase have been identified.

Clinical Pharmacology: Two large placebo-controlled studies conducted with a 60 minute IV infusion of 1,500,000 IU of streptokinase for acute myocardial infarction within 6 hours of the onset of symptoms have reported reductions in acute mortality from 20% to 25%.

In the GISSI study, the reduction in mortality was time dependent; there was a 47% reduction in mortality among patients treated within 1 hour of the onset of chest pain, a 23% reduction among patients treated within 3 hours, and a 17% reduction among patients treated between 3 and 6 hours.

The rate of reocclusion of the infarct-related vessel has been reported to be approximately 20%. The rate of reocclusion depends on dosage, additional anticoagulant therapy and residual stenosis. When the reinfarctions were evaluated in studies involving 8,800 streptokinase-treated patients, the overall rate was 3.8% (range 2% to 15%). In over 8,500 control patients, the rate of reinfarction was 2.4%.

Streptokinase, administered by the intracoronary route has resulted in thrombolysis usually within 1 hour and ensuing reperfusion results in limitation of infarct size, improvement of cardiac function, and reduction of mortality. Spontaneous reperfusion is known to occur. Data from one study show that 73% of the streptokinase-treated patients and 47% of the placebo-allocated patients reperfused during hospitalization.

Studies with thrombolytic therapy for pulmonary embolism show no significant difference in lung perfusion scan between the thrombolysis group and the heparin group at 1 year follow-up. However, measurements of pulmonary capillary blood volumes and diffusing capacities at 2 weeks and 1 year after therapy indicate that a more complete resolution of thrombolic obstruction and normalization of pulmonary physiology was achieved with thrombolytic therapy, thus preventing the long-term sequelae of pulmonary hypertension and pulmonary failure.

For deep vein thrombosis (DVT), the combined results of five randomized studies show no residual thrombotic material in 60% to 75% of patients treated with streptokinase versus 10% treated with heparin. Thrombolytic therapy also generally preserves venous valve function, avoiding the pathology that produces the clinical post-phlebitic syndrome which occurs in 90% of the DVT patients treated with heparin.

Indications:

Urokinase:

Pulmonary emboli

Coronary artery thrombosis

IV catheter clearance – To restore patency to IV catheters, including central venous catheters, obstructed by clotted blood or fibrin.

Streptokinase:

Acute evolving transmural myocardial infarction by either the IV or intracoronary route. Earlier administration is correlated with greater clinical benefit.

Deep vein thrombosis

Arterial thrombosis and embolism – Streptokinase is not indicated for arterial emboli originating from the left side of the heart due to the risk of new embolic phenomena, such as cerebral embolism.

Occluded AV cannulae – An alternative to surgical revision for clearing totally or partially occluded arteriovenous cannulae.

Contraindications:

Active internal bleeding; recent (within 2 months) cerebrovascular accident; intracranial or intraspinal surgery; intracranial neoplasm.

Streptokinase: Severe uncontrolled hypertension; patients having experienced severe allergic reaction to the product.

(Continued on following page)

Warnings:

Bleeding can be placed into two broad categories: Superficial or surface bleeding observed mainly at invaded or disturbed sites (eg, venous cutdowns, arterial punctures, sites of recent surgical intervention); and internal bleeding, involving the GI tract, GU tract or vagina, or occurring IM, retroperitoneal or intracerebral sites.

Minor bleeding occurs often, mainly at invaded or disturbed sites. Do not reduce dose when lytic therapy is continued; use local measures to control minor bleeding (apply pressure for at least 30 minutes, then apply a pressure dressing).

Several fatalities due to cerebral and other serious internal hemorrhages have occurred. Should uncontrollable bleeding occur, immediately discontinue infusion. Slowing the rate of administration will not help correct the bleeding and may make it worse. If necessary, manage blood loss and reverse the bleeding tendency with whole blood (fresh blood preferable), packed red blood cells and cryoprecipitate or fresh frozen plasma. Do not use dextran. Although the use of aminocaproic acid (p. 313) as an antidote in humans has not been documented, consider it in an emergency.

Streptokinase will cause lysis of hemostatic fibrin deposits such as those occurring at sites of needle punctures, and bleeding may occur. In order to minimize the risk of bleeding during treatment venipunctures and physical handling of the patient should be performed carefully and as infrequently as possible; avoid intramuscular injections.

Avoid arterial invasive procedures before and during treatment. Should an arterial puncture be necessary, upper extremity vessels are preferable.

High risk patients: Recent (within 10 days) major surgery, obstetrical delivery, organ biopsy, previous puncture of noncompressible vessels; recent (within 10 days) serious GI bleeding; recent trauma including cardiopulmonary resuscitation; severe uncontrolled arterial hypertension or likelihood of a left heart thrombus (eg, mitral stenosis with atrial fibrillation); subacute bacterial endocarditis; hemostatic defects including those secondary to severe hepatic or renal disease; pregnancy; age $\geq$ 75 years; cerebrovascular disease; diabetic hemorrhagic retinopathy; septic thrombophlebitis or occluded AV cannula at seriously infected site; other conditions in which bleeding might be hazardous or difficult to manage.

IV catheter clearance: If catheters are occluded by substances other than blood fibrin clots, such as drug precipitates, urokinase is not effective. Avoid excessive pressure when urokinase is injected into the catheter. Force could rupture the catheter or expel the clot into the circulation.

Arrhythmias: Rapid lysis of coronary thrombi may cause atrial or ventricular dysrhythmias, due to reperfusion, requiring immediate treatment. Reperfusion of the right coronary artery may carry a higher risk. Carefully monitor for arrhythmias during and immediately following intracoronary administration.

Hypotension, sometimes severe, not secondary to bleeding or anaphylaxis may occur during IV streptokinase (1% to 10%). Monitor patients and, should symptomatic or alarming hypotension occur, administer appropriate treatment. This may include a decrease in the IV streptokinase infusion rate. Smaller hypotensive effects are common and have not required treatment.

Non-cardiogenic pulmonary edema has been reported rarely in patients treated with streptokinase. The risk of this appears greater in patients who have large myocardial infarctions and are undergoing thrombolytic therapy by the intracoronary route.

Polyneuropathy has been temporally related to the use of streptokinase.

Should *pulmonary embolism* or recurrent pulmonary embolism occur during streptokinase therapy, complete the planned course of treatment in an attempt to lyse the embolus. While pulmonary embolism may occasionally occur during streptokinase treatment, the incidence is no greater than when patients are treated with heparin alone.

Hypersensitivity: Anaphylactic and anaphylactoid reactions have been observed rarely in patients treated with IV streptokinase. Anaphylactic shock was reported in one study with an incidence rate of 0.1%.

Skin testing may identify patients at risk for immediate-type allergic reactions to streptokinase. Manage mild or moderate reactions with concomitant antihistamine or corticosteroid therapy.

(Continued on following page)

Warnings (Cont.):

Usage in Pregnancy: (Category B – Urokinase). Safety for use during pregnancy has not been established. Use only when clearly needed and when the potential benefits outweigh the potential hazards to the fetus.

(Category C – Streptokinase). It is not known whether streptokinase can cause fetal harm when administered to a pregnant woman or can affect reproduction capacity. Streptokinase should be given to a pregnant woman only if clearly needed.

Usage in Lactation: Urokinase – It is not known whether this drug is excreted in breast milk. Exercise caution when administering to a nursing woman.

Usage in Children: Safety and efficacy for use in children have not been established.

Precautions:

Because of the increased likelihood of resistance, due to antistreptokinase antibody, streptokinase may not be effective if administered between 5 days and 6 months of prior streptokinase administration or streptococcal infections, ie, pharyngitis, acute rheumatic fever, or acute glomerulonephritis secondary to a streptococcal infection.

Monitoring: Before therapy, determine hematocrit, platelet count, thrombin time (TT), activated partial thromboplastin time (APTT), prothrombin time (PT), fibrinogen levels, and a hematocrit and platelet count. If heparin has been given, discontinue it. The TT or APTT should be less than twice the normal control value before therapy. Following the infusion, before (re)instituting heparin, the TT or APTT should be less than twice normal.

IV infusion: During infusion, decreases in the plasminogen and fibrinogen level and an increase in the FDP level (the latter two prolong the clotting times of coagulation tests) will generally confirm the existence of lysis. Results do not, however, reliably predict either efficacy or risk of bleeding. Frequently observe the clinical response and check the vital signs (ie, pulse, temperature, respiratory rate and blood pressure) at least every 4 hours. Do not take the blood pressure in the lower extremities to avoid dislodgment of possible deep vein thrombi. Monitor therapy by performing the TT, PT, APTT or fibrinogen approximately 4 hours after initiation of therapy.

Intracoronary artery infusion: During studies, laboratory monitoring of hemostatic parameters during intracoronary artery infusion showed minimal changes, if any. Heparin was continued or instituted following therapy and monitored accordingly.

Drug Interactions:

Anticoagulants and **antiplatelet agents**: Thrombolytic enzymes, alone or in combination with these agents, may cause bleeding complications; carefully monitor.

Drug/Lab Tests: IV administration of streptokinase will cause marked decreases in plasminogen and fibrinogen and increases in thrombin time (TT), activated partial thromboplastin time (APTT), and prothrombin time (PT). These changes may also occur in some patients with intracoronary administration of streptokinase.

Adverse Reactions:

Bleeding is of two types: *Minor* (superficial or surface bleeding) and *major* (internal, severe bleeding; incidence – 0% to 16%). The overall incidence of major bleeding with high dose IV infusion is 1.2%. See Warnings.

Allergic reactions:

Urokinase is a protein of human origin; there is no evidence of induced antibody formation. Relatively mild allergic reactions (eg, bronchospasm and skin rash) are reported rarely and usually respond to conventional therapy.

Streptokinase – Minor breathing difficulty, bronchospasm, periorbital swelling, angioneurotic edema, urticaria, itching, flushing, nausea, headache, musculoskeletal pain, and delayed hypersensitivity reactions (eg, vasculitis and interstitial nephritis). See Warnings.

Fever: Urokinase (2% to 3%) – A cause and effect relationship has not been established.

Streptokinase (0% to 28%) – Occurs in patients treated intravenously with streptokinase. Symptomatic treatment is usually sufficient. Use acetaminophen rather than aspirin.

Guillain-Barré Syndrome: Although a cause and effect relationship has not been established, several case reports suggest that streptokinase induces immunological responses that may initiate this syndrome.

(Products listed on following pages)

Complete prescribing information for these products begins on page 295

UROKINASE

Administration and Dosage:

IV infusion: Administer via a constant infusion pump capable of delivering a total volume of 195 ml.

Give a priming dose of 2000 units/lb (4400 units/kg) as an admixture of urokinase with either 0.9% Sodium Chloride Injection or 5% Dextrose Injection at a rate of 90 ml/hour over 10 minutes. Follow by continuous infusion of 2000 units/lb/hr (4400 units/kg/hr) at a rate of 15 ml/hour for 12 hours. Some admixture will remain in the tubing at the end of an infusion pump delivery cycle; therefore, perform the following flush procedure to ensure administration of the total dose: Administer a solution of 0.9% Sodium Chloride Injection or 5% Dextrose Injection, approximately equal in amount to the volume of the tubing in the infusion set, via the pump to flush the admixture from the entire length of the infusion set. Pump the flush solution at the continuous infusion rate of 15 ml/hour.

At the end of urokinase therapy, treat with continuous heparin IV infusion. Do not begin heparin until TT has decreased to less than twice the normal control value (approximately 3 to 4 hours after completing infusion).

Lysis of coronary artery thrombi: Prior to the infusion of urokinase, administer a bolus dose of heparin ranging from 2500 to 10,000 units IV. Consider prior heparin administration when calculating the heparin dose for this procedure. Following the bolus dose of heparin, infuse the prepared solution into the occluded artery at a rate of 4 ml/minute (6000 IU/minute) for periods up to 2 hours. In a clinical study, the average total dose of urokinase used for lysis of coronary artery thrombi was 500,000 IU.

Continue therapy until the artery is maximally opened, usually 15 to 30 minutes after the initial opening. Following the infusion, determine coagulation parameters. It is advisable to continue heparin therapy after the artery is opened.

IV catheter clearance: When the following procedure is used to clear a central venous catheter, instruct the patient to exhale and hold his breath any time the catheter is not connected to IV tubing or a syringe, to prevent air from entering the open catheter.

Disconnect the IV tubing connection at the catheter hub and attach an empty 10 ml syringe. Determine occlusion of the catheter by gently attempting to aspirate blood from the catheter with the 10 ml syringe. If aspiration is not possible, remove the syringe and attach a 1 ml tuberculin syringe filled with prepared urokinase to the catheter. Slowly and gently inject an amount of solution equal to the volume of the catheter. Remove the tuberculin syringe and connect an empty 5 ml syringe to the catheter. Wait at least 5 minutes before attempting to aspirate the drug and residual clot with the 5 ml syringe. Repeat aspiration attempts every 5 minutes. If the catheter is not open within 30 minutes, cap the catheter; allow urokinase to remain in the catheter 30 to 60 minutes before again attempting to aspirate. A second injection of urokinase may be necessary in resistant cases.

When patency is restored, aspirate 4 to 5 ml of blood to ensure removal of all drug and residual clot. Remove the blood filled syringe and replace it with a 10 ml syringe filled with 0.9% Sodium Chloride Injection. Gently irrigate the catheter with this solution to ensure patency of the catheter. Remove the 10 ml syringe and reconnect sterile IV tubing to the catheter hub.

Preparation of solution: Reconstitute vial with 5.2 ml Sterile Water for Injection. It is important to reconstitute only with Sterile Water for Injection without preservatives. Do not use Bacteriostatic Water for Injection. For further dilution procedures, consult manufacturer's literature. To minimize formation of filaments, avoid shaking the vial during reconstitution. Roll and tilt the vial to enhance reconstitution. The solution may be terminally filtered (ie, through a 0.45 micron or smaller cellulose membrane filter). Do not add other medications to this solution. Because urokinase contains no preservatives, do not reconstitute until immediately before use. Discard any unused portion of the reconstituted material.

Storage: Refrigerate vials at 2° to 8°C (35° to 47°F). The reconstituted solution is stable for 24 hours at room temperature (15° to 30°C) and under refrigeration (2° to 8°C).

Rx	**Abbokinase** (Abbott)	**Powder for Injection:** 250,000 IU per vial[1]	In 5 ml vials.
Rx	**Abbokinase Open-Cath** (Abbott)	**Powder for Reconstitution:** 5000 IU per ml after reconstitution[2]	In 1 ml Univials.

[1] With 25 mg mannitol.

[2] With 5 mg gelatin and 15 mg mannitol per ml when reconstituted.

Complete prescribing information for these products begins on page 295

STREPTOKINASE

Administration and Dosage:

Acute Evolving Transmural MI: Administer as soon as possible after symptom onset.

IV infusion: Use the 1,500,000 IU vial diluted to a total volume of 45 ml. Administer a total dose of 1,500,000 IU within 60 minutes.

Intracoronary infusion: Use the 250,000 IU vial diluted to a total volume of 125 ml. Administer 20,000 IU (10 ml) by bolus followed by 2,000 IU per minute for 60 minutes (60 ml/hr) for a total dose of 140,000 IU.

Pulmonary Embolism, DVT, Arterial Thrombosis or Embolism:

IV infusion: Use the 1,500,000 vial diluted to a total volume of 90 ml. Institute treatment as soon as possible after onset of thrombotic event, preferably within 7 days. A loading dose of 250,000 IU infused into a peripheral vein over 30 minutes has been found appropriate in over 90% of patients; follow with 100,000 IU/hour (6 ml/hr) for 24 to 72 hr for arterial thrombosis or embolism; 72 hr for DVT; and 24 hr for pulmonary embolism (72 hr if concurrent DVT is suspected). If the thrombin time or any other parameter of lysis after 4 hours of therapy is not significantly different from the normal control level, discontinue streptokinase because excessive resistance is present.

Intracoronary infusion: Same as for IV infusion; however, use the 1,500,000 infusion bottle diluted to a total volume of 45 ml, and infuse at a rate of 15 ml/hr for 30 minutes (loading dose) followed by 3 ml/hr (maintenance dose).

Continuous IV infusion of heparin, without a loading dose, has been recommended following termination of streptokinase infusion for treatment of pulmonary embolism or DVT to prevent rethrombosis. The effect of streptokinase on TT and APTT will usually diminish within 3 to 4 hours after therapy, and heparin therapy without a loading dose can be initiated when the TT or the APTT is less than twice the normal control value.

Arteriovenous Cannulae Occlusion: Before using, try to clear the cannula by careful syringe technique, using heparinized saline solution. If adequate flow is not reestablished, streptokinase may be used. Allow effect of pretreatment anticoagulants to diminish. Instill 250,000 IU in 2 ml solution into each occluded limb of the cannula slowly. Clamp off cannula limb(s) for 2 hrs. Observe closely for adverse effects. After treatment, aspirate contents of infused cannula limb(s), flush with saline, reconnect cannula.

Reconstitution/Dilution: Slight flocculation (thin translucent fibers) of reconstituted streptokinase occur occasionally but do not interfere with the safe use of the solution. Slowly add 5 ml Sodium Chloride Injection or Dextrose 5% Injection to the vial or bottle, directing the diluent at the side of the bottle or vial rather than into the drug powder. Roll and tilt gently to reconstitute. Avoid shaking.

Vial – Withdraw the entire reconstituted contents of the vial; slowly and carefully dilute further to a total volume as recommended for the specific indication. (If necessary, total volume may be increased to a maximum of 500 ml in glass or 50 ml in plastic containers; adjust infusion pump rate accordingly.) To facilitate setting the infusion pump, a total volume of 45 ml or a multiple thereof, is recommended.

Bottle – Add an additional 40 ml of diluent to the bottle, avoiding shaking and agitation. (Total Volume = 45 ml.) Administer by infusion pump. The reconstituted solution can be filtered through a 0.8 μm or larger pore size filter.

For Use in Arteriovenous Cannulae: Slowly reconstitute the contents of the 250,000 IU, vacuum-packed vial with 2 ml Sodium Chloride Injection or Dextrose 5% Injection.

Storage/Stability: Store unopened vials at controlled room temperature (15° to 30° C or 59° to 86°F). Because streptokinase contains no preservatives, it should be reconstituted immediately before use. The solution may be used for direct IV administration within 8 hours following reconstitution if stored at 2° to 8° C (36° to 46°F). Unused reconstituted drug should be discarded. Do not add other medication to streptokinase.

Rx	**Kabikinase** (Kabivitrum)	**Powder for Injection:** 250,000 IU, 600,000 IU or 750,000 IU per vial	In 5 ml vials.[1]
Rx	**Streptase** (Hoechst-Roussel)	**Powder for Injection**[2]: 250,000 IU or 750,000 IU	In 6.5 ml vials.
		1,500,000 IU	In 6.5 ml vials and 50 ml infusion bottle.

[1] With 11 mg sodium l-glutamate and 14.5 mg albumin (human)/100,000 IU streptokinase.

[2] With 25 mg cross-linked gelatin polypeptides, 25 mg sodium l-glutamate and 100 mg normal serum albumin (human).

PENTOXIFYLLINE

Actions:

Pharmacology: Pentoxifylline, a dimethylxanthine derivative, and its metabolites improve blood flow by decreasing blood viscosity. It produces dose-related hemorheologic effects, lowering blood viscosity and improving erythrocyte flexibility. In patients with chronic peripheral arterial disease, this increases blood flow to the affected microcirculation and enhances tissue oxygenation. Although the precise mechanism of action is unknown, pentoxifylline: 1) Improves RBC deformability by increasing cellular ATP content via a membrane stabilizing action, thus reducing RBC aggregation and local hyperviscosity. 2) Stimulates prostacyclin formation and release; inhibits phosphodiesterase degradation of platelet cAMP. The increase of cAMP levels decreases the synthesis of thromboxane A_2; the net result is reducing platelet aggregation. 3) Increases blood fibrinolytic activity; decreases fibrinogen concentration.

Pharmacokinetics: After administration, pentoxifylline is extensively absorbed. It undergoes a first-pass effect and the various metabolites appear in plasma very soon after dosing. Plasma levels of the parent drug peak within 1 hour. Pentoxifylline undergoes a first-pass effect. The major metabolites are Metabolite I and Metabolite V with plasma levels 5 and 8 times greater, respectively, than the parent drug. Plasma half-lives of pentoxifylline and its metabolites are 0.4 to 0.8 hours and 1 to 1.6 hours, respectively. There is no evidence of accumulation or enzyme induction. Excretion is primarily urinary. Less than 4% of the dose is recovered in feces.

Indications:

Intermittent claudication on the basis of chronic occlusive arterial disease of the limbs. It improves function and symptoms but does not replace definitive therapy.

Unlabeled Uses: Pentoxifylline was found superior to placebo in improving psychopathological symptoms in patients with cerebrovascular insufficiency. The drug has also been studied in diabetic angiopathies and neuropathies, transient ischemic attacks, leg ulcers, sickle cell thalassemias, strokes, high-altitude sickness, asthenozoospermia, acute and chronic hearing disorders, eye circulation disorders and Raynaud's phenomenon.

Contraindications:

Intolerance to pentoxifylline or methylxanthines (ie, caffeine, theophylline, theobromine).

Warnings:

Usage in impaired renal function: The clearance of pentoxifylline is reduced in patients with renal impairment, possibly resulting in toxicity. A lower dosage may be necessary in these patients.

Usage in Pregnancy: Category C. Animal studies showed no fetal malformation. Increased resorption was seen in rats at 25 times the maximum recommended human dose. No adequate studies exist in pregnant women. Use only if clearly needed.

Usage in Lactation: Pentoxifylline and its metabolites are excreted in breast milk. Because of the potential for tumorigenicity seen in rats, decide whether to discontinue nursing or discontinue the drug, taking into account the importance of the drug to the mother.

Usage in Children: Safety and efficacy for use in children less than 18 years of age are not established.

Precautions:

Patients with chronic occlusive arterial disease of the limbs frequently show other manifestations of arteriosclerotic disease. There have been occasional reports of angina, hypotension and arrhythmia. Periodic systemic blood pressure monitoring is recommended, especially in patients receiving concomitant antihypertensive therapy.

Drug Interactions:

Warfarin: Although a causal relationship has not been established, there have been reports of bleeding and prolonged prothrombin time (PT) in patients receiving pentoxifylline with or without anticoagulants or platelet aggregation inhibitors. Frequently monitor PT in patients on warfarin. Patients with other risk factors complicated by hemorrhage (eg, recent surgery, peptic ulceration) should have periodic exams for bleeding including hematocrit or hemoglobin.

(Continued on following page)

PENTOXIFYLLINE (Cont.)

Adverse Reactions:

Cardiovascular: Angina/chest pain (0.3%), edema, hypotension, dyspnea (< 1%).

GI: Dyspepsia (2.8%), nausea (2.2%), vomiting (1.2%), belching/flatus/bloating (0.6%), anorexia, cholecystitis, constipation, dry mouth/thirst (< 1%).

CNS: Dizziness (1.9%), headache (1.2%); tremor (0.3%), anxiety, confusion (< 1%).

Respiratory: Epistaxis, flu-like symptoms, laryngitis, nasal congestion, (< 1%).

Dermatologic: Brittle fingernails, pruritus, rash, urticaria (< 1%).

Ophthalmologic: Blurred vision, conjunctivitis, scotomata (< 1%).

Other: Earache, bad taste, excessive salivation, leukopenia, malaise, sore throat/swollen neck glands, weight change (< 1%).

Rare (causal relationship unknown): Arrhythmia, tachycardia, hepatitis, jaundice, decreased serum fibrinogen, pancytopenia, purpura, thrombocytopenia.

Overdosage:

Symptoms, apparently dose-related, usually occur 4 to 5 hours after ingestion and last about 12 hours. Flushing, hypotension, nervousness, agitation, tremors, convulsions, somnolence, loss of consciousness, fever and agitation have occurred. Bradycardia (30 to 40 beats/min) with first and second degree AV block occurred after 2 hours in a patient who ingested 4 to 6 g; first degree AV block persisted until 16 hours after admission.

Treatment: Treat with gastric lavage and administer activated charcoal. Monitor ECG and blood pressure. In addition to symptomatic treatment, support respiration, maintain blood pressure, treat cardiac arrhythmias and control seizures as required.

Administration and Dosage:

Take 400 mg 3 times daily with meals. If GI and CNS side effects occur, decrease to 400 mg twice daily. If side effects persist, discontinue. While therapeutic effects may be seen within 2 to 4 weeks, continue treatment for at least 8 weeks.

Rx	**Trental** (Hoechst-Roussel)	**Tablets, controlled release**: 400 mg	(#Trental). Pink. Film coated. In 100s and UD 100s.

Product identification code.

ANTITHROMBIN III (HUMAN)

Actions:

Antithrombin III (human), produced from pooled human plasma from healthy donors, is a glycoprotein of molecular weight 58,000 and consists of 425 amino acids in a single polypeptide chain crosslinked by three disulfide bridges. Antithrombin III is identical with heparin cofactor I, a factor in plasma necessary for heparin to exert its anticoagulant effect. The quantity of antithrombin III in 1 ml of normal pooled human plasma is conventionally taken as one unit. The potency assignment has been determined with a standard calibrated against a World Health Organization (WHO) Antithrombin III Reference Preparation.

Each unit of plasma used in the manufacture of this product has been tested and found nonreactive for hepatitis B surface antigen (HBsAg) and negative for antibody to human immunodeficiency virus (HIV) by FDA-approved tests. In addition, antithrombin III has been heat-treated in solution at 60°C ± 0.5°C for not less than 10 hours.

Pharmacology: Antithrombin III is a major coagulation inhibitor in blood. It inactivates thrombin and the activated forms of Factors IX, X, XI and XII, ie, all coagulation enzymes except Factor VIIa and Factor XIII. The concentration of antithrombin III in normal plasma has been estimated from 0.1 to 0.2 g/L. Antithrombin III levels are usually expressed as a percentage of a reference plasma.

In subjects with hereditary antithrombin III deficiency, the levels of antithrombin III are found to be about 50% of the level in normal human plasma. These subjects have a high risk of thromboembolic disease even at an early age. Surgery and pregnancy are significant factors precipitating venous thrombosis in antithrombin III deficient patients. Antithrombin III (human) is given as replacement treatment to patients with hereditary antithrombin III deficiency in connection with surgical or obstetrical procedures or when they suffer from thromboembolism.

Pharmacokinetics: The mean biological half-life in three patients with hereditary antithrombin III deficiency and one healthy subject was found to be 3 days. The half-life of antithrombin III is decreased by concurrent heparin treatment (see Drug Interactions).

Clinical trials: In clinical studies, 39 patients with hereditary antithrombin III deficiency were treated with antithrombin III on 60 separate occasions. In each case antithrombin III was given prophylactically or therapeutically. In 68% of the treatments the doses were between 30 and 50 IU/kg/day, and the duration of therapy was 2 to 8 days (range, 1 day to 20 weeks). Twenty women were given 47 prophylactic treatments during delivery and postpartum; 12 had previous thromboembolic complications. Further, seven women were treated during abortion; all these patients had at least two previous incidences of thromboembolism. In all cases treated with antithrombin there was no incidence of thrombosis. The same results were obtained when nine surgical patients were treated (13 operations). There was no thrombosis in connection with treatment, although seven patients had previous thrombosis. Additionally, 11 patients were treated for acute thrombosis. Five patients were treated with heparin alone without disappearance of soreness, swelling and pain. Addition of antithrombin III to the regimen reduced the thrombotic signs. The remaining six patients were treated with antithrombin III in combination with oral anticoagulants or heparin. In all cases but one, the clinical signs of acute thrombosis were reduced or eliminated after the combined treatment.

Indications:

Treatment of patients with hereditary antithrombin III deficiency in connection with surgical or obstetrical procedures or when they suffer from thromboembolism. Determine dosage so that the antithrombin III level in plasma is maintained higher than 80%. (See Precautions and Administration and Dosage sections.)

Warnings:

HBsAg and HIV: This product is prepared from pooled units of human plasma. Each unit of plasma used in the manufacture of this product has been tested and found nonreactive for HBsAg and negative for antibody to HIV by FDA-approved tests. These testing procedures are used to eliminate high-risk plasma donors, and a heat treatment step (60°C [140°F] for 10 hours in solution) in the manufacturing process is designed to reduce the risk of transmitting viral infections. However, test methods are not sensitive enough to detect all units of potentially infectious plasma, and treatment methods have not been shown to be totally effective in eliminating viral infectivity from this product.

Individuals who receive multiple infusions of blood or plasma products may develop signs or symptoms of some viral infections, particularly non-A, non-B hepatitis.

(Warnings continued on following page)

ANTITHROMBIN III (HUMAN) (Cont.)

Warnings (Cont.):

Neonatal thromboembolism: Measure the antithrombin III level in neonates of parents with hereditary antithrombin III deficiency immediately after birth. Fatal neonatal thromboembolism, such as aortic thrombi in children of women with hereditary antithrombin III deficiency has occurred. It is recommended that testing and treatment with antithrombin III of such neonates be discussed with an expert on coagulation.

Pregnancy: Category C. It is not known whether antithrombin III can cause fetal harm when administered to a pregnant woman or can affect reproduction capacity. Give to a pregnant woman only if clearly needed. Studies in pregnant women have not shown that antithrombin III increases the risk of fetal abnormalities if administered during the third trimester of pregnancy. Antithrombin III concentrates have been used in 23 full-term pregnancies; all resulted in deliveries with no neonatal complications and with healthy children.

Children: Only a few neonates and children have been treated with antithrombin III. Safety and efficacy in children have not yet been established.

Precautions:

Thrombosis: Inform subjects with antithrombin III deficiency about the risk of thrombosis in connection with pregnancy and surgery, and about the inheritance of the disease.

Recommended rate of infusion is 50 IU per minute (1 ml/min); do not exceed 100 IU per minute (2 ml/min). One healthy subject became dyspneic after a rapid IV injection (1500 IU in 5 minutes), and his blood pressure increased.

Antithrombin III deficiency diagnosis: Base the diagnosis of hereditary antithrombin III deficiency on a clear family history of venous thrombosis as well as decreased plasma antithrombin III levels, and the exclusion of acquired deficiency. Monitor antithrombin III plasma levels during the treatment period.

Antithrombin III in plasma may be measured with amidolytic assays by using synthetic chromogenic substrates or with clotting assays or with immunoassays. The latter does not detect all congenital antithrombin III deficiencies.

Drug Interactions:

Heparin: The anticoagulant effect of heparin is enhanced by concurrent antithrombin III in patients with hereditary antithrombin III deficiency. Thus, in order to avoid bleeding, reduced heparin dosage is recommended during antithrombin III treatment.

Adverse Reactions:

No adverse reactions occurred in conjunction with clinical trials in hereditary antithrombin III deficient patients. However, 2 of 65 patients, with acquired antithrombin III deficiency with severe disseminated intravascular coagulation, exhibited diuretic and vasodilatory effects. In one case, the recorded decrease in arterial systolic blood pressure was 25 mm Hg. The other decrease was not recorded.

Overdosage:

Antithrombin III levels of 150% to 210% have been found in a few patients, and no signs or symptoms of complications have been identified.

Administration and Dosage:

Each bottle of antithrombin III (human) is labeled with antithrombin III (AT-III) content expressed in International Units (IU). The quantity of antithrombin III in 1 ml of normal pooled human plasma is conventionally taken as one unit. The potency assignment has been determined with a standard calibrated against a World Health Organization (WHO) Antithrombin III Reference Preparation.

The amount of antithrombin III required to restore the recipient to a normal level varies with the circumstances and patient. Individualize dosage according to the needs of the patient. Consider the weight of the patient, the degree of the deficiency and the desired level of antithrombin III to be achieved. Base the dose on the medical judgment of the physician and on laboratory control values.

After the first dose the antithrombin III level should increase to about 120% of normal. Thereafter, maintain at levels > 80%. In general, this may be achieved by administration of maintenance doses once every 24 hours. Initially and until the patient is stabilized, measure the antithrombin III level at least twice a day, thereafter once a day, and always immediately before the next infusion.

(Administration and Dosage continued on following page)

ANTITHROMBIN III (HUMAN) (Cont.)

Administration and Dosage (Cont.):

The administration of one IU/kg raises the level of AT-III by 1% to 2.1% depending on the condition of the patient. Thus, an initial loading dose may be calculated from the following formula (assuming a plasma volume of 40 ml/kg).

$$\text{Dosage Units} = \frac{[\text{desired AT-III level (\%)} - \text{baseline AT-III level (\%)}] \times \text{body weight (kg)}}{1\%/(\text{IU/kg})}$$

Thus, if a 70 kg individual has a baseline AT-III level of 57%, the initial dose would be (120% – 57%) x 70/1 = 4410 IU.

Measure plasma AT-III levels preceding and 30 minutes after the dose, and calculate the in vivo recovery. If the recovery differs from an anticipated rise of 1% for each IU/kg administered, modify the formula accordingly. For example, if in the above example, the plasma level measured 30 minutes after the infusion is 147%, then the increases in AT-III measured per each 1 IU/kg administered is (147% – 57%) x 70 kg/4410 units = 1.43% rise for each IU/kg.

The above recommendations for dosing are provided only as a general guideline for therapy. Individualize the exact loading and maintenance dosages and dosing intervals for each subject based on the individual clinical conditions, response to therapy and actual plasma AT-III levels achieved. Perform laboratory tests to assure that the desired levels are achieved.

When an infusion of antithrombin III is indicated for a patient with hereditary deficiency to control an acute thrombotic episode or to prevent thrombosis following surgical or obstetrical procedures, raise the antithrombin III level to normal and maintain this level for 2 to 8 days depending on the indication for treatment, type and extensiveness of surgery, the patient's medical condition and history and the physician's judgment. Base concomitant administration of heparin in each of these situations on the medical judgment of the physician.

Reconstitution: Dissolve the powder in 10 ml Sterile Water for Injection, USP. Gently swirl the vial to dissolve the powder. Do not shake. Bring the solution to room temperature, and administer within 3 hours following reconstitution. Antithrombin III may be infused over 5 to 10 minutes. Administer IV.

Alternately, reconstitute with 0.9% Sodium Chloride Injection, USP, or 5% Dextrose Injection, USP. After reconstitution, antithrombin III may be further diluted with the same diluent.

Rx	**ATnativ** (Hyland)	**Powder for injection, lyophilized:** 500 IU of antithrombin III (human)	In 50 ml bottle with 10 ml Sterile Water for Injection.

ANTIHEMOPHILIC FACTOR (Factor VIII; AHF)

Actions:

Antihemophilic factor (AHF) is a protein found in normal plasma which is necessary for clot formation. The administration of AHF can temporarily correct the coagulation defect of patients with classical hemophilia (Hemophilia A). It is needed for the transformation of prothrombin (Factor II) to thrombin by the intrinsic pathway.

After infusion of AHF, an instantaneous rise in the coagulant level is followed by a rapid decrease in activity. The half-life of AHF administered to hemophiliacs is 9 to 15 hours.

Indications:

Classical Hemophilia (Hemophilia A), in which there is a deficiency of the plasma clotting factor, Factor VIII. Provides a means of temporarily replacing the missing clotting factor to correct or prevent bleeding episodes or perform surgery.

Not effective in controlling the bleeding of patients with von Willebrand's disease.

Contraindications:

Monoclonal antibody-derived Factor VIII: Hypersensitivity to mouse protein.

Warnings:

Hepatitis: AHF is prepared from human plasma; consequently, the risk of transmitting hepatitis is present. The individual units of plasma are nonreactive when tested for hepatitis B surface antigen. In addition, these products are heated during manufacturing to reduce the risk of hepatitis transmission (including some non-A, non-B hepatitis).

Patients who have not received multiple infusions of blood or plasma products are very likely to develop signs or symptoms of some viral infections, especially non-A, non-B hepatitis, after introduction of clotting factor concentrates. For such patients, especially those with mild hemophilia, use single donor products. For patients with moderate or severe hemophilia who have received numerous infusions of blood or blood products, the risk of hepatitis is small. Clotting factor concentrates have so greatly improved the management of severe hemophilia that these products should not be denied to appropriate patients.

AIDS: Hemophiliacs comprise approximately 1.6% of the victims of Acquired Immune Deficiency Syndrome (AIDS). Transmission through blood products is possible.

Human T-lymphocyte virus type III/lymphadenopathy-associated virus (HIV) is the virus believed to cause AIDS. Donor screening tests for antibodies to HIV are available and are used to screen donated blood. Positive tests are further screened. Antibodies develop in infected individuals within 2 to 3 months of infection.

Usage in Pregnancy: Category C. Animal reproductive studies have not been performed. Safety for use during pregnancy has not been established. Use only if clearly needed.

Precautions:

Factor VIII inhibitor: Approximately 10% of patients with hemophilia develop inhibitors to Factor VIII. In patients with inhibitors, the response to AHF may be greatly reduced, and patients with high inhibitor levels may not respond to AHF. Anti-inhibitor complex is available (see page 308).

Hemolysis: AHF contains naturally occurring blood group specific antibodies (Anti-A and Anti-B isoagglutinins). When large or frequently repeated doses are needed in patients of blood group A, B or AB, intravascular hemolysis may occur; monitor the hematocrit and Direct Coombs' test. Correct hemolytic anemia with compatible group O red blood cells.

Monoclonal antibody-derived Factor VIII: Formation of Antibodies to Mouse Protein – Although no hypersensitivity reactions have been observed, they may possibly occur due to trace amounts of mouse protein (less than 50 ng per 100 AHF activity units).

Pre-existing antibody to mouse protein was detected in some patients prior to treatment. In the assay used, people with rheumatoid factor may test falsely positive and other proteins may also show cross-reactivity.

Laboratory Tests: Assure that adequate AHF levels have been reached and are maintained. If the AHF level fails to reach expected levels or if bleeding is not controlled after apparently adequate dosage, inhibitors may be present. The presence of inhibitors can be demonstrated and quantitated in terms of AHF units neutralized by each ml of plasma or by the total estimated plasma volume. After sufficient dosage to neutralize inhibitor, additional dosage produces predicted clinical response.

(Continued on following page)

ANTIHEMOPHILIC FACTOR (Factor VIII; AHF) (Cont.)

Adverse Reactions:

Allergic reactions: Hives, fever, urticaria, mild chills, nausea, stinging at the infusion site, tightness of the chest, wheezing, hypotension and anaphylaxis may occur.

Patient Information:

Monoclonal antibody derived Factor VIII: Inform patient of early signs of hypersensitivity reactions (ie, hives, generalized urticaria, tightness of the chest, wheezing, hypotension and anaphylaxis). Discontinue use and contact physician if these symptoms occur.

Administration and Dosage:

One AHF unit is defined as the activity present in 1 ml normal pooled human plasma.

Administer IV only. Use a plastic syringe; solutions may stick to the surface of glass.

Individualize dosage. The dose depends on patient weight, severity of the deficiency, severity of hemorrhage, presence of inhibitors and the Factor VIII level desired. Clinical effect on the patient is the most important factor of therapy. When inhibitors are present, dosage requirements are extremely variable; determine by clinical response. It may be necessary to administer more AHF to obtain the desired result.

There is a linear dose-response relation with an approximate yield of 2% rise in Factor VIII activity for each unit of Factor VIII/kg transfused. The following formulas provide a guide for dosage calculations:

$$\text{Expected Factor VIII increase (in \% of normal)} = \frac{\text{AHF/IU administered} \times 2}{\text{body weight (in kg)}}$$

$$\text{AHF/IU required} = \text{body weight (kg)} \times \text{desired Factor VIII increase (\% normal)} \times 0.5$$

Follow therapy with Factor VIII level assays. It may be dangerous to assume any certain level has been reached without direct evidence.

Prophylaxis of spontaneous hemorrhage: The level of Factor VIII required to prevent spontaneous hemorrhage is approximately 5% of normal; 30% of normal is the minimum required for hemostasis following trauma and surgery. Mild superficial or early hemorrhages may respond to a single dose of 10 AHF/IU/kg, leading to a rise of approximately 20% Factor VIII level. In patients with early hemarthrosis (mild pain, minimal or no swelling, erythema, warmth and minimal or no joint limitation), if treated promptly, even smaller doses may be adequate.

Mild hemorrhage: Do not repeat therapy unless further bleeding occurs. Minor episodes generally subside with a single infusion if a level of 30% of normal or more is attained.

Moderate hemorrhage and minor surgery require plasma Factor VIII level to be raised to 30% to 50% of normal for optimum hemostasis. This usually requires an initial dose of 15 to 25 AHF/IU/kg; if further therapy is required, administer a maintenance dose of 10 to 15 AHF/IU/kg every 8 to 12 hours.

Severe hemorrhage: For life-threatening bleeding, or hemorrhage involving vital structures (CNS, retropharyngeal and retroperitoneal spaces, iliopsoas sheath), raise the Factor VIII level to 80% to 100% of normal. Administer an initial AHF dose of 40 to 50 AHF/IU/kg and a maintenance dose of 20 to 25 AHF/IU/kg every 8 to 12 hours.

Major surgery procedures require a dose of AHF sufficient to achieve a level of 80% to 100% of normal; give an hour before the procedure. Check the Factor VIII level prior to surgery to assure the level is achieved. Give a second dose half the size of the priming dose about 5 hours after the first dose. Maintain the Factor VIII level at a daily minimum of at least 30% of normal for a healing period of 10 to 14 days. Close laboratory control is recommended.

Rate of Administration: Administer preparations IV at a rate of ≈ 2 ml/minute. Can be given at up to 10 ml/min. As a precaution, determine the pulse rate before and during administration of the AHF concentrate. Should a significant increase of pulse rate occur, reduce the rate of administration or discontinue.

(Administration and Dosage continued on following page)

ANTIHEMOPHILIC FACTOR (Factor VIII; AHF) (Cont.)

Administration and Dosage (Cont.):

Storage: Refrigerate between 2° to 8°C (35° to 46°F). Do not freeze. After reconstitution, do not refrigerate; give within 3 hours.

Rx	**Antihemophilic Factor (Porcine) Hyate:C** (Porton)	A freeze-dried concentrate of Antihemophilic Factor VIII:C. Each vial contains between 400 and 700 porcine units	In vials.
Rx	**Hemofil M** (Hyland Therapeutic)	A stable dried preparation of Antihemophilic Factor in concentrated form. When reconstituted, contains ≈ 12.5 mg/ml albumin (human). Method M (monoclonal purified)	In 10, 20 and 30 ml with diluent.[1,2]
Rx	**Humate-P** (Armour)	A pasteurized, purified lyophilized concentrate of antihemophilic factor (human)	In single dose vials with diluent.[1,3]
Rx	**Koate HP** (Miles, Inc.)	A stable dried concentrate of Antihemophilic Factor. When reconstituted, contains ≤ 5 U/ml heparin, ≤ 1500 ppm PEG, ≤ 0.05 M glycine, ≤ 25 ppm polysorbate 80, ≤ 5 ppm TNBP, ≤ 3 mM calcium chloride, ≤ 1 ppm aluminum, ≤ 0.06 M histadine, ≤ 10 mg/ml albumin (human)	Includes Sterile Water for Injection, double-ended, transfer needle, filter needle, and administration set. In bottles of 250, 500, 1000 and 1500 IU Factor VIII activity (approximate).
Rx	**Koāte-HS** (Cutter)	A stable dried concentrate of Antihemophilic Factor. Heated in aqueous solution	In single dose vials with diluent.[1,4]
Rx	**Koāte-HT** (Cutter)	A stable dried concentrate of Antihemophilic Factor. Heat-treated	In single dose vials with diluent.[1]
Rx	**Monoclate** (Armour)	Monoclonal antibody derived stable lyophilized concentrate of Factor VIII:C and reduced amounts of Factor VIII:R. Heat-treated. With 1% to 2% Albumin (Human), 0.8% mannitol and 1.2 mM histadine	In 1 ml single dose vial with diluent.[1,5]
Rx	**Monoclate-P** (Armour)	A stable concentrate of Factor VIII: C. When reconstituted, contains ≈ 300 to 450 mmol sodium ions and ≈ 2 to 5 mmol calcium (as chloride per L, ≈ 1% to 2% albumin (human), 0.8% mannitol, 1.2 mmol histadine and < 50 ng/100 AHF activity units mouse protein	With diluent, double-ended needle, vented filter spike, winged infusion set and alcohol swabs.
Rx	**Profilate HP** (Alpha Therapeutic)	A stable freeze-dried concentrate of Antihemophilic Factor VIII:C (human) that has been suspended in heptane and heated	In single dose vials with 10 or 25 ml sterile water for injection.

[1] Actual number of AHF units are indicated on the vials.
[2] When reconstituted, contains 1.5 mg/ml PEG 3350, 0.055 M histidine, 0.03 M glycine and less than 10 ng/100 AHF activity units of mouse protein.
[3] Each 100 IU contains 60 to 100 mg glycine, 14 to 28 mg sodium citrate, 8 to 16 mg sodium chloride, 16 to 24 mg albumin (human), 4 to 20 mg of other proteins and 20 to 44 mg total proteins.
[4] With not more than 10 units/mL heparin and not more than 1500 ppm polyethylene glycol.
[5] Purified of extraneous plasma-derived protein by use of affinity chromatography.

ANTI-INHIBITOR COAGULANT COMPLEX

Actions:

Anti-Inhibitor Coagulant Complex is prepared from pooled human plasma and contains variable amounts of activated and precursor clotting factors. Kinin generating system factors are also present; it is standardized by its ability to correct the clotting time of Factor VIII deficient plasma or Factor VIII deficient plasma which contains inhibitors to Factor VIII.

Approximately 10% of individuals with hemophilia (ie, Hemophilia A; Factor VIII deficiency) have laboratory-measurable inhibitors to Factor VIII. The treatment depends upon the existing level of inhibitor, whether or not the patient responds to infusions of Antihemophilic Factor (AHF) with increased inhibitor levels (anamnestic rise in Factor VIII antibody) and the severity of the bleeding episode.

Indications:

Patients with Factor VIII inhibitors who are bleeding or who are to undergo surgery.

Treat patients whose present Factor VIII inhibitor levels are *greater than 10 Bethesda Units,* and whose inhibitor levels are known to rise to greater than 10 Bethesda Units following treatment with AHF, with Anti-Inhibitor Coagulant Complex.

Patients whose present Factor VIII inhibitor levels are *between 2 and 10 Bethesda Units* and whose inhibitor levels remain in this range following treatment with AHF may be treated with either AHF or Anti-Inhibitor Coagulant Complex, depending on the patient's clinical history and severity of the bleeding episode.

Patients with Factor VIII inhibitor levels of *less than 2 Bethesda Units* whose inhibitor levels are known to remain at 2 Bethesda Units or less following treatment with AHF may be treated with appropriate doses of AHF.

For patients who have low levels of Factor VIII inhibitor and whose history does not include adequate laboratory indications of an anamnestic response to AHF, base the treatment of choice on clinical judgment. In patients having noncritical or minor bleeding episodes, the use of Anti-Inhibitor Coagulant Complex will maintain the inhibitor at a low level and allow the use of other coagulant therapeutic agents in subsequent major emergencies.

Contraindications:

Signs of fibrinolysis; disseminated intravascular coagulation (DIC); patients with a normal coagulation mechanism.

Warnings:

Infectious disease transmission: Products are prepared from large pools of human plasma. Such plasma may contain the causative agents of viral hepatitis, AIDS or other viral diseases. Each unit of source plasma used in preparation is nonreactive for hepatitis B surface antigen (HBsAg) and HIV antibody by FDA approved tests. In addition, *Feiba VH Immuno* has been subjected to a vapor heat-treatment during the manufacturing process to reduce the risk of transmitting viral infections. However, no procedure is totally effective in eliminating viral infectivity.

Individuals who have not received multiple infusions of blood or plasma products are very likely to develop signs or symptoms of certain viral infections, especially non A, non B hepatitis.

Anamnestic responses with rise in Factor VIII inhibitor titer occurred in 20% of cases.

Tests used to control efficacy such as APTT, WBCT and TEG do not correlate with clinical improvement. Attempts at normalizing these values by increasing the dose of Anti-Inhibitor Coagulant Complex may not be successful and are strongly discouraged because of the potential hazard of producing DIC by overdosage.

Acute Hypersensitivity Reaction: Have epinephrine 1:1000 immediately available. Refer to Management of Acute Hypersensitivity Reactions on p. 2897

Usage in Pregnancy: Category C. Animal reproduction studies have not been performed. It is also not known whether the drug can cause fetal harm when administered to a pregnant woman or can affect reproduction capacity. Use only if clearly needed.

Usage in Children: No data are available regarding use in newborns for *Feiba VH Immuno*. For *Autoplex T*, give special caution and consideration to use in newborns. A higher morbidity and mortality may be associated with hepatitis.

Precautions:

Disseminated intravascular coagulation (DIC): If signs occur, including changes in blood pressure and pulse rate, respiratory distress, chest pain and cough, stop the infusion and monitor the patient. Laboratory indications include prolonged thrombin time, prothrombin time and partial thromboplastin time tests, decreased fibrinogen concentration, decreased platelet count or the presence of fibrin split products.

(Precautions continued on following page)

ANTI-INHIBITOR COAGULANT COMPLEX (Cont.)

Precautions (Cont.):

Identification of the clotting deficiency as caused by the presence of Factor VIII inhibitors is essential before initiating the administration of Anti-Inhibitor Coagulant Complex.

Usage in impaired hepatic function: Give special caution and consideration to the use of *Autoplex T* in individuals with preexisting liver disease.

If the infusion of the concentrate occurs more than 1 hour following reconstitution, there may be increased prekallikrein activator (PKA) with consequent hypotension.

Laboratory Tests: Activated partial thromboplastin time test may not correlate with clinical response. The appearance of hemostatic improvement may occur without a reduction of partial thromboplastin time. However, expect the prothrombin time to be shortened.

Drug Interactions:

Epsilon-aminocaproic acid (EACA) or **tranexamic acid**: The concomitant use of Anti-Inhibitor Coagulant Complex with such agents is not recommended since only limited data are available on the administration of these highly activated prothrombin complex products and antifibrinolytic agents.

Adverse Reactions:

Hypersensitivity: Fever and chills, indications of protein sensitivity, signs and symptoms of high prekallikrein activity (changes in blood pressure or pulse rate). Allergic reactions ranging from mild, short-term urticarial rashes to severe anaphylactoid reactions may occur.

A rapid rate of infusion may cause headache, flushing and changes in pulse rate and blood pressure. Stopping the infusion allows the symptoms to disappear promptly. With all but the most reactive individuals, infusion may be resumed at a slower rate.

Laboratory and clinical signs of DIC have occasionally been observed following high doses (single infusion of $>$ 100 U/kg and daily doses of 200 U/kg). Monitor patients on these doses carefully. See Precautions.

Administration and Dosage:

One unit of Factor VIII Correctional Activity is the quantity of activated prothrombin complex which, upon addition to an equal volume of Factor VIII deficient or inhibitor plasma, will correct the clotting time (ellagic acid-activated partial thromboplastin time) to 35 seconds (normal).

Administer by IV injection or drip only.

Dosage range: 25 to 100 Factor VIII correctional units/kg, depending upon the severity of hemorrhage. If no hemostatic improvement is observed at approximately 6 hours following the initial administration, repeat the dosage. Adjust subsequent dosages and administration intervals according to the patient's clinical response.

Joint hemorrhage: 50 to 100 U/kg at 12 hour intervals. Continue treatment until clear signs of clinical improvement appear (eg, relief of pain, reduction of swelling or mobilization of the joint).

Mucous membrane bleeding: 50 U/kg at 6 hour intervals under careful monitoring of visible bleeding site with repeated measurements of the patient's hematocrit. If hemorrhage does not stop, may increase to 100 U/kg at 6 hour intervals; do not exceed 200 U/kg/day.

Soft tissue hemorrhage: For serious soft tissue bleeding, such as retroperitoneal bleeding, 100 U/kg at 12 hour intervals. Do not exceed 200 U/kg/day.

Other severe hemorrhages, such as CNS bleeding, have been effectively treated with doses of 100 U/kg at 12 hour intervals. Anti-Inhibitor Coagulant Complex may be indicated at 6 hour intervals until clear clinical improvement is achieved.

Rate of administration: May be infused at rates as fast as 10 ml/minute; however, if headache, flushing, changes in pulse rate or blood pressure appear, stop the infusion until symptoms disappear, then reinitiate infusion at a rate of $\approx$ 2 ml per minute.

Children: Determine fibrinogen levels prior to the initial infusion and monitor during the course of treatment.

Storage: Refrigerate the unreconstituted complex between 2° to 8°C (35° to 46°F). Avoid freezing. Do not refrigerate after reconstitution. Complete administration within 1 hour *(Autoplex T)* to 3 hours *(Feiba VH Immuno)* after reconstitution.

Rx	**Autoplex T** (Hyland Therapeutic)	Dried anti-inhibitor coagulant complex. With a maximum of 2 units heparin and 2 mg polyethylene glycol per ml reconstituted material. Heat treated	In vials with diluent and needles. Each bottle is labeled with the units of Factor VIII correctional activity it contains.
Rx	**Feiba VH Immuno** (Immuno-U.S.)	Freeze-dried anti-inhibitor coagulant complex. Heparin free. Vapor heated	In vials with diluent and needles. Each bottle is labeled with the units of Factor VIII inhibitor bypassing activity it contains.

FACTOR IX COMPLEX (HUMAN)

Actions:

Pharmacology: The human Factor IX complex consists of stable dried purified plasma fractions. Factor IX Complex (plasma thromboplastin component) is involved in the intrinsic pathway of blood coagulation. The vitamin K-dependent coagulation Factors II, VII, IX, X and small amounts of other plasma proteins are synthesized in the liver.

Factor IX Complex raises Factor IX plasma levels and restores hemostasis in patients with Factor IX deficiency. Generally, a Factor IX level $< 5\%$ of normal will give rise to spontaneous hemorrhage while levels $> 20\%$ of normal will lead to satisfactory hemostasis even after trauma or surgery.

Factor IX Complex causes an increase in blood levels of Factors II, VII, IX and X. Congenital deficiencies of each of the four factors occur and may result in a bleeding tendency. Naturally low levels of the vitamin K-dependent factors may also be found in vitamin K deficiency and in severe liver disease.

Pharmacokinetics: Biological activity of infused Factor IX disappears from the plasma with a half-life of ≈ 24 hours; 30% to 50% of the Factor IX activity can be detected in a Hemophilia B recipient's plasma immediately after infusion.

The half-life of Factor VII in non-treated Factor IX Complex administered to Factor VII deficient patients ranges from 3 to 6 hours.

The half-life of Factor IX in non-treated Factor IX Complex administered to Factor IX deficient patients ranges from 24 to 32 hours.

Indications:

For Factor IX deficiency (Hemophilia B, Christmas disease) to prevent or control bleeding episodes. Do not use in mild Factor IX deficiency if fresh frozen plasma is effective.

For bleeding episodes in patients with inhibitors to Factor VIII.

For reversal of coumarin anticoagulant-induced hemorrhage. When prompt reversal is required (before emergency surgery, trauma), consider using fresh, frozen plasma initially.

Proplex T only – For prevention or control of bleeding episodes in patients with Factor VII deficiency.

Contraindications:

Not for use in the treatment of Factor VII deficiencies (except for Proplex T).

Liver disease with signs of intravascular coagulation or fibrinolysis.

Warnings:

Hepatitis and AIDS: These products are prepared from pooled units of plasma which have been individually tested and found nonreactive for hepatitis B surface antigen (HBsAg) and Human Immunodeficiency Virus (HIV) antibody by FDA-approved tests. Other screening procedures are used to eliminate high-risk plasma donors; a heat-treatment step in manufacturing is designed to reduce the risk of transmitting viral infections. However, since testing and treatment methods are not totally effective in eliminating viral infectivity, assume that hepatitis viruses are present.

Individuals who have not received multiple blood or plasma product infusions are likely to develop signs or symptoms of a viral infection, especially non-A, non-B hepatitis. Single donor fresh plasma may be appropriate.

Thrombosis is a well known risk of the postoperative period. Until more conclusive studies are available, do not use Factor IX in patients undergoing elective surgery, unless benefits outweigh risk of thrombosis, especially in those predisposed to thrombosis.

Reconstitution of Factor IX with heparin may reduce the risk of thrombosis. However, thrombosis can occur, even in the presence of heparin.

Intravascular coagulation: If signs of disseminated intravascular coagulation (DIC) occur, stop the infusion promptly. To reduce the risk of enhancing intravascular coagulation, do not attempt to raise Factor IX or Factor VII levels to more than about 50% of normal. If the need exists to raise the patient's Factor IX or Factor VII level higher than 50% of normal, monitor infusion to detect signs and symptoms of DIC. Do not use in known liver disease when there is any suspicion of DIC or fibrinolysis.

Usage in Pregnancy: Category C. Animal reproduction studies have not been conducted. It is also not known whether Factor IX can cause fetal harm when administered to a pregnant woman. Give to a pregnant woman only if clearly needed.

(Continued on following page)

FACTOR IX COMPLEX (HUMAN) (Cont.)

Drug Interactions:

Aminocaproic Acid: Do not coadminister; this may increase the risk of thrombosis.

Drug/Lab Tests: Since the dosage of Factor IX is calculated on the basis of its potency, frequent laboratory tests to monitor the effectiveness of treatment usually are unnecessary. This is particularly true for single dose treatment of an uncomplicated hemarthrosis. However, if a major bleeding episode is being treated in the hospital, or if adequate hemostatic levels of Factor VII or Factor IX are needed to permit performance of surgery, perform Factor VII or Factor IX assays at least once a day, prior to infusion, to ensure that the daily dose of Factor IX Complex is sufficient to maintain adequate levels of the desired clotting factor.

Continually monitor patients receiving Factor IX for prolonged periods at least for levels of Factors II, IX and X.

Adverse Reactions:

Thrombosis or DIC has occurred (see Warnings).

Pyrogenic reactions: Chills and fever (particularly when large doses are used).

Rapid infusion rate: Headache, flushing, changes in blood pressure, transient fever, chills, tingling, urticaria, nausea and vomiting may occur. Symptoms disappear promptly upon discontinuation. Except in the most reactive individuals, the infusion may be resumed at a slower rate.

The use of high doses of prothrombin complex concentrates may be associated with myocardial infarction, DIC, venous thrombosis and pulmonary embolism.

Administration and Dosage:

For IV use only. One unit is defined as the activity present in 1 ml of average normal fresh plasma. The potency is standardized in terms of Factor IX content.

When reconstitution of Factor IX Complex is complete, its infusion should commence within 3 hours. However, begin the infusion as promptly as is practical. Discard solution if not used immediately.

The amount of Factor IX Complex required to restore normal hemostasis varies with circumstances and patient. Administer sufficient drug to achieve and maintain a plasma level of at least 20% until hemostasis is achieved. Only 30% to 50% of the infused Factor IX activity can be detected in the hemophilia B recipient's plasma immediately after infusion, and there is no such inexplicable loss in the in vivo recovery of Factors II, VII and X. Dosage depends on degree of deficiency and desired hemostatic level of the deficient factor. To calculate dosage, use the following formula:

Units required to raise blood level percentages:

1 unit/kg × body weight (kg) × desired increase (% of normal).

If a 70 kg (154 lb) patient with a Factor IX level of 0% needs to be elevated to 25%, give 1 unit/kg × 70 kg × 25 = 1750 units.

The preceding formula is a reference and guide. Determine exact dosage based on the physician's judgment of circumstances, patient condition, degree of deficiency and the desired level of Factor IX to be achieved. If inhibitors to Factor IX appear, use sufficient additional dosage to overcome the inhibitors.

In preparation for and following surgery, maintain levels > 25% for at least a week. Use laboratory control to assure such levels. To maintain levels > 25% for a reasonable time, calculate each dose to raise level to 40% to 60% of normal.

(Administration and Dosage continued on following page)

FACTOR IX COMPLEX (HUMAN) (Cont.)

Administration and Dosage (Cont.):

To maintain an elevated level of the deficient factor, repeat dosage as needed. Clinical studies suggest relatively high levels may be maintained by daily or twice daily doses, while the lower effective levels may require injections only once every 2 or 3 days. A single dose may stop a minor bleeding episode.

Factor VII Deficiency: Units required to raise blood level percentages:

0.5 unit/kg × body weight (in kg) × desired increase (% of normal)

Repeat dose every 4 to 6 hours as needed.

If a 70 kg (154 lb) patient with a Factor VII level of 0% needs to be elevated to 25%, give 0.5 unit/kg × 70 kg × 25 = 875 units.

Dosage guidelines may be derived from the following table:

Pharmacology of Vitamin K-Dependent Coagulation Factors

Factor	Hemostatic Level† > % Normal		Dosage/kg		Half-life (hrs)	% Increase in Plasma Level/Dose of 1 U/kg
	Minor Spontaneous Hemorrhage	Major Trauma or Surgery	Initial (loading)	Maintenance (daily)		
IX	10-15	20-25	40-60 IU	10-20 IU	20-30	≈ 1
II	10-15	20-40	40 U	15-20 U	50-80	-
VII	5-10	10-20	5-10 U	5 U qid	5	1.2-2.7
X	5-10	15-20	10-15 U	10 U	25-60	1.9

† In general, 25% is the minimal hemostatic level for patients during surgery or severe accidental trauma. The range of values in normal clinical practice is likely to be much wider than those shown above. This is due to differences between patients, clinical condition and type of assay employed.

Hemarthroses occurring in hemophiliacs with inhibitors to Factor VIII: Employ dosage levels approximating 75 IU/kg. Give a second dose after 12 hours, if needed.

Anti-Inhibitor Coagulant Complex is recommended when hemarthroses occurring in hemophiliacs with inhibitors to Factor VII cannot be resolved by administration of Factor IX Complex, and in other types of bleeding episodes in Factor VII-inhibitor patients.

Maintenance Dose: Administer according to clinical response and Factor IX level achieved. Dose is usually 10 to 20 IU/kg/day.

Inhibitor Patients: For bleeding in Hemophilia A patients with inhibitors to Factor VIII, administer 75 IU/kg. Give a second dose after 12 hours, if needed.

Prophylaxis is the ideal treatment for proven congenital deficiency of the pro-coagulants. A dosage of 10 to 20 IU/kg once or twice/week may prevent spontaneous bleeding in Hemophilia B patients. Individualize maintenance dose. Administer additional Factor IX Complex when the patient is exposed to trauma or surgery.

Rate of administration varies with the individual product; adapt to response of the patient. Infuse slowly. Rates of ≈ 100 U/min and 2 to 3 ml/min have been suggested. Do not exceed 3 ml/min. If headache, flushing, changes in pulse rate or blood pressure appear, stop the infusion until symptoms subside, then resume at a slower rate.

Storage: Refrigerate between 2° to 8°C (35° to 46°F). Do not freeze.

Rx	**AlphaNine** (Alpha Therapeutic)	Dried plasma fraction of coagulation Factors II, VII, IX and X.[1] Heat-treated	In single dose vials w/ diluent, needle and filter.[2]
Rx	**Konȳne-80** (Cutter)	Dried plasma fraction of coagulation Factors II, VII, IX and X.[1] Heparin free. Heat-treated	In 10 & 20 ml vials w/ diluent.
Rx	**Profilnine Heat-Treated** (Alpha Therapeutic)	Dried plasma fraction of coagulation Factors II, VII, IX and X.[1] Heparin free. Heat-treated	In single dose vials w/ diluent.
Rx	**Proplex T** (Hyland)	Dried plasma fraction of coagulation Factors II, VII, IX and X.[1] Heat-treated	In vials with diluent and needles.[2]
Rx	**Proplex SX-T** (Hyland)	Dried plasma fraction of coagulation Factors II, VII, IX and X (less Factor VII).[1] Heat-treated	In vials with diluent and needles.[2]

[1] Actual number of units shown on each bottle. [2] Contains heparin.

AMINOCAPROIC ACID

Actions:

Pharmacology: Inhibits fibrinolysis via inhibition of plasminogen activator substances and, to a lesser degree, through antiplasmin activity.

Pharmacokinetics: The drug is absorbed rapidly following oral administration. Peak plasma levels occur 2 hours after an oral dose. A single IV dose has a duration of action less than 3 hours. After prolonged administration, it distributes throughout both the extravascular and intravascular compartments and readily penetrates red blood and other tissue cells.

A major portion of the compound is recovered unmetabolized in the urine. Renal clearance is high (about 75% of the creatinine clearance).

Indications:

Treatment of excessive bleeding resulting from systemic hyperfibrinolysis and urinary fibrinolysis. In life-threatening situations, fresh whole blood transfusions, fibrinogen infusions and other emergency measures may be required.

Unlabeled Uses: Oral or IV aminocaproic acid, 36 g/day in six divided doses, has been used to prevent recurrence of subarachnoid hemorrhage (SAH). In the management of amegakaryocytic thrombocytopenia, the need for platelet transfusion may be decreased by use of aminocaproic acid 8 to 24 g/day for 3 days to 13 months. The drug has also been used to abort and prevent attacks of hereditary angioneurotic edema. Aminocaproic acid has also been used in patients with acute promyelocytic leukemia who develop coagulopathy associated with low levels of alpha-2-plasmin inhibitor.

Contraindications:

Evidence of an active intravascular clotting process.

Disseminated intravascular coagulation (DIC): It is important to differentiate between hyperfibrinolysis and DIC because aminocaproic acid administered to a patient with DIC may produce potentially fatal thrombus formation. Criteria which may characterize hyperfibrinolysis include platelet count (normal), protamine paracoagulation (negative) and euglobulin clot lysis (reduced). Do not use aminocaproic acid in the presence of DIC without concomitant heparin.

Injectable not for use in newborns. Benzyl alcohol, a preservative used in these products, has been associated with toxicity in newborns.

Warnings:

Upper urinary tract bleeding: Administration may cause intrarenal obstruction in the form of glomerular capillary thrombosis, or clots in the renal pelvis and ureters. Do not use in hematuria of upper urinary tract origin, unless possible benefits outweigh risks.

Usage in Pregnancy: Animal data have demonstrated teratogenicity. Safety for use during pregnancy has not been established. Use in women of childbearing potential and particularly during early pregnancy only when clearly needed and when the potential benefits outweigh the potential hazards to the fetus.

Precautions:

Impairment of fertility consistent with the antifibrinolytic activity of aminocaproic acid has been suggested in some rodent studies.

Hyperfibrinolysis: Aminocaproic acid inhibits both plasminogen activator substances and, to a lesser degree, plasmin activity. Do not administer without a definite diagnosis or laboratory findings indicative of hyperfibrinolysis (hyperplasminemia).

Usage in cardiac, hepatic or renal disease: Administer with caution to these patients. Animal pathology has shown endocardial hemorrhages, myocardial fat degeneration and kidney concretions. Skeletal muscle weakness with necrosis of muscle fibers has been reported rarely. Consider the possibility of cardiac muscle damage when skeletal myopathy occurs. Monitor CPK levels in patients on long-term therapy; discontinue use if a rise in CPK is noted. Restrict use to patients in whom the potential benefits outweigh the potential hazards.

One case of cardiac and hepatic lesions occurred following 2 g of aminocaproic acid every 6 hours for a total dose of 26 g. Death was due to continued cerebral vascular hemorrhage. Necrotic changes in the heart and liver were noted at autopsy.

Clotting: Fibrinolysis is a normal process, presumably active at all times to ensure the fluidity of blood. Inhibition of fibrinolysis by aminocaproic acid may theoretically result in clotting or thrombosis. In the few reported cases, it appears that such intravascular clotting was more likely due to the patient's preexisting condition (eg, the presence of DIC), rather than to aminocaproic acid.

Extravascular clots formed in vivo may not undergo spontaneous lysis as do normal clots.

(Continued on following page)

AMINOCAPROIC ACID (Cont.)

Drug Interactions:

Oral contraceptives or **estrogens:** An increase in clotting factors leading to a hypercoagulable state may be produced by coadministration.

Drug/Lab Tests: Serum **potassium** may be elevated by aminocaproic acid, especially in impaired renal function.

Adverse Reactions:

GI: Nausea; cramps; diarrhea.

Cardiovascular: Hypotension.

Muscular: Malaise. Myopathy characterized by weakness, fatigue, elevated serum enzymes such as creatinine phosphokinase (CPK), rhabdomyolysis associated with myoglobinuria and renal failure have been reported.

CNS: Dizziness; tinnitus; headache; delirium; auditory, visual and kinesthetic hallucinations; weakness, dizziness and headache preceding a grand mal seizure. Two cases of convulsions following IV administration have been reported.

An isolated case of restlessness and loss of contact with surroundings has also been reported.

Miscellaneous: Conjunctival suffusion; nasal stuffiness; skin rash; reversible acute renal failure; thrombophlebitis.

There have also been some reports of dry ejaculation during the period of treatment. This occurred only in hemophilia patients who received the drug after undergoing dental surgical procedures. Symptoms resolved in all patients within 24 to 48 hours of completion of therapy.

There have been reports of an increased incidence of certain neurological deficits (eg, hydrocephalus, cerebral ischemia, cerebral vasospasm) associated with use of fibrinolytic agents in the treatment of SAH. All of these events have also been described as part of the natural course of SAH, or as a consequence of diagnostic procedures such as angiography. Drug relatedness remains unclear.

Administration and Dosage:

Plasma levels: An initial dose of 5 g orally or IV, followed by 1 to 1.25 g hourly, should achieve and sustain drug plasma levels at 0.13 mg/ml. This is the concentration apparently necessary for inhibition of fibrinolysis. Administration of more than 30 g/24 hours is not recommended.

IV: Administer by infusion, using compatible IV vehicles (eg, Sterile Water for Injection, Normal Saline, 5% Dextrose, or Ringer's Solution). Rapid IV injection undiluted into a vein is not recommended; hypotension, bradycardia or arrhythmias may result. For treatment of acute bleeding syndromes, give 4 to 5 g in 250 ml of diluent by infusion during the first hour, followed by continuous infusion at the rate of 1 to 1.25 g/hour in 50 ml of diluent. Continue for 8 hours or until bleeding is controlled.

Oral: If the patient is able to take oral medications, follow an identical dosage regimen.

For the treatment of acute bleeding syndromes due to elevated fibrinolytic activity, administer 5 g orally during the first hour of treatment, followed by a continuing rate of 1 to 1.25 g per hour. Continue this method of treatment for about 8 hours or until bleeding has been controlled.

Rx	**Aminocaproic Acid** (Various)	**Injection:** 250 mg per ml	In 20, 96 and 100 ml vials.
Rx	**Amicar** (Lederle)	**Injection:** 250 mg per ml	In 20 ml (5 g) vials and 96 ml (24 g) vials.[1]
		Tablets: 500 mg	(#LL A10). White, scored. In 100s.
		Syrup: 250 mg per ml	Saccharin and sorbitol. Raspberry flavor. In pt.

\# Product identification code.

[1] With 0.9% benzyl alcohol.

TRANEXAMIC ACID

Actions:

Pharmacology: Tranexamic acid is a competitive inhibitor of plasminogen activation, and at much higher concentrations, a noncompetitive inhibitor of plasmin. It has actions similar to aminocaproic acid. Tranexamic acid is about 10 times more potent in vitro than aminocaproic acid.

Tranexamic acid in a concentration of 1 mg/ml blood does not aggregate platelets in vitro; concentrations up to 10 mg/ml have no influence on platelet count, coagulation time or various coagulation factors in whole blood or citrated blood. On the other hand, tranexamic acid in concentrations of 1 and 10 mg/ml blood prolongs thrombin time.

Pharmacokinetics: Absorption/Distribution – Absorption of tranexamic acid after oral use is ≈ 30% to 50%; bioavailability is not affected by food. The peak plasma level 3 hours after 1 g orally is 8 mg/L and after 2 g, 15 mg/L. An antifibrinolytic concentration of drug remains in different tissues for about 17 hours, and in serum up to 7 or 8 hours.

Tranexamic acid diffuses rapidly into joint fluid and the synovial membrane. In the joint fluid, the same concentration is obtained as in the serum. The biological half-life in the joint fluid is about 3 hours.

The concentration of tranexamic acid in a number of other tissues is lower than in blood. Tranexamic acid concentration in cerebrospinal fluid is about 10% that of plasma. The drug passes into the aqueous humor where the concentration is about 10% of the plasma concentration.

Tranexamic acid has been detected in semen where it inhibits fibrinolytic activity but does not influence sperm migration.

The protein binding of tranexamic acid to plasminogen is about 3% at therapeutic plasma levels. It does not bind to serum albumin.

Metabolism/Elimination – After an IV dose of 1 g, the plasma concentration time curve shows a triexponential decay with a half-life of about 2 hours for the terminal elimination phase. The initial volume of distribution is about 9 to 12 L. Urinary excretion is the main route of elimination via glomerular filtration. Overall renal clearance is equal to overall plasma clearance (110 to 116 ml/min) and more than 95% of the dose is excreted unchanged in the urine. Excretion of tranexamic acid is about 90% at 24 hours after IV administration of 10 mg/kg. After oral administration of 10 to 15 mg/kg, the cumulative urinary excretion at 24 and 48 hours is 39% and 41% of the ingested dose, respectively, or 78% and 82% of the absorbed material, respectively. Only a small fraction is metabolized. After oral administration, 1% of the dicarboxylic acid and 0.5% of the acetylated compound are excreted.

Indications:

For short-term use (2 to 8 days) in hemophilia patients to reduce or prevent hemorrhage and to reduce the need for replacement therapy during and following tooth extraction.

Unlabeled Uses: Tranexamic acid has been used for many hemostatic purposes including prevention of bleeding after surgery or trauma (eg, tonsillectomy and adenoidectomy, prostatic surgery, ocular trauma and cervical conisation), and to prevent rebleeding of subarachnoid hemorrhage, spontaneous bleeding in hemophilia and spontaneous or postoperative corneal edema. It has also been used to treat primary or IUD-induced menorrhagia, gastric and intestinal hemorrhage, recurrent epistaxis and hereditary angioneurotic edema. The drug also inhibits induced hyperfibrinolysis during thrombolytic treatment with plasminogen activators.

Contraindications:

Acquired defective color vision: Prohibits measuring one endpoint of toxicity (see Warnings).

Subarachnoid hemorrhage: Cerebral edema and cerebral infarction may be caused by tranexamic acid in patients with subarachnoid hemorrhage.

Warnings:

Retinal changes: No retinal changes have been reported in patients treated with tranexamic acid for weeks to months in clinical trials. However, focal areas of retinal degeneration have developed in cats, dogs, rabbits and rats following oral or IV tranexamic acid at doses between 126 and 1600 mg/kg/day (3 to 40 times the recommended human dose) from 6 days to 1 year. The incidence of such lesions has varied from 25% to 100% and was dose-related. At lower doses, some lesions are reversible.

(Warnings continued on following page)

TRANEXAMIC ACID (Cont.)

Warnings (Cont.):

Visual abnormalities, often poorly characterized, are the most frequently reported post-marketing adverse reaction in Sweden. For patients who are to be treated for longer than several days, perform an ophthalmological examination (including visual acuity, color vision, eyeground and visual fields) before and at regular intervals during treatment. Discontinue tranexamic acid if changes are found.

Usage in Pregnancy: Category B. Reproduction studies in mice, rats and rabbits have not revealed any evidence of impaired fertility or adverse effects on the fetus. There are no adequate and well controlled studies in pregnant women. However, tranexamic acid passes the placenta and appears in cord blood at concentrations approximately equal to maternal concentrations. Use only if clearly needed.

Usage in Lactation: Tranexamic acid is present in breast milk at 1% of the corresponding serum levels. Exercise caution when administering to nursing women.

Usage in Children: The drug has had limited use in children, principally in connection with tooth extraction. Limited data suggest that dosing instructions for adults can be used for children needing tranexamic acid therapy.

Precautions:

Renal effects: Reduce dose in patients with renal insufficiency because of accumulation.

Carcinogenesis: Leukemia in male mice receiving tranexamic acid up to 5 g/kg/day may have been related to treatment.

Hyperplasia of the biliary tract and cholangioma and adenocarcinoma of the intrahepatic biliary system have been reported in one strain of rats after dietary administration exceeding the maximum tolerated dose for 22 months. Subsequent similar studies in a different strain of rat have failed to show hyperplastic/neoplastic changes in the liver.

Adverse Reactions:

GI: Nausea, vomiting and diarrhea occur, but disappear when dosage is reduced.

Giddiness has been reported occasionally.

Hypotension has been observed when IV injection is too rapid. Do not inject more rapidly than 1 ml/minute; this reaction has not been reported with oral use.

Overdosage:

There is no known case of overdosage. Treatment includes usual supportive measures. Refer to General Management of Acute Overdosage on p. 2895

Administration and Dosage:

For dental extraction in patients with hemophilia: Immediately before surgery, substitution therapy is given with tranexamic acid, 10 mg/kg IV. After surgery, give 25 mg/kg orally 3 to 4 times daily for 2 to 8 days.

Alternative: Give 25 mg/kg orally, 3 to 4 times/day beginning 1 day prior to surgery.

Parenteral: 10 mg/kg 3 to 4 times daily for patients unable to take oral medication.

Impaired renal function (moderate to severe:) The following dosages are recommended:

	Tranexamic Acid Dosage	
Serum Creatinine (μmol/L)	IV Dose	Tablets
120-250 (1.36-2.83 mg/dl)	10 mg/kg bid	15 mg/kg bid
250-500 (2.83-5.66 mg/dl)	10 mg/kg/day	15 mg/kg/day
> 500 (> 5.66 mg/dl)	10 mg/kg every 48 hours or 5 mg/kg every 24 hours	15 mg/kg every 48 hours or 7.5 mg/kg every 24 hours

Preparation of Solution: For IV infusion, tranexamic acid may be mixed with most solutions for infusion such as electrolyte, carbohydrate, amino acid and dextran solutions. Prepare mixture the same day solution is to be used. Heparin may be added to solution for injection. Do NOT mix with blood. The drug is a synthetic amino acid; do NOT mix with solutions containing penicillin.

Rx	**Cyklokapron** (KabiVitrum)	**Tablets:** 500 mg	(#CY). White. In 100s.
		Injection: 100 mg per ml	In 10 ml amps.

\# Product identification code.

THROMBIN, TOPICAL

Actions:

Thrombin directly converts fibrinogen to fibrin, requiring no intermediate physiological agent for its action. Commercially available thrombin is derived from bovine sources. Blood fails to clot in the rare case where the primary clotting defect is absence of fibrinogen itself. The speed with which thrombin clots blood depends on its concentration. For example, the contents of a 5000 United States (NIH) unit vial dissolved in 5 ml of saline diluent is capable of clotting an equal volume of blood in less than a second, or 1000 ml in less than a minute.

Indications:

As an aid in hemostasis wherever oozing blood and minor bleeding from capillaries and small venules is accessible.

In conjunction with absorbable gelatin sponges for hemostasis in various types of surgery.

Contraindications:

Sensitivity to any of its components or to material of bovine origin.

Warnings:

Thrombin must not be injected or otherwise allowed to enter large blood vessels. Extensive intravascular clotting and even death may result.

Acute Hypersensitivity Reaction: Thrombin is an antigenic substance and has caused sensitivity and allergic reactions when injected into animals. Have epinephrine 1:1000 immediately available. Refer to Management of Acute Hypersensitivity Reactions on p. 2897

Usage in Pregnancy: Category C. It is not known whether the drug can cause fetal harm when administered to a pregnant woman or can affect reproduction capacity. Safety for use during pregnancy has not been established. Use only when clearly needed and when the potential benefits outweigh the potential hazards to the fetus.

Usage in Children: Safety and efficacy for use in children have not been established.

Adverse Reactions:

An allergic type reaction following use for treatment of epistaxis has been reported. Febrile reactions have also been observed following the use of thrombin in certain surgical procedures, but no cause-effect relationship has been established.

Administration and Dosage:

Preparation of solution: Prepare in Sterile Distilled Water or Isotonic Saline. The intended use determines the strength of the solution. For general use in plastic surgery, dental extractions, skin grafting, neurosurgery, etc, solutions containing ≈ 100 units/ml are frequently used. Where bleeding is profuse, as from cut surfaces of liver and spleen, concentrations as high as 1000 to 2000 units/ml may be required. It may often be advantageous to use thrombin in dry form on oozing surfaces.

Topical use: The recipient surface should be sponged (not wiped) free of blood before thrombin is applied. A spray may be used or the surface may be flooded using a sterile syringe and small gauge needle. The most effective hemostasis results when the thrombin mixes freely with the blood as soon as it reaches the surface. In instances where thrombin in dry form is needed, the vial is opened and the dried thrombin is then broken up into a powder. Avoid sponging of treated surfaces to ensure that the clot remains securely in place.

Use in conjunction with absorbable gelatin sponge: Immerse sponge strips in the thrombin solution. Knead the sponge strips vigorously to remove trapped air, thereby facilitating saturation of the sponge. Apply saturated sponge to bleeding area. Hold in place for 10 to 15 seconds with a pledget of cotton or a small gauze sponge.

Stability and Storage: Use solutions immediately upon reconstitution. If necessary, refrigerate at approximately 5°C for up to 3 hours. Discard partially used vials.

Rx	**Thrombinar** (Jones Medical)	**Powder**	Preservative free. In 1,000,[1] 5,000,[2] 10,000,[2] 20,000[2] or 50,000[1] unit vials.
Rx	**Thrombogen** (J & J-Merck)	**Powder**	In 1,000, 5,000,[3] 10,000[4] or 20,000[4] unit vials.
Rx	**Thrombostat** (Parke-Davis)	**Powder**	In 1,000, 5,000,[5] 10,000[5] or 20,000[5] unit vials.

[1] With 50% mannitol and 45% sodium chloride.
[2] With 50% mannitol, 45% sodium chloride and Sterile Water for Injection diluent.
[3] With Isotonic Saline diluent and transfer needle.
[4] With Isotonic Saline diluent and transfer needle. Available in spray kit.
[5] With Isotonic Saline diluent containing benzethonium chloride.

MICROFIBRILLAR COLLAGEN HEMOSTAT

Actions:

Microfibrillar collagen hemostat (MCH) is an absorbable topical hemostatic agent prepared as a dry, sterile, fibrous, water insoluble, partial hydrochloric acid salt of purified bovine corium collagen.

In contact with a bleeding surface, MCH attracts platelets which adhere to the fibrils and undergo the release phenomenon to trigger aggregation of platelets into thrombi in the interstices of the fibrous mass. The effect on platelet adhesion and aggregation is not inhibited by heparin in vitro. Platelets of patients with clinical thrombasthenia do not adhere to the hemostat in vitro. However, in clinical trials, it was effective in 50 of 68 patients receiving aspirin. It cannot control bleeding due to systemic coagulation disorders. Institute appropriate therapy to correct the underlying coagulopathy prior to use of the drug. It is tenaciously adherent to surfaces wet with blood, but excess material not involved in the hemostatic clot may be removed by teasing or irrigation, usually without restarting bleeding.

MCH stimulates a mild, chronic cellular inflammatory response. When implanted in animal tissues, it is absorbed in less than 84 days and does not predispose to stenosis at vascular anastomotic sites. These findings have not been confirmed in human use. In human studies of hemostasis in osteotomy cuts, it does not interfere with bone regeneration or healing.

Indications:

Used in surgical procedures as an adjunct to hemostasis when control of bleeding by ligature or conventional procedures is ineffective or impractical.

Contraindications:

Do not use in closure of skin incisions; it may interfere with the healing of the skin edges due to simple mechanical interposition of dry collagen.

Do not use on bone surfaces to which prosthetic materials are to be attached with methylmethacrylate adhesives. By filling porosities of cancellous bone, MCH may significantly reduce the bond strength of methylmethacrylate adhesives.

Warnings:

Sterilization: MCH is inactivated by autoclaving. Ethylene oxide reacts with bound hydrochloric acid to form ethylene chlorohydrin.

Usage in infection: The presence of the hemostat does not enhance or initiate experimental staphylococcus wound infections to a greater or lesser extent than control agents. The effects on experimental wounds contaminated with a gram-negative aerobic rod and an anaerobic non-spore-forming bacteria are currently under investigation. Use in contaminated wounds may enhance infection.

Usage in Pregnancy: There are no well controlled studies in pregnant women. Safety for use during pregnancy has not been established. Use only when clearly needed and when the potential benefits outweigh the potential hazards to the fetus.

Precautions:

After several minutes, remove excess material; this is usually possible without the reinitiation of active bleeding. Failure to remove excess material may result in bowel adhesion or mechanical pressure sufficient to compromise the ureter. In otolaryngological surgery, precautions against aspiration should include removal of all excess dry material and thorough irrigation of the pharynx.

Contains a low level of intercalated bovine serum protein which reacts immunologically as does beef serum albumin (BSA). Increases in anti-BSA titer have been observed following treatment. About two-thirds of individuals exhibit antibody titers because of ingestion of food products of bovine origin. Intradermal skin tests have occasionally shown weak positive reactions to BSA or MCH, but these have not been correlated with IgG titers to BSA. Tests have failed to demonstrate clinically significant elicitation of antibodies of the IgE class against BSA following therapy.

Fragments of MCH may pass through filters of blood scavenging systems. Therefore, avoid reintroduction of blood from operative sites treated with MCH.

MCH should not be used in conjunction with autologous blood salvage circuits.

Avoid spillage on nonbleeding surfaces, particularly in abdominal or thoracic viscera.

Adverse Reactions:

Most serious: Potentiation of infection (including abscess formation, hematoma, wound dehiscence and mediastinitis).

Miscellaneous: Adhesion formation; allergic reaction; foreign body reaction; subgaleal seroma (single case).

The use of MCH in dental extraction sockets increases the incidence of alveolalgia. Transient laryngospasm due to aspiration of dry materials has been reported following use in tonsillectomy.

(Continued on following page)

MICROFIBRILLAR COLLAGEN HEMOSTAT (Cont.)

Administration and Dosage:

This product should not be resterilized. It is not for injection or intraocular use. Moistening or wetting with saline or thrombin impairs its hemostatic efficacy. It should be used dry. Discard any unused portion.

Fibrous form: Must be applied directly to the source of bleeding. Because of its adhesiveness, it may seal over the exit site of deeper hemorrhage and conceal an underlying hematoma as in penetrating liver wounds.

Surface preparation – Compress with dry sponges immediately prior to application of the dry product, then apply pressure over the hemostat with a dry sponge; the length of time varies with the force and severity of bleeding. A minute may suffice for capillary bleeding (eg, skin graft donor sites, dermatologic curettage), but 3 to 5 or more minutes may be required for brisk bleeding (eg, splenic tears) or high pressure leaks in major artery suture holes.

Control of oozing from cancellous bone – Pack firmly into the spongy bone surface. After 5 to 10 minutes, tease excess away; this can usually be accomplished with blunt forceps and is facilitated by wetting with sterile 0.9% saline solution and irrigation. If breakthrough bleeding occurs in areas of thin application, apply additional hemostat. The amount required depends on the severity of bleeding.

Capillary bleeding – 1 g is usually sufficient for a 50 cm^2 area. Thicker coverage is required for more brisk bleeding.

Application – Will adhere to wet gloves, instruments or tissue surfaces. To facilitate handling, use dry smooth forceps. Do not use gloved fingers to apply pressure.

Non-woven web form: In neurosurgical and other procedures, apply small squares to bleeding areas; then cover the sites with moist cottonoid "patties". To prevent wetting of the MCH, and to apply needed pressure, hold a suction tip against the cottonoid for one to several minutes, depending on the briskness of bleeding. After 5 to 10 minutes, remove excess MCH by teasing and irrigation.

Rx	**Avitene** (MedChem)	**Fibrous form**	In 1 and 5 g sterile jars.
		Non-woven web form: 70 mm x 70 mm x 1 mm and 70 mm x 35 mm x 1 mm	In sterile blister packs.
Rx	**Helistat** (Marion Merrell Dow)	**Sponge:** 1" x 2"	In 10s.
		3" x 4"	In 10s.
		9" x 10"	In 5s.
Rx	**Hemotene** (Astra)	**Absorbable collagen hemostat:** 1 g	In dispenser pack of 5.

ABSORBABLE GELATIN SPONGE

Actions:

A sterile, pliable surgical sponge prepared from purified gelatin solution and capable of absorbing and holding many times its weight of whole blood.

When implanted into tissues, it is absorbed completely within 4 to 6 weeks without inducing excessive scar tissue formation. When applied to bleeding areas of nasal, rectal or vaginal mucosa, it completely liquefies within 2 to 5 days.

Indications:

Surgical procedures as an adjunct to hemostasis when control of bleeding by ligature or conventional procedures is ineffective or impractical.

Also used in oral and dental surgery as an aid in providing hemostasis.

In open prostatic surgery, insertion into the prostatic cavity provides hemostasis.

Contraindications:

Do not use in the closure of skin incisions; may interfere with the healing of skin edges.

Warnings:

Sterilization: Do not resterilize by heat, since heating may change absorption time. Ethylene oxide is not recommended for resterilization; it may be trapped in the interstices of the foam and may cause burns or irritation to tissue in trace amounts.

Precautions:

Usage in infection: Not recommended in the presence of infection. If signs of infection or abscess develop in the area where the sponge has been placed, reoperation may be necessary to remove the infected material and allow drainage.

Do not use for controlling postpartum bleeding or menorrhagia.

By absorbing fluid, the sponge may expand and impinge on neighboring structures. Therefore, when placed into cavities or closed tissue spaces, use minimal preliminary compression and avoid overpacking.

Adverse Reactions:

The sponge may form a nidus of infection and abscess formation. Giant cell granuloma formation in the brain has been reported at the site of implantation, as well as compression of the brain and spinal cord as a result of accumulation of sterile fluid. Excessive fibrosis and prolonged fixation of the tendon were seen when the sponge was used about a tendon juncture in the repair of severed tendons.

Administration and Dosage:

Hemostasis: Apply dry or saturated with sodium chloride injection. When bleeding is controlled, leave the pieces in place. Since the sponge causes little more cellular infiltration than the blood clot, the wound may be closed over it. When applied to bleeding mucosa, the sponge will stay in place until it liquefies. When applied dry, compress the pieces before application to bleeding surface, then hold in place with moderate pressure for 10 to 15 seconds. When used with saline solutions, immerse in the solution, then withdraw, squeeze to remove the air bubbles present, and replace in the solution where it will swell to its original size. If it does not swell, remove and knead vigorously until all air is expelled. The piece is then left wet, or blotted to dampness on gauze, and applied to bleeding point. Hold in place for 10 to 15 seconds with a cotton pledget or small gauze sponge.

Dentistry: When used in the dry state, roll between the fingers and lightly compress to the diameter of the cavity or socket to be filled. Following insertion, apply light finger pressure for 1 or 2 minutes. When used moist, immerse in sodium chloride solution, then remove, squeeze thoroughly to remove air bubbles, and replace in the solution where it will swell to its original size. Take from the solution, blot on sterile gauze to remove the excess fluid and place in the cavity or wound.

Prostatectomy cones are designed for use with the Foley bag catheter.

Storage: Once the package is opened, the contents are subject to contamination.

Rx	**Gelfoam** (Upjohn)	**Sponges:** Size 12 – 3 mm (20 mm x 60 mm x 3 mm)	In 4s.
		Size 12 – 7 mm (20 mm x 60 mm x 7 mm)	In 4s and 12s.
		Size 50 – (80 mm x 62.5 mm x 10 mm)	In 4s.
		Size 100 – (80 mm x 125 mm x 10 mm)	In 6s.
		Size 200 – (80 mm x 250 mm x 10 mm)	In 6s.
		Size 100, compressed – (80 mm x 125 mm)	In 6s.
		Packs: Size 2 cm – (40 cm x 2 cm)	In single jars.
		Size 6 cm – (40 cm x 6 cm)	In 6s.
		Dental Packs: Size 2 – (10 mm x 20 mm x 7 mm)	In 15s.
		Size 4 – (20 mm x 20 mm x 7 mm)	In 15s.
		Prostatectomy Cones: Size 13 cm – [13 cm (5") in diameter]	In 6s.
		Size 18 cm – [18 cm (7") in diameter]	In 6s.

ABSORBABLE GELATIN FILM, STERILE

Actions:

A sterile, absorbable gelatin film for use in neurosurgery, thoracic and ocular surgery.

In the dry state, it has the appearance and texture of cellophane of equivalent thickness; when moistened, it assumes a rubbery consistency and can then be cut to desired size and fitted to rounded or irregular surfaces. The rate of absorption after implantation ranges from 1 to 6 months, depending upon the size of the implant and the site of implantation. Pleural and muscle implants are completely absorbed in 8 to 14 days; dural and ocular implants usually require at least 2 to 5 months for complete absorption. The absence of undue tissue reactions, with the consequent decreased likelihood of developing adhesions, has been of particular value in the case of dural and ocular implants.

Indications:

Neurosurgery: As a dural substitute; absorbable gelatin film is nonconducive to undue inflammatory reaction and absorbable at a rate sufficiently slow to permit dural regeneration and healing of the arachnoid layer. Its use in patients undergoing craniotomies reportedly prevented the development of meningocerebral adhesions, thereby reducing risk of postoperative sequelae.

Thoracic surgery: In the repair of pleural defects in connection with thoracotomies, thoracoplasties and extrapleural procedures, implantation has been followed by minimal tissue reaction and subsequent closure of the defect by ingrowth of regenerating pleural and fibrous tissue across the gradually resorbed implant.

Ocular surgery: In glaucoma filtration operations (ie, iridencleisis and trephination), extraocular muscle surgery and diathermy or scleral "buckling" operations for retinal detachment. There is a remarkable lack of cellular reaction to the film implanted subconjunctivally or used as a seton into the anterior chamber. Evidence shows that implants help prevent formation of adhesions between contiguous ocular structures.

Contraindications:

Since the rate of absorption is likely to be increased in the presence of purulent exudation, do not implant in grossly contaminated or infected surgical wounds.

Administration and Dosage:

Preparation: Immerse in sterile saline solution; soak until quite pliable; cut to the desired size and shape; apply as follows:

Covering dural defects: Place over the surface of the brain. Tuck the edges of the implant beneath the dura; then close the wound in the usual manner. If desired, the film can be sutured loosely to the dura. The moist film tears easily.

Covering pleural defects: Place over the defect and anchor in place by means of small interrupted sutures.

As a seton in iridencleisis: Place a small piece (≈ 4 mm x 10 mm) over the prolapsed iris pillar parallel to the limbus; Tenon's capsule and the conjunctiva are then closed with continuous absorbable sutures closely spaced to assure tight wound closure.

Diathermy or scleral "buckling" operations: Place film over the sclera, then suture the muscle and the conjunctiva over the underlying film.

Extraocular muscle surgery: Place film over and beneath the muscle before Tenon's capsule and the conjunctiva are closed in layers.

Storage: To insure sterility, use immediately after withdrawal from the envelope.

Rx	**Gelfilm** (Upjohn)	100 mm x 125 mm	In 1s.
Rx	**Gelfilm Ophthalmic** (Upjohn)	25 mm x 50 mm	In 6s.

ABSORBABLE GELATIN POWDER, STERILE

Actions:

Possesses hemostatic properties. When implanted in tissues, it is absorbed completely in 4 to 6 weeks without excessive scar tissue formation. When applied to bleeding areas of skin or nasal, rectal or vaginal mucosa, it completely liquefies within 2 to 5 days and is nonirritating.

Indications:

Hemostasis: Gelatin powder, made into a paste by the addition of sterile saline solution, is indicated in the control of bleeding from cancellous bone when ligatures or other conventional procedures are ineffective or impractical.

Unlabeled Use: Gelatin powder has been used to stimulate granulation in the treatment of small ulcers, chronic leg ulcers, decubitus ulcers or other oozing lesions.

Contraindications:

Do not use in the closure of skin incisions; it may interfere with the healing of skin edges.

Warnings:

Sterilization: Do not resterilize by heat, since heating may change its absorption time. Ethylene oxide is not recommended for resterilization, since it may be trapped in the interstices of the foam.

Precautions:

Usage in infection: Use is not recommended in the presence of infection. If signs of infection or abscess develop in an area where gelatin powder has been placed, reoperation may be necessary to remove the infected material and allow drainage.

Not recommended as the sole hemostatic agent in patients with blood dyscrasias characterized by abnormal bleeding. Employ concurrent therapeutic measures.

Do not use for controlling postpartum bleeding or menorrhagia.

Adverse Reactions:

The powder may act as a nidus for infection and abscess formation. Giant cell granuloma in the brain has been reported at the site of implantation, as well as compression of the brain and spinal cord as a result of accumulation of sterile fluid.

Excessive fibrosis and prolonged fixation of the tendon were seen when gelatin powder was used about the tendon juncture in the repair of severed tendons.

Administration and Dosage:

Hemostasis: Open jar and pour contents (1 g) carefully into a sterile beaker. A putty-like paste is prepared by adding a total of approximately 3 to 4 ml of sterile saline to the powder. Avoid dispersion of the powder by compressing with gloved fingers into the bottom of the beaker, and then kneading to the desired consistency. The paste may then be smeared or pressed against the cut surface of cancellous bone. When bleeding stops, remove excess.

Storage: Does not deteriorate under normal storage conditions. Use as soon as the package is opened and discard the unused contents.

Rx	**Gelfoam** (Upjohn)	**Powder**	In 1 g jars.

OXIDIZED CELLULOSE

Actions:

Pharmacology: An absorbable hemostatic agent prepared from cellulose by a special process that converts it into polyanhydroglucuronic acid (cellulosic acid). Oxidation of cellulose yields an absorbable product of known acidity, soluble in alkali.

Provides hemostatic action when applied to sites of bleeding. The mechanism of action is not completely understood, but it appears to be a physical effect rather than any alteration of the normal physiologic clotting mechanism. On contact with blood, oxidized cellulose becomes a dark reddish-brown or almost black, tenacious, adhesive mass. It conforms and adheres readily to the bleeding surface. After 24 to 48 hours, it becomes gelatinous and can be removed, usually without causing additional bleeding. If left in situ, absorption depends on several factors, including the amount used, degree of saturation with blood and the tissue bed.

Oxidized cellulose swells upon contact with blood; the resultant pressure adds to its hemostatic action. It does not enter the normal clotting mechanism; however, within a few minutes of contact with blood, it forms an artificially produced clot in the bleeding area.

Bactericidal effects – The hemostat is bactericidal in vitro against many gram-positive and gram-negative organisms including aerobes and anaerobes: *Staphylococcus aureus, S epidermidis, Micrococcus luteus, Streptococcus pyogenes* Group A and B, *S salivarius, Bacillus subtilis, Proteus vulgaris, Corynebacterium xerosis, Mycobacterium phlei, Clostridium tetani, Branhamella catarrhalis, Escherichia coli, Klebsiella aerogenes, Lactobacillus* sp, *Salmonella enteritidis, Shigella dysenteriae, Serratia marcescens, C perfringens, Bacteroides fragilis, Enterococcus, Enterobacter cloacae, Pseudomonas aeruginosa, P stutzeri* and *Proteus mirabilis.* In contrast to other hemostatic agents, it does not tend to enhance experimental infection.

Indications:

Used adjunctively in surgical procedures to assist in the control of capillary, venous and small arterial hemorrhage when ligation or other conventional methods of control are impractical or ineffective. Also indicated for use in oral surgery and exodontia.

Contraindications:

Do not apply as packing or wadding as a hemostatic agent.

Do not use for packing or implantation in fractures or laminectomies; it interferes with bone regeneration and can cause cyst formation.

Do not use to control hemorrhage from large arteries or on nonhemorrhagic serous oozing surfaces, since body fluids other than whole blood (eg, serum) do not react with oxidized cellulose to produce satisfactory hemostatic effects.

Do not use around the optic nerve and chiasm.

Warnings:

Sterilization: Do not autoclave; autoclaving causes physical breakdown.

Not intended as a substitute for careful surgery and proper use of sutures and ligatures.

Closing oxidized cellulose in a contaminated wound without drainage may lead to complications and should be avoided.

The hemostatic effect is greater when applied dry; therefore, do not moisten with water or saline. Do not impregnate with materials such as buffering or hemostatic substances. Its hemostatic effect is not enhanced by the addition of thrombin; the activity of thrombin is destroyed by the low pH of the product.

Usage in infections: Although it is bactericidal against a wide range of pathogenic microorganisms, it is not a substitute for systemic antimicrobial agents to control or prevent postoperative infections. Do not impregnate with anti-infective agents.

May be left in situ when necessary, but remove it once hemostasis is achieved.

Oxidized cellulose must always be removed from the site of application after use in laminectomy procedures, around the optic nerve and chiasm and from foramina in bone when hemostasis is obtained; by swelling, it may cause nerve damage by pressure in a bony confine. Paralysis has been reported when used around the spinal cord, particularly in surgery for herniated intervertebral disc.

Usage in vascular surgery: When used as a wrap during vascular surgery, do not apply too tightly.

There have been two reports of stenotic effect after use as a wrap during vascular surgery. Although it has not been established that the stenosis was directly related to the use of the hemostat, be cautious and avoid applying the material tightly as a wrapping. Use as a wrap during vascular surgery is controversial.

(Continued on following page)

OXIDIZED CELLULOSE (Cont.)

Precautions:

Apply by loosely packing against the bleeding surface. Avoid wadding or packing tightly, especially within the bony enclosure of the CNS and within other relatively rigid cavities, where swelling may interfere with normal function or possibly cause necrosis.

Use sparingly to control bleeding in open reduction of fractures and in cancellous bone. To minimize the possibility of interference with callus formation and the theoretical chance of cyst formation, remove any excess after bleeding is controlled.

Urological procedures: Use minimal amounts and exercise care to prevent plugging of the urethra, ureter or catheter.

Since absorption is prevented in chemically cauterized areas, its use should not be preceded by application of silver nitrate or any other escharotic chemicals.

If used temporarily to line the cavity of large open wounds, place so as not to overlap the skin edges. Remove from open wounds by forceps or by irrigation with sterile water or saline solution after bleeding has stopped.

Otorhinolaryngologic surgery: Exercise care so that none of the material is aspirated by the patient (eg, controlling hemorrhage after tonsillectomy; controlling epistaxis).

Adverse Reactions:

Encapsulation of fluid and foreign body reactions, with or without infection, have been reported.

Possible prolongation of drainage in cholecystectomies and difficulty passing urine per urethra after prostatectomy have been reported. There has been one report of a blocked ureter after kidney resection.

Burning has been reported when applied after nasal polyp removal and after hemorrhoidectomy. Headache, burning, stinging and sneezing in epistaxis and other rhinological procedures, and stinging when applied on surface wounds (varicose ulcerations, dermabrasions and donor sites) also have been reported. These are believed to be due to the low pH of the product.

Intestinal obstruction has occurred, due to transmigration of a bolus of oxidized cellulose from gallbladder bed to terminal ileum or to adhesions in a loop of denuded intestine to which oxidized cellulose had been applied.

Miscellaneous: Necrosis of nasal mucous membrane or perforation of nasal septum due to tight packing; urethral obstruction following retropubic prostatectomy and introduction of oxidized cellulose within enucleated prostatic capsule.

Administration and Dosage:

Withdraw hemostat from the container with dry sterile forceps. Minimal amounts of an appropriate size are laid on the bleeding site or held firmly against the tissues until hemostasis is obtained.

Storage: Discard opened, unused oxidized cellulose. It cannot be resterilized.

Rx	**Oxycel** (Becton-Dickinson)	**Pads:** 3″ x 3″, 8 ply	In 10s.
		Pledgets: 2″ x 1″ x 1″	In 10s.
		Strips: 18″ x 2″, 4 ply	
		5″ x ½″, 4 ply	
		36″ x ½″, 4 ply	
Rx	**Surgicel** (Johnson & Johnson)	**Strips:** 2″ x 14″	
		4″ x 8″	
		2″ x 3″	
		½″ x 2″	

Actions:

The plasma protein fractions include Plasma Protein Fraction 5% (88% albumin with alpha and beta globulins), Normal Serum Albumin 5% and Normal Serum Albumin 25%.

The albumin fraction of human blood has two known functions: Maintenance of plasma colloid osmotic pressure and carrier of intermediate metabolites in the transport and exchange of tissue products. It comprises about 50% to 60% of the plasma proteins, and provides approximately 85% of their colloid osmotic pressure. Thus, it is important in regulating the volume of circulating blood; its loss is critical, particularly in shock with hemorrhage or reduced plasma volume. When plasma volume is reduced, an adequate amount of albumin quickly restores the volume in most instances. Twenty-five grams of albumin is the osmotic equivalent of approximately 2 units (500 ml) of fresh frozen plasma; or 100 ml of Normal Serum Albumin 25% provides about as much plasma protein as does 500 ml of plasma or 2 pints of whole blood. Normal Serum Albumin 5% is osmotically equivalent to an approximately equal volume of citrated plasma. The 25% albumin solution is osmotically equivalent to 5 times the volume of citrated plasma.

Plasma Protein Fraction is effective in the maintenance of a normal blood volume, but has not been proven effective to maintain oncotic pressure. When the circulating blood volume has been depleted, the hemodilution following albumin administration persists for many hours. In individuals with normal blood volume, it usually lasts only a few hours.

There is no indication that normal serum albumin (human) interferes with normal coagulation mechanisms. Antibodies, especially isoagglutinins, have been removed, enabling the product to be used without regard to the patient's blood group or blood factors.

Unlike whole blood or plasma, plasma protein fractions are free of the danger of homologous serum hepatitis, since these solutions are heat-treated at 60°C for 10 hours; thus the possibility of transmitting serum hepatitis is reduced to a minimum. No crossmatching is required and the absence of cellular elements removes the risk of sensitization with repeated infusions.

Indications:

Unless the condition responsible for the hypoproteinemia can be corrected, albumin in any form can provide only symptomatic relief or supportive treatment.

Shock due to burns, trauma, surgery and infections; in the treatment of injuries of such severity that shock, although not immediately present, is likely to ensue; in other similar conditions where the restoration of blood volume is urgent.

In cases in which there has been a considerable loss of red blood cells, transfusion with whole blood or red blood cells is indicated.

For the earliest emergency treatment of shock, it may be more convenient to have 25% Normal Serum Albumin available because it is so highly concentrated. However, the concentrated solution depends for its maximum osmotic effect on holding in the circulation additional fluids which are drawn from the tissues or administered separately, and if the patient is dehydrated, maximum effect cannot be obtained without additional fluids. Therefore, for routine hospital use, Normal Serum Albumin 5% may be preferred, since maximum osmotic effect is obtained with no additional fluids.

Albumin 25% with appropriate crystalloids may offer therapeutic advantages in oncotic deficits or in long-standing shock where treatment has been delayed. Removal of ascitic fluid from the patient with cirrhosis may cause changes in cardiovascular function and even result in hypovolemic shock.

Burns: Albumin 5% or plasma protein 5% may be used in conjunction with adequate infusions of crystalloid to prevent hemoconcentration and to combat the water, protein and electrolyte losses which usually follow serious burns. Beyond 24 hours, albumin 25% can be used to maintain plasma colloid osmotic pressure.

Hypoproteinemia: In clinical situations usually associated with a low concentration of plasma protein and, consequently, a reduced volume of circulating blood.

Normal Serum Albumin 5% or Plasma Protein Fraction 5% may be used in hypoproteinemic patients, providing sodium restriction is not a problem. If sodium restriction is imperative, use 25% Normal Serum Albumin.

Adult respiratory distress syndrome (ARDS): Characterized by deficient oxygenation caused by pulmonary interstitial edema complicating shock and postsurgical conditions. When clinical signs are those of hypoproteinemia with a fluid volume overload, albumin 25%, together with a diuretic may play a role in therapy.

Cardiopulmonary bypass: Preoperative dilution of the blood using albumin and crystalloid is safe and well tolerated. Although the limit to which the hematocrit and plasma protein concentration can be safely lowered has not been defined, it is common to achieve a hematocrit of 20% and a plasma albumin concentration of 2.5 g per 100 ml.

(Indications continued on following page)

Indications (Cont.):

Acute liver failure with or without coma: Administration of albumin may serve the double purpose of supporting the colloid osmotic pressure of the plasma as well as binding excess plasma bilirubin.

Sequestration of protein rich fluids: This occurs in such conditions as acute peritonitis, pancreatitis, mediastinitis and extensive cellulitis. The magnitude of loss into the third space may require treatment of reduced volume or oncotic activity with albumin.

Erythrocyte resuspension: Albumin may be required to avoid excessive hypoproteinemia during certain types of exchange transfusion or with the use of very large volumes of previously frozen or washed red cells.

Acute nephrosis: Certain patients may not respond to cyclophosphamide or steroid therapy. A loop diuretic and albumin 25% may help control the edema and the patient may then respond to steroid treatment.

Renal dialysis: Albumin 25% may be of value in the treatment of shock or hypotension.

Hyperbilirubinemia and erythroblastosis fetalis: Albumin can be a useful adjunct in exchange transfusions, because it reduces the necessity for reexchange and increases the amount of bilirubin removed with each transfusion, lessening risk of kernicterus.

Contraindications:

A history of allergic reactions to albumin; severe anemia; cardiac failure; renal insufficiency; presence of normal or increased intravascular volume.

In chronic nephrosis, infused albumin is promptly excreted by the kidneys with no relief of the chronic edema or effect on the underlying renal lesion. It is of occasional use in the rapid "priming" diuresis of nephrosis. Similarly, in hypoproteinemic states associated with chronic cirrhosis, malabsorption, protein losing enteropathies, pancreatic insufficiency and undernutrition, the infusion of albumin as a source of protein nutrition is not justified.

Patients on cardiopulmonary bypass.

Warnings:

Usage in Pregnancy: Category C. Safety for use has not been established. Use only when clearly needed and when potential benefits outweigh potential hazards to the fetus.

Precautions:

Concomitant blood administration: Administration of large quantities of albumin should be supplemented with or replaced by whole blood to combat the relative anemia.

Not a substitute for whole blood in situations where the oxygen carrying capacity of whole blood is required in addition to plasma volume expansion. Contains no recognized blood coagulating factors and should not be used for control of hemorrhage due to deficiencies or defects in the clotting mechanism.

Hypotension: Rapid infusion ($\triangleright$ 10 ml/min) may produce hypotension. Monitor blood pressure during use and slow or discontinue infusion if hypotension occurs.

Hemorrhage: Supplement albumin with hemodilution. When circulating blood volume has been reduced, hemodilution following the administration of albumin persists for many hours. In patients with a normal blood volume, hemodilution lasts for a much shorter period.

Usage in shock: In the treatment of shock, monitor blood pressure frequently. Widening of the pulse pressure is correlated with an increase in stroke volume or cardiac output.

Usage in dehydration: Patients with marked dehydration require additional fluids.

Special risk patients: Use with caution in patients with hepatic or renal failure because of the added protein load.

Certain patients (eg, congestive cardiac failure, renal insufficiency, stabilized chronic anemia) are at risk of developing circulatory overload. Rapid infusion may cause vascular overload with resultant pulmonary edema. Monitor for signs of increased venous pressure.

Use caution in patients with low cardiac reserve or with no albumin deficiency. A rapid increase in plasma volume may cause circulatory embarrassment or pulmonary edema.

The quick rise in blood pressure which may follow administration of albumin after injuries or surgery necessitates observation of the injured patient to detect bleeding points which failed to bleed at the lower blood pressure; otherwise, new hemorrhage and shock may occur.

(Continued on following page)

Adverse Reactions:

Cardiovascular: Hypotension may result following rapid infusion or intra-arterial administration to patients on cardiopulmonary bypass. In addition, rapid administration may result in vascular overload, dyspnea and pulmonary edema.

Allergic or pyrogenic reactions: Characterized primarily by fever and chills. Flushing, urticaria, back pain, headache, rash, nausea, vomiting, increased salivation and febrile reactions, tachycardia, hypotension, and changes in respiration, pulse and blood pressure have also been reported. If such reactions occur, discontinue the infusion and institute appropriate therapy (eg, antihistamines). If the patient requires additional plasma protein fraction, use material from a different lot.

PLASMA PROTEIN FRACTION

Administration and Dosage:

Contains 130 to 160 mEq/L sodium.

Administer by IV infusion; preferably through an area of skin at some distance from any site of infection or trauma.

Do not give more than 250 g in 48 hours. When there is an indication that more than this is required, the patient probably needs whole blood or plasma rather than additional albumin.

Hypovolemic shock: The initial dose may be 250 or 500 ml. The rate of infusion and volume of total dose depend on the patient's condition and response. Infusion at rates exceeding 10 ml/min may result in hypotension. Monitor blood pressure during administration; slow or stop infusion if sudden hypotension occurs.

In infants and young children, it may be used in the initial therapy of shock due to dehydration or infection. Infuse a dose of 10 to 15 ml/lb (20 to 30 ml/kg), at a rate not exceeding 10 ml per minute. It may be repeated, depending upon the patient's condition and response.

Hypoproteinemia: Daily doses of 1000 to 1500 ml (50 to 75 g of protein) are appropriate; larger doses may be necessary in severe hypoproteinemia with continuing loss of plasma proteins. In these and other normovolemic patients, the rate of administration should not exceed 5 to 8 ml per minute; monitor such patients for signs of hypervolemia, which include dyspnea, pulmonary edema, abnormal rise in blood pressure and central venous pressure.

Adjust the rate of infusion in accordance with the clinical response.

If edema is present or if large amounts of protein are continuously lost, it may be preferable to use concentrated (25%) Normal Serum Albumin because of the greater amount of protein in a given volume. However, unless the pathology responsible for the hypoproteinemia can be corrected (as by proper diet in malnutrition), plasma derivatives can provide only symptomatic relief or supportive treatment.

Preparation: Ready for use without further preparation; may be administered without regard to the recipient's blood group or type.

Storage: Store at room temperature, not exceeding 30°C (86°F). Do not use if the solution is turbid or has been frozen, if there is a sediment in the bottle or if more than 4 hours have elapsed after the container has been entered. Contains no preservative, so the contents of each bottle should be used on one occasion only. Destroy unused portions to prevent the possibility of use of contaminated solutions.

Admixture compatibility: The solution is compatible with the usual IV solutions of carbohydrates or electrolytes, as well as with whole blood and packed red cells. However, certain solutions containing protein hydrolysates, amino acid solutions or alcohol must not be infused through the same administration set, since these combinations may cause the proteins to precipitate.

				C.I.*
Rx	**Plasmanate** (Cutter)	**Injection:** 5%	In 50 ml vials without injection set and 250 and 500 ml vials w/injection set.	377
Rx	**Plasma-Plex** (Armour)		In 250 and 500 ml vials w/injection set.	600
Rx	**Plasmatein** (Alpha Therapeutic)		In 250 and 500 ml vials w/injection set.	392
Rx	**Protenate** (Hyland)		In 250 and 500 ml vials w/injection set.	448

* Cost Index based on cost per gram albumin.

Complete prescribing information for these products begins on page 326

ALBUMIN HUMAN (Normal Serum Albumin), 5%

Administration and Dosage:

Contains 130 to 160 mEq/L sodium.

Administer by IV infusion and without further dilution.

Infusion rate: Since albumin in this concentration provides additional fluid for plasma volume expansion when used in patients with normal blood volume, infusion rate should be slow enough to prevent too rapid expansion of plasma volume.

Shock: In the treatment of a patient in shock with greatly reduced blood volume, albumin 5% may be given as rapidly as necessary to improve clinical condition and restore normal blood volume. In adults, an initial dose of 500 ml of the 5% albumin solution is given as rapidly as tolerated. If response within 30 minutes is inadequate, an additional 500 ml of 5% albumin solution may be given. The 50 ml dosage form would be appropriate for pediatric use. In neonates and infants, albumin 5% may be given in large amounts. The recommended dose is 10 to 20 ml/kg. Guide therapy by the clinical response, blood pressure and assessment of relative anemia. If more than 1000 ml are given, or if hemorrhage has occurred, the administration of whole blood or red blood cells may be desirable.

In patients with slightly low or normal blood volume, give at a rate of 2 to 4 ml/min. Usual administration rate for children is one-quarter to one-half the adult rate.

Burns: After a burn injury (usually beyond 24 hours), there is a correlation between the amount of albumin infused and the resultant increase in plasma colloid osmotic pressure. In severe burns, immediate therapy usually includes large volumes of crystalloid, with lesser amounts of 5% albumin solution to maintain an adequate plasma volume. After the first 24 hours, the ratio of albumin to crystalloid may be increased to establish and maintain a plasma albumin level of about 2.5 g $\pm$ 0.5 g/100 ml or a total serum protein level of about 5.2 g/100 ml. However, an optimal regimen for severe burns is not established. Duration of therapy is decided by loss of protein from burned areas and in urine. Do not consider albumin as a source of nutrition.

Hypoproteinemia: The infusion of albumin as a nutrient in the treatment of chronic hypoproteinemia is not recommended. In acute hypoproteinemia, 5% albumin may be used in replacing the protein lost in hypoproteinemic conditions. However, if edema is present or if large amounts of albumin are lost, albumin 25% is preferred because of the greater amount of protein in the concentrated solution.

Preparation for administration: Swab stopper top immediately after removing seal with suitable antiseptic prior to entering vial. Inspect visually for particulate matter and discoloration.

Storage: Store at room temperature not exceeding 30°C (86°F). Do not freeze.

				C.I.*
Rx	**Albuminar-5** (Armour)	**Injection:** 5%	In 50, 250, 500 and 1000 ml vials w/IV set.	600
Rx	**Albutein 5%** (Alpha Therapeutic)		In 250 and 500 ml vials w/IV set.	440
Rx	**Buminate 5%** (Hyland)		In 250 and 500 ml vials w/IV set.	448
Rx	**Normal Serum Albumin (Human) 5% Solution** (Immuno-US)		In 250 ml vials.	445
Rx	**Plasbumin-5** (Cutter)		In 50 ml vials and 250 and 500 ml vials w/IV set.	426

* Cost Index based on cost per gram albumin.

Complete prescribing information for these products begins on page 326

ALBUMIN HUMAN (Normal Serum Albumin), 25%

Administration and Dosage:

Contains 130 to 160 mEq/L sodium. Administer by IV infusion.

Preparation: May be given undiluted or diluted in normal saline. If sodium restriction is required, administer either undiluted or diluted in a sodium free carbohydrate solution such as 5% Dextrose in Water.

Hypoproteinemia with or without edema: Unless the underlying pathology responsible for the hypoproteinemia can be corrected, IV use of albumin 25% is purely symptomatic or supportive. The usual daily dose of albumin for adults is 50 to 75 g and for children 25 g. Patients with severe hypoproteinemia who continue to lose albumin may require larger quantities. Since hypoproteinemic patients usually have approximately normal blood volumes, administration rate should not exceed 2 ml/minute, as more rapid injection may precipitate circulatory embarrassment and pulmonary edema.

Burns: After a burn injury (usually beyond 24 hours) there is a correlation between the amount of albumin infused and the resultant increase in plasma colloid osmotic pressure. The aim should be to maintain the plasma albumin concentration in the region of 2.5 ± 0.5 g/100 ml, with a plasma oncotic pressure of 20 mm Hg (equivalent to a total plasma protein concentration of 5.2 g/100 ml). This can be achieved by the IV administration of albumin 25%. The duration of therapy is decided by the loss of protein from the burned areas and in the urine. In addition, oral or parenteral feeding with amino acids should be initiated, as albumin should not be considered as a source of nutrition.

Duration of treatment varies, depending upon the extent of protein loss through renal excretion, denuded areas of skin and decreased albumin synthesis. Attempts to raise the albumin level above 4 g/100 ml may result only in an increased rate of catabolism.

Shock: Determine initial dose by the patient's condition and response to treatment. Guide therapy by degree of venous and pulmonary congestion or hematocrit measurements.

Greatly reduced blood volume – Administer as rapidly as desired. If the initial response is inadequate, (ie, if pulse rate remains above 100/min, the blood pressure below 10 cm water, or if acrocyanosis or cold sweat is present) additional albumin may be given 15 to 30 minutes following the first dose.

Slightly low or normal blood volume – The rate of administration should be 1 ml/minute. If there is continued loss of protein, it may be desirable to give whole blood or other blood fractions.

Erythrocyte resuspension: About 25 g of albumin per liter of erythrocytes is commonly used, although the requirements in preexistent hypoproteinemia or hepatic impairment can be greater. Albumin 25% is added to the isotonic suspension of washed red cells immediately prior to transfusion.

Acute nephrosis: A loop diuretic and 100 ml albumin 25% repeated daily for 7 to 10 days may help control the edema and the patient may then respond to steroid treatment.

Renal dialysis: The usual volume administered is about 100 ml; avoid fluid overload. These patients cannot tolerate substantial volumes of salt solution.

Hyperbilirubinemia and erythroblastosis fetalis: The use of albumin in exchange transfusions reduces the necessity for reexchange and increases the amount of bilirubin removed with each transfusion. Administer 1 g/kg 1 to 2 hours before transfusion.

Storage: Store at room temperature not exceeding 30°C (86°F). Do not freeze.

	Product	Form	Package	C.I.*
Rx	**Albuminar-25** (Armour)	**Injection:** 25%	In 20 ml vials and 50 and 100 ml vials w/IV set.	600
Rx	**Albutein 25%** (Alpha Therapeutic)		In 50 ml vials w/IV set.	440
Rx	**Buminate 25%** (Hyland)		In 20 ml vials and 50 and 100 ml vials w/IV set.	470
Rx	**Normal Serum Albumin (Human) 25% Solution** (Immuno-US)		In 10 ml vials and 50 ml vials.	468
Rx	**Plasbumin-25** (Cutter)		In 20 ml vials and 50 and 100 ml vials w/IV set.	382

* Cost Index based on cost per gram albumin.

DEXTRAN 1

Actions:

Pharmacology: Although clinical dextran is not antigenic, its structure is similar to other antigenic polysaccharides. Some of the polysaccharide-reacting antibodies may cross-react with clinical dextran, forming antibody-antigen complexes. These large immune complexes can trigger an anaphylactic reaction. Therefore, anaphylactic reactions may occur in patients who have never received clinical dextran, but who have dextran-reacting antibodies (DRA) in numbers sufficient to form large immune complexes.

Dextran 1, a monovalent hapten, binds to only one of the two available sites on the DRA. It reacts with dextran-reactive immunoglobulin (IgG) without bridge formation and with no tendency for the formation of large immune complexes. A molar excess of monovalent hapten, given just prior to the IV administration of a clinical dextran solution, competitively prevents the formation of immune complexes with the polyvalent clinical dextrans and impedes occurrence of anaphylaxis. During the initial phase of a clinical dextran infusion, protection is effected by hapten inhibition.

During the later phase and on the following day, protection is exerted by the dextran molecules in clinical dextran solutions due to the fact that an antigen excess develops in the circulation and only small nonanaphylactogenic immune complexes can be found. An additional injection of dextran 1 is therefore recommended if 48 hours or more have elapsed since the previous infusion of clinical dextran.

Dextran-induced anaphylactic reactions have an incidence range of 0.002% to 0.025% per unit used (0.002% to 0.013% for Dextran 40 and 0.017% to 0.025% for Dextran 60/75). By means of hapten inhibition, the incidence is 15 to 20 times lower.

Pharmacokinetics: Because of its low molecular weight (MW = 1000), dextran 1 is rapidly and completely excreted by glomerular filtration. After IV injection of a single dose of 20 ml, about 50% is cleared from the blood within 30 minutes. Mean urinary elimination half-life was 41 ± 11 minutes in 12 normal healthy individuals.

Indications:

Prophylaxis of serious anaphylactic reactions to IV infusion of clinical dextran.

Mild dextran-induced anaphylactic (allergic) reactions are *not* prevented by dextran 1.

Contraindications:

Do not give dextran 1 if the IV administration of clinical dextran solutions is contraindicated. This includes marked hemostatic defects of all types or hemorrhagic tendencies, marked cardiac decompensation and renal disease with severe oliguria or anuria.

Warnings:

Cardiac effects: Severe hypotension and bradycardia have been reported.

Usage in Pregnancy: Category B. Reproduction studies in mice revealed no evidence of impaired fertility or fetal harm. In rabbits, doses 35 to 70 times the human dose resulted in increased incidence of fetal resorption, post-implantation fetal loss, retardation of fetal long-bone ossification and marginal fetal growth retardation. There are no adequate and well controlled studies in pregnant women. Use during pregnancy only if clearly needed.

Usage in Lactation: It is not known whether dextran 1 is excreted in human milk. Exercise caution when administering to nursing women.

Precautions:

If any reaction occurs, do not administer clinical dextran solutions.

Adverse Reactions:

Cutaneous reactions (0.016%); moderate hypotension (systolic BP > 60 mm Hg; 0.014%); bradycardia (< 60 bpm) and moderate hypotension (0.013%); nausea, pallor and shivering (0.011%); bradycardia alone (0.004%); bradycardia and severe hypotension (systolic BP < 60 mm Hg; 0.001%). Do not give a subsequent infusion if adverse reactions occur.

Overdosage:

Human data are not available. The drug is rapidly cleared by renal excretion. Any overdosage, therefore, should be of short duration and of minimal consequence.

Administration and Dosage:

For IV use only. Do NOT dilute or admix with clinical dextran.

Adults: 20 ml (150 mg/ml) IV rapidly, 1 to 2 min before IV infusion of clinical dextran.

Children: 0.3 ml/kg in a corresponding manner.

The time interval between administration of dextran 1 and clinical dextran solutions should not exceed 15 minutes; if a longer period elapses, repeat dextran 1 dose.

Repeat injection of dextran 1 if more than 48 hours have elapsed since the last infusion of clinical dextran. Administer 1 to 2 minutes before every IV clinical dextran infusion.

May give IV through a Y injection site if there is minimal dilution with primary solution. Do not give through an IV set used to infuse clinical dextran. May give through heparin lock.

Storage: Do not exceed 25°C (77°F). Protect from freezing.

Rx	**Promit** (Pharmacia)	**Injection:** 150 mg per ml	In 20 ml vials.

HETASTARCH (Hydroxyethyl Starch; HES)

Actions:

Pharmacology: Hetastarch (HES) is a complex mixture of ethoxylated amylopectin molecules of various molecular sizes; average molecular weight (MW) is 450,000 (range, 10,000 to > 1 million). The colloidal properties of 6% HES approximate those of human albumin. After IV infusion, plasma volume expands slightly in excess of the volume infused, which decreases over 24 to 36 hrs. Hemodynamic status may improve for 24 hrs or longer. Adding HES to whole blood increases the erythrocyte sedimentation rate and improves the efficiency of granulocyte collection by centrifugal means.

Pharmacokinetics: Hetastarch molecules below 50,000 MW are rapidly eliminated renally; ≈ 40% appear in the urine in 24 hours. Larger molecules are broken down to smaller ones. Approximately 90% of the dose is eliminated from the body with an average half-life of 17 days; the remainder has a half-life of 48 days. The hydroxyethyl group is not cleaved, but remains intact and attached to glucose units when excreted.

Indications:

Adjunct for plasma volume expansion in shock due to hemorrhage, burns, surgery, sepsis or other trauma.

Adjunct in leukapheresis to improve harvesting and increase the yield of granulocytes.

Contraindications:

Severe bleeding disorders; severe cardiac failure; renal failure with oliguria or anuria.

Warnings:

Because it does not have oxygen-carrying capacity or contain plasma proteins such as coagulation factors, hetastarch is not a substitute for blood or plasma.

Coagulation effects: Large volumes may alter coagulation and result in transient prolongation of prothrombin time (PT), partial thromboplastin time (PTT), bleeding and clotting times and decreased hematocrit and excessive dilution of plasma proteins.

Usage in leukapheresis: Significant declines in platelet count and hemoglobin levels have been observed in donors undergoing repeated leukapheresis procedures due to the volume expanding effects of hetastarch. Hemoglobin levels usually return to normal within 24 hours. Hemodilution by hetastarch and saline may also result in 24 hour declines of total protein, albumin, calcium and fibrinogen values.

Usage in Pregnancy: Do not use in pregnancy, particularly during early pregnancy, unless the benefits outweigh the hazards to the fetus.

Usage in Children: No data are available pertaining to use in children.

Precautions:

Special risk patients: The possibility of circulatory overload exists. Take special care in patients with impaired renal clearance and when the risk of pulmonary edema or congestive heart failure is increased.

Lab test alterations: Indirect bilirubin levels increased in two subjects receiving multiple infusions; levels returned to normal by 96 hours after infusion. Total bilirubin remained normal. Observe caution in liver disease.

Monitoring: During leukapheresis, monitor CBC, total leukocyte and platelet counts, leukocyte differential count, hemoglobin, hematocrit, PT and PTT.

Adverse Reactions:

Vomiting; mild temperature elevation; chills; itching; submaxillary and parotid glandular enlargement; mild influenza-like symptoms; headache; muscle pain; peripheral edema of the lower extremities.

Allergic or sensitivity reactions: Anaphylactoid reactions (periorbital edema, urticaria, wheezing) have been reported. If these occur, discontinue the drug. If necessary, give antihistamines. See also Management of Acute Hypersensitivity Reactions on p. viii.

Administration and Dosage:

Administer by IV infusion only. Total dosage and rate of infusion depend upon the amount of blood lost and the resultant hemoconcentration.

Plasma volume expansion: The usual amount is 500 to 1000 ml. Total dosage does not usually exceed 1500 ml/day (20 ml/kg). In acute hemorrhagic shock, rates approaching 20 ml/kg/hour may be used; in burn or septic shock, administer at slower rates.

Leukapheresis: In continuous flow centrifugation (CFC) procedures, 250 to 700 ml hetastarch is typically infused at a constant fixed ratio, usually 1:8, to venous whole blood.

Multiple CFC procedures using hetastarch of up to 2 per week and a total of 7 to 10 have been safe and effective; the safety of more frequent or a greater number of procedures is not established.

Store at room temperature not exceeding 40°C (104°F). Do not freeze. Do not use if solution is turbid deep brown or if crystalline precipitate forms.

Rx	**Hespan** (DuPont Critical Care)	**Injection:** 6 g per 100 ml in 0.9% sodium chloride	In 500 ml IV infusion bottle.

DEXTRAN, LOW MOLECULAR WEIGHT (Dextran 40)

Actions:

Dextran 40 is a branched polysaccharide plasma-volume expander with an average molecular weight of 40,000 (range 10,000 to 90,000). A 2.5% solution of dextran 40 is equivalent in colloid osmotic pressure to normal plasma. Generally, plasma volume is increased onefold to twofold over the volume of dextran 40 infused. The extent and duration of volume expansion produced will depend on the pre-existing blood volume, rate of infusion and rate of dextran clearance by the kidneys.

Pharmacokinetics: Dextran 40 is evenly distributed in the vascular system. Its distribution according to molecular weight shifts toward higher molecular weights as the smaller molecules are excreted by the kidney. Approximately 50% administered to a normovolemic subject is excreted in the urine within 3 hours, 60% within 6 hours and 75% within 24 hours. The remaining 25% is partly hydrolyzed and excreted in the urine, partly excreted in the feces and partly oxidized. Unexcreted dextran molecules diffuse into the extravascular compartment and are temporarily taken up by the reticuloendothelial system. Some of these molecules are returned to the intravascular compartment via the lymphatics. Dextran is slowly degraded by the enzyme dextranase to glucose.

Adjunctive therapy in shock: Enhances blood flow, particularly in the microcirculation, by a combination of the following mechanisms: Increases blood volume, venous return and cardiac output; decreases blood viscosity and peripheral vascular resistance; reduces aggregation of erythrocytes and other cellular elements of blood by coating them and maintaining their electronegative charges.

Administration to a patient in shock usually increases blood volume, central venous pressure, cardiac output, stroke volume, arterial blood pressure, pulse pressure, capillary perfusion, venous return, central venous pressure and urinary output; it also decreases blood viscosity, heart rate, peripheral resistance and mean transit time and prevents or reverses cellular aggregation. Hematocrit is lowered in proportion to the infusion volume.

The intense but relatively short-lived plasma expansion volume produced by dextran 40 is advantageous in the treatment of early shock, since it acts rapidly to correct hypovolemia while allowing control of the plasma volume. If overexpansion occurs, the discontinuation of the infusion will result in a decline in plasma volume due to loss of dextran from the intravascular space.

Priming solution for extracorporeal circulation: Its advantages over homologous blood and other priming fluids include: Decreased destruction of erythrocytes and platelets; reduced intravascular hemagglutination; maintenance of electronegativity of erythrocytes and platelets.

Prophylaxis against venous thrombosis and thromboembolism: The infusion of dextran 40 during and after surgical trauma reduces the incidence of deep venous thrombosis (DVT) and pulmonary embolism (PE) in surgical patients subject to procedures with a high incidence of thromboembolic complications. Dextran 40 simultaneously inhibits mechanisms essential to thrombus formation such as vascular stasis and platelet adhesiveness, and alters the structure and lysability of fibrin clots.

Dextran 40 increases cardiac output, arterial, venous and microcirculatory flow and reduces mean transit time, chiefly by expanding plasma volume and by reducing blood viscosity, through hemodilution and by reducing red cell aggregation.

Indications:

Adjunctive treatment of shock or impending shock due to hemorrhage, burns, surgery or other trauma. The solution is for emergency treatment when whole blood products are not available; it is not a substitute for whole blood or plasma proteins.

As a priming fluid, either as the sole primer or as an additive, in pump oxygenators during extracorporeal circulation.

Prophylaxis against DVT and PE in patients undergoing procedures associated with a high incidence of thromboembolic complications, such as hip surgery.

Contraindications:

Hypersensitivity to dextran; marked hemostatic defects of all types (thrombocytopenia, hypofibrinogenemia, etc), including those caused by drugs (heparin, warfarin, etc); marked cardiac decompensation; renal disease with severe oliguria or anuria.

Decreased urinary output, secondary to shock, is not a contraindication unless there is no improvement in urine output after the initial dose.

If administration of sodium or chloride could be clinically detrimental, 10% Dextran in 0.9% Sodium Chloride Injection is contraindicated.

(Continued on following page)

DEXTRAN, LOW MOLECULAR WEIGHT (Dextran 40) (Cont.)

Warnings:

Anaphylaxis: Antigenicity of dextrans is directly related to their degree of branching. Since dextran 40 has a very low degree of branching, it is relatively free of antigenic effect. Hypersensitivity reactions have, however, been reported (see Adverse Reactions). Infrequently, severe and fatal anaphylactoid reactions (eg, marked hypotension, cardiac and respiratory arrest) have been reported. Most of these reactions occurred early in the infusion period in patients not previously exposed to IV dextran, and have appeared after administration of as little as 10 ml. Stop infusion immediately if an anaphylactoid reaction is imminent. Refer to Management of Acute Hypersensitivity Reactions on p. 2713. In circulatory collapse due to anaphylaxis, institute rapid volume substitution with an agent other than dextran. Dextran 1 is indicated for prophylaxis of serious anaphylactic reactions to dextran infusions.

Fluid imbalance: These products are colloid hypertonic solutions and will attract water from the extravascular space. Poorly hydrated patients will need additional fluid therapy. If given in excess, vascular overload could occur. This can be avoided by monitoring central venous pressure.

Administration of dextran IV can cause fluid or solute overloading, resulting in dilution of serum electrolyte concentrations, overhydration, congested states or pulmonary edema. The risk of dilutional states is inversely proportional to electrolyte concentrations of administered parenteral solutions.

Renal effects: Renal excretion causes elevation of the specific gravity of the urine. In the presence of adequate urine flow, only minor elevations occur, but in patients with diminished urine flow, urine viscosity and specific gravity can be increased markedly. As osmolarity is only slightly increased by the presence of dextran molecules, assess a patient's state of hydration by determination of urine or serum osmolarity. If signs of dehydration are noted, administer additional fluids. An osmotic diuretic such as mannitol is useful in maintaining adequate urine flow.

Renal failure, sometimes irreversible, has been reported. While the preexisting clinical condition of these patients could account for the oliguria or anuria, it is possible that dextran use may have contributed to its development. Evidence of tubular vacuolization (osmotic nephrosis) has been found following administration. The exact clinical significance is unknown.

In patients with diminished renal function, use of solutions containing sodium ions may result in sodium retention. Excessive doses may precipitate renal failure.

Usage in hemorrhage: Use with caution in patients with active hemorrhage; the increase in perfusion pressure and improved microcirculatory flow may result in additional blood loss.

Avoid administering infusions that exceed the recommended dose, since a dose-related increase in the incidence of wound hematoma, wound seroma, wound bleeding, distant bleeding (hematuria and melena), and pulmonary edema has been observed.

Hematologic effects: Use with caution in patients with thrombocytopenia. Hematocrit should not be depressed below 30% by volume. When large volumes of dextran are administered, plasma protein levels will be decreased. Do not give dextran 40 to patients with marked thrombocytopenia or hypofibrinogenemia.

In individuals with normal hemostasis, dosages of up to 15 ml/kg or > 1000 ml may prolong bleeding time, increase bleeding tendency and depress platelet function. Dosages in this range also markedly decrease factor VIII; they also decrease factors V and IX to a greater degree than would be expected from hemodilution alone. Since these changes tend to be more pronounced following trauma or major surgery, observe all patients for early signs of bleeding complications.

Special risk patients: Use solutions containing sodium ions with great care, if at all, in patients with congestive heart failure, severe renal insufficiency, in clinical states in which edema exists with sodium retention (particularly in postoperative or elderly patients) and in patients receiving corticosteroids.

Use dextrose-containing solutions with caution in overt or known subclinical diabetes mellitus.

Usage in Pregnancy: Category C. Safety for use during pregnancy has not been established. Use only when clearly needed and when the potential benefits outweigh the potential hazards to the fetus.

Usage in Lactation: It is not known whether this drug is excreted in human milk. Exercise caution when dextran 40 is administered to a nursing woman.

(Continued on following page)

DEXTRAN, LOW MOLECULAR WEIGHT (Dextran 40) (Cont.)

Precautions:

Urine output should be carefully monitored. Usually, an increase in urine output occurs in oliguric patients after administration. If no increase is observed after the infusion of 500 ml, discontinue the drug until adequate diuresis develops spontaneously or can be induced by other means.

Exercise care to prevent a depression of the hematocrit below 30%.

Infusion of dextran may lead to excessive dilution of red blood cells and plasma proteins, dilution of other blood constituents (platelets, fibrinogen), or dilutional acidosis caused by dilution of the bicarbonate ion.

Observe patients for early signs of bleeding complications, particularly following surgery, major trauma or if anticoagulant drugs are being administered.

Drug Interactions:

Laboratory test alterations: **Blood sugar** determinations that employ high concentrations of acid (acetic or sulfuric) may cause hydrolysis of dextran; falsely elevated glucose assays may be reported in patients receiving dextran. In other laboratory tests, the presence of dextran may result in the development of turbidity, which can interfere with **bilirubin** assays in which alcohol has been employed, in **total protein** assays employing biuret reagent and in **blood sugar** determinations with the ortho-toluidine method. Consider withdrawal of blood for chemical laboratory tests prior to initiating therapy.

Blood typing and **crossmatching** procedures employing enzyme techniques may give unreliable readings if the samples are taken after infusion. Other blood typing and crossmatching procedures are not affected. Draw blood samples for the above determinations prior to initiating infusion or, alternatively, inform the laboratory that the patient has received dextran so that suitable assay methods can be applied.

Occasional abnormal **renal** and **hepatic** function values have been reported following IV use. The specific effect on renal and hepatic function could not be determined, since most of these patients had also undergone surgery or cardiac catheterization.

Adverse Reactions:

Hypersensitivity: Mild cutaneous eruptions, generalized urticaria, hypotension, nausea, vomiting, headache, dyspnea, fever, tightness of the chest, bronchospasm, wheezing, and, rarely, anaphylactoid (allergic) shock (see Warnings).

Miscellaneous: Reactions which may occur because of the solution or the technique of administration include febrile response, infection at the injection site, venous thrombosis or phlebitis extending from the injection site, extravasation and hypervolemia.

Hypernatremia may be associated with edema and exacerbation of congestive heart failure due to the retention of water, resulting in expanded extracellular fluid volume.

If solutions containing sodium chloride are infused in large volumes, chloride ions may cause a loss of bicarbonate ions, resulting in an acidifying effect.

(Continued on following page)

DEXTRAN, LOW MOLECULAR WEIGHT (Dextran 40) (Cont.)

Administration and Dosage:

For IV use only.

Adjunctive therapy in shock: Total dosage during the first 24 hours should not exceed 20 ml/kg. The first 10 ml/kg should be infused rapidly, with the remaining dose being administered more slowly. Monitor the central venous pressure frequently during the initial infusion. Should therapy continue beyond 24 hours, total daily dosage should not exceed 10 ml/kg and therapy should not continue beyond 5 days.

Hemodiluent in extracorporeal circulation: The dosage employed in the priming fluid will vary with the volume of pump oxygenator employed. It may be added as sole primer or as an additive. Generally, 10 to 20 ml/kg are added to the perfusion circuit. Do not exceed total dosage of 20 ml/kg; this can be limited and controlled by adding other priming fluids.

Prophylactic therapy of venous thrombosis and thromboembolism: Select dosage according to the risk of thromboembolic complications (eg, type of surgery and duration of immobilization). In general, initiate treatment during surgery. Administer 500 to 1000 ml (approximately 10 ml/kg) on the day of the operation. Continue treatment at a dose of 500 ml/day for an additional 2 to 3 days. Thereafter, and according to the risk of complications, 500 ml may be administered every second or third day during the period of risk, for up to 2 weeks.

In children the best guide is the body weight or surface area, and the total dosage should not exceed 20 ml/kg.

Storage: Store at a constant temperature, between 15°C (59°F) to 30°C (86°F). Protect from freezing.

	Product	Form	Package	C.I.*
Rx	**Dextran 40** (Kendall McGaw)	**Injection:** 10% dextran 40 in 0.9% sodium chloride	In 500 ml.	11
Rx	**Gentran 40** (Baxter)		In 500 ml.	8
Rx	**10% LMD** (Abbott)		In 500 ml.	4
Rx	**Rheomacrodex** (Pharmacia)		In 500 ml.	6
Rx	**Dextran 40** (Kendall McGaw)	**Injection:** 10% dextran 40 in 5% dextrose	In 500 ml.	11
Rx	**Gentran 40** (Baxter)		In 500 ml.	8
Rx	**10% LMD** (Abbott)		In 500 ml.	4
Rx	**Rheomacrodex** (Pharmacia)		In 500 ml.	6

* Cost Index based on cost per ml.

DEXTRAN, HIGH MOLECULAR WEIGHT (Dextran 70)

Actions:

Pharmacology: Dextrans are synthetic polysaccharides used to approximate the colloidal properties of albumin. Dextran 70 has an average molecular weight (MW) of 70,000 (range 20,000 to 200,000) and dextran 75 has an average MW of 75,000. Dextran 70 improves blood pressure, pulse rate, respiratory exchange and renal function in patients with hypovolemia or hypotensive shock. IV infusion results in an expansion of plasma volume slightly in excess of volume infused and decreases from this maximum over the next 24 hours. This plasma volume expansion improves hemodynamic status for ≥ 24 hours.

Pharmacokinetics: Dextran molecules below 50,000 molecular weight are eliminated by renal excretion, with approximately 50% appearing in the urine in 24 hours in the normovolemic patient. The remaining dextran is enzymatically degraded to glucose at a rate of about 70 to 90 mg/kg/day. This is a variable process.

Indications:

Treatment of shock or impending shock due to surgery or other trauma, hemorrhage or burns. Intended for emergency treatment only when whole blood or blood products are not available; do not regard as a substitute for whole blood or plasma proteins. It should not replace other forms of therapy known to be of value in the treatment of shock.

Contraindications:

Hypersensitivity to dextran; marked hemostatic defects of all types (thrombocytopenia, hypofibrinogenemia, etc), including those induced by drugs; marked cardiac decompensation; renal disease with severe oliguria or anuria; hypervolemic conditions and severe bleeding disorders.

Where use of sodium or chloride could be clinically detrimental.

Warnings:

Anaphylaxis: Severe and fatal anaphylactoid reactions (eg, marked hypotension, cardiac and respiratory arrest) have been reported. These reactions occurred early in the infusion period in patients not previously exposed to IV dextran. Stop infusion immediately if an anaphylactoid reaction is imminent. Refer to Management of Acute Hypersensitivity Reactions on p. viii. In circulatory collapse due to anaphylaxis, institute rapid volume substitution with an agent other than dextran. Dextran 1 is indicated for prophylaxis of serious anaphylactic reactions associated with dextran infusions.

Hematologic effects: In individuals with normal hemostasis, dosages approximating 15 ml/kg or > 1000 ml prolong bleeding time, increase bleeding tendency and depress platelet function; use with caution in patients with thrombocytopenia. Dosages in this range also markedly decrease factor VIII, and decrease factor V and factor IX to a greater extent than that expected from hemodilution alone. Since these changes tend to be more pronounced following trauma or major surgery, observe patients for early signs of bleeding complications. Transient prolongation of bleeding time may occur following doses > 1000 ml, particularly if the patient is on concomitant anticoagulation therapy. Take care to prevent depression of hematocrit below 30% by volume. When large volumes of dextran are given, plasma protein level will be decreased.

Special risk patients: Use solutions containing sodium ions with great care, if at all, in patients with congestive heart failure, pulmonary edema, severe renal insufficiency, patients receiving corticosteroids or corticotropin, and in clinical states in which edema exists with sodium retention. Circulatory overload may occur. Exercise special care in patients with impaired renal clearance or chronic liver disease.

Exercise care in patients with pathological abdominal conditions and to those undergoing bowel surgery.

Fluid imbalance: Fluid or solute overloading may occur, resulting in dilution of serum electrolyte concentrations, overhydration, congested states (CHF), and peripheral or pulmonary edema. The risk of dilutional states is inversely proportional to the electrolyte concentration of administered parenteral solutions.

The risk of solute overload causing congested states with peripheral and pulmonary edema is directly proportional to the electrolyte concentrations of such solutions.

Monitoring central venous blood pressure is recommended as a means for detecting overexpansion of blood volume. When signs of overexpansion appear, discontinuing IV infusion allows blood volume to readjust and decline, primarily by loss of fluid to urine.

Usage in Pregnancy: Category C. Safety for use during pregnancy has not been established. There are no adequate and well controlled studies in pregnant women. Use only when clearly needed and when potential benefits outweigh potential hazards.

Usage in Lactation: It is not known whether this drug is excreted in human milk. Exercise caution when administering to a nursing woman.

(Continued on following page)

DEXTRAN, HIGH MOLECULAR WEIGHT (Dextran 70) (Cont.)

Precautions:

Urine output should be carefully observed. An increase in urine output usually occurs in oliguric patients after the administration of dextran. If no increase is observed after the infusion of 500 ml of dextran, discontinue the drug until adequate diuresis develops spontaneously or can be provoked by other means.

Observe patients for early signs of bleeding complications, particularly following surgery or major trauma, or if anticoagulant drugs are being administered.

Drug Interactions:

Laboratory test alterations: **Blood sugar** determinations that employ high concentrations of acid (acetic or sulfuric) may cause hydrolysis of dextran; falsely elevated glucose assays may be reported in patients receiving dextran. In other laboratory tests, the presence of dextran may result in the development of turbidity, which can interfere with **bilirubin** assays in which alcohol has been employed, in **total protein** assays employing biuret reagent and in **blood sugar** determinations with the ortho-toluidine method.

Blood typing and **crossmatching** procedures employing enzyme techniques may give unreliable readings if the samples are taken after infusion. If blood is drawn after the infusion, the saline-agglutination and indirect antiglobulin methods may be used for typing and crossmatching. Draw blood samples for the above determinations prior to initiating infusion or, alternatively, inform the laboratory that the patient has received dextran so that suitable assay methods can be applied.

Adverse Reactions:

Hypersensitivity: Allergic reactions include urticaria, nasal congestion, wheezing, tightness of the chest, dyspnea, mild hypotension and, rarely, anaphylactoid (allergic) shock (see Warnings). Antihistamines may be effective in relieving these symptoms.

Miscellaneous: Sudden marked hypotension; nausea; vomiting; fever; joint pains.

Hypernatremia may be associated with edema and exacerbation of congestive heart failure due to retention of water, resulting in an expanded extracellular fluid volume.

If solutions containing sodium chloride are infused in large volumes, chloride ions may cause a loss of bicarbonate ions, resulting in an acidifying effect.

Infusion technique: Reactions which may occur because of the solution or the technique of administration include febrile response, infection at the injection site, venous thrombosis or phlebitis extending from the injection site, extravasation and hypervolemia. If a reaction develops, discontinue use and treat accordingly.

Administration and Dosage:

Administer by IV infusion only. Total dose and rate of infusion depend upon the magnitude of fluid loss and the resultant hemoconcentration. It is suggested that total dosage not exceed 20 ml/kg during the first 24 hours.

Adults: The amount usually administered is 500 to 1000 ml, which may be given at a rate of from 20 to 40 ml/minute in an emergency.

Children: The best guide to dosage is the body weight or surface area of the patient; total dosage should not exceed 20 ml/kg.

No additives should be delivered via plasma volume expanders.

Stability and storage: The solution has no bacteriostat; therefore, discard partially used containers. Do not use unless solution is clear. Store at a constant temperature not exceeding 25°C (77°F).

	Product	Formulation	Package	C.I.*
Rx	**Dextran 75** (Abbott)	**Injection:** 6% dextran 75 in 0.9% sodium chloride	In 500 ml.	11
Rx	**Gentran 75** (Baxter)		In 500 ml.	5
Rx	**Dextran 70** (Kendall McGaw)	**Injection:** 6% dextran 70 in 0.9% sodium chloride	In 500 ml.	2
Rx	**Gentran 70** (Baxter)		In 500 ml.	3
Rx	**Macrodex** (Pharmacia)		In 500 ml.	4
Rx	**Dextran 75** (Abbott)	**Injection:** 6% dextran 75 in 5% dextrose	In 500 ml.	11
Rx	**Macrodex** (Pharmacia)	**Injection:** 6% dextran 70 in 5% dextrose	In 500 ml.	4

* Cost Index based on cost per ml.

INTRAVASCULAR PERFLUOROCHEMICAL EMULSION, 20%

Actions:

Pharmacology: Intravascular perfluorochemical emulsion, 20%, is a stable emulsion of perfluorochemicals in Water for Injection. The perfluorochemical phase of the emulsion dissolves oxygen and carbon dioxide. The formulation is a sterile, nonpyrogenic fluid for intracoronary administration only during percutaneous transluminal coronary angioplasty.

Intravascular perfluorochemical emulsion has an osmolarity of approximately 410 mOsmol/L and contains emulsified perfluorochemical particles with a mean particle diameter of < 270 nm. The content of particles > 400 nm is < 10%. The pH of the emulsion when prepared for administration is approximately 7.3; fluoride ion content is < 2 ppm. It is less viscous than whole blood at 37°C and physiological shear rates.

Perfluorodecalin and perfluorotri-n-propylamine are the active oxygen carrying components of intravascular perfluorochemical emulsion. They are synthetic perfluorochemicals. Intravascular perfluorochemical emulsion, carries oxygen preferentially dissolved in the perfluorochemical emulsion particles. When the emulsion is oxygenated and injected transluminally through a coronary angioplasty balloon catheter, it will deliver oxygen to the myocardium distal to the point of balloon inflation.

Pharmacokinetics: The primary route of elimination of the perfluorochemicals is via the lung in expiratory gases. Perfluorodecalin and perfluorotri-n-propylamine, are taken up by the reticuloendothelial system, primarily in the liver, spleen and bone marrow. No perfluorochemicals have been detected in the brain. The molecules are excreted intact.

The half-life of perfluorochemicals in circulation and in organs is dose dependent. In a group of severely anemic hemorrhagic shock patients receiving intravascular perfluorochemical emulsion for transfusion therapy at a dose of 10 ml/kg, the half-life in circulation was about 8 hours. Four days following administration, 3.6% of the total perfluorodecalin dose and 5.7% of the total perfluorotri-n-propylamine dose were retained in the liver, while the spleen retained 1.2% of the perfluorodecalin and 2.2% of the perfluorotri-n-propylamine.

After a single dose of 10 ml/kg, trace amounts of perfluorochemicals will be present in the liver and spleen for up to 80 days, and in fat, bone marrow, adrenal, kidney and lung for lesser periods. In one patient given a single dose of 22 ml/kg for severe anemia, 0.62% of the injected dose of perfluorotri-n-propylamine was present in the liver 141 days after administration. Perfluorodecalin was not found in the liver after 141 days. At the 10 ml/kg dose, perfluorochemicals were not found after 210 days.

Accumulation of perfluorochemicals will result from repeated dosage, therefore intravascular perfluorochemical emulsion should not be given more than one time in 6 months (see Administration and Dosage).

Clinical trials: In controlled clinical trials, the use of oxygenated intravascular perfluorochemical emulsion perfusion preserves ventricular wall motion and global left ventricular ejection fraction during percutaneous transluminal coronary angioplasty (PTCA).

Echocardiographic studies from four randomized, blinded, controlled trials have shown that ventricular wall motion was preserved in patients who received oxygenated intravascular perfluorochemical emulsion perfusion compared to patients who received oxygenated Lactated Ringer's perfusion, nonoxygenated intravascular perfluorochemical emulsion perfusion, or no perfusion. Baseline values for global left ventricular ejection fraction were preserved in patients undergoing angioplasty with oxygenated intravascular perfluorochemical emulsion perfusion in comparison with significant declines in the control groups during balloon inflation times up to 90 seconds.

In a double-blind, randomized trial, patients undergoing angioplasty with oxygenated intravascular perfluorochemical emulsion perfusion had significantly less ST segment deviation at the end of balloon inflation; the number of patients experiencing severe angina was significantly less during oxygenated intravascular perfluorochemical emulsion perfusion than during routine PTCA (20.5% vs 33.7%).

In other double-blinded, randomized trials of a crossover design, patients had a longer time to onset of angina (61 vs 48.9 seconds). No improvements in complications of angioplasty or mortality were seen in these studies. Longer term effects of perfusion with intravascular perfluorochemical emulsion have not been studied.

In a multicenter, single-blind, crossover trial in selected subjects at high risk of ischemic complications, distal perfusion with oxygenated intravascular perfluorochemical emulsion preserved ventricular function during angioplasty. Cardiac output, systolic function, anginal pain, and ST segment changes were all significantly improved during balloon inflations with oxygenated intravascular perfluorochemical emulsion perfusion compared to routine, unprotected angioplasty. Reduction of ischemia in patients at high risk of such complications was demonstrated.

(Continued on following page)

INTRAVASCULAR PERFLUOROCHEMICAL EMULSION, 20% (Cont.)

Indications:

To prevent or diminish myocardial ischemia, as manifested by decreased ventricular wall motion and global ejection fraction, occurring during percutaneous transluminal coronary angioplasty in patients at high risk of ischemic complications of angioplasty such as patients with: 1) low baseline ejection fraction (< 45%); 2) large areas of the myocardium at risk; 3) recent myocardial infarction; or 4) unstable angina or refractory angina requiring hospitalization.

Contraindications:

Functionally critical secondary stenosis in the dilated and perfused vessel distal to the treated lesion; hypersensitivity to any of the constituents in the product.

Warnings:

Oxygenated intravascular perfluorochemical emulsion must be warmed to approximately 37°C prior to administration. Intracoronary infusion of ambient temperature emulsion (room temperature in the cardiac catheterization laboratory) has been associated with ventricular fibrillation requiring cardioversion.

Cardiovascular: Any coronary angioplasty procedure carries some degree of risk of coronary arterial dissection with occlusion, coronary artery spasm and vasospastic angina, myocardial infarction, distal intraluminal thrombus, arrhythmia, tachycardia, bradycardia and ventricular fibrillation requiring cardioversion. Supportive procedures and personnel must be available to handle these procedural complications.

Pregnancy: Category B. There are no adequate and well controlled studies in pregnant women. Use during pregnancy only if clearly needed.

Lactation: One day after peripheral IV infusion of 20 ml/kg of intravascular perfluorochemical emulsion when the fluorocrit was 0.5%, 0.58 mg/ml perfluorodecalin was detected in the breast milk; no perfluorotri-n-propylamine was detected. After administration of intravascular perfluorochemical emulsion, nursing mothers should not breastfeed the baby, even though the perfluorochemicals will not be absorbed orally.

Children: Safety and efficacy in children have not been established.

Precautions:

Percutaneous transluminal coronary angioplasty considerations: Undertake with or without oxygenated intravascular perfluorochemical emulsion perfusion only in accordance with institutional policy regarding surgical standby for emergency coronary artery bypass graft surgery.

If the balloon catheter occludes side branches which will not receive oxygenated intravascular perfluorochemical emulsion, ischemic ST segment changes, angina and creatinine kinase elevation may result. Be aware of potential complications of coronary angioplasty which may occur in spite of oxygenated intravascular perfluorochemical emulsion perfusion. Verify proper positioning of the balloon catheter before proceeding.

A characteristic ECG pattern of ST segment elevation, reaching a plateau at 30 to 45 seconds of balloon inflation with an amplitude of 1 to 2 mm, has been observed in many patients receiving distal perfusion with oxygenated intravascular perfluorochemical emulsion. The pattern of the ST changes was distinctly different from ischemic ST elevations in control patients which continue to rise after balloon inflation. The phenomenon appears to be a non-ischemic mechanical artifact of perfusion.

Perform perfusion with oxygenated intravascular perfluorochemical emulsion only with lumened catheters and guidewire systems which permit pressure monitoring or contrast agent delivery with the guidewire in place.

Monitor for signs of ischemia, including ECG monitoring.

Asplenia: Because the perfluorochemicals are deposited in the spleen, the half-life of perfluorochemical emulsion particles in circulation may be increased in asplenic patients, and the liver and other tissues may accumulate a larger proportion of the perfluorochemicals than would otherwise be expected.

(Continued on following page)

INTRAVASCULAR PERFLUOROCHEMICAL EMULSION, 20% (Cont.)

Drug Interactions:

Anesthetics: Administration of intravascular perfluorochemical emulsion may prolong the action of lipid soluble anesthetics. In animals the hepatotoxic effects of carbon tetrachloride were enhanced by the presence of retained perfluorochemicals.

Drug/Laboratory test interactions: Centrifuged blood samples containing intravascular perfluorochemical emulsion may contain a layer of perfluorochemicals at the bottom of the tube. Packed red blood cells are above the layer of perfluorochemicals and plasma is at the top. The volume percent of perfluorochemicals in the sample is the fluorocrit.

At high concentrations in blood (well above those expected in angioplasty perfusion), intravascular perfluorochemical emulsion may cause an upward displacement of the standard curve in some radioimmunoassays. Additionally, at high concentrations intravascular perfluorochemical emulsion may interfere with some spectrophotometric tests due to turbidity.

Adverse Reactions:

Procedure complications: Adverse reactions occurring during oxygenated intravascular perfluorochemical emulsion perfusion in angioplasty may be difficult to separate from complications attributable to the procedure itself. Some level of ischemia, evidenced by angina and ST segment elevation, may occur. A transient increase in pulmonary artery wedge pressure above baseline levels was observed in some patients receiving multiple balloon inflations with intravascular perfluorochemical emulsion perfusion. Wedge pressure returned to near baseline levels within 3 to 5 minutes after the procedure.

Potential adverse reactions to perfusion occurred in 2.1% (6/289) of patients; 0.7% (2/289) who received a perfusion of intravascular perfluorochemical emulsion at 37°C and 1.4% (4/289) who experienced arrhythmias related to perfusion at ambient temperatures. Although properly warmed oxygenated intravascular perfluorochemical emulsion has not been associated with cardiac rhythm disturbances, perfusion with oxygenated intravascular perfluorochemical emulsion at ambient temperatures in cardiac catheterization laboratories has been associated with ventricular fibrillation (see Warnings).

Cardiac: Ventricular tachycardia or ventricular fibrillation; bradycardia; chest discomfort; hypotension.

Respiratory: Dyspnea; increased respiratory rate; coughing.

Dermatologic: Mild pruritus.

Test dose reaction: In clinical trials, 1.2% (4/335) of patients reacted to a 0.5 ml IV test dose of intravascular perfluorochemical emulsion. If the patient experiences an adverse reaction (mild generalized pruritus, mild chills, nausea, vomiting, urticaria or mild back pain) after receiving the test dose, intravascular perfluorochemical emulsion should not be administered; treat the patient by an alternative procedure such as angioplasty without distal perfusion or coronary artery bypass graft surgery. IV diphenhydramine or methylprednisolone may be given to treat reactions to the IV test dose.

(Continued on following page)

INTRAVASCULAR PERFLUOROCHEMICAL EMULSION, 20% (Cont.)

Administration:

Administer oxygenated intravascular perfluorochemical emulsion only via intracoronary perfusion during balloon angioplasty by means of an angiographic power injector. Intravascular perfluorochemical emulsion consists of 3 separate parts which must be mixed prior to use: (1) The intravascular perfluorochemical emulsion; (2) Solution 1 (sodium bicarbonate, potassium chloride and Water for Injection, USP); and (3) Solution 2 (sodium chloride, anhydrous dextrose, magnesium chloride, calcium chloride and Water for Injection, USP). The additive solutions serve to adjust pH, ionic strength, and osmotic pressure in the final 20% emulsion, and must be added separately and sequentially prior to administration.

When the intravascular perfluorochemical emulsion and the two solutions are mixed for administration the resultant composition is as follows:

Composition of Intravascular Perfluorochemical Emulsion, 20% When Prepared for Administration

Ingredient	g/dl
Perfluorodecalin	14
Perfluorotri-n-propylamine	6
Poloxamer 188	2.72
Glycerin USP	0.8
Sodium Chloride USP	0.6
Egg Yolk Phospholipids	0.4
Sodium Bicarbonate USP	0.21
Dextrose USP, Anhydrous	0.18
Magnesium Chloride • $6H_2O$ USP	0.043
Calcium Chloride • $2H_2O$ USP	0.036
Potassium Chloride USP	0.034
Potassium Oleate	0.032
Water for Injection USP	qs

Electrolyte Concentration

Electrolyte	mEq/L	mmol/L
Sodium (Na^+)	127.6	127.6
Potassium (K^+)	5.5	5.5
Calcium (Ca^{++})	4.8	2.4
Magnesium (Mg^{++})	4.2	2.1
Chloride (Cl^-)	116.2	116.2
Bicarbonate (HCO_3^-)	25	25

The intravascular perfluorochemical emulsion must be thawed and mixed with Solutions 1 and 2 prior to administration. The thawed and reconstituted emulsion must be oxygenated to $>$ 600 mm Hg partial pressure of oxygen prior to use. The oxygenation procedure should be done with "Carbogen" (95% O_2/5% CO_2). Do not oxygenate the emulsion with 100% O_2 as this will adversely affect the pH of the emulsion. Refer to the "Directions for Use" which are packaged with the Continuous Oxygenation Kit which provides detailed preparation instructions.

Thaw intravascular perfluorochemical emulsion in a water bath at 37°C. After mixing and oxygenation are complete, fill the prepared product into an angiographic power injector and keep warm by means of a warming jacket on the injector. Administer the oxygenated intravascular perfluorochemical emulsion via an angiographic power injector through the central lumen of the angioplasty balloon catheter without removing the guidewire.

(Continued on following page)

INTRAVASCULAR PERFLUOROCHEMICAL EMULSION, 20% (Cont.)

Dosage:

Intravascular perfluorochemical emulsion should not be administered more than one time in 6 months. Prior to administration give a 0.5 ml IV test dose, especially in patients with hypersensitivity to angiographic contrast media.

Test dose: The 0.5 ml test dose should be withdrawn from the container of intravascular perfluorochemical emulsion prepared for administration and injected into a peripheral vein. The test dose may be performed with or without prior oxygenation of the intravascular perfluorochemical emulsion. Observe the patient for 10 minutes after receiving the test dose and if no untoward events occur, the intracoronary administration may proceed.

Adverse reactions to the test dose are rare. If it occurs intravascular perfluorochemical emulsion should not be administered; treat the patient by an alternative procedure, such as angioplasty without distal perfusion or coronary artery bypass graft surgery. IV diphenhydramine or methylprednisolone may be given to treat reactions to the test dose.

> Oxygenated intravascular perfluorochemical emulsion is to be injected at a rate of 60 to 90 ml/min at approximately 37°C during the period of balloon inflation depending on the size of the distal vessel bed.

It may be helpful to initiate oxygenated intravascular perfluorochemical emulsion perfusion shortly before balloon inflation and to continue momentarily after balloon deflation. Limit balloon inflation time by the patient's tolerance and by the physician's judgment of clinical status and desired therapeutic result. An angiographic power injector reservoir, filled with 260 ml of oxygenated intravascular perfluorochemical emulsion, will allow more than 4 minutes of perfusion time at a flow rate of 60 ml/minute (1 ml/second). Perfusion rates > 120 ml/minute and total intracoronary perfusion volumes > 500 ml have not been studied.

The selection of an angioplasty balloon catheter and guidewire can affect the perfusion of oxygenated intravascular perfluorochemical emulsion. A minimum lumen diameter of 0.004 inch with the guidewire in place is adequate to allow perfusion.

Compatibility: Additives other than Solution 1, Solution 2 and Carbogen gas must not be made to the container of intravascular perfluorochemical emulsion.

Filters should not be used as this may disturb the emulsion.

Do not administer the contents of any container in which there appears to be a separation of the emulsion.

Storage: The 400 ml container of intravascular perfluorochemical emulsion must be stored in the frozen state between –5°C and –30°C (23°F and –22°F). Do not use any container in which there is evidence that the emulsion has thawed prior to thawing at the time of use.

Solutions 1 and 2 may be stored at room temperature not exceeding 30°C (86°F). Do not freeze Solutions 1 and 2.

Do not thaw the emulsion in a microwave oven. This may cause uneven warming and localized overheating. Thaw the frozen emulsion in a water bath or warming cabinet at 37°C (98.6°F). About 30 minutes are required to liquify the emulsion and warm it to 37°C. Do not refreeze the emulsion.

Intravascular perfluorochemical emulsion must be administered within 8 hours of thawing the emulsion. Intravascular perfluorochemical emulsion is for single dose use only; any unused contents must be discarded and should not be stored or resterilized for later use.

Rx	**Fluosol** (Alpha Therapeutic)	**Emulsion:** Perfluorochemicals, 20%	Emulsion in 400 ml flexible plastic bag. Additive Solutions 1 and 2 supplied in separate continuous oxygenation kit including accessories for effecting oxygenation.[1]

[1] Includes Solution 1 (30 ml partial fill in 50 ml vial); Solution 2 (70 ml partial fill in 100 ml vial); 16 gauge, 8 inch oxygenation catheter with 14 gauge needle; two 0.2 mcm filters; 84 inch oxygen source tubing; 18 gauge needle; 3-way stopcock; protective plastic bag.

HEMIN

> **Warning:**
> Hemin for injection should only be used by physicians experienced in the management of porphyrias in hospitals where the recommended clinical and laboratory diagnostic and monitoring techniques are available.
> Consider hemin therapy after an appropriate period of alternate therapy (ie, 400 g glucose/day for 1 to 2 days).

Actions:

Hemin for injection is an enzyme inhibitor derived from processed red blood cells. It was known previously as hematin. The term hematin has been used to describe the chemical reaction product of hemin and sodium carbonate solution. Hemin is an iron-containing metalloporphyrin.

Pharmacology: Porphyrias are rare metabolic disorders that, as a group, represent disturbances of heme synthesis and are differentiated on the basis of specific enzymatic defects. Porphyrias are characterized clinically by neurologic (psychoses, seizures, paresis) or cutaneous (photosensitivity) manifestations, and chemically by overproduction of porphyrins or their precursors. Porphyrins are byproducts of heme synthesis; heme is the iron-containing constituent of hemoglobin and respiratory pigments and is produced and required by nearly every body tissue. Heme acts to limit the hepatic or marrow synthesis of porphyrin which is likely due to inhibition of delta-aminolevulinic acid synthetase, the enzyme which limits the rate of porphyrin/heme biosynthetic pathway. However, the exact mechanism by which hematin produces symptomatic improvement in patients with acute episodes of the hepatic porphyrias has not been elucidated.

Pharmacokinetics: Following IV administration of hematin in non-jaundiced patients, an increase in fecal urobilinogen can be observed which is roughly proportional to the amount of hematin administered. This suggests an enterohepatic pathway as at least one route of elimination. Bilirubin metabolites are also excreted in the urine following hematin injections.

Clinical pharmacology: Hemin therapy for the acute porphyrias is not curative. After discontinuation of treatment, symptoms generally return, although remission may be prolonged. Some neurological symptoms have improved weeks to months after therapy, although little or no response was noted at the time of treatment.

Indications:

For the amelioration of recurrent attacks of acute intermittent porphyria temporally related to the menstrual cycle in susceptible women. Manifestations such as pain, hypertension, tachycardia, abnormal mental status, and mild to progressive neurologic signs may be controlled in selected patients with this disorder.

Similar findings have been reported in other patients with acute intermittent porphyria, porphyria variegata and hereditary coproporphyria.

Contraindications:

Hypersensitivity to hemin; porphyria cutanea tarda.

Warnings:

Pregnancy: Category C. Safety for use during pregnancy has not been established. Use only when clearly needed and when the potential benefits outweigh the potential hazards to the fetus.

Lactation: It is not known whether hemin for injection is excreted in breast milk. Safety for use in the nursing mother has not been established.

Children: Safety and efficacy for use in children have not been established.

Precautions:

Neuronal damage: Clinical benefit depends on prompt administration. Attacks of porphyria may progress to irreversible neuronal damage. Hemin therapy is intended to prevent an attack from reaching the critical stage of neuronal degeneration. This agent is not effective in repairing neuronal damage.

Renal effects: Reversible renal shutdown has been observed where an excessive hematin dose (12.2 mg/kg) was administered in a single infusion. Oliguria and increased nitrogen retention occurred, although the patient remained asymptomatic. No worsening of renal function has been seen with use of recommended dosages of hematin.

Diagnostic tests: Before therapy is begun, diagnose the presence of acute porphyria using the following criteria: Presence of clinical symptoms and positive Watson-Schwartz or Hoesch test.

Clinical monitoring: Drug effect will be demonstrated by a decrease in urinary concentration of one or more of the following compounds: ALA (delta-aminolevulinic acid); UPG (uroporphyrinogen); PBG (porphobilinogen coproporphyrin).

(Continued on following page)

HEMIN (Cont.)

Drug Interactions:

Anticoagulants: Hemin has exhibited transient, mild anticoagulant effects during clinical studies; therefore, avoid concurrent anticoagulant therapy. The extent and duration of the hypocoagulable state has not been established.

Barbiturates, estrogens and **steroid metabolites** increase the activity of delta-aminolevulinic acid synthetase. Since hemin therapy limits the rate of porphyria/heme biosynthesis, possibly by inhibiting the enzyme delta-aminolevulinic acid synthetase, avoid use of these agents.

Adverse Reactions:

Phlebitis with or without leukocytosis and with or without mild pyrexia has occurred after administration of hematin through small arm veins.

There has been one report of coagulopathy. This patient exhibited prolonged prothrombin time, partial thromboplastin time, thrombocytopenia, mild hypofibrinogenemia, mild elevation of fibrin split products, and a 10% fall in hematocrit.

Overdosage:

Reversible renal shutdown has been observed in a case where an excessive hematin dose (12.2 mg/kg) was administered in a single infusion. Treatment of this case consisted of ethacrynic acid and mannitol.

Administration and Dosage:

For IV use only. Use a large arm vein or a central venous catheter to avoid the possibility of phlebitis.

Before administering hemin for injection, consider alternate therapy (ie, 400 g glucose/day for 1 to 2 days). If improvement is unsatisfactory for the treatment of acute attacks of porphyria, administer an IV infusion containing a dose of 1 to 4 mg/kg/day of hematin over a period of 10 to 15 minutes for 3 to 14 days, based on the clinical signs. In more severe cases, this dose may be repeated no earlier than every 12 hours. Give no more than 6 mg/kg in any 24 hour period.

Preparation of Solution: Reconstitute by adding 43 ml of Sterile Water for Injection to the dispensing vial. Shake well for a period of 2 to 3 minutes to aid dissolution.

After reconstitution, each ml contains the equivalent of approximately 7 mg of hematin (313 mg hemin/43 ml), 5 mg sodium carbonate (215 mg/43 ml) and 7 mg sorbitol (300 mg/43 ml). The drug may be administered directly from the vial.

Hemin Dosage Calculation Table
1 mg hematin equivalent = 0.14 ml
2 mg hematin equivalent = 0.28 ml
3 mg hematin equivalent = 0.42 ml
4 mg hematin equivalent = 0.56 ml

Since reconstituted hemin is not transparent, any undissolved particulate matter is difficult to see; therefore, terminal filtration through a sterile 0.45 micron or smaller filter is recommended.

Compatibility: Do not add any drug or chemical agent fluid admixture unless its effect on the chemical and physical stability has first been determined.

Stability and storage: Because this product contains no preservative and undergoes rapid chemical decomposition in solution, do not reconstitute until immediately before use.

Store lyophilized powder frozen until time of use. Discard any unused portion.

Rx	**Panhematin** (Abbott)	**Powder for Injection:** 313 mg hemin per vial[1] (equivalent to 7 mg hematin per ml) after reconstitution with 43 ml Sterile Water for Injection. Preservative free

[1] With 300 mg sorbitol.

chapter 3

hormones

For estrogens recommended for their antineoplastic action in prostatic carcinoma, refer to the estrogen section in the antineoplastics chapter.

This general discussion applies to all estrogens; consider when using any of these products.

Warning:

Estrogens have been reported to increase the risk of endometrial carcinoma.

Three independent studies have shown an increased risk of endometrial cancer in postmenopausal women exposed to exogenous estrogens for prolonged periods. This risk was independent of the other known risk factors. Incidence rates of endometrial cancer have increased sharply since 1969, which may relate to the rapidly expanding use of estrogens during the last decade.

The risk of endometrial cancer in estrogen users was 4.5 to 13.9 times greater than in nonusers and appears to depend on duration of treatment and dose. Therefore, when estrogens are used for the treatment of menopausal symptoms, use the lowest dose and discontinue medication as soon as possible. When prolonged treatment is indicated, reassess the patient at least semiannually to determine the need for continued therapy. *Cyclic administration of low doses of estrogen may carry less risk than continuous administration.*

Close clinical surveillance of all women taking estrogens is important. In undiagnosed persistent or recurring abnormal vaginal bleeding, exclude malignancy.

There is no evidence that "natural" estrogens are more or less hazardous than "synthetic" estrogens at equiestrogenic doses.

Do not use estrogens during pregnancy.

The use of female sex hormones (both estrogens and progestins) during early pregnancy may seriously damage the offspring. Females exposed *in utero* to diethylstilbestrol (DES) have an increased risk of developing vaginal or cervical cancer, estimated at not greater than 4 per 1000 exposures. Furthermore, a high percentage of such exposed women (30% to 90%) have vaginal adenosis (epithelial changes of the vagina and cervix). Although these changes are histologically benign, it is not known if they are precursors of malignancy. Similar data are not available for other estrogens, but it cannot be presumed that they would not induce similar changes.

There have also been congenital anomalies reported in male offspring whose mothers ingested the drug. The primary abnormalities have been related to structural problems of the genitourinary tract and to abnormal semen quality. The effect of these lesions on carcinoma development and fertility is yet to be determined.

Several reports suggest an association between intrauterine exposure to female sex hormones and congenital anomalies, including congenital heart defects and limb reduction defects. One study estimated a 4.7-fold increased risk of limb reduction defects in infants exposed *in utero* to sex hormones (oral contraceptives, hormone withdrawal tests for pregnancy or attempted treatment for threatened abortion). Some of these exposures involved only a few days of treatment. The risk of limb reduction defects in exposed fetuses is somewhat less than 1 per 1000.

Female sex hormones have been used during pregnancy to treat threatened or habitual abortion. There is considerable evidence that estrogens are ineffective for these indications and no evidence that progestins are effective.

If estrogens are used during pregnancy, or if the patient becomes pregnant while taking estrogens, inform her of the potential risks to the fetus.

Actions:

Although six different natural estrogens have been isolated from the human female, only three are present in significant quantities: Estradiol, estrone and estriol. The most potent and major secretory product of the ovary is estradiol; it is rapidly oxidized to estrone. Hydration of estrone produces estriol, which is much weaker. The estrogenic potency of estradiol is 12 times that of estrone and 80 times that of estriol.

Equipotent doses of estrogens produce similar pharmacological effects and side effects. Approximate equivalent doses of some estrogens are: Conjugated estrogens 5 mg, diethylstilbestrol 5 mg, mestranol 80 mcg, estradiol 50 mcg and ethinyl estradiol 50 mcg.

Pharmacology: Estrogens are important in the development and maintenance of the female reproductive system and secondary sex characteristics. They promote growth and development of the vagina, uterus, fallopian tubes and breasts. Estrogens also affect the release of pituitary gonadotropins and cause capillary dilatation, fluid retention, protein anabolism and thin cervical mucus; they inhibit ovulation and prevent postpartum breast discomfort. Indirectly, estrogens contribute to: The shaping of the skeleton (estrogens conserve calcium and phosphorus and encourage bone formation); maintenance of tone and elasticity of urogenital structures; changes in the epiphyses of the long bones that allow for the pubertal growth spurt and its termination; growth of axillary and pubic hair; and pigmentation of the nipples and genitals.

(Actions continued on following page)

Actions (Cont.)

Pharmacology (Cont.):

Estrogens induce proliferation in the epithelium of the fallopian tubes, endometrium, cervix and vagina and increase vascularity. Estrogens are responsible for vaginal acidity caused by the deposition of glycogen in vaginal epithelium. They encourage cornification of superficial vaginal cells to give a characteristic vaginal smear.

Estrogens do not induce ovulation. However, in the preovulatory phase, they produce changes in the tubular mucosa and stimulate the contraction and motility of the fallopian tubes to promote the ovum transport. Estrogens restore the endometrium, including its coiled arteries, after menstruation, but do not induce the glands to secrete. An endometrium suddenly deprived of estrogen breaks down and bleeds. The growth and secretory activity of cervical epithelium are determined in part by estrogens which also modify the physical and chemical properties of cervical mucus.

Menstruation - Decline of estrogenic activity at the end of the menstrual cycle can induce menstruation, although cessation of progesterone secretion is the most important factor in the mature ovulatory cycle. However, in the preovulatory or nonovulatory cycle, estrogen is the primary determinant of the onset of menstruation.

Menopause - The cessation of cyclic function is the basic ovarian event in the menopause. Functional changes can be attributed to depletion of follicles, although a few follicles persist as long as 5 years after the last menses.

The beginning of menopause is marked by decreasing frequency of ovulation, associated with irregular menses or variable periods of amenorrhea and later by decreasing estrogen secretion. Estrogen production, first to appear at menarche, is last to decline at menopause. The declining estrogen secretion is accompanied by signs and symptoms of hormone deficits in the estrogen-dependent organs, including pituitary, uterus, cervix, vagina and breasts. Pituitary gonadotropin secretion rises, reflected by increased quantities of gonadotropin in blood and urine. The endometrium becomes atrophic, myometrial mass decreases and the vaginal epithelium becomes thin as, deficient in glycogen, it fails to become keratinized.

Coronary heart disease: Several studies support the hypothesis that the postmenopausal use of estrogen reduces the risk of severe coronary heart disease. However, other reports conflict. An estrogen-induced change in HDL levels may play a role.

Pharmacokinetics:

Absorption/Distribution - Absorption of most natural estrogens and their derivatives from the GI tract is complete. The limited oral effectiveness of natural estrogens and their esters is due to their metabolism. In estrogen-responsive tissues (female genital organs, breasts, hypothalamus, pituitary), estrogen binds to tissue-specific receptor proteins in the cytoplasm. The resulting estrogen-protein complex penetrates the nuclear membrane and ultimately binds to materials in the cell nucleus. This activates increased synthesis of DNA, RNA and various proteins that in turn affect characteristic changes in responsive tissues. About 80% of estradiol is bound to sex hormone binding globulin; most of the rest is loosely bound to albumin and about 2% is unbound. Estrone is 50% to 80% bound to protein as it circulates in the blood, primarily as a conjugate with sulfate.

Transdermal System: In contrast to oral administration of estradiol, the skin metabolizes estradiol via the transdermal system only to a small extent. Therefore, transdermal administration produces therapeutic serum levels of estradiol with lower circulating levels of estrone and estrone conjugates, and requires smaller total doses. Transdermal use produces mean serum estradiol concentrations comparable to those produced by daily oral administration at about 20 times the daily transdermal dose.

Metabolism/Excretion - Metabolism and inactivation occur primarily in the liver. During cyclic passage through the liver, estrogens are degraded to less active estrogenic compounds conjugated with sulfuric and glucuronic acids. Some estrogens are excreted into the bile, then reabsorbed from the intestine and returned to the liver through the portal venous system. Water soluble estrogen conjugates are strongly acidic and are ionized in body fluids, which favor excretion in the urine; tubular reabsorption is minimal.

Indications:

Moderate to severe vasomotor symptoms associated with menopause: There is no evidence that estrogens are effective for nervous symptoms or depression, without associated vasomotor symptoms, which might occur during menopause; do not use them to treat these conditions.

Atrophic vaginitis; kraurosis vulvae.

Female hypogonadism; female castration; primary ovarian failure.

Breast cancer: Palliation only in selected women and men or those with metastatic disease.

Prostatic carcinoma: Palliative therapy of advanced disease.

(Indications continued on following page)

Indications (Cont.):

Postpartum breast engorgement: The incidence of significant painful engorgement is low and usually responds to analgesic or other supportive therapy. Weigh the benefits of estrogen therapy against the increased risk of puerperal thromboembolism associated with large estrogen doses.

Osteoporosis: **Conjugated estrogens** are indicated in postmenopausal women, with evidence of loss or deficiency of bone mass, to retard further bone loss and estrogen-deficiency-induced osteoporosis. Use conjugated estrogens with other important measures such as diet, calcium and physiotherapy. A more favorable benefit/risk ratio exists if women have had a hysterectomy; there is no risk of endometrial carcinoma.

Bone loss is increased in many women following menopause, but there is no clear way to identify those women who will develop osteoporotic fractures. Estrogens can reduce rate of bone loss in postmenopausal women but substantial evidence is lacking that estrogens decrease the incidence of osteoporotic bone fractures. However, a retrospective cohort study involving 2873 women supports the hypothesis that estrogens protect against hip fracture in postmenopausal women. Women who have had an early surgical menopause (oophorectomy) appear to be at increased risk for osteoporosis development.

The FDA has also approved the use of the other oral short-acting estrogens (DES, esterified estrogens, estradiol, ethinyl estradiol and estropipate) in the treatment of osteoporosis; however, labeling changes may not yet be reflective of this ruling.

Abnormal uterine bleeding due to hormonal imbalance in the absence of organic pathology (**conjugated estrogens, parenteral**).

Unlabeled Uses: Oral DES is an effective postcoital contraceptive when given in doses of 25 mg twice daily for 5 days if therapy is started no later than 72 hours after intercourse. Although the FDA has indicated that use of DES as an emergency treatment (not as a routine method of birth control) is approvable, no manufacturer currently holds an approved NDA for this use. Ethinyl estradiol, conjugated estrogens and other estrogens have also been evaluated for postcoital contraception.

Ethinyl estradiol: A 5 mcg tablet is being investigated for use in the treatment of Turner's syndrome. Gynex received orphan status for this product in July 1988.

Contraindications:

Breast cancer, except in appropriately selected patients being treated for metastatic disease; estrogen-dependent neoplasia; undiagnosed abnormal genital bleeding; active thrombophlebitis or thromboembolic disorders; history of thrombophlebitis, thrombosis or thromboembolic disorders associated with previous estrogen use (except when used in treatment of breast or prostatic malignancy); known or suspected pregnancy.

Warnings:

Induction of malignant neoplasms: Estrogens may increase the risk of endometrial carcinoma (see Warning Box). Long-term continuous administration of estrogens in some animals increased the frequency of carcinomas of the breast, cervix, vagina, kidney and liver. There is now evidence that estrogens increase the risk of carcinoma of the endometrium in humans. Closely monitor patients with an intact uterus for signs of endometrial cancer, and take appropriate diagnostic measures to rule out malignancy in the event of persistent or recurring abnormal vaginal bleeding.

There is no evidence that estrogens given to postmenopausal women increase the risk of breast cancer, although a recent report has raised this possibility. A prospective study of 23,244 women ≥ 35 years of age reported the relative risk of breast cancer increased 10% in women receiving estrogens for menopausal symptoms. The study concluded that ≥ 9 years of estrogen replacement treatment, use of estradiol, or estrogen-progestin combinations were associated with an increased risk. Other studies conflict. Because of animal data, use with caution in women who have a strong family history of breast cancer or who have breast nodules, fibrocystic disease or abnormal mammograms.

Gallbladder disease: There is a twofold to threefold increase in risk of gallbladder disease in women receiving postmenopausal estrogens.

Effects similar to those caused by estrogen-progestin oral contraceptives (OCs): Most of the serious adverse effects of OCs have NOT been documented as consequences of postmenopausal estrogen therapy. This may reflect the comparatively low doses of estrogen used in postmenopausal women. There is an increased risk of thrombosis in men receiving estrogens for prostatic cancer and in women receiving estrogens for postpartum breast engorgement, presumably because large doses are used in therapy. Consider the following effects noted in OC users as potential risks of estrogen use:

Hepatic adenoma - Although benign and rare, these may rupture and cause death through intra-abdominal hemorrhage. Consider such lesions in estrogen users having abdominal pain and tenderness, abdominal mass or hypovolemic shock. Hepatocellular carcinoma has also been reported; the relationship to these drugs is unknown.

Elevated blood pressure is common, but is seen less frequently with estrogen replacement therapy than with OC use; monitor the patient, especially if high doses are used.

(Warnings continued on following page)

Warnings (Cont.):

Effects similar to those caused by estrogen-progestin oral contraceptives (cont.):

Thromboembolic disease - OC users have an increased risk of thromboembolic and thrombotic vascular diseases, including thrombophlebitis, pulmonary embolism, stroke and myocardial infarction. Cases of retinal thrombosis, mesenteric thrombosis and optic neuritis have been reported. The risk of several of these adverse reactions is dose-related. An increased risk of postsurgical thromboembolic complications has also been reported. If feasible, discontinue estrogens at least 4 weeks before surgery associated with an increased risk of thromboembolism or during prolonged immobilization.

An increased rate of thromboembolic and thrombotic disease in postmenopausal users of estrogens has not been found, but such an increase may be present in some subgroups of women or in those receiving relatively large doses. Therefore, do not use in persons with active thrombophlebitis or thromboembolic disorders or in persons with a history of such disorders associated with estrogen use (except in treatment of malignancy). Use with caution in patients with cerebrovascular or coronary artery disease and only when estrogens are clearly needed. Cigarette smoking increases the risk of serious cardiovascular side effects from OCs. Risk increases with age and with heavy smoking (≥ 15 cigarettes per day) and is quite marked in women > 35 years of age.

Large doses (conjugated estrogens 5 mg/day), comparable to those used to treat prostate and breast cancer, have increased risk of nonfatal MI, pulmonary embolism and thrombophlebitis in men. When such estrogen doses are used, the thromboembolic and thrombotic adverse effects associated with OC use are a clear risk.

Glucose tolerance - Decreased glucose tolerance has been observed in a significant percentage of patients on OCs; observe diabetic patients carefully.

Hypercalcemia: Estrogens may lead to severe hypercalcemia in patients with breast cancer and bone metastases. If this occurs, discontinue the drug and take appropriate measures to reduce the serum calcium level.

Photosensitivity: Photosensitization may occur; therefore, caution patients to take protective measures (ie, sunscreens, protective clothing) against exposure to ultraviolet light or sunlight until tolerance is determined.

Pregnancy: Category X. See Warning Box.

Lactation: Estrogens are excreted in breast milk. Administer only when clearly needed.

Children: Safety and efficacy are not established. Because of effects on epiphyseal closure, use judiciously in young patients in whom bone growth is incomplete.

Precautions:

History/physical exam: Before initiating estrogen therapy, take a complete medical and family history. Pretreatment and periodic history and physical examinations every 6 to 12 months should include blood pressure, breasts, abdomen, pelvic organs and a Papanicolaou smear. Generally, do not prescribe estrogens for > 1 year between physical examinations.

Estropipate vaginal cream: Rule out gonorrhea or neoplasia before prescribing. Treat trichomonal, monilial or bacterial infection with appropriate anti-microbial therapy.

Excessive estrogenic stimulation: Certain patients may develop undesirable manifestations of excessive estrogenic stimulation (eg, abnormal or excessive uterine bleeding, mastodynia). Preexisting uterine leiomyoma may increase in size during estrogen use. Advise the pathologist of estrogen therapy when relevant specimens are submitted.

Fluid retention: Estrogens may cause some degree of fluid retention; conditions which might be influenced by this factor (eg, asthma, epilepsy, migraine and cardiac or renal dysfunction) require careful observation.

Mental depression: OCs appear to be associated with an increased incidence of mental depression. It is not clear whether this is due to the estrogenic or progestogenic component; observe patients with a history of depression.

Hepatic function impairment: Patients with a history of jaundice during pregnancy have an increased risk of recurrence while on estrogen-containing OCs. If jaundice develops in any patient on estrogen, discontinue the medication and investigate the cause. Estrogens may be poorly metabolized in impaired liver function; use with caution.

Calcium and phosphorus metabolism is influenced by estrogens; use caution in patients with metabolic bone diseases associated with hypercalcemia or in renal insufficiency.

Prolonged use of unopposed estrogen therapy may increase risk of endometrial hyperplasia.

Acute intermittent porphyria may be precipitated by estrogens.

Tartrazine sensitivity: Some of these products contain tartrazine which may cause allergic-type reactions (including bronchial asthma) in susceptible individuals. Although the incidence of sensitivity is low, it is frequently seen in patients who also have aspirin hypersensitivity. Specific products containing tartrazine are identified in the product listings.

(Continued on following page)

Drug Interactions:

Anticoagulants, oral: Estrogens may theoretically reduce the hypoprothrombinemic effect of anticoagulants.

Antidepressants, tricyclic: Pharmacologic effects of these agents may be altered by estrogens; the effects of this interaction may depend on the dose of the estrogen. An increased incidence of toxic reactions may also occur.

Barbiturates, rifampin and other agents that induce hepatic microsomal enzymes with concomitant estrogens may produce lower estrogen levels than expected.

Corticosteroids: Estrogen coadministration may reduce the clearance and increase the elimination half-life of corticosteroids.

Dantrolene: While a definite drug interaction with dantrolene has not yet been established, observe caution if the two drugs are given concomitantly. Hepatotoxicity has occurred more often in women > 35 years of age receiving dantrolene and estrogen therapy.

Drug/Lab Test Interactions: Certain endocrine and liver function tests may be affected by estrogen-containing OCs. Expect these similar changes with larger estrogen doses:

Increased **sulfobromophthalein retention**.

Increased **prothrombin** and **factors VII, VIII, IX** and **X**; decreased **antithrombin III**; increased norepinephrine-induced **platelet aggregability**.

Increased **thyroid binding globulin (TBG)** leading to increased circulating total thyroid hormone, as measured by **PBI, T_4** by column or **T_4** by radioimmunoassay. **Free T_3 resin uptake** is decreased, reflecting the elevated TBG; **free T_4** concentration is unaltered.

Impaired **glucose tolerance**; decreased **pregnanediol excretion**; reduced response to **metyrapone test**; reduced **serum folate** concentration; increased **serum triglyceride** and **phospholipid** concentration.

Adverse Reactions:

See Warnings regarding induction of neoplasia, adverse effects on the fetus, increased incidence of gallbladder disease and adverse effects similar to those of OCs.

GU: Breakthrough bleeding; spotting, change in menstrual flow; dysmenorrhea; premenstrual-like syndrome; amenorrhea during and after treatment; increase in size of uterine fibromyomata; vaginal candidiasis; change in cervical erosion and degree of cervical secretion; cystitis-like syndrome; hemolytic uremic syndrome; endometrial cystic hyperplasia.

GI: Nausea; vomiting; abdominal cramps; bloating; cholestatic jaundice; colitis; acute pancreatitis.

Dermatologic: Chloasma or melasma (may persist when drug is discontinued); erythema nodosum/multiforme; hemorrhagic eruption; scalp hair loss; hirsutism; urticaria; dermatitis.

Ophthalmic: Steepening of corneal curvature; intolerance to contact lenses.

CNS: Headache; migraine; dizziness; mental depression; chorea; convulsions.

Local: Pain at injection site; sterile abscess; postinjection flare; redness and irritation at application site with the **estradiol transdermal system** (17%) and rash (rare).

Miscellaneous: Increase or decrease in weight; reduced carbohydrate tolerance; aggravation of porphyria; edema; changes in libido; breast tenderness, enlargement or secretion.

Overdosage:

Serious ill effects have not been reported following ingestion of large doses of estrogen-containing OCs by young children. Overdosage of estrogen may cause nausea; withdrawal bleeding may occur in females.

Patient Information:

Patient package insert is available with products.

Diabetic patients: Glucose tolerance may be decreased; monitor urine sugar or serum glucose closely and report abnormalities to physician.

Notify physician if any of the following occur: Pain in the groin or calves of the legs; sharp chest pain or sudden shortness of breath; abnormal vaginal bleeding; missed menstrual period or suspected pregnancy; lumps in the breast; sudden severe headache, dizziness or fainting; vision or speech disturbance; weakness or numbness in an arm or leg; severe abdominal pain; yellowing of the skin or eyes; severe depression.

Administration:

Given cyclically for short-term use only: For treatment of moderate to severe vasomotor symptoms, atrophic vaginitis or kraurosis vulvae associated with the menopause, administer the lowest effective dose; discontinue medication as promptly as possible. Administration should be cyclic (eg, 3 weeks on and 1 week off). Attempt to discontinue or taper medication at 3 to 6 month intervals.

Cyclical: Female hypogonadism; female castration; primary ovarian failure; osteoporosis.

Short-term administration: Prevention of postpartum breast engorgement.

Chronic: Inoperable progressing prostatic cancer, inoperable progressing breast cancer in appropriately selected men and postmenopausal women (see Indications).

(Administration continued on following page)

Complete prescribing information for these products begins on page 350

Administration (Cont.):

Continued therapy with estrogen alone may induce functional uterine bleeding.

Concomitant progestin therapy: Addition of a progestin for 7 or more days of a cycle of estrogen has lowered the incidence of endometrial hyperplasia. Morphological and biochemical studies of endometrium suggest that 10 to 13 days of progestin are needed to provide maximal maturation of the endometrium and to eliminate any hyperplastic changes. It is not clearly established whether this will provide protection from endometrial carcinoma. There may be additional risks with the inclusion of progestin in estrogen replacement regimens, including adverse effects on carbohydrate and lipid metabolism. Choice of progestin and dosage may be important in minimizing these adverse effects.

Refer to product listings for dosages of individual agents.

ESTRONE

Administration and Dosage:

Administer IM only. Shake vial and syringe well prior to withdrawal and injection (using a 21 to 23 gauge needle) to properly suspend medication.

Cyclically:

Replacement therapy of estrogen deficiency associated conditions (eg, hypogonadism, female castration, primary ovarian failure) – Initial relief of symptoms may be achieved through the administration of 0.1 to 1 mg of estrone weekly in single or divided doses. Some patients may require 0.5 to 2 mg weekly.

Senile vaginitis and kraurosis vulvae – Generally, 0.1 to 0.5 mg estrone 2 or 3 times weekly.

Abnormal uterine bleeding due to hormone imbalance – May respond to brief courses of intensive estrogen therapy. Usual dose range is 2 to 5 mg daily for several days.

Chronically:

Inoperable progressing prostatic cancer – For palliation in prostatic cancer, estrone may be employed at a dosage level of 2 to 4 mg, 2 or 3 times weekly. If a response to estrogen therapy is going to occur, it should be apparent within 3 months of the beginning of therapy. If a response does occur, continue the hormone until the disease is again progressive.

Inoperable progressing breast cancer in appropriately selected men and postmenopausal women: Usual dose is 5 mg 3 or more times weekly according to severity of pain.

ESTRONE AQUEOUS SUSPENSION

	Product	Strength	Packaging	C.I.*
Rx	**Estrone Aqueous** (Various, eg, Balan, Geneva, Interstate, Keene, Major, Moore, Rugby, Steris, URL, Vortech)	**Injection:** 2 mg per ml	In 10 and 30 ml vials.	45+
Rx	**Aquest** (Dunhall)		In 10 ml vials.	NA
Rx	**Estronol** (Central)		In 10 ml vials.[1]	273
Rx	**Theelin Aqueous** (Parke-Davis)		In 10 ml Steri-vials[2]	526
Rx	**Estrone Aqueous** (Various, eg, Balan, Keene, Major, Moore, Pasadena, Rugby, Steris, Towne Paulsen, URL, Vortech)	**Injection:** 5 mg per ml	In 10 ml vials.	34+
Rx	**Estrone 5** (Keene)		In 10 ml vials.[1]	66
Rx	**Kestrone 5** (Hyrex)		In 10 ml vials.[1]	104

ESTROGENIC SUBSTANCE OR ESTROGENS (mainly estrone) AQUEOUS SUSPENSION

	Product	Strength	Packaging	C.I.*
Rx	**Estrogenic Substance Aqueous** (Various, eg, Century, Goldline, Ortega, Texas Drug, Towne Paulsen, Veratex, Wyeth-Ayerst)	**Injection:** 2 mg per ml	In 10 and 30 ml vials.	88+
Rx	**Estroject-2** (Mayrand)		In 10 ml vials.[1]	153
Rx	**Gynogen** (Forest)		In 10 ml vials.[1]	250
Rx	**Kestrin Aqueous** (Hyrex)		In 10 ml vials.[1]	183
Rx	**Wehgen** (Hauck)		In 10 ml vials.[1]	100

* Cost Index based on cost per 1 mg estrone.

[1] With sodium carboxymethylcellulose, povidone, benzyl alcohol and methyl and propyl parabens.

[2] With benzethonium chloride and benzyl alcohol.

Complete prescribing information for these products begins on page 350

ESTRADIOL ORAL

Administration and Dosage:

Moderate to severe vasomotor symptoms, atrophic vaginitis, kraurosis vulvae, female hypogonadism, female castration or primary ovarian failure: Initiate treatment with 1 or 2 mg daily; adjust to control presenting symptoms. Titrate to determine the minimal effective dose for maintenance therapy. Cyclic therapy is recommended. The usual regimen consists of 3 weeks on drug followed by 1 week off. Use short-term therapy only for relief of vasomotor symptoms, atrophic vaginitis or kraurosis vulvae.

Prostatic cancer (inoperable, progressing): Administer chronically, 1 to 2 mg 3 times daily. Judge the effectiveness of therapy by phosphatase determinations and by symptomatic improvement of the patient.

Breast cancer (inoperable, progressing): Given chronically in appropriately selected men and women, the usual dose is 10 mg 3 times daily for at least 3 months. **C.I.***

	Product	Form	How Supplied	C.I.
Rx	**Estrace** (Mead Johnson Labs)	**Tablets:** 1 mg micronized estradiol	Lavender, scored. In 100s and compact 25s.	141
		2 mg micronized estradiol	Tartrazine. Turquoise, scored. In 100s and compact 25s.	103

ESTRADIOL TRANSDERMAL SYSTEM

Indications:

Moderate to severe vasomotor symptoms associated with menopause; female hypogonadism; female castration; primary ovarian failure; atrophic conditions caused by deficient endogenous estrogen production, such as atrophic vaginitis and kraurosis vulvae; prevention of osteoporosis (loss of bone mass).

Administration and Dosage:

Initiation of therapy: Treatment of menopausal symptoms – Start with the 0.05 mg system applied to the skin twice weekly. Adjust dose as necessary to control symptoms. Use the lowest dosage necessary to control symptoms, especially in women with an intact uterus. Make attempts to taper or discontinue the drug at 3 to 6 month intervals.

Prophylactic therapy to prevent postmenopausal bone loss – Initiate with 0.05 mg/day as soon as possible after menopause. Adjust the dosage if necessary to control concurrent menopausal symptoms. Discontinuation of therapy may reestablish the natural rate of bone loss.

In women who are not taking oral estrogens, start treatment immediately. In women who are currently taking oral estrogens, start treatment 1 week after withdrawal of oral therapy or sooner if symptoms reappear in $<$ 1 week.

Therapeutic regimen: Therapy may be given continuously in patients who do not have an intact uterus. In patients with an intact uterus, therapy may be given on a cyclic schedule (eg, 3 weeks therapy followed by 1 week off).

Studies of the addition of a progestin for 7 or more days of a cycle of estrogen administration have reported a lowered incidence of endometrial hyperplasia. Morphological and biochemical studies of endometrium suggest that 12 to 13 days of progestin are needed to provide maximal maturation of the endometrium and to eliminate any hyperplastic changes. Whether this will provide protection from endometrial carcinoma has not been clearly established. Additional risks, including adverse effects on carbohydrate and lipid metabolism, may be associated with the inclusion of progestin in estrogen replacement regimens. The choice of progestin and dosage may be important in minimizing these adverse effects.

Application of system: Place adhesive side of the system on a clean, dry area of the skin on the trunk of the body, preferably the abdomen. Do not apply to the breasts. Rotate the application site with an interval of at least 1 week between applications to a particular site. The area selected should not be oily, damaged or irritated. Avoid the waistline, since tight clothing may rub the system off. Apply the system immediately after opening the pouch and removing the protective liner. Press firmly in place with the palm of the hand for about 10 seconds. Make sure there is good contact, especially around the edges. In the unlikely event that a system should fall off, the same system may be reapplied. If necessary, apply a new system. In either case, continue the original treatment schedule.

	Product/ Distributor	Release rate (mg/24 hr)	Surface area (cm^2)	Total estradiol content (mg)	How Supplied	C.I.*
Rx	**Estraderm** (Ciba)	0.05	10	4	Calendar Packs (8 and 24 systems).	1029
		0.1	20	8	Calendar Packs (8 and 24 systems).	1029

* Cost Index based on cost per mg estradiol or transdermal system.

Complete prescribing information for these products begins on page 350

ESTRADIOL VALERATE IN OIL

Provides 2 to 3 weeks of estrogenic effect from a single IM injection.

Administration and Dosage:

For IM injection only.

Moderate to severe vasomotor symptoms, atrophic vaginitis or kraurosis vulvae associated with menopause, female hypogonadism, female castration or primary ovarian failure: 10 to 20 mg every 4 weeks.

Prevention of postpartum breast engorgement: 10 to 25 mg, as a single injection, at the end of the first stage of labor.

Prostatic carcinoma: 30 mg or more every 1 or 2 weeks.

	Product	Strength	How supplied	C.I.*
Rx	**Estradiol Valerate** (Various, eg, Baxter, Major, Moore, Schein, Steris, URL)	**Injection:** 10 mg per ml	In 5 and 10 ml vials.	22+
Rx	**Delestrogen** (Mead Johnson)		In 5 ml vials.[1]	255
Rx	**Duragen-10** (Hauck)		In 10 ml vials.[1]	48
Rx	**Gynogen L.A. "10"** (Forest)		In 10 ml vials.[1]	60
Rx	**Valergen 10** (Hyrex)		In 10 ml vials.[1]	55
Rx	**Estradiol Valerate** (Various, eg, Baxter, Goldline, Major, Moore, Schein, Steris)	**Injection:** 20 mg per ml	In 10 ml vials.	14+
Rx	**Delestrogen** (Mead Johnson)		In 5 ml vials and 1 ml Unimatic Single Dose syringe.	183
Rx	**Dioval XX** (Keene)		In 10 ml vials.	25
Rx	**Duragen-20** (Hauck)		In 10 ml vials.[2]	31
Rx	**Estra-L 20** (Pasadena)		In 10 ml vials.[2]	27
Rx	**Gynogen L.A. "20"** (Forest)		In 10 ml vials.[2]	40
Rx	**L.A.E. 20** (Seatrace)		In 10 ml vials.[2]	30
Rx	**Valergen 20** (Hyrex)		In 10 ml vials.[2]	46
Rx	**Estradiol Valerate** (Various, eg, Baxter, Major, Moore, Schein, Steris)	**Injection:** 40 mg per ml	In 10 ml vials.	10+
Rx	**Deladiol-40** (Dunhall)		In 10 ml vials.[2]	20
Rx	**Delestrogen** (Mead Johnson)		In 5 ml vials.[2]	109
Rx	**Dioval 40** (Keene)		In 10 ml vials.	18
Rx	**Duragen-40** (Hauck)		In 10 ml vials.[2]	19
Rx	**Estra-L 40** (Pasadena)		In 10 ml vials.[2]	20
Rx	**Gynogen L.A. "40"** (Forest)		In 10 ml vials.[2]	28
Rx	**Valergen 40** (Hyrex)		In 10 ml vials.[2]	39

* Cost Index based on cost per mg.

[1] In sesame oil with chlorobutanol.

[2] In castor oil with benzyl benzoate and benzyl alcohol.

Complete prescribing information for these products begins on page 350

CONJUGATED ESTROGENS, ORAL

Contains 50% to 65% sodium estrone sulfate and 20% to 35% sodium equilin sulfate.

Administration and Dosage:

Administer cyclically (3 weeks of daily estrogen and 1 week off) for all indications except selected cases of carcinoma and prevention of postpartum breast engorgement.

Moderate to severe vasomotor symptoms associated with menopause: 1.25 mg/day. If the patient has not menstruated in 2 months or more, administration is started arbitrarily. If the patient is menstruating, begin administration on day 5 of bleeding.

Atrophic vaginitis and kraurosis vulvae associated with menopause: 0.3 to 1.25 mg or more daily, depending on tissue response of the patient.

Female hypogonadism: 2.5 to 7.5 mg daily, in divided doses for 20 days, followed by a rest period of 10 days. If bleeding does not occur by the end of this period, repeat dosage schedule. The number of courses of estrogen therapy necessary to produce bleeding may vary, depending on the responsiveness of the endometrium.

If bleeding occurs before the end of the 10 day period, begin a 20 day estrogen-progestin cyclic regimen with estrogen, 2.5 to 7.5 mg daily in divided doses. During the last 5 days of estrogen therapy, give an oral progestin. If bleeding occurs before this regimen is concluded, discontinue therapy and resume on the fifth day of bleeding.

Female castration and primary ovarian failure: 1.25 mg/day. Adjust according to severity of symptoms and patient response. For maintenance, adjust to lowest effective level.

Osteoporosis: 0.625 mg/day, cyclically.

Mammary carcinoma (for palliation): 10 mg 3 times daily for at least 3 months.

Prostatic carcinoma (for palliation): 1.25 to 2.5 mg 3 times daily. Effectiveness can be judged by phosphatase determinations as well as by symptomatic improvement.

Prevention of postpartum breast engorgement: 3.75 mg every 4 hours for 5 doses, or 1.25 mg every 4 hours for 5 days.

	Product	Strength	Description/Packaging	C.I.*
Rx	**Conjugated Estrogens** (Various, eg, Geneva, Goldline, Parmed, Purepac, Rugby, Zenith)	**Tablets:** 0.3 mg	In 100s and 1000s.	61+
Rx	**Premarin** (Wyeth-Ayerst)		(Premarin 0.3 868). Green. Oval. In 100s and 1000s.	257
Rx	**Conjugated Estrogens** (Various, eg, Geneva, Goldline, Parmed, Purepac, Rugby, Zenith)	**Tablets:** 0.625 mg	In 100s, 1000s and UD 100s.	35+
Rx	**Premarin** (Wyeth-Ayerst)		(Premarin 0.625 867). Maroon. Oval. In 100s, 1000s, 5000s, UD 100s and 25 tablet cycle packs.	171
Rx	**Premarin** (Wyeth-Ayerst)	**Tablets:** 0.9 mg	(Premarin 0.9 864). White. Oval. In 100s & 25 tablet cycle packs.	141
Rx	**Conjugated Estrogens** (Various, eg, Geneva, Goldline, Parmed, Purepac, Rugby, Zenith)	**Tablets:** 1.25 mg	In 100s, 1000s and UD 100s.	23+
Rx	**Premarin** (Wyeth-Ayerst)		(Premarin 1.25 866). Yellow. Oval. In 100s, 1000s, 5000s, UD 100s and 25 tablet cycle packs.	117
Rx	**Conjugated Estrogens** (Various, eg, Geneva, Goldline, Parmed, Purepac, Rugby, Zenith)	**Tablets:** 2.5 mg	In 100s, 1000s and UD 100s.	21+
Rx	**Premarin** (Wyeth-Ayerst)		(Premarin 2.5 865). Purple. Oval. In 100s and 1000s.	102

* Cost Index based on cost per 0.625 mg.

Complete prescribing information for these products begins on page 350

CONJUGATED ESTROGENS, PARENTERAL

Administration and Dosage:

Treatment of abnormal uterine bleeding due to hormonal imbalance in the absence of organic pathology. Administration IV produces a more rapid response and is preferred. Usual dose is one 25 mg injection IV or IM. Repeat in 6 to 12 hours if necessary. Inject slowly to obviate the occurrence of flushes.

Compatibility: Infusion of conjugated estrogens with other agents is not recommended. In emergencies, however, when an infusion has already been started, make the injection into the tubing just distal to the infusion needle. Solution is compatible with normal saline, dextrose and invert sugar solutions. It is not compatible with protein hydrolysate, ascorbic acid or any solution with an acid pH.

Storage: Before reconstitution, refrigerate at 2° to 8°C (36° to 46°F). Use the reconstituted solution within a few hours. Refrigerated reconstituted solution is stable for 60 days. Do not use if darkening or precipitation occurs. **C.I.***

Rx	**Premarin Intravenous** (Wyeth-Ayerst)	**Injection:** 25 mg conjugated estrogens	In Secules[1] (vials), each with 5 ml sterile diluent.[2]	139

ESTERIFIED ESTROGENS

These products contain 75% to 85% sodium estrone sulfate and 6% to 15% sodium equilin sulfate, in such proportion that the total of these two components is not less than 90% of the total esterified estrogens content.

Administration and Dosage:

Moderate to severe vasomotor symptoms, atrophic vaginitis or kraurosis vulvae associated with menopause: Cyclic therapy for short-term use. Average dose is 0.3 to 1.25 mg daily. Adjust dosage to lowest effective level and discontinue as soon as possible.

Female hypogonadism: Administer 2.5 to 7.5 mg daily in divided doses for 20 days followed by a 10 day rest period. If bleeding does not occur by the end of this period, repeat the same dosage schedule. The number of courses of estrogen therapy necessary to produce bleeding varies, depending on endometrial responsiveness.

If bleeding occurs before the end of the 10 day period, begin a 20 day estrogen-progestin cyclic regimen of 2.5 to 7.5 mg daily in divided doses for 20 days. During the last 5 days of estrogen therapy, give an oral progestin. If bleeding occurs before this regimen is concluded, discontinue therapy and resume on the fifth day of bleeding.

Female castration and primary ovarian failure: Give 1.25 mg daily, cyclically.

Prostatic carcinoma (inoperable, progressing): 1.25 to 2.5 mg, 3 times a day. Judge effectiveness of therapy by symptomatic response and phosphatase determinations.

Breast cancer (inoperable, progressing): In appropriately selected men and postmenopausal women, give 10 mg, 3 times a day for at least 3 months. **C.I.***

Rx	**Estratab** (Solvay Pharm.)	**Tablets:** 0.3 mg	(#RR 1014). Blue. Sugar coated. In 100s.	172
Rx	**Menest** (Beecham Labs)		Yellow. Film coated. In 100s.	130
Rx	**Estratab** (Solvay Pharm.)	**Tablets:** 0.625 mg	(#RR 1022). Yellow. Sugar coated. In 100s and 1000s.	114
Rx	**Menest** (Beecham Labs)		Orange-red. Film coated. In 100s.	88
Rx	**Estratab** (Solvay Pharm.)	**Tablets:** 1.25 mg	(#RR 1024). Orange. Sugar coated. In 100s and 1000s.	79
Rx	**Menest** (Beecham Labs)		Green. Film coated. In 100s and 1000s.	74
Rx	**Estratab** (Solvay Pharm.)	**Tablets:** 2.5 mg	(#RR 1025). Pink. Sugar coated. In 100s.	68
Rx	**Menest** (Beecham Labs)		Pink. Film coated. In 50s.	69

* Cost Index based on cost per 25 mg parenteral conjugated estrogens or 0.625 mg esterified estrogens.

\# Product identification code.

[1] With 200 mg lactose, 0.2 mg simethicone and 12.5 mg sodium citrate.

[2] With 2% benzyl alcohol.

Complete prescribing information for these products begins on page 350

ESTROPIPATE (Piperazine Estrone Sulfate)

Crystalline estrone solubilized as the sulfate and stabilized with piperazine.

Administration and Dosage: *Moderate to severe vasomotor symptoms, atrophic vaginitis or kraurosis vulvae associated with menopause:* Give cyclically for short-term use. Usual dosage range is 0.625 to 5 mg/day.

Female hypogonadism, female castration or primary ovarian failure: Administer cyclically, 1.25 to 7.5 mg/day for the first 3 weeks, followed by a rest period of 8 to 10 days. Repeat if bleeding does not occur by the end of the rest period. The duration of therapy necessary to produce withdrawal bleeding will vary according to the responsiveness of the endometrium. If satisfactory withdrawal bleeding does not occur, give an oral progestin in addition to estrogen during the third week of the cycle. **C.I.***

	Product	Form	Description	C.I.*
Rx	**Ogen** (Abbott)	**Tablets:** 0.625 mg (equiv. to 0.75 mg estropipate)	Yellow, scored. In 100s.	175
Rx	**Estropipate** (Various, eg, Harber, Major, Moore)	**Tablets:** 1.25 mg (equiv. to 1.5 mg estropipate)	In 100s and 500s.	52+
Rx	**Ogen** (Abbott)		Peach, scored. In 100s.	119
Rx	**Estropipate** (Various, eg, Harber, Major, Moore)	**Tablets:** 2.5 mg (equiv. to 3 mg estropipate)	In 100s.	45+
Rx	**Ogen** (Abbott)		Blue, scored. In 100s.	124
Rx	**Ogen** (Abbott)	**Tablets:** 5 mg (equiv. to 6 mg estropipate)	Light green, scored. In 100s.	98

ETHINYL ESTRADIOL

Administration and Dosage:

Moderate to severe vasomotor symptoms associated with menopause: Cyclical short-term use. Usual dosage range is 0.02 to 1.5 mg/day. The effective dose may be as low as 0.02 mg every other day. Dosage schedule for early menopause, while spontaneous menstruation continues, is 0.05 mg once/day for 21 days followed by a 7 day rest period. May add a progestational agent during the latter part of the cycle.

For initial treatment of late menopause, the same regimen is indicated with 0.02 mg for the first few cycles, after which the 0.05 mg dosage may be substituted. In more severe cases, such as those due to surgical and roentgenologic castration, give 0.05 mg, 3 times daily at the start of treatment. With adequate clinical improvement, usually obtainable in a few weeks, dosage may be reduced to 0.05 mg/day. A progestational agent may be added during the latter part of a planned cycle.

Female hypogonadism: 0.05 mg 1 to 3 times daily during the first 2 weeks of a theoretical menstrual cycle. Follow with progesterone during the last half of the arbitrary cycle. Continue for 3 to 6 months. The patient is then untreated for 2 months. Prescribe additional therapy if the cycle cannot be maintained without hormonal therapy.

Cancer of the female breast (inoperable, progressing): In appropriately selected postmenopausal women, 1 mg 3 times daily given chronically for palliation.

Prostatic carcinoma (inoperable, progressing): 0.15 to 2 mg/day given chronically for palliation. **C.I.***

	Product	Form	Description	C.I.*
Rx	**Estinyl** (Schering)	**Tablets:** 0.02 mg	(#Schering ER or 298). Beige. Sugar coated. In 100s and 250s.	122
Rx	**Estinyl** (Schering)	**Tablets:** 0.05 mg	(#Schering EM or 070). Pink. Sugar coated. In 100s and 250s.	82
Rx	**Feminone** (Upjohn)		(#Feminone). Pink, scored. In 100s.	19
Rx	**Estinyl** (Schering)	**Tablets:** 0.5 mg	(#Schering EP or 150). Peach, scored. In 100s.	17

QUINESTROL

Administration and Dosage: Quinestrol is stored in body fat, slowly released over several days and metabolized to ethinyl estradiol.

Moderate to severe vasomotor symptoms associated with menopause, atrophic vaginitis, kraurosis vulvae, female hypogonadism, female castration and primary ovarian failure: Initially, 100 mcg daily for 7 days; follow with 100 mcg once weekly for maintenance starting 2 weeks after treatment begins. Increase dosage to 200 mcg per week if the therapeutic response is not desirable or optimal. **C.I.***

	Product	Form	Description	C.I.*
Rx	**Estrovis** (P-D)	**Tablets:** 100 mcg	In 100s.	510

* Cost Index based on cost per 0.75 mg estropipate, 0.02 mg ethinyl estradiol or 100 mcg quinestrol.
# Product identification code.

Complete prescribing information for these products begins on page 350

DIETHYLSTILBESTROL (DES)

Administration and Dosage:

Prostatic carcinoma (inoperable, progressing): Given chronically, the usual dosage is 1 to 3 mg/day initially, increased in advanced cases; dosage may later be reduced to an average of 1 mg/day.

Breast cancer (inoperable, progressing): Given chronically in appropriately selected men and postmenopausal women, the usual dosage is 15 mg/day.

				C.I.*
Rx	**Diethylstilbestrol** (Various, eg, Allscripts, Lilly)	**Tablets:** 1 mg	In 20s, 100s and 1000s.	9+
Rx	**Diethylstilbestrol** (Lannett)	**Tablets:** 2.5 mg	In 1000s.	4
Rx	**Diethylstilbestrol** (Various, eg, Allscripts, Lilly)	**Tablets:** 5 mg	In 100s.	5+

CHLOROTRIANISENE

Administration and Dosage:

Postpartum breast engorgement: The usual dose is 12 mg 4 times/day for 7 days, or 50 mg every 6 hours for 6 doses. Give first dose within 8 hours after delivery.

Moderate to severe vasomotor symptoms associated with menopause: 12 to 25 mg/day given cyclically for 30 days; one or more courses may be prescribed.

Atrophic vaginitis and kraurosis vulvae: 12 to 25 mg/day cyclically for 30 to 60 days.

Female hypogonadism: 12 to 25 mg/day given cyclically for 21 days. May be followed immediately by 100 mg progesterone IM or by an oral progestin during the last 5 days of therapy. Next course may begin on the fifth day of induced uterine bleeding.

Prostatic carcinoma (inoperable, progressing): Given chronically, the usual dose is 12 to 25 mg/day.

				C.I.*
Rx	**Tace** (Merrell Dow)	**Capsules:** 12 mg	Tartrazine. (#Merrell 690). Green. In 100s.	410
		25 mg	Tartrazine. (#Merrell 691). Two-tone green. In 60s.	379
		72 mg[1]	Tartrazine. (#Merrell 692). Green and yellow. In 48s.	451

ESTRADIOL CYPIONATE IN OIL

Administration and Dosage:

Moderate to severe vasomotor symptoms associated with menopause: Usual dosage range is 1 to 5 mg IM, every 3 to 4 weeks.

Female hypogonadism: 1.5 to 2 mg IM at monthly intervals.

				C.I.*
Rx	**Depo-Estradiol Cypionate** (Upjohn)	**Injection:** 1 mg per ml	In 10 ml vials.[2]	605
Rx	**Estradiol Cypionate** (Various, eg, Balan, Bioline, Goldine, Major, Moore, Quad, Rugby, Schein, Steris, Texas Drug)	**Injection:** 5 mg per ml	In 10 ml vials.	33+
Rx	**depGynogen** (Forest)		In 10 ml vials.[2]	120
Rx	**Depo-Estradiol Cypionate** (Upjohn)		In 5 ml vials.[2]	379
Rx	**Depogen** (Hyrex)		In 10 ml vials.[2]	96
Rx	**Dura-Estrin** (Hauck)		In 10 ml vials.[2]	96
Rx	**Estra-D** (Seatrace)		In 10 ml vials.[2]	106
Rx	**Estro-Cyp** (Keene)		In 10 ml vials.[2]	63
Rx	**Estroject-L.A.** (Mayrand)		In 10 ml vials.[2]	105
Rx	**Estronol-LA** (Central)		In 10 ml vials.[2]	112

* Cost Index based on cost per 0.25 mg diethylstilbestrol, 12 mg chlorotrianisene or 1 mg estradiol.
# Product identification code.
[1] This strength is only for prevention of postpartum breast engorgement.
[2] In cottonseed oil with chlorobutanol.

Oral Combinations

ESTROGENS are used to alleviate symptoms associated with the menopausal syndrome. For complete prescribing information, see group monograph.

MEPROBAMATE and *CHLORDIAZEPOXIDE* are antianxiety agents used to treat concomitant symptoms of anxiety (see individual monographs).

Dose: 1 tablet 3 times a day in 21 day courses followed by a 1 week rest period.				**C.I.***
Rx	**PMB 200** (Wyeth-Ayerst)	**Tablets:** 0.45 mg conjugated estrogens and 200 mg meprobamate	Green. Oblong.In 60s.	395
Rx	**PMB 400** (Wyeth-Ayerst)	**Tablets:** 0.45 mg conjugated estrogens and 400 mg meprobamate	Pink. Oblong. In 60s.	468
Rx	**Menrium 5-2** (Roche)	**Tablets:** 0.2 mg esterified estrogens and 5 mg chlordiazepoxide	Light green. In 100s.	267
Rx	**Menrium 5-4** (Roche)	**Tablets:** 0.4 mg esterified estrogens and 5 mg chlordiazepoxide	Dark green. In 100s.	292
Rx	**Menrium 10-4** (Roche)	**Tablets:** 0.4 mg esterified estrogens and 10 mg chlordiazepoxide	Purple. In 100s.	364

Vaginal

Actions:

Depletion of endogenous estrogens occurs postmenopausally from a decline in ovarian function and may cause symptomatic vulvovaginal epithelial atrophy (atrophic vaginitis). The signs and symptoms of these atrophic changes may be alleviated by the topical application of an estrogenic hormone.

Indications:

Treatment of atrophic vaginitis and kraurosis vulvae associated with the menopause.

Warnings:

Vaginal bleeding: Since there is a possibility of absorption through the vaginal mucosa, uterine bleeding might be provoked by excessive administration in menopausal women. Cytologic study or D and C may be required to differentiate this uterine bleeding from carcinoma. Breast tenderness and vaginal discharge due to mucus hypersecretion may result from excessive estrogenic stimulation; endometrial withdrawal bleeding may occur if use is suddenly discontinued. Such reactions indicate overdosage.

May cause serious bleeding in sterilized women with endometriosis because the remaining foci of endometrium could be activated.

Patient Information:

Patient package insert is available with product.

Insert high into the vagina (≈ ⅔ the length of the applicator) with the applicator provided.

Administration and Dosage:

Treatment of atrophic vaginitis, kraurosis vulvae associated with the menopause. Choose the lower dose that will control symptoms and discontinue medication as promptly as possible. Make attempts to discontinue or taper medication at 3 to 6 month intervals.

Estropipate and conjugated estrogens – Administer cyclically; 3 weeks on and 1 week off. Give 2 to 4 g daily intravaginally depending on severity of condition.

Estradiol – 2 to 4 g daily for 2 weeks. Gradually reduce to one-half initial dosage for a similar period. A maintenance dose of 1 g 1 to 3 times a week may be used after restoration of the vaginal mucosa has been achieved.

Dienestrol – Usual dosage is 1 applicatorful once or twice daily for 1 or 2 weeks, then reduce to ½ initial dosage for a similar period. A maintenance dosage of 1 applicatorful 1 to 3 times a week may be used after restoration of vaginal mucosa has been achieved. **C.I.***

				C.I.*
Rx	**Ogen** (Abbott)	**Cream:** 1.5 mg estropipate per g	In 42.5 g with applicator.	141
Rx	**Estrace** (Mead Johnson)	**Cream:** 0.1 mg estradiol per g in a nonliquefying base	In 42.5 g with applicator.	116
Rx	**Premarin** (Wyeth-Ayerst)	**Cream:** 0.625 mg conjugated estrogens per g in a nonliquefying base	In 42.5 g with or w/o calibrated applicator.	126
Rx	**Ortho Dienestrol** (Ortho Pharm.)	**Cream:** 0.01% dienestrol	In 78 g with or w/o applicator.	78
Rx	**DV** (Merrell Dow)	**Cream:** 0.01% dienestrol with lactose in a water miscible base	In 30 g w/applicator.	87

* Cost Index based on cost per g cream or per tablet.

For progestins recommended only for their antineoplastic action in endometrial carcinoma, refer to the discussion of megestrol acetate and medroxyprogesterone acetate in the Antineoplastic section.

Warning:

Progestins have been used beginning with the first trimester of pregnancy to prevent habitual abortion or treat threatened abortion; however, there is no adequate evidence that such use is effective. There is evidence of potential harm to the fetus when given during the first 4 months of pregnancy. Therefore, the use of such drugs during the first 4 months of pregnancy is not recommended.

The cause of abortion is generally a defective ovum, which progestational agents could not be expected to influence. In addition, progestational agents have uterine relaxant properties that may cause a delay in spontaneous abortion when given to patients with fertilized defective ova.

Several reports suggest an association between intrauterine exposure to progestational drugs in the first trimester of pregnancy and genital abnormalities in male and female fetuses. The risk of hypospadias, 5 to 8 per 1,000 male births in the general population, may be approximately doubled with exposure to these drugs. There are insufficient data to quantify the risk to exposed female fetuses, but because some of these drugs induce mild virilization of the external genitalia of the female fetus, and because of the increased association of hypospadias in the male fetus, it is prudent to avoid use of these drugs during the first trimester of pregnancy.

If the patient is exposed to progestational drugs during the first 4 months of pregnancy or if she becomes pregnant while taking this drug she should be apprised of the potential risks to the fetus.

Actions:

Pharmacology: Progesterone, a principle of corpus luteum, is the primary endogenous progestational substance. Progestins (progesterone and derivatives) transform proliferative endometrium into secretory endometrium. They inhibit (at the usual dose range) the secretion of pituitary gonadotropins, which in turn prevents follicular maturation and ovulation. They also inhibit spontaneous uterine contraction. Progestins may demonstrate some estrogenic, anabolic or androgenic activity.

Pharmacokinetics: Absorption of oral tablets and parenteral oily solutions of progestins is rapid; however, the hormone undergoes prompt hepatic transformation.

Indications:

Amenorrhea; abnormal uterine bleeding; endometriosis. Refer to the product listings for specific indications of individual agents.

Unlabeled Uses: Medroxyprogesterone acetate (10 mg/day) has been used in the treatment of menopausal symptoms and to stimulate respiration in obstructive sleep apnea and other forms of chronic hypoventilation.

Addition of progestin for 7 or more days of a cycle of estrogen replacement therapy for menopause has lowered the incidence of endometrial hyperplasia. Morphological and biochemical studies of endometrium suggest that 10 to 13 days of progestin are needed to provide maximal maturation of the endometrium and to eliminate any hyperplastic changes. It is not clearly established whether this will provide protection from endometrial carcinoma. There may be additional risks with the inclusion of progestin in estrogen replacement regimens, including adverse effects on carbohydrate and lipid metabolism. Choice of progestin and dosage may be important in minimizing these adverse effects.

Progesterone suppositories (rectal or vaginal, 200 to 400 mg twice daily) have been used in the treatment of premenstrual syndrome (PMS). Some studies have reported no improvements in PMS symptoms with progesterone suppositories when compared to placebo; however, these studies may have had methodologic flaws. One controlled trial suggested that oral progesterone (100 mg in the morning, 200 mg at night for 10 days during the luteal phase) improved PMS symptoms. Further controlled studies are needed.

Progesterone has been used successfully in the treatment of premature labor in the late stages of pregnancy. Progesterone suppositories have also been used during the luteal phase to the end of the first trimester to decrease spontaneous abortions in previous aborters and in ovulatory women receiving clomiphene citrate or human menopausal gonadotropins, and in the treatment of luteal phase defects to improve fertility. However, see Warning Box.

Norethindrone (5 mg/day) appears to be effective in the treatment of hyperparathyroidism associated with mild hypercalcemia in postmenopausal women.

Contraindications:

Hypersensitivity to progestins; thrombophlebitis, thromboembolic disorders, cerebral hemorrhage or patients with a history of these conditions; impaired liver function or disease; carcinoma of the breast; undiagnosed vaginal bleeding; missed abortion; as a diagnostic test for pregnancy.

(Continued on following page)

Warnings:

Ophthalmologic effects: Discontinue medication pending examination if there is a sudden partial or complete loss of vision, or if there is sudden onset of proptosis, diplopia or migraine. If papilledema or retinal vascular lesions are present, discontinue use.

Thrombotic disorders (thrombophlebitis, cerebrovascular disorders, retinal thrombosis, pulmonary embolism) occasionally occur in patients taking progestins; be alert to the earliest manifestations of the disease. If these occur or are suspected, discontinue the drug immediately.

Pregnancy: Use is not recommended. See Warning Box.

Lactation: Detectable amounts of progestins enter the milk of mothers receiving these agents. The effect on the nursing infant has not been determined.

Medroxyprogesterone does not adversely affect lactation and may increase milk production and duration of lactation if given in the puerperium.

Precautions:

Pretreatment physical examination should include breasts and pelvic organs, as well as Papanicolaou smear. Advise the pathologist of progestin therapy when relevant specimens are submitted. In cases of irregular vaginal bleeding, consider nonfunctional causes. Adequately diagnose all cases of vaginal bleeding.

Fluid retention may occur; therefore, conditions influenced by this factor (epilepsy, migraine, asthma, cardiac or renal dysfunction) require careful observation.

Depression: Observe patients who have a history of psychic depression and discontinue the drug if the depression recurs to a serious degree.

Menopause: The age of the patient constitutes no absolute limiting factor, although treatment with progestins may mask the onset of the climacteric.

Photosensitivity: Photosensitization (photoallergy or phototoxicity) may occur; therefore, caution patients to take protective measures (ie, sunscreens, protective clothing) against exposure to ultraviolet light or sunlight until tolerance is determined.

Drug Interactions:

Aminoglutethimide may increase the hepatic metabolism of medproxyprogesterone, possibly decreasing its therapeutic effects.

Rifampin may reduce the plasma levels of norethindrone via hepatic microsomal enzyme induction, possibly decreasing its pharmacologic effects.

Drug/Lab Test Interactions: Laboratory test results of **hepatic function,** coagulation tests (increase in prothrombin, Factors VII, VIII, IX and X), thyroid, metyrapone test and **endocrine functions**, may be affected by progestins or estrogens.

A decrease in **glucose tolerance** has been observed in a small percentage of patients on estrogen-progestin combination drugs. The mechanism is obscure; observe diabetic patients who are receiving progestin therapy.

Pregnanediol determination may be altered by the use of progestins.

Adverse Reactions:

Breakthrough bleeding; spotting; change in menstrual flow; amenorrhea; changes in cervical erosion and cervical secretions; breast changes (tenderness); masculinization of the female fetus; edema; changes in weight (increase or decrease); cholestatic jaundice; rash (allergic) with and without pruritus; acne; melasma or chloasma; mental depression. A small percentage of patients have local reactions at the site of injection. Progesterone is irritating at the injection site whether the oil or aqueous vehicle is used; however, the aqueous preparation is particularly painful.

Medroxyprogesterone acetate: Thromboembolic phenomena including thrombophlebitis and pulmonary embolism; sensitivity reactions ranging from pruritus and urticaria to generalized rash; alopecia; hirsutism.

For information concerning adverse reactions associated with combined estrogen-progestin therapy, refer to the Oral Contraceptives group monograph.

Patient Information:

Patient package insert is available with product (not required to be dispensed to cancer patients).

If GI upset occurs, take with food.

Diabetic patients: Glucose tolerance may be decreased; monitor urine sugar closely and report any abnormalities to physician.

Notify physician if pregnancy is suspected or if any of the following occurs: Pain in the calves accompanied by swelling, warmth and redness; sudden severe headache; visual disturbance; numbness in an arm or leg.

(Products listed on following pages)

Complete prescribing information for these products begins on page 363.

ESTROGENS AND PROGESTINS COMBINED

This dual hormone therapy is indicated for the treatment of endometriosis and hypermenorrhea and for the production of cyclic withdrawal bleeding.

Consider the information given for Oral Contraceptives (see group monograph) when using these products.

Administration and Dosage:

Endometriosis – 5 to 10 mg daily for 2 weeks, beginning on day 5 of menstrual cycle. Administer this daily dose continuously (without cyclic interruption); increase by 5 or 10 mg increments at 2 week intervals, up to 20 mg/day. Continue this dose for 6 to 9 months. Increase further (up to 40 mg/day) if breakthrough bleeding occurs.

Hypermenorrhea – For emergency control of severe cases: 20 to 30 mg/day until bleeding is controlled, then reduce to 10 mg and continue through day 24 of cycle. Withdrawal flow usually will begin 2 or 3 days later. Cyclic withdrawal flow may be produced after treatment by giving 5 to 10 mg/day from day 5 through day 24 of the next 2 or 3 cycles.

	Oral Preparations			C.I.*
Rx	**Enovid 10 mg** (Searle)	**Tablets:** 150 mcg mestranol and 9.85 mg norethynodrel	(#Searle 10 101). Coral. In 50s.	513
Rx	**Enovid 5 mg** (Searle)	**Tablets:** 75 mcg mestranol and 5 mg norethynodrel	(#Searle 5 51). Pink. In 6 Calendar-pak 20s and bottles of 100.	270

* Cost Index based on cost per combination tablet.
# Product identification code.

Actions:

Oral contraceptives (OCs) include estrogen-progestin combos and progestin-only products.

Progestin-only: The mechanism by which progestin-only contraceptives prevent conception is not known, but they alter the cervical mucus, exert a progestational effect on the endometrium (interfering with implantation) and, in some patients, suppress ovulation.

Combination OCs inhibit ovulation by suppressing the gonadotropins, follicle-stimulating hormone (FSH) and luteinizing hormone (LH). Additionally, alterations in the genital tract, including cervical mucus (which inhibits sperm penetration) and the endometrium (which inhibits implantation), may contribute to contraceptive effectiveness.

These products differ both in the potency of the components and in the relative predominance of estrogenic or progestational activity. The two estrogens, mestranol and ethinyl estradiol, are generally considered to be equivalent in activity; 50 mcg of ethinyl estradiol is equivalent in ovulation suppression potency to 80 mcg mestranol.

Progestins may modify the effects of estrogens; these effects depend on the type or amount of progestin present and the ratio of progestin to estrogen. Dosage, potency, length of administration and concomitant estrogen administration contribute to total progestational potency, making it difficult to establish equivalent doses of progestins. Clinical observations indicate 0.5 mg norgestrel has a greater potency than 1 mg norethindrone, but less than 2 mg norethindrone. Norgestrel 0.5 mg is equivalent to 1 mg ethynodiol diacetate. Levonorgestrel is the active isomer; norgestrel, the racemate, has one-half the potency of levonorgestrel. Norethynodrel has estrogenic effects; norethindrone and ethynodiol diacetate have minor estrogenic effects at low doses, but may be antagonists at high doses. Norgestrel has antiestrogenic effects. Thus, the total estrogenic potency of an OC is based on the combined effects of the estrogen and the estrogenic/antiestrogenic effect of the progestin. The table on page 377 summarizes the effects of the various progestins.

There are three types of combination OCs: Monophasic, biphasic and triphasic.

Monophasic – Provides a fixed dosage of estrogen to progestin throughout the cycle.

Biphasic – Amount of estrogen remains the same throughout cycle. Decreased progestin:estrogen ratio in first half of cycle allows endometrial proliferation. Increased ratio in second half provides adequate secretory development.

Triphasic – Estrogen amount remains the same or varies throughout cycle. Progestin amount varies. *Ortho 7/7/7:* Estrogen amount remains the same; progestin dose increases. *Tri-Norinyl:* Estrogen amount remains the same; progestin first increases, then decreases. *Triphasil:* Estrogen amount first increases, then decreases; progestin progressively increases.

The biphasic and triphasic OCs are intended to deliver hormones in a fashion similar to physiologic processes. Long-term use of these OCs requires further evaluation.

Contraceptive efficacy: The following table gives pregnancy rates reported for various means of contraception. Efficacy (except the IUD) depends greatly upon degree of compliance.

Pregnancy Rates for Various Means of Contraception

Method of Contraception	Pregnancies/100 Woman Years
Oral Contraceptives	
35 mcg or more ethinyl estradiol	< 1
50 mcg or more mestranol	< 1
35 mcg or less ethinyl estradiol	> 1
Progestin-only	3
Mechanical/Chemical	
IUD	< 1 to 6
Levonorgestrel implants	< 1
Diaphragm (with spermicidal cream or gel)	2 to 20
Vaginal sponge	9 to 27[1]
Aerosol foams	2 to 29
Condoms	3 to 36
Gels and creams	4 to 36
Rhythm (all types)	< 1 to 47
Calendar method	14 to 47
Temperature method	1 to 20
Temperature method (intercourse only in postovulatory phase)	< 1 to 7
Mucus method	1 to 25
No contraception	60 to 80

[1] Highest failure rate in parous women.

(Actions continued on following page)

Actions (Cont.):

Noncontraceptive health benefits: The following health benefits related to the use of combination OCs are supported by epidemiological studies that largely utilized OC formulations containing estrogen doses exceeding 35 mcg.

Effects on menses: Increased menstrual cycle regularity; decreased blood loss and decreased incidence of iron deficiency anemia; decreased incidence of dysmenorrhea.

Effects related to inhibition of ovulation: Decreased incidence of functional ovarian cysts and ectopic pregnancies.

Other effects: Decreased incidence: Fibroadenomas and fibrocystic disease of the breast; acute pelvic inflammatory disease; endometrial cancer; ovarian cancer.

Pharmacokinetics: *Estrogens* – Ethinyl estradiol is rapidly absorbed with peak concentrations attained in 1 to 2 hours. It undergoes considerable first-pass elimination. Mestranol is demethylated to ethinyl estradiol. Ethinyl estradiol is approximately 98% bound to plasma albumin. Half-life varies from 6 to 20 hours. It is excreted in bile and urine as conjugates, and undergoes some enterohepatic recirculation.

Progestins – Peak concentrations of norethindrone occur 0.5 to 4 hours after oral administration; it undergoes first-pass metabolism with an overall bioavailability around 65%. Levonorgestrel reaches peak concentrations between 0.5 to 2 hours, does not undergo a first-pass effect and is completely bioavailable. Progestins are bound both to albumin and to sex hormone binding globulin. Both norethynodrel and ethynodiol diacetate are converted to norethindrone. Norethindrone and levonorgestrel are chiefly metabolized by reduction followed by conjugation. Terminal half-life of norethindrone varies from 5 to 14 hours and that of levonorgestrel from 11 to 45 hours.

Indications:

For the prevention of pregnancy. *Because of the positive association between estrogen dose and the risk of thromboembolism, minimize estrogen exposure by prescribing a product with the least estrogen activity which is compatible with an acceptable pregnancy rate and patient acceptance.*

Unlabeled use: Ovral (50 mcg ethinyl estradiol and 0.5 mg norgestrel) in high doses has been used successfully as a postcoital contraceptive or "morning after" pill. Patients are given 2 tablets at the initial visit and 2 tablets 12 hours later.

Contraindications:

Thrombophlebitis; thromboembolic disorders; history of deep vein thrombophlebitis; cerebral vascular disease; myocardial infarction; coronary artery disease; known or suspected breast carcinoma or estrogen-dependent neoplasia; past or present benign or malignant liver tumors that developed during use of estrogen-containing products (see Warnings); past or present angina pectoris; undiagnosed abnormal genital bleeding; known or suspected pregnancy (see Warnings); cholestatic jaundice of pregnancy/jaundice with prior pill use.

Warnings:

Cigarette smoking increases the risk of cardiovascular side effects from OCs. This risk increases with age and with heavy smoking (≥ 15 cigarettes per day) and is quite marked in women > 35 years of age. Women who use OCs should not smoke.

The use of OCs is associated with increased risk of venous and arterial thromboembolism, thrombotic and hemorrhagic stroke, MI, hypertension, visual disorders, hepatic adenomas and tumors, gallbladder disease and fetal abnormalities.

Mortality associated with all methods of birth control is low and below that associated with childbirth, with the exception of OC use in women ≥ 35 who smoke and ≥ 40 who do not smoke. The following table lists the annual number of birth-related or method related deaths associated with control of fertility according to age.

Estimated Annual Number of Deaths[1] due to Various Contraceptive Methods or to Pregnancy if Method Fails

	Age					
Method	15-19	20-24	25-29	30-34	35-39	40-44
No fertility control †	7	7.4	9.1	14.8	25.7	28.2
OCs, non-smoker ††	0.3	0.5	0.9	1.9	13.8	31.6
OCs, smoker ††	2.2	3.4	6.6	13.5	51.1	117.2
IUD ††	0.8	0.8	1	1	1.4	1.4
Condom †	1.1	1.6	0.7	0.2	0.3	0.4
Diaphragm/ Spermicide†	1.9	1.2	1.2	1.3	2.2	2.8
Periodic Abstinence †	2.5	1.6	1.6	1.7	2.9	3.6

[1] Among 100,000 nonsterile women, within 1 year of use.

† Deaths are birth-related. †† Deaths are method-related.

(Warnings continued on following page)

Warnings (Cont.):

Thromboembolic and cardiovascular problems: Be alert to the earliest symptoms of thromboembolic and thrombotic disorders. Should any of these occur or be suspected, discontinue the drug immediately. OC users are 1.9 to 11 times more likely to develop thromboembolic and thrombotic disease. The incidence of deep vein thrombosis appears lower in white patients with type O blood (there is no causal relationship established). Overall excess mortality due to pulmonary embolism or stroke is 1.3 to 3.4 deaths annually per 100,000 users, increasing with age. The estimated risk of hemorrhagic stroke is 2 times greater in OC users; the risk of thrombotic stroke is 4 to 9.5 times greater.

Risk of thromboembolism, including coronary thrombosis, is directly related to estrogen dose (and in some cases, progestin) used; however, estrogen quantity may not be the sole factor involved. Risk is not related to length of OC use.

Myocardial infarction (MI) risk associated with OC use is increased. The greater the number of underlying risk factors for coronary artery disease (cigarette smoking, hypertension, hypercholesterolemia, obesity, diabetes, history of pre-eclamptic toxemia), the higher the risk of developing MI; OC use is an additional risk factor. The risk is very low in women < 30 years of age. It is estimated that OC users who do not smoke are about twice as likely to have a fatal MI as nonusers who do not smoke.

Long-term use: Preliminary data suggest that the increased risk of MI persists after discontinuation of long-term use of OCs; the highest risk group includes women 40 to 49 years old who used OCs for > 10 years.

Smoking: OC users who also smoke have about a fivefold increased risk of fatal infarction compared to nonsmoking users, but a 10- to 12-fold increased risk compared to nonusers who do not smoke.

Cerebrovascular diseases: OCs increase the risks of cerebrovascular events (thrombotic and hemorrhagic strokes), although, in general, the risk is greatest in hypertensive women > 35 years of age who also smoke. Relative risk of thrombotic strokes ranges from 3 (normotensive users) to 14 (severe hypertensive users). Relative risk of hemorrhagic stroke is 1.2 for nonsmokers, 7.6 for smokers, 1.8 for normotensives, and 25.7 for severe hypertensives.

Vascular disease: A positive association is observed between the amount of estrogen and progestin in OCs and the risk of vascular disease. A decline in serum high density lipoproteins (HDL) has occurred with progestins. Because estrogens increase HDL cholesterol, the net effect depends on a balance achieved between doses of estrogen and progestin and the activity of the progestin.

Age: The risk of thromboembolic and thrombotic disease associated with OCs increases after approximately age 30. The risk of MI in OC users is substantially increased in women ≥ 35 years of age, especially those with other risk factors (eg, smoking, hypertension, hypercholesterolemia, obesity, diabetes, history of pre-eclamptic toxemia). The use of OCs in women in this age group is not recommended.

Postsurgical thromboembolism risk is increased 4- to 7-fold. If possible, discontinue OCs at least 2 to 4 weeks before and 2 weeks after surgery as OCs are associated with an increased risk of thromboembolism or prolonged immobilization. The decision as to when to resume OC use following major surgery or bed rest should balance the recognized risks of postsurgical thrombotic complications with the need to reinstate contraceptive practices.

Subarachnoid hemorrhage has been increased by OC use. Smoking alone increases the incidence of these accidents; smoking and OC use appear to work together to produce a combined risk greater than either alone.

Varicose veins substantially increase the risk of superficial venous thrombosis of the leg, depending on the severity of the varicosities. This has been correlated to the progestin dose. Varicose veins seem to have little effect on deep vein thrombosis.

Factor XII deficiency – Patients with Hageman Factor (Factor XII) deficiency may be at increased risk of developing thromboembolism.

Progestin-only products are not free of risk. Thromboembolic risk associated with these products has not been studied. Cases of thromboembolic disease have been reported.

Persistence of risk – An increased risk may persist for at least 6 years after discontinuation of OC use for cerebrovascular disease and at least 9 years for MI in users 40 to 49 years of age who had used OCs ≥ 5 years. A prospective study suggested the persistence of risk for subarachnoid hemorrhage also. There may also be an increased risk for nonrheumatic heart disease, cerebral thrombosis, transient ischemic attacks and cerebrovascular disease.

NOTE – The associations between OCs and cardiovascular disease are based on epidemiological studies whose conclusions have been criticized for several reasons: National trends of cardiovascular mortality are incompatible with these risk estimates; excess deaths may not be attributable entirely to smoking; the clinical diagnosis of thromboembolism is often unreliable. Also, new data concerning risks to ex-users of OCs have further confounded these analyses.

(Warnings continued on following page)

Adverse Reactions:

Serious: See Warnings. Thrombophlebitis and thrombosis; pulmonary embolism; coronary thrombosis; MI; cerebral thrombosis; Raynaud's disease; arterial thromboembolism; renal artery thrombosis; cerebral hemorrhage; hypertension; gallbladder disease; congenital anomalies; liver tumors and other hepatic lesions, with or without intra-abdominal bleeding; hepatocellular carcinoma.

There is evidence of an association between the following conditions and the use of OCs: Mesenteric thrombosis; Budd-Chiari syndrome; neuro-ocular lesions (eg, retinal thrombosis and optic neuritis).

GI: Nausea and vomiting (occurring in approximately 10% of patients during the first cycle); abdominal cramps; bloating; cholestatic jaundice.

Gynecologic: Breakthrough bleeding; spotting; change in menstrual flow; dysmenorrhea; amenorrhea during and after treatment; temporary infertility after discontinuation; change in cervical erosion and cervical secretions; endocervical hyperplasia; increased size of uterine leiomyomata; vaginal candidiasis.

Breast changes: Tenderness; enlargement; secretion; possible diminution in lactation when given immediately postpartum.

Dermatologic: Melasma; rash (allergic).

CNS: Migraine; mental depression.

Ophthalmic: Changes in corneal curvature (steepening); contact lens intolerance.

Miscellaneous: Edema; weight change (increase or decrease); reduced carbohydrate tolerance; prolactin-secreting pituitary tumors; chilblains; prevalence of cervical chlamydia trachomatis is increased several fold.

The following associations have been neither confirmed nor refuted: Premenstrual-like syndrome; cataracts; changes in libido; chorea; changes in appetite; cystitis-like syndrome; headache; nervousness; dizziness; hirsutism; loss of scalp hair; erythema multiforme; erythema nodosum; hemorrhagic eruption; vaginitis; renal function impairment; malignant nephrosclerosis (hemolytic uremic syndrome); porphyria; paresthesia; auditory disturbances; rhinitis; fatigue; backache; itching; anemia; pancreatitis; hepatitis; colitis; gingivitis; dry socket; lupus erythematosus; rheumatoid arthritis; malignant melanoma; endometrial, cervical and breast carcinoma; herpes gestationis; acute renal failure (sometimes irreversible); thrombotic thrombocytopenic purpura; malignant hypertension; premature ventricular contractions; pulmonary hypertension; Crohn's disease; pituitary tumors; ECG abnormalities; bile duct carcinoma; acne.

Overdosage:

Serious ill effects have not been reported following acute overdosage of OCs in young children. Overdosage may cause nausea. Withdrawal bleeding may occur in females.

Patient Information:

Patient package insert available with product.

To achieve maximum contraceptive effectiveness, take OCs exactly as directed at intervals not exceeding 24 hours. Take tablets regularly with a meal or at bedtime. Efficacy depends on strict adherence to the dosage schedule.

May cause spotting or breakthrough bleeding during the first few months of therapy; if it continues past the second month, notify physician.

Use an additional method of birth control until after the first week of administration in the initial cycle.

Missed doses: See Administration and Dosage.

(Continued on following page)

Complete prescribing information for these products begins on page 368

Combination Therapy Tablets

Administration and Dosage:

Sunday-Start Packaging: If the instructions recommend starting the regimen on Sunday, take the first tablet on the first Sunday after menstruation begins. If menstruation begins on Sunday, take the first tablet on that day.

21-Day regimen: Day 1 of the cycle is the first day of menstrual bleeding. Take 1 tablet daily for 21 days, according to number of tablets supplied for 1 cycle, beginning on day 5 of cycle. No tablets are taken for 7 days; whether bleeding has stopped or not, start a new course of 21 days. Withdrawal flow will normally occur 2 or 3 days after the last tablet is taken. Follow the schedule whether flow occurs as expected, or whether spotting or BTB occurs during the cycle.

28-Day regimen: To eliminate the need for patients to count the days between cycles, some products contain 7 inert or iron-containing tablets to permit continuous daily dosage during the entire 28-day cycle. Take 7 inert or iron tablets on the last 7 days of the cycle.

Biphasic and triphasic OCs: Ortho-Novum 10/11 – Take 1 white tablet daily for 10 days, then 1 peach tablet daily for 11 days for the 21-day regimen; no tablets are taken for the next 7 days. For the 28-day regimen, take 1 green tablet daily for the last 7 days.

Ortho-Novum 7/7/7 – Take 1 white tablet daily for 7 days, then 1 light peach tablet daily for 7 days, then 1 peach tablet daily for 7 days for the 21-day regimen; no tablets are taken for the next 7 days. For the 28-day regimen, take 1 green tablet for the last 7 days.

Tri-Norinyl – Take 1 blue tablet daily for 7 days, then 1 green tablet daily for 9 days, then 1 blue tablet daily for 5 days; no tablets are taken for the next 7 days for the 21-day regimen. For the 28-day regimen, take 1 orange tablet for the last 7 days.

Triphasil and Tri-Levlen – During the first cycle, begin on day 1 of the menstrual cycle. Take 1 brown tablet daily for 6 days, then 1 white tablet daily for 5 days, then 1 yellow tablet daily for 10 days; no tablets are taken for the next 7 days for the 21-day regimen. For the 28-day regimen, take 1 green tablet for the last 7 days.

Missed dose: While there is little likelihood of ovulation occurring if only 1 tablet is missed, the possibility of spotting or bleeding is increased. The possibility of ovulation occurring increases with each successive day that scheduled tablets are missed. This is particularly likely to occur if $\geq$ 2 consecutive tablets are missed. Any time $\geq$ 1 active tablets have been missed, use another method of contraception until tablets have been taken for 7 consecutive days. If a patient forgets to take 1 or more tablets, the following is suggested:

One tablet – Take it as soon as remembered, or take 2 tablets the next day; alternatively take 1 tablet, discard the other missed tablet, continue as scheduled and use another form of contraception until menses.

Two consecutive tablets – Take 2 tablets as soon as remembered with the next pill at the usual time, or take 2 tablets daily for the next 2 days, then resume the regular schedule. Use an additional form of contraception for the remainder of the cycle.

Three consecutive tablets – Begin a new compact of tablets, starting on day one of the cycle after the last pill was taken or starting 7 days after the last tablet was taken. Use an additional form of birth control until pills have been taken for 7 consecutive days.

Bleeding that resembles menstruation occurs rarely. Discontinue medication and begin taking tablets from a new compact on day 5 (or next Sunday). Persistent bleeding not controlled by this method indicates the need for re-examination of the patient; consider nonfunctional causes.

Missed menstrual period:

1. If the patient has not adhered to the prescribed dosage regimen, consider possible pregnancy after the first missed period; withhold OCs until ruling out pregnancy.
2. If the patient has adhered to the prescribed regimen and misses 2 consecutive periods, rule out pregnancy before continuing the contraceptive regimen.

After several months of treatment, menstrual flow may reduce to a point of virtual absence. This reduced flow may occur as a result of medication, and is not indicative of pregnancy.

Postpartum administration in non-nursing mothers may begin at the first postpartum examination (4 to 6 weeks), regardless of whether spontaneous menstruation has occurred. Immediate postpartum use is associated with increased risk of thromboembolism. Nursing mothers should defer taking OCs until the infant is weaned (see Warnings).

Dosage Adjustments:

Side effects noted during the initial cycles may be transient; if they continue, dosage adjustments may be indicated. Many side effects are related to the potency of the estrogen or progestin in the products. Some effects may be related to the relative dominance of either the estrogenic or progestational component. The following table summarizes these dose-related side effects.

(Dosage Adjustments continued on following page)

Combination Therapy Tablets (Cont.)

Dosage Adjustments (Cont.):

Achieving Proper Hormonal Balance In An Oral Contraceptive			
Estrogen		Progestin	
Excess	Deficiency	Excess	Deficiency
Nausea, bloating Cervical mucorrhea, polyposis Melasma Hypertension Migraine headache Breast fullness or tenderness Edema	Early or midcycle breakthrough bleeding Increased spotting Hypomenorrhea	Increased appetite Weight gain Tiredness, fatigue Hypomenorrhea Acne, oily scalp* Hair loss, hirsutism* Depression Monilial vaginitis Breast regression	Late breakthrough bleeding Amenorrhea Hypermenorrhea

* Result of androgenic activity of progestins.

Pharmacological Effects of Progestins Used in Oral Contraceptives	Progestin	Estrogen	Antiestrogen	Androgen
Norgestrel/levonorgestrel	+++	0	++	+++
Ethynodiol diacetate	++	+[1]	+[1]	+
Norethindrone acetate	+	+	+++	+
Norethindrone	+	+[1]	+[1]	+
Norethynodrel	+	+++	0	0

[1] Has estrogenic effect at low doses; may have antiestrogenic effect at higher doses.
Symbol Key: +++ *pronounced effect* ++ *moderate effect* + *slight effect* 0 *no effect*

Minimize the above effects by adjusting the estrogen/progestin balance or dosage. The following table categorizes products by both their estrogenic and progestational potencies. Because overall activity is influenced by the interaction of components, it is difficult to precisely classify products; placement in the table is only approximate. Differences between products within a group are probably not clinically significant.

Estimated Relative Oral Contraceptive Estrogen/Progestin Potency				
← PROGESTINS →	ESTROGENS: Low		ESTROGENS: Intermediate	
High			Ovral	
Intermediate	Demulen 1/35 Levlen	Lo/Ovral Nordette	Demulin 1/50 Norlestrin 2.5/50	Norlestrin Fe 2.5/50
Low	*Monophasic* Brevicon Genora 0.5/35 Genora 1/35 Genora 1/50 Loestrin 1/20 Loestrin Fe 1/20 Loestrin 1.5/30 Loestrin Fe 1.5/30 Modicon N.E.E. 1/35 E Nelova 0.5/35 E Nelova 1/35 E *Biphasic* Nelova 10/11 *Triphasic* Ortho-Novum 7/7/7 Tri-Levlen	 Nelova 1/50 M Norcept-E 1/35 Norethin 1/35 E Norethin 1/50 M Norinyl 1 + 35 Norinyl 1 + 50 Ortho-Novum 1/35 Ortho-Novum 1/50 Ovcon-35 Ortho-Novum 10/11 Tri-Norinyl Triphasil	*Monophasic* Norlestrin 1/50 Norlestrin Fe 1/50 Ovcon-50	

Durand JL, Bressler R. *Adv Intern Med* 1979;24:97. Dickey RP. *Int J Gynaecol Obstet* 1979;16:547.
Dickey RP, Stone SC. *Obstet Gynecol* 1976;47:106. Chihal HJW, Peppler RD, Dickey RP. *Am J Obstet Gynecol* 1975;121:75.

(Products listed on following page)

Refer to the general discussion of these products beginning on page 368.

Combination Therapy Tablets (Cont.)

The combination therapy products are listed in order of decreasing estrogen content.

Monophasic Oral Contraceptives

	Product & Distributor	Estrogen (mcg)	Progestin (mg)	How Supplied	C.I.*
Rx	**Genora 1/50** (Rugby)	50 mestranol	1 norethindrone	White or pale blue. In 21s and 28s. With 7 peach inert tablets in the 28s.	122
Rx	**Nelova 1/50M** (Warner Chilcott)			(#WC 942). Light blue. In 6 packs of 21s & 28s. With 7 white inert tablets (#WC 937) in the 28s.	108
Rx	**Norethin 1/50M** (Schiapparelli Searle)			(#Searle 431). In 21s and 28s. White with 7 blue inert tablets (#Searle P) in the 28s.	91
Rx	**Norinyl 1 + 50** (Syntex)			White. In Wallette 21s and 28s. With 7 orange inert tablets in the 28s.	179
Rx	**Ortho-Novum 1/50** (Ortho Pharm.)			(#Ortho 150). Yellow. In Dialpak 21s and 28s. With 7 green inert tablets in the 28s.	163
Rx	**Ovcon-50** (Mead Johnson Labs)	50 ethinyl estradiol	1 norethindrone	Yellow. In individual compacts and 6 compact cartons of 21s and 28s. With 7 green inert tablets in the 28s.	209
Rx	**Norlestrin 1/50** (Parke-Davis)	50 ethinyl estradiol	1 norethindrone acetate	Yellow. In 5 packs of 21s and 28s. With 7 white inert tablets in the 28s.	185
Rx	**Norlestrin Fe 1/50** (Parke-Davis)			Yellow with 7 brown tablets (75 mg ferrous fumarate/tab). In 5 packs of 28s.	185
Rx	**Demulen 1/50** (Searle)	50 ethinyl estradiol	1 ethynodiol diacetate	(#Searle 71). White. In 6 and 24 Compack 21s and 28s and 12 refill 21s and 28s. With 7 pink inert tablets (# Searle P) in the 28s.	214
Rx	**Norlestrin 21 2.5/50** (Parke-Davis)	50 ethinyl estradiol	2.5 norethindrone acetate	Pink. In 5 packs of 21s.	186
Rx	**Norlestrin Fe 2.5/50** (Parke-Davis)			(#P-D 901). Pink with 7 brown tablets (75 mg ferrous fumarate/tab). In 5 packs of 28s.	192
Rx	**Ovral** (Wyeth-Ayerst)	50 ethinyl estradiol	0.5 norgestrel	(#Wyeth 56). White. In 6 Pilpak 21s and 28s. With 7 pink inert tablets (#Wyeth 445) in the 28s.	165

* Cost Index based on cost per cycle. # Product identification code.

(Continued on following page)

The combination therapy products are listed in order of decreasing estrogen content.

Combination Therapy Tablets (Cont.)

Monophasic Oral Contraceptives (Cont.)

	Product & Distributor	Estrogen (mcg)	Progestin (mg)	How Supplied	C.I.*
Rx	**Genora 1/35** (Rugby)	35 ethinyl estradiol	1 norethindrone	Blue. In 21s or 28s. With 7 peach inert tablets in the 28s.	122
Rx	**GenCept 1/35** (Gencon)			In 21s and 28s (7 inert tablets).	NA
Rx	**N.E.E. 1/35** (Lexis)			Yellow. In 6 packs of 21s and 28s. With 7 peach inert tablets in the 28s.	81
Rx	**Nelova 1/35E** (Warner Chilcott)			(WC 930). Dark yellow. In 6 packs of 21s and 28s. With 7 white inert tablets (#WC 937) in the 28s.	109
Rx	**Norcept-E 1/35** (Gynopharma)			White. In 6 blister packs of 21s and 28s. With 7 green inert tablets in the 28s.	88
Rx	**Norethin 1/35E** (Schiapparelli Searle)			(Searle 221). White. In 6 packs of 21s and 28s. With 7 blue inert tablets (#Searle P) in the 28s.	91
Rx	**Norinyl 1+35** (Syntex)			Green. In Wallette 21s and 28s. With 7 orange inert tablets in the 28s.	181
Rx	**Ortho-Novum 1/35** (Ortho Pharm.)			(Ortho 135). Peach. In Dialpak 21s and 28s. With 7 green inert tablets in the 28s.	163
Rx	**Brevicon** (Syntex)	35 ethinyl estradiol	0.5 norethindrone	Blue. In Wallette 21s and 28s. With 7 orange inert tablets in the 28s.	187
Rx	**GenCept 0.5/35** (Gencon)			In 21s and 28s (7 inert tablets).	NA
Rx	**Genora 0.5/35** (Rugby)			White. In 21s and 28s. With 7 peach inert tablets in the 28s.	79
Rx	**Modicon** (Ortho Pharm.)			(Ortho 535). White. In Dialpak 21s and 28s. With 7 green inert tablets in the 28s.	184
Rx	**Nelova 0.5/35E** (Warner Chilcott)			(WC 929). Light yellow. In 6 packs of 21s and 28s. With 7 white inert tablets in the 28s.	109
Rx	**Ovcon-35** (Mead Johnson Labs)	35 ethinyl estradiol	0.4 norethindrone	(MJ). Peach. In individual packs and 6 packs of 21s and 28s. With 7 green inert tablets in the 28s.	190
Rx	**Demulen 1/35** (Searle)	35 ethinyl estradiol	1 ethynodiol diacetate	(Searle 151). White. In 6 and 24 Compack 21s and 28s and 12 and 24 refill 21s and 28s. With 7 blue inert tablets (#Searle P) in the 28s.	191
Rx	**Nelulen 1/35E** (Watson Labs)			In 21s and 28s.	NA
Rx	**Nelulen 1/50E** (Watson Labs)	50 ethinyl estradiol	1 ethynodiol diacetate	In 21s and 28s.	NA

* Cost Index based on cost per cycle.

(Continued on following page)

The combination therapy products are listed in order of decreasing estrogen content.

Combination Therapy Tablets (Cont.)

Monophasic Oral Contraceptives (Cont.)

	Product & Distributor	Estrogen (mcg)	Progestin (mg)	How Supplied	C.I.*
Rx	**Loestrin 21 1.5/30** (P-D)	30 ethinyl estradiol	1.5 norethindrone acetate	Green. In 5 packs of 21s.	186
Rx	**Loestrin Fe 1.5/30** (P-D)			Green with 7 brown tablets (75 mg ferrous fumarate/tab). In 5 packs of 28s.	186
Rx	**Lo/Ovral** (Wyeth-Ayerst)	30 ethinyl estradiol	0.3 norgestrel	(Wyeth 78). White. In 6 Pilpak 21s and 28s. With 7 pink inert tablets (Wyeth 486) in the 28s.	214
Rx	**Levlen** (Berlex)	30 ethinyl estradiol	0.15 levonorgestrel	(B 21). Orange. In 3 slidecase dispenser 21s and 28s. With 7 pink inert tablets (B 28) in the 28s.	160
Rx	**Nordette** (Wyeth-Ayerst)			(Wyeth 75). Light orange. In 6 Pilpak 21s and 28s. With 7 pink inert tablets (Wyeth 486) in the 28s.	161
Rx	**Loestrin 21 1/20** (P-D)	20 ethinyl estradiol	1 norethindrone acetate	White. In 5 packs of 21s.	186
Rx	**Loestrin Fe 1/20** (P-D)			White with 7 brown tablets (75 mg ferrous fumarate/tab). In 5 packs of 28s.	186

Biphasic Oral Contraceptives

	Product & Distributor	Composition	How Supplied	C.I.*
Rx	**Jenest-28** (Organon)	*Phase 1:* 7 Tablets (white), 0.5 mg norethindrone, 35 mcg ethinyl estradiol *Phase 2:* 14 Tablets (peach), 1 mg norethindrone, 35 mcg ethinyl estradiol	White = (ORG 07). Peach = (ORG 14). Green = (ORG). In cyclic dispensers of 28 tablets.	NA
Rx	**GenCept 10/11** (Gencon)	*Phase 1:* 10 Tablets 0.5 mg norethindrone, 35 mcg ethinyl estradiol *Phase 2:* 11 Tablets 1 mg norethindrone, 35 mcg ethinyl estradiol	With 7 inert tablets. In 21s and 28s.	
Rx	**Nelova 10/11** (Warner Chilcott)	*Phase 1:* 10 Tablets (light yellow), 0.5 mg norethindrone, 35 mcg ethinyl estradiol *Phase 2:* 11 Tablets (dark yellow), 1mg norethindrone, 35 mcg ethinyl estradiol	Light yellow = (WC 929). Dark yellow = (WC 930). In 6 packs of 21s and 28s. With 7 white inert tablets (WC 937) in the 28s.	109
Rx	**Ortho-Novum 10/11** (Ortho Pharm.)	*Phase 1:* 10 Tablets (white), 0.5 mg norethindrone, 35 mcg ethinyl estradiol *Phase 2:* 11 Tablets (peach), 1 mg norethindrone, 35 mcg ethinyl estradiol	White = (Ortho 535). Peach = (Ortho 135). In Dialpak 21s and 28s. With 7 green inert tablets in the 28s.	184

* Cost Index based on cost per cycle.

The combination therapy products are listed in order of decreasing estrogen content.

Combination Therapy Tablets (Cont.)

Triphasic Oral Contraceptives

	Product	*Phase 1*	*Phase 2*	*Phase 3*	How Supplied	C.I.*
Rx	**Tri-Norinyl** (Syntex)	0.5 mg norethindrone, 35 mcg ethinyl estradiol (7 blue tablets)	1 mg norethindrone, 35 mcg ethinyl estradiol (9 green tablets)	0.5 mg norethindrone, 35 mcg ethinyl estradiol (5 blue tablets)	28 day has 7 orange inert tabs. In 21s and 28s.	166
Rx	**Ortho Novum 7/7/7** (Ortho Pharm.)	0.5 mg norethindrone, 35 mcg ethinyl estradiol (7 white tablets)	0.75 mg norethindrone, 35 mcg ethinyl estradiol, (7 light peach tablets)	1 mg norethindrone, 35 mcg ethinyl estradiol, (7 peach tablets)	(#Ortho). White = (#535). Lt. peach = (#75). Peach = (#135). 28 day has 7 green inert tablets. In Dialpak 21s and 28s.	184
Rx	**Tri-Levlen** (Berlex)	0.05 mg levonorgestrel, 30 mcg ethinyl estradiol, (6 brown tablets)	0.075 mg levonorgestrel, 40 mcg ethinyl estradiol (5 white tablets)	0.125 mg levonorgestrel, 30 mcg ethinyl estradiol (10 yellow tablets)	Brown = (#B 95). White = (#B 96). Yellow = (#B 97). 28 day has 7 green placebo tablets (#B 11). In 3 slide case dispenser 21s & 28s.	153
Rx	**Triphasil** (Wyeth-Ayerst)				(#W). Brown = (#641). White = (#642). Yellow = (#643). 28 day has 7 light green inert tabs (#W 650). In 3 and 6 packs of compact and refill 21s and 28s.	187

Progestin-Only Products

Administration and Dosage:

Administer daily, starting on the first day of menstruation. Take one tablet at the same time each day, every day of the year.

Postpartum administration: May be initiated 2 weeks postpartum; however, consider the increased risk of thromboembolic disease associated with the postpartum period.

Missed dose:

One tablet – Take as soon as remembered, then take next tablet at regular time.

Two consecutive tablets – Take 1 of the missed tablets, discard the other and take daily tablet at usual time.

Three consecutive tablets – Discontinue immediately.

Use an additional method of contraception if 2 or more tablets are missed until menses appears or pregnancy is ruled out. If menses does not occur within 45 days, regardless of circumstances, discontinue drug, use a nonhormonal method of contraception and rule out pregnancy. Because of the slightly higher failure rate of the progestin-only products, a more conservative approach is to discontinue the regimen if only 1 tablet is missed and use other contraceptive methods until menses occurs or pregnancy is ruled out.

	Product		How Supplied	C.I.*
Rx	**Micronor** (Ortho Pharm.)	**Tablets:** 0.35 mg norethindrone	(#Ortho 0.35). Lime. In Dialpak 28s.	211
Rx	**Nor-Q.D.** (Syntex)		Yellow. In dispenser 42s.	220
Rx	**Ovrette** (Wyeth-Ayerst)	**Tablets:** 0.075 mg norgestrel	Tartrazine. (#Wyeth 62). Yellow. In 6 Pilpak 28s.	155

* Cost Index based on cost per cycle.

\# Product identification code.

LEVONORGESTREL IMPLANTS

Actions:

Pharmacology: Levonorgestrel implants are a set of six flexible closed capsules made of *Silastic* (dimethylsiloxane/methylvinylsiloxane copolymer), each containing 36 mg of the progestin levonorgestrel contained in an insertion kit to facilitate implantation. The capsules are sealed with *Silastic* adhesive (polydimethylsiloxane) and sterilized.

The dose of levonorgestrel is initially about 85 mcg/day, followed by a decline to about 50 mcg/day by 9 months, and to about 35 mcg/day by 18 months, with a further decline thereafter to about 30 mcg/day. The levonorgestrel implant is a progestin-only product and does not contain estrogen. Levonorgestrel is a totally synthetic and biologically active progestin which exhibits no significant estrogenic activity and is highly progestational. For further information, refer to the Progestins group monograph.

Diffusion of levonorgestrel through the wall of each capsule provides a continuous low dose of the progestin. Resulting blood levels are substantially below those generally observed among users of combination oral contraceptives containing the progestins norgestrel or levonorgestrel. Because of the range of variability in blood levels and variation in individual response, blood levels alone are not predictive of the risk of pregnancy in an individual woman.

Pharmacokinetics: Levonorgestrel concentrations among women show considerable variation. Levonorgestrel concentrations reach a maximum, or near maximum, within 24 hours after placement with mean values of 1600 ± 1100 pg/ml. They decline rapidly over the first month partially due to a circulating protein, SHBG, that binds levonorgestrel and which is depressed by the presence of levonorgestrel. Mean levels decline to values of around 400 pg/ml at 3 months to 258 ± 95 pg/ml at 60 months.

Concentrations decreased with increasing body weight by a mean of 3.3 pg/ml/kg. After capsule removal, mean concentrations drop to < 100 pg/ml by 96 hours and to below assay sensitivity (50 pg/ml) by 5 to 14 days. Fertility rates return to levels comparable to those seen in the general population of women using no method of contraception. Circulating concentrations can be used to forecast the risk of pregnancy only in a general statistical sense. Mean concentrations associated with pregnancy have been 210 ± 60 pg/ml. However, in clinical studies, 20% of women had one or more values below 200 pg/ml but an average annual gross pregnancy rate of < 1 per 100 women through 5 years.

Contraceptive efficacy:

Annual and 5 Year Cumulative Pregnancy Rates Per 100 Levonorgestrel Implant Users by Weight						
	Year					
Weight	1	2	3	4	5	Cumulative
< 50 kg (< 110 lbs)	0.2	0	0	0	0	0.2
50-59 kg (110-130 lbs)	0.2	0.5	0.4	2	0.4	3.4
60-69 kg (131-153 lbs)	0.4	0.5	1.6	1.7	0.8	5
≥ 70 kg (≥ 154 lbs)	0	1.1	5.1	2.5	0	8.5
All	0.2	0.5	1.2	1.6	0.4	3.9

The lowest expected failure rate for levonorgestrel implants during the first year of use is < 1. The efficacy of the implant does not depend on patient compliance. For pregnancy rates for various other means of contraception, see the Oral Contraceptives Group Monograph.

Indications:

Prevention of pregnancy. The implant system is a long-term (up to 5 years) reversible contraceptive system. Remove the capsules by the end of the 5th year; new capsules may be inserted at that time if continuing contraceptive protection is desired.

Contraindications:

Active thrombophlebitis or thromboembolic disorders; undiagnosed abnormal genital bleeding; known or suspected pregnancy; acute liver disease; benign or malignant liver tumors; known or suspected carcinoma of the breast.

(Continued on following page)

LEVONORGESTREL IMPLANTS (Cont.)

Warnings:

The following warnings are based on experience with levonorgestrel implants. For other warnings, refer to the Oral Contraceptives group monograph.

Bleeding irregularities: Most women can expect some variation in menstrual bleeding patterns. Irregular menstrual bleeding, intermenstrual spotting, prolonged episodes of bleeding and spotting, and amenorrhea occur in some women. Irregular bleeding patterns could mask symptoms of cervical or endometrial cancer. Overall, these irregularities diminish with continuing use. Since some users experience periods of amenorrhea, missed menstrual periods cannot serve as the only means of identifying early pregnancy. Perform pregnancy tests whenever a pregnancy is suspected. After a pattern of regular menses, ≥ 6 weeks of amenorrhea may signal pregnancy. If pregnancy occurs, the capsules must be removed.

Although bleeding irregularities have occurred in clinical trials, proportionately more women had increases rather than decreases in hemoglobin concentrations, a difference that was highly statistically significant. This finding generally indicates that reduced menstrual blood loss is associated with the use of levonorgestrel implants. In rare instances, blood loss did result in hemoglobin values consistent with anemia.

Delayed follicular atresia: If follicular development occurs, atresia of the follicle is sometimes delayed and the follicle may continue to grow beyond the size it would attain in a normal cycle. These enlarged follicles cannot be distinguished clinically from ovarian cysts. In the majority of women, enlarged follicles will spontaneously disappear and should not require surgery. Rarely, they may twist or rupture, sometimes causing abdominal pain; surgical intervention may be required.

Ectopic pregnancies have occurred among levonorgestrel implant users, although clinical studies have shown no increase in the rate of ectopic pregnancies per year among users as compared with users of no method or of IUDs. The incidence among users was 1.3 per 1000 woman-years, a rate significantly below the rate that has been estimated for non-contraceptive users in the US (2.7 to 3 per 1000 woman-years). The risk of ectopic pregnancy may increase with the duration of use and, possibly, with increased weight of the user. Any patient who presents with lower abdominal pain must be evaluated to rule out ectopic pregnancy.

Ocular lesions: There have been clinical case reports of retinal thrombosis associated with the use of oral contraceptives. Although it is believed that this adverse reaction is related to the estrogen component of oral contraceptives, remove the capsules if there is unexplained partial or complete loss of vision, onset of proptosis or diplopia, papilledema or retinal vascular lesions. Undertake appropriate diagnostic and therapeutic measures immediately.

Foreign body carcinogenesis: Rarely, cancers have occurred at the site of foreign body intrusions or old scars. None has been reported in levonorgestrel implant clinical trials. In rodents highly susceptible to such cancers, the incidence decreases with decreasing size of the foreign body. Because of the resistance of human beings to these cancers and because of the small size of the capsules, the risk to users is judged to be minimal.

Thromboembolic disorders: Patients who develop active thrombophlebitis or thromboembolic disease should have the levonorgestrel capsules removed. Also consider removal in women who will be immobilized for a prolonged period due to surgery or other illnesses.

Lactation: Steroids are not the contraceptives of first choice for lactating women. Levonorgestrel has been identified in breast milk. No significant effects were observed on the growth or health of infants whose mothers used the implants beginning 6 weeks after parturition in comparative studies with mothers using IUDs or barrier methods.

Precautions:

Physical examination and follow-up: Take a complete medical history and physical examination prior to the implantation or re-implantation of levonorestrel implants and at least annually during its use. These physical examinations should include special reference to the implant site, blood pressure, breasts, abdomen and pelvic organs, including cervical cytology and relevant laboratory tests. In case of undiagnosed, persistent or recurrent abnormal vaginal bleeding, conduct appropriate diagnostic measures to rule out malignancy. Carefully monitor women with a strong family history of breast cancer or who have breast nodules.

(Precautions continued on following page)

LEVONORGESTREL IMPLANTS (Cont.)

Precautions (Cont.):

Carbohydrate and lipid metabolism: An altered glucose tolerance characterized by decreased insulin sensitivity following glucose loading has been found in some users of combination and progestin-only oral contraceptives. The effects of the levonorgestrel implants on carbohydrate metabolism appear to be minimal. In a study in which pretreatment serum glucose levels were compared with levels after 1 and 2 years of use, no statistically significant differences in mean serum glucose levels were evident 2 hours after glucose loading. The clinical significance of these findings is unknown but carefully observe diabetic and prediabetic patients.

Closely follow women who are being treated for hyperlipidemias. Some progestins may elevate LDL levels and render the control of hyperlipidemias more difficult. Although lipoprotein levels were altered in several clinical studies with the levonorgestrel implants, the long-term clinical effects of these changes have not been determined. A decrease in total cholesterol levels has occurred in all lipoprotein studies and reached statistical significance in several. Both increases and decreases in HDL levels have been reported in clinical trials. LDL and triglyceride levels also decreased from pretreatment values.

Liver function: If jaundice develops consider removing the capsules. Steroid hormones may be poorly metabolized in patients with impaired liver function.

Fluid retention: Steroid contraceptives may cause some degree of fluid retention. Prescribe with caution, and only with careful monitoring, in patients with conditions which might be aggravated by fluid retention.

Emotional disorders: Consider removing the capsules in women who become significantly depressed since the symptom may be drug-related. Carefully observe women with a history of depression and consider removal if depression recurs to a serious degree.

Contact lens wearers who develop changes in vision or in lens tolerance should be assessed by an ophthalmologist.

Insertion and removal: To be sure that the woman is not pregnant at the time of capsule placement and to assure contraceptive efficacy during the first cycle of use, insert the capsules during the first 7 days of the cycle or immediately following an abortion. Insertion is not recommended before 6 weeks postpartum in breastfeeding women.

Insertion and removal are not difficult procedures but instructions must be followed closely. It is strongly advised that all health care professionals who insert and remove the capsules be instructed in the procedures before they attempt them. A proper insertion just under the skin will facilitate removals. Proper insertion and removal should result in minimal scarring. If the capsules are placed too deeply, they can be harder to remove. If all capsules cannot be removed at the first attempt, try removal later when the site has healed. Bruising may occur at the implant site during insertion or removal. In some women, hyperpigmentation occurs over the implantation site but is usually reversible following removal.

Infection at the implant site has been uncommon (0.7%). Attention to aseptic technique and proper insertion and removal of the capsules reduces the possibility of infection. If infection occurs, institute suitable treatment. If infection persists, remove the capsules.

Expulsion of capsules is uncommon. It occurs more frequently when placement of the capsules is extremely shallow, too close to the incision, or when infection is present. Replacement of an expelled capsule must be accomplished using a new sterile capsule. If infection is present, treat and cure before replacement. Contraceptive efficacy may be inadequate with $<$ 6 capsules.

Provisions for removal: Advise women that the capsules will be removed at any time for any reason. The removal should be done on such request or at the end of 5 years of usage by personnel instructed in the removal technique.

Drug Interactions:

Carbamazepine and **phenytoin:** Reduced efficacy (pregnancy) has occurred. Warn users of the possibility of decreased efficacy with use of any related drugs.

Drug/Lab test interactions: Certain endocrine tests may be affected by levonorgestrel implants: Sex hormone binding globulin concentrations are decreased; thyroxine concentrations may be slightly decreased and triiodothyronine uptake increased.

(Continued on following page)

LEVONORGESTREL IMPLANTS (Cont.)

Adverse Reactions:

Gross annual discontinuation and continuation rates of levonorgestrel implant users are summarized in the following table:

Annual and 5 Year Cumulative Discontinuation/Continuation Rates Per 100 Levonorgestrel Implant Users

Parameter	Year 1	2	3	4	5	Cumulative
Pregnancy	0.2	0.5	1.2	1.6	0.4	3.9
Bleeding irregularities	9.1	7.9	4.9	3.3	2.9	25.1
Medical (excluding bleeding irregularities)	6	5.6	4.1	4	5.1	22.4
Personal	4.6	7.7	11.7	10.7	11.7	38.7
Continuation	81	77.4	79.2	76.7	77.6	29.5

Levonorgestrel Implant Adverse Reactions During First Year of Use

Adverse Reaction	Incidence (%)
Many bleeding days or prolonged bleeding	27.6
Spotting	17.1
Amenorrhea	9.4
Irregular (onsets of) bleeding	7.6
Frequent bleeding onsets	7
Removal difficulties affecting subjects (based on 849 removals)	6.2
Scanty bleeding	5.2
Breast discharge	≥ 5
Cervicitis	≥ 5
Musculoskeletal pain	≥ 5
Abdominal discomfort	≥ 5
Leukorrhea	≥ 5
Vaginitis	≥ 5
Pain or itching near implant site (usually transient)	3.7
Infection at implant site	0.7

Other: Headache; nervousness; nausea; dizziness; adnexal enlargement; dermatitis; acne; change of appetite; mastalgia; weight gain; hirsutism; hypertrichosis; scalp hair loss.

Overdosage:

Overdosage can result if > 6 capsules are in situ. Remove all implanted capsules before inserting a new set. Overdosage may cause fluid retention with its associated effects and uterine bleeding irregularities.

Patient Information:

Provide the patient with a copy of the patient labeling to help describe the characteristics of the system. Advise the patient that the prescribing information is available to them at their request. It is recommended that prospective users be fully informed about the risks and benefits associated with the use of the system, with other forms of contraception, and with no contraception at all. It is also recommended that prospective users be fully informed about the insertion and removal procedures. Health care providers may wish to obtain informed consent from all patients in light of the techniques involved with insertion and removal.

Administration and Dosage:

Levonorgestrel implants consist of six *Silastic* capsules; each capsule is 2.4 mm in diameter and 34 mm in length and each contains 36 mg levonorgestrel. The total administered (implanted) dose is 216 mg. Perform implantation of all six capsules during the first 7 days of the onset of menses. Insertion is subdermal in the mid-portion of the upper arm about 8 to 10 cm above the elbow crease. Distribute capsules in a fan-like pattern, about 15° apart, for a total of 75°. Proper insertion will facilitate later removal. (See section on Insertion/Removal under Precautions and in the package literature included with the product.)

Rx	**Norplant System** (Wyeth-Ayerst)	**Kit:** Set of 6 capsules each containing 36 mg levonorgestrel	Also includes trocar, scalpel, forceps, syringe, 2 syringe needles, pkg of skin closures, 3 pkgs of gauze sponges, stretch bandages and surgical drapes.

Actions:

The *Progestasert* system, a T-shaped unit that contains a reservoir of 38 mg progesterone, is indicated for intrauterine contraception. The mechanism of action has not been demonstrated. Hypotheses include progesterone-induced inhibition of sperm capacitation or survival and alteration of the uterine milieu to prevent nidation. During use of the system, the endometrium shows progestational influence. Progesterone from the system suppresses proliferation of the endometrial tissue (an antiestrogenic effect). Following removal of the system, the endometrium rapidly returns to its normal cyclic pattern and can support pregnancy.

Contraceptive effectiveness is enhanced by continuous release of progesterone into the uterine cavity at an average rate of 65 mcg/day for 1 year. The mechanism is local, not systemic. The concentrations of luteinizing hormone, estradiol and progesterone in systemic venous plasma follow regular cyclic patterns, indicative of ovulation during use of the system. For pregnancy rates for various means of contraception, refer to the Oral Contraceptives group monograph.

Indications:

Intrauterine contraception in women who have had at least one child, are in a stable, mutually monogamous relationship, and have no history of pelvic inflammatory disease (PID).

Unlabeled use: This system has been used in the treatment of menorrhagia.

Contraindications:

Pregnancy or suspected pregnancy; previous ectopic pregnancy; presence or history of PID; patient or partner has multiple sexual partners; sexually transmitted disease; postpartum endometritis or infected abortion; pelvic surgery; abnormalities which result in uterine distortion or uteri that measure < 6 cm or > 10 cm by sounding; uterine or cervical malignancy, including an unresolved abnormal Pap smear; genital bleeding of unknown etiology; vaginitis or cervicitis unless infection has been completely controlled and is non-gonococcal and non-chlamydial; incomplete involution of the uterus following abortion or childbirth; previously inserted intrauterine device (IUD) still in place; genital actinomycosis; conditions or treatments associated with increased susceptibility to infections with microorganisms (eg, leukemia, diabetes, AIDS); IV drug abuse.

Warnings:

Pregnancy: Long-term effects on the fetus are unknown.

Septic abortion may be increased, associated in some instances with septicemia, septic shock and death in patients becoming pregnant with an IUD in place, usually in the second trimester. If pregnancy occurs with a system in situ, remove it if the thread is visible or, if removal is difficult, consider termination of the pregnancy.

Continuation of pregnancy: If pregnancy is maintained and the system remains in situ, warn the patient of the increased risk of spontaneous abortion and sepsis, including death, and premature labor and delivery. Advise her to report immediately all abnormal symptoms, such as flu-like syndrome, fever, chills, abdominal cramping and pain, bleeding or vaginal discharge; generalized symptoms of septicemia may be insidious.

Congenital anomalies: Systemically administered sex steroids, including progestational agents, have been associated with an increased risk of congenital anomalies. It is not known whether there is an increased risk of such anomalies when pregnancy is continued with this system in place.

Ectopic pregnancy: The *Progestasert* system acts in the uterus to prevent uterine pregnancy, but it does not prevent either ovulation or ectopic pregnancy. Therefore, a pregnancy that occurs while a patient is using an IUD is much more likely to be ectopic. Determine whether ectopic pregnancy has occurred in patients with delayed menses or unilateral pelvic pain.

In clinical trials of the progesterone system, 1 of 3.6 pregnancies in parous women and 1 of 6.2 pregnancies in nulliparous women were ectopic. The per-year risk of ectopic pregnancy in progesterone system users is ≈ 1 ectopic pregnancy in 200 users per year. This risk is approximately the same as in noncontracepting, sexually active women.

In two clinical studies, for the first year the risk of ectopic pregnancy was approximately 6 times higher among women using progesterone systems than among women using copper systems. Over 2 years, the risk of an ectopic pregnancy with the progesterone-releasing IUD was about 10 times higher than that with copper-releasing IUDs.

Women who have previously had acute PID subsequently have an eightfold to tenfold greater than normal risk of ectopic pregnancy (see Pelvic Infection). Multiple sexual partners or a partner with multiple sexual partners, previous pelvic surgery, endometritis, endometriosis and retrograde menstruation have also been recognized as risk factors for ectopic pregnancy.

(Warnings continued on following page)

Warnings (Cont.):

Pelvic infection: An increased risk of PID associated with IUD use has been reported; the highest rate occurs shortly after insertion and up to 4 months thereafter. Teach patients to recognize the symptoms of PID and ectopic pregnancy. Pelvic infection may occur with an IUD in situ, and may result in tubo-ovarian abscesses or general peritonitis. If this occurs, remove the IUD and institute appropriate antibiotic treatment. PID can result in tubal damage and occlusion, threatening future fertility or predisposing to ectopic pregnancy. PID may be asymptomatic but still result in tubal damage and its sequelae.

Following diagnosis of PID, initiate antibiotic therapy promptly and remove the progesterone IUD. Guidelines for treatment are available from the CDC.

Genital actinomycosis has been associated primarily with long-term IUD use.

Embedment: Partial penetration or lodging of an IUD in the endometrium can result in difficult removal. In some cases, this can result in IUD fragmentation, necessitating surgical removal.

Perforation, partial or total, of the uterine wall or cervix may occur. If perforation occurs, remove the device. Adhesions, foreign body reactions, peritonitis, cystic masses in the pelvis, intestinal penetrations, local inflammatory reaction with abscess formation and erosion of adjacent viscera and intestinal obstruction may result if the IUD is left in the peritoneal cavity.

Mortality risks: Refer to the Oral Contraceptives group monograph for risk of death associated with various methods of contraception.

Precautions:

Prior to insertion, complete a medical and social history, and determine risk of ectopic pregnancy because of previous PID. Perform pelvic examination, Pap smear, gonorrhea and chlamydia culture and, if indicated, tests for other sexually transmitted diseases. Carefully sound the uterus prior to insertion to determine the degree of patency of the endocervical canal and the internal os, and the direction and depth of the uterine cavity. Occasionally, severe cervical stenosis may be encountered. The uterus should sound to a depth of 6 to 10 cm. Inserting the system into a uterine cavity measuring < 6.5 cm may increase the incidence of expulsion, bleeding and pain.

To reduce the possibility of insertion in the presence of an undetermined pregnancy, insert during or shortly following menstruation.

Cervicitis or vaginitis: Postpone use in these patients until infection has cleared and until the cervicitis has been shown not to be due to gonorrhea or chlamydia.

Involution of uterus: Do not insert postpartum or postabortion until involution of the uterus is completed. Incidence of perforation (see Warnings) and expulsion is greater if involution is not completed. Involution may be delayed in nursing mothers.

Anemia: Use cautiously in those who have anemia or history of menorrhagia or hypermenorrhea. Patients experiencing menorrhagia or metrorrhagia following IUD insertion may be at risk of developing hypochromic microcytic anemia.

Syncope, bradycardia or other neurovascular episodes may occur during insertion or removal, especially in patients previously disposed to these conditions or cervical stenosis.

Valvular or congenital heart disease patients are more prone to develop subacute bacterial endocarditis. The use of the IUD may represent a potential source of septic emboli.

Reexamine patient shortly after the first postinsertion menses, since an IUD may be expelled or displaced, but definitely within 3 months after insertion. Thereafter, perform an annual examination.

Replace the device every 12 months, since the level of contraceptive efficacy after this time decreases.

Remove the device for the following reasons: Menorrhagia/metrorrhagia-producing anemia; pelvic infection; endometritis; genital actinomycosis; intractable pelvic pain; dyspareunia; pregnancy; endometrial or cervical malignancy; uterine or cervical perforation; increase of length of the threads extending from the cervix or any other indication of partial expulsion. If retrieval threads are not visible, they may have retracted into the uterus or have been broken; therefore, consider the system displaced and remove. After menstrual period, determine that the threads still protrude from the cervix. Caution patients not to pull on the threads. If partial expulsion occurs, removal is indicated and a new system may be inserted.

Bleeding and cramps may occur during the first few weeks after insertion; if symptoms continue or are severe, consult physician.

Prophylactic antibiotics may be considered prior to IUD insertion to decrease the risk of PID; however, the utility of this treatment is still under evaluation. Regimens include doxycycline 200 mg orally 1 hour before insertion or erythromycin 500 mg orally 1 hour before and 6 hours after insertion.

(Continued on following page)

Drug Interactions:

Anticoagulants: Use IUDs with caution in patients receiving anticoagulants or having a coagulopathy.

Adverse Reactions:

Endometritis; spontaneous abortion; septic abortion; septicemia; perforation of uterus and cervix; pelvic infection; cervical erosion; vaginitis; leukorrhea; pregnancy; ectopic pregnancy; uterine embedment; difficult removal; complete or partial expulsion; intermenstrual spotting; prolongation of menstrual flow; anemia; amenorrhea or delayed menses; pain and cramping; dysmenorrhea; backaches; dyspareunia; neurovascular episodes including bradycardia and syncope secondary to insertion; fragmentation of IUD; tubo-ovarian abscess; tubal damage; fetal damage and congenital anomalies. Perforation into the abdomen followed by peritonitis, abdominal adhesions, intestinal penetration, intestinal obstruction, local inflammatory reaction, abscess formation and erosion of adjacent viscera, and cystic masses in the pelvis have occurred. Some of these adverse reactions can lead to loss of fertility, partial or total removal of reproductive organs, hormonal imbalance or death.

Patient Information:

Patient package insert and patient instructions available with product. The patient must read and initial each section of the Patient Information Leaflet, and the Informed Choice Statement must be signed by the patient and by the physician.

Notify physician if any of the following occurs: Abnormal or excessive bleeding; severe cramping; abnormal or odorous vaginal discharge; fever or flu-like syndrome; pain; genital lesions or sores; missed period.

Administration and Dosage:

Insert a single system into the uterine cavity. Contraceptive effectiveness is retained for 1 year, and the system must be replaced 1 year after insertion. See manufacturer's literature for insertion and removal instructions.

Rx	**Progestasert** (Alza)	**Intrauterine System:** T-shaped unit containing a reservoir of 38 mg progesterone with barium sulfate dispersed in medical grade silicone fluid.	In 6s w/inserters.

Warnings (Cont.):

Edema, with or without congestive heart failure, may be a serious complication in patients with preexisting cardiac, renal or hepatic disease. Use with caution in epilepsy, migraine or other conditions that may be aggravated by fluid retention. In addition to discontinuation of the drug, diuretic therapy may be required. If the administration of testosterone enanthate is restarted, use a lower dose.

Gynecomastia frequently develops and occasionally persists in patients being treated for hypogonadism. Use with caution in patients with preexisting gynecomastia.

Bone maturation: Use androgens cautiously in healthy males with delayed puberty. Monitor bone maturation by assessing bone age of the wrist and hand every 6 months.

Carcinogenesis: Testosterone has induced cervical-uterine tumors in mice; these tumors metastasized in some cases. Injection of testosterone into some strains of female mice may increase their susceptibility to hepatoma. There are rare reports of hepatocellular carcinoma in patients receiving long-term therapy with androgens in high doses. Withdrawal of the drugs did not lead to regression of the tumors in all cases.

Elderly males treated with androgens may be at an increased risk of developing prostatic hypertrophy and prostatic carcinoma. Marked increase in libido may occur.

Pregnancy: Category X. Androgens are contraindicated in women who are or who may become pregnant. They cause virilization of the external genitalia of the female fetus (eg, clitoromegaly, abnormal vaginal development and fusion of genital folds to form a scrotal-like structure). The degree of masculinization is related to the amount of drug given and the age of the fetus. Masculinization is most likely to occur in the female fetus when androgens are given in the first trimester. If the patient becomes pregnant while taking these drugs, apprise her of the potential hazards to the fetus.

Lactation: It is not known whether androgens are excreted in breast milk. Decide whether to discontinue nursing or to discontinue the drug, taking into account the importance of the drug to the mother.

Children: Use androgens very cautiously in children; the drugs should only be given by specialists who are aware of the adverse effects on bone maturation.

Androgens may accelerate bone maturation without producing compensatory gain in linear growth. This adverse effect may result in compromised adult stature. The younger the child, the greater the risk of compromising final mature height.

Benzyl alcohol-containing products have been associated with a fatal "gasping syndrome" in premature infants. Refer to product listings.

Precautions:

Virilization: Observe women for signs of virilization (deepening voice, hirsutism, acne, clitoromegaly and menstrual irregularities). Discontinue therapy at the time of evidence of mild virilism to prevent irreversible virilization. Virilization is usual following high-dose androgens and is not prevented by concomitant use of estrogens. Some virilization should be tolerated during treatment for breast carcinoma.

Patients with benign prostatic hypertrophy may develop acute urethral obstruction. Priapism or excessive sexual stimulation may develop. Oligospermia may occur after prolonged administration or excessive dosage. If any of these effects appear, stop administration. If restarted, use a lower dosage. Avoid stimulation to the point of increasing nervous, mental and physical activities beyond the patient's cardiovascular capacity.

Monitoring: Frequently determine urine and serum calcium levels during the course of therapy in women with disseminated breast carcinoma.

Because of the hepatotoxicity associated with the use of methyltestosterone and fluoxymesterone, periodically perform liver function tests.

Make periodic (every 6 months) x-ray examinations of bone age during treatment of prepubertal males to determine the rate of bone maturation and the effects of the androgen therapy on the epiphyseal centers.

Check hemoglobin and hematocrit periodically for polycythemia in patients who are receiving high doses of androgens.

Acute intermittent porphyria: Androgens have precipitated attacks of acute intermittent porphyria; use cautiously in patients known to have this condition.

Hypercholesterolemia: Serum cholesterol may be altered during therapy; thus, use with caution in patients with a history of myocardial infarction or coronary artery disease. Perform serial determinations of serum cholesterol and adjust therapy accordingly.

Tartrazine sensitivity: Some of these products contain tartrazine, which may cause allergic-type reactions (including bronchial asthma) in susceptible individuals. Although the incidence of tartrazine sensitivity in the general population is low, it is frequently seen in patients who also have aspirin hypersensitivity. Specific products containing tartrazine are identified in the product listings.

(Continued on following page)

Drug Interactions:

Anticoagulants: The anticoagulant effect may be potentiated by 17-alkyl testosterone derivatives (eg, fluoxymesterone, methyltestosterone). Although the non-17-alkylated agent (testosterone) appears safer, at least one case report described a similar interaction. Avoid the combination with 17-alkyl derivatives if possible.

Imipramine: Coadministration with methyltestosterone resulted in a dramatic paranoid response in four of five patients.

Drug/Lab test interactions: Thyroid function tests – Decreased levels of thyroxine-binding globulin, resulting in decreased total T_4 serum levels and increased resin uptake of T_3 and T_4. Free thyroid hormone levels remain unchanged, and there is no clinical evidence of thyroid dysfunction.

Adverse Reactions:

Female: Most common – Amenorrhea and other menstrual irregularities; inhibition of gonadotropin secretion and virilization, including deepening voice and clitoral enlargement. The latter usually is not reversible after androgens are discontinued. When administered to a pregnant woman, androgens cause virilization of external genitalia of the female fetus.

Male: Gynecomastia; excessive frequency and duration of penile erections; decreased ejaculatory volume. Oligospermia may occur at high dosages.

Skin and appendages: Hirsutism; male pattern baldness; acne; seborrhea.

Fluid and electrolyte disturbances: Retention of sodium, chloride, water, potassium, calcium and inorganic phosphates. Hypercalcemia may occur, particularly in immobile patients and in those patients with metastatic breast carcinoma.

GI: Nausea; cholestatic jaundice; alterations in liver function tests; rarely, hepatocellular neoplasms, peliosis hepatis.

Hematologic: Suppression of clotting factors II, V, VII and X; polycythemia.

CNS: Increased or decreased libido; headache; anxiety; depression; generalized paresthesia; sleep apnea syndrome.

Hypersensitivity: Skin manifestations; rarely, anaphylactoid reactions; rash.

Miscellaneous: Inflammation and pain at the site of IM injection; stomatitis with buccal preparations; increased serum cholesterol.

Patient Information:

Oral tablets: May cause GI upset.

Buccal tablets: Do not swallow; allow to dissolve between the gum and cheek; avoid eating, drinking or smoking while tablet is in place.

Notify physician if nausea, vomiting, swelling of the extremities (edema), priapism or jaundice occurs.

Females: Notify physician if hoarseness, deepening of the voice, male-pattern baldness, hirsutism, acne or menstrual irregularities occur.

(Products listed on following pages)

Complete prescribing information for these products begins on page 389.

Short-Acting

TESTOSTERONE AND TESTOSTERONE PROPIONATE

Administration and Dosage:

For IM use only. Administer deep in the gluteal muscle. Do not inject IV. Shake well.

The suggested dosage for androgens varies depending on age, sex and diagnosis of the patient. Adjust dosage according to response and appearance of adverse reactions.

Androgen replacement therapy: The guideline dose is 25 to 50 mg 2 to 3 times weekly.

Delayed puberty: Dosages are generally in the lower ranges and for a limited duration (eg, 4 to 6 months). Various regimens have been used to induce pubertal changes in hypogonadal males. Some experts advocate lower initial doses, gradually increasing the dose as puberty progresses, with or without a decrease to maintenance levels. Other experts emphasize that higher dosages are needed to induce pubertal changes and lower dosages can be used for maintenance after puberty. Consider the chronological and skeletal ages when determining initial dose and adjusting dose.

Other suggested doses are as follows (injection in oil):

Growth stimulation in Turner syndrome or constitutional delay of puberty – 40 to 50 mg/m²/dose monthly for 6 months.

Male hypogonadism – Initiation of pubertal growth, 40 to 50 mg/m²/dose monthly until the growth rate falls to prepubertal levels (approximately 5 cm/year); during terminal growth phase, 100 mg/m²/dose monthly until growth ceases; maintenance virilizing dose, 100 mg/m²/dose twice monthly or 50 to 400 mg/dose every 2 to 4 weeks.

Palliation of mammary cancer: Usual dose is 50 to 100 mg, 3 times a week. Follow women with metastatic breast carcinoma closely because androgen therapy occasionally appears to accelerate the disease. Thus, many experts prefer to use the shorter-acting androgen preparations rather than those with prolonged activity for treating breast carcinoma, particularly during the early stages of androgen therapy.

Postpartum breast engorgement (testosterone propionate): 25 to 50 mg for 3 to 4 days, starting at the time of delivery.

	TESTOSTERONE (IN AQUEOUS SUSPENSION)			C.I.*
c-III	**Testosterone Aqueous** (Various)	**Injection:** 25 mg per ml	In 10 ml vials.	18+
c-III	**Testosterone Aqueous** (Various)	**Injection:** 50 mg per ml	In 10 and 30 ml vials.	13+
c-III	**Histerone 50** (Hauck)		In 10 ml vials.	7.3
c-III	**Testosterone Aqueous** (Various, eg, Goldline, Major)	**Injection:** 100 mg per ml	In 10 and 30 ml vials.	6.1+
c-III	**Andro 100** (Forest)		In 10 ml vials.[1]	7.4
c-III	**Histerone 100** (Hauck)		In 10 ml vials.[1]	7.4
c-III	**Tesamone** (Dunhall)		In 10 ml vials.[1]	NA
	TESTOSTERONE PROPIONATE (IN OIL)			
c-III	**Testosterone Propionate** (Various, eg, Geneva, Major, Schein)	**Injection:** 100 mg per ml	In 10 and 30 ml vials.	5.4+
c-III	**Testex** (Pasadena)		In 10 ml vials.[2]	5.9

* Cost Index based on cost per 25 mg.

[1] With sodium carboxymethylcellulose, methylcellulose, povidone, DSS and thimerosal.

[2] In sesame oil with benzyl alcohol.

Complete prescribing information for these products begins on page 389.

Long-Acting

The enanthate and cypionate esters provide therapeutic effects for about 4 weeks.

Administration and Dosage: For IM use only. Individualize dosage. In general, more than 400 mg/month is not required because of the prolonged action of the preparation.

Male hypogonadism: Replacement therapy (eunuchism) – 50 to 400 mg every 2 to 4 weeks.

Males with delayed puberty: 50 to 200 mg every 2 to 4 weeks for a limited duration.

Palliation of inoperable breast cancer in women: 200 to 400 mg every 2 to 4 weeks. Androgen therapy occasionally appears to accelerate metastatic breast carcinoma.

NOTE: Use of a wet needle or wet syringe may cause the solution to become cloudy; however, this does not affect the potency of the material.

Storage: Warming and shaking vial redissolves crystals that may have formed.

	TESTOSTERONE ENANTHATE (IN OIL)			C.I.*
c-III	**Testosterone Enanthate** (Various, eg, Schein)	**Injection:** 100 mg per ml	In 10 ml vials.	4+
c-III	**Delatest** (Dunhall)		In 10 ml vials.[1]	NA
c-III	**Everone 100** (Hyrex)		In 10 ml vials.[1]	7.1
c-III	**Testone LA 100** (Ortega)		In 10 ml vials.[1]	NA
c-III	**Testosterone Enanthate** (Various, eg, Geneva, Schein)	**Injection:** 200 mg per ml	In 10 ml vials.	3.8+
c-III	**Andro L.A. 200** (Forest)		In 10 ml vials.[1]	6
c-III	**Andropository-200** (Rugby)		In 10 ml vials.	7.5
c-III	**Delatestryl** (Mead Johnson Labs)		In 5 ml vials and 1 ml single dose syringes.[1]	32
c-III	**Durathate-200** (Hauck)		In 10 ml vials.[1]	4.9
c-III	**Everone 200** (Hyrex)		In 10 ml vials.[1]	5.3
c-III	**Testone LA 200** (Ortega)		In 10 ml vials.[1]	NA
c-III	**Testrin PA** (Pasadena)		In 10 ml vials.[1]	5.2

	TESTOSTERONE CYPIONATE (IN OIL)			
c-III	**Testosterone Cypionate** (Various, eg, Geneva, Goldline, Schein)	**Injection:** 100 mg per ml	In 10 ml vials.	5+
c-III	**Andro-Cyp 100** (Keene)		In 10 ml vials.[2]	5.1
c-III	**Andronate 100** (Pasadena)		In 10 ml vials.[2]	5.5
c-III	**depAndro 100** (Forest)		In 10 ml vials.[2]	7.4
c-III	**Depotest 100** (Hyrex)		In 10 ml vials.[2]	7
c-III	**Depo-Testosterone** (Upjohn)		In 10 ml vials.[3]	25
c-III	**Duratest-100** (Hauck)		In 10 ml vials.[2]	5.8
c-III	**Testosterone Cypionate** (Various, eg, Geneva, Goldline, Schein)	**Injection:** 200 mg per ml	In 10 ml vials.	3.9+
c-III	**Andro-Cyp 200** (Keene)		In 10 ml vials.[3]	4.3
c-III	**Andronate 200** (Pasadena)		In 10 ml vials.[3]	5.2
c-III	**depAndro 200** (Forest)		In 10 ml vials.[3]	6
c-III	**Depotest 200** (Hyrex)		In 10 ml vials.[3]	5
c-III	**Depo-Testosterone** (Upjohn)		In 1 and 10 ml vials.[3]	23
c-III	**Duratest-200** (Hauck)		In 10 ml vials.[3]	4.9
c-III	**Testred Cypionate** (ICN Pharm)		In 10 ml vials.	9.4

* Cost Index based on cost per 25 mg.
[1] In sesame oil with chlorobutanol.
[2] In cottonseed oil with benzyl alcohol.
[3] In cottonseed oil with benzyl benzoate and benzyl alcohol.

Complete prescribing information for these products begins on page 389.

METHYLTESTOSTERONE

Absorption through buccal mucosa into systemic circulation provides twice the androgenic activity of oral tablets.

Administration and Dosage:

Males: Hypogonadism, male climacteric and impotence – 10 to 40 mg/day orally.
Androgen deficiency – 10 to 50 mg/day orally (5 to 25 mg buccal).
Postpubertal cryptorchidism – 30 mg/day orally.

Females: Postpartum breast pain and engorgement – 80 mg/day orally for 3 to 5 days.
Breast cancer – 50 to 200 mg/day orally (25 to 100 mg buccal).

	Product	Form	Description	C.I.*
c-III	**Methyltestosterone** (Various, eg, Goldline, Major, Schein)	**Tablets:** 10 mg	In 100s and 1000s.	1.4+
c-III	**Android-10** (ICN Pharm)		(BP 958). Green. In 100s.	12
c-III	**Oreton Methyl** (Schering)		Lactose. (Schering 311). White. In 100s.	17
c-III	**Methyltestosterone** (Various, eg, Goldline, Major, Rugby, Schein)	**Tablets:** 25 mg	In 100s and 1000s.	1+
c-III	**Android-25** (ICN Pharm)		(BP 996). Yellow. In 100s.	13
c-III	**Methyltestosterone** (Various, eg, Major)	**Tablets (Buccal):** 10 mg	In 100s and 1000s.	2.6+
c-III	**Oreton Methyl** (Schering)		(Schering 970). Lavender. Oval. In 100s.	8.4
c-III	**Testred** (ICN Pharm)	**Capsules:** 10 mg	(ICN 0901). Red. In 100s.	15
c-III	**Virilon** (Star)		(Virilon 10 mg). Black and clear. In 100s & 1000s.	11

FLUOXYMESTERONE

Administration and Dosage:

Males: Hypogonadism – 5 to 20 mg daily.

Females: Inoperable breast carcinoma – 10 to 40 mg daily in divided doses. Continue for 1 month for a subjective response and 2 to 3 months for an objective response.
Prevention of postpartum breast pain and engorgement – 2.5 mg shortly after delivery. Then administer 5 to 10 mg daily in divided doses for 4 to 5 days.

	Product	Form	Description	C.I.*
c-III	**Halotestin** (Upjohn)	**Tablets:** 2 mg	Tartrazine, lactose, sucrose. (Halotestin 2). Peach, scored. In 100s.	11
c-III	**Halotestin** (Upjohn)	**Tablets:** 5 mg	Tartrazine, lactose, sucrose. (Upjohn 19). Lt. green, scored. In 100s.	11
c-III	**Fluoxymesterone** (Various, eg, Geneva, Major, Parmed, Rugby, Schein)	**Tablets:** 10 mg	In 100s.	2.5+
c-III	**Halotestin** (Upjohn)		Tartrazine, lactose, sucrose. (Halotestin 10). Green, scored. In 30s & 100s.	8.1

* Cost Index based on cost per 10 mg methyltestosterone oral, 5 mg methyltestosterone buccal or 2 mg fluoxymesterone.

FINASTERIDE

Actions:

Pharmacology: Finasteride, a synthetic 4-azasteroid compound, is a competitive and specific inhibitor of steroid 5α-reductase, an intracellular enzyme that converts testosterone into the potent androgen 5α-dihydrotestosterone (DHT). It has no affinity for the androgen receptor. The 5α-reduced steroid metabolites in blood and urine are decreased after administration of finasteride.

Progressive enlargement of the prostate gland is often associated with urinary symptoms and a decrease in urine flow, although a precise correlation between increased gland size and symptoms has not been demonstrated. Benign prostatic hyperplasia (BPH) produces symptoms in the majority of men > 50 years of age and its prevalence increases with age.

The development of the prostate gland is dependent on the potent androgen DHT. The enzyme 5α-reductase metabolizes testosterone to DHT in the prostate gland, liver and skin. DHT induces androgenic effects by binding to androgen receptors in the cell nuclei of these organs.

A single 5 mg oral dose produces a rapid reduction in serum DHT concentration, with maximum effect observed 8 hours after the first dose. The suppression of DHT is maintained throughout the 24 hour dosing interval and with continued treatment. Daily dosing at 5 mg/day for up to 24 months reduces the serum DHT concentration by approximately 70%. The median circulating level of testosterone increases by 10% but remains within the physiologic range.

Adult males with genetically inherited 5α-reductase deficiency also have decreased levels of DHT. Except for the associated urogenital defects present at birth, no other clinical abnormalities related to 5α-reductase deficiency have been observed in these individuals. These individuals have a small prostate gland throughout life and do not develop BPH.

In patients with BPH treated with finasteride (1 to 100 mg/day) for 7 to 10 days prior to prostatectomy, an approximate 80% lower DHT content was measured in prostatic tissue removed at surgery compared to placebo; testosterone tissue concentration was increased up to 10 times over pretreatment levels. Intraprostatic content of prostate-specific antigen (PSA) was also decreased. In healthy male volunteers treated with finasteride for 14 days, discontinuation of therapy resulted in a return of DHT levels to pretreatment levels in approximately 2 weeks.

In patients with BPH, finasteride had no effect on circulating levels of cortisol, estradiol, prolactin, thyroid-stimulating hormone or thyroxine, nor did it affect the plasma lipid profile. Increases of about 10% were observed in luteinizing hormone (LH), follicle-stimulating hormone (FSH) and testosterone levels in patients receiving finasteride, but levels remained within the normal range. In healthy volunteers the hypothalamic-pituitary-testicular axis was not affected.

Pharmacokinetics: Following an oral dose, a mean of 39% was excreted in the urine in the form of metabolites; 57% was excreted in the feces. The major compound isolated from urine was the monocarboxylic acid metabolite; virtually no unchanged drug was recovered. The t-butyl side chain monohydroxylated metabolite has been isolated from plasma. These metabolites possess no more than 20% of the 5α-reductase inhibitory activity of finasteride.

In a study in 15 healthy male subjects, the mean bioavailability of a 5 mg tablet was 63%. Maximum finasteride plasma concentration averaged 37 ng/ml and was reached 1 to 2 hours postdose. The mean plasma elimination half-life was 6 hours (range, 3 to 16 hours). Following an IV infusion, mean plasma clearance was 165 ml/min and mean steady-state volume of distribution was 76 L. The bioavailability of finasteride was not affected by food. Approximately 90% is bound to plasma proteins. Finasteride crosses the blood-brain barrier.

There is a slow accumulation phase after multiple dosing. After dosing with 5 mg/day for 17 days, plasma concentrations were 47% and 54% higher than after the first dose in men 45 to 60 years old (n = 12) and ≥ 70 years old (n = 12), respectively; mean trough concentrations were 6.2 and 8.1 ng/ml, respectively. Although steady state was not reached in this study, mean trough plasma concentration in another study in patients with BPH (mean age, 65 years) receiving 5 mg/day was 9.4 ng/ml after > 1 year of dosing.

(Actions continued on following page)

FINASTERIDE (Cont.)

Actions (Cont.):

Pharmacokinetics (Cont.):

The elimination rate of finasteride is decreased in the elderly, but no dosage adjustment is necessary. The mean terminal half-life in subjects ≥ 70 years of age was approximately 8 hours (range, 6 to 15 hours) compared to 6 hours (range, 4 to 12 hours) in subjects 45 to 60 years of age. As a result, mean AUC (0 to 24 hr) after 17 days of dosing was 15% higher in subjects ≥ 70 years of age.

No dosage adjustment is necessary in patients with renal insufficiency. Urinary excretion of metabolites was decreased in patients with renal impairment. This decrease was associated with an increase in fecal excretion of metabolites. Plasma concentrations of metabolites were significantly higher in patients with renal impairment. However, finasteride has been well tolerated in BPH patients with normal renal function receiving up to 80 mg/day for 12 weeks where exposure of these patients to metabolites would presumably be much greater.

In 16 subjects receiving 5 mg/day, concentrations in semen ranged from undetectable (< 1 ng/ml) to 21 ng/ml. Based on a 5 ml ejaculate volume, the amount of finasteride in ejaculate was estimated to be < 1/50 of the dose of finasteride (5 mcg) that had no effect on circulating DHT levels in adults.

Clinical trials: In two double-blind, placebo controlled, 12 month studies in patients with BPH treated with 5 mg/day, statistically significant regression of the enlarged prostate gland was noted at the first evaluation at 3 months and was maintained during the studies. In both studies, the maximum urinary flow rates showed statistically significant increases from baseline in patients treated from week 2 throughout the 12 month studies.

Median % Change in Prostate Volume from Baseline Following Finasteride (5 mg/day)

Evaluation period	North American study		International study	
	Finasteride (n = 297)	Placebo (n = 300)	Finasteride (n = 246)	Placebo (n = 255)
Month 3	- 12.1%	- 2.4%	- 19.1%	- 6%
Month 6	- 17.4%	- 2.8%	- 21.9%	- 5.5%
Month 12	- 19.2%	- 3%	- 24%	- 6.1%

Mean Increase in Maximum Urinary Flow Rate (ml/sec) from Baseline Following Finasteride (5 mg/day)

Evaluation period	North American study		International study	
	Finasteride (n = 297)	Placebo (n = 300)	Finasteride (n = 246)	Placebo (n = 255)
Week 2	0.5	- 0.2	0.6	0.2
Month 1	0.5	0.2	0.7	0.3
Month 2	0.9	0.3	1.1	0.6
Month 3	0.8	0.3	0.8	0.2
Month 4	1	0.4	1	0.6
Month 5	1	0.2	0.9	0.8
Month 6	0.8	0.1	1.1	0.7
Month 7	1.2	0.4	1.3	0.4
Month 8	1.4	0.3	1.3	0.5
Month 9	1.3	0.3	1.2	0.4
Month 10	1.5	0.5	1.3	0.7
Month 11	1.4	0.3	1.5	0.4
Month 12	1.6	0.2	1.3	0.4

(Actions continued on following page)

FINASTERIDE (Cont.)

Actions (Cont.):

Clinical trials (Cont.):

Symptomatic improvement was also evaluated in these multicenter studies. The obstructive symptoms evaluated were hesitancy, feeling of incomplete bladder emptying, interruption of urinary stream, impairment of size and force of urinary stream and terminal urinary dribbling. The total symptom score also included straining to start urinary flow, dysuria, frequency of clothes wetting and urgency to urinate. On a scale of 0 (absence of all symptoms) to 36 (worst response for all symptoms), the mean baseline total symptom scores for the two studies were 10.1 and 10.6. From week 2 the scores of the patients treated with finasteride were numerically lower than those of placebo and remained so throughout the 12 month study.

In both of these 12 month studies, patients treated with finasteride 5 mg had progressively decreasing prostate volumes, increasing maximum urinary flow rates and improvement of symptoms associated with BPH, suggesting an arrest in the disease process.

In long-term uncontrolled extensions of these studies in approximately 300 patients receiving finasteride 5 mg/day for 24 months, prostate volume was reduced by a median of 25.5%, maximum flow rate increased by a mean of 2.2 ml/sec and the total symptom score improved by a mean of 3.4 points. In addition, regression of the enlarged prostate gland and a decrease in PSA levels were maintained in approximately 50 patients who were treated for 36 months.

Indications:

Treatment of symptomatic benign prostatic hyperplasia (BPH).

Although there is a rapid regression of the enlarged prostate gland in most treated patients, < 50% of patients experience an increase in urinary flow and improvement in symtoms of BPH when treated for 12 months.

Unlabeled use: Finasteride is being investigated as adjuvant monotherapy following radical prostatectomy. Other potential uses include prevention of the progression of first-stage prostate cancer, treatment of male pattern baldness, acne and hirsutism; however, studies are needed to assess these uses.

Contraindications:

Hypersensitivity to finasteride or any component of this product; pregnancy, lactation, children (see Warnings).

Warnings:

Duration of therapy: A minimum of 6 months of treatment may be necessary to determine whether an individual will respond to finasteride. It is not possible to identify prospectively those patients who will respond.

Patient evaluation: Prior to initiating therapy, perform appropriate evaluation to identify other conditions that might mimic BPH, such as infection, prostate cancer, stricture disease, hypotonic bladder or other neurogenic disorders.

Hepatic function impairment: Use caution in those patients with liver function abnormalities since finasteride is metabolized extensively in the liver.

Carcinogenesis, mutagenesis, impairment of fertility: In a 19 month carcinogenicity study in mice, a statistically significant increase in the incidence of testicular Leydig cell adenomas was observed at a dose of 250 mg/kg/day (228 times the human exposure). In mice and rats at a dose of 25 to ≥ 40 mg/kg/day (23 to 39 times the human exposure) an increase in the incidence of Leydig cell hyperplasia was observed. A positive correlation between the proliferative changes in the Leydig cells and an increase in serum LH levels (two- to threefold above control) has been demonstrated in both rodent species treated with high doses of finasteride.

In an in vitro chromosome aberration assay, when Chinese hamster ovary cells were treated with high concentrations of finasteride, there was a slight increase in chromosome aberrations. However, the concentrations used in vitro are not achievable in a biological system.

In sexually mature male rats treated with 80 mg/kg/day (61 times the human exposure) for up to 24 or 30 weeks, there was an apparent decrease in fertility, fecundity and an associated significant decrease in the weights of the seminal vesicles and prostate. All these effects were reversible within 6 weeks of discontinuation of treatment. This decrease in fertility in finasteride-treated rats is secondary to its effect on accessory sex organs (prostate and seminal vesicles) resulting in failure to form a seminal plug. The seminal plug is essential for normal fertility in rats and is not relevant in man.

(Warnings continued on following page)

FINASTERIDE (Cont.)

Warnings (Cont.):

Pregnancy: Category X. Finasteride is not indicated for use in women.

Administration of finasteride to pregnant rats at doses ranging from 100 to 1000 mg/kg/day (1 to 1000 times the recommended human dose) resulted in dose-dependent development of hypospadias in 3.6% to 100% of male offspring. Pregnant rats produced male offspring with decreased prostatic and seminal vesicular weights, delayed preputial separation and transient nipple development when given finasteride at ≥ 30 mcg/kg/day (≥ 3/10 of the recommended human dose) and decreased anogenital distance when given finasteride at ≥ 3 mcg/kg/day (≥ 3/100 of the recommended human dose). The critical period during which these effects can be induced in male rats is days 16 to 17 of gestation. The changes described above are expected pharmacological effects. Administration of finasteride at 3 mg/kg/day (30 times the recommended human dose) during the late gestation and lactation period resulted in slightly decreased fertility in F_1 male rat offspring.

Finasteride is contraindicated in women who are or may become pregnant. Because of the ability of 5α-reductase inhibitors to inhibit the conversion of testosterone to DHT, finasteride may cause abnormalities of the external genitalia of a male fetus of a pregnant woman who receives finasteride. If this drug is used during pregnancy, or if pregnancy occurs while taking this drug, apprise the woman of the potential hazard to the male fetus.

It is not known whether the amount of finasteride that could potentially be absorbed by a pregnant woman through either direct contact with crushed finasteride tablets or from the semen of a patient taking finasteride can adversely affect a developing male fetus. Therefore, because of the potential risk to a male fetus, a woman who is pregnant or who may become pregnant should not handle crushed finasteride tablets. In addition, when the male patient's sexual partner is or may become pregnant, the patient should either avoid exposure of his partner to semen or he should discontinue finasteride.

Lactation: It is not known whether finasteride is excreted in breast milk; however, finasteride is not indicated for use in women.

Children: Safety and efficacy in children have not been established; however, finasteride is not indicated for use in children.

Precautions:

Prostate cancer evaluation: Perform digital rectal examinations, as well as other evaluations for prostate cancer, on patients with BPH prior to initiating therapy and periodically thereafter. Although currently not indicated for this purpose, serum PSA is being increasingly used as one of the components of the screening process to detect prostate cancer. Generally, a baseline PSA > 10 ng/ml *(Hybritech)* prompts further evaluation and consideration of biopsy; for PSA levels between 4 and 10 ng/ml, further evaluation is generally considered advisable. A baseline PSA < 4 ng/ml does not exclude the diagnosis of prostate cancer.

Finasteride causes a decrease in serum PSA levels in patients with BPH even in the presence of prostate cancer. Consider this reduction of PSA levels when evaluating PSA laboratory data; it does not suggest a beneficial effect of finasteride on prostate cancer. In controlled clinical trials, finasteride did not appear to alter the rate of prostate cancer detection.

Carefully evaluate any sustained increases in PSA levels while on finasteride, including consideration of non-compliance to therapy.

Obstructive uropathy: Since not all patients demonstrate a response to finasteride, carefully monitor patients with a large residual urinary volume or severely diminished urinary flow for obstructive uropathy. These patients may not be candidates for this therapy.

Drug Interactions:

Theophylline: In 12 healthy volunteers, finasteride 5 mg/day for 8 days significantly increased theophylline clearance by 7% and decreased its half-life by 10% after IV aminophylline administration. These changes were not clinically significant.

Drug/Lab test interactions: When PSA laboratory determinations are evaluated, give consideration to the fact that PSA levels are decreased in patients treated with finasteride. In controlled clinical trials in patients with BPH treated with finasteride, PSA levels decreased from baseline by a median of 41% and 48% at months 6 and 12, respectively.

(Continued on following page)

FINASTERIDE (Cont.)

Adverse Reactions:

Finasteride is generally well tolerated; adverse reactions usually have been mild and transient. The following reactions have occurred: Impotence (3.7%); decreased libido (3.3%); decreased volume of ejaculate (2.8%).

In North American and international clinical trials, 1.3% of patients were discontinued due to adverse experiences; only 1 of these patients (0.2%) discontinued therapy because of a sexual adverse experience.

Overdosage:

Patients have received single doses up to 400 mg and multiple doses up to 80 mg/day for 3 months without adverse effects.

Significant lethality was observed in male and female mice at single oral doses of 1500 mg/m² (500 mg/kg) and in female and male rats at single oral doses of 2360 mg/m² (400 mg/kg) and 5900 mg/m² (1000 mg/kg), respectively.

Patient Information:

Crushed finasteride tablets should not be handled by a woman who is pregnant or who may become pregnant because of the potential for absorption of finasteride and the subsequent potential risk to the male fetus. Similarly, when the male patient's sexual partner is or may become pregnant, the patient should either avoid exposure of his partner to semen or he should discontinue finasteride.

Inform patients that the volume of ejaculate may be decreased in some patients during treatment. This decrease does not appear to interfere with normal sexual function. However, impotence and decreased libido may occur.

Administration and Dosage:

Approved by the FDA on June 19, 1992.

The recommended dose is 5 mg once a day, with or without meals.

Although early improvement may be seen, at least 6 to 12 months of therapy may be necessary in some patients to assess whether a beneficial response has been achieved. Perform periodic follow-up evaluations to determine whether a clinical response has occurred.

Renal function impairment/elderly: No dosage adjustment is necessary.

Rx	**Proscar** (MSD)	**Tablets:** 5 mg	Lactose. (MSD 72 Proscar). Blue. Film coated. Apple shape. In unit-of-use 30s and 100s and UD 100s.

These agents are derived from, or are closely related to, the androgen testosterone (see Androgens group monograph); they have androgenic as well as anabolic activity. Although these products possess a high-anabolic, low-androgenic activity ratio, the dissociation of anabolic from androgenic effects is incomplete and variable. Effective February 27, 1991, these agents were switched to a c-*III* status by the DEA because of their abuse potential.

Warning:

Peliosis hepatis, a condition in which liver and sometimes splenic tissue is replaced with blood-filled cysts, has occurred in patients receiving androgenic anabolic steroid therapy. These cysts are sometimes present with minimal hepatic dysfunction, but they have been associated with liver failure. They are often not recognized until life-threatening liver failure or intra-abdominal hemorrhage develops. Withdrawal of drug usually results in complete disappearance of lesions.

Liver cell tumors: Most often these tumors are benign and androgen-dependent, but fatal malignant tumors have occurred. Withdrawal of drug often results in regression or cessation of tumor progression. However, hepatic tumors associated with androgens or anabolic steroids are much more vascular than other hepatic tumors and may be silent until life-threatening intra-abdominal hemorrhage develops.

Blood lipid changes associated with increased risk of atherosclerosis are seen in patients treated with androgens and anabolic steroids. These changes include decreased high-density lipoprotein and sometimes increased low-density lipoprotein. The changes may be very marked and could have a serious impact on the risk of atherosclerosis and coronary artery disease.

Actions:

Pharmacology: Anabolic steroids promote body tissue-building processes and reverse catabolic or tissue depleting processes. Administer adequate calories and protein to achieve positive nitrogen balance. Whether this positive nitrogen balance is of primary benefit in the utilization of protein-building dietary substances is not established.

During exogenous administration of anabolic androgens, endogenous testosterone release is inhibited through inhibition of pituitary luteinizing hormone (LH). At large doses, spermatogenesis may be suppressed through feedback inhibition of pituitary follicle-stimulating hormone (FSH).

The androgenic properties of anabolic agents may cause serious disturbances of growth and sexual development when given to young children. They suppress the gonadotropic functions of the pituitary and may exert a direct effect on the testes.

Indications:

Refer to individual product monographs for approved indications of specific products.

Anemia: Androgens stimulate erythropoiesis and may be of value in the treatment of certain types of anemia.

Hereditary angioedema: Prophylactic use may decrease frequency and severity of attacks.

Metastatic breast cancer: For control of metastatic breast cancer in women.

Contraindications:

Hypersensitivity to anabolic steroids; male patients with prostate or breast carcinoma; carcinoma of the breast in females with hypercalcemia; nephrosis; the nephrotic phase of nephritis; pregnancy (see Warnings); to enhance physical appearance or athletic performance (see Warnings).

Warnings:

Athletic performance is questionably modified by these agents and studies yield equivocal results. The athlete's motivation to use these steroids includes 1) increased muscle mass and strength; 2) decreased muscle recovery time allowing more frequent weight training; 3) decreased healing time after muscle injury; 4) increased aggressiveness. The increase in muscle size and weight gain is partially attributed to the increased sodium and water retention. Evidence suggests that if anabolic steroids increase lean muscle mass, the muscle tissue may be deficient in phosphate and structurally flawed. Although some athletes, previously trained in weight lifting, who continue intensive weight training and maintain a high-protein, high-calorie diet during steroid use may derive some benefit such as increased strength (due to reaching a chronic catabolic state), the serious health hazards associated with anabolic steroids minimize any real or perceived gain in performance. Effects of these agents may persist for up to 6 months after the last dose. Adverse effects may be serious and irreversible.

(Warnings continued on following page)

Warnings (Cont.):

Athletic performance (Cont.):

Steroid regimens used are often referred to as "stacking", "pyramiding" or "cycling". "Stacking", or "stacking the pyramid", describes the concurrent use of two or more agents at the same time, either using high doses or varying the dosage, possibly including both oral and injectable forms. This regimen is tapered upward, then downward, generally over 4 to 18 weeks, followed by a drug-free period over several months. "Pyramiding" follows the same concept but generally involves the use of a single agent. "Cycling" refers to the drug-free period which is used to aid in the preparation of an upcoming event in the hopes that the athlete will peak at the time of the contest. These regimens are used to achieve an optimal anabolic effect while minimizing side effects and detection during competition. Dosages used may be as high as 40 times the therapeutic amounts.

An abuse or addiction syndrome is now being recognized with the chronic use of these drugs. Long-term use can lead to a preoccupation with drug use, difficulty stopping despite side effects and drug craving. A type of withdrawal syndrome may be noted as well when drug levels fluctuate, with symptoms that are similar to those seen with alcohol, cocaine and narcotic withdrawal. To detect steroid use or abuse, be aware of physical, psychological and behavioral changes. Aggressive behavior is common in abusers.

In addition, athletes may ingest other drugs in an attempt to counteract short-term side effects of the steroids (eg, diuretics to minimize sodium and fluid retention).

Elderly: Geriatric patients treated with anabolic steroids may be at increased risk for the development of prostatic hypertrophy and prostatic carcinoma.

Pregnancy: Category X. Contraindicated because of possible fetal masculinization.

Lactation: It is not known whether anabolic steroids are excreted in breast milk. Because of the potential for serious adverse reactions in nursing infants, decide whether to discontinue nursing or to discontinue the drug.

Children: The adverse consequences of giving androgens to young children are not fully understood, but the possibility of causing serious disturbances does exist; weigh the possible benefits before instituting therapy in young children.

Anabolic agents may accelerate epiphyseal maturation more rapidly than linear growth in children, and the effect may continue for 6 months after the drug has been stopped. Therefore, monitor therapy by x-ray studies at 6 month intervals to avoid the risk of compromising adult height.

Safety and efficacy in children with hereditary angioedema or metastatic breast cancer (rarely found) have not been established.

Benzyl alcohol-containing products have been associated with a fatal "gasping syndrome" in premature infants. Refer to product listings.

Precautions:

Virilization in the female may occur. If amenorrhea or menstrual irregularities develop during treatment, discontinue the drug until etiology is determined.

Leukemia has been observed in patients with aplastic anemia treated with **oxymetholone,** but the role of oxymetholone is unclear.

Edema, with or without congestive heart failure, may occur. Concomitant administration of an adrenal steroid or ACTH may increase the edema. Use caution in patients with cardiac, renal or hepatic disease, epilepsy, migraine or other conditions that may be aggravated by fluid retention.

Hypercalcemia may develop both spontaneously and as a result of hormonal therapy in women with disseminated breast carcinoma. Perform frequent urine and serum calcium level examinations. If hypercalcemia occurs, discontinue the drug.

Diabetics: Monitor carefully. Tolerance to glucose may be altered. Monitor urine or blood sugar closely.

Seizure disorders: Patients may note an increase in seizure frequency.

(Continued on following page)

Drug Interactions:

Anticoagulants: The anticoagulant effect may be potentiated by 17-alkyl testosterone derivatives (eg, anabolic steroids). Avoid this combination if possible.

Sulfonylureas: The hypoglycemic action may be enhanced by methandrostenolone. Monitor blood glucose and observe patients for signs of hypoglycemia.

Drug/Lab test interactions: Glucose tests – Anabolic steroids have altered glucose tolerance tests. Monitor diabetics closely and adjust the insulin or oral hypoglycemic dosage accordingly.

Thyroid function tests – Decrease in protein-bound iodine (PBI), thyroxine-binding capacity, radioactive iodine uptake and an increase in T_3 uptake by resin; free thyroxine levels remain normal.

Miscellaneous – Altered metyrapone test.

Adverse Reactions:

GI: Nausea; vomiting; diarrhea; cholestatic jaundice; hepatic necrosis; death; hepatocellular neoplasms and peliosis hepatis (long-term therapy; see Warning Box).

CNS: Excitation; insomnia; habituation; depression.

Endocrine: Virilization is the most common undesirable effect. Acne occurs especially in women and prepubertal males. Anabolic steroids inhibit gonadotropin secretion.

Prepubertal males – The first signs of virilization are phallic enlargement and an increase in frequency of erections.

Postpubertal males – Acne; inhibition of testicular function with oligospermia; gynecomastia; testicular atrophy; chronic priapism; epididymitis; bladder irritability; change in libido; impotence.

Females – Hirsutism; acne; hoarseness or deepening of the voice; clitoral enlargement; change in libido; menstrual irregularities; male-pattern baldness. Voice changes, hirsutism and clitoral enlargement are usually not reversible even after prompt discontinuation. The use of estrogens with androgens will not prevent virilization in females. Masculinization of the fetus has occurred.

Fluid and electrolyte imbalance: Retention of sodium, chloride, water, potassium, phosphates and calcium; ankle swelling; decreased glucose tolerance.

Laboratory test abnormalities: Liver function tests – BSP retention; increased AST, serum bilirubin and alkaline phosphatase.

Blood coagulation tests – May suppress clotting factors II, V, VII and X and increase prothrombin time.

Miscellaneous – Increased creatinine and creatine excretion; increased serum cholesterol.

Miscellaneous: Premature closure of epiphyses in children; choreiform movement; increased serum cholesterol; increased serum levels of low-density lipoproteins and decreased levels of high-density lipoproteins.

Patient Information:

Diabetic patients: Glucose tolerance may be altered; monitor urine sugar closely and report abnormalities to physician.

Female patients: Notify physician if hoarseness, deepening of the voice, male-pattern baldness, hirsutism, menstrual irregularities or acne occurs.

May cause nausea or GI upset.

Notify physician if nausea, vomiting, changes in skin color or ankle swelling occurs.

(Products listed on following pages)

Complete prescribing information for these products begins on page 401

OXYMETHOLONE

Indications:

Anemias caused by deficient red cell production, acquired or congenital aplastic anemia, myelofibrosis and hypoplastic anemias due to the administration of myelotoxic drugs.

Administration and Dosage:

Anemias: 1 to 5 mg/kg/day. The usual effective dose is 1 to 2 mg/kg/day. Individualize dosage. Response is not often immediate; give for a minimum trial of 3 to 6 months. Following remission, some patients may be maintained without the drug, while others may be maintained on an established lower daily dosage. Continuous maintenance is usually necessary in patients with congenital aplastic anemia. **C.I.***

c-III	**Anadrol-50** (Syntex)	**Tablets:** 50 mg	Lactose. (Syntex 2902). White, scored. In 100s.	24

STANOZOLOL

Indications:

Hereditary angioedema: Prophylactic use to decrease frequency and severity of attacks.

Administration and Dosage:

Individualize dosage. Initial dosage is 2 mg 3 times a day. After a favorable response is obtained in terms of prevention of edematous attacks, decrease dosage at intervals of 1 to 3 months to a maintenance dosage of 2 mg/day. Some patients may be successfully managed on a 2 mg alternate day schedule. During the dose adjusting phase, closely monitor patient response, particularly if there is a history of airway involvement.

The prophylactic dose to be used prior to dental extraction, or other traumatic or stressful situations, has not been established and may be substantially larger.

Attacks of hereditary angioedema are generally infrequent in childhood, and the risks from stanozolol administration are substantially increased. Therefore, long-term prophylactic therapy is generally not recommended in children; consider the benefits and risks involved. **C.I.***

c-III	**Winstrol** (Winthrop Pharm.)	**Tablets:** 2 mg	Lactose. (W 53). Pink, scored. In 100s.	39

OXANDROLONE

Indications:

Adjunctive therapy to promote weight gain after weight loss following extensive surgery, chronic infections, or severe trauma, and in some patients who, without definite pathophysiologic reasons, fail to gain or to maintain normal weight; to offset the protein catabolism associated with prolonged administration of corticosteroids; for relief of the bone pain frequently accompanying osteoporosis.

Unlabeled uses:

Alcoholic hepatitis.

Orphan drug designation – Short stature associated with Turner syndrome; HIV wasting syndrome and HIV-associated muscle weakness.

Treatment IND – Constitutional delay of growth and puberty, which commonly is diagnosed when the height, pubertal development and bone age of an otherwise healthy adolescent are significantly below average for their chronological age.

Administration and Dosage:

Individualize dosage. Use intermittent therapy.

Adults: 2.5 mg 2 to 4 times daily. However, since the response of individuals to anabolic steroids varies, a daily dosage of as little as 2.5 mg or as much as 20 mg may be required to achieve the desired response. A course of therapy of 2 to 4 weeks is usually adequate. This may be repeated intermittently as indicated.

Children: Total daily dosage is $\leq$ 0.1 mg/kg or $\leq$ 0.045 mg/lb. this may be repeated intermittently as indicated.

c-III	**Oxandrin** (Gynex)	**Tablets:** 2.5 mg	Lactose. (Gynex 1111). White, oval, scored. In 100s.	NA

* Cost Index based on cost per 50 mg oxymetholone or 6 mg stanozolol.

Complete prescribing information for these products begins on page 401

NANDROLONE PHENPROPIONATE

Indications:

Control of metastatic breast cancer in women.

Administration and Dosage:

Inject deeply IM, preferably into the gluteal muscle.

If possible, therapy should be intermittent. Duration of therapy depends on patient response and adverse reactions.

Adults: 50 to 100 mg weekly, based on therapeutic response.

	Product	Form	Package	C.I.*
c-III	**Nandrolone Phenpropionate** (Various, eg, Lyphomed, Major)	**Injection (In Oil):** 25 mg per ml	In 5 ml vials.	71+
c-III	**Durabolin** (Organon)		In 5 ml vials.[1]	231
c-III	**Nandrobolic** (Forest)		In 5 ml vials.[1]	83
c-III	**Nandrolone Phenpropionate** (Various, eg, Keene, Major, Rugby)	**Injection (In Oil):** 50 mg per ml	In 2 ml vials.	78+
c-III	**Durabolin** (Organon)		In 2 ml vials.[1]	251
c-III	**Hybolin Improved** (Hyrex)		In 2 ml vials.[1]	93

NANDROLONE DECANOATE

Indications:

Management of the anemia of renal insufficiency. This drug increases hemoglobin and red cell mass. Surgically induced anephric patients may be less responsive.

Administration and Dosage:

If possible, therapy should be intermittent. Duration of therapy depends on response of the condition and appearance of adverse reactions.

Inject deeply IM, preferably into the gluteal muscle.

Anemia of renal disease:

Women – 50 to 100 mg per week.

Men – 100 to 200 mg per week.

Children (2 to 13 years) – Average dose is 25 to 50 mg every 3 to 4 weeks.

	Product	Form	Package	C.I.*
c-III	**Nandrolone Decanoate** (Various, eg, Goldline, Rugby, Schein)	**Injection (In Oil):** 50 mg per ml	In 2 ml vials.	51+
c-III	**Deca-Durabolin** (Organon)		In 2 ml vials[1] and 1 ml syringes.[1]	210
c-III	**Hybolin Decanoate-50** (Hyrex)		In 2 ml vials.[1]	99
c-III	**Neo-Durabolic** (Hauck)		In 2 ml vials.[1]	109
c-III	**Nandrolone Decanoate** (Various, eg, Goldline, Lyphomed, Major, Rugby, Schein, URL)	**Injection (In Oil):** 100 mg per ml	In 2 ml vials.	52+
c-III	**Deca-Durabolin** (Organon)		In 2 ml vials[1] and 1 ml syringes.[1]	179
c-III	**Hybolin Decanoate-100** (Hyrex)		In 2 ml vials.[1]	85
c-III	**Nandrolone Decanoate** (Various, eg, Lyphomed, Major, Schein)	**Injection (In Oil):** 200 mg per ml	In 1 ml vials.	50+
c-III	**Androlone-D 200** (Keene)		In 1 ml vials.[1]	67
c-III	**Deca-Durabolin** (Organon)		In 1 ml vials[1] and 1 ml syringes.[1]	172
c-III	**Neo-Durabolic** (Hauck)		In 1 ml vials.[1]	94

* Cost Index based on cost per 50 mg.

[1] In sesame oil with benzyl alcohol.

Refer to group monographs on Androgens and Estrogens for complete prescribing information.

Indications:

Moderate to severe vasomotor symptoms associated with menopause in patients not improved with estrogens alone.

There is no evidence that estrogens are effective for nervousness or depression which may occur during menopause; do not use to treat these conditions.

Postpartum breast engorgement: Although estrogens have been widely used to prevent postpartum breast engorgement, controlled studies indicate the incidence of significant painful engorgement is low and usually responsive to analgesic or other supportive therapy. Because of the potential increased risk of puerperal thromboembolism associated with large doses of estrogens, carefully weigh the benefits to be derived from their use.

In June 1989, the FDA's Fertility and Maternal Health Drugs Advisory Committee unanimously recommended that these agents should not be used for prevention of postpartum breast engorgement.

		Parenteral		C.I.*
Rx	**Testosterone Cypionate and Estradiol Cypionate** (Schein)	**Injection (In Oil):** 2 mg estradiol cypionate and 50 mg testosterone cypionate per ml	In 10 ml vials.	19
Rx	**Andro/Fem** (Pasadena)		In 10 ml vials.[1]	12
Rx	**De-Comberol** (Schein)		In 10 ml vials.	NA
Rx	**depAndrogyn** (Forest)		In 10 ml vials.	16
Rx	**Depo-Testadiol** (Upjohn)		In 1 & 10 ml vials.[1]	41
Rx	**Depotestogen** (Hyrex)		In 10 ml vials.[1]	12
Rx	**Duo-Cyp** (Keene)		In 10 ml vials.[1]	11
Rx	**Duratestrin** (Hauck)		In 10 ml vials.[1]	NA
Rx	**Test-Estro Cypionates** (Rugby)		In 10 ml vials.[1]	12
Rx	**Testosterone Enanthate and Estradiol Valerate** (Schein)	**Injection (In Oil):** 4 mg estradiol valerate and 90 mg testosterone enanthate per ml	In 10 ml vials.	9.6
Rx	**Androgyn L.A.** (Forest)		In 10 ml vials.[2]	9.6
Rx	**Deladumone** (Bristol-Myers Squibb)		In 5 ml vials.[2]	68
Rx	**Estra-Testrin** (Pasadena)		In 10 ml vials.[2]	7.1
Rx	**Valertest No. 1** (Hyrex)		In 10 ml vials.[2]	6.8

		Oral		C.I.*
Rx	**Halodrin** (Upjohn)	**Tablets:** 0.02 mg ethinyl estradiol and 1 mg fluoxymesterone	Lactose, sucrose. (Halodrin 38). Pink, scored. In 100s.	9.3
Rx	**Premarin with Methyltestosterone** (Wyeth-Ayerst)	**Tablets:** 1.25 mg conjugated estrogens and 10 mg methyltestosterone	(Ayerst 879). Yellow. In 100s.	20
Rx	**Premarin with Methyltestosterone** (Wyeth-Ayerst)	**Tablets:** 0.625 mg conjugated estrogens and 5 mg methyltestosterone	(Ayerst 878). Maroon. In 100s.	35
Rx	**Estratest** (Solvay Pharm.)	**Tablets:** 1.25 mg esterified estrogens and 2.5 mg methyltestosterone	Lactose, sucrose. (RR 1026). Dark green. Sugar coated. Capsule shape. In 100s and 1000s.	16
Rx	**Estratest H.S.** (Solvay Pharm.)	**Tablets:** 0.625 mg esterified estrogens and 1.25 mg methyltestosterone	Lactose, sucrose. (RR 1023). Light green. Sugar coated. Capsule shape. In 100s.	12

* Cost Index based on cost per mg estradiol (inj) or per tablet.
[1] With chlorobutanol in cottonseed oil.
[2] With chlorobutanol in sesame oil.
[3] With benzyl alcohol in sesame oil.

UROFOLLITROPIN (Cont.)

Precautions:

Selection of patients: Give careful attention to diagnosis in candidates for therapy. Before treatment is instituted, perform a thorough gynecologic and endocrinologic evaluation including a hysterosalpingogram (to rule out uterine and tubal pathology) and documentation of anovulation by means of basal body temperature, serial vaginal smears, examination of cervical mucus, determination of urinary pregnanediol and endometrial biopsy. Exclude primary ovarian failure by the determination of gonadotropin levels. Make careful examination to rule out early pregnancy. Patients in late reproductive life have a greater predilection to endometrial carcinoma and a higher incidence of anovulatory disorders. Perform cervical dilation and curettage for diagnosis before starting therapy. Evaluate the partner's fertility potential.

Treatment results in follicular growth and maturation to effect ovulation in the absence of an endogenous LH surge. HCG is given following the administration of urofollitropin when clinical assessment indicates sufficient follicular maturation has occurred. This is indirectly estimated by the estrogenic effect upon the target organs. With serum or urinary estrogen determinations and ultrasonography, the estrogenic effect is an acceptable means for monitoring the growth and development of follicles, timing HCG administration and minimizing the risk of hyperstimulation. Clinically confirm ovulation, with the exception of pregnancy, by indirect indices of progesterone production.

Adverse Reactions:

Reported in approximately 10% of patients: Hyperstimulation syndrome (see Warnings); mild to moderate ovarian enlargement; abdominal pain; pain, rash, swelling or irritation at injection site.

Reported in < 2% of patients: Nausea; vomiting; diarrhea; abdominal cramps; bloating; headache; breast tenderness; ectopic pregnancy. Febrile reactions accompanied by chills, musculoskeletal aches or pain, malaise and fatigue have occurred. It is not clear whether these are pyrogenic responses or possible allergic reactions. Dermatologic symptoms (dry skin, rash, hair loss, hives) have been reported.

Arterial thromboembolism (see Warnings) and hemoperitoneum have been reported with menotropins therapy and, therefore, may also occur during urofollitropin therapy.

Overdosage:

Aside from possible hyperstimulation and multiple gestations (see Warnings), little is known concerning the consequences of acute overdosage.

Patient Information:

Prior to therapy, inform patients of the following: Duration of treatment and monitoring required; possible adverse reactions; risk of multiple births.

Administration and Dosage:

Individualize dosage.

Initial dose: 75 IU/day IM urofollitropin, for 7 to 12 days followed by 5,000 to 10,000 U of HCG, one day after the last urofollitropin dose. Administration of urofollitropin may exceed 12 days if inadequate follicle development is indicated by estrogen or ultrasound measurement. Treat the patient until estrogenic activity is equivalent to or greater than that of a normal individual. If the ovaries are abnormally enlarged on the last day of therapy, do not give HCG in this course of therapy; this reduces the chances of developing hyperstimulation syndrome. If there is evidence of ovulation but no pregnancy, repeat this dosage regimen for at least two more courses before increasing the dose to 150 IU of FSH per day for 7 to 12 days. Follow this dose with 5,000 to 10,000 U of HCG one day after the last urofollitropin dose. If evidence of ovulation is present, but pregnancy does not ensue, repeat the same dose for two more courses. Larger doses are not recommended.

During treatment with urofollitropin and HCG and during a 2 week posttreatment period, examine patients at least every other day for signs of excessive ovarian stimulation. Stop administration if the ovaries become abnormally enlarged or if abdominal pain occurs. Most ovarian hyperstimulation occurs after treatment discontinuation and reaches its maximum at 7 to 10 days postovulation.

Encourage the couple to have intercourse daily, beginning on the day prior to HCG administration until ovulation is apparent from determination of progestational activity.

Preparation of solution: Dissolve contents of 1 ampule in 1 to 2 ml sterile saline; administer IM immediately. Discard unused reconstituted material.

Storage: Store at 3° to 25°C (37° to 77°F). Protect from light. **C.I.***

Rx	**Metrodin** (Serono)	**Powder for Injection:** 0.83 mg (75 IU FSH activity) per amp[1] with 2 ml amp sodium chloride injection.

[1] With 10 mg lactose, in a lyophilized form.

MENOTROPINS

Actions:

Menotropins is a purified preparation of gonadotropins extracted from the urine of postmenopausal women. It is biologically standardized for follicle stimulating hormone (FSH) and luteinizing hormone (LH) activities.

Women: Produces ovarian follicular growth in women who do not have primary ovarian failure. Treatment results only in follicular growth and maturation. To effect ovulation, human chorionic gonadotropin (HCG) is given following menotropins when clinical assessment indicates sufficient follicular maturation.

Men: Menotropins administered concomitantly with HCG for at least 3 months induces spermatogenesis in men with primary or secondary pituitary hypofunction who have achieved adequate masculinization with prior HCG therapy.

Indications:

Women: Menotropins and HCG given sequentially are indicated for induction of ovulation and pregnancy in the anovulatory infertile patient, in whom the cause of anovulation is functional and not due to primary ovarian failure.

Men: Menotropins and concomitant HCG are indicated for stimulation of spermatogenesis in men with primary hypogonadotropic hypogonadism due to a congenital factor or prepubertal hypophysectomy and in men with secondary hypogonadotropic hypogonadism due to hypophysectomy, craniopharyngioma, cerebral aneurysm or chromophobe adenoma.

Contraindications:

Women: High gonadotropin level indicating primary ovarian failure; overt thyroid and adrenal dysfunction; any cause of infertility other than anovulation; abnormal bleeding of undetermined origin; ovarian cysts or enlargement not due to polycystic ovary syndrome; organic intracranial lesion such as pituitary tumor; pregnancy.

Men: Normal gonadotropin levels indicating normal pituitary function; elevated gonadotropin levels indicating primary testicular failure; infertility disorders other than hypogonadotropic hypogonadism.

Warnings:

This drug should be used only by physicians thoroughly familiar with infertility problems. Menotropins can cause mild to severe adverse reactions in women.

Precautions:

Diagnosis prior to therapy:

Women – Perform a thorough gynecologic and endocrinologic evaluation, including a hysterosalpingogram. Document anovulation. Rule out primary ovarian failure and early pregnancy. Patients in late reproductive life have a greater predilection to endometrial carcinoma and a higher incidence of anovulatory disorders. Perform a cervical dilation and curettage before starting therapy in such patients. Evaluate the partner's fertility potential.

Men – Document lack of pituitary function. Prior to therapy, patients have low testosterone levels and low or absent gonadotropin levels. Patients with primary hypogonadotropic hypogonadism will have subnormal development of masculinization; those with secondary hypogonadotropic hypogonadism will have decreased masculinization.

Overstimulation of the ovary: To minimize the hazard of abnormal ovarian enlargement, use the lowest effective dose. Mild to moderate uncomplicated ovarian enlargement, with or without abdominal distention or abdominal pain, occurs in approximately 20% of those treated with HCG and menotropins and generally regresses without treatment in 2 to 3 weeks. The hyperstimulation syndrome characterized by sudden ovarian enlargement and ascites, with or without pain or pleural effusion, occurs in approximately 0.4% of patients at recommended doses. The overall incidence of this syndrome is about 1.3%.

Hyperstimulation syndrome develops rapidly over 3 to 4 days and generally occurs within 2 weeks following treatment; if it occurs, discontinue treatment and hospitalize patient. Hemoconcentration associated with fluid loss in the abdominal cavity has occurred; thoroughly assess by daily determination of fluid intake and output, weight, hematocrit, serum and urinary electrolytes and urine specific gravity. Treatment is primarily symptomatic and consists of bedrest, fluid and electrolyte replacement and analgesics. Never remove ascitic fluid because of the potential for injury to the ovary. Hemoperitoneum may occur from ruptured ovarian cysts, usually as a result of pelvic examination. If bleeding requires surgery, partial resection of the enlarged ovary is generally adequate. Prohibit intercourse where significant ovarian enlargement occurs after ovulation.

(Precautions continued on following page)

MENOTROPINS (Cont.)

Precautions (Cont.):

Multiple births: Pregnancies following therapy with HCG and menotropins resulted in 80% single births; 15% resulted in twins, of which 93% were viable; and 5% of pregnancies produced 3 or more conceptuses, of which 20% were viable. Advise patient of the frequency and potential hazards of multiple pregnancy.

Adverse Reactions:

Women: Ovarian enlargement, hyperstimulation syndrome, hemoperitoneum, arterial thromboembolism, hypersensitivity, febrile reactions. Birth defects occurred in 5 of 287 pregnancies.

Men: Occasional gynecomastia. Erythrocytosis (Hct 50%, Hgb 17.8 g%) in one patient.

Administration and Dosage:

Women: Treatment results only in follicular growth and maturation. To effect ovulation, HCG must be given following menotropins when clinical assessment indicates sufficient follicular maturation. This is indirectly estimated by the estrogenic effect on target organs (ie, changes in the vaginal smear, appearance and volume of cervical mucus, spinnbarkeit, ferning of cervical mucus). Urinary excretion of estrogens is a more reliable index of follicular maturation.

The clinical confirmation of ovulation, with the exception of pregnancy, is by indirect indices of progesterone production. These include: Rise in basal temperature; change of cervical mucus from a "fern" pattern to a "cellular" pattern; vaginal cytology characteristic of the luteal phase of the cycle; increase in urinary pregnanediol; menstruation following a shift in basal temperature.

Initial dosage – Individualize dosage. Initial IM dose is 75 IU FSH/75 IU LH (1 amp) per day, for 9 to 12 days; follow by 10,000 IU HCG 1 day after the last dose of menotropins. Hyperstimulation syndrome does not occur following this dosage schedule. Do not exceed 12 days of menotropins administration. Treat the patient until indices of estrogenic activity are equal to or greater than those of the normal individual. Urinary estrogen determinations are useful as a guide to therapy. If the total estrogen excretion is less than 100 mcg/24 hours or if the estriol excretion is less than 50 mcg/24 hours prior to HCG administration, hyperstimulation syndrome is less likely to occur. If the estrogen values are greater than this, it is not advisable to administer HCG because the hyperstimulation syndrome is more likely to occur. If the ovaries are abnormally enlarged on the last day of menotropins therapy, do not administer HCG in this course.

The couple should have intercourse daily, beginning on the day prior to HCG administration, until ovulation occurs. Take care to ensure insemination.

Repeat dosage – If there is evidence of ovulation, but no pregnancy, repeat the regimen for at least 2 more courses before increasing the dose to 150 IU FSH/150 IU LH (2 amps) per day for 9 to 12 days. Follow by 10,000 IU HCG 1 day after the last dose of menotropins. Two amps of menotropins per day is the most effective dose. If evidence of ovulation is present, but pregnancy does not ensue, repeat the same dose for 2 more courses; larger doses are not recommended.

During treatment with menotropins and HCG and for 2 weeks posttreatment, examine patients at least every other day for signs of excessive ovarian stimulation. Stop treatment if the ovaries become abnormally enlarged or if abdominal pain occurs. Hyperstimulation usually occurs after treatment has been discontinued and reaches its maximum 7 to 10 days postovulation.

Men: Prior to therapy with menotropins and HCG, pretreat with HCG alone (5,000 IU 3 times a week). Continue HCG for a sufficient period to achieve serum testosterone levels within the normal range and masculinization (ie, appearance of secondary sex characteristics). Pretreatment may require 4 to 6 months. The recommended dose is 1 amp menotropins IM 3 times a week and HCG 2,000 IU twice a week. Continue therapy for a minimum of 4 months to ensure detecting spermatozoa in the ejaculate.

If the patient has not responded with increased spermatogenesis at the end of 4 months, continue treatment with 1 amp 3 times a week or increase dose to 2 amps (150 IU FSH/150 IU LH) 3 times a week, with the HCG dose unchanged.

Preparation of solution: Dissolve contents of 1 amp in 1 to 2 ml sterile saline. Administer IM immediately. Discard any unused portion.

Storage: Lyophilized powder may be refrigerated or stored at room temperature, 3° to 30°C (37° to 86°F).

Rx	**Pergonal** (Serono)	**Powder for Injection:** 75 IU FSH activity and 75 IU LH activity per amp.[1] In 2 ml amps. 150 I FSH activity and 150 IU LH activity per amp.[1] In 2 ml amps.

[1] With 10 mg lactose in a lyophilized form.

CHORIONIC GONADOTROPIN (HCG)

HCG has no known effect on fat mobilization, appetite, sense of hunger or body fat distribution. HCG has NOT been demonstrated to be effective adjunctive therapy in the treatment of obesity. There is no substantial evidence that it increases weight loss beyond that resulting from caloric restriction, that it causes a more attractive or "normal" distribution of fat or that it decreases the hunger and discomfort associated with calorie restricted diets.

Actions:

Human chorionic gonadotropin (HCG), a polypeptide hormone produced by the human placenta, is composed of an α and β subunit. The α subunit is essentially identical to the α subunits of the human pituitary gonadotropins, luteinizing hormone (LH) and follicle stimulating hormone (FSH), as well as to the α subunit of human thyroid stimulating hormone (TSH). The β subunits of these hormones differ in amino acid sequence.

The action of HCG is virtually identical to pituitary LH, although HCG appears to have a small degree of FSH activity as well. It stimulates production of gonadal steroid hormones by stimulating the interstitial cells (Leydig cells) of the testis to produce androgens, and the corpus luteum of the ovary to produce progesterone. Androgen stimulation in the male leads to the development of secondary sex characteristics and may stimulate testicular descent when no anatomical impediment to descent is present. This descent is usually reversible when HCG is discontinued. During the normal menstrual cycle, LH participates with FSH in the development and maturation of the normal ovarian follicle, and the mid-cycle LH surge triggers ovulation; HCG can substitute for LH in this function. During a normal pregnancy, HCG secreted by the placenta maintains the corpus luteum after LH secretion decreases, supporting continued secretion of estrogen and progesterone and preventing menstruation.

Indications:

Prepubertal cryptorchidism not due to anatomical obstruction. HCG is thought to induce testicular descent in situations when descent would have occurred at puberty. HCG may help predict whether orchiopexy will be needed in the future. In some cases, descent following HCG administration is permanent, but in most cases the response is temporary. Therapy is usually instituted between the ages of 4 and 9.

Selected cases of hypogonadotropic hypogonadism (hypogonadism secondary to a pituitary deficiency) in males.

Induction of ovulation in the anovulatory, infertile woman in whom the cause of anovulation is secondary and not due to primary ovarian failure, and who has been appropriately pretreated with human menotropins.

Contraindications:

Precocious puberty; prostatic carcinoma or other androgen-dependent neoplasm; prior allergic reaction to chorionic gonadotropin.

Warnings:

HCG should be used in conjunction with human menopausal gonadotropins only by physicians experienced with infertility problems. The principal serious adverse reactions experienced with this indication are: Ovarian hyperstimulation, a syndrome of sudden ovarian enlargement; ascites with or without pain and pleural effusion; rupture of ovarian cysts with resultant hemoperitoneum; multiple births; arterial thromboembolism.

Usage in Pregnancy: Category C. Animal reproduction studies have not been conducted. It is also not known whether HCG can cause fetal harm when administered to a pregnant woman. Not indicated for use in pregnancy.

Precautions:

Precocious puberty: Induction of androgen secretion by chorionic gonadotropin may induce precocious puberty in patients treated for cryptorchidism. Discontinue use if signs of precocious puberty occur.

Fluid retention: Since androgens may cause fluid retention, use HCG with caution in patients with epilepsy, migraine, asthma, cardiac or renal disease.

If hypogonadism due to pituitary dysfunction has existed over a period of several years, irreparable testicular damage may have occurred, and response to therapy with chorionic gonadotropin may be unsatisfactory. Stimulation therapy is not recommended in the treatment of hypogonadism of testicular origin.

Adverse Reactions:

Headache, irritability, restlessness, depression, fatigue, edema, precocious puberty, gynecomastia and pain at injection site.

(Continued on following page)

CHORIONIC GONADOTROPIN (HCG) (Cont.)

Overdosage:

No cases of overdosage have been reported.

Administration and Dosage:

For IM use only. There is a marked variance of opinion concerning dosage regimens. The regimen employed will depend on the indication, age and weight of the patient and the physician's preference. The following dosage regimens have been advocated.

Prepubertal cryptorchidism not due to anatomical obstruction:

1. 4,000 USP units, 3 times weekly for 3 weeks.
2. 5,000 USP units every second day for 4 injections.
3. 15 injections of 500 to 1,000 USP units over a period of 6 weeks.
4. 500 USP units, 3 times weekly for 4 to 6 weeks. If this course of treatment is not successful, start another course 1 month later, giving 1,000 USP units per injection.

Selected cases of hypogonadotropic hypogonadism in males:

1. 500 to 1,000 USP units 3 times a week for 3 weeks, followed by the same dose twice a week for 3 weeks.
2. 1,000 to 2,000 USP units, 3 times weekly.
3. 4,000 USP units 3 times weekly for 6 to 9 months; reduce dosage to 2,000 USP units 3 times weekly for an additional 3 months.

Use with menotropins: After pretreatment with HCG, menotropins may be administered to stimulate spermatogenesis (see Menotropins, p. 412). Recommended HCG dose is 5,000 IU, 3 times weekly for 4 to 6 months. With the beginning of menotropins therapy, the HCG dose is continued at 2,000 IU twice weekly.

Induction of ovulation and pregnancy: In the anovulatory, infertile woman in whom the cause of anovulation is secondary and not due to primary ovarian failure, and who has been appropriately pretreated with human menotropins (see prescribing information for menotropins, p. 115d) – 5,000 to 10,000 USP units 1 day following the last dose of menotropins.

The following products consist of lyophilized powder, with or without diluent, to prepare solutions for injection providing the indicated number of units of HCG. Refer to manufacturers' labeling for preparation and storage.

	Product (Manufacturer)	Form	Package	C.I.*
Rx	**Glukor** (Hyrex)	**Powder for Injection:** 200 units per ml after reconstitution	In 10 and 25 ml vials[1] w/diluent.	650
Rx	**Chorionic Gonadotropin** (Various)	**Powder for Injection:** 5,000 units per vial with 10 ml diluent (to make 500 units per ml)	In 10 ml vials.	108+
Rx	**A.P.L.** (Ayerst)		In 10 ml vials.[2]	652
Rx	**Chorex-5** (Hyrex)		In 10 ml vials.[1]	260
Rx	**Corgonject-5** (Mayrand)		In 10 ml vials.[1]	290
Rx	**Profasi HP** (Serono)		In 10 ml vials.[1]	280
Rx	**Chorionic Gonadotropin** (Various)	**Powder for Injection:** 10,000 units per vial with 10 ml diluent (to make 1000 units per ml)	In 10 ml vials.	94+
Rx	**A.P.L.** (Ayerst)		In 10 ml vials.[2]	609
Rx	**Chorex-10** (Hyrex)		In 10 ml vials.[1]	189
Rx	**Chorigon** (Dunhall)		In 10 ml vials.[1]	N/A
Rx	**Choron 10** (Forest Pharm.)		In 10 ml vials.[3]	200
Rx	**Follutein** (Squibb)		In 10 ml vials with or w/o diluent.[4]	753
Rx	**Gonic** (Hauck)		In 10 ml vials.[1]	150
Rx	**Pregnyl** (Organon)		In 10 ml vials.[1]	145
Rx	**Profasi HP** (Serono)		In 10 ml vials.[1]	273
Rx	**Chorionic Gonadotropin** (Various)	**Powder for Injection:** 20,000 units per vial with 10 ml diluent (to make 2000 units per ml)	In 10 ml vials.	88+
Rx	**A.P.L.** (Ayerst)		In 10 ml vials.[2]	620

* Cost Index based on cost per 1000 units.
[1] With mannitol and benzyl alcohol.
[2] With benzyl alcohol, phenol and lactose.
[3] With mannitol.
[4] With phenol.

GONADORELIN ACETATE

Actions:

Pharmacology: Gonadorelin acetate is used for the induction of ovulation in women with primary hypothalamic amenorrhea. Gonadorelin acetate is a synthetic decapeptide that is identical in amino acid sequence to endogenous gonadotropin-releasing hormone (GnRH) synthesized in the human hypothalamus and in various neurons terminating in the hypothalamus.

Under physiologic conditions, GnRH is released by the hypothalamus in a pulsatile fashion. The primary effect of GnRH is the synthesis and release of luteinizing hormone (LH) in the anterior pituitary gland. GnHR also stimulates the synthesis and release of follicle stimulating hormone (FSH), but this effect is less pronounced. LH and FSH subsequently stimulate the gonads to produce steroids which are instrumental in regulating reproductive hormonal status. Unlike human menopausal gonadotropin (hMG) which supplies pituitary hormones, pulsatile administration of gonadorelin replaces defective hypothalamic secretion of GnRH. The pulsatile administration of gonadorelin approximates the natural hormonal secretory pattern, causing pulsatile release of pituitary gonadotropins. Accordingly, gonadorelin is useful in treating conditions of infertility caused by defective GnRH stimulation from the hypothalamus.

Pharmacokinetics: Following IV injection of GnRH into healthy subjects or hypogonadotropic patients, plasma GnRH concentrations rapidly decline with initial and terminal half-lives of 2 to 10 min and 10 to 40 min, respectively. High clearance values (500 to 1500 L/day) and low volumes of distribution (10 to 15 L) were calculated. The pharmacokinetics of GnRH in healthy subjects and in hypogonadotropic patients were similar. GnRH was rapidly metabolized to various biologically inactive peptide fragments which are readily excreted in urine. Renal failure, but not hepatic disease, prolonged the half-life and reduced the clearance of GnRH.

Clinical trials: The following information summarizes clinical efficacy of gonadorelin acetate administered by pulsatile IV injection to 44 patients with primary hypothalamic amenorrhea: 93% (41/44) were ovulatory with gonadorelin acetate therapy, 62% (24/39) became pregnant (five did not desire pregnancy), and 100% (7/7) of those failing past attempts at ovulation induction by other methods were ovulatory on gonadorelin.

Indications:

Primary hypothalamic amenorrhea treatment.

Gonadorelin HCl *(Factrel),* a related polypeptide hormone, is indicated for evaluating the functional capacity and response of the gonadotropes of the anterior pituitary and for evaluating residual gonadotropic function of the pituitary following removal of a pituitary tumor by surgery or irradiation. See individual monograph in In Vivo Diagnostic Aids section.

Contraindications:

Women with any condition that could be exacerbated by pregnancy (eg, pituitary prolactinoma); sensitivity to gonadorelin acetate, gonadorelin HCl or any component of the product; patients who have ovarian cysts or causes of anovulation other than those of hypothalamic origin; any condition that may be worsened by reproductive hormones, such as a hormonally dependent tumor, since gonadorelin is intended to initiate events including the production of reproductive hormones (eg, estrogens and progestins).

Warnings:

Ovarian hyperstimulation, a syndrome of sudden ovarian enlargement, ascites with or without pain, or pleural effusion, has occurred (< 1%). This may be related to pulse dosage or concomitant use of other ovulation stimulators. Hyperstimulation may be a greater risk in patients where spontaneous variations in endogenous GnRH secretion occur.

Therapy with gonadorelin acetate should be conducted by physicians familiar with pulsatile GnRH delivery and the clinical ramifications of ovulation induction. If hyperstimulation should occur, discontinue therapy; spontaneous resolution can be expected. The preservation of the endogenous feedback mechanisms (pulsatile therapy) makes severe hyperstimulation (with ascites and pleural effusion) rare. However, be aware of the possibility and be alert for any evidence of ascites, pleural effusion, hemoconcentration, rupture of a cyst, fluid or electrolyte imbalance or sepsis.

Among 268 patients participating in clinical trials, one case of moderate hyperstimulation has been reported, but this cycle included the concomitant use of clomiphene citrate. In contrast, menotropins (hMG) with hCG have been variously reported to cause some degree of hyperstimulation in up to 50% of conception cycles, and severe hyperstimulation may occur in up to 1.3% of all cycles.

(Warnings continued on following page)

GONADORELIN ACETATE (Cont.)

Warnings (Cont.):

Multiple pregnancy is a possibility (12%); minimize by careful attention to the recommended doses and ultrasonographic monitoring of the ovarian response to therapy, including follicle formulation. Multiple follicle development and spontaneous termination of pregnancy have occurred. Following a baseline pelvic ultrasound, conduct follow-up studies at a minimum on day 7 and day 14 of the therapy.

Asepsis: As with any IV medication, scrupulous attention to asepsis is important. The infusion area must be monitored as with all indwelling parenteral approaches. Change the cannula and IV site at 48-hour intervals.

Pregnancy: Category B. Studies in pregnant women have shown that gonadorelin acetate does not increase the risk of abnormalities when administered during the first trimester of pregnancy. The possibility of fetal harm appears remote if the drug is used during pregnancy. In clinical studies, 47 pregnant patients have used gonadorelin acetate during the first trimester of pregnancy (51 pregnancies) and the drug had no apparent adverse effect on the course of pregnancy. Reports on infants born to these women reveal no adverse effects or complications attributable to gonadorelin acetate. Nevertheless, use during pregnancy only for maintenance of the corpus luteum in ovulation induction cycles.

Lactation: It is not known whether the drug is excreted in breast milk. There is no indication for use of gonadorelin acetate in a nursing woman.

Children: Safety and efficacy in children < 18 years of age have not been established.

Precautions:

Differential diagnosis: Proper diagnosis is critical for successful treatment with gonadorelin. It must be established that hypothalamic amenorrhea or hypogonadism is due to a deficiency in quantity or pulsing of endogenous GnRH. The diagnosis of hypothalamic amenorrhea or hypogonadism is based on the exclusion of other causes of the dysfunction, since there is no practical technique to directly assess hypothalamic function. Prior to initiation of therapy, rule out disorders of general health, reproductive organs, anterior pituitary and central nervous system, other than abnormalities of GnRH secretion.

Lutrepulse pump is required. Provide the patient with detailed oral and written instructions regarding infusion pump usage and potential sepsis in order to minimize the frequency of infusion pump malfunction and inflammation, infection, mild phlebitis or hematoma at the catheter site.

Monitoring: Following a diagnosis of primary hypothalamic amenorrhea, initiation of gonadorelin acetate therapy may be monitored by: Ovarian ultrasound – baseline, therapy day 7, therapy day 14; mid-luteal phase serum progesterone; clinical observation of infusion site at each visit as needed; physical examination including pelvic at regularly scheduled visits.

Drug Interactions:

Ovulation stimulators should not be used concomitantly with gonadorelin acetate.

Adverse Reactions:

Adverse reactions have been reported in approximately 10% of treatment regimens. Ten of 268 patients interrupted therapy because of an adverse reaction but subsequently resumed treatment. One other subject did not resume treatment.

Ovarian hyperstimulation: In clinical studies involving 268 women, one case of moderate ovarian hyperstimulation occurred (see Warnings).

Multiple pregnancy: In clinical studies, 11 of 89 pregnancies (12%) were multiple (10 sets of twins, 1 set of triplets). See Warnings.

Local (Use of the infusion pump): Inflammation; infection; mild phlebitis; hematoma at the catheter site.

Anaphylaxis (bronchospasm, tachycardia, flushing, urticaria, induration of injection site) has been reported with the related polypeptide hormone gonadorelin HCl *(Factrel)*. (See individual monograph in In Vivo Diagnostic Aids Section.)

Overdosage:

Continuous, non-pulsatile exposure to gonadorelin acetate could temporarily reduce pituitary responsiveness. If the pump should malfunction and deliver the entire contents of the 3.2 mg system, no harmful effects would be expected. Bolus doses as high as 3000 mcg of gonadorelin HCl have not been harmful. Pituitary hyperstimulation and multiple follicle development can be minimized by adhering to recommended doses and appropriate monitoring of follicle formation (see Warnings).

(Continued on following page)

GONADORELIN ACETATE (Cont.)

Patient Information:

Patient instructions included with kit; also includes physician package insert and pump manual.

Dosage:

Primary hypothalamic amenorrhea: 5 mcg every 90 minutes (range, 1 to 20 mcg). This is delivered by *Lutrepulse* pump using the 0.8 mg solution at 50 mcl per pulse (see physician pump manual); 68% of the 5 mcg every 90 minute regimens induced ovulation in patients with primary hypothalamic amenorrhea.

The *Lutrepulse* pump can deliver 2.5, 5, 10 or 20 mcg of gonadorelin acetate every 90 minutes. The recommended treatment interval is 21 days. Some may be refractory to this dose. It may be necessary to raise the dose cautiously, and in stepwise fashion if there is no response after three treatment intervals. Carefully monitor all dose changes for inappropriate response. Some women may require a reduction in the recommended dose of 5 mcg.

The following table can be used to individualize the dose per pulse:

Gonadorelin Acetate Dose per Pulse			
Vial	Diluent	Volume/pulse	Dose/pulse
0.8 mg	8 ml	25 mcl	2.5 mcg
0.8 mg	8 ml	50 mcl	5 mcg
3.2 mg	8 ml	25 mcl	10 mcg
3.2 mg	8 ml	50 mcl	20 mcg

The response to gonadorelin acetate usually occurs within 2 to 3 weeks after therapy initiation. When ovulation occurs with the *Lutrepulse* pump in place, continue therapy for another 2 weeks to maintain the corpus luteum. A comparison of gonadorelin acetate to hCG or hCG plus gonadorelin acetate for corpus luteum maintenance revealed the following information:

Corpus Luteum Maintenance with Gonadorelin Acetate			
	hCG (n = 63)	Gonadorelin (n = 26)	hCG plus Gonadorelin (n = 25)
Delivered	68%	73%	76%
Aborted	32%	27%	24%

Gonadorelin alone was able to maintain the corpus luteum during pregnancy.

Administration:

Gonadorelin is to be reconstituted aseptically with 8 ml of diluent for gonadorelin acetate immediately prior to use and transfered to the plastic reservoir. First withdraw 8 ml of the saline diluent and then inject it onto the lyophile (drug product) cake. Shake for a few seconds to produce a solution which should be clear, colorless, and free of particulate matter. If particulate matter or discoloration are present, the solution should not be used. A pre-sterilized reservoir (bag) with the infusion catheter set supplied with the kit is filled with the reconstituted solution and administered IV using the *Lutrepulse* pump. Set the pump to deliver 25 or 50 mcl of solution, based upon the dose selected, over a pulse period of 1 minute and at a pulse frequency of 90 minutes. The 8 ml of solution will supply 90 minute pulsatile doses for approximately 7 consecutive days.

Storage: Store at controlled room temperature (15° to 30° C; 59° to 86°F).

Rx	**Lutrepulse** (Ferring)	**Powder for Injection (lyophilized):** 0.8 and 3.2 mg	In 10 ml vials. In kits containing 10 ml diluent, catheter and tubing, four IV cannula units, syringe and needle, four alcohol swabs, elastic belt and 9V battery; also includes *Lutrepulse Pump* kit with pump, two 9V batteries, 3V lithium battery, physician pump manual and package insert.

NAFARELIN ACETATE

Actions:

Pharmacology: Nafarelin acetate is a potent agonistic analog of gonadotropin-releasing hormone (GnRH). At the onset of administration, nafarelin stimulates the release of the pituitary gonadotropins, LH and FSH, resulting in a temporary increase of ovarian steroidogenesis. Repeated dosing abolishes the stimulatory effect on the pituitary gland. Twice daily administration leads to decreased secretion of gonadal steroids by about 4 weeks; consequently, tissues and functions that depend on gonadal steroids for their maintenance become quiescent.

Pharmacokinetics: Absorption/Distribution – Nafarelin is rapidly absorbed into systemic circulation after intranasal administration. Maximum serum concentrations are achieved between 10 and 40 minutes. Following a single dose of 200 mcg base, the observed average peak concentration is 0.6 ng/ml, whereas following a single dose of 400 mcg base, the observed average peak concentration is 1.8 ng/ml. Bioavailability from a 400 mcg dose averaged 2.8%. The average serum half-life following intranasal administration is approximately 3 hours. About 80% is bound to plasma proteins.

Metabolism/Excretion – After SC administration, 44% to 55% of the dose was recovered in urine and 18.5% to 44.2% was recovered in feces. Approximately 3% of the dose appears unchanged in urine. The serum half-life of the metabolites is about 85.5 hours. The activity of the six identified metabolites, the metabolism of nafarelin by nasal mucosa, and the pharmacokinetics of the drug in patients with hepatic and renal impairment have not been determined.

Clinical trials: In controlled clinical studies, nafarelin at doses of 400 and 800 mcg/day for 6 months was comparable to danazol, 800 mg/day, in relieving the clinical symptoms of endometriosis (pelvic pain, dysmenorrhea and dyspareunia) and in reducing the size of endometrial implants as determined by laparoscopy.

Nafarelin 400 mcg daily induced amenorrhea in approximately 65%, 80% and 90% of the patients after 60, 90 and 120 days, respectively. Most of the remaining patients reported episodes of only light bleeding or spotting. In the first, second and third post-treatment months, normal menstrual cycles resumed in 4%, 82% and 100%, respectively, of those patients who did not become pregnant.

At the end of treatment, 60% of patients who received 400 mcg/day were symptom free, 32% had mild symptoms, 7% had moderate symptoms and 1% had severe symptoms. Of the 60% of patients who had complete symptom relief, 17% had moderate symptoms 6 months after treatment was discontinued, 33% had mild symptoms, 50% remained symptom free and no patient had severe symptoms.

There is no evidence that nafarelin enhances or adversely affects pregnancy rates.

Indications:

Endometriosis, including pain relief and reduction of endometriotic lesions. Experience has been limited to women ≥ 18 years of age treated for 6 months.

Contraindications:

Hypersensitivity to GnRH, GnRH-agonist analogs or any of the excipients in the product; undiagnosed abnormal vaginal bleeding; pregnancy and lactation (see Warnings).

Warnings:

Carcinogenesis and impairment of fertility: Carcinogenicity studies of nafarelin were conducted in rats (24 months) at doses up to 100 mcg/kg/day and mice (18 months) at doses up to 500 mcg/kg/day using IM doses (up to 110 times and 560 times the maximum recommended human intranasal dose, respectively). As seen with other GnRH agonists, nafarelin induced proliferative responses (hyperplasia or neoplasia) of endocrine organs. At 24 months, there was an increase in the incidence of pituitary tumors (adenoma/carcinoma) in high-dose female rats and a dose-related increase in male rats. There was an increase in pancreatic islet cell adenomas in both sexes, and in benign testicular and ovarian tumors in the treated groups. There was a dose-related increase in benign adrenal medullary tumors in treated female rats. In mice, there was a dose-related increase in Harderian gland tumors in males and an increase in pituitary adenomas in high-dose females. No metastases of these tumors were observed. It is known that tumorigenicity in rodents is particularly sensitive to hormonal stimulation.

In reproduction studies in male and female rats, full reversibility of fertility suppression occurred when drug treatment was discontinued after continuous administration for up to 6 months.

(Warnings continued on following page)

NAFARELIN ACETATE (Cont.)

Warnings (Cont.):

Hypersensitivity reactions have occurred in 0.2% of subjects or patients. Refer to Management of Acute Hypersensitivity Reactions.

Pregnancy: Category X. IM nafarelin was administered to rats throughout gestation at 0.4, 1.6 and 6.4 mcg/kg/day (about 0.5, 2 and 7 times the maximum recommended human intranasal dose). An increase in major fetal abnormalities was observed in 4/80 fetuses at the highest dose. A similar, repeat study at the same doses in rats, and studies in mice and rabbits at doses up to 600 mcg/kg/day and 0.18 mcg/kg/day, respectively, failed to demonstrate an increase in fetal abnormalities. In rats and rabbits, there was a dose-related increase in fetal mortality and a decrease in fetal weight with the highest dose. The effects on rat fetal mortality are expected consequences of the alterations in hormonal levels brought about by the drug.

Safe use of nafarelin in pregnancy has not been established clinically. Before starting treatment with nafarelin, pregnancy must be excluded. When used regularly at the recommended dose, nafarelin usually inhibits ovulation and stops menstruation. Contraception is not assured, however, by taking nafarelin, particularly if patients miss successive doses. Therefore, patients should use nonhormonal methods of contraception. Advise patients that if they miss successive doses of nafarelin, breakthrough bleeding or ovulation may occur with the potential for conception. They should see their physician if they believe they may be pregnant. If the drug is used during pregnancy or if a patient becomes pregnant during treatment, discontinue the drug and apprise the patient of the potential risk to the fetus.

Lactation: It is not known whether nafarelin is excreted in breast milk. Because the effects of nafarelin on lactation or the nursing infant have not been determined, do not give nafarelin to nursing mothers.

Children: Safety and efficacy in children have not been established.

Precautions:

Menstruation: Since menstruation should stop with effective doses of nafarelin, the patient should notify her physician if regular menstruation persists. Patients missing successive doses of nafarelin may experience breakthrough bleeding.

Bone density loss: The induced hypoestrogenic state results in a small loss in bone density over the course of treatment, some of which may not be reversible. During one 6 month treatment period, this bone loss should not be important. In patients with major risk factors for decreased bone mineral content such as chronic alcohol or tobacco use, strong family history of osteoporosis, or chronic use of drugs that can reduce bone mass such as anticonvulsants or corticosteroids, nafarelin therapy may pose an additional risk. Weigh the risks and benefits carefully before therapy with nafarelin is instituted. Repeated courses of treatment with GnRH analogs are not advisable in patients with major risk factors for loss of bone mineral content (see Adverse Reactions).

Intercurrent rhinitis patients should consult their physician for the use of a topical nasal decongestant. If the use of a topical nasal decongestant is required during treatment with nafarelin, the decongestant must be used at least 30 minutes after nafarelin dosing to decrease the possibility of reducing drug absorption.

Retreatment is not recommended since safety data beyond 6 months are not available.

Drug Interactions:

Drug/Lab test interactions: Administration of nafarelin in therapeutic doses results in suppression of the pituitary-gonadal system. Normal function is usually restored within 4 to 8 weeks after treatment is discontinued. Therefore, diagnostic tests of pituitary gonadotropic and gonadal functions conducted during treatment and up to 4 to 8 weeks after discontinuation of nafarelin therapy may be misleading.

(Continued on following page)

NAFARELIN ACETATE (Cont.)

Adverse Reactions:

As would be expected with a drug that lowers serum estradiol levels, the most frequently reported adverse reactions were those related to hypoestrogenism. In controlled studies comparing nafarelin (400 mcg/day) and danazol (600 or 800 mg/day), adverse reactions most frequently reported and thought to be drug-related are:

Adverse Reactions of Nafarelin Acetate vs Danazol (≈ %)		
Adverse Reaction	Nafarelin (n = 203)	Danazol (n = 147)
Hypoestrogenic:		
Hot flashes	90	69
Libido decrease	22	7
Vaginal dryness	19	7
Headaches	19	21
Emotional lability	15	18
Insomnia	8	4
Androgenic:		
Acne	13	20
Myalgia	10	23
Breast size reduced	10	16
Edema	8	23
Seborrhea	8	17
Weight gain	8	28
Hirsutism	2	6
Libido increased	1	6
Local:		
Nasal irritation	10	3
Miscellaneous:		
Depression	2	5
Weight loss	1	3

Other adverse reactions (< 1%): Paresthesia; palpitations; chloasma; maculopapular rash; eye pain; urticaria; asthenia; lactation; breast engorgement; arthralgia. In formal clinical trials, immediate hypersensitivity possibly or probably related to nafarelin occurred in 3 (0.2%) of 1509 patients or healthy subjects (see Warnings).

Bone density changes: After 6 months of nafarelin treatment, vertebral trabecular bone density and total vertebral bone mass decreased by an average of 8.7% and 4.3%, respectively, compared to pretreatment levels. There was partial recovery of bone density in the post-treatment period; the average trabecular bone density and total bone mass were 4.9% and 3.3% less than the pretreatment levels, respectively. Total vertebral bone mass decreased by a mean of 5.9% at the end of treatment. Mean total vertebral mass 6 months after post-treatment was 1.4% below pretreatment levels. There was little, if any, decrease in mineral content in compact bone of the distal radius and second metacarpal. Use for longer than 6 months or in the presence of other known risk factors for decreased bone mineral content may cause additional bone loss. See Precautions.

Laboratory test abnormalities: Plasma enzymes – AST and ALT levels were more than twice the upper limit of normal in only one patient each. There was no other clinical or laboratory evidence of abnormal liver function, and levels returned to normal in both patients after treatment was stopped.

Lipids – At enrollment, 9% of the patients in the nafarelin 400 mcg/day group and 2% of the patients in the danazol group had total cholesterol values > 250 mg/dl. These patients also had cholesterol values > 250 mg/dl at the end of treatment.

Of patients whose pretreatment cholesterol values were < 250 mg/dl, 6% on nafarelin and 18% on danazol had post-treatment values > 250 mg/dl.

Mean pretreatment values for total cholesterol from all patients were 191.8 mg/dl with nafarelin and 193.1 mg/dl with danazol. After treatment, mean total cholesterol values were 204.5 mg/dl with nafarelin and 207.7 mg/dl with danazol.

Triglycerides were increased above the upper limit of 150 mg/dl in 12% of the patients who received nafarelin and in 7% of the patients who received danazol.

At the end of treatment, no nafarelin patients had abnormally low HDL cholesterol fractions (< 30 mg/dl) vs 43% of danazol patients. No nafarelin patients had abnormally high LDL cholesterol fractions (> 190 mg/dl) vs 15% of those on danazol. There was no increase in the LDL/HDL ratio in nafarelin patients, but there was an approximate twofold increase in the LDL/HDL ratio in danazol patients.

Other changes (10% to 15%) – Nafarelin treatment was associated with elevations of plasma phosphorous and eosinophil counts, and decreases in serum calcium and WBC counts. Danazol therapy was associated with an increase in hematocrit and WBC.

(Continued on following page)

NAFARELIN ACETATE (Cont.)

Patient Information:

An information pamphlet for patients is included with the product.

Notify physician if regular menstruation persists. Breakthrough bleeding or ovulation may occur if successive doses are missed. Use a nonhormonal method of contraception during treatment.

Do not use if pregnant or breastfeeding, or if undiagnosed abnormal vaginal bleeding or allergies to any of the ingredients exist.

Patients with intercurrent rhinitis should consult their physician about use of a topical nasal decongestant. Use the decongestant at least 30 minutes after using nafarelin.

Administration and Dosage:

Approved by the FDA in 1990.

Endometriosis: 400 mcg/day. One spray (200 mcg) into one nostril in the morning and one spray into the other nostril in the evening. Start treatment between days 2 and 4 of the menstrual cycle.

For occasional patients with persistent regular menstruation after months of treatment, the dose of nafarelin may be increased to 800 mcg daily. The 800 mcg dose is administered as one spray into each nostril in the morning (a total of two sprays) and again in the evening.

The recommended duration of administration is 6 months. Retreatment is not recommended since safety data are not available. If symptoms of endometriosis recur after a course of therapy, and further treatment with nafarelin is contemplated, assess bone density before retreatment begins to ensure that values are within normal limits.

If the use of a topical decongestant is necessary during treatment with nafarelin, the decongestant should not be used until at least 30 minutes after nafarelin dosing.

At 400 mcg/day, a bottle of nafarelin provides a 30 day (about 60 sprays) supply. If the daily dose is increased, increase the supply to the patient to ensure uninterrupted treatment for the recommended duration of therapy.

Storage: Store upright at room temperature. Protect from light.

Rx	**Synarel** (Syntex)	**Nasal Solution:** 2 mg/ml (as nafarelin base)	In 10 ml bottle with metered spray pump.[1]

[1] With benzalkonium chloride, glacial acetic acid and sorbitol.

HISTRELIN ACETATE

Actions:

Pharmacology: Histrelin, a gonadotropin releasing hormone (GnRH or LHRH) agonist, is a potent inhibitor of gonadotropin secretion when administered daily in therapeutic doses. Histrelin contains a synthetic nonapeptide agonist of the naturally occurring gonadotropin releasing hormone. The analog possesses a greater potency than the natural sequence hormone. Following an initial stimulatory phase, chronic SC administration desensitizes responsiveness of the pituitary gonadotropin which, in turn, causes a reduction in ovarian and testicular steroidogenesis.

Although animal studies have shown that *acute* administration of histrelin results in stimulation of the reproductive system, *chronic* administration in the rat delays sexual development, inhibits estrous cyclicity and pregnancy, reduces reproductive organ weight and inhibits ovarian and testicular steroidogenesis in a reversible fashion. In the rabbit, chronic administration resulted in decreased reproductive organ weights.

In human studies, chronic administration controls the secretion of pituitary gonadotropins resulting in decreased sex steroid levels and in the regression of secondary sexual characteristics in children with precocious puberty. In girls, menses cease, serum estradiol levels are decreased to prepubertal levels, linear growth velocities decrease, skeletal maturation is slowed and adult height predictions increase. In boys, testicular steroidogenesis is inhibited and testicular volume is reduced.

Continuous administration to patients with central precocious puberty can be monitored by standard GnRH testing and by serial determinations of sex steroid levels. The decreases in LH, FSH and sex steroid levels are evident within 3 months of therapy initiation.

Indications:

For control of the biochemical and clinical manifestations of central precocious puberty. Only patients with centrally mediated precocious puberty (either idiopathic or neurogenic, and occurring before age 8 in girls or 9.5 years in boys) should receive treatment. Patients must be able to maintain compliance with a *daily* regimen of injections.

Contraindications:

Hypersensitivity to any components of the product; pregnancy, lactation (see Warnings).

Warnings:

Inadequate control: Non-compliance with drug regimen or inadequate dosing may result in inadequate control of the pubertal process. The consequences of poor control include the return of pubertal signs such as menses, breast development and testicular growth. The long-term consequences of inadequate control of gonadal steroid secretion are unknown, but may include a further compromise of adult stature.

Hypersensitivity: Serious hypersensitivity reactions (angioedema, urticaria) have been reported following histrelin administration. Clinical manifestations may include: Cardiovascular collapse; hypotension; tachycardia; loss of consciousness; angioedema; bronchospasm; dyspnea; urticaria; flushing; pruritus. If any allergic reaction occurs, discontinue therapy. Serious acute hypersensitivity reactions may require emergency medical treatment. Refer to Management of Acute Hypersensitivity Reactions.

Carcinogenesis/Impairment of fertility: Carcinogenicity studies were conducted in rats for 2 years at doses of 5, 25, or 150 mcg/kg/day (up to 15 times the human dose) and in mice for 18 months at doses of 20, 200, or 2000 mcg/kg/day (up to 200 times the human dose). As seen with other GnRH agonists, histrelin was associated with an increase in tumors of hormonally responsive tissues. There was a significant increase in pituitary adenomas in rats. There was an increase in pancreatic islet cell adenomas in treated female rats and a non-dose-related increase in testicular Leydig cell tumors (highest incidence in the low-dose group). In mice, there was a significant increase in mammary gland adenocarcinomas in all treated females. In addition, there were increases in stomach papillomas in male rats given high doses, and an increase in histiocytic sarcomas in female mice at the highest dose.

Fertility studies have been conducted in rats and monkeys given SC daily doses of histrelin up to 180 mcg/kg for 6 months and full reversibility of fertility suppression was demonstrated.

(Warnings continued on following page)

HISTRELIN ACETATE (Cont.)

Warnings (Cont.)

Pregnancy: Category X. Histrelin is contraindicated in women who are or may become pregnant while receiving the drug. There was increased fetal size and mortality in rats and increased fetal mortality in rabbits after histrelin administration. Other responses included dystocia, a greater incidence of unilateral hydroureter and incomplete ossification in rat fetuses. When administered to rabbits on days 6 to 18 of pregnancy at doses of 20 to 80 mcg/kg/day (2 to 8 times the human dose), histrelin produced early termination of pregnancy and increased fetal death. In rats given histrelin on days 7 to 20 of pregnancy at doses of 1 to 15 mcg/kg/day (0.1 to 1.5 times the human dose) there was an increase in fetal resorptions. The effects on fetal mortality are expected consequences of the alterations in hormonal levels brought about by the drug. If this drug is inadvertently used during pregnancy or in the rare event that a patient becomes pregnant while taking this drug, apprise the patient of the potential hazard to the fetus.

Lactation: It is not known if this drug is excreted in breast milk. Because of the potential for serious adverse reactions in nursing infants, do not give to nursing women.

Children: Safety and efficacy in children < 2 years of age have not been established.

Precautions:

Physical and endocrinologic evaluation: Before treatment is instituted, perform a thorough physical and endocrinologic evaluation which includes:

1. Height and weight as baseline for serial monitoring.
2. Hand and wrist x-ray for bone age determination, to document advanced skeletal age, and as baseline for serially monitoring predicted height.
3. Total sex steroid level (estradiol or testosterone).
4. Adrenal steroid level, to exclude congenital adrenal hyperplasia.
5. Beta-human chorionic gonadotropin level, to rule out a chorionic gonadotropin-secreting tumor.
6. GnRH stimulation test, to demonstrate activation of the hypothalamic-pituitary-gonadal (HPG) axis.
7. Pelvic/adrenal/testicular ultrasound, to rule out a steroid-secreting tumor and to document gonadal size for serial monitoring.
8. Computerized tomography of the head, to rule out previously undiagnosed intracranial tumor.

HGP axis reactivation: Studies in rats and monkeys have indicated that all of the known biochemical and antifertility effects of histrelin are reversible. Because children who have received histrelin have not been followed long enough to ensure reactivation of the HPG axis following long-term therapy, use histrelin only when the benefits to the patient outweigh the potential risks. In addition, advise the patient or guardian that hypogonadism may result if the HPG axis fails to reactivate after the drug is discontinued.

Monitoring: Perform an initial pelvic ultrasound to exclude other conditions before treating with histrelin. Monitor the patient carefully after 3 months and every 6 to 12 months thereafter by serial clinical evaluations, repeated height measurements, bone age determinations (yearly), and serial GnRH testing to document that gonadotropin responsiveness of the pituitary remains prepubertal while on therapy. During the initial agonistic phase of treatment, the patient may demonstrate transient increases in breast tissue, moodiness, vaginal secretions or testicular volume. After this initial agonistic phase (usually 1 to 3 weeks), control of the biochemical and physical manifestations of puberty should remain as long as chronic therapy is in effect. Discontinue treatment when the onset of puberty is desired. Following the discontinuation of treatment, document the onset of normal puberty. In addition, monitor patients to assess menstrual cyclicity, reproductive function and ultimate adult height.

Adverse Reactions:

At least one adverse experience was reported for 139 of the 183 (76%) children in clinical studies of central precocious puberty. Three of the 183 children (2%) stopped therapy due to a hypersensitivity reaction. The following reactions have occurred in patients treated for precocious puberty (n = 183) as well as various other indications (n = 196).

Cardiovascular: Vasodilation (35%); edema (2% to 3%); palpitations, tachycardia, epistaxis, hypertension, migraine headache, pallor (1% to 3%).

Endocrine: Vaginal dryness (12%); leukorrhea (2% to 6%); metrorrhagia, breast pain/edema (1% to 10%); breast discharge, decreased breast size, tenderness of female genitalia (2% to 3%); goiter, hyperlipidemia, anemia, glycosuria (1%).

GI: GI/abdominal pain, nausea, vomiting, diarrhea, flatulence, decreased appetite, dyspepsia (2% to 12%); GI cramps/distress, constipation, decreased appetite, thirst, gastritis (1% to 3%).

(Adverse Reactions continued on following page)

HISTRELIN ACETATE (Cont.)

Adverse Reactions (Cont.)

Musculoskeletal: Arthralgia, joint stiffness, muscle cramp (3% to 10%); muscle stiffness, myalgia (2% to 3%); pain, hypotonia (1%).

CNS: Headache (22%); mood changes, nervousness, dizziness, depression, libido changes, insomnia, anxiety (1% to 10%); paresthesia, cognitive changes, syncope, somnolence, lethargy, impaired consciousness, tremor, hyperkinesia, anxiety (1% to 3%); convulsions (increased frequency), hot flashes/flushes (2%); conduct disorder (1%).

Respiratory: Upper respiratory infection, pharyngitis, respiratory congestion, cough (1% to 10%); asthma, breathing disorder, rhinorrhea, bronchitis, sinusitis (2% to 3%); hyperventilation (1% to 3%).

Dermatologic: Reactions at medication site such as redness, swelling and itching (12% to 45%); acne, rash (3% to 10%); sweating (1% to 10%); urticaria (4%); keratoderma, pruritus, pain, dyschromia, alopecia (1% to 3%); erythema (1%).

Special senses: Visual disturbances (2% to 6%); ear congestion (2% to 3%); abnormal pupillary function, otalgia, hearing loss, polyopia, photophobia (1% to 3%).

GU: Vaginal bleeding (usually only one episode within 1 to 3 weeks of starting therapy lasting several days) (22%); irritation/odor/pruritus/infections/pain/hypertrophy of the female genitalia, vaginitis, dysmenorrhea (1% to 10%); dyspareunia, polyuria, dysuria, urinary frequency, incontinence, hematuria, nocturia (1% to 3%).

Miscellaneous: Pyrexia (3% to 14%); various body pains, weight gain, fatigue, viral infection (1% to 10%); chills, malaise, purpura (1% to 3%).

Hypersensitivity: Acute generalized hypersensitivity reactions (angioedema, urticaria) have occurred (see Warnings).

Overdosage:

Histrelin up to 200 mcg/kg (rats, rabbits) or 2000 mcg/kg (mice) resulted in no systemic toxicity. This represents 20 to 200 times the maximal recommended human dose of 10 mcg/kg/day.

Patient Information:

Patient information is provided in each 7 day kit.

Prior to therapy, inform patients and their families of the importance of complying with the schedule of single, *daily* injections, given at approximately the same time each day. If injections are not given daily, the pubertal process may be reactivated. Histrelin contains no preservative. Inform patients that vials are to be used once and any unused solution is to be discarded. Allow medication to reach room temperature before injecting. Rotate daily injections through different body sites (upper arms, thighs, abdomen).

Make patients aware of the required monitoring of their condition and of the potential risks of therapy. Within the first month of therapy, girls being treated with histrelin may experience a light menstrual flow. This menstrual flow is common and likely is related to the lower estrogen levels brought about by treatment, and the withdrawal of estrogen support from the endometrium.

Irritation, redness or swelling at the injection sites may occur. If these reactions are severe or do not go away, notify the physician.

Advise the patients and their families to discontinue the drug and seek medical attention at the first sign of skin rash, urticaria, rapid heartbeat, difficulty in swallowing and breathing, or any swelling which may suggest angioedema (see Warnings).

Administration and Dosage:

Approved by the FDA in December 1991.

Central precocious puberty: 10 mcg/kg given as a single, daily SC injection. If prepubertal levels of sex steroids or a prepubertal gonadotropin response to GnRH testing are not achieved within the first 3 months of treatment, reevaluate the patient. Doses > 10 mcg/kg/day have not been evaluated in clinical trials. Vary the injection site daily.

Storage/Stability: Histrelin contains no preservative. Vials are to be used once. Any unused solution is to be discarded. Store refrigerated at 2° to 8° C (36° to 46° F) and protect from light. Remove vial from packaging only at time of use. Allow vial to reach room temperature before injecting contents.

Rx	**Supprelin** (Ortho Pharm)	**Injection:** 120 mcg/0.6 ml (200 mcg/ml peptide base)	In 7 day kit of single use 0.6 ml vials.[1]
		300 mcg/0.6 ml (500 mcg/ml peptide base)	In 7 day kit of single use 0.6 ml vials.[1]
		600 mcg/0.6 ml (1000 mcg/ml peptide base)	In 7 day kit of single use 0.6 ml vials.[1]

[1] With 0.9% sodium chloride and 10% mannitol. Preservative free. With 7 syringes and needles.

DANAZOL

Actions:

Pharmacology: A synthetic androgen derived from ethisterone, danazol suppresses the pituitary-ovarian axis by inhibiting the output of pituitary gonadotropins. It also has weak, dose-related androgenic activity and is not estrogenic or progestational. Danazol depresses the output of both follicle stimulating hormone (FSH) and luteinizing hormone (LH). Danazol acts by direct enzymatic inhibition of sex steroid synthesis and competitively inhibits binding of steroids to their cytoplasmic receptors in target tissues. Generally, the pituitary suppressive action is reversible. Ovulation and cyclic bleeding usually return within 60 to 90 days after therapy is discontinued.

In endometriosis, danazol alters the normal and ectopic endometrial tissue so that it becomes inactive and atrophic. Complete resolution of endometrial lesions occurs in the majority of cases. Changes in vaginal cytology and cervical mucus reflect the suppressive effect of danazol on the pituitary-ovarian axis.

Hereditary angioedema – Danazol prevents attacks of the disease characterized by episodic edema of the abdominal viscera, extremities, face and airway. In addition, danazol partially or completely corrects the primary biochemical abnormality of hereditary angioedema. It increases the levels of the deficient C1 esterase inhibitor (C1EI), thereby increasing the serum levels of the C4 component of the complement system.

Pharmacokinetics: Blood levels of danazol do not increase proportionately with increases in dose. When the dose is doubled, plasma levels increase only about 35% to 40%.

Indications:

Endometriosis: For the treatment of endometriosis amenable to hormonal management.

Fibrocystic breast disease: Most cases of symptomatic fibrocystic breast disease may be treated by simple measures (eg, padded bras and analgesics). Pain and tenderness may be severe enough to warrant suppression of ovarian function. Danazol is usually effective in decreasing nodularity, pain and tenderness, but it alters hormone levels; recurrence of symptoms is very common after cessation of therapy.

Hereditary angioedema: For the prevention of attacks of angioedema (cutaneous, abdominal, laryngeal) in males and females.

Unlabeled Uses: Danazol has been used to treat precocious puberty, gynecomastia and menorrhagia. It has also been studied in the treatment of iodiopathic immune thrombocytopenia, lupus-associated thrombocytopenia and autoimmune hemolytic anemia.

Contraindications:

Undiagnosed abnormal genital bleeding; markedly impaired hepatic, renal or cardiac function.

Pregnancy and lactation.

Warnings:

Carcinoma of the breast should be excluded before initiating therapy for fibrocystic breast disease. Nodularity, pain and tenderness due to fibrocystic disease may prevent recognition of underlying carcinoma; therefore, if any nodule persists or enlarges during treatment, rule out carcinoma.

Long-term experience with danazol is limited. Long-term therapy with other steroids alkylated at the 17 position has been associated with serious toxicity (cholestatic jaundice, peliosis hepatis). Similar toxicity may develop after long-term danazol. Determine the lowest dose that will provide adequate protection. If the drug was begun for exacerbation of angioneurotic edema due to trauma, stress or other cause, consider decreasing or withdrawing therapy periodically.

Androgenic effects may not be reversible even when the drug is discontinued. Watch patients closely for signs of virilization.

Usage in Pregnancy: Use a nonhormonal method of contraception. If a patient becomes pregnant during treatment, discontinue use. Continuing treatment may result in androgenic effects in the fetus, which has been limited to clitoral hypertrophy and labial fusion of the external genitalia in the female fetus. If a patient becomes pregnant while taking danazol, apprise her of the potential risks to the fetus.

(Continued on following page)

DANAZOL (Cont.)

Precautions:

Fluid retention: Conditions influenced by edema (eg, epilepsy, migraine, cardiac or renal dysfunction) require careful observation.

Hepatic dysfunction has been reported; perform periodic liver function tests.

Semen should be checked for volume, viscosity, sperm count and motility every 3 to 4 months, especially in adolescents.

Drug Interactions:

Insulin requirements may increase in diabetics. Abnormal glucose tolerance tests may be seen.

Warfarin: Prolongation of prothrombin time has been reported with concomitant use.

Adverse Reactions:

Androgenic: Acne, edema, mild hirsutism, decrease in breast size, deepening of the voice, oily skin or hair, weight gain and rarely, clitoral hypertrophy or testicular atrophy.

Hypoestrogenic: Flushing, sweating, vaginitis (itching, dryness, burning and vaginal bleeding), nervousness and emotional lability.

Hepatic dysfunction (elevated serum enzymes or jaundice) has been reported in patients receiving 400 mg/day or more.

The following have been reported, but the causal relationship is not confirmed:

Allergic - Skin rashes and rare nasal congestion.

CNS - Dizziness, headache, sleep disorders, fatigue, tremor; rarely, paresthesia of extremities, visual disturbances, anxiety, depression and changes in appetite.

GI - Gastroenteritis; rarely, nausea, vomiting and constipation.

Musculoskeletal - Muscle cramps or spasms; joint lock-up, joint swelling; pain in back, neck or legs.

GU - Rarely, hematuria.

Other - Hair loss; change in libido; elevated blood pressure; chills; pelvic pain; carpal tunnel syndrome.

Patient Information:

Notify physician if masculinizing effects occur (eg, abnormal growth of facial or other fine body hair, deepening of the voice, etc).

Use nonhormonal contraceptive measures during therapy. Discontinue use if pregnancy is suspected.

Administration and Dosage:

Endometriosis: Begin therapy during menstruation or make sure the patient is not pregnant. Administer 800 mg/day in 2 divided doses to best achieve amenorrhea and rapid response to painful symptoms. Downward titration to a dose sufficient to maintain amenorrhea may be considered depending upon response. Initially, for mild cases, give 200 to 400 mg in 2 divided doses. Individualize dosage. Continue therapy uninterrupted for 3 to 6 months; may extend to 9 months. If symptoms recur after termination, treatment can be reinstituted.

Fibrocystic breast disease: Begin therapy during menstruation or make sure patient is not pregnant. Dosage ranges from 100 to 400 mg/day in 2 divided doses.

Breast pain and tenderness are usually relieved by the first month and eliminated in 2 to 3 months; elimination of nodularity requires 4 to 6 months of uninterrupted therapy. Regular or irregular menstrual patterns, and amenorrhea each occur in approximately ⅓ of patients treated with 100 mg and higher doses. Approximately 50% of patients may have recurring symptoms within 1 year; treatment may be reinstituted.

Hereditary angioedema: Individualize dosage. Recommended starting dose is 200 mg, 2 or 3 times a day. After a favorable initial response, determine continuing dosage by decreasing the dosage by 50% or less at intervals of 1 to 3 months or longer if frequency of attacks prior to treatment dictates. If an attack occurs, increase dosage by up to 200 mg/day. During the dose adjusting phase, monitor response closely, particularly if patient has a history of airway involvement.

Rx	**Danocrine** (Winthrop Pharm.)	**Capsules:** 50 mg	(#Winthrop D03 50 mg). Orange/white. In 100s.
		100 mg	(#Winthrop D04 100 mg). Yellow. In 100s.
Rx	**Danazol** (Various, eg, American Therapeutics, Geneva, Goldline, Major, Moore, Parmed, Rugby, Schein, URL)	**Capsules:** 200 mg	In 50s, 100s and 500s.
Rx	**Danocrine** (Winthrop Pharm.)		(#Danocrine Winthrop D05 200 mg). Orange. In 100s.

Product identification code.

Actions:

Somatrem and somatropin are purified polypeptide hormones of recombinant DNA origin. Somatrem contains the identical sequence of 191 amino acids constituting pituitary-derived human growth hormone plus an additional amino acid, methionine. Somatropin's amino acid sequence is identical to that of human growth hormone of pituitary origin.

Linear growth: The primary action is the stimulation of linear growth. This effect is demonstrated in patients lacking adequate endogenous growth hormone production. Somatrem and somatropin are therapeutically equivalent to endogenous growth hormone. Short-term clinical studies in normal adults show equivalent pharmacokinetics. Treatment of growth hormone deficient children results in an increase in growth rate and IGF-1 (Insulin-like Growth Factor/somatomedin-C) levels similar to that seen with human growth hormone (pituitary origin).

Skeletal growth: These agents stimulate skeletal growth in patients with growth hormone deficiency. The measurable increase in body length after administration of somatropin or human growth hormone results from its effect on the epiphyseal growth plates of long bones. Concentrations of IGF-1, which may play a role in skeletal growth, are low in the serum of growth hormone deficient children but increase during treatment. Elevations in mean serum alkaline phosphatase concentrations are seen.

Cell growths: The total number of skeletal muscle cells is markedly decreased in short-stature children lacking endogenous growth hormone compared with normal children. Treatment with growth hormone increases both the number and the size of muscle cells.

Organ growth: Growth hormone influences internal organ size and increases red cell mass.

Protein metabolism: Linear growth is facilitated in part by increased cellular protein synthesis. This is reflected by nitrogen retention as demonstrated by a decline in urinary nitrogen excretion and blood urea nitrogen (BUN) following the initiation of growth hormone therapy. Treatment with somatrem or somatropin results in a similar decline in BUN.

Carbohydrate metabolism: Children with hypopituitarism sometimes experience fasting hypoglycemia that is improved by somatropin therapy. Large doses of growth hormone may impair glucose tolerance. Administration of growth hormone to normal adults results in increased serum insulin levels. Although the precise mechanism by which these drugs induce insulin resistance is not known, it is attributed to a decrease in insulin sensitivity. An increase in serum glucose levels is observed during somatropin treatment.

Lipid metabolism: Administration of growth hormone results in reduction in body fat stores, lipid mobilization and increased plasma fatty acids.

Mineral metabolism: Retention of sodium, potassium and phosphorus induced by growth hormone administration is thought to be due to cell growth. Serum levels of inorganic phosphate increase in patients with growth hormone deficiency after somatropin or somatrem therapy due to metabolic activity associated with bone growth as well as increased tubular reabsorption of phosphate by the kidney. Serum calcium is not significantly altered. Although calcium excretion in the urine is increased, there is a simultaneous increase in calcium absorption from the intestine.

Connective tissue metabolism: Growth hormone stimulates the synthesis of chondroitin sulfate and collagen as well as the urinary excretion of hydroxyproline.

Indications:

Long-term treatment of children who have growth failure due to a lack of adequate endogenous growth hormone secretion.

Contraindications:

Subjects with closed epiphyses.

Evidence of tumor activity. Intracranial lesions must be inactive and antitumor therapy completed prior to instituting therapy. Discontinue if there is evidence of tumor activity or recurrent tumor growth.

Somatrem: Patients with sensitivity to benzyl alcohol.

Somatropin: Do not use supplied diluent in patients with sensitivity to m-cresol or glycerin (see Administration and Dosage).

Precautions:

Insulin resistance may be induced by growth hormone; observe for glucose intolerance.

Concomitant glucocorticoid therapy may inhibit growth-promoting effect. Carefully adjust the glucocorticoid replacement dose in patients with coexisting ACTH deficiency to avoid an inhibitory effect on growth.

Hypothyroidism may develop during therapy; untreated, it may prevent optimal response to therapy. Perform periodic thyroid function tests; use thyroid hormone when indicated.

Endocrine disorders (including growth hormone deficiency): Patients may develop slipped capital epiphyses more frequently. Evaluate any child with the onset of a limp or complaints of hip or knee pain during therapy.

(Continued on following page)

Adverse Reactions:

Somatrem: Approximately 30% to 40% of all patients developed persistent antibodies. In patients who had been previously treated with pituitary-derived growth hormone, one of 22 subjects developed persistent antibodies.

In general, growth hormone antibodies are not neutralizing and do not interfere with the growth response to somatrem. One of 84 subjects treated for 6 to 36 months developed antibodies associated with high binding capacities and failed to respond.

Somatropin: Approximately 2% of 481 patients developed antibodies. Nevertheless, they experienced increases in linear growth without any unusual adverse events. Although growth-limiting antibodies have been observed with other growth hormone preparations (including products of pituitary origin), antibodies in patients treated with somatropin have not limited growth.

Of the 232 patients receiving somatropin for ≥ 6 months, 4.7% had serum binding of radiolabeled growth hormone in excess of twice the binding observed in control sera. In comparison, 74.5% of 106 patients treated for ≥ 6 months with somatrem in a similar trial had serum binding of radiolabeled growth hormone of at least twice that of the binding observed in control sera.

In any patient who fails to respond to therapy, evaluate compliance with the treatment program and thyroid status, and test for antibodies to growth hormone.

Infrequent in healthy adults: Headache; localized muscle pain; weakness; mild hyperglycemia; glucosuria; mild, transient edema (2.5%) early during treatment.

Leukemia has occurred in a small number of children receiving human growth hormone, somatropin or somatrem; the relationship, however, is uncertain.

Overdosage:

Acute overdosage could lead initially to hypoglycemia and subsequently to hyperglycemia. Long-term overdosage could result in signs and symptoms of acromegaly consistent with the known effects of excess human growth hormone.

SOMATREM

Administration and Dosage:

Individualize dosage. Up to 0.1 mg/kg (0.26 IU/kg) SC or IM, 3 times per week is recommended. Because of potential side effects, do not exceed this dosage.

Preparation of Solution: Reconstitute each 5 mg vial with 1 to 5 ml of Bacteriostatic Water for Injection, USP (Benzyl Alcohol Preserved) only. *DO NOT SHAKE. Do not inject* if solution is cloudy. Use a small enough syringe so that the prescribed dose can be drawn from the vial with reasonable accuracy. Use a needle of sufficient length (≥ 1 inch) to ensure that the injection reaches the muscle layer.

Newborns – Benzyl alcohol as a preservative has been associated with toxicity. When administering to newborns, reconstitute with Water for Injection. Use only one dose per vial; discard the unused portion. The pH after reconstitution is ≈ 7.8.

Store at 2°-8°C (36°-46°F). Use reconstituted vials in 7 days. Avoid freezing.

Rx	**Protropin** (Genentech)	**Powder for Injection (lyophilized):** 5 mg (≈ 13 IU) per vial[1]	In cartons of 2 vials and a 10 ml vial of diluent.[2]
		10 mg (≈ 26 IU) per vial	In cartons of 2 vials and 2 10 ml vials of diluent.[2]

SOMATROPIN

Administration and Dosage:

Individualize dosage. Up to 0.06 mg/kg (0.16 IU/kg) SC or IM, 3 times/week is recommended.

Preparation of solution: Reconstitute each 5 mg vial with 1.5 to 5 ml of diluent. *DO NOT SHAKE. Do not inject* if solution is cloudy or contains particulate matter. After reconstitution, each vial contains ≈ 2 mg somatropin/ml solution. Use a small enough syringe so that the prescribed dose can be drawn from the vial with reasonable accuracy.

If sensitivity to the diluent occurs, the vials may be reconstituted with Sterile Water for Injection, USP. When reconstituted in this manner, (1) use only one reconstituted dose per vial, (2) refrigerate the solution (36° to 46°F; 2° to 8°C) if it is not used immediately after reconstitution, (3) use the reconstituted dose within 24 hours, and (4) discard the unused portion.

Storage: Before reconstitution – Vials and diluent are stable when refrigerated at 2° to 8°C (36° to 46°F). Avoid freezing the diluent.

After reconstitution – Reconstituted vials are stable for up to 14 days stored in a refrigerator at 2° to 8°C (36° to 46°F). Avoid freezing.

Rx	**Humatrope** (Lilly)	**Powder for Injection (lyophilized):** 5 mg (≈ 13 IU) per vial	In vials[3] with 5 ml diluent.[4]

[1] With 40 mg mannitol.
[2] Bacteriostatic Water for Injection with benzyl alcohol.
[3] With 25 mg mannitol and 5 mg glycine.
[4] Water for Injection with 0.3% m-cresol and 1.7% glycerin.

ARGININE HCl

Actions:

Infusion IV often induces a pronounced rise in the plasma level of human growth hormone (HGH) in subjects with intact pituitary function. This rise is usually diminished or absent in patients with impairment of this function.

Indications:

Indicated as an IV stimulant to the pituitary for the release of HGH in patients where the measurement of pituitary reserve for HGH can be of diagnostic usefulness. It can be used as a diagnostic aid in such conditions as panhypopituitarism, pituitary dwarfism, chromophobe adenoma, postsurgical craniopharyngioma, hypophysectomy, pituitary trauma, acromegaly, gigantism and problems of growth and stature.

If the insulin hypoglycemia test has indicated a deficiency of pituitary reserve for HGH, a test with arginine is advisable to confirm the negative response. As patients may not respond during the first test, the unresponsive patient should be tested again to confirm the negative result. A second test can be performed after a waiting period of 1 day. Some patients who respond to arginine do not respond to insulin and vice versa. The rate of false positive responses is approximately 32%, and the rate of false negatives is approximately 27%.

Contraindications:

Persons having highly allergic tendencies.

Warnings:

Always administer by IV injection because of arginine's hypertonicity.

Hypersensitivity: Have a suitable antihistaminic drug available in case of an allergic reaction. Refer to Management of Acute Hypersensitivity Reactions on p. 2897.

Arginine is a diagnostic aid and not intended for therapeutic use.

Precautions:

Excessive infusion rates may result in local irritation and flushing, nausea or vomiting. Inadequate dosing or prolongation of the infusion period may diminish the stimulus to the pituitary and nullify the test.

Arginine has a high content of metabolizable nitrogen; consider the temporary effect of a high load of nitrogen upon the kidneys when administered.

The chloride ion content is 47.5 mEq/100 ml of solution; consider the effect of infusing this amount of chloride into patients with electrolyte imbalance before the test is undertaken.

Invert and inspect each bottle before use to be sure that the contents are clear. Discard any flask in which the contents are not clear or which lacks a vacuum.

Basal and poststimulation levels of growth hormone are elevated in patients who are pregnant or who are taking oral contraceptives.

Adverse Reactions:

Approximately 3% of the patients reported nonspecific side effects consisting of nausea, vomiting, headache, flushing, numbness and local venous irritation.

One patient had an allergic reaction which was manifested as a confluent macular rash with reddening and swelling of the hands and face. The rash subsided rapidly after the infusion was terminated and 50 mg diphenhydramine was administered. One patient had an apparent decrease in platelet count from 150,000 to 60,000. One patient with a history of acrocyanosis had an exacerbation of this condition following infusion.

(Continued on following page)

ARGININE HCl (Cont.)

Administration and Dosage:

Administer IV.

Dose:

Adults – 300 ml.

Children – 5 ml/kg body weight.

Test procedure: For successful administration of the test for measurement of pituitary reserve of human growth hormone, clinical conditions and procedures should be as follows:

1. Schedule the test in the morning following a normal night's sleep, and the overnight fast should continue through the test period. Place patient at bed rest, and for at least 30 minutes before the infusion begins, take care to minimize apprehension and distress. This is particularly important in children.

2. Infuse through an indwelling needle or soft catheter placed in an antecubital vein or other suitable vein. Take blood samples by venipuncture from the contra-lateral arm. A desirable schedule for drawing blood samples is at –30, 0, 30, 60, 90, 120, and 150 minutes. Promptly centrifuge blood samples and store the plasma at –20° until assayed by one of the published radioimmunoassay procedures.

3. Infuse arginine beginning at zero time at a uniform rate which will permit the recommended dose to be administered in 30 minutes.

Interpretation of results:

Infusion IV often induces a pronounced rise in the plasma level of human growth hormone (HGH) in subjects with intact pituitary function. This rise is usually diminished or absent in patients with impairment of this function.

Expected Plasma Levels of HGH in ng/ml		
Patient	Control Range	Range of Peak Response to Arginine
Normal	0-6	10-30
Pituitary deficient	0-4	0-10

These ranges are based on the mean values of plasma HGH levels calculated from the data of several clinical investigators and reflect their experiences with various methods of radioimmunoassay. Upon gaining experience with this diagnostic test, each clinician will establish his own ranges for control and peak levels of HGH.

Diagnostic test results showing a deficiency of pituitary reserve for HGH should be confirmed by a second test with arginine, or confirmed with the insulin hypoglycemia test. A waiting period of 1 day is advised between tests.

Rx	**R-Gene 10** (KabiVitrum)	**Injection:** 10% arginine HCl (950 mOsm/L). In 500 ml.[1]

[1] With 47.5 mEq chloride ion per 100 ml.

OCTREOTIDE ACETATE

Actions:

Pharmacology: Octreotide acetate is a long-acting octapeptide with pharmacologic actions mimicking those of the natural hormone somatostatin. In normal subjects, octreotide acetate suppresses secretion of serotonin and the gastroenteropancreatic peptides: Gastrin, vasoactive intestinal peptide, insulin, glucagon, secretin, motilin and pancreatic polypeptide. In addition, octreotide acetate suppresses growth hormone. In animals, it is a more potent inhibitor of growth hormone, glucagon and insulin release than natural somatostatin with greater selectivity for growth hormone and glucagon suppression. Octreotide, like somatostatin, decreases splanchnic blood flow.

Pharmacokinetics: Absorption/Distribution – After SC injection, octreotide is absorbed rapidly and completely from the injection site. Peak concentrations of 5.5 ng/ml (100 mcg dose) were reached 0.4 hours after dosing. Relative to an equivalent IV dose, the bioavailability of an SC dose was 80% to 135%. Peak concentrations and area under the curve values were dose proportional both after SC or IV single doses up to 400 mcg and with multiple doses of 200 mcg 3 times daily (600 mcg/day). Clearance was reduced by about 66% suggesting nonlinear kinetics of the drug at daily doses of 600 mcg/day as compared to 150 mcg/day.

The distribution of octreotide from plasma was rapid (alpha half-life = 0.2 h) and the volume of distribution was estimated to be 13.6 L. In blood, the distribution into the erythrocytes was found to be negligible and about 65% was bound in the plasma in a concentration-independent manner. Binding was mainly to lipoprotein and, to a lesser extent, to albumin.

Metabolism/Excretion – The elimination of octreotide from plasma had an apparent half-life of 1.5 hours compared with 1 to 3 minutes with the natural hormone. The duration of action is variable but extends up to 12 hours depending upon the type of tumor. About 32% of the dose is excreted unchanged in the urine.

In patients with severe renal failure requiring dialysis, clearance was reduced to about half that found in normal subjects (from approximately 10 to 4.5 L/h). The effect of hepatic diseases on the disposition of octreotide is unknown.

Indications:

Carcinoid Tumors: Symptomatic treatment of patients with metastatic carcinoid tumors where it suppresses or inhibits the associated severe diarrhea and flushing episodes.

Vasoactive Intestinal Peptide Tumors (VIPomas): Treatment of the profuse watery diarrhea associated with VIP-secreting tumors. Significant improvement has been noted in the overall condition of these otherwise therapeutically unresponsive patients. Therapy with octreotide results in improvement in electrolyte abnormalities, (eg, hypokalemia), often enabling reduction of fluid and electrolyte support.

Data are insufficient to determine whether the drug decreases size, rate of growth, or development of metastases in patients with these tumors. Octreotide acetate was used in patients ranging in age from 1 month to 83 years without any drug limiting toxicity.

Contraindications:

Sensitivity to this drug or any of its components.

Warnings:

Cholelithiasis: Octreotide therapy, like the natural hormone, somatostatin, may be associated with cholelithiasis, presumably by altering fat absorption and possibly by decreasing the motility of the gallbladder. Because patients with somatostatinomas have been reported to be at risk for these dysfunctions, monitor patients periodically for gallbladder disease. Surgical intervention has been required in a few patients who developed severe, abdominal pain associated with cholelithiasis.

Evaluate patients on extended therapy with baseline and periodic ultrasound evaluations of the gallbladder and bile ducts.

Usage in renal impairment: In patients with severe renal failure requiring dialysis, the half-life of the drug may be increased, necessitating adjustment of the maintenance dosage.

Usage in Pregnancy: Category B. Reproduction studies have been performed in rats and rabbits at doses up to 30 times the highest human dose and have revealed no evidence of impaired fertility or harm to the fetus. There are, however, no adequate and well controlled studies in pregnant women. This drug should be used during pregnancy only if clearly needed.

Usage in Lactation: It is not known whether this drug is excreted in breast milk. Exercise caution when octreotide acetate is administered to a nursing woman.

Usage in Children: The youngest patient to receive the drug was 1 month old. Doses of 1 to 10 mcg/kg body weight were well tolerated in the young patients. A single case of an infant (nesidioblastosis) was complicated by a seizure thought to be independent of octreotide acetate therapy.

(Continued on following page)

Actions:

Posterior pituitary secretions include oxytocin and vasopressin, polypeptides containing eight amino acids. Oxytocin is formed primarily in the paraventricular nuclei and vasopressin in the supraoptic nuclei of the hypothalamus. They are then transported in combination with a carrier protein, neurophysin, down to nerve endings in the posterior pituitary gland where they accumulate. Under appropriate stimuli, the hormones are released from the nerve endings and are absorbed into adjacent capillaries.

Posterior Pituitary Injection has both oxytocic and vasopressor activity. Posterior pituitary powder is obtained from the clean, dried posterior lobe of the pituitary of domesticated animals used for food by man. It contains both antidiuretic hormone (ADH) and oxytocin.

Vasopressin exhibits its most marked activity on the renal tubular epithelium, where it promotes the resorption of water (antidiuretic hormone effect) and the contraction of smooth muscles throughout the vascular bed (vasopressor effects). Vasoconstriction is marked in the portal and splanchnic vessels, somewhat less in peripheral, coronary, cerebral, and pulmonary vessels, and slight in the intrahepatic vessels. Vasopressin, and to a lesser extent, oxytocin, tends to enhance GI motility and tone.

Neurogenic or central diabetes insipidus is a disorder of water metabolism that results from a partial or complete deficiency in the production and secretion of vasopressin from the neurohypophysis. Nephrogenic or peripheral diabetes insipidus results from an insensitivity of the renal tubules to the action of antidiuretic hormone. Vasopressin and its synthetic analogs are the principal treatment of neurogenic diabetes insipidus, but are ineffective in treating the nephrogenic variant.

Vasopressin is a purified form of the posterior pituitary, having only pressor and antidiuretic hormone (ADH) activity. Vasopressin may be obtained from natural sources or by chemical synthesis. The synthetic derivatives, lypressin and desmopressin, act principally as ADH, possessing little pressor activity, and are relatively free of oxytocic activity. Desmopressin has a longer duration of action.

Oxytocin exerts its most marked activity in inducing uterine muscle contraction and inducing contraction of the lacteal glands, which results in milk ejection in lactating women. Uterine motility is controlled by a variety of biochemical and regulatory processes including cAMP, calcium, prostaglandins and oxytocin. The mechanism of oxytocin-facilitated smooth muscle contraction is poorly understood. The sensitivity of the uterus to oxytocin increases gradually during gestation, then increases sharply before parturition.

Naturally derived oxytocin is no longer commercially available, having been replaced by synthetic oxytocin. Oxytocin is most frequently used to induce or improve uterine contractions in labor. The ergot derivatives (ergonovine and methylergonovine) are also used for their oxytocic effects on the uterine muscle. These agents are most appropriately used to prevent postpartum uterine atony and hemorrhage.

Individual products of this group are summarized in the following table:

	Indications	Route	Concentration
Posterior Pituitary	Postoperative ileus Surgical hemostatis Enuresis of Diabetes Insipidus	Parenteral	20 u/ml
Vasopressin Derivatives			
Vasopressin	Diabetes Insipidus Postop. abdominal distention	Parenteral	20 u/ml
Vasopressin tannate	Diabetes Insipidus	Parenteral	5 u/ml (oil)
Lypressin	Diabetes Insipidus	Nasal spray	0.185 mg/ml
Desmopressin	Diabetes Insipidus	Nasal Parenteral	0.1 mg/ml 4 mcg/ml
Oxytocics[1]			
Oxytocin	Initiate/augment labor 2nd trimester abortion Postpartum hemorrhage	Parenteral	10 u/ml
	Initial milk let-down	Nasal	40 u/ml
Ergonovine	Postpartum/postabortal hemorrhage Migraine headache	Oral Parenteral	0.2 mg 0.2 mg/ml
Methylergonovine	Postpartum/postabortal hemorrhage	Oral Parenteral	0.2 mg 0.2 mg/ml

[1] Other agents with oxytocic effects on the uterus used to induce abortion are discussed under Abortifacients.

Refer to the general discussion of these products on page 435.

POSTERIOR PITUITARY INJECTION

Indications:

To control postoperative ileus; stimulate expulsion of gas prior to pyelography.

In surgery, used as an aid to achieve hemostasis. In the presence of esophageal varices, this drug may promote hemostasis and adjunctively treat accompanying shock. Not suitable for routine use in the treatment of surgical shock.

May be useful in treating enuresis of diabetes insipidus, but such treatment is not curative.

Contraindications:

Toxemia of pregnancy; cardiac disease; hypertension; epilepsy; advanced arteriosclerosis.

Do not use as an oxytocic. Injection before or during labor carries a high risk of inducing severe fetal distress, asphyxia neonatorum or rupture of the uterus.

Warnings:

Anaphylaxis, angioneurotic edema and urticaria may occur.

Coronary insufficiency and cardiac arrhythmias may be induced by this drug; this risk is enhanced in patients under barbiturate sedation or cyclopropane anesthesia.

Precautions:

The pressor effects of this agent result from constriction of the vascular bed and increased peripheral resistance. This activity is accompanied by decreased cardiac output and diminished coronary blood flow; thus, the underlying condition responsible for shock may be aggravated.

Drug Interactions:

Carbamazepine and chlorpropamide, which are known to potentiate ADH, may potentiate the antidiuretic effects of posterior pituitary hormones.

Adverse Reactions:

Most common: Facial pallor; increased GI activity; uterine cramps.

Blindness, unconsciousness, tinnitus, anxiety, proteinuria, eclampsia, mydriasis and diarrhea have also occurred.

Administration and Dosage:

Administer by injection, preferably IM.

Usual dose – 10 units SC or IM (range: 5 to 20 units).

Rx	**Pituitrin (S)** (Parke-Davis)	**Injection:** 20 units/ml	In 1 ml ampuls.[1]

[1] With 0.5% chlorobutanol.

Refer to the general discussion of these products on page 435.

VASOPRESSIN (8-Arginine-Vasopressin)

Possesses vasopressor and antidiuretic hormone (ADH) activity. Following IM or SC injection, the duration of antidiuretic activity for vasopressin aqueous solution is 2 to 8 hours. When administered IM, vasopressin tannate has a duration of action of 48 to 96 hours. Most is metabolized and rapidly destroyed in liver and kidneys. Both vasopressin aqueous solution and vasopressin tannate have a plasma half-life of about 10 to 20 minutes. After 4 hours, about 5% of an SC dose is excreted unchanged in urine.

Indications:

Neurogenic diabetes insipidus.

Vasopressin aqueous solution is also used in the prevention and treatment of postoperative abdominal distention, and in abdominal roentgenography to dispel interfering gas shadows.

Unlabeled Use: Vasopressin infusions (IV or selective intraarterial) are used to manage bleeding esophageal varices using a dosage of 0.2 units/min initially, increased to 0.4 units/min if bleeding continues. Maximum recommended dose is 0.9 units/min.

Contraindications:

Anaphylaxis or hypersensitivity to vasopressin or its components.

Warnings:

Do not administer vasopressin tannate IV.

Use with extreme caution in patients with vascular disease (especially coronary artery disease) since even small doses may precipitate anginal pain; with larger doses, consider the possibility of MI.

Vasopressin may produce water intoxication. Early signs of drowsiness, listlessness and headaches precede terminal coma and convulsions.

Severe vasoconstriction and local tissue necrosis may result if vasopressin extravasates during IV infusion. Gangrene of the extremities, tongue necrosis and ischemic colitis may occur during vasopressin therapy of esophageal varices.

Chronic nephritis with nitrogen retention contraindicates use until reasonable nitrogen blood levels have been attained.

Hypersensitivity: Local or systemic allergic reactions may occur in hypersensitive individuals (see Adverse Reactions). Anaphylaxis (cardiac arrest or shock) has been observed shortly after injection. Refer to Management of Acute Hypersensitivity Reactions on p. viii.

Usage in Pregnancy: Category C. It is not known whether vasopressin causes fetal harm when administered to a pregnant woman or affects reproductive capacity. Administer to a pregnant woman only if clearly needed.

Usage in Labor and Delivery: Doses sufficient for an antidiuretic effect are not likely to produce tonic uterine contractions that could be harmful to fetus or threaten the continuation of the pregnancy.

Usage in Lactation: Exercise caution when giving to a nursing woman.

Precautions:

Use vasopressin cautiously in the presence of epilepsy, migraine, asthma, heart failure or any state in which a rapid increase in extracellular water may result in further compromise.

Electrocardiograms and fluid and electrolyte status determinations are recommended at intervals during therapy.

Carbamazepine and **chlorpropamide,** which are known to potentiate ADH, may potentiate the effects of vasopressin.

Adverse Reactions:

Allergic reactions: Tremor; sweating; vertigo; cardiac arrest; circumoral pallor; "pounding" in head; abdominal cramps; passage of gas; nausea; vomiting; urticaria and bronchial constriction (see Warnings).

Vasopressin tannate administration may cause sterile abscesses.

Overdosage:

Treat water intoxication with water restriction and temporary withdrawal of vasopressin until polyuria occurs.

Severe water intoxication may require osmotic diuresis with mannitol, hypertonic dextrose, or urea alone or with furosemide.

Patient Information:

Side effects such as skin blanching, abdominal cramps and nausea may be reduced by taking one or two glasses of water with dose. These side effects usually are not serious and will probably disappear within a few minutes.

(Continued on following page)

Refer to the general discussion of these products on page 435.

VASOPRESSIN (8-Arginine-Vasopressin) (Cont.)

Administration and Dosage:

May be given IM or SC.

Five to ten units usually elicit full physiologic response in adult patients. Give IM at 3 or 4 hour intervals as needed. Reduce dosage proportionately for children.

Diabetes insipidus: Intranasal – Administer intranasally on cotton pledgets, by nasal spray or dropper. Individualize dosage.

Parenteral – 5 to 10 units 2 or 3 times daily as needed.

Abdominal distention: To prevent or relieve postoperative distention, give 5 units initially; increase to 10 units at subsequent injections, if necessary. Give IM at 3 or 4 hour intervals. Reduce dosage proportionately for children. These recommendations also apply to distention complicating pneumonia or other acute toxemias.

Abdominal roentgenography: Administer 2 injections of 10 units each. Give 2 hours and half an hour, respectively, before films are exposed. An enema may be given prior to first dose.

Rx	**Pitressin Synthetic** (Parke-Davis)	**Injection:** 20 pressor units/ml	In 0.5 or 1 ml ampuls.[1]

VASOPRESSIN TANNATE

Administration and Dosage:

Never administer IV.

Shake ampul thoroughly before use to obtain a uniform suspension. Contents of the ampuls may show a cloudiness or colorless crystals of solid fats from the peanut oil vehicle. If this occurs, warm the ampuls to dissolve the solid fats. Warming will also facilitate transfer of product form ampul to syringe.

Administer 0.3 to 1 ml IM; repeat as required. The duration of action varies with the patient and condition, and ranges from 48 to 96 hours.

Rx	**Pitressin Tannate In Oil** (Parke-Davis)	**Injection:** 5 pressor units/ml	In 1 ml ampuls.[2]

[1] With 0.5% chlorobutanol.
[2] In peanut oil.

Refer to the general discussion of these products on page 435.

LYPRESSIN (8-Lysine Vasopressin)

A synthetic lysine vasopressin analog which possesses antidiuretic activity with little vasopressor or oxytocic effect. The onset of antidiuretic effect is prompt, peaks in 30 to 120 minutes, and has a duration of 3 to 8 hours.

Indications:

For the control or prevention of the symptoms and complications of neurogenic diabetes insipidus (including polydipsia, polyuria and dehydration). Useful in patients who have become unresponsive to other therapy or who experience local or systemic reactions, allergic reactions or other undesirable effects (eg, excessive fluid retention) from preparations of animal origin.

Warnings:

Pregnancy: Safety for use during pregnancy is not established. Use only when clearly needed and when potential benefits outweigh potential hazards to the fetus.

Precautions:

Cardiovascular pressor effects are minimal or absent when administered as a nasal spray in therapeutic doses. Nevertheless, use cautiously when such effects would be undesirable; mild blood pressure elevation has been noted in unanesthetized subjects who received IV lypressin. Large doses intranasally may cause coronary artery constriction; use caution in treating patients with coronary artery disease.

Effectiveness may decrease in the presence of nasal congestion, allergic rhinitis and upper respiratory infections because of decreased absorption by the nasal mucosa; larger doses or adjunctive therapy may be required.

Test patients with known sensitivity to antidiuretic hormones.

Drug Interactions:

Carbamazepine and **chlorpropamide,** which are known to potentiate ADH, may potentiate the antidiuretic effects of lypressin.

Adverse Reactions:

Reactions have been infrequent and mild.

Local: Rhinorrhea; nasal congestion; irritation and pruritus of the nasal passages; nasal ulceration; periorbital edema with itching.

Systemic: Headache; conjunctivitis; heartburn secondary to excessive intranasal administration; abdominal cramps and increased bowel movements. Inadvertent inhalation has resulted in substernal tightness, coughing and transient dyspnea. Overdosage has caused marked, but transient fluid retention. Tolerance or tachyphylaxis has not been reported. Hypersensitivity manifested by a positive skin test has occurred.

Patient Information:

Review administration technique with patient. Spray into nostril(s) as directed.

To ensure that a uniform, well diffused spray is delivered, the bottle should be held upright and the patient should be in a vertical position with head upright.

Notify physician if drowsiness, listlessness, headache, shortness of breath, heartburn, nausea, abdominal cramps, or severe nasal congestion or irritation occurs.

Administration and Dosage:

Administer 1 or 2 sprays to one or both nostrils whenever frequency of urination increases or significant thirst develops. One spray provides approximately 2 Posterior Pituitary (Pressor) Units. The usual dosage for adults and children is 1 or 2 sprays into each nostril 4 times daily. An additional bedtime dose helps eliminate nocturia not controlled with regular daily dosage. For patients requiring more than 2 sprays per nostril every 4 to 6 hours, reduce the time between doses rather than increase the number of sprays at each dose. More than 2 or 3 sprays in each nostril is usually wasted; the unabsorbed excess will drain posteriorly (by way of the nasopharynx) into the digestive tract where it will be inactivated.

The spray permits individualization of dosage necessary to control the symptoms of diabetes insipidus. Patients quickly learn to regulate dosage in accordance with their degree of polyuria and thirst; once determined, daily requirements remain fairly stable for months or years. Dosage has ranged from 1 spray per day at bedtime to 10 sprays into each nostril every 3 to 4 hours. Larger doses may represent greater severity of disease or other phenomena, such as poor nasal absorption. Large doses may also be due to the presence of mixed hypothalamic-hypophyseal and nephrogenic diabetes insipidus; the latter condition being unresponsive to administration of antidiuretic hormone.

Rx	**Diapid** (Sandoz)	**Nasal Spray:** 0.185 mg lypressin (equivalent to 50 USP Posterior Pituitary [Pressor] Units)/ml	In 8 ml bottles.[1]

[1] With methyl and propyl parabens, sorbitol solution, glycerin and chlorobutanol.

Refer to the general discussion of these products on page 435.

DESMOPRESSIN ACETATE (1-Deamino-8-D-Arginine Vasopressin)

A synthetic analog of arginine vasopressin, the naturally occurring human antidiuretic hormone (ADH). Provides a prompt onset of action with a long duration. The antidiuretic action is more specific and more prolonged than that of the natural hormone or lypressin. A single dose of desmopressin produces an antidiuretic effect that persists for 8 to 20 hours. Desmopressin acetate injection has an antidiuretic effect about 10 times that of an equivalent intranasal dose. Urine volume is reduced and urine osmolality is increased. Vasopressor and oxytocic activity are not noted at normal therapeutic dosages.

Desmopressin produces a dose-related increase in factor VIII levels. The increase is rapid, becoming evident within 30 minutes and peaking in 90 to 120 minutes. The factor VIII-related antigen and ristocetin cofactor activity are also increased to a smaller degree. Biphasic half-lives of desmopressin acetate are 7.8 and 75.5 minutes for the fast and slow phases, respectively, compared with 2.5 and 14.5 minutes for lypressin. Plasminogen activator activity increases rapidly after IV infusion, but clinically significant fibrinolysis has not occurred.

Indications:

DDAVP:

Primary nocturnal enuresis (intranasal only) – May be used alone or adjunctive to behavioral conditioning or other nonpharmacological intervention. It is effective in some cases that are refractory to conventional therapies.

Central cranial diabetes insipidus (intranasal and parenteral) – ADH replacement therapy in the management of central cranial (neurogenic) diabetes insipidus and for temporary polyuria and polydipsia following head trauma or surgery in the pituitary region. *Ineffective* for the treatment of nephrogenic diabetes insipidus.

Hemophilia A (parenteral only) with factor VIII levels > 5%. Desmopressin will often maintain hemostasis in patients with hemophilia A during surgery and postoperatively when administered 30 minutes prior to procedure. The drug will also stop bleeding in hemophilia A patients with episodes of spontaneous or trauma-induced injuries such as hemarthroses, IM hematomas or mucosal bleeding.

Not indicated for the treatment of hemophilia A with factor VIII levels ≤ 5%, for the treatment of hemophilia B or in patients who have factor VIII antibodies. Some patients with factor VIII levels between 2% to 5% may be treatable.

Von Willebrand's disease (Type I) (parenteral only) – Mild to moderate classic von Willebrand's disease (Type I) with factor VIII levels > 5%. Hemostasis in these patients can often be maintained during surgery and postoperatively when the drug is administered 30 minutes prior to the procedure. Episodes of spontaneous or trauma-induced injuries such as hemarthroses, IM hematomas or mucosal bleeding can usually be stopped.

Patients who are least likely to respond are those with severe homozygous von Willebrand's disease with factor VIII coagulant activity, factor VIII antigen and von Willebrand's factor (ristocetin cofactor) activities < 1%. Other patients may respond in a variable fashion, depending on the type of molecular defect.

Not indicated for the treatment of severe classic von Willebrand's disease (Type I) and when an abnormal molecular form of factor VIII antigen is evident.

Concentraid: For renal concentration capacity testing which is used to determine the capacity of the kidneys to concentrate urine.

The test records renal tubular function over time in patients with renal disease and those exposed to certain drugs that may reduce the renal concentrating ability of the kidney. The test provides an aid to the diagnosis of renal disease.

Unlabeled uses: Intranasal – Treatment of hemophilia A and in certain types of von Willebrand's disease; treatment of chronic autonomic failure (eg, nocturnal polyuria, overnight weight loss, morning postural hypotension).

Contraindications:

Hypersensitivity to desmopressin acetate.

Warnings:

Caution very young and elderly patients to ingest only enough fluid to satisfy thirst to decrease the potential occurrence of water intoxication and hyponatremia.

Do not use to treat Type IIB von Willebrand's disease; platelet aggregation may be induced.

Pregnancy: Category B. No studies have been performed in pregnant women. Safety and efficacy for use during pregnancy has not been established. Use only when clearly needed and when the potential benefits outweigh the hazards to the fetus.

Lactation: Safety for use in nursing mothers has not been established. In one patient, little if any change occurred in breast milk following a 10 mcg intranasal dose. Exercise caution when administering desmopressin to a nursing woman.

(Warnings continued on following page)

Refer to the general discussion of these products on page 435.

DESMOPRESSIN ACETATE (1-Deamino-8-D-Arginine Vasopressin) (Cont.)

Warnings (Cont.):

Children: Infants and children require careful fluid intake restriction to prevent possible hyponatremia and water intoxication. Do not use desmopressin injection in infants < 3 months old in the treatment of hemophilia A or von Willebrand's disease. Safety and efficacy of desmopressin have not been established in children < 12 years of age (parenteral) or < 3 months of age (intranasal) with diabetes insipidus.

Intranasal desmopressin has been used in children with diabetes insipidus. If intranasal desmopressin is used in the very young, adjust the dose individually, with attention to the danger of an extreme decrease in plasma osmolality with resulting convulsions. Initiate doses at ≤ 0.05 ml.

Precautions:

High dosage has infrequently produced a slight elevation of blood pressure which disappeared with dosage reduction. Use with caution in patients with coronary artery insufficiency or hypertensive cardiovascular disease.

Changes in the nasal mucosa (eg, scarring, edema, discharge, blockage, congestion, severe atrophic rhinitis), cranial surgery (eg, transphenoidal hypophysectomy) and nasal packing compromise intranasal delivery; consider administering IV.

Monitoring therapy:

Diabetes insipidus – Monitor urine volume and osmolality and plasma osmolality.

Hemophilia A – Determine factor VIII coagulant activity before injecting desmopressin for hemostasis; if the activity is $< 5\%$ of normal, do not rely on desmopressin. Other tests to assess patient status include levels of factor VIII coagulant, factor VIII antigen and ristocetin cofactor, and activated partial thromboplastin time (APTT).

Von Willebrand's disease – Assess levels of factor VIII coagulant, factor VIII antigen and ristocetin cofactor. Skin bleeding time may also be helpful.

Although desmopressin pressor activity is very low, use large intranasal doses or parenteral doses as large as 0.3 mcg/kg cautiously with other pressor agents.

There are reports of an occasional change in response to intranasal desmopressin with time, usually > 6 months. Some patients may show a decreased responsiveness, others a shortened duration of effect. There is no evidence this effect is due to the development of binding antibodies but may be due to a local inactivation of the peptide.

Drug Interactions:

Carbamazepine and **chlorpropamide,** which are known to potentiate ADH, may potentiate the antidiuretic effects of desmopressin.

Adverse Reactions:

DDAVP: High dosages have produced transient headache, rhinitis, nausea, mild abdominal cramps, vulval pain, slight elevation of blood pressure and facial flushing. These symptoms disappear with dosage reduction. Injection of desmopressin acetate has produced local erythema, swelling or burning pain.

Concentraid: Three cases of symmetrical convulsions due to water retention and resultant hyponatremia occurred in 200 infants administered the test without restricted fluid intake. These effects did not occur when fluid intake was restricted by 50%. An additional case of water intoxication occurred in an infant with a congenital heart defect. Headache, nausea, vomiting, palpitations, shortness of breath and yawning have occurred infrequently.

Overdosage:

Symptoms may include headache, abdominal cramps, nausea and facial flushing. Reduce the dosage, decrease the frequency of administration or withdraw the drug according to the severity of the condition. There is no known specific antidote.

Patient Information:

Patient instructions provided with intranasal product; review administration with patient.

Notify physician if headache, shortness of breath, heartburn, nausea, abdominal cramps or vulval pain occurs.

Administration and Dosage:

Primary nocturnal enuresis: Individualize dosage. Initial dose (≥ 6 years of age) – 20 mcg (0.2 ml) intranasally at bedtime. Adjustment up to 40 mcg is suggested if the patient does not respond. Some patients may respond to 10 mcg and adjustment to that lower dose may be done if the patient has shown a response to 20 mcg. It is recommended that one-half of the dose be administered per nostril. Adequately controlled studies have not been conducted beyond 4 to 8 weeks.

(Administration and Dosage continued on following page)

Refer to the general discussion of these products on page 435.

DESMOPRESSIN ACETATE (1-Deamino-8-D-Arginine Vasopressin) (Cont.)

Administation and Dosage (Cont.):

Central cranial diabetes insipidus: Intranasal – The nasal tube delivery system is supplied with a flexible calibrated plastic tube (rhinyle). Draw solution into the rhinyle. Insert one end of tube into nostril; blow on the other end to deposit solution deep into nasal cavity. The nasal spray pump may also be used.

Adults: Usual dosage range – 0.1 to 0.4 ml daily, either as a single dose or divided into 2 or 3 doses. Most adults require 0.2 ml daily in 2 divided doses. Adjust morning and evening doses separately for an adequate diurnal rhythm of water turnover.

Children (3 months to 12 years): Usual dosage range – 0.05 to 0.3 ml daily, either as a single dose or divided into 2 doses.

Parenteral – Administer SC or by direct IV injection.

Adults: Usual range – 0.5 to 1 ml daily, in 2 divided doses, adjusted separately for an adequate diurnal rhythm of water turnover. For patients switching from intranasal to IV, the comparable IV antidiuretic dose is about 1⁄10 the intranasal dose. Estimate response by adequate sleep duration and adequate, not excessive, water turnover.

Hemophilia A and von Willebrand's disease (Type I): Administer 0.3 mcg/kg diluted in sterile physiologic saline; infuse IV slowly over 15 to 30 minutes. In adults and children weighing > 10 kg, use 50 ml of diluent; in children weighing ≤ 10 kg, use 10 ml. Monitor blood pressure and pulse during infusion. If used preoperatively, administer 30 minutes prior to the procedure.

Determine the necessity for repeat dose or use of any blood products for hemostasis by laboratory response and patient's clinical condition. Consider the tendency toward tachyphylaxis with repeating dose more than every 48 hours.

The nasal spray pump can only deliver doses of 0.1 ml (10 mcg) or multiples of 0.1 ml. If doses other than these are required, the nasal tube delivery system may be used.

Renal concentration capacity testing:

Adults – The test can be given at any time during the day. The usual adult dose is 40 mcg of desmopressin acetate (20 mcg in each nostril). The urine voided within 1 hour after drug administration is discarded. The two subsequent urines collected within 8 hours after administration are saved and tested for osmolality. Tell patients to drink only small amounts of fluid during the test day.

Children (12 months to 12 years) – Restrict fluid intake in children undergoing this test to avoid water retention. The test is administered in the morning as 20 mcg of desmopressin acetate (contents of one pipet) intranasally. Osmolality or specific gravity is measured on the samples passed over the next 3 to 5 hours.

The reference level for normal urine osmolality after administration is 800 mOsm/kg for children, ages 3 to 12 years, and is age-related for young children, ages 1 to 3 years. The reference levels after administration in healthy adults has been determined with a more limited number of subjects and decreases with age. Urine osmolality following testing, even when combined with partial fluid restriction, may vary more than values obtained after more prolonged fluid restriction alone. When values obtained with the test are under the age-related reference level, repeat the test. A similar low result on repeat testing may suggest an impaired ability to concentrate urine; refer the patient for further examination to determine the underlying cause of the abnormality. Erratic absorption in subjects with or without evident changes in the condition of the nasal mucosa may compromise test results. From studies, a falsely abnormal test result may be obtained in up to 13% of cases.

Storage: Refrigerate both nasal solution and injection at 4°C (39°F). Nasal solution will maintain stability for up to 3 weeks when stored at room temperature (22°C; 72°F)

	Product	Form	Supply
Rx	**Concentraid** (Ferring Labs)	**Nasal Solution:** 0.1 mg per ml (0.1 mg equals 400 IU arginine vasopressin)	In disposable intranasal pipets containing 20 mcg per 2 ml.
Rx	**DDAVP** (Rorer)		*Nasal spray pump:* In 5 ml bottle[1] with spray pump (50 doses of 10 mcg each).
			Nasal tube delivery system: In 2.5 ml vials[1] with applicator tubes.
Rx	**DDAVP** (Rorer)	**Injection:** 4 mcg per ml	In 1 ml amps.[1]

[1] With 5 mg chlorobutanol per ml.

Refer to the general discussion of these products on page 435.

OXYTOCIN

Important Note:
Oxytocin is indicated for the medical rather than the elective induction of labor. Available data and information are inadequate to define the benefit-to-risk considerations in the use of oxytocin for elective induction.

Actions:

Pharmacology: Oxytocin, an endogenous hormone produced in the posterior pituitary gland, has uterine stimulant properties, especially on the gravid uterus, as well as vasopressive and antidiuretic effects. Its exact role in normal labor and medically-induced labor is not fully understood. However, it may act primarily on uterine myofibril activity, thus augmenting the number of contracting myofibrils. The sensitivity of the uterus to oxytocin increases gradually during gestation and increases sharply before parturition.

Oxytocin has weak antidiuretic effects, but has led to fatal water intoxication. It also has a definite but transient relaxing effect on vascular smooth muscle.

Pharmacokinetics: Oxytocin is given parenterally and intranasally; however, the latter may be erratically absorbed. The plasma half-life of synthetic oxytocin is 1 to 6 minutes, but this decreases in late pregnancy and lactation. Following IV administration, uterine response occurs almost immediately and subsides within 1 hour. Uterine response after IM injection is within 3 to 5 minutes and persists for 2 to 3 hours. Steady-state plasma levels and the maximum uterine contractile response are reached in approximately 40 minutes using doses in the therapeutic range. Elimination is through the liver, kidneys and functional mammary gland and by the enzyme oxytocinase.

Indications:

Oxytocin (parenteral):

Antepartum – To initiate or improve uterine contractions to achieve early vaginal delivery, for fetal or maternal reasons, such as Rh problems, maternal diabetes, preeclampsia at or near term, when delivery is in the best interest of mother and fetus, or when membranes are prematurely ruptured and delivery is indicated; stimulation or reinforcement of labor, as in selected cases of uterine inertia; management of inevitable or incomplete abortion. In the first trimester, curettage is generally considered primary therapy. In second trimester abortion, oxytocin infusion is often successful in emptying the uterus. Other means of therapy, however, may be required in such cases.

Postpartum – To produce uterine contractions during the third stage of labor and to control postpartum bleeding or hemorrhage.

Oxytocin (nasal): For initial milk let-down.

Unlabeled Uses: Antepartum fetal heart rate testing (oxytocin challenge test); breast engorgement.

Contraindications:

Significant cephalopelvic disproportion; unfavorable fetal positions or presentations which are undeliverable without conversion prior to delivery (eg, transverse lies); in obstetrical emergencies where the benefit-to-risk ratio for either the fetus or the mother favors surgical intervention; cases of fetal distress where delivery is not imminent; prolonged use in uterine inertia or severe toxemia; hypertonic or hyperactive uterine patterns; where adequate uterine activity fails to achieve satisfactory progress; induction or augmentation of labor where vaginal delivery is contraindicated, such as invasive cervical carcinoma, active herpes genitalis, cord presentation or prolapse, total placenta previa and vasa previa; hypersensitivity to the drug.

Oxytocin (nasal) is contraindicated in pregnancy.

Warnings:

When used for induction or stimulation of labor, administer oxytocin only by the IV route. All patients receiving IV oxytocin must be under continuous observation to identify complications. A qualified physician should be immediately available.

Except in unusual circumstances, do not administer oxytocin in the following conditions: Fetal distress; partial placenta previa; prematurity; borderline cephalopelvic disproportion; previous major surgery on the cervix or uterus including cesarean section; overdistention of the uterus; grand multiparity; history of uterine sepsis; traumatic delivery; invasive cervical carcinoma. The decision can only be made by weighing the potential benefits which oxytocin can provide in a given case against rare but definite potential for the drug to produce hypertonicity or tetanic spasm.

Cyclopropane anesthesia may modify oxytocin's cardiovascular effects, producing unexpected results such as hypotension. Concomitant use of oxytocin with cyclopropane anesthesia can cause maternal sinus bradycardia with abnormal atrioventricular rhythms.

(Warnings continued on following page)

OXYTOCIN (Cont.)

Warnings (Cont.)

Maternal deaths due to hypertensive episodes, subarachnoid hemorrhage, rupture of the uterus, *fetal deaths* due to various causes and *infant brain damage* have been associated with the use of parenteral oxytocic drugs for induction of labor or for augmentation in the first and second stages of labor.

Pregnancy: No known indications for use in the first trimester exist other than in relation to spontaneous or induced abortion. Oxytocin is not expected to present a risk of fetal abnormalities when used as indicated (see Adverse Reactions in the fetus).

Lactation: Oxytocin may be found in small quantities in breast milk. If a postpartum dosage is required to control severe bleeding, nursing should not commence until the day after oxytocin has been discontinued.

Children: Oxytocin is not intended for use in children.

Precautions:

Uterine contractions: When properly administered, oxytocin stimulates uterine contractions similar to those in normal labor. Overstimulation of the uterus can be hazardous to both mother and fetus. Even with proper administration and supervision, hypertonic contractions can occur in a patient whose uterus is hypersensitive to oxytocin.

Water intoxication: Oxytocin has an intrinsic antidiuretic effect, acting to increase water reabsorption from the glomerular filtrate. Consider the possibility of water intoxication, particularly when oxytocin is administered by continuous infusion and the patient is receiving fluids by mouth.

Evaluate pelvic adequacy and maternal and fetal conditions when using oxytocin for induction or reinforcement of already existent labor.

Drug Interactions:

Sympathomimetics: If used concurrently with oxytocic drugs, the pressor effect of the sympathomimetics may be increased, possibly resulting in postpartum hypertension.

Severe hypertension occurred when oxytocin was given 3 to 4 hours following prophylactic administration of a vasoconstrictor in conjunction with caudal block anesthesia.

Adverse Reactions:

Maternal: Anaphylactic reaction; postpartum hemorrhage; cardiac arrhythmia; fatal afibrinogenemia; nausea; vomiting; premature ventricular contractions; increased blood loss; pelvic hematoma. Excessive dosage or hypersensitivity to the drug may result in uterine hypertonicity, spasm, tetanic contraction or rupture of the uterus. Severe water intoxication with convulsions and coma has occurred, associated with a slow oxytocin infusion over a 24 hour period. Maternal death due to oxytocin-induced water intoxication has occurred.

Fetal: Bradycardia, premature ventricular contractions and other arrhythmias, permanent CNS or brain damage and death have been caused by uterine motility. Use of oxytocin in the mother has caused low Apgar scores at 5 minutes, and neonatal jaundice and retinal hemorrhage have occurred.

Overdosage:

Overdosage depends on uterine hyperactivity. Hyperstimulation with hypertonic or tetanic contractions, or a resting tone of $\geq$ 15 to 20 mm H_2O between contractions can lead to tumultuous labor, uterine rupture, cervical and vaginal lacerations, postpartum hemorrhage, uteroplacental hypoperfusion, and variable deceleration of fetal heart, fetal hypoxia, hypercapnia or death. Water intoxication with convulsions is a serious complication that may occur if large doses (40 to 50 ml/min) are infused for long periods. To treat, discontinue drug, restrict fluid intake, initiate diuresis, administer IV hypertonic saline solution, correct electrolyte imbalance, control convulsions with judicious use of a barbiturate and provide special nursing care for the comatose patient.

(Products listed on following pages)

Complete prescribing information for these products begins on page 443.

OXYTOCIN, PARENTERAL

Administration and Dosage:

Determine dosage by uterine response.

Induction or stimulation of labor:

IV infusion (drip method) – This is the only acceptable method of administration for the induction or stimulation of labor. Accurate control of infusion flow is essential. An infusion pump or other device and frequent monitoring of strength, frequency and duration of contractions, resting uterine tone and fetal heart rate are necessary. If uterine contractions become too powerful, the infusion can be abruptly stopped; oxytocic stimulation of the uterine musculature will soon wane.

Start an IV infusion of non-oxytocin-containing solution. Use physiologic electrolyte solution, except under unusual circumstances.

Dosage – The initial dose should be no more than 1 to 2 mU/min (0.001 to 0.002 units/min). Gradually increase the dose in increments of no more than 1 to 2 mU/min at 15 to 30 minute intervals until a contraction pattern has been established which is similar to normal labor. Maximum doses should rarely exceed 20 mU/minute.

Discontinue the oxytocin infusion immediately in the event of uterine hyperactivity or fetal distress and administer oxygen to the mother, who should be put in a lateral position.

Control of postpartum uterine bleeding:

IV infusion (drip method) – Add 10 to 40 units to a maximum of 40 units to 1000 ml of a nonhydrating diluent and run at a rate necessary to control uterine atony.

IM – Administer 10 units after delivery of the placenta.

Treatment of incomplete or inevitable abortion: IV infusion of 10 units of oxytocin with 500 ml physiologic saline solution, or 5% dextrose in physiologic saline solution infused at a rate of 10 to 20 mU (20 to 40 drops) per minute.

Reconstitution: Add 1 ml (10 units) to 1000 ml of 0.9% aqueous Sodium Chloride or other IV fluid. The solution contains 10 mU/ml (0.01 units/ml). Use a constant infusion pump to accurately control the rate of infusion. Do not exceed 30 units in a 12 hour period due to risk of water intoxication.

IV solution compatibility: At a concentration of 5 U/L, oxytocin is physically compatible with the most commonly used Dextrose, Sodium Chloride and Ringer's solutions, as well as combinations of these solutions.

Oxytocin is rapidly decomposed in the presence of sodium bisulfite.

	Product	Form	How supplied	C.I.*
Rx	**Oxytocin** (Various)	**Injection:** 10 units per ml	In 1 ml amps and 1 and 10 ml vials.	24+
Rx	**Oxytocin** (Wyeth)		In 1 ml Tubex.	78
Rx	**Pitocin** (Parke-Davis)		In 0.5 and 1 ml amps,[1] 1 ml Steri-Dose syringe[1] and 10 ml Steri-Vial.[1]	48
Rx	**Syntocinon** (Sandoz)		In 1 ml amps.[2]	68

OXYTOCIN, SYNTHETIC, NASAL

Administration and Dosage:

Initial milk let-down: One spray into one or both nostrils 2 to 3 minutes before nursing or pumping of breasts.

Hold the squeeze bottle upright when administering the drug to the nose; the patient should be sitting rather than lying down. If preferred, the solution can be instilled in drop form by inverting the squeeze bottle and exerting gentle pressure.

	Product	Form	How supplied	C.I.*
Rx	**Syntocinon** (Sandoz)	**Nasal Spray:** 40 units/ml	In 2 and 5 ml squeeze bottles.[3]	103

* Cost Index based on cost per 10 units.

[1] With 0.5% chlorobutanol.

[2] With 0.5% chlorobutanol and 0.61% alcohol.

[3] With glycerin, sorbitol solution, chlorobutanol and methyl and propyl parabens.

Refer to the general discussion of these products on page 435.

ERGONOVINE MALEATE

Actions:

Pharmacology: When used after placental delivery, ergonovine increases the strength, duration and frequency of uterine contractions and decreases uterine bleeding. It exerts its effects by acting as a partial agonist or antagonist at α-adrenergic, dopaminergic and tryptaminergic receptors.

Pharmacokinetics: Ergonovine has a rapid onset of action which varies with the route of administration: IV – 40 seconds; IM – 7 to 8 minutes; oral – 10 minutes. Uterine contractions continue for 3 or more hours after injection.

Indications:

Prevention and treatment of postpartum and postabortal hemorrhage due to uterine atony.

Unlabeled Uses: Used diagnostically to identify Prinzmetal's angina (variant angina). Doses of 0.05 to 0.2 mg IV during coronary arteriography provoke spontaneous coronary arterial spasms responsible for Prinzmetal's angina, reversible with nitroglycerin. Arrhythmias, ventricular tachycardia and myocardial infarction have been precipitated.

Administered parenterally, ergonovine is generally not as effective as ergotamine in the treatment of migraine headache; however, ergonovine may be more useful than ergotamine when use of ergotamine has caused paresthesias.

Contraindications:

Induction of labor; cases of threatened spontaneous abortion; previous allergic or idiosyncratic reactions to the drug.

Warnings:

Parenteral use: Patients have been injured, and some have died because of the injudicious use of oxytocic agents. Hyperstimulation of the uterus during labor may lead to uterine tetany with marked impairment of the uteroplacental blood flow, uterine rupture, cervical and perineal lacerations, amniotic fluid embolism and trauma to the infant (eg, hypoxia, intracranial hemorrhage).

In some calcium-deficient patients, the uterus may not respond to ergonovine. Responsiveness can be immediately restored by cautious IV injection of calcium salts. Do not give calcium IV to patients receiving digitalis.

Oxytoxic agents must be administered under meticulous observation.

Usage in Lactation: Ergonovine may lower prolactin levels, which may decrease lactation.

Precautions:

Because of the high uterine tone produced, ergonovine is not recommended for routine use prior to the delivery of the placenta, unless the surgeon is familiar with the technique described by Davis and others.

Avoid prolonged use. Discontinue if symptoms of ergotism appear.

Use cautiously in patients with hypertension, heart disease, venoatrial shunts, mitral-valve stenosis, obliterative vascular disease, sepsis, hepatic or renal impairment.

Observe the character and amount of vaginal bleeding.

Laboratory tests: Monitor blood pressure, pulse and uterine response. Note sudden changes in vital signs or frequent periods of uterine relaxation.

Adverse Reactions:

GI: Nausea and vomiting may occur, but are uncommon.

Allergic phenomena including shock.

Postpartum use of ergotrates has been associated with rare cases of myocardial infarction.

Ergotism (acute ergotism is described in Overdosage).

Blood pressure elevation (sometimes extreme) and headache appear in a small percentage of patients; this is most frequently associated with regional anesthesia (caudal or spinal), previous use of a vasoconstrictor, and the IV administration of the oxytocic, but it may occur in the absence of these factors. The mechanism of such hypertension is obscure. The elevations are no more frequent with ergonovine than with other oxytocics. They usually subside promptly following 15 mg IV chlorpromazine.

(Continued on following page)

ERGONOVINE MALEATE (Cont.)

Overdosage:

Symptoms: The principal manifestations of serious overdosage are convulsions (acute) and gangrene (chronic). Acute symptoms include: Nausea, vomiting, diarrhea, rise or fall in blood pressure, weak pulse, dyspnea, loss of consciousness, numbness and coldness of the extremities, tingling, chest pain, gangrene of the fingers and toes, hypercoagulability, confusion, excitement, delirium, hallucinations, convulsions and coma.

Treatment: Delay absorption of ingested drug by giving tap water, milk or activated charcoal, then remove by gastric lavage or emesis followed by catharsis. Treat convulsions. Control hypercoagulability by administering heparin, and maintain blood-clotting time at approximately three times normal; give a vasodilator as an antidote. Nitroglycerin (sublingual or IV) is used for coronary vasospasm. Intravenous or intraarterial nitroprusside is the drug of choice for severe vasospasm. Gangrene may require surgical amputation.

Patient Information:

May cause nausea, vomiting, dizziness, increased blood pressure, headache, ringing in the ears, chest pain or shortness of breath.

Administration and Dosage:

Parenteral: Intended primarily for IM injection. It usually produces a firm contraction of the uterus within a few minutes.

The usual IM (or emergency IV) dose is 0.2 mg. Severe uterine bleeding may require repeated doses, but rarely more than one injection per 2 to 4 hours.

Administration IV produces a quicker response. However, because of the higher incidence of side effects, confine the IV route to emergencies such as excessive uterine bleeding.

Oral: To minimize late postpartum bleeding, 1 or 2 tablets may be given every 6 to 12 hours until danger of uterine atony has passed, usually 48 hours. Severe cramping is evidence of effectiveness, but may justify reduction in dosage. Tablets may be administered sublingually.

				C.I.*
Rx	**Ergonovine Maleate** (Various)	**Tablets:** 0.2 mg	In 1000s.	1+
Rx	**Ergotrate Maleate** (Lilly)	**Injection:** 0.2 mg per ml[1]	In 1 ml ampuls.	60
		Tablets: 0.2 mg	In 100s, 1000s and UD 100s.	10

* Cost Index based on cost per 0.2 mg.
# Product identification code.
[1] With 0.1% ethyl lactate and 0.25% phenol.

Refer to the general discussion of these products on page 435.

METHYLERGONOVINE MALEATE

Actions:

Increases the strength, duration and frequency of uterine contractions and decreases uterine bleeding following placental delivery. It induces a rapid and sustained tetanic uterotonic effect which shortens the third stage of labor and reduces blood loss.

Pharmacokinetics: The onset of action after IV administration is immediate; after IM administration, 2 to 5 minutes, and after oral administration, 5 to 10 minutes.

A 0.2 mg IV injection is rapidly distributed from plasma to peripheral tissues within an α-phase half-life of $\leq$ 2 to 3 minutes. The β-phase elimination half-life is $\geq$ 20 to 30 minutes, but clinical effects continue for about 3 hours.

IM injection of 0.2 mg afforded peak plasma concentrations of over 3 mg/ml at time to reach maximum concentrations of 30 minutes. After 2 hours, total plasma clearance was 120 to 240 ml/min.

After oral administration, bioavailability was reported as 60% with no cumulation after repeated doses. Bioavailability increased to 78% during delivery with parenteral injection.

Excretion is rapid and appears to be partially renal and partially hepatic. Whether the drug is able to penetrate the blood/brain barrier has not been determined.

Indications:

Routine management after delivery of the placenta; postpartum atony and hemorrhage; subinvolution.

Under full obstetric supervision, it may be given in the second stage of labor following delivery of the anterior shoulder.

Contraindications:

Hypertension; toxemia; pregnancy; hypersensitivity.

Warnings:

This drug should not be routinely administered IV because it may induce sudden hypertension and cerebrovascular accidents. If IV administration is considered essential, give slowly over no less than 60 seconds, with careful blood pressure monitoring.

Usage in Pregnancy: Category C. It is not known whether methylergonovine maleate can cause fetal harm or affect reproductive capacity. Use is contraindicated during pregnancy (see Indications).

Usage in Labor and Delivery: The uterotonic effect of methylergonovine maleate is used after delivery to assist involution and decrease hemorrhage, shortening the third stage of labor. Also use with caution during the second stage of labor. The necessity for manual removal of a retained placenta should occur only rarely with proper technique and adequate allowance of time for its spontaneous separation.

Usage in Lactation: Methylergonovine maleate may be given orally for a maximum of 1 week postpartum to control uterine bleeding. Recommended dosage is one 0.2 mg tablet 3 or 4 times daily. At this dosage level, a small quantity of drug appears in the patient's milk. Adverse effects have not been described, but exercise caution when methylergonovine maleate is administered to a nursing woman.

Precautions:

Exercise caution in the presence of sepsis, obliterative vascular disease, hepatic or renal involvement.

Methylergonovine has not been shown to alter prolactin levels; however, consider this possibility.

Adverse Reactions:

Nausea; vomiting; hypertension; dizziness; headache; tinnitus; diaphoresis; palpitations; temporary chest pain; dyspnea.

(Continued on following page)

METHYLERGONOVINE MALEATE (Cont.)

Overdosage:

Symptoms: Acute overdose may include nausea, vomiting, abdominal pain, numbness, tingling of the extremities, rise in blood pressure. In severe cases, these are followed by hypotension, respiratory depression, hypothermia, convulsions and coma. Because reports of overdosage are infrequent, the lethal dose in humans has not been established. Several cases of accidental methylergonovine maleate injection in newborn infants have been reported, and in such cases 0.2 mg represents an overdose of great magnitude. However, recovery occurred in all but one case following a period of respiratory depression, hypothermia, hypertonicity with jerking movements, and, in one case, a single convulsion.

Also, several children 1 to 3 years of age have accidentally ingested up to ten tablets (2 mg) with no apparent ill effects. A postpartum patient took four tablets at one time in error and reported paresthesias and clamminess as her only symptoms.

Treatment of acute overdosage is symptomatic and includes the usual procedures of inducing emesis, gastric lavage, catharsis and supportive diuresis; maintaining adequate pulmonary ventilation, especially if convulsions or coma develop; correcting hypotension with pressor drugs as needed; controlling convulsions with standard anticonvulsant agents; controlling peripheral vasospasm with warmth to the extremities if needed.

Patient Information:

May cause nausea, vomiting, dizziness, increased blood pressure, headache, ringing in the ears, chest pain or shortness of breath.

Administration and Dosage:

IM: 0.2 mg after delivery of the placenta, after delivery of the anterior shoulder, or during the puerperium. Repeat as required, at intervals of 2 to 4 hours.

IV: (See Warnings). Dosage same as for IM use.

Orally: 0.2 mg 3 or 4 times/day in the puerperium for a maximum of 1 week.

				C.I.*
Rx	**Methergine** (Sandoz)	**Injection:** 0.2 mg per ml[1]	In 1 ml ampuls.	67
		Tablets: 0.2 mg	(#Sandoz 78-54). Orchid rose. In 100s, 1000s and UD 100s.	12

* Cost Index based on cost per 0.2 mg.
# Product identification code.
[1] With 0.25 mg tartaric acid.

RITODRINE HCl

Actions:

Pharmacology: Ritodrine is a β-receptor agonist, which exerts a preferential effect on β_2-adrenergic receptors such as those in the uterine smooth muscle. Stimulation of the β_2 receptors inhibits contractility of the uterine smooth muscle through the cycle of adenyl cyclase stimulation, which increases intracellular cyclic adenosine 3′-5′-monophosphate (cAMP); this leads to altering cellular calcium balance that affects smooth muscle contractility. In addition, ritodrine may directly affect the interaction between the actin and myosin of muscle through inhibition of myosin light-chain kinase.

Infusions of 0.05 to 0.3 mg/min IV or single oral doses of 10 to 20 mg decrease the intensity and frequency of uterine contractions. These effects are antagonized by β-adrenergic blocking compounds. Administration IV induces an immediate dose-related elevation of heart rate (maximum mean increase 19 to 40 beats/minute) and widening of the pulse pressure. The average increase in systolic blood pressure is 4 mm Hg, and the average decrease in diastolic pressure is 12.3 mm Hg. With oral intake, the increase in heart rate is mild and delayed.

During IV infusion, transient elevations of blood glucose, insulin and free fatty acids have been observed. Decreased serum potassium has also been found.

Pharmacokinetics: Food may inhibit the efficacy of ritodrine. The drug crosses the placenta at 20% to 100% of maternal serum concentrations. The remainder of ritodrine's pharmacokinetics (determined in nonpregnant volunteers) are summarized below:

Route	Bioavailability	Peak Serum Levels (ng/ml)	Time to Peak Serum Levels (minutes)	Half-life			Percent[1] Eliminated in Urine in 24 hours	Protein Binding
				Distribution Phase (minutes)	Second Phase (hours)	Elimination Phase (hours)		
IV[2]	100%	32-50		6-9	1.7-2.6	15-17	90	32%
Oral[3]	30%	5-15	20-60		1.3	12-20	71-90	

[1] Primarily as metabolites. [2] 60 minute infusion of 9 mg. [3] Oral dose of 10 mg.

Indications:

Management of preterm labor in suitable patients. Institute therapy as soon as the diagnosis of preterm labor is established and contraindications are ruled out in pregnancies of 20 or more weeks gestation. The safety and efficacy in advanced labor (cervical dilatation more than 4 cm or effacement more than 80%) have not been established.

Contraindications:

Before the 20th week of pregnancy and in those conditions in which continuation of pregnancy is hazardous to the mother or fetus. Specifically: Antepartum hemorrhage which demands immediate delivery; eclampsia and severe preeclampsia; intrauterine fetal death; chorioamnionitis; maternal cardiac disease; pulmonary hypertension; maternal hyperthyroidism; uncontrolled maternal diabetes mellitus.

Preexisting maternal medical conditions that would be seriously affected by the pharmacologic properties of a betamimetic drug. These include hypovolemia, cardiac arrhythmias associated with tachycardia or digitalis intoxication, uncontrolled hypertension, pheochromocytoma and bronchial asthma already treated by betamimetics or steroids.

Known hypersensitivity to any component of the product.

Warnings:

Mild to moderate preeclampsia, hypertension or diabetes: Do not administer to patients with these disorders unless the benefits clearly outweigh the risks.

Maternal pulmonary edema has been reported in patients treated with ritodrine, sometimes after delivery. It has occurred more often when patients were treated concomitantly with corticosteroids; however, maternal death from this condition has been reported with or without corticosteroids. Closely monitor patients and avoid fluid overload. Fluid loading IV may be aggravated by the use of betamimetics, with or without corticosteroids, and may result in circulatory overload with subsequent pulmonary edema. If pulmonary edema develops, discontinue use and manage edema by conventional means.

Cardiovascular responses are common and more pronounced during IV administration; monitor these effects, including maternal pulse rate and blood pressure, fetal heart rate and maternal signs and symptoms of pulmonary edema. A persistent tachycardia (over 140 beats/minute) or persistent tachypnea (respiratory rate over 20/minute) may be signs of impending pulmonary edema. Occult cardiac disease may be unmasked with the use of ritodrine. If the patient complains of chest pain or tightness of chest, temporarily discontinue the drug and perform an ECG.

(Warnings continued on following page)

RITODRINE HCl (Cont.)

Warnings (Cont.):

Usage in Pregnancy: Category B. There are no adequate and well controlled studies of the drug's effects in pregnant women before 20 weeks gestation; **therefore, do not use this drug before the 20th week of pregnancy.**

Ritodrine crosses the placenta and appears in cord blood at 20% to 100% of maternal serum levels, but studies of pregnant women from gestation week 20 have not shown increased risk of fetal abnormalities. Follow-up of children for up to 2 years has not shown harmful effects on growth, or developmental or functional maturation, but the possibility cannot be excluded. Use only when clearly indicated. Fetal adverse effects occur, including tachycardia (up to 200 bpm), hyperglycemia or hypoglycemia (depending on administration time before delivery) and ketoacidosis with fetal death.

Infants born before 36 weeks gestation make up less than 10% of all births, but account for as many as 75% of perinatal deaths and 50% of all neurologically handicapped infants. By delaying or preventing preterm labor, the drug should cause an overall increase in neonatal survival.

Precautions:

Migraine headache: Transient cerebral ischemia associated with β-sympathomimetic therapy has been reported in two patients with migraine headaches.

When used to manage preterm labor in a patient with premature rupture of membranes, balance benefits of delaying delivery against risk of developing chorioamnionitis.

Among low birth weight infants, $\approx$ 9% may be growth retarded for gestational age. Therefore, consider intrauterine growth retardation (IUGR) in the differential diagnosis of preterm labor, especially when the gestational age is in doubt. The decision to continue or reinitiate administration will depend on an assessment of fetal maturity.

Laboratory Tests: Administration of ritodrine IV elevates plasma **insulin** and **glucose** and decreases plasma **potassium** concentrations; monitor glucose and electrolyte levels during protracted infusions. Decrease of plasma potassium concentrations is usually transient, returning to normal within 24 hours. Pay special attention to biochemical variables when treating diabetic patients or those receiving potassium-depleting diuretics. Serial hemograms may be helpful as an index of state of hydration.

Baseline ECG should be performed to rule out occult maternal heart disease.

Sulfites: Sulfites may cause serious allergic-type reactions (eg, hives, itching, wheezing, anaphylaxis) in certain susceptible persons. Although the overall incidence of sulfite sensitivity in the general population is probably low, it is seen more frequently in asthmatics or in atopic nonasthmatic persons. Specific products containing sulfites are identified in the product listings.

Drug Interactions:

Corticosteroids used concomitantly may lead to pulmonary edema (see Warnings).

Sympathomimetic amines: The effects when administered with ritodrine may be additive or potentiated. A sufficient time interval should elapse prior to administration of another sympathomimetic drug.

Magnesium sulfate, diazoxide, meperidine and **potent general anesthetics:** Cardiovascular effects of ritodrine (especially cardiac arrythmias or hypotension) may be potentiated by concomitant use.

Atropine: Systemic hypertension may be exaggerated with parasympatholytics.

β-adrenergic blockers inhibit the action of ritodrine; avoid coadministration.

(Continued on following page)

RITODRINE HCl (Cont.)

Adverse Reactions:

Unwanted effects of ritodrine are usually controllable through dosage adjustment.

Parenteral:

Usual (80% to 100%) cardiovascular effects – Dose-related alterations in maternal and fetal heart rates and in maternal blood pressure. With a maximum infusion rate of 0.35 mg/min, the maximum maternal and fetal heart rates averaged, respectively, 130 (range 60 to 180) and 164 (range 130 to 200) beats/minute. The maximum maternal systolic blood pressures averaged an increase of 12 mm Hg from pretreatment levels. The minimum maternal diastolic blood pressures averaged a decrease of 23 mm Hg from pretreatment levels. In less than 1% of patients, persistent maternal tachycardia or decreased diastolic blood pressure required drug withdrawal. Persistent tachycardia (> 140 beats/minute) may indicate impending pulmonary edema (see Warnings).

Infusion is associated with transient elevation of *blood glucose* and *insulin,* which decreases to normal after 48 to 72 hours despite continued infusion. Elevation of free fatty acids and cAMP has been reported. Expect reduced *potassium* levels.

Frequent effects – Palpitations (33%), tremor, nausea, vomiting, headache or erythema (10% to 15%).

Occasional effects (5% to 6%) – Nervousness, jitteriness, restlessness, emotional upset, anxiety or malaise.

Infrequent effects (1% to 3%) – Cardiac symptoms including chest pain or tightness (rarely associated with ECG abnormalities) and arrhythmia (supraventricular tachycardia). Anaphylactic shock, rash, heart murmur, angina pectoris, myocardial ischemia, epigastric distress, ileus, bloating, constipation, diarrhea, dyspnea, hyperventilation, hemolytic icterus, glycosuria, lactic acidosis, sweating, chills, drowsiness and weakness occurred.

In addition, ritodrine administration may uncover previously unknown cardiac pathology. Sinus bradycardia may occur upon drug withdrawal.

Oral: Frequent effects (< 50%) – Small increases in maternal heart rate, but little or no effect on either maternal systolic or diastolic blood pressure or on fetal heart rate.

Other effects include palpitations or tremor (10% to 15%); nausea and jitteriness (5% to 8%); rash (3% to 4%); arrhythmia (about 1%).

Neonatal effects infrequently reported are hypoglycemia and ileus. Hypocalcemia and hypotension have been reported in neonates whose mothers were treated with other betamimetic agents.

Overdosage:

Symptoms: Excessive β-adrenergic stimulation including exaggeration of pharmacologic effects, the most prominent being tachycardia (maternal and fetal), palpitations, cardiac arrhythmia, hypotension, dyspnea, nervousness, tremor, nausea and vomiting.

Treatment includes usual supportive measures. Refer to General Management of Acute Overdosage on 2711 When symptoms occur as a result of IV use, discontinue the drug. Use an appropriate β-blocker as an antidote. Ritodrine is dialyzable.

(Continued on following page)

RITODRINE HCl (Cont.)

Administration and Dosage:

The initial IV treatment is usually followed by oral administration. The optimum dose of the drug is determined by a balance of uterine response and unwanted effects. Treat recurrences of unwanted preterm labor with repeated infusion of ritodrine.

IV therapy: Begin as soon as possible after diagnosis. To minimize risks of hypotension, keep patient in the left lateral position during infusion and pay careful attention to hydration. *Avoid circulatory fluid overload.* Frequently monitor maternal uterine contractions, heart rate, blood pressure and fetal heart rate; individualize dosage.

Use a controlled infusion device to adjust flow rate in drops/min. An IV microdrip chamber (60 drops/ml) provide a convenient range of infusion rates.

The initial dose is 0.1 mg/min (0.33 ml/min, or 20 drops/min using a microdrip chamber at the recommended dilution), to be gradually increased by 0.05 mg/min (10 drops/min) every 10 minutes until the desired result is attained. The usual effective dosage is between 0.15 and 0.35 mg/min (30 to 70 drops/min), continued for at least 12 hours after uterine contractions cease. With the recommended dilution, the maximum volume of fluid that might be administered after 12 hours at the highest dose (0.35 mg/min) will be approximately 840 ml.

If other drugs need to be given IV, the use of "piggyback" or another site of IV administration permits continued independent control of the infusion rate of ritodrine.

Oral maintenance: Give 10 mg approximately 30 minutes before the termination of IV therapy, then 10 mg every 2 hours for the first 24 hours. Thereafter, give 10 to 20 mg every 4 to 6 hours, depending on uterine activity and unwanted effects. Do not exceed 120 mg/day. Continue treatment as long as it is desirable to prolong pregnancy.

Preparation of solution: 150 mg ritodrine in 500 ml fluid yields a final concentration of 0.3 mg/ml. When fluid restriction is desirable, a more concentrated solution may be prepared. For IV infusion, dilute with 5% Dextrose Solution. Use promptly after preparation.

Because of the increased probability of pulmonary edema, saline diluents (0.9% Sodium Chloride; Ringer's) and Hartmann's Solution should be reserved for cases where Dextrose Solution is undesirable (eg, diabetes mellitus).

Stability and storage: Do not use if the solution is discolored or contains any precipitate or particulate matter. Do not use after 48 hours of preparation.

Store at room temperature, below 30°C (86°F). Protect from excessive heat.

Rx	**Ritodrine HCl** (Quad)	**Injection:** 10 mg per ml	In 5 ml flip-top vials.[1]
		15 mg per ml	In 10 ml flip-top vials.[1]
Rx	**Yutopar** (Astra)	**Injection:** 10 mg per ml	In 5 ml amps.[1]
		15 mg per ml	In 10 ml vials[1] and syringes.[1]
		Tablets: 10 mg	(#Yutopar). Yellow, scored. In 60s and UD 100s.

Product identification code.

[1] With sodium metabisulfite.

Prostaglandins

Actions:

Pharmacology: Prostaglandins stimulate the myometrium of the gravid uterus to contract in a manner that is similar to the contractions seen in the term uterus during labor. The mechanism of action has not been determined. The myometrial contractions induced are sufficient to produce uterine evacuation in the majority of cases. Postpartum, the resultant myometrial contractions provide hemostasis at the site of placentation.

These agents also stimulate the smooth muscle of the GI tract; this activity may be responsible for the vomiting or diarrhea that may occur with their use. Large doses of carboprost can elevate blood pressure, probably by contracting the vascular smooth muscle, but this has not been clinically significant with doses used for terminating pregnancy. In contrast, large doses of dinoprostone may lower blood pressure. Body temperature elevation may also occur with both drugs.

Pharmacokinetics: Carboprost – In five postpartum women treated with a single IM injection of 250 mcg, the mean peak plasma concentration occurred at 15 minutes. With multiple dosing, average peak concentrations were slightly higher following each successive injection but always decreased to levels less than the preceding peak values by 2 hours after each administration.

Six metabolites have been identified. The liver appears to be the primary site for oxidation. Less than 1% of the drug is excreted unchanged in the urine. Urinary excretion of metabolites is rapid and nearly complete 24 hours following IM administration. About 80% of the dose is excreted in the first 5 to 10 hours and an additional 5% in the next 20 hours.

Indications:

For the termination of pregnancy from the following gestational weeks as calculated from the first day of the last normal menstrual period:

Carboprost: 13 to 20 weeks
Dinoprostone: 12 to 20 weeks

Carboprost: Second trimester abortion characterized by failure of expulsion of the fetus during the course of treatment by another method; premature rupture of membranes in intrauterine methods with loss of drug and insufficient or absent uterine activity; requirement of a repeat intrauterine instillation of drug for expulsion of the fetus; inadvertent or spontaneous rupture of membranes in the presence of a previable fetus and absence of adequate activity for expulsion; postpartum hemorrhage due to uterine atony which has not responded to conventional management (prior treatment should include use of IV oxytocin, manipulative techniques such as uterine massage and, unless contraindicated, IM ergot preparations).

Dinoprostone: Evacuation of the uterine content in the management of missed abortion or intrauterine fetal death up to 28 weeks gestational age as calculated from the first day of the last normal menstrual period; management of nonmetastatic gestational trophoblastic disease (benign hydatidiform mole).

Unlabeled uses: Low dose dinoprostone vaginal suppositories (2 to 3 mg) or gel (0.25 to 1 mg intracervical; 2 to 5 mg intravaginal) have been used to induce labor and to initiate cervical ripening before labor induction. However, the manufacturer states that neither the suppository nor any extemporaneous formulation made from the suppository should be used for cervical ripening or any other indication at term pregnancy.

Contraindications:

Hypersensitivity to any of these agents; acute pelvic inflammatory disease; active cardiac, pulmonary, renal or hepatic disease.

Warnings:

Recommended dosages: Use only in recommended dosages and only by medical personnel. Use in a hospital which can provide immediate intensive care and acute surgical facilities.

Viable fetus: Prostaglandins are not indicated if the fetus in utero has reached the stage of viability; they are not feticidal agents. They do not appear to directly affect the fetoplacental unit. Therefore, a previable fetus aborted by these agents could exhibit transient life signs.

Pregnancy: Category C. These drugs are embryotoxic in animals and any dose that produces increased uterine tone could put the embryo or fetus at risk. Animal studies suggest that certain prostaglandins may have teratogenic potential. Therefore, complete any failed attempts at pregnancy termination with these drugs by some other means.

(Continued on following page)

Precautions:

Special risk patients: Use cautiously in patients with a history of asthma, hypotension or hypertension, cardiovascular, adrenal, renal or hepatic disease, anemia, jaundice, diabetes, epilepsy or a compromised (scarred) uterus.

Chorioamnionitis: Use carboprost with caution in patients with chorioamnionitis. During clinical trials, chorioamnionitis was a complication contributing to postpartum uterine atony and hemorrhage in 7% of cases, 3 of which failed to respond to carboprost. This complication during labor may inhibit the uterine response to carboprost, similar to that reported with other oxytocic agents.

Incomplete abortion: Prostaglandin-induced abortion may sometimes be incomplete (incidence with carboprost is about 20%). In such cases, take other measures to ensure complete abortion.

Intrauterine fetal death confirmation: When a pregnancy diagnosed as missed abortion is electively interrupted with intravaginal dinoprostone administration, confirm intrauterine fetal death with a negative pregnancy test for chorionic gonadotropic activity (UCG test or equivalent). When a pregnancy with late fetal intrauterine death is interrupted with intravaginal dinoprostone administration, confirm intrauterine fetal death prior to treatment.

Vaginal conditions: Use dinoprostone suppositories with caution in the presence of cervicitis, infected endocervical lesions or acute vaginitis.

Bone effects: High dose animal studies lasting several weeks have shown that prostaglandins of the E and F series can induce proliferation of bone. Such effects have also been noted in neonates who have received prostaglandin E_1 during prolonged treatment. There is no evidence that short-term administration can cause similar bone effects.

GI effects: The pretreatment or concurrent administration of antiemetic and antidiarrheal drugs decreases the incidence of GI effects. Their use is an integral part of the management of patients undergoing abortion.

Increased blood pressure: When used for postpartum hemorrhage, 4% of patients treated with carboprost had a moderate increase in blood pressure. It is not certain whether this hypertension was due to a direct effect of carboprost or a return to a status of pregnancy-associated hypertension manifested by the correction of hypovolemic shock.

Blood count: Leukocytosis and differential white cell counts do not distinguish between endometritis and prostaglandin hyperthermia, since total WBCs may increase during infection and transient leukocytosis may also be drug-induced.

Benzyl alcohol: Carboprost contains benzyl alcohol, which has been associated with a fatal "gasping syndrome" in premature infants.

Pyrexia: Transient pyrexia due to hypothalamic thermoregulation may be seen. Temperature elevations exceeding 1.1°C (2°F) were observed in approximately 12% of patients receiving carboprost and 50% of those receiving dinoprostone. Temperature returned to normal when therapy ended. Force fluids in patients with drug-induced fever and no clinical or bacteriological evidence of intrauterine infection.

Differentiation of postabortion endometritis from drug-induced temperature elevations is difficult; the distinctions are summarized in the following table.

Differentiation of Endometritis vs Prostaglandin-Induced Pyrexia		
Parameter	Endometritis pyrexia	Prostaglandin-induced pyrexia
Onset	Typically, on the third day after abortion (≥ 38°C; ≥ 102°F).	Within 1 to 16 hrs after the first injection of carboprost; within 15 to 45 min of dinoprostone suppository.
Duration	Untreated pyrexia and infection continue and may give rise to other pelvic infections.	Temperatures return to pretreatment levels after discontinuation of carboprost therapy (within 2 to 6 hours for dinoprostone).
Retention	Products of conception often retained in cervical os or uterine cavity.	Temperature elevation occurs whether or not tissue is retained.
Histology	Endometrium infiltrated with lymphocytes; some areas are necrotic and hemorrhagic.	Endometrial stroma may be edematous and vascular, but not inflamed.
Uterus	Remains boggy with tenderness over the fundus, pain on moving the cervix on bimanual examination.	Uterine involution normal. Uterus is not tender.
Discharge	Foul smelling lochia and leukorrhea.	Lochia normal.

(Continued on following page)

Drug Interactions:

Oxytocics: The activity of oxytocic agents may be augmented by the prostaglandins.

Adverse Reactions:

Prostaglandin Adverse Reactions		
Adverse reaction	Carboprost	Dinoprostone
GI		
Vomiting	✓[1]	66%
Diarrhea	✓[1]	40%
Nausea	33%	33%
CNS		
Headache	✓	10%
Flushing	7%	✓
Anxiety/Tension	✓	✓
Hot flashes	✓	✓
Paresthesia	✓	✓
Syncope/Dizziness	✓	✓
Weakness	✓	✓
Cardiovascular		
Arrhythmias	✓	✓
Chest pain/tightness	✓	✓
GU		
Endometritis	✓	✓
Uterine rupture	✓	✓
Uterine/Vaginal pain	✓	✓
Respiratory		
Coughing	✓	✓
Dyspnea/Wheezing	✓	✓
Other		
Chills/Shivering	✓	10%
Backache	✓	✓
Blurred vision	✓	✓
Breast tenderness	✓	✓
Diaphoresis	✓	✓
Eye pain	✓	✓
Muscle cramp/pain	✓	✓
Pyrexia/Fever	✓	✓
Rash	✓	✓
Leg cramps	✓	✓

✓ = Occurs, no incidence reported.

[1] Incidence may be decreased with pretreatment or concurrent use of antiemetics/antidiarrheals.

Other adverse reactions reported (not all clearly drug-related) include the following:

Carboprost (in decreasing order of frequency): Hiccoughing; drowsiness; dystonia; asthma; injection site pain; tinnitus; sleep disorders; posterior cervical perforation; epigastric pain; excessive thirst; twitching eyelids; gagging; retching; dry throat; choking sensation; thyroid storm; palpitations; vertigo; vasovagal syndrome; dry mouth; hyperventilation; respiratory distress; hematemesis; taste alterations; urinary tract infections; septic shock; torticollis; lethargy, endometritis from UCD; nosebleed; upper respiratory infection; retained placental fragments; shortness of breath; fullness of throat; uterine sacculation; faintness; lightheadedness; hypertension; perforated uterus; nervousness; pulmonary edema.

The most common complications when carboprost was used for abortion requiring additional treatment after hospital discharge were endometritis, retained placental fragments and excessive uterine bleeding, occurring in $\approx$ 2% of patients.

Dinoprostone (in decreasing order of frequency): Joint inflammation, new or exacerbated; arthralgia; vaginitis or vulvitis; stiff neck; dehydration; tremor; hearing impairment; urine retention; pharyngitis; laryngitis; skin discoloration; vaginismus; myocardial infarction (two cases in patients with a history of cardiovascular disease).

Approximately 10% of patients exhibited transient diastolic blood pressure decreases of $>$ 20 mm Hg.

(Products listed on following page)

Complete prescribing information for these products begins on page 454.

Prostaglandins (Cont.)

CARBOPROST TROMETHAMINE

Administration and Dosage:

Abortion: For IM use only. Administer an initial dose of 250 mcg (1 ml) by deep IM injection. Give subsequent doses of 250 mcg at 1.5 to 3.5 hour intervals, depending on uterine response. The dose may be increased to 500 mcg if uterine contractility is inadequate after several 250 mcg doses.

An optional test dose of 100 mcg (0.4 ml) may be administered initially.

Do not exceed a 12 mg total dose or continuous administration for > 2 days.

Refractory postpartum uterine bleeding: Give an initial dose of 250 mcg by deep IM injection. The majority of successful cases (73%) responded to single injections. In some cases, multiple dosing at 15 to 90 minute intervals was performed with successful outcome. Do not exceed a total dose of 2 mg (8 doses).

Storage/Stability: Refrigerate at 2° to 4°C (36° to 39°F). Stable for 9 days at room temperature (not exceeding 25°C; 77°F).

Rx	**Hemabate** (Upjohn)	**Injection:** 250 mcg carboprost and 83 mcg tromethamine per ml	In 1 ml amps.[1]

DINOPROSTONE (Prostaglandin E2)

Administration and Dosage:

Insert one suppository (20 mg) high into the vagina. The patient should remain supine for 10 minutes following insertion. Administer each subsequent suppository at 3 to 5 hour intervals until abortion occurs. Within the above recommended intervals, determine administration time by abortifacient progress, uterine contractility response and by patient tolerance. Continuous administration for > 2 days is not advisable.

Storage: Store in a freezer not above − 20°C (− 4°F); bring to room temperature just prior to use.

Unlabeled administration and dosage: Dinoprostone suppositories (2 to 3 mg) and gel (0.25 to 1 mg intracervically; 2 to 5 mg intravaginally) are successful in preinduction of cervical ripening. One method used to prepare the gel is by triturating the suppositories in ethanol and mixing in methylcellulose base; the gel must be used within 3 days. Another method is to mix the suppository with mineral oil (5 ml), triturate in hydroxyethylcellulose gel (55 ml), package in syringes and freeze; consider a 30 day expiration date. However, the manufacturer states that the suppository should not be used for extemporaneous preparation of any other dosage form, and that neither the suppository nor any extemporaneous formulation should be used for cervical ripening or any other indication at term pregnancy.

Rx	**Prostin E2** (Upjohn)	**Vaginal Suppository:** 20 mg	In containers of 1 each.

[1] With 9.45% benzyl alcohol and 9 mg sodium chloride per ml.

Cortisol, the major endogenous glucocorticoid produced in the body, is produced and secreted via the hypothalamic-anterior pituitary-adrenocortical (HPA) axis. The adrenal cortex synthesizes and secretes the steroid hormones which include mineralocorticoids (aldosterone), glucocorticoids, and to a minor extent, androgenic hormones. Aldosterone secretion is controlled mainly by potassium and the renin-angiotensin system; physiological regulation of glucocorticoid synthesis and secretion is mediated by corticotropin (ACTH), which is secreted by the anterior pituitary gland. In response to low plasma cortisol levels, ACTH is secreted; high plasma cortisol levels inhibit ACTH secretion. This relationship follows a diurnal pattern. Cholesterol and its esters are converted to pregnenolone by ACTH, which is further converted to cortisol and other intermediary products (eg, androgens). ACTH secretion is also stimulated by hypothalamic corticotropin-releasing factor, which is stimulated by serotonin, dopamine and other neurotransmitters in response to stress (emotional, physical or chemical). ACTH secretion at any given time is influenced by a negative feedback relationship from circulating glucocorticoids and the neural signals associated with stress response and the circadian pattern.

Primary adrenocortical insufficiency (Addison's disease) requires replacement therapy with physiologic doses of both mineralocorticoids and glucocorticoids. Secondary adrenocortical insufficiency due to inadequate ACTH secretion may be treated either with replacement steroid administration or with ACTH. Pharmacologic doses of exogenous glucocorticoids are used for their profound anti-inflammatory effects.

Excessive secretion of glucocorticoids (Cushing's syndrome) is due to excessive ACTH or a primary adrenal source (eg, benign adenoma, carcinoma) and is most effectively treated surgically; however, aminoglutethimide inhibits glucocorticoid synthesis and may be used to suppress excessive adrenal activity.

The agents discussed in this section are listed below:

Adrenocorticotropic hormone (corticotropin or ACTH), secreted by the anterior pituitary, stimulates the adrenal cortex to produce and secrete its natural steroids by activating adenyl cyclase in the cell membranes. ACTH is included in this section since the therapeutic effects of its administration are due to the activity of the liberated adrenal steroids. Adequate adrenal function is necessary for ACTH to elicit a pharmacologic response. *Cosyntropin*, a synthetic analog of ACTH, has similar corticotropic activity, but is devoid of the immunogenic properties of ACTH of porcine origin.

Mineralocorticoids: Fludrocortisone is used for partial replacement therapy in adrenocortical insufficiency and for the treatment of salt-losing adrenogenital syndrome.

Glucocorticoids cause profound and varied metabolic effects in addition to modifying the body's immune response to diverse stimuli. The naturally occurring glucocorticoids and many synthetic steroids have both glucocorticoid and mineralocorticoid activity. Other synthetic steroids have potent glucocorticoid activity without significant mineralocorticoid activity.

Glucocorticoid product listings are included in the following sections:

- Oral and parenteral
- Retention enemas
- Respiratory inhalant
- Intranasal
- Ophthalmic
- Topical

Adrenal steroid inhibitor – Aminoglutethimide inhibits the enzymatic biosynthesis of adrenal steroids. It is useful in suppressing excessive adrenosteroid production in Cushing's syndrome.

(Continued on following pages)

Refer to the introductory statement on page 458.

Corticotropin (ACTH)

Actions:

Corticotropin (adrenocorticotropic hormone, ACTH) is secreted by the anterior pituitary and stimulates the adrenal cortex to produce and secrete adrenocortical hormones. Adequate adrenal function is necessary for corticotropin to elicit a pharmacological response. ACTH secretion is regulated by a negative feedback mechanism, whereby elevated plasma corticosteroid levels suppress ACTH secretion. Chronic administration of exogenous corticosteroids will decrease ACTH stores and induce morphological changes in the pituitary. In the absence of ACTH stimulation, the adrenal cortex may atrophy.

Cosyntropin is a synthetic peptide corresponding to the amino acid residues 1 to 24 of human ACTH, which exhibits the full corticosteroidogenic activity of natural ACTH. A dose of 0.25 mg cosyntropin is pharmacologically equivalent to 25 units of natural ACTH. Cosyntropin is less allergenic than natural ACTH. Because it is unavailable in a repository form, it is not used therapeutically, only diagnostically.

Pharmacokinetics: ACTH injection has a rapid onset. Plasma half-life is about 15 minutes. After IM or rapid IV administration of 25 units, peak plasma concentrations are usually achieved within 1 hour and begin to decrease after 2 to 4 hours. Repository corticotropin contains ACTH incorporated in a gelatin menstruum designed to delay the absorption rate and increase the period of effectiveness. Corticotropin zinc hydroxide consists of ACTH adsorbed on zinc hydroxide which also delays the absorption rate. Repository corticotropin and corticotropin zinc hydroxide have a slower onset but may sustain effects for up to 3 days.

Indications:

ACTH and cosyntropin: Diagnostic testing of adrenocortical function. Cosyntropin is more potent and less allergenic than the exogenous ACTH preparations.

ACTH: Corticotropin has limited therapeutic value in conditions responsive to corticosteroid therapy; in such cases, corticosteroid therapy is the treatment of choice. Corticotropin may be used in the following disorders:

Endocrine – Nonsuppurative thyroiditis; hypercalcemia associated with cancer.

Nervous system diseases – Acute exacerbations of multiple sclerosis.

Miscellaneous – Tuberculous meningitis with subarachnoid block or impending block when accompanied by antituberculous chemotherapy; trichinosis with neurologic or myocardial involvement; rheumatic, collagen, dermatologic, allergic, ophthalmic, respiratory, hematologic, neoplastic, edematous, and GI diseases in the same manner as the glucocorticoids. Refer to the Glucocorticoids monograph for a listing of specific conditions responsive to therapy.

Unlabeled use: Treatment of infantile spasms (see Administration and Dosage).

Contraindications:

Scleroderma; osteoporosis; systemic fungal infections; ocular herpes simplex; recent surgery; history of or presence of peptic ulcer; congestive heart failure (CHF); hypertension; sensitivity to porcine proteins. IV administration (except in the treatment of idiopathic thrombocytopenic purpura). IV administration may be used for diagnostic testing of adrenocortical function. Treatment of conditions accompanied by primary adrenocortical insufficiency or adrenocortical hyperfunction.

Warnings:

Do not administer until adrenal responsiveness has been verified with the route of administration (IM or SC) which will be used during treatment. A rise in urinary and plasma corticosteroid values provides direct evidence of a stimulatory effect.

Chronic administration may lead to irreversible adverse effects. ACTH may suppress signs and symptoms of chronic disease without altering the natural course of the disease. Since complications with corticotropin use are dependent on the dose and duration of treatment, a risk to benefit decision must be made in each case.

Prolonged use increases the risk of hypersensitivity reactions and may produce posterior subcapsular cataracts and glaucoma with possible damage to the optic nerve.

Stress: Although the action of ACTH is similar to that of exogenous adrenocortical steroids, the quantity of adrenocorticoid secreted may be variable. In patients who receive prolonged corticotropin therapy, use additional rapidly acting corticosteroids before, during and after an unusually stressful situation.

Infection: ACTH may mask signs of infection including fungal or viral eye infections that may appear during its use. There may be decreased resistance and inability to localize infection. When infection is present, administer appropriate anti-infective therapy.

Tuberculosis – Observe patients with latent tuberculosis or tuberculin reactivity who receive ACTH, as reactivation of the disease may occur. During prolonged ACTH therapy, administer chemoprophylaxis.

(Warnings continued on following page)

Corticotropin (ACTH) (Cont.)

Warnings (Cont.):

Immunosuppression: Perform immunization procedures with caution, especially when high doses are administered, because of the possible hazards of neurological complications and lack of antibody response. Immunization with live vaccines is usually contraindicated in patients on ACTH or corticosteroid therapy.

Electrolytes: Corticotropin can elevate blood pressure, cause salt and water retention and increase potassium and calcium excretion. Dietary salt restriction and potassium supplementation may be necessary.

Hypersensitivity: Cosyntropin exhibits slight immunologic activity, does not contain foreign animal protein, and is less risky to use than natural ACTH. Most patients with a history of a previous hypersensitivity reaction to natural ACTH or a preexisting allergic disease will tolerate cosyntropin without incident; however, hypersensitivity reactions are possible. Refer to Management of Acute Hypersensitivity Reactions.

Pregnancy: Category C. ACTH has embryocidal effects. Fetal abnormalities have been observed in animals. Use in pregnancy only when clearly needed and when potential benefits outweigh potential hazards to the fetus. Monitor infants born of mothers who have received substantial doses during pregnancy for signs of hyperadrenalism.

Lactation: It is not known whether this drug is excreted in breast milk. Because of the potential for serious adverse reactions in nursing infants from ACTH, decide whether to discontinue nursing or to discontinue the drug.

Children: Prolonged use of corticotropin in children will inhibit skeletal growth. If use is necessary, give intermittently and carefully observe the child.

Precautions:

Concomitant therapy: Since maximal corticotropin stimulation of the adrenals may be limited during the first few days of treatment, administer a rapidly acting corticosteroid (eg, hydrocortisone) when an immediate therapeutic effect is desirable.

Administer for treatment only when disease is intractable to more conventional therapy; ACTH should be adjunctive and not the sole therapy.

Use the lowest possible dose to control the condition, and when reduction in dosage is possible, it should be gradual.

Sensitivity to porcine proteins: Perform skin testing prior to treatment in patients with suspected sensitivity to porcine proteins. During or following administration, observe for sensitivity reactions.

Adrenocortical insufficiency induced by prolonged ACTH therapy may be minimized by gradual reduction of dosage. Insufficiency may persist for months after therapy discontinuation; therefore, in any situation of stress during that period, reinstitute corticosteroid therapy.

Hypothyroidism and cirrhosis: An enhanced effect of corticotropin may occur.

Multiple sclerosis: Although ACTH may speed the resolution of acute exacerbations of multiple sclerosis, it does not affect the ultimate outcome or natural course of the disease. Relatively high doses of ACTH are necessary to demonstrate a significant effect.

Acute gouty arthritis: Limit treatment of acute gouty arthritis to a few days. Since rebound attacks may occur when corticotropin is discontinued, administer conventional concomitant therapy during corticotropin treatment and for several days after it is stopped.

Mental disturbances: Psychic derangements may appear, ranging from euphoria, insomnia, mood swings, personality changes, and depression to frank psychosis. Existing emotional instability or psychotic tendencies may be aggravated.

Use with caution in patients with diabetes, abscess, pyogenic infections, diverticulitis, renal insufficiency and myasthenia gravis.

Drug abuse/dependence: Although drug dependence does not occur, sudden withdrawal of corticotropin after prolonged use may lead to recurrent symptoms which make it difficult to stop. It may be necessary to taper the dose and increase the injection interval to gradually discontinue the medication.

Drug Interactions:

Amphotericin B depletes potassium and may enhance the potassium wasting effect of corticotropin; it may also decrease adrenocortical responsiveness to corticotropin. Closely monitor serum potassium.

Antidiabetic agents: Increased requirements for insulin or oral hypoglycemic agents in diabetes have occurred in patients taking ACTH, due to the intrinsic hyperglycemic activity of glucocorticoids.

Diuretics that deplete potassium may enhance the potassium wasting effect of corticotropin. Closely monitor serum potassium.

(Drug Interactions continued on following page)

Corticotropin (ACTH) (Cont.)

Drug Interactions (Cont.):

Salicylates, indomethacin: Because of its known ulcerogenic effects, use aspirin cautiously in conjunction with corticotropin, especially in hypoprothrombinemia. Corticosteroids may increase the renal clearance of salicylates. Increased serum levels of salicylates and salicylate toxicity may occur when steroid therapy is discontinued.

Drug/Lab test interactions: Corticotropin may decrease I^{131} uptake and may suppress reactions to skin tests. It may affect the method of Brown used for determination of urinary estradiol and estriol, causing falsely decreased concentrations of these estrogens. The drug may also interfere with colorimetric/fluorometric procedures for determination of urinary estrogens causing a falsely decreased concentration of urinary estrogens.

Adverse Reactions:

Fluid and electrolyte disturbances: Sodium and fluid retention; potassium and calcium loss; hypokalemic alkalosis.

Musculoskeletal: Muscle weakness; steroid myopathy; loss of muscle mass; osteoporosis; vertebral compression fractures; pathologic fracture of long bones; aseptic necrosis of femoral and humeral heads.

GI: Pancreatitis; ulcerative esophagitis; abdominal distention; peptic ulcer with possible perforation and hemorrhage has been associated with steroid therapy (this association has been disputed).

Dermatologic: Impaired wound healing; petechiae and ecchymoses; increased sweating; hyperpigmentation; thin fragile skin; facial erythema; acne; suppression of skin test reactions.

Cardiovascular: Hypertension; CHF; necrotizing angiitis.

Neurological: Convulsions; vertigo; headache; increased intracranial pressure with papilledema, pseudotumor cerebri, usually after treatment.

Infections: Pneumonia, abscess and septic infection, and GI and GU infections (more frequent with higher doses).

Endocrine: Menstrual irregularities; suppression of growth in children; hirsutism; development of Cushingoid state; manifestations of latent diabetes mellitus; decreased carbohydrate tolerance; increased requirements for insulin or oral hypoglycemic agents in diabetics; secondary adrenocortical and pituitary unresponsiveness, especially during stress.

Ophthalmic: Posterior subcapsular cataracts; increased intraocular pressure; glaucoma with possible damage to optic nerve; exophthalmos.

Metabolic: Negative nitrogen balance due to protein catabolism.

Allergic reactions: Dizziness; nausea; vomiting; shock; skin reactions.

Miscellaneous: Prolonged use may result in antibody production and subsequent loss of the stimulatory effect of ACTH.

Patient Information:

ACTH may mask signs of infection. There may be decreased resistance and inability to localize infection.

Avoid immunizations with live vaccines.

Diabetics may have increased requirements for insulin or oral hypoglycemics.

Notify physician if marked fluid retention, muscle weakness, abdominal pain, seizures, or headache occurs.

Administration and Dosage:

Standard tests for verification of adrenal responsiveness to corticotropin may utilize as much as 80 units as a single injection, or one or more injections of a lesser dosage. Perform verification tests prior to treatment with corticotropins. The test should utilize the route(s) of administration proposed for treatment. Following verification, individualize dosage. Attempt only gradual change in dosage schedules after full drug effects have become apparent.

In the short test (single injection) for the ACTH stimulation test, a normal response is plasma cortisol > 20 mcg/dl on any sample. A blunted response indicates primary or secondary adrenal insufficiency. In the long test (8 hour infusion on 3 consecutive days), an absent or subnormal rise in plasma cortisol and 17-OHCS indicates primary adrenal failure. Plasma cortisol > 20 mcg/dl and a two- to threefold urinary 17-OHCS increase over baseline on day 4 indicates ACTH deficiency.

(Administration and Dosage continued on following page)

Corticotropin (ACTH) (Cont.)

Administration and Dosage (Cont.):

For diagnostic purposes: 10 to 25 units dissolved in 500 ml of 5% Dextrose Injection infused IV over 8 hours.

The usual IM or SC dose is 20 units 4 times daily. Chronic administration of > 40 units/day may be associated with uncontrollable adverse effects.

When indicated, reduce dosage gradually by increasing the duration between injections or decreasing the quantity of corticotropin injected or both.

Acute exacerbations of multiple sclerosis: 80 to 120 units/day IM for 2 to 3 weeks.

Infantile spasms: 20 to 40 units daily or 80 units every other day IM for 3 months or 1 month after cessation of seizures has been recommended.

Repository corticotropin injection: 40 to 80 units IM or SC every 24 to 72 hours.

Preparation and storage: Reconstitute powder by dissolving in Sterile Water for Injection or Sodium Chloride Injection so that the individual dose will be contained in 1 to 2 ml of solution. Refrigerate reconstituted solution. Use within 24 hours.

CORTICOTROPIN INJECTION

Give IM or SC. May be given IV for diagnostic purposes.

	Product	Form	Package	C.I.*
Rx	**Acthar** (Rorer)	**Powder for Injection:** 25 units per vial	In vials.[1]	17
Rx	**Corticotropin** (Various, eg, Baxter, Schein, Steris)	**Powder for Injection:** 40 units per vial	In vials.	9+
Rx	**ACTH** (Parke-Davis)		In vials.[2]	7
Rx	**Acthar** (Rorer)		In vials.[3]	15

REPOSITORY CORTICOTROPIN INJECTION

Give IM or SC. Not for IV use.

	Product	Form	Package	C.I.*
Rx	**ACTH-40** (URL)	**Repository Injection:** 40 units per ml	In 5 ml vials.	1.2+
Rx	**H.P. Acthar Gel** (Rorer)		In 1 and 5 ml vials.[4]	1.7
Rx	**ACTH-80** (Various, eg, Balan, Hauck)	**Repository Injection:** 80 units per ml	In 5 ml vials.	1+
Rx	**H.P. Acthar Gel** (Rorer)		In 1 and 5 ml vials.[4]	1.7

COSYNTROPIN

Administration and Dosage:

Administer IM or IV as a rapid screening test of adrenal function. It may also be given as an IV infusion over 4 to 8 hours to provide a greater stimulus to the adrenal glands. Doses of 0.25 to 0.75 mg have been used and a maximal response noted with the smallest dose. The suggested dose is 0.25 mg dissolved in sterile saline injected IM.

Children (≤ 2 years old): 0.125 mg will often suffice.

IV infusion: Add 0.25 mg cosyntropin to dextrose or saline solutions and give at a rate of approximately 0.04 mg/hour over 6 hours.

For test procedure and interpretation of results, refer to manufacturer's insert.

	Product	Form	Package	C.I.*
Rx	**Cortrosyn** (Organon)	**Powder for Injection:** 0.25 mg	In vials[5] with diluent.	8

* Cost Index based on cost per 10 units corticotropin or 0.1 mg cosyntropin.

[1] With 9 mg hydrolyzed gelatin.

[2] With 5 mg aminoacetic acid.

[3] With 14 mg hydrolyzed gelatin.

[4] With 16% gelatin.

[5] With 10 mg mannitol.

Refer to the introductory statement on page 458.

Mineralocorticoids

FLUDROCORTISONE ACETATE

Actions:

Fludrocortisone is an adrenal cortical steroid with potent mineralocorticoid activity and high glucocorticoid activity (about 15 times as potent as hydrocortisone), but is used only for its mineralocorticoid effects. Because of the similarity of effects, refer to the discussion of Glucocorticoids.

Mechanism: Mineralocorticoids act on the renal distal tubules to enhance the reabsorption of sodium. They increase urinary excretion of both potassium and hydrogen ions. The consequence of these three primary effects together with similar actions on cation transport in other tissues appears to account for the spectrum of physiological activities characteristic of mineralocorticoids.

In small oral doses, fludrocortisone produces marked sodium retention and increased urinary potassium excretion. It also causes a rise in blood pressure, apparently because of these effects on electrolyte levels. In larger doses, fludrocortisone inhibits endogenous adrenal cortical secretion, thymic activity, and pituitary corticotropin excretion, it promotes the deposition of liver glycogen, and, unless protein intake is adequate, it induces negative nitrogen balance.

Pharmacokinetics: Fludrocortisone is readily absorbed from the GI tract with peak concentrations in 1.7 hours. Plasma half-life is approximately 3.5 hours, but biological half-life ranges from 18 to 36 hours.

Indications:

Partial replacement therapy for primary and secondary adrenocortical insufficiency in Addison's disease and for the treatment of salt-losing adrenogenital syndrome.

Unlabeled use: Fludrocortisone 100 to 400 mcg/day has been used in the management of severe orthostatic hypotension.

Contraindications:

Hypersensitivity to fludrocortisone; systemic fungal infections.

Warnings:

Supplemental measures: Use mineralocorticoid therapy preferably in conjunction with other supplemental measures (eg, glucocorticoids, control of electrolytes, control of infection).

Adrenal insufficiency: To avoid drug-induced adrenal insufficiency, supportive dosage may be required in times of stress (eg, trauma, surgery, severe illness), both during treatment with fludrocortisone and for a year afterwards.

Pregnancy: Category C. Safety for use during pregnancy has not been established. Use only when clearly needed and when the potential benefits outweigh the potential hazards to the fetus. If it is necessary to give steroids during pregnancy, observe the newborn infant for signs of adrenocortical insufficiency and institute appropriate therapy, if necessary.

Lactation: Corticosteroids are found in the breast milk of lactating women. Exercise caution when administering to nursing women.

Children: Safety and efficacy for use in children have not been established. Monitor growth and development of infants and children on prolonged therapy.

Precautions:

Addison's disease: Patients with Addison's disease are more sensitive to the action of the hormone and may exhibit side effects in an exaggerated degree. Closely monitor patients and stop treatment if a significant increase in weight or blood pressure, edema or cardiac enlargement occurs.

Sodium retention and potassium loss are accelerated by a high sodium intake. If edema occurs, restrict dietary sodium. Perform frequent blood electrolyte determinations; potassium supplementation may be necessary.

Infection: Monitor patients for evidence of intercurrent infection. Should this occur, initiate appropriate anti-infective therapy.

(Continued on following page)

FLUDROCORTISONE ACETATE (Cont.):

Adverse Reactions:

Side effects may occur if dosage is too high or prolonged or if withdrawal is too rapid. Because it possesses glucocorticoid activity, fludrocortisone may cause side effects similar to those of the glucocorticoids (refer to Glucocorticoid section).

Cardiac: Edema; hypertension; CHF; enlargement of the heart.

Dermatologic: Bruising; increased sweating; hives or allergic skin rash.

Other: Hypokalemic alkalosis.

Overdosage:

Symptoms: Hypertension; edema; hypokalemia; excessive weight gain; increase in heart size.

Treatment: Discontinue the drug; symptoms usually subside within several days. Resume subsequent treatment with reduced doses. Muscular weakness may develop due to excessive potassium loss; treat with potassium supplements. Monitor blood pressure and serum electrolytes regularly.

Patient Information:

Notify physician if dizziness, severe or continuing headaches, swelling of feet or lower legs, or unusual weight gain occurs.

Administration and Dosage:

Addison's disease: The usual dose is 0.1 mg/day (range 0.1 mg 3 times a week to 0.2 mg/day). If transient hypertension develops as a consequence of therapy, reduce the dose to 0.05 mg/day. Administration in conjunction with cortisone (10 to 37.5 mg/day) or hydrocortisone (10 to 30 mg/day) is preferable.

Children and adults – Another recommended dose is 0.05 to 0.1 mg/24 hours.

Infants – A recommended dose is 0.1 to 0.2 mg/24 hours.

Salt-losing adrenogenital syndrome: 0.1 to 0.2 mg/day.

Rx	**Florinef Acetate** (Apothecon)	**Tablets:** 0.1 mg	(429). Pink, scored. Biconvex. In 100s.

Refer to the introductory statement on page 458.

Glucocorticoids

Actions:

Pharmacology: The naturally occurring adrenal cortical steroids have both anti-inflammatory (glucocorticoid) and salt-retaining (mineralocorticoid) properties. Glucocorticoids cause profound and varied metabolic effects. In addition, they modify the body's immune responses to diverse stimuli.

These compounds, including hydrocortisone (cortisol) and cortisone, are used as replacement therapy in adrenocortical deficiency states and may be used for their anti-inflammatory effects. The synthetic steroid compounds prednisone, prednisolone and fludrocortisone also have both glucocorticoid and mineralocorticoid activity. Prednisone and prednisolone are used primarily for their glucocorticoid effects.

In addition, a group of synthetic compounds with marked glucocorticoid activity are distinguished by the absence of any significant salt-retaining activity. These include triamcinolone, dexamethasone, methylprednisolone and betamethasone. These agents are used for their potent anti-inflammatory effects.

Pharmacokinetics: Hydrocortisone and most of its congeners are readily absorbed from the GI tract; greatly altered onsets and durations are usually achieved with injections of suspensions and esters.

Distribution – Hydrocortisone is reversibly bound to corticosteroid-binding globulin (CBG or transcortin) and corticosteroid binding albumin (CBA). Exogenous glucocorticoids are bound to these proteins to a significantly lesser degree. In hypoproteinemic or dysproteinemic states, the total endogenous hydrocortisone levels are decreased. Conversely, with increased CBG (pregnancy, estrogen therapy), the total plasma hydrocortisone levels are elevated. These alterations are not of clinical significance because it is the unbound fraction of the hormone that is metabolically active. However, the administration of exogenous glucocorticoids to patients with altered protein binding capacities will result in significant differences in glucocorticoid pharmacological effects.

Metabolism/Excretion – Hydrocortisone is metabolized by the liver, which is the rate-limiting step in its clearance. The metabolism and excretion of the synthetic glucocorticoids generally parallel hydrocortisone. Induction of hepatic enzymes will increase the metabolic clearance of hydrocortisone and the synthetic glucocorticoids. Approximately 1% of its usual daily production, or about 200 mcg of the unchanged hormone is excreted in the urine daily. Renal clearance is increased when plasma levels are increased. Prednisone is inactive and must be metabolized to prednisolone

The following table summarizes the approximate dosage equivalencies (based on glucocorticoid properties) of the various glucocorticoid preparations and several of their pharmacokinetic parameters. The half-life values refer to the intrinsic activity of each agent; insoluble salts of these drugs are used as repository injections and have sustained effects due to delayed absorption from the injection site.

Glucocorticoid Equivalencies, Potencies and Half-Life

Glucocorticoid	Approximate equivalent dose (mg)	Relative anti-inflammatory (glucocorticoid) potency	Relative mineralocorticoid potency	Half-life	
				Plasma (min)	Biologic (hrs)
Short-acting					
Cortisone	25	0.8	2	30	8-12
Hydrocortisone	20	1	2	80-118	8-12
Intermediate-acting					
Prednisone	5	4	1	60	18-36
Prednisolone	5	4	1	115-212	18-36
Triamcinolone	4	5	0	200 +	18-36
Methylprednisolone	4	5	0	78-188	18-36
Long-acting					
Dexamethasone	0.75	20-30	0	110-210	36-54
Betamethasone	0.6-0.75	20-30	0	300 +	36-54

(Continued on following page)

Glucocorticoids (Cont.)

Indications:

Endocrine disorders: Primary or secondary adrenal cortical insufficiency (hydrocortisone or cortisone is the drug of choice; synthetic analogs may be used in conjunction with mineralocorticoids; in infancy, mineralocorticoid supplementation is important); congenital adrenal hyperplasia; nonsuppurative thyroiditis; hypercalcemia associated with cancer.

Parenteral use: Acute adrenal cortical insufficiency (hydrocortisone or cortisone is the drug of choice); preoperatively or in the event of serious trauma or illness with known adrenal insufficiency or when adrenal cortical reserve is doubtful; shock unresponsive to conventional therapy if adrenal cortical insufficiency exists or is suspected.

Rheumatic disorders: As adjunctive therapy for short-term administration (for acute episode or exacerbation) in: Ankylosing spondylitis; acute and subacute bursitis; acute nonspecific tenosynovitis; acute gouty arthritis; psoriatic arthritis; rheumatoid arthritis, including juvenile rheumatoid arthritis (selected cases may require low-dose maintenance therapy); posttraumatic osteoarthritis; synovitis of osteoarthritis; epicondylitis.

Collagen diseases: For exacerbation or maintenance therapy in selected cases of systemic lupus erythematosus, acute rheumatic carditis or systemic dermatomyositis (polymyositis).

Dermatologic diseases: Pemphigus; bullous dermatitis herpetiformis; severe erythema multiforme (Stevens-Johnson syndrome); mycosis fungoides; severe psoriasis; angioedema or urticaria; exfoliative, severe seborrheic, contact or atopic dermatitis.

Allergic states: Control of severe or incapacitating allergic conditions intractable to conventional treatment in serum sickness and drug hypersensitivity reactions.

Parenteral therapy is indicated for urticarial transfusion reactions and acute noninfectious laryngeal edema (epinephrine is the drug of first choice).

Ophthalmic: Severe acute and chronic allergic and inflammatory processes involving the eye and its adnexa such as: Allergic conjunctivitis; keratitis; allergic corneal marginal ulcers; herpes zoster ophthalmicus; iritis and iridocyclitis; chorioretinitis; diffuse posterior uveitis and choroiditis; optic neuritis; sympathetic ophthalmia and anterior segment inflammation.

Respiratory diseases: Symptomatic sarcoidosis; bronchial asthma (including status asthmaticus); Loeffler's syndrome not manageable by other means; berylliosis; fulminating or disseminated pulmonary tuberculosis when accompanied by appropriate antituberculous chemotherapy; aspiration pneumonitis; seasonal or perennial allergic rhinitis.

Hematologic disorders: Idiopathic thrombocytopenic purpura and secondary thrombocytopenia in adults (IV only; IM use is contraindicated); acquired (autoimmune) hemolytic anemia; erythroblastopenia (RBC anemia); congenital (erythroid) hypoplastic anemia.

Neoplastic diseases: For palliative management of leukemias and lymphomas in adults and acute leukemia of childhood.

Edematous states: To induce diuresis or remission of proteinuria in the nephrotic syndrome (without uremia) of the idiopathic type or that due to lupus erythematosus.

GI diseases: To tide the patient over a critical period of the disease in ulcerative colitis, regional enteritis (Crohn's disease) and intractable sprue.

Nervous system: Acute exacerbations of multiple sclerosis (see Precautions).

Miscellaneous: Tuberculous meningitis with subarachnoid block or impending block when accompanied by appropriate antituberculous chemotherapy; in trichinosis with neurologic or myocardial involvement.

Intra-articular or soft tissue administration: Short-term adjunctive therapy (to tide the patient over an acute episode) in synovitis of osteoarthritis; rheumatoid arthritis; acute and subacute bursitis; acute gouty arthritis; epicondylitis; acute nonspecific tenosynovitis; posttraumatic osteoarthritis.

Intralesional administration: Keloids; localized hypertrophic, infiltrated, inflammatory lesions of lichen planus, psoriatic plaques, granuloma annulare, lichen simplex chronicus (neurodermatitis); discoid lupus erythematosus; necrobiosis lipoidica diabeticorum; alopecia areata. May be useful in cystic tumors of an aponeurosis or tendon (ganglia).

Dexamethasone is also indicated for testing of adrenal cortical hyperfunction; cerebral edema associated with primary or metastatic brain tumor, craniotomy or head injury.

Triamcinolone is also indicated for the treatment of pulmonary emphysema where bronchospasm or bronchial edema plays a significant role, and diffuse interstitial pulmonary fibrosis (Hamman-Rich syndrome); in conjunction with diuretic agents to induce a diuresis in refractory congestive heart failure (CHF) and in cirrhosis of the liver with refractory ascites; and for postoperative dental inflammatory reactions.

(Indications continued on following page)

Glucocorticoids (Cont.)

Indications (Cont.):

Unlabeled uses:

Glucocorticoid Unlabeled Uses	
Use	Drug/Comment
Acute mountain sickness	Dexamethasone 4 mg q 6 h; prevention or treatment
Antiemetic	Dexamethasone most common, 16 to 20 mg
Bacterial meningitis	Dexamethasone 0.15 mg/kg q 6 h; to decrease incidence of hearing loss
Bronchopulmonary dysplasia in preterm infants	Dexamethasone 0.5 mg/kg, then taper.
COPD	Prednisone 30 to 60 mg/day for 1 to 2 weeks, then taper
Depression, diagnosis of	Dexamethasone 1 mg
Duchenne's muscular dystrophy	Prednisone 0.75 to 1.5 mg/kg/day; to improve strength and function
Graves ophthalmopathy	Prednisone 60 mg/day, taper to 20 mg/day
Hepatitis, severe alcoholic	Methylprednisolone 32 mg/day; to reduce mortality
Hirsutism	Dexamethasone 0.5 to 1 mg/day
Respiratory distress syndrome	Prevention in premature neonates (betamethasone most common); adults, methylprednisolone 30 mg/kg (controversial)
Septic shock	Methylprednisolone 30 mg/kg IV most common (very controversial)
Spinal cord injury, acute	Methylprednisolone IV within 8 hours of injury; to improve neurologic function
Tuberculous pleurisy	Prednisolone 0.75 mg/kg/day, then taper; concurrently with antituberculous therapy

Contraindications:

Systemic fungal infections; hypersensitivity to the drug; IM use in idiopathic thrombocytopenic purpura; administration of live virus vaccines (eg, smallpox) in patients receiving immunosuppressive corticosteroid doses (see Warnings).

Warnings:

Infections: Corticosteroids may mask signs of infection, and new infections may appear during their use. There may be decreased resistance and inability of the host defense mechanisms to prevent dissemination of the infection. If an infection occurs during therapy, it should be promptly controlled by suitable antimicrobial therapy.

Tuberculosis – Restrict use in active tuberculosis to those cases of fulminating or disseminated disease in which the corticosteroid is used for disease management with appropriate chemotherapy. If corticosteroids are indicated in patients with latent tuberculosis or tuberculin reactivity, observe closely as reactivation of disease may occur. During prolonged corticosteroid therapy, these patients should receive chemoprophylaxis.

Fungal – Corticosteroids may exacerbate systemic fungal infections; do not use in such infections, except to control drug reactions due to amphotericin B. Concomitant use of amphotericin B and hydrocortisone has been followed by cardiac enlargement and CHF.

Amebiasis – Corticosteroids may activate latent amebiasis. Rule out amebiasis before giving to a patient who has spent time in the tropics or has unexplained diarrhea.

Cerebral malaria – A double-blind trial has shown that corticosteroid use is associated with prolongation of coma and a higher incidence of pneumonia and GI bleeding.

Hepatitis: Although corticosteroids have been advocated for use in chronic active hepatitis, they may be harmful in chronic active hepatitis positive for hepatitis B surface antigen.

Ocular effects: Prolonged use may produce posterior subcapsular cataracts, glaucoma with possible damage to the optic nerves, and may enhance the establishment of secondary ocular infections due to fungi or viruses. Use cautiously in ocular herpes simplex because of possible corneal perforation.

Fluid and electrolyte balance: Average and large doses of hydrocortisone or cortisone can cause elevation of blood pressure, salt and water retention and increased excretion of potassium. These effects are less likely to occur with the synthetic derivatives except when used in large doses. Dietary salt restriction and potassium supplementation may be necessary. All corticosteroids increase calcium excretion.

(Warnings continued on following page)

Warnings (Cont.):

Renal function impairment: Edema may occur in the presence of renal disease with a fixed or decreased glomerular filtration rate. Use with caution in renal insufficiency, acute glomerulonephritis and chronic nephritis.

Peptic ulcer: The relationship between peptic ulceration and glucocorticoid therapy is unclear. Patients who appear to be at risk are those being treated for nephrotic syndrome or liver disease, or who are comatose postcraniotomy. Other predisposing factors include a total prednisone intake exceeding 1 g, a history of ulcer disease, concomitant use of known gastric irritants (as in arthritic patients) and stress. It may be desirable to use prophylactic antacids pending clarification of the relationship of glucocorticoids and ulcers.

Hypersensitivity: Anaphylactoid reactions have occurred rarely with corticosteroid therapy; take precautionary measures, especially in patients with a history of allergies. Refer to Management of Acute Hypersensitivity Reactions.

Immunosuppression: During therapy, do not use live virus vaccines (eg, smallpox). Do not undertake immunization procedures in patients who are receiving corticosteroids, especially on high doses, because of possible hazards of neurological complications and a lack of antibody response. This does not apply to patients who are receiving corticosteroids as replacement therapy. Corticosteroids may suppress reactions to skin tests.

Adrenal suppression: Prolonged therapy of pharmacologic doses may lead to hypothalamic-pituitary-adrenal suppression. The degree of adrenal suppression varies with the dosage, relative glucocorticoid aactivity, biological half-life and duration of glucocorticoid therapy within each individual. Adrenal suppression may be minimized by the use of intermediate-acting glucocorticoids (prednisone, prednisolone, methylprednisolone) on an alternate day schedule (see Administration).

Following prolonged therapy, abrupt discontinuation may result in a withdrawal syndrome without evidence of adrenal insufficiency. To minimize morbidity associated with adrenal insufficiency, discontinue exogenous corticosteroid therapy gradually. During withdrawal therapy, increased supplementation may be necessary during times of stress. Symptoms of adrenal insufficiency as a result of too rapid withdrawal include: Nausea; fatigue; anorexia; dyspnea; hypotension; hypoglycemia; myalgia; fever; malaise; arthralgia; dizziness; desquamation of skin; fainting. Continued supervision after therapy termination is essential; severe disease manifestations may reappear suddenly.

Stress: In patients receiving or recently withdrawn from corticosteroid therapy subjected to unusual stress, increased dosage of rapidly acting corticosteroids is indicated before, during and after stressful situations, except in patients on high-dose therapy. Relative adrenocortical insufficiency may persist for months after therapy ends; in any stress situation occurring during that period, reinstitute therapy. Since mineralocorticoid secretion may be impaired, administer salt or a mineralocorticoid concurrently.

Cardiovascular: Reports suggest an apparent association between corticosteroid use and left ventricular free wall rupture after a recent myocardial infarction. Use with great caution in these patients.

Elderly: Consider the risk/benefit factors of steroid use. Consider lower doses because of body changes caused by aging (ie, diminution of muscle mass and plasma volume). Monitor blood pressure, blood glucose and electrolytes at least every 6 months.

Pregnancy (Category C – Prednisolone sodium phosphate): Corticosteroids cross the placenta (prednisone has the poorest transport). In animal studies, large doses of cortisol administered early in pregnancy produced cleft palate, stillborn fetuses and decreased fetal size. Chronic maternal ingestion during the first trimester has shown a 1% incidence of cleft palate in humans. If used in pregnancy, or in women of childbearing potential, weigh benefits against the potential hazards to the mother and fetus. Carefully observe infants born of mothers who have received substantial corticosteroid doses during pregnancy for signs of hypoadrenalism.

Lactation: Corticosteroids appear in breast milk and could suppress growth, interfere with endogenous corticosteroid production or cause other unwanted effects in the nursing infant. Advise mothers taking pharmacologic corticosteroid doses not to nurse. However, several studies suggest that amounts excreted in breast milk are negligible with prednisone or prednisolone doses ≤ 20 mg/day or methylprednisolone doses ≤ 8 mg/day, and large doses for short periods may not harm the infant. Alternatives to consider include waiting 3 to 4 hours after the dose before breastfeeding and using prednisolone rather than prednisone (resulting in a lower corticosteroid dose to the infant).

Children: Carefully observe growth and development of infants and children on prolonged corticosteroid therapy. Some of these products contain benzyl alcohol which has been associated with a fatal "gasping syndrome" in premature infants.

(Continued on following page)

Precautions:

Use the lowest possible dose. Make a benefit/risk decision in each individual case as to the size of the dose, duration of treatment and the use of daily or intermittent therapy, since complications of treatment are dependent on these factors.

Monitoring: Observe patients for weight increase, edema, hypertension, and excessive potassium excretion, as well as for less obvious signs of adrenocortical steroid-induced untoward effects. Monitor for a negative nitrogen balance due to protein catabolism. A liberal protein intake is essential during prolonged therapy. Evaluate blood pressure and body weight, and do routine laboratory studies, including 2 hour postprandial blood glucose and serum potassium and a chest x-ray at regular intervals during prolonged therapy. Upper GI x-rays are desirable in patients with known or suspected peptic ulcer disease or significant dyspepsia or in patients complaining of gastric distress. Observe growth and development of infants and children on prolonged therapy.

Use with caution in: GI – Nonspecific ulcerative colitis if there is a probability of impending perforation, abscess or other pyogenic infection; diverticulitis; fresh intestinal anastomoses; active or latent peptic ulcer (see Warnings).

Cardiovascular – Hypertension; CHF; thromboembolitic tendencies; thrombophlebitis.

Miscellaneous – Osteoporosis; exanthema; Cushing's syndrome; antibiotic-resistant infections; convulsive disorders; metastatic carcinoma; myasthenia gravis; vaccinia; varicella; diabetes mellitus.; hypothyroidism, cirrhosis (enhanced effect of corticosteroids).

Steroid psychosis: Steroid psychosis is characterized by a delirious or toxic psychosis with clouded sensorium. Other symptoms may include euphoria, insomnia, mood swings, personality changes and severe depression. The onset of symptoms usually occurs within 15 to 30 days. Predisposing factors include doses > 40 mg prednisone equivalent, female predominance, and, possibly, a family history of psychiatric illness. A patient history of psychiatric problems does not correlate well with predisposition to steroid-induced psychosis. Incidence appears to correlate with dose. One study of 718 patients treated with prednisone revealed ≤ 40 mg/day = 1.3%; 41 to 80 mg/day = 4.6%; ≥ 80 mg/day = 18.4%. If the steroids cannot be discontinued, psychotropic medication is effective.

Multiple sclerosis: Although corticosteroids are effective in speeding the resolution of acute exacerbations of multiple sclerosis, they do not affect the ultimate outcome or natural history of the disease. Relatively high doses of corticosteroids are necessary to demonstrate a significant effect.

Tartrazine sensitivity: Some of these products contain tartrazine, which may cause allergic-type reactions (including bronchial asthma) in susceptible individuals. Although the incidence of tartrazine sensitivity in the general population is low, it is frequently seen in patients who also have aspirin hypersensitivity. Specific products containing tartrazine are identified in the product listings.

Sulfite sensitivity: Some of these products contain sodium bisulfite which may cause severe allergic reactions in certain susceptible individuals, particularly those with asthma. Anaphylactoid and hypersensitivity reactions have occurred. Do not use in patients allergic to sulfites. Specific products containing sulfites are identified in the product listings.

Repository injections: To minimize the likelihood and severity of atrophy, do not inject SC, avoid injection into the deltoid and avoid repeated IM injections into the same site, if possible. Repository injections are not recommended as initial therapy in acute situations.

Local injections: Intra-articular injection may produce systemic and local effects. A marked increase in pain accompanied by local swelling, further restriction of joint motion, fever and malaise is suggestive of septic arthritis. Appropriate examination of any joint fluid present is necessary. If a diagnosis of sepsis is confirmed, institute appropriate antimicrobial therapy. Avoid local injection into an infected site and into unstable joints.

Strongly impress patients with the importance of not overusing joints in which symptomatic benefit has been obtained as long as the inflammatory process remains active. *Frequent intra-articular injection may result in damage to joint tissues.*

Avoid overdistention of the joint capsule and deposition of steroid along the needle track in intra-articular injection, as it may lead to subcutaneous atrophy. While crystals of adrenal steroids in the dermis suppress inflammatory reactions, their presence may cause disintegration of the cellular elements and physiochemical changes in the ground substance of the connective tissue.

The resultant dermal or subdermal changes may form depressions in the skin at the injection site; the degree will vary with the amount of adrenal steroid injection. Regeneration is usually complete within a few months or after all crystals of the adrenal steroid have been absorbed. In order to minimize the incidence of dermal and subdermal atrophy, exercise care not to exceed recommended doses in injections. Make multiple small injections into the area of the lesion whenever possible.

(Continued on following page)

Drug Interactions:

Corticosteroid Drug Interactions			
Precipitant drug	Object drug*		Description
Aminoglutethimide	Dexamethasone	↓	Possible loss of dexamethasone-induced adrenal suppression.
Barbiturates	Corticosteroids	↓	Decreased pharmacologic effects of the corticosteroid may be observed.
Cholestyramine	Hydrocortisone	↓	The hydrocortisone AUC may be decreased.
Contraceptives, oral	Corticosteroids	↑	Corticosteroid half-life and concentration may be increased and clearance decreased.
Ephedrine	Dexamethasone	↓	A decreased half-life and increased clearance of dexamethasone may occur.
Estrogens	Corticosteroids	↑	Corticosteroid clearance may be decreased.
Hydantoins	Corticosteroids	↓	Corticosteroid clearance may be increased, resulting in reduced therapeutic effects.
Ketoconazole	Corticosteroids	↑	Corticosteroid clearance may be decreased and the AUC increased.
Macrolide antibiotics	Methylprednisolone	↑	A significant decrease in methylprednisolone clearance occurs. This has been utilized to decrease the methylprednisolone dose.
Rifampin	Corticosteroids	↓	Corticosteroid clearance may be increased resulting in decreased therapeutic effects.
Corticosteroids	Anticholinesterases	↓	Anticholinesterase effects may be antagonized in myasthenia gravis.
Corticosteroids	Anticoagulants, oral	↔	Anticoagulant dose requirements may be reduced. Conversely, corticosteroids may oppose the anticoagulant action.
Corticosteroids	Cyclosporine	↑	Although this combination is therapeutically beneficial for organ transplants, toxicity may be enhanced.
Corticosteroids	Digitalis glycosides	↑	Coadministration may enhance the possibility of digitalis toxicity associated with hypokalemia.
Corticosteroids	Isoniazid	↓	Isoniazid serum concentrations may be decreased.
Corticosteroids	Nondepolarizing muscle relaxants	↔	Corticosteroids may potentiate, counteract or have no effect on the neuromuscular blocking action.
Corticosteroids	Potassium-depleting agents (eg, diuretics)	↑	Observe patients for hypokalemia.
Corticosteroids	Salicylates	↓	Corticosteroids will reduce serum salicylate levels and may decrease their effectiveness.
Corticosteroids	Somatrem	↓	Growth-promoting effect of somatrem may be inhibited.
Corticosteroids	Theophyllines	↔	Alterations in the pharmacologic activity of either agent may occur.

* ↑ = Object drug increased. ↓ = Object drug decreased. ↔ = Undetermined effect.

(Drug Interactions continued on following page)

Drug Interactions (Cont.)

Drug/Lab test interactions: **Urine glucose** and **serum cholesterol** levels may be increased. Decreased serum levels of **potassium, triiodothyronine (T_3)**, and a minimal decrease of **thyroxine (T_4)** may occur. **Thyroid I^{131}** uptake may be decreased. False-negative results with the **nitroblue-tetrazolium test** for bacterial infection. **Dexamethasone,** given for cerebral edema, may alter the results of a brain scan (decreased uptake of radioactive material).

Adverse Reactions:

Fluid and electrolyte disturbances: Sodium and fluid retention; hypokalemia; hypokalemic alkalosis; metabolic alkalosis; hypocalcemia; CHF in susceptible patients; hypotension or shock-like reactions; hypertension (see Warnings).

Musculoskeletal: Muscle weakness; steroid myopathy; muscle mass loss; tendon rupture; osteoporosis; aseptic necrosis of femoral and humeral heads (1% to 37%); spontaneous fractures, including vertebral compression fractures and pathologic fracture of long bones.

Cardiovascular: Thromboembolism or fat embolism; thrombophlebitis; necrotizing angiitis; cardiac arrhythmias or ECG changes due to potassium deficiency; syncopal episodes; aggravation of hypertension; myocardial rupture following recent MI (see Warnings). There are reports of cardiac arrhythmias, fatal arrest or circulatory collapse following the rapid administration of large IV doses of **methylprednisolone** (0.5 to 1 g in $<$ 10 to 120 minutes). See Fluid and Electrolyte Disturbances.

GI: Pancreatitis; abdominal distension; ulcerative esophagitis; nausea; vomiting; increased appetite and weight gain. Peptic ulcer with perforation and hemorrhage (see Warnings). Perforation of the small and large bowel, particularly in inflammatory bowel disease.

Dermatologic: Impaired wound healing; thin fragile skin; petechiae and ecchymoses; erythema; lupus erythematosus-like lesions; suppression of skin test reactions; subcutaneous fat atrophy; purpura; striae; hirsutism; acneiform eruptions; other cutaneous reactions such as allergic dermatitis; urticaria; angioneurotic edema; perineal irritation.

Neurological: Convulsions; increased intracranial pressure with papilledema (pseudotumor cerebri), usually after stopping treatment; vertigo; headache; neuritis/paresthesias; aggravation of pre-existing psychiatric conditions; steroid psychoses (see Precautions).

Endocrine: Amenorrhea, postmenopausal bleeding and other menstrual irregularities; development of Cushingoid state (eg, moonface, buffalo hump, supraclavicular fat pad enlargement, central obesity); suppression of growth in children; secondary adrenocortical and pituitary unresponsiveness, particularly in times of stress (eg, trauma, surgery, illness); increased sweating; decreased carbohydrate tolerance; hyperglycemia; glycosuria; increased insulin or sulfonylurea requirements in diabetics; manifestations of latent diabetes mellitus; negative nitrogen balance due to protein catabolism; hirsutism.

Ophthalmic: Posterior subcapsular cataracts; increased IOP; glaucoma; exophthalmos.

Other: Anaphylactoid/hypersensitivity reactions, aggravation/masking of infections (see Warnings); malaise; leukocytosis (including neonates receiving dexamethasone via maternal injection); fatigue; insomnia; increased or decreased motility and number of spermatozoa.

Parenteral therapy: Rare instances of blindness associated with intralesional therapy around the face and head; hyperpigmentation or hypopigmentation; subcutaneous and cutaneous atrophy; sterile abscess; Charcot-like arthropathy; burning or tingling, especially in the perineal area (after IV injection); scarring, induration, inflammation, paresthesia, occasional irritation at the injection site or occasional brief increase in joint discomfort; transient or delayed pain or soreness; muscle twitching, ataxia, hiccoughs and nystagmus (low incidence following injection); anaphylactic reactions with or without circulatory collapse; cardiac arrest; bronchospasm; arachnoiditis after intrathecal use; foreign body granulomatous reactions involving the synovium with repeated injections.

Intra-articular - Osteonecrosis; tendon rupture; infection; skin atrophy; postinjection flare; hypersensitivity; facial flushing. Systemic reactions may also occur.

Intraspinal - Meningitis (tuberculous, bacterial, cryptococcal, aseptic, chemical); adhesive arachnoiditis; conus medullaris syndrome.

Overdosage:

Symptoms: There are two categories of toxic effects from therapeutic use of glucocorticoids:

Acute adrenal insufficiency due to too rapid withdrawal of corticosteroids after long-term use resulting in fever, myalgia, arthralgia, malaise, anorexia, nausea, desquamation of skin, orthostatic hypotension, dizziness, fainting, dyspnea and hypoglycemia.

Cushingoid changes from continued use of large doses resulting in moonface, central obesity, striae, hirsutism, acne, ecchymoses, hypertension, osteoporosis, myopathy, sexual dysfunction, diabetes, hyperlipidemia, peptic ulcer, increased susceptibility to infection and electrolyte and fluid imbalance. Reports of acute toxicity or death are rare.

(Overdosage continued on following page)

Overdosage (Cont.):

Treatment: Recovery of normal adrenal and pituitary function may require up to 9 months. Gradually taper the steroid under the supervision of a physician. Frequent lab tests are necessary. Supplementation is required during periods of stress (eg, illness, surgery, injury). Eventually reduce to the lowest dose that will control the symptoms or discontinue the corticosteroid completely. For large, acute overdoses, treatment includes gastric lavage or emesis and usual supportive measures. Refer to General Management of Acute Overdosage.

Patient Information:

May cause GI upset; take with meals or snacks. Take single daily or alternate day doses in the morning prior to 9 am. Take multiple doses at evenly spaced intervals throughout the day.

Patients on chronic steroid therapy should wear or carry identification to that effect.

Notify physician if unusual weight gain, swelling of the lower extremities, muscle weakness, black tarry stools, vomiting of blood, puffing of the face, menstrual irregularities, prolonged sore throat, fever, cold or infection occurs.

Signs of adrenal insufficiency include fatigue, anorexia, nausea, vomiting, diarrhea, weight loss, weakness, dizziness and low blood sugar. Notify physician promptly if these symptoms occur following dosage reduction or withdrawal of therapy.

High dose or long-term therapy: Avoid abrupt withdrawal of therapy.

Administration:

The maximal activity of the adrenal cortex is between 2 and 8 am, and it is minimal between 4 pm and midnight. Exogenous corticosteroids suppress adrenocortical activity the least when given at the time of maximal activity (am). Therefore, administer glucocorticoids in the morning prior to 9 am. When large doses are given, administer antacids between meals to help prevent peptic ulcers.

Initiation of therapy: The initial dosage depends on the specific disease entity being treated. Maintain or adjust the initial dosage until a satisfactory response is noted. If after a reasonable period of time there is a lack of satisfactory clinical response, discontinue the drug and transfer the patient to other appropriate therapy. *It should be emphasized that dosage requirements are variable and must be individualized.* For infants and children, the recommended dosage should be governed by the same considerations rather than by strict adherence to the ratio indicated by age or body weight.

Maintenance therapy: After a favorable response is observed, determine the maintenance dosage by decreasing the initial dosage in small amounts at intervals until the lowest dosage that will maintain an adequate clinical response is reached. Constant monitoring of drug dosage is required. Situations which may make dosage adjustments necessary are changes in the disease process, the patient's individual drug responsiveness, and the effect of patient exposure to stress; in this latter situation it may be necessary to increase the dosage for a period of time consistent with the patient's condition.

Withdrawal of therapy: If, after long-term therapy, the drug is to be stopped, it must be withdrawn gradually. If spontaneous remission occurs in a chronic condition, discontinue treatment gradually. Continued supervision of the patient after discontinuation of corticosteroids is essential, since there may be a sudden reappearance of severe manifestations of the disease.

Alternate day therapy is a dosing regimen in which twice the usual daily dose is administered every other morning. The purpose is to provide the patient requiring long-term treatment with the beneficial effects of corticosteroids while minimizing pituitary-adrenal suppression, the cushingoid state, withdrawal symptoms and growth suppression in children. *The benefits of alternate day therapy are only achieved by using the intermediate-acting agents.*

The rationale for this treatment schedule is based on two major premises: (a) The therapeutic effect of intermediate-acting corticosteroids persists longer than their physical presence and metabolic effects; (b) administration of the corticosteroid every other morning allows for reestablishment of a more normal hypothalamic-pituitary-adrenal (HPA) activity on the off-steroid day. Keep the following in mind when considering alternate day therapy:

1. Benefits of alternate day therapy do not encourage indiscriminate steroid use.
2. Alternate day therapy is primarily designed for patients in whom long-term corticosteroid therapy is anticipated.

(Administration continued on following page)

Administration (Cont.):

Alternate day therapy (Cont.):

3. In less severe disease processes, it may be possible to initiate treatment with alternate day therapy. More severe disease states usually require daily divided high-dose therapy for initial control. Continue the initial suppressive dose until satisfactory clinical response is obtained, usually 4 to 10 days in the case of many allergic and collagen diseases. Keep the period of initial suppressive dose as brief as possible, particularly when use of alternate day therapy is intended. Once control has been established, two courses are available: (a) Change to alternate day therapy, then gradually reduce the amount of corticosteroid given every other day or (b) reduce the daily dose of corticosteroid to the lowest effective level as rapidly as possible, then change over to an alternate day schedule. Theoretically, course (a) may be preferable.

4. Because of the advantages of alternate day therapy, it may be desirable to try patients on this form of therapy who have been on daily corticosteroids for long periods of time (eg, patients with rheumatoid arthritis). Since these patients may already have a suppressed HPA axis, establishing them on alternate day therapy may be difficult and not always successful; however, it is recommended that such regular attempts be made. It may be helpful to triple or even quadruple the daily maintenance dose and administer this every other day rather than just doubling the daily dose if difficulty is encountered. Once the patient is controlled, attempt to reduce this dose to a minimum.

5. Long-acting corticosteroids (eg, dexamethasone, betamethasone), due to their prolonged suppressive effect on adrenal activity, are not recommended for alternate day therapy.

6. It is important to individualize therapy. Complete control of symptoms will not be possible in all patients. An explanation of the benefits of alternate day therapy will help the patient to understand and tolerate the possible flare-up in symptoms which may occur in the latter part of the off-steroid day. Other therapy to relieve symptoms may be added or increased at this time if needed.

7. In the event of an acute flare-up of the disease process, it may be necessary to return to a full suppressive daily corticosteroid dose for control. Once control is established, alternate day therapy may be reinstituted.

Intra-articular injection: Dose depends on the joint size and varies with the severity of the condition. In chronic cases, injections may be repeated at intervals of 1 to 5 or more weeks depending upon the degree of relief obtained from the initial injection. Injection must be made into the synovial space. Do not inject unstable joints. Repeated intra-articular injection may result in joint instability. X-ray follow-up is suggested in selected cases to detect deterioration.

Suitable sites for injection are the knee, ankle, wrist, elbow, shoulder, hip and phalangeal joints. Since difficulty is frequently encountered in entering the hip joint, avoid any large blood vessels in the area. Joints *not* suitable for injection are those that are anatomically inaccessible and devoid of synovial space such as the spinal joints and the sacroiliac joints. Treatment failures frequently result from failure to enter the joint space; little or no benefit follows injection into surrounding tissue. If failures occur when injections into the synovial spaces are certain, as determined by aspiration of fluid, repeated injections are usually of no benefit. Local therapy does not alter the underlying disease process; whenever possible, employ comprehensive therapy including physiotherapy and orthopedic correction (see Precautions).

Miscellaneous (tendinitis, epicondylitis, ganglion): In the treatment of conditions such as tendinitis or tenosynovitis, inject into the tendon sheath rather than into the substance of the tendon. When treating conditions such as epicondylitis, outline the area of greatest tenderness and infiltrate the drug into the area. For ganglia of the tendon sheaths, inject the drug directly into the cyst. In many cases, a single injection markedly decreases size of the cystic tumor and may effect disappearance. The dose varies with the condition being treated. In recurrent or chronic conditions, repeated injections may be needed.

Injections for local effect in dermatologic conditions: Avoid injection of sufficient material to cause blanching, since this may be followed by a small slough. One to four injections are usually employed. The intervals between injections vary with the type of lesion being treated and the duration of improvement produced by the initial injection.

(Products listed on following pages)

Complete prescribing information for these products begins on page 465.

Glucocorticoids (Cont.)

CORTISONE

The drug is insoluble in water.

Dosage:

Initial dosage: 25 to 300 mg/day. In less severe diseases, lower doses may suffice.

	Product	Form	Description	C.I.*
Rx	**Cortisone Acetate** (Upjohn)	**Tablets:** 5 mg	(Upjohn 15). White, scored. In 50s.	35
Rx	**Cortisone Acetate** (Upjohn)	**Tablets:** 10 mg	(Upjohn 23). White, scored. In 100s.	33
Rx	**Cortisone Acetate** (Various, eg, Bioline, Dixon-Shane, Goldline, Major, Moore, Rugby, Schein)	**Tablets:** 25 mg	In 100s and 500s	4.3+
Rx	**Cortone Acetate** (MSD)		(MSD 219). White, scored. In 100s.	35

HYDROCORTISONE (Cortisol)

Cortisol suspension is insoluble in water.

Dosage:

Initial dosage: 20 to 240 mg/day.

	Product	Form	Description	C.I.*
Rx	**Cortef** (Upjohn)	**Tablets:** 5 mg	(Cortef 5). White, scored. In 50s.	24
Rx	**Hydrocortisone** (Major)	**Tablets:** 10 mg	In 100s.	7.1
Rx	**Cortef** (Upjohn)		(Cortef 10). White, scored. In 100s.	21
Rx	**Hydrocortone** (MSD)		(MSD 619). White, scored. Oval. In 100s.	23
Rx	**Hydrocortisone** (Various, eg, Major, Moore, Rugby, Schein, URL)	**Tablets:** 20 mg	In 100s.	4.3+
Rx	**Cortef** (Upjohn)		(Cortef 20). White, scored. In 100s.	20
Rx	**Hydrocortone** (MSD)		(MSD 625). White, scored. Oval. In 100s.	22

HYDROCORTISONE CYPIONATE

Dosage:

Initial dosage: 20 to 240 mg/day.

	Product	Form	Description	C.I.*
Rx	**Cortef** (Upjohn)	**Oral Suspension:** 10 mg per 5 ml hydrocortisone (as cypionate)	Sucrose. In 120 ml.	74

HYDROCORTISONE SODIUM PHOSPHATE

A water soluble salt with a rapid onset but short duration of action.

Dosage:

Administer by IV, IM or SC injection.

Initial dosage: 15 to 240 mg/day. Usually, ⅓ to ½ the oral dose every 12 hours.

Acute diseases: Doses higher than 240 mg may be required.

	Product	Form	Description	C.I.*
Rx	**Hydrocortone Phosphate** (MSD)	**Injection:** 50 mg/ml hydrocortisone (as sodium phosphate) solution	In 2 and 10 ml vials.[1]	114

* Cost Index based on cost per 25 mg cortisone or 20 mg hydrocortisone.

[1] With 3.2 mg sodium bisulfite, and 1.5 mg methylparaben and 0.2 mg propylparaben.

Complete prescribing information for these products begins on page 465.

Glucocorticoids (Cont.)

HYDROCORTISONE SODIUM SUCCINATE

A water soluble salt which is rapidly active.

Dosage:

May be administered IV or IM. The initial dose is 100 to 500 mg, and may be repeated at 2, 4 or 6 hour intervals depending on patient response and clinical condition.

	Product	Form	Packaging	C.I.*
Rx	**A-Hydrocort** (Abbott)	**Injection:** 100 mg hydrocortisone (as sodium succinate) per vial	In 2 ml Univials[1] and flip-top vials.	29
Rx	**Solu-Cortef** (Upjohn)		In vials and 2 ml Act-O-Vials.[1]	56
Rx	**A-Hydrocort** (Abbott)	**Injection:** 250 mg hydrocortisone (as sodium succinate) per vial	In 2 ml Univials[1] and flip-top vials.	26
Rx	**Solu-Cortef** (Upjohn)		In 2 ml Act-O-Vials.[1]	52
Rx	**A-Hydrocort** (Abbott)	**Injection:** 500 mg hydrocortisone (as sodium succinate) per vial	In 4 ml Univials[1] and flip-top vials.	26
Rx	**Solu-Cortef** (Upjohn)		In 4 ml Act-O-Vials.[1]	50
Rx	**A-Hydrocort** (Abbott)	**For Injection:** 1000 mg hydrocortisone (as sodium succinate) per vial	In 8 ml Univials[1] and flip-top vials.	26
Rx	**Solu-Cortef** (Upjohn)		In 8 ml Act-O-Vials.[1]	50

HYDROCORTISONE ACETATE

Hydrocortisone acetate has a slow onset but long duration of action when compared with more soluble preparations. Because of its insolubility, it is suitable for intra-articular, intralesional and soft tissue injection where its anti-inflammatory effects are confined mainly to the area in which it has been injected, although it is capable of producing systemic hormonal effects.

Dosage:

For intralesional, intra-articular or soft tissue injection only. Not for IV use.

Large joints (eg, knee) – 25 mg; occasionally, 37.5 mg.
Small joints (eg, interphalangeal, temporomandibular) – 10 to 25 mg.
Tendon sheaths – 5 to 12.5 mg.
Soft tissue infiltration – 25 to 50 mg; occasionally, 75 mg.
Bursae – 25 to 37.5 mg.
Ganglia – 12.5 to 25 mg.

If desired, a local anesthetic may be injected before hydrocortisone acetate or mixed in a syringe and given simultaneously.

If used prior to intra-articular injection of the steroid, inject most of the anesthetic into the soft tissues of the surrounding area and instill a small amount into the joint.

If given together, mix in the injection syringe by drawing the steroid in first, then the anesthetic. In this way, the anesthetic will not be introduced inadvertently into the vial of the steroid. *The mixture must be used immediately and any unused portion discarded.*

	Product	Form	Packaging	C.I.*
Rx	**Hydrocortisone Acetate** (Various, eg, Dixon-Shane, Major, Moore, Rugby, Schein, URL)	**Injection:** 25 mg per ml suspension	In 10 ml vials.	25+
Rx	**Hydrocortone Acetate** (MSD)		In 5 ml vials.[2]	159
Rx	**Hydrocortisone Acetate** (Various, eg, Major, Moore, Rugby, URL)	**Injection:** 50 mg per ml suspension	In 10 ml vials.	14+
Rx	**Hydrocortone Acetate** (MSD)		In 5 ml vials.[2]	152

* Cost Index based on cost per 25 mg.
[1] With benzyl alcohol.
[2] With 4 mg polysorbate 80, 5 mg sodium carboxymethylcellulose and 9 mg benzyl alcohol per ml.

Complete prescribing information for these products begins on page 465.

Glucocorticoids (Cont.)

PREDNISONE

Dosage:

Initial dosage varies from 5 to 60 mg/day. Prednisone is inactive and must be metabolized to prednisolone. This conversion may be impaired in patients with liver disease.

	Product	Form	Description	C.I.*
Rx	**Meticorten** (Schering)	**Tablets:** 1 mg	Lactose. (KEM or 843). White. In 100s.	34
Rx	**Orasone** (Solvay Pharm.)		Lactose. (RR 1). Pink, scored. In 100s and 1000s.	8.6
Rx	**Panasol-S** (Seatrace)		Pink, scored. In 100s and 1000s.	14
Rx	**Deltasone** (Upjohn)	**Tablets:** 2.5 mg	Lactose, sucrose. (Deltasone 2.5). Scored. In 100s.	3.6
Rx	**Prednisone** (Various, eg, Barr, Bioline, Geneva Marsam, Goldline, Major, Parmed, Rugby)	**Tablets:** 5 mg	In 100s, 500s, 1000s, 5000s and UD 100s.	2.3+
Rx	**Deltasone** (Upjohn)		Lactose, sucrose. (Deltasone 5). Scored. In 100s, 500s, UD 100s & Dosepak 21s.	2
Rx	**Orasone** (Solvay Pharm.)		Lactose. (RR 5). White, scored. In 100s and 1000s.	2.1
Rx	**Prednicen-M** (Central)		(131/07). Red. Film coated. In 100s, 1000s and unit pak 21s.	5.3
Rx	**Sterapred** (Mayrand)		(M/R). Blue. In Uni-Pak 21s.	15
Rx	**Prednisone** (Various, eg, Barr, Bioline, Geneva Marsam, Goldline, Major, Parmed, Rugby)	**Tablets:** 10 mg	In 100s, 1000s and UD 100s.	1.3+
Rx	**Deltasone** (Upjohn)		Lactose, sucrose. (Deltasone 10). Scored. In 100s, 500s and UD 100s.	1.3
Rx	**Orasone** (Solvay Pharm.)		Lactose. (RR 10). Blue, scored. In 100s and 1000s.	1.6
Rx	**Sterapred DS** (Mayrand)		(MP 0364). White, scored. In Uni-Pak 21s and 48s.	12
Rx	**Prednisone** (Various, eg, Barr, Bioline, Geneva Marsam, Goldline, Major, Parmed, Rugby)	**Tablets:** 20 mg	In 100s, 500s, 1000s and UD 100s.	1.1+
Rx	**Deltasone** (Upjohn)		Lactose, sucrose. (Deltasone 20). Scored. In 100s, 500s and UD 100s.	1.1
Rx	**Orasone** (Solvay Pharm.)		Lactose. (RR 20). Yellow, scored. In 100s and 1000s.	1.4
Rx	**Prednisone** (Various, eg, Geneva Marsam, Major, Rugby)	**Tablets:** 50 mg	In 100s and UD 100s.	1.3+
Rx	**Deltasone** (Upjohn)		Lactose, sucrose. (Deltasone 500). Scored. In 100s.	1
Rx	**Orasone** (Solvay Pharm.)		Lactose. (RR 50). White, scored. Film coated. In 100s.	1.2
Rx	**Prednisone** (Roxane)	**Oral Solution:** 5 mg per 5 ml	5% alcohol. Fructose, saccharin. Dye free. In 500 ml and UD 5 ml (40s).	10
Rx	**Prednisone Intensol Concentrate** (Roxane)	**Oral Solution:** 5 mg per ml	30% alcohol. In 30 ml.	25
Rx	**Liquid Pred** (Muro)	**Syrup:** 5 mg per 5 ml	5% alcohol. Saccharin, sorbitol and sucrose. In 120 and 240 ml.	17

* Cost Index based on cost per 5 mg.

Complete prescribing information for these products begins on page 465.

Glucocorticoids (Cont.)

PREDNISOLONE

Dosage:

Initial dosage: 5 to 60 mg/day.

Multiple sclerosis: In treatment of acute exacerbations of multiple sclerosis, 200 mg daily for a week followed by 80 mg every other day for 1 month.

	Product	Form	Description	C.I.*
Rx	**Prednisolone** (Various, eg, Bioline, Dixon-Shane, Geneva Marsam, Goldline, Major, Moore, Roxane, Rugby, Schein, URL)	**Tablets:** 5 mg	In 100s, 1000s and 5000s.	1.5+
Rx	**Delta-Cortef** (Upjohn)		Lactose, sucrose. White, scored. In 100s and 500s.	7.4
Rx	**Prelone** (Muro)	**Syrup:** 15 mg per 5 ml	5% alcohol. Saccharin, sucrose. Cherry flavor. In 240 ml.	10

PREDNISOLONE ACETATE

Relatively insoluble.

Dosage:

Systemic: Not for IV use. *Initial dosage* – 4 to 60 mg/day, IM.

Intralesional, intra-articular or soft tissue injection: 4 mg, up to 100 mg.

Multiple sclerosis: 200 mg daily for a week, followed by 80 mg every other day or 4 to 8 mg dexamethasone every other day for 1 month.

	Product	Form	Description	C.I.*
Rx	**Prednisolone Acetate** (Various, eg, Rugby, URL)	**Injection:** 25 mg per ml suspension	In 10 and 30 ml vials.	4.6+
Rx	**Key-Pred 25** (Hyrex)		In 10 and 30 ml vials.	6.1
Rx	**Predcor-25** (Hauck)		In 10 ml vials.[1]	6.4
Rx	**Prednisolone Acetate** (Various, eg, Geneva Marsam, Goldline, Major, Moore, Rugby, Schein, URL)	**Injection:** 50 mg per ml suspension	In 10 and 30 ml vials.	3.9+
Rx	**Articulose-50** (Seatrace)		In 10 ml vials.	4.2
Rx	**Key-Pred 50** (Hyrex)		In 10 ml vials.	4.4
Rx	**Predaject-50** (Mayrand)		In 10 ml vials.	9.2
Rx	**Predalone 50** (Forest)		In 10 ml vials.[1]	4.1
Rx	**Predcor-50** (Hauck)		In 10 ml vials.[1]	4.4
Rx	**Predicort-50** (Dunhall)		In 10 ml vials.[1]	5.7

PREDNISOLONE TEBUTATE

Slightly soluble with a slow onset and prolonged duration of action.

Dosage:

Intra-articular, intralesional or soft tissue administration:

Large joints (eg, knee) - 20 mg; occasionally, 30 mg. Doses > 40 mg are not recommended.

Small joints (eg, interphalangeal, temporomandibular) - 8 to 10 mg.

Bursae - 20 to 30 mg. *Tendon sheaths* - 4 to 10 mg. *Ganglia* - 10 to 20 mg.

	Product	Form	Description	C.I.*
Rx	**Prednisolone Tebutate** (Major)	**Injection:** 20 mg per ml suspension	In 10 ml vials.	13
Rx	**Hydeltra-T.B.A.** (MSD)		In 1 and 5 ml vials.[2]	74
Rx	**Predalone T.B.A.** (Forest)		In 10 ml vials.[2]	13
Rx	**Prednisol TBA** (Pasadena)		In 10 ml vials.[2]	11

* Cost Index based on cost per 5 mg.

[1] With polysorbate 80, carboxymethylcellulose and benzyl alcohol.

[2] With polysorbate 80, sorbitol and benzyl alcohol.

Complete prescribing information for these products begins on page 465.

Glucocorticoids (Cont.)

PREDNISOLONE SODIUM PHOSPHATE

Water soluble and rapid acting, but has a short duration of action.

Prednisolone sodium phosphate oral liquid produces a 20% higher peak plasma level of prednisolone which occurs approximately 15 minutes earlier than the peak seen with tablet formulations.

Dosage: *Parenteral:* For IV or IM use. *Initial dosage* – 4 to 60 mg/day.

Intra-articular, intralesional or soft tissue administration:

Large joints (eg, knee) – 10 to 20 mg.
Small joints (eg, interphalangeal, temporomandibular) – 4 to 5 mg.
Bursae – 10 to 15 mg.
Tendon sheaths – 2 to 5 mg.
Soft tissue infiltration – 10 to 30 mg.
Ganglia – 5 to 10 mg.

Oral: Initial dosage – 5 to 60 ml (5 to 60 mg base) per day.

Multiple sclerosis (acute exacerbations): 200 mg daily for a week, followed by 80 mg every other day or 4 to 8 mg dexamethasone every other day for 1 month.

	Product	Form	Description	C.I.*
Rx	**Hydeltrasol** (MSD)	**Injection:** 20 mg per ml prednisolone (as sodium phosphate) solution	In 2 and 5 ml vials.[1]	117
Rx	**Key-Pred-SP** (Hyrex)		In 10 ml vials.[1]	12
Rx sf	**Pediapred** (Fisons)	**Oral Liquid:** 5 mg prednisolone (as sodium phosphate) per 5 ml	Alcohol and dye free. Raspberry flavor. In 120 ml.	36

TRIAMCINOLONE, ORAL

Dosage: Initial daily dosage in specific disorders is:

Adrenocortical insufficiency – 4 to 12 mg, in addition to mineralocorticoid therapy.
Rheumatic and dermatological disorders and bronchial asthma – 8 to 16 mg.
Allergic states – 8 to 12 mg. *Ophthalmological diseases* – 12 to 40 mg.
Respiratory diseases – 16 to 48 mg. *Hematologic disorders* – 16 to 60 mg.
Tuberculous meningitis – 32 to 48 mg. *Acute rheumatic carditis* – 20 to 60 mg.
Acute leukemia and lymphoma (adults) – 16 to 40 mg. It may be necessary to give as much as 100 mg/day in leukemia; *acute leukemia (children)* – 1 to 2 mg/kg.
Edematous states – 16 to 20 mg (up to 48 mg) until diuresis occurs.
Systemic lupus erythematosus – 20 to 32 mg.

	Product	Form	Description	C.I.*
Rx	**Aristocort** (Fujisawa)	**Tablets:** 1 mg	Lactose. (LL A1). Yellow, scored. Oblong, flat. In 50s.	89
Rx	**Aristocort** (Fujisawa)	**Tablets:** 2 mg	Lactose. (LL A2). Pink, scored. Oblong. In 100s.	94
Rx	**Triamcinolone** (Various, eg, Dixon-Shane, Moore, Rugby, Schein, URL)	**Tablets:** 4 mg	In 100s and 500s.	3.8+
Rx	**Aristocort** (Fujisawa)		Lactose. (LL A4). White, scored. Oblong, flat. In 30s, 100s and Aristo-Pak 16s.	85
Rx	**Atolone** (Major)		White, scored. In 100s and Uni-Pak 16s.	73
Rx	**Kenacort** (Apothecon)		Lactose. In 100s.	56
Rx	**Aristocort** (Fujisawa)	**Tablets:** 8 mg	Lactose. (LL A8). Yellow, scored. Oblong, flat. In 50s.	70
Rx	**Kenacort** (Apothecon)		Lactose, tartrazine. In 50s.	48
Rx	**Kenacort** (Apothecon)	**Syrup:** 4 mg (as diacetate) per 5 ml	Sucrose. In 120 ml.	69

* Cost Index based on cost per 5 mg prednisolone phosphate or 4 mg triamcinolone.
[1] With niacinamide, EDTA, phenol and sodium bisulfite. *sf* – Sugar free.

Complete prescribing information for these products begins on page 465.

Glucocorticoids (Cont.)

TRIAMCINOLONE DIACETATE

Slightly soluble providing a prompt onset of action and a longer duration of effect.

Dosage:

Systemic: Not for IV use. May be administered IM for initial therapy; however, most clinicians prefer to adjust the dose orally until adequate control is attained. The average dose is 40 mg IM per week. In general, a single parenteral dose 4 to 7 times the oral daily dose controls the patient from 4 to 7 days, up to 3 to 4 weeks.

Intra-articular and intrasynovial: 5 to 40 mg.

Intralesional or sublesional: 5 to 48 mg. Do not use more than 12.5 mg per injection site. The usual average dose is 25 mg per lesion.

	Product	Form	Packaging	C.I.*
Rx	**Aristocort Intralesional** (Fujisawa)	**Injection:** 25 mg per ml suspension	In 5 ml vials.[1]	46
Rx	**Triamcinolone** (Various, eg, Major, Moore, Rugby, URL)	**Injection:** 40 mg per ml suspension	In 5 ml vials.	39+
Rx	**Trilone** (Hauck)		In 5 ml vials.	12
Rx	**Amcort** (Keene)		In 5 ml vials.[1]	8.1
Rx	**Aristocort Forte** (Fujisawa)		In 1 and 5 ml vials.[1]	33
Rx	**Articulose L.A.** (Seatrace)		In 5 ml vials.	14
Rx	**Cenocort Forte** (Central)		In 5 ml vials.[1]	20
Rx	**Triam Forte** (Hyrex)		In 5 ml vials.	11
Rx	**Triamolone 40** (Forest)		In 5 ml vials.[1]	13
Rx	**Tristoject** (Mayrand)		In 5 ml vials.	15

TRIAMCINOLONE HEXACETONIDE

Relatively insoluble, slowly absorbed and has a prolonged action.

Dosage: Not for IV use.

Intra-articular: 2 to 20 mg average. *Large joints* (eg, knee, hip, shoulder) – 10 to 20 mg; *small joints* (eg, interphalangeal, metacarpophalangeal) – 2 to 6 mg.

Intralesional or sublesional: Up to 0.5 mg per square inch of affected area.

	Product	Form	Packaging	C.I.*
Rx	**Aristospan Intralesional** (Fujisawa)	**Injection:** 5 mg per ml suspension	In 5 ml vials.[2]	124
Rx	**Aristospan Intra-articular** (Fujisawa)	**Injection:** 20 mg per ml suspension	In 1 and 5 ml vials.[2]	78

* Cost Index based on cost per 4 mg.

[1] With polysorbate 80, polyethylene glycol and benzyl alcohol.

[2] With polysorbate 80, sorbitol and benzyl alcohol.

Complete prescribing information for these products begins on page 465.

Glucocorticoids (Cont.)

TRIAMCINOLONE ACETONIDE

Relatively insoluble. Has an extended duration which may be permanent or sustained for several weeks.

Dosage: *Systemic: Initial IM dose* – 2.5 to 60 mg/day. Not for IV use.

Intra-articular or intrabursal administration and for injection into tendon sheaths: Initial dose – 2.5 to 5 mg for smaller joints and 5 to 15 mg for larger joints. For adults, doses up to 10 mg for smaller areas and up to 40 mg for larger areas are usually sufficient.

Intradermal: Use only the 3 mg/ml or 10 mg/ml strength. The initial dose varies, but limit to 1 mg per injection site.

Clumping results from exposure to freezing temperatures; do not use.

	Product	Form	Supplied	C.I.*
Rx	**Tac-3** (Herbert)	**Injection:** 3 mg per ml suspension	In 5 ml vials.[1]	143
Rx	**Kenalog-10** (Westwood-Squibb)	**Injection:** 10 mg per ml suspension	In 5 ml vials.[1]	33
Rx	**Triamcinolone Acetonide** (Various, eg, Bioline, Dixon-Shane, Geneva Marsam, Goldline, Moore, Schein, URL)	**Injection:** 40 mg per ml suspension	In 1 and 5 ml vials.	8.6+
Rx	**Cenocort A-40** (Central)		In 5 ml vials.[1]	23
Rx	**Kenaject-40** (Mayrand)		In 5 ml vials.	26
Rx	**Kenalog-40** (Westwood-Squibb)		In 1, 5 and 10 ml vials.[1]	28
Rx	**Tac-40** (Parnell)		In 5 ml vials.	NA
Rx	**Triam-A** (Hyrex)		In 5 ml vials.	11
Rx	**Triamonide 40** (Forest)		In 5 ml vials.[1]	13
Rx	**Tri-Kort** (Keene)		In 5 ml vials.[1]	9.9
Rx	**Trilog** (Hauck)		In 5 ml vials.[1]	13

METHYLPREDNISOLONE

Dosage: *Initial dose* – 4 to 48 mg/day; adjust until a satisfactory response is noted. Individualize dosage. Determine maintenance dose by decreasing initial dose in small decrements at appropriate intervals until reaching the lowest effective dose.

Dosepak 21 therapy: Follow manufacturer's directions.

Alternate day therapy (ADT): Twice the usual dose is administered every other morning. The patient on long-term treatment receives the beneficial effects of corticosteroids while minimizing certain undesirable effects. In less severe diseases requiring long-term therapy, treatment may be initiated with ADT.

	Product	Form	Supplied	C.I.*
Rx	**Methylprednisolone** (Various, eg, Bioline, Geneva Marsam, Major, Moore, Parmed, Rugby)	**Tablets:** 4 mg	In 21s and 100s.	12+
Rx	**Methylprednisolone** (Various, eg, Bioline, Rugby, URL)	**Tablets:** 16 mg	In 50s.	14
Rx	**Medrol** (Upjohn)	**Tablets:** 2 mg[2]	Pink, scored. Elliptical. In 100s.	34
		4 mg[2]	White, scored. Elliptical. In 30s, 100s, 500s, UD 100s and Dosepak 21s.	32
		8 mg[2]	Peach, scored. Elliptical. In 25s.	23
		16 mg[2]	White, scored. Elliptical. In 50s and ADT Pak 14s.	18
		24 mg[2]	Tartrazine. Yellow, scored. Elliptical. In 25s.	14
		32 mg[2]	Peach, scored. Elliptical. In 25s.	13

* Cost Index based on cost per 4 mg.

[1] With polysorbate 80, carboxymethylcellulose and benzyl alcohol.

[2] With lactose and sucrose.

Complete prescribing information for these products begins on page 465.

Glucocorticoids (Cont.)

METHYLPREDNISOLONE SODIUM SUCCINATE

Highly soluble; has rapid effect by IV or IM routes.

Dosage: *Initial dose* – 10 to 40 mg IV, administered over 1 to several minutes. Give subsequent doses IV or IM. *Infants and children* – Not less than 0.5 mg/kg/24 hours.

For high dose therapy, give 30 mg/kg IV, infused over 10 to 20 minutes. May repeat every 4 to 6 hours, not beyond 48 to 72 hours.

	Product	Form	Packaging	C.I.*
Rx	**Methylprednisolone Sodium Succinate** (Various, eg, Elkins Sinn, Lyphomed)	**Powder for Injection:** 40 mg per vial	In 1 and 3 ml vials.	21+
Rx	**A-Methapred** (Abbott)		In 1 ml Univial.[1]	13
Rx	**Solu-Medrol** (Upjohn)		In 1 ml Act-O-Vial.[1]	14
Rx	**Methylprednisolone Sodium Succinate** (Various, eg, Elkins Sinn, Lyphomed)	**Powder for Injection:** 125 mg per vial	In 2 and 5 ml vials.	19+
Rx	**A-Methapred** (Abbott)		In 2 ml Univial.[2]	11
Rx	**Solu-Medrol** (Upjohn)		In 2 ml Act-O-Vial.[2]	9.7
Rx	**Methylprednisolone Sodium Succinate** (Various, eg, Elkins Sinn, Lyphomed)	**Powder for Injection:** 500 mg per vial	In 1, 4 and 20 ml vials.	21+
Rx	**A-Methapred** (Abbott)		In 4 ml Univial and 500 mg ADD-Vantage vials.[3]	11
Rx	**Solu-Medrol** (Upjohn)		In 8 ml vials and 8 ml vials w/diluent.[3]	8.1
Rx	**Methylprednisolone Sodium Succinate** (Various, eg, Elkins Sinn, Lyphomed)	**Powder for Injection:** 1 g per vial	In 1, 8 and 50 ml vials.	18+
Rx	**A-Methapred** (Abbott)		In 8 ml Univial and 500 mg ADD-Vantage vials.[4]	9.4
Rx	**Solu-Medrol** (Upjohn)		In 1 g vials, 1 g vials w/ diluent and 8 ml Act-O-Vial.[4]	6.9
Rx	**Solu-Medrol** (Upjohn)	**Powder for Injection:** 2 g per vial	In 2 g vials w/diluent.	6.3

* Cost Index based on cost per 4 mg.

[1] With sodium phosphate anhydrous (1.6 mg monobasic, 17.5 mg dibasic), 25 mg lactose and 9 mg benzyl alcohol.

[2] With sodium phosphate anhydrous (1.6 mg monobasic, 17.4 mg dibasic), ≈ 18 mg benzyl alcohol.

[3] With sodium phosphate anhydrous (6.4 mg monobasic, 69.6 mg dibasic). May contain 36 to 70.2 mg benzyl alcohol.

[4] With sodium phosphate anhydrous (12.8 mg monobasic, 139.2 mg dibasic). May contain 66.8 to 141 mg benzyl alcohol.

[5] With sodium phosphate anhydrous (25.6 mg monobasic, 278 mg dibasic), 273 mg benzyl alcohol.

Complete prescribing information for these products begins on page 465.

Glucocorticoids (Cont.)

METHYLPREDNISOLONE ACETATE

Because of its low solubility, methylprednisolone acetate has a sustained effect.

Dosage: *Systemic:* Not for IV use. As a temporary substitute for oral therapy, administer the total daily dose as a single IM injection. For prolonged effect, give a single weekly dose.

Adrenogenital syndrome – A single 40 mg injection IM every 2 weeks.

Rheumatoid arthritis – Weekly IM maintenance dose varies from 40 to 120 mg.

Dermatologic lesions – 40 to 120 mg IM weekly for 1 to 4 weeks. In severe dermatitis (eg, poison ivy), relief may result within 8 to 12 hours of a single dose of 80 to 120 mg IM. In chronic contact dermatitis, repeated injections every 5 to 10 days may be necessary. In seborrheic dermatitis, a weekly dose of 80 mg IM may be adequate.

Asthma and allergic rhinitis – 80 to 120 mg IM.

Intra-articular and soft tissue: Large joints – 20 to 80 mg; *medium joints* – 10 to 40 mg; *small joints* – 4 to 10 mg; *ganglion, tendinitis, epicondylitis and bursitis* – 4 to 30 mg.

Intralesional: 20 to 60 mg.

	Product	Form	Packaging	C.I.*
Rx	**Methylprednisolone Acetate** (Various, eg, Rugby, Schein)	**Injection:** 20 mg per ml suspension	In 5 and 10 ml vials.	7.5+
Rx	**Depo-Medrol** (Upjohn)		In 5 ml vials.[1]	15
Rx	**Methylprednisolone Acetate** (Various, eg, Dixon-Shane, Goldline, Major, Moore, Rugby, Schein, URL)	**Injection:** 40 mg per ml suspension	In 5 and 10 ml vials.	6.1+
Rx	**depMedalone 40** (Forest)		In 5 ml vials.[1]	13
Rx	**Depoject** (Mayrand)		In 10 ml vials.[1]	14
Rx	**Depo-Medrol** (Upjohn)		In 1, 5 and 10 ml vials.[1]	28
Rx	**Depopred-40** (Hyrex)		In 5 and 10 ml vials.	11
Rx	**Duralone-40** (Hauck)		In 10 ml vials.[1]	9.3
Rx	**Medralone 40** (Keene)		In 5 ml vials.[1]	7.7
Rx	**M-Prednisol-40** (Pasadena)		In 5 ml vials.	10
Rx	**Rep-Pred 40** (Central)		In 5 ml vials.[1]	19
Rx	**Methylprednisolone Acetate** (Various, Dixon-Shane, Goldline, Moore, Rugby, Schein, URL)	**Injection:** 80 mg per ml suspension	In 5 ml vials.	6.2+
Rx	**depMedalone 80** (Forest)		In 5 ml vials.[1]	11
Rx	**Depoject** (Mayrand)		In 5 ml vials.[1]	14
Rx	**Depo-Medrol** (Upjohn)		In 1 and 5 ml vials.[1]	25
Rx	**Depopred-80** (Hyrex)		In 5 ml vials.	11
Rx	**D-Med 80** (Ortega)		In 5 ml vials.[1]	NA
Rx	**Duralone-80** (Hauck)		In 5 ml vials.[1]	9.3
Rx	**Medralone 80** (Keene)		In 5 ml vials.[1]	6.1
Rx	**M-Prednisol-80** (Pasadena)		In 5 ml vials.	8.4
Rx	**Rep-Pred 80** (Central)		In 5 ml vials.[1]	8.1

* Cost Index based on cost per 4 mg.

[1] With polyethylene glycol and myristyl-gamma-picolinium chloride.

Complete prescribing information for these products begins on page 465

Glucocorticoids (Cont.)

DEXAMETHASONE, ORAL

Dosage:

Initial dosage: 0.75 to 9 mg/day.

In acute, self-limited allergic disorders or acute exacerbations of chronic allergic disorders, the following dosage schedule combining parenteral and oral therapy (0.75 mg tablets) is suggested: Dexamethasone sodium phosphate injection, 4 mg/ml: *First day* – 1 or 2 ml IM. *Second day* – 4 tablets in 2 divided doses. *Third day* – 4 tablets in 2 divided doses. *Fourth day* – 2 tablets in 2 divided doses. *Fifth day* – *1 tablet. Sixth day* – 1 tablet. *Seventh day* – No treatment. *Eighth day* - Follow-up visit.

Suppression tests:

For Cushing's syndrome – Give 1 mg at 11 pm. Draw blood for plasma cortisol determination the following day at 8 am. For greater accuracy, give 0.5 mg every 6 hours for 48 hours. Collect 24 hour urine to determine 17-hydroxycorticosteroid excretion.

Test to distinguish Cushing's syndrome due to pituitary ACTH excess from Cushing's syndrome due to other causes – Give 2 mg every 6 hours for 48 hours. Collect 24 hour urine to determine 17-hydroxycorticosteroid excretion.

Unlabeled uses: The dexamethasone suppression test has been used for the detection, diagnosis and management of depression; however, pending further evaluation and research, its value is unproven.

	Product	Form	Description	C.I.*
Rx	**Dexamethasone** (Various, eg, Major, Rugby)	**Tablets:** 0.25 mg	In 100s.	7.6+
Rx	**Decadron** (MSD)		Lactose. (MSD 20). Orange, scored. Pentagonal. In 100s.	49
Rx	**Dexamethasone** (Various, eg, Bioline, Goldline, Roxane, Rugby)	**Tablets:** 0.5 mg	In 100s.	4.9+
Rx	**Decadron** (MSD)		Lactose. (MSD 41). Yellow, scored. Pentagonal. In 100s and UD 100s.	44
Rx	**Dexameth** (Major)		In 100s.	6.4
Rx	**Dexone** (Solvay Pharm.)		Lactose. (RR 3205). Yellow, scored. In 100s and UD 100s.	7.3
Rx	**Dexamethasone** (Various, eg, Bioline, Goldline, Parmed, Roxane, Rugby)	**Tablets:** 0.75 mg	In 100s and 1000s.	3.2+
Rx	**Decadron** (MSD)		Lactose. (MSD 63). Bluish-green, scored. Pentagonal. In 12s, 100s and UD 100s.	36
Rx	**Dexameth** (Major)		In 100s and Unipak 12s.	4.8
Rx	**Dexone** (Solvay Pharm.)		Lactose. (RR 3210). Green, scored. In 100s and UD 100s.	5.4
Rx	**Dexamethasone** (Roxane)	**Tablets:** 1 mg	(54 489). Yellow, scored. In 100s, 1000s and UD 100s.	9.3
Rx	**Dexamethasone** (Various, eg, Bioline, Goldline, Roxane, Rugby)	**Tablets:** 1.5 mg	In 50s and 100s.	2.9+
Rx	**Decadron** (MSD)		Lactose. (MSD 95). Pink, scored. Pentagonal. In 50s and UD 100s.	33
Rx	**Dexameth** (Major)		In 100s.	5.7
Rx	**Dexone** (Solvay Pharm.)		Lactose. (RR 3215). Pink, scored. In 100s and UD 100s.	4.9
Rx	**Hexadrol** (Organon)		Peach, scored. In 100s.	9.8
Rx	**Dexamethasone** (Roxane)	**Tablets:** 2 mg	(54 662). White, scored. In 100s and UD 100s.	9.1

* Cost Index based on cost per 0.75 mg.

(Continued on following page)

Complete prescribing information for these products begins on page 465.

Glucocorticoids (Cont.)

DEXAMETHASONE, ORAL (Cont.)				C.I.*
Rx	**Dexamethasone** (Various, eg, Bioline, Goldline, Rugby)	**Tablets:** 4 mg	In 50s and 100s.	2.8+
Rx	**Decadron** (MSD)		Lactose. (MSD 97). White, scored. Pentagonal. In 50s & UD 100s.	20
Rx	**Dexameth** (Major)		In 100s.	3
Rx	**Dexone** (Solvay Pharm.)		Lactose. (RR 3220). White, scored. In 100s and UD 100s.	3.9
Rx	**Hexadrol** (Organon)		Green, scored. In 100s.	7.6
Rx	**Dexamethasone** (Goldline)	**Tablets:** 6 mg	In 50s and 100s.	2.6
Rx	**Decadron** (MSD)		Lactose. (MSD 147). Green, scored. Pentagonal. In 50s and UD 100s.	20
Rx	**Hexadrol** (Organon)	**Tablets:** Therapeutic Pack	Six 1.5 mg tablets (peach, scored) and eight 0.75 mg tablets (white, scored).	NA
Rx	**Dexamethasone** (Various, eg, Bioline, Geneva Marsam, Goldline, Major, PBI, Roxane, Rugby)	**Elixir:** 0.5 mg per 5 ml	In 100, 120, 240 and 500 ml, and UD 5 and 20 ml.	28+
Rx	**Decadron** (MSD)		5% alcohol. Saccharin. In 100 and 237 ml.	72
Rx	**Hexadrol** (Organon)		5% alcohol. Sorbitol. Cherry flavor. In 120 ml.	36
Rx *sf*	**Dexamethasone** (Roxane)	**Oral Solution:** 0.5 mg per 5 ml	Dye free. Sorbitol. In 500 ml and UD 5 & 20 ml (100s).	15
Rx	**Dexamethasone Intensol** (Roxane)	**Oral Solution:** 0.5 mg per 0.5 ml	30% alcohol. In 30 ml w/dropper.	78

DEXAMETHASONE ACETATE

A long-acting repository preparation with prompt onset of action.

Dosage: Not for IV use. *Systemic:* 8 to 16 mg IM, may repeat in 1 to 3 weeks. *Intralesional:* 0.8 to 1.6 mg. *Intra-articular and soft tissue:* 4 to 16 mg; may repeat at 1 to 3 week intervals.

				C.I.*
Rx	**Dexamethasone Acetate** (Various, eg, Bioline, Dixon-Shane, Goldline, Major, Moore, Rugby, URL)	**Injection:** 8 mg per ml (as acetate) suspension. Not for IV use.	In 5 ml vials.	11+
Rx	**Dalalone L.A.** (Forest)		In 5 ml vials.[1]	12
Rx	**Decadron-LA** (MSD)		In 1 and 5 ml vials.[1]	50
Rx	**Decaject-L.A.** (Mayrand)		In 5 ml vials.	27
Rx	**Dexacen LA-8** (Central)		In 5 ml vials.[1]	13
Rx	**Dexasone L.A.** (Hauck)		In 5 ml vials.[1]	17
Rx	**Dexone LA** (Keene)		In 5 ml vials.[1]	12
Rx	**Solurex LA** (Hyrex)		In 5 ml vials.	13
Rx	**Dalalone D.P.** (Forest)	**Injection:** 16 mg per ml (as acetate) suspension. Not for IV or intralesional use.	In 1 and 5 ml vials.[1]	11

* Cost Index based on cost per 0.75 mg.

[1] With creatinine, polysorbate 80, carboxymethylcellulose, sodium bisulfite, EDTA and benzyl alcohol.

Complete prescribing information for these products begins on page 465.

Glucocorticoids (Cont.)

DEXAMETHASONE SODIUM PHOSPHATE

Has a rapid onset and short duration of action when compared to less soluble preparations.

Dosage:

Systemic: Initial dosage – 0.5 to 9 mg daily. Usual dose ranges are ⅓ to ½ the oral dose given every 12 hours. However, in certain acute, life-threatening situations, dosages exceeding the usual may be justified and may be in multiples of the oral dosages.

Cerebral edema – In adults, administer an initial IV dose of 10 mg, followed by 4 mg IM every 6 hours until maximum response has been noted. Response is usually noted within 12 to 24 hours. Dosage may be reduced after 2 to 4 days and gradually discontinued over 5 to 7 days. For palliative management of patients with recurrent or inoperable brain tumors, maintenance therapy with either the injection or tablets in a dosage of 2 mg 2 or 3 times daily may be effective.

Unresponsive shock – Reported regimens range from 1 to 6 mg/kg as a single IV injection, to 40 mg initially followed by repeated IV injections every 2 to 6 hours while shock persists.

Intra-articular, intralesional or soft tissue:

Large joints – 2 to 4 mg.
Small joints – 0.8 to 1 mg.
Bursae – 2 to 3 mg.
Tendon sheaths – 0.4 to 1 mg.
Soft tissue infiltration – 2 to 6 mg.
Ganglia – 1 to 2 mg.

	Product	Formulation	Packaging	C.I.*
Rx	**Dexamethasone Sodium Phosphate** (Various, eg, Bioline, Dixon-Shane, Elkins Sinn, Geneva Marsam, Kendall McGaw, Lyphomed, Major, Moore, Rugby, URL)	**Injection:** 4 mg per ml dexamethasone phosphate (as sodium phosphate) solution	In 1, 5, 10 and 30 ml vials, 1 ml disp. syringe and 1 ml fill in 2 ml vials.	2.9+
Rx	**Dalalone** (Forest)		In 5 ml vials.[1]	12
Rx	**Decadron Phosphate** (MSD)		In 1, 5 and 25 ml vials and 2.5 ml syringes.[2]	62
Rx	**Decaject** (Mayrand)		In 5 and 10 ml vials.	15
Rx	**Dexacen-4** (Central)		In 10 ml vials.[1]	13
Rx	**Dexasone** (Hauck)		In 5, 10 and 30 ml vials.[3]	8.7
Rx	**Dexone** (Keene)		In 5 and 10 ml vials.[1]	13
Rx	**Hexadrol Phosphate** (Organon)		In 1 and 5 ml vials and 1 ml disp. syringe.[1]	13
Rx	**Solurex** (Hyrex)		In 5, 10 and 30 ml vials.	8.6
Rx	**Dexamethasone Sodium Phosphate** (Various, eg, Elkins-Sinn, Lyphomed, Schein)	**Injection:** 10 mg per ml dexamethasone phosphate (as sodium phosphate) solution	In 1 and 10 ml vials and 1 ml disp. syringe.	7.9+
Rx	**Hexadrol Phosphate** (Organon)		In 10 ml (IV or IM) vials and 1 ml disp. syringe.[1]	14
Rx	**Hexadrol Phosphate** (Organon)	**Injection:** 20 mg per ml dexamethasone phosphate (as sodium phosphate solution)	In 5 ml vials (IV).[1]	20
Rx	**Decadron Phosphate** (MSD)	**Injection:** 24 mg/ml dexamethasone phosphate (as sodium phosphate) solution. For IV use only	In 5 and 10 ml vials.[4]	40

* Cost Index based on cost per 0.75 mg.
[1] With sodium sulfite and benzyl alcohol.
[2] With methyl and propyl parabens and sodium bisulfite.
[3] With sodium metabisulfite, EDTA and methyl and propyl parabens.
[4] With EDTA, methyl and propyl parabens and sodium bisulfite.

Complete prescribing information for these products begins on page 465.

Glucocorticoids (Cont.)

DEXAMETHASONE SODIUM PHOSPHATE WITH LIDOCAINE HCl

Dexamethasone sodium phosphate provides prompt activity. Lidocaine HCl is a local anesthetic with a rapid onset and a duration of 45 minutes to 1 hour (see Local Anesthetics monograph). Steroid activity usually begins by the time the anesthesia wears off.

Dosage:

Soft tissue injection: Acute and subacute bursitis – 0.5 to 0.75 ml.
Acute and subacute nonspecific tenosynovitis – 0.1 to 0.25 ml.

	Product	Form	Packaging	C.I.*
Rx	**Decadron w/Xylocaine** (MSD)	**Injection:** 4 mg dexamethasone sodium phosphate and 10 mg lidocaine HCl per ml solution	In 5 ml vials.[1]	67

BETAMETHASONE

Dosage:

Initial dosage: 0.6 to 7.2 mg/day.

	Product	Form	Packaging	C.I.*
Rx	**Celestone** (Schering)	**Tablets:** 0.6 mg	(Schering BDA or 011). Pink, scored. In 100s and 500s and UD 21s (6 day).	66
		Syrup: 0.6 mg per 5 ml	< 1% alcohol. Sorbitol, sugar. In 118 ml.	69

BETAMETHASONE SODIUM PHOSPHATE

Betamethasone phosphate is highly soluble, has a prompt onset and may be given IV.

Dosage:

Systemic and local: The initial dosage may vary up to 9 mg/day.

	Product	Form	Packaging	C.I.*
Rx	**Betamethasone Sodium Phosphate** (Various, eg, Dixon-Shane, Major, Moore, Rugby, Schein)	**Injection:** 4 mg betamethasone sodium phosphate (equivalent to 3 mg betamethasone alcohol) per ml solution	In 5 ml vials.	14+
Rx	**Celestone Phosphate** (Schering)		In 5 ml vials.[2]	27
Rx	**Cel-U-Jec** (Hauck)		In 5 ml vials.[2]	15
Rx	**Selestoject** (Mayrand)		In 5 ml vials.	31

BETAMETHASONE SODIUM PHOSPHATE AND BETAMETHASONE ACETATE

Betamethasone sodium phosphate provides prompt activity, while betamethasone acetate is only slightly soluble and affords sustained activity.

Dosage:

Systemic: Not for IV use. *Initial dose* – 0.5 to 9 mg/day. Dosage ranges are ⅓ to ½ the oral dose given every 12 hours. In certain acute, life-threatening situations, dosages exceeding the usual may be justified and may be in multiples of oral dosages.

Intrabursal, intra-articular, intradermal and intralesional:

Bursitis, tenosynovitis, peritendinitis – 1 ml.

Rheumatoid arthritis and osteoarthritis – 0.5 to 2 ml.

Very large joints: 1 to 2 ml. Medium joints: 0.5 to 1 ml.
Large joints: 1 ml. Small joints: 0.25 to 0.5 ml.

Dermatologic conditions – 0.2 ml/cm² intradermally. *Maximum dose:* 1 ml/week.

Foot disorders – The following doses are recommended at 3 to 7 day intervals:

Bursitis: Under heloma durum or heloma molle – 0.25 to 0.5 ml. Under calcaneal spur – 0.5 ml. Over hallux rigidus or digiti quinti varus – 0.5 ml.

Tenosynovitis, periostitis of cuboid: 0.5 ml.

Acute gouty arthritis: 0.5 to 1 ml.

	Product	Form	Packaging	C.I.*
Rx	**Betamethasone Sodium Phosphate and Betamethasone Acetate** (Major)	**Injection:** 3 mg betamethasone acetate and 3 mg betamethasone sodium phosphate per ml suspension	In 5 ml vials.	41
Rx	**Celestone Soluspan** (Schering)		In 5 ml vials.[3]	20

* Cost Index based on cost per 0.75 mg dexamethasone phosphate or 0.6 mg betamethasone.
[1] With EDTA, parabens and sodium bisulfite.
[2] With EDTA, phenol and sodium bisulfite.
[3] With EDTA and benzalkonium chloride.

Refer to the general discussion of these products beginning on page 465.

For information on corticosteroid-containing preparations for anorectal use, refer to the Topicals section.

Glucocorticoid Retention Enemas

Actions:

Hydrocortisone is partially absorbed following rectal administration. Ulcerative colitis patients have absorbed up to 50% of hydrocortisone administered by enema.

Indications:

Adjunctive therapy in the treatment of ulcerative colitis, including ulcerative proctitis, ulcerative proctosigmoiditis and left-sided ulcerative colitis. It has proved useful in some cases involving the transverse and ascending colons.

Contraindications:

Systemic fungal infections; ileocolostomy during immediate or early postoperative period.

Warnings:

If improvement fails to occur within 2 or 3 weeks, discontinue therapy. Symptomatic improvement may be misleading and should not be used as the sole criterion in judging efficacy. Sigmoidoscopic examination and x-ray visualization are essential for adequate monitoring.

Precautions:

Use with caution where there is a probability of impending perforation or abscess; pyogenic infections; intestinal anastomoses; obstruction; extensive fistulas and sinus tracts.

Adverse Reactions:

Local pain or burning; rectal bleeding; apparent exacerbations or sensitivity reactions.

HYDROCORTISONE RETENTION ENEMA

Administration and Dosage:

Usual course of therapy is 100 mg nightly for 21 days, or until clinical and proctological remission occurs. Clinical symptoms usually subside in 3 to 5 days. Improvement in mucosal appearance may lag behind clinical improvement. Difficult cases may require 2 or 3 months of treatment. If therapy exceeds 21 days, discontinue gradually. **C.I.***

			C.I.*
Rx	**Cortenema** (Solvay Pharm.)	**Retention Enema:** 100 mg per 60 ml unit.[1]	32

Glucocorticoid Intrarectal Foam

HYDROCORTISONE ACETATE INTRARECTAL FOAM

Indications:

Adjunctive therapy in the treatment of ulcerative proctitis of the distal portion of the rectum in patients who cannot retain corticosteroid enemas.

Contraindications:

Obstruction; abscess; perforation; peritonitis; recent intestinal anastomoses; extensive fistulas and sinus tracts.

Warnings:

Because the foam is not expelled, systemic hydrocortisone absorption may be greater than with corticosteroid enema formulations.

If no clinical or proctologic improvement occurs within 2 or 3 weeks, or if the patient's condition worsens, discontinue use.

Administer with caution to patients with severe ulcerative disease because these patients are predisposed to perforation of the bowel wall.

Administration and Dosage:

Usual dose is 1 applicatorful once or twice daily for 2 or 3 weeks, and every second day thereafter. Do not insert any part of the aerosol container into the anus. Satisfactory response usually occurs within 5 to 7 days. Sigmoidoscopy is recommended to judge dosage adjustment, duration of therapy and rate of improvement. **C.I.***

				C.I.*
Rx	**Cortifoam** (Reed & C)	**Aerosol:** 90 mg/applicatorful	In 20 g (14 applications).	134

* Cost Index based on cost per 100 mg hydrocortisone, or 1 applicatorful hydrocortisone foam.

[1] In aqueous solution with carboxypolymethylene, polysorbate 80 and methylparaben.

TRILOSTANE

Actions:

Trilostane reversibly lowers elevated circulating levels of glucocorticoids by inhibiting the enzyme system essential for their production in the adrenal gland. It does not possess inherent hormonal activity.

After 2 to 12 weeks of therapy in patients with Cushing's syndrome, there was at least a 25% reduction in urinary free and plasma cortisol in over 70% of patients. Because of its mode of action, trilostane also causes an increase in the urinary levels of 17-ketosteroids.

The reduction in cortisol and increase in 17-ketosteroids becomes apparent during the first few days of treatment with effective doses. Patient response to any one dose may not be uniform and individualization of dosage is required.

Indications:

For the amelioration of adrenal cortical hyperfunction in Cushing's syndrome (hypercortisolism). Trilostane does not cure the underlying disease process. Reserve use for cases where definitive therapy is not appropriate or as a temporary measure until more definitive measures such as surgery or radiation (pituitary) can be undertaken. In clinical trials, only small numbers of patients with Cushing's syndrome were treated for longer than 3 months; accordingly, data are insufficient to support the safety of the drug beyond that period.

Contraindications:

Adrenal insufficiency; severe renal or hepatic disease.

Pregnancy: Category X (see Warnings).

Warnings:

Trilostane alone may cause adrenal cortical hypofunction, especially under conditions of stress such as surgery, trauma or acute illness. Gonadal function may also be depressed during therapy.

Concomitant therapy: Use cautiously and with close monitoring of adrenal status in patients receiving other drugs that suppress adrenal function. Only patients who remain unequivocally hyperadrenal on one agent should be given a second.

Usage in Pregnancy: Category X. Trilostane can cause fetal harm when administered to a pregnant woman. It has been reported to reduce circulating progesterone, produce cervical dilation and terminate pregnancy in some women.

Trilostane has been shown to be teratogenic and to terminate pregnancy in rats when given in doses approximately 13 times the recommended human dose. Concurrent administration of progesterone reduced or eliminated the interceptive effect and skeletal abnormalities produced by trilostane alone.

Trilostane inhibits adrenal, ovarian and placental steroidogenesis when given to rhesus monkeys. In pregnant monkeys, it reduces circulating levels of progesterone and has an interceptive action. Concurrent administration of progesterone prevents this interceptive effect.

Exclude pregnancy before starting treatment. Use nonhormonal contraceptive measures during treatment. If the drug is used during pregnancy or if the patient becomes pregnant while taking the drug, apprise her of the potential hazards to the fetus.

Usage in Lactation: It is not known whether this drug is excreted in breast milk. Because of the potential for serious adverse effects from trilostane on the adrenal glands of nursing infants, decide whether to discontinue nursing or to discontinue the drug, taking into account the importance of the drug to the mother.

Usage in Children: Safety and efficacy for use in children have not been established.

Precautions:

Stress: Although trilostane will not irreversibly block adrenal function, it may prevent a maximal response to ACTH in a stress situation. Therefore, if patients develop a severe illness or need surgery, discontinuance of drug, monitoring of circulating corticosteroid and electrolyte levels, or exogenous corticosteroid therapy may be indicated. In patients with Cushing's syndrome, initiate therapy in the hospital.

Monitoring: During therapy, monitor the therapeutic response by measuring circulating corticosteroids and plasma electrolytes at appropriate intervals.

Carcinogenesis, mutagenesis, impairment of fertility: In an 18 month study in rats, an increased incidence of adrenal adenomas was noted at the 250 mg/kg/day dosage level. Studies in hypophysectomized rats and in rats given dexamethasone concurrently with trilostane indicate that adrenal hypertrophy and adenoma formation associated with trilostane are due to compensatory ACTH stimulation and not directly to the action of trilostane. Trilostane was not mutagenic when evaluated by standard tests.

Orthostatic Hypotension: Trilostane may cause orthostatic hypotension by suppressing aldosterone production in the adrenal cortex. Monitor blood pressure in all patients.

(Continued on following page)

TRILOSTANE (Cont.)

Drug Interactions:

Aminoglutethimide or **mitotane** (o,p'-DDD): In Cushing's syndrome, concurrent use of trilostane may cause severe adrenocortical hypofunction.

Given concurrently with **thiazide** or **loop diuretics**, trilostane's effect of inhibiting aldosterone production reduces the loss of potassium ion in the urine usually observed with these diuretics.

Adverse Reactions:

Adverse reactions have been reported in about one in four patients, occurring more frequently in patients treated with high initial doses (≥ 250 mg/day).

GI (most common): Diarrhea (≈ 17%); abdominal pain, discomfort, cramps and upset stomach (16%); nausea, flatulence, belching and bloating (5%).

Other reactions reported were burning of oral or nasal membranes (≈ 8%), flushing (5%) and headache (4%).

Less frequent reactions were muscle or joint pains, nasal stuffiness, rhinorrhea or lacrimation, skin rash, erythema, numbness or tingling, fever and fatigue or fainting.

Adrenal insufficiency was reported in two patients but only documented in one patient who had received mitotane immediately prior to the initiation of trilostane therapy. In both cases, trilostane was reinstituted without further incidence. In a few patients, therapy was discontinued due to adverse reactions.

Overdosage:

Remove the drug from the stomach by emesis or gastric lavage as soon as possible after ingestion. Monitor circulating levels of adrenal steroids and watch the patient closely for several days for evidence of adrenal insufficiency. Replacement therapy with adrenal steroids may be required.

Patient Information:

Therapy with trilostane requires close and frequent laboratory monitoring.

This drug does not cure the underlying disease process.

Notify physician if any of the following occurs or persists: Diarrhea, nausea, skin rash, headache, fever or fatigue.

In times of stress, such as severe illness or surgery, therapy with corticosteroids may be indicated.

Administration and Dosage:

Institute treatment in a hospital until a stable dosage regimen is achieved.

Initiate therapy with 30 mg, 4 times a day and gradually increase at intervals of 3 to 4 days with careful monitoring of plasma or urinary hormones and electrolyte levels. The majority of patients demonstrated favorable therapeutic response at a dose less than 360 mg per day. Doses above 480 mg per day are not recommended.

If a patient fails to demonstrate an appropriate therapeutic response to an escalating dose within 2 weeks, discontinue therapy.

Rx	**Modrastane** (Winthrop Pharm.)	**Capsules:** 30 mg	(#W M-91 30 mg). Pink. In 100s.
		60 mg	(#W M-90 60 mg). Pink and black. In 100s.

Product identification code.

AMINOGLUTETHIMIDE

Actions:

Pharmacology: Aminoglutethimide inhibits the enzymatic conversion of cholesterol to Δ^5-pregnenolone, thereby reducing the synthesis of adrenal glucocorticoids, mineralocorticoids, estrogens and androgens. Aminoglutethimide blocks several other steps in steroid synthesis, including the hydroxylations required for the aromatization of androgens to estrogens.

Pharmacokinetics: Aminoglutethimide is effectively absorbed orally and is minimally bound to plasma protein. Its half-life is 11 to 16 hours initially, but decreases after 1 to 2 weeks to 5 to 9 hours. Approximately 50% is excreted unchanged in the urine and 20% to 50% is excreted as the acetylated metabolite (less than one-fifth as active as the parent compound). The acetylation mechanism is genetically controlled.

Indications:

For the suppression of adrenal function in selected patients with Cushing's syndrome.

Because aminoglutethimide does not affect the underlying disease process, it has been used primarily until more definitive therapy (ie, surgery) can be undertaken, or in cases where such therapy is not appropriate. Only a small number of patients have been treated for longer than 3 months. A decreased effect or escape from a favorable effect occurs more frequently in pituitary-dependent Cushing's syndrome, probably because of increasing ACTH levels in response to decreasing glucocorticoid levels.

Unlabeled Uses: Has been used successfully in postmenopausal patients with advanced breast carcinoma and in patients with metastatic prostate carcinoma.

Contraindications:

Hypersensitivity to glutethimide or aminoglutethimide.

Warnings:

Cortical hypofunction: May cause adrenal cortical hypofunction, especially under conditions of stress such as surgery, trauma or acute illness. Monitor patients carefully and give hydrocortisone and mineralocorticoid supplements as indicated. Do not use dexamethasone. (See Drug Interactions.)

Hypotension: Aminoglutethimide may suppress aldosterone production by the adrenal cortex and may cause orthostatic or persistent hypotension. Monitor blood pressure in all patients at appropriate intervals.

Usage in Pregnancy: Category D. Aminoglutethimide can cause fetal harm when administered to pregnant women. In about 5000 patients, two cases of pseudohermaphroditism were reported in female infants whose mothers took aminoglutethimide and concomitant anticonvulsants. Normal pregnancies have also occurred during the administration of the drug. When administered to rats at doses ½ to 3 times the maximum human dose, aminoglutethimide caused a decrease in fetal implantation, and increased fetal deaths, teratogenic effects and pseudohermaphroditism. If this drug must be used during pregnancy, or if the patient becomes pregnant while taking the drug, apprise her of the potential hazard to the fetus.

Usage in Lactation: It is not known whether this drug is excreted in breast milk. Decide whether to discontinue nursing or to discontinue the drug, taking into account the importance of the drug to the mother.

Usage in Children: Safety and efficacy have not been established.

Precautions:

Laboratory tests: Hypothyroidism may occur. Make appropriate clinical observations and perform thyroid function studies as indicated. Supplementary thyroid hormone may be required.

Hematologic abnormalities have been reported. Elevations in SGOT, alkaline phosphatase and bilirubin have been reported. Perform appropriate clinical observations and regular laboratory studies before and during therapy. Determine serum electrolytes periodically.

Drug Interactions:

Dexamethasone metabolism is accelerated by aminoglutethimide. If glucocorticoid replacement is needed, prescribe hydrocortisone.

Coumarin and **warfarin** effects are diminished by aminoglutethimide.

Alcohol administered with aminoglutethimide may potentiate the effects of the drug.

Oral anticoagulants, theophylline, digitoxin and **medroxyprogesterone**: Pharmacologic effects of these drugs may be decreased due the induction of hepatic microsomal enzymes by aminoglutethimide. Doses may have to be increased.

(Continued on following page)

AMINOGLUTETHIMIDE (Cont.)

Adverse Reactions:

Untoward effects have been reported in 50% to 67% of patients treated for four or more weeks in Cushing's syndrome. The most frequent effects are: Drowsiness, morbilliform skin rash (17%), nausea and anorexia (≈ 10% to 13%). These are reversible and often disappear spontaneously within 1 or 2 weeks of continued therapy.

Hematologic abnormalities: In 4 of 27 patients with adrenal carcinoma who were treated for at least 4 weeks, there were single occurrences of neutropenia, leukopenia (patient received mitotane concomitantly) and pancytopenia. One patient with adrenal hyperplasia showed decreased hemoglobin and hematocrit during the course of treatment. In 1214 non-Cushingoid patients, transient leukopenia was reported once. Coombs-negative hemolytic anemia was reported in one patient. In approximately 300 patients with nonadrenal malignancy, 10 to 12 cases showed some degree of anemia and two developed pancytopenia. Thrombocytopenia and agranulocytosis have also occurred.

Endocrine: Adrenal insufficiency occurred during 4 or more weeks of therapy in 3% of patients with Cushing's syndrome. Hypothyroidism, occasionally associated with thyroid enlargement, may be detected early or confirmed by measuring the plasma levels of the thyroid hormones. Masculinization and hirsutism in females and precocious sex development in males have occasionally occurred.

CNS: Headache and dizziness, possibly caused by decreased vascular resistance or orthostasis (5%).

Cardiovascular: Hypotension, occasionally orthostatic (3%); tachycardia (2.5%).

GI and hepatic: Vomiting (3%); isolated instances of abnormal liver function tests; suspected hepatotoxicity (less than 1 in 1000); cholestatic jaundice (hypersensitivity mechanism suspected).

Dermatologic: Rash (17%, often reversible on continued therapy); pruritus (5%). These may be allergic or hypersensitivity reactions. Urticaria has occurred rarely.

Miscellaneous: Myalgia (3%). Fever, possibly related to therapy, has been reported in several patients receiving aminoglutethimide for less than 4 weeks when administered with other drugs.

Overdosage:

Symptoms: Overdosage has caused ataxia, somnolence, lethargy, dizziness, fatigue, coma, hyperventilation, respiratory depression, hypovolemic shock due to dehydration and hypotension. Extreme weakness has been reported with divided doses of 3 g/day. No reports of death following doses estimated as large as 7 g.

The signs and symptoms of acute overdosage with aminoglutethimide may be aggravated or modified if alcohol, hypnotics, tranquilizers or tricyclic antidepressants have been taken at the same time.

Treatment: Gastric lavage and supportive treatment have been employed. Full consciousness following deep coma was regained 40 hours or less after ingestion of 3 or 4 g without lavage. No evidence of hematologic, renal or hepatic effects were subsequently found. Consider dialysis in severe intoxication. Treatment includes usual supportive measures. Refer to General Management of Acute Overdosage on p. 2895

Patient Information:

May produce drowsiness or dizziness; patients should observe caution while driving or performing other tasks requiring alertness.

May cause rash, fainting, weakness or headache; notify physician if these become pronounced.

Nausea and loss of appetite may occur during the first 2 weeks of therapy; notify physician if these persist or become pronounced.

Administration and Dosage:

Institute treatment in a hospital until a stable dosage regimen is achieved.

Give 250 mg 4 times daily, preferably at 6 hour intervals. Follow adrenal cortical response by careful monitoring of plasma cortisol until the desired level of suppression is achieved. If cortisol suppression is inadequate, the dosage may be increased in increments of 250 mg daily at intervals of 1 to 2 weeks to a total daily dose of 2 g.

Dose reduction or temporary discontinuation may be required in the event of adverse responses (ie, extreme drowsiness, severe skin rash or excessively low cortisol levels). If skin rash persists for longer than 5 to 8 days, or becomes severe, discontinue the drug. It may be possible to reinstate therapy at a lower dosage following the disappearance of a mild or moderate rash.

Mineralocorticoid replacement therapy (ie, fludrocortisone) may be necessary. If glucocorticoid replacement therapy is needed, 20 to 30 mg hydrocortisone orally in the morning will replace endogenous secretion.

Rx	**Cytadren** (Ciba)	**Tablets:** 250 mg	(#Ciba 24). White, scored. In 100s.

\# Product identification code.

METYRAPONE

Actions:

Metyrapone inhibits endogenous adrenal corticosteroid synthesis. It reduces cortisol and corticosterone production by inhibiting the 11-β-hydroxylation reaction in the adrenal cortex. In the normal person, an increase in ACTH production by the pituitary and an increase in the adrenocortical secretion of the immediate precursors, 11-deoxycortisol and desoxycorticosterone occur, leading to an elevation of these steroids in plasma and of their metabolites in urine. Metyrapone may also suppress biosynthesis of aldosterone, resulting in a mild natriuresis.

Pharmacokinetics: Metyrapone is rapidly and well absorbed; plasma concentrations during the treatment period are 0.5 to 1 mcg/ml. Peak steroid excretion occurs during the 24 hours following administration. Elimination half-life averages 1 to 2.5 hours. Within 2 days after initiation, 40% of the dose is excreted in urine, mostly as glucuronides.

Indications:

Diagnostic test drug for hypothalamic-pituitary ACTH function.

Unlabeled Uses: Metyrapone is used in Cushing's syndrome to control cortisol secretion.

Contraindications:

Adrenal cortical insufficiency; hypersensitivity to metyrapone.

Warnings:

Usage in Pregnancy: Category C. A subnormal response may occur in pregnant women. Animal reproduction studies have not been conducted. The metyrapone test was administered to 20 pregnant women in their second and third trimesters of pregnancy and the fetal pituitary responded to the enzymatic block. It is not known if metyrapone can affect reproduction capacity. Give to a pregnant woman only if clearly needed.

Usage in Lactation: It is not known whether this drug is excreted in breast milk. Decide whether a woman undergoing the test should discontinue nursing for the duration of the test.

Precautions:

Demonstrate ability of adrenals to respond to exogenous ACTH before employing metyrapone as a test. In the presence of hypothyroidism or hyperthyroidism, the test response may be subnormal. Metyrapone may induce acute adrenal insufficiency in patients with reduced adrenal secretory capacity. Monitor adrenal function.

Drug Interactions:

Cyproheptadine or **phenytoin**: Erroneous test results in pituitary function may occur in patients taking these drugs within the previous 2 weeks. Metyrapone metabolism is accelerated by phenytoin. A subnormal response may also occur in patients on **estrogen** therapy.

Adverse Reactions:

Nausea, abdominal discomfort, dizziness, headache, sedation, allergic rash.

Overdosage:

A 6-year-old girl died after ingesting 2 g metyrapone.

Symptoms are characterized by GI upset and signs of acute adrenocortical insufficiency.

Cardiovascular: Cardiac arrhythmias, hypotension, dehydration.

CNS: Anxiety, confusion, weakness, impaired consciousness.

GI: Nausea, vomiting, epigastric pain, diarrhea.

Laboratory tests: Hyponatremia, hypochloremia, hyperkalemia.

In patients under treatment with insulin or oral antidiabetics, the signs and symptoms of acute metyrapone poisoning may be aggravated or modified.

Treatment: Besides general measures to eliminate the drug and reduce absorption, immediately administer a large dose of hydrocortisone, together with saline and glucose infusions. Monitor blood pressure and fluid and electrolyte balance for a few days. Refer to General Management of Acute Overdosage on p. 2895

(Continued on following page)

METYRAPONE (Cont.)

Administration and Dosage:

Discontinue all corticosteroid therapy prior to and during testing.

Day 1: Control period – Collect 24 hour urine to measure 17-hydroxycorticosteroids (17-OHCS) or 17-ketogenic steroids (17-KGS).

Day 2: ACTH test – Standard ACTH test (ie, administer 50 units ACTH by infusion over 8 hours and measure 24 hour urinary steroids). If results indicate adequate response, proceed with the test.

Days 3 to 4: Rest period.

Day 5: Administer metyrapone, preferably with milk or a snack.

Adults – 750 mg every 4 hours for 6 doses. A single dose is approximately equivalent to 15 mg/kg.

Children – 15 mg/kg every 4 hours for 6 doses. Use a minimal 250 mg single dose.

Day 6: Determine 24 hour urinary steroids for effect.

Interpretation:

ACTH: The normal 24 hour urinary excretion of 17-OHCS is 3 to 12 mg. Following ACTH, it increases to 15 to 45 mg/24 hours.

Metyrapone: Normal response – In patients with a normally functioning pituitary, metyrapone induces a twofold to fourfold increase of 17-OHCS excretion or doubling of 17-KGS excretion.

Subnormal response in patients without adrenal insufficiency indicates some degree of impaired pituitary function, either panhypopituitarism or partial hypopituitarism (limited pituitary reserve).

Panhypopituitarism is readily diagnosed by clinical and chemical evidence of hypogonadism, hypothyroidism and hypoadrenocorticism. These patients usually have subnormal basal urinary steroid levels. Depending upon the duration of the disease and the degree of adrenal atrophy, they may fail to respond to exogenous ACTH. Metyrapone administration is not essential in the diagnosis, but, if given, it will not induce an appreciable increase in urinary steroids.

Partial hypopituitarism or limited pituitary reserve is the more difficult diagnosis as these patients do not present the classical signs and symptoms of hypopituitarism. The response to exogenous ACTH is usually normal. The response to metyrapone is subnormal; no significant increase in 17-OHCS or 17-KGS excretion occurs which may be interpreted as evidence of impaired pituitary-adrenal reserve.

Cushing's syndrome: Subnormal response in patients with Cushing's syndrome suggests either autonomous adrenal tumors that suppress the ACTH-releasing capacity of the pituitary or nonendocrine ACTH-secreting tumors.

Excessive response – An excessive excretion of 17-OHCS or 17-KGS after metyrapone administration suggests Cushing's syndrome associated with adrenal hyperplasia. These patients have an elevated excretion of urinary corticosteroids under basal conditions and often show a "supernormal" response to ACTH and also to metyrapone, excreting more than 35 mg per 24 hours of either 17-OHCS or 17-KGS.

Rx	**Metopirone** (Ciba)	**Tablets:** 250 mg	(#Ciba 130). White, scored. In 18s.

Product identification code.

Actions:

Insulin, secreted by the beta cells of the pancreas, is the principal hormone required for proper glucose use in normal metabolic processes. It is composed of two amino acid chains, A (acidic) and B (basic), joined together by disulfide linkages. Insulin preparations are commonly extracted from either beef or pork pancreas. Human insulin has minor but significant differences from animal insulin with respect to the amino acid sequence on the B-chain (see below). It is derived from a bio-synthetic process with strains of *E coli* (recombinant DNA; rDNA) or from a semisynthetic process in which pork insulin is enzymatically converted at the B-30 terminal amino acid to human insulin.

Insulin Amino Acids			
Source	A-Chain		B-Chain
	Position 8	Position 10	Position 30
Beef	Alanine	Valine	Alanine
Pork	Threonine	Isoleucine	Alanine
Human	Threonine	Isoleucine	Threonine

Human insulin may have a more rapid onset and shorter duration of action than pork insulin in some patients. However, the bioavailability of the insulins is identical when given SC. The human insulins are slightly less antigenic than either pork or beef insulins. Consider the potential for flocculation with human insulin. Human insulin is also the insulin of choice for patients with insulin allergy, insulin resistance, all pregnant patients with diabetes and any patient who uses insulin intermittently.

Insulin preparations are divided into three categories according to promptness, duration and intensity of action following SC administration: Rapid, intermediate or long-acting.

Crystalline regular insulin is prepared by precipitation in the presence of zinc chloride. Regular insulins available in the US are prepared at neutral pH; this improves stability. Modified forms have been developed to alter the pattern of activity.

PZI: Insulin and zinc react with the basic protein, protamine, to form a protein complex. When injected, it dissolves slowly and insulin is absorbed at a slow but steady rate.

Isophane (NPH): A modified, crystalline protamine zinc insulin. Its effects are comparable to a mixture of 2 to 3 parts regular insulin and 1 part protamine zinc insulin.

Extended insulin zinc suspension (Ultralente): Large crystals of insulin with high zinc content are collected and resuspended in a sodium acetate/sodium chloride solution. This relatively insoluble insulin is formed without a modifying protein.

Prompt insulin zinc suspension (Semilente): Amorphous (noncrystalline) insulin precipitated at a high pH.

Insulin zinc suspension (Lente): Stable mixture of 70% ultralente and 30% semilente.

Individual response to insulin varies and is affected by diet, exercise, concomitant drug therapy and other factors. Characteristics of various insulins given SC are compared below:

Pharmacokinetics and Compatibility of Various Insulins						
	Insulin Preparations	Onset (hrs)	Peak (hrs)	Duration (hrs)	Compatible mixed with
Rapid-Acting	Insulin Injection (Regular)	½ to 1		6 to 8	All
	Prompt Insulin Zinc Suspension (Semilente)	1 to 1½	5 to 10	12 to 16	Lente
Intermediate-Acting	Isophane Insulin Suspension (NPH)	1 to 1½	4 to 12	24	Regular
	Insulin Zinc Suspension (Lente)	1 to 2½	7 to 15	24	Regular, semilente
Long-Acting	Protamine Zinc Insulin Suspension (PZI)	4 to 8	14 to 24	36	Regular
	Extended Insulin Zinc Suspension (Ultralente)	4 to 8	10 to 30	>36	Regular, semilente

(Actions continued on following page)

Actions (Cont.):

Purified insulins: The beta cells form insulin from a single-chain precursor, proinsulin. Commercial preparations may contain small amounts of proinsulin and other related molecules due to incomplete conversion of the prohormone. These contaminants may contribute to adverse immunogenic responses including local or systemic allergic reactions, lipodystrophy and antibody formation. Chromatographic purification techniques significantly reduce the amount of proinsulin and other protein contaminants. All commercially available insulins in the US contain no more than 25 parts per million (ppm) proinsulin. "Improved single peak" insulin contains ≤ 20 ppm proinsulin and "purified" insulin contains ≤ 10 ppm proinsulin. Purified pork insulins have ≈ 1 ppm and human insulins (recombinant DNA and semisynthetic) have 0 and 1 ppm, respectively. These three are the least immunogenic insulins available. Internal specifications and the amount of zinc, excess protamine and preservatives vary per manufacturer.

Indications:

Diabetes mellitus type I (insulin-dependent).

Diabetes mellitus type II (non-insulin-dependent) that cannot be properly controlled by diet, exercise and weight reduction.

In hyperkalemia, infusion of glucose and insulin produces a shift of potassium into cells and lowers serum potassium levels.

Insulin injection (regular insulin) may be given IV or IM for rapid effect in severe ketoacidosis or diabetic coma.

Highly purified (single component) and human insulins: Local insulin allergy, immunologic insulin resistance, lipodystrophy at injection site; temporary insulin administration (ie, surgery, acute stress type II diabetes, gestational diabetes); newly diagnosed diabetics.

Warnings:

Change insulins cautiously and under medical supervision. Changes in purity, strength, brand, type or species source may result in need for dosage adjustment. Teach patients using insulin to self monitor blood glucose levels and keep daily records of results.

Pregnancy: Pregnancy may make the management of diabetes more difficult. Insulin is the drug of choice for the control of diabetes in pregnancy. Keep patients under close medical supervision. Rigid control of serum glucose and avoidance of ketoacidosis are desired throughout pregnancy. Following delivery, insulin requirements may drop for 24 to 72 hours, rising towards the normal pre-pregnancy dose during the next 6 weeks.

Lactation: Insulin does not pass into breast milk. Breastfeeding may decrease insulin requirements despite the increase in necessary caloric intake.

Precautions:

Insulin resistance occurs rarely. Insulin resistant patients require > 200 units of insulin/day for > 2 days in the absence of ketoacidosis or acute infection. Sometimes, the resistance is due to high levels of IgG antibodies to insulin. Insulin resistance may also occur in obese patients, patients with acanthosis nigricans and patients with insulin receptor defects; insulin resistance during infection may be due to a postreceptor defect. The hyperglycemia may be managed by changing the insulin species source (ie, beef or mixed beef-pork to pork or human insulin). Corticosteroids may be administered if changing the insulin is not effective. Corticosteroids may decrease IgG production or decrease insulin binding to the antibody. Monitor closely for signs of hyperglycemia and for the adverse effects of high-dose corticosteroids. Highly concentrated insulin (U-500) may also be administered to insulin-resistant patients. Use with caution to avoid hypoglycemia. Some Type II patients with insulin resistance have been treated with a combination of glyburide plus insulin (see Administration and Dosage).

Hypoglycemia may result from excessive insulin dose or may be due to: Increased work or exercise without eating; food not being absorbed in the usual manner because of postponement or omission of a meal or in illness with vomiting, fever or diarrhea; when insulin requirements decline.

Eating sugar or a sugar-sweetened product will often correct the condition and prevent more serious symptoms. Commercial products containing 40% glucose are also available; glucagon may be used and IV dextrose may be necessary (see individual monographs). If hypoglycemic symptoms occur, notify a physician promptly.

In acute, usually suicidal overdoses of insulin, successful management has included excision of the injection site.

Symptoms of hypoglycemia are less pronounced with the use of human insulin than with animal-based products. Warn patients using human insulin of this possibility.

Diabetic ketoacidosis is a potentially life-threatening condition requiring prompt diagnosis and treatment. Hyperglucagonemia, hyperglycemia and ketoacidosis may result. Diabetic ketoacidosis may result from stress, illness or insulin omission, or may develop slowly after a long period of poor insulin control. Treatment involves fluids, correction of acidosis and hypotension, and low-dose regular insulin IM or IV infusion.

(Precautions continued on following page)

Precautions (Cont.):

Symptoms of Hypoglycemia vs Ketoacidosis							
		Urine glucose/	Symptoms				
Reaction	Onset	acetone	CNS	Respiration	Mouth/GI	Skin	Miscellaneous
Hypoglycemic reaction (insulin reaction)	sudden	0/0	fatigue weakness nervousness confusion headache diplopia convulsions psychoses dizziness unconsciousness	rapid shallow	numb tingling hunger nausea	pallor moist shallow or dry	normal or non-characteristic pulse eyeballs normal
Ketoacidosis (diabetic coma)	gradual (hours or days)	+/+	drowsiness dim vision	air hunger	thirst acetone breath nausea vomiting abdominal pain loss of appetite	dry flushed	rapid pulse soft eyeballs

Insulin allergy: Local – Occasionally, redness, swelling and itching at the injection site may develop. This occurs if the injection is not properly made, if the skin is sensitive to the cleansing solution or if the patient is allergic to insulin or insulin additives (ie, preservatives). The condition usually resolves in a few days to a few weeks. A change in the type or species source of insulin may be tried.

Systemic reactions, less common, may present as a rash, shortness of breath, fast pulse, sweating, a drop in blood pressure, anaphylaxis or angioedema and may be life-threatening. Perform a skin test on patients with severe systemic reactions with each new preparation prior to initiating therapy with that preparation.

Lipodystrophy: Lipoatrophy is the breakdown of adipose tissue at the insulin injection site causing a depression in the skin. It may be the result of an immune response or when less pure insulins are administered. Injection of human or purified pork insulins into the site over a 2 to 4 week period may result in SC fat accumulation.

Lipohypertrophy is the result of repeated insulin injection into the same site. It is the accumulation of SC fat and it may interfere with insulin absorption from the site. This condition may be avoided by rotating the injection site.

Diet: Patients must follow a prescribed diet and exercise regularly. Determine the time, number and amount of individual doses and distribution of food among the meals of the day. Do not change this regimen unless prescribed otherwise.

Drug Interactions:

Decrease Hypoglycemic Effect of Insulin		Increase Hypoglycemic Effect of Insulin	
Contraceptives, oral	Epinephrine	Alcohol	MAO inhibitors
Corticosteroids	Smoking	Anabolic steroids	Phenylbutazone
Dextrothyroxine	Thiazide diuretics	Beta-blockers[1]	Salicylates
Diltiazem	Thyroid hormone	Clofibrate	Sulfinpyrazone
Dobutamine		Fenfluramine	Tetracyclines
		Guanethidine	

[1] Nonselective beta blockers may delay recovery from hypoglycemic episodes and mask signs/symptoms of hypoglycemia. Cardioselective agents may be alternatives.

Patient Information:

Use the same type and brand of syringe unit to avoid dosage errors. Rotate administration sites to prevent lipodystrophy. If using a "pen-filled" device, follow the information for proper use in the insert.

Do not change the order of mixing insulins (if applicable) or change the brand, strength, type, species or dose without your physician's knowledge.

Insulin requirements may change in patients who become ill, especially with vomiting or fever. Consult a physician.

See your dentist twice yearly; see an ophthalmologist regularly.

(Patient Information continued on following page)

Patient Information (Cont.):

Patient information inserts are available with products; read and understand all aspects of insulin use. Patients must receive complete instructions about the nature of diabetes. Strict adherence to prescribed diet, an exercise program and personal hygiene are essential.

Patients should wear diabetic identification (Medic-Alert) so appropriate treatment can be given if complications occur away from home.

Monitor blood glucose and urine for glucose and ketones as prescribed; monitor blood pressure regularly.

Administration and Dosage:

The number and size of daily doses, time of administration and diet and exercise require continuous medical supervision. Dosage adjustment may be necessary when changing types of insulin, particularly when changing from single-peak to the more purified animal or human insulins.

For insulin suspensions, ensure uniform dispersion by rolling the vial gently between hands. Avoid vigorous shaking that may result in the formation of air bubbles or foam. Regular insulin should be a clear solution.

Administer maintenance doses SC. Rotate administration sites to prevent lipodystrophy. A general rule is to not administer within 1 inch of the same site for 1 month. The rate of absorption is more rapid when the injection is in the abdomen (possibly > 50% faster), followed by the upper arm, thigh and buttocks. Therefore, it may be best to rotate sites within an area rather than rotating areas. Give regular insulin IV or IM in severe ketoacidosis or diabetic coma.

Dosage guidelines: Doses must be individualized and monitored closely in patients with diabetes mellitus; however, the following dosage guidelines may be considered.

Children and adults – 0.5 to 1 U/kg/day.

Adolescents (during growth spurt) – 0.8 to 1.2 U/kg/day.

Adjust doses to achieve premeal and bedtime blood glucose levels of 80 to 140 mg/dl (children < 5 years of age, 100 to 200 mg/dl).

Storage: Proper storage is critical. Insulin preparations being used are generally stable if stored at room temperature (and not exposed to extreme temperatures or direct sunlight). Discard partially filled bottles if the insulin has not been used for several weeks. Always store extra bottles in the refrigerator; do not freeze.

Insulin prefilled in plastic or glass syringes is stable for 1 week under refrigeration according to one manufacturer. However, there is some documentation that insulin in plastic syringes is stable for at least 14 days. Further studies are needed.

Insulin mixtures: When mixing 2 types of insulin, always draw the clear regular insulin into the syringe first. Patients stabilized on such mixtures should have a consistent response if the mixing is standardized. An unexpected response is most likely to occur when switching from separate injections to use of a mixture or vice versa. To avoid dosage error, do not alter the order of mixing insulins or change the model or brand of syringe or needle. Each different type of insulin used to prepare insulin mixtures must be of the same concentration (units/ml).

NPH/regular mixtures of insulin are now available from the manufacturer in pre-mixed formulations of 70% NPH and 30% regular. A 50/50 combination will also be available soon. NPH/regular combinations of insulin are stable and are absorbed as if injected separately. In mixtures of regular and lente insulins, binding is detectable 5 minutes to 24 hours after mixing. If the regular/lente mixtures are not administered within the first 5 minutes after mixing, the effect of the regular insulin is diminished. The excess zinc binds with the regular and forms a lente type insulin. It is thus critical that mixtures of regular with the lente insulins be mixed and injected immediately.

These mixtures remain stable for 1 month at room temperature or for 3 months under refrigeration. These mixtures can also be stored in prefilled plastic or glass syringes for 1 week to possibly 14 days under refrigeration. Keep filled syringes in a vertical or oblique position with the needle pointing upward to avoid plugging problems. Prior to injection, pull back the plunger, and tip the syringe back and forth and slightly agitate to remix the insulins. Check for normal appearance.

Semilente, ultralente and lente insulins may be mixed in any ratio; they are chemically identical and differ only in size and structure of insulin particles in suspension. These mixtures are also stable for 1 month at room temperature or 3 months under refrigeration.

Insulin adsorption onto plastic IV infusion sets has been reported to remove up to 80% of a dose; however, 20% to 30% is more common. The percent adsorbed is inversely proportional to the concentration of insulin; it takes place within 30 to 60 minutes. Because this phenomenon cannot be accurately predicted, patient monitoring is essential.

Concomitant sulfonylurea therapy: Insulin and oral sulfonylurea coadministration has been used with some success in type II diabetic patients who are difficult to control with diet and sulfonylurea therapy alone. Further study is needed, however.

(Products listed on following pages)

Complete prescribing information for these products begins on page 494.

INSULIN INJECTION				C.I.*
otc	**Regular Iletin** I (Lilly)	**Injection:** 40 or 100 units per ml Beef and pork.	In 10 ml bottles.	1.2
otc	**Regular Insulin** (Novo Nordisk)	**Injection:** 100 units per ml Pork.	In 10 ml vials.	1.1
otc	**Beef Regular Iletin** II (Lilly)	**Injection:** 100 units per ml Purified beef.	In 10 ml bottles.	1.6
otc	**Pork Regular Iletin** II (Lilly)	**Injection:** 100 units per ml Purified pork.	In 10 ml bottles.	1.9
otc	**Regular Purified Pork Insulin** (Novo Nordisk)		In 10 ml vials.	1.7
otc	**Velosulin** (Novo Nordisk)		In 10 ml vials.	1.7
otc	**Humulin R** (Lilly)	**Injection:** 100 units per ml Human insulin (rDNA).	In 10 ml bottles.	1.5
otc	**Humulin BR** (Lilly)	**Injection:** 100 units per ml Buffered human insulin (rDNA).	In 10 ml bottles.[1]	1.8
otc	**Novolin R** (Novo Nordisk)	**Injection:** 100 units per ml Human insulin (semisynthetic).	In 10 ml vials.	1.5
otc	**Velosulin** (Novo Nordisk)		In 10 ml vials.	1.5
otc	**Novolin R PenFill** (Novo Nordisk)	**Cartridges:** 100 units per ml Human insulin (semisynthetic). For use with *NovoPen*	In 1.5 ml.	3

INSULIN ZINC SUSPENSION, PROMPT (SEMILENTE)
Small particles of zinc insulin in suspension.

otc	**Semilente Iletin** I (Lilly)	**Injection:** 40 or 100 units per ml Beef and pork.	In 10 ml bottles.	1.2
otc	**Semilente Insulin** (Novo Nordisk)	**Injection:** 100 units per ml Beef.	In 10 ml vials.	1.1

ISOPHANE INSULIN SUSPENSION (NPH)
Insulin combined with protamine and zinc.

otc	**NPH Iletin** I (Lilly)	**Injection:** 40 or 100 units per ml Beef and pork.	In 10 ml bottles.	1.2
otc	**NPH Insulin** (Novo Nordisk)	**Injection:** 100 units per ml Beef.	In 10 ml vials.	1.1
otc	**Beef NPH Iletin** II (Lilly)	**Injection:** 100 units per ml Purified beef.	In 10 ml bottles.	1.6
otc	**NPH Purified** (Novo Nordisk)	**Injection:** 100 units per ml Purified pork.	In 10 ml vials.	1.7
otc	**Pork NPH Iletin** II (Lilly)		In 10 ml bottles.	1.9
otc	**Insulatard NPH** (Novo Nordisk)		In 10 ml vials.	1.7
otc	**Humulin N** (Lilly)	**Injection:** 100 units per ml Human insulin (rDNA).	In 10 ml bottles.	1.5
otc	**Insulatard NPH** (Novo Nordisk)	**Injection:** 100 units per ml Human insulin (semisynthetic).	In 10 ml vials.	1.5
otc	**Novolin N** (Novo Nordisk)		In 10 ml vials.	1.5
otc	**Novolin N PenFill** (Novo Nordisk)	**Cartridges:** 100 units per ml Human insulin (semisynthetic). For use with *NovoPen*	In 1.5 ml	3

* Cost Index based on cost per 100 units or 150 unit cartridge.
[1] For use only in external insulin pumps.

Complete prescribing information for these products begins on page 494.

ISOPHANE INSULIN SUSPENSION AND INSULIN INJECTION

70% isophane insulin and 30% insulin injection. Provides rapid activity (onset ½ hour) with a duration of up to 24 hours. Maximal effect is within 4 to 8 hours. **C.I.***

	Product	Description	Packaging	C.I.*
otc	**Humulin 70/30** (Lilly)	**Injection:** 100 units per ml Human insulin (rDNA).	In 10 ml bottles.	1.8
otc	**Mixtard** (Novo Nordisk)	**Injection:** 100 units per ml Purified pork.	In 10 ml vials.	1.7
otc	**Mixtard Human 70/30** (Novo Nordisk)	**Injection:** 100 units per ml Human insulin (semisynthetic).	In 10 ml vials.	1.5
otc	**Novolin 70/30** (Novo Nordisk)		In 10 ml vials.	1.5
otc	**Novolin 70/30 PenFill** (Novo Nordisk)	**Cartridges:** 100 units per ml Human insulin (semisynthetic). For use with *NovoPen*	In 1.5 ml.	3

ISOPHANE INSULIN SUSPENSION AND INSULIN INJECTION

50% isophane insulin and 50% insulin injection. **C.I.***

	Product	Description	Packaging	C.I.*
otc	**Humulin 50/50** (Lilly)	**Injection:** 100 units per ml Human Insulin (rDNA).	In 10 ml vials.	NA

INSULIN ZINC SUSPENSION (LENTE)

70% crystalline and 30% amorphous insulin suspension. Has an intermediate duration of activity; duration of effect is approximately 24 hours. **C.I.***

	Product	Description	Packaging	C.I.*
otc	**Lente Iletin** I (Lilly)	**Injection:** 40 and 100 units per ml Beef and pork.	In 10 ml bottles.	1.2
otc	**Lente Insulin** (Novo Nordisk)	**Injection:** 100 units per ml Beef.	In 10 ml vials.	1.1
otc	**Lente Iletin** II (Lilly)	**Injection:** 100 units per ml Purified beef.	In 10 ml bottles.	1.6
otc	**Lente Iletin** II (Lilly)	**Injection:** 100 units per ml Purified pork.	In 10 ml bottles.	1.9
otc	**Lente Purified Pork Insulin** (Novo Nordisk)		In 10 ml vials.	1.7
otc	**Humulin L** (Lilly)	**Injection:** 100 units per ml Human insulin (rDNA).	In 10 ml bottles.	1.5
otc	**Novolin L** (Novo Nordisk)	**Injection:** 100 units per ml Human insulin (semisynthetic).	In 10 ml vials.	1.5

PROTAMINE ZINC INSULIN SUSPENSION (PZI)

Takes effect gradually; duration of activity is about 36 hours. **C.I.***

	Product	Description	Packaging	C.I.*
otc	**Protamine, Zinc & Iletin** I (Lilly)	**Injection:** 40 and 100 units per ml Beef and pork.	In 10 ml bottles.	1.2
otc	**Protamine, Zinc & Iletin** II **(Beef)** (Lilly)	**Injection:** 100 units per ml Purified beef.	In 10 ml bottles.	2
otc	**Protamine, Zinc & Iletin** II **(Pork)** (Lilly)	**Injection:** 100 units per ml Purified pork.	In 10 ml bottles.	1.9

INSULIN ZINC SUSPENSION, EXTENDED (ULTRALENTE)

Takes effect 4 to 8 hours after injection; activity lasts more than 36 hours. **C.I.***

	Product	Description	Packaging	C.I.*
otc	**Ultralente Iletin** I (Lilly)	**Injection:** 40 and 100 units per ml Beef and pork.	In 10 ml bottles.	1.2
otc	**Ultralente Insulin** (Novo Nordisk)	**Injection:** 100 units per ml Beef.	In 10 ml vials.	1.1
otc	**Humulin U Ultralente** (Lilly)	**Injection:** 100 units per ml Human insulin (rDNA).	In 10 ml bottles.	1.8

* Cost Index based on cost per 100 units or 150 unit cartridge.

Refer to the general discussion of these products beginning on page 494.

High Potency Insulin

INSULIN INJECTION CONCENTRATED

Actions:

Insulin resistance: Diabetes can usually be controlled with daily insulin doses of 40 to 60 units or less; however, an occasional patient develops such resistance or becomes so unresponsive to the effect of insulin that daily doses of several hundred or even several thousand units are required. Patients who require doses in excess of 300 to 500 units daily usually have impaired insulin receptor function.

Occasionally, the cause of insulin resistance can be found (eg, hemochromatosis, cirrhosis of the liver, some complicating disease of the endocrine glands other than the pancreas, obesity, allergy, infection), but in other cases, no cause can be determined.

Concentrated insulin injection is not modified by any agent that might prolong its action. It frequently has a duration similar to repository insulin; a single dose demonstrates activity for 24 hours. This has been credited to the high concentration of the preparation.

Indications:

Treatment of diabetic patients with marked insulin resistance (requirements > 200 units/day). A large dose may be administered SC in a reasonable volume.

Contraindications:

Patients with a history of systemic allergic reactions to pork or mixed beef/pork insulin should not receive the product unless they have been successfully desensitized.

Warnings:

Dosage adjustments: Most patients will show a "tolerance" to insulin, so that minor variations in dosage will not result in the development of untoward symptoms of insulin shock. It is not possible to identify which patients will require a dosage reduction to avoid hypoglycemia. However, a small number of patients may require dosage adjustments. Adjustment may be needed with the first dose or may be required over a period of several weeks. Symptoms of either hypoglycemia or hyperglycemia may occur.

Insulin shock: Observe extreme caution in the measurement of dosage; inadvertent overdose may result in irreversible insulin shock. Serious consequences may result if not used under constant medical supervision.

Hypersensitivity: Less common than local allergic reactions (see Adverse Reactions), but potentially more serious, is systemic allergy to insulin, which may cause generalized urticaria, dyspnea or wheezing and may, on continued administration of the insulin, progress to anaphylaxis. Do not use IV injection since allergic or anaphylactoid reactions may develop.

If a severe allergic reaction occurs, discontinue the drug and treat the patient with the usual agents (eg, epinephrine, antihistamines, corticosteroids). In such patients, perform a skin test with another insulin preparation before its initiation. Desensitization procedures may permit resumption of insulin administration. Refer to Management of Acute Hypersensitivity Reactions.

Precautions:

Insulin resistance: Patients with immunologic insulin resistance to beef insulin (this diagnosis is usually confirmed by the finding of increased serum antibody titers) may require an immediate dosage reduction of 20% to 50% when treated with pork or human insulin. Insulin resistance is frequently self-limited; after several weeks or months of high dosage, responsiveness may be regained and dosage can be reduced.

Monitor blood glucose closely and often until dosage is established. Some may require only one dose daily, others may require two or three injections per day.

Adverse Reactions:

Hypoglycemic reactions may occur. However, secondary hypoglycemic reactions may develop 18 to 24 hours after injection. Consequently, observe patients carefully, and initiate prompt treatment with glucagon injections, glucose by IV injection or gavage.

Allergic reactions: Erythema, swelling or pruritus may occur at injection sites. Such localized allergic manifestations usually resolve within a few days or weeks (see Warnings).

Administration and Dosage:

Administer SC or IM. Do not inject IV (allergic or anaphylactoid reactions may develop).

Use a tuberculin syringe for dosage measurement. Dosage variations are frequent in the insulin-resistant patient, since the individual is unresponsive to the pharmacologic effect of the insulin. Nevertheless, encourage accuracy of measurement because of the potential danger of the preparations.

Storage: Keep in a cold place, preferably in a refrigerator. Avoid freezing.

				C.I.*
Rx	**Regular (Concentrated) Iletin II U-500** (Lilly)	**Injection:** 500 units per ml purified pork.	In 20 ml vials.[1]	1

* Cost Index based on cost per 100 units.

[1] With 0.25% m-cresol and 1.6% glycerin.

The sulfonylurea hypoglycemic agents are sulfonamide derivatives, but are devoid of antibacterial activity. These agents are divided into two groups: First generation (acetohexamide, chlorpropamide, tolazamide, tolbutamide) and second generation (glipizide, glyburide). They are used as adjuncts to diet and exercise in the treatment of non-insulin-dependent diabetes mellitus (NIDDM). NIDDM has also been referred to as adult-onset or maturity-onset diabetes, ketosis-resistant diabetes and Type II diabetes.

NIDDM is characterized by insulin resistance and defects in insulin secretion.

Guidelines for oral hypoglycemic therapy in NIDDM patients may include:

- Onset of diabetes at ≥ 40 years of age
- Obese or normal body weight
- Duration of diabetes < 5 years
- Absence of ketoacidosis
- Fasting serum glucose ≤ 200 mg/dl
- Insulin requirement < 40 units/day
- Absence of renal or hepatic dysfunction

Actions:

Pharmacology: The sulfonylurea hypoglycemic agents appear to lower blood glucose by stimulating insulin release from beta cells in the pancreatic islets possibly due to increased intracellular cAMP. These agents are only effective in patients with some capacity for endogenous insulin production. They may improve the binding between insulin and insulin receptors or increase the number of insulin receptors. Hypoglycemic effects seem to be due to improved beta cell sensitivity or extrapancreatic effects (suppression of glucagon release and hepatic glucose production) occurring in the liver, and on insulin sensitivity of peripheral tissues.

Other pharmacologic activity includes: Potentiation of the effect of antidiuretic hormone (ADH); tolazamide, acetohexamide, glyburide and glipizide may produce a mild diuresis; acetohexamide has significant uricosuric activity.

Pharmacokinetics: The sulfonylureas are well absorbed after oral administration. All sulfonylureas except glipizide can be taken with food. Absorption of glipizide is delayed by food; it is more effective when taken about 30 minutes before a meal. Tolazamide is absorbed more slowly than the other sulfonylureas. They are metabolized in the liver to active and inactive metabolites and are excreted primarily in the urine. Glyburide is excreted as metabolites in the bile and urine, approximately 50% by each route. The hypoglycemic effects of sulfonylureas may be prolonged in severe liver disease due to decreased metabolism.

Although the mechanisms of action and maximal hypoglycemic effects are similar, the second and first generation sulfonylureas differ. Second generation compounds possess a more nonpolar or lipophilic side chain. Therapeutically effective doses and serum concentrations of the second generation sulfonylureas are lower, due to their higher intrinsic potency. All sulfonylureas are strongly bound to plasma proteins, primarily albumin. Protein binding of the first generation sulfonylureas is ionic; that of the second generation agents is predominantly nonionic. The clinical therapeutic significance of this difference is unknown; however, because they are bound to albumin by ionic bindings, the first generation agents may be more likely to be displaced by drugs which competitively bind to proteins (eg, warfarin, phenylbutazone). Displacement of sulfonylurea agents from protein would result in greater hypoglycemic response (see Drug Interactions).

Differences exist among the sulfonylureas in the duration of hypoglycemic effects (see following table). Tolbutamide is short-acting because it is rapidly metabolized to an inactive metabolite; it may be useful in patients with kidney disease. The active metabolite of acetohexamide is 2.5 times as potent as the parent compound. Because the metabolite is excreted in the urine, the duration of action of acetohexamide is prolonged in renal disease. Tolazamide has two active metabolites which are less potent than the parent compound. The renal elimination of chlorpropamide may be sensitive to changes in urinary pH; urinary alkalinization increases its excretion in the urine. When the urine pH is < 6, urinary excretion decreases and hepatic metabolism is the primary route of elimination. The half-life of chlorpropamide is prolonged in renal disease.

(Actions continued on following page)

Actions: (Cont.):

Pharmacokinetics (Cont.):

Major Pharmacokinetic Parameters of the Sulfonylureas						
Sulfonylureas	Equivalent doses (mg)	Doses/ day	Serum t½ (hrs)	Onset (hrs)	Duration (hrs)	Metabolism
First generation						
Acetohexamide	500	1-2	6-8 (parent drug + metabolite)	1	12-24	Reduced in liver to potent active metabolite
Chlorpropamide	250	1	36	1	Up to 60	80% metabolized in liver; metabolite activity unknown
Tolazamide	250	1	7	4-6	12-24	Several mildly active metabolites
Tolbutamide	1000	2-3	4.5-6.5	1	6-12	Oxidized in liver to inactive metabolites
Second generation						
Glipizide	10	1-2	2-4	1-1.5	10-16	Liver metabolism to inactive metabolites
Glyburide Nonmicronized	5	1-2	10	2-4	24	Liver metabolism to weakly active metabolites
Micronized	3	1-2	≈ 4	1	24	

Indications:

As an adjunct to diet to lower the blood glucose in patients with non-insulin-dependent diabetes mellitus (Type II) whose hyperglycemia cannot be controlled by diet alone.

Unlabeled uses: **Chlorpropamide** in doses of 200 to 500 mg/day has been used in the treatment of neurogenic diabetes insipidus.

Sulfonylureas have been used as temporary adjuncts to insulin therapy in selected NIDDM patients to improve diabetic control (see Administration and Dosage).

Contraindications:

Hypersensitivity to sulfonylureas; diabetes complicated by ketoacidosis, with or without coma; sole therapy of insulin-dependent (Type I) diabetes mellitus; diabetes when complicated by pregnancy.

Warnings:

The administration of oral hypoglycemic drugs has been associated with increased cardiovascular mortality as compared to treatment with diet alone or diet plus insulin. Despite controversy regarding its interpretation, this warning is based on the study conducted by the University Group Diabetes Program (UGDP). This long-term prospective clinical trial involving 823 patients evaluated the effectiveness of glucose-lowering drugs in preventing or delaying vascular complications in patients with non-insulin-dependent diabetes. (*Diabetes* 1970;19[Suppl 2]:747-830.)

Patients treated for 5 to 8 years with diet plus tolbutamide (1.5 g/day) had a rate of cardiovascular mortality approximately 2.5 times that of patients treated with diet alone. A significant increase in total mortality was not observed. Consider this for other sulfonylureas as well.

Inform the patient of potential risks, advantages and alternative modes of therapy.

Bioavailability: Micronized glyburide 3 mg tablets provide serum concentrations that are *not* bioequivalent to those from the conventional formulation (nonmicronized) 5 mg tablets. Therefore, retitrate patients when transferring patients from any hypoglycemic agent to micronized glyburide.

Hepatic and renal function impairment: Oral hypoglycemic agents are metabolized in the liver. The drugs and most of their metabolites are excreted by the kidneys. Hepatic impairment may result in inadequate release of glucose in response to hypoglycemia. Renal impairment may cause decreased elimination of sulfonylureas leading to accumulation producing hypoglycemia. Therefore, use these agents with caution in NIDDM patients with renal or hepatic impairment, and monitor renal and liver function frequently.

Elderly: Elderly and debilitated patients are particularly susceptible to the hypoglycemic action of the sulfonylureas. Hypoglycemia may be difficult to recognize in the elderly. Use with caution.

(Warnings continued on following page)

Warnings (Cont.):

Pregnancy: (Category C. Category B – Glyburide). Sulfonylureas (except glyburide) are teratogenic in animals. There are no adequate studies in pregnant women. Use during pregnancy only if clearly needed. In general, avoid the sulfonylurea agents in pregnancy since they will not provide good control in patients who cannot be controlled by diet alone.

Because abnormal blood glucose levels during pregnancy may be associated with a higher incidence of congenital abnormalities, insulin is recommended to maintain blood glucose levels as close to normal as possible. However, fetal mortality and major congenital anomalies generally occur 3 to 4 times more often in offspring of diabetic mothers.

Labor and delivery: Prolonged severe hypoglycemia (4 to 10 days) has occurred in neonates born to mothers who were receiving a sulfonylurea at the time of delivery. This has been reported more frequently with agents with prolonged half-lives. If sulfonylureas are used during pregnancy, discontinue at least 2 days to 4 weeks before the expected delivery date.

Lactation: Chlorpropamide and tolbutamide are excreted in breast milk. A chlorpropamide breast milk concentration of 5 mcg/ml has been detected following a 500 mg dose (normal peak blood level after 250 mg is 30 mcg/ml). It is not known if the other sulfonylureas are excreted in breast milk. Because of the potential for hypoglycemia in nursing infants, decide whether to discontinue nursing or to discontinue the drug.

Children: Safety and efficacy in children have not been established.

Precautions:

Diet and exercise remain the primary considerations of diabetic patient management. Caloric restriction and weight loss are essential in the obese diabetic. These drugs are an adjunct to, not a substitute for, dietary regulation. Also, loss of blood glucose control on diet alone may be transient, thus requiring only short-term sulfonylurea therapy. Identify cardiovascular risk factors and take corrective measures where possible.

Monitoring: Keep patients under continuous medical supervision. During the initial test period, the patient should communicate with the physician daily, and report at least weekly for the first month for physical examination and evaluation of diabetic control. After the first month, examine at monthly intervals or as indicated. Uncooperative individuals may be unsuitable for treatment with oral agents.

During the transitional period, test the urine for glucose and acetone at least three times daily and have the results reviewed by a physician frequently. Measurement of glycosylated hemoglobin is also useful. It is important that patients be taught to correctly and frequently self-monitor blood glucose.

Hyperglycemia is a major risk factor in the development of diabetic complications. Maintaining blood glucose levels helps prevent the progression of nephropathy, neuropathy and retinopathy. Hyperglycemia is also associated with the risk factors of atherosclerosis.

Hypoglycemia: All sulfonylureas may produce severe hypoglycemia. Proper patient selection, dosage and instructions are important to avoid hypoglycemic episodes. Renal or hepatic insufficiency may elevate drug blood levels and the latter may also diminish gluconeogenic capacity, both of which increase the risk of serious hypoglycemic reactions. Elderly, debilitated or malnourished patients, and those with adrenal or pituitary insufficiency are particularly susceptible to the hypoglycemic action of glucose-lowering drugs. Hypoglycemia may be difficult to recognize in the elderly, and in patients taking β-adrenergic blocking drugs. Hypoglycemia is more likely to occur when caloric intake is deficient, after severe or prolonged exercise, when alcohol is ingested or when more than one glucose-lowering drug is used.

Because of the long half-life of chlorpropamide, patients who become hypoglycemic during therapy require careful supervision of the dose and frequent feedings for at least 3 to 5 days. Hospitalization and IV glucose may be necessary.

Asymptomatic patients: Controlling blood glucose in NIDDM with sulfonylureas has not been definitely established to be effective in preventing the long-term cardiovascular or neural complications of diabetes.

Loss of blood glucose control: When a patient stabilized on any diabetic regimen is exposed to stress such as fever, trauma, infection or surgery, a loss of control may occur. At such times, it may be necessary to discontinue the drug and administer insulin.

The effectiveness of any oral hypoglycemic in lowering blood glucose to a desired level decreases in many patients over time (secondary failure); this may be due to progression of the severity of the diabetes or to diminished drug responsiveness. Adequately adjust dose and assess adherence to diet before classifying a patient as a secondary failure. Primary failure occurs when the drug is ineffective in a patient when first given. Certain patients who demonstrate an inadequate response or true primary or secondary failure to one sulfonylurea may benefit from a transfer to another sulfonylurea.

(Continued on following page)

Precautions (Cont.)

Disulfiram-like syndrome: A sulfonylurea-induced facial flushing reaction may occur when some sulfonylureas are administered with alcohol. This syndrome is characterized by facial flushing and occasional breathlessness but without the nausea, vomiting and hypotension seen with a true alcohol-disulfiram reaction. The facial flushing reaction occurs in approximately 33% of NIDDM patients taking chlorpropamide and alcohol. It is uncertain whether glyburide and glipizide can cause the facial flushing reaction.

Syndrome of inappropriate secretion of antidiuretic hormone (SIADH): Water retention and dilutional hyponatremia have occurred after administration of sulfonylureas to NIDDM patients, especially those with congestive heart failure or hepatic cirrhosis. The drugs stimulate antidiuretic hormone (ADH) release, augmenting hypothalamic-pituitary release of ADH. The result is excessive water retention, hyponatremia, low serum osmolality and high urine osmolality.

Glipizide, acetohexamide, tolazamide and glyburide are mildly diuretic.

Drug Interactions:

Sulfonylurea Drug Interactions			
Precipitant drug	Object drug*		Description
Androgens Anticoagulants Chloramphenicol Clofibrate Fenfluramine Fluconazole Gemfibrozil Histamine H_2 antagonists Magnesium salts Methyldopa MAO inhibitors Phenylbutazone Probenecid Salicylates Sulfinpyrazone Sulfonamides Tricyclic antidepressants Urinary acidifiers	Sulfonylureas	↑	The hypoglycemic effect of the sulfonylureas may be enhanced due to various mechanisms (eg, decreased hepatic metabolism, inhibition of renal excretion, displacement from protein binding sites, decreased blood glucose or alteration of carbohydrate metabolism).
Beta blockers Cholestyramine Diazoxide Hydantoins Rifampin Thiazide diuretics Urinary alkalinizers	Sulfonylureas	↓	The hypoglycemic effect of the sulfonylureas may be decreased due to various mechanisms (eg, increased hepatic metabolism, decreased insulin release, increased renal excretion).
Charcoal	Sulfonylureas	↓	Charcoal can reduce the absorption of the sulfonylureas; depending on the clinical situation, this will reduce their efficacy or toxicity.
Ethanol	Sulfonylureas	↔	Ethanol may prolong but not augment glipizide-induced reductions in blood glucose. Chronic ethanol use may decrease the half-life of tolbutamide. Ethanol ingestion by patients taking chlorpropamide may result in a disulfiram-like reaction (see Precautions).
Sulfonylureas	Digitalis glycosides	↑	Concurrent administration may result in increased digitalis serum levels.

* ↓ = Object drug increased ↑ = Object drug decreased ↔ = Undetermined effect

Drug/Food interaction: Absorption of glipizide is delayed by about 40 minutes when taken with food; the drug is more effective when given approximately 30 minutes before a meal. The other sulfonylureas may be taken with food.

Drug/Lab test interaction: A metabolite of tolbutamide in the urine may give a false-positive reaction for **albumin** if measured by the acidification-after-boiling test, which causes the metabolite to precipitate. There is no interference with the sulfosalicylic acid test.

(Continued on following page)

Adverse Reactions:

Hypoglycemia: See Precautions.

GI: GI disturbances (eg, nausea, epigastric fullness, heartburn) are the most common reactions. They tend to be dose-related and may disappear when dosage is reduced. Diarrhea (glipizide); taste alteration (tolbutamide); cholestatic jaundice (rare, discontinue the drug if this occurs).

Dermatologic: Allergic skin reactions; eczema; pruritus; erythema; urticaria; morbilliform or maculopapular eruptions; lichenoid reactions. These may be transient and may disappear despite continued use of the drug; if skin reactions persist, discontinue the drug. Porphyria cutanea tarda; photosensitivity reactions.

Hematologic: Leukopenia; thrombocytopenia; aplastic anemia; agranulocytosis; hemolytic anemia; pancytopenia; hepatic porphyria.

Endocrine: Reactions identical to the syndrome of inappropriate secretion of antidiuretic hormone (SIADH). See Precautions.

Miscellaneous: Disulfiram-like reactions (see Precautions); weakness; paresthesia; tinnitus; fatigue; dizziness; vertigo; malaise; headache (infrequent).

Lab test abnormalities: Elevated liver function tests; occasional mild to moderate elevations in BUN and creatinine.

Overdosage:

Symptoms: Overdosage can produce hypoglycemia. In order of general appearance, the signs and symptoms associated with hypoglycemia include: Tingling of lips and tongue; nausea; diminished cerebral function (lethargy, yawning, confusion, agitation, nervousness); increased sympathetic activity (tachycardia, sweating, tremor, hunger) and ultimately, convulsions, stupor and coma.

Treatment: Treat mild hypoglycemia without loss of consciousness or neurologic findings aggressively with oral glucose and adjustments in drug dosage or meal patterns. Continue close monitoring until the patient is stabilized. Severe hypoglycemic reactions occur infrequently, but require immediate hospitalization. If hypoglycemic coma is suspected, rapidly inject concentrated (50%) dextrose IV. Follow by a continuous infusion of more dilute (10%) dextrose at a rate that will maintain the blood glucose at a level of about 100 mg/dl. Closely monitor for a minimum of 24 to 48 hours since hypoglycemia may recur after apparent clinical recovery. Because of the long half-life of **chlorpropamide,** patients who become hypoglycemic from this drug require close supervision for a minimum of 3 to 5 days.

In one patient with renal failure on hemodialysis, charcoal hemoperfusion shortened the half-life of chlorpropamide following an overdose. Charcoal administration also reduces the absorption of the sulfonylureas and may reduce their toxicity.

Patient Information:

Patients must receive full and complete instructions about the nature of diabetes. Strict adherence to prescribed diet, an exercise program, personal hygiene and avoidance of infection are essential. It is important to teach patients to self-monitor blood glucose.

Do not discontinue medication except on the advice of a physician.

May cause GI upset; may be taken with food. Take glipizide ≈ 30 minutes before a meal to increase effectiveness.

Avoid alcohol (disulfiram reaction and interference with blood sugar control) and salicylates except on professional advice.

Monitor urine for glucose and ketones as prescribed; monitor blood glucose as prescribed.

Notify physician if any of the following occurs:

Hypoglycemia: Fatigue, excessive hunger, profuse sweating, numbness of extremities.
Hyperglycemia: Excessive thirst or urination, urinary glucose or ketones.
Other: Fever, sore throat, rash, unusual bruising or bleeding.

(Continued on following page)

Administration:

Institution of therapy: Individualize therapy. Selection of an individual agent is influenced by the drug's potency, duration of action, metabolism, adverse reactions and the patient's personal preference.

Short-term administration of sulfonylureas may be sufficient during periods of transient loss of control in patients usually well controlled on diet.

Transfer from other hypoglycemic agents:

Sulfonylureas – When transferring patients from one oral hypoglycemic agent to another, no transitional period and no initial or priming dose is necessary. However, when transferring patients from chlorpropamide, exercise particular care during the first 2 weeks because the prolonged retention of chlorpropamide in the body and subsequent overlapping drug effects may provoke hypoglycemia.

Insulin – During insulin withdrawal period, test blood for glucose and urine for ketones 3 times daily and report results to physician daily. The following may be used as a guide to determine daily insulin requirement.

Insulin Requirement When Instituting Sulfonylurea Therapy	
Insulin dose	Insulin requirement
< 20 units	Start directly on oral agent and discontinue insulin abruptly.
20-40 units	Initiate oral therapy with concurrent 25% to 50% reduction in insulin dose. Further reduce insulin as response is observed. With glyburide, insulin may be discontinued immediately.
> 40 units	Initiate oral therapy with concurrent 20% to 50% reduction in insulin dose. Further reduce insulin as response is observed.

Elderly patients may be particularly sensitive to these agents; therefore, start with a lower initial dose before breakfast, and check blood and urine glucose during the first 24 hours of therapy. If control is satisfactory, continue or gradually increase dose. If there is a tendency toward hypoglycemia, reduce dose or discontinue the drug.

Acute complications: During the course of intercurrent complications (eg, ketoacidosis, severe trauma, major surgery, infections, severe diarrhea, nausea, vomiting), supportive therapy with insulin may be necessary. Continue or withdraw sulfonylurea therapy while insulin is used. Insulin is indispensable in managing acute complications; carefully instruct all diabetics in its use.

Combination insulin therapy: Concurrent administration of insulin and an oral sulfonylurea (generally glipizide or glyburide) has been used with some success in Type II diabetic patients who are difficult to control with diet and sulfonylurea therapy alone. One proposed method is referred to as the BIDS system: Bedtime insulin, usually NPH, in combination with a daytime (morning only or morning and evening) sulfonylurea, usually glyburide.

CHLORPROPAMIDE

Dosage:

Initial dose: 250 mg/day in the mild to moderately severe, middle-aged, stable diabetic patient; use 100 to 125 mg/day in older patients.

Maintenance therapy: ≤ 100 to 250 mg/day. Severe diabetics may require 500 mg/day. Avoid doses > 750 mg/day.

	Product	Form	Description	C.I.*
Rx	**Chlorpropramide** (Various, eg, Geneva, Major, Mylan, Parmed, Rugby)	**Tablets:** 100 mg	In 100s, 250s, 500s, 1000s and UD 100s.	2+
Rx	**Diabinese** (Pfizer)		(393). Blue, scored. D-shaped. In 100s, 500s and UD 100s.	15
Rx	**Chlorpropamide** (Various, eg, Geneva, Goldline, Major, Mylan, Parmed, Rugby, Schein)	**Tablets:** 250 mg	In 100s, 500s, 1000s and UD 100s.	1+
Rx	**Diabinese** (Pfizer)		(394) Blue, scored. D-shaped. In 100s, 250s, 1000s and UD 100s.	17

* Cost Index based on cost per 100 mg chlorpropamide.

Complete prescribing information for these products begins on page 501.

TOLBUTAMIDE

Dosage:

Initial dose: 1 to 2 g/day (range, 0.25 to 3 g). A maintenance dose > 2 g/day is seldom required. Total dose may be taken in the morning, but divided doses may allow increased GI tolerance.

	Product	Form	Description	C.I.*
Rx	**Orinase** (Upjohn)	**Tablets:** 250 mg	White, scored. In unit-of-use 100s.	12
Rx	**Tolbutamide** (Various, eg, Barr, Geneva, Major, Mylan, Parmed, Rugby, Schein, Vitarine)	**Tablets:** 500 mg	In 100s, 500s and 1000s.	2.4+
Rx	**Orinase** (Upjohn)		White, scored. In 200s, 500s, 1000s, UD 100s and unit-of-use 100s.	12

ACETOHEXAMIDE

Dosage:

Initial dose: 250 mg to 1.5 g/day. Patients on ≤ 1 g daily can be controlled with once-daily dosage. Those receiving 1.5 g/day usually benefit from twice-daily dosage before morning and evening meals. Doses > 1.5 g/day are not recommended.

	Product	Form	Description	C.I.*
Rx	**Acetohexamide** (Various, eg, Barr, Major, Rugby, Schein)	**Tablets:** 250 mg	In 100s, 200s and 1000s.	8.9+
Rx	**Dymelor** (Lilly)		White, scored. In 50s, 200s and 500s.	7.1
Rx	**Acetohexamide** (Various, eg, Barr, Geneva, Major, Rugby, Schein)	**Tablets:** 500 mg	In 50s, 100s, 200s, 500s and 1000s.	7.2+
Rx	**Dymelor** (Lilly)		Yellow, scored. In 50s, 200s and 500s.	12

TOLAZAMIDE

Dosage:

Initial dose: 100 to 250 mg/day with breakfast or the first main meal. If fasting blood sugar (FBS) is < 200 mg/dl, use 100 mg/day, or 250 mg/day if FBS is > 200 mg/dl. If patients are malnourished, underweight, elderly or not eating properly, use 100 mg once a day. Adjust dose to response. If > 500 mg/day is required, give in divided doses twice daily. Doses > 1 g/day are not likely to improve control.

	Product	Form	Description	C.I.*
Rx	**Tolazamide** (Various, eg, Geneva, Major, Parmed, Rugby, Schein, Zenith)	**Tablets:** 100 mg	In 100s, 250s and 500s.	3.8+
Rx	**Tolinase** (Upjohn)		White, scored. In unit-of-use 100s.	12
Rx	**Tolazamide** (Various, eg, Geneva, Mylan, Parmed, Rugby, Schein, Zenith)	**Tablets:** 250 mg	In 100s, 200s, 250s, 500s and 1000s.	3.7+
Rx	**Tolinase** (Upjohn)		White, scored. In 200s, 1000s, UD 100s and unit-of-use 100s.	9.9
Rx	**Tolazamide** (Various, eg, Geneva, Mylan, Parmed, Rugby, Schein, Zenith)	**Tablets:** 500 mg	In 100s, 250s, 500s and 1000s.	2.3+
Rx	**Tolinase** (Upjohn)		White, scored. In unit-of-use 100s.	9.5

* Cost Index based on cost per 500 mg tolbutamide, 250 mg acetohexamide or 100 mg tolazamide.

Complete prescribing information for these products begins on page 501.

GLIPIZIDE

Dosage:

Give approximately 30 minutes before a meal to achieve the greatest reduction in postprandial hyperglycemia.

Initial dose: 5 mg, given ≈ 30 minutes before breakfast. Geriatric patients or those with liver disease may be started on 2.5 mg.

Adjust dosage in 2.5 to 5 mg increments, as determined by blood glucose response. Several days should elapse between titration steps. If response to a single dose is not satisfactory, dividing that dose may prove effective. The maximum recommended once daily dose is 15 mg. The maximum recommended total daily dose is 40 mg.

Maintenance dose: Some patients may be controlled on a once-a-day regimen, while others show better response with divided dosing. Divide total daily doses > 15 mg and give before meals of adequate caloric content. Total daily doses > 30 mg have been safely given on a twice-daily basis to long-term patients. **C.I.***

	Product	Form/Strength	Description	C.I.
Rx	**Glucotrol** (Roerig)	**Tablets:** 5 mg	Lactose. (Pfizer 411). Dye free. White, scored. Diamond shape. In 100s, 500s and UD 100s.	14
		10 mg	Lactose. (Pfizer 412). Dye free. White, scored. Diamond shape. In 100s, 500s and UD 100s.	13

GLYBURIDE (Glibenclamide)

Dosage:

DiaBeta/Micronase: Initial dose – 2.5 to 5 mg daily, administered with breakfast or the first main meal. For patients who may be more sensitive to hypoglycemic drugs, start at 1.25 mg daily.

Maintenance dose: 1.25 to 20 mg daily. Give as a single dose or in divided doses. Increase in increments of no more than 2.5 mg at weekly intervals based on the patient's blood glucose response. Daily doses > 20 mg are not recommended.

Glynase: Initial dose – 1.5 to 3 mg/day, administered with breakfast or the first main meal. For patients who may be more sensitive to hypoglycemic drugs, start at 0.75 mg/day.

Maintenance dose – 0.75 to 12 mg/day. Give as a single dose or in divided doses; some patients, particularly those receiving > 6 mg/day, may have a more satisfactory response with twice-daily dosing. Increase in increments of no more than 1.5 mg at weekly intervals based on the patient's blood glucose response. Daily doses > 12 mg are not recommended. **C.I.***

	Product	Form/Strength	Description	C.I.
Rx	**DiaBeta** (Hoechst-Roussel)	**Tablets:** 1.25 mg	(Dia β). White, scored. Oblong. In 50s.	15
Rx	**Micronase** (Upjohn)		White, scored. In 100s.	19
Rx	**Glynase PresTab** (Upjohn)	**Tablets, micronized:** 1.5 mg	Lactose. White, scored. Oval. In 30s, 60s, 100s, 500s, 1000s and UD 100s.	NA
Rx	**DiaBeta** (Hoechst-Roussel)	**Tablets:** 2.5 mg	(Dia β). Pink, scored. Oblong. In 30s, 60s, 100s, 500s and UD 100s.	13
Rx	**Micronase** (Upjohn)		Pink, scored. In 30s, 60s, 100s and UD 100s.	15
Rx	**Glynase PresTab** (Upjohn)	**Tablets, micronized:** 3 mg	Lactose. Blue, scored. Oval. In 30s, 60s, 90s, 100s, 500s, 1000s and UD 100s.	NA
Rx	**DiaBeta** (Hoechst-Roussel)	**Tablets:** 5 mg	(Dia β). Green, scored. In 30s, 60s, 100s, 500s, 1000s and UD 100s.	11
Rx	**Micronase** (Upjohn)		Blue, scored. In 30s, 60s, 90s, 100s, 500s, 1000s and UD 100s.	13

* Cost Index based on cost per 5 mg glipizide or 2.5 mg glyburide.

GLUCAGON

Actions:

Pharmacology: Glucagon, a polypeptide hormone produced by the alpha cells of the pancreas, accelerates liver glycogenolysis by stimulating cyclic AMP synthesis and increasing phosphorylase kinase activity. Increased breakdown of glycogen to glucose, and inhibition of glycogen synthetase results in blood glucose elevation. Additionally, glucagon stimulates hepatic gluconeogenesis by promoting the uptake of amino acids and converting them to glucose precursors. Lipolysis in the liver and adipose tissue is enhanced (via adenyl cyclase activation), providing free fatty acids and glycerol to further stimulate ketogenesis and gluconeogenesis.

Parenteral administration of glucagon produces relaxation of the smooth muscle of the GI tract. It also decreases gastric and pancreatic secretions in the GI tract and increases myocardial contractility.

Pharmacokinetics: Parenteral administration to comatose hypoglycemic patients (with normal liver glycogen stores) usually produces a return to consciousness within 5 to 20 minutes. Glucagon is degraded in the liver and kidney, in plasma, and at its tissue receptor sites in plasma membranes. Plasma half-life is 3 to 6 minutes.

Indications:

Hypoglycemia: Counteracts severe hypoglycemic reactions in diabetic patients or during insulin shock therapy in psychiatric patients. Glucagon is helpful in hypoglycemia only if liver glycogen is available. It is of little or no help in states of starvation, adrenal insufficiency or chronic hypoglycemia.

In Type I (juvenile diabetics), blood glucose levels do not respond as well as in adult stable diabetics; give supplementary carbohydrates as soon as possible.

Diagnostic aid in the radiologic examination of the stomach, duodenum, small bowel and colon when a hypotonic state is advantageous.

Unlabeled Uses: Glucagon has been used in the treatment of propranolol overdose, cardiovascular emergencies and GI disturbances associated with spasms.

Contraindications:

Hypersensitivity to glucagon.

Warnings:

Insulinoma/pheochromocytoma: Administer cautiously to patients with a history of insulinoma or pheochromocytoma. In patients with insulinoma, IV glucagon will produce an initial increase in blood glucose but, because of its insulin-releasing effect, may subsequently cause hypoglycemia. It also stimulates catecholamine release, causing a marked increase in blood pressure in patients with pheochromocytoma.

Usage in Pregnancy: Category B. Reproduction studies performed in rats at 90 to 120 times the human dose have revealed no evidence of harm to the fetus. There are no adequate and well controlled studies in pregnant women. Use during pregnancy only if clearly needed.

Usage in Lactation: It it not known whether this drug is excreted in breast milk. Exercise caution when administering to a nursing mother.

Precautions:

Hypoglycemia: Although glucagon may be used for emergency treatment of hypoglycemia, notify the physician when hypoglycemic reactions occur so that the insulin dose may be adjusted.

Drug Interactions:

Oral anticoagulants: The hypoprothrombinemic effects may be increased, possibly with bleeding. The interaction may occur after several days of therapy and appears to be dose-related. Monitor prothrombin time and adjust oral anticoagulant dose accordingly.

Adverse Reactions:

Occasional nausea and vomiting; this may also occur with hypoglycemia.

Generalized allergic reactions including urticaria, respiratory distress and hypotension have been reported.

Overdosage:

There have been no reports of overdosage in humans. Treatment should be symptomatic, primarily for nausea, vomiting and possible hypokalemia.

(Continued on following page)

GLUCAGON (Cont.)

Administration and Dosage:

Patient instructions are provided with product.

Hypoglycemia: 0.5 to 1 mg SC, IM or IV usually produces a response in 5 to 20 minutes. If the response is delayed, administer 1 or 2 additional doses. Arouse the patient as quickly as possible. In view of the deleterious effects of cerebral hypoglycemia, give glucose IV if the patient fails to respond to glucagon.

When the patient responds, give supplemental carbohydrate to restore the liver glycogen and prevent secondary hypoglycemia.

Insulin shock therapy: After 1 hour of coma, inject 0.5 to 1 mg or more, if desired, SC, IM or IV. The patient will usually awaken in 10 to 25 minutes. If no response occurs, repeat the dose. Upon awakening, feed the patient orally, as soon as possible, and follow the usual dietary regimen.

In a very deep state of coma give glucose IV in addition to glucagon for a more immediate response.

Diagnostic aid: Administer the doses in the following chart for relaxation of the stomach, duodenum and small bowel, depending on the time of onset of action and the duration of effect required. Since the stomach is less sensitive to the effect of glucagon, 0.5 mg IV or 2 mg IM are recommended.

Dose	Route	Onset (min)	Duration (min)
0.25 to 0.5 mg (0.25-0.5 unit)	IV	1	9-17
1 mg (1 unit)	IM	8-10	12-27
2 mg (2 units)*	IV	1	22-25
2 mg (2 units)*	IM	4-7	21-32

* 2 mg doses produces a higher incidence of nausea and vomiting.

For examination of the colon, administer 2 mg IM approximately 10 minutes prior to initiation of the procedure.

Stability: Store at room temperature prior to reconstitution. After reconstitution, use immediately. May be kept at 5°C (41°F) for up to 48 hrs, if necessary.

If given in doses higher than 2 mg, reconstitute with Sterile Water for Injection and use immediately.

Rx	**Glucagon** (Lilly)	**Powder for Injection (lyophilized):** 1 mg (1 unit) vials[1] with 1 ml diluent.[2] 10 mg (10 units) vials[1] with 10 ml diluent.[2]

[1] With lactose.

[2] With 1.6% glycerin and 0.2% phenol.

DIAZOXIDE, ORAL

Parenteral diazoxide is used for hypertensive emergencies; see page 841.

Actions:

Pharmacology: Diazoxide is a benzothiadiazine derivative related to the thiazide diuretics. Oral diazoxide produces a prompt dose-related increase in the blood glucose by inhibiting pancreatic insulin release, and also by an extrapancreatic effect. The hyperglycemic effect begins within an hour and generally lasts no more than 8 hours with normal renal function.

Diazoxide decreases sodium chloride and water excretion, resulting in fluid retention. The blood pressure effects are usually not marked with the oral preparation.

Other actions include: Increased pulse rate; increased serum uric acid levels due to decreased excretion; increased serum levels of free fatty acids; decreased para-aminohippuric acid (PAH) clearance with little effect on glomerular filtration rate.

Insulin or tolbutamide reverses diazoxide-induced hyperglycemia.

Pharmacokinetics: Diazoxide is extensively bound (90%) to serum proteins. The plasma half-life is 28 $\pm$ 8.3 hours. In four children, the plasma half-life varied from 9.5 to 24 hours. The half-life may be prolonged following overdosage, and in patients with impaired renal function. Diazoxide is excreted by the kidneys.

Indications:

Management of hypoglycemia due to hyperinsulinism in the following:

Adults – Inoperable islet cell adenoma or carcinoma, or extrapancreatic malignancy.

Infants and children – Leucine sensitivity, islet cell hyperplasia, nesidioblastosis, extrapancreatic malignancy, islet cell adenoma or adenomatosis. May be used preoperatively as a temporary measure, and postoperatively if hypoglycemia persists.

Contraindications:

Functional hypoglycemia. Do not use in patients hypersensitive to diazoxide or to other thiazides unless the potential benefits outweigh the possible risks.

Warnings:

Fluid retention in patients with compromised cardiac reserve may precipitate CHF. Fluid retention will respond to conventional diuretic therapy.

Ketoacidosis and nonketotic hyperosmolar coma have occurred with recommended doses, usually during intercurrent illness. Prompt recognition and treatment are essential (see Overdosage), and prolonged surveillance following the acute episode is necessary because of the long half-life. The patient must monitor the urine for glucose and ketones and promptly report abnormal findings and unusual symptoms.

Cataracts: Transient cataracts occurred in association with hyperosmolar coma in an infant, and subsided on correction of the hyperosmolarity.

Usage in Pregnancy: Category C. Reproduction studies in rats and rabbits have revealed increased fetal resorptions, delayed parturition and fetal skeletal and cardiac anomalies. In animals, the drug causes degeneration of fetal pancreatic beta cells. Since there are no adequate human data, safety for use during pregnancy has not been established. Use only when clearly needed and when the potential benefits outweigh the unknown potential hazards to the fetus.

Diazoxide crosses the placenta. When given to the mother prior to delivery, the drug may produce fetal or neonatal hyperbilirubinemia, thrombocytopenia, altered carbohydrate metabolism or other side effects that have occurred in adults. Alopecia and hypertrichosis lanuginosa have occurred in infants whose mothers received oral diazoxide the last 19 to 60 days of pregnancy.

Labor and Delivery: Administration IV during labor may cause cessation of uterine contractions. Oxytocic agents may be required to reinstate labor; use caution.

Precautions:

Monitoring: Observe patients closely when treatment is initiated. Monitor clinical response and blood glucose until the patient's condition has stabilized, usually several days. If not effective after 2 or 3 weeks, discontinue the drug.

Prolonged treatment requires regular monitoring of the urine for glucose and ketones, especially under stress conditions. Monitor blood glucose levels periodically to determine the need for dose adjustment.

Serum uric acid levels might be elevated, particularly in patients with hyperuricemia or a history of gout.

Higher blood levels have been observed with the liquid than with the capsule formulation. Adjust dosage as necessary when changing formulations.

Use in impaired renal function: Decreased protein binding is seen in patients with renal failure. The higher level of free drug corresponds to an increase in hypotensive effect.

(Continued on following page)

DIAZOXIDE, ORAL (Cont.)

Drug Interactions:

Alpha-adrenergic blocking agents: Inhibition of insulin release by diazoxide is antagonized by these agents.

Sulfonylureas: When diazoxide is administered concurrently, the pharmacologic effects of both drugs may be decreased.

Bilirubin or **coumarin** and its derivatives: Diazoxide is highly bound to serum protein and may displace other agents resulting in higher blood levels of these substances.

Thiazide diuretics: Concomitant administration may potentiate diazoxide's hyperglycemic and hyperuricemic effects. Hypotension may occur.

Antihypertensive agents: Diazoxide may enhance the effect of these agents.

Phenytoin: Concomitant administration may result in a loss of seizure control, possibly due to increased hepatic metabolism of phenytoin.

Phenothiazines: Concomitant use may cause an increase in the pharmacologic effects of diazoxide. Hyperglycemia may result.

Adverse Reactions:

Frequent and serious: Sodium and fluid retention is most common in infants and adults; may precipitate CHF in patients with compromised cardiac reserve (see Warnings).

Infrequent but serious: Hyperglycemia or glycosuria may require dosage reduction to avoid progression to ketoacidosis or hyperosmolar coma. Diabetic ketoacidosis and hyperosmolar nonketotic coma may develop very rapidly (see Overdosage).

GI: Anorexia, nausea, vomiting, abdominal pain, ileus, diarrhea, transient loss of taste; acute pancreatitis/pancreatic necrosis.

Cardiovascular: Tachycardia, palpitations; occasional hypotension; transient hypertension; chest pain (rare).

Hematologic: Frequent – Thrombocytopenia with or without purpura may require discontinuation of the drug. Transient neutropenia is not associated with increased susceptibility to infection and ordinarily does not require discontinuance.

Eosinophilia; decreased hemoglobin/hematocrit; excessive bleeding; decreased IgG.

Hepato-Renal: Increased serum uric acid; increased AST and alkaline phosphatase; azotemia; decreased creatinine clearance; reversible nephrotic syndrome; decreased urinary output; hematuria; albuminuria.

CNS: Headache, weakness, malaise; anxiety; dizziness; insomnia; polyneuritis; paresthesia; extrapyramidal signs.

Ophthalmologic: Transient cataracts; subconjunctival hemorrhage; ring scotoma; blurred vision; diplopia; lacrimation.

Dermatologic: Hirsutism of the lanugo type mainly on the forehead, back and limbs, subsides on discontinuation of the drug.

Skin rash; pruritus; monilial dermatitis; herpes; loss of scalp hair.

Other: Gout; advance in bone age; galactorrhea; enlargement of lump in breast; fever.

Overdosage:

Symptoms: Marked hyperglycemia which may be associated with ketoacidosis.

Treatment: Promptly administer insulin and restore fluid and electrolyte balance. Because of the drug's long half-life, symptoms require prolonged surveillance for up to 7 days, until the blood sugar level stabilizes within the normal range. Successful lowering of diazoxide blood levels by peritoneal dialysis and by hemodialysis in two patients has been reported.

Treatment includes usual supportive measures. Refer to General Management of Acute Overdosage on p. vi.

Patient Information:

Monitor urine regularly for glucose and ketones; report any abnormalities to physician.

Administration and Dosage:

Individualize dosage. Assure accuracy of dosage in infants and young children.

Adults and children: 3 to 8 mg/kg/day, in 2 or 3 equal doses every 8 or 12 hours. Patients with refractory hypoglycemia may require higher dosages.

Infants and newborns: 8 to 15 mg/kg/day, in 2 or 3 equal doses every 8 or 12 hours.

Storage: Protect **suspension** from light.

Rx	**Proglycem** (Medical Market Specialties)	**Capsules:** 50 mg	(#MMS PBA or 830). Orange and clear. In 100s.
		Oral Suspension: 50 mg per ml	Chocolate-mint flavor. In 30 ml with calibrated dropper.

Product identification code.

Parenteral dextrose (d-glucose) is also used in the treatment of acute hypoglycemia. See page 122

GLUCOSE

Actions:

Glucose, a monosaccharide, is absorbed from the intestine after administration and then used, distributed and stored by the tissues. Direct absorption takes place, resulting in a rapid increased blood glucose concentration. Therefore, it is effective in small doses; no evidence of toxicity has been reported. Glucose provides 4 calories/gram.

Indications:

Management of hypoglycemia.

Adverse Reactions:

Isolated reports of nausea, which may also occur with hypoglycemia.

Administration and Dosage:

Administer 10 to 20 g orally; repeat in 10 minutes if necessary. Response should occur in 10 minutes.

Glucose is not absorbed from the buccal cavity; it must be swallowed to be effective. While swallowing reflexes may be preserved in the unconscious patient, the lack of normal gag reflexes may lead to aspiration. When possible, use other methods of treating hypoglycemia in unconscious patients.

Children: Do not give to children under 2 years of age, unless directed by a physician.

otc	**Glutose** (Paddock)	**Gel:** Liquid glucose (40% dextrose)	Dye free. In 80 g bottle and 25 g tube.
otc	**Insta-Glucose** (ICN)		Cherry flavor. In UD 30.8 g tubes.
otc	**Insulin Reaction** (Sherwood)		Lime flavor. In UD 25 g tubes.
otc	**B-D Glucose** (Becton Dickinson)	**Tablets, chewable:** 5 g	In 36s.

ALGLUCERASE (Glucocerebrosidase-beta-glucosidase)

Actions:

Alglucerase was approved by the FDA in April 1991. Alglucerase is a modified form of the enzyme beta-glucocerebrosidase used for the treatment of Gaucher's disease; it is prepared by modification of the oligosaccharide chains of human beta-glucocerebrosidase. The modification alters the sugar residues at the nonreducing ends of the oligosaccharide chains of the glycoprotein so that they are predominantly terminated with mannose residues (specifically recognized by carbohydrate receptors on macrophage cells).

Alglucerase is purified from a large pool of human placental tissue collected from selected donors. The risk of viral contamination has been reduced; however, no procedure is totally effective in removing viral infectivity (see Precautions). Each lot of product has been tested and found negative for hepatitis B surface antigen (HBsAg) and for antigens of the human immunodeficiency virus (HIV-1).

Pharmacology: Alglucerase catalyzes the hydrolysis of the glycolipid glucocerebroside to glucose and ceramide as part of the normal degradation pathway for membrane lipids. Glucocerebroside is primarily derived from hematological cell turnover.

Gaucher's disease is characterized by a functional deficiency in beta-glucocerebrosidase enzymatic activity and the resultant accumulation of lipid glucocerebroside in tissue macrophages which become engorged and are termed Gaucher's cells. Gaucher's cells are typically found in liver, spleen and bone marrow and, occasionally, in lung, kidney and intestine. Secondary hematologic sequelae include severe anemia and thrombocytopenia in addition to the characteristic progressive hepatosplenomegaly. Skeletal complications, including osteonecrosis and osteopenia with secondary pathological fractures, are a common feature of Gaucher's disease.

Pharmacokinetics: Following an IV infusion of different doses (between 0.6 and 234 U/kg) over a 4 hour period, steady-state enzymatic activity was achieved by 60 minutes. Individual steady-state enzymatic activity and area under the curve of the activity increased linearly with the infused dose (0.6 to 121 U/kg). Following infusion termination, plasma enzymatic activity declined rapidly with elimination half-life ranging between 3.6 and 10.4 minutes. Plasma clearance calculated from plasma enzymatic activity was variable and ranged between 6.34 and 25.39 ml/min/kg, whereas the volume of distribution ranged from 49.4 to 282.1 ml/kg. Within the dosage range of 0.6 and 121 U/kg, elimination half-life, plasma clearance and volume of distribution values appear to be independent of the infused dose.

Clinical trials: Chronic administration of alglucerase in 13 patients with Type 1 Gaucher's disease induced the following effects:

Splenomegaly and hepatomegaly were significantly reduced, presumably by disruption of the lysosomal storage sites and metabolism of glucocerebroside in Gaucher's cells. This effect was demonstrated within 6 months of therapy initiation.

Hematologic deficiencies in hemoglobin, hematocrit, erythrocyte and platelet counts were significantly improved. In most patients, a change in hemoglobin was the first observable effect. In some patients, hemoglobin levels were normalized after 6 months of therapy.

Improved mineralization occurred in four patients after prolonged treatment as a result of a reduction in the osteolytic actions of lipid-laden Gaucher's cells in the marrow.

Cachexia and wasting in children were reduced.

Indications:

Long-term enzyme replacement therapy for patients with a confirmed diagnosis of Type 1 Gaucher's disease who exhibit signs and symptoms severe enough to result in one or more of the following conditions: Moderate-to-severe anemia; thrombocytopenia with bleeding tendency; bone disease; significant hepatomegaly or splenomegaly.

Contraindications:

Hypersensitivity to the product.

Warnings:

Pregnancy: Category C. It is not known whether alglucerase can cause fetal harm when administered to a pregnant woman, or can affect reproductive capacity. Use in pregnancy only if clearly needed.

Lactation: It is not known whether this drug is excreted in breast milk. Exercise caution when administering to a nursing woman.

(Continued on following page)

ALGLUCERASE (Glucocerebrosidase-beta-glucosidase) (Cont.)

Precautions:

Viral infectious agents: Alglucerase is prepared from pooled human placental tissue that may contain the causative agents of some viral diseases. Manufacturing steps have been designed to reduce the risk of transmitting viral infectious agents. These steps have demonstrated in vitro inactivation of a panel of model viruses, including human immunodeficiency virus (HIV-1). The risk of contamination from slowly acting or latent viruses, including the Creutzfeldt-Jacob disease agent, is believed to be remote but has not been tested. Accordingly, assess benefits and risks of treatment with this product prior to use.

Adverse Reactions:

During clinical studies involving 31 patients, 28 adverse experiences occurred that were possibly related to alglucerase. Seven of these were related to the route of administration and included discomfort, burning and swelling at the site of venipuncture. The remaining 21 experiences (of which ≈ 75% were reported by 2 patients) consisted of slight fever, chills, abdominal discomfort, nausea or vomiting. None of these events were judged to require medical intervention.

Most patients treated on a chronic basis have not formed detectable antibodies. Six months after therapy initiation, a 72-year-old patient demonstrated a positive response in testing procedures designed to detect antibodies to alglucerase. Close monitoring indicated no diminution of clinical response, and therapy has been continued.

Overdosage:

No obvious toxicity was detected after single doses up to 234 U/kg. There is no experience with higher doses.

Administration and Dosage:

Administer by IV infusion over 1 to 2 hours. Individualize dosage. An initial dosage up to 60 U/kg per infusion may be used. The usual frequency of infusion is once every 2 weeks, but disease severity and patient convenience may dictate administration as often as once every other day or as infrequently as once every 4 weeks. After patient response is well established, dosage may be adjusted downward for maintenance therapy. Dosage can be progressively lowered at intervals of 3 to 6 months while closely monitoring response parameters. Ultrastructural evidence suggests that glucocerebroside lipid storage may respond to doses as low as 1 U/kg.

On the day of use, the appropriate amount of alglucerase for each patient is diluted with normal saline to a final volume not to exceed 100 ml. The use of an in-line particulate filter is recommended for the infusion apparatus.

Relatively low toxicity, combined with the extended time course of response, allows small dosage adjustments to be made occasionally to avoid discarding partially used bottles. Thus, the dosage administered in individual infusions may be slightly increased or decreased to fully utilize each bottle as long as the monthly administered dosage remains substantially unaltered.

Storage/stability: Do not shake; shaking may denature the glycoprotein, rendering it biologically inactive. Store at 4°C (39°F). Do not use any bottles exhibiting particulate matter or discoloration. Do not use after the expiration date on the bottle. Alglucerase does not contain any preservative; after opening, do not store for subsequent use.

Rx	**Ceredase** (Genzyme[1])	**Injection:** 80 IU/ml[2]	In 5 ml bottles.[3]

[1] Genzyme Corporation, One Kendall Square, Cambridge, MA 02139. (617) 252-7500.
[2] An international enzyme unit is defined as the amount of enzyme required to hydrolyze 1 micromole of the synthetic substrate.
[3] With 1% albumin (human), 53 mM citrate and 143 mM sodium.

Thyroid Hormones

Preparations: Thyroid hormones include both natural and synthetic derivatives. The natural products, desiccated thyroid and thyroglobulin, are derived from beef or pork. Although these preparations are most economical, standardization by iodine content or bioassay is inexact; synthetic derivatives are generally preferred because of more uniform standardization of potency.

Synthetic derivatives include levothyroxine (T_4), liothyronine (T_3) and liotrix (a 4 to 1 mixture of T_4 and T_3).

Actions:

Physiological effects: The mechanisms by which thyroid hormones exert their physiologic action are not well understood; however, it is believed that most of their effects are exerted through control of DNA transcription and protein synthesis. The principal effect of thyroid hormones is to increase the metabolic rate of body tissues noted by increases in the following: Oxygen consumption; respiratory rate; body temperature; cardiac output; heart rate; blood volume; rate of fat, protein and carbohydrate metabolism; enzyme system activity; growth and maturation. Thyroid hormones exert a profound influence on every organ system in the body and are particularly important in CNS development.

Thyroid hormones are also concerned with growth and differentiation of tissues. In deficiency states in the young, there is growth retardation and failure of maturation of the skeletal and other body systems, especially in failure of ossification in the epiphyses and in brain growth and development.

Regulation of thyroid secretion – Thyroid hormone synthesis is controlled by thyrotropin (Thyroid Stimulating Hormone; TSH) secreted by the anterior pituitary. TSH secretion is, in turn, controlled by a feedback mechanism effected by the thyroid hormones and by thyrotropin releasing hormone (TRH), a tripeptide of hypothalamic origin. Endogenous thyroid hormone secretion is suppressed when exogenous thyroid hormones are administered to euthyroid individuals in excess of the normal gland's secretion.

Pharmacology: Thyroid administration increases basal metabolic rate. The effect develops slowly, but is prolonged. It begins within 48 hours and reaches a maximum in 8 to 10 days, although full effects of continued administration may not be evident for several weeks.

The primary effect of the thyroid hormones is the result of T_3 activity. The normal thyroid gland contains, per gram of gland, approximately 200 mcg of T_4 and 15 mcg of T_3. The ratio of these two hormones in the circulation does not represent the ratio in the thyroid gland, since about 80% of peripheral T_3 comes from monodeiodination of T_4. Peripheral monodeiodination of T_4 also results in the formation of reverse triiodothyronine (rT_3), which is calorigenically inactive. These facts seem to advocate T_4 as the treatment of choice for the hypothyroid patient and to caution against the administration of hormone combinations which, while normalizing thyroxine levels, may produce T_3 levels in the thyrotoxic range.

"Low triiodothyronine syndrome" – The T_3 level is low in the fetus and newborn, in the elderly and in cases of chronic caloric deprivation, hepatic cirrhosis, renal failure, surgical stress and chronic illnesses.

Pharmacokinetics:

Absorption – Absorption of T_4 from the GI tract varies from 48% to 79% of the dose administered; fasting increases absorption; malabsorption syndromes cause excessive fecal loss. In 4 hours, T_3 is 95% absorbed. The hormones in natural preparations are absorbed in a manner similar to the synthetic hormones.

Protein binding - More than 99% of circulating hormones are bound to serum proteins, including thyroid binding globulin (TBg), thyroid binding prealbumin (TBPA) and albumin (TBa), whose capacities and affinities vary for the hormones. The higher affinity of T_4 for both TBg and TBPA as compared to T_3 partially explains the higher serum levels and longer half-life of T_4. Both protein-bound hormones exist in reverse equilibrium with minute amounts of free hormone.

Metabolism – Under normal circumstances, the ratio of T_4 to T_3 released from the thyroid gland is 20:1. Approximately 35% of T_4 is converted in the periphery to T_3. Thus, 80% of T_3 comes from monodeiodination of T_4. Deiodination of T_4 occurs at a number of sites, including liver, kidney and other tissues. The conjugated hormone, in the form of glucuronide or sulfate, is found in the bile and gut where it may complete an enterohepatic circulation. Eighty-five percent of T_4 metabolized daily is deiodinated.

(Actions continued on following page)

Actions (Cont.):

Pharmacokinetics (Cont.):

Various Pharmacokinetic Parameters of Thyroid Hormones				
Hormone	Ratio released from thyroid gland	Biologic potency	Half-life (days)	Protein binding (%)[2]
Levothyroxine (T_4)	20	1	6-7[1]	99+
Liothyronine (T_3)	1	4	≤2	99+

[1] 3 to 4 days in hyperthyroidism, 9 to 10 days in myxedema.
[2] Includes TBg, TBPA and TBa.

Indications:

Hypothyroidism: As replacement or supplemental therapy in hypothyroidism of any etiology, except transient hypothyroidism during the recovery phase of subacute thyroiditis. Specific indications include: Cretinism, myxedema, non-toxic goiter and ordinary hypothyroidism; primary hypothyroidism resulting from functional deficiency, primary atrophy, partial or total absence of thyroid gland, or the effects of surgery, radiation or drugs, with or without the presence of goiter; secondary (pituitary) or tertiary (hypothalamic) hypothyroidism.

Pituitary TSH suppressants: In the treatment or prevention of various types of euthyroid goiters, including thyroid nodules, subacute or chronic lymphocytic thyroiditis (Hashimoto's), multinodular goiter and in the management of thyroid cancer.

Thyrotoxicosis: May be used with antithyroid drugs to treat thyrotoxicosis, to prevent goitrogenesis and hypothyroidism and thyrotoxicosis during pregnancy.

Diagnostic use in suppression tests to differentiate suspected hyperthyroidism from euthyroidism.

Unlabeled uses: Thyroid hormones have been used to treat obesity; however, they are ineffective and should not be used for this condition. See Warnings.

Contraindications:

Acute myocardial infarction and thyrotoxicosis uncomplicated by hypothyroidism. However, when hypothyroidism is a complicating or causative factor in myocardial infarction or heart disease, consider the judicious use of small doses of thyroid.

Where hypothyroidism and hypoadrenalism (Addison's disease) coexist, unless treatment of hypoadrenalism with adrenocortical steroids precedes the initiation of thyroid therapy (see Warnings).

Hypersensitivity to active or extraneous constituents.

Warnings:

Obesity has been treated with thyroid hormones. In euthyroid patients, hormonal replacement doses are ineffective for weight reduction. Larger doses may produce serious or even life-threatening toxicity, particularly when given with sympathomimetic amines such as anorexiants.

Infertility: Thyroid hormone therapy is unjustified for the treatment of male or female infertility, unless the condition is accompanied by hypothyroidism.

Cardiovascular disease: Use caution when the integrity of the cardiovascular system, particularly the coronary arteries, is suspect. This includes patients with angina or the elderly, in whom there is a greater likelihood of occult cardiac disease. In these patients, initiate therapy with low doses, ie, 25 to 50 mcg T_4 or its equivalent. When, in such patients, a euthyroid state can only be reached at the expense of an aggravation of the cardiovascular disease, reduce thyroid hormone dosage. The development of chest pain or other worsening of cardiovascular disease requires a decrease in dosage.

Observe patients with coronary artery disease during surgery, since the possibility of precipitating cardiac arrhythmias may be greater in those treated with thyroid hormones.

(Warnings continued on following page)

Warnings (Cont.):

Endocrine disorders: Thyroid hormone therapy in patients with concomitant diabetes mellitus or insipidus or adrenal insufficiency (Addison's disease) exacerbates the intensity of their symptoms. Appropriate adjustments in the therapy of these concomitant endocrine diseases are required.

Severe and prolonged hypothyroidism can lead to a decreased level of adrenocortical activity commensurate with the lowered metabolic state. When thyroid replacement therapy is administered, the metabolism increases at a greater rate than adrenocortical activity, which can precipitate adrenocortical insufficiency. Therefore, supplemental adrenocortical steroids may be necessary. The therapy of myxedema coma requires simultaneous administration of glucocorticoids.

In patients whose hypothyroidism is secondary to hypopituitarism, adrenal insufficiency will probably be present; correct adrenal insufficiency with corticosteroids before administering thyroid hormones.

Morphologic hypogonadism and nephrosis: Rule out prior to initiating therapy.

Myxedema: Patients with myxedema are particularly sensitive to thyroid preparations. Begin treatment with small doses and gradual increments.

Hyperthyroid effects: In rare instances the administration of thyroid hormone may precipitate a hyperthyroid state or may aggravate existing hyperthyroidism.

Pregnancy: Category A. Thyroid hormones do not readily cross the placenta. Clinical experience does not indicate any adverse effect on the fetus when thyroid hormones are administered to a pregnant woman. Do not discontinue thyroid replacement therapy in hypothyroid women during pregnancy.

Lactation: Minimal amounts of thyroid hormones are excreted in breast milk. Thyroid is not associated with serious adverse reactions. However, exercise caution when thyroid is administered to a nursing woman.

Children: Congenital hypothyroidism – Pregnant women provide little or no thyroid hormone to the fetus. The incidence of congenital hypothyroidism is relatively high (1:4000) and the hypothyroid fetus would not benefit from the small amounts of hormone crossing the placenta. Routine determinations of serum T_4 or TSH are strongly advised in neonates in view of the deleterious effects of thyroid deficiency on growth and development.

Initiate treatment immediately upon diagnosis, and maintain for life, unless transient hypothyroidism is suspected; in this case, therapy may be interrupted for 2 to 8 weeks after the age of 3 years to reassess the condition. Cessation of therapy is justified in patients who have maintained a normal TSH during those 2 to 8 weeks.

In infants, excessive doses of thyroid hormone preparations may produce craniosynostosis.

In children, partial loss of hair may be experienced in the first few months of thyroid therapy; this is usually a transient phenomenon that results in later recovery.

Precautions:

Monitoring: Treatment of patients with thyroid hormones requires the periodic assessment of thyroid status by means of appropriate laboratory tests. The TSH suppression test can be used to test the effectiveness of any thyroid preparation, keeping in mind the relative insensitivity of the infant pituitary to the negative feedback effect of thyroid hormones. Serum T_4 levels can be used to test the effectiveness of all thyroid medications except T_3. When the total serum T_4 is low but TSH is normal, a test specific to assess unbound (free) T_4 levels is warranted. Specific measurements of T_4 and T_3 by competitive protein binding or radioimmunoassay are not influenced by blood levels of organic or inorganic iodine and have essentially replaced older tests (ie, PBI, BEI and T_4 by column). See Administration and Dosage.

Persistent clinical and laboratory evidence of hypothyroidism in spite of adequate dosage replacement indicates poor patient compliance, poor absorption, excessive fecal loss or inactivity of the preparation. Intracellular resistance to thyroid hormone is rare.

Decreased bone density: Long-term levothyroxine therapy has been associated with decreased bone density in the hip and spine in pre- and postmenopausal women. These effects may be avoided by using levothyroxine only after appropriate clinical evaluation, gradually increasing the dose until the appropriate serum level is reached using the minimal dose required and periodically monitoring the patient. It may be beneficial to obtain a basal bone density measurement, then monitor closely for osteoporosis development.

Tartrazine sensitivity: Some of these products contain tartrazine, which may cause allergic-type reactions (including bronchial asthma) in susceptible individuals. Although the incidence of tartrazine sensitivity in the general population is low, it is frequently seen in patients who also have aspirin hypersensitivity. Specific products containing tartrazine are identified in the product listings.

(Continued on following page)

Drug Interactions:

Thyroid Hormone Drug Interactions			
Precipitant Drug	Object Drug*		Description
Cholestyramine and colestipol	Thyroid hormones	⬇	Loss of efficacy of thyroid hormone and potential hypothyroidism. Administer 4 to 6 hours apart.
Estrogens	Thyroid hormones	⬇	Estrogens increase TBg and may therefore decrease the response to thyroid hormone therapy in patients with a nonfunctioning thyroid gland. This is based on theoretical considerations.
Thyroid hormones	Anticoagulants	⬆	The anticoagulant action is increased; a decreased dose may be necessary.
Thyroid hormones	Beta blockers	⬇	The actions of particular beta blockers may be impaired when the hypothyroid patient is converted to the euthyroid state.
Thyroid hormones	Digitalis glycosides	⬇	Serum digitalis glycoside levels are reduced in hyperthyroidism or when the hypothyroid patient is converted to the euthyroid state. Therapeutic effects of digitalis glycosides may be reduced.
Thyroid hormones	Theophyllines	⬆	Decreased theophylline clearance can be expected in hypothyroid patients; clearance returns to normal when euthyroid state is achieved.

* ⬆ = Object drug increased ⬇ = Object drug decreased.

Drug/Food interactions: Fasting increases the absorption of T_4 from the GI tract.

Drug/Lab test interactions: Consider changes in TBg concentration when interpreting T_4 and T_3 values. In such cases, measure the unbound (free) hormone. Pregnancy, infectious hepatitis, estrogens and estrogen-containing oral contraceptives increase TBg concentrations. Decreases in TBg concentrations are observed in nephrosis, acromegaly and after androgen or corticosteroid therapy. Familial hyper- or hypothyroxine binding globulinemias have been described. The incidence of TBg deficiency approximates 1 in 9000.

Medicinal or dietary iodine interferes with all in vivo tests of radioiodine uptake, producing low uptakes which may not reflect a true decrease in hormone synthesis.

(Drug Interactions continued on following page)

Thyroid Hormones (Cont.)

Drug Interactions (Cont.):

Effects of Drugs on Thyroid Function Tests

↑ Increased
⇧ Slightly increased
↓ Decreased
⇩ Slightly decreased
0 No effect
blank space signifies no data

Drug	Free T_4	Serum T_4	T_3 uptake resin	Free thyroxine index (FTI)	Serum T_3	Serum TSH
p-aminosalicylic acid		↓		↓		
Aminoglutethimide		↓				↑
Amiodarone	0/↑	↑		↑	↓	↑
Anabolic steroids/androgens	0	↓	↑	0	↓	0
Antithyroid (PTU, methimazole)	0	0	↓	0	↓	0
Asparaginase		↓	↑	0	↓	0
Barbiturates	0	↓	0/⇧	↓	0	0
Carbamazepine	0/↓	↓	0/↑	↓	0/↑	0/↑
Chloral hydrate		↓	0/⇧	0	↓	0
Cholestiramine	0	↓		↓	0/↑	0
Clofibrate	0	↑	↓	0	↑	0
Colestipol	0	↓		↓	0/↑	0/↑
Contraceptives, oral	0	↑	↓	0	↑	0
Corticosteroids	0	↓	↑	0	↓	0/↓
Danazol	0	↓	↑	0	↓	0
Diazepam		↓		⇩		
Estrogens	0	↑	↓	0/⇧	↑	0
Ethionamide		↓				
Fluorouracil		↓	0/⇧	0	↓	0
Heparin (IV)		↓	0/↑	↑	0	
Insulin		↑				
Lithium carbonate		0/↓	0/↓	0/↓	0/↓	0/↑
Methadone		↑	↓	0	↑	0
Mitotane		↓	0/⇧	0	↓	0
Nitroprusside		↓				
Oxyphenbutazone/phenylbutazone		↓	0/⇧	0	↓	0
Perphenazine		↑	↓	↓	↑	
Phenytoin	0/↓	↓	0/⇧	↓	0/↑	0/↑
Propranolol	0	0/↓	0/↑	0/↓	0/↓	0
Resorcinol (excessive topical use)		↓	↓	↓	↓	↑
Salicylates (large doses)	0	↓	0/⇧	0	↓	0
Sulfonylureas		↓	0	0		
Thiazides		0			↑	

Adverse Reactions:

Adverse reactions other than those indicating hyperthyroidism due to therapeutic overdosage, either initially or during the maintenance period, are rare.

If symptoms of excessive dosage appear, discontinue medication for several days and reinstitute at a lower dosage. Symptoms of overdosage include:

Cardiac – Palpitations; tachycardia; cardiac arrhythmias; angina pectoris; cardiac arrest.

CNS – Tremors; headache; nervousness; insomnia. Pseudotumor cerebri occurred in two children after initiation of thyroxine for autoimmune thyroiditis.

GI – Diarrhea; vomiting. Gastric intolerance may occur rarely in patients highly sensitive to beef or pork products or corn.

Hypersensitivity – Allergic skin reactions (rare).

Miscellaneous – Weight loss; menstrual irregularities; sweating; heat intolerance; fever.

(Continued on following page)

Overdosage:

These agents rarely result in clinical toxicity.

Chronic excessive dosage may produce signs and symptoms of hyperthyroidism (eg, headache, irritability, nervousness, sweating, tachycardia, increased bowel motility, menstrual irregularities, palpitations, vomiting, psychosis, seizure, fever). Angina pectoris or CHF may be induced or aggravated. Shock may develop. Complications may include cardiac failure and arrhythmias, which could be fatal. Massive overdosage may result in symptoms resembling thyroid storm.

Reduce dosage or temporarily discontinue therapy. Reinstitute treatment at a lower dosage. In healthy individuals, normal hypothalamic-pituitary-thyroid axis function is restored in 6 to 8 weeks after thyroid suppression. Therapeutic regimens are not justified in asymptomatic patients.

Serum T_4 levels do not appear to correlate with the severity of toxicity. Some patients with high T_4 concentrations remain asymptomatic. In five children, T_4 levels were 12.2 to 22.9 mcg/dl (normal 4 to 12 mcg/dl) but the children were asymptomatic. T_4 ingestion also appears to be less toxic than T_3 ingestion, and symptoms may be delayed due to the metabolic conversion time from T_4 to T_3.

Acute massive overdosage: Treatment is aimed at reducing GI absorption of the drug and counteracting central and peripheral effects, mainly those of increased sympathetic activity. Refer to General Management of Acute Overdosage. Cardiac glycosides may be indicated if CHF develops. Control fever, hypoglycemia or fluid loss, if needed. Antiadrenergic agents, particularly propranolol (1 to 3 mg IV over 10 minutes or 80 to 160 mg orally per day), have been used to treat increased sympathetic activity. Consider treatment of unrecognized adrenal insufficiency. Acetaminophen may be useful for fever control.

Patient Information:

Replacement therapy is to be taken for life, except in cases of transient hypothyroidism, usually associated with thyroiditis, and in those patients receiving a trial of the drug.

Take as a single daily dose, preferably before breakfast.

Brand interchange: Do not change from one brand of this drug to another without consulting your pharmacist or physician. Products manufactured by different companies may not be equally effective.

Do not discontinue medication except on advice of a physician.

Notify physician if headache, nervousness, diarrhea, excessive sweating, heat intolerance, chest pain, increased pulse rate, palpitations (symptoms of hyperthyroidism) or any unusual event occurs.

Partial loss of hair may be experienced by children in the first few months of thyroid therapy, but this is usually a transient phenomenon that results in later recovery.

These agents should not be used as primary or adjunctive therapy in a weight control program.

If levothyroxine is taken on an empty stomach, absorption is increased.

Administration and Dosage:

Individualize dosage to approximate the deficit in the patient's thyroid secretion. Determine patient response by clinical judgment in conjunction with laboratory findings.

Generally, institute thyroid therapy at relatively low doses and slowly increase in small increments until the desired response is obtained. Administer thyroid as a single daily dose, preferably before breakfast.

Treatment of choice for hypothyroidism is T_4 under most circumstances because of its consistent potency, restoration of normal constant serum levels of T_4 and T_3 and its prolonged duration of action. However, it has a slow onset of action and its effects are cumulative over several weeks.

The rapid onset and dissipation of action of T_3, as compared with T_4, have led some clinicians to prefer its use in patients who might be more susceptible to the untoward effects of thyroid medication. However, the wide swings in serum T_3 levels following administration and the possibility of more pronounced cardiovascular side effects tend to offset the stated advantages. If there is a need for rapidly correcting the hypothyroid state, the administration of T_3 is preferable because of its rapid onset and dissipation of action.

T_3 may be used in preference to T_4 during radioisotope scanning procedures, since induction of hypothyroidism in those cases is more abrupt and can be of shorter duration. It may also be preferred when impaired peripheral conversion of T_4 and T_3 is suspected.

(Administration and Dosage continued on following page)

Administration and Dosage (Cont.):

Thyroid cancer: Exogenous thyroid hormone may produce regression of metastases from follicular and papillary carcinoma of the thyroid and is used as ancillary therapy of these conditions with radioactive iodine. Amounts larger than those used for replacement therapy are required. Medullary carcinoma of the thyroid is usually unresponsive.

Laboratory tests useful in the diagnosis and evaluation of thyroid function are listed in the following table, indicating the alterations noted in various thyroid disorders.

Laboratory Tests for Diagnosis and Evaluation of Thyroid Function

↑ = Increased ↓ = Decreased N = Normal	Normal	Pregnancy	Primary hypothyroid	Secondary hypothyroid	Hyperthyroid	T_3 thyrotoxicosis	Normal values
Free T_4 (unbound)	N	N	↓	↓	↑	N	
Total T_4	N	↑	↓	↓	↑	N	5-11 mcg/dl
Serum T_3	N	↑	↓	↓	↑	↑	85-185 ng/dl
T_3 resin uptake (RT_3U)	N	↓	↓	↓	↑		25%-35%
Free thyroxine index (FT_4I)	N	N	↓	↓	↑		1.3-4.2
TSH	N	N	↑	↓	N/↓[1]		0.4-4.8 mcU/ml

[1] When tested using the more sensitive immunometric assays.

Serum free T_4 and TSH values are usually sufficient to diagnose thyroid status; however, serum TSH is more sensitive. FT_4 appears to be a better indicator of thyroid status than total T_4 since total T_4 levels can vary drastically in the absence of thyroid dysfunction; total T_4 is therefore not reliable and is not an adequate first-line test. Total T_4 may be useful in some special comprehensive situations. All FT_4 immunoassays are 90% to 100% accurate in diagnosing patients with simple thyroid disease. FT_4I is a crude estimate for serum FT_4 and is calculated from the results of total T_4 and the thyroid hormone binding ratio (THBR, formerly T_3 or T_4 uptake). Newer methods for FT_4I have not been fully evaluated. Free T_3 assays have not been fully evaluated at this time but may be a more useful measurement than serum T_3. Serum T_3/FT_3 are adjunctive second-line tests that may be useful in confirming less common forms of hyperthyroidism and diagnosing T_3 thyrotoxicosis, but they should not be used for diagnosing hypothyroidism. In summary, serum TSH by a sensitive immunometric assay is the best general test, followed by FT_4.

Drug effects on thyroid laboratory tests must also be considered; see Drug Interactions.

Thyrotropin (TSH) may be utilized to determine subclinical hypothyroidism and to differentiate primary and secondary hypothyroidism. Refer to individual monograph.

Protirelin (thyrotropin releasing hormone) may be useful in the differentiation of primary, secondary and tertiary hypothyroidism. Refer to individual monograph.

Dosage equivalents of thyroid products: In changing from one thyroid product to another, the following dosage equivalents may be used. However, each patient may still require fine dosage adjustments because these equivalents are only estimates.

Dosage Equivalents of Thyroid Products

Preparation	Composition ratio T_4	Composition ratio T_3	Dosage equivalents
Crude hormone			
Thyroid USP	2 to 5	1	60 mg (1 grain)
Thyroglobulin	2.5	1	60 mg
Thyroid Strong	3.1	1	45 mg
Synthetic hormone			
Levothyroxine	1	0	0.05 to 0.06 mg[1]
Liothyronine	0	1	15 to 37.5 mcg
Liotrix	4	1	50 to 60 mcg T_4 and 12.5 to 15 mcg T_3

[1] Previously considered to be 0.1 mg.

(Products listed on following pages)

Complete prescribing information for these products begins on page 516.

Thyroid Hormones (Cont.)

THYROID DESICCATED

Thyroid USP is composed of desiccated animal thyroid glands. The active thyroid hormones (T_4 and T_3) are available in their natural state and ratio. These preparations are standardized by iodine content; some manufacturers also use biological methods of standardization.

Administration and Dosage:

Optimal dosage is determined by the patient's clinical response and laboratory findings.

Hypothyroidism: Initial dosage – Institute therapy using low doses, with increments that depend on cardiovascular status. Usual starting dose is 30 mg, with increments of 15 mg every 2 to 3 weeks. Use 15 mg/day in patients with long-standing mxyedema, particularly if cardiovascular impairment is suspected. Reduce dosage if angina occurs.

Maintenance dosage – 60 to 120 mg/day; failure to respond to 180 mg doses suggests lack of compliance or malabsorption.

Readjust dosage within the first 4 weeks of therapy after proper clinical and laboratory evaluations.

Thyroid cancer: Larger amounts of thyroid hormone than those used for replacement therapy are required.

Children: Follow the recommendations in the following table. In infants with congenital hypothyroidism, instutite therapy with full doses as soon as diagnosis has been made.

Recommended Pediatric Dosage for Congenital Hypothyroidism		
Age	Dose per day (mg)	Daily dose per kg (mg)
0 to 6 mos	15 to 30	4.8 to 6
6 to 12 mos	30 to 45	3.6 to 4.8
1 to 5 yrs	45 to 60	3 to 3.6
6 to 12 yrs	60 to 90	2.4 to 3
> 12 yrs	> 90	1.2 to 1.8

	Product	Dosage form		C.I.*
Rx	**Thyroid USP** (Various, eg, Lannett)	**Tablets:** 15 mg (¼ grain)	In 1000s.	15+
Rx	**Armour Thyroid** (Rhone-Poulenc Rorer)		Dextrose. In 100s and 1000s.	53
Rx	**Thyroid USP** (Various, eg, Major, Rugby, Schein)	**Tablets:** 30 mg (½ grain)	In 1000s.	7+
Rx	**Armour Thyroid** (Rhone-Poulenc Rorer)		Dextrose. In 100s, 1000s, 5000s and UD 100s.	28
Rx	**Thyroid USP** (Various, eg, Goldline, Major, Moore, Parmed, Rugby, Schein)	**Tablets:** 60 mg (1 grain)	In 100s, 1000s and 5000s.	4+
Rx	**Armour Thyroid** (Rhone-Poulenc Rorer)		Dextrose. In 100s, 1000s, 5000s and UD 100s.	16
Rx	**Armour Thyroid** (Rhone-Poulenc Rorer)	**Tablets:** 90 mg (1½ grain)	(TJ). In 100s.	16
Rx	**Thyroid USP** (Various, eg, Goldline, Major, Moore, Parmed, Rugby)	**Tablets:** 120 mg (2 grain)	In 100s, 1000s and 5000s.	3+
Rx	**Armour Thyroid** (Rhone-Poulenc Rorer)		Dextrose. (TF). In 100s, 1000s, 2500s and UD 100s.	14

* Cost Index based on cost per 60 mg (1 grain) thyroid.

(Continued on following page)

Complete prescribing information for these products begins on page 516.

Thyroid Hormones (Cont.)

THYROID DESICCATED (Cont.)				C.I.*
Rx	**Thyroid USP** (Various, eg, Major, Parmed, Rugby)	**Tablets:** 180 mg (3 grain)	In 1000s.	5+
Rx	**Armour Thyroid** (Rhone-Poulenc Rorer)		Dextrose. (TG). In 100s and 1000s.	15
Rx	**Armour Thyroid** (Rhone-Poulenc Rorer)	**Tablets:** 240 mg (4 grain)	Dextrose. (TH). In 100s.	17
Rx	**Thyroid USP** (Various, eg, Lannett)	**Tablets:** 300 mg (5 grain)	In 500s and 1000s.	1+
Rx	**Armour Thyroid** (Rhone-Poulenc Rorer)		Dextrose. (TI). In 100s.	17
Rx	**Thyroid Strong** (Jones Medical)	50% stronger than thyroid USP. Each grain is eqivalent to 1½ grains of thyroid USP.		
		Tablets: 30 mg (½ grain)	(JMI 686). In 100s and 1000s.	17
		60 mg (1 grain)	(JMI 674). In 100s and 1000s.	12
		120 mg (2 grain)	(JMI 675). In 100s and 1000s.	9
		Tablets, sugar coated:		
		30 mg (½ grain)	(JMI 626). In 100s.	24
		60 mg (1 grain)	(JMI 627). In 100s and 1000s.	13
		120 mg (2 grain)	(JMI 628). In 100s.	11
		180 mg (3 grain)	(JMI 629). In 100s.	9
Rx	**Thyrar** (Rhone-Poulenc Rorer)	Bovine thyroid.		
		Tablets: 30 mg (½ grain)	In 100s.	184
		60 mg (1 grain)	In 100s.	108
		120 mg (2 grain)	In 100s.	66
Rx	**S-P-T** (Fleming)	Pork thyroid suspended in soybean oil.		
		Capsules: 60 mg (1 grain)	Green. In 100s and 1000s.	17
		120 mg (2 grain)	Brown. In 100s and 1000s.	11
		180 mg (3 grain)	Red. In 100s and 1000s.	9
		300 mg (5 grain)	Black. In 100s and 1000s.	7

THYROGLOBULIN

Contains T_4 and T_3 in an approximate ratio of 2.5 to 1.

Administration and Dosage:

See Thyroid Desiccated Administration and Dosage.

Not recommended for suppression therapy.

				C.I.*
Rx	**Proloid** (Parke-Davis)	**Tablets:** 30 mg (½ grain)	Gray. In 100s.	32
		60 mg (1 grain)	Gray, scored. In 100s and 1000s.	17
		90 mg (1½ grain)	Gray. In 100s.	14
		120 mg (2 grain)	Gray, scored. In 100s.	15
		180 mg (3 grain)	Gray. In 100s.	13

* Cost Index based on cost per 60 mg (1 grain) thyroid.

Complete prescribing information for these products begins on page 516.

Thyroid Hormones (Cont.)

LEVOTHYROXINE SODIUM (T_4; L-thyroxine)

An active principle of the thyroid gland, prepared synthetically in pure crystalline form.

Dosage equivalence: 0.05 to 0.06 mg equals approximately 60 mg (1 grain) thyroid (previously considered to be 0.1 mg levothyroxine equals 60 mg thyroid).

Bioavailability: Bioequivalence problems have been documented in the past for levothyroxine products marketed by different manufacturers. However, studies using high pressure liquid chromatography (HPLC) methods have shown bioequivalence; also, studies in patients have shown no difference in clinical efficacy between brands based on thyroid function tests. Brand interchange is not recommended unless comparative bioavailability data which provide evidence of therapeutic equivalence are available.

Administration and Dosage:

Optimal dosage is determined by the patient's clinical response and laboratory findings.

Hypothyroidism: Initial dosage – Institute therapy using low doses, with increments that depend on cardiovascular status. Usual starting dose is 0.05 mg, with increments of 0.025 mg every 2 to 3 weeks. Use $\leq$ 0.025 mg/day in patients with long-standing hypothyroidism, particularly if cardiovascular impairment is suspected. Reduce dosage if angina occurs.

Maintenance dosage – Most patients require no more than 0.2 mg/day; failure to respond to 0.3 mg doses suggests lack of compliance or malabsorption. Readjust dosage within the first 4 weeks of therapy after proper evaluations.

IV or IM injection can be substituted for the oral dosage form when oral ingestion is precluded for long periods of time. The initial parenteral dosage should be approximately one-half of the previously established oral dosage.

Myxedema coma: Consider a medical emergency. Levothyroxine may be administered via a nasogastric tube but the IV route is preferred. A starting dose of 0.4 mg given rapidly is usually well tolerated, even in the elderly. Sudden administration of such large doses is not without cardiovascular risks; therefore, do not undertake IV therapy without weighing the alternative risks. Clinical judgment may dictate smaller IV doses.

The initial dose is followed by daily supplements of 0.1 to 0.2 mg IV. Normal T_4 levels are achieved in 24 hours followed in 3 days by threefold elevation of T_3. Maintain continued daily IV administration of lesser amounts until the patient is fully capable of accepting a daily oral dose.

A daily maintenace dose of 0.05 to 0.1 mg parenterally should suffice to maintain the euthyroid state, once established. Resume oral therapy as soon as the clinical situation has been stabilized and the patient is able to take oral medication.

TSH suppression in thyroid cancer, nodules and euthyroid goiters: Larger amounts of thyroid hormone than those used for replacement therapy are required. This therapy is also used in treating nontoxic solitary nodules and multi-nodular goiters, and to prevent thyroid enlargement in chronic (Hashimoto's) thyroiditis.

Thyroid suppression therapy: 2.6 mcg/kg/day for 7 to 10 days. These doses usually yield normal serum T_4 and T_3 levels and lack of response to TSH.

Children: Follow the recommendations in the following table: In infants with congenital hypothyroidism, institute therapy with full doses as soon as diagnosis has been made.

Levothyroxine tablets may be given to infants and children who cannot swallow intact tablets. Crush the proper dose tablet and suspend the freshly crushed tablet in a small amount of formula or water. The suspension can be given by spoon or dropper. Do NOT store the suspension for any period of time. The crushed tablet may also be sprinkled over a small amount of food such as cooked cereal or applesauce.

Recommended Pediatric Dosage for Congenital Hypothyroidism		
Age	Dose per day (mcg)	Daily dose per kg (mcg)
0 to 6 months	25 to 50	8 to 10
6 to 12 months	50 to 75	6 to 8
1 to 5 years	75 to 100	5 to 6
6 to 12 years	100 to 150	4 to 5
> 12 years	> 150	2 to 3

Alternative suggested doses include: 0 to 1 year, 8 to 10 mcg/kg/day; 1 to 5 years, 4 to 6 mcg/kg/day; > 5 years to adolescence, 3 to 4 mcg/kg/day.

Preparation of injectable solution: Reconstitute by adding 5 ml 0.9% Sodium Chloride Injection, USP or Bacteriostatic Sodium Chloride Injection, USP with Benzyl Alcohol only. Shake the vial to ensure complete mixing. Use immediately after reconstitution. Do not add to other IV fluids. Discard any unused portion.

(Products listed on following page)

Thyroid Hormones (Cont.)

LEVOTHYROXINE SODIUM (T_4; L-thyroxine) (Cont.)

	Product	Dosage	Description	C.I.*
Rx	**Levothroid** (R-P Rorer)	**Tablets:** 0.025 mg	(LK). Orange. In 100s.	76
Rx	**Levoxine** (Daniels)		Orange, oval. In 100s, 1000s and UD 100s.	32
Rx	**Synthroid** (Boots)		(Flint 25). Orange, scored. In 100s and 1000s.[1]	50
Rx	**Levothroid** (R-P Rorer)	**Tablets:** 0.05 mg	(LL). White. In 100s and UD 100s.	42
Rx	**Levoxine** (Daniels)		White, oval. In 100s, 1000s and UD 100s.	18
Rx	**Synthroid** (Boots)		(Flint 50). White, scored. In 100s, 1000s and UD 100s.[1]	38
Rx	**Levothroid** (R-P Rorer)	**Tablets:** 0.075 mg	(LT). Gray. In 100s.	30
Rx	**Levoxine** (Daniels)		Purple, oval. In 100s, 1000s and UD 100s.	12
Rx	**Synthroid** (Boots)		(Flint 75). Violet, scored. In 100s, 1000s and UD 100s.[1]	28
Rx	**Levoxine** (Daniels)	**Tablets:** 0.088 mg	Olive, oval. In 100s, 1000s and UD 100s.	12
Rx	**Synthroid** (Boots)		(Flint 88). Olive, scored. In 100s.[1]	38
Rx	**Levothyroxine Sodium** (Various, eg, Lederle, Major, Moore, PBI, Rugby, Schein, URL, Vangard)	**Tablets:** 0.1 mg	In 100s, 1000s and UD 100s.	15+
Rx	**Levothroid** (R-P Rorer)		(LM). Yellow. In 100s and UD 100s.	24
Rx	**Levoxine** (Daniels)		Yellow, oval. In 100s, 1000s and UD 100s.	10
Rx	**Synthroid** (Boots)		(Flint 100). Yellow, scored. In 100s, 1000s and UD 100s.[1]	22
Rx	**Levoxine** (Daniels)	**Tablets:** 0.112 mg	Rose, oval. In 100s, 1000s and UD 100s.	10
Rx	**Synthroid** (Boots)		(Flint 112). Rose, scored. In 100s, 1000s and UD 100s[1].	34
Rx	**Levothroid** (R-P Rorer)	**Tablets:** 0.125 mg	(LH). Purple. In 100s.	22
Rx	**Levoxine** (Daniels)		Brown, oval. In 100s, 1000s and UD 100s.	10
Rx	**Synthroid** (Boots)		(Flint 125). Brown, scored. In 100s, 1000s and UD 100s.[1]	20
Rx	**Levothyroxine Sodium** (Various, eg, Lederle, Major, PBI, Rugby, Schein, URL, Vangard)	**Tablets:** 0.15 mg	In 100s, 1000s and UD 100s.	NA
Rx	**Levothroid** (R-P Rorer)		(LN). Blue. In 100s and UD 100s.	20
Rx	**Levoxine** (Daniels)		Blue, oval. In 100s, 1000s and UD 100s.	8
Rx	**Synthroid** (Boots)		(Flint 150). Blue, scored. In 100s, 1000s and UD 100s.[1]	18
Rx	**Levothroid** (R-P Rorer)	**Tablets:** 0.175 mg	(1¾ LP). Turquoise. In 100s.	20
Rx	**Levoxine** (Daniels)		Turquoise, oval. In 100s, 1000s and UD 100s.	28
Rx	**Synthroid** (Boots)		(Flint 175). Lilac, scored. In 100s.[1]	NA

* Cost Index based on cost per 0.1 mg.

[1] With lactose and sugar.

(Products continued on following page)

Thyroid Hormones (Cont.)

LEVOTHYROXINE SODIUM (T_4; L-thyroxine) (Cont.)

	Product	Form	Description	C.I.*
Rx	**Levothyroxine Sodium** (Various, eg, Lederle, Major, Moore, Rugby, Schein, URL, Vangard)	**Tablets:** 0.2 mg	In 100s, 1000s and UD 100s.	1+
Rx	**Levothroid** (R-P Rorer)		(LR). Pink. In 100s and UD 100s.	18
Rx	**Levoxine** (Daniels)		Pink, oval. In 100s, 1000s and UD 100s.	8
Rx	**Synthroid** (Boots)		(Flint 200). Pink, scored. In 100s, 1000s and UD 100s.[1]	16
Rx	**Levothyroxine Sodium** (Various, eg, Lederle, Major, Moore, PBI, Rugby, Schein, URL)	**Tablets:** 0.3 mg	In 100s, 1000s and UD 100s.	4+
Rx	**Levothroid** (R-P Rorer)		(LS). Green. In 100s and UD 100s.	16
Rx	**Levoxine** (Daniels)		Green, oval. In 100s, 1000s and UD 100s.	6
Rx	**Synthroid** (Boots)		(Flint 300). Green, scored. In 100s, 1000s and UD 100s.[1]	14
Rx	**Levothyroxine** (Various, eg, Loch, Quad, Schein)	**Powder for injection, lyophilized:** 200 mcg per vial	In 6 ml vials & 10 ml vials.	1726+
Rx	**Levothroid** (R-P Rorer)		In 6 ml vials.[2]	3688
Rx	**Synthroid** (Boots)		In 10 ml vials.[3]	2086
Rx	**Levothyroxine** (Various, eg, Loch, McGuff, Quad, Schein)	**Powder for injection, lyophilized:** 500 mcg per vial	In vials.	700+
Rx	**Levothroid** (R-P Rorer)		In 6 ml vials.[2]	2110
Rx	**Synthroid** (Boots)		In 10 ml vials.[3]	918

* Cost Index based on cost per 0.1 mg.
[1] With lactose and sugar.
[2] With 15 mg mannitol per vial.
[3] With 10 mg mannitol per vial.

LIOTHYRONINE SODIUM (T_3)

A synthetic form of the natural thyroid hormone T_3, with pharmacologic activities of the natural substance. It has a short duration of activity which permits quick dosage adjustment and facilitates control of overdosage, should it occur. It can be used in patients allergic to desiccated thyroid or thyroid extract derived from pork or beef.

Dosage equivalents: 15 to 37.5 mcg equals ≈ 60 mg (1 grain) desiccated thyroid.

Administration and Dosage:

Administer cautiously to patients in whom there is a strong suspicion of thyroid gland autonomy; exogenous hormone effects will be additive to the endogenous source.

Mild hypothyroidism: Starting dose is 25 mcg/day. Daily dosage may then be increased by 12.5 or 25 mcg every 1 or 2 weeks. Usual maintenance dose is 25 to 75 mcg/day. Smaller doses may be fully effective in some patients, while dosages of 100 mcg/day may be required in others.

Congenital hypothyroidism: Starting dose is 5 mcg/day, with a 5 mcg increment every 3 to 4 days until the desired response is achieved. Infants a few months old may require only 20 mcg/day for maintenance. At 1 year of age, 50 mcg/day may be required. Above 3 years, full adult dosage may be necessary.

Simple (nontoxic) goiter: Starting dose is 5 mcg/day. Dosage may be increased every 1 to 2 weeks by 5 or 10 mcg. When 25 mcg/day is reached, dosage may be increased every 1 to 2 weeks by 12.5 or 25 mcg. Usual maintenance dosage is 75 mcg/day.

T_3 suppression test: 75 to 100 mcg daily for 7 days, then repeat I^{131} Thyroid Uptake test. A ≥ 50% suppression of uptake indicates a normal thyroid-pituitary axis and thus rules out thyroid gland autonomy.

(Administration and Dosage continued on following page)

Complete prescribing information for these products begins on page 516.

Thyroid Hormones (Cont.)

LIOTHYRONINE SODIUM (T_3) (Cont.)

Administration and Dosage (Cont.):

Myxedema: Starting dose is 5 mcg/day. This may be increased by 5 to 10 mcg/day every 1 to 2 weeks. When 25 mcg/day is reached, dosage may often be increased by 12.5 or 25 mcg every 1 or 2 weeks. Usual maintenance dose is 50 to 100 mcg/day.

Myxedema coma/precoma (injectable only), usually precipitated in the hypothyroid patient of long standing by intercurrent illness or drugs such as sedatives and anesthetics, is a medical emergency. Direct therapy at the correction of electrolyte disturbances, possible infection or other intercurrent illness in addition to IV liothyronine administration. Simultaneous glucocorticoids are required.

Liothyronine injection is for IV use only; do not give IM or SC. Proper administration of an adequate dose is important in determining clinical outcome. Base initial and subsequent doses on continuous monitoring of the patient's clinical status and response. Administer doses at least 4 hours, and no more than 12 hours, apart. Administration of at least 65 mcg/day in initial days of therapy is associated with lower mortality. There is limited clinical experience with doses > 100 mg/day.

An initial IV dose ranging from 25 to 50 mcg is recommended in the emergency treatment of myxedema complications in adults. In patients with known or suspected cardiovascular disease, an initial dose of 10 to 20 mcg is suggested. However, base doses on continuous monitoring of the condition and response to therapy. Exercise caution in adjusting the dose due to the potential of large changes to precipitate adverse cardiovascular events.

Switching to oral therapy – Resume oral therapy as soon as the clinical situation has been stabilized and the patient is able to take oral medication. When switching to tablets, discontinue the injectable, initiate oral therapy at a low dosage and increase gradually according to response. If levothyroxine is used as oral therapy, keep in mind that there is a delay of several days in the onset of activity; therefore discontinue IV therapy gradually.

Elderly or children: Start therapy with 5 mcg/day; increase only by 5 mcg increments at the recommended intervals.

Exchange therapy: When switching a patient to T_3 from thyroid, T_4 or thyroglobulin, discontinue the other medication, initiate T_3 at a low dosage and increase gradually according to the patient's response. When selecting a starting dosage, keep in mind that T_3 has a rapid onset of action, and that residual effects of the other thyroid preparation may persist for the first several weeks of therapy.

Storage: Injection – Store between 2° and 8°C (36° to 46°F).

	Product	Form	Description	C.I.*
Rx	**Cytomel** (SK-Beecham)	**Tablets:** 5 mcg	(SKF D14). White. In 100s.	96
Rx	**Liothyronine Sodium** (Various, eg, Geneva, Rugby)	**Tablets:** 25 mcg	In 100s.	8+
Rx	**Cytomel** (SK-Beecham)		(SKF D16). White, scored. In 100s.	24
Rx	**Cytomel** (SK-Beecham)	**Tablets:** 50 mcg	(SKF D17). White, scored. In 100s.	18
Rx	**Triostat** (SK-Beecham)	**Injection:** 10 mcg/ml	In 1 ml vials.[1]	NA

* Cost Index based on cost per 25 mcg.

[1] With 6.8% alcohol, 2.19 mg ammonia as ammonium hydroxide.

Complete prescribing information for these products begins on page 516.

Thyroid Hormones (Cont.)

LIOTRIX

A uniform mixture of synthetic T_4 and T_3 in a 4 to 1 ratio by weight.

Dosage equivalents: As shown in the product listings below, manufacturers differ on approximate equivalents to 1 grain thyroid. In patients previously rendered euthyroid with another thyroid product, each 60 mg liotrix tablet will usually replace 60 mg (1 grain) of desiccated thyroid, 0.05 to 0.06 mg T_4 or 12.5 to 15 mcg T_3.

Administration and Dosage:

Optimal dosage is determined by the patient's clinical response and laboratory findings.

Hypothyroidism: Initial dosage – Institute therapy using low doses, with increments that depend on cardiovascular status. Usual starting dose is 30 mg liotrix with increments of 15 mg every 2 to 3 weeks. Use 15 mg/day in patients with long-standing hypothyroidism, particularly if cardiovascular impairment is suspected. Reduce dosage if angina occurs.

Maintenance dosage – Most patients require 60 to 120 mg/day; failure to respond to 180 mg doses suggests lack of compliance or malabsorption.

Readjust dosage within the first 4 weeks of therapy after proper clinical and laboratory evaluations.

Thyroid cancer: Larger amounts of thyroid hormone than those used for replacement therapy are required.

Children: Follow the recommendations in the following table. In infants with congenital hypothyroidism, institute therapy with full doses as soon as diagnosis has been made.

Recommended Pediatric Dosage for Congenital Hypothyroidism		
	Tetraiodothyronine (T_4, levothyroxine) sodium	
Age	Dose per day	Daily dose per kg of body weight
0-6 mos	25-50 mcg	8-10 mcg
6-12 mos	50-75 mcg	6-8 mcg
1-5 yrs	75-100 mcg	5-6 mcg
6-12 yrs	100-150 mcg	4-5 mcg
over 12 yrs	over 150 mcg	2-3 mcg

	Product and Distributor	Tablet strength (grain)	Content (mcg) T_4	Content (mcg) T_3	Thyroid equivalent (mg)	How Supplied	C.I.*
Rx	**Euthroid** (Parke-Davis)	½	30	7.5	30	Tartrazine, mannitol. (P-D 0260). Orange. In 100s.	5
		1	60	15	60	Tartrazine, mannitol. (P-D 0261). Brown. In 100s.	3
		2	120	30	120	Mannitol. (P-D 0262). Violet. In 100s.	2
		3	180	45	180	Tartrazine, mannitol. (P-D 0263). Gray. In 100s.	1.5
Rx	**Thyrolar** (Rhone-Poulenc Rorer)	¼	12.5	3.1	15	Lactose. (YC). Violet/white. Layered. In 100s.	15
		½	25	6.25	30	Lactose. (YD). Peach/white. Layered. In 100s.	8.3
		1	50	12.5	60	Lactose. (YE). Pink/white. Layered. In 100s.	5.2
		2	100	25	120	Lactose. (YF). Green/white. Layered. In 100s.	3
		3	150	37.5	180	Lactose. (YH). Yellow/white. Layered. In 100s.	2.5

* Cost Index based on cost per 1 grain thyroid equivalent.

Iodine Products

Actions:

Pharmacology: An adequate intake of iodine is necessary for normal thyroid function and the synthesis of thyroid hormones.

Elemental iodine (from the diet or as medication) is reduced in the GI tract and enters the circulation in the form of iodide, which is actively transported and concentrated by the thyroid gland. Hormone synthesis requires the oxidation of iodide and iodination of tyrosyl residues in thyroglobulin to form iodotyrosine precursors. These precursors undergo a "coupling reaction" to yield the active thyroid hormones T_3 and T_4. High concentrations of iodide greatly influence iodine metabolism by the thyroid gland. Large doses of iodides can inhibit T_4 and T_3 synthesis and rapidly inhibit proteolysis of colloid and the release of T_4 and T_3 into the bloodstream.

The effects of iodides are evident within 24 hours; maximum effects are attained after 10 to 15 days of continuous therapy. If administered chronically, therapeutic effects may persist for up to 6 weeks after the crisis has abated.

Indications:

Used adjunctively with an antithyroid drug in hyperthyroid patients in preparation for thyroidectomy and to treat thyrotoxic crisis or neonatal thyrotoxicosis.

Thyroid blocking in a radiation emergency.

For use of potassium iodide as an expectorant and for other respiratory tract conditions, see the Iodine Products monograph in the Expectorant section.

Unlabeled uses: Potassium iodide (60 mg 3 times daily) has been used effectively in a limited number of patients for Sweet's syndrome (acute febrile neutrophilic dermatosis) in combination with a potent topical steroid, as an alternative to systemic corticosteroids.

Also effective for the treatment of lymphocutaneous sporotrichosis (a dimorphic fungus that typically infects the skin and lymphatic system).

Contraindications:

Hypersensitivity to iodides.

Warnings:

Pregnancy: Category D (potassium iodide). Iodides readily cross the placenta and may cause hypothyroidism and goiter in the fetus or newborn when used long-term or close to term; short-term use (eg, 10 days) may not carry this risk. Administer to pregnant women only if clearly needed.

Lactation: Iodide is excreted in breast milk; however, the significance to the infant is not known. According to the American Academy of Pediatrics, these agents are not contraindicated in breastfeeding.

Drug Interactions:

Lithium carbonate and iodide preparations may have synergistic hypothyroid activity; concomitant use may result in hypothyroidism.

Adverse Reactions:

Possible side effects of potassium iodide include: Skin rashes; swelling of the salivary glands; "iodism" (metallic taste, burning mouth and throat, sore teeth and gums, symptoms of a head cold and sometimes stomach upset and diarrhea); allergic reactions (ie, fever and joint pains, swelling of parts of the face and body and, at times, severe shortness of breath requiring immediate medical attention). Overactivity or underactivity of the thyroid gland or enlargement of the thyroid gland (goiter) may occur rarely.

Overdosage:

Acute poisoning: Symptoms – Iodine is corrosive, and toxic symptoms are mainly the result of local GI tract irritation. Gastroenteritis, abdominal pain and diarrhea (sometimes bloody) may be seen. Fatalities may occur from circulatory collapse due to shock, corrosive gastritis or asphyxiation from swelling of the glottis or larynx.

Treatment – Gastric lavage with a soluble starch solution (15 g cornstarch or flour in 500 ml water) is recommended for removing iodine from the stomach. A 1% oral solution of sodium thiosulfate is a specific antidote, as it will reduce iodine to iodide. Milk may help relieve gastric irritation. Correct fluid and electrolyte imbalance, and treat shock if necessary.

Chronic poisoning: Discontinue use of iodine or iodides. High sodium chloride intake will speed recovery. For iodism characterized by skin or mucous membrane reactions, give cortisone or equivalent corticosteroid 25 to 100 mg every 6 hours orally until symptoms abate.

(Continued on following page)

Iodine Products (Cont.)

Patient Information:

Strong iodine solution: Dilute with water or fruit juice to improve taste.

Discontinue use and notify physician if fever, skin rash, metallic taste, swelling of the throat, burning of the mouth and throat, sore gums and teeth, head cold symptoms, severe GI distress or enlargement of the thyroid gland (goiter) occurs.

Administration and Dosage:

Recommended dietary allowances (RDAs): The RDA for iodine is 150 mcg for adults.

To prepare hyperthyroid patients for thyroidectomy, administer 2 to 6 drops strong iodine solution 3 times daily for 10 days prior to surgery.

For thyroid blocking in a radiation emergency: Use only as directed by state or local public health authorities in the event of a radiation emergency. Take for 10 days unless directed otherwise by state or local public health authorities.

Adults and children (> 1 year) – One tablet (130 mg) daily (crush tablets for small children).

Infants (< 1 year) – ½ crushed tablet (65 mg) daily.

Rx	**Strong Iodine Solution (Lugol's Solution)** (Various, eg, Lannett)	**Solution:** 5% iodine and 10% potassium iodide	In 120 ml, pt and gal.
Rx	**Thyro-Block**[1] (Wallace)	**Tablets:** 130 mg potassium iodide	White, scored. In 14s.

[1] Available only to State and Federal agencies.

Antithyroid Agents

Actions:

Pharmacology: Propylthiouracil (PTU) and methimazole inhibit the synthesis of thyroid hormones and, thus, are effective in the treatment of hyperthyroidism. They do not inactivate existing thyroxine (T_4) and triiodothyronine (T_3) which are stored in the thyroid or which circulate in the blood, nor do they interfere with the effectiveness of exogenous thyroid hormones. PTU partially inhibits the peripheral conversion of T_4 to T_3.

Both drugs are concentrated in the thyroid gland. Pharmacokinetic data are summarized in the following table:

Various Pharmacokinetic Parameters of Antithyroid Agents						
Antithyroid agent	Bioavailability (%)	Protein binding (%)	Transplacental passage	Breast milk levels (M:P)[1]	Half-life (hrs)	Excreted in urine (%)
Propylthiouracil	80-95	75-80	Low	Low (0.1)	1-2	35
Methimazole	80-95	0	High	High (1)	6-13	< 10

[1] Approximate milk:plasma ratio.

Indications:

Hyperthyroidism: Long-term therapy may lead to disease remission. Also used to ameliorate hyperthyroidism in preparation for subtotal thyroidectomy or radioactive iodine therapy. PTU is also used when thyroidectomy is contraindicated or not advisable.

Unlabeled use: PTU (300 mg/day) may be useful in reducing the mortality due to alcoholic liver disease by reducing the hepatic hypermetabolic state induced by alcohol.

Contraindications:

Hypersensitivity to antithyroid drugs; nursing mothers (see Warnings).

Warnings:

Agranulocytosis is potentially the most serious side effect of therapy. Instruct patients to report any symptoms of agranulocytosis, such as hay fever, sore throat, skin eruptions, fever, headache or general malaise. In such cases, white blood cell and differential counts should be made to determine whether agranulocytosis has developed. Exercise particular care with patients receiving additional drugs known to cause agranulocytosis. Leukopenia, thrombocytopenia and aplastic anemia (pancytopenia) may also occur. Discontinue the drug in the presence of agranulocytosis, aplastic anemia, hepatitis, fever or exfoliative dermatitis. Monitor the patient's bone marrow function.

One report recommends routine monitoring of the WBC count for at least the first 3 months of therapy, thereby potentially detecting agranulocytosis prior to becoming evident by infection.

Carcinogenesis: Laboratory animals treated with PTU for > 1 year have demonstrated thyroid hyperplasia and carcinoma formation. Such animal findings are seen with continuous suppression of thyroid function by sufficient doses of a variety of antithyroid agents, as well as in dietary iodine deficiency, subtotal thyroidectomy, and implantation of autonomous thyrotropic hormone-secreting pituitary tumors. Pituitary adenomas have also been described.

Pregnancy: Category D. These agents, used judiciously, are effective drugs in hyperthyroidism complicated by pregnancy. Because they readily cross the placenta and can induce goiter and even cretinism in the developing fetus, it is important that a sufficient, but not excessive, dose be given. In many pregnant women, the thyroid dysfunction diminishes as the pregnancy proceeds, thus making a reduction of dose possible. In some instances, these products can be withdrawn 2 or 3 weeks before delivery. PTU can cause fetal harm when administered to a pregnant woman. Approximately 10% will develop neonatal goiter. However, if an antithyroid agent is needed, PTU is preferred because it is less likely than methimazole to cross the placenta and induce fetal/neonatal complications (eg, aplasia cutis).

Lactation: Postpartum patients receiving antithyroid preparations should not nurse their babies. However, if necessary, the preferred drug is PTU.

Children: In several case reports, PTU hepatotoxicity has occurred in pediatric patients. Discontinue the drug immediately if signs and symptoms of hepatic dysfunction develop.

(Continued on following page)

Precautions:

Hemorrhagic effects: Because PTU may cause hypoprothrombinemia and bleeding, monitor prothrombin time during therapy, especially before surgical procedures.

Monitoring: Monitor thyroid function tests periodically during therapy. Once clinical evidence of hyperthyroidism has resolved, the finding of an elevated serum TSH indicates that a lower maintenance dose of PTU should be used.

Drug Interactions:

Anticoagulants: The activity of oral anticoagulants may be potentiated by the anti-vitamin K activity attributed to PTU.

Adverse Reactions:

Adverse reactions probably occur in < 1% of patients.

Agranulocytosis is the most serious effect.

CNS: Paresthesias; neuritis; headache; vertigo; drowsiness; neuropathies; CNS stimulation; depression.

GI: Nausea and vomiting; epigastric distress; loss of taste; sialadenopathy.

Dermatologic: Skin rash; urticaria; pruritis; erythema nodosum; skin pigmentation; exfoliative dermatitis; lupus-like syndrome, including splenomegaly, hepatitis, periarteritis and hypoprothrombinemia and bleeding.

Hematologic: Inhibition of myelopoiesis (agranulocytosis, granulocytopenia and thrombocytopenia); aplastic anemia; hypoprothrombinemia; periarteritis. About 10% of patients with untreated hyperthyroidism have leukopenia (WBC count < 4000 per mm^3), often with relative granulocytopenia.

Hepatic: Jaundice (which may persist for several weeks after discontinuance); hepatitis.

Renal: Nephritis.

Other: Abnormal hair loss; arthralgia; myalgia; edema; lymphadenopathy; drug fever; interstitial pneumonitis insulin autoimmune syndrome (may result in hypoglycemic coma).

Overdosage:

Symptoms: Nausea; vomiting; epigastric distress; headache; fever; arthralgia; pruritus; edema; pancytopenia. Agranulocytosis is the most serious effect. Rarely, exfoliative dermatitis, hepatitis, neuropathies or CNS stimulation or depression may occur.

Treatment: Protect the patient's airway and support ventilation and perfusion. Meticulously monitor and maintain, within acceptable limits, the patient's vital signs, blood gases, serum electrolytes, etc. Monitor the patient's bone marrow function. Refer to General Management of Acute Overdosage.

Forced diuresis, peritoneal dialysis, hemodialysis or charcoal hemoperfusion have not been established as beneficial for an overdose of propylthiouracil.

Patient Information:

Take at regular intervals around the clock (usually every 8 hours), unless directed otherwise by physician.

Notify physician if fever, sore throat, unusual bleeding or bruising, headache, rash, yellowing of the skin or vomiting occurs.

Administration and Dosage:

In one study, the rate of remission and time to relapse of Grave's disease was significantly increased when antithyroid therapy was given for a prolonged duration (18 months) vs short-term (6 month) treatment. However, the monitoring of thyroid stimulating antibody values may be a useful guide for shortening the duration of treatment in some patients.

One small study reported that single and divided daily doses of methimazole were equally effective in hyperthyroid patients. Traditionally administered in divided doses, it was suggested that a single daily dose would be effective since methimazole is present in the thyroid for 20 hours and is active for 40 hours despite a serum half-life of 6 to 13 hours. Further study is needed.

(Continued on following page)

PROPYLTHIOURACIL (PTU)

Administration and Dosage:

Usually administered in 3 equal doses at approximately 8 hour intervals.

Adults: Initial – 300 mg/day. In patients with severe hyperthyroidism, very large goiters, or both, the initial dosage is usually 400 mg/day; an occasional patient will require 600 to 900 mg/day initially.

Maintenance – Usually, 100 to 150 mg daily.

Children: 6 to 10 years – Initial dose is 50 to 150 mg/day.

≥ 10 years – Initial dose is 150 to 300 mg/day.

Maintenance – Determined by patient response.

Another suggested dosage for children is as follows:

Initial: 5 to 7 mg/kg/day or 150 to 200 mg/m²/day in divided doses every 8 hours.

Maintenance: ⅓ to ⅔ the intial dose beginning when the patient is euthyroid.

				C.I.*
Rx	**Propylthiouracil** (Various, eg, Barr, Dixon-Shane, Geneva Marsam, Major, Rugby, Schein)	**Tablets:** 50 mg	In 100s and 1000s.	2.3+

METHIMAZOLE

Administration and Dosage:

Usually administered in 3 equal doses at approximately 8 hour intervals.

Adults: Initial – 15 mg daily for mild hyperthyroidism, 30 to 40 mg/day for moderately severe hyperthyroidism and 60 mg/day for severe hyperthyroidism.

Maintenance – 5 to 15 mg/day.

Children: Initial – 0.4 mg/kg daily.

Maintenance – Approximately one-half the initial dose.

Another suggested dosage for children is as follows:

Initial: 0.5 to 0.7 mg/kg/day or 15 to 20 mg/m²/day in 3 divided doses.

Maintenance: ⅓ to ⅔ of intial dose beginning when the patient is euthyroid.

Maximum: 30 mg/24 hours.

				C.I.*
Rx	**Tapazole** (Lilly)	**Tablets:** 5 mg	(Lilly J94). White, scored. In 100s.	25
		10 mg	(Lilly J95). White, scored. In 100s.	20

* Cost Index based on cost per 50 mg propylthiouracil or 5 mg methimazole.

SODIUM IODIDE I 131

Actions:

Pharmacokinetics: Sodium iodide I 131 is readily absorbed from the GI tract. Following absorption, the iodide is primarily distributed within the extracellular fluid of the body. It is trapped and rapidly converted to protein-bound iodine by the thyroid; it is concentrated, but not protein-bound, by the stomach and salivary glands. It is promptly excreted by the kidneys. About 90% of the local irradiation is caused by beta radiation and 10% by gamma radiation.

Iodine 131 decays by beta and gamma emissions with a physical half-life of 8.04 days. Following oral administration, about 40% of the activity has an effective half-life of 0.34 days and 60% has an effective half-life of 7.61 days. Consult product literature for specific calibration and dosimetry information.

Indications:

Treatment of hyperthyroidism and selected cases of thyroid carcinoma. Palliative effects may be seen in patients with papillary or follicular carcinoma of the thyroid. Thyrotropin may effect stimulation of radioiodide uptake. (Radioiodide will not be taken up by giant cell and spindle cell carcinoma of the thyroid or by amyloid solid carcinomas.)

Contraindications:

Preexisting vomiting and diarrhea; pregnancy (see Warnings).

Warnings:

Patients < 30 years old: Sodium iodide I 131 is not usually used for the treatment of hyperthyroidism in patients < 30 years old unless circumstances preclude other treatment.

Pregnancy: Category X. Sodium iodide I 131 can cause fetal harm when administered to a pregnant woman. Permanent damage to the fetal thyroid can occur. The drug is contraindicated in women who are or may become pregnant. If it is used during pregnancy, or if the patient becomes pregnant while taking this drug, inform her of the potential hazard to the fetus.

Lactation: Since iodine is excreted in breast milk, substitute with formula feedings.

(Continued on following page)

SODIUM IODIDE I 131 (Cont.)

Precautions:

Antithyroid therapy of a severely hyperthyroid patient is usually discontinued for 3 to 4 days before administration of radioiodide.

Drug Interactions:

Stable iodine (any form), thyroid, antithyroid agents: The uptake of iodine 131 will be affected by recent intake of these agents. Question the patient regarding previous medication and procedures involving radiographic contrast media.

Adverse Reactions:

The immediate adverse reactions following treatment of hyperthyroidism are usually mild, but following the larger doses used in thyroid carcinoma, may be much more severe.

Hematologic: Depression of the hematopoietic system (large doses); bone marrow depression; acute leukemia; anemia; blood dyscrasias; leukopenia; thrombocytopenia.

Other: Radiation sickness (some degree of nausea and vomiting); chest pain; tachycardia; itching skin; rash; hives; increase in clinical symptoms; acute thyroid crises; severe sialoadenitis; chromosomal abnormalities; death.

Tenderness and swelling of the neck, pain on swallowing, sore throat and cough may occur around the third day after treatment and are usually amenable to analgesics.

Temporary thinning of the hair may occur 2 to 3 months after treatment.

Allergic type reactions have been reported infrequently following the administration of iodine-containing radiopharmaceuticals.

Overdosage:

In the treatment of hyperthyroidism, overdosage may result in hypothyroidism, the onset of which may be delayed. Appropriate replacement therapy is recommended if hypothyroidism occurs.

Administration and Dosage:

Measure the dose by a radioactivity calibration system just prior to administration. Consult product literature for specific calibration and dosimetry information.

Hyperthyroidism: The total amount needed to achieve a clinical remission without destruction of the entire thyroid varies widely; the usual dose range is 4 to 10 millicuries (mCi). Toxic nodular goiter and other special situations will require larger doses.

Thyroid carcinoma: Individualize dosage. The usual dose for ablation of normal thyroid tissue is 50 mCi, with subsequent therapeutic doses usually 100 to 150 mCi.

Preparation of oral solution: To prepare stock solution, dilute oral solution with Purified Water, USP containing 0.2% sodium thiosulfate as a reducing agent. Acidic diluents may cause a pH drop below 7.5 and may stimulate volatilization of iodine 131-hydriodic acid.

Rx	**Iodotope** (Squibb Diagnostics)	**Capsules:** Radioactivity range is 8, 15, 30, 50 or 100 mCi per capsule at time of calibration	Blue/buff. In 5s, 10s,15s and 20s.
		Oral Solution:[1] Radioactivity concentration of 7.05 mCi per ml at time of calibration	In vials containing approximately 7, 14, 28, 70 or 106 mCi at time of calibration.
Rx	**Sodium Iodide I 131 Therapeutic** (Mallinckrodt)	**Capsules:** Radioactivity range is 0.75 to 100 mCi per capsule. **Oral Solution:** Radioactivity range is 3.5 to 150 mCi per vial.	

[1] With 1 mg EDTA per ml.

CALCITONIN

Actions:

Calcitonins are polypeptide hormones secreted by parafollicular cells of the thyroid in mammals. Calcitonin has a role in the regulation of calcium and bone metabolism, and has direct renal effects and actions on the GI tract. Calcitonin-salmon appears essentially identical to mammalian calcitonins, but its potency per mg and duration of action are greater. Calcitonin-human is a synthetic hormone consisting of 32 amino acids in the same linear sequence as found in naturally occurring human calcitonin.

Bone: Single injections of calcitonin transiently inhibit bone resorption. With prolonged use, there is a persistent, smaller decrease in the rate of bone resorption, associated with decreased resorptive activity and number of osteoclasts. Osteocytic resorption may also be decreased.

Endogenous calcitonin, with parathyroid hormone (PTH), regulates blood calcium. High blood calcium levels increase secretion of calcitonin which inhibits bone resorption. In normal adults, the administration of exogenous calcitonin results in only a slight decrease in serum calcium. In normal children and in patients with generalized Paget's disease, bone resorption is more rapid and decreases in serum calcium are more pronounced in response to calcitonin.

Paget's disease of bone (osteitis deformans) is characterized by abnormal and accelerated bone formation and resorption in one or more bones. Active Paget's disease involving a large bone mass may increase the urinary hydroxyproline excretion (reflecting breakdown of collagen-containing bone matrix) and serum alkaline phosphatase (reflecting increased bone formation).

Calcitonin, presumably by blocking bone resorption, improves the biochemical abnormalities ($>$ 30% reduction). It decreases the rate of bone turnover with a resultant fall in the serum alkaline phosphatase and urinary hydroxyproline excretion in approximately two-thirds of patients. These biochemical changes appear to correspond to more normal bone, as evidenced by: 1) Radiologic regression of Pagetic lesions; 2) improvement of impaired auditory nerves (infrequent) and other neurologic functions, including improvement in the basilar compression syndrome, spinal cord and spinal nerve lesions; 3) decreases in abnormally elevated cardiac output. Improvements occur rarely and spontaneously; they cannot be predicted.

Some patients with Paget's disease who have good biochemical or symptomatic responses initially, later relapse. Explanations remain incomplete.

Hypercalcemia: Calcitonin salmon lowers elevated serum calcium in patients with carcinoma, multiple myeloma or primary hyperparathyroidism (lesser response). Patients with higher serum calcium tend to show greater reduction. The decrease in calcium occurs about 2 hours after injection and lasts for 6 to 8 hours. Given every 12 hours, the drug lowered calcium for 5 to 8 days. Average reduction of 8 hour postinjection serum calcium was about 9%.

Kidney: Calcitonin increases the excretion of filtered phosphate, calcium and sodium by decreasing tubular reabsorption. In some patients, the inhibition of bone resorption is of such magnitude that the consequent reduction of filtered calcium load more than compensates for the decrease in tubular reabsorption of calcium. This decreases rather than increases urinary calcium. Transient increases in sodium and water excretion may occur after the initial injection, but these changes usually return to pretreatment levels with continued therapy.

GI: Short-term administration of calcitonin results in marked transient decreases in the volume and acidity of gastric juice and in the volume of trypsin and amylase content of pancreatic juice. Whether these effects continue during chronic therapy has not been investigated.

Metabolism: Animal studies suggest that calcitonin is rapidly converted to smaller inactive fragments, primarily in the kidneys, but also in the blood and peripheral tissues. A small amount of unchanged hormone and its inactive metabolites are excreted in the urine.

The metabolic clearance rate of exogenously administered immunoreactive calcitonin-human in normal subjects has been determined to be 8.4 $\pm$ 1.1 ml/kg/min. The half-life is 1.02 hours after single 0.5 mg SC doses.

(Continued on following page)

CALCITONIN (Cont.)

Indications:

For patients with moderate to severe Paget's disease characterized by polyostotic involvement with elevated serum alkaline phosphatase and urinary hydroxyproline excretion.

There is no evidence that the prophylactic use is beneficial in asymptomatic patients. Treatment may be considered in cases in which there is extensive involvement of the skull or spinal cord with the possibility of irreversible neurologic damage. Base treatment on the demonstrated effect of calcitonin on Pagetic bone.

Calcitonin-salmon: Postmenopausal osteoporosis in conjunction with an adequate calcium and vitamin D intake to prevent the progressive loss of bone mass.

Hypercalcemia – Early treatment of hypercalcemic emergencies, along with other appropriate agents, when a rapid decrease in serum calcium is required, until more specific treatment can be accomplished. It may also be added to existing therapeutic regimens for hypercalcemia.

Contraindications: Clinical allergy to synthetic calcitonin-salmon.

Warnings:

Antibody Formation: Circulating antibodies to **calcitonin-salmon** occur after 2 to 18 months of treatment in about half the treated Paget's disease patients, but calcitonin treatment remained effective in many of these cases. Occasionally, patients with high antibody titers are found. These patients usually will have suffered a biochemical relapse of Paget's disease and are unresponsive to the acute hypocalcemic effects of calcitonin.

The risk of diminishing efficacy due to antibody formation or hypersensitivity reactions is less with **calcitonin-human.** Calcitonin-human has been effective in patients who have developed resistance to nonhuman calcitonins.

Osteogenic sarcoma is known to increase in Paget's disease. Pagetic lesions, with or without therapy, may appear by x-ray to progress markedly, possibly with some loss of definition of periosteal margins. Evaluate such lesions carefully to differentiate them from osteogenic sarcoma.

Usage in Pregnancy: Category C. Calcitonin-salmon has decreased fetal birth weights in rabbits when given in doses 14 to 56 times the recommended human dose. Since calcitonin does not cross the placenta, this may be due to metabolic effects of calcitonin on the pregnant animal. There are no studies in pregnant women. Animal studies have not been conducted with calcitonin-human. Use these agents only if the potential benefits outweigh the unknown potential hazards to the fetus.

Usage in Lactation: Calcitonin-salmon inhibits lactation in animals; however, it is not known whether the drug is excreted in breast milk. Safety for use in the nursing mother has not been established.

Usage in Children: Disorders of bone in children (juvenile Paget's disease) have been reported rarely. No adequate data support usage in children.

Precautions:

Allergy: Because calcitonin is a protein, the possibility of a systemic allergic reaction exists. Make provisions for emergency treatment. Have epinephrine 1:1000 immediately available. Refer to Management of Acute Hypersensitivity Reactions on p. viii. Consider skin testing prior to treatment with calcitonin, particularly for patients with suspected sensitivity. (See Administration and Dosage).

Hypocalcemic tetany could occur with calcitonin, although no cases have been reported. Have parenteral calcium available during the first several doses.

Periodically examine urine sediment of patients on chronic therapy. Coarse granular casts and renal tubular epithelial cell casts were reported in young adult volunteers at bed rest who were given calcitonin-salmon to study the effect on immobilization osteoporosis. There was no other evidence of renal abnormality and the urine sediment became normal after calcitonin was stopped.

Adverse Reactions:

GI: Nausea with or without vomiting (salmon: 10%; human: 14% to 21%) is most evident when treatment is initiated and tends to decrease with continued administration. Anorexia, diarrhea, epigastric discomfort, abdominal pain and salty taste may occur.

Dermatologic: Inflammatory reactions at the injection site (salmon: 10%); flushing of face or hands (salmon: 2% to 5%; human: 16% to 21%); pruritus of ear lobes; edema of feet; skin rashes.

Other: Nocturia; feverish sensation; eye pain.

In addition, the following have been reported with calcitonin-human:

GU – Increased urinary frequency (5% to 10%) .

Metabolic – Mild tetanic symptoms (rare); asymptomatic mild hypercalcemia (rare).

Other – Chills, chest pressure, weakness, headache, tender palms and soles, dizziness, nasal congestion, shortness of breath, metallic taste, paresthesia.

(Continued on following page)

CALCITONIN (Cont.)

Overdosage:

A dose of 1000 IU SC may produce nausea and vomiting as the only adverse effects. Doses of 32 units/kg/day for 1 or 2 days demonstrate no other adverse effects. Data on chronic high dose administration are insufficient to judge toxicity.

CALCITONIN-SALMON

Administration and Dosage:

Skin testing: Prepare a dilution at 10 IU per ml by withdrawing 0.05 ml of the 200 IU/ml solution or 0.1 ml of the 100 IU/ml solution in a tuberculin syringe and filling it to 1 ml with sodium chloride injection. Mix well, discard 0.9 ml and inject intracutaneously 0.1 ml (approximately 1 IU), on the inner aspect of the forearm. Observe the injection site 15 minutes after injection. The appearance of more than mild erythema or wheal constitutes a positive response.

Paget's disease: Starting dose – 100 IU per day SC (preferred for outpatient self-administration) or IM. Monitor by periodic measurement of serum alkaline phosphatase and 24 hour urinary hydroxyproline and evaluation of symptoms. Normalization of biochemical abnormalities and decreased bone pain is usually seen, if it is going to occur, within the first few months. Improvement of neurologic lesions requires a longer period, often more than 1 year.

Doses of 50 IU per day or every other day are usually sufficient to maintain biochemical and clinical improvement. Data are insufficient to determine whether this dose will have the same effect as the higher dose on forming more normal bone structure. Maintain the higher dose in any patient with serious deformity or neurological involvement.

In any patient with a good response initially who later relapses (clinically or biochemically), investigate for antibody formation. The patient may be tested for antibodies by an appropriate specialized test or evaluated for the possibility of antibody formation by critical clinical evaluation. Also assess patient compliance in the event of relapse. In patients who relapse, whether because of antibodies or for unexplained reasons, a dosage increase beyond 100 IU/day does not elicit an improved response.

Postmenopausal osteoporosis: 100 IU/day SC or IM. Patients also receive supplemental calcium such as calcium carbonate 1.5 g daily and an adequate vitamin D intake (400 units daily). An adequate diet is also essential.

Hypercalcemia: Starting dose – 4 IU/kg every 12 hours, SC or IM. If response is not satisfactory after 1 or 2 days, increase to 8 IU/kg every 12 hours. If the response remains unsatisfactory after 2 more days, the dose may be further increased to a maximum of 8 IU/kg every 6 hours. If the volume to be injected exceeds 2 ml, IM injection is preferable and multiple sites of injection should be used.

Storage: Refrigerate between 2° to 6° C (36° to 43° F).

Rx	**Calcimar** (Rorer)	**Injection:** 200 IU per ml solution. In 2 ml vials.[1]
Rx	**Miacalcin** (Sandoz)	**Injection:** 200 IU per ml. In 2 ml vials.[2]
Rx	**Miacalcin** (Sandoz)	**Injection:** 100 IU per ml. In 1 ml amps.

CALCITONIN-HUMAN

Administration and Dosage:

Paget's disease: Starting dose is 0.5 mg/day, SC. Some patients may improve at 0.5 mg, 2 or 3 times weekly or 0.25 mg/day. Nausea and flushing may be minimized by administration at bedtime.

More severe cases (eg, mechanically weak bones with osteolytic lesions) may require doses up to 1 mg/day (0.5 mg twice/day). Continue treatment for 6 months. If symptoms have been relieved, discontinue therapy until symptoms or radiologic signs recur.

Determine serum alkaline phosphatase and urinary hydroxyproline excretion prior to therapy, during the first 3 months and every 3 to 6 months during chronic therapy.

Use reconstituted material within 6 hours.

Storage: Store below 25°C (77°F); protect from light.

Rx	**Cibacalcin** (Ciba)	**Injection:** 0.5 mg per vial. In double chambered vials.[3]

[1] With 0.5% phenol.
[2] With 2.25 mg acetic acid, 5 mg phenol, 2 mg sodium acetate trihydrate and 7.5 mg sodium Cl.
[3] With mannitol.

Actions:

Etidronate disodium (EHDP) and pamidronate disodium (APD) are biphosphonates that act primarily on bone. Their major pharmacologic action is the inhibition of normal and abnormal bone resorption. Secondarily, etidronate reduces bone formation since formation is coupled to resorption; pamidronate inhibits bone resorption apparently without inhibiting bone formation and mineralization.

The reduction of abnormal bone resorption is responsible for the therapeutic benefit in hypercalcemia. The antiresorptive action has been demonstrated under a variety of conditions. Although the exact mechanism(s) is not fully understood, it may be related to the drug's inhibition of hydroxyapatite crystal dissolution or its action on bone resorbing cells. Pamidronate inhibits the accelerated bone resorption that results from osteoclast hyperactivity induced by various tumors in animals. The number of osteoclasts in active bone turnover sites is substantially reduced after etidronate therapy. Etidronate can also inhibit the formation and growth of hydroxyapatite crystals and their amorphous precursors at concentrations in excess of those required to inhibit crystal dissolution.

Etidronate does not appear to alter renal tubular reabsorption of calcium, and does not affect hypercalcemia in patients with hyperparathyroidism where increased calcium reabsorption may be a factor in the hypercalcemia. Hyperphosphatemia has been observed in etidronate patients, usually with doses of 10 to 20 mg/kg/day; no adverse effects have been noted and its occurrence is not a contraindication. It is apparently due to drug-related increased phosphate tubular reabsorption by the kidneys. Serum phosphate levels generally return to normal 2 to 4 weeks post-therapy. Hyperphosphatemia occurs less frequently with IV medication of patients with hypercalcemia of malignancy.

Pamidronate therapy has resulted in decreased serum phosphate levels, presumably due to decreased release of phosphate from bone and increased renal excretion as parathyroid hormone levels (which are usually suppressed in hypercalcemia associated with malignancy) return towards normal. Phosphate therapy was administered in 30% of patients; phosphate levels usually returned towards normal within 7 to 10 days. Urinary calcium/creatinine and urinary hydroxyproline/creatinine ratios decrease and usually return to within or below normal after treatment. These changes occur within the first week, as do decreases in serum calcium levels.

Pharmacokinetics: Etidronate is not metabolized. Absorption averages about 1% of an oral dose of 5 mg/kg/day. This increases to about 2.5% at 10 mg/kg/day and 6% at 20 mg/kg/day. Absorption is complete within 2 hours and may be reduced by foods or other preparations containing divalent cations. Most of the absorbed drug is cleared from the blood within 6 hours. Within 24 hours, about half of the absorbed dose is excreted in the urine. The remainder is chemically adsorbed to bone, especially to areas of elevated osteogenesis, and is slowly eliminated. Unabsorbed drug is excreted intact in the feces.

A large fraction of the infused dose is excreted rapidly and unchanged in the urine. The mean residence time in the exchangeable pool is approximately 8.7 $\pm$ 1 hours. The mean volume of distribution at steady state in healthy subjects is 1370 $\pm$ 203 ml/kg while the plasma half-life is 6 $\pm$ 0.7 hours. In these same subjects, nonrenal clearance from the exchangeable pool amounts to 30% to 50% of the infused dose. This nonrenal clearance is due to uptake by bone; subsequently, the drug is slowly eliminated through bone turnover. The half-life on bone is $>$ 90 days.

Pamidronate – In cancer patients who had minimal or no bony involvement who were given an IV infusion of 60 mg over 4 or 24 hours, a mean of 51% (32% to 80%) was excreted unchanged in the urine within 72 hours. Body retention during this period was calculated to be a mean of 49% (range, 20% to 68%) of the dose, or 29.3 mg (12 to 41 mg). The urinary excretion rate profile after administration of 60 mg over 4 hours exhibited biphasic disposition characteristics with an alpha half-life of 1.6 hours and a beta half-life of 27.2 hours. The rate of elimination from bone has not been determined.

After IV administration in rats, $\approx$ 50% to 60% was rapidly adsorbed by bone and slowly eliminated from the body by the kidneys. In rats given 10 mg/kg bolus injections, $\approx$ 30% of the compound was found in the liver shortly after administration and was then redistributed to bone or eliminated by the kidneys over 24 to 48 hours. The drug was rapidly cleared from the circulation and taken up mainly by bones, liver, spleen, teeth and tracheal cartilage. Bone uptake occurred preferentially in areas of high bone turnover. The terminal phase of elimination half-life in bone was estimated to be $\approx$ 300 days.

Clinical trials: Paget's disease – Etidronate slows accelerated bone turnover (resorption and accretion) in pagetic lesions and, to a lesser extent, in normal bone. Reduced bone turnover is often accompanied by symptomatic improvement, including reduced bone pain. The incidence of pagetic fractures may be reduced, and elevated cardiac output and other vascular disorders may be improved. In many patients, the disease process will be suppressed for at least 1 year following cessation of therapy. Etidronate treatment in patients with asymptomatic Paget's disease may be warranted if extensive involvement threatens irreversible neurologic damage, major joints or major weight-bearing bones.

(Actions continued on following page)

Actions (Cont.):

Clinical trials (Cont.):

Hypercalcemia of malignancy is usually related to increased bone resorption due to osteoclastic hyperactivity associated with the presence of neoplastic tissue. It occurs in 8% to 20% of patients with malignant disease. Whereas hypercalcemia is more often seen in patients with demonstrable osteolytic, osteoblastic or mixed metastatic tumors in bone, discrete skeletal lesions cannot be demonstrated in at least 30% of patients.

As hypercalcemia of malignancy evolves, the renal tubules develop a diminished capacity to concentrate urine. The resultant polyuria and nocturia decrease the extracellular fluid volume. Thus, the ability of the kidney to eliminate excess calcium is compromised. Renal impairment can eventually cause nitrogen retention, acidosis, renal failure and a further decrease in excretion of calcium. Infusion of biphosphonates, by inhibiting excessive bone resorption, interrupts this process. Adequate fluid administration to correct volume deficits is also essential. Salt loading and use of "high ceiling" or "loop" diuretics may be used to promote calcium excretion, because the rate of renal calcium excretion is directly related to the rate of sodium excretion.

Etidronate – Patients with elevated calcium levels (10.1 to 17.4 mg/dl) were treated simultaneously with daily IV administration over a 3 day period and up to 3000 ml saline and a loop diuretic. In terms of total serum calcium changes, 88% of patients had reductions of serum calcium of ≥ 1 mg/dl. Total serum calcium returned to normal in 63% of patients within 7 days compared to 33% of patients treated with hydration alone. Reductions in urinary calcium excretion, which accompany reductions in excessive bone resorption, became apparent after 24 hours. This was accompanied or followed by maximum decreases in serum calcium which were observed, most frequently, 72 hours after the first infusion.

When the total serum calcium values were adjusted for serum albumin levels, there was a return of normocalcemia in 24% of etidronate-treated patients and in 7% of patients treated with saline infusion alone. Of patients receiving etidronate, 87% vs 67% of patients on saline had albumin-adjusted serum calcium levels that returned to normal or were reduced by at least 1 mg/dl. Reductions in urinary calcium excretion, which accompany reductions in excessive bone resorption, became apparent after 24 hours. Decreases in serum calcium became maximal on the third day in most patients.

A second 3 day course of IV etidronate was tried in 14 patients who had a recurrence of hypercalcemia following an initial response to a 3 day infusion. All patients showed a decrease in total serum calcium of at least 1 mg/dl. Normalization of total serum calcium occurred in 11 patients.

Continuation of etidronate therapy with oral tablets may maintain clinically acceptable serum calcium levels and prolong normocalcemia.

Pamidronate – Patients who had hypercalcemia of malignancy received either 30, 60 or 90 mg as a single 24 hour IV infusion if their corrected serum calcium levels were ≥ 12 mg/dl after 48 hours of saline hydration. The majority of patients (64%) had decreases in albumin-corrected serum calcium levels by 24 hours after initiation of treatment. Mean-corrected serum calcium levels at days 2 to 7 after treatment initiation were significantly reduced from baseline in all three dosage groups. As a result, by 7 days after initiation of treatment, 40%, 61% and 100% of the patients receiving 30, 60 and 90 mg, respectively, had normal corrected serum calcium levels. Many patients (33% to 53%) in the 60 and 90 mg dosage groups continued to have normal-corrected serum calcium levels, or a partial response (≥ 15% decrease of corrected serum calcium from baseline), at day 14.

Etidronate vs pamidronate – Cancer patients who had corrected serum calcium levels of ≥ 12 mg/dl after at least 24 hours of saline hydration were randomized to receive either 60 mg pamidronate (n = 30) as a single 24 hour IV infusion or 7.5 mg/kg etidronate (n = 35) as a 2 hour IV infusion daily for 3 days. By day 7, 70% of the patients in the pamidronate group and 41% in the etidronate group had normal corrected serum calcium levels. When partial responders (≥ 15% decrease of serum calcium from baseline) were also included, the response rates were 97% for pamidronate and 65% for etidronate. Mean corrected serum calcium for the pamidronate and etidronate groups decreased from baseline values (14.6 and 13.8 mg/dl, respectively) to 10.4 and 11.2 mg/dl, respectively, on day 7. At day 14, 43% on pamidronate and 18% on etidronate still had normal corrected serum calcium levels, or maintenance of a partial response. For responders in pamidronate and etidronate groups, the median duration of response was similar (7 and 5 days, respectively). Pamidronate patients had similar response rates in the presence or absence of bone metastases.

Twenty-five patients who had recurrent or refractory hypercalcemia of malignancy were given a second course of 60 mg pamidronate. Of these, 40% showed a complete response and 20% showed a partial response to the retreatment, and these responders had about a 3 mg/dl decrease in mean corrected serum calcium levels 7 days after treatment.

(Actions continued on following page)

Actions (Cont.):

Clinical trials (Cont.)

Heterotopic ossification: Etidronate is effective in heterotopic ossification following total hip replacement or due to spinal cord injury. There is no evidence that etidronate affects mature heterotopic bone. Etidronate reduces the incidence of clinically important heterotopic bone by about two-thirds and retards the progression of immature lesions and reduces the severity by at least half. Follow-up data (at least 9 months) suggest these benefits persist.

Total hip replacement: Etidronate does not promote loosening of the prosthesis or impede trochanteric reattachment.

Spinal cord injury: Etidronate does not inhibit fracture healing or spinal stabilization.

Indications:

Etidronate: Symptomatic Paget's disease of bone (oral) – Etidronate arrests or impedes the disease process.

Prevention and treatment of heterotopic ossification (oral) following total hip replacement or due to spinal injury.

Hypercalcemia of malignancy inadequately managed by dietary modification or oral hydration (parenteral): Initiate rehydration with saline together with "high ceiling" or "loop" diuretics if indicated to restore urine output. This also increases the renal excretion of calcium and initiates a reduction in serum calcium. Concurrent therapy with etidronate is recommended as soon as there is a restoration of urine output.

Hypercalcemia of malignancy which persists after adequate hydration has been restored (parenteral): Patients with and without metastases and with a variety of tumors have been responsive to treatment. Maintain adequate hydration, but avoid overhydration in aged patients and in those with cardiac failure.

Pamidronate: Hypercalcemia of malignancy – In conjunction with adequate hydration for the treatment of moderate or severe hypercalcemia associated with malignancy, with or without bone metastases. Patients who have either epidermoid or non-epidermoid tumors respond to treatment. Initiate vigorous saline hydration (an integral part of hypercalcemia therapy) promptly and attempt to restore the urine output to about 2 L/day throughout treatment. Mild or asymptomatic hypercalcemia may be treated with conservative measures (ie, saline hydration, with or without loop diuretics). Hydrate patients adequately throughout the treatment, but avoid overhydation, especially in those patients who have cardiac failure. Do not use diuretic therapy prior to correction of hypovolemia.

Unlabeled uses: Etidronate has been used to treat postmenopausal osteoporosis (intermittent cyclical therapy of 400 mg/day usually followed by calcium). Spinal bone mass is increased and the incidence of new vertebral fractures is reduced. An NDA has been filed for this indication; however, approval has not been recommended since a follow-up study showed a 50% increase in new vertebral fractures during the third year of treatment. Further study is needed.

Pamidronate may be useful in the treatment of Paget's disease of bone (60 mg as a 24 hour infusion, followed by 20 mg/day for 10 days). Other potential uses for pamidronate include: Postmenopausal osteoporosis; bone metastases from breast cancer to prevent further development of tumor-related hypercalcemia and reduce the incidence of pathological fractures and severe bone pain; hyperparathyroidism; to prevent glucocorticoid-induced osteoporosis; to reduce bone pain in patients with prostatic carcinoma and multiple myeloma osteolytic lesions; immobilization-related hypercalcemia.

Contraindications:

Hypersensitivity to biphosphonates.

Etidronate: Patients with Class Dc and higher renal functional impairment (serum creatinine > 5 mg/dl).

Warnings:

Paget's disease (etidronate): Response to therapy may be slow and may continue for months after treatment has been discontinued. Do not increase dosage prematurely or resume treatment before there is evidence of reactivation of the disease process. Do not initiate retreatment until the patient has had at least a 90 day drug-free interval.

Renal effects: Occasional mild to moderate abnormalities in renal function (elevated BUN or serum creatinine) have been observed when etidronate was given as directed to patients with hypercalcemia of malignancy. These changes were reversible or remained stable, without worsening, after completion of therapy. In some patients with pre-existing renal impairment or in those who had received potentially nephrotoxic drugs, further depression of renal function was sometimes seen. Monitor renal function.

Normal renal function is adequate to handle not only the increased fluid load but also the excretion of etidronate itself. In patients with underlying renal disease, use only after a careful assessment of renal status or potential risks and potential benefits.

(Warnings continued on following page)

Warnings (Cont.):

Renal effects (Cont.):

Reduction of the etidronate dose, if used at all, may be advisable in Class Cc (Classification of Renal Functional Impairment, American Heart Association. *Ann Intern Med* 1971;75:251-52) renal functional impairment (serum creatinine 2.5 to 4.9 mg/dl). Use only if the potential benefit of hypercalcemia correction will substantially exceed the potential for worsening of renal function. In patients with Class Dc and higher renal functional impairment (serum creatinine > 5 mg/dl), withhold etidronate.

In animals, nephropathy has been associated with IV bolus pamidronate. A 3 month study in rats found cortical tubular changes including epithelial degeneration with IV doses ≥ 5 mg/kg given once every 2 weeks. Following a recovery period (1 month), the degenerative changes were completely reversed. Focal fibrosis of renal tubules was partially reversed. In two studies in dogs, pamidronate was given as a bolus IV injection either daily for 1 month or once a week for 3 months. In the 1 month study, tubulointerstitial nephritis, tubular degeneration and dilation occurred at 2 mg/kg. At recovery (1 month), the severity of these lesions was minimal or trace. Similar lesions (slight to marked severity) were noted in the 3 month study at ≥ 3 mg/kg. However, no improvement of the lesions was observed following the 1 month recovery period.

Patients with hypercalcemia who receive an IV infusion of pamidronate should have periodic evaluations of standard laboratory and clinical parameters of renal function.

Pamidronate has not been tested in patients who have Class Dc renal impairment (creatinine > 5 mg/dl). Use clinical judgment to determine whether the potential benefit outweighs the potential risk in such patients.

Carcinogenesis, impairment of fertility: In a 104 week carcinogenicity study (daily oral pamidronate administration) in rats, there was a positive dose response relationship for benign adrenal pheochromocytoma in males.

In rats, decreased fertility occurred in first-generation offspring of parents who had received 150 mg/kg oral pamidronate; however, this occurred only when animals were mated with members of the same dose group.

Pregnancy: Category B (oral etidronate). Editronate has caused skeletal abnormalities in rats when given at oral dose levels of 300 mg/ml (15 to 60 times the human dose). Other effects on the offspring (including decreased live births) are at dosages that cause significant toxicity in the parent generation and are 25 to 200 times the human dose. The skeletal effects are thought to be the result of the pharmacological effects of the drug on bone. There are no adequate and well controlled studies in pregnant women. Use only when clearly needed and when potential benefits outweigh potential hazards to the fetus.

Category C (parenteral). Pamidronate increases the length of gestation and parturition in rats resulting in an increase in pup mortality when given orally at daily doses of 60 and 150 mg/kg/day from before pregnancy until after parturition. When corrected for oral bioavailability, each daily dose is approximately 0.7 to 1.7 times the highest recommended human dose for a single IV infusion. It is not known if IV pamidronate can cause fetal harm when administered to pregnant women or if it can affect reproduction capacity. There are no adequate and well controlled studies in pregnant women. Use during pregnancy only if the potential benefit justifies the potential risk to the fetus.

Lactation: It is not known whether these drugs are excreted in breast milk. Exercise caution when administering to a nursing mother.

Children: Safety and efficacy for use in children have not been established.

Children have been treated with etidronate at doses recommended for adults, to prevent heterotopic ossifications or soft tissue calcifications. A rachitic syndrome has been reported infrequently at doses of ≥ 10 mg/kg/day and for prolonged periods approaching or exceeding a year. The epiphyseal radiologic changes associated with retarded mineralization of new osteoid and cartilage, and occasional symptoms reported, have been reversible when medication is discontinued.

Precautions:

Nutrition: Patients should maintain adequate nutrition, particularly an adequate intake of calcium and vitamin D.

Enterocolitis: Etidronate therapy has been withheld from patients with enterocolitis because diarrhea is seen in some patients, particularly at higher doses.

Osteoid: Etidronate suppresses bone turnover and may retard mineralization of osteoid laid down during the bone accretion process. These effects are dose- and time-dependent. Osteoid, which may accumulate noticeably at doses of 10 to 20 mg/kg/day, mineralizes normally post-therapy. In patients with fractures, especially of long bones, it may be advisable to delay or interrupt treatment until callus is evident.

(Precautions continued on following page)

Precautions (Cont.):

Fracture: In Paget's patients, treatment regimens of etidronate exceeding the recommended daily maximum dose of 20 mg/kg or continuous administration for periods > 6 months may be associated with an increased risk of fracture.

Long bones predominantly affected by lytic lesions, particularly in those patients unresponsive to therapy may be especially prone to fracture. Radiographically and biochemically monitor patients with predominantly lytic lesions to permit termination of etidronate in those patients unresponsive to treatment.

Hypocalcemia: In animal studies, administration of etidronate in amounts or at rates in excess of those recommended produced transient hypocalcemia or induced proximal renal tubular damage.

In one trial, 33 of 185 patients (18%) treated one or more times had serum calcium values below the lower limits of normal. When adjusted for levels of reduced serum albumin, < 1% of the 185 patients are estimated to have hypocalcemic ionized serum calcium levels. No adverse effects have been traced to this hypocalcemia.

The hypercalcemia of hyperparathyroidism is refractory to etidronate. It is possible for this disease to coexist in patients with malignancy.

Hypocalcemia (6% to 12%) has occurred with pamidronate therapy. One case of hypocalcemia with symptomatic tetany occurred during oral pamidronate treatment. If hypocalcemia occurs, consider short-term calcium therapy.

Monitoring: Carefully monitor standard hypercalcemia-related metabolic parameters, such as serum levels of calcium, phosphate, magnesium and potassium following initiation of pamidronate therapy. Cases of asymptomatic hypophosphatemia (16%), hypokalemia (9%), hypomagnesemia (12%) and hypocalcemia (6% to 12%) have occurred.

Closely monitor serum calcium, electrolytes, phosphate, magnesium and creatinine as well as CBC, differential and hematocrit/hemoglobin in patients treated with pamidronate. Carefully monitor patients who have pre-existing anemia, leukopenia or thrombocytopenia in the first 2 weeks following treatment.

Adverse Reactions:

Etidronate: The incidence of GI complaints (diarrhea, nausea) is the same at 5 mg/kg/day as for placebo (about 6.7%). At 10 to 20 mg/kg/day, this may increase to 20% or 30%. These complaints are often alleviated by dividing the total daily dose.

Hypersensitivity reactions including angioedema, urticaria, rash and pruritus have been reported rarely.

Paget's disease – Increased or recurrent bone pain at pagetic sites, or the onset of pain at previously asymptomatic sites has occurred. At 5 mg/kg/day, about 10% (vs 6.7% with placebo) report these phenomena. At higher doses, the incidence rises to about 20%. When the therapy continues, pain resolves in some patients but persists in others. Focal osteomalacia has occurred.

Hypercalcemia of malignancy is frequently associated with abnormal elevations of serum creatinine and BUN which improve in some patients or remain unchanged in most. However, in ≈ 10% of patients, occasional mild to moderate abnormalities in renal function (increases of > 0.5 mg/dl serum creatinine) were observed during or immediately after treatment. The possibility that etidronate contributed to these changes cannot be excluded.

A metallic, altered or loss of taste, which usually disappeared within hours, occurred during or shortly after etidronate in 5% of patients.

Pamidronate: Transient mild elevation of temperature by at least 1°C was noted 24 to 48 hours after administration in 27% of patients.

Drug-related local soft tissue symptoms (redness, swelling or induration and pain on palpation) at the site of catheter insertion were most common (18%) in patients treated with 90 mg. When all on-therapy events are considered, that rate rises to 41%. Symptomatic treatment resulted in rapid resolution in all patients.

Uveitis occurred in one patient who had hypercalcemia of malignancy; another patient who had Paget's disease of bone developed mild iritis that was responsive to indomethacin and topical steroid.

Four of 82 patients (4.9%) had seizures; two had pre-existing seizure disorders. None of the seizures were considered to be drug-related. However, a possible relationship between the drug and the occurrence of seizures cannot be ruled out.

At least 15% of patients treated with pamidronate for hypercalcemia of malignancy also experienced the following adverse events during a clinical trial:

General: Fluid overload; generalized pain.
Cardiovascular: Hypertension.
GI: Abdominal pain; anorexia; constipation; nausea; vomiting.
GU: Urinary tract infection.
Musculoskeletal: Bone pain.
Lab test abnormalities: Anemia; hypokalemia; hypomagnesemia; hypophosphatemia.

(Adverse Reactions continued on following page)

Adverse Reactions (Cont.):

Biphosphonate Adverse Reactions: Etidronate vs Pamidronate (%)

Adverse reaction	Pamidronate (n = 67)		Etidronate (n = 35)
	60 mg	90 mg	7.5 mg/kg x 3 days
General			
Fever	20	18	9
Infusion site reaction	6	18	0
Fatigue	0	12	0
Moniliasis	0	6	0
Fluid overload	0	0	6
GI			
Nausea	0	18	6
Anorexia	2	12	0
Constipation	0	6	3
GI hemorrhage	0	6	0
Abdominal pain	2	0	0
Ulcerative stomatitis	0	0	3
Respiratory			
Rales	0	6	0
Rhinitis	0	6	0
Upper respiratory infection	2	0	0
Dyspnea	0	0	3

Adverse reaction	Pamidronate (n = 67)		Etidronate (n = 35)
	60 mg	90 mg	7.5 mg/kg x 3 days
CNS			
Somnolence	2	6	0
Insomnia	2	0	0
Abnormal vision	2	0	0
Convulsions	0	0	3
Taste perversion	0	0	3
Cardiovascular			
Atrial fibrillation	0	6	0
Hypertension	0	6	0
Syncope	0	6	0
Tachycardia	0	6	0
Other			
Hypothyroidism	0	6	0
Anemia	0	6	0
Lab abnormalities			
Hypophosphatemia	14	18	3
Hypokalemia	4	18	0
Hypomagnesemia	8	12	3
Hypocalcemia	2	12	0
Abnormal hepatic function	0	0	3

Overdosage:

Oral etidronate: Symptoms – Clinical experience with etidronate overdosage is extremely limited. Decreases in serum calcium following substantial overdosage may be expected in some patients. Signs and symptoms of hypocalcemia may also occur. In one event, an 18-year-old female who ingested an estimated single dose of 4,000 to 6,000 mg (67 to 100 mg/kg) was mildly hypocalcemic (7.52 mg/dl) and experienced paresthesia of the fingers. Some patients may develop vomiting and expel the drug.

Treatment – Gastric lavage may remove unabsorbed drug. Standard procedures for treating hypocalcemia, including the administration of calcium IV, would be expected to restore physiologic amounts of ionized calcium and relieve signs and symptoms of hypocalcemia. Such treatment has been effective.

Parenteral: Rapid IV administration of etidronate at doses > 27 mg/kg has produced ECG changes and bleeding problems in animals. These abnormalities are probably related to marked or rapid decreases in ionized calcium levels in blood and tissue fluids. They are thought to be due to chelation of calcium by massive amounts of the diphosphonate. These abnormalities have been reversible in animal studies by use of ionizable calcium salts. Similar problems are not expected to occur in humans treated with etidronate as recommended. Moreover, signs and symptoms of hypocalcemia such as paresthesias and carpopedal spasms have not been reported with either agent. The chelation effects of the diphosphonate, should they occur, should be reversible with IV calcium gluconate.

Administration of IV etidronate at doses and possibly at rates in excess of those recommended has been associated with renal insufficiency.

One obese woman (95 kg) who was treated with pamidronate 285 mg/day for 3 days experienced high fever (39.5°C), hypotension and transient taste perversion, noted about 6 hours after the first infusion. Fever and hypotension were rapidly corrected with steroids.

(Products listed on following pages)

ETIDRONATE DISODIUM (ORAL)

Patient Information:

Take on an empty stomach 2 hours before meals.

May cause GI upset (nausea, diarrhea).

Administration and Dosage:

Administer as a single dose. However, if GI discomfort occurs, divide the dose. To maximize absorption, avoid the following within 2 hours of dosing:

1) Food, especially items high in calcium, such as milk or milk products.

2) Vitamins with mineral supplements or antacids high in metals (eg, calcium, iron, magnesium or aluminum.

Paget's disease:

Initial treatment – 5 to 10 mg/kg/day, not to exceed 6 months or 11 to 20 mg/kg/day, not to exceed 3 months. Reserve doses above 10 mg/kg/day for use when lower doses are ineffective, when there is an overriding requirement for suppression of increased bone turnover or when prompt reduction of elevated cardiac output is required. Doses in excess of 20 mg/kg/day are not recommended.

Retreatment – Initiate only after an etidronate-free period of at least 90 days and if there is biochemical, symptomatic or other evidence of active disease process. Monitor patients every 3 to 6 months, although some patients may go drug free for extended periods. Retreatment regimens are the same as for initial treatment. For most patients, the original dose will be adequate for retreatment. If not, consider increasing the dose within the recommended guidelines.

Heterotopic ossification due to spinal cord injury: 20 mg/kg/day for 2 weeks, followed by 10 mg/kg/day for 10 weeks; total treatment period is 12 weeks. Institute as soon as feasible following the injury, preferably prior to evidence of heterotopic ossification.

Heterotopic ossification complicating total hip replacement: 20 mg/kg/day for 1 month preoperatively, followed by 20 mg/kg/day for 3 months postoperatively; total treatment period is 4 months.

Rx	**Didronel** (Procter & Gamble Pharm.)	**Tablets:** 200 mg	(P&G 402). White. In 60s.
		400 mg	(NE 406). White, scored. In 60s.

ETIDRONATE DISODIUM (PARENTERAL)

Administration and Dosage:

Recommended dose is 7.5 mg/kg/day for 3 successive days. This daily dose must be diluted in at least 250 ml of sterile normal saline. The diluted solution stored at controlled room temperature (15° to 30°C; 59° to 86°F) shows no drug loss for 48 hours.

Infusion time: Administer the diluted dose IV over a period of at least 2 hours. Infusion may be added to volumes of fluid > 250 ml when convenient.

Regardless of the volume of solution in which etidronate IV infusion is diluted, slow infusion is important. Observe the minimum infusion time of 2 hours at the recommended dose, or smaller doses. The usual course of treatment is one infusion of 7.5 mg/kg/day on each of 3 consecutive days, but some patients have been treated for up to 7 days. When patients are treated for > 3 days, there may be an increased possibility of hypocalcemia.

Retreatment may be appropriate if hypercalcemia recurs. There should be at least a 7 day interval between courses of treatment. The dose and manner of retreatment is the same as that for initial treatment. Retreatment for more than 3 days has not been adequately studied. The safety and efficacy of more than two courses of therapy have not been studied. In the presence of renal impairment, dose reduction may be advisable.

Oral editronate may be started on the day after the last infusion. The recommended oral dose for patients who have had hypercalcemia is 20 mg/kg/day for 30 days. If serum calcium levels remain normal or clinically acceptable, treatment may be extended. Use for > 90 days is not adequately studied and is not recommended.

Storage: Avoid excessive heat (> 40°C; 104°F).

Rx	**Didronel IV** (MGI Pharma)	**Injection:** 300 mg per amp	In 6 ml amps.

PAMIDRONATE DISODIUM

Pamidronate was approved by the FDA in October 1991.

Administration and Dosage:

Give consideration to both the severity and the symptoms of hypercalcemia. The recommended dose in moderate hypercalcemia (corrected serum calcium of approximately 12 to 13.5 mg/dl) is 60 to 90 mg, and in severe hypercalcemia (corrected serum calcium $>$ 13.5 mg/dl) is 90 mg. Give as an initial single-dose IV infusion over 24 hours.

Vigorous saline hydration alone may be sufficient for treating mild, asymptomatic hypercalcemia. Avoid overhydration in patients who have potential for cardiac failure. In hypercalcemia associated with hematologic malignancies, the use of glucocorticoid therapy may be helpful.

Consider retreatment if hypercalcemia recurs; allow a minimum of 7 days to elapse before retreatment to allow for full response to the initial dose. The dose and manner of retreatment are identical to that of the initial therapy.

Preparation of solution: Reconstitute by adding 10 ml Sterile Water for Injection, USP, to each vial, resulting in a solution of 30 mg/10 ml. The pH of the reconstituted solution is 6 to 7.4. Allow drug to dissolve before withdrawing. Administer as an IV infusion over 24 hours. Dilute in 1000 ml sterile 0.45% or 0.9% Sodium Chloride, USP, or 5% Dextrose Injection, USP.

Storage/Stability: The infusion solution is stable for up to 24 hours at room temperature. Pamidronate reconstituted with Sterile Water for Injection may be stored under refrigeration at 2° to 8°C (36° to 46°F) for up to 24 hours.

Incompatibility: Do not mix with calcium-containing infusion solutions, such as Ringer's solution.

Rx	**Aredia** (Ciba)	**Injection, lyophilized:** 30 mg	In vials.[1]

[1] With 470 mg mannitol.

GALLIUM NITRATE

Warning:

Concurrent use of gallium nitrate with other potentially nephrotoxic drugs (eg, aminoglycosides, amphotericin B) may increase the risk for developing severe renal insufficiency in patients with cancer-related hypercalcemia. If use of a potentially nephrotoxic drug is indicated during therapy, discontinue gallium nitrate and continue hydration for several days after administering the potentially nephrotoxic drug. Closely monitor serum creatinine and urine output during and after this period. Discontinue gallium nitrate therapy if the serum creatinine level exceeds 2.5 mg/dl.

Actions:

Gallium nitrate was approved by the FDA in January 1991.

Pharmacology: Gallium nitrate is a hydrated nitrate salt of the group IIIa element, gallium. Gallium nitrate exerts a hypocalcemic effect by inhibiting calcium resorption from bone, possibly by reducing increased bone turnover. The precise mechanism has not been determined. No cytotoxic effects were observed on bone cells in animals.

Cancer-related hypercalcemia is a common problem in hospitalized patients with malignancy. It may affect 10% to 20% of patients with cancer. A higher incidence of hypercalcemia has been observed in patients with non-small-cell lung cancer, breast cancer, multiple myeloma, kidney cancer and cancer of the head and neck. Hypercalcemia of malignancy seems to result from an imbalance between the net resorption of bone and urinary excretion of calcium. Hypercalcemia may produce signs and symptoms including: Anorexia; lethargy; fatigue; nausea; vomiting; constipation; dehydration; renal insufficiency; impaired mental status; coma; cardiac arrest. A rapid rise in serum calcium may cause more severe symptoms for a given level of hypercalcemia.

Pharmacokinetics: Gallium nitrate was infused at a daily dose of 200 mg/m² for 5 (n = 2) or 7 (n = 10) consecutive days to 12 cancer patients. Apparent steady state is generally achieved in 24 to 48 hours. The range of average steady-state plasma levels of gallium observed among 7 patients was between 1134 and 2399 ng/ml. The average plasma clearance following daily infusion at a dose of 200 mg/m² for 5 or 7 days was 0.15 L/hr/kg (range, 0.12 to 0.2 L/hr/kg). In one patient who received daily infusion doses of 100, 150 and 200 mg/m², the apparent steady-state gallium levels did not increase proportionally with a dose increase. Gallium nitrate is not metabolized either by the liver or the kidney and appears to be significantly excreted via the kidney.

Clinical trials: A randomized double-blind clinical study comparing gallium nitrate with calcitonin was conducted in patients with a serum calcium concentration (corrected for albumin) ≥ 12 mg/dl following 2 days of hydration. Gallium nitrate was given as a continuous 200 mg/m²/day IV infusion for 5 days and calcitonin 8 IU/kg IM was given every 6 hours for 5 days. Elevated serum calcium (corrected for albumin) was normalized in 75% (18 of 24) of the patients receiving gallium nitrate and in 27% (7 of 26) of the patients receiving calcitonin. The time-course of effect on serum calcium (corrected for albumin) is summarized in the following table.

Change in Serum Calcium by Gallium Nitrate vs Calcitonin		
	Mean change in serum calcium (mg/dl)[2]	
Time period[1] (hours)	Gallium nitrate	Calcitonin
24	-0.4	-1.6
48	-0.9	-1.4
72	-1.5	-1.1
96	-2.9	-1.1
120	-3.3	-1.3

[1] Time after initiation of therapy in hours.
[2] Change from baseline in serum calcium (corrected for albumin).

The median duration of normocalcemia/hypocalcemia was 7.5 days for patients treated with gallium nitrate and 1 day for patients treated with calcitonin. A total of 92% of patients treated with gallium nitrate had a decrease in serum calcium (corrected for albumin) ≥ 2 mg/dl vs 54% of patients treated with calcitonin.

(Actions continued on following page)

GALLIUM NITRATE (Cont.)

Actions (Cont.):

Clinical trials (Cont.):

An open-label, non-randomized study was conducted to examine a range of doses and dosing schedules of gallium nitrate for control of cancer-related hypercalcemia. The principal dosing regimens were 100 and 200 mg/m²/day, administered as continuous IV infusions for 5 days. A dose of 200 mg/m²/day for 5 days normalized elevated serum calcium levels (corrected for albumin) in 83% of patients vs 50% of patients receiving 100 mg/m²/day for 5 days. A decrease in serum calcium (corrected for albumin) ≥ 2 mg/dl was observed in 83% and 94% of patients at dosages of 100 and 200 mg/m²/day for 5 days, respectively.

Indications:

Cancer-related hypercalcemia (clearly symptomatic) unresponsive to adequate hydration.

In general, patients with a serum calcium (corrected for albumin) < 12 mg/dl would not be expected to be symptomatic. Mild or asymptomatic hypercalcemia may be treated with conservative measures (eg, saline hydration, with or without diuretics). In the treatment of cancer-related hypercalcemia, it is important first to establish adequate hydration, preferably with IV saline, in order to increase the renal excretion of calcium and correct dehydration caused by hypercalcemia.

Contraindications:

Severe renal impairment (serum creatinine > 2.5 mg/dl).

Warnings:

Renal function impairment: Hypercalcemia in cancer patients is commonly associated with impaired renal function (elevated BUN or serum creatinine). It is strongly recommended that serum creatinine be monitored during therapy. It is important that such patients be adequately hydrated with oral or IV fluids (preferably saline) and that a satisfactory urine output (2 L/day is recommended) be established before therapy is started. Maintain adequate hydration throughout the treatment period, with careful attention to avoid overhydration in patients with compromised cardiovascular status. Do not use diuretic therapy prior to correction of hypovolemia. Discontinue gallium nitrate therapy if the serum creatinine level exceeds 2.5 mg/dl.

The use of gallium nitrate in patients with marked renal insufficiency (serum creatinine > 2.5 mg/dl) has not been systematically examined. If therapy is undertaken in patients with moderately impaired renal function (serum creatinine 2 to 2.5 mg/dl), frequent monitoring of the patient's renal status is recommended. Discontinue treatment if the serum creatinine level exceeds 2.5 mg/dl.

Pregnancy: Category C. It is not known whether gallium nitrate can cause fetal harm when administered to a pregnant woman or can affect reproductive capacity. Administer to a pregnant woman only if clearly needed.

Lactation: It is not known whether gallium nitrate is excreted in breast milk. Because of the potential for serious adverse reactions in nursing infants, decide whether to discontinue nursing or discontinue the drug, taking into account the importance of the drug to the mother.

Children: The safety and efficacy of gallium nitrate have not been established.

Precautions:

Asymptomatic or mild to moderate hypocalcemia (6.5 to 8 mg/dl, corrected for serum albumin) occurred in approximately 38% of patients in the controlled clinical trial. One patient exhibited a positive Chvostek's sign. If hypocalcemia occurs, stop gallium nitrate therapy; short-term calcium therapy may be necessary.

Visual and auditory disturbances: A small proportion (< 1%) of patients treated with multiple high doses of gallium nitrate combined with other investigational anticancer drugs, have developed acute optic neuritis. While these patients were critically ill and had received multiple drugs, a reaction to high-dose gallium nitrate is possible. Most patients had full visual recovery; however, at least one case of persistent visual impairment has occurred. One patient with cancer-related hypercalcemia developed a hearing loss following gallium nitrate administration. Due to the patient's underlying condition and concurrent therapies, the relationship of this event to gallium nitrate administration is unclear. Tinnitus and partial loss of auditory acuity have occurred rarely (< 1%) in patients who received high-dose gallium nitrate as anticancer treatment.

Monitoring: Renal function (serum creatinine and BUN) and serum calcium must be closely monitored during gallium nitrate therapy. In addition to baseline assessment, the suggested frequency of calcium and phosphorous determinations is daily and twice weekly, respectively. Discontinue gallium nitrate if the serum creatinine exceeds 2.5 mg/dl.

(Continued on following page)

GALLIUM NITRATE (Cont.)

Drug Interactions:

Nephrotoxic drugs (eg, aminoglycosides, amphotericin B): Combined use of gallium nitrate with other potentially nephrotoxic drugs may increase the risk for developing renal insufficiency in patients with cancer-related hypercalcemia (see Warning box).

Adverse Reactions:

Renal: Adverse renal effects, as demonstrated by rising BUN and creatinine, have occurred in about 12.5% of patients.

Two patients receiving gallium nitrate developed acute renal failure, but the relationship of these events to the drug was unclear (see Warnings).

Metabolic: Hypocalcemia may occur after treatment (see Precautions).

Transient hypophosphatemia of mild-to-moderate degree may occur in up to 79% of hypercalcemic patients following treatment. In a controlled clinical trial, 33% of patients had at least one serum phosphorous measurement between 1.5 to 2.4 mg/dl, while 46% of patients had at least one serum phosphorous value < 1.5 mg/dl. Patients who develop hypophosphatemia may require oral phosphorous therapy.

Decreased serum bicarbonate, possibly secondary to mild respiratory alkalosis, occurred in 40% to 50% of cancer patients treated with gallium nitrate. The cause was not clear. This effect has been asymptomatic and has not required specific treatment.

Hematologic: The use of very high doses (up to 1400 mg/m^2) has been associated with anemia, and several patients have received red blood cell transfusions. Due to the serious nature of the underlying illness, it is uncertain that the anemia was caused by gallium nitrate. Also, leukopenia has occurred.

Cardiovascular: Tachycardia; lower extremity edema (causal relationship unknown).

Blood pressure: A decrease in mean systolic and diastolic blood pressure was observed several days after treatment with gallium nitrate in a controlled clinical trial. The decrease in blood pressure was asymptomatic and did not require specific treatment.

Special senses: Acute optic neuritis; visual impairment, decreased hearing (see Precautions).

Respiratory (causal relationship unknown): Dyspnea; rales and rhonchi; pleural effusion; pulmonary infiltrates.

GI (causal relationship unknown): Nausea or vomiting; diarrhea; constipation.

Miscellaneous: Other clinical events reported in association with gallium nitrate treatment for cancer as well as cancer-related hypercalcemia include: Lethargy; confusion; hypothermia; fever; paresthesia; skin rash. Due to the serious nature of the underlying condition of these patients, the relationship of these events to therapy with gallium nitrate is unknown.

Overdosage:

Symptoms: Rapid IV infusion of gallium nitrate or use of doses higher than recommended (200 mg/m^2) may cause nausea and vomiting and a substantially increased risk of renal insufficiency.

Treatment: Discontinue further drug administration and monitor serum calcium. Administer vigorous IV hydration, with or without diuretics, for 2 to 3 days. During this time, carefully monitor renal function and urinary output for balanced fluid intake and output.

Administration and Dosage:

Usual dose: 200 mg/m^2 daily for 5 consecutive days. In patients with mild hypercalcemia and few symptoms, a lower dosage of 100 mg/m^2/day for 5 days may be considered. If serum calcium levels are lowered into the normal range in < 5 days, treatment may be discontinued early. The daily dose must be given as an IV infusion over 24 hours.

Dilute the daily dose, preferably in 1 L 0.9% Sodium Chloride Injection, USP or 5% Dextrose Injection, USP, for administration as an IV infusion over 24 hours. Maintain adequate hydration throughout the treatment period, with careful attention to avoid overhydration in patients with compromised cardiovascular status. Controlled studies have not been undertaken to evaluate the safety and efficacy of retreatment with gallium nitrate.

Storage/Stability: When gallium nitrate is added to either 0.9% Sodium Chloride Injection, USP or 5% Dextrose Injection, USP, it is stable for at least 48 hours at room temperature (15° to 30°C; 59° to 86°F) and for 7 days if stored under refrigeration (2° to 8°C; 36° to 46°F). Contains no preservative; discard unused portion.

Rx	**Ganite** (Fujisawa)	**Injection:** 25 mg/ml	In 20 ml flip-top vials.

chapter 4

diuretics and cardiovasculars

Actions:

Pharmacology: These agents are nonbacteriostatic sulfonamides that noncompetitively inhibit the enzyme carbonic anhydrase. This action reduces the rate of aqueous humor formation, resulting in decreased intraocular pressure (IOP). This action is independent of systemic acid-base balance.

By inhibiting hydrogen ion secretion by the renal tubule, these agents cause increased excretion of sodium, potassium, bicarbonate and water, thus producing an alkaline diuresis. Carbonic anhydrase inhibitors cause some decrease in renal blood flow and glomerular filtration rate. Redistribution of flow to the renal cortex occurs. These changes are mild and unrelated to diuretic activity.

Pharmacokinetics of these agents are summarized in the table below:

Carbonic Anhydrase Inhibitor	IOP Lowering Effects			Relative Inhibitor Potency
	Onset (Hours)	Peak Effect (Hours)	Duration (Hours)	
Dichlorphenamide	within 1	2 to 4	6 to 12	30
Acetazolamide				1
Tablets	1 to 1½	2 to 4	8 to 12	
Sustained Release Capsules	2	8 to 12	18 to 24	
Injection (IV)	2 min	15 min	4 to 5	
Methazolamide	2 to 4	6 to 8	10 to 18	†

† Quantitative data not available; reported to be more active than acetazolamide.

Indications:

Glaucoma: For adjunctive treatment of chronic simple (open-angle) glaucoma and secondary glaucoma; preoperatively in acute angle-closure glaucoma when delay of surgery is desired to lower IOP.

Acetazolamide *(tablets, sustained release capsules and injection)* is also indicated for the prevention or amelioration of symptoms associated with acute mountain sickness in climbers attempting rapid ascent and in those who are susceptible to acute mountain sickness despite gradual ascent.

Acetazolamide *(tablets and injection only)* is for adjunctive treatment of edema due to CHF, drug-induced edema and centrencephalic epilepsy (petit mal, unlocalized seizures).

Unlabeled Uses: Treatment of hyperkalemic and hypokalemic periodic paralysis.

Contraindications:

Hypersensitivity to these agents.

Depressed sodium or potassium serum levels, marked kidney and liver disease or dysfunction, hyperchloremic acidosis, electrolyte imbalance, adrenocortical insufficiency/failure.

Severe pulmonary obstruction with inability to increase alveolar ventilation since acidosis may be increased.

Long-term use in chronic noncongestive angle-closure glaucoma, since organic closure of the angle may occur while worsening glaucoma is masked by lowered IOP; severe or absolute glaucoma.

Warnings:

Usage in Pregnancy: Animal studies with some of these drugs have demonstrated teratogenic (skeletal anomalies) and embryocidal effects at high doses. While there is no evidence of increased fetal risk in humans, do not use during pregnancy, especially during the first trimester, unless the potential benefits outweigh the potential hazards.

Usage in Lactation: Safety for use in the nursing mother has not been established. Acetazolamide appeared in breast milk of a patient taking 500 mg twice/day. However, the infant ingested only 0.06% of the dose, an amount unlikely to cause adverse effects.

Precautions:

Increasing the dose does not increase diuresis and may increase drowsiness or paresthesia; it often results in decreased diuresis. However, very large doses have been given with other diuretics to promote diuresis in complete refractory failure.

Electrolyte imbalance: Adequate and balanced electrolyte intake is essential in all patients whose clinical condition may cause electrolyte imbalance.

Hypokalemia may develop when severe cirrhosis is present, during concomitant use of **steroids** or **ACTH**, and with interference with adequate oral electrolyte intake. Hypokalemia can sensitize or exaggerate the response of the heart to the toxic effects of **digitalis** (eg, increased ventricular irritability). Hypokalemia may be avoided or treated with potassium supplements or foods with a high potassium content.

Usage in impaired hepatic function could precipitate hepatic coma.

(Precautions continued on following page)

Precautions (Cont.):

Pulmonary: Use with caution in patients with severe degrees of respiratory acidosis. These drugs may precipitate or aggravate acidosis. Use with caution in patients with pulmonary obstruction or emphysema when alveolar ventilation may be impaired.

Monitor for hematologic reactions common to sulfonamides. Obtain baseline CBC and platelet counts before initiating therapy and at regular intervals during therapy.

Cross-sensitivity between antibacterial sulfonamides and sulfonamide derivative diuretics, including acetazolamide and various thiazides, has been reported.

Drug Interactions:

Amphetamines, ephedrine, flecainide, pseudoephedrine, quinidine: Since carbonic anhydrase inhibitors alkalinize the urine, the renal excretion of these agents may be decreased, increasing their pharmacologic effects. However, long-term consequences of concurrent administration are unclear. Also, since **methenamine** requires an acid urine to be effective, acetazolamide may decrease its efficacy.

Digitalis: Carbonic anhydrase inhibitors may induce hypokalemia, which sensitizes the patient to digitalis toxicity.

Primidone: When given concurrently, oral acetazolamide may delay primidone absorption. Exact incidence and clinical significance is unknown.

Salicylates: Combined therapy may result in severe metabolic acidosis, increasing potential for salicylate toxicity (eg, drowsiness, confusion, lethargy, hyperventilation, tinnitus, anorexia). Acetazolamide toxicity may also occur due to displacement from protein binding sites and decreased clearance by salicylates.

Drug/Lab tests: Acetazolamide may interfere with diagnostic tests for **urinary protein** causing possible false-positive results due to alkalinization of urine.

Adverse Reactions:

Sulfonamide-type adverse reactions may occur (see p.1900).

GI: Melena, anorexia, nausea, vomiting, constipation.

Renal: Hematuria, glycosuria, urinary frequency, renal colic, renal calculi, crystalluria, polyuria.

Hepatic: Hepatic insufficiency.

CNS: Convulsions, weakness, malaise, fatigue, nervousness, sedation, drowsiness, depression, dizziness, disorientation, confusion, ataxia, tremor, tinnitus, globus hystericus, headache, vertigo, flaccid paralysis. Paresthesias of the extremities, tongue or at the mucocutaneous junction of the lips, mouth or anus.

Ophthalmic: Transient myopia that subsides upon drug diminution or discontinuance.

Hematologic: Bone marrow depression, thrombocytopenia, thrombocytopenic purpura, hemolytic anemia, leukopenia, pancytopenia, agranulocytosis.

Dermatologic: Urticaria, pruritus, skin eruptions, rash (including erythema multiforme, Stevens-Johnson syndrome, toxic epidermal necrolysis); photosensitivity (rare).

Miscellaneous: Weight loss; fever; acidosis (usually corrected by administering bicarbonate).

Patient Information:

If GI upset occurs, take with food.

May cause drowsiness; observe caution while driving or performing other tasks requiring alertness.

Notify physician if sore throat, fever, unusual bleeding or bruising, tingling or tremors in the hands or feet, flank or loin pain, or skin rash occurs.

Bioavailability: Bioequivalence problems have been documented for carbonic anhydrase inhibitors marketed by different manufacturers. Brand interchange is not recommended unless comparative bioavailability data provide evidence of therapeutic equivalence.

DICHLORPHENAMIDE

Administration and Dosage:

Glaucoma: Most effective when given with miotics. In acute angle-closure glaucoma, dichlorphenamide may be used with miotics and osmotic agents to rapidly reduce intraocular tension. If quick relief does not occur, surgery may be mandatory.

Adults: Individualize dosage. *Initial dose* - 100 to 200 mg, followed by 100 mg every 12 hours, until the desired response is obtained.

Maintenance dosage - 25 to 50 mg, 1 to 3 times daily.

				C.I.*
Rx	**Daranide** (MSD)	**Tablets:** 50 mg	(#MSD 49). Yellow, scored. In 100s.	34

* Cost Index based on cost per 50 mg dichlorphenamide.

Product identification code.

Complete prescribing information for these products begins on page 554.

ACETAZOLAMIDE

Administration and Dosage:

Chronic simple (open-angle) glaucoma: Adults – 250 mg to 1 g/day, usually in divided doses for amounts over 250 mg. Dosage in excess of 1 g daily does not usually increase the effect.

Secondary glaucoma and preoperative treatment of acute congestive (closed-angle) glaucoma: Adults – Short-term therapy: 250 mg every 4 hours or 250 mg twice daily.
Acute cases: 500 mg followed by 125 or 250 mg every 4 hours.

IV therapy may be used for rapid relief of increased intraocular pressure. A complementary effect occurs when acetazolamide is used with miotics or mydriatics.

Children – 5 to 10 mg/kg/dose, IM or IV, every 6 hours or 10 to 15 mg/kg/day, orally, in divided doses, every 6 to 8 hours.

Diuresis in congestive heart failure: Adults – Initially, 250 to 375 mg (5 mg/kg) once daily in the morning. If, after an initial response, the patient stops losing edema fluid, do not increase the dose; allow for kidney recovery by skipping medication for a day. Best diuretic results occur when given on alternate days, or for 2 days alternating with a day of rest. Failures in therapy may result from overdosage or from too frequent dosages.

Drug-induced edema: Most effective if given every other day or for 2 days alternating with a day of rest. *Adults* – 250 to 375 mg once daily for 1 or 2 days.

Children – 5 mg/kg/dose, oral or IV, once daily in the morning.

Epilepsy: Adults and Children – 8 to 30 mg/kg/day in divided doses. The optimum range is 375 to 1000 mg daily. When given in combination with other anticonvulsants, the starting dose is 250 mg once daily.

Acute mountain sickness: 500 to 1000 mg/day, in divided doses of tablets or sustained release capsules. For rapid ascent (ie, in rescue or military operations), use the higher dose (1000 mg). If possible, initiate dosing 24 to 48 hours before ascent and continue for 48 hours while at high altitude, or longer as needed to control symptoms.

Sustained release: May be used twice daily, but is only indicated for use in glaucoma and acute mountain sickness.

Parenteral: Direct IV administration is preferred; IM administration is painful because of the alkaline pH of the solution.

Preparation and storage of parenteral solution: Reconstitute each 500 mg vial with at least 5 ml of Sterile Water for Injection. Reconstituted solutions retain potency for 1 week if refrigerated. However, since this product contains no preservative, use within 24 hours of reconstitution.

If an *oral liquid dosage form* is required, acetazolamide tablets may be crushed and suspended in a cherry, chocolate, raspberry or other sweet syrup. Do not use a vehicle with alcohol or glycerin. Alternatively, one tablet can be submerged in 10 ml of hot water and added to 10 ml of honey or syrup.

	Product	Form	Description	C.I.*
Rx	**Acetazolamide** (Mutual)	**Tablets:** 125 mg	(MP/65). White, scored. In 50s, 100s, 250s, 500s and 1000s.	NA
Rx	**Diamox** (Lederle)		(Diamox 125, D1/LL). White, scored. In 100s.	33
Rx	**Acetazolamide** (Various)	**Tablets:** 250 mg	In 100s, 1000s and UD 100s.	4+
Rx	**Ak-Zol** (Akorn)		In 100s and 1000s.	9
Rx	**Dazamide** (Major)		In 100s, 250s, 1000s and UD 100s.	8
Rx	**Diamox** (Lederle)		(Diamox 250 D2/LL). White, scored. In 100s, 1000s and UD 100s.	24
Rx	**Storzolamide** (Storz)		(S19 Storz). White, scored in quarters. In 100s.	NA
Rx	**Diamox Sequels** (Lederle)	**Capsules, sustained release:** 500 mg	(Diamox D3). Orange. In 30s and 100s.	29
Rx	**Diamox** (Lederle)	**Injection:** 500 mg (as sodium) per vial.		874

METHAZOLAMIDE

Administration and Dosage:

Glaucoma: 50 to 100 mg, 2 or 3 times daily. May be used with miotic and osmotic agents.

	Product	Form	Description	C.I.*
Rx	**Neptazane** (Lederle)	**Tablets:** 25 mg	In 100s.	71
		50 mg	(N1). White, scored. In 100s.	43

* Cost Index based on cost per 250 mg acetazolamide or 50 mg methazolamide.

Actions:

Pharmacology: Thiazide diuretics increase the renal excretion of sodium and chloride in approximately equivalent amounts. They inhibit tubular reabsorption of sodium and chloride by direct action on the distal segment. All of these compounds possess some degree of carbonic anhydrase inhibition activity due to the sulfonamide moiety. Other common actions include: Increased potassium excretion, decreased calcium excretion and uric acid retention. At maximal therapeutic dosages all thiazides are approximately equal in diuretic efficacy, but metolazone may be more effective in patients with impaired renal function. Metolazone and quinethazone (quinazoline derivatives), chlorthalidone (a phthalimidine derivative) and indapamide (an indoline) are included here because of their structural and pharmacological similarities to the thiazides.

The exact antihypertensive mechanism of the thiazides is unknown, although it may result from an altered sodium balance. During initial therapy, cardiac output decreases and blood volume diminishes. With chronic therapy, cardiac output normalizes, peripheral vascular resistance falls, and there is a persistent small reduction in extracellular water and plasma volume.

In hypertensive patients, daily doses of indapamide have no appreciable cardiac inotropic or chronotropic effect, and little or no effect on glomerular filtration rate or renal plasma flow. The drug decreases peripheral resistance, with little or no effect on cardiac output, rate or rhythm. Indapamide had an antihypertensive effect in patients with varying degrees of renal impairment, although in general, diuretic effects declined as renal function decreased.

Pharmacokinetics: The onset, peak and duration of diuretic action, approximate equivalent dose and available pharmacokinetic data for these agents are listed below. The antihypertensive action requires several days to produce effects. Administration for up to 3 to 4 weeks is usually required for optimal therapeutic effect. The duration of the antihypertensive effect of the thiazides is sufficiently long to adequately control blood pressure with a single daily dose. Despite extensive use of diuretics, pharmacokinetic data are limited. It is important to emphasize the lack of relationship between plasma levels and diuretic effect.

THIAZIDES AND RELATED DIURETICS

Diuretic	Onset (hours)	Peak (hours)	Duration (hours)	Equivalent Dose (mg)	% absorbed	t½ (hours)
Chlorothiazide	1 to 2	4	6 to 12	500	10 to 21*	1 to 2
Hydrochlorothiazide	2	4 to 6	6 to 12	50	65 to 75	5.6 to 14.8
Bendroflumethiazide	2	4	6 to 12	5	≈ 100	3 to 3.9
Cyclothiazide	within 6	7 to 12	18 to 24	2		
Methyclothiazide	2	4 to 6	24	5		
Benzthiazide	2	4 to 6	6 to 12	50		
Hydroflumethiazide	2	4	6 to 12	50	50	17
Trichlormethiazide	2	6	24	2		2.3 to 7.3
Polythiazide	2	6	24 to 48	2		25.7
Quinethazone	2	6	18 to 24	50		
Metolazone[1]	1	2	12 to 24	5	64	8
Chlorthalidone	2	2 to 6	24 to 72	50	64*	40
Indapamide	1 to 2	within 2	up to 36	2.5	≈ 100	14
Flumethiazide	2	4 to 6	12 to 18	500		

* Bioavailability may be dose-dependent.

[1] *Microx:* Peak plasma concentrations reached in 2 to 4 hrs, t½ ≈ 14 hrs.

(Continued on following page)

Indications:

Edema: Adjunctive therapy in edema associated with congestive heart failure (CHF), hepatic cirrhosis and corticosteroid and estrogen therapy. Useful in edema due to renal dysfunction (ie, nephrotic syndrome, acute glomerulonephritis and chronic renal failure).

Indapamide alone is indicated for edema associated with CHF.

Hypertension: As the sole therapeutic agent or to enhance other antihypertensive drugs.

Unlabeled uses: Thiazide diuretics have been used alone and in combination with amiloride or allopurinol to prevent formation and recurrence of *calcium nephrolithiasis* in hypercalciuric and normal calciuric patients. Thiazides correct hypercalciuria, reduce urinary saturation, enhance inhibitor activity against spontaneous nucleation of both calcium oxalate and brushite, and restore normal parathyroid function and intestinal calcium absorption. Doses of hydrochlorothiazide 50 mg, one or two times daily, trichloromethiazide 4 mg/day, chlorthalidone 50 mg/day, metolazone 2.5 to 10 mg/day, and indapamide 2.5 mg/day have been used.

Thiazide diuretics may be useful in reducing the incidence of *osteoporosis* in postmenopausal women, either alone or in combination with calcium or estrogen. Further studies are necessary to confirm this use.

In *diabetes insipidus,* thiazide diuretics reduce urine volume by 30% to 50%. Although these agents play an adjuvant role in neurogenic diabetes insipidus, they constitute the only drug therapy available for nephrogenic diabetes insipidus.

Contraindications:

Anuria, renal decompensation; hypersensitivity to thiazides, any individual agent or sulfonamides.

Metolazone: Hepatic coma or precoma.

Warnings:

Parenteral use: Use IV **chlorothiazide** only when patients are unable to take oral medication or in an emergency. In infants and children, IV use has been limited and is not recommended.

Avoid simultaneous administration of chlorothiazide with whole blood or its derivatives.

Usage in impaired renal function: Use with caution in severe renal disease since these agents may precipitate azotemia. Cumulative effects of the drug may develop in patients with impaired renal function. If progressive renal impairment becomes evident, indicated by a rising nonprotein nitrogen (NPN) or BUN, withhold or discontinue therapy. If the patient has a creatinine clearance less than 40 to 50 ml/min, a glomerular filtration rate less than 25 ml/min or is not responsive to thiazides, a loop diuretic may be more effective.

Usage in impaired hepatic function or progressive liver disease: Use with caution since minor alterations of fluid and electrolyte balance may precipitate hepatic coma.

Hypersensitivity reactions may occur in patients with or without a history of allergy or bronchial asthma; cross-sensitivity with sulfonamides may also occur. Have epinephrine 1:1000 immediately available. Refer to Management of Acute Hypersensitivity Reactions on p. viii.

Lupus erythematosus exacerbation or activation has been reported.

Usage in Pregnancy: (Category B – Indapamide, Metolazone. Category C – Cyclothiazide, Trichlormethiazide. Category D – Hydroflumethiazide.) Routine use during normal pregnancy is inappropriate. Diuretics decrease plasma volume and can decrease placental perfusion. Diuretics do not prevent development of preeclampsia toxemia, nor are they useful in the treatment of preeclampsia.

Thiazides are indicated in pregnancy when edema is due to pathologic causes, just as they are in the absence of pregnancy. Dependent edema in pregnancy, resulting from restriction of venous return by the gravid uterus, is not properly treated by the use of diuretics. In rare instances, hypervolemia during normal pregnancy results in edema that may cause extreme discomfort that is not relieved by rest; a short course of diuretics may provide relief.

Thiazides cross the placental barrier and appear in cord blood. Use only when clearly needed and when potential benefits outweigh the potential hazards to the fetus. These hazards include fetal or neonatal jaundice, thrombocytopenia, hemolytic anemia, electrolyte imbalances and hypoglycemia.

Usage in Lactation: Thiazides appear in breast milk. Chlorthalidone has a low milk to plasma ratio of 0.05. If thiazide diuretics are necessary, the patient should stop nursing.

Usage in Children: Cyclothiazide, Hydroflumethiazide, Trichlormethiazide – Safety and efficacy have not been established. Until additional data are obtained, **metolazone** is not recommended for use in children.

(Continued on following page)

Precautions:

Monitor fluid/electrolyte balance: Perform periodic determinations of serum electrolytes, BUN, uric acid and glucose. Observe patients for clinical signs of fluid or electrolyte imbalance (eg, hyponatremia, hypochloremic alkalosis, hypokalemia, hypomagnesemia, changes in serum and urinary calcium). Serum and urine electrolyte determinations are particularly important in patients vomiting excessively or receiving parenteral fluids, in patients subject to electrolyte imbalance (including those with heart failure, kidney disease and cirrhosis), and in patients on a salt restricted diet. Warning signs of imbalance include: Dry mouth, thirst, weakness, fatigue, lethargy, drowsiness, restlessness, muscle pains or cramps, muscular fatigue, hypotension, oliguria, tachycardia and GI disturbances.

Hypokalemia may develop (with consequent weakness, cramps and cardiac dysrhythmias) during concomitant use of **corticosteroids, ACTH** or after prolonged therapy, especially with brisk diuresis in severe cirrhosis. Inadequate oral electrolyte intake will also contribute to hypokalemia. Hypokalemia can sensitize or exaggerate the response of the heart to the toxic effects of **digitalis** (eg, increased ventricular irritability). Avoid or treat hypokalemia by using a potassium-sparing diuretic, potassium supplements or foods with a high potassium content.

Sodium and chloride - A chloride deficit is generally mild and does not require specific treatment, except in extraordinary circumstances (as in liver or renal disease). However, treatment of metabolic or hypochloremic alkalosis may require chloride replacement. Dilutional hyponatremia may occur in edematous patients in hot weather; appropriate therapy is water restriction, rather than salt administration, except in rare life-threatening instances. Thiazide-induced hyponatremia is associated with death and neurologic damage in elderly patients. CNS manifestations include seizures, coma and extensor-plantar response.

Calcium excretion is decreased by diuretics. Thiazides may cause a slight intermittent elevation of serum calcium in the absence of calcium metabolism disorders. Pathologic changes in the parathyroid glands with hypercalcemia and hypophosphatemia may occur in a few patients on prolonged thiazide therapy. Marked hypercalcemia may be evidence of hidden hyperparathyroidism. Common complications of hyperparathyroidism such as renal lithiasis, bone resorption and peptic ulceration are not seen. Discontinue thiazides before performing parathyroid function tests.

Hypercalcemia induced by thiazides has aggravated manic-depressive episodes previously controlled with lithium.

Hyperuricemia with infrequent gouty attacks may occur in patients with a history of gout. Monitor serum uric acid concentrations periodically during treatment. One report suggests that it is not necessary to lower uric acid levels with pharmacologic measures in patients receiving thiazide diuretics who are without renal damage or gout symptoms.

Serum uric acid increased by an average of 1 mg/dl in patients on **indapamide**.

Glucose tolerance: Insulin requirements in diabetic patients may be altered. Latent diabetes mellitus may become manifest during diuretic administration; diabetic complications may occur. Monitor serum glucose concentrations.

Antihypertensive effects may be enhanced in the postsympathectomy patient.

Tartrazine sensitivity: Some of these products contain tartrazine, which may cause allergic-type reactions (including bronchial asthma) in certain susceptible individuals. Although the overall incidence of tartrazine sensitivity in the general population is low, it is frequently seen in patients who also have aspirin hypersensitivity. Specific products containing tartrazine are identified in the product listings.

Drug Interactions:

Cholestyramine and **colestipol** decrease the absorption of thiazides.

Diazoxide: Coadministration with thiazide diuretics results in additive pharmacologic activity; hyperglycemia, hyperuricemia and hypotension may occur.

(Drug Interactions continued on following page)

Drug Interactions (Cont.):

Digitalis glycosides: Diuretic-induced hypokalemia may precipitate **digitalis** toxicity.

Lithium: Thiazide diuretics may increase the therapeutic and toxic effects (eg, GI symptoms, polyuria, muscular weakness, lethargy, tremor) of lithium by decreasing its renal excretion. Monitor lithium levels as a lower dose may be necessary.

Furosemide: Profound diuresis and a greater than predicted electrolyte loss may occur when metolazone and furosemide are administered concurrently. This synergistic effect has been employed in patients refractory to furosemide. The mechanism may be related to the ability of metolazone to block proximal tubular sodium reabsorption. This effect has been reported with other thiazide diuretics. Weight, urine output, blood pressure and BUN should be closely monitored.

Nondepolarizing Muscle Relaxants: Neuromuscular blocking effects may be increased by thiazide diuretics, probably due to hypokalemia. Prolonged respiration with extended periods of apnea may occur.

Sulfonylureas: Hypoglycemic effects may be decreased due to thiazide-induced glucose intolerance. Hyponatremia has occurred with **chlorpropamide** and thiazides.

Adverse Reactions:

Whenever adverse reactions are moderate or severe, thiazide dosage should be reduced or therapy withdrawn.

GI: Anorexia, gastric irritation, nausea; vomiting, abdominal pain, bloating, diarrhea; constipation, jaundice (intrahepatic and cholestatic), hepatitis, pancreatitis, sialadenitis, dry mouth, bitter taste, cholecystitis.

GU: Frequent urination, nocturia, polyuria. Hematuria (one case following IV use), impotence, reduced libido.

CNS: Dizziness (**metolazone** 10%); vertigo, headache (**metolazone** 9%), paresthesias, xanthopsia, weakness, restlessness (sometimes resulting in insomnia), syncope, drowsiness, fatigue (**metolazone** 4%); anxiety, depression, nervousness, neuropathy.

Indapamide (> 5%) – Headache; dizziness; fatigue; weakness; loss of energy; lethargy; tiredness; malaise; muscle cramps or spasm; numbness of the extremities; nervousness; tension; anxiety; irritability; agitation.

Indapamide (< 5%) – Lightheadedness; drowsiness; vertigo; insomnia; depression; blurred vision; tingling of extremities.

Hematologic: Leukopenia, thrombocytopenia, agranulocytosis, aplastic anemia, hemolytic anemia, neutropenia.

Respiratory: Respiratory distress (including pneumonitis), cough, epistaxis, sinus congestion, sore throat.

Cardiovascular: Orthostatic hypotension (may be aggravated by alcohol, barbiturates or narcotics), venous thrombosis, excessive volume depletion, hemoconcentration, palpitations, chest pain (**metolazone** 3%), premature ventricular contractions, irregular heartbeat, cold extremities, allergic myocarditis.

Hypersensitivity/Dermatologic: Purpura, photosensitivity, rash, urticaria, vasculitis, necrotizing angitis (vasculitis, cutaneous vasculitis), fever. Respiratory distress including pneumonitis and pulmonary edema; anaphylactic reactions, hives, pruritus, dry skin.

Metabolic: Hyperglycemia, glycosuria, hyperuricemia, electrolyte imbalance.

Musculoskeletal: Muscle cramps or spasm, joint pain, swelling (**metolazone** 3%).

Miscellaneous: Acute gouty attacks, transient blurred vision, chills, rhinorrhea, flushing, weight loss, dyspnea, photosensitivity, rash.

Clinical laboratory test findings: Hypercalcemia, metabolic acidosis in diabetic patients, hypokalemia, hyponatremia, hypomagnesemia, hypochloremia, hypochloremic alkalosis, hypophosphatemia, hyperuricemia, increase in BUN. Elevation of creatinine, hyperglycemia, glycosuria, decreased serum PBI levels.

Clinical hypokalemia occurred in 3% and 7% of patients given **indapamide** 2.5 mg and 5 mg, respectively.

Increases in plasma levels of total cholesterol, triglycerides and LDL cholesterol (but not HDL cholesterol) have been associated with thiazide diuretics, but appear to return to pretreatment levels with long-term therapy. **Indapamide** does not appear to increase serum cholesterol.

Fluid/electrolyte imbalance - There are isolated reports of nonedematous individuals developing severe fluid and electrolyte derangements after only brief exposure to normal doses. This condition is usually manifested as severe dilutional hyponatremia, hypokalemia and hypochloremia. It may be due to inappropriately increased ADH secretion and appears to be idiosyncratic. Potassium replacement is apparently the most important therapy along with removal of the offending drug.

(Continued on following page)

Overdosage:

Symptoms: Electrolyte imbalance; signs of potassium deficiency (eg, confusion, dizziness, muscular weakness, and GI disturbances); nausea; vomiting. In severe instances, hypotension and depressed respiration may occur. Lethargy of varying degrees may progress to coma within a few hours, with minimal depression of respiration and cardiovascular function and without significant serum electrolyte changes or dehydration. GI irritation and hypermotility may also occur. Temporary BUN elevation and seizures have also been reported.

Treatment: Perform gastric lavage or induce emesis; give activated charcoal. Prevent aspiration. GI effects are usually of short duration, but may require symptomatic treatment. Maintain hydration, electrolyte balance, respiration and cardiovascular-renal function. Asymptomatic hyperuricemia usually responds to fluids, but if clinical gout is suspected, indomethacin may be started. Support respiration and cardiac circulation if hypotension and depressed respiration occur. Refer to General Management of Acute Overdosage on p. 2895

Patient Information:

May cause GI upset; may be taken with food or milk.

Drug will increase urination; take early during the day.

Notify physician if muscle weakness or cramps, nausea, vomiting, diarrhea or dizziness occurs.

May increase blood sugar levels in diabetics.

Do not take other medications without physician's approval; this includes nonprescription medicines for appetite control, asthma, colds, cough, hay fever or sinus.

Administration and Dosage:

Edema: Intermittent therapy may be advantageous. With administration every other day, or on a 3 to 5 day per week schedule, electrolyte imbalance is less likely to occur.

Hypertension: Reduce dosage of other agents as soon as thiazides are added to the regimen to prevent excessive hypotension. As blood pressure falls, a further reduction in dosage may be necessary.

Renal impairment: Metolazone is the only thiazide-like diuretic that may have significant activity if serum creatinine is $>$ 2 mg/dl. If the patient has a creatinine clearance less than 40 to 50 ml/min, a glomerular filtration rate less than 25 ml/min or is not responsive to thiazides, a loop diuretic may be more effective.

Concomitant administration: Concurrent metolazone and furosemide have been used in the management of patients refractory to furosemide due to their synergistic effect on diuresis (see Drug Interactions). Metolazone 2.5 to 10 mg is added to the therapy, and the dose is doubled every 24 hours until the desired response is achieved. Decrease the furosemide dose if synergism occurs with the first dose of metolazone. Hydrochlorothiazide (50 mg) may be used and may be safer because of its shorter action.

(Products listed on following pages)

CHLOROTHIAZIDE

Administration and Dosage:

Bioavailability studies demonstrate that saturable absorption of chlorothiazide occurs. Doses greater than 250 mg do not increase effect. Chlorothiazide 250 mg every 6 or 12 hours produces a greater diuresis than doses > 250 mg administered at one time.

Adults: Edema – 0.5 to 2 g once or twice a day, orally or IV. Reserve IV route for patients unable to take oral medication or for emergency situations.

Many patients with edema respond to intermittent therapy (administration on alternate days or on 3 to 5 days each week). With an intermittent schedule, excessive response and undesirable electrolyte imbalance are less likely to occur.

Hypertension (oral forms only) – Starting dose is 0.5 to 2 g daily as a single or divided dose. Adjust dosage according to the blood pressure response. Rarely, some patients may require up to 2 g/day in divided doses.

Infants and Children: Oral – 10 mg/lb/day (22 mg/kg/day) in two doses. Infants under 6 months may require up to 15 mg/lb/day (33 mg/kg/day) in two doses.

On this basis, infants up to 2 years of age may be given 125 to 375 mg daily in 2 doses. Children from 2 to 12 years of age may be given 375 mg to 1 g daily in two doses.

IV use is not generally recommended.

Preparation of parenteral solution: Add 18 ml of Sterile Water for Injection to the vial to prepare an isotonic solution. Discard unused solution after 24 hours. The solution is compatible with dextrose or sodium chloride solutions for IV infusion. Avoid simultaneous administration with whole blood or its derivatives.

	Product	Form	Description	**C.I.***
Rx	**Chlorothiazide** (Various)	**Tablets:** 250 mg	In 100s, 1000s and UD 100s.	5+
Rx	**Diachlor** (Major)		In 100s, 250s and 1000s and UD 100s.	10
Rx	**Diurigen** (Goldline)		In 100s and 1000s.	9
Rx	**Diuril** (MSD)		(#MSD 214). White, scored. In 100s and 1000s.	18
Rx	**Chlorothiazide** (Various)	**Tablets:** 500 mg	In 100s, 500s, 1000s and UD 100s.	4+
Rx	**Diachlor** (Major)		In 100s, 250s, 1000s and UD 100s.	7
Rx	**Diurigen** (Goldline)		In 100s and 1000s.	7
Rx	**Diuril** (MSD)		(#MSD 432). White, scored. In 100s, 1000s and UD 100s.	14
Rx	**Diuril** (MSD)	**Oral Suspension:** 250 mg per 5 ml	0.5% alcohol. Saccharin. In 237 ml.	27
Rx	**Diuril Sodium** (MSD)	**Powder for Injection:** 500 mg (as sodium)	In 20 ml vials.[1]	594

* Cost Index based on cost per 500 mg.

\# Product identification code.

[1] With 0.25 g mannitol and 0.4 mg thimerosal.

Complete prescribing information for these products begins on page 557.

HYDROCHLOROTHIAZIDE

Dosage:

Edema: Initial – 25 to 200 mg daily for several days, or until dry weight is attained.
Maintenance – 25 to 100 mg daily or intermittently. Refractory patients may require up to 200 mg daily.

Hypertension: Initial – 50 to 100 mg daily as a single or divided dose.
Maintenance – 25 to 100 mg daily. Rarely, patients require up to 200 mg/day in divided doses.

Infants and Children: Usual dosage is 1 mg/lb (2.2 mg/kg) daily in two doses.
Infants under 6 months – Up to 1.5 mg/lb (3.3 mg/kg) daily in two doses.
Infants up to 2 years of age – 12.5 to 37.5 mg daily in two doses.
Children from 2 to 12 years – 37.5 to 100 mg daily in two doses.

	Product	Form	Description	C.I.*
Rx	**Hydrochlorothiazide** (Various)	**Tablets:** 25 mg	In 30s, 100s, 500s, 1000s, UD 32s and UD 100s.	2+
Rx	**Esidrix** (Ciba)		(Ciba 22). Pink, scored. In 100s, 1000s and Accu-Pak 100s.	15
Rx	**HydroDIURIL** (MSD)		(MSD 42). Peach, scored. In 100s and 1000s.	18
Rx	**Hydro-T** (Major)		In 100s, 1000s and UD 100s.	4
Rx	**Oretic** (Abbott)		White. In 100s, 1000s and UD 100s.	8
Rx	**Thiuretic** (Warner-Chilcott)		(W-C/702). White, scored. In 100s.	5
Rx	**Hydrochlorothiazide** (Various)	**Tablets:** 50 mg	In 30s, 100s, 500s, 1000s and UD 100s.	2+
Rx	**Diaqua** (Hauck)		(Diaqua Hauck 038). Peach, scored. In 100s and 1000s.	5
Rx	**Esidrix** (Ciba)		(Ciba 46). Yellow, scored. In 100s, 360s, 720s and 1000s and UD 100s.	12
Rx	**Ezide** (Econo Med)		In 100s and 1000s.	4
Rx	**Hydro-Chlor** (Vortech)		In 1000s.	4
Rx	**HydroDIURIL** (MSD)		(MSD 105). Peach, scored. In 100s, 1000s and UD 100s.	14
Rx	**Hydromal** (Hauck)		In 1000s.	2
Rx	**Hydro-T** (Major)		In 100s, 1000s and UD 100s.	2
Rx	**Hydro-Z-50** (Mayrand)		In 100s and 1000s.	4
Rx	**Hydrozide-50** (T.E. Williams)		In 100s.	6
Rx	**Oretic** (Abbott)		White, scored. In 100s, 1000s and UD 100s.	6
Rx	**Thiuretic** (Warner-Chilcott)		(W-C/710). White, scored. In 100s, 1000s and UD 100s.	3
Rx	**Hydrochlorothiazide** (Various)	**Tablets:** 100 mg	In 30s, 100s, 500s, 1000s and UD 100s.	1+
Rx	**Esidrix** (Ciba)		(Ciba 192). Blue, scored. In 100s.	11
Rx	**HydroDIURIL** (MSD)		(MSD 410). Peach, scored. In 100s.	13
Rx	**Hydro-T** (Major)		In 100s, 250s, 1000s and UD 100s.	1
Rx	**Hydrochlorothiazide** (Roxane)	**Solution:** 50 mg per 5 ml	In 5 ml unit dose cups and 500 ml.	8
Rx	**Hydrochlorothiazide** (Roxane)	**Intensol Solution:** 100 mg per ml	In 30 ml w/dropper.	9

* Cost Index based on cost per 50 mg.

Complete prescribing information for these products begins on page 557.

BENDROFLUMETHIAZIDE

Dosage:

Edema: 5 mg once daily, preferably in the morning. *Initial* – Up to 20 mg once daily or divided into 2 doses. *Maintenance* – 2.5 to 5 mg daily.

Hypertension: Initial – 5 to 20 mg daily. *Maintenance* –2.5 to 15 mg/day. **C.I.***

	Product	Form/Strength	Description	C.I.*
Rx	**Naturetin** (Princeton)	**Tablets:** 5 mg	(#606). Green, scored. In 100s and 1000s.	36
		10 mg	(#618). Orange, scored. In 100s.	27

METHYCLOTHIAZIDE

Dosage:

Edema: Adults – 2.5 to 10 mg once daily. Maximum effective single dose is 10 mg.

Hypertension: Adults – 2.5 to 5 mg once daily. If control of blood pressure is not satisfactory after 8 to 12 weeks of therapy with 5 mg once daily, add another antihypertensive drug. **C.I.***

	Product	Form/Strength	Description	C.I.*
Rx	**Methyclothiazide** (Various)	**Tablets:** 2.5 mg	In 100s, 500s and 1000s.	9+
Rx	**Enduron** (Abbott)		(#a Enduron). Orange, scored. In 100s and 1000s.	34
Rx	**Ethon** (Major)		In 100s.	17
Rx	**Methyclothiazide** (Various)	**Tablets:** 5 mg	In 30s, 100s, 500s, 1000s and UD 100s.	3+
Rx	**Aquatensen** (Wallace)		(#Wallace 153). Peach, scored. In 100s and 500s.	37
Rx	**Enduron** (Abbott)		(#a Enduron). Salmon, scored. In 100s, 1000s and Abbo-Pac 100s.	22
Rx	**Ethon** (Major)		In 100s and 1000s.	11

BENZTHIAZIDE

Dosage:

Edema:

Initial –50 to 200 mg daily for several days, or until dry weight is attained. If dosages exceed 100 mg daily, administer in 2 doses, following morning and evening meal.

Maintenance – 50 to 150 mg daily.

Hypertension:

Initial – 50 to 100 mg daily. Give in 2 doses of 25 or 50 mg each, after breakfast and after lunch. Continue until a therapeutic drop in blood pressure occurs.

Maintenance – Individualize dosage; maximal effective dose is 200 mg daily. **C.I.***

	Product	Form/Strength	Description	C.I.*
Rx	**Aquatag** (Solvay Pharm.)	**Tablets:** 50 mg	Tartrazine. (#RPL 1234). Aqua, scored. In 100s.	13
Rx	**Exna** (Robins)		Tartrazine. (AHR 5449). Yellow, scored. In 100s.	11
Rx	**Hydrex** (Trimen)		White, scored. In 100s.	10
Rx	**Marazide** (Vortech)		In 100s.	7
Rx	**Proaqua** (Solvay Pharm.)		Tartrazine. (#RPL 1040). Aqua, scored. In 100s.	13

* Cost Index based on cost per 5 mg bendroflumethiazide, 5 mg methyclothiazide or 50 mg benzthiazide.

Product identification code.

Complete prescribing information for these products begins on page 557.

HYDROFLUMETHIAZIDE

Dosage:

Edema: Initial – 50 mg once or twice a day.
Maintenance – 25 mg to 200 mg daily. Administer in divided doses when dosage exceeds 100 mg daily.

Hypertension: Initial – 50 mg twice daily.
Maintenance – 50 to 100 mg/day. Do not exceed 200 mg/day.

	Product	Form/Strength	Description	C.I.*
Rx	**Hydroflumethiazide** (Various)	**Tablets:** 50 mg	In 100s, 500s and 1000s.	8+
Rx	**Diucardin** (Ayerst)		(#Diucardin 50). White, scored. In 100s.	18
Rx	**Saluron** (Bristol Labs.)		(#BL S2). Scored. In 100s.	27

TRICHLORMETHIAZIDE

Dosage:

Edema: 1 to 4 mg daily.

Hypertension: 2 to 4 mg daily.

	Product	Form/Strength	Description	C.I.*
Rx	**Trichlormethiazide** (Various)	**Tablets:** 2 mg	In 100s and 1000s.	2+
Rx	**Metahydrin** (Merrell Dow)		Tartrazine. (#Merrell 62). Pink. In 100s.	21
Rx	**Naqua** (Schering)		(#S AHG or 822). Pink. In 100s.	19
Rx	**Trichlormethiazide** (Various)	**Tablets:** 4 mg	In 100s and 1000s.	1+
Rx	**Diurese** (American Urologicals)		(#AU). Blue, scored. In 100s and 1000s.	7
Rx	**Metahydrin** (Merrell Dow)		Tartrazine. (#Merrell 63). Aqua. In 100s.	16
Rx	**Naqua** (Schering)		(#S AHH or 547). Aqua. In 100s and 1000s.	15
Rx	**Niazide** (Major)		In 100s and 1000s.	1
Rx	**Trichlorex** (Lannett)		Blue, scored. In 100s and 1000s.	2

POLYTHIAZIDE

Dosage:

Edema: 1 to 4 mg daily.

Hypertension: 2 to 4 mg daily.

	Product	Form/Strength	Description	C.I.*
Rx	**Renese** (Pfizer)	**Tablets:** 1 mg	(#375). White, scored. In 100s and 1000s.	44
		2 mg	(#376). Yellow, scored. In 100s and 1000s.	29
		4 mg	(#377). White, scored. In 100s and 1000s.	24

QUINETHAZONE

Dosage:

Adults: 50 to 100 mg once daily. Occasionally, 50 mg twice daily; 150 to 200 mg daily may be necessary infrequently.

	Product	Form/Strength	Description	C.I.*
Rx	**Hydromox** (Lederle)	**Tablets:** 50 mg	(#LL H1). White, scored. In 100s and 500s.	54

* Cost Index based on cost per 50 mg hydroflumethiazide, 2 mg trichlormethiazide, 2 mg polythiazide or 50 mg quinethazone.

Product identification code.

Complete prescribing information for these products begins on page 557.

METOLAZONE

Dosage: Individualize dosage.

Diulo and Zaroxolyn:

Mild to moderate essential hypertension – 2.5 to 5 mg once daily.

Edema of renal disease – 5 to 20 mg once daily.

Edema of cardiac failure – 5 to 10 mg once daily.

For patients with congestive failure and paroxysmal nocturnal dyspnea, employ a dosage near the upper end of the range to ensure action for 24 hours.

Mykrox: Mild to moderate hypertension – 0.5 mg as a single daily dose taken in the morning. If response is inadequate, increase the dose to 1 mg daily.

Do not increase dosage if blood pressure is not controlled with 1 mg Mykrox. Rather, add another antihypertensive agent with a different mechanism of action.

	Product	Form	Description	C.I.*
Rx	**Diulo** (Schiapparelli Searle)	**Tablets:** 2.5 mg	(Searle 501). Pink. In 100s.	34
		5 mg	(Searle 511). Blue. In 100s.	19
		10 mg	(Searle 521). Yellow. In 100s.	11
Rx	**Zaroxolyn** (Fisons)	**Tablets:** 2.5 mg	(2½). Pink. In 100s & UD 100s.	21
		5 mg	(5). Blue. In 100s, 500s, 1000s and UD 100s.	26
		10 mg	(10). Yellow. In 100s, 500s, 1000s and UD 100s.	12
Rx	**Mykrox** (Fisons)	**Tablets:** 0.5 mg	(Mykrox ½). In 100s, 500s & 1000s.	24

CHLORTHALIDONE

Dosage: Individualize dosage. Initiate therapy at lowest possible dose. Give a single dose with food in the morning. Maintenance doses may be lower than initial doses.

Edema: Initiate therapy with 50 to 100 mg daily, or 100 mg on alternate days. Some patients may require 150 or 200 mg at these intervals.

Hypertension: Initiate therapy with a single dose of 25 mg/day. If response is insufficient after a suitable trial, increase to 50 mg. For additional control, increase dosage to 100 mg once daily or add a second antihypertensive. Increases in serum uric acid and decreases in serum potassium are dose-related over the 25 to 100 mg/day range.

Note – Doses above 25 mg/day are likely to potentiate potassium excretion, but provide no further benefit in sodium excretion or blood pressure reduction.

	Product	Form	Description	C.I.*
Rx	**Thalitone** (Horus Therapeutics)	**Tablets:** 15 mg	Lactose. (HT1/77). In 100s.	NA
Rx	**Chlorthalidone** (Various)	**Tablets:** 25 mg	30s, 100s, 500s, 1000s, UD 100s.	6+
Rx	**Hygroton** (Rorer)		In 100s, 1000s and UD 100s.	52
Rx	**Hylidone** (Major)		In 100s, 250s, 1000s & UD 100s.	12
Rx	**Thalitone** (Horus Therapeutics)		Lactose. (HT1/76). In 100s.	NA
Rx	**Chlorthalidone** (Various)	**Tablets:** 50 mg	30s, 100s, 500s, 1000s, UD 100s.	4+
Rx	**Hygroton** (Rorer)		In 100s, 1000s and UD 100s.	32
Rx	**Hylidone** (Major)		In 100s, 250s, 1000s & UD 100s.	7
Rx	**Chlorthalidone** (Various)	**Tablets:** 100 mg	In 30s, 100s and UD 100s.	3+
Rx	**Hygroton** (Rorer)		In 100s, 1000s and UD 100s.	27
Rx	**Hylidone** (Major)		In 100s, 250s, 500s & 1000s.	4

INDAPAMIDE

Dosage: *Hypertension and edema of congestive heart failure: Adults* – 2.5 mg as a single daily dose taken in the morning. If the response is not satisfactory after 1 week (edema) to 4 weeks (hypertension), increase the dose to 5 mg once daily.

If the antihypertensive response is insufficient, combine with other antihypertensives. Reduce the usual dose of other agents by 50% during initial combination therapy. Further dosage adjustments may be necessary.

In general, doses of 5 mg and greater have not provided additional effects on blood pressure or heart failure, but are associated with a greater degree of hypokalemia. There is little experience with doses greater than 5 mg once daily.

	Product	Form	Description	C.I.*
Rx	**Lozol** (Rorer)	**Tablets:** 2.5 mg	White, film coated. In 100s, 1000s and UD 100s.	37

* Cost Index based on cost per 5 mg metolazone (0.5 mg *Mykrox*), 50 mg chlorthalidone or 2.5 mg indapamide.

Warning:
These are potent diuretics; excess amounts can lead to a profound diuresis with water and electrolyte depletion. Careful medical supervision is required and dosage must be individualized.

Actions:

Pharmacology: These agents inhibit the reabsorption of sodium and chloride, not only in the proximal and distal tubules, but also in the loop of Henle. Their high degree of efficacy is largely due to this unique site of action. The action on the distal tubule is independent of any inhibitory effect on carbonic anhydrase or aldosterone.

In contrast, bumetanide is more chloruretic than natriuretic and may have an additional action in the proximal tubule. It does not appear to act on the distal tubule.

Because ethacrynic acid inhibits the reabsorption to a much greater proportion of filtered sodium than most other diuretics, it may be effective in many patients with significant degrees of renal insufficiency.

Pharmacokinetics: All three drugs are metabolized and excreted primarily through the urine. Protein binding of these agents exceeds 90%. Furosemide is metabolized approximately 30% to 40%, and its urinary excretion is 60% to 70%. Significantly more furosemide is excreted in urine after IV injection than after the tablet or oral solution. Recent evidence suggests that furosemide glucuronide is the only, or at least the major, biotransformation product of furosemide.

Oral administration of bumetanide revealed that 81% was excreted in urine, 45% of it as unchanged drug. Bumetanide increases potassium excretion in a dose-related fashion; it also decreases uric acid excretion and increases serum uric acid. Urinary and biliary metabolites are formed by oxidation of the N-butyl side chain. Biliary excretion of bumetanide amounted to only 2% of the administered dose.

Pharmacokinetic variables of the loop diuretics are summarized below:

Diuretic	Bioavailability (%)	t½ (min)	Onset of action (min)	Peak (min)	Duration of action (hr)	Dosage (mg)	Relative potency	Frequency of administration (doses/day)
Furosemide (PO) (IV)	60-64[1]	≈ 120[2]	within 60 within 5	60-120[3] 30	6-8 2	20-80 20-40	1	1-2
Ethacrynic Acid (PO) (IV)	≈100	60	within 30 within 5	120 15-30	6-8 2	50-100 50	0.6-0.8	1-2 1
Bumetanide (PO) (IV)	72-96	60-90[4]	30-60 within minutes	60-120 15-45	4-6	0.5-2 0.5-1	40-60	1 1-3

[1] Decreased in uremia and nephrosis.
[2] Prolonged in renal failure, uremia, congestive heart failure (CHF), and in neonates.
[3] Decreased in CHF.
[4] Prolonged in renal disease.

Indications:

Edema associated with CHF, hepatic cirrhosis and renal disease, including the nephrotic syndrome. Particularly useful when greater diuretic potential is desired.

IV administration is indicated when a rapid onset of diuresis is desired (eg, acute pulmonary edema), when GI absorption is impaired or when oral medication is not practical.

Oral furosemide is also used to treat *hypertension,* alone or in combination with other antihypertensive drugs. Hypertensive patients who are inadequately controlled with thiazides may not be adequately controlled with furosemide alone. Also used as adjunctive therapy in acute pulmonary edema.

Ethacrynic acid is also indicated for short-term management of *ascites* due to malignancy, idiopathic edema and lymphedema, and for short-term management of hospitalized pediatric patients, other than infants, with *congenital heart disease.*

(Continued on following page)

Contraindications:

Anuria; history of hypersensitivity to these compounds.

Bumetanide is contraindicated in patients with hepatic coma or in states of severe electrolyte depletion until the condition is improved or corrected.

Do not treat infants with **ethacrynic acid**.

Warnings:

Dehydration: Excessive diuresis may result in dehydration and reduction in blood volume with circulatory collapse and the possibility of vascular thrombosis and embolism, particularly in elderly patients.

Hepatic cirrhosis and ascites: In these patients, initiate therapy in the hospital.

In hepatic coma and states of electrolyte depletion, do not institute therapy until the basic condition is improved. Sudden alterations of fluid and electrolyte balance in patients with cirrhosis may precipitate hepatic encephalopathy, coma and death; therefore, strict observation is necessary during the period of diuresis. Supplemental potassium chloride and, if required, an aldosterone antagonist are helpful in preventing hypokalemia and metabolic alkalosis.

Usage in impaired renal function: If increasing azotemia, oliguria or marked increases in BUN or creatinine occur during treatment of severe progressive renal disease, discontinue therapy.

If high dose parenteral **furosemide** therapy is used in patients with severely impaired renal function, controlled IV infusion is advisable. For adults, an infusion rate not exceeding 4 mg/min has been used.

Ototoxicity: Tinnitus, reversible hearing impairment, deafness and vertigo with a sense of fullness in the ears have been reported. Deafness is usually reversible and of short duration (1 to 24 hours); however, irreversible hearing impairment has occurred. Usually, ototoxicity is associated with rapid injection, with severe renal impairment, with doses several times the usual dose and with concurrent use with other ototoxic drugs.

Observe for blood dyscrasias, liver damage or idiosyncratic reactions.

Systemic lupus erythematosus may be exacerbated or activated.

Hypersensitivity: Patients with known sulfonamide sensitivity may show allergic reactions to **furosemide** or **bumetanide**. Bumetanide use following instances of allergic reactions to furosemide suggests a lack of cross-sensitivity. Have epinephrine 1:1000 immediately available. Refer to Management of Acute Hypersensitivity Reactions on p. 2897

Diarrhea: In a few patients, **ethacrynic acid** has produced severe, watery diarrhea. If this occurs, the drug should be discontinued and not readministered.

Because of the amount of sorbitol present in the vehicle of the **furosemide solution,** the possibility of diarrhea, especially in children, exists when higher dosages are given.

Usage in Pregnancy: Category B – Ethacrynic acid; Category C – Furosemide and bumetanide: There are no adequate and well controlled studies in pregnant women. Use only when clearly needed and when the potential benefits outweigh the potential hazards to the fetus.

Furosemide caused unexplained maternal deaths and abortions in rabbits when 25 to 100 mg/kg (2 to 8 times the maximum recommended human dose) was administered. No pregnant rabbits survived a dose of 100 mg/kg. Data indicate that fetal lethality can preceed maternal deaths. Studies in mice and rabbits showed an increased incidence of fetal hydronephrosis.

Bumetanide appears to be nonteratogenic, but has a slight embryocidal effect in rats when given in doses of 3400 times the maximum human therapeutic dose and in rabbits at doses of 3.4 times the maximum human therapeutic dose. In rabbits, a decrease in litter size and an increase in resorption rate were noted at oral doses 3.4 to 10 times the maximum human therapeutic dose.

Usage in Lactation: Furosemide appears in breast milk; such transfer of ethacrynic acid and bumetanide is unknown. Because of the potential for adverse reactions in nursing infants, decide whether to discontinue nursing or to discontinue the drug, taking into account the importance of the drug to the mother.

Usage in Children and Infants: Safety and efficacy for use of **bumetanide** or **IV ethacrynic acid** in children under 18 have not been established. Safety and efficacy of oral **ethacrynic acid** in infants have not been established (see Contraindications). **Furosemide** stimulates renal synthesis of prostaglandin E_2 and may increase the incidence of patent ductus arteriosus when given to premature infants with respiratory-distress syndrome.

Renal calcifications (from barely visible on x-ray to staghorn) have occurred in some severely premature infants treated with IV **furosemide** for edema due to patent ductus arteriosus and hyaline membrane disease. Concurrent use of chlorothiazide has reportedly decreased hypercalciuria and dissolved some calculi.

(Continued on following page)

Precautions:

Cardiovascular effects: Too vigorous a diuresis, as evidenced by rapid and excessive weight loss, may induce an acute hypotensive episode. In elderly cardiac patients, avoid rapid contraction of plasma volume and the resultant hemoconcentration to prevent thromboembolic episodes, such as cerebral vascular thromboses and pulmonary emboli.

Electrolyte imbalance may occur, especially in patients receiving high doses with restricted salt intake. Perform periodic determinations of serum electrolytes. Observe patients for signs of fluid or electrolyte imbalance (eg, hyponatremia, hypochloremic alkalosis and hypokalemia). Digitalis therapy may exaggerate metabolic effects of hypokalemia with reference to myocardial activity. Serum and urine electrolyte determinations are important in patients who are vomiting excessively, in patients who are receiving parenteral fluids, during brisk diuresis or when cirrhosis is present. Warning signs are dryness of mouth, thirst, anorexia, weakness, lethargy, drowsiness, restlessness, paresthesias, muscle pains or cramps, muscle fatigue, tetany (rarely), hypotension, oliguria, tachycardia, arrhythmia and GI disturbances (ie, nausea and vomiting).

Profound electrolyte and water loss may be avoided by weighing the patient periodically, adjusting dosage, initiating treatment with small doses and using the drugs intermittently. When excessive diuresis occurs, withdraw the drugs until homeostasis is restored. If excessive electrolyte loss occurs, reduce dosage or withdraw drug temporarily.

Hypokalemia prevention requires particular attention in patients receiving digitalis and diuretics for CHF, hepatic cirrhosis and ascites; in aldosterone excess with normal renal function; potassium-losing nephropathy; certain diarrheal states; or where hypokalemia is an added risk to the patient (eg, history of ventricular arrhythmias).

Possible drug-related deaths occurred with **ethacrynic acid** in critically ill patients refractory to other diuretics. There are two categories: Patients with severe myocardial disease who received digitalis and developed acute hypokalemia with fatal arrhythmia; or patients with severely decompensated hepatic cirrhosis with ascites, with or without encephalopathy, who had electrolyte imbalances and died because of intensification of the electrolyte defect. Liberalization of salt intake and supplementary potassium are often necessary.

Hypomagnesemia – Loop diuretics increase the urinary excretion of magnesium.

Laboratory tests: Asymptomatic hyperuricemia can occur, and rarely, gout may be precipitated. Reversible elevations of BUN may be seen, usually in association with dehydration, particularly in patients with renal insufficiency.

May lower serum calcium levels; rare cases of tetany have been reported.

Hypoproteinemia may reduce response to **ethacrynic acid**; consider the use of 25% normal serum albumin.

Increases in blood glucose and alterations in glucose tolerance tests (fasting and 2 hour postprandial sugar) have been observed. Rare cases of precipitation of diabetes mellitus have been reported. Although these effects have not been reported with **bumetanide**, the possibility of an effect on glucose metabolism exists.

Perform frequent serum electrolyte, calcium, glucose, uric acid, CO_2 and BUN determinations during the first few months of therapy and periodically thereafter.

Photosensitivity: Photosensitization (photoallergy and/or phototoxicity) may occur; therefore, caution patients to take protective measures (ie, sunscreens, protective clothing) against exposure to ultraviolet light or sunlight until tolerance is determined.

Drug Interactions:

Aminoglycoside antibiotics (parenteral): Coadministration of loop diuretics increases potential for ototoxicity. In impaired renal function, avoid excessive use.

Cisplatin: Coadministration with loop diuretics may increase potential for ototoxicity.

Digitalis glycosides: Diuretic-induced potassium loss may precipitate digitalis toxicity, possibly increasing the frequency of cardiac arrhythmias.

Indomethacin: Coadministration may reduce natriuretic and antihypertensive effects of loop diuretics due to inhibition of prostaglandin synthesis by indomethacin. Whether these effects are sustained during long-term administration has not been firmly established. **Sulindac** has a similar effect on bumetanide.

Lithium: Loop diuretics may increase the therapeutic and toxic effects (eg, GI symptoms, polyuria, muscular weakness, lethargy, tremor) of lithium. Monitor lithium levels and lower the dose if necessary.

(Drug Interactions continued on following page)

Drug Interactions (Cont.)

Metolazone: Profound diuresis and a greater than predicted electrolyte loss may occur when metolazone and furosemide are coadministered. This synergistic effect has been used in management of patients refractory to furosemide. The mechanism may be related to the ability of metolazone to block proximal tubular sodium reabsorption. This effect has been reported with other thiazide diuretics.

Nondepolarizing muscle relaxants: Furosemide causes increases and decreases in neuromuscular blocking effects of these agents. Action of **succinylcholine**, a depolarizing agent, and **tubocurarine** may be potentiated by low doses, reversed with high doses.

Warfarin: Ethacrynic acid may increase the hypoprothrombinemic effect of warfarin. Furosemide and bumetanide do not appear to interact.

Drug/Food: The bioavailability of furosemide is decreased and its degree of diuresis reduced when administered with food.

Adverse Reactions:

GI: Anorexia, nausea, vomiting, diarrhea, acute pancreatitis, jaundice, pain.

CNS: Vertigo, headache, blurred vision, tinnitus, irreversible hearing loss, dizziness.

Hematologic: Thrombocytopenia and agranulocytosis.

Other: Rash; occasionally, local irritation and pain have occurred with parenteral use.

Laboratory abnormalities: Hyperuricemia; hypochloremia; hypokalemia; azotemia; hyponatremia; increased serum creatinine; hyperglycemia; variations in phosphorus, CO_2 content, bicarbonate and calcium.

Furosemide:

GI – Oral and gastric irritation, constipation.

CNS – Paresthesia; xanthopsia; restlessness.

Hematologic – Anemia, leukopenia and purpura. Rarely, aplastic anemia.

Dermatologic/Hypersensitivity – Photosensitivity, urticaria, pruritus, necrotizing angiitis (vasculitis, cutaneous vasculitis), exfoliative dermatitis, erythema multiforme.

Cardiovascular – Orthostatic hypotension may occur and be aggravated by alcohol, barbiturates or narcotics; thrombophlebitis; chronic aortitis.

Other – Glycosuria, muscle spasm, weakness, urinary bladder spasm.

Ethacrynic acid:

GI – Sudden watery, profuse diarrhea; GI bleeding; dysphagia.

Metabolic – Acute symptomatic hypoglycemia with convulsions occurred in two uremic patients who received doses above those recommended.

Hematologic – Severe neutropenia has been reported in a few critically ill patients also receiving agents known to produce this effect. Rare instances of Henoch-Schönlein purpura have been reported in patients with rheumatic heart disease receiving many drugs, including ethacrynic acid.

Other – Fever, chills, hematuria, apprehension, confusion, fatigue, malaise, acute gout and sense of fullness in the ears. Abnormal liver function tests occur rarely in seriously ill patients on multiple drug therapy that included ethacrynic acid.

Bumetanide:

CNS – Asterixis; encephalopathy with preexisting liver disease; impaired hearing; ear discomfort.

GI – Upset stomach; dry mouth.

GU – Premature ejaculation; difficulty maintaining erection; renal failure.

Musculoskeletal – Weakness; arthritic pain; pain; muscle cramps; fatigue.

Cardiovascular – Hypotension; ECG changes; chest pain.

Other – Hives; pruritus; dehydration; sweating; hyperventilation; nipple tenderness.

Lab abnormalities – Diuresis rarely ($\leq$ 1%) accompanied by changes in LDH, total serum bilirubin, serum proteins, AST, ALT, alkaline phosphatase, cholesterol and creatinine clearance. Also, deviations in hemoglobin, prothrombin time, hematocrit, WBC, platelet counts and differential counts; also increases in urinary glucose and protein.

Overdosage:

Symptoms: Acute profound water loss, volume and electrolyte depletion, dehydration, reduction of blood volume, and circulatory collapse with a possibility of vascular thrombosis and embolism. Electrolyte depletion may be manifested by weakness, dizziness, mental confusion, anorexia, lethargy, vomiting and cramps.

Treatment: Replace fluid and electrolyte losses by careful monitoring of the urine and electrolyte output and serum electrolyte levels. Assure adequate drainage in patients with urinary bladder outlet obstruction (such as prostatic hypertrophy). Hemodialysis does not accelerate furosemide elimination. Induce emesis or perform gastric lavage. If required, give oxygen or artificial respiration. Treatment includes supportive measures. Refer to General Management of Acute Overdosage on p. 2895

(Continued on following page)

Patient Information:

May cause GI upset; take with food or milk (see Drug Interactions).

Drug will increase urination; take early in the day.

Notify physician if muscle weakness, cramps, nausea or dizziness occurs.

Postural hypotension may occur; get up slowly.

Diabetes mellitus patients: May increase blood glucose levels, affecting urine glucose tests.

Photosensitivity may occur in some patients.

Hypertensive patients should avoid medications that may increase blood pressure, including *otc* products for appetite suppression and cold symptoms.

Administration:

Individualize therapy. Reserve parenteral use for patients in whom oral medication is not practical or in emergency situations. Replace with oral therapy as soon as practical.

Concomitant administration: Concurrent metolazone and furosemide have been used in the management of patients refractory to furosemide due to their synergistic effect on diuresis (see Drug Interactions). Metolazone 2.5 to 10 mg is added to the therapy, and the dose is doubled every 24 hours until the desired response is achieved. Decrease the furosemide dose if the synergism occurs with the first dose of metolazone. Hydrochlorothiazide (50 mg) may be used and may be safer because of its shorter action.

FUROSEMIDE

Dosage:

Oral:

Edema – Initial dose: 20 to 80 mg/day as a single dose. Ordinarily, prompt diuresis ensues. Depending on response, administer a second dose 6 to 8 hours later. If response is not satisfactory, increase by increments of 20 or 40 mg, no sooner than 6 to 8 hours after previous dose, until desired diuresis occurs. This dose should then be given once or twice daily (eg, at 8 am and 2 pm). Dosage may be titrated up to 600 mg/day in patients with severe edema.

Mobilization of edema may be most efficiently and safely accomplished with an intermittent dosage schedule; drug is given 2 to 4 consecutive days each week. With doses exceeding 80 mg/day, clinical and laboratory observations are advisable.

Hypertension – Initial dose: 40 mg twice a day; adjust according to response. If the patient does not respond, add other antihypertensive agents. Observe blood pressure changes when used with other antihypertensives, especially during initial therapy. Reduce dosage of other agents by at least 50% as soon as furosemide is added, to prevent excessive drop in blood pressure. As blood pressure falls, reduce dose or discontinue other antihypertensives.

Infants and children – Initial dose: 2 mg/kg. If diuresis is unsatisfactory, increase by 1 or 2 mg/kg, no sooner than 6 to 8 hours after previous dose. Doses > 6 mg/kg are not recommended. For maintenance therapy, adjust dose to the minimum effective level.

Parenteral:

Edema – Initial dose: 20 to 40 mg IM or IV. Give the IV injection slowly (1 to 2 minutes); ordinarily, prompt diuresis ensues. If needed, another dose may be given in the same manner 2 hours later. The dose may be raised by 20 mg and given no sooner than 2 hours after previous dose, until desired diuretic effect is obtained. This dose should then be given once or twice daily. Administer high dose parenteral therapy as a controlled infusion at a rate not exceeding 4 mg/min.

Acute pulmonary edema – The usual initial dose is 40 mg IV (over 1 to 2 minutes). If response is not satisfactory within 1 hour, increase to 80 mg IV (over 1 to 2 minutes). Additional therapy (eg, digitalis, oxygen) may be administered concomitantly.

Infants and children – Initial dose (IV or IM): 1 mg/kg given slowly under close supervision. If diuretic response after the initial dose is not satisfactory, increase dosage by 1 mg/kg, no sooner than 2 hours after previous dose, until desired effect is obtained. Doses greater than 6 mg/kg are not recommended.

IV incompatibility – Furosemide is a mildly buffered alkaline solution; do not mix with highly acidic solutions of pH below 5.5. Isotonic saline, Lactated Ringer's Injection and 5% Dextrose Injection have been used after pH has been adjusted when necessary. Freshly prepare mixtures and use within 24 hours. A precipitate formed when furosemide was admixed with gentamicin or netilmicin in 5% Dextrose or 0.9% Sodium Chloride, but not with amikacin, kanamycin or tobramycin.

Stability: Exposure to light may cause slight discoloration; do not dispense discolored tablets or use discolored injection. Store injection and oral solution at room temperature (59°F-86°F).

(Products listed on following page)

Complete prescribing information for these products begins on page 567.

FUROSEMIDE (Cont.)				C.I.*
Rx	**Furosemide** (Various)	**Tablets:** 20 mg	In 30s, 100s, 500s, 1000s and UD 32s and 100s.	3+
Rx	**Fumide** (Everett)		In 100s and 1000s.	16
Rx	**Lasix** (Hoechst-Roussel)		(#Lasix/Hoechst). White. In 100s, 500s, 1000s and UD 100s.	18
Rx	**Luramide** (Major)		In 100s, 1000s and UD 100s.	8
Rx	**Furosemide** (Various)	**Tablets:** 40 mg	In 30s, 100s, 500s, 1000s and UD 32s and 100s.	2+
Rx	**Fumide** (Everett)		In 100s and 1000s.	12
Rx	**Lasix** (Hoechst-Roussel)		(#Lasix 40). White, scored. In 30s, 60s, 100s, 500s, 1000s and UD 100s.	11
Rx	**Luramide** (Major)		In 100s, 500s, 1000s and UD 100s.	5
Rx	**Furosemide** (Various)	**Tablets:** 80 mg	In 50s, 100s, 500s and UD 100s.	4+
Rx	**Lasix** (Hoechst-Roussel)		(#Lasix 80). White. In 50s, 500s and UD 100s.	10
Rx	**Luramide** (Major)		In 100s, 500s and UD 100s.	8
Rx *sf*	**Furosemide** (Roxane)	**Oral Solution:** 10 mg per ml	Sorbitol, 0.02% alcohol. Sodium free. Orange flavor. In 60 ml.	42
Rx	**Lasix** (Hoechst-Roussel)		Sorbitol, 11.5% alcohol. Orange flavor. In 60 and 120 ml.	50
Rx *sf*	**Furosemide** (Roxane)	**Oral Solution:** 40 mg per 5 ml	Sorbitol, 0.2% alcohol. Sodium free. Pineapple/peach flavor. In 5, 10 and 500 ml.	18
Rx	**Furosemide** (Various)	**Injection:** 10 mg per ml	In 2, 4 and 10 ml amps; 2, 4, 8 and 10 ml vials and 2, 4, 5, 6, 8, 10 and 12 ml syringes.	23+
Rx	**Furomide M.D.** (Hyrex)		In 10 ml multiple-dose vials.	356
Rx	**Lasix** (Hoechst-Roussel)		In 2, 4 and 10 ml amps, syringes and vials.	202

* Cost Index based on cost per 40 mg.
# Product identification code.
sf – Sugar free.

Complete prescribing information for these products begins on page 567.

ETHACRYNIC ACID

Administration and Dosage:

Oral initial therapy: Give minimally effective dose (usually, 50 to 200 mg daily) on a continuous or intermittent dosage schedule to produce gradual weight loss (1 to 2 lbs/day). Adjust dose in 25 to 50 mg increments. Higher doses, up to 200 mg twice daily, achieved gradually, are most often required in patients with severe, refractory edema.

Children – Initial dose is 25 mg. Make careful increments of 25 mg to achieve maintenance. Dosage for infants has not been established.

Oral maintenance therapy: Administer intermittently after an effective diuresis is obtained using an alternate daily schedule or more prolonged periods of diuretic therapy interspersed with rest periods. This allows time to correct any electrolyte imbalance and may provide a more efficient diuretic response. The chloruretic effect may cause retention of bicarbonate and metabolic alkalosis. Correct by giving chloride (ammonium chloride or arginine chloride). Do not give ammonium chloride to cirrhotic patients.

Concomitant diuretic therapy – Ethacrynic acid has additive effects when used with other diuretics; therefore, the initial dose should be 25 mg and changes in dose should be in 25 mg increments to avoid electrolyte depletion.

Parenteral: Do not give SC or IM because of local pain and irritation. The usual IV dose for the average adult is 50 mg, or 0.5 to 1 mg/kg. Give slowly through the tubing of a running infusion or by direct IV injection over several minutes. Usually, only one dose is necessary; occasionally, a second dose may be required; use a new injection site to avoid thrombophlebitis. A single IV dose, not exceeding 100 mg, has been used. Insufficient pediatric experience precludes recommendation for this age group.

Preparation of solution: Add 50 ml of 5% Dextrose Injection or Sodium Chloride Injection to vial. 5% Dextrose Injection solutions may have a low pH (< 5); the resulting solution may be hazy or opalescent. Use of such a solution is not recommended. Do not mix this solution with whole blood or its derivatives. Discard unused reconstituted solution after 24 hours. **C.I.***

Rx	**Edecrin** (MSD)	**Tablets:** 25 mg	(#MSD 65). White, scored. In 100s.	41
		50 mg	(#MSD 90). Green, scored. In 100s.	29
Rx	**Edecrin Sodium** (MSD)	**Powder for Injection:** 50 mg (as ethacrynate sodium) per vial	In 50 ml vials for reconstitution.[1]	1295

BUMETANIDE

Administration and Dosage:

Because cross-sensitivity with furosemide is rare, bumetanide can be substituted at about a 1:40 ratio of bumetanide to furosemide in patients allergic to furosemide.

Oral: 0.5 to 2 mg/day, given as a single dose. If diuretic response is not adequate, give a second or third dose at 4 to 5 hour intervals, up to a maximum daily dose of 10 mg. An intermittent dose schedule, given on alternate days or for 3 to 4 days with rest periods of 1 to 2 days in between, is the safest and most effective method for the continued control of edema. In patients with hepatic failure, keep the dose to a minimum, and if necessary, increase the dose carefully.

Parenteral: Reserve for patients in whom GI absorption may be impaired or in whom oral administration is not practical.

Initially, 0.5 to 1 mg IV or IM. Administer IV over a period of 1 to 2 minutes. If the initial response is insufficient, give a second or third dose at intervals of 2 to 3 hours; do not exceed a daily dosage of 10 mg. End parenteral treatment and start oral treatment as soon as possible.

Stability: Bumetanide injection with 5% Dextrose in Water, 0.9% Sodium Chloride and Lactated Ringer's Solution in glass and plasticized PVC *(Viaflex)* containers have no significant absorption effects or loss due to drug degradation. However, freshly prepare solutions and use within 24 hours. **C.I.***

Rx	**Bumex** (Roche)	**Tablets:** 0.5 mg	(#Roche Bumex 0.5). Green, scored. In 30s, 100s, 500s and UD 100s.	15
		1 mg	(#Roche Bumex 1). Yellow, scored. In 30s, 100s, 500s and UD 100s.	10
		2 mg	(#Roche Bumex 2). In 100s and UD 100s.	9
		Injection: 0.25 mg per ml	In 2 ml amps[2] & 2, 4, 10 ml vials.[2]	132

* Cost Index based on cost per 50 mg ethacrynic acid or 0.5 mg bumetanide.
\# Product identification code.
[1] With 62.5 mg mannitol and 0.1 mg thimerosal. [2] With 0.01% EDTA and 1% benzyl alcohol.

In the kidney, potassium is filtered at the glomerulus and then absorbed parallel to sodium throughout the proximal tubule and thick ascending limb of the loop of Henle, so that only minor amounts reach the distal convoluted tubule. As a result, potassium appearing in urine is secreted at the distal tubule and collecting duct. The potassium sparing diuretics interfere with sodium reabsorption at the distal tubule, thus decreasing potassium secretion. They exert a weak diuretic and antihypertensive effect when used alone. Their major use is to enhance the action and counteract the kaliuretic effect of thiazides and loop diuretics.

Spironolactone, a competitive inhibitor of aldosterone, binds to aldosterone receptors of the distal tubule and prevents the formation of a protein important in sodium transport. The dose of spironolactone required to produce an effect varies according to the amount of aldosterone present. It is effective in both primary and secondary hyperaldosteronism. Spironolactone is effective in lowering systolic and diastolic blood pressure in both primary hyperaldosteronism and essential hypertension, although aldosterone secretion may be normal in benign essential hypertension. In addition, spironolactone interferes with testosterone synthesis and may increase peripheral conversion of testosterone to estradiol. This action may be responsible for endocrine abnormalities occasionally noted with therapy.

Amiloride and **triamterene** not only inhibit sodium reabsorption induced by aldosterone, but also inhibit basal sodium reabsorption. They are not aldosterone antagonists, but act directly on the renal distal tubule. They induce a reversal of polarity of the transtubular electrical-potential difference and inhibit active transport of sodium and potassium. Amiloride may inhibit sodium and potassium-ATPase. Amiloride decreases the enhanced urinary excretion of magnesium which occurs when a thiazide or loop diuretic is used alone.

The pharmacological and pharmacokinetic properties of the potassium sparing diuretics are summarized in the following table:

Potassium-Sparing Diuretics

Parameters	Diuretics		
	Amiloride	**Spironolactone**	**Triamterene**
Pharmacology:			
Tubular site of action	Proximal + distal	Distal	Distal
Mechanism of action	Na^+; K^+-ATPase inhibition	Aldosterone antagonism	Membrane effect
Action:			
Onset (hours)	2	24 to 48	2 to 4
Peak (hours)	6 to 10	48 to 72	6 to 8
Duration (hours)	24	48 to 72	12 to 16
Pharmacokinetics:			
Bioavailability	15% to 25%	> 90%	30% to 70%
Protein Binding	23%	98 +%[1]	50% to 67%
Half-life (hours)	6 to 9	20[2]	3
Active metabolites	none	canrenone	hydroxytriamterene sulfate
Peak plasma levels (hours)	3 to 4	canrenone: 2 to 4[3]	—
Excreted unchanged in urine	50%[4]	†	≈ 20%
Daily dose (mg)	5 to 20	25 to 200	200 to 300

[1] canrenone > 90%.
[2] 10 to 35 hours for canrenone.
[3] 1st phase of decline – 3 to 12 hours.
2nd phase of decline – 12 to 96 hours.
[4] 40% excreted in stool within 72 hours.
† metabolites primarily excreted in urine, but also in bile.

(Products listed on following pages)

Refer to the general discussion of these agents beginning on page 574.

AMILORIDE HCl

Indications:

Adjunctive treatment with thiazide or loop diuretics in congestive heart failure (CHF) or hypertension to: Help restore normal serum potassium in patients who develop hypokalemia on the kaliuretic diuretic; prevent hypokalemia in patients who would be at particular risk if hypokalemia were to develop (eg, digitalized patients or patients with significant cardiac arrhythmias).

Contraindications:

Hypersensitivity to amiloride.

Hyperkalemia: Do not use if serum potassium is greater than 5.5 mEq/L.

Antikaliuretic therapy or potassium supplementation: Do not give to patients receiving spironolactone or triamterene. Do not use potassium supplementation (medication or a potassium rich diet) with amiloride, except in severe or refractory cases of hypokalemia. Such concomitant therapy can be associated with rapid increases in serum potassium levels. If potassium supplementation is used, monitor serum potassium.

Impaired renal function: Anuria, acute or chronic renal insufficiency and evidence of diabetic nephropathy are contraindications because potassium retention is accentuated and may result in the rapid development of hyperkalemia. Do not give to patients with evidence of renal impairment (BUN > 30 mg/dl or serum creatinine > 1.5 mg/dl) or diabetes mellitus without continuous monitoring of serum electrolytes, creatinine and BUN levels.

Warnings:

Hyperkalemia: Amiloride may cause hyperkalemia which, if uncorrected, is potentially fatal. Hyperkalemia occurs commonly (about 10%) when amiloride is used alone. This incidence is greater in patients with renal impairment, diabetes mellitus (with or without recognized renal insufficiency) and in the elderly. When amiloride is used concomitantly with a thiazide diuretic in patients without these complications, the risk of hyperkalemia is reduced to about 1% to 2%. Monitor serum potassium carefully, particularly when amiloride is first introduced, at the time of diuretic dosage adjustments and during any illness that could affect renal function.

Symptoms of hyperkalemia include paresthesias, muscular weakness, fatigue, flaccid paralysis of the extremities, bradycardia, shock, and ECG abnormalities. The ECG in hyperkalemia is characterized primarily by tall, peaked T waves or elevations from previous tracings. There may also be lowering of the R wave, increased depth of the S wave, widening or disappearance of the P wave, progressive widening of the QRS complex, prolongation of the PR interval, and ST depression. Mild hyperkalemia is not usually associated with an abnormal ECG.

Treatment - Discontinue the drug immediately. Monitor ECG and serum potassium levels. If serum potassium exceeds 6.5 mEq/L, take active measures to reduce it, including IV sodium bicarbonate solution or oral or parenteral glucose with rapid-acting insulin. If needed, give sodium polystyrene sulfonate orally or by enema. Persistent hyperkalemia may require dialysis.

Diabetes mellitus: Hyperkalemia has been reported with the use of amiloride, even in patients without evidence of diabetic nephropathy. If possible, avoid use of amiloride in diabetic patients. If it is used, monitor serum electrolytes and renal function frequently. Discontinue use at least 3 days before glucose tolerance testing.

Metabolic or respiratory acidosis: Cautiously institute amiloride in severely ill patients in whom respiratory or metabolic acidosis may occur, such as patients with cardiopulmonary disease or poorly controlled diabetes. Monitor acid-base balance frequently. Shifts in acid-base balance alter the ratio of extracellular/intracellular potassium; the development of acidosis may be associated with rapid increases in serum potassium.

Usage in Pregnancy: Category B. There are no adequate and well controlled studies in pregnant women. Safety for use during pregnancy has not been established. Use only when clearly needed and when the potential benefits outweigh the unknown hazards to the fetus. See also discussion of thiazide diuretic use during pregnancy.

Usage in Lactation: Safety for use in the nursing mother has not been established. Studies in rats have shown that amiloride is excreted in milk in concentrations higher than those found in blood. It is not known whether it is excreted in breast milk. Because of the potential for serious adverse reactions in nursing infants, a decision should be made whether to discontinue nursing or to discontinue the drug, taking into account the importance of the drug to the mother.

Usage in Children: Safety and efficacy for use in children have not been established.

(Continued on following page)

AMILORIDE HCl (Cont.)

Precautions:

Electrolyte imbalance and BUN increases: Hyponatremia and hypochloremia may occur when amiloride is used with other diuretics. Increases in BUN levels usually accompany vigorous fluid elimination, especially when diuretic therapy is used in seriously ill patients, such as those who have hepatic cirrhosis with ascites and metabolic alkalosis, or those with resistant edema. Carefully monitor serum electrolytes and BUN levels. In patients with preexisting severe liver disease, hepatic encephalopathy, manifested by tremors, confusion and coma, and increased jaundice, may occur in association with amiloride.

Because amiloride is not metabolized by the liver, drug accumulation is not anticipated in patients with hepatic dysfunction, but accumulation can occur if hepatorenal syndrome develops.

Drug Interactions:

Angiotensin-converting enzyme inhibitors decrease aldosterone production which may result in an elevation of serum potassium. Concurrent use with amiloride may lead to significant hyperkalemia.

Digoxin: A study in six healthy subjects showed that amiloride increased the renal clearance and decreased the nonrenal clearance of digoxin. It also appeared to decrease the inotropic effect of digoxin. The clinical significance of these findings in patients with congestive heart failure is unknown.

Lithium generally should not be given with diuretics because they reduce its renal clearance and add a high risk of lithium toxicity.

Potassium preparations: Coadministration with amiloride may result in hyperkalemia, possibly with cardiac arrhythmias or cardiac arrest. Avoid coadministration especially in patients with impaired renal function.

Adverse Reactions:

CNS: Headache (3% to 8%), dizziness and encephalopathy ($>$ 1%); paresthesia, tremors, vertigo, nervousness, mental confusion, insomnia, decreased libido, depression, somnolence ($\leq$ 1%).

GI: Nausea, anorexia, diarrhea, and vomiting (3% to 8%); abdominal pain, gas pain, appetite changes, constipation ($>$ 1%); jaundice, GI bleeding, abdominal fullness, thirst, dry mouth, heartburn, flatulence, dyspepsia ($\leq$ 1%).

Metabolic: Elevated serum potassium levels ($>$ 5.5 mEq/L), ($>$ 1%).

Musculoskeletal: Weakness, fatigue, muscle cramps ($>$ 1%); joint pain, back pain, chest pain, neck or shoulder ache, pain of the extremities ($\leq$ 1%).

Respiratory: Cough and dyspnea ($>$ 1%). Shortness of breath ($\leq$ 1%).

GU: Impotence ($>$ 1%); polyuria, dysuria, urinary frequency, and bladder spasms ($\leq$ 1%).

Cardiovascular: Angina, orthostatic hypotension, arrhythmia and palpitations.

Dermatologic: Skin rash, itching, pruritus and alopecia.

Special senses: Visual disturbances, nasal congestion, tinnitus and increased intraocular pressure.

(Continued on following page)

AMILORIDE HCl (Cont.)

Overdosage:

Symptoms: The most likely signs are dehydration and electrolyte imbalance.

Treatment: Discontinue therapy and observe patient closely. Induce emesis or perform gastric lavage. Treatment is symptomatic and supportive. Refer to General Management of Acute Overdosage on **2895** If hyperkalemia occurs, reduce the serum potassium levels (see Warnings). It is not known whether amiloride is dialyzable.

Patient Information:

May cause GI upset; take with food.

Notify physician if any of the following occurs: Muscular weakness, fatigue, muscle cramps or weakness.

May cause dizziness, headache or visual disturbances; observe caution while driving or performing other tasks requiring alertness.

Avoid large quantities of potassium rich food.

Administration and Dosage:

Administer with food.

Concomitant therapy: Add amiloride 5 mg/day to the usual antihypertensive or diuretic dosage of a kaliuretic diuretic. Increase dosage to 10 mg/day, if necessary. If persistent hypokalemia is documented with 10 mg, increase the dose to 15 mg, then 20 mg, with careful titration of the dose and careful monitoring of electrolytes.

In patients with CHF, potassium loss may decrease after an initial diuresis; reevaluate the need or dosage for amiloride. Maintenance therapy may be intermittent.

Single drug therapy (see Warnings): The starting dose is 5 mg/day. Increase to 10 mg/day, if necessary. If persistent hypokalemia is documented with 10 mg, increase the dose to 15 mg, then 20 mg, with careful monitoring of electrolytes.

	Product	Form	Description	**C.I.***
Rx	**Amiloride HCl** (Various)	**Tablets:** 5 mg	In 100s, 500s and 1000s.	16+
Rx	**Midamor** (MSD)		(#MSD 92). Yellow. In 100s.	31

* Cost Index based on cost per 5 mg.
# Product identification code.

Refer to the general discussion of these agents beginning on page 574.

SPIRONOLACTONE

> **Warning:**
> Spironolactone has been shown to be a tumorigen in chronic toxicity studies in rats (see Warnings). Use only in those conditions described in the Indications section.

Indications:

Primary hyperaldosteronism: Diagnosis of primary hyperaldosteronism.

Short-term preoperative treatment of patients with primary hyperaldosteronism.

Long-term maintenance therapy for patients with discrete aldosterone-producing adrenal adenomas who are poor operative risks, or who decline surgery.

Long-term maintenance therapy for patients with bilateral micronodular or macronodular adrenal hyperplasia (idiopathic hyperaldosteronism).

Edematous conditions when other therapies are inappropriate or inadequate:

CHF – Management of edema and sodium retention; also indicated with digitalis.

Cirrhosis of the liver accompanied by edema or ascites for maintenance therapy in conjunction with bed rest and the restriction of fluid and sodium.

Nephrotic syndrome.

Essential hypertension, usually in combination with other drugs.

Hypokalemia and the prophylaxis of hypokalemia in patients taking digitalis.

Unlabeled Uses: Spironolactone has been used in the treatment of hirsutism (50 to 200 mg/day) due to its antiandrogenic properties. One study suggested that a lower dosage (50 mg twice daily on days 4 through 21 of the menstrual cycle) may help minimize the risk of menorrhagia that occurs with higher doses.

Symptoms of premenstrual syndrome (PMS) have been relieved at a dosage of 25 mg 4 times daily beginning on day 14 of the menstrual cycle.

Contraindications:

Anuria; acute renal insufficiency; significant impairment of renal function; hyperkalemia.

Warnings:

Carcinogenicity: Spironolactone has been shown to be a tumorigen in chronic toxicity studies in rats. At 25 to 250 times the usual human dose, there was a dose-related increase in benign adenomas of the thyroid and testes, in malignant mammary tumors and in proliferative changes in the liver. At 500 mg/kg, the effects included hepatocytomegaly, hyperplastic liver nodules and hepatocellular carcinoma. A dose-related (above 20 mg/kg/day) incidence of myelocytic leukemia was observed in rats fed daily doses of potassium canrenoate. In the rat, myelocytic leukemia and hepatic, thyroid, testicular and mammary tumors were observed.

Usage in Pregnancy: Spironolactone or its metabolites may cross the placental barrier. Feminization occurs in male rat fetuses. Weigh anticipated benefit against possible hazard to the fetus. See also discussion of thiazide diuretic use during pregnancy.

Usage in Lactation: Canrenone, a metabolite of spironolactone, appears in breast milk. If use of spironolactone is essential, institute an alternative method of infant feeding.

Precautions:

Hyperkalemia: Carefully evaluate patients for possible fluid and electrolyte balance disturbances. Hyperkalemia may occur in patients with impaired renal function or excessive potassium intake and can cause cardiac arrhythmias which may be fatal. No potassium supplement should ordinarily be given with spironolactone.

Treat hyperkalemia promptly by IV glucose (20% to 50%) and regular insulin, using 0.25 to 0.5 units of insulin/g of glucose. This is a temporary measure to be repeated as required. Treatment of hyperkalemia may also include: IV calcium to antagonize effects on the heart; bicarbonate if patient is acidotic; or sodium polystyrene sulfonate exchange resin to remove potassium. Discontinue spironolactone and restrict potassium intake (including dietary potassium).

Hyponatremia may be caused or aggravated by spironolactone, especially in combination with other diuretics. Symptoms include dry mouth, thirst, lethargy and drowsiness.

Gynecomastia may develop and appears to be related to both dosage and duration of therapy. It is normally reversible when therapy is discontinued; however, in rare instances, some breast enlargement may persist.

Usage in impaired renal function may cause a transient elevation of BUN, especially in patients with preexisting renal impairment. The drug may cause mild acidosis.

Reversible hyperchloremic metabolic acidosis, usually in association with hyperkalemia, occurs in some patients with decompensated hepatic cirrhosis, even in the presence of normal renal function.

(Continued on following page)

SPIRONOLACTONE (Cont.)

Drug Interactions:

Angiotensin converting enzyme inhibitors decrease aldosterone production, which may result in an elevation of serum potassium. Concurrent use with spironolactone may lead to significant hyperkalemia.

Digitalis glycosides: The interaction between spironolactone and digitalis glycosides is complex and difficult to predict. Spironolactone increases the half-life of **digoxin** and can decrease digoxin clearance. This may result in increased serum digoxin levels and subsequent digitalis toxicity. Reduce maintenance and digitalization doses if necessary when spironolactone is administered. Carefully monitor the patient to avoid over- or underdigitalization. In addition, spironolactone may blunt the inotropic action of digoxin. Spironolactone both decreases and increases the elimination half-life of **digitoxin.** Further studies are needed.

Mitotane: One patient failed to respond to mitotane while receiving concurrent spironolactone. The patient developed mitotane toxicity when spironolactone was discontinued.

Potassium preparations: Coadministration with spironolactone may result in hyperkalemia, possibly with cardiac arrhythmias or cardiac arrest. Avoid coadministration, especially in patients with impaired renal function.

Salicylates: The diuretic effect of spironolactone may be decreased by concurrent salicylate use, possibly due to reduced tubular secretion of canrenone; this interaction is dose-dependent. The antihypertensive action does not appear altered.

Drug/Food: The administration of spironolactone with food appears to increase its absorption. In one study, the AUC and maximum serum concentration of spironolactone were significantly increased by food.

Drug/Lab Tests: Spironolactone and its metabolites can interfere with the radioimmunoassay for measuring **digoxin**, resulting in falsely elevated serum digoxin values.

Adverse Reactions:

Adverse reactions are usually reversible upon discontinuation of the drug and include:

GI: Cramping, diarrhea, gastric bleeding, ulceration, gastritis and vomiting.

CNS: Drowsiness, lethargy, headache, mental confusion, ataxia.

Endocrine: Inability to achieve or maintain erection; gynecomastia; irregular menses or amenorrhea; postmenopausal bleeding; hirsutism; deepening of the voice.

Dermatologic: Maculopapular or erythematous cutaneous eruptions; urticaria.

Other: Drug fever; hyperchloremic metabolic acidosis in decompensated hepatic cirrhosis; carcinoma of the breast (cause and effect relationship not established); agranulocytosis.

Patient Information:

May produce drowsiness, ataxia and mental confusion; observe caution while driving or performing other tasks requiring alertness.

May cause GI cramping, diarrhea, lethargy, thirst, headache, skin rash, menstrual abnormalities, deepening of the voice and breast enlargement. Notify physician if these effects occur.

(Continued on following page)

SPIRONOLACTONE (Cont.)

Administration and Dosage:

Spironolactone may be administered in single or divided doses.

Diagnosis of primary hyperaldosteronism: As an initial diagnostic measure to provide presumptive evidence of primary hyperaldosteronism in patients on normal diets, as follows:

Long test – 400 mg/day for 3 to 4 weeks. Correction of hypokalemia and hypertension provides presumptive evidence for the diagnosis of primary hyperaldosteronism.

Short test – 400 mg/day for 4 days. If serum potassium increases, but decreases when spironolactone is discontinued, consider a presumptive diagnosis of primary hyperaldosteronism.

Maintenance therapy for hyperaldosteronism: 100 to 400 mg daily in preparation for surgery. For patients unsuitable for surgery, employ the drug for long-term maintenance therapy at lowest possible dose.

Edema:

Adults (CHF, hepatic cirrhosis, nephrotic syndrome) – Initially, 100 mg/day (range 25 to 200 mg/day). When given as the sole diuretic agent, continue for at least 5 days at the initial dosage level, then adjust to the optimal level. If after 5 days an adequate diuretic response has not occurred, add a second diuretic, which acts more proximally in the renal tubule. Because of the additive effect of spironolactone with such diuretics, an enhanced diuresis usually begins on the first day of combined treatment; combined therapy is indicated when more rapid diuresis is desired. The dosage of spironolactone should remain unchanged when other diuretic therapy is added.

Children – 1.5 mg/lb/day (3.3 mg/kg/day).

For *small children,* tablets may be pulverized and administered as a suspension in cherry syrup, NF. When refrigerated, this suspension is stable for 1 month.

Essential hypertension:

Adults – Initially, 50 to 100 mg/day. May also be combined with diuretics, which act more proximally, and with other antihypertensive agents. Continue treatment for at least 2 weeks since the maximal response may not occur sooner. Individualize dosage.

Hypokalemia: 25 to 100 mg/day. Useful in treating diuretic-induced hypokalemia when oral potassium supplements or other potassium-sparing regimens are considered inappropriate.

				C.I.*
Rx	**Spironolactone** (Various)	**Tablets:** 25 mg	In 60s, 100s, 250s, 500s, 1000s and UD 35s, 100s and 600s.	6+
Rx	**Alatone** (Major)		In 100s, 250s, 500s, 1000s and UD 100s.	11
Rx	**Aldactone** (Searle)		(#Searle 1001 on one side; Aldactone 25 on other side). Film coated. Yellow. In 100s, 500s, 1000s and UD 100s.	45
Rx	**Aldactone** (Searle)	**Tablets:** 50 mg	(#Searle 1041 on one side; Aldactone 50 on other side). Film coated. Orange, scored. In 100s and UD 100s.	40
Rx	**Aldactone** (Searle)	**Tablets:** 100 mg	(#Searle 1031 on one side; Aldactone 100 on other side). Film coated. Peach, scored. In 100s and UD 100s.	34

* Cost Index based on cost per 50 mg.
# Product identification code.

Refer to the general discussion of these agents beginning on page 574.

TRIAMTERENE

Indications:

Edema associated with congestive heart failure (CHF), hepatic cirrhosis and the nephrotic syndrome; also in steroid-induced edema, idiopathic edema and edema due to secondary hyperaldosteronism.

May be used alone or with other diuretics, either for additive diuretic effect or antikaliuretic effect. It promotes increased diuresis in patients resistant or only partially responsive to other diuretics because of secondary hyperaldosteronism.

Contraindications:

Do not give triamterene to patients receiving spironolactone or amiloride.

Anuria; severe hepatic disease; hyperkalemia; hypersensitivity to triamterene. Severe or progressive kidney disease or dysfunction, with the possible exception of nephrosis.

Do not use in patients with preexisting elevated serum potassium (impaired renal function, azotemia) or patients who develop hyperkalemia while on triamterene.

Warnings:

Monitor patients regularly for blood dyscrasias, liver damage or other idiosyncratic reactions. Blood dyscrasias have been reported in patients receiving triamterene.

Use in impaired renal function: Perform periodic BUN and serum potassium determinations to check kidney function, especially in patients with suspected or confirmed renal insufficiency and in elderly or diabetic patients; diabetic patients with nephropathy are especially prone to develop hyperkalemia.

Use in impaired hepatic function: Triamterene is extensively metabolized in the liver. One study showed that the clearance of triamterene is markedly decreased in patients with cirrhosis and ascites. However, the overall diuretic response may not be affected.

Usage in Pregnancy: Category B. Triamterene crosses the placental barrier and appears in the cord blood of animals; this may occur in humans. No congenital defects have been noted when used during pregnancy. There are no adequate and well controlled studies in pregnant women. Use only when clearly needed and when the potential benefits outweigh the potential hazards to the fetus. See also discussion of thiazide diuretic use during pregnancy.

Usage in Lactation: Triamterene appears in the milk of animals receiving the drug; this may occur in humans. If the drug is essential, the patient should stop nursing.

Usage in Children: Safety and efficacy have not been established.

Precautions:

Hyperkalemia may occur, especially in patients with renal insufficiency, in those receiving potassium supplementation and in diabetic nephropathy, and is associated with cardiac irregularities. Hyperkalemia rarely occurs in patients with adequate urinary output, but is possible if large doses are used for long periods of time; if it occurs, withdraw triamterene. Normal adult serum potassium range is 3.5 to 5 mEq/L. Treat levels persistently above 6 mEq/L. Neonate levels are higher than adult levels. Serum potassium levels do not necessarily indicate true body potassium concentration. A rise in plasma pH may cause a decrease in plasma potassium concentration and an increase in the intracellular potassium concentration. Patients who receve intensive or prolonged therapy may experience a rebound kaliuresis upon abrupt withdrawal. Gradually withdraw triamterene in such patients.

When triamterene is added to other diuretic therapy, or when patients are switched to triamterene from other diuretics, discontinue potassium supplementation.

If hyperkalemia is present or suspected, obtain an ECG. If the ECG shows no widening of the QRS or arrhythmia in the presence of hyperkalemia, discontinue triamterene and any potassium supplementation and substitute a thiazide alone. Sodium polystyrene sulfonate may be administered to enhance excess potassium excretion. The presence of a widened QRS complex or arrhythmia in association with hyperkalemia requires prompt additional therapy. For tachyarrhythmia, infuse 44 mEq of sodium bicarbonate or 10 ml of 10% calcium gluconate or calcium chloride over several minutes. For asystole, bradycardia or AV block, transvenous pacing is also recommended.

The effect of calcium and sodium bicarbonate is transient. Repeat as required. Remove excess K^+ by dialysis or oral or rectal administration of sodium polystyrene sulfonate. Infusion of glucose and insulin are also used to treat hyperkalemia.

The following agents, given with triamterene, may cause hyperkalemia especially in patients with renal insufficiency: Blood from blood bank (may contain up to 30 mEq of potassium per liter of plasma or up to 65 mEq per liter of whole blood when stored for more than 10 days); low-salt milk (may contain up to 60 mEq of potassium per liter); potassium-containing medications (such as parenteral penicillin G potassium); salt substitutes (most contain substantial amounts of potassium).

(Precautions continued on following page)

TRIAMTERENE (Cont.)

Precautions (Cont.)

Electrolyte imbalance: In CHF, renal disease or cirrhosis, electrolyte imbalance may be aggravated or caused by diuretics. The use of full doses of a diuretic when salt intake is restricted can result in a low salt syndrome.

Triamterene can cause mild nitrogen retention which is reversible upon withdrawal; this is seldom observed with intermittent therapy.

Renal stones: Triamterene has been found in renal stones with other usual calculus components. Therefore, use cautiously in patients with histories of stone formation.

Triamterene is a weak *folic acid antagonist.* Since cirrhotics with splenomegaly may have marked variations in hematological status, it may contribute to the appearance of megaloblastosis in cases where folic acid stores have been depleted. Perform periodic blood studies in these patients.

Triamterene may cause decreasing alkali reserve with a possibility of metabolic acidosis.

Drug Interactions:

Amantadine: Triamterene may increase the toxic effects (ataxia, agitation) of amantadine, possibly by decreasing its renal excretion.

Angiotensin converting enzyme inhibitors decrease aldosterone production, which may elevate serum potassium. Concurrent use with triamterene may lead to significant hyperkalemia.

Indomethacin: Concomitant triamterene administration may produce an unexpectedly high incidence of nephrotoxicity. Anuric renal failure has also been reported in one patient.

Potassium preparations: Concurrent administration with triamterene may result in hyperkalemia, possibly with cardiac arrhythmias or cardiac arrest. Avoid coadministration, especially in patients with impaired renal function.

Drug/lab tests: Triamterene and **quinidine** have similar fluorescence spectra; thus, triamterene will interfere with the fluorescent measurement of quinidine serum levels.

Adverse Reactions:

GI: Diarrhea, nausea, vomiting and jaundice or liver enzyme abnormalities. Nausea can usually be prevented by giving the drug after meals.

Renal: Azotemia, elevated BUN and creatinine. Triamterene has been found in renal stones (see Precautions).

Interstitial nephritis has been reported rarely in patients on a hydrochlorothiazide/triamterene combination and with triamterene alone. Onset was immediate to 10 weeks after initiation of therapy; resolution began upon discontinuation of the drug.

In patients predisposed to gouty arthritis, serum uric acid levels may increase.

Hematologic: Thrombocytopenia, megaloblastic anemia.

Electrolyte imbalance and hyperkalemia (see Precautions).

Miscellaneous: Weakness, fatigue, dizziness, hypokalemia, headache, dry mouth, anaphylaxis, photosensitivity and rash.

Overdosage:

Symptoms: Electrolyte imbalance is the major concern, particularly hyperkalemia. Other symptoms may include nausea, vomiting, other GI disturbances and weakness. Hypotension may occur. Triamterene may induce reversible acute renal failure.

Treatment: Induce immediate evacuation of the stomach through emesis and gastric lavage. Carefully evaluate electrolyte and fluid balance. Dialysis may be of some benefit. Treatment includes usual supportive measures. Refer to General Management of Acute Overdosage on p. 2895

Patient Information:

May cause GI upset; take after meals.

May cause weakness, headache, nausea, vomiting, and dry mouth; notify physician if these become severe or persistent.

Notify physician if fever, sore throat, mouth sores, or unusual bleeding or bruising occurs.

Avoid prolonged exposure to sunlight; photosensitivity may occur.

If single daily dose is prescribed, take in morning to minimize effect of increased frequency of urination on nighttime sleep.

If dose is missed, do not take more than prescribed dose at next dosing interval.

Administration and Dosage:

Individualize dosage.

When used alone, the usual starting dose is 100 mg twice/day after meals. When combined with other diuretics or antihypertensives, decrease the total daily dosage of each agent initially, and then adjust to the patient's needs. Do not exceed 300 mg/day. **C.I.***

Rx	**Dyrenium**	**Capsules:** 50 mg	(#Dyrenium SKF 50). Red. In 100s and UD 100s.	45
	(SKF)	100 mg	(#Dyrenium SKF 100). Red. In 100s, 1000s & UD 100s.	28

* Cost Index based on cost per 100 mg. # Product identification code.

Fixed dose combination drugs are not indicated for initial therapy of edema or hypertension; they require therapy titrated to the individual patient. If the fixed combination represents the determined dosage, its use may be more convenient in patient management. The treatment of hypertension and edema is not static; reevaluate as conditions in each patient warrant.

The combination of a thiazide and a potassium sparing diuretic provides additive diuretic activity and antihypertensive effects through different mechanisms of action and also minimizes the potassium depletion characteristics of thiazides.

Bioavailability of triamterene/hydrochlorothiazide combinations: Use caution when changing a patient from optimally bioavailable hydrochlorothiazide tablets to combination products or when changing the patient from one triamterene/hydrochlorothiazide combination product to another. The combination products are not equivalent.

The triamterene 75 mg/hydrochlorothiazide 50 mg tablet delivers the same amount of hydrochlorothiazide as a 50 mg hydrochlorothiazide tablet. Two triamterene 50 mg/hydrochlorothiazide 25 mg capsules deliver approximately 25 mg of hydrochlorothiazide to the bloodstream.

For complete information concerning the components of the combined diuretic products, consult the appropriate drug monographs as indicated below.

HYDROCHLOROTHIAZIDE, p. 563
AMILORIDE HCl, p. 575
SPIRONOLACTONE, p. 578
TRIAMTERENE, p. 581

	Product	Formulation	Packaging	C.I.*
Rx	**Amiloride w/Hydrochlorothiazide** (Various, eg, Bioline, Geneva Marsam, Goldline, Lederle, Major, Moore, Parmed, Rugby, Schein, Warner Chilcott)	**Tablets:** 5 mg amiloride HCl and 50 mg hydrochlorothiazide *Dose:* 1 to 2 daily, with meals.	In 100s, 500s and 1000s.	20+
Rx	**Moduretic** (MSD)		(MSD 917). Peach, scored. In 100s, UD 100s.	33
Rx	**Spironolactone w/ Hydrochlorothiazide** (Various)	**Tablets:** 25 mg spironolactone and 25 mg hydrochlorothiazide *Dose:* 1 to 8 daily.	In 30s, 60s, 100s, 250s, 500s, 1000s and UD 32s and 100s.	3+
Rx	**Alazide** (Major)		In 100s, 250s, 1000s and UD 100s.	7
Rx	**Aldactazide** (Searle)		(Searle 1011/Aldactazide 25). Tan. Film coated. In 100s, 500s, 1000s and UD 100s.	24
Rx	**Spironazide** (Schein)		(bp 0129). In 100s, 1000s.	4
Rx	**Spirozide** (Rugby)		In 100s, 500s, 1000s.	5
Rx	**Aldactazide** (Searle)	**Tablets:** 50 mg spironolactone and 50 mg hydrochlorothiazide *Dose:* 1 to 4 daily.	(Searle 1021/Aldactazide 50). Tan, scored. Film coated. In 100s, UD 100s.	43
Rx	**Maxzide-25MG** (Lederle)	**Tablets:** 37.5 mg triamterene and 25 mg hydrochlorothiazide *Dose:* 1 or 2 daily.	(Maxzide/LL M9). Lt. green, scored. In 100s and UD 100s.	20
Rx	**Triamterene w/ Hydrochlorothiazide** (Various)	**Capsules:** 50 mg triamterene and 25 mg hydrochlorothiazide *Dose:* 1 or 2 twice daily, after meals.	In 100s, 500s and 1000s.	18
Rx	**Dyazide** (SmithKline Beecham)		(SKF Dyazide). Red and white. In 1000s, unit-of-use 100s and UD 100s.	29
Rx	**Triamterene w/ Hydrochlorothiazide** (Various)	**Tablets:** 75 mg triamterene and 50 mg hydrochlorothiazide *Dose:* 1 daily.	In 30s, 100s, 500s and 1000s.	23
Rx	**Maxzide** (Lederle)		(Maxzide/LL M8). Lt yellow, scored. In 100s, 500s and UD 100s.	35

* Cost Index based on cost per capsule or tablet.

Osmotic agents induce diuresis by elevating the osmolarity of the glomerular filtrate, thereby hindering the tubular reabsorption of water. Excretion of sodium and chloride is increased. These agents are: Freely filtered at the glomerulus; poorly reabsorbed by the renal tubule; relatively pharmacologically inert; usually resistant to metabolic alteration (except glycerin). Activity in the kidneys depends on the concentration of osmotically active particles in solution.

The main indication for osmotic diuretics (primarily mannitol) is prophylaxis of acute renal failure in conditions in which glomerular filtration is greatly reduced (ie, severe trauma, cardiovascular operations). By maintaining a flow of dilute urine, damage to the nephron by high concentrations of toxic solute does not occur. They are also employed to reduce intracranial pressure and elevated intraocular pressure. In the eyes, these agents act by creating an osmotic gradient between the plasma and ocular fluids.

Mannitol is the most widely used osmotic diuretic. The other agents include urea, glycerin and isosorbide. For specific approved indications, refer to individual drug monographs.

Pharmacokinetics: **Mannitol** is only slightly metabolized, while the rest is freely filtered by the glomeruli and excreted intact in the urine. About 7% is reabsorbed by the renal tubules. Approximately 90% of an injected dose is recovered in the urine after 24 hours. In severe renal insufficiency, the rate of mannitol excretion is greatly reduced; retained mannitol may increase extracellular tonicity, expand the extracellular fluid and induce an apparent hyponatremia with increased serum osmolality.

Comparative pharmacokinetic data of osmotic diuretics are summarized in the table below:

OSMOTIC DIURETICS

Diuretic	Route	Onset (min)	Peak (hrs)	Duration (hrs)	Half-life	Metabolized (%)	Ocular Penetration	Distribution
Mannitol	IV	30-60	1	6-8	15-100 minutes	7-10	very poor	E[1]
Urea	IV	30-45	1	5-6	—	—	good	TBW[2]
Glycerin	PO	10-30	1-1.5	4-5	30-45 minutes	80	poor	E[1]
Isosorbide	PO	10-30	1-1.5	5-6	5-9.5 hrs	0	good	TBW[2]

[1] E = extracellular water
[2] TBW = total body water

(Products listed on following pages)

Refer to the general discussion of these agents on page 584.

MANNITOL

Indications:

Therapeutic: To promote diuresis in the prevention or treatment of the oliguric phase of acute renal failure before irreversible renal failure becomes established.

Reduction of intracranial pressure and treatment of cerebral edema.

Reduction of elevated intraocular pressure when the pressure cannot be lowered by other means.

To promote urinary excretion of toxic substances and urinary irrigation.

Diagnostic: Measurement of glomerular filtration rate.

Contraindications:

Anuria due to severe renal disease; severe pulmonary congestion or frank pulmonary edema; active intracranial bleeding except during craniotomy; severe dehydration; progressive renal damage or dysfunction after instituting mannitol therapy, including increasing oliguria and azotemia; progressive heart failure or pulmonary congestion after mannitol therapy.

Warnings:

Usage in impaired renal function: Use a test dose (see Administration and Dosage); try a second test dose if there is an inadequate response, but do not attempt more than two test doses.

If urine output continues to decline during infusion, closely review the patient's clinical status and suspend mannitol infusion, if necessary. Accumulation of mannitol may result in overexpansion of the extracellular fluid which may intensify existing or latent congestive heart failure and pulmonary edema.

Osmotic nephrosis may proceed to severe irreversible nephrosis.

Fluid and electrolyte imbalance: By sustaining diuresis, mannitol may obscure and intensify inadequate hydration or hypovolemia. Excessive loss of water and electrolytes may lead to serious imbalances. Loss of water in excess of electrolytes can cause hypernatremia. Shift of sodium free intracellular fluid into the extracellular compartment following mannitol infusion may lower serum sodium concentration and aggravate preexisting hyponatremia. Also, movement of potassium ions from intracellular to extracellular space may cause hyperkalemia. Electrolyte measurements, including sodium and potassium, are therefore of vital importance in monitoring mannitol infusion.

Usage in Pregnancy: Category C. Safety for use during pregnancy has not been established. Do not use in women of childbearing potential unless the potential benefits outweigh the possible hazards.

Usage in Lactation: It is not known whether this drug is excreted in breast milk, exercise caution when administering to a nursing woman.

Usage in Children: Dosage for patients $\leq$ 12 years of age has not been established.

Precautions:

Carefully evaluate the patient's cardiovascular status before rapid administration of mannitol since sudden expansion of the extracellular fluid may lead to fulminating congestive heart failure.

Do not give electrolyte free mannitol solutions with blood. If blood is given simultaneously, add at least 20 mEq of sodium chloride to each liter of mannitol solution to avoid pseudoagglutination.

The obligatory diuretic response following rapid infusion of 15%, 20% or 25% mannitol may further aggravate preexisting hemoconcentration.

Adverse Reactions:

Isolated cases reported during or following mannitol infusion include:

Cardiovascular: Edema; thrombophlebitis; hypotension; hypertension; tachycardia; angina-like chest pains.

CNS: Headache; blurred vision; convulsions; dizziness.

GI: Nausea; vomiting; diarrhea.

GU: Marked diuresis; urinary retention.

Metabolic: Fluid and electrolyte imbalance; acidosis; electrolyte loss; dehydration.

Pulmonary: Pulmonary congestion.

Other: Dry mouth; thirst; rhinitis; arm pain; skin necrosis; chills; urticaria; fever.

(Continued on following page)

MANNITOL (Cont.)

Overdosage:

Symptoms: Larger than recommended doses may result in increased electrolyte excretion, particularly sodium, chloride and potassium. Sodium depletion can result in orthostatic tachycardia or hypotension and decreased central venous pressure. Chloride metabolism closely follows that of sodium. Potassium deficit can impair neuromuscular function and cause intestinal dilation and ileus. If urine flow is inadequate, pulmonary edema or water intoxication may occur. Other symptoms include hypotension, polyuria that rapidly converts to oliguria, stupor, convulsions, hyperosmolality, hyponatremia.

Treatment: Discontinue infusion immediately. Institute supportive measures to correct fluid and electrolyte imbalances. Hemodialysis is beneficial to clear mannitol and reduce serum osmolality.

Administration and Dosage:

Administer by IV infusion only. Individualize concentration and rate of administration. The usual adult dose ranges from 50 to 200 g/24 hours; in most instances, an adequate response will be achieved with 100 g/24 hours. Adjust the administration rate to maintain a urine flow of at least 30 to 50 ml/hour.

Test dose: For patients with marked oliguria or inadequate renal function, give 0.2 g/kg (about 50 ml of a 25% solution, 75 ml of a 20% solution, or 100 ml of a 15% solution) infused over 3 to 5 minutes. If urine flow does not increase, administer a second test dose. If response is inadequate, reevaluate the patient.

Prevention of acute renal failure (oliguria): Adults – 50 to 100 g as a 5% to 25% solution during cardiovascular and other types of surgery.

Treatment of oliguria: Adults – 300 to 400 mg/kg of a 20% or 25% solution, or up to 100 g of a 15% or 20% solution.

Reduction of intracranial pressure and brain mass: 1.5 to 2 g/kg as a 15% to 25% solution, infused over 30 to 60 minutes, to reduce brain mass before or after neurosurgery. Evaluate the circulatory and renal reserve, fluid and electrolyte balance, body weight, and total input and output before and after mannitol infusion. Reduced cerebral spinal fluid pressure must be observed within 15 minutes after starting infusion.

Reduction of intraocular pressure: 1.5 to 2 g/kg as a 20% or 25% solution (6 to 8 ml/kg), as a 20% solution (7.5 to 10 ml/kg) or as a 15% solution (10 to 13 ml/kg) over a period as short as 30 minutes. When used preoperatively, administer 1 to 1½ hours before surgery to achieve maximal effect.

Adjunctive therapy to promote diuresis in intoxications: The concentration depends upon the fluid requirement and urinary output of the patient. Give IV fluids and electrolytes to replace losses. If benefits are not seen after 200 g mannitol, discontinue the infusion.

Measurement of glomerular filtration rate (GFR): Dilute 100 ml of a 20% solution (20 g) with 180 ml of Sodium Chloride Injection (normal saline). Infuse the resulting 280 ml of 7.2% solution at a rate of 20 ml/minute. Collect the urine by catheter for a specific time period and analyze for mannitol excreted in mg per minute. Draw a blood sample at the start and at the end of the time period and determine the concentration of mannitol in mg/ml of plasma.

Urologic Irrigation: Use 2.5% solution. The use of 2.5% mannitol solution minimizes hemolytic effect of water alone, the entrance of hemolyzed blood into the circulation, and the resulting hemoglobinemia which is considered a major factor in producing serious renal complications.

Dilution of Mannitol: Add contents of two 50 ml vials (25% mannitol) to 900 ml sterile water for injection.

Preparation of solution: When exposed to low temperatures, mannitol solution may crystallize. Concentrations greater than 15% have a greater tendency to crystallize. If crystals are observed, warm the bottle in a hot water bath or autoclave, then cool to body temperature before administering.

When infusing concentrated mannitol, the administration set should include a filter.

Rx	**Mannitol** (Various)	**Injection:** 5%	In 1000 ml.
		10%	In 1000 ml.
		15%	In 150 and 500 ml.
		20%	In 250 and 500 ml.
		25%	In 50 ml.
Rx	**Osmitrol** (Baxter)	**Injection:** 5%	In 1000 ml.
		10%	In 500 and 1000 ml.
		15%	In 150 and 500 ml.
		20%	In 250 and 500 ml.

Refer to the general discussion of these agents beginning on page 584.

UREA

Indications:

The 30% solution is used to reduce intracranial pressure (in the control of cerebral edema) and intraocular pressure.

Unlabeled Use: Intra-amniotic injection has been used to induce abortion.

Contraindications:

Severely impaired renal function; active intracranial bleeding; marked dehydration; frank liver failure.

Do not infuse in veins of the lower extremities of elderly patients, phlebitis and thrombosis of superficial and deep veins may occur.

Warnings:

Electrolyte imbalance: Urea may cause depletion of electrolytes that can result in hyponatremia and hypokalemia.

Extravasation of the solution at the injection site may cause local reactions ranging from mild irritation to tissue necrosis.

Usage in hepatic impairment: Administer with caution in patients with liver impairment, since there may be a significant rise in blood ammonia levels.

Usage in Pregnancy: Category C. Safety for use during pregnancy has not been established. Use only when clearly needed and when the potential benefits outweigh the potential hazards to the fetus.

Usage in Lactation: It is not known whether this drug is excreted in breast milk. Exercise caution when administering to a nursing mother.

Precautions:

Intracranial bleeding: Arterial oozing has been reported when intracranial surgery is performed on patients following treatment with urea; however, this has not been a significant problem. Do not use in the presence of active intracranial bleeding unless such use is preliminary to prompt surgical intervention to control hemorrhage. Reduction of brain edema induced by urea may result in reactivation of intracranial bleeding.

Usage in renal impairment: Administer with caution. Mild elevation of BUN does not preclude its use. Perform frequent laboratory studies, determine if renal function is adequate to eliminate the infused urea and that produced endogenously.

Patients exhibiting a temporary reduction in urine volume are generally able to maintain a satisfactory elimination of urea. However, if diuresis does not follow the injection of urea in such patients within 6 to 12 hours, withdraw the drug pending further evaluation of renal function.

To ensure bladder emptying, use an indwelling urethral catheter in comatose patients.

Rapid IV administration of hypertonic solutions of urea may be associated with hemolysis as well as a direct effect on the cerebral vasomotor centers that may result in increased capillary bleeding. Do not exceed an infusion rate of 4 ml/minute.

Blood loss: Urea may temporarily maintain circulatory volume and blood pressure in spite of considerable blood loss. Consequently, when excessive blood loss occurs within a short period of time, blood replacement should be adequate and simultaneous with the infusion of urea. Do not administer urea through the same administration set that blood is being infused. Hypothermia, when used with urea infusion, may increase the risk of venous thrombosis and hemoglobinuria.

Drug Interactions:

Lithium: Urea may increase the renal excretion of lithium, thereby decreasing its effects. A higher dose of lithium may be required. This interaction may be clinically useful in treating lithium overdose.

Adverse Reactions:

No serious reactions have been noted when solutions are infused slowly, provided renal function is not seriously impaired and there is no active intracranial bleeding. If an adverse reaction occurs, discontinue the infusion, evaluate the patient and institute appropriate therapy; save the remainder of the fluid for examination.

Headaches (similar to those following lumbar puncture), nausea and vomiting, and occasionally, syncope and disorientation. *Less frequent:* Transient agitated confusional state. *Infrequent:* Chemical phlebitis and thrombosis near the injection site.

Reactions that may occur because of the reconstituted solution or the technique of administration include febrile response, infection at the injection site, venous thrombosis or phlebitis extending from the injection site, extravasation and hypervolemia.

(Continued on following page)

UREA (Cont.)

Overdosage:

In the event of overdosage, as reflected by unusually elevated blood urea nitrogen (BUN) levels, discontinue the drug, evaluate the patient and institute corrective measures.

Administration and Dosage:

Administer as a 30% solution by slow IV infusion, at a rate not to exceed 4 ml/minute.

An isosmotic concentration of dextrose or invert sugar is administered with urea to prevent the hemolysis produced by pure solutions of urea.

Do not exceed 120 g/day.

Adults: 1 to 1.5 g/kg (0.45 to 0.68 g/lb).

Children: 0.5 to 1.5 g/kg. In children up to 2 years of age, as little as 0.1 g/kg may be adequate.

Preparation of solution: For 135 ml of a 30% solution of sterile urea, mix the contents of one 40 g vial with 105 ml of 5% or 10% Dextrose Injection or 10% Invert Sugar in Water. Each ml of a 30% solution provides 300 mg of urea. Use fresh solution; discard any unused portion within 24 hours after reconstitution.

Rx	**Ureaphil** (Abbott)	**Injection:** 40 g per 150 ml single dose container.

GLYCERIN (Glycerol)

Actions:

An oral osmotic agent for reducing intraocular pressure. It adds to the tonicity of the blood until metabolized and eliminated by the kidneys. Maximal reduction of intraocular pressure will occur 1 hour after glycerin administration. The effect will last approximately 5 hours.

Indications:

Glaucoma to interrupt acute attacks, and when a temporary drop in pressure is required but cannot be otherwise attained.

Prior to ocular surgery performed under local anesthesia (ie, glaucoma surgery, cataract surgery) where preoperative reduction of intraocular pressure is indicated.

Unlabeled Use: Glycerin has also been given by the IV route (with proper preparation) to lower intraocular and intracranial pressure.

Contraindications:

Well established anuria; severe dehydration; frank or impending acute pulmonary edema; severe cardiac decompensation.

Hypersensitivity to any of the ingredients.

Warnings:

For oral use only; not for injection.

Usage in Pregnancy: Category C. Safety for use during pregnancy has not been established. Use only when clearly needed and when the potential benefits outweigh the potential hazards to the fetus.

Usage in Lactation: It is not known whether this drug is excreted in breast milk. Exercise caution when administering to a nursing woman.

Usage in Children: Safety and efficacy for use in children have not been established.

Precautions:

Use cautiously in hypervolemia, confused mental states, congestive heart disease, as well as in the elderly, senile and diabetic patients and severely dehydrated individuals. Avoid acute urinary retention in the preoperative period. Continued use may result in weight gain.

Adverse Reactions:

Nausea, vomiting, headache, confusion and disorientation may occur. Severe dehydration, cardiac arrhythmias or hyperosmolar nonketotic coma which can result in death have been reported.

Administration and Dosage:

1 to 1.5 g/kg, 1 to 1½ hours prior to surgery.

				C.I.*
Rx	**Glyrol** (Iolab Pharm.)	**Solution:** 75% (0.94 g glycerin/ml)[1]	In 120 ml.	248
Rx	**Osmoglyn** (Alcon)	**Solution:** 50% (0.6 g glycerin/ml)	Lime flavor. In 220 ml.	355

* Cost Index based on cost per 30 ml glycerin.

[1] Not USP; pH may differ from USP.

Refer to the general discussion of these agents beginning on page 584.

ISOSORBIDE

Indications:

For the short-term reduction of intraocular pressure prior to and after intraocular surgery.

May be used to interrupt an acute attack of glaucoma. Use where less risk of nausea and vomiting than that posed by other oral hyperosmotic agents is needed.

Contraindications:

Well established anuria due to severe renal disease; severe dehydration; frank or impending acute pulmonary edema; severe cardiac decompensation.

Hypersensitivity to any component of this preparation.

Warnings:

With repeated doses, maintain adequate fluid and electrolyte balance.

If urinary output continues to decrease, closely review the patient's clinical status. Accumulation may result in overexpansion of the extracellular fluid.

Pregnancy: Category B. Reproduction studies in animals have shown no evidence of harm to the fetus. There is no adequate information on whether this drug affects fertility in humans or has a teratogenic potential or other adverse fetal effect. Use during pregnancy only if clearly needed.

Precautions:

Use repetitive doses with caution, particularly in patients with diseases associated with salt retention. Ensure that the patient's bladder has been emptied prior to surgery.

Adverse Reactions:

Nausea, vomiting, headache, confusion and disorientation may occur. Very rarely gastric discomfort, thirst, hiccoughs, hypernatremia, hyperosmolarity, rash, irritability, syncope, lethargy, vertigo, dizziness and lightheadedness have occurred.

Administration and Dosage:

For oral use only.

Initial dose: 1.5 g/kg (equivalent to 1.5 ml/lb).

Dose range: 1 to 3 g/kg 2 to 4 times a day as indicated.

Palatability may be improved if the medication is poured over cracked ice and sipped.

Rx	**Ismotic** (Alcon)	**Solution:** 45% (100 g per 220 ml)	With 4.6 mEq sodium and 0.9 mEq potassium per 220 ml. Alcohol. Saccharin, sorbitol. Vanilla-mint flavor. In 220 ml.

Nonprescription diuretic products are promoted for the alleviation of menstrual discomfort. When taken 5 to 6 days before onset of menses, *otc* diuretics may help relieve symptoms related to water retention. These include: Excess water weight, bloating, swelling, painful breasts, cramps and tension.

The most frequently used *otc* diuretic agents are pamabrom, ammonium chloride and caffeine. These agents are classified as Category I (generally recognized as safe and effective and not misbranded).

PAMABROM, a theophylline derivative, has weak diuretic properties when taken alone. It is often combined with analgesics and antihistamines to relieve premenstrual syndrome. Daily doses should not exceed 200 mg.

AMMONIUM CHLORIDE, an acid-forming salt, has limited value in promoting diuresis (4 to 5 days). Its use in combination with caffeine is effective in water weight reduction. Doses up to 3 g/day may be given in divided doses 3 to 4 times daily for up to 6 days. Large doses (4 to 12 g/day) may cause GI symptoms including nausea and vomiting. CNS toxicity including headache, hyperventilation, drowsiness and mental confusion may also occur. Ammonium chloride is contraindicated in patients with impaired renal and liver function; metabolic acidosis may occur.

CAFFEINE, a xanthine derivative, promotes diuresis through inhibition of renal tubular reabsorption of sodium and chloride. It may alleviate the mental and physical fatigue associated with water retention. Caffeine is effective for relief of premenstrual and menstrual symptoms in doses of 100 to 200 mg every 3 to 4 hours. Doses above 100 mg may cause GI irritation. Advise patients that caffeine-containing products taken within 4 hours of bedtime may cause sleeplessness. Consider this when drinking coffee, tea, hot chocolate or colas, and when taking other caffeine-containing products.

	Product	Composition / Dose	Supplied	**C.I.***
otc	**Fluidex with Pamabrom** (O'Connor)	**Capsules:** 50 mg pamabrom *Dose:* 1 every 6 hours.	In 12s and 24s.	7
otc	**Aqua•Ban** (Thompson Medical)	**Tablets, enteric coated:** 325 mg ammonium chloride and 100 mg caffeine *Dose:* 2 tablets 3 times daily after meals. Start 4 to 5 days before menstruation.	Blue. In 60s.	4
otc	**Aqua•Ban Plus** (Thompson Medical)	**Tablets, enteric coated:** 650 mg ammonium chloride, 200 mg caffeine and 6 mg iron (as ferrous sulfate) *Dose:* 1 tablet 3 times daily after meals. Start 5 to 6 days before menstruation.	Blue. In 30s.	10
otc	**Tri-Aqua** (Pfeiffer)	**Tablets:** 100 mg caffeine, extracts of buchu, uva ursi, zea and triticum *Dose:* One tablet with liquid at each meal.	In 50s and 100s.	2
otc	**Aqua-Rid** (Goldline)	**Tablets:** 65 mg powdered buchu, 65 mg powdered couch grass, 32.5 mg powdered corn silk and 32.5 mg powdered hydrangea *Dose:* One tablet before each meal and at bedtime with water. May be continued for 10 days.	In 100s.	3
otc	**Fluidex** (O'Connor)	**Tablets:** 65 mg powdered buchu, 65 mg powdered couch grass, 32.5 mg corn silk and 32.5 mg powdered hydrangea *Dose:* One tablet after meals with a full glass of water.	In 36s.	NA

* Cost Index based on cost per capsule or tablet.

The cardiac (or digitalis) glycosides include: Digitoxin, derived from *Digitalis purpurea;* and deslanoside and digoxin, derived from *Digitalis lanata.* Although these glycosides differ pharmacokinetically, their therapeutic effects on the heart are qualitatively similar.

Actions:

Pharmacology: The influence of the digitalis glycosides on the myocardium is dose-related, and involves both a direct action on cardiac muscle and the specialized conduction system, and indirect actions on the cardiovascular system mediated by the autonomic nervous system. These indirect actions involve a vagomimetic action, which is responsible for the depression of the sinoatrial (SA) node and the prolonged conduction to the atrioventricular (AV) node; and also a baroreceptor sensitization which results in increased carotid sinus nerve activity and enhanced sympathetic withdrawal for any given increment in mean arterial pressure.

Direct effects include increasing the force and velocity of myocardial systolic contraction (positive inotropic action), increasing the refractory period of the AV node and increasing total peripheral resistance. In higher doses, digitalis increases sympathetic outflow from the CNS to both cardiac and peripheral sympathetic nerves, which may increase atrial or ventricular rate. This increase in sympathetic activity may be an important factor in digitalis cardiac toxicity. Most of the extracardiac manifestations of digitalis toxicity are also mediated by the CNS.

Mechanism – The cellular basis for the inotropic effects of the digitalis glycosides appears to be inhibition of sodium, potassium-ATPase in the sarcolemal membrane, which alters excitation-contraction coupling. In the myocardium, calcium enters the cell by the slow calcium channel during the action potential, which triggers the release of calcium from intracellular binding sites on the sarcoplasmic reticulum. The digitalis glycosides, by inhibiting sodium, potassium-ATPase, make more calcium available to activate the contractile proteins actin and myosin, thereby enhancing the force of myocardial contraction.

Pharmacokinetics:

Pharmacokinetic Parameters of Digitalis Glycosides							
Digitalis Glycoside	**Route**	**Onset (Minutes)**	**Peak (Hours)**	**Plasma $t_{1/2}$ (Hours)**	**% GI Absorption**	**% Protein Binding**	**Major Route of Elimination**
Deslanoside	IV	10-30	2-3	≈36	—	25	Renal
Digoxin	PO IV	30-120 5-30	2-6 1-5	30-40[1]	55-90	20-25	Renal
Digitoxin	PO	60-240	8-12	168-192	90-100	90-97	Hepatic 50%-70%; Renal (metabolites)

[1] In anuric patients: 100+hours.

Absorption – Absorption following oral administration is a function of polarity; only digitoxin is highly lipid soluble and almost completely absorbed. Digoxin tablets are absorbed 60% to 80%; the elixir is absorbed 70% to 85% and a solution-filled capsule is 90% to 100%. When oral digoxin is taken after meals, the rate of absorption is slowed but total amount absorbed is usually unchanged. However, when taken with meals high in bran fiber, the amount absorbed may be reduced.

In some patients, orally administered digoxin is converted to cardioinactive reduction products (eg, dihydrodigoxin) by colonic bacteria in the gut thereby reducing its bioavailability. Although inactivation of these bacteria by antibiotics is rapid, serum digoxin concentration will rise at a rate consistent with elimination half-life of digoxin. Magnitude of rise in serum digoxin concentration relates to extent of bacterial inactivation, and may be as much as two-fold in some cases. This interaction is significantly reduced if digoxin is given as digoxin solution in capsules. Data suggest that one in ten patients treated with digoxin tablets will degrade 40% or more of the ingested dose.

Distribution – Cardiac glycosides are widely distributed in tissues; high concentrations are found in the myocardium, skeletal muscle, liver and kidneys. Digoxin crosses both the blood-brain barrier and the placenta. At delivery, serum digoxin concentration in the newborn is similar to the serum level in the mother. Serum digoxin concentrations are not significantly altered by large changes in fat tissue weight, so that distribution space correlates best with lean (ideal) body weight.

(Actions continued on following page)

Actions (Cont.):

Pharmacokinetics (Cont.): Elimination – Digitoxin is inactivated by hepatic degradation, 50% to 70% to inactive metabolites (excreted by the kidneys). About 8% is converted to digoxin; 30% to 50% is excreted unchanged in the urine and feces. Digoxin and deslanoside are excreted by the kidneys largely as parent drug and active metabolites. In patients with impaired renal function, significant accumulation may occur, except with digitoxin.

Because of the long half-lives of these agents, clinical effects do not fully develop until steady state plasma levels are achieved. Conversely, several days are required for complete dissipation of effects following therapy discontinuation (ie, 6 to 8 days for digoxin and 3 to 5 weeks for digitoxin). Digoxin is not effectively removed by dialysis, exchange transfusion or during cardiopulmonary bypass, since most is found in tissue rather than circulating in the blood. Digitoxin is not effectively removed by peritoneal or hemodialysis, probably because of its high degree of plasma-protein binding.

Glycoside serum levels – The relationship of serum digitalis glycoside levels to signs or symptoms of intoxication varies significantly from patient to patient; therefore, the value and limitations of this test must be recognized. It is difficult to establish normal glycoside levels that would accurately define toxicity.

Digitalis Glycoside Serum Levels		
Digitalis Glycoside	Drug Serum Levels (ng/ml)	
	Therapeutic	Toxic
Digitoxin	14 to 26	>35
Digoxin	0.5 to 2	>2.5

Indications:

Congestive heart failure (CHF) all degrees: Increased cardiac output results in diuresis and general amelioration of disturbances characteristic of right heart failure (venous congestion, edema) and left heart failure (dyspnea, orthopnea, cardiac asthma). Digitalis is generally most effective in "low-output" failure and less effective in "high-output" failure (bronchopulmonary insufficiency, arteriovenous fistula, anemia, infection, hyperthyroidism). The drug is generally continued after heart failure is abolished unless some other known precipitating factor is corrected. However, a number of studies suggest many patients with normal sinus rhythm stabilized on chronic therapy (including diuretics, vasodilators, etc) can discontinue digitalis without exacerbation of CHF. Hemodynamic effects can be demonstrated in almost all patients, but corresponding improvement in signs and symptoms of heart failure is not necessarily apparent. In patients in whom digoxin may be difficult to regulate, or in whom risk of toxicity may be great (eg, patients with unstable renal function or whose potassium levels tend to fluctuate), consider a cautious withdrawal of digoxin. If digoxin is discontinued, regularly monitor for clinical evidence of recurrent heart failure.

Atrial fibrillation, especially when the ventricular rate is elevated. Digitalis rapidly reduces ventricular rates and eliminates the pulse deficit. Palpitation, precordial distress or weakness are relieved and concomitant congestive failure ameliorated. Continue digitalis in doses necessary to maintain the desired ventricular rate, both at rest and in response to exercise and other clinical effects.

Atrial flutter: Digitalis slows the heart; normal sinus rhythm may appear. Often, flutter is converted to atrial fibrillation with a slow ventricular rate. Stopping treatment at this point may restore sinus rhythm, especially if the flutter was paroxysmal. It is preferable to continue digitalis if failure ensues or if atrial flutter occurs often (electrical cardioversion is often the treatment of choice for atrial flutter).

Paroxysmal atrial tachycardia (PAT): Digitalis may be used, especially if tachycardia is resistant to lesser measures. Depending on urgency, a more rapid-acting parenteral preparation may be used to initiate digitalization. If heart failure has ensued or paroxysms recur often, maintain digitalis by oral route. Digitalis is not indicated in sinus tachycardia or premature systoles in absence of heart failure. In infants, continue digoxin for 3 to 6 months after a single PAT episode to prevent recurrence.

Cardiogenic shock: The value of these drugs has not been established; however, they are often employed when the condition is accompanied by pulmonary edema. Digitalis may adversely affect shock due to infections.

(Continued on following page)

Contraindications:

Ventricular fibrillation; ventricular tachycardia, unless congestive failure supervenes after protracted episode not due to digitalis; presence of digitalis toxicity; beriberi heart disease, hypersensitivity to digoxin; some cases of hypersensitive carotid sinus syndrome. Allergy, though rare, may occur (may not extend to all cardiac glycosides; another may be tried).

Warnings:

Obesity: Digitalis alone or with other drugs has been promoted for use in the treatment of obesity. Potentially fatal arrhythmias or other adverse effects make the use of these drugs in treating obesity dangerous and unwarranted.

Digitalis toxicity: Many of the arrhythmias for which digitalis is indicated are identical with those reflecting digitalis intoxication. If digitalis intoxication cannot be excluded, cardiac glycosides should be withheld temporarily, if the clinical situation permits. Determination of drug serum levels may be helpful.

Since symptoms of anorexia, nausea and vomiting may be associated with digitalis intoxication and CHF, a clinical determination of their cause must be made before further administration of the drug.

When the risk of digitalis intoxication is great, use a relatively short-acting, rapidly eliminated glycoside, such as digoxin. Although intoxication cannot always be prevented by the selection of one glycoside over another, certain glycosides may be preferred in patients who have fixed disabilities (eg, liver impairment, drug intolerance). Digitoxin can be used in patients with impaired renal function.

Cardiovascular disease: Electrical conversion of arrhythmias may require reduction of dosage to avoid induction of ventricular arrhythmias. However, consider the consequences of rapid increase in ventricular response to atrial fibrillation if digoxin is withheld 1 to 2 days prior to cardioversion. If digitalis toxicity might exist, delay elective cardioversion. If it is not prudent to delay cardioversion, select a minimal energy level at first and carefully increase to avoid precipitating ventricular arrhythmias.

Exercise great caution when giving digitalis to patients still experiencing effects from previous digitalis preparations.

Patients with incomplete AV block, especially those subject to Stokes-Adams attacks, may develop advanced or complete heart block if digitalis is given. Heart failure in these patients can usually be controlled by increasing the heart rate and other measures.

In patients with acute or unstable chronic atrial fibrillation, digitalis may not normalize the ventricular rate even when the serum concentration exceeds the usual therapeutic level. Although these patients may be less sensitive to the toxic effects of digitalis than patients with normal sinus rhythm, do not increase dosage to potentially toxic levels.

Patients with acute myocardial infarction (MI), severe pulmonary disease, severe carditis (eg, carditis associated with rheumatic fever or viral myocarditis) or advanced heart failure may be more sensitive to digitalis and more prone to disturbances of rhythm. If heart failure develops, digitalization may be tried with relatively low doses and cautiously increased until a beneficial effect is obtained. If a therapeutic trial does not result in improvement, discontinue drug. Patients with chronic constrictive pericarditis may fail to respond to digitalis. In addition, slowing of the heart rate by digoxin in some patients may further decrease cardiac output.

Cases of idiopathic hypertrophic subaortic stenosis must be managed with extreme care (outflow obstruction may worsen). Unless cardiac failure is severe, it is doubtful that digitalis should be employed.

In patients with Wolff-Parkinson-White Syndrome and atrial fibrillation, digoxin can enhance transmission of impulses through the accessory pathway. This may result in extremely rapid ventricular rates and even ventricular fibrillation.

In some patients with sinus node disease (ie, Sick Sinus syndrome), digoxin may worsen sinus bradycardia or sinoatrial block.

Patients with heart failure from amyloid heart disease or constrictive cardiomyopathies respond poorly to treatment with digoxin.

Impaired renal function: Renal insufficiency delays excretion of all glycosides except digitoxin; adjust dosage in patients with renal disease. Digitoxin may be given in usual doses. However, these differences do not necessarily dictate a choice of glycosides; clinical judgment is important. Digoxin toxicity also develops more frequently and lasts longer in patients with renal impairment because of decreased digoxin excretion.

The presence of acute glomerulonephritis accompanied by CHF requires extreme care in digitalization. A relatively low total dose, administered in divided doses, and concomitant use of antihypertensive agents has been recommended. Constant ECG monitoring is essential. Discontinue digitalis as soon as possible.

Dialysis (peritoneal and hemodialysis) has little effect on any of these glycosides.

Combined renal and hepatic failure may prolong digoxin elimination more than normally expected.

Impaired hepatic function does not appear to significantly alter transformation or effects of deslanoside and digoxin; however, reduction in digitoxin dosage may be necessary.

(Warnings continued on following page)

Warnings (Cont.):

Usage in Pregnancy: Category C – Digoxin, Digitoxin. Animal studies have not demonstrated teratogenic effects, and no reports of congenital defects have been reported for the various digitalis glycosides. However, both digoxin and digitoxin rapidly pass into the fetus in a concentration of 50% to 83% of maternal serum. Maternally administered digoxin has been used to treat fetal tachycardia and CHF; fetal toxicity and neonatal death have been a consequence of maternal overdosage. The dosing and control of digoxin in pregnancy may be less predictable than in nonpregnant patients. It is not known whether cardiac glycosides cause fetal harm when administered to a pregnant woman or affect reproduction capacity. Use only when clearly needed and when the potential benefits outweigh the potential hazards to the fetus.

Usage in Lactation: **Digoxin** is excreted into breast milk at a milk:plasma ratio of 0.6 to 0.9. The amount the infant receives is very small and no infant adverse effects have been reported. Safety for use in the nursing mother has not been established. It is not known whether **digitoxin** is excreted in breast milk; exercise caution when administering to a nursing woman.

Usage in Children: Newborn infants display considerable variability in tolerance. Premature and immature infants are particularly sensitive; dosage must be reduced and digitalization should be even more individualized according to infant's degree of maturity. Digitalis glycosides are an important cause of accidental poisoning in children. Impaired renal function must also be taken into consideration.

Carefully titrate dosage and consider differences in the bioavailability of parenteral preparations, capsules, elixirs, and tablets when switching from one preparation to another. ECG monitoring may be necessary to avoid intoxication.

Usage in the Elderly: Exercise special care in elderly patients because their body mass tends to be small and renal clearance is likely to be reduced.

Precautions:

Electrolyte imbalance:

Potassium – Hypokalemia sensitizes the myocardium to digitalis and may reduce the positive inotropic effect of digitalis. Toxicity may develop even with "normal" serum glycoside levels. Therefore, it is desirable to maintain normal serum potassium levels. Potassium wastage may result from diuretic or corticosteroid therapy, hemodialysis or from suction of GI secretions. It may accompany malnutrition, diarrhea, prolonged vomiting, old age, or long-standing CHF. Also, infusion of carbohydrate solution may lower serum potassium by causing an intracellular shift of potassium. In general, avoid rapid changes in serum potassium or other electrolytes; reserve treatment of CHF with IV potassium for special circumstances (see Treatment of Toxicity).

Calcium – Calcium affects cardiac contractility and excitability in a manner similar to digitalis. Calcium, particularly when administered rapidly IV, may produce serious arrhythmias in digitalized patients. Hypercalcemia from any cause predisposes the patient to digitalis toxicity. However, hypocalcemia can nullify the effects of digoxin; thus, digoxin may be ineffective until serum calcium is restored to normal.

Magnesium – Hypomagnesemia may predispose to digitalis toxicity. If low magnesium levels are detected in a patient receiving digoxin, institute replacement therapy.

Thyroid dysfunction: The plasma levels of cardiac glycosides are inversely related to thyroid status. In myxedema, digitalis requirements are less because excretion rate is decreased. In thyrotoxic patients with heart failure, larger doses of the glycoside may be necessary. Results may not be satisfactory until the hyperthyroidism is corrected.

Atrial arrhythmias associated with hypermetabolic states are particularly resistant to digitalis treatment; avoid toxicity if digitalis is used to treat these arrhythmias. Digoxin requirements are reduced in hypothyroidism; digoxin responses in patients with compensated thyroid disease are normal.

Laboratory monitoring tests: Perform periodic determinations of heart rate, electrolytes (especially potassium), ECG and renal function (BUN or serum creatinine). Digoxin may produce false positive ST-T changes in the ECG during exercise testing.

Serum digoxin concentrations - It may also be useful to measure glycoside serum concentrations periodically, especially if digitalis intoxication is suspected.

The relationship of serum glycoside levels to signs or symptoms of intoxication varies significantly from patient to patient; therefore, the value and limitations of this test must be recognized. It is difficult to establish normal glycoside levels that would accurately define toxicity.

To allow adequate time for equilibration of digoxin between serum and tissue, sample serum concentrations at least 6 to 8 hours after the last dose. Ideally, sampling for assessment of steady-state concentrations should be done just before the next dose. Interpret the serum concentration data in the overall clinical context; do not use an isolated serum concentration value alone as a basis for increasing or decreasing digoxin dosage.

(Continued on following page)

Drug Interactions:

Increased digoxin serum levels: The following agents may increase digoxin serum levels, possibly increasing its therapeutic and toxic effects:

Agent	Mechanism
Aminoglycosides, oral[1]	Alteration in GI flora
Amiodarone	Decreased systemic clearance, increased bioavailability
Anticholinergics	Increased GI absorption
Benzodiazepines	Unknown
Captopril	Decreased renal clearance
Diltiazem[2]	Decreased renal clearance
Erythromycin[1]	Alteration in GI flora
Esmolol	Unknown
Flecainide	Unknown
Hydroxychloroquine	Unknown
Ibuprofen	Unknown; possible decreased renal elimination
Indomethacin	Unknown; possible decreased renal elimination
Nifedipine[3]	Decreased renal clearance
Quinidine[2,3]	Decreased distribution and renal and nonrenal clearance
Quinine	Inhibition of nonrenal clearance
Tetracycline[1]	Alteration in GI flora
Tolbutamide	Unknown
Verapamil[2]	Decreased total body clearance, renal and extrarenal elimination

[1] Occurs in < 10% of patients. [2] Though not as well established, digitoxin data appear similar.
[3] Despite increased levels, positive inotropic effect of digoxin may be diminished.

Decreased GI absorption of digitalis glycosides may be caused by the following agents, possibly decreasing the serum levels and therapeutic effects:

- Aminoglycosides, oral
- Aminosalicylic acid
- Antacids (aluminum or magnesium salts)
- Antineoplastics, combination (bleomycin, carmustine, cyclophosphamide, cytarabine, doxorubicin, methotrexate, procarbazine, vincristine)†
- Cholestyramine†
- Colestipol
- Kaolin/pectin
- Metoclopramide†
- Sulfasalazine

† The absorption of the gelatin capsule and elixir formulations of digoxin may not be affected to as great an extent.

Aminoglutethimide, barbiturates, hydantoins, phenylbutazone, and **rifampin** induce the microsomal enzymes that metabolize digitoxin. When these drugs are discontinued, digitoxin toxicity may occur. Monitor digitoxin serum levels; adjust the dose as necessary.

Disopyramide may alter pharmacologic effects of digoxin, although one study suggests a beneficial pharmacodynamic interaction occurs.

Nondepolarizing muscle relaxants and **succinylcholine:** When administered with digitalis glycosides, toxicity (cardiac arrhythmias) of either agent may be increased.

Penicillamine may decrease pharmacologic effects of digoxin, despite administration route.

Potassium-sparing diuretics: Spironolactone may increase or decrease toxic effects of digitalis glycosides; changes cannot be predicted; monitoring is required. Spironolactone may interfere with some digoxin assays. **Amiloride** may decrease inotropic effects of digoxin; **triamterene** may increase its pharmacologic effects.

Thiazide and **loop diuretics** increase urinary loss of potassium; hypokalemia may increase effects and toxicity of digitalis glycosides. Magnesium excretion is also increased and possibly sensitizes myocardium to effects of digitalis glycosides. Observe patients for clinical signs of fluid or electrolyte imbalance; replace electrolytes as appropriate.

Thyroid hormones and **thioamines:** Thyroid hormones may decrease therapeutic effectiveness of digitalis glycosides; thioamines may increase their therapeutic and toxic effects. Euthyroid patients usually require no dosage adjustment of the digitalis glycoside. However, when converting a patient from hypothyroid or hyperthyroid state to euthyroid state, dosage adjustment may be necessary (see Precautions).

(Continued on following page)

Adverse Reactions:

The frequency and severity of adverse reactions to digoxin depend on dose and route of administration, and on the patient's underlying disease or concomitant therapy. Overall incidence of adverse reactions is 5% to 20%, with 15% to 20% considered serious (1% to 4% of patients receiving digoxin). Evidence suggests that the incidence of toxicity has decreased since the introduction of serum digoxin assay and improved standardization of digoxin tablets. Cardiac toxicity accounts for about one-half, GI disturbances for about one-fourth, and CNS and other toxicity for about one-fourth of these adverse reactions.

Anorexia, nausea and vomiting may occur. These effects are central in origin, but following large oral doses, there is also a local emetic action. Abdominal discomfort or pain and diarrhea may also occur. Gynecomastia, allergy, skin rash, eosinophilia and thrombocytopenia can occur, but are rare.

Digitalis Toxicity:

GI: Most common early symptoms are anorexia, nausea, vomiting and diarrhea. However, uncontrolled heart failure may also produce such symptoms. Abdominal discomfort or pain often accompanies GI symptoms. Digitalis toxicity very rarely may cause hemorrhagic necrosis of the intestines.

CNS: Headache, weakness, apathy, drowsiness, visual disturbances (blurred, yellow or green vision, and halo effect), mental depression, confusion, restlessness, disorientation, seizures, EEG abnormalities, delirium, hallucinations, neuralgia and psychosis.

Cardiac disturbances: Ventricular tachycardia may result from digitalis toxicity. Unifocal or multiform premature ventricular contractions (PVCs), especially in bigeminal or trigeminal patterns, are the most common toxic arrhythmias. Paroxysmal and nonparoxysmal nodal rhythms, AV dissociation, accelerated junctional (nodal) rhythm and PAT with block are also common. Excessive slowing of the pulse is a clinical sign of overdosage. AV block of increasing degree may proceed to complete heart block. Atrial fibrillation can occur following large doses of digitalis. Ventricular fibrillation is the most common cause of death from digitalis poisoning. The ECG is fundamental in determining the presence and nature of these cardiac disturbances. Other ECG changes (PR prolongations, the ST depression) provide no measure of the degree of digitalization.

Alterations in cardiac rate and rhythm occurring in digitalis poisoning may simulate almost any known type of arrhythmia seen clinically. Extrasystoles are probably the most frequent effect. An ECG is necessary to aid in differentiation of arrhythmia due to digitalis poisoning from that due to heart disease. Older patients, particularly those with disease of the coronary arteries and impaired myocardial blood supply, are more susceptible to these untoward effects. Sinus arrhythmia may occur early as a minor toxic effect. Paroxysmal atrial and ventricular tachycardia call for immediate cessation of the drug.

Children: Toxicity differs from the adult in a number of respects. Anorexia, nausea, vomiting, diarrhea, neurologic and visual disturbances are rarely seen as initial signs of digitalis toxicity in children. Visual disturbances (blurred or yellow vision), headache, weakness, apathy and psychosis may occur but may be difficult to recognize in infants and children. Cardiac arrhythmias are more frequent and reliable signs of toxicity. Digoxin in children may produce any arrhythmia. Common manifestations of digitalis toxicity in children include conduction disturbances or supraventricular tachyarrhythmias, such as AV block (Wenckebach), atrial tachycardia with or without block and junctional (nodal) tachycardia. Ventricular arrhythmias such as unifocal or multiform ventricular premature contractions, especially in bigeminal or trigeminal patterns are less common. Ventricular tachycardia may result from digitalis toxicity. Sinus bradycardia may also be a sign of impending digoxin intoxication, especially in infants, even in the absence of first degree heart block. Any arrhythmia or alteration in cardiac conduction that develops in a child taking digoxin should initially be assumed to be a consequence of digoxin intoxication.

(Continued on following page)

Treatment of Toxicity:

Adults: Discontinue digitalis until all signs of toxicity are abolished. This may be all that is necessary if toxic manifestations are not severe and appear after peak effect of the drug.

Potassium salts are commonly used, particularly if hypokalemia is present. Potassium chloride in divided oral doses totaling 3 to 6 g (40 to 80 mEq) for adults may be given, provided renal function is adequate. When correction of arrhythmia is urgent and serum potassium level is low to normal, give potassium IV in 5% dextrose injection. For adults, give a total of 40 to 80 mEq (diluted to a concentration of 40 mEq per 500 ml) at a rate not exceeding 20 mEq per hour, or slower if limited by pain due to local irritation. Give additional amounts if arrhythmia is uncontrolled and potassium and fluid volume are well tolerated. Since the action of potassium ion lasts only minutes after infusion is discontinued, give oral potassium for prolonged suppression of arrhythmias. Monitor the ECG to avoid potassium toxicity (eg, peaking of T waves) and to observe the arrhythmia so that infusion may be stopped when desired effect is achieved.

Caution: Do not use potassium when severe or complete heart block is due to digitalis and not related to tachycardia. Potassium is contraindicated in the presence of renal failure.

Phenytoin – For atrial and ventricular arrhythmias unresponsive to potassium, administer phenytoin 0.5 mg/kg, at a rate not exceeding 50 mg/min, at 1 to 2 hour intervals; the maximum dose should not exceed 10 mg/kg/day.

Lidocaine – 1 mg/kg over 5 minutes, then infusing 15 to 50 mcg/kg/min to maintain normal cardiac rhythm may be an alternative.

Cholestyramine, colestipol or activated charcoal may be useful in digitalis toxicity by binding the glycoside in the intestine, thus preventing enterohepatic recirculation.

Atropine – Severe sinus bradycardia or a slow ventricular rate due to secondary AV block may be symptomatically treated with atropine (0.01 mg/kg, IV).

Other agents used for the treatment of digitalis toxicity include quinidine, procainamide and propranolol. Other antiarrhythmics appear less successful or more hazardous. In advanced heart block, temporary ventricular pacing may be beneficial.

Countershock – Interruption of life-threatening arrhythmias by direct-current countershock is considered hazardous in digitalis overdosage and should be the last resort. If countershock is required, begin therapy at low voltage levels.

Digoxin immune FAB – A new treatment of digitalis intoxication is digoxin immune FAB (p. 2689). Given in approximate equimolar quantities as digoxin, it generally reverses all signs and symptoms of toxicity and leads to total recovery in over 80% of treated cases. Improvement usually begins within half an hour of administration.

Children: Potassium preparations may be given orally in divided doses totaling 1 to 1.5 mEq/kg. When correction of the arrhythmia is urgent, give approximately 0.5 mEq/kg/hr of potassium, with careful ECG monitoring. The potassium IV solution should be dilute enough to avoid local irritation; however, take care to avoid IV fluid overload, especially in infants. Digoxin immune FAB may also be used in infants and children.

Patient Information:

Do not discontinue medication without first checking with a physician.

Avoid *otc* antacids, cough, cold, allergy and diet drugs, except on professional advice.

Notify physician if loss of appetite, lower stomach pain, nausea, vomiting, diarrhea, unusual tiredness or weakness, drowsiness, headache, blurred or yellow vision, skin rash or hives, or mental depression occurs.

Administration:

Loading doses: The use of initial large loading doses rapidly establishes effective plasma levels, but also increases risks of toxicity because of its narrow toxic-therapeutic ratio. Administration of small daily maintenance doses are then given to replace daily losses due to metabolism and excretion. Without a loading dose, slow digitalization may be achieved within 1 week with digoxin and in 10 to 14 days with digitoxin, with a much lower risk of toxicity than when giving a loading dose. For a rapid effect in acutely ill patients, parenteral administration of deslanoside or digoxin can be used. Use parenterally only when the drug cannot be taken orally or rapid digitalization is urgent.

Maintenance therapy: Maintenance dosage is determined tentatively by the amount necessary to sustain the desired therapeutic effect. Recommended dosages are practical average figures which may require considerable modification as dictated by individual sensitivity or associated conditions. Diminished renal function is the most important factor requiring modification of recommended doses of digoxin.

(Products listed on following pages)

Complete prescribing information for these products begins on page 591.

DIGITOXIN

Administration and Dosage:

Loading dose:

Rapid – 0.6 mg initially, followed by 0.4 mg, then 0.2 mg at intervals of 4 to 6 hours.

Slow – 0.2 mg twice daily for a period of 4 days, followed by maintenance dosage.

Maintenance: Ranges from 0.05 to 0.3 mg daily, the most common dose being 0.15 mg daily.

Children (loading dose): Individualize dosage. Monitor ECG to avoid toxic doses.

Generally, premature and immature infants are particularly sensitive and require a reduced dosage that must be determined by careful adjustment. Divide the total dose into 3, 4 or more portions, with 6 hours or more between doses.

After the neonatal period, the recommended digitalizing dose is as follows:

Under one year of age – 0.045 mg/kg.

One to two years of age – 0.04 mg/kg.

Over two years of age – 0.03 mg/kg (0.75 mg/m²).

Children (maintenance dose): Administer one-tenth (10%) of the digitalizing dose.

				C.I.*
Rx	**Digitoxin** (Various)	**Tablets:** 0.1 mg	In 1000s.	4+
Rx	**Digitoxin** (Various)	**Tablets:** 0.2 mg	In 1000s.	3+

DESLANOSIDE (Desacetyl-Lanatoside C)

Administration and Dosage:

Use parenteral administration only when the drug cannot be taken orally, or rapid digitalization is very urgent.

Loading dose: Rapid results can be obtained within 12 hours by giving 1.6 mg IM or IV.

IV – May be given as one injection or in portions of 0.8 mg each.

IM – Inject 0.8 mg at each of 2 sites.

Maintenance: May be accomplished by starting administration of an oral preparation within 12 hours.

				C.I.*
Rx	**Cedilanid-D** (Sandoz)	**Injection:** 0.2 mg per ml.[1]	In 2 ml ampuls.	638

* Cost Index based on cost per 0.1 mg.

[1] With 15% glycerin and 9.8% alcohol.

Complete prescribing information for these products begins on page 591 .

DIGOXIN

Administration:

Parenteral administration: The IV digitalizing dose is ≈ 20% less than an oral dose. Intramuscular injection offers no advantages and can cause severe pain at injection site; IV administration is preferred. Give injections over 5 minutes or longer, undiluted or diluted with a fourfold or greater volume of Sterile Water for Injection, 0.9% Sodium Chloride Injection, 5% Dextrose Injection or Lactated Ringer's Injection. Use of less diluent could lead to digoxin precipitation. Use diluted product immediately.

Dosage:

Adults:

Rapid digitalization with a loading dose – Peak body digoxin stores of 8 to 12 mcg/kg should provide therapeutic effect. Larger stores (10 to 15 mcg/kg) are often required for control of ventricular rate in patients with atrial flutter or fibrillation. Use conservative projected peak body stores for patients with renal insufficiency (ie, 6 to 10 mcg/kg). Base the loading dose on the projected peak body stores and administer in several portions with roughly half the total given as the first dose. Give additional fractions at 4 to 8 hour intervals IV or orally, with careful assessment of clinical response before each additional dose.

In undigitalized patients, a single initial IV dose of 400 to 600 mcg (0.4 to 0.6 mg) usually produces a detectable effect in 5 to 30 minutes that becomes maximal in 1 to 4 hours. The usual parenteral amount for a 70 kg patient to achieve 8 to 15 mcg/kg peak body stores is 600 to 1000 mcg (0.6 to 1 mg). A single initial oral dose of 500 to 750 mcg (0.5 to 0.75 mg) usually produces a detectable effect in 0.5 to 2 hours that becomes maximal in 2 to 6 hours. The usual oral amount required for a 70 kg patient to achieve 8 to 15 mcg/kg peak body stores is 750 to 1250 mcg (0.75 to 1.25 mg).

Base the maintenance dose upon the percentage of the peak body stores lost each day through elimination. The following formula has wide clinical use:

$$\text{Maintenance Dose} = \text{Peak Body Stores (ie, Loading Dose)} \times \frac{\text{\% Daily Loss}}{100} \text{ (ie, 14 + Ccr/5)}$$

Ccr is creatinine clearance, corrected to 70 kg body weight or 1.73 m^2 body surface area.

Gradual digitalization with a maintenance dose – The following table provides average oral (tablet) daily maintenance dose requirements for patients with heart failure based upon lean body weight and renal function:

Usual Digoxin Tablet Daily Maintenance Dose Requirements (mcg) For Estimated Peak Body Stores of 10 mcg/kg							
Corrected Ccr (ml/min/70 kg)	Lean Body Weight (kg/lbs)						Number of Days Before Steady-State Achieved
	50/110	60/132	70/154	80/176	90/198	100/220	
0	63*†	125	125	125	188††	188	22
10	125	125	125	188	188	188	19
20	125	125	188	188	188	250	16
30	125	188	188	188	250	250	14
40	125	188	188	250	250	250	13
50	188	188	250	250	250	250	12
60	188	188	250	250	250	375	11
70	188	250	250	250	250	375	10
80	188	250	250	250	375	375	9
90	188	250	250	250	375	500	8
100	250	250	250	375	375	500	7

* 63 mcg = 0.063 mg.

† ½ of 125 mcg tablet or 125 mcg every other day.

†† 1½ of 125 mcg tablet.

Example – A patient with an estimated lean body weight of 70 kg and a Ccr of 60 ml/min should be given a 250 mcg (0.25 mg) tablet each day. Steady-state serum concentrations should not be anticipated before 11 days.

(Dosage continued on following page)

DIGOXIN (Cont.)

Dosage (Cont.):

Infants and children: Individualize dosage. Divided daily dosing is recommended for infants and young children under 10 years of age. Children over 10 require adult dosages in proportion to their body weight.

Rapid digitalization with a loading dose – Digitalizing and daily maintenance doses for each age group are given below. Larger doses are often required for adequate control of ventricular rate in patients with atrial flutter or fibrillation.

Administer loading dose in several portions, give roughly half the total as the first dose. Give additional fractions of total dose at 6 to 8 hr intervals (oral) or 4 to 8 hr intervals (parenteral). Carefully assess clinical response before each additional dose.

Usual Digitalizing and Maintenance Dosages with Normal Renal Function Based on Lean Body Weight

Age	Digitalizing Dose† (mcg/kg)		Daily Maintenance Dose (mcg/kg)
	Oral	IV	
Premature	20-30	15-25	20%-30% of the loading dose††
Full term	25-35	20-30	25%-35% of the loading dose††
1-24 months	35-60	30-50	
2-5 years	30-40	25-35	
5-10 years	20-35	15-30	
Over 10 years	10-15	8-12	

† IV digitalizing doses are 80% of oral digitalizing doses.
†† Projected or actual digitalizing dose providing desired clinical response.

Gradual digitalization is accomplished by beginning an appropriate maintenance dose. The range of percentages provided above can be used in calculating this dose. *Both the adult and pediatric dosage guidelines provided are based upon average patient response; substantial individual variation can be expected.*

Adjust maintenance dose in previously digitalized patients at steady-state in proportion to the ratio of desired vs measured serum concentration (ie, doubling the dose results in doubling the serum concentration).

Lanoxicaps (gelatin capsules) have greater bioavailability than standard tablets. Therefore, the 0.2 mg capsule is equivalent to 0.25 mg tablets; the 0.1 mg capsule is equivalent to 0.125 mg tablets; and the 0.05 mg capsule is equivalent to 0.0625 mg.

Use in the elderly: Since digoxin is eliminated by the kidneys, a decreased clearance may occur in elderly patients with decreased renal function. Therefore, a lower maintenance dose of digoxin may be necessary. Adjust the dose accordingly.

Bioequivalence: Bioavailability differences have been documented. Current requirements for FDA approved products should minimize such problems; however, monitor patients being changed from one product to another for changes in clinical response.

	Product	Form	Description	C.I.*
Rx	**Lanoxicaps** (Burroughs Wellcome)	**Capsules:** 0.05 mg	(#A2C). Red. In 100s.	753
		0.1 mg	(#B2C). Yellow. In 100s.	412
		0.2 mg	(#C2C). Green. In 100s.	240
Rx	**Digoxin** (Vangard)	**Tablets:** 0.125 mg	In UD 32s.	144
Rx	**Lanoxin** (B-W)		(#Lanoxin Y3B). In 100s, 1000s.	264
Rx	**Digoxin** (Various)	**Tablets:** 0.25 mg	In 100s, 1000s and UD 32s.	18+
Rx	**Lanoxin** (Burroughs Wellcome)		(#Lanoxin X3A). White. In 100s, 1000s, UD 100s and u-of-u 30s.	132
Rx	**Lanoxin** (B-W)	**Tablets:** 0.5 mg	(#Lanoxin T9A). Green. In 100s.	96
Rx	**Digoxin** (Pharmafair)	**Elixir, pediatric:** 0.05 mg per ml	10% alcohol. Lime flavor.	644
Rx	**Digoxin** (Roxane)		10% alcohol. In 60 ml and UD 2.5 and 5 ml.	700
Rx	**Lanoxin** (Burroughs Wellcome)		10% alcohol. Lime flavor. In 60 ml with dropper.	493
Rx	**Digoxin** (Elkins-Sinn)	**Injection:** 0.25 mg per ml	In 2 ml amps.[1]	988
Rx	**Digoxin** (Wyeth)		In 1 and 2 ml Tubex.[2]	2283
Rx	**Lanoxin** (B-W)		In 2 ml amps.[2]	1100
Rx	**Lanoxin** (Burroughs Wellcome)	**Injection, pediatric:** 0.1 mg per ml	In 1 ml amps.[2]	5267

* Cost Index based on cost per 0.25 mg.
\# Product identification code.
[1] With 0.1 ml alcohol.
[2] With 40% propylene glycol and 10% alcohol.

AMRINONE LACTATE

Actions:

Pharmacology: Amrinone is a positive inotropic agent with vasodilator activity, different in structure and mode of action from either digitalis glycosides or catecholamines. Its mechanism has not been fully elucidated.

Amrinone is not a β-adrenergic agonist. It inhibits myocardial cyclic adenosine monophosphate (c-AMP) phosphodiesterase activity and increases cellular levels of c-AMP. It does not inhibit sodium-potassium ATPase activity.

Amrinone reduces afterload and preload by its direct relaxant effect on vascular smooth muscle. In patients with depressed myocardial function, amrinone produces a prompt increase in cardiac output due to its inotropic and vasodilator actions.

Improvement in left ventricular function and relief of congestive heart failure (CHF) in patients with ischemic heart disease have been observed without inducing symptoms or electrocardiographic signs of myocardial ischemia.

Amrinone produces hemodynamic and symptomatic benefits to patients not satisfactorily controlled by conventional therapy with diuretics and cardiac glycosides.

Pharmacokinetics:

Distribution – Amrinone has a volume of distribution of 1.2 liters/kg and a distribution half-life of about 4.6 minutes. It is 10% to 49% protein bound. In CHF patients, after a loading bolus dose, steady-state plasma levels of about 2.4 mcg/ml are maintained by an infusion of 5 to 10 mcg/kg/min. With associated compromised renal and hepatic perfusion, plasma levels may rise.

Metabolism/Excretion – Amrinone is metabolized by conjugative pathways. Mean elimination half-life is about 3.6 hours. In patients with CHF, the mean elimination half-life is about 5.8 hours (range 3 to 15 hours).

The primary route of excretion is via the urine as both amrinone and metabolites. Approximately 63% of an oral dose is excreted in the urine over 96 hours. Approximately 18% is excreted in the feces in 72 hours. In a 24 hour IV amrinone study, 10% to 40% was excreted unchanged in the urine.

Onset/Duration/Effect – Dose-related maximum increases in cardiac output occur; the peak effect occurs within 10 minutes at all doses. The duration of effect depends upon the dose, lasting about one-half hour at 0.75 mg/kg and approximately 2 hours at 3 mg/kg. Increases in cardiac index show a linear relationship to plasma concentration at a range of 0.5 to 7 mcg/ml.

Pulmonary capillary wedge pressure (PCWP) and total peripheral resistance show dose-related decreases. At doses up to 3 mg/kg, dose-related decreases in diastolic pressure (up to 13%) have been observed. Mean arterial pressure decreases (9.7%) at a dose of 3 mg/kg. Heart rate is generally unchanged.

Indications:

For the short-term management of CHF. Use only in patients who can be closely monitored and who have not responded adequately to digitalis, diuretics or vasodilators. Duration of therapy depends on patient responsiveness.

Contraindications:

Hypersensitivity to amrinone or bisulfites.

Warnings:

Amrinone's inotropic effects are additive to those of digitalis. In cases of atrial flutter/fibrillation, amrinone may increase ventricular response rate because of its slight enhancement of atrioventricular (AV) conduction. In these cases, prior treatment with digitalis is recommended.

Hypersensitivity occurred in patients treated for about 2 weeks with oral amrinone (see Adverse Reactions). Consider hypersensitivity reactions in any patient maintained for a prolonged period on amrinone. Refer to Management of Acute Hypersensitivity Reactions on p. viii.

Carcinogenesis, mutagenesis, impairment of fertility: Dystocia occurred in rats receiving 100 mg/kg/day, resulting in increased numbers of stillbirths, decreased litter size and poor pup survival.

Usage in Pregnancy: Category C. Animal studies (15 to 50 mg/kg) are conflicting. There are no adequate and well-controlled studies in pregnant women. Use during pregnancy only if the potential benefit justifies the potential risk to the fetus.

Usage in Lactation: It is not known whether amrinone is secreted in breast milk. Exercise caution when administering to nursing women.

Usage in Children: Safety and efficacy in children have not been established. In a preterm infant, the short-term use of amrinone (5 mg/kg/min) was effective in the management of the infant's CHF.

(Continued on following page)

AMRINONE LACTATE (Cont.)

Precautions:

Do not use amrinone in patients with severe aortic or pulmonic valvular disease in lieu of surgical relief of the obstruction. It may aggravate outflow tract obstruction in hypertrophic subaortic stenosis.

Arrhythmias, supraventricular and ventricular, have been observed in the very high-risk population treated. While amrinone per se is not arrhythmogenic, the potential for arrhythmia present in CHF itself may be increased by any drug or drug combination.

Thrombocytopenia is more common in patients receiving prolonged therapy. In patients whose platelet counts were not allowed to remain depressed, no bleeding occurred.

Platelet reduction is dose-dependent and appears to be due to a decreased platelet survival time. Bone marrow examinations were normal. There is no evidence of immune response or a platelet-activating factor.

Usage in acute myocardial infarction: No clinical trials have been carried out in patients in the acute phase of postmyocardial infarction. Therefore, amrinone is not recommended in these cases.

Hepatotoxicity: If acute marked alterations in liver enzymes occur together with clinical symptoms, discontinue amrinone. If less than marked enzyme alterations occur without clinical symptoms, continue amrinone, reduce dosage or discontinue the drug based on benefit-to-risk considerations.

Fluid Balance: Patients who have received vigorous diuretic therapy may have insufficient cardiac filling pressure to respond adequately to amrinone; cautious liberalization of fluid and electrolyte intake may be indicated.

Monitoring: Fluids and Electrolytes – Monitor fluid and electrolyte changes and renal function during amrinone therapy; improvement in cardiac output with resultant diuresis may necessitate a reduction in the dose of diuretic. Potassium loss due to excessive diuresis may predispose digitalized patients to arrhythmias. Therefore, correct hypokalemia by potassium supplementation in advance of or during amrinone use.

Monitor blood pressure and heart rate and slow or stop the infusion rate in patients showing excessive decreases in blood pressure.

Patient improvement may be reflected by increases in cardiac output, cardiac index, reduction in pulmonary capillary wedge pressure and such clinical responses as a lessening of dyspnea, orthopnea and fatigue.

Monitoring central venous pressure (CVP) may be valuable in assessing hypotension and fluid balance management. Also, measure urine output and body weight.

Sulfite Sensitivity: This product contains sodium metabisulfite, a sulfite that may cause allergic-type reactions (including anaphylactic symptoms and life-threatening or less severe asthmatic episodes) in certain susceptible people. The overall prevalence of sulfite sensitivity in the general population is unknown and probably low. Sulfite sensitivity is seen more frequently in asthmatic people.

Adverse Reactions:

Thrombocytopenia, (< 100,000/cu mm), has occurred in 2.4% of patients (see Precautions).

GI: Nausea (1.7%); vomiting (0.9%); abdominal pain (0.4%); anorexia (0.4%); hepatotoxicity (0.2%) (see Precautions). Should severe or debilitating GI effects occur, reduce dosage or discontinue the drug based on the usual benefit-to-risk considerations.

Cardiovascular: Arrhythmia (3%) and hypotension (1.3%).

Hypersensitivity: Pericarditis, pleuritis and ascites (fatal in 1 case), myositis with interstitial shadowing on chest x-ray and elevated sedimentation rate (1 case) and vasculitis with nodular pulmonary densities, hypoxemia and jaundice with oral amrinone (see Warnings).

Miscellaneous: Fever (0.9%); chest pain (0.2%); burning at the injection site (0.2%).

Management of adverse reactions: Platelet count reductions – Asymptomatic platelet count reduction (to < 150,000/cu mm) may be reversed within 1 week of a decrease in drug dosage. Further, with no change in drug dosage, the count may stabilize at lower than pre-drug levels without any clinical sequelae. Pre-drug platelet counts and frequent platelet counts during therapy are recommended. If a platelet count less than 150,000/cu mm occurs, consider the following:

- Maintain total daily dose unchanged
- Decrease total daily dose
- Discontinue if risk exceeds the potential benefit

(Continued on following page)

AMRINONE LACTATE (Cont.)

Overdosage:

A death has occurred with a massive accidental overdose, although causal relationship is uncertain. Exercise diligence during product preparation and administration.

Amrinone's vasodilator effect may produce hypotension. If this occurs, reduce or discontinue administration. Institute general measures for circulatory support. Refer to Management of Acute Overdosage.

Administration and Dosage:

Administer as supplied or dilute in normal or one-half normal saline solution to a concentration of 1 to 3 mg/ml. Use diluted solutions within 24 hours.

Initial therapy: 0.75 mg/kg IV bolus slowly over 2 to 3 minutes.

Maintenance infusion: 5 to 10 mcg/kg/min.

An additional bolus of 0.75 mg/kg may be given 30 minutes after initiating therapy.

Do not exceed a total daily dose (including loading doses) of 10 mg/kg. A limited number of patients studied at higher doses support a dosage regimen of up to 18 mg/kg/day for shortened durations of therapy.

Adjust rate of administration and duration of therapy according to patient response.

The above dosing regimen creates plasma concentration of ≈ 3 mcg/ml.

Incompatibilities: A chemical interaction occurs slowly over a 24 hour period when amrinone is mixed *directly* with dextrose-containing solutions. Therefore, do NOT dilute with dextrose-containing solutions prior to injection. Amrinone may be injected into a running dextrose infusion through a Y-connector or directly into the tubing where preferable.

When furosemide is injected into an IV line of amrinone infusion, a precipitate immediately forms. Do not administer furosemide in IV lines containing amrinone.

Storage: Protect ampuls from light.

Rx	**Inocor** (Winthrop Pharm.)	**Injection:** 5 mg/ml (as lactate)	In 20 ml amps.[1]

[1] With 0.25 mg sodium metabisulfite.

Antianginal agents include rapid-acting nitrates used to relieve the pain of acute angina and long-acting preparations used for prophylaxis or to decrease the severity of angina pectoris. Dipyridamole, β-adrenergic blocking agents and the calcium channel blockers are also used in the prophylaxis of chronic angina. Refer to individual monographs.

NITRATES

Actions:

Pharmacology: Relaxation of vascular smooth muscle via stimulation of intracellular cyclic guanosine monophosphate production is the principal pharmacologic action of nitrates. Although venous effects predominate, nitroglycerin produces a dose-dependent dilation of both arterial and venous beds. Dilation of the postcapillary vessels, including large veins, promotes peripheral pooling of blood and decreases venous return to the heart, reducing left ventricular end-diastolic pressure (preload). Arteriolar relaxation reduces systemic vascular resistance and arterial pressure (afterload). Myocardial oxygen consumption or demand (as measured by the pressure-rate product, tension-time index and stroke-work index) is decreased by both arterial and venous effects of nitroglycerin, and a more favorable supply-demand ratio is achieved. In coronary circulation, the nitrates redistribute circulating blood flow along collateral channels, improving perfusion to the ischemic myocardium. While the large epicardial coronary arteries are also dilated by nitroglycerin, the extent to which this action contributes to relief of exertional angina is unclear.

Therapeutic doses reduce systolic, diastolic and mean arterial blood pressure. Effective coronary perfusion pressure is usually maintained, but can be compromised if blood pressure falls excessively or increased heart rate decreases diastolic filling time. Elevated central venous and pulmonary capillary wedge pressures (PCWP), pulmonary vascular resistance and systemic vascular resistance are also reduced. Reflex tachycardia may occur, presumably in response to decreased blood pressure. Cardiac index may be increased, decreased or unchanged. Patients with elevated left ventricular filling pressure and systemic vascular resistance values with a depressed cardiac index are likely to have improved cardiac index. When filling pressures and cardiac index are normal, cardiac index may be slightly reduced by nitrates.

Pharmacokinetics:

Doseform, Onset and Duration of Available Nitrates			
Nitrates	Dosage form	Onset (minutes)	Duration
Amyl nitrite	Inhalant	0.5	3 to 5 min
Nitroglycerin	IV	1 to 2	3 to 5 min
	Sublingual	1 to 3	30 to 60 min
	Translingual spray	2	30 to 60 min
	Transmucosal tablet	1 to 2	3 to 5 hours[1]
	Oral, sustained release	20 to 45	3 to 8 hours
	Topical ointment	30 to 60	2 to 12 hours[2]
	Transdermal	30 to 60	up to 24 hours[3]
Isosorbide dinitrate	Sublingual	2 to 5	1 to 3 hours
	Oral	20 to 40	4 to 6 hours
	Oral, sustained release	up to 4 hours	6 to 8 hours
Isosorbide mononitrate	Oral	30 to 60	nd
Erythrityl tetranitrate	Sublingual & chewable	5	3 hours
	Oral	15 to 30	6 hours
Pentaerythritol tetranitrate	Oral	20 to 60	≈ 5 hours
	Oral, sustained release	30	up to 12 hours

nd = No data.

[1] A significant antianginal effect can persist for 5 hours if the tablet has not completely dissolved by this time.

[2] Depends on total amount used per unit of surface area.

[3] Tolerance may develop after 12 hours (see Precautions and Administration and Dosage).

(Actions continued on following page)

NITRATES (Cont.)

Actions (Cont.):

Pharmacokinetics (Cont.): Nitroglycerin, isosorbide dinitrate and erythrityl tetranitrate are readily absorbed from the sublingual mucosa. Nitroglycerin is also absorbed through the skin. Nitroglycerin ointments and transdermal systems provide a gradual release of the drug which reaches target organs before hepatic inactivation.

Nitroglycerin has a short half-life, estimated at 1 to 4 minutes, resulting in a low plasma concentration after IV infusion. At plasma concentrations between 50 and 500 ng/ml, plasma protein binding of nitroglycerin is approximately 60%.

Nitrates are metabolized in the liver by nitrate reductase. Although less potent as vasodilators, the two active major metabolites, 1,2 and 1,3 dinitroglycerols, have longer plasma half-lives than the parent compound and appear in substantial concentration; therefore, they may be responsible for some of the pharmacologic activity. Dinitrates are further metabolized to inactive mononitrates. Isosorbide dinitrate, however, is metabolized to 2- and 5-mononitrates, which are both active and accumulate more than the parent drug with long-term therapy, and ultimately to glycerol and CO_2. Since isosorbide mononitrate is a major active metabolite of isosorbide dinitrate, and since most of the clinical activity of the dinitrate is attributable to the mononitrate, isosorbide mononitrate is now available as a single entity product.

Extensive first-pass deactivation follows GI absorption. Hepatic reductase activity may be saturated by some oral nitroglycerin doses, resulting in prolonged pharmacologic effects.

Approximately one-third of an inhaled dose of amyl nitrite is excreted in the urine.

Indications:

Acute angina (nitroglycerin-sublingual, transmucosal or translingual spray; isosorbide dinitrate-sublingual; amyl nitrite): For relief of acute anginal episodes; prophylaxis prior to events likely to provoke an attack. Because of the more rapid relief of chest pain with sublingual nitroglycerin, limit the use of sublingual isosorbide dinitrate for aborting an acute anginal attack to patients intolerant or unresponsive to sublingual nitroglycerin.

Angina prophylaxis (nitroglycerin-topical, transdermal, translingual spray, transmucosal and oral sustained release; isosorbide dinitrate; isosorbide mononitrate; erythrityl tetranitrate; pentaerythritol tetranitrate): Prophylaxis and long-term management of recurrent angina.

Nitroglycerin IV: Control of blood pressure in perioperative hypertension associated with surgical procedures, especially cardiovascular procedures, such as endotracheal intubation, anesthesia, skin incision, sternotomy, cardiac bypass and in the immediate post-surgical period.

Congestive heart failure (CHF) associated with acute myocardial infarction (MI); treatment of angina pectoris unresponsive to organic nitrates or β-blockers; production of controlled hypotension during surgical procedures.

Unlabeled uses: Sublingual and topical nitroglycerin and oral nitrates have been used to reduce cardiac workload in patients with acute MI and in CHF.

Nitroglycerin ointment has been used as adjunctive treatment of Raynaud's disease and other peripheral vascular diseases. A synergistic effect (reduced platelet deposition and increased platelet survival) occurred when isosorbide dinitrate (40 mg/day) and prostaglandin E_1 (5 ng/kg/min for 6 hours) were used in patients with peripheral vascular disease. It may also be beneficial as an aid to venous cannulation in children < 1 year of age using a dose of 0.4 to 0.8 mg.

IV nitroglycerin (5 to 100 mcg/min infusion) may be used in the treatment of hypertensive crisis, specifically in patients who have hypertension with angina or MI.

Refer to individual drug monographs on the following pages for FDA labeled indications.

Contraindications:

Hypersensitivity or idiosyncrasy to nitrates; severe anemia; closed angle glaucoma; postural hypotension; early MI (sublingual nitroglycerin); head trauma or cerebral hemorrhage (since these drugs may increase intracranial pressure); allergy to adhesives (transdermal).

Amyl nitrite: Pregnancy (see Warnings).

Nitroglycerin IV: Hypotension or uncorrected hypovolemia, since IV use in such states could produce severe hypotension or shock; inadequate cerebral circulation; increased intracranial pressure; constrictive pericarditis; pericardial tamponade.

(Continued on following page)

NITRATES (Cont.)

Warnings:

MI: Data supporting the use of nitrates during the early days of the acute phase of MI are insufficient to establish safety. In acute MI, use nitrates only under close clinical observation and with hemodynamic monitoring. In general, a long-acting form should not be used because its effects are difficult to terminate rapidly should excessive hypotension or tachycardia develop. The effects of isosorbide mononitrate are difficult to terminate rapidly; avoid use in patients with acute MI or CHF.

Arcing: A cardioverter/defibrillator should not be discharged through a paddle electrode that overlies a transdermal nitroglycerin system. The arcing that may be seen in this situation is harmless in itself, but it may be associated with local current concentration that can cause damage to the paddles and burns to the patient.

Postural hypotension may occur, even with small doses. Transient episodes of dizziness, weakness, syncope or other signs of cerebral ischemia due to postural hypotension may develop following administration, particularly if the patient is standing immobile. Alcohol accentuates this reaction. Use measures which facilitate venous return (eg, head-low posture, deep breathing, movements of the extremities) to hasten recovery. Fatalities have occurred.

Angina: Nitrates may aggravate angina caused by hypertrophic cardiomyopathy.

Nitroglycerin IV: The available preparations differ in concentration or volume per vial or ampul. When switching from one product to another, pay attention to the dilution, dosage and administration instructions. Some of these products contain alcohol and propylene glycol; safety for intracoronary injection has not been established.

Absorption – Nitroglycerin readily migrates into many plastics. To avoid absorption of nitroglycerin into plastic parenteral solution containers, dilute and store only in glass parenteral solution bottles. Since some filters also absorb nitroglycerin, avoid if possible (see IV Administration and Dosage).

Hepatic or renal disease, severe: Use with caution.

Hypotension – Avoid excessive prolonged hypotension, because of possible deleterious effects on the brain, heart, liver and kidney from poor perfusion and the attendant risk of ischemia, thrombosis and altered organ function. Paradoxical bradycardia and increased angina pectoris may accompany nitroglycerin-induced hypotension. Use with caution in subjects who may have volume depletion from diuretics or in those with low systolic blood pressure (eg, < 90 mmHg). Patients with normal or low PCWP are especially sensitive to the hypotensive effects of IV nitroglycerin. A fall in PCWP precedes the onset of arterial hypotension; the PCWP is thus a useful guide to safe titration of the drug.

Alcohol intoxication has developed in patients receiving high doses of IV nitroglycerin. Consider this complication when administering high doses for prolonged periods.

Sublingual nitroglycerin: Absorption is dependent on salivary secretion. Dry mouth (including drug-induced dry mouth) decreases absorption.

Transdermal nitroglycerin is not for immediate relief of anginal attacks.

Pregnancy: Category C. Safety for use during pregnancy has not been established. Use only when clearly needed and when the potential benefits outweigh the potential hazards to the fetus.

Category X (amyl nitrite). Because it markedly reduces systemic blood pressure and blood flow on the maternal side of the placenta, amyl nitrite can cause harm to the fetus when it is administered to a pregnant woman.

Lactation: It is not known whether nitrates are excreted in breast milk. Exercise caution when administering to a nursing woman.

Because of the potential for serious adverse reactions in nursing infants from **amyl nitrite,** decide whether to discontinue nursing or to discontinue the drug, taking into account the importance of the drug to the mother.

Children: Safety and efficacy for use in children have not been established.

Precautions:

Glaucoma: Intraocular pressure may be increased; therefore, caution is required in administering to patients with glaucoma.

Excessive dosage may produce severe headache. Lowering the dose and using analgesics will help control the headaches, which diminish or disappear as therapy continues. Discontinue the drug if blurred vision or dry mouth occurs.

Volume depletion/hypotension: Severe hypotension (particularly with upright posture) may occur with even small doses of isosorbide mononitrate. Exercise caution in patients who may be volume depleted or hypotensive for any reason. Hypotension may be accompanied by paradoxical bradycardia and increased angina pectoris.

(Precautions continued on following page)

Complete prescribing information for these products begins on page 604.

AMYL NITRITE

Indications:

Relief of angina pectoris.

Administration and Dosage:

Usual adult dose is 0.3 ml by inhalation, as required.

Crush the capsule and wave under the nose; 1 to 6 inhalations from one capsule are usually sufficient to produce the desired effect. May repeat in 3 to 5 minutes.

Storage: Protect from light. Store in a cool place, 15° to 30°C (59° to 86°F).

				C.I.*
Rx	**Amyl Nitrite** (Various, eg, Goldline, Moore)	**Inhalant:** 0.3 ml	In 12s.	54+
Rx	**Amyl Nitrite Aspirols** (Lilly)		In 12s.	27
Rx	**Amyl Nitrite Vaporole** (B-W)		In 12s.	47

NITROGLYCERIN, SUBLINGUAL

Indications:

Prophylaxis, treatment and management of angina pectoris.

Administration and Dosage:

Dissolve 1 tablet under tongue or in buccal pouch (between cheek and gum) at first sign of an acute anginal attack. Repeat approximately every 5 minutes until relief is obtained. Take no more than 3 tablets in 15 minutes. If pain continues, notify physician immediately. May be used prophylactically 5 to 10 minutes prior to activities which might precipitate an acute attack.

Storage: Dispense in the original container; store at room temperature. Protect from moisture. The stabilized sublingual tablets are less subject to potency loss than the previous conventional sublingual tablets; *Nitrostat* carries a 5 year expiration date, under proper storage conditions in the unopened container. Traditionally, unused tablets should be discarded 6 months after the original bottle is opened.

				C.I.*
Rx	**Nitrostat** (Parke-Davis)	**Tablets, sublingual:** 0.15 mg (1/400 gr)	In 100s and unit-of-use 100s.	8.9
		0.3 mg (1/200 gr)	In 100s and unit-of-use 100s.	4.4
		0.4 mg (1/150 gr)	In 100s and unit-of-use 100s.	3.3
		0.6 mg (1/100 gr)	In 100s and unit-of-use 100s.	2.1

NITROGLYCERIN, TRANSLINGUAL

Indications:

Acute relief of an attack or prophylaxis of angina pectoris due to coronary artery disease.

Administration and Dosage:

At the onset of attack, spray 1 or 2 metered doses onto or under the tongue. No more than 3 metered doses are recommended within 15 minutes. If chest pain persists, seek prompt medical attention. May use prophylactically 5 to 10 minutes prior to engaging in activities which might precipitate an acute attack. Do not inhale spray.

				C.I.*
Rx	**Nitrolingual** (Rhone-Poulenc Rorer)	**Spray:** 0.4 mg per metered dose	In 14.49 g containing 200 metered doses per canister.	8.7

NITROGLYCERIN, TRANSMUCOSAL

Indications:

Treatment and prevention of angina pectoris due to coronary artery disease.

Administration and Dosage: 1 mg every 3 to 5 hours during waking hours. Place tablet between lip and gum above incisors, or between cheek and gum.

				C.I.*
Rx	**Nitrogard** (Forest)	**Tablets, buccal, controlled release:** 1 mg	(1). Off-white. In 100s and UD 100s.	20
		2 mg	(2). Off-white. In 100s and UD 100s.	11
		3 mg	(3). Off-white. In 100s and UD 100s.	7.7

* Cost Index based on cost per 0.3 ml amyl nitrite, 0.3 mg sublingual nitroglycerin, 0.4 mg translingual nitroglycerin or 1 mg transmucosal nitroglycerin.

Complete prescribing information for these products begins on page 604.

NITROGLYCERIN, SUSTAINED RELEASE

Indications:

Prevention of angina pectoris. "Possibly effective" for the management, prophylaxis or treatment of anginal attacks.

Administration and Dosage:

The usual starting dose is 2.5 or 2.6 mg, 3 or 4 times daily. Titrate upward to an effective dose until side effects limit the dose. The dose generally may be increased by 2.5 or 2.6 mg increments 2 to 4 times daily over a period of days or weeks. Doses as high as 26 mg given 4 times daily have been reported effective.

Give the smallest effective dose 2 to 4 times daily. Monitor blood pressure at initiation of therapy or dosage change.

Tolerance may develop. Consider administering on a reduced schedule (once or twice daily). See Precautions.

Capsules must be swallowed; not for chewing or sublingual use.

	Product	Form	Description	C.I.*
Rx	**Nitrong** (R-P Rorer)	**Tablets, sustained release:** 2.6 mg	Light green granules. Scored. In 100s.	NA
Rx	**Nitrong** (R-P Rorer)	**Tablets, sustained release:** 6.5 mg	Light orange granules. Scored. In 100s.	NA
Rx	**Nitrong** (R-P Rorer)	**Tablets, sustained release:** 9 mg	Blue granules. Scored. In 60s and 500s.	NA
Rx	**Nitroglycerin** (Various, eg, Dixon-Shane, Geneva Marsam, Goldline, Major, Moore, Purepac, Rugby, Schein, URL, Vitarine)	**Capsules, sustained release:** 2.5 mg	In 60s, 100s and UD 60s and 100s.	2+
Rx	**Nitro-Bid Plateau Caps** (Marion Merrell Dow)		Lactose, sucrose. (Marion/ 1550). Lt. purple/clear, white beads. In 60s and 100s.	9
Rx	**Nitrocine Timecaps** (Schwarz Pharma Kremers Urban)		Lactose, sucrose. (Kremers Urban 320). Violet/clear, white beads. In 100s.	6
Rx	**Nitroglyn** (Kenwood)		In 100s.	2.1
Rx	**Nitroglycerin** (Various, eg, Dixon-Shane, Geneva Marsam, Goldline, Major, Moore, Purepac, Rugby, Schein, URL, Vitarine)	**Capsules, sustained release:** 6.5 mg	In 60s, 100s and UD 100s.	1+
Rx	**Nitro-Bid Plateau Caps** (Marion Merrell Dow)		Lactose, sucrose. (Marion/ 1551). Dk. blue/yellow. In 60s and 100s.	4.6
Rx	**Nitrocine Timecaps** (Schwarz Pharma Kremers Urban)		Lactose, sucrose. (Kremers Urban 330). Dk. blue/orange. In 100s.	2.1
Rx	**Nitroglyn** (Kenwood)		In 100s.	1
Rx	**Nitroglycerin** (Various, eg, Dixon-Shane, Geneva Marsam, Goldline, Major, Moore, Rugby, Schein, URL, Vitarine)	**Capsules, sustained release:** 9 mg	In 30s, 60s, 100s and UD 100s.	1+
Rx	**Nitro-Bid Plateau Caps** (Marion Merrell Dow)		Lactose, sucrose. (Marion/ 1553). Green/yellow. In 60s and 100s.	3.8
Rx	**Nitrocine Timecaps** (Schwarz Pharma Kremers Urban)		Lactose, sucrose. (Kremers Urban 340). Clear, white beads. In 100s.	1.7
Rx	**Nitroglyn** (Kenwood)		In 100s.	1.4
Rx	**Nitroglyn** (Kenwood)	**Capsules, sustained-release:** 13 mg	In 100s.	NA

* Cost Index based on cost per mg.

Complete prescribing information for these products begins on page 604.

NITROGLYCERIN TRANSDERMAL SYSTEMS

When a pad is applied to the skin, nitroglycerin is continuously absorbed into the systemic circulation.

Nitrate tolerance may be more likely with higher dosages, longer acting products or more frequent dosing. Transdermal systems release nitroglycerin at a constant rate and maintain steady-state plasma concentration; thus, tolerance may occur (see Precautions and Starting Dose in Administration and Dosage).

Indications: Prevention of angina pectoris due to coronary artery disease.

Administration and Dosage: Patient instructions for application are provided with products.

Apply pad once each day to a skin site free of hair and not subject to excessive movement. Do not apply to the distal parts of the extremities. Avoid areas with cuts or irritations.

Individualize dosage. Titrate dose as needed for optimum effect.

Starting dose: 0.2 to 0.4 mg/hr. Doses between 0.4 and 0.8 mg/hr have shown continued effectiveness for 10 to 12 hours daily for at least 1 month of intermittent administration. Although the minimum nitrate-free interval has not been defined, data show that a nitrate-free interval of 10 to 12 hours is sufficient. Thus, an appropriate dosing schedule would include a daily "patch-on" period of 12 to 14 hours and a "patch-off" period of 10 to 12 hours. Tolerance is a major factor limiting efficacy when the system is used continuously for > 12 hours each day.

These products differ in delivery system mechanism. The most important common denominator is amount of drug released per hour. However, a wide range of patient variability has been seen in bioavailability studies. The skin is a major factor influencing absorption rate; physical exercise and elevated ambient temperatures (eg, sauna) may increase the absorption. Other factors are related to the patient's preference and product differences: Ease of application and removal, adhesiveness, comfort, size and appearance.

	Product/Distributor	Release Rate (mg/hr)	Surface Area (cm^2)	Total NTG Content (mg)	How Supplied	C.I.*
Rx	**Minitran** (3M Pharm.)	0.1	3.3	9	In 33s.	243
Rx	**Nitro-Dur** (Key)	0.1	5	20	In 30s and 100s.	340
Rx	**Transderm-Nitro** (Summit)	0.1	5	12.5	In 30s.	337
Rx	**Nitroglycerin Transdermal** (Various, eg, Dixon-Shane, Major)	0.2	10	62.5	In 30s.	146+
Rx	**Minitran** (3M Pharm.)	0.2	6.7	18	In 33s.	127
Rx	**Nitrodisc** (Searle)	0.2	8	16	In 30s and 100s.	181
Rx	**Nitro-Dur** (Key)	0.2	10	40	In 30s and 100s.	147
Rx	**Transderm-Nitro** (Summit)	0.2	10	25	In 30s.	169
Rx	**Deponit** (Schwarz Pharma K-U)	0.2	16	16	In 30s.	140
Rx	**Nitrodisc** (Searle)	0.3	12	24	In 30s and 100s.	127
Rx	**Nitro-Dur** (Key)	0.3	15	60	In 30s and 100s.	116
Rx	**Nitroglycerin Transdermal** (Various, eg, Dixon-Shane, Major)	0.4	20	125	In 30s.	91+
Rx	**Minitran** (3M Pharm.)	0.4	13.3	36	In 33s.	70
Rx	**Nitrodisc** (Searle)	0.4	16	32	In 30s and 100s.	100
Rx	**Nitro-Dur** (Key)	0.4	20	80	In 30s and 100s.	94
Rx	**Transderm-Nitro** (Summit)	0.4	20	50	In 30s.	95
Rx	**Deponit** (Schwarz Pharma K-U)	0.4	32	32	In 30s.	72
Rx	**Minitran** (3M Pharm.)	0.6	20	54	In 33s.	52
Rx	**Nitrocine** (Schwarz Pharma K-U)	0.6	30	187.5	In 30s.	44
Rx	**Nitro-Dur** (Key)	0.6	30	120	In 30s and 100s.	69
Rx	**Transderm-Nitro** (Summit)	0.6	30	75	In 30s.	71

* Cost Index based on cost per 0.2 mg/hr transdermal system.

Complete prescribing information for these products begins on page 604.

NITROGLYCERIN, TOPICAL

Indications:

Prevention and treatment of angina pectoris due to coronary artery disease.

Administration and Dosage:

Usual therapeutic dose: 1 to 2 inches (25 to 50 mm) every 8 hours, up to 4 to 5 inches (100 to 125 mm) or application every 4 hours. Start with ½ inch (12.5 mm) every 8 hours; increase by ½ inch with each application to achieve desired effects. The greatest attainable decrease in resting blood pressure not associated with clinical hypotension, especially during orthostasis, indicates optimal dosage.

When applying ointment, spread with the applicator or dose-measuring paper over at least a 2¼ x 3½ inch area in a thin uniform layer. The ointment may be applied to the chest or back.

One inch (25 mm) of ointment contains ≈ 15 mg nitroglycerin.

	Product	Form	Supply	C.I.*
Rx	**Nitroglycerin** (Various, eg, Dixon-Shane, Fougera, Major, Schein)	**Ointment:** 2% in a lanolin-petrolatum base	In 30 and 60 g tubes.	14+
Rx	**Nitro-Bid** (Marion Merrell Dow)		In 20 & 60 g tubes & UD 1 g (100s).	14
Rx	**Nitrol** (Adria)		In 30 & 60 g tubes with and without applicator & UD 3 g (50s).	25

ISOSORBIDE DINITRATE, SUBLINGUAL AND CHEWABLE

Indications:

Treatment and prevention of angina pectoris.

Administration and Dosage:

Angina pectoris: Usual starting dose is 2.5 to 5 mg for sublingual tablets and 5 mg for chewable tablets. Titrate upward until angina is relieved or side effects limit the dose.

Acute prophylaxis: 5 to 10 mg sublingual or chewable tablets every 2 to 3 hours. Limit use of sublingual or chewable isosorbide dinitrate for aborting an acute anginal attack to patients intolerant of or unresponsive to sublingual nitroglycerin.

Do not crush or chew sublingual tablets; do not crush chewable tablets before administering.

	Product	Form	Supply	C.I.*
Rx	**Isosorbide Dinitrate** (Various, eg, Barr, Geneva Marsam, Goldline, Major, Moore, Schein, URL)	**Tablets, sublingual:** 2.5 mg	In 100s, 500s, 1000s and UD 100s.	12+
Rx	**Isordil** (Wyeth-Ayerst)		Lactose. Yellow. In 100s, 500s & UD 100s.	38
Rx	**Sorbitrate** (ICI Pharma)		(S 853). White. In 100s & UD 100s.	36
Rx	**Isosorbide Dinitrate** (Various, eg, Barr, Geneva Marsam, Goldline, Major, Moore, Rugby, Schein, URL)	**Tablets, sublingual:** 5 mg	In 100s, 1000s and UD 100s.	6.2+
Rx	**Isordil** (Wyeth-Ayerst)		Lactose. Pink. In 100s, 500s & UD 100s.	41
Rx	**Sorbitrate** (ICI Pharma)		(S 760). Pink. In 100s & UD 100s.	44
Rx	**Isordil** (Wyeth-Ayerst)	**Tablets, sublingual:** 10 mg	Lactose. White. In 100s.	24
Rx	**Sorbitrate** (ICI Pharma)		(S 761). Yellow. In 100s & UD 100s.	22
Rx	**Sorbitrate** (ICI Pharma)	**Tablets, chewable:** 5 mg	(S 810). Green, scored. In 100s, 500s and UD 100s.	36
Rx	**Sorbitrate** (ICI Pharma)	**Tablets, chewable:** 10 mg	(S 815). Yellow, scored. In 100s & UD 100s.	22

* Cost Index based on cost per 1 g nitroglycerin ointment or 10 mg isosorbide dinitrate.

Complete prescribing information for these products begins on page 604.

ISOSORBIDE DINITRATE, ORAL

Indications:

Treatment and prevention of angina pectoris; not to abort acute anginal episodes.

Administration and Dosage:

Tablets: Initial dose is 5 to 20 mg; maintenance dose is 10 to 40 mg every 6 hours.

Sustained release: The initial dose is 40 mg; maintenance controlled release dose is 40 to 80 mg every 8 to 12 hours. Do not crush or chew these preparations.

Tolerance to these agents may develop. Consider administering the short-acting preparations 2 or 3 times daily (last dose no later than 7 pm) and the sustained release preparations once daily or twice daily at 8 am and 2 pm. See Precautions.

	Product	Form/Strength	Description	C.I.*
Rx	**Isosorbide Dinitrate** (Various, eg, Barr, Danbury, Geneva Marsam, Goldline, Major, Parmed, Rugby, URL, Vangard)	**Tablets:** 5 mg	In 100s, 1000s and UD 100s.	6+
Rx	**Isordil Titradose** (Wyeth-Ayerst)		Pink, scored. In 100s, 500s, 1000s and UD 100s.[1]	41
Rx	**Sorbitrate** (ICI Pharma)		(S 770). Green, scored. Oval. In 100s, 500s and UD 100s.[1]	39
Rx	**Isosorbide Dinitrate** (Various, eg, Barr, Danbury, Geneva Marsam, Goldline, Major, Moore, Parmed, Rugby, Schein, URL, Vangard)	**Tablets:** 10 mg	In 100s, 500s, 1000s and UD 100s.	1+
Rx	**Isordil Titradose** (Wyeth-Ayerst)		White, scored. In 100s, 500s, 1000s and UD 100s.[1]	24
Rx	**Sorbitrate** (ICI Pharma)		(S 780). Yellow, scored. Oval. In 100s, 500s and UD 100s.	22
Rx	**Isosorbide Dinitrate** (Various, eg, Goldline, Major, Moore, Schein, URL, Vangard)	**Tablets:** 20 mg	In 1000s and UD 100s.	1.8+
Rx	**Isordil Titradose** (Wyeth-Ayerst)		Green, scored. In 100s, 500s and UD 100s.[1]	15
Rx	**Sorbitrate** (ICI Pharma)		(S 820). Blue, scored. Oval. In 100s and UD 100s.[1]	18
Rx	**Isosorbide Dinitrate** (Various, eg, Barr, Major, Rugby, URL)	**Tablets:** 30 mg	In 100s and 1000s.	1.8+
Rx	**Isordil Titradose** (Wyeth-Ayerst)		Blue, scored. In 100s, 500s and UD 100s.[1]	15
Rx	**Sorbitrate** (ICI Pharma)		(S 773). White, scored. Oval. In 100s and UD 100s.[1]	13
Rx	**Isosorbide Dinitrate** (Various, eg, Geneva Marsam, Major)	**Tablets:** 40 mg	In 100s and 1000s.	1.9+
Rx	**Isordil Titradose** (Wyeth-Ayerst)		Light green, scored. In 100s and UD 100s.[1]	12
Rx	**Sorbitrate** (ICI Pharma)		(S 774). Light blue, scored. Oval. In 100s & UD 100s.[1]	10
Rx	**Isosorbide Dinitrate** (Various, eg, Major, Moore, Rugby, Schein, URL)	**Tablets, sustained release:** 40 mg	In 100s and 1000s.	1.2+
Rx	**Isordil Tembids** (Wyeth-Ayerst)		Green, scored. In 100s, 500s and 1000s.[1]	12
Rx	**Sorbitrate SA** (ICI Pharma)		(S 880). Yellow. In 100s & UD 100s.[1]	10

* Cost Index based on cost per 10 mg.

[1] Contains lactose.

(Continued on following page)

Complete prescribing information for these products begins on page 604.

ISOSORBIDE DINITRATE, ORAL (Cont.)

	Product	Form	Description	C.I.*
Rx	**Isosorbide Dinitrate** (Various, eg, Parmed, Rugby, URL)	**Capsules, sustained release:** 40 mg	In 100s and 1000s.	1.9+
Rx	**Dilatrate-SR** (Reed & Carnrick)		Pink/clear. In 100s.	9.9
Rx	**Iso-Bid** (Geriatric Pharm.)		In 100s and 500s.	8.9
Rx	**Isordil Tembids** (Wyeth-Ayerst)		Sugar. Blue/clear. In 100s & 500s.	12.4
Rx	**Isotrate Timecelles** (Hauck)		In 100s and 500s.	7.4

ERYTHRITYL TETRANITRATE

Indications:

Prophylaxis and long-term treatment of frequent or recurrent anginal pain and reduced exercise tolerance associated with angina pectoris.

Administration and Dosage:

Initiate therapy with 5 to 10 mg sublingually prior to anticipated physical or emotional stress. If oral administration is preferred, initiate therapy with 10 mg before each meal, as well as mid-morning and mid-afternoon, if needed. Administer additional doses at bedtime for patients subject to nocturnal attacks. Adjust the dose as needed. Dosage titrations up to 100 mg daily are well tolerated, but temporary headache is more apt to occur with increasing doses. When headache occurs, reduce the dose for a few days. If headache is troublesome during dosage adjustment, administer an analgesic.

	Product	Form	Description	C.I.*
Rx	**Cardilate** (Burroughs Wellcome)	**Tablets, oral or sublingual:** 10 mg	(Cardilate X7A). White, scored. Square. In 100s.	51

PENTAERYTHRITOL TETRANITRATE (P.E.T.N.)

Indications:

"Possibly effective" for relief and prophylaxis of angina pectoris (pain associated with coronary artery disease). Not intended to abort the acute anginal episode.

Administration and Dosage:

Oral: Initially, 10 or 20 mg, 3 to 4 times daily. Titrate to 40 mg, 4 times daily, ½ hour before or 1 hour after meals and at bedtime. Give in individualized doses up to 160 mg/day.

Sustained release: One capsule or tablet every 12 hours on an empty stomach. Do not crush or chew sustained release preparations.

	Product	Form	Description	C.I.*
Rx	**Peritrate SA** (Parke-Davis)	**Tablets, sustained release:** 80 mg	(P-D 004). Two-tone green, layered. In 100s, 1000s and UD 100s.	5.7
Rx	**Pentylan** (Lannett)	**Tablets:** 10 mg	Light green. In 500s & 1000s.	8
Rx	**Peritrate** (Parke-Davis)		Lactose. (P-D 013). Light green. In 100s and 1000s.	14
Rx	**Pentylan** (Lannett)	**Tablets:** 20 mg	Green. In 100s, 500s & 1000s.	7.1
Rx	**Peritrate** (Parke-Davis)		Lactose. (P-D 001). Light green, scored. In 100s, 1000s & UD 100s.	9.6
Rx	**Peritrate** (Parke-Davis)	**Tablets:** 40 mg	Lactose, sugar. (P-D 008). Coral, scored. In 100s.	8.4
Rx	**Duotrate** (Jones Medical)	**Capsules, sustained release:** 30 mg	(JMI/Duotrate 30 mg). Black/clear, white pellets. In 100s.	18
Rx	**Duotrate 45** (Jones Medical)	**Capsules, sustained release:** 45 mg	(JMI/Duotrate 45 mg). Black/blue. In 100s.	14

* Cost Index based on cost per 10 mg isosorbide dinitrate, erythrityl tetranitrate or P.E.T.N.

DIPYRIDAMOLE

The FDA has announced a plan to revoke the temporary exemption which allowed dipyridamole-containing products to remain on the market beyond the time limit established by the Drug Efficacy Study Implementation (DESI) program. It has also proposed withdrawal of approval for long-term therapy of chronic angina. Pharmaceutical manufacturers have requested hearings to submit data supporting the effectiveness of dipyridamole for long-term therapy of angina. Pending the outcome of the hearings, dipyridamole products may remain on the market.

Persantine (Boehringer Ingelheim) has been approved by the FDA for use as an adjunct to coumarin anticoagulants in the prevention of postoperative thromboembolic complications of cardiac valve replacement. See individual monograph in Antiplatelet Agents section. Some generic companies have received approval for this indication; others have submitted ANDA supplements for this indication.

Actions:

Dipyridamole increases coronary blood flow primarily by a selective dilation of the coronary arteries. In therapeutic doses, it usually produces no significant alteration of systemic blood pressure or of blood flow in peripheral arteries.

Dipyridamole injection is also available as an in vivo diagnostic aid as an alternative to exercise in thallium myocardial perfusion imaging for evaluation of coronary artery disease. See individual monograph.

Indications:

"Possibly effective" for long-term therapy of chronic angina pectoris. Prolonged therapy may reduce the frequency of or eliminate anginal episodes, improve exercise tolerance and reduce nitroglycerin requirements. Not intended to abort the acute anginal attack.

Administration and Dosage:

Differences in bioavailability of dipyridamole products have been demonstrated.

Administer 50 mg 3 times a day, at least 1 hour before meals. Higher doses may be necessary, but increased dosage is associated with an increased incidence of side effects. Clinical response may not be evident before the second or third month of continuous therapy.

Dispense in tight, light resistant containers.

				C.I.*
Rx	**Dipyridamole** (Various, eg, Geneva, Goldline, Lederle, Major, Moore, Parmed, Rugby, Schein, URL)	**Tablets:** 25 mg	In 100s, 500s, 1000s, 2500s and UD 100s.	1+
Rx	**Dipyridamole** (Various, eg, Geneva, Goldline, Lederle, Major, Moore, Parmed, Rugby, Schein, URL)	**Tablets:** 50 mg	In 100s, 500s, 1000s and UD 100s and 1000s.	1+
Rx	**Dipyridamole** (Various, eg, Geneva, Goldline, Lederle, Major, Moore, Parmed, Rugby, Schein, URL)	**Tablets:** 75 mg	In 100s, 250s, 500s, 1000s and UD 100s.	2+

* Cost Index based on cost per 25 mg.

Optimal therapy of cardiac arrhythmias requires documentation, accurate diagnosis and modification of precipitating causes, and if indicated, proper selection and use of antiarrhythmic drugs. Comprehensive information on individual agents is presented on the following pages.

These drugs are classified according to their effects on the action potential of cardiac cells and their presumed mechanism of action. Although drugs within the same group are similar, that does not imply that another agent within the group would not be more effective or safer in an individual patient.

Group I: Local anesthetics or membrane-stabilizing agents that depress phase 0.

IA (quinidine, procainamide, disopyramide): Depress phase 0 and prolong the action potential duration.

IB (tocainide, lidocaine, phenytoin, mexiletine): Depress phase 0 slightly and may shorten the action potential duration. Although arrhythmia is not a labeled indication for *phenytoin,* it is commonly used in treatment of digitalis-induced arrhythmias.

IC (flecainide, encainide, propafenone): Marked depression of phase 0. Slight effect on repolarization. Profound slowing of conduction. *Encainide* was voluntarily withdrawn from the market, but is still available on a limited basis.

Moricizine is a Group I agent that shares some of the characteristics of the Group IA, B and C agents.

Group II (propranolol, esmolol, acebutolol): Depress phase 4 depolarization.

Group III (bretylium, amiodarone): Produce a prolongation of phase 3 (repolarization).

Group IV (verapamil): Depress phase 4 depolarization and lengthen phases 1 and 2 of repolarization.

Digitalis glycosides (digoxin) cause a decrease in maximal diastolic potential and action potential duration and increase the slope of phase 4 depolarization.

Adenosine slows conduction time through the AV node and can interrupt the reentry pathways through the AV node.

Serum drug levels: Some antiarrhythmic drugs (eg, quinidine) can produce toxic effects which can be easily confused with the symptoms for which the drug has been prescribed. Drug serum levels are important in evaluating toxic or subtherapeutic dosage regimens of most of the antiarrhythmic drugs. They are also aids in monitoring active metabolites (eg, procainamide/NAPA), suspected drug interactions and subtherapeutic response due to drug failure, noncompliance, altered clearance or altered absorption.

Proarrhythmic effects: Antiarrhythmic agents may cause new or worsened arrhythmias. Such proarrhythmic effects range from an increase in frequency of PVCs to the development of more severe ventricular tachycardia, ventricular fibrillation or torsade de pointes (ie, tachycardia that is more sustained or more rapid), which may lead to fatal consequences. It is often not possible to distinguish a proarrhythmic effect from the patient's underlying rhythm disorder. It is therefore essential that each patient be evaluated electrocardiographically and clinically prior to and during therapy to determine whether the response to the drug supports continued treatment.

Cardiac Arrhythmia Suppression Trial (CAST): In the National Heart, Lung and Blood Institute's Cardiac Arrhythmia Suppression Trial (CAST), a long-term, multicenter, randomized, double-blind study in patients with asymptomatic non-life-threatening ventricular ectopy who had a myocardial infarction (MI) > 6 days but < 2 years previously, and demonstrated mild to moderate left ventricular dysfunction, an excessive mortality or non-fatal cardiac arrest rate was seen in patients treated with encainide or flecainide (56/730) compared with that seen in patients assigned to carefully matched placebo-treated groups (22/725). This led to discontinuation of those two arms of the trial. The average duration of treatment with encainide or flecainide in this study was 10 months.

The moricizine and placebo arms of the trial were continued in CAST II. In this randomized, double-blind trial, patients with asymptomatic non-life-threatening arrhythmias who had an MI within 4 to 90 days and left ventricular ejection fraction ≤ 0.4 prior to enrollment were evaluated. The average duration of moricizine treatment was 18 months. The study was discontinued because there was no possibility of demonstrating a benefit toward improved survival with moricizine and because of an evolving adverse trend after long-term treatment.

The applicability of these results to other populations (eg, those without recent MI) and to other antiarrhythmic drugs is uncertain, but at present it is prudent (1) to consider any IC agent (especially one documented to provoke new serious arrhythmias) to have a similar risk and (2) to consider the risks of Class IC agents, coupled with the lack of any evidence of improved survival, generally unacceptable in patients without life-threatening ventricular arrhythmias, even if the patients are experiencing unpleasant, but not life-threatening symptoms or signs.

(Continued on following page)

Pharmacokinetics: The information in the pharmacokinetics table together with clinical data and observation can be a valuable tool. However, the information must be used rationally and the data obtained properly (ie, obtaining and analyzing serum level data) to be effective. See individual monographs for more detailed explanations.

Antiarrhythmic Electrophysiology/Electrocardiogram Effects

Antiarrhythmic		Electrophysiology[1] Automaticity		Electrophysiology[1] Conduction velocity			Electrophysiology[1] Refractory period					ECG changes[1]				
Group	Drug	SA node	Ectopic pacemaker	Atrium	AV node	His-Purkinje	Atrium	AV node	His-Purkinje	Ventricle	Accessory pathways[2]	Heart rate	PR interval	QRS complex	QT_c interval	JT interval
I	Moricizine[3]	0	↓	0	↓	↓	±	0	0	0-↑	↑	0-↑	↑	↑	0	↓
A	Quinidine	±	↓	↓	±	↓	↑↑	0-↑[4]	↑↑	↑	↑	±	±	↑	↑	↑
A	Procainamide	±	↓	↓	±	↓	↑	0-↑[4]	↑↑	↑	↑↑	±	±	↑	↑	↑
A	Disopyramide	±	↓	↓	0-↑	↓	↑↑	0-↑[4]	↑↑	↑	↑	±	±	↑	↑	↑
B	Lidocaine	0	↓	—	0-↑	0-↑	—	±	±	±	↑-↓	0	0	0	0-↓	0
B	Phenytoin	↓-0	↓	—	0-↑	0-↑	—	±	±	±	—	±	0-↓	0	↓	0
B	Tocainide	0-↓	↓	0	0	0	↓	↓	±	↓	↑	0	0	0	0-↓	0
B	Mexiletine	↓	↓	0	0	0	0	±	↑	↑	↑	—	0	0	0	0
C	Flecainide	↓	↓	↓↓	↓	↓↓	0	0	↑	↑	↑↑	0	↑[5]	↑↑[5]	0-↑[5]	0
C	Encainide[6]	0-↓	↓	↓↓	↓	↓↓	0-↑	0-↑	↑	↑	↑↑	0	↑[5]	↑↑[5]	0-↑[5]	0
C	Propafenone	0	↓	0	↓	↓	0	↑	↑	↑	↑	0	↑[5]	↑[5]	0-↑[5]	—
II	Propranolol	↓	↓	±	↓	0-↓	±	↑	0	0	0-↑	↓	0-↑	0	0-↓	0
II	Esmolol	↓	↓	±	↓	0-↑	±	↑	0	0	0-↑	↓	0-↑	0	0-↓	0
II	Acebutolol	↓	↓	±	↓	0-↑	±	↑	0	0	0-↑	↓	0-↑	0	0-↓	0
III	Bretylium	↑	↑	0	0	0-↑	0	↓-0-↑[7]	↑	0-↑	±	0	0	0	0	↑
III	Amiodarone	↓	↓	↓	↓	↓	↑	↑	↑	↑	↑	↓	↑	↑	↑↑	↑↑
IV	Verapamil	↓	↓	0	↓	0	0	↑	0	0	0	↓	↑	0	0	0
—	Digoxin	0-↓	↑	±	↓	0-↓	±	↑	0	↓	↓-↑	↓	↑	0	↓	↓
—	Adenosine	↓	↓	0	↓	0	0	↑	0	0	0	↑	↑	0	0	—

[1] These values assume therapeutic levels.
[2] Accessory pathways occur in Wolff-Parkinson-White syndrome (preexcitation phenomena) and possibly other abnormal conditions.
[3] Does not belong to any of the 3 subclasses (A, B or C), but does have some properties of each.
[4] Retrograde AV node RP↑; antegrade RP not affected.
[5] Dose-related increases.
[6] Withdrawn from the market; however, available on a limited basis.
[7] Due to a complex balance of direct and indirect autonomic effects.

Antiarrhythmic Pharmacokinetics

Group	Drug	Onset (hrs) (oral)[1]	Duration (hrs)	Half-life (hrs)	Protein binding (%)	Excreted unchanged (%)	Therapeutic serum levels (mcg/ml)	Toxic serum levels (mcg/ml)
I	Moricizine	2	10-24	1.5-3.5[2]	95	< 1	not applicable	—
A	Quinidine	0.5	6-8	6-7	80-90	10-50	2-6	> 8
A	Procainamide	0.5	3+	2.5-4.7	14-23	40-70	4-8	> 16
A	Disopyramide	0.5	6-7	4-10	20-60[3]	40-60	2-8	> 9
B	Lidocaine	—	0.25[4]	1-2	40-80	< 3	1.5-6	> 7
B	Phenytoin	0.5-1	24+	22-36[5]	87-93	< 5	10-20	> 20
B	Tocainide	—	—	11-15	10-20	28-55	4-10	> 10
B	Mexiletine	—	—	10-12	50-60	10	0.5-2	> 2
C	Flecainide	—	—	12-27	40	30	0.2-1	> 1
C	Encainide[6]	—	—	1-2[7]	75-85	< 5[8]	not applicable	—
C	MODE[9]			6-12	92		wide range	—
C	ODE[9]			3-4	75-85		0.1-0.3	—
C	Propafenone	—	—	2-10[10]	97	< 1	0.06-1	—
II	Propranolol	0.5	3-5	2-3	90-95	< 1	0.05-0.1	—
II	Esmolol	< 5 min	very short	0.15	55	< 2	—	—
II	Acebutolol	—	24-30	3-4	26	15-20	—	—
III	Bretylium	—	6-8	5-10	0-8	> 80	0.5-1.5	—
III	Amiodarone	1-3 wks[11]	weeks to months	26-107 days	96	negligible	0.5-2.5	> 2.5
IV	Verapamil	0.5	6	3-7	90	3-4	0.08-0.3	—
—	Digoxin	0.5-2	24+	30-40	20-25	60	0.5-2 ng/ml	> 2.5 ng/ml
—	Adenosine	— (34 sec IV)	1-2 min	< 10 sec	—	0 (enters body pool)	Not applicable	—

[1] Within 1 to 5 minutes with IV use.
[2] Half-life may be prolonged in patients after multiple dosing.
[3] Protein binding is concentration-dependent.
[4] Very short after discontinuation of IV infusion.
[5] Half-life increases with increasing dosage.
[6] Withdrawn from the market; however, available on a limited basis.
[7] Half-life 6 to 11 hours in < 10% of patients (poor metabolizers).
[8] > 50% in poor metabolizers.
[9] MODE (3-methoxy-O-demethyl encainide) and ODE (O-demethyl encainide), metabolites more active than encainide on a per mg basis.
[10] Half-life 10 to 32 hours in < 10% of patients (slow metabolizers).
[11] Onset of action may occur in 2 to 3 days.

MORICIZINE HCl (Cont.)

Warnings (Cont.):

Proarrhythmic effects: Like other antiarrhythmic drugs, moricizine can provoke new rhythm disturbances or make existing arrhythmias worse. These proarrhythmic effects can range from an increase in the frequency of VPDs to the development of new or more severe ventricular tachycardia (eg, tachycardia that is more sustained or more resistant to conversion to sinus rhythm, with potentially fatal consequences). It is often not possible to distinguish a proarrhythmic effect from the patient's underlying rhythm disorder; therefore, consider the occurrence rates that follow approximations. Note also that drug-induced arrhythmias can generally be identified only when they occur early after starting the drug and when the rhythm can be identified, usually because the patient is being monitored. It is clear from the CAST study that some antiarrhythmic drugs can cause increased sudden death mortality, presumably due to new arrhythmias or asystole that do not appear early after treatment but that represent a sustained increased risk.

Domestic pre-marketing trials included 1072 patients given moricizine; 397 had baseline lethal arrhythmias (sustained VT or VF and non-sustained VT with hemodynamic symptoms) and 576 had potentially lethal arrhythmias (increased VPDs or NSVT in patients with known structural heart disease, active ischemia, CHF or an LVEF $< 40\%$ or CI < 2 L/min/m^2). In this population there were 40 (3.7%) identified proarrhythmic events, 26 (2.5%) of which were serious, either fatal (6), new hemodynamically significant sustained VT or VF (4), new sustained VT that was not hemodynamically significant (11) or sustained VT that became syncopal/presyncopal when it had not been before (5).

In general, serious proarrhythmic effects were equally common in patients with more and less severe arrhythmias, 2.5% in the patients with baseline lethal arrhythmias vs 2.8% in patients with potentially lethal arrhythmias, although the patients with serious effects were more likely to have a history of sustained VT (38% vs 23%).

Five of the six fatal proarrhythmic events were in patients with baseline lethal arrhythmias; four had prior cardiac arrests. Rates and severity of proarrhythmic events were similar in patients given 600 to 900 mg/day and those given higher doses. Patients with proarrhythmic events were more likely than the overall population to have coronary artery disease (85% vs 67%), history of acute MI (75% vs 53%), CHF (60% vs 43%) and cardiomegaly (55% vs 33%). All of the six proarrhythmic deaths were in patients with coronary artery disease; five of six each had documented acute MI, CHF and cardiomegaly.

In two recent studies, moricizine (400 to 1000 mg/day) was ineffective in patients with refractory sustained ventricular arrhythmias (failed therapy with other class I agents) and carried a considerable risk for life threatening proarrhythmia. In one study, seven of 26 patients (27%) developed proarrhythmia during moricizine loading, and in the other study four of 21 patients (19%) had a probable proarrhythmic response.

Electrolyte disturbances: Hypokalemia, hyperkalemia or hypomagnesemia may alter the effects of Class I antiarrhythmic drugs. Correct electrolyte imbalances before administration of moricizine.

Sick sinus syndrome: Use with extreme caution in patients with sick sinus syndrome since it may cause sinus bradycardia, sinus pause or sinus arrest.

Hepatic function impairment: Patients with significant liver dysfunction have reduced plasma clearance and an increased half-life of moricizine. Although the precise relationship of moricizine levels to effect is not clear, treat hepatic disease patients with lower doses and closely monitor for excessive pharmacological effects, including ECG intervals, before dosage adjustment. Administer with particular care to patients with severe liver disease, if at all (see Administration and Dosage).

Renal function impairment: Plasma levels of intact moricizine are unchanged in hemodialysis patients, but a significant portion (39%) is metabolized and excreted in the urine. Although no identified active metabolite is known to increase in people with renal failure, metabolites of unrecognized importance could be affected. Administer cautiously. Start patients with significant renal dysfunction on lower doses and monitor for excessive pharmacologic effects, including ECG intervals, before dosage adjustment (see Administration and Dosage).

(Warnings continued on following page)

MORICIZINE HCl (Cont.)

Warnings (Cont.):

Carcinogenesis: In a 24 month mouse study in which moricizine was administered to provide up to 320 mg/kg/day, ovarian tubular adenomas and granulosa cell tumors were limited to moricizine-treated animals.

In a 24 month study in which moricizine was administered to rats at doses of 25, 50 and 100 mg/kg/day, Zymbal's Gland Carcinoma was observed in one mid-dose and two high-dose males. The rats also showed a dose-related increase in hepatocellular cholangioma in both sexes, along with fatty metamorphosis, possibly due to disruption of hepatic choline utilization for phospholipid biosynthesis.

Pregnancy: Category B. In a study in which rats were dosed with moricizine prior to and during mating, and throughout gestation and lactation, dose levels 3.4 and 6.7 times the maximum recommended human daily dose produced a dose-related decrease in pup and maternal weight gain, possibly related to a larger litter size. In a study in which dosing was begun on day 15 of gestation, moricizine, at a level 6.7 times the maximum recommended human daily dose, produced a retardation in maternal weight gain but no effect on pup growth. There are no adequate and well controlled studies in pregnant women. Use during pregnancy only if clearly needed.

Lactation: Moricizine is excreted in the milk of animals and is present in human breast milk. Because of the potential for serious adverse reactions in nursing infants, decide whether to discontinue nursing or to discontinue the drug, taking into account the importance of the drug to the mother.

Children: Safety and efficacy in children $<$ 18 years of age have not been established.

Precautions:

ECG changes/Conduction abnormalities: Moricizine slows AV nodal and intraventricular conduction, producing dose-related increases in PR and QRS intervals. In clinical trials, the average increase in PR interval was 12% and QRS interval was 14%. Although the QT_c interval is increased, this is due to QRS prolongation; the JT interval is shortened, indicating absence of significant slowing of ventricular repolarization. The degree of lengthening of PR and QRS intervals does not predict efficacy.

In controlled clinical trials and in open studies, the overall incidence of delayed ventricular conduction, including new bundle branch block pattern, was $\approx$ 9.4%. In patients without baseline conduction abnormalities, the frequency of second-degree AV block was 0.2% and third-degree AV block did not occur. In patients with baseline conduction abnormalities, the frequencies of second-degree AV block and third-degree AV block were 0.9% and 1.4%, respectively.

Therapy was discontinued in 1.6% of patients due to ECG changes (0.6% due to sinus pause or asystole, 0.2% to AV block, 0.2% to junctional rhythm, 0.4% to intraventricular conduction delay and 0.2% to wide QRS or PR interval).

In patients with pre-existing conduction abnormalities, initiate therapy cautiously. If second- or third-degree AV block occurs, discontinue therapy unless a ventricular pacemaker is in place. When changing the dose or adding concomitant medications which may also affect cardiac conduction, monitor ECG.

Congestive heart failure: Most patients with CHF have tolerated the recommended daily doses without unusual toxicity or change in effect. Pharmacokinetic differences between patients with and without CHF were not apparent (see Hepatic function impairment). In some cases, worsened heart failure has been attributed to moricizine. Carefully watch patients with pre-existing heart failure when therapy is initiated.

Effects on pacemaker threshold: Since the effect of moricizine on the sensing and pacing thresholds of artificial pacemakers has not been sufficiently studied, monitor pacing parameters if moricizine is used.

Drug fever: Three patients developed rechallenge-confirmed drug fever, with one patient experiencing an elevation above 39.5° to 40.6°C (103° to 105°F) with rigors. Fevers occurred at about 2 weeks in two cases, and after 21 weeks in the third. Fevers resolved within 48 hours after discontinuation of moricizine.

(Continued on following page)

MORICIZINE HCl (Cont.)

Drug Interactions:

Moricizine Drug Interactions			
Precipitant Drug	Object Drug*		Comments
Cimetidine	Moricizine	↑	1.4 fold increase in moricizine plasma levels, 49% decrease in clearance. Initiate moricizine at low doses (not > 600 mg/day).
Digoxin	Moricizine	↑	Additive prolongation of the PR interval, but not with a significant increase in the rate of second- or third-degree AV block. Little change in serum digoxin levels or pharmacokinetics.
Propranolol	Moricizine	↑	Small additive increase in PR interval; no changes in overall ECG intervals.
Moricizine	Theophylline	↓	Theophylline clearance increased 44% to 66% and plasma half-life decreased 19% to 33% (conventional and sustained-release theophylline).

* ↑ = Object drug increased ↓ = Object drug decreased

Drug/Food interaction: Administration of moricizine 30 minutes after a meal delays the rate of absorption, resulting in lower peak plasma concentrations, but the extent of absorption is not altered.

Adverse Reactions:

The most serious adverse reaction reported is proarrhythmia (see Warnings). This occurred in 3.7% of 1072 patients with ventricular arrhythmias who received a wide range of doses under a variety of circumstances. In addition, in controlled clinical trials and in open studies, adverse reactions led to discontinuation of moricizine in 7% of 1105 patients with ventricular and supraventricular arrhythmias, including: Nausea (3.2%); ECG abnormalities (1.6%; principally conduction defects, sinus pause, junctional rhythm or AV block); CHF (1%); dizziness, anxiety, drug fever, urinary retention, blurred vision, GI upset, rash, laboratory abnormalities (0.3% to 0.4%).

Cardiovascular: Palpitations (5.8%); sustained ventricular tachycardia, cardiac chest pain, CHF, cardiac death (2% to < 5%); hypotension, hypertension, syncope, supraventricular arrhythmias (including atrial fibrillations/flutter), cardiac arrest, bradycardia, pulmonary embolism, MI, vasodilation, cerebrovascular events, thrombophlebitis (< 2%).

CNS: Dizziness (15.1%); headache (8%); fatigue (5.9%); hypesthesias, asthenia, nervousness, paresthesias, sleep disorders (2% to < 5%); tremor, anxiety, depression, euphoria, confusion, somnolence, agitation, seizure, coma, abnormal gait, hallucinations, nystagmus, diplopia, speech disorder, akathisia, memory loss, ataxia, abnormal coordination, dyskinesia, vertigo, tinnitus (< 2%).

Dizziness appears to be related to the size of each dose. In a comparison of 900 mg/day given at 450 mg twice daily or 300 mg 3 times daily, > 20% of patients experienced dizziness on the twice daily regimen vs 12% on the 3 times daily regimen.

GU: Urinary retention or frequency, dysuria, urinary incontinence, kidney pain, impotence, decreased libido (< 2%).

Respiratory: Dyspnea (5.7%); hyperventilation, apnea, asthma, pharyngitis, cough, sinusitis (< 2%).

GI: Nausea (9.6%); abdominal pain, dyspepsia, vomiting, diarrhea (2% to < 5%); anorexia, bitter taste, dysphagia, flatulence, ileus (< 2%).

Other: Sweating, musculoskeletal pain, dry mouth, blurred vision (2% to < 5%); drug fever, hypothermia, temperature intolerance, eye pain, rash, pruritus, dry skin, urticaria, swelling of the lips and tongue, periorbital edema (< 2%).

Two patients developed thrombocytopenia that may have been drug-related. Clinically significant elevations in liver function tests (bilirubin, serum transaminases) and jaundice consistent with hepatitis occurred rarely. Although a cause-and-effect relationship has not been established, caution is advised in patients who develop unexplained signs of hepatic dysfunction; consider discontinuing therapy.

Elderly: Adverse reactions were generally similar in patients > 65 years old (n = 375) and < age 65 (n = 697), although discontinuation of therapy for reasons other than proarrhythmia was more common in older patients (13.9% vs 7.7%). Overall mortality was greater in older patients (9.3% vs 3.9%), but those were not deaths attributed to treatment, and the older patients had more serious underlying heart disease.

(Continued on following page)

MORICIZINE HCl (Cont.)

Overdosage:

Symptoms: Emesis; lethargy; coma; syncope; hypotension; conduction disturbances; exacerbation of CHF; MI; sinus arrest; arrhythmias (including junctional bradycardia, ventricular tachycardia, ventricular fibrillation and asystole); respiratory failure. Deaths have occurred after accidental or intentional overdoses of 2250 and 10,000 mg, respectively. Accidental introduction of moricizine into the lungs of monkeys resulted in rapid arrhythmic death.

Treatment should be supportive. Hospitalize patients and monitor for cardiac, respiratory and CNS changes. Provide advanced life support systems, including an intracardiac pacing catheter where necessary. Treat acute overdosage with appropriate gastric evacuation, and with special care to avoid aspiration. Refer to General Management of Acute Overdosage.

Patient Information:

Take exactly as prescribed. Dosage changes must be supervised by the physician.

Contact the physician immediately if chest pain or discomfort, pounding in the chest (palpitations), irregular heartbeat or fever occur.

Hospitalization is required when starting on this medication.

Administration and Dosage:

Approved by the FDA on June 26, 1990.

Individualize dosage. Clinical, cardiac rhythm monitoring, ECG intervals, exercise testing, or programmed electrical stimulation testing may be used to guide antiarrhythmic response and dosage adjustment. In general, the patients will be at high risk; hospitalize for the initiation of therapy.

Usual adult dosage is between 600 and 900 mg/day, given every 8 hours in three equally divided doses. Within this range, the dosage can be adjusted as tolerated, in increments of 150 mg/day at 3 day intervals, until the desired effect is obtained. Patients with life-threatening arrhythmias who exhibit a beneficial response as judged by objective criteria (eg, Holter monitoring, programmed electrical stimulation, exercise testing) can be maintained on chronic moricizine therapy. As the antiarrhythmic effect of moricizine persists for > 12 hours, some patients whose arrhythmias are well controlled on an every 8 hour regimen may be given the same total daily dose in an every 12 hour regimen to increase convenience and help assure compliance. When higher doses are used, patients may experience more dizziness and nausea on the every 12 hour regimen.

Hepatic or renal function impairment: Start at ≤ 600 mg/day and monitor closely, including measurement of ECG intervals, before dosage adjustment.

Transfer from another antiarrhythmic: Recommendations for transferring patients from another antiarrhythmic to moricizine can be given based on theoretical considerations. Withdraw previous antiarrhythmic therapy for 1 to 2 plasma half-lives before starting moricizine at the recommended dosages. In patients in whom withdrawal of a previous antiarrhythmic is likely to produce life-threatening arrhythmias, hospitalize.

Transferring to Moricizine from Another Antiarrhythmic	
Agent transferred from	Start moricizine
Quinidine, disopyramide	6 to 12 hours after last dose
Procainamide	3 to 6 hours after last dose
Encainide, mexiletine, propafenone or tocainide	8 to 12 hours after last dose
Flecainide	12 to 24 hours after last dose

Rx	**Ethmozine** (DuPont)	**Tablets:** 200 mg	Lactose. Light green. Film coated. Oval, convex. In 100s and UD 100s.
		250 mg	Lactose. Light orange. Film coated. Oval, convex. In 100s and UD 100s.
		300 mg	Lactose. Light blue. Film coated. Oval, convex. In 100s and UD 100s.

Refer to the general discussion concerning these products on page 618.

QUINIDINE

Actions:

Pharmacology: Quinidine, a class IA antiarrhythmic, depresses myocardial excitability, conduction velocity and contractility. Therapeutically, it prolongs the effective refractory period and increases conduction time, thereby preventing the reentry phenomenon. In addition, quinidine exerts an indirect anticholinergic effect; it decreases vagal tone and may facilitate conduction in the atrioventricular junction.

Pharmacokinetics:

Absorption/Distribution – There are differences in the anhydrous quinidine alkaloid content among the various salts. See table below:

Anhydrous Quinidine Alkaloid Content in Various Salts			
	Quinidine content		Time to peak plasma levels (hours)
Quinidine salts	Active drug	Absorbed	
Quinidine Sulfate	83%	73%	1 to 3[1]
Quinidine Gluconate	62%	70%	3-5
Quinidine Polygalacturonate	80%	—	6

[1] 3 to 5 hours for sustained release form.

Quinidine is rapidly absorbed from the GI tract. Maximum effects of quinidine gluconate occur 30 to 90 minutes after IM administration; onset is more rapid after IV administration. Activity persists for 6 to 8 hours or more. The average therapeutic serum levels are reported to be 2 to 7 mcg/ml. Toxic reactions may occur at levels from 5 to ≥ 8 mcg/ml. Quinidine is 80% to 90% bound to plasma proteins; the unbound fraction may be significantly increased in patients with hepatic insufficiency. Accumulation occurs in most tissues, except the brain. The polygalacturonate salt slows ionization of the drug and protects the GI tract by its demulcent effect.

Metabolism/Excretion – From 60% to 80% of a dose is metabolized via the liver into several metabolites; the primary metabolites are 3-hydroxyquinidine and 2-oxoquinidinone. Whether or not these or other metabolites have antiarrhythmic activity is unclear and controversial. Quinidine is excreted unchanged (10% to 50%) in the urine within 24 hours. The elimination half-life ranges from 4 to 10 hours in healthy patients, with a mean of 6 to 7 hours. Urinary acidification facilitates quinidine elimination, and alkalinization retards it. In patients with cirrhosis, the elimination half-life may be prolonged and the volume of distribution increased. In congestive heart failure (CHF), total clearance and volume of distribution are decreased. In the elderly, the elimination half-life may be increased. The influence of renal dysfunction on the disposition of quinidine is controversial; volume of distribution and renal clearance may be reduced.

Indications:

Oral: Premature atrial, AV junctional and ventricular contractions; paroxysmal atrial (supraventricular) tachycardia; paroxysmal AV junctional rhythm; atrial flutter; paroxysmal and chronic atrial fibrillation; established atrial fibrillation when therapy is appropriate; paroxysmal ventricular tachycardia not associated with complete heart block; maintenance therapy after electrical conversion of atrial fibrillation or flutter.

Parenteral: When oral therapy is not feasible or when rapid therapeutic effect is required.

Quinidine gluconate – Life-threatening *Plasmodium falciparum* malaria: Unless impossible, start therapy in an intensive care setting with continuous ECG monitoring, frequent blood pressure monitoring and periodic monitoring of parasitemia.

Contraindications:

Hypersensitivity or idiosyncrasy to quinidine or other cinchona derivatives manifested by thrombocytopenia, skin eruption or febrile reactions; myasthenia gravis; history of thrombocytopenic purpura associated with quinidine administration; digitalis intoxication manifested by arrhythmias or AV conduction disorders; complete heart block; left bundle branch block or other severe intraventricular conduction defects exhibiting marked QRS widening or bizarre complexes; complete AV block with an AV nodal or idioventricular pacemaker; aberrant ectopic impulses and abnormal rhythms due to escape mechanisms; history of drug-induced torsade de pointes; history of long QT syndrome.

(Continued on following page)

QUINIDINE (Cont.)

Warnings:

Hepatotoxicity (including granulomatous hepatitis) due to quinidine hypersensitivity has occurred. Unexplained fever or elevation of hepatic enzymes, particularly in the early stages of therapy, warrants consideration. Monitor liver function during the first 4 to 8 weeks of therapy. Discontinuation of quinidine usually results in resolution of toxicity.

Atrial flutter or fibrillation: Reversion to sinus rhythm may be preceded by a progressive reduction in the degree of AV block to a 1:1 ratio, which results in an extremely rapid ventricular rate. Prior to use in atrial flutter, pretreat the patient with a digitalis preparation.

Although quinidine reduces recurrences of atrial fibrillation after cardioversion, it may be associated with an increase in mortality.

Cardiotoxicity (eg, increased PR and QT intervals, 50% widening of QRS complex, ventricular tachyarrhythmias, frequent ventricular ectopic beats or tachycardia) dictates immediate discontinuation of quinidine; closely monitor the ECG. Some specialists recommend quinidine therapy be initiated only in hospitalized patients with ECG monitoring. However, this is generally reserved for patients receiving large doses or who are at high risk.

In susceptible individuals (ie, marginally compensated cardiovascular disease), quinidine may produce clinically important depression of cardiac function such as hypotension, bradycardia or heartblock.

Large oral doses may reduce the arterial pressure by means of peripheral vasodilation. Serious hypotension is more likely with parenteral use.

Use quinidine with extreme caution in incomplete AV block, since complete block and asystole may result. The drug may cause unpredictable dysrhythmias in digitalized patients; use with caution in the presence of digitalis intoxication. Use cautiously in patients with partial bundle branch block, severe CHF and hypotensive states due to the depressant effects of quinidine on myocardial contractility and arterial pressure; usefulness of quinidine is limited unless these conditions are due to or aggravated by the arrhythmia. Consider the potential disadvantages and benefits.

Parenteral therapy: The dangers of parenteral use of quinidine are increased in the presence of AV block or in the absence of atrial activity. Administration is more hazardous in patients with extensive myocardial damage. The use of quinidine in a digitalis-induced cardiac arrhythmia is extremely dangerous because the cardiac glycoside may already have caused serious impairment of the intracardiac conduction system. Too rapid IV administration of as little as 200 mg may precipitate a fall of 40 to 50 mm Hg in arterial pressure. Inject slowly (see Administration and Dosage).

Syncope occasionally occurs in patients on long-term quinidine therapy, usually resulting from ventricular tachycardia or fibrillation. It is manifested by sudden loss of consciousness and by polymorphic ventricular tachycardia. This syndrome does not appear to be related to dose or plasma levels but occurs more often with prolonged QT intervals. Syncopal episodes frequently terminate spontaneously or respond to treatment, but are sometimes fatal. Torsade de pointes is often the cause.

Hypersensitivity: Asthma, muscle weakness and infection with fever prior to quinidine administration may mask hypersensitivity reactions to the drug.

Test dose – Administer a single 200 mg tablet of quinidine sulfate or 200 mg IM quinidine gluconate prior to the initiation of treatment to determine whether the patient has an idiosyncrasy to quinidine.

During the first weeks of therapy, although rare, consider hypersensitivity to quinidine including anaphylactoid reactions (eg, angioedema, purpura, acute asthmatic episode, vascular collapse). Refer to Management of Acute Hypersensitivity Reactions.

Renal, hepatic or cardiac insufficiency: Use with caution in patients with renal (especially renal tubular acidosis), cardiac or hepatic insufficiency because of potential toxicity.

Pregnancy: Category C. Quinidine crosses the placenta and achieves fetal serum levels similar to maternal levels. Neonatal thrombocytopenia has been reported after maternal use. Safety for use during pregnancy has not been established. Use only when clearly needed and when the potential benefits outweigh the potential hazards to the fetus.

Oxytocic properties are reported with quinidine, as with quinine; clinical significance is not known.

Lactation: Safety for use in the nursing mother has not been established. Quinidine is excreted into breast milk with a milk:serum ratio of approximately 0.71. Use caution when quinidine is administered to a nursing woman. The American Academy of Pediatrics considers quinidine to be compatible with breast feeding.

Children: Safety and efficacy have not been established.

(Continued on following page)

QUINIDINE (Cont.)

Precautions:

Vagolytic effects: Because quinidine has vagolytic activity on the atrium and the AV node, the administration of cholinergic drugs or the use of any other procedure to enhance vagal activity may fail to terminate paroxysmal supraventricular tachycardia.

Potassium balance: The effect of quinidine is enhanced by potassium and reduced if hypokalemia is present. The risk of drug-induced torsade de pointes is increased by concomitant hypokalemia.

Malaria (P falciparum): Dosing schedules known to be effective have been associated with hypotension, increased QRS and corrected QT intervals and cinchonism. Closely monitor ECG and blood pressure.

Monitoring: Perform periodic blood counts and liver and kidney function tests. Discontinue use if blood dyscrasias or signs of hepatic or renal disorders occur. Initiate therapy in the hospital and continuously monitor ECG and check quinidine levels. This is generally done when large doses are used or the patient is at increased risk. Frequently measure arterial blood pressure during IV use; discontinue if blood pressure falls significantly.

Drug Interactions:

Quinidine Drug Interactions

Precipitant drug	Object drug*		Description
Amiodarone	Quinidine	↑	Increased quinidine levels may occur with possible production of potentially fatal cardiac dysrhythmias.
Antacids	Quinidine	↑	Certain antacids may increase serum quinidine levels, which may result in toxicity.
Barbiturates	Quinidine	↓	Quinidine serum levels and elimination half-life may be decreased.
Cholinergic drugs	Quinidine	↓	Since quinidine antagonizes the effect of vagal excitation upon the atrium and AV node, concurrent cholinergic agents may result in failure to terminate paroxysmal supraventricular tachycardia.
Cimetidine	Quinidine	↑	Quinidine serum levels may be increased.
Hydantoins	Quinidine	↓	A decrease in the therapeutic effect of quinidine may occur.
Nifedipine	Quinidine	↓	Serum levels and actions of quinidine may be lower than predicted by the dosage.
Rifampin	Quinidine	↓	Increased metabolism of quinidine which may be associated with a reduction in its therapeutic effects.
Sucralfate	Quinidine	↓	Serum quinidine levels may be reduced, decreasing the therapeutic effects.
Urinary alkalinizers	Quinidine	↑	Urinary elimination of quinidine is reduced. Serum quinidine levels may be increased accompanied by increased pharmacologic effects.
Verapamil	Quinidine	↑	Quinidine clearance may be reduced and its half-life prolonged, resulting in hypotension, bradycardia, ventricular tachycardia, AV block and pulmonary edema.
Quinidine	Anticholinergics	↑	Quinidine exhibits a distinct anticholinergic activity in the myocardial tissues. Concurrent use may cause an additive vagolytic effect.
Quinidine	Anticoagulants	↑	Anticoagulation may be potentiated; hemorrhage could occur.
Quinidine	Beta blockers	↑	Effects of metoprolol or propranolol may be increased in "extensive metabolizers."
Quinidine	Cardiac glycosides (digitoxin, digoxin)	↑	Plasma levels of the cardiac glycosides are markedly increased. Pharmacologic effects are increased and toxicity may occur.

* ↑ = Object drug increased. ↓ = Object drug decreased.

(Drug Interactions continued on following page)

QUINIDINE (Cont.)

Drug Interactions (Cont.):

Quinidine Drug Interactions (Cont.)			
Precipitant drug	Object drug*		Description
Quinidine	Disopyramide	↑	Increased disopyramide levels or decreased quinidine levels may occur.
Disopyramide	Quinidine	↓	
Quinidine	Nondepolarizing neuromuscular blockers	↑	Nondepolarizing neuromuscular blocker effects may be enhanced.
Quinidine	Procainamide	↑	Pharmacologic effects of procainamide may be increased; elevated procainamide and NAPA (major metabolite) plasma levels with toxicity may occur.
Quinidine	Propafenone	↑	Serum propafenone levels may be increased in rapid extensive metabolizers of the drug (≈ 90% of patients), increasing the pharmacologic effects.
Quinidine	Succinylcholine	↑	The neuromuscular blockade produced by succinylcholine may be prolonged.
Quinidine	Tricyclic antidepressants	↑	The clearance of the tricyclic antidepressants may be reduced, possibly resulting in increased pharmacologic effects.

* ↑ = Object drug increased. ↓ = Object drug decreased.

Drug/Lab test interaction: **Triamterene** and quinidine have similar fluorescence spectra; thus, triamterene will interfere with the fluorescent measurement of quinidine serum levels.

Adverse Reactions:

Cinchonism: Ringing in the ears; hearing loss; headache; nausea; dizziness; vertigo; lightheadedness; disturbed vision. These may appear after a single dose.

Cardiovascular: Widening of QRS complex; cardiac asystole; ventricular ectopy; idioventricular rhythms (including ventricular tachycardia and fibrillation and torsade de pointes in some instances); paradoxical tachycardia; arterial embolism; hypotension; ventricular extrasystoles occurring at the rate of one or more every 6 normal beats; prolonged QT interval; complete AV block; ventricular flutter.

Stop use if any of these occur: Increase of > 25% in duration of QRS complex; disappearance of P waves; restoration of sinus rhythm; decrease in heart rate to 120 bpm in the ECG.

GI effects, the most common reactions seen with quinidine, include: Nausea; vomiting; abdominal pain; diarrhea; anorexia. These may be preceded by fever.

Rarely, oral quinidine has been associated with esophageal disorders, primarily esophagitis.

Renal/Hepatic: Lupus nephritis; hepatic toxicity including granulomatous hepatitis; hepatitis.

Hematologic: Acute hemolytic anemia; hypoprothrombinemia; thrombocytopenic purpura; agranulocytosis; drug-induced hypoprothrombinemic hemorrhage in patients on chronic anticoagulant therapy (see Drug Interactions); thrombocytopenia; leukocytosis; shift to left in WBC differential; neutropenia.

CNS: Headache; fever; vertigo; apprehension; excitement; confusion; delirium; syncope; dementia; ataxia; depression.

Ophthalmic: Mydriasis; blurred vision; disturbed color perception; reduced vision field; photophobia; diplopia; night blindness; scotomata; optic neuritis.

Dermatologic: Rash; urticaria; cutaneous flushing with intense pruritus; photosensitivity; eczema; exfoliative eruptions; psoriasis; abnormalities of pigmentation.

Lupus erythematosus has occurred. Symptoms include hepatosplenomegaly/lymphadenopathy and a positive antinuclear antibody test. Symptoms resolve after withdrawal of the drug.

Hypersensitivity reactions: Angioedema; acute asthma; vascular collapse; respiratory arrest; hepatic dysfunction including granulomatous hepatitis; hepatic toxicity; purpura; vasculitis. See Warnings.

Miscellaneous: Arthralgia; myalgia; increase in serum skeletal muscle creatine phosphokinase; disturbed hearing (tinnitus, decreased auditory acuity).

(Continued on following page)

QUINIDINE (Cont.)

Overdosage:

Severe quinidine intoxication may be associated with depressed mental function, even in hemodynamically stable patients. The patient progresses from lethargy to coma, including respiratory arrest; recurrent generalized motor seizures may occur. The onset of CNS manifestations may be substantially delayed beyond the onset of cardiovascular toxicity; conversely, recovery from coma is often delayed.

Symptoms:

CNS – Lethargy; confusion; coma; respiratory depression or arrest; seizures; headache; parasthesia; vertigo.

GI – Vomiting; abdominal pain; diarrhea; nausea.

Cardiovascular – Tachyarrhythmias (sinus tachycardia, ventricular tachycardia, ventricular fibrillation, torsade de pointes); depressed automaticity and conduction (QRS and QT_c prolongation, bundle branch block, sinus bradycardia, sinoatrial block, sinus arrest, AV block, ST depression, T inversion); hypotension (depressed contractility and cardiac output, vasodilation); syncope; heart failure.

Other – Cinchonism; hypokalemia; visual/auditory disturbances; tinnitus; acidosis.

Treatment: If ingestion of quinidine is recent, gastric lavage, emesis or administration of activated charcoal may reduce absorption. Management of overdosage includes: Symptomatic treatment; ECG, blood gases, serum electrolytes and blood pressure monitoring; cardiac pacing if indicated; acidification of the urine. Avoid alkalinization of the urine. Mechanical ventilation and other supportive measures may be required.

IV infusion of ⅙ molar sodium lactate reportedly reduces the cardiotoxic effects of quinidine. Since marked CNS depression may occur even in the presence of convulsions, do not give CNS depressants. Hypotension may be treated, if necessary, with metaraminol or norepinephrine after adequate fluid volume replacement. Tachydysrhythmias should respond to phenytoin or lidocaine. Hemodialysis has been effective in overdosage, but is rarely warranted.

Patient Information:

Do not discontinue therapy unless instructed by physician.

May cause GI upset; take with food.

Notify physician if ringing in the ears, visual disturbances, dizziness, headache, nausea, skin rash or breathing difficulty occurs.

Do not crush or chew sustained release tablets.

Administration and Dosage:

Test dose: Administer a single 200 mg tablet of quinidine sulfate or 200 mg IM quinidine gluconate to determine whether the patient has an idiosyncratic reaction. Continuously monitor ECG when quinidine is used in large doses.

Adjust the dosage to maintain the plasma concentration between 2 to 6 mcg/ml.

Oral:

Premature atrial and ventricular contractions – 200 to 300 mg 3 or 4 times daily.

Paroxysmal supraventricular tachycardias – 400 to 600 mg every 2 or 3 hours until the paroxysm is terminated.

Atrial flutter – Administer quinidine after digitalization. Individualize dosage.

Conversion of atrial fibrillation – 200 mg every 2 or 3 hours for 5 to 8 doses, with subsequent daily increases until sinus rhythm is restored or toxic effects occur. Do not exceed a total daily dose of 3 to 4 g in any regimen. Prior to quinidine administration, control the ventricular rate and CHF (if present) with digoxin.

Maintenance therapy – 200 to 300 mg 3 or 4 times daily. Other patients may require larger doses or more frequent administration than the usually recommended schedule. However, institute such an increased dosage only after careful evaluation of the patient, including ECG and quinidine serum level monitoring.

Sustained release forms – 300 to 600 mg every 8 or 12 hours. Since the rate of absorption from the various sustained release formulations may be markedly different, and since the anhydrous quinidine content is different, do not consider them interchangeable.

(Administration and Dosage continued on following page)

Complete prescribing information for these products begins on page 629.

QUINIDINE (Cont.)

Administration and Dosage (Cont.):

Parenteral: The patient must be under close clinical, ECG and blood pressure monitoring, especially during IV administration to detect any change in rate or rhythm. If the patient's condition is not critical, give quinidine gluconate IM. On the other hand, extreme palpitation, dyspnea, vomiting, and a shocklike state in patients with ventricular tachycardia are signs that IV administration may be required as a lifesaving measure when D-C cardioversion is not available.

IM – In the treatment of acute tachycardia, the initial dose is 600 mg quinidine gluconate. Subsequently, 400 mg quinidine gluconate can be repeated as often as every 2 hours. Determine successive doses by the effect of the preceding dose.

IV – In about 50% of patients who respond successfully to quinidine, the arrhythmia can be terminated by $\leq$ 330 mg quinidine gluconate (or its equivalent in other salts); as much as 500 to 750 mg may be required. Inject slowly. Dilute 10 ml (800 mg) of quinidine gluconate injection to 50 ml with 5% Dextrose Injection, USP. Inject the diluted solution slowly at a rate of 1 ml/min for maximum safety.

Quinidine gluconate – P falciparum malaria: Two regimens have been empirically shown to be effective, with or without concomitant exchange transfusions. As soon as practical, institute standard oral antiplasmodial therapy.

1) *Loading,* 15 mg/kg in 250 ml normal saline infused over 4 hours followed by: *Maintenance,* beginning 24 hours after the beginning of the loading dose, 7.5 mg/kg infused over 4 hours, every 8 hours for 7 days or until oral therapy can be instituted.

2) *Loading,* 10 mg/kg in 250 ml normal saline infused over 1 to 2 hours, followed immediately by: *Maintenance,* 0.02 mg/kg/min for up to 72 hours or until parasitemia decreases to $<$ 1% or oral therapy can be instituted.

Children: The following doses have been suggested – *Oral* (quinidine sulfate): 30 mg/kg/24 hours or 900 mg/m^2/24 hours in 5 divided doses. *IV* (quinidine gluconate): 2 to 10 mg/kg/dose every 3 to 6 hours as needed; however this route is not recommended.

(Products listed on following page)

Complete prescribing information for these products begins on page 629.

QUINIDINE SULFATE

Contains 83% anhydrous quinidine alkaloid.

	Product	Form	Description	C.I.*
Rx	**Quinidine Sulfate** (Various, eg, Danbury, Goldline, Major, Parmed, Rugby, Schein, Vangard, Warner Chilcott)	**Tablets:** 200 mg	In 90s, 100s, 120s, 200s, 1000s, UD 100s.	12+
Rx	**Quinidine Sulfate** (Various, eg, Danbury, Major, Rugby, Schein)	**Tablets:** 300 mg	In 100s, 500s, 1000s and UD 100s.	16+
Rx	**Quinora** (Key Pharm.)		(Quinora 300). White. Convex. In 100s.	25
Rx	**Quinidex Extentabs** (Robins)	**Tablets, sustained release:** 300 mg	Sucrose. (Quinidex AHR). White. Sugar coated. In 100s, 250s and UD 100s.	59

QUINIDINE GLUCONATE

Contains 62% anhydrous quinidine alkaloid.

	Product	Form	Description	C.I.*
Rx	**Quinidine Gluconate** (Various, eg, Geneva, Goldline, Major, Parmed, Rugby, Schein, Warner Chilcott)	**Tablets, sustained release:** 324 mg	In 100s, 250s, 500s, 1000s and UD 100s.	33+
Rx	**Quinaglute Dura-Tabs** (Berlex)		Sugar. White. In 100s, 250s, 500s and UD 100s.	74
Rx	**Quinalan** (Lannett)		(Q). Off-white, scored. Convex. In 100s, 250s and 500s.	NA
Rx	**Quinidine Gluconate** (Lilly)	**Injection:** 80 mg/ml (50 mg/ml quinidine)	In 10 ml vials.[1]	862

QUINIDINE POLYGALACTURONATE

Contains 80% anhydrous quinidine alkaloid.

	Product	Form	Description	C.I.*
Rx	**Cardioquin** (Purdue Frederick)	**Tablets:** 275 mg (equiv. to 200 mg sulfate)	Lactose. (PF C275). Scored. In 100s and 500s.	97

* Cost Index based on cost per 200 mg quinidine sulfate, 324 mg quinidine gluconate or 275 mg quinidine polygalacturonate.

[1] With 0.005% EDTA and 0.25% phenol.

Refer to the general discussion concerning these products on page 618.

PROCAINAMIDE HCl

Warning:
The prolonged administration of procainamide often leads to the development of a positive antinuclear antibody (ANA) test, with or without symptoms of a lupus erythematosus-like syndrome. If a positive ANA titer develops, assess the benefit/risk ratio related to continued procainamide therapy.

Actions:

Pharmacology: Procainamide, a class IA antiarrhythmic, increases the effective refractory period of the atria, and to a lesser extent the bundle of His-Purkinje system and ventricles of the heart. It reduces impulse conduction velocity in the atria, His-Purkinje fibers, and ventricular muscle, but has variable effects on the atrioventricular (AV) node, a direct slowing action and a weaker vagolytic effect which may speed AV conduction slightly.

Myocardial excitability is reduced in the atria, Purkinje fibers, papillary muscles, and ventricles by an increase in the threshold for excitation, combined with inhibition of ectopic pacemaker activity by retardation of the slow phase of diastolic depolarization, thus decreasing automaticity especially in ectopic sites. Contractility of the undamaged heart is usually not affected by therapeutic concentrations, although slight reduction of cardiac output may occur, and may be significant in the presence of myocardial damage. Therapeutic levels of procainamide may exert vagolytic effects and produce slight acceleration of heart rate, while high or toxic concentrations may prolong AV conduction time or induce AV block, or even cause abnormal automaticity and spontaneous firing, by unknown mechanisms.

Electrophysiology – The ECG may reflect these effects by showing slight sinus tachycardia (due to the anticholinergic action) and widened QRS complexes and, less regularly, prolonged QT and PR intervals (due to longer systole and slower conduction), as well as some decrease in QRS and T wave amplitude. These direct effects on electrical activity, conduction, responsiveness, excitability and automaticity are characteristic of a group IA antiarrhythmic agent, the prototype for which is quinidine; procainamide effects are very similar. However, procainamide has weaker vagal blocking action than does quinidine, does not induce alpha-adrenergic blockade, and is less depressing to cardiac contractility.

Pharmacokinetics: Absorption/Distribution – Oral procainamide is resistant to digestive hydrolysis, and the drug is well absorbed from the entire small intestinal surface, but individual patients vary in their completeness of absorption. Following oral administration, plasma levels reach about 50% of peak in 30 minutes, 90% at 1 hour and peak at about 90 to 120 minutes. Following IM injection, absorption into the bloodstream is rapid; plasma levels peak in 15 to 60 minutes, considerably faster than oral administration. IV use can produce therapeutic plasma levels within minutes after an infusion is started. About 15% to 20% is reversibly bound to plasma proteins, and considerable amounts are more slowly and reversibly bound to tissues of the heart, liver, lung and kidney. The apparent volume of distribution eventually reaches about 2 L/kg with a half-life of approximately 5 minutes. While procainamide crosses the blood-brain barrier in the dog, it did not concentrate in the brain at levels higher than in plasma. Plasma esterases are far less active in hydrolysis of procainamide than of procaine.

Metabolism/Excretion – A significant fraction of the circulating procainamide may be metabolized in hepatocytes to N-acetylprocainamide (NAPA), ranging from 16% to 21% of an administered dose in "slow acetylators" to 24% to 33% in "fast acetylators". Since NAPA also has significant antiarrhythmic activity and somewhat slower renal clearance than procainamide, both hepatic acetylation rate capability and renal function, as well as age, have significant effects on the effective biologic half-life of therapeutic action of administered procainamide and the NAPA derivative. The elimination half-life of procainamide is 3 to 4 hours in patients with normal renal function, but reduced creatinine clearance (Ccr) and advancing age each prolong the elimination half-life. Half-life and renal clearance are also reduced in infants. Trace amounts may be excreted in the urine as free and conjugated p-aminobenzoic acid, 30% to 60% as unchanged procainamide, and 6% to 52% as the NAPA derivative. Both procainamide and NAPA are eliminated by active tubular secretion as well as by glomerular filtration. Action of procainamide on the CNS is not prominent, but high plasma concentrations may cause tremors.

(Actions continued on following page)

PROCAINAMIDE HCl (Cont.)

Actions (Cont.)

Pharmacokinetics: Metabolism/Excretion (Cont.) –

While therapeutic plasma levels for procainamide have been reported to be 3 to 10 mcg/ml, certain patients such as those with sustained ventricular tachycardia may need higher levels for adequate control. This may justify the increased risk of toxicity (see Overdosage). Where programmed ventricular stimulation has been used to evaluate efficacy of procainamide in preventing recurrent ventricular tachyarrhythmias, higher plasma levels (mean, 13.6 mcg/ml) were found necessary for adequate control. Plasma levels of NAPA that produce arrhythmia suppression range from 10 to 30 mcg/ml. Toxicity may occur with levels > 30 mcg/ml, although there appears to be overlap between the therapeutic and toxic ranges.

Indications:

Treatment of documented ventricular arrhythmias, such as sustained ventricular tachycardia, that are judged to be life-threatening. Because of the proarrhythmic effects, use with lesser arrhythmias is generally not recommended.

Because procainamide has the potential to produce serious hematologic disorders (0.5%), particularly leukopenia or agranulocytosis (sometimes fatal), reserve its use for patients in whom the benefits of treatment clearly outweigh the risks (see Warnings).

Contraindications:

Complete heart block; idiosyncratic hypersensitivity; lupus erythematosus; torsade de pointes (see Warnings).

Warnings:

Blood dyscrasias: Agranulocytosis, bone marrow depression, neutropenia, hypoplastic anemia and thrombocytopenia in patients receiving procainamide have been reported at a rate of approximately 0.5%. Most of these patients received procainamide within the recommended dosage range. Fatalities have occurred (with approximately 20% to 25% mortality in reported cases of agranulocytosis). Since most of these events have been noted during the first 12 weeks of therapy, it is recommended that complete blood counts including white cell, differential and platelet counts be performed at weekly intervals for the first 3 months of therapy, and periodically thereafter. Perform complete blood counts promptly if the patient develops any signs of infection (eg, fever, chills, sore throat, stomatitis), bruising or bleeding. If any of these hematologic disorders are identified, discontinue therapy. Blood counts usually return to normal within 1 month of discontinuation. Use caution in patients with preexisting marrow failure or cytopenia of any type (see Adverse Reactions).

Mortality: In the National Heart, Lung and Blood Institute's Cardiac Arrhythmia Suppression Trial (CAST), a long-term, multicentered, randomized, double-blind study in patients with asymptomatic non-life-threatening ventricular arrhythmias who had had myocardial infarctions (MI) > 6 days but < 2 years previously, an excessive mortality or nonfatal cardiac arrest rate was seen in patients treated with encainide or flecainide (56/730) compared with that seen in patients assigned to matched placebo-treated groups (22/725). The average duration of treatment with encainide or flecainide in this study was 10 months.

The applicability of these results to other populations (eg, those without recent MIs) or to other antiarrhythmic drugs is uncertain, but at present it is prudent to consider any antiarrhythmic agent to have a significant risk in patients with structural heart disease.

Survival: Antiarrhythmic drugs have not been shown to enhance survival in patients with ventricular arrhythmias.

Complete heart block: Do not administer to patients with complete heart block because of its effects in suppressing nodal or ventricular pacemakers and the hazard of asystole. It may be difficult to recognize complete heart block in patients with ventricular tachycardia, but if significant slowing of ventricular rate occurs during treatment without evidence of AV conduction appearing, stop procainamide. In cases of second-degree AV block or various types of hemiblock, avoid or discontinue procainamide because of the possibility of increased severity of block, unless the ventricular rate is controlled by an electrical pacemaker.

Torsade de pointes: In the unusual ventricular arrhythmia called "les torsade de pointes" (twistings of the points), characterized by alternation of one or more ventricular premature beats in the directions of the QRS complexes on ECG in persons with prolonged QT and often enhanced U waves, group IA antiarrhythmic drugs are contraindicated. Administration of procainamide in such cases may aggravate this special type of ventricular extrasystole or tachycardia instead of suppressing it.

(Warnings continued on following page)

PROCAINAMIDE HCl (Cont.)

Warnings (Cont.):

Lupus erythematosus: An established diagnosis of systemic lupus erythematosus is a contraindication to procainamide therapy, since aggravation of symptoms is highly likely. If the lupus erythematosus-like syndrome develops in a patient with recurrent life-threatening arrhythmias not controlled by other agents, corticosteroid suppressive therapy may be used concomitantly with procainamide. Since the procainamide-induced lupoid syndrome rarely includes the dangerous pathologic renal changes, therapy may not necessarily have to be stopped unless the symptoms of serositis and the possibility of further lupoid effects are of greater risk than the benefit of procainamide in controlling arrhythmias. Patients with rapid acetylation capability are less likely to develop the lupoid syndrome after prolonged procainamide therapy.

Asymptomatic ventricular premature contractions: Avoid treatment of patients with this condition.

Digitalis intoxication: Exercise caution in the use of procainamide in arrhythmias associated with digitalis intoxication. Procainamide can suppress digitalis-induced arrhythmias; however, if there is concomitant marked disturbance of AV conduction, additional depression of conduction and ventricular asystole or fibrillation may result. Therefore, consider use of procainamide only if discontinuation of digitalis, and therapy with potassium, lidocaine or phenytoin, are ineffective.

First-degree heart block: Exercise caution if the patient exhibits or develops first-degree heart block while taking procainamide; dosage reduction is advised in such cases. If the block persists despite dosage reduction, continuation of procainamide must be evaluated on the basis of current benefit vs risk of increased heart block.

Predigitalization for atrial flutter or fibrillation: Cardiovert or digitalize patients with atrial flutter or fibrillation prior to procainamide administration to avoid enhancement of AV conduction which may result in ventricular rate acceleration beyond tolerable limits. Adequate digitalization reduces but does not eliminate the possibility of sudden increase in ventricular rate as the atrial rate is slowed by procainamide in these arrhythmias.

Congestive heart failure (CHF): Use with caution in patients with CHF and in those with acute ischemic heart disease or cardiomyopathy since even slight depression of myocardial contractility may further reduce cardiac output of the damaged heart.

Concurrent antiarrhythmic agents: Concurrent use of procainamide with other group IA antiarrhythmic agents (eg, quinidine, disopyramide) may produce enhanced prolongation of conduction or depression of contractility and hypotension, especially in patients with cardiac decompensation. Reserve such use for patients with serious arrhythmias unresponsive to a single drug and use only if close observation is possible (see Drug Interactions).

Myasthenia gravis: Patients may show worsening of symptoms from procainamide due to its procaine-like effect on diminishing acetylcholine release at skeletal muscle motor nerve endings. Procainamide administration may be hazardous without optimal adjustment of anticholinesterase medications and other precautions. Immediately after initiation of therapy, closely observe patients for muscular weakness if myasthenia gravis is a possibility.

Hypersensitivity, idiosyncratic: In patients sensitive to procaine or other ester-type local anesthetics, cross-sensitivity to procainamide is unlikely; however, consider the possibility. Do not use procainamide if it produces acute allergic dermatitis, asthma or anaphylactic symptoms.

Renal insufficiency may lead to accumulation of high plasma levels from conventional oral doses of procainamide, with effects similar to those of overdosage (see Overdosage), unless dosage is adjusted for the individual patient.

Pregnancy: Category C. Procainamide crosses the placenta. It is not known whether procainamide can cause fetal harm when administered to a pregnant woman or can affect reproduction capacity. Give to a pregnant woman only if clearly needed.

Lactation: Both procainamide and NAPA are excreted in breast milk and absorbed by the nursing infant. Because of the potential for serious adverse reactions in nursing infants, decide whether to discontinue nursing or the drug, taking into account the importance of the drug to the mother.

Children: Safety and efficacy have not been established. However, see Administration and Dosage.

(Continued on following page)

PROCAINAMIDE HCl (Cont.)

Precautions:

Embolization: In conversion of atrial fibrillation to normal sinus rhythm by any means, dislodgement of mural thrombi may lead to embolization.

Monitoring: After achieving and maintaining therapeutic plasma concentrations and satisfactory ECG and clinical responses, continue frequent periodic monitoring of vital signs and ECG. If evidence of QRS widening of > 25% or marked prolongation of the QT interval occurs, concern for overdosage is appropriate; reduction in dosage is advisable if a 50% increase occurs. Elevated serum creatinine or urea nitrogen, reduced Ccr or history of renal insufficiency, as well as use in older patients (over age 50), provide grounds to anticipate that less than the usual dosage and longer time intervals between doses may suffice, since the urinary elimination of procainamide and NAPA may be reduced, leading to gradual accumulation beyond normally predicted amounts. If facilities are available for measurement of plasma procainamide and NAPA levels or acetylation capability, individual dose adjustment for optimal therapeutic levels may be easier, but close observation of clinical effectiveness is the most important criterion.

In the longer term, periodic complete blood counts are useful to detect possible idiosyncratic hematologic effects of procainamide on neutrophil, platelet or red cell homeostasis; agranulocytosis may occur occasionally in patients on long-term therapy. A rising titer of serum ANA may precede clinical symptoms of the lupoid syndrome. Laboratory tests such as ECG and serum creatinine or urea nitrogen may be indicated, depending on the clinical situation.

Tartrazine: Some of these products contain tartrazine which may cause allergic-type reactions (including bronchial asthma) in certain susceptible individuals. Although the overall incidence of tartrazine sensitivity in the general population is low, it is frequently seen in patients who also have aspirin hypersensitivity.

Sulfites: Some of these products contain sulfites that may cause allergic-type reactions including anaphylactic symptoms and life-threatening or less severe asthmatic episodes in certain susceptible persons. The overall prevalance of sulfite sensitivity in the general population is unknown and probably low. It is seen more frequently in asthmatic or atopic nonasthmatic persons.

Drug Interactions:

Procainamide Drug Interactions

Precipitant drug	Object drug*		Description
Beta blockers	Procainamide	↑	Propranolol may increase procainamide serum levels.
Ethanol	Procainamide	↔	The actions of procainamide could be altered, but because the main metabolite (NAPA) is also an antiarrhythmic, specific effects are unclear.
Histamine H_2 antagonists	Procainamide	↑	Cimetidine and ranitidine appear to increase the bioavailability of both procainamide and NAPA.
Quinidine	Procainamide	↑	Pharmacologic effects of procainamide may be increased. Elevated procainamide and NAPA plasma levels with toxicity may occur.
Trimethoprim	Procainamide	↑	Elevated procainamide and NAPA serum levels may occur, possibly resulting in increased pharmacologic effects.
Procainamide	Lidocaine	↑	Additive cardiodepressant action may occur with the potential for conduction abnormalities.
Procainamide	Succinylcholine	↑	The succinylcholine neuromuscular blockade may be potentiated.

* ↑ = Object drug increased. ↔ = Undetermined effect.

Drug/Lab test interactions: Suprapharmacologic concentrations of lidocaine and meprobamate may inhibit fluorescence of procainamide and NAPA, and propranolol shows a native fluorescence close to the procainamide/NAPA peak wavelengths; therefore, tests that depend on fluorescence measurement may be affected.

(Continued on following page)

PROCAINAMIDE HCl (Cont.)

Adverse Reactions:

Cardiovascular: Hypotension following oral administration is rare. Hypotension and serious disturbances of cardiorhythm such as ventricular asystole or fibrillation are more common after IV administration (see Overdosage and Warnings). Second-degree heart block has been reported in 2 of almost 500 patients taking procainamide orally.

Lupus erythematosus: A lupus erythematosus-like syndrome of arthralgia, pleural or abdominal pain, and sometimes arthritis, pleural effusion, pericarditis, fever, chills, myalgia and possibly related hematologic or skin lesions is fairly common after prolonged administration, perhaps more often in patients who are slow acetylators (see Warnings). While some studies have reported the syndrome in $<$ 1 in 500, others have reported it in up to 30% of patients on long-term oral therapy. If discontinuation does not reverse the lupoid symptoms, corticosteroid treatment may be effective.

Hematologic: Neutropenia; thrombocytopenia; hemolytic anemia (rare). Agranulocytosis has occurred after repeated use of procainamide; deaths have occurred (see Warnings).

Skin: Angioneurotic edema; urticaria; pruritus; flushing; maculopapular rash.

GI: Anorexia, nausea, vomiting, abdominal pain, bitter taste, diarrhea (3% to 4%; oral). Hepatomegaly with increased serum aminotransferase activity has occurred after a single oral dose.

CNS: Dizziness; giddiness; weakness; mental depression; psychosis with hallucinations.

Overdosage:

Symptoms: Progressive widening of the QRS complex, prolonged QT and PR intervals, lowering of the R and T waves, as well as increasing AV block, may be seen with doses which are excessive for a given patient. Increased ventricular extrasystoles, or even ventricular tachycardia or fibrillation may occur. After IV administration but seldom after oral therapy, transient high plasma levels may induce hypotension, affecting systolic more than diastolic pressures, especially in hypertensive patients. Such high levels may also produce CNS depression, tremor and even respiratory depression.

Plasma levels $>$ 10 mcg/ml are increasingly associated with toxic findings, which are seen occasionally in the 10 to 12 mcg/ml range, more often in the 12 to 15 mcg/ml range and commonly in patients with plasma levels $>$ 15 mcg/ml. Overdosage symptoms may result following a single 2 g dose, while 3 g may be dangerous, especially if the patient is a slow acetylator and has decreased renal function or underlying organic heart disease.

Treatment includes general supportive measures, close observation, monitoring of vital signs and possibly IV pressor agents and mechanical cardiorespiratory support. Refer to General Management of Acute Overdosage. If available, procainamide and NAPA plasma levels may be helpful in assessing the potential degree of toxicity and response to therapy. Both procainamide and NAPA are removed from the circulation by hemodialysis but not peritoneal dialysis. No specific antidote for procainamide is known.

Patient Information:

Close cooperation in adhering to the prescribed dosage schedule is of great importance in safely controlling the cardiac arrhythmia. More medication is not necessarily better and may be dangerous; skipping doses or increasing intervals between doses to suit personal convenience may lead to loss of control of the heart problem, and "making up" missed doses by doubling up later may be hazardous.

The patient should disclose any history of drug sensitivity, especially to procaine, other local anesthetic agents or aspirin, and to report any history of kidney disease, congestive heart failure, myasthenia gravis, liver disease or lupus erythematosus.

The patient should report promptly any symptoms of arthralgia, myalgia, fever, chills, skin rash, easy bruising, sore throat or sore mouth, infections, dark urine or icterus, wheezing, muscular weakness, chest or abdominal pain, palpitations, nausea, vomiting, anorexia, diarrhea, hallucinations, dizziness or depression.

(Continued on following page)

PROCAINAMIDE HCl (Cont.)

Administration and Dosage:

Oral: Oral dosage forms are preferable for less urgent arrhythmias as well as for long-term maintenance after initial parenteral therapy. Individualize dosage based on clinical assessment of the degree of underlying myocardial disease, the patient's age and renal function.

As a general guide, for younger adult patients with normal renal function, an initial total daily oral dose of up to 50 mg/kg may be used, given in divided doses every 3 hours, to maintain therapeutic blood levels. For older patients, especially those > 50 years of age, or for patients with renal, hepatic or cardiac insufficiency, lesser amounts or longer intervals may produce adequate blood levels and decrease the probability of occurrence of dose-related adverse reactions. Administer the total daily dose in divided doses at 3, 4 or 6 hour intervals and adjust according to the patient's response.

Guidelines to Provide up to 50 mg/kg/day Procainamide			
Weight		Dose every 3 hours (standard formulation)	Dose every 6 hours (sustained release)
lb	kg		
88-110	40-50	250 mg	500 mg
132-154	60-70	375 mg	750 mg
176-198	80-90	500 mg	1 g
> 220	> 100	625 mg	1.25 g

[1] Initial dosage schedule guide only, to be adjusted for each patient individually, based on age, cardiorenal function, blood level (if available) and clinical response.

Parenteral: Useful for arrhythmias that require immediate suppression and for maintenance of arrhythmia control. IV therapy allows most rapid control of serious arrhythmias, including those following MI; use in circumstances where close observation and monitoring of the patient are possible, such as in hospital or emergency facilities. IM administration is less apt to produce temporary high plasma levels but therapeutic plasma levels are not obtained as rapidly as with IV administration.

IM administration may be used as an alternative to the oral route for patients with less threatening arrhythmias but who are nauseated or vomiting, who are ordered to receive nothing by mouth preoperatively, or who may have malabsorptive problems. An initial daily dose of 50 mg/kg may be estimated. Divide this amount into fractional doses of ⅛ to ¼ to be injected IM every 3 to 6 hours until oral therapy is possible. If > 3 injections are given, assess patient factors such as age and renal function, clinical response and, if available, blood levels of procainamide and NAPA in adjusting further doses for that individual. For treatment of arrhythmias associated with anesthesia or surgery, the suggested dose is 100 to 500 mg by IM injection.

IV –

Dilutions and Rates for IV Infusions of Procainamide				
Infusion	Final concentration	Infusion volume[1]	Procainamide to be added	Infusion rate
Initial loading infusion	20 mg/ml	50 ml	1000 mg	1 ml/min (for up to 25 to 30 min)
Maintenance infusion[2]	2 mg/ml	500 ml	1000 mg	1 to 3 ml/min
	or 4 mg/ml	250 ml	1000 mg	0.5 to 1.5 ml/min

[1] All infusions should be made up to final volume with 5% Dextrose Injection, USP.

[2] The maintenance infusion rates are calculated to deliver 2 to 6 mg/min depending on body weight, renal elimination rate and steady-state plasma level needed to maintain control of the arrhythmia. The 4 mg/ml maintenance concentration may be preferred if total infused volume must be limited.

(Administration and Dosage continued on following page)

PROCAINAMIDE HCl (Cont.)

Administration and Dosage (Cont.):

Parenteral (Cont.):

Cautiously administer the IV injection to avoid a possible hypotensive response. Initial arrhythmia control, under blood pressure and ECG monitoring, may usually be accomplished safely within 30 minutes by either of the two methods that follow:

1) Slowly direct injection into a vein or into tubing of an established infusion line at a rate not to exceed 50 mg/min. It is advisable to dilute either the 100 or the 500 mg/ml concentrations prior to IV injection to facilitate control of dosage rate. Doses of 100 mg may be administered every 5 minutes at this rate until the arrhythmia is suppressed or until 500 mg has been administered, after which it is advisable to wait ≥ 10 minutes to allow for more distribution into tissues before resuming.

2) Alternatively, a loading infusion containing 20 mg/ml (1 g diluted to 50 ml with 5% Dextrose Injection, USP) may be administered at a constant rate of 1 ml/min for 25 to 30 minutes to deliver 500 to 600 mg. Some effects may be seen after infusion of the first 100 or 200 mg; it is unusual to require > 600 mg to achieve satisfactory antiarrhythmic effects.

The maximum advisable dosage to be given either by repeated bolus injections or such loading infusion is 1 g.

To maintain therapeutic levels, a more dilute IV infusion at a concentration of 2 mg/ml is convenient (1 g in 500 ml 5% Dextrose Injection, USP), and may be administered at 1 to 3 ml/min. If daily total fluid intake must be limited, a 4 mg/ml concentration (1 g in 250 ml of 5% Dextrose Injection, USP) administered at 0.5 to 1.5 ml/min will deliver an equivalent 2 to 6 mg/min. Assess the amount needed in a given patient to maintain the therapeutic level principally from the clinical response. This will depend on the patient's weight and age, renal elimination, hepatic acetylation rate and cardiac status, but adjust for each patient based on close observation. A maintenance infusion rate of 50 mcg/kg/min to a person with a normal renal procainamide elimination half-life of 3 hours should to produce a plasma level of approximately 6.5 mcg/ml.

Since the principal route for elimination of procainamide and NAPA is renal excretion, reduced excretion will prolong the half-life of elimination and lower the dose rate needed to maintain therapeutic levels. Advancing age reduces the renal excretion of procainamide and NAPA independently of reductions in Ccr; compared to normal young adults, there is an ≈ 25% reduction at age 50 and a 50% reduction at age 75.

Terminate IV therapy if persistent conduction disturbances or hypotension develop. As soon as the patient's basic cardiac rhythm appears to be stabilized, oral antiarrhythmic maintenance therapy is preferable (if indicated and possible). A period of about 3 to 4 hours (one half-life for renal elimination, ordinarily) should elapse after the last IV dose before administering the first dose of oral procainamide.

Children: The following doses have been suggested.

Oral – 15 to 50 mg/kg/day divided every 3 to 6 hours; maximum 4 g/day.

IM – 20 to 30 mg/kg/day divided every 4 to 6 hours; maximum 4 g/day.

IV – *Loading dose,* 3 to 6 mg/kg/dose over 5 minutes. *Maintenance,* 20 to 80 mcg/kg/min continuous infusion. Maximum 100 mg/dose or 2 g/day.

				C.I.*
Rx	**Procainamide HCl** (Rugby)	**Tablets:** 250 mg	In 100s, 120s and 500s.	20
Rx	**Pronestyl** (Princeton Pharm.)		Tartrazine. (431). Yellow. Filmlok. In 100s.	43
Rx	**Pronestyl** (Princeton Pharm.)	**Tablets:** 375 mg	Tartrazine. (434). Filmlok. Orange. In 100s.	40
Rx	**Pronestyl** (Princeton Pharm.)	**Tablets:** 500 mg	Tartrazine. (438). Red. Filmlok. In 100s.	38
Rx	**Procainamide HCl** (Various, eg, Goldline, Major, Parmed, Rugby, Schein, Zenith)	**Capsules:** 250 mg	In 100s, 250s and 1000s.	6.7+
Rx	**Pronestyl** (Princeton Pharm.)		Lactose. (758). Yellow. In 100s, 1000s and UD 100s.	43
Rx	**Procainamide HCl** (Various, eg, Major, Parmed, Rugby, Schein, Zenith)	**Capsules:** 375 mg	In 100s and 1000s.	6.7+
Rx	**Pronestyl** (Princeton Pharm.)		Lactose. (756). White/orange. In 100s and UD 100s.	70

* Cost Index based on cost per 250 mg.

(Continued on following page)

PROCAINAMIDE HCl (Cont.)

	Product	Form	Description	C.I.*
Rx	**Procainamide HCl** (Various, eg, Major, Parmed, Rugby, Schein, Zenith)	**Capsules:** 500 mg	In 100s, 250s and 1000s.	6+
Rx	**Pronestyl** (Princeton Pharm.)		(757). Yellow/orange. In 100s, 1000s and UD 100s.	38
Rx	**Procainamide HCl** (Various, eg, Abbott, Elkins Sinn, IMS, Quad, Solopak)	**Injection:** 100 mg/ml	In 10 ml.	398
Rx	**Pronestyl** (Princeton Pharm.)		In 10 ml vials.[1]	1267
Rx	**Procainamide HCl** (Various, eg, Abbott, Elkins Sinn, IMS, Quad, Sanofi Winthrop, Solopak)	**Injection:** 500 mg/ml	In 2 ml vials and 2 and 4 ml disp. syringes.	179+
Rx	**Pronestyl** (Princeton Pharm.)		In 2 ml vials.[2]	1267

PROCAINAMIDE SUSTAINED RELEASE

Sustained release products are not recommended for initial therapy. Total dosage (50 mg/kg/day) may be given in divided doses every 6 hours.

	Product	Form	Description	C.I.*
Rx	**Procainamide HCl** (Various, eg, Geneva, Goldline, Major, Parmed, Rugby, Sidmak)	**Tablets, sustained release:** 250 mg	In 100s, 250s, 500s, 1000s and UD 100s.	16+
Rx	**Procan SR** (Parke-Davis)		Lactose. (P-D 202). Green. Elliptical. Film coated. In 100s, 120s & UD 100s.	20
Rx	**Procainamide HCl** (Various, eg, Geneva, Goldline, Major, Parmed, Rugby, Schein, Sidmak)	**Tablets, sustained release:** 500 mg	In 100s, 250s, 500s and 1000s.	11+
Rx	**Procan SR** (Parke-Davis)		Sucrose. (PD 204). Yellow, scored. Elliptical. Film coated. In 100s, 120s, 500s and UD 100s.	27
Rx	**Pronestyl-SR** (Princeton Pharm.)		(775). Green-yellow. Biconvex, oval. Filmlok. In 100s.	27
Rx	**Procainamide HCl** (Various, eg, Geneva, Goldline, Major, Parmed, Rugby, Schein)	**Tablets, sustained release:** 750 mg	In 100s, 250s and 500s.	16+
Rx	**Procan SR** (Parke-Davis)		(PD 205). Orange, scored. Elliptical. Film coated. In 100s, 120s, 500s and UD 100s.	27
Rx	**Procan SR** (Parke-Davis)	**Tablets, sustained release:** 1000 mg	(PD 207). Red, scored. Elliptical. Film coated. In 100s and 120s.	18

* Cost Index based on cost per 250 mg.

[1] With 0.9% benzyl alcohol and ≤ 0.09% sodium bisulfite.

[2] With 0.1% methylparaben and ≤ 0.2% sodium bisulfite.

Refer to the general discussion concerning these products on page 618.

DISOPYRAMIDE

Actions:

Pharmacology:

Mechanism of action – Disopyramide is a class IA antiarrhythmic agent pharmacologically similar to, but chemically unrelated to, procainamide and quinidine. It decreases the rate of diastolic depolarization (phase 4), decreases the upstroke velocity (phase 0), increases the action potential duration of normal cardiac cells and prolongs the refractory period (phases 2 and 3). It also decreases the disparity in refractoriness between infarcted and adjacent normally perfused myocardium and does not affect alpha- or beta-adrenergic receptors.

Electrophysiology – Disopyramide shortens sinus node recovery time and lengthens atrial and ventricular refractoriness. The effects on AV nodal conduction and refractoriness and sinus node function vary due to a depressant effect that is counteracted by a vagolytic action. The principal metabolite, mono-N-dealkyldisopyramide (MND), exhibits little antiarrhythmic activity, but is 20 to 30 times more anticholinergic than the parent drug. Little effect has been shown on the AV nodal and His-Purkinje conduction times or on QRS duration, but conduction in accessory pathways is prolonged.

Hemodynamics – At recommended oral doses, disopyramide rarely produces significant alterations of blood pressure in patients without congestive heart failure (see Warnings). With IV disopyramide (dosage form not available in US), either increases in systolic/diastolic or decreases in systolic blood pressure have occurred depending on the infusion rate and the patient population. IV disopyramide may cause cardiac depression with an approximate mean 10% reduction of cardiac output, which is more pronounced in patients with cardiac dysfunction.

Anticholinergic activity – In vitro anticholinergic activity is approximately 0.06% that of atropine; the usual dose of 150 mg every 6 hours or 300 mg controlled release every 12 hours compares to approximately 0.4 to 0.6 mg of atropine.

Pharmacokinetics: Absorption/Distribution – Following oral administration of immediate release disopyramide, the drug is rapidly and almost completely (≈ 90%) absorbed. Peak plasma levels usually occur within 2 hours. Therapeutic plasma levels of disopyramide are 2 to 4 mcg/ml. Protein binding is concentration-dependent and varies from 50% to 65%; it is difficult to predict the concentration of the free drug when total drug is measured. After the oral administration of 200 mg disopyramide to 10 cardiac patients with borderline to moderate heart failure, the time to peak serum concentration of 2.3 ± 1.5 hours was increased, and the mean peak serum concentration of 4.8 ± 1.6 mcg/ml was higher than in healthy volunteers.

Metabolism/Excretion – About 50% is excreted in the urine as the unchanged drug and 30% as metabolites (20% MND). The plasma concentration of MND is ≈ one tenth that of disopyramide. The mean plasma half-life is 6.7 hours (range, 4 to 10 hours).

In impaired renal function (creatinine clearance [Ccr] < 40 ml/min), half-life values ranged from 8 to 18 hours. Therefore, decrease the dose in renal failure to avoid drug accumulation (see Administration and Dosage). Altering urinary pH does not affect plasma half-life.

Dialysis: A preliminary report of three patients on long-term hemodialysis revealed a 45% to 72% reduction in disopyramide half-life during dialysis. In contrast, another study in patients on chronic hemodialysis demonstrated little difference in disopyramide half-life without dialysis (16.8 vs 16.1 hours). Resin and charcoal hemoperfusion were effective in rapidly decreasing disopyramide plasma levels in acute overdosage (see Overdosage).

Immediate release vs controlled release: In a crossover study in healthy subjects, the bioavailability of the controlled release form was similar to that from the immediate release capsules. With a single 300 mg oral dose, peak disopyramide plasma concentrations of 3.23 ± 0.75 mcg/ml at 2.5 ± 2.3 hours were obtained with two 150 mg immediate release capsules and 2.22 ± 0.47 mcg/ml at 4.9 ± 1.4 hours with two 150 mg controlled release capsules. The elimination half-life was 8.31 ± 1.83 hours with the immediate release capsules and 11.65 ± 4.72 hours with controlled release capsules. The amount of disopyramide and MND excreted in the urine in 48 hours was 128 and 48 mg, respectively, with the immediate release capsules and 112 and 33 mg, respectively, with controlled release capsules.

Following multiple doses, steady-state plasma levels of between 2 and 4 mcg/ml were attained following either 150 mg every 6 hours with immediate release capsules or 300 mg every 12 hours with controlled release capsules.

(Continued on following page)

DISOPYRAMIDE (Cont.)

Indications:

Treatment of documented ventricular arrhythmias (eg, sustained ventricular tachycardia) considered to be life-threatening.

Unlabeled use: Disopyramide may be beneficial in the treatment of paroxysmal supraventricular tachycardia.

Contraindications:

Cardiogenic shock; preexisting second- or third-degree AV block (if no pacemaker is present); congenital QT prolongation; sick sinus syndrome; hypersensitivity to disopyramide.

Warnings:

Proarrhythmic effects: Because of the proarrhythmic effects, use with lesser arrhythmias is generally not recommended.

Asymptomatic ventricular premature contractions: Avoid treatment of patients with this condition.

Survival: Antiarrhythmic drugs have not been shown to enhance survival in patients with ventricular arrhythmias.

Negative inotropic properties: Heart failure/hypotension – May cause or aggravate CHF or produce severe hypotension, especially in patients with depressed systolic function. Do not use in patients with uncompensated or marginally compensated CHF or hypotension unless secondary to cardiac arrhythmia. Treat patients with a history of heart failure with careful attention to the maintenance of cardiac function, including optimal digitalization. If hypotension occurs or CHF worsens, discontinue use; restart at a lower dosage after adequate cardiac compensation has been established.

Do not give a loading dose to patients with myocarditis or other cardiomyopathy; closely monitor initial dosage and subsequent adjustments.

QRS widening (> 25%), although unusual, may occur; discontinue use in such cases.

QT_C prolongation and worsening of the arrhythmia, including ventricular tachycardia and fibrillation, may occur. Patients who have QT prolongation in response to quinidine may be at particular risk. As with other Type IA antiarrhythmics, disopyramide has been associated with torsade de pointes. If QT prolongation > 25% is observed and if ectopy continues, monitor closely and consider discontinuing the drug.

Atrial tachyarrhythmias: Digitalize patients with atrial flutter or fibrillation prior to administration to ensure that enhancement of AV conduction does not increase ventricular rate beyond acceptable limits.

Conduction abnormalities: Use caution in patients with sick sinus syndrome, Wolff-Parkinson-White (WPW) syndrome or bundle branch block.

Heart block: If first degree heart block develops, reduce dosage. If the block persists, drug continuation must depend upon the benefit compared to the risk of higher degrees of heart block. Development of second- or third-degree AV block or unifascicular, bifascicular or trifascicular block requires discontinuation of therapy, unless ventricular rate is controlled by a ventricular pacemaker.

Concomitant antiarrhythmic therapy: Reserve concomitant use of disopyramide with other class IA antiarrhythmics or propranolol for life-threatening arrhythmias unresponsive to a single agent. Such use may produce serious negative inotropic effects or may excessively prolong conduction, particularly in patients with cardiac decompensation.

Hypoglycemia has been reported in rare instances. Monitor blood glucose levels in patients with CHF, chronic malnutrition, hepatic disease and in those taking drugs which could compromise normal glucoregulatory mechanisms in the absence of food (eg, beta-adrenoceptor blockers, alcohol).

Anticholinergic activity: Do not use in patients with urinary retention, glaucoma or myasthenia gravis unless adequate overriding measures are taken. Urinary retention may occur in patients of either sex, but males with benign prostatic hypertrophy are at particular risk. In patients with a family history of glaucoma, measure intraocular pressure before initiating therapy. Use with special care in patients with myasthenia gravis, since disopyramide could precipitate a myasthenic crisis.

Renal function impairment: Reduce dosage in impaired renal function. Carefully monitor ECG for prolongation of PR interval, evidence of QRS widening or other signs of overdosage (see Overdosage). The controlled release form is not recommended for patients with severe renal insufficiency (Ccr ≤ 40 ml/min).

Hepatic function impairment increases plasma half-life; therefore, reduce dosage in such patients. Carefully monitor the ECG. Patients with cardiac dysfunction have a higher potential for hepatic impairment.

(Warnings continued on following page)

DISOPYRAMIDE (Cont.)

Warnings (Cont.)

Pregnancy: Category C. Disopyramide was associated with decreased numbers of implantation sites and decreased growth and survival of pups when administered to pregnant rats at 250 mg/kg/day (≥ 20 times the usual daily human dose), a level at which weight gain and food consumption of dams were also reduced. Increased resorption rates were reported in rabbits at 60 mg/kg/day (≥ 5 times the usual daily human dose). At a maternal concentration of 2.3 mg/L disopyramide, the fetal cord concentration is 0.9 mg/L. Well controlled studies have not been performed in pregnant women and experience is limited. Use only when clearly needed and when the potential benefits outweigh the potential hazards to the fetus. Disopyramide has been found in human fetal blood. Disopyramide may stimulate contractions of the pregnant uterus.

Lactation: Disopyramide has been detected in breast milk at a concentration not exceeding that in maternal plasma. Therefore, decide whether to discontinue nursing or to discontinue the drug taking into account the importance of the drug to the mother.

Precautions:

Potassium imbalance: Disopyramide may be ineffective in *hypo*kalemia and its toxic effects may be enhanced in *hyper*kalemia. Correct any potassium deficit before instituting therapy.

Drug Interactions:

Disopyramide Drug Interactions			
Precipitant drug	Object drug*		Description
Antiarrhythmics	Disopyramide	↑	Other antiarrhythmics (eg, procainamide, lidocaine) have been used with disopyramide; however, widening of the QRS complex or QT prolongation may occur.
Beta blockers	Disopyramide	↔	This interaction is difficult to predict. Disopyramide clearance may be decreased; other adverse effects (eg, sinus bradycardia, hypotension) may occur. Others report no occurrence of synergistic or additive negative inotropic effects.
Erythromycin	Disopyramide	↑	Increased disopyramide plasma levels may occur. Arrhythmias and increased QTc intervals have occurred.
Hydantoins	Disopyramide	↓	Disopyramide serum levels, half-life and bioavailability may be decreased; anticholinergic effects may be enhanced. Effects may persist for several days after hydantoin withdrawal.
Quinidine	Disopyramide	↑	Concurrent use may result in increased disopyramide serum levels or decreased quinidine levels. This may result in disopyramide toxicity or decreased response to quinidine.
Disopyramide	Quinidine	↓	
Rifampin	Disopyramide	↓	Disopyramide serum levels may be decreased.
Disopyramide	Anticoagulants	↓	Decreased prothrombin time after disopyramide discontinuation may occur. However, this may be due to a hemodynamic effect and not an interaction.
Disopyramide	Digoxin	↑	Although serum digoxin levels may be increased, a clinically significant interaction appears unlikely. A beneficial interaction has also been suggested.

* ↑ = Object drug increased. ↓ = Object drug decreased. ↔ = Undetermined effect.

Adverse Reactions:

The most serious adverse reactions are hypotension and CHF. The most common reactions are anticholinergic and dose-dependent. These may be transitory, but may be persistent or severe. Urinary retention is the most serious anticholinergic effect.

Anticholinergic: Dry mouth (32%); urinary hesitancy (14%); constipation (11%); blurred vision, dry nose, eyes and throat (3% to 9%).

GU: Urinary retention, frequency and urgency (3% to 9%); impotence (1% to 3%); dysuria, elevated creatinine (< 1%).

(Adverse Reactions continued on following page)

DISOPYRAMIDE (Cont.)

Adverse Reactions (Cont.)

Cardiovascular: Hypotension with or without CHF, increased CHF, edema, weight gain, cardiac conduction disturbances, shortness of breath, syncope, chest pain (1% to 3%); AV block (< 1%). There have been reports of severe myocardial depression (with hypotension and an increase in venous pressure) and unexplained severe epigastric pain following standard oral doses.

Hematologic: Decreased hemoglobin, hematocrit (< 1%); thrombocytopenia, reversible agranulocytosis (rare).

CNS: Dizziness, fatigue, headache (3% to 9%); nervousness (1% to 3%); depression, insomnia (< 1%); acute psychosis (rare, prompt reversal when therapy discontinued).

GI: Nausea, pain, bloating, gas (3% to 9%); anorexia, diarrhea, vomiting (1% to 3%); elevated liver enzymes (< 1%); reversible cholestatic jaundice.

Dermatologic: Generalized rash, dermatoses, itching (1% to 3%).

Miscellaneous: Muscle weakness, malaise, aches/pain (3% to 9%); hypokalemia, elevated cholesterol and triglycerides (1% to 3%); numbness, tingling, elevated BUN (< 1%); hypoglycemia; fever and respiratory difficulty; gynecomastia (rare); anaphylactoid reactions; lupus erythematosus symptoms (most cases occurred in patients who had been switched to disopyramide from procainamide following the development of symptoms).

Overdosage:

Symptoms: Overdose may be followed by apnea, loss of consciousness, cardiac arrhythmias, loss of spontaneous respiration and death. Toxic plasma levels produce excessive widening of the QRS complex and QT interval, worsening of CHF, hypotension, varying conduction disturbances, bradycardia, and finally, asystole. Anticholinergic effects may also be observed.

Treatment: Prompt, vigorous treatment is necessary even in the absence of symptoms. Such treatment may be lifesaving and may include emesis, gastric lavage or a cathartic followed by activated charcoal by mouth or stomach tube.

Administration of isoproterenol, dopamine, cardiac glycosides, diuretics, intra-aortic balloon counterpulsation, mechanical ventilation, hemodialysis or charcoal hemoperfusion may be used. Monitor ECG.

If progressive AV block develops, implement endocardial pacing. In case of impaired renal function, measures to increase the GFR may reduce the toxicity. Altering urinary pH does not affect plasma half-life or the amount of disopyramide excreted in the urine.

Anticholinergic effects can be reversed with neostigmine.

Refer also to General Management of Acute Overdosage.

Patient Information:

May cause dry mouth, difficult urination, dizziness, breathing difficulty, constipation or blurred vision. Notify physician if symptoms persist, but do not discontinue unless instructed to do so by physician.

Do not break or chew sustained release capsules.

Administration and Dosage:

Approved by the FDA in 1977.

Individualize dosage. Initiate treatment in the hospital.

Adults: 400 to 800 mg/day. The recommended dosage for most adults is 600 mg/day. For patients < 50 kg (110 pounds), give 400 mg/day. Divide the total daily dose and administer every 6 hours in the immediate release form or every 12 hours in the controlled release form.

Children: Divide daily dosage and administer equal doses every 6 hours or at intervals according to patient needs. Closely monitor plasma levels and therapeutic response. Hospitalize patients during initial treatment and start dose titration at the lower end of the ranges provided below:

Suggested Total Daily Disopyramide Dosage in Children[1]	
Age (years)	Disopyramide (mg/kg/day)
< 1	10 to 30
1 to 4	10 to 20
4 to 12	10 to 15
12 to 18	6 to 15

[1] Prepare a 1 to 10 mg/ml suspension by adding contents of the immediate release capsule to cherry syrup, NF. The resulting suspension, when refrigerated, is stable for 1 month; shake thoroughly before measuring dose. Dispense in an amber glass bottle. Do not use the controlled release form to prepare the solution.

(Administration and Dosage listed on following page)

DISOPYRAMIDE (Cont.)

Administration and Dosage (Cont.)

Initial loading dose: For rapid control of ventricular arrhythmia, give an initial loading dose of 300 mg immediate release (200 mg for patients < 50 kg [110 lbs]). Therapeutic effects are attained in 30 minutes to 3 hours. If there is no response or no evidence of toxicity within 6 hours of the loading dose, 200 mg every 6 hours may be administered instead of the usual 150 mg. If there is no response within 48 hours, discontinue the drug or carefully monitor subsequent doses of 250 or 300 mg every 6 hours.

Do not use the controlled release form initially if rapid plasma levels are desired.

Severe refractory ventricular tachycardia: A limited number of patients have tolerated up to 1600 mg/day (400 mg every 6 hours), resulting in plasma levels up to 9 mcg/ml. Hospitalize patients for close evaluation and continuous monitoring.

Cardiomyopathy or possible cardiac decompensation: Do not administer a loading dose, and limit the initial dosage to 100 mg immediate release every 6 to 8 hours. Make subsequent dosage adjustments gradually.

Renal/hepatic failure: For patients with moderate renal insufficiency (Ccr > 40 ml/min) or hepatic insufficiency, the recommended dosage is 400 mg/day given in divided doses (either 100 mg every 6 hours for immediate release or 200 mg every 12 hours for controlled release).

In severe renal insufficiency (Ccr ≤ 40 ml/min), the recommended dosage is 100 mg of the immediate release form given at the intervals shown in the table below, with or without an initial loading dose of 150 mg.

Disopyramide Dosage in Renal Impairment

Creatinine clearance (ml/min)	Loading dose (mg)	Dose (mg)	Dosage interval (hours)
40-30	150	100	8
30-15	150	100	12
< 15	150	100	24

Transfer to disopyramide: Use the regular maintenance schedule, without a loading dose, 6 to 12 hours after the last dose of quinidine or 3 to 6 hours after the last dose of procainamide. Where withdrawal of quinidine or procainamide is likely to produce life-threatening arrhythmias, consider hospitalization.

When transferring from immediate to controlled release, start maintenance schedule of controlled release 6 hours after the last dose of immediate release.

	Product	Form	Description	C.I.*
Rx	**Disopyramide Phosphate** (Various, eg, Barr, Major, Rugby, Schein, Zenith)	**Capsules:** 100 mg (as phosphate)	In 100s, 500s, 1000s and UD 100s.	26+
Rx	**Norpace** (Searle)		Lactose. (Searle 2752 Norpace 100 mg). White and orange. In 100s, 500s, 1000s and UD 100s.	67
Rx	**Disopyramide Phosphate** (Various, eg, Barr, Major, Rugby, Schein, Zenith)	**Capsules:** 150 mg (as phosphate)	In 100s, 500s, 1000s and UD 100s.	21+
Rx	**Norpace** (Searle)		Lactose. (Searle 2762 Norpace 150 mg). Brown and orange. In 100s, 500s, 1000s and UD 100s.	40
Rx	**Disopyramide Phosphate** (Various, eg, Ethex, Goldline, Schein)	**Capsules, extended release:** 100 mg (as phosphate)	In 100s.	53+
Rx	**Norpace CR** (Searle)		Sucrose. (Searle 2732 Norpace CR 100 mg). White and light green. In 100s, 500s and UD 100s.	81
Rx	**Disopyramide Phosphate** (Various, eg, Barr, Ethex, Geneva, Goldline, Schein, Warner Chilcott)	**Capsules, extended release:** 150 mg (as phosphate)	In 100s, 500s and UD 100s.	23+
Rx	**Norpace CR** (Searle)		Sucrose. (Searle 2742 Norpace CR 150 mg). Brown and light green. In 100s, 500s and UD 100s.	64

* Cost Index based on cost per 100 mg.

Refer to the general discussion concerning these products on page 618.

LIDOCAINE HCl

Actions:

Pharmacology: Therapeutic concentrations of lidocaine attenuate phase 4 diastolic depolarization, decrease automaticity and cause a decrease or no change in excitability and membrane responsiveness. Action potential duration and effective refractory period (ERP) of Purkinje fibers and ventricular muscle are decreased, while the ratio of ERP to action potential duration is increased. The AV node ERP may increase, decrease or remain unchanged, and atrial ERP is unchanged. Lidocaine raises the ventricular fibrillation threshold. Lidocaine has little or no effect on the autonomic tone.

Clinical electrophysiological studies have demonstrated no change in sinus node recovery time or sinoatrial conduction time. AV nodal conduction time is unchanged or shortened, and His-Purkinje conduction time is unchanged. Lidocaine increases the electrical stimulation threshold of the ventricle during diastole. In therapeutic doses, lidocaine produces no change in myocardial contractility, systolic arterial blood pressure or absolute refractory period.

Pharmacokinetics: Absorption/Distribution – Lidocaine is ineffective orally; 60% to 70% of an oral dose is metabolized by the liver before reaching the systemic circulation. It is most commonly administered IV with an immediate onset (within minutes) and brief duration (10 to 20 minutes) of action following a bolus dose. Continuous IV infusion of lidocaine (1 to 4 mg/min) is necessary to maintain antiarrhythmic effects. Following IM administration, therapeutic serum levels are achieved in 5 to 15 minutes and may persist for up to 2 hours. Higher and more rapid serum levels are achieved by injection into the deltoid muscle, which is preferred over the gluteus or vastus lateralis. Therapeutic serum levels are 1.5 to 6 mcg/ml; serum levels $>$ 6 to 10 mcg/ml are usually toxic. Lidocaine is about 50% protein bound (concentration dependent).

Metabolism/Excretion – Extensive biotransformation in the liver ($\approx$ 90%) results in at least two active metabolites, monoethylglycinexylidide (MEGX) and glycinexylidide (GX). These metabolites exhibit both antiarrhythmic and convulsant properties. The hepatic extraction ratio is between 62% and 81%. Lidocaine exhibits a biphasic half-life. The distribution phase (half-life $\approx$ 10 minutes) accounts for the short duration of action following IV bolus administration. The elimination half-life is 1.5 to 2 hours; half-life may be $\geq$ 3 hours following infusions of $>$ 24 hours. Because of the rapid rate at which lidocaine is metabolized, any condition that alters liver function, including changes in liver blood flow, which could result from severe congestive heart failure (CHF) or shock, may alter lidocaine kinetics. Less than 10% of the parent drug is excreted unchanged in the urine. Renal elimination plays an important role in the elimination of the metabolites. Accumulation of GX in patients with severely impaired renal function on prolonged infusions may contribute to lidocaine toxicity.

Indications:

IV: Acute management of ventricular arrhythmias occurring during cardiac manipulation, such as cardiac surgery or in relation to acute myocardial infarction (MI).

IM: Single doses are justified in the following exceptional circumstances: When ECG equipment is not available to verify the diagnosis but the potential benefits outweigh the possible risks; when facilities for IV administration are not readily available; by the patient in the prehospital phase of suspected acute MI, directed by qualified medical personnel viewing the transmitted ECG.

Unlabeled uses: In pediatric patients with cardiac arrest, $<$ 10% develop ventricular fibrillation, and others develop ventricular tachycardia; the hemodynamically compromised child may develop ventricular couplets or frequent premature ventricular beats. In these cases, lidocaine 1 mg/kg should be administered by the IV, intraosseous or endotracheal route. A second 1 mg/kg dose may be given in 10 to 15 minutes. Start a lidocaine infusion if the second dose is required; a third bolus may be needed in 10 to 15 minutes to maintain therapeutic levels.

Contraindications:

Hypersensitivity to amide local anesthetics; Stokes-Adams syndrome; Wolff-Parkinson-White syndrome; severe degrees of sinoatrial, atrioventricular (AV) or intraventricular block in the absence of an artificial pacemaker.

Warnings:

Survival: Prophylactic single dose lidocaine administered in a monitored environment does not appear to affect mortality in the earliest phase of acute MI, and may actually be harmful to some patients who are later shown not to have suffered an acute MI.

Constant ECG monitoring is essential for proper administration. Have emergency resuscitative equipment and drugs immediately available to manage adverse reactions involving the cardiovascular, respiratory or central nervous systems.

(Warnings continued on following page)

LIDOCAINE HCl (Cont.)

Warnings (Cont.):

IV use: Signs of excessive depression of cardiac conductivity, such as sinus node dysfunction, prolongation of PR interval, widening of the QRS complex, and the appearance or aggravation of arrhythmias, should be followed by dosage reduction and, if necessary, prompt cessation of IV infusion.

IM use: May increase creatine phosphokinase (CPK) levels. Use of the enzyme determination without isoenzyme separation, as a diagnostic test for acute MI, may be compromised.

Cardiac effects: Use with caution and in lower doses in patients with CHF, reduced cardiac output, digitalis toxicity accompanied by AV block and in the elderly.

In sinus bradycardia or incomplete heart block, lidocaine administration for the elimination of ventricular ectopy without prior acceleration in heart rate (eg, by atropine, isoproterenol or electric pacing) may promote more frequent and serious ventricular arrhythmias or complete heart block (see Contraindications). Use with caution in patients with hypovolemia and shock, and all forms of heart block.

Acceleration of ventricular rate may occur when administered to patients with atrial flutter or fibrillation.

Hypersensitivity reactions may occur (see Adverse Reactions). Refer to Management of Acute Hypersensitivity Reactions.

Renal or hepatic function impairment: Lidocaine is metabolized mainly in the liver and excreted by the kidney. Use caution with repeated or prolonged use in patients with liver or renal disease due to possible toxic accumulation of lidocaine or its metabolites.

Pregnancy: Category B. Lidocaine readily crosses the placental barrier. However, there are no adequate and well controlled studies in pregnant women; therefore use during pregnancy only when clearly needed.

Lactation: In a single case report, lidocaine was excreted into breast milk at concentrations 40% of serum levels. At this level, an infant might ingest up to 1.5 mg, a very small amount that would not be expected to lead to significant accumulation. However, exercise caution when administering to a nursing woman.

Children: Safety and efficacy have not been established; reduce dosage. The IM auto-injector device is not recommended in children < 50 kg (110 lbs).

Precautions:

Malignant hyperthermia: Amide local anesthetic administration has been associated with acute onset of fulminant hypermetabolism of skeletal muscle known as malignant hyperthermic crisis. Recognition of early unexplained signs of tachycardia, tachypnea, labile blood pressure and metabolic acidosis may precede temperature elevation. Successful outcome depends on early diagnosis, prompt discontinuance of the triggering agent and institution of treatment, including oxygen, supportive measures and IV dantrolene sodium (see individual monograph).

The safety of amide local anesthetics in patients with genetic predisposition of malignant hyperthermia has not been fully assessed; use lidocaine with caution in such patients. In hospitals where triggering agents for malignant hyperthermia are administered, a standard protocol for management should be available.

Drug Interactions:

Lidocaine Drug Interactions			
Precipitant drug	Object drug*		Description
Beta blockers	Lidocaine	↑	Increased lidocaine levels may occur, possibly resulting in toxicity.
Cimetidine	Lidocaine	↑	Decreased lidocaine clearance with possible toxicity. Ranitidine, and perhaps other H_2 antagonists, do not appear to interact.
Procainamide	Lidocaine	↑	Additive cardiodepressant action may occur with potential for conduction abnormalities.
Tocainide	Lidocaine	↑	Since these agents are pharmacologically similar, concomitant use may cause an increased incidence of adverse reactions.
Lidocaine	Succinylcholine	↑	Prolongation of neuromuscular blockade may occur.

* ↑ = Object drug increased

(Continued on following page)

LIDOCAINE HCl (Cont.)

Adverse Reactions:

CNS: Lightheadedness; nervousness; drowsiness; dizziness; apprehension; confusion; mood changes; "doom anxiety"; hallucinations; euphoria; tinnitus; blurred or double vision; sensation of heat, cold or numbness; twitching; tremors; convulsions; unconsciousness.

Cardiovascular: Hypotension; bradycardia; cardiovascular collapse, which may lead to cardiac arrest.

Hypersensitivity: Infrequent allergic reactions may occur, characterized by cutaneous lesions, urticaria, edema or anaphylactoid reactions. Skin testing has doubtful value. See Warnings.

Other: Occasional soreness at the IM injection site; febrile response; infection at the injection site; venous thrombosis or phlebitis extending from the site of injection; extravasation; vomiting; respiratory depression and arrest.

Toxicity:

Symptoms: Lidocaine blood concentrations may correlate with CNS toxicity (see Adverse Reactions). Mild CNS symptoms (drowsiness, dizziness, transient paresthesias) quickly resolve. General guidelines are provided in the table below:

Lidocaine Plasma[1] Concentrations and Effects

Concentration (mcg/ml)	Toxicity[2]
< 1.5	Idiosyncratic
1.5 to 4	Mild CNS and cardiovascular effects
4 to 6	Mild CNS effects common; cardiovascular in those with concomitant disease
6 to 8	Significant risk of CNS and cardiovascular depression
> 8	Seizures, obtundation, hypotension, respiratory depression, decreased cardiac output, coma

1 Whole blood concentrations may be 10% to 30% lower.

2 Patients with significant conduction system abnormalities or marginal hemodynamic status may develop apparent toxicity even at very low lidocaine concentrations. Metabolites also can contribute to toxicity even with modest lidocaine plasma concentrations.

Treatment: In the case of severe reaction, discontinue the drug. Institute emergency resuscitative procedures and supportive treatment. For severe convulsions, use small increments of diazepam or an ultra-short-acting barbiturate (thiopental or thiamylal); if those are not available, use a short-acting barbiturate (pentobarbital or secobarbital). If the patient is under anesthesia, succinylcholine may be given IV. Assure a patent airway and adequate ventilation. If circulatory depression occurs, administer vasopressors and, if necessary, institute CPR.

Administration and Dosage:

IM: 300 mg. The deltoid muscle is preferred. Avoid intravascular injection. Use only the 10% solution for IM injection.

The *LidoPen Auto-Injector* unit is for self-administration into the deltoid muscle or the anterolateral aspect of the thigh. Patient instructions are provided with the product.

Replacement therapy – As soon as possible, change patient to IV lidocaine or to an oral antiarrhythmic preparation for maintenance therapy. However, if necessary, an additional IM injection may be administered after 60 to 90 minutes.

IV: Use only lidocaine injection without preservatives, clearly labeled for IV use. Monitor ECG constantly to avoid potential overdosage and toxicity.

IV bolus is used to establish rapid therapeutic blood levels. Continuous IV infusion is necessary to maintain antiarrhythmic effects. The usual dose is 50 to 100 mg, given at a rate of 25 to 50 mg/minute. If the initial injection does not produce the desired clinical response, give a second bolus dose after 5 minutes. Give no more than 200 to 300 mg/hour.

Reduce loading (bolus) doses in patients with CHF or reduced cardiac output and in the elderly. However, some investigators recommend the usual loading dose be administered and only the maintenance dosage be reduced.

(Administration and Dosage continued on following page)

LIDOCAINE HCl (Cont.)

Administration and Dosage (Cont.):

IV continuous infusion is used to maintain therapeutic plasma levels following loading doses in patients in whom arrhythmias tend to recur and who cannot receive oral antiarrhythmic drugs. Administer at a rate of 1 to 4 mg/min (20 to 50 mcg/kg/min). Reduce maintenance doses in patients with heart failure or liver disease, or who are also receiving other drugs known to decrease clearance of lidocaine or decrease liver blood flow (see Drug Interactions) and in patients > 70 years of age. Reassess the rate of infusion as soon as the cardiac rhythm stabilizes or at the earliest signs of toxicity. Change patients to oral antiarrhythmic agents for maintenance therapy as soon as possible. It is rarely necessary to continue IV infusions for prolonged periods. Use a precision volume control IV set for continuous IV infusion.

Children – The American Heart Association's Standards and Guidelines recommend a bolus dose of 1 mg/kg, followed by an infusion of 30 mcg/kg/min. The following dosage has also been suggested:

Loading dose, 1 mg/kg/dose given IV or intratracheally every 5 to 10 min to desired effect, maximum total dose 5 mg/kg; *maintenance,* 20 to 50 mcg/kg/min.

Preparation of infusion – Add 1 or 2 g lidocaine to 1 L of 5% Dextrose in Water to prepare a 0.1% to 0.2% solution; each ml will contain ≈ 1 to 2 mg lidocaine. Therefore, 1 to 4 ml/min (of a 1 mg/ml solution) will provide 1 to 4 mg lidocaine/minute. If fluid restriction is desirable, prepare a more concentrated solution.

Storage/stability – Lidocaine is stable for 24 hours after dilution in 5% Dextrose in Water.

				C.I.*
		For IM Administration		
Rx	**LidoPen Auto-Injector** (Survival Technology)	**Injection:** 300 mg/3 ml automatic injection device.[1]		1400
		For Direct IV Administration		
Rx	**Lidocaine HCl for Cardiac Arrhythmias** (Abbott)	**Injection:** 1% (10 mg/ml)	In 5 ml amps, 20, 30 and 50 ml vials and 5 ml Abboject syringes.	NA
Rx	**Xylocaine HCl IV for Cardiac Arrhythmias** (Astra)		In 5 ml (50 mg) disp. syringes.	1007
Rx	**Lidocaine HCl for Cardiac Arrhythmias** (Various, eg, Abbott, Lyphomed)	**Injection:** 2% (20 mg/ml)	In 5, 10, 20, 30 and 50 ml vials and 5 ml syringes.	NA
Rx	**Xylocaine HCl IV for Cardiac Arrhythmias** (Astra)		In 5 ml amps and 5 ml disp. syringes.	277
		For IV Admixtures		
Rx	**Lidocaine HCl for Cardiac Arrhythmias** (Various, eg, Abbott, Lyphomed)	**Injection:** 4% (40 mg/ml)	In 5 ml amps and 25 and 50 ml vials.	NA
Rx	**Xylocaine HCl IV for Cardiac Arrhythmias** (Astra)		In 25 ml (1 g) and 50 ml (2 g) single dose vials and additive syringes.	273
Rx	**Lidocaine HCl for Cardiac Arrhythmias** (Abbott)	**Injection:** 10% (100 mg/ml)	In 10 ml additive vials.	NA
Rx	**Lidocaine HCl for Cardiac Arrhythmias** (Abbott)	**Injection:** 20% (200 mg/ml)	In 5 and 10 ml syringes and 10 ml vials.	NA
Rx	**Xylocaine HCl IV for Cardiac Arrhythmias** (Astra)		In 5 ml (1 g) and 10 ml (2 g) additive syringes.	52
		For IV Infusion		
Rx	**Lidocaine HCl in 5% Dextrose** (Various, eg, Baxter, McGaw)	**Injection:** 0.2% (2 mg/ml)	In 500 and 1000 ml.	NA
		0.4% (4 mg/ml)	In 250 and 500 ml.	NA
		0.8% (8 mg/ml)	In 250 and 500 ml.	NA

* Cost Index based on cost per 100 mg.

[1] With EDTA and methylparaben.

Refer to the general discussion concerning these products on page 618.

TOCAINIDE HCl

Warnings:

Blood dyscrasias: Agranulocytosis, bone marrow depression, leukopenia, neutropenia, aplastic/hypoplastic anemia, thrombocytopenia and sequelae such as septicemia and septic shock have occurred in patients receiving tocainide, most within the recommended dosage range. Fatalities have occurred (with approximately 25% mortality in reported agranulocytosis cases). Since most of these events have been noted during the first 12 weeks of therapy, perform complete blood counts, including white cell, differential and platelet counts, optimally, at weekly intervals for the first 3 months of therapy, and frequently thereafter. Perform complete blood counts promptly if the patient develops any signs of infection (eg, fever, chills, sore throat, stomatitis), bruising or bleeding. If any of these hematologic disorders is identified, discontinue tocainide and institute appropriate treatment if necessary. Blood counts usually return to normal within 1 month of discontinuation. Use with caution in patients with preexisting bone marrow failure or cytopenia of any type.

Pulmonary fibrosis, interstitial pneumonitis, fibrosing alveolitis, pulmonary edema and pneumonia have occurred in patients receiving tocainide. Many of these events occurred in patients who were seriously ill. Fatalities have occurred. The experiences are usually characterized by bilateral infiltrates on x-ray and are frequently associated with dyspnea and cough. Fever may be present. Instruct patients to promptly report any pulmonary symptoms (eg, exertional dyspnea, cough, wheezing). Chest x-rays are advisable at that time. If these pulmonary disorders develop, discontinue tocainide.

Actions:

Pharmacology: Tocainide, like lidocaine, produces dose-dependent decreases in sodium and potassium conductance, thereby decreasing the excitability of myocardial cells. Most patients who respond to lidocaine also respond to tocainide. Failure to respond to lidocaine usually predicts failure to respond to tocainide, but there are exceptions.

Electrophysiology – Tocainide is a Class IB antiarrhythmic with electrophysiologic properties similar to those of lidocaine. In patients with cardiac disease, tocainide produces no clinically significant changes in sinus nodal function, effective refractory periods or intracardiac conduction times. Tocainide does not prolong QRS duration or QT intervals. Theoretically, it may be useful for ventricular arrhythmias associated with a prolonged QT interval.

Hemodynamics – Tocainide usually produces a small degree of depression of left ventricular function and left ventricular end diastolic pressure. Usually no changes in cardiac output or increasing CHF occur in the well compensated patient. Small significant increases in aortic and pulmonary arterial pressures observed are probably related to small increases in vascular resistance. Used concomitantly with a β-adrenergic blocking drug, tocainide further reduces cardiac index and left ventricular dP/dt and further increases pulmonary wedge pressure.

No clinically significant changes in heart rate, blood pressure or signs of myocardial depression were observed in post-MI patients receiving long-term therapy. Tocainide has been used safely in patients with acute MI and various degrees of CHF. However, a small negative inotropic effect can increase peripheral resistance slightly.

Pharmacokinetics: Absorption/Distribution – Following oral administration the bioavailability of tocainide approaches 100%; peak serum concentrations are attained in 0.5 to 2 hours. The extent of its bioavailability is unaffected by food. Unlike lidocaine, tocainide undergoes negligible first-pass hepatic degradation. Approximately 10% to 20% is plasma protein bound. The therapeutic range is 4 to 10 mcg/ml.

Metabolism/Excretion – Inactivated via conjugation in the liver. The average plasma half-life is approximately 15 hours. About 40% is excreted unchanged in urine; alkalinization of urine reduces the percent of drug excreted unchanged, yet acidification causes no alterations. The pharmacokinetics did not differ significantly in patients with MI compared with healthy subjects. Half-life increased in severe renal dysfunction.

Indications:

Treatment of life-threatening ventricular arrhythmias (see Warning box).

Unlabeled uses: Tocainide may be beneficial in the treatment of myotonic dystrophy (800 to 1200 mg/day) and trigeminal neuralgia (20 mg/kg/day in 3 divided doses). Further study is needed.

Contraindications:

Hypersensitivity to tocainide or to amide-type local anesthetics; patients with second- or third-degree AV block in the absence of an artificial ventricular pacemaker.

(Continued on following page)

TOCAINIDE (Cont.)

Adverse Reactions (Cont.):

Hematologic: Leukopenia, neutropenia, agranulocytosis, bone marrow depression, hypoplastic/aplastic anemia and thrombocytopenia (0.18%). These hematologic disorders usually manifest during the first 12 weeks of therapy and fatalities have occurred (see Warning box). Hemolytic anemia; anemia; eosinophilia.

Cardiovascular: Ventricular fibrillation; extension of acute MI; cardiogenic shock; angina; AV block; hypertension; increased QRS duration; pericarditis; prolonged QT interval; right bundle branch block; syncope; vaso-vagal episodes; cardiomegaly; sinus arrest; vasculitis; orthostatic hypotension.

Pulmonary: Respiratory arrest; pulmonary edema; pulmonary embolism; fibrosing alveolitis; pneumonia; interstitial pneumonitis; dyspnea; pleurisy; pulmonary fibrosis (0.11%). Symptoms of pulmonary disorders or x-ray changes usually occurred following 3 to 18 weeks of therapy; fatalities have occurred. See Warning box.

Special senses: Diplopia; earache; taste perversion/smell perversion.

Other: Increased ANA; urinary retention; polyuria, increased diuresis; cinchonism; claudication; cold extremities; edema; fever; hiccoughs; muscle cramps; muscle twitching/spasm; neck pain, pain radiating from neck; pressure on shoulder; yawning; pancreatitis; septicemia; septic shock; chills; asthenia.

Lab test abnormalities: Abnormal liver function tests, particularly in early stages of therapy, have occurred. Consider periodic monitoring of liver function.

Overdosage:

Symptoms: The initial and most important signs and symptoms of overdosage are usually related to the CNS. Tremor may indicate that the maximum dose is being approached. Other adverse reactions, such as GI disturbances (see Adverse Reactions), may follow. One patient died after ingesting a large quantity of tocainide; the serum level was 68 mg/L (≈ 7 times the upper recommended therapeutic level). This patient presented with ventricular tachyarrhythmias with coma, indicating that high levels of tocainide may have primary myocardiotoxicity in addition to CNS effects.

Treatment: If convulsions or respiratory depression or arrest develop, immediately assure the patency of the airway and adequacy of ventilation. Gastric lavage and administration of charcoal may be useful. If seizures persist despite ventilatory therapy with oxygen, give small increments of an anticonvulsant IV. Examples of such agents include a benzodiazepine (eg, diazepam), an ultra short-acting barbiturate (eg, thiopental, thiamylal) or a short-acting barbiturate (eg, pentobarbital, secobarbital).

Hemodialysis clearance of tocainide is approximately equivalent to its renal clearance.

Patient Information:

Notify physician if any of the following occurs: Exertional dyspnea, cough, wheezing, tremor, palpitations, rash, easy bruising or bleeding, fever, sore throat, soreness and ulcers in the mouth, or chills.

May cause drowsiness or dizziness. Observe caution while driving or performing other tasks requiring alertness, coordination or physical dexterity.

May cause nausea, vomiting or diarrhea. Notify physician if these become severe.

Administration and Dosage:

Approved by the FDA in 1984.

Individualize dosage. Guide dosage titration by clinical and ECG evaluation. Dose-related adverse effects tend to occur early in treatment, and they usually decrease in severity and frequency with time. These effects may be minimized by taking tocainide with food or by taking smaller, more frequent doses.

Initial dose: 400 mg every 8 hours. Range is 1200 to 1800 mg/day given in 3 divided doses. Doses > 2400 mg/day have been administered infrequently. Patients who tolerate the three times daily regimen may be tried on a twice-daily regimen with careful monitoring.

Some patients, particularly those with renal or hepatic impairment, may be adequately treated with < 1200 mg/day.

				C.I.*
Rx	**Tonocard** (MSD)	**Tablets:** 400 mg	(MSD 707). Yellow, scored. Film coated. Oval. In 100s and UD 100s.	78
		600 mg	(MSD 709). Yellow, scored. Film coated. Oblong. In 100s and UD 100s.	67

* Cost Index based on cost per 400 mg.

Refer to the general discussion concerning these products on page 618.

MEXILETINE HCl

Actions:

Pharmacology: Mechanism – Like lidocaine, mexiletine inhibits the inward sodium current, thus reducing the rate of rise of the action potential, Phase O. Mexiletine decreases the effective refractory period (ERP) in Purkinje fibers. The decrease in ERP is of lesser magnitude than the decrease in action potential duration (APD), with a resulting increase in ERP/APD ratio.

Electrophysiology – Mexiletine is a local anesthetic and a Class IB antiarrhythmic compound with electrophysiologic properties similar to lidocaine. In patients with normal conduction systems, mexiletine has minimal effect on cardiac impulse generation and propagation. In clinical trials, no development of second-degree or third-degree AV block was observed. It did not prolong ventricular depolarization (QRS duration) or repolarization (QT intervals). Theoretically, mexiletine may be useful in the treatment of ventricular arrhythmias associated with a prolonged QT interval. In patients with preexisting conduction defects, depression of the sinus rate, prolongation of sinus node recovery time, decreased conduction velocity and increased ERP of the intraventricular conduction system have occasionally been observed.

Among the patients entered into studies, about 30% in each treatment group had a ≥ 70% reduction in PVC count, and about 40% failed to complete the 3 month studies because of adverse effects. Follow-up of patients has demonstrated continued effectiveness in long-term use.

Hemodynamics – Small decreases in cardiac output and increases in systemic vascular resistance have occurred, with no significant negative inotropic effect. Blood pressure and pulse rate remain essentially unchanged. Mild depression of myocardial function has been observed following IV mexiletine (dosage form not available in the US) in patients with cardiac disease.

Pharmacokinetics: Absorption/Distribution – Mexiletine is well absorbed (≈ 90%) from the GI tract. The absorption rate is reduced in clinical situations in which gastric emptying time is increased. Narcotics, atropine and magnesium-aluminum hydroxide may slow absorption; metoclopramide may accelerate absorption (see Drug Interactions). The first-pass metabolism of mexiletine is low.

Peak blood levels are reached in 2 to 3 hours. The therapeutic range is approximately 0.5 to 2 mcg/ml. An increase in the frequency of CNS adverse effects has been observed when plasma levels exceed 2 mcg/ml. Plasma levels within the therapeutic range can be attained with either 2 or 3 times daily dosing, but peak to trough differences are greater with the twice-daily regimen. It is 50% to 60% bound to plasma protein with a volume of distribution of 5 to 7 L/kg.

Metabolism/Excretion – Mexiletine is metabolized in the liver. The most active minor metabolite is N-methylmexiletine, which is < 20% as potent as mexiletine. The urinary excretion of N-methylmexiletine is < 0.5%.

In healthy subjects, the elimination half-life is 10 to 12 hours. Hepatic impairment prolongs it to a mean of 25 hours. Little change in half-life occurs with reduced renal function. In eight patients with creatinine clearance < 10 ml/min, the mean plasma elimination half-life was 15.7 hours; in seven patients with creatinine clearance between 11 and 40 ml/min, the mean half-life was 13.4 hours.

Approximately 10% is excreted unchanged by the kidney. Urinary acidification accelerates excretion, while alkalinization retards it (see Drug Interactions).

Indications:

Treatment of documented, life-threatening ventricular arrhythmias, such as sustained ventricular tachycardia. Because of the proarrhythmic effects of mexiletine, use with lesser arrhythmias is generally not recommended.

Unlabeled uses: The use of prophylactic mexiletine may significantly reduce the incidence of ventricular tachycardia and other ventricular arrhythmias in the acute phase of myocardial infarction (MI). However, mortality may not be reduced.

Mexiletine (150 mg/day for 3 days, then 300 mg/day for 3 days followed by 10 mg/kg/day) may be beneficial in reducing pain, dysesthesia and paresthesia associated with diabetic neuropathy.

Contraindications:

Cardiogenic shock; preexisting second- or third-degree AV block (if pacemaker not present).

Warnings:

Proarrhythmia: Mexiletine can worsen arrhythmias; it is uncommon in patients with less serious arrhythmias (frequent premature beats or nonsustained ventricular tachycardia) but is of greater concern in patients with life-threatening arrhythmias, such as sustained ventricular tachycardia.

Survival: Antiarrhythmic drugs have not been shown to enhance survival in patients with ventricular arrhythmias.

(Warnings continued on following page)

MEXILETINE HCl (Cont.)

Warnings (Cont.):

Initial therapy: As with other antiarrhythmics, initiate mexiletine therapy in the hospital.

Mortality: In the National Heart, Lung and Blood Institute's Cardiac Arrhythmia Suppression Trial (CAST), a long-term, multicentered, randomized, double-blind study in patients with asymptomatic non-life-threatening ventricular arrhythmias who had experienced MIs > 6 days but < 2 years previously, an excessive mortality or non-fatal cardiac arrest rate was seen in patients treated with encainide or flecainide (56/730) compared with patients assigned to matched placebo-treated groups (22/725). The average duration of treatment with encainide or flecainide in this study was 10 months.

The applicability of these results to other populations (eg, those without recent MI) or to other antiarrhythmic drugs is uncertain, but at present it is prudent to consider any antiarrhythmic agent to have a significant risk in patients with structural heart disease.

Hepatic function impairment: Since mexiletine is metabolized in the liver, and hepatic impairment prolongs the elimination half-life, carefully monitor patients with liver disease. Observe caution in patients with hepatic dysfunction secondary to CHF.

Pregnancy: Category C. Mexiletine freely crosses the placenta. There are no adequate and well controlled studies in pregnant women. Use during pregnancy only if the potential benefits outweigh the potential hazards to the fetus.

Lactation: Mexiletine appears in breast milk in concentrations similar to or higher than those in plasma. If mexiletine is essential, consider alternative infant feeding.

Children: Safety and efficacy in children have not been established.

Precautions:

Cardiovascular effects: If a ventricular pacemaker is operative, patients with second- or third-degree heart block may be treated with mexiletine if continuously monitored. Some patients with preexisting first-degree AV block were treated with mexiletine; none developed second- or third-degree AV block. Exercise caution in such patients or in patients with preexisting sinus node dysfunction or intraventricular conduction abnormalities.

Use with caution in patients with hypotension and severe CHF.

Hepatic effects: Abnormal liver function tests have been reported, some in the first few weeks of therapy with mexiletine. Most have occurred along with CHF or ischemia; their relationship to mexiletine has not been established.

AST elevation and liver injury – Elevations of AST > 3 times the upper limit of normal occurred in about 1% of both mexiletine-treated and control patients. Approximately 2% of patients in the mexiletine compassionate use program had elevations of AST ≥ 3 times the upper limit of normal. These elevations were frequently associated with CHF, acute MI, blood transfusions and other medications. These elevations were often asymptomatic and transient and usually not associated with elevated bilirubin levels and usually did not require discontinuation of therapy. Marked elevations of AST (> 1000 U/L) were seen before death in four patients with end-stage cardiac disease (severe CHF, cardiogenic shock).

Rare instances of severe liver injury, including hepatic necrosis, have been reported in foreign markets. Carefully evaluate patients in whom an abnormal liver test has occurred, or who have signs or symptoms suggesting liver dysfunction. If persistent or worsening elevation of hepatic enzymes is detected, consider discontinuing therapy.

Hematologic effects: Among 10,867 patients treated with mexiletine in the compassionate use program, marked leukopenia (neutrophils < 1000/mm^3) or agranulocytosis were seen in 0.06%; milder depressions of leukocytes were seen in 0.08% and thrombocytopenia was observed in 0.16%. Many of these patients were seriously ill and were receiving concomitant medications. Rechallenge with mexiletine in several cases was negative. If significant hematologic changes are observed, carefully evaluate the patient and, if warranted, discontinue mexiletine. Blood counts usually return to normal within 1 month of discontinuation.

CNS effects: Convulsions occurred in about 2 of 1000 patients. Of these patients, 28% discontinued therapy. Convulsions occurred in patients with and without a history of seizures. Use with caution in patients with a known seizure disorder.

Urinary pH: Avoid concurrent drugs or diets which may markedly alter urinary pH. Minor fluctuations in urinary pH associated with normal diet do not affect mexiletine excretion. See Drug Interactions.

(Continued on following page)

MEXILETINE HCl (Cont.)

Drug Interactions:

Mexiletine Drug Interactions			
Precipitant drug	Object drug*		Description
Aluminum-Magnesium Hydroxide Atropine Narcotics	Mexiletine	↓	Mexiletine absorption may be slowed.
Cimetidine	Mexiletine	↔	Cimetidine may increase or decrease mexiletine plasma levels.
Hydantoins	Mexiletine	↓	Increased mexiletine clearance leading to lower steady-state plasma levels may occur.
Metoclopramide	Mexiletine	↑	Mexiletine absorption may be accelerated.
Rifampin	Mexiletine	↓	Increased mexiletine clearance leading to lower steady-state plasma levels may occur.
Urinary acidifiers	Mexiletine	↓	Renal clearance of mexiletine is related to urinary pH. In acidic urine, mexiletine clearance may be increased.
Urinary alkalinizers	Mexiletine	↑	Renal clearance of mexiletine is related to urinary pH. In alkaline urine, mexiletine clearance may be decreased.
Mexiletine	Caffeine	↓	Clearance of caffeine may be decreased by 50%
Mexiletine	Theophylline	↑	Serum theophylline levels may be increased; increased pharmacologic and toxic effects may occur.

* ↑ = Object drug increased ↓ = Object drug decreased ↔ = Undetermined effect

Adverse Reactions:

Dosages in controlled studies ranged from 600 to 1200 mg/day; some patients (8%) in the compassionate use program were treated with 1600 to 3200 mg/day. In the controlled trials, the most frequent adverse reactions were upper GI distress (41%), tremor (12.6%), lightheadedness (10.5%) and coordination difficulties (10.2%). These reactions were generally not serious. They were dose-related and were reversible if the dosage was reduced, if the drug was taken with food or antacids or if it was discontinued. However, they still led to therapy discontinuation in 40%.

Cardiovascular: Palpitations (4.3% to 7.5%); chest pain (2.6% to 7.5%); increased ventricular arrhythmias/PVCs (1% to 1.9%); angina/angina-like pain (0.3% to 1.7%); CHF (< 1%); syncope, hypotension (0.6%); bradycardia (0.4%); edema, AV block/conduction disturbances, hot flashes (0.2%); atrial arrhythmias, hypertension, cardiogenic shock (0.1%).

GI: Nausea/vomiting/heartburn (≈ 40%); diarrhea (5.2%); constipation (4%); dry mouth (2.8%); changes in appetite (2.6%); abdominal pain/cramps/discomfort (1.2%); pharyngitis (< 1%); altered taste (0.5%); salivary changes (0.4%); dysphagia (0.2%); oral mucous membrane changes (0.1%); peptic ulcer (0.08%); upper GI bleeding (0.07%); esophageal ulceration (0.01%).

CNS: Dizziness/lightheadedness (18.9% to 26.4%); tremor (13.2%); nervousness (5% to 11.3%); coordination difficulties (≈ 9.7%); changes in sleep habits (≈ 7.5%); headache, blurred vision/visual disturbances (5.7% to 7.5%); paresthesias/numbness (2.4% to 3.8%); weakness (1.9% to 5%); fatigue (1.9% to 3.8%); speech difficulties (2.6%); confusion/clouded sensorium (1.9% to 2.6%); tinnitus (1.9% to 2.4%); depression (2.4%); short-term memory loss (0.9%); hallucinations and other psychological changes, malaise (0.3%); psychosis and convulsions/seizures (0.2%); loss of consciousness (0.06%).

(Adverse Reactions continued on following page)

MEXILETINE HCl (Cont.)

Adverse Reactions (Cont.):

Other: Rash (3.8% to 4.2%); nonspecific edema (3.8%); dyspnea/respiratory (3.3% to 5.7%); arthralgia (1.7%); fever (1.2%); diaphoresis (0.6%); hair loss, impotence/decreased libido (0.4%); urinary hesitancy/retention (0.2%); hiccoughs, dry skin, laryngeal/pharyngeal changes (0.1%); SLE syndrome (0.04%).

Myelofibrosis was reported in two patients; one was receiving long-term thiotepa therapy and the other had pretreatment myeloid abnormalities.

Rare cases of exfoliative dermatitis and Stevens-Johnson syndrome have occurred.

Lab test abnormalities: Abnormal liver function tests (0.5%); positive ANA, thrombocytopenia (0.2%); leukopenia, including neutropenia and agranulocytosis (0.1%); myelofibrosis (0.02%).

Overdosage:

Symptoms: Nine cases of mexiletine overdosage have been reported; two were fatal.

CNS symptoms almost always precede serious cardiovascular effects.

Symptoms may include dizziness, drowsiness, nausea, hypotension, sinus bradycardia, paresthesia, seizures, intermittent left bundle branch block and temporary asystole. With massive overdoses, coma and respiratory arrest may occur.

Treatment includes usual supportive measures. Refer to General Management of Acute Overdosage. Acidification of the urine may be useful. Treatment may include the administration of atropine if hypotension or bradycardia occurs.

Patient Information:

Take medication with food or an antacid.

Adverse effects such as nausea, vomiting, heartburn, diarrhea, constipation, dizziness, tremor, nervousness, coordination difficulties, changes in sleep habits, headache, visual disturbances, tingling/numbness, weakness, ringing in the ears and palpitations/chest pain may occur. Notify physician if they become bothersome.

Notify physician if signs of liver injury or blood cell damage occur, such as unexplained general tiredness, jaundice, fever or sore throat.

Avoid changes in diet that could drastically acidify or alkalinize the urine.

Administration and Dosage:

Approved by the FDA on December 30, 1985.

Individualize dosage. Administer with food or antacids.

Perform clinical and ECG evaluation as needed to determine whether the desired antiarrhythmic effect has been obtained and to guide titration and dose adjustment.

Initial dose: 200 mg every 8 hours when rapid control of arrhythmia is not essential, with a minimum of 2 to 3 days between adjustments. Adjust dose in 50 or 100 mg increments.

Control can be achieved in most patients with 200 to 300 mg given every 8 hours. If satisfactory response is not achieved at 300 mg every 8 hours, and the patient tolerates mexiletine well, try 400 mg every 8 hours. The severity of CNS side effects increases with total daily dose; do not exceed 1200 mg/day.

Renal/hepatic function impairment: In general, patients with renal failure will require the usual doses of mexiletine. Patients with severe liver disease, however, may require lower doses and must be monitored closely. Similarly, marked right-sided CHF can reduce hepatic metabolism and reduce the dose needed.

Loading dose: When rapid control of ventricular arrhythmia is essential, administer an initial loading dose of 400 mg, followed by a 200 mg dose in 8 hours. Onset of therapeutic effect is usually observed within 30 minutes to 2 hours.

Twice-daily dosage: If adequate suppression is achieved on a dose of ≤ 300 mg every 8 hours, the same total daily dose may be given in divided doses every 12 hours with monitoring. The dose may be adjusted to a maximum of 450 mg every 12 hours.

Transferring to mexiletine: Based on theoretical considerations, initiate with a 200 mg dose, and titrate to response as described above, 6 to 12 hours after the last dose of quinidine sulfate, 3 to 6 hours after the last dose of procainamide, 6 to 12 hours after the last dose of disopyramide or 8 to 12 hours after the last dose of tocainide.

Hospitalize patients in whom withdrawal of the previous antiarrhythmic agent is likely to produce life-threatening arrhythmias.

When transferring from lidocaine to mexiletine, stop the lidocaine infusion when the first oral dose of mexiletine is administered. Maintain the IV line until suppression of the arrhythmia appears satisfactory. Consider the similarity of adverse effects of lidocaine and mexiletine and the additive potential.

				C.I.*
Rx	**Mexitil** (Boehringer Ingelheim)	**Capsules:** 150 mg	(BI 66). Red and caramel. In 100s and UD 100s.	112
		200 mg	(BI 67). Red. In 100s and UD 100s.	100
		250 mg	(BI 68). Red and aqua. In 100s and UD 100s.	93

* Cost Index based on cost per 200 mg.

Refer to the general discussion of these products on page 618.

ENCAINIDE HCl

Encainide has been voluntarily withdrawn from the market by the manufacturer because of continuing uncertainty about the implications of the Cardiac Arrhythmia Suppression Trial (CAST). However, the drug will be available on a limited basis for those patients effectively controlled on encainide for life-threatening ventricular arrhythmias, and who according to the patient's physician should not be switched to another agent. The *Enkaid* Continuing Patient Access Program will be available only to those patients who received encainide on or prior to September 16, 1991. For further information, contact Bristol-Myers Squibb at (800) 527-6741.

Actions:

Pharmacology: Mechanisms of action of the antiarrhythmic effects are unknown but probably are the result of encainide's ability to slow conduction, reduce membrane responsiveness, inhibit automaticity and increase the ratio of the effective refractory period to action potential duration. Encainide produces a differentially greater effect on the ischemic zone as compared with normal cells in the myocardium. This could eliminate the disparity in the electrophysiologic properties between these two zones and eliminate pathways of abnormal impulse conduction, development of boundary currents or sites of abnormal impulse generation.

Electrophysiology – Encainide, a Class IC antiarrhythmic agent, blocks the sodium channel of Purkinje fibers and the myocardium. Its electrophysiologic profile is characterized by a dose-related slowing of phase 0 depolarization and little effect on either the action potential duration or repolarization.

The electrophysiologic effects are a result of encainide and of two metabolites present in most patients (> 90%) at therapeutic levels. Encainide and its metabolites produce a dose-related decrease in intracardiac conduction in all parts of the heart; with slowing of conduction in the His-Purkinje system and AV node and an increase in the refractoriness in accessory atrioventricular pathways and in the AV node.

Hemodynamics – In oral studies, encainide had no effect on measurements of cardiac performance such as cardiac or stroke volume index, pulmonary capillary wedge pressure or peripheral blood pressure either at rest or during exercise. In noninvasive studies that included both geriatric patients and younger patients with impaired left ventricular function (New York Heart Association Class III & IV), there were no detrimental effects on ejection fractions acutely or after > 12 months of therapy. Doses of 75 to 300 mg/day, which reduced the incidence of premature ventricular complexes by at least 80%, did not adversely affect exercise tolerance, and were well tolerated by patients with markedly impaired left ventricular function. In a few instances, however, apparent new or worsened congestive heart failure (CHF) developed.

Pharmacokinetics: Absorption/Distribution – Absorption after oral administration is nearly complete with peak plasma levels present 30 to 90 minutes after dosing. Encainide and its two active metabolites, O-demethyl encainide (ODE) and 3-methoxy-O-demethyl encainide (MODE), follow a nonlinear pharmacokinetic disposition. Absorption is delayed by food, but the overall bioavailability is not altered.

Encainide and ODE are bound moderately to plasma proteins (75% to 85%), while MODE binding is somewhat greater (92%).

Metabolism/Elimination – There are two major genetically determined patterns of encainide metabolism. In > 90% of patients, the drug is rapidly and extensively metabolized with an elimination half-life of 1 to 2 hours. These patients convert encainide to the two active metabolites, ODE and MODE, that are more active (on a per mg basis) than encainide. These metabolites are eliminated more slowly than encainide, with half-lives of 3 to 4 hours for ODE and 6 to 12 hours for MODE. A major urinary metabolite is ODE, with lesser amounts of encainide and MODE present.

In < 10% of patients, metabolism of encainide is slower and the estimated encainide elimination half-life is 6 to 11 hours. The renal excretion of encainide is a major route of elimination, and little metabolite is present in plasma.

Despite the differences in pharmacogenetics, 3 to 5 days of dosing are required in all patients to achieve steady-state conditions. The recommended dosage regimen is appropriate for all patients.

Hepatic disease – The clearance of encainide and conversion to active metabolites is reduced, but serum concentrations of ODE and MODE are similar to those in normal patients. There is insufficient experience to determine the need for alteration in the normal dose or dosing interval, but increase doses cautiously.

Renal disease – The clearance of encainide is reduced, and plasma levels of the active metabolites ODE and MODE are increased in patients with significant renal impairment; reduce dosage.

(Continued on following page)

ENCAINIDE HCl (Cont.)

Indications:

For the treatment of documented life-threatening arrhythmias (eg, sustained ventricular tachycardia).

Contraindications:

Symptomatic nonsustained ventricular arrhythmias and frequent premature ventricular complexes.

Patients with preexisting second-degree or third-degree AV block, or with right bundle branch block when associated with a left hemiblock (bifascicular block), unless a pacemaker is present to sustain the cardiac rhythm should complete heart block occur.

Cardiogenic shock.

Hypersensitivity to encainide.

Warnings:

Proarrhythmia: Encainide can cause new or worsened arrhythmias. Effects range from an increase in frequency of PVCs to the development of more severe ventricular tachycardia. In patients with malignant arrhythmias, it is often difficult to distinguish a spontaneous variation in the patient's underlying rhythm disorder from drug-induced worsening, so the following occurrence rates are approximations:

In clinical trials, about 10% of all patients had proarrhythmic events. About 6% of them represented new or worsened ventricular tachycardia; these occurred most frequently in patients who had a history of sustained ventricular tachycardia (12% of such patients), cardiomyopathy (10%), CHF (12%) or sustained ventricular tachycardia with cardiomyopathy or CHF (17%). The incidence of proarrhythmic events in patients without ventricular tachycardia or overt clinical heart disease ranged from 3% to 4%. Proarrhythmia occurred least frequently in patients with no known structural heart disease.

A review of deaths in clinical trials indicates that about 1% of patients might have died of a possible proarrhythmic effect of encainide; virtually all of them had a history of ventricular tachycardia. In most cases, patients had a history of sustained ventricular tachycardia or ventricular fibrillation. Proarrhythmic events occurred most commonly during the first week of therapy and were much more common when doses exceeded 200 mg/day. Initiating therapy at 75 mg/day combined with gradual dose adjustment reduced the risk of proarrhythmia.

Congestive heart failure: New or worsened CHF occurred infrequently (< 1%); use cautiously in patients with CHF or congestive cardiomyopathy.

Electrolyte disturbances: Hypokalemia or hyperkalemia may alter the effects of Class I antiarrhythmic drugs. Correct preexisting hypokalemia or hyperkalemia before administration of encainide.

Sick sinus syndrome (bradycardia-tachycardia syndrome): Use only with extreme caution because encainide may cause sinus bradycardia, sinus pause or sinus arrest.

(Warnings continued on following page)

ENCAINIDE HCl (Cont.)

Warnings (Cont.):

Electrocardiographic changes: Encainide produces dose-related changes in the PR and QRS interval linearly from 30 to 225 mg/day. There is no consistent change in JT. The QTc interval is increased, but only to the extent of the increase in QRS interval.

Encainide-Induced Changes in ECG Intervals*						
	Total daily dose					
	75 mg		150 mg		200 mg	
	sec	(%)	sec	(%)	sec	(%)
PR	0.02	(12)	0.04	(21)	0.04	(24)
QRS	0.01	(12)	0.02	(23)	0.02	(26)

*Percent change based on mean baseline values: PR = 0.169 and QRS = 0.088 (n = 504).

Unlike the changes in the PR, QRS and QTc intervals observed with the Class IA drugs, the ECG changes induced by encainide are not indications of effectiveness, toxicity or overdosage, nor can they routinely be used to predict efficacy.

Clinically significant changes in cardiac conduction have been observed. Sinus bradycardia, sinus pause or sinus arrest occurred in 1% of the patients and prolongation of QRS interval to ≥ 0.2 sec developed in about 7% of the patients. The incidence of second-degree or third-degree AV block was less, 0.5% and 0.2%, respectively.

Hepatic function impairment: Hepatic impairment significantly reduces the elimination rate of encainide. The need for alterations in the dose or dosing interval is uncertain, but it is prudent to increase doses cautiously.

Renal function impairment: Limited data suggest that reduction in the elimination of encainide and its active metabolites in patients with serum creatinine > 3.5 mg/dl or creatinine clearance < 20 ml/min results in significant accumulation of metabolites and, to a lesser degree, encainide. Initiate therapy with a single daily dose of 25 mg. The dose may be increased to 25 mg twice daily after 7 days, and again to 25 mg, 3 times a day after an additional 7 days. Doses > 150 mg/day are not recommended. Consider reducing dosage if renal function deteriorates significantly.

Pregnancy: Category B. There are no adequate and well controlled studies in pregnant women. Use during pregnancy only if clearly needed.

Lactation: Encainide appears in breast milk. However, the potential for serious adverse reactions in nursing infants is unknown. Decide whether to discontinue nursing or to discontinue the drug, taking into account the importance of the drug to the mother.

Children: Safety and efficacy in children < 18 years of age have not been established.

Drug Interactions:

Diuretics/cardiovasculars: Because of possible additive pharmacologic effects, use caution when encainide is used with any other drug that affects cardiac conduction.

Cimetidine increases plasma concentrations of encainide and its metabolites. Although no clinically significant consequences have been reported, use caution when the two drugs are administered simultaneously. If cimetidine is given, reduce encainide dosage.

Adverse Reactions:

Most serious: Provocation or aggravation of ventricular arrhythmias (see Warnings), occurring in about 10% of patients. In some cases, this resulted in sustained ventricular tachycardia or ventricular fibrillation.

Most frequent: Dizziness; blurred or abnormal vision; headache.

Adverse events caused discontinuation in about 7% of patients in clinical trials.

Only 0.4% of patients discontinued therapy due to CHF or related causes. Second-degree or third-degree AV block developed in 0.5% and 0.2%, respectively. Sinus bradycardia, sinus pause or sinus arrest occurred in 1%. There have been rare reports of elevated serum liver enzymes, hepatitis and jaundice, and of elevated blood glucose levels or increased insulin requirements in diabetic patients. If unexplained jaundice or signs of hepatic dysfunction or hyperglycemia occurs, consider discontinuing therapy.

(Adverse Reactions continued on following page)

ENCAINIDE HCl (Cont.)

Adverse Reactions (Cont.):

The following table gives the incidence of the most common adverse events during clinical trials involving 749 patients with ventricular arrhythmias and includes all adverse events regardless of relationship to drug therapy. The "Other trials" column includes reports from 2 multicenter trials not reported in the dose-response trials.

Incidence (%) of the Most Common Encainide Adverse Reactions at Various Doses

Adverse reaction	Daily doses			
	75 mg (n = 298)	150 mg (n = 260)	> 200 mg (n = 208)	Other trials (n = 241)
Body as a whole				
Asthenia	4	5	9	6.5 to 14.8
Chest pain	5	2	6	8.5 to 10.2
Death				1.3 to 3.4
Headache	3	5	12	5.7 to 8.5
Upper/Lower extremity pain	< 1	1	2 to 3	2 to 5.7
Pain	< 1	< 1	< 1	
Paresthesia	1	< 1	2	
Cardiovascular				
Congestive heart failure	< 1	1	2	
Palpitations	4	3	8	7.2 to 12.5
Peripheral edema				1.3 to 2.3
PVCs	< 1	< 1	3	
QRS interval prolonged > 0.2 seconds	< 1	3	4	
Syncope	< 1	1	5	
Ventricular tachycardia	3	3	8	
GI				
Abdominal pain	2	2	3	1.1 to 3.3
Constipation	< 1	< 1	2	2.2 to 4.6
Diarrhea	< 1	< 1	2	0 to 9.2
Dry mouth				0 to 3.9
Dyspepsia	< 1	< 1	3	1.3 to 4.5
Nausea	2	2	6	2.3 to 8.5
Vomiting				0.7 to 2.3
CNS				
Anorexia				1.1 to 2
Dizziness	6	10	18	15.7 to 15.9
Insomnia				2 to 3.4
Nervousness				1.1 to 2
Somnolence				0 to 3.9
Tremor	< 1	< 1	2	
Respiratory				
Dyspnea	2	5	4	3.9 to 8
Increased cough	< 1	1	2	
Skin and appendages				
Rash	< 1	< 1	4	1.1 to 2
Special senses				
Abnormal/blurred vision	4	8	26	3.4 to 11.1
Taste perversion	1	2	1	
Tinnitus				0 to 3.9

Other events occurring in < 1% of patients include: Malaise; decreased or increased blood pressure; confusion; ataxia; abnormal gait; abnormal sensation; abnormal dreams; diplopia; photophobia; periorbital edema.

(Continued on following page)

ENCAINIDE HCl (Cont.)

Overdosage:

Symptoms: Overdosages have resulted in death. Overdosage may produce excessive widening of the QRS complex and QT interval and AV dissociation. Hypotension, bradycardia and asystole may develop. Conduction disturbances may be observed. Convulsions occurred in one case of intentional overdosage.

Treatment: Provide cardiac monitoring and advanced life support systems. One report suggested that hypertonic sodium bicarbonate may be useful in managing the cardiac toxicity. Treat acute overdosages by gastric lavage followed by activated charcoal and usual supportive measures. Refer to General Management of Acute Overdosage.

Administration and Dosage:

For sustained ventricular tachycardia, initiate therapy in the hospital. Hospitalization is advisable for patients with a high risk of proarrhythmia (ie, symptomatic CHF, cardiomyopathy or nonsustained ventricular tachycardia), depending on their cardiac status and underlying cardiac disease. Also, hospitalize patients at the time of a dose increase to ≥ 200 mg/day.

Individualize dosage.

Initial dose: Adults – 25 mg every 8 hours. After 3 to 5 days, increase the dosage to 35 mg 3 times a day if necessary. If the desired therapeutic response is not achieved after an additional 3 to 5 days, the dose may be adjusted to 50 mg 3 times a day. Avoid rapid dose escalation.

Hepatic or renal impairment patients may require dose or dosing interval adjustment.

Dosage adjustment: Adjust gradually, allowing 3 to 5 days between dosing increments to achieve steady-state blood levels of encainide and its active metabolites before increasing the dose. Gradual dose adjustments will help prevent the use of higher than necessary doses which may increase the risk of proarrhythmic events.

In an occasional patient with ventricular ectopic activity, the dosage may have to be increased to 50 mg 4 times a day . Higher doses are not normally recommended. However, after careful dose titration has failed, patients with documented life-threatening arrhythmias may be treated with up to 75 mg 4 times a day. Once the desired therapeutic response is achieved, many patients can be maintained on chronic therapy at lower doses.

Patients with malignant arrhythmias who exhibit a beneficial response as judged by objective criteria (eg, Holter monitoring, programmed electrical stimulation, exercise testing) can be maintained on chronic therapy.

Some patients whose arrhythmias are well controlled by dosages of 50 mg 3 times a day or less may be transferred to a 12 hour dosage regimen to increase convenience and compliance. The total daily dose may be given in two equally divided doses at approximately 12 hour intervals; carefully monitor the patient. The maximum single dose is 75 mg.

Loading dose is not recommended. Use of higher initial doses and more rapid dosage adjustments have resulted in an increased incidence of proarrhythmic events, particularly during the first few days of dosing.

Concomitant therapy: Although limited experience with the concomitant use of encainide and IV lidocaine has revealed no adverse effects, no formal studies demonstrate the utility of such combined therapy. Clinical experience on transferring patients to encainide from another antiarrhythmic is also limited. As a general principle, withdraw antiarrhythmic therapy for 2 to 4 plasma half-lives before starting encainide. If withdrawing antiarrhythmic therapy is potentially life-threatening, consider hospitalization. Digoxin/encainide therapy has been administered without adverse effects (see Drug Interactions). No clinical evidence of arrhythmia exacerbation or "rebound" has been noted following discontinuation.

Rx	**Enkaid**[1] (Bristol-Myers Squibb)	**Capsules:** 25 mg	(Enkaid 25 mg Bristol 732). Green and yellow. In 100s and UD 100s.
		35 mg	(Enkaid 35 mg Bristol 734). Green and orange. In 100s and UD 100s.
		50 mg	(Enkaid 50 mg Bristol 735). Green and brown. In 100s and UD 100s.

[1] Voluntarily withdrawn from the market by the manufacturer. Still available on a limited basis through the *Enkaid* Continuing Patient Access Program. For further information contact Bristol-Myers Squibb at (800) 527-6741.

Refer to the general discussion concerning these products on page 618.

PROPAFENONE HCl

Actions:

Pharmacology: Propafenone is a Class IC antiarrhythmic drug with local anesthetic effects and a direct stabilizing action on myocardial membranes. The electrophysiological effect of propafenone manifests itself in a reduction of upstroke velocity (Phase 0) of the monophasic action potential. In Purkinje fibers, and to a lesser extent myocardial fibers, propafenone reduces the fast inward current carried by sodium ions. Diastolic excitability threshold is increased and effective refractory period prolonged. Propafenone reduces spontaneous automaticity and depresses triggered activity.

Propafenone has beta-sympatholytic activity at about 1/50 the potency of propranolol in animals and a beta-adrenergic blocking potency (per mg) about 1/40 that of propranolol in man. In clinical trials, resting heart rate decreases of about 8% were noted at the higher end of the therapeutic plasma concentration range. At very high concentrations in vitro, propafenone can inhibit the slow inward current carried by calcium but this calcium antagonist effect probably does not contribute to antiarrhythmic efficacy. Propafenone has local anesthetic activity approximately equal to procaine.

Propafenone causes a dose- and concentration-related decrease in the rate of single and multiple PVCs and can suppress recurrence of ventricular tachycardia. Based on the percent of patients attaining substantial (80% to 90%) suppression of ventricular ectopic activity, it appears that trough levels of 0.2 to 1.5 mcg/ml can provide good suppression, with higher concentrations giving a greater rate of good response.

Electrophysiology – In electrophysiology studies in patients with ventricular tachycardia, propafenone prolongs atrioventricular (AV) conduction while having little or no effect on sinus node function. Both AV nodal conduction time (AH interval) and His Purkinje conduction time (HV interval) are prolonged. Propafenone has little or no effect on the atrial functional refractory period, but AV nodal functional and effective refractory periods are prolonged. In patients with WPW, propafenone reduces conduction and increases the effective refractory period of the accessory pathway in both directions. Propafenone slows conduction and consequently produces dose-related changes in the PR interval and QRS duration. QT_C interval does not change.

Mean Changes in ECG Intervals Produced by Propafenone[1]

	Total daily dose							
	337.5 mg		450 mg		675 mg		900 mg	
Interval	msec	%	msec	%	msec	%	msec	%
RR	−14.5	−1.8	30.6	3.8	31.5	3.9	41.7	5.1
PR	3.6	2.1	19.1	11.6	28.9	17.8	35.6	21.9
QRS	5.6	6.4	5.5	6.1	7.7	8.4	15.6	17.3
QT_C	2.7	0.7	−7.5	−1.8	5	1.2	14.7	3.7

[1] In any individual patient, ECG changes in the table cannot be readily used to predict either efficacy or plasma concentration.

Hemodynamics – Sympathetic stimulation may be a vital component supporting circulatory function in patients with congestive heart failure (CHF), and its inhibition by the beta blockade produced by propafenone may in itself aggravate CHF.

Additionally, like other Class IC antiarrhythmic drugs, propafenone exerts a negative inotropic effect on the myocardium. Cardiac catheterization studies in patients with moderately impaired ventricular function (mean CI = 2.61 L/min/m²) utilizing IV propafenone infusions (2 mg/kg over 10 min plus 2 mg/min for 30 min) that gave mean plasma concentrations of 3 mcg/ml (well above the therapeutic range of 0.2 to 1.5 mcg/ml) showed significant increases in pulmonary capillary wedge pressure, systemic and pulmonary vascular resistances and depression of cardiac output and index.

Pharmacokinetics: Absorption/Distribution – Propafenone is nearly completely absorbed after oral administration with peak plasma levels occurring approximately 3.5 hours after administration in most individuals. It exhibits extensive first-pass metabolism resulting in a dose-dependent and dosage-form-dependent absolute bioavailability (eg, a 150 mg tablet had absolute bioavailability of 3.4%, a 300 mg tablet 10.6% and 300 mg solution 21.4%). Bioavailability increases further at doses above those recommended and with decreased liver function. The clearance of propafenone is reduced and the elimination half-life increased in patients with significant hepatic dysfunction (see Warnings). Propafenone follows a nonlinear pharmacokinetic disposition presumably due to saturation of first-pass hepatic metabolism as the liver is exposed to higher concentrations of propafenone and shows a very high degree of interindividual variability. For example, for a threefold increase in daily dose from 300 to 900 mg/day, there is a tenfold increase in steady-state plasma concentration.

(Actions continued on following page)

PROPAFENONE HCl (Cont.)

Actions (Cont.):

Pharmacokinetics (Cont.):

Metabolism/Excretion – There are two genetically determined patterns of propafenone metabolism. In > 90% of patients, the drug is rapidly and extensively metabolized with an elimination half-life of 2 to 10 hours. These patients metabolize propafenone into two active metabolites: 5-hydroxypropafenone and N-depropylpropafenone. In vitro, these metabolites have antiarrhythmic activity comparable to propafenone, but in man they both are usually present in concentrations < 20% of propafenone. Nine additional metabolites have been identified, most in only trace amounts. The saturable hydroxylation pathway is responsible for the nonlinear pharmacokinetic disposition.

In < 10% of patients, metabolism of propafenone is slower because the 5-hydroxy metabolite is not formed or is minimally formed. The estimated propafenone elimination half-life ranges from 10 to 32 hours. In these patients, the N-depropylpropafenone is present in quantities comparable to the levels measured in extensive metabolizers. In slow metabolizers, propafenone pharmacokinetics are linear.

There are significant differences in plasma concentrations of propafenone in slow and extensive metabolizers, the former achieving concentrations 1.5 to 2 times those of the extensive metabolizers at daily doses of 675 to 900 mg/day. At low doses the differences are greater, with slow metabolizers attaining concentrations > 5 times those of extensive metabolizers. Because the difference decreases at high doses and is mitigated by the lack of the active 5-hydroxy metabolite in the slow metabolizers, and because steady-state conditions are achieved after 4 to 5 days of dosing in all patients, the recommended dosing regimen is the same for all patients. Titrate dosage carefully with close attention paid to clinical and ECG evidence of toxicity. In addition, the beta-blocking action of propafenone appears to be enhanced in slow metabolizers.

Indications:

Treatment of documented life-threatening ventricular arrhythmias, such as sustained ventricular tachycardia.

Because of the proarrhythmic effects of propafenone, reserve its use for patients in whom the benefits of treatment outweigh the risks. The use of propafenone is not recommended in patients with less severe ventricular arrhythmias, even if the patients are symptomatic.

Unlabeled uses: Propafenone appears to be effective in the treatment of supraventricular tachycardias including atrial fibrillation and flutter and arrhythmias associated with Wolff-Parkinson-White syndrome.

Contraindications:

Uncontrolled CHF; cardiogenic shock; sinoatrial, AV and intraventricular disorders of impulse generation or conduction (eg, sick sinus node syndrome, AV block) in the absence of an artificial pacemaker; bradycardia; marked hypotension; bronchospastic disorders; manifest electrolyte imbalance; hypersensitivity to the drug.

Warnings:

Mortality: In the National Heart, Lung and Blood Institute's Cardiac Arrhythmia Suppression Trial (CAST), a long-term, multicenter, randomized, double-blind study in patients with asymptomatic non-life-threatening ventricular ectopy who had a myocardial infarction (MI) > 6 days but < 2 years previously, and demonstrated mild to moderate left ventricular dysfunction, an excessive mortality or non-fatal cardiac arrest rate was seen in patients treated with encainide or flecainide (56/730) compared with that seen in patients assigned to carefully matched placebo-treated groups (22/725). The average duration of treatment with encainide or flecainide in this study was 10 months.

The applicability of these results to other populations (eg, those without recent MI) and to other antiarrhythmic drugs is uncertain, but at present it is prudent (1) to consider any IC agent (especially one documented to provoke new serious arrhythmias) to have a similar risk and (2) to consider the risks of Class IC agents, coupled with the lack of any evidence of improved survival, generally unacceptable in patients without life-threatening ventricular arrhythmias, even if the patients are experiencing unpleasant, but not life-threatening symptoms or signs.

(Warnings continued on following page)

PROPAFENONE HCl (Cont.)

Warnings (Cont.):

Proarrhythmic effects: Propafenone, like other antiarrhythmic agents, may cause new or worsened arrhythmias. Such proarrhythmic effects range from an increase in frequency of PVCs to the development of more severe ventricular tachycardia, ventricular fibrillation or torsade de pointes (ie, tachycardia that is more sustained or more rapid), which may lead to fatal consequences. It is therefore essential that each patient be evaluated electrocardiographically and clinically prior to, and during therapy to determine whether the response to propafenone supports continued treatment.

Overall in clinical trials, 4.7% of all patients had new or worsened ventricular arrhythmia possibly representing a proarrhythmic event. Of the patients who had worsening of VT (4%), 92% had a history of VT or VT/VF, 71% had coronary artery disease and 68% had a prior MI. The incidence of proarrhythmia in patients with less serious or benign arrhythmias, which include patients with an increase in frequency of PVCs, was 1.6%. Although most proarrhythmic events occurred during the first week of therapy, late events also were seen and the CAST study (see Warnings) suggests that an increased risk is present throughout treatment.

Non-life-threatening arrhythmias: Use of propafenone is not recommended in patients with less severe ventricular arrhythmias, even if the patients are symptomatic.

Survival: There is no evidence from controlled trials that the use of propafenone favorably affects survival or the incidence of sudden death.

Nonallergic bronchospasm (eg, chronic bronchitis, emphysema): In general, these patients should not receive propafenone or other agents with beta-adrenergic blocking activity.

Congestive heart failure: New or worsened CHF has occurred in 3.7% of patients; of those, 0.9% were probably or definitely related to propafenone. Of the patients with CHF probably related to propafenone, 80% had preexisting heart failure and 85% had coronary artery disease. CHF attributable to propafenone developed rarely (< 0.2%) in patients who had no previous history of CHF.

As propafenone exerts both beta blockade and a (dose-related) negative inotropic effect on cardiac muscle, patients with CHF should be fully compensated before receiving propafenone. If CHF worsens, discontinue propafenone unless CHF is due to the cardiac arrhythmia and, if indicated, restart at a lower dosage only after adequate cardiac compensation has been established.

Conduction disturbances: Propafenone slows AV conduction and also causes first degree AV block. Average PR interval prolongation and increases in QRS duration are closely correlated with dosage increases and concomitant increases in propafenone plasma concentrations. The incidence of first-, second- and third-degree AV block observed in 2127 patients was 2.5%, 0.6% and 0.2%, respectively. Development of second- or third-degree AV block requires a reduction in dosage or discontinuation of propafenone. Bundle branch block (1.2%) and intraventricular conduction delay (1.1%) have occurred in patients receiving propafenone. Bradycardia has also occurred (1.5%). Experience in patients with sick sinus node syndrome is limited and these patients should not be treated with propafenone.

Effects on pacemaker threshold: Pacing and sensing thresholds of artificial pacemakers may be altered. Monitor and program pacemakers accordingly during therapy.

Hematologic disturbances: One case of agranulocytosis with fever and sepsis occurred. The agranulocytosis appeared after 8 weeks of therapy. Propafenone therapy was stopped, and the white count had normalized by 14 days; the patient recovered. In the course of > 800,000 patient years of exposure during marketing outside the US since 1978, seven additional cases have occurred. Unexplained fever or decrease in white cell count, particularly during the first 3 months of therapy, warrants consideration of possible agranulocytosis/granulocytopenia. Instruct patients to promptly report the development of any signs of infection such as fever, sore throat or chills.

Hepatic function impairment: Propafenone is highly metabolized by the liver; administer cautiously to patients with impaired hepatic function. Severe liver dysfunction increases the bioavailability of propafenone to approximately 70%, compared to 3% to 40% for patients with normal liver function; the mean half-life is approximately 9 hours. The dose of propafenone should be approximately 20% to 30% of the dose given to patients with normal hepatic function. Carefully monitor for excessive pharmacological effects.

Renal function impairment: A considerable percentage of propafenone metabolites (18.5% to 38% of the dose/48 hours) are excreted in the urine. Administer cautiously to patients with impaired renal function. Carefully monitor for signs of overdosage.

(Warnings continued on following page)

PROPAFENONE HCl (Cont.)

Warnings (Cont.):

Fertility impairment: IV propafenone decreases spermatogenesis in rabbits, dogs and monkeys. These effects were reversible, were not found following oral dosing and were seen only at lethal or sublethal dose levels.

Elderly: Because of the possible increased risk of impaired hepatic or renal function in this age group, use with caution. The effective dose may be lower in these patients.

Pregnancy: Category C. Propafenone is embryotoxic in rabbits and rats when given in doses 10 and 40 times, respectively, the maximum recommended human dose. In a perinatal and postnatal study in rats, propafenone (at ≥ 6 times the maximum recommended human dose) produced dose-dependent increases in maternal and neonatal mortality, decreased maternal and pup body weight gain and reduced neonatal physiological development. There are no adequate and well controlled studies in pregnant women. Use during pregnancy only if the potential benefit justifies the potential risk to the fetus.

Lactation: It is not known whether this drug is excreted in breast milk. Decide whether to discontinue nursing or to discontinue the drug, taking into account the importance of the drug to the mother.

Children: The safety and efficacy of propafenone in children have not been established.

Precautions:

Elevated ANA titers: Positive ANA titers have occurred. They have been reversible upon cessation of treatment and may disappear even with continued therapy. These laboratory findings were usually not associated with clinical symptoms, but there is one case of drug-induced lupus erythematosus (positive rechallenge); it resolved completely upon therapy discontinuation. Carefully evaluate patients who develop an abnormal ANA test and, if persistent or worsening elevation of ANA titers is detected, consider discontinuing therapy.

Renal/hepatic changes: Renal changes have been observed in the rat following 6 months of oral administration of propafenone at doses of 180 and 360 mg/kg/day (12 to 24 times the maximum recommended human dose). Both inflammatory and non-inflammatory changes in the renal tubules with accompanying interstitial nephritis were observed. These lesions were reversible in that they were not found in rats treated at these dosage levels and allowed to recover for 6 weeks. Fatty degenerative changes of the liver were found in rats following chronic administration of propafenone at dose levels 19 times the maximum recommended human dose.

Drug Interactions:

Propafenone Drug Interactions

Precipitant drug	Object drug *		Description
Anesthetics, local	Propafenone	↑	Concurrent use (ie, during pacemaker implantations, surgery or dental use) may increase the risks of CNS side effects.
Cimetidine	Propafenone	↑	The maximum propafenone concentration may be increased, possibly resulting in increased pharmacologic effects.
Quinidine	Propafenone	↑	Serum propafenone levels may be increased in rapid, extensive metabolizers of the drug, possibly increasing the pharmacologic effects.
Rifampin	Propafenone	↓	Increased propafenone clearance may occur, resulting in decreased plasma levels and a possible loss of therapeutic effect.
Propafenone	Anticoagulants	↑	Increased warfarin plasma levels and prothrombin time may occur.
Propafenone	Beta blockers	↑	The plasma levels and pharmacologic effects of beta blockers metabolized by the liver may be increased.
Propafenone	Cyclosporine	↑	Increased whole blood cyclosporine trough levels and decreased renal function may occur.
Propafenone	Digoxin	↑	Serum digoxin levels may be increased, resulting in toxicity.

* ↑ = Object drug increased. ↓ = Object drug decreased.

Drug/Food interaction: Although food increased the peak blood level and bioavailability of propafenone in a single dose study, food did not change bioavailability significantly during multiple dose administration.

(Continued on following page)

Refer to the general discussion concerning these products on page 618.

FLECAINIDE ACETATE

Actions:

Pharmacology: Flecainide has local anesthetic activity and belongs to the membrane stabilizing (Class I) group of antiarrhythmic agents; it has electrophysiologic effects characteristic of the IC class of antiarrhythmics.

Electrophysiology – Flecainide produces a dose-related decrease in intracardiac conduction in all parts of the heart, with the greatest effect on the His-Purkinje system (H-V conduction). Effects upon atrioventricular (AV) nodal conduction time and intra-atrial conduction times are less pronounced than those on the ventricle. Significant effects on refractory periods were observed only in the ventricle. Sinus node recovery times (corrected) are somewhat increased; this may be significant in sinus node dysfunction (see Warnings).

Flecainide causes a dose-related and plasma level-related decrease in single and multiple PVCs and can suppress recurrence of ventricular tachycardia. Plasma levels of 0.2 to 1 mcg/ml may be needed to obtain the maximal therapeutic effect; trough plasma levels in patients successfully treated for recurrent ventricular tachycardia were between 0.2 and 1 mcg/ml. Plasma levels > 0.7 to 1 mcg/ml are associated with a higher rate of cardiac adverse experiences (ie, conduction defects or bradycardia). The relationship of plasma levels to proarrhythmic events is not established, but dose reduction appears to lead to a reduced frequency and severity of such events.

Hemodynamics – Flecainide does not usually alter heart rate, although bradycardia and tachycardia have been reported occasionally.

Decreases in ejection fraction, consistent with a negative inotropic effect, have been observed after a single dose of 200 to 250 mg; both increases and decreases in ejection fraction have been encountered during multidose therapy at usual therapeutic doses (see Warnings).

Pharmacokinetics: Absorption/Distribution – Oral absorption is nearly complete. Peak plasma levels are attained at about 3 hours (range, 1 to 6 hours). Flecainide does not undergo significant first-pass effect. Food or antacids do not affect absorption.

The plasma half-life averages 20 hours (range, 12 to 27 hours) after multiple oral doses. Steady-state levels are approached in 3 to 5 days; once at steady-state, no accumulation occurs during chronic therapy. Over the usual therapeutic range, plasma levels are approximately proportional to dose.

In patients with congestive heart failure (CHF; NYHA class III), the rate of flecainide elimination from plasma (mean half-life, 19 hours) is moderately slower than for healthy subjects (mean half-life, 14 hours).

Plasma protein binding is about 40% and is independent of plasma drug level over the range of 0.015 to about 3.4 mcg/ml.

Metabolism/Excretion – About 30% of a single oral dose (range, 10% to 50%) is excreted in urine unchanged. The two major urinary metabolites are meta-O-dealkylated flecainide (active, but about 1/5 as potent) and the meta-O-dealkylated lactam (inactive). These two metabolites (primarily conjugated) account for most of the remaining portion of the dose. Several minor metabolites (≤ 3%) are also found in urine; 5% is excreted in feces.

Flecainide elimination depends on renal function. With increasing renal impairment, the extent of unchanged drug in urine is reduced and the half-life is prolonged. There is no simple relationship between creatinine clearance and the rate of flecainide elimination from plasma.

Hemodialysis removes only about 1% of an oral dose as unchanged flecainide.

Indications:

For the prevention of paroxysmal atrial fibrillation/flutter (PAF) associated with disabling symptoms and paroxysmal supraventricular tachycardias (PSVT), including atrioventricular nodal reentrant tachycardia, atrioventricular reentrant tachycardia and other supraventricular tachycardias of unspecified mechanism associated with disabling symptoms in patients without structural heart disease.

Prevention of documented life-threatening ventricular arrhythmias, such as sustained ventricular tachycardia.

Not recommended in patients with less severe ventricular arrhythmias even if the patients are symptomatic (see Warnings). Because of proarrhythmic effects of flecainide (see Warnings), reserve use for patients in whom benefits outweigh risks.

Contraindications:

Preexisting second- or third-degree AV block, right bundle branch block when associated with a left hemiblock (bifascicular block), unless a pacemaker is present to sustain the cardiac rhythm if complete heart block occurs; recent myocardial infarction (MI) (see Warnings); presence of cardiogenic shock; hypersensitivity to the drug.

(Continued on following page)

FLECAINIDE ACETATE (Cont.)

Warnings:

Mortality: Flecainide was included in the National Heart Lung and Blood Institute's Cardiac Arrhythmia Suppression Trial (CAST), a long-term multi-center, randomized, double-blind study in patients with asymptomatic non-life-threatening ventricular arrhythmias who had an MI > 6 days, but < 2 years previously. An excessive mortality or non-fatal cardiac arrest rate was seen in patients treated with flecainide compared with that seen in a carefully matched placebo-treated group. This rate was 16/315 (5.1%) for flecainide and 7/309 (2.3%) for its matched placebo. The average duration of treatment was 10 months.

Ventricular pro-arrhythmic effects in patients with atrial fibrillation/flutter: A review of the world literature revealed reports of 568 patients treated with oral flecainide for paroxysmal atrial fibrillation/flutter (PAF). Ventricular tachycardia was experienced in 0.4% (2/568) of these patients. Of 19 patients in the literature with chronic atrial fibrillation (CAF), 10.5% (2) experienced VT or VF. Flecainide is not recommended for use in patients with chronic atrial fibrillation. Case reports of ventricular proarrhythmic effects in patients treated with flecainide for atrial fibrillation/flutter have included increased PVCs, VT, VF and death.

As with other class I agents, patients treated with flecainide for atrial flutter have been reported with 1:1 atrioventricular conduction due to slowing the atrial rate. A paradoxical increase in the ventricular rate also may occur in patients with atrial fibrillation who receive flecainide. Concomitant negative chronotropic therapy such as digoxin or beta-blockers may lower the risk of this complication.

Survival: As with other antiarrhythmics, there is no evidence that flecainide favorably affects survival or the incidence of sudden death.

Non-life-threatening ventricular arrhythmias: The applicability of the CAST results to other populations (eg, those without recent infarction) is uncertain, but at present it is prudent to consider the risks of Class IC agents, coupled with the lack of any evidence of improved survival, generally unacceptable in patients whose ventricular arrhythmias are not life-threatening, even if the patients are experiencing unpleasant but not life-threatening symptoms or signs.

Proarrhythmic effects: Flecainide can cause new or worsened arrhythmias. Such proarrhythmic effects range from an increase in frequency of PVCs to the development of more severe ventricular tachycardia. Three-fourths of proarrhythmic events were new or worsened ventricular tachyarrhythmias, the remainder being increased frequency of PVCs or new supraventricular arrhythmias.

In patients treated with flecainide for sustained ventricular tachycardia, 80% of proarrhythmic events occurred within 14 days of the onset of therapy. In studies of 225 patients with supraventricular arrhythmia, there were 9 (4%) proarrhythmic events, 8 of them in patients with paroxysmal atrial fibrillation. Of the 9, 7 were exacerbations of supraventricular arrhythmias, while 2 were ventricular arrhythmias, including one fatal case of VT/VF and one wide complex VT, both in patients with paroxysmal atrial fibrillation and known coronary artery disease.

It is uncertain if flecainide's risk of proarrhythmia is exaggerated in patients CAF, high ventricular rate or exercise. Wide complex tachycardia and ventricular fibrillation have been reported in two of 12 CAF patients undergoing maximal exercise tolerance testing. In patients with complex arrhythmias, it is difficult to distinguish a spontaneous variation in the underlying rhythm disorder from drug-induced worsening. As a result, the occurrence rates are approximations.

Among patients treated for *sustained* ventricular tachycardia (who frequently also had heart failure, a low ejection fraction, a history of MI or cardiac arrest), the incidence of proarrhythmic events was 13% when dosage was initiated at 200 mg/day with slow upward titration, without exceeding 300 mg/day. In patients with *sustained* ventricular tachycardia using a higher initial dose (400 mg/day) the incidence of proarrhythmic events was 26%; moreover, in about 10%, proarrhythmic events were fatal. With lower initial doses, the incidence of fatal proarrhythmic events decreased to 0.5%.

The relatively high frequency of proarrhythmic events in patients with sustained ventricular tachycardia and serious underlying heart disease, and the need for titration and monitoring, requires that therapy of patients with sustained ventricular tachycardia be started in the hospital.

Sick sinus syndrome: Use only with extreme caution; the drug may cause sinus bradycardia, sinus pause or sinus arrest. The frequency probably increases with higher trough plasma levels, especially when they exceed 1 mcg/ml.

(Warnings continued on following page)

FLECAINIDE ACETATE (Cont.)

Warnings (Cont.):

Heart failure: Flecainide has a negative inotropic effect and may cause or worsen CHF, particularly in patients with cardiomyopathy, preexisting severe heart failure (NYHA functional class III or IV) or low ejection fractions (< 30%). In patients with supraventricular arrhythmias, new or worsened CHF developed in 0.4% of patients. In patients with sustained ventricular tachycardia during a mean duration of 7.9 months of flecainide therapy, 6.3% developed new CHF. In patients with sustained ventricular tachycardia and a history of CHF in a mean duration of 5.4 months of therapy, 25.7% developed worsened CHF. Exacerbation of preexisting CHF occurred more commonly in studies including patients with Class III or IV failure than in studies which excluded such patients. Use cautiously in patients with a history of CHF or myocardial dysfunction. The initial dosage should be no more than 100 mg twice daily; monitor patients carefully. Give close attention to maintenance of cardiac function, including optimal digitalis, diuretic or other therapy. Where CHF has developed or worsened during treatment, the time of onset has ranged from a few hours to several months after starting therapy. Some patients who develop reduced myocardial function while on flecainide can continue with adjustment of digitalis or diuretics; others may require dosage reduction or discontinuation of flecainide. When feasible, monitor plasma flecainide levels. Keep trough plasma levels < 1 mcg/ml.

Cardiac conduction: Flecainide slows cardiac conduction in most patients to produce dose-related increases in PR, QRS and QT intervals.

The PR interval increases an average of 25% (0.04 seconds) and as much as 118%. Approximately one-third of patients may develop new first-degree AV heart block (PR interval ≥ 0.2 seconds). The QRS complex increases an average of 25% (0.02 seconds) and as much as 150%. Many patients develop QRS complexes with a duration of ≥ 0.12 seconds. In one study, 4% of patients developed new bundle branch block. The degree of lengthening of PR and QRS intervals does not predict either efficacy or the development of cardiac adverse effects. In clinical trials, it was unusual for PR intervals to increase to ≥ 0.3 seconds, or for QRS intervals to increase to ≥ 0.18 seconds; thus, use caution and consider dose reductions. The QT interval widens about 8% but most (about 60% to 90%) is due to widening of the QRS duration. The JT interval (QT minus QRS) only widens about 4% on the average. Significant JT prolongation occurs in < 2% of patients. Rare cases of torsade de pointes-type arrhythmias have occurred.

Clinically significant conduction changes have been observed at these rates: Sinus node dysfunction such as sinus pause, sinus arrest and symptomatic bradycardia (1.2%), second-degree AV block (0.5%), and third-degree AV block (0.4%). If second- or third-degree AV block, or right bundle branch block associated with a left hemiblock occurs, discontinue therapy unless a ventricular pacemaker is in place to ensure an adequate ventricular rate.

Electrolyte disturbance: Hypokalemia or hyperkalemia may alter the effects of Class I antiarrhythmic drugs. Correct preexisting hypokalemia or hyperkalemia before administration.

Effects on pacemaker thresholds: Flecainide increases endocardial pacing thresholds and may suppress ventricular escape rhythms. These effects are reversible if flecainide is discontinued. Use with caution in patients with permanent pacemakers or temporary pacing electrodes. Do not administer to patients with existing poor thresholds or nonprogrammable pacemakers unless suitable pacing rescue is available.

Determine the pacing threshold in patients with pacemakers prior to instituting therapy, after 1 week of administration and at regular intervals thereafter. Generally, threshold changes are within the range of multiprogrammable pacemakers, and a doubling of either voltage or pulse width is usually sufficient to regain capture.

Urinary pH alters flecainide elimination; alkalinization (as may occur in rare conditions such as renal tubular acidosis or strict vegetarian diet) decreases, and acidification increases, flecainide renal excretion. These alterations in pH (outside a range of pH 5 to 7) may produce toxic or subtherapeutic plasma levels. See Drug Interactions.

Hepatic function impairment: Since flecainide elimination from plasma can be markedly slower in patients with significant hepatic impairment, do not use in such patients unless the potential benefits outweigh the risks. If used, frequent and early plasma level monitoring is required to guide dosage (see Plasma level monitoring in the Administration and Dosage section); make dosage increases very cautiously when plasma levels have plateaued (after > 4 days).

Elderly: From age 20 to 80, plasma levels are only slightly higher with advancing age; flecainide elimination from plasma is somewhat slower in elderly subjects than in younger subjects. Patients up to age 80 and above have been safely treated with usual doses.

(Warnings continued on following page)

FLECAINIDE ACETATE (Cont.)

Warnings (Cont.):

Pregnancy: Category C. Flecainide had teratogenic and embryotoxic effects in one breed of rabbit when given in doses up to 35 mg/kg/day. There are no adequate and well controlled studies in pregnant women. Use during pregnancy only if potential benefits outweigh potential hazards to the fetus.

Lactation: Flecainide is excreted in breast milk in concentrations as high as 4 times (with average levels about 2.5 times) corresponding plasma levels; assuming a maternal plasma level at the top of the therapeutic range (1 mcg/ml), the calculated daily dose to a nursing infant (assuming about 700 ml breast milk over 24 hours) would be < 3 mg. Because of the drug's potential for serious adverse effects in infants, determine whether to discontinue nursing or discontinue the drug, taking into account the importance of the drug to the mother.

Children: Safety and efficacy for use in children < 18 years of age have not been established.

Based on several studies flecainide appears to be beneficial in treating supraventricular and ventricular arrhythmias in children. Clearance of flecainide is similar to that of adults, but elimination half-life is shorter and volume of distribution is smaller.

Drug Interactions:

Flecainide Drug Interactions

Precipitant drug	Object drug*		Description
Amiodarone	Flecainide	↑	Flecainide plasma levels may be increased.
Cimetidine	Flecainide	↑	Flecainide bioavailability and total renal excretion may be increased.
Disopyramide	Flecainide	↑	Disopyramide has negative inotropic properties; do not use with flecainide unless benefits outweigh risks.
Propranolol	Flecainide	↑	Flecainide and propranolol levels were increased in healthy subjects. Negative inotropic effects were additive; effects on PR interval were less than additive.
Flecainide	Propranolol	↑	
Smoking	Flecainide	↓	Compared to nonsmokers, smokers have a greater plasma clearance of flecainide. An increased flecainide dose may be necessary.
Urinary acidifiers	Flecainide	↓	Alterations in urinary excretion and plasma elimination of flecainide occur with changes in urinary pH (acidic urine increases elimination and decreases bioavailability; alkaline urine decreases elimination and increases bioavailability). See Warnings.
Urinary alkalinizers	Flecainide	↑	
Verapamil	Flecainide	↑	Verapamil has negative inotropic properties; do not use with flecainide unless benefits outweigh risks.
Flecainide	Digoxin	↑	Digoxin's absorption, peak concentration and bioavailability may be increased.

* ↑ = Object drug increased ↓ = Object drug decreased

Adverse Reactions:

Most frequent: Dizziness (18.9%), including lightheadedness, faintness, unsteadiness and near syncope; dyspnea (10.3%); headache (9.6%); nausea (8.9%); fatigue (7.7%); palpitation (6.1%); chest pain (5.4%); asthenia (4.9%); tremor (4.7%); constipation (4.4%); edema (3.5%); abdominal pain (3.3%).

GI: Vomiting, diarrhea, dyspepsia, anorexia (1% to 3%); flatulence, change in taste, dry mouth (< 1%).

CNS: Hypoesthesia, paresthesia, paresis, ataxia, flushing, increased sweating, vertigo, syncope, somnolence, tinnitus, anxiety, insomnia, depression, malaise (1% to 3%); twitching, weakness, convulsions, neuropathy, speech disorder, stupor, amnesia, confusion, euphoria, depersonalization, morbid dreams, apathy (< 1%).

(Adverse Reactions continued on following page)

FLECAINIDE ACETATE (Cont.)

Adverse Reactions (Cont.):

Cardiovascular: New or worsened arrhythmias (see Warnings); episodes of unresuscitatable VT or ventricular fibrillation (cardiac arrest); new or worsened CHF (see Warnings); second-degree (0.5%) or third-degree (0.4%) AV block; sinus bradycardia, sinus pause or sinus arrest (1.2%) (see Warnings); tachycardia (1% to 3%); angina pectoris, bradycardia, hypertension, hypotension (< 1%).

In post-MI patients with asymptomatic PVCs and non-sustained ventricular tachycardia, flecainide therapy was associated with a 5.1% rate of death and non-fatal cardiac arrest, compared with a 2.3% rate in a matched placebo group (see Warnings).

Ophthalmic: Visual disturbances including blurred vision, difficulty in focusing, spots before eyes (15.9%); diplopia (1% to 3%); eye pain/irritation, photophobia, nystagmus (< 1%).

Hematologic: Leukopenia, thrombocytopenia (< 1%).

GU: Impotence, decreased libido, polyuria, urinary retention (< 1%).

Skin: Rash (1% to 3%); urticaria, exfoliative dermatitis, pruritus, alopecia (< 1%).

Other: Fever (1% to 3%); swollen lips, tongue and mouth, arthralgia, bronchospasm, myalgia (< 1%).

Overdosage:

Symptoms: Animal studies suggest that the following events might occur with overdosage: Lengthening of the PR interval; increase in the QRS duration, QT interval and amplitude of the T wave; reduction in heart rate and myocardial contractility; conduction disturbances; hypotension; death from respiratory failure or asystole.

Treatment should be supportive and may include the following: Removal of unabsorbed drug from the GI tract (charcoal instillation appears to be effective in lowering flecainide plasma concentrations, even after an interval of 90 minutes from ingestion of flecainide); inotropic agents or cardiac stimulants such as dopamine, dobutamine or isoproterenol; mechanical ventilation; circulatory assists such as intra-aortic balloon pumping; transvenous pacing in the event of conduction block. Because of the drug's long plasma half-life (12 to 27 hours) and the possibility of nonlinear elimination kinetics at very high doses, these supportive treatments may need to be continued for extended periods of time. Since flecainide elimination is much slower when urine is very alkaline (pH ≥ 8), theoretically, acidification of urine to promote drug excretion may be beneficial in overdose cases with very alkaline urine. There is no evidence that acidification from normal urinary pH increases excretion. Hemodialysis is not effective. Refer to General Management of Acute Overdosage.

Patient Information:

Take as prescribed; serious heart disturbances can result from missing doses, and serious side effects can result from increasing or decreasing doses without supervision.

Administration and Dosage:

Approved by the FDA in 1985.

For patients with sustained ventricular tachycardia, initiate therapy in the hospital and monitor rhythm.

Flecainide has a long half-life (12 to 27 hours). Steady-state plasma levels in normal renal and hepatic function may not be achieved until 3 to 5 days of therapy at a given dose. Therefore, do not increase dosage more frequently than once every 4 days, since optimal effect may not be achieved during the first 2 to 3 days of therapy.

An occasional patient not adequately controlled by (or intolerant of) a dose given at 12 hour intervals may be dosed at 8 hour intervals.

Once the arrhythmia is controlled, it may be possible to reduce the dose, as necessary, to minimize side effects or effects on conduction.

PSVT and PAF: The recommended starting dose is 50 mg every 12 hours. Doses may be increased in increments of 50 mg twice daily every 4 days until efficacy is achieved. For PAF patients, a substantial increase in efficacy without a substantial increase in discontinuation for adverse experiences may be achieved by increasing the flecainide dose from 50 to 100 mg twice daily. The maximum recommended dose for patients with paroxysmal supraventricular arrhythmias is 300 mg/day.

Sustained ventricular tachycardia: Initial dose – 100 mg every 12 hours. Increase in 50 mg increments twice daily every 4 days until effective. Most patients do not require > 150 mg every 12 hours (300 mg/day). Maximum dose is 400 mg/day.

Use of higher initial doses and more rapid dosage adjustments have resulted in an increased incidence of proarrhythmic events and CHF, particularly during the first few days of dosing (see Warnings). Therefore, a loading dose is not recommended.

CHF or MI: Use cautiously in patients with a history of CHF or myocardial dysfunction (see Warnings).

(Administration and Dosage continued on following page)

FLECAINIDE ACETATE (Cont.)

Administration and Dosage (Cont.):

Renal impairment: In severe renal impairment (Ccr ≤ 35 ml/min/1.73 m²), the initial dosage is 100 mg once daily (or 50 mg twice daily). Frequent plasma level monitoring is required to guide dosage adjustments. In patients with less severe renal disease, initial dosage is 100 mg every 12 hours. Increase dosage cautiously at intervals > 4 days, observing the patient closely for signs of adverse cardiac effects or other toxicity. It may take > 4 days before a new steady-state plasma level is reached following a dosage change. Monitor plasma levels to guide dosage adjustments (see below).

Transfer to flecainide: Theoretically, when transferring patients from another antiarrhythmic to flecainide, allow at least 2 to 4 plasma half-lives to elapse for the drug being discontinued before starting flecainide at the usual dosage. Consider hospitalization of patients in whom withdrawal of a previous antiarrhythmic is likely to produce life-threatening arrhythmias.

Plasma level monitoring: The majority of patients treated successfully had trough plasma levels between 0.2 and 1 mcg/ml. The probability of adverse experiences, especially cardiac, may increase with higher trough plasma levels, especially levels > 1 mcg/ml. Monitor trough plasma levels periodically, especially in patients with severe or moderate chronic renal failure or severe hepatic disease and CHF, as drug elimination may be slower.

				C.I.*
Rx	**Tambocor** (3M Pharm.)	**Tablets:** 50 mg	(Riker TR 50). White. In 100s and UD 100s.	63
		100 mg	(Riker TR 100). White, scored. In 100s and UD 100s.	84
		150 mg	(Riker TR 150). White, scored. Oval. In 100s.	158

* Cost Index based on cost per 100 mg.

Refer to the general discussion concerning these products on page 618.

BRETYLIUM TOSYLATE

Actions:

Pharmacology: Bretylium tosylate inhibits norepinephrine release by depressing adrenergic nerve terminal excitability, inducing a chemical sympathectomy-like state. Catecholamine stores are not depleted, but the drug causes an early release of norepinephrine from the adrenergic postganglionic nerve terminals. Therefore, transient catecholamine effects on the myocardium (tachycardia) and on peripheral vascular resistance (rise in blood pressure) are often seen shortly after administration. Subsequently, bretylium blocks the release of norepinephrine in response to neuron stimulation. Peripheral adrenergic blockade causes orthostatic hypotension but has less effect on supine blood pressure. It has a positive inotropic effect on the myocardium.

Electrophysiology – The mechanisms of action are not established. The following actions have been demonstrated in animals: (1) Increase in ventricular fibrillation threshold; (2) increase in action potential duration and effective refractory period without changes in heart rate; (3) little effect on the rate of rise or amplitude of the cardiac action potential (Phase 0) or in resting membrane potential (Phase 4) in normal myocardium. However, when cell injury slows the rate of rise, decreases amplitude and lowers resting membrane potential, bretylium transiently restores these parameters toward normal; (4) decrease in the disparity in action potential duration between normal and infarcted regions; (5) increase in impulse formation and spontaneous firing rate of pacemaker tissue, and in ventricular conduction velocity.

The restoration of injured myocardial cell electrophysiology toward normal, as well as the increase of the action potential duration and effective refractory period, without changing their ratio, may help suppress reentry of aberrant impulses and decrease induced dispersion of local excitable states.

Hemodynamic effects – The mild increase in arterial pressure, followed by a modest decrease, remain within normal limits. Pulmonary artery pressure, pulmonary capillary wedge pressure, right atrial pressure, cardiac index, stroke volume index and stroke work index are not significantly changed.

Pharmacokinetics: Peak plasma concentration and peak hypotensive effects are seen within 1 hour of IM administration. However, suppression of premature ventricular beats is not maximal until 6 to 9 hours after dosing, when mean plasma concentration declines to less than one half of peak level. Antifibrillatory effects occur within minutes of an IV injection. Suppression of ventricular tachycardia and other ventricular arrhythmias develops more slowly, usually 20 min to 2 hours after parenteral administration.

The terminal half-life ranges from 6.9 to 8.1 hours. In two patients with creatinine clearances of 1 and 21 ml/min, half-lives were 31.5 and 16 hours, respectively. During dialysis, a twofold increase in clearance occurs. The drug is eliminated intact by the kidneys. Approximately 70% to 80% of an IM dose is excreted in the urine during the first 24 hours, with an additional 10% excreted over the next 3 days.

Indications:

For prophylaxis and therapy of ventricular fibrillation.

In the treatment of life-threatening ventricular arrhythmias (ie, ventricular tachycardia) which have failed to respond to first-line antiarrhythmic agents (eg, lidocaine).

Unlabeled uses: Bretylium is a second-line agent following lidocaine in the protocol for advanced cardiac life support during CPR. For resistant VF and VT (after lidocaine, defibrillation and procainamide failures), administer bretylium 5 to 10 mg/kg IV, and repeat as needed up to 30 mg/kg; use a bolus every 15 to 30 minutes, infusion 1 to 2 mg/min. For life-threatening arrhythmia use an undiluted infusion of 1 g/250 ml.

Warnings:

Limit use to intensive care units, coronary care units or other facilities with equipment and personnel for constant cardiac and blood pressure monitoring.

Hypotension (postural) occurs regularly in about 50% of patients while they are supine, manifested by dizziness, lightheadedness, vertigo or faintness. Hypotension may occur at doses lower than those needed to suppress arrhythmias. Keep patients supine until tolerance develops. Tolerance occurs unpredictably but may be present after several days. Hypotension with supine systolic pressure > 75 mm Hg need not be treated unless symptomatic. If supine systolic pressure falls below 75 mm Hg, infuse dopamine or norepinephrine to increase blood pressure; use dilute solution and monitor blood pressure closely because pressor effects are enhanced by bretylium. Perform volume expansion with blood or plasma and correct dehydration where appropriate.

Transient hypertension and increased frequency of arrhythmias may occur due to initial release of norepinephrine from adrenergic postganglionic nerve terminals.

Renal function impairment: Since the drug is excreted principally via the kidney, increase the dosage interval in patients with impaired renal function.

(Warnings continued on following page)

BRETYLIUM TOSYLATE (Cont.)

Warnings (Cont.)

Fixed cardiac output: Avoid use in patients with fixed cardiac output (ie, severe aortic stenosis or severe pulmonary hypertension) since severe hypotension may result from a fall in peripheral resistance without a compensatory increase in cardiac output. If survival is threatened by the arrhythmia, the drug may be used, but administer vasoconstrictive catecholamines (eg, norepinephrine) promptly if severe hypotension occurs.

Pregnancy: Category C. Reduced uterine blood flow with fetal hypoxia (bradycardia) is a potential risk. It is not known whether bretylium tosylate can cause harm when administered to a pregnant woman or can affect reproduction capacity. Give to a pregnant woman only if clearly needed.

Children: Safety and efficacy for use in children have not been established. It has been administered to a limited number of pediatric patients, but such use has been inadequate to define proper dosage and limitations. See Administration and Dosage.

Drug Interactions:

Bretylium Drug Interactions			
Precipitant drug	Object drug *		Description
Bretylium	Catecholamines	↑	The pressor effects of catecholamines (eg, dopamine, norepinephrine) are enhanced by bretylium. When catecholamines are administered, use dilute solutions and closely monitor blood pressure (see Warnings).
Bretylium	Digoxin	↑	Digitalis toxicity may be aggravated by the initial release of norepinephrine caused by bretylium. When a life-threatening cardiac arrhythmia occurs, use bretylium only if the etiology of the arrhythmia does not appear to be digitalis toxicity and if other antiarrhythmic drugs are not effective. Avoid simultaneous initiation of therapy.

* ↑ = Object drug increased

Adverse Reactions:

Cardiovascular: Hypotension and postural hypotension (most frequent; see Warnings); bradycardia, increased premature ventricular contractions, transient hypertension, initial increase in arrhythmias, precipitation of angina, sensation of substernal pressure (0.1% to 0.2%).

GI: Nausea and vomiting, primarily after rapid IV administration (3%).

CNS: Vertigo, dizziness, lightheadedness, syncope (0.7%).

Drug relationship not clearly established: Renal dysfunction, diarrhea, abdominal pain, hiccoughs, erythematous macular rash, flushing, hyperthermia, confusion, paranoid psychosis, emotional lability, lethargy, generalized tenderness, anxiety, shortness of breath, diaphoresis, nasal stuffiness, mild conjunctivitis (0.1%).

Overdosage:

Symptoms: In the presence of life-threatening arrhythmias, underdosing with bretylium probably presents a greater risk to the patient than potential overdosage. However, one case of accidental overdose has been reported in which a rapidly injected IV bolus of 30 mg/kg was given instead of an intended 10 mg/kg dose during an episode of ventricular tachycardia. Marked hypertension resulted, followed by protracted refractory hypotension. The patient died 18 hours later in asystole, complicated by renal failure and aspiration pneumonitis. Bretylium serum levels were 8000 ng/ml.

The exaggerated hemodynamic response was attributed to the rapid injection of a very large dose while some effective circulation was still present. Neither the total dose nor the serum levels observed in this patient are in themselves associated with toxicity. Total doses of 30 mg/kg are not unusual and do not cause toxicity when given incrementally during cardio-pulmonary resuscitation procedures. Similarly, patients maintained on chronic bretylium tosylate therapy have had documented serum levels of 12,000 ng/ml. These levels were achieved after sequential dosage increases over time with no apparent ill effects.

Treatment: If bretylium tosylate is overdosed and symptoms of toxicity develop, administer nitroprusside or consider another short-acting IV antihypertensive agent. Do not use long-acting drugs that might potentiate the subsequent hypotensive effects of bretylium. Treat hypotension with appropriate fluid therapy and pressor agents such as dopamine or norepinephrine. Dialysis is probably not useful in the treatment of bretylium overdose.

(Continued on following page)

BRETYLIUM TOSYLATE (Cont.)

Administration and Dosage:

For short-term use only.

Keep patient supine during therapy or closely observe for postural hypotension. The optimal dose has not been determined. Dosages > 40 mg/kg/day have been used without apparent adverse effect. As soon as possible, and when indicated, change patient to an oral antiarrhythmic agent for maintenance therapy.

Immediate life-threatening ventricular arrhythmias (eg, ventricular fibrillation, hemodynamically unstable ventricular tachycardia): Administer undiluted, 5 mg/kg by rapid IV injection. If ventricular fibrillation persists, increase dosage to 10 mg/kg and repeat as necessary.

Maintenance – For continuous suppression, administer the diluted solution by continuous IV infusion at 1 to 2 mg/minute. Alternatively, infuse the diluted solution at a dosage of 5 to 10 mg/kg over > 8 minutes, every 6 hours. More rapid infusion may cause nausea and vomiting.

Other ventricular arrhythmias:

IV – Dilute before administration. Administer 5 to 10 mg/kg by IV infusion over > 8 minutes. More rapid infusion may cause nausea and vomiting. Give subsequent doses at 1 to 2 hour intervals if the arrhythmia persists. For maintenance therapy, the same dosage may be administered every 6 hours, or a constant infusion of 1 to 2 mg/min may be given.

IM – 5 to 10 mg/kg undiluted. Do not dilute prior to injection. Give subsequent doses at 1 to 2 hour intervals if the arrhythmia persists. Thereafter, maintain with same dosage every 6 to 8 hours.

Do not give > 5 ml in any one site. Do not inject into or near a major nerve; vary injection sites. Repeated injection into the same site may cause atrophy and necrosis of muscle tissue, fibrosis, vascular degeneration and inflammatory changes.

Children: The following dosages have been suggested.

Acute ventricular fibrillation – 5 mg/kg/dose IV, followed by 10 mg/kg at 15 to 30 minute intervals, maximum total dose 30 mg/kg; *maintenance,* 5 to 10 mg/kg/dose every 6 hours.

Other ventricular arrhythmias – 5 to 10 mg/kg/dose every 6 hours.

Dilution and administration rates for continuous infusion: Dilute bretylium using the following table and administer as a constant infusion of 1 to 2 g/min.

Administration Rates for Continuous Infusion Maintenance Bretylium Therapy

Preparation				Administration		
Amount of bretylium	Volume of IV fluid[1] (ml)	Final volume (ml)	Final conc. (mg/ml)	Dose (mg/min)	Microdrops per min	ml/hr
500 mg (10 ml)[2]	50[2]	60[2]	8.3[2]	1	7	7
				1.5	11	11
				2	14	14
2 g (40 ml)	500	540	3.7	1	16	16
1 g (20 ml)	250	270	3.7	1.5	24	24
				2	32	32
1 g (20 ml)	500	520	1.9	1	32	32
500 mg (10 ml)	250	260	1.9	1.5	47	47
				2	63	63

[1] May be either Dextrose or Sodium Chloride Injection, USP. [2] For fluid restricted patients.

IV compatibility: Bretylium is compatible with the following IV solutions and additives: 5% Dextrose Injection; 5% Dextrose in 0.45% Sodium Chloride; 5% Dextrose in 0.9% Sodium Chloride; 5% Dextrose in Lactated Ringer's; 0.9% Sodium Chloride; 5% Sodium Bicarbonate; 20% Mannitol; ⅙ M Sodium Lactate; Lactated Ringer's; Calcium Chloride (54.4 mEq/L) in 5% Dextrose; Potassium Chloride (40 mEq/L) in 5% Dextrose.

				C.I.*
Rx	**Bretylium Tosylate** (Various, eg, Abbott, American Regent, Astra, Elkins-Sinn)	**Injection:** 50 mg per ml	In 10 ml amps, vials and syringes.	417+
Rx	**Bretylol** (DuPont Critical Care)		In 10 ml amps, disp. syringes and single use vials and 20 ml single use vials.	422

* Cost Index based on cost per 50 mg.

Refer to the general discussion concerning these products on page 618.

AMIODARONE HCl

Actions:

Pharmacology: Amiodarone has predominantly Class III antiarrhythmic effects. The antiarrhythmic effect may be due to at least two major properties: A prolongation of the myocardial cell-action potential duration and refractory period, and noncompetitive α- and β-adrenergic inhibition.

Electrophysiology – Amiodarone increases the cardiac refractory period without influencing resting membrane potential, except in automatic cells where the slope of the prepotential is reduced, generally reducing automaticity. These electrophysiologic effects are reflected in a decreased sinus rate of 15% to 20%, increased PR and QT intervals of about 10%, the development of U waves, and changes in T wave contour. These changes should not require discontinuation, although amiodarone can cause marked sinus bradycardia or sinus arrest and heart block. On rare occasions, QT prolongation has been associated with worsening of arrhythmia (see Warnings).

Electrophysiologic effects, such as prolongation of QTc, can be seen within hours after a parenteral dose. However, effects on abnormal rhythms are not seen before 2 to 3 days and usually require 1 to 3 weeks, even when a loading dose is used. There is evidence that the time to effect is shorter when a loading-dose regimen is used.

Hemodynamics – After IV administration (dosage form not available in US), amiodarone relaxes vascular smooth muscle, reduces peripheral vascular resistance (afterload) and slightly increases cardiac index. After oral dosing, however, it produces no significant change in left ventricular ejection fraction (LVEF), even in patients with depressed LVEF. After acute IV dosing, the drug may have a mild negative inotropic effect.

Pharmacokinetics: Absorption – Following oral administration, amiodarone is slowly and variably absorbed; bioavailability is approximately 50% (between 35% and 65%). Maximum plasma concentrations are attained 3 to 7 hours after a single dose. Despite this, the onset of action may occur in 2 to 3 days, but more commonly takes 1 to 3 weeks, even with loading doses. Plasma concentrations with chronic dosing at 100 to 600 mg/day are approximately dose-proportional, with a mean 0.5 mg/L increase for each 100 mg/day. These means, however, include considerable individual variability.

Distribution – Amiodarone has a very large but variable volume of distribution, averaging about 60 L/kg, because of extensive accumulation in various sites, especially adipose tissue and highly perfused organs (eg, liver, lung, spleen). One major metabolite, desethylamiodarone, accumulates to an even greater extent in almost all tissues. The pharmacological activity of this metabolite is not known. The plasma ratio of metabolite to parent compound is approximately one. Amiodarone and its metabolite have a limited transplacental transfer (10% to 50%). They have been detected in breast milk (see Warnings). The drug is highly protein bound ($\approx$ 96%).

Metabolism – The main route of elimination is via hepatic excretion into bile; some enterohepatic recirculation may occur. The drug has a very low plasma clearance with negligible renal excretion, so that it does not appear necessary to modify the dose in patients with renal failure. Neither amiodarone nor its metabolite is dialyzable.

Elimination – Following discontinuation of chronic oral therapy, amiodarone has a biphasic elimination with an initial one-half reduction of plasma levels after 2.5 to 10 days. A much slower terminal plasma elimination phase shows a half-life of the parent compound ranging from 26 to 107 days (mean 53 days), with most patients in the 40 to 55 day range. Steady-state plasma concentrations would therefore be reached between 130 and 535 days (average 265 days). For the metabolite, mean plasma elimination half-life was $\approx$ 61 days. The considerable intersubject variation requires attention to individual responses. Antiarrhythmic effects persist for weeks or months after the drug is discontinued. In general, when the drug is resumed after recurrence of the arrhythmia, control is established rapidly compared to the initial response, presumably because tissue stores were not depleted at the time of recurrence.

Clinical pharmacology: Pharmacodynamics – There is no well established relationship of plasma concentration to effectiveness, but concentrations much below 1 mcg/ml are often ineffective and levels $>$ 2.5 mcg/ml are generally not needed. Plasma concentration measurements can be used to identify patients whose levels are unusually low, and who might benefit from a dose increase, or unusually high, and who might have dosage reduction in the hope of minimizing side effects. Some observations suggest a plasma concentration, dose or dose/duration relationship for side effects such as pulmonary fibrosis, liver enzyme elevations, corneal deposits, facial pigmentation, peripheral neuropathy and GI and CNS effects.

Monitoring – Predicting efficacy of any antiarrhythmic is difficult and controversial.

1. If a patient with a history of cardiac arrest does not manifest a hemodynamically unstable arrhythmia during ECG monitoring prior to treatment, assessment of the effectiveness of amiodarone requires some provocative approach, either exercise or programmed electrical stimulation (PES).

(Actions continued on following page)

AMIODARONE HCl (Cont.)

Warnings (Cont.):

Carcinogenesis/fertility impairment: Amiodarone caused a statistically significant, dose-related increase in the incidence of thyroid tumors (follicular adenoma or carcinoma) in rats. It also reduced fertility of male and female rats at a dose of 90 mg/kg/day (8 times the highest recommended human maintenance dose).

Pregnancy: Category D. Amiodarone has been embryotoxic (increased fetal resorption and growth retardation) in the rat when given orally at a dose of 200 mg/kg/day (18 times the maximum recommended maintenance dose). Amiodarone can cause fetal harm when administered to a pregnant woman. Amiodarone concentrations in the infant at birth are approximately 25% of maternal levels, 10% for the metabolite. Although its use is uncommon, there have been a small number of reports of congenital goiter/hypothyroidism and hyperthyroidism. If amiodarone is used during pregnancy or if the patient becomes pregnant while taking amiodarone, apprise the patient of the potential hazard to the fetus. Use only if the potential benefits outweigh the potential hazards to the fetus.

Lactation: Amiodarone is excreted in breast milk. Nursing offspring of lactating rats administered amiodarone are less viable and have reduced body-weight gains. Therefore, when amiodarone therapy is indicated, advise the mother to discontinue nursing.

Children: Safety and efficacy for use in children have not been established.

Precautions:

Ophthalmologic effects: Asymptomatic corneal microdeposits appear in the majority of adults treated with amiodarone > 6 months. They are usually discernible only by slit-lamp examination, but give rise to symptoms such as visual halos or blurred vision in as many as 10% of patients. Corneal microdeposits are reversible upon reduction of dose or drug discontinuation. Asymptomatic microdeposits are not a reason to reduce dose or stop treatment. Some patients develop photophobia and dry eyes. Vision is rarely affected and drug discontinuation is rarely indicated.

Thyroid abnormalities: Amiodarone inhibits peripheral conversion of thyroxine (T_4) to triiodothyronine (T_3), prompting increased T_4 levels, increased levels of inactive reverse T_3 and decreased levels of T_3. It is also a potential source of large amounts of inorganic iodine. It can cause hypothyroidism or hyperthyroidism. Monitor thyroid function at baseline and periodically during therapy, particularly in the elderly and in any patient with a history of thyroid nodules, goiter or other thyroid dysfunction. Because of the slow elimination of amiodarone and its metabolites, high plasma iodide levels, altered thyroid function, and abnormal thyroid function tests may persist for several weeks or even months following amiodarone withdrawal.

Hypothyroidism has been reported in 2% to 10% of patients. It is probably best diagnosed by relevant clinical symptoms and particularly by elevated TSH. In some clinically hypothyroid amiodarone-treated patients, free thyroxine index values may be normal. Hypothyroidism is best managed by dose reduction or thyroid hormone supplement. However, therapy must be individualized, and it may be necessary to discontinue amiodarone in some patients.

Hyperthyroidism occurs in about 2% of patients receiving amiodarone, but the incidence may be higher among patients with prior inadequate dietary iodine intake. Amiodarone-induced hyperthyroidism usually poses a greater hazard to the patient than hypothyroidism because of the possibility of arrhythmia breakthrough or aggravation. In fact, if any new signs of arrhythmia appear, consider the possibility of hyperthyroidism. Hyperthyroidism is best identified by relevant clinical symptoms and signs, accompanied usually by abnormally elevated levels of serum T_3 RIA, and further elevations of serum T_4, and a subnormal serum TSH level. Since arrhythmia breakthroughs may accompany amiodarone-induced hyperthyroidism, aggressive medical treatment is indicated, including, if possible, dose reduction or withdrawal of amiodarone. The institution of antithyroid drugs, beta-adrenergic blockers or temporary corticosteroid therapy may be necessary. The action of antithyroid drugs may be especially delayed in amiodarone-induced thyrotoxicosis because of substantial quantities of preformed thyroid hormones stored in the gland. Radioactive iodine therapy is contraindicated because of the low radioiodine uptake associated with amiodarone-induced hyperthyroidism. Experience with thyroid surgery in this setting is extremely limited, and this form of therapy runs the theoretical risk of inducing thyroid storm. Amiodarone-induced hyperthyroidism may be followed by a transient period of hypothyroidism.

Post-bypass hypotension occurs rarely upon discontinuation of cardiopulmonary bypass during open heart surgery in patients receiving amiodarone. Causal relationship is unknown.

(Precautions continued on following page)

AMIODARONE HCl (Cont.)

Precautions (Cont.):

Electrolyte disturbances: Antiarrhythmics may be ineffective or arrhythmogenic in patients with hypokalemia; correct potassium or magnesium deficiency before therapy begins.

Adult respiratory distress syndrome (ARDS): Postoperatively, rare occurrences of ARDS have been reported in patients receiving amiodarone therapy who have undergone either cardiac or noncardiac surgery. Although patients usually respond well to vigorous respiratory therapy, in rare instances the outcome has been fatal. One possible mechanism of this deleterious effect may be the generation of super oxide radicals during oxygenation; therefore keep the postoperative FiO_2 as close to room air as possible.

Photosensitivity: Amiodarone has induced photosensitization in about 10% of patients; some protection may be afforded by sun barrier creams or protective clothing. During long-term treatment, a blue-gray discoloration of the exposed skin may occur. The risk may be increased in patients of fair complexion or those with excessive sun exposure, and may be related to cumulative dose and duration of therapy. This is slowly and occasionally incompletely reversible on discontinuation of drug but is of cosmetic importance only.

Drug Interactions:

Amiodarone Drug Interactions			
Precipitant drug	Object drug*		Description
Amiodarone	Anticoagulants	↑	Hypoprothrombinemic effect of anticoagulants is augmented. A 30% to 50% reduction in dose is typically required. The effect may persist for months after amiodarone discontinuation.
Amiodarone	Beta blockers	↑	Pharmacologic effects of metoprolol and possibly other beta blockers eliminated by hepatic metabolism may be increased.
Amiodarone	Digoxin	↑	Serum levels of digoxin are increased; actions may be enhanced, perhaps to the point of toxicity.
Amiodarone	Flecainide	↑	Increased flecainide plasma levels may occur.
Amiodarone	Hydantoins	↑	Increased hydantoin concentrations with symptoms of toxicity may occur. Also, amiodarone serum levels may be decreased.
Hydantoins	Amiodarone	↓	
Amiodarone	Procainamide	↑	Procainamide serum levels may be increased.
Amiodarone	Quinidine	↑	Quinidine serum levels may be increased, possibly producing potentially fatal cardiac arrhythmias.
Amiodarone	Theophylline	↑	Increased theophylline levels with toxicity may occur. Effects may not be seen for ≥ 1 week of concomitant therapy and may persist for an extended period after amiodarone discontinuation.

* ↑ = Object drug increased ↓ = Object drug decreased

Drug/Lab test interactions: Amiodarone alters the results of thyroid function tests, causing an increase in serum T_4 and serum reverse T_3 levels and a decline in serum T_3 levels. Despite these biochemical changes, most patients remain clinically euthyroid. See Precautions.

(Continued on following page)

AMIODARONE HCl (Cont.)

Adverse Reactions:

Adverse reactions, common with ≥ 400 mg/day, occur in about 75% of patients and cause discontinuation in 7% to 18%. Most effects appear more frequently with treatment beyond 6 months, though rates appear relatively constant beyond 1 year.

Reactions requiring discontinuation include: Pulmonary infiltrates or fibrosis, paroxysmal ventricular tachycardia, CHF, elevation of liver enzymes. Other symptoms causing discontinuation less often include: Visual disturbances, solar dermatitis, blue discoloration of skin, hyperthyroidism, hypothyroidism.

CNS: Neurologic problems (20% to 40%) are rarely a reason to stop therapy and may respond to dose reductions. The following have been reported: Malaise, fatigue, tremor/abnormal involuntary movements, lack of coordination, abnormal gait/ataxia, dizziness, paresthesias (4% to 9%); decreased libido, insomnia, headache, sleep disturbances, abnormal smell (1% to 3%); peripheral neuropathy.

GI complaints occur in about 25% of patients but rarely require discontinuation of drug. These commonly occur during high-dose administration (ie, loading dose) and usually respond to dose reduction or divided doses. Nausea, vomiting (10% to 33%); constipation, anorexia (4% to 9%); abdominal pain, abnormal taste, abnormal salivation, (1% to 3%).

Ophthalmologic: Visual disturbances (4% to 9%); optic neuritis (< 1%). See Precautions.

Dermatologic reactions occur in about 15% of patients; photosensitivity is most common (10%; see Precautions). Other reactions include: Solar dermatitis (4% to 9%); blue discoloration of skin (see Precautions), rash, spontaneous ecchymosis, alopecia (< 1%).

Cardiovascular reactions, other than exacerbation of arrhythmias (see Warnings), include CHF (3%) and bradycardia. Bradycardia usually responds to dosage reduction but may require a pacemaker. Rarely, CHF requires drug discontinuation. Cardiac conduction abnormalities are infrequent and are reversible on drug discontinuation. The following have also been reported: Cardiac arrhythmias, SA node dysfunction, flushing (1% to 3%); hypotension, cardiac conduction abnormalities (< 1%).

Hepatic: Abnormal liver function tests (4% to 9%; see Warnings); nonspecific hepatic disorders (1% to 3%); hepatitis, cholestatic hepatitis, cirrhosis (rare).

Other: Pulmonary inflammation or fibrosis (4% to 9%; see Warnings); hypothyroidism and hyperthyroidism (see Precautions), edema, coagulation abnormalities (1% to 3%); epididymitis, vasculitis, pseudotumor cerebri, thrombocytopenia (< 1%).

Overdosage:

There have been a few reported cases of overdose in which 3 to 8 g of the drug were taken. There were no deaths or permanent sequelae.

Treatment includes usual supportive measures. Refer to General Management of Acute Overdosage. In addition, monitor the patient's cardiac rhythm and blood pressure; if bradycardia occurs, use a β-adrenergic agonist or a pacemaker. Treat hypotension with inadequate tissue perfusion, by using positive inotropic or vasopressor agents. Neither amiodarone nor its metabolite is dialyzable. Results from a small number of patients suggest that cholestyramine may be useful in accelerating the reversal of side effects of amiodarone by enhancing drug elimination; it is not known if this is beneficial in an overdose situation.

(Continued on following page)

AMIODARONE HCl (Cont.)

Administration and Dosage:

Approved by the FDA on December 27, 1985.

Because of the unique pharmacokinetic properties, difficult dosing schedule and severity of side effects, amiodarone should be administered only by physicians with experience with life-threatening arrhythmia treatment who are thoroughly familiar with the risks and benefits of amiodarone therapy and have access to laboratory facilities capable of adequately monitoring effectiveness and side effects.

In order to ensure that an antiarrhythmic effect will be observed without waiting several months, loading doses are required. Individual patient titration is suggested.

For life-threatening ventricular arrhythmias, such as ventricular fibrillation or hemodynamically unstable ventricular tachycardia, administer the loading dose in a hospital. Loading doses of 800 to 1600 mg/day are required for 1 to 3 weeks (occasionally longer) until initial therapeutic response occurs. Administer in divided doses with meals for total daily doses of ≥ 1000 mg, or when GI intolerance occurs. If side effects become excessive, reduce the dose. Elimination of recurrence of ventricular fibrillation and tachycardia usually occurs within 1 to 3 weeks, along with reduction in complex and total ventricular ectopic beats.

Upon starting amiodarone therapy, attempt to gradually discontinue prior antiarrhythmic drugs (see concurrent antiarrhythmic drugs). When adequate arrhythmia control is achieved, or if side effects become prominent, reduce dose to 600 to 800 mg/day for 1 month and then to the maintenance dose, usually 400 mg/day. Some patients may require larger maintenance doses, up to 600 mg/day, and some can be controlled on lower doses. May be administered as a single daily dose, or in patients with severe GI intolerance, as a twice daily dose. In each patient, determine the chronic maintenance dose according to antiarrhythmic effect as assessed by symptoms, Holter recordings or programmed electrical stimulation and by patient tolerance. Plasma concentrations may be helpful in evaluating nonresponsiveness or unexpectedly severe toxicity.

Use the lowest effective dose to prevent the occurrence of side effects. In all instances, be guided by the severity of the patient's arrhythmia and response to therapy. When dosage adjustments are necessary, closely monitor the patient for an extended time because of the long and variable half-life and the difficulty in predicting the time required to attain a new steady-state drug level. Dosage suggestions are summarized below:

Suggested Amiodarone Dosing in Ventricular Arrhythmias

Loading dose (daily) For 1 to 3 weeks	Adjustment and maintenance dose (daily)	
	For ≈ 1 month	Usual maintenance
800 to 1600 mg	600 to 800 mg	400 mg

Concurrent antiarrhythmic agents: In general, reserve the combination of amiodarone with other antiarrhythmic therapy for patients with life-threatening arrhythmias who are incompletely responsive to a single agent or incompletely responsive to amiodarone. During transfer to amiodarone, reduce the dose levels of previously administered agents by 30% to 50% several days after the addition of amiodarone when arrhythmia suppression should be beginning. Review the continued need for the other antiarrhythmic agent after the effects of amiodarone have been established, and attempt discontinuation. If the treatment is continued, carefully monitor these patients for adverse effects, especially conduction disturbances and exacerbation of tachyarrhythmias, as amiodarone is continued. In amiodarone-treated patients who require additional antiarrhythmic therapy, the initial dose of such agents should be approximately half of the usual recommended dose.

				C.I.*
Rx	**Cordarone** (Wyeth-Ayerst)	**Tablets:** 200 mg	(C 200 Wyeth 4188). Pink, scored. Convex. In 60s and UD 100s.	187

* Cost Index based on cost per 200 mg.

Refer to the general discussion concerning these products on page 618.

ADENOSINE

Actions:

Pharmacology: Adenosine is an endogenous nucleoside occurring in all cells of the body. It is not chemically related to other antiarrhythmic agents. Adenosine slows conduction time through the AV node, can interrupt the reentry pathways through the AV node and can restore normal sinus rhythm in patients with paroxysmal supraventricular tachycardia (PSVT), including PSVT associated with Wolff-Parkinson-White (WPW) Syndrome.

The drug is antagonized competitively by methylxanthines such as caffeine and theophylline and potentiated by blockers of nucleoside transport such as dipyridamole (see Drug Interactions). Adenosine is not blocked by atropine.

Hemodynamics – The usual IV bolus dose of 6 or 12 mg will not have systemic hemodynamic effects. When larger doses are given by infusion, adenosine decreases blood pressure by decreasing peripheral resistance.

Pharmacokinetics: IV adenosine is removed from the circulation very rapidly. Following an IV bolus, adenosine is taken up by erythrocytes and vascular endothelial cells. The half-life of adenosine is estimated to be < 10 seconds. Adenosine enters the body pool and is primarily metabolized to inosine and adenosine monophosphate (AMP).

Clinical trials: In controlled studies, bolus doses of 3, 6, 9 and 12 mg were studied. A cumulative 60% of patients with PSVT had converted to normal sinus rhythm within 1 minute after an IV bolus dose of 6 mg (some converted on 3 mg and failures were given 6 mg), and a cumulative 92% converted after a bolus dose of 12 mg. From 7% to 16% of patients converted after 1 to 4 placebo bolus injections.

Similar responses were seen in a variety of patient subsets, including those using or not using digoxin, those with WPW Syndrome, males, females, blacks, Caucasians and Hispanics.

Indications:

Conversion to sinus rhythm of paroxysmal supraventricular tachycardia, including that associated with accessory bypass tracts (WPW Syndrome). When clinically advisable, attempt appropriate vagal maneuvers (eg, Valsalva maneuver) prior to administration.

Unlabeled use: Adenosine has been used in the noninvasive assessment of patients with suspected coronary artery disease in conjunction with ^{201}thallium tomography; results are similar to assessment with exercise stress test or IV dipyridamole.

Adenosine phosphate is used for the symptomatic relief of varicose vein complications with stasis dermatitis (see Adenosine Phosphate monograph in the Miscellaneous section).

Contraindications:

Second- or third-degree AV block or sick sinus syndrome (except in patients with a functioning artificial pacemaker); atrial flutter, atrial fibrillation and ventricular tachycardia (the drug is not effective in converting these arrhythmias to normal sinus rhythm; see Warnings); hypersensitivity to adenosine.

Warnings:

Systemic circulation: It is important to be sure the solution actually reaches the systemic circulation (see Administration and Dosage).

Heart block: Adenosine decreases conduction through the AV node and may produce a short lasting first-, second- or third-degree heart block. In extreme cases, transient asystole may result (one case has been reported in a patient with atrial flutter who was receiving carbamazepine). Institute appropriate therapy as needed. Patients who develop high-level block on one dose of adenosine should not be given additional doses. Because of the very short half-life, these effects are generally self-limiting.

Arrhythmias at time of conversion: At the time of conversion to normal sinus rhythm, a variety of new rhythms may appear on the ECG. They generally last only a few seconds without intervention, and may take the form of premature ventricular contractions, atrial premature contractions, sinus bradycardia, sinus tachycardia, skipped beats and varying degrees of AV nodal block. Such findings were seen in 55% of patients.

Treatment of other arrhythmias: Adenosine is not effective in converting rhythms other than PSVT, such as atrial flutter, atrial fibrillation or ventricular tachycardia to normal sinus rhythm. To date, administration of adenosine to such patients did not result in adverse consequences.

Ventricular response: In the presence of atrial flutter or atrial fibrillation, a transient modest slowing of ventricular response may occur immediately following administration.

Hepatic and renal failure: Hepatic and renal failure should have no effect on the activity of a bolus adenosine injection. Since the drug has a direct action, hepatic and renal function are not required for the activity or the metabolism of a bolus adenosine injection.

(Warnings continued on following page)

ADENOSINE (Cont.)

Warnings (Cont.):

Mutagenesis: Adenosine, like other nucleosides at millimolar concentrations present for several doubling times of cells in culture, is known to produce a variety of chromosomal alterations. In rats and mice, adenosine administered intraperitoneally once a day for 5 days at 50, 100 and 150 mg/kg caused decreased spermatogenesis and increased numbers of abnormal sperm, a reflection of the ability of adenosine to produce chromosomal damage.

Pregnancy: Category C. As adenosine is a naturally occurring material, widely dispersed throughout the body, no fetal effects would be anticipated. However, since it is not known whether the drug can cause fetal harm when administered to pregnant women, use during pregnancy only if clearly needed.

Precautions:

Asthma: A limited number of patients with asthma have received adenosine and have not experienced exacerbation of their asthma. However, inhaled adenosine induces bronchoconstriction in asthmatic patients but not in healthy individuals. Be alert to the possibility that adenosine could produce bronchoconstriction in patients with asthma.

Drug Interactions:

Adenosine Drug Interactions

Precipitant drug	Object drug*		Description
Carbamazepine	Adenosine	↑	Carbamazepine increases the degree of heart block produced by other agents. As the primary effect of adenosine is to decrease conduction through the AV node, higher degrees of heart block may be produced in the presence of carbamazepine.
Dipyridamole	Adenosine	↑	The effects of adenosine are potentiated. Thus, smaller doses of adenosine may be effective in the presence of dipyridamole.
Methylxanthines (eg, caffeine, theophylline)	Adenosine	↓	The effects of adenosine are antagonized. In the presence of methylxanthines, larger doses of adenosine may be required or adenosine may not be effective.

* ↑ = Object drug increased ↓ = Object drug decreased

Adverse Reactions:

Cardiovascular: Facial flushing (18%); headache (2%); sweating, palpitations, chest pain, hypotension (< 1%).

Respiratory: Shortness of breath/dyspnea (12%); chest pressure (7%); hyperventilation, head pressure (< 1%).

CNS: Lightheadedness (2%); dizziness, tingling in arms, numbness (1%); apprehension, blurred vision, burning sensation, heaviness in arms, neck and back pain (< 1%).

GI: Nausea (3%); metallic taste, tightness in throat, pressure in groin (< 1%).

Overdosage:

The half-life of adenosine is < 10 seconds. Thus, adverse effects are generally rapidly self-limiting. Individualize treatment of any prolonged adverse effects and direct toward the specific effect. Methylxanthines (eg, caffeine, theophylline) are competitive antagonists of adenosine (see Drug Interactions). Refer to General Management of Acute Overdosage.

Administration and Dosage:

For rapid bolus IV use only. To be certain the solution reaches the systemic circulation, administer either directly into a vein or, if given into an IV line, as proximal as possible and follow with a rapid saline flush.

Initial dose: 6 mg as a rapid IV bolus (administered over a 1 to 2 second period).

Repeat administration: If first dose does not result in elimination of the supraventricular tachycardia within 1 to 2 minutes, give 12 mg as a rapid IV bolus. This 12 mg dose may be repeated a second time if required.

Doses > 12 mg are not recommended.

Storage/Stability: Store at controlled room temperature 15° to 30°C (59° to 86°F). Do not refrigerate as crystallization may occur. If crystallization has occurred, dissolve crystals by warming to room temperature. The solution must be clear at the time of use. Contains no preservatives. Discard unused portion.

Rx	**Adenocard** (Fujisawa)	**Injection:** 6 mg/2 ml	Preservative free. In 2 ml vials.

Actions:

Pharmacology: In specialized automatic and conducting cells in the heart, calcium is involved in genesis of action potential. In contractile cells of the myocardium, it links excitation to contraction and controls energy storage and use. Systemic and coronary arteries are influenced by movement of calcium across cell membranes of vascular smooth muscle. Contractile processes of cardiac and vascular smooth muscle depend upon movement of extracellular calcium ions into these cells through specific ion channels.

The calcium channel blocking agents, also referred to as slow channel blockers or calcium antagonists, share the ability to inhibit movement of calcium ions across the cell membrane. The resultant pharmacological effects on the cardiovascular system include depression of mechanical contraction of myocardial and smooth muscle, and depression of both impulse formation (automaticity) and conduction velocity. Bepridil also inhibits fast sodium inward channels. The calcium channel blockers are classified by structure as follows: Diphenylalkylamines – verapamil; benzothiazepines – diltiazem; dihydropyridines – felodipine, isradipine, nicardipine, nifedipine, nimodipine.

Although these agents are similar in that they all act on the slow (calcium) channel, they have different degrees of selectivity in their effects on vascular smooth muscle, myocardium or specialized conduction and pacemaker tissues. The resulting clinical effects depend on the direct activity of the drug, reflex physiological responses (primarily β-adrenergic response to vasodilation) and the patient's cardiovascular status. This heterogeneity of the calcium blockers, in part, determines their clinical application and the different side effects produced by each agent.

In animal studies, nimodipine had a greater effect on cerebral arteries than on other arteries, possibly because it is highly lipophilic, allowing it to cross the blood-brain barrier. Concentrations as high as 12.5 ng/ml were detected in the cerebrospinal fluid of patients with subarachnoid hemorrhage (SAH). It was hoped that nimodipine would prevent arterial spasm in SAH patients. While clinical studies demonstrate a favorable effect on the severity of neurological deficits caused by cerebral vasospasm following SAH, there is no arteriographic evidence that the drug either prevents or relieves spasm of these arteries. Therefore, the actual mechanism of action is unknown.

Hemodynamics (see Pharmacology/Pharmacokinetics table): These agents dilate the coronary arteries and arterioles, both in normal and ischemic regions, and inhibit coronary artery spasm. This increases myocardial oxygen delivery in patients with vasospastic (Prinzmetal's or variant) angina. Whether this mechanism plays any role in their effectiveness for treatment of classical angina is not clear.

Calcium channel blockers reduce arterial blood pressure at rest and with exercise by dilating peripheral arterioles and reducing total peripheral resistance (afterload) against which the heart works. This reduces myocardial energy consumption and oxygen requirements and probably accounts for their effectiveness in chronic stable angina.

Although these agents exhibit a negative inotropic effect, this is rarely seen clinically because of reflex responses to the vasodilation. In patients with normal ventricular function, there may be a small increase in cardiac index without major effects on ejection fraction, left ventricular end diastolic pressure or volume (LVEDP or LVEDV). Usual doses of **IV verapamil** may slightly increase left ventricular filling pressure. A worsening of heart failure may be seen when **verapamil** is given to patients with moderate to severe cardiac dysfunction. When **nifedipine** was administered to patients with decreased ventricular function, there was some increase in ejection fraction and decrease in LVEDP. **Nicardipine** administration to patients with normal or moderately abnormal left ventricular function resulted in significant increases in ejection fraction and cardiac output with no significant change or a small decrease in LVEDP.

Electrophysiology (see Pharmacology/Pharmacokinetics table): **Verapamil** slows AV conduction and prolongs the ERP within the AV node in a rate-related manner, thus reducing elevated ventricular rate due to atrial flutter or atrial fibrillation. By interrupting reentry at the AV node, verapamil can restore normal sinus rhythm in patients with paroxysmal supraventricular tachycardias (PSVT), including Wolff-Parkinson-White (W-P-W) syndrome. It can interfere with sinus node impulse generation and induce sinus arrest in patients with sick sinus syndrome; it can also induce AV block, although this is rare clinically. Verapamil may shorten the antegrade ERP of the accessory bypass tracts. It does not alter the normal atrial action potential or intraventricular conduction time, but it depresses amplitude, velocity of depolarization and conduction in depressed atrial fibers.

About 60% to 80% of patients with supraventricular tachycardia convert to normal sinus rhythm within 10 minutes after IV verapamil. About 70% of patients with atrial flutter or fibrillation with a fast ventricular rate respond with a decrease in heart rate of at least 20%. Conversion of atrial flutter or fibrillation to sinus rhythm is uncommon ($\approx$ 10%) after verapamil and may reflect the spontaneous conversion rate. The effect of a single injection lasts for 30 to 60 minutes when conversion to sinus rhythm does not occur.

(Actions continued on following page)

Actions (Cont.):

Pharmacokinetics: Although these agents are well absorbed (80% to 90%) following oral administration, they are subject to extensive first-pass effects, resulting in an absolute bioavailability that is considerably less.

Calcium Channel Blocking Agents: Pharmacology/Pharmacokinetics

	Parameters	Nifedipine/SR	Verapamil	Diltiazem/SR	Nicardipine
Pharmacokinetics	Extent of absorption (%)	90	90	80-90	≈ 100
	Absolute bioavailability (%)	45-70/86	20-35	40-67	35
	Onset of action – oral (min)	20	30[1]	30-60	20
	Time of peak plasma levels (hrs)	0.5/6	1-2.2	2-3/6-11	0.5-2
	Protein binding (%)	92-98	83-92	70-80	> 95
	Therapeutic serum levels (ng/ml)	25-100	80-300	50-200	28-50
	Metabolite	Acid or lactone[2]	Norverapamil[3]	Desacetyl-diltiazem[4]	Glucuronide conjugates
	Excreted unchanged in urine (%)	1-2	3-4	2-4	< 1
	Half-life, elimination (hrs)	2-5	3-7[6]	3.5-6/5-7	2-4
Electrophysiology	Effective refractory period Atrium	0	0	0	0
	AV node	±	↑↑	↑	↑↓
	His-Purkinje	0	0	0	↓
	Ventricle	0	0	0	0
	Accessory pathway	0	±	?	0
	SA node automaticity[7]	0	↓↓	↓	0
	AV node conduction[7]	±	↓↓↓	↓↓	0-↑
	Sinus node recovery time	0	0[8]	0[8]	0
ECG Changes	Heart rate	↑	↑↓	↓-0	↑
	QRS complex	0	0	0	0
	PR interval	0	↑	↑	nd
	QT interval	nd	nd	nd	↑
Hemodynamics	Myocardial contractility[7]	↓	↓↓	↓	0
	Cardiac output	↑↑	↑↓	0-↑	↑↑
	Peripheral vascular resistance	↓↓↓	↓↓	↓	↓↓↓
	Negative inotropic effect ratio[10]	1	0.1	0.02	nd
	Arterial dilatation ratio[10]	1	0.1	0.05	nd
	Antianginal dose ratio[10]	1	6-10	6-10	2

↑↑↑ or ↓↓↓ = pronounced effect
↑↑ or ↓↓ = moderate effect
↑ or ↓ = slight effect
± = negligible effect
0 = no effect
nd = no data
na = not applicable

[1] Peak therapeutic effects occur within 3 to 5 minutes after IV administration.
[2] Inactive.
[3] Pharmacologic activity 20% of verapamil.
[4] Pharmacologic activity 25% to 50% of diltiazem; plasma levels 10% to 20% of parent drug.
[5] Of 6 metabolites identified, account for > 75%.
[6] 4.5 to 12 hours with multiple dosing; may be prolonged in elderly.
[7] Direct effects may be counteracted by reflex activity.
[8] Prolonged in sick sinus syndrome.
[9] Dose-related.
[10] Ratio as compared with nifedipine as 1.
[11] Attenuates over time.

(Actions continued on following page)

Actions (Cont.):

Calcium Channel Blocking Agents: Pharmacology/Pharmacokinetics					
Nimodipine	Isradipine	Bepridil	Felodipine	Parameters	
nd	90-95	≈ 100	≈ 100	Extent of absorption (%)	Pharmacokinetics
13	15-24	59	20	Absolute bioavailability (%)	
nd	120	60	120-300	Onset of action – oral (min)	
≤ 1	1.5	2-3	2.5-5	Time of peak plasma levels (hrs)	
> 95	95	> 99	> 99	Protein binding (%)	
nd	nd	1-2	nd	Therapeutic serum levels (ng/ml)	
Unknown[2]	Monoacids and cyclic lactone[5]	4-OH-N-phenylbepridil	Six identified[2]	Metabolite	
< 1	0	±	< 0.5	Excreted unchanged in urine (%)	
1-2	8	24	11-16	Half-life, elimination (hrs)	
na				Effective refractory period	Electrophysiology
	0	↑	nd	Atrium	
	0	↑	nd	AV node	
	0	↑	nd	His-Purkinje	
	0	↑	nd	Ventricle	
	nd	↑	nd	Accessory pathway	
	0	↓	nd	SA node automaticity[7]	
	0	↓	0	AV node conduction[7]	
	±	nd	nd	Sinus node recovery time	
	±	↓	↑[11]	Heart rate	ECG Changes
	0	0	nd	QRS complex	
	0	↑	0	PR interval	
	↑	↑↑[9]	nd	QT interval	
	0	↓	↑	Myocardial contractility[7]	Hemodynamics
	↑	0	↑	Cardiac output	
	↓↓↓	↓	↓↓↓	Peripheral vascular resistance	
	nd	nd	nd	Negative inotropic effect ratio[10]	
	nd	nd	nd	Arterial dilatation ratio[10]	
	nd	nd	nd	Antianginal dose ratio[10]	

↑↑↑ or ↓↓↓ = pronounced effect
↑↑ or ↓↓ = moderate effect
↑ or ↓ = slight effect

± = negligible effect
0 = no effect

nd = no data
na = not applicable

[1] Peak therapeutic effects occur within 3 to 5 minutes after IV administration.
[2] Inactive.
[3] Pharmacologic activity 20% of verapamil.
[4] Pharmacologic activity 25% to 50% of diltiazem; plasma levels 10% to 20% of parent drug.
[5] Of 6 metabolites identified, account for > 75%.
[6] 4.5 to 12 hours with multiple dosing; may be prolonged in elderly.
[7] Direct effects may be counteracted by reflex activity.
[8] Prolonged in sick sinus syndrome.
[9] Dose-related.
[10] Ratio as compared with nifedipine as 1.
[11] Attenuates over time

(Continued on following page)

Indications:

Calcium Channel Blocking Agents – Summary of Indications[1]												
Indications	Bepridil	Diltiazem	Diltiazem SR	Felodipine	Isradipine	Nicardipine	Nifedipine	Nifedipine SR	Nimodipine	Verapamil	Verapamil SR	Verapamil IV
Angina pectoris												
Vasospastic		✓					✓	✓		✓		
Chronic stable	✓	✓				✓	✓	✓		✓		
Unstable										✓		
Hypertension, essential			✓	✓	✓	✓		✓		✓	✓	
Arrhythmias										✓		
Supraventricular tachyarrhythmias												✓
Subarachnoid hemorrhage									✓			
Unlabeled uses												
Migraine headache							✓		✓	✓		
Raynaud's syndrome		✓					✓					
Congestive heart failure						✓	✓					
Cardiomyopathy							✓			✓		

[1] Refer to following section for further information on indications and additional unlabeled uses.

Vasospastic (Prinzmetal's variant) angina (nifedipine, sustained release nifedipine, oral verapamil, diltiazem): Treatment of spontaneous coronary artery spasm presenting as Prinzmetal's variant angina (resting angina with ST segment elevation during attacks).

Chronic stable (classic effort-associated) angina (nifedipine, sustained release nifedipine, oral verapamil, diltiazem, nicardipine, bepridil): In patients who cannot tolerate β-adrenergic blockers or nitrates, or who remain symptomatic despite adequate doses of these agents. Diltiazem and nifedipine have been effective in short-term controlled trials in reducing angina frequency and increasing exercise tolerance, but confirmation of sustained efficacy is incomplete.

Unstable (crescendo, preinfarction) angina: Oral verapamil.

Essential hypertension (oral verapamil, sustained release diltiazem, nicardipine, sustained release nifedipine, isradipine, felodipine): Sustained release verapamil and diltiazem are *only* indicated for essential hypertension.

Arrhythmias (oral verapamil): In association with digitalis, to control ventricular rate at rest and during stress in chronic atrial flutter or atrial fibrillation (see Warnings).

Also for prophylaxis of repetitive paroxysmal supraventricular tachycardia.

Supraventricular tachyarrhythmias (parenteral verapamil) including: Rapid conversion to sinus rhythm of PSVT, including those associated with accessory bypass tracts such as W-P-W and Lown-Ganong-Levine (L-G-L) syndromes. When clinically advisable, attempt appropriate vagal maneuvers (eg, Valsalva) prior to use.

Also for temporary control of rapid ventricular rate in atrial flutter/fibrillation.

Subarachnoid hemorrhage (nimodipine): Improvement of neurological deficits due to spasm following SAH from ruptured congenital intracranial aneurysms in patients who are in good neurological condition post-ictus (eg, Hunt and Hess Grades I-III). Begin therapy within 96 hours of the SAH and continue for 21 days.

Unlabeled uses: Nifedipine 10 to 20 mg (children: 2.5 mg for weight $<$ 10 kg, 5 mg for weight of 10 to 20 kg) administered orally, sublingually (puncture capsules and squeeze contents under the tongue), chewed (puncture $\approx$ 10 times, then chew) or rectally has been used to lower blood pressure in hypertensive emergencies. One study indicated that biting the capsule and swallowing the contents results in faster absorption and higher plasma levels compared to sublingual administration, and therefore is preferable in treating cardiovascular emergencies. Preliminary studies suggest nifedipine may also be useful for prophylaxis in migraine headache and in the treatment of primary pulmonary hypertension, asthma, preterm labor, severe pregnancy-associated hypertension, esophageal disorders, biliary and renal colic, cardiomyopathy, to reduce progression of coronary artery disease, CHF and Raynaud's syndrome.

(Indications continued on following page)

Warnings (Cont.):

Antiplatelet effects: Calcium channel blockers, alone and with aspirin, have caused inhibition of platelet function. Episodes of bruising, petechiae and bleeding have occurred.

Nifedipine decreases platelet aggregation in vitro. Limited clinical studies have demonstrated a moderate but statistically significant decrease in platelet aggregation and increase in bleeding time in some patients. This is thought to be a function of inhibition of calcium transport across the platelet membrane.

Withdrawal syndrome: Abrupt withdrawal of calcium channel blockers may cause increased frequency and duration of chest pain. The rebound angina is probably the result of the increased flow of calcium into cells causing coronary arteries to spasm. Gradually taper the dose under medical supervision. Results of other studies do not support the occurrence of a withdrawal syndrome; however, caution is still warranted when discontinuing these agents.

β-blocker withdrawal/nifedipine: Patients recently withdrawn from β-blockers may develop a withdrawal syndrome with increased angina, probably related to increased sensitivity to catecholamines. Initiation of nifedipine will not prevent this occurrence and might exacerbate it by provoking reflex catecholamine release. Taper β-blockers rather than stopping them abruptly before beginning nifedipine.

Nicardipine – Gradually reduce β-blocker dose over 8 to 10 days with coadministration.

Agranulocytosis: In US clinical trials of > 800 patients treated with **bepridil** for up to 5 years, two cases of marked leukopenia and neutropenia were reported. Both patients were diabetic and elderly. One died with overwhelming gram-negative sepsis, itself a possible cause of marked leukopenia. The other recovered rapidly when bepridil was stopped.

Hepatic function impairment: The pharmacokinetics, bioavailability and patient response to **verapamil** and **nifedipine** may be significantly affected by hepatic cirrhosis. With IV verapamil, clearance is greatly reduced, half-life is increased fourfold and volume of distribution is doubled. Peak plasma concentration is higher and occurs earlier; bioavailability is doubled with oral verapamil in cirrhosis. Severe liver dysfunction prolongs **verapamil's** elimination half-life to about 14 to 16 hours; therefore, give ≈ 30% of the normal dose. Bioavailability of nifedipine is increased in hepatic cirrhosis. With IV nifedipine, half-life and volume of distribution are increased and plasma protein binding is decreased. Carefully monitor for abnormal prolongation of the PR interval and other signs of excessive pharmacologic effects.

Since **diltiazem, nicardipine, bepridil, felodipine** and **nimodipine** are extensively metabolized by the liver, use with caution in patients with impaired hepatic function or reduced hepatic blood flow. In patients with severe liver disease, elevated nicardipine blood levels (four-fold increase in AUC) and prolonged half-life (19 hours) occurred; patients receiving nimodipine had substantially reduced clearance and an approximately doubled maximum concentration of the drug. Consider decreasing the dose of calcium channel blockers, and monitor drug response (ie, blood pressure and PR interval) in cirrhosis patients.

Renal function impairment: The pharmacokinetics of **diltiazem** and **verapamil** in patients with impaired renal function are similar to the pharmacokinetic profile of patients with normal renal function. However, caution is still advised. About 70% of a dose of **verapamil** is excreted as metabolites in the urine. Administer verapamil cautiously to patients with impaired renal function. Effects of single IV doses should not increase, although duration may be prolonged.

Nifedipine's plasma concentration is slightly increased in patients with renal impairment. One study showed a significant increase in half-life and volume of distribution at steady state with IV nifedipine. Total body clearance remained the same. Hemodialysis and peritoneal dialysis do not significantly affect nifedipine pharmacokinetics. Although nifedipine has been used safely in patients with renal dysfunction and has exerted a beneficial effect in certain cases, rare, reversible elevations in BUN and serum creatinine have occurred in patients with preexisting chronic renal insufficiency. The relationship to therapy is uncertain in most cases.

Nicardipine's mean plasma concentrations, AUC and maximum concentration were approximately twofold higher in patients with mild renal impairment. Doses must be adjusted. However, one study suggested nicardipine can be used without any dosage adjustment in hypertensive patients with advanced chronic renal failure.

Use **bepridil** with caution in patients with serious renal disorders since the metabolites of bepridil are excreted primarily in the urine.

Increased angina: Occasional patients have increased frequency, duration or severity of angina on starting **nifedipine** or **nicardipine** or at the time of dosage increases. The mechanism of this response is not established.

(Warnings continued on following page)

Warnings (Cont.):

Duchenne's muscular dystrophy: **Verapamil** may decrease neuromuscular transmission in patients with Duchenne's muscular dystrophy, and prolong recovery from the neuromuscular blocking agent vecuronium. It may be necessary to decrease dosage of verapamil when administering it to patients with attenuated neuromuscular transmission. IV verapamil can precipitate respiratory muscle failure in these patients; therefore, use with caution.

Increased intracranial pressure: **IV verapamil** has increased intracranial pressure in patients with supratentorial tumors at the time of anesthesia induction. Use with caution and perform appropriate monitoring.

Carcinogenesis: Rats treated with **nicardipine** showed a dose-dependent increase in thyroid hyperplasia and neoplasia (follicular adenoma carcinoma), possibly linked to a nicardipine-induced reduction in plasma thyroxine levels with a consequent increase in TSH plasma levels. In rats given **nimodipine,** a higher incidence of adenocarcinoma of the uterus and Leydig-cell adenoma of testes occurred. Unilateral follicular adenomas of the thyroid were observed in rats following lifetime high dose **bepridil**. In rats given **isradipine** or **felodipine**, there were dose-dependent increases in benign Leydig cell tumors and testicular hyperplasia.

Elderly: **Verapamil, nifedipine** and **felodipine** may cause a greater hypotensive effect than that seen in younger patients, probably due to age-related changes in drug disposition. With felodipine, monitor blood pressure closely during dosage adjustment; rarely are doses > 10 mg required.

Pregnancy: Category C. Teratogenic and embryotoxic effects have been demonstrated in small animals, usually at doses higher than the usual human dosage. There are no well controlled studies in pregnant women. Use during pregnancy only when clearly needed and when potential benefits outweigh potential hazards to the fetus.

Diltiazem given at 5 to 10 times the human dose resulted in fetal death and skeletal abnormalities; incidence of stillbirths was increased at ≥ 20 times the human dose.

Verapamil, oral in animals with doses 1.5 and 6 times the human dose revealed no evidence of teratogenicity. However, in rats the multiple dose was embryocidal and retarded fetal growth and development, probably due to reduced weight gains in dams. Verapamil crosses the placenta and can be detected in umbilical vein blood at delivery.

Nifedipine has been used in severe pregnancy-associated hypertension, and no adverse fetal effects were determined.

Nicardipine was embryocidal in animals at 75 times, but not 25 to 50 times the human dose. However, dystocia, reduced birth weights, reduced neonatal survival and reduced neonatal weight gain occurred at 50 times the human dose.

Nimodipine in animals has resulted in malformations and stunted fetuses at doses of 1 to 10 mg/kg/day, but not at 3 mg/kg/day in one study. Doses of 30 to 100 mg/kg/day resulted in resorption, stunted growth, stillbirths and higher incidences of skeletal variation.

Bepridil, in rats administered doses 37 times the maximum daily recommended dosage, resulted in reduced litter size at birth.

Isradipine produced a significant reduction in maternal weight gain in rats with a dose 150 times the human dose. Decrements in maternal body weight gain and increased fetal resorptions occurred in rabbits following doses 7.5 and 25 times the human dose. Also, reduced maternal body weight gain during late pregnancy in rats was associated with reduced birth weights and decreased peri and postnatal pup survival.

Felodipine in rabbits at doses 0.4 to 4 times the maximum dosage resulted in digital anomalies (dose-related) in the fetuses, and a prolongation of parturition with difficult labor and increased frequency of fetal and early postnatal deaths occurred in rats. Significant enlargement of the mammary glands also occurred in pregnant rabbits.

Lactation: **Verapamil, diltiazem** and **bepridil** are excreted in breast milk. One report suggests that diltiazem concentrations in breast milk may approximate serum levels. Bepridil is estimated to reach about one third the concentration in serum. Significant concentrations of **nicardipine** and **nimodipine** appear in maternal milk of rats. An insignificant amount of **nifedipine** is transferred into breast milk (over 24 hours, < 5% of a dose). It is not known if **isradipine** or **felodipine** are excreted in breast milk. Decide whether to discontinue nursing or discontinue the drug while these agents are being used, taking into account the importance of the drug to the mother.

Children: Safety and efficacy of **diltiazem, bepridil, felodipine** and **isradipine** have not been established.

Controlled studies of **IV verapamil** have not been conducted in pediatric patients, but uncontrolled experience indicates that results of treatment are similar to those in adults. Patients < 6 months of age may not respond to IV verapamil; this resistance may be related to a developmental difference of AV node responsiveness. However, in rare instances, severe hemodynamic side effects have occurred following IV verapamil administration in neonates and infants (see Administration and Dosage).

(Continued on following page)

Precautions:

Acute hepatic injury: In rare instances, symptoms consistent with acute hepatic injury, as well as significant elevations in enzymes such as alkaline phosphatase, CPK, LDH, AST and ALT have occurred with **diltiazem** and **nifedipine**. These were reversible on drug discontinuation. Drug relationship was uncertain in most cases, but probable in some. These laboratory abnormalities have rarely been associated with clinical symptoms; however, cholestasis with or without jaundice has occurred with **nifedipine**. Rare instances of allergic hepatitis also occurred with **nifedipine**.

Elevations of transaminases with and without concomitant elevations in alkaline phosphatase and bilirubin have occurred with **verapamil**. Elevations have been transient and may disappear with continued verapamil treatment. Several cases of hepatocellular injury related to verapamil have been proven by rechallenge; half of these cases had clinical symptoms (malaise, fever or right upper quadrant pain) in addition to elevations of AST, ALT and alkaline phosphatase. Periodically monitor liver function in patients treated with verapamil.

Isolated cases of elevated LDH, alkaline phosphatase and ALT levels have occurred rarely with **nimodipine.**

Clinically significant transaminase elevations have occurred in approximately 1% of patients receiving **bepridil;** however, no patient became clinically symptomatic or jaundiced, and values returned to normal when the drug was stopped.

Edema, mild to moderate, typically associated with arterial vasodilation and not due to left ventricular dysfunction, occurs in 10% of patients receiving **nifedipine**. It occurs primarily in the lower extremities and usually responds to diuretics. In patients with CHF, differentiate this peripheral edema from the effects of decreasing left ventricular function.

Peripheral edema, generally mild and not associated with generalized fluid retention, may occur with **felodipine** within 2 to 3 weeks of therapy initiation. The incidence is both age- and dose-dependent, with frequency ranging from 10% in patients < 50 years of age taking 5 mg/day to 30% in patients > 60 years of age taking 20 mg/day.

Drug Interactions:

Calcium Channel Blocker Drug Interactions			
Precipitant drug	Object drug*		Description
Barbiturates	Calcium blockers – Verapamil	↓	Verapamil bioavailability may be decreased.
Calcium salts	Calcium blockers – Verapamil	↓	Clinical effects and toxicities of verapamil may be reversed.
Histamine H_2 antagonists	Calcium blockers – Diltiazem, felodipine, nicardipine, nifedipine, verapamil	↑	Cimetidine and ranitidine may increase the bioavailability of diltiazem, felodipine (≈ 50%), nifedipine and nicardipine. Cimetidine may increase verapamil's bioavailability, although this has been refuted.
Quinidine	Calcium blockers – Verapamil, nifedipine	↔	Hypotension, bradycardia, ventricular tachycardia, AV block and pulmonary edema may occur. Use concomitantly only when no other alternatives exist. Serum quinidine levels may also be decreased by nifedipine.
Rifampin	Calcium blockers – Verapamil, oral	↓	Loss of clinical effectiveness of oral verapamil may occur; IV verapamil may circumvent the interaction.
Sulfinpyrazone	Calcium blockers – Verapamil	↓	The clearance of verapamil may be increased.
Vitamin D	Calcium blockers – Verapamil	↓	The therapeutic efficacy of verapamil may be reduced.
Calcium blockers – Nifedipine	Anticoagulants	↑	Rare reports of increased prothrombin time.
Calcium blockers – all	Beta blockers	↑	Although advantageous in some patients, coadministration may also result in increased adverse effects due to depressant effects on myocardial contractility or AV conduction (see Warnings).

* ↑ = Object drug increased. ↓ = Object drug decreased. ↔ = Undetermined effect.

(Drug Interactions continued on following page)

Drug Interactions (Cont.):

Calcium Channel Blockers Drug Interactions (Cont.)			
Precipitant drug	Object drug*		Description
Calcium blockers – Diltiazem, verapamil	Carbamazepine	↑	Increased carbamazepine serum levels with possible toxicity may occur. Nifedipine does not appear to interact.
Calcium blockers – Diltiazem, nicardipine, verapamil	Cyclosporine	↑	Increased cyclosporine levels with possible toxicity may occur. However, verapamil may be nephroprotective when given before cyclosporine. Monitor cyclosporine levels. Nifedipine does not appear to interact.
Calcium blockers – Bepridil, diltiazem, felodipine, nifedipine, verapamil	Digitalis glycosides	↑	Serum digoxin levels may be increased; however, some studies suggest no significant interaction occurs with bepridil, diltiazem or nifedipine. Isradipine and nicardipine do not appear to interact. Verapamil may also increase digitoxin levels.
Calcium blockers – Verapamil	Etomidate	↑	The anesthetic effect of etomidate may be increased with prolonged respiratory depression and apnea.
Calcium blockers – all	Fentanyl	↑	Severe hypotension or increased fluid volume requirements have occurred in patients receiving nifedipine; however, consider for all calcium blockers.
Calcium blockers – Verapamil	Lithium	↔	Both a reduction in lithium levels causing decreased antimanic control and lithium toxicity have occurred.
Calcium blockers – Nifedipine	Magnesium sulfate, parenteral	↑	Neuromuscular blockade and hypotension have occurred with coadministration.
Calcium blockers – Verapamil	Nondepolarizing muscle relaxants	↑	Muscle relaxant effects may be enhanced, respiratory depression may be prolonged.
Calcium blockers – Verapamil	Prazosin	↑	Prazosin serum concentrations may be increased which may increase the sensitivity to prazosin-induced postural hypotension.
Calcium blockers – Diltiazem, nifedipine, verapamil	Theophyllines	↑	The pharmacologic actions of theophyllines may be enhanced, particularly drug intoxication.

* ↑ = Object drug increased. ↓ = Object drug decreased. ↔ = Undetermined effect.

Drug/Food interactions: Food (specifically a low-fat meal) may slow the rate but not extent of **nifedipine** absorption; therefore, nifedipine may be administered without regard to meals.

When **nicardipine** was given 1 or 3 hours after a high-fat meal, the mean maximum concentration and AUC were 20% to 30% lower compared to fasting subjects.

Administration of **bepridil** after a meal results in a clinically insignificant delay in time to peak concentration, but neither peak plasma levels nor the extent of absorption was changed.

Administration of **isradipine** with food significantly increases the time to peak by about an hour, but has no effect on the total bioavailability of the drug.

The administration of sustained release **verapamil** with food increases the time to reach maximum plasma levels of the parent drug as well as the metabolite norverapamil; however, the bioavailability is not appreciably affected; therefore, it may be administered without regard to meals.

Bioavailability of **felodipine** is not affected by food. However, felodipine bioavailability increased more than two fold when taken with doubly concentrated grapefruit juice compared to water or orange juice.

(Continued on following page)

Adverse Reactions:

Generally not serious; rarely require discontinuation of therapy or dosage adjustment.

Adverse Reactions of Calcium Channel Blockers (%)

	Adverse Reactions	Nifedipine[1]	Verapamil Oral (IV)	Diltiazem[1]	Nicardipine	Nimodipine	Bepridil	Isradipine	Felodipine
Cardiovascular	Peripheral edema	10-30	2.1	2.4-9	7.1-8	0.4-1.2	≤ 2	7.2	22.3
	Hypotension	≤ 1-5	2.5 (1.5)	1	< 0.4	1.2-8.1		≤ 1	≤ 1.5
	Palpitations	≤ 2-7	< 1	< 1	3.3-4.1	< 1	0-6.5	4[2]	1.8
	Syncope	≤ 1	< 1	< 1	0.8			≤ 1	≤ 1.5
	AV block (1°, 2° or 3°)		0.8-1.2	0.6-7.6	< 0.4				≤ 1.5
	Bradycardia		1.4 (1.2)	1.5-6		0.6-1	≤ 2		
	Congestive heart failure	2-6.7	1.8	< 1		< 1		≤ 1	
	Myocardial infarction	4-6.7	< 1		< 0.4			≤ 1	≤ 1.5
	Arrhythmia (unspecified)	≤ 1		< 1					≤ 1.5
	Pulmonary edema	7	1.8						
	Angina	≤ 1		<1	5.6			2.4	≤ 1.5
	Tachycardia	≤ 1	(1)	< 1	0.8-3.4	1	≤ 2	1.5	≤ 1.5
	Abnormal ECG			4.1	0.6	0.6-1.4			
	Ventricular extrasystoles			< 1	†				
Central Nervous System	Dizziness/lightheadedness	4.1-27	3.5 (1.2)	1.5-7	4-6.9	< 1	11.6-27	7.3	5.8
	Drowsiness						≥ 7	≤ 1	
	Nervousness	≤ 2-7		< 1	0.6		7.4-11.6	≤ 1	≤ 1.5
	Sleep disturbances	≤ 2	< 0.5	< 1					
	Psychiatric disturbances (depression, amnesia, paranoia, psychosis, hallucinations)	†	< 1 (†)	< 1	†	1.4	≤ 2	≤ 1	≤ 1.5
	Blurred vision/equilibrium disturbances	≤ 2	< 0.5		†		≤ 2	≤ 1	
	Headache	10-23	2.2 (1.2)	2.1-12	6.4-8.2	1.4-4.1	6.9-13.6	13.7	18.6
	Weakness/shakiness/jitteriness	≤ 2-12	< 1	1.2	0.6			1.2	
	Paresthesia	< 3	< 1	<1	1		2.5	≤ 1	2.5
	Somnolence	< 3	< 1	1.3	1.1-1.4				≤ 1.5
	Asthenia	< 3	1.7	2.8-5	4.2-5.8		6.5-14		4.7
	Insomnia	< 3		1	0.6		2.7	≤ 1	≤ 1.5
	Abnormal dreams	≤ 1		< 1	0.4				
	Confusion		< 1		†				
	Tinnitus	≤ 1		< 1	†		0-6.5		
	Malaise	≤ 1			0.6				
	Anxiety	≤ 1			†		≤ 2		≤ 1.5
Gastrointestinal	Nausea	3.3-11	2.7 (0.9)	1.6-1.9	1.9-2.2	0.6-1.4	7-26	1.8	1.9
	Diarrhea	< 3	< 1	< 1		1.7-4.2	0-10.9	1.1	1.6
	Constipation	≤ 3.3	7.3	1.6	0.6		2.8	≤ 1	1.6
	Hepatitis/hepatotoxicity	< 0.5	†			< 1			
	Abdominal discomfort/cramps/dyspepsia	≤ 3	< 1 (0.6)	1.3	0.8-1.5	2	3-6.8	1.7	1.8-2.3
	Dysgeusia	≤ 1		< 1					
	Vomiting	≤ 1		< 1	0.4	< 1		1.1	≤ 1.5
	Dry mouth	< 3	< 1	< 1	0.4-1.4		3.4	≤ 1	≤ 1.5
	Flatulence	≤ 3					≤ 2		≤ 1.5

[1] Includes data for sustained release form.
[2] Appears to be dose-related.
† Occurs, no incidence reported.

(Adverse Reactions continued on following page)

Adverse Reactions (Cont.):

Adverse Reactions of Calcium Channel Blockers (%) (Cont.)									
	Adverse Reactions	Nifedipine[1]	Verapamil Oral (IV)	Diltiazem[1]	Nicardipine	Nimodipine	Bepridil	Isradipine	Felodipine
Dermatologic	Dermatitis/rash	≤ 3	1.2	1-1.5	0.4-1.2	0.6-2.4	≤ 2	1.5	1.5
	Pruritus/urticaria	≤ 3	< 1 (†)	< 1		< 1		≤ 1	≤ 1.5
	Hair loss	≤ 1	< 0.5	†					
	Photosensitivity	†		< 1					
	Erythema multiforme	†	< 1	†					
	Stevens-Johnson syndrome	†	< 1	†					
Hematologic	Anemia	< 0.5				< 1			≤ 1.5
	Leukopenia	< 0.5		†				≤ 1	
	Thrombocytopenia	< 0.5				< 1			
	Petechiae/ecchymosis/ purpura/bruising/ hematoma	< 0.5	< 1	< 1		< 1			
Other	Flushing	< 3-25	< 1	1.7-3	5.6-9.7	1-2.1		2.6	6.4
	Nasal/chest congestion/ rhinitis/sinusitis	≤ 2-6	†	< 1	†		≤ 2		≤ 1.5
	Gingival hyperplasia	≤ 1	†	†					< 0.5
	Polyuria/nocturia	< 3	< 1	1.3	0.4			≤ 1	
	Sweating	≤ 2	1 (†)			< 1	≤ 2	≤ 1	
	Sexual difficulties	≤ 3	< 1	< 1	†		≤ 2	≤ 1	≤ 1.5
	Shortness of breath/ dyspnea/wheezing	≤ 2-8	1.4	< 1	0.6	1.2	0-8.7	1.8	≤ 1.5
	Muscle cramps/inflamma- tion/pain	≤ 2-8	< 1			0.2-1.4			≤ 1.9
	Joint stiffness/pain/ arthritis	≤ 3		< 1	†				
	Gynecomastia	†	†	†					
	Hyperglycemia	†		< 1					
	Weight gain	≤ 1		< 1					
	Epistaxis	≤ 1		< 1					≤ 1.5
	Cough	6					≤ 2	≤ 1	2.9
	Anorexia			< 1			≤ 7		
	Respiratory infection	≤ 1					2.8		≤ 5.5

[1] Includes data for sustained release form. † Occurs, no incidence reported.

In addition to the adverse effects listed in the table, the following have been reported:

Nifedipine: Giddiness (27%); fever, chills (≤ 3%); facial and periorbital edema, ataxia, hypertonia, hypoesthesia, migraine, gastroesophageal reflux, melena, gout, respiratory disorder, abnormal lacrimation, breast pain, dysuria, eructation, hematuria (≤ 1%); transient blindness, erythromelalgia (< 0.5%); neuromuscular effects (myoclonic dystonia); dysosmia; hypokalemia.

Verapamil: Claudication, hyperkeratosis, spotty menstruation, atrioventricular dissociation, cerebrovascular accident (< 1%); rotary nystagmus; tachyphylaxis, hyperprolactinemia with galactorrhea (one case).

Diltiazem: Gait abnormality, tremor, amblyopia, eye irritation, bundle branch block, amnesia, thirst (< 1%).

Nicardipine: Infection; allergic reaction; atypical chest pain; peripheral vascular disease; sore throat; hyperkinesia.

Nimodipine: Acne (1%); GI hemorrhage, rebound vasospasm, jaundice, hypertension, hyponatremia, disseminated intravascular coagulation, deep vein thrombosis (< 1%).

Bepridil: Hand tremor (≤ 9.3%); GI distress, tremor (≤ 7%); flu syndrome (2%); fever, pain, myalgic asthenia, superinfection, hypertension, vasodilation, ventricular premature contractions, prolonged QT interval (see Warnings), pharyngitis, gastritis, appetite increase, arthritis, fainting, akathisia, adverse behavior effect, skin irritation, taste change (≤ 2%).

(Adverse Reactions continued on following page)

Refer to general discussion of these agents on page 688.

NICARDIPINE HCl

Indications:

Oral: Immediate release only – Chronic stable (effort-associated) angina. Use alone or with beta-blockers.

Immediate and sustained release – Management of essential hypertension alone or with other antihypertensives. Be aware of the relatively large peak to trough differences in blood pressure effect.

IV: Short-term treatment of hypertension when oral therapy is not feasible or not desirable. For prolonged control of blood pressure, transfer patients to oral therapy as soon as their clinical condition permits.

Administration and Dosage:

Approved by the FDA in December 1988.

Oral: Angina (immediate release only) – Individualize dosage. Usual initial dose is 20 mg 3 times/day (range, 20 to 40 mg 3 times/day). Allow at least 3 days before increasing dose to ensure achievement of steady-state plasma drug concentrations.

Hypertension – Individualize dosage.

Immediate release: Initial dose is 20 mg 3 times daily (range, 20 to 40 mg 3 times daily). The maximum blood pressure-lowering effect occurs ≈ 1 to 2 hours after dosing. To assess adequacy of blood pressure response, measure blood pressure 8 hours after dosing. Because of nicardipine's prominent peak effects, measure blood pressure 1 to 2 hours after dosing, particularly during initiation of therapy. Allow at least 3 days before increasing dose to ensure achievement of steady-state plasma drug concentrations.

Sustained release: Initial dose is 30 mg twice daily. Effective doses have ranged from 30 to 60 mg twice daily. The maximum blood pressure lowering effect at steady state is sustained from 2 until 6 hours after dosing. When initiating therapy or increasing the dose, measure blood pressure 2 to 4 hours after the first dose or dose increase, as well as at the end of a dosing interval.

The total daily dose of immediate release nicardipine may not be a useful guide in judging the effective dose of the sustained release form. Titrate patients currently receiving the immediate release form with the sustained release form starting at their current daily dose of immediate release, then reexamine to assess adequacy of blood pressure control.

Renal impairment – Titrate dose beginning with 20 mg 3 times a day (immediate release) or 30 mg twice daily (sustained release).

Hepatic impairment – Starting dose is 20 mg twice a day (immediate release) with individual titration.

IV: For IV use only. Individualize dosage. Monitor blood pressure during and after the infusion; avoid too rapid or excessive reduction in either systolic or diastolic blood pressure during treatment.

Preparation – Warning: Amps must be diluted before infusion.

Dilution: Dilute each amp with 240 ml of one of the following compatible IV fluids, resulting in 250 ml of solution containing 0.1 mg/ml.

IV compatibilities and incompatibilities: Nicardipine is compatible and stable in glass or polyvinyl chloride containers for 24 hours at controlled room temperature with the following – 5% Dextrose, USP; 5% Dextrose and 0.45% NaCl, USP; 5% Dextrose and 0.9% NaCl, USP; 5% Dextrose with 40 mEq Potassium, USP; 0.45% and 0.9% NaCl, USP.

Nicardipine IV is incompatible with 5% Sodium Bicarbonate, USP and Lactated Ringer's, USP.

Dosage – Substitute for oral nicardipine therapy: The IV infusion rate required to produce an average plasma concentration equivalent to a given oral dose at steady state is as follows:

Equivalent IV Nicardipine Dose to Oral Therapy	
Oral dose	Equivalent IV infusion
20 mg every 8 hrs	0.5 mg/hr
30 mg every 8 hrs	1.2 mg/hr
40 mg every 8 hrs	2.2 mg/hr

(Administration and Dosage continued on following page)

Refer to general discussion of these agents on page 688.

NICARDIPINE HCl

Administration and Dosage (Cont.):

IV: Dosage – (Cont.):

Initiation of therapy in a drug free patient: The time course of blood pressure decrease is dependent on the initial rate of infusion and the frequency of dosage adjustment. Administer by slow continuous infusion at a concentration of 0.1 mg/ml. Blood pressure begins to fall within minutes. It reaches about 50% of its ultimate decrease in about 45 minutes and does not reach final steady state for about 50 hours. When treating acute hypertensive episodes in patients with chronic hypertension, discontinuation of infusion is followed by a 50% offset of action in 30 ± 7 minutes but plasma levels and gradually decreasing effects exist for about 50 hours.

Titration – For gradual blood pressure reduction, initiate at 50 ml/hr (5 mg/hr). The infusion rate may be increased to 25 ml/hr (2.5 mg/hr) every 15 minutes to a maximum of 150 ml/hr (15 mg/hr) until the desired effect is achieved.

For more rapid reduction, initiate at 50 ml/hr. Increase infusion rate by 25 ml/hr every 5 minutes to a maximum of 150 ml/hr until the desired effect is achieved. Once the blood pressure goal is achieved, decrease the rate to 30 ml/hr (3 mg/hr).

Maintenance – Adjust the rate of infusion as needed to maintain the desired response.

Conditions requiring infusion adjustment – Hypotension or tachycardia: Discontinue the infusion if there is impending concern of hypotension or tachycardia. When blood pressure has stabilized, infusion may be restarted at low doses (eg, 30 to 50 ml/hr) and adjusted as necessary.

Infusion site change: Continue as long as blood pressure control is needed. Change the infusion site every 12 hours if administered via a peripheral vein.

Cardiac, hepatic or renal function impairment: Use caution when titrating nicardipine IV in patients with these conditions.

Transfer to oral antihypertensive agents – If transfer is to an oral agent other than nicardipine, initiate therapy upon discontinuation of the infusion. If oral nicardipine is to be used, administer the first dose 1 hour prior to infusion discontinuation.

Storage/Stability – Store at controlled room temperature (15° to 30°C; 59° to 86°F). Avoid exposure to elevated temperatures. Freezing does not adversely affect the product. Protect from light; store amps in carton until used. The diluted solution is stable for 24 hours at room temperature.

	Product	Dosage form	Description	C.I.*
Rx	**Cardene** (Syntex)	**Capsules:** 20 mg	(Cardene 20 mg/Syntex 2437). White. In 100s, 500s and UD 100s.	142
		30 mg	(Cardene 30 mg/Syntex 2438). Blue. In 100s, 500s and UD 100s.	149
Rx	**Cardene SR** (Syntex)	**Capsules, sustained release:** 30 mg[1]	(Cardene SR 30 mg Syntex 2440). Pink. In 60s, 200s and UD 100s.	NA
		45 mg[1]	(Cardene SR 45 mg Syntex 2441). Powder blue. In 60s, 200s and UD 100s.	NA
		60 mg[1]	(Cardene SR 60 mg Syntex 2442). Light blue/white. In 60s, 200s and UD 100s.	NA
Rx	**Cardene IV** (DuPont Pharm)	**Injection:** 25 mg (2.5 mg/ml)	In 10 ml amps.[2]	NA

* Cost Index based on cost per 60 mg nicardipine.

[1] With lactose.

[2] With Water for Injection, USP, 48 mg sorbitol, 0.525 mg citric acid monohydrate and 0.09 mg sodium hydroxide.

Refer to general discussion of these agents on page 688.

BEPRIDIL HCl

Indications:

Treatment of chronic stable angina (classic effort-associated angina). Because bepridil has caused serious ventricular arrhythmias, including torsade de pointes type ventricular tachycardia, and the occurrence of agranulocytosis associated with its use, reserve for patients who have failed to respond optimally to, or are intolerant of, other antianginals.

Bepridil may be used alone or with beta blockers or nitrates. An added effect occurs when administered to patients already receiving propranolol.

Administration and Dosage:

Approved by the FDA in December 1990.

Individualize dosage. Usual initial dose is 200 mg/day. After 10 days, dosage may be adjusted upward depending on response. Most patients are maintained at 300 mg. Maximum daily dose is 400 mg; minimum effective dose is 200 mg.

Elderly: Starting dose does not differ from that for younger patients; however, after therapeutic response is demonstrated, the elderly may require more frequent monitoring.

Rx	**Vascor** (McNeil)	**Tablets:** 200 mg[1]	(Vascor 200). Light blue, scored. Film coated. In 30s & UD 100s.
		300 mg[1]	(Vascor 300). Blue. Film coated. In 30s and UD 100s.
		400 mg[1]	(Vascor 400). Dark blue. Film coated. In 30s and UD 100s.

ISRADIPINE

Indications:

Management of hypertension, alone or concurrently with thiazide-type diuretics.

Administration and Dosage:

Approved by the FDA in December 1990.

Individualize dosage. Recommended initial dose is 2.5 mg twice daily. An antihypertensive response usually occurs within 2 to 3 hours; maximal response may require 2 to 4 weeks. If a satisfactory response does not occur after this period, the dose may be adjusted in increments of 5 mg/day at 2 to 4 week intervals up to a maximum of 20 mg/day. However, most patients show no additional response to doses > 10 mg/day, and adverse effects are increased in frequency above 10 mg/day.

Rx	**DynaCirc** (Sandoz)	**Capsules:** 2.5 mg	(DynaCirc 2.5). White. In 60s, 100s and UD 100s.
		5 mg	(DynaCirc 5). Light pink. In 60s, 100s and UD 100s.

NIMODIPINE

Indications:

Improvement of neurological deficits due to spasm following subarachnoid hemorrhage (SAH) from ruptured congenital intracranial aneurysms in patients who are in good neurological condition post-ictus (eg, Hunt and Hess Grades I-III).

Administration and Dosage:

Approved by the FDA in December 1988.

Commence therapy within 96 hours of the SAH, using 60 mg every 4 hours for 21 consecutive days.

If the capsule cannot be swallowed (eg, time of surgery, unconscious patient), make a hole in both ends of the capsule with an 18 gauge needle and extract the contents into a syringe. Empty the contents into the patient's in situ naso-gastric tube and wash down the tube with 30 ml normal saline.

				C.I.*
Rx	**Nimotop** (Miles Inc.)	**Capsules, liquid:** 30 mg	(Miles 855). Ivory. In UD 100s.	800

* Cost Index based on cost per 300 mg nimodipine.

[1] With lactose.

Refer to the general discussion of these agents on page 688.

FELODIPINE

Indications:

Treatment of hypertension, alone or concurrently with other antihypertensives.

Administration and Dosage:

Approved by the FDA in August 1991.

Individualize dosage. Initial dose is 5 mg once daily. Adjust according to response, generally at intervals of not less than 2 weeks. Usual dosage range is 5 to 10 mg once daily. Maximum dosage is 20 mg once daily; this dose results in an increased blood pressure response as well as a large increase in the rate of peripheral edema and other vasodilatory adverse reactions. Closely monitor blood pressure in elderly patients > 65 years of age and in patients with impaired hepatic function during dosage adjustment; generally, do not consider doses > 10 mg.

Swallow whole; do not crush or chew.

Rx	**Plendil** (MSD)	**Tablets, extended release:** 5 mg[1]	(Plendil MSD 451). Light red-brown, convex. In 30s, 100s and UD 100s.
		10 mg[1]	(Plendil MSD 452). Red-brown, convex. In 30s, 100s and UD 100s.

[1] With lactose.

Refer to the general discussion of these agents on page 688.

DILTIAZEM HCl

Indications:

Oral: Angina pectoris due to coronary artery spasm.
Chronic stable angina (classic effort-associated angina).
Sustained release – Only for management of essential hypertension.

Parenteral: Atrial fibrillation or flutter.
Paroxysmal supraventricular tachycardia.

Administration and Dosage:

Approved by the FDA in 1982.

Oral: Individualize dosage.

Tablets – Start with 30 mg 4 times/day, before meals and at bedtime; gradually increase dosage to 180 to 360 mg (given in divided doses 3 or 4 times/day) at 1 to 2 day intervals until optimum response is obtained.

Sustained release – Cardizem SR: Start with 60 to 120 mg twice daily. Adjust dosage when maximum antihypertensive effect is achieved (usually by 14 days chronic therapy). Optimum dosage range is 240 to 360 mg/day, but some patients may respond to lower doses.

Cardizem CD: 180 to 240 mg once daily; some patients may respond to lower doses. Maximum antihypertensive effect is usually achieved by 14 days chronic therapy; therefore, adjust dosage accordingly. Usual range is 240 to 360 mg once daily; experience with doses > 360 mg is limited.

Dilacor XR: 180 to 240 mg once daily; adjust dose as needed. Usual range is 180 to 480 mg once daily. Although current clinical experience with the 540 mg dose is limited, the dose may be increased to 540 mg with little or no increased risk of adverse reactions. Do not open, chew or crush the capsules; swallow whole.

Parenteral: Direct IV single injections (bolus) – The initial dose is 0.25 mg/kg as a bolus administered over 2 minutes (20 mg is a reasonable dose for the average patient). If response is inadequate, a second dose may be administered after 15 minutes. The second bolus dose should be 0.35 mg/kg administered over 2 minutes (25 mg is a reasonable dose for the average patient). Individualize subsequent IV bolus doses. Dose patients with low body weights on a mg/kg basis. Some patients may respond to an initial dose of 0.15 mg/kg, although duration of action may be shorter.

Continuous IV infusion – For continued reduction of the heart rate (up to 24 hours) in patients with atrial fibrillation or atrial flutter, an IV infusion may be administered. Immediately following bolus administration of 20 mg (0.25 mg/kg) or 25 mg (0.35 mg/kg) and reduction of heart rate, begin an IV infusion. The recommended initial infusion rate is 10 mg/hr. Some patients may maintain response to an initial rate of 5 mg/hr. The infusion rate may be increased in 5 mg/hr increments up to 15 mg/hr as needed, if further reduction in heart rate is required. The infusion may be maintained for up to 24 hours. Therefore, infusion duration longer than 24 hours and infusion rates > 15 mg/hr are not recommended.

Dilution – For continuous IV infusion, aseptically transfer the appropriate quantity (see table) to the desired volume of either Normal Saline, D5W, or D5W/0.45% NaCl. Mix thoroughly. Use within 24 hours. Keep refrigerated until use.

Dilution of Diltiazem Injection

Diluent volume (ml)	Quantity of diltiazem injection	Final concentration (mg/ml)	Administration	
			Dose[1] (mg/hr)	Infusion rate (ml/hr)
100	125 mg (25 ml)	1	10 15	10 15
250	250 mg (50 ml)	0.83	10 15	12 18
500	250 mg (50 ml)	0.45	10 15	22 33

[1] 5 mg/hr may be appropriate for some patients.

Admixture compatibility/incompatibility – Diltiazem is physically compatible and chemically stable in the following parenteral solutions for at least 24 hours when stored in glass or PVC bags at controlled room temperature (15° to 30°C; 59° to 86°F) or refrigerated (2° to 8°C; 36° to 46°F): 5% Dextrose Injection, USP; 0.9% Sodium Chloride Injection, USP; 5% Dextrose and 0.45% Sodium Chloride Injection, USP.

Diltiazem is incompatible when mixed directly with furosemide solution.

(Administration and Dosage continued on following page)

Refer to the general discussion of these agents on page 688.

DILTIAZEM HCl (Cont.)

Administration and Dosage (Cont.):

Concomitant therapy with β-blockers or digitalis is usually well tolerated, but the effects of coadministration cannot be predicted, especially in patients with left ventricular dysfunction or cardiac conduction abnormalities. Use caution in titrating dosages for impaired renal or hepatic function patients, since dosage requirements are not available.

Sublingual nitroglycerin may be taken as required to abort acute anginal attacks. Diltiazem may be safely used with short-acting and long-acting nitrates, but no controlled studies have evaluated the antianginal efficacy of this combination.

An additive antihypertensive effect occurs when diltiazem is coadministered with other antihypertensives. Adjust the dose of diltiazem or the concomitant antihypertensive accordingly.

Storage/Stability: Store injection under refrigeration at 2° to 8°C (36° to 46°F). Do not freeze. May be stored at room temperature for up to 1 month; destroy after 1 month at room temperature. Discard unused portion of single-use containers.

	Product	Dosage form	Description	C.I.*
Rx	**Cardizem** (Marion Merrell Dow)	**Tablets:** 30 mg	(Marion 1771). Green. In 100s, 500s and UD 100s.	181
		60 mg	(Marion 1772). Yellow, scored. In 90s, 100s, 500s and UD 100s.	148
		90 mg	(Cardizem 90 mg). Green, scored. In 90s, 100s and UD 100s.	155
		120 mg	(Cardizem 120 mg). Yellow, scored. In 100s and UD 100s.	140
Rx	**Cardizem SR** (Marion Merrell Dow)	**Capsules, sustained release:** 60 mg	(Cardizem SR 60 mg). Ivory and brown. In 100s and UD 100s.	161
		90 mg	(Cardizem SR 90 mg). Gold and brown. In 100s and UD 100s.	156
		120 mg	(Cardizem SR 120 mg). Caramel and brown. In 100s and UD 100s.	152
Rx	**Cardizem CD** (Marion Merrell Dow)	**Capsules, sustained release:** 180 mg	Sucrose. (1796 180 mg). Turquoise/blue. In 30, 90s and UD 100s.	NA
		240 mg	Sucrose. (1797 240 mg). Blue. In 30s, 90s and UD 100s.	NA
		300 mg	Sucrose. (1798 300 mg). Gray/blue. In 30s, 90s and UD 100s.	NA
Rx	**Dilacor XR** (Rhone-Poulenc Rorer)	**Capsules, sustained release:** 180 mg	(Dilacor XR 180 mg 0251). Orange/white. In 100s and UD 100s.	NA
		240 mg	(Dilacor XR 240 mg 0252). Brown/white. In 100s and UD 100s.	NA
Rx	**Cardizem** (Marion Merrell Dow)	**Injection:** 25 mg (5 mg/ml)	In 5 ml vials.[1]	NA
		50 mg (5 mg/ml)	In 10 ml vials.[2]	NA

* Cost Index based on cost per 120 mg diltiazem.

[1] With 3.75 mg citric acid, 3.25 mg sodium citrate dihydrate and 357 mg sorbitol solution.

[2] With 7.5 mg citric acid, 6.5 mg sodium citrate dihydrate and 714 mg sorbitol solution.

Refer to general discussion of these agents on page 688.

VERAPAMIL HCl

Indications:

Oral: Angina. Treatment of vasospastic (Prinzmetal's variant), chronic stable (classic effort-associated) and unstable (crescendo, preinfarction) angina.

Arrhythmias. With digitalis to control ventricular rate at rest and during stress in chronic atrial flutter or fibrillation. May use for prophylaxis of repetitive paroxysmal supraventricular tachycardia (PSVT).

Essential hypertension.

Sustained release – Only for management of essential hypertension.

Parenteral: Treatment of supraventricular tachyarrhythmias.

Temporary control of rapid ventricular rate in atrial flutter or atrial fibrillation.

Administration and Dosage:

If heart failure is not severe or rate-related, use digitalis and diuretics, as appropriate, *before* verapamil. In moderately severe to severe cardiac dysfunction (PCWP > 20 mm Hg, ejection fraction < 30%), acute worsening of heart failure may occur.

Individualize dosage. Do not exceed 480 mg/day; safety and efficacy are not established. Half-life increases during chronic use; maximum response may be delayed.

Oral: Angina at rest and chronic stable angina – Usual initial dose is 80 to 120 mg 3 times a day. However, 40 mg 3 times a day may be warranted if patients may have increased response to verapamil (eg, decreased hepatic function, elderly). Base upward titration on safety and efficacy evaluated ≈ 8 hours after dosing. Increase dosage daily (eg, unstable angina) or weekly until optimum clinical response is obtained.

Arrhythmias – Dosage range in digitalized patients with chronic atrial fibrillation is 240 to 320 mg/day in divided doses 3 or 4 times a day. Dosage range for prophylaxis of PSVT (non-digitalized patients) is 240 to 480 mg/day in divided doses 3 or 4 times/day. In general, maximum effects will be apparent during the first 48 hours of therapy.

Essential hypertension – The usual initial monotherapy dose is 80 mg 3 times/day (240 mg/day). Daily dosages of 360 and 480 mg have been used, but there is no evidence that dosages > 360 mg provide added effect. Consider beginning titration at 40 mg 3 times/day in patients who might respond to lower doses, (eg, elderly or people of small stature). Antihypertensive effects are evident within the first week of therapy. Base upward titration on therapeutic efficacy, assessed at the end of the dosing interval.

Sustained release (essential hypertension) – Give with food. Usual daily dose is 240 mg/day, in the morning. However, 120 mg/day may be warranted in patients who may have increased response (eg, elderly or people of small stature). Base upward titration on safety and efficacy evaluated ≈ 24 hours after dosing. If adequate response is not obtained, titrate upward to 240 mg/morning and 120 mg/evening, then 240 mg every 12 hours, if needed. When switching from immediate release tablets, total daily dose (in mg) may remain the same. Antihypertensive effects are evident within the first week.

Parenteral (supraventricular tachyarrhythmias): For IV use only. Give as slow IV injection over at least 2 min under continuous ECG and blood pressure monitoring. A small fraction (< 1%) of patients may have life-threatening adverse responses (rapid ventricular rate in atrial flutter/fibrillation, marked hypotension or extreme bradycardia/asystole); monitor initial use of IV verapamil and have resuscitation facilities available. An IV infusion has been used (5 mg/hour); precede the infusion with an IV loading dose.

Initial dose – 5 to 10 mg (0.075 to 0.15 mg/kg) as IV bolus over 2 minutes.

Repeat dose – 10 mg (0.15 mg/kg) 30 minutes after the first dose if the initial response is not adequate.

Older patients – Give over at least 3 min to minimize risk of untoward drug effects.

Children – ≤ 1 year: 0.1 to 0.2 mg/kg (usual single dose range, 0.75 to 2 mg) as an IV bolus over 2 minutes (under continuous ECG monitoring).

1 to 15 years: 0.1 to 0.3 mg/kg (usual single dose range, 2 to 5 mg) IV over 2 minutes. Do not exceed 5 mg.

Repeat dose: Repeat above dose 30 minutes after the first dose if the initial response is not adequate (under continuous ECG monitoring). Do not exceed a single dose of 10 mg in patients 1 to 15 years of age.

Incompatibility: A crystalline precipitate immediately forms when verapamil is administered into an infusion line containing 0.45% sodium chloride with sodium bicarbonate. A milky white precipitate forms when verapamil is given by IV push into the same line being used for nafcillin infusion.

For stability reasons this product is not recommended for dilution with sodium lactate injection in polyvinyl chloride bags. Avoid admixing IV verapamil with albumin, amphotericin B, hydralazine HCl, aminophylline and trimethoprim/sulfamethoxazole. Verapamil will precipitate in any solution with a pH above 6.

Storage: Protect IV solution from light. Discard any unused amount of solution.

(Continued on following page)

VERAPAMIL HCl (Cont.)

	Product	Form/Strength	Description	C.I.*
Rx	**Verapamil HCl** (Rugby)	**Tablets:** 40 mg	In 100s.	NA
Rx	**Calan** (Searle)		(Calan 40). Pink. Film coated. In 100s.	203
Rx	**Isoptin** (Knoll)		Scored. Film coated. In 100s and UD 100s.	203
Rx	**Verapamil HCl** (Various, eg, Barr, Bioline, Geneva, Lederle, Moore, Parmed, Rugby, Schein, URL)	**Tablets:** 80 mg	In 100s, 250s, 500s, 1000s and UD 100s.	47+
Rx	**Calan** (Searle)		(Calan 80). Peach, scored. Oval. Film coated. In 100s, 500s, 1000s and UD 100s.	146
Rx	**Isoptin** (Knoll)		(Knoll Isoptin 80). Yellow, scored. Film coated. In 100s, 500s, 1000s and UD 100s.	139
Rx	**Verapamil HCl** (Various, eg, Barr, Bioline, Geneva, Lederle, Moore, Parmed, Rugby, Schein, URL)	**Tablets:** 120 mg	In 100s, 250s, 500s, 1000s and UD 100s.	42+
Rx	**Calan** (Searle)		(Calan 120). Brown, scored. Oval. Film coated. In 100s, 500s, 1000s and UD 100s.	131
Rx	**Isoptin** (Knoll)		(Knoll Isoptin 120). White, scored. Film coated. In 100s, 500s, 1000s and UD 100s.	131
Rx	**Calan SR** (Searle)	**Tablets, sustained release:** 120 mg	(Calan SR 120). Light violet. Film coated. Oval. In 100s and UD 100s.	NA
Rx	**Isoptin SR** (Knoll)		(Knoll 120 SR). Light violet. Film coated. Oval. In 100s and UD 100s.	NA
Rx	**Calan SR** (Searle)	**Tablets, sustained release:** 180 mg	Light pink, scored. Oval. Film coated. In 100s and UD 100s.	NA
Rx	**Isoptin SR** (Knoll)		(Isoptin SR 180 mg). Light pink, scored. Film coated. Oval. In 100s and UD 100s.	NA
Rx	**Calan SR** (Searle)	**Tablets, sustained release:** 240 mg	(Calan SR 240). Light green, scored. Capsule shape. Film coated. In 100s, 500s and UD 100s.	129
Rx	**Isoptin SR** (Knoll)		(Isoptin SR). Light green, scored. Film coated. Capsule shape. In 100s, 500s and UD 100s.	129
Rx	**Verelan** (Lederle)	**Capsules, sustained release:** 120 mg	(Lederle V8 Verelan 120 mg). Yellow. In 100s.	NA
		180 mg	In 100s.	NA
		240 mg	(Lederle V9 Verelan 240 mg). Blue/yellow. In 100s.	NA
Rx	**Verapamil HCl** (Various, eg, Abbott, American Regent, IMS, Lyphomed, Quad, Solopak)	**Injection:** 5 mg/2 ml	In 2 and 4 ml vials, amps and syringes and 4 ml fill in 5 ml vials.	420+
Rx	**Isoptin** (Knoll)		In 2 and 4 ml amps, vials and disp. syringes.	2041

* Cost Index based on cost per 240 mg oral or 5 mg parenteral verapamil.

CYCLANDELATE

Actions:

Cyclandelate is a musculotropic, direct-acting vascular smooth muscle relaxant with no significant adrenergic stimulating or blocking actions. Drug activity measured by pharmacological tests against various types of smooth muscle spasm produced by acetylcholine, histamine and barium chloride, exceeds that of papaverine, particularly in regard to the neurotropic component produced by acetylcholine. Cyclandelate is also a mild calcium entry blocker and is active in calcium overload situations; this mechanism may be responsible for the improved blood flow properties and inhibition of platelet aggregation that occur with cyclandelate.

Indications:

"Possibly effective" for adjunctive therapy in intermittent claudication; arteriosclerosis obliterans; thrombophlebitis (to control associated vasospasm and muscular ischemia); nocturnal leg cramps; Raynaud's phenomenon; selected cases of ischemic cerebral vascular disease.

Unlabeled Uses: Cyclandelate (1200 to 1600 mg/day) has been used in the treatment of dementia of cerebrovascular origin and multi-infarct dementia, various memory disorders, migraine prophylaxis, vertigo of circulatory origin, tinnitus and visual disturbances attributable to chronic cerebrovascular insufficiency and diabetic peripheral polyneuropathy.

Contraindications:

Hypersensitivity to cyclandelate.

Warnings:

Use with extreme caution in patients with severe obliterative coronary artery or cerebral vascular disease; these diseased areas may be compromised by vasodilatory effects of the drug elsewhere.

Although prolongation of bleeding time did not occur with therapeutic dosages, it occurred in animals at very large doses. Consider this hazard when administering cyclandelate to a patient with active bleeding or a bleeding tendency.

Pregnancy: Safety for use during pregnancy has not been established. Use only when clearly needed and when the potential benefits outweigh the potential hazards to the fetus.

Lactation: Safety for use in nursing has not been established. Use only when clearly needed and when potential benefits outweigh potential hazards to the nursing infant.

Precautions:

Use with caution in patients with glaucoma.

Adverse Reactions:

GI: Heartburn, pain and eructation (infrequent, mild).

Miscellaneous: Mild flushing, headache, feeling of weakness or tachycardia may occur, especially during the first weeks of administration.

Patient Information: Take medication with meals or antacids to reduce GI distress.

Administration and Dosage:

Although objective signs of therapeutic benefit may be rapid and dramatic, improvement usually occurs gradually over weeks of therapy. Prolonged use may be necessary. Short-term use is rarely beneficial or permanent.

Initial therapy: 1.2 to 1.6 g/day in divided doses before meals and at bedtime. When a clinical response is noted, decrease dosage in 200 mg decrements until the maintenance dosage is reached.

Maintenance therapy: 400 to 800 mg/day in 2 to 4 divided doses.

	Product	Form/Strength	Package	C.I.*
Rx	**Cyclandelate** (Various)	**Tablets:** 200 mg	In 100s, 1000s and UD 100s.	19+
Rx	**Cyclandelate** (Various)	**Tablets:** 400 mg	In 100s, 1000s and UD 100s.	13+
Rx	**Cyclandelate** (Various)	**Capsules:** 200 mg	In 60s, 100s, 500s, 1000s and UD 100s.	18+
Rx	**Cyclan** (Major)		In 100s, 1000s and UD 100s.	34
Rx	**Cyclospasmol** (Wyeth-Ayerst)		(#Wyeth 4124). Blue. In 100s.	194
Rx	**Cyclandelate** (Various)	**Capsules:** 400 mg	In 60s, 100s, 500s, 1000s and UD 100s.	13+
Rx	**Cyclan** (Major)		In 100s, 250s, 1000s, UD 100s.	21
Rx	**Cyclospasmol** (Wyeth-Ayerst)		(#Wyeth 4148). Blue and red. In 100s.	175

* Cost Index based on cost per 100 mg. # Product identification code.

ISOXSUPRINE HCl

Actions:

A vasodilator acting primarily on blood vessels within skeletal muscle. In normal subjects, resting blood flow in skeletal muscle is increased; cutaneous blood flow is usually not affected. Isoxsuprine is an α-adrenoreceptor antagonist with β-adrenoreceptor stimulating properties; however, vasodilatation is not blocked by propranolol. Isoxsuprine may act directly on vascular smooth muscle. The drug also causes cardiac stimulation (increased contractility, heart rate and cardiac output) and uterine relaxation. At high doses, it lowers blood viscosity and inhibits platelet aggregation.

Indications:

"Possibly effective" for relief of symptoms associated with cerebral vascular insufficiency; in peripheral vascular disease of arteriosclerosis obliterans, thromboangiitis obliterans (Buerger's disease) and Raynaud's disease.

Unlabeled Uses: Isoxsuprine has been used in the treatment of dysmenorrhea and threatened premature labor (see Warnings), but efficacy has not been established.

Contraindications:

Do not give immediately postpartum or in the presence of arterial bleeding.

Warnings:

Pregnancy: Isoxsuprine crosses the placenta (maternal serum concentration is approximately equivalent to cord serum concentrations) and may cause hypotension in the newborn. Safety for use in pregnancy has not been established.

Isoxsuprine has been used to inhibit preterm labor. Maternal and fetal tachycardia may occur under such use. Hypocalcemia, hypoglycemia, hypotension and ileus have occurred in infants whose mothers received isoxsuprine. Pulmonary edema has been reported in mothers treated with β-stimulants. Isoxsuprine is neither approved nor recommended for use in the treatment of premature labor; more selective agents are available (see ritodrine).

Adverse Reactions:

Hypotension; tachycardia; chest pain; nausea; vomiting; dizziness; weakness; abdominal distress; severe rash. If rash appears, discontinue use. A causal relationship is not established.

Patient Information:

May cause palpitations or skin rash. Notify physician if these symptoms become particularly bothersome.

If dizziness (orthostatic hypotension) occurs, avoid sudden changes in posture.

Administration and Dosage:

10 to 20 mg, 3 or 4 times daily.

	Product	Form	Packaging	C.I.*
Rx	**Isoxsuprine HCl** (Various)	**Tablets:** 10 mg	In 60s, 100s, 500s, 1000s and UD 100s.	28+
Rx	**Vasodilan** (Mead Johnson)		In 100s, 1000s and UD 100s.	436
Rx	**Voxsuprine** (Major)		In 100s, 250s, 1000s and UD 100s.	59
Rx	**Isoxsuprine HCl** (Various)	**Tablets:** 20 mg	In 60s, 100s, 500s, 1000s and UD 100s.	21+
Rx	**Vasodilan** (Mead Johnson)		In 100s, 500s, 1000s and UD 100s.	349
Rx	**Voxsuprine** (Major)		In 100s, 250s, 1000s and UD 100s.	41

* Cost Index based on cost per 10 mg.

NYLIDRIN HCl

Actions:

Nylidrin acts by β-adrenergic stimulation to dilate arterioles in skeletal muscle and increase cardiac output. It may also have a direct action on vascular smooth muscle. Effects on cutaneous blood flow are negligible.

Pharmacokinetics: Nylidrin is readily absorbed from the GI tract. Pharmacologic effects begin in about 10 minutes, peak in about 30 minutes and last about 2 hours.

Indications:

"Possibly effective" whenever an increase in blood supply is desirable in vasospastic disorders such as:

Peripheral vascular disease - Arteriosclerosis obliterans; thromboangiitis obliterans (Buerger's disease); diabetic vascular disease; night leg cramps; Raynaud's phenomenon and disease; ischemic ulcer; frostbite; acrocyanosis; acroparesthesia; thrombophlebitis; cold feet, legs and hands.

Circulatory disturbances of the inner ear - Primary cochlear cell ischemia; cochlear stria vascular ischemia; macular or ampullar ischemia; other disturbances due to labyrinthine artery spasm or obstruction.

Unlabeled Use: Elderly patients with cognitive, emotional and physical impairment may show improvement in symptoms with nylidrin therapy (6 to 24 mg/day).

Contraindications:

Acute myocardial infarction; paroxysmal tachycardia; progressive angina pectoris; thyrotoxicosis.

Warnings:

Cardiac disease: In patients with tachyarrhythmias or uncompensated congestive heart failure, weigh the benefit/risk ratio prior to therapy and reconsider at intervals during treatment.

Pregnancy: Maternal hyperglycemia has been reported with use during the last trimester of pregnancy; increases are more marked in diabetic women. Safety for use in pregnancy has not been established.

Adverse Reactions:

CNS: Trembling; nervousness; weakness; dizziness (not associated with labyrinthine artery insufficiency).

GI: Nausea; vomiting.

Cardiovascular: Postural hypotension; palpitations.

Patient Information:

May cause dizziness (orthostatic hypotension); avoid sudden changes in posture. Observe caution while driving or performing other tasks requiring alertness.

May cause trembling, nervousness, weakness, nausea or vomiting. Notify physician if these symptoms become severe or if palpitations occur.

Administration and Dosage:

3 to 12 mg 3 or 4 times daily.

	Product	Form	Packaging	C.I.*
Rx	**Nylidrin HCl** (Various)	**Tablets:** 6 mg	In 100s, 1000s and UD 100s.	30+
Rx	**Adrin** (Major)		In 100s and 1000s.	49
Rx	**Arlidin** (Rorer)		(#45/USV). White, scored. In 100s and 1000s.	1179
Rx	**Nylidrin HCl** (Various)	**Tablets:** 12 mg	In 100s, 1000s and UD 100s.	15+
Rx	**Adrin** (Major)		In 100s and 1000s.	33
Rx	**Arlidin** (Rorer)		(#46/USV). White, scored. In 100s and 1000s.	888

NICOTINIC ACID

The weak vasodilating action of nicotinic acid (niacin) is well documented; however, its therapeutic value as a vasodilating agent has not been well established.

For complete information on nicotinic acid, and for product listings, see the Niacin monograph in the Vitamins section.

* Cost Index based on cost per 6 mg.

Product identification code.

PAPAVERINE HCl

Actions:

Papaverine is an alkaloid originally derived from crude opium; it has no narcotic properties.

Pharmacology: Papaverine directly relaxes the tonus of all smooth muscle, especially when it has been spasmodically contracted. Vasodilatation may be related to its ability to inhibit cyclic nucleotide phosphodiesterase, thus increasing levels of intracellular cyclic AMP. This relaxation is noted in the vascular system, bronchial musculature and in the gastrointestinal, biliary and urinary tracts. During administration, the muscle cell is not paralyzed and still responds to drugs and other stimuli causing contraction. The antispasmodic effect is direct and unrelated to muscle innervation. It has little effect on the CNS, although very large doses tend to produce some sedation and sleepiness. In certain circumstances, mild respiratory stimulation can be observed due to stimulation of carotid and aortic body chemoreceptors.

Possibly due to its direct vasodilating action on cerebral blood vessels, papaverine increases cerebral blood flow and decreases cerebral vascular resistance in normal subjects; oxygen consumption is unaltered. These effects have been used to explain the reported benefits in cerebral vascular encephalopathy.

Large doses of papaverine depress AV nodal and intraventricular conduction by suppressing myocardial excitability, thus prolonging the refractory period of the myocardium. Its action as a coronary vasodilator may be an additional factor when these arrhythmias are secondary to coronary insufficiency or occlusion.

Experimentally in dogs, the alkaloid has caused fairly marked and long-lasting coronary vasodilation and an increase in coronary blood flow. However, it also appears to have a direct inotropic effect and, when increased mechanical activity coincides with decreased systemic pressure, increases in coronary blood flow may not be sufficient to prevent brief periods of hypoxic myocardial depression.

Pharmacokinetics: Absorption/Distribution – Papaverine is effective by all routes of administration. Oral bioavailability is about 54%. Peak plasma levels occur 1 to 2 hours after an oral dose. Sustained release preparations may be poorly and erratically absorbed. A considerable fraction of the drug localizes in fat depots and in the liver, with the remainder being distributed throughout the body. About 90% of the drug is bound to plasma protein.

Metabolism/Excretion – Papaverine is metabolized in the liver. Although estimates of its biologic half-life vary widely, reasonably constant plasma levels can be maintained with oral administration at 6 hour intervals. The drug is excreted in the urine in an inactive form.

Indications:

Although papaverine has been used for many years for a number of conditions, there is insufficient objective evidence of any therapeutic value.

Oral: As a smooth muscle relaxant. For relief of cerebral and peripheral ischemia associated with arterial spasm and myocardial ischemia complicated by arrhythmias.

Parenteral: Used in various conditions accompanied by muscle spasm, such as: Vascular spasm associated with acute myocardial infarction (coronary occlusion); angina pectoris; peripheral and pulmonary embolism; peripheral vascular disease in which there is a vasospastic element; certain cerebral angiospastic states; visceral spasm as in ureteral, biliary and GI colic.

Unlabeled Use: Papaverine (2.5 to 60 mg) has been used alone or in combination with phentolamine as an intracavernous injection for impotence.

Contraindications:

Complete AV heart block.

Warnings:

Cardiac: Large doses can depress AV and intraventricular conduction and thereby produce serious arrhythmias. When conduction is depressed, it may produce transient ectopy of ventricular origin, either premature beats or paroxysmal tachycardia.

Pregnancy: Category C. Safety for use during pregnancy has not been established. Use only when clearly needed and when the potential benefits outweigh the unknown potential hazards to the fetus.

Lactation: It is not known whether this drug is excreted in breast milk. Safety for use in the nursing mother has not been established.

Children: Safety and efficacy for use in children have not been established.

(Continued on following page)

PAPAVERINE HCl (Cont.)

Precautions:

Glaucoma: Use with caution in patients with glaucoma.

Hepatic hypersensitivity has been reported with GI symptoms, jaundice, eosinophilia and altered liver function tests. Discontinue medication if these symptoms occur.

Drug abuse and dependence resulting from the abuse of many of the selective depressants, including papaverine, have been reported.

Drug Interactions:

Levodopa: The antiparkinson effectiveness may be decreased by concomitant administration of papaverine, due to possible blockade of dopamine receptors.

Adverse Reactions:

GI: Nausea; abdominal distress; anorexia; constipation; diarrhea. Hepatic hypersensitivity, resulting in jaundice, eosinophilia and altered liver function tests.

CNS: Vertigo; drowsiness; excessive sedation; headache.

Cardiovascular: Increase in heart rate and depth of respiration; slight increase in blood pressure.

Miscellaneous: Sweating; flushing of face; skin rash; malaise.

Hepatitis, probably related to an immune mechanism, occurs infrequently. Rarely, it has progressed to cirrhosis.

Overdosage:

Ingestion of more than ten times the usual therapeutic dose has not resulted in untoward effects; however, a single dose of 0.1 to 0.5 g/kg could be fatal to an adult.

Acute poisoning:

Symptoms – Drowsiness, weakness, nystagmus, diplopia, incoordination and lassitude, progressing to coma with cyanosis and respiratory depression.

Treatment – To delay drug absorption, give tap water, milk or activated charcoal; then evacuate stomach contents by gastric lavage or emesis, followed by catharsis. If coma and respiratory depression occur, take appropriate measures. Hemodialysis has been suggested. Maintain blood pressure. Avoid concurrent administration of other depressant drugs.

Chronic poisoning:

Symptoms – Drowsiness, depression, weakness, anxiety, ataxia, headache, blurred vision, gastric upset and pruritic skin rashes characterized by urticaria or erythematous macular eruptions. Any of the formed elements of the blood may be decreased in number.

Treatment – Discontinue medication at the onset of any unusual symptoms or abnormal hematologic findings. Severe hypotension may occur when any depressant, including papaverine, is used. Recovery should occur, except in patients with aplastic anemia.

Parenteral symptoms often result from vasomotor instability and include nausea, vomiting, weakness, central nervous system depression, nystagmus, diplopia, diaphoresis, flushing, dizziness and sinus tachycardia. In large overdoses, papaverine is a potent inhibitor of cellular respiration and a weak calcium antagonist. Following an oral overdose of 15 g, metabolic acidosis with hyperventilation, hyperglycemia and hypokalemia have been reported. Following IV overdosing in animals, seizures, tachyarrhythmias and ventricular fibrillations have occurred.

Treatment – Consider the possibility of multiple drug overdoses, interaction among drugs, and unusual drug kinetics. Protect the patient's airway and support ventilation and perfusion. Meticulously monitor vital signs, blood gases, blood chemistry values and other variables.

If convulsions occur, consider diazepam, phenytoin or phenobarbital. If the seizures are refractory, general anesthesia with thiopental or halothane and paralysis with a neuromuscular blocking agent may be necessary.

For hypotension, consider IV fluids, elevation of the legs and an inotropic vasopressor, such as dopamine or norepinephrine. Theoretically, calcium gluconate may be helpful in treating some of papaverine's toxic cardiovascular effects; monitor the ECG and plasma calcium concentrations.

The benefits of forced diuresis, peritoneal dialysis, hemodialysis or charcoal hemoperfusion have not been established.

Patient Information:

May cause dizziness (hypotension) or drowsiness; use caution when driving or performing other tasks requiring alertness. Alcohol may intensify these effects.

May cause flushing, sweating, headache, tiredness, jaundice, skin rash, nausea, anorexia, abdominal distress, constipation or diarrhea. Notify physician if these effects become pronounced.

(Products listed on following pages)

PAPAVERINE HCl (Cont.)

Administration and Dosage:

Oral: 100 to 300 mg, 3 to 5 times daily.

Oral, timed release: 150 mg every 12 hours. In difficult cases, increase to 150 mg every 8 hours, or 300 mg every 12 hours.

Parenteral: Administer 30 to 120 mg every 3 hours as indicated. For cardiac extrasystoles, give 2 doses 10 minutes apart IV or IM. The IV route is recommended when an immediate effect is desired; inject slowly over 1 or 2 minutes.

Incompatibility: Do not add to Lactated Ringer's Injection because precipitation will result.

				C.I.*
Rx	**Papaverine HCl** (Various)	**Capsules, timed release:** 150 mg	In 60s, 100s, 250s, 500s, 1000s and UD 32s and 100s.	49+
Rx	**Cerespan** (Rorer)		(#115/USV). In 100s.	1209
Rx	**Genabid** (Goldline)		In 100s and 1000s.	99
Rx	**Pavabid Plateau Caps** (Marion Merrell Dow)		(#Marion/1555). In 100s, 250s, 1000s and UD 100s.	303
Rx	**Pavarine Spancaps** (Vortech)		In 100s.	124
Rx	**Pavased** (Hauck)		In 100s and 1000s.	165
Rx	**Pavatine** (Major)		In 100s, 1000s and UD 100s.	88
Rx	**Pavatym** (Everett)		In 100s, 1000s and UD 100s.	225
Rx	**Paverolan Lanacaps** (Lannett)		Brown and clear. In 100s and 1000s.	100
Rx	**Papaverine HCl** (Lannett)	**Tablets:** 30 mg	In 100s.	233
Rx	**Papaverine HCl** (Various)	**Tablets:** 60 mg	In 100s, 500s and 1000s.	73+
Rx	**Papaverine HCl** (Various)	**Tablets:** 100 mg	In 100s, 500s and 1000s.	54+
Rx	**Papaverine HCl** (Genetco)	**Tablets:** 150 mg	In 100s.	120
Rx	**Papaverine HCl** (Various)	**Tablets:** 200 mg	In 100s, 500s and 1000s.	53+
Rx	**Pavasule** (Misemer)	**Tablets, timed release:** 200 mg	In 100s.	200
Rx	**Papaverine HCl** (Various)	**Tablets:** 300 mg	In 60s and 100s.	58+
Rx	**Pavabid HP Capsulets** (Marion Merrell Dow)		(#Marion Pavabid HP). Light orange. In 60s.	229
Rx	**Papaverine HCl** (Lilly)	**Injection:** 30 mg per ml	In 2 and 10 ml amps.[1]	1733

* Cost Index based on cost per 150 mg.
# Product identification code.
[1] With EDTA.

ETHAVERINE HCl

Actions:

Ethaverine is closely related to papaverine and has similar actions and uses (see papaverine monograph).

Indications:

Peripheral and cerebral vascular insufficiency associated with arterial spasm; as a smooth muscle spasmolytic in spastic conditions of the GI and GU tracts. Data are not conclusive to show ethaverine to be effective in the conditions for which it is presently labeled.

Contraindications:

Complete atrioventricular dissociation.

Warnings:

Pregnancy: Safety for use during pregnancy has not been established. Do not use in pregnant women unless essential to the welfare of the patient.

Lactation: Safety for use in the nursing mother has not been established. Do not use in women of childbearing age unless essential to the welfare of the patient.

Precautions:

Glaucoma: Administer with caution to patients with glaucoma.

Adverse Reactions:

Nausea; anorexia; abdominal distress; dryness of the throat; hypotension; malaise; vertigo; headache; lassitude; drowsiness; flushing; sweating; respiratory depression; cardiac depression; cardiac arrhythmia.

Patient Information:

May cause dizziness (hypotension) or drowsiness; use caution when driving or performing other tasks requiring alertness.

May cause flushing, sweating, headache, tiredness, rash, nausea, anorexia, abdominal distress or diarrhea. Notify physician if these symptoms become pronounced.

Administration and Dosage:

100 mg 3 times daily. May be increased to 200 mg 3 times daily. It is most effective when given early in course of vascular disorder. Long-term therapy is required.

	Product	Form	Description	C.I.*
Rx	**Ethaquin** (Ascher)	**Tablets:** 100 mg	In 100s, 500s and 1000s.	582
Rx	**Ethatab** (Whitby)		(Glaxo 281). Yellow. In 100s and UD 100s.	670
Rx	**Ethavex-100** (Econo Med)		(Ethavex). Scored. In 100s and 1000s.	299
Rx	**Isovex** (U.S. Pharm.)	**Capsules:** 100 mg	In 100s and 1000s.	472

PERIPHERAL VASODILATOR COMBINATIONS

In these combinations: *NIACIN* (see Vitamins monograph) is used for its vasodilating action.

				C.I.*
Rx	**Lipo-Nicin/100 mg** (ICN Pharm)	**Tablets:** 100 mg niacin, 75 mg niacinamide, 150 mg vitamin C, 25 mg B_1, 2 mg B_2 and 10 mg B_6. *Dose:* 1 tablet daily.	Blue. In 100s.	197
Rx	**Lipo-Nicin/250 mg** (ICN Pharm)	**Tablets**: 250 mg niacin, 75 mg niacinamide, 150 mg vitamin C, 25 mg B_1, 2 mg B_2 and 10 mg B_6. *Dose:* 1 tablet daily.	Yellow. In 100s.	100
Rx	**Lipo-Nicin/300 mg** (ICN Pharm)	**Capsules, timed release:** 300 mg niacin, 150 mg vitamin C, 25 mg B_1, 2 mg B_2 and 10 mg B_6. *Dose:* 1 capsule daily.	Clear. In 100s.	107

* Cost Index based on cost per 150 mg ethaverine or 100 mg niacin.

Shock is a state of inadequate tissue perfusion. It can be caused by, or cause, a decreased supply of, or an increased demand for, oxygen and nutrients. The imbalance between supply and demand interferes with normal cellular function. Widespread cellular dysfunction can result in death. Inadequate tissue perfusion can occur even if cardiac output, peripheral resistance and other factors which determine blood pressure (eg, blood volume) are normal or elevated. Therefore, hypotension need not be present for the patient to be in shock.

Shock produces various physiologic responses. Some, such as lactic acidosis, occur as a direct result of tissue hypoperfusion. Others, such as catecholamine release, also serve to compensate for the absolute or relative reduction in tissue perfusion. The systemic responses to shock can be beneficial in the early stages and classically consist of an increase in circulating catecholamines, vasodilation and increased vascular permeability. These early responses produce a "hyperdynamic" state which may be referred to as "warm" shock, so named because blood flow to the skin and extremities is still maintained. If left uncorrected, however, these responses become counterproductive, and contribute to the relentless progression of the shock state. Profound vascular decompensation occurs, which is associated with a further loss of blood flow to the vital organs, skin and extremities. Thus, more advanced shock is "cold" shock.

Clinical manifestations of shock are variable and non-specific. In addition, underlying or concurrent disease states, drug therapy and patient age may alter the response to hypoperfusion. Signs and symptoms of shock include:

Skin – pallor, cyanosis, cold and clammy, sweating
CNS – agitation, confusion, disorientation, coma
Cardiovascular – tachycardia, arrhythmias, wide pulse pressure, gallop rhythm, hypotension
Pulmonary – tachypnea, pulmonary edema
Renal – oliguria (<0.5 ml/kg/hr)
Metabolic – acidosis, hypoglycemia or hyperglycemia

Causes of shock are varied. Despite the etiology, advanced shock tends to follow a common clinical course. However, identifying the underlying cause may assist in the selection of general supportive therapy and is essential for selecting specific therapy.

Types of shock:

Hypovolemic shock occurs when intravascular volume is reduced by > 15% to 25%. The volume loss can be absolute (eg, hemorrhage, fluid loss due to burns, diarrhea or vomiting, excess diuresis, diabetes) or relative (eg, sequestration of body fluids, capillary leak).

Cardiogenic shock occurs when the heart is unable to deliver an adequate cardiac output to maintain vital organ perfusion. This can be caused by an acute myocardial infarction, sustained ventricular arrhythmias, severe cardiomyopathy or congestive heart failure.

Septic shock occurs as a result of circulatory insufficiency associated with overwhelming infection.

Obstructive shock occurs when obstruction to blood flow results in inadequate tissue perfusion. Massive pulmonary embolism, pericardial tamponade, restrictive pericarditis, and severe cardiac valve dysfunction can reduce blood flow enough to produce shock.

Neurogenic shock is an uncommon form of shock which occurs as a result of blockade of neurohumoral outflow. The neurohumoral blockade may be induced by pharmacologic agents (eg, spinal anesthesia) or by direct injury to the spinal cord.

Other causes of shock include anaphylaxis, hypoglycemia, hypothyroidism and hypoadrenalism (ie, Addison's disease).

Management of shock is aimed at providing basic life support (airway, breathing and circulation) while attempting to correct the underlying cause. Antibiotics, inotropes, hormones (eg, insulin, thyroid) and other agents may be used to treat the underlying disease states in the shock patient. However, initial pharmacologic interventions are primarily aimed at supporting the circulation.

Blood pressure is a function of the peripheral vascular resistance and the cardiac output. Cardiac output is determined by the heart rate and stroke volume. The stroke volume is a function of the contractile state of the heart and the volume of blood in the ventricle available to be pumped out (ie, preload). Manipulation of any of these parameters can produce a change in blood pressure.

(Continued on following page)

Management (Cont.):

Fluids: Relative or absolute volume depletion occurs in most shock states, especially in the early or "warm" phase in which vasodilation is prominent. Adequate volume repletion is necessary to maintain cardiac output, urine flow, and the integrity of the microcirculation. Attempts to support the circulation with vasopressors or inotropes will be unsuccessful if the intravascular volume is depleted.

The choice of fluids is probably irrelevant in the early stages. Although whole blood might be preferred for the patient with hemorrhagic shock, the delay in availability of blood products often negates any advantage. There is no clear superiority of crystalloids or colloids in emergency fluid resuscitation. Hydroxyethyl starch and the dextrans are also suitable plasma volume expanders.

Vasopressors: Sympathomimetic agents are used in shock to treat hypoperfusion in normovolemic patients and in patients unresponsive to whole blood or plasma volume expanders. These agents increase myocardial contractility, constrict capacitance vessels and dilate resistance vessels. In cardiogenic shock or advanced shock from other causes associated with a low cardiac output, they may be combined with vasodilators (eg, nitroprusside or nitroglycerin) to maintain blood pressure while the vasodilator improves myocardial performance. Nitroprusside is used to reduce preload and afterload and improve cardiac output. Nitroglycerin directly relaxes the venous vasculature and decreases preload.

Pharmacology: Sympathomimetic agents produce α-adrenergic stimulation (vasoconstriction), β_1-adrenergic stimulation (increase myocardial contractility, heart rate, automaticity and AV conduction), and β_2-adrenergic activity (peripheral vasodilation). Dopamine also causes vasodilation of the renal and mesenteric, cerebral and coronary beds by dopaminergic receptor activation. Adrenergic agents are useful in improving hemodynamic status by improving myocardial contractility and increasing heart rate, which results in increased cardiac output. Peripheral resistance is increased by vasoconstriction. Increased cardiac output and increased peripheral resistance increase blood pressure. The relative activity and predominance of these actions result in a number of hemodynamic responses which may affect coronary perfusion, renal perfusion, cardiac output, total peripheral resistance and blood pressure. These actions are summarized in the table on the following page. The actual response of an individual patient will depend largely on clinical status at time of administration.

Other drugs: A number of other drug classes have been used as supportive therapy in shock patients. However, with the exception of vasodilator treatment of cardiogenic shock, none of these treatments appear superior to vasopressor therapy. These drugs include: Opiate antagonists, prostaglandin inhibitors, corticosteroids and thyrotropin-releasing hormone.

Monitoring shock patients and their response to drugs requires special vigilance. Monitor heart rate, blood pressure and ECG continuously. Record urine output and fluid intake frequently. Due to rapid and life-threatening changes that can occur in the hemodynamically unstable patient, optimal drug selection, dose titration and management is probably best achieved with the use of invasive hemodynamic monitoring. Monitoring of central venous pressures via a central venous catheter will provide an estimation of the patient's fluid status by approximating the diastolic pressure of the right ventricle. When warranted, additional hemodynamic data can be obtained through the use of a pulmonary artery catheter (ie, Swan-Ganz). Changes in the pulmonary artery wedge pressure (a measure of left ventricular end diastolic volume), cardiac output and peripheral vascular resistance can be monitored and therapy adjusted accordingly.

Administration should only be via the IV route using a large-bore, free flowing IV in the antecubital vein or a central vein due to unpredictable absorption. Small IVs in the extremities are both unreliable and unsafe for vasopressor administration. Frequent monitoring of the IV sites for extravasation injury is essential when vasopressor agents are being used.

Prolonged, high-dose therapy can produce cyanosis and tissue necrosis of distal extremities. The principle of using the lowest dose which produces an adequate response for the shortest period of time is very important when using these agents.

Plasma volume depletion: Prolonged use of vasopressors may result in plasma volume depletion; this should be corrected by appropriate fluid and electrolyte replacement therapy. If plasma volumes are not corrected, hypotension may recur when these drugs are discontinued. Blood pressure may be maintained at the risk of severe peripheral vasoconstriction with diminution in blood flow and tissue perfusion.

Acidosis lessens the response to vasopressors; therefore, correct acidosis if it exists or develops during the course of vasopressor therapy.

Avoid continuous IV therapy: Acute tolerance develops during continuous IV administration. High concentration/low volume (250 ml) vasopressor solutions administered with the aid of an infusion control device allows for maximum dosing flexibility since fluids and drugs can be regulated independently, and the development of tolerance is minimized.

(Continued on following page)

Symbol key:
- +++ *pronounced effect*
- ++ *moderate effect*
- + *slight effect*
- 0 *no effect*
- ↑ *increase*
- ↓ *decrease*

		SITES OF ACTION				HEMODYNAMIC RESPONSE			
		HEART		BLOOD VESSELS					
Class	Drug	Contractility (Inotropic) β_1	SA Node Rate (Chronotropic) β_1	Vasoconstriction α	Vasodilatation β_2	Renal Perfusion	Cardiac Output	Total Peripheral Resistance	Blood Pressure
Inotropic	Isoproterenol	+ + +	+ + +	0	+ + +	↑[1] or ↓[2]	↑	↓	↑[3]↓[4]
Inotropic	Dobutamine	+ + +	0 to +[5]	0 to +[5]	+	0	↑	↓	↑
Inotropic	Dopamine	+ + +	+ to + +[5]	+ to + +[5]	0 to +[6]	↑[5]	↑	↓[5] or ↑	0 to ↑
Mixed	Epinephrine	+ + +	+ + +	+ +[5]	+ +[5]	↓	↑	↓	↑[3]↓[4]
Mixed	Norepinephrine	+ +	+ +[7]	+ + +	0	↓	0 or ↓	↑	↑
Mixed	Ephedrine	+ +	+ +	+	0 to +	↓	↑	↑ or ↓	↑
Mixed	Mephentermine	+	+	+	+ +	↑ or ↓	↑	0 to ↑	↑
Pressors	Metaraminol	+	+	+ +	0	↓	↓	↑	↑
Pressors	Methoxamine	0	0[7]	+ + +	0	↓	0 or ↓	↑	↑
Pressors	Phenylephrine	0	0[7]	+ + +	0	↓	↓	↑	↑

[1] Cardiogenic or septicemic shock.
[2] Normotensive patient.
[3] Systolic effect.
[4] Diastolic effect.
[5] Effects are dose dependent.
[6] Dilates renal and splanchnic beds via dopaminergic effect at doses $<$ 10 mcg/kg/min.
[7] Decreased heart rate may result from reflex mechanisms.

Common Dilutions and Infusion Rates for Selected Drugs Used in Shock

Drug	Usual Dilution for IV Infusion	Infusion Rate
Isoproterenol	2 mg (10 ml) in 500 ml D5W (4 mcg/ml) or 1 mg (5 ml) in 250 ml D5W	5 mcg/min
Dobutamine	250 mg in 250 to 500 ml NS or D5W (500 to 1000 mcg/ml)	2.5 to 15 mcg/kg/min
Dopamine	200 to 800 mg in 250 to 500 ml NS or D5W (400 to 3200 mcg/ml)	Low dose – 2.5 to 10 mcg/kg/min High dose – 20 to 50 mcg/kg/min
Norepinephrine	4 mg in 250 ml of D5W (16 mcg/ml)	Initial: 8 to 12 mcg/min Maintenance: 2 to 4 mcg/min

ISOPROTERENOL HCl (Cont.)

Administration and Dosage (Cont.):

Dosage for Adults with Heart Block, Adams-Stokes Attacks and Cardiac Arrest			
Route	Dilution	Initial Dose	Subsequent Dose Range
IV injection	Dilute 1 ml of 1:5000 solution (0.2 mg) to 10 ml with Sodium Chloride or 5% Dextrose Injection	0.02 to 0.06 mg (1 to 3 ml of diluted solution)	0.01 to 0.2 mg (0.5 to 10 ml of diluted solution)
IV infusion	Dilute 10 ml of 1:5000 solution (2 mg) in 500 ml of D5W or dilute 5 ml of 1:5000 solution (1 mg) in 250 ml of D5W	5 mcg/min (1.25 ml/min of diluted solution)	
IM	Undiluted 1:5000 solution	0.2 mg (1 ml)	0.02 to 1 mg (0.1 to 5 ml)
SC	Undiluted 1:5000 solution	0.2 mg (1 ml)	0.15 to 0.2 mg (0.75 to 1 ml)
Intracardiac	Undiluted 1:5000 solution	0.02 mg (0.1 ml)	

Sublingual or rectal:

The usual route of administration of isoproterenol in emergency treatment of patients with severe heart block is IV injection or infusion. If time is not of utmost importance, initial therapy by IM or SC injection may be used. If further maintenance therapy is necessary, glossets may be administered sublingually. Always monitor the ECG.

The glossets form of isoproterenol is usually administered sublingually.

Heart block and certain ventricular arrhythmias - Sublingual or rectal administration is effective in the control of mild stabilized symptomatic heart block and ventricular arrhythmias. However, in acute symptomatic heart block, particularly in patients with postcardiac surgery block, electrical pacing is the preferred method of treatment for maintenance of an adequate ventricular rate. Moreover, in ventricular arrhythmias, electroshock may have to be used, and is usually the treatment of choice.

If given in acute symptomatic heart block, IV administration, with constant monitoring, is preferred. This avoids the irregular absorption which is possible with the sublingual and rectal routes of administration. Rectal administration is more satisfactory for long-term therapy because the effect is produced within 30 minutes and lasts for 2 to 4 hours. Sinus rhythm sometimes occurs and persists for a variable period, but often relapses again into complete block. In other cases, isoproterenol merely maintains an acceptable heart rate somewhere above 90 to 100 beats/minute. The table below summarizes the dosage regimen suggested for adults.

Suggested Isoproterenol Dosage For Heart Block In Adults		
Route of Administration	Initial Dose	Subsequent Dose Range
Sublingual	10 mg	5 to 50 mg
Rectal	5 mg	5 to 15 mg

Storage: Store in a cool place between 8° to 15°C (46° to 59°F). Do not use if solution is pinkish to brownish in color.

				C.I.*
Rx	**Isoproterenol** (Various)	**Injection:** 1:5000 solution (0.2 mg per ml)[1]	In 5 and 10 ml vials and 5 ml amps.	119+
Rx	**Isuprel** (Winthrop Pharm.)		In 1 and 5 ml amps.	497
Rx	**Isuprel** (Winthrop Pharm.)	**Glossets**[2] 10 mg	Saccharin. In 50s.	89
		15 mg	Saccharin. In 50s.	106

* Cost Index based on cost per glosset or ml.

Product identification code.

[1] With sodium metabisulfite.

[2] For sublingual or rectal use. Contains 2 mg sodium metabisulfite.

Refer to the general discussion of these products on page 717.

DOBUTAMINE

Actions:

Pharmacology: Dobutamine is chemically related to dopamine. Its primary activity results from stimulation of the $beta_1$ receptors of the heart while producing comparatively mild chronotropic, hypertensive, arrhythmogenic and vasodilative effects. It has minor alpha (vasoconstrictor) and $beta_2$ (vasodilator) effects. It does not cause the release of endogenous norepinephrine, as does dopamine.

Hemodynamics – In patients with depressed cardiac function, both dobutamine and isoproterenol increase the cardiac output to a similar degree. With dobutamine, this increase is usually not accompanied by marked increases in heart rate (although tachycardia is occasionally observed), and the cardiac stroke volume is usually increased. In contrast, isoproterenol increases the cardiac index primarily by increasing the heart rate while stroke volume changes little or declines. Dobutamine produces less increase in heart rate and less decrease in peripheral vascular resistance for a given inotropic effect than does isoproterenol.

Facilitation of atrioventricular conduction has been observed in human electrophysiologic studies and in patients with atrial fibrillation.

Systemic vascular resistance is usually decreased; occasionally, minimal vasoconstriction has been observed.

Pharmacokinetics: Onset – The onset of action is within 1 to 2 minutes; however, as much as 10 minutes may be required to obtain the peak effect of a particular infusion rate. The therapeutic plasma level is 40 to 190 ng/ml.

Metabolism/Excretion – The principal routes of metabolism are methylation of the catechol and conjugation. The plasma half-life of dobutamine is two minutes. In urine, the major excretion products are the conjugates of dobutamine and the inactive 3-O-methyl dobutamine.

Clinical Pharmacology: Most clinical experience with dobutamine is short-term, up to several hours in duration. In the limited number of patients who were studied for 24, 48 and 72 hours, a persistent increase in cardiac output occurred in some, whereas the output of others returned toward baseline values.

Alteration of synaptic concentrations of catecholamines with either reserpine or tricyclic antidepressants does not alter the actions of dobutamine in animals, which indicates that the actions of dobutamine are not dependent on presynaptic mechanisms.

Indications:

Inotropic support in the short-term treatment of adults with cardiac decompensation due to depressed contractility, resulting either from organic heart disease or from cardiac surgical procedures.

In patients who have atrial fibrillation with rapid ventricular response, use a digitalis preparation prior to instituting therapy with dobutamine.

Unlabeled Uses: Doses of dobutamine 2 and 7.75 mcg/kg/min infused for 10 minutes each have been used investigationally in 12 children with congenital heart disease undergoing diagnostic cardiac catheterization. The drug appears effective in augmenting cardiovascular function in children, and no adverse effects were noted.

Contraindications:

Idiopathic hypertrophic subaortic stenosis (IHSS). Patients hypersensitive to dobutamine.

Warnings:

Increase in heart rate or blood pressure: Dobutamine may cause a marked increase in heart rate or blood pressure, especially systolic pressure. Approximately 10% of patients in clinical studies have had rate increases of 30 beats/min or more, and about 7.5% have had a 50 mm Hg or greater increase in systolic pressure. Usually, reduction of dosage promptly reverses these effects. Because the drug facilitates atrioventricular conduction, patients with atrial fibrillation are at risk of developing rapid ventricular response. Patients with preexisting hypertension appear to face an increased risk of developing an exaggerated pressor response.

Ectopic Activity: Dobutamine may precipitate or exacerbate ventricular ectopic activity, but it rarely has caused ventricular tachycardia.

Hypersensitivity reactions, including skin rash, fever, eosinophilia and bronchospasm, may occur occasionally with dobutamine.

Usage in Pregnancy: Dobutamine has not been administered to pregnant women; use only when clearly needed and when the potential benefits outweigh the potential hazards to the fetus.

Usage in Children: Safety and efficacy for use in children have not been established.

(Continued on following page)

DOBUTAMINE (Cont.)

Precautions:

Monitoring: Continuously monitor ECG and blood pressure. Monitor pulmonary wedge pressure and cardiac output whenever possible.

Hypovolemia: Use is not a substitute for the replacement of blood, plasma, fluids and electrolytes, which should be restored promptly when loss has occurred.

Correct hypovolemia with suitable volume expanders before treatment is instituted.

No improvement may be observed in the presence of marked mechanical obstruction, such as severe valvular aortic stenosis.

Usage following acute myocardial infarction: Clinical experience following myocardial infarction has been insufficient to establish the safety of the drug for this use. Any agent which increases contractile force and heart rate may increase the size of an infarction by intensifying ischemia.

Sulfite sensitivity: This product contains sulfites which may cause allergic-type reactions including anaphylactic symptoms and life-threatening or less severe asthmatic episodes in certain susceptible persons. The overall prevalence of sulfite sensitivity in the general population is unknown and probably low. Sulfite sensitivity is seen more frequently in asthmatic or atopic nonasthmatic persons.

Drug Interactions:

Bretylium may potentiate the action of vasopressors on adrenergic receptors, possibly resulting in arrhythmias.

Guanethidine may increase the pressor response of the direct-acting vasopressors, possibly resulting in severe hypertension.

Halogenated hydrocarbon anesthetics may sensitize the myocardium to the effects of catecholamines. Use of vasopressors may lead to serious arrhythmias; use with extreme caution.

Oxytocic drugs: In obstetrics, if vasopressor drugs are used either to correct hypotension or added to local anesthetic solutions, some oxytocic drugs may cause severe persistent hypertension.

Tricyclic antidepressants: The pressor response of the direct-acting vasopressors may be potentiated by these agents; use with caution.

Adverse Reactions:

Increased heart rate, blood pressure and ventricular ectopic activity: A 10 to 20 mm Hg increase in systolic blood pressure and an increase in heart rate of 5 to 15 beats per minute have been noted in most patients. (See Warnings regarding exaggerated chronotropic and pressor effects.) Approximately 5% of patients have had increased premature ventricular beats during infusions. These effects are dose-related.

Reactions at injection site: Phlebitis has occurred occasionally, and local inflammatory changes have occurred following inadvertent infiltration.

Miscellaneous (uncommon, 1% to 3%): Nausea; headache; anginal pain; nonspecific chest pain; palpitations; shortness of breath.

Long-term safety: Infusions of up to 72 hours have revealed no adverse effects other than those seen with infusions of shorter duration.

Overdosage:

Symptoms: Excessive alteration of blood pressure or tachycardia.

Treatment: Reduce the rate of administration or temporarily discontinue until condition stabilizes. Because the duration of action is short, usually no additional remedial measures are necessary.

(Continued on following page)

DOBUTAMINE (Cont.)

Administration and Dosage:

Rate of administration: The rate of infusion needed to increase cardiac output usually ranges from 2.5 to 10 mcg/kg/min. On rare occasions, infusion rates up to 40 mcg/kg/min have been required. A metering device is recommended for controlling the rate of drug administration.

Adjust the rate of administration and the duration of therapy according to patient response, as determined by heart rate, presence of ectopic activity, blood pressure, urine flow, and, whenever possible, measurement of central venous or pulmonary wedge pressure and cardiac output.

Concentrations up to 5000 mcg/ml have been administered (250 mg/50 ml). Determine the final volume administered by the fluid requirements of the patient.

Infusion Rates of Various Dilutions of Dobutamine

Desired Delivery Rate (mcg/kg/min)	Infusion Rate (ml/kg/min)		
	250 mcg/ml[1]	500 mcg/ml[2]	1000 mcg/ml[3]
2.5	0.01	0.005	0.0025
5.0	0.02	0.01	0.005
7.5	0.03	0.015	0.0075
10.0	0.04	0.02	0.01
12.5	0.05	0.025	0.0125
15.0	0.06	0.03	0.015

[1] 250 mg per liter of diluent.
[2] 500 mg per liter or 250 mg per 500 ml of diluent.
[3] 1000 mg per liter or 250 mg per 250 ml of diluent.

Admixture incompatibility: Incompatible with alkaline solutions; do not mix with products such as 5% Sodium Bicarbonate Injection. Do not use dobutamine in conjunction with other agents or diluents containing both sodium bisulfite and ethanol. Dobutamine is also physically incompatible with hydrocortisone sodium succinate; cefazolin; cefamandole; neutral cephalothin; penicillin; sodium ethacrynate; sodium heparin.

Admixture compatibility: Dobutamine is compatible when administered through common tubing with dopamine, lidocaine, tobramycin, nitroprusside, potassium chloride and protamine sulfate.

Preparation and storage of solution: Store the reconstituted solution under refrigeration for 48 hours or at room temperature for 6 hours.

Reconstituted solution must be further diluted to at least 50 ml prior to administration in 5% Dextrose Injection, 5% Dextrose and 0.45% Sodium Chloride Injection, 5% Dextrose and 0.9% Sodium Chloride Injection, 10% Dextrose Injection, *Isolyte M* with 5% Dextrose Injection, Lactated Ringer's Injection, 5% Dextrose in Lactated Ringer's Injection, *Normosol-M* in D5-W, 20% *Osmitrol* in Water for Injection, 0.9% Sodium Chloride Injection or Sodium Lactate Injection. After dilution (in glass or Viaflex containers), the solution is stable for 24 hours at room temperature. Use IV solutions within 24 hours.

Freezing is not recommended due to possible crystallization.

Stability: Solutions containing dobutamine may exhibit a pink color that, if present, will increase with time. This color change is due to slight oxidation of the drug, but there is no significant loss of potency during the time periods stated above.

				C.I.*
Rx	**Dobutrex** (Lilly)	**Injection:** 250 mg (as HCl) per vial	In 20 ml vials.[1]	491

* Cost Index based on cost per ml.
[1] With 0.24 mg sodium bisulfite.

Refer to the general discussion of these products on page 717.

DOPAMINE HCl

Actions:

Pharmacology: Dopamine is an endogenous catecholamine and a precursor of norepinephrine. It acts both directly and indirectly (releases norepinephrine stores) on alpha and $beta_1$ receptors and has dopaminergic effects.

$Beta_1$ actions produce an inotropic effect on the myocardium resulting in increased cardiac output. Dopamine causes less increase in myocardial oxygen consumption than isoproterenol and is usually not associated with a tachyarrhythmia. Systolic and pulse pressure usually increases with either no effect or a slight increase in diastolic pressure.

Total peripheral resistance (α effects) at low and intermediate therapeutic doses is usually unchanged. Blood flow to peripheral vascular beds may decrease while mesenteric flow increases. Dopamine dilates the renal and mesenteric vasculature presumptively by activation of a dopaminergic receptor. This action is accompanied by increases in GFR, renal blood flow, and sodium excretion. An increase in urinary output produced by dopamine is usually not associated with a decrease in osmolality of the urine. The dopaminergic effect is overridden by alpha-adrenergic activity at higher doses of dopamine ($>$ 10 mcg/kg/min).

Organ perfusion – Urine flow appears to be one of the better monitoring parameters of vital organ perfusion. Also, observe the patient for signs of reversal of confusion or comatose condition. Loss of pallor, increase in toe temperature or adequacy of nail bed capillary filling may also be used as indices of adequate dosage.

Renal function – When dopamine is administered before urine flow has decreased to levels approximately 0.3 ml/minute, prognosis is more favorable. Nevertheless, in oliguric or anuric patients, administration has resulted in an increase in urine flow which has reached normal levels. Dopamine may also increase urine flow in patients whose output is within normal limits, thus reducing preexisting fluid accumulation. Above those optimal doses, urine flow may decrease, necessitating dosage reduction. Coadministration of dopamine and diuretic agents may produce an additive or potentiating effect.

Cardiac output – Increased cardiac output is related to dopamine's direct inotropic effect on the myocardium, and at low or moderate doses appears to be related to a favorable prognosis. Increase in cardiac output has been associated with either static or decreased systemic vascular resistance (SVR). Low or moderate increments in cardiac output is believed to be a reflection of differential effects on specific vascular beds, with increased resistance in peripheral vascular beds (eg, femoral) and concomitant decreases in mesenteric and renal vascular beds. Redistribution of blood flow parallels these changes so that an increase in cardiac output is accompanied by an increase in mesenteric and renal blood flow; often the renal fraction of the total cardiac output has been found to increase. Increase in cardiac output produced by dopamine is not associated with substantial decreases in SVR.

Blood pressure – Manage hypotension due to inadequate cardiac output with low to moderate doses, which have little effect on SVR. At high doses, alpha-adrenergic activity is more prominent and may correct hypotension due to diminished SVR.

As in other circulatory decompensation states, prognosis is better in patients whose blood pressure and urine flow have not undergone extreme deterioration. Administer dopamine as soon as a definite trend toward decreased systolic and diastolic pressure becomes apparent.

Pharmacokinetics: Dopamine has an onset of action within 5 minutes, a plasma half-life of about 2 minutes and a duration of action of less than 10 minutes. The drug is widely distributed in the body but does not cross the blood-brain barrier.

Metabolism/Excretion – Dopamine is metabolized in the liver, kidney and plasma by MAO and catechol-O-methyltransferase to inactive compounds. About 25% of the dose is taken up into specialized neurosecretory vesicles (the adrenergic nerve terminals), where it is hydroxylated to form norepinephrine. About 80% of the drug is excreted in the urine within 24 hours, primarily as HVA and its sulfate and glucuronide conjugates and as 3,4-dihydroxy-phenylacetic acid. A very small portion is excreted unchanged.

Indications:

Correction of hemodynamic imbalances present in the shock syndrome due to myocardial infarction, trauma, endotoxic septicemia, open heart surgery, renal failure, and chronic cardiac decompensation as in refractory congestive failure.

Patients most likely to respond adequately are those in whom physiological parameters such as urine flow, myocardial function and blood pressure have not profoundly deteriorated. The shorter the time between onset of signs and symptoms of shock and initiation of therapy with volume correction and dopamine, the better the prognosis.

(Continued on following page)

EPINEPHRINE (Cont.)

Contraindications:

Hypersensitivity to the drug or any component. Narrow-angle (congestive) glaucoma; shock (nonanaphylactic); during general anesthesia with halogenated hydrocarbons or cyclopropane; individuals with cerebral arteriosclerosis or organic brain damage; with local anesthesia of certain areas (eg, fingers, toes) because of the danger of vasoconstriction producing sloughing of tissue; in labor because it may delay the second stage; in cardiac dilatation and coronary insufficiency; to counteract circulatory collapse or hypotension due to phenothiazines, since such agents may reverse the pressor effect of epinephrine, leading to a further lowering of blood pressure.

Warnings:

Initially, epinephrine administered parenterally may produce constriction of renal blood vessels and decrease urine formation.

Use with caution in the following: Elderly patients; cardiovascular disease; hypertension; diabetes; hyperthyroidism; psychoneurotic individuals; bronchial asthma and emphysema with degenerative heart disease; thyrotoxicosis.

Cardiovascular effects: Inadvertently induced high arterial blood pressure may result in angina pectoris (especially when coronary insufficiency is present), or aortic rupture.

Epinephrine may induce potentially serious cardiac arrhythmias in patients not suffering from heart disease. In patients with organic heart disease or who are receiving drugs that sensitize the myocardium, arrhythmias, including fatal ventricular fibrillation may occur. Closely monitor patients. Epinephrine causes changes in the ECG, even in normal patients, including a decrease in amplitude of the T-wave.

Cerebrovascular hemorrhage may occur from overdosage or inadvertent IV injection of epinephrine resulting from the sharp rise in blood pressure.

Pulmonary edema may result in fatalities because of the peripheral constriction and cardiac stimulation produced.

Usage in Pregnancy: Category C. Epinephrine is teratogenic in small animals when given in doses about 25 times the human dose. Epinephrine crosses the placenta. Use during pregnancy may cause anoxia. There are no adequate and well controlled studies in pregnant women. Use during pregnancy only if the potential benefit justifies the potential risk to the fetus.

Usage in Labor and Delivery: Parenteral administration of epinephrine, if used to support blood pressure during low or other spinal anesthesia for delivery, can cause acceleration of fetal heart rate and should not be used in obstetrics when maternal blood pressure exceeds 130/80 mm Hg. If administered during labor, epinephrine may delay the second stage. If administered in a dosage sufficiently high to reduce uterine contractions, it may cause prolonged uterine atony with hemorrhage.

Usage in Lactation: Epinephrine is excreted in breast milk. Because of the potential for serious adverse effects in nursing infants, decide whether to discontinue nursing or to discontinue the drug, taking into account the importance of the drug to the mother.

Usage in Children: Administer with caution to infants and children. Syncope has occurred following the administration of epinephrine to asthmatic children.

Precautions:

Although epinephrine can produce ventricular fibrillation, its actions in restoring electrical activity in asystole and in enhancing defibrillation are well documented. However, use with caution in patients with ventricular fibrillation.

In patients with prefibrillatory rhythm, IV epinephrine must be used with extreme caution because of its excitatory action on the heart. Since the myocardium is sensitized to the drug by many anesthetic agents, epinephrine may convert asystole to ventricular fibrillation if used in the treatment of anesthetic cardiac accidents.

Diabetic patients receiving epinephrine may require an increase in dosage of insulin or oral hypoglycemic agents.

Parkinson's disease: Epinephrine may temporarily increase rigidity and tremor.

Tolerance may occur with prolonged use of epinephrine.

Psychiatric effects: Epinephrine may induce or aggravate psychomotor agitation, disorientation, impairment of memory, assaultive behavior, panic, hallucinations, suicidal or homicidal tendencies, and schizophrenic-type thought disorder or paranoid delusions.

Hypovolemia: Use is not a substitute for the replacement of blood, plasma, fluids and electrolytes, which should be restored promptly when loss has occurred.

(Precautions continued on following page)

EPINEPHRINE (Cont.)

Precautions (Cont.):

Sulfite Sensitivity: Sulfites may cause allergic-type reactions (eg, hives, itching, wheezing, anaphylaxis) in certain susceptible persons. Although the overall prevalence of sulfite sensitivity in the general population is probably low, it is seen more frequently in asthmatics or in atopic nonasthmatic persons. Specific products containing sulfites are identified in the product listings.

Drug Interactions:

Beta-adrenergic blockers, nonspecific, administered concomitantly with epinephrine may block the beta-adrenergic effects of epinephrine, causing hypertension.

Bretylium may potentiate the action of vasopressors on adrenergic receptors, possibly resulting in arrhythmias.

Guanethidine may increase the pressor response of the direct-acting vasopressors, possibly resulting in severe hypertension.

Halogenated hydrocarbon anesthetics may sensitize the myocardium to the effects of catecholamines. Use of vasopressors may lead to serious arrhythmias; use with extreme caution.

Oxytocic drugs: In obstetrics, if vasopressor drugs are used either to correct hypotension or added to the local anesthetic solution, some oxytocic drugs may cause severe persistent hypertension.

Tricyclic antidepressants: The pressor response of the direct-acting vasopressors may be potentiated by these agents; use with caution.

Laboratory tests: After prolonged use or epinephrine overdosage, elevated serum lactic acid levels with severe metabolic acidosis may occur. Transient elevations of blood glucose may be associated with epinephrine administration.

Adverse Reactions:

Transient and minor: Anxiety, headache, fear and palpitations often occur with therapeutic doses, especially in hyperthyroid and hypertensive individuals.

Cardiac arrhythmias and excessive rise in blood pressure may occur with therapeutic doses or inadvertent overdosage.

Local: Urticaria, wheal and hemorrhage may occur at the site of injection. Repeated local injections can result in necrosis from vascular constriction at injection sites.

Systemic: Cerebral hemorrhage; hemiplegia; subarachnoid hemorrhage; anginal pain in patients with angina pectoris; anxiety; restlessness; throbbing headache; tremor; weakness; dizziness; pallor; respiratory difficulty; palpitations; apprehensiveness; sweating; nausea; vomiting; "epinephrine-fastness" with prolonged use; syncope in children.

Overdosage:

Symptoms: Erroneous administration of large doses of epinephrine may lead to precordial distress, vomiting, headache, dyspnea, and unusually elevated blood pressure.

Epinephrine overdosage may produce: Extremely elevated arterial pressure, which may result in cerebrovascular hemorrhage, particularly in elderly patients; severe peripheral constriction and cardiac stimulation, resulting in pulmonary arterial hypertension and potentially fatal pulmonary edema; and ventricular hyperirritability, which may result in death from ventricular fibrillation.

Epinephrine overdosage can also cause transient bradycardia followed by tachycardia; these may be accompanied by potentially fatal cardiac arrhythmias. Ventricular premature contractions may appear within 1 minute after injection and may be followed by multifocal ventricular tachycardia (prefibrillation rhythm). Subsidence of the ventricular effects may be followed by atrial tachycardia, and occasionally, by atrioventricular block.

The lethal dose is highly variable and appears to depend to a significant extent on patient factors that enhance susceptibility to serious toxicity. Subarachnoid hemorrhage has followed an SC dose of 0.5 mg. While doses of $\leq$ 10 mg IV have been fatal, survival has followed doses as high as 30 mg IV or 110 mg SC.

Overdosage sometimes results in extreme pallor and coldness of the skin, metabolic acidosis and kidney failure. Take suitable corrective measures.

Treatment: Most toxic effects can be counteracted by injection of an α-adrenergic blocker and a β-adrenergic blocker. In the event of a sharp rise in blood pressure, rapid acting vasodilators such as the nitrites, or α-adrenergic blocking agents can counteract the marked pressor effects. If prolonged hypotension follows, it may be necessary to administer another pressor drug, such as norepinephrine.

If an epinephrine overdose induces pulmonary edema that interferes with respiration, treatment consists of a rapidly acting α-adrenergic blocking drug such as phentolamine or intermittent positive pressure respiration.

Treat cardiac arrhythmias with a β-blocker (eg, propranolol).

(Continued on following page)

EPINEPHRINE (Cont.)

Administration and Dosage:

Administer by IV injection or in cardiac arrest by an endotracheal tube or intracardiac injection into the left ventricular chamber.

Cardiac arrest: 0.5 to 1 mg (5 to 10 ml of 1:10,000 solution). A dose of 0.5 ml may be diluted to 10 ml with sodium chloride injection. During a resuscitation effort, administer 0.5 to 1 mg (5 to 10 ml) IV every 5 minutes.

Intracardiac injection should only be administered by personnel well trained in the technique, if there has not been sufficient time to establish an IV route. Follow intracardial administration with external cardiac massage to permit the drug to enter coronary circulation. Use epinephrine secondarily to unsuccessful attempts with physical or electromechanical methods.

The intracardiac dose usually ranges from 0.3 to 0.5 mg (3 to 5 ml of 1:10,000 solution).

Cardiopulmonary resuscitation for cardiac arrest (Wyeth): IV or intracardiac administration of 1 to 10 ml of a 1:10,000 dilution is recommended. This emergency measure is generally adopted only if other measures (artificial ventilation, internal or external cardiac compression, administration of sodium bicarbonate) have failed. Artificial ventilation and cardiac compression must be continued. Doses of 1 to 10 ml of the 1:10,000 dilution may be repeated every 5 minutes as required. The IV route may be preferred since it need not interrupt cardiac compression.

Intravenous infusion: 1 mg in 250 ml of 5% Dextrose in Water (4 mcg/ml) to run at 1 to 4 mcg/min (15 to 60 ml/hour) has been recommended.

Intraspinal use: Usual dose is 0.2 to 0.4 ml of a 1:1000 solution added to anesthetic spinal fluid mixture (may prolong anesthetic action by limiting absorption).

Endotracheal tube: If IV access is not available, the drug may be injected via the endotracheal tube. Perform five rapid insufflations; forcefully expel 10 ml containing 1 mg epinephrine (0.1 mg/ml) directly into the endotracheal tube; follow with five quick insufflations.

Concomitant administration with local anesthetic: Epinephrine 1:100,000 to 1:20,000 is the usual concentration employed with local anesthetics.

Compatibility: If epinephrine and sodium bicarbonate are to be coadministered, inject individually at separate sites. Epinephrine is unstable in alkaline solution.

Stability and storage: Protect the solution from light, extreme heat and freezing. Do not use the injection if it is brown or contains a precipitate. Do not administer unless solution is clear and seal is intact. Do not remove ampuls or syringes from carton until ready to use. Discard unused portion.

	Product	Solution	Packaging	C.I.*
Rx	**Epinephrine HCl** (Various)	**Solution:** 1:1000 (1 mg/ml as the HCl)	In 1 ml amps, 1 ml vials, 1 ml syringes and 30 ml vials.	13+
Rx	**Epinephrine** (Abbott)		In 1 ml amps[1]	183
Rx	**Epinephrine HCl** (Elkins-Sinn)		In 1 ml Dosette amps.	126
Rx	**Epinephrine HCl** (Wyeth)		In 1 ml Tubex.[2]	513
Rx	**Epinephrine HCl** (Hollister-Stier)		In 2 ml syringe.[2]	750
Rx	**Adrenalin Chloride** (Parke-Davis)		In 1 ml amps[3] and 30 ml Steri-vials.[2]	558
Rx	**Epinephrine** (Various)	**Solution:** 1:10,000 (0.1 mg/ml)	In 3 and 10 ml syringes.	1437
Rx	**Epinephrine** (Abbott)	**Solution:** 1:10,000 (0.1 mg/ml as the HCl)	In 10 ml Abboject.[4]	2517
Rx	**Epinephrine HCl** (LyphoMed)		In 10 ml Bristoject.[5]	1937
Rx	**Epinephrine Pediatric** (Abbott)	**Solution:** 1:100,000 (0.01 mg/ml)	In 5 ml Abboject.[4]	39533

* Cost Index based on cost per 1 mg.
[1] With 0.9 mg sodium metabisulfite per ml.
[2] With not more than 5 mg chlorobutanol and 1.5 mg sodium bisulfite per ml.
[3] With not more than 0.1% sodium bisulfite.
[4] With 0.46 mg sodium metabisulfite per ml.
[5] With 0.5 mg sodium bisulfite.

Refer to the general discussion of these products on page 717.

NOREPINEPHRINE (Levarterenol)

Actions:

A powerful peripheral vasoconstrictor acting on both arterial and venous beds (α-adrenergic action) and as a potent inotropic stimulator of the heart (β_1 action). Coronary vasodilation occurs secondary to enhanced myocardial contractility. These actions result in an increase in systemic blood pressure and coronary artery blood flow. Cardiac output will vary in response to systemic hypertension, but is usually increased in hypotension when the blood pressure is raised to an optimal level. Venous return is increased and the heart tends to resume a more normal rate and rhythm than in the hypotensive state.

In hypotension that persists after correction of blood volume deficits, norepinephrine helps raise the blood pressure to an optimal level and establish a more adequate circulation.

Pharmacokinetics: Norepinephrine is ineffective orally; SC absorption is poor. It is rapidly inactivated by catechol-O-methyltransferase and monoamine oxidase. Negligible amounts are normally found in urine. When given by IV infusion, the onset is rapid; duration is 1 to 2 minutes following discontinuation of infusion.

Indications:

Restoration of blood pressure in controlling certain acute hypotensive states (eg, pheochromocytomectomy, sympathectomy, poliomyelitis, spinal anesthesia, myocardial infarction (MI), septicemia, blood transfusion, and drug reactions), and as an adjunct in the treatment of cardiac arrest and profound hypotension.

Contraindications:

Do not give to patients who are hypotensive from blood volume deficits, except as an emergency measure to maintain coronary and cerebral artery perfusion until blood volume replacement therapy can be completed. If continuously administered to maintain blood pressure in the absence of blood volume replacement, the following may occur: Severe peripheral and visceral vasoconstriction, decreased renal perfusion and urine output, poor systemic blood flow despite "normal" blood pressure, tissue hypoxia, and lactic acidosis.

Do not give to patients with mesenteric or peripheral vascular thrombosis (because of the risk of increasing ischemia and extending the area of infarction) unless administration is necessary as a life saving procedure.

Use of norepinephrine during cyclopropane and halothane anesthesia is generally considered contraindicated because of the risk of producing ventricular tachycardia or fibrillation. The same type of cardiac arrhythmias may result from use in patients with profound hypoxia or hypercarbia.

Precautions:

Hypovolemia: Use is not a substitute for the replacement of blood, plasma, fluids and electrolytes, which should be restored promptly when loss has occurred.

Avoid hypertension: Because of its potency and varying response to pressor substances, dangerously high blood pressure may be produced with overdoses. Monitor the blood pressure every 2 minutes from the time administration is started until the desired blood pressure is obtained, then every 5 minutes if administration is to be continued. Constantly watch flow rate. Never leave patient unattended during infusion. Headache may be a symptom of hypertension due to overdosage.

Infusion site: Whenever possible, infuse into a large vein, particularly an antecubital vein, to minimize necrosis of the overlying skin from prolonged vasoconstriction. The femoral vein may also be an acceptable route of administration. Avoid a catheter tie-in technique, if possible, since the obstruction to blood flow around the tubing may cause stasis and increased local concentration of the drug. Occlusive vascular diseases (ie, atherosclerosis, arteriosclerosis, diabetic endarteritis, Buerger's disease) are more likely to occur in the lower extremity; therefore, avoid the veins of the leg in elderly patients or in those suffering from such disorders.

(Precautions continued on following page)

EPHEDRINE (Cont.)

Overdosage:

Symptoms: The principal manifestation of ephedrine poisoning is convulsions. The following have occurred in acute poisoning: Nausea, vomiting, chills, cyanosis, irritability, nervousness, fever, suicidal behavior, tachycardia, dilated pupils, blurred vision, opisthotonos, spasms, convulsions, pulmonary edema, gasping respirations, coma and respiratory failure. Initially, the patient may have marked hypertension, followed later by hypotension accompanied by anuria. Large doses may lead to personality changes, with a psychological craving for the drug. Chronic use of ephedrine can also cause symptoms of tension and anxiety progressing to psychosis.

Treatment: Discontinue the drug. Remove the drug from the stomach by ipecac emesis, followed by activated charcoal or airway protected gastric lavage in depressed or hyperactive patients. If respirations are shallow or cyanosis is present, administer artificial respiration. Vasopressors are contraindicated. In cardiovascular collapse, maintain blood pressure.

For hypertension, 5 mg phentolamine mesylate diluted in saline may be administered slowly IV, or 100 mg may be given orally. Convulsions may be controlled by diazepam or paraldehyde. Cool applications and dexamethasone, 1 mg/kg, administered slowly IV, will control pyrexia. Recovery is likely if the patient survives the first 6 hours.

Administration and Dosage:

May be adminstered SC, IM or slow IV.

Adults: The usual dose is 25 to 50 mg. Absorption by the IM route is more rapid (onset within 10 to 20 minutes) than by SC injection. The IV route may be used if an immediate effect is desired. Also, 10 to 25 mg may be administered slow IV push. Additional doses may be given at 5 to 10 minute intervals, not to exceed 150 mg in 24 hours.

Pediatric dose: 3 mg/kg/day or 25 to 100 mg/m^2/day IV or SC divided into 4 to 6 doses.

Labor: Administer only sufficient dosage to maintain blood pressure at or below 130/80 mm Hg.

Acute attacks of asthma: Administer the smallest effective dose (0.25 to 0.5 ml).

Stability and storage: Ephedrine is subject to oxidation. Protect against exposure to light. Do not administer unless solution is clear. Discard unused portion.

	Product	Form	Packaging	C.I.*
Rx	**Ephedrine Sulfate** (Lilly)	**Injection:** 25 mg/ml	In 1 ml amps.	289
Rx	**Ephedrine Sulfate** (Various)	**Injection:** 50 mg/ml	In 1 ml amps.	150+
Rx	**Ephedrine Sulfate** (Abbott)		In 1 ml amps.	323
Rx	**Ephedrine Sulfate** (Lilly)		In 1 ml amps.	290
Rx	**Ephedrine** (LyphoMed)	**Injection:** 50 mg/ml	Preservative free. In 1 ml amps and 10 ml Bristoject.	325

* Cost Index based on cost per ml.

Refer to the general discussion of these products on page 717.

MEPHENTERMINE SULFATE

Actions:

Pharmacology: Mephentermine sulfate is a mixed-acting sympathomimetic amine that acts both directly and indirectly (ie, releases norepinephrine). The increase in blood pressure produced by mephentermine is probably due primarily to an increase in cardiac output resulting from enhanced cardiac contraction; to a lesser degree, an increase in peripheral resistance due to peripheral vasoconstriction may also contribute to the elevation in blood pressure.

Pharmacokinetics: The duration of action is prolonged. Pressor response is evident 5 to 15 minutes after IM injection and has a duration of 1 to 2 hours. Following IV administration, the pressor response is almost immediate and persists for 15 to 30 minutes after the drug is discontinued.

Indications:

Treatment of hypotension secondary to ganglionic blockade and that occurring with spinal anesthesia.

Although not recommended as corrective therapy for shock of hypotension secondary to hemorrhage, it may be used as an emergency measure to maintain blood pressure until blood or blood substitutes become available.

Contraindications:

Hypersensitivity to the drug; hypotension induced by chlorpromazine, since the sympathomimetic amines will act to potentiate, rather than correct, the hypotension secondary to the adrenolytic effects of chlorpromazine; in combination with any MAO inhibitor (see Drug Interactions).

Warnings:

Use mephentermine with caution in patients with known cardiovascular disease, and in chronically ill patients, since the drug's action on the cardiovascular system may be profound.

Persistent hypotension during or after surgery usually indicates hypovolemia. Treat by replacing blood volume.

Usage in Pregnancy and Lactation: Safety for use during pregnancy, in the nursing mother, or in women of childbearing potential has not been established. Use only when clearly needed and when the potential benefits outweigh the potential hazards to the fetus or to the nursing infant.

Precautions:

Hypovolemia: Use is not a substitute for the replacement of blood, plasma, fluids and electrolytes, which should be restored promptly when loss has occurred (ie, during or after surgery).

Hemorrhagic shock: Use with caution in treatment of shock secondary to hemorrhage. For effective emergency treatment, infuse 300 to 600 mg mephentermine in D5W. This will maintain blood pressure until volume replacement is accomplished.

Usage in hyperthyroidism: Increased responsiveness to vasopressor agents may be seen.

Usage in hypertensive patients: Administer with care to known hypertensives.

Drug Interactions:

Guanethidine: The antihypertensive effects of guanethidine may be partially or totally reversed by the mixed-acting sympathomimetics.

Halogenated hydrocarbon anesthetics may sensitize the myocardium to the effects of catecholamines. Use of vasopressors may lead to serious arrhythmias; use with extreme caution.

Monoamine oxidase (MAO) inhibitors increase the pressor response to mixed-acting vasopressors. Possible hypertensive crisis and intracranial hemorrhage may occur. This interaction may also occur with **furazolidone**, an antimicrobial with MAO inhibitor activity. Avoid this combination; if given inadvertently and hypertension occurs, administer phentolamine.

Oxytocic drugs: In obstetrics, if vasopressor drugs are used either to correct hypotension or are added to the local anesthetic solution, some oxytocics may cause severe persistent hypertension.

Tricyclic antidepressants: The pressor response of the mixed-acting vasopressors may be decreased by these agents; a higher dose of the sympathomimetic may be necessary.

Adverse Reactions:

Side effects following administration are minimal and result from the central stimulatory effects. Following recommended doses, an occasional patient may display signs of anxiety. Cardiac arrhythmias may be produced and blood pressure may be raised excessively, particularly in patients with heart disease.

(Continued on following page)

MEPHENTERMINE SULFATE (Cont.)

Administration and Dosage:

Can be administered IM without irritation or abnormal tissue reaction. Injection of an undiluted parenteral solution containing 30 mg/ml, or a continuous infusion of a 1 mg/ml solution in 5% Dextrose in Water, directly into the vein, is the preferable route for treatment of shock. IV administration of undiluted mephentermine does not produce vascular irritation and no untoward tissue reaction will develop should extravasation occur.

Dosage used in treatment of shock and hypotension is based on experimental observation that 0.5 mg/kg produces a positive inotropic action.

Prevention of hypotension attendant to spinal anesthesia: Administer 30 to 45 mg IM 10 to 20 minutes prior to anesthesia, operation or termination of the operative procedure.

Hypotension following spinal anesthesia: Administer 30 to 45 mg IV in a single injection. Repeat doses of 30 mg as necessary to maintain blood pressure. An immediate response and maintenance of blood pressure can be accomplished by the continuous IV infusion of a 0.1% solution of mephentermine in 5% Dextrose in Water (1 mg/ml). Regulate flow and duration of therapy according to the response of the patient.

Hypotension secondary to spinal anesthesia in the obstetrical patient undergoing cesarean section, who is known to be sensitive to drugs: Administer an initial dose of 15 mg of mephentermine IV. This dose may be repeated if the response is not adequate.

Treatment of shock following hemorrhage: Although not recommended, the continuous IV infusion of a 0.1% solution of mephentermine in 5% Dextrose in Water may be useful in maintaining blood pressure until whole blood replacement can be accomplished.

Preparation of IV solution: The 0.1% solution can be prepared in the approximate concentration (0.115%) by adding 10 or 20 ml of mephentermine, 30 mg/ml, to 250 or 500 ml of 5% Dextrose in Water, respectively.

				C.I.*
Rx	**Wyamine Sulfate** (Wyeth)	**Injection:** 15 mg per ml[1]	In 10 ml vials and 2 ml amps.	252
		30 mg per ml[1]	In 10 ml vials.	400

* Cost Index based on cost per ml.

[1] With 1.8 mg methylparaben and 0.2 mg propylparaben.

Refer to the general discussion of these products on page 717.

METARAMINOL

Actions:

Pharmacology: A potent sympathomimetic amine that increases both systolic and diastolic blood pressure, primarily by vasoconstriction; this effect is usually accompanied by a marked reflex bradycardia. Metaraminol has a direct effect on alpha-adrenergic receptors. It does not depend on release of norepinephrine but it has indirect activity. Prolonged infusions can deplete norepinephrine from sympathetic nerve endings. Repeated use may result in an overall diminution of sympathetic activity.

Renal, coronary and cerebral blood flow are a function of perfusion pressure and regional resistance. In most instances of cardiogenic shock, the beneficial effect of sympathomimetic amines is their positive inotropic effect. In patients with insufficient or failing vasoconstriction, there is additional advantage to the peripheral action of metaraminol, but in most patients with shock, vasoconstriction is adequate and any further increase is unnecessary. Therefore, blood flow to vital organs may decrease with metaraminol if regional resistance increases excessively. It increases cardiac output in hypotensive patients.

Metaraminol increases venous tone, causes pulmonary vasoconstriction and elevates pulmonary pressure even when cardiac output is reduced.

Pressor effect is decreased, but not reversed, by alpha-adrenergic blocking agents. When pressor responses are due primarily to vasoconstriction, cardiac stimulation may play a small role. Although uncommon, tachyphylaxis and a fall in blood pressure may occur with repeated use.

Pharmacokinetics: The pressor effect begins 1 to 2 minutes after IV infusion, about 10 minutes after IM injection, and 5 to 20 minutes after SC injection. The effect lasts from about 20 minutes to 1 hour.

Indications:

Prevention and treatment of the acute hypotensive state occurring with spinal anesthesia; adjunctive treatment of hypotension due to hemorrhage; reactions to medications; surgical complications; shock associated with brain damage due to trauma or tumor.

"Probably effective" as an adjunct in the treatment of hypotension due to cardiogenic shock or septicemia.

Contraindications:

Avoid use with cyclopropane or halothane anesthesia, unless clinical circumstances demand such use (see Drug Interactions); hypersensitivity to metaraminol.

Warnings:

Cardiac effects: Metaraminol may cause cardiac arrhythmias. This may be particularly dangerous in patients with MI or in patients who have received anesthetics which sensitize the heart to catecholamines (ie, cyclopropane, halothane, etc).

Prolonged administration may reduce the venous return and cardiac output and increase the work load of the heart. Metabolic acidosis may ensue.

(Continued on following page)

METARAMINOL (Cont.)

Precautions:

Use with caution in heart or thyroid disease, hypertension or diabetes.

Hypovolemia: Use is not a substitute for the replacement of blood, plasma, fluids and electrolytes, which should be restored promptly when loss has occurred.

Vasoconstriction: When vasopressor amines are used for long periods, the resulting vasoconstriction may prevent adequate expansion of circulating volume and may perpetuate the shock state. Measurement of central venous pressure is useful in assessment of plasma volume. Therefore, employ blood or plasma volume expanders when circulating volume is decreased.

Hypertension: Avoid excessive blood pressure response. Rapidly induced hypertensive responses have been reported to cause acute pulmonary edema, arrhythmias and cardiac arrest.

Usage in cirrhosis: Treat patients with cirrhosis cautiously and with adequate restoration of electrolytes if diuresis ensues. Fatal ventricular arrhythmia has been reported in one patient with Laennec's cirrhosis while receiving the drug. In several instances, ventricular extrasystoles that appeared during infusion subsided promptly when the rate of infusion was reduced.

Cumulative effects: Because of its prolonged action, a cumulative effect is possible, and with an excessive vasopressor response there may be a prolonged elevation of blood pressure, even with discontinuation. It is important to make frequent assessments of the blood pressure, particularly when administering IV.

Extravasation: Exercise care when selecting the site of administration of this drug, particularly when given by the IV route. The use of larger veins (the antecubital fossa or the thigh) is preferred. Avoid those of the ankle or dorsum of the hand, especially in patients with peripheral vascular disease, diabetes mellitus, Buerger's disease or hypercoagulability states. Extravasation may cause abscess formation, tissue necrosis and sloughing of surrounding tissue. Monitor the infusion site closely for free flow. Discontinue the infusion immediately if infiltration or thrombosis occurs.

Antidote for extravasation - To prevent sloughing and necrosis in ischemic areas, infiltrate area as soon as possible with 10 to 15 ml saline solution containing 5 to 10 mg phentolamine. Use a syringe with a fine hypodermic needle and infiltrate liberally throughout the ischemic area. Sympathetic blockade with phentolamine causes immediate and conspicuous local hyperemic changes if the area is infiltrated within 12 hours.

Malaria: Sympathomimetic amines may provoke a relapse in patients with a history of malaria.

Sulfite Sensitivity: Sulfites may cause allergic-type reactions (eg, hives, itching, wheezing, anaphylaxis) in certain susceptible persons. Although the overall prevalence of sulfite sensitivity in the general population is probably low, it is seen more frequently in asthmatics or in atopic nonasthmatic persons. Specific products containing sulfites are identified in the product listings.

Drug Interactions:

Guanethidine: The antihypertensive effects of guanethidine may be partially or totally reversed by the mixed-acting sympathomimetics.

Halogenated hydrocarbon anesthetics may sensitize the myocardium to the effects of catecholamines. Use of vasopressors may lead to serious arrhythmias; use with extreme caution.

Monoamine oxidase (MAO) inhibitors increase the pressor response to mixed-acting vasopressors. Possible hypertensive crisis and intracranial hemorrhage may occur. This interaction may also occur with **furazolidone**, an antimicrobial with MAO inhibitor activity. Avoid this combination; if given inadvertently and hypertension occurs, administer phentolamine.

Oxytocic drugs: If vasopressor drugs are used in obstetrics to correct hypotension or added to the local anesthetic solution, some oxytocic drugs may cause severe persistent hypertension.

Tricyclic antidepressants: The pressor response of the mixed-acting vasopressors may be decreased by these agents; a higher dose of the sympathomimetic may be necessary.

(Continued on following page)

METARAMINOL (Cont.)

Adverse Reactions:

Cardiovascular: Sympathomimetic amines may cause sinus or ventricular tachycardia, or other arrhythmias, especially in patients with MI. Hypertension, hypotension following cessation of the drug, cardiac arrhythmias, cardiac arrest and palpitation have occurred.

Miscellaneous: Headache; flushing; sweating; tremors; dizziness; nausea; apprehension; abscess formation; tissue necrosis; sloughing at injection site.

Overdosage:

Overdosage with metaraminol may cause convulsions, cerebral hemorrhage or cardiac arrhythmias. Patients with hyperthyroidism or hypertension are particularly sensitive to these effects.

Administration and Dosage:

May be given IM, SC or IV, although the IM and SC routes are rarely used. Because the maximum effect is not immediately apparent, allow at least 10 minutes to elapse before increasing the dose. When the vasopressor is discontinued, observe the patient carefully so that therapy can be reinitiated promptly if the blood pressure falls too rapidly. The response to vasopressors may be poor in patients with coexistent shock and acidosis. Established methods of shock management and other measures directed to the specific cause of the shock state should also be employed.

IM or SC injection (prevention of hypotension): The recommended dose is 2 to 10 mg. Wait at least 10 minutes before evaluating the effects of the initial dose prior to readministration.

IV infusion (adjunctive treatment of hypotension): The recommended dose is 15 to 100 mg in 250 or 500 ml of Sodium Chloride Injection or 5% Dextrose Injection; adjust the rate of infusion to maintain the blood pressure at the desired level. Higher concentrations, 150 to 500 mg/250 or 500 ml of infusion fluid, have been used. The concentration of drug in the infusion fluid may be adjusted depending on the patient's need for fluid replacement.

Direct IV injection: In severe shock, give by direct IV injection. The suggested dose is 0.5 to 5 mg, followed by an infusion of 15 to 100 mg in 250 to 500 ml of infusion fluid, as described previously.

Unlabeled route of administration:

Endotracheal tube – If IV access is not available, the drug may be injected via the endotracheal tube. Perform five rapid insufflations; forcefully expel 5 mg diluted to a volume of 10 ml into the endotracheal tube; follow with five quick insufflations.

Children: 0.01 mg/kg as a single dose or a solution of 1 mg/25 ml in dextrose or saline.

Compatibility: In addition to Sodium Chloride Injection and 5% Dextrose Injection, the following infusion solutions were found physically and chemically compatible with metaraminol when 5 ml (10 mg/ml) was added to 500 ml of infusion solution: Ringer's Injection, Lactated Ringer's Injection, 6% Dextran in Saline, *Normosol-R* pH 7.4, *Normosol-M* in D5-W.

Stability: Infusion solutions should be used within 24 hours.

				C.I.*
Rx	**Metaraminol Bitartrate** (LyphoMed)	**Injection:** 10 mg per ml (1%, as bitartrate)	In 10 ml Bristoject.	337
Rx	**Aramine** (MSD)		In 10 ml vials.[1]	262

* Cost Index based on cost per ml.

[1] With 0.15% methylparaben, 0.02% propylparaben and 0.2% sodium bisulfite.

Refer to the general discussion of these products on page 717.

METHOXAMINE HCl

Actions:

Pharmacology: A vasopressor that produces a prompt and prolonged rise in blood pressure by increasing peripheral resistance (α effect). It is especially useful for maintaining blood pressure during operations under spinal anesthesia. It may also be used during general anesthesia.

Provides potent, prolonged pressor action. There is no increase in cardiac rate; occasionally, a decrease in rate develops as the blood pressure increases. This bradycardia is apparently caused by a carotid sinus reflex; this is abolished by atropine.

Indications:

For supporting, restoring or maintaining blood pressure during anesthesia (including cyclopropane anesthesia); for terminating some episodes of supraventricular tachycardia.

Contraindications:

Severe hypertension; hypersensitivity to methoxamine.

Warnings:

Usage in Pregnancy: Category C. Methoxamine decreases uterine blood flow, decreases fetal heart rate and adversely affects the fetal acid-base status in pregnant ewes and monkeys at doses comparable to those used in humans. There are no adequate and well controlled studies in pregnant women. There has been one report of a fetal death; the mother received methoxamine concomitantly with several other drugs. A direct causal relationship to methoxamine was not established. Use during pregnancy only if the potential benefit justifies the potential risk to the fetus.

Usage in Lactation: It is not known whether methoxamine is excreted in breast milk. Exercise caution when administering methoxamine to a nursing woman.

Usage in Children: Safety and efficacy in children have not been established.

Precautions:

Hypovolemia: Use is not a substitute for the replacement of blood, plasma, fluids and electrolytes, which should be restored promptly when loss has occurred.

Extravasation: When infused, large veins of the antecubital fossa are preferred to veins in the hand or ankle to prevent extravasation. Extravasation may cause necrosis and sloughing of surrounding tissue. Monitor the infusion site closely for free flow.

Antidote for extravasation – To prevent sloughing and necrosis in ischemic areas, infiltrate as soon as possible with 10 to 15 ml saline solution containing 5 to 10 mg phentolamine. Use a fine hypodermic needle and infiltrate liberally throughout the ischemic area. Sympathetic blockade with phentolamine causes immediate and conspicuous local hyperemic changes if area is infiltrated within 12 hours.

Use with care in patients with hyperthyroidism, bradycardia, partial heart block, myocardial disease or severe arteriosclerosis.

Sulfite Sensitivity: Sulfites may cause allergic-type reactions (eg, hives, itching, wheezing, anaphylaxis) in certain susceptible persons. Although the overall prevalence of sulfite sensitivity in the general population is probably low, it is more frequent in asthmatics or in atopic nonasthmatic persons. Specific products containing sulfites are identified in the product listings.

Drug Interactions:

Bretylium may potentiate the action of vasopressors on adrenergic receptors, possibly resulting in arrhythmias.

Guanethidine may increase the pressor response of the direct-acting vasopressors, possibly resulting in severe hypertension.

Halogenated hydrocarbon anesthetics may sensitize the myocardium to the effects of catecholamines. Use of vasopressors may lead to serious arrhythmias; use with extreme caution.

Oxytocic drugs: If vasopressors are used in obstetrics to correct hypotension or are added to the local anesthetic solution, some oxytocics may cause severe persistent hypertension.

Tricyclic antidepressants: The pressor response of the direct-acting vasopressors may be potentiated by these agents; use with caution.

Drug/Lab Tests: Methoxamine may increase plasma cortisol and ACTH levels. Exercise caution when interpreting plasma cortisol and ACTH levels in patients receiving methoxamine.

(Continued on following page)

METHOXAMINE HCl (Cont.)

Adverse Reactions:

Cardiovascular: Excessive blood pressure elevations particularly with high dosage, ventricular ectopic beats.

GI: Nausea, vomiting (often projectile).

CNS: Headache (often severe), anxiety.

Integumentary: Sweating, pilomotor response.

GU: Uterine hypertonus, fetal bradycardia, urinary urgency.

Overdosage:

Symptoms: Undesirably high blood pressure or excessive bradycardia. Clinically significant elevations of blood pressure may be reversed with an α-adrenergic blocking agent (eg, phentolamine). Bradycardia may be abolished with atropine.

Administration and Dosage:

Emergencies: 3 to 5 mg IV injected slowly. IV injection may be supplemented by IM injections to provide a prolonged effect.

Spinal anesthesia - Usual IM dose is 10 to 15 mg shortly before or with spinal anesthesia to prevent hypotension. A 10 mg dose may be adequate at lower levels; 15 to 20 mg may be required at high levels of spinal anesthesia. Repeat doses if necessary, but allow time for the previous dose to act (about 15 minutes).

Correcting a fall in blood pressure - 10 to 15 mg IM, depending on degree of decrease. Where systolic pressure falls below 60 mm Hg or when an emergency exists, give 3 to 5 mg IV. This may be accompanied by 10 to 15 mg IM for prolonged effect or a continuous infusion starting at 5 mcg/min (40 mg in 250 ml 5% Dextrose in Water).

Pre- and postoperative use (moderate hypotension): 5 to 10 mg IM may be adequate.

Supraventricular tachycardia: Average dose, 10 mg IV injected slowly.

				C.I.*
Rx	**Vasoxyl** (Burroughs Wellcome)	**Injection:** 20 mg/ml	In 1 ml amps.[1]	358

* Cost Index based on cost per ml.

[1] With 0.1% potassium metabisulfite.

Refer to the general discussion of these products on page 717.

PHENYLEPHRINE HCl

Actions:

Pharmacology: Phenylephrine is a powerful postsynaptic alpha-receptor stimulant with little effect on the beta receptors of the heart.

The predominant actions of phenylephrine are on the cardiovascular system. Parenteral administration causes a rise in systolic and diastolic pressures due to peripheral vasoconstriction. Accompanying the pressor response to phenylephrine is a marked reflex bradycardia that can be blocked by atropine; after atropine, large doses of the drug increase the heart rate only slightly. Cardiac output is slightly decreased and peripheral resistance is considerably increased. Circulation time is slightly prolonged, and venous pressure is slightly increased; venous constriction is not marked. Most vascular beds are constricted; renal, splanchnic, cutaneous and limb blood flows are reduced, but coronary blood flow is increased. Pulmonary vessels are constricted, and pulmonary arterial pressure is raised.

The drug is a powerful vasoconstrictor, with properties very similar to those of norepinephrine, but almost completely lacking the chronotropic and inotropic actions on the heart. Cardiac irregularities are seen only very rarely, even with large doses. In contrast to epinephrine and ephedrine, phenylephrine produces longer lasting vasoconstriction, a reflex bradycardia and increases the stroke output, producing no disturbance in the rhythm of the pulse.

In therapeutic doses, it produces little if any stimulation of either the spinal cord or cerebrum. An advantage is that repeated injections produce comparable effects.

Indications:

Treatment of vascular failure in shock, shock-like states, drug-induced hypotension, or hypersensitivity; to overcome paroxysmal supraventricular tachycardia; to prolong spinal anesthesia; as a vasoconstrictor in regional analgesia; to maintain an adequate level of blood pressure during spinal and inhalation anesthesia.

Contraindications:

Hypersensitivity to the drug; severe hypertension; ventricular tachycardia.

Warnings:

Usage in Pregnancy: Category C. Safety for use during pregnancy has not been established. Use only when clearly needed and when the potential benefits outweigh the potential hazards to the fetus.

Labor and Delivery: If used in conjunction with **oxytocic drugs**, the pressor effect of sympathomimetic pressor amines is potentiated.

Usage in Lactation: It is not known whether this drug is excreted in breast milk. Safety for use in the nursing mother has not been established. Because many drugs are excreted in breast milk, exercise caution when administering to a nursing woman.

Precautions:

Use with extreme caution in elderly patients, patients with hyperthyroidism, bradycardia, partial heart block, myocardial disease or severe arteriosclerosis.

Hypovolemia: Use is not a substitute for the replacement of blood, plasma, fluids and electrolytes, which should be restored promptly when loss has occurred.

Extravasation: When infused, large veins of the antecubital fossa are preferred to veins in the hand or ankle to prevent extravasation. Extravasation may cause necrosis and sloughing of surrounding tissue. Monitor the infusion site closely for free flow.

Antidote for extravasation – To prevent sloughing and necrosis in ischemic areas, infiltrate area as soon as possible with 10 to 15 ml saline solution containing 5 to 10 mg phentolamine. Use a syringe with a fine hypodermic needle and infiltrate liberally throughout the ischemic area. Sympathetic blockade with phentolamine causes immediate and conspicuous local hyperemic changes if the area is infiltrated within 12 hours.

Sulfite Sensitivity: Sulfites may cause allergic-type reactions (eg, hives, itching, wheezing, anaphylaxis) in certain susceptible persons. Although the overall prevalence of sulfite sensitivity in the general population is probably low, it is seen more frequently in asthmatics or in atopic nonasthmatic persons. Specific products containing sulfites are identified in the product listings.

(Continued on following page)

PHENYLEPHRINE HCl (Cont.)

Drug Interactions:

Bretylium may potentiate the action of vasopressors on adrenergic receptors, possibly resulting in arrhythmias.

Guanethidine may increase the pressor response of the direct-acting vasopressors, possibly resulting in severe hypertension.

Halogenated hydrocarbon anesthetics may sensitize the myocardium to the effects of catecholamines. Use of vasopressors may lead to serious arrhythmias; use with extreme caution.

Monoamine oxidase (MAO) inhibitors may significantly enhance the adrenergic effects of phenylephrine, and its pressor response may be increased twofold to threefold. Phenylephrine is metabolized by gut and liver MAO. This interaction may also occur with **furazolidone,** an antimicrobial with MAO inhibitor activity. Avoid this combination; if given inadvertently and hypertension occurs, administer phentolamine.

Oxytocic drugs: If vasopressors are used in obstetrics to correct hypotension or are added to the local anesthetic solution, some oxytocics may cause severe persistent hypertension.

Tricyclic antidepressants have both increased and decreased the sensitivity to IV phenylephrine.

Adverse Reactions:

Headache; reflex bradycardia; excitability; restlessness; rarely, arrhythmias.

Overdosage:

Symptoms: Ventricular extrasystoles; short paroxysms of ventricular tachycardia; sensation of fullness in the head; tingling of the extremities.

Treatment: Relieve an excessive elevation of blood pressure by an α-adrenergic blocking agent (ie, phentolamine).

Administration and Dosage:

Inject SC, IM, slow IV, or in dilute solution as a continuous IV infusion. In patients with paroxysmal supraventricular tachycardia and, if indicated, in case of emergency, administer directly IV. Adjust dose according to the pressor response.

Phenylephrine Dosage Calculations

Dose Required (mg)	0.1	0.2	0.5	1	5	10
Phenylephrine 1% (ml)	—	—	—	0.1	0.5	1
Diluted Phenylephrine[1] 0.1% (ml)	0.1	0.2	0.5	—	—	—

[1] For convenience in intermittent IV administration, dilute 1 ml phenylephrine 1% with 9 ml Sterile Water for Injection, USP.

(Administration and Dosage continued on following page)

PHENYLEPHRINE HCl (Cont.)

Administration and Dosage (Cont.):

Mild or moderate hypotension:

SC or IM – 2 to 5 mg (range, 1 to 10 mg). Do not exceed an initial dose of 5 mg. A 5 mg IM dose should raise blood pressure for 1 to 2 hours.

IV – 0.2 mg (range, 0.1 to 0.5 mg). Do not exceed an initial dose of 0.5 mg. Do not repeat injections more often than every 10 to 15 minutes. A 0.5 mg IV dose should elevate the pressure for about 15 minutes.

To prepare a 0.1% solution of phenylephrine (0.1 mg/0.1 ml), dilute 1 ml of 1% solution with 9 ml Sterile Water for Injection.

Severe hypotension and shock including drug-related hypotension: Correct blood volume depletion as completely as possible before any vasopressor is administered. When intraaortic pressures must be maintained as an emergency measure to prevent cerebral or coronary artery ischemia, phenylephrine can be administered before and concurrently with blood volume replacement.

Hypotension and occasionally severe shock may result from overdosage or idiosyncratic reactions following administration of certain drugs, especially adrenergic and ganglionic blocking agents, rauwolfia, veratrum alkaloids and phenothiazine derivatives. Patients who receive a phenothiazine as preoperative medication are especially susceptible. As an adjunct in the management of such episodes, phenylephrine is a suitable agent for restoring blood pressure.

Higher initial and maintenance doses are required in patients with persistent or untreated severe hypotension or shock. Hypotension produced by powerful peripheral adrenergic blocking agents (chlorpromazine) or pheochromocytomectomy may also require more intensive therapy.

Continuous infusion – Add 10 mg to 250 or 500 ml of Dextrose Injection or Sodium Chloride Injection (providing a 1:25,000 or 1:50,000 dilution). To raise the blood pressure rapidly, start the infusion at about 100 to 180 mcg per minute (based on 20 drops per ml, this would be 50 to 90 or 100 to 180 drops per minute). When the blood pressure is stabilized (at a low normal level for the individual), a maintenance rate of 40 to 60 mcg per minute usually suffices (based on 20 drops per ml, this would be 20 to 30 or 40 to 60 drops per minute). If the drop size of the infusion system varies from 20 drops per ml, adjust the dose accordingly.

If a prompt initial vasopressor response is not obtained, add additional increments of the drug (10 mg or more) to the infusion bottle. Adjust the flow rate until the desired blood pressure level is obtained. (A more potent vasopressor, such as norepinephrine, may be required.) Avoid hypertension. Check blood pressure frequently. Headache or bradycardia may indicate hypertension. Arrhythmias are rare.

Spinal anesthesia: Hypotension – Administer SC or IM 3 or 4 minutes before injection of the spinal anesthetic. The total requirement for high anesthetic levels is usually 3 mg, and for lower levels, 2 mg. For hypotensive emergencies during spinal anesthesia, phenylephrine may be injected IV beginning with a dose of 0.2 mg. Any subsequent dose should not exceed the previous dose by more than 0.1 to 0.2 mg; do not administer more than 0.5 mg in a single dose.

Pediatric dose: To combat hypotension during spinal anesthesia in children, administer 0.5 to 1 mg per 25 lbs, SC or IM.

Prolongation of spinal anesthesia: The addition of 2 to 5 mg phenylephrine to the anesthetic solution increases the duration of motor block by as much as 50% without an increase in the incidence of complications (eg, nausea, vomiting or blood pressure disturbances).

Vasoconstrictor for regional analgesia: Concentrations about 10 times those of epinephrine are recommended. The optimum strength is 1:20,000 (made by adding 1 mg phenylephrine to every 20 ml of local anesthetic solution). Some pressor responses may be expected when 2 mg or more are injected.

Paroxysmal supraventricular tachycardia: Rapid IV injection (within 20 to 30 seconds) is recommended; do not exceed an initial dose of 0.5 mg. Subsequent doses, which are determined by the initial blood pressure response, should not exceed the preceding dose by more than 0.1 to 0.2 mg, and should never exceed 1 mg.

IV compatibility: Phenylephrine at a concentration of 1 mg/L was found to be physically compatible with the following IV solutions: Dextrose-Ringer's combinations; Dextrose-Lactated Ringer's combinations; Dextrose-saline combinations; Dextrose 2½%, 5% and 10% in Water; Ringer's Injection; Lactated Ringer's Injection; 0.45% and 0.9% Sodium Chloride Injection; ⅙ M Sodium Lactate Injection.

				C.I.*
Rx	**Neo-Synephrine** (Winthrop Pharm.)	**Injection:** 1% (10 mg per ml)	In 1 ml Uni-Nest amps.[1]	973

* Cost Index based on cost per ml.

[1] With sodium bisulfite.

Actions:

Pharmacology: Beta-adrenergic receptor blocking agents compete with beta-adrenergic agonists for available beta receptor sites. Propranolol, nadolol, timolol, penbutolol, carteolol and pindolol inhibit both the β_1 receptors (located chiefly in cardiac muscle) and β_2 receptors (located chiefly in the bronchial and vascular musculature), inhibiting the chronotropic, inotropic and vasodilator responses to β-adrenergic stimulation. Metoprolol, acebutolol, esmolol, betaxolol and atenolol are cardioselective and preferentially inhibit β_1 receptors.

Propranolol and, to a lesser extent, acebutolol, betaxolol and pindolol, exert a quinidine-like (anesthetic) membrane action (membrane stabilizing activity; MSA) which affects cardiac action potential. Nadolol, carteolol, atenolol and timolol do not have MSA and have little direct myocardial depressant activity. The MSA was once considered to be responsible for the antiarrhythmic effectiveness of these agents; however, MSA appears to occur only with doses that far exceed those used in the treatment of arrhythmias. Pindolol, carteolol, penbutolol and acebutolol have intrinsic sympathomimetic activity (ISA) in therapeutic dosage ranges. The ISA or partial agonist activity is mediated directly at adrenergic receptor sites and may be blocked by other β antagonists. ISA is manifested by a smaller reduction in resting cardiac output and a smaller reduction in the resting heart rate (4 to 8 bpm) than is seen with drugs lacking ISA; clinical significance has not been evaluated and there is no evidence that exercise cardiac output is less affected by pindolol.

Pharmacologic/Pharmacokinetic Properties of Beta-Adrenergic Blocking Agents

Drug	Adrenergic receptor blocking activity	Membrane stabilizing activity	Intrinsic sympathomimetic activity	Lipid solubility	Extent of absorption (%)	Absolute oral bioavailability (%)	Half-life (hrs)	Protein binding (%)	Metabolism/Excretion
Acebutolol	β_1[1]	+	+	Low	90	20-60	3-4	26	hepatic; renal excretion 30% to 40%; non-renal excretion 50% to 60% (bile; intestinal wall)
Atenolol	β_1[1]	0	0	Low	50	50-60	6-9	6-16	≈ 50% excreted unchanged in feces
Betaxolol	β_1[1]	+	0	Low	≈ 100	89	14-22	≈ 50	hepatic; > 80% recovered in urine, 15% unchanged
Esmolol	β_1[1]	0	0	Low	na	na	0.15	55	Rapid metabolism by esterases in cytosol of red blood cells
Metoprolol	β_1[1]	0[2]	0	Moderate	95	40-50	3-7	12	hepatic; renal excretion
Carteolol	β_1 β_2	0	++	Low	80	85	6	23-30	50% to 70% excreted unchanged in urine
Nadolol	β_1 β_2	0	0	Low	30	30-50	20-24	30	urine, unchanged
Penbutolol	β_1 β_2	0	+	High	≈100	≈100	5	80-98	hepatic (conjugation and oxidation); renal excretion of metabolites (17% as conjugate)
Pindolol	β_1 β_2	+	+++	Moderate	95	≈100	3-4[3]	40	urinary excretion of metabolites (60% to 65%) and unchanged drug (35% to 40%)
Propranolol	β_1 β_2	++	0	High	90	30	3-5	90	hepatic; < 1% excreted unchanged in urine
Propranolol, long-acting						9-18	8-11		
Timolol	β_1 β_2	0	0	Low to moderate	90	75	4	10	hepatic; urinary excretion of metabolites and unchanged drug
Labetalol[4]	β_1 β_2 α_1	0	0	Moderate	100	30-40	5.5-8	50	55% to 60% excreted in urine as conjugates or unchanged drug

[1] Inhibits β_2 receptors (bronchial and vascular) at higher doses.
[2] Detectable only at doses much greater than required for beta blockade.
[3] In elderly hypertensive patients with normal renal function, t½ variable: 7 to 15 hours.
[4] See labetalol monograph. na = Not applicable (available IV only).

(Actions continued on following page)

Actions (Cont.):

Pharmacokinetics:

Absorption –Systemic bioavailability following oral administration of metoprolol, acebutolol, timolol and propranolol is low because of significant first-pass hepatic metabolism. Pindolol and carteolol have no significant first-pass effect. Ingestion with food enhances the bioavailability of propranolol and metoprolol; this effect is not noted with nadolol, carteolol, pindolol or betaxolol.

Distribution –There is no simple correlation between dose or plasma level and therapeutic effect; the dose-sensitivity range observed in clinical practice is wide because sympathetic tone varies widely among individuals. There is no reliable test to estimate sympathetic tone or to determine whether total β blockade has been achieved; proper dosage requires titration. Inhibition of maximal exercise tachycardia is a reasonable index of total β blockade; isoproterenol sensitivity testing may also be used. There appear to be significant correlations between **acebutolol** plasma levels and both the reduction in resting heart rate and the percent of β blockade of exercise-induced tachycardia.

Metoprolol and propranolol readily enter the CNS. Because of their high water solubility, acebutolol, carteolol, nadolol and atenolol do not pass the blood brain barrier; these drugs may have a lower incidence of CNS side effects.

Clinical Pharmacology: Clinical response to β blockade includes slowing of sinus heart rate, depressed AV conduction, decreased cardiac output at rest and on exercise, reduction of systolic and diastolic blood pressure at rest and on exercise, reduction of both supine and standing blood pressure, inhibition of isoproterenol-induced tachycardia and reduction of reflex orthostatic tachycardia. β-adrenergic receptor blockade is useful in conditions (angina, hypertension) in which, because of pathologic or functional changes, sympathetic activity is detrimental to the patient. Also, in some situations, sympathetic stimulation is vital. In patients with severely damaged hearts, adequate ventricular function is maintained by virtue of sympathetic drive which should be preserved. β-adrenergic blockade may worsen AV block by preventing necessary facilitating effects of sympathetic activity on conduction.

β_2-adrenergic blockade results in passive bronchial constriction by interfering with endogenous adrenergic bronchodilator activity in patients subject to bronchospasm and may also interfere with exogenous bronchodilators. Although pindolol does not eliminate sympathetic tone entirely, there is no controlled evidence that it is safer than other agents or is less likely to cause such conditions as heart failure, heart block or bronchospasm.

Hypertension – β-blockers decrease standing and supine blood pressure. They are effective antihypertensives when used alone or with other antihypertensives.

Although not established, several mechanisms have been proposed which include: Competitive antagonism of catecholamines at peripheral (non-CNS) adrenergic neuron sites (especially cardiac) leading to decreased cardiac output; a central effect leading to reduced sympathetic outflow to the periphery; and by blockade of the beta-adrenergic receptors responsible for renin release from the kidneys. These mechanisms appear less likely for **pindolol** than other β-blockers in view of the modest effect on resting cardiac output and its inconsistent effect on plasma renin activity. Although total peripheral resistance may increase initially, it readjusts to the pretreatment level, or lower, with chronic usage. Effects on plasma volume appear to be minor and somewhat variable. **Propranolol** may cause a small increase in serum potassium concentration when used in the treatment of hypertensive patients.

Angina – **Propranolol** and **nadolol** may reduce myocardial oxygen requirements by blocking catecholamine-induced increases in heart rate, systolic blood pressure and the velocity and extent of myocardial contraction. Oxygen requirements may be increased by increasing left ventricular fiber length, end diastolic pressure and systolic ejection period. The net physiologic effect of β-adrenergic blockade is advantageous and is manifested during exercise by delayed onset of pain and increased work capacity.

Arrhythmias – **Propranolol** and **acebutolol** exert antiarrhythmic effects in concentrations associated with β-adrenergic blockade. The significance of the MSA in the treatment of arrhythmias is uncertain. Propranolol and acebutolol prolong the effective refractory period of the AV node, and slow AV conduction.

Myocardial infarction (MI) – **Timolol, propranolol, metoprolol** and **atenolol** are labeled for use in the prevention of reinfarction. The mechanism is unknown, but the protective effect is consistent regardless of age, sex or site of infarction. The effect is clearest in patients with a first infarction who were at high risk of dying, defined as those with one or more of the following characteristics during the acute phase: Transient left ventricular failure, cardiomegaly, new atrial fibrillation or flutter, systolic hypotension or AST levels greater than 4 times the upper normal limit. The incidence of nonfatal reinfarction is also reduced.

Migraine – The mechanism of **propranolol's** antimigraine effect has not been established. Beta-adrenergic receptors have been demonstrated in the pial vessels of the brain.

Antitremor – The specific mechanism of **propranolol's** antitremor effects has not been established, but β_2 receptors may be involved. A central effect is also possible.

(Continued on following page)

Indications:

Beta-Adrenergic Blocking Agents – Summary of Indications[1]

Indications ✓ = labeled × = unlabeled	Acebutolol	Atenolol	Betaxolol	Carteolol	Esmolol	Metoprolol	Nadolol	Penbutolol	Pindolol	Propranolol	Timolol	Labetalol
Hypertension	✓	✓	✓	✓		✓	✓	✓	✓	✓	✓	✓
Angina pectoris		✓		×		✓	✓			✓		
Hypertrophic subaortic stenosis										✓		
Cardiac arrhythmias												
Supraventricular arrhythmias/ tachycardias		×			✓					✓		
Sinus tachycardia					✓							
Ventricular arrhythmias/ tachycardias		×				×	×		×	✓	×	
PVCs	✓									✓		
Digitalis-induced tachyarrhythmias										✓		
Resistant tachyarrhythmias (catecholamine/anesthesia)										✓		
Atrial ectopy						×						
Myocardial infarction		✓				✓				✓	✓	
Pheochromocytoma										✓		×
Migraine prophylaxis		×				×	×			✓	✓	
Tremors												
Essential						×	×			✓	×	
Lithium-induced							×					
Parkinsonism							×			×		
Alcohol withdrawal syndrome		×								×		
Aggressive behavior						×	×			×		
Antipsychotic-induced akathisia							×		×	×		
Esophageal varices rebleeding							×			×		
Situational anxiety		×					×		×	×		
Enhanced cognitive performance						×						
Schizophrenia										×		
Acute panic										×		
Gastric bleeding in portal hypertension										×		
Vaginal contraceptive										×		
Decrease intraocular pressure							×					
Anxiety										×		

[1] See Indications on the following pages, and individual monographs, for more detailed information.

(Indications continued on following page)

Indications (Cont.):

Hypertension (except esmolol): Used alone as a Step 1 agent or in combination with other drugs, particularly a thiazide diuretic. Not indicated for treatment of hypertensive emergencies.

Angina pectoris **(nadolol, propranolol, atenolol, metoprolol):** For long-term management of patients with angina pectoris.

Hypertrophic subaortic stenosis **(propranolol):** Useful in managing exertional or other stress-induced angina, palpitations and syncope. Improves exercise performance. Effectiveness appears to be due to reduction of elevated outflow pressure gradient which is exacerbated by beta receptor stimulation. Clinical improvement may be temporary.

Cardiac arrhythmias **(acebutolol, esmolol, propranolol):** Use acebutolol for the management of ventricular premature beats only.

Supraventricular arrhythmias – Paroxysmal atrial tachycardias, particularly those arrhythmias induced by catecholamines or digitalis or associated with the Wolff-Parkinson-White syndrome (see Warnings). Persistent sinus tachycardia which is noncompensatory and impairs the well-being of the patient.

Tachycardias and arrhythmias due to thyrotoxicosis when they cause distress or increased hazard and when immediate effect is necessary as adjunctive, short-term (2 to 4 weeks) therapy. May be used with, but not in place of, specific therapy.

Persistent atrial extrasystoles which impair the well-being of the patient and do not respond to conventional measures. Atrial flutter and fibrillation when ventricular rate cannot be controlled by digitalis alone, or when digitalis is contraindicated.

Supraventricular tachycardia (esmolol) – Indicated for the rapid control of ventricular rate in patients with atrial fibrillation or atrial flutter in perioperative, postoperative or other emergent circumstances where short term control of ventricular rate with a short-acting agent is desirable.

Sinus tachycardia (esmolol) – Indicated in noncompensatory sinus tachycardia where, in the physician's judgment, the rapid heart rate requires intervention. Esmolol is not intended for use in chronic settings where transfer to another agent is anticipated.

Ventricular tachycardias – In ventricular tachycardias, with the exception of those induced by catecholamines or digitalis, propranolol is not the drug of first choice. In critical situations when cardioversion techniques or other drugs are not indicated or are ineffective, propranolol may be considered.

Persistent premature ventricular extrasystoles which impair the well-being of the patient and do not respond to conventional measures.

Tachyarrhythmias of digitalis intoxication, if persistent following discontinuation of digitalis and correction of electrolyte abnormalities, are usually reversible with oral propranolol. Severe bradycardia may occur. Reserve IV propranolol for life-threatening arrhythmias. Temporary maintenance with oral therapy may be indicated.

Resistant tachyarrhythmias due to excessive catecholamine action during anesthesia – All general inhalation anesthetics produce some degree of myocardial depression; therefore, use propranolol with extreme caution.

Myocardial infarction (**timolol** and **propranolol**): Indicated in clinically stable patients who have survived the acute phase of an MI to reduce cardiovascular mortality and risk of reinfarction. Initiate treatment within 1 to 4 weeks after infarction.

Metoprolol and **atenolol** are also indicated in the treatment of hemodynamically stable patients with definite or suspected acute MI. Treatment can be initiated as soon as the patient's clinical condition allows or within 3 to 10 days of the acute event.

Pheochromocytoma (**propranolol**): After primary treatment with an alpha-adrenergic blocking agent has been instituted, propranolol may be useful as adjunctive therapy if the control of tachycardia becomes necessary before or during surgery.

With inoperable or metastatic pheochromocytoma, propranolol may be useful as an adjunct to the management of symptoms due to excessive beta receptor stimulation.

Migraine (**propranolol** and **timolol**): For the prophylaxis of common migraine headache.

Essential tremor **(propranolol):** For the management of familial or hereditary essential tremor consisting of involuntary, rhythmic and oscillatory movements. Propranolol causes a reduction in the tremor amplitude but not in the tremor frequency. It is not indicated for the treatment of tremor associated with Parkinsonism.

(Indications continued on following page)

Indications (Cont.):

Unlabeled Uses: The agents listed have been evaluated for use in the following conditions:

Alcohol withdrawal syndrome – Atenolol (50 to 100 mg/day) and propranolol.

Aggressive behavior – Metoprolol (200 to 300 mg/day), nadolol (40 to 160 mg/day) and propranolol (80 to 300 mg/day).

Antipsychotic-induced akathisia – Nadolol (40 to 80 mg/day), pindolol (5 mg/day) and propranolol (20 to 80 mg/day).

Essential tremor – Metoprolol (50 to 300 mg/day), nadolol (120 to 240 mg/day) and timolol (10 mg/day). Nadolol (20 to 40 mg/day) has also been used to treat lithium-induced tremor, and both nadolol (80 to 320 mg/day) and propranolol (160 mg/day) have been investigated for the treatment of tremors associated with Parkinson's disease.

Migraine prophylaxis – Atenolol (50 to 100 mg/day), metoprolol (50 to 100 mg twice daily) and nadolol (40 to 80 mg/day).

Rebleeding from esophageal varices in cirrhotic patients – Nadolol (40 to 160 mg/day) and propranolol (20 to 180 mg twice daily).

Situational anxiety (eg, stage fright) – Nadolol (20 mg) and propranolol (40 mg); the timing of administration should be based on the drug's onset of action. Atenolol and pindolol may also be useful in this condition.

Ventricular arrhythmias – Atenolol (50 to 100 mg/day), metoprolol (200 mg/day), nadolol (10 to 640 mg/day), timolol and pindolol.

In addition, atenolol, carteolol, nadolol, metoprolol and propranolol have been investigated for use in several other conditions:

Atenolol – 50 mg/day, started 72 hours before coronary artery bypass operations, appears effective in reducing the incidence of supraventricular arrhythmias.

Carteolol – A dose of 10 mg/day has reduced the frequency of anginal attacks.

Nadolol – A dose of 10 to 20 mg twice daily has significantly reduced intraocular pressure.

Metoprolol – Enhancement of cognitive performance in elderly patients; suppression of atrial ectopy in patients with chronic obstructive pulmonary disease.

Propranolol – Schizophrenia (300 to 5000 mg/day); acute panic symptoms (40 to 320 mg/day); anxiety (80 to 320 mg/day); intermittent explosive disorder (50 to 1600 mg/day); management of nonvariceal gastric bleeding in portal hypertension (24 to 480 mg/day). Preliminary findings suggest propranolol may be an effective vaginal contraceptive; however, systemic absorption may occur.

Contraindications:

Sinus bradycardia; greater than first degree heart block; cardiogenic shock; congestive heart failure (CHF) unless secondary to a tachyarrhythmia treatable with β-blockers; overt cardiac failure; hypersensitivity to β-blocking agents.

Acebutolol and **carteolol** in persistently severe bradycardia.

Propranolol, nadolol, timolol, penbutolol, carteolol and **pindolol** are contraindicated in patients with bronchial asthma or bronchospasm, including severe chronic obstructive pulmonary disease.

Metoprolol is contraindicated in the treatment of MI in patients with a heart rate < 45 beats/min; significant heart block greater than first degree (PR interval ≥ 0.24 sec); systolic blood pressure < 100 mm Hg; moderate to severe cardiac failure.

Warnings:

Cardiac failure: Sympathetic stimulation is a vital component supporting circulatory function in CHF, and β blockade carries the potential hazard of further depressing myocardial contractility and precipitating more severe failure. Administer cautiously in hypertensive patients who have CHF controlled by digitalis and diuretics. β-blockers do not abolish the inotropic action of digitalis on heart muscle. Digitalis and β-blockers both slow AV conduction. If cardiac failure persists, withdraw β-blocker therapy.

Although cardiac failure rarely occurs in properly selected patients, advise patients to consult a physician at the first sign or symptom of impending CHF or unexplained respiratory symptoms.

In patients without a history of cardiac failure, continued myocardial depression can lead to cardiac failure. At the first sign or symptom of impending cardiac failure, fully digitalize patients or treat with diuretics and closely observe the response. If cardiac failure continues, withdraw therapy (gradually, if possible).

In patients with Wolff-Parkinson-White syndrome, several cases have been reported in which, after **propranolol** administration with as little as 5 mg, the tachycardia was replaced by a severe bradycardia requiring a demand pacemaker.

(Warnings continued on following page)

Warnings (Cont.):

Abrupt withdrawal: The occurrence of a β-blocker withdrawal syndrome is controversial. However, hypersensitivity to catecholamines has been observed in patients withdrawn from β-blocker therapy. Exacerbation of angina, MI, ventricular arrhythmias and death have occurred after abrupt discontinuation of therapy. When discontinuing chronically administered β-blocking agents, particularly in patients with ischemic heart disease, reduce dosage gradually over 1 to 2 weeks and carefully monitor the patient. If therapy with an alternative β-adrenergic blocker is desired, the patient may be transferred directly to comparable doses of another agent without interrupting β-blocking therapy. If angina markedly worsens or acute coronary insufficiency develops, reinstitute administration promptly, at least temporarily, and employ other measures to manage unstable angina.

Because coronary artery disease may be unrecognized, do not discontinue therapy abruptly, even in patients treated only for hypertension, as abrupt withdrawal may result in transient symptoms (eg, tremulousness, sweating, palpitations, headache and malaise).

It has been suggested that β-adrenergic blockers may be discontinued abruptly during acute MI if indicated since the withdrawal phenomenon is not a major clinical problem in these patients.

Peripheral vascular disease: Treatment with β-antagonists reduces cardiac output and can precipitate or aggravate the symptoms of arterial insufficiency in patients with peripheral or mesenteric vascular disease. Caution should be exercised with such patients and they should be observed closely for evidence of progression of arterial obstruction.

Pheochromocytoma: It is hazardous to use **propranolol** unless α-adrenergic blocking drugs are already in use, since this would predispose to serious blood pressure elevation. Blocking only the peripheral dilator (β) action of epinephrine leaves its constrictor (α) action unopposed. In the event of hemorrhage or shock, there is a disadvantage in having both β and α blockade, since the combination prevents the increase in heart rate and peripheral vasoconstriction needed to maintain blood pressure.

Nonallergic bronchospasm (eg, chronic bronchitis, emphysema): In general, do not administer β-blockers to patients with bronchospastic diseases. Administer nadolol, timolol, penbutolol, propranolol and pindolol with caution, since they may block bronchodilation produced by endogenous or exogenous catecholamine stimulation of β_2 receptors.

Because of their relative β_1 selectivity, low doses of metoprolol, acebutolol and atenolol may be used with caution in patients with bronchospastic disease who do not respond to, or cannot tolerate, other antihypertensive treatment. Since β_1 selectivity is not absolute, a β_2-stimulating agent should be used. It may be advisable initially to administer in smaller divided doses, instead of larger doses twice daily, to avoid the higher plasma levels associated with the longer dosing interval. Esmolol may also be used with caution in patients with asthma if an IV agent is required.

Because it is unknown to what extent β_2-stimulating agents may exacerbate myocardial ischemia and the extent of infarction, β-blockers should not be used prophylactically. If bronchospasm not related to CHF occurs, discontinue β-blockers. A theophylline derivative or a β_2 agonist may be administered cautiously, depending on the clinical condition of the patient. Both theophylline derivatives and β_2 agonists may produce serious cardiac arrhythmias.

Bradycardia: Metoprolol produces a decrease in sinus heart rate in most patients; this decrease is greatest among patients with high initial heart rates and least among patients with low initial heart rates. Acute MI (particularly inferior infarction) may in itself produce significant lowering of the sinus rate. If the sinus rate decreases to < 40 beats/min, particularly if associated with lowered cardiac output, give IV atropine (0.25 to 0.5 mg). If treatment with atropine is not successful, discontinue metoprolol and consider cautious administration of isoproterenol or installation of a cardiac pacemaker.

AV block: Metoprolol slows AV conduction and may produce significant first (PR interval $\geq$ 0.26 sec), second, or third-degree heart block. Acute myocardial infarction also produces heart block.

If heart block occurs, discontinue metoprolol and give IV atropine (0.25 to 0.5 mg). If treatment with atropine is not successful, consider cautious administration of isoproterenol or installation of a cardiac pacemaker.

(Warnings continued on following page)

Warnings (Cont.)

Hypotension: If hypotension (systolic blood pressure ≤ 90 mm Hg) occurs, discontinue the drug and carefully assess the hemodynamic status of the patient and the extent of myocardial damage. Invasive monitoring of central venous, pulmonary capillary wedge, and arterial pressures may be required. Institute appropriate therapy with fluids, positive inotropic agents, balloon counterpulsation, or other treatment modalities. If hypotension is associated with sinus bradycardia or AV block, direct treatment at reversing these.

In clinical trials, 20% to 50% of patients treated with esmolol have had hypotension, generally defined as systolic pressure less than 90 mm Hg or diastolic pressure less than 50 mm Hg. About 12% of the patients have been symptomatic (mainly diaphoresis or dizziness). Hypotension can occur at any dose but is dose-related, therefore doses beyond 200 mcg/kg/min are not recommended. Patients should be closely monitored, especially if pretreatment blood pressure is low. Decrease of dose or termination of infusion reverses hypotension, usually within 30 minutes.

Anaphylaxis has occurred and may include symptoms such as profound hypotension, bradycardia with or without AV nodal block, severe sustained bronchospasm, hives and angioedema. Deaths have occurred. Refer to Management of Acute Hypersensitivity Reactions on 2713. However, patients have been resistant to conventional therapy, especially epinephrine. Aggressive therapy may be required.

Anesthesia and major surgery: The necessity, or desirability, of withdrawal of β-blocking therapy prior to major surgery is controversial. β blockade impairs the ability of the heart to respond to β-adrenergically mediated reflex stimuli. While this might be of benefit in preventing arrhythmic response, the risk of excessive myocardial depression during general anesthesia may be enhanced, and difficulty in restarting and maintaining the heart beat also occurred. If β-blockers are withdrawn, allow 48 hours to elapse between the last dose and anesthesia. If treatment is continued, take particular care when using anesthetic agents which depress the myocardium, such as ether, cyclopropane and trichlorethylene; use the lowest possible doses of a β-blocking agent. Others may recommend withdrawal of β-blockers well before surgery takes place.

In the event of emergency surgery, effects of β-adrenergic blocking agents can be reversed by administration of β receptor agonists (eg, isoproterenol, dopamine, dobutamine or norepinephrine).

Pregnancy: (Category C: Atenolol, labetalol, esmolol, metoprolol, nadolol, timolol, propranolol, penbutolol, carteolol). Embryotoxic effects have been demonstrated in animals at doses 5 to 50 times higher than the maximum recommended doses in humans.

(*Category B:* Acebutolol, pindolol). Doses exceeding the maximum human recommended dose revealed no embryotoxicity or teratogenicity in rats and rabbits, although studies show that acebutolol and its major metabolite, diacetolol, cross the placenta. Safety for use during pregnancy has not been established. Use only when clearly needed and when the potential benefits outweigh the potential hazards to the fetus.

Although cases of teratogenicity in humans have not been reported, problems have occurred during delivery. These include: Neonatal bradycardia, hypoglycemia and apnea, low Apgar scores, maternal and fetal bradycardia, hypothermia, oliguria, poor peripheral perfusion and small birth weight infants (due to chronic therapy). Some of the effects on the neonate may last up to 72 hours postpartum.

Other studies suggest these agents are relatively safe when used during pregnancy with little risk to the fetus. However, several guidelines have been suggested until further data are available: Avoid use during the first trimester; use the lowest possible dose; discontinue at least 2 to 3 days prior to delivery (if possible); use those agents with β_1 selectivity, intrinsic sympathomimetic activity or α-blocking activity.

Lactation: Propranolol is excreted in breast milk but in a concentration too low to have any significant effect. Pindolol, timolol and nadolol are excreted in breast milk. Acebutolol and diacetolol (its major metabolite) appear in breast milk with a milk:plasma ratio of 7.1 and 12.2, respectively. Metoprolol is excreted in breast milk in very small quantities; an infant consuming 1 liter of breast milk would receive a dose of less than 1 mg of the drug. Atenolol is excreted in breast milk at a ratio of 1.5 to 6.8. In one patient, the peak atenolol milk:plasma ratio was 3.6 and the estimated infant dose (maternal dose, 100 mg/day) was 0.13 mg/feeding (75 ml). Another infant developed cyanosis and two incidences of bradycardia following maternal atenolol ingestion (100 mg/day). It is not known if penbutolol or carteolol are excreted in breast milk. Although adverse effects in the infant have not been demonstrated, in general, nursing should not be undertaken by mothers receiving these drugs.

Children: Safety and efficacy for use in children have not been established.

IV administration of propranolol is not recommended in children; however, oral propranolol has been used (see Administration and Dosage).

(Continued on following page)

Precautions:

Diabetes and hypoglycemia: β-adrenergic blockade may blunt premonitory signs and symptoms (eg, tachycardia and blood pressure changes) of acute hypoglycemia. Nonselective β-blockers may potentiate insulin-induced hypoglycemia. Atenolol does not potentiate insulin-induced hypoglycemia and, unlike nonselective β-blockers, does not delay recovery of blood glucose to normal levels.

Use with caution in diabetic patients, especially those with labile diabetes. β blockade reduces the release of insulin in response to hyperglycemia; it may be necessary to adjust the dose of antidiabetic drugs.

Thyrotoxicosis: β-adrenergic blockers may mask clinical signs (eg, tachycardia) of developing or continuing hyperthyroidism. Abrupt withdrawal may exacerbate symptoms of hyperthyroidism, including thyroid storm; therefore, monitor closely and withdraw the drug slowly.

Serum lipid concentrations: Although study results conflict, β-blockers may alter serum lipids including an increase in the concentration of total triglycerides, total cholesterol and LDL and VLDL cholesterol, and a decrease in the concentration of HDL cholesterol. Other studies suggest pindolol does not significantly alter serum lipid concentrations and acebutolol actually lowers total and LDL cholesterol levels; carteolol did not significantly alter total cholesterol and triglycerides. Further studies are needed.

Hepatic or renal function impairment: Use with caution. Timolol's half-life is essentially unchanged in moderate renal insufficiency; however, marked hypotensive responses have been seen in patients with marked renal impairment undergoing dialysis. Dosage reduction may be necessary in patients with impaired renal or hepatic function.

Because nadolol, carteolol and atenolol are eliminated primarily by the kidneys, half-life increases in renal failure; dosage adjustments are necessary (see Administration and Dosage). Although acebutolol is excreted through the GI tract, the active metabolite, diacetolol, is eliminated primarily by the kidneys; reduce the daily dose of acebutolol (see Administration and Dosage). Administer esmolol with caution to patients with impaired renal function because the acid metabolite of esmolol is primarily excreted unchanged by the kidneys. The elimination half-life of the acid metabolite was prolonged ten-fold and the plasma level was considerably elevated in patients with end-stage renal disease. Poor renal function has only minor effects on pindolol clearance, but poor hepatic function may cause blood levels of pindolol to increase substantially. Accumulation of penbutolol conjugate may be expected upon multiple dosing in renal insufficiency. The systemic availability and half-life of metoprolol in patients with renal failure do not differ significantly from those in normal subjects; consequently, reduction in dosage is usually not needed.

Muscle weakness: β-blockade has potentiated muscle weakness consistent with certain myasthenic symptoms (eg, diplopia, ptosis, generalized weakness). Timolol rarely increased muscle weakness in some patients with myasthenia gravis or myasthenic symptoms.

Drug Interactions:

Agents that increase β-adrenergic blocking agent effects:

Cimetidine may increase metoprolol plasma levels. Cimetidine appears to inhibit hepatic enzymes responsible for propranolol first-pass metabolism, leading to increased propranolol bioavailability. Reduced hepatic blood flow or extraction may also be responsible.

Contraceptives, oral may increase the pharmacologic effects of metoprolol.

Morphine – Administration IV may increase esmolol steady-state levels by 46%.

Quinidine – Pharmacologic effects of metoprolol may be increased. Orthostatic hypotension has occurred during concurrent atenolol or propranolol therapy.

Rifampin and **phenobarbital** may decrease propranolol and metoprolol plasma levels due to hepatic enzyme induction.

Agents that decrease β-adrenergic blocking agent effects:

Nonsteroidal anti-inflammatory agents and **salicylates** may decrease antihypertensive action of β-blockers due to possible inhibition of endogenous prostaglandin synthesis.

Smoking may reduce serum levels and increase the clearance of propranolol in patients receiving long-term propranolol.

Sympathomimetics – Effects of β-blockers can be reversed by **isoproterenol, norepinephrine, dopamine** or **dobutamine**. However, patients on these drugs may be subject to protracted severe hypotension. **IV epinephrine** use in patients on propranolol can result in a rapid blood pressure increase, as well as a significant fall in heart rate. The β-adrenergic activity of epinephrine is blocked while α-adrenergic effects are unopposed.

Thyroid hormones may decrease pharmacologic effects of metoprolol and propranolol. Euthyroid patients usually require no dosage adjustment. However, when converting a patient from a *hypothyroid* to euthyroid state, the β-blocker dosage may need to be increased. When converting a patient from a *hyperthyroid* to a euthyroid state with **methimazole** or **propylthiouracil**, the β-blocker dosage may need to be decreased.

(Drug Interactions continued on following page)

Drug Interactions (Cont.):

β-adrenergic blocking agents increase effects of the following agents:

Digoxin – Concomitant esmolol may increase digoxin blood levels 10% to 20%.

Insulin's hypoglycemic effects may be prolonged by noncardioselective β-blockers.

Lidocaine – β-blockers may increase the effects of lidocaine. Elevated plasma levels with toxicity characterized by lethargy, confusion and other CNS and cardiovascular symptoms may occur.

Miscellaneous drug interactions:

Calcium channel blockers – **Oral verapamil** and β-blockers coadministered may be beneficial in patients with chronic stable angina; information is not sufficient to predict the effects of concurrent treatment, especially in patients with left ventricular dysfunction or cardiac conduction abnormalities. There may be adverse effects on cardiac function. Because experience is limited, it is preferable to use verapamil alone. If combined therapy is used, clinically evaluate the patient and periodically reassess use. Avoid combined therapy in patients with AV conduction abnormalities or with depressed left ventricular function.

IV verapamil has been administered to patients receiving oral β-blockers without serious effects. However, since both drugs may depress myocardial contractility or AV conduction, consider the possibility of an untoward response. Rarely, the concomitant administration of IV β-blockers and IV verapamil has resulted in serious adverse reactions, especially in patients with severe cardiomyopathy, CHF or recent MI.

Nifedipine and β-blocking agents used concomitantly are usually well tolerated. Occasional reports have suggested that this combination may increase the likelihood of CHF, severe hypotension or exacerbation of angina.

Catecholamine depleting drugs (eg, reserpine) may have an additive effect with β-blocking agents. Closely observe patients for evidence of excessive reduction of sympathetic tone which may produce vertigo, syncope or postural hypotension.

Clonidine – The severity of rebound hypertension caused by abrupt discontinuation of clonidine may be enhanced in patients taking β-blocking agents. Also, this combination has uncommonly caused paradoxical hypertension.

Disopyramide – Pharmacologic effects of both drugs may be increased during concurrent β-blocker therapy. Atenolol has increased disopyramide serum levels.

Haloperidol and propranolol coadministration has resulted in severe hypotension.

Hydralazine – Pharmacologic effects of both agents may be increased during administration of propranolol or metoprolol.

Neuromuscular blockers, nondepolarizing – Both enhancement of, and resistance to, the neuromuscular blocking effects of these agents has occurred during propranolol coadministration.

Phenothiazines – Chlorpromazine and thioridazine have increased the plasma levels of propranolol; however, chlorpromazine and thioridazine levels have also increased.

Prazosin – β-blocking agents may increase the "first dose response" (acute postural hypotension) which often occurs following initiation of prazosin therapy.

Theophylline – Nonselective β-blockers antagonize the bronchodilating action of theophylline, and may decrease theophylline clearance; this effect is notable in patients who have increased theophylline clearance induced by cigarette smoking.

Drug/Food Interactions: Food enhances the bioavailability of **metoprolol** and **propranolol**; this effect is not noted with **nadolol** or **pindolol.** The rate of **carteolol** and **penbutolol** absorption is slowed by the presence of food; however, extent of absorption is not appreciably affected.

Drug/Lab Test Interactions: These agents may produce hypoglycemia and interfere with **glucose** or **insulin** tolerance tests. Propranolol may interfere with the glaucoma screening test due to a reduction in intraocular pressure.

(Continued on following page)

Complete prescribing information for these products begins on page 750

ESMOLOL HCl

Indications:

Supraventricular tachycardia: For rapid control of ventricular rate in patients with atrial fibrillation or atrial flutter in perioperative, postoperative or other emergent circumstances where short-term control of ventricular rate with a short-acting agent is desirable.

Noncompensatory sinus tachycardia when heart rate requires specific intervention.

Dosage:

Supraventricular tachycardia: 50 to 200 mcg/kg/min; average dose is 100 mcg/kg/min although dosages as low as 25 mcg/kg/min have been adequate. Dosages as high as 300 mcg/kg/min provide little added effect and an increased rate of adverse effects, and are not recommended. Individualize dosage by titration in which each step consists of a loading dose followed by a maintenance dose.

To initiate treatment, administer a loading dose infusion of 500 mcg/kg/min for 1 minute followed by a 4 minute maintenance infusion of 50 mcg/kg/min. If an adequate therapeutic effect is not observed within 5 minutes, repeat the loading dose and follow with a maintenance infusion increased to 100 mcg/kg/min. Continue titration procedure, repeating loading infusion, increasing maintenance infusion by increments of 50 mcg/kg/min (for 4 minutes). As the desired heart rate or a safety end-point (eg, lowered blood pressure) is approached, omit the loading infusion and reduce incremental dose in maintenance infusion from 50 mcg/kg/min to 25 mcg/kg/min or lower. Also, if desired, increase interval between titration steps from 5 to 10 minutes.

Dosage in Supraventricular Tachycardia								
		1 minute loading infusion (mcg/kg/min)	4 minute maintenance infusion (mcg/kg/min)					
		500	50	100	150	200	250	300
Suggested Administration for Supraventricular Tachycardia • Drug dilution: 5 g esmolol in 500 ml diluent = 10 mg/ml								
Patient wt		Infusion rates (ml/min)	Infusion rates (ml/hr)					
lbs	kg							
110	50	2.5	15	30	45	60	75	90
121	55	2.75	16.5	33	49.5	66	82.5	99
132	60	3	18	36	54	72	90	108
143	65	3.25	19.5	39	59.5	78	98.5	117
154	70	3.5	21	42	63	84	105	126
165	75	3.75	22.5	45	67.5	90	112.5	135
176	80	4	24	48	72	96	120	144
187	85	4.25	25.5	51	76.5	102	127.5	153
198	90	4.5	27	54	81	108	135	162
209	95	4.75	28.5	57	85.5	114	142.5	171
220	100	5	30	60	90	120	150	180
231	105	5.25	31.5	63	94.5	126	157.5	189
242	110	5.5	33	66	99	132	165	198

This specific dosage regimen has not been intraoperatively studied. Because of the time required for titration, it may not be optimal for intraoperative use.

Maintenance dosages > 200 mcg/kg/min do not significantly increase benefits. The safety of dosages > 300 mcg/kg/min has not been studied.

In the event of an adverse reaction, reduce dosage or discontinue the drug. If a local infusion site reaction develops, use an alternative site. Avoid butterfly needles.

Transfer to alternative agents: After achieving adequate heart rate control and stable clinical status, transition to alternative antiarrhythmic agents (eg, propranolol, digoxin, verapamil) may be accomplished. A recommended dosage guideline is propranolol 10 to 20 mg every 4 to 6 hours, digoxin 0.125 to 0.5 mg every 6 hours (orally or IV) or verapamil 80 mg every 6 hours. However, consider labeling instructions for the agent selected.

Reduce the dosage of esmolol as follows: One-half hour after the first dose of the alternative agent, reduce esmolol infusion rate by 50%. Following the second dose of the alternative agent, monitor patient's response and, if satisfactory control is maintained for the first hour, discontinue esmolol infusion.

(Dosage continued on following page)

ESMOLOL HCl (Cont.)

Dosage (Cont.):

Withdrawal effects may occur with abrupt withdrawal of β-blockers following chronic use in patients with coronary artery disease (see Warnings), but these have not been reported with esmolol. However, use caution when abruptly discontinuing esmolol infusions.

The use of esmolol infusions up to 24 hours has been well documented. Limited data indicate that esmolol is well tolerated up to 48 hours.

Administration:

The 250 mg/ml strength is not for direct IV injection. This strength is concentrated; dilute prior to infusion. Do not mix with sodium bicarbonate. Do not mix with other drugs prior to dilution in a suitable IV fluid. The 10 mg/ml vial is ready to use.

Venous irritation and thrombophlebitis are associated more often with infusion concentrations of 20 rather than 10 mg/ml. Avoid concentrations greater than 10 mg/ml.

Preparation of solution (10 ml amp): Remove 20 ml from a 500 ml bottle of one of the IV fluids listed below (see Compatibility and Stability), and add the contents of two ampuls (each containing 2.5 g esmolol). This yields a final concentration of 10 mg/ml. The diluted solution is stable for at least 24 hours at room temperature. Esmolol has been well tolerated when administered via a central vein.

Compatibility and stability: Esmolol, at a final concentration of 10 mg/ml, is compatible with the following solutions and was stable for at least 24 hours at controlled room temperatures or under refrigeration: 5% Dextrose Injection; 5% Dextrose in Lactated Ringer's Injection; 5% Dextrose in Ringer's Injection; 5% Dextrose and 0.9% or 0.45% Sodium Chloride Injection; Lactated Ringer's Injection; Potassium Chloride (40 mEq/L) in 5% Dextrose Injection; 0.9% or 0.45% Sodium Chloride Injection.

Esmolol is NOT compatible with 5% Sodium Bicarbonate Injection.

				C.I.*
Rx	**Brevibloc** (DuPont Critical Care)	**Injection:** 10 mg/ml	In 10 ml vials.[1]	NA
		250 mg/ml	In 10 ml amps.[1]	3855

BETAXOLOL HCl

Indications:

Management of hypertension, used alone or concomitantly with other antihypertensive agents, particularly thiazide-type diuretics.

For a complete discussion of indications, refer to page 752.

Administration and Dosage:

Initial dose: 10 mg once daily, alone or added to diuretic therapy. The full antihypertensive effect is usually seen within 7 to 14 days; if the desired response is not achieved the dose can be doubled. Increasing the dose beyond 20 mg has not produced a statistically significant additional hypertensive effect; however, the 40 mg dose is well tolerated. Anticipate an increased effect (reduction) on heart rate with increasing dosage. To discontinue treatment, gradually withdraw betaxolol over 2 weeks.

Elderly: Consider reducing the starting dose to 5 mg.

				C.I.*
Rx	**Kerlone** (Searle)	**Tablets:** 10 mg	(Kerlone 10). White, scored. Film coated. In 100s and UD 100s.	NA
		20 mg	(Kerlone 20β). White. Film coated. In 100s and UD 100s.	NA

PINDOLOL

Indications:

Management of hypertension, used alone or with other antihypertensive agents, particularly with a thiazide-type diuretic.

For a complete discussion of indications, refer to page 752

Administration and Dosage:

Individualize dosage.

Initial dose: 5 mg twice daily, alone or with other antihypertensive agents. The antihypertensive response usually occurs within the first week of treatment. Maximal response, however, may occur within 2 weeks or, occasionally, longer. If a satisfactory reduction in blood pressure does not occur within 3 to 4 weeks, adjust the dose in increments of 10 mg/day at 3 to 4 week intervals, to a maximum of 60 mg/day.

				C.I.*
Rx	**Visken** (Sandoz)	**Tablets:** 5 mg	(Visken 5/78-111). White, scored. In 100s.	1196
		10 mg	(Visken 10/78-73). White, scored. In 100s.	763

* Cost index based on cost per 250 mg esmolol or 10 mg pindolol.

[1] With 25% propylene glycol.

Complete prescribing information for these products begins on page 750

ACEBUTOLOL HCl

Indications:

Hypertension; ventricular arrhythmias.

For a complete discussion of indications, refer to page 752

Administration and Dosage:

Hypertension: Initial dose – 400 mg in uncomplicated mild to moderate hypertension. May be given in a single daily dose, but 200 mg twice daily may be required for adequate control. Optimal response usually occurs with 400 to 800 mg/day (range, 200 to 1200 mg/day given twice daily). The drug may be combined with another antihypertensive agent. As dosage is increased, β_1-selectivity diminishes.

Ventricular arrhythmia: Initial dose – 400 mg (200 mg twice daily). Increase dosage gradually until optimal response is obtained, usually 600 to 1200 mg/day. To discontinue treatment, gradually reduce dosage over 2 weeks.

Older patients: Since bioavailability increases about twofold, older patients may require lower maintenance doses. Avoid doses above 800 mg per day.

Renal and hepatic function impairment: Reduce the daily dose by 50% when creatinine clearance is < 50 ml/min/1.73 m². Reduce by 75% when it is < 25 ml/min/1.73 m². Use cautiously in impaired hepatic function.

	Product	Form/Strength	Description	C.I.*
Rx	**Sectral** (Wyeth-Ayerst)	**Capsules:** 200 mg	(Wyeth 4177 Sectral 200). Purple and orange. In 100s and UD 100s.	1596
		400 mg	(Wyeth 4179 Sectral 400). Brown and orange. In 100s and UD 100s.	1061

NADOLOL

Indications:

Long-term management of angina pectoris; hypertension.

For a complete discussion of indications, refer to page 752

Administration and Dosage:

Individualize dosage. May be given without regard to meals.

Angina pectoris: Initial – 40 mg/day. Gradually increase dosage in 40 to 80 mg increments at 3 to 7 day intervals until optimum clinical response is obtained or there is pronounced slowing of the heart rate. *Maintenance dose* – Usual dose is 40 to 80 mg/day. Up to 160 to 240 mg/day may be needed.

The safety and efficacy of dosages exceeding 240 mg/day have not been established. To discontinue, reduce dosage gradually over 1 to 2 weeks.

Hypertension: Initial – 40 mg once daily, alone or in addition to diuretic therapy. Gradually increase dosage in 40 to 80 mg increments until optimum blood pressure reduction is achieved. *Maintenance dose* – Usual dose is 40 to 80 mg once daily. Up to 240 to 320 mg once daily may be needed.

Renal failure: Nadolol is excreted principally by the kidneys and, although nonrenal elimination does occur, dosage adjustments are necessary in patients with renal impairment. The following dosage intervals are recommended:

Nadolol Dosage Adjustment in Renal Failure

Creatinine clearance (ml/min/1.73 m²)	Dosage interval (hours)
> 50	24
31-50	24-36
10-30	24-48
< 10	40-60

	Product	Form/Strength	Description	C.I.*
Rx	**Corgard** (Bristol Myers Squibb)	**Tablets:** 20 mg	(232). Scored. In 100s and Unimatic 100s.	1548
		40 mg	(Squibb 207). Scored. In 100s, 1000s and Unimatic 100s.	908
		80 mg	(Squibb 241). Scored. In 100s, 1000s and Unimatic 100s.	622
		120 mg	(208). Scored. In 100s and 1000s.	541
		160 mg	(246). Scored. In 100s.	451

* Cost Index based on cost per 400 mg acebutolol or 40 mg nadolol .

Complete prescribing information for these products begins on page 750

TIMOLOL MALEATE

Indications:

Hypertension, used alone or with other antihypertensive agents, especially thiazide-type diuretics. Myocardial infarction, for clinically stable survivors of acute MI, to reduce cardiovascular mortality and the risk of reinfarction. Migraine prophylaxis.

For a complete discussion of indications, refer to page 752

Administration and Dosage:

Hypertension: Initial dosage – 10 mg twice daily used alone or added to a diuretic. *Maintenance dosage* – 20 to 40 mg/day. Titrate, depending on blood pressure and heart rate. Increases to a maximum of 60 mg/day divided into 2 doses may be necessary. There should be an interval of at least 7 days between dosage increases.

Myocardial infarction (long-term prophylactic use in patients who have survived the acute phase of a MI): 10 mg twice daily.

Migraine: Initial dosage is 10 mg twice daily. During maintenance therapy the 20 mg daily dosage may be given as a single dose. Total daily dosage may be increased to a maximum of 30 mg in divided doses or decreased to 10 mg once daily depending on clinical response and tolerability. Discontinue if a satisfactory response is not obtained after 6 to 8 weeks of the maximum daily dosage.

	Product	Form	Description	C.I.*
Rx	**Timolol Maleate** (Various, eg, Geneva Marsam, Goldline, Major, Moore, Parmed, PBI, Rugby, URL)	**Tablets:** 5 mg	In 100s.	600+
		10 mg	In 100s.	475+
		20 mg	In 100s.	420+
Rx	**Blocadren** (MSD)	**Tablets:** 5 mg	(MSD 59 Blocadren). Light blue. In 100s.	954
		10 mg	(MSD 136 Blocadren). Light blue, scored. In 100s and UD 100s.	590
		20 mg	(MSD 437 Blocadren). Lt. blue, scored. In 100s.	544

PROPRANOLOL HCl

Indications:

Cardiac arrhythmias; MI; hypertrophic subaortic stenosis; pheochromocytoma; hypertension; migraine prophylaxis; angina pectoris due to coronary atherosclerosis; essential tremor.

For a complete discussion of indications, refer to page 752

Administration and Dosage:

Propranolol Dosage Based on Indication

Indication	Initial dosage	Usual range	Maximum daily dose
Arrhythmias		10-30 mg tid-qid (given ac-hs)	
Hypertension	40 mg bid or 80 mg once daily (SR)	120-240 mg/day (given bid-tid) or 120-160 mg once daily (SR)	640 mg
Angina	80-320 mg bid, tid, qid or 80 mg once daily (SR)	160 mg once daily (SR)	320 mg
MI		180-240 mg/day (given tid-qid)	240 mg
IHSS		20-40 mg tid-qid (given ac-hs) or 80-160 mg once daily (SR)	
Pheochromocytoma		60 mg/day × 3 days preoperatively (in divided doses)	
Inoperable tumor		30 mg/day (in divided doses)	
Migraine	80 mg/day once daily (SR) or in divided doses	160-240 mg/day (in divided doses)	
Essential tremor	40 mg bid	120 mg/day	320 mg

* Cost Index based on cost per 10 mg timolol.

(Administration and Dosage continued on following page)

LABETALOL HCl (Cont.)

Drug Interactions (Cont.):

Halothane: Synergistic adverse effects on cardiovascular hemodynamics may occur with concurrent halothane and IV labetalol, resulting in significant myocardial depression. During controlled hypotensive anesthesia, do not use high concentrations (3% or above) of halothane. If an interaction occurs, a reduction in halothane dose will rapidly reverse the symptoms.

Nitroglycerin: Labetalol blunts the reflex tachycardia that may be produced by nitroglycerin without preventing its hypotensive effect; additional antihypertensive effects may occur.

Drug/Lab Tests: Presence of a labetalol metabolite in urine may falsely increase urinary catecholamine levels when measured by a nonspecific trihydroxyindole reaction. In screening patients for pheochromocytoma who are on labetalol, use specific radioenzymatic or high performance liquid chromatography assay techniques.

There have been reversible increases of serum transaminases in 4% of patients treated with labetalol and tested, and more rarely, reversible increases in blood urea.

Adverse Reactions:

Labetalol is usually well tolerated. Most adverse effects have been mild and transient. With oral labetalol, most occur early in the course of treatment. Discontinuation was required in 7% of all patients in controlled clinical trials.

Oral: CNS – Fatigue; headache; drowsiness; paresthesias; rare instances of syncope.

GU – Ejaculation failure; impotence; priapism; difficulty in micturition; acute urinary bladder retention; Peyronie's disease.

GI/hepatic/biliary – Diarrhea; cholestasis with or without jaundice; reversible increases in serum transaminases.

Respiratory – Dyspnea; bronchospasm.

Musculoskeletal – Asthenia; muscle cramps; toxic myopathy.

Dermatologic – Rashes such as generalized maculopapular, lichenoid, urticarial; bullous lichen planus; psoriaform; facial erythema; reversible alopecia.

Other – Systemic lupus erythematosus; positive antinuclear factor (ANF); antimitochondrial antibodies; edema; nasal stuffiness; fever; vision abnormality; dry eyes.

Parenteral: CNS – Hypoesthesia (numbness); somnolence/yawning.

Cardiovascular – Ventricular arrhythmias.

Renal – Transient increases in BUN and serum creatinine, associated with drops in BP, generally in patients with prior renal insufficiency.

Other – Pruritus; flushing; wheezing.

Oral and parenteral: GI – Nausea; vomiting; dyspepsia; taste distortion.

CNS – Dizziness; tingling of scalp/skin; vertigo.

Other – Postural hypotension; increased sweating.

Adverse effects not listed above have been reported with other β-adrenergic blockers:

CNS – Mental depression progressing to catatonia; an acute reversible syndrome characterized by disorientation for time/place, short-term memory loss, emotional lability, clouded sensorium and decreased performance on neuropsychometrics.

Cardiovascular – Intensification of AV block. See Contraindications.

Allergic – Fever with aching and sore throat; laryngospasm; respiratory distress.

Hematologic – Agranulocytosis; thrombocytopenic or nonthrombocytopenic purpura.

Gastrointestinal – Mesenteric artery thrombosis; ischemic colitis.

Overdosage:

Symptoms: Excessive hypotension which is posture-sensitive; excessive bradycardia.

Treatment: Institute gastric lavage or induce emesis to remove the drug after oral ingestion. Place patients in supine position and raise legs, if necessary. Employ the following if necessary:

Excessive bradycardia – Administer atropine or epinephrine.

Cardiac failure – Administer a digitalis glycoside and a diuretic. Dopamine or dobutamine may also be useful.

Hypotension – Administer vasopressors. Norepinephrine may be the drug of choice.

Bronchospasm – Administer epinephrine or an aerosolized β_2-agonist.

Seizures – Administer diazepam.

In severe β-blocker overdose resulting in hypotension or bradycardia, glucagon has been effective in large doses (5 to 10 mg rapidly over 30 seconds, followed by continuous infusion of 5 mg/hr that can be reduced as the patient improves).

Neither hemodialysis nor peritoneal dialysis removes a significant amount of labetalol from the general circulation ($< 1\%$).

Patient Information:

Do not discontinue medication except on advice from physician.

Consult physician at any sign of impending cardiac failure.

Transient scalp tingling may occur, especially when treatment is initiated.

(Continued on following page)

LABETALOL HCl (Cont.)

Administration and Dosage:

Oral: Initial dose – Individualize dosage. 100 mg twice daily, alone or added to a diuretic. After 2 or 3 days, using standing BP as an indicator, titrate dosage in increments of 100 mg twice daily, every 2 or 3 days. The full antihypertensive effect of labetalol is usually seen within the first 1 to 3 hours of the initial dose or dose increment.

Maintenance dose – 200 to 400 mg twice daily. Patients with severe hypertension may require 1.2 to 2.4 g/day. Should side effects (principally nausea or dizziness) occur with twice daily dosing, the same total daily dose administered 3 times a day may improve tolerability. Titration increments should not exceed 200 mg twice a day.

When transferring patients from other antihypertensive drugs, introduce labetalol and progressively decrease the dosage of the existing therapy.

Parenteral: For IV use. Individualize dosage. Keep patients supine during injection. Establish the patient's ability to tolerate an upright position before permitting ambulation.

Repeated IV injection – Initially, 20 mg (0.25 mg/kg for an 80 kg patient) slowly over 2 minutes. Measure supine BP immediately before and at 5 and 10 minutes after injection. Additional injections of 40 or 80 mg can be given at 10 minute intervals until a desired supine BP is achieved or a total of 300 mg has been injected. The maximum effect usually occurs within 5 minutes of each injection.

Slow continuous infusion – Dilute contents with IV fluids listed below. Two methods are: Add 200 mg to 160 ml of IV fluid to prepare 1 mg/ml solution at a rate of 2 ml/min (2 mg/min). Or, add 200 mg to 250 ml of an IV fluid to prepare 2 mg/3 ml solution; give at a rate of 3 ml/min (2 mg/min). Adjust infusion rate according to BP response. Use a controlled administration device. Continue infusion until satisfactory response is obtained; then discontinue infusion and start oral labetalol. Effective IV dose range is 50 to 200 mg, up to 300 mg.

Transfer to oral dosing (hospitalized patients): Begin oral dosing when supine diastolic BP begins to rise. Recommended initial dose is 200 mg, then 200 or 400 mg, 6 to 12 hours later, depending on BP response. Thereafter, titration may proceed as follows:

Inpatient Titration Instructions	
Regimen	Daily Dose*
200 mg bid	400 mg
400 mg bid	800 mg
800 mg bid	1600 mg
1200 mg bid	2400 mg

* Total daily dose may be given in 3 divided doses.

While in the hospital, the dosage of labetalol may be increased at one day intervals to achieve the desired blood pressure reduction.

IV compatibility: At final concentrations of 1.25 to 3.75 mg/ml, labetalol is compatible and stable for 24 hours with the following parenteral solutions: Ringer's; Lactated Ringer's; 5% Dextrose and Ringer's; 5% Lactated Ringer's and 5% Dextrose; 5% Dextrose; 0.9% Sodium Chloride; 5% Dextrose and 0.2% Sodium Chloride; 2.5% Dextrose and 0.45% Sodium Chloride; 5% Dextrose and 0.9% Sodium Chloride; and 5% Dextrose and 0.33% Sodium Chloride.

Labetalol is NOT compatible with 5% Sodium Bicarbonate Injection.

Storage: Store between 2° and 30°C (36° and 86°F). Protect unit dose boxes from excessive moisture. *Injection* – Do not freeze. Protect from light.

Rx	**Normodyne** (Schering)	**Tablets:** 100 mg	(#Schering 244 Normodyne 100). Light brown, scored. Film coated. In 100s, 500s and UD 100s.
		200 mg	(#Schering 752 Normodyne 200). White, scored. Film coated. In 100s, 500s & UD 100s.
		300 mg	(#Schering 438 Normodyne 300). Blue. Film coated. In 100s, 500s and UD 100s.
		Injection: 5 mg per ml[1]	In 20 ml amps & 40 & 60 ml multidose vials.
Rx	**Trandate** (Allen & Hanburys)	**Tablets:** 100 mg	(#Trandate 100 Glaxo). Light orange, scored. Film coated. In 100s, 500s and UD 100s.
		200 mg	(#Trandate 200 Glaxo). White, scored. Film coated. In 100s, 500s and UD 100s.
		300 mg	(#Trandate 300 Glaxo). Peach, scored. Film coated. In 100s, 500s and UD 100s.
		Injection: 5 mg per ml[1]	In 20 and 40 ml multidose vials.

\# Product identification code. [1] With 0.1 mg EDTA and 0.8 mg methyl and 0.1 mg propyl paraben.

Agents used in hypertension therapy are listed in the table below:

Pharmacological Effects of Antihypertensive Agents

↑ = increase
⇧ = slight increase
0 = no change
⇩ = slight decrease
↓ = decrease

	Onset (min)	Peak effect[1] (hrs)	Duration of action[2] (hrs)	Plasma volume	Plasma renin activity	RBF GFR[3]	Peripheral resistance	Cardiac output	Heart rate
Diuretics									
Thiazides and derivatives	60-120	4	6-48	↓	↑	↓	↓	↓	0
Loop diuretics	within 60	1-2	4-8	↓	↑	↑	↓	↓	0
Amiloride	120	6-10	24	↓	↑	0	↓	↓	0
Spironolactone	24-48 hr	48-72	48-72	↓	↑	0	↓	0	0
Triamterene	2-4 hr	6-8	12-16						
Antiadrenergic Agents - Centrally Acting									
Methyldopa	120	4-6	12-24	↑	⇩/0	⇩/0	↓	⇩/0	⇩/0
Clonidine	30-60	2-4	12-24	↑	⇩	⇩/0	↓	⇩/0	↓
Guanabenz	60	2-4	6-12	0	↓	0	↓	0	↓
Guanfacine		1-4	24	⇩/0	↓		↓	0	⇩
Antiadrenergic Agents - Peripherally Acting									
Reserpine	days	6-12	6-24	↑	⇩/0	⇩/0	↓	0/↓	↓
Guanethidine		6-8	24-48	↑	⇩/0	⇩/0	↓	0/↓	↓
Guanadrel	30-120	4-6	9-14	↑		0	↓	0	↓
Prazosin	120-130	1-3	6-12	0/⇧	⇩/0	0	↓	0/⇧	0/⇧
Terazosin	15	1-2	12-24	0	0	0	↓	⇧	⇧
Antiadrenergic Agents - Beta-Adrenergic Blockers									
Metoprolol		1.5	13-19	⇩/0	↓	⇩/0	0/↓	↓	↓
Atenolol		2-4	24 +	⇩/0	↓	↓/0	0	↓	↓
Acebutolol		3-8	24-30				⇩	↓	↓
Nadolol		3-4	17-24	⇩/0	↓	0	0	↓	↓
Pindolol		1	24 +		0	0	↓	⇩	⇩
Timolol		1-3	12	⇩/0	↓		0	↓	↓
Propranolol		2-4	8-12	⇩/0	↓	↓	⇩/0	↓	↓
Penbutolol		1.5-3	20 +		↓	⇩	0	↓	↓
Antiadrenergic Agent - Alpha/Beta-Adrenergic Blocker									
Labetalol		2-3	8-12	↑	↓	0/↑	↓	0	↓
Angiotensin Converting Enzyme (ACE) Inhibitors									
Captopril	15-30	1-1.5	6-12	⇧	↑	RBF ↑ GFR 0	↓	0/↑	0
Enalapril Maleate	60	4-6	24	0/⇧	↑	RBF ↑ GFR 0	↓	↑	0
Lisinopril	60	≈ 7	24		↑	RBF ⇧ GFR 0	↓	0	0
Calcium Channel Blocking Agents									
Verapamil	30	1-2.2			0/⇧	0	↓	↑/↓	↑/↓
Nicardipine	20	0.5-2			⇧/↑	⇧	↓	↑	↑

[1] Peak clinical effect following a single oral dose, except where indicated.
[2] Duration of action is frequently dose-dependent. [3] Renal blood flow and glomerular filtration rate.

(Continued on following page)

Agents used in hypertension therapy are listed in the table below:

Pharmacological Effects of Antihypertensive Agents (Cont.)

↑ = increase
⇧ = slight increase
0 = no change
⇩ = slight decrease
↓ = decrease

	Onset (min)	Peak effect[1] (hrs)	Duration of action[2] (hrs)	Plasma volume	Plasma renin activity	RBF GFR[3]	Peripheral resistance	Cardiac output	Heart rate
Vasodilators									
Hydralazine	45	0.5-2	6-8	↑	↑	↑	↓	↑	↑
Minoxidil	30	2-3	24-72	↑	↑	0	↓	↑	↑
Agents For Pheochromocytoma									
Phentolamine	immed.		5-10 min	⇧	↑	↑	↓	0/↑	↑
Phenoxybenzamine		2-3	24 +	⇧	↑	↑	↓	↑	↑
Metyrosine		6 +	2-3 days				↓		↓
Agents For Hypertensive Emergencies									
Nitroprusside	0.5-1		3-5 min	↑	↑	0	↓	⇩	⇧
Diazoxide	1-2	5 min	< 12	↑	↑	↑	↓	↑	↑
Trimethaphan Camsylate	1-2		10-15 min	↑	↓	0	↓	↓	↓
Nitroglycerin (IV)	immed.		transient	0	0		↓	↑	↑
Miscellaneous Agents									
Mecamylamine	30-120		6-12 +	↑	↓	↓	↓	↓	↓
Pargyline		4-21 days	3 weeks			↓	↓	0	0

[1] Peak clinical effect following a single oral dose, except where indicated.
[2] Duration of action is frequently dose-dependent. [3] Renal blood flow and glomerular filtration rate.

METHYLDOPA AND METHYLDOPATE HCl (Cont.)

Drug Interactions:

Haloperidol and concomitant methyldopa may produce adverse mental symptoms (dementia) and a high incidence of sedation.

Levodopa: Methyldopa may potentiate the effects of levodopa. Additive or synergistic hypotensive effects have also been described.

Lithium toxicity characterized by GI symptoms, polyuria, muscular weakness, lethargy and tremor has been reported following methyldopa coadministration.

Propranolol and methyldopa may cause paradoxical hypertension rarely.

Sympathomimetics: Methyldopa may potentiate the pressor effects of sympathomimetics and lead to hypertension.

Tolbutamide metabolism may be impaired by methyldopa, resulting in enhanced hypoglycemic effects.

Drug/Lab Tests: Methyldopa may interfere with tests for: **Urinary uric acid** by phosphotungstate method; **serum creatinine** by alkaline picrate method; **AST** by colorimetric methods. Interference with spectrophotometry for AST analysis is not reported.

Since methyldopa causes fluorescence in urine samples at the same wave lengths as catecholamines, falsely high levels of **urinary catecholamines** may occur and will interfere with the diagnosis of pheochromocytoma. Methyldopa does not interfere with measurement of vanillylmandelic acid (VMA) by methods converting VMA to vanillin.

Adverse Reactions:

CNS: Sedation, usually transient, may occur during initial therapy or whenever the dose is increased; headache, asthenia or weakness (may be early, transient symptoms); dizziness; lightheadedness; symptoms of cerebrovascular insufficiency; paresthesias; parkinsonism; Bell's palsy; decreased mental acuity; involuntary choreoathetotic movements; psychic disturbances including nightmares and reversible mild psychoses or depression; verbal memory impairment.

Cardiovascular: Bradycardia; prolonged carotid sinus hypersensitivity; aggravation of angina pectoris; paradoxical pressor response; pericarditis; myocarditis (fatal); orthostatic hypotension; edema (and weight gain) usually relieved by a diuretic. Discontinue methyldopa if edema progresses or signs of heart failure appear.

GI: Nausea; vomiting; distention; constipation; flatus; diarrhea; colitis; mild dry mouth; sore or "black" tongue; pancreatitis; sialadenitis.

Hepatic: Abnormal liver function tests; jaundice; hepatitis, liver disorders (see Warnings).

Hematologic: Positive Coombs' test, hemolytic anemia (see Warnings); bone marrow depression; leukopenia; granulocytopenia; thrombocytopenia; positive tests for antinuclear antibody, LE cells and rheumatoid factor.

Dermatologic: Rash as in eczema or lichenoid eruption; toxic epidermal necrolysis.

Allergic: Fever; lupus-like syndrome.

Endocrine: Breast enlargement; gynecomastia; lactation; hyperprolactinemia; amenorrhea; galactorrhea.

GU: Impotence; failure to ejaculate; decreased libido.

Other: Nasal stuffiness; rise in BUN; mild arthralgia; myalgia; septic shock-like syndrome.

Overdosage:

Symptoms: Sedation; coma; acute hypotension; weakness; bradycardia; dizziness; lightheadedness; constipation; distention; flatus; diarrhea; nausea; vomiting and other responses attributable to brain and gastrointestinal malfunction. Atrioventricular conduction may be impaired. Delayed absorption from the gut may delay onset of maximum hypotension.

Treatment: Employ gastric evacuation and general supportive measures when ingestion is recent. When ingestion has been earlier, infusions may be helpful to promote urinary excretion. Otherwise, management includes special attention to cardiac rate and output, blood volume, electrolyte imbalance, paralytic ileus, urinary function and cerebral activity. Refer to General Management of Acute Overdosage on 2711 Place patient in Trendelenburg position. Sympathomimetic drugs (eg, norepinephrine, epinephrine, metaraminol bitartrate) may be indicated. In severe cases consider hemodialysis.

(Continued on following page)

METHYLDOPA AND METHYLDOPATE HCl (Cont.)

Patient Information:

When urine is exposed to air after voiding, it may darken.

Notify physician of unexplained prolonged general tiredness, fever or jaundice.

Administration and Dosage:

Use in impaired renal function: Methyldopa is largely excreted by the kidneys; patients with impaired renal function may respond to smaller doses.

Use in the elderly: Syncope in older patients may be related to an increased sensitivity and advanced arteriosclerotic vascular disease. This may be avoided by lower doses.

Adults: Initial therapy – 250 mg, 2 or 3 times a day in the first 48 hours. Adjust dosage at intervals of not less than 2 days until an adequate response is achieved. To minimize sedation, increase dosage in the evening. By adjustment of dosage, morning hypotension may be prevented without sacrificing control of afternoon blood pressure.

Maintenance therapy – 500 mg to 3 g daily in 2 to 4 doses. Methyldopa is usually administered in 2 divided doses; some patients may be controlled with a single daily dose given at bedtime.

Concomitant drug therapy – When methyldopa is given with antihypertensives other than thiazides, limit the initial dosage to 500 mg/day in divided doses; when added to a thiazide, the dosage of thiazide need not be changed.

Children: Individualize dosage. Initial oral dosage is based on 10 mg/kg/day in 2 to 4 doses. The maximum daily dosage is 65 mg/kg or 3 g, whichever is less.

Tolerance may occur, usually between the second and third month of therapy. Adding a diuretic or increasing the dosage of methyldopa frequently restores blood pressure control. A thiazide is recommended if therapy was not started with a thiazide or if effective control of blood pressure cannot be maintained on 2 g methyldopa daily.

Discontinuation: Methyldopa has a relatively short duration of action; therefore, withdrawal is followed by return of hypertension, usually within 48 hours. This is not complicated by an overshoot of blood pressure above pretreatment levels.

IV: Add the dose to 100 ml of 5% Dextrose or give in 5% Dextrose in Water in a concentration of 10 mg/ml. Administer over 30 to 60 minutes. When control has been obtained, substitute oral therapy starting with the same parenteral dosage schedule.

Adults – 250 to 500 mg every 6 hours as required (maximum: 1 g every 6 hours).

Children – 20 to 40 mg/kg/day in divided doses every 6 hours. The maximum daily dosage is 65 mg/kg or 3 g, whichever is less.

	Product	Dosage form	Packaging	C.I.*
Rx	**Methyldopa** (Various)	**Tablets:** 125 mg methyldopa	In 100s, 500s, 1000s & UD 100s.	49+
Rx	**Aldomet** (MSD)		(#MSD 135). Yellow. Film coated. In 100s.	132
Rx	**Amodopa** (Major)		In 100s and UD 100s.	70
Rx	**Methyldopa** (Various)	**Tablets:** 250 mg methyldopa	In 40s, 42s, 50s, 60s, 100s, 500s, 1000s & UD 32s, 100s and 300s.	24+
Rx	**Aldomet** (MSD)		(#MSD 401). Yellow. Film coated. In 100s, 1000s and UD 100s.	84
Rx	**Amodopa** (Major)		In 100s, 1000s and UD 100s.	55
Rx	**Methyldopa** (Various)	**Tablets:** 500 mg methyldopa	In 30s, 50s, 60s, 100s, 500s, 720s, 1000s & UD 32s & 100s.	26+
Rx	**Aldomet** (MSD)		(#MSD 516). Yellow. Film coated. In 100s, 500s and UD 100s, unit-of-use 60s.	76
Rx	**Amodopa** (Major)		In 100s, 500s and UD 100s.	49
Rx	**Methyldopa** (Various)	**Oral Suspension:** 250 mg methyldopa per 5 ml	In 5 ml (UD 100s).	344+
Rx	**Aldomet** (MSD)[1]		1% alcohol. Orange-pineapple flavor. In 473 ml.	156
Rx	**Methyldopate HCl** (Various)	**Injection:** 250 mg methyldopate HCl per 5 ml	In 5 and 10 ml vials.	1663+
Rx	**Aldomet** (MSD)[2]		In 5 ml vials.	3070

* Cost Index based on cost per 250 mg.

\# Product identification code.

[1] With 0.2% sodium bisulfite. Avoid light and freezing.

[2] With 2.5 mg EDTA, 7.5 mg methylparaben, 1 mg propylparaben and 16 mg sodium bisulfite.

Refer to the general discussion of these products beginning on page 773.

CLONIDINE HCl

Actions:

Pharmacology: Clonidine, an imidazoline derivative, is a central α-adrenergic stimulant that inhibits sympathetic cardioaccelerator and vasoconstrictor centers. Initially, clonidine stimulates peripheral α-adrenergic receptors producing transient vasoconstriction. Stimulation of alpha-adrenergic in the brain stem results in reduced sympathetic outflow from the CNS and a decrease in peripheral resistance, renal vascular resistance, heart rate and blood pressure. Renal blood flow and glomerular filtration rate remain essentially unchanged.

Orthostatic effects are mild and infrequent since supine pressure is reduced to essentially the same extent as standing pressure. The drug does not alter normal hemodynamic responses to exercise. Acute studies have demonstrated a moderate reduction (15% to 20%) of cardiac output in the supine position with no change in the peripheral resistance, while at a 45° tilt there is a smaller reduction in cardiac output and a decrease of peripheral resistance. During long-term therapy, cardiac output tends to return to control values, while peripheral resistance remains decreased. The coadministration of a diuretic enhances the antihypertensive efficacy of clonidine.

Plasma renin activity and excretion of aldosterone and catecholamines is reduced. Clonidine acutely stimulates growth hormone release in both children and adults, but does not produce a chronic elevation of growth hormone with long-term use.

Pharmacokinetics: Blood pressure declines within 30 to 60 minutes after an oral dose. The peak plasma level occurs in approximately 3 to 5 hours with a plasma half-life of 12 to 16 hours. About 50% of the absorbed dose is metabolized in the liver. In patients with impaired renal function, half-life increases to 30 to 40 hours. Clonidine and its metabolites are excreted mainly in the urine. About 40% to 60% of the absorbed dose is recovered in the urine as unchanged drug in 24 hours.

Transdermal System: The system, a 0.2 mm thick film with four layers, contains a drug reservoir of clonidine, released at an approximately constant rate for 7 days. A microporous polypropylene membrane controls the rate of delivery from the system to the skin surface.

Therapeutic plasma levels, which are achieved 2 to 3 days after initial application are lower than during oral therapy with equipotent doses. Application of a new system at weekly intervals continuously maintains therapeutic plasma concentrations. When the system is removed (and not replaced), therapeutic plasma clonidine levels will persist for about 8 hours and then decline slowly over several days; blood pressure returns gradually to pretreatment levels. The elimination half-life is approximately 19 hours.

Indications:

Hypertension.

Unlabeled Uses: Clonidine has been evaluated for use in the following conditions:

Clonidine Unlabeled Uses	
Use	**Dosage**[1]
Alcohol withdrawal	0.3 to 0.6 mg every 6 hours
Constitutional growth delay in children	0.0375 to 0.15 mg/m²/day
Diabetic diarrhea	0.15 to 1.2 mg/day or 0.3 mg/24 hr patch (1 to 2 patches/week)
Gilles de la Tourette syndrome	0.15 to 0.2 mg/day
Hypertensive "urgencies" (diastolic > 120 mm Hg)	initially 0.1 to 0.2 mg, followed by 0.05 to 0.1 mg every hour to a maximum of 0.8 mg
Menopausal flushing	0.1 to 0.4 mg/day or 0.1 mg/24 hr patch
Methadone/opiate detoxification	15 to 16 mcg/kg/day
Pheochromocytoma diagnosis (overnight clonidine suppression test)	0.3 mg
Postherpetic neuralgia	0.2 mg/day
Reduction of allergen-induced inflammatory reactions in patients with extrinsic asthma	0.15 mg for 3 days
Smoking cessation facilitation	0.15 to 0.4 mg/day or 0.2 mg/24 hour patch
Ulcerative colitis	0.3 mg 3 times a day

[1] Dosage given as oral unless otherwise specified.

(Continued on following page)

CLONIDINE HCl (Cont.)

Contraindications:

Hypersensitivity to clonidine or any component of adhesive layer of transdermal system.

Warnings:

Use with caution in patients with severe coronary insufficiency, recent myocardial infarction (MI), cerebrovascular disease or chronic renal failure.

Tolerance may develop, necessitating a reevaluation of therapy.

Usage in Pregnancy: Category C. Embryotoxicity was evident in animal studies at doses as low as 1.2 times the maximum recommended dose. However, there are no adequate and well controlled studies in pregnant women. Because animal reproduction studies are not always predictive of human response, clonidine should be used in pregnancy only if clearly needed. Clonidine crosses the placenta, resulting in cord concentrations that are equal to maternal serum concentrations, and amniotic fluid concentrations that are up to four times that found in serum. Also, the plasma levels in the newborn are approximately half of the maternal levels.

Usage in Lactation: Clonidine is excreted in breast milk; following a 0.15 mg oral dose, milk concentrations of 1.5 ng/ml may be achieved (milk:plasma ratio 1.5). Clinical significance is unknown. Exercise caution when administering to a nursing woman.

Usage in Children: Safety and efficacy for use in children have not been established.

Precautions:

Rebound hypertension: Do not discontinue therapy without consulting a physician (see also p. 775 Discontinue therapy by reducing the dose gradually over 2 to 4 days to avoid a rapid rise in blood pressure. Abrupt withdrawal of clonidine may result in subjective symptoms such as nervousness, agitation, headache and elevated catecholamine concentrations in the plasma, but such occurrences have usually been associated with previous administration of high oral doses (exceeding 1.2 mg/day) or with continuation of concomitant β-blocker therapy. Tachycardia, rebound hypertension, flushing, nausea, vomiting and cardiac arrhythmias have also occurred. The risk may be dose-related, and the risk may be increased with multiple drug therapy. Rare instances of hypertensive encephalopathy and death have been reported after abrupt cessation of therapy.

If an excessive rise in blood pressure occurs, it can be reversed by resumption of therapy or by IV phentolamine, phenoxybenzamine or prazosin. Direct vasodilators and captopril have also been used. If therapy is to be discontinued in patients receiving β-blockers and clonidine concurrently, β-blockers should be discontinued several days before the gradual withdrawal of clonidine.

Rebound hypertension has also occurred following discontinuation of the transdermal patch. In one case this occurred when a patient was switched from oral to transdermal therapy.

Ophthalmologic effects: Perform periodic eye examinations, since retinal degeneration has been noted in animal studies.

Perioperative use: Continue administration of clonidine to within 4 hours of surgery and resume as soon as possible thereafter. Carefully monitor blood pressure and institute appropriate measures to control it as necessary. If transdermal therapy is started during the perioperative period, note that therapeutic plasma levels are not achieved until 2 to 3 days after initial application.

Sensitization to transdermal clonidine: In patients who have developed localized contact sensitization to transdermal clonidine, substitution of oral clonidine HCl therapy may be associated with development of a generalized skin rash. In patients who develop an allergic reaction to transdermal clonidine that extends beyond the local patch site (such as generalized skin rash, urticaria, or angioedema) oral clonidine HCl substitution may elicit a similar reaction.

Drug Interactions:

Beta-adrenergic blocking agents: The severity of withdrawal hypertension caused by abrupt discontinuation of clonidine may be greater in patients taking beta-adrenergic blocking agents, possibly due to unopposed α-adrenergic stimulation. Also, this combination has uncommonly caused paradoxical hypertension.

Tricyclic antidepressants may block antihypertensive effects of clonidine.

(Continued on following page)

CLONIDINE HCl (Cont.)

Adverse Reactions:

Most common: Dry mouth (40%); drowsiness (33%); dizziness (16%); sedation and constipation (10%). Constipation, dizziness, headache and fatigue tend to diminish within 4 to 6 weeks.

GI: Anorexia; malaise; nausea and vomiting; parotid pain and rarely, parotitis; mild transient abnormalities in liver function tests.

Metabolic: Weight gain; transient elevation of blood glucose or serum creatine phosphokinase (rare); gynecomastia.

Cardiovascular: Congestive heart failure; orthostatic symptoms; palpitations, tachycardia and bradycardia; Raynaud's phenomenon; ECG abnormalities manifested as Wenckebach period or ventricular trigeminy; conduction disturbances, arrhythmias, sinus bradycardia and atrioventricular block (rare).

CNS: Dreams or nightmares; insomnia; hallucinations; delirium; nervousness; agitation; restlessness; anxiety; depression; headache.

Dermatologic: Rash, angioneurotic edema, hives, urticaria; hair thinning and alopecia; pruritus not associated with rash.

GU: Impotence; decreased sexual activity/loss of libido; nocturia, difficulty in micturition and urinary retention.

Musculoskeletal: Weakness; fatigue; muscle or joint pain; cramps of the lower limbs.

Other: Increased sensitivity to alcohol; dryness, itching or burning of the eyes; dryness of the nasal mucosa; pallor; fever; weakly positive Coombs' test.

Transdermal system: The most frequent systemic reactions were dry mouth and drowsiness. The following have also been reported:

GI – Constipation; nausea; change in taste; dry throat.

CNS – Fatigue; headache; lethargy; sedation; insomnia; nervousness; dizziness.

GU – Impotence/sexual dysfunction.

Dermatologic – Transient localized skin reactions; pruritus; erythema, allergic contact sensitization and contact dermatitis; localized vesiculation; hyperpigmentation; edema; excoriation; burning; papules; throbbing; blanching; generalized macular rash.

Causal relationship not established – Maculopapular skin rash; urticaria; angioedema of the face and tongue.

Overdosage:

Symptoms: Bradycardia; hypotension; CNS depression; respiratory depression; apnea; hypothermia; miosis; seizures; lethargy; agitation; irritability; vomiting; diarrhea; hypoventilation; reversible cardiac conduction defects; arrhythmias; transient hypertension. Profound hypotension, weakness, somnolence, diminished or absent reflexes and vomiting followed accidental ingestion by several children between the ages of 9 months to 5 years.

In a patient who ingested 100 mg clonidine, plasma levels were 60 ng/ml (1 hour), 190 ng/ml (1.5 hours), 370 ng/ml (2 hours) and 120 ng/ml (5.5 and 6.5 hours). The patient developed hypertension followed by hypotension, bradycardia, apnea, hallucinations, semicoma and premature ventricular contractions. The patient fully recovered after intensive treatment.

Profound hypotension occurred in a 9-month-old infant after sucking on a discarded transdermal clonidine patch. The child recovered following dopamine infusion.

Treatment: Induction of emesis is usually contraindicated because of the rapid onset of CNS depression. Establish respiration if necessary, perform gastric lavage and administer activated charcoal. A saline cathartic (magnesium sulfate) will increase the rate of transport through the GI tract. Routine hemodialysis is of limited benefit, since a maximum of 5% of circulating clonidine is removed.

Atropine sulfate (0.6 mg for adults; 0.01 mg/kg in children) given IV may be useful for treatment of persistent bradycardia. Epinephrine, dopamine or tolazoline have also been used. Treat hypotension by administering IV fluids and elevating the legs; dopamine (2 to 20 mcg/kg/min) or tolazoline IV (1 mg/kg/dose, maximum 10 mg/dose) may be used if hypotension is unresponsive.

Hypertension has been treated with IV furosemide or diazoxide, or α-blocking agents such as phentolamine. Tolazoline, an α-blocker, in IV doses of 10 mg at 30 minute intervals may reverse clonidine's effects if other efforts fail.

(Continued on following page)

Antiadrenergic Agents – Centrally Acting (Cont.)

CLONIDINE HCl (Cont.)

Administration and Dosage – Oral:

Individualize dosage.

Initial dose: 0.1 mg twice daily. Elderly patients may benefit from a lower initial dose.

Maintenance dose: Increments of 0.1 or 0.2 mg/day may be made until desired response is achieved; most common range is 0.2 to 0.8 mg/day given in divided doses. The maximum dose is 2.4 mg/day. Minimize sedative effects by slowly increasing the daily dosage and giving the majority of the daily dose at bedtime.

Children: 5 to 25 mcg/kg/day in divided doses every 6 hours; increase at 5 to 7 day intervals.

Unlabeled route of administration: Sublingual clonidine, using a dosage of 0.2 to 0.4 mg/day, may be effective in hypertensive patients unable to take oral medication. The onset occurs within 30 to 60 minutes and blood pressure appears to be maintained on a twice daily regimen.

Renal Impairment: Adjust dosage according to degree of renal impairment and carefully monitor patients. Since only a minimal amount of clonidine is removed during hemodialysis, there is no need to give supplemental clonidine following dialysis.

	Product (Distributor)	Dosage form	How Supplied	C.I.*
Rx	**Clonidine** (Various)	**Tablets:** 0.1 mg	In 30s, 56s, 100s, 500s, 1000s and UD 100s.	8+
Rx	**Catapres** (Boehringer-Ingelheim)		(#B-I 6). Tan, scored. In 100s, 1000s and UD 100s.	100
Rx	**Clonidine** (Various)	**Tablets:** 0.2 mg	In 30s, 36s, 60s, 100s, 500s, 1000s and UD 32s and 100s.	5+
Rx	**Catapres** (Boehringer-Ingelheim)		(#B-I 7). Orange, scored. In 100s, 1000s and UD 100s.	77
Rx	**Clonidine** (Various)	**Tablets:** 0.3 mg	In 56s, 100s, 500s, 1000s and UD 100s.	5+
Rx	**Catapres** (Boehringer-Ingelheim)		(#B-I 11). Peach, scored. In 100s.	58

Administration and Dosage – Transdermal:

Apply to a hairless area of intact skin on upper arm or torso, once every 7 days. Use a different skin site from the previous application. If the system loosens during the 7 day wearing, apply the adhesive overlay directly over the system to ensure good adhesion.

For initial therapy, start with the 0.1 mg system. If, after 1 or 2 weeks, desired blood pressure reduction is not achieved, add another 0.1 mg system or use a larger system. Dosage > two 0.3 mg systems usually does not improve efficacy. Note that the antihypertensive effect of the system may not commence until 2 to 3 days after application. Therefore, when substituting the transdermal system in patients on prior antihypertensive therapy, a gradual reduction of prior drug dosage is advised. Previous antihypertensive treatment may have to be continued, particularly in patients with severe hypertension.

	Product/Distributor	Release Rate (mg/24 hr)	Surface Area (cm^2)	Total Clonidine Content (mg)	How Supplied	C.I.*
Rx	**Catapres-TTS-1**	0.1	3.5	2.5	In 12s.	1456
	Catapres-TTS-2	0.2	7	5	In 12s.	1226
	Catapres-TTS-3 (Boehringer-Ingelheim)	0.3	10.5	7.5	In 4s.	1132

* Cost Index based on cost per 0.1 mg tablet or patch release rate. # Product identification code.

Refer to the general discussion of these products beginning on page 773

GUANFACINE HCl

Actions:

Pharmacology: Guanfacine HCl is a centrally acting oral antihypertensive with α_2-adrenoreceptor agonist properties. Its principal mechanism of action appears to be stimulation of central α_2-adrenergic receptors. Guanfacine reduces sympathetic nerve impulses from the vasomotor center to the heart and blood vessels, resulting in a decrease in peripheral vascular resistance and a reduction in heart rate.

Controlled clinical trials in patients with mild to moderate hypertension receiving a thiazide-type diuretic have defined the dose-response relationship for blood pressure response of guanfacine and have shown that the response can persist for 24 hours after a single dose. In the dose-response study, patients were randomized to placebo or to doses of 0.5, 1, 2 and 3 mg guanfacine, each given at bedtime. The observed mean changes from baseline, tabulated below, indicate the similarity of response for placebo and the 0.5 mg dose. Doses of 1, 2, and 3 mg resulted in decreased blood pressure in the sitting position with no real differences among the three doses. In the standing position, there was some increase in response with dose.

Mean Decrease in Seated and Standing Blood Pressure (BP) by Guanfacine Dosage Group (in mm Hg)

Vital Sign	Placebo n = 63	0.5 mg n = 63	1 mg n = 64	2 mg n = 58	3 mg n = 59
Change in Systolic BP (seated)	– 5	– 5	– 14	– 12	– 16
Change in Diastolic BP (seated)	– 7	– 6	– 13	– 13	– 13
Change in Systolic BP (standing)	– 3	– 5	– 11	– 9	– 15
Change in Diastolic BP (standing)	– 5	– 4	– 9	– 10	– 12

While most of guanfacine's effectiveness was present at 1 mg, adverse reactions at this dose were not clearly distinguishable from those associated with placebo. Adverse reactions were clearly present at 2 and 3 mg (see Adverse Reactions).

In a placebo controlled study of guanfacine, a significant decrease in blood pressure was maintained for a full 24 hours after dosing. While there was no significant difference between the 12 and 24 hour blood pressure readings, the fall in blood pressure at 24 hours was numerically smaller, suggesting possible escape of blood pressure in some patients and the need for individualization of therapy.

In a double-blind, randomized trial, either guanfacine or clonidine was given at recommended doses with 25 mg chlorthalidone for 24 weeks and then abruptly discontinued. Results showed equal degrees of blood pressure reduction with the two drugs; there was no tendency for blood pressure to increase despite maintenance of the same daily dose of the two drugs. Signs and symptoms of rebound phenomena were infrequent upon discontinuation of either drug. Abrupt withdrawal of clonidine produced a rapid return of diastolic and, especially, systolic blood pressure to approximately pretreatment levels, with occasional values significantly greater than baseline. Guanfacine withdrawal produced a more gradual increase to pretreatment levels, but also with occasional values significantly greater than baseline.

Hemodynamic studies in man showed that the decrease in blood pressure observed after single dose or long-term oral treatment with guanfacine was accompanied by a significant decrease in peripheral resistance and a slight reduction in heart rate (5 beats/min). Cardiac output under conditions of rest or exercise was not altered by guanfacine.

Guanfacine lowered elevated plasma renin activity and plasma catecholamine levels in hypertensive patients, but this does not correlate with individual blood pressure responses. Growth hormone secretion was stimulated with single oral doses of 2 and 4 mg. Long-term use had no effect on growth hormone levels.

Guanfacine had no effect on plasma aldosterone. A slight but insignificant decrease in plasma volume occurred after 1 month of guanfacine therapy. There were no changes in mean body weight or electrolytes.

(Actions continued on following page)

GUANFACINE HCl (Cont.)

Actions (Cont.):

Pharmacokinetics: Absorption/Distribution – Relative to a 3 mg IV dose, the absolute oral bioavailability of guanfacine is about 80%. Peak plasma concentrations occur from 1 to 4 hours with an average of 2.6 hours after single oral doses or at steady-state. The area under the concentration time curve (AUC) increases linearly with the dose.

The drug is approximately 70% bound to plasma proteins, independent of drug concentration. The whole body volume of distribution is high (a mean of 6.3 L/kg), which suggests a high distribution of drug to the tissues.

Metabolism/Excretion – In individuals with normal renal function, the average elimination half-life is approximately 17 hours (range 10 to 30 hours). Younger patients tend to have shorter elimination half-lives (13 to 14 hours) while older patients tend to have half-lives at the upper end of the range. Steady-state blood levels were attained within 4 days in most subjects. Guanfacine and its metabolites are excreted primarily in the urine. Approximately 50% (30% to 75%) of the dose is eliminated in the urine as unchanged drug; the remainder is eliminated mostly as conjugates of metabolites produced by oxidative metabolism of the aromatic ring. The guanfacine to creatinine clearance ratio is greater than 1, suggesting that tubular secretion of drug occurs.

Indications:

Management of hypertension. Dosing has been established in the presence of a thiazide-type diuretic. Use in patients who are already receiving a thiazide-type diuretic.

Unlabeled Use: Guanfacine (0.03 to 1.5 mg/day) may be beneficial in ameliorating withdrawal symptoms in patients discontinuing heroin usage.

Contraindications:

Patients with known hypersensitivity to guanfacine.

Warnings:

Usage in impaired renal function: Guanfacine clearance in patients with varying degrees of renal insufficiency is reduced, but drug plasma levels are only slightly increased compared to patients with normal renal function. When prescribing for patients with renal impairment, use the low end of the dosing range. Patients on dialysis can be given usual doses of guanfacine, since the drug is poorly dialyzed.

Usage in Pregnancy: Category B. Administration to rats and rabbits at doses 200 and 100 times the maximum recommended human dose, respectively, were associated with reduced fetal survival and maternal toxicity. Rat experiments have shown that guanfacine crosses the placenta. There are no adequate and well controlled studies in pregnant women. Use during pregnancy only if clearly needed.

Labor and Delivery – Not recommended in the treatment of acute hypertension associated with preeclampsia.

Usage in Lactation: Experiments with rats show that guanfacine is excreted in milk. It is not known whether guanfacine is excreted in human breast milk. Use caution when administering to a nursing mother.

Usage in Children: Safety and efficacy in children less than 12 years of age have not been demonstrated. Therefore, use in this age group is not recommended.

Precautions:

General: Like other antihypertensives, use guanfacine with caution in patients with severe coronary insufficiency, recent myocardial infarction, cerebrovascular disease, or chronic renal or hepatic failure.

Sedation: Like other orally active central α_2-adrenergic agonists, guanfacine causes sedation or drowsiness, especially when beginning therapy. These symptoms are dose-related. When used with other centrally active depressants (such as phenothiazines, barbiturates or benzodiazepines), consider the potential for additive sedative effects.

Rebound: Abrupt cessation of therapy with orally active central α_2-adrenergic agonists may be associated with increases in plasma and urinary catecholamines, symptoms of nervousness and anxiety and, less commonly, increases in blood pressure to levels significantly greater than those prior to therapy.

The frequency of rebound hypertension is low, but when rebound occurs, it does so after 2 to 4 days, which is delayed compared with clonidine HCl. This is consistent with guanfacine's longer half-life. In most cases, after abrupt withdrawal of guanfacine, blood pressure returns to pretreatment levels slowly (in 2 to 4 days) without ill effects.

(Continued on following page)

Refer to the general discu...on of these products beginning on page 773

...adrenergic Agents – Peripherally Acting

RAUWOLFIA DERIVA...S

The rauwolfia deri... includ... whole root rauwolfia, alseroxylon (an extraction of alkaloids) and the r... alkaloids reserpine, rescinnamine and deserpidine.

Actions:

Pharmac... ...wolfia alkaloids probably exert their antihypertensive effects through deple...ue stores of catecholamines (epinephrine and norepinephrine) from pe.... Reserpine depletes stores of catecholamines and 5-hydroxytryptamine ...s, including the brain and adrenal medulla. Most of its pharmacological ...been attributed to this action. Depletion is slower and less complete in the ...ulla than in other tissues.

...ession of sympathetic nerve function results in a decreased heart rate and a ...f arterial blood pressure. The sedative and tranquilizing properties may be ...depletion of catecholamines and 5-hydroxytryptamine from the brain.

...ntihypertensive effect is often accompanied by bradycardia. The carotid sinus ... inhibited, but postural hypotension is rarely seen. Both the cardiovascular and ...fects may persist following withdrawal of these drugs.

...cokinetics: Rauwolfia alkaloids are characterized by slow onset of action and sus-...d effect.

...ollowing absorption from the GI tract, rauwolfia alkaloids concentrate in tissues ...h high lipid content. Rauwolfia crosses the blood brain barrier and the placenta.

Mean maximum plasma levels of 1.54 ng/ml were attained after a median of 3.5 hours in six normal subjects receiving a single oral dose of four 0.25 mg reserpine tablets. Bioavailability was approximately 50% that of a corresponding IV dose. Plasma levels of reserpine after IV administration declined with a mean half-life of 33 hours. Reserpine is extensively bound (96%) to plasma proteins.

Rauwolfia alkaloids are metabolized in the liver to inactive compounds that are excreted primarily in the urine. Unchanged alkaloids are excreted primarily in the feces.

Indications:

Mild essential hypertension. Adjunctive therapy with other antihypertensive agents for treatment of severe hypertension.

Relief of symptoms in agitated psychotic states, eg, schizophrenia, (rauwolfia, reserpine and deserpidine), primarily in those with a phenothiazine derivative intolerance or who also require antihypertensive medication.

Refer to individual product listings for specific indications.

Contraindications:

Hypersensitivity to rauwolfia derivatives; mental depression (especially with suicidal tendencies); active peptic ulcer; ulcerative colitis; electroconvulsive therapy.

Warnings:

Depression: Reserpine may cause mental depression. Exercise extreme caution in patients with a history of mental depression. Recognition of depression may be difficult because this condition may often be disguised by somatic complaints (masked depression). Use higher doses of rauwolfia derivatives cautiously as serious mental depression and other side effects may increase considerably. Discontinue the drug at first sign of despondency, early morning insomnia, loss of appetite, impotence or self-deprecation. Drug-induced depression may persist for several months after withdrawal and may be severe enough to result in suicide.

Carcinogenicity: Rodent studies have shown that reserpine at about 100 to 300 times the usual human dose caused an increased incidence of mammary fibroadenomas in female mice, malignant tumors of the seminal vesicles in male mice and malignant adrenal medullary tumors in male rats. The breast neoplasms are thought to be related to reserpine's prolactin-elevating effect.

Risk to humans is uncertain. Tissue culture experiments show that about one-third of human breast tumors are prolactin-dependent in vitro, very important if use of the drug is contemplated in a patient with previously detected breast cancer. An increased risk of breast cancer in reserpine users has been studied extensively with conflicting results. Although a few epidemiologic studies suggest a slightly increased risk (generally less than twofold) in women who have used reserpine, other studies have not confirmed this. While long-term clinical observation has not suggested such an association, the available evidence is too limited to be conclusive.

(Warnings continued on following page)

RAUWOLFIA DERIVATIVES (Cont.)

Warnings (Cont.):

Usage in Pregnancy: Category C (rauwolfia, reserpine, alseroxylon). ... *for use during* pregnancy is not established. Use only when clearly needed and ... potential benef- its outweigh potential hazards to the fetus. Rauwolfia alkaloids cross ... enta and appear in cord blood; use near term has resulted in increased respir... ns, nasal congestion, hypothermia, cyanosis, retractions, lethargy and an... neonate.

Usage in Lactation: Rauwolfia alkaloids are excreted in breast milk. Increas... tract secretions, nasal congestion, cyanosis and anorexia may occur in bre... infants. Because of the potential for serious adverse reactions in nursing in... tumorigenicity shown in animal studies, either discontinue nursing or discon... drug, taking into account importance of the drug to the mother.

Usage in Children: Safety and efficacy for use in children have not been establishe... Because of adverse effects such as emotional depression and lability, sedation an... stuffy nose, reserpine is not usually recommended as a step-2 drug in the treatmen... hypertensive children, although reserpine has been administered. (See Administratio... and Dosage p. 794)

Usage in the Elderly: Geriatric patients may show increased sensitivity to alseroxylon's hypotensive effects; low dosages may be necessary.

Precautions:

Electroshock therapy: Discontinue reserpine 7 days before electroshock therapy.

Usage in GI distress: Rauwolfia preparations increase GI motility and secretion; therefore, use cautiously in patients with a history of peptic ulcer, ulcerative colitis or gallstones (biliary colic may be precipitated). Observe patients on high dosage carefully to detect possible reactivation of peptic ulcer.

Use in impaired renal function: Exercise caution when treating hypertensive patients with renal insufficiency since they adjust poorly to lowered blood pressure levels.

Preoperative withdrawal of rauwolfia alkaloids does not assure circulatory stability; hypotension has occurred in patients receiving rauwolfia. Anticholinergic or adrenergic drugs (metaraminol, norepinephrine) have been used to treat adverse vagocirculatory effects.

Patient's drug intake: The anesthesiologist must be aware of the patient's drug intake and consider this in the overall management since hypotension has occurred in patients receiving rauwolfia preparations.

Acute hypersensitivity reactions may occur in patients with or without a history of allergy or bronchial asthma. Have epinephrine 1:1000 immediately available. Refer to Management of Acute Hypersensitivity Reactions on p. 2897

Tartrazine sensitivity: Some of these products contain tartrazine, which may cause allergic-type reactions (including bronchial asthma) in susceptible individuals. Although the incidence of tartrazine sensitivity in the general population is low, it is frequently seen in patients who also have aspirin hypersensitivity. Specific products containing tartrazine are identified in the product listings.

Drug Interactions:

Alkaloids of the rauwolfia class: Do not administer two or more rauwolfia alkaloids together.

Antihypertensives/diuretics: Antihypertensive effects may be potentiated.

Digitalis and **quinidine:** Use cautiously since cardiac arrhythmias have occurred with rauwolfia preparations.

Ephedrine or **mephentermine:** Hypertension may occur following direct-acting sympathomimetics, while the effects of mixed-acting sympathomimetics may be decreased.

General anesthesia has been associated with hypotension and bradycardia in patients taking rauwolfia alkaloids.

Levodopa: Exacerbation of Parkinsonian signs and symptoms may result with reserpine coadministration. Effects of levodopa may be inhibited (whole root rauwolfia).

MAO inhibitors and concomitant reserpine may result in a hypertensive reaction. Coadministration should be avoided or used with extreme caution.

Methotrimeprazine: Administration with rauwolfia alkaloids may result in excessive excitation, hypertension and sympathetic response.

Sympathomimetics: *Direct acting* – rauwolfia alkaloids may prolong sympathomimetic effects. *Indirect acting* – rauwolfia alkaloids may inhibit sympathomimetic effects.

(Drug Interactions continued on following page)

Refer to the general discussion of these products beginning on page 773.

Antiadrenergic Agents – Peripherally Acting (Cont.)

GUANADREL SULFATE

Actions:

Pharmacology: Guanadrel, structurally and pharmacologically similar to guanethidine, inhibits sympathetic vasoconstriction by inhibiting norepinephrine release from neuronal storage sites in response to nerve stimulation. Depletion of norepinephrine causes a relaxation of vascular smooth muscle which decreases total peripheral resistance and venous return. A hypotensive effect results, greater in the standing than in the supine position by about 10 mm Hg systolic and 3.5 mm Hg diastolic. The drug does not inhibit parasympathetic nerve function nor does it enter the CNS.

Guanadrel begins to decrease blood pressure within 2 hours and produces maximal decreases in 4 to 6 hours. No significant change in cardiac output accompanies the blood pressure decline in normal individuals. Heart rate is also decreased by about 5 beats/minute. Fluid retention occurs, particularly when guanadrel is not accompanied by a diuretic.

Guanadrel causes increased sensitivity to circulating norepinephrine, probably by preventing uptake of norepinephrine by adrenergic neurons. Thus it is dangerous in the presence of excess norepinephrine, eg, pheochromocytoma.

Clinical Pharmacology: Patients with initial supine blood pressures averaging 160 to 170/105 to 110 mm Hg have decreases in blood pressure of 20 to 25/15 to 20 mm Hg in the standing position. Guanethidine and guanadrel are similar in effectiveness while methyldopa has a larger effect on supine systolic pressure. Side effects of guanadrel and guanethidine are generally similar while methyldopa has more CNS effects (depression, drowsiness) but fewer orthostatic effects and less diarrhea.

Pharmacokinetics: Absorption – It is rapidly absorbed after oral administration. Plasma concentrations peak 1.5 to 2 hours after ingestion. Protein binding is less than 20%.

Metabolism/Excretion – The half-life is about 10 hours, but individual variability is great. Approximately 85% of the drug is eliminated in the urine. Urinary excretion is about 85% complete within 24 hours; about 40% of a dose is excreted unchanged.

Indications:

Treatment of hypertension Step 2 therapy in patients not responding adequately to a thiazide-type diuretic. Add to a diuretic regimen for optimum blood pressure control.

Contraindications:

Known or suspected pheochromocytoma; concurrently with, or within 1 week of MAOIs; hypersensitivity to guanadrel; frank congestive heart failure (CHF).

Warnings:

Orthostatic hypotension and its consequences (dizziness and weakness) are frequent. Rarely, fainting upon standing or exercise occurs. Careful instructions to the patient can minimize symptoms; supine blood pressure is not an adequate assessment of guanadrel's effects. Patients with known regional vascular disease (cerebral, coronary) are at particular risk from marked orthostatic hypotension; avoid hypotensive episodes even if this requires a poorer degree of blood pressure control.

Surgery: To reduce the possibility of vascular collapse during anesthesia, discontinue guanadrel 48 to 72 hours before elective surgery. If emergency surgery is required, administer preanesthetic and anesthetic agents cautiously in reduced dosage. Use vasopressors cautiously, as guanadrel can enhance the pressor response and increase arrhythmogenicity.

Asthma: Special care is needed in patients with bronchial asthma, as it may be aggravated by catecholamine depletion and sympathomimetic amines may interfere with the hypotensive effect of guanadrel.

Usage in Pregnancy: Category B. Safety for use during pregnancy has not been established. Use only when clearly needed and when the potential benefits outweigh the potential hazards to the fetus.

Usage in Lactation: Safety for use in the nursing mother has not been established. Because of the potential for serious adverse reactions in the nursing infant, decide whether to discontinue nursing or to discontinue the drug, taking into account the importance of the drug to the mother.

Usage in Children: Safety and efficacy for use in children have not been established.

(Continued on following page)

GUANADREL SULFATE (Cont.)

Precautions:

Salt and water retention may occur. Patients with CHF have not been studied, but guanadrel could interfere with the adrenergic mechanisms.

Peptic ulcer: Use guanadrel cautiously in patients with a history of peptic ulcer, which could be aggravated by a relative increase in parasympathetic tone.

Tricyclic antidepressants block the norepinephrine-depleting effect and the blood pressure lowering effect of guanadrel in animals. Presume inhibition of the antihypertensive effects of guanadrel by tricyclic antidepressants in humans. Use caution if guanadrel sulfate and a tricyclic antidepressant are used concomitantly. If the tricyclic antidepressant is discontinued abruptly, an enhanced effect of guanadrel may occur.

Drug Interactions:

Tricyclic antidepressants (see Precautions) and **indirect-acting sympathomimetics** such as ephedrine or phenylpropanolamine, and possibly **phenothiazines,** can reverse the effects of neuronal blocking agents.

Direct-acting sympathomimetics: Guanadrel enhances the activity of these drugs (ie, norepinephrine) by blocking neuronal uptake.

Alpha- or **beta-adrenergic blocking agents** and **reserpine** affect the adrenergic response by the same or other mechanisms and may potentiate the effects of guanadrel, causing excessive postural hypotension and bradycardia.

Vasodilators: Use with guanadrel is not generally recommended because concomitant use may increase the potential for symptomatic orthostatic hypotension. The possibility of this interaction has not been adequately studied.

Adverse Reactions:

The following table displays the frequency of side effects which are generally higher during the first 8 weeks of therapy. Approximately 3.6% of patients withdrew from guanadrel therapy because of untoward effects.

	Drug (No. patients treated) Event	*Guanadrel* (1544) (%)	*Methyldopa* (743) (%)	*Guanethidine* (330) (%)
Cardiovascular/ Respiratory	Shortness of breath on exertion	46	53	49
	Palpitations	30	35	25
	Chest pain	28	37	27
	Coughing	27	36	22
	Shortness of breath at rest	18	22	17
Central Nervous System	Fatigue	64	76	57
	Headache	58	69	50
	Faintness (orthostatic/other)	47-49	41-46	45-48
	Drowsiness	45	64	29
	Visual disturbances	29	35	26
	Paresthesias	25	35	16
	Confusion	15	23	11
	Psychological problems	4	5	4
	Depression	2	4	2
	Sleep disorders	2	2	3
	Syncope	< 1	< 1	2
Gastrointestinal	Increased bowel movements	31	28	36
	Gas pain/indigestion	24-32	31-40	19-29
	Constipation	21	29	20
	Anorexia	19	23	18
	Glossitis	8	11	5
	Nausea/vomiting	4	5	4
	Dry mouth, dry throat	2	4	< 1
	Abdominal distress or pain	2	2	2
Genitourinary	Nocturia	48	52	42
	Urination urgency or frequency	34	40	28
	Peripheral edema	29	37	23
	Ejaculation disturbances	18	21	22
	Impotence	5	12	7
	Hematuria	2	4	2
Musculoskeletal/ Miscellaneous	Excessive weight gain/loss	42-44	51-54	42
	Aching limbs	43	52	34
	Leg cramps - nighttime	26	33	21
	Leg cramps - daytime	21	26	20
	Backache or neckache	2	1	2
	Joint pain or inflammation	2	2	2

(Continued on following page)

Antiadrenergic Agents – Peripherally Acting (Cont.)

GUANADREL SULFATE (Cont.)

Overdosage:

Symptoms: Marked dizziness and blurred vision related to postural hypotension progressing to syncope on standing. The patient should lie down until these symptoms subside.

Treatment: If excessive hypotension occurs and persists despite conservative treatment, a vasoconstrictor such as phenylephrine may be needed, but use carefully because patients may be hypersensitive to such agents.

Patient Information:

The medication may cause orthostatic hypotension; sit or lie down immediately at the onset of dizziness or weakness to prevent loss of consciousness. Postural hypotension is worst in the morning and upon arising, and may be exaggerated by alcohol, fever, hot weather, prolonged standing or exercise.

Do not take any prescription or over-the-counter medications, especially medications for treatment of colds, allergy or asthma, without physician's advice.

Administration and Dosage:

Individualize dosage. The usual starting dosage is 10 mg/day, which can be given as 5 mg, 2 times daily by breaking the 10 mg tablet. Most patients will require a daily dosage of 20 to 75 mg, usually in twice daily doses. For larger doses, 3 or 4 times daily dosing may be needed. Adjust the dosage weekly or monthly until blood pressure is controlled.

With long-term therapy, some tolerance may occur and the dosage may have to be increased. Because guanadrel has a substantial orthostatic effect, monitor both supine and standing pressures, especially while adjusting dosage.

				C.I.*
Rx	**Hylorel** (Pennwalt)	**Tablets:** 10 mg	(#Hylorel 10). Light orange, scored. In 100s.	442
		25 mg	(#Hylorel 25). White, scored. In 100s.	274

* Cost Index based on cost per 10 mg.

Product identification code.

Refer to the general discussion of these products beginning on page 773.

Antiadrenergic Agents – Peripherally Acting (Cont.)

ALPHA-1-ADRENERGIC BLOCKERS

Actions:

Pharmacology: Prazosin, terazosin and doxazosin selectively block postsynaptic α-1-adrenergic receptors. These drugs dilate both resistance (arterioles) and capacitance (veins) vessels. Both supine and standing blood pressure are lowered. This effect is most pronounced on the diastolic blood pressure. Terazosin decreases blood pressure gradually within 15 minutes following oral administration. Unlike conventional α-blockers, the antihypertensive actions of prazosin and terazosin are usually not accompanied by reflex tachycardia. With doxazosin, maximum reductions in blood pressure usually occur 2 to 6 hours after dosing and are associated with a small increase in standing heart rate. Tolerance to the antihypertensive effect of these agents has not been observed.

Prazosin does not appear to increase renin release as do the direct-acting vasodilators; a decrease in plasma renin activity has occurred during therapy. Plasma renin activity was unchanged by terazosin.

Use of prazosin as a single antihypertensive agent is limited by its tendency to cause sodium and water retention and increased plasma volume.

Clinical studies of terazosin used once-daily (the great majority) and twice-daily regimens. Total doses usually ranged from 5 to 20 mg/day in patients with mild (about 77%, diastolic pressure 95 to 105 mm Hg) or moderate (23%, diastolic pressure 105 to 115 mm Hg) hypertension. Blood pressure responses persisted throughout the interval, with the usual supine responses 5 to 10 mm Hg systolic and 3.5 to 8 mm Hg diastolic greater than placebo. The responses in the standing position tended to be somewhat larger, by 1 to 3 mm Hg. The magnitude of the blood pressure responses was similar to prazosin and less than hydrochlorothiazide (in a single study). In measurements 24 hours after dosing, heart rate was unchanged.

Doxazosin has a greater effect on blood pressure and heart rate in the standing position. In placebo controlled studies at doses of 1 to 16 mg given once daily, blood pressure was lowered at 24 hours by about 10/8 mm Hg compared to placebo in the standing position and about 9/5 mm Hg in the supine position. There was no apparent difference in the blood pressure response of Caucasians and Blacks or of patients above and below age 65.

Pharmacokinetics: Prazosin is extensively metabolized. The metabolites of prazosin are active. Duration of antihypertensive effect is 10 hours. Elimination is slower in patients with congestive heart failure (CHF) than in normal subjects. The pharmacokinetics may be altered in chronic renal failure (eg, elimination half-life prolonged, protein binding decreased and peak plasma concentrations increased).

Terazosin undergoes minimal hepatic first-pass metabolism; nearly all of the circulating dose is in the form of parent drug. Approximately 10% of an oral dose is excreted as parent drug in the urine, and approximately 20% is excreted in the feces. The remainder is eliminated as metabolites.

Doxazosin is extensively metabolized in the liver, mainly by O-demethylation or hydroxylation. Approximately 4.8% is excreted in the feces as unchanged drug, with only a trace in the urine. Enterohepatic recycling is suggested by secondary peaking of plasma doxazosin concentrations. Although several active metabolites have been identified, their pharmacokinetics have not been characterized. The low plasma concentrations of the known active and inactive metabolites compared to the parent drug indicate that the contribution of even the most potent compound to the antihypertensive efficacy is probably small.

Pharmacokinetics of Alpha-1-Adrenergic Blockers

Parameters	Prazosin	Terazosin	Doxazosin
Oral bioavailability	48% to 68%	90%	65%
Affected by food	No	No	nd
Peak plasma level, time	1 to 3 hrs	1 to 2 hrs	2 to 3 hrs
Protein binding	92% to 97%	90% to 94%	98%
Half-life	2 to 3 hrs	9 to 12 hrs	22 hrs
Excretion: Bile/feces	< 90%	60%	63%
Urine	< 10%	40%	9%

nd = no data

(Continued on following page)

ALPHA-1-ADRENERGIC BLOCKERS (Cont.)

Indications:

For the treatment of hypertension, alone or in combination with other antihypertensive agents (eg, diuretics or β-adrenergic blocking agents).

Unlabeled uses: Prazosin has been used in refractory CHF. It decreases cardiac afterload (left ventricular systolic wall tension) and preload (left ventricular end-diastolic volume or pressure). By reducing aortic impedance and venous return, prazosin helps improve reduced cardiac output and relieve pulmonary congestion. It has produced improvement in the clinical symptoms, exercise tolerance and functional class (NYHA classification) of CHF in short-term studies.

Prazosin has been effective in the management of Raynaud's vasospasm and in the treatment of prostatic outflow obstruction.

Contraindications:

Hypersensitivity to quinazolines (eg, doxazosin, prazosin, terazosin).

Warnings:

"First-dose" effect: Prazosin, terazosin and doxazosin, like other α-adrenergic blocking agents, can cause marked hypotension (especially postural hypotension) and syncope with sudden loss of consciousness with the first few doses. Anticipate a similar effect if therapy is interrupted for more than a few doses, if dosage is increased rapidly, or if another antihypertensive drug is introduced. Syncope is due to an excessive postural hypotensive effect, although the syncopal episode has occasionally been preceded by severe supraventricular tachycardia with heart rates of 120 to 160 beats per minute.

The "first-dose" phenomenon may be minimized by limiting the initial dose to 1 mg of terazosin or prazosin (given at bedtime) or doxazosin. The 2, 5 and 10 mg terazosin tablets or 2 and 5 mg prazosin capsules or 2, 4 and 8 mg doxazosin tablets are not indicated as initial therapy. Slowly increase dosage of these drugs with increases in dose every 2 weeks. Add additional antihypertensives with caution. Caution patients to avoid situations where injury could result should syncope occur during initiation of therapy. Hypotension may develop in patients also receiving a β-adrenergic blocker.

If syncope occurs, place patient in recumbent position and treat supportively. This effect is self-limiting and in most cases does not recur after the initial period of therapy or during subsequent dosage adjustments. More common than loss of consciousness are dizziness and lightheadedness.

Syncopal episodes have usually ocurred within 30 to 90 minutes of the initial dose of prazosin; the incidence is ≈ 1% with an initial dose of ≥ 2 mg. Syncope occurred in about 1% of terazosin patients, was in no case severe or prolonged, and was not necessarily associated with early doses. There is evidence that the orthostatic effect of terazosin is greater, even in chronic use, shortly after dosing. Syncope occurred in 0.7% of doxazosin patients; none of these events were reported at the starting dose of 1 mg and 1.2% occurred at 16 mg/day. Other symptoms of lowered blood pressure, such as dizziness, lightheadedness and palpitations, are more common, occurring in approximately 28% of terazosin patients and up to 23% of doxazosin patients (≈ 2% of doxazosin patients discontinued therapy). This may present an occupational hazard to some patients. Treat these patients with caution and advise them as to what measures to take if symptoms develop.

Hepatic function impairment: Administer doxazosin with caution to patients with evidence of impaired hepatic function or to patients receiving drugs known to influence hepatic metabolism.

Fertility impairment: Reduced fertility occurred in male rats treated with doxazosin 20 mg/kg/day (about 75 times the maximum recommended human dose). The effect was reversible within 2 weeks of drug withdrawal. Nine of 39 male rats failed to sire a litter after terazosin 30 to 120 mg/kg/day. Testicular atrophy has also occurred in rats and dogs receiving terazosin or prazosin.

Elderly: There was no apparent difference in the blood pressure response of patients above and below age 65 receiving doxazosin.

(Warnings continued on following page)

ALPHA-1-ADRENERGIC BLOCKERS (Cont.)

Warnings (Cont.):

Pregnancy: Category C (prazosin, terazosin); *Category B* (doxazosin). There are no adequate and well controlled studies in pregnant women. Safety for use during pregnancy has not been established. Use only when clearly needed and when the potential benefits outweigh the potential hazards to the fetus.

In peri- and postnatal studies in rats, postnatal development at maternal doses of 40 or 50 mg/kg/day of doxazosin was delayed as evidenced by slower body weight gain and a slightly later appearance of anatomical features and reflexes. Also, significantly more rat pups died following maternal terazosin doses of 120 mg/kg/day compared to placebo.

Lactation: Doxazosin accumulates in breast milk of lactating rats following a single 1 mg/kg dose, with a maximum concentration about 20 times greater than the maternal plasma concentration. It is not known whether terazosin is excreted in breast milk. Prazosin is excreted in small amounts in breast milk. Exercise caution when administering these drugs to a nursing woman.

Children: Safety and efficacy for use in children have not been established.

Precautions:

Hemodilution: Small but statistically significant decreases in hematocrit, hemoglobin, white blood cells, total protein and albumin were observed in controlled clinical trials with terazosin. The magnitude of the decreases did not worsen with time. These laboratory findings suggested the possibility of hemodilution.

In patients receiving doxazosin, mean WBC and neutrophil counts were decreased by 2.4% and 1%, respectively, compared to placebo. No patients became symptomatic, and WBC and neutrophil counts returned to normal following doxazosin withdrawal.

Weight gain: There was a tendency for patients to gain weight during terazosin therapy. In placebo controlled monotherapy trials, male and female patients receiving terazosin gained a mean of 1.7 and 2.2 pounds, respectively, compared to losses of 0.2 and 1.2 pounds, respectively, in the placebo group.

Cholesterol: During controlled clinical studies, patients receiving terazosin monotherapy had a small but statistically significant decrease (3%) in total cholesterol and the combined LDL and VLDL fractions. No significant changes were observed in HDL fraction and triglycerides. Prazosin therapy has also been associated with a decrease in total cholesterol levels and an increase in HDL. Other studies have shown no change in serum lipids in patients receiving terazosin or prazosin. In clinical trials involving normocholesterolemic patients, doxazosin reduced total serum cholesterol by 2% to 3% and LDL by 4%, and increased HDL to total cholesterol ratio by 4%. The clinical significance is unknown.

Cardiotoxicity: An increased incidence of myocardial necrosis or fibrosis occurred in rats and mice following 6 to 18 months of doxazosin 40 to 80 mg/kg/day. There is no evidence that similar lesions occur in humans.

Ethnic differences: There was no apparent difference in the blood pressure response of Caucasians and blacks receiving doxazosin.

Drug Interactions:

Beta-adrenergic blocking agents may enhance the acute postural hypotensive reaction following the first dose of prazosin; terazosin and doxazosin have been combined with beta blockers with no adverse reaction.

Indomethacin: The antihypertensive action of prazosin may be decreased, possibly due to inhibition of prostaglandin synthesis. No interaction occurred in patients receiving doxazosin and nonsteroidal anti-inflammatory agents.

Nitroglycerin: One case of syncope occurred from an interaction between prazosin and nitroglycerin.

Verapamil and nifedipine: Coadministration with prazosin may produce an acute hypotensive effect which is greater than when either drug is taken alone.

Drug/Lab test interactions: In a study of five patients given prazosin 12 to 24 mg/day for 10 to 14 days, there was an average increase of 42% in the urinary metabolite of norepinephrine and an average increase in urinary VMA of 17%. Therefore, false-positive results may occur in screening tests for pheochromocytoma in patients who are being treated with prazosin. If an elevated VMA is found, discontinue prazosin and retest the patient after a month.

(Continued on following page)

Antiadrenergic Agents – Peripherally Acting (Cont.)

ALPHA-1-ADRENERGIC BLOCKERS (Cont.)

Adverse Reactions:

Alpha-1-Adrenergic Blocker Adverse Reactions			
Adverse Reaction	Prazosin	Terazosin	Doxazosin
Cardiovascular			
Palpitations	5.3%	4.3%	2%
Postural hypotension/hypotension	✓	1.3%	0.3%-1%
Tachycardia	✓	1.9%	0.3%
Arrhythmia, chest pain	no report	1%	1%-2%
Vasodilation	no report	1%	no report
GI			
Nausea	4.9%	4.4%	3%
Vomiting, dry mouth	✓	1%	≤ 2%
Diarrhea, constipation	✓	1%	1%-2%
Abdominal discomfort/pain	✓	1%	1%
Flatulence	no report	1%	1%
Respiratory			
Dyspnea	✓	3.1%	1%
Nasal congestion	✓	5.9%	no report
Sinusitis	no report	2.6%	< 0.5%
Bronchitis/cold symptoms/ bronchospasm	no report	1%	< 0.5%
Epistaxis	✓	1%	1%
Flu symptoms/increased cough	no report	1%	< 0.5%
Pharyngitis/rhinitis	no report	1%	3%
Musculoskeletal			
Shoulder/neck/back/extremity pain	no report	1%-3.5%	< 0.5%-2%
Arthritis, joint/muscle pain, gout	no report	1%	1%
Arthralgia	✓	1%	1%
Special senses			
Blurred vision	✓	1.6%	no report
Abnormal vision	no report	1%	2%
Conjunctivitis, reddened sclera	✓	1%	1%
Tinnitus	✓	1%	1%
Vertigo	no report	no report	2%
CNS			
Depression	✓	< 1%	1%
Dizziness	10.3%	19.3%	19%
Decreased libido/sexual dysfunction	no report	< 1%	2%
Nervousness	✓	2.3%	2%
Paresthesia	✓	2.9%	1%
Somnolence	no report	5.4%	5%
Anxiety/insomnia	no report	1%	1%
Asthenia †	≈ 7%	11.3%	1%-12%
Drowsiness	7.6%	✓	✓
Ataxia	no report	no report	1%
Hypertonia	no report	no report	1%
GU			
Impotence	✓	1.2%	no report
Urinary frequency	✓	1%	0%
Urinary tract infection	no report	1%	no report
Incontinence	✓	no report	1%
Polyuria	no report	no report	2%
Priapism	✓	no report	no report
Dermatologic			
Pruritis/rash/sweating	✓	1%	1%
Alopecia/lichen planus	✓	no report	< 0.5%
Miscellaneous			
Headache	7.8%	16.2%	14%
Edema	✓	< 1%	4%
Peripheral edema	no report	5.5%	no report
Weight gain	no report	< 1%	0.5%-1%
Facial edema	no report	1%	1%
Fever	✓	1%	< 0.5%
Flushing	no report	no report	1%

✓ Reactions associated with the drug, incidence unknown.
† Includes weakness, tiredness, lassitude and fatigue.

(Continued on following page)

ALPHA-1-ADRENERGIC BLOCKERS (Cont.)

Overdosage:

Symptoms: Accidental ingestion of at least 50 mg prazosin in a 2-year-old child produced profound drowsiness and depressed reflexes. No decrease in blood pressure was noted. Recovery was uneventful.

Treatment: Restore blood pressure and normalize heart rate by keeping the patient supine. Treat shock with volume expanders. If necessary, use vasopressors, and monitor and support renal function. These drugs are highly protein bound; dialysis may not be of benefit. Refer to General Management of Acute Overdosage.

Patient Information:

Inform patients of the possibility of syncopal and orthostatic symptoms, especially at the initiation of therapy. Avoid driving or hazardous tasks for 12 to 24 hours after the first dose, after a dosage increase, and after interruption of therapy when treatment is resumed. Use caution when rising from a sitting or lying position. If dizziness or palpitations are bothersome, report to the physician so that dose adjustment can be considered.

Drowsiness or somnolence can occur. Use caution when driving or operating heavy machinery.

Prazosin and terazosin: Take the first dose at bedtime.

PRAZOSIN

Administration and Dosage:

Individualize dosage.

Initial dose: 1 mg 2 or 3 times daily. When increasing dosages, give the first dose of each increment at bedtime to reduce syncopal episodes.

Maintenance dose: 6 to 15 mg/day in divided doses. Doses > 20 mg usually do not increase efficacy; however, a few patients may benefit from up to 40 mg/day. After initial adjustment, some patients can be maintained on a twice-daily regimen.

Concomitant therapy: When adding a diuretic or other antihypertensive agent, reduce dosage to 1 or 2 mg 3 times a day and then retitrate.

				C.I.*
Rx	**Prazosin** (Various, eg, Balan, Geneva, Goldline, Lederle, Major, Moore, Rugby, Schein, Squibb Mark, Zenith)	**Capsules:** 1 mg	In 60s, 100s, 250s, 500s, 1000s and UD 100s.	2.2+
Rx	**Minipress** (Pfizer)		(Pfizer 431 Minipress). White. In 250s, 1000s and UD 100s	10.2
Rx	**Prazosin** (Various, eg, Balan, Geneva, Goldline, Lederle, Major, Moore, Rugby, Schein, Squibb Mark, Zenith)	**Capsules:** 2 mg	In 60s, 100s, 250s, 500s, 1000s and UD 100s.	1.5+
Rx	**Minipress** (Pfizer)		(Pfizer 437 Minipress). Pink and white. In 250s, 1000s and UD 100s.	4.9
Rx	**Prazosin** (Various, eg, Balan, Geneva, Goldline, Lederle, Major, Moore, Rugby, Schein, Squibb Mark, Zenith)	**Capsules:** 5 mg	In 60s, 100s, 250s, 500s, 1000s and UD 100s.	1+
Rx	**Minipress** (Pfizer)		(Pfizer 438 Minipress). Blue and white. In 250s, 500s and UD 100s.	4.8

* Cost Index based on cost per 1 mg prazosin.

Antiadrenergic Agents – Peripherally Acting (Cont.)

TERAZOSIN

Administration and Dosage:

Adjust dose and the dose interval (12 or 24 hours) individually. The following is a guide.

Initial dose – 1 mg at bedtime for all patients. Do not exceed this dose. Strictly observe this initial dosing regimen to avoid severe hypotensive effects.

Subsequent doses – Slowly increase the dose to achieve the desired blood pressure response. The recommended dose range is 1 to 5 mg daily; however, some patients may benefit from doses as high as 20 mg/day. Doses over 20 mg do not appear to provide further blood pressure effect, and doses over 40 mg have not been studied. Monitor blood pressure at the end of the dosing interval to be sure control is maintained. Measure blood pressure 2 to 3 hours after dosing to see if the maximum and minimum responses are similar, and to evaluate symptoms such as dizziness or palpitations. If response is substantially diminished at 24 hours, consider an increased dose or a twice daily regimen. If terazosin is discontinued for several days or longer, reinstitute therapy using the initial dosing regimen. In clinical trials, except for the initial dose, the dose was given in the morning.

Concomitant therapy: Observe caution when terazosin is administered concomitantly with other antihypertensive agents (eg, calcium antagonists) to avoid the possibility of significant hypotension. When adding a diuretic or other antihypertensive agent, dosage reduction and retitration may be necessary.

Rx	**Hytrin** (Abbott/Burroughs Wellcome)	**Tablets:** 1 mg	(DF). White. In 100s, 500s and UD 100s.	24
		2 mg	(DH). Orange. In 100s, 500s and UD 100s.	12
		5 mg	(DJ). Tan. In 100s, 500s and UD 100s.	4.8
		10 mg	(DI). Green. In 100s and UD 100s.	2.4

DOXAZOSIN MESYLATE

Administration and Dosage:

Individualize dosage.

Initial dose: 1 mg once daily. Postural effects are most likely to occur between 2 and 6 hours after a dose; therefore take blood pressure measurements during this time period after the first dose and with each increase.

Maintenance dose: Depending on standing blood pressure response, dosage may be increased to 2 mg and thereafter, if necessary, to 4, 8 and 16 mg to achieve the desired reduction in blood pressure. Increases in dose beyond 4 mg increase the likelihood of excessive postural effects.

Rx	**Cardura** (Roerig)	**Tablets:** 1 mg	White. In 100s.	NA
		2 mg	Yellow. In 100s.	NA
		4 mg	Orange. In 100s.	NA
		8 mg	Green. In 100s.	NA

* Cost Index based on cost per 1 mg.

Refer to the general discussion of these products beginning on page 773.

Vasodilators

HYDRALAZINE HCl

Actions:

Pharmacology: Hydralazine exerts a peripheral vasodilating effect through a direct relaxation of vascular smooth muscle, with little effect on the venous capacitance vessels. Hydralazine, by altering cellular calcium metabolism, interferes with the calcium movements within the vascular smooth muscle that are responsible for initiating or maintaining the contractile state.

The peripheral vasodilating effect of hydralazine results in decreased arterial blood pressure (diastolic more than systolic); decreased peripheral vascular resistance; and an increased heart rate, stroke volume and cardiac output. The preferential dilatation of arterioles, as compared to veins, minimizes postural hypotension and promotes the increase in cardiac output. Hydralazine usually increases the renin activity in plasma, presumably as a result of increased secretion of renin by the renal juxtaglomerular cells in response to reflex sympathetic discharge. This increase in renin activity leads to the production of angiotensin II, which then causes stimulation of aldosterone and consequent sodium reabsorption. The drug also maintains or increases renal and cerebral blood flow. Because of the reflex increases in cardiac function, hydralazine is commonly used in combination with a drug which inhibits sympathetic activity (ie, beta-adrenergic blockers, clonidine or methyldopa).

Pharmacokinetics: Hydralazine is rapidly absorbed after oral use. Half-life is 3 to 7 hours. Protein binding is 87%, and bioavailability is 30% to 50%. Plasma levels vary widely among individuals. Peak plasma concentrations occur 30 to 120 min after ingestion; duration of action is 6 to 8 hours. Hypotensive effects are seen 10 to 20 min after parenteral use and last 2 to 4 hours. Hydralazine is subject to polymorphic acetylation; slow acetylators generally have higher plasma levels of hydralazine and require lower doses to maintain control of blood pressure. Hydralazine undergoes extensive hepatic metabolism; it is excreted in the urine as active drug (12% to 14%) and metabolites.

Indications:

Oral: Essential hypertension, alone or in combination with other agents.

Parenteral: Severe essential hypertension when the drug cannot be given orally or when the need to lower blood pressure is urgent.

Unlabeled Use: Hydralazine in doses up to 800 mg, 3 times daily has been effective in reducing afterload in the treatment of congestive heart failure (CHF), severe aortic insufficiency and after valve replacement.

Contraindications:

Hypersensitivity to hydralazine; coronary artery disease; mitral valvular rheumatic heart disease.

Warnings:

Lupus erythematosus: Hydralazine may produce a clinical picture simulating acute systemic lupus erythematosus (eg, arthralgia, myalgia, dermatoses, fever, anemia, splenomegaly and rarely, cutaneous necrotizing vasculitis) including glomerulonephritis. Symptoms usually regress when the drug is discontinued, but residual effects have been detected years later. Long-term treatment with steroids may be necessary. Lupus occurs more frequently in "slow acetylators". Although hydralazine-induced lupus may develop in patients on low doses ($\leq$ 200 mg/day), the likelihood increases with large doses and with long duration of therapy; 10% to 20% of patients on prolonged therapy with hydralazine at doses exceeding 400 mg/day develop lupus.

Perform complete blood counts, LE cell preparations and antinuclear antibody (ANA) titer determinations before and during prolonged therapy, even in the asymptomatic patient. These studies are also indicated if the patient develops arthralgia, fever, chest pain, continued malaise or other unexplained signs or symptoms. If ANA titer or LE cell reaction is positive, carefully weigh benefits to be derived from hydralazine.

Usage in Pregnancy: Category C. Animal studies indicate that high doses of hydralazine are teratogenic (cleft palate and facial and cranial bone malformations) in mice. Safety for use during pregnancy has not been established. Use only when clearly needed and when the potential benefits outweigh potential hazards to the fetus.

Thrombocytopenia, leukopenia, petechial bleeding and hematomas have been reported in newborns of females taking hydralazine. Symptoms resolved spontaneously within 1 to 3 weeks.

Usage in Lactation: It is not known if hydralazine is excreted in breast milk. Exercise caution when administering to a nursing woman.

Usage in Children: Safety and efficacy for use in children have not been established in controlled clinical trials, although there is experience with use in children.

(Continued on following page)

HYDRALAZINE HCl (Cont.)

Precautions:

Cardiovascular: The "hyperdynamic" circulation caused by hydralazine may accentuate cardiovascular inadequacies (eg, increased pulmonary artery pressure in patients with mitral valvular disease). It may reduce the pressor responses to epinephrine. Postural hypotension may result. Use with caution in patients with cerebral vascular accidents.

Coronary artery disease – Myocardial stimulation produced by hydralazine can cause anginal attacks and ECG changes of myocardial ischemia. The drug has been implicated in the production of myocardial infarction. Use with caution in patients with suspected coronary artery disease.

Pulmonary hypertension – Use hydralazine with caution in patients with pulmonary hypertension. Severe hypotension may result. Monitor carefully.

Withdrawal: In patients with marked reduction in blood pressure, withdraw hydralazine gradually to avoid a possible sudden rise in blood pressure.

Dosage increase: In patients with more severe forms of hypertension, and with uremia, too rapid an increase of dosage may produce a marked fall in blood pressure. Certain cerebral symptoms, from mild anxiety or depression to acute anxiety or severe depression and coma may appear.

Renal function: May improve where control values were below normal prior to administration. Use with caution in patients with advanced renal damage.

Peripheral neuritis, evidenced by paresthesias, numbness and tingling, has been observed. Evidence suggests an antipyridoxine effect; add pyridoxine to the regimen if symptoms develop.

Hematologic effects: Blood dyscrasias consisting of reduction in hemoglobin and red cell count, leukopenia, agranulocytosis and purpura have been reported. If such abnormalities develop, discontinue therapy. Periodic blood counts are advised.

Tartrazine sensitivity: Some of these products contain tartrazine, which may cause allergic-type reactions (including bronchial asthma) in susceptible individuals. Although the incidence of tartrazine sensitivity in the general population is low, it is frequently seen in patients who also have aspirin hypersensitivity. Specific products containing tartrazine are identified in the product listings.

Drug Interactions:

MAO inhibitors: Use with caution in patients receiving hydralazine.

Sympathomimetics: Hydralazine alone may induce tachycardia and angina; use these agents with great caution.

Propranolol, metoprolol and oxprenolol: Oral bioavailability of certain high clearance lipophilic β-blockers may be increased by coadministration with hydralazine.

Parenteral antihypertensive drugs (eg, diazoxide): When other potent parenteral antihypertensive agents are used in combination with hydralazine, observe patients continuously for several hours for any excessive fall in blood pressure. Profound hypotensive episodes may occur.

Adverse Reactions:

Adverse reactions with hydralazine are usually reversible when dosage is reduced. However, it may be necessary to discontinue the drug.

Most common: Headache; anorexia; nausea; vomiting; diarrhea; palpitations; tachycardia; angina pectoris. The incidence of toxic reactions, particularly the LE cell syndrome, is high in the group of patients receiving large doses of hydralazine. (See Warnings.)

Ophthalmic: Lacrimation; conjunctivitis.

Neurological: Peripheral neuritis evidenced by paresthesia, numbness and tingling (see Precautions); dizziness; tremors; psychotic reactions characterized by depression, disorientation or anxiety.

Hypersensitivity: Rash; urticaria; pruritus; fever; chills; arthralgia; eosinophilia; and rarely hepatitis and obstructive jaundice.

GI and GU: Constipation; paralytic ileus; difficulty in micturition; impotence.

Hematologic: Blood dyscrasias, consisting of reduction in hemoglobin and RBC; leukopenia; agranulocytosis and purpura (see Precautions); lymphadenopathy; splenomegaly.

Miscellaneous: Nasal congestion; flushing; edema; muscle cramps; hypotension; paradoxical pressor response; dyspnea and lupus-like syndrome. Hoarseness due to drug-induced lupus.

(Continued on following page)

HYDRALAZINE HCl (Cont.)

Overdosage:

No deaths due to acute poisoning have been reported. Highest known dose survived: Adults, 10 g orally.

Symptoms: Hypotension, tachycardia, headache and generalized skin flushing are to be expected. Myocardial ischemia and subsequent myocardial infarction, and cardiac arrhythmias can develop; profound shock can occur in severe overdosage.

Treatment: There is no specific antidote. Evacuate gastric contents, prevent aspiration and protect the airway; instill activated charcoal slurry, if possible. These manipulations may have to be omitted or carried out after cardiovascular status has been stabilized, since they might precipitate cardiac arrhythmias or increase the depth of shock.

Cardiovascular support is of primary importance. Treat shock with volume expanders without vasopressors. If necessary, use a vasopressor that is least likely to precipitate or aggravate tachycardia and cardiac arrhythmias. Digitalization may be necessary. Monitor renal function and support as required.

No experience has been reported with extracorporeal or peritoneal dialysis.

Patient Information:

Take with meals.

Notify physician of any unexplained prolonged general tiredness or fever, muscle or joint aching or chest pain (angina).

Administration and Dosage:

The bioavailability of hydralazine tablets is enhanced by the concurrent ingestion of food.

Initiate therapy in gradually increasing dosages; individualize dosage. Start with 10 mg 4 times daily for the first 2 to 4 days, increase to 25 mg 4 times daily for the balance of the first week.

Second and subsequent weeks: Increase dosage to 50 mg 4 times daily.

Maintenance: Adjust dosage to lowest effective level. During chronic administration, tolerance may develop and higher dosages may be required. Twice daily dosage may be adequate. In some patients, up to 300 mg/day may be required.

Children: Initial – 0.75 mg/kg/day in 4 divided doses. Dosage may be increased gradually over the next 3 to 4 weeks to a maximum of 7.5 mg/kg or 200 mg daily.

Parenteral: Therapy in the hospitalized patient may be initiated IV or IM. Use parenterally only when the drug cannot be given orally. Usual dose is 20 to 40 mg, repeated as necessary. Certain patients (especially those with marked renal damage) may require a lower dose. Check blood pressure frequently; it may begin to fall within a few minutes after injection; average maximal decrease occurs in 10 to 80 minutes. Where there is a previously existing increased intracranial pressure, lowering the blood pressure may increase cerebral ischemia. Most patients can transfer to the oral form in 24 to 48 hrs.

Children – 0.1 to 0.2 mg/kg/dose every 4 to 6 hours as needed.

Stability: Use hydralazine injection as quickly as possible after drawing through a needle into a syringe. Hydralazine changes color after contact with a metal filter.

(Products listed on following page)

Vasodilators (Cont.)

HYDRALAZINE HCl (Cont.)

	Product	Dosage form	Package	C.I.*
Rx	**Hydralazine** (Various)	**Tablets:** 10 mg	In 100s, 1000s and UD 32s, 100s and 1000s.	53+
Rx	**Alazine** (Major)		In 100s and 1000s.	150
Rx	**Apresoline** (Ciba)		(#Ciba 37). Yellow. In 100s and 1000s.	328
Rx	**Hydralazine** (Various)	**Tablets:** 25 mg	In 100s, 120s, 500s, 1000s and UD 32s, 100s and 1000s.	22+
Rx	**Alazine** (Major)		In 100s and 1000s.	66
Rx	**Apresoline** (Ciba)		(#Ciba 39). Blue. In 100s, 500s and 1000s.	188
Rx	**Hydralazine** (Various)	**Tablets:** 50 mg	In 100s, 500s, 1000s and UD 100s and 1000s.	17+
Rx	**Alazine** (Major)		In 100s and 1000s.	45
Rx	**Apresoline** (Ciba)		(#Ciba 73). Light blue. In 100s, 500s and 1000s.	144
Rx	**Hydralazine** (Various)	**Tablets:** 100 mg	In 100s and 1000s.	16+
Rx	**Apresoline** (Ciba)		Tartrazine. (#Ciba 101). Peach. In 100s.	99
Rx	**Hydralazine** (Various)	**Injection:** 20 mg per ml	In 1 ml amps and vials.	3645+
Rx	**Apresoline** (Ciba)		In 1 ml amps.[1]	4896

* Cost Index based on cost per 25 mg.
# Product identification code.
[1] With propylene glycol and methyl and propyl parabens.

Refer to the general discussion of these products beginning on page 773

MINOXIDIL

Warnings:

Minoxidil may produce serious adverse effects. It can cause pericardial effusion, occasionally progressing to tamponade, and it can exacerbate angina pectoris. Reserve for severely hypertensive patients who do not respond adequately to maximum therapeutic doses of a diuretic and two other antihypertensive agents.

In experimental animals, minoxidil caused several kinds of myocardial lesions and other adverse cardiac effects (see Warnings).

Administer under close supervision, usually concomitantly with a beta-adrenergic blocking agent, to prevent tachycardia and increased myocardial workload. Usually, it must be given with a diuretic, frequently a high-ceiling agent, to prevent serious fluid accumulation. When first administering minoxidil, hospitalize and monitor patients with malignant hypertension and those already receiving guanethidine (see Drug Interactions) to avoid too rapid or large orthostatic decreases in blood pressure.

Actions:

Pharmacology: The exact mechanism of action on the vascular smooth muscle is unknown. Minoxidil, an antihypertensive peripheral vasodilator, does not interfere with vasomotor reflexes, therefore, it does not produce orthostatic hypotension. The drug does not affect CNS function in man. It appears to block calcium uptake through the cell membrane.

Antihypertensive effects – Minoxidil, a direct-acting peripheral vasodilator, reduces elevated systolic and diastolic blood pressure by decreasing peripheral vascular resistance. The blood pressure response to minoxidil is dose-related and proportional to the extent of hypertension. In man, forearm and renal vascular resistance decline; forearm blood flow increases while renal blood flow and glomerular filtration rate (GFR) are preserved.

When used in severely hypertensive patients resistant to other therapy, frequently with an accompanying diuretic and β-adrenergic blocker, minoxidil decreased the blood pressure and reversed encephalopathy and retinopathy. The drug reduced supine diastolic blood pressure by 20 mm Hg, or to 90 mm Hg or less in approximately 75% of the patients studied.

Hemodynamic effects – Because it causes peripheral vasodilation, minoxidil elicits a reduction of peripheral arteriolar resistance. This action, with the associated fall in blood pressure, triggers sympathetic, vagal inhibitory and renal homeostatic mechanisms, including an increase in renin secretion, that leads to increased cardiac rate and output, and salt and water retention. These adverse effects can usually be minimized by coadministration of a diuretic and a β-adrenergic blocking agent or other sympathetic nervous system suppressant.

Pharmacokinetics:

Absorption/Distribution – Minoxidil is at least 90% absorbed from the GI tract. Plasma levels of the parent drug reach a maximum within the first hour and decline rapidly thereafter. Minoxidil is not protein bound; it concentrates in arteriolar smooth muscle.

Metabolism/Excretion – Approximately 90% is metabolized, predominantly by conjugation with glucuronic acid. Metabolites exert much less pharmacologic effect than minoxidil itself; all are excreted principally in the urine. Renal clearance corresponds to the GFR. Minoxidil and its metabolites are hemodialyzable. Average plasma half-life is 4.2 hours.

Onset/Duration of Action – The extent and time course of blood pressure reduction by minoxidil do not correspond closely to its plasma concentration. After an effective single oral dose, blood pressure usually starts to decline within ½ hour, reaches a minimum between 2 and 3 hours and recovers at a linear rate of about 30% per day. The total duration of effect is approximately 75 hours.

When minoxidil is administered chronically, once or twice a day, the time required to achieve maximum effect on blood pressure is inversely related to the size of the dose. Thus, maximum effect is achieved on 10 mg/day within 7 days, on 20 mg/day within 5 days and on 40 mg/day within 3 days.

(Continued on following page)

MINOXIDIL (Cont.)

Indications:

Severe hypertension that is symptomatic or associated with target organ damage, and is not manageable with maximum therapeutic doses of a diuretic plus two other antihypertensives. Due to potential for serious adverse effects, use in milder degrees of hypertension is not recommended; benefit-risk relationship in such patients is not defined.

Topical: Treatment of male pattern baldness (alopecia androgenetica) of the vertex of the scalp (see Minoxidil topical solution, *Rogaine*).

Contraindications:

Pheochromocytoma, because the drug may stimulate secretion of catecholamines from the tumor through its antihypertensive action.

Acute myocardial infarction; dissecting aortic aneurysm.

Warnings:

Cardiac Lesions:

Animal toxicology – Minoxidil has produced cardiac lesions in nonprimate species, including grossly visible hemorrhagic lesions of the atrium, epicardium, endocardium and walls of small arteries and arterioles; necrosis of papillary muscles and subendocardial areas of left ventricle. Cardiac hypertrophy and dilation occurred but was partly reversed by diuretics in monkeys, suggesting increased heart weight may be related to fluid overload. In a 1 year dog study serosanguinous pericardial fluid was noted.

Human toxicology – Autopsies of 79 patients who died from various causes and who had received minoxidil did not reveal right atrial or other hemorrhagic pathology of the kind seen in dogs. Instances of necrotic areas in papillary muscles were seen, but occurred in presence of known preexisting ischemic heart disease and did not appear different from or more common than lesions in patients never exposed to minoxidil. Studies cannot exclude the possibility that minoxidil may cause cardiac damage in humans.

Fluid and electrolyte balance; congestive heart failure (CHF): Monitor fluid and electrolyte balance and body weight. Give with a diuretic to prevent fluid retention and possible CHF; a loop diuretic is usually required. If used without a diuretic, retention of several hundred mEq salt and corresponding volumes of water can occur in a few days, leading to increased plasma and interstitial fluid volume and local or generalized edema. Diuretics alone, or with restricted salt intake, usually minimize fluid retention, but reversible edema developed in ≈ 10% of nondialysis patients so treated. Ascites has also occurred. Diuretic effectiveness is limited by impaired renal function. Condition of patients with preexisting CHF occasionally deteriorates due to fluid retention, but because of the fall in blood pressure (afterload reduction), more than twice as many improve than worsen.

Refractory fluid retention rarely may require discontinuation of minoxidil. Under close medical supervision, it may be possible to resolve refractory salt retention by discontinuing the drug for 1 or 2 days, and then resuming treatment in conjunction with vigorous diuretic therapy.

Tachycardia: Minoxidil increases heart rate; this can be prevented by concomitant administration of a β-adrenergic blocking drug or other sympathetic nervous system suppressants (eg, clonidine or methyldopa). The ability of β-adrenergic blocking agents to minimize papillary muscle lesions in animals is further reason for such concomitant use.

In addition, angina may worsen or appear for the first time during treatment, probably because of the increased oxygen demands associated with increased heart rate and cardiac output. This can usually be prevented by sympathetic blockade.

Pericardial effusion, occasionally with tamponade, has occurred in about 3% of treated patients not on dialysis, especially those with inadequate or compromised renal function. Many cases were associated with connective tissue disease, the uremic syndrome, CHF or fluid retention, but were instances in which these potential causes of effusion were not present. Observe patients closely for signs of pericardial disorder.

Perform echocardiographic studies if suspicion arises. More vigorous diuretic therapy, dialysis, pericardiocentesis or surgery may be required. If the effusion persists, consider drug withdrawal.

Hazard of rapid control of blood pressure: In patients with very severe blood pressure elevation, too rapid control of blood pressure can precipitate syncope, cerebrovascular accidents, myocardial infarction and ischemia of special sense organs with resulting decrease or loss of vision or hearing. Patients with compromised circulation or cryoglobulinemia may also suffer ischemic episodes of affected organs. Although such events have not been unequivocally associated with minoxidil use, experience is limited.

Hospitalize any patient with malignant hypertension during initial treatment to assure that blood pressure is not falling more rapidly than intended.

(Warnings continued on following page)

MINOXIDIL (Cont.)

Warnings (Cont.):

Hypersensitivity manifested as a skin rash occurs in less than 1% of patients; whether the drug should be discontinued depends on treatment alternatives.

Usage in impaired renal function: Renal failure or dialysis patients may require smaller doses; closely supervise to prevent cardiac failure or exacerbation of renal failure.

Pericardial effusion: Observe for signs and symptoms of pericardial effusion.

Usage in Pregnancy: Category C. Minoxidil reduced conception rate and increased fetal absorption in small animals when administered at 5 times the human dose. There is no evidence of teratogenic effects in small animals. There are no adequate and well controlled studies in pregnant women. Use only when clearly needed and when potential benefits outweigh potential hazards to the fetus.

Usage in Lactation: Safety for use in the nursing mother has not been established. Minoxidil is excreted in breast milk; do not nurse while taking minoxidil.

Usage in Children: Use in children is limited, particularly in infants. The recommendations under Administration and Dosage are only a rough guide; careful titration is essential.

Precautions:

Use after myocardial infarction: Minoxidil has not been used in patients who have had a myocardial infarction within the preceding month. A reduction in arterial pressure with the drug might further limit blood flow to the myocardium, although this might be compensated by decreased oxygen demand because of lower blood pressure.

Laboratory tests: Repeat tests that are abnormal at initiation of minoxidil therapy, (eg, urinalysis, renal function tests, ECG, chest x-ray, echocardiogram) to ascertain whether improvement or deterioration is occurring under therapy. Initially, perform such tests frequently, at 1 to 3 month intervals; and as stabilization occurs, at 6 to 12 month intervals.

Drug Interactions:

Guanethidine: Although minoxidil does not cause orthostatic hypotension, use in patients on guanethidine can result in profound orthostatic effects. If possible, discontinue guanethidine well before minoxidil is instituted. If this is not possible, start minoxidil in the hospital and institutionalize the patient until severe orthostatic effects are no longer present or the patient has learned to avoid activities that provoke them.

Adverse Reactions:

Fluid and electrolyte balance: Temporary edema developed in 7% of patients.

Hypertrichosis: Elongation, thickening and enhanced pigmentation of fine body hair develops within 3 to 6 weeks after starting therapy in approximately 80% of patients. It is usually first noticed on the temples, between the eyebrows, between the hairline and the eyebrows or in the sideburn area of the upper lateral cheek, later extending to the back, arms, legs and scalp. Upon discontinuation of the drug, new hair growth stops, but 1 to 6 months may be required for restoration to pretreatment appearance.

No endocrine abnormalities have been found to explain the abnormal hair growth; thus, it is hypertrichosis without virilism. Inform patients (especially children and women) about this effect before therapy is begun.

Allergic: Rashes including bullous eruptions (rare) and Stevens-Johnson syndrome.

Cardiovascular: Pericardial effusion and tamponade (see Warnings). Changes in direction and magnitude of T waves occur (60%). Rarely, a large negative amplitude of the T wave may encroach upon the ST segment, but the ST segment is not independently altered. These changes usually disappear with continuance of treatment and revert to the pretreatment state if therapy is discontinued. No symptoms, alterations in blood cell counts or plasma enzyme concentrations, or signs of myocardial damage have been noted. Long-term treatment of patients manifesting such changes has provided no evidence of deteriorating cardiac function. At present, the changes appear to be nonspecific and without identifiable clinical significance.

Rebound hypertension following gradual withdrawal has occurred in children.

Hematologic: Initially, hematocrit, hemoglobin and erythrocyte count usually fall about 7%, and then recover to pretreatment levels. Thrombocytopenia and leukopenia (WBC $< 3000/mm^3$) have been reported rarely.

GI: Nausea and vomiting. In clinical trials, the incidence of nausea and vomiting associated with the underlying disease has decreased from pretrial levels.

Miscellaneous: Breast tenderness (< 1%), fatigue, headache and darkening of the skin.

Altered laboratory findings: Alkaline phosphatase increased varyingly without other evidence of liver or bone abnormality. Serum creatinine increased an average of 6% and BUN slightly more, but later declined to pretreatment levels. An isolated case of elevated antinuclear antibody (ANA) level occurred.

(Continued on following page)

MINOXIDIL (Cont.)

Overdosage:

Symptoms: Exaggerated hypotension is likely in association with residual sympathetic nervous system blockade from previous therapy (guanethidine-like effects or alpha-adrenergic blockade), which prevents compensatory maintenance of blood pressure.

Treatment: Administer normal saline IV to maintain blood pressure and facilitate urine formation. Avoid sympathomimetics (eg, norepinephrine, epinephrine) with excessive cardiac stimulating action. Phenylephrine, angiotensin II, vasopressin and dopamine reverse hypotension due to minoxidil, but use only in underperfusion of a vital organ.

Radioimmunoassay can determine plasma concentration. However, due to blood level variations, it is difficult to establish a warning level. At 100 mg/day, peak blood levels of 1641 and 2441 ng/ml were seen in two patients, respectively. Regard an increase > 2000 ng/ml as overdosage, unless the patient has taken no more than the max dose.

Patient Information:

Patient package insert is available with product.

Minoxidil is usually taken with at least two other antihypertensive medications. Take all medications as prescribed; do not discontinue any except on advice of physician.

Enhanced growth and darkening of fine body hair (≈ 80% of patients) may occur; however, do not stop medication without consulting physician.

Notify physician if any of the following occur: Heart rate of ≥ 20 bpm over normal; rapid weight gain of > 5 pounds (2.3 kg); unusual swelling of extremities, face or abdomen; breathing difficulty, especially when lying down; new or aggravated angina symptoms (chest, arm or shoulder pain); severe indigestion; dizziness, lightheadedness or fainting.

Nausea or vomiting may occur.

Administration and Dosage:

Adults (≥ 12 years): Initial dosage is 5 mg/day as a single dose. Daily dosage can be increased to 10, 20, then 40 mg in single or divided doses if required. Effective range is usually 10 to 40 mg/day. Maximum dosage is 100 mg/day.

Children (< 12 years): Initial dosage is 0.2 mg/kg/day as a single dose. May be increased in 50% to 100% increments until optimum blood pressure control is achieved. Effective range is usually 0.25 to 1 mg/kg/day. Maximum dosage is 50 mg daily. (Experience in children is limited; monitor closely; titrate carefully for optimal effects.)

Dose frequency: The magnitude of within-day fluctuation of arterial pressure during therapy is directly proportional to the extent of pressure reduction. If supine diastolic pressure has been reduced less than 30 mm Hg, administer the drug only once a day; if reduced more than 30 mm Hg, divide the daily dosage into 2 equal parts.

Dosage adjustment intervals, which must be carefully titrated, should be at least 3 days because the full response to a given dose is not obtained until then. If more rapid management is required, adjustments can be made every 6 hours with careful monitoring.

Concomitant drug therapy: Diuretics – Use minoxidil with a diuretic in patients relying on renal function for maintaining salt and water balance. Diuretics have been used at the following dosages when starting therapy with minoxidil: Hydrochlorothiazide (50 mg twice daily) or other thiazides at equieffective doses; chlorthalidone (50 to 100 mg once daily); furosemide (40 mg twice daily). If excessive salt and water retention results in a weight gain > 5 lb (2.3 kg), change diuretic therapy to furosemide. In furosemide-treated patients, increase dosage in accordance with their requirements.

Beta-blockers or other sympathetic nervous system suppressants - When therapy is begun, the β-blocker dosage should be equal to 80 to 160 mg/day propranolol in divided doses. If β-blockers are contraindicated, use methyldopa, 250 to 750 mg twice daily; give for at least 24 hours before starting minoxidil due to delay in onset. Clonidine may also be used; usual dosage is 0.1 to 0.2 mg twice daily.

Sympathetic nervous system suppressants may not completely prevent a heart rate increase, but usually prevent tachycardia. Typically, patients receiving a β-blocker prior to minoxidil have a bradycardia; expect an increase in heart rate toward normal when minoxidil is added. Simultaneous treatment with minoxidil and a β-blocker or other sympathetic nervous system suppressant causes little change in heart rate, since their opposing cardiac effects usually nullify each other.

				C.I.*
Rx	**Minoxidil** (Various)	**Tablets:** 2.5 mg	In 100s, 500s and 1000s.	515+
		10 mg	In 100s, 500s and 1000s.	219+
Rx	**Loniten** (Upjohn)	**Tablets:** 2.5 mg	(#U 121/2½). White, scored. In 100s.	920
		10 mg	(#U 137/Loniten 10). White, scored. In 100s.	506
Rx	**Minodyl** (Quantum)	**Tablets:** 2.5 mg	(#QPL/243). White, scored. In 100s and 500s.	678
		10 mg	(#QPL/228 10). In 100s and 500s.	293

* Cost Index based on cost per 5 mg. # Product identification code.

Refer to the general discussion of these products beginning on page 773.

Angiotensin Converting Enzyme Inhibitors

Actions:

Pharmacology: The angiotensin converting enzyme inhibitors (ACEIs) appear to act primarily through suppression of the renin-angiotensin-aldosterone system; however, no consistent correlation has been described between renin levels and drug response.

Synthesized by the kidneys, renin is released into the circulation where it acts on a plasma globulin substrate to produce angiotensin I, a relatively inactive decapeptide. Angiotensin I is then converted by angiotensin converting enzyme (ACE) to angiotensin II, a potent endogenous vasoconstrictor that also stimulates aldosterone secretion from the adrenal cortex, contributing to sodium and fluid retention. These agents prevent the conversion of angiotensin I to angiotensin II by inhibiting ACE; they do not alter pressor responses to other agents. ACEIs may also inhibit local angiotensin II at vascular and renal sites and attenuate the release of catecholamines from adrenegic nerve endings.

Inhibiting ACE results in decreased plasma angiotensin II and increased plasma renin activity (PRA), the latter resulting from loss of negative feedback on renin release caused by reduction in angiotensin II. This leads to decreased aldosterone secretion, resulting in small increases in serum potassium ($\approx$ 0.2 mEq/L with enalapril, 0.07 mmol/L with quinapril), and sodium and fluid loss.

Increased prostaglandin synthesis may also play a role in the antihypertensive action of captopril. Single doses of captopril increase urinary excretion of prostaglandin E_2 and plasma levels of PGE_2 and $PGE_{2\alpha}$ metabolites. The antihypertensive effects persist longer than does demonstrable inhibition of circulating ACE.

Pharmacokinetics of ACEIs

ACEI	Onset/ Duration (hrs)	Time to peak serum levels (hrs)	Percent absorbed	Active metabolite	t½ Normal renal function	t½ Impaired renal function	Elimination 24 hr Total	Elimination 24 hr Unchanged
Benazepril	1/24	0.5 to 1	37%[1]	Benazeprilat	10 to 11[2]	Prolonged	nd	trace
Captopril	0.25/ dose-related	0.5 to 1.5	75%[3]		< 2 hr	3.5 to 32 hr	> 95%	40% to 50% in urine
Enalapril	1/24	0.5 to 1.5 (enalaprilat 3 to 4)	60%[1]	Enalaprilat	1.3 hr	nd	94% urine and feces	54% in urine (40% enalaprilat)
Enalaprilat	0.25/ ≈ 6	na	na		11 hr	Prolonged[4]	nd	> 90% (urine)
Fosinopril	1/24	≈ 3	36%[1]	Fosinoprilat	12 hr (fosinoprilat IV)	Prolonged	50% urine, 50% feces	negligible
Lisinopril	1/24	≈ 7	25%[1]		12 hr	Prolonged[4]	nd	urine, 100%[5]
Quinapril	1/24	1	60%[3]	Quinaprilat	2 hr (quinaprilat)	Prolonged	≈ 60% urine, ≈ 37% feces	trace
Ramipril	1 to 2/ 24	1 (ramiprilat 2 to 4)	50% to 60%[3]	Ramiprilat	13-17 hr (ramiprilat)	Prolonged	60% urine, 40% feces	< 2%[5]

[1] Absorption not influenced by food.
[2] Effective t½ of accumulation of metabolite following multiple dosing.
[3] Absorption reduced by food (see Drug Interactions)
[4] At glomerular filtration rate ≤ 30 ml/min.
[5] Time frame undefined.
nd – No data.
na – Not applicable (available IV only).

Clinical pharmacology: The ACEIs produce a reduction of peripheral arterial resistance in hypertensive patients, and either no change or an increase in cardiac output. Renal blood flow increases, but glomerular filtration rate (GFR) is usually unchanged.

Blood pressure reduction may be progressive; to achieve maximal effects, several weeks of therapy may be required. Blood pressure-lowering effects of ACEIs and thiazide-type diuretics are additive, but captopril and β-blockers have a less than additive effect. Standing and supine blood pressures are lowered to about the same extent. Orthostatic effects and tachycardia are infrequent, but may occur in volume or salt-depleted patients. Abrupt withdrawal is not associated with a rapid increase in blood pressure.

Enalapril: Peak blood pressure reduction is achieved by 4 to 6 hours. Enalaprilat is dialyzable (62 ml/min).

(Actions continued on following page)

Angiotensin Converting Enzyme Inhibitors (Cont.)

Actions (Cont.):

Clinical pharmacology (Cont.):

Captopril's blood pressure reduction is maximal 60 to 90 minutes after oral administration. Captopril is 25% to 30% protein bound and is dialyzable.

Lisinopril: Peak reduction of blood pressure occurs by 6 hours. Although an antihypertensive effect may occur 24 hours after single daily doses, the effect is more consistent and mean effect larger with doses of $\geq$ 20 mg. At all doses, mean effect is substantially smaller 24 hours vs 6 hours after dosing. Lisinopril is dialyzable.

Ramipril: Peak reduction of blood pressure occurs 3 to 6 hours after dosing. Ramiprilat, the active metabolite, has about 6 times the ACE inhibitory activity of ramipril. Protein binding is $\approx$ 73% and 56% for ramipril and ramiprilat, respectively.

Fosinopril: Peak reduction of blood pressure occurs 2 to 6 hours after dosing. Fosinoprilat is highly protein bound ($\approx$ 95%) and is not well dialyzed.

Benazepril: Peak reduction of blood pressure occurs 2 to 4 hours after dosing. Benazepril and benazeprilat are highly protein bound ($>$ 95%). Benazeprilat is dialyzable.

Quinapril: Peak reduction of blood pressure occurs by 2 to 4 hours after dosing; most of the antihypertensive effect of a given dose is obtained in 1 to 2 weeks. Quinapril and quinaprilat are approximately 97% bound to plasma proteins. Dialysis has little effect on the elimination of quinapril and quinaprilat.

The ACE inhibitors are antihypertensive even in low-renin hypertensives. They are antihypertensive in all races studied, but black hypertensives (usually low-renin hypertensives) show a smaller average response to monotherapy than non-blacks.

In patients with heart failure, captopril and enalapril significantly decreased peripheral resistance, blood pressure (afterload), pulmonary capillary wedge pressure (preload), pulmonary vascular resistance and heart size, and increased cardiac output and exercise tolerance time. These effects occur after the first dose and persist for the duration of therapy. Quinapril reduces total peripheral resistance and renal vascular resistance with little or no change in heart rate or cardiac index.

Indications:

Hypertension: The ACEIs are effective alone and in combination with other antihypertensive agents, especially thiazide-type diuretics. Blood pressure-lowering effects of ACEIs and thiazides are approximately additive.

Captopril may be used as initial therapy in patients with normal renal function in whom risk is relatively low. In patients with impaired renal function, particularly those with collagen vascular disease, reserve captopril for patients who develop unacceptable side effects on other drugs or who do not respond to drug combinations.

Enalaprilat is indicated when oral therapy is not practical.

Heart failure: Captopril, enalapril – For patients who have not responded adequately to, or cannot be controlled by, conventional diuretic and digitalis therapy. Use with diuretics and digitalis, except when digitalis use is poorly tolerated or otherwise not feasible.

Unlabeled uses:

Captopril – Management of hypertensive crises (25 mg initially, 100 mg 90 to 120 minutes later, 200 to 300 mg/day for 2 to 5 days, then adjusted). Sublingual captopril 25 mg has also been used effectively.

Diabetic nephropathy (reduction of proteinuria, albuminuria and glomerular hypertension). See Warnings.

Neonatal and childhood hypertension. For neonates, the use of a solution of captopril in water (used immediately) is effective.

Rheumatoid arthritis (75 to 150 mg/day in divided doses).

Diagnosis of anatomic renal artery stenosis ("captopril test").

Hypertension related to scleroderma renal crisis.

Diagnosis of primary aldosteronism.

Idiopathic edema.

Bartter's syndrome (improves potassium metabolism and corrects hypokalemia).

Raynaud's syndrome (symptomatic relief).

Hypertension of Takayasu's disease.

Prevention of left ventricular dysfunction following MI (50 to 100 mg/day).

Enalapril – Diabetic nephropathy (reduction of proteinuria, albuminuria and glomerular hypertension). See Warnings.

Childhood hypertension and hypertension related to scleroderma renal crisis.

Enalaprilat – May be used for hypertensive emergencies (1.25 to 5 mg every 6 hours), but the effects are often variable.

Lisinopril, quinapril, ramipril – Congestive heart failure.

Contraindications:

Hypersensitivity to these products (eg, patients with a history of angioedema related to previous treatment with an ACEI).

(Continued on following page)

Angiotensin Converting Enzyme Inhibitors (Cont.)

Warnings:

Neutropenia/Agranulocytosis: Neutropenia ($< 1000/mm^3$) with myeloid hypoplasia resulted from use of captopril. About half of the neutropenic patients developed systemic or oral cavity infections or other features of agranulocytosis. The risk of neutropenia is dependent on the patient's clinical status.

In hypertensive patients with normal renal function (serum creatinine $<$ 1.6 mg/dl, no collagen vascular disease), neutropenia occurred in one patient of $>$ 8600 exposed.

In patients with some degree of renal failure (serum creatinine $\geq$ 1.6 mg/dl) but no collagen vascular disease, the risk of neutropenia was about 1 per 500. Daily doses of captopril were relatively high. Concomitant **allopurinol** and captopril have been associated with neutropenia (see Drug Interactions).

In patients with collagen vascular diseases (eg, systemic lupus erythematosus, scleroderma) and impaired renal function, neutropenia has occurred in 3.7% of patients.

In heart failure, the same risk factors for neutropenia appear present; $\approx$ ½ of cases had serum creatinine $\geq$ 1.6 mg/dl, and $>$ 75% were also on procainamide.

Neutropenia has been detected within 3 months after captopril initiation. Bone marrow examinations consistently showed myeloid hypoplasia, frequently accompanied by erythroid hypoplasia and decreased numbers of megakaryocytes (eg, hypoplastic bone marrow and pancytopenia); anemia and thrombocytopenia were sometimes seen.

In general, neutrophils returned to normal $\approx$ 2 weeks after captopril was discontinued; serious infections were limited to clinically complex patients. About 13% of neutropenia cases were fatal, but almost all were in patients with serious illness having collagen vascular disease, renal failure, heart failure, immunosuppressant therapy or a combination of these factors.

Discontinuation of captopril has generally led to prompt return of the normal WBC count; upon confirmation of neutropenia, withdraw the drug and closely observe patient.

Neutropenia/agranulocytosis has occurred rarely with enalapril or lisinopril and in one patient on quinapril; a causal relationship cannot be excluded. Data are insufficient to show that ramipril, quinapril or fosinopril do not cause agranulocytosis at similar rates. Periodically monitor WBC counts.

Angioedema has occurred in patients treated with ACEIs. It may occur especially following the first dose of enalapril (0.2%), captopril (0.1%), lisinopril (0.1%) or quinapril (0.1%). Angioedema of face, extremities, lips, mucous membranes, tongue, glottis or larynx has occurred. In instances where swelling has been confined to the face and lips, the condition has generally resolved without treatment, although antihistamines have been useful in relieving symptoms (enalaprilat). Angioedema associated with laryngeal edema may be fatal. If laryngeal stridor or angioedema of the face, tongue, larynx or glottis occurs and appears likely to cause airway obstruction, discontinue treatment and institute appropriate therapy (eg, epinephrine solution 1:1000 SC) immediately. Use with extreme caution in patients with hereditary angioedema (caused by a deficiency of C1 esterase inhibitor).

Renal function impairment: Some hypertensive patients with renal disease, particularly those with severe renal artery stenosis, have developed increases in BUN and serum creatinine after reduction of blood pressure (20% of patients with enalapril). Monitor renal function in such patients during the first few weeks of therapy. Dosage reduction or discontinuation of the diuretic may be required. For some patients, it may not be possible to normalize blood pressure and maintain adequate renal perfusion.

About 20% of heart failure patients develop stable elevations of BUN and serum creatinine $>$ 20% above normal or baseline with long-term captopril. Less than 5% of patients, generally those with severe preexisting renal disease, require discontinuation of treatment; subsequent improvement probably relies on the severity of underlying renal disease.

In patients with severe CHF whose renal function may depend on the activity of the renin-angiotensin-aldosterone system, treatment with ACEIs may be associated with oliguria or progressive azotemia and, rarely, with acute renal failure or death.

Some hypertensive patients with no apparent preexisting renal vascular disease have developed increases in BUN and serum creatinine, usually minor and transient, especially when enalapril, lisinopril or ramipril has been given with a diuretic. Dosage reduction of enalapril, lisinopril or ramipril, or discontinuation of the diuretic may be required. However, to confuse the situation, captopril and enalapril have shown renal protective effects in hypertensive patients with some renal dysfunction.

Impaired renal function decreases lisinopril elimination, which is excreted principally through the kidneys, but this decrease becomes clinically important only when the glomerular filtration rate is $<$ 30 ml/min. The elimination half-life of quinaprilat increases as Ccr decreases. Dosage adjustment may be necessary for quinapril, benazepril, ramipril and lisinopril. Impaired renal function decreases total clearance of fosinoprilat and approximately doubles AUC. In general, however, no dosing adjustment is needed.

(Warnings continued on following page)

Warnings (Cont.):

Hepatic function impairment: Since ramipril and fosinopril are primarily metabolized to their active metabolites, patients with impaired liver function could develop markedly elevated plasma levels of unchanged fosinopril or ramipril. No formal kinetic studies with ramipril have been done in hypertensive patients with impaired liver function. In patients with alcoholic or biliary cirrhosis, the rate, but not extent of fosinopril hydrolysis was reduced; the total body clearance of fosinoprilat was decreased and AUC approximately doubled. Quinaprilat concentrations are reduced in patients with alcoholic cirrhosis due to impaired deesterification of quinapril.

Proteinuria: Total urinary proteins > 1 g/day were seen in 0.7% of captopril patients. Nephrotic syndrome occurred in about 20% of these cases. About 90% of affected patients showed evidence of prior renal disease or received relatively high doses of captopril (> 150 mg/day) or both. In most cases, proteinuria cleared within 6 months, regardless of whether captopril was continued. Creatinine and BUN were seldom altered.

Since most cases of proteinuria occur by the eighth month of therapy, estimate urinary protein (dip-stick on first morning urine) prior to therapy and periodically thereafter. However, in patients with diabetic nephropathy, captopril has improved renal hemodynamics and associated proteinuria (see Unlabeled uses).

Hypotension: First dose effect – ACE inhibitors may cause a profound fall in blood pressure following the first dose. Excessive hypotension is rare in hypertensive patients, but is possible with ACEI use in severely salt/volume depleted persons (eg, those treated vigorously with diuretics or patients on dialysis) and in those with CHF; it may be associated with oliguria, progressive azotemia, and rarely with acute renal failure and death. Excessive perspiration, dehydration, vomiting or diarrhea may lead to an excessive fall in blood pressure because of reduction in fluid volume.

In heart failure, where the blood pressure was either normal or low, transient decreases in mean blood pressure > 20% occurred in about half of the patients. Transient hypotension may occur after the first several doses. This effect is usually well tolerated, is asymptomatic or produces brief, mild lightheadedness, although it has been associated with arrhythmia or conduction defects. Hypotension forced drug discontinuation in 3.6% of patients with heart failure.

Start therapy under close medical supervision. Follow patients closely for the first 2 weeks and whenever the dose of ACEI or diuretic is increased. Apply similar considerations to patients with ischemic heart or cerebrovascular disease in whom an excessive fall in blood pressure could result in myocardial infarction or cerebrovascular accident.

Minimize the possibility of hypotension by either discontinuing the diuretic or increasing salt intake approximately 1 week prior to initiating ACEIs, or initiate with small doses. Alternatively, provide medical supervision for at least 2 hours after the initial dose and until blood pressure has stabilized for at least an additional hour.

Hypotension is not a reason to discontinue captopril. Some decrease in systemic blood pressure is common and desirable in heart failure. The magnitude of the decrease is greatest early in treatment, stabilizes within 1 to 2 weeks, and generally returns to pretreatment levels without a decrease in efficacy within 2 months.

A transient hypotensive response is not a contraindication to further doses of these agents, which usually can be given without difficulty once the blood pressure has increased after volume expansion. If hypotension occurs, place patient in supine position and, if necessary, give IV normal saline.

Elderly patients may have higher lisinopril blood levels and area under plasma concentration-time curve (AUC), and higher peak ramiprilat and quinaprilat levels and AUC than younger patients. This may relate to decreased renal function rather than to age itself. No overall differences in effectiveness or safety were observed between elderly patients receiving fosinopril or benazepril and younger patients; however, greater sensitivity of some older individuals cannot be ruled out.

Pregnancy: (Category C – Captopril; Category D – Benazepril, enalapril, fosinopril, lisinopril, quinapril, ramipril). These drugs cross the placenta. ACE inhibitors can cause fetal and neonatal morbidity and mortality when administered to pregnant women. When ACE inhibitors have been used during the second and third trimesters of pregnancy, there have been reports of neonatal hypotension, renal failure, skull hypoplasia and death. Oligohydramnios has also occurred, presumably resulting from decreased fetal renal function; oligohydramnios has been associated with fetal limb contractures, craniofacial malformations, hypoplastic lung development and intrauterine growth retardation. Prematurity and patent ductus arteriosus have been reported, although it is not clear whether these occurrences were due to the ACE inhibitor exposure or to the mother's underlying disease.

(Warnings continued on following page)

Warnings (Cont.):

Pregnancy: (Cont.)

It is not known whether exposure limited to the first trimester can adversely affect fetal outcome. Apprise the patient who becomes pregnant while taking ACE inhibitors, or who takes ACE inhibitors when already pregnant, of the potential hazard to the fetus. If she continues to receive ACE inhibitors during the second or third trimester of pregnancy, perform frequent ultrasound examinations to look for oligohydramnios. When oligohydramnios is found, generally discontinue the ACE inhibitor. Closely observe infants with histories of in utero exposure to ACE inhibitors for hypotension, oliguria and hypokalemia. If oliguria occurs, direct attention toward support of blood pressure and renal perfusion.

Captopril – Two cases of fetal abnormality have occurred with captopril use during pregnancy. One report involved fetal malformation discovered following a first trimester abortion. The second report involved intrauterine growth retardation and the presence of a patent ductus arteriosus. In both reports, other factors (abortion procedure, other drugs or the severity of maternal disease) may have contributed to the reported malformation. However, captopril was embryocidal and reduced neonatal survival in animal studies. Fatal neonatal anuria and a fetal death possibly related to captopril have also occurred.

Enalapril – Conflicting animal data are reported of maternal and fetal toxicity at dosages ranging from 1 to 1200 mg/kg/day. Reversible acute renal failure occurred in a premature newborn following the administration of enalapril 20 mg/day for 17 days to a pregnant woman.

Fosinopril was embryocidal in rabbits at 10 and 40 mg/kg/day, and slight reductions in placental weights, degree of skeletal ossification and fetal body weights were observed in rats at 25 to 400 mg/kg/day.

Lisinopril – In mice, there was an increase in fetal resorptions at doses of 100 mg/kg. In rats, there was an increased incidence in pup deaths and a lower average body weight of pups. Fetotoxicity was demonstrated in rabbits by an increased incidence of fetal resorptions at a dose of 1 mg/kg/day and by an increased incidence of incomplete ossification at the lowest dose tested (0.1 mg/kg/day).

Quinapril – In rats, reduced offspring body weight was seen at maternal doses > 25 mg/kg/day; changes in renal histology occurred at 150 mg/kg/day. Maternal toxicity and embryotoxicity occurred in rabbits at quinapril doses of 0.5 mg/kg/day (the recommended human dose) and 1 mg/kg/day, respectively.

Ramipril increases the incidence of dilated renal pelvises in rat fetuses, retards birth weights in mice and is toxic to pregnant rabbits and monkeys. On a mg/kg basis, doses used in these studies were 2 to 2500 times the maximum recommended human dose.

Lactation: Ingestion of 20 mg/day fosinopril resulted in detectable fosinoprilat levels in breast milk; do not administer to nursing mothers. Concentrations of captopril in breast milk are approximately 1% of those in maternal blood. Benazepril, enalapril and enalaprilat are detected in breast milk in trace amounts; a newborn would receive < 0.1% of the mg/kg maternal dose of benazepril and benazeprilat. The effect on the nursing infant has not been determined. Exercise caution when these drugs are administered to nursing women. It is not known whether lisinopril, quinapril or ramipril is excreted in breast milk; quinapril is excreted to a limited extent in the milk of lactating rats (≤ 5% of plasma concentration). Decide whether to discontinue nursing or discontinue the drug, taking into account the importance of the drug to the mother.

Children: Safety and efficacy have not been established. However, there is limited experience with the use of captopril in children. Dosage, on a weight basis, was comparable to or less than that used in adults. Infants, especially newborns, may be more susceptible to the adverse hemodynamic effects of captopril. Excessive, prolonged and unpredictable decreases in blood pressure and associated complications, including oliguria and seizures, have occurred. Use captopril in children only when other measures for controlling blood pressure have not been effective.

In one study, 11 neonates (five premature) with severe hypertension were effectively treated with captopril 0.01 to 0.5 mg/kg/day. The potency and duration are greater in this age group. Use the lowest possible effective maintenance dose. Other infants, however, have developed neurologic complications following captopril therapy. Caution is warranted.

Precautions:

Valvular stenosis: Theoretically, patients with aortic stenosis might be at risk of decreased coronary perfusion when treated with vasodilators, because they do not develop as much afterload reduction as others.

(Precautions continued on following page)

Angiotensin Converting Enzyme Inhibitors (Cont.)

Adverse Reactions (Cont.):

Adverse reactions	Adverse reactions shared by the ACEIs[1] (%)						
	Benazepril	Captopril	Enalapril	Fosinopril	Lisinopril	Quinapril	Ramipril
Respiratory							
Asthma	< 1		≤ 1				
Bronchitis	< 1		1.3		≤ 1	0.5-1	
Bronchospasm		✓	≤ 1	≤ 1			
Cough†	1.9-3.4	0.5-2	1.3-2.2	2.2	2.9	2	12
Dyspnea	< 1	0.5-2	1.3		1.1		< 1
Upper respiratory infection			≤ 1				✓
Sinusitis	< 1			≤ 1	≤ 1	0.5-1	
Dermatologic							
Alopecia		0.5-2	≤ 1				
Diaphoresis/Increased sweating	< 1		≤ 1	≤ 1	≤ 1	0.5-1	< 1
Erythema multiforme		✓	≤ 1				
Exfoliative dermatitis		✓	≤ 1			0.5-1	
Flushing	< 1		≤ 1	≤ 1	≤ 1		
Photosensitivity		✓	✓	≤ 1		0.5-1	< 1
Pruritus	✓	2	≤ 1	≤ 1	≤ 1	0.5-1	✓
Rash	✓	4-7	1.3-1.4	≤ 1	1.5		✓
Stevens-Johnson syndrome		✓	≤ 1				
Urticaria			≤ 1	≤ 1	≤ 1		
Miscellaneous							
Angioedema†	0.5	0.1	0.2	≤ 1	0.1	0.1	0.3
Impotence	< 1	✓	≤ 1		0.7		< 1
Decreased libido	< 1			≤ 1	≤ 1		
Muscle cramps				≤ 1	≤ 1		0.6
Asthenia	< 1	✓	1.1-1.6		1.3		2
Syncope	0.1	✓	2.2	≤ 1	0.1-1	0.5-1	< 1
Anemia		✓[2]			✓		
Blurred vision		✓	≤ 1		≤ 1		
Fever		✓	✓		≤ 1		✓
Myalgia	< 1	✓	✓	≤ 1	✓		< 1
Tinnitus			≤ 1	≤ 1			< 1
Arthralgia	< 1	✓	✓	≤ 1	✓		< 1
Arthritis	< 1		✓		✓		< 1
Eosinophilia		✓	✓				
Vasculitis		✓	✓		≤ 1		
Renal†	Transient elevation (reversible) of BUN and creatinine may occur, especially in patients with volume depletion or renovascular hypertension. Rapid reduction of long-standing or severely elevated blood pressure may transiently decrease GFR, resulting in transient rises in creatinine and BUN. Small increases in serum potassium concentrations frequently occur, especially in patients with renal impairment. Renal failure has occurred.						

[1] Data included for both hypertension and heart failure indications.
[2] Including aplastic or hemolytic.

† See Warnings or Precautions.
✓ Reported. No incidence given.

(Adverse Reactions continued on following page)

Angiotensin Converting Enzyme Inhibitors (Cont.)

Adverse Reactions (Cont.):

Renal: Captopril – Proteinuria (1%); renal insufficiency, nephrotic syndrome, polyuria, urinary frequency (0.1% to 0.2%); interstitial nephritis.

Enalapril – Renal dysfunction (≤ 1%).

Lisinopril – Progressive azotemia (≤ 1%).

Hematologic: Captopril – Neutropenia/agranulocytosis (see Warnings); thrombocytopenia; pancytopenia.

Enalapril – Decreased hemoglobin (0.3 g/dl) and hematocrit (1%) occur frequently in hypertensive or CHF patients but are rarely of clinical importance unless another cause of anemia coexists. Discontinuation resulted in < 0.1% of patients. Rarely, bone marrow depression, neutropenia and thrombocytopenia. A few cases of hemolysis have occurred in patients with G-6-PD deficiency.

Lisinopril – Small decreases in hemoglobin (≈ 0.4 g/dl) and hematocrit (≈ 1.3%) occurred frequently but are rarely of clinical importance in patients without some other cause of anemia. In clinical trials, < 0.1% of patients discontinued therapy due to anemia. Rarely, neutropenia and bone marrow depression.

Ramipril – Decreases in hemoglobin or hematocrit (a low value and a decrease of 5 g/dl or 5%, respectively) were rare, occurring in 0.4% of patients on ramipril alone and 1.5% of those on ramipril plus a diuretic. Occasional leukopenia, eosinophilia and proteinuria.

Fosinopril – Mean hemoglobin decrease of 0.1 g/dl. Decreases in hemoglobin or hematocrit were usually transient, small and not associated with symptoms. Occasional neutropenia, leukopenia and eosinophilia.

Benazepril – Decreased hemoglobin (a low value and a decrease of 5 g/dl; rare). Occasional leukopenia, eosinophilia and proteinuria.

Quinapril – Agranulocytosis, thrombocytopenia (0.5% to 1%).

Dermatologic: Captopril – Rash, often with pruritus (and sometimes fever, arthralgia and eosinophilia) occurs usually during the first 4 weeks of therapy. The rash is usually maculopapular, rarely urticarial, mild and disappears within a few days of dosage reduction, short-term antihistamine treatment or discontinuation of therapy. Remission may occur even if captopril is continued. Between 7% and 10% of patients with skin rash have shown eosinophilia or positive ANA titers.

Reversible pemphigoid-like lesions; bullous pemphigus; scalded mouth sensation; onycholysis; flushing, pallor (0.2% to 0.5%).

Ramipril – Apparent hypersensitivity reactions (manifested by dermatitis, pruritus or rash with or without fever); purpura (< 1%).

Benazepril – Apparent hypersensitivity reactions (manifested by dermatitis, pruritus or rash).

Cardiovascular: Captopril – Raynaud's syndrome, CHF (0.2% to 0.3%).

Enalapril – Pulmonary embolism and infarction, pulmonary edema, atrial fibrillation, bradycardia (≤ 1%).

Ramipril – Arrhythmia (< 1%).

Fosinopril – Hypertensive crisis, claudication (≤ 1%).

Quinapril – Vasodilation, heart failure, hypertensive crisis (0.5% to 1%).

GI: Captopril – Gastric irritation, aphthous ulcers, peptic ulcer (0.5% to 2%). Dysgeusia is reversible and usually self-limiting, even with continued therapy (2 to 3 months). Weight loss may be associated with taste loss. Jaundice, cholestasis.

Enalapril – Ileus, stomatitis (≤ 1%).

Fosinopril – Dysphagia, abdominal distention, flatulence, heartburn, appetite/weight change (≤ 1%).

Lisinopril – Flatulence (≤ 1%).

Quinapril – GI hemorrhage (0.5% to 1%).

Ramipril – Abdominal pain occurs, sometimes with enzyme changes suggesting pancreatitis. Dysphagia, gastroenteritis, increased salivation (< 1%).

CNS: Fosinopril – Memory disturbance, tremor, mood change, drowsiness (≤ 1%).

Lisinopril – Stroke (≤ 1%).

Ramipril – Amnesia, convulsions, hearing loss, neuralgia, neuropathy, tremor, vision disturbances (< 1%).

Electrolytes: Hyperkalemia (see Warnings); hyponatremia (benazepril; captopril, particularly in patients on a low sodium diet or concomitant diuretics).

Lab test abnormalities: Elevated liver enzymes, serum bilirubin, uric acid and blood glucose.

Benazepril – ECG changes.

(Adverse Reactions continued on following page)

Angiotensin Converting Enzyme Inhibitors (Cont.)

Adverse Reactions (Cont.):

Miscellaneous: Benazepril – Hypertonia, infection (< 1%).

Captopril – Eosinophilic pneumonitis; gynecomastia; myasthenia; rhinitis.

Enalapril – Pneumonia, anosmia, rhinorrhea, sore throat, hoarseness, toxic epidermal necrolysis, herpes zoster, conjunctivitis, dry eyes, tearing, hearing loss (≤ 1%).

Fosinopril – Edema, weakness, sexual dysfunction, gout, lymphadenopathy, musculoskeletal pain, pharyngitis, rhinitis, laryngitis, epistaxis, vision/taste disturbance, eye irritation, renal insufficiency, urinary frequency (≤ 1%).

Lisinopril – Upper respiratory symptoms (3%); pharyngeal pain, back/joint/shoulder pain, nasal congestion, gout, chest discomfort (≤ 1%).

Quinapril – Back pain, amblyopia, pharyngitis (0.5% to 1%).

Ramipril – Flu syndrome; edema, epistaxis, weight gain (< 1%).

A symptom complex has occurred and may include: Positive ANA, elevated erythrocyte sedimentation rate, arthralgia, arthritis, myalgia, fever, interstitial nephritis, vasculitis, rash, eosinophilia, serositis, leukocytosis, photosensitivity, other dermatologic manifestations.

Overdosage:

Symptoms: The most common symptom is hypotension. Systolic blood pressures of 95 and 80 mm Hg have occurred following lisinopril and captopril overdoses, respectively.

Treatment includes usual supportive measures. Refer to General Management of Acute Overdosage. The primary concern is correction of hypotension. Volume expansion with an IV infusion of normal saline is the treatment of choice to restore blood pressure.

Captopril, enalaprilat and lisinopril may be removed by hemodialysis. Enalaprilat has been removed from neonatal circulation by peritoneal dialysis. Benazeprilat can be removed by dialysis, but this intervention should rarely, if ever, be required. It is not known if ramipril or ramiprilat are removed by hemodialysis. Hemodialysis and peritoneal dialysis have little effect on the elimination of quinapril and quinaprilat.

Patient Information:

Take 1 hour before meals (captopril).

Do not interrupt or discontinue medication without consulting physician.

Notify physician if any of the following occurs: Sore throat, fever, swelling of hands or feet, irregular heartbeat, chest pains, signs of angioedema (swelling of face, eyes, lips, tongue, difficulty swallowing or breathing, hoarseness). Excessive perspiration, dehydration, vomiting and diarrhea may lead to a fall in blood pressure.

May cause dizziness, fainting or lightheadedness, especially during the first days of therapy; avoid sudden changes in posture. If actual syncope occurs, discontinue drug until consulting physician. Heart failure patients should avoid rapid increases in physical activity.

May cause skin rash or impaired taste perception. Notify physician if these persist.

Do not use salt substitutes containing potassium without consulting a physician.

A persistent dry cough may occur and usually does not subside unless the medication is stopped. If this effect becomes bothersome, consult a physician.

(Products listed on following pages)

Refer to the general discussion of these products on page 773.

Angiotensin Converting Enzyme Inhibitors (Cont.)

QUINAPRIL HCl

Quinapril was approved by the FDA in November 1991.

Indications:

Treatment of hypertension, alone or in combination with thiazide diuretics.

Administration and Dosage:

Initial dose: 10 mg once daily. Adjust according to blood pressure response at peak (2 to 6 hours) and trough (predose) blood levels. Adjust dosage at intervals of at least 2 weeks.

Maintenance dosage: Most patients require 20, 40 or 80 mg/day as a single dose or in two equally divided doses. In some patients treated with once-daily dosing, the antihypertensive effect may diminish toward the end of the dosing interval. In general, doses of 40 to 80 mg and divided doses give a somewhat greater effect at the end of the dosing interval.

Patients taking diuretics: Symptomatic hypotension may occur following the initial dose of quinapril. To reduce the likelihood of this effect, discontinue the diuretic 2 to 3 days prior to quinapril therapy if possible. If blood pressure is not controlled, resume diuretic therapy. If diuretic cannot be discontinued, use an initial dose of 5 mg quinapril.

Renal function impairment: Initial dose is 10 mg with Ccr > 60 ml/min, 5 mg with Ccr 30 to 60 ml/min and 2.5 mg with Ccr 10 to 30 ml/min.

	Product	Form	Description	C.I.*
Rx	**Accupril** (Parke-Davis)	**Tablets:** 5 mg[1]	Lactose. (PD 527 5). Brown, scored. Elliptical. Film coated. In 90s.	26
		10 mg[1]	Lactose. (PD 530 10). Brown, scored. Triangular. Film coated. In 90s and UD 100s.	13
		20 mg[1]	Lactose. (PD 532 20). Brown, scored. Film coated. In 90s and UD 100s.	6.5
		40 mg	Lactose. (P 535 40). Brown, scored. Elliptical. In 90s and UD 100s.	3.3

* Cost Index based on cost per 20 mg quinapril.
[1] With magnesium carbonate and stearate.

CAPTOPRIL

Administration and Dosage:

Individualize dosage. Administer 1 hour before meals. If possible, discontinue previous antihypertensive drug regimen 1 week before starting captopril.

Hypertension: Initial – 25 mg 2 or 3 times/day. If satisfactory blood pressure reduction is not achieved after 1 or 2 weeks, increase to 50 mg 2 or 3 times/day. If blood pressure is not controlled after 1 or 2 weeks at this dose (and patient is not already on a diuretic), add a modest dose of a thiazide diuretic (eg, hydrochlorothiazide 25 mg/day). May increase diuretic dose at 1 to 2 week intervals until its highest usual antihypertensive dose is reached. Concomitant sodium restriction may be beneficial when captopril is used alone.

If further blood pressure reduction is required, increase to 100 mg captopril 2 or 3 times/day and then, if necessary, to 150 mg 2 or 3 times/day (while continuing diuretic). Usual dose is 25 to 150 mg 2 or 3 times/day. Do not exceed daily dose of 450 mg.

Accelerated or malignant hypertension – When temporary discontinuation of current antihypertensive therapy is not practical, or when prompt titration of blood pressure is indicated, continue diuretic but stop current medication and promptly initiate captopril at 25 mg 2 or 3 times daily under close supervision. Increase dose every 24 hours until a satisfactory response is obtained or the maximum dose is reached. In this regimen, a more potent diuretic (eg, furosemide) may be indicated. Beta-blockers may be used with captopril, but the effects are less than additive.

Heart failure: Consider recent diuretic therapy and the possibility of severe salt/volume depletion. In patients with normal or low blood pressure who have been vigorously treated with diuretics and who may be hyponatremic or hypovolemic, a starting dose of 6.25 or 12.5 mg 3 times daily may minimize the magnitude or duration of the hypotensive effect. Titrate to the usual daily dosage within the next several days.

Usual initial dosage is 25 mg 3 times daily. After 50 mg 3 times daily is reached, delay further dosage increases, where possible, for at least 2 weeks to determine if a satisfactory response occurs. Most patients have had a satisfactory clinical improvement at 50 or 100 mg 3 times daily. Do not exceed a daily dose of 450 mg.

Use in conjunction with a diuretic and digitalis. Initiate captopril therapy under very close medical supervision (see Drug Interactions).

(Continued on following page)

Refer to the general discussion of these products beginning on page 773.

Angiotensin Converting Enzyme Inhibitors (Cont.)

CAPTOPRIL (Cont.)

Administration and Dosage (Cont.):

Renal impairment: Excretion is reduced in patients with impaired renal function; these patients may respond to smaller or less frequent doses. Accordingly, reduce initial dosage and use smaller increments for titration, which should be quite slow (1 to 2 week intervals). After the desired therapeutic effect is achieved, slowly back-titrate to the minimal effective dose. When diuretic therapy is required, a loop diuretic (eg, furosemide) is preferred in patients with severe renal impairment.

				C.I.*
Rx	**Capoten** (Bristol-Myers Squibb)	**Tablets:** 12.5 mg	Lactose. (Squibb 450). White, scored. Oval. In 100s, 1000s and UD 100s.	5.4
		25 mg	Lactose. (Squibb 452). White, scored. Biconvex rounded square. In 100s, 1000s & UD 100s.	3
		50 mg	Lactose. (Squibb 482). White, scored. Biconvex oval. In 100s, 1000s and UD 100s.	2.5
		100 mg	Lactose. (Squibb 485). White, scored. Biconvex oval. In 100s and UD 100s.	1.8

RAMIPRIL

Ramipril was approved by the FDA in 1991.

Indications:

Treatment of hypertension, alone or in combination with thiazide diuretics.

Administration and Dosage:

Initial dose: 2.5 mg once daily in patients not receiving a diuretic. Adjust according to blood pressure response.

Maintenance dosage: 2.5 to 20 mg/day as a single dose or in two equally divided doses. If the antihypertensive effect diminishes at the end of the dosing interval in patients treated once daily, consider twice daily administration or an increase in dosage.

Patients taking diuretics: Symptomatic hypotension may occur following the initial dose of ramipril. To reduce the likelihood of this effect, discontinue the diuretic 2 to 3 days prior to beginning ramipril therapy if possible. If blood pressure is not controlled, resume diuretic therapy. If diuretic cannot be discontinued, use an initial dose of 1.25 mg ramipril.

Renal function impairment: 1.25 mg once daily in patients with Ccr of < 40 ml/min/1.73 m^2 (serum creatinine > 2.5 mg/dl). Dosage may be titrated upward until blood pressure is controlled or to a maximum of 5 mg/day.

				C.I.*
Rx	**Altace** (Hoechst-Roussel/Upjohn)	**Capsules:** 1.25 mg	Yellow. In 100s and UD 100s.	3
		2.5 mg	Orange. In 100s and UD 100s.	6
		5 mg	Red. In 100s and UD 100s.	3.2
		10 mg	Blue. In 100s.	NA

FOSINOPRIL SODIUM

Fosinopril was approved by the FDA in 1991.

Indications:

Treatment of hypertension, alone or in combination with thiazide diuretics.

Administration and Dosage:

Initial dose: 10 mg once daily. Adjust according to blood pressure response at peak (2 to 6 hours) and trough (about 24 hours after dosing) blood levels.

Maintenance dosage: Usual range needed to maintain a response is 20 to 40 mg/day but some patients appear to have a further response to 80 mg. In some patients treated with once daily dosing, the antihypertensive effect may diminish toward the end of the dosing interval. If trough response is inadequate, consider dividing the daily dose.

Patients taking diuretics: Symptomatic hypotension may occur following the initial dose of fosinopril. To reduce the likelihood of this effect, discontinue the diuretic 2 to 3 days prior to beginning fosinopril if possible. If blood pressure is not controlled, resume diuretic therapy. If diuretic cannot be discontinued, use an initial dose of 10 mg fosinopril.

Renal function impairment: Total body clearance of fosinoprilat does not differ appreciably with any degree of renal insufficiency. Therefore, use the usual dose of fosinopril.

				C.I.*
Rx	**Monopril** (Mead Johnson)	**Tablets:** 10 mg	Lactose. (158 Squibb M). White to off-white. Biconvex, diamond shaped. In 100s and UD 100s.	12
		20 mg	Lactose. (609 Squibb M). White to off-white. Oval. In 100s and UD 100s.	6

* Cost Index based on cost per 25 mg captopril, 2.5 mg ramipril or 20 mg fosinopril.

Refer to the general discussion of these products beginning on page 773.

Angiotensin Converting Enzyme Inhibitors (Cont.)

BENAZEPRIL HCl

Benazepril was approved by the FDA in June 1991.

Indications:

Hypertension, alone or in combination with thiazide diuretics.

Administration and Dosage:

Initial dose: 10 mg once daily.

Maintenance dosage: 20 to 40 mg/day as a single dose or two divided doses. The divided regimen is more effective in controlling trough (pre-dosing) blood pressure. Base dosage adjustment on peak (2 to 6 hours after dosing) and trough responses. If a once daily regimen does not give adequate trough response, consider an increase in dosage or divided administration. A dose of 80 mg gives an increased response, but experience is limited; total daily doses > 80 mg have not been evaluated.

Patients taking diuretics: Symptomatic hypotension may occur following the initial dose of benazepril. To reduce this likelihood, discontinue the diuretic 2 to 3 days prior to beginning benazepril therapy. If blood pressure is not controlled, resume diuretic therapy. If the diuretic cannot be discontinued, use an initial dose of 5 mg benazepril.

Renal function impairment: 5 mg once daily in patients with Ccr of < 30 ml/min/1.73 m^2 (serum creatinine > 3 mg/dl). Dosage may be titrated upward until blood pressure is controlled or to a maximum of 40 mg/day.

				C.I.*
Rx	**Lotensin** (Ciba)	**Tablets:** 5 mg	Lactose. (Lotensin 5). Light yellow. In 100s and UD 100s.	22
		10 mg	Lactose. (Lotensin 10). Dark yellow. In 100s and UD 100s.	11
		20 mg	Lactose. (Lotensin 20). Tan. In 100s and UD 100s.	5.5
		40 mg	Lactose. (Lotensin 40). Dark rose. In 100s and UD 100s.	2.8

* Cost Index based on cost per 20 mg.

ENALAPRIL MALEATE

Administration and Dosage:

Oral: Hypertension – Patients taking diuretics: Symptomatic hypotension occasionally may occur following the initial dose of enalapril. Discontinue the diuretic, if possible, for 2 to 3 days before beginning enalapril to reduce the likelihood of hypotension. If blood pressure is not controlled with enalapril alone, diuretics may be resumed.

If the diuretic cannot be discontinued, give an initial dose of 2.5 mg. Keep patient under medical supervision for at least 2 hours and until blood pressure has stabilized for at least an additional hour.

Patients not taking diuretics: Initial dose is 5 mg once a day. Adjust dosage according to blood pressure response. The usual dosage range is 10 to 40 mg/day as a single dose or in 2 divided doses. In some patients treated once daily, the antihypertensive effect may diminish toward the end of the dosing interval. In such patients, consider an increase in dosage or twice daily administration. If blood pressure is not controlled with enalapril alone, a diuretic may be added.

Impaired renal function: Titrate the dosage upward until blood pressure is controlled or until a maximum dose of 40 mg/day is reached. Use initial dose of 5 mg/day in normal renal function and mild impairment (creatinine clearance [Ccr] 30 to 80 ml/min, serum creatinine < 3 mg/dl); 2.5 mg/day in moderate to severe renal impairment (Ccr ≤ 30 ml/min, serum creatinine ≥ 3 mg/dl) and in dialysis patients on dialysis days (adjust dosage on nondialysis days based on blood pressure response).

Oral: Heart failure – As adjunctive therapy with diuretics and digitalis, the recommended starting dose is 2.5 mg once or twice daily. After the initial dose, observe the patient for at least 2 hours and until blood pressure has stabilized for at least an additional hour. If possible, reduce the dose of the diuretic; this may diminish the likelihood of hypotension. The appearance of hypotension after the initial dose of enalapril does not preclude subsequent careful dose titration with the drug, following effective management of the hypotension. The usual therapeutic dosing range for the treatment of heart failure is 5 to 20 mg/day given in two divided doses. The maximum daily dose is 40 mg. Once-daily dosing has been effective in a controlled study, but nearly all patients in this study were given 40 mg, the maximum recommended daily dose, and there has been much more experience with twice-daily dosing. In addition, patients in the mortality trial received therapy twice daily. Dosage may be adjusted depending upon clinical or hemodynamic response.

(Administration and Dosage continued on following page)

ENALAPRIL MALEATE (Cont.)

Administration and Dosage (Cont.)

Oral: Heart failure (Cont.) –

In a placebo controlled study which demonstrated reduced mortality in patients with severe heart failure (NYHA Class IV), patients were treated with 2.5 to 40 mg/day enalapril, almost always administered in two divided doses.

Renal impairment or hyponatremia – (Serum sodium < 130 mEq/L or with serum creatinine > 1.6 mg/dl): Initiate therapy at 2.5 mg/day under close medical supervision. The dose may be increased to 2.5 mg twice daily, then 5 mg twice daily and higher as needed, usually at intervals of 4 days or more if, at the time of dosage adjustment, there is not excessive hypotension or significant deterioration of renal function. The maximum daily dose is 40 mg.

Parenteral (enalaprilat): For IV administration only.

Hypertension – 1.25 mg every 6 hours IV over 5 minutes. A clinical response is usually seen within 15 minutes. Peak effects after the first dose may not occur for up to 4 hours. The peak effects of subsequent doses may exceed those of the first.

No dosage regimen for enalaprilat has been clearly shown to be more effective in treating hypertension than 1.25 mg every 6 hours. However, doses as high as 5 mg every 6 hours were well tolerated for up to 36 hours. There is inadequate experience with doses > 20 mg/day. Patients have received enalaprilat for as long as 7 days.

The dose for patients being converted to IV from oral therapy is 1.25 mg every 6 hours. For conversion from IV to oral therapy, the recommended initial dose of tablets is 5 mg once a day with subsequent dosage adjustments as necessary.

Patients taking diuretics – Starting dose for hypertension is 0.625 mg IV over 5 minutes. Clinical response is usually seen within 15 minutes. Peak effects after the first dose may not occur for up to 4 hours, although most of the effect is usually apparent within the first hour. If there is inadequate clinical response after 1 hour, repeat the 0.625 mg dose. Give additional doses of 1.25 mg at 6 hour intervals.

For conversion from IV to oral therapy, the recommended initial dose of enalapril maleate tablets for patients who have responded to 0.625 mg enalaprilat every 6 hours is 2.5 mg once a day with subsequent dosage adjustment as necessary.

Renal function impairment – Administer 1.25 mg enalaprilat every 6 hours for patients with Ccr > 30 ml/min (serum creatinine < 3 mg/dl). For patients with Ccr ≤ 30 ml/min (serum creatinine ≥ 3 mg/dl), initial dose is 0.625 mg. If there is inadequate clinical response after 1 hour, the 0.625 mg dose may be repeated. May give additional 1.25 mg doses at 6 hour intervals. For dialysis patients, initial dose is 0.625 mg every 6 hours.

For conversion from IV to oral therapy, the recommended initial dose is 5 mg once a day for patients with Ccr > 30 ml/min and 2.5 mg once daily for patients with Ccr ≤ 30 ml/min. Adjust dosage according to blood pressure response.

Administration – Give as a slow IV infusion, as indicated above, over at least 5 minutes. It may be used as provided or diluted with up to 50 ml of a compatible diluent.

Compatibility and stability – Enalaprilat as supplied and mixed with the following IV diluents has been found to maintain full activity for 24 hours at room temperature: 5% Dextrose Injection; 0.9% Sodium Chloride Injection; 0.9% Sodium Chloride Injection in 5% Dextrose; 5% Dextrose in Lactated Ringer's Injection; *Isolyte E.*

				C.I.*
Rx	**Vasotec** (MSD)	**Tablets:** 2.5 mg	Lactose. (Vasotec MSD 014). Yellow, scored. Biconvex, barrel shaped. In 100s and UD 100s.	2.8
		5 mg	Lactose. (Vasotec MSD 712). White, scored. Barrel shaped. In 100s and UD 100s.	6.2
		10 mg	Lactose. (Vasotec MSD 713). Salmon. Barrel shaped. In 100s and UD 100s.	3.3
		20 mg	Lactose. (Vasotec MSD 714). Peach. Barrel shaped. In 100s and UD 100s.	2.3
Rx	**Vasotec I.V.** (MSD)	**Injection:** 1.25 mg enalaprilat per ml	In 1 and 2 ml vials.[1]	351

* Cost Index based on cost per 5 mg.

[1] With 9 mg benzyl alcohol.

Refer to the general discussion of these products beginning on page 773.

Angiotensin Converting Enzyme Inhibitors (Cont.)

LISINOPRIL

Administration and Dosage:

Initial therapy: 10 mg once/day in patients with uncomplicated essential hypertension not on diuretic therapy. The usual dosage range is 20 to 40 mg/day as a single daily dose. The antihypertensive effect may diminish toward the end of the dosing interval, but most commonly with a dose of 10 mg daily. Evaluate by measuring blood pressure just prior to dosing to determine whether satisfactory control is being maintained for 24 hours. If it is not, consider an increase in dose. Doses up to 80 mg have been used but do not appear to give a greater effect. If blood pressure is not controlled with lisinopril alone, a low dose of a diuretic may be added (eg, hydrochlorothiazide 12.5 mg). After addition of a diuretic, it may be possible to reduce the dose of lisinopril.

Diuretic-treated patients: Symptomatic hypotension may occur occasionally following the initial dose of lisinopril. Discontinue diuretic, if possible, for 2 to 3 days before beginning therapy with lisinopril to reduce the likelihood of hypotension (see Warnings). If patient's blood pressure is not controlled with lisinopril alone, resume diuretic therapy as above.

If the diuretic cannot be discontinued, use an initial dose of 5 mg under medical supervision for at least 2 hours and until blood pressure has stabilized for at least an additional hour.

Elderly: In general, blood pressure response and adverse experiences are similar in younger and older patients given similar doses of lisinopril. However, maximum blood levels and area under the plasma concentration-time curve (AUC) are doubled in older patients. Make dosage adjustments with particular caution.

Dosage adjustment in renal impairment: Initiate lisinopril daily dosage according to the following chart. Titrate dosage upward until blood pressure is controlled or to a maximum of 40 mg daily.

Lisinopril Dosage in Renal Impairment

Renal status	Creatinine clearance (ml/min)	Serum creatinine (mg/dl)	Initial dose (mg/day)
Normal function to mild impairment	> 30	≤ 3	10 mg
Moderate to severe impairment	$\geq 10 \leq 30$	≥ 3	5 mg
Dialysis patients	< 10	—	2.5 mg*

* Adjust dosage or dosing interval depending on the blood pressure response.

	Product	Strength	Description	C.I.*
Rx	**Prinivil** (MSD)	**Tablets:** 5 mg	(MSD 19 Prinivil). White, scored. Shield shaped. In 100s and UD 100s.	5.6
Rx	**Zestril** (Stuart)		(Zestril 5 130). Pink, scored. In 100s and UD 100s.	5.3
Rx	**Prinivil** (MSD)	**Tablets:** 10 mg	(MSD 106 Prinivil). Light yellow. Shield shaped. In 30s, 100s and UD 100s.	2.9
Rx	**Zestril** (Stuart)		(Zestril 10 131). Pink. In 100s and UD 100s.	2.7
Rx	**Prinivil** (MSD)	**Tablets:** 20 mg	(MSD 207 Prinivil). Peach. Shield shaped. In 30s, 100s and UD 100s.	1.4
Rx	**Zestril** (Stuart)		(Zestril 20 132). Red. In 100s and UD 100s.	1.5
Rx	**Prinivil** (MSD)	**Tablets:** 40 mg	(MSD 237 Prinivil). Rose red. Shield shaped. In 100s.	1
Rx	**Zestril** (Stuart)		(Zestril 40 134). Yellow. In 100s and UD 100s.	1.2

* Cost Index based on cost per 5 mg.

Refer to the general discussion of these products beginning on page 773.

Agents for Pheochromocytoma

PHENTOLAMINE

Actions:

Pharmacology: Phentolamine, an α-adrenergic blocking agent, blocks presynaptic (α_2) and postsynaptic (α_1) α-adrenergic receptors. It is a competitive antagonist of endogenous and exogenous α-active agents. It also acts on both the arterial tree and venous bed. Thus, total peripheral resistance is lowered and venous return to the heart is diminished. Phentolamine also causes cardiac stimulation.

Phentolamine has an immediate onset and short duration of action.

Indications:

Pheochromocytoma: Prevention or control of hypertensive episodes that may occur in a patient with pheochromocytoma as a result of stress or manipulation during preoperative preparation and surgical excision.

Pharmacological test for pheochromocytoma (not the method of choice – see Warnings).

Prevention and treatment of dermal necrosis and sloughing following IV administration or extravasation of norepinephrine or dopamine.

Unlabeled uses: Phentolamine has been used to treat hypertensive crises secondary to MAO inhibitor/sympathomimetic amine interactions and rebound hypertension on withdrawal of clonidine, propranolol or other antihypertensive agents. It has also been used in combination with papaverine as an intracavernous injection for impotence.

Contraindications:

Myocardial infarction, coronary insufficiency, angina or other evidence suggestive of coronary artery disease. Hypersensitivity to phentolamine or related compounds.

Warnings:

Myocardial infarction, cerebrovascular spasm and cerebrovascular occlusion have followed phentolamine administration, usually in association with marked hypotensive episodes with shock-like states which occasionally follow parenteral use.

For screening tests in patients with hypertension, the generally available urinary assay of catecholamines or other biochemical assays have largely supplanted phentolamine and other pharmacological tests. None of the chemical or pharmacological tests are infallible in the diagnosis of pheochromocytoma. The phentolamine test is not the procedure of choice; reserve for cases in which additional confirmatory evidence is necessary and consider the risks involved.

Pregnancy and Lactation: Safety for use during pregnancy or lactation has not been established. Use only when clearly needed and when the potential benefits outweigh the potential hazards to the fetus or nursing infant.

Precautions:

Tachycardia and cardiac arrhythmias may occur with phentolamine use. When possible, defer administration of cardiac glycosides until cardiac rhythm returns to normal.

Drug Interactions:

Epinephrine and **ephedrine:** The vasoconstricting and hypertensive effects of these drugs are antagonized by phentolamine.

Adverse Reactions:

Acute and prolonged hypotensive episodes, tachycardia and cardiac arrhythmias.

Weakness; dizziness; flushing; orthostatic hypotension; nasal stuffiness; nausea; vomiting and diarrhea.

Overdosage:

If blood pressure drops to a dangerous level or other evidence of shock occurs, treat vigorously and promptly. Include IV infusion of norepinephrine, titrated to maintain normal blood pressure. Epinephrine is contraindicated because it stimulates both α- and β-receptors; since α-receptors are blocked, the net effect of epinephrine administration is vasodilation and a further drop in blood pressure (epinephrine reversal).

(Continued on following page)

PHENTOLAMINE (Cont.)

Administration and Dosage:

Prevention or control of hypertensive episodes in pheochromocytoma: For use in preoperative reduction of elevated blood pressure, inject 5 mg (1 mg for children) IV or IM 1 or 2 hours before surgery. Repeat if necessary. During surgery, administer 5 mg for adults (1 mg for children) IV as indicated to help prevent or control paroxysms of hypertension, tachycardia, respiratory depression, convulsions or other effects of epinephrine intoxication.

Postoperatively, norepinephrine may be given to control hypotension which may follow complete removal of a pheochromocytoma.

Prevention and treatment of dermal necrosis and sloughing following IV administration or extravasation of norepinephrine: For prevention, add 10 mg to each liter of solution containing norepinephrine. The pressor effect of norepinephrine is not affected. For treatment, inject 5 to 10 mg in 10 ml saline into the area of extravasation within 12 hours. For children, use 0.1 to 0.2 mg/kg up to a maximum of 10 mg.

Diagnosis of pheochromocytoma (phentolamine blocking test): Withhold sedatives, analgesics and all other medication not considered essential for at least 24 hours (preferably 48 to 72 hours) prior to the test. Withhold antihypertensive drugs until blood pressure returns to the untreated, hypertensive level. Do not perform the test on normotensive patients. Keep patient at rest in supine position throughout the test, preferably in a quiet, darkened room. Delay injection until blood pressure is stabilized, as evidenced by blood pressure readings taken every 10 minutes for at least 30 minutes.

IV test – Although a 5 mg test dose (1 mg for children) has been recommended, a 2.5 mg test dose will produce fewer false-positive tests and may minimize dangerous drops in blood pressure in patients with pheochromocytoma. If the 2.5 mg dose is negative, perform a 5 mg test before considering the test negative. Dissolve 5 mg phentolamine mesylate in 1 ml Sterile Water for Injection. Insert the syringe needle into a vein and delay injection until pressor response to venipuncture has subsided. Inject rapidly. Record blood pressure immediately, at 30 second intervals for the first 3 minutes, then at 60 second intervals for the next 7 minutes.

Positive response, suggestive of pheochromocytoma, is indicated by a drop in blood pressure of more than 35 mm Hg systolic and 25 mm Hg diastolic pressure. A typical positive response is a pressure reduction of 60 mm Hg systolic and 25 mm Hg diastolic. Maximal decrease in pressure is usually evident within 2 minutes after injection. Return to preinjection pressure commonly occurs within 15 to 30 minutes, but may return more rapidly. If blood pressure falls to a dangerous level, treat patient as outlined in the Overdosage section. Always confirm a positive response by other diagnostic procedures, preferably the measurement of urinary catecholamines or their metabolites.

Negative response is indicated when the blood pressure is unchanged, elevated or is reduced less than 35 mm Hg systolic and 25 mm Hg diastolic after injection. A negative response may not exclude the diagnosis of pheochromocytoma, especially in patients with paroxysmal hypertension in whom the incidence of false-negative response is high.

IM test – Preparation is the same as for the IV test. Adult dosage is 5 mg IM; for children it is 3 mg. Record blood pressure every 5 minutes for 30 to 45 minutes following IM injection. Positive response is indicated by a drop in blood pressure of 35 mm Hg systolic and 25 mm Hg diastolic or greater within 20 minutes following injection.

Reliability – The test is most reliable in patients with sustained hypertension and least reliable in those with paroxysmal hypertension. False-positive tests may occur in patients with hypertension without pheochromocytoma.

Storage: Store between 15° to 30°C (59° to 86°F). Use reconstituted solution upon preparation; do not store.

				C.I.*
Rx	**Regitine** (Ciba Pharm.)	**Injection:** 5 mg (as mesylate) per vial.[1]	In 1 ml vials.	34,350

* Cost Index based on cost per 5 mg.

[1] With 25 mg sterile, lyophilized mannitol.

Refer to the general discussion of these products beginning on page 773.

Agents for Pheochromocytoma (Cont.)

PHENOXYBENZAMINE HCl

Actions:

Pharmacology: An irreversible alpha-adrenergic receptor (both presynaptic and postsynaptic) blocking agent which can produce and maintain "chemical sympathectomy." It increases blood flow to the skin, mucosa and abdominal viscera, and lowers both supine and standing blood pressures. It has no effect on the parasympathetic system.

Pharmacokinetics: Absorption from the GI tract is incomplete (20% to 30%).

Indications:

Pheochromocytoma, to control episodes of hypertension and sweating. If tachycardia is excessive, it may also be necessary to use a beta-blocker concomitantly.

Unlabeled Use: Phenoxybenzamine (5 to 60 mg/day) has shown efficacy in micturition disorders resulting from neurogenic bladder, functional outlet obstruction and partial prostatic obstruction.

Contraindications: Conditions where a fall in blood pressure may be undesirable.

Warnings:

Concomitant therapy: Phenoxybenzamine-induced alpha-adrenergic blockade leaves beta-adrenergic receptors unopposed. Compounds that stimulate both types of receptors (ie, epinephrine) may produce an exaggerated hypotensive response and tachycardia.

Carcinogenesis and mutagenesis: Phenoxybenzamine has shown in vitro mutagenic activity in the Ames test and in the mouse lymphoma assay. In animals, repeated intraperitoneal phenoxybenzamine resulted in peritoneal sarcomas; chronic oral dosing produced malignant GI tract tumors. Clinical significance is not established. Nevertheless, consider these results in determining benefit-to-risk ratio.

Precautions:

Administer with caution to patients with marked cerebral or coronary arteriosclerosis or renal damage. Adrenergic blocking effects may aggravate respiratory infections.

Adverse Reactions:

Nasal congestion, miosis, postural hypotension, tachycardia and inhibition of ejaculation may occur. These vary according to the degree of adrenergic blockade, and tend to decrease as therapy continues. GI irritation, drowsiness and fatigue have also occurred.

Overdosage:

Symptoms may include postural hypotension resulting in dizziness or fainting; tachycardia, particularly postural; vomiting; lethargy; shock. These are largely due to block of the sympathetic nervous system and of the circulating epinephrine.

Treatment: Discontinue the drug. Treat circulatory failure, if present. In mild overdosage, recumbent position with legs elevated usually restores cerebral circulation. In more severe cases, institute measures to combat shock. Usual pressor agents are not effective. Do not use epinephrine (see Warnings). The patient may have to be kept flat 24 hours or more as drug's effect is prolonged. Leg bandages and an abdominal binder may shorten the disability period. Norepinephrine IV may be used to combat severe hypotension because it primarily stimulates alpha receptors. Although phenoxybenzamine is an alpha-blocker, sufficient norepinephrine will overcome this effect.

Patient Information:

Avoid alcoholic beverages.

If dizziness (postural hypotension) occurs, avoid sudden changes in posture.

Medication may cause nasal congestion and constricted pupils. Inhibition of ejaculation may occur, but generally decreases with continued therapy.

Avoid cough, cold or allergy medications containing sympathomimetics, except on professional recommendation.

Administration and Dosage:

Individualize dosage. Slowly increase small initial doses until the desired effect is obtained or side effects become troublesome. Observe the patient before increasing dosage. Increase dosage to a point where symptomatic relief or objective improvement are obtained, but not so high that blockade side effects become troublesome.

Initially, give 10 mg twice a day. Increase dosage every other day until an optimal dosage is obtained as judged by blood pressure control. The usual dosage range is 20 to 40 mg, 2 or 3 times daily. In children, give 1 to 2 mg/kg/day, divided every 6 to 8 hours.

				C.I.*
Rx	**Dibenzyline** (SKF)	**Capsules:** 10 mg.	(#SKF E33). Red. In 100s.	617

* Cost Index based on cost per 10 mg. # Product identification code.

Refer to the general discussion of these products beginning on page 773.

Agents for Pheochromocytoma (Cont.)

METYROSINE

Actions:

Pharmacology: Metyrosine inhibits tyrosine hydroxylase, which catalyzes the first transformation in catecholamine biosynthesis, ie, the conversion of tyrosine to dihydroxyphenylalanine (DOPA). Because this is the rate-limiting step, hydroxylase blockade results in decreased endogenous levels of catecholamines, usually measured as decreased urinary excretion of catecholamines and their metabolites.

In patients with pheochromocytoma who produce excessive amounts of norepinephrine and epinephrine, 1 to 4 g/day has reduced catecholamine biosynthesis from about 35% to 80%, as measured by the total excretion of catecholamines and their metabolites (metanephrine and vanillylmandelic acid). The maximum biochemical effect usually occurs within 2 to 3 days; the urinary concentration of catecholamines and their metabolites usually returns to pretreatment levels within 3 to 4 days after discontinuation. In some patients, the total excretion of catecholamines and catecholamine metabolites may be lowered to normal or near normal levels (< 10 mg/24 hours). In most patients treatment duration has been 2 to 8 weeks, but several patients have received metyrosine for periods of 1 to 10 years.

Most patients treated with metyrosine experience decreased frequency and severity of hypertensive attacks with associated headache, nausea, sweating and tachycardia. In patients who respond, blood pressure decreases progressively during the first 2 days of therapy; after withdrawal, it usually increases gradually to pretreatment values within 2 to 3 days.

Pharmacokinetics: Metyrosine is well absorbed from the GI tract. Approximately 53% to 88% (mean 69%) is recovered in the urine as unchanged drug following maintenance oral dosages of 600 to 4000 mg/24 hours. Less than 1% of administered drug is recovered as catechol metabolites. These metabolites are probably not present in sufficient amounts to contribute to the biochemical effects of metyrosine. The quantities excreted, however, are sufficient to interfere with accurate determination of urinary catecholamines determined by routine techniques.

The plasma half-life over 8 hours after single oral doses was 3.4 to 3.7 hours in three patients.

Indications:

Pheochromocytoma: Preoperative preparation of patients for surgery; management when surgery is contraindicated; chronic treatment of malignant pheochromocytoma.

Not recommended for the control of essential hypertension.

Contraindications: Hypersensitivity to metyrosine.

Warnings:

Maintain fluid volume during and after surgery: When metyrosine is used preoperatively, especially in combination with alpha-adrenergic blocking drugs, maintain adequate intravascular volume intraoperatively (especially after tumor removal) and postoperatively to avoid hypotension and decreased perfusion of vital organs resulting from vasodilatation and expanded volume capacity. Following tumor removal, large volumes of plasma may be needed to maintain blood pressure and central venous pressure.

Life-threatening arrhythmias may occur during anesthesia and surgery and may require treatment with a beta-blocker or lidocaine. During surgery, monitor blood pressure and ECG continuously.

Intraoperative effects: While the preoperative use of metyrosine is thought to decrease intraoperative problems with blood pressure control, it does not eliminate the danger of hypertensive crises or arrhythmias during manipulation of the tumor. Phentolamine, an alpha-adrenergic blocking drug, may be needed.

Usage in impaired hepatic/renal function: Use with caution.

Usage in Pregnancy: Category C. Safety for use during pregnancy has not been established. Use only when clearly needed and when the potential benefits outweigh the potential hazards to the fetus.

Usage in Lactation: It is not known whether metyrosine is excreted in breast milk. Safety for use in the nursing mother has not been established.

Usage in Children: Safety and efficacy for use in children under 12 years of age have not been established.

Precautions:

Long-term use: Human experience is limited and chronic animal studies have not been performed. Therefore, perform laboratory tests periodically in patients requiring prolonged metyrosine use, and observe caution with patients with impaired hepatic or renal function.

(Precautions continued on following page)

METYROSINE (Cont.)

Precautions (Cont.):

Metyrosine crystalluria and urolithiasis have been found in dogs treated at doses similar to those used in humans; crystalluria has also been observed in a few patients. To minimize this risk, maintain sufficient water intake to achieve a daily urine volume of 2000 ml or more, particularly with doses greater than 2 g/day. Routinely examine the urine. Metyrosine will crystallize as needles or rods. If crystalluria occurs, further increase fluid intake; if it persists, reduce dosage or discontinue use.

Drug Interactions:

Phenothiazines or **haloperidol:** Extrapyramidal effects of these drugs may be potentiated due to inhibition of catecholamine synthesis by metyrosine.

Drug/Lab tests: Spurious increases in urinary catecholamines may be observed due to the presence of metyrosine metabolites.

Adverse Reactions:

CNS: Sedation is most common, moderate to severe at low and high dosages. Sedative effects begin within the first 24 hours of therapy, are maximal after 2 to 3 days and tend to wane during the next few days. Sedation usually is not obvious after 1 week unless the dosage is increased, but at dosages greater than 2 g/day, some degree of sedation or fatigue may persist.

In most patients who experience sedation, temporary changes in sleep pattern (insomnia lasting 2 or 3 days; feelings of increased alertness and ambition) occur following drug withdrawal. Even those not experiencing sedation may report symptoms of psychic stimulation when the drug is discontinued.

Headache is reported infrequently.

Extrapyramidal signs – Drooling, speech difficulty and tremor (10%), occasionally accompanied by trismus and frank parkinsonism.

Anxiety and psychic disturbances – Depression, hallucinations, disorientation and confusion may be dose-dependent and may disappear with dosage reduction.

GI: Diarrhea (10%) may be severe. Antidiarrheals may be needed if metyrosine is continued. Infrequent – Decreased salivation, dry mouth, nausea, vomiting, abdominal pain.

GU: Infrequent – Impotence or failure to ejaculate. Crystalluria, transient dysuria and hematuria.

Miscellaneous: Infrequent – Slight breast swelling, galactorrhea, nasal stuffiness, eosinophilia, anemia, thrombocytopenia, thrombocytosis, increased AST, peripheral edema; hypersensitivity reactions such as urticaria and pharyngeal edema (rare).

Overdosage:

Signs of metyrosine overdosage include those central nervous system effects observed in some patients even at low dosages.

At doses exceeding 2 g/day, some degree of sedation or feeling of fatigue may persist. Doses 2 to 4 g/day can result in anxiety or agitated depression, neuromuscular effects (including fine tremor of the hands, gross tremor of the trunk, tightening of the jaw with trismus), diarrhea and decreased salivation with dry mouth.

Reducing dose or discontinuing treatment causes these symptoms to disappear.

Patient Information:

Maintain a daily liberal fluid intake.

Avoid alcohol or other CNS depressants.

May cause drowsiness; use caution while driving or performing tasks requiring alertness.

Notify physician if any of the following occur: Drooling, speech difficulty, tremors, disorientation, diarrhea, painful urination.

Administration and Dosage:

Adults and children over 12: Initial dosage is 250 mg 4 times daily. This may be increased by 250 to 500 mg every day to a maximum of 4 g/day in divided doses. When used for preoperative preparation, give the optimally effective dosage for at least 5 to 7 days (between 2 and 3 g/day); titrate by monitoring clinical symptoms and catecholamine excretion. In hypertensive patients, titrate dosage to achieve normal blood pressure and control of clinical symptoms. In normotensive patients, titrate dosage to reduce urinary metanephrines or vanillylmandelic acid by 50% or more.

Use in children under 12 years of age is limited and a dosage schedule cannot be given.

If patients are not adequately controlled by metyrosine, add an alpha-adrenergic blocker (phenoxybenzamine).

				C.I.*
Rx	**Demser** (MSD)	**Capsules:** 250 mg	(#MSD 690 Demser). Two-tone blue. In 100s.	1674

* Cost Index based on cost per 250 mg. # Product identification code.

Refer to the general discussion of these products beginning on page 773.

Agents for Hypertensive Emergencies

In addition to the agents listed in this section, parenteral forms of methyldopa and hydralazine are also indicated for use in malignant hypertension.

NITROPRUSSIDE SODIUM

Warning:

After reconstitution, nitroprusside is not suitable for direct injection. The reconstituted solution must be further diluted in sterile 5% Dextrose Injection before infusion (see Administration and Dosage).

Nitroprusside can cause precipitous decreases in blood pressure (see Administration and Dosage). In patients not properly monitored, these decreases can lead to irreversible ischemic injuries or death. Use only when available equipment and personnel allow blood pressure to be continuously monitored.

Except when used briefly or at low (< 2 mcg/kg/min) infusion rates, nitroprusside injection gives rise to important quantities of cyanide ion, which can reach toxic, potentially lethal levels (see Warnings). The usual dose rate is 0.5 to 10 mcg/kg/min, but infusion at the maximum dose rates should never last > 10 minutes. If blood pressure has not been adequately controlled after 10 minutes of infusion at the maximum rate, terminate administration immediately.

Although acid-base balance and venous oxygen concentration should be monitored and may indicate cyanide toxicity, these laboratory tests provide imperfect guidance.

Actions:

Pharmacology: Nitroprusside is a potent IV antihypertensive agent. The principal pharmacological action of nitroprusside is relaxation of vascular smooth muscle and consequent dilation of peripheral arteries and veins. Other smooth muscle (eg, uterus, duodenum) is not affected. Nitroprusside is more active on veins than on arteries, but this selectivity is much less marked than that of nitroglycerin. Dilation of the veins promotes peripheral pooling of blood and decreases venous return to the heart, thereby reducing left ventricular end-diastolic pressure and pulmonary capillary wedge pressure (preload). Arteriolar relaxation reduces systemic vascular resistance, systolic arterial pressure and mean arterial pressure (afterload). Dilation of the coronary arteries also occurs.

In association with the decrease in blood pressure, nitroprusside administered IV to hypertensive and normotensive patients produces slight increases in heart rate and a variable effect on cardiac output. In hypertensive patients, moderate doses induce renal vasodilation roughly proportional to the decrease in systemic blood pressure, so there is no appreciable change in renal blood flow or glomerular filtration rate.

In normotensive subjects, acute reduction of mean arterial pressure to 60 to 75 mm Hg by infusion of nitroprusside caused a significant increase in renin activity. In the same study, ten renovascular-hypertensive patients given nitroprusside had significant increases in renin release from the involved kidney at mean arterial pressures of 90 to 137 mm Hg.

The hypotensive effect of nitroprusside is seen within 1 to 2 minutes after the start of an adequate infusion, and it dissipates almost as rapidly after an infusion is discontinued. The effect is augmented by ganglionic blocking agents and inhaled anesthetics.

Pharmacokinetics: Infused nitroprusside is rapidly distributed to a volume that is approximately coextensive with the extracellular space. The drug is cleared from this volume by intraerythrocytic reaction with hemoglobin (HgB), and nitroprusside's resulting circulatory half-life is about 2 minutes.

The products of the nitroprusside/HgB reaction are cyanmethemoglobin (cyanmetHgB) and cyanide ion (CN^-). Safe use of nitroprusside injection must be guided by knowledge of the further metabolism of these products. The essential features of nitroprusside metabolism are: One molecule of nitroprusside is metabolized by combination with HgB to produce one molecule of cyanmetHgB and four CN^- ions; methemoglobin, obtained from HgB, can sequester cyanide as cyanmetHgB; thiosulfate reacts with cyanide to produce thiocyanate (SCN^-); thiocyanate is eliminated in the urine; cyanide not otherwise removed binds to cytochromes; cyanide is much more toxic than methemoglobin or thiocyanate.

(Actions continued on following page)

NITROPRUSSIDE SODIUM (Cont.)

Actions (Cont.):

Pharmacokinetics (Cont.): When the Fe^{+++} of cytochromes is bound to cyanide, the cytochromes are unable to participate in oxidative metabolism. In this situation, cells may be able to provide for their energy needs by utilizing anaerobic pathways, but they thereby generate an increasing body burden of lactic acid. Other cells may be unable to utilize these alternate pathways, and they may die hypoxic deaths.

When CN^- is infused or generated within the bloodstream, essentially all of it is bound to methemoglobin until intraerythrocytic methemoglobin has been saturated. At healthy steady state, most people have < 1% of their HgB in the form of methemoglobin. Nitroprusside metabolism can lead to methemoglobin formation (a) through dissociation of cyanmetHgB formed in the original reaction of nitroprusside with HgB and (b) by direct oxidation of HgB by the released nitroso group. Relatively large quantities of nitroprusside, however, are required to produce significant methemoglobinemia.

When thiosulfate is supplied only by normal physiologic mechanisms, conversion of CN^- to SCN^- generally proceeds at about 1 mcg/kg/min. This rate of CN^- clearance corresponds to steady-state processing of a nitroprusside infusion of slightly > 2 mcg/kg/min. CN^- begins to accumulate when nitroprusside infusions exceed this rate.

In patients with normal renal function, clearance of SCN^- is primarily renal, with a half-life of about 3 days. In renal failure, the half-life can be doubled or tripled.

Clinical trials: Nitroprusside has a prompt hypotensive effect, at least initially, in all populations. With increasing rates of infusion, nitroprusside lowers blood pressure without an observed limit of effect. The hypotensive effect of nitroprusside is also associated with reduced blood loss in a variety of major surgical procedures.

Many trials have verified the clinical significance of the metabolic pathways described above. In patients receiving unopposed infusions of nitroprusside, cyanide and thiocyanate levels have increased with increasing rates of nitroprusside infusion. Mild to moderate metabolic acidosis has usually accompanied higher cyanide levels, but peak base deficits have lagged behind the peak cyanide levels by ≥ 1 hour.

Progressive tachyphylaxis to the hypotensive effects of nitroprusside has occurred in several trials and numerous case reports. This tachyphylaxis has frequently been attributed to concomitant cyanide toxicity; however, this is unproven and the mechanism of tachyphylaxis to nitroprusside remains unknown.

Indications:

Immediate reduction of blood pressure of patients in hypertensive crises. Administer concomitant longer-acting antihypertensive medication so that the duration of treatment with nitroprusside can be minimized.

Production of controlled hypotension in order to reduce bleeding during surgery.

Unlabeled uses: Nitroprusside, either alone or in combination with dopamine, has been used in patients with severe refractory congestive heart failure. Coadministration of these two agents has also been used in patients with acute myocardial infarction.

Contraindications:

Treatment of compensatory hypertension, where the primary hemodynamic lesion is aortic coarctation or arteriovenous shunting; to produce hypotension during surgery in patients with known inadequate cerebral circulation or in moribund patients (A.S.A. Class 5E) coming to emergency surgery; patients with congenital (Leber's) optic atrophy or with tobacco amblyopia (these rare conditions are probably associated with defective or absent rhodanase and patients with unusually high cyanide/thiocyanate ratios).

Warnings:

Excessive hypotension: Small transient excesses in the infusion rate of nitroprusside can result in excessive hypotension, sometimes to levels so low as to compromise the perfusion of vital organs. These hemodynamic changes may lead to a variety of associated symptoms (see Adverse Reactions). Nitroprusside-induced hypotension will be self-limited within 1 to 10 minutes after discontinuation of the infusion; during these few minutes, it may be helpful to put the patient into a head-down (Trendelenburg) position to maximize venous return. If hypotension persists more than a few minutes after discontinuation of the infusion, nitroprusside is not the cause, and the true cause must be sought.

(Warnings continued on following page)

NITROPRUSSIDE SODIUM (Cont.)

Warnings (Cont.):

Cyanide toxicity: Nitroprusside infusions at rates > 2 mcg/kg/min generate CN^- faster than the body can normally dispose of it. (When sodium thiosulfate is given, the body's capacity for CN^- elimination is greatly increased.) Methemoglobin normally present in the body can buffer a certain amount of CN^-, but the capacity of this system is exhausted by the CN^- produced from about 500 mcg/kg nitroprusside. This amount of nitroprusside is administered in < 1 hour when the drug is administered at 10 mcg/kg/min (the maximum recommended rate). Thereafter, the toxic effects of CN^- may be rapid, serious and even lethal.

The true rates of clinically important cyanide toxicity cannot be assessed from spontaneous reports or published data. Most patients reported to have experienced such toxicity have received relatively prolonged infusions, and the only patients whose deaths have been unequivocally attributed to nitroprusside-induced cyanide toxicity have been patients who had received nitroprusside infusions at rates much greater than those now recommended (30 to 120 mcg/kg/min). Elevated cyanide levels, metabolic acidosis, and marked clinical deterioration, however, have occasionally been reported in patients who received infusions at recommended rates for only a few hours and even, in one case, for only 35 minutes. In some of these cases, infusion of sodium thiosulfate caused dramatic clinical improvement, supporting the diagnosis of cyanide toxicity.

Cyanide toxicity may manifest itself as venous hyperoxemia with bright red venous blood, as cells become unable to extract the oxygen delivered to them; metabolic (lactic) acidosis; air hunger; confusion; death. Cyanide toxicity due to causes other than nitroprusside has been associated with angina pectoris and myocardial infarction, ataxia, seizures and stroke, and other diffuse ischemic damage.

Hypertensive patients and patients concomitantly receiving other antihypertensive medications may be more sensitive to the effects of nitroprusside.

Methemoglobinemia: Nitroprusside infusions can cause sequestration of hemoglobin as methemoglobin. The back-conversion process is normally rapid, and clinically significant methemoglobinemia (> 10%) is seen only rarely. Even patients congenitally incapable of back-converting methemoglobin should demonstrate 10% methemoglobinemia only after they have received about 10 mg/kg nitroprusside; a patient receiving nitroprusside at the maximum recommended rate (10 mcg/kg/min) would take > 16 hours to reach this total accumulated dose.

Methemoglobin levels can be measured by most clinical laboratories. Suspect the diagnosis in patients who have received > 10 mg/kg of nitroprusside and who exhibit signs of impaired oxygen delivery despite adequate cardiac output and adequate arterial pO_2. Classically, methemoglobinemic blood is described as chocolate brown, without color change on exposure to air.

When methemoglobinemia is diagnosed, the treatment of choice is 1 to 2 mg/kg of methylene blue, administered IV over several minutes. In patients likely to have substantial amounts of cyanide bound to methemoglobin as cyanmetHgB, treatment of methemoglobinemia with methylene blue must be undertaken with extreme caution.

Thiocyanate toxicity: Most of the cyanide produced during metabolism of nitroprusside is eliminated in the form of thiocyanate. When cyanide elimination is accelerated by the co-infusion of thiosulfate, thiocyanate production is increased. Thiocyanate is mildly neurotoxic (eg, tinnitus, miosis, hyperreflexia) at serum levels of 1 mmol/L (60 mg/L). Thiocyanate toxicity is life-threatening when levels are 3 or 4 times higher (200 mg/L).

The steady-state thiocyanate level after prolonged infusions of nitroprusside is increased with increased infusion rate, and the half-time of accumulation is 3 to 4 days. To keep the steady-state thiocyanate level < 1 mmol/L, a prolonged infusion should not be more rapid than 3 mcg/kg/min; in anuric patients, the corresponding limit is just 1 mcg/kg/min. When prolonged infusions are more rapid than these, measure thiocyanate levels daily.

Physiologic maneuvers (eg, those that alter the pH of the urine) are not known to increase the elimination of thiocyanate. Thiocyanate clearance rates during dialysis, on the other hand, can approach the blood flow rate of the dialyzer.

Thiocyanate interferes with iodine uptake by the thyroid.

Hepatic insufficiency: Since cyanide is metabolized by hepatic enzymes, it may accumulate in patients with severe liver impairment. Therefore, use with caution in patients with hepatic insufficiency.

(Warnings continued on following page)

NITROPRUSSIDE SODIUM (Cont.)

Warnings (Cont.):

Pregnancy: Category C. In three studies in pregnant ewes, nitroprusside crossed the placental barrier. Fetal cyanide levels were dose-related to maternal levels of nitroprusside. The metabolic transformation of nitroprusside given to pregnant ewes led to fatal levels of cyanide in the fetuses. The infusion of 25 mcg/kg/min nitroprusside for 1 hour in pregnant ewes resulted in the death of all fetuses. There are no adequate or well controlled studies in pregnant women. It is not known whether nitroprusside can cause fetal harm when administered to a pregnant woman or can affect reproductive capacity. Give to a pregnant woman only if clearly needed. Nitroprusside has been used in pregnant women and neither the mother nor the fetus demonstrated evidence of cyanide intoxication.

The effects of administering sodium thiosulfate in pregnancy, either by itself or as a co-infusion with sodium nitroprusside, are completely unknown.

Lactation: It is not known whether nitroprusside and its metabolites are excreted in breast milk. Because of the potential for serious adverse reactions in nursing infants, decide whether to discontinue nursing or to discontinue the drug, taking into account the importance of the drug to the mother.

Children: See Administration and Dosage.

Precautions:

Intracranial pressure: Like other vasodilators, nitroprusside can cause increases in intracranial pressure. In patients whose intracranial pressure is already elevated, use only with extreme caution.

Anesthesia: When nitroprusside (or any other vasodilator) is used for controlled hypotension during anesthesia, the patient's capacity to compensate for anemia and hypovolemia may be diminished. If possible, correct pre-existing anemia and hypovolemia prior to administration.

Hypotensive anesthetic techniques may also cause abnormalities of the pulmonary ventilation/perfusion ratio. Patients intolerant of these abnormalities may require a higher fraction of inspired oxygen.

Exercise extreme caution in patients who are especially poor surgical risks (A.S.A. Classes 4 and 4E).

Monitoring: The cyanide-level assay is technically difficult, and cyanide levels in body fluids other than packed red blood cells are difficult to interpret. Cyanide toxicity will lead to lactic acidosis and venous hyperoxemia, but these findings may not be present until $\geq$ 1 hour after the cyanide capacity of the body's red-cell mass has been exhausted.

Adverse Reactions:

Rapid blood pressure reduction: Abdominal pain, apprehension, diaphoresis, dizziness, headache, muscle twitching, nausea, palpitations, restlessness, retching, and retrosternal discomfort have been noted when the blood pressure was reduced too rapidly. These symptoms quickly disappeared when the infusion was slowed or discontinued, and they did not reappear with a continued (or resumed) slower infusion.

Cardiovascular: Bradycardia; ECG changes; tachycardia.

Hematologic: Decreased platelet aggregation; methemoglobinemia (see Warnings).

Miscellaneous: Thiocyanate toxicity (see Warnings); flushing; venous streaking; irritation at the infusion site; rash; hypothyroidism; ileus; increased intracranial pressure (see Precautions).

Overdosage:

Symptoms: Toxicity has occurred at doses well below the recommended maximum infusion rate of 10 mcg/kg/min. Overdosage of nitroprusside can be manifested as excessive hypotension, cyanide toxicity or as thiocyanate toxicity (see Warnings).

The acute IV mean lethal doses (LD_{50}) of nitroprusside in rabbits, dogs, mice and rats are 2.8, 5, 8.4 and 11.2 mg/kg, respectively.

(Overdosage continued on following page)

NITROPRUSSIDE SODIUM (Cont.)

Overdosage (Cont.):

Treatment of cyanide toxicity: Measure cyanide levels and blood gases for venous hyperoxemia or acidosis. Acidosis may not appear until > 1 hour after the appearance of dangerous cyanide levels; do not wait for laboratory tests. Reasonable suspicion of cyanide toxicity is adequate grounds for initiation of treatment.

Treatment of cyanide toxicity consists of: Discontinuing the administration of nitroprusside; providing a buffer for cyanide by using sodium nitrite to convert as much HgB into methemoglobin as the patient can safely tolerate; and then infusing sodium thiosulfate in sufficient quantity to convert the cyanide into thiocyanate.

The necessary medications for this treatment are contained in commercially available Cyanide Antidote Kits. Alternatively, discrete stocks of medications can be used. Hemodialysis is ineffective in removal of cyanide, but it will eliminate most thiocyanate.

Cyanide Antidote Kits contain both amyl nitrite and sodium nitrite for induction of methemoglobinemia. The amyl nitrite is supplied in the form of inhalant ampuls, for use where IV administration of sodium nitrite may be delayed. In a patient who already has a patent IV line, use of amyl nitrite confers no benefit that is not provided by infusion of sodium nitrite.

Sodium nitrite is available in a 3% solution; inject 4 to 6 mg/kg (about 0.2 ml/kg) over 2 to 4 minutes. This dose converts about 10% of the patient's HgB into methemoglobin; this level of methemoglobinemia is not associated with any important hazard of its own. The nitrite infusion may cause transient vasodilation and hypotension, and this hypotension must, if it occurs, be routinely managed.

Immediately after infusion of the sodium nitrite, infuse sodium thiosulfate. This agent is available in 10% and 25% solutions, and the recommended dose is 150 to 200 mg/kg; a typical adult dose is 50 ml of the 25% solution. Thiosulfate treatment of an acutely cyanide-toxic patient will raise thiocyanate levels, but not to a dangerous degree.

The nitrite-thiosulfate regimen may be repeated, at half the original doses, after 2 hours.

Administration and Dosage:

Solution of the powder: Dissolve the contents of a 50 mg vial in 2 to 3 ml Dextrose in Water. No other diluent should be used.

Dilution to proper strength for infusion: Depending on the desired concentration, the initially reconstituted solution containing 50 mg must be further diluted in 250 to 1000 ml sterile 5% Dextrose Injection. Protect the diluted solution from light by promptly wrapping with aluminum foil or other opaque material. It is not necessary to cover the infusion drip chamber or the tubing.

Verification of the chemical integrity of the product: Nitroprusside solution can be inactivated by reactions with trace contaminants. The products of these reactions are often blue, green or red, much brighter than the faint brownish color of unreacted nitroprusside. Do not use discolored solutions, or solutions in which particulate matter is visible. If properly protected from light, the freshly reconstituted and diluted solution is stable for 24 hours.

Incompatibility: Do not administer other drugs in the same solution with nitroprusside.

Avoidance of excessive hypotension: While the average effective rate in adults and children is about 3 mcg/kg/min, some patients will become dangerously hypotensive when they receive nitroprusside at this rate. Therefore, start at a very low rate (0.3 mcg/kg/min), with gradual upward titration every few minutes until the desired effect is achieved or the maximum recommended infusion rate (10 mcg/kg/min) has been reached.

Because nitroprusside's hypotensive effect is very rapid in onset and in dissipation, small variations in infusion rate can lead to wide, undesirable variations in blood pressure. Do not infuse through ordinary IV apparatus regulated only by gravity and mechanical clamps. Use only an infusion pump, preferably a volumetric pump.

Because nitroprusside can induce essentially unlimited blood pressure reduction, the blood pressure of a patient receiving this drug must be continuously monitored, using either a continually reinflated sphygmomanometer or (preferably) an intra-arterial pressure sensor. Use special caution in elderly patients since they may be more sensitive to the hypotensive effects of the drug.

(Administration and Dosage continued on following page)

Agents for Hypertensive Emergencies (Cont.)

NITROPRUSSIDE SODIUM (Cont.)

Administration and Dosage (Cont.):

Infusion rates: The table below shows the infusion rates for adults and children of various weights corresponding to the recommended initial and maximal doses (0.3 mcg/kg/min and 10 mcg/kg/min, respectively). Some of the listed infusion rates are so slow or so rapid as to be impractical, and these practicalities must be considered when the concentration to be used is selected. Note that when the concentration used in a given patient is changed, the tubing is still filled with a solution at the previous concentration.

Infusion Rates to Achieve Initial (0.3 mcg/kg/min) and Maximal (10 mcg/kg/min) Dosing of Nitroprusside

Patient weight		Nitroprusside concentration					
		200 mcg/ml		100 mcg/ml		50 mcg/ml	
		Infusion rate (ml/hr)		Infusion rate (ml/hr)		Infusion rate (ml/hr)	
kg	lbs	Initial	Maximal	Initial	Maximal	Initial	Maximal
10	22	1	30	2	60	4	120
20	44	2	60	4	120	7	240
30	66	3	90	5	180	11	360
40	88	4	120	7	240	14	480
50	110	5	150	9	300	18	600
60	132	5	180	11	360	22	720
70	154	6	210	13	420	25	840
80	176	7	240	14	480	29	960
90	198	8	270	16	540	32	1080
100	220	9	300	18	600	36	1200

Avoidance of cyanide toxicity: When > 500 mcg/kg nitroprusside is administered faster than 2 mcg/kg/min, cyanide is generated faster than the unaided patient can eliminate it. Administration of sodium thiosulfate increases the rate of cyanide processing, reducing the hazard of cyanide toxicity. Although toxic reactions to sodium thiosulfate have not been reported, the co-infusion regimen has not been extensively studied and it cannot be recommended without reservation. In one study, sodium thiosulfate appeared to potentiate the hypotensive effects of nitroprusside.

Co-infusions of sodium thiosulfate have been administered at rates of 5 to 10 times that of nitroprusside. Care must be taken to avoid the indiscriminate use of prolonged or high doses of nitroprusside with sodium thiosulfate as this may result in thiocyanate toxicity and hypovolemia. Incautious administration of nitroprusside must still be avoided, and all of the precautions concerning nitroprusside administration must still be observed.

Consideration of methemoglobinemia and thiocyanate toxicity: Rare patients receiving > 10 mg/kg of nitroprusside will develop methemoglobinemia; other patients, especially those with impaired renal function, will predictably develop thiocyanate toxicity after prolonged, rapid infusions. Test patients with suggestive findings for these toxicities.

	Product	Form	Packaging	C.I.*
Rx	**Sodium Nitroprusside** (Elkins-Sinn)	**Powder for Injection:** 50 mg per vial	In single-dose 5 ml vials.	5750
Rx	**Nipride** (Roche Labs)		In 5 ml vials.	20450
Rx	**Nitropress** (Abbott)		In vials, *ADD-Vantage* vials and single-dose 2 ml *Univials*.	8533

* Cost Index based on cost per 50 mg.

Refer to the general discussion of these products beginning on page 773.

Agents for Hypertensive Emergencies (Cont.)

DIAZOXIDE, PARENTERAL

Oral diazoxide is used to increase blood glucose levels in hyperinsulinism; see page 511

Actions:

Pharmacology: Diazoxide, a nondiuretic antihypertensive, is structurally related to the thiazides. It promptly reduces blood pressure by relaxing smooth muscle in the peripheral arterioles. Increases in heart rate and in cardiac output occur as blood pressure is reduced. Coronary blood flow is maintained. Renal blood flow is increased after an initial decrease. Transient hyperglycemia occurs in the majority of patients treated.

Pharmacokinetics: Diazoxide is extensively bound to serum protein (> 90%) and may therefore displace other highly protein bound agents. The plasma half-life is 28 ± 8.3 hours. The duration of antihypertensive effect varies, but is generally < 12 hours.

Generally, hypotensive effects begin within 1 min., maximum effects occurring within 2 to 5 min. Blood pressure increases gradually over the next 20 minutes, and then more slowly over the next 3 to 15 hours, rarely exceeding pretreatment level.

Indications:

Emergency reduction of blood pressure, short-term use in severe, nonmalignant and malignant hypertension in hospitalized adults, and in acute severe hypertension in hospitalized children when urgent decrease of diastolic pressure is required. Institute treatment with oral agents as soon as the hypertensive emergency is controlled.

Contraindications:

Treatment of compensatory hypertension, such as that associated with aortic coarctation or arteriovenous shunt; dissecting aortic aneurysm; hypersensitivity to diazoxide, thiazides or to other sulfonamide derivatives.

Diazoxide is ineffective against hypertension due to pheochromocytoma.

Warnings:

Myocardial lesions in animals: Diazoxide IV in dogs induces subendocardial necrosis and necrosis of papillary muscles. These lesions, which are also produced by other vasodilators (ie, hydralazine, minoxidil) and catecholamines, are presumed to be related to anoxia from reflex tachycardia and decreased blood pressure.

Rapid decrease in blood pressure: Observe caution when reducing severely elevated blood pressure. Use only the 150 mg minibolus. The 300 mg IV dose of diazoxide is less predictable and less controllable and has been associated with angina and with myocardial and cerebral infarction. Optic nerve infarction was reported when a 100 mm Hg reduction in diastolic pressure occurred over 10 minutes following a single 300 mg bolus. In one prospective trial conducted in patients with severe hypertension and coexistent coronary artery disease, a 50% incidence of ischemic changes in the ECG was observed following single 300 mg bolus injections of diazoxide. Achieve the desired blood pressure over as long a period of time as is compatible with the patient's status. At least several hours and preferably 1 or 2 days is tentatively recommended.

Improved safety with equal efficacy can be achieved by administering diazoxide as a minibolus dose (see Administration and Dosage) until a diastolic blood pressure below 100 mm Hg is achieved. If hypotension severe enough to require therapy results from the reduction in blood pressure, it will usually respond to the Trendelenberg maneuver. If necessary, administer sympathomimetic agents such as dopamine or norepinephrine. Special attention is required for patients with diabetes mellitus and those in whom retention of salt and water may present serious problems.

Transient hyperglycemia occurs in the majority of patients, but usually requires treatment only in patients with diabetes mellitus; it will respond to the usual management including insulin. Monitor blood glucose levels, especially in patients with diabetes and in those requiring multiple injections of diazoxide. Cataracts have been observed in a few animals receiving repeated daily doses of IV diazoxide.

Fluid and electrolyte balance: Diazoxide causes sodium retention; repeat injections may precipitate edema and CHF. This retention responds to diuretic agents if adequate renal function exists. Coadministered thiazides may potentiate diazoxide's antihypertensive, hyperglycemic and hyperuricemic actions (see Drug Interactions). Increased extracellular fluid volume may cause treatment failure in nonresponsive patients.

Usage in Pregnancy: Category C. Safety for use during pregnancy has not been established. Diazoxide crosses the placenta and appears in cord blood. Diazoxide has been shown to reduce fetal or pup survival, and to reduce fetal growth in rats, rabbits, and dogs at daily doses of 30, 21 or 10 mg/kg, respectively. In rats treated at term, diazoxide at doses of 10 mg/kg and above prolonged parturition.

When given prior to delivery, it may produce fetal or neonatal hyperbilirubinemia, thrombocytopenia, altered carbohydrate metabolism and other adverse reactions.

(Warnings continued on following page)

DIAZOXIDE, PARENTERAL (Cont.)

Warnings (Cont.):

Usage in Labor and Delivery: Not for use during pregnancy. Administration IV during labor may stop uterine contractions, requiring administration of an oxytocic agent. An episode of maternal hypotension and fetal bradycardia occurred in a patient in labor who received both reserpine and hydralazine prior to administration of diazoxide. Neonatal hyperglycemia following intrapartum administration of diazoxide IV occurred.

Usage in Lactation: Information is not available concerning the passage of diazoxide in breast milk. Decide whether to discontinue nursing or to discontinue the drug, taking into account the importance of the drug to the mother.

Precautions:

Diazoxide requires close and frequent blood pressure monitoring; it may cause hypotension requiring treatment with sympathomimetic drugs. Use diazoxide primarily in the hospital and where facilities exist to treat such untoward reactions.

Use with care in patients with impaired cerebral or cardiac circulation, in whom abrupt reductions in blood pressure might be detrimental or in whom mild tachycardia or decreased blood perfusion may be deleterious. Avoid prolonged hypotension so as not to aggravate preexisting renal failure.

Monitoring: Perform appropriate diagnostic laboratory tests prior to, during and following diazoxide injection. Tests include: Hematologic (hematocrit, hemoglobin, white blood cell and platelet counts); metabolic (glucose, uric acid, total protein, albumin); electrolyte (sodium, potassium) and osmolality; renal function (creatinine, urine-protein); ECG.

Drug Interactions:

Hydantoins: Hepatic metabolism may be increased by diazoxide. Reduced hydantoin plasma levels, possibly with a suboptimal therapeutic response, may occur.

Sulfonylureas: Diazoxide appears to inhibit insulin release from pancreatic islet cells. Antagonism may occur when administered to patients on sulfonylureas, decreasing the pharmacologic effects of both drugs.

Thiazide diuretics: The coadministration of diazoxide with these agents may potentiate the hyperuricemic and antihypertensive effects of diazoxide.

Drug/Lab Tests: Hyperglycemic and hyperuricemic effects of diazoxide preclude assessment of these metabolic states. Increased renin secretion, IgG concentrations and decreased cortisol secretion have occurred. Diazoxide inhibits glucagon-stimulated insulin release and will cause a false-negative insulin response to glucagon.

Adverse Reactions:

The following adverse reactions were reported with rapid IV bolus administration of 300 mg diazoxide. The currently recommended minibolus dosing regimen may result in similar adverse effects, but with less frequency and severity. The most common adverse reactions were: Hypotension (7%); nausea and vomiting (4%); dizziness and weakness (2%). Additional adverse reactions were as follows:

Cardiovascular – Sodium and water retention after repeated injections, especially important in patients with impaired cardiac reserve; hypotension to shock levels; myocardial ischemia, usually transient and manifested by angina, atrial and ventricular arrhythmias and marked ECG changes, but occasionally leading to myocardial infarction; optic nerve infarction following too rapid decrease in severely elevated blood pressure; supraventricular tachycardia, palpitations; bradycardia; chest discomfort or nonanginal "chest tightness."

(Adverse Reactions continued on following page)

DIAZOXIDE, PARENTERAL (Cont.)

Adverse Reactions (Cont.):

CNS – Cerebral ischemia, usually transient, but occasionally leading to infarction and manifested by unconsciousness, convulsions, paralysis, confusion or focal neurological deficit such as numbness of the hands; vasodilative phenomena (eg, orthostatic hypotension), sweating, flushing and generalized or localized sensations of warmth; transient neurological findings secondary to alteration in regional blood flow to the brain, such as headache (sometimes throbbing), dizziness, lightheadedness, sleepiness (also reported as lethargy, somnolence or drowsiness), euphoria or "funny feeling," ringing in the ears and momentary hearing loss; weakness of short duration; apprehension; anxiety; malaise; blurred vision.

GI – Acute pancreatitis (rare); nausea; vomiting; abdominal discomfort; anorexia; alterations in taste; parotid swelling; salivation; dry mouth; ileus; constipation; diarrhea.

Other – Hyperglycemia in diabetic patients, especially after repeated injections; hyperosmolar coma in an infant; transient hyperglycemia in nondiabetic patients; transient retention of nitrogenous wastes; respiratory findings secondary to smooth muscle relaxation, such as dyspnea, cough and choking sensation; warmth or pain along the injected vein; cellulitis without sloughing or phlebitis at the injection site of extravasation; back pain and increased nocturia; lacrimation; hypersensitivity reactions (rash, leukopenia and fever); papilledema induced by plasma volume expansion secondary to the administration of diazoxide in a patient who had received 11 injections (300 mg/dose) over a 22 day period; transient cataract in an infant; hirsutism; decreased libido.

Overdosage:

Overdosage may cause undesirable hypotension that usually can be controlled with the Trendelenberg maneuver. If necessary, sympathomimetic agents, such as dopamine or norepinephrine, may be administered. Failure of blood pressure to rise in response to such agents suggests that the hypotension may not have been caused by diazoxide. Excessive hyperglycemia resulting from overdosage will respond to conventional therapy of hyperglycemia.

Diazoxide may be removed from the blood by hemodialysis.

Administration and Dosage:

During and immediately following injection, the patient should remain supine. Administer only into a peripheral vein. The dose is given IV in 30 seconds or less. Do not give IM, SC or into body cavities. The solution's alkalinity is irritating to tissue; avoid extravasation. Subcutaneous administration has produced inflammation and pain without subsequent necrosis. If SC leakage occurs, treat with warm compresses and rest.

Adults: Administer undiluted and rapidly by IV injections of 1 to 3 mg/kg, up to a maximum of 150 mg in a single injection. This dose may be repeated at 5 to 15 minute intervals until a satisfactory reduction in blood pressure has been achieved (diastolic pressure below 100 mm Hg).

This method of administration of diazoxide is as effective as bolus administration of 300 mg, but usually reduces blood pressure more gradually, perhaps lessening the circulatory and neurological risks associated with acute hypotension.

Repeated administration at intervals of 4 to 24 hours will usually maintain the blood pressure below pretreatment levels until oral antihypertensive medication can be instituted. Adjust the interval between injections by the duration of the response to each injection. It is usually unnecessary to continue treatment for more than 4 to 5 days; do not use for longer than 10 days.

Monitor the blood pressure closely until it has stabilized. Thereafter, hourly measurements will indicate any unusual response. Further decreases in blood pressure at 30 minutes or more after injection may be due to causes other than diazoxide. Have the patient remain recumbent for at least 1 hour after injection. In ambulatory patients, measure the blood pressure with the patient standing before ending surveillance.

Concomitant diuretic therapy: Since repeated administration can lead to sodium and water retention, a diuretic may be necessary for maximal blood pressure reduction and to avoid congestive failure.

Storage: Protect from light and freezing. Store between 2° to 30°C (36° to 86°F).

	Product	Form	Packaging	C.I.*
Rx	**Diazoxide Injection, USP** (Quad)	**Injection:** 15 mg/ml	In single dose flip-top vials.	35967
Rx	**Diazoxide Injection, USP** (Various)	**Injection:** 300 mg/20 ml	In single dose vials.	35342
Rx	**Hyperstat IV** (Schering)		In amps.	45050

* Cost Index based on cost per 150 mg.

Refer to the general discussion of these products beginning on page 773.

TRIMETHAPHAN CAMSYLATE

Actions:

Pharmacology: A short-acting ganglionic blocking agent, trimethaphan blocks transmission in autonomic (both sympathetic and parasympathetic) ganglia without producing any preceding or concomitant change in membrane potentials. It does not modify impulse conduction in the preganglionic or postganglionic neurons, or prevent acetylcholine release by preganglionic impulses. It occupies ganglion receptors and stabilizes postsynaptic membranes against the action of acetylcholine liberated from the presynaptic nerve endings.

Trimethaphan also exerts a direct peripheral vasodilator effect. Pooling of blood in the dependent periphery and the splanchnic system occurs, resulting in a lowering of the blood pressure. The drug liberates histamine.

Pharmacokinetics: Trimethaphan has a rapid onset and brief duration of action (10 to 30 minutes) after IV infusion. Tachyphylaxis may occur, requiring increasing doses to maintain effect. Action of the drug is enhanced by placing the patient in a reversed Trendelenburg position.

Indications:

For the production of controlled hypotension during surgery; for the short-term acute control of blood pressure in hypertensive emergencies; in the emergency treatment of pulmonary edema in patients with pulmonary hypertension associated with systemic hypertension.

Unlabeled Use: Trimethaphan has been used in patients with dissecting aortic aneurysm or in ischemic heart disease when other agents cannot be used.

Contraindications:

Where hypotension may subject the patient to undue risk, eg, uncorrected anemia, hypovolemia, shock (both incipient and frank), asphyxia or uncorrected respiratory insufficiency. Unavailability of fluids and inability to replace blood may also constitute contraindications.

Warnings:

Use of trimethaphan to produce hypotension in surgical or medical indications should be limited to physicians with proper training in this technique. Adequate facilities, equipment and personnel must be available for vigilant monitoring of the circulation. Dilute before use. Assure adequate oxygenation during treatment, particularly with regard to coronary and cerebral circulation. Use extreme caution in patients with arteriosclerosis, cardiac disease, hepatic or renal disease, degenerative CNS disease, Addison's disease, diabetes and in patients who are taking steroids.

Usage in Pregnancy: Induced hypotension may have serious consequences to the fetus. Trimethaphan is not effective in the control of hypertension in preeclamptic patients.

Usage in Children: Use with great caution.

Usage in Elderly: Use with great caution in elderly or debilitated patients.

Precautions:

Allergic individuals: Because this drug liberates histamine, use with caution.

Pupillary dilation does not necessarily indicate anoxia or the depth of anesthesia, since the drug appears to have a specific effect on the pupil.

Respiratory effects: Animal studies indicate that aggressive dosage may result in respiratory arrest. Rare cases of respiratory arrest have occurred in humans, although a causal relationship has not been established. Monitor respiratory status closely.

Drug Interactions:

Anesthetic agents: Use with caution with anesthetic agents, especially spinal anesthetics, which may produce hypotension.

Neuromuscular blocking agents: Trimethaphan may potentiate the neuromuscular blocking action of the nondepolarizing agents and succinylcholine.

(Continued on following page)

Refer to the general discussion of these products beginning on page 773.

Agents for Hypertensive Emergencies (Cont.)

TRIMETHAPHAN CAMSYLATE (Cont.)

Overdosage:

Vasopressor agents may be used to correct undesirable low pressures during surgery or to effect a more rapid return to normotensive levels. Use phenylephrine HCl or mephentermine sulfate initially; reserve norepinephrine for refractory cases.

Administration and Dosage:

Administer by IV infusion. Dilute 500 mg (10 ml) of trimethaphan to 500 ml (1 mg/ml, or 0.1%) in 5% Dextrose Injection. Other diluents are not recommended. Freshly prepare solution; discard unused portion. Do not use the infusion fluid as a vehicle for simultaneous administration of other drugs.

Position patient to avoid cerebral anoxia. When using trimethaphan in surgery, establish adequate anesthesia. Start IV drip at a rate of 3 to 4 ml/min (3 to 4 mg/min), then individualize. A marked variation in individual responses to the drug occurs; rates of administration vary from 0.3 to 6 ml/min (0.3 to 6 mg/min). Determine blood pressure frequently.

Children: 50 to 150 mcg/kg/min.

Surgical use: Stop administration prior to wound closure to permit blood pressure to return to normal. A systolic pressure of 100 mm Hg will usually be attained within 10 minutes after discontinuation.

Storage: Refrigerate; do not freeze.

				C.I.*
Rx	**Arfonad** (Roche)	**Injection:** 50 mg per ml	In 10 ml amps.	10700

* Cost Index based on cost per 500 mg.

Refer to the general discussion of these products beginning on page 773.

Miscellaneous Agents

MECAMYLAMINE HCl

Actions:

Pharmacology: Mecamylamine is a potent, oral ganglionic blocker. Although the antihypertensive effect is predominantly orthostatic, the supine blood pressure is also significantly reduced. Because of the many side effects, ganglionic blockers are infrequently used.

Pharmacokinetics: Mecamylamine is almost completely absorbed from the GI tract. It has a gradual onset of action (0.5 to 2 hours) and a long-lasting effect (6 to 12 hours or more). It crosses the placenta and the blood-brain barrier. It is slowly excreted unchanged in the urine. The rate of renal elimination is markedly influenced by urinary pH. Alkalinization of urine reduces and acidification promotes renal excretion of mecamylamine.

Indications:

For moderately severe to severe essential hypertension; uncomplicated malignant hypertension.

Contraindications:

Coronary insufficiency or recent myocardial infarction.

Contraindicated in uremia. Do not treat patients receiving antibiotics and sulfonamides with ganglionic blockers.

Glaucoma, organic pyloric stenosis or hypersensitivity to mecamylamine.

Mild, moderate or labile hypertension; uncooperative patients.

Warnings:

CNS effects: Mecamylamine readily penetrates into the brain and may produce CNS effects. Tremor, choreiform movements, mental aberrations, and convulsions occur rarely, but most often with large doses, especially in patients with cerebral or renal insufficiency.

Discontinuation of therapy: When mecamylamine is discontinued suddenly, hypertension returns. In patients with malignant hypertension and others, this may occur abruptly and may cause fatal cerebral vascular accidents or acute congestive heart failure. Withdraw drug gradually and substitute other antihypertensive therapy. The effects of mecamylamine can last from hours to days after therapy is discontinued.

Usage in Pregnancy: Category C. Mecamylamine crosses the placenta. Safety for use in pregnancy has not been established. Use only when clearly needed and when the potential benefits outweigh the potential hazards to the fetus.

Usage in Lactation: Because of the potential for serious adverse reactions in nursing infants, either discontinue nursing or discontinue the drug, taking into account the importance of the drug to the mother.

Precautions:

Evaluate the patient's condition, particularly renal and cardiovascular function. Give with great discretion when renal insufficiency is manifested by a rising or elevated BUN. When renal, cerebral or coronary blood flow is deficient, avoid any additional impairment which might result from hypotension. Use with caution in patients with marked cerebral and coronary arteriosclerosis or after a recent cerebral vascular accident.

The action of mecamylamine may be potentiated by: Excessive heat; fever; infection; hemorrhage; pregnancy; anesthesia; surgery; vigorous exercise; other antihypertensive drugs; alcohol; salt depletion resulting from diminished intake or increased excretion due to diarrhea, vomiting, excessive sweating or diuretics. During therapy, do not restrict sodium intake; if necessary, adjust the dosage.

Urinary retention may occur; use caution in patients with prostatic hypertrophy, bladder neck obstruction and urethral stricture.

Adverse Reactions:

GI: Anorexia; dry mouth; glossitis; nausea; vomiting; constipation (sometimes preceded by small, frequent, liquid stools); ileus.

Frequent loose bowel movements with abdominal distention and decreased borborygmi may be the first signs of paralytic ileus. Discontinue the drug immediately and take remedial steps.

Cardiovascular: Orthostatic dizziness; syncope.

Respiratory: Interstitial pulmonary edema; fibrosis; postural hypotension.

CNS: Weakness; fatigue; sedation; dilated pupils; blurred vision; paresthesia. Rarely, tremor; choreiform movements; mental aberrations; convulsions.

GU: Decreased libido; impotence; urinary retention.

(Continued on following page)

MECAMYLAMINE HCl (Cont.)

Overdosage:

Signs of overdosage include: Hypotension (which may progress to peripheral vascular collapse); postural hypotension; nausea; vomiting; diarrhea; constipation; paralytic ileus; urinary retention; dizziness; anxiety; dry mouth; mydriasis; blurred vision or palpitations. A rise in intraocular pressure may occur.

Pressor amines may be used to counteract excessive hypotension. Since patients treated with ganglion blockers are more than normally reactive to pressor amines, use small doses to avoid excessive response.

Patient Information:

Take after meals. Timing of doses in relation to meals should be consistent.

Notify physician if tremor or signs of ileus occur.

Mecamylamine may cause dizziness, lightheadedness or fainting, especially when rising from a lying or sitting position. This effect may be increased by alcoholic beverages, exercise or hot weather. Arising slowly may alleviate such symptoms.

Administration and Dosage:

Start with 2.5 mg twice daily. Adjust dosage in increments of 2.5 mg at intervals of not less than 2 days until the desired blood pressure response occurs (a dosage just under that which causes signs of mild postural hypotension).

The average total daily dosage is 25 mg, usually in 3 divided doses. However, as little as 2.5 mg/day may be sufficient. A range of 2 to 4 or more doses may be required in severe cases when smooth control is difficult to obtain. In severe or urgent cases, larger increments at shorter intervals may be needed. Partial tolerance may develop, requiring an increase in dosage.

Administration after meals may cause a more gradual absorption and smoother control of blood pressure. The timing of doses in relation to meals should be consistent. Since blood pressure response is increased in the early morning, give the larger dose at noontime and in the evening. The morning dose should be relatively small or may be omitted.

Blood pressure monitoring: Determine the initial and maintenance dosage by blood pressure readings in the erect position at the time of maximal drug effect, as well as by other signs and symptoms of orthostatic hypertension.

Limit the effective maintenance dose to that which causes slight faintness or dizziness in the erect posture. If the patient or a relative can use a sphygmomanometer, instructions may be given to reduce or omit a dose if readings fall below a designated level or if faintness or lightheadedness occurs. However, do not institute any changes without consulting a physician.

Close supervision, patient education and critical dosage adjustment are essential to successful therapy.

Concomitant antihypertensive therapy: Reduce the dosage of other agents, as well as that of mecamylamine, to avoid excessive hypotension. However, continue thiazides in usual dosage while decreasing mecamylamine by at least 50%.

				C.I.*
Rx	**Inversine** (MSD)	**Tablets:** 2.5 mg	(#MSD 52). Yellow, scored. In 100s.	144

* Cost Index based on cost per 2.5 mg.

\# Product identification code.

TOLAZOLINE HCl

Actions:

Pharmacology: Tolazoline is a direct peripheral vasodilator with moderate competitive alpha-adrenergic blocking activity. It decreases peripheral resistance and increases venous capacitance. It has the following actions: (1) Sympathomimetic, including cardiac stimulation; (2) parasympathomimetic, including GI tract stimulation that is blocked by atropine; and (3) histamine-like, including stimulation of gastric secretion and peripheral vasodilatation. Tolazoline given IV produces vasodilatation, primarily due to a direct effect on vascular smooth muscle and cardiac stimulation; blood pressure response depends on the relative contributions of the two effects. Tolazoline usually reduces pulmonary arterial pressure and vascular resistance.

In neonates, half-life ranges from 3 to 10 hours.

Indications:

Persistent pulmonary hypertension of the newborn ("persistent fetal circulation") when systemic arterial oxygenation cannot be satisfactorily maintained by usual supportive care (supplemental oxygen or mechanical ventilation).

Contraindications:

Hypersensitivity to tolazoline.

Warnings:

Gastric secretion is stimulated by tolazoline which may activate stress ulcers. Through this mechanism, it can produce significant hypochloremic alkalosis. Pretreatment of infants with antacids may prevent GI bleeding.

Hypotension: Observe closely for signs of systemic hypotension. Institute supportive therapy if needed.

Usage in mitral stenosis: May produce either a fall or a rise in pulmonary artery pressure and total pulmonary resistance. Use with caution in known or suspected mitral stenosis.

Usage in Pregnancy: Category C. Safety for use during pregnancy has not been established. Use only when clearly needed and when the potential benefits outweigh the potential hazards to the fetus.

Usage in Lactation: It is not known whether this drug is excreted in breast milk. Safety for use in the nursing mother has not been established. Exercise caution when administering to a nursing woman.

Precautions:

Use tolazoline in a highly supervised setting, where vital signs, oxygenation, acid-base status and fluid and electrolytes can be monitored and maintained.

The effects of tolazoline on pulmonary vessels may be pH-dependent. Acidosis may decrease the effect.

Drug Interactions:

Epinephrine administration with large doses of tolazoline may cause "epinephrine reversal" (further reduction in blood pressure followed by exaggerated rebound).

Adverse Reactions:

Cardiovascular: Hypotension; tachycardia; cardiac arrhythmias; hypertension; pulmonary hemorrhage.

GI: GI hemorrhage; nausea; vomiting; diarrhea; hepatitis.

Dermatologic: Flushing; increased pilomotor activity with tingling or chilliness; rash.

Hematologic: Thrombocytopenia; leukopenia.

Renal: Edema; oliguria; hematuria.

Overdosage:

Symptoms: Increased pilomotor activity, peripheral vasodilatation and skin flushing, and in rare instances, hypotension and shock.

Treatment: In treating hypotension, place the patient in the Trendelenburg position and administer IV fluids. Do not use epinephrine since large doses of tolazoline may cause "epinephrine reversal."

Administration and Dosage:

Initial dose: 1 to 2 mg/kg, via scalp vein over 10 minutes. Follow by an infusion of 1 to 2 mg/kg/hour to significantly increase arterial oxygen. There is very little experience with infusions lasting beyond 36 to 48 hours. Response, if it occurs, can be expected within 30 minutes after the initial dose.

Storage: Store between 15° to 30°C (59° to 86°F). Protect from light.

				C.I.*
Rx	**Priscoline HCl** (Ciba)	**Injection:** 25 mg per ml	In 4 ml amps.[1]	14054

* Cost Index based on cost per 25 mg.

[1] With 0.65% tartaric acid, 0.5% anhydrous chlorobutanol and 0.65% hydrous sodium citrate.

Effective management of many hypertensive patients frequently requires concomitant administration of two or more antihypertensive agents when adequate control is not achieved by a single drug. Synergistic effects are achieved by administration of antihypertensive drugs which act by different mechanisms; therefore, dose-related side effects may be minimized.

The following fixed combination drugs are not indicated for initial therapy of hypertension. Establish proper therapy by adjusting the dosage of each agent to patient response. Periodically reevaluate antihypertensive therapy as conditions in each patient warrant. If a fixed combination product represents a satisfactory dosage determined for the patient, its use may be more convenient.

For complete information concerning the components of the antihypertensive combination products, consult the appropriate drug monographs as indicated below:

THIAZIDE and RELATED DIURETICS:
- Bendroflumethiazide
- Chlorothiazide
- Chlorthalidone
- Flumethiazide
- Hydrochlorothiazide
- Hydroflumethiazide
- Methyclothiazide
- Polythiazide
- Quinethazone
- Trichlormethiazide

BETA-ADRENERGIC BLOCKING AGENTS:
- Atenolol
- Labetalol
- Nadolol
- Propranolol
- Timolol

ANTIADRENERGIC AGENTS:
- Clonidine
- Guanethidine
- Methyldopa
- Prazosin

RAUWOLFIA DERIVATIVES:
- Deserpidine
- Rauwolfia Serpentina
- Reserpine

ANGIOTENSIN CONVERTING ENZYME INHIBITORS:
- Captopril
- Enalapril

MISCELLANEOUS:
- Cryptenamine
- Hydralazine
- Pargyline
- Potassium Chloride

(Products listed on following pages)

ANTIHYPERTENSIVE COMBINATIONS (Cont.)

Refer to the general discussion of these products on page 850.

	Product and Distributor	Diuretic	Other Content	How Supplied	C.I.*
Rx	**Corzide Tablets 80/5** (Princeton Pharmaceuticals)	5 mg bendroflumethiazide	80 mg nadolol	(#284). White and blue mottled. Scored. In 100s.	1494
Rx	**Corzide Tablets 40/5** (Princeton Pharmaceuticals)	5 mg bendroflumethiazide	40 mg nadolol	(#283). White and blue mottled. Scored. In 100s.	1132
Rx	**Timolide 10-25 Tablets** (MSD)	25 mg hydrochlorothiazide	10 mg timolol maleate	(#Timolide MSD 67). Lt. blue. In 100s.	701
Rx	**Inderide LA 160/50 Capsules** (Wyeth-Ayerst)	50 mg hydrochlorothiazide	160 mg propranolol HCl	Long-acting. (#Inderide LA 160/50). Brown with gold bands. In 100s.	1314
Rx	**Inderide LA 120/50 Capsules** (Wyeth-Ayerst)	50 mg hydrochlorothiazide	120 mg propranolol HCl	Long-acting. (#Inderide LA 120/50). Beige brown with gold bands. In 100s.	1124
Rx	**Inderide LA 80/50 Capsules** (Wyeth-Ayerst)	50 mg hydrochlorothiazide	80 mg propranolol HCl	Long-acting. (#Inderide LA 80/50). Beige with gold bands. In 100s.	942
Rx	**Propranolol and Hydrochlorothiazide Tablets** (Various)	25 mg hydrochlorothiazide	80 mg propranolol HCl	In 100s, 500s and 1000s.	239+
Rx	**Inderide 80/25 Tablets** (Wyeth-Ayerst)			(#Inderide 80/25). Off-white, scored. In 100s, 1000s and UD 100s.	947
Rx	**Propranolol and HCTZ Tablets** (Various)	25 mg hydrochlorothiazide	40 mg propranolol HCl	In 30s, 100s, 500s, 1000s and UD 100s.	165+
Rx	**Inderide 40/25 Tablets** (Wyeth-Ayerst)			(#Inderide 40/25). Off-white, scored. In 30s, 100s, 1000s & UD 100s.	679
Rx	**Normozide Tablets** (Schering)	25 mg hydrochlorothiazide	300 mg labetalol HCl	(#Normozide 391). Blue, scored. Film coated. In 100s.	882
Rx	**Trandate HCT Tablets** (Allen & Hanburys)			(#Glaxo 373). Peach. Film coated. In 100s, 500s and UD 100s.	774
Rx	**Normozide Tablets** (Schering)	25 mg hydrochlorothiazide	200 mg labetalol HCl	(#Normozide 227). White, scored. Film coated. In 100s.	663
Rx	**Trandate HCT Tablets** (Allen & Hanburys)			(#Glaxo 372). White. Film coated. In 100s, 500s and UD 100s.	582

* Cost Index based on cost per capsule or tablet.
# Product identification code.

(Continued on following page)

ANTIHYPERTENSIVE COMBINATIONS (Cont.)

Refer to the general discussion of these products on page 850.

	Product and Distributor	Diuretic	Other Content	How Supplied	C.I.*
Rx	**Normozide Tablets** (Schering)	25 mg hydrochlorothiazide	100 mg labetalol HCl	(#Normozide 235). Light brown, scored. Film coated. In 100s.	452
Rx	**Trandate HCT Tablets** (Allen & Hanburys)			(#Glaxo 371). Peach. Film coated. In 100s, 500s and UD 100s	397
Rx	**Methyldopa and Hydrochlorothiazide Tablets** (Various)	50 mg hydrochlorothiazide	500 mg methyldopa	In 100s, 250s and 500s.	535+
Rx	**Aldoril D50 Tablets** (MSD)			(#MSD 935). White. Film coated. In 100s.	1016
Rx	**Methyldopa and Hydrochlorothiazide Tablets** (Various)	30 mg hydrochlorothiazide	500 mg methyldopa	In 100s, 250s and 500s.	521+
Rx	**Aldoril D30 Tablets** (MSD)			(#MSD 694). Salmon. Film coated. In 100s.	945
Rx	**Aldoclor-250 Tablets** (MSD)	250 mg chlorothiazide	250 mg methyldopa	(#MSD 634). Green. Film coated. In 100s.	595
Rx	**Aldoclor-150 Tablets** (MSD)	150 mg chlorothiazide	250 mg methyldopa	(#MSD 612). Beige. Film coated. In 100s.	525
Rx	**Methyldopa and Hydrochlorothiazide Tablets** (Various)	25 mg hydrochlorothiazide	250 mg methyldopa	In 60s, 100s, 500s and 1000s.	259+
Rx	**Aldoril-25 Tablets** (MSD)			(#MSD 456). White. Film coated. In 100s, 1000s and UD 100s.	595
Rx	**Alodopa-25 Tablets** (Major)			In 100s	250
Rx	**Methyldopa and HCTZ Tablets** (Various)	15 mg hydrochlorothiazide	250 mg methyldopa	In 100s, 500s and 1000s.	247+
Rx	**Aldoril-15 Tablets** (MSD)			(#MSD 423). Salmon. Film coated. In 100s, 1000s and UD 100s.	525
Rx	**Alodopa-15 Tablets** (Major)			In 100s.	230
Rx	**Lopressor HCT 100/50 Tablets** (Geigy)	50 mg hydrochlorothiazide	100 mg metoprolol tartrate	(#Geigy 73 73). White and yellow, scored. In 100s.	1039
Rx	**Lopressor HCT 100/25 Tablets** (Geigy)	25 mg hydrochlorothiazide	100 mg metoprolol tartrate	(#Geigy 53 53). White and pink, scored. In 100s.	980
Rx	**Lopressor HCT 50/25 Tablets** (Geigy)	25 mg hydrochlorothiazide	50 mg metoprolol tartrate	(#Geigy 35 35). White and blue, scored. In 100s.	629

* Cost Index based on cost per tablet.

\# Product identification code.

(Continued on following page)

ANTIHYPERTENSIVE COMBINATIONS (Cont.)

Refer to the general discussion of these products on page 850 .

	Product and Distributor	Diuretic	Other Content	How Supplied	C.I.*
Rx	**Capozide 50/25 Tablets** (Squibb)	25 mg hydrochlorothiazide	50 mg captopril	(#390). Peach, scored. In 100s.	1156
Rx	**Capozide 25/25 Tablets** (Squibb)	25 mg hydrochlorothiazide	25 mg captopril	(#349). Peach, scored. In 100s.	702
Rx	**Capozide 50/15 Tablets** (Squibb)	15 mg hydrochlorothiazide	50 mg captopril	(#384). White/orange. In 100s.	1141
Rx	**Capozide 25/15 Tablets** (Squibb)	15 mg hydrochlorothiazide	25 mg captopril	(#338). White/orange. In 100s.	687
Rx	**Vaseretic 10-25 Tablets** (MSD)	25 mg hydrochlorothiazide	10 mg enalapril maleate	(# Vaseretic MSD 720). Red. In 100s.	1265
Rx	**Prinzide 25 Tablets** (MSD)	25 mg hydrochlorothiazide	20 mg lisinopril	(#MSD 142 Prinzide). In 30s and 100s.	1236
Rx	**Zestoretic Tablets** (Stuart)			(#Stuart 145). Peach. In 100s.	N/A
Rx	**Prinzide 12.5 Tablets** (MSD)	12.5 mg hydrochlorothiazide	20 mg lisinopril	(#MSD 140 Prinzide). In 30s and 100s.	1221
Rx	**Zestoretic Tablets** (Stuart)			(#Stuart 142). White. In 100s.	N/A
Rx	**Clonidine HCl and Chlorthalidone Tablets** (Various)	15 mg chlorthalidone	0.3 mg clonidine HCl	In 100s.	591+
Rx	**Combipres 0.3 Tablets (Boehringer Ingelheim)**			(#BI 10). White, scored. In 100s.	1028
Rx	**Clonidine HCl and Chlorthalidone Tablets** (Various)	15 mg chlorthalidone	0.2 mg clonidine HCl	In 100s, 500s and 1000s.	350+
Rx	**Combipres 0.2 Tablets** (BI)			(#BI 9). Blue, scored. In 100s & 1000s.	518
Rx	**Clonidine HCl and Chlorthalidone Tablets** (Various)	15 mg chlorthalidone	0.1 mg clonidine HCl	In 100s, 500s and 1000s.	350+
Rx	**Combipres 0.1 Tablets** (BI)			(#BI 8). Pink, scored. In 100s, 1000s.	636
Rx	**Minizide 5 Capsules** (Pfizer)	0.5 mg polythiazide	5 mg prazosin HCl	(#Pfizer Minizide 436). Blue-green and blue. In 100s.	1109
Rx	**Minizide 2 Capsules** (Pfizer)	0.5 mg polythiazide	2 mg prazosin HCl	(#Pfizer Minizide 432). Blue-green and pink. In 100s.	753
Rx	**Minizide 1 Capsules** (Pfizer)	0.5 mg polythiazide	1 mg prazosin HCl	(#Pfizer Minizide 430). Blue-green. In 100s.	598
Rx	**Esimil Tablets** (Ciba)	25 mg hydrochlorothiazide	10 mg guanethidine monosulfate	(#Ciba 47). White, scored. In 100s.	780
Rx	**Eutron Filmtabs** (Abbott)	5 mg methyclothiazide	25 mg pargyline HCl	(#Abbott NK). Light purple. In 100s.	6705
Rx	**Diutensen Tablets** (Wallace)	2.5 mg methyclothiazide	2 mg cryptenamine (as tannate)	White-blue mottled. In 100s and 500s.	1081

* Cost Index based on cost per capsule or tablet. # Product identification code.

SODIUM POLYSTYRENE SULFONATE

Actions:

Sodium polystyrene sulfonate is a cation exchange resin used for the reduction of elevated potassium levels. As the resin passes along the intestine, or is retained in the colon after administration by enema, the sodium ions are partially released and are replaced by potassium ions. This action occurs primarily in the large intestine. The efficiency of this process is limited and unpredictable. Although the exchange capacity in vitro approximates 3.1 mEq potassium per gram, in vivo it is approximately 33%, or 1 mEq potassium per gram; however, the range is so large that electrolyte balance must be monitored. Onset of action after oral administration ranges from 2 to 12 hours, and is longer after rectal administration.

Indications:

Treatment of hyperkalemia.

Warnings:

Severe hyperkalemia: Since effective lowering of serum potassium may take hours to days, treatment with this drug alone may be insufficient to rapidly correct severe hyperkalemia associated with states of rapid tissue breakdown (eg, burns and renal failure) or hyperkalemia so marked as to constitute a medical emergency. Consider other definitive measures, including the use of IV calcium to antagonize the effects of hyperkalemia on the heart, IV sodium bicarbonate or glucose and insulin to cause an intracellular shift of potassium, or dialysis.

Hypokalemia: Serious potassium deficiency can occur. Carefully control by frequent serum potassium determinations within each 24 hour period. Since intracellular potassium deficiency is not always reflected by serum potassium levels, determine the level at which treatment should be discontinued based on the patient's clinical condition and ECG. Early clinical signs of severe hypokalemia include irritable confusion and delayed thought processes. It is often associated with a lengthened QT interval, widening, flattening or inversion of the T wave and prominent U waves. Cardiac arrhythmias may occur, such as premature atrial, nodal and ventricular contractions, and supraventricular and ventricular tachycardias. Toxic effects of digitalis are likely to be exaggerated. Severe muscle weakness, at times extending into paralysis, may also occur.

Electrolyte imbalance: Sodium polystyrene sulfonate is not totally selective for potassium, and small amounts of other cations (magnesium and calcium) can also be lost during treatment. Accordingly, monitor patients for all applicable electrolyte disturbances.

Precautions:

Sodium: Use caution when administering to patients who cannot tolerate even a small increase in sodium loads (ie, severe congestive heart failure, severe hypertension or marked edema). One gram contains 100 mg (4.1 mEq) sodium, with about one-third being delivered to the body. Compensatory restriction of sodium intake from other sources may be indicated.

Constipation, if it occurs, is treated with 10 to 20 ml of 70% sorbitol every 2 hours or as needed to produce one or two watery stools daily. This measure also reduces any tendency toward fecal impaction.

Drug Interactions:

Nonabsorbable cation donating antacids and **laxatives** (eg, magnesium hydroxide, aluminum carbonate): Systemic alkalosis has been reported after cation-exchange resins were administered orally in combination with these drugs. Do not administer **magnesium hydroxide** with sodium polystyrene sulfonate. A grand mal seizure has been reported in one patient with chronic hypocalcemia of renal failure who was given sodium polystyrene sulfonate with magnesium hydroxide as a laxative. The simultaneous oral administration of sodium polystyrene sulfonate with these drugs may reduce the resin's potassium exchange capability. The effects of this interaction have only been demonstrated in patients with renal failure.

Adverse Reactions:

GI: Gastric irritation; anorexia, nausea, vomiting and constipation may occur, especially with high doses. Occasionally, diarrhea develops. Large doses in elderly individuals may cause fecal impaction, which may be obviated through use of the resin in enemas. Intestinal obstruction, due to concretions of aluminum hydroxide when used in combination with sodium polystyrene sulfonate, has been reported.

Electrolyte balance: Hypokalemia, hypocalcemia and sodium retention.

(Continued on following page)

Overdosage:

Overzealous instillation may result in unnecessary dilatation of the myocardial vasculature and leakage into the perivascular myocardium, possibly causing tissue edema.

Administration and Dosage:

The following information is a guide:

Following institution of cardiopulmonary bypass at perfusate temperatures of 28° to 30°C, (82° to 86°F) and cross-clamping of the ascending aorta, administer the buffered solution by rapid infusion into the aortic root. The initial rate of infusion may be 300 ml/m²/minute (about 540 ml/min in a 1.8 meter, 70 kg adult with 1.8 square meters of surface area) given for 2 to 4 minutes. Concurrent external cooling (regional hypothermia of the pericardium) may be accomplished by instilling a refrigerated (4°C) physiologic solution such as *Normosol-R* (balanced electrolyte replacement solution) or Ringer's Injection into the chest cavity. If myocardial electromechanical activity persists or recurs, the solution may be reinfused at a rate of 300 ml/m²/min for 2 minutes. Repeat every 20 to 30 minutes or sooner if myocardial temperature rises above 15° to 20°C or returning cardiac activity is observed. The regional hypothermia solution around the heart also may be replenished continuously or periodically in order to maintain adequate hypothermia. Suction may be used to remove warmed infusates. An implanted thermistor probe may be used to monitor myocardial temperature.

The volumes of solution instilled into the aortic root may vary depending on the duration or type of open heart surgical procedure.

Preparation of solution: The solution contains no preservatives and is intended only for a single operative procedure. After adjusting pH with sodium bicarbonate, extemporaneous alternative buffering is not recommended. Discard the unused portion.

Add 10 ml (840 mg) of 8.4% Sodium Bicarbonate Injection (10 mEq each of sodium and bicarbonate) to each 1000 ml of the cardioplegic solution just prior to administration to adjust pH to approximately 7.8 when measured at room temperature. Use of any other Sodium Bicarbonate Injection may not achieve this pH due to the varying pH's of Sodium Bicarbonate Injections. Cool the buffered solution with added sodium bicarbonate to 4°C prior to administration and use within 24 hours of mixing.

Admixture incompatibility: Additives may be incompatible. Consult with pharmacist, if possible. When introducing additives, use aseptic technique, mix thoroughly and do not store.

Storage: Store at 25°C (77°F); however, brief exposure up to 40°C (104°F) does not adversely affect the product. Protect from freezing and extreme heat.

Rx	**Plegisol** (Abbott)	**Solution:** 17.6 mg calcium chloride dihydrate, 325.3 mg magnesium chloride hexahydrate, 119.3 mg potassium chloride and 643 mg sodium chloride per 100 ml (approx. 260 mOsm/L)	In single dose 1000 ml flexible plastic container.

Food seasoning to be used as a substitute for salt (NaCl) at the table or in cooking to help regulate dietary sodium intake. Appropriate for persons on low sodium diets (ie, persons whose sodium intake has been restricted for medical reasons).

For normal healthy people. Persons having diabetes, heart or kidney disease or persons receiving medical treatment should consult a physician before using a salt substitute or alternative.

Contraindications:

Hyperkalemia, oliguria and severe kidney disease.

Caution:

Evaluate the potassium intake of persons receiving potassium-sparing diuretics or potassium supplementation. Use with extreme caution in these patients.

Excessive sodium depletion may lead to symptoms such as weakness, nausea and muscle cramps; in severe cases, uremia may follow. On the appearance of early symptoms, liberalize sodium intake.

Salt substitutes contain a significant amount of potassium and other electrolytes. Excessive use could result in hyperkalemia.

	Product and Distributor	Contents	Sodium Content[1]		Potassium Content[1]		How Supplied
			mg/5 g	mEq/5 g	mg/5 g	mEq/5 g	
otc	**Adolph's Salt Substitute** (Adolph's)	potassium chloride, silicon dioxide and tartaric acid	0	0	2480	64	In 99.2 g.
otc	**Morton Salt Substitute** (Morton Salt)	potassium chloride, fumaric acid, tricalcium phosphate and monocalcium phosphate	<0.5	<0.02	2515	64	In 88.6 g.
otc	**Adolph's Seasoned Salt Substitute** (Adolph's)	potassium chloride, silicon dioxide, tartaric acid, sugar, paprika, garlic and onion powder, cottonseed and soybean oil	0	0	1360	35	In 92.1 g.
otc	**Morton Seasoned Salt Substitute** (Morton Salt)	potassium chloride, spices, sugar, fumaric acid, tricalcium phosphate, monocalcium phosphate	<1	<0.04	2165	56	In 85.1 g.
otc	**NoSalt Seasoned** (Norcliff Thayer)	potassium chloride, dextrose, onion and garlic, spices, lactose, cream of tartar, paprika, silica, disodium inosinate, disodium guanylate, turmeric and extractives of paprika	<5	<0.2	1328	34	In 240 g.
otc	**NoSalt** (Norcliff Thayer)	potassium chloride, potassium bitartrate, adipic acid, mineral oil and fumaric acid	<10	<0.43	2502	64	In 330 g.
otc	**Nu-Salt** (Cumberland Pkg.)	potassium chloride, potassium bitartrate, calcium silicate, natural flavor derived from yeast	0.85	<0.04	2640	68	In 100 g.

[1] The amounts of sodium and potassium given are approximate values.

EDETATE DISODIUM (EDTA)

> **Warning:** Use of this drug is recommended only when the severity of the clinical condition justifies the aggressive measures associated with this type of therapy.

Actions:

Edetate disodium (EDTA) forms chelates with many divalent and trivalent metals. Because of its affinity for calcium, EDTA will lower serum calcium levels during IV infusion. Slow infusion may cause mobilization of extracirculatory calcium stores. The chelate formed is excreted in the urine. EDTA exerts a negative inotropic effect on the heart.

Additionally, EDTA forms chelates with other polyvalent metals, thus increasing urinary excretion of magnesium, zinc and other trace elements. It does not chelate with potassium, but may reduce the serum level; increased potassium excretion may occur.

Indications:

Emergency treatment of hypercalcemia.

Control of ventricular arrhythmias associated with digitalis toxicity.

See also Edetate Calcium Disodium.

Unlabeled Uses: Chelation treatment is not indicated for atherosclerotic vascular diseases. Although it has been advocated for these diseases (eg, coronary artery disease, cerebrovascular disease, peripheral vascular disease) based on the theory of decalcification of atherosclerotic plaques, both the proposed explanations of pathogenesis and mechanism of action are suspect. In addition, EDTA is not innocuous. The medical community generally agrees that chelation therapy is not an acceptable treatment for atherosclerotic vascular diseases.

Contraindications:

Anuria. Hypersensitivity to any component of the preparation.

Warnings:

Rapid IV infusion or a high serum concentration of EDTA may cause a precipitous drop in serum calcium and may result in death. Toxicity depends on total dosage and rate of administration. Do not exceed recommended dosage and rates of administration.

Dilution before infusion is necessary because of its irritant effect on the tissues and because of the danger of serious side effects.

Renal function: Prior to treatment, assess renal excretory function; perform periodic BUN and creatinine determinations and daily urinalysis during treatment.

Monitoring: Because of the possibility of inducing an electrolyte imbalance during treatment, perform appropriate laboratory determinations to evaluate cardiac status. Repeat as often as clinically indicated, particularly in patients with ventricular arrhythmia and those with a history of seizures or intracranial lesions. If clinical evidence suggests any disturbance of liver function during treatment, perform appropriate laboratory determinations; withdraw drug if required.

Calcium – The oxalate method of determining serum calcium tends to give low readings in the presence of EDTA; modification (ie, acidifying the sample) or use of a different method may be required for accuracy. The least interference will be noted immediately before a subsequent dose is administered.

Hypokalemia – Use with caution in patients with clinical or subclinical potassium deficiency; monitor serum potassium levels and ECG changes.

Hypomagnesemia should be kept in mind during prolonged therapy.

Blood sugar and insulin requirements may be lower in insulin-dependent diabetics.

Usage in Pregnancy: Category C. Safety for use during pregnancy has not been established. Use only when clearly needed and when the potential benefits outweigh the potential hazards to the fetus.

Usage in Lactation: Safety for use in the nursing mother has not been established.

Precautions:

After infusion, have the patient remain supine for a short time because of the possibility of postural hypotension.

Cardiac effects: Consider the possibility of an adverse effect on myocardial contractility when administering the drug to patients with heart disease. Use this drug cautiously in patients with limited cardiac reserve or incipient congestive failure.

(Continued on following page)

EDETATE DISODIUM (EDTA) (Cont.)

Adverse Reactions:

GI: Nausea, vomiting and diarrhea (fairly common).

CNS: Transient circumoral paresthesia, numbness and headache.

Other: Transient drop in systolic and diastolic blood pressure; thrombophlebitis, febrile reactions; hyperuricemia; anemia; exfoliative dermatitis; other toxic skin and mucous membrane reactions. Nephrotoxicity and damage to the reticuloendothelial system with hemorrhagic tendencies have been reported with excessive dosages.

Overdosage:

Because EDTA may produce a precipitous drop in the serum calcium, have an IV calcium salt (such as calcium gluconate) available. Exercise extreme caution in the use of IV calcium in the treatment of tetany, especially in digitalized patients, because the action of the drug and the replacement of calcium ions may produce a reversal of the desired digitalis effect.

Administration and Dosage:

Adults: Administer 50 mg/kg/day to a maximum dose of 3 g in 24 hours. Dissolve dose in 500 ml of 5% Dextrose Injection or 0.9% Sodium Chloride Injection. Infuse over 3 or more hours and do not exceed the patient's cardiac reserve. A suggested regimen includes 5 consecutive daily doses followed by 2 days without medication, with repeated courses, as necessary, to a total of 15 doses.

Children: Administer 40 mg/kg/day (18 mg/lb) to a maximum dose of 70 mg/kg/day. Another source has recommended a range of 15 to 50 mg/kg/day to a maximum of 3 g/day, allowing 5 days between courses. Dissolve in a sufficient volume of 5% Dextrose Injection or 0.9% Sodium Chloride Injection to bring the final concentration to not more than 3%. Infuse over 3 or more hours; do not exceed the patient's cardiac reserve.

Storage: Store at room temperature. Brief exposures up to 40°C (104°F) do not adversely affect the product.

	Product	Form	Package	**C.I.***
Rx	**Edetate Disodium** (Various)	**Injection:** 150 mg per ml	In 20 ml vials.	5+
Rx	**Chealamide** (Vortech)		In 20 ml vials.	10
Rx	**Disotate** (Forest)		In 20 ml vials.	10
Rx	**Endrate** (Abbott)		In 20 ml amps.	53

* Cost Index based on cost per 50 mg.

Treatment of hyperlipidemia is based on the assumption that lowering serum lipids decreases morbidity and mortality of atherosclerotic cardiovascular disease. Hyperlipidemia, particularly elevated serum cholesterol and low density lipoprotein (LDL) levels, is a risk factor in the development of atherosclerotic cardiovascular disease. The National Heart, Lung and Blood Institute Type II Coronary Intervention Study demonstrated that cholestyramine and diet therapy decreased total cholesterol and LDL levels and retarded the progression of coronary artery disease (assessed by angiography) in patients with Type II hyperlipoproteinemia (*Circulation* 1984;69:313-37). The Lipid Research Clinics Coronary Primary Prevention Trial demonstrated that cholestyramine and diet therapy decreased LDL cholesterol in Type II hyperlipoproteinemia and was associated with a significant reduction (19%) in the risk of coronary heart disease (deaths and nonfatal infarcts) (*JAMA* 1984;251:351-64).

Individually assess potential benefits and risks of therapy. The cornerstone of treatment in primary hyperlipidemia is diet restriction and weight reduction. Limit or eliminate alcohol intake. Use drug therapy in conjunction with diet, and after maximal efforts to control serum lipids by diet alone prove unsatisfactory, when tolerance to or compliance with diet is poor or when hyperlipidemia is severe and risk of complications is high. Treat contributory diseases such as hypothyroidism or diabetes mellitus.

Elevated blood cholesterol levels are a major cause of coronary artery disease. Lowering these levels (specifically, LDL cholesterol) will reduce the risk of heart attacks caused by coronary heart disease (CHD). Risk factors for CHD include: Male sex, family history of premature CHD, smoking, hypertension, low HDL-cholesterol, diabetes mellitus, definite cerebrovascular or peripheral vascular disease and severe obesity. All Americans (except children < 2 years old) should adopt a diet that reduces total dietary fat, decreases intake of saturated fat, increases intake of polyunsaturated fat and reduces daily cholesterol intake to 250 to 300 mg or less. The National Cholesterol Education Program of the National Heart, Lung and Blood Institute has provided guidelines for the treatment of high blood cholesterol in adults ≥ 20 years of age (*Arch Intern Med 1988;148:36-69)*:

Classification of Total Cholesterol Levels	
Level (mg/dl)	Classification
< 200	desirable
200-239	borderline-high
≥ 240	high

1. Level < 200 mg/dl: Give general dietary and risk reduction education materials, repeat serum cholesterol test within 5 years.
2. Level > 200 mg/dl: Confirm level with repeat test; use average of two tests as guide for subsequent treatment.
3. Level 200 to 239 mg/dl without definite CHD or two other risk factors: Provide dietary information and recheck annually.
4. Level 200 to 239 mg/dl with CHD or two other risk factors, or level > 240 mg/dl: Complete lipoprotein analysis. Base further action on LDL-cholesterol level as follows:

Classification of LDL-Cholesterol Levels	
Level (mg/dl)	Classification
< 130	desirable
130-159	borderline-high
≥ 160	high

1. Level ≥ 160 mg/dl without CHD or two other risk factors, or level ≥ 130 mg/dl with CHD or two other risk factors: Dietary treatment.
2. Level ≥ 190 mg/dl without CHD or two other risk factors, or level ≥ 160 mg/dl with CHD or two other risk factors: Drug treatment.

(Continued on following page)

Hyperlipidemias: Elevation of serum cholesterol, triglycerides or both is characteristic of hyperlipidemias. Differentiation of the specific biochemical abnormality requires identification of specific lipoprotein fractions in the serum. Lipoproteins transport serum lipids and are identified by their density and electrophoretic mobility. Chylomicrons are the largest and least dense of the lipoproteins, followed in order of increasing density and decreasing size by very low density lipoproteins (VLDL or pre-β), intermediate low density lipoproteins (ILDL or broad-β), low density lipoproteins (LDL or β) and high density lipoproteins (HDL or α). Triglycerides are transported primarily by chylomicrons and VLDL; the predominant cholesterol transporting lipoprotein is LDL.

Elevations and treatment associated with each type of hyperlipidemia follow:

HYPERLIPIDEMIAS AND THEIR TREATMENT

Hyperlipidemia Type	I	IIa	IIb	III	IV	V
Lipids						
Cholesterol	N-⇧	↑	↑	N-↑	N-⇧	N-↑
Triglycerides	↑	N	↑	N-↑	↑	↑
Lipoproteins						
Chylomicrons	↑	N	N	N	N	↑
VLDL (pre-β)	N-⇧	N-↓	↑	N-⇧	↑	↑
ILDL (broad-β)[1]				↑		
LDL (β)	↓	↑	↑	↑	N-⇩	↓
HDL (α)	↓	N	N	N	N-⇩	↓
Treatment	Diet	Diet Cholestyramine Colestipol Dextrothyroxine Nicotinic acid Probucol Lovastatin	Diet Cholestyramine[2] Colestipol[2] Probucol[2] Clofibrate[3] Gemfibrozil[4] Nicotinic acid Lovastatin	Diet Clofibrate Nicotinic acid	Diet Clofibrate Gemfibrozil Nicotinic acid	Diet Clofibrate Gemfibrozil Nicotinic acid[5]

N = normal ↑ = increase ↓ = decrease ⇧ = slight increase ⇩ = slight decrease

[1] An abnormal lipoprotein. [2] Particularly useful if hypercholesterolemia predominates.

[3] With high serum triglyceride levels and moderately elevated cholesterol.

[4] In patients with inadequate response to weight loss, bile acid sequestrants and nicotinic acid.

[5] Norethindrone acetate (women) and oxandrolone (men) are effective, but use is not FDA-approved.

Dietary Treatment: Reducing elevated cholesterol levels and maintaining adequate nutrition is the aim of dietary therapy. Step-One and Step-Two diets are specifically designed to progressively reduce saturated fatty acids and cholesterol intake and promote weight loss in overweight individuals.

Step-One: Total fat intake < 30% of calories; saturated fatty acid intake < 10% of calories; cholesterol intake < 300 mg/day. Measure serum total cholesterol and adherence to diet at 4 to 6 weeks and at 3 months. If cholesterol and LDL level goals are met, monitor quarterly the first year and twice yearly thereafter. If response is insufficient, proceed to Step-Two.

Step-Two: Saturated fatty acid intake < 7% of calories; cholesterol intake < 200 mg/day. Measure serum total cholesterol and adherence to diet at 4 to 6 weeks and at 3 months. Begin long-term monitoring if goal has been met. Consider drug therapy if goal has not been attained. Carry out intensive diet therapy and counseling before starting drug therapy. Continue dietary treatment during drug treatment.

(Continued on following page)

Drug Treatment:

Cholestyramine, colestipol, probucol and dextrothyroxine are used to lower cholesterol. Clofibrate, gemfibrozil lovastatin and nicotinic acid are used to lower both cholesterol and triglycerides. Serum triglycerides are lowered much more effectively by clofibrate and gemfibrozil, than are cholesterol levels. When both cholesterol and triglycerides are elevated, treatment of the hypertriglyceridemia should take precedence. When hypercholesterolemia is treated first, an exacerbation of the hypertriglyceridemia may occur. Serum cholesterol often falls to normal levels without specific therapy following treatment of the hypertriglyceridemia.

Drugs of first choice include cholestyramine, colestipol or nicotinic acid. In patients with concurrent hypertriglyceridemia, nicotinic acid is preferred. Second-line agents include lovastatin and gemfibrozil. Lovastatin's long-term safety and effects on CHD have not been established, therefore it is not a drug of first choice. Measure LDL-cholesterol levels at 4 to 6 weeks and at 3 months. If the response is adequate, monitor every 4 months; if inadequate, switch to another agent or use a combination of two drugs. Refer patients who fail to respond to combination therapy to a lipid disorder specialist.

Combination therapy: Since drug therapy of different hyperlipoproteinemias involves different mechanisms and different pharmacologic actions, it is reasonable to consider a combined drug regimen in stubborn cases. Experience with combination therapy is, however, limited. The coadministration of a bile acid sequestrant with either nicotinic acid or lovastatin can lower LDL-cholesterol levels by 40% to 50% or more. Clofibrate added to a diet-colestipol regimen reduced total serum cholesterol 28% compared with 16% to 25% by diet plus colestipol. When cholestyramine was added to diet plus probucol, the average decrease in serum cholesterol was raised from 7.7% to 18.2%. Clofibrate and nicotinic acid also decrease elevated serum triglyceride levels caused by bile acid sequestrants. Do not use lovastatin and gemfibrozil concomitantly due to risks of myopathy, rhabdomyolysis and acute renal failure.

The following table summarizes the effects of the various antihyperlipidemic drugs on serum lipids and lipoproteins:

Antihyperlipidemic Drug Effects

Drug	Lipids		Lipoproteins		
	Cholesterol	Triglycerides	VLDL (pre-β)	LDL (β)	HDL
Cholestyramine	↓	→↑	→↑	↓	→↑
Colestipol	↓	→↑	↑	↓	→↑
Probucol	↓	→	↑↓	↓	↓
Dextrothyroxine	↓	→	→	↓	→
Clofibrate	↓	↓	↓	→↓	→↑
Gemfibrozil	↓	↓	↓	→↓	↑
Nicotinic Acid	↓	↓	↓	↓	↑
Lovastatin	↓	↓	↓	↓	↑

↓ = decrease
↑ = increase
→ = unchanged

General Considerations:

1. Define the type of hyperlipoproteinemia and establish baseline serum cholesterol and triglyceride levels.
2. Institute a trial of diet and weight reduction. Remind patients to restrict their dietary intake of cholesterol and saturated fats and adhere to prescribed dietary regimens. Drug therapy does not reduce the importance of adhering to diet.
3. Carefully monitor the patient during treatment, including serum cholesterol and triglyceride levels.
4. Consider failure of cholesterol to fall, or a significant rise in triglyceride level, as indications to discontinue medication.

(Products listed on following pages)

Refer to the general discussion of these products beginning on page 865.

Bile Acid Sequestrants

Actions:

Cholesterol is the major (and probably the sole) precursor of bile acids. During normal digestion, bile acids are secreted via the bile from the liver and gall bladder into the intestines to emulsify the fat and lipid materials in food, thus facilitating absorption. A major portion of the bile acids secreted is reabsorbed from the intestines and returned via the portal circulation to the liver, thus completing the enterohepatic cycle.

Bile acid sequestering resins bind bile acids in the intestine to form an insoluble complex which is excreted in the feces. This results in a partial removal of bile acids from the enterohepatic circulation, preventing their absorption. Since these agents are anion-exchange resins, the chloride anions of the resin are replaced by other anions. These agents are hydrophilic, but insoluble in water. They remain unchanged in the GI tract and are not absorbed. The lipid-lowering effect of 4 g cholestyramine equals 5 g colestipol.

The increased fecal loss of bile acids leads to an increased oxidation of cholesterol to bile acids and a decrease in low density lipoproteins (LDL) and serum cholesterol levels. In humans, these drugs increase the hepatic synthesis of cholesterol, but plasma cholesterol levels fall secondary to an increased rate of clearance of cholesterol-rich lipoproteins from the plasma. Serum triglyceride levels may increase 5% to 20% the first weeks of therapy, decreasing gradually to pretreatment values within 4 weeks.

The fall in LDL concentration is apparent in 4 to 7 days. Treatment with anion-exchange resins may result in a 20% reduction in LDL. The decline in serum cholesterol is usually evident by 1 month. When the resins are discontinued, serum cholesterol usually returns to baseline within 1 month. Cholesterol may rise even with continued use; determine serum levels periodically.

When bile secretion is partially blocked, serum bile acid concentration rises. In patients with partial biliary obstruction, reduction of serum bile acid levels by cholestyramine reduces bile acid deposits in the dermal tissues with resultant decrease in pruritus.

Clinical Pharmacology: Colestipol is more effective than clofibrate in lowering total serum cholesterol and LDL in Type IIa hyperlipoproteinemia without affecting high density lipoprotein (HDL) cholesterol. In patients with heterozygous familial hypercholesterolemia who do not respond optimally to colestipol alone, adding nicotinic acid effectively lowers serum cholesterol, triglyceride and LDL cholesterol, and increases HDL cholesterol values significantly. In many such patients, it is possible to normalize serum lipid values.

In a large, multiclinic study, hypercholesterolemic subjects treated with cholestyramine had significant reductions in total and low-density lipoprotein cholesterol. Over the 7 year study period, the cholestyramine group experienced a 19% reduction in the combined rate of coronary heart disease death plus non-fatal MI (cumulative incidences of 7% cholestyramine and 8.6% placebo). The subjects included in the study were middle-aged men (age 35 to 59) with serum cholesterol levels above 265 mg/dl and no previous history of heart disease. It is not clear to what extent these findings can be extrapolated to other segments of the hypercholesterolemic population.

Indications:

Hyperlipoproteinemia – (**Cholestyramine** and **colestipol**): Adjunctive therapy for the reduction of elevated serum cholesterol in patients with primary hypercholesterolemia (elevated LDL).

These agents may lower elevated cholesterol in patients who also have hypertriglyceridemia, but they are not indicated where hypertriglyceridemia is the abnormality of most concern.

Biliary obstruction-(**Cholestyramine**): Relief of pruritus associated with partial biliary obstruction.

Unlabeled Uses: Cholestyramine in vitro binds the toxin produced by *Clostridium difficile,* the causative organism of antibiotic-induced pseudomembranous colitis, with variable success. It is also effective in bile salt-mediated diarrhea and postvagotomy diarrhea.

Cholestyramine has been used in the treatment of chlordecone *(Kepone)* pesticide poisoning. By binding chlordecone in the intestine, cholestyramine inhibits its enterohepatic recirculation, increases fecal excretion and accelerates elimination from the body.

Cholestyramine and colestipol have been used in the treatment of digitalis toxicity (see Cardiac Glycosides).

Contraindications:

Hypersensitivity to bile acid sequestering resins; complete biliary obstruction.

(Continued on following page)

Bile Acid Sequestrants (Cont.)

Warnings:

To avoid accidental inhalation or esophageal distress, do not take dry. Mix with fluids.

Carcinogenesis: The incidence of intestinal tumors in studies was greater in cholestyramine-treated rats than in controls. The relevance of this observation is not known. The total incidence of fatal and nonfatal neoplasms was similar in both treatment groups. Various alimentary system cancers were more prevalent with cholestyramine. The small numbers and the multiple categories prevent conclusions from being drawn.

Usage in Pregnancy: Safety for use during pregnancy has not been established. Use only when clearly needed and when the potential benefits outweigh the potential hazards.

Since **cholestyramine** is not absorbed systemically, it is not expected to cause fetal harm when given during pregnancy in recommended dosages. However, its interference with fat-soluble vitamin absorption may be detrimental even with supplementation.

Usage in Lactation: Exercise caution when administering to a nursing woman. The possible lack of proper vitamin absorption may have an effect on nursing infants.

Usage in Children: Dosage schedules have not been established. The effects of long-term administration and effectiveness in maintaining lowered cholesterol levels are unknown.

Precautions:

Diet: Before instituting therapy, a vigorous attempt should be made to control serum cholesterol by an appropriate dietary regimen and weight reduction.

Investigate and treat diseases contributing to increased blood cholesterol before starting therapy (eg, hypothyroidism, diabetes mellitus, nephrotic syndrome, dysproteinemias and obstructive liver disease). Cholesterol reduction should occur during the first month of therapy. Continue therapy to sustain cholesterol reduction. If adequate reduction is not attained, discontinue therapy.

Malabsorption: Because they sequester bile acids, these resins may interfere with normal fat absorption and digestion and may prevent absorption of fat-soluble vitamins such as A, D, E and K. With long-term therapy, supplemental vitamins A and D may be given in a water-miscible form or administered parenterally.

Chronic use of resins may be associated with increased bleeding tendency due to hypoprothrombinemia associated with vitamin K deficiency. This will usually respond promptly to parenteral vitamin K_1; prevent recurrences by administering oral vitamin K_1.

Reduction of serum or red cell folate has been reported over long-term administration of cholestyramine. Consider supplementation with folic acid.

Determine serum cholesterol levels frequently during the first few months of therapy and periodically thereafter. Periodically measure serum triglyceride levels to detect significant changes.

These drugs are chloride anion-exchange resins. Prolonged use may cause hyperchloremic acidosis, especially in younger and smaller patients where relative dosage may be higher.

Constipation: These agents may produce or severely worsen preexisting constipation. Fecal impaction may occur and hemorrhoids may be aggravated. Avoid constipation in patients with symptomatic coronary artery disease. Most instances of constipation are mild, transient and controlled with standard treatment. Some patients require decreased dosage or discontinuation of therapy. Predisposing factors are high dose and age > 60 years. A laxative, stool softener or increased fluid intake may be helpful.

Drug Interactions:

These resins may delay or reduce the absorption of concomitant oral medication by binding the drugs in the gut. Take other drugs at least 1 hour before or 4 to 6 hours after these agents. Discontinuance of these resins could pose a hazard if a potentially toxic drug that is significantly bound to the resin has been titrated to a maintenance level while the patient was taking the resin.

Absorption of the following agents may be reduced by coadministration of cholestyramine:

Acetaminophen	Naproxen	Thyroid
Amiodarone	Phenylbutazone	Ursodiol
Corticosteroids	Piroxicam	Warfarin
Digitalis glycosides[1]	Propranolol	
Methotrexate	Thiazide diuretics	

[1] The enterohepatic recycling of these agents may also be affected.

(Drug Interactions continued on following page)

Drug Interactions (Cont.)

Colestipol reduces absorption of **digitalis glycosides, propranolol, thiazide diuretics** and **ursodiol** and may also interact with the other agents listed; further studies are necessary.

Iopanoic acid: Coadministration of cholestyramine resulted in abnormal cholecystography. Cholestyramine has an apparent high affinity for iopanoic acid.

Fat-soluble vitamins A, D, E and K: Malabsorption may occur during administration of the bile acid sequestrants (see Precautions). When cholestyramine is administered for long periods of time, consider concomitant supplementation with water-miscible (or parenteral) forms of vitamins A and D.

Adverse Reactions:

GI: Most common – Constipation at times is severe and is occasionally accompanied by fecal impaction. Hemorrhoids may be aggravated.

Less frequent – Abdominal pain and distention; GI bleeding; belching; flatulence; nausea; vomiting; diarrhea; heartburn; anorexia; steatorrhea.

Other: Bleeding tendencies due to hypoprothrombinemia (vitamin K deficiency); vitamin A (one case of night blindness) and D deficiencies; rash and irritation of the skin, tongue and perianal area; hyperchloremic acidosis in children; osteoporosis.

A 10-month-old baby with biliary atresia had an impaction presumed to be due to cholestyramine after 3 days administration of 9 g daily. She died of acute intestinal sepsis.

Calcified material has been observed in the biliary tree and the gall bladder; however, this may be due to liver disease and may not be drug-related. One patient experienced biliary colic on each of three occasions on which he took cholestyramine. Another patient, diagnosed as having an acute abdominal symptom complex, showed a "pasty mass" in the transverse colon on x-ray.

Other reactions (not necessarily drug-related) include:

GI: Rectal bleeding and pain; black stools; hemorrhoidal bleeding; bleeding duodenal ulcer; peptic ulceration; GI irritation and bleeding; dysphagia; dental bleeding; hiccoughs; sour taste; pancreatitis; diverticulitis; cholecystitis; cholelithiasis.

Hematologic: Increased prothrombin time; ecchymosis; anemia.

Hypersensitivity: Urticaria; dermatitis; asthma; wheezing.

Musculoskeletal: Backache; muscle and joint pains; arthritis; osteoporosis.

Neurologic: Headache; anxiety; vertigo; dizziness; fatigue; tinnitus; syncope; drowsiness; femoral nerve pain; paresthesia.

Renal: Hematuria; dysuria; burnt odor to urine; diuresis.

Miscellaneous: Uveitis; anorexia; fatigue; weight loss or gain; increased libido; swollen glands; edema; weakness; shortness of breath.

Altered laboratory findings: Transient and modest elevations of AST and alkaline phosphatase were observed in patients treated with colestipol. Some patients have an increase in serum phosphorus and chloride with a decrease in sodium and potassium.

Overdosage:

Overdosage has not been reported, but the chief potential harm would be GI tract obstruction. Location and degree of obstruction and status of gut motility determine treatment.

Patient Information:

Medication is usually taken before meals. Do not take the powder in dry form; mix with beverages, highly fluid soups, cereals or pulpy fruits (see Dosage section).

Chew each cholestyramine bar thoroughly. Drink plenty of fluids.

Medication may interfere with absorption of other drugs taken simultaneously. Take other drugs 1 hour before or 4 to 6 hours after cholestyramine or colestipol.

Constipation, flatulence, nausea and heartburn may occur and may disappear with continued therapy. Notify physician if these effects become bothersome or if unusual bleeding (eg, from the gums or rectum) occurs.

(Continued on following page)

Bile Acid Sequestrants (Cont.)

Administration:

Although generally given 3 to 4 times daily, there appears to be no advantage to dosing more frequently than twice daily.

Concomitant therapy: Preliminary evidence suggests that the cholesterol-lowering effects of these agents and lovastatin are additive. In addition, this combined effect may be useful in treating severe and refractory forms of hypercholesterolemia.

CHOLESTYRAMINE

Dosage:

Adults: 4 g 1 to 6 times daily. Individualize dosage.

Preparation: Mix the contents of one powder packet or one level scoopful with 2 to 6 fl oz (60 to 180 ml) water or noncarbonated beverage. Do not take in dry form. Always mix with water or other fluids, highly fluid soups or pulpy fruits, such as applesauce or crushed pineapple.

Bar – Chew thoroughly and drink plenty of fluids.

				C.I.*
Rx	**Cholybar** (Parke-Davis)	**Bar:** 4 g anhydrous cholestyramine resin per bar	Sorbitol, fructose. Chewable. Caramel (50 calories/bar) or raspberry (60 calories/bar) flavor. In 25s.	193
Rx	**Questran** (Bristol Labs)	**Powder:** 4 g anhydrous cholestyramine resin per 9 g powder	Sucrose. In 378 g cans and 9 g single dose packets (60s).	134
Rx	**Questran Light** (Bristol Labs)	**Powder for Oral Suspension:** 4 g anhydrous cholestyramine resin per 5 g powder.	Sucrose, aspartame. 16.8 mg phenylalamine/5 g dose. 1.6 calories per packet or scoop. In 210 g cans (42 doses) and cartons of 5 g packets (60s).	134

COLESTIPOL HCl

Dosage:

Adults: 5 to 30 g/day given once or in divided doses. The starting dose should be 5 g once or twice daily with a daily increment of 5 g at 1 or 2 month intervals.

Preparation: Mix in liquids, soups, cereals or pulpy fruits. Do not take dry. Add the prescribed amount to a glassful (≥ 90 ml) of liquid; stir until completely mixed. Colestipol will not dissolve. May also mix with carbonated beverages, slowly stirred in a large glass. Rinse glass with a small amount of additional beverage to ensure that all the medication is taken.

				C.I.*
Rx	**Colestid** (Upjohn)	**Granules**	In 300 and 500 g bottles and 5 g packets (30s and 90s).	125

* Cost Index based on cost per minimum daily dose (4 g cholestyramine or 5 g colestipol).

Refer to the general discussion of these products beginning on page 864.

HMG-CoA Reductase Inhibitors

Actions:

Pharmacology: These agents specifically competitively inhibit 3-hydroxy-3-methylglutaryl-coenzyme A (HMG-CoA) reductase, the enzyme which catalyzes the early rate-limiting step in cholesterol biosynthesis, conversion of HMG-CoA to mevalonate. HMG-CoA reductase inhibitors increase HDL cholesterol and decrease LDL cholesterol, VLDL cholesterol and plasma triglycerides. The effect of these induced changes in lipoprotein levels on cardiovascular morbidity or mortality has not been established.

The mechanism of the LDL-lowering effect may involve both reduction of VLDL cholesterol concentration and induction of the LDL receptor, leading to reduced production or increased catabolism of LDL cholesterol.

These agents are highly effective in reducing total and LDL cholesterol in heterozygous familial and non-familial forms of hypercholesterolemia. A marked response was seen within 1 to 2 weeks, and the maximum therapeutic response occurred within 4 to 6 weeks. The response was maintained during therapy. In the studies of some agents, single daily doses given in the evening were more effective than the same dose given in the morning, perhaps because cholesterol is synthesized mainly at night.

In multicenter, double-blind studies in patients with familial or non-familial hypercholesterolemia, lovastatin (20 to 80 mg), pravastatin (10 to 40 mg), and simvastatin (5 to 40 mg) consistently and significantly decreased total plasma cholesterol, LDL cholesterol, total cholesterol/HDL cholesterol ratio and LDL cholesterol/HDL cholesterol ratio. In addition, they increased total HDL and decreased VLDL and plasma triglycerides.

Lovastatin was compared to cholestyramine in a randomized open parallel study and to probucol in a double-blind parallel study. At all dosage levels tested, lovastatin produced a significantly greater reduction of total plasma cholesterol and total cholesterol/HDL cholesterol ratio when compared to cholestyramine or probucol. The increase in HDL cholesterol was also significantly greater with lovastatin than with probucol, but not cholestyramine.

Simvastatin was compared to cholestyramine or probucol in double-blind parallel studies. At all dosage levels, simvastatin produced significantly greater reductions in total plasma cholesterol, LDL cholesterol, VLDL cholesterol, triglycerides, and total cholesterol/HDL cholesterol ratio. Effect on HDL was significantly different when comparing simvastatin with probucol, but not cholestyramine.

Patients treated with pravastatin in combination with cholestyramine had $\geq$ 50% reductions in LDL cholesterol. Pravastatin attenuated cholestyramine-induced increases in triglyceride levels, which are of unknown clinical significance.

Pharmacokinetics:

Pharmacokinetics of HMG-CoA Reductase Inhibitors			
Parameter	Lovastatin	Pravastatin	Simvastatin
Bioavailability	$\approx$ 35% absorbed; extensive first-pass hepatic extraction (liver is primary site of action); < 5% of oral dose reaches general circulation as active inhibitors	$\approx$ 34% absorbed; absolute bioavailability 17%; extensive first-pass hepatic extraction; plasma levels may not correlate with lipid-lowering efficacy	$\approx$ 85% absorbed; extensive first-pass hepatic extraction; < 5% of oral dose reaches general circulation as active inhibitors
T_{max}	2 to 4 hours	1 to 1.5 hours	1.3 to 2.4 hours
Excretion	10% in urine 83% in feces	20% in urine 70% in feces	13% in urine 60% in feces
Elimination $t_{1/2}$	nd	77 hours	nd
Major metabolites	Beta-hydroxyacid; 6′-hydroxyderivative; two additional metabolites	Major degradation product: 3α-hydroxy isomeric metabolite	Beta-hydroxyacid; 6′-hydroxy, 6′-hydroxymethyl, 6′-exomethylene derivatives
Protein binding	> 95%	$\approx$ 50%	$\approx$ 95%
Effect of food	Plasma concentrations $\approx$ 2/3 lower when given under fasting conditions; administer with food	Lipid-lowering effects similar when given with or without food; administer without regard to meals	Plasma profile of inhibitors not affected by food; administer without regard to meals
Effects of renal/hepatic impairment		Mean AUC varied 18-fold in cirrhotic patients and peak values varied 47-fold	Higher systemic exposure may occur in severe renal insufficiency

(Continued on following page)

Indications:

Adjunct to diet for the reduction of elevated total and LDL cholesterol levels in patients with primary hypercholesterolemia (Types IIa and IIb), when the response to diet and other nonpharmacological measures alone has been inadequate.

Unlabeled uses: Lovastatin may be useful in diabetic dyslipidemia, nephrotic hyperlipidemia, familial dysbetalipoproteinemia and familial combined hyperlipidemia. Until further studies are done, limit such use to high-risk patients not responding to other therapies.

Although lovastatin may be useful in reducing elevated LDL cholesterol levels in patients with combined hypercholesterolemia and hypertriglyceridemia where hypercholesterolemia is the major abnormality (Type IIb hyperlipoproteinemia), it has not been studied in conditions where the major abnormality is elevation of chylomicrons, VLDL or intermediate density lipoprotein (IDL) (ie, hyperlipoproteinemia types I, III, IV or V).

Pravastatin can significantly lower elevated cholesterol levels in patients with: Heterozygous familial hypercholesterolemia; familial combined hyperlipidemia; diabetic dyslipidemia in non-insulin dependent diabetics; hypercholesterolemia secondary to the nephrotic syndrome; homozygous familial hypercholesterolemia in patients who are not completely devoid of LDL receptors but have a reduced level of LDL receptor activity.

Simvastatin – Trials suggest that simvastatin can signficantly lower elevated cholesterol levels in patients with heterozygous familial hypercholesterolemia, familial combined hyperlipidemia, diabetic dyslipidemia in non-insulin dependent diabetics, hyperlipidemia secondary to the nephrotic syndrome and homozygous familial hypercholesterolemia in patients who have defective, rather than absent, LDL receptors.

Contraindications:

Hypersensitivity to any component of these products; active liver disease or unexplained persistent elevations of liver function tests; pregnancy, lactation (see Warnings).

Warnings:

Liver dysfunction: Use with caution in patients who consume substantial quantities of alcohol or who have a history of liver disease.

Marked persistent increases (to > 3 times the upper limit of normal) in serum transaminases occurred in 1.9% of adult patients who received lovastatin for at least 1 year, in 1.3% of pravastatin-treated patients over an average period of 18 months, and in 1% of simvastatin-treated patients in clinical trials. When the drug was interrupted or discontinued, transaminase levels usually fell slowly to pretreatment levels. The increases usually appeared 3 to 12 months after the start of lovastatin therapy, and were not associated with jaundice or other clinical signs or symptoms in lovastatin- and pravastatin-treated patients. In pravastatin-treated patients, abnormalities did not appear to be related to treatment duration and were not associated with cholestasis.

Perform liver function tests every 4 to 6 weeks during the first 3 months of therapy, every 6 to 8 weeks during the next 12 months and periodically thereafter (≈ 6 month intervals). Pay special attention to patients who develop elevated serum transaminase levels; repeat measurements promptly and perform tests more frequently. If transaminase levels progress, particularly if they rise to 3 times the upper limit of normal and are persistent, discontinue the drug. Consider liver biopsy if elevations persist beyond drug discontinuation.

Skeletal muscle effects: Rhabdomyolysis with renal dysfunction secondary to myoglobinuria has occurred. Myalgia has occurred with lovastatin. Transient, mildly elevated creatine phosphokinase (CPK) levels are commonly seen. In clinical trials of lovastatin, ≈ 0.5% of patients developed a myopathy (ie, myalgia or muscle weakness associated with markedly elevated CPK levels). Myopathy was reported as possibly due to pravastatin in only one patient. In clinical trials, and since lovastatin was marketed, severe rhabdomyolysis (rare) has precipitated acute renal failure, especially in cardiac transplant patients on immunosuppressive therapy including cyclosporine. Most patients who developed myopathy while taking lovastatin were receiving concomitant therapy with cyclosporine, erythromycin, gemfibrozil or nicotinic acid (see Drug Interactions). In clinical trials, about 30% of patients on concomitant immunosuppressive therapy including cyclosporine developed myopathy; the corresponding percentages for gemfibrozil and nicotinic acid were ≈ 5% and 2%, respectively. Carefully consider benefits and risks of using lovastatin concomitantly with these agents.

In six cardiac transplant patients on both immunosuppressants (including cyclosporine) and lovastatin 20 mg/day, average plasma level of active metabolites of lovastatin was elevated to ≈ 4 times the expected levels. Because of an apparent relationship between increased plasma levels of active metabolites of HMG-CoA reductase inhibitors and myopathy, do not exceed 20 mg/day lovastatin or 10 mg/day simvastatin in patients on immunosuppressants. Even at this dosage, carefully consider benefits and risks in patients on immunosuppressants.

(Warnings continued on following page)

Warnings (Cont.):

Skeletal muscle effects (Cont.):

Myopathy was not observed in small numbers of patients treated with pravastatin together with niacin. A small trial of combined therapy with pravastatin and gemfibrozil showed a trend toward more frequent CPK elevations and patient withdrawals due to musculoskeletal symptoms, compared with placebo, gemfibrozil alone or pravastatin alone; myopathy was not reported. One patient developed myopathy when clofibrate was added to a previously well tolerated pravastatin regimen; myopathy resolved when clofibrate therapy was stopped. Since the use of fibrates alone may occasionally be associated with myopathy, avoid combined use of HMG-CoA reductase inhibitors and fibrates.

Consider myopathy in any patient with diffuse myalgias, muscle tenderness or weakness, or marked elevation of CPK. Advise patients to report promptly unexplained muscle pain, tenderness or weakness, particularly with malaise or fever. Discontinue these agents if markedly elevated CPK levels occur or if myopathy is diagnosed.

Consider temporarily withholding or discontinuing drug therapy in any patient with a risk factor predisposing to the development of renal failure secondary to rhabdomyolysis, including: Severe acute infection; hypotension; major surgery; trauma; severe metabolic, endocrine or electrolyte disorders; uncontrolled seizures.

Cardiovascular morbidity/mortality: The effect of HMG-CoA reductase inhibitor-induced changes in lipoprotein levels, including reduction of serum cholesterol, on cardiovascular morbidity or mortality has not been established.

Endocrine effects: Although cholesterol is the precursor of all steroid hormones, lovastatin has shown no effect on steroidogenesis. Pravastatin showed inconsistent results with regard to possible effects on basal steroid hormone levels; simvastatin did not reduce basal plasma cortisol concentration or basal plasma testosterone concentration, or impair adrenal reserve. Appropriately evaluate patients who display clinical evidence of endocrine dysfunction. Exercise caution when administering HMG-CoA reductase inhibitors with drugs that affect steroid levels or activity.

CNS: In dogs, CNS vascular lesions, characterized by perivascular hemorrhage and edema and mononuclear cell infiltration of perivascular spaces, were seen at doses of 25 mg/kg/day pravastatin (which produced plasma drug levels about 50 times higher than the mean drug level in humans receiving 40 mg/day). Similar CNS vascular lesions have been observed with other drugs in this class.

Renal function impairment: A single 20 mg dose of pravastatin was administered to 24 patients with varying degrees of renal impairment. Although no effect on the pharmacokinetics of pravastatin or its 3α-hydroxy isomeric metabolite was observed, a small increase in mean AUC values and half-life was seen for the inactive hydroxylation metabolite. Closely monitor patients with renal impairment who are receiving pravastatin. Higher systemic exposure of simvastatin may occur in severe renal insufficiency.

Carcinogenesis/Fertility impairment: In a 21 month study in mice, a statistically significant increase in the incidence of hepatocellular carcinomas and adenomas was observed at lovastatin doses of 500 mg/kg/day (312 times the maximum recommended human dose). In addition, an increase in the incidence of papilloma in nonglandular stomach mucosa was seen in mice on 100 and 500 mg/kg/day (62.5 and 312 times the maximum recommended human dose).

A 2 year study in rats given pravastatin doses of 10, 30 or 100 mg/kg showed an increased incidence of hepatocellular carcinomas in males at the highest dose (up to 125 times the human dose but with serum drug levels only 6 to 10 times higher than in humans receiving the maximum recommended dose). Oral administration in mice of 10, 30 or 100 mg/kg for 22 months resulted in a significant increase in the incidence of malignant lymphomas in treated females.

In mice receiving simvastatin (25, 100 and 400 mg/kg/day) for 72 weeks, liver carcinoma incidence was significantly increased in high-dose females and mid- and high-dose males, and liver adenoma incidence was significantly increased in mid- and high-dose females. The incidence of lung adenomas was significantly increased in mid- and high-dose males and females. In a 2 year study in rats receiving simvastatin at levels $\approx$ 45 times higher than the maximum recommended human dose, there was a statistically significant increase in the incidence of thyroid follicular adenomas in the females.

Drug-related testicular atrophy, decreased spermatogenesis, spermatocytic degeneration and giant cell formation were seen in dogs given lovastatin 20 mg/kg/day (12.5 times maximum recommended human dose) and in dogs given simvastatin 10 mg/kg/day.

There was decreased fertility in male rats treated with simvastatin 25 mg/kg for 34 weeks. In simvastatin-treated humans, there was a small decrease in the mean percentage of vital sperm and a small increase in the mean percentage of abnormal forms; these changes reached statistical significance at week 14. There was no effect on numbers or concentration of motile sperm.

(Warnings continued on following page)

Warnings (Cont.):

Pregnancy: Category X. Contraindicated during pregnancy. Skeletal malformations have occurred in animals following lovastatin administration. There are no data in pregnant women. However, because HMG-CoA reductase inhibitors can decrease synthesis of cholesterol and possibly other products of the cholesterol biosynthesis pathway, they may cause fetal harm when given to pregnant women. Give to women of childbearing age only if they are highly unlikely to conceive. If a patient becomes pregnant while on this drug, discontinue the drug and apprise her of the potential hazard to the fetus.

Lactation: Lovastatin is excreted in milk of rats; it is not known whether lovastatin and simvastatin are excreted in human breast milk; a small amount of pravastatin is excreted in human breast milk. Because of the potential for serious adverse reactions in nursing infants, caution women taking these drugs not to nurse their infants.

Children: Safety and efficacy in individuals < 18 years old have not been established. Because children are not likely to benefit from cholesterol lowering for at least a decade and because experience with this drug is limited, do not use in children.

Precautions:

Diet: Before instituting therapy, attempt to control hypercholesterolemia with appropriate diet, exercise, and weight reduction in obese patients. Treat underlying medical problems.

Ophthalmologic effects: There was a high prevalence of baseline lenticular opacities in the patient population included in the early clinical trials with lovastatin. During these trials the appearance of new opacities was noted in both the lovastatin and placebo groups. There was no clinically significant change in visual acuity in the patients who had new opacities reported nor was any patient, including those with opacities noted at baseline, discontinued from therapy because of a decrease in visual acuity.

An interim analysis was performed at 2 years in 192 hypercholesterolemic patients who participated in a placebo controlled, parallel, double-blind study to assess the effect of lovastatin on the human lens. There were no clinically significant differences between lovastatin and placebo groups in the incidence, type or progression of lenticular opacities.

Optic nerve degeneration occurred in dogs treated with simvastatin 180 mg/kg/day.

Homozygous familial hypercholesterolemia: Lovastatin and simvastatin are less effective in patients with the rare homozygous familial hypercholesterolemia, possibly because these patients have no functional LDL receptors. Pravastatin may be useful in these patients who are not completely devoid of LDL receptors but have a reduced level of LDL receptor activity. Lovastatin appears to increase the risk of elevated serum transaminases (see Warnings) in these homozygous patients.

Drug Interactions:

HMG-CoA Reductase Inhibitor Drug Interactions			
Precipitant drug	Object drug *		Description
HMG-CoA reductase inhibitors	Warfarin	⬆	The anticoagulant effect of warfarin may be increased. Monitor prothrombin time.
Bile acid sequestrants	Pravastatin	⬇	A 40% to 50% decrease in pravastatin bioavailability may occur. Take pravastatin 1 hour before or 4 hours after the bile acid sequestrant.
Cyclosporine	Lovastatin	⬆	Severe myopathy or rhabdomyolysis may occur with coadministration.
Erythromycin	Lovastatin	⬆	Severe myopathy or rhabdomyolysis may occur with coadministration.
Gemfibrozil	HMG-CoA reductase inhibitors	⬆	Severe myopathy or rhabdomyolysis may occur; this has been reported with lovastatin. The urinary excretion and protein binding of pravastatin may be decreased by gemfibrozil. Avoid coadministration.
Niacin	Lovastatin	⬆	Severe myopathy or rhabdomyolysis may occur with coadministration.

* ⬆ = Object drug increased. ⬇ = Object drug decreased.

(Drug Interactions continued on following page)

Drug Interactions (Cont.):

Drug/Food interactions: When lovastatin is given under fasting conditions, plasma concentrations are about two-thirds of those found when it is administered immediately after meals; take lovastatin with meals.

The presence of food reduces systemic bioavailability of pravastatin, but the lipid-lowering effects of the drug are similar whether taken with or 1 hour prior to meals; pravastatin may be taken without regard to meals.

When simvastatin is given under fasting conditions, the plasma profile of inhibitors is similar to that seen when administered with food; simvastatin may be taken without regard to meals.

Adverse Reactions:

These agents are generally well tolerated; adverse reactions usually have been mild and transient. About 2% of patients were discontinued from all studies with lovastatin due to adverse experiences; about one-third of these patients discontinued therapy due to increases in serum transaminases.

In 4-month long placebo controlled trials, 1.7% of pravastatin-treated patients and 1.2% of placebo treated patients were discontinued from treatment because of adverse events; in long-term studies, the most common reasons for discontinuation were asymptomatic serum transaminase increases and mild, non-specific GI complaints.

HMG-CoA Reductase Inhibitor Adverse Reactions (%)

Adverse reaction	Lovastatin (n = 613)	Pravastatin (n = 900)	Simvastatin (n = 1583)
GI			
Nausea/Vomiting	4.7	7.3	1.3
Diarrhea	5.5	6.2	1.9
Abdominal pain	5.7	5.4	3.2
Constipation	4.9	4	2.3
Flatulence	6.4	3.3	1.9
Heartburn	1.6	2.9	—
Dyspepsia	3.9	—	1.1
Musculoskeletal			
Localized pain	—	10	—
Myalgia	2.4	2.7	—
Muscle cramps	1.1	—	—
CNS			
Headache	9.3	6.2	3.5
Dizziness	2	3.3	—
Respiratory			
Upper respiratory infection	—	—	2.1
Common cold	—	7	—
Rhinitis	—	4	—
Cough	—	2.6	—
Other			
Rash/Pruritus	5.2	4	—
Cardiac chest pain	—	4	—
Fatigue	—	3.8	—
Influenza	—	2.4	—
Urinary abnormality	—	2.4	—
Blurred vision	1.5	—	—
Dysgeusia	0.8	—	—
Asthenia	—	—	1.6

The following adverse effects have been reported with drugs in this class:

Skeletal: Myopathy; rhabdomyolysis (see Warnings); arthralgias.

Neurological: Dysfunction of certain cranial nerves (including alteration of taste, impairment of extra-ocular movement, facial paresis); tremor; vertigo; memory loss; paresthesia; peripheral neuropathy; peripheral nerve palsy; anxiety; insomnia; depression.

Hypersensitivity reactions: An apparent hypersensitivity syndrome has been reported rarely which has included one or more of the following features: Anaphylaxis; angioedema; lupus erythematous-like syndrome; polymyalgia rheumatica; vasculitis; purpura; thrombocytopenia; leukopenia; hemolytic anemia; positive ANA; ESR increase; arthritis; arthralgia; urticaria; asthenia; photosensitivity; fever; chills; flushing; malaise; dyspnea; toxic epidermal necrolysis; erythema multiforme, including Stevens-Johnson syndrome.

(Adverse Reactions continued on following page)

Adverse Reactions (Cont.):

GI: Pancreatitis; hepatitis, including chronic active hepatitis; cholestatic jaundice; fatty change in liver; cirrhosis; fulminant hepatic necrosis; hepatoma; anorexia; vomiting; stomatitis.

Reproductive: Gynecomastia; loss of libido; erectile dysfunction.

Ophthalmologic: Progression of cataracts (lens opacities; see Precautions); ophthalmoplegia.

CNS: Psychic disturbances (including anxiety); paresthesia.

Hematologic: Transient asymptomatic eosinophilia; anemia; thrombocytopenia; leukopenia.

Other: Alopecia; edema.

Lab test abnormalities: Increased serum transaminases (AST, ALT), CPK (11% with lovastatin, levels at least twice normal), alkaline phosphatase (lovastatin) and bilirubin (lovastatin); thyroid function test abnormalities (lovastatin).

Overdosage:

Five healthy volunteers received up to 200 mg lovastatin as a single dose without clinically significant adverse experiences. A few cases of accidental overdosage have been reported; no patients had any specific symptoms, and all recovered without sequelae. The maximum dose taken was fifty-two 20 mg tablets (1.04 g). The dialyzability of lovastatin and its metabolites is not known.

There are no reports of overdoses with pravastatin or simvastatin. Treat symptomatically and institute supportive measures as required.

Patient Information:

Promptly report unexplained muscle pain, tenderness or weakness, especially if accompanied by fever or malaise.

Follow dietary recommendations.

Take lovastatin with meals; pravastatin and simvastatin may be taken without regard to meals.

(Products listed on following page)

HMG-CoA Reductase Inhibitors (Cont.)

LOVASTATIN (Mevinolin)

Lovastatin was approved by the FDA in 1989.

Administration and Dosage:

Place the patient on a standard cholesterol-lowering diet before starting lovastatin and continue on this diet during treatment. Give lovastatin with meals.

Individualize dosage.

Initial dose: 20 mg/day with the evening meal.

For those patients with severely elevated serum cholesterol levels (ie, > 300 mg/dl [7.8 mmol/L] on diet), initiate dosage at 40 mg/day.

Dose range: 20 to 80 mg/day in single or divided doses.

Maximum dose: 80 mg/day. Adjust at intervals of at least 4 weeks.

Monitor cholesterol levels periodically and consider reducing the dosage if cholesterol levels fall below the targeted range.

Immunosuppressive therapy – In patients taking immunosuppressive drugs concomitantly with lovastatin, maximum recommended dosage is 20 mg/day (see Warnings).

				C.I.*
Rx	**Mevacor** (MSD)	**Tablets:** 10 mg	(MSD 730). Peach. Octagonal. In UD 60s.	NA
		20 mg	(MSD 731). Light blue. Octagonal. In UD 60s and 100s.	318
		40 mg	(MSD 732). Green. Octagonal. In UD 60s.	281

PRAVASTATIN SODIUM

Pravastatin was approved by the FDA in October 1991.

Administration and Dosage:

Place the patient on a standard cholesterol-lowering diet for at least 3 to 6 months before starting pravastatin and continue on this diet during treatment. May give without regard to meals.

Individualize dosage.

Initial dose: 10 to 20 mg once daily at bedtime. *Elderly:* 10 mg once daily at bedtime.

Dose range: 10 to 40 mg once daily at bedtime.

Rx	**Pravachol** (Bristol-Myers Squibb)	**Tablets:** 10 mg	(154). White to off white, biconvex. In 100s & UD 100s.
		20 mg	(178). White to off white, biconvex. In 100s & UD 100s.

SIMVASTATIN

Simvastatin was approved by the FDA in December 1991.

Administration and Dosage:

Place the patient on a standard cholesterol-lowering diet for at least 3 to 6 months before starting simvastatin and continue on this diet during treatment. May give without regard to meals.

Individualize dosage. Consider reducing dose if cholesterol falls below targeted range.

Initial dose: 5 to 10 mg once daily in the evening. Consider starting dose of 5 mg/day for patients with LDL ≤ 190 mg/dl; 10 mg/day for patients with LDL > 190 mg/dl.

Elderly: Consider starting dose of 5 mg/day; maximum LDL reductions may be achieved with ≤ 20 mg/day.

Dose range: 5 to 40 mg/day as single dose in the evening. Adjust dose at intervals of at least 4 weeks.

Rx	**Zocor** (MSD)	**Tablets:** 5 mg[1]	(MSD 726). Buff. Shield-shaped. In 60s and 90s.
		10 mg[1]	(MSD 735). Peach. Shield-shaped. In 60s, 90s and UD 100s.
		20 mg[1]	(MSD 740). Tan. Shield-shaped. In 60s.
		40 mg[1]	(MSD 749). Brick-red. Shield-shaped. In 60s.

* Cost Index based on cost per 20 mg lovastatin.

[1] With lactose.

Refer to the general discussion of these products beginning on page 864.

PROBUCOL

Actions:

Pharmacology: Probucol lowers serum cholesterol with relatively little effect on serum triglycerides. Patients responding to probucol exhibit a decrease in low density lipoprotein (LDL) cholesterol. Cholesterol is reduced not only in the LDL fraction, but also in some high density lipoprotein (HDL) fractions with proportionately greater effect on the HDL portion in some patients. Epidemiological studies have shown that low HDL cholesterol and high LDL cholesterol are independent risk factors for coronary heart disease. The risk of lowering HDL cholesterol while lowering LDL cholesterol is unknown. Little or no effect is reported on very low density lipoprotein (VLDL).

Probucol increases the fractional rate of LDL catabolism. This effect may be linked to the increased excretion of fecal bile acids. Probucol also inhibits early stages of cholesterol synthesis and slightly inhibits absorption of dietary cholesterol. There is no increase in the cyclic precursors of cholesterol; hence, probucol does not appear to affect later stages of cholesterol biosynthesis. An animal study suggests that probucol prevents atherosclerotic lesions independently of its effect on cholesterol, possibly by inhibition of LDL oxidation.

Plasma levels of LDL are lowered 10% to 15% when probucol is used in conjunction with proper diet. The maximum effect on plasma cholesterol will occur in 1 to 3 months.

Pharmacokinetics: Absorption/Distribution – Absorption from the GI tract is limited (< 10%) and variable. When administered with food, peak blood levels are higher and less variable. With administration of 500 mg twice daily, blood levels gradually increase over the first 3 to 4 months, then remain fairly constant. In patients treated for 3 months to 1 year, mean blood level was 23.6 ± 17.2 mcg/ml (± SD) ranging to 78.3 mcg/ml.

Probucol is lipid soluble and accumulates slowly in adipose tissue, persisting in fat and blood for 6 months or longer after the last dose. In one study, 6 weeks after cessation of therapy, the average blood level had fallen by 60%; after 6 months it had fallen by 80%. The cholesterol-lowering effects of probucol disappear long before tissue levels decrease.

Metabolism/Excretion – The major pathway of elimination is via the bile and feces.

Indications:

For reduction of elevated serum cholesterol in patients with primary hypercholesterolemia (elevated LDL) who have not responded to diet, weight reduction and control of diabetes mellitus. May be useful to lower elevated cholesterol that occurs with combined hypercholesterolemia and hypertriglyceridemia, but it is not indicated when hypertriglyceridemia is the major concern.

Selection of therapy: Do not use therapy for the routine treatment of elevated blood lipids to prevent coronary heart disease. Dietary therapy is the initial treatment of choice. Consider excess body weight prior to any drug therapy. Treat contributory diseases such as hypothyroidism or diabetes mellitus.

Contraindications:

Hypersensitivity to probucol. Evidence of recent or progressive myocardial damage or findings suggestive of serious ventricular arrhythmias or with unexplained syncope or syncope of cardiovascular origin. Patients with an abnormally long QT interval.

Warnings:

Cardiovascular: Prolongation of the QT interval can occur in patients on probucol. Serious arrhythmias have occurred in association with an abnormally long QT interval in patients on probucol alone and in patients on probucol and a concomitant antiarrhythmic. Perform a baseline, 6 month and 1 year repeat ECG tracing. If marked prolongation of the QT interval occurs, consider possible benefits and risks before continuing administration.

(Warnings continued on following page)

PROBUCOL (Cont.)

Warnings (Cont.):

Cardiovascular (Cont.):

Probucol therapy should be discontinued or not started if the QT interval at an observed heart rate on a resting ECG is persistently more than one of the values listed below:

Observed Heart Rate (beats/min)	QT Interval in Sec (15% Above the Upper Limit of Normal)*	
	Males	Females
40	0.56	0.58
50	0.52	0.53
60	0.49	0.50
70	0.45	0.47
80	0.43	0.44
86	0.42	0.43
92	0.40	0.41
100	0.39	0.40
109	0.37	0.38
120	0.36	0.36
133	0.34	0.35

* Values calculated from Burch GE, Winsor T. A primer of electrocardiography. Philadelphia, PA: Lea and Febiger;1958:p. 272 (Table 6).

Drugs that prolong the QT interval are more likely to be associated with ventricular tachycardia after an increase in the dose of the drug; addition of a second drug that prolongs the QT interval (including tricyclic antidepressants, class I and III antiarrhythmics, and phenothiazines); hypokalemia or hypomagnesemia; severe bradycardia due to intrinsic heart disease or drug effects on the atrial rate (beta-blockers) or AV block (digoxin); development of recent or acute myocardial infarction, ischemia or inflammation. Base the use of probucol in patients receiving any of these drugs on the conclusion that alternate methods of hypocholesterolemic therapy are either ineffective or not tolerated, and the potential benefits of cholesterol lowering outweigh the risk of serious arrhythmia.

In patients developing unexplained syncope or syncope of cardiovascular origin, discontinue probucol and perform ECG surveillance.

Usage in Pregnancy: Category B. Because there are no adequate studies in pregnant women, use only if clearly needed. If a patient wishes to become pregnant, withdraw the drug and use birth control for at least 6 months due to the prolonged persistence of the drug in the body.

Usage in Lactation: It is not known if this drug is excreted in breast milk; excretion has been shown in animals. Nursing is not recommended during probucol use.

Usage in Children: Safety and efficacy for use in children have not been established.

Precautions:

The following conditions should be resolved or corrected prior to initiation of probucol therapy: Hypokalemia; hypomagnesemia; severe bradycardia due to intrinsic heart disease or drug effects on the atrial rate (beta-blockers) or AV block (digoxin); recent or acute myocardial infarction, ischemia or inflammation.

Monitoring: Perform adequate baseline studies to determine the patient has persistently elevated total and LDL cholesterol levels representing a primary lipid disorder, and that the increased cholesterol is not due to secondary conditions (ie, hypothyroidism, poorly controlled diabetes mellitus, obstructive liver disease, nephrotic syndromes or dysproteinemias).

Determine serum lipid levels, including HDL cholesterol: After an overnight fast before treatment; during an adequate trial of diet and weight reduction therapy prior to addition of drug therapy; and periodically during combined diet and drug therapy, including assessment during the first several months of drug treatment. A favorable trend in cholesterol reduction should occur in the first 3 to 4 months of administration. If satisfactory lipid alteration is not achieved, discontinue therapy.

(Continued on following page)

PROBUCOL (Cont.)

Adverse Reactions:

Cardiovascular: Prolongation of the QT interval on the ECG; syncope; ventricular arrhythmias (ventricular tachycardia, torsades de pointes, ventricular fibrillation); sudden death.

GI: Diarrhea or loose stools; flatulence; abdominal pain; nausea; vomiting; indigestion; GI bleeding.

Idiosyncratic reactions (observed with initiation of therapy) characterized by dizziness, palpitations, syncope, nausea, vomiting and chest pain have occurred.

CNS: Headache; dizziness; paresthesia; insomnia; tinnitus; peripheral neuritis.

Hematologic: Eosinophilia; low hemoglobin or hematocrit; thrombocytopenia.

Dermatologic: Rash; pruritis; ecchymosis; petechiae; hyperhidrosis; fetid sweat.

GU: Impotence; nocturia.

Ophthalmic: Conjunctivitis; tearing; blurred vision.

Endocrine: Enlargement of multinodular goiter.

Other: Diminished sense of taste and smell; anorexia; angioneurotic edema.

Altered laboratory findings: Transient elevations of the serum transaminases (AST, ALT), bilirubin, alkaline phosphatase, creatine phosphokinase, uric acid, BUN and blood glucose have been seen. If abnormal lab tests persist or worsen, or if systemic manifestations occur, discontinue the drug.

Overdosage:

A 15 kg, 3-year-old child ingested 5 g probucol. Following induced emesis, the child remained well, apart from a brief episode of loose stools and flatulence. Probucol is not dialyzable. Treatment is symptomatic and supportive. See General Management of Acute Overdosage on p. 2895

Patient Information:

Take with meals.

Medication may cause diarrhea, flatulence, abdominal pain, nausea or vomiting. Notify physician if they persist.

Administration and Dosage:

Adults: 500 mg twice daily with morning and evening meals. Once daily administration of 500 mg may be as effective as a twice daily regimen.

Concomitant therapy: Addition of clofibrate to probucol is not recommended, since the lowering effect on mean serum levels of either LDL or total cholesterol is generally not significantly additive and, in some patients, there may be pronounced lowering of HDL cholesterol.

				C.I.*
Rx	**Lorelco** (Merrell Dow)	**Tablets:** 250 mg	(#Dow 51 or Lorelco 250). White. Film coated. In 120s.	303
		500 mg	(#Lorelco 500). White. Film coated. In 100s.	293

* Cost Index based on cost per daily dose (1 gram).

Product identification code.

Refer to the general discussion of these products beginning on page 864.

DEXTROTHYROXINE SODIUM

Actions:

Dextrothyroxine sodium stimulates the liver to increase catabolism and excretion of cholesterol and its degradation products via the biliary route into the feces. Cholesterol synthesis is not inhibited, and abnormal metabolic end products do not accumulate in the blood. The predominant effect is reduction of serum cholesterol and low density lipoprotein (LDL) levels in hyperlipidemic patients. Elevated β lipoprotein and triglyceride fractions may also be reduced.

Indications:

As an adjunct to diet and other measures for reduction of elevated serum cholesterol (LDL) in euthyroid patients with no known evidence of organic heart disease.

Contraindications:

Euthyroid patients with one or more of the following conditions: Organic heart disease, including angina pectoris; history of myocardial infarction; history of cardiac arrhythmia, including tachycardia; rheumatic heart disease; history of congestive heart failure; decompensated or borderline compensated cardiac status; hypertension (other than mild, labile systolic hypertension); advanced liver or kidney disease; history of iodism.

Contraindicated in pregnancy and in lactation (see Warnings).

Warnings:

Obesity: Drugs with thyroid hormone activity have been used to treat obesity. In euthyroid patients, daily hormonal requirement doses are ineffective for weight reduction. Larger doses may produce serious or life-threatening toxicity, particularly when given with sympathomimetic amines used for their anorectic effects.

Surgery: Since the possibility of precipitating cardiac arrhythmias during surgery may be greater in patients treated with thyroid hormones, discontinue dextrothyroxine in euthyroid patients at least 2 weeks prior to an elective operation. Observe patients carefully during emergency surgery.

Use in impaired renal/hepatic function: When either or both are present, weigh advantages of dextrothyroxine therapy against possible deleterious results.

Usage in Pregnancy: Contraindicated in pregnancy and in nursing mothers. Women of childbearing age with familial hypercholesterolemia or hyperlipemia should not be deprived of use of this drug; it can be given to patients exercising strict birth control. Administer only after weighing possible risk to the fetus against possible benefits to the mother. Teratogenic studies in two animal species have resulted in no abnormalities in the offspring.

Usage in Children: A few children with familial hypercholesterolemia have been treated for periods of 1 year or longer with no adverse effects on growth. However, continue the drug in children only if a significant serum cholesterol-lowering effect is observed.

Precautions:

Serum levels: Increased serum thyroxine levels are evidence of absorption and transport of the drug, and should not be interpreted as evidence of hypermetabolism. Therefore, they may not be used for titrating the effective dose. Thyroxine values in the range of 10 to 25 mcg% in treated patients are common. If signs or symptoms of iodism develop during therapy, discontinue use.

Tartrazine sensitivity: Some of these products contain tartrazine, which may cause allergic-type reactions (including bronchial asthma) in susceptible individuals. Although the incidence of sensitivity is low, it is frequently seen in patients who also have aspirin hypersensitivity. Specific products containing tartrazine are identified in the product listings.

(Continued on following page)

DEXTROTHYROXINE SODIUM (Cont.)

Drug Interactions:

Anticoagulants, oral: Dextrothyroxine may potentiate the hypoprothrombinemic effects. Reduce the dosage of anticoagulants when initiating dextrothyroxine therapy and readjust on the basis of prothrombin time; monitor weekly during the first few weeks of therapy. Consider withdrawal of the drug 2 weeks prior to surgery if the use of anticoagulants during surgery is contemplated.

Beta-adrenergic blockers: Pharmacologic effects may be decreased by dextrothyroxine.

Cholestyramine may decrease the GI absorption of dextrothyroxine.

Digitalis glycosides: Therapeutic effectiveness of digitalis glycosides may be decreased by concurrent dextrothyroxine, with possible exacerbation of cardiac arrhythmias or congestive heart failure. Effects of this interaction may occur up to several days after the discontinuation of dextrothyroxine.

Insulin or **sulfonylureas:** Dextrothyroxine in diabetic patients can increase blood sugar levels with a resultant increase in dosage requirements of hypoglycemic agents.

Thyroid hormones: Consider the dosage when used concomitantly with dextrothyroxine. As with all thyroactive drugs, hypothyroid patients are more sensitive to a given dose of dextrothyroxine than euthyroid patients.

Tricyclic antidepressants: Dextrothyroxine given concomitantly may produce CNS stimulation, nervousness, tachycardia and other cardiac arrhythmias.

Adverse Reactions:

Side effects are mainly due to increased metabolism, and may be minimized by following the recommended dosage schedule. Adverse effects are least commonly seen in euthyroid patients with no signs or symptoms of organic heart disease.

Cardiovascular: Angina pectoris, arrhythmias (extrasystoles, ectopic beats or supraventricular tachycardia), ECG evidence of ischemic myocardial changes and increase in heart size. Myocardial infarctions, both fatal and nonfatal, have occurred, but these are not unexpected in untreated patients in the age groups studied. Drug relationship is unknown.

CNS: Insomnia; nervousness; tremors; headache; tinnitis; dizziness; psychic changes; decreased sensorium; paresthesia.

GI: Dyspepsia; nausea; vomiting; constipation; diarrhea; decrease in appetite; weight loss. Gallstones and cholestatic jaundice have occurred (relationship to therapy not established).

Dermatologic: Hair loss; skin rashes; itching.

Ophthalmic: Visual disturbances; exophthalmos; retinopathy; lid lag.

Other: Sweating; flushing; hyperthermia; diuresis; menstrual irregularities; changes in libido; hoarseness; peripheral edema; malaise; tiredness; muscle pain; worsening of peripheral vascular disease.

Patient Information:

Notify physician of chest pain, palpitations, sweating, diarrhea, headache or skin rash.

Administration and Dosage:

Adults:

Initial dose – 1 to 2 mg/day; increase by 1 to 2 mg at intervals of not less than 1 month to a maximum of 4 to 8 mg daily.

Maintenance dose – 4 to 8 mg daily.

Children:

Initial dose – 0.05 mg/kg/day; increase in up to 0.05 mg/kg/day increments at monthly intervals to a maximum of 0.4 mg/kg/day or 4 mg/day.

Maintenance dose – 0.1 mg/kg/day.

If signs or symptoms of cardiac disease develop during therapy, discontinue use.

				C.I.*
Rx	**Choloxin** (Flint)	**Tablets:** 1 mg	(#1). Orange, scored. In 100s.	595
		2 mg	Tartrazine. (#2). Yellow, scored. In 100s and 250s.	311
		4 mg	(#4). White, scored. In 100s and 250s.	191
		6 mg	Tartrazine. (#6). Green, scored. In 100s.	147

* Cost Index based on cost per minimum daily maintenance dose (4 mg).
# Product identification code.

Refer to the general discussion of these products beginning on page 864.

CLOFIBRATE

Actions:

Pharmacology: Clofibrate predominantly lowers serum triglycerides and very low density lipoprotein (VLDL) levels; serum cholesterol and low density lipoproteins (LDL) are lowered less predictably and effectively.

The mechanism of action is not established; the triglyceride-lowering effect appears to be due to accelerated catabolism of VLDL to LDL and decreased hepatic synthesis of VLDL. Cholesterol formation is inhibited early in the biosynthetic chain, and the excretion of neutral sterols is increased.

Clofibrate also has a platelet-inhibiting effect.

Pharmacokinetics: Absorption/Distribution – Clofibrate is hydrolyzed to p-chlorophenoxyisobutyric acid (CPIB), the active form of the drug. The parent compound is not detectable in the plasma. Absorption of CPIB is complete; peak plasma levels occur in 3 to 6 hours. Plasma protein binding of CPIB is 92% to 97%; it decreases with increasing plasma concentration of CPIB and is reduced in the nephrotic syndrome, renal failure and decreased albumin-concentrations and cirrhosis.

Metabolism/Excretion – 40% to 70% of the drug is recovered in the urine as a glucuronide ester of CPIB. The plasma elimination half-life is approximately 15 hours; half-lives of 30 to 110 hours have been reported in patients with renal impairment.

Indications:

For primary dysbetalipoproteinemia (type III hyperlipidemia) not responding to diet.

May be considered for the treatment of adults with very high serum triglyceride levels (types IV and V hyperlipidemia) who present a risk of abdominal pain and pancreatitis and who do not respond to diet. Patients with triglyceride levels > 750 mg/dl are likely to present such risk. Clofibrate is not useful for the hypertriglyceridemia of type I hyperlipidemia.

Contraindications:

Clinically significant hepatic or renal dysfunction; primary biliary cirrhosis, since clofibrate may raise the already elevated cholesterol in these cases.

Contraindicated in pregnancy and lactation (see Warnings).

Warnings:

Because of the hepatic tumorigenicity of clofibrate in rodents and the possible increased risk of malignancy and cholelithiasis in humans, use this drug only as indicated; discontinue if significant lipid response is not obtained. No evidence substantiates a beneficial effect from clofibrate on cardiovascular mortality.

Based on two large prospective studies and other studies, consider the following:

1. Clofibrate, in general, causes a relatively modest reduction of serum cholesterol and a somewhat greater reduction of serum triglycerides. In type III hyperlipidemia, however, substantial reductions of both cholesterol and triglycerides can occur.
2. No study shows a convincing reduction in incidence of *fatal* myocardial infarction.
3. Clofibrate users have twice the risk of developing cholelithiasis and cholecystitis requiring surgery as do nonusers. Anticipate an increase in morbidity from this complication and mortality from cholecystectomy during clofibrate treatment.
4. A 36% increase in incidence of noncardiovascular deaths was reported in one study. An increase in cardiac arrhythmias and intermittent claudication and in definite or suspected thromboembolic events and angina was reported in another.
5. Administration of clofibrate (5 to 8 times the human dose) to mice and rats in long-term studies resulted in a higher incidence of benign and malignant liver tumors.

Usage in Pregnancy: No reports link the use of clofibrate with congenital defects. Animal studies demonstrate placental transfer of the drug. The drug is metabolized by glucuronide conjugation; since this system is immature in the neonate, accumulation may occur. Strict birth control procedures must be exercised by women of childbearing potential. In patients who plan to become pregnant, withdraw clofibrate several months before conception. Weigh the possible benefits of the drug to the patient against possible hazards to the fetus.

Usage in Lactation: Animal studies suggest drug excretion into breast milk; thus, clofibrate is contraindicated in nursing women.

Usage in Children: Safety and efficacy for use in children have not been established.

(Continued on following page)

CLOFIBRATE (Cont.)

Precautions:

Response to therapy: Clofibrate has little effect on the elevated cholesterol levels of most subjects with hypercholesterolemia. A minority of subjects show a more pronounced response. Be very selective and confine clofibrate treatment to patients with clearly defined risk due to severe hypercholesterolemia (eg, individuals with familial hypercholesterolemia starting in childhood) who inadequately respond to diet and more effective cholesterol-lowering drugs.

Do not use drug therapy for routine treatment of elevated blood lipids for the prevention of coronary heart disease. Dietary therapy specific for the type of hyperlipidemia is the initial treatment of choice. Excess body weight and alcohol intake may be important factors in hypertriglyceridemia and should be addressed prior to any drug therapy. Physical exercise can be an important ancillary measure. Diagnose and adequately treat contributory diseases such as hypothyroidism or diabetes mellitus. Consider drug therapy only when reasonable attempts have been made to obtain satisfactory results with nondrug methods. If the decision ultimately is to use drugs, instruct the patient that this does not reduce the importance of adhering to diet.

Because clofibrate is associated with certain serious adverse findings reported in two large clinical trials, agents other than clofibrate may be more suitable for a particular patient.

Monitoring: Perform adequate baseline studies. Obtain *serum lipid* determinations frequently during the first few months, and periodically thereafter. Withdraw the drug after 3 months if response is inadequate. However, in the case of xanthoma tuberosum, use the drug for longer periods (up to 1 year) provided there is a reduction in the size or number of the xanthomata.

Obtain subsequent serum lipid determinations to detect a paradoxical rise in serum cholesterol or triglycerides. Clofibrate will not alter the seasonal variations of serum cholesterol peak elevations in midwinter and late summer and decreases in fall and spring. If the drug is discontinued, maintain the patient on diet and monitor serum lipids until stabilized; a rise to or above the original baseline value may occur.

Hepatic – During therapy, perform frequent serum transaminase determinations and other liver function tests. Abnormalities are usually reversible when the drug is discontinued. Hepatic biopsies are usually normal. If the hepatic function tests rise steadily or show excessive abnormalities, withdraw the drug. Use with caution in those patients with a history of jaundice or hepatic disease.

Cholelithiasis is a possible side effect of clofibrate therapy; perform appropriate diagnostic procedures if signs and symptoms related to biliary disease occur.

"Flu-like" symptoms (muscular aching, soreness, cramping) may occur. The physician should differentiate this from actual viral or bacterial disease.

Perform complete blood counts periodically since anemia, and, more frequently, leukopenia have been reported in patients taking clofibrate.

Various cardiac arrhythmias have occurred with the use of clofibrate.

Atherogenesis: Clofibrate may produce a decrease in cholesterol linoleate but an increase in palmitoleate and oleate, the latter being considered atherogenic in experimental animals. The significance of this finding is unknown.

Peptic ulcer: Use with caution in patients with peptic ulcer since reactivation has been reported; whether this is drug-related is unknown.

(Continued on following page)

CLOFIBRATE (Cont.)

Drug Interactions:

Anticoagulants, oral: The hypoprothrombinemic effects of these agents may be increased by concurrent clofibrate. Reduce the dosage of the anticoagulant if necessary to maintain the prothrombin time at the desired level to prevent bleeding complications. Use caution during coadministration; obtain frequent prothrombin determinations until the prothrombin level stabilizes.

Insulin and **sulfonylureas:** The pharmacologic effects of these agents may be increased by concurrent administration of clofibrate, resulting in hypoglycemia. Monitor blood glucose and reduce the dose of the insulin or sulfonylurea as necessary.

Probenecid may increase the therapeutic and toxic effects of clofibrate by impairing its renal and metabolic clearance. A lower dose of clofibrate may be necessary.

Adverse Reactions:

GI: Most common – Nausea. Less common – Vomiting; diarrhea; loose stools; dyspepsia; flatulence; bloating; abdominal distress; hepatomegaly (not associated with hepatotoxicity); stomatitis; gastritis. Studies indicate an increase in the incidence of gallstones in long-term therapy.

Cardiovascular: Increased or decreased angina, cardiac arrhythmias, swelling and phlebitis at xanthoma site.

Dermatologic: Skin rash; alopecia; dry skin; dry brittle hair; pruritus; allergic reactions, including urticaria.

Genitourinary: Impotence; decreased libido; renal dysfunction as evidenced by dysuria, hematuria, proteinuria and decreased urine output. One patient's renal biopsy suggested "allergic reaction".

Hematologic: Leukopenia; anemia; eosinophilia.

Musculoskeletal: Myalgia (muscle cramps, aches, weakness); "flu-like" symptoms; arthralgia.

CNS: Fatigue; weakness; drowsiness; dizziness; headache.

Miscellaneous: Weight gain; polyphagia.

Other (drug relationship not established): Peptic ulcer; GI hemorrhage; rheumatoid arthritis; tremors; increased perspiration; systemic lupus erythematosus; blurred vision; gynecomastia; thrombocytopenic purpura.

Altered laboratory findings: Increased transaminase (AST and ALT); BSP retention; proteinuria; increased thymol turbidity; increased creatine phosphokinase.

Overdosage:

Institute symptomatic supportive measures. Refer to General Management of Acute Overdosage on p. 2895

Patient Information:

Patient package insert available with product.

If GI upset occurs, may be taken with food.

Notify physician if any of the following effects occur: Chest pain; shortness of breath; irregular heartbeat; severe stomach pain with nausea and vomiting; fever and chills or sore throat; blood in the urine; decrease in urination; swelling of lower extremities; weight gain.

Administration and Dosage:

Adults: 2 g daily in divided doses. Some patients may respond to lower dosage.

Maintenance: Same as initial dose.

				C.I.*
Rx	**Clofibrate** (Various)	**Capsules:** 500 mg	In 100s.	120+
Rx	**Atromid-S** (Wyeth-Ayerst)		(#Atromid-S 500). In 100s.	295

* Cost Index based on cost per daily dose (2 g).

Product identification code.

Refer to the general discussion of these products beginning on page 865.

GEMFIBROZIL

Actions:

Pharmacology: Gemfibrozil is a lipid regulating agent which decreases serum triglycerides and very low density lipoprotein (VLDL) cholesterol, and increases high density lipoprotein (HDL) cholesterol. While modest decreases in total and low density lipoprotein (LDL) cholesterol may be observed with gemfibrozil therapy, treatment of patients with elevated triglycerides due to Type IV hyperlipoproteinemia often results in a rise in LDL-cholesterol. LDL-cholesterol levels in Type IIb patients with elevations of both serum LDL-cholesterol and triglycerides are, in general, minimally affected by gemfibrozil treatment; however, it usually raises HDL-cholesterol significantly in this group.

Gemfibrozil inhibits peripheral lipolysis and decreases the hepatic extraction of free fatty acids, thus reducing hepatic triglyceride production. Gemfibrozil also inhibits synthesis of VLDL carrier apolipoprotein B, leading to a decrease in VLDL production. How gemfibrozil raises HDL concentration is not known.

The drug may, in addition to elevating HDL cholesterol, reduce incorporation of long-chain fatty acids into newly formed triglycerides, accelerate turnover and removal of cholesterol from the liver and increase excretion of cholesterol in the feces.

Clinical Pharmacology: In the Helsinki Heart Study, a large, randomized, double-blind, placebo controlled, primary prevention trial in 4081 male patients between the ages of 40 and 55, gemfibrozil therapy was associated with significant reductions in total plasma triglycerides and a significant increase in HDL-cholesterol. Moderate reductions in total plasma cholesterol and LDL-cholesterol were observed for the gemfibrozil treatment group as a whole. The study involved subjects with serum non-HDL-cholesterol of over 200 mg/dl and no previous history of coronary heart disease. Over the 5-year study period, the gemfibrozil group experienced a 34% reduction in serious coronary events (sudden cardiac deaths plus fatal and nonfatal myocardial infarctions) compared to placebo. There was a 37% reduction in nonfatal myocardial infarction. The greatest reduction in the incidence of serious coronary events occurred in Type IIb patients who had elevations of both LDL-cholesterol and total plasma triglycerides. The mean increase in HDL-cholesterol among the Type IIb patients in this study was 12.6% compared to placebo.

Pharmacokinetics: Absorption/Distribution – Gemfibrozil is well absorbed from the GI tract. Peak plasma levels occur in 1 to 2 hours. Plasma levels appear proportional to the dose and do not accumulate following multiple doses.

Metabolism/Excretion – Gemfibrozil mainly undergoes oxidation to form a hydroxymethyl and a carboxyl metabolite. It has a plasma half-life of 1.5 hours following multiple doses. Biological half-life is considerably longer, as some of the drug undergoes enterohepatic circulation and is reabsorbed in the GI tract. Approximately 70% is excreted in the urine, mostly as the glucuronide conjugate, with less than 2% excreted as unchanged drug; 6% is accounted for in the feces.

Indications:

Hypertriglyceridemia in adult patients (Types IV and V hyperlipidemia) who present a risk of pancreatitis and who do not respond to diet. Consider therapy for those with triglyceride elevations between 1000 and 2000 mg/dl,and who have a history of pancreatitis or of recurrent abdominal pain typical of pancreatitis.

Reducing coronary heart disease risk: First consider bile acid sequestrants and nicotinic acid. Consider gemfibrozil therapy in those Type IIb patients who have low HDL-cholesterol levels in addition to elevated LDL-cholesterol and triglycerides and who have not responded to weight loss, dietary therapy, exercise and other pharmacologic agents.

Gemfibrozil is not useful for the hypertriglyceridemia of Type I hyperlipidemia.

Contraindications:

Hepatic or severe renal dysfunction, including primary biliary cirrhosis; preexisting gallbladder disease; hypersensitivity to gemfibrozil.

(Continued on following page)

GEMFIBROZIL (Cont.)

Warnings:

Clofibrate and gemfibrozil have pharmacological similarities; the adverse findings with clofibrate may also apply to gemfibrozil.

Cholelithiasis: Gemfibrozil may increase cholesterol excretion into the bile leading to cholelithiasis. If cholelithiasis is suspected, perform gallbladder studies. Discontinue therapy if gallstones are found.

Concomitant therapy with gemfibrozil and lovastatin has been associated with rhabdomyolysis, markedly elevated creatine kinase (CK) levels and myoglobinuria, leading in a high proportion of cases to acute renal failure (see Drug Interactions). In most subjects who have had an unsatisfactory lipid response to either drug alone, the possible benefit of combined therapy does not outweigh the risks. The use of fibrates alone, including gemfibrozil, may occasionally be associated with myositis. Promptly evaluate patients complaining of muscle pain, tenderness or weakness for myositis, including serum CK level determination. However, there is no assurance that periodic monitoring of CK will prevent the occurrence of severe myopathy and kidney damage. If myositis is suspected or diagnosed, withdraw therapy.

Carcinogenesis, Mutagenesis, Impairment of fertility: Long-term administration of high doses (1 and 10 times the human dose) of gemfibrozil in rats was associated with an increased incidence of benign liver nodules, liver carcinomas and benign Leydig cell tumors; subcapsular unilateral and bilateral cataracts also occurred. Administration of ≈ 3 and 10 times the human dose to male rats for 10 weeks resulted in a dose-related decrease of fertility. This effect was reversed after a drug-free period of about 8 weeks, and it was not transmitted to their offspring.

Usage in Pregnancy: Category B. There are no studies in pregnant women. Because gemfibrozil is tumorigenic in male rats, use during pregnancy only when the benefit clearly outweighs the possible risk to the patient or fetus.

Usage in Lactation: Because of the potential for tumorigenicity shown in rats, decide whether to discontinue nursing or discontinue the drug, taking into account the importance of the drug to the mother.

Usage in Children: Safety and efficacy in children have not been established.

Precautions:

Estrogen therapy is sometimes associated with massive rises in plasma triglycerides, especially in subjects with familial hypertriglyceridemia. In such cases, discontinuation of estrogen may obviate the need for specific drug therapy of hypertriglyceridemia.

Contributory diseases such as hypothyroidism or diabetes mellitus should be adequately treated. Consider the use of drugs only when reasonable attempts have been made to obtain satisfactory results with nondrug methods.

Monitoring therapy: Perform adequate pretreatment laboratory studies. Obtain periodic determinations of serum lipids during administration. Withdraw the drug after 3 months if response is inadequate.

Hematologic – Mild hemoglobin, hematocrit and white blood cell decreases have been observed. However, these levels stabilized during long-term administration. Rarely, severe anemia, leukopenia, thrombocytopenia and bone marrow hypoplasia may occur. Perform periodic blood counts during the first 12 months of administration.

Liver function – Abnormal elevations of AST, ALT, LDH, bilirubin and alkaline phosphatase have occurred, and are usually reversible on drug discontinuation. Perform periodic liver function studies and terminate therapy if abnormalities persist.

Blood glucose – Gemfibrozil has a moderate hyperglycemic effect. Carefully monitor blood glucose levels during therapy.

Drug Interactions:

Anticoagulants, oral: Gemfibrozil may enhance the pharmacologic effect of these agents. Adjust anticoagulant dosage to maintain prothrombin time at desired level to prevent bleeding complications. Frequently determine prothrombin time.

Lovastatin: Rhabdomyolysis has occurred with combined gemfibrozil and lovastatin therapy. It may be seen as early as 3 weeks after initiation of combined therapy or after several months (see Warnings).

(Continued on following page)

GEMFIBROZIL (Cont.)

Adverse Reactions:

GI: Dyspepsia (19.6%); abdominal pain (9.8%); diarrhea (7.2%); nausea/vomiting (2.5%); constipation (1.4%); acute appendicitis (1.2%).

CNS: Fatigue (3.8%); vertigo (1.5%); headache (1.2%); paresthesia; hypesthesia.

Dermatologic: Eczema (1.9%); rash (1.7%).

Cardiovascular: Atrial fibrillation (0.7%).

Special senses: Taste perversion.

Other (drug relationship probable or not established):

GI – Cholestatic jaundice; pancreatitis, hepatoma; colitis.

CNS – Dizziness; somnolence; peripheral neuritis; decreased libido; depression; headache; confusion; convulsions; syncope.

Cardiovascular – Intracerebral hemorrhage; peripheral vascular disease; extrasystole.

Special senses – Blurred vision; retinal edema; cataracts.

Musculoskeletal – Myopathy; myasthenia; myalgia; painful extremities; arthralgia; synovitis; rhabdomyolysis.

Hematopoietic – Anemia; leukopenia; bone marrow hypoplasia; eosinophilia; thrombocytopenia.

Immunologic – Angioedema; laryngeal edema; urticaria; anaphylaxis; lupus-like syndrome; vasculitis.

GU – Impotence; decreased male fertility.

Dermatologic: Exfoliative dermatitis; dermatitis; pruritus; alopecia.

Miscellaneous – Weight loss; viral and bacterial infection (common cold, cough and urinary tract infections).

Altered laboratory findings – Liver function abnormalities (increased AST, ALT, LDH, CPK, bilirubin, alkaline phosphatase); positive antinuclear antibody; mild decreases in hemoglobin, hematocrit and white blood cells (see Precautions).

Overdosage:

Institute symptomatic supportive measures. Refer to General Management of Acute Overdosage on p. 2895

Patient Information:

May cause dizziness or blurred vision; patients should observe caution while driving or performing other tasks requiring alertness.

Medication may cause abdominal or epigastric pain, diarrhea, nausea or vomiting. Notify physician if these become pronounced.

Administration and Dosage:

Adults: 1200 mg/day in 2 divided doses, 30 minutes before the morning and evening meals.

				C.I.*
Rx	**Lopid** (Parke-Davis)	**Capsules:** 300 mg	(#P-D Lopid 669). White and maroon. In 100s & 500s.	278
		Tablets: 600 mg	(#P-D 737). White, scored. Film coated. In 60s.	297

* Cost Index based on cost per daily dose (1200 mg). # Product identification code.

Refer to the general discussion of these products beginning on page 864.

NICOTINIC ACID (Niacin)

The following is an abbreviated monograph for nicotinic acid. For complete prescribing information, see page 19

Actions:

Pharmacology: Pharmacologic doses of nicotinic acid reduce serum cholesterol and triglyceride levels in Types II, III, IV and V hyperlipoproteinemia. Triglycerides and very low density lipoproteins (VLDL) are reduced by 20% to 40% in 1 to 4 days. Low density lipoprotein (LDL) reduction may be seen in 5 to 7 days. The effect on LDL concentration is dose-dependent. The maximal effect will be seen in 3 to 5 weeks. The decrease in LDL will be greater if niacin is used with a bile acid-binding resin (40% to 60%). High density lipoproteins (HDL) are increased by 20%. The exact mechanism of action is unknown. It is known that nicotinic acid inhibits lipolysis in adipose tissue, decreases esterification of triglyceride in the liver and increases lipoprotein lipase activity. Niacinamide does NOT have hypolipemic effects.

Pharmacokinetics: The drug is rapidly and nearly completely absorbed in the intestines. Peak plasma levels are reached in 45 minutes. Urinary recovery of a 3 g dose is 88%.

Indications:

Adjunctive therapy in patients with significant hyperlipidemia (elevated cholesterol or triglycerides) who do not respond adequately to diet and weight loss.

Contraindications:

Hepatic dysfunction; active peptic ulcer; severe hypotension; hemorrhaging.

Patient Information:

Cutaneous flushing and a sensation of warmth, especially of the face and upper body, may occur. Itching or tingling and headache may also occur. These effects are transient and usually subside with continued therapy.

In patients for whom flushing is distressing or persistent, 300 mg of aspirin given 30 minutes before each scheduled dose of nicotinic acid or slow upward adjustment of dose may help ameliorate this reaction.

May cause GI upset; take with meals.

If dizziness occurs, avoid sudden changes in posture.

Administration and Dosage:

Administer dosages of 1 to 2 g, 3 times per day, with or following meals. The usual maximum dose is 8 g/day.

Concomitant therapy: In one study, the triple combination of nicotinic acid, colestipol and lovastatin was more effective in reducing LDL than nicotinic acid in combination with either colestipol or lovastatin.

For complete listing of available products, see page 21.

Sympathomimetics

Actions:

These agents are used to produce bronchodilation. They relieve reversible bronchospasm by relaxing the smooth muscles of the bronchioles in conditions associated with asthma, bronchitis, emphysema or bronchiectasis. Bronchodilation may additionally facilitate expectoration. Some agents are also used for other purposes. See monographs for Vasopressors Used in Shock, Nasal Decongestants and Ophthalmic Vasoconstrictors/ Mydriatics.

Pharmacology: The pharmacologic actions of these agents include: Alpha-adrenergic stimulation (vasoconstriction, nasal decongestion, pressor effects); β_1-adrenergic stimulation (increased myocardial contractility and conduction); and β_2-adrenergic stimulation (bronchial dilation and vasodilation). Beta-adrenergic drugs stimulate adenyl cyclase, the enzyme which catalyzes the formation of cyclic-3′5′ adenosine monophosphate (cyclic AMP) from adenosine triphosphate (ATP). The cyclic AMP that is formed mediates the cellular responses.

In addition to the cardiovascular/pulmonary effects, other adrenergic actions include alpha receptor-mediated contraction of GI and urinary sphincters; α and β receptor-mediated lipolysis; and α and β receptor-mediated decrease in GI tone, and changes in renin secretion, uterine relaxation, hepatic glycogenolysis/gluconeogenesis and pancreatic beta cell secretion.

The relative selectivity of action of sympathomimetic agents is the primary determinant of clinical usefulness; it can predict the most likely side effects. The β_2 selective agents provide the greatest benefit with minimal side effects. Direct administration via inhalation provides prompt effects and minimizes systemic activity. These drugs also inhibit histamine release from mast cells, produce vasodilation and increase ciliary motility. Bitolterol functions as a prodrug which must first be hydrolyzed by esterases in tissue and blood to its active moiety, colterol. Isoproterenol is one of the most potent bronchodilators available.

Sympathomimetic Bronchodilators: Pharmacologic Effects and Pharmacokinetic Properties

Sympathomimetic	Adrenergic receptor activity	Route	Onset (minutes)	Duration (hrs)
Albuterol[1]	$\beta_1 < \beta_2$	PO Inh[2]	within 30 within 5	4-8 3-8
Bitolterol[1]	$\beta_1 < \beta_2$	Inh	3-4	5-$\geq$8
Isoetharine[1]	$\beta_1 < \beta_2$	Inh[2]	within 5	1-3
Metaproterenol[1]	$\beta_1 < \beta_2$	PO Inh[2]	$\approx$ 30 5-30	4 2-6
Pirbuterol[1]	$\beta_1 < \beta_2$	Inh	within 5	5
Terbutaline[1]	$\beta_1 < \beta_2$	PO SC Inh	30 5-15 5-30	4-8 1.5-4 3-6
Isoproterenol	β_1 β_2	SL IV Inh[2]	$\approx$ 30 immediate 2-5	1-2 $<$1 0.5-2
Ethylnorepinephrine	$\alpha < \beta_1$ β_2	SC IM	5-10 5-10	1-2 1-2
Ephedrine	α β_1 β_2	PO SC IM IV	within 60 $>$20 10-20 —	3-5 $\leq$1 $\leq$1 —
Epinephrine	α β_1 β_2	SC IM Inh[2]	5-15 — 1-5	1-4 1-4 1-3

[1] These agents all have minor β_1 activity.

[2] May be administered via aerosol nebulizer, bulb nebulizer or IPPB administration.

(Continued on following page)

Indications:

Relief of reversible bronchospasm associated with acute and chronic bronchial asthma, exercise-induced bronchospasm, bronchitis, emphysema, bronchiectasis or other obstructive pulmonary diseases.

According to the National Heart, Lung and Blood Institute, inhaled beta agonists are recommended for mild acute asthma; inhaled or oral beta agonists plus an anti-inflammatory for moderate asthma; and beta agonists plus an oral corticosteroid for severe asthma.

Refer to individual monographs for indications of specific agents.

Contraindications:

Hypersensitivity to any component (allergic reactions are rare); cardiac arrhythmias associated with tachycardia; tachycardia or heart block caused by digitalis intoxication, angina (isoproterenol); narrow angle glaucoma, shock, during general anesthesia with halogenated agents or cyclopropane, organic brain damage (epinephrine).

Warnings:

Special risk patients: Administer with caution to individuals with – Diabetes mellitus; hyperthyroidism; prostatic hypertrophy (ephedrine); history of seizures; elderly patients, psychoneurotic individuals, patients with long-standing bronchial asthma and emphysema who have developed degenerative heart disease (epinephrine).

In patients with status asthmaticus and abnormal blood gas tensions, improvement in vital capacity and blood gas tensions may not accompany apparent relief of bronchospasm following isoproterenol. Facilities for administering oxygen and ventilatory assistance are necessary.

Diabetes – Large doses of **IV albuterol** may aggravate preexisting diabetes mellitus and ketoacidosis. Relevance to the use of oral or inhaled albuterol is unknown. Diabetic patients receiving any of these agents may require an increase in dosage of insulin or oral hypoglycemic agents.

Cardiovascular effects: Use with caution in patients with cardiovascular disorders including coronary insufficiency, ischemic heart disease, history of stroke, coronary artery disease, cardiac arrhythmias, CHF and hypertension. These agents may cause toxic symptoms through idiosyncratic response or overdosage. If cardiac rate increases sharply, patients with angina pectoris may experience anginal pain until the cardiac rate decreases.

Closely monitor patients receiving **epinephrine**. Inadvertently induced high arterial blood pressure may result in angina pectoris, aortic rupture or cerebral hemorrhage. Cardiac arrhythmias develop in some individuals even after therapeutic doses. Epinephrine causes changes in the ECG even in healthy persons, including a decrease in amplitude of the T wave.

Ephedrine may cause hypertension resulting in intracranial hemorrhage. It may induce anginal pain in patients with coronary insufficiency or ischemic heart disease.

Significant changes in systolic and diastolic blood pressure can occur in some patients after use of any beta-adrenergic aerosol bronchodilator.

Excessive use of inhalants: Occasional patients have developed severe paradoxical airway resistance with repeated, excessive use of inhalation preparations; the cause is unknown. Discontinue the drug immediately and institute alternative therapy, since patients may not respond to other therapy until the drug is withdrawn.

Deaths have been reported; the exact cause is unknown, but cardiac arrest following an unexpected severe acute asthmatic crisis and subsequent hypoxia is suspected.

Usual dose response: Advise patients to contact a physician if they do not respond to their usual dose of a sympathomimetic amine.

Reduce epinephrine dose if bronchial irritation, nervousness, restlessness or sleeplessness occurs. Do not continue to use epinephrine inhalation, but seek medical assistance immediately, if symptoms are not relieved within 20 minutes or become worse.

CNS effects: Sympathomimetics may produce CNS stimulation.

Long-term use: Prolonged use of **ephedrine** may produce a syndrome resembling an anxiety state and many patients develop nervousness; a sedative may be needed to relieve symptoms. After prolonged use or overdosage of **epinephrine,** elevated serum lactic acid levels with severe metabolic acidosis have occurred, as have transient blood glucose elevations.

Morbidity/Mortality: An increased risk of death or near death from asthma may be associated with the regular use of inhaled beta agonists. Further study is needed.

Overdosage or inadvertent IV injection of conventional SC **epinephrine** doses may cause severe or fatal hypertension or cerebrovascular hemorrhage resulting from the sharp rise in blood pressure. Fatalities may also occur from pulmonary edema resulting from peripheral constriction and cardiac stimulation. The marked pressor effects may be counteracted by use of rapidly acting vasodilators (eg, nitrites, α blockers).

(Warnings continued on following page)

Warnings (Cont.):

Respiratory depression: When compressed oxygen is used as the aerosol propellant, determine the percentage of oxygen by the patient's individual requirements to avoid depression of respiratory drive.

Hypersensitivity (allergic) reactions can occur after administration of **bitolterol, albuterol, metaproterenol, terbutaline, ephedrine** and possibly other bronchodilators. See Management of Acute Hypersensitivity Reactions.

Carcinogenesis: A significant increase in the incidence of leiomyomas of the mesovarium has been demonstrated with **albuterol** and **terbutaline** in animal studies.

Elderly: Lower doses may be required due to increased sympathomimetic sensitivity.

Pregnancy: Category B (terbutaline). *Category C* (albuterol, bitolterol, ephedrine, epinephrine, ethylnorepinephrine, isoetharine, isoproterenol, metaproterenol). Several of these agents are teratogenic and embryocidal in animal studies. There are no adequate and well controlled studies in pregnant women. Use only when clearly needed and when potential benefits outweigh potential hazards to the fetus.

Labor and delivery: Use of β_2 active sympathomimetics inhibits uterine contractions (see Terbutaline monograph). Other reactions include increased heart rate, transient hyperglycemia, hypokalemia, cardiac arrhythmias, pulmonary edema, cerebral and myocardial ischemia and increased fetal heart rate and hypoglycemia in the neonate. Although these effects are unlikely with aerosol use, consider the potential for untoward effects.

Oral **albuterol** and **terbutaline** have delayed preterm labor. There are no well controlled studies which demonstrate that they stop preterm labor or prevent labor at term. Therefore, use cautiously in pregnant patients when given for relief of bronchospasm to avoid interference with uterine contractility. Maternal death has been reported with terbutaline and other drugs in this class.

Lactation: **Terbutaline** and **epinephrine** are excreted in breast milk. It is not known whether other agents are excreted in breast milk. Decide whether to discontinue nursing or to discontinue the drug, taking into account the drug's importance to the mother.

Children:

Inhalation – Safety and efficacy for use of **bitolterol, pirbuterol, isoetharine, isoproterenol, terbutaline** and **albuterol** in children $\leq$ 12 years of age (*Ventolin* – $<$ 4 years) have not been established. **Metaproterenol** may be used in children $\geq$ 6 years of age.

Injection – Parenteral **terbutaline** is not recommended for use in children $<$ 12 years old. Administer **epinephrine** with caution to infants and children. Syncope has occurred following administration to asthmatic children.

Oral – **Metaproterenol** is not recommended for use in children $<$ 6 years old. **Terbutaline** is not recommended for use in children $<$ 12 years old. **Albuterol:** Safety and efficacy have not been established for children $<$ 2 years (syrup), $<$ 6 years (tablets) and $<$ 12 years (tablets, timed release).

In children, **ephedrine** is effective in the oral therapy of asthma. Because of its CNS-stimulating effect, it is rarely used alone. This effect is usually countered by an appropriate sedative; however, its rationale has been questioned.

Precautions:

Tolerance may occur with prolonged use of sympathomimetic agents, but temporary cessation of the drug restores its original effectiveness.

Hypokalemia: Decreases in serum potassium levels have occurred, possibly through intracellular shunting which can produce adverse cardiovascular effects. The decrease is usually transient, not requiring supplementation.

Parkinson's disease: **Epinephrine** may temporarily increase rigidity and tremor.

Drug abuse/dependence: Prolonged abuse of **ephedrine** can lead to symptoms of paranoid schizophrenia. Patients exhibit such signs as tachycardia, poor nutrition and hygiene, fever, cold sweat and dilated pupils. Some measure of tolerance develops, but addiction does not occur. With all sympathomimetic aerosols, cardiac arrest and even death may be associated with abuse.

Parenteral use: Avoid intraneural or intravascular injection of **ethylnorepinephrine**.

Administer **epinephrine** with great caution and in carefully circumscribed quantities in areas of the body served by end arteries or with otherwise limited blood supply (eg, fingers, toes, nose, ears, genitals) or if peripheral vascular disease is present to avoid vasoconstriction-induced tissue sloughing.

Combined therapy: Concomitant use with other sympathomimetic agents is not recommended, as it may lead to deleterious cardiovascular effects. This does not preclude the judicious use of an adrenergic stimulant aerosol bronchodilator in patients receiving tablets. Do not give on a routine basis. If regular coadministration is required, consider alternative therapy.

(Precautions continued on following page)

Sympathomimetics (Cont.)

Precautions (Cont.):

Sulfites: Some products contain sulfites that may cause allergic-type reactions including anaphylactic symptoms and life-threatening/less severe asthmatic episodes in susceptible persons. The overall prevalence in the general population is unknown and probably low. It is seen more frequently in asthmatic or atopic nonasthmatic persons.

Drug Interactions:

Most interactions listed apply to sympathomimetics when used as vasopressors; however, consider the interaction when using the bronchodilator sympathomimetics.

Sympathomimetic Bronchodilator Drug Interactions			
Precipitant drug	Object drug*		Description
Beta blockers	Epinephrine	↑	An initial hypertensive episode followed by bradycardia may occur.
Furazolidine	Sympathomimetics	↑	The pressor sensitivity to mixed-acting sympathomimetics (eg, ephedrine) may be increased. Direct-acting agents (eg, epinephrine) are not affected.
Guanethidine	Sympathomimetics		Guanethidine potentiates the effects of the direct-acting sympathomimetics (eg, epinephrine) and inhibits the effects of the mixed-acting agents (eg, ephedrine). Guanethidine hypotensive action may also be reversed.
	Direct	↑	
	Mixed	↓	
Sympathomimetics	Guanethidine	↓	
Lithium	Sympathomimetics	↓	The pressor sensitivity of direct-acting sympathomimetics (eg, epinephrine) may be decreased.
Methyldopa	Sympathomimetics	↑	Concurrent administration may result in an increased pressor response.
MAO inhibitors	Sympathomimetics	↑	Coadministration of MAO inhibitors and mixed-acting sympathomimetics (eg, ephedrine) may result in severe headache, hypertension and hyperpyrexia, possibly resulting in hypertensive crisis. Direct-acting agents (eg, epinephrine) interact minimally, if at all.
Oxytocic drugs (eg, ergonovine)	Sympathomimetics	↑	Concurrent administration may result in hypertension.
Rauwolfia alkaloids	Sympathomimetics		Reserpine potentiates the pressor response of the direct-acting sympathomimetics (eg, epinephrine) which may result in hypertension. The pressor response of the mixed-acting agents (eg, ephedrine) is decreased.
	Direct	↑	
	Mixed	↓	
Tricyclic antidepressants (TCAs)	Sympathomimetics		TCAs potentiate the pressor response of direct-acting sympathomimetics (eg, epinephrine); dysrhythmias have occurred. The pressor response of mixed-acting agents (eg, ephedrine) is decreased.
	Direct	↑	
	Mixed	↓	
Albuterol	Digoxin	↓	Digoxin serum levels may be decreased.
Sympathomimetics	Theophylline	↔	Enhanced toxicity, particularly cardiotoxicity, has been noted. Decreased theophylline levels may occur. Ephedrine may cause theophylline toxicity.
Epinephrine	Insulin or oral hypoglycemic agents	↓	Diabetics may require an increased dose of the hypoglycemic agent.

* ↑ = Object drug increased ↓ = Object drug decreased ↔ = Undetermined effect

Drug/Lab test interactions: **Isoproterenol** causes false elevations of bilirubin as measured in vitro by a sequential multiple analyzer. Isoproterenol inhalation may result in enough absorption of the drug to produce elevated urinary epinephrine values. Although small with standard doses, the effect is likely to increase with larger doses.

(Continued on following page)

Sympathomimetics (Cont.)

Adverse Reactions:

Sympathomimetic Bronchodilator Adverse Reactions (%)[1]											
	Adverse reaction	Albuterol	Bitolterol	Ephedrine	Epinephrine	Ethylnorepinephrine	Isoetharine	Isoproterenol	Metaproterenol	Pirbuterol	Terbutaline
Cardiovascular	Palpitations	1-10	1.5-3	✓	7.8-30	✓	✓	5-22	0.3-4	1.3-1.7	7.8-23
	Tachycardia	1-10	<1	✓	≤2.6		✓	2-10	<17	1.3	1.3-3
	Blood pressure changes/ hypertension	3.1-5			✓	✓	✓	2-5	0.3		<1
	Chest tightness/pain/discomfort, angina	<1	<1		≤2.6			✓		1.3	1.5
	PVCs, arrhythmias, skipped beats		0.5	✓	✓			1-3		<1	≈4
CNS	Tremor	1-20	9-14		16-18		✓	<15	3.3-33	1.3-6	5-38
	Dizziness/ vertigo	1-7	1-3	✓	3.3-7.8	✓	✓	1.5-5	1-4	0.6-1.2	1.3-10
	Shakiness/ nervousness/ tension	1-20	1.5-5	✓	8.5-31		✓	<15	2.6-14	4.5-7	5-31
	Weakness	<2			1.6-2.6		✓	✓	1.3	<1	≤1.3
	Drowsiness	<1			8.2-14			<5	0.7		5-11.7
	Restlessness	<1			✓		✓	✓			
	Hyperactivity/ Hyperkinesia, excitement	1-20	<1				✓	✓		<1	
	Headache	2-7	≈4	✓	3.3-10	✓	✓	1.5-10	≤4	1.3-2	7.8-10
	Insomnia	1-3.1	<1	✓	✓		✓	1.5		<1	✓
GI	Nausea/ Vomiting	2-15	≤3	✓	1-11.5	✓	✓	<15	<14	≤1.7	1.3-10
	Heartburn/GI distress/ disorder	≤5						5-10	≤4		<10
	Diarrhea	≤1							0.7	<1.3	
	Dry mouth	<1							1.3	<1.3	
Respiratory	Cough	1-5	4.1					1-5	≤4	1.2	
	Wheezing	≤1.5						1.5			✓
	Dyspnea	1.5	≤1		≤2			≤1.5			≤2
	Bronchospasm	1-15.4	≤1					≤18			✓
	Throat dryness/irritation, pharyngitis	≤6	3-5					3.1	≤4	<1	✓
Other	Flushing	<1	rare		≤1.3			✓		<1	≤2.4
	Sweating	<1		✓	✓			✓			≤2.4
	Anorexia/ Appetite loss	1		✓	✓					<1	
	Unusual/bad taste or taste/ smell change	2							0.3	<1	✓

✓ Reported; no incidence given.
[1] Data pooled for all routes of administration and all age groups.

(Adverse Reactions continued on following page)

Adverse Reactions (Cont.):

Adverse reactions are generally transient, and no cumulative effects have been reported. It is usually not necessary to discontinue treatment; however, in selected cases temporarily reduce dosage. After the reaction has subsided, increase dosage in small increments to optimal dosage.

Other adverse reactions:

Albuterol: CNS – CNS stimulation; malaise (1.5%); emotional lability, fatigue, nightmares, aggressive behavior (1%); lightheadedness, disturbed sleep, irritability (< 1%).

Respiratory – Bronchitis (1.5% to 4%); nasal congestion (1% to 2%); sputum increase (1.5%); epistaxis (1% to 3%); hoarseness (rare in adults; 2% in children 4 to 12 years old).

Miscellaneous – Increased appetite (3%); muscle cramps (1% to 3%); pallor, conjunctivitis, anorexia, teeth discoloration (1%); dilated pupils, epigastric pain, micturition difficulty, muscle spasm, voice changes (< 1%); urticaria, angioedema, rash, bronchospasm, oropharyngeal edema (rare with inhaled albuterol).

Bitolterol: Lightheadedness (3%). Elevations of AST, decrease in platelets and WBC counts and proteinuria (rare); clinical relevance or relationship unknown. The overall incidence of cardiovascular effects was ≈ 5%.

Ephedrine: Precordial pain; contact dermatitis after topical application. *Parenteral* – Vesical sphincter spasm may result in difficult and painful urination; urinary retention may develop in males with prostatism. Confusion, delirium and hallucinations have been reported; excessive doses may cause a sharp rise in blood pressure sufficient to produce cerebral hemorrhage.

Epinephrine: Anxiety, fear, pallor. *Parenteral* – Cerebral hemorrhage caused by rapid rises in blood pressure, particularly in elderly patients with cerebrovascular disease. Parenteral use may induce or aggravate psychomotor agitation, disorientation, impairment of memory, assaultive behavior, panic, hallucinations, suicidal or homicidal tendencies, schizophrenic-type thought disorders or paranoid delusions, hemiplegia and subarachnoid and cerebral hemorrhage. Initially parenteral epinephrine may produce constriction of renal blood vessels and decreased urine formation. Syncope has occurred in children. Patients with Parkinson's disease may experience a temporary increase in rigidity and tremor. Fatal ventricular fibrillation, occlusion of the central retinal artery and shock have occurred. Urticaria, wheal and hemorrhage at injection site; pain at injection site (1.6% to 2.6%). Repeated injections at the same site may result in necrosis from vascular constriction.

Ethylnorepinephrine: Elevated pulse rate.

Isoetharine: Anxiety.

Isoproterenol: Cardiac – Adams-Stokes attacks, cardiac arrest, hypotension, precordial ache/distress. In a few patients, presumably with organic disease of the AV node and its branches, isoproterenol has precipitated Adams-Stokes seizures during normal sinus rhythm or transient heart block.

Respiratory – Bronchitis (5%); sputum increase (1.5%); bronchial edema and inflammation, ECG evidence of coronary insufficiency; paradoxical airway resistance; pulmonary edema.

Miscellaneous – Swelling of the parotid glands with prolonged use.

Metaproterenol: Respiratory – Asthma exacerbation (1% to 4%); hoarseness, nasal congestion (0.7%).

Miscellaneous – Rash (1.3%); backache, fatigue, skin reaction (0.7%).

Pirbuterol: CNS – Anxiety, confusion, depression, fatigue, syncope (< 1%).

Dermatologic – Alopecia, edema, pruritus, rash (< 1%); bruising (≤ 1%).

GI – Abdominal pain/cramps, glossitis, stomatitis (< 1%).

Miscellaneous – Hypotension, numbness in extremities, weight gain (< 1%).

Terbutaline: ECG changes such as sinus pause, atrial premature beats, AV block, ventricular premature beats, ST-T-wave depression, T-wave inversion, sinus bradycardia and atrial escape beat with aberrant conduction; increased heart rate; muscle cramps; central stimulation; pain at injection site (0.5% to 2.6%); elevations in liver enzymes and hypersensitivity vasculitis (rare).

Overdosage:

Inhalation:

Symptoms – Exaggeration of the effects listed under Adverse Reactions can occur. Seizures, hypokalemia, anginal pain and hypertension may result.

Treatment includes general supportive measures. Sedatives (barbiturates) may be given for restlessness. The judicious use of a cardioselective β-receptor blocker (ie, metoprolol, atenolol) is suggested, bearing in mind the danger of inducing an asthmatic attack. Dialysis is not appropriate.

(Overdosage continued on following page)

Overdosage (Cont.):

Systemic:

Symptoms – Palpitations; tachycardia; bradycardia; extrasystoles; heart block; chest pain; hypokalemia; elevated blood pressure; fever; chills; cold perspiration; blanching of the skin; nausea; vomiting; mydriasis. Central actions produce insomnia, anxiety and tremor. Delirium, convulsions, collapse and coma may occur.

Treatment – Discontinuation or reduction in dosage will generally control toxicity. Emesis, gastric lavage or charcoal may be useful following overdosage with oral agents. If pronounced, a β-adrenergic blocker (propranolol) may be used, but consider the possibility of aggravation of airway obstruction; phentolamine may be used to block strong α-adrenergic actions. Treatment includes usual supportive measures. Refer to General Management of Acute Overdosage.

Patient Information:

Inhalation:

Patient instructions are available with products. Many patients do not use metered-dose inhalers correctly, even after repeated instructions. Do not assume the patient understands the use of inhaled drugs and the proper administration technique. Use verbal instructions as well as an actual demonstration if possible. Repeat instructions at follow-up visits.

Have patient tilt head back and keep the metered dose inhaler mouthpiece ≈ 2 inches (or 2 finger widths) from open mouth or place the mouthpiece between open lips. Spacer devices are also available to aid the patient in proper administration of the drug. The patient should press down on the canister, breathe in slowly, hold their breath for at least 10 seconds or as long as comfortable, then exhale. Administer pressurized inhalation during the second half of inspiration as the airways are open wider and the aerosol distribution is more extensive.

Do not exceed recommended dosage; excessive use may lead to adverse effects or loss of effectiveness. Do not stop or adjust the dose.

Do not change from one brand to another without consulting the physician or pharmacist.

If more than one inhalation per dose is necessary, wait at least one full minute between inhalations (administer second inhalation at 3 to 5 minutes for isoproterenol and epinephrine, 10 minutes for metaproterenol.)

Notify physician of failure to respond to usual dosage or of dizziness or chest pain.

Isoproterenol may cause the patient's saliva to turn pinkish-red.

Oral:

Do not exceed prescribed dosage. If GI upset occurs, take with food.

Sublingual tablets *(Isuprel):* Do not swallow; allow to dissolve under tongue.

May cause nervousness, restlessness, insomnia (especially ephedrine); if these effects continue after reducing dosage, notify physician.

Notify physician if palpitations, tachycardia, chest pain, muscle tremors, dizziness, headache, flushing or difficult urination (ephedrine) occurs, or if breathing difficulty persists.

(Products listed on following pages)

Complete prescribing information for these products begins on page 894.

Sympathomimetics (Cont.)

ALBUTEROL

Indications:

Relief and prevention of bronchospasm in patients with reversible obstructive airway disease; prevention of exercise-induced bronchospasm.

Unlabeled use: In a small number of patients on hemodialysis, nebulized albuterol therapy (10 or 20 mg) significantly decreased potassium concentrations and therefore may be useful as an adjunct in treating serious acute hyperkalemia in hemodialysis patients.

Administration and Dosage:

Inhalation aerosol: Adults and children ≥ 12 years (Ventolin – Adults and children ≥ 4 years) – 2 inhalations repeated every 4 to 6 hours. In some patients, 1 inhalation every 4 hours may be sufficient. More frequent administration or a larger number of inhalations is not recommended. If a previously effective dosage fails to provide the relief, seek medical advice immediately; this is often a sign of seriously worsening asthma which requires reassessment of therapy.

Prevention of exercise-induced bronchospasm: Adults and children ≥ 12 years – 2 inhalations 15 minutes prior to exercise.

Inhalation solution: Adults and children ≥ 12 years – 2.5 mg 3 to 4 times daily by nebulization. Dilute 0.5 ml of the 0.5% solution with 2.5 ml sterile normal saline solution. Deliver over approximately 5 to 15 minutes.

Inhalation capsules: Adults and children ≥ 4 years – Usual dose is 200 mcg inhaled every 4 to 6 hours using a Rotahaler inhalation device. In some patients, 400 mcg every 4 to 6 hours may be necessary.

Prevention of exercise-induced bronchospasm: Adults and children ≥ 12 years – 200 mcg inhaled using a Rotahaler inhalation device 15 minutes before exercise.

Tablets: Adults and children ≥ 12 years – Usual starting dosage is 2 or 4 mg 3 or 4 times daily. Do not exceed a total daily dose of 32 mg. Use doses > 4 mg 4 times daily only when the patient fails to respond. If a favorable response does not occur, cautiously increase stepwise, up to a maximum of 8 mg 4 times daily, as tolerated.

Children 6 to 12 years – Usual starting dosage is 2 mg 3 to 4 times/day. For those who fail to respond to the initial starting dosage, cautiously increase stepwise, but do not exceed 24 mg/day in divided doses.

Elderly patients and those sensitive to β-adrenergic stimulants – Start with 2 mg 3 or 4 times daily. If adequate bronchodilation is not obtained, increase dosage gradually to as much as 8 mg 3 or 4 times daily.

Tablets, extended release: Adults and children ≥ 12 years – Usual starting dosage is 4 or 8 mg every 12 hours. Use doses > 8 mg twice/day only when the patient fails to respond. If a favorable response does not occur with the 4 mg initial dosage, cautiously increase stepwise up to a maximum of 16 mg twice a day. Do not exceed 32 mg/day.

Switching to extended release tablets – Patients maintained on regular release albuterol can be switched to *Proventil Repetabs.* A 4 mg extended release tablet every 12 hours is equivalent to a regular 2 mg tablet every 6 hours. Multiples of this regimen up to the maximum recommended dose also apply.

Syrup: Adults and children > 14 years – Usual dose is 2 or 4 mg 3 or 4 times/day. Give doses > 4 mg 4 times/day only when patient fails to respond. If a favorable response does not occur, cautiously increase, but do not exceed 8 mg 4 times/day.

Children (6 to 14) – Usual starting dose is 2 mg 3 or 4 times/day. If patient does not respond to 2 mg 4 times/day, cautiously increase step-wise. Do not exceed 24 mg/day in divided doses.

Children (2 to 6) – Initiate at 0.1 mg/kg 3 times daily. Do not exceed 2 mg 3 times daily. If the patient does not respond to the initial dose, increase step-wise to 0.2 mg/kg 3 times a day. Do not exceed 4 mg 3 times a day.

Elderly patients and those sensitive to β-adrenergic stimulation: Restrict initial dose to 2 mg 3 or 4 times daily. Individualize dosage thereafter.

				C.I.*
Rx	**Albuterol** (Various, eg, Biocraft, Geneva, Goldline, Lederle, Moore, Mutual, Parmed, UDL, URL, Warner Chilcott)	**Tablets:** 2 mg (as sulfate)	In 24s, 100s, 250s, 500s, 1000s and UD 100s.	11+
Rx	**Proventil** (Schering)		Lactose. (Proventil 2 252). White. In 100s and 500s.	23
Rx	**Ventolin** (Glaxo)		Lactose. (Glaxo Ventolin 2). White. In 100s and 500s.	28

* Cost Index based on cost per 2 mg.

(Continued on following page)

Complete prescribing information for these products begins on page 894.

Sympathomimetics (Cont.)

ALBUTEROL (Cont.)

	Product (Manufacturer)	Form/Strength	Description/Packaging	Cost Index*
Rx	**Albuterol** (Various, eg, Biocraft, Geneva, Goldline, Lederle, Moore, Mutual, Parmed, UDL, URL, Warner Chilcott)	**Tablets:** 4 mg (as sulfate)	In 100s, 250s, 500s, 1000s and UD 100s.	9+
Rx	**Proventil** (Schering)		Lactose. (Proventil 4 573). White. In 100s and 500s.	18
Rx	**Ventolin** (Glaxo)		Lactose. (Glaxo Ventolin 4). White. In 100s and 500s.	13
Rx	**Proventil Repetabs** (Schering)	**Tablets, extended release:** 4 mg (as sulfate)	Lactose, sugar. (431). White. In 100s and UD 100s.	17
Rx	**Albuterol** (Lemmon)	**Syrup:** 2 mg (as sulfate) per 5 ml	Sorbitol. Strawberry flavor. In 480 ml.	NA
Rx	**Proventil** (Schering)		Saccharin. Strawberry flavor. In 480 ml.	22
Rx	**Ventolin** (Glaxo)		Saccharin. Strawberry flavor. In 480 ml.	17
Rx	**Proventil** (Schering)	**Aerosol:** Each actuation delivers 90 mcg albuterol	In 17 g (≈ 200 inhalations).	7.3
Rx	**Ventolin** (Glaxo)		In 17 g (200 inhalations).	5.6
Rx	**Albuterol** (Dey)	**Solution for Inhalation:** 0.083% (as sulfate)	In UD 3 ml.	NA
Rx	**Proventil** (Schering)		In 3 ml.	17
Rx	**Albuterol** (Copley)	**Solution for Inhalation:** 0.5% (as sulfate)	In 20 ml with dropper.	31
Rx	**Proventil** (Schering)		In 20 ml with dropper.	NA
Rx	**Ventolin** (Glaxo)		In 20 ml with dropper.	24
Rx	**Ventolin Rotacaps** (Glaxo)	**Capsules for Inhalation:** 200 mcg microfine (as sulfate)	Lactose. (Ventolin 200 Glaxo). Lt. blue/clear. In UD 24s and 96s with Rotahaler inhalation device.	16

* Cost Index based on cost per 90 mcg aerosol, 2 mg tablet or syrup, or 0.5 ml solution.

METAPROTERENOL SULFATE

Indications:

For bronchial asthma and reversible bronchospasm; treatment of acute asthmatic attacks in children ≥ 6 years of age (*Alupent* solution for inhalation *only*).

Administration and Dosage:

Metered dose inhaler: 2 to 3 inhalations every 3 to 4 hours. Do not exceed 12 inhalations/day. Not recommended for children < 12 years of age.

Inhalant solutions: Usually, treatment need not be repeated more often than every 4 hours to relieve acute bronchospasm attacks. In chronic bronchospastic pulmonary diseases, give 3 to 4 times a day. A single dose of nebulized metaproterenol in the treatment of an acute attack of asthma may not completely abort an attack. Not recommended for children < 12 years of age.

Dosage and Dilution for Metaproterenol Inhalant Solutions			
Administration	Usual dose	Range	Dilution
Hand bulb nebulizer	10 inhalations	5-15 inhalations	No dilution
IPPB	0.3 ml	0.2-0.3 ml	In ≈ 2.5 ml saline or other diluent

Administer the unit dose vial by oral inhalation using an IPPB device. The usual adult dose is one vial per nebulization treatment. Each 0.4% vial is equivalent to 0.2 ml of the 5% solution diluted to 2.5 ml with normal saline. Each 0.6% vial is equivalent to 0.3 ml of the 5% solution diluted to 2.5 ml with normal saline.

Oral: Adults and children (> 9 years or > 60 lbs) – 20 mg 3 or 4 times a day.

Children (> 6 to 9 years or < 60 lbs) – 10 mg 3 or 4 times a day.

Children (< 6 years) – Doses of ≈ 1.3 to 2.6 mg/kg/day in divided doses of syrup were well tolerated in 78 children. Tablets are not recommended for this age group.

Storage: Store inhalant solution at 25° C (77° F). Protect from light. Do not use solution if it is brown or darker than slightly yellow, pinkish or if it contains a precipitate.

(Products listed on following page)

Complete prescribing information for these products begins on page 894.

Sympathomimetics (Cont.)

METAPROTERENOL (Cont.):

	Product	Form	Description	C.I.*
Rx	**Metaproterenol Sulfate** (Various, eg, Goldline, Major, Moore, Par, Parmed, PBI, Qualitest, Rugby, Schein, URL)	**Tablets:** 10 mg	In 100s and 1000s.	28+
Rx	**Alupent** (Boehringer-Ingelheim)		(BI/74). White, scored. In 100s.[1]	45
Rx	**Metaprel** (Sandoz)		(78-212 10) White, scored. In 100s.[1]	22
Rx	**Metaproterenol Sulfate** (Various, eg, IDE, Major, Moore, Par, Parmed, PBI, Qualitest, Rugby, Schein, URL)	**Tablets:** 20 mg	In 100s and 1000s.	18+
Rx	**Alupent** (Boehringer-Ingelheim)		(BI/72). White, scored. In 100s.[1]	29
Rx	**Metaprel** (Sandoz)		(78-213 20). White, scored. In 100s.[1]	14
Rx	**Metaproterenol Sulfate** (Various, eg, Copley, Genetco, Geneva, IDE, Major, Moore, PBI, Qualitest, Rugby, Schein)	**Syrup:** 10 mg per 5 ml	In 480 ml.	22+
Rx	**Alupent** (Boehringer-Ingelheim)		Saccharin, sorbitol. Cherry flavor. In 480 ml.	49
Rx	**Metaprel** (Sandoz)		Saccharin, sorbitol. Cherry flavor. In 480 ml.	24
Rx	**Alupent** (Boehringer Ingelheim)	**Aerosol:** 75 mg as micronized powder in inert propellant (100 inhalations). Each dose delivers 0.65 mg	In 5 ml inhaler.	NA
Rx	**Alupent** (Boehringer Ingelheim)	**Aerosol:** 150 mg as micronized powder in inert propellant (200 inhalations). Each dose delivers 0.65 mg	In 10 ml inhaler or 10 ml refill.	NA
Rx	**Metaprel** (Sandoz)		In 10 ml inhaler or 10 ml refill.	21
Rx	**Metaproterenol Sulfate** (Various, eg, Dey, Par)	**Solution for Inhalation:** 0.4%	In 2.5 ml.	NA
Rx	**Alupent** (B-I)		In 2.5 ml UD vials.[2]	NA
Rx	**Arm-a-Med Metaproterenol Sulfate** (Astra)		In 2.5 ml vials.[2]	55
Rx	**Metaproterenol Sulfate** (Various, eg, Dey, Major, Moore, Par)	**Solution for Inhalation:** 0.6%	In 2.5 ml.	32+
Rx	**Alupent** (B-I)		In 2.5 ml UD vials.[2]	32
Rx	**Arm-a-Med Metaproterenol Sulfate** (Astra)		In 2.5 ml vials.[2]	24
Rx	**Metaproterenol Sulfate** (Various, eg, Dey, Goldline, IDE, Moore, PBI, Qualitest, Rugby)	**Solution for Inhalation:** 5%	In 0.3 and 30 ml vials.	NA
Rx	**Alupent** (Boehringer-Ingelheim)		In 10 or 30 ml w/ dropper.	60
Rx	**Metaprel** (Sandoz)		In 10 ml w/dropper.	66

* Cost Index based on cost per 650 mcg aerosol inhalation, 15 mg nebulization or 20 mg oral.
[1] Contains lactose. [2] For use with an IPPB device.

Complete prescribing information for these products begins on page 894.

Sympathomimetics (Cont.)

ISOETHARINE HCl

Indications:

For bronchial asthma and reversible bronchospasm that occurs with bronchitis and emphysema.

Administration and Dosage:

Individualize dosage. Pediatric dosage has not been established.

Isoetharine Doses (Volume) Based on Strength of Solution		
Solution strength	Usual dose (IPPB[1] or oxygen aerosolization[2])	Equivalent isoetharine 1% dose
1%	0.25 to 1 ml (IPPB) or 0.25 to 0.5 ml (O_2 aerosolization) diluted 1:3 with saline or other diluent	same
0.25%	2 ml	0.5 ml
0.2%	1.25 to 2.5 ml	0.25 to 0.5 ml
0.17%	3 ml	0.5 ml
0.167%	3 ml	0.25 to 0.5 ml
0.125%	2 to 4 ml	0.25 to 0.5 ml
0.1%	2.5 to 5 ml	0.25 to 0.5 ml
0.08%	3 ml	0.25 ml
0.062%	4 ml	0.25 ml

[1] Usually an inspiratory flow rate of 15 L/min at a cycling pressure of 15 cm H_2O; may adjust flow rate to 6 to 30 L/min, cycling pressure to 10 to 15 cm H_2O.

[2] When given with oxygen, adjust flow to 4 to 6 L/min over 15 to 20 minutes.

Hand nebulizer: 3 to 7 inhalations undiluted.

Aerosol nebulizer: 1 or 2 inhalations. Occasionally, more may be required; however, wait 1 full minute after the initial dose to be certain another dose is necessary.

Usually, treatment need not be repeated more often than every 4 hours, although in severe cases more frequent administration may be necessary.

Storage/Stability: Do not use if solution is discolored or contains a precipitate. Protect from light.

	Product	Dosage form	How supplied	C.I.*
Rx	**Arm-a-Med Isoetharine HCl** (Astra)	**Solution for inhalation:** 0.062%	In single use 4 ml vials.[1]	22
Rx	**Isoetharine HCl** (Various, eg, Dey)	**Solution for inhalation:** 0.08%	In 3 ml vials.[2]	37+
Rx	**Isoetharine HCl** (Various, eg, Dey, Roxane)	**Solution for inhalation:** 0.1%	In single use 2.5 and 5 ml vials.	30+
Rx	**Isoetharine HCl** (Roxane)	**Solution for inhalation:** 0.125%	In single use 4 ml vials.[3]	15
Rx	**Arm-a-Med Isoetharine HCl** (Astra)		In single use 4 ml vials.[1]	11
Rx	**Isoetharine HCl** (Various, eg, Roxane)	**Solution for inhalation:** 0.167%	In single use 3 ml vials.[3]	15+
Rx	**Arm-a-Med Isoetharine HCl** (Astra)		In single use 3 ml vials.[1]	11
Rx	**Isoetharine HCl** (Various, eg, Dey)	**Solution for inhalation:** 0.17%	In single use 3 ml vials.[2]	18+
Rx	**Isoetharine HCl** (Various, eg, Roxane)	**Solution for inhalation:** 0.2%	In single use 2.5 ml vials.[3]	15+
Rx	**Arm-a-Med Isoetharine HCl** (Astra)		In single use 2.5 ml vials.[1]	11

* Cost Index based on cost per mg.

[1] With sodium metabisulfite and glycerin.

[2] With glycerin and EDTA.

[3] With glycerin, EDTA, sodium sulfite and sodium bisulfite.

(Continued on following page)

Complete prescribing information for these products begins on page 894.

Sympathomimetics (Cont.)

ISOETHARINE HCl (Cont.)

				C.I.*
Rx	**Isoetharine HCl** (Various, eg, Dey, Roxane)	**Solution for inhalation:** 0.25%	In single use 2 ml vials.	15+
Rx	**Arm-a-Med Isoetharine HCl** (Astra)		In single use 2 ml vials.[1]	11
Rx	**Isoetharine HCl** (Various, eg, Dey, Roxane)	**Solution for inhalation:** 1%	In UD 0.25 and 0.5 ml vials.	6.5+
Rx	**Beta-2** (Nephron)		In 10 and 30 ml with dropper.[2]	5
Rx	**Bronkosol** (Winthrop)		In 10 and 30 ml.[2]	10
Rx	**Bronkometer** (Winthrop)	**Aerosol:** 0.61% (as mesylate). Delivers 340 mcg isoetharine per metered dose	In 10 and 15 ml with oral nebulizer (≈ 20 doses/ml).[3]	19

TERBUTALINE SULFATE

Indications:

A bronchodilator for bronchial asthma and for reversible bronchospasm which may occur with bronchitis and emphysema.

Unlabeled use: Oral and IV terbutaline have successfully inhibited premature labor. Initiate IV administration at 10 mcg/minute; titrate upward to a maximum dose of 80 mcg/minute. Maintain IV dosage at the minimum effective dose for 4 hours. Oral doses of 2.5 mg every 4 to 6 hours have been used as maintenance therapy until term.

Administration and Dosage:

Inhalation: Adults and children ≥ 12 years – 2 inhalations separated by 60 seconds every 4 to 6 hours. Do not repeat more often than every 4 to 6 hours.

Oral: Adults and children > 15 years – 5 mg, given at 6 hour intervals, 3 times daily during waking hours. If side effects are pronounced, dose may be reduced to 2.5 mg 3 times daily. Do not exceed 15 mg in 24 hours.

Children (12 to 15 years) – 2.5 mg 3 times daily. Do not exceed 7.5 mg in 24 hours. Not recommended for children < 12 years of age.

Parenteral: Usual dose is 0.25 mg SC into the lateral deltoid area. If significant improvement does not occur in 15 to 30 minutes, administer a second 0.25 mg dose. Do not exceed a total dose of 0.5 mg in 4 hours. If a patient fails to respond to a second 0.25 mg dose within 15 to 30 minutes, consider other therapeutic measures.

				C.I.*
Rx	**Brethine** (Geigy)	**Tablets:** 2.5 mg	Lactose. (Geigy 72). White, scored. Oval. In 100s, 1000s, UD 100s and Gy-Pak 100s.	21
Rx	**Bricanyl** (Marion Merrell Dow)		Lactose. (Bricanyl 2½). White. In 100s and 1000s.	18
Rx	**Brethine** (Geigy)	**Tablets:** 5 mg	Lactose. (Geigy 105). White, scored. In 100s, 1000s, UD 100s and Gy-Pak 100s.	15
Rx	**Bricanyl** (Marion Merrell Dow)		Lactose. (Bricanyl 5). White, scored. Square. In 100s and 1000s.	13
Rx	**Brethaire** (Geigy)	**Aerosol:** 0.2 mg per actuation	In 10.5 g cans (≥ 300 inhalations).	5.8
Rx	**Brethine** (Geigy)	**Injection:** 1 mg/ml	In 2 ml amp with 1 ml fill.	21
Rx	**Bricanyl** (Marion Merrell Dow)		In 2 ml amp with 1 ml fill.	20

* Cost Index based on cost per 1 mg isoetharine HCl, 340 mcg isoetharine mesylate or 5 mg oral, 0.2 mg aerosol or 0.25 mg parenteral terbutaline.

[1] With glycerin and sodium metabisulfite.

[2] With glycerin, sodium bisulfite and parabens.

[3] With saccharin, menthol and alcohol.

Complete prescribing information for these products begins on page 894.

Sympathomimetics (Cont.)

ETHYLNOREPINEPHRINE HCl

Indications:

A bronchodilator for bronchial asthma and for reversible bronchospasm that may occur with bronchitis and emphysema.

Administration and Dosage:

Adults: The usual dose by SC or IM injection is 0.5 to 1 ml. Depending on severity of the asthmatic attack, smaller doses (0.3 to 0.5 ml) may suffice.

Children: Dosage varies according to age and weight; usual dose is 0.1 to 0.5 ml.

Storage: Protect from light.

				C.I.*
Rx	**Bronkephrine** (Winthrop Pharm.)	**Injection:** 2 mg/ml	In 1 ml amps.[1]	433

* Cost Index based on cost per 2 mg.

[1] With sodium bisulfite.

ISOPROTERENOL

Indications:

Inhalation: Treatment of bronchospasm associated with acute and chronic bronchial asthma, pulmonary emphysema, bronchitis and bronchiectasis.

Injection: Management of bronchospasm during anesthesia.

Sublingual: Management of patients with bronchopulmonary disease.

Isoproterenol is also used as a vasopressor in shock. Refer to Vasopressors Used in Shock in the Cardiovascular section.

Administration and Dosage:

Inhalation:

Acute bronchial asthma -

Hand bulb nebulizer: In adults and children, administer the 1:200 solution in a dosage of 5 to 15 deep inhalations. In adults, the 1:100 solution may be used if a stronger solution seems indicated. The dose is 3 to 7 deep inhalations. If no relief is evident after 5 to 10 minutes, repeat doses one more time. If acute attack recurs, repeat treatment up to 5 times daily if necessary.

Metered dose inhaler: The usual dose is 1 to 2 inhalations. Start with 1 inhalation. If no relief is evident after 2 to 5 minutes, a second inhalation may be taken. For daily maintenance, use 1 to 2 inhalations 4 to 6 times daily. Do not take more than 2 inhalations at any one time, nor more than 6 inhalations per hour.

Bronchospasm in chronic obstructive lung disease -

Hand bulb nebulizer: Usually 5 to 15 deep inhalations using the 1:200 solution. Some patients with severe attacks may require 3 to 7 inhalations using the 1:100 solution. Do not use at less than 3 to 4 hour intervals.

Nebulization by compressed air or oxygen: 0.5 ml of a 1:200 solution is diluted to 2 to 2.5 ml with appropriate diluent for a concentration of 1:800 to 1:1000. Deliver the solution over 10 to 20 minutes. May repeat up to 5 times daily.

IPPB: 0.5 ml of a 1:200 solution diluted to 2 to 2.5 ml with water or isotonic saline. Deliver over 15 to 20 minutes. May repeat up to 5 times daily.

Metered dose inhaler: 1 or 2 inhalations; repeat at no less than 3 to 4 hour intervals (4 to 6 times daily).

Children - Administration is similar to that of adults, since children's smaller ventilatory exchange capacity automatically provides proportionally smaller aerosol intake. The 1:200 solution is recommended for an acute attack of bronchospasm. Do not use more than 0.25 ml of the 1:200 solution for each 10 to 15 minute programmed treatment.

Injection: For the management of bronchospasm during anesthesia, dilute 1 ml of a 1:5000 solution to 10 ml with Sodium Chloride Injection or 5% Dextrose Injection. Administer an initial dose of 0.01 to 0.02 mg IV and repeat when necessary.

Sublingual: The average adult dose is 10 mg (15 to 20 mg may be required) depending on patient response. However, do not exceed a total of 60 mg/day. For children, the dose is from 5 to 10 mg, not exceeding a total of 30 mg/day.

Allow tablets to disintegrate under the tongue. Do not crush or chew sublingual tablets. Instruct patients not to swallow saliva until absorption has taken place. Do not repeat treatment more often than every 3 or 4 hours, or $>$ 3 times daily.

(Products listed on following page)

Complete prescribing information for these products begins on page 894.

Sympathomimetics (Cont.)

ISOPROTERENOL (Cont.)

	Product	Form	Package	C.I.*
Rx	**Isuprel Glossets** (Winthrop Pharm.)	**Sublingual tablets:** 10 mg	Lactose, saccharin. In 50s.[1]	37
		15 mg	Lactose, saccharin. In 50s.[1]	50
Rx	**Isoproterenol HCl** (Various, eg, Goldline, Moore)	**Solution for inhalation:** 0.25% (1:400)	In 15 ml.	NA
Rx	**Dispos-a-Med Isoproterenol HCl** (Parke-Davis)		In 0.5 ml.[2] (Use only with Dispos-a-vial solutions.)	57
Rx	**Isoproterenol HCl** (Various, eg, Dey)	**Solution for inhalation:** 0.5% (1:200)	In 0.5 ml single use vials.[3]	26+
Rx	**Dispos-a-Med Isoproterenol HCl** (Parke-Davis)		In 0.5 ml.[2] (Use only with Dispos-a-vial solutions.)	29
Rx	**Isuprel** (Winthrop Pharm.)		In 10 and 60 ml.[4]	2.1
Rx	**Isuprel** (Winthrop Pharm.)	**Solution for inhalation:** 1% (1:100) isoproterenol HCl	In 10 ml.[5]	2.6
Rx	**Isoproterenol HCl** (Various, eg, Schein)	**Aerosol:** 0.25% (1:400)	In 15 ml.	NA
Rx	**Isuprel Mistometer** (Winthrop Pharm.)	**Aerosol:** Delivers 131 mcg isoproterenol HCl solution/dose in fine mist	In 10 and 15 ml and 15 ml refill.	13
Rx	**Medihaler-Iso** (3M)	**Aerosol:** 0.2% isoproterenol sulfate. Delivers 80 mcg/measured dose	In 15 ml (≈ 300 doses) or 22.5 ml (≈ 450 doses) w/adapter and 15 ml refill.	43
Rx	**Isoproterenol HCl** (Various, eg, Elkins-Sinn)	**Injection:** (1:5000 solution) 0.2 mg/ml	In 5 ml amps.	NA
Rx	**Isuprel** (Winthrop Pharm.)		In 1 and 5 ml amps.[6]	295

ISOPROTERENOL HCl AND PHENYLEPHRINE BITARTRATE

Indications:

Treatment of bronchospasm associated with acute and chronic asthma, and reversible bronchospasm which may be associated with emphysema or chronic bronchitis.

Administration and Dosage:

Relief of dyspnea: Acute episode, 1 to 2 inhalations. Start with one inhalation; if not relieved in 2 to 5 minutes, administer a second. *Daily maintenance* – 1 to 2 inhalations, 4 to 6 times daily. Do not take > 2 inhalations at any one time or > 6 in any 1 hour within 24 hours.

	Product	Form	Package	C.I.*
Rx	**Duo-Medihaler** (3M)	**Aerosol:** Each valve actuation releases 0.16 mg isoproterenol HCl and 0.24 mg phenylephrine bitartrate	In 15 ml (≈ 300 metered doses) or 22.5 ml (≈ 450 metered doses) medihalers or 15 and 22.5 ml refills.	5.9

* Cost Index based on cost per 10 mg sublingual, 125 mcg inhalation or 0.2 mg parenteral isoproterenol or per dose of isoproterenol HCl/phenylephrine bitartrate.

[1] With 2 mg sodium metabisulfite.
[2] With glycerin and sodium bisulfites.
[3] With sodium metabisulfite and parabens.
[4] With chlorobutanol, sodium metabisulfite and glycerin.
[5] With chlorobutanol, sodium metabisulfite and saccharin.
[6] With sodium metabisulfite.

Complete prescribing information for these products begins on page 894.

Sympathomimetics (Cont.)

BITOLTEROL MESYLATE

Indications:

Prophylaxis and treatment of bronchial asthma and reversible bronchospasm. May be used with or without concurrent theophylline or steroid therapy.

Administration and Dosage:

Bronchospasm: Adults and children > 12 years of age – 2 inhalations at an interval of at least 1 to 3 minutes, followed by a third inhalation if needed.

Prevention of bronchospasm: 2 inhalations every 8 hours.

Do not exceed 3 inhalations every 6 hours or 2 inhalations every 4 hours.

				C.I.*
Rx	**Tornalate** (Winthrop)	**Aerosol:** 0.8%. Delivers 0.37 mg/actuation	In 15 ml metered dose inhaler[1] (≥ 300 inhalations) and 15 ml refill.	16

* Cost Index based on cost per 0.37 mg bitolterol.
[1] With saccharin, menthol and alcohol.

EPINEPHRINE

Indications:

Inhalation: Temporary relief from acute paroxysms (eg, shortness of breath, tightness of chest, wheezing) of bronchial asthma; treatment of postintubation and infectious croup.

MicroNefrin – Chronic obstructive lung disease, chronic bronchitis, broncheolitis, bronchial asthma and other peripheral airway diseases.

Injection: To relieve respiratory distress in bronchial asthma or during acute asthma attacks and for reversible bronchospasm in patients with chronic bronchitis, emphysema and other obstructive pulmonary diseases.

Treatment of hypersensitivity reactions to drugs, sera, insect stings or other allergens, including such symptoms as bronchospasm, urticaria, pruritus, angioneurotic edema, or swelling of the lips, eyelids, tongue and nasal mucosa.

Epinephrine is also used as a vasopressor in shock (refer to Vasopressors Used in Shock in the Cardiovascular section) and for infiltration of tissue to delay absorption of drugs such as local anesthetics.

Administration and Dosage:

Refer to specific product labeling for detailed administration and dosage information.

Inhalation aerosol: Start treatment at the first symptoms of bronchospasm. Individualize dosage. Wait 1 to 5 minutes between inhalations.

Nebulization: Place 8 to 15 drops into the nebulizer reservoir. Place the nebulizer nozzle into the partially opened mouth. Squeeze the bulb 1 to 3 times. Inhale deeply. If relief does not occur within 5 minutes, administer 2 to 3 additional inhalations. Nebulizer use, 4 to 6 times daily, is usually sufficient to maintain comfort.

IPPB – Add 0.5 ml epinephrine to 20 ml water just prior to treatment. Administer for 15 minutes every 3 to 4 hours.

Injection:

Solution (1:1000) - The initial adult SC or IM dose is 0.3 to 0.5 ml (0.3 to 0.5 mg); repeat every 20 minutes to 4 hours. *For infants and children* (except premature infants and full-term newborns), give 0.01 ml/kg or 0.3 ml/m² (0.01 mg/kg or 0.3 mg/m²) SC. Do not exceed 0.5 ml (0.5 mg) in a single pediatric dose. Repeat every 20 minutes to 4 hours or more often if necessary.

Suspension (1:200) - For SC use only. Administer subsequent doses only when necessary and not more often than every 6 hours.

Adults – 0.1 to 0.3 ml (0.5 to 1.5 mg) SC.

Infants and children (1 month to 12 years) – 0.005 ml/kg (0.025 mg/kg) SC.

Children ≤ 30 kg – The maximum single dose is 0.15 ml (0.75 mg).

Repeated local injections can result in necrosis at injection sites from vascular constriction. Tolerance can occur with prolonged use.

Storage – Refrigerate the suspension; do not freeze. Do not expose to temperatures > 30°C (86°F). Shake well before using.

Alkalies and oxidizers (eg, oxygen, chlorine, bromine, iodine, permanganates, chromates, nitrites and salts of easily reducible metals, especially iron) destroy epinephrine.

(Products listed on following page)

Complete prescribing information for these products begins on page 894.

Sympathomimetics (Cont.)

EPINEPHRINE (Cont.)

	Product	Form	Packaging	C.I.*
otc	**Adrenalin Chloride** (Parke-Davis)	**Solution for inhalation:** 1:100 solution epinephrine HCl	In 7.5 ml.[1]	111
otc	**AsthmaNefrin** (Menley & James)	**Solution for inhalation:** 2.25% racepinephrine HCl (equivalent to 1.125% epinephrine base)	In 15 and 30 ml and complete nebulizer.[2]	NA
otc	**microNefrin** (Bird)		In 15 and 30 ml.[3]	400
otc	**Nephron** (Nephron)		In 7.5 and 15 ml.	NA
Rx	**Racepinephrine** (Dey)		In 0.25 ml single use vials.	37
otc	**S-2** (Nephron)		In 15 ml.[3]	95
otc	**Vaponefrin** (Fisons)	**Solution for inhalation:** 2% racepinephrine base (equivalent to 1% epinephrine base)	In 15 and 30 ml.[4]	54
otc	**AsthmaHaler Mist** (Menley & James)	**Aerosol:** 0.3 mg epinephrine bitartrate (equivalent to 0.16 mg epinephrine base per spray)	Alcohol free. In 15 ml w/adapter or 15 ml refill.	32
otc	**Bronitin Mist** (Whitehall)		In 15 ml or 15 ml refills.	56
otc	**Medihaler-Epi** (3M)		In 15 ml w/adapter or 15 ml refills.	51
otc	**Primatene Mist Suspension** (Whitehall)		In 10 ml, 15 ml w/mouthpiece or 15 and 22.5 ml refills.	NA
otc	**Bronkaid Mist** (Winthrop Pharm.)	**Aerosol:** 0.5% epinephrine (as nitrate and HCl, equivalent to 0.25 mg epinephrine per spray)	33% alcohol. In 10 ml and 15 ml (≥ 300 doses) w/actuator or 15 and 22.5 ml refills.	62
otc	**Primatene Mist** (Whitehall)	**Aerosol:** 0.2 mg epinephrine per spray	34% alcohol. In 15 ml w/mouthpiece or 15 and 22.5 ml refills.	105
Rx	**Epinephrine** (Various, eg, Abbott, American Regent, Elkins-Sinn, IMS, Lyphomed, Wyeth-Ayerst)	**Injection:** 1:1000 (1 mg/ml as HCl) solution	In 1 ml amps.	NA
Rx	**Adrenalin Chloride Solution** (Parke-Davis)		In 1 ml amps[5] and 30 ml Steri-vials.[6]	206
Rx	**Sus-Phrine** (Forest)	**Injection:** 1:200 (5 mg/ml) suspension	In 0.3 ml amps[7] and 5 ml vials.[7]	598

* Cost Index based on cost per mg.
[1] With benzethonium chloride and 0.2% sodium bisulfite.
[2] With benzoic acid, chlorobutanol, glycerin and sodium bisulfite.
[3] With sodium bisulfite, potassium metabisulfite, chlorobutanol, benzoic acid and propylene glycol.
[4] With chlorobutanol and sodium metabisulfite.
[5] With sodium bisulfite.
[6] With sodium bisulfite and chlorobutanol.
[7] With thioglycolic acid, phenol and glycerin.

Complete prescribing information for these products begins on page 894.

Sympathomimetics (Cont.)

EPHEDRINE SULFATE

Ephedrine sulfate is a sympathomimetic alkaloid which stimulates alpha and beta receptors as well as the CNS. It is effective both orally and parenterally. It is longer acting but less potent than epinephrine.

Indications:

Treatment of allergic disorders, such as bronchial asthma, and for local treatment of nasal congestion in acute coryza, vasomotor rhinitis, acute sinusitis and hay fever.

Parenteral ephedrine is sometimes used to relieve acute bronchospasm, but it is less effective than epinephrine for this purpose and has been given as a CNS stimulant in narcolepsy and depressive states.

Ephedrine is also used as a vasopressor in shock. Refer to Vasopressors Used in Shock in the Cardiovascular section.

Administration and Dosage:

Adults: The usual oral dose is 25 to 50 mg, 2 or 3 times a day. The usual parenteral dose is 25 to 50 mg, administered SC, IM or slowly IV.

Children: 3 mg/kg/day or 100 mg/m²/day divided into 4 to 6 doses by the oral, SC or IV route.

				C.I.*
otc	**Ephedrine Sulfate** (Various, eg, Goldline, IDE, Lannett, Major, Moore, Schein, URL, West-Ward)	**Capsules:** 25 mg	In 100s, 500s, 1000s and UD 100s.	33+
Rx	**Ephedrine Sulfate** (Various, eg, Rugby)	**Capsules:** 50 mg	In 1000s.	1+
Rx	**Ephedrine Sulfate** (Lilly)	**Injection:** 25 mg/ml	In 1 ml amps.	NA
Rx	**Ephedrine Sulfate** (Various, eg, Abbott, Lilly, Lyphomed)	**Injection:** 50 mg/ml	In 1 ml amps, 10 ml vials and 10 ml disp. syringes.	NA

PIRBUTEROL ACETATE

Indications:

Prevention and reversal of bronchospasm in patients with reversible bronchospasm including asthma. Use with or without concurrent theophylline or steroid therapy.

Administration and Dosage:

Adults and children ≥ 12 years of age: 2 inhalations (0.4 mg) repeated every 4 to 6 hours. One inhalation (0.2 mg) may be sufficient for some patients.

Do not exceed a total daily dose of 12 inhalations.

If previously effective dosage regimen fails to provide the usual relief, seek medical advice immediately as this is often a sign of seriously worsening asthma which would require reassessment of therapy.

Rx	**Maxair** (3M Pharm.)	**Aerosol:** Delivers 0.2 mg/ actuation	In 25.6 g metered dose inhaler (≥ 300 inhalations).	25

Diluents

SODIUM CHLORIDE

Indications:

To dilute bronchodilator solutions for inhalation. Also for tracheal lavage.

otc	**Sodium Chloride 0.45%** (Dey)	**Solution:** 0.45% sodium chloride	Preservative free. In single-use 3 and 5 ml vials.
otc	**Sodium Chloride 0.9%** (Dey)	**Solution:** 0.9% sodium chloride	Preservative free. In 1, 3, 5, 10 & 15 ml Dey-Paks & 3, 5, 10 & 20 ml Dey-Vials.
otc	**Broncho Saline** (Blairex)		In 90 and 240 ml with metered dispensing valve.

* Cost Index based on cost per 25 mg ephedrine or 0.2 mg pirbuterol.

Xanthine Derivatives

Actions:

Pharmacology: The methylxanthines (theophylline, its soluble salts and derivatives) directly relax the smooth muscle of the bronchi and pulmonary blood vessels, stimulate the CNS, induce diuresis, increase gastric acid secretion, reduce lower esophageal sphincter pressure and inhibit uterine contractions. Theophylline is also a central respiratory stimulant. Aminophylline has a potent effect on diaphragmatic contractility in healthy persons and may then be capable of reducing fatigability and thereby improve contractility in patients with chronic obstructive airways disease. The exact mode of action is unclear.

For many years, the proposed main mechanism of action of the xanthines was inhibition of phosphodiesterase, which results in an increase in cyclic adenosine monophosphate (cAMP). However, this effect is negligible at therapeutic concentrations. Other effects that appear to occur at therapeutic concentrations and may collectively play a role in the mechanism of the xanthines include: Inhibition of extracellular adenosine (which causes bronchoconstriction), although it is unlikely that this is a main mechanism; stimulation of endogenous catecholamines, although this also does not appear to be a major mechanism; antagonism of prostaglandins PGE_2 and $PGF_{2\alpha}$; direct effect on mobilization of intracellular calcium resulting in smooth muscle relaxation; beta-adrenergic agonist activity on the airways. None of these mechanisms has been proven.

Pharmacokinetics: Absorption – Theophylline is well absorbed from oral liquids and from uncoated plain tablets; maximal plasma concentrations are reached in 2 hours. Since rectal absorption from suppositories is slow and erratic, the oral route is generally preferred. Enteric coated tablets and some sustained release dosage forms may be unreliably absorbed. Food may alter the bioavailability and absorption pattern of some sustained release theophylline preparations; close monitoring is advised (see Drug Interactions).

Distribution – Average volume of distribution is 0.45 L/kg (range, 0.3 to 0.7 L/kg). Theophylline does not distribute into fatty tissue, but readily crosses the placenta and is excreted into breast milk. Approximately 40% is bound to plasma protein. Therapeutic serum levels generally range from 10 to 20 mcg/ml. Although some bronchodilatory effect occurs at lower concentrations, stabilization of hyperreactive airways is most evident at levels $>$ 10 mcg/ml, and adverse effects are uncommon at levels $<$ 20 mcg/ml. Once a patient is stabilized, serum levels tend to remain constant with the same dosage.

Metabolism/Excretion – Xanthines are biotransformed in the liver (85% to 90%) to 1, 3-dimethyluric acid, 3-methylxanthine and 1-methyluric acid; 3-methylxanthine accumulates in concentrations approximately 25% of those of theophylline.

Excretion is by the kidneys; $<$ 15% of the drug is excreted unchanged. Elimination kinetics vary greatly. The plasma elimination half-life of theophylline averages about 3 to 15 hours in adult nonsmokers, 4 to 5 hours in adult smokers (1 to 2 packs per day), 1 to 9 hours in children and 20 to 30 hours for premature neonates. In the neonate, theophylline is metabolized partially to caffeine. The premature neonate excretes about 50% unchanged theophylline and may accumulate the caffeine metabolite.

A prolonged half-life may occur in patients with congestive heart failure, liver dysfunction, alcoholism, respiratory infections and in patients receiving certain other drugs (see Drug Interactions). Total theophylline clearance appears relatively unaffected by renal failure.

Equivalent dose: Because of differing theophylline content, the various salts and derivatives are not equivalent on a weight basis. The table below indicates the percentage of anhydrous theophylline and the approximate equivalent dose of each compound. Product listings include anhydrous theophylline dosage equivalents.

Theophylline Content and Equivalent Dose of Various Theophylline Salts

Theophylline salts	Theophylline %	Equivalent dose
Theophylline anhydrous	100	100 mg
Theophylline monohydrate	91	110 mg
Aminophylline anhydrous	86	116 mg
Aminophylline dihydrate	79	127 mg
Oxtriphylline	64	156 mg

Dyphylline, a chemical derivative of theophylline, is not a theophylline salt as are the other agents. It is about one-tenth as potent as theophylline. Following oral administration, dyphylline is 68% to 82% bioavailable. Peak plasma concentrations are reached within 1 hour, and its half-life is 2 hours. The minimal effective therapeutic concentration is 12 mcg/ml. It is not metabolized to theophylline and 83% $\pm$ 5% is excreted unchanged in the urine.

(Continued on following page)

Indications:

Symptomatic relief or prevention of bronchial asthma and reversible bronchospasm associated with chronic bronchitis and emphysema.

Unlabeled uses: Treatment of apnea and bradycardia of prematurity. Doses of 2 mg/kg/day have been used to maintain serum concentrations between 3 and 5 mcg/ml.

Theophylline 300 mg/day was effective in reducing essential tremor in one study of 20 patients.

Theophylline 10 mg/kg/day may significantly improve pulmonary function and dyspnea in patients with chronic obstructive pulmonary disease.

Contraindications:

Hypersensitivity to any xanthine; peptic ulcer; underlying seizure disorders (unless receiving appropriate anticonvulsant medication).

Aminophylline: Hypersensitivity to ethylenediamine.

Aminophylline rectal suppositories: In the presence of irritation or infection of the rectum or lower colon.

Warnings:

Status asthmaticus is a medical emergency and is not rapidly responsive to usual doses of conventional bronchodilators. Optimal therapy frequently requires both parenteral medication and close monitoring, preferably in an intensive care setting. Oral theophylline products alone are not appropriate treatment for status asthmaticus.

Toxicity: Excessive doses may cause severe toxicity; monitor serum levels to assure maximum benefit with minimum risk. Incidence of toxicity increases significantly at serum levels > 20 mcg/ml (in 75% of patients with serum levels > 25 mcg/ml). Serum levels > 20 mcg/ml are rarely found after appropriate administration of recommended doses. However, in patients in whom theophylline plasma clearance is reduced for any reason (eg, hepatic function impairment; patients > 55 years of age, particularly males and those with chronic lung disease; cardiac failure; sustained high fever; infants < 1 year of age), even conventional doses may result in increased serum levels and potential toxicity. Frequently, such patients have markedly prolonged levels following drug discontinuation.

Serious side effects such as ventricular arrhythmias, convulsions or even death may appear as the first sign of toxicity without any previous warning. Less serious signs of toxicity (eg, nausea, restlessness) may occur frequently when initiating therapy, but are usually transient; when such signs are persistent during maintenance therapy, they are often associated with serum concentrations > 20 mcg/ml. Serious toxicity is not reliably preceded by less severe side effects.

Cardiac effects: Theophylline may cause dysrhythmias or worsen pre-existing arrhythmias. Any significant change in cardiac rate or rhythm warrants monitoring and further investigation. Many patients who require theophylline may exhibit tachycardia due to their underlying disease process so that the relationship to elevated serum theophylline concentrations may not be appreciated. Ventricular arrhythmias respond to lidocaine.

Pregnancy: Category C. It is not known whether theophylline can cause fetal harm when administered to a pregnant woman or can affect reproduction capacity. Give to a pregnant woman only if clearly needed. Theophylline has been found in cord serum and crosses the placental barrier; newborns may have therapeutic serum levels. Apnea has been associated with theophylline withdrawal in a neonate. Theophylline-related human congenital defects or malformations have not been reported.

Lactation: Theophylline distributes readily into breast milk with a milk:plasma ratio of 0.7 and may cause irritability or other signs of toxicity in nursing infants. Decide whether to discontinue nursing or to discontinue the drug, taking into account the importance of the drug to the mother.

Children: Sufficient numbers of infants < 1 year of age have not been studied in clinical trials to support use in this age group; however, there is evidence that the use of dosage recommendations for older infants and young children may result in the development of toxic serum levels. Consequently, carefully consider associated benefits and risks of use of the drug in this age group. (See Administration and Dosage and Unlabeled uses.)

Precautions:

Use with caution in: Cardiac disease; hypoxemia; hepatic disease; hypertension; congestive heart failure (CHF); alcoholism; the elderly (particularly males) and neonates.

GI effects: Use cautiously in patients with peptic ulcer. Local irritation may occur; centrally mediated GI effects may occur with serum levels > 20 mcg/ml. Reduced lower esophageal pressure may cause reflux, aspiration and worsening of airway obstruction.

Alcohol: The addition of alcohol in liquid formulations is not necessary for absorption and may be potentially harmful.

(Continued on following page)

Xanthine Derivatives (Cont.)

Drug Interactions:

Agents that Decrease Theophylline Levels		
Aminoglutethimide	Rifampin	Carbamazepine[1]
Barbiturates	Smoking (cigarettes and marijuana)	Isoniazid[1]
Charcoal	Sulfinpyrazone	Loop diuretics[1]
Hydantoins[2]	Sympathomimetics (β-agonists)	
Ketoconazole	Thioamines[3]	

Agents that Increase Theophylline Levels		
Allopurinol	Disulfiram	Quinolones
Beta blockers (non-selective)	Ephedrine	Thiabendazole
Calcium channel blockers	Influenza virus vaccine	Thyroid hormones[4]
Cimetidine	Interferon	
Contraceptives, oral	Macrolides	Carbamazepine[1]
Corticosteroids	Mexiletine	Isoniazid[1]
		Loop diuretics[1]

[1] May increase or decrease theophylline levels.
[2] Decreased hydantoin levels may also occur.
[3] Increased theophylline clearance in hyperthyroid patients.
[4] Decreased theophylline clearance in hypothyroid patients.

Miscellaneous interactions:

Benzodiazepines: The sedative effects of benzodiazepines may be antagonized by theophyllines, although their pharmacokinetics do not appear to be altered. Coadministration may be beneficial in reversing sedation produced by benzodiazepines.

Beta-agonists and theophylline act synergistically in vitro; an additive effect has also been demonstrated in vivo.

Halothane and theophylline coadministration has resulted in catecholamine-induced arrhythmias.

Ketamine and theophylline coadministration has resulted in extensor-type seizures.

Lithium plasma levels may be reduced by theophyllines.

Nondepolarizing muscle relaxants: A dose-dependent reversal of neuromuscular blockade by theophyllines may occur.

Probenecid may increase the pharmacologic effects of dyphylline due to decreased dyphylline renal excretion.

Propofol: Theophyllines may antagonize the sedative effects of propofol.

Ranitidine: Case reports suggest that theophylline plasma levels may be increased by ranitidine, possibly increasing pharmacologic and toxic effcts. However, several controlled studies indicate that an interaction does not occur. It appears that if this interaction occurs, it is rare.

Tetracyclines: The incidence of theophylline adverse reactions may possibly be enhanced by concurrent tetracyclines.

Drug/Food interaction: Theophylline elimination is increased (half-life shortened) by a low carbohydrate, high protein diet and charcoal broiled beef (due to a high polycyclic carbon content). Conversely, elimination is decreased (prolonged half-life) by a high carbohydrate low protein diet. Food may alter the bioavailability and absorption pattern of certain sustained release preparations. Some sustained release preparations may be subject to rapid release of their contents when taken with food, resulting in toxicity. It appears that consistent administration in the fasting state allows predictability of effects.

Drug/Lab test interactions: Currently available analytical methods for measuring serum theophylline levels are specific, and metabolites and other drugs generally do not affect the results. However, be aware of the specific laboratory method used and whether other factors will interfere with the assay for theophylline.

Adverse Reactions:

Adverse reactions/toxicity are uncommon at serum theophylline levels < 20 mcg/ml.

Levels > 20 mcg/ml: 75% of patients experience adverse reactions (eg, nausea, vomiting, diarrhea, headache, insomnia, irritability).

Levels > 35 mcg/ml: Hyperglycemia; hypotension; cardiac arrhythmias; tachycardia (> 10 mcg/ml in premature newborns); seizures; brain damage; death.

CNS: Irritability; restlessness; headache; insomnia; reflex hyperexcitability; muscle twitching; convulsions.

(Adverse Reactions continued on following page)

Adverse Reactions (Cont.):

GI: Nausea; vomiting; epigastric pain; hematemesis; diarrhea; rectal irritation or bleeding (aminophylline suppositories). Therapeutic doses of theophylline may induce gastroesophageal reflux during sleep or while recumbent, increasing the potential for aspiration which can aggravate bronchospasm.

Cardiovascular: Palpitations; tachycardia; extrasystoles; hypotension; circulatory failure; life-threatening ventricular arrhythmias.

Respiratory: Tachypnea; respiratory arrest.

Renal: Proteinuria; potentiation of diuresis.

Other: Fever; flushing; hyperglycemia; inappropriate antidiuretic hormone syndrome; rash; alopecia. Ethylenediamine in aminophylline can cause sensitivity reactions, including exfoliative dermatitis and urticaria.

Overdosage:

Symptoms: Anorexia; nausea; vomiting; nervousness; insomnia; agitation; irritability; headache; tachycardia; extrasystoles; tachypnea; fasciculation; tonic/clonic convulsions. Convulsions or ventricular arrhythmias may be the first signs of toxicity. Hyperamylasemia, simulating pancreatitis, has also been noted. Other symptoms of intoxication are listed under Adverse Reactions.

Serious adverse effects are rare at serum theophylline concentrations < 20 mcg/ml. Between 20 and 40 mcg/ml, sinus tachycardia and cardiac arrhythmias occur. Above 40 mcg/ml, seizures and cardiorespiratory arrest can occur. However, convulsions and death have been reported at concentrations as low as 25 mcg/ml.

Acute overdosage appears to be better tolerated with the more serious reactions (eg, seizures) occurring with chronic overdosage (levels > 40 mcg/ml), but rarely in the acute situation unless levels exceed 100 mcg/ml. Also, symptoms such as hypokalemia, hypercalcemia, hyperglycemia and decreased serum bicarbonate concentrations occur more frequently with acute overdosage.

Overdosage with sustained release preparations may cause a dramatic increase in serum theophylline concentrations much later (≥ 12 hours) than the increases that occur with other preparations. Early treatment will help but not prevent these delayed elevated levels.

Treatment if seizure has not occurred: Induce vomiting, even if emesis has occurred spontaneously; ipecac syrup is preferred. However, do not induce emesis in patients with impaired consciousness. Take precautions against aspiration, especially in infants and children. If vomiting is unsuccessful or contraindicated, perform gastric lavage (of no value ≥ 1 hour post-ingestion). Administer a cathartic (particularly for sustained-release preparations; sorbitol may be useful) and activated charcoal. Prophylactic phenobarbital may increase the seizure threshold.

If seizure occurs: Establish an airway and administer oxygen. Administer IV diazepam 0.1 to 0.3 mg/kg, up to 10 mg. Monitor vital signs, maintain blood pressure and provide adequate hydration.

Post-seizure coma: Maintain airway and oxygenation. Perform intubation and lavage instead of inducing emesis. Introduce the cathartic and activated charcoal via a large bore gastric lavage tube. Provide full supportive care and adequate hydration while the drug is metabolized. If repeated oral activated charcoal is ineffective, charcoal hemoperfusion may be indicated.

Supportive care: Employ usual supportive measures. Refer to General Management of Acute Overdosage. Do not use stimulants (analeptic agents). Continuously monitor cardiac function. Verapamil has been used to treat atrial arrhythmias; lidocaine or procainamide may be used for ventricular arrhythmias. May need IV fluids to treat dehydration, acid-base imbalance and hypotension; the latter may also be treated with vasopressors. Apnea will require ventilatory support. Treat hyperpyrexia, especially in children, with tepid water sponge baths or a hypothermic blanket.

Monitor theophylline serum level until it falls below 20 mcg/ml because secondary rises of plasma theophylline may occur from redistribution, delayed absorption, etc; this has been reported with sustained release products.

Dialysis: Charcoal hemoperfusion rapidly removes theophylline and may be indicated when the serum concentration is > 60 mcg/ml, even in the absence of obvious toxicity. Forced diuresis, peritoneal dialysis and extracorporeal methods are inadequate. However, hemodialysis appears capable of removing ≈ 36% to 40% of serum theophylline.

"Gastric dialysis" with oral activated charcoal, 20 to 40 g every 4 hours until serum level is < 20 mcg/ml, may shorten the half-life and speed removal, regardless of the route. Mechanism may include enhancing the drug concentration gradient into the GI lumen, a disruption of an enterohepatic recycling process or binding unabsorbed drug.

(Continued on following page)

Patient Information:

If GI upset occurs with liquid preparations or non-sustained release forms, take with food.

Do NOT chew or crush enteric coated or sustained release tablets or capsules.

Take at the same time, with or without food, each day.

Notify physician if nausea, vomiting, insomnia, jitteriness, headache, rash, severe GI pain, restlessness, convulsions or irregular heartbeat occurs.

Avoid large amounts of caffeine-containing beverages, such as tea, coffee, cocoa and cola drinks or large amounts of chocolate; these products may increase side effects.

Brand interchange: Do not change from one brand to another without consulting your pharmacist or physician. Products manufactured by different companies may not be equally effective.

Individual doses are determined by response (decrease in symptoms). Blood levels must be checked regularly to avoid underdosing and overdosing. Do not change the dose of your medication without consulting your physician.

Administration and Dosage:

Parenteral administration: See theophylline and dextrose and aminophylline.

Individualize dosage. Base dosage adjustments on clinical response and improvement in pulmonary function with careful monitoring of serum levels. If possible, monitor serum levels to maintain levels in the therapeutic range of 10 to 20 mcg/ml. Levels > 20 mcg/ml may produce toxicity, and it may even occur with levels between 15 to 20 mcg/ml, particularly when factors known to reduce theophylline clearance are present (see Warnings). Once stabilized on a dosage, serum levels tend to remain constant. Data are available that indicate that the serum theophylline concentrations required to produce maximum physiologic benefit may fluctuate with the degree of bronchospasm present and are variable.

Calculate dosages on the basis of lean body weight, since theophylline does not distribute into fatty tissue. Regardless of salt used, dosages should be equivalent based on anhydrous theophylline content.

Individualize frequency of dosing. With immediate release products, dosing every 6 hours is generally required, especially in children; intervals up to 8 hours may be satisfactory in adults. Some children and adults requiring higher than average doses (those having rapid rates of clearance; eg, half-lives < 6 hours) may be more effectively controlled during chronic therapy with sustained release products. Determine dosage intervals to produce minimal fluctuations between peak and trough serum theophylline concentrations. Consider the absorption profile and the elimination rate. When converting from an immediate release to a sustained release product, the total daily dose should remain the same, and only the dosing interval adjusted.

Acute symptoms requiring rapid theophyllinization in patients not receiving theophylline: To achieve a rapid effect, an initial loading dose is required. Dosage recommendations are for theophylline anhydrous.

Dosage Guidelines for Rapid Theophyllinization[1]

Patient Group	Oral loading	Maintenance
Children 1 to 9 years	5 mg/kg	4 mg/kg q 6 h
Children 9 to 16 and young adult smokers	5 mg/kg	3 mg/kg q 6 h
Otherwise healthy non-smoking adults	5 mg/kg	3 mg/kg q 8 h
Older patients and patients with cor pulmonale	5 mg/kg	2 mg/kg q 8 h
Patients with congestive heart failure	5 mg/kg	1-2 mg/kg q 12 h

[1] In patients not receiving theophylline.

Infants (preterm to < 1 year):

Theophylline Dosage Guidelines for Infants

Age	Initial maintenance dose
Premature infants ≤ 24 days postnatal > 24 days postnatal	 1 mg/kg q 12 h 1.5 mg/kg q 12 h
Infants (6 to 52 weeks) Up to 26 weeks 26 to 52 weeks	[(0.2 x age in weeks) + 5] x kg = 24 hr dose in mg Divide into q 8 h dosing Divide into q 6 h dosing

Guide final dosage by serum concentration after a steady state has been achieved.

(Administration and Dosage continued on following page)

Administration and Dosage (Cont.):

Acute symptoms requiring rapid theophyllinization in patients receiving theophylline: Each 0.5 mg/kg theophylline administered as a loading dose will increase the serum theophylline concentration by approximately 1 mcg/ml. Ideally, defer the loading dose if a serum theophylline concentration can be obtained rapidly.

If this is not possible, exercise clinical judgment. When there is sufficient respiratory distress to warrant a small risk, then 2.5 mg/kg of theophylline administered in rapidly absorbed form is likely to increase serum concentration by approximately 5 mcg/ml. If the patient is not experiencing theophylline toxicity, this is unlikely to result in dangerous adverse effects. Maintenance doses are in the Dosage Guidelines table.

Chronic therapy: Slow clinical titration is generally preferred.

Initial dose – 16 mg/kg/24 hours or 400 mg/24 hours, whichever is less, of anhydrous theophylline in divided doses at 6 or 8 hour intervals.

Increasing dose – The above dosage may be increased in approximately 25% increments at 3 day intervals so long as the drug is tolerated or until the maximum dose (indicated below) is reached.

Maximum dose (where the serum concentration is not measured): Do not attempt to maintain any dose that is not tolerated.

Maximum Daily Theophylline Dose Based on Age	
Age	Maximum daily dose[1]
1 to 9 years	24 mg/kg/day
9 to 12 years	20 mg/kg/day
12 to 16 years	18 mg/kg/day
> 16 years	13 mg/kg/day

[1] Not to exceed listed dose or 900 mg, whichever is less.

Exercise caution in younger children who cannot complain of minor side effects. Older adults and those with cor pulmonale, CHF or liver disease may have unusually low dosage requirements; they may experience toxicity at the maximal dosages recommended.

Measurement of serum theophylline concentrations during chronic therapy is recommended. Obtain the serum sample at the time of peak absorption, 1 to 2 hours after administration for immediate release products and 5 to 9 hours after the morning dose for most sustained release formulations. The patient must not miss doses during the previous 48 hours, and dosing intervals must have been reasonably typical during that period of time. The table below provides guidance to dosage adjustments based on serum theophylline level determinations:

Dosage Adjustment After Serum Theophylline Measurement		
If serum theophylline is:		Directions
Too low	5 to 10 mcg/ml	Increase dose by about 25% at 3 day intervals until either the desired clinical response or serum concentration is achieved.[1]
Within desired range	10 to 20 mcg/ml	Maintain dosage if tolerated. Recheck serum theophylline concentration at 6 to 12 month intervals.[2]
Too high	20 to 25 mcg/ml	Decrease doses by about 10%. Recheck serum theophylline concentration after 3 days.[2]
	25 to 30 mcg/ml	Skip next dose and decrease subsequent doses by about 25%. Recheck serum theophylline after 3 days.
	> 30 mcg/ml	Skip next 2 doses and decrease subsequent doses by 50%. Recheck serum theophylline after 3 days.

[1] The total daily dose may need to be administered at more frequent intervals if asthma symptoms occur repeatedly at the end of a dosing interval.

[2] Finer adjustments in dosage may be needed for some patients.

(Products listed on following pages)

Complete prescribing information for these products begins on page 911.

Xanthine Derivatives (Cont.)

THEOPHYLLINE

	Immediate Release Capsules and Tablets			C.I.*
Rx	**Theophylline** (Various, eg, Schein)	**Tablets:** 100 mg	In 100s.	12+
Rx	**Slo-Phyllin** (Rhone-Poulenc Rorer)		Dye free. (WHR 351). White, scored. In 100s & UD 100s.	11
Rx	**Theolair** (3M Pharmaceuticals)	**Tablets:** 125 mg	(Riker 342). White, scored. In 100s.	16
Rx	**Theophylline** (Various, eg, Schein)	**Tablets:** 200 mg	In 100s and 500s.	8+
Rx	**Slo-Phyllin** (Rhone-Poulenc Rorer)		Dye free. (WHR 352). White, scored. In 100s & UD 100s.	7
Rx	**Theolair** (3M Pharmaceuticals)	**Tablets:** 250 mg	(Riker/Theolair 250). White, scored. Capsule shape. In 100s.	12
Rx	**Theophylline** (Various, eg, Schein)	**Tablets:** 300 mg	In 100s, 500s and 1000s.	7+
Rx	**Quibron-T Dividose** (Bristol Labs)		(BL 512). Ivory. Triple scored. In 100s and 500s.	6
Rx	**Bronkodyl** (Winthrop)	**Capsules:** 100 mg	Brown and white. In 100s.	22
Rx	**Elixophyllin** (Forest)		Dye free. (Forest 642). In 100s.	27
Rx	**Bronkodyl** (Winthrop)	**Capsules:** 200 mg	Green and white. In 100s.	15
Rx	**Elixophyllin** (Forest)		Dye free. (Forest 643). In 100s and 500s.	18

* Cost Index based on cost per 100 mg.

(Continued on following page)

Complete prescribing information for these products begins on page 911 .

Xanthine Derivatives (Cont.)

THEOPHYLLINE (Cont.)

	Product	Liquids		C.I.*
Rx	**Aquaphyllin** (Ferndale)	**Syrup:** 80 mg per 15 ml (26.7 mg per 5 ml)	Alcohol free. Dye free. In 120 ml, pt, gal and UD 5, 15 and 30 ml.	28
Rx *sf*	**Slo-Phyllin** (Rhone-Poulenc Rorer)		Alcohol free.[1] In pt.	47
Rx *sf*	**Theoclear-80** (Central)		Alcohol free. Dye free. Saccharin, sorbitol. Cherry flavor. In pt and gal.	42
Rx	**Theostat 80** (Laser)		1% alcohol. Sugar. In pt and gal.	37
Rx	**Accurbron** (Marion Merrell Dow)	**Syrup:** 150 mg per 15 ml (50 mg per 5 ml)	7.5% alcohol. Dye free. Saccharin, sorbitol, sugar. In pt.	111
Rx	**Theophylline** (Various, eg, Balan, Barre National, Bioline, Geneva, Goldline, Moore, Rugby, Schein, URL)	**Elixir:** 80 mg per 15 ml (26.7 mg per 5 ml)	In pt and gal and UD 15 and 30 ml.	10+
Rx	**Asmalix** (Century)		20% alcohol. In gal.	6
Rx	**Elixomin** (Cenci)		20% alcohol. Orange raspberry flavor. In pt.	14
Rx	**Elixophyllin** (Forest)		20% alcohol. Saccharin. Mixed fruit flavor. In pt, qt and gal.	119
Rx *sf*	**Lanophyllin** (Lannett)		20% alcohol. In pt and gal.	8
Rx *sf*	**Theophylline Oral** (Roxane)	**Solution:** 80 mg per 15 ml (26.7 mg per 5 ml)	0.4% alcohol. Dye free. Saccharin, sorbitol. In 500 ml & UD 15 and 18.75 & 30 ml.	21
Rx	**Theolair** (3M Pharmaceuticals)		Alcohol free. Sorbitol, sucrose.[1] In pt.	6
Rx *sf*	**Aerolate** (Fleming)	**Oral Solution:** 150 mg per 15 ml (50 mg per 5 ml)	Alcohol free. Tangerine flavor. In pt.	29

* Cost Index based on cost per 100 mg.
sf – Sugar free.
[1] With parabens.

(Continued on following page)

Complete prescribing information for these products begins on page 911 .

Xanthine Derivatives (Cont.)

THEOPHYLLINE (Cont.)

Timed Release Capsules

These dosage forms gradually release the active medication so that the total daily dosage may be administered in 1 to 3 doses divided by 8 to 24 hours, depending on the patient's pharmacokinetic profile, thus reducing the number of daily doses required. In the following product listings, the manufacturer's recommended average dosing intervals are presented in parentheses. Nevertheless, frequency of dosing must be individualized, based on the absorption profile of the drug and the rate of elimination of the drug from the patient. These products are not necessarily interchangeable. If patients are switched from one brand to another, closely monitor their theophylline serum levels; serum concentrations may vary greatly following brand interchange.

	Product	Dosage form	Strength	Description	C.I.*
Rx	**Aerolate** (Fleming)	**Capsules, timed release (8 to 12 hours):**	III: 65 mg	(III/III). Red and clear. In 100s.	14
			JR: 130 mg	(JR./JR.). Red and clear. In 100s.	9
			SR: 260 mg	(SR./SR.). Red and clear. In 100s.	5
Rx	**Elixophyllin SR** (Forest)	**Capsules, timed release (8 to 12 hours):**	125 mg	Dye free. (Forest 646). White. In 100s, 1000s and UD 100s.	27
			250 mg	Dye free. (Forest 647). Clear. In 100s, 1000s, and UD 100s.	16
Rx	**Slo-bid Gyrocaps** (Rhone-Poulenc Rorer)	**Capsules, timed release (8 to 12 hours):**	50 mg	Dye free. (50). White/clear. In 100s, 1000s & UD 100s.	29
			75 mg	Dye free. (75). White and clear. In 100s and UD 100s.	21
			100 mg	Dye free. (100). Clear. In 100s, 1000s and UD 100s.	18
			125 mg	Dye free. (125). White. In 100s and UD 100s.	18
			200 mg	Dye free. (200). White and clear. In 100s, 1000s and UD 100s.	13
			300 mg	Dye free. (300). White. In 100s, 1000s and UD 100s.	11
Rx	**Slo-Phyllin Gyrocaps** (Rhone-Poulenc Rorer)	**Capsules, timed release (8 to 12 hours):**	60 mg	Sucrose. (WHR 1354). White. In 100s.	23
			125 mg	Sucrose. (WHR 1355). Brown. In 100s, 1000s and UD 100s.	17
			250 mg	Sucrose. (WHR 1356). Purple. In 100s, 1000s and UD 100s.	10

* Cost Index based on cost per 100 mg.

(Continued on following page)

Complete prescribing information for these products begins on page 911 .

Xanthine Derivatives (Cont.)

THEOPHYLLINE (Cont.)

		Timed Release Capsules (Cont.)		C.I.*
Rx	**Theo-24** (Searle)	**Capsules, timed release (24 hours):** 100 mg	(Theo-24 100 mg Searle 2832). Gold and clear. In 100s and UD 100s.	15
		200 mg	(Theo-24 200 mg Searle 2842). Orange and clear. In 100s, 500s and UD 100s.	11
		300 mg	(Theo-24 300 mg Searle 2852). Red and clear. In 100s, 500s and UD 100s.	9
		Note: Patients receiving once daily doses ≥ 13 mg/kg or ≥ 900 mg (whichever is less) should avoid eating a high-fat-content morning meal or take medication at least 1 hour before eating. If patient cannot comply with this regimen, place on alternative therapy.		
Rx	**Theobid Jr. Duracaps** (Russ)	**Capsules, timed release (12 hours):** 130 mg	(Theobid 130). Clear. In 60s.	12
Rx	**Theobid Duracaps** (Russ)	**Capsules, timed release (12 hours):** 260 mg	(Theobid 260). Clear. In 60s and 500s.	8
Rx	**Theoclear L.A.** (Central)	**Capsules, timed release (12 hours):** 130 mg	(130 mg). Clear. In 100s & 1000s.	11
		260 mg	(260 mg). Clear. In 100s & 1000s.	7
Rx	**Theo-Dur Sprinkle** (Key)	**Capsules, timed release (12 hours):** 50 mg	(Theo-Dur Sprinkle 50 mg). White and clear. In 100s.	23
		75 mg	(Theo-Dur Sprinkle 75 mg). White and clear. In 100s.	17
		125 mg	(Theo-Dur Sprinkle 125 mg). White and clear. In 100s.	12
		200 mg	(Theo-Dur Sprinkle 200 mg). White and clear. In 100s.	8
		Note: May be administered whole or by sprinkling the beads on a spoonful of soft food (eg, applesauce, pudding). Swallow immediately with water or juice; do not chew. Do not subdivide contents of capsule.		
Rx	**Theospan-SR** (Laser)	**Capsules, timed release (12 hours):** 130 mg	Sucrose. (Laser 0161 Theospan SR 130). White/clear. In 100s & 1000s.	1
		260 mg	Sucrose. (Theospan SR 260). White and clear. In 100s and 1000s.	6
Rx	**Theovent** (Schering)	**Capsules, timed release (12 hours):** 125 mg	(Schering 402). Green and yellow. In 100s.	21
		250 mg	(Schering 753). Green and clear. In 100s.	13

* Cost Index based on cost per 100 mg.

(Continued on following page)

Complete prescribing information for these products begins on page 911 .

Xanthine Derivatives (Cont.)

THEOPHYLLINE (Cont.)

	Timed Release Tablets			C.I.*
Rx	**Theophylline SR** (Various)	**Tablets, timed release (12 to 24 hours):** 100 mg	In 100s and 500s.	10+
		200 mg	In 100s, 500s, 1000s, UD 100s.	5+
		300 mg	In 100s, 500s, 1000s, UD 100s.	4.7+
		450 mg	In 100s, 250s and 500s.	4+
Rx	**Constant-T** (Geigy)	**Tablets, timed release (8 to 12 hours):** 200 mg	(Geigy 42). Pink, scored. Oval. In 100s and UD 100s.	7
		300 mg	(Geigy 57). In 100s and UD 100s.	6
Rx	**Quibron-T/SR Dividose** (Bristol)	**Tablets, timed release (8 to 12 hours):** 300 mg	White. Triple scored. In 100s & 500s.	6
Rx	**Respbid** (Boehringer-Ingelheim)	**Tablets, timed release (8 to 12 hours):** 250 mg	(BI 48). White, scored. In 100s.	8
		500 mg	(BI 49). White, scored. In 100s.	6
Rx	**Sustaire** (Pfizer Labs)	**Tablets, sustained release (8 to 12 hours):** 100 mg	Dye free. Sucrose. Scored. In 100s.	11
		300 mg	Dye free. Sucrose. Scored. In 100s.	6
Rx	**Theochron** (Inwood)	**Tablets, timed release (12 to 24 hours):** 100 mg	Dye free. (IL/3584). White scored. Convex. In 100s, 500s, 1000s.	NA
		200 mg	Dye free. (IL/3583). White, scored. Oval. In 100s, 500s, 1000s.	6
		300 mg	Dye free. (IL/3581). In 100s, 500s and 1000s.	5
Rx	**Theo-Dur** (Key)	**Tablets, timed release (8 to 24 hours):** 100 mg	Dye free. (Theo-Dur 100). In 100s, 500s, 1000s, UD 100s.	12
		200 mg	Dye free. (Theo-Dur 200). In 100s, 500s, 1000s, UD 100s.	9
		300 mg	Dye free. (Theo-Dur 300). In 100s, 500s, 1000s, UD 100s.	7
		450 mg	Dye free. (Theo-Dur 450). White, scored. In 100s and UD 100s.	NA
Rx	**Theolair-SR** (3M Pharmaceuticals)	**Tablets, timed release (8 to 12 hours):** 200 mg	(Riker SR 200). White, scored. In 100s and 1000s.	8
		250 mg	(Riker SR 250). White, scored. In 100s and 250s.	8
		300 mg	(Riker SR 300). White, scored. Oval. In 100s and 1000s.	7
		500 mg	(Riker SR 500). White, scored. Capsule shape. In 100s & 250s.	6
Rx	**Theo-Sav** (Savage)	**Tablets, timed release (8 to 24 hours):** 100 mg	(S 168). White, scored. In 100s.	8
		200 mg	(S 169). White, scored. Oval. In 100s, 500s and 1000s.	4.6
		300 mg	(S 170). White, scored. Capsule shape. In 100s, 500s and 1000s.	4.8
Rx	**Theox** (Carnrick)	**Tablets, controlled release (12 to 24 hours):** 100 mg	(C 8631). White, scored. In 100s and 500s.	NA
		200 mg	(C 8632). In 100s, 500s, 1000s.	NA
		300 mg	(C 8633). In 100s, 500s, 1000s.	NA
Rx	**T-Phyl** (Purdue Frederick)	**Tablets, timed release (8 to 12 hours):** 200 mg	(T200). Scored. In 100s.	8
Rx	**Uniphyl** (Purdue Frederick)	**Tablets, timed release (24 hours):** 400 mg	(PF U400). White, scored. In 100s, 500s and UD 100s.	7

* Cost Index based on cost per 100 mg.

Complete prescribing information for these products begins on page 911 .

Xanthine Derivatives (Cont.)

OXTRIPHYLLINE (Choline Theophyllinate) – 64% theophylline

Dosage: *Adults:* 4.7 mg/kg every 8 hours.

Children (9 to 16 years) and adult smokers: 4.7 mg/kg every 6 hours.

Children (1 to 9 years): 6.2 mg/kg every 6 hours.

Sustained action: If total daily maintenance dosage is established at approximately 800 or 1200 mg, 1 sustained action tablet every 12 hours may be substituted.

	Product	Form	Description	C.I.*
Rx	**Oxtriphylline** (Various, eg, Bolar, Genetco, Goldline, Interstate, Major, Rugby)	**Tablets:** 100 mg (equiv. to 64 mg theophylline)	In 100s and 500s.	11+
Rx	**Choledyl** (Parke-Davis)		Sucrose. (PD 210). Red. Enteric and sugar coated. In 100s.	19
Rx	**Oxtriphylline** (Various, eg, Balan, Bioline, Bolar, Interstate, Major, Parmed, Rugby)	**Tablets:** 200 mg (equiv. to 127 mg theophylline)	In 100s, 500s and 1000s.	5.5+
Rx	**Choledyl** (Parke-Davis)		Sucrose. (PD 211). Yellow. Enteric and sugar coated. In 100s, 1000s and UD 100s.	13
Rx	**Choledyl SA** (Parke-Davis)	**Tablets, sustained action:** 400 mg (equiv. to 254 mg theophylline)	Sugar. Pink. Film coated. In 100s and UD 100s.	7.3
		600 mg (equiv. to 382 mg theophylline)	Sugar. Tan. Film coated. In 100s and UD 100s.	5.9
Rx	**Oxtriphylline** (Various, eg, Moore, PBI)	**Syrup, pediatric:** 50 mg (equiv. to 32 mg theophylline) per 5 ml	In pt.	14+
Rx	**Choledyl** (Parke-Davis)		Menthol, saccharin, sorbitol, sugar. Vanilla-mint flavor. In 474 ml.	40
Rx	**Oxtriphylline** (Various, eg, PBI, Schein, UDL)	**Elixir:** 100 mg (equiv. to 64 mg theophylline) per 5 ml	In pt and UD 5 and 10 ml.	10+
Rx	**Choledyl** (Parke-Davis)		20% alcohol. Saccharin, sorbitol, sucrose. Sherry flavor. In 474 ml.	21

THEOPHYLLINE AND DEXTROSE

Substitute oral therapy for IV theophylline as soon as adequate improvement is achieved.

See also aminophylline for parenteral administration guidelines, noting the difference of theophylline content.

The following may be incompatible when mixed with theophylline in IV fluids:

Anileridine; ascorbic acid; chlorpromazine; codeine phosphate; corticotropin; dimenhydrinate; epinephrine HCl; erythromycin gluceptate; hydralazine; hydroxyzine HCl; insulin; levorphanol tartrate; meperidine; methadone; methicillin sodium; morphine sulfate; norepinephrine bitartrate; oxytetracycline; papaverine; penicillin G potassium; phenobarbital sodium; phenytoin sodium; procaine; prochlorperazine maleate; promazine; promethazine; tetracycline; vancomycin; vitamin B complex with C.

Children: Due to marked variation in theophylline metabolism, use this drug only if clearly needed in infants $<$ 6 months of age.

	Product	Form	Description	C.I.*
Rx	**Theophylline and 5% Dextrose** (Abbott and Baxter)	**Injection:** 200 mg/container	In 50 ml (4 mg/ml) and 100 ml (2 mg/ml).	NA
		400 mg/container	In 100 ml (4 mg/ml), 250 ml (1.6 mg/ml), 500 ml (0.8 mg/ml) and 1000 ml (0.4 mg/ml).	NA
		800 mg/container	In 250 ml (3.2 mg/ml), 500 ml (1.6 mg/ml) and 1000 ml (0.8 mg/ml).	NA

* Cost Index based on cost per 100 mg theophylline equivalent.

Complete prescribing information for these products begins on page 911 .

Xanthine Derivatives (Cont.)

AMINOPHYLLINE (Theophylline Ethylenediamine) – 79% theophylline

Dosage:

For oral and rectal dosage refer to the Equivalent Dosage table in Actions and to the Administration section.

For dosage in infants from preterm up to 8-week-old term infants, see Administration section.

IV: The loading dose may be infused into 100 to 200 ml of 5% Dextrose Injection or 0.9% Sodium Chloride Injection. Do not exceed 25 mg/min infusion rate.

Parenteral administration: Inject aminophylline slowly, not more than 25 mg/min, when given IV. Substitute oral therapy for IV aminophylline as soon as adequate improvement is achieved.

Loading dose –

In patients currently not receiving theophylline products: 6 mg/kg.

In patients currently receiving theophylline products: If possible, determine the time, amount, route of administration and form of last dose and defer loading dose if a serum concentration can be rapidly obtained. Each 0.5 mg/kg theophylline (0.6 mg/kg aminophylline) will increase the serum theophylline concentration by approximately 1 mcg/ml. When respiratory distress warrants a small risk, 2.5 mg/kg theophylline (3.1 mg aminophylline IV) increases serum concentration by approximately 5 mcg/ml. If the patient is not experiencing theophylline toxicity, this is unlikely to result in dangerous side effects. The proper time to obtain blood to measure the peak serum level of theophylline after an IV loading dose is 15 to 30 minutes.

Maintenance infusions – Administer by a large volume infusion to deliver the desired amount of drug each hour. Aminophylline is compatible with most common IV solutions. Monitor serum theophylline concentrations to accurately maintain therapeutic concentrations and guide dosage adjustments.

Aminophylline Maintenance Infusion Rates (mg/kg/hr)		
Patient Group	First 12 hours	Beyond 12 hours
Neonates to infants < 6 months	Not recommended	
Children 6 months to 9 years	1.2	1
Children ages 9 to 16 and young adult smokers	1	0.8
Otherwise healthy nonsmoking adults	0.7	0.5
Older patients and those with cor pulmonale	0.6	0.3
Patients with CHF, liver disease	0.5	0.1-0.2

Compatibility: Do not mix the following solutions with aminophylline in IV fluids: Anileridine HCl; ascorbic acid; chlorpromazine; codeine phosphate; dimenhydrinate; dobutamine HCl; epinephrine; erythromycin gluceptate; hydralazine; insulin; levorphanol tartrate; meperidine; methadone; methicillin; morphine sulfate; norepinephrine bitartrate; oxytetracycline; penicillin G potassium; phenobarbital; phenytoin; prochlorperazine; promazine; promethazine; tetracycline; vancomycin; verapamil; vitamin B complex with C.

(Products listed on following page)

Complete prescribing information for these products begins on page 911 .

Xanthine Derivatives (Cont.)

AMINOPHYLLINE (Theophylline Ethylenediamine) (Cont.)				C.I.*
Rx	**Aminophylline** (Various, eg, Balan, Bioline, Geneva-Marsam, Goldline, Major, Roxane, Rugby, Schein, Searle, URL)	**Tablets:** 100 mg (equiv. to 79 mg theophylline)	Plain or enteric coated. In 100s, 1000s and UD 100s.	3+
Rx	**Aminophylline** (Various, eg, Balan, Bioline, Geneva-Marsam, Goldline, Major, Moore, Roxane, Rugby, Searle, URL)	**Tablets:** 200 mg (equiv. to 158 mg theophylline)	Plain or enteric coated. In 100s, 1000s and UD 100s.	3+
Rx	**Phyllocontin** (Purdue Frederick)	**Tablets, controlled release (12 hours):** 225 mg (equiv. to 178 mg theophylline)	Scored. In 100s.	13
Rx	**Aminophylline** (Various, eg, Balan, Barre, Bioline, Major, PBI, Roxane, Rugby, URL)	**Oral Liquid:** 105 mg (equiv. to 90 mg theophylline) per 5 ml	In 240 and 500 ml.	15+
Rx	**Aminophylline** (Various, eg, Abbott, American Regent, Elkins-Sinn, Lyphomed, Moore, Solopak)	**Injection:** 250 mg (equiv. to 197 mg theophylline) per 10 ml For IV use.	In 10 and 20 ml amps & vials & syringes.	60+
Rx	**Aminophylline** (Various, eg, Baxter, Rugby, Schein)	**Suppositories:** 250 mg (equiv. to 197.5 mg theophylline)	In 10s and 25s.	14+
Rx	**Truphylline** (G & W)		In UD 10s and 25s.	22
Rx	**Aminophylline** (Various, eg, Baxter, Parmed, Rugby, Schein)	**Suppositories:** 500 mg (equiv. to 395 mg theophylline)	In 10s and 25s.	3+
Rx	**Truphylline** (G & W)		In UD 10s, 25s and 50s.	3

* Cost Index based on cost per 100 mg theophylline equivalent.

Complete prescribing information for these products begins on page 911 .

Xanthine Derivatives (Cont.)

DYPHYLLINE (Dihydroxypropyl Theophyllline)

Dyphylline is a derivative of theophylline; it is not a theophylline salt, and is not metabolized to theophylline in vivo. Although dyphylline is 70% theophylline by molecular weight ratio, the amount of dyphylline equivalent to a given amount of theophylline is not known. Dyphylline may result in fewer side effects than theophylline salts, but blood levels and possibly activity are lower. Specific dyphylline serum levels may be used to monitor therapy; serum theophylline levels will NOT measure dyphylline. The minimal effective therapeutic concentration is 12 mcg/ml.

Dosage:

Oral: Adults – Up to 15 mg/kg every 6 hours.

IM: (Not for IV administration.)

Adults – 250 to 500 mg injected slowly every 6 hours. Do not exceed 15 mg/kg every 6 hours.

Children – Safety and efficacy have not been established.

	Product	Form	Description	C.I.*
Rx	**Dyphylline** (Various, eg, Balan, Major)	**Tablets:** 200 mg	In 100s and 1000s.	1.8+
Rx	**Dilor** (Savage)		Blue, scored. In 100s, 1000s and UD 100s.	2.7
Rx	**Dyflex-200** (Econo Med)		(EM). In 100s and 1000s.	1
Rx	**Lufyllin** (Wallace)		(Wallace 521). White. Rectangular. In 100s, 1000s and UD 100s.	6
Rx	**Neothylline** (Lemmon)		(Lemmon 30). White, scored. In 100s.	2.1
Rx	**Dyphylline** (Various, eg, Balan, Major, URL)	**Tablets:** 400 mg	In 100s and 1000s.	1+
Rx	**Dilor-400** (Savage)		In 100s, 1000s and UD 100s.	1.9
Rx	**Dyflex-400** (Econo Med)		In 100s and 500s.	NA
Rx	**Lufyllin-400** (Wallace)		(Wallace 731). White. Capsule shape. In 100s, 1000s and UD 100s.	4.5
Rx	**Neothylline** (Lemmon)		(Lemmon 37). White, scored. Oblong. In 100s.	1.3
Rx	**Lufyllin** (Wallace)	**Elixir:** 100 mg per 15 ml (33.3 mg/5 ml)	20% alcohol. White port wine, saccharin. In pt and gal.	24
Rx	**Dilor** (Savage)	**Elixir:** 160 mg per 15 ml (53.3 mg/5 ml)	18% alcohol. Saccharin, sorbitol, sucrose. Mint flavor. In pt.	11
Rx	**Dilor** (Savage)	**Injection:** 250 mg per ml	In 2 ml amps.	16
Rx	**Lufyllin** (Wallace)		In 2 ml amps.	40

* Cost Index based on cost per 300 mg.

Refer to the general discussion of Systemic Glucocorticoids on page 465 .

Corticosteroids

Actions:

Pharmacology: These agents are synthetic adrenocortical steroids with basic glucocorticoid actions and effects. The mechanism responsible for the potent anti-inflammatory activity and the precise mechanism of action of the aerosolized drug in the lung is unknown. Glucocorticoids may decrease the number and activity of inflammatory cells, enhance the effect of beta-adrenergic drugs on cyclic AMP production, inhibit bronchoconstrictor mechanisms or produce direct smooth muscle relaxation. Use of the inhaler makes it possible to provide effective local steroid activity with minimal systemic effect.

Pharmacokinetics:

Beclomethasone dipropionate – Systemic absorption occurs rapidly with all routes of administration. There is no evidence of tissue storage of beclomethasone or its metabolites. Lung slices can metabolize beclomethasone dipropionate rapidly to beclomethasone 17-monopropionate, and more slowly to free beclomethasone. The principal route of excretion of drug and metabolites is via the feces; $<$ 10% is excreted in the urine.

Dexamethasone sodium phosphate – Because of the high water solubility of dexamethasone sodium phosphate, the aerosolized particles dissolve readily in bronchial and bronchiolar mucous membrane secretions. On a regimen of 12 inhalations daily, the patient absorbs $\approx$ 0.4 to 0.6 mg dexamethasone (about 40% to 60% absorption) or 3 to 4 mg or 11 to 16 mg prednisone or hydrocortisone equivalent, respectively.

Triamcinolone acetonide – Studies demonstrate rapid disappearance from the lungs. Peak blood levels occur in 1 to 2 hours. Three metabolites have been identified; the major portion of the dose is eliminated in the feces.

Flunisolide – After inhalation of 1 mg flunisolide, systemic availability was 40%. The absorbed flunisolide is rapidly and extensively metabolized during the first pass through the liver. Plasma half-life is approximately 1.8 hours.

Indications:

For control of bronchial asthma in patients requiring chronic treatment with corticosteroids. Such patients include those already receiving systemic corticosteroids, and those inadequately controlled on a nonsteroid regimen in whom steroid therapy has been withheld because of concern over potential adverse effects.

For related corticosteroid-responsive bronchospastic states intractable to adequate trial of conventional therapy.

NOT indicated for relief of asthma which can be controlled by bronchodilators and other nonsteroid medications, in patients who require systemic corticosteroid treatment infrequently, or in the treatment of nonasthmatic bronchitis.

Contraindications:

Primary treatment of status asthmaticus or other acute episodes of asthma when intensive measures are required; hypersensitivity to any ingredient; systemic fungal infections; persistently positive sputum cultures for *Candida albicans*.

Warnings:

Adrenal insufficiency: Deaths due to adrenal insufficiency have occurred in asthmatic patients during and after transfer from systemic corticosteroids to aerosol steroids. After withdrawal from systemic corticosteroids, several months are required for recovery of hypothalamic-pituitary-adrenal (HPA) function. During this period of HPA suppression, patients may exhibit symptoms of adrenal insufficiency when exposed to trauma, surgery or infections, particularly gastroenteritis. Although aerosolized glucocorticoids may control asthmatic symptoms during these episodes, they do NOT provide the systemic steroid necessary for the treatment of these emergencies.

Stress/Severe asthma attack: During periods of stress or a severe asthmatic attack, patients withdrawn from systemic corticosteroids should resume them (in large doses) immediately and contact their physician. Patients should carry a warning card indicating they may need supplementary systemic steroids during these periods.

Infections: Localized fungal infections with *Candida albicans* or *Aspergillus niger* have occurred in the mouth, pharynx and occasionally in the larynx. Positive cultures for oral *Candida* may be present in up to 75% of patients. The incidence of clinically apparent infection is low, and may require treatment with appropriate antifungal therapy or discontinuance of aerosol steroid treatment.

Acute asthma: These products are not bronchodilators and are not indicated for rapid relief of bronchospasm. Patients should contact a physician immediately when episodes of asthma are not responsive to bronchodilators. Patients may require systemic corticosteroids.

There is no evidence that control of asthma can be achieved by administration of inhaled corticosteroids in amounts greater than recommended doses.

(Warnings continued on following page)

Corticosteroids (Cont.)

Warnings (Cont.):

Replacement therapy: Transfer from systemic steroid therapy may unmask allergic conditions previously suppressed (eg, rhinitis, conjunctivitis, eczema). During withdrawal from oral steroids, some patients may experience withdrawal symptoms (eg, joint or muscular pain, lassitude, depression) despite maintenance or improvement of respiratory function.

Hypersensitivity reactions have occurred following beclomethasone use (see Adverse Reactions). Refer to Management of Acute Hypersensitivity Reactions.

Pregnancy (Triamcinolone – Category D. Flunisolide – Category C). Glucocorticoids are teratogenic in rodent species. Findings include cleft palate, internal hydrocephaly and skeletal defects. There are no well controlled studies in pregnant women. Use these agents during pregnancy only if the benefit clearly justifies the potential risk to the fetus. Observe infants born of mothers who received substantial doses during pregnancy for adrenal insufficiency.

Lactation: Glucocorticoids are excreted in breast milk. It is not known whether inhaled corticosteroids are excreted in breast milk, but it is likely. Decide whether to discontinue nursing or to discontinue the drug.

Children: Insufficient information is available to warrant use in children < 6 years of age.

Precautions:

Adrenal effects: In responsive patients, inhaled corticosteroids may permit control of asthmatic symptoms without HPA suppression. Since these agents are absorbed and can be systemically active, the beneficial effects in minimizing or preventing HPA dysfunction may be expected only when recommended dosages are not exceeded.

Long-term effects of inhaled glucocorticoids are unknown; although there is no clinical evidence of adverse effects, the local effects on developmental or immunologic processes in the mouth, pharynx, trachea and lung are unknown.

There is also no information about effects on pulmonary infection (including active or quiescent tuberculosis), or effects of long-term administration on lung or other tissues.

Pulmonary infiltrates with eosinophilia may occur with beclomethasone or flunisolide. Although this may become manifest due to systemic steroid withdrawal when inhalational agents are used, a causative role for either agent or its vehicle cannot be ruled out.

Dysphonia: A relatively common occurrence, intermittent dysphonia has occurred in $\leq 50\%$ of patients and may be due to laryngeal candidiasis or a bilateral adductor vocal cord deformity induced by the corticosteroid. This symptom may be dose-related.

Coughing and wheezing may be more common with the use of beclomethasone and appears to be due to the dispersant rather than the drug. An alternative agent may diminish these effects. Also, pretreatment with an aerosol bronchodilator is effective in reducing coughing and wheezing in some patients.

Adverse Reactions:

Local: Throat irritation; hoarseness/dysphonia, coughing (see Precautions); dry mouth; rash; wheezing; facial edema. Laryngeal/pharyngeal fungal infections have responded promptly to discontinuation of therapy and institution of antifungal treatment.

Systemic: Suppression of HPA function has occurred in adults who used beclomethasone 1600 mcg/day for 1 month and 4000 mcg/day triamcinolone or recommended doses for 6 to 12 weeks. Deaths due to adrenal insufficiency have occurred during and after transfer from systemic to aerosol corticosteroids. (See Warnings.)

Beclomethasone: Rare cases of immediate and delayed hypersensitivity reactions, including urticaria, angioedema, rash and bronchospasm have occurred. See Warnings.

For complete information on the systemic effects of glucocorticoids, refer to the glucocorticoid section of the Adrenal Cortical Steroids group monograph.

Patient Information:

Patient instructions are available with product.

Medication is for preventive therapy only; do NOT use to abort an acute asthmatic attack; use at regularly scheduled intervals as prescribed.

Advise patients receiving bronchodilators (eg, isoproterenol, metaproterenol, epinephrine) by inhalation to use the bronchodilator several minutes *before* the corticosteroid aerosol to enhance penetration of the steroid into the bronchial tree.

Notify physician if sore throat or sore mouth occurs.

Administration technique: The success of these agents is a function of proper administration technique. Therefore, the following guidelines may be useful: Thoroughly shake the inhaler; take a drink of water to moisten the throat; place the inhaler mouthpiece two finger-widths away from the mouth; tilt head back slightly; while activating the inhaler, take a slow, deep breath for 3 to 5 seconds, hold the breath for ≈ 10 seconds and breathe out slowly; allow at least 1 minute between inhalations (puffs); rinse the mouth with water or mouthwash after each use to help reduce dry mouth and hoarseness.

(Continued on following page)

Corticosteroids (Cont.)

Administration:

Patients receiving concomitant systemic steroids: Transfer to steroid inhalant and subsequent management may be more difficult because of slow HPA function recovery which may last up to 12 months. These agents may be effective and may permit replacement or significant reduction in corticosteroid dosage.

Stabilize the patient's asthma before treatment is started. Initially, use aerosol concurrently with usual maintenance dose of systemic steroid. After approximately 1 week, start gradual withdrawal of the systemic steroid by reducing the daily or alternate daily dose. Make the next reduction after 1 to 2 weeks, depending on response. These decrements should not exceed 2.5 mg prednisone or equivalent. A slow rate of withdrawal cannot be overemphasized.

During withdrawal, some patients may experience symptoms of steroid withdrawal despite maintenance or even improvement of respiratory function. Encourage continuance with the inhaler, but observe for objective signs of adrenal insufficiency. If adrenal insufficiency occurs, increase the systemic steroid dose temporarily and continue further withdrawal more slowly.

During periods of stress or severe asthma attack, transfer patients will require supplementary systemic steroids. See Warnings.

BECLOMETHASONE DIPROPIONATE

Administration and Dosage:

50 mcg released at the valve delivers approximately 42 mcg to the patient.

Adults: 2 inhalations (84 mcg) 3 or 4 times daily. Alternatively, 4 inhalations (168 mcg) given twice daily has been effective in some patients. In patients with severe asthma, start with 12 to 16 inhalations a day and adjust dosage downward according to response. Do not exceed 20 inhalations (840 mcg) daily.

Children (6 to 12 years of age): 1 or 2 inhalations (42 to 84 mcg) 3 or 4 times daily according to response. Alternatively, 2 to 4 inhalations (84 to 168 mcg) given twice daily has been effective in some patients. Do not exceed 10 inhalations (420 mcg) daily. Clinical data are insufficient with respect to administration in children < 6 years if age.

Patients not receiving systemic steroids: Follow above directions. In responsive patients, pulmonary function usually improves within 1 to 4 weeks.

Concomitant systemic steroid therapy: See Administration section.

	Product	Form	Package	C.I.*
Rx	**Beclovent** (Allen & Hanburys)	**Aerosol:** Each actuation delivers approx. 42 mcg	In 16.8 g inhaler w/adapter and 16.8 g refill. (200 metered doses per inhaler.)	1.2
Rx	**Vanceril** (Schering)			1.2

DEXAMETHASONE SODIUM PHOSPHATE

Administration and Dosage:

Recommended initial dosage:

Adults – 3 inhalations 3 or 4 times per day; maximum 12 inhalations/day.

Children – 2 inhalations 3 or 4 times per day; maximum 8 inhalations/day.

Concomitant systemic steroid therapy: See Administration section.

	Product	Form	Package	C.I.*
Rx	**Decadron Phosphate Respihaler** (MSD)	**Aerosol:** Each activation releases dexamethasone sodium phosphate equivalent to approximately 84 mcg dexamethasone	In 12.6 g container.[1] (170 metered doses per inhaler.)	1

* Cost Index based on cost per inhalation (42 mcg beclomethasone or 84 mcg dexamethasone).

[1] With 2% alcohol.

Corticosteroids (Cont.)

TRIAMCINOLONE ACETONIDE

Administration and Dosage:

200 mcg released with each actuation delivers approximately 100 mcg to the patient.

Adults: The usual dosage is 2 inhalations (approximately 200 mcg) 3 to 4 times a day. Do not exceed a maximum daily intake of 16 inhalations (1600 mcg). Higher initial doses (12 to 16 inhalations per day) may be advisable in patients with more severe asthma, the dosage then being adjusted downward according to patient response. In some patients, maintenance can be accomplished when the total daily dose is administered twice a day.

Children (6 to 12 years): The usual dosage is 1 or 2 inhalations (100 to 200 mcg) 3 to 4 times a day. Do not exceed a maximum daily intake of 12 inhalations (1200 mcg). Clinical data are insufficient with respect to use in children < 6 years of age.

Patients not receiving systemic steroids: Follow above directions. In responsive patients, an improvement in pulmonary function is usually apparent within 1 to 2 weeks.

Concomitant systemic steroid therapy: See Administration section.

	Product	Form	Package	C.I.*
Rx	**Azmacort** (Rhone-Poulenc Rorer)	**Aerosol:** Each actuation delivers approx. 100 mcg. Contains 60 mg triamcinolone acetonide	In 20 g inhaler w/adapter.[1] (240 metered doses per inhaler.)	1.4

FLUNISOLIDE

Administration and Dosage:

Each actuation delivers approximately 250 mcg flunisolide to the patient.

Adults: 2 inhalations (500 mcg) twice daily, morning and evening (total daily dose 1000 mcg). Do not exceed 4 inhalations twice daily (2000 mcg).

Children (6 to 15 years): 2 inhalations twice daily, morning and evening (total daily dose 1000 mcg). Higher doses have not been studied. Safety and efficacy for use in children < 6 years have not been established. With chronic use, monitor children for growth as well as for effects on the HPA axis.

Patients not receiving systemic steroids: In responsive patients, pulmonary function usually improves within 1 to 4 weeks.

Concomitant systemic steroid therapy: See Administration section.

	Product	Form	Package	C.I.*
Rx	**AeroBid** (Forest)	**Aerosol:** Each actuation delivers approx. 250 mcg	In 7 g canister with mouthpiece. (100 metered doses per inhaler.)	1.3

* Cost Index based on cost per dose (200 mcg triamcinolone or 500 mcg flunisolide).

[1] With 1% alcohol.

Mucolytics

ACETYLCYSTEINE (N-Acetylcysteine)

Actions:

The viscosity of pulmonary mucus secretions depends on the concentration of mucoprotein in the secretory fluid, the presence of disulfide bonds between these macromolecules and, to a lesser extent, DNA. The mucolytic action of acetylcysteine is related to the sulfhydryl group in the molecule, which acts directly to split disulfide linkages between mucoprotein molecular complexes, resulting in depolymerization and a decrease in mucus viscosity. Its action is unaffected by the presence of DNA. The mucolytic activity of acetylcysteine increases with increasing pH. Significant mucolysis occurs between pH 7 and 9.

Acetylcysteine reduces the extent of liver injury following acetaminophen overdose. It is thought that acetylcysteine protects the liver by maintaining or restoring glutathione levels, or by acting as an alternate substrate for conjugation with, and thus, detoxification of, the reactive metabolite of acetaminophen.

Indications:

Mucolytic: Adjuvant therapy for abnormal, viscid or inspissated mucus secretions in chronic bronchopulmonary disease (chronic emphysema, emphysema with bronchitis, chronic asthmatic bronchitis, tuberculosis, bronchiectasis, primary amyloidosis of the lung); acute bronchopulmonary disease (pneumonia, bronchitis, tracheobronchitis); pulmonary complications of cystic fibrosis; tracheostomy care; pulmonary complications associated with surgery; use during anesthesia; posttraumatic chest conditions; atelectasis due to mucus obstruction; diagnostic bronchial studies (bronchograms, bronchospirometry, bronchial wedge catheterization).

Antidote: To prevent or lessen hepatic injury which may occur following ingestion of a potentially hepatotoxic quantity of acetaminophen. Initiate treatment as soon as possible after overdose and, in any case, within 24 hours of ingestion.

Unlabeled uses: As an ophthalmic solution to treat keratoconjunctivitis sicca (dry eye). It has been used as an enema to treat bowel obstruction due to meconium ileus or its equivalent.

Contraindications:

Hypersensitivity to acetylcysteine.

There are no contraindications for use as an antidote.

Warnings:

An increased volume of liquefied bronchial secretions may occur; when cough is inadequate, maintain an open airway by mechanical suction if necessary. When there is a large mechanical block due to a foreign body or local accumulation, clear the airway by endotracheal aspiration, with or without bronchoscopy.

Observe asthmatics under treatment with acetylcysteine carefully. If bronchospasm progresses, discontinue medication immediately.

Antidotal use:

Allergic effects – Generalized urticaria has been observed rarely. If this or other allergic symptoms appear, discontinue treatment unless it is deemed essential and the allergic symptoms can be otherwise controlled.

Hepatic effects – If encephalopathy due to hepatic failure occurs, discontinue treatment to avoid further administration of nitrogenous substances. No data indicate that acetylcysteine adversely influences hepatic failure, but this is theoretically possible.

Vomiting, occasionally severe and persistent, occurs as a symptom of acute acetaminophen overdose. Treatment with oral acetylcysteine may aggravate this. Evaluate patients at risk of gastric hemorrhage (eg, esophageal varices, peptic ulcers) concerning the risk of upper GI hemorrhage versus the risk of developing hepatic toxicity. Diluting acetylcysteine minimizes its propensity to aggravate vomiting.

Precautions:

Administration may initially produce a slight disagreeable odor which soon disappears. A face mask may cause stickiness on the face after nebulization; remove with water.

Solution color may change in the opened bottle, but does not significantly impair the drug's safety or efficacy.

Continued nebulization of acetylcysteine with a dry gas results in concentration of drug in the nebulizer due to evaporation. Extreme concentration may impede nebulization and drug delivery. Dilute with Sterile Water for Injection as concentration occurs.

Incompatibility: Tetracycline, chlortetracycline, oxytetracycline, erythromycin lactobionate, amphotericin B and sodium ampicillin are incompatible when mixed in the same solution with acetylcysteine. Administer from separate solutions. Also incompatible are iodized oil, chymotrypsin, trypsin and hydrogen peroxide.

(Continued on following page)

ACETYLCYSTEINE (N-Acetylcysteine) (Cont.)

Adverse Reactions:

Sensitivity reactions and sensitization have been reported very rarely.

Bronchospasm of varying degrees may occur in a few susceptible patients, particularly asthmatics. Most patients are quickly relieved by a nebulized bronchodilator.

Miscellaneous: Stomatitis, nausea and rhinorrhea.

Antidotal use: Large doses of oral acetylcysteine may result in nausea, vomiting and other GI symptoms. Rash, with or without mild fever, has been observed rarely.

Administration and Dosage:

Nebulization (face mask, mouth piece, tracheostomy): 1 to 10 ml of the 20% solution or 2 to 20 ml of the 10% solution every 2 to 6 hours; the dose for most patients is 3 to 5 ml of the 20% solution or 6 to 10 ml of the 10% solution 3 to 4 times a day.

Nebulization (tent, croupette): Very large volumes are required, occasionally up to 300 ml during a treatment period. The dose is the volume of solution that will maintain a very heavy mist in the tent or croupette for the desired period. Administration for intermittent or continuous prolonged periods, including overnight, may be desirable.

Instillation: Direct – 1 to 2 ml of a 10% to 20% solution as often as every hour.

Tracheostomy – 1 to 2 ml of a 10% to 20% solution every 1 to 4 hours by instillation into the tracheostomy.

May be introduced directly into a particular segment of the bronchopulmonary tree by inserting (under local anesthesia and direct vision) a plastic catheter into the trachea. Instill 2 to 5 ml of the 20% solution by a syringe connected to the catheter.

Percutaneous intratracheal catheter – 1 to 2 ml of the 20% solution or 2 to 4 ml of the 10% solution every 1 to 4 hours by a syringe attached to the catheter.

Diagnostic bronchograms: 2 or 3 administrations of 1 to 2 ml of the 20% solution or 2 to 4 ml of the 10% solution by nebulization or by instillation intratracheally, prior to the procedure.

Preparation of solution: The 20% solution may be diluted with either normal saline or Water for Injection. The 10% solution may be used undiluted. Refrigerate unused, undiluted solution and use within 96 hours.

Equipment compatibility: Certain materials in nebulization equipment react with acetylcysteine, especially certain metals (notably iron and copper) and rubber. Where materials may come into contact with acetylcysteine solution, use parts made of the following materials: Glass, plastic, aluminum, anodized aluminum, chromed metal, tantalum, sterling silver or stainless steel. Silver may become tarnished after exposure, but this is not harmful to the drug action or to the patient.

Acetaminophen overdosage: Administer acetylcysteine immediately if 24 hours or less have elapsed from the reported time of acetaminophen ingestion. Do not await results of assays for acetaminophen level before initiating treatment. The following procedures are recommended:

1. Empty the stomach promptly by lavage or by inducing emesis with syrup of ipecac. Repeat the dose of ipecac if emesis does not occur in 20 minutes.
2. If activated charcoal has been administered, lavage before administering acetylcysteine. Activated charcoal may adsorb acetylcysteine, thereby reducing its effectiveness.
3. Draw blood for acetaminophen plasma assay and for baseline SGOT, SGPT, bilirubin, prothrombin time, creatinine, BUN, blood sugar and electrolytes. If an assay cannot be obtained or if the acetaminophen level is clearly in the toxic range, continue acetylcysteine for the full course of therapy. Monitor hepatic and renal function and electrolyte and fluid balance.
4. Administer a 140 mg/kg loading dose of acetylcysteine.
5. Administer the first maintenance dose (70 mg/kg) 4 hours after the loading dose. Repeat the maintenance dose at 4 hour intervals for a total of 17 doses unless the acetaminophen assay reveals a nontoxic level.
6. If the patient vomits the loading dose or any maintenance dose within 1 hour of administration, repeat that dose.
7. If the patient is persistently unable to retain the orally administered acetylcysteine, administer by duodenal intubation.
8. Repeat SGOT, SGPT, bilirubin, prothrombin time, creatinine, BUN, blood sugar and electrolytes daily if the acetaminophen plasma level is in the potentially toxic range.

(Administration and Dosage continued on following page)

ACETYLCYSTEINE (N-Acetylcysteine) (Cont.)

Administration and Dosage (Cont.):

Acetaminophen overdosage (Cont.):

Preparation of oral solution – Dilute the 20% solution with cola drinks or other soft drinks, to a final concentration of 5% (see table on page 934). If administered via gastric tube or Miller-Abbott tube, water may be used as the diluent. Prepare fresh dilutions and use within 1 hour. Remaining undiluted solutions in opened vials can be refrigerated up to 96 hours.

Acetaminophen assays – The acute ingestion of acetaminophen in quantities of 150 mg/kg or greater may result in hepatic toxicity. However, the reported history of the quantity of a drug ingested as an overdose is often inaccurate and is not a reliable guide to antidotal therapy. Therefore, determine plasma or serum acetaminophen concentrations as early as possible, but no sooner than 4 hours following an acute overdose to assess the potential risk of hepatotoxicity. If an acetaminophen assay cannot be obtained, assume that the overdose is potentially toxic.

Interpretation of acetaminophen assays – When results of the plasma acetaminophen assay are available, refer to the nomogram on page 933 . Values above the solid line connecting 200 mcg/ml at 4 hours with 50 mcg/ml at 12 hours are associated with a possibility of hepatic toxicity if an antidote is not administered. (Do not wait for assay results to begin treatment.)

If the plasma level is above the broken line, continue with maintenance doses of acetylcysteine. It is better to err on the safe side; thus, the broken line is plotted 25% below the solid line which defines possible toxicity.

If the plasma level is below the broken line described above, there is minimal risk of hepatic toxicity and acetylcysteine treatment can be discontinued.

(Administration and Dosage continued on following page)

ACETYLCYSTEINE (N-Acetylcysteine) (Cont.)

Administration and Dosage (Cont.):

Acetaminophen overdosage (Cont.):

Estimating potential for hepatotoxicity – The following nomogram estimates the probability that plasma levels in relation to intervals postingestion will result in hepatotoxicity.

Plasma or Serum Acetaminophen Concentration vs Time Postingestion of Acetaminophen*

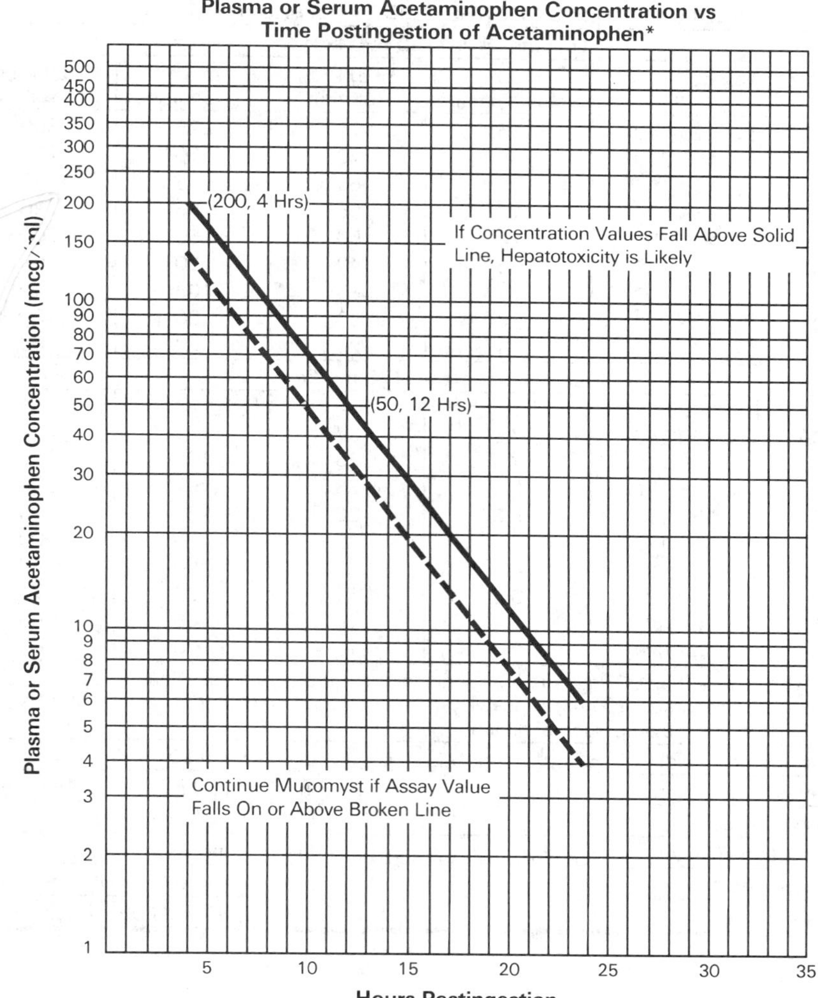

* Adapted from Rumack and Matthews, *Pediatrics* 55:871-876, 1975.

(Administration and Dosage continued on following page)

Mucolytics (Cont.)

ACETYLCYSTEINE (N-Acetylcysteine) (Cont.)

Administration and Dosage (Cont.):

Supportive treatment: Maintain fluid and electrolyte balance. Treat as necessary for hypoglycemia. Administer vitamin K_1 if prothrombin time ratio exceeds 1.5; administer fresh frozen plasma if the prothrombin time ratio exceeds 3. Avoid diuretics and forced diuresis.

ACETYLCYSTEINE DOSAGE GUIDE AND PREPARATION					
Loading Dose (140 mg/kg)†					
Body Weight (kg)	(lb)	**grams Acetylcysteine**	**ml of 20% Solution**	**ml of Diluent**	**Total ml of 5% Solution**
100-109	220-240	15	75	225	300
90-99	198-218	14	70	210	280
80-89	176-196	13	65	195	260
70-79	154-174	11	55	165	220
60-69	132-152	10	50	150	200
50-59	110-130	8	40	120	160
40-49	88-108	7	35	105	140
30-39	66-86	6	30	90	120
20-29	44-64	4	20	60	80
Maintenance Dose† (70 mg/kg)					
(kg)	(lb)				
100-109	220-240	7.5	37	113	150
90-99	198-218	7	35	105	140
80-89	176-196	6.5	33	97	130
70-79	154-174	5.5	28	82	110
60-69	132-152	5	25	75	100
50-59	110-130	4	20	60	80
40-49	88-108	3.5	18	52	70
30-39	66-86	3	15	45	60
20-29	44-64	2	10	30	40

† If patient weighs less than 20 kg (usually patients younger than 6 years), calculate the dose. Each ml of 20% solution contains 200 mg of acetylcysteine. Add 3 ml of diluent to each ml of 20% solution. Do not decrease the proportion of diluent.

Rx	**Acetylcysteine** (Quad)	**Solution:** 10% (as sodium)	In 4, 10 and 30 ml vials.
Rx	**Mucomyst** (Apothecon)		In 10 and 30 ml and UD 4 ml vials.
Rx	**Mucosol** (Dey Labs)		In 4, 10 and 30 ml vials.
Rx	**Acetylcysteine** (Quad)	**Solution:** 20% (as sodium)	In 4, 10 and 30 ml vials.
Rx	**Mucomyst** (Apothecon)		In 10 and 30 ml and UD 4 ml vials.
Rx	**Mucosol** (Dey Labs)		In 4, 10, 30 and 100 ml vials.

IPRATROPIUM BROMIDE

Actions:

Ipratropium br for oral inhalation is a synthetic quaternary ammonium compound chemically related to atropine.

Pharmacology: Ipratropium br is an anticholinergic (parasympatholytic) which appears to inhibit vagally mediated reflexes by antagonizing the action of acetylcholine. Anticholinergics prevent the increases in intracellular concentration of cyclic guanosine monophosphate (cyclic GMP) which are caused by interaction of acetylcholine with the muscarinic receptor on bronchial smooth muscle.

The bronchodilation following inhalation is primarily a local, site-specific effect, not a systemic one. Much of an inhaled dose is swallowed as shown by fecal excretion studies. Ipratropium is not readily absorbed into the systemic circulation either from the surface of the lung or from the GI tract as confirmed by blood levels and renal excretion studies.

Pharmacokinetics: The elimination half-life is about 2 hours after inhalation or IV administration. Autoradiographic studies in rats have shown that ipratropium does not penetrate the blood-brain barrier.

Clinical Pharmacology: In controlled 90 day studies in patients with bronchospasm associated with chronic obstructive pulmonary disease (chronic bronchitis and emphysema), significant improvements in pulmonary function (FEV_1 and $FEF_{25\% \text{ to } 75\%}$ increases of 15% or more) occurred within 15 minutes, reached a peak in 1 to 2 hours and persisted for 3 to 4 hours in the majority of patients and up to 6 hours in some patients. In addition, significant increases in Forced Vital Capacity (FVC) have been demonstrated.

Controlled clinical studies have demonstrated that ipratropium does not alter either mucociliary clearance or the volume or viscosity of respiratory secretions. In studies without a positive control, it did not alter pupil size, accomodation or visual acuity.

Ventilation/perfusion studies have shown no clinically significant effects on pulmonary gas exchange or arterial oxygen tension. The drug does not produce clinically significant changes in pulse rate or blood pressure.

Indications:

As a bronchodilator for maintenance treatment of bronchospasm associated with chronic obstructive pulmonary disease, including chronic bronchitis and emphysema.

Contraindications:

Hypersensitivity to atropine or its derivatives.

Warnings:

Not indicated for the initial treatment of acute episodes of bronchospasm where rapid response is required.

Use with caution in patients with narrow-angle glaucoma, prostatic hypertrophy or bladder neck obstruction.

Usage in Pregnancy: Category B. Oral reproduction studies in animals (at doses approximately 2,000 to 200,000 times the maximum recommended daily human dose) and inhalation reproduction studies in rats and rabbits (at doses approximately 312 and 375 times the maximum recommended human daily dose, respectively) have demonstrated no evidence of teratogenic effects. However, no adequate and well controlled studies have been conducted in pregnant women. Use during pregnancy only if clearly needed.

Usage in Lactation: It is not known whether this drug is excreted in breast milk. Although lipid-insoluble quaternary bases pass into breast milk, it is unlikely that ipratropium would reach the infant to an important extent especially when taken by aerosol. However, exercise caution when administering to a nursing mother.

Usage in Children: Safety and efficacy for use in children less than 12 years of age have not been established.

Drug Interactions:

Ipratropium has been used concomitantly with other drugs, including sympathomimetic bronchodilators, methylxanthines, steroids and cromolyn sodium, commonly used in the treatment of chronic obstructive pulmonary disease, without adverse drug reactions. There are no formal studies fully evaluating the interactive effects of ipratropium and these drugs with respect to effectiveness.

(Continued on following page)

IPRATROPIUM BROMIDE (Cont.)

Adverse Reactions:

Adverse reactions occurring in > 1% of patients in the 90 day controlled clinical trials (n = 254) include:

CNS: Nervousness (3.1%); dizziness and headache (2.4%).
GI: Nausea (2.8%); GI distress (2.4%).
EENT: Blurred vision (1.2%); dry mouth (2.4%); irritation from aerosol (1.6%).
Respiratory: Cough (5.9%); exacerbation of symptoms (2.4%).
Other: Palpitations (1.8%); rash (1.2%).

Additional adverse reactions reported in < 1% of patients (possibly due to ipratropium) include urinary difficulty, fatigue, insomnia and hoarseness.

Of the 2301 patients treated in a large uncontrolled study and in clinical trials other than the 90 day studies, the most common adverse reactions reported were:

Dryness of the oropharynx (5%); cough, exacerbation of symptoms and irritation from aerosol (each 3%); headache (2%); nausea, dizziness, blurred vision/difficulty in accommodation, and drying of secretions (each 1%). Less frequently reported adverse reactions that were possibly due to ipratropium include tachycardia, paresthesias, drowsiness, coordination difficulty, itching, hives, flushing, alopecia, constipation, tremor and mucosal ulcers.

Cases of precipitation or worsening or narrow-angle glaucoma, acute eye pain and hypotension have been reported.

One case of giant urticaria with positive rechallenge has been reported from the foreign marketing experience.

Overdosage:

Acute overdosage by inhalation is unlikely since ipratropium is not well absorbed systemically after aerosol or oral administration.

Patient Information:

Temporary blurred vision may result if aerosol is sprayed into eyes.

Administation and Dosage:

The usual dose is 2 inhalations (36 mcg) 4 times a day. Patients may take additional inhalations as required; however, do not exceed 12 inhalations in 24 hours.

Storage: Store below 30°C (86°F); avoid excessive humidity.

Rx	**Atrovent** (Boehringer Ingelheim)	**Aerosol**: Each actuation delivers 18 mcg	In 14 g metered dose inhaler w/ mouthpiece (200 inhalations).

For information on cromolyn ophthalmic solution, refer to page 2208.

Miscellaneous

CROMOLYN SODIUM (Disodium Cromoglycate)

Actions:

Pharmacology: Cromolyn is an antiasthmatic, antiallergic and mast cell stabilizer. It has no intrinsic bronchodilator, antihistaminic, anticholinergic, vasoconstrictor or anti-inflammatory activity.

In animal studies, cromolyn inhibits the degranulation of sensitized and nonsensitized mast cells which occurs after exposure to specific antigens. The drug inhibits the release of histamine and SRS-A (the slow-reacting substance of anaphylaxis, a leukotriene) from the mast cell. Bronchial asthma or rhinitis induced by the inhalation of antigens can be inhibited to varying degrees by pretreatment with cromolyn.

Cromolyn acts locally on the lung to which it is directly applied. The Spinhaler (inhalation capsule) route delivers more drug to the lungs compared to nebulization of the solution, but there is no difference in effectiveness.

Pharmacokinetics: After inhalation, about 7% to 8% is absorbed from the lung and is rapidly excreted unchanged in bile and urine. The remainder is either exhaled, or deposited in the oropharynx, swallowed and excreted via the alimentary tract.

Cromolyn is poorly absorbed from the GI tract. No more than 1% of an administered dose is absorbed after oral administration, the remainder being excreted in the feces. Very little absorption of cromolyn was seen after oral administration of 500 mg to each of 12 volunteers. From 0.25% to 0.5% of the administered dose was recovered in the first 24 hours of urinary excretion in 3 subjects. The mean urinary excretion over 24 hours in the remaining 9 subjects was 0.45%.

Clinical trials: Cromolyn nebulization solution vs theophylline – Cromolyn solution 20 mg 4 times daily was compared to theophylline and to a combination of both drugs in asthmatic children. Cromolyn solution was at least as effective in controlling the symptoms of chronic asthma as oral theophylline in the 1 to 6 year age group, without side effects. The combination of cromolyn with theophylline gave no additional benefits.

Indications:

Severe bronchial asthma (nebulization solution, inhalation capsules, aerosol): Prophylactic management of severe bronchial asthma where the frequency, intensity and predictability of episodes indicate the continued use of symptomatic medication. Such patients must have a significant bronchodilator-reversible component to their airway obstruction as demonstrated by pulmonary function tests.

Improvement ordinarily occurs within the first 4 weeks of administration, manifested by a decrease in the severity of clinical symptoms, or the need for concomitant therapy, or both. Long-term administration is justified if the drug produces a significant reduction in the severity of the symptoms of asthma, permits a significant reduction in, or elimination of, steroid dosage, or improves management of patients who have intolerable side effects to sympathomimetic agents or methylxanthines.

Prevention of exercise-induced bronchospasm (nebulization solution, capsules, aerosol).

Prevention of acute bronchospasm induced by toluene diisocyanate, environmental pollutants and known antigens (aerosol).

Allergic rhinitis (nasal solution): Prevention and treatment of allergic rhinitis.

Mastocytosis (oral):– Improves diarrhea, flushing, headaches, vomiting, urticaria, abdominal pain, nausea and itching in some patients.

Unlabeled uses: Oral use is being evaluated in patients with food allergies to prevent GI and systemic reactions. Also being evaluated for use in eczema, dermatitis, ulcerations, urticaria pigmentosa, chronic urticaria, hay fever and postexercise bronchospasm.

Contraindications:

Hypersensitivity to cromolyn or to any ingredient contained in these products.

Warnings:

Acute asthma: Cromolyn has no role in the treatment of acute asthma, especially status asthmaticus, because it is a prophylactic drug with no benefit for acute situations.

Hypersensitivity: Severe anaphylactic reactions may occur rarely with oral cromolyn. Refer to General Management of Acute Hypersensitivity Reactions.

Hepatic or renal function impairment: In view of the biliary and renal routes of excretion, decrease the dose or discontinue the drug in impaired renal or hepatic function.

Pregnancy: Category B. Safety for use during pregnancy has not been established. Use only when clearly needed and when the potential benefits outweigh the unknown potential hazards to the fetus.

Animal studies have demonstrated adverse fetal effects (increased resorptions, decreased fetal weight) only at very high parenteral doses (38 to 338 times the human dose) in combination with isoproterenol at high doses (90 times the human dose).

(Warnings continued on following page)

CROMOLYN SODIUM (Disodium Cromoglycate) (Cont.)

Warnings (Cont.)

Lactation: Safety for use in the nursing mother has not been established. Exercise caution when the drug is administered to a nursing mother.

Children: Inhalation capsules – Clinical experience in children < 5 years of age is limited due to administration by inhalation. Capsule use is not recommended.

Aerosol – Safety and efficacy in children < 5 years old are not established.

Nebulizer solution – Safety and efficacy in children < 2 years old are not established.

Nasal solution – Safety and efficacy in children < 6 years old are not established.

Oral capsule – Animal studies suggest increased risk of toxicity in premature animals when given in doses much higher than clinically recommended. In term infants up to 6 months of age, data suggest the dose not exceed 20 mg/kg/day. Reserve use in children < 2 years for patients with severe disease in which potential benefits clearly outweigh risks.

Precautions:

Bronchospasm: Occasionally, patients experience cough or bronchospasm following inhalation and, at times, may not be able to continue treatment despite prior bronchodilator administration. Very severe bronchospasm has occurred rarely.

Asthma symptoms may recur if drug is reduced below recommended dosage or discontinued.

Eosinophilic pneumonia (pulmonary infiltrates with eosinophilia): If this occurs during the course of therapy, discontinue the drug.

Nasal stinging or sneezing may be experienced by some patients immediately following instillation of the **nasal solution.** This has rarely caused discontinuation of therapy.

Aerosol: Because of the propellants in this preparation, use with caution in patients with coronary artery disease or cardiac arrhythmias.

Drug Interaction:

Isoproterenol and cromolyn sodium: See Pregnancy.

Adverse Reactions:

Inhalation capsules and aerosol:

EENT –Lacrimation; swollen parotid gland.

GU – Dysuria; urinary frequency.

CNS – Dizziness; headache.

Allergic – Rash; urticaria; angioedema.

Miscellaneous – Joint swelling and pain; nausea.

Causal relationship unknown or rare – Anaphylaxis; anemia; exfoliative dermatitis; hemoptysis; hoarseness; myalgia; nephrosis; periarteric vasculitis; pericarditis; peripheral neuritis; photodermatitis; polymyositis; pulmonary infiltrates with eosinophilia; vertigo; nasal itching, bleeding or burning; sneezing; serum sickness; liver disease.

Adverse effects related to the cromolyn inhalation capsule delivery system are inhalation of gelatin particles, mouthpiece or propeller.

Additional effects reported with the aerosol include: Dry or irritated throat; bad taste; cough; wheezing; substernal burning and myopathy (rare).

Nebulizer solution: Cough; nasal congestion; wheezing; sneezing; nasal itching; epistaxis; nose burning; abdominal pain.

Nasal solution: Sneezing (10%); nasal stinging (5%); nasal burning (4%); nasal irritation (2.5%); headaches, bad taste in mouth (2%); epistaxis, postnasal drip, rash (< 1%).

Oral capsules: Most of the adverse events reported in mastocytosis patients have been transient and could represent symptoms of the disease. The most frequently reported adverse events in mastocytosis patients who have received cromolyn during clinical studies were headache and diarrhea. Each occurred in 4 of 87 patients. Pruritis, nausea and myalgia were each reported in 3 patients and abdominal pain, rash and irritability in 2 patients each. One report of malaise was also recorded.

A generally similar profile of adverse events has been reported during studies in other clinical conditions. Additional reports that have been received during the course of these studies and spontaneous reports during foreign marketing include:

CNS: Dizziness; fatigue; paresthesia; migraine; psychosis; anxiety; depression; insomnia; behavior change; hallucinations; postprandial lightheadedness; lethargy.

Dermatologic: Flushing; urticaria/angioedema; skin erythema and burning.

GI: Taste perversion; esophagospasm; flatulence; dysphagia; hepatic function test abnormality; burning mouth and throat.

Miscellaneous: Arthralgia; edema; dyspnea; polycythemia; neutropenia; dysuria; stiffness and weakness of the legs. These events are infrequent, the majority representing only a single report; in many cases, causal relationship to cromolyn is uncertain.

(Continued on following page)

Miscellaneous (Cont.)

CROMOLYN SODIUM (Disodium Cromoglycate) (Cont.)

Overdosage:

No action other than medical observation should be necessary.

Patient Information:

Inhalation or nasal: Do not discontinue therapy abruptly except on advice of physician.

For inhalation use only; do not swallow capsule.

Notify physician if coughing or wheezing occurs.

Patient instructions for use of Spinhaler device and Nasalmatic device accompany each product.

Oral: The effect of therapy depends upon administration at regular intervals as directed.

Take at least one-half hour before meals. Do not mix with fruit juice, milk or foods.

Drink all of the liquid.

Administration and Dosage:

Nebulizer solution and inhalation capsules: Adults and children (≤ 5 years for capsules; ≥ 2 years for nebulizer solution) – Initially, 20 mg inhaled 4 times daily at regular intervals. Carefully instruct patients in the use of the inhaler. The effectiveness of therapy depends upon administration at regular intervals.

Administer solution from a power operated nebulizer having an adequate flow rate and equipped with a suitable face mask. *Hand operated nebulizers are not suitable.*

Introduce cromolyn into the patient's therapeutic regimen when the acute episode has been controlled and the patient is able to inhale adequately.

Prevention of exercise-induced bronchospasm: Inhale one 20 mg capsule or 20 mg of the nebulizer solution no more than 1 hour before anticipated exercise. The drug's protective effect will be stronger the shorter the interval between inhalation and exercise. Repeat inhalation as required for protection during prolonged exercise.

Concomitant corticosteroid treatment and bronchodilators should be continued following the introduction of cromolyn. If the patient improves, attempt to decrease corticosteroid dosage. Even if the steroid-dependent patient fails to improve following cromolyn use, attempt gradual tapering of steroid dosage while maintaining close patient supervision. Consider reinstituting steroid therapy for a patient subjected to significant stress (a severe asthmatic attack, surgery, trauma or severe illness) while being treated or within 1 year (occasionally up to 2 years) after steroid treatment has been terminated, in case of adrenocortical insufficiency. When the inhalation of cromolyn is impaired, a temporary increase in the amount of steroids or other agents may be required.

Cautiously withdraw cromolyn in cases where its use has permitted a reduction in the maintenance dose of steroids as there may be a sudden reappearance of asthma which will require immediate therapy and possible reintroduction of corticosteroids.

Aerosol: For management of bronchial asthma in adults and children ≥ 5 years of age, the usual starting dose is two metered sprays inhaled 4 times daily at regular intervals. Do not exceed this dose. Not all patients will respond to the recommended dose, and a lower dose may provide efficacy in younger patients.

Advise patients with chronic asthma that the effect of therapy is dependent upon its administration at regular intervals, as directed. Introduce therapy into the patient's therapeutic regimen when the acute episode has been controlled, the airway has been cleared and the patient is able to inhale adequately.

For the prevention of acute bronchospasm which follows exercise, exposure to cold dry air or environmental agents, the usual dose is inhalation of two metered dose sprays shortly, (ie, 10 to 15 minutes but not more than 60 minutes), before exposure to the precipitating factor.

Nasal solution: Adults and children ≥ 6 years – One spray in each nostril 3 to 6 times daily at regular intervals. Clear the nasal passages before administering the spray and inhale through the nose during administration.

Seasonal (pollenotic) rhinitis, and for prevention of rhinitis caused by exposure to other types of specific inhalant allergens – Treatment will be more effective if started prior to contact with the allergen. Continue treatment throughout exposure period.

Perennial allergic rhinitis – Effects of treatment may require 2 to 4 weeks of treatment. Concomitant use of antihistamines or nasal decongestants may be necessary during the initial phase of treatment, but the need for this medication should diminish and may be eliminated when the full benefit of therapy is achieved.

Use with Nasalmatic metered spray device. Replace pump device every 6 months.

(Administration and Dosage continued on following page)

CROMOLYN SODIUM (Disodium Cromoglycate) (Cont.)

Administration and Dosage (Cont):

Oral: Adults – Two capsules 4 times daily one-half hour before meals and at bedtime.

Children: Premature to term infants – Not recommended.

Term to 2 years – 20 mg/kg/day in four divided doses. Use of this product in children < 2 years is not recommended and should be attempted only in those patients with severe incapacitating diseases where benefits clearly outweigh risks.

2 to 12 years – One capsule 4 times daily one-half hour before meals and bedtime.

If satisfactory control of symptoms is not achieved within 2 to 3 weeks, the dosage may be increased but should not exceed 40 mg/kg/day (30 mg/kg/day for children 6 months to 2 years)

The effect of therapy is dependent upon its administration at regular intervals as directed.

Maintenance: Once a therapeutic response has been achieved the dose may be reduced to the minimum required to maintain the patient with a lower degree of symptomatology. To prevent relapses, maintain the dosage.

Administer as a solution in water at least one-half hour before meals after preparation according to the following directions.

1. Open capsule(s) and pour powder contents into one-half glass of hot water.
2. Stir until completely dissolved (clear solution).
3. Add equal quantity of cold water while stirring.
4. Do not mix with fruit juice, milk or foods.
5. Drink all of the liquid.

Each capsule contains a precisely measured dose. The capsules are intentionally oversized to prevent the powder from spilling when the capsule is opened.

Oral capsules are not for inhalation.

Compatibility: Cromolyn **nebulizer solution** is compatible with metaproterenol sulfate, isoproterenol HCl, 0.25% isoetharine HCl, epinephrine HCl, terbutaline sulfate and 20% acetylcysteine solution for at least 1 hour after their admixture.

Storage: Store the **nebulizer solution** below 30°C (86°F); protect from direct light.

				C.I.*
Rx	**Intal** (Fisons)	**Capsules (for inhalation only)**[1]: 20 mg[2]	In 60s and 120s.	97
		Solution (for nebulizer only): 20 mg	In 2 ml amps.	113
		Aerosol Spray: Each actuation delivers 800 mcg.	In 8.1 g (112 metered sprays) and 14.2 g (200 metered sprays).	60
Rx	**Nasalcrom** (Fisons)	**Nasal Solution:** 40 mg/ml.[3] Each actuation delivers 5.2 mg.	In 13 ml metered spray device or refill (≈ 100 sprays).	29
Rx	**Gastrocrom** (Fisons)	**Capsules (Oral):** 100 mg	In oversized 100s.	N/A

* Cost Index based on cost per 20 mg inhalation capsules, 800 mcg aerosol actuation or 5.2 mg solution actuation.

[1] To be used with Spinhaler turbo-inhaler.

[2] With 20 mg lactose.

[3] With 0.01% benzalkonium chloride and 0.01% EDTA.

Actions:

Decongestants are sympathomimetic amines administered directly to swollen membranes (spray, drops, etc) or systemically via the oral route. They are used in such acute conditions as hay fever, allergic rhinitis, vasomotor rhinitis, acute coryza, sinusitis and the common cold to relieve membrane congestion.

Pharmacology: Decongestants stimulate α-adrenergic receptors of vascular smooth muscle (vasoconstriction, pressor effects, nasal decongestion), although some retain β-adrenergic properties (ie, ephedrine, pseudoephedrine). Other alpha effects include contraction of the GI and urinary sphincters, mydriasis and decreased pancreatic beta cell secretion. The α-adrenergic effects cause intense vasoconstriction when applied directly to mucous membranes; systemically, the products have similar muted effects and decongestion occurs without drastic changes in blood pressure, vascular redistribution or cardiac stimulation. Constriction in the mucous membranes results in their shrinkage; this promotes drainage, thus improving ventilation and the stuffy feeling.

Oral agents are not as effective as topical products, especially on an immediate basis, but generally have a longer duration of action, cause less local irritation and are not associated with rebound congestion (rhinitis medicamentosa).

Available Routes, Doses and Strengths of the Nasal Decongestants

	Drug and Route	*Usual Adult Dose*	*Strengths*
Arylalkylamines	Phenylpropanolamine – Oral	25 mg q 4 hrs; 50 mg q 8 hrs	25 mg, 50 mg
	Phenylpropanolamine – Oral-SR	75 mg q 12 hrs	75 mg
	Pseudoephedrine – Oral	60 mg q 4 to 6 hrs	30 mg, 60 mg, 7.5 mg/0.8 ml, 15 mg/5 ml, 30 mg/5 ml, 30 mg/ml
	Pseudoephedrine – Oral-SR	120 mg q 12 hrs	120 mg
	Phenylephrine – Topical	1 to 2 sprays or a few drops q 3 to 4 hrs	0.125%, 0.16%, 0.2%, 0.25%, 0.5%, 1%, 0.5% jelly
	Epinephrine – Topical	Maximum 1 ml/15 min[1]	0.1%
	Ephedrine – Topical	2 to 3 drops q 4 hrs	0.5%, 0.6% jelly
	Desoxyephedrine – Topical	Inhale twice q 2 hrs	50 mg inhaler
Imidazolines	Naphazoline – Topical	2 drops q 3 hrs	0.05%
	Oxymetazoline – Topical	2 to 3 drops twice daily	0.025%, 0.05%
	Tetrahydrozoline – Topical	2 to 4 drops q 3 hrs	0.05%, 0.1%
	Xylometazoline – Topical	2 to 3 drops q 8 to 10 hrs	0.05%, 0.1%
Cycloalkylamine	Propylhexedrine – Topical	2 inhalations through each nostril. Use as needed, but avoid excessive use	250 mg inhaler

[1] Refer to manufacturer's directions.

Indications:

Oral: For temporary relief of nasal congestion due to the common cold, hay fever or other upper respiratory allergies, and nasal congestion associated with sinusitis; to promote nasal or sinus drainage; for relief of eustachian tube congestion.

Topical: Symptomatic relief of nasal and nasopharyngeal mucosal congestion due to the common cold, sinusitis, hay fever or other upper respiratory allergies.

Adjunctive therapy of middle ear infections by decreasing congestion around the eustachian ostia. Nasal inhalers may relieve ear block and pressure pain in air travel.

Contraindications:

Monoamine oxidase inhibitor (MAOI) therapy; hypersensitivity or idiosyncrasy to sympathomimetic amines manifested by insomnia, dizziness, weakness, tremor or arrhythmias.

Oral: Severe hypertension and coronary artery disease.

Phenylpropanolamine – Nursing mothers.

Phenylpropanolamine, sustained release – Children under 12.

Topical: Systemic effects are less likely from topical use, but use caution in the above conditions. Adverse reactions are more likely with excessive use, in the elderly and in children.

Tetrahydrozoline – 0.1% solution is contraindicated in children under 6 years of age. The 0.05% solution is not to be used for infants under 2 years of age.

Naphazoline – Glaucoma.

(Continued on following page)

Warnings:

Administer with caution to patients with hypertension, hyperthyroidism, diabetes mellitus, cardiovascular disease, coronary artery disease, ischemic heart disease, increased intraocular pressure or prostatic hypertrophy. Sympathomimetics may cause CNS stimulation and convulsions or cardiovascular collapse with hypotension.

Hypertensive patients should use these products only with medical advice, as they may experience a change in blood pressure because of the added vasoconstriction. Studies suggest pseudoephedrine is the drug of choice and that phenylpropanolamine should be avoided. Sustained action preparations may affect the cardiovascular system less.

Excessive use of decongestants may cause systemic effects (nervousness, dizziness, sleeplessness) which are more likely in infants and in the elderly. Habituation and toxic psychosis have followed long-term high dose therapy.

Rebound congestion (rhinitis medicamentosa) following topical application may occur after the vasoconstriction subsides. Patients may increase the amount of drug and frequency of use, producing toxicity and perpetuating the rebound congestion.

Treatment – A simple but uncomfortable solution is to completely withdraw the topical medication. A more acceptable method is to gradually withdraw therapy by initially discontinuing the medication in one nostril, followed by total withdrawal. Substituting an oral decongestant for a topical one may also be useful.

Usage in the Elderly: Patients 60 years and older are more likely to experience adverse reactions to sympathomimetics. Overdosage may cause hallucinations, convulsions, CNS depression and death. Demonstrate safe use of a short-acting sympathomimetic before use of a sustained action formulation in elderly patients.

Usage in Pregnancy: (Category C – tetrahydrozoline). It is not known whether these agents can cause fetal harm or affect reproduction capacity. Give only when clearly needed.

Usage in Lactation: Oral phenylpropanolamine is contraindicated in the nursing mother because of the higher than usual risks to infants from sympathomimetic agents.

Other oral preparations – Consult a physician before using.

Topical – It is not known if these agents are excreted in breast milk. Exercise caution when administering to a nursing woman.

Usage in Children: Do not administer sustained release phenylpropanolamine preparations to children under 12.

Precautions:

Use topical decongestants only in acute states and not longer than 3 to 5 days. Use sparingly (especially the imidazolines) in all patients, particularly infants, children and patients with cardiovascular disease.

Some individuals may experience a mild, transient stinging sensation after topical application. This often disappears after a few applications.

Drug Interactions:

Beta-adrenergic blockers: Blockade of the beta effects of **epinephrine** results in unopposed alpha activity. Increased blood pressure and bradycardia may occur. Cardioselective β_1 blockers may cause less hypertension and bradycardia.

Guanethidine: The antihypertensive effects of guanethidine may be partially or totally reversed by the mixed-acting sympathomimetics, and it may increase the pressor response of the direct-acting agents.

Methyldopa may potentiate the α-adrenergic (pressor) effects of sympathomimetics and may lead to hypertension.

Monoamine oxidase (MAO) inhibitors increase the pressor response to mixed-acting vasopressors. Possible hypertensive crisis and intracranial hemorrhage may occur. This may also occur with **furazolidone,** an antimicrobial with MAO inhibitor activity. Avoid this combination; if given inadvertently and hypertension occurs, give phentolamine.

Phenothiazines may block the α-adrenergic effects of **epinephrine,** producing hypotension and tachycardia. One fatality due to ventricular arrhythmias has been attributed to **thioridazine** and a nasal decongestant containing **phenylpropanolamine**.

Theophylline: Concomitant use with **ephedrine** has been associated with increased incidence of GI discomfort (nausea, vomiting) and CNS symptoms (hyperactivity, nervousness, insomnia). The dose of one or both drugs may need to be decreased.

Tricyclic antidepressants may potentiate the response of the direct-acting sympathomimetics and decrease the response of the mixed-acting agents.

Urinary alkalinization may increase the pharmacologic and toxic effects of ephedrine and pseudoephedrine.

(Continued on following page)

Adverse Reactions:

CNS: Fear; anxiety; tenseness; restlessness; headache; lightheadedness; dizziness; drowsiness; tremor; insomnia; hallucinations; psychological disturbances; prolonged psychosis (paranoia, terror, delusions); convulsions; CNS depression; weakness.

Cardiovascular: Arrhythmias and cardiovascular collapse with hypotension; palpitations; tachycardia; precordial pain; transient hypertension; bradycardia.

Ocular: Blepharospasm (ocular irritation, tearing, photophobia).

GI: Nausea; vomiting; anorexia.

GU: Difficult or painful urination.

Miscellaneous: Pallor; respiratory difficulty; orofacial dystonia; sweating.

Topical use: Burning; stinging; sneezing; dryness; local irritation; rebound congestion.

Overdosage:

Symptoms: Somnolence, sedation or coma may occur. Sedation may be accompanied by profuse sweating, hypotension or shock. With marked overdosage, CNS depression is accompanied by hypertension, bradycardia and rebound hypotension.

Treatment: Treatment is supportive; in severe cases, IV phentolamine may be used. See General Management of Acute Overdosage on p. 2895

Tetrahydrozoline – There is no known antidote. The use of stimulants is contraindicated. If respiratory rate drops to 10 or below, administer oxygen and assist respiration. Monitor blood pressure to prevent hypotensive crisis.

Patient Information:

Topical: Notify physician of insomnia, dizziness, weakness, tremor or irregular heart beat.

Do not exceed recommended dosage and do not use longer than 3 to 5 days.

Stinging, burning or drying of the nasal mucosa may occur.

Oral: Do not exceed recommended dosage; higher doses may cause nervousness, dizziness or sleeplessness.

If symptoms do not improve within 7 days or are accompanied by a high fever, consult physician before continuing use.

Patients with hypertension or other cardiovascular diseases, hyperthyroidism, diabetes mellitus or prostatic hypertrophy should use these products only with medical advice.

PHENYLPROPANOLAMINE HCl

Also used as an *otc* anorexiant (see Nonprescription Diet Aids).

Administration and Dosage:

Adults: 25 mg every 4 hours or 50 mg every 8 hours, not to exceed 150 mg/day (or 75 mg sustained release every 12 hours).

Children (6 to 12 years): 12.5 mg every 4 hours. Do not exceed 75 mg/day.

Children (2 to 6 years): 6.25 mg every 4 hours.

				C.I.*
otc	**Phenylpropanolamine HCl** (Various)	**Tablets:** 25 mg	In 1000s.	2+
otc	**Propagest** (Carnrick)		(C). White, scored. In 100s.	23
otc	**Phenylpropanolamine HCl** (Various)	**Tablets:** 50 mg	In 1000s.	1+
otc	**Phenylpropanolamine HCl** (Various)	**Capsules, timed release:** 75 mg	In 100s and 1000s.	2+
Rx	**Rhindecon** (McGregor)		(MCG 215). In 60s.	18

PSEUDOEPHEDRINE SULFATE

Administration and Dosage:

Adults and children 12 years and over: 120 mg every 12 hours.

Do not crush or chew sustained release preparations.

				C.I.*
otc	**Afrinol Repetabs** (Schering)	**Tablets, extended release:** 120 mg (60 mg immediate release/60 mg delayed release)	(Afrinol). In 12s and 100s.	62
otc	**Drixoral Non-Drowsy Formula** (Schering)		Sugar, lactose. In 10s and 20s.	NA

* Cost Index based on cost per 25 mg phenylpropanolamine or 120 mg pseudoephedrine sulfate.

Complete prescribing information for these products begins on page 941.

PSEUDOEPHEDRINE HCl (d-Isoephedrine HCl)

Administration and Dosage:

Adults: 60 mg every 4 to 6 hours (120 mg sustained release every 12 hours). Do not exceed 240 mg in 24 hours.

Children (6 to 12): 30 mg every 6 hours. Do not exceed 120 mg in 24 hours.

(2 to 5): 15 mg every 6 hours (as syrup). Do not exceed 60 mg in 24 hours.

				C.I.*
otc	**Pseudoephedrine HCl** (Various)	**Tablets:** 30 mg	In 12s, 24s, 100s, 1000s and UD 24s and 100s.	9+
otc	**Cenafed** (Century Pharm.)		In 100s and 1000s.	13
otc	**Genaphed** (Goldline)		In 24s and 100s.	23
otc	**Halofed** (Halsey)		In 100s and 1000s.	10
otc	**Pseudogest** (Major)		In 24s.	46
otc	**Sudafed** (Burroughs Wellcome)		Red. Sugar coated. In 24s, 48s, 100s and 1000s.	56
otc	**Sudrin** (JMI-Canton Pharm.)		White. In 100s and 1000s.	10
otc	**Pseudoephedrine HCl** (Various)	**Tablets:** 60 mg	In 12s, 15s, 21s, 24s, 100s, 1000s and UD 100s.	6+
otc	**Cenafed** (Century Pharm.)		In 100s and 1000s.	9
otc	**DeFed-60** (Ferndale)		In 1000s.	11
otc	**Halofed Adult Strength** (Halsey)		Sugar coated. In 100s and 1000s.	13
otc	**Neofed** (Pal-Pak)		Green, scored. In 100s and 1000s.	12
otc	**Pseudogest** (Major)		In 100s and 1000s.	10
otc	**Sudafed** (Burroughs Wellcome)		In 100s and 1000s.	45
otc	**Sudrin** (JMI-Canton Pharm.)		White. In 100s and 1000s.	8
otc	**AlleRid** (Murdock)	**Capsules:** 60 mg	In 30s.	NA
otc	**SinuStat** (Murdock)		In 30s.	NA
otc	**Sudafed** (Burroughs Wellcome)	**Tablets:** 120 mg	Coated. In 10s and 20s.	NA
Rx	**Novafed** (Lakeside)	**Capsules, timed release:** 120 mg	(Dow 104 or Novafed). Brown and orange. In 100s.	27
otc	**Dorcol Children's Decongestant** (Sandoz)	**Liquid:** 15 mg per 5 ml	Sorbitol. In 120 ml.	152
otc	**Pseudoephedrine HCl** (Various)	**Liquid:** 30 mg per 5 ml	In 120 ml, 480 ml and 10 ml (UD 100s).	55+
otc	**Decofed Syrup** (Various)		In pt and gal.	20+
otc	**Cenafed Syrup** (Century Pharm.)		In 120 ml, pt and gal.	13
otc	**Children's Sudafed** (Burroughs Wellcome)		In 120 ml.	94
otc	**Halofed Syrup** (Halsey)		In 120 & 240 ml, pt, gal.	24
otc	**Myfedrine** (Pharmaceutical Basics)		In 473 ml.	63
otc	**Pseudo Syrup** (Major)		In 120 ml, pt and gal.	50
otc	**PediaCare Infants' Decongestant** (McNeil)	**Drops:** 7.5 mg per 0.8 ml	Cherry flavor. In 15 ml w/dropper.	469

Miscellaneous Nasal Decongestants

				C.I.*
Rx	**No-Hist** (Dunhall)	**Capsules:** 5 mg phenylephrine HCl, 40 mg phenylpropanolamine HCl and 40 mg pseudoephedrine HCl	Caramel and buff. In 100s.	60

* Cost Index based on cost per 60 mg pseudoephedrine or 5 mg phenylephrine.

Complete prescribing information for these products begins on page 941.

PHENYLEPHRINE HCl

Administration and Dosage:

Adults: 0.25% (1 to 2 sprays) in each nostril every 4 hours. The 0.5% to 1% solution may be needed in resistant cases.

Children (6 years): 0.25% (1 to 2 sprays) in each nostril every 3 to 4 hours.

Children (2 to 6 years): 0.125% to 0.2% (1 drop) in each nostril every 2 to 4 hrs.

	Product	Form	How supplied	C.I.*
otc	**Neo-Synephrine** (Winthrop Consumer)	**Solution:** 0.125%	In 30 ml dropper bottle.[1]	171
otc	**St. Joseph Measured Dose** (Plough)		In 15 ml.[2]	197
otc	**Alconefrin 12** (Webcon)	**Solution:** 0.16%	In 30 ml dropper bottle.	109
otc	**Rhinall-10** (Scherer)	**Solution:** 0.2%	In 30 ml dropper bottle.[3]	54
otc	**Phenylephrine HCl** (Various)	**Solution:** 0.25%	In 30 ml, pt and gal.	11+
otc	**Alconefrin 25** (Webcon)		**Drops:** In 30 ml. **Spray:** In 30 ml.	70 90
otc	**Doktors** (Scherer)		**Drops:** In 30 ml dropper bottle.[3] **Spray:** In 30 ml.[3]	44 44
otc	**Neo-Synephrine** (Winthrop Consumer)		**Drops:** In 15 and 480 ml.[1] **Spray:** In 15 ml.[1]	109 120
otc	**Nōstril** (Boehringer-I)		In 15 ml pump, spray.[4]	125
otc	**Rhinall** (Scherer)		**Drops:** In 30 ml.[3] **Spray:** In 30 ml.[3]	44 44
otc	**Alconefrin 50** (Webcon)	**Solution:** 0.5%	In 30 ml dropper bottle.	45
otc	**Duration** (Plough)		In 15 ml spray.[5]	58
otc	**Neo-Synephrine** (Winthrop Consumer)		**Drops:** In 15 ml.[1] **Spray (regular):** In 15, 30 ml.[1] **Spray (menthol):** In 15 ml.[1,6]	58 58 65
otc	**Nōstril** (Boehringer-I)		In 15 ml pump spray.[4]	62
otc	**Sinex** (Vicks Health Care)		In 15 and 30 ml spray.[6,7]	60
otc	**Phenylephrine HCl** (Various)	**Solution:** 1%	In pt and gal.	1+
otc	**Neo-Synephrine** (Winthrop Consumer)		**Drops:** In 15 and 480 ml.[1] **Spray:** In 15 ml.[1]	33 37
otc	**Neo-Synephrine** (Winthrop Consumer)	**Jelly:** 0.5%	In 18.75 g.	26

EPINEPHRINE HCl

Administration and Dosage:

Adults and children (≥ 6 years): Apply locally as drops or spray, or with a sterile swab, as required. Do not use in children under 6, except on physician's advice.

	Product	Form	How supplied	C.I.*
otc	**Adrenalin Chloride** (Parke-Davis)	**Solution:** 0.1%	In 30 ml dropper bottle.[8]	69

EPHEDRINE

Administration and Dosage:

Adults and children (≥ 6 years): Instill every 4 hours, or apply a small amount of jelly, in each nostril. Do not use for more than 3 or 4 consecutive days. Do not use in children under 6, unless directed by physician.

	Product	Form	How supplied	C.I.*
otc	**Vatronol Nose Drops** (Vicks Health Care)	**Solution:** 0.5% ephedrine sulfate	In 15 and 30 ml dropper bottles.[6,9]	75
otc	**Efedron Nasal** (Hyrex)	**Jelly:** 0.6% ephedrine HCl	In 20 g.[6,10]	64

* Cost Index based on cost per 5 mg phenylephrine, 1 mg epinephrine or 10 mg ephedrine.

[1] With benzalkonium chloride and thimerosal.

[2] With phenylmercuric acetate, sorbitol, cetylpyridinium chloride and EDTA.

[3] With chlorobutanol, sodium bisulfite and benzalkonium chloride.

[4] With benzalkonium chloride and boric acid.

[5] With cetylpyridinium chloride and sorbitol.

[6] With aromatics (ie, menthol, camphor, eucalyptol).

[7] With cetylpyridinium chloride and thimerosal.

[8] With chlorobutanol and sodium bisulfite.

[9] With thimerosal.

[10] With chlorobutanol.

Complete prescribing information for these products begins on page 941.

NAPHAZOLINE HCl

Administration and Dosage:

Adults and children (≥ 12 years): 2 drops or sprays in each nostril as needed, no more than every 3 hours (drops) or 4 to 6 hours (spray). Do not use in children < 12, unless directed by physician.

	Product	Solution	Package	C.I.*
otc	**Privine** (Ciba Consumer)	**Solution:** 0.05%	**Drops:** In 20 ml with dropper.[1] **Spray:** In 15 ml.[1]	42 64

OXYMETAZOLINE HCl

Administration and Dosage:

Adults and children (≥ 6): 2 or 3 sprays or 2 to 3 drops of 0.05% solution in each nostril twice daily, morning and evening.

Children (2 to 5 years): 2 or 3 drops of 0.025% solution in each nostril twice daily, morning and evening.

	Product	Solution	Package	C.I.*
otc	**Afrin Children's Nose Drops** (Schering)	**Solution:** 0.025%	In 20 ml dropper bottle.[2]	82
otc	**Oxymetazoline HCl** (Various)	**Solution:** 0.05%	In 15 ml spray.	28+
otc	**Afrin** (Schering)		**Drops:** In 20 ml.[2] **Spray (regular):** In 15 and 30 ml.[2] **Spray (menthol):** In 15 ml.[2,3]	59 77 77
otc	**Allerest 12-Hour Nasal** (Pharmacraft)		In 15 ml spray.	60
otc	**Chlorphed-LA** (Hauck)		In 15 ml spray.[4]	50
otc	**Coricidin Nasal Mist** (Schering)		In 20 ml spray.[2]	51
otc	**Dristan Long Lasting** (Whitehall)		**Spray (regular):** In 15 and 30 ml.[5] **Spray (menthol):** In 15 ml.[3,5]	64 64
otc	**Duramist Plus** (Pfeiffer)		In 15 ml spray.[6]	37
otc	**Duration** (Plough)		**Spray (regular):** In 15 and 30 ml[4] and 15 ml pump spray.[2] **Spray (menthol):** In 15 ml.[3,4]	56 56
otc	**4-Way Long Acting Nasal** (Bristol-Myers)		In 15 ml spray.[2]	62
otc	**Genasal** (Goldline)		In 15 and 30 ml.[4]	49
otc	**Neo-Synephrine 12 Hour** (Winthrop Consumer)		**Drops:** In 30 ml.[2] **Spray (regular):** In 15 ml and 15 ml pump spray.[2] **Spray (menthol):** In 15 ml.[2,3]	36 72 72
otc	**Nōstrilla** (Boehringer-I)		In 15 ml pump spray.[7]	70
otc	**NTZ Long Acting Nasal** (Winthrop Consumer)		**Drops:** In 15 ml.[2] **Spray:** In 15 ml.[2]	60 53
otc	**Sinarest 12-Hour** (Pharmacraft)		In 15 ml spray.	54
otc	**Sinex Long-Acting** (Vicks Health Care)		In 15 and 30 ml spray.[3,6]	65
otc	**Twice-A-Day** (Major)		In 15 and 30 ml.	33

* Cost Index based on cost per 0.5 mg naphazoline or 0.5 mg oxymetazoline.
[1] With benzalkonium chloride, EDTA, hydrochloric acid and chloramine-T.
[2] With benzalkonium chloride, glycine, phenylmercuric acetate and sorbitol.
[3] With aromatics (ie, menthol, camphor, eucalyptol).
[4] With phenylmercuric acetate.
[5] With benzalkonium chloride and thimerosal.
[6] With thimerosal.
[7] With benzalkonium chloride, glycine and sorbitol.

Complete prescribing information for these products begins on page 941.

TETRAHYDROZOLINE HCl

Administration and Dosage:

Adults and children (≥ 6 years): 2 to 4 drops of 0.1% solution in each nostril as needed, no more than every 3 hours.

Children (2 to 6 years): 2 to 3 drops of 0.05% solution in each nostril every 4 to 6 hours, no more often than every 3 hours.

	Product	Form	Packaging	C.I.*
Rx	**Tyzine Pediatric Drops** (Kenwood Labs)	**Solution:** 0.05%	In 15 ml.[1]	170
Rx	**Tyzine Drops** (Kenwood Labs)	**Solution:** 0.1%	In 30 and 473 ml.[1]	59

XYLOMETAZOLINE HCl

Administration and Dosage:

Adults (≥ 12 years): 2 to 3 drops or 2 to 3 sprays (0.1%) in each nostril every 8 to 10 hours.

Children (2 to 12 years): 2 to 3 drops (0.05%) in each nostril every 8 to 10 hrs.

	Product	Form	Packaging	C.I.*
otc	**Otrivin Pediatric Nasal Drops** (Ciba Consumer)	**Solution:** 0.05%	In 20 ml dropper bottle.[2]	131
otc	**Xylometazoline HCl** (Various)	**Solution:** 0.1%	In 15 and 20 ml spray.	19+
otc	**Otrivin** (Ciba Consumer)		**Drops:** In 20 ml.[2] **Spray:** In 15 ml.[2]	76 80

Inhalers

Inhale through each nostril while blocking the other. Use as needed; avoid excessive use.

Abuse: Propylhexedrine has been extracted from inhalers and injected IV as an amphetamine substitute. It has also been ingested by soaking the fibrous interior in hot water. Chronic abuse has caused cardiomyopathy (severe left and right ventricular failure), pulmonary hypertension, foreign body granuloma (emboli), dyspnea and sudden death.

otc	**Benzedrex** (SmithKline Consumer)	**Inhaler:** 250 mg propylhexedrine	In single plastic tubes.[3]
otc	**Dristan Decongestant** (Whitehall)		In single plastic tubes.[4]
otc	**Vicks Inhaler** (Vicks Health Care)	**Inhaler:** 50 mg l-desoxyephedrine	In single plastic inhalers.[4]

* Cost Index based on cost per 1 mg tetrahydrozoline or 1 mg xylometazoline.

[1] With benzalkonium chloride, EDTA and hydrochloric acid.

[2] With benzalkonium chloride.

[3] With menthol.

[4] With aromatics (eg, menthol, camphor, eucalyptol).

In these combinations: *PHENYLEPHRINE HCl* and *NAPHAZOLINE HCl* are decongestants. *PYRILAMINE MALEATE and PHENIRAMINE MALEATE* are antihistamines.

Solutions

	Product	Content	Supplied	C.I.*
otc	**Myci-Spray** (Misemer)	**Solution:** 0.25% phenylephrine HCl, 0.15% pyrilamine maleate	In 20 ml spray.	32
otc	**Dristan Nasal** (Whitehall)	**Solution:** 0.5% phenylephrine HCl and 0.2% pheniramine maleate	**Spray (regular):** In 15 and 30 ml.[1]	62
			Spray (menthol): In 15 ml.[2,3]	67
otc	**4-Way Fast Acting** (Bristol-Myers)	**Solution:** 0.5% phenylephrine HCl, 0.05% naphazoline HCl and 0.2% pyrilamine maleate	**Spray (regular):** In 15 and 30 ml.[4]	55
			Spray (menthol): In 15 and 30 ml.[2,4]	55

Miscellaneous Nasal Products

To restore moisture and relieve dry, crusted and inflamed nasal membranes due to colds, low humidity, nasal decongestant overuse, allergies, nose bleeds and other irritations.

	Product	Content	Supplied	C.I.*
otc	**Salinex** (Muro)	**Solution:** 0.4% sodium chloride	**Drops:** In 15 ml.[5]	81
			Spray: In 50 ml.[5]	33
otc	**Pretz** (Parnell)	**Solution:** 0.6% sodium chloride	In 15 ml.[5]	54
otc	**Ayr Saline** (Ascher)	**Solution:** 0.65% sodium chloride	**Drops:** In 20 ml.[4]	39
			Spray: In 50 ml.[4]	17
otc	**HuMIST Saline Nasal Mist** (Scherer)		In 45 ml spray.[6]	13
otc	**NāSal Saline Nasal** (Winthrop Consumer)		**Drops:** Alcohol free. In 15 ml.[4]	37
			Spray: Alcohol free. In 15 ml.[4]	44
otc	**Ocean Mist** (Fleming)		In 45 ml spray and pt.[7]	15

* Cost Index based on cost per 5 mg phenylephrine or 6.5 mg sodium chloride.
[1] With 0.4% alcohol, benzalkonium chloride, eucalyptol, menthol, thimerosal.
[2] With aromatics (eg, menthol, camphor, eucalyptol).
[3] With benzalkonium chloride, methyl salicylate, thimerosal.
[4] With benzalkonium chloride and thimerosal.
[5] With EDTA and benzalkonium chloride.
[6] With chlorobutanol.
[7] With benzyl alcohol.

For a discussion of the physiological and pharmacological effects of corticosteroids, refer to the systemic Adrenal Cortical Steroids (glucocorticoids) monograph.

Actions:

Pharmacology: These drugs have potent glucocorticoid and weak mineralocorticoid activity. The mechanisms responsible for the anti-inflammatory action of corticosteroids on the nasal mucosa are unknown. These agents, when administered topically in recommended doses, exert local anti-inflammatory effects with minimal systemic effects. Exceeding the recommended dose may result in systemic effects, including hypothalamic-pituitary-adrenal (HPA) function suppression.

Clinical trials: A study in ≈ 100 patients compared the recommended dose of **flunisolide** nasal solution with an oral dose providing equivalent systemic amounts of flunisolide. Results show the clinical effectiveness, when used topically as recommended, is due to direct local effect and not to an indirect effect through systemic absorption.

One study compared the intranasal and IM formulations of **triamcinolone acetonide** with doses chosen to deliver comparable total amounts to determine if systemic absorption played a role in the response to the intranasal route. Evidence suggests that the intranasal formulation, at least to some degree, acts by a systemic mechanism.

Indications:

See individual product listings for specific labeled indications.

Contraindications:

Untreated localized infections involving the nasal mucosa.

Hypersensitivity to the drug or any component of the product.

Warnings:

Systemic corticosteroids: The combined administration of alternate day systemic prednisone with these products may increase the likelihood of HPA suppression. Therefore, use with caution in patients already on alternate day prednisone.

Withdrawal: During withdrawal from oral corticosteroids, some patients may experience symptoms (eg, joint or muscular pain, lassitude, depression). Carefully monitor patients previously treated for prolonged periods with systemic corticosteroids and transferred to intranasal steroids to avoid acute adrenal insufficiency in response to stress. This is particularly important in patients who have asthma or other conditions where too rapid a decrease in systemic corticosteroids may cause a severe exacerbation of their symptoms.

Excessive doses/sensitivity: If recommended doses of intranasal beclomethasone are exceeded or if individuals are particularly sensitive or predisposed by virtue of recent systemic steroid therapy, symptoms of hypercorticism may occur, including, very rarely, menstrual irregularities, acneiform lesions and cushingoid features. If such changes occur, discontinue slowly, consistent with accepted procedures for discontinuing oral steroids.

Hypersensitivity: Rare cases of immediate and delayed hypersensitivity reactions, including angioedema and bronchospasm, have occurred. Have epinephrine 1:1000 immediately available. Refer to Management of Acute Hypersensitivity Reactions.

Pregnancy: Category C. In animals, systemic administration of large doses produced teratogenic, fetotoxic and embryocidal effects. Topical administration of recommended doses is unlikely to achieve significant systemic levels; however, use these agents during pregnancy only if the potential benefits outweigh the potential hazards to the fetus.

Carefully observe infants born of mothers who have received substantial doses of corticosteroids during pregnancy for signs of adrenal insufficiency.

Lactation: Advise mothers taking pharmacologic doses not to nurse. **Dexamethasone** appears in breast milk and could suppress growth, interfere with endogenous corticosteroid production or cause other unwanted effects.

Beclomethasone, flunisolide, triamcinolone: It is not known whether these drugs are excreted in breast milk. Use caution when administering to nursing women.

Children: Safety and efficacy for use in children $<$ 6 years or $<$ 12 years (**triamcinolone**) have not been established. Use in children $<$ 6 years is not recommended; carefully follow growth and development if prolonged therapy is used.

Precautions:

Infections: Localized infections of the nose and pharynx with *Candida albicans* have developed only rarely. When such an infection occurs, it may require treatment with appropriate local therapy or discontinuation of steroid treatment.

When steroids are used in the presence of infection, use proper anti-infective therapy.

Use with caution in patients with active or quiescent tuberculosis infections of the respiratory tract, or in untreated fungal, bacterial or systemic viral infections or ocular herpes simplex.

Wound healing: Because of the inhibitory effect of corticosteroids on wound healing in patients who have experienced recent nasal septal ulcers, recurrent epistaxis, nasal surgery or trauma, use nasal steroids with caution until healing has occurred.

(Precautions continued on following page)

Precautions (Cont.)

Vasoconstrictors: In the presence of excessive nasal mucosa secretion or edema of the nasal mucosa, the drug may fail to reach the site of intended action. In such cases, use a nasal vasoconstrictor during the first 2 to 3 days of therapy.

Systemic effects: Although systemic absorption is low when used in recommended dosage, HPA suppression and other systemic effects may occur, especially with excessive doses.

Long-term treatment: Examine patients periodically over several months or longer for possible changes in the nasal mucosa.

Adverse Reactions:

Most common: Mild nasopharyngeal irritation; nasal irritation; burning; stinging; dryness; headache.

Other: Lightheadedness; nausea; epistaxis (transient episodes) or bloody mucus; rebound congestion; bronchial asthma; occasional sneezing attacks (may be more common in children); rhinorrhea; anosmia; loss of sense of taste; throat discomfort.

Rare: Ulceration of the nasal mucosa; watery eyes; sore throat; vomiting; immediate and delayed hypersensitivity reactions (urticaria, angioedema, rash, bronchospasm; see Warnings); localized infections of nose and pharynx with *C albicans* (see Precautions); wheezing, nasal septum perforation and increased intraocular pressure (extremely rare); signs of adrenal hypercorticism (ie, Cushing's syndrome), especially with overdosage.

Patient Information:

Patient instructions provided with products.

Do not exceed recommended dosage.

May cause irritation and drying of nasal mucosa. Contact physician if symptoms do not improve, if the condition worsens or if sneezing or nasal irritation occurs.

Clear nasal passages of secretions prior to use. If nasal passages are blocked, use a decongestant just before administration to ensure adequate penetration of the spray.

Effects are not immediate. Benefit requires regular use and usually occurs in a few days.

DEXAMETHASONE SODIUM PHOSPHATE

Indications: Allergic or inflammatory nasal conditions; nasal polyps (excluding polyps originating within the sinuses).

Administration and Dosage:

Adults: 2 sprays (168 mcg) into each nostril 2 or 3 times a day. Maximum daily dose is 12 sprays (1008 mcg).

Children (6 to 12 years): 1 or 2 sprays (84 to 168 mcg) into each nostril 2 times a day. Maximum daily dose is 8 sprays (672 mcg).

When improvement occurs, reduce dosage. Some patients will be symptom free on 1 spray into each nostril 2 times a day. Do not exceed the recommended dosage. Discontinue therapy as soon as feasible. Reinstitute if symptoms recur. **C.I.***

Rx	**Decadron Phosphate Turbinaire** (MSD)	**Aerosol:** Each metered spray delivers dexamethasone sodium phosphate equivalent to ≈ 84 mcg dexamethasone (170 sprays per cartridge)	With 2% alcohol. In 12.6 g with adapter or 12.6 g refill.	40

FLUNISOLIDE

Indications: Relief of the symptoms of seasonal or perennial rhinitis when effectiveness of or tolerance to conventional treatment is unsatisfactory.

Administration and Dosage:

Adults: Starting dose is 2 sprays (50 mcg) in each nostril 2 times a day (total dose 200 mcg/day). May increase to 2 sprays in each nostril 3 times a day (total dose 300 mcg/day). Maximum daily dose is 8 sprays in each nostril (400 mcg/day).

Children (6 to 14 years): Starting dose is 1 spray (25 mcg) in each nostril 3 times a day or 2 sprays (50 mcg) in each nostril 2 times a day (total dose 150 to 200 mcg/day). Maximum daily dose is 4 sprays in each nostril (200 mcg/day).

Improvement in symptoms usually becomes apparent within a few days. However, relief may not occur in some patients for as long as 3 weeks. Do not continue beyond 3 weeks in absence of significant symptomatic improvement.

Maintenance dose: After desired clinical effect is obtained, reduce maintenance dose to smallest amount necessary to control symptoms. Approximately 15% of patients with perennial rhinitis may be maintained on 1 spray in each nostril per day. **C.I.***

Rx	**Nasalide** (Syntex)	**Spray:** Each actuation delivers approximately 25 mcg flunisolide (≥ 200 sprays per bottle)	In 25 ml[1] bottle with pump unit.	30

* Cost Index based on cost per single spray (84 mcg dexamethasone or 25 mg flunisolide).

[1] With propylene glycol, polyethylene glycol 3350, benzalkonium chloride, EDTA.

BECLOMETHASONE DIPROPIONATE

Indications: Relief of the symptoms of seasonal or perennial rhinitis in those cases poorly responsive to conventional treatment.

Prevention of recurrence of nasal polyps following surgical removal.

Spray formulations – For nonallergic (vasomotor) rhinitis.

Administration and Dosage:

Adults and children ≥ 12 years: 1 inhalation (42 mcg) in each nostril 2 to 4 times a day (total dose 168 to 336 mcg/day). Patients can often be maintained on a maximum dose of 1 inhalation in each nostril 3 times a day (252 mcg/day).

Children 6 to 12 years of age: 1 inhalation in each nostril 3 times a day (252 mcg/day). Not recommended for children < 6 years of age since safety and efficacy studies have not been conducted in this age group.

Improvement in symptoms usually becomes apparent within a few days. Results from two clinical trials showed significant symptomatic relief within 3 days. Relief may not occur in some patients for as long as 2 weeks. Do not continue therapy beyond 3 weeks in the absence of symptomatic improvement.

Nasal polyps: Treatment may have to be continued for several weeks or more before a therapeutic result can be fully assessed. Recurrence of symptoms due to polyps can occur after stopping treatment, depending on the severity of the disease.

Storage: Therapeutic effect may decrease when aerosol canister is cold. Shake well before using.

				C.I.*
Rx	**Beconase Inhalation** (Allen & Hanburys)	**Aerosol:** Each actuation delivers 42 mcg beclomethasone dipropionate (200 metered doses per canister)	In 16.8 g canisters[1] with adapter or 16.8 g refills.[1]	34
Rx	**Vancenase Nasal Inhaler** (Schering)		In 16.8 g canisters[1] with adapter.	34
Rx	**Beconase AQ Nasal** (Allen & Hanburys)	**Spray:** 0.042% beclomethasone dipropionate, monohydrate (≥ 200 metered doses per bottle)	In 25 g bottles[2] w/ metering atomizing pump & nasal adapter.	36
Rx	**Vancenase AQ Nasal** (Schering)		In 25 g bottles[2] w/ metered pump & nasal adapter.	36

TRIAMCINOLONE ACETONIDE

Indications:

Treatment of seasonal and perennial allergic rhinitis symptoms.

Administration and Dosage:

Adults and children > 12 years: Individual patients will experience a variable time to onset and degree of symptom relief. Starting dose is 2 sprays (110 mcg) in each nostril once a day (total dose 220 mcg/day). Assess the effect in 4 to 7 days; some relief can be expected in approximately two-thirds of patients within that time. May increase to 440 mcg/day either as once a day dosage or divided up to 4 times a day (ie, twice a day [2 sprays/nostril] or 4 times a day [1 spray/nostril]). The degree of relief does not seem to be significantly different when comparing 2 or 4 times a day dosing with once a day dosing. After desired effect is obtained, some patients (≈ 50%) may be maintained on as little as 1 spray in each nostril once a day.

A dose-response between 110 and 440 mcg/day is not clearly discernible. In general, the highest dose tends to provide relief sooner. This suggests an alternative approach to starting therapy: Start treatment with 440 mcg (4 sprays/nostril/day), and then, depending on response, decrease the dose by 1 spray per day every 4 to 7 days.

A decrease in symptoms may occur as soon as 12 hours after starting steroid therapy and generally can be expected to occur within a few days of initiating therapy in allergic rhinitis. If improvement is not evident after 2 to 3 weeks, re-evaluate the patient.

				C.I.*
Rx	**Nasacort** (Rhone-Poulenc Rorer)	**Spray:** Each actuation delivers approximately 55 mcg triamcinolone acetonide (100 sprays per canister)	In 15 mg canister with nasal adapter.	NA

* Cost Index based on cost per single spray (42 mcg beclomethasone or 55 mcg triamcinolone).

[1] With propellants.

[2] With benzalkonium chloride and 0.25% v/w phenylethyl alcohol.

ALPHA$_1$-PROTEINASE INHIBITOR (HUMAN) (Alpha$_1$-PI)

Actions:

Alpha$_1$-proteinase inhibitor (alpha$_1$-PI; alpha$_1$-antitrypsin) is a sterile, stable, lyophilized preparation of purified human alpha$_1$-proteinase inhibitor used in patients with panacinar emphysema who have alpha$_1$-antitrypsin deficiency. It is prepared from pooled human plasma of normal donors. Each unit of plasma has been tested and found nonreactive for HIV antibody and hepatitis B surface antigen (HBsAg). See Warnings.

The specific activity of alpha$_1$-proteinase inhibitor is $\geq$ 0.35 mg functional alpha$_1$-PI/mg protein. When reconstituted, alpha$_1$-PI has a concentration of $\geq$ 20 mg/ml, a pH of 6.6 to 7.4, a sodium content of 100 to 210 mEq/L, a chloride content of 60 to 180 mEq/L, a sodium phosphate content of 0.015 to 0.025 M, a polyethylene glycol content of NMT 5 ppm and NMT 0.1% sucrose; contains small amounts of other plasma proteins.

Pharmacology: Alpha$_1$-antitrypsin deficiency is a chronic hereditary, usually fatal, autosomal recessive disorder in which a low concentration of alpha$_1$-PI is associated with slowly progressive, severe, panacinar emphysema that most often manifests itself in the third to fourth decades of life. Although the terms "alpha$_1$-proteinase inhibitor" and "alpha$_1$-antitrypsin" are used interchangeably in the scientific literature, the hereditary disorder associated with a reduction in the serum level of alpha$_1$-PI is conventionally referred to as "alpha$_1$-antitrypsin deficiency" while the deficient protein is referred to as "alpha$_1$-proteinase inhibitor".

The pathogenesis is not well understood. It is believed to be due to a chronic biochemical imbalance between elastase (an enzyme capable of degrading elastin tissues, released by inflammatory cells, primarily neutrophils, in the lower respiratory tract) and alpha$_1$-PI (the principal inhibitor of neutrophil elastase). As a result, alveolar structures are unprotected from chronic exposure to elastase resulting in progressive degradation of elastin tissues. The eventual outcome is emphysema. Neonatal hepatitis with cholestatic jaundice appears in $\approx$ 10% of newborns with alpha$_1$-antitrypsin deficiency. In some adults, alpha$_1$-antitrypsin deficiency is complicated by cirrhosis.

Clinical Pharmacology/Pharmacokinetics: In clinical studies of alpha$_1$-PI in 23 subjects with the PiZZ variant of congenital deficiency of alpha$_1$-antitrypsin deficiency and documented destructive lung disease, the mean in vivo recovery of alpha$_1$-PI was 4.2 mg (immunologic)/dl/mg (functional)/kg administered. Half-life of alpha$_1$-PI in vivo was $\approx$ 4.5 days. Nineteen of the subjects received alpha$_1$-PI replacement therapy, 60 mg/kg, once weekly for up to 26 weeks (avg 24 wks). Blood levels of alpha$_1$-PI were maintained above 80 mg/dl. Within a few weeks, bronchoalveolar lavage studies demonstrated significantly increased levels of alpha$_1$-PI and functional antineutrophil elastase capacity in the epithelial lining fluid of the lower respiratory tract of the lungs.

Indications:

Congenital alpha$_1$-antitrypsin deficiency: For chronic replacement in individuals with clinically demonstrable panacinar emphysema. Only those with early evidence of such disease should be considered for chronic replacement therapy with alpha$_1$-PI. Subjects with the PiMZ or PiMS phenotypes of alpha$_1$-antitrypsin deficiency should not be considered for such treatment as they appear to be at small risk for panacinar emphysema. Only adult subjects have received alpha$_1$-PI to date.

Alpha$_1$-proteinase inhibitor is not indicated for use in patients other than those with PiZZ, PiZ(null) or Pi(null)(null) phenotypes.

Warnings:

Infectious transmission: Alpha$_1$-PI is purified from large pools of fresh human plasma obtained from many paid donors. Although each unit of plasma has been found nonreactive for hepatitis B surface antigen (HBsAg) using an FDA approved test, the presence of hepatitis viruses in such pools must be assumed.

Alpha$_1$-PI is heat-treated to reduce potential for transmission of infectious agents. No procedure has been totally effective in removing viral infectivity from plasma products. No cases of hepatitis, either hepatitis B or non-A, non-B were recorded in individuals on alpha$_1$-PI. However, all individuals received prophylaxis against hepatitis B.

Monitoring: The "threshold" level of alpha$_1$-PI in serum believed to provide adequate antielastase activity in lungs of individuals with alpha$_1$-antitrypsin deficiency is 80 mg/dl (based on commercial standards for alpha$_1$-PI immunologic assay). However, assays based on commercial standards measure antigenic activity of alpha$_1$-PI whereas labeled potency value is expressed as actual functional activity (ie, actual capacity to neutralize porcine pancreatic elastase). As functional activity may be less than antigenic activity, serum levels determined by commercial immunologic assays may not accurately reflect actual functional alpha$_1$-PI levels. Therefore, although it may help to monitor serum levels using currently available commercial assays of antigenic activity, do not use results of these assays to determine required dosage.

(Warnings continued on following page)

ALPHA$_1$-PROTEINASE INHIBITOR (HUMAN) (Alpha$_1$-PI) (Cont.)

Warnings (Cont.):

Pregnancy: Category C. It is not known whether this drug can cause fetal harm when administered to a pregnant woman or can affect reproduction capacity. Use only when clearly needed and when the potential benefits outweigh the potential hazards to the fetus.

Children: Safety and efficacy in children have not been established.

Precautions:

A number of factors could reduce the efficacy of this product or even result in an ill effect, including improper storage and handling of the product, diagnosis, dosage, method of administration and biological differences in patients. It is important that this product be stored properly, that the directions be followed carefully, and that the risk of transmitting viruses be carefully weighed before the product is prescribed.

Circulatory overload: As with any colloid solution, there will be an increase in plasma volume following IV administration of alpha$_1$-PI. Exercise caution in patients at risk for circulatory overload.

Hepatitis B immunization: In preparation for receiving alpha$_1$-PI, recipients should be immunized against hepatitis B using a licensed Hepatitis B Vaccine. Should it become necessary to treat an individual with alpha$_1$-PI, and time is insufficient for adequate antibody response to vaccination, administer a single dose of Hepatitis B Immune Globulin (Human), 0.06 ml/kg IM, at the time of administration of the initial dose of Hepatitis B Vaccine.

Adverse Reactions:

Delayed fever (maximum temperature rise 38.9°C, resolving spontaneously over 24 hours) occurring up to 12 hours following treatment (0.77%); lightheadedness (0.19%); dizziness (0.19%). Mild transient leukocytosis several hours after infusion also occurred.

Administration and Dosage:

For IV use only. May be given at a rate of 0.08 ml/kg/min or greater.

IV Administration of Alpha$_1$-Proteinase Inhibitor

Body Weight (Approx lb/kg)	Dosage[1] (mg)	IV Administration Rate[2] (ml/min)
75/34	2,040	2.7
90/41	2,460	3.3
105/48	2,880	3.8
120/55	3,300	4.4
135/61	3,660	4.9
150/68	4,080	5.5
165/75	4,500	6.0
180/82	4,920	6.5
195/89	5,340	7.1
210/96	5,760	7.6
225/102	6,120	8.2
240/109	6,540	8.7

[1] Based on 60 mg/kg.
[2] Based on 0.08 ml/kg/min.

Dosage: 60 mg/kg once weekly to increase and maintain a level of functional alpha$_1$-PI in the epithelial lining of the lower respiratory tract providing adequate anti-elastase activity in the lungs of individuals with alpha$_1$-antitrypsin deficiency.

Stability: Administer within 3 hours after reconstitution. Give alone, without mixing other agents or diluting solutions. If required, alpha$_1$-PI may be diluted with normal saline.

Storage: Refrigerate at 2° to 8°C (35° to 46°F). Avoid freezing. Do not refrigerate after reconstitution. Discard unused solution.

Rx	**Prolastin** (Cutter)	**Injection:** $\geq$ 20 mg alpha$_1$-PI per ml when reconstituted	Preservative free. In $\approx$ 500 mg activity/single dose vials[3] w/20 ml sterile water or $\approx$ 1000 mg activity/single dose vial[3] w/40 ml sterile water.

[3] With polyethylene glycol, sucrose and small amounts of other plasma proteins. With total alpha$_1$-PI functional activity in mg stated on the label of each vial.

COLFOSCERIL PALMITATE (Synthetic Lung Surfactant; Dipalmitoylphosphatidylcholine; DPPC)

Actions:

Pharmacology: Surfactant deficiency is an important factor in the development of the neonatal respiratory distress syndrome (RDS). Thus, surfactant replacement therapy early in the course of RDS should ameliorate the disease and improve symptoms. Natural surfactant, a combination of lipids and apoproteins, exhibits not only surface tension reducing properties (conferred by the lipids), but also rapid spreading and adsorption (conferred by the apoproteins). The major fraction of the lipid component of natural surfactant is dipalmitoylphosphatidylcholine (DPPC), which comprises up to 70% of natural surfactant by weight.

Although DPPC reduces surface tension, DPPC alone is ineffective in RDS because it spreads and adsorbs poorly. In colfosceril, which is protein-free, cetyl alcohol acts as the spreading agent for the DPPC on the air-fluid interface. Tyloxapol, a polymeric long-chain repeating alcohol, is a nonionic surfactant which acts to disperse both DPPC and cetyl alcohol. Sodium chloride is added to adjust osmolality.

Pharmacokinetics: Colfosceril is administered directly into the trachea. DPPC can be absorbed from the alveolus into lung tissue where it can be catabolized extensively and reutilized for further phospholipid synthesis and secretion. In the developing rabbit, 90% of alveolar phospholipids are recycled. In premature rabbits, the alveolar half-life of intratracheally administered phosphatidylcholine is approximately 12 hours.

Clinical trials:

Prophylactic treatment – The efficacy of a single dose of colfosceril in prophylactic treatment of infants at risk of developing RDS was examined in three double-blind, placebo controlled studies, one involving 215 infants weighing 500 to 700 g, one involving 385 infants weighing 700 to 1350 g, and one involving 446 infants weighing 700 to 1100 g (see following table). The infants were intubated and placed on mechanical ventilation, and received 5 ml/kg or placebo (air) within 30 minutes of birth.

The efficacy of one vs three doses of colfosceril in prophylactic treatment of infants at risk of developing RDS was examined in a double-blind, placebo controlled study of 823 infants weighing 700 to 1100 g (see following table). The infants were intubated and placed on mechanical ventilation, and received a first 5 ml/kg dose within 30 minutes. Repeat 5 ml/kg doses of colfosceril or placebo (air) were given to all infants who remained on mechanical ventilation at approximately 12 and 24 hours of age.

Prophylactic Colfosceril Treatment — Efficacy Assessment

	Number of doses (birth weight range)							
	Single dose (500 to 700 g)		Single dose (700 to 1350 g)		Single dose (700 to 1100 g)		One vs three doses (700 to 1100 g)	
Parameter	Placebo (n = 106)	Colfosceril (n = 109)	Placebo (n = 185)	Colfosceril (n = 176)	Placebo (n = 222)	Colfosceril (n= 224)	One dose (n = 356)	Three doses (n = 360)
Death ≤ day 28	53%	50%	11%	6%	21%	15%	16%	9%
Death through 1 year	59%	60%	14%	11%	30%	20%	17%	12%
Death from RDS	25%	13%	4%	3%	10%	5%	3%	2%
Intact cardiopulmonary survival[1]	29%	25%	69%	78%	65%	68%	74%	78%
Bronchopulmonary dysplasia	43%	44%	23%	18%	19%	21%	8%	12%
RDS incidence	73%	81%	46%	42%	55%	55%	63%	68%

[1] Defined by survival through 28 days of life without bronchopulmonary dysplasia.

Rescue treatment: The efficacy of colfosceril in the rescue treatment of infants with RDS was examined in two double-blind, placebo controlled studies (see following table). One study enrolled 419 infants weighing 700 to 1350 g; the second enrolled 1237 infants weighing ≥ 1250 g. Infants received an initial dose (5 ml/kg) of colfosceril or placebo (air) between 2 and 24 hours of life followed by a second dose (5 ml/kg) approximately 12 hours later to infants who remained on mechanical ventilation.

(Actions continued on following page)

COLFOSCERIL PALMITATE (Synthetic Lung Surfactant; Dipalmitoylphosphatidylcholine; DPPC) (Cont.)

Actions (Cont.):

Clinical trials (Cont.):

Rescue Colfosceril Treatment – Efficacy Assessments				
	Number of doses (birth weight range)			
	Two doses (700 to 1350 g)		Two doses (≥ 1250 g)	
Parameter	Placebo (n = 213)	Colfosceril (n = 206)	Placebo (n = 623)	Colfosceril (n = 614)
Death ≤ day 28	23%	11%	7%	4%
Death through 1 year	27%	15%	9%	6%
Death from RDS	10%	3%	3%	1%
Intact cardiopulmonary survival[1]	62%	75%	88%	93%
Bronchopulmonary dysplasia	18%	15%	6%	3%

[1] Defined by survival through 28 days of life without bronchopulmonary dysplasia.

Results: In these six controlled clinical studies, infants in the colfosceril group showed significant improvements in fraction of inspired oxygen (FiO_2) and ventilator settings which persisted for at least 7 days. Pulmonary air leaks were significantly reduced in each study. Five of these studies also showed a significant reduction in death from RDS. Further, overall mortality was reduced for all infants weighing > 700 g. The one vs three dose prophylactic treatment study in 700 to 1100 g infants showed a further reduction in overall mortality with two additional doses. Various forms of pulmonary air leak and use of pancuronium were reduced in infants receiving colfosceril in all six studies. Follow-up data at 1 year adjusted age are available on 1094 of 2470 surviving infants. Growth and development of infants who received colfosceril in this sample were comparable to infants who received placebo.

Indications:

Prophylactic treatment: Infants with birth weights < 1350 g at risk of developing RDS. Infants with birth weights > 1350 g who have evidence of pulmonary immaturity.

Rescue treatment: Infants who have developed RDS.

For *prophylactic* treatment, administer the first dose as soon as possible after birth (see Administration and Dosage).

Infants considered as candidates for *rescue* treatment with colfosceril should be on mechanical ventilation and have a diagnosis of RDS by both of the following criteria:

1. Respiratory distress not attributable to causes other than RDS, based on clinical and laboratory assessments.
2. Chest radiographic findings consistent with the diagnosis of RDS.

Warnings:

Intratracheal administration: Administer only by instillation into the trachea (see Administration and Dosage).

The use of colfosceril requires expert clinical care by experienced neonatologists and other clinicians accomplished at neonatal intubation and ventilatory management. Adequate personnel, facilities, equipment and medications are required to optimize perinatal outcome in premature infants.

Instillation of colfosceril should be performed only by trained medical personnel experienced in airway and clinical management of unstable premature infants. Give vigilant clinical attention to all infants prior to, during and after administration.

Pulmonary effects: Colfosceril can rapidly affect oxygenation and lung compliance.

Lung compliance – If chest expansion improves substantially after dosing, reduce peak ventilator inspiratory pressures immediately, without waiting for confirmation of respiratory improvement by blood gas assessment. Failure to reduce inspiratory ventilator pressures rapidly can result in lung overdistention and fatal pulmonary air leak.

Hyperoxia – If the infant becomes pink, and transcutaneous oxygen saturation is in excess of 95%, reduce FiO_2 in small but repeated steps (until saturation is 90% to 95%) without waiting for confirmation of elevated arterial pO_2 by blood gas assessment. Failure to reduce FiO_2 in such instances can result in hyperoxia.

Hypocarbia – If arterial or transcutaneous CO_2 measurements are < 30 torr, reduce the ventilator rate at once. Failure to reduce ventilator rates in such instances can result in marked hypocarbia, which is known to reduce brain blood flow.

(Warnings continued on following page)

COLFOSCERIL PALMITATE (Synthetic Lung Surfactant; Dipalmitoylphosphatidylcholine; DPPC) (Cont.)

Warnings (Cont.):

Pulmonary hemorrhage: In the single study conducted in infants weighing < 700 g at birth, the incidence of pulmonary hemorrhage was significantly increased in the colfosceril group (10% vs 2% in the placebo group). None of the five studies involving infants with birth weights > 700 g showed a significant increase in pulmonary hemorrhage in the colfosceril group. In an analysis of these five studies, pulmonary hemorrhage was reported for 1% (14/1420) of infants in the placebo group and 2% (27/1411) of infants in the colfosceril group. Fatal pulmonary hemorrhage occurred in three infants, two in the colfosceril group and one in the placebo group. Mortality from all causes among infants who developed pulmonary hemorrhage was 43% in the placebo group and 37% in the colfosceril group.

Pulmonary hemorrhage in both colfosceril and placebo infants was more frequent in infants who were younger, smaller, male or who had a patent ductus arteriosus. Pulmonary hemorrhage typically occurred in the first 2 days of life in both treatment groups.

In > 7700 infants in the open, uncontrolled study, pulmonary hemorrhage occurred in 4%, but fatal pulmonary hemorrhage was reported rarely (0.4%).

In the controlled clinical studies, colfosceril-treated infants who received steroids > 24 hours prior to delivery or indomethacin postnatally had a lower rate of pulmonary hemorrhage than other colfosceril-treated infants. Pay attention to early and aggressive diagnosis and treatment (unless contraindicated) of patent ductus arteriosus during the first 2 days of life (while the ductus arteriosus is often clinically silent). Other potentially protective measures include attempting to decrease FiO_2 preferentially over ventilator pressures during the first 24 to 48 hours after dosing, and attempting to decrease positive end-expiratory pressure (PEEP) minimally for at least 48 hours after dosing.

Mucous plugs: Infants whose ventilation becomes markedly impaired during or shortly after dosing may have mucous plugging of the endotracheal tube, particularly if pulmonary secretions were prominent prior to drug administration. Suctioning of all infants prior to dosing may lessen the chance of mucous plugs obstructing the endotracheal tube. If endotracheal tube obstruction is suspected, and suctioning is unsuccessful in removing the obstruction, replace the blocked endotracheal tube immediately.

Precautions:

Congenital anomalies: In controlled clinical studies, infants known prenatally or postnatally to have major congenital anomalies, or who were suspected of having congenital infection, were excluded from entry. However, these disorders cannot be recognized early in life in all cases, and a few infants with these conditions were entered. The benefits of colfosceril in the affected infants who received the drug appeared to be similar to the benefits observed in infants without anomalies or occult infection.

Prophylactic treatment: Infants < 700 g – In infants weighing 500 to 700 g, a single prophylactic dose of colfosceril significantly improved FiO_2 and ventilator settings, reduced pneumothorax, and reduced death from RDS, but increased pulmonary hemorrhage (see Warnings). Overall mortality did not differ significantly between the placebo and colfosceril groups. Data on multiple doses in infants in this weight class are not yet available. Accordingly, clinicians should carefully evaluate the potential risks and benefits of administration in these infants.

Rescue treatment: Number of doses – A small number of infants with RDS have received more than two doses of colfosceril as rescue treatment. Definitive data on the safety and efficacy of these additional doses are not available.

Adverse Reactions:

Premature birth is associated with a high incidence of morbidity and mortality. Despite significant reductions in overall mortality associated with colfosceril, some infants who received colfosceril developed severe complications and either survived with permanent handicaps or died.

In controlled clinical studies evaluating the safety and efficacy of colfosceril, numerous safety assessments were made. In infants receiving colfosceril, pulmonary hemorrhage, apnea and use of methylxanthines were increased. A number of other adverse events were significantly reduced in the colfosceril group, particularly various forms of pulmonary air leak and use of pancuronium.

(Adverse Reactions continued on following page)

COLFOSCERIL PALMITATE (Synthetic Lung Surfactant; Dipalmitoylphosphatidylcholine; DPPC) (Cont.)

Adverse Reactions (Cont.):

Cofosceril Adverse Reactions (%)[1]				
	Prophylactic treatment (1 to 3 doses)		Rescue treatment (2 doses)	
Adverse reaction	Colfosceril (n = 883)	Placebo (n = 878)	Colfosceril (n = 821)	Placebo (n = 835)
Intraventricular hemorrhage				
Overall	27-57	31-51	18-52	23-48
Severe	8-25	9-26	4-9	5-13
Pulmonary air leak				
Overall	11-48	16-52	18-34	30-54
Pneumothorax	6-12	5-23	10-20	20-29
Pneumopericardium	0-4	< 1-2	1-2	1-4
Pneumomediastinum	1-3	2-7	2-4	5-8
Pulmonary interstitial emphysema	7-44	13-43	13-25	24-48
Death	< 1-6	< 1-4	1-3	< 1-7
Patent ductus arteriosus	53-70	49-66	45-57	54-66
Necrotizing enterocolitis	2-13	2-11	2-3	1-3
Pulmonary hemorrhage	4-10	1-4	1	< 1-3
Congenital pneumonia	1-4	1-4	2-3	2
Nosocomial pneumonia	4-15	2-14	2-7	2-5
Non-pulmonary infections	29-39	28-35	13-22	13-19
Sepsis	24-34	23-30	8-17	8-15
Death from sepsis	2-4	1-4	≤ 1	< 1
Meningitis	1-6	1-4	< 1	1
Other infections	3-11	5-10	6-8	5
Major anomalies	1-4	2-7	3-4	3-4
Hypotension	47-77	52-70	39-57	50-62
Hyperbilirubinemia	21-61	20-63	10-19	12-17
Exchange transfusion	1-3	1-4	2-4	1-3
Thrombocytopenia[2]	8-25	9-21	< 1-11	4-10
Persistent fetal circulation	< 1-2	0-1	1-2	1-6
Seizures	2-9	2-11	3-10	6-10
Apnea	33-73	34-76	44-65	37-48
Additional drug therapy required				
Antibiotics	96-99	96-> 99	98-99	98-100
Anticonvulsants	8-24	9-23	5-17	10-17
Diuretics	37-65	39-64	34-65	45-60
Inotropes	20-40	20-46	16-31	27-36
Methylxanthines	43-82	38-77	53-74	49-62
Pancuronium	11-14	15-22	15-17	33-34
Sedatives	52-71	52-65	64-68	72-76

[1] Data pooled from several birth weight ranges.
[2] Thrombocytopenia requiring platelet transfusion.

Pulmonary hemorrhage: See Warnings.

Abnormal laboratory values are common in critically ill, mechanically ventilated, premature infants. A higher incidence of abnormal laboratory values in the colfosceril group was not reported.

Reflux of colfosceril into the endotracheal tube during dosing has been observed and may be associated with rapid drug administration. If reflux occurs, stop drug administration and, if necessary, increase peak inspiratory pressure on the ventilator by 4 to 5 cm H_2O until the endotracheal tube clears.

Drop in transcutaneous oxygen saturation (> 20%): If transcutaneous oxygen saturation declines during dosing, stop drug administration and, if necessary, increase peak inspiratory pressure on the ventilator by 4 to 5 cm H_2O for 1 to 2 minutes. In addition, increases of FiO_2 may be required for 1 to 2 minutes.

Mucous plugs: See Warnings.

(Adverse Reactions continued on following page)

COLFOSCERIL PALMITATE (Synthetic Lung Surfactant; Dipalmitoylphosphatidylcholine; DPPC) (Cont.)

Adverse Reactions (Cont.):

Colfosceril Adverse Reactions During the Open, Uncontrolled Study (%)[1]		
Adverse reaction	Prophylactic treatment (n = 1127)	Rescue treatment (n = 7711)
Reflux of colfosceril	20	31
Drop in O_2 saturation ($\geq$ 20%)	6	22
Rise in O_2 saturation ($\geq$ 10%)	5	6
Drop in transcutaneous pO_2 ($\geq$ 20 mm Hg)	1	8
Rise in transcutaneous pO_2 ($\geq$ 20 mm Hg)	2	5
Drop in transcutaneous pCO_2 ($\geq$ 20 mm Hg)	$<$ 1	1
Rise in transcutaneous pCO_2 ($\geq$ 20 mm Hg)	1	3
Bradycardia ($<$ 60 beats/min)	1	3
Tachycardia ($>$ 200 beats/min)	$<$ 1	$<$ 1
Gagging	1	5
Mucous plugs	$<$ 1	$<$ 1

[1] Infants may have experienced more than one event. Investigators were prohibited from adjusting FiO_2 or ventilator settings during dosing unless significant clinical deterioration occurred.

Administration and Dosage:

Preparation of suspension: Colfosceril is best reconstituted immediately before use because it does not contain antibacterial preservatives. Solutions containing buffers or preservatives should not be used for reconstitution. Do not use Bacteriostatic Water for Injection, USP. Reconstitute each vial with 8 ml of the accompanying diluent (preservative-free Sterile Water for Injection) as follows:

1) Fill a 10 or 12 ml syringe with 8 ml preservative-free Sterile Water for Injection using an 18 or 19 gauge needle.

2) Allow the vacuum in the vial to draw the sterile water into the vial.

3) Aspirate as much as possible of the 8 ml out of the vial into the syringe (while maintaining the vacuum), then suddenly release the syringe plunger.

Repeat Step 3 three or four times to assure adequate mixing of the vial contents. If vacuum is not present, the vial of colfosceril should not be used.

Draw the appropriate dosage volume for the entire dose (5 ml/kg) into syringe from below the froth in the vial (again maintaining vacuum). If the infant weighs $<$ 1600 g, unused suspension will remain in the vial after the entire dose is drawn into syringe. If the infant weighs $>$ 1600 g, at least two vials will be required for each dose.

Reconstituted colfosceril is a milky white suspension with a total volume of 8 ml per vial. If the suspension separates, gently shake or swirl the vial to resuspend the preparation. Inspect the reconstituted product visually for homogeneity immediately before administration; if persistent large flakes or particulates are present, do not use the vial.

Dosage: Accurate determination of weight at birth is the key to accurate dosing.

Prophylactic treatment: Administer the first dose as a single 5 ml/kg dose as soon as possible after birth. Administer second and third doses approximately 12 and 24 hours later to all infants who remain on mechanical ventilation at those times.

Rescue treatment: Administer in two 5 ml/kg doses. Administer the initial dose as soon as possible after the diagnosis of RDS is confirmed. Administer the second dose approximately 12 hours following the first dose, provided the infant remains on mechanical ventilation. A small number of infants with RDS have received more than two doses of colfosceril as rescue treatment. Definitive data on the safety and efficacy of these additional doses are not available (see Precautions).

Use of special endotracheal tube adapter: With each vial of colfosceril, five different-sized endotracheal tube adapters each with a special right-angle Luer-lock sideport are supplied. The adapters are clean but not sterile. Use the adapters as follows:

1) Select an adapter size that corresponds to the inside diameter of the endotracheal tube.

2) Insert the adapter into the endotracheal tube with a firm push-twist motion.

3) Connect the breathing circuit wye to the adapter.

4) Remove the cap from the sideport on the adapter. Attach the syringe containing drug to the sideport.

5) After completion of dosing, remove the syringe and recap the sideport.

(Administration and Dosage continued on following page)

COLFOSCERIL PALMITATE (Synthetic Lung Surfactant; Dipalmitoylphosphatidylcholine; DPPC) (Cont.)

Administration and Dosage (Cont.):

Administration: Suction the infant prior to administration, but do not suction for 2 hours after colfosceril is administered, except when clinically necessary.

Colfosceril suspension is administered via the sideport on the special endotracheal tube adapter without interrupting mechanical ventilation.

Each dose is administered in two 2.5 ml/kg half-doses. Each half-dose is instilled slowly over 1 to 2 minutes (30 to 50 mechanical breaths) in small bursts timed with inspiration. After the first 2.5 ml/kg half-dose is administered in the midline position, the infant's head and torso are turned 45° to the right for 30 seconds while mechanical ventilation is continued. After the infant is returned to the midline position, the second 2.5 ml/kg half-dose is given in an identical fashion over another 1 to 2 minutes. The infant's head and torso are then turned 45° to the left for 30 seconds while mechanical ventilation is continued, and the infant is then turned back to the midline position. These maneuvers allow gravity to assist in the lung distribution of colfosceril.

During dosing, monitor heart rate, color, chest expansion, facial expressions, the oximeter and endotracheal tube patency and position. If heart rate slows, the infant becomes dusky or agitated, transcutaneous oxygen saturation falls $>$ 15% or colfosceril backs up in the endotracheal tube, slow or halt dosing and, if necessary, turn up peak inspiratory pressure, ventilator rate or FiO_2. On the other hand, rapid improvements in lung function may require immediate reductions in peak inspiratory pressure, ventilator rate or FiO_2. (See Warnings and below for additional administration information.)

General guidelines for administration: Administration of colfosceril should not take precedence over clinical assessment and stabilization of critically ill infants.

Intubation: Prior to dosing with colfosceril, it is important to ensure that the endotracheal tube tip is in the trachea and not in the esophagus or right or left mainstem bronchus. Confirm brisk and symmetrical chest movement with each mechanical inspiration prior to dosing, as well as equal breath sounds in the two axillae. In prophylactic treatment, dosing with colfosceril need not be delayed for radiographic confirmation of the endotracheal tube tip position. In rescue treatment, bedside confirmation of endotracheal tube tip position is usually sufficient, if at least one chest radiograph subsequent to the last intubation confirmed proper position of the endotracheal tube tip. Some lung areas will remain undosed if the endotracheal tube tip is too low.

Monitoring: Continuous ECG and transcutaneous oxygen saturation monitoring during dosing are essential. In most infants treated prophylactically, initiate such monitoring prior to administration of the first dose of colfosceril. For subsequent prophylactic and all rescue doses, arterial blood pressure monitoring during dosing is also highly desirable. After both prophylactic and rescue dosing, frequent arterial blood gas sampling is required to prevent post-dosing hyperoxia and hypocarbia (see Warnings).

Ventilatory support during dosing: The 5 ml/kg dosage volume may cause transient impairment of gas exchange by physical blockage of the airway, particularly in infants on low ventilator settings. As a result, infants may exhibit a drop in oxygen saturation during dosing, especially if they are on low ventilator settings prior to dosing. These transient effects are easily overcome by increasing peak inspiratory pressure on the ventilator by 4 to 5 cm H_2O for 1 to 2 minutes during dosing. FiO_2 can also be increased if necessary. In infants particularly fragile or reactive to external stimuli, increasing peak inspiratory pressure by 4 to 5 cm H_2O or FiO_2 20% just prior to dosing may minimize any transient deterioration in oxygenation. However, in virtually all cases it should be possible to return the infant to pre-dose settings within a very short time of dose completion.

Post-Dosing: At the end of dosing, confirm endotracheal tube position by listening for equal breath sounds in the two axillae. Pay attention to chest expansion, color, transcutaneous saturation and arterial blood gases. Some infants on colfosceril and other surfactants have rapid improvements in pulmonary compliance, minute ventilation and gas exchange (see Warnings). Constant bedside attention for at least 30 minutes after dosing and frequent blood gas sampling are absolutely essential. Rapid lung function changes require immediate changes in peak inspiratory pressure, ventilator rate or FiO_2.

Educational material: A videotape on dosing is available from Burroughs Wellcome. This videotape demonstrates techniques for safe administration of colfosceril and should be viewed by health care professionals who will administer the drug.

Storage: Store at 15° to 30°C (59° to 86°F) in a dry place.

Rx	**Exosurf Neonatal** (Burroughs Wellcome)	**Lyophilized Powder for Injection:** 108 mg colfosceril palmitate[1]	In 10 ml vials with 10 ml Sterile Water for Injection and 2.5, 3, 3.5, 4 and 4.5 mm endotracheal tube adapters.

[1] With 12 mg cetyl alcohol and 8 mg tyloxapol. When reconstituted to a total volume of 8 ml per vial, each 1 ml contains 13.5 mg colfosceril, 1.5 mg cetyl alcohol, 1 mg tyloxapol and sodium chloride to provide a 0.1 N concentration.

BERACTANT (Natural Lung Surfactant)

Actions:

Pharmacology: Beractant is a sterile, non-pyrogenic pulmonary surfactant intended for intratracheal use only. It is a natural bovine lung extract containing phospholipids, neutral lipids, fatty acids and surfactant-associated proteins to which colfosceril palmitate (dipalmitoylphosphatidylcholine; DPPC), palmitic acid and tripalmitin are added to standardize the composition and to mimic surface-tension lowering properties of natural lung surfactant. Its protein content consists of two hydrophobic, low molecular weight, surfactant-associated proteins commonly known as SP-B and SP-C. It does not contain the hydrophilic, large molecular weight surfactant-associated protein known as SP-A.

Endogenous pulmonary surfactant lowers surface tension on alveolar surfaces during respiration and stabilizes the alveoli against collapse at resting transpulmonary pressures. Deficiency of pulmonary surfactant causes respiratory distress syndrome (RDS) in premature infants. Beractant replenishes surfactant and restores surface activity to the lungs of these infants.

Beractant reproducibly lowers minimum surface tension to < 8 dynes/cm in vitro, restores pulmonary compliance to excised rat lungs artifically made surfactant-deficient in situ, and improves lung pressure-volume measurements, lung compliance, and oxygenation in premature rabbits and sheep in vivo.

Pharmacokinetics: Beractant is administered directly to the target organ, the lungs, where biophysical effects occur at the alveolar surface. In surfactant-deficient premature rabbits and lambs, alveolar clearance of the lipid components is rapid. Most of the dose becomes lung-associated within hours of administration, and the lipids enter endogenous surfactant pathways of reutilization and recycling. In surfactant-sufficient adult animals, clearance is more rapid than in premature and young animals. There is less reutilization and recycling of surfactant in adult animals.

Clinical trials: Each dose in all studies was 100 mg phospholipids/kg birth weight.

Prevention studies – In infants of 600 to 1250 g birth weight and 23 to 29 weeks estimated gestational age, a dose of beractant was given within 15 minutes of birth to prevent the development of RDS. Up to three additional doses in the first 48 hours, as often as every 6 hours, were given if RDS subsequently developed and infants required mechanical ventilation with an $FiO_2 \geq 0.3$.

Rescue studies – In infants of 600 to 1750 g birth weight with RDS requiring mechanical ventilation and an $FiO_2 \geq 0.4$, the initial dose of beractant was given after RDS developed and before 8 hours of age. Infants could receive up to three additional doses in the first 48 hours, as often as every 6 hours, if they required mechanical ventilation and an $FiO_2 \geq 0.3$.

Prevention/Rescue Studies with Beractant				
	Prevention studies[1]		Rescue studies[1]	
Parameter	Beractant (n = 210)	Control (n = 220)	Beractant (n = 402)	Control (n = 396)
Incidence of RDS (%)	27.6 – 28.6	48.3 – 63.5	na	na
Death due to RDS (%)	1.1 – 2.5	10.5 – 19.5	6.4 – 11.6	18.1 – 22.3
Death or BPD due to RDS (%)	27.5 – 48.7	44.2 – 52.8	43.6 – 59.1	63.4 – 66.8
Death due to any cause (%)	7.6 – 16.5[3]	13.7 – 22.8	15.2 – 21.7	26.4 – 28.2
Air leaks[2] (%)	5.9 – 14.5	19.6 – 21.7	11.2 – 11.8	22.2 – 29.5
Pulmonary interstitial emphysema (%)	20.8 – 26.5	33.2 – 40	16.3 – 20.8	34 – 44.4

[1] Data pooled from two studies

[2] Pneumothorax or pneumopericardium.

[3] In one study, no cause of death in the beractant group was significantly increased; the higher number of deaths in this group was due to the sum of all causes.

na = Not applicable.

Marked improvements in oxygenation may occur within minutes of administration.

Significant improvements in the arterial-alveolar oxygen ratio (a/APO_2), FiO_2 and mean airway pressure (MAP) were sustained for 48 to 72 hours in beractant-treated infants in four single-dose and two multiple-dose rescue studies and in two multiple-dose prevention studies. In the single-dose prevention studies, the FiO_2 improved significantly.

Multiple-dose studies – In 605 (333 treated) of 916 surviving infants, there are trends for decreased cerebral palsy and need for supplemental oxygen in beractant infants. Wheezing at the time of examination tended to be more frequent among beractant infants, although there was no difference in bronchodilator therapy.

(Continued on following page)

BERACTANT (Natural Lung Surfactant) (Cont.)

Indications:

Prevention and treatment ("rescue") of RDS (hyaline membrane disease) in premature infants. Beractant significantly reduces the incidence of RDS, mortality due to RDS and air leak complications.

Prevention: In premature infants < 1250 g birth weight or with evidence of surfactant deficiency, give beractant as soon as possible, preferably within 15 minutes of birth.

Rescue: To treat infants with RDS confirmed by x-ray and requiring mechanical ventilation, give beractant as soon as possible, preferably by 8 hours of age.

Warnings:

Intratracheal administration: Administer only by instillation into the trachea (see Administration and Dosage).

Oxygenation/lung compliance: Beractant can rapidly affect oxygenation and lung compliance. Therefore, restrict its use to a highly supervised clinical setting with immediate availability of clinicians experienced with intubation, ventilator management and general care of premature infants. Frequently monitor infants receiving beractant with arterial or transcutaneous measurement of systemic oxygen and CO_2.

Transient episodes of bradycardia and decreased oxygen saturation have occurred during dosing. If these occur, stop the dosing procedure and initiate appropriate measures to alleviate the condition. After stabilization, resume the dosing procedure.

Precautions:

Rales and moist breath sounds can occur transiently after administration. Endotracheal suctioning or other remedial action is not necessary unless clear-cut signs of airway obstruction are present.

Nosocomial sepsis: Increased probability of post-treatment nosocomial sepsis in beractant-treated infants was observed in controlled clinical trials. The increased risk for sepsis was not associated with increased mortality among these infants. The causative organisms were similar in treated and control infants.

Adverse Reactions:

The most commonly reported adverse experiences were associated with the dosing procedure. In the multiple-dose controlled clinical trials, transient bradycardia occurred with 11.9% of doses. Oxygen desaturation occurred with 9.8% of doses.

Other reactions during the dosing procedure occurred with < 1% of doses and included: Endotracheal tube reflux; pallor; vasoconstriction; hypotension; endotracheal tube blockage; hypertension; hypocarbia; hypercarbia; apnea. No deaths occurred during the dosing procedure, and all reactions resolved with symptomatic treatment.

The occurrence of concurrent illnesses common in premature infants was evaluated in the controlled trials.

Concurrent Illnesses During Beractant Treatment (%)

Concurrent event	Beractant	Control
Patent ductus arteriosus	46.9	47.1
Intracranial hemorrhage	48.1	45.2
Severe intracranial hemorrhage	24.1	23.3
Pulmonary air leaks	10.9	24.7
Pulmonary interstitial emphysema	20.2	38.4
Necrotizing enterocolitis	6.1	5.3
Apnea	65.4	59.6
Severe apnea	46.1	42.5
Post-treatment sepsis	20.7	16.1
Post-treatment infection	10.2	9.1
Pulmonary hemorrhage	7.2	5.3

When all controlled studies were pooled, there was no difference in intracranial hemorrhage. However, in one of the single-dose rescue studies and one of the multiple-dose prevention studies, the rate of intracranial hemorrhage was significantly higher in beractant patients than control patients (63.3% vs 30.8% and 48.8% vs 34.2%, respectively).

Overdosage:

Symptoms: Based on animal data, overdosage might result in acute airway obstruction. Rales and moist breath sounds can transiently occur after beractant is given, and do not indicate overdosage. Endotracheal suctioning or other remedial action is not required unless clear-cut signs of airway obstruction are present.

Treatment should be symptomatic and supportive. Refer to General Management of Acute Overdosage.

(Continued on following page)

BERACTANT (Natural Lung Surfactant) (Cont.)

Administration and Dosage:

For intratracheal administration only.

Marked improvements in oxygenation may occur within minutes of administration of beractant. Therefore, frequent and careful clinical observation and monitoring of systemic oxygenation are essential to avoid hyperoxia.

Dosage:

Each dose of beractant is 100 mg of phospholipids/kg birth weight (4 ml/kg). The following table shows the total dosage for a range of birth weights.

Beractant Dosing Chart			
Weight (g)	Total dose (ml)	Weight (g)	Total dose (ml)
600-650	2.6	1301-1350	5.4
651-700	2.8	1351-1400	5.6
701-750	3	1401-1450	5.8
751-800	3.2	1451-1500	6
801-850	3.4	1501-1550	6.2
851-900	3.6	1551-1600	6.4
901-950	3.8	1601-1650	6.6
951-1000	4	1651-1700	6.8
1001-1050	4.2	1701-1750	7
1051-1100	4.4	1751-1800	7.2
1101-1150	4.6	1801-1850	7.4
1151-1200	4.8	1851-1900	7.6
1201-1250	5	1901-1950	7.8
1251-1300	5.2	1951-2000	8

Four doses can be administered in the first 48 hours of life; give doses no more frequently than every 6 hours.

Preparation: Inspect visually for discoloration prior to administration. The color of beractant is off-white to light brown. If settling occurs during storage, swirl the vial gently (do not shake) to redisperse. Some foaming at the surface may occur during handling and is inherent in the nature of the product.

Beractant is to be refrigerated (2° to 8°C; 36° to 46°F). Before administration, warm by standing at room temperature for at least 20 minutes or warm in the hand for at least 8 minutes. Artificial warming methods should not be used. If a prevention dose is to be given, begin preparation before the infant's birth.

Unopened, unused vials that have been warmed to room temperature may be returned to the refrigerator within 8 hours of warming and stored for future use. The drug should not be warmed and returned to the refrigerator more than once. Enter each single-use vial of beractant only once. Discard used vials with residual drug. Beractant does not require reconstitution or sonication before use.

Dosing procedures: Beractant is administered intratracheally by instillation through a 5 French end-hole catheter inserted into the infant's endotracheal tube with the tip of the catheter protruding just beyond the end of the endotracheal tube above the infant's carina. Before inserting the catheter through the endotracheal tube, shorten the length of the catheter. Beractant should not be instilled into a main-stem bronchus.

It is important to ensure homogenous distribution of beractant throughout the lungs. In the controlled clinical trials, each dose was divided into four quarterdoses. Each quarter-dose was administered with the infant in a different position. The sequence of positions was: Head and body inclined slightly down, head turned to the right; head and body inclined slightly down, head turned to the left; head and body inclined slightly up, head turned to the right; head and body inclined slightly up, head turned to the left.

First dose: Determine the total dose based on the infant's birth weight. Slowly withdraw the entire contents of the vial into a plastic syringe through a large-gauge needle (eg, at least 20 gauge). Do not filter beractant and avoid shaking.

Attach the premeasured 5 French end-hole catheter to the syringe. Fill the catheter with beractant and discard any excess through the catheter so that only the total dose to be given remains in the syringe.

Before administering beractant, assure proper placement and patency of the endotracheal tube. The endotracheal tube may be suctioned before administering beractant. Allow the infant to stabilize before proceeding with dosing.

(Administration and Dosage continued on following page)

BERACTANT (Natural Lung Surfactant) (Cont.)

Administration and Dosage (Cont.)

First dose (Cont.):

Prevention strategy: Weigh, intubate and stabilize the infant. Administer the dose as soon as possible after birth, preferably within 15 minutes. Position the infant appropriately and gently inject the first quarter-dose through the catheter over 2 to 3 seconds.

After administration of the first quarter-dose, remove the catheter from the endotracheal tube. Manually ventilate with a hand-bag with sufficient oxygen to prevent cyanosis, at a rate of 60 breaths/minute, and sufficient positive pressure to provide adequate air exchange and chest wall excursion.

Rescue strategy: Give the first dose as soon as possible after the infant is placed on a ventilator for management of RDS. In the clinical trials, immediately before instilling the first quarter-dose, the infant's ventilator settings were changed to a rate of 60/minute, inspiratory time 0.5 second and FiO_2 1.

Position the infant appropriately and gently inject the first quarter-dose through the catheter over 2 to 3 seconds. After administration of the first quarter-dose, remove the catheter from the endotracheal tube. Return the infant to the mechanical ventilator.

Both strategies: Ventilate the infant for at least 30 seconds or until stable. Reposition the infant for instillation of the next quarter-dose.

Instill the remaining quarter-doses using the same procedures. After instillation of each quarter-dose, remove the catheter and ventilate for at least 30 seconds or until the infant is stabilized. After instillation of the final quarter-dose, remove the catheter without flushing it. Do not suction the infant for 1 hour after dosing unless signs of significant airway obstruction occur.

After completion of the dosing procedure, resume usual ventilator management and clinical care.

Repeat doses: The dosage is also 100 mg phospholipids/kg and is based on the infant's birth weight. The infant should not be reweighed for determination of the dosage.

The need for additional doses is determined by evidence of continuing respiratory distress. Significant reductions in mortality due to RDS were observed in multiple-dose trials. Administer dose no sooner than 6 hours after the preceding dose if the infant remains intubated and requires at least 30% inspired oxygen to maintain a $PaO_2 \leq 80$ torr.

Obtain radiographic confirmation of RDS before administering additional doses to those who received a prevention dose.

Prepare beractant and position the infant for administration of each quarter-dose as previously described. After instillation of each quarter-dose, remove the dosing catheter from the endotracheal tube and ventilate the infant for at least 30 seconds or until stable.

In clinical studies, ventilator settings used to administer repeat doses were different than those used for the first dose. For repeat doses, the FiO_2 was increased by 0.2 or an amount sufficient to prevent cyanosis. The ventilator delivered a rate of 30/minute with an inspiratory time < 1 second. If the infant's pretreatment rate was ≥ 30 it was left unchanged during instillation.

Manual hand-bag ventilation should not be used to administer repeat doses. During the dosing procedure, ventilatory settings may be adjusted at the discretion of the clinician to maintain appropriate oxygenation and ventilation. After completion of the dosing procedure, resume usual ventilator management and clinical care.

Educational material: Review of audiovisual instructional materials describing dosage and administration procedures is recommended before using beractant. Materials are available on request from Ross Laboratories.

Storage: Store unopened vials under refrigeration (2° to 8°C; 36° to 46°F). Protect from light. Store vials in carton until ready for use. Vials are for single use only. Upon opening, discard unused drug. **C.I.***

Rx	**Survanta** (Ross Laboratories)	**Suspension:** 25 mg phospholipids per ml suspended in 0.9% sodium chloride solution.[1]	In single use vials containing 8 ml suspension.

[1] With 0.5 to 1.75 mg triglycerides, 1.4 to 3.5 mg free fatty acids and < 1 mg protein per ml.

Actions:

Pharmacology: Antihistamines competitively antagonize histamine at the H_1 receptor site, but do not bind with histamine to inactivate it. Terfenadine and astemizole, the most specific H_1 antagonists available, bind preferentially to peripheral rather than central H_1 receptors. Antihistamines do not block histamine release, antibody production or antigen-antibody interactions. They antagonize in varying degrees most of the pharmacological effects of histamine. They also have anticholinergic (drying), antipruritic and sedative effects; terfenadine and astemizole have little or no anticholinergic and sedative effects. Antihistamines with predominant sedative effects are used as nonprescription sleep aids (see monograph). Cyproheptadine and azatadine also have antiserotonin activity. Antihistamines with antiemetic effects are useful in the management of nausea, vomiting and motion sickness (see Antiemetic/Antivertigo agents). Conversely, GI upset is a frequent side effect of the ethylenediamines.

Although symptoms of the common cold might be modified with antihistamine use, the drugs do not prevent or cure colds, nor do they shorten the course of the disease.

Switching from one class of antihistamine to another may restore responsiveness when a patient becomes refractory to the effects of a particular antihistaminic agent.

ANTIHISTAMINES: DOSAGE AND EFFECTS

Antihistamine	Dose[1] (mg)	Dosing Interval[2] (hrs)	Sedative Effects[3]	Antihistaminic Activity[3]	Anticholinergic Activity[3]	Antiemetic Effects[3]
ETHANOLAMINES						
Diphenhydramine	25 to 50	6 to 8	+ + +	+ to + +	+ + +	+ + to + + +
Carbinoxamine	4 to 8	6 to 8	+ +	+ to + +	+ + +	+ + to + + +
Clemastine	1	12	+ +	+ to + +	+ + +	+ + to + + +
ETHYLENEDIAMINES						
Tripelennamine	25 to 50	4 to 6	+ +	+ to + +	±	—
Pyrilamine	25 to 50	6 to 8	+	+ to + +	±	—
ALKYLAMINES						
Chlorpheniramine	4	4 to 6	+	+ +	+ +	—
Dexchlorpheniramine	2	4 to 6	+	+ + +	+ +	—
Brompheniramine	4	4 to 6	+	+ + +	+ +	—
Triprolidine	2.5	4 to 6	+	+ + to + + +	+ +	—
PHENOTHIAZINES						
Promethazine	12.5 to 25	6 to 24	+ + +	+ + +	+ + +	+ + + +
Trimeprazine	2.5	6	+ +	+ + to + + +	+ + +	+ + + +
Methdilazine	8	6 to 12	+	+ + to + + +	+ + +	+ + + +
PIPERIDINES						
Cyproheptadine	4	8	+	+ +	+ +	—
Azatadine	1 to 2	12	+ +	+ +	+ +	—
Diphenylpyraline	5[4]	12[4]	+	+ +	+ +	—
Phenindamine	25	4 to 6	—[5]	+ +	+ +	—
MISCELLANEOUS						
Terfenadine	60	12	±	+ + to + + +	±	—
Astemizole	10	24	±	+ + to + + +	±	—

[1] Usual single oral adult dose.
[2] For conventional dosage forms.
[3] + + + + = very high, + + + = high, + + = moderate, + = low, ± = low to none.
[4] Available only in timed release form.
[5] Stimulation possible.

(Actions continued on following page)

Precautions:

Hematologic: Use **promethazine** with caution in bone marrow depression. Leukopenia and agranulocytosis have been reported, usually when used with other toxic agents.

Hazardous tasks: May cause drowsiness and reduce mental alertness; patients should not drive or perform other tasks requiring alertness. Astemizole and terfenadine appear to cause less sedation. Supervise children who are taking antihistamines when they engage in potentially hazardous activities (eg, bicycle riding).

Anticholinergic effects: Antihistamines have varying degrees of atropine-like actions; use with caution in patients with a predisposition to urinary retention, history of bronchial asthma, increased intraocular pressure, hyperthyroidism, cardiovascular disease or hypertension. Antihistamines may thicken bronchial secretions due to anticholinergic (drying) properties and may inhibit expectoration and sinus drainage. Astemizole and terfenadine appear to have less anticholinergic effects.

Use **phenothiazines** with caution in patients with cardiovascular disease, liver dysfunction or ulcer disease. Promethazine has been associated with cholestatic jaundice.

Use cautiously in persons with acute or chronic respiratory impairment, particularly children, since phenothiazines may suppress the cough reflex. If hypotension occurs, epinephrine is not recommended since phenothiazines may reverse its usual pressor effect and cause a paradoxical further lowering of blood pressure. Since these drugs have an antiemetic action, they may obscure signs of intestinal obstruction, brain tumor or overdosage of toxic drugs.

Phenothiazines elevate prolactin levels which persist through chronic administration. Approximately one-third of breast cancers are prolactin-dependent in vitro, an important factor if these drugs are prescribed for a patient with a history of breast cancer. Although galactorrhea, amenorrhea, gynecomastia and impotence have been reported, the clinical significance of elevated serum prolactin levels is unknown.

Discontinue phenothiazines at least 48 hours before myelography and do not resume for at least 24 hours postprocedure. Do not use phenothiazines to control nausea and vomiting before or after myelography.

Usage in impaired hepatic and renal function: Use caution in patients with cirrhosis or other liver diseases.

Parenteral: Do not give **promethazine** intra-arterially because of possible severe arteriospasm and resultant gangrene. Do not give SC; chemical irritation and necrotic lesions have resulted.

Sulfite sensitivity: Some of these products contain sulfites, which may cause allergic-type reactions (eg, hives, itching, wheezing, anaphylaxis) in certain susceptible persons. Although the overall prevalence of sulfite sensitivity in the general population is probably low, it is seen more frequently in asthmatics or in atopic nonasthmatic persons. Specific products containing sulfites are identified in the product listings.

Drug Interactions:

Alcohol and **other CNS depressants** (hypnotics, sedatives, tranquilizers, antianxiety agents, narcotic analgesics) may have additive effects with antihistamines. Dosage adjustment of CNS depressants may be necessary to avoid profound CNS depression. This may be less likely to occur with astemizole and terfenadine.

MAO inhibitors prolong and intensify the anticholinergic (drying) effects of antihistamines; use with **phenothiazines** may cause hypotension and extrapyramidal reactions. **Dexchlorpheniramine** may cause severe hypotension when given with an MAOI.

See the Antipsychotic Agents monograph for a complete discussion of the drug interactions that relate to the three phenothiazine antihistamines: Promethazine, trimeprazine and methdilazine.

Drug/Lab Tests: **Diagnostic pregnancy tests** based on immunological reactions between HCG and anti-HCG may result in false-negative or false-positive interpretations in patients on promethazine. Increased **blood glucose** has occurred in promethazine patients.

In patients on phenothiazines, the following have occurred: Increased **serum cholesterol, blood glucose, spinal fluid protein** and **urinary urobilinogen levels;** decreased **protein bound iodine (PBI)**; false-positive **urine bilirubin tests;** interference with **urinary ketone determinations, pregnancy tests** and **steroid determinations.**

Discontinue antihistamines about 4 days prior to **skin testing procedures;** these drugs may prevent or diminish otherwise positive reactions to dermal reactivity indicators.

Drug/Food Interaction: **Astemizole** absorption is reduced by 60% when taken with food. Take at least 2 hours after a meal, with no food for 1 hour after taking the drug.

(Continued on following page)

Adverse Reactions:

Allergic reactions: Peripheral, angioneurotic and laryngeal edema; dermatitis; asthma; lupus erythematosus-like syndrome; urticaria drug rash; anaphylactic shock; photosensitivity.

Cardiovascular: Postural hypotension; palpitations; bradycardia; tachycardia; reflex tachycardia; extrasystoles; faintness; increases and decreases in blood pressure; venous thrombosis at injection site following IV promethazine; cardiac arrest; ECG changes, including blunting of T waves and prolongation of the Q-T interval.

CNS: Most frequent – Drowsiness (often transient); sedation; dizziness; faintness; disturbed coordination.

Other – Fatigue; lassitude; confusion; restlessness; excitation; nervousness; tremor; grand mal seizures; headache; irritability; insomnia; euphoria; paresthesias; blurred vision; oculogyric crisis; torticollis; catatonic-like states; hallucinations; disorientation; tongue protrusion (usually in association with IV administration or excessive dosage); disturbing dreams/nightmares; pseudoschizophrenia; weakness; diplopia; vertigo; tinnitus; acute labyrinthitis; hysteria; neuritis; convulsions. paradoxical excitation, especially in children and in the elderly. Extrapyramidal reactions, including opisthotonos, dystonia, akathisia, dyskinesia and parkinsonism may occur with high doses; these are usually responsive to a reduction in dosage. CNS stimulation is possible with **phenindamine.**

GI: Most frequent – Epigastric distress (especially **ethylenediamines**). *Other* – Anorexia; increased appetite and weight gain; nausea; vomiting; diarrhea; constipation; change in bowel habits.

GU: Urinary frequency; dysuria; urinary retention; early menses; induced lactation; gynecomastia; inhibition of ejaculation; decreased libido; impotence.

Hematologic: Hemolytic anemia; hypoplastic anemia; aplastic anemia; thrombocytopenia; leukopenia; agranulocytosis; pancytopenia.

Respiratory: Most frequent – Thickening of bronchial secretions. *Other* – Chest tightness; wheezing; nasal stuffiness; dry mouth, nose and throat; sore throat; respiratory depression.

Other: Tingling, heaviness and weakness of the hands; thrombocytopenic purpura; obstructive jaundice (usually reversible upon drug discontinuation); tissue necrosis following SC administration of IV promethazine; erythema; stomatitis; high or prolonged glucose tolerance curves; glycosuria; elevated spinal fluid proteins; elevation of plasma cholesterol levels; excessive perspiration; chills.

Terfenadine adverse reactions: Alopecia; arrhythmia; visual disturbances; angioedema; skin eruption and itching; urticaria; rash; bronchospasm; cough; depression; galactorrhea; menstrual disorders (eg, dysmenorrhea); musculoskeletal pain; nightmares; mild or moderate transaminase elevations. Terfenadine may cause less drowsiness than **chlorpheniramine** or **clemastine.**

Isolated reports of jaundice, cholestatic hepatitis and hepatitis have occurred; a causal relationship of liver abnormalities to terfenadine is unclear.

Astemizole adverse reactions: Headache (6.7%); appetite increase (3.9%); weight gain (3.6%, average gain 3.2 kg); nausea (2.5%); nervousness (2.1%); dizziness (2%); diarrhea (1.8%); pharyngitis (1.7%); abdominal pain (1.4%); conjunctivitis, arthralgia (1.2%); angioedema; bronchospasm; depression; edema; epistaxis; myalgia; palpitation; photosensitivity; pruritus; rash. Astemizole caused less drowsiness, fatigue and dry mouth than **chlorpheniramine, clemastine, pheniramine** and **dexchlorpheniramine.**

Phenothiazine antihistamines infrequently cause typical phenothiazine adverse effects. See the Antipsychotic Agents monograph for a complete discussion of the phenothiazine adverse reactions.

Overdosage:

Symptoms: Effects may vary from mild CNS depression (sedation, apnea, diminished mental alertness) and cardiovascular collapse to stimulation (insomnia, hallucinations, tremors or convulsions), especially in children and geriatric patients. Profound hypotension, respiratory depression, unconsciousness, coma and death may occur, particularly in infants and children. Convulsions rarely occur. The convulsant dose lies near the lethal dose. Convulsions indicate a poor prognosis.

Toxic effects are seen within 30 minutes to 2 hours and result in drowsiness, dizziness, ataxia, tinnitus, blurred vision and hypotension. Anticholinergic effects result in fixed dilated pupils, flushing, dry mouth, hyperthermia (especially likely in children) and fever. GI symptoms may also occur. Hyperpyrexia to 41.8°C (107°F) and acute oral and facial dystonic reactions have been reported.

(Overdosage continued on following page)

Overdosage (Cont.):

Symptoms (Cont.)

Children often manifest CNS stimulation and may have hallucinations, toxic psychosis, delirium tremens, excitement, ataxia, incoordination, muscle twitching, athetosis, hyperthermia, cyanosis convulsions and hyperreflexia followed by post-ictal depression and cardiorespiratory arrest. Seizures resistant to therapy may follow and may be preceded by mild depression. A paradoxical reaction has been reported in children receiving single doses of 75 to 125 mg oral **promethazine,** characterized by hyperexcitability and nightmares. CNS stimulation in adults usually manifests as seizures. Marked cerebral irritation, resulting in jerking of muscles and possible convulsions, may be followed by deep stupor. Occasionally, a latent period is followed by respiratory depression, cardiovascular collapse and death.

Less common findings include ECG changes, such as wandering pacemaker, prolonged QT interval and nonspecific ST-T wave changes that disappear quickly. The EEG may show general cerebral dysrhythmia and diffuse delta wave activity that can persist after clinical recovery. Serious ventricular arrhythmias, including Torsades de pointes, have occurred following **astemizole** doses of greater than 200 mg; however, no ill effects have occurred with doses up to 500 mg.

Several cases of **terfenadine** overdosage have occurred. Generally, signs and symptoms were absent or mild (eg, headache, nausea, confusion). However, severe ventricular arrhythmias (Torsades de pointes) developed 15 hours after ingestion of 56 tablets (3360 mg) of terfenadine, 14 capsules (7000 mg) of cephalexin and 2 tablets (1200 mg) of ibuprofen. This progressed to ventricular fibrillation that responded well to defibrillation and lidocaine. Therefore, cardiac monitoring for at least 24 hours is recommended along with standard measures to remove any unabsorbed drug.

Single doses as high as ten times (600 mg) the recommended therapeutic dose in adults have been well tolerated.

Treatment: Induce emesis even if emesis has occurred spontaneously, using syrup of ipecac, except with **phenothiazine** antihistamines (see the Antipsychotic Agents monograph for management of phenothiazine overdosage). Following emesis, administer activated charcoal as a slurry with water and a cathartic to minimize absorption. Oral sodium or magnesium sulfate may be given; saline cathartics (eg, milk of magnesia) draw water into the bowel by osmosis and, therefore, are valuable for their action in rapid dilution of bowel content. Correct acidosis and electrolyte imbalances. Do not induce emesis in unconscious patients. If vomiting is unsuccessful, gastric lavage is indicated within 3 hours after ingestion and even later if large amounts of milk or cream were given. Early gastric lavage may be beneficial if **promethazine** has been taken orally. Isotonic or ½ isotonic saline is the lavage of choice, particularly in children. In adults, tap water can be used. Continue therapy directed at reversing the effects of timed-release medication and at supporting the patient for as long as symptoms remain. Treatment includes usual supportive measures. Refer to General Management of Acute Overdosage.

Hypotension is an early sign of impending cardiovascular collapse; treat it vigorously using general supportive measures or specific treatment with a vasopressor (norepinephrine, phenylephrine, dopamine). Avoid epinephrine because it may worsen hypotension. Propranolol can be used for refractory ventricular arrhythmias.

Use only short-acting depressants (eg, diazepam) to treat convulsions; repeat as necessary. IV physostigmine can be used to control centrally-mediated convulsions. Avoid analeptics because they may cause convulsions. Note that any depressant effects of **promethazine** are not reversed by naloxone.

Ice packs and cooling sponge baths, not alcohol, can aid in reducing the fever commonly seen in children.

Hemoperfusion may be used in severe cases.

Astemizole does not appear to be dialyzable. It is not known if **terfenadine** is dialyzable.

Patient Information:

Inform physician of a history of glaucoma, peptic ulcer, urinary retention or pregnancy before starting antihistamine therapy.

May cause nervousness and insomnia.

May cause drowsiness or dizziness (except astemizole and terfenadine); patients should observe caution while driving or performing other tasks requiring alertness. Avoid alcohol and other CNS depressants (sedatives, hypnotics, tranquilizers, etc).

May cause dry mouth.

May cause GI upset; take with food. Take astemizole on an empty stomach, at least 2 hours after a meal; do not eat food for 1 hour after taking the drug.

Do not crush or chew sustained release preparations.

Phenothiazines: Patients should report any involuntary muscle movements or unusual sensitivity to sunlight.

(Products listed on following pages)

Complete prescribing information for these products begins on page 964

Ethanolamines

DIPHENHYDRAMINE HCl

Indications: In addition to the general uses discussed in the group monograph, diphenhydramine is indicated for active and prophylactic treatment of motion sickness; as a nighttime sleep aid; for parkinsonism (including drug-induced) in the elderly intolerant of more potent agents, for mild cases in other age groups and in combination with centrally-acting anticholinergics. As a nonnarcotic cough suppressant; however, only the "syrup" formulations are labeled for this indication.

Administration and Dosage:

Individualize dosage.

Oral: Adults – 25 to 50 mg, every 6 to 8 hours.

Children (over 10 kg) – 12.5 to 25 mg, 3 or 4 times daily or 5 mg/kg/day or 150 mg/m²/day. Maximum daily dosage is 300 mg.

In motion sickness, give full dosage for prophylactic use; give the first dose 30 minutes before exposure to motion and similar doses before meals and at bedtime for the duration of exposure.

Nighttime sleep aid: Adults – 50 mg at bedtime.

Parenteral: Administer IV or deeply IM.

Adults – 10 to 50 mg; 100 mg if required; maximum daily dosage is 400 mg.

Children – 5 mg/kg/day or 150 mg/m²/day. Maximum daily dosage is 300 mg divided into 4 doses.

NOTE: The syrup formulations may include ammonium chloride and sodium citrate as expectorants, although there is inadequate evidence of their clinical value. Therapeutic claims for these components have been deleted, although they remain in the product formulation as inactive ingredients.

	Product	Form	Description	C.I.*
otc/ Rx[1]	**Diphenhydramine HCl** (Various)	**Capsules:** 25 mg	In 20s, 24s, 30s, 100s, 250s, 500s, 1000s and UD 100s.	9+
otc	**Banophen** (Major)		In 100s, 1000s and UD 100s.	19
Rx	**Benadryl** (Parke-Davis)		(P-D 471). Pink/white. In 100s, 1000s and UD 100s.	112
otc	**Benadryl 25** (Parke-Davis Consumer)		In 24s and 48s.	83
Rx	**Genahist** (Goldline)		In 24s.	66
Rx	**Nordryl** (Vortech)		In 1000s.	16
otc/ Rx[1]	**Diphenhydramine HCl** (Various)	**Capsules:** 50 mg	In 15s, 24s, 30s, 100s, 250s, 500s, 1000s & UD 32s, 100s.	5+
Rx	**Banophen** (Major)		In 100s, 250s, 1000s.	10
Rx	**Benadryl Kapseals** (Parke-Davis)		(P-D 373). Pink/white. In 100s, 1000s and UD 100s.	56
Rx	**Nordryl** (Vortech)		In 1000s.	13
otc/ Rx[1]	**Diphenhydramine HCl** (Various)	**Tablets:** 25 mg	In 24s, 30s, 100s and 1000s.	14+
otc	**AllerMax Caplets** (Pfeiffer)		In 24s.	53
otc	**Banophen Caplets** (Major)		In 24s and 100s.	49
otc	**Benadryl 25** (Parke-Davis Consumer)		Film coated. In 24s.	64
otc	**Diphenhist Captabs** (Rugby)		Capsule shaped. In 100s and UD 24s.	NA
Rx	**Genahist** (Goldline)		In 24s.	62
Rx	**Diphenhydramine HCl** (Various)	**Tablets:** 50 mg	In 30s, 50s, 100s and 1000s.	9+
otc	**AllerMax Caplets** (Pfeiffer)		In 24s.	35
otc	**Dormarex 2** (Republic)		In 16s and 32s.	58
otc sf	**Scot-Tussin Allergy** (Scot-Tussin)	**Liquid:** 12.5 mg/5 ml	Dye free. Parabens, menthol. In 120 ml.	NA
otc	**Diphenhist** (Rugby)	**Elixir:** 12.5 mg/5 ml	In 120 ml, pt and gal.	NA

* Cost Index based on cost per 50 mg.

[1] Products are available *otc* or *Rx,* depending on product labeling.

(Continued on following page)

Ethanolamines (Cont.)

DIPHENHYDRAMINE HCl (Cont.)				C.I.*
otc/ Rx[1]	**Diphenhydramine HCl** (Various)	**Elixir:** 12.5 mg per 5 ml	In 120 ml, pt, gal and UD 5, 10 and 20 ml (100s).	43+
otc sf	**Belix** (Halsey)		14% alcohol, sorbitol. In 118 ml, pt and gal.	40
Rx	**Benadryl** (Parke-Davis Consumer)		14% alcohol. In 120 ml, pt, gal and UD 5 ml (100s).	236
otc	**Genahist** (Goldline)		14% alcohol. In 120 ml.	124
Rx	**Hydramine** (Goldline)		In 120 ml, pt and gal.	62
otc	**Nidryl** (Geneva Generics)		14% alcohol. In 120 ml.	74
Rx	**Nordryl** (Vortech)		14% alcohol. In 120 ml, gal.	128
otc	**Phendry** (LuChem)		14% alcohol. In pt and gal.	115
otc	**Phendry Children's Allergy Medicine** (LuChem)		14% alcohol. In 120 ml.	134
otc/ Rx[1]	**Diphenhydramine HCl** (Various)	**Syrup:** 12.5 mg per 5 ml	In 4, 120 and 240 ml, pt, gal and UD 5 ml.	56
otc	**Benylin Cough** (Parke-Davis Consumer)		5% alcohol, saccharin. In 120 & 240 ml, pt and gal.	158
otc	**Bydramine Cough** (Major)		5% alcohol. In 118 ml, pt, gal.	106
otc	**Diphen Cough** (Pharmaceutical Basics)		In 120 ml, pt and gal.	37
otc	**Gen-D-phen** (Goldline)		5% alcohol. In 120 ml.	25
otc	**Hydramine Cough** (Goldline)		5% alcohol. In 120 and 240 ml, pt and gal.	112
Rx	**Hydramyn** (LuChem)		5% alcohol. In pt.	140
otc	**Nordryl Cough** (Vortech)		5% alcohol. In 120 ml, gal.	147
Rx	**Tusstat** (Century Pharm.)		5% alcohol. In 120 ml, pt and gal.	33
Rx	**Diphenhydramine HCl** (Various)	**Injection:** 10 mg per ml	In 10 and 30 ml vials.	33+
Rx	**Bena-D 10** (Seatrace)		In 30 ml vials.[2]	101
Rx	**Benadryl** (Parke-Davis)		In 10 and 30 ml Steri-vials.[3]	219
Rx	**Benahist 10** (Keene)		In 30 ml vials.[3]	89
Rx	**Benoject-10** (Mayrand)		In 30 ml vials.[2]	136
Rx	**Nordryl** (Vortech)		In 30 ml vials.[2]	138
Rx	**Diphenhydramine HCl** (Various)	**Injection:** 50 mg per ml	In 1 and 10 ml vials and 1 ml amps.	22+
Rx	**Bena-D 50** (Seatrace)		In 10 ml vials.[2]	54
Rx	**Benadryl** (Parke-Davis)		In 1 ml amps, 10 ml Steri-vials, 1 ml Steri-dose syringe.[3]	158
Rx	**Benahist-50** (Keene)		In 10 ml vials.[3]	83
Rx	**Ben-Allergin-50** (Dunhall)		In 10 ml vials.[2]	50
Rx	**Benoject-50** (Mayrand)		In 10 ml vials.[2]	83
Rx	**Dihydrex** (Kay Pharm.)		In 10 ml vials.[2]	40
Rx	**Diphenacen-50** (Central)		In 10 ml vials.[3]	86
Rx	**Hyrexin-50** (Hyrex)		In 10 ml multi-dose vials.[2]	93
Rx	**Nordryl** (Vortech)		In 10 ml vials.[2]	81
Rx	**Wehdryl** (Hauck)		In 10 ml vials.[2]	93

* Cost Index based on cost per 50 mg oral or 25 mg parenteral.
sf – Sugar free.
[1] Products are available *otc* or *Rx*, depending on product labeling.
[2] With chlorobutanol.
[3] With benzethonium chloride.

Complete prescribing information for these products begins on page 964.

Ethanolamines (Cont.)

CLEMASTINE FUMARATE

Administration and Dosage:

Adults and children (over 12): 1.34 mg twice daily to 2.68 mg 3 times daily. Do not exceed 8.04 mg/day. For dermatologic conditions, use the 2.68 mg dosage level only.

Children (under 12 years): Safety and efficacy for use have not been established.

	Product	Form/Strength	Description	C.I.*
Rx	**Clemastine Fumarate** (Various, eg, Lemmon, Schein)	**Tablets:** 1.34 mg	White, scored. In 100s.	NA
Rx	**Tavist-1** (Sandoz)		(Tavist 1 78/75). White, scored. In 100s.	284
Rx	**Clemastine Fumarate** (Various, eg, Lemmon, Schein)	**Tablets:** 2.68 mg	White, scored. In 100s.	NA
Rx	**Tavist** (Sandoz)		(Tavist 78/72). White, scored. In 100s.	177
Rx	**Tavist** (Sandoz)	**Syrup:** 0.67 mg (equiv. to 0.5 mg base) per 5 ml	5.5% alcohol, saccharin and sorbitol. Citrus flavor. In 120 ml.	723

Ethylenediamines

TRIPELENNAMINE HCl

Administration and Dosage:

Tablets and elixir:

Adults – 25 to 50 mg every 4 to 6 hours. As little as 25 mg may control symptoms; as much as 600 mg daily may be given in divided doses.

Children and infants – 5 mg/kg/day or 150 mg/m²/day divided into 4 to 6 doses. Maximum total dose is 300 mg/day.

Sustained release tablets:

Adults – 100 mg in the morning and evening. In difficult cases, 100 mg every 8 hours may be required.

Children – Do not use in children.

	Product	Form/Strength	Description	C.I.*
Rx	**PBZ** (Geigy)	**Tablets:** 25 mg	(Geigy 111). White, scored. In 100s.	35
Rx	**Tripelennamine HCl** (Various)	**Tablets:** 50 mg	In 100s and 1000s.	2+
Rx	**PBZ** (Geigy)		(Geigy 117). White, scored. In 100s & 1000s.	27
Rx	**Pelamine** (Major)		In 1000s.	2
Rx	**PBZ-SR** (Geigy)	**Tablets, sustained release:** 100 mg	(Geigy 48). Lavender. In 100s.	22
Rx	**PBZ** (Geigy)	**Elixir:** 37.5 mg tripelennamine citrate (equiv. to 25 mg HCl) per 5 ml	Cinnamon flavor. In 473 ml.	34

PYRILAMINE MALEATE

Administration and Dosage:

Adults: 25 to 50 mg, 3 or 4 times daily.

	Product	Form/Strength	Description	C.I.*
otc	**Pyrilamine Maleate** (Rugby)	**Tablets:** 25 mg	In 1000s.	3
Rx	**Nisaval** (Vale)		In 1000s.	5

* Cost Index based on cost per 4 mg carbinoxamine, 2.68 mg clemastine, 25 mg tripelennamine or 25 mg pyrilamine.

Complete prescribing information for these products begins on page 964.

Alkylamines

CHLORPHENIRAMINE MALEATE

Administration and Dosage:

Tablets or syrup:

Adults and children over 12 – 4 mg every 4 to 6 hours. Do not exceed 24 mg in 24 hours.

Children (6 to 12) – 2 mg every 4 to 6 hours. Do not exceed 12 mg in 24 hours.

(2 to 6) – 1 mg every 4 to 6 hours. Do not exceed 4 mg in 24 hours.

Administration with food delays absorption, but does not affect bioavailability.

Sustained release forms:

Adults (12 years and older) – 8 to 12 mg at bedtime or every 8 to 12 hours during the day. Do not exceed 24 mg in 24 hours.

Children (6 to 12) – 8 mg at bedtime or during the day, as indicated.

(< 6) – Not recommended for this age group.

Parenteral: The 10 mg/ml injection is intended for IV, IM or SC administration. The 100 mg/ml injection is intended for IM or SC use only.

Allergic reactions to blood or plasma – 10 to 20 mg as a single dose. The maximum recommended dose is 40 mg per 24 hours.

Anaphylaxis – 10 to 20 mg IV as a single dose.

Uncomplicated allergic conditions – 5 to 20 mg as a single dose.

	Product	Form	Description	C.I.*
otc	**Chlo-Amine** (Hollister-Stier)	**Tablets, chewable:** 2 mg	Orange. In 96s.	69
otc/ Rx[1]	**Chlorpheniramine Maleate** (Various)	**Tablets:** 4 mg	In 24s, 100s, 1000s and UD 24s, 100s and 1000s.	2+
otc	**Aller-chlor** (Rugby)		In 24s, 100s & 1000s.	9
otc	**Allergy** (Parmed)		In 24s and 100s.	NA
otc	**Chlorate** (Major)		In 24s and 100s.	6
Rx	**Chlortab-4** (Vortech)		In 1000s.	3
otc	**Chlor-Trimeton** (Schering)		(Schering TW or 080). Yellow, scored. In 24s, 96s and 100s.	29
otc	**Pfeiffer's Allergy** (Pfeiffer)		Dye free. In 24s.	3
Rx	**Phenetron** (Lannett)		In 1000s.	2
otc	**Chlorpheniramine Maleate** (Various)	**Tablets:** 8 mg	In 100s and 1000s.	16+
otc Rx[1]	**Chlorpheniramine Maleate** (Various)	**Tablets, timed release:** 8 mg	In 100s and 1000s.	7+
Rx	**Chlortab-8** (Vortech)		In 1000s.	4
otc	**Chlor-Trimeton Repetabs** (Schering)		(Schering CC or 374). Yellow, sugar coated. In 24s, 48s and 100s.	8
otc/ Rx[1]	**Chlorpheniramine Maleate** (Various)	**Capsules, timed release:** 8 mg	In 100s, 250s and 1000s.	34+
Rx	**Telachlor** (Major)		In 100s and 1000s.	7
otc/ Rx[1]	**Chlorpheniramine Maleate** (Various)	**Tablets:** 12 mg	In 100s and 1000s.	4+
Rx	**Chlorpheniramine Maleate** (Various)	**Tablets, timed release:** 12 mg	In 100s.	5+
otc	**Chlor-Trimeton Repetabs** (Schering)		(Schering AAE or 009). Sugar coated. Orange. In 12s, 24s and 100s.	26

* Cost Index based on cost per 4 mg.

[1] Products are available *otc* or *Rx*, depending on product labeling.

(Continued on following page)

Complete prescribing information for these products begins on page 964.

Alkylamines (Cont.)

CHLORPHENIRAMINE MALEATE (Cont.)

				C.I.*
otc	**Chlorpheniramine Maleate** (Various)	**Capsules:** 12 mg	In 100s.	5+
otc/ Rx[1]	**Chlorpheniramine Maleate** (Various)	**Capsules, timed release:** 12 mg	In 100s, 250s and 1000s.	1+
Rx	**Chlorspan-12** (Vortech)		In 1000s.	4
Rx	**Telachlor** (Major)		In 100s, 250s and 1000s.	3
otc	**Teldrin** (SmithKline Consumer)		In 12s, 24s and 48s.	31
otc	**Pedia Care Allergy Formula** (McNeil-CPC)	**Liquid:** 1 mg per 5 ml	Alcohol free. Sorbitol, sucrose. Grape flavor. In 120 ml.	N/A
otc/ Rx[1]	**Chlorpheniramine Maleate** (Various)	**Syrup:** 2 mg per 5 ml	In 120 ml, pt and gal.	13+
otc	**Aller-Chlor** (Rugby)		In 120 ml, pt and gal.	31
otc	**Chlor-Trimeton** (Schering)		7% alcohol. In 120 ml.	88
Rx	**Phenetron** (Lannett)		In pt and gal.	10
Rx	**Chlorpheniramine Maleate** (Various)	**Injection:** 10 mg per ml	In 30 ml vials.	6+
Rx	**Chlor-Pro 10** (Schein)		In 30 ml vials.[2]	8
Rx	**Chlor-Trimeton** (Schering)		In 1 ml amps.	223
Rx	**Chlorpheniramine Maleate** (Various)	**Injection:** 100 mg per ml	In 10 ml vials.	2+
Rx	**Chlor-100** (Vortech)		In 10 ml vials.[2]	50
Rx	**Chlor-Pro** (Schein)		In 10 ml vials.[2]	3

DEXCHLORPHENIRAMINE MALEATE

Administration and Dosage:

Adults: 2 mg every 4 to 6 hours, or 4 to 6 mg timed release tablets at bedtime, or every 8 to 10 hours during the day.

Children: 6 to 11 years – 1 mg every 4 to 6 hours or a 4 mg timed release tablet once daily at bedtime. *2 to 5 years* – 0.5 mg every 4 to 6 hours. Do not use timed release form.

				C.I.*
Rx	**Polaramine** (Schering)	**Tablets:** 2 mg	(#Schering AGT or 820). Red. In 100s.	68
Rx	**Dexchlorpheniramine Maleate** (Various)	**Tablets, timed release:** 4 mg	In 100s.	7+
Rx	**Dexchlor** (Schein)		In 100s.	7
Rx	**Poladex** (Major)		In 100s and 1000s.	7
Rx	**Polaramine** (Schering)		(#Schering AGA or 095). Light red. Sugar coated. In 100s.	58
Rx	**Polargen** (Goldline)		In 100s.	8
Rx	**Dexchlorpheniramine Maleate** (Various)	**Tablets, timed release:** 6 mg	In 100s and 1000s.	6+
Rx	**Dexchlor** (Schein)		In 100s and 1000s.	7
Rx	**Poladex** (Major)		In 100s and 1000s.	7
Rx	**Polaramine** (Schering)		(#Schering AGB or 148). Red. Sugar coated. In 100s and 1000s.	29
Rx	**Polargen** (Goldline)		In 100s and 1000s.	8
Rx	**Polaramine** (Schering)	**Syrup:** 2 mg/5 ml	6% alcohol. Sorbitol, menthol. Orange flavor. In 480 ml.	83

* Cost Index based on cost per 4 mg chlorpheniramine or 2 mg dexchlorpheniramine.

Product identification code.

[1] Products are available *otc* or *Rx*, depending on product labeling. [2] With benzyl alcohol.

Complete prescribing information for these products begins on page 964.

Alkylamines (Cont.)

BROMPHENIRAMINE MALEATE

Administration and Dosage:

Oral: Adults (12 and older) – 4 mg every 4 to 6 hours, or 8 or 12 mg of the sustained release form every 8 to 12 hours. Do not exceed 24 mg in 24 hours.

Children (6 to 12) – 2 mg every 4 to 6 hours. Do not exceed 12 mg in 24 hours. Administer sustained release preparations only as directed by a physician.

Children (< 6 years) – Use only as directed by a physician.

Parenteral: Give IM or SC, the 10 mg/ml concentration without dilution. Give IV, either undiluted or diluted 1 to 10 with Sterile Saline for Injection. Administer slowly, preferably to recumbent patient. May add to normal saline, 5% glucose or whole blood for IV use.

Adults – Usual dose, 10 mg (range 5 to 20 mg). Duration of action, 3 to 12 hours; twice daily administration is usually sufficient. Maximum dose is 40 mg/24 hours.

Children (< 12) – 0.5 mg/kg/day or 15 mg/m²/day, in 3 or 4 divided doses.

	Product	Form	Description	C.I.*
otc/ Rx[1]	**Brompheniramine** (Various)	**Tablets:** 4 mg	In 100s and 1000s.	4+
otc	**Dimetane** (Robins)		(#AHR 1857). Peach, scored. In 24s, 100s and 500s.	23
Rx	**Veltane** (Lannett)		Scored. In 100s and 1000s.	5
Rx	**Brompheniramine** (Various)	**Tablets:** 8 mg	In 100s and 1000s.	2+
Rx	**Diamine T.D.** (Major)	**Tablets, timed release:** 8 mg	In 100s, 250s and 1000s.	5
otc	**Dimetane Extentabs** (Robins)		(#AHR 1868). Rose. In 12s, 100s and 500s.	22
Rx	**Brompheniramine** (Various)	**Tablets:** 12 mg	In 100s.	3+
Rx	**Diamine T.D.** (Major)	**Tablets, timed release:** 12 mg	In 100s.	3
otc	**Dimetane Extentabs** (Robins)		(#AHR 1843). Peach. In 12s, 100s and 500s.	21
otc/ Rx[1]	**Brompheniramine** (Various)	**Elixir:** 2 mg per 5 ml	In 120 ml, pt and gal.	10+
otc/ Rx[1]	**Bromphen** (Various)		In 120 ml, pt & gal.	21+
otc	**Dimetane** (Robins)		3% alcohol. Saccharin. In 120 & 480 ml.	54
Rx	**Codimal-A** (Central)	**Injection:** 10 mg per ml	In 10 ml vials.[2]	114
Rx	**Cophene-B** (Dunhall)		In 10 ml vials.[2]	53
Rx	**Dehist** (Forest)		In 10 ml vials.[2]	61
Rx	**Histaject** (Mayrand)		In 10 ml vials.[2]	113
Rx	**Nasahist B** (Keene)		In 10 ml vials.[2]	73
Rx	**ND Stat** (Hyrex)		In 10 ml vials.[2]	75
Rx	**Oraminic II** (Vortech)		In 10 ml multi-dose vials.[2]	73
Rx	**Sinusol-B** (Kay Pharm.)		In 10 ml vials.[2]	41

TRIPROLIDINE HCl

Administration and Dosage:

Adults (12 and older): 2.5 mg every 4 to 6 hours.

Children (6 to 12 years): 1.25 mg every 4 to 6 hours. *Children < 6:* Consult physician. Do not exceed 4 doses in 24 hours.

	Product	Form	Description	C.I.*
otc	**Actidil** (Burroughs W)	**Tablets:** 2.5 mg	Scored. In 100s.	36
Rx	**Triprolidine HCl** (Various)	**Syrup:** 1.25 mg per 5 ml	In 120 ml, pt and gal.	18+
otc	**Actidil** (Burroughs W)		4% alcohol. Sorbitol. In 473 ml.	79
Rx	**Myidyl** (Pharmaceutical Basics)		In 120 ml, pt, gal.	13

* Cost Index based on cost per 4 mg brompheniramine or 2.5 mg triprolidine.

Product identification code.

[1] Products are available *otc* or *Rx*, depending on product labeling.

[2] With methyl and propyl parabens.

Complete prescribing information for these products begins on page 964.

Phenothiazines

PROMETHAZINE HCl

Indications:

In addition to uses discussed in the general monograph, promethazine is indicated for: Active and prophylactic treatment of motion sickness; preoperative, postoperative or obstetric sedation; prevention and control of nausea and vomiting associated with anesthesia and surgery; an adjunct to analgesics for control of postoperative pain; sedation and relief of apprehension, and to produce light sleep; antiemetic effect in postoperative patients.

Intravenous: Special surgical situations such as repeated bronchoscopy, ophthalmic surgery, poor risk patients and with reduced amounts of meperidine or other narcotic analgesics as an adjunct to anesthesia and analgesia.

Administration and Dosage:

Oral and Rectal:

Tablets and suppositories are not recommended for children less than 2 years of age.

Allergy – Average dose is 25 mg at bedtime. Give 12.5 mg before meals and at bedtime, if necessary. Children may be given 25 mg at bedtime or 6.25 to 12.5 mg 3 times daily. When the oral route is not feasible, use 25 mg suppositories. Repeat dose in 2 hours if necessary, but resume oral therapy when circumstances permit. Promethazine in 25 mg doses will control minor allergic transfusion reactions.

Motion sickness – 25 mg twice daily. Take initial dose ½ to 1 hour before travel; repeat in 8 to 12 hours, if necessary. Thereafter, give 25 mg doses on arising and before the evening meal. For children, 12.5 to 25 mg twice daily, oral or rectal.

Nausea and vomiting – 25 mg orally. Repeat doses of 12.5 to 25 mg, as necessary, at 4 to 6 hour intervals. When oral medication cannot be tolerated, administer parenterally or rectally. For prophylaxis of nausea and vomiting (as during surgery and the postoperative period) the average dose is 25 mg every 4 to 6 hours. For children, adjust the dose to the age and weight of the patient (0.5 mg/lb or 1 mg/kg).

Sedation – Adults: 25 to 50 mg. Children: 12.5 to 25 mg orally or rectally.

Preoperative use – 12.5 to 25 mg for children and 50 mg for adults, given the night before surgery. Children – 0.5 mg/lb (1 mg/kg) in combination with an equal dose of meperidine and the appropriate dose of an atropine-like drug. Adults - 50 mg with an equal amount of meperidine and the required amount of belladonna alkaloid.

Postoperative sedation and adjunctive use with analgesics – 25 to 50 mg in adults and 12.5 to 25 mg in children.

Parenteral: The preferred route is deep IM injection. Proper IV administration is well tolerated, but not without hazard. Injection SC is contraindicated as it may result in tissue necrosis. Do not administer by intra-arterial injection due to the likelihood of arteriospasm and the possibility of resultant gangrene.

Administer promethazine IV in a concentration no greater than 25 mg/ml and at a rate not to exceed 25 mg/minute.

Reduce the dose of barbiturates by at least one-half and the dose of narcotics by one-quarter to one-half when given concomitantly with promethazine.

Adults -

Allergy (including allergic reactions to blood or plasma): 25 mg, repeated within 2 hours if necessary.

Nausea and vomiting: 12.5 to 25 mg, not to be repeated more frequently than every 4 hours. When used for control of postoperative nausea and vomiting, reduce dosage of analgesics and barbiturates accordingly.

Nighttime sedation: 25 to 50 mg.

Preoperative and postoperative use: 25 to 50 mg in adults may be combined with appropriately reduced doses of analgesics and anticholinergics.

Labor: 50 mg in early stages of labor. When labor is established, give 25 to 75 mg IM or IV with a reduced dose of narcotic. Administer amnesic agents as needed. If necessary, give with a reduced dose of analgesic; this may be repeated once or twice, at 4 hour intervals. A maximum total dose in 24 hours is 100 mg.

Children (< 12 years) – Dosage should not exceed one-half the adult dose. As an adjunct to premedication, the dose is 0.5 mg/lb (1 mg/kg) in combination with a narcotic or barbiturate and the appropriate dose of an anticholinergic drug.

Do not use antiemetics in vomiting of unknown etiology.

(Products listed on following page)

Phenothiazines (Cont.)

PROMETHAZINE HCl (Cont.)				C.I.*
Rx	**Promethazine HCl** (Various)	**Tablets:** 12.5 mg	In 100s and 1000s.	8+
Rx	**Phenergan** (Wyeth-Ayerst)		Saccharin. (#Wyeth 19). Orange, scored. In 100s.	66
Rx	**Promethazine HCl** (Various)	**Tablets:** 25 mg	In 10s, 20s, 30s, 100s, 1000s and UD 100s.	3+
Rx	**Phenameth** (Major)		In 100s and 1000s.	7
Rx	**Phenergan** (Wyeth-Ayerst)		Saccharin. (#Wyeth 27). White, scored. In 100s and UD 100s.	59
Rx	**Promethazine HCl** (Various)	**Tablets:** 50 mg	In 100s and 1000s.	3+
Rx	**Phenergan** (Wyeth-Ayerst)		(#Wyeth 227). Pink. In 100s.	45
Rx	**Promethazine HCl** (Various)	**Syrup:** 6.25 mg per 5 ml	In 120 ml, pt, gal and UD 5 ml.	24+
Rx	**Phenergan Plain** (Wyeth-Ayerst)		7% alcohol. Saccharin. In 120, 180 & 240 ml, pt & gal.	141
Rx	**Prothazine Plain** (Vortech)		7% alcohol. In 118 ml.	133
Rx	**Promethazine HCl** (Various)	**Syrup:** 25 mg per 5 ml	In 120 ml, pt and gal.	27+
Rx	**Phenergan Fortis** (Wyeth-Ayerst)		1.5% alcohol. Saccharin. In 480 ml.	87
Rx	**Phenergan** (Wyeth-Ayerst)	**Suppositories:** 12.5 mg	(#498). In 12s.	759
Rx	**Phenergan** (Wyeth-Ayerst)	**Suppositories:** 25 mg	(#212). In 12s & UD 25s.	436
Rx	**Promethazine HCl** (Various)	**Suppositories:** 50 mg	In 12s and 25s.	200+
Rx	**Phenergan** (Wyeth-Ayerst)		(#229). In 12s & UD 25s.	290
Rx	**Promethazine HCl** (Various)	**Injection:** 25 mg per ml	In 1 ml amps and 1 and 10 ml vials.	29+
Rx	**Anergan 25** (Forest)		In 10 ml vials.[1]	167
Rx	**Phenazine 25** (Keene)		In 10 ml vials.[1]	87
Rx	**Phenergan** (Wyeth-Ayerst)		In 1 ml amps.[2]	207
Rx	**Prorex-25** (Hyrex)		In 10 ml vials.[1]	93
Rx	**Prothazine** (Vortech)		In 10 ml vials.[1]	132
Rx	**V-Gan 25** (Hauck)		In 10 ml vials.[1]	93
Rx	**Promethazine HCl** (Various)	**Injection:** 50 mg per ml (For IM use only)	In 1 ml amps and 10 ml vials.	18+
Rx	**Anergan 50** (Forest)		In 10 ml vials.[2]	108
Rx	**K-Phen-50** (Kay Pharm.)		In 10 ml vials.[2]	41
Rx	**Pentazine** (Century Pharm.)		In 10 ml vials.[2]	43
Rx	**Phenazine 50** (Keene)		In 10 ml vials.[2]	64
Rx	**Phencen-50** (Central)		In 10 ml vials.[2]	80
Rx	**Phenergan** (Wyeth-Ayerst)		In 1 ml amps.[2]	127
Rx	**Phenoject-50** (Mayrand)		In 10 ml vials.[2]	84
Rx	**Pro-50** (Dunhall)		In 10 ml vials.[2]	50
Rx	**Prometh-50** (Seatrace)		In 10 ml vials.[2]	49
Rx	**Prorex-50** (Hyrex)		In 10 ml vials.[2]	65
Rx	**Prothazine** (Vortech)		In 10 ml vials.[2]	81
Rx	**V-Gan 50** (Hauck)		In 10 ml vials.[2]	74

* Cost Index based on cost per 25 mg. # Product identification code.

[1] With EDTA, benzyl alcohol and sodium metabisulfite.

[2] With EDTA, phenol and sodium metabisulfite.

Complete prescribing information for these products begins on page 964

Phenothiazines (Cont.)

TRIMEPRAZINE

Administration and Dosage:

Tablets and syrup:

Adults – 2.5 mg, 4 times daily.

Children (over 3 years) – 2.5 mg at bedtime or 3 times daily, if needed.

Children (6 months to 3 years) – 1.25 mg at bedtime or 3 times daily, if needed.

Sustained release capsules:

Adults – 5 mg every 12 hours.

Children (≥ 6 years) – 5 mg per day.

	Product	Form	Description	C.I.*
Rx	**Temaril** (Herbert Labs)	**Tablets:** 2.5 mg (as tartrate)	(#HL T41). Gray. In 100s, 1000s and UD 100s.	123
		Spansules (sustained release capsules): 5 mg (as tartrate)	(#HL T50). Gray and clear. In 50s and UD 100s.	112
Rx	**Temaril** (Herbert Labs)	**Syrup:** 2.5 mg per 5 ml (as tartrate)	5.7% alcohol. Saccharin. Raspberry/strawberry flavor. In 120 ml.	178

METHDILAZINE HCl

Administration and Dosage:

Adults: 8 mg, 2 to 4 times daily.

Children (over 3 years): 4 mg, 2 to 4 times daily.

	Product	Form	Description	C.I.*
Rx	**Tacaryl** (Westwood)	**Tablets, chewable:** 4 mg	(#W 7300). Saccharin. Pink. In 100s.	255
		Tablets: 8 mg	(#W 7400). Peach, scored. In 100s.	135
		Syrup: 4 mg per 5 ml	7.37% alcohol. Menthol. Sorbitol. In pt.[1]	274

Piperidines

CYPROHEPTADINE HCl

Indications:

In addition to the general uses discussed in the antihistamine monograph, cyproheptadine is also indicated for cold urticaria.

Unlabeled Uses: Cyproheptadine has antihistaminic, anticholinergic, antiserotonin and appetite-stimulating properties. Cyproheptadine has been used with variable success to stimulate appetite in underweight patients and in those with anorexia nervosa. It has also been used to treat vascular cluster headaches.

Administration and Dosage:

Individualize dosage.

Adults: 4 to 20 mg daily. Initiate therapy with 4 mg 3 times daily. A majority of patients require 12 to 16 mg per day and occasionally as much as 32 mg per day. Do not exceed 0.5 mg/kg/day (0.23 mg/lb/day).

Children: Calculate total daily dosage as approximately 0.25 mg/kg (0.11 mg/lb) or 8 mg/m^2.

Children (2 to 7 years) – 2 mg 2 or 3 times daily. Do not exceed 12 mg/day.

Children (7 to 14 years) – 4 mg 2 or 3 times daily. Do not exceed 16 mg/day.

	Product	Form	Description	C.I.*
Rx	**Cyproheptadine HCl** (Various)	**Tablets:** 4 mg	In 20s, 30s, 60s, 100s, 500s, 1000s and UD 100s.	5+
Rx	**Periactin** (MSD)		(#MSD 62). White, scored. In 100s.	100
Rx	**Cyproheptadine HCl** (Various)	**Syrup:** 2 mg per 5 ml	In 120 ml, pt and gal.	30+

* Cost Index based on cost per 2.5 mg trimeprazine, 8 mg methdilazine or 4 mg cyproheptadine.

\# Product identification code.

[1] With sodium bisulfite.

Complete prescribing information for these products begins on page 964

Piperidines (Cont.)

AZATADINE MALEATE

Administration and Dosage:

Individualize dosage.

Adults: 1 or 2 mg twice a day.

Children: Not intended for use in children less than 12 years old.

				C.I.*
Rx	**Optimine** (Schering)	**Tablets:** 1 mg	(#Schering 282). White, scored. In 100s.	163

DIPHENYLPYRALINE HCl

Administration and Dosage:

Individualize dosage.

Adults: 5 mg every 12 hours.

Children (6 to 12 years): 5 mg/day. Not recommended for children < 6 years old.

				C.I.*
Rx	**Hispril Spansules** (SKF)	**Capsules, timed release:** 5 mg	(#SKF Hispril). In 50s.	89

PHENINDAMINE TARTRATE

Administration and Dosage:

Adults: 25 mg every 4 to 6 hours. Do not exceed 150 mg in 24 hours.

Children (6 to < 12 years): 12.5 mg every 4 to 6 hours. Do not exceed 75 mg in 24 hours.

Children (under 6 years): As directed by physician.

				C.I.*
otc	**Nolahist** (Carnrick)	**Tablets:** 25 mg	(#C 8652). White, scored. In 100s.	37

MISCELLANEOUS ANTIHISTAMINES

ASTEMIZOLE

Administration and Dosage:

Adults and children ≥ 12 years: The recommended maintenance dosage is 10 mg/day. Pharmacokinetics are dose proportional following single doses of 10 to 30 mg. To reduce time to steady-state concentration, a single dose of 30 mg may be given on the first day, then 20 mg on the second day, followed by 10 mg daily.

Take on an empty stomach at least 2 hours after a meal. There should be no additional food intake for at least 1 hour post-dosing.

Children < 12 years: Safety and efficacy are not established.

				C.I.*
Rx	**Hismanal** (Janssen)	**Tablets:** 10 mg	(#Janssen AST/10). White, scored. In 100s and UD 100s.	N/A

TERFENADINE

Indications:

Unlabeled Uses: Terfenadine may be useful in some lower respiratory conditions such as histamine-induced bronchoconstriction in asthmatics and exercise and hyperventilation-induced bronchospasm.

Administration and Dosage:

Adults and children ≥ 12 years: 60 mg twice daily.

Children: The following doses have been suggested:

(6 to 12 years) – 30 to 60 mg twice daily.

(3 to 6 years) – 15 mg twice daily.

				C.I.*
Rx	**Seldane** (Merrell Dow)	**Tablets:** 60 mg	(#Seldane). White. In 100s.	181

COMBINED ANTIHISTAMINE PREPARATIONS

Administration and Dosage:

Adults: 10 ml every 4 hours.

Children (6 to 12 years): 5 ml every 4 hours.

Children (2 to 6 years): 2.5 ml every 4 hours.

Children (< 2 years): As directed by physician.

				C.I.*
Rx	**Poly-Histine** (Bock)	**Elixir:** 4 mg pheniramine maleate, 4 mg pyrilamine maleate and 4 mg phenyltoloxamine citrate per 5 ml	4% alcohol. In pt.	506

* Cost Index based on cost per 1 mg azatadine, 5 mg diphenylpyraline, 25 mg phenindamine tartrate, 60 mg terfenadine or minimum daily adult dose antihistamine combination.

Product identification code.

The following is an abbreviated monograph covering the primary considerations in the use of codeine as an antitussive. For complete information on opiates, some having antitussive properties, refer to the Narcotic Agonist Analgesics monograph.

CODEINE

Actions:

Codeine has good antitussive activity; side effects are infrequent at the usual antitussive dose. The dose required to suppress coughing is lower than the dose required for analgesia.

Pharmacokinetics: Codeine and its salts are well absorbed. Codeine is metabolized primarily in the liver and is excreted primarily in the urine within 24 hours, 5% to 15% as unchanged codeine and the remainder as the products of glucuronide conjugation and metabolites. The plasma half-life of codeine is about 2.9 hours.

Indications:

For suppression of cough induced by chemical or mechanical respiratory tract irritation.

Relief of mild to moderate pain (see Narcotic Agonist Analgesics monograph).

Contraindications:

Hypersensitivity to the drug; premature infants or during labor when delivery of a premature infant is anticipated (see Warnings).

Warnings:

Head injury and increased intracranial pressure: The respiratory depressant effects of the opiates and their capacity to elevate cerebrospinal fluid pressure may be markedly exaggerated in the presence of head injury, intracranial lesions or a preexisting increase in intracranial pressure. Usual oral doses of codeine produce little respiratory depression; however, exercise caution, particularly with larger doses. Furthermore, opiates may produce adverse reactions which may obscure the clinical course of patients with head injuries.

Asthma and other respiratory conditions: Use with extreme caution in patients having an acute asthmatic attack, patients with chronic obstructive pulmonary disease or cor pulmonale, patients having a substantially decreased respiratory reserve and patients with preexisting respiratory depression, hypoxia or hypercapnia. Usual therapeutic doses may decrease respiratory drive while simultaneously increasing airway resistance to the point of apnea. In asthma and pulmonary emphysema, codeine may, due to its drying action on the respiratory mucosa, precipitate insufficiency resulting from increased viscosity of the bronchial secretions and suppression of the cough reflex.

Acute abdominal conditions: Administration of codeine or other opiates may obscure the diagnosis or clinical course in patients with acute abdominal conditions.

Pregnancy: Category C. Dependence has been reported in newborns whose mothers took opiates regularly during pregnancy. Withdrawal signs include irritability, excessive crying, tremors, hyperreflexia, fever, vomiting and diarrhea. Signs usually appear during the first few days of life. Use during pregnancy only if the potential benefits outweigh the potential hazards to the fetus.

Labor and delivery: Opiates cross the placental barrier. The closer to delivery and the larger the dose used, the greater the possibility of respiratory depression in the newborn. Avoid use during labor if a premature infant is anticipated. If the mother has received opiates during labor, closely observe newborn for signs of respiratory depression. Resuscitation and, in severe depression, naloxone may be required. Codeine may also prolong labor.

Lactation: Exercise caution. Some studies have reported detectable amounts of codeine in breast milk. The levels are probably not clinically significant after usual therapeutic dosage. Clinically important amounts may be excreted in breast milk in individuals abusing codeine.

Children: Do not use opiates, including codeine, in premature infants. Opiates cross the immature blood-brain barrier to a greater extent, producing disproportionate respiratory depression. Give opiates to infants and small children only with great caution and carefully monitor dosage. Safety and efficacy of codeine in newborn infants have not been established.

(Continued on following page)

CODEINE (Cont.)

Precautions:

Administer with caution, and reduce the initial dose in patients with acute abdominal conditions, convulsive disorders, significant hepatic or renal impairment, fever, hypothyroidism, Addison's disease, ulcerative colitis, prostatic hypertrophy, urethral stricture, patients with recent GI or urinary tract surgery and in very young, elderly or debilitated patients.

Drug Interactions:

CNS depressants (eg, other opiates, general anesthetics, phenothiazines, tricyclic antidepressants, tranquilizers) and **alcohol:** Use codeine cautiously and in reduced dosage to avoid additive effects when given concomitantly.

Drug/Lab test interaction: Because opiates may increase biliary tract pressure, with resultant increases in plasma amylase or lipase levels, determination of these enzyme levels may be unreliable for 24 hours after an opiate has been given.

Adverse Reactions:

In usual oral antitussive doses, codeine has minimal side effects. Nausea, vomiting, sedation, dizziness and constipation are most common.

CNS: CNS depression, particularly respiratory depression, and to a lesser extent, circulatory depression; respiratory arrest, shock and cardiac arrest, particularly in overdosage or with rapid IV administration. Other effects include: Lightheadedness; dizziness; sedation; euphoria; dysphoria; weakness; headache; hallucinations; disorientation; visual disturbances; convulsions. These effects are more common with larger parenteral doses, in ambulatory patients and in those who are not experiencing severe pain. Some reactions in ambulatory patients may be alleviated by lying down.

GI: Nausea; vomiting; constipation; biliary tract spasm. Patients with ulcerative colitis may experience increased colonic motility or toxic dilation.

Cardiovascular: Tachycardia; bradycardia; palpitation; faintness; syncope; orthostatic hypotension.

GU: Oliguria; urinary retention; antidiuretic effect.

Allergic reactions to opiates occur infrequently; pruritus, giant urticaria, angioneurotic edema and laryngeal edema have occurred following IV administration.

Overdosage:

The lethal oral dose of codeine in an adult is in the range of 0.5 to 1 g. Infants and children are relatively more sensitive to opiates on a body weight basis. Elderly patients are also comparatively intolerant.

For a description of opiate overdosage and treatment, see the Narcotic Agonist Analgesics monograph. Refer also to General Management of Acute Overdosage.

Drug Abuse and Dependence:

Abuse: The abuse potential of codeine is less than that of heroin or morphine.

Most patients who receive opiates for medical indications do not develop drug-seeking behavior or compulsive drug use. However, give under close supervision to patients with a history of drug abuse or dependence.

Dependence: Psychological dependence, physical dependence and tolerance may occur.

The severity of the abstinence syndrome is related to degree of dependence, abruptness of withdrawal and the drug used. If the syndrome is precipitated by a narcotic antagonist, symptoms appear in a few minutes and are maximal within 30 minutes.

While codeine can partially suppress the symptoms of morphine withdrawal, the codeine withdrawal syndrome (after 1.2 to 1.8 g codeine/day), though similar to that seen with morphine, is less intense. Withdrawal symptoms in patients dependent on codeine include yawning, sweating, lacrimation, rhinorrhea, a restless sleep, dilated pupils, gooseflesh, irritability, tremor, nausea, vomiting and diarrhea. Treatment is primarily symptomatic and supportive, including maintenance of proper fluid and electrolyte balance.

(Continued on following page)

CODEINE (Cont.)

Patient Information:

May impair the mental or physical abilities required for the performance of potentially hazardous tasks. Observe caution while driving or performing other tasks requiring alertness, coordination or physical dexterity.

The concomitant use of alcohol or other CNS depressants, including sedatives, hypnotics, antidepressants, tranquilizers, phenothiazines and antihistamines, may have an additive effect.

May produce orthostatic hypotension (dizziness, lightheadedness when rising quickly from a sitting or lying position) in some ambulatory patients.

Do not take for persistent or chronic cough, such as occurs with smoking, asthma or emphysema; or where cough is accompanied by excessive secretions, except under supervision of physician.

May cause dry mouth or constipation.

May cause GI upset; take with food or milk.

Administration and Dosage:

Adults: 10 to 20 mg every 4 to 6 hours. Maximum 120 mg/day.

Children:

6 to 12 years – 5 to 10 mg every 4 to 6 hours. Maximum 60 mg/day.
2 to 6 years – 2.5 to 5 mg every 4 to 6 hours. Maximum 30 mg/day.

Infants: Do not use in premature infants. Safety and efficacy in newborn infants have not been established.

Codeine is also available in many multi-ingredient respiratory preparations as an antitussive. Refer to the Upper Respiratory Combinations.

				C.I.*
c-II	**Codeine Sulfate** (Various, eg, Halsey, Knoll, Lilly, Roxane)	**Tablets:** 15 mg	In 100s and UD 100s.	3+
		30 mg	In 100s, 1000s and UD 100s.	1.3+
		60 mg	In 100s and UD 100s.	1.1+

* Cost Index based on cost per 15 mg.

DEXTROMETHORPHAN HBr

Dextromethorphan is the d-isomer of the codeine analog of levorphanol; it lacks analgesic and addictive properties. Its cough suppressant action is due to a central action on the cough center in the medulla. Dextromethorphan 15 to 30 mg equals 8 to 15 mg codeine as an antitussive.

Indications:

To control nonproductive cough.

Contraindications:

Hypersensitivity to any component.

Warnings:

Do not use for persistent or chronic cough (eg, smoking, asthma, emphysema) or where cough is accompanied by excessive secretions. Persons with a high fever, rash, persistent headache, nausea or vomiting should use only under medical supervision.

Drug Abuse and Dependence:

Anecdotal reports of abuse of dextromethorphan-containing cough/cold products has increased, especially among teenagers. The FDA Drug Abuse Advisory Committee states that additional data is needed before determining the abuse and dependency potential of dextromethorphan.

Drug Interactions:

MAO inhibitors: Patients may develop hypotension, hyperpyrexia, nausea, myoclonic leg jerks and coma following coadministration.

Overdosage:

Symptoms: Children – Ataxia, respiratory depression; convulsions.

Adults – Altered sensory perception; ataxia; slurred speech; dysphoria.

Administration and Dosage:

Liquid, lozenges and syrup:

Adults and children (> 12 years of age) – 10 to 30 mg every 4 to 8 hours. Do not exceed 120 mg in 24 hours.

Children (6 to 12 years) – 5 to 10 mg every 4 hours or 15 mg every 6 to 8 hours. Do not exceed 60 mg in 24 hours.

Children (2 to 6 years) – *Syrup:* 2.5 to 7.5 mg every 4 to 8 hours. Do not exceed 30 mg in 24 hours.

Children (< 2 years) – Use only as directed by a physician.

Sustained action liquid: Adults – 60 mg every 12 hours.

Children (6 to 12 years) – 30 mg every 12 hours.

Children (2 to 5 years) – 15 mg every 12 hours.

	Product	Form	Description	C.I.*
otc sf	**Scot-Tussin DM Cough Chasers** (Scot-Tussin)	**Lozenges:** 2.5 mg	Dye free. Sorbitol. In 20s.	16
otc	**Children's Hold** (Menley & James)	**Lozenges:** 5 mg	Sucrose, corn syrup. In 10s.	8
otc	**Hold DM** (Menley & James)		Corn syrup, sucrose. In 10s.	8
otc	**Robitussin Cough Calmers** (Robins)		Corn syrup, sucrose. (AHR). Square. Cherry flavor. In 16s.	NA
otc	**Sucrets Cough Control** (SK-Beecham)		Corn syrup, sucrose. In 24s.	6.3
otc	**Suppress** (Ferndale)	**Lozenges:** 7.5 mg	In 1000s.	NA
otc	**Trocal** (Hauck)		In 500s.	2.4
otc	**Creo-Terpin** (Medtech)	**Liquid:** 10 mg per 15 ml (3.33 mg/5 ml)	Tartrazine, 25% alcohol, creosote, corn syrup, saccharin. In 120 ml.	NA
otc	**Pertussin CS** (Pertussin)	**Liquid:** 3.5 mg per 5 ml	Alcohol free. Sorbitol, sucrose. Wild berry flavor. In 120 ml.	2
otc sf	**Robitussin Pediatric** (Robins)	**Liquid:** 7.5 mg per 5 ml	Alcohol free. Saccharin, sorbitol. Cherry flavor. In 120 & 240 ml.	1.6
otc	**St. Joseph Cough Suppressant** (Schering-Plough)		Alcohol free. Sucrose. Cherry flavor. In 60 and 120 ml.	3.9

* Cost Index based on cost per 15 mg dextromethorphan.

sf – Sugar free.

(Continued on following page)

DEXTROMETHORPHAN HBr (Cont.)

	Product	Dosage form	Description	C.I.*
otc	**Pertussin ES** (Pertussin)	**Liquid:** 15 mg per 5 ml	9.5% alcohol. Sugar, sorbitol. In 120 ml.	1.6
otc	**Vicks Formula 44** (Richardson-Vicks)		10% alcohol. Sugar. In 120 and 240 ml.	5.4
otc	**Vicks Formula 44 Pediatric Formula** (Richardson-Vicks)	**Syrup:** 15 mg per 15 ml (1 mg/ml)	Alcohol free. Sorbitol, sucrose. Cherry flavor. In 120 ml.	5.4
otc	**Dextromethorphan** (Various, eg, PBI, Rugby)	**Syrup:** 10 mg per 5 ml	Alcohol. In 120 ml & gal.	1.5+
otc	**Benylin DM** (Parke-Davis)		5% alcohol. Glucose, menthol, sucrose. In 118 ml.	3
otc	**Delsym** (Fisons)	**Liquid, sustained action:** Dextromethorphan polistirex equivalent to 30 mg dextromethorphan HBr/5 ml.	Alcohol free. Corn syrup, sucrose. Orange flavor. In 89 ml.	2

DIPHENHYDRAMINE HCl

Refer to the Antihistamines group monograph for complete prescribing information.

Indications:

For the control of cough due to colds or allergy.

Administration and Dosage:

Adults: 25 mg every 4 hours, not to exceed 150 mg in 24 hours.

Children (6 to 12 years): 12.5 mg every 4 hours, not to exceed 75 mg in 24 hours.

Children (2 to 6 years): 6.25 mg every 4 hours, not to exceed 25 mg in 24 hours.

Note: These formulations may contain ammonium chloride and sodium citrate. Although these ingredients have been used as expectorants, there is inadequate evidence of their clinical value; they have not been approved by the FDA as *otc* expectorants. Products currently on the market have deleted any therapeutic claims for these components. They remain in the product formulation and are listed only as inactive ingredients.

	Product	Dosage form	Description	C.I.*
otc/ Rx[1]	**Diphenhydramine HCl Cough** (Various, eg, IDE, Major, URL)	**Syrup:** 12.5 mg per 5 ml	In 120 and 240 ml, pt and gal.[2]	4+
otc	**Benylin Cough** (Parke-Davis)		Ammonium chloride, sodium citrate, 5% alcohol, menthol, glucose, sucrose, saccharin. In 118 and 240 ml.	8
otc	**Bydramine** (Major)		5% alcohol. In 118 ml.	3.6
otc	**Diphen Cough** (PBI)		Ammonium chloride, sodium citrate, 5% alcohol, sugar, menthol, sorbitol, sucrose. Raspberry flavor. In 120 ml, pt and gal.	3.8
otc	**Silphen Cough** (Silarx)		Menthol, sucrose, 5% alcohol. Strawberry flavor. In 118 ml.	NA
Rx	**Tusstat** (Century)		5% alcohol. In 30 and 120 ml, pt and gal.	1.7
otc	**Uni-Bent Cough** (URL)		5% alcohol. In 118 ml.	1

* Cost Index based on cost per 15 mg dextromethorphan or 50 mg diphenhydramine.

[1] Products are available *otc* or *Rx,* depending on product labeling.

[2] May contain sodium citrate.

BENZONATATE

Actions:

Benzonatate is related to tetracaine. It anesthetizes the stretch receptors in the respiratory passages, lungs and pleura, dampening their activity, and reducing the cough reflex at its source. It has no inhibitory effect on the respiratory center in recommended dosage. Onset of action occurs in 15 to 20 minutes; effects last for 3 to 8 hours.

Indications:

Symptomatic relief of cough.

Contraindications:

Hypersensitivity to benzonatate or related compounds (eg, tetracaine).

Warnings:

Pregnancy: Category C. It is not known whether the drug can cause fetal harm or can affect reproduction capacity. Give to a pregnant woman only if clearly needed.

Lactation: It is not known whether this drug is excreted in breast milk. Exercise caution when administering to a nursing woman.

Precautions:

Local anesthesia: Release of benzonatate in the mouth can produce a temporary local anesthesia of the oral mucosa. Swallow the capsules without chewing.

Adverse Reactions:

Sedation; headache; mild dizziness; constipation; nausea; GI upset; pruritus; skin eruptions; nasal congestion; sensation of burning in the eyes; a vague "chilly" sensation; chest numbness; hypersensitivity.

Overdosage:

Symptoms: If capsules are chewed or dissolved in the mouth, oropharyngeal anesthesia will develop rapidly. CNS stimulation may cause restlessness and tremors which may proceed to clonic convulsions followed by profound CNS depression.

Treatment includes usual supportive measures. Refer to General Management of Acute Overdosage. Even in the conscious patient, cough and gag reflexes may be so depressed as to necessitate protection against aspiration of gastric contents.

Treat convulsions with an IV short-acting barbiturate. Employ intensive support of respiration and cardiovascular-renal function if required. Do not use CNS stimulants.

Patient Information:

Do not chew or break capsules; swallow whole.

Administration and Dosage:

Adults and children (> 10 years): 100 mg 3 times daily, up to 600 mg/day.

				C.I.*
Rx	**Tessalon Perles** (Forest)	**Capsules:** 100 mg	Yellow. In 100s and 500s.	7.8

DEXTROMETHORPHAN HBr and BENZOCAINE

Administration and Dosage:

Vicks Formula 44: Adults and children ≥ 12 years – 2 lozenges dissolved in mouth, one at a time, every 4 hours. Do not exceed 12 lozenges in 24 hours.

Children 3 to 12 years – 1 lozenge every 4 hours. Do not exceed 6 lozenges in 24 hours.

Children < 3 years – Use only as directed by physician.

Vicks Cough Silencers: Adults and children ≥ 12 years – 4 lozenges dissolved in mouth, one at a time, every 4 hours. Do not exceed 48 lozenges in 24 hours.

Children 6 to < 12 years – 2 to 4 lozenges every 4 hours. Do not exceed 24 lozenges in 24 hours.

Children 2 to < 6 years – 1 to 2 lozenges every 4 hours. Do not exceed 12 lozenges in 24 hours.

Children < 2 – Use only as directed by physician.

Spec-T: Adults and children ≥ 6 years – 1 lozenge every 3 hours. Do not exceed 6 lozenges in 24 hours.

Children < 6 years – Use only as directed.

				C.I.*
otc	**Spec-T** (Apothecon)	**Lozenges:** 10 mg dextromethorphan HBr and 10 mg benzocaine	Tartrazine, sucrose, dextrose, glucose. In 10s.	2.7
otc	**Vicks Formula 44 Cough Control Discs** (Richardson-Vicks)	**Lozenges:** 5 mg dextromethorphan HBr and 1.25 mg benzocaine	4.3 mg menthol, sucrose. (F 44). In 24s.	6.3
otc	**Vicks Cough Silencers** (Richardson-Vicks)	**Lozenges:** 2.5 mg dextromethorphan HBr, 1 mg benzocaine	Tartrazine, menthol, anethole, corn syrup, sucrose. In 14s.	4

* Cost Index based on cost per 15 mg dextromethorphan or 100 mg benzonatate.

GUAIFENESIN (Glyceryl Guaiacolate)

Actions:

Guaifenesin is claimed to enhance the output of respiratory tract fluid by reducing adhesiveness and surface tension facilitating the removal of viscous mucus. As a result, nonproductive coughs become more productive and less frequent. There is a lack of convincing studies to document efficacy.

Indications:

For the symptomatic relief of respiratory conditions characterized by dry, nonproductive cough and in the presence of mucus in the respiratory tract.

Contraindications:

Hypersensitivity to guaifenesin.

Warnings:

Not for persistent cough such as occurs with smoking, asthma or emphysema, or where cough is accompanied by excessive secretions.

Precautions:

Persistent cough may indicate a serious condition. If cough persists for more than 1 week, tends to recur, or is accompanied by high fever, rash or persistent headache, consult physician. Excessive dosage may cause nausea and vomiting.

Drug Interactions:

Drug/Lab test interactions: May cause a color interference with certain laboratory determinations of 5-hydroxyindoleacetic acid (5-HIAA) and vanillylmandelic acid (VMA).

Adverse Reactions:

Nausea, vomiting (most common); dizziness; headache; rash (including urticaria).

Administration and Dosage:

Adults and children (≥ 12): 100 to 400 mg every 4 hours. Do not exceed 2.4 g/day.
Children (6 to 12): 100 to 200 mg every 4 hours. Do not exceed 1.2 g/day.
Children (2 to 6): 50 to 100 mg every 4 hours. Do not exceed 600 mg/day.

	Product	Form	Description	C.I.*
otc	**Guaifenesin** (Various, eg, Lederle, Major, Roxane, UDL)	**Syrup:** 100 mg per 5 ml	In 120 and 240 ml, pt, gal and UD 5, 10 and 15 ml.	5.5+
otc	**Guiatuss** (Various, eg, Barre-National, Genetco, Goldline, Moore)		In 120 and 240 ml, pt and gal.	1+
otc	**Anti-Tuss** (Century)		3.5% alcohol. In 120 ml and gal.	5.6
otc	**Genatuss** (Goldline)		3.5% alcohol. In 120 ml.	6.3
otc	**Glyate** (Geneva)		3.5% alcohol. In 118 & 480 ml.	NA
otc	**Halotussin** (Halsey)		3.5% alcohol. In 120 and 240 ml, pt and gal.	2.8
otc	**Malotuss** (Hauck)		3.5% alcohol. In 118 ml.	7.2
otc	**Mytussin** (PBI)		3.5% alcohol. Sugar, menthol. Raspberry flavor. In 120 ml, pt & gal.	3.1
otc	**Robitussin** (Robins Consumer)		3.5% alcohol, glucose, corn syrup, saccharin. In 30, 60, 120 & 240 ml, pt, gal & UD 5, 10 & 15 ml.	20
otc sf	**Scot-tussin Expectorant** (Scot-Tussin)		3.5% alcohol, saccharin, menthol, sorbitol. Dye free. In 120 ml, pt and gal.	12
otc	**Uni-tussin** (URL)		3.5% alcohol. In 118 ml.	NA
otc sf	**Naldecon Senior EX** (Apothecon)	**Liquid:** 200 mg per 5 ml	Saccharin, sorbitol. In 118 and 480 ml.	13
otc	**Breonesin** (Winthrop)	**Capsules:** 200 mg	(Breon). Red. Sugar coated. In 100s.	10
otc	**GG-Cen** (Central)		Purple and white. In 24s & 100s.	5.6
otc sf	**Hytuss 2X** (Hyrex)		(Hyrex). Maroon and white. In 50s, 100s and 1000s.	3.5
Rx	**Humibid Sprinkle** (Adams Labs)	**Capsules, sustained release:** 300 mg	(Adams/0018). Green and clear. In 100s.	10

* Cost Index based on cost per 100 mg. *sf* – Sugar free.

(Continued on following page)

Ingredients (Cont.):

Sympathomimetics are used for their α-adrenergic (vasoconstrictor/decongestant) or β_2-adrenergic (bronchodilator) effects.

Decongestants (see individual monograph): Used for temporary relief of nasal congestion due to colds or allergy. Given orally, they are less effective than topical nasal decongestants, and they have a potential for systemic side effects. Frequent or prolonged topical use may lead to local irritation and rebound congestion.

Bronchodilators (see individual monograph): Ephedrine is common in these combinations; however, it stimulates cardiac (β_1) receptors. Bronchodilation is weaker than with the catecholamines; α-adrenergic effects may decrease congestion of mucous membranes. Other β-active agents are effective bronchodilators, but pseudoephedrine is not.

Narcotic antitussives: The antitussive dose is lower than that required for analgesia. Consider general precautions for the use of narcotics, including the potential for abuse, when using these products. See Narcotic Antitussive monograph for complete prescribing information. See also the Narcotic Agonist Analgesics monograph for complete information on the narcotics.

Codeine – 10 to 20 mg every 4 to 6 hours.
Hydrocodone (dihydrocodeinone) – 5 to 10 mg every 6 to 8 hours.
Hydromorphone HCl – 2 mg every 4 hours.

Nonnarcotic antitussives decrease the cough reflex without inducing many of the common characteristics of narcotic preparations.

Dextromethorphan – 10 to 30 mg every 4 to 8 hours.
Diphenhydramine – 25 mg every 4 hours.
Carbetapentane has atropine-like and local anesthetic actions and suppresses cough reflex through selective depression of the medullary cough center.
Dose: 15 to 30 mg, 3 or 4 times daily.
Caramiphen edisylate – A weak anticholinergic and centrally acting antitussive.
Dose: Adults – 10 to 20 mg every 4 to 6 hours.
Children (6 to 12) – 5 to 10 mg q 4 to 6 h; *(2 to 6)* – 2.5 to 5 mg q 4 to 6 h.

Expectorants: In the FDA's final monograph for *otc* expectorants, guaifenesin (see individual monograph) is the only agent approved for use as an expectorant. Guaifenesin may help loosen phlegm and thin bronchial secretions to rid the bronchial passageways of bothersome mucus, drain bronchial tubes or make coughs more productive. Humidification of room air and adequate fluid intake (6 to 8 glasses/day) are important therapeutic measures as well.

Dose: Adults – 200 to 400 mg every 4 hours, not to exceed 2400 mg in 24 hours.
Children – Lower dosages are specified on labeling. Consult a physician for children < 2 years of age.

Other ingredients not upgraded by the FDA include: Ammonium chloride, beechwood creosote, benzoin preparations, camphor, eucalyptol/eucalyptus oil, iodines, ipecac syrup, menthol/peppermint oil, pine tar preparations, potassium guaiacolsulfonate, sodium citrate, squill preparations, terpin hydrate preparations, tolu preparations and turpentine oil. Products containing these ingredients must be reformulated.

Analgesics (eg, acetaminophen, aspirin, ibuprofen, sodium salicylate) are frequently included for symptoms of headache, fever, muscle aches and pain. See individual monographs.

Anticholinertics (see individual monograph) are included for their drying effects on mucous secretions. This action may be beneficial in acute rhinorrhea; however, drying of respiratory secretions may lead to obstruction. Traditionally, anticholinergics have been avoided in patients with asthma or chronic obstructive pulmonary disease (COPD); however, some patients respond well to these agents. Caution is still advised in this group.

An anticholinergic for oral inhalation is available as a bronchodilator for maintenance of bronchospasm associated with COPD, including chronic bronchitis and emphysema (see Ipratropium monograph).

The FDA has ruled that no anticholinergic product for *otc* use is recognized as safe and effective. Therefore, the products must be reapproved by new drug application (NDA) before November 10, 1986, or be regarded as misbranded (*Federal Register* 1985 Nov 8; 50:46582-87).

Papaverine HCl (see individual monograph) relaxes the smooth muscle of the bronchial tree.

Barbiturates (see individual monograph) are included for their sedative effects as "correctives" in combination with xanthines or sympathomimetics which may cause CNS stimulation. The sedative efficacy of low doses (eg, 8 mg phenobarbital) is questionable.

Caffeine (see individual monograph) is included in some combinations for CNS stimulation to counteract antihistamine depression and to enhance concomitant analgesics.

(Products listed on following pages)

ANTIASTHMATIC COMBINATIONS

Refer to the general discussion of these products beginning on page 990
Content given per capsule or tablet.

Xanthine Combinations, Capsules and Tablets

	Product & Distributor	Xanthine[1]	Expectorant	Other	Average Adult Dose	How Supplied	C.I.*
Rx	**Quibron-300 Capsules** (Bristol-Myers Squibb)	300 mg theophylline	180 mg guaifenesin		1 q 6 to 8 h	Yellow and white. In 100s.	16
Rx	**Bronchial Capsules** (Various, eg, Geneva Marsam, Moore)	150 mg theophylline	90 mg guaifenesin		1 or 2/day	In 100s.	2.5+
Rx	**Glyceryl-T Capsules** (Rugby)[2]				1 or 2 bid or tid	In 100s and 1000s.	1.5
Rx	**Lanophyllin-GG Capsules** (Lannett)				1 q 6 h	In 100s and 500s.	2
Rx	**Quibron Capsules** (Bristol-Myers Squibb)				1 or 2 q 6 to 8 h	Yellow. In 100s, 1000s and UD 100s.	10
Rx	**Theo-G Capsules** (Dixon-Shane)					In 100s and 1000s.	2.5
Rx	**Slo-Phyllin GG Capsules** (Rhone-Poulenc Rorer)			Sorbitol	16 mg/kg/day, in divided doses, q 6 to 8 h	In 100s.	8.5
Rx	**Asbron G Inlay-Tabs** (Sandoz)	150 mg theophylline (300 mg theophylline sodium glycinate)	100 mg guaifenesin	Sucrose	1 or 2 tid or qid	(Asbron G 78-202). Green and white. In 100s.	19

* Cost Index based on cost per capsule or tablet.
[1] Theophylline content given as anhydrous unless otherwise specified.
[2] Form of theophylline unknown.

(Continued on following page)

ANTIASTHMATIC COMBINATIONS (Cont.)

Refer to the general discussion of these products beginning on page 990
Content given per tablet.

Xanthine Combinations, Capsules and Tablets (Cont.)

	Product & Distributor	Xanthine[1]	Expectorant	Other	Average Adult Dose	How Supplied	C.I.*
Rx	**Mudrane GG-2 Tablets** (Poythress)	111 mg theophylline (130 mg aminophylline anhydrous)	100 mg guaifenesin		1 tid or qid	(GG 9533). Green, mottled. In 100s.	7
Rx	**Mudrane-2 Tablets** (Poythress)	111 mg theophylline (130 mg aminophylline anhydrous)	195 mg potassium iodide		1 tid or qid	(9532). White, scored. In 100s.	7
Rx	**Dilor-G Tablets** (Savage)	200 mg dyphylline	200 mg guaifenesin		1 tid or qid	In 100s, 1000s, UD 100s.	14
Rx	**Dyflex-G Tablets** (Econo Med)				1 or 2 qid up to 15 mg/kg (5/dose)	Scored. In 100s and 1000s.	6
Rx	**Dyline-GG Tablets** (Seatrace)				1 tid or qid	In 100s and 1000s.	5.5
Rx	**Lufyllin-GG Tablets** (Wallace)				1 qid	(Wallace 541). Yellow, scored. In 100s, 1000s and UD 100s.	31
Rx	**Neothylline-GG Tablets** (Lemmon)			Lactose	1 qid	(Lemmon 128-128). White, scored. In 100s.	7.5
Rx	**Brondecon Tablets** (Parke-Davis)	128 mg theophylline (200 mg oxtriphylline)	100 mg guaifenesin	Lactose, saccharin, sucrose	1 qid	Salmon pink. In 100s.	16

* Cost Index based on cost per tablet.
[1] Theophylline content given as anhydrous unless otherwise specified.

ANTIASTHMATIC COMBINATIONS (Cont.)

Refer to the general discussion of these products beginning on page 990.
Content given per 15 ml.

Xanthine Combinations, Liquids

	Product & Distributor	Xanthine[1]	Expectorant	Other	Average Adult Dose	How Supplied	C.I.*
Rx	**Theolate Liquid** (Various, eg, Barre, Dixon-Shane, Genetco, Moore, Quali-test, Schein)	150 mg theophylline	90 mg guaifenesin		15 to 30 ml q 6 to 8 h	In 118 ml, pt and gal.	5.5+
Rx	**Glyceryl-T Liquid** (Rugby)					Alcohol and dye free. In pt.	4.5
Rx	**Q.B. Liquid** (Major)					In pt.	6
Rx	**Quibron Liquid** (Bristol-Myers Squibb)			Sorbitol, sucrose	15 to 30 ml q 6 to 8 h	Alcohol and dye free. In pt and gal.	30
Rx	**Slo-Phyllin GG Syrup** (Rhone-Poulenc Rorer)			Saccharin, sorbitol, sucrose	16 mg/kg/day in divided doses, q 6 to 8 h	Alcohol and dye free. Lemon-vanilla flavor. In 480 ml.	34
Rx	**Asbron G Elixir** (Sandoz)	150 mg theophylline (300 mg theophylline sodium glycinate)	100 mg guaifenesin	15% alcohol. Saccharin, sorbitol, sucrose	15 to 30 ml tid or qid	Citrus flavor. In 480 ml.	56
Rx	**Synophylate-GG Syrup** (Central)			10% alcohol. Saccharin, sorbitol, sucrose	3 mg/kg q 8 h	In pt & gal.	27
Rx sf	**Elixophyllin GG Liquid** (Forest)	100 mg theophylline	100 mg guaifenesin	Sorbitol	3 mg/kg q 8 h	Alcohol and dye free. Cherry-berry flavor. In 237 and 473 ml.	46

* Cost Index based on cost per 15 ml.
sf – Sugar free.
[1] Theophylline content given as anhydrous unless otherwise specified.

(Continued on following page)

ANTIASTHMATIC COMBINATIONS (Cont.)

Refer to the general discussion of these products beginning on page 990.
Content given per 15 ml.

Xanthine Combinations, Liquids (Cont.)

	Product & Distributor	Xanthine[1]	Expectorant	Other	Average Adult Dose	How Supplied	C.I.*
Rx	**Theophylline KI Elixir** (Various, eg, Barre, Geneva Marsam, Major, Moore, PBI, Qualitest, Rugby, Schein)	80 mg theophylline	130 mg potassium iodide	Alcohol	30 ml tid	In pt and gal.	4+
Rx	**Elixophyllin-KI Elixir** (Forest)			10% alcohol. Saccharin, sodium bisulfite, sucrose	3 mg/kg q 8 h	In 240 ml.	102
Rx	**Iophylline Elixir** (Various, eg, Dixon-Shane, Major)	120 mg theophylline	30 mg iodinated glycerol	15% alcohol	15 to 30 ml tid	In pt.	17+
Rx	**Theo-Organidin Elixir** (Wallace)			15% alcohol. Saccharin	15 to 30 ml tid q 6 to 8 h	In pt and gal.	65
Rx	**Theo-R-Gen Elixir** (Goldline)			15% alcohol	15 to 30 ml tid	Wine flavor. In pt.	21
Rx	**Dilor-G Liquid** (Savage)	300 mg dyphylline	300 mg guaifenesin	Saccharin, sorbitol, sucrose	5 or 10 ml tid or qid	Mint flavor. Alcohol free. In pt.	33
Rx	**Dyline-GG Liquid** (Seatrace)				5 or 10 ml tid or qid	Alcohol free. In pt.	17
Rx	**Lufyllin-GG Elixir** (Wallace)	100 mg dyphylline	100 mg guaifenesin	17% alcohol. Saccharin, sucrose	30 ml qid	Wine flavor. In pt and gal.	56
Rx	**Brondelate Elixir** (Various, eg, Barre, Dixon-Shane, Major, Moore, Schein)	192 mg theophylline (300 mg oxtriphylline)	150 mg guaifenesin	Alcohol	10 ml qid	In pt and gal.	13+
Rx	**Brondecon Elixir** (Parke-Davis)			20% alcohol. Saccharin, sucrose	10 ml qid	Cherry flavor. In 237 and 474 ml.	35

* Cost Index based on cost per 15 ml.
[1] Theophylline content given as anhydrous unless otherwise specified.

Refer to the general discussion of these products beginning on page 990.
Content given per capsule or tablet.

Xanthine-Sympathomimetic Combinations, Capsules and Tablets

	Product & Distributor	Xanthine[1]	Sympathomimetic	Expectorant	Other	Average Adult Dose	How Supplied	C.I.*
Rx	**Tedral SA Tablets** (Parke-Davis)	180 mg theophylline	48 mg ephedrine HCl		25 mg phenobarbital, sucrose, lactose	1 q 12 h	Sustained action. Coral/mottled white, layered. In 100s.	21
otc	**Theodrine Tablets** (Rugby)	125 mg theophylline[2]	25 mg ephedrine HCl		8 mg phenobarbital[3], lactose	1 to 2 q 4 h up to 3 doses/day	In 100s and 1000s.	2
otc	**Theotal Tablets** (Major)					1 q 4 h up to 3/day	In 1000s.	1.7
otc	**Tedrigen Tablets** (Goldline)				8 mg phenobarbital[3]	1 q 4 h up to 3 doses/day	White. In 100s.	2
otc	**Tedral Tablets** (Parke-Davis)	118 mg theophylline	24 mg ephedrine HCl		8 mg phenobarbital[3], lactose	1 or 2 q 4 h	In 24s and 100s.	1.3
otc	**Primatene Tablets** (Whitehall)	130 mg theophylline	24 mg ephedrine HCl			1 or 2 initially, then 1 q 4 h up to 6/day	In 24s and 60s.	8.5
otc	**T.E.P. Tablets** (Geneva)	130 mg theophylline	24 mg ephedrine HCl		8 mg phenobarbital		White. In 100s.	NA
otc	**Amesec Capsules** (Whitby[4])	104 mg theophylline[2] (130 mg aminophylline)	25 mg ephedrine HCl			1 q 6 h	Orange and blue. In 100s.	8.5
otc	**Bronkaid Tablets** (Winthrop)	100 mg theophylline[2]	24 mg ephedrine sulfate	100 mg guaifenesin		1 q 4 h up to 5/day	(D). In 24s and 60s.	7

* Cost Index based on cost per capsule or tablet.
[1] Theophylline content given as anhydrous unless otherwise specified.
[2] Form of theophylline unknown.
[3] Limited availability according to state laws.
[4] Whitby Research Inc., 2801 Reserve Street, P.O. Box 27426, Richmond, VA 23261-7426 (804) 254-4400

(Continued on following page)

ANTIASTHMATIC COMBINATIONS (Cont.)

Refer to the general discussion of these products beginning on page 990 Content given per capsule or tablet.

Xanthine-Sympathomimetic Combinations, Capsules and Tablets (Cont.)

	Product & Distributor	Xanthine[1]	Sympathomimetic	Expectorant	Other	Average Adult Dose	How Supplied	C.I.*
Rx	**Hydrophed Tablets**[2] (Rugby)	130 mg theophylline	25 mg ephedrine sulfate		10 mg hydroxyzine HCl	1 bid to qid	White. In 100s, 500s and 1000s.	1.5
Rx	**Marax Tablets**[2] (Roerig)						(254). Dye free. Scored. In 100s and 500s.	16
Rx	**Moxy Compound Tablets** (Major)						In 100s.	1
Rx	**T.E.H. Tablets** (Geneva Marsam)						White. In 100s and 500s.	4.5
Rx	**Quibron Plus Capsules** (Bristol-Myers Squibb)	150 mg theophylline	25 mg ephedrine HCl	100 mg guaifenesin	20 mg butabarbital	1 to 2 bid or tid	Green. In 100s.	17
otc	**Bronitin Tablets** (Whitehall)	118 mg theophylline (130 mg theophylline hydrous)	24.3 mg ephedrine HCl	100 mg guaifenesin	16.6 mg pyrilamine maleate	1 q 4 h	In 24s and 60s.	7
otc	**Bronkotabs Tablets** (Winthrop)	100 mg theophylline[2]	24 mg ephedrine sulfate	100 mg guaifenesin	8 mg phenobarbital[3]	1 q 3 or 4 h 4 to 5 times/day	Scored. In 100s.	14
Rx	**Mudrane GG Tablets** (Poythress)	112 mg theophylline (130 mg aminophylline anhydrous)	16 mg ephedrine HCl	100 mg guaifenesin	8 mg phenobarbital	1 tid or qid	(GG). Yellow, mottled. In 100s.	7
Rx	**Mudrane Tablets** (Poythress)	112 mg theophylline (130 mg aminophylline anhydrous)	16 mg ephedrine HCl	195 mg potassium iodide	8 mg phenobarbital	1 tid or qid	Yellow. Scored. In 100s.	7
Rx	**Quadrinal Tablets** (Knoll)	65 mg theophylline (130 mg theophylline calcium salicylate)	24 mg ephedrine HCl	320 mg potassium iodide	24 mg phenobarbital	1 tid or qid	(14). White, scored. Biconvex. In 100s.	16
Rx	**Lufyllin-EPG Tablets** (Wallace)	100 mg dyphylline	16 mg ephedrine HCl	200 mg guaifenesin	16 mg phenobarbital, lactose	1 to 2 q 6 h	(Wallace 561). Pink, scored. In 100s.	35

* Cost Index based on cost per capsule or tablet.
[1] Theophylline content given as anhydrous unless otherwise specified.
[2] Form of theophylline unknown.
[3] Limited availability according to state laws.

ANTIASTHMATIC COMBINATIONS (Cont.)

Refer to the general discussion of these products beginning on page 990 Content given per 15 ml.

Xanthine-Sympathomimetic Combinations, Liquids

	Product & Distributor	Xanthine[1]	Sympathomimetic	Expectorant	Other	Average Adult Dose	How Supplied	C.I.*
otc	**Tedral Suspension** (Parke-Davis)	177.3 mg theophylline	36 mg ephedrine HCl		12 mg phenobarbital[2]. Saccharin, sugar	10 to 20 ml q 4 h	In 237 ml.	35
Rx	**Quibron Plus Elixir** (B-M Squibb)	150 mg theophylline	25 mg ephedrine HCl	100 mg guaifenesin	20 mg butabarbital. 15% alcohol	15 to 30 ml bid or tid	In pt.	NA
Rx sf	**Mudrane GG Elixir** (Poythress)	60 mg theophylline	12 mg ephedrine HCl	78 mg guaifenesin	7.5 mg phenobarbital, 20% alcohol	15 ml tid or qid	In pt and half gal.	26
otc	**Bronkolixir Elixir** (Winthrop)	45 mg theophylline[3]	36 mg ephedrine sulfate	150 mg guaifenesin	12 mg phenobarbital[2], 19% alcohol. Saccharin, sucrose	10 ml q 3 or 4 h up to 4 times/day	In 480 ml.	41
otc	**Guiaphed Elixir** (Goldline)	45 mg theophylline[3]	36 mg ephedrine sulfate	150 mg guaifenesin	12 mg phenobarbital[2]	10 ml q 3 or 4 h	In 480 ml.	11
Rx	**Lufyllin-EPG Elixir** (Wallace)	150 mg dyphylline	24 mg ephedrine HCl	300 mg guaifenesin	24 mg phenobarbital, 5.5% alcohol. Saccharin, sucrose	10 to 20 ml q 6 h	Fruit flavor. In 480 ml.	82

Pediatric Xanthine-Sympathomimetic Combinations

	Product & Distributor	Xanthine[1]	Sympathomimetic	Expectorant	Other	Average Adult Dose	How Supplied	C.I.*
Rx	**Theomax DF** (Barre)	32.5 mg theophylline	6.25 mg ephedrine sulfate		2.5 mg hydroxyzine HCl per 5 ml. 5% alcohol	*Children (> 5 yrs)* – 5 ml tid or qid *(2 to 5 yrs)* – 2.5 to 5 ml tid or qid	Cherry flavor. In pt and gal.	NA
Rx	**Marax-DF Syrup** (Roerig)	97.5 mg theophylline	18.75 mg ephedrine sulfate		7.5 mg hydroxyzine HCl, 5% alcohol. Sucrose	*Children (2 to > 5 yrs)* – 2.5 to 5 ml tid or qid	Cherry flavor. In pt and gal.	43

* Cost Index based on cost per 15 ml.
[1] Theophylline content given as anhydrous unless otherwise specified.
[2] Limited availability according to state laws.
[3] Form of theophylline unknown.
sf – Sugar free.

UPPER RESPIRATORY COMBINATIONS

Refer to the general discussion of these products beginning on page 990.
Content given per tablet.

Decongestant Combinations

	Product & Distributor	Decongestant	Other	Average Adult Dose	How Supplied	C.I.*
otc	**Contac Non-Drowsy Formula Sinus Caplets** (SK-Beecham)	30 mg pseudoephedrine HCl	500 mg acetaminophen	2 q 6 h	(Contac-S). In 24s.	NA
otc	**No Drowsiness Dristan Cold Caplets** (Whitehall)				In 20s.	7.5
otc	**Maximum Stength Ornex Caplets** (Menley & James)			2 q 4 h up to 8/day	(Ornex Max). In 24s, 30s and 48s.	NA
otc	**Maximum Strength Sine-Aid Tablets and Caplets** (McNeil-CPC)			2 q 4 to 6 h up to 8/24 h	**Tablets:** In 24s and 100s. **Caplets:** (Sine-Aid). In 24s and 50s.	6
otc	**Maximum Strength Sinutab Without Drowsiness Tablets and Caplets** (Parke-Davis)			2 q 6 h	**Tablets:** In 24s and 50s. **Caplets:** White. In 24s.	7 7
otc	**Sudafed Sinus Tablets and Caplets** (Burroughs Wellcome)				**Tablets:** (Sudafed Sinus). In 24s and 48s. **Caplets:** (Sudafed Sinus). In 24s and 48s.	8.5 8
otc	**Maximum Strength Tylenol Sinus Tablets, Caplets and Gelcaps** (McNeil-CPC)			2 q 4 to 6 h up to 8/24 h	**Tablets:** (Tylenol Sinus). In 24s and 50s. **Caplets:** (Tylenol Sinus). In 24s and 50s. **Gelcaps:** Capsule shape. In 20s and 40s.	6 6 8.5
otc	**No Drowsiness Sinarest Tablets** (Fisons)			2 q 6 h	(Sinarest). In 20s.	7.5
otc	**Sine-Off Maximum Strength No Drowsiness Formula Caplets** (SK-Beecham)				(Sine-Off). In 24s.	8
otc	**Sinus Excedrin Tablets and Caplets** (Bristol-Myers Squibb)				(Sinus Excedrin). Orange. In 24s and 50s.	7

* Cost Index based on cost per tablet.

(Continued on following page)

UPPER RESPIRATORY COMBINATIONS (Cont.)

Refer to the general discussion of these products beginning on page 990.
Content given per capsule, tablet or packet.

Decongestant Combinations (Cont.)

	Product & Distributor	Decongestant	Other	Average Adult Dose	How Supplied	C.I.*
otc	**Coldrine Tablets** (Hauck)	30 mg pseudoephedrine HCl	325 mg acetaminophen	2 q 6 h	In 1000s and Sani-Pak 1000s.	3
otc	**No-Drowsiness Allerest Tablets** (Fisons)			2 q 4 to 6 h up to 8/day	In 20s.	17
otc	**Ornex Caplets** (Menley & James)			2 q 4 h up to 8/day	(Ornex). In 24s and 48s.	NA
otc	**Sinus-Relief Tablets** (Major)			2 q 4 to 6 h up to 8/day	In 24s.	NA
otc	**Sinutab Without Drowsiness Tablets** (Parke-Davis)			2 q 4 h up to 8/day	In 12, 24s and 100s.	8.7
otc	**BC Cold Powder Non-Drowsy Formula** (Block)	25 mg phenylpropanolamine HCl	650 mg aspirin, lactose	1 dose q 4 h up to qid	In 6 and 24 packets.	126
otc	**Ursinus Inlay-Tabs** (Sandoz)	30 mg pseudoephedrine HCl	325 mg aspirin, lactose	2 q 4 h up to 8/day	In 24s.	19
otc	**Advil Cold & Sinus** (Whitehall)	30 mg pseudoephedrine HCl	200 mg ibuprofen	1 to 2 q 4 to 6 h up to 6/day	In 20s, 48s and 100s.	17
otc	**Dristan Sinus Caplets** (Whitehall)			1 to 2 q 4 to 6 h up to 6/day	In 20s and 40s.	18
otc	**Genex Capsules** (Goldline)	18 mg phenylpropanolamine HCl	325 mg acetaminophen	2 q 4 h up to 8/day	Blue/white. In 100s.	4

* Cost Index based on cost per capsule, tablet or packet.

(Continued on following page)

UPPER RESPIRATORY COMBINATIONS (Cont.)

Refer to the general discussion of these products beginning on page 990. Content given per capsule, tablet or lozenge.

Decongestant Combinations (Cont.)

	Product & Distributor	Decongestant	Other	Average Adult Dose	How Supplied	C.I.*
otc	**Rhinocaps Capsules** (Ferndale)	20 mg phenylpropanolamine HCl	162 mg acetaminophen, 162 mg aspirin	2 q 4 to 6 h up to 6/day	In 100s.	7.3
otc	**Saleto-D Capsules** (Hauck)	18 mg phenylpropanolamine HCl	240 mg acetaminophen, 120 mg salicylamide, 16 mg caffeine	2 q 4 h	Maroon and pink. In 1000s and Sani-Pak 500s.	4
otc	**Spec-T Sore Throat/Decongestant Lozenges** (Apothecon)	10.5 mg phenylpropanolamine HCl, 5 mg phenylephrine HCl	10 mg benzocaine, tartrazine, dextrose, glucose, sucrose	1 q 3 h up to 6/day	In 10s.	10

Pediatric Decongestant Combinations

	Product & Distributor	Decongestant	Other	Average Dose	How Supplied	C.I.*
otc *sf*	**St. Joseph Aspirin-Free Cold Tablets for Children** (Schering-Plough)	3.125 mg phenylpropanolamine HCl	80 mg acetaminophen	*Children* – 2 to 8 q 4 h up to 4 doses/day	Chewable. Fruit flavor. In 30s.	5
otc	**Congespirin for Children Tablets** (Bristol-Myers Squibb)	1.25 mg phenylephrine HCl	81 mg acetaminophen, saccharin, sucrose	*Children* – 2 to 8 q 4 h up to 4 doses/day	Chewable. (C). Orange, scored. In 24s.	9.5

Antihistamine and Analgesic Combinations

	Product & Distributor	Antihistamine	Analgesic	Other	Average Adult Dose	How Supplied	C.I.*
otc	**Coricidin Tablets** (Schering-Plough)	2 mg chlorpheniramine maleate	325 mg acetaminophen	Sugar, lactose	2 q 4 h	(522). In 12s, 24s, 48s and 100s.	17
otc	**Phenetron Compound Tablets** (Lannett)	2 mg chlorpheniramine maleate	390 mg aspirin	30 mg caffeine	1 pc and hs	Red. Sugar coated. In 100s and 1000s.	1
otc	**Aceta-Gesic Tablets** (Rugby)	30 mg phenyltoloxamine citrate	325 mg acetaminophen		1 or 2 q 4 h up to 8/day	In 24s, 100s and 1000s.	5.4
otc	**Major-gesic Tablets** (Major)	30 mg phenyltoloxamine citrate	325 mg acetaminophen		1 or 2 q 4 h up to 8/day	Scored. In 100s.	3.3
otc	**Percogesic Tablets** (Richardson-Vicks)	30 mg phenyltoloxamine citrate	325 mg acetaminophen	Sucrose	1 or 2 q 4 h up to 8/day	In 24s, 50s and 90s.	18
otc	**Phenylgesic Tablets** (Goldline)	30 mg phenyltoloxamine citrate	325 mg acetaminophen		1 or 2 q 4 h up to 8/day	Orange. In 100s and 1000s.	3

* Cost Index based on cost per capsule, tablet or lozenge.

sf – Sugar free.

UPPER RESPIRATORY COMBINATIONS (Cont.)

Refer to the general discussion of these products beginning on page 990. Content given per capsule.

Decongestants and Antihistamines, Sustained Release

	Product & Distributor	Decongestant	Antihistamine	Average Adult Dose	Other Content & How Supplied	C.I.*
Rx	**Cophene No. 2 Capsules** (Dunhall)	120 mg pseudoephedrine HCl	12 mg chlorpheniramine maleate	1 q 12 h	In 100s and 500s.	14
otc	**Dallergy-D Capsules** (Laser)				Sucrose. (Laser 175 Dallergy-D). Red & clear. In 12s and 100s.	12
otc	**T-Dry Capsules** (Jones Medical)				In 100s.	16
Rx	**Anamine T.D. Capsules** (Mayrand)	120 mg pseudoephedrine HCl	8 mg chlorpheniramine maleate	1 q 8 to 12 h	(M/R). In 100s.	10
Rx	**Brexin-L.A. Capsules** (Savage)			1 q 12 h	Red and clear. In 100s.	12
Rx	**Chlorafed Timecelles (Capsules)** (Hauck)				Dye free. Clear. In 100s, 500s and UD 50s.	13
Rx	**Chlordrine S.R. Capsules** (Rugby)				In 100s.	10
Rx	**Codimal-L.A. Capsules** (Central)				In 100s and 1000s.	1.5
Rx	**Colfed-A Capsules** (Parmed)				In 100s.	8.5
Rx	**Deconamine SR Capsules** (Berlex)				Sucrose. Blue and yellow. In 100s and 500s.	19
Rx	**Chlorpheniramine Maleate and Pseudoephedrine HCl Capsules** (Vitarine)				Sucrose. (PP-1304). Dk. blue/clear. In 100s and 1000s.	10
Rx	**Duralex Capsules** (American Urologicals)				In 100s and 1000s.	12
Rx	**Fedahist Timecaps (Capsules)** (Schwarz Pharma Kremers Urban)				Sucrose. (Kremers Urban 055). Clear. In 100s.	15
otc	**Isoclor Timesules (Capsules)** (Fisons)				Sugar. Dye free. In 10s, 20s, 100s and 500s.	20
Rx	**Klerist-D Capsules** (Nutripharm)				Dye free. In 100s and 500s.	6

* Cost Index based on cost per capsule.

(Continued on following page)

UPPER RESPIRATORY COMBINATIONS (Cont.)

Refer to the general discussion of these products beginning on page 990.
Content given per capsule or tablet.

Decongestants and Antihistamines, Sustained Release (Cont.)

	Product & Distributor	Decongestant	Antihistamine	Average Adult Dose	How Supplied	C.I.*
Rx	**Kronofed-A Capsules** (Ferndale)	120 mg pseudoephedrine HCl	8 mg chlorpheniramine maleate	1 q 12 h	Dye free. White/clear. In 100s and 500s.	9
Rx	**N D Clear Capsules** (Seatrace)				(N D Clear/1-AM/PM). Clear. In 100s.	7
Rx	**Novafed A Capsules** (Marion Merrell Dow)				Sucrose. (106 or Novafed A). Red and orange. In 100s.	19
Rx	**Pseudo-Chlor Capsules** (Major)				Sucrose. In 250s.	7
Rx	**Rinade B.I.D. Capsules** (Econo Med)	120 mg d-isoephedrine HCl	8 mg chlorpheniramine maleate	1 q 12 h	In 100s.	9
otc	**Chlor-Trimeton 12 Hour Relief Tablets** (Schering-Plough)	120 mg pseudoephedrine sulfate	8 mg chlorpheniramine maleate	1 q 12 h	Lactose. (LA CTM D). In 12s and 36s.	6
Rx	**Fedahist Gyrocaps (Capsules)** (Schwarz Pharma Kremers Urban)	65 mg pseudoephedrine HCl	10 mg chlorpheniramine maleate	1 q 12 h	Sucrose. (Kremers Urban 053). White and yellow. In 100s.	13
Rx	**Chlorafed HS Timecelles (Capsules)** (Hauck)	60 mg pseudoephedrine HCl	4 mg chlorpheniramine maleate	2 q 12 h	Dye free. Clear. In 100s, 500s and UD 50s.	11
Rx	**Codimal-L.A. Half Capsules** (Central)				Sucrose. In 100s.	NA

* Cost Index based on cost per capsule or tablet.

(Continued on following page)

UPPER RESPIRATORY COMBINATIONS (Cont.)

Refer to the general discussion of these products beginning on page 990.
Content given per capsule or tablet.

Decongestants and Antihistamines, Sustained Release (Cont.)

	Product & Distributor	Decongestant	Antihistamine	Average Adult Dose	How Supplied	C.I.*
Rx	**Phenylpropanolamine HCl and Chlorpheniramine Maleate Caps** (Vitarine)	75 mg phenylpropanolamine HCl	12 mg chlorpheniramine maleate	1 q 12 h	(PP-256). Blue & clear. In 100s, 250s, 500s and 1000s.	7.5
otc	**Allerest 12 Hour Caplets** (Fisons)				(Allerest 12). In 10s.	16
Rx	**CPA TR Caps** (Schein)				In 100s and 1000s.	4.3
Rx	**Condrin-LA Capsules** (Hauck)			1 or 2 q 12 h	In 1000s.	3
otc	**Contac Maximum Strength 12 Hour Caplets** (SmithKline Beecham)			1 q 12 h	Lactose. (Contac). White. In 20s.	12
Rx	**Drize Capsules** (Ascher)				Dye free. Sugar. (225-405). Clear. In 100s.	14
Rx	**Oragest SR Caps** (Major)				In 100s and 1000s.	4.6
Rx	**Ordrine S.R. Capsules** (Vitarine)				In 100s, 250s, 500s and 1000s.	NA
Rx	**Ornade Spansules** (SmithKline Beecham)				Sucrose. (Ornade). Red & natural. In 50s, 500s & UD 100s.	23
Rx	**Parhist SR Capsules** (Parmed)				In 100s and 1000s.	4.9
Rx	**Resaid Capsules** (Geneva)				In 100s and 1000s.	11
Rx	**Rhinolar-EX 12 Capsules** (McGregor)				Dye free. Sucrose. In 60s.	11
Rx	**Ru-Tuss II Capsules** (Boots)				Dye free. Sucrose. (Ru-Tuss II 31 Boots 31). Green/clear. In 100s.	14
otc	**Triaminic-12 Tabs** (Sandoz)				Lactose. In 10s and 20s.	13

* Cost Index based on cost per capsule or tablet.

(Continued on following page)

UPPER RESPIRATORY COMBINATIONS (Cont.)

Refer to the general discussion of these products beginning on page 990.
Content given per capsule or tablet.

Decongestants and Antihistamines, Sustained Release (Cont.)

	Product & Distributor	Decongestant	Antihistamine	Average Adult Dose	How Supplied	C.I.*
Rx	**Dura-Vent/A Capsules** (Dura)	75 mg phenylpropanolamine HCl	10 mg chlorpheniramine maleate	1 q 12 h	(Dura-Vent/A 51479002). Clear. In 100s.	12
otc	**Contac 12 Hour Capsules** (SmithKline Beecham)	75 mg phenylpropanolamine HCl	8 mg chlorpheniramine maleate	1 q 12 h	Sucrose (Contac). In 10s.	18
otc	**Dehist Capsules** (Forest)				Sucrose. In 100s & 1000s.	7.5
otc	**Gencold Capsules** (Goldline)				Sucrose. Reddish orange/clear. In 10s.	11
Rx	**Rhinolar-EX Capsules** (McGregor)				Dye free. Sucrose. In 60s.	10
otc	**12 Hour Cold Capsules** (Hudson)	75 mg phenylpropanolamine HCl	4 mg chlorpheniramine maleate	1 q am and hs	In 10s.	5.3
otc	**Demazin Tablets** (Schering-Plough)	25 mg phenylpropanolamine HCl	4 mg chlorpheniramine maleate	2 q 8 h	Sugar. In 24s and 100s.	12
Rx	**Alersule Capsules** (Misemer)	20 mg phenylephrine HCl	8 mg chlorpheniramine maleate	1 q 12 h	Black/clear. In 100s.	12
Rx	**Allent Capsules** (Ascher)	120 mg pseudoephedrine HCl	12 mg brompheniramine maleate	1 q 12 h	Dye free. (225-480). Clear. In 100s.	15
Rx	**Bromfed Capsules** (Muro)				Sucrose. (Bromfed Muro 12-120). Lt. green/clear. In 100s & 500s.	19
Rx	**Endafed Capsules** (UAD)				In 100s.	17

* Cost Index based on cost per capsule or tablet.

(Continued on following page)

Refer to the general discussion of these products beginning on page 990.
Content given per tablet.

Decongestants and Antihistamines, Sustained Release (Cont.)

	Product & Distributor	Decongestant	Antihistamine	Average Adult Dose	How Supplied	C.I.*
Rx[1]	**Bromatapp Extended Release Tablets** (Various, eg, Copley, Moore)	75 mg phenylpropanolamine HCl	12 mg brompheniramine maleate	1 q 12 h	In 12s, 24s, 30s, 100s and 1000s.	NA
otc	**Dimaphen Release-Tabs (Tablets)** (Major)				Lactose. In 12s and 24s.	12
otc	**Dimetapp Extentabs (Tablets)** (Robins)				Sucrose. (Dimetapp AHR). Pale blue. Sugar coated. In 12s, 24s, 48s, 100s, 500s and UD 100s.	15
otc	**Allergy Formula Sinutab Tablets** (Parke-Davis)	120 mg pseudoephedrine sulfate	6 mg dexbrompheniramine maleate	1 q 12 h	Sugar, sucrose. In 10s and 20s.	17
Rx	**Disobrom Tablets** (Geneva)			1 q am and hs	In 100s and 1000s.	8.5
Rx[1]	**Dexaphen S.A. Tablets** (Major)			1 q 12 h	In 10s, 20s, 40s, 100s and 500s.	1.5
otc	**Disophrol Chronotabs (Tablets)** (Schering-Plough)				Sugar, lactose. In 100s.	19
otc	**Drixoral Sustained-Action Tablets** (Schering-Plough)				Sugar, lactose. In 10s, 20s and 40s.	18
otc	**Histodrix Tablets** (Rugby)				Blue. Sugar coated. In 20s.	8.5
Rx	**Par-Drix Tablets** (Parmed)			1 q am and hs	Green. In 1000s.	4
otc	**Resporal Tablets** (Pioneer Pharm.)			1 q 12 h	In 10s, 20s, 30s, 50s, 100s and 1000s.	17
otc	**12 Hour Antihistamine Nasal Decongestant Tablets** (URL)				Sugar, sucrose. In 10s.	18

* Cost Index based on cost per tablet.

[1] Products available *otc* or *Rx*, depending on product labeling.

(Continued on following page)

UPPER RESPIRATORY COMBINATIONS (Cont.)

Refer to the general discussion of these products beginning on page 990
Content given per capsule or tablet.

Decongestants and Antihistamines, Sustained Release (Cont.)

	Product & Distributor	Decongestant	Antihistamine	Average Adult Dose	How Supplied	C.I.*
otc	**Actifed 12-Hour Capsules** (Burroughs Wellcome)	120 mg pseudoephedrine HCl	5 mg triprolidine HCl	1 q 12 h	Sucrose. (Actifed 12-Hour). In 10s & 20s.	15
Rx	**Tavist-D Tablets** (Sandoz)	75 mg phenylpropanolamine HCl	1.34 mg clemastine fumarate	1 q 12 h	Lactose. (Tavist D). White. Film coated. In 100s.	34
Rx	**Carbiset-TR Tablet** (Nutripharm)	120 mg pseudoephedrine HCl	8 mg carbinoxamine maleate	1 q 12 h	Dye free. (512). In 100s.	7.3
Rx	**Carbodec TR Tabs** (Rugby)			1 bid	Film coated. In 100s.	12
Rx	**Rondec-TR Tablets** (Ross)			1 bid	Sugar, lactose. (6240). Blue. Film coated. In 100s.	27
Rx	**Trinalin Repetabs (Tablets)** (Schering)	120 mg pseudoephedrine sulfate	1 mg azatadine maleate	1 bid	Sugar, lactose. (Schering or Trinalin 703). Coral. In 100s.	25
Rx	**Seldane-D Tablets** (Marion Merrell Dow)	120 mg pseudoephedrine HCl	60 mg terfenadine	1 q am and hs	Lactose. (Seldane-D). White to off-white. Capsule shape. In 100s.	49
Rx	**Atrohist Sprinkle Capsules** (Adams)	10 mg phenylephrine HCl	2 mg brompheniramine maleate, 25 mg phenyltoloxamine citrate	3 q 12 h	(Adams/022). Yellow and clear. In 100s.	18
Rx	**Comhist LA Capsules** (Procter & Gamble Pharm.)	20 mg phenylephrine HCl	4 mg chlorpheniramine maleate, 50 mg phenyltoloxamine citrate	1 q 8 to 12 h	Sugar. (Comhist LA 0149 0446). Yellow and clear. In 100s.	20
Rx	**Nolamine Tablets** (Carnrick)	50 mg phenylpropanolamine HCl	4 mg chlorpheniramine maleate, 24 mg phenindamine tartrate	1 q 8 h	(C 86204). Pink. In 100s & 250s.	11
Rx	**Panadyl Tablets** (Misemer)	50 mg phenylpropanolamine HCl	25 mg pyrilamine maleate, 25 mg pheniramine maleate	1 tid	In 100s and 1000s.	11
Rx	**Triaminic TR Tablets** (Sandoz)				Lactose, sucrose. (Dorsey Triaminic TR). Yellow. Coated. In 100s.	15
Rx	**Poly-Histine-D Capsules** (Bock)	50 mg phenylpropanolamine HCl	16 mg phenyltoloxamine citrate, 16 mg pyrilamine maleate, 16 mg pheniramine maleate	1 q 8 to 12 h	In 100s.	20
Rx	**Panadyl Forte Tablets** (Misemer)	50 mg phenylpropanolamine HCl, 25 mg phenylephrine HCl	8 mg chlorpheniramine maleate	1 q 12 h	Yellow. In 100s.	10

* Cost Index based on cost per capsule or tablet.

(Continued on following page)

UPPER RESPIRATORY COMBINATIONS (Cont.)

Refer to the general discussion of these products beginning on page 990
Content given per capsule or tablet.

Decongestants and Antihistamines, Sustained Release (Cont.)

	Product & Distributor	Decongestant	Antihistamine	Average Adult Dose	How Supplied	C.I.*
Rx	**Nasahist Capsules** (Keene)	40 mg phenylpropanolamine HCl, 10 mg phenylephrine HCl	12 mg chlorpheniramine maleate	1 q 12 h	Orange and clear. In 100s.	2.5
Rx	**Bromatapp Extended Tablets** (Moore)	15 mg phenylpropanolamine HCl, 15 mg phenylephrine HCl	12 mg brompheniramine maleate	1 q 12 h	In 100s.	2.5
Rx	**Bromophen T.D. Tablets** (Rugby)			1 q am and hs	In 1000s.	3.5
Rx	**Dimaphen S.A. Tabs** (Major)			1 bid	Light blue. In 100s and 1000s.	3.5
	Partapp TD Tablets (Parmed)			1 q am and hs	In 1000s.	1.5
Rx	**Tamine S.R. Tablets** (Geneva)			1 q am and hs or 1 q 8 h	Blue. In 100s and 1000s.	12
Rx	**Veltap Lanatabs** (Lannett)			1 q 12 h	In 100s, 500s and 1000s.	2
Rx	**Decongestabs Tablets** (Various, eg, Dixon-Shane, Geneva, Moore, Parmed)	40 mg phenylpropanolamine HCl, 10 mg phenylephrine HCl	5 mg chlorpheniramine maleate, 15 mg phenyltoloxamine citrate	1 tid	In 100s, 500s and 1000s.	1.5+
Rx	**Decongestant Tablets** (Various, eg, Geneva, Moore)				In 100s and 1000s.	1+
Rx	**Naldecon Tablets** (Bristol Labs)				Lactose, sucrose. In 100s and 500s.	202
Rx	**Nalgest Tablets** (Major)				In 100s and 1000s.	2
Rx	**New Decongestant Tablets** (Goldline)				Blue specks. In 100s and 1000s.	2
Rx	**Par Decon Tablets** (Par)				In 100s, 500s and 1000s.	NA
Rx	**Quadra-Hist Tablets** (Schein)				In 100s and 1000s.	2
Rx	**Tri-Phen-Chlor T.R. Tablets** (Rugby)				In 1000s.	1.5
Rx	**Uni-Decon Tablets** (URL)				In 100s & 1000s.	2

* Cost Index based on cost per capsule or tablet.

UPPER RESPIRATORY COMBINATIONS (Cont.)

Refer to the general discussion of these products beginning on page 990
Content given per capsule.

Pediatric Decongestants and Antihistamines, Sustained Release

	Product & Distributor	Decongestant	Antihistamine	Average Dose	How Supplied	C.I.*
Rx	**Kronofed-A Jr. Kronocaps** (Ferndale)	60 mg pseudoephedrine HCl	4 mg chlorpheniramine maleate	*Children (6 to 12 years)* – 1 q 12 h	Dye free. White/clear. In 100s and 500s.	8
Rx	**Bromfed-PD Capsules** (Muro)	60 mg pseudoephedrine HCl	6 mg brompheniramine maleate	*Children (6 to 12 years)* – 1 q 12 h	Sucrose. (Bromfed-PD Muro 6-60). Green/clear. In 100s & 500s.	17
Rx	**Dallergy-JR. Capsules** (Laser)				(Dallergy-Jr Laser 176). Maize/clear. In 100s and 1000s.	11
Rx	**Poly-Histine-D Ped Caps** (Bock)	25 mg phenylpropanolamine HCl	8 mg phenyltoloxamine citrate, 8 mg pyrilamine maleate, 8 mg pheniramine maleate	*Children (6 to 12 years)* – 1 q 8 to 12 h	In 100s.	17

* Cost Index based on cost per capsule.

UPPER RESPIRATORY COMBINATIONS (Cont.)

Refer to the general discussion of these products beginning on page 990
Content given per capsule or tablet.

Decongestants and Antihistamines, Capsules and Tablets

	Product & Distributor	Decongestant	Antihistamine	Average Adult Dose	How Supplied	C.I.*
Rx	**Bromfed Tablets** (Muro)	60 mg pseudoephedrine HCl	4 mg brompheniramine maleate	1 q 4 h	(Muro 4060). White, scored. In 100s.	8.8
otc	**Dristan Allergy Caplets** (Whitehall)			1 q 4 to 6 h up to 4/day	In 20s.	NA
otc	**Co-Pyronil 2 Pulvules** (Dista)	60 mg pseudoephedrine HCl	4 mg chlorpheniramine maleate	1 q 6 h	In 100s.	17
Rx	**Deconamine Tablets** (Berlex)			1 tid or qid	Dye free. (Berlex 184). White, scored. In 100s.	12
Rx	**Dura-Tap/PD Capsules** (Dura)			2 q 12 h	(51479-007). Blue and clear. In 100s.	14
otc	**Fedahist Tablets** (Schwarz Pharma Kremers Urban)			1 q 4 to 6 h up to 4/day	Lactose. Scored. In 100s.	8.2
otc	**Isoclor Tablets** (Fisons)				In 100s.	12
Rx	**Klerist-D Tablets** (Nutripharm)			1 tid or qid	Dye free. In 24s and 100s.	4
otc	**Napril Tablets** (Randob)			1 q 4 to 6 h up to 4/day	Lactose. Scored. In 30s.	NA
otc	**Pseudo-gest Plus Tablets** (Major)				In 24s and 100s.	2.5
otc	**Sudafed Plus Tablets** (Burroughs Wellcome)				Lactose. White, scored. In 24s and 48s.	9.1
otc	**Chlor-Trimeton 4 Hour Relief Tablets** (Schering-Plough)	60 mg pseudoephedrine sulfate	4 mg chlorpheniramine maleate	1 q 4 to 6 h up to 4/day	Lactose. (901). In 24s and 48s.	8.9
otc	**Allerest Maximum Strength Tablets** (Fisons)	30 mg pseudoephedrine	2 mg chlorpheniramine maleate	2 q 4 to 6 h up to 8/day	(Allerest). In 24s, 48s and 72s.	8.7
otc	**Conex D.A. Tablets** (Forest)	37.5 mg phenylpropanolamine HCl	4 mg chlorpheniramine maleate	1 q 4 to 6 h	In 100s and 1000s.	2.2

* Cost Index based on cost per capsule or tablet.

(Continued on following page)

UPPER RESPIRATORY COMBINATIONS (Cont.)

Refer to the general discussion of these products beginning on page 990 Content given per tablet or capsule.

Decongestants and Antihistamines, Capsules and Tablets (Cont.)

	Product & Distributor	Decongestant	Antihistamine	Average Adult Dose	How Supplied	C.I.*
otc	**Allergy Relief Medicine Tablets** (Rugby)	25 mg phenylpropanolamine HCl	4 mg chlorpheniramine maleate	1 q 4 h up to 4/day	In 20s.	5.1
otc	**A.R.M. Caplets** (SK-Beecham)			1 q 4 h	(ARM). In 20s and 40s.	11
otc	**Triaminic Allergy Tablets** (Sandoz)				In 24s.	11
otc	**Tri•Nefrin Extra Strength Tablets** (Pfeiffer)				Lactose. In 24s.	6.8
otc	**Chlor-Rest Tablets** (Rugby)	18.7 mg phenylpropanolamine HCl	2 mg chlorpheniramine maleate	2 q 4 h up to 8/day	In 100s.	1.8
otc	**Triaminic Cold Tablets** (Sandoz)	12.5 mg phenylpropanolamine HCl	2 mg chlorpheniramine maleate	2 q 4 h	Lactose, saccharin. In 24s.	7.8
otc	**Histatab Plus Tablets** (Century)	5 mg phenylephrine HCl	2 mg chlorpheniramine maleate	2 initially then 1 q 4 h	In 100s and 1000s.	1
otc	**Bromatapp Tablets** (Moore)	25 mg phenylpropanolamine HCl	4 mg brompheniramine maleate	1 q 4 h	In 24s, 100s and 1000s.	1.6
otc	**Dimaphen OTC Tabs** (Major)			1 q 4 to 6 h	In 24s.	4.8
otc	**Dimetapp Tablets** (Robins)			1 q 4 h	(AHR 2254). Blue, scored. In 24s.	10
otc	**Dimetane Decongestant Caplets** (Robins)	10 mg phenylephrine HCl	4 mg brompheniramine maleate	1 q 4 h	(AHR 2117). Light blue, scored. Capsule shape. In 24s and 48s.	7.9
otc	**Disophrol Tablets** (Schering-Plough)	60 mg pseudoephedrine sulfate	2 mg dexbrompheniramine maleate	1 q 4 to 6 h	Sugar. (WBS). In 100s.	12
otc	**Benadryl Decongestant Kapseals and Tablets** (P-D)	60 mg pseudoephedrine HCl	25 mg diphenhydramine HCl	1 q 4 to 6 h, up to 4/day	**Kapseals:** Lactose. In 24s. **Tablets:** Film coated. In 24s.	3.4 3.4
Rx	**Carbiset Tablets** (Nutripharm)	60 mg pseudoephedrine HCl	4 mg carbinoxamine maleate	1 qid	Dye free. (NPL 510). In 100s, 500s.	6.2
Rx	**Carbodec Tablets** (Rugby)				In 100s.	6.9
Rx	**Rondec Tablets** (Ross)				Lactose. (5726). Orange. Film coated. In 100s and 500s.	15

* Cost Index based on cost per tablet or capsule.

(Continued on following page)

UPPER RESPIRATORY COMBINATIONS (Cont.)

Refer to the general discussion of these products beginning on page 990   Content given per tablet.

Decongestants and Antihistamines, Capsules and Tablets (Cont.)

	Product & Distributor	Decongestant	Antihistamine	Average Adult Dose	How Supplied	C.I.*
Rx	**Comhist Tablets** (Procter & Gamble Pharm.)	10 mg phenylephrine HCl	2 mg chlorpheniramine maleate, 25 mg phenyltoloxamine citrate	1 or 2 tid (q 8 h)	Sugar. (Comhist 0149 0444). Yellow, scored. In 100s.	19
Rx	**R-Tannate Tablets** (Various, eg, Copley, Schein, Warner-C)	25 mg phenylephrine tannate	8 mg chlorpheniramine tannate, 25 mg pyrilamine tannate	1 or 2 q 12 h	In 100s.	16+
Rx	**Decotan Tablets** (Sidmak)				(SL/520). Orange, scored. Capsule shape. In 100s, 500s and 1000s.	21
Rx	**Rhinatate Tablets** (Major)				In 100s and 250s.	21
Rx	**R-Tannamine Tablets** (Qualitest)				In 100s.	21
Rx	**Tanoral Tablets** (Parmed)				In 100s.	26
Rx	**Triotann Tablets** (Duramed)				(INV 234). Buff, scored. Capsule shape. In 100s and 500s.	NA
Rx	**Tri-Tannate Tablets** (Rugby)				In 100s and 250s.	19
Rx	**Rynatan Tablets** (Wallace)				(Wallace 713). Buff. Capsule shape. In 100s and 500s.	38
Rx	**Tritan Tablets** (Vitarine)	25 mg phenylephrine tannate	8 mg chlorpheniramine tannate, 25 mg pyrilamine maleate	1 or 2 q 12 h	Lactose. Tan, scored. In 100s and 1000s.	NA
Rx	**Hista-Vadrin Decongestant Tablets** (Scherer)	40 mg phenylpropanolamine HCl, 5 mg phenylephrine HCl	6 mg chlorpheniramine maleate	1 q 6 h	In 100s.	19
Rx	**Histalet Forte Tablets** (Solvay)	50 mg phenylpropanolamine HCl, 10 mg phenylephrine HCl	4 mg chlorpheniramine maleate, 25 mg pyrilamine maleate	1 bid or tid	Lactose, sugar. (Solvay 1039). White with blue dots, scored. Capsule shape. In 100s and 250s.	35
Rx	**Histatime Forte Caplets** (Major)				In 100s.	14
Rx	**Vanex Forte Caplets** (Abana)				(A/A). Pink. Film coated. In 100s.	27

* Cost Index based on cost per tablet.

(Continued on following page)

UPPER RESPIRATORY COMBINATIONS (Cont.)

Refer to the general discussion of these products beginning on page 990. Content given per capsule or tablet.

Decongestants and Antihistamines, Capsules and Tablets (Cont.)

	Product & Distributor	Decongestant	Antihistamine	Average Adult Dose	How Supplied	C.I.*
Rx[1]	**Pseudoephedrine HCl and Triprolidine HCl Tablets** (Various, eg, Major, Purepac, UDL, West-Ward)	60 mg pseudoephedrine HCl	2.5 mg triprolidine HCl	1 q 4 to 6 h up to 4/day	In 24s, 100s and 1000s.	1.2+
otc	**Actagen Tablets** (Goldline)			1 q 4 to 6 h up to 4/day	White. In 100s and 1000s.	2.4
otc	**Actifed** (Burroughs Wellcome)				**Capsules:** (Actifed). In 10s & 20s.	15
					Tablets: Sucrose, lactose. (Actifed M2A). White. In 12s, 24s, 48s and 100s.	7.9
otc	**Allercon Tablets** (Parmed)				In 100s and 1000s.	3.1
otc	**Allerfrin Tablets** (Rugby)				In 24s, 100s and 1000s.	4.9
otc	**Allergy Cold Tablets** (Geneva)				Scored. In 100s.	2.3
otc	**Aprodine Tablets** (Major)				In 1000s.	1.1
otc	**Atrofed Tablets** (Genetco)				Scored. In 1000s.	1.8
otc	**Cenafed Plus Tabs** (Century)				In 100s and 1000s.	6.6
otc	**Genac Tablets** (Goldline)				White. In 24s and 100s.	6.6
otc	**Triafed Tablets** (Schein)				Lactose. Scored. In 24s, 100s and 1000s.	1.8
Rx	**Trifed Tablets** (Geneva)			1 tid or qid	(GG 25). White, scored. In 100s and 1000s.	5.6
otc	**Triposed Tablets** (Halsey)			1 q 4 to 6 h up to 4/day	Lactose. White, scored. In 24s, 30s, 100s and 1000s.	3.9

* Cost Index based on cost per capsule or tablet.

[1] Products available *otc* or *Rx*, depending on product labeling.

UPPER RESPIRATORY COMBINATIONS (Cont.)

Refer to the general discussion of these products beginning on page 990 .
Content given per 5 ml.

Decongestants and Antihistamines, Liquids

	Product & Distributor	Decongestant	Antihistamine	Other	Average Adult Dose	How Supplied	C.I.*
otc	**Rhinosyn Syrup** (Great Southern)	60 mg pseudo-ephedrine HCl	4 mg chlorpheniramine maleate	0.45% alcohol, sucrose	5 ml q 4 h	In 120 ml and pt.	8.6
Rx	**Histalet Syrup** (Solvay)	45 mg pseudo-ephedrine HCl	3 mg chlorpheniramine maleate	Saccharin, sorbitol, sugar	10 ml qid	In pt.	17
Rx *sf*	**Anamine Syrup** (Mayrand)	30 mg pseudo-ephedrine HCl	2 mg chlorpheniramine maleate		10 ml q 4 to 6 h	Alcohol and dye free. In pt.	7.6
otc *sf*	**Chlorafed Liquid** (Hauck)					Alcohol and dye free. In 120 and 480 ml.	9.3
Rx	**Deconamine Syrup** (Berlex)			Sorbitol, sucrose	5 to 10 ml tid or qid	Alcohol and dye free. Grape flavor. In pt.	11
otc	**Fedahist Decongestant Syrup** (Schwarz Pharma Kremers Urban)			Saccharin, sorbitol, sucrose	10 ml q 4 to 6 h up to 40 ml/day	Alcohol free. In 120 ml.	9.9
otc *sf*	**Hayfebrol Liquid** (Scot-Tussin)				10 ml q 6 h	Alcohol and dye free. In 118 ml.	14
otc	**Isoclor Liquid** (Fisons)			Sorbitol	10 ml q 4 to 6 h up to 40 ml/day	In pt.	10
otc	**Myfedrine Plus Liquid** (PBI)				10 ml q 4 to 6 h up to 40 ml/day	Lemon flavor. In 120 ml.	NA
otc	**Rhinosyn-PD Syrup** (Great Southern)			1.2% alcohol, sucrose	10 ml q 4 h	In 120 ml.	7.3
otc *sf*	**Ryna Liquid** (Wallace)			Sorbitol	10 ml q 6 h	Alcohol and dye free. In 118 and 473 ml.	19
otc	**Sudafed Plus Liquid** (Burroughs Wellcome)			Sucrose	10 ml q 4 to 6 h up to 40 ml/day	Lemon flavor. In 118 ml.	11

* Cost Index based on cost per 5 ml.
sf – Sugar free.

(Continued on following page)

UPPER RESPIRATORY COMBINATIONS (Cont.)

Refer to the general discussion of these products beginning on page 990.
Content given per 5 ml.

Decongestants and Antihistamines, Liquids (Cont.)

	Product & Distributor	Decongestant	Antihistamine	Other	Average Adult Dose	How Supplied	C.I.*
otc	**Demazin Syrup** (Schering-Plough)	12.5 mg phenylpropanolamine HCl	2 mg chlorpheniramine maleate	7.5% alcohol, menthol, sugar	10 ml q 4 to 6 h	In 118 ml.	11
otc	**Genamin Cold Syrup** (Goldline)				10 ml q 4 h	Alcohol free. In 120 ml.	5.6
otc	**Myminic Syrup** (PBI)					Pineapple-orange flavor. In 120 & 240 ml, pt and gal.	4.2
otc	**Triaminic Syrup** (Sandoz)			Sorbitol, sucrose	10 ml q 4 h	Alcohol free. In 120 ml.	9.1
otc *sf*	**Trind Liquid** (Mead Johnson Nutritional)			5% alcohol	10 ml q 4 h	Orange flavor. In 150 ml.	12
otc	**Tripalgen Cold Syrup** (Barre)				10 ml q 4 to 6 hr	Orange flavor. In 120, 240 and 480 ml.	NA
otc	**Triphenyl Syrup** (Rugby)			Sorbitol, sucrose	10 ml q 4 h	In 118 ml and pt.	4.5
otc	**Children's NyQuil Nighttime Head Cold, Allergy Formula Liquid** (Richardson-Vicks)	10 mg pseudoephedrine HCl	0.67 mg chlorpheniramine maleate	Sorbitol, sucrose	15 to 30 ml at bedtime	Alcohol free. Grape flavor. In 120 ml.	NA
Rx	**Tussanil Plain Syrup** (Misemer)	10 mg phenylephrine HCl	4 mg chlorpheniramine maleate	5% alcohol	5 ml tid or qid	Grape flavor. In 480 ml.	9.4

* Cost Index based on cost per 5 ml.
sf – Sugar free.

(Continued on following page)

UPPER RESPIRATORY COMBINATIONS (Cont.)

Refer to the general discussion of these products beginning on page 990.
Content given per 5 ml.

Decongestants and Antihistamines, Liquids (Cont.)

	Product & Distributor	Decongestant	Antihistamine	Other	Average Adult Dose	How Supplied	C.I.*
otc	**Dallergy-D Syrup** (Laser)	5 mg phenylephrine HCl	2 mg chlorpheniramine maleate	Sugar	10 ml q 4 h	Alcohol free. Raspberry-vanilla flavor. In 118 ml.	7.7
otc	**Dihistine Elixir** (Various, eg, Barre, Goldline, Moore)				10 ml q 4 h	In 120 ml, pt and gal.	7.4+
Rx	**Histor-D Syrup** (Hauck)			2% alcohol	5 to 10 ml q 4 to 6 h	In 480 ml.	7.1
otc *sf*	**Decohistine Elixir** (PBI)			5% alcohol	10 ml q 4 h	Fruit flavor. In 120 ml, pt and gal.	3.6
otc *sf*	**Novahistine Elixir** (Marion Merrell Dow)			5% alcohol, sorbitol	10 ml q 4 h	In 120 ml.	11
otc	**Ru-Tuss Liquid** (Boots)			5% alcohol, saccharin, glucose, menthol	10 ml q 4 to 6 h	In 473 ml.	7.5
otc	**Bromaline Elixir** (Rugby)	12.5 mg phenylpropanolamine HCl	2 mg brompheniramine maleate	2.3% alcohol, saccharin, sorbitol	10 ml q 4 to 6 h	Grape flavor. In 118 ml, pt and gal.	4.9
otc *sf*	**Bromatap Elixir** (Goldline)				10 ml q 4 h	Grape flavor. In 120 and 240 ml, pt and gal.	2.9
otc *sf*	**Bromphen Elixir** (Schein)					Grape flavor. In 118 and 237 ml and pt.	5.6
otc	**Dimaphen Elixir** (Major)			2.5% alcohol, saccharin, sorbitol	10 ml q 4 to 6 h	Grape flavor. In 120 and 240 ml, pt and gal.	4.4
otc	**Dimetapp Elixir** (Robins)				10 ml q 4 h	Grape flavor. In 120, 240 and 360 ml, pt, gal and UD 5 ml.	28
otc	**Genatap Elixir** (Goldline)					Grape flavor. In 118 ml.	5.2
otc *sf*	**Partapp Elixir** (Parmed)					Grape flavor. In 118 ml.	4.4
otc	**Myphetapp Elixir** (PBI)			2.3% alcohol	10 ml q 4 h	Grape flavor. In 118 ml, pt.	1.9

* Cost Index based on cost per 5 ml. *sf* – Sugar free.

(Continued on following page)

UPPER RESPIRATORY COMBINATIONS (Cont.)

Refer to the general discussion of these products beginning on page 990.
Content given per 5 ml.

Decongestants and Antihistamines, Liquids (Cont.)

	Product & Distributor	Decongestant	Antihistamine	Other	Average Adult Dose	How Supplied	C.I.*
otc	**Bromfed Syrup** (Muro)	30 mg pseudo-ephedrine HCl	2 mg brompheniramine maleate	Saccharin, sorbitol, sucrose	10 ml q 4 to 6 h up to 40 ml/day	Orange-lemon flavor. Alcohol free. In 120 and 480 ml.	11
otc	**Drixoral Syrup** (Schering-Plough)	30 mg pseudo-ephedrine sulfate	2 mg brompheniramine maleate	Sorbitol, sugar	10 ml q 4 to 6 h up to 40 ml/day	Alcohol free. In 118 ml.	11
otc	**Dimetane Decongestant Elixir** (Robins)	5 mg phenylephrine HCl	2 mg brompheniramine maleate	2.3% alcohol, sorbitol	10 ml q 4 h	Grape flavor. In 120 ml.	9.4
otc	**Benylin Decongestant Liquid** (Parke-Davis)	30 mg pseudo-ephedrine HCl	12.5 mg diphen-hydramine HCl	5% alcohol, saccharin, sucrose, menthol, glucose	10 ml q 4 h up to 40 ml/day	In 118 ml.	NA
otc	**Benadryl Decongestant Elixir** (Parke-Davis)				10 ml q 4 to 6 h up to 40 ml/day	In 118 ml.	11
Rx	**Promethazine VC Syrup** (Various, eg, Cenci, Dixon-Shane, Geneva, Lederle, PBI, Qualitest, Rugby, Schein, URL)	5 mg phenylephrine HCl	6.25 mg promethazine HCl	Alcohol	5 ml q 4 to 6 h	In 120 ml, pt and gal.	4.3+
Rx	**Prometh VC Plain Liquid** (Various, eg, Barre-National, Goldline, Moore)			Alcohol	5 ml q 4 to 6 h	In 120 ml, pt and gal.	4.2+
Rx	**Promethazine DC Plain Syrup** (Lannett)			7% alcohol	5 ml q 4 to 6 h	In 120 ml, pt and gal.	1.9
Rx	**Pherazine VC Syrup** (Halsey)			7% alcohol, sorbitol, sugar	5 ml q 4 to 6 h	In 120 ml, pt and gal.	1.9
Rx	**Phenergan VC Syrup** (Wyeth-Ayerst)			7% alcohol, saccharin	5 ml q 4 to 6 h	In 118 ml and pt.	6.9

* Cost Index based on cost per 5 ml.

(Continued on following page)

UPPER RESPIRATORY COMBINATIONS (Cont.)

Refer to the general discussion of these products beginning on page 990.
Content given per 5 ml.

Decongestants and Antihistamines, Liquids (Cont.)

	Product & Distributor	Decongestant	Antihistamine	Other	Average Adult Dose	How Supplied	C.I.*
Rx	**Carbodec Syrup** (Rugby)	60 mg pseudo-ephedrine HCl	4 mg carbinoxamine maleate		5 ml qid	In 473 ml.	4
Rx	**Cardec-S Syrup** (Barre-National)					In pt.	5.5
Rx *sf*	**Rondec Syrup** (Ross)			Sorbitol	5 ml qid	Alcohol free. Berry flavor. In 120 and 480 ml.	14
Rx[1]	**Triprolidine HCl w/Pseudo-ephedrine HCl Syrup** (Various, eg, Cenci, Major)	30 mg pseudo-ephedrine HCl	1.25 mg triprolidine HCl		10 ml q 4 to 6 h up to 40 ml/day	In 120 and 240 ml, pt and gal.	5.6+
otc	**Actagen Syrup** (Goldline)					Pineapple flavor. In 118 ml.	7.1
otc	**Actifed Syrup** (Burroughs Wellcome)			Sorbitol	10 ml q 4 to 6 h up to 40 ml/day	In 118 and 473 ml.	10
otc	**Allerfrin OTC Syrup** (Rugby)				10 ml q 4 to 6 h up to 40 ml/day	In pt.	5.3
otc	**Allerphed Syrup** (Great Southern)					In 120 ml.	6.3
otc	**Triofed Syrup** (Barre-National)					In 120 ml, pt and gal.	4.7
otc	**Triposed Syrup** (Halsey)			Sucrose	10 ml q 4 to 6 h up to 40 ml/day	In 236 ml, pt and gal.	5.4

* Cost Index based on cost per 5 ml.
[1] Products available *otc* or *Rx,* depending on product labeling.
sf – Sugar free.

(Continued on following page)

UPPER RESPIRATORY COMBINATIONS (Cont.)

Refer to the general discussion of these products beginning on page 990.
Content given per 5 ml.

Decongestants and Antihistamines, Liquids (Cont.)

	Product & Distributor	Decongestant	Antihistamine	Other	Average Adult Dose	How Supplied	C.I.*
Rx	**Poly-Histine-D Elixir** (Bock)	12.5 mg phenylpropanolamine HCl	4 mg pyrilamine maleate, 4 mg phenyltoloxamine citrate, 4 mg pheniramine maleate	4% alcohol	10 ml q 4 h	In 120 and 480 ml.	11
Rx	**Veltap Elixir** (Lannett)	5 mg phenylpropanolamine HCl, 5 mg phenylephrine HCl	4 mg brompheniramine maleate	3% alcohol	5 to 10 ml tid or qid	In pt and gal.	1.6
Rx	**Naldelate Syrup** (Various, eg, Barre-National, Qualitest, URL)	20 mg phenylpropanolamine HCl, 5 mg phenylephrine HCl	2.5 mg chlorpheniramine maleate, 7.5 mg phenyltoloxamine citrate		5 ml q 3 to 4 h up to 20 ml/day	In pt and gal.	5.3+
Rx	**Nalgest Syrup** (Major)					In pt and gal.	4.4
Rx	**Nalspan Syrup** (PBI)					Alcohol free. Strawberry flavor. In pt.	4.3
Rx	**Naldecon Syrup** (Bristol Labs)			Sorbitol		In 480 ml.	13
Rx	**New Decongest Syrup** (Goldline)				5 ml q 4 h up to 20 ml/day	Grape flavor. In pt.	5.4
Rx	**Quadra-Hist ER Syrup** (Schein)					In pt.	4.3
Rx	**Tri-Phen-Chlor Syrup** (Rugby)					In pt.	3.1

* Cost Index based on cost per 5 ml.

UPPER RESPIRATORY COMBINATIONS (Cont.)

Refer to the general discussion of these products beginning on page 990
Content given per 5 ml liquid, 1 ml drops, pack or tablet.

Pediatric Decongestants and Antihistamines

	Product & Distributor	Decongestant	Antihistamine	Other	Average Dose	How Supplied	C.I.*
otc	**Children's Allerest Tablets** (Fisons)	9.4 mg phenylpropanolamine HCl	1 mg chlorpheniramine maleate	Saccharin, sorbitol	*Children (6 to ≤ 12 yrs)* – 2 q 4 h up to 8/day	Chewable. (C Allerest). In 24s.	8.3
otc	**Snaplets-D Granules** (Baker Cummins)	6.25 mg phenylpropanolamine HCl	1 mg chlorpheniramine maleate		*6 to < 12 yrs* – 2 packs q 4 h	Taste free. In 30s.	NA
otc	**Triaminic Chewable Tablets** (Sandoz)	6.25 mg phenylpropanolamine HCl	0.5 mg chlorpheniramine maleate	Saccharin, sucrose.	*Children (6 to 12 yrs)* – 2 q 4 h	In 24s.	6.1
Rx *sf*	**Rondec Oral Drops** (Ross)	25 mg pseudoephedrine HCl per ml	2 mg carbinoxamine maleate per ml	Sorbitol	*Infants* – 0.25 to 1 ml qid	Alcohol free. Berry flavor. In 30 ml w/dropper.	3.1
otc	**Dorcol Pediatric Cold Formula Liquid** (Sandoz)	15 mg pseudoephedrine HCl	1 mg chlorpheniramine maleate	Sorbitol, sucrose	*Children (6 to < 12)* – 10 ml q 4 to 6 h up to 40 ml/day	Alcohol free. In 120 ml.	9.1
otc	**Coltab Children's Tablets** (Hauck)	2.5 mg phenylephrine HCl	1 mg chlorpheniramine maleate		*Children (> 2 yrs)* – 1 to 2 tid	Chewable. In 1000s.	5.4
Rx	**R-Tannate Pediatric Suspension** (Various)	5 mg phenylephrine tannate	2 mg chlorpheniramine tannate, 12.5 mg pyrilamine tannate		*Children (> 6 yrs)* – 5 to 10 ml q 12 h *(2 to 6 yrs)* – 2.5 to 5 ml q 12 h *(< 2 yrs)* – Titrate individually	In 480 ml.	14+
Rx	**R-Tannamine Pediatric Suspension** (Qualitest)					In pt.	NA
Rx	**Rynatan Pediatric Suspension** (Wallace)			Saccharin, sucrose		Strawberry-currant flavor. In 120 and 480 ml.	31
Rx	**Triotann Pediatric Suspension** (Various, eg, Duramed, Parmed)					In pt.	19+
Rx	**Tritann Pediatric Suspension** (Geneva)			Saccharin, sucrose, kaolin, parabens		In 473 ml.	NA
Rx	**Tri-Tannate Pediatric Suspension** (Rugby)					In 473 ml.	16

* Cost Index based on cost per 5 ml liquid, 1 ml drops, pack or tablet.

sf – Sugar free.

(Continued on following page)

UPPER RESPIRATORY COMBINATIONS (Cont.)

Refer to the general discussion of these products beginning on page 990 .
Content given per 5 ml liquid or 1 ml drops.

Pediatric Decongestants and Antihistamines (Cont.)

	Product & Distributor	Decongestant	Antihistamine	Other	Average Dose	How Supplied	C.I.*
Rx	**Triaminic Oral Infant Drops** (Sandoz)	20 mg phenylpropanolamine HCl per ml	10 mg pyrilamine maleate and 10 mg pheniramine maleate per ml	Sorbitol, sucrose, saccharin	*Infants* – 1 drop/2 lbs qid	In 15 ml dropper bottle (≈ 24 drops/ml).	33
Rx	**Naldelate Pediatric Syrup** (Various, eg, Barre-National, URL)	5 mg phenylpropanolamine HCl, 1.25 mg phenylephrine HCl	0.5 mg chlorpheniramine maleate, 2 mg phenyltoloxamine citrate		*Children (6 to 12 mos)* – 2.5 ml q 3 to 4 h *(1 to 6 yrs)* – 5 ml q 3 to 4 h *(6 to 12 yrs)* – 10 ml q 3 to 4 h up to 4 doses/day	In 120 ml, pt and gal.	3.1+
Rx	**Naldecon Pediatric Syrup** (Bristol Labs)			Sorbitol		In 480 ml.	12
Rx	**Nalgest Pediatric Syrup** (Major)					In pt and gal.	4.4
Rx *sf*	**New Decongest Pediatric Syrup** (Goldline)					Strawberry flavor. In pt.	4.7
Rx	**Tri-Phen-Chlor Pediatric Syrup** (Rugby)					In pt and gal.	3.1
Rx	**Naldecon Pediatric Drops** (Bristol Labs)			Sorbitol	*Children (3 to 6 mos)* – 0.25 ml q 3 to 4 h *(6 to 12 mos)* – 0.5 ml q 3 to 4 h *(1 to 6 yrs)* – 1 ml q 3 to 4 h up to 4 doses/day	In 30 ml.	16
Rx	**Nalgest Pediatric Dops** (Major)					In 30 ml.	20
Rx *sf*	**New Decongest Pediatric Drops** (Goldline)					Strawberry flavor. In 30 ml.	26
Rx *sf*	**Tri-Phen-Chlor Pediatric Drops** (Rugby)					In 30 ml with dropper.	16

* Cost Index based on cost per 5 ml liquid or 1 ml drops.
sf – Sugar free.

UPPER RESPIRATORY COMBINATIONS (Cont.)

Refer to the general discussion of these products beginning on page 990. Content given per capsule, tablet or pack.

Decongestant, Antihistamine and Analgesic Combinations

	Product & Distributor	Decongestant	Antihistamine	Analgesic/Other	Average Adult Dose	How Supplied	C.I.*
Rx	**Phenate T.D. Tablets** (Hauck)	40 mg phenylpropanolamine HCl	4 mg chlorpheniramine maleate	325 mg acetaminophen	1 q 6 to 8 h	Timed release. In 100s and 1000s.	4.7
otc	**Allerest Sinus Pain Formula Tablets** (Fisons)	30 mg pseudoephedrine HCl	2 mg chlorpheniramine maleate	500 mg acetaminophen	2 q 6 h	In 20s.	5.7
otc	**Maximum Strength Tylenol Allergy Sinus** (McNeil-CPC)					**Caplets:** In 24s and 50s. **Gelcaps:** In 20s and 40s.	5.7 6.7
otc	**Sinarest Extra Strength Tablets** (Fisons)	30 mg pseudoephedrine HCl	2 mg chlorpheniramine maleate	500 mg acetaminophen	2 q 6 h	In 24s.	5.1
otc	**Allerest Headache Strength Tablets** (Fisons)	30 mg pseudoephedrine HCl	2 mg chlorpheniramine maleate	325 mg acetaminophen	2 q 4 h up to 8/day	In 24s.	4.7
otc	**Sinarest Tablets** (Fisons)	30 mg pseudoephedrine HCl	2 mg chlorpheniramine maleate	325 mg acetaminophen	2 q 4 h up to 8/day	In 20s, 40s and 80s.	4.9
otc	**Sinulin Tablets** (Carnrick)	25 mg phenylpropanolamine HCl	4 mg chlorpheniramine maleate	650 mg acetaminophen	1 q 4 to 6 h	In 20s, 100s and UD 168s.	6.7
otc	**Triaminicin Tablets** (Sandoz)			650 mg acetaminophen, lactose	1 q 4 h	In 12s, 24s, 48s, 100s and UD 200s.	6
Rx	**Alumadrine Tablets** (Fleming)	25 mg phenylpropanolamine HCl	4 mg chlorpheniramine maleate	500 mg acetaminophen	2 q 4 to 6 h	Purple, scored. In 100s and 1000s.	2.3
otc	**Pyrroxate Capsules** (Roberts)				1 q 4 h	In 24s and 500s.	4.7
otc	**Conex Plus Tablets** (Forest)	25 mg phenylpropanolamine HCl	4 mg chlorpheniramine maleate	325 mg acetaminophen	1 q 4 h	In 1000s.	1
otc	**BC Multi Symptom Cold Powder Packets** (Block)	25 mg phenylpropanolamine HCl	4 mg chlorpheniramine maleate	650 mg aspirin, lactose	1 dose dissolved in water q 4 h up to 4/day	In 6 and 24s.	28

* Cost Index based on cost per capsule, tablet or pack.

(Continued on following page)

UPPER RESPIRATORY COMBINATIONS (Cont.)

Refer to the general discussion of these products beginning on page 990. Content given per capsule or tablet.

Decongestant, Antihistamine and Anticholinergic Combinations, Sustained Release

	Product & Distributor	Decongestant	Antihistamine	Anticholinergic	Average Adult Dose	Other Content & How Supplied	C.I.*
Rx	**Rhinolar Capsules** (McGregor)	75 mg phenylpropanolamine HCl	8 mg chlorpheniramine maleate	2.5 mg methscopolamine nitrate	1 q 12 h	Dye free. Sucrose. In 60s.	2
Rx	**Alersule Forte Capsules** (Misemer)	20 mg phenylephrine HCl	8 mg chlorpheniramine maleate	2.5 mg methscopolamine nitrate	1 q 12 h	In 100s.	2.1
Rx	**Dallergy Capsules** (Laser)					(Dallergy). Pink and clear. In 100s and 1000s.	2.3
Rx	**Dura-Vent/DA Tablets** (Dura)					(Dura DA). Light brown, scored. In 100s.	1.8
Rx	**Extendryl SR Capsules** (Fleming)					In 100s and 1000s.	NA
Rx	**Histor-D Timecelles (Capsules)** (Hauck)					Black/clear. In 100s and 500s.	2.5
Rx	**Atrohist L.A. Tablets** (Adams)	120 mg pseudoephedrine HCl	4 mg brompheniramine maleate, 50 mg phenyltoloxamine citrate	0.0242 mg atropine sulfate (for immediate release)	1 q 12 h	(Adams/0021). Yellow, scored. In 100s.	3.3
Rx	**Ru-Tuss Tablets** (Boots)	50 mg phenylpropanolamine HCl, 25 mg phenylephrine HCl	8 mg chlorpheniramine maleate	0.19 mg hyoscyamine sulfate, 0.04 mg atropine sulfate, 0.01 mg scopolamine HBr	1 bid	(58). Green, scored. Elongated. In 100s and 500s.	2.2
Rx	**Stahist Tablets** (Huckaby)					Lactose. Light green, scored. In 100s.	
Rx	**Phenahist-TR Tablets** (T.E. Williams)	50 mg phenylpropanolamine HCl, 25 mg phenylephrine HCl	8 mg chlorpheniramine maleate	0.1936 mg hyoscyamine sulfate, 0.0362 mg atropine sulfate, 0.0121 mg scopolamine HBr	1 q 8 to 12 h	Green. In 100s.	1.7
Rx	**Phenchlor SHA Tablets** (Rugby)	50 mg phenylpropanolamine HCl, 25 mg phenylephrine HCl	8 mg chlorpheniramine maleate	0.19 mg hyoscyamine sulfate, 0.04 mg atropine sulfate, 0.01 mg scopolamine HBr	1 bid	In 100s and 500s.	1

* Cost Index based on cost per capsule or tablet.

UPPER RESPIRATORY COMBINATIONS (Cont.)

Refer to the general discussion of these products beginning on page 990.
Content given per tablet, capsule or 5 ml.

Decongestant, Antihistamine and Anticholinergic Combinations, Miscellaneous

	Product & Distributor	Decongestant	Antihistamine	Anticholinergic	Average Adult Dose	How Supplied	C.I.*
Rx	**Dallergy Tablets** (Laser)	10 mg phenylephrine HCl	4 mg chlorpheniramine maleate	1.25 mg methscopolamine nitrate	1 q 4 to 6 h	(Dallergy Laser). White, scored. In 100s and 1000s.	1.8
Rx	**D.A. Chewable Tablets** (Dura)	10 mg phenylephrine HCl	2 mg chlorpheniramine maleate	1.25 mg methscopolamine nitrate	1 or 2 q 4 h	(Dura DA JR). Orange, scored. Orange flavor. In 100s.	4
Rx	**Extendryl Chewable Tablets** (Fleming)					Rootbeer flavor. In 100s.	1.3
Rx	**Extendryl Syrup** (Fleming)				10 ml q 4 h	Rootbeer flavor. In pt.	1
Rx	**Dallergy Syrup** (Laser)	10 mg phenylephrine HCl	2 mg chlorpheniramine maleate	0.625 mg methscopolamine nitrate	5 or 10 ml q 4 to 6 h	In pt and gal.	1.8

Pediatric Decongestant, Antihistamine and Anticholinergic Combinations

	Product & Distributor	Decongestant	Antihistamine	Anticholinergic	Average Adult Dose	How Supplied	C.I.*
otc	**Extendryl JR Capsules** (Fleming)	10 mg phenylephrine HCl	4 mg chlorpheniramine maleate	1.25 mg methscopolamine nitrate	*Children (6 to 12 yrs)* – 1 q 12 h	Sustained release. In 100s and 1000s.	1.3

* Cost Index based on cost per tablet, capsule or 5 ml.

COUGH PREPARATIONS

Refer to the general discussion of these products beginning on page 990. Content given per capsule or tablet.

Antitussive Combinations, Capsules and Tablets

	Product & Distributor	Decongestant	Antihistamine	Antitussive	Other	Average Adult Dose	How Supplied	C.I.*
c-III	**Hycodan Tablets** (Du Pont)			5 mg hydrocodone bitartrate	1.5 mg homatropine MBr, lactose	1 q 4 to 6 h	(Hycodan Du Pont). White. In 100s, 500s.	3
c-III	**Tussigon Tablets** (Daniels)				1.5 mg homatropine MBr	1 q 4 to 6 h	Blue, scored. In 100s and 500s.	1.8
c-III	**Nucofed Capsules** (SK-Beecham)	60 mg pseudoephedrine HCl		20 mg codeine phosphate	Lactose	1 q 6 h	Green/clear. In 60s.	3
Rx	**Ordrine AT Extended-Release Capsules** (Vitarine)	75 mg phenylpropanolamine HCl		40 mg caramiphen edisylate	Sucrose	1 q 12 h	(PP-345). White/clear. In 50s, 100s and 500s.	6.3
Rx	**Rescaps-D S.R. Capsules** (Geneva)					1 q 12 h	Prolonged release. (PP 2002). Clear. In 100s.	3.4
Rx	**Tuss-Allergine Modified T.D. Caps** (Rugby)						In 100s, 500s and 1000s.	1
Rx	**Tuss-Genade Modified Capsules** (Goldline)						Sustained release. In 100s.	1.5
Rx	**Tussogest Extended-Release Caps** (Major)						Timed release. In 100s, 500s.	1.4
Rx	**Tuss-Ornade Spansules** (SK-Beecham)						Sustained release. (Tuss-Ornade). Blue/natural. In 50s and 500s.	9.4
otc	**Sudafed Severe Cold Formula Tablets** (B-W)	30 mg pseudoephedrine HCl		15 mg dextromethorphan HBr	500 mg acetaminophen	2 q 6 h	(Sudafed SCF). In 10s and 20s.	2.3
otc	**Tylenol No Drowsiness Cold Caplets** (McNeil-CPC)	30 mg pseudoephedrine HCl		15 mg dextromethorphan HBr	325 mg acetaminophen	2 q 6 h	White. Capsule shape. In 24s and 50s.	1.5

* Cost Index based on cost per capsule or tablet.

(Continued on following page)

COUGH PREPARATIONS (Cont.)

Refer to the general discussion of these products beginning on page 990. Content given per capsule, tablet or packet.

Antitussive Combinations, Capsules and Tablets (Cont.)

	Product & Distributor	Decongestant	Antihistamine	Antitussive	Other	Average Adult Dose	How Supplied	C.I.*
otc	**Dondril Tablets** (Whitehall)	5 mg phenylephrine HCl	1 mg chlorphenir-amine maleate	10 mg dextromethor-phan HBr		2 q 4 h up to 8/day	In 24s.	3
otc	**Triaminicol Multi-Symptom Cold Tablets** (Sandoz)	12.5 mg phenylpro-panolamine HCl	2 mg chlorphenir-amine maleate	10 mg dextromethor-phan HBr	Lactose	2 q 4 h	In 24s.	3.6
Rx	**Rynatuss Tablets** (Wallace)	10 mg phenylephrine tannate, 10 mg ephedrine tannate	5 mg chlorphenir-amine tannate	60 mg carbetapen-tane tannate		1 to 2 q 12 h	Mauve. Capsule shaped. In 100s and 500s.	17
otc	**Remcol-C Capsules** (Shionogi)		2 mg chlorphenir-amine maleate	15 mg dextromethor-phan HBr	300 mg acetamino-phen, lactose	1 q 4 h up to 4/day	In 24s.	2.3
c-III	**Hycomine Compound Tablets** (Du Pont)	10 mg phenylephrine HCl	2 mg chlorphenir-amine maleate	5 mg hydrocodone bitartrate	250 mg acetamino-phen, 30 mg caffeine (anhydrous)	1 q 4 h up to 4/day	Coral pink, scored. In 100s and 500s.	9.9
otc	**Medi-Flu Caplets** (Parke-Davis)	30 mg pseudoephed-rine HCl	2 mg chlorphenir-amine maleate	15 mg dextromethor-phan HBr	500 mg acetamino-phen	2 q 6 h	(Medi Flu). In 16s.	2.7
otc	**Viro-Med Tablets** (Whitehall)						In 20s and 48s.	3.4
otc	**Tylenol Cold & Flu Medication Powder** (McNeil-CPC)	60 mg pseudoephed-rine HCl	4 mg chlorphenir-amine maleate	30 mg dextromethor-phan HBr	650 mg acetamino-phen, aspartame, sucrose, 11 mg phenylalanine	1 packet dis-solved in 6 oz water q 6 h up to 4 doses/day	Lemon flavor. In 6 and 12 packs.	11
otc	**Contac Severe Cold & Flu Hot Medicine Powder** (SK-Beecham)	60 mg pseudoephed-rine HCl	4 mg chlorphenir-amine maleate	20 mg dextromethor-phan HBr	650 mg acetamino-phen, sucrose	1 packet in 6 oz hot water q 4 to 6 h up to 4 doses/day	Lemon flavor. In 6 packs.	12
otc	**TheraFlu Flu, Cold & Cough Medicine Powder** (Sandoz)					1 packet in 6 oz water q 4 h up to 4 doses/day	Lemon flavor. In 6 packs.	13

* Cost Index based on cost per capsule, tablet or packet.

(Continued on following page)

COUGH PREPARATIONS (Cont.)

Refer to the general discussion of these products beginning on page 990.
Content given per capsule, tablet or packet.

Antitussive Combinations, Capsules and Tablets (Cont.)

	Product & Distributor	Decongestant	Antihistamine	Antitussive	Other	Average Adult Dose	How Supplied	C.I.*
otc	**Dristan Cold & Flu Powder** (Whitehall)	60 mg pseudoephedrine HCl	4 mg chlorphenir-amine	20 mg dextromethorphan HBr	500 mg acetaminophen, ascorbic acid, corn syrup, sucrose	1 packet dissolved in 6 oz hot water q 4 h up to 4 doses/day	Lemon flavor. In 6 packs.	NA
otc	**Flu, Cold & Cough Medicine Powder** (Major)				500 mg acetaminophen, sucrose	1 packet dissolved in water q 4 h up to 4 doses/day	Lemon flavor. In 6 packs.	7.6
otc	**Contact Day & Night Cold & Flu Caplets** (SK-Beecham)	60 mg pseudoephedrine HCl	50 mg diphenhydramine HCl	30 mg dextromethorphan HBr	650 mg acetaminophen	*Day* – 1 yellow caplet q 6 h. *Night* – 1 blue caplet q 6 h. No more than 4 in any combination, per 24 h	(C-Night). Blue. In 5s (night).	NA
		60 mg pseudoephedrine HCl		30 mg dextromethorphan HBr	650 mg acetaminophen		(C-Day). Yellow. In 15s (day).	
otc	**NyQuil LiquiCaps (Capsules)** (Richardson-Vicks)	30 mg pseudoephedrine HCl	25 mg diphenhydramine HCl	15 mg dextromethorphan HBr	250 mg acetaminophen	2 at bedtime	In 20s.	NA
otc	**Co-Apap Tablets** (Various, eg, Rugby, Schein)	30 mg pseudoephedrine HCl	2 mg chlorphenir-amine maleate	15 mg dextromethorphan HBr	325 mg acetaminophen	2 q 6 h up to 8/day	In 24s, 50s, 100s and 1000s.	1+
otc	**Tylenol Cold Tablets and Caplets** (McNeil-CPC)						**Tablets:** (Tylenol Cold). Yellow. In 24s and 50s.	3.6
							Caplets: (Tylenol Cold). Light yellow. In 24s and 50s.	3.6
otc	**Ty-Cold Tablets** (Major)						In 24s.	2.7

* Cost Index based on cost per capsule, tablet or packet.

(Continued on following page)

COUGH PREPARATIONS (Cont.)

Refer to the general discussion of these products beginning on page 990.
Content given per capsule or tablet.

Antitussive Combinations, Capsules and Tablets (Cont.)

	Product & Distributor	Decongestant	Antihistamine	Antitussive	Other	Average Adult Dose	How Supplied	C.I.*
otc	**Comtrex Tablets and Caplets** (Bristol-Myers)	30 mg pseudoephedrine HCl	2 mg chlorpheniramine maleate	10 mg dextromethorphan HBr	325 mg acetaminophen	2 q 4 h up to 8/day	**Tablets:** (C). Yellow. In 10s, 50s and UD 24s.	3
							Caplets: (Comtrex). Yellow. In 50s and UD 24s.	4.4
otc	**Kolephrin/DM Caplets** (Pfeiffer)					2 q 4 to 6 h up to 8/day	In 30s.	2.4
otc	**Day-Night Comtrex** (Bristol-Myers)	30 mg pseudoephedrine HCl	2 mg chlorpheniramine maleate	10 mg dextromethorphan HBr	325 mg acetaminophen	*Night* – 2 at bedtime not sooner than 4 h after last daytime dose	*Night Tablets* – (C). Yellow. In 6s.	NA
		30 mg pseudoephedrine HCl		10 mg dextromethorphan HBr	325 mg acetaminophen	*Day* – 2 q 4 h up to 6/day	*Day Caplets* – (C). Orange. In 18s.	
otc	**Contac Severe Cold Formula Caplets** (SK-Beecham)	12.5 mg phenylpropanolamine HCl	2 mg chlorpheniramine maleate	15 mg dextromethorphan HBr	500 mg acetaminophen	2 q 6 h up to 8/day	(SCF). In 10s and 20s.	7
otc	**Extreme Cold Formula Caplets** (Major)						In 10s.	NA
otc	**Cold Relief Tablets** (Rugby)	12.5 mg phenylpropanolamine HCl	2 mg chlorpheniramine maleate	10 mg dextromethorphan HBr	325 mg acetaminophen	2 q 4 h up to 12/day	In 50s.	1.4
otc	**Comtrex Liqui-Gels (Capsules)** (Bristol-Myers)						Sorbitol. (Comtrex). Yellow. In UD 24s and 50s.	NA
otc	**Genacol Tablets** (Goldline)						In 50s.	NA

* Cost Index based on cost per capsule or tablet.

COUGH PREPARATIONS (Cont.)

Refer to the general discussion of these products beginning on page 990. Content given per 5 ml.

Antitussive Combinations, Liquids

	Product & Distributor	Decongestant	Antihistamine	Antitussive	Other	Average Adult Dose	How Supplied	C.I.*
c-III	**Hydrocodone Compound Syrup** (Various, eg, Geneva, Moore, PBI)			5 mg hydrocodone bitartrate	1.5 mg homatropine MBr	5 ml q 4 to 6 h	In 120 ml, pt and gal.	NA
c-III	**Hycodan Syrup** (Du Pont)				1.5 mg homatropine MBr, sorbitol, sugar		Cherry flavor. In pt and gal.	11
c-III	**Hydromet Syrup** (Barre-National)				1.5 mg homatropine MBr		In pt and gal.	3.4
c-III	**Hydropane Syrup** (Halsey)					5 to 15 ml pc and hs (not less than q 4 h)	Cherry flavor. In pt and gal.	3.6
c-III	**Detussin Liquid** (Various, eg, Barre-National, Dixon-Shane, Major, PBI, Qualitest, Schein)	60 mg pseudoephedrine HCl		5 mg hydrocodone bitartrate	Alcohol	5 ml qid	In 480 ml.	3.5+
c-III	**Tussgen Liquid** (Goldline)				5% alcohol		Fruit flavor. In 480 ml.	4
c-III *sf*	**Entuss-D Liquid** (Hauck)	30 mg pseudoephedrine HCl		5 mg hydrocodone bitartrate		5 to 7.5 ml pc and hs (not less than q 4 h)	Alcohol and dye free. In 480 ml.	9.3

* Cost Index based on cost per 5 ml.
sf – Sugar free.

(Continued on following page)

COUGH PREPARATIONS (Cont.)

Refer to the general discussion of these products beginning on page 990. Content given per 5 ml.

Antitussive Combinations, Liquids (Cont.)

	Product & Distributor	Decongestant	Antihistamine	Antitussive	Other	Average Adult Dose	How Supplied	C.I.*
c-III	**Codamine Syrup** (Various, eg, Barre-National, Dixon-Shane, Goldline, Major, Qualitest)	25 mg phenylpropanolamine HCl		5 mg hydrocodone bitartrate		5 ml pc and hs (not less than 4 hours apart)	In pt and gal.	3.6+
c-III	**Hycomine Syrup** (Du Pont)				Saccharin, sorbitol	5 ml q 4 h	Cherry flavor. In pt and gal.	11
c-III	**Phenylpropanolamine HCl and Hydrocodone Syrup** (PBI)					5 ml pc and hs (not less than 4 hours apart)	In 480 ml.	3.5
otc	**Vicks Formula 44D Liquid** (Richardson-Vicks)	20 mg pseudoephedrine HCl		10 mg dextromethorphan HBr	10% alcohol, saccharin, sucrose	15 ml q 6 h	In 120, 240 and 360 ml.	1.8
c-III	**Nucofed Syrup** (SK-Beecham)	60 mg pseudoephedrine HCl		20 mg codeine phosphate	Sorbitol, sucrose	5 ml q 6 h	Alcohol free. Mint flavor. In 480 ml.	9.7
otc	**Triaminic-DM Syrup** (Sandoz)	12.5 mg phenylpropanolamine HCl		10 mg dextromethorphan HBr	Sorbitol, sucrose	10 ml q 4 h	Alcohol free. In 120 and 240 ml.	3.5
Rx	**Tuss-Ornade Liquid** (SK-Beecham)	12.5 mg phenylpropanolamine HCl		6.7 mg caramiphen edisylate	5% alcohol, menthol, sorbitol	10 ml q 4 h	Fruit flavor. In 480 ml.	12
c-III	**Tussionex Extended-Release Suspension** (Fisons)		8 mg chlorpheniramine (as polistirex)	10 mg hydrocodone (as polistirex)	Sucrose, corn syrup	5 ml q 12 h	Alcohol free. In 480 and 900 ml.	9

* Cost Index based on cost per 5 ml. *sf* – Sugar free.

(Continued on following page)

COUGH PREPARATIONS (Cont.)

Refer to the general discussion of these products beginning on page 990. Content given per 5 ml.

Antitussive Combinations, Liquids (Cont.)

	Product & Distributor	Decongestant	Antihistamine	Antitussive	Other	Average Adult Dose	How Supplied	C.I.*
c-v	**Bromanyl Syrup** (Various, eg, Barre-National, Dixon-Shane, Moore, Schein)		12.5 mg bromodiphenhydramine HCl	10 mg codeine phosphate	Alcohol	5 or 10 ml q 4 to 6 h	In 120 ml, pt and gal.	2.7+
c-v	**Ambenyl Cough Syrup** (Forest)				5% alcohol, glucose, sucrose, menthol		In 118 ml, pt and gal.	18
c-v	**Amgenal Cough Syrup** (Goldline)				5% alcohol		In pt and gal.	3.5
c-v	**Bromotuss w/Codeine Syrup** (Rugby)						In 480 ml.	2.5
c-v	**Bromodiphenhydramine HCl and Codeine Cough Syrup** (PBI)						In 480 ml.	2.7
c-v	**Promethazine HCl w/Codeine Liquid** (Various, eg, Dixon-Shane, Geneva, Halsey, Major, Moore, Purepac, Schein, URL)		6.25 mg promethazine HCl	10 mg codeine phosphate	Alcohol	5 ml q 4 to 6 h	In 120 ml, pt and gal.	1.8+
c-v	**Prometh w/Codeine Syrup** (Various, eg, Barre-National, Goldline, Moore)						In 120 ml, pt and gal.	2+
c-v	**Phenergan with Codeine Syrup** (Wyeth-Ayerst)				7% alcohol, saccharin		In 118 and 480 ml.	6.3
c-v	**Pherazine w/Codeine Syrup** (Halsey)				7% alcohol, sorbitol, sucrose		Cherry flavor. In 120 ml, pt and gal.	3.2

* Cost Index based on cost per 5 ml.

(Continued on following page)

COUGH PREPARATIONS (Cont.)

Refer to the general discussion of these products beginning on page 990. Content given per 5 ml.

Antitussive Combinations, Liquids (Cont.)

	Product & Distributor	Decongestant	Antihistamine	Antitussive	Other	Average Adult Dose	How Supplied	C.I.*
c-v	**Tricodene Cough and Cold Liquid** (Pfeiffer)		12.5 mg pyrilamine maleate	8.2 mg codeine phosphate	Menthol, honey, glucose, sucrose	10 ml q 4 to 6 h	In 120 ml.	5.2
otc	**Effective Strength Cough Formula Liquid** (Barre-National)		2 mg chlorpheniramine maleate	15 mg dextromethorphan HBr	10% alcohol	10 ml q 6 h	Menthol flavor. In 240 ml.	2.9
otc	**Primatuss Cough Mixture 4 Liquid** (Rugby)				10% alcohol, sorbitol, sucrose	10 ml q 8 h	In 118 ml.	2
otc *sf*	**Scot-Tussin DM Liquid** (Scot-Tussin)					5 ml q 4 h or 10 ml q 6 to 8 h	Alcohol free. In 118 ml.	4.3
otc *sf*	**Tycodene Sugar Free Liquid** (Pfeiffer)		2 mg chlorpheniramine maleate	10 mg dextromethorphan HBr	Menthol, saccharin, sorbitol	10 ml q 4 h	Alcohol free. In 120 ml.	2.9
Rx	**Promethazine DM Syrup** (Various, eg, Dixon-Shane, Geneva, Lannett, Moore, PBI, Qualitest, Rugby, Schein)		6.25 mg promethazine HCl	15 mg dextromethorphan HBr	Alcohol	5 ml q 4 to 6 h	In 120 ml, pt and gal.	1.2+
Rx	**Phenameth DM Syrup** (Major)						In 120 ml.	2.4
Rx	**Phenergan w/Dextromethorphan Syrup** (Wyeth-Ayerst)				7% alcohol, saccharin		In 118 and 480 ml.	4.5
Rx	**Pherazine DM Syrup** (Halsey)				7% alcohol, sorbitol, sucrose		In 120 ml, pt and gal.	1.3
Rx	**Prometh w/Dextromethorphan Syrup** (Barre-National)				7% alcohol		In 118 ml, pt and gal.	1.6

* Cost Index based on cost per 5 ml.
sf – Sugar free

(Continued on following page)

COUGH PREPARATIONS (Cont.)

Refer to the general discussion of these products beginning on page 990.
Content given per 5 ml.

Antitussive Combinations, Liquids (Cont.)

	Product & Distributor	Decongestant	Antihistamine	Antitussive	Other	Average Adult Dose	How Supplied	C.I.*
Rx	**Cardec DM Syrup** (Various, eg, Barre-National, Dixon-Shane, Goldline, Moore, Schein, URL)	60 mg pseudoephedrine HCl	4 mg carbinoxamine maleate	15 mg dextromethorphan HBr	Alcohol	5 ml qid	In 120 ml, pt and gal.	2.6+
Rx	**Carbinoxamine Compound Syrup** (PBI)				< 0.6% alcohol		Grape flavor. In 120 ml, pt and gal.	NA
Rx	**Carbodec DM Syrup** (Various, eg, Rugby, Schein)						In 118 ml, pt and gal.	1.9+
Rx	**Pseudo-Car DM Syrup** (Geneva)						Grape flavor. In pt and gal.	3.5
Rx *sf*	**Rondec-DM Syrup** (Ross)				Menthol, sorbitol		Alcohol free. Grape flavor. In 120 & 480 ml.	11
Rx	**Tussafed Syrup** (Everett)				< 0.6% alcohol		In 118 & 480 ml.	6.7
otc *sf*	**Cerose-DM Liquid** (Wyeth-Ayerst)	10 mg phenylephrine HCl	4 mg chlorpheniramine maleate	15 mg dextromethorphan HBr	2.4% alcohol, saccharin	5 to 10 ml qid	In 118 and 480 ml.	5.5
otc	**Rhinosyn-DM Liquid** (Great Southern)	30 mg pseudoephedrine HCl	2 mg chlorpheniramine maleate	15 mg dextromethorphan HBr	1.4% alcohol, sucrose	10 ml q 6 h	In 120 ml.	4
otc	**Tussar DM Cough Syrup** (Rhone-Poulenc Rorer)				Sucrose, glucose	10 ml q 6 h	Alcohol free. In 473 ml.	9.1
otc *sf*	**Trimedine Liquid** (Trimen)	5 mg phenylephrine HCl	1 mg chlorpheniramine maleate	15 mg dextromethorphan HBr	Sorbitol	10 ml qid	Cherry flavor. In pt and gal.	4
otc *sf*	**Codimal DM Syrup** (Central)	5 mg phenylephrine HCl	8.33 mg pyrilamine maleate	10 mg dextromethorphan HBr	4% alcohol, menthol, saccharin, sorbitol	5 to 10 ml q 4 h	In 120 ml, pt and gal.	5.9

* Cost Index based on cost per 5 ml. *sf* – Sugar free.

(Continued on following page)

COUGH PREPARATIONS (Cont.)

Refer to the general discussion of these products beginning on page 990. Content given per 5 ml.

Antitussive Combinations, Liquids (Cont.)

	Product & Distributor	Decongestant	Antihistamine	Antitussive	Other	Average Adult Dose	How Supplied	C.I.*
Rx	**Poly-Histine DM Syrup** (Bock)	12.5 mg phenylpropanolamine HCl	2 mg brompheniramine maleate	10 mg dextromethorphan HBr		10 ml q 4 h	Alcohol free. Raspberry flavor. In 120 & 480 ml.	6.3
otc	**Kophane Cough & Cold Formula Liquid** (Pfeiffer)	12.5 mg phenylpropanolamine HCl	2 mg chlorpheniramine maleate	10 mg dextromethorphan HBr	Menthol, sucrose	10 ml q 4 h	Alcohol free. In 120 ml.	2.9
otc	**Myminicol Liquid** (PBI)						Alcohol free. Raspberry-cherry flavor. In 120 ml, pt and gal.	2.4
otc	**Threamine DM Syrup** (Barre-National)				Saccharin, sorbitol, sucrose	10 ml q 4 to 6 h	Cherry flavor. In pt and gal.	2.4
otc	**Triaminicol Multi-Symptom Relief Liquid** (Sandoz)				Sorbitol, sucrose	10 ml q 4 h	Alcohol free. In 120, 240 ml.	4.5
otc	**Tricodene Forte Liquid** (Pfeiffer)						Alcohol free. In 120 ml.	3.8
otc	**Tricodene NN Liquid** (Pfeiffer)				Menthol, sucrose		Alcohol free. In 120 ml.	2.9
otc	**Triminol Cough Syrup** (Rugby)				Saccharin, sorbitol, sugar		In 118 ml.	2.4
otc sf	**Trind DM Liquid** (Mead-J)	12.5 mg phenylpropanolamine HCl	2 mg chlorpheniramine maleate	7.5 mg dextromethorphan HBr	5% alcohol	10 ml q 4 h	Fruit flavor. In 150 ml.	6.9
otc	**Cheracol Plus Liquid** (Roberts)	8.3 mg phenylpropanolamine HCl	1.3 mg chlorpheniramine maleate	6.7 mg dextromethorphan HBr	8% alcohol, sorbitol	15 ml q 4 h	In 120 and 180 ml.	3.5
otc	**Orthoxicol Cough Syrup** (Roberts)						In 60, 120 and 480 ml.	4.1
otc	**Dimetapp DM Elixir** (Robins)	12.5 mg phenylpropanolamine HCl	2 mg brompheniramine maleate	10 mg dextromethorphan HBr	2.3% alcohol, saccharin, sorbitol	10 ml q 4 h	Grape flavor. In 120 and 240 ml.	4.6

* Cost Index based on cost per 5 ml. *sf* – Sugar free.

(Continued on following page)

COUGH PREPARATIONS (Cont.)

Refer to the general discussion of these products beginning on page 990. Content given per 5 ml.

Antitussive Combinations, Liquids (Cont.)

	Product & Distributor	Decongestant	Antihistamine	Antitussive	Other	Average Adult Dose	How Supplied	C.I.*
otc	**All-Nite Cold Formula Liquid** (Major)	10 mg pseudoephedrine HCl	1.25 mg doxylamine succinate	5 mg dextromethorphan HBr	167 mg acetaminophen, 25% alcohol, sucrose	30 ml hs or 30 ml q 6 h	Mint and cherry flavors. In 180 and 300 ml.	2.3
otc	**Genite Liquid** (Goldline)				167 mg acetaminophen, 25% alcohol, tartrazine		Anise flavor. In 177 ml.	2.7
otc	**Nite Time Cold Formula Liquid** (Barre-National)				167 mg acetaminophen, 25% alcohol		Licorice and cherry flavor. In 180 and 300 ml.	NA
otc	**NyQuil Nighttime Cold/Flu Medicine Liquid** (Richardson-Vicks)				167 mg acetaminophen, 25% alcohol, sucrose; saccharin (cherry flavor); tartrazine (regular flavor)		Regular and cherry flavor. In 180, 300 and 420 ml.	3.3
otc	**Nytcold Medicine Liquid** (Rugby)				167 mg acetaminophen, 25% alcohol, glucose, saccharin, sucrose		Cherry flavor. In 177 ml.	2.1
otc	**Pertussin PM Liquid** (Pertussin Labs)				167 mg acetaminophen, 25% alcohol, saccharin, sucrose		Cherry flavor. In 240 ml.	3.2
otc	**Tylenol Cold Night Time Liquid** (McNeil-CPC)	10 mg pseudoephedrine HCl	8.3 mg diphenhydramine HCl	5 mg dextromethorphan HBr	108.3 mg acetaminophen, 10% alcohol, sucrose	30 ml q 6 h	Cherry flavor. In 150 ml.	NA
otc	**Vicks Formula 44M Cough and Cold Liquid** (Richardson-Vicks)	15 mg pseudoephedrine HCl	1 mg chlorpheniramine maleate	7.5 mg dextromethorphan HBr	125 mg acetaminophen, 20% alcohol, saccharin, sucrose	20 ml q 6 h	In 120 and 240 ml.	4.1

* Cost Index based on cost per 5 ml.

(Continued on following page)

COUGH PREPARATIONS (Cont.)

Refer to the general discussion of these products beginning on page 990 .
Content given per 5 ml.

Antitussive Combinations, Liquids (Cont.)

	Product & Distributor	Decongestant	Antihistamine	Antitussive	Other	Average Adult Dose	How Supplied	C.I.*
otc	**Contac Severe Cold & Flu Nighttime Liquid** (SK-Beecham)	10 mg pseudoephedrine HCl	0.67 mg chlorphenir-amine maleate	5 mg dextromethor-phan HBr	167 mg acetamino-phen, 18.5% alcohol, saccharin, sorbitol, glucose	30 ml q 6 h	In 180 ml.	3.5
otc	**Medi-Flu Liquid** (Parke-Davis)				167 mg acetamino-phen, 19% alcohol, saccharin, sorbitol, sugar		In 180 ml.	NA
otc	**Robitussin Night Relief Liquid** (Robins)	1.67 mg phenyl-ephrine HCl	8.3 mg pyrilamine maleate	5 mg dextromethor-phan HBr	108.3 mg acetamino-phen, saccharin, sorbitol	30 ml hs or 30 ml q 6 h	In 120 and 240 ml.	3.6
otc	**Tylenol Cough with Decongestant Liquid** (McNeil-CPC)	15 mg pseudoephed-rine HCl		7.5 mg dextromethor-phan HBr	250 mg acetamino-phen, 10% alcohol, saccharin, sorbitol, sucrose	20 ml q 6 to 8 h	In 120 and 240 ml.	NA
otc	**Comtrex Liquid** (Bristol-Myers)	10 mg pseudo-ephedrine HCl	0.67 mg chlorphenir-amine maleate	3.3 mg dextromethor-phan HBr	108.3 mg acetamino-phen, 20% alcohol, sucrose	30 ml q 4 h up to 120 ml/day	Cherry flavor. In 180 ml.	3.8
Rx	**Tusquelin Syrup** (Circle)	5 mg phenylpro-panolamine, 5 mg phenylephrine HCl	2 mg chlorphenir-amine maleate	15 mg dextromethor-phan HBr	5% alcohol, 0.17 min fluid-extract ipecac, potassium guaiacol-sulfonate	5 or 10 ml qid	In 480 ml.	2.6

* Cost Index based on cost per 5 ml.

(Continued on following page)

COUGH PREPARATIONS (Cont.)

Refer to the general discussion of these products beginning on page 990.
Content given per 5 ml.

Antitussive Combinations, Liquids (Cont.)

	Product & Distributor	Decongestant	Antihistamine	Antitussive	Other	Average Adult Dose	How Supplied	C.I.*
c-III	**Rolatuss with Hydrocodone Liquid** (Major)	3.3 mg phenylpropanolamine HCl, 5 mg phenylephrine HCl	3.3 mg pyrilamine maleate, 3.3 mg pheniramine maleate	1.67 mg hydrocodone bitartrate		10 ml qid	In 480 ml.	4.1
c-III	**Ru-Tuss w/Hydrocodone Liquid** (Boots)				5% alcohol, glucose, menthol, saccharin, sorbitol	10 ml q 4 to 6 h up to 40 ml/day	In 473 ml.	6.4
c-v	**T-Koff Liquid** (T.E. Williams)	20 mg phenylpropanolamine HCl, 20 mg phenylephrine HCl	5 mg chlorpheniramine maleate	10 mg codeine phosphate	Menthol, saccharin, sorbitol, sucrose, glucose	5 ml q 4 to 6 h	Grape flavor. In 480 ml.	5.7
otc	**Tylenol Cough Liquid** (McNeil-CPC)			7.5 mg dextromethorphan HBr	250 mg acetaminophen, saccharin, sorbitol, sucrose	20 ml q 6 to 8 h	In 120 ml	NA
otc sf	**Contac Cough & Sore Throat Liquid** (SK-Beecham)			5 mg dextromethorphan HBr	125 mg acetaminophen, 10% alcohol, saccharin, sorbitol	20 ml q 4 to 6 h up to 80 ml/day	In 120 ml.	4.2

* Cost Index based on cost per 5 ml.

COUGH PREPARATIONS (Cont.)

Refer to the general discussion of these products beginning on page 990. Content given per 5 ml or pack.

Pediatric Antitussive Combinations

	Product & Distributor	Decongestant	Antihistamine	Antitussive	Other	Average Dose	How Supplied	C.I.*
c-III	**Codamine Pediatric Syrup** (Various, eg, Barre-National, Dixon-Shane, Goldline, Major)	12.5 mg phenylpropanolamine HCl		2.5 mg hydrocodone bitartrate		*6 to 12 yrs* – 5 ml q 4 h	In 480 ml.	1.2+
c-III	**Hycomine Pediatric Syrup** (Du Pont)				Saccharin, sorbitol		Cherry flavor. In 480 ml.	3.3
c-III	**Hydrocodone Bitartrate and Phenylpropanolamine HCl Pediatric Syrup** (PBI)					*6 to 12 yrs* – 5 ml pc & hs q 4 h	Fruit flavor. In 118 ml, pt and gal.	1.1
otc	**Tricodene Pediatric Liquid** (Pfeiffer)	12.5 mg phenylpropanolamine HCl		10 mg dextromethorphan HBr	Sucrose	*2 to 12 yrs* – 2.5 to 5 ml q 4 h	Alcohol free. Cherry flavor. In 120 ml.	1.2
otc	**Snaplets-DM Granules** (Baker Cummins)	6.25 mg phenylpropanolamine HCl		5 mg dextromethorphan HBr		*6 to < 12 yrs* – 2 packs q 4 h *2 to < 6 yrs* – 1 pack q 4 h	Taste free. In 30s.	NA
otc	**Robitussin Pediatric Cough & Cold Formula** (Robins)	15 mg pseudoephedrine HCl		7.5 mg dextromethorphan HBr	Saccharin, sorbitol	*2 to 6 yrs* – 5 ml q 6 to 8 h *6 to 12 yrs* – 10 ml q 6 to 8 h	Cherry flavor. In 120 and 240 ml.	NA
otc *sf*	**Contac Jr. Non-Drowsy Cold Liquid** (SK-Beecham)	15 mg pseudoephedrine HCl		5 mg dextromethorphan HBr	160 mg acetaminophen, saccharin, sorbitol	*31 to > 85 lbs* – 2.5 to 10 ml q 4 to 6 h	Alcohol free. Berry flavor. With dose cup. In 120 ml.	2

* Cost Index based on cost per 5 ml or pack. *sf* – Sugar free.

(Continued on following page)

COUGH PREPARATIONS (Cont.)

Refer to the general discussion of these products beginning on page 990. Content given per tablet or 5 ml.

Pediatric Antitussive Combinations (Cont.)

	Product & Distributor	Decongestant	Antihistamine	Antitussive	Other	Average Dose	How Supplied	C.I.*
otc	**Pedia Care NightRest Liquid** (McNeil-CPC)	15 mg pseudoephedrine HCl	1 mg chlorphenir-amine maleate	7.5 mg dextromethor-phan HBr	Sorbitol, sucrose	*6 to 11 yrs* – 10 ml q 6 to 8 h	Alcohol free. Cherry flavor. In 120 ml.	1.4
otc	**Triaminic Nite Light Liquid** (Sandoz)					*6 to < 12 yrs* – 10 ml q 6 h	Alcohol free. Grape flavor. In 120 and 240 ml.	2
otc	**Aspirin-Free St. Joseph Complete Nighttime Cold Relief Liquid** (Schering-Plough)	15 mg pseudoephedrine HCl	1 mg chlorphenir-amine maleate	5 mg dextromethor-phan HBr	160 mg acetamino-phen, sucrose	*6 to 12 yrs* – 10 to 15 ml q 4 to 6 h up to 3 doses/day	Alcohol free. Cherry flavor. In 120 ml.	1.8
otc	**Pedia Care Cough-Cold Liquid** (McNeil-CPC)				Sorbitol, sucrose	*6 to 11 yrs* – 10 ml q 4 to 6 h up to 40 ml/day	Alcohol free. Cherry flavor. In 120 ml.	1.7
otc	**Children's NyQuil Cold/Cough Liquid** (Richardson-Vicks)	10 mg pseudoephedrine HCl	0.67 mg chlorpheni-ramine maleate	5 mg dextromethor-phan HBr	Sucrose	*6 to 11 yrs* – 15 ml q 6 h	Alcohol free. Cherry flavor. In 120 ml.	1.5
otc	**Pedia Care Cough-Cold Chewable Tablets** (McNeil-CPC)	7.5 mg pseudoephedrine HCl	0.5 mg chlorphenir-amine maleate	2.5 mg dextromethor-phan HBr	Aspartame (3 mg phenylalanine), dextrose, sucrose	*6 to 11 yrs* – 4 q 4 to 6 h up to 16/day	Fruit flavor. In 24s.	1.1

* Cost Index based on cost per tablet or 5 ml.

(Continued on following page)

COUGH PREPARATIONS (Cont.)

Refer to the general discussion of these products beginning on page 990.
Content given per 5 ml liquid, 1 ml drops or pack.

Pediatric Antitussive Combinations (Cont.)

	Product & Distributor	Decongestant	Antihistamine	Antitussive	Other	Average Dose	How Supplied	C.I.*
Rx	**Cardec DM Drops** (Various, eg, Barre-National, Schein)	25 mg pseudo-ephedrine HCl per ml	2 mg carbinoxamine maleate per ml	4 mg dextromethor-phan HBr per ml	Alcohol	*1 to 18 mos.* – 0.25 to 1 ml qid	In 30 ml.	1.4+
Rx	**Carbodec DM Drops** (Various, eg, Rugby, Schein)				< 0.6% alcohol	0.25 to 1 ml qid	In 30 ml.	1+
Rx	**Carbinoxamine Compound Drops** (PBI)					*1 to 18 mos* – 0.25 to 1 ml qid	Grape flavor. In 30 ml.	1.4
Rx	**Rondamine-DM Drops** (Major)					0.25 to 1 ml qid	In 30 ml.	1.4
Rx *sf*	**Rondec-DM Drops** (Ross)				Menthol, sorbitol	*1 to 18 mos.* – 0.25 to 1 ml qid	Alcohol free. Grape flavor. In 30 ml w/ dropper.	5.7
Rx	**Tussafed Drops** (Everett)				< 0.6% alcohol	0.25 to 1 ml qid	In 30 ml.	3.3
otc	**Snaplets-Multi Granules** (Baker Cummins)	6.25 mg phenylpro-panolamine HCl	1 mg chlorphenir-amine maleate	5 mg dextromethor-phan HBr		*6 to < 12 yrs* – 2 packs q 4 h *2 to < 6 yrs* – 1 pack q 4 h	Taste free. In 30s.	NA
Rx	**Rentamine Pediatric Suspension** (Major)	5 mg phenylephrine tannate, 5 mg ephedrine tannate	4 mg chlorphenir-amine tannate	30 mg carbeta-pentane tannate	Saccharin, sucrose	*2 to > 6 yrs* – 2.5 to 10 ml q 12 h	In pt.	6.1
Rx	**Rynatuss Pediatric Suspension** (Wallace)				Tartrazine, saccharin, sucrose		Strawberry-currant flavor. In 237 and 473 ml.	9.2
Rx	**Tri-Tannate Plus Pediatric Suspension** (Rugby)				Saccharin, sucrose		In 480 ml.	4.9

* Cost Index based on cost per 5 ml liquid, 1 ml drops or pack. *sf* – Sugar free.

COUGH PREPARATIONS (Cont.)

Refer to the general discussion of these products beginning on page 990   Content given per capsule or tablet.

Expectorant Combinations, Capsules and Tablets (Cont.)

	Product & Distributor	Decongestant	Antihistamine	Expectorant	Average Adult Dose	How Supplied	C.I.*
Rx	**Phenylpropanolamine HCl and Guaifenesin Tablets** (Various)	75 mg phenylpropanolamine HCl		400 mg guaifenesin	1 bid	Long-acting. Plain or film coated. In 100s and 500s.	2.4+
Rx	**Ami-Tex LA Tablets** (Amide)					Long-acting. Blue, scored. In 100s, 500s and 1000s.	1.9
Rx	**Despec Capsules** (Inter. Ethical Labs)					Long-acting. (Intetlab/Despec). Dark/light green. In 100s.	15
Rx	**Entex LA Tablets** (Procter & Gamble Pharm.)					Sugar. Long-acting. (Entex LA 0149 0436). Orange, scored. In 100s and 500s.	13
Rx	**Gentab-LA Caplets** (Genetco)					Long-acting. In 100s and 500s.	1.9
Rx	**Guaipax Tablets** (Vitarine)					Long-acting. (PP-745). Lt. blue, scored. In 100s, 500s and 1000s.	1.5
Rx	**Nolex LA Tablets** (Carnrick)					Long-acting. (8673 C). White, blue specks, scored. Oval. In 100s, 500s.	9.5
Rx	**Partuss LA Tablets** (Parmed)					Long-acting. Capsule shape. In 100s and 500s.	2.2
Rx	**Phenylfenesin L.A. Tablets** (Goldline)					Long-acting. Blue, oval. In 100s and 500s.	2.8
Rx	**Rymed-TR Caplets** (Edwards)					Long-acting. In 100s.	6.2
Rx	**Stamoist LA Tablets** (Huckaby)					Yellow, scored. Film coated. In 100s.	NA
Rx	**ULR-LA Tablets** (Geneva)					Long-acting. White, scored. In 100s.	5
Rx	**Vanex-LA Tablets** (Abana)					Long-acting. (Abana 400/75). Green, scored. In 100s.	6.6

* Cost Index based on cost per capsule or tablet.

(Continued on following page)

COUGH PREPARATIONS (Cont.)

Refer to the general discussion of these products beginning on page 990. Content given per capsule or tablet.

Expectorant Combinations, Capsules and Tablets (Cont.)

	Product & Distributor	Decongestant	Antihistamine	Expectorant	Average Adult Dose	How Supplied	**C.I.***
Rx	**Dura-Gest Capsules** (Dura)	45 mg phenylpropanolamine HCl, 5 mg phenylephrine HCl		200 mg guaifenesin	1 qid (q 6 h)	(Dura-Gest 51479005). Gray/white. In 100s and 500s.	3.1
Rx	**Enomine Capsules** (Major)					In 500s.	3.3
Rx	**Entex Capsules** (Procter & Gamble Pharm.)					(Entex 0149 0412). Orange/white. In 100s & 500s.	7.9
Rx	**Respinol-G Tablets** (Misemer)				1 qid	Pink. Film coated. In 100s.	4.5

* Cost Index based on cost per capsule or tablet.

COUGH PREPARATIONS (Cont.)

Refer to the general discussion of these products beginning on page 990. Content given per 5 ml.

Expectorant Combinations, Liquids

	Product & Distributor	Decongestant	Antihistamine	Expectorant	Other	Average Adult Dose	How Supplied	C.I.*
otc	**Cheralin Expectorant Liquid** (Lannett)			88 mg potassium guaiacolsulfonate, 88 mg ammonium chloride, 1 mg antimony potassium tartrate	3% alcohol	5 to 10 ml q 4 h up to 40 ml/day	In pt and gal.	1
Rx	**Broncholate Syrup** (Bock)	6.25 mg ephedrine HCl		100 mg guaifenesin	Saccharin, sucrose	10 to 20 ml q 4 h	In 480 ml.	2.9
Rx	**KIE Syrup** (Laser)	8 mg ephedrine HCl		150 mg potassium iodide		15 to 20 ml q 4 to 6 h	Cherry flavor. In pt and gal.	3.8
Rx	**Norisodrine w/Calcium Iodide Syrup** (Abbott)			150 mg anhydrous calcium iodide	3 mg isoproterenol sulfate, 6% alcohol, sucrose, glucose	5 to 10 ml q 4 to 6 h	In 480 ml.	5.5
Rx	**Histalet X Syrup** (Solvay)	45 mg pseudoephedrine HCl		200 mg guaifenesin	15% alcohol, fructose, saccharin, sorbitol, sucrose	10 ml qid	In 473 ml.	6.9
otc *sf*	**Fedahist Expectorant Syrup** (Schwarz Pharma Kremers Urban)	30 mg pseudoephedrine HCl		200 mg guaifenesin	Saccharin, sorbitol	10 ml q 4 to 6 h up to 40 ml/day	Alcohol free. In 120 ml.	4.3
otc	**Guaifed Syrup** (Muro)				Saccharin, sorbitol, sucrose		Alcohol free. In 120 and 480 ml.	6.6
otc	**Guiatuss PE Liquid** (Barre-National)	30 mg pseudoephedrine HCl		100 mg guaifenesin	1.4% alcohol	10 ml q 4 h up to 40 ml/day	Fruit-mint flavor. In 120 ml.	2.1
otc	**Robitussin-PE Syrup** (Robins)				1.4% alcohol, high fructose corn syrup, glucose, saccharin		In 120, 240 and 480 ml.	2.7
otc	**Rymed Liquid** (Edwards)				1.4% alcohol	10 ml q 4 h	In 480 ml.	3.2
otc	**Codimal Expectorant Liquid** (Central)	25 mg phenylpropanolamine HCl		100 mg guaifenesin	Menthol, sucrose	5 ml q 4 h	Alcohol free. In 120 ml.	3.6

* Cost Index based on cost per 5 ml. *sf* – Sugar free.

(Continued on following page)

COUGH PREPARATIONS (Cont.)

Refer to the general discussion of these products beginning on page 990. Content given per 5 ml.

Expectorant Combinations, Liquids (Cont.)

	Product & Distributor	Decongestant	Antihistamine	Expectorant	Other	Average Adult Dose	How Supplied	C.I.*
otc	**Conex Syrup** (Forest)	12.5 mg phenylpropanolamine HCl		100 mg guaifenesin		5 to 10 ml q 4 h up to 50 ml/d	In 118 ml.	2.8
otc	**Myminic Expectorant Liquid** (PBI)				5% alcohol	10 ml q 4 h	Fruit punch flavor. In 120 and 240 ml, pt, gal.	1.3
otc	**Triaminic Expectorant Liquid** (Sandoz)				Sorbitol, sucrose		Alcohol free. In 120 and 240 ml.	3.8
otc	**Theramine Expectorant** (Major)						In 118 and 240 ml.	2.3
otc	**Triphenyl Expectorant Liquid** (Rugby)				5% alcohol, saccharin, sorbitol, sucrose		In 118 ml.	2.1
Rx	**Contuss Liquid** (Parmed)	20 mg phenylpropanolamine HCl, 5 mg phenylephrine HCl		100 mg guaifenesin	5% alcohol, saccharin, sorbitol, sucrose	10 ml qid	In 480 ml.	4.4
Rx	**Despec Liquid** (Inter. Ethical Labs)				5% alcohol	10 ml q 6 h	Pineapple flavor. In 118 ml.	6.1
Rx	**Entex Liquid** (Procter & Gamble Pharm.)				5% alcohol, saccharin, sorbitol, sucrose		In 480 ml.	5.2
otc sf	**Lanatuss Expectorant Liquid** (Lannett)	5 mg phenylpropanolamine HCl	2 mg chlorpheniramine maleate	100 mg guaifenesin	Saccharin, sorbitol	5 ml tid or qid up to 40 ml/day	In 118 ml, pt and gal.	1
Rx	**Bronkotuss Expectorant Liquid** (Hyrex)	8.2 mg ephedrine sulfate	4 mg chlorpheniramine maleate	100 mg guaifenesin, 1.67 ml hydriodic acid syrup	5% alcohol, dextrose, saccharin, sucrose	5 ml q 3 to 4 h	Licorice flavor. In pt and gal.	3.5
Rx	**Polaramine Expectorant Liquid** (Schering)	20 mg pseudoephedrine sulfate	2 mg dexchlorpheniramine maleate	100 mg guaifenesin	7.2% alcohol, menthol, sorbitol, sugar	5 to 10 ml tid or qid	In 473 ml.	8.4

* Cost Index based on cost per 5 ml.   *sf* – Sugar free.

COUGH PREPARATIONS (Cont.)

Refer to the general discussion of these products beginning on page 990.
Content given per 5 ml liquid, 1 ml drops or pack.

Pediatric Expectorant Combinations

	Product & Distributor	Decongestant	Antihistamine	Expectorant	Other	Average Dose	How Supplied	C.I.*
otc	**Fedahist Expectorant Pediatric Drops** (Schwarz Pharma Kremers Urban)	7.5 mg pseudoephedrine HCl per ml		40 mg guaifenesin per ml	Saccharin, sorbitol	*6 to < 12 yrs* – 4 ml q 4 to 6 h up to 16 ml/day *2 to < 6 yrs* – 2 ml q 4 to 6 h up to 8 ml/day	In 30 ml w/dropper.	1.2
otc sf	**Naldecon EX Children's Syrup** (Apothecon)	6.25 mg phenylpropanolamine HCl		100 mg guaifenesin	5% alcohol, saccharin, sorbitol	*2 to < 12 yrs* – 5 to 10 ml q 4 h	Fruit flavor. In 118 ml.	1
otc	**Snaplets-EX Granules** (Baker Cummins)	6.25 mg phenylpropanolamine HCl		50 mg guaifenesin		*6 to < 12 yrs* – 2 packs q 4 h *2 to < 6 yrs* – 1 pack q 4 h	Taste free. In 30s.	NA
otc sf	**Naldecon EX Pediatric Drops** (Apothecon)	6.25 mg phenylpropanolamine HCl per ml		50 mg guaifenesin per ml	Saccharin, sorbitol	*2 to < 6 yrs* – 1 ml q 4 h	Fruit flavor. In 30 ml w/dropper.	1.3
Rx	**Donatussin Drops** (Laser)	2 mg phenylephrine HCl per ml	1 mg chlorpheniramine maleate per ml	20 mg guaifenesin per ml		*< 3 mos* – 2 to 3 drops per month of age q 4 to 6 h *3 mos to 2 yrs* – 0.3 to 2 ml q 4 to 6 h	Peach flavor. In 30 ml.	1.4

* Cost Index based on cost per 5 ml liquid, 1 ml drops or pack. *sf* – Sugar free.

COUGH PREPARATIONS (Cont.)

Refer to the general discussion of these products beginning on page 990.
Content given per 5 ml.

Narcotic Antitussives with Expectorants

	Product & Distributor	Antitussive	Expectorant	Other	Average Adult Dose	How Supplied	C.I.*
c-v	**Cheracol Syrup** (Roberts)	10 mg codeine phosphate	100 mg guaifenesin	4.75% alcohol, fructose, sucrose	10 ml q 4 to 6 h up to 6 doses/day	In 60, 120 and 480 ml.	3.5
c-v	**Guiatuss AC Syrup** (Various, eg, Barre-National, Goldline, Moore, Schein)			Alcohol	10 ml q 4 h	In 120 ml, pt and gal.	1.1+
c-v	**Guiatussin w/Codeine Expectorant Liquid** (Rugby)			3.5% alcohol		In 120 ml, pt and gal.	1
c-v	**Mytussin AC Cough Syrup** (PBI)			3.5% alcohol, menthol, sorbitol, sugar	5 to 10 ml q 4 to 6 h	In 480 ml.	1.2
c-v *sf*	**Robitussin A-C Syrup** (Robins)			3.5% alcohol, saccharin, sorbitol	10 ml q 4 h	In 60 and 120 ml, pt and gal.	4.9
c-v	**Iophen-C Liquid** (Various, eg, Barre-National, Dixon-Shane, Major, Moore, Qualitest, Rugby, Schein, URL)	10 mg codeine phosphate	30 mg iodinated glycerol		5 to 10 ml q 4 h	In 120 ml, pt and gal.	1.5+
c-v	**Iodinated Glycerol and Codeine Phosphate Liquid** (Geneva)					Raspberry flavor. In pt.	1.9
c-v	**IoTuss Liquid** (Muro)			Saccharin, sorbitol		Cherry flavor. In 480 ml.	4.9
c-v	**Par Glycerol C Liquid** (Par)					Cherry flavor. In pt and gal.	2.2
c-v[1] *sf*	**Tussi-Organidin Liquid** (Wallace)					Alcohol free. In pt and gal.	5.9
c-v *sf*	**Tussi-R-Gen Liquid** (Goldline)				5 to 10 ml q 4 h	Alcohol free. In pt and gal.	2.4

* Cost Index based on cost per 5 ml. *sf* – Sugar free. [1] Available Rx only.

(Continued on following page)

COUGH PREPARATIONS (Cont.)

Refer to the general discussion of these products beginning on page 990
Content given per tablet or 5 ml.

Narcotic Antitussives with Expectorants (Cont.)

	Product & Distributor	Antitussive	Expectorant	Other	Average Adult Dose	How Supplied	C.I.*
c-v	**Terpin Hydrate and Codeine Elixir** (Various, eg, Parmed)	10 mg codeine	85 mg terpin hydrate	>40% alcohol	5 ml q 2 to 4 h	In 118 ml, pt & gal.	1.6+
c-v	**Cheralin w/Codeine Liquid** (Lannett)	10 mg codeine phosphate	80 mg potassium guaiacol-sulfonate, 80 mg ammonium Cl, 5 mg antimony potassium tartrate		5 to 10 ml q 4 h	In pt and gal.	1.3
c-v	**Calcidrine Syrup** (Abbott)	8.4 mg codeine	152 mg calcium iodide anhydrous	6% alcohol, glucose, sucrose	5 to 10 ml q 4 h	In 480 ml.	4.7
c-III sf	**Entuss Expectorant Tablets** (Hauck)	5 mg hydrocodone bitartrate	300 mg guaifenesin		1 to 1.5 q 4 h pc & hs up to qid	In 100s.	5.1
c-III sf	**Codiclear DH Syrup** (Central)	5 mg hydrocodone bitartrate	100 mg guaifenesin		5 ml q 4 h pc & hs up to 30 ml/day	Alcohol and dye free. In 120 and 480 ml.	5.8
c-III	**Hycotuss Expectorant Syrup** (Du Pont)			10% alcohol, saccharin, sorbitol, sugar	5 ml q 4 h pc & hs	Butterscotch flavor. In 480 ml.	6.2
c-III sf	**Kwelcof Liquid** (Ascher)			Menthol, saccharin, sorbitol		Alcohol & dye free. Fruit flavor. In 480 ml.	5.3
c-III sf	**Entuss Expectorant Liquid** (Hauck)	5 mg hydrocodone bitartrate	300 mg potassium guaiacolsulfonate		5 to 7.5 ml q 4 h pc & hs up to qid	Alcohol free. In 120 & 480 ml.	6.2
c-II	**Dilaudid Cough Syrup** (Knoll)	1 mg hydromorphone HCl	100 mg guaifenesin	5% alcohol, tartrazine	5 ml q 3 to 4 h	Peach flavor. In 480 ml.	5.3

* Cost Index based on cost per tablet or 5 ml. *sf* – Sugar free.

COUGH PREPARATIONS (Cont.)

Refer to the general discussion of these products beginning on page 990
Content given per 5 ml.

Pediatric Narcotic Antitussives with Expectorants Combinations

	Product & Distributor	Decongestant	Antihistamine	Antitussive	Expectorant	Other & Average Dose	How Supplied	C.I.*
c-v	**Nucofed Pediatric Expectorant Syrup** (SK-Beecham)	30 mg pseudoephedrine HCl		10 mg codeine phosphate	100 mg guaifenesin	6% alcohol, saccharin, sucrose. *2 to < 12 yrs* – 2.5 to 5 ml q 6 h	Strawberry flavor. In 480 ml.	1.2
c-v	**Nucotuss Pediatric Expectorant Liquid** (Barre-National)					6% alcohol. *2 to < 12 yrs* – 2.5 to 5 ml q 6 h	Strawberry flavor. In 480 ml.	1.1
c-v	**Pediacof Syrup** (Winthrop)	2.5 phenylephrine HCl	0.75 mg chlorpheniramine maleate	5 mg codeine phosphate	75 mg potassium iodide	5% alcohol, glucose, saccharin. *6 mo to 12 yrs* – 1.25 to 10 ml q 4 to 6 h	Raspberry flavor. In 480 ml.	1.4
c-v	**Pedituss Cough Syrup** (Major)					5% alcohol, saccharin, sorbitol, sucrose. *6 mos to 12 yrs* – 1.25 to 10 ml q 4 to 6 h	In pt and gal.	1

* Cost Index based on cost per 5 ml.

COUGH PREPARATIONS (Cont.)

Refer to the general discussion of these products beginning on page 990. Content given per tablet or 5 ml.

Nonnarcotic Antitussives with Expectorants

	Product & Distributor	Antitussive	Expectorant	Other	Average Adult Dose	How Supplied	C.I.*
Rx	**Humibid DM Tablets** (Adams)	30 mg dextromethorphan HBr	600 mg guaifenesin		1 or 2 q 12 h	Long-acting. (Adams/030). Dark green, scored. In 100s.	15
otc *sf*	**Naldecon Senior DX Liquid** (Apothecon)	15 mg dextromethorphan HBr	200 mg guaifenesin	Saccharin, sorbitol	10 ml q 6 to 8 h	Alcohol free. In 118 and 480 ml.	5.3
otc	**Extra Action Cough Syrup** (Rugby)	15 mg dextromethorphan HBr	100 mg guaifenesin	1.4% alcohol, corn syrup, saccharin, sucrose	10 ml q 6 to 8 h	In 118 ml.	2.3
otc	**Guiatussin with Dextromethorphan Liquid** (Rugby)			1.4% alcohol		In 480 ml.	1.3
otc	**Halotussin-DM Syrup** (Halsey)			1.4% alcohol, corn syrup, menthol, saccharin, sugar		Cherry and raspberry flavor. In 120 & 240 ml, pt and gal.	2.3
otc *sf*	**Halotussin-DM Sugar Free Liquid** (Halsey)			Saccharin, sorbitol		In 120, 240 and 480 ml.	2.3
otc	**Queltuss Tablets** (Forest)				2 q 6 to 8 h	In 1000s.	1
otc	**Rhinosyn-DMX Syrup** (Great Southern)				10 ml q 6 h	In 120 ml.	4
otc	**Uni-tussin DM Syrup** (URL)			1.4% alcohol	10 ml q 6 to 8 h	In 118 ml.	2
otc *sf*	**Tuss-DM Tablets** (Hyrex)	10 mg dextromethorphan HBr	200 mg guaifenesin	—	1 or 2 q 4 h up to 12/day	Dye free. In 100s and 1000s.	2.7

* Cost Index based on cost per tablet or 5 ml. *sf* – Sugar free.

(Continued on following page)

COUGH PREPARATIONS (Cont.)

Refer to the general discussion of these products beginning on page 990. Content given per tablet or 5 ml.

Nonnarcotic Antitussives with Expectorants (Cont.)

	Product & Distributor	Antitussive	Expectorant	Other	Average Adult Dose	How Supplied	C.I.*
otc	**Kolephrin GG/DM Liquid** (Pfeiffer)	10 mg dextromethorphan HBr	150 mg guaifenesin	Glucose, saccharin, sucrose	10 ml q 4 h	Alcohol free. Cherry flavor. In 120 ml.	3.3
otc	**Cheracol D Cough Liquid** (Roberts)	10 mg dextromethorphan HBr	100 mg guaifenesin	4.75% alcohol, fructose, sucrose	10 ml q 4 h	In 60, 120 and 180 ml.	4
otc	**Genatuss DM Syrup** (Goldline)			1.4% alcohol, glucose, saccharin, sucrose	10 ml q 4 h	Fruit/mint flavor. In 120 ml, pt and gal.	3
otc	**Guiatuss-DM Liquid** (Various)				10 ml q 4 h	In 120, 240 ml, pt, gal.	2.3+
otc	**Glycotuss-dM Tablets** (Pal-Pak)				1 to 2 q 4 h	In 100s and 1000s.	2.7
otc	**Mytussin DM Liquid** (PBI)			1.4% alcohol	5 to 10 ml q 4 h	Cherry flavor. In 120 and 240 ml, pt & gal.	2.7
otc	**Robafen DM Syrup** (Major)			1.4% alcohol, sugar, menthol, sorbitol	5 to 10 ml q 4 h	In 473 ml.	NA
otc	**Robitussin-DM Liquid** (Robins)			Saccharin, glucose, high fructose corn syrup	10 ml q 4 h	In 120, 240 and 360 ml, pt, gal, UD 10 ml and Dis-Co Pack 5 & 10 ml.	4.3
otc *sf*	**Tolu-Sed DM Liquid** (Scherer)			10% alcohol	5 to 10 ml q 4 h or 15 ml q 6 to 8 h	In 120 ml.	3.3
otc	**Contac Cough Formula Liquid** (SK-Beecham)	10 mg dextromethorphan HBr	67 mg guaifenesin	Menthol, saccharin, sugar	15 ml q 6 to 8 h	Alcohol free. Cherry flavor. In 120 ml.	4
otc *sf*	**Medatussin Cough Syrup** (Dal-Med)	10 mg dextromethorphan HBr	100 mg glyceryl guaiacolate, 85 mg potassium citrate, 35 mg citric acid		10 ml q 3 to 4 h	Alcohol free. In 120 and 240 ml and pt.	4.3
otc *sf*	**Phanatuss Cough Syrup** (Pharmakon Labs)	10 mg dextromethorphan HBr	85 mg glyceryl guaiacolate, 75 mg potassium citrate, 35 mg citric acid	Menthol, saccharin, sorbitol	10 ml q 3 to 4 h	Alcohol free. In 118 ml.	5.7

* Cost Index based on cost per tablet or 5 ml. *sf* – Sugar free.

(Continued on following page)

COUGH PREPARATIONS (Cont.)

Refer to the general discussion of these products beginning on page 990.
Content given per tablet or 5 ml.

Antitussive and Expectorant Combinations (Cont.)

	Product & Distributor	Decongestant	Antitussive	Expectorant	Other	Adult Dose	How Supplied	C.I.*
otc	**Pertussin AM Liquid** (Pertussin Labs)	20 mg pseudo-ephedrine HCl	6.7 mg dextro-methorphan HBr	67 mg guaifenesin	10% alcohol, saccharin, sucrose	15 ml q 4 h up to 60 ml/day	Cherry flavor. In 240 ml.	1.4
otc	**Cough Formula Comtrex Liquid** (Bristol-Myers)	15 mg pseudo-ephedrine HCl	7.5 mg dextromethor-phan HBr	50 mg guaifenesin	125 mg aceta-minophen, 20% alcohol, men-thol, saccharin, sucrose	20 ml q 4 h up to 80 ml/day	Raspberry fla-vor. In 120 and 240 ml.	2.4
otc *sf*	**Contac Cough & Chest Cold Liquid** (SK-Beecham)	15 mg pseudo-ephedrine HCl	5 mg dextro-methorphan HBr	50 mg guaifenesin	125 mg aceta-minophen, 10% alcohol, sac-charin, sorbitol	20 ml q 4 to 6 h up to 80 ml/day	In 120 ml.	2.6
otc	**DayCare Liquid** (Richardson-Vicks)	10 mg pseudo-ephedrine HCl	3.3 mg dextro-methorphan HBr	33.3 mg guaifenesin	108.3 mg ace-taminophen, 10% alcohol, saccharin, sucrose	30 ml q 4 h up to 120 ml/day	In 180 and 300 ml.	2.1
otc *sf*	**Anatuss Syrup** (Mayrand)	25 mg phenyl-propanolamine HCl	15 mg dextro-methorphan HBr	100 mg guaifenesin		10 ml q 6 h	Alcohol free. In 120 & 473 ml.	3.4
Rx	**Anatuss Tablets** (Mayrand)				325 mg aceta-minophen	2 q 4 to 6 h up to 8/day	Green. Film coated. In 100s.	4.2
otc	**Phanacōl Cough Syrup** (Pharmakon)	25 mg phenyl-propanolamine HCl	10 mg dextro-methorphan HBr	100 mg guaifenesin	325 mg aceta-minophen, sugar	10 ml q 4 to 8 h up to 30 ml/day	Cherry flavor. In 118 and 236 ml.	NA
c-III	**Tussanil DH Tablets** (Misemer)	25 mg phenyl-propanolamine HCl	1.66 mg hydrocodone bitartrate	100 mg guaifenesin	300 mg salicyl-amide	1 to 2 q 4 to 6 h	Purple. Capsule shape. In 100s.	4.3

* Cost Index based on cost per tablet or 5 ml.
sf – Sugar free.

(Continued on following page)

COUGH PREPARATIONS (Cont.)

Refer to the general discussion of these products beginning on page 990.
Content given per capsule or 5 ml.

Antitussive and Expectorant Combinations (Cont.)

	Product & Distributor	Decongestant	Antitussive	Expectorant	Other	Adult Dose	How Supplied	C.I.*
otc	**Sudafed Cough Syrup** (Burroughs Wellcome)	15 mg pseudo-ephedrine HCl	5 mg dextro-methorphan HBr	100 mg guaifenesin	2.4% alcohol, saccharin, sucrose	20 ml q 4 h up to 80 ml/day	Fruity mint flavor. In 118 ml.	2.3
otc	**Naldecon DX Adult Liquid** (Apothecon)	12.5 mg phenyl-propanolamine HCl	10 mg dextro-methorphan HBr	200 mg guaifenesin	0.06% alcohol	10 ml q 4 h	In 118 and 480 ml.	2.6
otc	**Guiatuss CF Liquid** (Barre-National)	12.5 mg phenyl-propanolamine HCl	10 mg dextro-methorphan HBr	100 mg guaifenesin	4.75% alcohol	10 ml q 4 h	Cherry flavor. In 120 ml.	1.6
otc	**Robafen CF Liquid** (Major)						In 118 ml.	2.2
otc	**Robitussin-CF Syrup** (Robins)				4.75% alcohol, saccharin, sorbitol		In 120, 240, 360 and 480 ml.	2.6
Rx	**Cophene-X Capsules** (Dunhall)	10 mg phenyl-ephrine HCl, 10 mg phenyl-propanolamine HCl		20 mg carbeta-pentane citrate	45 mg potassium guaiacolsulfonate	1 or 2 tid or qid	In 100s.	3.6

* Cost Index based on cost per capsule or 5 ml.

(Continued on following page)

chapter 6

central nervous system

CAFFEINE

Actions:

Pharmacology: Caffeine, a methylxanthine, exerts its pharmacological effects by increasing calcium permeability in sarcoplasmic reticulum, inhibiting phosphodiesterase promoting accumulation of cyclic AMP, and competitively blocking adenosine receptors. It is a potent stimulant of the CNS. It also produces cardiac stimulation, dilatation of coronary and peripheral blood vessels, constriction of cerebral blood vessels, skeletal muscle stimulation, augmentation of gastric acid secretion and diuretic activity. Low concentrations of caffeine produce a small decrease in heart rate; higher concentrations produce tachycardia or premature ventricular contractions.

Because of its CNS stimulating effects and constriction of cerebral blood vessels, caffeine is frequently used as an analgesic adjuvant. In various studies, the addition of ≥ 65 mg per tablet (≤ 600 mg/day) increased the analgesic effects and decreased time to onset of aspirin, acetaminophen and combinations. It also increased absorption of ergot alkaloids.

Tolerance to the cardiovascular, CNS and diuretic effects may develop. Differences in effects of caffeine on various organ systems may be observed in nonusers of caffeine vs habitual consumers. Acute ingestion of caffeine produces increases in systolic blood pressure, plasma catecholamines, plasma renin activity and heart rate; chronic ingestion has little or no effect on these hemodynamic variables, nor is caffeine arrhythmogenic. The amount of caffeine derived from dietary sources is given in the following table:

Caffeine Content from Various Dietary Sources[1]

Dietary source	Range of caffeine content
Coffee – Regular: Brewed	40-180 mg/5 to 8 oz
Instant	30-120 mg/5 to 8 oz
Coffee – Decaffeinated: Brewed	2-5 mg/5 to 8 oz
Instant	1-5 mg/5 to 8 oz
Tea: Brewed	20-110 mg/5 to 8 oz
Instant	25-50 mg/5 to 8 oz
Iced	≈ 70 mg/12 oz
Other: Soft drinks	0-54 mg/12 oz
Cocoa	2-50 mg/5 to 8 oz
Chocolate milk	2-7 mg/5 oz
Milk chocolate	1-15 mg/1 oz
Bakers chocolate	25-35 mg/1 oz

[1] Depending on strength of brew and product.

Pharmacokinetics: Absorption/Distribution – Caffeine is well absorbed orally (99%). Peak plasma levels of 5 to 25 mcg/ml are achieved 15 to 45 minutes after 250 mg. Protein binding is 15% to 17%. Caffeine readily crosses the blood brain barrier and placenta. Therapeutic plasma concentrations are ≈ 6 to 13 mcg/ml; those > 20 mcg/ml produce adverse effects. The lethal concentration is > 100 mcg/ml.

Metabolism/Excretion – Caffeine is metabolized in the liver; 0.5% to 3.5% is excreted unchanged in the urine. Clearance is decreased in alcoholic liver disease. In the adult, plasma half-life ranges from 3 to 7.5 hours (average 3.5 hours). Half-life is prolonged in pregnancy (up to 18 hours) and with concomitant use of some drugs (see Drug Interactions).

In neonates, caffeine is eliminated almost entirely by excretion of unchanged drug in the urine. Preterm infants at birth exhibit half-lives of 65 to 103 hours; term infants at birth, 82 hours; 3 to 4½-month-old infants, 14.4 hours; and 5- to 6-month-old infants, 2.6 hours. In newborns, plasma and cerebrospinal fluid levels are nearly identical.

Indications:

Oral: As an aid in staying awake and restoring mental alertness.

As an adjuvant in analgesic formulations.

Parenteral: IM – As an analeptic in conjunction with supportive measures to treat respiratory depression associated with overdosage with CNS depressants (eg, narcotic analgesics, alcohol). However, because of questionable benefit and transient action, most authorities believe caffeine and other analeptics should not be used in these conditions and recommend other supportive therapy.

(Indications continued on following page)

CAFFEINE (Cont.)

Indications (Cont.):

Unlabeled uses: Neonatal apnea – An initial dose of 10 mg/kg caffeine followed by a maintenance dose of 2.5 mg/kg/day. Control is associated with plasma concentrations of 5 to 20 mcg/ml. Do not use products containing sodium benzoate in neonates.

Atopic dermatitis – Topical treatment with 30% caffeine in a hydrophilic base or in a hydrocortisone cream produces improvement in pruritus, erythema, scaling, lichenification, oozing and dermatitis. This may be related to caffeine's property of liberating water from epidermal and subcutaneous tissues, similar to urea.

Headache – To alleviate headaches following spinal puncture (500 mg).

Alcohol – For the treatment of excited or comatose alcoholic patients.

Asthma – Although potentially beneficial at higher doses, caffeine offers no advantage over theophylline.

Orthostatic hypotension due to autonomic failure was attenuated, especially in the postprandial state, by 250 mg caffeine in a small number of patients.

Warnings:

Depression: Too vigorous treatment with parenteral caffeine can produce further depression in the already depressed patient; therefore, do not exceed 1 g as a single dose of caffeine and sodium benzoate.

GI effects: Large quantities of caffeine-containing products may reactivate duodenal ulcers.

Pregnancy: Category C. Safety for use in pregnancy has not been established; pregnant women should consume sparingly or avoid caffeine-containing food and drugs. Caffeine crosses the placenta and achieves fetal blood and tissue levels similar to maternal concentrations. Excessive caffeine intake has been weakly associated with increased fetal loss, low birth weight and premature deliveries; however, when used in moderation there is no association with these effects or congenital malformations. Caffeine causes birth defects in animals.

Lactation: Caffeine appears in the breast milk of nursing mothers. Milk:plasma ratios of 0.5 have been reported. Approximately 1.5 to 3.1 mg of caffeine would be ingested by a nursing infant whose mother had one cup of coffee.

Precautions:

Hyperglycemic effects: Higher blood glucose levels may result from caffeine use.

Drug Interactions:

Caffeine Drug Interactions

Precipitant drug	Object drug*		Description
Cimetidine Contraceptives, oral Disulfiram Fluoroquinolones – ciprofloxacin enoxacin	Caffeine	↑	Caffeine metabolism may be impaired, resulting in decreased clearance and increased half-life. Excessive CNS effects may occur.
Phenylpropanolamine	Caffeine	↑	Serum caffeine levels may be increased, resulting in an increase in pharmacologic and toxic effects.
Smoking	Caffeine	↓	Elimination of caffeine may be enhanced.

* ↑ = Object drug increased ↓ = Object drug decreased

Drug/Lab test interactions: Caffeine produces false positive elevations of serum urate as measured by the Bittner method. Caffeine also produces slight increases in urine levels of VMA, catecholamines and 5-hydroxyindoleacetic acid. Because high urine levels of VMA or catecholamines may result in false positive diagnosis of pheochromocytoma or neuroblastoma, avoid caffeine intake during tests for these disorders.

Drug/Food interaction: **Coffee** and **tea** consumed with a meal or 1 hour after a meal significantly inhibits the absorption of dietary **iron**. Clinical significance has not been determined.

Adverse Reactions:

CNS: Insomnia; restlessness; excitement; nervousness; tinnitus; scintillating scotoma; muscular tremor; headaches; lightheadedness.

Anxiety neurosis – Large doses of caffeine may produce symptoms mimicking anxiety neurosis (eg, tremulousness, muscle twitching, sensory disturbances, irritability, flushing, tachypnea, palpitations, arrhythmias, GI disturbances, diuresis).

(Adverse Reactions continued on following page)

CAFFEINE (Cont.)

Adverse Reactions (Cont.):

GI: Nausea; vomiting; diarrhea; stomach pain.

Cardiac: Tachycardia; extrasystoles; palpitations.

GU: Diuresis.

Withdrawal: Headache, anxiety and muscle tension may occur following abrupt cessation of the drug after regular consumption of 500 to 600 mg/day. Symptoms usually start between 12 to 18 hours after the last caffeine ingestion.

Overdosage:

Symptoms: Toxic symptoms can be produced in the adult with $\geq$ 1 g oral caffeine. Deaths have occurred after the IV and oral administration of caffeine and rectal administration of coffee. The acute lethal dose of caffeine ranges from 5 to 10 g IV or oral.

Adults – Initially, insomnia, dyspnea, mild delirium. Alternating states of consciousness and muscle twitching may appear. Diuresis, arrhythmias and hyperglycemia have occurred. The terminal event is usually seizures.

Infants – Caffeine overdosage has been reported in newborns given a single dose of caffeine, 36 to 94 mg/kg, at birth. Symptoms included hypertonicity alternating with hypotonicity, opisthotonic posturing, coarse tremors, bradycardia, hypotension and severe acidosis. Intracranial hemorrhage has also occurred.

Treatment: Symptomatic and supportive. Gastric lavage followed by activated charcoal may be useful. Control seizures with diazepam or phenobarbital.

Patient Information:

Do not exceed recommended dosage.

Discontinue use if increased or abnormal heart rate, dizziness or palpitations occur.

If fatigue persists or recurs, consult physician.

Not intended for use as a substitute for normal sleep.

Administration and Dosage:

Oral: 100 to 200 mg every 3 to 4 hours, as needed. Not recommended for children.

Timed release – 200 mg every 3 to 4 hours.

An oral solution of caffeine may be prepared as follows – Dissolve 10 g caffeine citrate powder in 250 ml Sterile Water for Irrigation, USP, qs to 500 ml with 2 parts simple syrup to 1 part cherry syrup. Final concentration is 10 mg/ml caffeine base (20 mg/ml caffeine citrate). Stable for at least 3 months.

Parenteral: Sodium benzoate increases caffeine's solubility in aqueous solutions.

Adults – 500 mg (250 mg caffeine) IM (or slow IV injection in emergency respiratory failure) or a maximum single dose of 1 g (500 mg caffeine). The usual and maximum safe dose is 500 mg. The total dose in 24 hours should *rarely* exceed 2.5 g.

Analeptic use of caffeine is strongly discouraged by most clinicians.

Alternative parenteral formulation – An IV formulation of caffeine may be prepared by one of the two following methods:

1) Dissolve 10 g caffeine citrate powder in 250 ml Sterile Water for Injection, USP, qs to 500 ml, filter, and autoclave. Final concentration is 10 mg/ml caffeine base (20 mg/ml caffeine citrate). Stable for at least 3 months.
2) Dissolve 10 g caffeine powder and 10.94 g citric acid powder in Bacteriostatic Water for Injection, USP, qs to 1 L. Sterilize by filtration.

	Product	Form	Description	C.I.*
otc	**NoDoz** (Bristol-Myers)	**Tablets:** 100 mg	Sucrose. (NoDoz). White. In 15s, 16s, 36s and 60s.	NA
otc	**Tirend** (SK-Beecham)		Lactose. Lemon flavor. In 12s, 30s and 60s.	30
otc	**Quick Pep** (Thompson)	**Tablets:** 150 mg	Dextrose, sucrose. In 32s.	20
otc	**Vivarin** (SK-Beecham)	**Tablets:** 200 mg	Dextrose. Capsule shape. In 16s, 24s, 40s and 80s.	37
otc	**Caffedrine** (Thompson)	**Tablets, timed release:** 200 mg anhydrous caffeine	Lactose. Capsule shape. In 20s.	20
otc	**Coffee Break Caplets** (Columbia)		Capsule shape. In 20s.	25
otc	**Caffedrine** (Thompson)	**Capsules, timed release:** 200 mg anhydrous caffeine	Sucrose. (Caffedrine). Clear w/purple band. In 16s.	20
Rx	**Caffeine and Sodium Benzoate** (Pasadena)	**Injection:** 250 mg per ml (equal parts caffeine and sodium benzoate)	In 2 ml amps.	NA

* Cost Index based on cost per 100 mg caffeine.

DOXAPRAM HCl

Actions:

Pharmacology: Produces respiratory stimulation by activating the peripheral carotid chemoreceptors. The respiratory stimulant action is manifested by an increase in tidal volume associated with a slight increase in respiratory rate. As the dosage is increased, the medullary respiratory centers are stimulated with progressive stimulation of other parts of the brain and spinal cord.

A pressor response due to improved cardiac output rather than peripheral vasoconstriction may occur. If there is no cardiac impairment, the pressor effect is greater in hypovolemic than in normovolemic states. Following administration, an increased release of catecholamines has occurred.

Although opiate-induced respiratory depression is antagonized by doxapram, the analgesia is not affected.

Pharmacokinetics: The onset of respiratory stimulation following the recommended single IV injection usually occurs in 20 to 40 seconds, with peak effect at 1 to 2 minutes. The duration of effect varies from 5 to 12 minutes. Doxapram is rapidly metabolized (up to 99%) and metabolites are excreted in urine. The plasma half-life ranges from 2.4 to 4.1 hours.

Indications:

Postanesthesia: To stimulate respiration in patients with drug-induced postanesthesia respiratory depression or apnea other than that due to muscle relaxants.

May also be used with simultaneous administration of oxygen to pharmacologically stimulate deep breathing in the "stir-up" regimen in the postoperative patient.

Drug-induced CNS depression: To stimulate respiration, hasten arousal and encourage return of laryngopharyngeal reflexes in patients with mild to moderate respiratory and CNS depression due to overdosage. Exercise care to prevent vomiting and aspiration.

Controlled ventilation and standard supportive care for respiratory depression due to CNS overdose is safer, more reliable and more effective than doxapram.

Chronic pulmonary disease associated with acute hypercapnia: As a temporary measure in hospitalized patients with acute respiratory insufficiency superimposed on chronic obstructive pulmonary disease. Use for a short period of time (approximately 2 hours) to prevent elevation of arterial CO_2 tension during the administration of oxygen. Do not use in conjunction with mechanical ventilation.

Unlabeled Use: Low dose doxapram has been studied in the treatment of apnea of prematurity when methylxanthines have failed. (See Contraindications.)

Contraindications:

This product contains benzyl alcohol; do not use in newborns.

Epilepsy or other convulsive states; incompetence of the ventilatory mechanism due to muscle paresis; flail chest; hypersensitivity to doxapram; head injury.

Pulmonary disease: Pneumothorax, acute bronchial asthma, pulmonary fibrosis; other conditions resulting in restriction of chest wall, muscles of respiration or alveolar expansion.

Cardiovascular disease: Severe hypertension or cerebrovascular accidents; significant cardiovascular impairment.

Warnings:

Postanesthetic use: Doxapram is neither an antagonist to muscle relaxant drugs nor a specific narcotic antagonist. Assure adequacy of airway and oxygenation prior to use. Administer carefully to patients with hyperthyroidism or pheochromocytoma.

Since narcosis may recur after stimulation with doxapram, maintain close observation until patient has been fully alert for 30 minutes to 1 hour.

Drug-induced CNS and respiratory depression: Doxapram alone may not stimulate adequate spontaneous breathing or provide sufficient arousal in patients who are severely depressed either due to respiratory failure or to CNS depressant drugs. Use as an adjunct to established supportive measures and resuscitative techniques.

Chronic obstructive pulmonary disease: In an attempt to lower pCO_2, do not increase rate of infusion in severely ill patients because of the associated increased work in breathing. Do not use in conjunction with mechanical ventilation.

Usage in Pregnancy: Category B. Safety for use during pregnancy has not been established. Use during pregnancy only when clearly needed.

Usage in Lactation: It is not known whether this drug is excreted in breast milk. Exercise caution when administering to a nursing mother.

Usage in Children: Safety and efficacy for use in children under 12 years of age have not been established. The use of benzyl alcohol in newborns has been associated with metabolic, CNS, respiratory, circulatory and renal dysfunction.

(Continued on following page)

DOXAPRAM HCl (Cont.)

Precautions:

Avoid extravasation or use of a single injection site over an extended period; thrombophlebitis or local skin irritation may occur. Rapid infusion may result in hemolysis.

Monitor blood pressure and deep tendon reflexes to prevent overdosage.

Have short-acting IV barbiturates, oxygen and resuscitative equipment readily available to manage overdosage manifested by excessive CNS stimulation. Slow administration and careful observation of the patient during and following administration are advisable to assure that the protective reflexes have been restored and to prevent possible posthyperventilation hypoventilation. (See Overdosage.)

Blood pressure increases are generally modest, but significant increases have occurred. Not recommended for use in severe hypertension. If sudden hypotension or dyspnea develops, discontinue use.

Chronic obstructive pulmonary disease: In some patients, arrhythmias in acute respiratory failure secondary to chronic obstructive pulmonary disease are probably the result of hypoxia. Use with caution in these patients.

Measure arterial blood gases prior to the initiation of doxapram infusion and oxygen administration, then at least every ½ hour. Doxapram administration does not diminish the need for careful patient monitoring or the need for supplemental oxygen in acute respiratory failure. Discontinue use if the arterial blood gases deteriorate and initiate mechanical ventilation.

Lowered pCO_2 induced by hyperventilation produces cerebral vasoconstriction and slowing of the cerebral circulation.

Drug Interactions:

Sympathomimetics or **monoamine oxidase inhibitors:** Administer cautiously to patients receiving these drugs since an additive pressor effect may occur.

Halothane, cyclopropane and **enflurane:** Since an increase in epinephrine release has been noted with doxapram, delay initiation of therapy for at least 10 minutes following discontinuance of anesthetics known to sensitize the myocardium to catecholamines.

Muscle relaxants: Doxapram may temporarily mask residual effects of muscle relaxants.

Adverse Reactions:

Central and autonomic nervous systems: Headache; dizziness; apprehension; disorientation; pupillary dilatation; hyperactivity; convulsions; bilateral Babinski; involuntary movements; muscle spasticity; increased deep tendon reflexes; clonus; pyrexia; flushing; sweating; pruritus and paresthesia such as a feeling of warmth, burning or hot sensation, especially in the area of the genitalia and perineum.

Respiratory: Cough; dyspnea; tachypnea; laryngospasm; bronchospasm; hiccoughs; rebound hypoventilation.

Hematologic: A decrease in hemoglobin, hematocrit or red blood cell count has occurred in postoperative patients. In the presence of preexisting leukopenia, a further decrease in WBC has occurred following anesthesia and treatment with doxapram. Elevation of BUN has also occurred. A cause and effect relationship has not been determined.

Cardiovascular: Phlebitis; variations in heart rate; lowered T waves; arrhythmias; chest pain; tightness in chest. A mild to moderate increase in blood pressure is commonly noted and may be of concern in patients with severe cardiovascular diseases.

GI: Nausea; vomiting; diarrhea; desire to defecate.

GU: Urinary retention; spontaneous voiding; proteinuria.

Overdosage:

Symptoms: Excessive pressor effect, tachycardia, skeletal muscle hyperactivity and enhanced deep tendon reflexes may be early signs of overdosage. Evaluate blood pressure, pulse rate and deep tendon reflexes periodically and adjust dosage or infusion rate accordingly.

Treatment: There is no specific antidote. Treatment is supportive. Refer to General Management of Acute Overdosage on p. vi. Convulsive seizures are unlikely at recommended dosages, but IV barbiturates, oxygen and resuscitative equipment should be available. There is no evidence that doxapram is dialyzable. Due to the half-life of doxapram, it is unlikely that dialysis would be appropriate treatment for overdosage.

(Continued on following page)

Complete prescribing information for these products begins on page 1084

AMPHETAMINE SULFATE (Racemic Amphetamine Sulfate)

Administration and Dosage:

Narcolepsy: 5 to 60 mg/day in divided doses.

Children (6 to 12 years) – Narcolepsy seldom occurs in children under 12. When it does, initial dose is 5 mg daily; increase in increments of 5 mg at weekly intervals until optimal response is obtained (maximum 60 mg/day).

Adults (12 years and older) – Start with 10 mg daily; raise in increments of 10 mg/day at weekly intervals. If adverse reactions appear (eg, insomnia or anorexia), reduce dose. Long-acting forms may be used for once-a-day dosage. With tablets or elixir, give first dose on awakening; additional doses (1 or 2) at intervals of 4 to 6 hours.

Attention deficit disorder in children:

Not recommended for children under 3 years of age.

Children (3 to 5 years) – 2.5 mg daily; increase in increments of 2.5 mg/day at weekly intervals until optimal response is obtained. Usual range is 0.1 to 0.5 mg/kg/dose every morning.

Children (6 years and older) – 5 mg once or twice daily; increase in increments of 5 mg/day at weekly intervals until optimal response is obtained. Dosage will rarely exceed 40 mg/day. Usual range is 0.1 to 0.5 mg/kg/dose every morning.

Long-acting forms may be used for once-a-day dosage. With tablets or elixir, give first dose on awakening; additional doses (1 or 2) may be given at intervals of 4 to 6 hours.

Exogenous obesity: 5 to 30 mg daily in divided doses of 5 to 10 mg, 30 to 60 minutes before meals. Long-acting form: 10 or 15 mg in the morning. Not recommended for children under 12 years of age.

				C.I.*
c-II	**Amphetamine Sulfate** (Lannett)	**Tablets:** 5 mg	In 1000s.	13
		10 mg	In 1000s.	8

DEXTROAMPHETAMINE SULFATE

Administration and Dosage:

See amphetamine sulfate above.

				C.I.*
c-II	**Dextroamphetamine Sulfate** (Various)	**Tablets:** 5 mg	In 500s and 1000s.	9+
c-II	**Dexedrine** (SKF)		Tartrazine. (#SKF E19). Orange, scored. In 100s and 1000s.	60
c-II	**Ferndex** (Ferndale)		Blue, scored. In 100s.	22
c-II	**Dextroamphetamine Sulfate** (Various)	**Tablets:** 10 mg	In 500s and 1000s.	14+
c-II	**Oxydess II** (Vortech)		In 100s.	20
c-II	**Dexedrine Spansules** (SKF)	**Capsules, sustained release:** 5 mg	Tartrazine. (#SKF E12). Natural and brown. In 50s.	129
c-II	**Dexedrine Spansules** (SKF)	**Capsules, sustained release:** 10 mg	Tartrazine. (#SKF E13). Natural and brown. In 50s and 500s.	161
c-II	**Dextroamphetamine Sulfate** (Various)	**Capsules, sustained release:** 15 mg	In 250s.	16+
c-II	**Dexedrine Spansules** (SKF)		Tartrazine. (#SKF E14). Natural and brown. In 50s and 500s.	68
c-II	**Spancap No. 1** (Vortech)		In 1000s.	12
c-II	**Dexedrine** (SKF)	**Elixir:** 5 mg per 5 ml	Tartrazine. 10% alcohol. Orange flavor. In 480 ml.	63

* Cost Index based on cost per 5 mg amphetamine or dextroamphetamine.
# Product identification code.

Complete prescribing information for these products begins on page 1084

METHAMPHETAMINE HCl (Desoxyephedrine HCl)

Administration and Dosage:

Attention deficit disorder in children: Initially, 5 mg once or twice a day; increase in increments of 5 mg/day at weekly intervals until an optimum response is achieved. Usual effective dose is 20 to 25 mg daily.

Total daily dose may be given as conventional tablets in 2 divided doses, or once daily using the long-acting form. Do not use the long-acting form for initiation of dosage or until the titrated daily dose is equal to or greater than the dosage provided in a long-acting tablet. Where possible, interrupt drug administration to determine if there is a recurrence of behavioral symptoms sufficient to require continued therapy.

Obesity: 5 mg, 30 minutes before each meal. *Long-acting form* – 10 to 15 mg in the morning. Treatment duration should not exceed a few weeks. Do not use in children under 12 years old.

				C.I.*
c-II	**Desoxyn** (Abbott)	**Tablets:** 5 mg	White. In 100s.	140
c-II	**Desoxyn Gradumets** (Abbott)	**Tablets, long-acting:** 5 mg	(#MC). White. In 100s.	375
		10 mg	(#ME). Orange. In 100s and 500s.	252
		15 mg	Tartrazine. (#MF). Yellow. In 100s and 500s.	214

AMPHETAMINE COMPLEX

Resin complex of amphetamine and dextroamphetamine.

Administration and Dosage:

Attention deficit disorder in children: Begin therapy with dextroamphetamine to determine appropriate dosage. Once the optimal response dosage level has been established, use amphetamine complex for once-a-day dosage wherever convenient.

Obesity: One capsule daily, 10 to 14 hours before retiring; adjust dose to individual requirements.

				C.I.*
c-II	**Biphetamine 12½** (Fisons)	**Capsules:** 6.25 mg dextroamphetamine and 6.25 mg amphetamine (equivalent to 10 mg dextroamphetamine)	(#Biphet 12½). Black and white. In 100s.	166
c-II	**Biphetamine 20** (Fisons)	**Capsules:** 10 mg dextroamphetamine and 10 mg amphetamine (equivalent to 15 mg dextroamphetamine)	(#Biphet 20). Black. In 100s.	119

AMPHETAMINE MIXTURES

These mixtures contain various salts of amphetamine and dextroamphetamine.

Administration and Dosage:

See amphetamine sulfate, page 1087

				C.I.*
c-II	**Obetrol-10** (Obetrol Pharm)	**Tablets:** 2.5 mg dextroamphetamine sulfate, 2.5 mg dextroamphetamine saccharate, 2.5 mg amphetamine aspartate and 2.5 mg amphetamine sulfate	(#OP-32). Blue, scored. In 100s, 500s and 1000s.	28
c-II	**Obetrol-20** (Obetrol Pharm)	**Tablets:** 5 mg dextroamphetamine sulfate, 5 mg dextroamphetamine saccharate, 5 mg amphetamine aspartate and 5 mg amphetamine sulfate	(#OP-33). Orange, scored. In 100s, 500s and 1000s.	20

* Cost Index based on cost per 5 mg methamphetamine, 5 mg amphetamine complex or 5 mg total amphetamine content.

Product identification code.

In addition to the nonamphetamine anorexiants included in this section, amphetamines are also used for short-term obesity therapy.

Actions:

Pharmacology: The nonamphetamine anorexiants, commonly known as "anorectics" or "anorexigenics", are indirect-acting sympathomimetic amines. Except for mazindol (an imidazoline), phenmetrazine and phendimetrazine (morpholines), all are phenethylamine (amphetamine-like) analogs, and are pharmacologically similar to the amphetamines.

Although the exact mechanism of action has not been established, it is thought that appetite suppression is produced by a direct stimulant effect on the satiety center in the hypothalamic and limbic regions. Diethylpropion and phentermine act primarily on adrenergic pathways; mazindol acts on both adrenergic and dopaminergic pathways; fenfluramine influences serotonin pathways. Secondary actions include CNS stimulation and blood pressure elevation. Fenfluramine differs from other drugs of this class since it produces CNS depression. Fenfluramine's mechanism of action may be related to brain levels (or turnover rates) of serotonin or to increased glucose utilization.

Pharmacokinetics:

Absorption – After oral administration, the immediate release dosage forms generally exert their effects for 4 to 6 hours, except for mazindol (8 to 15 hours).

Fenfluramine is well absorbed from the GI tract and a maximal anorectic effect generally occurs in 2 to 4 hours.

Distribution – Fenfluramine is widely distributed in body tissues. It is lipid soluble and crosses the blood-brain barrier. Diethylpropion and its active metabolites cross the blood brain barrier and the placenta.

Excretion – Most of the drug and metabolites are excreted via the kidneys. The elimination rate of fenfluramine is pH-dependent; much smaller amounts appear in an alkaline urine than in an acid urine.

The half-life of fenfluramine is about 20 hours compared with 5 hours for amphetamines and from 1.9 to 9.8 hours for phendimetrazine tartrate. Fenfluramine's half-life can be reduced to 11 hours if urinary excretion is rapid and the pH is acidic ($<$ pH 5). Fenfluramine reaches steady-state concentrations in plasma within 3 to 4 days following chronic dosage.

Clinical Pharmacology: Short-term clinical trials report greater weight loss in adult obese subjects treated with dietary management and anorexiants vs those treated with diet and placebo. The rate of weight loss is greatest in the first weeks of therapy and decreases in succeeding weeks. The amount of weight loss varies from trial to trial, and appears to be related, in part, to variables other than the drug prescribed, such as the investigator, the population treated and the diet prescribed.

Clinical studies demonstrate that anorexiants with behavior therapy produce better weight loss in obese patients than either therapy alone; however, better weight loss maintenance is achieved with behavior therapy alone.

Factors influencing successful treatment and anorexiant use include: Weight loss during diet alone; eating habits; motivation; personality; obesity characteristics; and adherence to treatment.

Indications:

Exogenous obesity: As a short-term (8 to 12 weeks) adjunct in a regimen of weight reduction based on caloric restriction. Measure the limited usefulness of these agents against their inherent risks.

Unlabeled Use: Preliminary studies suggest **fenfluramine** may be useful in treating autistic children with elevated serotonin levels. Adverse effects have occurred when used in autistic children without elevated serotonin levels.

Contraindications:

Advanced arteriosclerosis; symptomatic cardiovascular disease; moderate to severe hypertension; hyperthyroidism; known hypersensitivity or idiosyncrasy to sympathomimetic amines; glaucoma; agitated states; history of drug abuse; during or within 14 days following the administration of MAO inhibitors (hypertensive crises may result); coadministration with other CNS stimulants.

Do not administer **fenfluramine** to alcoholics, since psychiatric symptoms (paranoia, depression, psychosis) have been reported in a few such patients.

Pregnancy: Category X. **Benzphetamine HCl** is contraindicated during pregnancy (see Warnings).

(Continued on following page)

Warnings:

Concomitant surgical anesthesia: A fatal cardiac arrest occurred shortly after the induction of anesthesia in a patient who had been taking **fenfluramine** prior to surgery. Fenfluramine may have a catecholamine-depleting effect when administered for prolonged periods; administer potent anesthetics cautiously to patients taking fenfluramine. Full cardiac monitoring and facilities for resuscitative measures are necessary.

Tolerance to the anorectic effects may develop within a few weeks; cross tolerance is almost universal. Discontinue the drug rather than increase the dosage. It has been suggested that therapy may be continued past 12 weeks if the patient continues to lose weight, does not develop dependence or side effects, and does not require an increased dosage. However, patients should be closely monitored and therapy should not exceed 6 months duration.

Drug dependence: These drugs are chemically and pharmacologically related to the amphetamines, and have abuse potential. Intense psychological or physical dependence and severe social dysfunction may be associated with long-term therapy or abuse. If this occurs, gradually reduce the dosage to avoid withdrawal symptoms (eg, extreme fatigue, sleep EEG changes and mental depression). Chronic intoxication is manifested by severe dermatoses, marked insomnia, irritability, hyperactivity and personality changes. Psychosis, often clinically indistinguishable from schizophrenia, is the most severe manifestation.

Fenfluramine's abuse potential appears qualitatively different. Doses of 80 to 400 mg were associated with euphoria, derealization and perceptual changes.

Usage in Pregnancy: (*Category X* – Benzphetamine HCl. *Category C* – Fenfluramine. *Category B* – Diethylpropion.) Safety for use during pregnancy has not been established. Use in women who are or who may become pregnant (especially those in the first trimester) only when clearly needed and when the potential benefits outweigh the potential hazards to the fetus.

In animal studies with relatively high doses of **mazindol**, neonatal mortality and incidence of rib anomalies were increased; with **phenmetrazine**, conception rate was adversely affected, as well as survival and body weight of pups. Congenital malformations are associated with phenmetrazine use, but a causal relationship has not been proven. **Fenfluramine** produced questionable embryotoxic effects in rats and a reduced conception rate when given in doses 20 times the human dose. Other studies were negative. Animal and clinical studies have not shown a teratogenic potential for **diethylpropion**. Abuse of diethylpropion during pregnancy may result in withdrawal symptoms in the human neonate.

Usage in Lactation: Safety for use in the nursing mother has not been established.

Diethylpropion and its metabolites are excreted in breast milk. Exercise caution when administering to a nursing woman.

Usage in Children: Not recommended for use in children under 12 years of age.

Precautions:

Potentially hazardous tasks: May produce dizziness, extreme fatigue and depression after abrupt cessation of prolonged high dosage therapy; patients should observe caution while driving or performing other tasks requiring alertness.

Psychological disturbances occurred in patients who received an anorectic agent together with a restrictive diet.

Cardiovascular disease: Use with caution and monitor blood pressure in patients with mild hypertension. Not recommended for patients with symptomatic cardiovascular disease, including arrhythmias.

Pulmonary hypertension occurred in two females taking **fenfluramine** (120 to 160 mg/day) for over 8 months. Symptoms disappeared 3 to 6 weeks after drug discontinuation. In one patient, pulmonary hypertension recurred on rechallenge (80 mg daily for 6 weeks). Advise patients to immediately report any deterioration in exercise tolerance.

Convulsions may increase in some epileptics receiving **diethylpropion**. Dose titration or drug discontinuance may be necessary.

Depression: **Fenfluramine's** central effects are mediated by 5-hydroxytryptamine (5-HT) in the brain stem. A rapid reduction in 5-HT in the brain can lead to depression. This commonly occurs immediately following abrupt withdrawal of fenfluramine; therefore, do not discontinue abruptly. Depression may be provoked while the patient is taking fenfluramine or following abrupt withdrawal, especially in those with a history of mental depression. Control symptoms of depression by reinstituting therapy; follow by gradual withdrawal.

Blood glucose levels: **Mazindol** and **fenfluramine** moderately lower blood glucose levels independent of appetite suppressant effects by increasing glucose uptake in human skeletal muscle.

(Precautions continued on following page)

Precautions (Cont.):

Tartrazine sensitivity: Some of these products contain tartrazine, which may cause allergic-type reactions (including bronchial asthma) in susceptible individuals. Although the incidence of tartrazine sensitivity in the general population is low, it is frequently seen in patients who also have aspirin hypersensitivity. Specific products containing tartrazine are identified in the product listings.

Drug Interactions:

Guanethidine: Anorexiants may decrease the hypotensive effect of guanethidine.

Insulin and **sulfonylureas:** Hypoglycemic effects may be increased due to increased skeletal muscle uptake of glucose by fenfluramine. Monitor blood glucose and adjust the insulin or sulfonylurea dose as necessary.

Monoamine oxidase (MAO) inhibitors may increase the pressor response to the anorexiants. Possible hypertensive crisis and intracranial hemorrhage may occur. This interaction may also occur with **furazolidone**, an antimicrobial with MAO inhibitor activity. Avoid this combination; if given inadvertently and hypertension occurs, administer phentolamine.

Tricyclic antidepressants may decrease the effects of the anorexiants. An increased dose may be necessary.

Adverse Reactions:

Cardiovascular: Palpitations; tachycardia; arrhythmias; hypertension or hypotension; fainting; precordial pain; pulmonary hypertension. ECG changes with **diethylpropion**.

CNS: Overstimulation; nervousness; restlessness; dizziness; insomnia; weakness or fatigue; malaise; anxiety; tension; euphoria; elevated mood; drowsiness; depression; agitation; dysphoria; tremor; dyskinesia; dysarthria; confusion; incoordination; tremor; headache; change in libido; rarely, psychotic episodes. An increase in convulsive episodes occurred in a few epileptics.

Fenfluramine may cause CNS depression, drowsiness and impotence. Withdrawal symptoms (ataxia, tremor, disturbed concentration and memory, loss of sense of reality, visual hallucinations, inverted visual field, depression, suicidal feelings) have been reported following discontinuation of a 1 month course of fenfluramine, 60 mg/day.

GI: Dry mouth; unpleasant taste; nausea; vomiting; abdominal discomfort; diarrhea; constipation; stomach pain.

Allergic: Urticaria; rash; erythema; burning sensation.

Ocular: Mydriasis; eye irritation; blurred vision.

GU: Dysuria; polyuria; urinary frequency; impotence; menstrual upset. Testicular pain has been reported with **mazindol**.

Hematopoietic: Bone marrow depression; agranulocytosis; leukopenia.

Miscellaneous: Hair loss; ecchymosis; muscle pain; chest pain; excessive sweating; clamminess; chills; flushing; fever; myalgia; gynecomastia.

Overdosage:

Symptoms: CNS – Restlessness; tremor; hyperreflexia; rapid respiration; hyperpyrexia; tachypnea; dizziness; confusion; belligerence; assaultiveness; hallucinations; panic states. Depression and fatigue usually follow central stimulation.

Cardiovascular – Arrhythmias (tachycardia); hypertension or hypotension; circulatory collapse.

GI – Nausea; vomiting; diarrhea; abdominal cramps.

Convulsions, coma and death may result.

Fenfluramine – Frequent: Agitation and drowsiness; confusion; flushing; tremor (or shivering); fever; sweating; abdominal pain; hyperventilation; rotary nystagmus; dilated nonreactive pupils. Reflexes may be either exaggerated or depressed. Tachycardia may be present; blood pressure may be normal or only slightly elevated. Convulsions, coma and ventricular extrasystoles, culminating in ventricular fibrillation and cardiac arrest, may occur at higher dosage; death has occurred.

Doses less than 5 mg/kg are toxic; 5 to 10 mg/kg may produce coma and convulsions. Reported single overdoses have ranged from 300 to 2000 mg; the lowest reported fatal dose was a few hundred milligrams in a small child and the highest reported nonfatal dose was 1800 mg in an adult. Most deaths were due to respiratory failure and cardiac arrest.

Toxic effects appear within 30 to 60 minutes and may progress rapidly to potentially fatal complications in 1.5 to 4 hours. Symptoms may persist for extended periods depending upon amount ingested.

(Overdosage continued on following page)

Overdosage (Cont.):

Treatment includes symptomatic and supportive therapy. Refer to Management of Acute Overdosage on p. 2895

Sedate patient with a barbiturate, maintain respiratory exchange and cardiac monitoring. Chlorpromazine may antagonize the CNS effects when excess CNS stimulation is present. If an anticholinergic drug has been taken recently, administer an antipsychotic without prominent anticholinergic actions (eg, haloperidol). IV phentolamine, a nitrite or a rapidly acting alpha receptor blocking agent may be useful in treating acute, severe hypertension.

Experience with hemodialysis or peritoneal dialysis is inadequate to permit recommendations. Acidification of urine increases excretion.

Fenfluramine – Do not induce emesis because the patient may become unconscious at an early stage. If gastric lavage is not feasible due to trismus, perform endotracheal intubation after administration of muscle relaxants; then induce gastric evacuation. Administer activated charcoal after emesis or lavage. If necessary, institute mechanical respiration, defibrillation or cardioversion. Administer diazepam or phenobarbital for convulsions or muscular hyperactivity; propranolol for extreme tachycardia; lidocaine for ventricular extrasystoles; chlorpromazine for hyperpyrexia. After overdosage, only a small percentage of fenfluramine is excreted in the urine. Forced acid diuresis has been recommended only in extreme cases in which the patient survives the early hours of intoxication but fails to show decisive improvement from other measures.

Since fenfluramine has a slight lowering effect on blood sugar, hypoglycemia may occur; however, this effect has not been reported in clinical overdosage cases.

Patient Information:

May cause insomnia; avoid taking medication late in the day.

Weight reduction requires strict adherence to dietary restriction.

Do not take more frequently than prescribed.

Notify physician if palpitations, nervousness or dizziness occurs.

Medication may cause dry mouth and constipation; notify physician if these become pronounced.

May produce dizziness or blurred vision; observe caution while driving or performing other tasks requiring alertness.

Fenfluramine may cause drowsiness. Avoid concomitant consumption of alcohol.

These drugs should generally be taken on an empty stomach; *mazindol* may be taken with meals to reduce GI irritation.

Do not crush or chew sustained release products.

Administration:

Intermittent or interrupted courses of therapy may be useful in the treatment of obesity. A 3 to 6 week course of therapy followed by a discontinuation period of half the original treatment length has been suggested.

(Products listed on following pages)

Complete prescribing information for these products begins on page 1089

PHENTERMINE HCl

Administration and Dosage:

Take 8 mg 3 times daily, one-half hour before meals, or 15 to 37.5 mg as a single daily dose before breakfast or 10 to 14 hours before retiring.

	Product	Dosage form	Description / Packaging	C.I.*
c-IV	**Phentermine HCl** (Various)	**Tablets:** 8 mg (equivalent to 6.4 mg base)	In 100s and 1000s.	38+
c-IV	**Phentrol** (Vortech)		In 100s.	74
c-IV	**Phentermine HCl** (Various)	**Capsules:** 15 mg (equivalent to 12 mg base)	In 100s and 1000s.	119+
c-IV	**Phentermine HCl** (Camall)	**Capsules:** 18.75 mg (equivalent to 15 mg base)	(CC 18.75). Gray and yellow. In 100s, 500s and 1000s.	119
c-IV	**Phentermine HCl** (Various)	**Tablets:** 30 mg (equivalent to 24 mg base)	In 100s and 1000s.	16+
c-IV	**Phentermine HCl** (Various)	**Capsules:** 30 mg (equivalent to 24 mg base)	In 7s, 30s, 100s and 1000s.	13+
c-IV	**Anoxine-AM** (Hauck)		In 100s.	159
c-IV	**Fastin** (Beecham Labs.)		(Beecham/Fastin). Blue and clear. In 100s, 450s, and UD 150s.	249
c-IV	**Obephen** (Hauck)		Yellow. In 1000s.	13
c-IV	**Obermine** (Forest)		(0832/G536C). In 1000s.	22
c-IV	**Obestin-30** (Ferndale)		Blue and clear. In 100s.	58
c-IV	**Parmine** (Parmed)		Black. In 100s.	100
c-IV	**Phentrol 2** (Vortech)		In 1000s.	32
c-IV	**Phentrol 4** (Vortech)		In 1000s.	31
c-IV	**Phentrol 5** (Vortech)		In 1000s.	25
c-IV	**Zantryl** (Ion)		In 100s.	NA
c-IV	**Phentermine HCl** (Various)	**Tablets:** 37.5 mg (equivalent to 30 mg base)	In 30s, 100s, 500s, 1000s.	24+
c-IV	**Adipex-P** (Lemmon)		(Lemmon 9). Blue and white, scored. In 100s, 400s and 1000s.	134
c-IV	**Phentermine HCl** (Camall)	**Capsules:** 37.5 mg (equivalent to 30 mg base)	In 100s, 500s and 1000s.	48+
c-IV	**Adipex-P** (Lemmon)		(Adipex-P 37.5). Blue and white. In 100s, 400s and 1000s.	192
c-IV	**Dapex-37.5** (Ferndale)		Blue and clear. In 100s.	53
c-IV	**Obe-Nix 30** (Holloway)		In 100s.	80
c-IV	**Phentermine Resin** (Various)	**Capsules:** 15 mg (as resin complex)	In 100s.	121+
c-IV	**Ionamin** (Pennwalt)		(Ionamin 15). Yellow and gray. In 100s and 400s.	356
c-IV	**Phentermine Resin** (Various)	**Capsules:** 30 mg (as resin complex)	In 100s and 400s.	152+
c-IV	**Ionamin** (Pennwalt)		(Ionamin 30). Yellow. In 100s and 400s.	248

BENZPHETAMINE HCl

Administration and Dosage:

Initiate dosage with 25 to 50 mg once daily; increase according to response. Dosage ranges from 25 to 50 mg, 1 to 3 times daily.

	Product	Dosage form	Description / Packaging	C.I.*
c-III	**Didrex** (Upjohn)	**Tablets:** 25 mg	Sorbitol; tartrazine. (Upjohn 18). Yellow. In 100s.	231
		50 mg	Sorbitol. (Didrex 50). Peach, scored. In 100s and 500s.	224

* Cost Index based on cost per 24 mg phentermine or 75 mg benzphetamine.

Complete prescribing information for these products begins on page 1089

PHENMETRAZINE HCl

Administration and Dosage:

Maximum adult dose is 75 mg per day.

Sustained release tablets: 75 mg once daily. Provides appetite suppression for ≈ 12 hrs, determine administration time by the period of day anorectic effect is desired. **C.I.***

	Product	Form	Description	C.I.*
c-II	**Preludin** (Boehringer-Ingelheim)	**Tablets, sustained release:** 75 mg	Tartrazine. (#BI 62). Pink. In 100s.	404

PHENDIMETRAZINE TARTRATE

Administration and Dosage:

Tablets and capsules: 35 mg 2 or 3 times daily, 1 hour before meals.

Sustained release capsules: 105 mg once daily in the morning before breakfast. **C.I.***

	Product	Form	Description	C.I.*
c-III	**Phendimetrazine Tartrate** (Various)	**Tablets:** 35 mg	In 100s and 1000s.	3+
c-III	**Adphen** (Ferndale)		Orange, scored. In 100s.	40
c-III	**Bacarate** (Solvay Pharm.)		(#RR 1654). Pink, scored. In 100s and 1000s.	100
c-III	**Bontril PDM** (Carnrick)		(#C 8648). Green, white and yellow layered. Scored. In 100s and 1000s.	44
c-III	**Melfiat** (Solvay Pharm.)		(#RR 1079). Peach, scored. In 100s and 1000s.	101
c-III	**Metra** (Forest)		Green, scored. In 1000s.	10
c-III	**Obalan** (Lannett)		In 1000s.	10
c-III	**Obeval** (Vale)		Tartrazine. Yellow. In 100s and 1000s.	16
c-III	**Phenzine** (Hauck)		Green, scored. In 1000s.	8
c-III	**Plegine** (Ayerst)		(#Plegine 35). Scored. In 100s and 1000s.	144
c-III	**Statobex** (Lemmon)		Tartrazine. (#Lemmon 71-71). Green and white, scored. In 100s and 1000s.	66
c-III	**Trimstat** (Laser)		(#Laser 35). Orange. In 100s and 1000s.	53
c-III	**Trimtabs** (Mayrand)		(#M/R). Lavender, scored. In 100s and 500s.	47
c-III	**Weightrol** (Vortech)		In 100s.	20
c-III	**Phendimetrazine Tartrate** (Various)	**Capsules:** 35 mg	In 1000s.	8+
c-III	**Anorex** (Dunhall)		Blue. In 100s.	75
c-III	**Weh-less** (Hauck)		(#053). Pink and burgundy. In 100s and 1000s.	79

* Cost Index based on cost per 75 mg phenmetrazine or 35 mg phendimetrazine.
# Product identification code.

(Continued on following page)

Actions (Cont.):

Pharmacokinetic profiles are summarized in the table below using morphine as the standard. Data based on IM administration unless otherwise noted.

Pharmacokinetics of Narcotic Agonist Analgesics						
Drug	Onset (minutes)	Peak (hours)	Duration[1] (hours)	t½ (hours)	Equianalgesic Doses[2]	
					IM (mg)	Oral (mg)
Alfentanil	immediate	nd	nd	1-2[8]	nd	na
Codeine	10 to 30	0.5 to 1	4 to 6	3	120	200
Fentanyl	7 to 8	nd	1 to 2	1.5 to 6	0.1	na
Hydrocodone	nd	nd	4 to 8	3.3 to 4.5	nd	nd
Hydromorphone	15 to 30	0.5 to 1	4 to 5	2 to 3	1.5	7.5
Levorphanol	30 to 90	0.5 to 1	6 to 8	12 to 16	2	4
Meperidine	10 to 45	0.5 to 1	2 to 4	3 to 4	75	300
Methadone	30 to 60	0.5 to 1	4 to 6[4]	15 to 30	10	20
Morphine	15 to 60[5]	0.5 to 1	3 to 7	1.5 to 2	10	60
Oxycodone (PO)	15 to 30	1	4 to 6	nd	na	30
Oxymorphone	5 to 10	0.5 to 1	3 to 6	nd	1	10[3]
Propoxyphene (PO)	30 to 60	2 to 2.5	4 to 6	6 to 12	nd	130[6]/200[7]
Sufentanil	1.3 to 3[8]	nd	nd	2.5	0.02	na

nd – No data available. na – Not applicable.

[1] After IV administration, peak effects may be more pronounced but duration is shorter. Duration of action may be longer with the oral route.

[2] Based on acute, short-term use. Chronic administration may alter pharmacokinetics and decrease the oral: parenteral dose ratio. The morphine oral-parenteral ratio decreases to ≈ 1.5 to 2.5:1 upon chronic dosing.

[3] Rectal.

[4] Duration and half-life increase with repeated use due to cumulative effects.

[5] Data based on intrathecal or epidural administration.

[6] HCl salt.

[7] Napsylate salt. [8] Data based on IV administration.

Administration IV is most reliable and rapid; IM or SC use may delay absorption and peak effect, especially with impaired tissue perfusion. Many agents undergo a significant first-pass effect. All are metabolized by the liver and excreted primarily in urine. Meperidine is metabolized to normeperidine, a metabolite with significant pharmacologic activity. The half-life of normeperidine is 15 to 30 hours and accumulates with chronic dosing, especially in patients with renal dysfunction. The accumulation of this metabolite may lead to CNS excitation (eg, tremors, twitches, seizures).

Indications:

Relief of moderate to severe pain; preoperative medication; as analgesic adjuncts during anesthesia. Some agents are also used for their antitussive (see Narcotic Antitussives) and antidiarrheal (see Antidiarrheal Combination Products) effects. Methadone is also indicated for detoxification treatment of narcotic addiction and temporary maintenance treatment of narcotic addiction. Refer to individual product listings for specific indications.

Contraindications:

Hypersensitivity to narcotics; diarrhea caused by poisoning until the toxic material has been eliminated; acute bronchial asthma; upper airway obstruction.

Morphine: *Epidural or intrathecal* – Presence of infection at injection site; anticoagulant therapy; bleeding diathesis; parenterally administered corticosteroids within a 2 week period or other concomitant drug therapy or medical condition that would contraindicate the technique of epidural or intrathecal analgesia.

Levorphanol: Acute alcoholism; bronchial asthma; increased intracranial pressure; respiratory depression; anoxia.

Meperidine: In patients taking monoamine oxidase inhibitors (MAOIs) or in those who have received such agents within 14 days.

Hydromorphone injection: In patients not already receiving large amounts of parenteral narcotics; patients with respiratory depression in the absence of resuscitative equipment; status asthmaticus; use as obstetrical analgesia.

Warnings:

Drug dependence: Narcotic analgesics have abuse potential. Psychological dependence and physical tolerance and dependence may develop upon repeated use. However, most patients who receive opiates for medical reasons do not develop dependence syndromes (see Physical Dependence).

(Warnings continued on following page)

Warnings (Cont.):

Suicide: Do not prescribe **propoxyphene** for patients who are suicidal or addiction-prone. Many of the propoxyphene-related deaths have occurred in patients with previous histories of emotional disturbances or suicide attempts as well as misuse of tranquilizers, alcohol and other CNS-active drugs. Some deaths were accidental, or a consequence of accidental ingestion of excessive quantities of propoxyphene alone or in combination with other drugs. Warn patients not to exceed dosage recommended by physician.

Head injury and increased intracranial pressure: Narcotics may obscure the clinical course of patients with head injuries. The respiratory depressant effects and the capacity to elevate cerebrospinal fluid pressure may be markedly exaggerated in the presence of head injury, brain tumor, other intracranial lesions or a preexisting elevated intracranial pressure. Use with extreme caution and only if deemed essential.

Parenteral therapy: Give by very slow IV injection, preferably as a diluted solution. The patient should be lying down. Rapid IV injection increases the incidence of adverse reactions; respiratory depression, hypotension, apnea, circulatory collapse, cardiac arrest and anaphylactoid reactions have occurred. Do not administer IV unless a narcotic antagonist and facilities for assisted or controlled respiration are available. Use caution when injecting SC or IM in chilled areas or in patients with hypotension or shock, since impaired perfusion may prevent complete absorption; with repeated injections, an excessive amount may be suddenly absorbed if normal circulation is reestablished.

Limit epidural or intrathecal administration of **morphine** to the lumbar area.

Smooth muscle hypertonicity may result in biliary colic, difficulty in urination and possible urinary retention requiring catheterization. Give consideration to inherent risks in urethral catherization (eg, sepsis) when epidural or intrathecal administration is considered, especially in the perioperative period.

Hydrochlorides of opium alkaloids – Do not administer IV.

Asthma and other respiratory conditions: Use with extreme caution in patients with acute asthma, bronchial asthma, chronic obstructive pulmonary disease or cor pulmonale, a substantially decreased respiratory reserve, and with preexisting respiratory depression, hypoxia or hypercapnia. Even therapeutic doses of narcotics may decrease respiratory drive while simultaneously increasing airway resistance to the point of apnea. Reserve use for those whose conditions require endotracheal intubation and respiratory support or control of ventilation.

Hypotensive effect: Narcotic analgesics may cause severe hypotension in individuals whose ability to maintain blood pressure has been compromised by a depleted blood volume, or coadministration of drugs such as phenothiazines or general anesthetics. In ambulatory patients, orthostatic hypotension may occur.

Administer with caution to patients in circulatory shock, since vasodilation produced by the drug may further reduce cardiac output and blood pressure.

Renal and hepatic dysfunction may cause a prolonged duration and cumulative effect; smaller doses may be necessary.

Meperidine: In patients with renal dysfunction, normeperidine (an active metabolite of meperidine) may accumulate, resulting in increased CNS adverse reactions.

Pregnancy: Category C. Safety for use during pregnancy has not been established.

The placental transfer of narcotics is rapid. Maternal addiction and neonatal withdrawal occurs following illicit use. Withdrawal symptoms include irritability, excessive crying, yawning, sneezing, increased respiratory rate, tremors, hyperreflexia, fever, vomiting, increased stools and diarrhea. Symptoms usually appear during the first days of life.

Some association between congenital defects and first trimester exposure to **codeine** has been reported. **Alfentanil** and **sufentanil** have an embryocidal effect in rats and rabbits when given in doses 2.5 times the upper human dose for 10 days to over 30 days. **Fentanyl** has been shown to impair fertility and to have an embryocidal effect in rats at doses 0.3 times the upper human dose for 12 days.

Labor: Narcotics cross the placental barrier and can produce depression of respiration and psycho-physiologic effects in the neonate. Resuscitation may be required; have naloxone available. The use of **alfentanyl, sufentanil** and **fentanyl** is not recommended. Do not use **methadone** for obstetrical analgesia. Its long duration of action increases the probability of neonatal respiratory depression. It has also been associated with low infant birth weight and subsequent development of SIDS.

Therapeutic doses of **morphine** and **codeine** have increased the duration of labor.

(Warnings continued on following page)

Warnings (Cont.):

Lactation: Most of these agents appear in breast milk; however, the effects on the infant may not be significant. Some recommend waiting 4 to 6 hours after administration before nursing.

Methadone enters breast milk in concentrations (range, 0.17 to 5.6 mcg/ml) approaching plasma levels and may prevent withdrawal symptoms in addicted infants. **Meperidine** achieves an average milk:plasma ratio of about 1 (peak milk levels of 0.13 mcg/ml occur 2 hours after a 50 mg IM dose). Significant levels of **alfentanil** were found in breast milk 4 hours after administration of 60 mcg/kg. No detectable levels were found after 28 hours. Use caution when administering alfentanil to nursing women.

Children: Safety and efficacy of **sufentanil** in children < 2 years undergoing cardiovascular surgery have been documented in a limited number of cases. Safety and efficacy of **fentanyl** in children < 2 years is not established. Methemoglobinemia has occurred rarely in premature neonates undergoing emergency anesthesia and surgery including combined use of fentanyl, pancuronium and atropine; cause and effect relationship has not been established. Hypotension has occurred in neonates with respiratory distress syndrome receiving **alfentanil** 20 mcg/kg.

Do not use **oxycodone** in children; **propoxyphene** use is not recommended in children. **Methadone** is not recommended for use as an analgesic in children because documented clinical experience is insufficient to establish suitable dosage regimens. The safe use of **oxymorphone** is not established in children. The safety and efficacy of **hydromorphone** use in children is not established.

Precautions:

Acute abdominal conditions: Diagnosis or clinical course may be obscured by narcotics.

Special risk patients: Exercise caution in elderly and debilitated patients and in those suffering from conditions accompanied by hypoxia or hypercapnia when even moderate therapeutic doses may dangerously decrease pulmonary ventilation. Also exercise caution in patients sensitive to CNS depressants, including those with cardiovascular disease; myxedema; convulsive disorders; increased ocular pressure; acute alcoholism; delirium tremens; cerebral arteriosclerosis; ulcerative colitis; fever; decreased respiratory reserve (eg, emphysema, severe obesity); hypothyroidism; kyphoscoliosis; Addison's disease; prostatic hypertrophy or urethral stricture; CNS depression or coma; gallbladder disease; recent GI or GU tract surgery; toxic psychosis.

In obese patients (> 20% above ideal body weight), determine the **alfentanil** and **sufentanil** dosage on the basis of ideal body weight.

Fentanyl and **alfentanil** may produce bradycardia which may be treated with atropine. Use caution when administering to patients with bradyarrhythmias.

Supraventricular tachycardias: Use with caution in atrial flutter and other supraventricular tachycardias; vagolytic action may increase the ventricular response rate.

Seizures may be aggravated or may occur in individuals without a history of convulsive disorders if dosage is substantially increased because of tolerance. Observe closely patients with known seizure disorders for **morphine**-induced seizure activity.

Cough reflex is suppressed. Exercise caution when using narcotic analgesics postoperatively and in patients with pulmonary disease.

Tolerance: Some patients develop tolerance to the narcotic analgesic. This may occur after days or months of continuous therapy. The dose generally needs to be increased to obtain adequate analgesia.

Cross-tolerance among these agents is not complete. Switching to another narcotic agonist, starting with one-half the predicted equianalgesic dose, may circumvent the cross-tolerance.

Sulfite sensitivity: May cause allergic-type reactions (eg, hives, itching, wheezing, anaphylaxis) in certain susceptible persons. Although the overall prevalence of sulfite sensitivity in the general population is probably low, it is seen more frequently in asthmatics or in atopic nonasthmatic persons. Specific products containing sulfites are identified in the product listings.

Potentially hazardous tasks: May produce drowsiness or dizziness; patients should observe caution while driving or performing other tasks requiring alertness or physical dexterity.

Drug Interactions:

Anticoagulants: The anticoagulant effect of warfarin may be potentiated by propoxyphene.

Barbiturate anesthetics may increase the respiratory and CNS depressive effects of the narcotics due to additive pharmacologic activity.

Carbamazepine: Pharmacologic effects may be increased when used concurrently with propoxyphene. Monitor serum carbamazepine levels and the patient for symptoms of toxicity.

Chlorpromazine: Although the analgesic effect of narcotics may be potentiated, a higher incidence of toxic effects may occur.

(Drug Interactions continued on following page)

Drug Interactions (Cont.):

Cimetidine: Case reports have described CNS toxicity (confusion, disorientation, respiratory depression, apnea, seizures) following coadministration with narcotic analgesics; no clear-cut cause and effect relationship was established.

Diazepam may produce cardiovascular depression when given with high doses of fentanyl and alfentanil. Administration prior to or following high doses of alfentanil decreases blood pressure secondary to vasodilation; recovery may be prolonged.

Droperidol and fentanyl may cause hypotension and decrease pulmonary arterial pressure.

Hydantoins may decrease the pharmacologic effects of meperidine and methadone, possibly due to increased hepatic metabolism of the narcotic.

Monoamine oxidase inhibitors (MAOIs) and **furazolidone**: Meperidine has precipitated unpredictable and occasionally fatal reactions in those concurrently receiving or those who have received such agents within 14 days. The mechanism is unclear, but may be related to a pre-existing hyperphenylalaninemia. Some reactions have been characterized by coma, respiratory depression, cyanosis and hypotension; in others, hyperexcitability, convulsions, tachycardia, hyperpyrexia and hypertension have occurred. Use caution.

If a narcotic is needed, perform a sensitivity test. Hydrocortisone IV or prednisolone is used to treat severe reactions; use IV chlorpromazine in those exhibiting hypertension and hyperpyrexia. The value of narcotic antagonists for these reactions is unknown.

Nitrous oxide may cause cardiovascular depression with high dose sufentanil and fentanyl.

Rifampin may reduce methadone plasma levels to a degree sufficient to produce withdrawal symptoms. The mechanism may be due to increased hepatic metabolism of methadone.

Drug/Food Interaction: In one study, the administration of morphine oral solution following a high-fat meal resulted in a 34% increase in morphine's area under the curve compared to morphine administration in the fasting state.

Drug/Lab Interaction: Narcotics may increase biliary tract pressure with resultant increases in plasma **amylase** or **lipase;** therefore, determinations of these levels may be unreliable for 24 hours after narcotic administration.

Adverse Reactions:

Major hazards: Respiratory depression; apnea; circulatory depression; respiratory arrest; coma; shock; cardiac arrest.

Most frequent: Lightheadedness; dizziness; sedation; nausea; vomiting; sweating. More prominent in ambulatory patients and in those without severe pain. Use lower doses.

CNS: Euphoria; dysphoria; delirium; insomnia; agitation; anxiety; fear; hallucinations; disorientation; drowsiness; sedation; lethargy; impairment of mental and physical performance; skeletal or uncoordinated movements; coma; mood changes; weakness; headache; mental cloudiness; blurred vision; visual disturbances; diplopia; miosis; tremor; convulsions; psychic dependence; toxic psychoses; depression; increased intracranial pressure; miosis. Injection near a nerve trunk may result in sensory-motor paralysis which is usually transitory.

Choreic movements have been induced by **methadone.** Seizures have occurred following **fentanyl** administration.

GI: Nausea; vomiting; diarrhea; cramps; abdominal pain; taste alterations; dry mouth; anorexia; constipation; biliary tract spasm. Patients with chronic ulcerative colitis may experience increased colonic motility; toxic dilatation occurred in patients with acute ulcerative colitis.

Coadministration of anthraquinone laxatives (especially senna compounds) in an approximate dose of 187 mg senna concentrate per 120 mg codeine equivalent may counteract narcotic-induced constipation.

Cardiovascular: Facial flushing; chills; faintness; peripheral circulatory collapse; tachycardia; bradycardia; arrhythmia; palpitations; chest wall rigidity; hypertension; hypotension; orthostatic hypotension; syncope; asystole hypercarbia (**alfentanil**) and phlebitis following IV injection.

GU: Ureteral spasm and spasm of vesical sphincters; urinary retention or hesitancy; oliguria; antidiuretic effect; reduced libido or potency.

Allergic: Pruritus; urticaria; other skin rashes; diaphoresis; laryngospasm; edema; hemorrhagic urticaria (rare). Wheal and flare over the vein with IV injection may occur. Anaphylactoid reactions have occurred following IV administration. A case of **morphine**-induced thrombocytopenia has occurred.

Other: Bronchospasm; depression of cough reflex; interference with thermal regulation; laryngospasm; muscular rigidity; paresthesia; pain at injection site; local tissue irritation and induration following SC injection, particularly when repeated; diaphoresis (**fentanyl**); reversible jaundice (**propoxyphene**); nystagmus (**hydromorphone**). **Sufentanil** may cause erythema, chills and intraoperative muscle movement. Postoperative confusion, blurred vision, shivering and hypercapnia have occurred with **alfentanil**.

Laboratory test abnormalities: Abnormal liver function tests with **propoxyphene.**

(Continued on following page)

Complete prescribing information for these products begins on page 1098

MORPHINE SULFATE

Morphine is the principal opium alkaloid.

Indications: Relief of moderate to severe acute and chronic pain. Preoperatively to sedate patient, allay apprehension, facilitate induction of anesthesia, reduce anesthetic dosage.

Unlabeled uses: Dyspnea associated w/acute left ventricular failure and pulmonary edema.

Administration and Dosage:

Morphine sulfate is less potent orally because of first-pass metabolism. Oral administration is ⅓ to ⅙ as effective as parenteral administration.

Oral: 10 to 30 mg every 4 hours or as directed by physician.

Controlled release – 30 mg every 8 to 12 hours or as directed by physician. Do not crush or chew.

Medication may suppress respiration in the elderly, the very ill and those patients with respiratory problems; therefore, lower doses may be required.

SC/IM: Adults – 10 mg (5 to 20 mg)/70 kg every 4 hours. *Children* – 0.1 to 0.2 mg/kg (up to 15 mg) every 4 hours.

IV: Adults – 2.5 to 15 mg/70 kg in 4 to 5 ml of Water for Injection, administered over 4 to 5 minutes. Rapid IV use increases the incidence of adverse reactions (see Warnings). Do not administer IV unless a narcotic antagonist is immediately available.

Continuous IV infusion: 0.1 to 1 mg/ml in 5% Dextrose in Water by controlled-infusion device; higher concentrations have been used.

Rectal: 10 to 20 mg every 4 hours or as directed by physician.

Epidural: Adults – Initial injection of 5 mg in the lumbar region may provide satisfactory pain relief for up to 24 hours. If adequate pain relief is not achieved within 1 hour, carefully administer incremental doses of 1 to 2 mg at intervals sufficient to assess effectiveness. Give no more than 10 mg/24 hr.

For continuous infusion, an initial dose of 2 to 4 mg/24 hours is recommended. Further doses of 1 to 2 mg may be given if pain relief is not achieved initially.

Aged or debilitated patients – Administer with extreme caution (see Precautions). Doses < 5 mg may provide satisfactory pain relief for up to 24 hours.

Intrathecal: Adult – Intrathecal dosage is usually 1/10 that of epidural dosage. A single injection of 0.2 to 1 mg may provide satisfactory pain relief for up to 24 hours. Caution: This is only 0.4 to 2 ml of the 5 mg/10 ml ampul or 0.2 to 1 ml of the 10 mg/10 ml ampul. Do not inject intrathecally > 2 ml of the 5 mg/10 ml ampul or 1 ml of the 10 mg/10 ml ampul. Use in the lumbar area only is recommended. Repeated intrathecal injections are not recommended. A constant IV infusion of naloxone, 0.6 mg/hr, for 24 hours after intrathecal injection may reduce incidence of potential side effects.

Aged or debilitated – Use extreme caution. A lower dosage is usually satisfactory.

Repeat dosage – If pain recurs, consider alternative administration routes, since experience with repeated doses by this route is limited.

Intraventricular: Currently available data indicate that this route of administration is effective in select patients with intractable pain and short life expectancy. One to two doses per day are generally administered.

	Product	Form	Packaging	C.I.*
c-II	**Morphine Sulfate** (Abbott)	**Injection:** 0.5 mg/ml	In 10 ml amps.	2674
c-II	**Astramorph PF**[1] (Astra)		In 2, 10 ml amps, 10 ml vials.	2571
c-II	**Duramorph**[1] (Elkins-Sinn)		In 10 ml amps.	2300
c-II	**Morphine Sulfate** (Various, eg, Abbott, Baxter)	**Injection:** 1 mg/ml	In 10 ml amps and 30 and 60 ml amps.	1425+
c-II	**Astramorph PF**[1] (Astra)		In 2 and 10 ml amps and 10 ml vials.	1371
c-II	**Duramorph**[1] (Elkins-Sinn)		In 10 ml amps.	1233
c-II	**Morphine Sulfate** (Various, eg, Baxter, Winthrop)	**Injection:** 2 mg/ml	In 60 ml vials and 1 and 2 ml disp. syringes.	204+
c-II	**Morphine Sulfate** (Baxter)	**Injection:** 3 mg/ml	In 50 ml vials.	221
c-II	**Morphine Sulfate** (Various)	**Injection:** 4 mg/ml	In 1 and 2 ml disp. syringes.	121+
c-II	**Morphine Sulfate** (Various)	**Injection:** 5 mg/ml	In 1 and 30 ml vials.	148+
c-II	**Morphine Sulfate** (Various)	**Injection:** 8 mg/ml	In 1 ml vials, amps, syringes.	93+
c-II	**Morphine Sulfate** (Various)	**Injection:** 10 mg/ml	1 ml vials, amps, 10 ml vials.	53+
c-II	**Infumorph 200** (Elkins-Sinn)		Preservative free. In 20 ml ampuls.	NA

* Cost Index based on cost per 10 mg morphine.

[1] Preservative free.

(Products continued on following page)

MORPHINE SULFATE (Cont.)

	Product	Form/Strength	Packaging	C.I.*
c-II	**Morphine Sulfate** (Various, eg, Elkins-Sinn, Lilly)	**Injection:** 15 mg/ml	In 1 ml amps and vials, 20 ml amps and vials.	51+
c-II	**Morphine Sulfate** (IMS)	**Injection:** 25 mg/ml	In 4, 10, 20 and 40 ml *Select-A-Jet* syringe systems.	NA
c-II	**Infamorph 500** (Elkins-Sinn)		Preservative free. In 20 ml ampuls.	NA
c-II	**Morphine Sulfate** (IMS)	**Injection:** 50 mg/ml	In 20, 20 and 40 ml *Select-A-Jet* syringe systems.	NA
c-II	**Morphine Sulfate** (Lilly)	**Soluble Tablets:** 10 mg	In 100s.	24
		15 mg	In 100s and 500s.	21
		30 mg	In 100s and 500s.	17
c-II	**Morphine Sulfate** (Roxane)	**Tablets:** 15 mg	(54 733). In 100s and UD 100s.	13
c-II	**MSIR** (Purdue Frederick)		(PF MI 30). In 50s.	13
c-II	**MS Contin** (Purdue-Frederick)	**Tablets, controlled release:** 15 mg	(PF M15). Blue. In 100s and UD 100s.	149
c-II	**Morphine Sulfate** (Roxane)	**Tablets:** 30 mg	(54 2262). In 100s, UD 100s.	11
c-II	**MSIR** (Purdue Frederick)		(PF MI 30). In 50s.	11
c-II	**MS Contin** (Purdue Frederick)	**Tablets, controlled release:** 30 mg	In 50s, 100s, 250s, 500s and UD 25s, 100s and 300s.	41
c-II	**Roxanol SR** (Roxane)		In 50s, 250s and UD 100s.	23
c-II	**Oramorph SR** (Roxane)	**Tablets, controlled release:** 30 mg	Lactose. White. In 50s, 100s, 250s and UD 100s.	NA
		60 mg	Lactose. In 100s, UD 25s.	NA
		100 mg	Lactose. In 100s, UD 25s.	NA
c-II	**MS Contin** (Purdue Frederick)	**Tablets, controlled release:** 60 mg	(PF M 60). Orange. In 100s and UD 25s, 100s and 300s.	35
c-II	**MS Contin** (Purdue-Frederick)	**Tablets, controlled release:** 100 mg	(PF 100). Gray. In 100s and UD 100s.	134
c-II	**Morphine Sulfate** (Roxane)	**Solution:** 10 mg/5 ml	In 100, 500 ml, UD 5, 10 ml.	33
c-II	**MSIR** (Purdue Frederick)		In 120, 500 ml and UD 5 ml.	9
c-II	**Roxanol Rescudose** (Roxane)	**Solution:** 10 mg/ 2.5 ml	In UD 2.5 ml.	NA
c-II	**Morphine Sulfate** (Roxane)	**Solution:** 20 mg/5 ml	In 100 and 500 ml.	34
c-II	**MSIR** (Purdue Frederick)		In 120, 500 ml and UD 5 ml.	6
c-II	**MSIR** (Purdue Frederick)	**Solution:** 20 mg/ml	In 30 and 120 ml.	27
c-II	**OMS Concentrate** (Upsher Smith)		In 30 and 120 ml w/dropper.	82
c-II	**Roxanol** (Roxane)		In 30 and 120 ml.	31
c-II	**Roxanol UD** (Roxane)		In UD 1 ml and 1.5 ml vials.	105
c-II	**Roxanol 100** (Roxane)	**Solution:** 100 mg/5 ml	In 240 ml.	23
c-II	**Morphine Sulfate** (Various)	**Rectal Suppositories:** 5 mg	In UD 12s and 50s.	169+
c-II	**RMS** (Upsher-Smith)		In UD 12s.	292
c-II	**Roxanol** (Roxane)		In UD 12s.	513
c-II	**Morphine Sulfate** (Various)	**Rectal Suppositories:** 10 mg	In UD 12s and 50s.	94+
c-II	**RMS** (Upsher-Smith)		In UD 12s.	172
c-II	**Roxanol** (Roxane)		In UD 12s.	295
c-II	**Morphine Sulfate** (Various)	**Rectal Suppositories:** 20 mg	In UD 12s and 50s.	51+
c-II	**RMS** (Upsher-Smith)		In UD 12s.	104
c-II	**Roxanol** (Roxane)		In UD 12s.	175
c-II	**Morphine Sulfate** (Various)	**Rectal Suppositories:** 30 mg	In UD 12s and 50s.	54+
c-II	**RMS** (Upsher-Smith)		In UD 12s.	97
c-II	**Roxanol** (Roxane)		In UD 12s.	149

* Cost Index based on cost per 10 mg morphine.

Complete prescribing information for these products begins on page 1098

CODEINE

Codeine is a narcotic analgesic and antitussive that resembles morphine pharmacologically but with milder actions. It is a less potent antitussive than morphine on a weight basis; however, it is widely used as a cough suppressant because of its low incidence of adverse reactions at the usual antitussive dose. Codeine is ⅔ as effective orally as parenterally.

Indications:

Relief of mild to moderate pain and for coughing induced by chemical or mechanical irritation of the respiratory system.

Administration and Dosage:

Analgesic:

Adults – 15 to 60 mg every 4 to 6 hours, orally, IM, IV or SC. Usual dose is 30 mg. Do not exceed 360 mg in 24 hours.

Children (≥ 1 year of age) – 0.5 mg/kg or 15 m² of body surface every 4 to 6 hours SC, IM or orally. Do not use IV in children.

Antitussive: (See also Narcotic Antitussive Monograph).

Adults – 10 to 20 mg every 4 to 6 hours. Do not exceed 120 mg in 24 hours.

Children (6 to 12 years) – 5 to 10 mg orally every 4 to 6 hours. Do not exceed 60 mg in 24 hours.

(2 to 6 years) – 2.5 to 5 mg orally every 4 to 6 hours. Do not exceed 30 mg in 24 hours.

Storage: Protect from light (injection).

				C.I.*
C-II	**Codeine Sulfate** (Various, eg, Lilly, Roxane)	**Tablets:** 15 mg	In 100s and UD 100s.	131+
C-II	**Codeine Sulfate** (Various, eg, Halsey, Knoll, Lilly, Roxane, Wyeth-Ayerst)	**Tablets:** 30 mg	In 25s, 100s, 250s, 1000s and UD 100s.	64+
C-II	**Codeine Sulfate** (Various, eg, Knoll, Lilly, Roxane)	**Tablets:** 60 mg	In 100s, 1000s and UD 100s.	61+
C-II	**Codeine Sulfate** (Lilly)	**Tablets, Soluble:** 15 mg	In 100s.	120
		30 mg	In 100s.	119
		60 mg	In 100s.	114
C-II	**Codeine Phosphate** (Various, eg, Elkins-Sinn, Winthrop, Wyeth-Ayerst[1])	**Injection:** 30 mg	In 1 ml vials, 1 and 2 ml syringes and 1 ml Tubex.	173+
C-II	**Codeine Phosphate** (Various, eg, Elkins-Sinn, Winthrop, Wyeth-Ayerst[2])	**Injection:** 60 mg	In 1 ml vials, 1 and 2 ml syringes and 1 ml Tubex.	100+
C-II	**Codeine Phosphate** (Lilly)	**Tablets, Soluble:** 30 mg	In 100s.	130
		60 mg	In 100s and 500s.	124

OXYCODONE HCl

Indications:

Relief of moderate to moderately severe pain.

Administration and Dosage:

Adults: 5 mg or 5 ml every 6 hours as needed. Individualize dosage.

Children: Not recommended for use in children.

C-II	**Roxicodone** (Roxane)	**Tablets:** 5 mg	(54 582). White, scored. In 100s and UD 100s.	112
		Oral Solution: 5 mg/5 ml	Sorbitol. Burgundy cherry flavor. In 500 ml.	62
C-II	**Roxicodone Intensol** (Roxane)	**Solution, concentrate:** 20 mg/ml	In 30 ml w/dropper.	54

* Cost Index based on cost per 30 mg codeine or 5 mg oxycodone.
[1] With ≤ 1.5 mg sodium metabisulfite.
[2] With ≤ 2 mg sodium metabisulfite.

Complete prescribing information for these products begins on page 1098

PROPOXYPHENE (Dextropropoxyphene)

Actions:

Pharmacology: Propoxyphene is a centrally-acting narcotic analgesic structurally related to methadone; its analgesic effect resides in the dextrorotatory isomer. Propoxyphene is ½ to ⅔ as potent as codeine. Propoxyphene alone in usual analgesic doses (32 to 65 mg of the hydrochloride or 50 to 100 mg of the napsylate salt), is no more and possibly less effective than 30 to 60 mg codeine or 600 mg aspirin. Propoxyphene combined with other analgesics (eg, codeine, aspirin) is more effective than propoxyphene or other analgesics alone.

Pharmacokinetics: Absorption/Distribution – Water soluble hydrochloride (HCl) salt is absorbed more rapidly than the relatively water insoluble napsylate salt; peak plasma concentrations for the HCl are achieved in 2 to 2.5 hours. In equimolar doses (100 mg of napsylate equals 65 mg of HCl), the two salts achieve similar peak plasma concentrations (great intersubject variation). A 65 mg oral dose of propoxyphene HCl achieves peak plasma levels of 0.05 to 0.1 mcg/ml. Bioavailability is reduced to 30% to 70% due to extensive first-pass biotransformation. Approximately 80% of propoxyphene and its metabolites are bound to plasma proteins. Highly lipid soluble, the drug is stored in fatty tissue in large quantities. Propoxyphene crosses the placenta and appears in breast milk.

Metabolism/Excretion – Propoxyphene is metabolized in the liver with a half-life of 6 to 12 hours. The major metabolite, norpropoxyphene, has a half-life of 30 to 36 hours. Propoxyphene is excreted in the urine primarily as metabolites. Norpropoxyphene has substantially less CNS depressant effects than propoxyphene, but a greater local anesthetic effect similar to that of amitriptyline and antiarrhythmic agents, such as lidocaine and quinidine.

Indications:

Relief of mild to moderate pain.

Contraindications:

Hypersensitivity to propoxyphene.

Warnings:

Fatalities: Propoxyphene products in excessive doses, either alone or in combination with other CNS depressants (including alcohol), are a major cause of drug-related deaths. In a survey conducted in 1975, in approximately 20% of the fatal cases, death occurred within the first hour (5% within 15 minutes). Judicious prescribing of propoxyphene is essential for safety. Consider nonnarcotic analgesics for depressed or suicidal patients. Do not prescribe propoxyphene for suicidal or addiction-prone patients. Because of added CNS depressant effects, cautiously prescribe with concomitant sedatives, tranquilizers, muscle relaxants, antidepressants or other CNS depressant drugs. Advise patients of the additive depressant effects of these combinations with alcohol.

Many propoxyphene-related deaths have occurred in patients with histories of emotional disturbances, suicidal ideation or attempts, or misuse of tranquilizers, alcohol and other CNS active drugs. Do not exceed the recommended dosage.

Drug dependence: In higher than recommended doses over long time periods, propoxyphene can produce drug dependence characterized by psychic dependence and, less frequently, physical dependence and tolerance. Propoxyphene will only partially suppress the withdrawal syndrome in individuals physically dependent on other narcotics. Abuse liability is similar to that of codeine.

Hepatic or renal function impairment: Administer propoxyphene with caution since higher serum concentrations or delayed elimination may occur. Consider reduction of total daily doses for these patients.

Pregnancy: Safety for use during pregnancy has not been established. In 2914 exposures to propoxyphene during pregnancy, 46 (1.6%) possible associations of congenital defects were observed: Clubfoot (18), benign tumors (12), microcephaly (6), ductus arteriosus persistens (5) and cataract (5). Confirmation is required.

Neonatal withdrawal following heavy maternal ingestion has been reported. Use only when the potential benefits outweigh the potential hazards to the fetus.

Lactation: Low levels have been detected in breast milk. No adverse effects have been noted in nursing infants.

Children: Not recommended for use in children.

(Continued on following page)

PROPOXYPHENE (Dextropropoxyphene) (Cont.)

Precautions:

Potentially hazardous tasks: May impair mental or physical abilities required to perform potentially hazardous tasks; observe caution while driving or performing other tasks requiring alertness.

Drug Interactions:

Barbiturate anesthetics may increase respiratory and CNS depressive effects of propoxyphene due to additive pharmacologic activity. The CNS depressant effects are additive.

Carbamazepine: Concomitant administration of propoxyphene may increase carbamazepine levels and produce dizziness, ataxia and nausea.

Charcoal decreases the GI absorption of propoxyphene.

Cigarette smoking may induce liver enzymes responsible for the metabolism of propoxyphene; efficacy is reportedly decreased in smokers. Patients may increase the dosage to obtain adequate pain relief.

Cimetidine: Case reports have described CNS toxicity (confusion, disorientation, respiratory depression, apnea, seizures) following coadministration with narcotic analgesics; no clear-cut cause and effect relationship was established.

Warfarin: Potentiation of the hypoprothrombinemic effect of warfarin by propoxyphene may occur.

Adverse Reactions:

Less than 1% of hospitalized patients taking propoxyphene HCl at recommended doses experience side effects.

Most frequent: Dizziness; sedation; nausea; vomiting.

Other: Constipation; abdominal pain; skin rashes; lightheadedness; headache; weakness; euphoria; dysphoria; minor visual disturbances; abnormal liver function; reversible jaundice (rare).

Overdosage:

Symptoms: The patient is usually somnolent, but may be stuporous or comatose and convulsing. Respiratory depression is characteristic; ventilatory rate or tidal volume is decreased, resulting in cyanosis and hypoxia. Pupils, initially pinpoint, may dilate as hypoxia increases. Cheyne-Stokes respiration and apnea may occur. Blood pressure falls and cardiac performance deteriorates, resulting in pulmonary edema and circulatory collapse, unless corrected promptly. Cardiac arrhythmias and conduction delay may be present. A combined respiratory-metabolic acidosis occurs due to hypercapnia and lactic acid formation. Death may occur.

Treatment: Promptly initiate resuscitative measures. Treatment includes usual supportive measures. Refer to General Management of Acute Overdosage. Induction of emesis may be hazardous; it might coincide with seizures. Naloxone (see individual monograph) will markedly reduce the degree of respiratory depression; administer 0.4 to 2 mg IV promptly, and carefully repeat at 2 to 3 minute intervals, as necessary. Due to the short duration of action of naloxone and the long half-life of propoxyphene and its metabolites, repeated dosages of naloxone may be necessary. Naloxone may also be given by continuous IV infusion. If no response is observed after administration of 10 mg naloxone, question the diagnosis of propoxyphene toxicity.

Monitor blood gases, pH and electrolytes; promptly correct acidosis and electrolyte disturbance. Ventricular fibrillation or cardiac arrest may occur. Respiratory acidosis rapidly subsides as ventilation is restored and carbon dioxide is eliminated, but lactic acidosis may require IV bicarbonate.

Dialysis is of little value.

Patient Information:

May cause drowsiness, dizziness or blurring of vision; use caution while driving or performing other tasks requiring alertness.

Avoid alcohol and other sedative or drowsiness-causing drugs.

May cause nausea, vomiting or constipation; notify physician if these become prominent.

If GI upset occurs, these agents may be taken with food.

Notify physician if shortness of breath or difficulty in breathing occurs.

(Products listed on following page)

Refer to the general discussion of these products on page 1112

PROPOXYPHENE HCl (Cont.)

Administration and Dosage:

Usual dose: 65 mg every 4 hours as needed. Do not exceed 390 mg per day.

In hepatic or renal impairment, consider reducing total daily dosage.

	Product	Form	Packaging	C.I.*
c-IV	**Darvon Pulvules** (Lilly)	**Capsules:** 32 mg	In 100s and 500s.	90
c-IV	**Propoxyphene HCl** (Various, eg, Balan, Geneva, Goldline, Halsey, Lannett, Lemmon, Moore, Roxane, Rugby, Schein)	**Capsules:** 65 mg	In 20s, 100s, 500s, 1000s and UD 100s.	6+
c-IV	**Darvon Pulvules** (Lilly)		In 100s, 500s and UD 100s and 500s.	80
c-IV	**Dolene** (Lederle)		(#Lederle D36). Pink. In 100s and 500s.	20

PROPOXYPHENE NAPSYLATE

Because of differences in molecular weight, 100 mg of propoxyphene napsylate is required to supply propoxyphene equivalent to 65 mg of the HCl. In hepatic or renal impairment, consider reducing total daily dosage.

Administration and Dosage:

Usual dose: 100 mg every 4 hours as needed. Do not exceed 600 mg per day.

Storage: Avoid freezing the suspension.

	Product	Form	Packaging	C.I.*
c-IV	**Darvon-N** (Lilly)	**Tablets:** 100 mg	Buff. In 100s, 500s and UD 100s.	117
		Suspension: 10 mg/ml	In 480 ml.	166

* Cost Index based on cost per single dose (65 mg propoxyphene HCl or 100 mg propoxyphene napsylate).

\# Product identification code.

Complete prescribing information for these products begins on page 1098

ALFENTANIL HCl

Indications:

As an analgesic adjunct given in incremental doses in the maintenance of anesthesia with barbiturate/nitrous oxide/oxygen.

As an analgesic administered by continuous infusion with nitrous oxide/oxygen in the maintenance of general anesthesia.

As a primary anesthetic for induction of anesthesia in general surgery when endotracheal intubation and mechanical ventilation are required.

Administration and Dosage:

Individualize dosage. In obese patients (> 20% above ideal total body weight), determine dosage on the basis of lean body weight. Reduce dose in elderly or debilitated patients.

Monitor vital signs routinely.

Children < 12 years of age: Use is not recommended.

Premedication: Individualize the selection of preanesthetic medications.

Neuromuscular blocking agents should be compatible with the patient's condition.

In patients administered anesthetic (induction) dosages, qualified personnel and adequate facilities are essential for the management of intraoperative and postoperative respiratory depression.

For administering small volumes of alfentanil accurately, use a tuberculin syringe or equivalent.

Alfentanil Dosage Range

Indication	≈ Duration of Anesthesia	Induction (Initial Dose)	Maintenance (Increments/Infusion)	Total Dose	Effects
Incremental Injection	≤ 30 min	8-20 mcg/kg	3-5 mcg/kg or 0.5-1 mcg/kg/min	8-40 mcg/kg	Spontaneously breathing or assisted ventilation when required.
Incremental Injection	30-60 min	20-50 mcg/kg	5-15 mcg/kg	up to 75 mcg/kg	Assisted or controlled ventilation required. Attenuation of response to laryngoscopy and intubation.
Anesthetic induction	> 45 min	130-245 mcg/kg	0.5-1.5 mcg/kg/min or general anesthetic	dependent on duration of procedure	Assisted or controlled ventilation required. Give slowly (over 3 min). Reduce concentration of inhalation agents by 30%-50% for initial hour.
Continuous Infusion*	> 45 min	50-75 mcg/kg	0.5-3 mcg/kg/min Average Infusion Rate 1-1.5 mcg/kg/min	dependent on duration of procedure	Assisted or controlled ventilation required. Some attenuation of response to intubation and incision, with intraoperative stability.

*0.5-3 mcg/kg/min administered with nitrous oxide/oxygen in patients undergoing general surgery. Following an anesthetic induction dose, reduce infusion rate requirements by 30% to 50% for the first hour of maintenance.

Changes in vital signs that indicate a response to surgical stress or lightening of anesthesia may be controlled by increasing the rate to a maximum of 4 mcg/kg/min or administering bolus doses of 7 mcg/kg. If changes are not controlled after three bolus doses given over 5 minutes, use a barbiturate, vasodilator or inhalation agent. Always adjust infusion rates downward in the absence of these signs until there is some response to surgical stimulation.

Rather than an increase in infusion rate, administer 7 mcg/kg bolus doses of alfentanil or a potent inhalation agent in response to signs of lightening of anesthesia within the last 15 minutes of surgery. Discontinue infusion at least 10 to 15 minutes prior to the end of surgery.

Preparation of solution: The physical and chemical compatibilities of alfentanil have been demonstrated in solution (concentration range, 25 to 80 mcg/ml) with Normal Saline, 5% Dextrose in Normal Saline, 5% Dextrose in Water and Lactated Ringers.

As an example of the preparation for infusion, 20 ml alfentanil added to 230 ml diluent provides a 40 mcg/ml solution.

				C.I.*
c-II	**Alfenta**[1] (Janssen)	**Injection:** 500 mcg (as HCl) per ml	In 2, 5, 10 and 20 ml amps.	83

* Cost index based on cost per ml.

[1] Preservative free.

NARCOTIC ANALGESIC COMBINATIONS

Components of these combinations include (see individual monographs):

NARCOTIC ANALGESICS: Codeine, hydrocodone bitartrate, dihydrocodeine bitartrate, opium, oxycodone HCl, oxycodone terephthalate, meperidine HCl, propoxyphene HCl and propoxyphene napsylate.

NONNARCOTIC ANALGESICS: Acetaminophen; salicylates; salicylamide.

CAFFEINE, a traditional component of many analgesic formulations, may be beneficial in certain vascular headaches.

MAGNESIUM-ALUMINUM HYDROXIDES and *CALCIUM CARBONATE,* used as buffers.

BARBITURATES, ACETYLCARBROMAL, CARBROMAL and BROMISOVALUM, are used for their sedative effects.

PROMETHAZINE HCl (a phenothiazine derivative with antihistaminic properties), used for its sedative effect.

BELLADONNA ALKALOIDS, used as antispasmodics.

Content given per tablet or 5 ml liquid.

	Product and Distributor	Narcotic	Acetaminophen	Aspirin	Caffeine	Other Content	How Supplied	C.I.*
c-III	**Tylenol w/Codeine No. 1 Tablets** (McNeil-CPC)	7.5 mg codeine phosphate	300 mg			Sodium metabisulfite	(#McNeil Tylenol Codeine 1). White. In 100s.	64
c-v	**Acetaminophen w/Codeine Elixir** (Various, eg, Balan, Bioline, Geneva, Goldline, Moore, PBI, Roxane, Rugby, Schein, URL)	12 mg codeine phosphate	120 mg				In 120 and 500 ml, pt, gal and UD 5, 10, 12.5 and 15 ml (100s).	30+
c-v	**Capital w/Codeine Suspension** (Carnrick)						Fruit punch flavor. In pt.	73
c-v	**Tylenol w/Codeine Elixir** (McNeil-CPC)					7% alcohol, saccharin, sucrose	Cherry flavor. In pt and UD 5 and 15 ml.	167
c-III	**Acetaminophen w/Codeine Tablets** (Various, eg, Balan, Bioline, Geneva, Lemmon, Moore, Purepac, Rugby, Schein, URL, Warner Chilcott)	15 mg codeine phosphate	300 mg				In 30s, 50s, 100s, 500s and 1000s.	19+
c-III	**Tylenol w/Codeine No. 2 Tablets** (McNeil-CPC)					Sodium metabisulfite	(#McNeil Tylenol Codeine 2). White. In 100s, 500s and UD 500s (20 x 25s).	89

* Cost Index based on cost per tablet or 5 ml. # Product identification code.

(Continued on following page)

NARCOTIC ANALGESIC COMBINATIONS (Cont.)

Refer to the general discussion of these products on page1120. Content given per capsule or tablet.

	Product and Distributor	Narcotic	Acetaminophen	Aspirin	Caffeine	Other Content	How Supplied	C.I.*
c-III	**Phenaphen w/Codeine No. 2 Capsules** (Robins)	15 mg codeine phosphate	325 mg				(AHR 6242). Black and yellow. In 100s.	66
c-III	**Aceta w/Codeine Tablets** (Century)	30 mg codeine phosphate	325 mg				Scored. In 100s and 1000s.	33
c-III	**Phenaphen w/Codeine No. 3 Capsules** (Robins)	30 mg codeine phosphate	325 mg				(AHR 6257). Black and green. In 100s, 500s & Dis-Co Pack 100s.	92
c-III	**Acetaminophen w/Codeine Tablets** (Various, eg, Geneva, Goldline, Lannett, Lederle, Lemmon, Moore, Roxane, Rugby, Warner Chilcott, Zenith)	30 mg codeine phosphate	300 mg				In 15s, 30s, 50s, 100s, 500s, 1000s and UD 100s.	25+
c-III	**Papadeine #3 Tablets** (Vangard)						(465/3 #3). White. In 100s and 1000s.	68
c-III	**Tylenol w/Codeine No. 3 Tablets** (McNeil-CPC)						(McNeil Tylenol Codeine 3). White. In 100s, 500s, 1000s and UD Dispensit 500s.	97
c-III	**Codaphen Tablets** (Roxane)	30 mg codeine phosphate	500 mg				In 100s and UD 100s.	121
c-III	**Phenaphen-650 w/Codeine Tablets** (Robins)	30 mg codeine phosphate	650 mg			Sodium bisulfite	(AHR 6251). White, scored. In 50s.	113
c-III	**Acetaminophen w/Codeine Tablets** (Various, eg, Geneva, Goldline, Lederle, Lemmon, Moore, Roxane, Rugby, Schein, Warner Chilcott, Zenith)	60 mg codeine phosphate	300 mg				In 50s, 100s, 500s, 1000s and UD 100s.	48+
c-III	**Tylenol w/Codeine No. 4 Tablets** (McNeil-CPC)						(McNeil Tylenol Codeine 4). White. In 100s, 500s and UD 500s.	171
c-III	**Phenaphen w/Codeine No. 4 Capsules** (Robins)	60 mg codeine phosphate	325 mg				(AHR 6274). Green and white. In 100s, 500s and Dis-Co Pak 100s (4 x 25s).	158

* Cost Index based on cost per capsule or tablet.

(Continued on following page)

NARCOTIC ANALGESIC COMBINATIONS (Cont.)

Refer to the general discussion of these products on page 1120

Content given per tablet.

	Product and Distributor	Narcotic	Acetaminophen	Aspirin	Caffeine	Other Content	How Supplied	C.I.*
c-III	**Aspirin w/Codeine Tablets No. 2** (Various, eg, Balan, Barr, Baxter, Harber, Halsey, Moore, Qualitest, Rugby, URL, Warner Chilcott)	15 mg codeine phosphate		325 mg			In 100s, 500s and 1000s.	21+
c-III	**Empirin w/Codeine No. 2 Tablets** (Burroughs Wellcome)						(#Empirin 2). White. In 100s and 1000s.	80
c-III	**Aspirin w/Codeine Tablets No. 3** (Various, eg, Barr, Baxter, Geneva, Goldline, Moore, Rugby, Schein, URL, Warner Chilcott, Zenith)	30 mg codeine phosphate		325 mg			In 12s, 15s, 20s, 30s, 100s, 500s and 1000s.	22+
c-III	**Empirin w/Codeine No. 3 Tablets** (Burroughs Wellcome)						(#Empirin 3). White. In 100s, 500s, 1000s and Dispenser-pak 25s.	96
c-III	**Aspirin w/Codeine Tablets No. 4** (Various, eg, Barr, Baxter, Geneva, Goldline, Moore, Rugby, Schein, URL, Warner Chilcott, Zenith)	60 mg codeine phosphate		325 mg			In 15s, 30s, 50s, 100s, 500s and 1000s.	91+
c-III	**Empirin w/Codeine No. 4 Tablets** (Burroughs Wellcome)						(#Empirin 4). White. In 100s, 500s, 1000s and Dispenser-pak 25s.	257

* Cost Index based on cost per tablet.
# Product identification code.

(Continued on following page)

NARCOTIC ANALGESIC COMBINATIONS (Cont.)

Refer to the general discussion of these products on page 1120

Content given per capsule, tablet or 5 ml liquid.

	Product and Distributor	Narcotic	Acetaminophen	Aspirin	Caffeine	Other Content	How Supplied	C.I.*
c-III	**Dolprn #3 Tablets** (Bock)	30 mg codeine phosphate	400 mg	250 mg		60 mg magnesium hydroxide, 60 mg aluminum hydroxide	(#Bock 3). Green, layered. Oval. In 100s.	103
c-II	**Codalan No. 1 Tablets** (Lannett)	8 mg codeine phosphate	150 mg	230 mg	30 mg		Orange. In 100s, 500s and 1000s.	22
c-II	**Codalan No. 2 Tablets** (Lannett)	15 mg codeine phosphate	150 mg	230 mg	30 mg		White. In 100s, 500s and 1000s.	26
c-II	**Codalan No. 3 Tablets** (Lannett)	30 mg codeine phosphate	150 mg	230 mg	30 mg		Green. In 100s, 500s and 1000s.	42
c-III	**Amaphen w/Codeine #3 Capsules** (Trimen)	30 mg codeine phosphate	325 mg		40 mg	50 mg butalbital	(#Trimen). Pink and maroon. In 100s.	75
c-III	**Esgic w/Codeine Capsules** (Forest)						(#Forest 677). Black and blue. In 100s.	191
c-III	**Valdeine Tablets** (Pal-Pak)	16.2 mg codeine phosphate		389 mg	32.4 mg		In 1000s.	N/A
c-III	**Fiorinal w/Codeine No. 3 Capsules** (Sandoz)	30 mg codeine phosphate		325 mg	40 mg	50 mg butalbital	(#S F-C #3 Sandoz 78-107). Blue and yellow. In 100s and Control-Pak 25s.	316
c-V	**Rid-A-Pain w/Codeine Tablets** (Pfeiffer)	1 mg codeine phosphate	97.2 mg	226.8 mg	32.4 mg	32.4 mg salicylamide	In 24s and 48s.	46
c-III	**Lortab Liquid** (Russ)	2.5 mg hydrocodone bitartrate	120 mg				In pt.	135
c-III	**Lortab Tablets** (Russ)	2.5 mg hydrocodone bitartrate	500 mg				White and pink, mottled. Scored. In 100s.	117

* Cost Index based on cost per capsule, tablet or 5 ml.
# Product identification code.

(Continued on following page)

NARCOTIC ANALGESIC COMBINATIONS (Cont.)

Refer to the general discussion of these products on page 1120
Content given per capsule or tablet.

	Product and Distributor	Narcotic	Acetaminophen	Aspirin	Caffeine	Other Content	How Supplied	C.I.*
c-III	**Amacodone Tablets** (Trimen)	5 mg hydrocodone bitartrate	500 mg				(Trimen). White/blue specks, scored. Capsule shape. In 100s.	85
c-III	**Anodynos DHC Tablets** (Forest)						(Forest 416). Green, scored. In 100s.	168
c-III	**Bancap HC Capsules** (Forest)						(Forest 610). Black and red. In 100s and 500s.	191
c-III	**Co-Gesic Tablets** (Central)						(500/5 Central). White, scored, oval. In 100s & 500s.	103
c-III	**Dolfen Tablets** (Pharmics)						In 500s.	NA
c-III	**Duocet Tablets** (Mason)						(M D-C). Blue. In 100s.	119
c-III	**Dolacet Capsules** (Hauck)						Black and red. In 100s and 500s.	129
c-III	**Duradyne DHC Tablets** (Forest)						In 100s and 1000s.	174
c-III	**Hydrocet Capsules** (Carnrick)						Blue and white. In 100s and UD 100s.	91
c-III	**Hydrocodone Bitartrate and Acetaminophen Capsules** (Various, eg, LuChem, Major)						In 100s and 500s.	33
c-III	**Hydrocodone Bitartrate and Acetaminophen Tablets** (Watson)						(Watson 349). White, scored. Capsule shape. In 30s, 100s and 500s.	NA
c-III	**Hydrogesic Capsules** (Edwards)						(Hydrogesic E). White. In 100s.	83
c-III	**Hy-Phen Tablets** (Ascher)						(Ascher 225-450). White, scored. Capsule shape. In 100s, 500s & UD 100s.	95

* Cost Index based on cost per capsule or tablet.

(Continued on following page)

NARCOTIC ANALGESIC COMBINATIONS (Cont.)

Refer to the general discussion of these products on page 1120
Content given per capsule or tablet.

	Product and Distributor	Narcotic	Acetaminophen	Aspirin	Caffeine	Other Content	How Supplied	C.I.*
c-III	**Lorcet Tablets** (UAD)	5 mg hydrocodone bitartrate	500 mg				White, scored. In 500s.	NA
c-III	**Lorcet-HD Capsules** (UAD)						(1120). Maroon. In 100s.	NA
c-III	**Lortab 5 Tablets** (Russ)						White, blue specks, scored. In 100s, 500s and UD 100s.	125
c-III	**Anexsia 5/500 Tablets** (Beecham Labs)						(BMP 207). White, scored. In 100s.	111
c-III	**Norcet Capsules** (Abana)						(Norcet). White, blue specks, scored. Capsule shape. In 100s and 500s.	75
c-III	**T-Gesic Capsules** (T.E. Williams)						In 100s.	105
c-III	**Vicodin Tablets** (Knoll)						(Vicodin). White, scored. In 100s, 500s, UD 100s.	139
c-III	**Zydone Capsules** (DuPont)						(Zydone). White. In 100s.	94
c-III	**Lortab 7/500 Tablets** (Russ)	7.5 mg hydrocodone bitartrate	500 mg				White, green specks, scored. In 100s, UD 100s.	144
c-III	**Anexsia 7.5/650 Tablets** (Beecham Labs)	7.5 mg hydrocodone bitartrate	650 mg				(BMP 188). Peach, scored. Capsule shape. In 100s.	156
c-III	**Lorcet Plus Tablets** (UAD)						(U U201). In 100s.	NA
c-III	**Norcet 7 Tablets** (Abana)						In 100s.	120
c-III	**Vicodin ES Tablets** (Knoll)	7.5 mg hydrocodone bitartrate	750 mg				(Vicodin ES). White. In 100s & UD 100s.	130
c-III	**Azdone Tablets** (Central)	5 mg hydrocodone bitartrate		500 mg			(21 Central). Pink, scored. In 100s & 1000s.	95
c-III	**Damason-P Tablets** (Mason)						(M D-P). Pink. In 100s and 1000s.	NA
c-III	**Lortab ASA Tablets** (Russ)						Pink. In 100s.	135

* Cost Index based on cost per capsule or tablet.

(Continued on following page)

NARCOTIC ANALGESIC COMBINATIONS (Cont.)

Refer to the general discussion of these products on page 1120
Content given per capsule, tablet, suppository or 5 ml.

	Product and Distributor	Narcotic	Acetaminophen	Aspirin	Caffeine	Other Content	How Supplied	C.I.*
c-III	**Dihydrocodeine Compound Capsules** (Gen-King)	16 mg dihydrocodeine bitartrate		356.4 mg	30 mg		In 100s and 500s.	48
c-III	**Synalgos-DC Capsules** (Wyeth-Ayerst)						In 100s and 500s.	233
c-II	**B & O Supprettes No. 15A Suppositories** (Webcon)	30 mg powdered opium				15 mg powdered belladonna extract	Scored. In 12s.	833
c-II	**Opium and Belladonna Suppositories** (Wyeth-Ayerst)	60 mg powdered opium				15 mg belladonna extract	In 20s.	768
c-II	**B & O Supprettes No. 16A Suppositories** (Webcon)	60 mg powdered opium				15 mg powdered belladonna extract	Scored. In 12s.	938
c-II	**Acetaminophen with Oxycodone Tablets** (Halsey)	5 mg oxycodone HCl	325 mg				(G20C 879). White, scored. In 100s, 500s, 1000s and UD 25s.	45
c-II	**Percocet Tablets** (DuPont)						(Percocet DuPont). White, scored. In 100s and 500s.	117
c-II	**Roxicet Tablets** (Roxane)						(54 543). White, scored. In 100s, 500s and UD 100s.	61
c-II	**Roxicet Oral Solution** (Roxane)					0.4% alcohol, saccharin	In 500 ml and UD 5 ml.	93

* Cost Index based on cost per capsule, tablet, suppository or 5 ml.

(Continued on following page)

NARCOTIC ANALGESIC COMBINATIONS (Cont.)

Refer to the general discussion of these products on page 1120

Content given per capsule.

	Product and Distributor	Narcotic	Acetaminophen	Aspirin	Caffeine	Other Content	How Supplied	C.I.*
c-IV	**Darvon w/A.S.A. Pulvules** (Lilly)	65 mg propoxyphene HCl		325 mg			Pink and red. In 100s.	142
c-IV	**Darvon Compound Pulvules** (Lilly)	32 mg propoxyphene HCl		389 mg	32.4 mg		Pink and gray. In 100s and 500s.	76
c-IV	**Propoxyphene HCl Compound Capsules** (Various, eg, Balan, Dixon-Shane, Harber, Lannett, Moore, Parmed, Qualitest, Schein, URL, Zenith)	65 mg propoxyphene HCl		389 mg	32.4 mg		In 100s, 500s and 1000s.	15+
c-IV	**Bexophene Capsules** (Hauck)						In 500s.	36
c-IV	**Darvon Compound-65 Pulvules** (Lilly)						Red/gray. In 100s, 500s and UD 100s.	139

* Cost Index based on cost per capsule.

Narcotic agonist-antagonist analgesics compete with other substances at the mu (μ) receptor. The μ receptors mediate morphine-like supraspinal analgesia, euphoria and respiratory and physical depression. Refer to the Narcotic Agonist Analgesic introduction for further information on the action of the narcotics in general. There are two types of narcotic agonist-antagonists: 1) Drugs which are antagonists at the μ receptor and are agonists at other receptors (ie, pentazocine), 2) Partial agonists (ie, buprenorphine) which have limited agonist activity at the μ receptor.

The narcotic agonist-antagonist analgesics are potent analgesic agents with a lower abuse potential than pure narcotic agonists. Because of their narcotic antagonist activity, these agents may precipitate withdrawal symptoms in those with opiate dependence.

Narcotic Agonist-Antagonist Pharmacokinetics

Agonist/Antagonist		Onset (min)	Peak (min)	Duration (hrs)	t½ (hrs)	Equivalent Dose[1] (mg)	Relative Antagonist Activity
Buprenorphine	IM	15	60	6	2-3	0.3	Equipotent with Naloxone
	IV[2]						
Butorphanol	IM	< 10	30-60	3-4	2.5-4	2-3	30x Pentazocine or 1/40 Naloxone
Dezocine	IM	≤ 30	30-150	2-4[3]	nd	10	Greater than Pentazocine
	IV	≤ 15			2.4[4]		
Nalbuphine	IM	< 15[5]	60	3-6	5	10	10x Pentazocine
	IV	2-3	30				
Pentazocine	IM	15-20[2]	15-60	3	2-3	30	Weak
	IV	2-3	nd				
	Oral	15-30	60-180				

[1] Parenteral dose equivalent to 10 mg morphine.
[2] Time to onset and peak effect shorter.
[3] Dose related.
[4] For 10 or 20 mg dose; 1.7 hr for 5 mg dose.
[5] Also for subcutaneous administration.
nd – no data

DEZOCINE

Actions:

Dezocine is a strong synthetic opioid agonist-antagonist parenteral analgesic of the aminotetralin series. Its analgesic potency, onset and duration of action in the relief of postoperative pain are comparable to morphine.

Pharmacokinetics: Absorption/Distribution – Dezocine is completely and rapidly absorbed following IM injection in healthy volunteers, with an average peak serum concentration of 19 ng/ml (range, 10 to 38 ng/ml) occurring between 10 and 90 minutes after a 10 mg IM injection. Following a 10 mg IV infusion over 5 minutes, the average terminal half-life of dezocine is 2.4 hours (range, 1.2 to 7.4 hours). The average volume of distribution is 10.1 L/kg (range, 4.7 to 20.1 L/kg), and the average total body clearance is 3.3 L/hr/kg (range, 1.7 to 7.2 L/hr/kg). There is evidence of nonlinear (dose-dependent) pharmacokinetics at doses > 10 mg: In a study where 5, 10 and 20 mg IV doses of dezocine were given (n = 12), dose-proportional serum levels were observed after 5 and 10 mg injections, but the area under the serum concentration-time curve for the 20 mg dose was about 25% greater, and the total body clearance was about 20% lower when compared to the 5 and 10 mg doses. The pharmacokinetics of dezocine following chronic administration (steady-state pharmacokinetics) are predicted to yield serum levels for 5 and 15 mg IM doses given every 4 hours of 6 to 9 ng/ml and 240 to 310 ng/ml, respectively. Pain relief in patients with postoperative pain is clinically evident when steady-state serum levels exceed 5 to 9 ng/ml. The side effects listed in Adverse Reactions were observed in patients whose average peak levels were < 45 ng/ml. Peak analgesic effect lags peak serum levels by 20 to 60 minutes.

Metabolism/Excretion – Approximately two-thirds of a dose is recovered in the urine with about 1% being excreted as unchanged dezocine and the remainder as the glucuronide conjugate.

Mean (Range) Pharmacokinetic Parameters of Dezocine in Healthy Volunteers

Route/Parameter	Dose: 5 mg (n = 12)	10 mg (n = 36)	20 mg (n = 12)
Intravenous			
Clearance (L/hr/kg)	3.52 (2.1-6.2)	3.33 (1.7-7.2)	2.76 (1.7-4.1)
Volume of distribution (L/kg)	10.7 (6.4-15.5)	10.1 (4.7-20.1)	8.8 (5.8-13.5)
Half-life (hr)	1.7 (0.6-4.4)	2.4 (1.2-7.4)	2.4 (1.4-5.2)
Intramuscular		(n = 24)	
Bioavailability		100%	
Peak plasma concentration (ng/ml)		10-38	
Time-to-peak plasma concentration (min)		10-90	

Hepatic insufficiency did not alter total body clearance in one study of 7 patients with cirrhosis. The volume of distribution and consequently the half-life, however, were increased by 30% to 50% relative to healthy volunteers following a 10 mg IV dose.

Use cautiously with reduced doses in patients with renal dysfunction because the primary elimination of dezocine is through the urine as a glucuronide.

Narcotic antagonist activity: Dezocine is a mixed opioid agonist-antagonist analgesic. Its opioid antagonist activity is less than that of nalorphine but greater than that of pentazocine when measured by antagonism of morphine-induced narcosis in rats.

Effect on respiration: Decozine and morphine produce a similar degree of respiratory depression when given in the usual analgesic doses. The effect is dose-dependent and may be reversed by naloxone. As the dose of dezocine is increased, there appears to be an upper limit to the magnitude of the respiratory depression produced by the drug in both animals and healthy human volunteers. Dezocine, like other mixed agonist-antagonist analgesics, may offer increased safety over pure agonist drugs such as morphine.

Cardiovascular effects: Dezocine is not associated with significant changes in mean systemic artery pressure, mean pulmonary artery pressure, pulmonary capillary wedge pressure, cardiac output, stroke index and left ventricular stroke work index.

(Actions continued on following page)

DEZOCINE (Cont.)

Actions (Cont.):

Clinical trials: Postoperative analgesia – The analgesic efficacy of dezocine was investigated in randomized controlled clinical trials in postoperative general surgical pain (orthopedic, gynecologic, abdominal). The studies were primarily double-blind, single-dose, parallel trials in which IV doses of 2.5 to 10 mg (85 to 160 patients per treatment group) or IM doses of 5 to 20 mg (39 to 221 patients per treatment group) was compared to 5 to 10 mg of morphine or 1 mg of IV butorphanol in patients with moderate-to-severe pain.

The onset of analgesic action was similar for dezocine, morphine and butorphanol, occurring within 15 minutes of IV and 30 minutes of IM administration of the drug. Doses of 10 mg IM produced analgesia similar to that produced by 10 mg of IM morphine while 5 mg IV was equivalent to 1 mg of IV butorphanol.

The peak analgesic effect and duration of analgesia were comparable for both routes of administration. Half of the patients remedicated within 2 hours after 5 mg of dezocine or 1 mg of butorphanol IV, 3 hours after 10 mg of dezocine or morphine IM and 4 hours after 15 mg of dezocine IM.

Pain relief was proportional to the dose of dezocine for single doses < 20 mg. Some data suggest that the maximally effective dose of dezocine in postoperative pain may be 15 mg due to dezocine's mixed agonist-antagonist pharmacology.

Chronic pain states – Data has been gathered in trials of burn patients (n = 16) and cancer pain (n = 88). The daily dose for most patients has ranged between 20 and 60 mg/day, although doses as large as 90 to 140 mg/day have been used. Dezocine has not been adequately studied in the management of chronic pain. It is not recommended for use in patients who may have developed significant tolerance to opioid drugs from long-term use because of the risk of precipitating acute withdrawal symptoms.

Indications:

Management of pain when the use of an opioid analgesic is appropriate.

Contraindications:

Hypersensitivity to the drug.

Warnings:

Drug dependence/abuse: Because of its opioid antagonist properties, dezocine is not recommended for patients physically dependent on narcotics. Patients who have recently taken substantial amounts of narcotics may experience withdrawal symptoms. Because of the difficulty in assessing dependence in patients who have previously received substantial amounts of narcotics, use caution in the administration of dezocine to such patients. To avoid precipitating an acute narcotic abstinence reaction, allow a sufficient period of withdrawal from opioids before administering dezocine.

Use of dezocine in combination with alcohol or other CNS depressant drugs will result in increased risk to the patient. Use with caution in individuals with active drug or alcohol addiction who are not in a medically controlled environment. Self-administration of any strong opioid may increase the relapse rate in populations recovering from addiction in abstinence-based recovery programs.

Dezocine has shown no evidence of abuse in clinical use during drug development. Mixed opioid agonist-antagonists of this type generally have less potential for abuse than pure agonists such as morphine or meperidine, but all such drugs have abuse potential, especially in those individuals with a history of opioid drug abuse or dependence.

Hepatic or renal function impairment: Dezocine undergoes extensive hepatic metabolism and renal excretion of the glucuronide metabolite (see Pharmacokinetics). Give cautiously with reduced doses to patients with hepatic or renal dysfunction.

Elderly: Like all strong, mixed opioid agonist-antagonist analgesics, dezocine can depress respiration and reduce ventilatory drive to a clinically significant extent. It also can alter mental status or induce delirium in elderly patients. Dezocine has not undergone sufficient clinical testing in the geriatric population to assess its relative risk compared to other opioid analgesics, but reduce the initial dose of all drugs of this class in the geriatric patient and individualize subsequent doses.

(Warnings continued on following page)

DEZOCINE (Cont.)

Warnings (Cont.):

Pregnancy: Category C. Dezocine caused a dose-related suppression of body weight and food consumption of the parental generation in rats receiving either IV or IM doses. Pup body weight was suppressed in a dose-related fashion. There are no adequate and well controlled studies in pregnant women. Use during pregnancy only if the potential benefit justifies the potential risk to the fetus.

Labor and delivery: Safety to the mother and fetus after dezocine administration during labor is unknown. Use in labor and delivery only when its use is essential to the welfare of the mother and infant.

Lactation: The use of dezocine in nursing mothers is not recommended since it is not known whether this drug is excreted in breast milk.

Children: Safety and efficacy in patients < 18 years old have not been established.

Precautions:

Head injury and increased intracranial pressure: Although there is no clinical experience in patients with head injury, the possible respiratory depressant effect and the potential of strong analgesics to elevate cerebrospinal fluid pressure (resulting from vasodilation following CO_2 retention) may be markedly exaggerated in the presence of head injury, intracranial lesions, or a preexisting increase in intracranial pressure. Strong analgesics can produce effects that may obscure the clinical course of patients with head injuries. Use only when essential and with extreme caution.

Chronic obstructive pulmonary disease: Because strong opioids cause some respiratory depression, administer only with caution and in low doses to patients with preexisting respiratory depression (eg, from other medication, uremia, severe infection), severely limited respiratory reserve, bronchial asthma, obstructive respiratory conditions or cyanosis. Respiratory depression induced by dezocine can be reversed by naloxone.

Biliary surgery: Although there is no evidence that dezocine alters the tonic pressure within the common bile duct, therapeutic doses of other opioid analgesics can significantly increase pressure within the common bile duct. Therefore, use with caution in such settings.

Ambulatory patients: Strong opioid analgesics impair the mental or physical abilities required for the performance of potentially dangerous tasks such as driving a car or operating machinery. Patients who have been given dezocine should not drive or operate dangerous machinery until the effects of the drug are no longer present.

Sulfite sensitivity: This product contains sodium metabisulfite, a sulfite that may cause allergic-type reactions including anaphylactic symptoms and life-threatening or less severe asthmatic episodes in certain susceptible people. The overall prevalence of sulfite sensitivity in the general population is unknown and probably low. Sulfite sensitivity is seen more frequently in asthmatic than in nonasthmatic people.

Drug Interactions:

CNS depressants: Opioid analgesics, general anesthetics, sedatives, tranquilizers, hypnotics or other CNS depressants (including alcohol) administered concomitantly with dezocine may have an additive effect. When such combined therapy is contemplated, reduce the dose of one or both agents.

Adverse Reactions:

A total of 2192 patients have received dezocine on an acute or chronic basis in the initial clinical trials. In nearly all cases, the type and incidence of side effects were those expected of a strong analgesic, and no unforeseen or unusual toxicity occurred. There is, as yet, limited information on the use of dezocine for periods longer than 48 to 72 hours, but there was no evidence of hepatic, hematologic or renal toxicity in 73 patients who received the drug for > 7 days.

Body as a whole: Sweating, chills, flushing, low hemoglobin, edema (< 1%).

Cardiovascular: Hypotension, heart or pulse irregularity, hypertension, chest pain, pallor, thrombophlebitis (< 1%).

GI: Nausea, vomiting (3% to 9%); dry mouth, constipation, diarrhea, abdominal pain/distress/disorder (< 1%); increased alkaline phosphatase and AST (< 1%, causal relationship unknown).

(Adverse Reactions continued on following page)

DEZOCINE (Cont.)

Adverse Reactions (Cont.):

Musculoskeletal: Cramps/aching/pain (< 1%).

CNS: Sedation (3% to 9%); dizziness/vertigo (1% to 3%); anxiety, confusion, crying, delusions, sleep disturbance, headache, delirium, depression (< 1%).

Respiratory: Respiratory depression, respiratory symptoms, atelectasis (< 1%); hiccups (< 1%, causal relationship unknown).

Skin: Injection site reactions (3% to 9%); pruritus, rash, erythema (< 1%).

Special senses: Diplopia, slurred speech, blurred vision (< 1%); congestion in ears, tinnitus (< 1%, causal relationship unknown).

GU: Urinary frequency, hesitancy and retention (< 1%).

Overdosage:

Symptoms: Based on preclinical pharmacology, overdosage will produce acute respiratory depression, cardiovascular compromise and delirium. The largest dose of dezocine given to nontolerant healthy volunteers without toxicity has been 30 mg/70 kg.

Treatment: Administer naloxone IV. Evaluate the respiratory and cardiac status of the patient constantly and institute appropriate supportive measures, such as oxygen, IV fluids, vasopressors and assisted or controlled respiration. Refer to General Management of Acute Overdosage.

Administration and Dosage:

Adults:

IM – Single dose of 5 to 20 mg (usual, 10 mg). Adjust dosage according to the patient's weight, age, severity of pain, physical status and other medications that the patient may be receiving. Repeat every 3 to 6 hours as necessary.

Maximum dose – 20 mg; probable upper limit of 120 mg/day. There is insufficient information regarding the risk of chronic use of dezocine to establish limits for the maximum recommended duration of treatment with the drug.

IV – 2.5 to 10 mg repeated every 2 to 4 hours. The usual initial IV dose is 5 mg.

SC – Not recommended. Repeated injection of dezocine at a single site has been associated with subcutaneous inflammation, vascular irritation and venous thrombosis in animals. The significance for patients is unknown, although injection site reactions occurred in 4% of patients treated with dezocine in clinical trials.

Children: Not recommended for patients < 18 years old.

Storage: Store at room temperature and protect from light. Do not use if the solution contains a precipitate.

Rx	**Dalgan** (Astra)	**Injection:** 5 mg/ml	In 2 ml[1] single-dose vials and 2 ml[1] Tubex syringes.
		10 mg/ml	In 2 ml[1] single-dose vials, 10 ml multiple-dose vials and 2 ml[1] Tubex syringes.
		15 mg/ml	In 2 ml[1] single-dose vials and 2 ml[1] Tubex syringes.

[1] 1 ml fill in 2 ml.

PENTAZOCINE

Warnings:

Talwin Nx is intended for oral use only. Severe, potentially lethal reactions (eg, pulmonary emboli, vascular occlusion, ulceration and abscesses, withdrawal symptoms in narcotic-dependent individuals) may result from misuse of this drug by injection or in combination with other substances.

Actions:

Pharmacology: Pentazocine, a potent analgesic, weakly antagonizes the effects of morphine, meperidine and other opiates at the μ-opioid receptor. Pentazocine, presumed to exert its agonistic actions at the kappa (κ) and sigma (σ) opioid receptors, may precipitate withdrawal symptoms in patients taking narcotic analgesics regularly. In addition, it produces incomplete reversal of cardiovascular, respiratory and behavioral depression induced by morphine and meperidine. Pentazocine also has sedative activity. Parenterally, 30 mg is usually as effective an analgesic as 10 mg morphine or 75 to 100 mg meperidine. Orally, a 50 mg dose is equivalent to 60 mg codeine.

Talwin NX tablets, which contain naloxone, produce analgesic effects when administered orally because naloxone has poor bioavailability. Injected IV (an unintended use), naloxone will block the pharmacologic effects of pentazocine, producing withdrawal symptoms in opioid-dependent individuals.

Pharmacokinetics: Pentazocine is well absorbed from the GI tract and from SC and IM sites. However, it undergoes extensive first-pass hepatic metabolism. Oral bioavailability is $< 20\%$, and was increased threefold in cirrhotic patients. Concentrations in plasma coincide closely with onset, intensity and duration of analgesia. Pentazocine is excreted via the kidney, $< 5\%$ unchanged. Pentazocine passes into the fetal circulation.

Indications:

Oral and parenteral: Relief of moderate to severe pain.

Parenteral: For preoperative or preanesthetic medication; supplement to surgical anesthesia.

Contraindications:

Hypersensitivity to pentazocine, naloxone (in *Talwin NX*) or any product component.

Warnings:

Drug dependence: Exercise special care in prescribing to emotionally unstable patients and to those with a history of drug abuse; closely supervise them when therapy exceeds 4 or 5 days. Psychological and physical dependence have occurred in such patients and, rarely, in patients without a history of drug abuse. Abrupt discontinuation following extended use of pentazocine has resulted in withdrawal symptoms. If more than minor difficulty is encountered, reinstitute parenteral pentazocine with gradual withdrawal. Avoid substituting methadone or other narcotics for pentazocine in pentazocine abstinence syndrome.

"Ts and Blues": Injection IV of oral preparations of **pentazocine** (*Talwin,* "Ts") and **tripelennamine** (PBZ, "Blues"), an H_1-blocking antihistamine has become a common form of drug abuse. The combination is used as a "substitute" for heroin. The tablets are dissolved in tap water, filtered and injected IV.

The most frequent and serious complication of IV "Ts and Blues" addiction is pulmonary disease, due to occlusion of pulmonary arteries and arterioles with unsterile particles of cellulose and talc used as tablet binders. The occlusion leads to granulomatous foreign body reactions, infections, increased pulmonary artery resistance and pulmonary hypertension. Neurologic complications from IV injection of "Ts and Blues" include seizures, strokes and CNS infections. The replacement of oral pentazocine with the pentazocine/naloxone combination may decrease the popularity of this mixture. A few cases of abuse involving pentazocine/naloxone combination and tripelennamine have been reported, however.

Tissue damage: Severe sclerosis of the skin, subcutaneous tissues and underlying muscle has occurred at the injection sites of patients who have received multiple doses of pentazocine lactate. Rotate injection sites; IM may be tolerated better than SC.

Head injury and increased intracranial pressure: Pentazocine can produce effects which may obscure the clinical course of head injury patients. The potential for elevating cerebrospinal fluid pressure may be attributed to CO_2 retention due to the respiratory depressant effects of the drug. These effects may be exaggerated in the presence of head injury, other intracranial lesions or a preexisting increase in intracranial pressure. Use with extreme caution and only if essential.

Myocardial infarction (MI): Exercise caution in the IV use of pentazocine for patients with acute MI accompanied by hypertension or left ventricular failure. Pentazocine IV elevates systemic and pulmonary arterial pressure, systemic vascular resistance and left ventricular end-diastolic pressure, causing increased cardiac workload. Use the oral form with caution in MI patients who have nausea or vomiting.

(Warnings continued on following page)

PENTAZOCINE (Cont.)

Warnings (Cont.):

Acute CNS manifestations: Patients receiving therapeutic doses have experienced hallucinations (usually visual), disorientation and confusion which have cleared spontaneously. If the drug is reinstituted, acute CNS manifestations may recur.

Seizures have occurred with the use of pentazocine.

Renal/Hepatic function impairment: Because the drug is metabolized in the liver and excreted by the kidney, administer with caution to patients with such impairment. Extensive liver disease predisposes to greater side effects (eg, marked apprehension, anxiety, dizziness, drowsiness), and may be the result of decreased drug metabolism.

Pregnancy: Category C. Pentazocine rapidly crosses the placenta with cord blood levels 40% to 70% of maternal serum levels. Chronic maternal ingestion of pentazocine may result in neonatal withdrawal symptoms. Mothers addicted to "Ts and Blues" have lower birth weight infants who have problems similar to infants born of other narcotic addicted mothers. Safe use during pregnancy has not been established. Administer only when the benefits outweigh the hazards.

Labor: Patients receiving pentazocine during labor have experienced no adverse effects other than those that occur with commonly used analgesics. Use with caution in women delivering premature infants.

Lactation: Safety for use in the nursing mother has not been established.

Children: Safety and efficacy in children < 12 years old have not been established.

Precautions:

Respiratory conditions: Use caution and low dosage in patients with respiratory depression (eg, from other medication, uremia, severe infection), severely limited respiratory reserve, severe bronchial asthma, obstructive respiratory conditions, cyanosis.

Biliary tract pressure elevation generally occurs for varying periods following narcotic use. Some evidence suggests pentazocine may differ in this respect (ie, it causes little or no elevation in biliary tract pressures). The clinical significance of these findings is unknown.

Patients receiving narcotics: Pentazocine is a mild narcotic antagonist. Some patients previously given narcotics, including methadone for the daily treatment of narcotic dependence, have experienced withdrawal symptoms after receiving pentazocine.

Sulfite sensitivity: May cause allergic-type reactions (eg, hives, itching, wheezing, anaphylaxis) in certain susceptible persons. Although the overall prevalence of sulfite sensitivity in the general population is probably low, it is seen more frequently in asthmatics or in atopic nonasthmatic persons.

Potentially hazardous tasks: May produce sedation, dizziness and occasional euphoria; observe caution while driving or performing other tasks requiring alertness, coordination or physical dexterity.

Drug Interactions:

Alcohol: Due to the potential for increased CNS depressant effects, use cautiously in patients currently receiving pentazocine.

Barbiturate anesthetics may increase the respiratory and CNS depression of pentazocine because of additive pharmacologic activity.

Adverse Reactions:

Most common: Nausea; dizziness or lightheadedness; vomiting; euphoria.

GI: Constipation; cramps; abdominal distress; anorexia; diarrhea; dry mouth; taste alteration.

CNS: Sedation; headache; weakness or faintness; depression; disturbed dreams; insomnia; syncope; hallucinations; tremor; irritability; excitement; tinnitus; disorientation; confusion (see Warnings).

Ophthalmic: Blurred vision; focusing difficulty; nystagmus; diplopia; miosis.

Allergic: Edema of the face; sweating; anaphylactic reaction; rash; urticaria.

Dermatologic: Soft tissue induration; nodules; cutaneous depression; ulceration (sloughing); severe sclerosis of the skin, subcutaneous tissues and, rarely, underlying muscle at the injection site; diaphoresis; stinging on injection; flushed skin; dermatitis; pruritus; toxic epidermal necrolysis.

Cardiovascular: Hypotension; decrease in blood pressure; tachycardia; circulatory depression; shock; hypertension.

Respiratory: Respiratory depression; dyspnea; transient apnea in newborns whose mothers received parenteral pentazocine during labor.

Hematologic: Depression of white blood cells (especially granulocytes), usually reversible; moderate transient eosinophilia.

Other: Urinary retention; paresthesia; chills; neuromuscular and psychiatric muscle tremors; alterations in rate or strength of uterine contractions during labor (parenteral form).

(Continued on following page)

BUPRENORPHINE HCl

Actions:

Pharmacology: Buprenorphine is a semisynthetic centrally-acting opioid analgesic derived from thebaine; a 0.3 mg dose is approximately equivalent to 10 mg morphine in analgesic effects. Buprenorphine exerts its analgesic effect via high affinity binding of CNS opiate receptors. It has a high affinity for the μ receptors and dissociates from them slowly, which may contribute to its long duration of action and low physical dependence.

Its narcotic antagonist activity is approximately equipotent to naloxone.

Cardiovascular – Buprenorphine may cause a decrease or, rarely, an increase in pulse rate and blood pressure in some patients.

Respiratory effects – A therapeutic dose of 0.3 mg buprenorphine can decrease respiratory rate similarly to an equianalgesic dose of morphine (10 mg).

Pharmacokinetics: Onset of analgesic effect occurs 15 minutes after IM injection, peaks in about 1 hour, and persists up to 6 hours. When given IV, the time to onset and peak is shortened.

Plasma protein binding is about 96%. Buprenorphine is metabolized by the liver and its clearance is related to hepatic blood flow. Terminal half-life is 2 to 3 hours. The drug is excreted predominantly in the feces as free buprenorphine with traces of the N-dealkyl metabolite.

Indications:

Relief of moderate to severe pain.

Contraindications:

Hypersensitivity to buprenorphine.

Warnings:

Narcotic-dependent patients: Because of the narcotic antagonist activity of buprenorphine, use in physically dependent individuals may result in withdrawal effects. Buprenorphine, a partial agonist, has opioid properties which may lead to psychic dependence due to a euphoric component of the drug. Direct dependence studies have shown little physical dependence when the drug is withdrawn. The drug may not be substituted in acutely dependent narcotic addicts due to its antagonist component.

Respiratory effects: There have been occasional reports of clinically significant respiratory depression associated with buprenorphine. Use with caution in patients with compromised respiratory function and those given other respiratory depressants. In such cases, reduce the dose by one half. The use of assisted or controlled ventilation may be necessary.

Head injury/increased intracranial pressure: Buprenorphine may elevate cerebrospinal fluid (CSF) pressure; use with caution in head injury, intracranial lesions and other states where CSF pressure may be increased. Buprenorphine can produce miosis and changes in consciousness levels which may interfere with patient evaluation.

Hepatic function impairment: Buprenorphine is metabolized by the liver; the activity may be altered in those individuals with impaired hepatic function.

Pregnancy: Category C. In animals, buprenorphine produced mild post-implantation losses and early fetal deaths at 10 and 100 times the human dose. In rabbits, buprenorphine produced a dose-related trend for extra rib formation at 1000 times the human dose.

There are no adequate and well controlled studies in pregnant women. Use only if the potential benefits outweigh the potential hazards to the fetus.

Labor and Delivery: Safety has not been established.

Lactation: It is not known whether buprenorphine is excreted in breast milk. Exercise caution when administering to a nursing mother.

Children: Safety and efficacy for use in children have not been established.

(Continued on following page)

BUPRENORPHINE HCl (Cont.)

Precautions:

Use with caution in the following: Elderly or debilitated; severe impairment of hepatic, pulmonary or renal function; myxedema or hypothyroidism; adrenal cortical insufficiency (eg, Addison's disease); CNS depression or coma; toxic psychoses; prostatic hypertrophy or urethral stricture; acute alcoholism; delirium tremens or kyphoscoliosis. Naloxone may not be effective in reversing respiratory depression.

Biliary tract dysfunction: Buprenorphine increases intracholedochal pressure to a similar degree as other opiates; administer with caution.

Potentially hazardous tasks: May cause dizziness or drowsiness; observe caution while driving or performing other tasks requiring alertness.

Drug Interactions:

Barbiturate anesthetics may increase the respiratory and CNS depression of buprenorphine because of additive pharmacologic activity.

Diazepam: Respiratory and cardiovascular collapse was reported in a patient who received therapeutic doses of buprenorphine and this drug.

Adverse Reactions:

CNS: Sedation (66%); dizziness/vertigo (5% to 10%); headache (1% to 5%); confusion, dreaming, psychosis, euphoria, weakness/fatigue, nervousness, slurred speech, paresthesia, depression (< 1%); malaise, hallucinations, depersonalization, coma, tremor (infrequent); dysphoria/agitation, convulsions/lack of muscle coordination (rare).

Cardiovascular: Hypotension (1% to 5%); hypertension, tachycardia, bradycardia, Wenckebach block (< 1%).

GI: Nausea/vomiting (1% to 5%); constipation, dry mouth (< 1%); dyspepsia, flatulence (infrequent); loss of appetite, diarrhea (rare).

Respiratory: Hypoventilation (1% to 5%); dyspnea, cyanosis (< 1%); apnea (infrequent).

Ophthalmologic: Miosis (1% to 5%); blurred vision, diplopia, conjunctivitis, visual abnormalities (< 1%); amblyopia (infrequent).

Dermatologic: Sweating (1% to 5%); pruritus, injection site reaction (< 1%); rash, pallor (infrequent); urticaria (rare).

Other: Urinary retention; flushing/warmth; chills/cold; tinnitus.

Overdosage:

Symptoms: Although the antagonist activity of buprenorphine may become manifest at doses somewhat above the recommended therapeutic range, doses in the recommended therapeutic range may produce clinically significant respiratory depression in certain circumstances (see Warnings).

Treatment: Carefully monitor cardiac and respiratory status. Establish a patent airway and institute assisted or controlled ventilation. Employ oxygen, IV fluids, vasopressors and other supportive measures as indicated. Refer to General Management of Acute Overdosage. The primary management of overdose is mechanical assistance of respiration. Naloxone may be of value in managing overdose; doxapram has also been used.

Patient Information:

May cause dizziness or drowsiness; observe caution while driving or performing other tasks requiring alertness.

Do not exceed prescribed dosage. Avoid alcohol and benzodiazepines.

Administration and Dosage:

Patients ≥ 13 years of age: 0.3 mg IM or slow IV, every 6 hours, as needed. Repeat once (up to 0.3 mg) if required, 30 to 60 minutes after initial dosage, giving consideration to previous dose pharmacokinetics; use thereafter only as needed. In high-risk patients (eg, elderly, debilitated, presence of respiratory disease) or in patients where other CNS depressants are present, such as in the immediate postoperative period, reduce dose by approximately one-half. Exercise extra caution with the IV route of administration, particularly with the initial dose.

Occasionally, it may be necessary to give up to 0.6 mg. Data are insufficient to recommend single IM doses > 0.6 mg for long-term use.

IV compatibility: Buprenorphine is compatible with: Isotonic saline, Lactated Ringer's Solution, 5% Dextrose and 0.9% Saline, 5% Dextrose, scopolamine HBr, haloperidol, glycopyrrolate, droperidol and hydroxyzine HCl.

IV incompatibility: Buprenorphine is incompatible with diazepam and lorazepam.

Storage: Avoid excessive heat (> 40°C or 104°F) and light.

				C.I.*
c-v	**Buprenex** (Procter & Gamble Pharm.)	**Injection:** 0.324 mg (equiv. to 0.3 mg buprenorphine) per ml	In 1 ml amps.[1]	600

* Cost Index based on cost per single dose (0.3 mg).

[1] With 50 mg anhydrous dextrose.

This agent acts by central mechanisms and is therefore distinct from the salicylates and other nonsteroidal anti-inflammatory agents which act peripherally.

METHOTRIMEPRAZINE

Actions:

Pharmacology: A phenothiazine derivative and potent CNS depressant which produces suppression of sensory impulses, reduction of motor activity, sedation and tranquilization. Methotrimeprazine raises the pain threshold and produces amnesia. It also has antihistaminic, anticholinergic and antiadrenergic effects.

It produces an analgesic effect comparable to morphine and meperidine with a marked sedative effect. Respiratory depression in the patient or in the newborn during or following preanesthetic or obstetrical use occurs infrequently. The drug does not appear to affect the cough reflex. Its use has not been reported to result in addiction, dependence or withdrawal symptoms even with large doses or with prolonged administration.

Pharmacokinetics: Peak plasma concentrations occur 30 to 90 minutes after injection. Maximum analgesic effect usually occurs within 20 to 40 minutes after IM injection and is maintained for about 4 hours. Methotrimeprazine is metabolized into sulfoxides and glucuronic conjugates and largely excreted in the urine as such. Elimination half-life is 15 to 30 hours. Small amounts of unchanged drug are excreted in the feces and in the urine (1%). Elimination into the urine usually continues for several days after IM administration is discontinued.

Indications:

Relief of moderate to marked pain in nonambulatory patients.

For obstetrical analgesia and sedation where respiratory depression is to be avoided.

Preanesthetic for producing sedation, somnolence and relief of apprehension and anxiety.

Contraindications:

Concurrent administration with antihypertensive agents including MAO inhibitors; history of phenothiazine hypersensitivity; presence of overdosage of CNS depressants or comatose states; severe myocardial, renal or hepatic disease; clinically significant hypotension; patients < 12 years of age.

Warnings:

Following administration, orthostatic hypotension, sedation, fainting or dizziness may occur. Avoid or carefully supervise ambulation for at least 6 hours following the initial dose. Once this effect is tolerated, it will usually be maintained unless more than several days elapse between subsequent doses. Therapy with vasopressors has been required very rarely. Phenylephrine and methoxamine are suitable vasopressors; however, do not use epinephrine since a paradoxical decrease in blood pressure may result. Reserve norepinephrine for hypotension not reversed by other vasopressors.

Pregnancy: Use with caution in women of childbearing potential and during early pregnancy. There is no evidence of adverse developmental effects when administered during late pregnancy and labor.

Children: Do not use in children < 12 years of age since safety and efficacy have not been established.

Elderly and debilitated: Elderly and debilitated patients with heart disease are more sensitive to phenothiazine effects. Therefore, give a low initial dose and individualize dosage thereafter. Monitor pulse, blood pressure and general circulatory status until dosage requirements and response are stabilized.

Precautions:

Prolonged administration for > 30 days is usually unnecessary, and is only advised when narcotic drugs are contraindicated or in terminal illnesses. When long-term use is anticipated, perform periodic blood counts and liver function studies.

Sulfite sensitivity: May cause allergic-type reactions (eg, hives, itching, wheezing, anaphylaxis) in certain susceptible persons. Although the overall prevalence of sulfite sensitivity in the general population is probably low, it is seen more frequently in asthmatics or in atopic nonasthmatic persons.

Drug Interactions:

CNS depressant drugs (eg, **narcotics, barbiturates, general anesthetics**) exert CNS additive effects. Individualize each drug regimen.

Atropine, scopolamine and **succinylcholine:** Use cautiously. Tachycardia and fall in blood pressure may occur, and undesirable CNS effects such as stimulation, delirium and extrapyramidal symptoms may be aggravated.

(Continued on following page)

METHOTRIMEPRAZINE (Cont.)

Adverse Reactions:

Most of these effects have occurred only with long-term, high dosage administration. Some of these effects have been reported with users of methotrimeprazine with dosages not within the recommended range.

Cardiovascular: The most important side effects are associated with orthostatic hypotension, and include fainting or syncope and weakness. Avoid by keeping the patient supine for about 6 to 12 hours after injection. Blood pressure (usually within physiological range) often drops, beginning within 10 to 20 minutes following IM injection, and may last 4 to 6 hours (up to 12 hours); it usually diminishes or disappears with continued or intermittent administration. Occasionally, fall in blood pressure may be profound and may require immediate restorative measures.

CNS: Disorientation; dizziness; excessive sedation; weakness; slurring of speech.

GI: Abdominal discomfort; nausea; vomiting.

GU: Difficult urination; rarely, uterine inertia.

Allergic: Local inflammation; swelling.

Hematologic: Agranulocytosis with long-term, high dosage.

Hepatic: Jaundice with long-term, high dosage.

Miscellaneous: Chills; dry mouth; nasal congestion; pain at injection site.

Refer to the phenothiazine group monograph for a complete discussion of adverse effects related to use of phenothiazines.

Administration and Dosage:

Administer by deep IM injection into a large muscle mass. Rotate injection sites. Do not administer SC, as local irritation may occur. Do not administer IV.

Analgesia (adult): 10 to 20 mg (0.5 to 1 ml) IM every 4 to 6 hours as required (range, 5 to 40 mg [0.5 to 2 ml] at intervals of 1 to 24 hours). A flexible dosage schedule and initial dose of 10 mg are advisable until individual patient response and tolerance have been determined.

Elderly patients sensitive to phenothiazine effects: Initial dose of 5 to 10 mg (0.25 to 0.5 ml). Gradually increase subsequent doses if needed.

Analgesia for acute or intractable pain: Initially, 10 to 20 mg, with adjustment of subsequent doses every 4 to 6 hours for pain relief.

Obstetrical analgesia: During labor, an initial dose of 15 to 20 mg may be repeated or adjusted as needed.

Preanesthetic medication: Administer 2 to 20 mg 45 minutes to 3 hours before surgery. A dose of 10 mg is often satisfactory, and 15 to 20 mg may be used for more sedation. Atropine sulfate or scopolamine HBr may be used concurrently in lower than usual doses.

Postoperative analgesia: In the immediate postoperative period, give an initial dosage of 2.5 to 7.5 mg, since residual effects of anesthetic agents and other medications may be additive. Administer at intervals of 4 to 6 hours as needed. Supervise ambulation.

IV admixture incompatibilities: May be given IM in the same syringe with either atropine sulfate or scopolamine HBr. Do NOT mix in the same syringe with other drugs. **C.I.***

Rx	**Levoprome** (Lederle)	**Injection:** 20 mg (as HCl) per ml[1]	In 10 ml vials.	2656

* Cost Index based on cost per single adult dose (10 mg).

[1] With 0.9% benzyl alcohol, 0.065% EDTA and 0.3% sodium metabisulfite.

ACETAMINOPHEN (N-Acetyl-P-Aminophenol, APAP)

Actions:

Pharmacology: Acetaminophen (APAP) is the principal active metabolite of phenacetin and acetanilid, but is associated with less toxicity in usual recommended dosages.

The site and mechanism of the analgesic effect is unclear. APAP reduces fever by a direct action on the hypothalamic heat-regulating centers, which increases dissipation of body heat (via vasodilatation and sweating). The action of endogenous pyrogen on heat-regulating centers is inhibited. APAP is almost as potent as aspirin in inhibiting prostaglandin synthetase in the CNS, but its peripheral inhibition of prostaglandin synthesis is minimal, which may account for its lack of clinically significant antirheumatic or anti-inflammatory effects.

Generally, the antipyretic and analgesic effects of APAP and aspirin are comparable. Aspirin is clearly superior to APAP for treating pain of inflammatory origin. APAP does not inhibit platelet aggregation, affect prothrombin response or produce GI ulceration.

Pharmacokinetics: Absorption of acetaminophen is rapid and almost complete from the GI tract. Peak plasma concentrations occur within 0.5 to 2 hours, with slightly faster absorption of liquid preparations. With overdosage, absorption is complete in 4 hours. The rate and extent of acetaminophen absorption from suppositories varies.

Distribution – Usual analgesic doses produce total serum concentrations of 5 to 20 mcg/ml; a good correlation between serum concentration and analgesic effect has not been found. Serum protein binding varies from 20% to 50% at toxic serum concentrations.

Metabolism/Excretion – Acetaminophen is extensively metabolized and excreted in the urine primarily as inactive glucuronate and sulfate conjugates (94%). Approximately 4% is metabolized via cytochrome P-450 oxidase to a toxic metabolite which is normally detoxified by preferential conjugation with hepatic glutathione and excreted in the urine as conjugates of cysteine and mercapturic acid. When acetaminophen is used chronically or taken acutely in large doses, glutathione stores are depleted and hepatic necrosis may occur; 2% to 4% is excreted unchanged. The average elimination half-life is 1 to 3 hours; half-life is slightly prolonged in neonates (2.2 to 5 hours) and in cirrhotics.

Indications:

An analgesic-antipyretic in the presence of aspirin allergy, hemostatic disturbances (including anticoagulant therapy), bleeding diatheses (eg, hemophilia), upper GI disease (eg, ulcer, gastritis, hiatus hernia) and gouty arthritis; variety of arthritic and rheumatic conditions involving musculoskeletal pain, as well as in other painful disorders; diseases accompanied by discomfort and fever such as the common cold, "flu" and other bacterial or viral infections.

Unlabeled use: The prophylactic administration of APAP to children receiving a DTP vaccination appears to decrease the incidence of fever and pain at the injection site. A dose immediately following the vaccination and every 4 to 6 hours thereafter for 48 to 72 hours has been suggested.

Contraindications:

Hypersensitivity to acetaminophen.

Warnings:

Do not exceed the recommended dosage. Consult physician for use in children < 3 years of age, or for oral use longer than 5 days (children), 10 days (adults) or 3 days for fever.

Hepatic function impairment: Hepatotoxicity and severe hepatic failure occurred in chronic alcoholics following therapeutic doses. The hepatotoxicity is believed to be caused by induction of hepatic microsomal enzymes resulting in an increase in toxic metabolites, or by the reduced amount of glutathione responsible for conjugating toxic metabolites. The dose which can safely be administered to a chronic alcohol abuser has not been determined. Caution chronic alcoholics to limit acetaminophen intake to ≤ 2 g/day.

Pregnancy: Acetaminophen crosses the placenta. It is routinely used during all stages of pregnancy; when used in therapeutic doses, it appears safe for short-term use. Continuous high daily dosage caused severe anemia in a mother, and the neonate had fatal kidney disease. Although there is no evidence of a relationship between acetaminophen ingestion and congenital malformations, three cases of congenital hip dislocation may have been associated with acetaminophen.

Lactation: Acetaminophen is excreted in breast milk in low concentrations with reported milk:plasma ratios of 0.91 to 1.42 at 1 and 12 hours, respectively. No adverse effects in nursing infants were reported.

(Continued on following page)

ACETAMINOPHEN (N-Acetyl-P-Aminophenol, APAP) (Cont.)

Precautions:

If a sensitivity reaction occurs, discontinue use.

Severe or recurrent pain or high or continued fever may indicate serious illness. If pain persists for more than 5 days, if redness is present or in arthritic and rheumatic conditions affecting children < 12 years old, consult physician immediately.

Drug Interactions:

The potential hepatotoxicity of APAP may be increased by large doses or long-term administration of the following agents due to hepatic microsomal enzyme induction. The therapeutic effects of APAP may also be decreased.

Barbiturates	**Hydantoins**	**Sulfinpyrazone**
Carbamazepine	**Rifampin**	

Alcohol, ethyl: Chronic, excessive ingestion apparently increases the toxicity of larger therapeutic doses or overdoses of APAP.

Charcoal, activated, administered immediately, reduces acetaminophen absorption.

Drug/Lab test interaction: Acetaminophen may interfere with *Chemstrip bG, Dextrostix* and *Visidex* II home blood glucose measurement systems; decreases of $> 20\%$ in mean glucose values may be noted. This effect appears to be drug, concentration and system dependent.

Adverse Reactions:

Used as directed, acetaminophen rarely causes severe toxicity or side effects.

Hematologic: Hemolytic anemia; neutropenia; leukopenia; pancytopenia; thrombocytopenia.

Allergic: Skin eruptions; urticarial and erythematous skin reactions; fever.

Other: Hypoglycemia; jaundice.

Overdosage:

Symptoms: Acute poisoning may be manifested by nausea, vomiting, drowsiness, confusion, liver tenderness, low blood pressure, cardiac arrhythmias, jaundice and acute hepatic and renal failure. Death has occurred due to liver necrosis. Often, however, there are no specific early symptoms or signs.

The course of APAP poisoning is divided into 4 clinical stages (postingestion time):

Stage I: (12-24 hours) – Nausea, vomiting, diaphoresis, anorexia;
Stage 2: (24-48 hours) – Clinically improved; AST, ALT, bilirubin and prothrombin levels begin to rise;
Stage 3: (72-96 hours) – Peak hepatotoxicity; AST of 20,000 not unusual;
Stage 4: (7-8 days) – Recovery.

Hepatotoxicity may result. The minimal toxic dose is 10 g (140 mg/kg), but liver damage has occurred with a single 5.85 g dose. The minimum lethal dose is 15 g (200 mg/kg). Children appear less susceptible to toxicity than adults. Initial signs of toxicity may include nausea, vomiting, anorexia, malaise, diaphoresis, abdominal pain and diarrhea. Clinical and laboratory evidence of hepatotoxicity usually is not apparent for 48 to 72 hours. If an acute dose of ≥ 150 mg/kg was ingested, or if the dose cannot be determined, obtain a serum acetaminophen assay as early as possible, but no sooner than 4 hours following ingestion. If in the toxic range, obtain liver function studies and repeat at 24 hour intervals. Hepatic failure may lead to encephalopathy, coma and death.

Plasma acetaminophen levels greater than 300 mcg/ml at 4 hours postingestion are always associated with hepatic damage; minimal hepatic damage is anticipated if plasma levels at 4 hours are below 120 mcg/ml. Hepatotoxicity is also likely if plasma levels at 12 hours are greater than 50 mcg/ml. In addition, if the half-life is greater than 4 hours, hepatic necrosis is probable; if greater than 12 hours, hepatic coma is probable. (See nomogram on page 933.)

Chronic daily ingestions of 5 to 8 g acetaminophen over several weeks, or 3 to 4 g/day for 1 year have also resulted in liver damage. The kidneys may undergo tubular necrosis; the myocardium may be acutely damaged.

Treatment: Refer also to General Management of Acute Overdosage.

Oral *N-acetylcysteine* is a specific antidote for APAP toxicity. Administration IV can cause anaphylaxis. If patient vomits within 1 hour of administration of *N-acetylcysteine* the dose should be repeated. Refer to page 930 to 934 for complete prescribing information and for a specific nomogram to guide treatment.

Patient Information:

Severe or recurrent pain or high or continued fever may indicate serious illness. If pain persists for more than 5 days, if redness is present or in arthritic and rheumatic conditions affecting children < 12 years old, consult physician immediately.

Do not exceed the recommended dosage. Consult physician for use in children < 3 years of age, or for oral use > 5 days (children), 10 days (adults) or 3 days for fever.

(Continued on following page)

ACETAMINOPHEN (N-Acetyl-P-Aminophenol, APAP) (Cont.)

Administration and Dosage:

Oral: Adults – 325-650 mg every 4 to 6 hrs, or 1 g 3-4 times/day. Do not exceed 4 g/day.

Children – May repeat doses 4 or 5 times daily; do not exceed 5 doses in 24 hours.

Acetaminophen Dosage for Children			
Age (years)	Dosage (mg)	Age (years)	Dosage (mg)
0-3 months	40	4-5	240
4-11 months	80	6-8	320
1-2	120	9-10	400
2-3	160	11	480

A 10 mg/kg/dose schedule has also been recommended.

Suppositories: Adults – 650 mg every 4 to 6 hrs. Give no more than 6 in 24 hours.

Children (6 to 12) – 325 mg every 4 to 6 hours. Give no more than 2.6 g in 24 hours.

Children (3 to 6) – 120 mg every 4 to 6 hours. Give no more than 720 mg in 24 hrs.

Children (< 3) – Consult physician.

Storage: Store suppositories below 27°C (80°F) or refrigerate.

	Product	Form	Packaging	C.I.*
otc	**Acetaminophen** (Various, eg, Balan, Bioline, Dixon-Shane, Goldline, Harber, Major, Moore, Roxane, Rugby, Schein)	**Suppositories:** 120 mg	In 12s, 50s, 100s and UD 12s, 50s, 100s, 500s and 1000s.	401+
otc	**Acetaminophen Uniserts** (Upsher-Smith)		In UD 12s and 50s.	542
otc	**Acephen** (G & W Labs)		In 12s, 50s and 100s.	464
otc	**Feverall, Children's** (Upsher-Smith)		In 6s.	310
otc	**Suppap-120** (Raway)		In 12s, 50s, 100s, 500s, 1000s.	446
otc	**Neopap** (Webcon)	**Suppositories**: 125 mg	In 12s.	975
otc	**Acetaminophen** (Harber)	**Suppositories:** 300 mg	In 12s.	237
otc	**Acetaminophen** (Various, eg, Balan, Baxter, Rugby)	**Suppositories:** 325 mg	In 12s and 100s.	188+
otc	**Acetaminophen Uniserts** (Upsher-Smith)		In UD 12s and 50s.	219
otc	**Acephen** (G & W Labs)		In 12s, 50s and 100s.	175
otc	**Feverall, Junior Strength** (Upsher-Smith)		In 6s.	123
otc	**Suppap-325** (Raway)		In 100s.	100
otc	**Acetaminophen** (Various, eg, Balan, Bioline, Goldline, Harber, Lannett, Major, Roxane, Rugby, Schein, Vangard)	**Suppositories:** 650 mg	In 10s, 12s, 50s, 100s, 500s and UD 12s, 50s, 100s, 500s and 1000s.	82+
otc	**Acetaminophen Uniserts** (Upsher-Smith)		In 12s, 50s and 500s.	117
otc	**Acephen** (G & W Labs)		In 12s, 50s, 100s and 500s.	89
otc	**Suppap-650** (Raway)		In 50s, 100s, 500s and 1000s.	75
otc	**Acetaminophen** (Various, eg, Balan, Dixon-Shane, Gen-King, Major, Mason, Moore, Rugby, Schein)	**Tablets, chewable:** 80 mg	In 30s, 50s, 100s and 1000s.	81
otc	**Apacet** (Parmed)		In 100s.	30
otc	**Anacin-3, Children's** (Whitehall)		Scored. Cherry flavor. In 30s.	183
otc	**Genapap, Children's** (Goldline)		Pink. In 30s.	175
otc *sf*	**Panadol, Children's** (Glenbrook)		(#P). Scored. Fruit flavor. In 30s.	159

* Cost Index based on cost per 325 mg. # Product identification code. *sf* – Sugar free.

(Continued on following page)

ACETAMINOPHEN (N-Acetyl-P-Aminophenol, APAP) (Cont.)				C.I.*
otc	**St. Joseph Aspirin-Free for Children** (Plough)	**Tablets, chewable:** 80 mg	Fruit flavor. In 30s.	131
otc	**Tempra** (Mead Johnson Nutritional)		In 30s.	173
otc	**Tylenol, Children's** (McNeil-CPC)		(Tylenol 80). Scored. Fruit or grape flavor. In 30s and 48s.	178
otc	**Feverall Sprinkle Caps** (Upsher-Smith)	**Capsules:** 80 mg	Taste free. In 20s.	221
otc	**Snaplets-FR Granules** (Baker Cummins)	**Granules:** 80 mg	In 32 premeasured packs.	NA
otc	**Tylenol Junior Strength** (McNeil-CPC)	**Tablets:** 160 mg	In 30s.	119
otc	**Tempra** (Mead-J)		Chewable. In 30s.	92
otc	**Feverall Sprinkle Caps** (Upsher-Smith)	**Capsules:** 160 mg	Taste free. In 20s.	122
otc	**Acetaminophen** (Various, eg, Balan, Geneva, Lannett, Lederle, Lemmon, Major, Moore, Roxane, Rugby, Schein)	**Tablets:** 325 mg	In 15s, 20s, 24s, 30s, 60s, 100s, 120s, 200s, 250s, 1000s, 5000s and UD 64s, 100s, 200s and 500s.	3+
otc	**Aceta** (Century)		In 100s and 1000s.	7
otc	**Anacin-3** (Whitehall)		In 24s, 50s and 100s.	21
otc	**Aspirin Free Pain Relief** (Hudson)		In 100s.	11
otc	**Dapa** (Ferndale)		In 100s, 1000s and UD 1000s.	15
otc	**Genebs** (Goldline)		White. In 100s and 1000s.	10
otc	**Halenol** (Halsey)		In 100s and 1000s.	4
otc	**Meda Tab** (Circle)		In 100s.	16
otc	**Panex** (Hauck)		In 100s and 1000s.	12
otc	**Phenaphen Caplets** (Robins)		In 100s.	22
otc	**Tylenol Caplets** (McNeil-CPC)		In 24s, 50s and 100s.	24
otc	**Tylenol Regular Strength Tablets** (McNeil-CPC)		In 24s, 50s, 100s and 200s.	26
otc	**Valadol** (Squibb Mark)		In 100s.	18
otc	**Acetaminophen** (Various, eg, Dixon-Shane, Genetco, Lannett, Lederle, Major, Moore, Murray, URL)	**Capsules:** 500 mg	In 50s, 100s, 500s, 1000s and UD 100s.	3+
otc	**Dapa Extra Strength** (Ferndale)		In 100s, 1000s and UD 1000s.	28
otc	**Meda Cap** (Circle)		In 25s, 60s and 100s.	13
otc	**Acetaminophen** (Various, eg, Balan, Baxter, Geneva, Lederle, Major, Moore, Roxane, Rugby, Schein, Warner Chilcott)	**Tablets:** 500 mg	In 24s, 30s, 50s, 60s, 100s, 125s, 200s, 250s, 500s, 1000s and UD 100s and 200s.	4+
otc	**Aceta** (Century)		In 100s and 1000s.	12
otc	**Anacin-3 Maximum Strength** (Whitehall)		**Caplets:** In 30s, 60s, 100s. **Tablets:** In 12s, 30s, 60s, 100s.	36 18
otc	**Arthritis Pain Formula Aspirin Free** (Whitehall)		In 30s and 75s.	23
otc	**Aspirin Free Pain Relief** (Hudson)		**Caplets:** Capsule shape. In 100s. **Tablets:** In 100s.	9 NA
otc	**Banesin** (Forest)		In 1000s.	10

* Cost Index based on cost per 325 mg.

(Continued on following page)

ACETAMINOPHEN (N-Acetyl-P-Aminophenol, APAP) (Cont.)

	Product	Dosage	Description	C.I.*
otc	**Datril Extra Strength** (Bristol-Myers)	**Tablets:** 500 mg	(Datril). White. In 30s, 60s and 100s.	16
otc	**Genapap Extra Strength** (Goldline)		**Caplets:** White. Oblong. In 50s and 100s.	13
			Tablets: White. In 30s, 60s and 100s.	12
otc	**Genebs Extra Strength** (Goldline)		**Caplets:** White. In 100s and 1000s.	12
			Tablets: White. In 100s and 1000s.	4
otc	**Halenol Extra Strength** (Halsey)		**Caplets:** Coated. In 50s, 100s and 1000s.	1
			Tablets: In 100s and 1000s.	5
otc	**Panadol** (Glenbrook)		**Caplets:** (Panadol 500). In 24s and 50s.	24
			Tablets: (Panadol 500). In 30s and 60s.	21
otc	**Panex 500** (Hauck)		In 1000s.	12
otc	**Redutemp** (Inter. Ethical Labs)		In 60s.	NA
otc	**Tapanol Extra Strength** (Republic)		**Caplets:** In 50s and 100s.	NA
			Tablets: In 100s.	15
otc	**Tylenol Extra Strength** (McNeil-CPC)		**Caplets:** (Tylenol). White. Capsule shape. In 24s, 50s, 100s and 175s.	23
			Gelcaps: Yellow/red. Gelatin coated. In 24s, 50s and 100s.	25
			Tablets: (Tylenol). White. In 10s, 30s, 60s, 100s and 200s.	22
otc	**Acetaminophen** (Roxane)	**Tablets:** 650 mg	In 1000s and UD 100s.	8
otc *sf*	**Dolanex** (Lannett)	**Elixir:** 325 mg per 5 ml	23% alcohol. In pt and gal.	25
otc	**Acetaminophen** (Various, eg, Balan, Bioline, Goldline, Lederle, Major, Purepac, Roxane, Rugby, Schein)	**Elixir:** 160 mg per 5 ml	In 120, 240 and 500 ml, pt, gal and UD 5, 10, 10.15, 20 and 20.3 ml (100s).	44+
otc	**Aceta** (Century)		7% alcohol. In 120 ml and gal.	51
otc	**Genapap Children's** (Goldline)		Alcohol free. Cherry flavor. In 120 ml.	110
otc	**Liquiprin Elixir** (Beecham)		Dextrose, fructose, sucrose. Cherry flavor. In 120 ml.	138
otc	**Tylenol Children's** (McNeil-CPC)		Alcohol free. Sorbitol, sucrose. Cherry or grape flavor. In 60 and 120 ml.	199
otc	**Acetaminophen** (Various, eg, Denison, Lannett, Pharm. Assoc. Inc)	**Elixir:** 120 mg per 5 ml	In 120 ml, pt and gal and UD 5 and 10, 13.5, 25 and 27 ml (100s).	30+
otc	**Oraphen-PD** (Great Southern)		5% alcohol. Cherry flavor. In 120 ml.	186

* Cost Index based on cost per 325 mg.
sf – Sugar free.

(Continued on following page)

ACETAMINOPHEN (N-Acetyl-P-Aminophenol, APAP) (Cont.)

	Product	Form/Strength	Description	C.I.*
otc	**Acetaminophen** (UDL Labs)	**Liquid:** 160 mg/5 ml	Alcohol free. In 120 and 480 ml and UD 2.5 and 5 ml (50s).	63
otc	**Anacin-3 Children's** (Whitehall)		Alcohol free. Cherry flavor. In 60 and 120 ml.	183
otc	**Dorcol Children's Fever and Pain Reducer** (Sandoz)		Sucrose. In 120 ml.	102
otc	**Halenol Children's** (Halsey)		Alcohol free. Cherry flavor. In 120, 240 and 480 ml and pt.	33
otc *sf*	**Panadol, Children's** (Glenbrook)		Alcohol free. Saccharin, sorbitol. Fruit flavor. In 60 and 120 ml.	179
otc *sf*	**St. Joseph Aspirin-Free Fever Reducer for Children** (Plough)		Alcohol free. Saccharin, sorbitol. Cherry flavor. In 60 and 120 ml.	203
otc	**Tempra Syrup** (Mead Johnson Nutritional)		Alcohol free. Cherry flavor. In 120 and 480 ml.	191
otc	**Acetaminophen** (UDL Labs)	**Elixir:** 130 mg/5 ml	In UD 12.5 and 25 ml (100s).	522
otc	**Tylenol Extra Strength** (McNeil-CPC)	**Liquid:** 500 mg/ 15 ml	7% alcohol. Sorbitol, sucrose. Mint flavor. In 240 ml with dosage cup.	83
otc	**Acetaminophen Drops** (Various, eg, Barre-National, Bioline, Moore, Schein)	**Solution:** 100 mg/ml	In 15 ml.	184+
otc	**Anacin-3, Infants' Drops** (Whitehall)		Alcohol free. Saccharin, sorbitol. Fruit flavor. In 15 ml with 0.8 ml dropper.	397
otc	**Genapap, Infants' Drops** (Goldline)		Alcohol free. Fruit flavor. In 15 ml with 0.8 ml dropper.	324
otc *sf*	**Myapap Drops** (Gen-King)		Alcohol free. In 15 ml with 0.8 ml dropper.	143
otc *sf*	**Panadol, Infants' Drops** (Glenbrook)		Alcohol free. Saccharin. Fruit flavor. In 15 ml with 0.8 ml dropper.	338
otc *sf*	**St. Joseph Aspirin-Free Infant Drops** (Plough)		Alcohol free. Saccharin. Fruit flavor. In 15 ml with 0.8 ml dropper.	332
otc	**Tempra Drops** (Mead Johnson Nutritional)		Alcohol free. Grape flavor. In 15 ml with 0.8 ml dropper.	378
otc	**Tylenol, Infants' Drops** (McNeil-CPC)		Alcohol free. Saccharin. Fruit flavor. In 15 ml with 0.8 ml dropper.	390
otc	**Uni-Ace, Infants' Drops** (URL)		Alcohol free. Fruit flavor. In 15 ml with dropper.	N/A
otc	**Liquiprin Infants' Drops** (Beecham)	**Solution:** 120 mg/ 2.5 ml	Alcohol free. Fruit flavor. In 35 ml with dropper.	242

ACETAMINOPHEN, BUFFERED

	Product	Form/Strength	Description	C.I.*
otc	**Bromo Seltzer** (Warner-Lambert)	**Effervescent Granules:** 325 mg with 2.781 g sodium bicarbonate and 2.224 g citric acid per dosage measure	With 761 mg sodium. In 78.75, 127.5 and 270 g and UD 48s.	

* Cost Index based on cost per 325 mg acetaminophen.

sf – Sugar free.

The salicylates have analgesic, antipyretic and anti-inflammatory effects. Aspirin and other salicylic acid derivatives are hydrolyzed to salicylic acid. Salicylamide and diflunisal are structurally related, but are not true salicylates since they are not hydrolyzed to salicylic acid.

Salicylic Acid Derivatives

Warning:
Children and teenagers should not use salicylates for chickenpox or flu symptoms before a doctor is consulted about Reye's syndrome, a rare but serious illness.

Actions:

Pharmacology: Salicylates have analgesic, antipyretic, anti-inflammatory and antirheumatic effects. The pharmacological effects of these agents are qualitatively similar. Salicylates lower elevated body temperature through vasodilation of peripheral vessels, thus enhancing dissipation of excess heat. The anti-inflammatory and analgesic activity may be mediated through inhibition of the prostaglandin synthetase enzyme complex.

Aspirin differs from the other agents in this group in that it more potently inhibits prostaglandin synthesis, has greater anti-inflammatory effects and irreversibly inhibits platelet aggregation. The acetyl group of the aspirin molecule is believed to account for these differences. Aspirin inhibits the production of prostaglandins by acetylating cyclo-oxygenase, the initial enzyme in the prostaglandin biosynthesis pathway.

Irreversible inhibition of platelet aggregation (aspirin) – Single analgesic aspirin doses prolong bleeding time. Acetylation of platelet cyclo-oxygenase prevents synthesis of thromboxane A_2, a prostaglandin derivative, which is a potent vasoconstrictor and inducer of platelet aggregation and platelet release reaction. Aspirin, but not other salicylates, inhibits platelet aggregation for the life of the platelet (7 to 10 days).

Aspirin has shown some success as an antiplatelet agent in patients with thromboembolic disease. Low doses of aspirin inhibit platelet aggregation and may be more effective than higher doses. Larger doses inhibit cyclo-oxygenase in arterial walls, interfering with prostacyclin production, a potent vasodilator and inhibitor of platelet aggregation. Combinations of dipyridamole or sulfinpyrazone with aspirin have been recommended for antithrombotic action for prophylaxis in various high risk situations (ie, coronary bypass graft patency and total hip replacement).

Myocardial infarction – Aspirin therapy in MI patients was associated with an $\approx$ 20% reduction in risk of subsequent death and nonfatal reinfarction, a median absolute decrease of 3% from the 12% to 22% event rates in the placebo groups. Daily aspirin dosage in the post-MI studies was 300 mg in one study and 900 to 1500 mg in five. In aspirin-treated unstable angina patients (325 mg/day), the reduction in risk was about 50%, a reduction in event rate of 5% from the 10% rate in the placebo group over the 12 week study.

In the Aspirin Myocardial Infarction Study (AMIS) trial, 1000 mg per day was associated with small increases in systolic BP (average 1.5 to 2.1 mm Hg) and diastolic BP (0.5 to 0.6 mm Hg). Uric acid levels and BUN were also increased, but by $<$ 1 mg%.

In the Second International Study of Infarct Survival (ISIS-2) trial, patients who received a combination of aspirin (160 mg/day) and streptokinase after the onset of suspected acute MI had significantly fewer reinfarctions, strokes and deaths than those patients who received placebo. Also, the combination was significantly better than either drug alone, and their separate effects on vascular deaths appeared additive.

Other pharmacological actions – Inhibition of prothrombin synthesis and prolonged prothrombin time are clinically significant only after large doses ($\geq$ 6 g/day). Doses $>$ 3 to 5 g/day have a uricosuric effect; low doses ($<$ 2 g/day) decrease uric acid secretion.

Pharmacokinetics: Absorption/Distribution – Salicylates are rapidly and completely absorbed after oral use. Bioavailability is dependent on the dosage form, presence of food, gastric emptying time, gastric pH, presence of antacids or buffering agents and particle size. Bioavailability of some enteric coated products may be erratic. Food slows the absorption of salicylates. Absorption from rectal suppositories is slower, resulting in lower salicylate levels. Aspirin is partially hydrolyzed to salicylic acid during absorption and is distributed to all body tissues and fluids, including fetal tissues, breast milk and CNS. Highest concentrations are found in plasma, liver, renal cortex, heart and lungs. Protein binding of salicylates is concentration-dependent. At low therapeutic concentrations (100 mcg/ml), about 90% is bound; at higher plasma concentrations (400 mcg/ml), 76% is bound. Signs of salicylism (eg, tinnitus) occur at serum levels $>$ 200 mcg/ml; severe toxic effects may occur at levels $>$ 400 mcg/ml (see Adverse Reactions).

(Actions continued on following page)

Actions (Cont.):

Metabolism/Elimination – Salicylic acid is eliminated by renal excretion of salicylic acid and by oxidation and conjugation of metabolites. Aspirin has a half-life of ≈ 15 to 20 minutes. Salicylic acid has a half-life of 2 to 3 hours at low doses; at higher doses, it may exceed 20 hours. In therapeutic anti-inflammatory doses, half-life ranges from 6 to 12 hrs. Plasma salicylate levels increase disproportionately as salicylate dosage is increased. Elimination is determined by zero order kinetics. Renal excretion of unchanged drug depends upon urine pH. As urinary pH changes from 5 to 8, renal clearance of free ionized salicylate increases from 2% to 3% of the amount excreted to more than 80%.

Indications:

Mild to moderate pain; fever; various inflammatory conditions such as rheumatic fever, rheumatoid arthritis and osteoarthritis.

Aspirin, for reducing the risk of recurrent transient ischemic attacks (TIAs) or stroke in men who have had transient ischemia of the brain due to fibrin platelet emboli. It has not been effective in women and is of no benefit for completed strokes.

Aspirin, to reduce the risk of death or nonfatal myocardial infarction (MI) in patients with previous infarction or unstable angina pectoris.

Unlabeled Uses: The possible protective effect of long-term use of aspirin-like analgesics against cataract formation is being studied. Although dipyridamole is often added to aspirin to prevent MI and stroke, data do not show improved antithrombotic efficacy of aspirin during coadministration. Low-dose aspirin may be useful in preventing toxemia of pregnancy. It may also be beneficial in pregnant women with inadequate uteroplacental blood flow (eg, systemic lupus erythematosus). Further studies are needed. See Warnings.

Contraindications:

Hypersensitivity to salicylates or nonsteroidal anti-inflammatory drugs (NSAIDs). Give with extreme caution to any patient with a history of adverse reactions to salicylates. Cross-sensitivity may exist between aspirin and other NSAIDs which inhibit prostaglandin synthesis, and between aspirin and tartrazine dye. Aspirin cross-sensitivity does not appear to occur with sodium salicylate, salicylamide or choline salicylate. Aspirin hypersensitivity is more prevalent in patients with asthma, nasal polyposis or chronic urticaria.

In hemophilia, bleeding ulcers and hemorrhagic states.

Magnesium salicylate in advanced chronic renal insufficiency due to magnesium retention.

Warnings:

Reye's syndrome: Salicylate association – Use of salicylates, particularly aspirin, in children or teenagers with influenza or chickenpox may be associated with the development of Reye's syndrome. This rare, acute, life-threatening condition is characterized by vomiting, lethargy and belligerence that may progress to delirium and coma. The mortality rate is 20% to 30% and permanent brain damage has been reported in survivors.

A causal relationship to salicylates is controversial, but the CDC, the FDA, the American Academy of Pediatrics' Committee on Infectious Diseases and the Surgeon General advise against use of salicylates in children and teenagers with influenza or chickenpox. (See Warning Box.)

Otic effects: Discontinue use if dizziness, ringing in ears (tinnitus) or impaired hearing occurs. Tinnitus probably represents blood salicylic acid levels reaching or exceeding the upper limit of the therapeutic range. It is a helpful guide to dose titration. Temporary hearing loss disappears gradually upon discontinuation of the drug.

Use in surgical patients: Avoid aspirin, if possible, for 1 week prior to surgery because of the possibility of postoperative bleeding.

Usage in impaired hepatic function: Use with caution in liver damage, preexisting hypoprothrombinemia and vitamin K deficiency. Reversible hepatic encephalopathy occurred in a chronic alcoholic with cirrhosis who took ASA 5 g/day for osteoarthritis. Aspirin-induced hepatotoxicity occurred after therapeutic doses for rheumatoid arthritis.

Hypersensitivity: Aspirin intolerance, manifested by acute bronchospasm, generalized urticaria/angioedema, severe rhinitis or shock occurs in 4% to 19% of asthmatics. Symptoms occur within 3 hours after ingestion. The aspirin triad consists of the association of asthma, nasal polyps and aspirin intolerance. Have epinephrine 1:1000 immediately available. Refer to Management of Acute Hypersensitivity Reactions on p. 2897

Foods containing salicylate may contribute to a reaction. Some foods with 6 mg/100 g salicylate include curry powder, paprika, licorice, Benedictine liqueur, prunes, raisins, tea and gherkins. A typical American diet contains 10 to 200 mg/day salicylate.

Desensitization has been successfully induced and maintained. It should be done in a hospital; it is generally maintained with one aspirin/day. Any NSAID can maintain desensitization. However, if maintenance is interrupted, sensitivity will reappear (2 to 5 days).

(Warnings continued on following page)

Complete prescribing information for these products begins on page 1153

Salicylic Acid Derivatives (Cont.)

ASPIRIN (Acetylsalicylic Acid; ASA) (Cont.)

	Product	Form/Strength	Description/Packaging	C.I.*
otc	**Aspirin** (URL)	**Tablets:** 500 mg	In 100s.	4+
otc	**Maximum Bayer Aspirin Tablets and Caplets** (Glenbrook)		**Tablets:** Film coated. In 30s, 60s and 100s.	33
			Caplets: Film coated. In 30s and 60s.	33
otc	**Norwich Extra-Strength** (Procter & Gamble Pharm.)		In 150s.	7
otc	**Aspirin** (Various, eg, Geneva, Major, Moore, Parmed, Rugby, URL)	**Tablets, enteric coated:** 325 mg	In 30s, 60s, 90s, 100s, 1000s and UD 100s.	3+
otc	**Ecotrin Tablets and Caplets** (SmithKline Beecham)		**Tablets:** (Ecotrin Reg). In 100s, 250s and 1000s.	25
			Caplets: (Ecotrin Reg). In 100s.	25
otc	**Therapy Bayer Caplets** (Glenbrook)		Delayed release. In 50s and 100s.	NA
otc	**Ecotrin Maximum Strength Tablets and Caplets** (SK Beecham)	**Tablets, enteric coated:** 500 mg	**Tablets:** (Ecotrin Max). In 60s and 150s.	30
			Caplets: (Ecotrin Max). In 60s.	30
otc	**Aspirin** (Various, eg, Goldline, Moore, Rugby)	**Tablets, enteric coated:** 650 mg	In 100s and 1000s.	6+
Rx	**Aspirin** (Rugby)	**Tablets, enteric coated:** 975 mg	In 100s.	NA
Rx	**Easprin** (Parke-Davis)		Delayed release. (P-D 490). In 100s.	32
otc	**8-Hour Bayer Timed-Release Caplets** (Glenbrook)	**Tablets, timed release:** 650 mg	White, scored. In 30s, 72s and 125s.	24
Rx	**ZORprin** (Boots)	**Tablets, controlled release:** 800 mg	(BA57). White. Elongated. In 100s.	28
otc	**Aspirin** (Various, eg, Goldline, Moore, Rugby, URL)	**Suppositories**[1]: 120 mg	In 12s.	NA
		200 mg	In 12s.	NA
		300 mg	In 12s.	NA
		600 mg	In 12s and 100s.	NA

ASPIRIN (Acetylsalicylic Acid; ASA), BUFFERED

The addition of small amounts of antacids may decrease GI irritation and increase the dissolution and absorption rates of these products.

	Product	Form/Strength	Description/Packaging	C.I.*
otc	**Tri-Buffered Bufferin Tablets and Caplets** (Bristol-Myers Squibb)	**Tablets:** 325 mg with calcium carbonate, magnesium oxide and magnesium carbonate	**Tablets:** (B). White. In 12s, 36s, 60s, 100s, 200s, 275s, 1000s.	27
			Caplets: (B). White, scored. In 36s, 60s and 100s.	NA
otc	**Buffered Aspirin** (Various, eg, Geneva, Goldline, Major, Moore, Rugby, UDL, URL)	**Tablets:** 325 mg with buffers	In 100s, 500s, 1000s and UD 100s and 200s.	7+
otc	**Buffex** (Hauck)	**Tablets:** 325 mg with aluminum glycinate and magnesium carbonate	In 1000s and Sani-Pak 1000s.	7
otc	**Wesprin Buffered** (Wesley)	**Tablets:** 325 mg with aluminum and magnesium hydroxides	Peach, oval. In 1000s.	8

* Cost Index based on cost per 325 mg.

[1] Refrigerate.

(Continued on following page)

Complete prescribing information for these products begins on page 1153

Salicylic Acid Derivatives (Cont.)

	ASPIRIN (Acetylsalicylic Acid; ASA), BUFFERED (Cont.)			C.I.*
otc	**Magnaprin** (Rugby)	**Tablets, coated:** 325 mg with 50 mg magnesium hydroxide, 50 mg aluminum hydroxide and calcium carbonate	Film coated. In 100s and 500s.	11
otc	**Regular Strength Ascriptin** (Rhone Poulenc Rorer)		In 60s.	19
otc	**Ascriptin A/D** (Rorer)	**Tablets, coated:** 325 mg with 75 mg magnesium hydroxide, 75 mg aluminum hydroxide and calcium carbonate	Capsule shape. In 225s.	32
otc	**Magnaprin Arthritis Strength Captabs** (Rugby)		Capsule shape. In 100s and 500s.	13
otc	**Bufferin** (Bristol-Myers)	**Tablets, coated:** 325 mg with 158 mg calcium carbonate, 63 mg magnesium oxide and 34 mg magnesium carbonate	**Tablets:** (B). In 12s, 36s, 60s, 100s, 200s and UD 150s.	22
			Caplets: (B/B). Coated, scored. In 36s, 60s and 100s.	22
otc	**Arthritis Strength Bufferin** (Bristol-Myers)	**Tablets:** 500 mg with magnesium carbonate and aluminum glycinate	White. In 40s and 100s.	20
otc	**Bufferin Extra Strength** (Bristol-Myers)	**Tablets:** 500 mg with magnesium carbonate and aluminum glycinate	**Coated:** (ES Bufferin). White. In 30s, 60s, 100s.	20
			Uncoated: (ESB). White. In 30s, 60s, 100s.	20
otc	**Extra Strength Bayer Plus Caplets** (Glenbrook)	**Tablets:** 500 mg with calcium carbonate, magnesium carbonate and magnesium oxide	In 30s and 60s.	NA
otc	**Ascriptin Extra Strength** (Rhone-Poulenc Rorer)	**Tablets, coated:** 500 mg with 80 mg magnesium hydroxide, 80 mg aluminum hydroxide and calcium carbonate	Capsule shape. In 50s.	26
otc	**Cama Arthritis Pain Reliever** (Sandoz Consumer)	**Tablets:** 500 mg with 150 mg magnesium oxide and 150 mg aluminum hydroxide	(Dorsey Cama 500). White w/salmon inlay. In 100s and 250s.	15
otc	**Arthritis Pain Formula** (Whitehall)	**Tablets:** 500 mg with 100 mg magnesium hydroxide and 27 mg aluminum hydroxide	Capsule shape. In 40s, 100s and 175s.	24
otc	**Alka-Seltzer with Aspirin** (Miles Inc)	**Tablets, effervescent:** 325 mg with 1.9 g sodium bicarbonate and 1 g citric acid per dry tablet, 567 mg sodium/tablet	In 12s, 24s, 36s, 72s, 96s and 100s.	40
otc	**Alka-Seltzer with Aspirin (Flavored)** (Miles Inc)	**Tablets, effervescent:** 325 mg with 1.7 g sodium bicarbonate and 1.2 g citric acid per dry tablet, 506 mg sodium/tablet	Saccharin and flavoring. In 12s, 24s and 36s.	40
otc	**Alka-Seltzer Extra Strength with Aspirin** (Miles)	**Tablet, effervescent:** 500 mg with 1.9 g sodium bicarbonate and 1 g citric acid	In 12s and 24s.	50

* Cost Index based on cost per 325 mg aspirin.

Complete prescribing information for these products begins on page 1153

Salicylic Acid Derivatives (Cont.)

SALSALATE (Salicylsalicylic Acid)

After absorption, the drug is partially hydrolyzed into two molecules of salicylic acid. Insoluble in gastric secretions, it is not absorbed until it reaches the small intestine.

Administration and Dosage:

Usual adult dose is 3000 mg/day given in divided doses.

	Product	Form	Description	C.I.*
Rx	**Amigesic** (Amide)	**Capsules:** 500 mg	White and green. In 100s and 500s.	NA
Rx	**Disalcid** (3M)		(Riker Disalcid). Aqua and white. In 100s.	84
Rx	**Salsalate** (Various, eg, Copley, Geneva, Goldline, Major, Moore, Rugby, Schein, URL, Vitarine)	**Tablets:** 500 mg	In 100s, 500s and UD 100s.	23+
Rx	**Amigesic** (Amide)		Yellow or blue. Film coated. In 100s and 500s.	NA
Rx	**Argesic-SA** (Econo Med)		In 100s.	NA
Rx	**Disalcid** (3M)		(Riker Disalcid). Aqua, scored. Film coated. In 100s, 500s and UD 100s.	80
Rx	**Salflex** (Carnrick)		Dye free. (C 8671). White. Film coated. In 100s.	60
Rx	**Salsitab** (Upsher-Smith)		(500). Blue. Film coated. In 100s, 500s and UD 100s.	32
Rx	**Salsalate** (Various, eg, Copley, Geneva, Goldline, Major, Moore, Rugby, Schein, URL, Vitarine)	**Tablets:** 750 mg	In 100s, 500s and UD 100s.	17+
Rx	**Amigesic Caplets** (Amide)		Yellow or blue, scored. Film coated. Capsule shaped. In 100s and 500s.	NA
Rx	**Artha-G** (T.E. Williams)		(Artha-G). Lavender, scored. In 120s.	40
Rx	**Disalcid** (3M)		(Riker Disalcid 750). Aqua, scored. Film coated. In 100s, 500s and UD 100s.	68
Rx	**Mono-Gesic** (Central)		(Central 750 mg). Pink, scored. Film coated. In 100s and 500s.	42
Rx	**Salsitab** (Upsher-Smith)		(750). Blue, scored. Film coated. In 100s, 500s and UD 100s.	30
Rx	**Salflex** (Carnrick)		Dye free. (C 8672) White, scored. Film coated. In 100s and 500s.	52

SODIUM SALICYLATE

Less effective than an equal dose of aspirin in reducing pain or fever. Patients hypersensitive to aspirin may be able to tolerate sodium salicylate. Platelets are not affected; however, prothrombin time is increased. Each gram contains 6.25 mEq sodium.

Administration and Dosage:

325 to 650 mg every 4 hours.

	Product	Form	Description	C.I.*
otc	**Sodium Salicylate** (Various, eg, Moore, Rugby)	**Tablets, enteric coated:** 325 mg	In 1000s.	6+
otc	**Sodium Salicylate** (Various, eg, Moore, Rugby)	**Tablets, enteric coated:** 650 mg	In 100s, 500s and 1000s.	6+

* Cost Index based on cost per 325 mg salsalate or 325 mg sodium salicylate.

Complete prescribing information for these products begins on page 1153

Salicylic Acid Derivatives (Cont.)

SODIUM THIOSALICYLATE

Administration and Dosage: Intramuscular administration is preferred.

Acute gout: 100 mg every 3 to 4 hours for 2 days, then 100 mg/day until the patient is asymptomatic.

Muscular pain and musculoskeletal disturbances: 50 to 100 mg/day or on alternate days.

Rheumatic fever: 100 to 150 mg every 4 to 8 hours for 3 days, then reduce to 100 mg twice daily. Continue until patient is asymptomatic. **C.I.***

	Product	Form	Description	C.I.*
Rx	**Sodium Thiosalicylate** (Various)	**Injection:** 50 mg per ml	In 30 ml vials and 2 ml amps.	53+
Rx	**Asproject** (Mayrand)		In 30 ml vials.	218
Rx	**Rexolate** (Hyrex)		In 30 ml vials.	180
Rx	**Tusal** (Hauck)		In 30 ml vials.[1]	157

CHOLINE SALICYLATE

Has fewer GI side effects than aspirin.

Administration and Dosage:

Adults and children (over 12 years): 870 mg every 3 to 4 hours; maximum 6 times/day. Rheumatoid arthritis patients may start with 5 to 10 ml, up to 4 times/day. **C.I.***

	Product	Form	Description	C.I.*
otc	**Arthropan** (Purdue Frederick)	**Liquid:** 870 mg per 5 ml[2]	Mint flavor. In 240 and 480 ml.	53

MAGNESIUM SALICYLATE

A sodium free salicylate derivative that may have a low incidence of GI upset. The product labeling and dosage are expressed as magnesium salicylate anhydrous. The possibility of magnesium toxicity exists in persons with renal insufficiency.

Administration and Dosage:

Usual dose is 650 mg every 4 hours or 1090 mg, 3 times a day. May increase to 3.6 to 4.8 g/day in 3 or 4 divided doses.

Safety and efficacy for use in children have not been established. **C.I.***

	Product	Form	Description	C.I.*
otc	**Original Doan's** (Ciba Consumer)	**Caplets:** 325 mg	In 24s and 48s.	59
otc	**Extra Strength Doan's** (Ciba Consumer)	**Caplets:** 500 mg	In 24s and 48s.	48
Rx	**Magan** (Adria)	**Tablets:** 545 mg	(Adria 412). Pink. In 100s and 500s.	77
Rx	**Mobidin** (Ascher)	**Tablets:** 600 mg	(0310). Yellow, scored. In 100s and 500s.	39

SALICYLATE COMBINATIONS

	Product	Form	Description	C.I.*
Rx	**Choline Magnesium Trisalicylate** (Sidmark)	**Tablets:** 500 mg salicylate (as 293 mg choline salicylate and 362 mg Mg salicylate)	(SL 528). Yellow, scored. In 100s and 500s.	NA
Rx	**Tricosal** (URL)		Yellow. Film coated. In 100s.	NA
Rx	**Trilisate** (Purdue Frederick)		(PF/T500). Pink, scored. In 100s and UD 100s.	142
Rx	**Choline Magnesium Trisalicylate** (Sidmark)	**Tablets:** 750 mg salicylate (as 440 mg choline salicylate and 544 mg Mg salicylate)	(SL 529). Blue, scored. Film coated. Capsule shape. In 100s and 500s.	NA
Rx	**Tricosal** (URL)		Blue. Film coated. In 100s.	NA
Rx	**Trilisate** (Purdue Frederick)		(PF/T750). White, scored. In 100s, UD 100s.	176
Rx	**Choline Magnesium Trisalicylate** (Sidmark)	**Tablets:** 1000 mg salicylate (as 587 mg choline salicylate and 725 mg Mg salicylate)	(SL 530). Pink, scored. In 100s and 500s.	NA
Rx	**Trilisate** (Purdue Frederick)		(PF/T1000). Red, scored. Film coated. In 60s.	240
Rx	**Trilisate** (Purdue Frederick)	**Liquid:** 500 mg salicylate (as 293 mg choline salicylate and 362 mg Mg salicylate) per 5 ml	Cherry-cordial flavor. In 237 ml.	139

* Cost Index based on cost per 50 mg sodium thiosalicylate, 435 mg choline salicylate, 300 mg magnesium salicylate (anhydrous) or per tablet or 5 ml combination.

[1] With 2% benzyl alcohol. [2] Contains menthol.

DIFLUNISAL

Actions:

Diflunisal, a salicylic acid derivative, is a nonsteroidal, peripherally-acting, nonnarcotic analgesic with anti-inflammatory and antipyretic properties. Chemically, it differs from aspirin and is not metabolized to salicylic acid. Its mechanisms are unknown. Diflunisal is a prostaglandin synthetase inhibitor.

Pharmacokinetics: Absorption/Distribution – Diflunisal is rapidly and completely absorbed following oral administration; peak plasma concentrations occur between 2 to 3 hours, producing significant analgesia within 1 hour and maximum analgesia within 2 to 3 hours. The first dose tends to have a slower onset of pain relief than other drugs achieving comparable peak effects. Time required to achieve steady-state increases with dosage, from 3 to 4 days with 125 mg twice daily to 7 to 9 days with 500 mg twice daily, because of its long half-life and nonlinear pharmacokinetics. An initial loading dose shortens the time to reach steady-state levels; 2 to 3 days of observation are necessary for evaluating changes in treatment regimens if a loading dose is not used. More than 99% is bound to plasma proteins.

Metabolism/Elimination – Concentration-dependent pharmacokinetics prevail; doubling the dosage more than doubles drug accumulation. The plasma half-life of diflunisal is 8 to 12 hours; it increases in renal impairment. The drug is excreted in the urine as glucuronide conjugates which account for about 90% of the dose. Less than 5% is recovered in the feces.

Clinical Pharmacology: Diflunisal 500 mg is comparable in analgesic efficacy but produces longer lasting responses than aspirin 650 mg, acetaminophen 600 to 650 mg and acetaminophen 650 mg with propoxyphene napsylate 100 mg. Diflunisal 1 g is comparable in analgesic efficacy to acetaminophen 600 mg with codeine 60 mg. Patients treated with diflunisal generally continue to have a good analgesic effect 8 to 12 hours after dosing.

Osteoarthritis – Diflunisal 500 or 750 mg daily was as effective as aspirin 2 or 3 g daily, and produced a lower overall incidence of GI disturbances, dizziness, edema and tinnitus.

Rheumatoid arthritis – In controlled clinical trials, diflunisal's effectiveness was established for both acute exacerbations and long-term management of rheumatoid arthritis. Activity was demonstrated by clinical improvement in the signs and symptoms of disease activity.

Diflunisal has been compared to aspirin in several controlled trials. Diflunisal dosages of 500 mg to 1 g daily have been comparable to aspirin dosages of 2 to 4 g daily for 8 to 12 weeks (up to 52 weeks in open-label extensions). Patients also generally experienced less GI effects, tinnitus, hearing loss and dyspepsia with diflunisal.

In two double-blind multicenter studies of 12 weeks' duration, diflunisal 500 or 750 mg daily was compared to ibuprofen 1.6 or 2.4 g daily or naproxen 750 mg daily; they were comparable in effectiveness and tolerability. The naproxen study was extended to 48 weeks on an open-label basis; diflunisal continued to be effective and generally well tolerated.

In patients with rheumatoid arthritis, diflunisal and gold salts may be used in combination at their usual dosage levels. The combination does not alter the course of the underlying disease but usually results in additional symptomatic relief.

Antipyretic activity – Diflunisal is not recommended for use as an antipyretic agent. In single 250, 500 or 750 mg doses, the drug produced measurable, but not clinically useful, decreases in temperature in patients with fever; however, it may mask fever in some patients, particularly with chronic or high doses.

Uricosuric effect – An increase in the renal clearance of uric acid and a decrease in serum uric acid occurred with diflunisal doses of 500 or 750 mg daily. Patients on long-term diflunisal therapy, 500 mg or 1 g daily, showed prompt and consistent reduction in mean serum uric acid levels, as much as 1.4 mg%. It is not known whether diflunisal interferes with the activity of other uricosuric agents.

(Actions continued on following page)

DIFLUNISAL (Cont.)

Actions (Cont.):

Clinical Pharmacology (Cont.):

Effect on platelet function – As an inhibitor of prostaglandin synthetase, diflunisal has a dose-related effect on platelet function and bleeding time. At 2 g daily, diflunisal inhibits platelet function. In contrast to aspirin, these effects were reversible because of the absence of the acetyl group. Bleeding time was only slightly increased at 1 g daily; at 2 g daily, a greater increase occurred.

Effect on fecal blood loss was not significantly different from placebo at a dose of 1 g daily. Diflunisal 2 g daily caused a statistically significant increase in fecal blood loss, but only one-half that associated with aspirin 2.6 g daily.

Indications:

Acute or long-term symptomatic treatment of mild to moderate pain, rheumatoid arthritis and osteoarthritis.

Contraindications:

Hypersensitivity to diflunisal.

Patients in whom acute asthmatic attacks, urticaria or rhinitis are precipitated by aspirin or other nonsteroidal anti-inflammatory drugs.

Warnings:

Peptic ulceration and GI bleeding have been reported. Fatalities occurred rarely. In patients with active GI bleeding or an active peptic ulcer, weigh the benefits of therapy against possible hazards; institute an appropriate ulcer treatment regimen and monitor progress. When administered to patients with a history of GI disease, monitor closely.

Usage in Pregnancy: Category C. Safety for use during pregnancy has not been established. Use during the first two trimesters only if the potential benefits outweigh the unknown potential hazards to the fetus. Because of the known effect of this drug class on the fetal cardiovascular system (closure of ductus arteriosus), use during the third trimester is not recommended.

Usage in Lactation: Diflunisal is excreted in breast milk in concentrations 2% to 7% of that in plasma. Because of the potential for adverse reactions in nursing infants, discontinue either nursing or the drug.

Usage in Children below 12 years of age is not recommended. Safety and efficacy in infants and children have not been established.

Precautions:

Platelet function and bleeding time are inhibited by diflunisal at higher doses.

Ophthalmologic effects have been reported with these agents; perform ophthalmologic studies in patients who develop eye complaints during treatment.

Impaired renal function: Since diflunisal is eliminated primarily by the kidneys, monitor patients with significantly impaired renal function; use a lower daily dosage.

Peripheral edema has been observed. Use with caution in patients with compromised cardiac function, hypertension or other conditions predisposing to fluid retention.

Acetylsalicylic acid has been associated with Reye's syndrome. Since diflunisal is a salicylic acid derivative, the possibility of its association with Reye's syndrome cannot be excluded.

Laboratory tests: Borderline elevations of **liver tests** may occur in up to 15% of patients. These abnormalities may progress, may remain essentially unchanged or may be transient with continued therapy. Meaningful (3 times the upper limit of normal) elevations of ALT or AST occurred in less than 1% of patients.

A patient with signs or symptoms suggesting liver dysfunction, or with an abnormal liver test, should be evaluated for evidence of development of more severe hepatic reactions. Severe hepatic reactions, including jaundice, have occurred with diflunisal and other NSAIDs. Although such reactions are rare, if abnormal liver tests persist or worsen, if clinical signs and symptoms consistent with liver disease develop, or if systemic manifestations occur (eg, eosinophilia, rash), discontinue drug; liver reactions can be fatal.

Drug Interactions:

Acetaminophen: Administration of diflunisal resulted in ≈ 50% increased acetaminophen plasma levels. Acetaminophen had no effect on diflunisal plasma levels.

Anticoagulants, oral: Coadministration of diflunisal may increase hypoprothrombinemic effects of anticoagulants. Diflunisal competitively displaces coumarins from protein-binding sites. Monitor prothrombin time during and for several days after coadministration. Adjust dosage of oral anticoagulants as required.

Hydrochlorothiazide: Coadministration of diflunisal resulted in significantly increased plasma levels of hydrochlorothiazide. Diflunisal decreased the hyperuricemic effects of hydrochlorothiazide.

(Drug Interactions continued on following page)

DIFLUNISAL (Cont.)

Drug Interactions (Cont.):

Indomethacin: Administration of diflunisal decreased renal clearance and significantly increased plasma levels of indomethacin. The combined use has also been associated with fatal GI hemorrhage.

Sulindac: Administration of diflunisal resulted in lowering of the plasma levels of the active sulindac sulfide metabolite by approximately one-third.

Adverse Reactions:

Listed below are adverse reactions reported in 1314 patients who received long-term treatment (24 to 96 weeks). In general, the adverse reactions listed below were 2 to 14 times less frequent in 1113 patients who received short-term treatment.

Incidence < 1% to 9% (causal relationship known):

GI – Nausea, dyspepsia, GI pain, diarrhea (3% to 9%); vomiting, constipation, flatulence (1% to 3%); peptic ulcer, GI bleeding/perforation, anorexia, eructation, cholestasis, jaundice (sometimes with fever), gastritis, hepatitis, abnormal liver function tests (< 1%).

GU – Dysuria, renal impairment (including renal failure), interstitial nephritis, hematuria, proteinuria (< 1%).

CNS – Headache (3% to 9%); dizziness, somnolence, insomnia (1% to 3%); vertigo, nervousness, depression, hallucinations, confusion, disorientation, lightheadedness, paresthesias (< 1%).

Hypersensitivity (< 1%) – Acute anaphylactic reaction with bronchospasm. A potentially life-threatening apparent hypersensitivity syndrome was reported. This multisystem syndrome includes constitutional symptoms (fever, chills) and cutaneous findings. It may include involvement of major organs (changes in liver function, jaundice, leukopenia, thrombocytopenia, eosinophilia, renal impairment including renal failure) and less specific findings (adenitis, arthralgia, arthritis, malaise, anorexia, disorientation).

Dermatologic – Rash (3% to 9%); pruritus, sweating, dry mucous membranes, stomatitis, erythema multiforme, Stevens-Johnson syndrome, toxic epidermal necrolysis, exfoliative dermatitis, photosensitivity, urticaria (< 1%).

Miscellaneous – Fatigue/tiredness, tinnitus (1% to 3%); asthenia, edema, thrombocytopenia, agranulocytosis (rare), transient visual disturbances including blurred vision (< 1%).

Incidence < 1% (causal relationship unknown):

Cardiovascular – Palpitations; syncope; chest pain.

Miscellaneous – Dyspnea; muscle cramps.

Overdosage:

Symptoms: Cases of overdosage have occurred and deaths have been reported. Most patients recovered without permanent sequelae. The most common signs and symptoms were drowsiness, vomiting, nausea, diarrhea, hyperventilation, tachycardia, sweating, tinnitus, disorientation, stupor and coma. Diminished urine output and cardiorespiratory arrest have also been reported.

The lowest fatal dosage was 15 g without any other drugs. In a mixed drug overdose, ingestion of 7.5 g diflunisal resulted in death.

Treatment is symptomatic and supportive. Empty the stomach by inducing vomiting or by gastric lavage. Refer to General Management of Acute Overdosage on2895 Because of the high degree of protein binding, hemodialysis may not be effective.

Patient Information:

May cause GI upset; may be taken with water, milk or meals.

Do not take **aspirin** or **acetaminophen** with diflunisal, except on professional advice.

Swallow tablets whole; do not crush or chew.

Administration and Dosage:

Mild to moderate pain: Initially, 1 g, followed by 500 mg every 8 to 12 hours. A lower dosage may be appropriate; for example, 500 mg initially, followed by 250 mg every 8 to 12 hours.

Osteoarthritis/rheumatoid arthritis: 500 mg to 1 g daily in 2 divided doses. Individualize dosage. Do not exceed maintenance doses higher than 1.5 g daily.

				C.I.*
Rx	**Dolobid** (MSD)	**Tablets:** 250 mg	(#MSD 675). Peach. Film coated. In unit-of-use 60s and UD 100s.	628
		500 mg	(#MSD 697). Orange. Film coated. In UD 100s and unit-of-use 60s.	393

* Cost Index based on cost per 500 mg.

\# Product identification code.

NONNARCOTIC ANALGESIC COMBINATIONS

Components of these combinations include:

NONNARCOTIC ANALGESICS: Acetaminophen, 1147 ; Salicylates, 1153 ; Salsalate, p 1161 ; Salicylamide, 1162 .

BARBITURATES (1398), *MEPROBAMATE* (1252) and *ANTIHISTAMINES* (964) are used for their sedative effects.

ANTACIDS (p 1564) are used to minimize gastric upset from salicylates.

CAFFEINE (1078), a traditional component of many analgesic formulations, may be beneficial in certain vascular headaches.

BELLADONNA ALKALOIDS (1582) are used as antispasmodics.

PAMABROM (590) is used as a diuretic.

CINNAMEDRINE, a sympathomimetic amine, claimed to have a relaxant effect on the uterus, is used in products for premenstrual syndrome. Its real value has not been established.

AMINOBENZOATE retards the conjugation of salicylic acid and prolongs the action of salicylates.

Other components listed, but not contributing to the analgesic properties of these products include: Calcium gluconate, ipecac and camphor.

Dose: The average adult dose is 1 or 2 capsules or tablets or 1 powder packet, every 2 to 6 hours as needed for pain.

Content given per capsule or tablet.

	Product and Distributor	Acetaminophen	Aspirin	Other Analgesics	Caffeine	Other Content	How Supplied	C.I.*
otc	**Saleto Tablets** (Hauck)	115 mg	210 mg	65 mg salicylamide	16 mg		Pink. In 50s, 100s, 1000s and sani-pak 1000s.	15
otc	**Salocol Tablets** (Hauck)						Mottled. In 1000s.	11
otc	**Presalin Tablets** (Hauck)	120 mg	260 mg	120 mg salicylamide		100 mg aluminum hydroxide	Mottled. In 50s.	26
otc	**Trigesic Tablets** (Squibb)	125 mg	230 mg		30 mg		In 100s.	27
otc	**Gelpirin** (Alra)	125 mg	240 mg		32 mg		Buffered. In 100s and 1000s.	NA
otc	**Salatin Capsules** (Ferndale)	129.6 mg	259.2 mg		16.2 mg		Red and blue. In 100s.	25
otc	**Valesin Tablets** (Vale)	150 mg	150 mg	150 mg salicylamide			In 1000s.	76
otc	**S-A-C Tablets** (Lannett)	150 mg		230 mg salicylamide	30 mg		Orange. In 36s, 100s and 1000s.	7
otc	**Supac Tablets** (Mission)	160 mg	230 mg		33 mg	60 mg calcium gluconate	White, scored. In 100s and 1000s.	16
otc	**Tri-Pain Tablets** (Ferndale)	162 mg	162 mg	162 mg salicylamide	16.2 mg		In 100s.	23
otc	**Buffets II Tablets** (JMI)	162 mg	226.8 mg		32.4 mg	50 mg aluminum hydroxide	In 1000s.	9
otc	**Duradyne Tablets** (Forest)	180 mg	230 mg		15 mg		In 1000s.	11

* Cost Index based on cost per capsule or tablet.

(Continued on following page)

NONNARCOTIC ANALGESIC COMBINATIONS (Cont.)

Refer to the general discussion of these products on page 250. Content given per capsule or tablet.

	Product and Distributor	Acetaminophen	Aspirin	Other Analgesics	Caffeine	Other Content	How Supplied	C.I.*
otc	**Vanquish Caplets** (Glenbrook)	194 mg	227 mg		33 mg	50 mg magnesium hydroxide, 25 mg aluminum hydroxide	White. In 15s, 30s, 60s and 100s.	22
otc	**Pain Reliever Tabs** (Rugby)	250 mg	250 mg		65 mg		In 100s and 1000s.	12
otc	**Extra Strength Excedrin Caplets and Tablets** (Bristol-Myers USP)						**Caplets:** In 24s, 50s and 80s.	41
							Tablets: (E). White. In 12s, 30s, 60s, 100s, 165s, 225s.	30
otc	**Tenol-Plus Tablets** (Vortech)						In 1000s.	9
otc	**Gemnisyn Tablets** (Kremers-U)	325 mg	325 mg				In 100s.	34
otc	**Menoplex Tablets** (Fiske)	325 mg				30 mg phenyltoloxamine citrate	In 20s.	75
otc	**Regular Strength Midol Multi-Symptom Formula Caplets** (Glenbrook)	325 mg				12.5 mg pyrilamine maleate	In 30s.	NA
otc	**Pamprin, Extra Strength Multi-Symptom Relief Formula Tablets** (Chattem)	400 mg				25 mg pamabrom, 15 mg pyrilamine maleate	In 24s and 48s.	34
otc	**Aspirin Free Excedrin Caplets** (B-M Products)	500 mg			65 mg		Saccharin. In 24s, 50s and 100s.	NA
otc	**Excedrin P.M. Caplets and Tablets** (Bristol-Myers USP)	500 mg				38 mg diphenhydramine citrate	**Caplets:** (Excedrin P.M.). Blue. In 30s and 50s.	NA
							Tablets: (PM). Blue-green. In 10s, 30s, 50s and 80s.	42
otc	**Midol PMS Caps** (Glenbrook)	500 mg				25 mg pamabrom, 15 mg pyrilamine maleate	Red/white. In 8s, 16s, 32s.	58
otc	**Pamprin Maximum Cramp Relief Capsules** (Chattem)						In 8s, 16s and 32s.	51
otc	**Prēmsyn PMS Caps** (Chattem)						In 20s and 40s.	48
otc	**Lurline PMS Tablets** (Fielding)	500 mg				25 mg pamabrom, 50 mg pyridoxine	In 24s and 50s.	NA

* Cost Index based on cost per capsule or tablet.

(Continued on following page)

NONNARCOTIC ANALGESIC COMBINATIONS (Cont.)

Refer to the general discussion of these products on page 250.

Content given per capsule, tablet or 30 ml.

	Product and Distributor	Acetaminophen	Aspirin	Other Analgesics	Caffeine	Other Content	How Supplied	C.I.*
otc	**Pamprin Maximum Cramp Relief Caplets** (Chattem)	500 mg				25 mg pamabrom, 15 mg pyrilamine maleate	In 16s and 32s.	48
otc	**Prēmsyn PMS Caplets** (Chattem)						In 20s and 40s.	58
otc	**Maximum Strength Midol Multi-Symptom Formula Caplets** (Glenbrook)	500 mg				15 mg pyrilamine maleate	In 32s.	68
otc	**Excedrin P.M. Liquid** (Bristol-Myers)	1000 mg				50 mg diphenhydramine HCl, 10% alcohol, sucrose	Wild berry flavor. In 180 ml.	NA
otc	**Dasin Capsules** (Beecham Labs)		130 mg		8 mg	0.13 mg atropine sulfate, 3 mg ipecac, 15 mg camphor	(BMP 112). Yellow. In 100s and 500s.	32
otc	**BC Tablets** (Block)		325 mg	95 mg salicylamide	16 mg		In 12s, 50s and 100s.	16
c-IV	**Meprobamate and Aspirin Tablets** (Various)		325 mg			200 mg meprobamate	In 100s and 500s.	37+
c-IV	**Epromate Tablets** (Major)						In 100s and 500s.	52
c-IV	**Equagesic Tablets** (Wyeth)						(Wyeth 91). Pink and yellow. Layered, scored. In 100s and UD 100s.	179
c-IV	**Equazine M Tablets** (Rugby)					200 mg meprobamate, tartrazine	In 100s and 500s.	41
c-IV	**Meprogesic Q Tablets** (Various)					200 mg meprobamate	In 100s and 500s.	42+
c-IV	**Micrainin Tablets** (Wallace)						In 100s.	217
otc	**Anacin Caplets and Tablets** (Whitehall)		400 mg		32 mg		**Caplets:** In 30s, 50s, 100s.	25
							Tablets: White. In 12s, 30s, 50s, 100s and 200s.	25
otc	**Gensan Tablets** (Goldline)						In 100s.	13
otc	**P-A-C Tablets** (Upjohn)					Tartrazine	In 100s and 1000s.	14

* Cost Index based on cost per capsule, tablet or 30 ml.

(Continued on following page)

NONNARCOTIC ANALGESIC COMBINATIONS (Cont.)

Refer to the general discussion of these products on page 1166

Content given per tablet or powder packet.

	Product and Distributor	Acetaminophen	Aspirin	Other Analgesics	Caffeine	Other Content	How Supplied	C.I.*
otc	**Anodynos Tablets** (Buffington)		420.6 mg	34.4 mg salicylamide	34.4 mg		In 100s, 500s and unit-of-use 200s and 500s.	18
otc	**Cope Tablets** (Mentholatum)		421 mg		32 mg	50 mg magnesium hydroxide, 25 mg aluminum hydroxide	In 36s and 60s.	22
otc	**Midol Caplets** (Glenbrook)		454 mg		32.4 mg	14.9 mg cinnamedrine HCl	White. In 12s, 30s and 60s.	33
otc	**Anacin Maximum Strength Tablets** (Whitehall)		500 mg		32 mg		(#500, A-3). White. In 12s, 20s, 24s, 40s, 72s, 75s & 150s.	33
otc	**Midol For Cramps Caplets** (Glenbrook)		500 mg		32.4 mg	14.9 mg cinnamedrine HCl	White. In 8s, 16s and 32s.	50
otc	**Momentum Caplets** (Whitehall)		500 mg			15 mg phenyltoloxamine citrate	(#M). White. In 24s and 48s.	61
otc	**BC Powder** (Block)		650 mg	195 mg salicylamide	32 mg		In 2s, 6s, 24s and 50s.	27
otc	**Arthritis Strength BC Powder** (Block)		742 mg	222 mg salicylamide	36 mg		In 6s, 24s and 50s.	28
Rx	**Pabalate-SF Enteric Coated Tablets** (Robins)			300 mg potassium salicylate		300 mg potassium amino-benzoate (3.4 mEq potassium per tablet)	(#AHR 5883). Rose. In 100s and 500s.	32
otc	**Pabalate Enteric Coated Tablets** (Robins)			300 mg sodium salicylate		300 mg sodium aminobenzoate	(#AHR 5816). Yellow. In 100s and 500s.	32
otc	**Mobigesic Tablets** (Ascher)			325 mg magnesium salicylate		30 mg phenyltoloxamine citrate	In 18s, 50s and 100s.	29
Rx	**Magsal Tablets** (U.S. Pharm.)			600 mg magnesium salicylate		25 mg phenyltoloxamine citrate	In 100s.	120

* Cost Index based on cost per tablet or powder packet.
# Product identification code.

Refer to the general discussion of these products on page 1166

Nonnarcotic Analgesics with Barbiturates

Dose: *Adults* – 1 or 2 every 4 hours, as needed.

	Product	Content	Description	C.I.*
Rx	**Butalbital, Acetaminophen and Caffeine Tablet** (Various, eg, Balan, Geneva, Goldline, Halsey, Major, Moore, Parmed, Qualitest, Schein, Texas Drug)	**Tablets:** 325 mg acetaminophen, 40 mg caffeine, 50 mg butalbital	In 100s and 500s.	24+
Rx	**Arcet** (Econo Med)		In 100s.	NA
Rx	**Esgic** (Forest)		(Forest 630). White, scored. In 100s and 500s.	118
Rx	**Fioricet** (Sandoz)		(S Fioricet). Light blue. In 100s, 500s and UD 100s.	124
Rx	**Isocet** (Rugby)		In 100s.	NA
Rx	**Repan** (Everett)		(Everett 162). White. In 100s.	83
Rx	**Amaphen** (Trimen)	**Capsules:** 325 mg acetaminophen, 40 mg caffeine, 50 mg butalbital	(Trimen/Trimen). White and pink. In 100s.	55
Rx	**Anoquan** (Hauck)		In 100s and 1000s.	28
Rx	**Butace** (American Urologicals)		(AUI). Clear. In 100s.	83
Rx	**Endolor** (Keene)		(Keene 7777). Pink and white. In 100s.	68
Rx	**Esgic** (Forest)		(Forest 631). White. In 100s.	126
Rx	**Femcet** (Russ Pharmaceuticals)		(Russ/702). Lavender. In 100s.	63
Rx	**Medigesic** (U.S. Pharm.)		(US-US). Gray and maroon. In 100s.	90
Rx	**Repan** (Everett)		Two-tone blue. In 100s.	93
Rx	**Tencet** (Hauck)		(244-03). Dark/Lt blue. In 100s and 1000s.	56
Rx	**Triad** (UAD)		In 100s.	NA
Rx	**Two-Dyne** (Hyrex)		(Hyrex/Hyrex) Red. In 100s and 1000s.	60
Rx	**Phrenilin** (Carnrick)	**Tablets:** 325 mg acetaminophen, 50 mg butalbital	(C 8650). Violet, scored. In 100s.	55
Rx	**Bancap** (Forest)	**Capsules:** 325 mg acetaminophen, 50 mg butalbital	(Forest 546) Red and white. In 100s and 500s.	63
Rx	**Triaprin** (Dunhall)		(Dunhall 2811). Orange and white. In 100s and 500s.	90
Rx	**Esgic-Plus** (Forest)	**Tablets:** 500 mg acetaminophen, 40 mg caffeine, 50 mg butalbital	(Forest 678). White, scored. Capsule shaped. In 100s and 500s.	NA
Rx	**Sedapap-10** (Mayrand)	**Tablets:** 650 mg acetaminophen, 50 mg butalbital	(M/R). White, scored. In 100s.	93
Rx	**Bucet** (UAD)	**Capsules:** 650 mg acetaminophen, 50 mg butalbital	In 100s.	NA
Rx	**Phrenilin Forte** (Carnrick)		(C 8656). Amethyst. In 100s.	66
Rx	**Tencon** (Inter. Ethical Labs)		(Tencon). Gray. In 100s.	NA

* Cost Index based on cost per capsule or tablet.

(Continued on following page)

Nonnarcotic Analgesics with Barbiturates (Cont.)

Product	Form/Strength	Description/Packaging	C.I.*
c-III **Butalbital, Aspirin and Caffeine Tablets** (Various, eg, Gen-King, Goldline, Halsey, Harber, Pharmafair, Scripts, Towne Paulsen, VHA Supply, Veratex, West-Ward)	**Tablets:** 325 mg aspirin, 40 mg caffeine, 50 mg butalbital	In 20s, 100s, 1000s and UD 100s.	14+
c-III **Butalbital Compound** (Various, eg, Dixon-Shane, General, Lemmon, Parmed, Purepac, Schein, Texas Drug, Zenith)		In 15s, 30s, 100s, 500s and 1000s.	13+
c-III **Fiorgen PF** (Goldline)		White. In 100s and 1000s.	29
c-III **Fiorinal** (Sandoz)		(#Fiorinal/Sandoz). White. In 100s, 1000s and UD 100s.	124
c-III **Isollyl Improved** (Rugby)		In 100s and 1000s.	15
c-III **Lanorinal** (Lannett)		(#0527/1043). White. In 1000s.	60
c-III **Marnal** (Vortech)		In 100s.	16
c-III **Butalbital, Aspirin and Caffeine Capsules** (Various, eg, Dixon-Shane, Harber, Regal)	**Capsules:** 325 mg aspirin, 40 mg caffeine, 50 mg butalbital	In 100s and 1000s.	27+
c-III **Butalbital Compound** (Various, eg, Parmed, Purepac, Qualitest, Redi-Med)		In 24s, 30s, 100s and 1000s.	11+
c-III **Fiorinal** (Sandoz)		(#Fiorinal 78-103). Two-tone green. In 100s, 500s & UD 25s.	124
c-III **Isollyl Improved** (Rugby)		In 100s and 1000s.	50
c-III **Lanorinal** (Lannett)		(#0527/1552). Green/Lt green. In 100s & 1000s.	25
c-III **Marnal** (Vortech)		In 100s and 1000s.	38
Rx **B-A-C** (Mayrand)	**Tablets:** 650 mg aspirin, 40 mg caffeine, 50 mg butalbital	(#M/R). Yellow, white. Scored. In 100s.	93
Rx **Axotal** (Adria)	**Tablets:** 650 mg aspirin, 50 mg butalbital	(#Adria 130). White. In 100s and 500s.	140

* Cost Index based on cost per capsule or tablet.
# Product identification code.

Actions:

Clinically, there are no clear guidelines to assist in selecting the most appropriate agent for a patient. Base selection on clinical experience, patient convenience, side effects and cost.

Pharmacology: Nonsteroidal anti-inflammatory drugs (NSAIDs) have analgesic and antipyretic activities. Although the exact mode of action is not known, the major mechanism of action is believed to be inhibition of cyclooxygenase activity and prostaglandin synthesis; however, other mechanisms may exist as well, such as inhibition of lipoxygenase, leukotriene synthesis, lysosomal enzyme release, neutrophil aggregation and various cell-membrane functions. These agents may also suppress production of rheumatoid factor.

Although most NSAIDs are primarily used for their anti-inflammatory effects, they are effective analgesics and are useful for relief of mild to moderate pain (eg, post-extraction dental pain, postsurgical episiotomy pain, soft tissue athletic injuries, primary dysmenorrhea). These agents do not alter the course of the underlying disease.

Pharmacokinetics:

Absorption/Distribution – NSAIDs are rapidly and almost completely absorbed; naproxen sodium is used as an analgesic because it is more rapidly absorbed. In general, food delays absorption but does not significantly affect the total amount absorbed. Administer these agents with meals to minimize GI effects. Some NSAIDs can be administered with an aluminum and magnesium hydroxide antacid, which does not affect absorption. All NSAIDs are highly protein bound (> 90%). Since diclofenac is an enteric coated preparation, its time to peak levels are delayed despite its relatively short half-life.

Metabolism/Elimination – Elimination of the NSAIDs depends largely on hepatic biotransformation. Excretion is via the kidney, primarily as metabolites. Sulindac and nabumetone are inactive prodrugs converted by the liver to the active metabolites.

Naproxen may exhibit an increase in unbound fraction and a reduced clearance of free drug in cirrhotic liver patients, suggesting an increased potential for toxicity in this group; the dose may need to be reduced. Also, the sulindac AUC may be increased in patients with cirrhosis due to alterations in sulfide formation/metabolism. The disposition of total and free etodolac is not altered in patients with compensated hepatic cirrhosis. The effects of hepatic disease on other NSAIDs is unknown.

Pharmacokinetic Parameters/Maximum Dosage Recommendations of NSAIDS

NSAID	Time to peak levels (hrs)[1]	Half-life (hrs)	Analgesic action		Antirheumatic action		Maximum recommended daily dose (mg)
			Onset (hrs)	Duration (hrs)	Onset (days)	Peak (weeks)	
Propionic acids							
Fenoprofen	1 to 2	2 to 3	—	—	2	2 to 3	3200
Flurbiprofen	1.5	5.7	—	—	—	—	300
Ibuprofen	1 to 2	1.8 to 2.5	0.5	4 to 6	within 7	1 to 2	3200
Ketoprofen	0.5 to 2	2 to 4	—	—	—	—	300
Naproxen	2 to 4	12 to 15	1	up to 7	within 14	2 to 4	1500
Naproxen sodium	1 to 2	12 to 13	1	up to 7	within 14	2 to 4	1375
Acetic acids							
Diclofenac sodium	2 to 3	1 to 2	—	—	—	—	200
Etodolac	1 to 2	7.3	0.5	4 to 12	—	—	1200
Indomethacin	1 to 2 SR: 2 to 4	4.5 SR: 4.5 to 6	0.5	4 to 6	within 7	1 to 2	200 SR: 150
Ketorolac	0.5 to 1	2.4 to 8.6	IM: 10 min	IM: up to 6	—	—	IM: 120[4] Oral: 40
Nabumetone	2.5 to 4	22.5 to 30[2]	—	—	—	—	2000
Sulindac	2 to 4	7.8 (16.4)[2]	—	—	within 7	2 to 3	400
Tolmetin	0.5 to 1	1 to 1.5	—	—	within 7	1 to 2	2000
Fenamates (anthranilic acids)							
Meclofenamate	0.5 to 1	2 (3.3)[3]	—	—	few days	2 to 3	400
Mefenamic acid	2 to 4	2 to 4	—	—	—	—	1000
Oxicams							
Piroxicam	3 to 5	30 to 86	1	48 to 72	7 to 12	2 to 3	20

[1] Food decreases the rate of absorption and may delay the time to peak levels.
[2] Half-life of active metabolite.
[3] Half-life with multiple doses.
[4] 150 mg on the first day.

(Actions continued on following page)

Actions (Cont.):

Clinical pharmacology: In rheumatoid arthritis and osteoarthritis, NSAIDs are comparable to aspirin in controlling signs and symptoms and some agents may be associated with a significant reduction in milder GI side effects. However, long-term use of oral ketorolac 10 mg is associated with more GI tract adverse effects than aspirin 650 mg 4 times a day. NSAIDs may be well tolerated in some who experience GI side effects with aspirin, but carefully follow such patients for signs and symptoms of ulceration and bleeding. Information is insufficient to further differentiate these agents on the basis of side effects.

Rheumatoid arthritis – Anti-inflammatory activity is shown by reduced joint swelling, pain, duration of morning stiffness and disease activity, increased mobility and by enhanced functional capacity (demonstrated by an increase in grip strength, delay in time to onset of fatigue and a decrease in time to walk 50 feet).

Osteoarthritis – Improvement is demonstrated by reduced tenderness with pressure, pain in motion and at rest, night pain, stiffness and swelling, overall disease activity, by increased range of motion, and other symptoms of allergic or anaphylactoid reactions.

Acute gouty arthritis, ankylosing spondylitis – Relief of pain, reduced fever, swelling, redness and tenderness, and increased range of motion have occurred.

Dysmenorrhea – Excess prostaglandins may produce uterine hyperactivity. These agents reduce elevated prostaglandin levels in menstrual fluid and reduce resting and active intrauterine pressure, as well as frequency of uterine contractions. Probable mechanism of action is to inhibit prostaglandin synthesis rather than provide analgesia.

Indications:

See individual product listings for specific labeled indications.

NSAIDs: Summary of Indications

Indications ✓ – Labeled × – Unlabeled	Diclofenac	Etodolac	Fenoprofen	Flurbiprofen	Ibuprofen	Indomethacin / SR	Ketoprofen	Ketorolac	Meclofenamate	Mefenamic acid	Nabumetone	Naproxen / Naproxen Sod.	Piroxicam	Sulindac	Tolmetin
Rheumatoid arthritis	✓	×	✓	✓	✓	✓	✓		✓		✓	✓	✓	✓	✓
Osteoarthritis	✓	✓	✓	✓	✓	✓	✓		✓		✓	✓	✓	✓	✓
Ankylosing spondylitis	✓	×		×		✓						✓		✓	
Mild to moderate pain	×	✓	✓	×	✓		✓	✓	✓	✓[1]		✓			
Primary dysmenorrhea				×	✓	×	✓			✓		✓	×		
Juvenile rheumatoid arthritis	×		×		×		×					✓ |	×	×	✓
Tendinitis		×		×		✓						✓		✓	
Bursitis		×		×		✓						✓		✓	
Acute painful shoulder	×	×		×		✓								✓	
Acute gout		×		×		✓ |						✓		✓	
Fever					✓							×			
Sunburn	×		×	×	×	×[2]	×		×	×		×	×	×	×
Migraine Abortive (acute attack)				×					×	×		| ×			
Prophylactic			×			× |	×					×			
Menstrual			×				×		×	×		×			
Cluster headache						× |								
Polyhydramnios						× |								
Acne vulgaris, resistant					×[3]										
Menorrhagia									×						
Premenstrual syndrome										×		| ×			
Cystoid macular edema						×[4]									
Closure of persistent patent ductus arteriosus						×[5]									

[1] If therapy will be ≤ 1 week.
[2] Topical indomethacin may prevent and treat sunburn.
[3] With tetracycline.
[4] Topical eye drops 0.5% to 1%.
[5] Indomethacin IV approved for this indication (see Agents for Patent Ductus Arteriosus).

(Indications continued on following page)

Indications (Cont.):

Rheumatoid arthritis (except etodolac, ketorolac and mefenamic acid) *and osteoarthritis* (except ketorolac and mefenamic acid): Relief of signs and symptoms; treatment of acute flares and exacerbation; long-term management.

Concomitant therapy with other second-line drugs (eg, gold salts) demonstrates additional therapeutic benefit. Whether they can be used with partially effective doses of corticosteroids for a "steroid-sparing" effect and result in greater improvement is not established.

Use with salicylates is not recommended; greater benefit is not achieved, and the potential for adverse reactions is increased. The use of aspirin with NSAIDs may cause a decrease in blood levels of the nonaspirin drug.

Juvenile rheumatoid arthritis (tolmetin, naproxen).

Mild to moderate pain (etodolac, fenoprofen, ibuprofen, ketoprofen, ketorolac, meclofenamate, mefenamic acid, naproxen, naproxen sodium, nabumetone): Post-extraction dental pain, postsurgical episiotomy pain and soft tissue athletic injuries.

Primary dysmenorrhea (ibuprofen, ketoprofen, mefenamic acid, naproxen, naproxen sodium).

Unlabeled uses: Selected NSAIDs have been used in the treatment of juvenile rheumatoid arthritis, symptomatic treatment of sunburn and for various migraine headaches. For other uses, refer to the Summary of Indications table.

Contraindications:

NSAID hypersensitivity: Because of potential cross-sensitivity to other NSAIDs, do not give these agents to patients in whom aspirin, iodides or other NSAIDs have induced symptoms of asthma, rhinitis, urticaria, nasal polyps, angioedema, bronchospasm and other symptoms of allergic or anaphylactoid reactions.

Fenoprofen or *mefenamic acid:* Preexisting renal disease.

Mefenamic acid: Active ulceration or chronic inflammation of either the upper or lower GI tract.

Indomethacin suppositories: History of proctitis or recent rectal bleeding.

Warnings:

GI effects: Serious GI toxicity such as bleeding, ulceration and perforation can occur at any time, with or without warning symptoms, in patients treated chronically with NSAID therapy. Although minor upper GI problems (eg, dyspepsia) are common, usually developing early in therapy, remain alert for ulceration and bleeding in patients treated chronically with NSAIDs even in the absence of previous GI tract symptoms. In patients observed in clinical trials of several months to 2 years duration, symptomatic upper GI ulcers, gross bleeding or perforation occurred in approximately 1% of patients treated for 3 to 6 months, and in about 2% to 4% of patients treated for 1 year; in patients receiving nabumetone, the incidence of peptic ulcers was 0.3% at 3 to 6 months, 0.5% at 1 year and 0.8% at 2 years. Inform patients about the signs or symptoms of serious GI toxicity and what steps to take if they occur.

Studies have not identified any subset of patients not at risk of developing peptic ulceration and bleeding. Except for a history of serious GI events and other risk factors associated with peptic ulcer disease (eg, alcoholism, smoking) no factors (eg, age, sex) are associated with increased risk. Elderly or debilitated patients seem to tolerate ulceration or bleeding less than other individuals and account for most spontaneous reports of fatal GI events. Studies are inconclusive concerning the relative risk of NSAIDs in causing such reactions. High dose NSAIDs probably carry a greater risk of these reactions, although controlled clinical trials generally do not show this. In considering the use of relatively large doses (within the recommended dosage range), sufficient benefit should offset the potential increased risk of GI toxicity.

In patients with active peptic ulcer and active rheumatoid arthritis, attempt to treat the arthritis with nonulcerogenic drugs.

Do not give **indomethacin** or **sulindac** to patients with active GI lesions or a history of recurrent GI lesions, unless the very high risk is warranted and patients can be monitored very closely. To reduce GI effects, give NSAIDs after meals, with food or with antacids (does not apply to enteric-coated **diclofenac**).

If diarrhea occurs with **mefenamic acid** or **meclofenamate**, reduce dosage or temporarily discontinue use. Some patients may be unable to tolerate further therapy with these agents.

CNS effects: **Indomethacin** may aggravate depression or other psychiatric disturbances, epilepsy and parkinsonism; use with considerable caution. If severe CNS adverse reactions develop, discontinue the drug. Some of these agents may also cause headaches (highest incidence with fenoprofen, indomethacin and ketorolac). If headache persists despite dosage reduction, discontinue use.

(Warnings continued on following page)

Adverse Reactions (Cont.):

CNS: Dizziness (3% to 9%; **flurbiprofen** and **diclofenac** 1% to 3%); headache (see Warnings; **ketorolac** 17%; **fenoprofen** 15%; **indomethacin** 11%; **diclofenac, flurbiprofen, meclofenamate, nabumetone, naproxen** and **tolmetin** 3% to 9%; **ketoprofen** > 3%); somnolence/drowsiness (**fenoprofen** 15%; **naproxen** 3% to 9%); lightheadedness; vertigo; nervousness; excitation; paresthesia; peripheral neuropathy; tremor; convulsions; aggravation of epilepsy and parkinsonism; myalgia; muscle weakness; asthenia; somnolence; malaise; fatigue; insomnia; confusion; inability to concentrate; depression; emotional lability; psychic disturbances, including psychotic episodes; hallucinations; depersonalization; migraine; aseptic meningitis with fever and coma; akathisia; syncope; amnesia; coma; anxiety; mental confusion; involuntary muscle movements; dyspnea; muzziness.

Cardiovascular: Congestive heart failure; exacerbation of angiitis; hypotension; hypertension; palpitations; arrhythmias; tachycardia; vasodilation; peripheral edema and fluid retention (see Precautions); chest pain; sinus bradycardia; peripheral vascular disease.

Renal: Hematuria; cystitis; urinary tract infection; azotemia; nocturia; proteinuria; elevated BUN; increased serum creatinine; decreased creatinine clearance; polyuria; dysuria; urinary frequency; pyuria; oliguria; anuria; renal insufficiency, including renal failure; acute renal failure in patients with impaired renal function; renal papillary necrosis; nephrosis; nephrotic syndrome; glomerular and interstitial nephritis; urinary casts. (See Warnings.)

Hematologic: Neutropenia; eosinophilia; leukopenia; pancytopenia; thrombocytopenia; agranulocytosis; granulocytopenia; aplastic anemia; hemolytic anemia; decreases in hemoglobin and hematocrit; anemia secondary to obvious or occult bleeding; hypocoagulability; epistaxis; menometrorrhagia; menorrhagia; hemorrhage; bruising; bone marrow depression; mild hepatic toxicity (see Precautions).

Cases of autoimmune hemolytic anemia are associated with continuous use of **mefenamic acid** for 12 months or longer. In such cases, Coombs test results are positive with evidence of both accelerated RBC production and destruction. The process is reversible upon drug discontinuation.

Special senses: Visual disturbances; blurred vision; photophobia; amblyopia; scotomata; swollen, dry or irritated eyes; corneal deposits; retinal degeneration; retinal hemorrhage and pigmentation change; conjunctivitis; iritis; reversible loss of color vision (see Precautions); hearing disturbances or loss (see Precautions); deafness; ear pain; change in taste (metallic or bitter); diplopia; optic neuritis; cataracts; tinnitus; parosmia.

Hypersensitivity: Asthma; anaphylaxis; acute respiratory distress; rapid fall in blood pressure resembling a shock-like state; angioedema; dyspnea; angiitis. (See Warnings.)

Respiratory: Dyspnea; hemoptysis; pharyngitis; bronchospasm; laryngeal edema; rhinitis; shortness of breath; eosinophilic pneumonitis; pulmonary infiltrates (**naproxen**).

Dermatologic: Rash; erythema; urticaria; desquamation; vesiculobullous eruptions; cutaneous vasculitis; toxic epidermal necrolysis; exfoliative dermatitis; erythema multiforme; Stevens-Johnson syndrome; erythema nodosum; angioneurotic edema; ecchymosis; petechiae; purpura; alopecia; pruritus; eczema; skin discoloration; hyperpigmentation; onycholysis; photosensitivity; skin irritation; peeling. Rash/dermatitis, including maculopapular type (3% to 9%; **ibuprofen, sulindac** and **meclofenamate**).

Metabolic/Endocrine: Decreased or increased appetite; weight decrease or increase (3% to 9% with **tolmetin**); glycosuria; hyperglycemia; hypoglycemia; hyperkalemia; hyponatremia; flushing or sweating; menstrual disorders; impotence; vaginal bleeding; diabetes mellitus.

Miscellaneous: Thirst; pyrexia (fever and chills); sweating; breast changes; gynecomastia; muscle cramps; facial edema; serum sickness; pain; aseptic meningitis.

Causal relationship unknown: Aphthous ulceration of buccal mucosa; fever; pseudotumor cerebri; disorientation; dysphoria; dream abnormalities; trigeminal neuralgia; libido changes; personality changes; pulmonary edema; ECG changes; atrial fibrillation; supraventricular tachycardia; myocardial infarction; burning tongue; lupus erythematosus; acute tubulopathy; Henoch-Schönlein vasculitis; acidosis; mastodynia; lymphadenopathy; septicemia; shock; leukemia; vesicular exanthema; nail disorders; aphasia; impaired consciousness; nystagmus; cerebrovascular accident; blepharitis; renal calculi; lens opacities; puffy or twitching eyelids; respiratory infections; bronchitis; sinusitis; pulmonary thromboembolism; hematuria; leukorrhea; renal calculus.

(Continued on following page)

Overdosage:

Symptoms may include: Drowsiness; dizziness; mental confusion; disorientation; lethargy; paresthesia; numbness; vomiting; gastric irritation; nausea; abdominal pain; intense headache; tinnitus; sweating; convulsions; blurred vision; elevations in serum creatinine and BUN; acute renal failure, coma, grand mal seizures and muscle twitching (**mefenamic acid**); hypotension and tachycardia (acute ingestion of **fenoprofen**); stupor, coma, diminished urine output and hypotension (**sulindac**; deaths have occurred); metabolic acidosis (acute **ibuprofen** overdosage); acute renal failure (**diclofenac** 2.5 g).

Treatment includes general supportive measures. Refer to General Management of Acute Overdosage. Because these agents are acidic and are excreted in the urine, it is theoretically beneficial to administer alkali and induce diuresis. NSAIDs are strongly bound to plasma proteins; hemodialysis and peritoneal dialysis may be of little value.

Ketoprofen is dialyzable; hemodialysis may be useful to remove circulating drug and to assist in renal failure.

Meclofenamate: Dialysis may be required to correct serious azotemia or electrolyte imbalance.

Patient Information:

Side effects of NSAIDs can cause discomfort and, rarely, more serious side effects such as GI bleeding which may result in hospitalization and even fatalities. NSAIDs are often essential in the management of arthritis and have a major role in treating pain, but they also may be commonly employed for less serious conditions. Apprise patients of potential risks.

Avoid aspirin and alcoholic beverages while taking medication.

If GI upset occurs, take with food, milk or antacids. For GI upset with **tolmetin**, use antacids other than sodium bicarbonate; bioavailability is affected by food and milk. If GI symptoms persist, notify physician.

May cause drowsiness, dizziness or blurred vision; patients should observe caution while driving or performing other tasks requiring alertness.

Notify physician if skin rash, itching, visual disturbances, weight gain, edema, black stools or persistent headache occurs.

Mefenamic acid and meclofenamate: If rash, diarrhea or other digestive problems occur, discontinue use and consult a physician.

Ibuprofen (otc use): Do not take for > 3 days for fever, or 10 days for pain. If these symptoms persist, worsen or if new symptoms develop, contact a physician.

(Products listed on following pages)

Complete prescribing information for these agents begins on page 1172

FLURBIPROFEN

Indications:

Acute or long-term treatment of the signs and symptoms of rheumatoid arthritis and osteoarthritis.

Administration and Dosage:

Rheumatoid arthritis and osteoarthritis: Initial recommended total daily dose is 200 to 300 mg; administer in divided doses 2, 3 or 4 times daily. Most experience with rheumatoid arthritis has been with dosage 3 or 4 times per day. The largest recommended single dose in a multiple-dose daily regimen is 100 mg. Tailor the dose to each patient according to the severity of the symptoms and the response to therapy.

Although a few patients have received higher doses, doses > 300 mg per day are not recommended until more clinical experience is obtained.

				C.I.*
Rx	**Ansaid** (Upjohn)	**Tablets:** 50 mg	(Ansaid 50 mg). White. In 100s, 500s and UD 100s.	23
		100 mg	(Ansaid 100 mg). Blue. In 100s, 500s and UD 100s.	21

FENOPROFEN CALCIUM

Indications:

Relief of the signs and symptoms of rheumatoid arthritis and osteoarthritis (in acute flares and exacerbations and long-term management); relief of mild to moderate pain.

Administration and Dosage:

Do not exceed 3.2 g/day. If GI upset occurs, take with meals or milk.

Rheumatoid arthritis and osteoarthritis: 300 to 600 mg 3 or 4 times daily. Individualize dosage. Improvement may occur in a few days, but 2 to 3 weeks may be required.

Mild to moderate pain: 200 mg every 4 to 6 hours, as needed.

				C.I.*
Rx	**Fenoprofen** (Various, eg, Dixon-Shane, Geneva, Halsey, Major, Par, Parmed, Qualitest, Rugby)	**Capsules:** 200 mg	In 100s.	10+
Rx	**Nalfon Pulvules** (Dista)		(H76). White/ocher. In Rx pak 100s.	21
Rx	**Fenoprofen** (Various, eg, Dixon-Shane, Major, Par, Parmed, Rugby, Warner Chilcott)	**Capsules:** 300 mg	In 100s.	8.5+
Rx	**Nalfon Pulvules** (Dista)		(H77). Yellow & ocher. In 500s, Rx pak 100s.	16
Rx	**Fenoprofen** (Various, eg, Dixon-Shane, Geneva, Major, Rugby, Schein, Warner Chilcott, Zenith)	**Tablets:** 600 mg	In 100s and 500s,	6.2+
Rx	**Nalfon** (Dista)		(Dista Nalfon). Yellow, scored. In 500s, Rx pak 100s.	11

NABUMETONE

Indications:

For acute and chronic treatment of signs and symptoms of osteoarthritis and rheumatoid arthritis.

Administration and Dosage:

Recommended starting dose is 1000 mg as a single dose with or without food. Some patients may obtain more symptomatic relief from 1500 to 2000 mg/day. Nabumetone can be given either once or twice daily. Dosages > 2000 mg/day have not been studied. Use the lowest effective dose for chronic treatment.

Rx	**Relafen** (SK-Beecham)	**Tablets:** 500 mg	(Relafen 500). White. Film coated. Oval shape. In 100s, 500s and UD 100s.
		750 mg	(Relafen 750). Beige. Film coated. Oval shape. In 100s, 500s and UD 100s.

* Cost Index based on cost per 300 mg flurbiprofen or 1200 mg fenoprofen.

Complete prescribing information for these agents begins on page 1172

IBUPROFEN

Indications:

Relief of signs and symptoms of rheumatoid arthritis and osteoarthritis; relief of mild to moderate pain; treatment of primary dysmenorrhea; reduction of fever.

Administration and Dosage:

Approved by the FDA in 1974.

Adults: Do not exceed 3.2 g/day. If GI upset occurs, take with meals or milk.

Rheumatoid arthritis and osteoarthritis – 1.2 to 3.2 g/day (300 mg 4 times daily or 400, 600 or 800 mg 3 or 4 times daily). Individualize dosage. Therapeutic response sometimes occurs in a few days to a week, but most often within 2 weeks. Rheumatoid arthritis patients seem to require higher doses than osteoarthritis patients.

Mild to moderate pain – 400 mg every 4 to 6 hours, as necessary.

Primary dysmenorrhea – 400 mg every 4 hours, as necessary.

Otc use (minor aches and pains, dysmenorrhea, fever reduction) – 200 mg every 4 to 6 hours while symptoms persist. If pain or fever do not respond to 200 mg, 400 mg may be used. Do not exceed 1.2 g in 24 hours. Do not take for pain for > 10 days or for fever for > 3 days, unless directed by physician.

Children: Juvenile arthritis: Usual dose is 30 to 40 mg/kg/day in 3 or 4 divided doses; 20 mg/kg/day may be adequate for milder disease.

Fever reduction in children 12 months to 12 years old – Adjust dosage on the basis of the initial temperature level. If the baseline temperature is ≤ 39.2°C (102.5°F), the recommended dose is 5 mg/kg; if the baseline temperature is > 39.2°C (102.5°F), the recommended dose is 10 mg/kg. The duration of fever reduction is generally 6 to 8 hours and is longer with the higher dose. The maximum daily dose is 40 mg/kg.

				C.I.*
otc	**Ibuprofen** (Various)	**Tablets:** 200 mg	In 24s, 50s, 100s, 250s and 1000s.	1.9+
otc	**Aches-N-Pain** (Lederle)		(I27). In 50s.	3.3
otc	**Advil Tablets and Caplets** (Whitehall)		**Tablets:** Lecithin, sucrose. In 8s, 24s, 50s, 100s, 165s, 250s. **Caplets:** Lecithin, sucrose. In 24s, 50s, 100s, 165s and 250s.	3.5 3.5
otc	**Excedrin IB Caplets and Tablets** (Bristol-Myers)		**Tablets:** White. In 24s. **Caplets:** White. In 24s.	NA NA
otc	**Genpril Tablets and Caplets** (Goldline)		**Tablets:** White. In 50s and 100s. **Caplets:** White. In 100s.	2.4 2.4
otc	**Haltran** (Roberts)		(Haltran). In 30s.	4.5
otc	**Ibuprin** (Thompson Medical)		In 50s and 100s.	NA
otc	**Ibuprohm Tablets and Caplets** (Ohm Labs)		**Tablets:** In 24s, 50s, 100s, 165s, 250s, 500s & 1000s. **Caplets:** In 24s, 50s, 100s and 250s.	NA NA
otc	**Ibu-Tab** (Alra)		(Alra 215). Orange. Film coated. In 30s, 60s, 100s and 250s.	NA
otc	**Medipren Tablets and Caplets** (McNeil-CPC)		**Tablets:** (Medipren). White. In 24s, 50s and 125s. **Caplets:** (Medipren). White. In 24s, 50s and 125s.	3.9 3.9
otc	**Menadol Tablets** (Rugby)		In 50s and 100s.	NA
otc	**Midol 200** (Glenbrook)		White. In 16s & 32s.	4.8
otc	**Motrin IB Tablets and Caplets** (Upjohn)		In 24s, 50s, 100s and 165s.	2.7
otc	**Nuprin Tablets and Caplets** (Bristol-Myers)		**Tablets:** (Nuprin). Yellow. In 8s, 24s, 50s, 100s, 150s and 225s. **Caplets:** (Nuprin). Yellow. In 24s, 50s and 100s.	NA NA
otc	**Pamprin-IB** (Chattem)		(IB). Coated. In 12s and 24s.	4.4
otc	**Saleto-200** (Hauck)		In 1000s and UD 500s.	1.2
otc	**Trendar** (Whitehall)		Lecithin, sucrose. In 20s & 40s.	3.8

* Cost Index based on cost per 1200 mg.

(Continued on following page)

Complete prescribing information for these agents begins on page 1172

INDOMETHACIN (Cont.)

	Product	Form	Description	C.I.*
Rx	**Indomethacin** (Various, eg, Barr, Dixon-Shane, Geneva Marsam, Lemmon, Major, Parmed, Rugby, Schein, Warner Chilcott, Zenith)	**Capsules:** 25 mg	In 60s, 100s, 500s, 1000s and UD 100s.	1.6+
Rx	**Indocin** (MSD)		Lactose, lecithin. (MSD 25). Blue and white. In 100s, 1000s, UD 100s and unit-of-use 100s.	10.7
Rx	**Indomethacin** (Various, eg, Barr, Dixon-Shane, Geneva Marsam, Lemmon, Major, Parmed, Rugby, Schein, Warner Chilcott, Zenith)	**Capsules:** 50 mg	In 90s, 100s, 250s, 500s and UD 100s.	1+
Rx	**Indocin** (MSD)		Lactose, lecithin. (MSD 50). Blue/white. In 100s and UD 100s.	8.8
Rx	**Indomethacin SR** (Various, eg, Dixon-Shane, Geneva Marsam, Inwood, Lemmon, Major, Parmed, Rugby, Schein, URL, Warner Chilcott)	**Capsules, sustained release:** 75 mg	In 60s and 100s.	4.4+
Rx	**Indocin SR** (MSD)		(MSD 693). Blue and clear. In unit-of-use 30s and 60s.	8.6
Rx	**Indomethacin** (Roxane)	**Oral Suspension:** 25 mg per 5 ml	Fruit mint flavor. In 500 ml.	10
Rx	**Indocin** (MSD)		1% alcohol, sorbitol. Pineapple coconut mint flavor. In 237 ml.	17
Rx	**Indocin** (MSD)	**Suppositories:** 50 mg	White. In 30s.	15

DICLOFENAC SODIUM

Indications:

Acute and chronic treatment of the signs and symptoms of rheumatoid arthritis, osteoarthritis and ankylosing spondylitis.

Administration and Dosage:

Osteoarthritis: 100 to 150 mg/day in divided doses.

Rheumatoid arthritis: 150 to 200 mg/day in divided doses.

Ankylosing spondylitis: 100 to 125 mg/day. Give as 25 mg 4 times/day, with an extra 25 mg dose at bedtime, if necessary.

	Product	Form	Description	C.I.*
Rx	**Voltaren** (Geigy)	**Tablets, enteric coated:** 25 mg	(Voltaren 25). Yellow. In 60s, 100s and UD 100s.	18
		50 mg	(Voltaren 50). Lt brown. In 60s, 100s, 1000s, UD 100s.	18
		75 mg	(Voltaren 75). White. In 60s, 100s, 1000s and UD 100s.	15

* Cost Index based on cost per 75 mg indomethacin or 150 mg diclofenac.

Complete prescribing information for these agents begins on page 1172

SULINDAC

Indications:

For acute or long-term use in the relief of signs and symptoms of the following: Osteoarthritis; rheumatoid arthritis; ankylosing spondylitis; acute painful shoulder (acute subacromial bursitis/supraspinatus tendinitis); acute gouty arthritis.

Administration and Dosage:

Administer twice a day with food. The usual maximum dosage is 400 mg/day. Dosages above 400 mg/day are not recommended.

Osteoarthritis, rheumatoid arthritis and ankylosing spondylitis: Initial dosage is 150 mg twice a day. Individualize dosage.

Response occurs within 1 week in about half of patients with osteoarthritis, ankylosing spondylitis and rheumatoid arthritis. Others may require longer to respond.

Acute painful shoulder (acute subacromial bursitis/supraspinatus tendinitis); acute gouty arthritis: 200 mg twice/day. After satisfactory response, reduce dosage accordingly.

In acute painful shoulder, therapy for 7 to 14 days is usually adequate. In acute gouty arthritis, therapy for 7 days is usually adequate.

Children: Safety and efficacy have not been established.

				C.I.*
Rx	**Sulindac** (Various, eg, Danbury, Dixon-Shane, Major, Parmed, Schein, UDL, Warner Chilcott)	**Tablets:** 150 mg	In 60s, 100s, 500s and UD 100s.	10.6+
Rx	**Clinoril** (MSD)		(MSD 941). Yellow. Hexagonal. In 100s, UD 100s and unit-of-use 60s and 100s.	13
Rx	**Sulindac** (Various, eg, Major, Schein, UDL, Warner Chilcott)	**Tablets:** 200 mg	In 60s, 100s and 500s.	9.8+
Rx	**Clinoril** (MSD)		(MSD 942). Yellow, scored. Hexagonal. In 100s, UD 100s & unit-of-use 60s and 100s.	10.1

TOLMETIN SODIUM

Indications:

Treatment of acute flares and long-term management of rheumatoid arthritis and osteoarthritis; treatment of juvenile rheumatoid arthritis.

Administration and Dosage:

Expect therapeutic response in a few days to a week. Anticipate progressive improvement during succeeding weeks of therapy. If GI symptoms occur, give with antacids other than sodium bicarbonate; bioavailability is affected by food or milk.

Adults: Rheumatoid arthritis and osteoarthritis – Initially, 400 mg 3 times/day; preferably include dose on arising and at bedtime. Control is usually achieved at doses of 600 to 1800 mg/day generally in 3 divided doses. Doses > 1800 mg/day have not been studied and are not recommended.

Children: (≥ 2 yrs) – Initially, 20 mg/kg/day in 3 or 4 divided doses. When control is achieved, usual dose ranges from 15 to 30 mg/kg/day. Doses > 30 mg/kg/day have not been studied and are not recommended.

				C.I.*
Rx	**Tolectin 200** (McNeil Pharm.)	**Tablets:** 200 mg tolmetin (as sodium)	18 mg sodium. (McNeil Tolectin 200). White, scored. In 100s.	2.5
Rx	**Tolmetin Sodium** (Various, eg, Mutual, URL)	**Tablets:** 200 mg **Capsules:** 400 mg	In 100s. In 100s and 500s.	NA NA
Rx	**Tolectin 600** (McNeil Pharm.)	**Tablets:** 600 mg tolmetin (as sodium)	54 mg sodium. (McNeil Tolectin 600). Orange. Film coated. In 100s and 500s.	2
Rx	**Tolectin DS** (McNeil Pharm.)	**Capsules:** 400 mg tolmetin (as sodium)	36 mg sodium. (McNeil Tolectin DS). Orange. In 100s, 500s and UD 100s.	2.1

* Cost Index based on cost per 300 mg sulindac or 200 mg tolmetin sodium.

Complete prescribing information for these agents begins on page 1172

MECLOFENAMATE SODIUM

Indications:

Relief of mild to moderate pain; treatment of primary dysmenorrhea; treatment of idiopathic heavy menstrual blood loss; acute and chronic rheumatoid arthritis and osteoarthritis: Use requires careful assessment of benefit/risk ratio.

Administration and Dosage:

Mild to moderate pain – 50 mg every 4 to 6 hours. Doses of 100 mg may be required for optimal pain relief. Do not exceed daily dosage of 400 mg.

Excessive menstrual blood loss and primary dysmenorrhea – 100 mg 3 times daily for up to 6 days, starting at the onset of menstrual flow.

Rheumatoid arthritis and osteoarthritis:

Usual dosage – 200 to 400 mg per day in 3 or 4 equal doses.

Initial dosage – Initiate at lower dosage; increase as needed to improve response. Individualize dosage. Do not exceed 400 mg/day. Improvement may occur in a few days; optimum benefit may not occur for 2 to 3 weeks.

Dosage adjustment – After satisfactory response is achieved, adjust as required. A lower dosage may suffice for long-term use. May give with meals or milk. If intolerance occurs, reduce dosage. Discontinue if severe adverse reactions occur.

Functional Class IV – Safety and efficacy are not established in this class of rheumatoid arthritis patients.

Children: Safety and efficacy in children < 14 years of age are not established.

				C.I.*
Rx	**Meclofenamate** (Various, eg, Bolar, Geneva Marsam, Goldline, Lederle, Lemmon, Major, Moore, PBI, Purepac, Rugby)	**Capsules:**[1] 50 mg	In 100s, 250s, 500s and UD 100s.	9.2+
Rx	**Meclomen** (Parke-Davis)		Lactose. In 100s & UD 100s.	13
Rx	**Meclofenamate** (Various, eg, Bolar, Geneva Marsam, Goldline, Lederle, Lemmon, Major, Moore, PBI, Purepac, Rugby)	**Capsules:**[1] 100 mg	In 100s, 250s, 500s and UD 100s.	4.8+
Rx	**Meclomen** (Parke-Davis)		Lactose. In 100s, 500s, UD 100s.	8.7

MEFENAMIC ACID

Indications:

Relief of moderate pain if therapy will be ≤ 1 week; primary dysmenorrhea.

Administration and Dosage:

Acute pain: Adults (> 14 yrs) – 500 mg, then 250 mg every 6 hours, as needed, usually not to exceed 1 week. Give with food.

Primary dysmenorrhea: 500 mg, then 250 mg every 6 hours. Start with onset of bleeding and associated symptoms. Treatment should not be necessary for more than 2 to 3 days.

Children: Safety and efficacy in children < 14 years have not been established.

				C.I.*
Rx	**Ponstel** (Parke-Davis)	**Capsules:** 250 mg	In 100s.	12

ETODOLAC

Indications:

Acute and long-term use in the management of signs and symptoms of osteoarthritis; management of pain.

Administration and Dosage:

Osteoarthritis: Initially 800 to 1200 mg/day in divided doses, followed by dosage adjustment within the range of 600 to 1200 mg/day in divided doses (400 mg 2 or 3 times daily; 300 mg 2, 3 or 4 times daily; 200 mg 3 or 4 times daily). Do not exceed 1200 mg/day.

Patients ≤ 60 kg – Do not exceed 20 mg/kg.

Analgesia: For acute pain, 200 to 400 mg every 6 to 8 hours as needed. Do not exceed 1200 mg/day.

Patients ≤ 60 kg – Do not exceed 20 mg/kg.

Rx	**Lodine** (Wyeth-Ayerst)	**Capsules:** 200 mg	Lactose. (Lodine 200). Two-tone gray w/red bands. In 100s, UD 100s.	NA
		300 mg	Lactose. (Lodine 300). Lt. gray w/red bands. In 100s and UD 100s.	NA

* Cost Index based on cost per 200 mg meclofenamate sodium or 750 mg mefenamic acid.

[1] Meclofenamic acid equivalent, as meclofenamate sodium.

KETOROLAC TROMETHAMINE

Ketorolac was approved by the FDA in November 1989.

Indications:

IM: Short-term (up to 5 days) management of pain.

Oral: Limited duration use, as needed, for management of pain.

Administration and Dosage:

IM: Ketorolac may be used on a regular schedule or as needed. For the short-term management of pain, the initial dose is 30 or 60 mg IM, as a loading dose, followed by half of the loading dose (eg, 15 or 30 mg) every 6 hours as long as needed to control pain. The rationale for the recommended loading dose and the maintenance dosages is based upon pharmacokinetic and pharmacodynamic considerations: 60 mg loading dose/30 mg maintenance dosages and 30 mg loading dose/15 mg maintenance dosages achieve average plasma levels of 1.5 and 0.8 mcg/ml, respectively, which lie within the therapeutic range of 0.3 to 5 mcg/ml. The recommended maximum total daily dose is 150 mg for the first day and 120 mg/day thereafter; limit to short-term therapy (not > 5 days).

If as needed management is elected, and since the half-life is ≈ 6 hours, base an assessment of the size of a repeat dose on the duration of pain relief from the previous dose. For example, if pain returns within 3 to 5 hours, the next dose could be increased by up to 50%. [Note: The recommended maximum total daily dose is 120 mg (150 mg on the first day)]. An alternative would be to use morphine or meperidine concomitantly. Alternatively, if pain does not return for 8 to 12 hours, the next dose could be decreased by as much as 50%, or the previous dose could be given every 8 to 12 hours.

The lower end of the recommended dosage range is recommended for patients under 50 kg (110 pounds), for patients > 65 years of age and for patients with reduced renal function.

Oral: Recommended dose – 10 mg as needed every 4 to 6 hours for limited duration. Do not use chronic doses of 10 mg 4 times daily.

Maximum dose – 40 mg daily.

Transition from IM to oral ketorolac: Do not exceed total combined dose of 120 mg on day of transition, including a maximum of 40 mg orally. Subsequent oral dosing should not exceed 40 mg daily.

Storage: Injection – Protect from light.

Rx	**Toradol** (Syntex)	**Tablets:** 10 mg	Lactose. (Toradol Syntex). White. Film coated. In 100s and UD 100s.
Rx	**Toradol** (Syntex)	**Injection:** 15 mg/ml	In 1 ml Cartrix or Tubex syringes.[1]
		30 mg/ml	In 1 and 2 ml Cartrix or Tubex syringes.[2]

[1] With 10% alcohol and 6.68 mg sodium chloride in sterile water.

[2] With 10% alcohol and 4.35 mg sodium chloride in sterile water.

Therapeutic alternatives in the treatment of rheumatoid arthritis and related conditions include a diverse array of agents ranging from aspirin and similarly acting nonsteroidal anti-inflammatory agents (NSAIDs), to the slow-acting and possibly disease modifying agents such as gold compounds and penicillamine. Because of their toxicity, the slow-acting agents are generally reserved for progressive disease unresponsive to more conservative therapy. Drugs and groups of drugs useful in the treatment of rheumatoid arthritis are listed below.

Anti-inflammatory Agents

GLUCOCORTICOIDS (page 465) provide dramatic anti-inflammatory effects by inhibiting the initiation of inflammatory reactions. However, because of the consequences of prolonged therapy, use chronically only in patients with uncontrollable rheumatoid arthritis who fail to respond to other measures. Short-term therapy can be used in acute flares until other agents have a chance to act.

SALICYLATES (page 1153 Aspirin, the most widely used NSAID, is generally considered the drug of first choice for rheumatoid arthritis. Adequate analgesia is usually achieved with 3 g/day of aspirin; 3 to 6 g/day are usually required for significant anti-inflammatory effects. At maximum doses, aspirin is as effective as any of the other NSAIDs. Gastro-intestinal intolerance is the most common side effect. Other salicylate derivatives may offer the advantage of fewer GI complaints without interfering with platelet aggregation at recommended doses; however, when comparing anti-inflammatory agents, nonaspirin salicylates have not been proven as effective as aspirin.

NONSTEROIDAL ANTI-INFLAMMATORY ANALGESICS (page 1172 have essentially the same therapeutic benefits as aspirin. With the exception of indomethacin, the newer non-steroidal agents may offer the advantage of a lower incidence of GI side effects.

PYRAZOLINE DERIVATIVES (page 1192) include phenylbutazone and its metabolite, oxy-phenbutazone. These agents have effective analgesic and anti-inflammatory effects. Because of the incidence of severe adverse reactions, these agents are generally reserved for short-term therapy of acute symptoms unresponsive to more conservative therapy.

Slow-Acting Antirheumatic Agents

HYDROXYCHLOROQUINE SULFATE (page 1196), an antimalarial agent, may be effective in moderate to severe rheumatoid arthritis unresponsive to conventional treatment. Up to 6 months may be required for a clinical response to this agent. Side effects are frequent.

GOLD COMPOUNDS (page 1200 are quite effective in the treatment of actively progressing rheumatoid arthritis. Prolonged therapy is required. Serious side effects may require dis-continuation of therapy.

PENICILLAMINE (page 2705 is used in severe rheumatoid arthritis unresponsive to conven-tional therapy. Response to therapy is slow (2 to 3 months); adverse effects may be severe.

AZATHIOPRINE (page 2767 is an immunosuppressive agent used in the treatment of severe, active and erosive disease not responsive to conventional therapy.

METHOTREXATE (page 2511 and *CAPTOPRIL* (page 822) have been used investigationally in the treatment of severe rheumatoid arthritis.

(Products listed on following pages)

PHENYLBUTAZONE AND OXYPHENBUTAZONE

The information that follows applies to both phenylbutazone and oxyphenbutazone.

Important Note:

Because of the increased risk of agranulocytosis and aplastic anemia, these drugs are not recommended as initial therapy. Use only after other nonsteroidal anti-inflammatory drugs (NSAIDs) have proven unsatisfactory. These drugs are not simple analgesics; never administer casually. Carefully evaluate patients before initiating treatment and keep under close supervision. Observe the following precautions:

Do not initiate therapy until a careful detailed history and complete physical and laboratory examination, including a complete hemogram and urinalysis, etc, have been made. Perform these examinations at regular, frequent intervals throughout the duration of therapy or if any signs of blood dyscrasia occur.

Carefully select patients, avoiding those in whom the drugs are contraindicated as well as those who will respond to ordinary therapeutic measures, or those who cannot be observed at frequent intervals.

Warn patients not to exceed the recommended dosage, since this may lead to toxic effects, and to discontinue therapy and immediately report any sign of: Fever, sore throat, mouth lesions, symptoms of anemia, unusual bleeding or bruising, dyspepsia, epigastric pain, black or tarry stools or other evidence of intestinal ulceration; skin rashes, significant weight gain or edema.

The risk of aplastic anemia is greater in women, in the elderly of both sexes and with chronic therapy, but even short-term exposure of healthy young persons can result in fatal aplastic anemia.

A trial period of 1 week of therapy is adequate to determine therapeutic effect. In the absence of a favorable response, discontinue use. In elderly patients (60 years and over), restrict use to short-term treatment: 1 week maximum if possible.

If long-term treatment is necessary, use the lowest possible effective dose; warn patients and monitor them closely.

Actions:

Phenylbutazone and its analog, oxyphenbutazone, are closely related chemically and pharmacologically to the pyrazolines, aminopyrine and antipyrine. These drugs have anti-inflammatory, antipyretic, analgesic and mild uricosuric actions resulting in symptomatic relief only; the disease process is unaltered.

The exact mechanism of the anti-inflammatory effect is unknown, but these agents inhibit factors believed to be involved in the inflammatory process, including prostaglandin synthesis, leukocyte migration and release and activity of lysosomal enzymes.

Pharmacokinetics: Absorption/Distribution - Both drugs are rapidly and completely absorbed after oral administration. About 98% is bound to serum albumin. After administration of 300 mg phenylbutazone, a peak plasma concentration of 43 mg/L is attained within 2.5 $\pm$ 1.4 hours. Steady-state plasma concentrations are about 4 times higher than the peak concentration after the first single dose.

Metabolism/Excretion - Elimination of oxyphenbutazone is mainly by biotransformation in the liver. The plasma elimination half-life is approximately 77 hours for phenylbutazone and approximately 72 hours for oxyphenbutazone. At steady-state, 61% of phenylbutazone is excreted in the urine and 27% in the feces.

The major metabolite of phenylbutazone is oxyphenbutazone; steady-state plasma levels are about 50% those of phenylbutazone. Less than 2% of the phenylbutazone dose appears in the urine as oxyphenbutazone.

Indications:

Phenylbutazone is for use only after other therapeutic measures, including other NSAIDs, have proven unsatisfactory.

Relief of symptoms of acute gouty arthritis, active rheumatoid arthritis and active ankylosing spondylitis; acute attacks of degenerative joint disease of the hips and knees; painful shoulder (peritendinitis, capsulitis, bursitis and acute arthritis of that joint).

Contraindications:

Children 14 years of age or under; senile patients; patients with a history or suggestion of prior toxicity, hypersensitivity or idiosyncrasy to phenylbutazone or oxyphenbutazone; patients who have a bronchospastic reaction to aspirin or other NSAIDs.

(Continued on following page)

PHENYLBUTAZONE AND OXYPHENBUTAZONE (Cont.)

Warnings:

Gastrointestinal effects: Perform upper GI diagnostic tests in patients with persistent or severe dyspepsia. Peptic ulceration, reactivation of latent peptic ulcer, perforation and GI bleeding, sometimes severe, have been reported.

Hematologic effects: Phenylbutazone can cause aplastic anemia and agranulocytosis. The reported incidence of deaths from these disorders was 2.2 per 100,000 exposures. There is increased risk with long-term use and use in elderly patients, especially women, with a rate of 6.5 deaths per 100,000 women over age 65. Perform frequent and regular hematologic evaluations on patients receiving the drug for over 1 week. If any signs or symptoms suggesting a blood cell dyscrasia develop, examine red cells, white cells and platelets. Significant change in the total white cell count, relative decrease in granulocytes, appearance of immature forms or fall in hematocrit or platelet count require immediate cessation of therapy and a complete hematologic investigation. Hematologic toxicity may occur suddenly or many days or weeks after cessation of treatment as manifested by anemia, leukopenia, thrombocytopenia or hemorrhagic diathesis.

Leukemia – There have been reports associating phenylbutazone with leukemia. However, a causal relationship to the drug has not been clearly established.

Renal Effects: Long-term administration of phenylbutazone to animals results in renal papillary necrosis and other abnormal renal pathology. In humans, acute interstitial nephritis with hematuria, proteinuria and occasionally nephrotic syndrome may occur.

A second form of renal toxicity may occur in patients with prerenal conditions leading to reduction in renal blood flow or blood volume, where the renal prostaglandins have a supportive role in maintenance of renal perfusion. In these patients, phenylbutazone may cause a dose-dependent reduction in prostaglandin formation and precipitate overt renal decompensation. Patients at greatest risk are those with impaired renal function, heart failure, liver dysfunction, those taking diuretics and the elderly. Discontinuation of phenylbutazone is typically followed by recovery to the pretreatment state.

Closely monitor a patient with significantly impaired renal function. Consider a lower daily dose to avoid excessive drug accumulation.

Hepatic: Borderline elevations of one or more liver test values may occur in up to 15% of patients. These abnormalities may progress, may remain unchanged or may be transient with continued therapy. Meaningful elevations (3 times the upper limit of normal) of SGPT (ALT) or SGOT (AST) have occurred in controlled clinical trials in less than 1% of patients. Evaluate any patient with symptoms or signs suggesting liver dysfunction, or in whom abnormal liver test results have occurred, for development of more severe hepatic reactions. Jaundice and fatal hepatitis have been reported. Although such reactions are rare, if abnormal liver tests persist or worsen, if clinical signs and symptoms consistent with liver disease develop or if systemic manifestations (eosinophilia, rash, etc) occur, discontinue therapy.

Blurred vision: Patients reporting visual disturbances during therapy should discontinue treatment and have an ophthalmologic examination (see Adverse Reactions).

Elderly: In patients 40 years and over, the possibility of adverse reactions appears to increase. In elderly patients (60 years and older), restrict treatment to 1 week. Use with greater care in the elderly and avoid use in the senile patient.

Respiratory: Like other drugs with prostaglandin synthetase inhibition activity, these drugs may precipitate acute episodes of asthmatic attacks.

Edema: These agents increase sodium retention. Use with caution when fluid retention would aggravate a condition such as severe cardiac or renal disease. Fluid retention in patients with a danger of cardiac decompensation is an indication to discontinue use.

Usage in Pregnancy: Category C. Animal reproduction studies with doses up to 16 times the maximum daily human dose have revealed no evidence of teratogenicity. However, slightly reduced litter sizes, an increase in stillbirths and a reduced offspring survival rate were observed in some rodent studies.

These and similar agents could cause constriction of the ductus arteriosus in utero, inhibit labor and prolong pregnancy.

There are no adequate and well controlled studies in pregnant women. Phenylbutazone may appear in cord blood. Use during pregnancy only if the potential benefits outweigh the potential hazards to the fetus.

Usage in Lactation: Phenylbutazone is excreted in breast milk in small quantities. Because of the potential for serious adverse reactions in nursing infants, decide whether to discontinue nursing or to discontinue the drug taking into account the importance of the drug to the mother.

Usage in Children: Safety and efficacy in children ≤ 14 years have not been established.

(Continued on following page)

PHENYLBUTAZONE AND OXYPHENBUTAZONE (Cont.)

Precautions:

Other medical conditions: Use with caution in patients with incipient cardiac failure, blood dyscrasias, pancreatitis, parotitis, stomatitis, polymyalgia rheumatica, temporal arteritis, senility or drug allergy. Also observe caution in the presence of severe renal, cardiac and hepatic disease, and in patients with a history of peptic ulcer disease or symptoms of GI inflammation or active ulceration. Serious adverse reactions or aggravation of existing medical problems can occur.

Concomitant medications: Do not use in patients receiving other drugs which accentuate or share similar toxicity. Do not administer with other potent drugs because of the increased possibility of toxic reactions (see Drug Interactions).

Potentially Hazardous Tasks: May cause drowsiness; patients should observe caution while driving or performing other tasks requiring alertness.

Sulfite Sensitivity: Sulfites may cause allergic-type reactions (eg, hives, itching, wheezing, anaphylaxis) in certain susceptible persons. Although the overall prevalence of sulfite sensitivity in the general population is probably low, it is seen more frequently in asthmatics or in atopic nonasthmatic persons. Specific products containing sulfites are identified in the product listings.

Mutagenesis: An increased incidence of chromosome anomalies has been reported in cultured leukocyte cells from patients receiving therapeutic doses of phenylbutazone.

Drug Interactions:

Alcohol coadministered with phenylbutazone and oxyphenbutazone may impair psychomotor skills.

Anti-inflammatory agents, oral anticoagulants, oral antidiabetics, sulfonamides, sodium valproate and **phenytoin** are competitively displaced by phenylbutazone from serum-binding sites. The activity, duration of effect and toxicity of the displaced drugs may be increased.

Barbiturates, promethazine, chlorpheniramine, rifampin and **corticosteroids,** inducers of hepatic microsomal enzymes, may decrease the half-life of phenylbutazone.

Cholestyramine reduces the enteral absorption of phenylbutazone.

Coumarin-type anticoagulants: Hypoprothrombinemic effects are accentuated by phenylbutazone and oxyphenbutazone; administered alone, prothrombin activity is not affected.

Dicumarol, digitoxin and **cortisone** may induce the hepatic microsomal metabolism of phenylbutazone. Conversely, phenylbutazone may inhibit the metabolism of **phenytoin.** Concomitant administration of phenylbutazone or oxyphenbutazone and phenytoin may increase serum levels and toxicity of phenytoin.

Methotrexate, insulin, sulfonylureas and **sulfonamide drugs:** Effects may be potentiated by phenylbutazone. Phenylbutazone increases the serum concentration of **lithium** by increasing tubular reabsorption, and it reduces the renal clearance of **sulfonylureas**.

Methylphenidate is reported to prolong the half-life of phenylbutazone and to increase the serum level of oxyphenbutazone.

Drug/Laboratory tests: These agents may reduce iodine uptake by the thyroid and may interfere with laboratory tests of thyroid function.

Adverse Reactions:

Aplastic anemia and agranulocytosis are the most serious adverse reactions that occur with phenylbutazone (see Warnings).

Most frequent: Abdominal discomfort and distress, edema and water retention (3% to 9%); nausea, dyspepsia (including indigestion and heartburn) and rash (> 1%).

The following have occurred in < 1% of patients:

GI: Vomiting; abdominal distention with flatulence; constipation; diarrhea; esophagitis; epigastric distress; gastritis; salivary gland enlargement; stomatitis, sometimes with ulceration; ulceration and perforation of the intestinal tract including acute and reactivated peptic ulcer with perforation, hemorrhage and hematemesis; anemia due to occult GI bleeding; hepatitis, both fatal and nonfatal, sometimes associated with evidence of cholestasis.

Hematologic: Anemia; leukopenia; thrombocytopenia with associated purpura, petechiae and hemorrhage; pancytopenia; aplastic anemia; bone marrow depression; agranulocytosis and agranulocytic anginal syndrome; hemolytic anemia.

Hypersensitivity: Urticaria; anaphylactic shock; arthralgia, drug fever or fever; hypersensitivity angiitis (polyarteritis) and vasculitis; Lyell's syndrome; serum sickness; Stevens-Johnson syndrome; activation of systemic lupus erythematosus; aggravation of temporal arteritis in patients with polymyalgia rheumatica.

Dermatologic: Pruritus; erythema nodosum and multiforme; nonthrombocytopenic purpura.

(Adverse Reactions continued on following page)

HYDROXYCHLOROQUINE SULFATE (Cont.)

Overdosage:

Symptoms: Toxic symptoms may occur within 30 minutes and consist of headache, drowsiness, visual disturbances, cardiovascular collapse and convulsions, followed by sudden and early respiratory and cardiac arrest. ECG may reveal atrial standstill, nodal rhythm, prolonged intraventricular conduction time and progressive bradycardia leading to ventricular fibrillation or arrest. Rarely, these symptoms occur with lower doses in hypersensitive patients.

Treatment is symptomatic and must be prompt, with immediate evacuation of the stomach. Treatment includes usual supportive measures. Refer to General Management of Acute Overdosage on p. vi. Activated charcoal, in a dose not less than 5 times the estimated dose ingested, may inhibit further intestinal absorption if introduced by stomach tube after lavage within 30 minutes after ingestion. Control convulsions before attempting gastric lavage. If due to cerebral stimulation, attempt cautious administration of an ultrashort-acting barbiturate; if due to anoxia, correct with oxygen, artificial respiration or, in shock with hypotension, use vasopressor therapy. Perform tracheal intubation or tracheostomy followed by gastric lavage if necessary. Exchange transfusions have been used to reduce the level of drug in the blood. Closely observe, for at least 6 hours, patients surviving the acute phase who are asymptomatic. Fluids may be forced. Sufficient ammonium chloride (8 g daily in divided doses for adults) administered for a few days will acidify the urine and help promote urinary excretion.

Patient Information:

May cause GI upset; take with food or milk.

Notify physician if any of the following occur: Blurring or other vision changes; ringing in the ears or hearing loss; fever, sore throat or unusual bleeding or bruising; unusual pigmentation (blue-black) of the skin or inside of mouth; skin rash or itching; unusual muscle weakness; bleaching or loss of hair; mood or mental changes.

Administration and Dosage:

Rheumatoid arthritis: Initial dosage - 400 to 600 mg daily, taken with a meal or a glass of milk. Side effects rarely require temporary reduction. Later (usually from 5 to 10 days), dose may gradually be increased to optimum response level, often without return of side effects.

Maintenance dosage - When a good response is obtained (usually in 4 to 12 weeks), reduce dosage by 50% and continue at a level of 200 to 400 mg daily. Incidence of retinopathy is higher when this dose is exceeded.

The compound is cumulative and requires several weeks to exert therapeutic effects; minor side effects may occur early. Maximum effects may not be obtained for several months. If objective improvement (reduced joint swelling, increased mobility) does not occur within 6 months, discontinue the drug. Safe use of hydroxychloroquine in the treatment of juvenile rheumatoid arthritis has not been established.

Should relapse occur after medication is withdrawn, resume therapy or continue on an intermittent schedule if there are no ocular contraindications.

Corticosteroids and salicylates may be used in conjunction with this compound; generally they can be gradually decreased or eliminated after hydroxychloroquine has been used for several weeks. When gradual reduction of steroid dosage is indicated, reduce (every 4 to 5 days) dose of cortisone by no more than 5 to 15 mg; hydrocortisone from 5 to 10 mg; prednisolone and prednisone from 1 to 2.5 mg; methylprednisolone and triamcinolone from 1 to 2 mg; or dexamethasone from 0.25 to 0.5 mg.

Lupus erythematosus: Initially, 400 mg once or twice daily, continued for several weeks or months, depending on response. For prolonged maintenance therapy, a smaller dose (200 to 400 mg daily) will frequently suffice. The incidence of retinopathy has reportedly been higher when maintenance dose is exceeded.

			C.I.*
Rx	**Plaquenil Sulfate** (Winthrop Pharm.)	**Tablets:** 200 mg (equivalent to 155 mg base). (# P61). Scored. In 100s.	606

* Cost Index based on cost per 400 mg.

Product identification code.

Gold Compounds

Warning:

Signs of gold toxicity include: Fall in hemoglobin, leukopenia $<$ 4000 WBC/cu mm, granulocytes $<$ 1500/cu mm, platelets $<$ 100,000 to 150,000/cu mm, proteinuria, hematuria, pruritus, rash, stomatitis or persistent diarrhea. Review recommended laboratory work results before instituting therapy and before each injection or written prescription for oral gold. See patient before each injection to determine presence or absence of adverse reactions; some of these can be severe or even fatal. Physicians planning to use gold compounds should be experienced with chrysotherapy and thoroughly familiar with both toxicity and benefits of gold.

Routinely explain the possibility of adverse reactions to patients before starting therapy. Advise patients to report promptly any symptoms of toxicity (see Patient Information).

Actions:

Pharmacology: Gold suppresses or prevents, but does not cure, arthritis and synovitis. Gold is taken up by macrophages; inhibition of phagocytosis and possible inhibition of lysosomal enzyme activity results. Gold also decreases concentrations of rheumatoid factor and immunoglobulins. The exact mode of action in rheumatoid arthritis is unknown. No substantial evidence exists that gold induces remission of rheumatoid arthritis.

Therapeutic effects from gold compounds occur slowly. Early improvement, often limited to reduction in morning stiffness, may begin after 6 to 8 weeks of treatment with gold sodium thiomalate, but beneficial effects may not be observed until after months of therapy. Therapeutic effects from auranofin may be seen after 3 to 4 months of treatment, but in some patients, not before 6 months.

Pharmacokinetics: Due to differences in administration routes (IM vs oral), dosage regimens (weekly vs daily) and actual quantity of gold administered to the patient, expect differences in the pharmacokinetic parameters of injectable gold and oral gold.

Parenteral gold compounds are water soluble but aurothioglucose is an oily suspension because the aqueous solution is unstable on long standing; suspension results in delayed IM absorption. Both compounds are similar in biologic and pharmacokinetic behavior.

Although parenteral gold is widely distributed in body tissues, highest concentrations occur in the reticuloendothelial system and in adrenal and renal cortices. Binding of gold to red blood cells from injectable gold compounds is lower compared to auranofin-derived gold. Blood to synovial fluid ratios are similar, ≈ 1.7:1, and synovial fluid levels are ≈ 50% of the blood concentrations. No correlation between blood-gold concentrations and safety or efficacy has been established.

Major differences of auranofin and injectable gold compounds are summarized below:

<table>
<tr><th>Drug</th><th>Gold content (%)</th><th>% Absorbed</th><th>Time to peak (hrs)</th><th>Mean steady-state plasma levels (mcg/ml)</th><th>Protein binding (%)</th><th>Plasma half-life (days)</th><th>% Excreted in urine</th><th>% Excreted in feces</th></tr>
<tr><td>Auranofin</td><td>29</td><td>25 (15-33)</td><td>1-2</td><td>0.3-1</td><td>60</td><td>26 (21-31)</td><td>60[1]</td><td>85-95</td></tr>
<tr><td>Aurothioglucose</td><td>50</td><td>nd</td><td>4-6</td><td rowspan="2">1-5</td><td rowspan="2">95-99</td><td>3-27 (single dose)</td><td rowspan="2">70</td><td rowspan="2">30</td></tr>
<tr><td>Gold Sodium Thiomalate</td><td>50</td><td>nd</td><td>2-6</td><td>14-40 (3rd dose)
up to 168 (11th dose)</td></tr>
</table>

[1] 60% of the absorbed gold (15% of administered dose). nd – No data.

Indications:

Parenteral: Active rheumatoid arthritis, both adult and juvenile types (cases not adequately controlled by other anti-inflammatory agents or conservative measures). Greatest benefit occurs in the early active stage. In late-stage illness, when cartilage and bone are damaged, gold only checks progression and prevents further joint damage. It cannot repair damage caused by previously active disease. Use only as one part of therapy program; alone, it is not a complete treatment.

Oral: Adult management of active classical or definite rheumatoid arthritis (ARA criteria) who show insufficient therapeutic response or intolerance to an adequate trial of one or more NSAIDs. Add auranofin to baseline program; include non-drug therapies.

Unlabeled Uses: Alternative or adjuvant to corticosteroids in treatment of pemphigus. For psoriatic arthritis in patients who do not tolerate or respond to NSAIDs.

(Continued on following page)

Contraindications:

Parenteral: Known hypersensitivity to any component; in uncontrolled diabetes mellitus; severe debilitation; renal disease; hepatic dysfunction or history of infectious hepatitis; marked hypertension; uncontrolled congestive heart failure; systemic lupus erythematosus; agranulocytosis or hemorrhagic diathesis; blood dyscrasias; patients recently radiated; those with severe toxicity from previous exposure to gold or other heavy metals; urticaria; eczema; colitis.

Gold therapy is usually contraindicated in pregnancy (see Warnings).

Oral: In patients with a history of any of the following gold-induced disorders: Anaphylactic reactions, necrotizing enterocolitis, pulmonary fibrosis, exfoliative dermatitis, bone marrow aplasia or other severe hematologic disorders.

Warnings:

Thrombocytopenia has occurred in 1% to 3% of patients treated with auranofin. It appears peripheral in origin and is usually reversible upon withdrawal. Onset is not related to duration of therapy; its course may be rapid. If signs and symptoms of thrombocytopenia (eg, purpura, ecchymoses or petechiae) occur, immediately withdraw auranofin and other therapies; obtain additional platelet counts. Do not reinstate auranofin unless thrombocytopenia resolves and studies show that it was not due to gold therapy.

Diabetes mellitus or CHF should be under control before gold therapy is instituted.

Extreme caution is indicated in patients with any of the following: History of blood dyscrasias such as granulocytopenia or anemia caused by drug sensitivity; allergy or hypersensitivity to medications; skin rash; previous kidney or liver disease; marked hypertension; compromised cerebral or cardiovascular circulation.

Weigh the potential benefits of using auranofin in patients with progressive renal disease, significant hepatocellular disease, inflammatory bowel disease, skin rash or history of bone marrow depression, against potential risks of gold toxicity on compromised organ systems and the difficulty in quickly detecting and correctly attributing the toxic effect.

Immediate effects following injection, or at any time during therapy, include: Anaphylactic shock, syncope, bradycardia, thickening of the tongue, dysphagia, dyspnea and angioneurotic edema. These effects may occur immediately after injection or as late as 10 minutes after injection. If such effects occur, discontinue treatment.

Carcinogenesis, mutagenesis and impairment of fertility: Renal adenomas developed in rats receiving injectable gold at doses higher and more frequent than recommended human doses. Sarcomas at the injection site occurred in some rats. Neither renal adenoma or sarcoma at the injection site in humans has been reported.

Studies demonstrated an increase in the frequency of renal tubular cell karyomegaly and cytomegaly, renal adenoma and malignant renal epithelial tumors in animals treated with auranofin and gold sodium thiomalate.

Usage in the Elderly: Tolerance to gold usually decreases with advancing age.

Usage in Pregnancy: Category C. Gold crosses the human placenta. The placenta showed numerous gold deposits and smaller amounts were detected in the fetal liver and kidneys.

Gold therapy is usually contraindicated in pregnant patients. Warn the patient about the hazards of becoming pregnant while on gold therapy. Rheumatoid arthritis frequently improves when the patient becomes pregnant. Do not superimpose the potential nephrotoxicity of gold on the increased renal burden which normally occurs in pregnancy. Discontinue gold therapy upon recognition of pregnancy, if possible. Consider the slow excretion of gold and its persistence in body tissues after discontinuing treatment when a woman being treated with gold plans to become pregnant.

Animals – Gold sodium thiomalate was teratogenic during the organogenic period in small animals when given in doses 140 to 175 times the usual human dose. Auranofin showed impaired food intake, decreased maternal and fetal weights, and increased resorptions, abortions and congenital abnormalities.

There are no adequate, well controlled studies in pregnant women. Use only when clearly needed and when potential benefits outweigh potential hazards to the fetus.

Usage in Lactation: Gold is excreted in breast milk. Trace amounts appear in the serum and red blood cells of nursing offspring. This may cause rashes, nephritis, hepatitis and hematologic aberrations in nursing infants. Decide whether to discontinue nursing or to discontinue parenteral gold, taking into account the importance of the drug to the mother. Nursing during auranofin therapy is not recommended.

Usage in Children: Safety and efficacy for use of aurothioglucose in children under 6 years of age have not been established. Auranofin is not recommended for use in children; safety and efficacy have not been established.

(Continued on following page)

Precautions:

Concomitant therapy: Use of salicylates, NSAIDs and systemic corticosteroids may be continued when parenteral gold therapy is instituted. After improvement begins, slowly discontinue analgesics and NSAIDs as symptoms permit.

Do not use **penicillamine** or **antimalarials** with gold salts. Safety of coadministration with **hydroxychloroquine, cytotoxic drugs** or **immunosuppressive agents** (eg, cyclophosphamide, azathioprine or methotrexate) other than corticosteroids is not established. Safety of auranofin with injectable gold or high doses of corticosteroids is not established.

Monitoring: Before instituting treatment, rule out pregnancy; perform CBC with differential, platelet count, urinalysis and renal and liver function tests. Perform urinalysis for protein and sediment changes prior to each injection. Perform complete blood counts (CBC) including platelet estimation before every second injection throughout treatment. Purpura or ecchymoses always require a platelet count. Inquire regarding pruritus, rash, sore mouth, metallic taste and indigestion before each injection. Monitor CBC, platelet count and urinalysis at least monthly. Observe patient at least 15 minutes after each injection.

Rapid reduction of hemoglobin, granulocytes < 1500/cu mm, leukopenia < 4000 WBC/cu mm, eosinophilia $> 5\%$, platelet $< 100{,}000$ to 150,000/cu mm, albuminuria, hematuria, dermatitis, pruritus, skin eruption, stomatitis, persistent diarrhea, jaundice or petechiae are signs of possible gold toxicity. Do not give additional therapy unless further studies show these abnormalities to be caused by conditions other than gold toxicity. Monitor patients with GI symptoms for GI bleeding.

Aurothioglucose – Patients with HLA-D locus histocompatibility antigens DRw2 and DRw3 may have a genetic predisposition to develop certain toxic reactions, such as proteinuria, during treatment with gold or D-penicillamine. Use aurothioglucose with caution in patients with compromised cardiovascular or cerebral circulation.

Nonvasomotor postinjection reaction: Arthralgia may occur for a day or two after injection; it usually subsides after the first few injections. The mechanism of the transient increase in rheumatic symptoms after gold injection is unknown. These reactions are usually mild, but occasionally may be so severe that treatment is stopped prematurely.

Drug Interactions:

One report suggests coadministration of auranofin and **phenytoin** may increase phenytoin blood levels.

Adverse Reactions:

Adverse reactions to gold therapy may occur during treatment or many months after discontinuation. Incidence of toxic reactions is apparently unrelated to gold plasma levels, but may relate to cumulative body content of gold. Higher than conventional dosages may increase occurrence and severity of toxicity. Adverse reactions are most frequent when cumulative dose is 400 to 800 mg (gold sodium thiomalate) or 300 to 500 mg (aurothioglucose). Auranofin use appears to result in fewer adverse reactions than injectable gold use; however, therapeutic efficacy may also be less.

Cutaneous: Dermatitis is the most common reaction to injectable gold and second most common to auranofin. Any eruption, especially pruritic, is a reaction to gold until proven otherwise. Rash, urticaria and angioedema may occur. Pruritus often exists before dermatitis appears, and is a warning of cutaneous reaction. Erythema, and occasionally more severe reactions, such as papular, vesicular and exfoliative dermatitis leading to alopecia and shedding of nails, may occur. Chrysiasis (gray-to-blue pigmentation caused by deposition of gold in the tissues) has been reported, especially on photoexposed areas. Gold dermatitis may be aggravated by exposure to sunlight or an actinic rash may develop.

Mucous membranes: Stomatitis, the second most common adverse reaction to injectable gold, is also seen with auranofin, and may be manifested by shallow ulcers on the buccal membranes, on the borders of the tongue and on the palate or in the pharynx. Diffuse glossitis or gingivitis may develop. A metallic taste may precede these reactions. Careful oral hygiene is important. Inflammation of the upper respiratory tract, pharyngitis, gastritis, colitis, tracheitis, vaginitis and rarely, conjunctivitis have been reported.

Pulmonary injury may be shown by gold bronchitis, interstitial pneumonitis and fibrosis. Fever, rash, cough, shortness of breath and mouth ulcers may indicate widespread interstitial and alveolar infiltrates. Chest x-ray and pulmonary function tests may be used to evaluate pulmonary injury. Pulmonary symptoms may not resolve after therapy is ended.

Renal: Gold may produce a nephrotic syndrome or glomerulitis with proteinuria and hematuria; these reactions are usually relatively mild and subside completely if recognized early and treatment is discontinued. They may become severe and chronic if treatment is continued after onset. Acute renal failure secondary to acute tubular necrosis, acute nephritis or degeneration of the proximal tubular epithelium may occur; perform regular urinalysis and discontinue treatment if proteinuria or hematuria develop.

(Adverse Reactions continued on following page)

In addition to the agents in this section, sulindac and indomethacin (see Nonsteroidal Anti-inflammatory Agents monograph) and phenylbutazone and oxyphenbutazone (see individual monograph) are indicated for the treatment of gout.

Uricosurics

PROBENECID

Actions:

Pharmacology: A uricosuric and renal tubular blocking agent, probenecid inhibits the tubular reabsorption of urate, thus increasing the urinary excretion of uric acid and decreasing serum uric acid levels. Effective uricosuria reduces the miscible urate pool, retards urate deposition and promotes resorption of urate deposits.

Probenecid also inhibits the tubular secretion of most penicillins and cephalosporins and usually increases plasma levels by any route the antibiotic is given. A twofold to fourfold plasma elevation has been demonstrated.

Pharmacokinetics: Probenecid is well absorbed after oral administration and produces peak plasma concentrations in 2 to 4 hours. It is highly protein bound (85% to 95%) to plasma albumin. The half-life is dose-dependent and varies from $<$ 5 to $>$ 8 hours. Probenecid is hydroxylated to active metabolites and is excreted in the urine primarily as metabolites.

Clinical pharmacology: Probenecid is most useful in gouty arthritis patients with reduced urinary excretion of uric acid ($<$ 800 mg/day) on an unrestricted diet. Allopurinol is more appropriate for patients with excessive uric acid synthesis as indicated by $>$ 800 mg uric acid urinary excretion daily on a purine free diet.

Indications:

Treatment of hyperuricemia associated with gout and gouty arthritis.

Adjuvant to therapy with penicillins or cephalosporins, for elevation and prolongation of plasma levels of the antibiotic.

Contraindications:

Hypersensitivity to probenecid; children $<$ 2 years of age; blood dyscrasias or uric acid kidney stones. Do not start therapy until an acute gouty attack has subsided.

Warnings:

Exacerbation of gout following therapy with probenecid may occur; in such cases, colchicine or other appropriate therapy is advisable.

Hypersensitivity: Rarely, severe allergic reactions and anaphylaxis have occurred. Most of these occur within several hours after readministration following prior use of the drug. The appearance of hypersensitivity reactions requires cessation of therapy. Refer to Management of Acute Hypersensitivity Reactions.

Renal function impairment: Dosage requirements may be increased in renal impairment. Probenecid may not be effective in chronic renal insufficiency, particularly when the glomerular filtration rate is $\leq$ 30 ml/minute. Probenecid is not recommended in conjunction with a penicillin in the presence of known renal impairment.

Pregnancy: Probenecid crosses the placenta and appears in cord blood. Use only when clearly needed and when potential benefits outweigh potential hazards to the fetus.

Children: Do not use in children $<$ 2 years of age.

Precautions:

Alkalinization of urine: Hematuria, renal colic, costovertebral pain and formation of urate stones associated with use in gouty patients may be prevented by alkalization of urine and liberal fluid intake; monitor acid-base balance. See Administration and Dosage.

Peptic ulcer history: Use with caution.

(Continued on following page)

PROBENECID

Drug Interactions:

Probenecid Drug Interactions			
Precipitant drug	Object drug*		Description
Probenecid	Acyclovir	⬆	Decreased acyclovir renal clearance and increased bioavailability following IV use may occur.
Probenecid	Allopurinol	⬆	A beneficial interaction; coadministration may increase the uric acid lowering effect.
Probenecid	Barbiturate	⬆	The anesthesia produced by thiopental may be extended or achieved at lower doses.
Probenecid	Benzodiazepines	⬆	A more rapid onset or more prolonged benzodiazepine effect may occur.
Probenecid	Clofibrate	⬆	Accumulation of clofibric acid (active metabolite of clofibrate) may occur, leading to higher steady-state serum concentrations.
Probenecid	Dapsone	⬆	Possible accumulation of dapsone and its metabolites.
Probenecid	Dyphylline	⬆	Increased half-life and decreased clearance of dyphylline may occur. This may be beneficial in extending the dyphylline dosing interval.
Probenecid	Methotrexate	⬆	Methotrexate's plasma levels, therapeutic effects and toxicity may be enhanced.
Probenecid	NSAIDs	⬆	NSAID plasma levels may be increased; toxicity may be enhanced.
Probenecid	Penicillamine	⬆	Pharmacologic effects of penicillamine may be attenuated.
Probenecid	Sulfonylureas	⬆	Half-life of sulfonylureas may be increased.
Probenecid	Zidovudine	⬆	Increased zidovudine bioavailability; cutaneous eruptions accompanied by systemic symptoms including malaise, myalgia or fever have occurred.
Salicylates	Probenecid	⬇	Coadministration may inhibit the uricosuric action of either drug alone.

* ⬆ = Object drug increased ⬇ = Object drug decreased

Drug/Lab test interactions: A reducing substance may appear in the urine during therapy. Although this disappears with discontinuation, a false diagnosis of glycosuria may be made. Confirm suspected glycosuria by using a test specific for glucose.

Falsely high determination of **theophylline** has occurred in vitro using the Schack and Waxler technique, when therapeutic concentrations of theophylline and probenecid were added to human plasma.

Probenecid may inhibit the renal excretion of: **Phenolsulfonphthalein (PSP), 17-ketosteroids** and **sulfobromophthalein (BSP)**.

Adverse Reactions:

Headache; anorexia; nausea; vomiting; urinary frequency; hypersensitivity reactions (including anaphylaxis, dermatitis, pruritus and fever; see Warnings); sore gums; flushing; dizziness; anemia; hemolytic anemia (possibly related to G-6-PD deficiency); nephrotic syndrome; hepatic necrosis; aplastic anemia; exacerbation of gout; uric acid stones with or without hematuria; renal colic or costovertebral pain.

Patient Information:

Avoid taking aspirin or other salicylates which may antagonize the effects of probenecid.

May cause GI upset; may be taken with food or antacids. If nausea, vomiting or loss of appetite persists, notify physician.

Drink plenty of water, at least 6 to 8 full (8 oz) glasses daily, to prevent development of kidney stones.

(Continued on following page)

PROBENECID (Cont.)

Administration and Dosage:

Gout: Do not start therapy until an acute gouty attack has subsided. However, if an acute attack is precipitated during therapy, probenecid may be continued. Give full therapeutic doses of colchicine or other appropriate therapy to control the acute attack.

Adults – 0.25 g twice daily for 1 week, followed by 0.5 g twice daily thereafter. Gastric intolerance may indicate overdosage, and may be reduced by decreasing dosage.

Renal impairment – Some degree of renal impairment may be present in patients with gout. A daily dosage of 1 g may be adequate. However, if necessary, the daily dosage may be increased by 0.5 g increments every 4 weeks within tolerance (usually not > 2 g/day) if symptoms of gouty arthritis are not controlled or the 24 hour urate excretion is not > 700 mg. Probenecid may not be effective in chronic renal insufficiency, particularly when the glomerular filtration rate is ≤ 30 ml/minute.

Urinary alkalinization – Urates tend to crystallize out of an acid urine; therefore, a liberal fluid intake is recommended, as well as sufficient sodium bicarbonate (3 to 7.5 g/day) or potassium citrate (7.5 g/day) to maintain an alkaline urine; continue alkalization until the serum uric acid level returns to normal limits and tophaceous deposits disappear. Thereafter, urinary alkalization and the restriction of purine-producing foods may be relaxed.

Maintenance therapy – Continue the dosage that maintains normal serum uric acid levels. When there have been no acute attacks for ≥ 6 months and serum uric acid levels have remained within normal limits, decrease the daily dosage by 0.5 g every 6 months. Do not reduce the maintenance dosage to the point where serum uric acid levels increase.

Penicillin or cephalosporin therapy: The PSP excretion test may be used to determine the effectiveness of probenecid in retarding penicillin excretion and maintaining therapeutic levels. The renal clearance of PSP is reduced to about 1/5 the normal rate when dosage of probenecid is adequate.

Adults – 2 g/day in divided doses. Reduce dosage in older patients in whom renal impairment may be present. Not recommended in conjunction with penicillin or a cephalosporin in the presence of known renal impairment.

Children (2 to 14 yrs) – Initial dose 25 mg/kg or 0.7 g/m^2. Maintenance dose 40 mg/kg/day or 1.2 g/m^2, divided into 4 doses. For children weighing > 50 kg (110 lb), use the adult dosage. Do not use in children < 2 years of age.

Gonorrhea (uncomplicated) – Give probenecid as a single 1 g dose 30 minutes before 4.8 million units penicillin G procaine, aqueous, divided into at least two doses.

Gonococcal infections (uncomplicated urethral, endocervical or rectal infection, alternative regimen) – Adults: If infection was acquired from a source proven not to have penicillin-resistant gonorrhea, a penicillin such as amoxicillin 3 g plus 1 g probenecid followed by doxycycline may be used.[1]

Neurosyphilis – Aqueous procaine penicillin G, 2 to 4 million units/day IM plus probenecid 500 mg 4 times daily, both for 10 to 14 days.[1]

	Product	Dosage form	Description	C.I.*
Rx	**Probenecid** (Various, eg, Danbury, Dixon-Shane, Geneva Marsam, Goldline, Moore, Parmed, Purepac, Schein, URL, Zenith)	**Tablets:** 0.5 g	In 100s and 1000s.	25+
Rx	**Benemid** (MSD)		(MSD 501). Yellow, scored. Film coated. Capsule shape. In 100s, 1000s & UD 100s.	79
Rx	**Probalan** (Lannett)		Scored. In 100s and 1000s.	23

* Cost Index based on cost per 500 mg.

[1] CDC 1989 Sexually Transmitted Diseases Treatment Guidelilnes. *Morbidity and Mortality Weekly Report* 1989 Sept 1;38 (No. S-8):1-43.

SULFINPYRAZONE

Actions:

Pharmacology: Sulfinpyrazone, a pyrazolidine derivative, is a potent uricosuric agent which also has antithrombotic and platelet inhibitory effects. It lacks anti-inflammatory and analgesic properties. Sulfinpyrazone inhibits renal tubular reabsorption of uric acid. It reduces renal tubular secretion of other organic anions (eg, PAH, salicylic acid) and displaces other organic anions bound extensively to plasma proteins (eg, sulfonamides, salicylates). It is not intended for the relief of an acute attack of gout.

Sulfinpyrazone competitively inhibits prostaglandin synthesis which prevents platelet aggregation.

Pharmacokinetics: Sulfinpyrazone is well absorbed after oral administration; 98% to 99% is bound to plasma proteins. The plasma half-life is about 2.2 to 3 hours. Approximately one-half of the administered dose appears in the urine unchanged.

Indications:

Treatment of chronic and intermittent gouty arthritis.

Unlabeled uses: The *Anturane* Reinfarction Trial reported that sulfinpyrazone 300 mg 4 times daily may decrease the incidence of sudden cardiac death when given to patients 1 to 6 months post-myocardial infarction. Because of criticisms of this multicenter trial, however, further studies are indicated. In the *Anturane* Reinfarction Italian Study, sulfinpyrazone 400 mg twice daily reduced the recurrence of myocardial infarction, but there was no difference in overall mortality when compared to placebo.

A placebo controlled study of 186 patients with rheumatic mitral stenosis suggested that sulfinpyrazone may decrease the frequency of systemic embolism.

Contraindications:

Active peptic ulcer or symptoms of GI inflammation or ulceration; hypersensitivity to phenylbutazone or other pyrazoles; blood dyscrasias.

Warnings:

Renal function impairment: Periodically assess renal function. Renal failure has occurred, but a cause and effect relationship has not always been clearly established.

Pregnancy: Use only when clearly needed and when the potential benefits outweigh the potential hazards to the fetus.

Precautions:

Monitoring: Keep patients under close medical supervision; perform periodic blood counts.

Healed peptic ulcer: Administer with care.

Alkalinization of urine: Because it is a potent uricosuric, sulfinpyrazone may precipitate acute gouty arthritis, urolithiasis and renal colic, especially in initial stages of therapy. Therefore, adequate fluid intake and alkalinization of the urine are recommended.

Drug Interactions:

Sulfinpyrazone Drug Interactions			
Precipitant drug	Object drug*		Description
Sulfinpyrazone	Acetaminophen	↔	Risk of acetaminophen hepatotoxicity may be increased. Also, therapeutic effects of acetaminophen may be reduced.
Sulfinpyrazone	Anticoagulants	↑	The anticoagulant activity of warfarin will likely be enhanced; hemorrhage could occur.
Sulfinpyrazone	Theophylline	↓	Plasma theophylline clearance may be increased, thus lowering plasma levels.
Sulfinpyrazone	Tolbutamide	↑	Decreased clearance and increased half-life of tolbutamide may occur; hypoglycemia may result. Glyburide was not affected in one study.
Sulfinpyrazone	Verapamil	↓	Increased clearance and decreased bioavailability of verapamil may occur.
Niacin	Sulfinpyrazone	↓	Sulfinpyrazone's uricosuric effect may be reduced.
Salicylates	Sulfinpyrazone	↓	The uricosuria produced by sulfinpyrazone may be suppressed.

* ↑ = Object drug increased ↓ = Object drug decreased ↔ = Undetermined effect

(Continued on following page)

SULFINPYRAZONE (Cont.)

Adverse Reactions:

Most frequent: Upper GI disturbances. Administer with food, milk or antacids; despite this precaution, the drug may aggravate or reactivate peptic ulcer.

Less frequent: Rash (in most instances did not necessitate discontinuing therapy); rare blood dyscrasias (eg, anemia, leukopenia, agranulocytosis, thrombocytopenia, aplastic anemia); bronchoconstriction in patients with aspirin-induced asthma.

Overdosage:

Symptoms: Nausea; vomiting; diarrhea; epigastric pain; ataxia; labored respiration; convulsions; coma. Possible symptoms, seen after overdosage with other pyrazolidine derivatives: Anemia, jaundice; ulceration.

Treatment: No specific antidote. Treatment includes usual supportive measures. Refer to General Management of Acute Overdosage.

Patient Information:

May cause GI upset; take with food, milk or antacids.

Avoid aspirin and other products containing salicylates which may antagonize the action of sulfinpyrazone.

Drink at least 10 to 12 glasses (8 ounces each) of fluid daily.

Administration and Dosage:

Initial: 200 to 400 mg daily in 2 divided doses, with meals or milk, gradually increasing when necessary to full maintenance dosage in 1 week.

Maintenance: 400 mg daily, given in 2 divided doses; may increase to 800 mg daily or reduce to as low as 200 mg daily after the blood urate level has been controlled. Continue treatment without interruption even in the presence of acute exacerbations, which can be concomitantly treated with phenylbutazone or colchicine. Patients previously controlled with other uricosuric therapy may be transferred to sulfinpyrazone at full maintenance dosage.

	Product	Form	Description	C.I.*
Rx	**Sulfinpyrazone** (Various, eg, Barr, Geneva Marsam, Goldline, Major, Rugby, Schein, Zenith)	**Tablets:** 100 mg	In 100s and 500s.	73+
Rx	**Anturane** (Ciba)		(Ciba 41). White, scored. In 100s.	186
Rx	**Sulfinpyrazone** (Various, eg, Barr, Geneva Marsam, Goldline, Major, Rugby, Schein, Zenith)	**Capsules:** 200 mg	In 100s, 500s and 1000s.	60+
Rx	**Anturane** (Ciba)		(Anturane 200 Ciba 168). Green. In 100s.	150

* Cost Index based on cost per 200 mg.

ALLOPURINOL

Actions:

Pharmacology: Allopurinol inhibits xanthine oxidase, the enzyme responsible for the conversion of hypoxanthine to xanthine to uric acid. Allopurinol is metabolized to oxipurinol (alloxanthine), which is also an inhibitor of xanthine oxidase. Allopurinol acts on purine catabolism, reducing the production of uric acid, without disrupting the biosynthesis of vital purines.

Reutilization of both hypoxanthine and xanthine for nucleotide and nucleic acid synthesis is markedly enhanced when their oxidation is inhibited by allopurinol. This reutilization does not disrupt normal nucleic acid anabolism, however, because feedback inhibition is an integral part of purine biosynthesis. The serum concentration of hypoxanthine plus xanthine in patients receiving allopurinol for hyperuricemia usually ranges from 0.3 to 0.4 mg/dl compared to a normal level of approximately 0.15 mg/dl. A maximum of 0.9 mg/dl of these oxypurines has been reported when the serum urate was lowered to $<$ 2 mg/dl. These values are far below the saturation levels at which point their precipitation would occur ($>$ 7 mg/dl).

Administration generally results in a fall in both serum and urinary uric acid within 2 to 3 days. The magnitude of this decrease is dose-dependent. One week or more of treatment may be required before the full effects of the drug are manifested; likewise, uric acid may return to pretreatment levels slowly following cessation of therapy. This reflects primarily the accumulation and slow clearance of oxipurinol. In some patients, a dramatic fall in urinary uric acid excretion may not occur, particularly in those with severe tophaceous gout. This may be due to the mobilization of urate from tissue deposits as the serum uric acid level begins to fall.

Pharmacokinetics: Allopurinol is approximately 90% absorbed from the GI tract. Peak plasma levels occur at 1.5 hours and 4.5 hours for allopurinol and oxipurinol, respectively. After a single 300 mg dose, maximum plasma levels of about 3 mcg/ml of allopurinol and 6.5 mcg/ml of oxipurinol are produced.

Allopurinol has a plasma half-life of about 1 to 2 hours. Oxipurinol, however, has a plasma half-life of approximately 15 hours. Therefore, effective xanthine oxidase inhibition is maintained over 24 hours with single daily doses. Allopurinol is cleared essentially by glomerular filtration; oxipurinol is reabsorbed in the kidney tubules in a manner similar to the reabsorption of uric acid. Approximately 20% is excreted in the feces.

The clearance of oxipurinol is increased by uricosuric drugs, and as a consequence, the addition of a uricosuric may reduce the degree of xanthine oxidase inhibition by oxipurinol and increase the urinary uric acid excretion. However, such combined therapy may achieve minimum serum uric acid levels, provided the total urinary uric acid load does not exceed the competence of the patient's renal function.

Clinical pharmacology: Hyperuricemia may be primary, as in gout, or secondary to diseases such as acute and chronic leukemia, polycythemia vera, multiple myeloma and psoriasis. It may occur with the use of diuretics, during renal dialysis, in the presence of renal damage, during starvation or reducing diets and in the treatment of neoplastic disease where rapid resolution of tissue masses may occur.

Allopurinol's action differs from that of uricosuric agents, which lower the serum uric acid level by increasing urinary uric acid excretion. Allopurinol reduces both the serum and urinary uric acid levels by inhibiting the formation of uric acid. The use of allopurinol to block the formation of urates avoids the hazard of increased renal uric acid excretion posed by uricosuric agents.

Allopurinol can substantially reduce serum and urinary uric acid levels in refractory patients even when renal damage renders uricosuric drugs virtually ineffective. Salicylates may be given concomitantly without compromising the action of allopurinol. In contrast, salicylates antagonize the effect of uricosuric drugs.

(Continued on following page)

ALLOPURINOL (Cont.)

Indications:

Gout: Management of signs and symptoms of primary or secondary gout (acute attacks, tophi, joint destruction, uric acid lithiasis or nephropathy).

Malignancies: Management of patients with leukemia, lymphoma and malignancies receiving therapy which causes elevations of serum and urinary uric acid. Discontinue allopurinol when the potential for overproduction of uric acid is no longer present.

Calcium oxalate calculi: Management of patients with recurrent calcium oxalate calculi whose daily uric acid excretion exceeds 800 mg/day (males) or 750 mg/day (females). Carefully assess therapy initially and periodically to determine that treatment is beneficial and that the benefits outweigh the risks.

Unlabeled uses: In a limited number of patients, the use of an allopurinol mouthwash (20 mg in 3% methylcellulose; 1 mg/ml) after fluorouracil administration prevented stomatitis, a major dose-limiting toxicity of fluorouracil. However, another report indicated that allopurinol mouthwash is not effective. Further study is needed.

In one study, allopurinol (600 mg/day) ameliorated the granulocyte suppressant effect of fluorouracil.

Contraindications:

Patients who have developed a severe reaction should not be restarted on the drug.

Warnings:

Asymptomatic hyperuricemia: This drug is not innocuous. Do not use to treat asymptomatic hyperuricemia.

Hypersensitivity: Discontinue at first appearance of skin rash or other signs of allergic reactions. In some instances, rash may be followed by more severe hypersensitivity reactions such as exfoliative, urticarial or purpuric lesions, or Stevens-Johnson syndrome (erythema multiforme exudativum), generalized vasculitis, irreversible hepatotoxicity and rarely, death. Refer to Management of Acute Hypersensitivity Reactions.

Hepatotoxicity: A few cases of reversible clinical hepatotoxicity have occurred; in some patients, asymptomatic rises in serum alkaline phosphatase or serum transaminase levels have been observed. If anorexia, weight loss or pruritis develop in patients on allopurinol, evaluation of liver function should be part of their diagnostic workup. Perform periodic liver function tests during early stages of therapy, particularly in patients with preexisting liver disease.

Renal function impairment: Some patients with preexisting renal disease or poor urate clearance have increased BUN during allopurinol administration. Although the mechanism has not been established, patients with impaired renal function require less drug and careful observation during the early stages of treatment; reduce dosage or discontinue therapy if increased abnormalities in renal function appear and persist.

Renal failure in association with allopurinol has been observed among patients with hyperuricemia secondary to neoplastic diseases. Concurrent conditions such as multiple myeloma and congestive myocardial disease were present. Renal failure is also frequently associated with gouty nephropathy and rarely with allopurinol-associated hypersensitivity reactions. Albuminuria has occurred among patients who developed clinical gout following chronic glomerulonephritis and chronic pyelonephritis.

In patients with severely impaired renal function or decreased urate clearance, the plasma half-life of oxipurinol is greatly prolonged. A dose of 100 mg/day or 300 mg twice a week, or less, may be sufficient to maintain adequate xanthine oxidase inhibition to reduce serum urate levels.

Pregnancy: Category C. There are no adequate and well controlled studies in pregnant women. Use only when clearly needed.

Lactation: Allopurinol and oxipurinol have been found in the breast milk of a mother who received allopurinol. Exercise caution when administering to a nursing woman.

Children: Allopurinol is rarely indicated for use in children, with the exception of those with hyperuricemia secondary to malignancy or to certain rare inborn errors of purine metabolism.

(Continued on following page)

ALLOPURINOL (Cont.)

Precautions:

Acute attacks of gout have increased during the early stages of allopurinol administration, even when normal or subnormal serum uric acid levels have been attained; in general, give maintenance doses of colchicine prophylactically when allopurinol is begun. In addition, start patient at a low dose of allopurinol (100 mg daily) and increase at weekly intervals by 100 mg until a serum uric acid level of ≤ 6 mg/dl is attained without exceeding the maximum recommended dose. The attacks usually become shorter and less severe after several months of therapy. A possible explanation for these episodes may be the mobilization of urates from tissue deposits which causes fluctuations in the serum uric acid level. Even with adequate therapy it may require several months to deplete the uric acid pool sufficiently to control acute episodes.

Fluid intake sufficient to yield a daily urinary output of at least 2 L and the maintenance of a neutral or slightly alkaline urine are desirable to avoid the theoretic possibility of formation of xanthine calculi under the influence of allopurinol therapy and to help prevent renal precipitation of urates in patients receiving concomitant uricosurics.

Drowsiness has occurred occasionally. Patients should observe caution while driving or performing other tasks requiring alertness, coordination or physical dexterity.

Bone marrow depression has occurred in patients receiving allopurinol, most of whom received concomitant drugs with the potential for causing this reaction. This has occurred as early as 6 weeks to as long as 6 years after the initiation of therapy. Rarely, a patient may develop varying degrees of bone marrow depression, affecting one or more cell lines, while receiving allopurinol alone.

Monitoring: Periodically determine liver and kidney function especially during the first few months of therapy. Perform BUN, serum creatinine or creatinine clearance and reassess the patient's dosage.

Drug Interactions:

Allopurinol Drug Interactions			
Precipitant drug	Object drug*		Description
Allopurinol	Ampicillin	↑	The rate of ampicillin-induced skin rash appears much higher with allopurinol coadministration than with either drug alone.
Allopurinol	Anticoagulants	↑	Data are conflicting. The anticoagulant action of some agents may be enhanced, but probably not that of warfarin.
Allopurinol	Cyclophosphamide	↑	Myelosuppressive effects of cyclophosphamide may be enhanced, possibly increasing the risk of bleeding or infection.
Allopurinol	Theophyllines	↑	Theophylline clearance may be decreased with large allopurinol doses (600 mg/day) leading to increased plasma theophylline levels and possible toxicity.
Allopurinol	Thiopurines	↑	Clinically significant increases in pharmacologic and toxic effects of oral thiopurines have occurred.
ACE Inhibitors	Allopurinol	↑	Possibly higher risk of hypersensitivity reaction when these agents are coadministered than when each drug is administered alone.
Aluminum salts	Allopurinol	↓	Pharmacologic effects of allopurinol may be decreased.
Thiazide diuretics	Allopurinol	↑	Coadministration may increase the incidence of hypersensitivity reactions to allopurinol.
Uricosuric agents	Allopurinol	↓	Uricosuric agents which increase the excretion of urate are also likely to increase the excretion of oxipurinol and thus lower the degree of inhibition of xanthine oxidase.

* ↑ = Object drug increased ↓ = Object drug decreased

(Continued on following page)

COLCHICINE (Cont.)

Administration and Dosage (Cont.):

Parenteral: For IV use only. Severe local irritation occurs if given SC or IM. If leakage into surrounding tissue or outside the vein should occur, considerable irritation and possible tissue damage may follow. There is no specific antidote. Local application of heat or cold, as well as use of analgesics, may afford relief.

Administer over 2 to 5 minutes. Do not dilute with 5% Dextrose in Water. If a decrease in concentration of colchicine is required, use 0.9% Sodium Chloride Injection which does not contain a bacteriostatic agent. Do not use solutions which have become turbid.

Treatment of acute gouty arthritis – Average initial dose is 2 mg. This may be followed by 0.5 mg every 6 hours until a satisfactory response is achieved. In general, do not exceed a total dosage of 4 mg for a 24 hour period. Do not exceed total dosage of 4 mg for one course of treatment. Some clinicians recommend a single IV dose of 3 mg, while others recommend not > 1 mg IV for the initial dose, followed by 0.5 mg once or twice daily if needed.

If pain recurs, it may be necessary to administer a daily dose of 1 to 2 mg for several days; however, do not give more colchicine by any route for at least 7 days after a full course of IV therapy (4 mg). Transfer to oral colchicine in a dose similar to that being given IV.

Prophylaxis or maintenance of recurrent or chronic gouty arthritis – 0.5 to 1 mg once or twice daily. Oral colchicine is preferable, usually in conjunction with a uricosuric agent.

				C.I.*
Rx	**Colchicine** (Abbott)	**Tablets:** 0.5 mg (1/120 gr)	Sugar, sucrose. Sugar coated granules. Yellow. In 100s.	96
Rx	**Colchicine** (Various, eg, Abbott, Goldline, Major, Zenith)	**Tablets:** 0.6 mg (1/100 gr)	In 100s, 250s, 1000s & UD 100s.	22+
Rx	**Colchicine** (Lilly)	**Injection:** 1 mg (1/60 gr)	In 2 ml amps.	118

PROBENECID AND COLCHICINE COMBINATIONS

Refer to prescribing information for probenecid and colchicine when using these products.

Indications:

Treatment of chronic gouty arthritis complicated by frequent, recurrent acute attacks.

Administration and Dosage:

Do not initiate therapy until an acute gouty attack has subsided. If an acute attack is precipitated during therapy, administer additional colchicine or other appropriate therapy to control the attack; do not alter the dose of probenecid.

Initial dosage: 1 tablet daily for 1 week, followed by 1 tablet twice daily thereafter. Gastric intolerance may indicate overdose; correct by decreasing dosage.

Fluid intake and urinary alkalinization: Maintain a liberal fluid intake as well as sufficient sodium bicarbonate (3 to 7.5 g daily) or potassium citrate (7.5 g daily) to maintain an alkaline urine. Alkalinize the urine until serum urate levels return to normal (maximum normal level in males 6 mg/dl, in females 5 mg/dl) and tophaceous deposits disappear (ie, when urinary excretion of urates is at a high level). Thereafter, urine alkalinization and the usual restriction of purine-producing foods may be somewhat relaxed.

Maintenance therapy: Continue therapy at the dosage needed to maintain normal serum urate levels. When there have been no acute attacks for ≥ 6 months and serum urate levels have remained normal, decrease daily dosage by 1 tablet every 6 months. Do not reduce dosage to the point where serum urate levels begin to rise.

Dosage in renal impairment: Some degree of renal impairment may be present in patients with gout. A daily dose of 2 tablets may be adequate for control. If necessary, increase the dose by 1 tablet every 4 weeks within tolerance (usually not > 4 tablets per day) if symptoms of gouty arthritis are not controlled or the 24 hour urate excretion is not > 700 mg. Probenecid may not be effective in chronic renal insufficiency, particularly when the glomerular filtration rate is ≤ 30 ml/min.

				C.I.*
Rx	**Probenecid w/ Colchicine** (Various, eg, Major, Zenith)	**Tablets:** 500 mg probenecid and 0.5 mg colchicine	In 100s, 1000s and unit-of-issue 100s.	63+
Rx	**ColBenemid** (MSD)		(MSD 614). White, scored. Capsule shape. In 100s.	185
Rx	**Col-Probenecid** (Various, eg, Goldline)		In 100s, 1000s and UD 100s.	75+
Rx	**Proben-C** (Rugby)		White. In 100s and 1000s.	54

* Cost Index based on cost per 1 mg colchicine or initial daily dose of the combination.

In addition to the agents listed, propranolol and timolol are indicated for migraine prophylaxis (see Beta-Adrenergic Blocking Agents monograph).

METHYSERGIDE MALEATE

Warning:

Retroperitoneal fibrosis, pleuropulmonary fibrosis and fibrotic thickening of cardiac valves may occur in patients receiving long-term methysergide therapy. Reserve this drug for prophylaxis in patients whose vascular headaches are frequent or severe and uncontrollable and who are under close medical supervision.

Actions:

Methysergide is a semisynthetic ergot derivative. It has no intrinsic vasoconstrictor properties and its mechanism of action has not been established. It inhibits or blocks the effects of serotonin, a substance which may be involved in the mechanism of vascular headaches. Serotonin has been described as a central neurohumoral agent or chemical mediator, as a "headache substance" acting directly or indirectly to lower pain threshold. Serotonin is also a potent vasoconstrictor. Plasma serotonin levels are elevated during the preheadache phase of classical migraine and decreased during an attack. Without serotonin, the extracranial arteries are dilated and distended, resulting in headache. Methysergide may displace serotonin on receptor pressor sites of the walls of cranial arteries during a migraine attack and thereby preserve the vasoconstriction afforded by serotonin.

Methysergide is a peripheral antagonist of serotonin, competitively blocking the serotonin receptor in the blood vessel. It also inhibits histamine release from mast cells and stabilizes platelets against spontaneous or induced release of serotonin. Centrally, methysergide may act as a serotonin agonist, especially in the midbrain. It has very weak uterotonic and emetic actions.

Allow 1 to 2 days for the protective effects to develop; following termination, 1 to 2 days are required before the effects subside.

Indications:

Vascular headache:

Prevention or reduction of intensity and frequency in patients suffering from one or more severe vascular headaches per week or from vascular headaches that are so severe that preventive therapy is indicated, regardless of the frequency of the attack.

Prophylaxis of vascular headache. Not for management of acute attacks.

Contraindications:

Pregnancy (see Warnings); peripheral vascular disease; severe arteriosclerosis; severe hypertension; coronary artery disease; phlebitis or cellulitis of the lower limbs; pulmonary disease; collagen diseases or fibrotic processes; impaired liver or renal function; valvular heart disease; debilitated states; serious infections.

Warnings:

Prolonged therapy: With long-term, uninterrupted administration, retroperitoneal fibrosis or related conditions (pleuropulmonary fibrosis and cardiovascular disorders with murmurs or vascular bruits) have occurred. Continuous administration should not exceed 6 months. There must be a drug free interval of 3 to 4 weeks after each 6 month treatment course. Reduce dosage gradually during the last 2 to 3 weeks of each treatment course to avoid "headache rebound."

Retroperitoneal fibrosis, a nonspecific fibrotic process, is usually confined to the retroperitoneal connective tissue above the pelvic brim and may present clinically with one or more symptoms such as general malaise, fatigue, weight loss, backache, low grade fever (elevated sedimentation rate), urinary obstruction (girdle or flank pain, dysuria, polyuria, oliguria, elevated BUN), or vascular insufficiency of the lower limbs (leg pain, Leriche syndrome, edema of legs, thrombophlebitis). The most useful diagnostic procedure is IV pyelography. Typical deviation and obstruction of one or both ureters may be observed.

Pleuropulmonary fibrosis, a similar nonspecific fibrotic process limited to pleural and immediately subjacent pulmonary tissues, usually presents with dyspnea, chest tightness/pain, pleural friction rubs and pleural effusion. Confirm by chest x-ray.

Cardiac fibrosis – Nonrheumatic fibrotic thickenings of the aortic root and of the aortic and mitral valves usually present clinically with cardiac murmurs and dyspnea.

Other fibrotic complications – Fibrotic plaques simulating Peyronie's disease.

Supervise and regularly examine patients for developing fibrotic or vascular complications. The manifestations of retroperitoneal fibrosis, pleuropulmonary fibrosis and vascular shutdown have shown a high incidence of regression once methysergide is withdrawn. Cardiac murmurs, which may indicate endocardial fibrosis, have shown varying degrees of regression, with complete disappearance in some and persistence in others.

(Warnings continued on following page)

METHYSERGIDE MALEATE (Cont.)

Warnings (Cont.):

Pregnancy: Contraindicated in pregnancy due to oxytocic properties.

Lactation: Ergot derivatives in the milk of nursing mothers have caused symptoms of ergotism (eg, vomiting, diarrhea) in the infant.

Children: Not recommended for use in children.

Precautions:

Tartrazine sensitivity: This product contains tartrazine, which may cause allergic-type reactions (including bronchial asthma) in susceptible individuals. Although the incidence of tartrazine sensitivity in the general population is low, it is frequently seen in patients who also have aspirin hypersensitivity.

Drug Interactions:

Beta blockers and concurent methysergide therapy may result in peripheral ischemia manifested by cold extremities with possible peripheral gangrene.

Adverse Reactions:

Adverse reactions occur in up to 30% to 50% of patients.

Fibrosis: See Warnings.

Cardiovascular: Encroachment of retroperitoneal fibrosis on the aorta, inferior vena cava and their common iliac branches may cause vascular insufficiency of the lower limbs.

Intrinsic vasoconstriction of large and small arteries, involving one or more vessels or vessel segments, may occur at any stage of therapy. Depending on the vessel, this complication may present with chest pain, abdominal pain or cold, numb, painful extremities with or without paresthesias and diminished or absent pulses. Progression to ischemic tissue damage is rare.

Postural hypotension and tachycardia have also been observed.

GI: Nausea, vomiting, diarrhea, heartburn and abdominal pain tend to appear early and can frequently be obviated by gradual introduction of the medication and by administration with meals. Constipation and elevation of gastric hydrochloric acid have occurred.

CNS: Insomnia; drowsiness; mild euphoria; dizziness; ataxia; weakness; lightheadedness; hyperesthesia; unworldly feelings (described as "dissociation" or "hallucinatory experiences"). Some symptoms may be unrelated to the drug.

Dermatologic: Facial flush, telangiectasia, nonspecific rashes (rare); increased hair loss (usually abates despite continued therapy).

Edema: Peripheral edema, and more rarely, localized brawny edema. Dependent edema has responded to lowered doses, salt restriction or diuretics.

Hematologic: Neutropenia; eosinophilia.

Miscellaneous: Arthralgia; myalgia; weight gain.

Patient Information:

May cause GI upset; take with food or milk.

Caution patients regarding their caloric intake.

May cause drowsiness; use caution when driving or performing other tasks requiring alertness, coordination or physical dexterity.

Continuous administration should not exceed 6 months. There must be a drug free interval of 3 to 4 weeks after each 6 month course of treatment. Do not stop taking suddenly; reduce dosage gradually during the last 2 to 3 weeks of each treatment course to avoid "headache rebound".

Notify physician of cold, numb or painful extremities, leg cramps when walking, girdle, flank or chest pain, painful urination or shortness of breath.

Administration and Dosage:

Adults: 4 to 8 mg daily; take with meals. There must be a drug free interval of 3 to 4 weeks after every 6 month course of treatment.

If, after a 3 week trial period, efficacy has not been demonstrated, continued administration is unlikely to be beneficial.

				C.I.*
Rx	**Sansert** (Sandoz)	**Tablets:** 2 mg	Tartrazine, lactose, sucrose. (Sandoz 78-58). In 100s.	12

* Cost Index based on cost per 4 mg.

ERGOTAMINE DERIVATIVES

Actions:

Pharmacology: Ergotamine has partial agonist or antagonist activity against tryptaminergic, dopaminergic and alpha-adrenergic receptors, depending upon their site; it is a highly active uterine stimulant. It constricts peripheral and cranial blood vessels and depresses central vasomotor centers.

Ergotamine reduces extracranial blood flow, causes a decline in the amplitude of pulsation in the cranial arteries and decreases hyperperfusion of the basilar artery territory. It does not reduce cerebral hemispheric blood flow. It may inhibit receptor reuptake of norepinephrine at sympathetic nerve endings, increasing the vasoconstrictive action. Ergotamine is a potent emetic that stimulates the chemoreceptor trigger zone. Small doses increase force and frequency of uterine contractions; larger doses increase resting uterine tone. The gravid uterus is more sensitive to these effects.

Dihydroergotamine, a hydrogenated derivative of ergotamine, differs mainly in its degree of activity. It has less vasoconstrictive action than ergotamine, is 12 times less active as an emetic and has less oxytocic effect.

Pharmacokinetics: Absorption/Distribution – GI absorption of ergotamine is incomplete and erratic; following oral administration, peak blood levels are reached in about 2 hours. Absorption by inhalation of the aerosol preparation appears rapid and complete. Absorption across the buccal mucosa is extremely poor. For patients who cannot tolerate or retain oral ergotamine, rectal suppositories may be beneficial (ergotamine is only available as a rectal dosage form in combination with other agents). Caffeine administered concurrently increases absorption rate and peak plasma levels of ergotamine; caffeine/ergotamine combination products are listed under Migraine Combinations.

Onset of action occurs in 15 to 30 minutes following IM administration of dihydroergotamine and persists for 3 to 4 hours. Repeat dosage at 1 hour intervals; up to 3 hours may be required to obtain maximal effect.

Metabolism/Excretion – Ergotamine is metabolized by the liver; 90% of the metabolites are excreted in the bile. Unmetabolized drug is erratically secreted in saliva, and only trace amounts of unmetabolized drug are excreted in the feces and urine. Although plasma half-life is about 2 hours, ergotamine has long-lasting effects which may be due to tissue storage.

Clinical pharmacology: Ergotamine effectively controls up to 70% of acute migraine attacks; thus, it is specific for this syndrome. Ergotamine constricts both arteries and veins. In doses used in vascular headaches, it usually produces only small increases in blood pressure, but it increases peripheral resistance and decreases blood flow in various organs.

Indications:

To abort or prevent vascular headaches such as migraine, migraine variant and cluster headache (histaminic cephalalgia).

Dihydroergotamine is used when rapid control is desired or when other routes of administration are not feasible.

Contraindications:

Pregnancy, women who may become pregnant (ergotamine's powerful uterine stimulant actions may cause fetal harm; see Warnings); hypersensitivity to ergot alkaloids; peripheral vascular disease (eg, thromboangiitis obliterans, leutic arteritis, severe arteriosclerosis, thrombophlebitis, Raynaud's disease); hepatic or renal impairment; severe pruritus; coronary artery disease; hypertension; sepsis; malnutrition.

Warnings:

Pregnancy: Category X. Although no specific teratogenic effects have been found, the fetus suffers if ergotamine is given to the mother. Retarded fetal growth, increased intrauterine death and resorption occurred in animals, possibly resulting from drug-induced uterine motility and increased vasoconstriction in the placental vascular bed.

Lactation: Ergotamine is secreted into breast milk and has caused symptoms of ergotism (eg, vomiting, diarrhea) in the infant. Exercise caution when administering to a nursing woman. Excessive dosing or prolonged administration may inhibit lactation.

Children: Safety and efficacy for use in children have not been established.

(Continued on following page)

ERGOTAMINE DERIVATIVES (Cont.)

Precautions:

Avoid prolonged administration or excessive dosage because of the danger of ergotism and gangrene.

Drug abuse and dependence: Patients who take ergotamine for extended periods of time may become dependent upon it and require progressively increasing doses for relief of vascular headaches and for prevention of dysphoric effects which follow withdrawal.

Drug Interactions:

Ergot Alkaloid Drug Interactions			
Precipitant drug	Object drug*		Description
Beta blockers	Ergot alkaloids	↑	Peripheral ischemia manifested by cold extremities, possible peripheral gangrene.
Macrolides	Ergot alkaloids	↑	Acute ergotism manifested as peripheral ischemia has occurred.
Dihydroergotamine	Nitrates	↓	Functional antagonism between these agents, decreasing the antianginal effects. Also, increased bioavailability of oral dihydroergotamine (dosage form not available in US) with resultant increase in mean standing systolic blood pressure.
Ergot alkaloids	Vasodilators	↑	The pressor effects of concurrent use can combine to cause dangerous hypertension.

* ↑ = Object drug increased ↓ = Object drug decreased

Adverse Reactions:

Side effects usually do not necessitate interruption of therapy; however, serious toxicity may occur (see Overdosage). Nausea and vomiting occur in up to 10% of patients and may be relieved by atropine or phenothiazine antiemetics.

Miscellaneous: Numbness and tingling of fingers and toes; muscle pain in the extremities; pulselessness; weakness in the legs; precordial distress and pain; transient tachycardia or bradycardia; localized edema; itching.

Large doses raise arterial pressure, produce coronary vasoconstriction and slow the heart by both a direct action and a vagal effect. Ergotamine has oxytocic and spasmolytic properties.

Overdosage:

Symptoms: Some cases of ergotamine poisoning have occurred in patients who have taken < 5 mg. Usually, however, toxicity is seen at doses in excess of about 15 mg in 24 hours or 40 mg in a few days. Overdosage causes nausea, vomiting, weakness of the legs, pain in limb muscles, numbness and tingling of fingers and toes, precordial pain, tachycardia or bradycardia, hypertension or hypotension, and localized edema and itching with signs and symptoms of ischemia due to vasoconstriction of peripheral arteries and arterioles. The feet and hands become cold, pale and numb. Muscle pain occurs while walking and later at rest also. Gangrene may ensue. Confusion, depression, drowsiness and convulsions are occasional signs of ergotamine toxicity. Overdosage is particularly likely to occur in patients with sepsis or impaired renal or hepatic function. Patients with peripheral vascular disease are especially at risk of developing peripheral ischemia following treatment with ergotamine.

Treatment consists of the withdrawal of the drug followed by symptomatic measures including attempts to maintain an adequate circulation in the affected parts. Anticoagulant drugs, low molecular weight dextran and potent vasodilator drugs may all be beneficial. IV infusion of sodium nitroprusside has been successful. Vasodilators must be used with special care in the presence of hypotension. Ergotamine is dialyzable.

(Continued on following page)

ERGOTAMINE DERIVATIVES (Cont.)

Patient Information:

A patient package insert is available with these products.

Initiate therapy at first sign of attack. Do NOT exceed recommended dosage.

Notify physician if any of the following occurs: Irregular heart beat, nausea, vomiting, numbness or tingling of fingers or toes, or pain or weakness of extremities.

Administration and Dosage:

Sublingual: Initiate therapy as soon as possible after the first symptoms of an attack. Place 1 tablet under the tongue; take subsequent doses at 30 minute intervals if necessary. Do not exceed 3 tablets/24 hours. Do not exceed 10 mg/week.

Inhalation: Start with 1 inhalation; repeat if not relieved in 5 minutes. Space additional inhalations at least 5 minutes apart. Do not exceed 6 inhalations in 24 hours or 15 inhalations/week.

ERGOTAMINE TARTRATE				C.I.*
Rx	**Ergostat** (Parke-Davis)	**Tablets, sublingual:** 2 mg	Lactose, saccharin. (P-D 111). Orange. In UD 24s.	1.9
Rx	**Medihaler Ergotamine** (3M)	**Aerosol:** 9 mg per ml (delivers 0.36 mg/dose)	In 2.5 ml vial with adapter. (≈ 62.5 doses.)	2.3

DIHYDROERGOTAMINE MESYLATE

Administration and Dosage:

IM: Inject 1 mg at first sign of headache; repeat at 1 hour intervals to a total of 3 mg. For optimal results, adjust the dose for several headaches to determine the minimal effective dose; use this dose at the onset of subsequent attacks.

IV: Where more rapid effect is desired, administer IV to a maximum of 2 mg. Do not exceed 6 mg/week.

				C.I.*
Rx	**D.H.E. 45** (Sandoz)	**Injection:** 1 mg per ml	In 1 ml amps.[1]	30

* Cost Index based on cost per 2 mg sublingual or 0.36 mg inhalation ergotamine tartrate or 1 mg dihydroergotamine mesylate.

[1] With methanesulfonic acid, 6.1% alcohol and 15% glycerin.

ISOMETHEPTENE MUCATE/DICHLORALPHENAZONE/ACETAMINOPHEN

Actions:

Isometheptene mucate is an unsaturated aliphatic amine with sympathomimetic properties. It acts by constricting dilated cranial and cerebral arterioles, thus reducing the stimuli that lead to vascular headaches.

Dichloralphenazone, a mild sedative, reduces the patient's emotional reaction to the pain of both vascular and tension headaches.

Acetaminophen raises the threshold to painful stimuli, thus exerting an analgesic effect against all types of headaches. Refer to individual monograph.

Indications:

For relief of tension and vascular headaches.

Based on a review of this drug (isometheptene mucate) by the National Academy of Sciences-National Research Council or other information, FDA has classified the other indication as "possibly" effective in the treatment of migraine headache. Final classification of the less-than-effective indication requires further investigation.

Contraindications:

Glaucoma; severe cases of renal disease; hypertension; organic heart disease; hepatic disease; MAO inhibitor therapy (see Drug Interactions).

Precautions:

Observe caution in hypertension, peripheral vascular disease and after recent cardiovascular attacks.

Drug Interactions:

MAO inhibitors: Since isometheptene has sympathomimetic properties, concurrent use may result in severe headache, hypertension and hyperpyrexia, possibly resulting in hypertensive crisis.

Adverse Reactions:

Transient dizziness and skin rash may appear in hypersensitive patients; this can usually be eliminated by reducing the dose.

Administration and Dosage:

Migraine headache: Usual dosage is 2 capsules at once followed by 1 capsule every hour until relieved, up to 5 capsules within a 12 hour period.

Tension headache: Usual dosage is 1 or 2 capsules every 4 hours, up to 8 capsules per day.

				C.I.*
Rx	**Isometheptene/Dichloralphenazone/Acetaminophen** (Various, eg, Goldline, URL)	**Capsules:** 65 mg isometheptene mucate, 100 mg dichloralphenazone, 325 mg APAP	In 100s.	1+
Rx	**Isocom** (Nutripharm)		In 50s, 100s and 250s.	NA
Rx	**Isopap** (Geneva Marsam)		Red/white. In 100s.	1
Rx	**Midchlor** (Schein)		In 100s.	1.1
Rx	**Midrin** (Carnrick)		(C 86120). Red with pink band. In 50s and 100s.	1.5
Rx	**Migratine** (Major)		In 100s and 250s.	1

* Cost Index based on cost per capsule.

MIGRAINE COMBINATIONS (Cont.)

For complete information on these ingredients, refer to the individual monographs.
ERGOTAMINE TARTRATE is used for its specific action against migraine.
CAFFEINE, a cranial vasoconstrictor, is added to ergotamine to enhance vasoconstrictive effects. It may enhance the absorption of ergotamine.
BARBITURATES are used for sedation.
BELLADONNA ALKALOIDS are used for their anticholinergic and antiemetic effects in individuals experiencing excessive nausea and vomiting during attacks.

	Product & Distributor	Ergotamine tartrate	Caffeine	Other content	Dosage	How supplied	C.I.*
Rx	**Cafergot Tablets** (Sandoz)	1 mg	100 mg		2 tablets at first sign of an attack; follow with 1 tablet every ½ hour, if needed. Maximum dose is 6 tablets/attack. Do not exceed 10 tablets/week.	(Cafergot). Pink. In 90s and 250s.	4
Rx	**Ercaf Tablets** (Geneva Marsam)					Beige. In 100s.	2.8
Rx	**Wigraine Tablets** (Organon)					Lactose. (Organon 542). White. In foil strip 20s and 100s.	2.6
Rx	**Cafatine-PB Tablets** (Major)	1 mg	100 mg	0.125 mg l-alkaloids of belladonna, 30 mg sodium pentobarbital	2 tablets at first sign of an attack; follow with 1 tablet every ½ hour, if needed. Maximum dose is 6 tablets/attack. Do not exceed 10 tablets/week.	In 90s.	3.7
Rx	**Cafatine Supps** (Major)	2 mg	100 mg		Maximum dose is 2/attack.	In 12s.	5.9
Rx	**Cafergot Supps** (Sandoz)			Cocoa butter		(Cafergot Suppository 78.33 Sandoz) In 12s.	NA
Rx	**Cafetrate Supps** (Schein)					In 12s.	6.1
Rx	**Wigraine Supps** (Organon)	2 mg	100 mg	21.5 mg tartaric acid	Maximum dose is 2/attack.	In 12s.	9

* Cost Index based on cost per tablet or suppository.

Antidopaminergics (Cont.)

PROCHLORPERAZINE (Cont.)

	Product	Dosage form	Packaging	C.I.*
Rx	**Prochlorperazine** (Various)	**Tablets:** 5 mg (as maleate)	In 12s, 30s, 100s, 1000s and UD 100s.	61+
Rx	**Compazine** (SKF)		(#SKF C66). Yellow-green. In 100s, 1000s and UD 100s.	333
Rx	**Prochlorperazine** (Various)	**Tablets:** 10 mg (as maleate)	In 20s, 30s, 100s, 1000s and UD 32s and 100s.	38+
Rx	**Compazine** (SKF)		(#SKF C67). Yellow-green. In 100s, 1000s and UD 100s.	250
Rx	**Prochlorperazine** (Various)	**Tablets:** 25 mg (as maleate)	In 100s, 1000s and UD 100s.	24+
Rx	**Compazine** (SKF)		(#SKF C69). Yellow-green. In 100s and 1000s.	126
Rx	**Compazine Spansules** (SKF)	**Capsules, sustained release:** 10 mg (as maleate)	(#SKF C44). Black/clear. In 50s, 500s, UD 100s.	316
Rx	**Compazine Spansules** (SKF)	**Capsules, sustained release:** 15 mg (as maleate)	(#SKF C46). Black/clear. In 50s, 500s, UD 100s.	313
Rx	**Compazine Spansules** (SKF)	**Capsules, sustained release:** 30 mg (as maleate)	(#SKF C47). Black and clear. In 50s, 500s and UD 100s.	190
Rx	**Compazine** (SKF)	**Syrup:** 5 mg/5 ml (as edisylate)	Fruit flavor. In 120 ml.	454
Rx	**Prochlorperazine** (Various)	**Injection:** 5 mg/ml	In 10 ml vials.	1046+
Rx	**Prochlorperazine** (Various)	**Injection:** 5 mg/ml (as edisylate)	In 2 ml amps and 2 and 10 ml vials.	700+
Rx	**Compazine** (SKF)		In 2 ml amps[1], 10 ml multi-dose vials[2] and 2 ml disp. syringes.[2]	1995
Rx	**Compazine** (SKF)	**Suppositories:** 2.5 mg	(#SKF C60). In 12s.	2425
		5 mg	(#SKF C61). In 12s.	1354
		25 mg	(#SKF C62). In 12s.	335

* Cost Index based on cost per 10 mg.
# Product identification code.
[1] With sodium sulfite and sodium bisulfite.
[2] With sodium saccharin and benzyl alcohol.

Refer to the general discussion of these products beginning on page 1227

Antidopaminergics (Cont.)

PROMETHAZINE HCl

This is an abbreviated monograph. For complete prescribing information refer to the Antihistamines monograph.

Indications:

Oral or rectal: Active and prophylactic treatment of motion sickness; prevention and control of nausea and vomiting associated with anesthesia and surgery; antiemetic in postoperative patients.

Parenteral: Treatment of motion sickness; prevention and control of nausea and vomiting associated with anesthesia and surgery.

Administration and Dosage:

Oral and rectal:

Motion sickness – The average adult dose is 25 mg twice daily. Take the initial dose ½ to 1 hour before travel, and repeat 8 to 12 hours later, if necessary. On succeeding days, administer 25 mg on arising and again before the evening meal. For children, administer 12.5 to 25 mg twice daily.

Nausea and vomiting – The average dose for active therapy in children or adults is 25 mg. Repeat as necessary in doses of 12.5 to 25 mg at 4 to 6 hour intervals.

Give children 0.25 to 0.5 mg/kg every 4 to 6 hours rectally, as needed. Do not use in children under 2 years. Adjust dose based on age, weight and severity of condition.

Parenteral: Administer preferably by deep IM injection. Proper IV administration is well tolerated, but hazardous. When used IV, give in a concentration no greater than 25 mg/ml, and at a rate not to exceed 25 mg/min; it is preferable to inject through an appropriate site in tubing of an IV infusion set.

Motion sickness – 12.5 to 25 mg; may repeat as necessary 3 or 4 times a day.

Nausea and vomiting – 12.5 to 25 mg; do not repeat more frequently than every 4 hours. For postoperative nausea and vomiting, administer IM or IV and reduce dosage of analgesics and barbiturates accordingly.

In children under the age of 12 years, do not exceed one-half the adult dose. As an adjunct to premedication, administer 0.5 mg/lb (1.1 mg/kg) in combination with an equal dose of narcotic or barbiturate and the appropriate dose of an atropine-like drug. Do not use in premature infants or neonates or in vomiting of unknown etiology in children.

Inadvertent intra-arterial injection can result in gangrene of the affected extremity. Subcutaneous injection is contraindicated as it may result in tissue necrosis.

For a complete listing of promethazine HCl products refer to the Antihistamine Product Pages.

THIETHYLPERAZINE MALEATE

This is an abbreviated monograph. For complete prescribing information, refer to the Antipsychotic Agents monograph.

Actions: Mechanism of action is unknown. However, animal experiments suggest a direct action on both the chemoreceptor trigger zone (CTZ) and the vomiting center (VC).

Indications: Relief of nausea and vomiting.

Contraindications:

Severe CNS depression; comatose states; hypersensitivity to phenothiazines; IV administration; pregnancy.

Administration and Dosage:

Do not use IV (may cause severe hypotension). Use of this drug has not been studied following intracardiac or intracranial surgery.

When used in the treatment of nausea or vomiting associated with anesthesia and surgery, administer by deep IM injection at, or shortly before, termination of anesthesia.

Adults: Oral and Rectal – 10 to 30 mg daily in divided doses.

IM – 2 ml, 1 to 3 times daily.

Children: Dosage has not been determined. Not for use in < 12.

Storage: Store suppositories below 25°C (77°F) in a tight container (eg, sealed foil).

	Product	Form		C.I.*
Rx	**Norzine** (Purdue Frederick)	**Tablets:** 10 mg	Tartrazine. Sorbitol. In 100s.	101
Rx	**Torecan** (Roxane)		Tartrazine. Sorbitol. In 100s.	117
Rx	**Norzine** (Purdue Frederick)	**Suppositories:** 10 mg	In 12s.	370
Rx	**Torecan** (Roxane)		In 12s.	409
Rx	**Norzine** (Purdue Frederick)	**Injection:** 5 mg per ml	In 2 ml amps.[1]	702
Rx	**Torecan** (Roxane)		In 2 ml amps.[1]	925

* Cost Index based on cost per 10 mg.

[1] With ascorbic acid, sodium metabisulfite and sorbitol.

Refer to the general discussion of these products beginning on page 1227

Antidopaminergics (Cont.)

METOCLOPRAMIDE

This is an abbreviated monograph. For complete prescribing information refer to the GI Stimulants monograph.

Indications:

Parenteral: Prevention of nausea and vomiting associated with emetogenic cancer chemotherapy.

Unlabeled Uses: Studies have indicated some potential value of metoclopramide (10 mg orally or IV 30 minutes before each meal and at bedtime) in nausea and vomiting of a variety of etiologies (uncontrolled studies report 80% to 90% efficacy), including emesis during pregnancy and labor (5 to 10 mg orally or 5 to 20 mg IV or IM, 3 times a day).

Administration and Dosage:

Prevention of chemotherapy-induced emesis: For doses in excess of 10 mg, dilute injection in 50 ml of a parenteral solution (Dextrose 5% in Water, Sodium Chloride Injection, Dextrose 5% in 0.45% Sodium Chloride, Ringer's or Lactated Ringer's Injection). Infuse slowly IV over not less than 15 minutes, 30 minutes before beginning cancer chemotherapy; repeat every 2 hours for 2 doses, then every 3 hours for 3 doses.

The initial 2 doses should be 2 mg/kg if highly emetogenic drugs such as cisplatin or dacarbazine are used alone or in combination. For less emetogenic regimens, 1 mg/kg/dose may be adequate.

If extrapyramidal symptoms occur, administer 50 mg diphenhydramine IM.

	Product (Manufacturer)	Dosage form	How supplied	C.I.*
Rx *sf*	**Reglan** (Robins)	**Syrup:** 5 mg/5 ml (as monohydrochloride monohydrate)	In pt and UD 10 ml (100s).	77
Rx	**Metoclopramide HCl** (Quad)	**Injection:** 5 mg/ml (as monohydrochloride monohydrate)	In 2, 10, 30, 50 and 100 ml vials.	292
Rx	**Reglan** (Robins)		In 2 and 10 ml amps and 2, 10 and 30 ml vials.	380
Rx	**Reglan** (Robins)	**Tablets:** 5 mg metoclopramide HCl	In 100s.	30
Rx	**Metoclopramide** (Various)	**Tablets:** 10 mg (as monohydrochloride monohydrate)	In 100s, 500s, 1000s and UD 100s.	12+
Rx	**Clopra** (Quantum)		(#QPL/217). White, scored. In 100s, 500s and 1000s.	27
Rx	**Maxolon** (Beecham)		(#BMP 192). Blue, scored. In 100s.	20
Rx	**Octamide** (Adria)		(#Adria 230). In 100s and 500s.	39
Rx	**Reclomide** (Major)		In 100s, 500s, 1000s and UD 100s.	37
Rx	**Reglan** (Robins)		(#Reglan AHR 10). Pink, scored. In 100s, 500s and UD 100s.	50

* Cost Index based on cost per 10 mg.
\# Product identification code.
sf – Sugar free.

Refer to the general discussion of these products beginning on page 1227

Anticholinergics

CYCLIZINE AND MECLIZINE

Actions:

Cyclizine and meclizine have antiemetic, anticholinergic and antihistaminic properties. They reduce the sensitivity of the labyrinthine apparatus. The action may be mediated through nerve pathways to the vomiting center (VC) from the chemoreceptor trigger zone (CTZ), peripheral nerve pathways, the VC or other CNS centers.

Cyclizine and meclizine have an onset of action of 30 to 60 minutes, depending on dosage; their duration of action is 4 to 6 hours and 12 to 24 hours, respectively.

Indications:

Prevention and treatment of nausea, vomiting and dizziness of motion sickness.

Meclizine is *"possibly effective"* for the management of vertigo associated with diseases affecting the vestibular system.

Contraindications:

Hypersensitivity to cyclizine or meclizine.

Warnings:

Pregnancy. Category B: Cyclizine and meclizine have been teratogenic in rodents, but large scale human studies have not demonstrated adverse fetal effects. Use only when clearly needed and when the potential benefits outweigh the potential hazards to the fetus. It has been suggested that, based on available data, meclizine presents the lowest risk of teratogenicity and is the drug of first choice in treating nausea and vomiting during pregnancy.

Lactation: Safety for use in the nursing mother has not been established.

Children: Safety and efficacy for use in children have not been established. Not recommended for use in children under 12 years of age.

Precautions:

Potentially hazardous tasks: May produce drowsiness; patients should observe caution while driving or performing other tasks requiring alertness.

Because of the anticholinergic action of these agents, use with caution and with appropriate monitoring in patients with glaucoma, obstructive disease of the GI or GU tract and in elderly males with possible prostatic hypertrophy. These drugs may have a hypotensive action, which may be confusing or dangerous in postoperative patients.

May have additive effects with alcohol and other CNS depressants (eg, hypnotics, sedatives, tranquilizers, antianxiety agents); use with caution.

Adverse Reactions:

CNS: Drowsiness; restlessness; excitation; nervousness; insomnia; euphoria; blurred vision; diplopia; vertigo; tinnitus; auditory and visual hallucinations (particularly when dosage recommendations are exceeded).

Dermatologic: Urticaria; rash.

GI: Dry mouth; anorexia; nausea; vomiting; diarrhea; constipation; cholestatic jaundice (cyclizine).

GU: Urinary frequency; difficult urination; urinary retention.

Cardiovascular: Hypotension; palpitations; tachycardia.

Other: Dry nose and throat.

Overdosage:

Symptoms: Moderate overdosage may cause hyperexcitability alternating with drowsiness. Massive overdosage may cause convulsions, hallucinations and respiratory paralysis.

Treatment includes appropriate supportive and symptomatic treatment. Refer to General Management of Acute Overdosage on 2895 Consider dialysis.

Caution: Do not use morphine or other respiratory depressants.

(Products listed on following page)

Refer to the general discussion of these products beginning on page 1227

Anticholinergics (Cont.)

TRIMETHOBENZAMIDE HCl

Actions: The mechanism of action is obscure, but may be mediated through the chemoreceptor trigger zone (CTZ); direct impulses to the vomiting center (VC) are not inhibited.

Indications: Control of nausea and vomiting.

Contraindications: Hypersensitivity to trimethobenzamide, benzocaine or similar local anesthetics; parenteral use in children; suppositories in premature infants or neonates.

Warnings:

Pregnancy: Safety for use has not been established. Use only when clearly needed and when the potential benefits outweigh the potential hazards to the fetus.

Lactation: Safety for use in the nursing mother has not been established.

Precautions: Encephalitides, gastroenteritis, dehydration, electrolyte imbalance (especially in children and the elderly or debilitated) and CNS reactions have occurred when used during acute febrile illness.

Exercise caution when giving the drug with alcohol and other CNS-acting agents such as phenothiazines, barbiturates and belladonna derivatives.

Adverse Reactions:

Hypersensitivity reactions; parkinson-like symptoms; hypotension or pain following IM injection; blood dyscrasias; blurred vision; coma; convulsions; depression; diarrhea; disorientation; dizziness; drowsiness; headache; jaundice; muscle cramps; opisthotonos; allergic-type skin reactions. If these occur, discontinue use. While these symptoms usually disappear spontaneously, symptomatic treatment may be indicated.

Administration and Dosage:

Oral: Adults – 250 mg, 3 or 4 times daily.

Children (30 to 90 lbs; 13.6 to 40.9 kg) – 100 to 200 mg, 3 or 4 times daily.

Rectal: Adults – 200 mg, 3 or 4 times daily.

Children (30 to 90 lbs; 13.6 to 40.9 kg) – 100 to 200 mg, 3 or 4 times daily.

(< 30 lbs) – 100 mg, 3 or 4 times daily. Do not use in premature or newborn infants.

Injection: For IM use only. *Adults* – 200 mg 3 or 4 times/day. Pain, stinging, burning, redness and swelling may develop at injection site.

	Product (Manufacturer)	Form/Strength	Package	C.I.*
Rx	**Tigan** (Beecham Labs.)	**Capsules:** 100 mg	(Tigan 100 mg). In 100s.	251
Rx	**Trimazide** (Major)		In 100s.	233
Rx	**Trimethobenzamide** (Various)	**Capsules:** 250 mg	In 100s and 500s.	61+
Rx	**Tigan** (Beecham Labs.)		(Tigan 250 mg). Blue. In 100s.	121
Rx	**Trimethobenzamide** (Various)	**Pediatric Suppositories:** 100 mg	In 10s.	319+
Rx	**Triban** (Great Southern)		In 10s.[1]	351
Rx	**Tebamide** (G&W Labs)		In 10s.[1]	402
Rx	**T-Gen** (Goldline)		In 10s.[1]	285
Rx	**Tigan** (Beecham Labs.)		In 10s.[1]	965
Rx	**Trimazide** (Major)		In 10s.	153
Rx	**Trimethobenzamide** (Various)	**Suppositories:** 200 mg	In 10s and 50s.	162+
Rx	**Tebamide** (G&W)		In 10s[1] and 50s.[1]	228
Rx	**T-Gen** (Goldline)		In 10s[1] and 50s.[1]	223
Rx	**Tigan** (Beecham Labs.)		In 10s[1] and 50s.[1]	517
Rx	**Triban** (Great Southern)		In 10s[1] and 50s.	279
Rx	**Trimazide** (Major)		In 10s.	452
Rx	**Trimethobenzamide HCl** (Various)	**Injection:** 100 mg per ml	In 2 ml amps and 20 ml vials.	218+
Rx	**Arrestin** (Vortech)		In 20 ml vials.[2]	543
Rx	**Ticon** (Hauck)		In 20 ml vials.[2]	445
Rx	**Tiject-20** (Mayrand)		In 20 ml vials.[2]	615
Rx	**Tigan** (Beecham Labs.)		In 2 ml amps[3], 20 ml vials[2] and 2 ml syringe.[4]	651

* Cost Index based on cost per 200 mg.
[1] With 2% benzocaine.
[2] With phenol.
[3] With methyl and propyl parabens.
[4] With phenol and EDTA.

Refer to the general discussion of these products beginning on page 1227

Anticholinergics (Cont.)

SCOPOLAMINE, TRANSDERMAL

Actions:

In addition to its systemic anticholinergic effects, scopolamine is effective in motion sickness. Refer to the Gastrointestinal Anticholinergic/Antispasmodics monograph.

Scopolamine is a belladonna alkaloid with well-known pharmacological properties. The drug has a long history of oral and parenteral use for central anticholinergic activity, including prophylaxis of motion sickness. The mechanism of action of scopolamine in the CNS is not definitely known but may include anticholinergic effects. The ability of scopolamine to prevent motion-induced nausea is believed to be associated with inhibition of vestibular input to the CNS, which results in inhibition of the vomiting reflex. In addition, scopolamine may have a direct action on the vomiting center within the reticular formation of the brain stem.

The transdermal system is a 0.2 mm thick film with four layers. It is 2.5 cm^2 in area and contains 1.5 mg scopolamine which is gradually released from an adhesive matrix of mineral oil and polyisobutylene following application to the postauricular skin. An initial priming dose released from the system's adhesive layer saturates the skin binding site for scopolamine and rapidly brings the plasma concentration to the required steady-state level. A continuous controlled release of scopolamine flows from the drug reservoir through the rate controlling membrane to maintain a constant plasma level. Antiemetic protection is produced within several hours following application behind the ear.

In clinical studies at sea or in a controlled motion environment, there was a 75% reduction in the incidence of motion-induced nausea and vomiting. The system provided significantly greater protection than that obtained with oral dimenhydrinate.

Indications:

Prevention of nausea and vomiting associated with motion sickness in adults.

Contraindications:

Hypersensitivity to scopolamine or any component of the product; glaucoma.

Warnings:

Potentially alarming idiosyncratic reactions may occur with therapeutic doses.

Pregnancy: Category C. Studies in rabbits at plasma levels approximately 100 times those achieved in humans using a transdermal system revealed a marginal embryotoxic effect. Use in pregnancy only if potential benefits justify potential risk to the fetus.

Lactation: It is not known whether scopolamine is excreted in breast milk. Exercise caution when administering to a nursing woman.

Children: Safety and efficacy have not been established. Children are particularly susceptible to the side effects of belladonna alkaloids. Do not use the transdermal system in children.

Precautions:

Use with caution in patients with pyloric obstruction, urinary bladder neck obstruction and in patients suspected of having intestinal obstruction. Use with special caution in the elderly or in individuals with impaired metabolic, liver or kidney functions because of the increased likelihood of CNS effects.

Potentially hazardous tasks: May produce drowsiness, disorientation and confusion. Warn patients against engaging in activities that require mental alertness, such as driving a motor vehicle or operating dangerous machinery.

In patients taking drugs which cause CNS effects, including alcohol, use scopolamine with care.

Drug Withdrawal: Dizziness, nausea, vomiting, headache and disturbances of equilibrium have been reported in a few patients following discontinuation of the use of the transdermal system. This occurred most often in patients who used the system for more than 3 days.

Adverse Reactions:

Most common: Dry mouth (67%); drowsiness ($<$ 17%); transient impairment of eye accommodation including blurred vision and dilation of the pupils. Unilateral fixed and dilated pupil has been reported, apparently from accidentally touching one eye after manipulation of the patch.

Infrequent: Disorientation; memory disturbances; dizziness; restlessness; hallucinations; confusion; difficulty urinating; rashes or erythema; acute narrow-angle glaucoma; dry, itchy or red eyes.

(Continued on following page)

SCOPOLAMINE, TRANSDERMAL (Cont.)

Overdosage:

Disorientation, memory disturbances, dizziness, restlessness, hallucinations or confusion. Remove the system immediately if these symptoms occur. Initiate appropriate parasympathomimetic therapy if symptoms are severe. Refer to General Management of Acute Overdosage on p. 2895

For information on overdosage with other dose forms, refer to the GI Anticholinergics/ Antispasmodics monograph.

Patient Information:

Patient package insert is available with the transdermal product.

Medication may cause dry mouth. May produce drowsiness or blurred vision; patients should observe caution while driving or performing other tasks requiring alertness. If eye pain, blurred vision, dizziness or rapid pulse occurs, discontinue use and consult physician.

Wash hands thoroughly after handling the transdermal disc. Temporary dilation of the pupils and blurred vision may occur if scopolamine comes in contact with the eyes.

Administration and Dosage:

Initiation of therapy: Apply one system to the postauricular skin (ie, behind the ear) at least 4 hours before the antiemetic effect is required. Scopolamine 0.5 mg will be delivered over 3 days. Wear only one disc at a time.

Handling: After applying the disc on dry skin behind the ear, wash hands thoroughly with soap and water, then dry them. Discard the removed disc and wash the hands and application site thoroughly with soap and water to prevent any traces of scopolamine from coming into direct contact with the eyes.

Continuation of Therapy: If the disc is displaced, discard it and place a fresh one on the hairless area behind the other ear. If therapy is required for longer than 3 days, discard the first disc and place a fresh one on the hairless area behind the other ear.

Rx	**Transderm-Scōp** (Ciba)	**Transdermal Therapeutic System:** 1.5 mg scopolamine (delivers 0.5 mg scopolamine in vivo over 3 days)	(#4345). In 4 unit blister packs.

* Cost Index based on cost per 0.25 mg oral scopolamine.
# Product identification code.

Refer to the general discussion of these products beginning on page 1227

Miscellaneous

DIPHENIDOL

Diphenidol may cause hallucinations, disorientation or confusion. Limit use to patients who are hospitalized or under comparable continuous, professional supervision. Carefully weigh benefits against possible risks and consider alternate therapeutic measures.

Actions:

Diphenidol exerts a specific antivertigo effect on the vestibular apparatus to control vertigo, and inhibits the chemoreceptor trigger zone (CTZ) to control nausea and vomiting.

Indications:

Peripheral (labyrinthine) vertigo and associated nausea and vomiting; Meniere's disease and middle and inner ear surgery (labyrinthitis).

Control of nausea and vomiting in postoperative states, malignant neoplasms and labyrinthine disturbances.

Contraindications:

Hypersensitivity to diphenidol; anuria (since approximately 90% of the drug is excreted in the urine, accumulation could occur); nausea and vomiting of pregnancy.

Warnings:

CNS effects: The incidence of auditory and visual hallucinations, disorientation and confusion appears to be < 0.5%, or approximately one in 350 patients. The reaction usually occurs within 3 days of starting the drug and subsides spontaneously, usually within 3 days after discontinuation. If such a reaction occurs, discontinue the drug.

Pregnancy: Safety for use during pregnancy has not been established. Use only when clearly needed and when the potential benefits outweigh the potential hazards to the fetus. Do not use diphenidol for nausea and vomiting of pregnancy.

Lactation: Safety for use in the nursing mother has not been established. Weigh benefits against potential hazards.

Children: Diphenidol is not recommended for use in children < 50 pounds.

Precautions:

The antiemetic action may mask signs of drug overdose or may obscure diagnosis of conditions such as intestinal obstruction and brain tumor.

Diphenidol has a weak peripheral anticholinergic effect; use with care in patients with glaucoma, obstructive lesions of the GI and GU tracts such as stenosing peptic ulcer, prostatic hypertrophy, pyloric and duodenal obstruction and organic cardiospasm.

Tartrazine sensitivity: This product contains tartrazine, which may cause allergic-type reactions (including bronchial asthma) in susceptible individuals. Although the incidence of tartrazine sensitivity in the general population is low, it is frequently seen in patients who also have aspirin hypersensitivity.

Adverse Reactions:

CNS: Auditory and visual hallucinations; disorientation; confusion; drowsiness; overstimulation; depression; sleep disturbance; blurred vision. Rarely: Slight dizziness, malaise, headache.

Cardiovascular: Slight, transient lowering of blood pressure.

GI: Dry mouth; nausea; indigestion; heartburn (rare).

Hepatic: Mild jaundice (relationship not established).

Miscellaneous: Skin rash.

Overdosage:

Treatment includes usual supportive measures. Refer to General Management of Acute Overdosage on 2895 Early gastric lavage may be indicated, depending on the amount of overdose and symptoms.

Administration and Dosage:

Adults: For vertigo or nausea and vomiting. The usual dose is 25 mg every 4 hours. Some patients may require 50 mg.

Children: For nausea and vomiting only. The usual dose is 0.4 mg/lb (0.88 mg/kg). The dosage for children 50 to 100 lbs is 25 mg. Do not give more often than every 4 hours. However, if symptoms persist after the first dose, repeat after 1 hour. Thereafter, administer every 4 hours, as needed. The total dose in 24 hours should not exceed 2.5 mg/lb (5.5 mg/kg).

				C.I.*
Rx	**Vontrol** (SKF)	**Tablets:** 25 mg (as HCl)	Tartrazine. (#SKF 25). Orange. In 100s.	94

* Cost Index based on cost per 25 mg. # Product identification code.

Miscellaneous (Cont.)

BENZQUINAMIDE HCl

Actions:

Benzquinamide HCl has antiemetic, antihistaminic, mild anticholinergic and sedative action in animals. The mechanism of action in humans is unknown.

Pharmacokinetics: The onset of antiemetic activity usually occurs within 15 minutes. Benzquinamide is about 58% plasma protein bound. Most of the drug undergoes metabolism in the liver; 5% to 10% of the drug is excreted unchanged in the urine. Elimination half-life is about 40 minutes.

Indications:

Prevention and treatment of nausea and vomiting associated with anesthesia and surgery. Restrict prophylactic use to those patients in whom emesis would endanger the surgical outcome or result in harm to the patient.

Contraindications:

Hypersensitivity to benzquinamide HCl.

Warnings:

Cardiovascular effects: Sudden increase in blood pressure and transient arrhythmias (premature ventricular and atrial contractions) have occurred following IV administration; thus, the IM route is preferable. Restrict IV route to patients without cardiovascular disease who are receiving no preanesthetic or concomitant cardiovascular drugs.

Benzquinamide may mask signs of drug overdosage or obscure such conditions as intestinal obstruction and brain tumor.

Pregnancy: Safety for use during pregnancy has not been established; usage in pregnancy is not recommended.

Children: Safety and efficacy for use in children have not been established.

Drug Interactions:

Pressor agents: Give benzquinamide in fractions of the normal dose. Monitor blood pressure, particularly in hypertensive patients.

Adverse Reactions:

Drowsiness appears to be the most common reaction.

Autonomic nervous system: Dry mouth; shivering; sweating; increased temperature; hiccoughs; flushing; salivation; blurred vision; chills.

CNS: Drowsiness; insomnia; fatigue; restlessness; dizziness; headache; excitement; nervousness.

Cardiovascular: Hypertension; hypotension; atrial fibrillation; premature atrial and ventricular contractions.

GI: Anorexia; nausea.

Musculoskeletal: Twitching; shaking/tremors; weakness.

Dermatologic: Hives/rash; allergic reaction (pyrexia and urticaria [one case]).

Overdosage:

Symptoms: Overdosage in humans may manifest itself as a combination of CNS stimulant and depressant effects.

Treatment includes usual supportive measures. There is no specific antidote for benzquinamide. Refer to General Management of Acute Overdosage. Atropine may be helpful. Dialysis is not likely to be of value since benzquinamide is extensively bound to plasma protein.

Patient Information:

Medication may cause dry mouth.

Administration and Dosage:

IM: 50 mg (0.5 to 1 mg/kg). Repeat first dose in 1 hour, then every 3 to 4 hours, as necessary. Use the deltoid area only if well developed. To prevent nausea and vomiting, give IM at least 15 minutes prior to emergence from anesthesia.

IV: 25 mg (0.2 to 0.4 mg/kg as a single dose) slowly (1 ml/0.5 to 1 minute). Give subsequent doses IM.

Restrict IV use to patients without cardiovascular disease (see Warnings). If used IV in the elderly or debilitated, administer cautiously and in the lower dose range.

Preparation and storage of solution: Reconstitute initially with 2.2 ml of Sterile Water or Bacteriostatic Water for Injection with benzyl alcohol or with methyl- and propylparaben. This yields 2 ml of a solution equivalent to 25 mg benzquinamide/ml; it is potent for 14 days at room temperature.

			C.I.*
Rx	**Emete-Con** (Roerig)	**Injection:** 50 mg per vial.	1837

* Cost Index based on cost per 50 mg.

Refer to the general discussion of these products beginning on page 1227

Miscellaneous (Cont.)

DRONABINOL

Actions:

Pharmacology: Dronabinol is the principal psychoactive substance present in *Cannabis sativa L* (marijuana). It is used in the treatment of nausea and vomiting associated with cancer chemotherapy. Nontherapeutic effects of dronabinol are identical to those of marijuana and other centrally active cannabinoids (see Warnings). The mechanism of action is unknown.

Cannabinoids have complex CNS effects. Patients may experience mood changes (eg, euphoria, detachment, depression, anxiety, panic, paranoia), decrements in cognitive performance and memory, a decreased ability to control drives and impulses, and alterations of reality (eg, distortions in perception of objects and sense of time, hallucinations). These latter phenomena are more common with larger doses; however, a full blown picture of psychosis (psychotic organic brain syndrome) may occur in patients receiving doses in the lower portion of the therapeutic range.

Dronabinol, within or slightly above the recommended dose range, increases heart rate and conjunctival injection. Blood pressure effects are inconsistent, but occasional subjects experience orthostatic hypotension or fainting upon standing. In one study, a slight but consistent decrease in oral temperature was recorded.

Pharmacokinetics: Absorption/Distribution – Following oral administration, dronabinol has a systemic bioavailability of 10% to 20%. The drug undergoes extensive first-pass metabolism. Numerous metabolites have been identified, including 11-hydroxy-THC, which is psychoactive. It appears in plasma in roughly the same quantities as the parent drug. The maximum plasma concentrations of dronabinol and 11-hydroxy-THC occur approximately 2 to 3 hours after oral dosing.

Metabolism/Excretion – Biliary excretion is the major route of elimination. Within 72 hours following oral administration, ≈ 50% of the dose is recovered in feces; another 10% to 15% appears in the urine either unchanged or as a metabolite. Renal clearance in healthy individuals is ≈ 10% of the glomerular filtration rate. The elimination phase of dronabinol exhibits biphasic kinetics with an alpha half-life of 4 hours and a terminal half-life of 25 to 36 hours. The terminal plasma half-life for 11-hydroxy-THC is ≈ 15 to 18 hours. Extended use at the recommended doses may cause accumulation of toxic amounts of dronabinol and its metabolites.

Indications:

Treatment of nausea and vomiting associated with cancer chemotherapy in patients who have failed to respond adequately to conventional antiemetic treatment.

Because dronabinol may alter the mental state, it is intended for use when the patient can be closely supervised.

Contraindications:

Nausea and vomiting from any cause other than cancer chemotherapy; hypersensitivity to dronabinol, marijuana or sesame oil.

Warnings:

Drug abuse and dependence: Dronabinol is highly abusable. Limit prescriptions to the amount necessary for a single cycle of chemotherapy.

It is not known what proportion of individuals exposed chronically to these drugs will develop either psychological or physical dependence. Long-term use of cannabinoids has been associated with disorders of motivation, judgment and cognition. It is not clear if this is a manifestation of the underlying personalities of chronic users of this class of drugs, or if cannabinoids are directly responsible.

Following 30 days of dronabinol, tolerance to the cardiovascular and subjective effects developed at doses up to 210 mg/day. An initial tachycardia induced by dronabinol was replaced successively by normal sinus rhythm and then bradycardia. A fall in supine blood pressure, made worse by standing, was also observed initially. Within days, these effects disappeared, indicating development of tolerance.

A withdrawal syndrome consisting of irritability, insomnia and restlessness was observed in some subjects within 12 hours following abrupt withdrawal of dronabinol. The syndrome reached its peak intensity at 24 hours when subjects exhibited hot flashes, sweating, rhinorrhea, loose stools, hiccoughs and anorexia. The syndrome was essentially complete within 96 hours. EEG changes following discontinuation were consistent with a withdrawal syndrome. Several subjects reported impressions of disturbed sleep for several weeks after discontinuing high doses.

(Warnings continued on following page)

DRONABINOL (Cont.)

Warnings (Cont):

Hazardous tasks: Because of its profound effects on mental status, warn patients not to drive, operate complex machinery or engage in any activity requiring sound judgment and unimpaired coordination while receiving treatment. Effects may persist for a variable and unpredictable period of time. Dronabinol is highly lipid soluble, and its metabolites may persist in tissues, including plasma, for days.

Patient supervision: Because of individual variation, determine clinically the period of patient supervision required. Closely observe patients receiving cannabinoids within an inpatient setting, if possible. This is especially important during treatment of patients with no prior experience with cannabis or dronabinol. However, even patients experienced with these agents may have serious untoward responses not predicted by prior uneventful exposures. Closely observe any patient who has a psychotic experience with dronabinol until the mental state returns to normal. Do not give additional doses until the patient has been examined and the circumstances evaluated. If the situation warrants it, give a lower dose under very close supervision.

Pregnancy: Category B. There are no adequate and well controlled studies in pregnant women. Use during pregnancy only if clearly needed.

Lactation: Dronabinol is concentrated and excreted in breast milk, and is absorbed by the nursing baby. Because the effects on the infant of chronic exposure to the drug and its metabolites are unknown, nursing mothers should not use dronabinol.

Precautions:

Use with caution in the following situations: Patients with hypertension or heart disease. since dronabinol may cause a general increase in central sympathomimetic activity.

Manic, depressive or schizophrenic patients; symptoms of these disease states may be unmasked by the use of cannabinoids.

Individuals receiving other psychoactive drugs (see Drug Interactions).

Drug Interactions:

Alcohol, sedatives, hypnotics or other **psychotomimetic substances:** Do not give dronabinol in combination with any CNS depressants. Effects of dronabinol on blood ethanol levels are complex. During subchronic dronabinol administration (60 mg/day) for 10 days, lower and delayed peak blood alcohol levels occurred. Ethanol metabolism increased in some subjects and decreased in others. The overall rate of ethanol disappearance was decreased by about 10%.

Adverse Reactions:

Dronabinol Adverse Reactions (%)

Body system/ adverse reaction	Dronabinol (n = 317)	Placebo (n = 68)	Body system/ adverse reaction	Dronabinol (n = 317)	Placebo (n = 68)
CNS			*CNS (cont.)*		
Drowsiness	48	49	Tinnitus	< 1	nd
High, heightened awareness, euphoria	24	nd	Nightmares	< 1	nd
Dizziness	21	1	*Autonomic nervous system*		
Anxiety	16	24	Dry mouth	3	1
Muddled thinking	12	1	Paresthesia	3	1
Perceptual difficulties	11	0	Visual distortions	3	0
Coordination impairment	9	10	Speech difficulty	< 1	nd
Irritability/weird feeling	7	0	Facial flushing	< 1	nd
Depression	7	15	Perspiring	< 1	nd
Weakness, sluggishness	6	1	*Cardiovascular*		
Headache	6	4	Tachycardia	1	0
Hallucinations	5	0	Postural hypotension	1	0
Memory lapse	5	0	Syncope	< 1	nd
Unsteadiness, ataxia	4	0	*Other*		
Paranoia	2	0	Diarrhea	< 1	nd
Depersonalization	2	0	Fecal incontinence	< 1	nd
Disorientation, confusion	1	2	Muscular pains	< 1	nd

nd = No data.

(Continued on following page)

DRONABINOL (Cont.)

Overdosage:

Signs and symptoms of overdosage are an extension of psychotomimetic and physiologic effects. The clinical picture may vary widely between patients. Overdosages are of two types: Those at therapeutic doses and those at higher, supratherapeutic doses.

Overdosage at prescribed dosages may produce disturbing psychiatric symptoms. Observe patient in a quiet environment and provide supportive measures, including reassurance. Withhold subsequent doses until the patient has returned to baseline mental status. If indicated, resume routine dosing at a lower dosage. Reactions spontaneously disappear within 24 hours without specific therapy.

Monitor vital signs; tachycardia, hypotension and hypertension are common adverse reactions. Treat, if necessary, in the usual manner.

Overdosage at multiples of prescribed dosages was not reported in controlled clinical studies. Few deaths have occurred from the use of dronabinol in any of its many forms (eg, hashish, marijuana). Two deaths following the ingestion of large overdoses of Indian hemp have occurred, while one death resulting from smoking cannabis herb or resin occurred. The estimated acute lethal IV dose of dronabinol is 1 to 2 g; this is a fivefold to tenfold multiple of the maximum oral dose recommended for dronabinol in 24 hours.

Treatment: If psychotic episodes occur, manage the patient conservatively, if possible. For moderate psychotic episodes and anxiety reactions, verbal support and comforting may be sufficient. Treatment for respiratory depression and comatose state consists of symptomatic and supportive therapy. Pay particular attention to the occurrence of hypothermia. Refer to General Management of Acute Overdosage.

Patient Information:

Avoid alcohol and barbiturates.

May cause dizziness or drowsiness; do not drive or perform hazardous tasks requiring alertness.

Apprise patients of possible changes in mood and other adverse behavioral effects of the drug so they will not panic in the event of such manifestations.

Patients should remain under supervision of a responsible adult.

Administration and Dosage:

Initially, give 5 mg/m², 1 to 3 hours prior to the administration of chemotherapy, then every 2 to 4 hours after chemotherapy is given, for a total of 4 to 6 doses/day. If the 5 mg/m² dose is ineffective, and there are no significant side effects, increase the dose by 2.5 mg/m² increments to a maximum of 15 mg/m² per dose. Use caution, however, as the incidence of disturbing psychiatric symptoms increases significantly at this maximum dose.

c-II	**Marinol** (Roxane)	**Gelatin Capsules**[1]: 2.5 mg	(RL). White. In 25s.
		5 mg	(RL). Brown. In 25s.
		10 mg	(RL). Orange. In 25s.

[1] In sesame oil.

PHOSPHORATED CARBOHYDRATE SOLUTION

Actions:

Hyperosmolar carbohydrate solutions with phosphoric acid relieve nausea and vomiting by a direct local action on the wall of the GI tract that reduces smooth muscle contraction and delays gastric emptying time in direct proportion to the amount used.

The data available do not appear sufficient to document effectiveness.

Indications:

Symptomatic relief of nausea and vomiting.

Precautions:

Nausea may signal a serious condition. If symptoms are not relieved or recur often, consult a physician.

Diabetic patients should avoid these preparations because they contain significant amounts of carbohydrates.

Hereditary fructose intolerance: Individuals with this condition should avoid these preparations.

Adverse Reactions:

Large doses of fructose can cause abdominal pain and diarrhea.

Administration and Dosage:

Do not dilute. Do not take oral fluids immediately before the dose, or for at least 15 minutes after the dose.

Epidemic and other functional vomiting, or nausea and vomiting due to psychogenic factors:

Infants and children – 5 or 10 ml at 15 minute intervals until vomiting ceases. Do not take for more than 1 hour (5 doses).

Adults – 15 or 30 ml in same manner. If first dose is rejected, resume same dosage schedule in 5 minutes.

Regurgitation in infants: 5 or 10 ml, 10 to 15 minutes before each feeding; in refractory cases, 10 or 15 ml, 30 minutes before feeding.

Morning sickness: 15 to 30 ml on arising; repeat every 3 hours or when nausea threatens.

Motion sickness and nausea and vomiting due to drug therapy or inhalation anesthesia: 5 ml doses for young children; 15 ml doses for older children and adults.

				C.I.*
otc	**Naus-A-Way** (Hauck)	**Solution:** Fructose, dextrose and orthophosphoric acid with controlled hydrogen ion concentration	In 473 ml.	93
otc	**Emetrol** (Bock)		Lemon-mint flavor. In 120 and 480 ml.	223
otc	**Nausetrol** (Various)		In 120 ml, pt and gal.	49+

* Cost Index based on cost per 15 ml.

MEPROBAMATE

Actions:

Pharmacology: Meprobamate, an antianxiety agent, is a carbamate derivative that has selective effects at multiple sites in the CNS, including the thalamus and limbic system. It also appears to inhibit multineuronal spinal reflexes. Meprobamate is mildly tranquilizing, and has some anticonvulsant and muscle relaxant properties.

Pharmacokinetics: Absorption/Distribution – Meprobamate is well absorbed from the GI tract; peak plasma concentrations are reached within 1 to 3 hours. During chronic administration of sedative doses, concentrations in blood range between 5 and 20 mcg/ml. Plasma protein binding is approximately 15%.

Metabolism/Excretion – The liver metabolizes 80% to 92% of the drug; the remainder is excreted unchanged in the urine. Following a single dose, the plasma half-life ranges from 6 to 17 hours, but during chronic administration, may be as long as 24 to 48 hours. Meprobamate can induce some hepatic microsomal enzymes, but it is not known whether it induces its own metabolism. Excretion is mainly renal (90%), with < 10% appearing in feces.

Indications:

Management of anxiety disorders or short-term relief of the symptoms of anxiety. Anxiety or tension associated with the stress of everyday life usually does not require treatment with an anxiolytic.

Effectiveness in long-term use (> 4 months) has not been assessed by systematic clinical studies. Periodically reassess usefulness of the drug for the individual patient.

Contraindications:

Acute intermittent porphyria; allergic or idiosyncratic reactions to meprobamate or related compounds (eg, carisoprodol).

Warnings:

Drug dependence: Physical and psychological dependence and abuse may occur. Avoid prolonged use, especially in alcoholics and addiction prone persons. Consider possibility of suicide attempts. Carefully supervise dose and amounts prescribed; dispense least amount of drug feasible at any one time.

Abrupt discontinuation after prolonged and excessive use may precipitate a recurrence of pre-existing symptoms or withdrawal syndrome characterized by anxiety, anorexia, insomnia, vomiting, ataxia, tremors, muscle twitching, confusional states and hallucinations. Generalized seizures occur in about 10% of cases and are more likely to occur in persons with CNS damage or preexistent or latent convulsive disorders. Onset of withdrawal symptoms usually occurs within 12 to 48 hours after drug discontinuation; symptoms usually cease in the next 12 to 48 hours.

When excessive dosage has continued for weeks or months, reduce gradually over a period of 1 or 2 weeks rather than stopping abruptly. Alternatively, a short-acting barbiturate may be substituted and then gradually withdrawn.

Hypersensitivity: Usually seen between the first to fourth dose in patients having no previous exposure to the drug. In case of allergic or idiosyncratic reactions, discontinue the drug and initiate approprate symptomatic therapy, which may include epinephrine, antihistamines and in severe cases, corticosteroids. In evaluating possible allergic reactions, also consider allergy to excipients. See Adverse Reactions. Refer to Management of Acute Hypersensitivity Reactions.

Renal and hepatic function impairment: Use with caution to avoid accumulation, since meprobamate is metabolized in the liver and excreted by the kidney.

Elderly or debilitated patients: To avoid oversedation, use lowest effective dose.

Pregnancy: Meprobamate passes the placental barrier. It is present in umbilical cord blood, at or near maternal plasma levels. An increased risk of congenital malformations is associated with its use during the first trimester of pregnancy. Since few indications exist for this drug in the pregnant woman, use with extreme caution, if at all, during pregnancy. Consider the possibility that a woman of childbearing potential may be pregnant at the time of institution of therapy.

Lactation: Meprobamate is excreted into breast milk at concentrations 2 to 4 times that of maternal plasma. The effect of this amount of drug on the nursing infant is unknown.

Children: Do not administer to children < 6 years of age since there is a lack of documented evidence of safety and efficacy. The 600 mg tablet is not intended for use in children.

Precautions:

Epilepsy: May precipitate seizures in epileptic patients.

Potentially hazardous tasks: May produce drowsiness, dizziness or blurred vision; patients should observe caution while driving or performing other tasks requiring alertness.

(Continued on following page)

MEPROBAMATE (Cont.)

Drug Interactions:

Alcohol: Acute ingestion may result in a decreased clearance of meprobamate through inhibition of hepatic metabolic systems; enhanced CNS depressant effects may occur. Tolerance may occur with chronic alcohol ingestion, presumably due to enhanced metabolic capacity.

CNS depressants (eg, barbiturates, narcotics): Anticipate additive CNS depressant effects.

Adverse Reactions:

CNS: Drowsiness; ataxia; dizziness; slurred speech; headache; vertigo; weakness; impairment of visual accommodation; euphoria; overstimulation; paradoxical excitement; fast EEG activity.

GI: Nausea; vomiting; diarrhea.

Cardiovascular: Palpitations; tachycardia; various arrhythmias; transient ECG changes; syncope and hypotensive crises (including one fatality).

Allergic or idiosyncratic: Usually seen between the first to fourth dose in patients having no previous exposure to the drug.

Milder reactions are characterized by an itchy, urticarial or erythematous maculopapular rash which may be generalized or confined to the groin. Other reactions have included leukopenia, acute nonthrombocytopenic purpura, petechiae, ecchymoses, eosinophilia, peripheral edema, adenopathy, fever, fixed drug eruption with cross reaction to **carisoprodol**.

More severe, rare hypersensitivity reactions include hyperpyrexia, chills, angioneurotic edema, bronchospasm, oliguria, anuria, anaphylaxis, erythema multiforme, exfoliative dermatitis, stomatitis and proctitis. Stevens-Johnson syndrome and bullous dermatitis have also occurred, including one fatal case of the latter after administration of meprobamate in combination with prednisolone (see Warnings).

Hematologic: Agranulocytosis and aplastic anemia (rarely fatal) have occurred, but no causal relationship has been established. Rarely, thrombocytopenic purpura.

Other: Exacerbation of porphyric symptoms; paresthesias.

Overdosage:

Symptoms: Acute intoxication produces drowsiness, lethargy, stupor, ataxia, coma, shock, vasomotor and respiratory collapse and death. Cardiovascular disturbances include arrhythmias, tachycardia, bradycardia and reduced venous return. Profound and persistent hypotension occurs and can appear unexpectedly in mildly comatose patients. Excessive oronasal secretion or relaxation of the pharyngeal wall may cause airway obstruction problems. The following data represent the usual ranges:

Acute simple overdose (meprobamate alone) – Death has occurred with ingestion of as little as 12 g and survival with as much as 40 g.

Blood levels –

0.5 to 3 mg/dl – Therapeutic range.
3 to 10 mg/dl – Mild to moderate overdosage; stupor, light coma.
10 to 20 mg/dl – Deeper coma requiring intensive therapy; some fatalities.
$>$ 20 mg/dl – $>$ 50% fatalities.

Acute combined overdose with other psychotropic drugs, other CNS depressants or alcohol renders the above values useless as a prognostic indicator.

Treatment: Since meprobamate is rapidly absorbed, gastric lavage (or emesis in a conscious patient) may be of value only if carried out shortly after ingestion. Ingestion of large amounts may form drug conglomerates in the stomach; continue gastric lavage. Gastroscopy may be indicated. Relapse and death after initial recovery have been attributed to incomplete gastric emptying and delayed absorption. Frequent measurements of vital signs cannot be overemphasized.

Provide symptomatic and supportive treatment. Hypotension may appear rapidly and become persistent unless blood volume is expanded. Avoid fluid overload; fatal pulmonary edema has occurred. Provide respiratory assistance when needed. Exercise care in the treatment of convulsions because of the combined effect of agents on CNS depression. Refer to General Management of Acute Overdosage.

If the patient's condition deteriorates despite assisted respiration, try forced diuresis and pressor agents, then institute hemodialysis. Meprobamate is dialyzable. Hemoperfusion (resin or charcoal) is more effective than hemodialysis. The half-life during hemoperfusion may be reduced more than threefold.

(Continued on following page)

MEPROBAMATE (Cont.)

Patient Information:

Advise patients that if they become pregnant during therapy or intend to become pregnant, they should consult with their physician about use of the drug.

May cause drowsiness, dizziness or blurred vision; use caution while driving or performing other tasks requiring alertness.

Avoid alcohol and other CNS depressants while taking this drug.

Notify physician if skin rash, sore throat or fever occurs.

Do not crush or chew tablets and sustained release capsules.

Administration and Dosage:

Adults: 1.2 to 1.6 g/day in 3 to 4 divided doses; do not exceed 2.4 g/day.
Sustained release – 400 to 800 mg in the morning and at bedtime.

Children (6 to 12 years): 100 to 200 mg 2 or 3 times daily.
Sustained release – 200 mg in the morning and at bedtime.

	Product	Dosage form	Description	C.I.*
c-IV	**Meprobamate** (Various, eg, Balan, Dixon-Shane, Geneva, Goldline, Lannett, Major, Moore, Rugby, Schein, Spencer Mead)	**Tablets:** 200 mg	In 20s, 100s and 1000s.	5+
c-IV	**Equanil** (Wyeth-Ayerst)		(Wyeth 2). White. In 100s.	72
c-IV	**Miltown** (Wallace)		(Wallace 37 1101). White. Sugar coated. In 100s.	258
c-IV	**Meprobamate** (Various, eg, Balan, Dixon-Shane, Geneva, Goldline, Lannett, Major, Moore, Rugby, Schein, Spencer Mead)	**Tablets:** 400 mg	In 20s, 100s, 500s, 1000s and UD 100s.	3+
c-IV	**Equanil** (Wyeth-Ayerst)		(Wyeth 1). White, scored. In 100s and 500s.	45
c-IV	**Miltown** (Wallace)		(Wallace 37 1001). White, scored. In 100s, 500s and 1000s.	158
c-IV	**Neuramate** (Halsey)		In 100s and 1000s.	8
c-IV	**Miltown 600** (Wallace)	**Tablets:** 600 mg	(Wallace 600 37 1601). White. Capsule shape. In 100s.	164
c-IV	**Meprospan** (Wallace)	**Capsules, sustained release:** 200 mg	(Wallace 200 37-1401). Yellow. In 100s.	490
c-IV	**Meprospan** (Wallace)	**Capsules, sustained release:** 400 mg	(Wallace 400 37-1301). Blue. In 100s.	387

* Cost Index based on cost per 200 mg.

Warnings (Cont.):

Dependence: Prolonged use of therapeutic doses can lead to dependence. Withdrawal syndrome has occurred after as little as 4 to 6 weeks of treatment. It is more likely if the drug was short-acting (eg, alprazolam), if it was taken regularly for > 3 months and if it was abruptly discontinued. Higher dosages may not be a factor affecting withdrawal.

After rapid decrease of dosage or abrupt discontinuation, withdrawal seizures were reported in alprazolam patients receiving recommended (or higher) doses for brief periods of time (1 week to 4 months).

Onset is within 1 to 10 days, depending on the rate of metabolism of the agent; duration of reaction may be 5 days to a month or more depending on agent, dose, etc. Symptoms generally begin with anxiety-like manifestations; the following may occur in ≥ 50% of cases: Increased anxiety; sensory disturbances (paresthesias, hypercusis, photophobia, hypersomnia, metallic taste); flu-like illness; concentration difficulties; fatigue; restlessness; anorexia; dizziness; sweating; vomiting; insomnia; irritability; nausea; headache; muscle tension/cramps; tremor; dysphoria. Major symptoms include: Confusion; abnormal perception of movement; depersonalization; muscle twitching; "psychosis;" paranoid delusions; hallucinations; memory impairment; seizures (grand mal).

Abrupt withdrawal of **clonazepam**, particularly in those patients on long-term, high dose therapy, may precipitate status epilepticus. While clonazepam is being gradually withdrawn, the simultaneous substitution of another anticonvulsant may be indicated. Other symptoms include vomiting, diarrhea and sweating. Keep addiction-prone individuals (drug addicts or alcoholics) under careful surveillance.

When discontinuing therapy in patients who have used these agents for prolonged periods, decrease dosage gradually over 4 to 8 weeks to avoid the possibility of withdrawal symptoms, especially in patients with a history of seizures or epilepsy, regardless of their concomitant anticonvulsant drug therapy. Patients on short-acting benzodiazepines may be switched to longer-acting drugs (eg, diazepam) which produce a gradual decrease in drug concentration and decrease the chance of withdrawal symptoms. Clonidine, propranolol and carbamazepine have been used as adjuncts in the treatment of benzodiazepine withdrawal symptoms.

Parenteral administration: Parenteral (IM or IV) therapy is indicated primarily in acute states. Keep patients under observation, preferably in bed, for up to 3 hours. Do not permit ambulatory patients to operate a vehicle following an injection.

Do not inject intra-arterially; may produce arteriospasm resulting in gangrene which may require amputation.

Administer parenterally with extreme care (particularly IV) to the elderly or very ill and to those with limited pulmonary reserve. Because of the possibility of apnea or cardiac arrest, resuscitative facilities should be available. Not recommended for obstetric use. Do not administer to patients in shock, coma or in acute alcohol intoxication.

Tonic status epilepticus has been precipitated in patients treated with IV **diazepam** for petit mal status or petit mal variant status. Laryngospasm, increased cough reflex, depressed respiration, dyspnea, hyperventilation, and pain in the throat or chest have been reported during peroral endoscopic procedures; use topical anesthetics. Hypotension or muscular weakness is possible, particularly when benzodiazepines are used with narcotics, barbiturates or alcohol.

Renal or hepatic function impairment: Observe usual precautions in the presence of impaired renal or hepatic function to avoid accumulation of these agents. Lorazepam injection is not recommended in these patients. Metabolites of **clonazepam** are excreted by the kidneys; to avoid excess accumulation, exercise caution in patients with impaired renal function. Also, clonazepam is contraindicated in patients with significant liver disease.

Elderly or debilitated patients: The initial dose should be small and dosage increments made gradually, in accordance with the response of the patient, to preclude ataxia or excessive sedation. Hypotension is rare; however, use with caution if cardiac complications may result from a drop in blood pressure.

Pregnancy: Category D (No category designation for clonazepam). Benzodiazepines and their metabolites freely cross the placenta and accumulate in the fetal circulation. An increased risk of congenital malformations associated with the use of minor tranquilizers during the first trimester of pregnancy has been suggested. Malformations reported include cleft lip or palate, microcephaly and retardation, and pyloric stenosis. Recent studies suggest diazepam use in the first trimester does not cause an increased risk of cleft lip or palate. Because use of these drugs is rarely a matter of urgency, avoid their use during this period. Consider the possibility that a woman of childbearing potential may be pregnant at the time of institution of therapy. Advise patients that if they become pregnant, or plan to become pregnant during therapy, they should discuss the desirability of discontinuing the drug.

(Warnings continued on following page)

Warnings (Cont.):

Labor and delivery: Benzodiazepines have been found in maternal and cord blood, indicating placental transfer of drug. Therefore, benzodiazepines are not recommended for obstetrical use.

Neonatal withdrawal consisting of severe tremulousness and irritability has been attributed to maternal ingestion of benzodiazepines as well as neonatal flaccidity and respiratory problems. Use during labor has resulted in a "floppy infant" syndrome, manifested by hypotonia, lethargy and sucking difficulties.

Prolonged CNS depression has been observed in neonates, apparently due to inability to biotransform **diazepam** into inactive metabolites.

Lactation: Benzodiazepines are excreted in breast milk (**lorazepam** not known). Since neonates metabolize benzodiazepines more slowly than adults, accumulation of the drug and its metabolites to toxic levels is possible. Chronic **diazepam** use in nursing mothers reportedly caused infants to become lethargic and to lose weight; do not give to nursing mothers.

Children: The initial dose should be small and dosage increments made gradually, in accordance with the response of the patient, to preclude ataxia or excessive sedation. Hypotension is rare; however, use with caution if cardiac complications may result from a drop in blood pressure.

Chlordiazepoxide is not recommended in children < 6 years (oral) or 12 years (injectable).

Halazepam, prazepam, alprazolam: Safety and efficacy for use in patients < 18 years old have not been established.

Lorazepam: Do not use in patients < 18 years old (injection); safety and efficacy for use in patients < 12 years old are not established (oral).

Clorazepate: Not recommended for use in patients < 9 years old.

Diazepam: Not for use in children < 6 months old (oral); safety and efficacy have not been established in the neonate (≤ 30 days old; injectable).

Precautions:

Suicide: In those patients in whom depression accompanies anxiety, suicidal tendencies may be present, and protective measures may be required. Dispense the least amount of drug feasible to the patient.

Potentially hazardous tasks: May produce drowsiness or dizziness; observe caution while driving or performing other tasks requiring alertness.

Monitoring: Because of isolated reports of neutropenia and jaundice, perform periodic blood counts and liver function tests during long-term therapy. There have been reports of abnormal liver and kidney function tests and of decrease in hematocrit.

Paradoxical reactions: Excitement, stimulation and acute rage have occurred in psychiatric patients and hyperactive aggressive children. These reactions may be secondary to relief of anxiety and usually appear in the first 2 weeks of therapy. Acute hyperexcited states, anxiety, hallucinations, increased muscle spasticity, insomnia and sleep disturbances have also occurred. Should these occur, discontinue the drug. Minor EEG changes, usually low voltage fast activity, have been observed during and after therapy and are of no known significance. Anger, hostility and episodes of mania and hypomania have been reported with **alprazolam**.

Multiple seizure type: When used in patients in whom several different types of seizure disorders coexist, **clonazepam** may increase the incidence or precipitate the onset of generalized tonic-clonic (grand mal) seizures. This may require the addition of other anticonvulsants or an increase in their dosage.

Diazepam – If use in patients with seizure disorders results in an increase in the frequency or severity of grand mal seizures, there may be a need to increase the dosage of standard anticonvulsant medication.

Chronic respiratory disease: **Clonazepam** may produce an increase in salivation. Use with caution in patients if increased salivation causes respiratory difficulty. Due to possibility of respiratory depression, use with caution in such patients.

Tartrazine sensitivity: Some of these products contain tartrazine, which may cause allergic-type reactions (including bronchial asthma) in susceptible individuals. Although the incidence of tartrazine sensitivity in the general population is low, it is frequently seen in patients who also have aspirin hypersensitivity. Specific products containing tartrazine are identified in the product listings.

(Continued on following page)

Drug Interactions:

The elimination of benzodiazepines that undergo oxidative hepatic metabolism (alprazolam, chlordiazepoxide, clorazepate, diazepam, halazepam, prazepam) may be decreased by the following drugs due to inhibition of hepatic metabolism. Pharmacologic effects of these benzodiazepines may be increased and excessive sedation/impaired psychomotor function may occur.

cimetidine	**isoniazid**	**propoxyphene**
contraceptives, oral	**ketoconazole**	**propranolol**
disulfiram	**metoprolol**	**valproic acid**
fluoxetine		

Alcohol and other **CNS depressants (eg, barbiturates, narcotics):** Increased CNS effects (eg, impaired psychomotor function, sedation) may occur.

Antacids may alter the rate but generally not the extent of GI absorption. Staggering administration times may help avoid possible interaction.

Contraceptives, oral: The clearance rate of benzodiazepines that undergo glucuronidation (lorazepam, oxazepam) may be increased.

Digoxin's serum concentrations may be increased. Toxicity characterized by GI and neuropsychiatric symptoms and cardiac arrhythmias may occur. Monitor digoxin serum levels.

Levodopa's antiparkinson efficacy may be decreased by coadministration of benzodiazepines.

Neuromuscular blocking agents: Benzodiazepines may potentiate, counteract or have no effect on the actions of these agents.

Phenytoin serum concentrations may be increased, resulting in toxicity, but data are conflicting. Phenytoin may increase oxazepam clearance.

Probenecid may interfere with benzodiazepine conjugation in the liver, possibly resulting in a more rapid onset or prolonged effect.

Ranitidine may reduce the GI absorption of diazepam.

Rifampin: The oxidative metabolism of benzodiazepines may be increased due to microsomal enzyme induction. Pharmacologic effects of some benzodiazepines may be decreased.

Scopolamine, used concomitantly with parenteral lorazepam, may increase the incidence of sedation, hallucinations and irrational behavior.

Theophyllines may antagonize the sedative effects of the benzodiazepines.

Adverse Reactions:

Discontinuation of therapy due to undesirable effects is rare. Transient mild drowsiness is commonly seen in the first few days of therapy. Drowsiness, ataxia and confusion have occurred, especially in the elderly and debilitated. If persistent, reduce dosage. Ataxia is rare with oxazepam and does not appear to be specifically related to dose or age. Other adverse reactions less frequently reported include:

CNS: Sedation and sleepiness; depression; lethargy; apathy; fatigue; hypoactivity; lightheadedness; memory impairment; disorientation; anterograde amnesia; restlessness; confusion; crying; sobbing; delirium; headache; slurred speech; aphonia; dysarthria; stupor; seizures; coma; syncope; rigidity; tremor; dystonia; vertigo; dizziness; euphoria; nervousness; irritability; difficulty in concentration; agitation; inability to perform complex mental functions; akathisia; hemiparesis; hypotonia; unsteadiness; ataxia; incoordination; weakness; vivid dreams; psychomotor retardation; "glassy-eyed" appearance; extrapyramidal symptoms; paradoxical reactions (see Precautions).

Psychiatric: Behavior problems; hysteria; psychosis; suicidal tendencies.

GI: Constipation; diarrhea; dry mouth; coated tongue; sore gums; nausea; anorexia; change in appetite; vomiting; difficulty in swallowing; increased salivation; gastritis.

GU: Incontinence; changes in libido; urinary retention; menstrual irregularities.

Cardiovascular: Bradycardia; tachycardia; cardiovascular collapse; hypertension; hypotension; palpitations; edema; phlebitis and thrombosis at IV sites. Decrease in systolic blood pressure has been observed.

(Adverse Reactions continued on following page)

Adverse Reactions (Cont.):

EENT: Visual disturbances; diplopia; nystagmus; depressed hearing; nasal congestion; auditory disturbances.

Skin: Urticaria; pruritus; skin rash, including morbilliform, urticarial and maculopapular; dermatitis; hair loss; hirsutism; ankle and facial edema.

Other: Hiccoughs; fever; diaphoresis; paresthesias; muscular disturbance; gynecomastia; galactorrhea; respiratory disturbances; elevations of LDH, alkaline phosphatase, ALT and AST; hepatic dysfunction (including hepatitis and jaundice); leukopenia; blood dyscrasias including agranulocytosis; anemia; thrombocytopenia; eosinophilia; increase or decrease in body weight; dehydration; lymphadenopathy; joint pain; pain, burning and redness following IM injection. Partial airway obstruction has occurred and is believed to be due to excessive sedation at time of procedure (lorazepam injection).

Overdosage:

There are no well documented fatal overdoses resulting from oral ingestion of benzodiazepines alone. Most fatalities implicate benzodiazepines only as a component in multiple drug ingestions.

Symptoms: Mild symptoms include drowsiness, confusion, somnolence, impaired coordination, diminished reflexes and lethargy. These agents rarely cause significant respiratory or circulatory depression, particularly when they are the sole agents ingested. Serious symptoms may include ataxia, hypotonia, hypotension, hypnosis, stages one to three coma, and rarely, death. Consider multiple drug ingestion.

Unlike oral ingestions, IV administration of diazepam is associated with 1.7% incidence of life-threatening reactions, including hypotension and respiratory or cardiac arrest.

Treatment: Induce vomiting if it has not occurred spontaneously. Employ general supportive measures, along with immediate gastric lavage or ipecac. Follow with activated charcoal administration and a saline cathartic. Monitor respiration, pulse and blood pressure. Administer IV fluids and maintain an adequate airway. Treat hypotension with norepinephrine or metaraminol. With normal kidney function, forced diuresis with osmotic diuretics, IV fluids and electrolytes may accelerate elimination of benzodiazepines. Dialysis is of limited value; however, in more critical situations, renal dialysis and exchange blood transfusions may be indicated. Refer to General Management of Acute Overdosage.

Infusion of 0.5 to 4 mg of physostigmine IV at the rate of 1 mg/minute may reverse symptoms suggestive of central anticholinergic overdose (eg, confusion, memory disturbance, visual disturbances, hallucinations, delirium); however, weigh the hazards associated with the use of physostigmine (eg, induction of seizures) against its possible clinical benefit.

There have been occasional reports of excitation in patients following overdosage with chlordiazepoxide; if this occurs, do not give barbiturates.

Patient Information:

May cause drowsiness; avoid driving or other tasks requiring alertness.

Avoid alcohol or other CNS depressants.

May be taken with food or water if stomach upset occurs.

Patients on long-term or high dosage therapy may experience withdrawal symptoms on abrupt cessation of therapy; do not discontinue therapy abruptly or change dosage except on advice of physician.

Concomitant ingestion with antacids may alter the rate of absorption of these drugs (documented with **diazepam** and **chlordiazepoxide**).

Clonazepam, clorazepate and diazepam: Patient should carry identification (Medic Alert) indicating medication usage and epilepsy.

(Products listed on following pages)

Complete prescribing information for these products begins on page 1255

Benzodiazepines (Cont.)

OXAZEPAM

Indications:

For the management of anxiety disorders or for the short-term relief of the symptoms of anxiety. Anxiety associated with depression is also responsive to oxazepam therapy.

For the management of anxiety, tension, agitation and irritability in older patients.

Alcoholics with acute tremulousness, inebriation or with anxiety associated with alcohol withdrawal are responsive to therapy.

Administration and Dosage:

Individualize dosage.

Mild to moderate anxiety, with associated tension, irritability, agitation or related symptoms of functional origin or secondary to organic disease: 10 to 15 mg 3 or 4 times daily.

Severe anxiety syndromes, agitation or anxiety associated with depression: 15 to 30 mg 3 or 4 times daily.

Older patients with anxiety, tension, irritability and agitation: Initial dosage is 10 mg 3 times daily. If necessary, increase cautiously to 15 mg 3 or 4 times daily.

Alcoholics with acute inebriation, tremulousness or anxiety on withdrawal: 15 to 30 mg 3 or 4 times daily.

Children (6 to 12 years): Dosage is not established.

	Product	Dosage form	Description	C.I.*
c-IV	**Oxazepam** (Various)	**Capsules:** 10 mg	In 100s, 250s, 500s and 1000s.	87+
c-IV	**Serax** (Wyeth-Ayerst)		(Wyeth 51). Pink and white. In 100s, 500s and Redipak 25s and 100s.	290
c-IV	**Oxazepam** (Various)	**Capsules:** 15 mg	In 100s, 500s, 1000s and UD 100s.	78+
c-IV	**Serax** (Wyeth-Ayerst)		(Wyeth 6). Red and white. In 100s, 500s and Redipak 25s and 100s.	250
c-IV	**Oxazepam** (Various)	**Capsules:** 30 mg	In 100s, 250s, 500s, 1000s and UD 100s.	55+
c-IV	**Serax** (Wyeth-Ayerst)		(Wyeth 52). Maroon and white. In 100s, 500s and Redipak 25s and 100s.	189
c-IV	**Oxazepam** (Various)	**Tablets:** 15 mg	In 100s, 500s and 1000s.	114+
c-IV	**Serax** (Wyeth-Ayerst)		Tartrazine. (Wyeth 317). Yellow. In 100s.	250

PRAZEPAM

Indications: Management of anxiety disorders; short-term relief of the symptoms of anxiety.

Administration and Dosage:

Individualize dosage.

The usual dose is 30 mg/day administered in divided doses. Adjust dosage gradually within the range of 20 to 60 mg/day in accordance with the response of the patient.

Elderly or debilitated patients: Initiate treatment at 10 to 15 mg/day in divided doses.

May also be administered as a single daily dose at bedtime. The starting dose is 20 mg/night. Adjust dosage to maximize the antianxiety effect with a minimum of daytime drowsiness. The optimum dose ranges from 20 to 40 mg.

	Product	Dosage form	Description	C.I.*
c-IV	**Prazepam** (Various)	**Capsules:** 5 mg	In 100s and 500s.	NA
c-IV	**Centrax** (Parke-Davis)		(Centrax P-D 552). In 100s and 500s.	351
c-IV	**Prazepam** (Various)	**Capsules:** 10 mg	In 100s and 500s.	NA
c-IV	**Centrax** (Parke-Davis)		(Centrax P-D 553). In 100s and 500s.	204
c-IV	**Centrax** (Parke-Davis)	**Capsules:** 20 mg	(Centrax P-D 554). In 100s.	167
c-IV	**Prazepam** (Various)	**Tablets:** 5 mg	In 100s and 500s.	NA
c-IV	**Prazepam** (Various)	**Tablets:** 10 mg	In 100s and 500s.	NA
c-IV	**Centrax** (Parke-Davis)		Blue, scored. In 100s and UD 100s.	204

* Cost Index based on cost per 15 mg oxazepam or 10 mg prazepam.

Complete prescribing information for these products begins on page 1255

Benzodiazepines (Cont.)

LORAZEPAM

Indications:

For the management of anxiety disorders or for the short-term relief of the symptoms of anxiety or anxiety associated with depressive symptoms.

Parenteral: In adults for preanesthetic medication, producing sedation, relief of anxiety and a decreased ability to recall events related to surgery.

Unlabeled uses: Lorazepam injection may help manage status epilepticus, chemotherapy-induced nausea and vomiting, acute alcohol withdrawal syndrome and psychogenic catatonia. Oral lorazepam appears useful for chronic insomnia.

Lorazepam given sublingually is absorbed more rapidly than after oral administration and compares favorably to IM administration.

Administration and Dosage:

Individualize dosage. Increase dosage gradually to minimize adverse effects. When higher dosage is indicated, increase the evening dose before the daytime doses.

Oral: 2 to 6 mg/day (varies from 1 to 10 mg/day) given in divided doses; take the largest dose before bedtime.

Anxiety – Initial dose, 2 to 3 mg/day given 2 or 3 times daily.

Insomnia due to anxiety or transient situational stress – 2 to 4 mg given at bedtime.

Elderly or debilitated patients – Initial dose, 1 to 2 mg/day in divided doses; adjust as needed and tolerated.

IM: 0.05 mg/kg up to a maximum of 4 mg. For optimum effect, administer at least 2 hours before operative procedure. Inject undiluted, deep into the muscle mass.

IV: Initial dose is 2 mg total or 0.044 mg/kg (0.02 mg/lb), whichever is smaller. This will sedate most adults; ordinarily, do not exceed in patients > 50 years old. If a greater lack of recall would be beneficial, doses as high as 0.05 mg/kg up to a total of 4 mg may be given. For optimum effect, administer 15 to 20 minutes before the procedure.

Immediately prior to IV use, lorazepam must be diluted with an equal volume of compatible solution (Sterile Water for Injection, Sodium Chloride Injection or 5% Dextrose Injection). Inject directly into a vein or into the tubing of an existing IV infusion. Do not exceed 2 mg per minute. Have equipment to maintain a patent airway available.

Children (< 18 years): Due to insufficient data, parenteral use is not recommended.

Storage and stability: Do not use if solution is discolored or contains a precipitate. Protect from light; refrigerate solution.

	Product	Form	Description	C.I.*
c-IV	**Lorazepam** (Various, eg, Elkins-Sinn, Lederle, Major, Rugby, Squibb Mark, Warner-C)	**Tablets:** 0.5 mg	In 30s, 100s, 250s, 500s, 1000s and UD 100s and 32s.	46+
c-IV	**Ativan** (Wyeth-Ayerst)		Lactose. (A Wyeth 81). White. Five sided. In 100s, 500s & Redipak 250s & 100s.	289
c-IV	**Lorazepam** (Various, eg, Elkins-Sinn, Geneva, Goldline, Lederle, Major, Moore, Rugby, Squibb Mark, Warner-C)	**Tablets:** 1 mg	In 20s, 30s, 100s, 500s, 1000s and UD 100s and 32s.	29+
c-IV	**Ativan** (Wyeth-Ayerst)		Lactose. (A Wyeth 64). White, scored. Five sided. In 100s, 500s, 1000s & Redipak 100s and 250s.	193
c-IV	**Lorazepam** (Various, eg, Elkins-Sinn, Lederle, Major, Rugby, Squibb Mark, Warner-C)	**Tablets:** 2 mg	In 20s, 30s, 100s, 250s, 500s, 1000s and UD 100s.	21+
c-IV	**Ativan** (Wyeth-Ayerst)		Lactose. (A Wyeth 65). White, scored. In 100s, 500s, 1000s & Redipak 100s & 250s.	145
c-IV	**Lorazepam Intensol** (Roxane)	**Concentrated oral solution:** 2 mg/ml	In 30 ml with dropper. Alcohol and dye free.	NA
c-IV	**Ativan** (Wyeth-Ayerst)	**Injection:** 2 mg/ml 4 mg/ml	In 1 and 10 ml vials[1] and 1 ml fill in 2 ml Tubex.[1]	1745

* Cost Index based on cost per 1 mg.

[1] With PEG 400, propylene glycol, 2% benzyl alcohol.

Complete prescribing information for these products begins on page 1255

Benzodiazepines (Cont.)

DIAZEPAM (Cont.)

	Product	Form/Strength	Description/Packaging	C.I.*
c-iv	**Valrelease** (Roche)	**Capsules, sustained release:** 15 mg	Yellow and blue. In 100s and Rx pak 30s.	156
c-iv	**Diazepam** (Roxane)	**Oral Solution:** 5 mg per 5 ml	Wintergreen-spice flavor. In 500 ml and 5 and 10 mg patient cups.	116
c-iv	**Diazepam Intensol** (Roxane)	**Oral Solution:** 5 mg per ml	In 30 ml with dropper.	206
c-iv	**Diazepam** (Various, eg, Elkins-Sinn, Geneva, Goldline, Lederle, Lemmon, Major, Roxane, Squibb Mark, Warner Chilcott, Zenith)	**Tablets:** 2 mg	In 30s, 100s, 500s, 1000s, 2500s and UD 32s, 100s and 500s.	28+
c-iv	**Valium** (Roche)		(Roche 2 Valium). White, scored. In 100s, 500s, UD 100s and RN 500s.	272
c-iv	**Diazepam** (Various, eg, Elkins-Sinn, Geneva, Goldline, Lederle, Lemmon, Major, Roxane, Squibb Mark, Warner Chilcott, Zenith)	**Tablets:** 5 mg	In 15s, 30s, 100s, 500s, 720s, 1000s, 1080s, 2500s and UD 32s and 100s.	27+
c-iv	**Valium** (Roche)		(Roche 5 Valium). Yellow, scored. In 100s, 500s, UD 100s and RN 500s.	169
c-iv	**Diazepam** (Various, eg, Elkins-Sinn, Geneva, Goldline, Lederle, Lemmon, Major, Roxane, Squibb Mark, Warner Chilcott, Zenith)	**Tablets:** 10 mg	In 15s, 30s, 100s, 500s, 720s, 1000s, 1080s and UD 100s.	10+
c-iv	**Valium** (Roche)		(Roche 10 Valium). Blue, scored. In 100s, 500s, UD 100s and RN 500s.	171
c-iv	**Diazepam** (Various, eg, Baxter, Elkins-Sinn, Goldline, Lederle, Lemmon, Lyphomed, Moore, Rugby, Schein, Warner Chilcott)	**Injection:** 5 mg per ml	In 2 ml amps & 1, 2 and 10 ml vials & 2 ml disposable syringes.	438+
c-iv	**Valium** (Roche)		In 2 ml amps, 10 ml vials and 2 ml Tel-E-Ject.[1]	744
c-iv	**Zetran** (Hauck)		In 10 ml vials.[1]	570

HALAZEPAM

Indications:

Management of anxiety disorders; short-term relief of the symptoms of anxiety.

Administration and Dosage:

Individualize dosage. Increase dosage cautiously to avoid adverse effects.

The usual dose is 20 to 40 mg 3 or 4 times a day.

The optimal dosage usually ranges from 80 to 160 mg daily. If side effects occur with the starting dose, lower the dose.

Elderly (≥ 70 years) or debilitated patients: 20 mg once or twice/day. Adjust dosage.

	Product	Form/Strength	Description/Packaging	C.I.*
c-iv	**Paxipam** (Schering)	**Tablets:** 20 mg	(Schering 251). Orange, scored. In 100s.	284
		40 mg	(Schering 538). White, scored. In 100s.	198

* Cost Index based on cost per 5 mg diazepam or 40 mg halazepam.

[1] With 40% propylene glycol, 10% ethyl alcohol, 5% sodium benzoate, benzoic acid and 1.5% benzyl alcohol.

Complete prescribing information for these products begins on page 1255

Benzodiazepines (Cont.)

CLORAZEPATE DIPOTASSIUM

Indications:

For management of anxiety disorders or short-term relief of symptoms of anxiety.

For the symptomatic relief of acute alcohol withdrawal.

As adjunctive therapy in the management of partial seizures (see Anticonvulsants section).

Administration and Dosage:

Symptomatic relief of anxiety: 30 mg/day in divided doses. Adjust gradually within the range of 15 to 60 mg/day. *Elderly or debilitated patients* – initiate treatment at a dose of 7.5 to 15 mg/day. Lower doses may be indicated.

May also be administered as a single daily dose at bedtime; the initial dose is 15 mg. After the initial dose, the patient may require adjustment of subsequent dosage. Drowsiness may occur at the initiation of treatment and with dosage increments.

Maintenance therapy – Give the 22.5 mg tablet in a single daily dose as an alternate dosage form for patients stabilized on 7.5 mg 3 times/day. Do not use to initiate therapy.

The 11.25 mg tablet may be administered as a single dose every 24 hours.

Symptomatic relief of acute alcohol withdrawal:

Day 1 – 30 mg initially; followed by 30 to 60 mg in divided doses.
Day 2 – 45 to 90 mg in divided doses.
Day 3 – 22.5 to 45 mg in divided doses.
Day 4 – 15 to 30 mg in divided doses.

Thereafter, gradually reduce the dose to 7.5 to 15 mg daily. Discontinue drug as soon as patient's condition is stable.

The maximum recommended total daily dose is 90 mg. Avoid excessive reductions in the total amount of drug administered on successive days.

				C.I.*
c-IV	**Clorazepate Dipotassium** (Various, eg, American Therapeutics, Geneva, Lederle, Martec, Moore, PBI, Rugby, Squibb Mark, URL)	**Capsules:** 3.75 mg	In 100s, 500s, 1000s and UD 100s.	100+
c-IV	**Clorazepate Dipotassium** (Various, eg, American Therapeutics, Geneva, Lederle, Martec, Moore, PBI, Rugby, Squibb Mark, URL)	**Capsules:** 7.5 mg	In 100s, 500s and 1000s.	70+
c-IV	**Clorazepate Dipotassium** (Various, eg, American Therapeutics, Geneva, Lederle, Martec, Moore, PBI, Rugby, Squibb Mark, URL)	**Capsules:** 15 mg	In 100s, 500s and 1000s.	50+

* Cost Index based on cost per 7.5 mg.

(Continued on following page)

Complete prescribing information for these products begins on page 1255

Benzodiazepines (Cont.)

CLORAZEPATE DIPOTASSIUM (Cont.):				C.I.*
c-IV	**Clorazepate Dipotassium** (Various, eg, American Therapeutics, Bioline, Goldline, Lederle, Major, Moore, Rugby, Schein, Squibb Mark, Warner Chilcott)	**Tablets:** 3.75 mg	In 100s, 500s, 1000s and UD 100s.	70+
c-IV	**Gen-Xene** (Alra)		(Alra GX). Gray, scored. In 30s, 100s, 500s and UD 100s.	70
c-IV	**Tranxene** (Abbott)		(TL). Blue, scored. In 100s, 500s and UD 100s.	550
c-IV	**Clorazepate Dipotassium** (Various, eg, American Therapeutics, Bioline, Goldline, Lederle, Major, Moore, Rugby, Schein, Squibb Mark, Warner Chilcott)	**Tablets:** 7.5 mg	In 20s, 100s, 500s, 1000s and UD 100s and 500s.	50+
c-IV	**Gen-Xene** (Alra)		(Alra GT). Yellow, scored. In 30s, 100s, 500s and UD 100s.	40
c-IV	**Tranxene** (Abbott)		(TM). Peach, scored. In 100s, 500s and UD 100s.	340
c-IV	**Clorazepate Dipotassium** (Various, eg, American Therapeutics, Bioline, Goldline, Lederle, Major, Moore, Rugby, Schein, Squibb Mark, Warner Chilcott)	**Tablets:** 15 mg	In 100s, 500s, 1000s and UD 100s.	30+
c-IV	**Gen-Xene** (Alra)		(Alra GN). Green, scored. In 30s, 100s, 500s and UD 100s.	30
c-IV	**Tranxene** (Abbott)		(TN). Lavender, scored. In 100s, 500s and UD 100s.	230
c-IV	**Tranxene-SD Half Strength** (Abbott)	**Tablets, single dose:** 11.25 mg	(TX). Blue. In 100s.	480
c-IV	**Tranxene-SD** (Abbott)	**Tablets, single dose:** 22.5 mg	(TY). Tan. In 100s.	310

* Cost Index based on cost per 7.5 mg.

Miscellaneous Agents

BUSPIRONE HCl

Actions:

Pharmacology: Buspirone HCl is an azaspirodecanedione agent not chemically or pharmacologically related to the benzodiazepines, barbiturates or other sedative/anxiolytic drugs. Mechanism of action is unknown. Buspirone differs from benzodiazepines in that it does not exert anticonvulsant or muscle relaxant effects. It also lacks prominent sedative effects associated with more typical anxiolytics. In vitro, buspirone has a high affinity for serotonin ($5\text{-}HT_{1A}$) receptors; it has no significant affinity for benzodiazepine receptors and does not affect GABA bindings. Buspirone has moderate affinity for brain D_2-dopamine receptors and appears to act as a presynaptic dopamine agonist. It also increases norepinephrine metabolism in the locus ceruleus.

Pharmacokinetics: A multiple dose study suggests that buspirone has nonlinear pharmacokinetics. Thus, dose increases and repeated dosing may lead to somewhat higher blood levels of unchanged buspirone than would be predicted from results of single dose studies.

Absorption – Buspirone is rapidly absorbed and undergoes extensive first-pass metabolism. Following oral administration, plasma concentrations of unchanged buspirone are very low and variable between subjects. Peak plasma levels of 1 to 6 ng/ml have been observed 40 to 90 minutes after single oral doses of 20 mg. The single dose bioavailability of unchanged buspirone from a tablet is about 90% of an equivalent dose of solution, but there is large variability.

Administration with food may decrease the rate of absorption, but it may increase the bioavailability by decreasing the first-pass metabolism. In one study, the AUC doubled when a 20 mg oral dose was administered with food.

Distribution – Approximately 95% of buspirone is plasma protein bound, but other highly bound drugs (eg, phenytoin, propranolol, warfarin) are not displaced in vitro; however, buspirone does displace digoxin.

Metabolism – Buspirone is metabolized primarily by oxidation, producing several hydroxylated derivatives and a pharmacologically active metabolite, 1-pyrimidinyl piperazine (1-PP). Blood samples from humans chronically exposed to buspirone do not exhibit high levels of 1-PP.

Elimination – In a single dose study, 29% to 63% of the dose was excreted in the urine within 24 hours, primarily as metabolites; fecal excretion accounted for 18% to 38% of the dose. The average elimination half-life of unchanged buspirone after single doses of 10 to 40 mg is about 2 to 3 hours (range, 2 to 11 hours).

Clinical trials: Although buspirone is for the short-term treatment of anxiety, there is no evidence that the effects differ when the drug is used in "longer-term" therapy, ie, > 4 weeks. In studies of patients receiving buspirone for up to 1 year, the dosage remained consistently near 20 mg, with efficacy maintained and no increase in side effects over time. No withdrawal syndrome or other significant adverse reactions were reported upon abrupt discontinuation after 1 year of therapy.

Patients on buspirone often show improvement within 7 to 10 days. However, as with many psychotropic drugs, optimal therapeutic results are generally achieved after 3 to 4 weeks of treatment. During initial stages of therapy, look for subtle improvement in anxious symptoms, interpersonal skills and overall patient functioning. Because the drug is not associated with the prominent sedative effects characteristic of benzodiazepines, advise patients of the need to adhere to the therapeutic regimen.

Indications:

Management of anxiety disorders or short-term relief of symptoms of anxiety.

Unlabeled use: Buspirone 25 mg/day may be useful in decreasing the symptoms (eg, aches, pains, fatigue, cramps, irritability) of premenstrual syndrome.

Contraindications:

Hypersensitivity to buspirone HCl.

(Continued on following page)

BUSPIRONE HCl (Cont.)

Warnings:

Buspirone has no established antipsychotic activity; it should not be employed in lieu of appropriate antipsychotic treatment.

Physical and psychological dependence: Buspirone has shown no potential for abuse or diversion and there is no evidence that it causes tolerance or physical or psychological dependence. However, it is difficult to predict from experiments the extent to which a CNS active drug will be misused, diverted or abused once marketed. Consequently, carefully evaluate patients for a history of drug abuse and follow such patients closely, observing them for signs of misuse or abuse (eg, tolerance, drug-seeking behavior).

Hepatic or renal function impairment: Since buspirone is metabolized by the liver and excreted by the kidneys, do not use in patients with severe hepatic or renal impairment.

Elderly: Buspirone has not been systematically evaluated in older patients; however, several hundred elderly patients have participated in clinical studies and no unusual adverse age-related phenomena have been identified.

Pregnancy: Category B. Adequate and well controlled studies have not been performed in pregnant women. Use during pregnancy only if clearly needed.

Lactation: The extent of the excretion in breast milk of buspirone or its metabolites is not known. In rats, however, buspirone and its metabolites are excreted in milk. Avoid administration to nursing women, if possible.

Children: Safety and efficacy for use in children < 18 years are not known.

Precautions:

Interference with cognitive and motor performance: Buspirone is less sedating than other anxiolytics and does not produce significant functional impairment. However, its CNS effect may not be predictable. Therefore, caution patients about driving or using complex machinery until they are certain that buspirone does not affect them adversely.

Withdrawal reactions: Buspirone does not exhibit cross-tolerance with benzodiazepines and other sedative/hypnotic drugs. It will not block the withdrawal syndrome often seen with cessation of therapy with these drugs. Therefore, withdraw patients from their prior treatment gradually before starting buspirone, especially patients who have been using a CNS depressant chronically. Rebound or withdrawal symptoms may occur over varying time periods, depending in part on the type of drug and its effective elimination half-life.

Dopamine receptor binding: Buspirone can bind to central dopamine receptors; a question has been raised about its potential to cause acute and chronic changes in dopamine-mediated neurological function (eg, dystonia, pseudoparkinsonism, akathisia, tardive dyskinesia). Clinical experience in controlled trials has failed to identify any significant neuroleptic-like activity; however, a syndrome of restlessness has appeared shortly after initiation of treatment in a small fraction of buspirone-treated patients. The syndrome may be explained in several ways. For example, buspirone may increase central noradrenergic activity. Alternatively, the effect may be attributable to dopaminergic effects (ie, may represent akathisia).

Monitoring: Effectiveness for more than 3 to 4 weeks has not been demonstrated in controlled trials. However, patients have been treated for several months without ill effect. If used for extended periods, periodically reassess the usefulness of the drug.

Drug Interactions:

Alcohol: Formal studies of the interaction of buspirone with alcohol indicate that buspirone does not increase alcohol-induced impairment in motor and mental performance, but it is prudent to avoid concomitant use.

Haloperidol and buspirone coadministration may result in increased serum haloperidol concentrations.

Monoamine oxidase inhibitors (MAOIs): There have been reports of elevated blood pressure when buspirone was added to a regimen including an MAOI. Therefore, do not use concomitantly.

Trazodone: One report suggests that concomitant use may have caused threefold to sixfold elevations of ALT in a few patients. In a similar study attempting to replicate this finding, no interactive effect on hepatic transaminases was identified.

Drug/Food interaction: Administration with food may decrease buspirone's rate of absorption, but food may increase its bioavailability by decreasing first-pass metabolism. In one study, the AUC doubled when a 20 mg oral dose was given with food.

(Continued on following page)

BUSPIRONE HCl (Cont.)

Adverse Reactions:

Most common: Dizziness; nausea; headache; nervousness; lightheadedness; excitement.

Approximately 10% of the 2200 patients in premarketing trials in anxiety disorders lasting 3 to 4 weeks discontinued treatment due to adverse events which included: CNS disturbances (3.4%), primarily dizziness, insomnia, nervousness, drowsiness and lightheadedness; GI disturbances (1.2%), primarily nausea; miscellaneous disturbances (1.1%), primarily headache and fatigue. In addition, 3.4% of patients had multiple complaints, none of which were primary.

Adverse Reactions of Buspirone HCl vs Placebo (%)

Adverse Reaction	Buspirone (n = 477)	Placebo (n = 464)
CNS		
Dizziness	12	3
Drowsiness	10	9
Nervousness	5	1
Insomnia	3	3
Lightheadedness	3	—
Decreased concentration	2	2
Excitement	2	—
Anger/Hostility	2	—
Confusion	2	—
Depression	2	2
GI		
Nausea	8	5
Dry mouth	3	4
Abdominal/Gastric distress	2	2
Diarrhea	2	—
Constipation	1	2
Vomiting	1	2
Neurological		
Numbness	2	—
Paresthesia	1	—
Incoordination	1	—
Tremor	1	—
Miscellaneous		
Headache	6	3
Fatigue	4	4
Weakness	2	—
Blurred vision	2	—
Tachycardia/Palpitations	1	1
Sweating/Clamminess	1	—
Musculoskeletal aches/Pains	1	—
Skin rash	1	—

— Incidence < 1%.

Cardiovascular: Nonspecific chest pain (≥ 1%); syncope, hypotension, hypertension (0.1% to 1%); cerebrovascular accident, congestive heart failure, myocardial infarction, cardiomyopathy, bradycardia (< 0.1%).

CNS: Dream disturbances (≥ 1%); depersonalization, dysphoria, noise intolerance, euphoria, akathisia, fearfulness, loss of interest, disassociative reaction, hallucinations, suicidal ideation, seizures (0.1% to 1%); feelings of claustrophobia, cold intolerance, stupor and slurred speech, psychosis (< 0.1%).

(Adverse Reactions continued on following page)

BUSPIRONE HCl (Cont.)

Adverse Reactions (Cont.):

EENT: Tinnitus, sore throat, nasal congestion (≥ 1%); redness and itching of the eyes, altered taste, altered smell, conjunctivitis (0.1% to 1%); inner ear abnormality, eye pain, photophobia, pressure on eyes (< 0.1%).

Endocrine: Galactorrhea, thyroid abnormality (< 0.1%).

GI: Flatulence, anorexia, increased appetite, salivation, irritable colon, rectal bleeding (0.1% to 1%); burning of the tongue (< 0.1%).

GU: Urinary frequency, urinary hesitancy, menstrual irregularity, spotting and dysuria (0.1% to 1%); amenorrhea, pelvic inflammatory disease, enuresis, nocturia (< 0.1%).

Musculoskeletal: Muscle cramps, muscle spasms, rigid/stiff muscles, arthralgias (0.1% to 1%).

Neurological: Involuntary movements, slowed reaction time (0.1% to 1%); muscle weakness (< 0.1%).

Respiratory: Hyperventilation, shortness of breath, chest congestion (0.1% to 1%); epistaxis (< 0.1%).

Sexual function: Decreased or increased libido (0.1% to 1%); delayed ejaculation, impotence (< 0.1%).

Dermatologic: Edema, pruritus, flushing, easy bruising, hair loss, dry skin, facial edema, blisters (0.1% to 1%); acne, thinning of nails (< 0.1%).

Miscellaneous: Weight gain, fever, roaring sensation in the head, weight loss, malaise (0.1% to 1%); alcohol abuse, bleeding disturbance, loss of voice, hiccoughs (< 0.1%).

Laboratory test abnormalities: Increases in hepatic aminotransferases (AST, ALT) (0.1% to 1%); eosinophilia, leukopenia, thrombocytopenia (< 0.1%).

Overdosage:

Symptoms: Doses as high as 375 mg/day were administered to healthy male volunteers. As this dose was approached, the following symptoms were observed: Nausea, vomiting, dizziness, drowsiness, miosis and gastric distress. No deaths have been reported.

Treatment: No specific antidote is known. Use general symptomatic and supportive measures along with immediate gastric lavage. Refer to General Management of Acute Overdosage. Dialyzability of buspirone has not been determined.

Patient Information:

Inform physician if any chronic abnormal movements occur (eg, motor restlessness, involuntary repetitive movements of facial or neck muscles).

May cause drowsiness and dizziness. Use caution while driving or performing other tasks requiring alertness. Avoid alcohol and use other CNS depressants with caution.

Inform physician if you are pregnant, become pregnant or are planning to become pregnant while taking buspirone or if you are breast-feeding.

Optimum results are generally achieved after 3 to 4 weeks of treatment. Some improvement will be seen in 7 to 10 days.

Administration and Dosage:

Initial dose: 15 mg daily (5 mg 3 times a day).

To achieve an optimal therapeutic response, increase the dosage 5 mg/day, at intervals of 2 to 3 days, as needed. Do not exceed 60 mg/day. Divided doses of 20 to 30 mg/day have been commonly used.

				C.I.*
Rx	**BuSpar** (Mead Johnson Pharm.)	**Tablets:** 5 mg	Lactose. (MJ 5 mg BuSpar). White, scored. Ovoid-rectangular. In 100s, 500s and UD 100s.	178
		10 mg	Lactose. (MJ 10 mg BuSpar). White, scored. Ovoid-rectangular. In 100s, 500s and UD 100s.	152

* Cost Index based on cost per 5 mg.

HYDROXYZINE

Actions:

Pharmacology: Hydroxyzine is a piperazine antihistamine. It is not a cortical depressant; its action may be due to a suppression of activity in the subcortical areas of the CNS.

Primary skeletal muscle relaxation has been demonstrated experimentally. Bronchodilator activity, antihistaminic and analgesic effects have been confirmed clinically. Hydroxyzine has antispasmodic properties, apparently mediated through interference with the mechanism that responds to spasmogenic agents such as serotonin, acetylcholine and histamine. An antiemetic effect has been demonstrated. Hydroxyzine in therapeutic dosage does not increase gastric secretion or acidity and in most cases provides mild antisecretory activity.

Pharmacokinetics: Oral hydroxyzine is rapidly absorbed from the GI tract; clinical effects are usually noted within 15 to 30 minutes after administration. Following a single 100 mg oral dose, peak levels of 82 ng/ml were reached in ≈ 3 hours. Mean elimination half-life is 3 hours; half-life may be longer in elderly patients. Hydroxyzine is mainly metabolized by the liver.

Indications:

Symptomatic relief of anxiety and tension associated with psychoneurosis and as an adjunct in organic disease states in which anxiety is manifest.

The efficacy of hydroxyzine as an antianxiety agent for long-term use (▷ 4 months) has not been assessed; periodically reevaluate its usefulness.

Management of pruritus due to allergic conditions such as chronic urticaria, atopic and contact dermatoses and in histamine-mediated pruritus.

As a sedative when used as premedication and following general anesthesia.

IM only: For the acutely disturbed or hysterical patient; the acute or chronic alcoholic with anxiety withdrawal symptoms or delirium tremens; as pre- and postoperative and pre- and postpartum adjunctive medication to permit reduction in narcotic dosage, allay anxiety and control emesis; adjunctive therapy in asthma.

Contraindications:

Hypersensitivity to hydroxyzine; early pregnancy, lactation (see Warnings).

Hydroxyzine injection is for IM use only. Do not inject SC, IV or intra-arterially. Tissue necrosis has been associated with SC or intra-arterial injection; hemolysis has occurred following IV administration.

Warnings:

Hypersensitivity reactions have occurred (see Adverse Reactions). Refer to Management of Acute Hypersensitivity Reactions.

Pregnancy: Clinical data in humans are inadequate to establish safety in early pregnancy. In doses substantially above the human therapeutic range, hydroxyzine has induced fetal abnormalities in animals. Do not use in pregnancy.

Lactation: It is not known whether this drug is excreted in breast milk; therefore, do not give hydroxyzine to nursing mothers.

Precautions:

Potentially hazardous tasks: May produce drowsiness; patients should observe caution while driving or performing other tasks requiring alertness.

IM use: Inject well within the body of a relatively large muscle. In adults, the preferred site is the upper outer quadrant of the buttock or the midlateral thigh. In children, inject into the midlateral muscles of the thigh. In infants and small children, use the periphery of the upper outer quadrant of the gluteal region only when necessary, such as in burn patients, in order to minimize the possibility of sciatic nerve damage.

Use the deltoid area only if well developed, and then only with caution to avoid radial nerve injury. Do not inject into the lower and mid-third of the upper arm.

Drug Interactions:

CNS depressants (eg, **narcotics, barbiturates**): Consider the potentiating action when used with hydroxyzine. When CNS depressants are given concomitantly with hydroxyzine, reduce their dosage by 50%. Cardiac arrest has occurred (rare).

(Continued on following page)

HYDROXYZINE (Cont.)

Adverse Reactions:

Dry mouth; drowsiness is usually transitory and may disappear after a few days of continued therapy or upon dosage reduction; involuntary motor activity, including rare instances of tremor and convulsions, usually with higher than recommended dosage; hypersensitivity reactions (wheezing, dyspnea, chest tightness) have occurred (see Warnings).

Overdosage:

Symptoms: The most common manifestation is oversedation. As in management of any overdosage, consider that multiple agents may have been ingested.

Treatment: Induce vomiting if it has not occurred spontaneously. Immediate gastric lavage is also recommended. General supportive care is indicated; frequently monitor vital signs and observe the patient. Control hypotension with IV fluids and norepinephrine or metaraminol. Do not use epinephrine; hydroxyzine counteracts its pressor action. There is no specific antidote. It is doubtful that hemodialysis would be of value. Refer also to General Management of Acute Overdosage.

Patient Information:

May produce drowsiness; patients should observe caution while driving or performing other tasks requiring alertness. Avoid alcoholic beverages and other CNS depressants; they may intensify this effect.

Administration and Dosage:

Start patients on IM therapy when indicated. Maintain on oral therapy whenever practicable. Adjust dosage according to patient's response.

Oral: Symptomatic relief of anxiety – Adults: 50 to 100 mg 4 times/day. Children (> 6): 50 to 100 mg/day in divided doses. Children (< 6): 50 mg/day in divided doses.

Management of pruritus – Adults: 25 mg 3 or 4 times daily. Children (> 6): 50 to 100 mg/day in divided doses. Children (< 6): 50 mg/day in divided doses.

Sedative (as premedication and following general anesthesia) – Adults: 50 to 100 mg. Children: 0.6 mg/kg.

IM: For adult psychiatric and emotional emergencies, including acute alcoholism – 50 to 100 mg immediately and every 4 to 6 hours as needed.

Nausea and vomiting – Adults: 25 to 100 mg. Children: 1.1 mg/kg (0.5 mg/lb).

Pre- and postoperative adjunctive medication – Adults: 25 to 100 mg. Children: 1.1 mg/kg (0.5 mg/lb).

Pre- and postpartum adjunctive therapy – 25 to 100 mg.

	Product	Form	Description	C.I.*
Rx	**Hydroxyzine HCl** (Various, eg, Baxter, Geneva, Goldline, Lannett, Lederle, Major, Moore, PBI, Rugby, Schein)	**Tablets:** 10 mg (as HCl)	In 20s, 30s, 50s, 100s, 250s, 500s, 1000s and UD 32s and 100s.	37+
Rx	**Atarax** (Roerig)		Orange. In 100s, 500s and UD 100s.	497
Rx	**Hydroxyzine HCl** (Various, eg, Baxter, Geneva, Goldline, Lannett, Lederle, Major, Moore, PBI, Rugby, Schein)	**Tablets:** 25 mg (as HCl)	In 12s, 15s, 20s, 24s, 30s, 40s, 50s, 60s, 100s, 250s, 500s, 1000s and UD 32s and 100s.	20+
Rx	**Anxanil** (Econo Med)		(ANX). Lt. green, scored. Film coated. In 100s and 500s.	40
Rx	**Atarax** (Roerig)		Green. In 100s, 500s and UD 100s.	292
Rx	**Hydroxyzine HCl** (Various, eg, Baxter, Geneva, Goldline, Lannett, Major, Moore, PBI, Rugby, Schein, Spencer Mead)	**Tablets:** 50 mg (as HCl)	In 30s and 100s.	20+
Rx	**Atarax** (Roerig)		Yellow. In 100s, 500s and UD 100s.	178
Rx	**Atarax 100** (Roerig)	**Tablets:** 100 mg (as HCl)	Red. In 100s and UD 100s.	219

* Cost Index based on cost per 25 mg.

(Continued on following page)

Miscellaneous Agents (Cont.)

HYDROXYZINE (Cont.)

	Product	Dosage form	Description	C.I.*
Rx	**Hydroxyzine HCl** (Various, eg, Baxter, Geneva, Goldline, Major, Moore, PBI, Rugby, Schein, UDL, Warner-C)	**Syrup:** 10 mg per 5 ml (as HCl)	In 16 and 120 ml, pt, gal and UD 5, 12.5 and 25 ml.	74+
Rx	**Atarax** (Roerig)		Sucrose and menthol. 0.5% alcohol. In 480 ml.	490
Rx	**Hydroxyzine Pamoate** (Various, eg, Baxter, Geneva, Goldline, Lannett, Major, Moore, Rugby, Schein, Spencer Mead, Zenith)	**Capsules:** 25 mg (as pamoate equivalent to HCl)	In 12s, 20s, 50s, 100s, 500s, 1000s and UD 32s and 100s.	19+
Rx	**Vistaril** (Pfizer)		Two-tone green. In 100s, 500s and UD 100s.	292
Rx	**Hydroxyzine Pamoate** (Various, eg, Baxter, Geneva, Goldline, Lannett, Major, Moore, Rugby, Schein, Spencer Mead, Zenith)	**Capsules:** 50 mg (as pamoate equivalent to HCl)	In 12s, 20s, 100s, 500s, 1000s and UD 32s and 100s.	12+
Rx	**Vistaril** (Pfizer)		Green and white. In 100s, 500s and UD 100s.	178
Rx	**Hydroxyzine Pamoate** (Various, eg, Barr, Baxter, Goldline, Lannett, Major, Moore, Rugby, Schein, Spencer Mead, URL)	**Capsules:** 100 mg (as pamoate equivalent to HCl)	In 100s, 500s, 1000s and UD 100s.	14+
Rx	**Vistaril** (Pfizer)		Green/gray. In 100s, 500s, UD 100s.	109
Rx	**Vistaril** (Pfizer)	**Oral Suspension:** 25 mg per 5 ml (as pamoate equiv. to HCl)	Sorbitol. Lemon flavor. In 120 and 480 ml.	464
Rx	**Hydroxyzine HCl** (Various, eg, American Regent, Balan, Goldline, Lyphomed, Major, Moore, Rugby, Schein, Solopak, Steris)	**Injection:** 25 mg/ml (as HCl)	In 2 ml syringes and 1 and 10 ml vials.	290+
Rx	**Hydroxyzine HCl** (Elkins-Sinn)		In 1 ml Dosette vials.	300
Rx	**Hydroxyzine HCl** (Winthrop Pharm.)		In 1 ml fill in 2 ml Carpuject syringe.[1]	310
Rx	**Vistaject-25** (Mayrand)		In 10 ml vials.[1]	290
Rx	**Vistaril** (Roerig)		In 10 ml vials.[1]	529

* Cost Index based on cost per 25 mg.

[1] With benzyl alcohol.

(Continued on following page)

Miscellaneous Agents (Cont.)

HYDROXYZINE (Cont.)

				C.I.*
Rx	**Hydroxyzine HCl** (Various, eg, Balan, Bioline, Goldline, Lyphomed, Major, Moore, Rugby, Schein, Solopak, Steris)	**Injection:** 50 mg/ml (as HCl)	In 2 ml amps, 1 and 2 ml syringes and 1, 2 and 10 ml vials.	290+
Rx	**Hydroxyzine HCl** (Elkins-Sinn)		In 1 and 2 ml Dosette vials and 10 ml vials.[1]	200
Rx	**Hydroxyzine HCl** (Winthrop Pharm.)		In 1 and 2 ml fill in 2 ml Carpuject syringes.[1]	180
Rx	**E-Vista** (Seatrace)		In 10 ml vials.[1]	119
Rx	**Hydroxacen** (Central)		In 10 ml vials.[1]	178
Rx	**Hyzine-50** (Hyrex)		In 10 ml vials.[1]	165
Rx	**Quiess** (Forest)		In 10 ml vials.[1]	181
Rx	**Vistacon** (Hauck)		In 10 ml vials.[1]	138
Rx	**Vistaject-50** (Mayrand)		In 10 ml vials.[1]	170
Rx	**Vistaquel 50** (Pasadena)		In 10 ml vials.[1]	48
Rx	**Vistaril** (Roerig)		In 10 ml vials[1], 1 & 2 ml UD vials.[1]	422
Rx	**Vistazine 50** (Keene)		In 10 ml vials.[1]	90

* Cost Index based on cost per 25 mg.

[1] With benzyl alcohol.

DOXEPIN HCl

Doxepin is a tricyclic antidepressant which also has antianxiety effects. The following is an abbreviated monograph for doxepin. For complete information, refer to the Tricyclic Antidepressants monograph.

Indications:

For the treatment of psychoneurotic patients with depression or anxiety; depression or anxiety associated with alcoholism or organic disease; psychotic depressive disorders with associated anxiety including involutional depression and manic-depressive disorders.

The target symptoms of psychoneurosis that respond to doxepin include anxiety, tension, depression, somatic symptoms and concerns, insomnia, guilt, lack of energy, fear, apprehension and worry.

Administration and Dosage:

Individualize dosage.

The total daily dosage may be given on a divided or once-a-day dosage schedule. If the once-a-day schedule is employed, the maximum recommended dose is 150 mg/day, given at bedtime.

Not recommended in children < 12 years old.

Mild to moderate severity: Start with 75 mg/day. The optimum dose range is 75 to 150 mg/day.

More severely ill: Gradual increase to 300 mg/day may be necessary. Additional therapeutic effect is rarely obtained by exceeding a dose of 300 mg/day.

Very mild symptoms or emotional symptoms accompanying organic disease: Some of these patients have been controlled on doses as low as 25 to 50 mg/day.

Dilute the oral concentrate with 120 ml of liquid (eg, water, milk and some fruit juices) just prior to administration; not compatible with a number of carbonated beverages. For patients on methadone maintenance taking oral doxepin, mix the concentrate with methadone and lemonade, orange juice, water, sugar water or powdered fruit drink. *Do not mix with grape juice.* Preparation and storage of bulk dilutions are not recommended.

(Products listed on following page)

Miscellaneous Agents (Cont.)

DOXEPIN HCl (Cont.):			C.I.*
Rx **Doxepin HCl** (Various, eg, Balan, Baxter, Elkins-Sinn, Geneva, Goldline, Lederle, Major, Moore, Rugby, Schein)	**Capsules:** 10 mg	In 100s, 500s, 1000s and UD 100s.	79+
Rx **Adapin** (Fisons)		(Adapin 10). Yellow-orange. In 100s, 1000s, & UD 100s.	289
Rx **Sinequan** (Roerig)		In 100s, 1000s and UD 100s.	298
Rx **Doxepin HCl** (Various, eg, Balan, Baxter, Bioline, Elkins-Sinn, Geneva, Goldline, Major, Moore, Rugby, Schein)	**Capsules:** 25 mg	In 30s, 50s, 100s, 360s, 500s, 1000s and UD 100s.	31+
Rx **Adapin** (Fisons)		(Adapin 25). Green. In 100s, 1000s and UD 100s.	149
Rx **Sinequan** (Roerig)		In 100s, 1000s, 5000s and UD 100s.	147
Rx **Doxepin HCl** (Various, eg, Balan, Baxter, Elkins-Sinn, Geneva, Goldline, Lederle, Major, Moore, Rugby, Schein)	**Capsules:** 50 mg	In 30s, 100s, 360s, 500s, 1000s and UD 100s.	21+
Rx **Adapin** (Fisons)		(Adapin 50). Green. In 100s, 1000s and UD 100s.	104
Rx **Sinequan** (Roerig)		In 100s, 1000s, 5000s and UD 100s.	108
Rx **Doxepin HCl** (Various, eg, Balan, Baxter, Elkins-Sinn, Geneva, Goldline, Lederle, Major, Moore, Rugby, Schein)	**Capsules:** 75 mg	In 30s, 100s, 500s, 1000s and UD 100s.	28+
Rx **Adapin** (Fisons)		(Adapin 75). White/orange. In 100s, 1000s and UD 100s.	117
Rx **Sinequan** (Roerig)		In 100s, 1000s and UD 100s.	120
Rx **Doxepin HCl** (Various, eg, Balan, Baxter, Bioline, Geneva, Goldline, Lederle, Major, Moore, Rugby, Schein)	**Capsules:** 100 mg	In 100s, 500s, 1000s and UD 100s.	18+
Rx **Adapin** (Fisons)		(Adapin 100). White/green. In 100s, 1000s and UD 100s.	95
Rx **Sinequan** (Roerig)		In 100s, 1000s and UD 100s.	98
Rx **Doxepin HCl** (Various, eg, Balan, Bioline, Dixon-Shane, Goldline, Lederle, Major, Martec, Par, Rugby)	**Capsules:** 150 mg	In 50s, 100s, 500s and UD 100s.	34+
Rx **Adapin** (Fisons)		Brown/beige. In 50s and UD 100s.	105
Rx **Sinequan** (Roerig)		In 50s, 500s and UD 100s.	108
Rx **Doxepin HCl** (Various, eg, Balan, Bioline, Geneva, Goldline, Harber, PBI, Rugby, Schein, Warner-C)	**Oral Concentrate:** 10 mg/ml	In 120 ml.	109+
Rx **Sinequan Concentrate** (Roerig)		In 120 ml.	191

* Cost Index based on cost per 25 mg.

Miscellaneous Agents (Cont.)

CHLORMEZANONE

Actions:

Pharmacology: Chlormezanone improves the emotional state by allaying mild anxiety, usually without impairing clarity of consciousness. The mechanism of action is unknown.

Pharmacokinetics: The relief of symptoms is often apparent 15 to 30 minutes after administration and may last 6 hours or longer. Peak plasma concentrations are attained within 1 to 2 hours; mean elimination half-life is 24 hours.

Indications:

Treatment of mild anxiety and tension states.

The effectiveness of chlormezanone in long-term use (> 4 months) has not been assessed by clinical studies. Periodically reassess the usefulness of the drug for the individual patient.

Contraindications:

Hypersensitivity to chlormezanone.

Warnings:

Pregnancy and lactation: Safety for use during pregnancy or lactation has not been established. Use only when clearly needed and when the potential benefits outweigh the potential hazards to the fetus.

Precautions:

Potentially hazardous tasks: Should drowsiness occur, reduce dose; patients should observe caution while driving or performing other tasks requiring alertness.

Drug Interactions:

Alcohol or other **CNS depressants** (eg, **barbiturates, narcotics**): Possible additive CNS effects may occur when taken with chlormezanone.

Adverse Reactions:

Drug rash; dizziness; flushing; nausea; drowsiness; depression; edema; inability to void; dry mouth; weakness; excitement; tremor; confusion; headache. Rare insances of erythema multiform, Stevens-Johnson syndrome and toxic epidermal necrolysis have occurred. Discontinue medication or adjust as the case demands. Cholestatic jaundice has occurred rarely, but was reversible upon discontinuance.

Overdosage:

Two patients ingested 7 g and 9 g; one patient became sleepy and vomited, the other was comatose with depressed reflexes. Neither exhibited disturbances of respiratory, renal or hepatic function. Both made uneventful recoveries. Five hours after ingesting 11 g of chlormezanone, a third patient alternated between periods of coma and excitement. He also experienced anticholinergic effects.

Patient Information:

This drug may impair the mental or physical abilities required for the performance of potentially hazardous tasks such as driving or operating machinery.

Avoid alcohol while taking this drug.

Notify physician if skin rash, sore throat or fever occurs.

Administration and Dosage:

Adults: 200 mg 3 or 4 times daily; in some patients 100 mg may suffice.

Children (5 to 12 years): 50 to 100 mg 3 or 4 times daily.

Since the effect of CNS acting drugs varies, treatment, particularly in children, should begin with the lowest dosage possible which may be increased as needed.

				C.I.*
Rx	**Trancopal Caplets** (Winthrop Pharm.)	**Tablets:** 100 mg	Saccharin. Peach, scored. In 100s.	473
		200 mg	Saccharin. Green, scored. In 100s and 1000s.	271

* Cost Index based on cost per 200 mg.

Drugs with clinically useful antidepressant effects include the tricyclic antidepressants (TCAs), maprotiline, trazodone, fluoxetine, bupropion and the monoamine oxidase inhibitors (MAOIs). The antidepressant agents all appear effective in the treatment of depression. "Major depressive episode" implies a prominent and relatively persistent (nearly every day for at least 2 weeks) depressed or dysphoric mood that usually interferes with daily functioning, and includes at least five of the following nine symptoms: Depressed mood; markedly diminished interest or pleasure in all, or almost all activities; significant weight loss or gain when not dieting or decrease or increase in appetite; insomnia or hypersomnia; psychomotor agitation or retardation; fatigue or loss of energy; feelings of worthlessness or excessive or inappropriate guilt; diminished ability to think or concentrate or indecisiveness; recurrent thoughts of death, suicidal ideation or suicide attempt.

Mechanism of action: Effective antidepressant activity has traditionally been associated with the "biogenic amine hypothesis of depression." The theory is that depression is due to reduced functional activity of one or more of the endogenous monoamines (norepinephrine, serotonin) in the brain. It was believed that certain types of depression were caused by brain neurotransmitter deficiency and that antidepressants relieve depression by inhibiting the reuptake of serotonin and norepinephrine, thereby correcting this deficiency and facilitating neurotransmission. This explanation is now being questioned for several reasons. First, several antidepressant agents lack any apparent effect on neurotransmitter reuptake. More importantly, the blockade of neurotransmitter reuptake occurs within minutes to hours of antidepressant drug initiation while the antidepressant effects usually take 1 to 4 weeks to become manifest.

The emphasis of research has shifted from acute reuptake effects to the slower adaptive changes in norepinephrine and serotonin receptor systems induced by chronic antidepressant therapy. Postsynaptic receptors participate in nerve impulse neurotransmission while the presynaptic receptors regulate neurotransmitter release and reuptake, an important mechanism of neurotransmitter inactivation. Long-term antidepressant treatment produces complex changes in the sensitivities of both presynaptic and postsynaptic receptor sites. The available antidepressant agents may increase the sensitivity of postsynaptic alpha (α_1) adrenergic and serotonin receptors and may decrease the sensitivity of presynaptic receptor sites. The net effect is the correction (re-regulation) of an abnormal receptor-neurotransmitter relationship. Clinically, this re-regulatory action speeds up the patient's natural recovery process from the depressive episode by normalizing neurotransmission efficacy.

Drug selection: The non-MAOIs (TCAs, maprotiline, trazodone, fluoxetine and bupropion) are used much more frequently than the MAOIs mainly because of (1) the perception that MAOIs are less effective than the non-MAOI antidepressants and (2) the risk of hypertensive crisis when the patient ingests foods containing tyramine or via drug interaction (eg, sympathomimetics) with the MAOIs. However, when MAOIs are used in therapeutic doses, they are probably equieffective to non-MAOIs for the treatment of depression.

Base antidepressant drug selection on the patient's past history of drug response (if any), the specific drug's side effect profile relative to patient medical conditions and other factors, and clinician familiarity with specific antidepressants. Nortriptyline and desipramine are preferred TCAs in a patient without a history of favorable response to a specific antidepressant because they cause less sedation and have less anticholinergic activity than tertiary TCAs such as amitriptyline and, in the case of nortriptyline, are less likely to cause orthostatic hypotension. Trazodone has less anticholinergic activity than TCAs and causes fewer problems than TCAs when taken in overdose. Fluoxetine generally lacks the adverse reactions (eg, sedation, anticholinergic effects) associated with TCAs, causes few cardiovascular side effects (including orthostasis), is associated with weight loss rather than weight gain as is the case with TCAs, and causes fewer problems than TCAs when taken in overdose. However, its use is associated with other side effects such as headache, nervousness and insomnia. Fluoxetine is recommended to be taken in the morning. Use maprotiline and bupropion only when other antidepressants have not proven effective.

(Continued on following page)

Actions:

The table below summarizes some of the important pharmacologic and pharmacokinetic data of these agents.

Antidepressant Pharmacologic and Pharmacokinetic Parameters

0 – none; + – slight; ++ – moderate; +++ – high; ++++ – very high; +++++ – highest	Major Side Effects			Amine Uptake Blocking Activity				
	Anticholinergic	Sedation	Orthostatic Hypotension	Norepinephrine	Serotonin	Half-life (hours)	Therapeutic Plasma Level (ng/ml)	Time to Reach Steady State (days)
Tertiary Amines								
Amitriptyline	++++	++++	++	++	++++	31-46	110-250[1]	4-10
Clomipramine	+++	+++	++	++	+++++	19-37	80-100	7-14
Doxepin	++	+++	++	+	++	8-24	100-200[1]	2-8
Imipramine	++	++	+++	++[2]	++++	11-25	200-350[1]	2-5
Trimipramine	++	+++	++	+	+	7-30	180[1]	2-6
Secondary Amines								
Amoxapine[3]	+++	++	+	+++	++	8[4]	200-500	2-7
Desipramine	+	+	+	++++	++	12-24	125-300	2-11
Nortriptyline	++	++	+	++	+++	18-44	50-150	4-19
Protriptyline	+++	+	+	++++	++	67-89	100-200	14-19
Tetracyclic								
Maprotiline	++	++	+	+++	0/+	21-25	200-300[1]	6-10
Triazolopyridine								
Trazodone	+	++	++	0	+++	4-9	800-1600	3-7
Bicyclic								
Fluoxetine	+	+/0	+	+	+++++	7-9 days	—	2-4 weeks
Aminoketone								
Bupropion[5]	++	++	+	+/0	+/0	8-24	—	1.5-5

[1] Parent compound plus active metabolite.
[2] Via desipramine, the major metabolite.
[3] Also blocks dopamine receptors.
[4] 30 hours for major metabolite 8-hydroxyamoxapine.
[5] Inhibits dopamine uptake.

Tricyclic Compounds

Maprotiline, a tetracyclic antidepressant, is included in this monograph because of pharmacologic and therapeutic similarities to the tricyclic agents.

Actions:

Pharmacology: The tricyclic antidepressants (TCAs), structurally related to the phenothiazine antipsychotic agents, possess three major pharmacologic actions in varying degrees: Blocking of the amine pump, sedation, and peripheral and central anticholinergic action. In contrast to the phenothiazines, which act on dopamine receptors, the TCAs act to inhibit the reuptake of norepinephrine or serotonin (5-hydroxytryptamine, 5-HT) at the presynaptic neuron. Amoxapine, a metabolite of loxapine, retains some of the postsynaptic dopamine receptor-blocking action of the neuroleptics.

Amine uptake inhibition: The amine hypothesis of depression proposes that a relationship exists between depression and levels of the CNS bioamines at the postsynaptic adrenergic receptors in the brain. TCAs can be characterized by their ability to inhibit presynaptic reuptake of norepinephrine and serotonin (see table in introduction).

Although amine pump blockade may be immediate, antidepressant response can take days to weeks.

Other pharmacological effects: Inhibition of histamine and acetylcholine activity. Clinical effects, in addition to antidepressant effects, include sedation, anticholinergic effects, mild peripheral vasodilator effects and possible "quinidine-like" actions.

Pharmacokinetics:

Absorption/Distribution – Although the TCAs are well absorbed from the GI tract with peak plasma concentrations occurring in 2 to 4 hours, they undergo a significant first-pass effect. They are highly bound (> 90%) to plasma proteins, are lipid soluble and are widely distributed in tissues, including the CNS. Although there is a suggested therapeutic range for many of the TCAs (see table in introduction), the association between plasma levels and therapeutic effect has not been adequately defined. Wide interpatient variation in steady-state plasma levels at a given dosage is due primarily to differences in the rate of metabolism or first-pass effect. Effective dosage levels vary greatly and must be individualized.

Metabolism/Excretion – Metabolism of TCAs occurs in the liver by demethylation, hydroxylation and glucuronidation, and it varies for each patient. Some intermediate active metabolites include:

Amitriptyline → nortriptyline
Amoxapine → 7 hydroxy and 8 hydroxyamoxapine
Clomipramine → desmethylclomipramine
Doxepin → desmethyldoxepin
Imipramine → desipramine

The TCAs are partially secreted into the hepatobiliary circulation and stomach and are reabsorbed and excreted in the urine.

Because of the long half-life, a single daily dose may be given. Up to 2 to 4 weeks may be required to achieve maximal clinical response.

Indications:

Relief of symptoms of depression (except clomipramine).

Agents with significant sedative action may be useful in depression associated with anxiety and sleep disturbances.

Doxepin: Anxiety.

Imipramine: Treatment of enuresis in children ≥ 6 years of age.

Clomipramine: Only for treatment of Obsessive – Compulsive Disorder (OCD).

Unlabeled uses:

Chronic pain (migraine, chronic tension headache, diabetic neuropathy, tic douloureux, cancer pain, peripheral neuropathy with pain, postherpetic neuralgia, arthritic pain): Amitriptyline (50 to 100 mg/day); doxepin (50 to 300 mg/day); imipramine (75 to 150 mg/day); clomipramine.

Pathologic laughing and weeping secondary to forebrain disease: Amitriptyline (25 to 75 mg).

Obstructive sleep apnea: Protriptyline.

Peptic ulcer disease: Trimipramine; doxepin.

Facilitation of cocaine withdrawal: Desipramine (50 to 200 mg/day).

Panic disorder: Imipramine; clomipramine; nortriptyline (25 to 75 mg/day). Other antidepressants may also be used.

Eating disorders (effective in bulimia nervosa): Imipramine; desipramine; amitriptyline.

Premenstrual depression: Nortriptyline (50 to 125 mg/day).

Dermatologic disorders (chronic urticaria and angioedema, nocturnal pruritis in atopic eczema): Doxepin (10 to 30 mg/day); trimipramine (50 mg/day); nortriptyline (75 mg/day).

(Continued on following page)

Contraindications:

Prior sensitivity to any tricyclic drug. Not recommended for use during the acute recovery phase following myocardial infarction. Concomitant use of monoamine oxidase inhibitors (MAOIs) is generally contraindicated (see Drug Interactions).

Doxepin: Patients with glaucoma or a tendency to urinary retention.

Maprotiline: Patients with known or suspected seizure disorder.

Warnings:

Tardive dyskinesia, a syndrome consisting of potentially irreversible, involuntary, dyskinetic movements may develop in patients treated with neuroleptics (eg, antipsychotics). **Amoxapine** is not an antipsychotic, but it has substantive neuroleptic activity. Although the syndrome appears most often among the elderly, especially elderly women, it is impossible to determine which patients will develop the syndrome. Whether neuroleptic drugs differ in their potential to cause tardive dyskinesia is unknown. For a more complete discussion of tardive dyskinesia, see the Antipsychotic Agents group monograph.

Neuroleptic malignant syndrome (NMS) is a potentially fatal condition reported in association with antipsychotic drugs and with **amoxapine**. Clinical manifestations of NMS are hyperpyrexia, muscle rigidity, altered mental status and evidence of autonomic instability (irregular pulse or blood pressure, tachycardia, diaphoresis and cardiac arrhythmias). The management of NMS should include: (1) Immediate discontinuation of antipsychotic drugs, amoxapine and other drugs not essential to concurrent therapy, (2) intensive symptomatic treatment and medical monitoring, and (3) treatment of any concomitant serious medical problems for which specific treatments are available. There is no general agreement about specific pharmacological treatment regimens for uncomplicated NMS.

Once the NMS is resolved, use a different antidepressant drug if the patient continues to require antidepressant treatment.

Hyperthermia has occurred with **clomipramine;** most cases occurred when it was used in combination with other drugs (eg, neuroleptics) and may be examples of a NMS.

Seizure disorders: Because TCAs lower the seizure threshold, use with caution in patients with a history of seizures. However, seizures have occurred both in patients with and without a history of seizure disorders. **Maprotiline** is associated with seizure occurrence in overdose and with therapeutic doses. Seizure was identified as the most significant risk of **clomipramine** use in premarket evaluation.

Anticholinergic effects: Use with caution in patients with a history of urinary retention, urethral or ureteral spasm; angle-closure glaucoma or increased intraocular pressure. In patients with angle-closure glaucoma, even average doses may precipitate an attack. In occasional susceptible patients or in those receiving anticholinergic drugs (including antiparkinson agents), the atropine-like effects may become more pronounced (eg, paralytic ileus). See table in introduction for relative anticholinergic actions.

Cardiovascular disorders: Use with extreme caution in patients with cardiovascular disorders (eg, severe coronary heart disease with ECG abnormalities, progressive heart failure, conduction disturbances, angina pectoris, paroxysmal tachycardia). In high doses, TCAs may produce arrhythmias, sinus tachycardia and prolong conduction time. Tachycardia may increase the frequency and severity of anginal attacks in the patient with coronary artery disease. Tachycardia and postural hypotension may occur more frequently with **protriptyline**. Orthostatic hypotension may occur in patients with decreased left ventricular performance (LVP). Myocardial infarction and stroke have occurred.

Hyperthyroid patients or those receiving thyroid medication require close supervision because of the possibility of cardiovascular toxicity, including arrhythmias.

Hazardous tasks: May impair mental or physical abilities required for the performance of potentially hazardous tasks; patients should observe caution while driving or performing other tasks requiring alertness, coordination or dexterity.

Renal or hepatic function impairment: Use with caution and in reduced doses in patients with hepatic impairment; metabolism may be impaired, leading to drug accumulation. Use with caution in patients with significantly impaired renal function.

Psychiatric patients: Schizophrenic or paranoid patients may exhibit a worsening of psychosis with TCA therapy, and manic-depressive patients may experience a shift to a hypomanic or manic phase; this may also occur when switching antidepressants and withdrawing them. In overactive or agitated patients, increased anxiety or agitation may occur. Paranoid delusions, with or without associated hostility, may be exaggerated. Reduction of TCA dosage and concomitant antipsychotic therapy may be necessary.

The possibility of suicide in depressed patients remains during treatment and until significant remission occurs. Patients should not have easy access to large quantities of the drug; prescribe small quantities of TCAs.

(Warnings continued on following page)

Warnings (Cont.):

Pregnancy (Category C: Amoxapine, trimipramine; *Category B:* Imipramine, maprotiline). Clinical experience is limited. These agents have demonstrated teratogenicity and embryotoxicity in dosages greater than maximum human doses. There have been clinical reports of congenital malformations associated with **imipramine.** Limb reduction anomalies have been reported with **amitriptyline** and **nortriptyline** and neonatal withdrawal symptoms have been seen with **clomipramine, desipramine** and **imipramine.** All are isolated reports.

Safety for use during pregnancy has not been established; use only when clearly needed and when the potential benefits outweigh the potential hazards to the fetus.

Lactation: These agents are excreted into breast milk in low concentrations (approximate milk:plasma ratio of 0.4 to 1.5). Exercise caution when administering these drugs to a nursing woman. At steady state, the concentrations of **maprotiline** in milk correspond closely to the concentrations in whole blood. The clinical effects of exposure are not known.

Children: Not recommended for patients < 12 years of age. Safety and efficacy are not established for **amoxapine** in children < 16 years old, **maprotiline** in children < 18 years old or **trazodone** or **clomipramine** in children < 10 years old. Safety and efficacy have not been established in the pediatric age group for **trimipramine, nortriptyline** and **protriptyline**.

Do not exceed 2.5 mg/kg/day of **imipramine**. ECG changes of unknown significance have occurred in pediatric patients with doses twice this amount. Effectiveness of imipramine in children for conditions other than nocturnal enuresis has not been established.

Precautions:

Monitor ECG prior to initiation of large doses of TCAs and at appropriate intervals thereafter. Patients with cardiovascular disease require cardiac surveillance at all dosage levels. Elderly patients and patients with cardiac disease or a history of cardiac disease are at special risk of developing cardiac abnormalities with TCAs.

Electroconvulsive therapy with coadministration of TCAs may increase the hazards of therapy.

Elective surgery: Discontinue therapy for as long as possible before elective surgery.

Blood sugar levels, both elevated and lowered, have occurred.

Monitoring: Perform baseline and periodic leukocyte and differential counts and liver function studies. Fever or sore throat may signal serious neutrophil depression; discontinue therapy if there is evidence of pathological neutropenia.

Sexual dysfuntion was markedly increased in male patients with OCD taking **clomipramine** (42% ejaculatory failure, 20% impotence) compared to placebo.

Weight changes: Weight gain occurred in 18% of patients receiving **clomipramine**. Some patients had weight gain in excess of 25% of their initial body weight.

Sulfite sensitivity: Some of the injectable antidepressant products contain sulfites that may cause allergic-type reactions including anaphylactic symptoms and life-threatening or less severe asthmatic episodes in certain susceptible people. The overall prevalence of sulfite sensitivity in the general population is unknown but is probably low. Sulfite sensitivity is seen more frequently in asthmatic than in non-asthmatic people. Products containing sulfites are identified in the product listings.

Tartrazine sensitivity: Some of these products contain tartrazine, which may cause allergic type reactions (including bronchial asthma) in susceptible individuals. Although the incidence of tartrazine sensitivity in the general population is low, it is frequently seen in patients who also have aspirin hypersensitivity. Specific products containing tartrazine are identified in the product listings.

Photosensitivity: Photosensitization (photoallergy or phototoxicity) may occur; therefore, caution patients to take protective measures (ie, sunscreens, protective clothing) against exposure to ultraviolet light or sunlight until tolerance is determined.

Drug Interactions:

Anticholinergics: The anticholinergic effects may be enhanced by the coadministration of certain TCAs.

Barbiturates may lower serum levels of TCAs; central and respiratory depressant effects may be additive.

Charcoal can prevent TCA absorption, thereby reducing their effectiveness or toxicity.

(Drug Interactions continued on following page)

Drug Interactions (Cont):

Cimetidine has increased serum TCA concentrations. Anticholinergic symptoms (eg, severe dry mouth, urinary retention, blurred vision) have been associated with elevated TCA serum levels when cimetidine therapy is initiated. Additionally, higher than expected TCA levels have occurred when they are begun in patients already taking cimetidine. Ranitidine may be an alternative.

Clonidine: Dangerous elevation in blood pressure and hypertensive crisis have occurred in patients receiving concurrent TCAs. Avoid coadministration.

Dicumarol: TCAs may increase the half-life or bioavailability of dicumarol, possibly resulting in increased anticoagulation effects.

Disulfiram and TCA coadministration may result in acute organic brain syndrome. The bioavailability of the antidepressant may also be increased.

Fluoxetine may increase the pharmacologic and toxic effects of TCAs; symptoms may persist for several weeks after the discontinuation of fluoxetine.

Guanethidine: TCAs may antagonize the antihypertensive action of guanethidine by inhibiting uptake into adrenergic neurons. Avoid this combination when possible; if concurrent therapy is required, monitor blood pressure. At dosages up to 150 mg/day, doxepin may be given with guanethidine without reducing the antihypertensive effect.

Haloperidol may increase serum concentrations of TCAs; a tonic-clonic seizure occurred in one patient.

Levodopa absorption may be delayed and its bioavailability decreased by TCAs. Hypertensive episodes have also occurred.

MAOIs should not be administered together with or immediately following TCAs. Such combinations can produce seizures, sweating, coma, hyperexcitability, hyperthermia, tachycardia, tachypnea, headache, mydriasis, flushing, confusion, hypotension, disseminated intravascular coagulation and death. At least 7 to 10 days should elapse between the discontinuation of MAOIs and the institution of the TCA. Some TCAs have been used safely and successfully in combination with MAOIs. Initiate the TCA cautiously with gradual dosage increase until achieving optimum response. **Furazolidone** may interact similarly with TCAs.

Oral contraceptives inhibit the hepatic metabolism of TCAs and may increase their plasma levels. **Estrogens** may increase or decrease the pharmacologic effect of TCAs depending on the estrogen dose.

Phenothiazines may increase serum levels of the TCAs by inhibition of hepatic metabolism.

Smoking may increase the metabolic biotransformation of TCAs.

Adverse Reactions:

Sedation and anticholinergic effects are reported most frequently. Tolerance to these effects develops, but side effects may be minimized by starting with a low dose and then gradually increasing the dose.

Cardiovascular: Orthostatic hypotension; hypertension; syncope; tachycardia; palpitations; myocardial infarction; arrhythmias; heart block; precipitation of CHF; stroke; ECG changes (most frequently with toxic doses); hypertensive episodes during surgery **(desipramine)**.

CNS: Confusion (especially in the elderly); disturbed concentration; hallucinations, disorientation; decrease in memory; feelings of unreality; delusions; anxiety; nervousness; restlessness; agitation; panic; insomnia; nightmares; hypomania; mania; exacerbation of psychosis; drowsiness; dizziness; weakness; fatigue; headache; depression, hypertonia, sleep disorder, psychosomatic disorder, yawning, abnormal dreaming, migraine, depersonalization, irritability, emotional lability, aggressive reaction **(clomipramine)**.

Neurological: Numbness; tingling; paresthesias of extremities; incoordination; motor hyperactivity; akathisia; ataxia; tremors; peripheral neuropathy; tardive dyskinesia **(amoxapine)**; extrapyramidal symptoms; seizures; alterations in EEG patterns; myoclonus, twitching, paresis, asthenia **(clomipramine)**.

Anticholinergic: Dry mouth and, rarely, associated sublingual adenitis; blurred vision; disturbance of accommodation, increased intraocular pressure and mydriasis; constipation; paralytic ileus; urinary retention; delayed micturition; dilation of the urinary tract.

Allergic: Skin rash; pruritus; vasculitis; petechiae, urticaria; photosensitization; itching; edema (general or of face and tongue); drug fever; dermatitis, acne, dry skin **(clomipramine)**.

Hematologic: Bone marrow depression including agranulocytosis; eosinophilia; purpura; thrombocytopenia; leukopenia; anemia **(clomipramine)**.

GI: Nausea and vomiting; anorexia; epigastric distress; diarrhea; flatulence; dysphagia; peculiar taste in mouth; increased salivation; stomatitis; glossitis; parotid swelling; abdominal cramps; pancreatitis; black tongue; dyspepsia, esophagitis, eructation **(clomipramine)**.

(Adverse Reactions continued on following page)

Tricyclic Compounds (Cont.)

Adverse Reactions (Cont.):

Hepatic: Rarely, hepatitis and jaundice. Elevation in transaminase; changes in alkaline phosphatase.

Endocrine: Gynecomastia and testicular swelling in the male; breast enlargement, menstrual irregularity and galactorrhea in the female; increased or decreased libido; painful ejaculation; impotence; nocturia; urinary frequency; urinary tract infection, dysuria, cystitis, dysmenorrhea, lactation (nonpuerperal), vaginitis, leukorrhea, breast pain, amenorrhea, ejaculation failure **(clomipramine)**.

Elevation or depression of blood sugar levels; elevation of prolactin levels; inappropriate ADH secretion.

Respiratory: Pharyngitis, rhinitis, sinusitis, coughing, bronchospasm, epistaxis, dyspnea, laryngitis **(clomipramine)**.

Special senses: Speech blockage; dysarthria; tinnitus; abnormal lacrimation; conjunctivitis, anisocoria, blepharospasm, otitis media, occular allergy, vestibular disorder **(clomipramine)**.

Other: Nasal congestion; excessive appetite; weight gain or loss; increased perspiration; hyperthermia; flushing; chills; alopecia; tooth disorder, abnormal skin odor, chest pain, fever, halitosis, thirst, myalgia, back pain, arthralgia, muscle weakness **(clomipramine)**.

Withdrawal symptoms: Although not indicative of addiction, abrupt cessation after prolonged therapy may produce nausea, headache, vertigo, nightmares and malaise. Gradual dosage reduction may produce, within 2 weeks, transient symptoms including irritability, restlessness, dreams and sleep disturbance. Rare instances of mania or hypomania occurring within 2 to 7 days following cessation of chronic therapy have occurred.

Enuretic children: Consider adverse reactions reported with adult use. Most common are nervousness, sleep disorders, tiredness and mild GI disturbances. These usually disappear with continued therapy or dosage reduction. Other reported reactions include: Constipation; convulsions; anxiety; emotional instability; syncope; collapse. Do not exceed 2.5 mg/kg/day of **imipramine**.

Overdosage:

Children are reportedly more sensitive than adults to acute overdose. Consider any overdose in infants or young children serious and potentially fatal.

Symptoms:

CNS: Early signs include confusion, agitation and hallucinations. Seizures are common, especially with **maprotiline** and **amoxapine,** and may begin within 12 hours after ingestion. Status epilepticus may develop. Physical examination may reveal clonus, choreoathetosis, hyperactive reflexes and a positive Babinski's sign. The patient may rapidly succumb to coma. Overdoses with amoxapine are particularly characterized by CNS toxicity. Maprotiline is associated with a high incidence of seizures (often with QRS intervals > 0.1 sec).

Anticholinergic: Flushing; dry mouth; dilated pupils; hyperpyrexia.

Cardiovascular: TCAs exert cardiotoxicity due to their anticholinergic activity and a quinidine-like effect that depresses myocardial contractility, heart rate and coronary blood flow. Cardiac arrhythmias include tachycardia, intraventricular blocks and complete AV block. With ingestions up to 20 mg/kg, re-entry ventricular arrhythmias, premature ventricular contractions, ventricular tachycardia or fibrillation may occur. Sudden cardiac arrest has been reported. Pulmonary edema and hypotension are common.

Renal: Renal failure may develop 2 to 5 days after toxic overdosage of **amoxapine** in patients who may appear otherwise recovered; acute tubular necrosis with rhabdomyolysis and myoglobinuria is most common. This reaction probably occurs in $< 5\%$ of overdose cases, and is typical in those who have experienced multiple seizures.

Treatment: Hospitalize and closely observe with ECG monitoring, even when the amount ingested is thought to be small or the initial degree of intoxication appears slight to moderate. Blood and urine levels are unreliable indicators for clinical management. Monitor patients with ECG abnormalities continuously for at least 3 to 5 days; observe closely until well after cardiac status returns to normal. A prolonged QRS interval may indicate the patient to be at higher risk for developing seizures, arrhythmias or hypotension. Relapses may occur after apparent recovery.

Maintain adequate respiratory exchange. Do not use respiratory stimulants. Use normal or half-normal saline to avoid water intoxication, especially in children. Instillation of activated charcoal slurry may help reduce absorption. Refer to General Management of Acute Overdosage.

(Overdosage continued on following page)

Complete prescribing information for these products begins on page 1282

Tricyclic Compounds (Cont.)

DOXEPIN HCl

Administration and Dosage:

Not recommended for use in children < 12 years old.

Mild to moderate anxiety or depression: Initially, 75 mg/day. Individualize dosage. Usual optimum dosage is 75 to 150 mg/day. Alternatively, the total daily dosage, up to 150 mg, may be given at bedtime.

Mild symptomatology or emotional symptoms accompanying organic disease: 25 to 50 mg/day is often effective.

More severe anxiety or depression: Higher doses (eg, 50 mg 3 times per day) may be required; if necessary, gradually increase to 300 mg/day. Additional effectiveness is rarely obtained by exceeding 300 mg/day.

Although optimal antidepressant response may not be evident for 2 to 3 weeks, anti-anxiety activity is rapidly apparent.

Dilute oral concentrate with approximately 120 ml of water, milk or fruit juice just prior to administration. Do not prepare or store bulk dilutions.

	Product	Form	Packaging	C.I.*
Rx	**Doxepin HCl** (Various, eg, Balan, Baxter, Elkins Sinn, Geneva, Goldline, Lederle, Major, Moore, Rugby, Schein)	**Capsules:** 10 mg	In 100s, 500s, 1000s and UD 100s.	21+
Rx	**Adapin** (Fisons)		In 100s, 1000s, and UD 100s.	49
Rx	**Sinequan** (Roerig)		In 100s, 1000s and UD 100s.	82
Rx	**Doxepin HCl** (Various, eg, Balan, Baxter, Bioline, Elkins Sinn, Geneva, Goldline, Major, Moore, Rugby, Schein)	**Capsules:** 25 mg	In 30s, 50s, 100s, 360s, 500s, 1000s and UD 100s.	9+
Rx	**Adapin** (Fisons)		In 100s, 1000s, 5000s and UD 100s.	25
Rx	**Sinequan** (Roerig)		In 100s, 1000s, 5000s and UD 100s & unit-of-use 90s.	42
Rx	**Doxepin HCl** (Various, eg, Balan, Baxter, Elkins Sinn, Geneva, Goldline, Lederle, Major, Moore, Rugby, Schein)	**Capsules:** 50 mg	In 30s, 100s, 360s, 500s, 1000s and UD 100s.	5+
Rx	**Adapin** (Fisons)		In 100s, 1000s, 5000s and UD 100s.	18
Rx	**Sinequan** (Roerig)		In 100s, 1000s, 5000s and UD 100s & unit-of-use 90s.	30
Rx	**Doxepin HCl** (Various, eg, Balan, Baxter, Elkins Sinn, Geneva, Goldline, Lederle, Major, Moore, Rugby, Schein)	**Capsules:** 75 mg	In 30s, 100s, 500s, 1000s and UD 100s.	6+
Rx	**Adapin** (Fisons)		In 100s, 1000s and UD 100s.	24
Rx	**Sinequan** (Roerig)		In 100s, 1000s and UD 100s.	33
Rx	**Doxepin HCl** (Various, eg, Balan, Baxter, Bioline, Geneva, Goldline, Lederle, Major, Moore, Rugby, Schein)	**Capsules:** 100 mg	In 100s, 500s, 1000s and UD 100s.	5+
Rx	**Adapin** (Fisons)		In 100s, 1000s and UD 100s.	19
Rx	**Sinequan** (Roerig)		In 100s, 1000s and UD 100s.	27

* Cost Index based on cost per 75 mg doxepin.
# Product identification code.

(Continued on following page)

Complete prescribing information for these products begins on page 1282

Tricyclic Compounds (Cont.)

	DOXEPIN HCl (Cont.)			**C.I.***
Rx	**Doxepin HCl** (Various, eg, Balan, Bioline, Dixon-Shane, Goldline, Lederle, Major, Martec, Par, Rugby)	**Capsules:** 150 mg	In 50s, 100s and 500s and UD 100s.	10+
Rx	**Adapin** (Fisons)		In 50s and UD 100s.	19
Rx	**Sinequan** (Roerig)		In 50s, 500s and UD 100s.	30
Rx	**Doxepin HCl** (Various, eg, Balan, Bioline, Geneva, Goldline, Harber, PBI, Rugby, Schein, Warner Chilcott)	**Oral Concentrate:** 10 mg/ml	In 120 ml.	33+
Rx	**Sinequan Concentrate** (Roerig)		In 120 ml.	53

TRIMIPRAMINE MALEATE

Administration and Dosage:

Not recommended for use in children.

Adult outpatients: Initially, 75 mg/day in divided doses; increase to 150 mg/day. Do not exceed 200 mg/day. The total dosage requirement may be given at bedtime.

Adult hospitalized patients: Initially, 100 mg/day in divided doses, increased gradually in a few days to 200 mg/day depending upon individual response and tolerance. If improvement does not occur in 2 to 3 weeks, increase to a maximum dose of 250 to 300 mg/day.

Adolescent and elderly patients: Initially, 50 mg/day, with gradual increments up to 100 mg/day.

Maintenance medication may be required at the lowest dose that will maintain remission (range 50 to 150 mg/day). Administer as a single bedtime dose. To minimize relapse, continue maintenance therapy for about 3 months.

				C.I.*
Rx	**Trimipramine Maleate** (Various, eg, Balan, Bioline, Dixon-Shane, Geneva, Goldline, Major, Moore, Parmed, Rugby, Schein)	**Capsules:** 25 mg	In 100s.	25+
Rx	**Surmontil** (Wyeth-Ayerst)		(Wyeth 4132). Blue and yellow. In 100s and Redipak 100s.	56
Rx	**Trimipramine Maleate** (Various, eg, Balan, Bioline, Dixon-Shane, Geneva, Goldline, Major, Moore, Parmed, Rugby, Schein)	**Capsules:** 50 mg	In 100s.	24+
Rx	**Surmontil** (Wyeth-Ayerst)		(Wyeth 4133). Blue and orange. In 100s and Redipak 100s.	46
Rx	**Trimipramine Maleate** (Various, eg, Balan, Best, Dixon-Shane, Major, Moore, Parmed, PBI, Rugby, Schein)	**Capsules:** 100 mg	In 100s.	24+
Rx	**Surmontil** (Wyeth-Ayerst)		(Wyeth 4158). Blue and white. In 100s.	34

* Cost Index based on cost per 75 mg doxepin or trimipramine.

Complete prescribing information for these products begins on page 1282

Tricyclic Compounds (Cont.)

AMOXAPINE

Administration and Dosage:

Amoxapine is not recommended for patients < 16 years old.

Usual effective dosage is 200 to 300 mg/day. Three weeks is an adequate trial period providing dosage has reached 300 mg/day (or a lower level of tolerance) for at least 2 weeks. If no response is seen at 300 mg, increase dosage, depending upon tolerance, to 400 mg/day. Hospitalized patients refractory to antidepressant therapy and who have no history of convulsive seizures may have dosage cautiously increased up to 600 mg/day in divided doses.

Adults: Initially, 50 mg 2 or 3 times daily. Depending upon tolerance, increase dosage to 100 mg 2 or 3 times daily by the end of the first week. (Initial dosage of 300 mg/day may cause sedation during the first few days of therapy.) Increase above 300 mg/day only if 300 mg/day has been ineffective for at least 2 weeks. Once an effective dosage is established, the drug may be given in a single bedtime dose (not to exceed 300 mg). If the total daily dosage exceeds 300 mg, give in divided doses.

Elderly patients: Initially, 25 mg 2 or 3 times a day. If tolerated, dosage may be increased by the end of the first week to 50 mg 2 or 3 times a day. Although 100 to 150 mg/day may be adequate for many elderly patients, some may require higher dosage; carefully increase up to 300 mg/day.

Maintenance dosage is the lowest dose that will maintain remission. If symptoms reappear, increase dosage to the earlier level until they are controlled.

	Product	Form	Description	C.I.*
Rx	**Amoxapine** (Various, eg, Bioline, Goldline, Major, Mason, Moore, Parmed, Qualitest, Rugby, Watson)	**Tablets:** 25 mg	In 100s.	103+
Rx	**Asendin** (Lederle)		(#25 LL A13). Off-white, scored. Heptagonal. In 100s.	117
Rx	**Amoxapine** (Various, eg, Bioline, Geneva, Goldline, Major, Mason, Moore, Parmed, Qualitest, Rugby, Watson)	**Tablets:** 50 mg	In 100s and 500s.	83+
Rx	**Asendin** (Lederle)		(#50 LL A15). Orange, scored. Heptagonal. In 100s, 500s and UD 100s.	95
Rx	**Amoxapine** (Various, eg, Bioline, Goldline, Major, Mason, Moore, Qualitest, Rugby, Watson)	**Tablets:** 100 mg	In 100s.	79+
Rx	**Asendin** (Lederle)		(#100 LL A17). Blue, scored. Heptagonal. In 100s and UD 100s.	80
Rx	**Amoxapine** (Various, eg, Goldline, Major, Mason, Moore, Qualitest, Rugby, Watson)	**Tablets:** 150 mg	In 30s and 100s.	84+
Rx	**Asendin** (Lederle)		(#150 LL A18). Peach, scored. Heptagonal. In 30s.	84

* Cost Index based on cost per 150 mg.
# Product identification code.

Complete prescribing information for these products begins on page 1282

Tricyclic Compounds (Cont.)

DESIPRAMINE HCl

Administration and Dosage:

Not recommended for use in children < 12 years of age.

Initial therapy may be given in divided doses or as a single daily dose. Maintenance therapy may be administered once daily. Continue a lower maintenance dosage for at least 2 months after a satisfactory response has been achieved.

Adults: 100 to 200 mg/day. In more severely ill patients, the dose may be gradually increased to 300 mg/day, if necessary. Do not exceed 300 mg/day. Treatment of patients requiring as much as 300 mg should generally be initiated in hospitals. Maintain continued therapy at the optimal dosage level during the active phase of depression. In cases of relapse due to premature withdrawal of the drug, a prompt response may be obtained by immediate resumption of treatment. Clinical symptoms of intolerance (eg, drowsiness, dizziness and postural hypotension) require dosage reduction.

Geriatrics and adolescents: 25 to 100 mg/day. Dosages > 150 mg not recommended. **C.I.***

	Product	Dosage form	Package	C.I.
Rx	**Desipramine HCl** (Various, eg, Balan, Bioline, Dixon-Shane, Geneva, Goldline, Harber, Major, Moore, Parmed, Rugby)	**Tablets:** 10 mg	In 100s and 1000s.	49+
Rx	**Norpramin** (Merrell Dow)		(#68-7). Blue. Film coated. In 100s.	108
Rx	**Desipramine HCl** (Various, eg, Balan, Bioline, Geneva, Goldline, Major, Moore, Rugby, Schein, Warner-C)	**Tablets:** 25 mg	In 30s, 100s, 500s, 1000s and UD 100s.	23+
Rx	**Norpramin** (Merrell Dow)		(#Merrell 11 or Norpramin 25). Yellow. Film coated. In 100s, 1000s and UD 100s.	52
Rx	**Desipramine HCl** (Various, eg, Balan, Bioline, Geneva, Goldline, Lemmon, Major, Moore, Rugby, Schein, Warner Chilcott)	**Tablets:** 50 mg	In 30s, 100s, 500s, 1000s and UD 100s.	20+
Rx	**Norpramin** (Merrell Dow)		(#Merrell 11 or Norpramin 25). Green. Film coated. In 100s, 1000s and UD 100s.	49
Rx	**Desipramine HCl** (Various, eg, Balan, Bioline, Geneva, Goldline, Lemmon, Major, Moore, Rugby, Schein, Warner Chilcott)	**Tablets:** 75 mg	In 30s, 100s, 500s, 1000s and UD 100s.	16+
Rx	**Norpramin** (Merrell Dow)		(#Merrell 19 or Norpramin 75) Orange. Film coated. In 100s.	41
Rx	**Desipramine HCl** (Various, eg, Balan, Bioline, Geneva, Goldline, Lemmon, Major, Moore, Rugby, Schein, Warner Chilcott)	**Tablets:** 100 mg	In 100s and 500s.	19+
Rx	**Norpramin** (Merrell Dow)		(#Merrell 20 or Norpramin 100). Peach. Film coated. In 100s.	41
Rx	**Desipramine HCl** (Various, eg, Balan, Bioline, Dixon-Shane, Geneva, Goldline, Harber, Major, Moore, Parmed, Rugby)	**Tablets:** 150 mg	In 50s and 100s.	18+
Rx	**Norpramin** (Merrell Dow)		(#Merrell 21 or Norpramin 150). White. Film coated. In 50s.	39
Rx	**Pertofrane** (Rorer)	**Capsules:** 25 mg	(#USV 160). Pink. In 100s.	92
		50 mg	(#USV 161). Maroon and pink. In 100s.	80

* Cost Index based on cost per 75 mg. # Product identification code.

Complete prescribing information for these products begins on page 1282

Tricyclic Compounds (Cont.)

PROTRIPTYLINE HCl

Administration and Dosage:

Not recommended for use in children.

Adults: 15 to 40 mg/day divided into 3 or 4 doses. May increase to 60 mg/day. Dosages above 60 mg/day are not recommended. Make any increases in the morning dose.

Adolescent and elderly patients: Initially, 5 mg 3 times/day; increase gradually, if necessary. In elderly patients, monitor the cardiovascular system closely if dose exceeds 20 mg/day.

				C.I.*
Rx	**Vivactil** (MSD)	**Tablets:** 5 mg	(#MSD 26). Orange. Film coated. Oval. In 100s.	49
		10 mg	(#MSD 47). Yellow. Film coated. Oval. In 100s and UD 100s.	36

CLOMIPRAMINE HCl

Indications:

Treatment of obsessions and compulsions in patients with Obsessive-Compulsive Disorder (OCD). The obsessions or compulsions must cause marked distress, be time-consuming or significantly interfere with social or occupational functioning, in order to meet the DSM-III-R (circa 1989) diagnosis of OCD.

Administration and Dosage:

Initial:

Adults – Initiate at 25 mg daily and gradually increase, as tolerated, to approximately 100 mg during the first 2 weeks. Administer in divided doses with meals to reduce GI side effects. Thereafter, the dosage may be increased gradually over the next several weeks to a maximum of 250 mg/day. After titration, the total daily dose may be given once daily at bedtime to minimize daytime sedation.

Children and adolescents – Initiate at 25 mg daily and gradually increase during the first 2 weeks, as tolerated, to a daily maximum of 3 mg/kg or 100 mg, whichever is smaller. Administer in divided doses with meals to reduce GI side effects. Thereafter, the dosage may be increased to a daily maximum of 3 mg/kg or 200 mg, whichever is smaller. After titration, the total daily dose may be given once daily at bedtime to minimize daytime sedation.

Maintenance:

Adults, adolescents and children – The efficacy of clomipramine after 10 weeks has not been documented in controlled trials. However, patients have continued therapy in double-blind studies for up to 1 year without loss of benefit. Adjust the dosage to maintain the patient on the lowest effective dosage and periodically reassess the patient to determine the need for treatment.

				C.I.*
Rx	**Anafranil** (Ciba)	**Capsules:** 25 mg	(#Anafranil 25 mg). Ivory and melon yellow. In 100s and UD 100s.	30
		50 mg	(#Anafranil 50 mg). Ivory and aqua blue. In 100s and UD 100s.	21
		75 mg	(#Anafranil 75 mg). Ivory and yellow. In 100s and UD 100s.	18

* Cost Index based on cost per 15 mg protriptyline or 25 mg clomipramine.

Product identification code.

Complete prescribing information for these products begins on page 1282

Tetracyclic Compounds

MAPROTILINE HCl

Maprotiline, a tetracyclic antidepressant, is included in this section because of pharmacologic and therapeutic similarities to the tricyclic agents.

Indications:

For the treatment of depressive illness in patients with depressive neurosis (dysthymic disorder) and manic-depressive illness, depressed type (major depressive disorder). Also effective for the relief of anxiety associated with depression.

Administration and Dosage:

May be given as a single daily dose or in divided doses. Therapeutic effects are sometimes seen within 3 to 7 days, although as long as 2 to 3 weeks are usually necessary before improvement is observed.

Initial adult dosage: Mild to moderate depression – An initial dose of 75 mg/day is suggested for outpatients. In some patients, especially the elderly, an initial dose of 25 mg daily may be used. Because of the long half-life of maprotiline, maintain initial dosage for 2 weeks. The dosage may then be increased gradually in 25 mg increments, as required and tolerated. Most patients respond to a dose of 150 mg/day, but doses as high as 225 mg/day may be required.

Severe depression – Give hospitalized patients an initial daily dose of 100 to 150 mg, which may be gradually increased, as required and tolerated. Most hospitalized patients with moderate to severe depression respond to a daily dosage of 150 mg, although dosages as high as 225 mg may be required. Do not exceed 225 mg/day.

Maintenance: Dosage during prolonged maintenance therapy should be kept at the lowest effective level. Dosage may be reduced to 75 to 150 mg/day with adjustment depending on therapeutic response.

Elderly patients: In general, lower doses are recommended for patients > 60 years of age. Doses of 50 to 75 mg/day are satisfactory as maintenance therapy for elderly patients who do not tolerate higher amounts.

Maprotiline is not recommended for patients < 18 years of age.

	Product	Form	Description	C.I.*
Rx	**Maprotiline HCl** (Various, eg, Balan, Geneva, Goldline, Major, Moore, Rugby, Schein, UDL, URL, Warner Chilcott)	**Tablets:** 25 mg	In 20s, 100s, 500s, 1000s and UD 100s.	25+
Rx	**Ludiomil** (Ciba)		(#Ciba 110). Orange, scored. Coated. Oval. In 100s and Accu-Pak 100s.	50
Rx	**Maprotiline HCl** (Various, eg, Balan, Geneva, Goldline, Major, Moore, Rugby, Schein, UDL, URL, Warner Chilcott)	**Tablets:** 50 mg	In 20s, 100s, 500s, 1000s and UD 100s.	19+
Rx	**Ludiomil** (Ciba)		(#Ciba 26). Orange, scored. Coated. Oval. In 100s and Accu-Pak 100s.	31
Rx	**Maprotiline HCl** (Various, eg, Balan, Geneva, Goldline, Major, Moore, Rugby, Schein, UDL, URL, Warner Chilcott)	**Tablets:** 75 mg	In 20s, 100s, 500s, 1000s and UD 100s.	17+
Rx	**Ludiomil** (Ciba)		(#Ciba 135). White, scored. Coated. Oval. In 100s and Accu-Pak 100s.	34

* Cost Index based on cost per 75 mg.

Product identification code.

TRAZODONE HCl

Actions:

Pharmacology: The mechanism of antidepressant action in humans is not fully understood. Trazodone is not a monoamine oxidase inhibitor and, unlike amphetamine-type drugs, does not stimulate the CNS. In animals, it selectively inhibits serotonin uptake by brain synaptosomes and potentiates the behavioral changes induced by the serotonin precursor, 5-hydroxytryptophan.

Cardiac conduction effects in the anesthetized dog are qualitatively dissimilar and quantitatively less pronounced than those seen with tricyclic antidepressants.

Pharmacokinetics: Absorption/Distribution – Trazodone is well absorbed after oral administration without selective localization in any tissue. When taken shortly after ingestion of food, there may be a slight increase in the amount of drug absorbed, a decrease in maximum concentration and a lengthening in the time to maximum concentration. Peak plasma levels occur in approximately 1 hour when taken on an empty stomach or in 2 hours when taken with food.

Metabolism/Excretion – Trazodone is extensively metabolized in the liver; < 1% is excreted unchanged in the urine and feces. Elimination is biphasic, with a half-life of 3 to 6 hours (mean, 4.4) and 5 to 9 hours (mean, 7 to 8), respectively, and is unaffected by food. Since the clearance of trazodone from the body is sufficiently variable, in some subjects it may accumulate in the plasma. The clearance of trazodone may be reduced in elderly male patients.

Onset of action – For those who responded to trazodone, one-third of the inpatients and one-half of the outpatients had a significant therapeutic response by the end of the first week of treatment. Three-fourths of all responders demonstrated a significant therapeutic effect by the end of the second week. One-fourth of responders required 2 to 4 weeks for a significant therapeutic response.

Indications:

Treatment of depression.

Unlabeled uses: Trazodone 50 mg twice daily and tryptophan 500 mg twice daily have been successful in the treatment of aggressive behavior. Dose adjustments were made until therapeutic response was achieved or unacceptable adverse effects developed. A dosage of 300 mg/day may also be useful for treatment of patients with panic disorder or agoraphobia with panic attacks.

Trazodone has also been used to treat cocaine withdrawal.

Contraindications:

Hypersensitivity to trazodone.

Warnings:

Preexisting cardiac disease: Not recommended for use during the initial recovery phase of myocardial infarction. Clinical studies and post-marketing reports in patients with preexisting cardiac disease indicate that trazodone may be arrhythmogenic in some patients. Arrhythmias identified include isolated PVCs, ventricular couplets and short episodes (3 to 4 beats) of ventricular tachycardia. Closely monitor patients with preexisting cardiac disease, particularly for cardiac arrhythmias.

Priapism has been reported in patients receiving trazodone. Patients with prolonged or inappropriate penile erection should discontinue use immediately and consult a physician. Injection of norepinephrine, epinephrine or dopamine may be successful in treating priapism. In approximately one-third of the cases reported, surgical intervention was required and, in a portion of these cases, permanent impairment of erectile function or impotence resulted.

Pregnancy: Category C. Trazodone has caused increased fetal resorption and congenital anomalies in the rat and rabbit fetus when given at approximately 15 to 50 times the maximum human dose. There are no adequate and well controlled studies in pregnant women. Use during pregnancy only if the potential benefit justifies the potential risk to the fetus.

Lactation: Trazodone and its metabolites have been found in the milk of rats, suggesting that the drug may be excreted in breast milk. Exercise caution when administering to a nursing mother.

Children: Safety and efficacy for use in children < 18 years of age are not established.

(Continued on following page)

TRAZODONE HCl (Cont.)

Precautions:

Suicide: The possibility of suicide in seriously depressed patients is inherent in the illness and may persist until significant remission occurs. Therefore, write prescriptions for the smallest number of tablets consistent with good patient management.

Hypotension, including orthostatic hypotension and syncope, has occurred.

Electroconvulsive therapy: Avoid concurrent administration with electroconvulsive therapy because of the absence of experience in this area.

Potentially hazardous tasks: May produce drowsiness, dizziness or blurred vision; patients should observe caution while driving or performing other tasks requiring alertness, coordination or dexterity.

Laboratory tests: Occasional low white blood cell and neutrophil counts have been noted, but were not considered clinically significant; however, discontinue the drug in any patient whose white blood cell count or absolute neutrophil count falls below normal levels. White blood cell and differential counts are recommended for patients who develop fever and sore throat (or other signs of infection) during therapy.

Drug Interactions:

Alcohol, barbiturates and other **CNS depressants:** Trazodone may enhance the CNS depressant response to these agents.

Digoxin serum levels were increased in a patient receiving concurrent trazodone.

Monoamine oxidase inhibitors: It is not known whether interactions will occur. If MAOIs are discontinued shortly before, or are to be given concomitantly with trazodone, initiate therapy cautiously.

Phenytoin serum levels were increased in a patient receiving trazodone.

Warfarin: In a single case report, trazodone coadministration with warfarin decreased prothrombin time and partial thromboplastin time. The hypoprothrombinemic effect of warfarin may be decreased.

Adverse Reactions:

Allergic: Skin conditions, edema (> 1%); allergic reaction; purpuric and maculopapular eruptions; rash; pruritis; urticaria.

Cardiovascular: Hypertension, hypotension, shortness of breath, syncope, tachycardia, palpitations (> 1%); chest pain; myocardial infarction; ventricular ectopic activity including ventricular tachycardia; vasodilation; conduction block; orthostatic hypotension; bradycardia; cardiac arrest; atrial fibrillation; arrhythmias. Occasional sinus bradycardia has occurred in long-term studies (see Warnings).

CNS: Anger, hostility, nightmares/vivid dreams, confusion, disorientation, decreased concentration, dizziness, lightheadedness, drowsiness, excitement, fatigue, headache, insomnia, impaired memory, nervousness, incoordination, paresthesia, tremors (> 1%); hallucinations; psychosis; vertigo; hypomania; mania; impaired speech; akathisia; numbness; delusions; agitation; weakness; grand mal seizures; extrapyramidal symptoms; tardive dyskinesia; stupor.

EENT: Tinnitus, blurred vision, red eyes (tired/itching), nasal/sinus congestion (> 1%); diplopia.

Endocrine: Decreased libido (> 1%); increased libido; impotence; priapism; retrograde ejaculation; early menses; missed periods; breast enlargement and engorgement; lactation.

GI: Abdominal/gastric disorder, bad taste in mouth, dry mouth, nausea, vomiting, diarrhea, constipation (> 1%); flatulence; hypersalivation; inappropriate ADH syndrome.

Hematologic: Anemia; hemolytic anemia; methemoglobinemia.

Hepatic: Liver enzyme alterations; intrahepatic cholestasis; hyperbilirubinemia; jaundice.

Musculoskeletal: Musculoskeletal aches and pains (> 1%); muscle twitches; ataxia.

Renal: Hematuria; delayed urine flow; increased urinary frequency; urinary incontinence/retention.

Other: Decreased appetite, sweating, clamminess, head (full/heavy), weight gain or loss, malaise (> 1%); increased appetite; apnea; alopecia; edema; leukonychia; unexplained death.

(Continued on following page)

TRAZODONE HCl (Cont.)

Overdosage:

Symptoms: Death from overdose has occurred in patients ingesting trazodone and other drugs concurrently (ie, alcohol, alcohol plus chloral hydrate plus diazepam, amobarbital, chlordiazepoxide or meprobamate).

The most severe reactions reported with overdose of trazodone alone have been priapism, respiratory arrest, seizures and ECG changes. Overdosage may cause an increase in incidence or severity of any of the reported adverse reactions.

Clinical manifestations of overdose may include any of those listed in Adverse Reactions, with drowsiness and vomiting reported most frequently.

Treatment: There is no specific antidote. Treatment should be symptomatic and supportive for hypotension or excessive sedation. Patients suspected of having taken an overdose should have their stomachs emptied by gastric lavage. Forced diuresis may be useful in elimination of the drug. Refer to General Management of Acute Overdosage.

Patient Information:

Take with food.

May produce drowsiness or dizziness; patients should observe caution while driving or performing other tasks requiring alertness, coordination or dexterity.

Notify physician of dizziness, lightheadedness, fainting or blood in urine.

Male patients with prolonged, inappropriate and painful erections should immediately discontinue the drug and consult their physician.

Medication may cause dry mouth, irregular heartbeat, shortness of breath, nausea and vomiting; notify physician if these become pronounced.

Avoid alcohol and other depressant drugs.

Administration and Dosage:

Initiate dosage at a low level and increase gradually. Drowsiness may require the administration of a major portion of the daily dose at bedtime or a reduced dosage. Take shortly after a meal or light snack. Symptomatic relief may be seen during the first week, with optimal effects typically evident within 2 weeks. Approximately 25% of those who respond to therapy require 2 to 4 weeks of drug administration.

Adults: An initial dose is 150 mg/day. This may be increased by 50 mg/day every 3 to 4 days. The maximum dose for outpatients usually should not exceed 400 mg/day in divided doses. Inpatients or more severely depressed subjects may be given up to, but not in excess of, 600 mg/day in divided doses.

Maintenance: Keep dosage at the lowest effective level. Once an adequate response has been achieved, dosage may be gradually reduced with subsequent adjustment depending on response.

	Product	Form	Description	C.I.*
Rx	**Trazodone HCl** (Various, eg, Balan, Elkins-Sinn, Geneva, Goldline, Lederle, Moore, Rugby, Schein, Squibb Mark, Warner-C)	**Tablets:** 50 mg	In 30s, 100s, 250s, 500s, 1000s and UD 100s.	33+
Rx	**Desyrel** (Mead Johnson Pharm.)		(#MJ 775 Desyrel). Orange, scored. Film coated. In 100s, 1000s and UD 100s.	67
Rx	**Trazodone HCl** (Various, eg, Balan, Elkins-Sinn, Geneva, Goldline, Lederle, Moore, Rugby, Schein, Squibb Mark, Warner-C)	**Tablets:** 100 mg	In 30s, 100s, 250s, 500s, 1000s and UD 100s.	10+
Rx	**Desyrel** (Mead Johnson Pharm.)		(#MJ 776 Desyrel). White, scored. Film coated. In 100s, 1000s and UD 100s.	58
Rx	**Trazodone HCl** (Various, eg, Balan, Bioline, Dixon-Shane, Goldline, Lederle, Major, Moore, Rugby, Schein, Warner-C)	**Tablets:** 150 mg	In 30s, 100s, 250s, 500s and 1000s.	14+
Rx	**Desyrel Dividose** (Mead Johnson Pharm.)		(#MJ 778 50). Orange, triple scored. In 100s and 500s.	37
Rx	**Desyrel Dividose** (Mead Johnson Pharm.)	**Tablets:** 300 mg	(#MJ 796 100). Yellow. Triple scored. In 100s.	27

* Cost Index based on cost per 100 mg.

Product identification code.

FLUOXETINE HCl

Actions:

Pharmacology: Fluoxetine is an oral antidepressant chemically unrelated to tricyclic, tetracyclic or other available antidepressants. The antidepressant action of fluoxetine is presumed to be linked to its inhibition of CNS neuronal uptake of serotonin. Studies have demonstrated fluoxetine blocks uptake of serotonin, but not of norepinephrine, into human platelets. Animal studies suggest fluoxetine is a much more potent uptake inhibitor of serotonin than of norepinephrine.

Antagonism of muscarinic, histaminergic and α_1-adrenergic receptors has been hypothesized to be associated with various anticholinergic, sedative and cardiovascular effects of tricyclic antidepressants. Fluoxetine binds to these and other membrane receptors from brain tissue much less potently in vitro than do the tricyclics.

Pharmacokinetics: Absorption/Distribution – Systemic bioavailability: Following a single oral 40 mg dose, peak plasma concentrations range from 15 to 55 ng/ml after 6 to 8 hours. Food does not appear to affect systemic bioavailability although it may delay absorption. Thus, fluoxetine may be administered with or without food. Over the concentration range (200 to 1000 ng/ml), approximately 94.5% of fluoxetine is bound in vitro to human serum proteins.

Metabolism – Fluoxetine is extensively metabolized in the liver to norfluoxetine (demethylation of fluoxetine) and other unidentified metabolites. In animal models, norfluoxetine's potency and selectivity as a serotonin uptake blocker are equivalent to fluoxetine's. The primary route of elimination appears to be hepatic metabolism to inactive metabolites excreted by the kidneys.

Elimination – The relatively slow elimination of fluoxetine (elimination half-life, 2 to 3 days) and norfluoxetine (elimination half-life, 7 to 9 days) assures significant accumulation in chronic use. After 30 days of dosing at 40 mg/day, plasma concentrations of fluoxetine range from 91 to 302 ng/ml and for norfluoxetine 72 to 258 ng/ml. Plasma concentrations of fluoxetine were higher than those predicted by single dose studies, presumably because fluoxetine's metabolism is not proportional to dose. Norfluoxetine, however, appears to have linear pharmacokinetics.

Thus, even if patients are given a fixed dose, steady-state plasma concentrations are only achieved after continuous dosing for approximately 4 or 5 weeks. Also, even when dosing is stopped, active drug substance will persist in the body for weeks. This is of potential consequence when drug discontinuation is required.

Indications:

Depression: The efficacy was established in depressed outpatients whose diagnoses corresponded most closely to the DSM-III category of major depressive disorder.

The effectiveness in long-term use, for > 5 to 6 weeks, has not been systematically evaluated. Therefore, periodically reevaluate the drug when used for extended periods.

Unlabeled uses: Fluoxetine (20 to 60 mg/day) has been investigated in the treatment of obesity (see Precautions). Fluoxetine may also be useful in the treatment of bulimia nervosa (60 to 80 mg/day) and obsessive-compulsive disorders.

Contraindications:

Hypersensitivity to the drug.

(Continued on following page)

FLUOXETINE HCl (Cont.)

Warnings:

Rash and accompanying events: Approximately 4% of patients have developed a rash or urticaria. Almost a third were withdrawn from treatment. Clinical findings reported in association with rash include: Fever, leukocytosis, arthralgias, edema, carpal tunnel syndrome, respiratory distress, lymphadenopathy, proteinuria and mild transaminase elevation. Most patients improved promptly with discontinuation of fluoxetine or adjunctive treatment with antihistamines or steroids, and all patients recovered completely.

Two patients developed a serious cutaneous systemic illness. Neither patient had an unequivocal diagnosis, but one had a leukocytoclastic vasculitis; the other had a severe desquamating syndrome that was considered variously to be vasculitis or erythema multiforme. Several other patients have had systemic syndromes suggestive of serum sickness.

Systemic events, possibly related to vasculitis, have developed in patients with rash. Although these events are rare, they may be serious, involving the lung, kidney or liver. Death has occurred in association with these systemic events.

Anaphylactoid events, including bronchospasm, angioedema and urticaria alone and in combination, have occurred.

Pulmonary events, including inflammatory processes of varying histopathology or fibrosis, have occurred rarely. These events have occurred with dyspnea as the only preceding symptom.

It is unknown whether the association of rash and other events constitutes a true fluoxetine-induced syndrome. No patient sustained lasting injury. Though almost two-thirds of patients developing a rash continued to take fluoxetine without any consequence, discontinue the drug upon appearance of rash.

Hepatic function impairment can affect the elimination of fluoxetine. The elimination half-life of fluoxetine was prolonged in a study of cirrhotic patients, with a mean of 7.6 days; norfluoxetine elimination was also delayed, with a mean duration of 12 days for cirrhotic patients. Use fluoxetine with caution in patients with liver disease. Use a lower or less frequent dose.

Renal function impairment: In single dose studies, the pharmacokinetics of fluoxetine and norfluoxetine were similar among subjects with all levels of impaired renal function, including anephric patients on chronic hemodialysis. However, with chronic administration, additional accumulation of fluoxetine or its metabolites may occur in patients with severely impaired renal function; use a lower or less frequent dose.

Elderly: The disposition of single doses of fluoxetine in healthy elderly subjects ($>$ 65 years of age) did not differ significantly from that in younger normal subjects. However, data are insufficient to rule out possible age-related differences during chronic use.

Pregnancy: Category B. There are no adequate and well controlled studies in pregnant women. Use during pregnancy only if clearly needed.

Lactation: Exercise caution when administering to a nursing woman. In one breast milk sample, the concentration of fluoxetine plus norfluoxetine was 70.4 ng/ml; the mother's plasma concentration was 259 ng/ml. No adverse effects on the infant occurred.

Children: Safety and efficacy have not been established.

Precautions:

Anxiety, nervousness and insomnia (10% to 15% of patients) led to drug discontinuation in 5% of patients.

Altered appetite and weight: Significant weight loss, especially in underweight depressed patients. Approximately 9% of patients experienced anorexia. A weight loss of $>$ 5% occurred in 13% of fluoxetine-treated patients compared to 4% of placebo and 3% of tricyclic antidepressant-treated patients. However, only rarely has the drug been discontinued because of weight loss.

Activation of mania/hypomania occurred in approximately 1%. Activation of mania/hypomania has also occurred in a small proportion of patients with Major Affective Disorder treated with other marketed antidepressants.

Seizures: Twelve patients among $>$ 6000 (0.2%) experienced convulsions (or events described as seizures). This appears similar to the rate associated with other antidepressants. Use with care in patients with a history of seizures.

Suicide: The possibility of a suicide attempt is inherent in depression and may persist until significant remission occurs. Closely supervise high-risk patients during initial drug therapy. Write prescriptions for smallest quantity of capsules consistent with good patient management to reduce risk of overdose.

(Precautions continued on following page)

FLUOXETINE HCl (Cont.)

Precautions (Cont.):

The long elimination half-life of fluoxetine and norfluoxetine means that changes in dose will not be fully reflected in plasma for several weeks, affecting titration to final dose and withdrawal from treatment.

Concomitant illness: Clinical experience is limited. Use caution in patients with diseases or conditions that could affect metabolism or hemodynamic responses.

Heart disease: Fluoxetine has not been evaluated or used to any appreciable extent in patients with a recent history of myocardial infarction or unstable heart disease. However, the ECGs of 312 patients were retrospectively evaluated; no conduction abnormalities that resulted in heart block were observed. The mean heart rate was reduced by approximately 3 beats/min.

Physical and psychological dependence: Premarketing clinical experience did not reveal any tendency for a withdrawal syndrome or any drug-seeking behavior. However, it is not possible to predict on the basis of this limited experience the extent to which a CNS active drug will be misused, diverted, or abused once marketed. Consequently, carefully evaluate patients for history of drug abuse and follow such patients closely, observing them for signs of misuse or abuse (eg, development of tolerance, incrementation of dose, drug-seeking behavior).

Hazardous tasks: May cause dizziness or drowsiness. Patient should observe caution while driving or performing tasks requiring alertness, coordination or dexterity.

Electroconvulsive therapy (ECT): There are no clinical studies establishing the benefit of the combined use of ECT and fluoxetine. A single report of a prolonged seizure in a patient on fluoxetine has occurred.

Hyponatremia: Several cases of hyponatremia (some with serum sodium < 110 mmol/L) have occurred. The hyponatremia appeared to be reversible when fluoxetine was discontinued. Although these cases were complex with varying possible etiologies, some were possibly due to the syndrome of inappropriate antidiuretic hormone secretion (SIADH). The majority of these occurrences have been in older patients and in patients taking diuretics or who were otherwise volume depleted.

Diabetes: Fluoxetine may alter glycemic control. Hypoglycemia has occurred during therapy, and hyperglycemia has developed following discontinuation of the drug. The dosage of insulin or the sulfonylurea may need to be adjusted when fluoxetine is started or discontinued.

Drug Interactions:

Diazepam: The half-life of coadministered diazepam may be prolonged.

Haloperidol: A patient developed severe extrapyramidal reactions during coadministration of haloperidol and fluoxetine.

Lithium serum levels may be increased with possible neurotoxicity during fluoxetine coadministration. Monitor lithium levels.

Monoamine oxidase inhibitors (MAOIs): Although limited clinical data are available on the effects of the combined use of fluoxetine and MAO inhibitors, it seems prudent to avoid their combined use. Based on experience with combined administration of MAOIs and tricyclics, at least 14 days should elapse between MAOI discontinuation and initiation of fluoxetine.

Because of the long half-lives of fluoxetine and its active metabolite, at least 5 weeks (approximately 5 half-lives of norfluoxetine) should elapse between discontinuation of fluoxetine and initiation of therapy with an MAOI. Administration of an MAOI within 5 weeks of discontinuation of fluoxetine may increase the risk of serious events. While a causal relationship to fluoxetine has not been established, death has occurred following the initiation of MAOI therapy shortly after discontinuation of fluoxetine.

Tricyclic antidepressants: The pharmacologic and toxic effects of these agents may be increased by fluoxetine.

L-tryptophan: Five patients receiving fluoxetine in combination with tryptophan experienced agitation, restlessness and GI distress.

Because fluoxetine is tightly bound to plasma protein, administration to a patient taking another drug which is tightly bound to protein (eg, warfarin, digitoxin) may cause a shift in plasma concentrations potentially resulting in an adverse effect. Conversely, adverse effects may result from displacement of protein-bound fluoxetine by other tightly bound drugs.

(Continued on following page)

SERTRALINE HCl (Cont.)

Warnings:

MAO inhibitors: In patients receiving another serotonin reuptake inhibitor drug in combination with an MAOI, there have been reports of serious, sometimes fatal, reactions including hyperthermia, rigidity, myoclonus, autonomic instability with possible rapid fluctuations of vital signs, and mental status changes that include extreme agitation progressing to delirium and coma. These reactions have also occurred in patients who have recently discontinued that drug and have been started on an MAOI. Some cases presented with features resembling neuroleptic malignant syndrome. Therefore, it is recommended that sertraline not be used in combination with an MAOI, or within 14 days of discontinuing treatment with an MAOI. Similarly, allow at least 14 days after stopping sertraline before starting an MAOI (see Drug Interactions).

Hepatic function impairment: Sertraline is extensively metabolized by the liver. Use with caution in patients with severe hepatic impairment.

Renal function impairment: Since sertraline is extensively metabolized, excretion of unchanged drug in urine is a minor route of elimination. However, use with caution in patients with severe renal impairment.

Carcinogenesis/Fertility impairment: There was a dose-related increase in the incidence of liver adenomas in male mice receiving sertraline at 10 to 40 mg/kg (10 times, on a mg/kg basis, the maximum recommended human dose). Liver adenomas have a variable rate of spontaneous occurrence in the CD-1 mouse and are of unknown significance to humans. There was an increase in follicular adenomas of the thyroid in female rats receiving sertraline at 40 mg/kg; this was not accompanied by thyroid hyperplasia. While there was an increase in uterine adenocarcinomas in rats receiving sertraline at 10 to 40 mg/kg compared to placebo controls, this effect was not clearly drug related.

A decrease in fertility was seen in one of two rat studies at a dose of 80 mg/kg (20 times the maximum human dose on a mg/kg basis).

Elderly: Several hundred elderly patients have participated in clinical studies with sertraline. The pattern of adverse reactions in the elderly was similar to that in younger patients. However, sertraline plasma clearance may be lower (see Pharmacokinetics).

Pregnancy: Category B. At doses ≈ 2.5 to 10 times the maximum daily human mg/kg dose, sertraline was associated with delayed ossification in fetuses of rats and rabbits, probably secondary to effects on the dams. There was also decreased neonatal survival following maternal administration of sertraline at doses as low as ≈ 5 times the maximum human mg/kg dose. The decrease in pup survival was shown to be most probably due to in utero exposure to sertraline.

There are no adequate and well controlled studies in pregnant women. Use during pregnancy only if clearly needed.

Lactation: It is not known whether sertraline or its metabolites are excreted in breast milk. Exercise caution when sertraline is administered to a nursing woman.

Children: Safety and efficacy in children have not been established.

Precautions:

Activation of mania/hypomania: During premarketing testing, hypomania or mania occurred in ≈ 0.4% of sertraline-treated patients. Activation of mania/hypomania has also occurred in a small number of patients with Major Affective Disorder treated with other marketed antidepressants.

Weight loss: Significant weight loss may be an undesirable result of treatment with sertraline for some patients, but on average, patients in controlled trials had minimal 1 to 2 pound weight loss versus smaller changes on placebo. Only rarely have sertraline patients been discontinued for weight loss.

Seizure: Sertraline has not been evaluated in patients with a seizure disorder. However, like other antidepressants, introduce sertraline with care in epileptic patients.

Suicide: The possibility of a suicide attempt is inherent in depression and may persist until significant remission occurs. Close supervision of high-risk patients should accompany initial drug therapy. Write prescriptions for the smallest quantity of tablets consistent with good patient management, in order to reduce the risk of overdose.

(Precautions continued on following page)

SERTRALINE HCl (Cont.)

Precautions (Cont.):

Uricosuric effect: Sertraline is associated with a mean decrease in serum uric acid of ≈ 7%. The clinical significance of this weak uricosuric effect is unknown, and there have been no reports of acute renal failure with sertraline.

Concomitant illness: Caution is advisable in using sertraline in patients with diseases or conditions that could affect metabolism or hemodynamic responses.

Drug abuse and dependence: Sertraline is not a controlled substance. However, carefully evaluate patients for history of drug abuse and follow such patients closely, observing them for signs of misuse or abuse (eg, development of tolerance, incrementation of dose, drug-seeking behavior).

Drug Interactions:

Drugs highly bound to plasma proteins: Because sertraline is highly bound to plasma protein, the administration of sertraline to a patient taking another drug which is highly bound to protein (eg, warfarin, digitoxin) may cause a shift in plasma concentrations potentially resulting in an adverse effect. Conversely, adverse effects may result from displacement of protein-bound sertraline by other highly bound drugs.

Microsomal enzyme induction: Preclinical studies have shown sertraline to induce hepatic microsomal enzymes. In clinical studies, sertraline induced hepatic enzymes minimally as determined by a small (5%) but statistically significant decrease in antipyrine half-life following administration of 200 mg/day for 21 days. This small change in antipyrine half-life reflects a clinically insignificant change in hepatic metabolism.

Sertraline Drug Interactions			
Precipitant drug	Object drug*		Description
MAO inhibitors	Sertraline	↑	Serious, sometimes fatal reactions may occur, including hyperthermia, rigidity, myoclonus, autonomic instability with possible rapid fluctuation of vital signs, and mental status changes that include extreme agitation progressing to delirium and coma (see Warnings).
Sertraline	Alcohol	↔	Although potentiation of cognitive and psychomotor effects of alcohol did not occur in healthy subjects, concurrent use is not recommended in depressed patients.
Sertraline	Diazepam	↑	In one study there was a 32% decrease in diazepam clearance with concurrent sertraline (vs 19% with placebo). Desmethyldiazepam T_{max} increased 23% (vs 20% decrease with placebo). Clinical significance is unknown.
Sertraline	Lithium	↔	In healthy volunteers sertraline did not affect lithium levels; however, monitor lithium levels following initiation of sertraline.
Sertraline	Tolbutamide	↑	In one study sertraline significantly decreased the clearance of tolbutamide (16%). Clinical significance is unknown.
Sertraline	Warfarin	↑	In one study concurrent sertraline and warfarin resulted in an 8% increase in prothrombin time (PT) (vs 1% decrease with placebo) and delayed normalization of PT. Clinical significance is unknown. Monitor PT.

* ↑ = Object drug increased. ↔ = Undetermined effect.

Drug/Food interaction: In one study following a single dose of sertraline with and without food, the sertraline AUC was slightly increased and the C_{max} was 25% greater. The time to reach peak plasma concentration decreased from 8 hours postdosing to 5.5 hours.

(Continued on following page)

SERTRALINE HCl (Cont.)

Adverse Reactions:

The most commonly observed adverse events associated with the use of sertraline and not seen at an equivalent incidence among placebo-treated patients were: GI complaints, including nausea, diarrhea/loose stools and dyspepsia; tremor; dizziness; insomnia; somnolence; increased sweating; dry mouth; male sexual dysfunction (primarily ejaculatory delay).

Of 2710 subjects who received sertraline in premarketing multiple dose clinical trials, 15% discontinued treatment due to an adverse event. The more common events (reported by at least 1% of subjects) associated with discontinuation included: Agitation; insomnia; male sexual dysfunction (primarily ejaculatory delay); somnolence; dizziness; headache; tremor; anorexia; diarrhea/loose stools; nausea; fatigue.

Sertraline Adverse Reactions		
Autonomic nervous system		
Dry mouth 16.3% Increased sweating 8.4% ***Infrequent (0.1% to 1%)*** Flushing	Mydriasis Increased saliva Cold/Clammy skin	***Rare (< 0.1%)*** Pallor
Cardiovascular		
Palpitations 3.5% Chest pain 1% ***Infrequent (0.1% to 1%)*** Postural dizziness Hypertension Hypotension	Postural hypotension Edema (dependent, periorbital, peripheral) Peripheral ischemia Syncope Tachycardia	***Rare (< 0.1%)*** Precordial/Substernal chest pain Aggravated hypertension Myocardial infarction Varicose veins
Central/Peripheral nervous system		
Headache 20.3% Dizziness 11.7% Tremor 10.7% Paresthesia 2% Hypoesthesia 1.7% Twitching 1.4% Hypertonia 1.3% Confusion 1%	***Infrequent (0.1% to 1%)*** Ataxia Abnormal coordination Abnormal gait Hyperesthesia Hyperkinesia Hypokinesia Migraine Nystagmus Vertigo	***Rare (< 0.1%)*** Local anesthesia Coma Convulsions Dyskinesia Dysphonia Hyporeflexia Hypotonia Ptosis
Dermatologic		
Rash 2.1% ***Infrequent (0.1% to 1%)*** Acne Alopecia Pruritus Erythematous rash Maculopapular rash Dry skin	***Rare (< 0.1%)*** Bullous eruption Dermatitis Erythema multiforme Abnormal hair texture Hypertrichosis Photosensitivity Follicular rash	Skin discoloration Abnormal skin odor Urticaria
GI		
Nausea 26.1% Diarrhea/Loose stools 17.7% Constipation 8.4% Dyspepsia 6% Vomiting 3.8% Flatulence 3.3% Anorexia 2.8% Abdominal pain 2.4% Increased appetite 1.3%	***Infrequent (0.1% to 1%)*** Dysphagia Eructation ***Rare (< 0.1%)*** Diverticulitis Fecal incontinence Gastritis Gastroenteritis Glossitis Gum hyperplasia	Hemorrhoids Hiccup Melena Hemorrhagic peptic ulcer Proctitis Stomatitis Ulcerative stomatitis Tenesmus Tongue edema/ulceration
Musculoskeletal		
Myalgia 1.7% ***Infrequent (0.1% to 1%)*** Arthralgia	Arthrosis Dystonia Muscle cramps/weakness	***Rare (< 0.1%)*** Hernia

(Adverse Reactions continued on following page)

SERTRALINE HCl (Cont.)

Adverse Reactions (Cont.):

Sertraline Adverse Reactions (Cont.)		
Psychiatric		
Insomnia 16.4%	***Infrequent (0.1% to 1%)***	Hallucination
Sexual dysfunction	Abnormal dreams	Neurosis
male 15.5%	Aggressive reaction	Paranoid reaction
female 1.7%	Amnesia	Suicide ideation/attempt
Somnolence 13.4%	Apathy	Teeth-grinding
Agitation 5.6%	Delusion	Abnormal thinking
Nervousness 3.4%	Depersonalization	***Rare (< 0.1%)***
Anxiety 2.6%	Depression	Hysteria
Yawning 1.9%	Aggravated depression	Somnambulism
Impaired concentration 1.3%	Emotional lability	Withdrawal syndrome
	Euphoria	
Reproductive		
Menstrual disorder 1%	***Rare (< 0.1%)***	Female breast pain
Infrequent (0.1% to 1%)	Amenorrhea	Leukorrhea
Dysmenorrhea	Balanoposthitis	Menorrhagia
Intermenstrual bleeding	Breast enlargement	Atrophic vaginitis
Respiratory		
Rhinitis 2%	Dyspnea	Sinusitis
Pharyngitis 1.2%	Epistaxis	Stridor
Infrequent (0.1% to 1%)	***Rare (< 0.1%)***	
Bronchospasm	Bradypnea	
Coughing	Hyperventilation	
Special senses		
Abnormal vision 4.2%	Conjunctivitis	***Rare (< 0.1%)***
Tinnitus 1.4%	Diplopia	Abnormal lacrimation
Taste perversion 1.2%	Earache	Photophobia
Infrequent (0.1% to 1%)	Eye pain	Visual field defect
Abnormal accommodation	Xerophthalmia	
GU		
Micturition frequency 2%	Face edema	***Rare (< 0.1%)***
Micturition disorder 1.4%	Nocturia	Oliguria
Infrequent (0.1% to 1%)	Polyuria	Renal pain
Dysuria	Urinary incontinence	Urinary retention
Miscellaneous		
Fatigue 10.6%	Rigors	Anemia
Hot flushes 2.2%	Weight decrease/increase	Anterior chamber eye hemorrhage
Fever 1.6%	Lymphadenopathy	
Back pain 1.5%	Purpura	Dehydration
Thirst 1.4%	***Rare (< 0.1%)***	Hypercholesterolemia
Asthenia 1%	Enlarged abdomen	Hypoglycemia
Infrequent (0.1% to 1%)	Halitosis	Exophthalmos
Malaise	Otitis media	Gynecomastia
Generalized edema	Aphthous stomatitis	

Laboratory test abnormalities: Asymptomatic elevations in serum transaminases (AST or ALT) have occurred infrequently (≈ 0.8%) in association with sertraline administration. These hepatic enzyme elevations usually occurred within the first 1 to 9 weeks of drug treatment and promptly diminished upon drug discontinuation.

Sertraline therapy was associated with small mean increases in total cholesterol (≈ 3%) and triglycerides (≈ 5%) and a small mean decrease in serum uric acid (≈ 7%) of no apparent clinical importance.

(Continued on following page)

BUPROPION HCl (Cont.)

Adverse Reactions (Cont.):

Most common: Agitation; dry mouth; insomnia; headache/migraine; nausea/vomiting; constipation; tremor.

Adverse reactions caused discontinuation in approximately 10% of 2400 patients and volunteers. The more common events causing discontinuation include: Neuropsychiatric disturbances, primarily agitation and abnormalities in mental status (3%); GI disturbances, primarily nausea and vomiting (2.1%); neurological disturbances, primarily seizures, headaches and sleep disturbances (1.7%); dermatologic problems, primarily rashes (1.4%). Many of these events occurred at doses that exceeded the recommended daily dose.

Causal relationship not established:

Cardiovascular: Edema (1%); ECG abnormalities (premature beats and nonspecific ST-T changes), chest pain, shortness of breath/dyspnea (0.1% to 1%); pallor, phlebitis, flushing, myocardial infarction (< 0.1%).

Dermatologic: Rashes (1%); alopecia, dry skin (0.1% to 1%); acne, hair color change, hirsutism (< 0.1%).

Endocrine: Gynecomastia (0.1% to 1%); glycosuria, hormone level change (< 0.1%).

GI: Dysphagia, thirst disturbance, liver damage/jaundice (0.1% to 1%); rectal complaints, colitis, GI bleeding, stomach ulcer, intestinal perforation (< 0.1%).

GU: Nocturia (1%); vaginal irritation, testicular swelling, urinary tract infection, painful erection, retarded ejaculation (0.1% to 1%); dysuria, enuresis, urinary incontinence, menopause, ovarian disorder, pelvic infection, cystitis, dyspareunia, painful ejaculation (< 0.1%).

Hematologic: Anemia, pancytopenia, lymphadenopathy (< 0.1%).

Neurologic (see Warnings): Ataxia/incoordination, seizure, myoclonus, dyskinesia, dystonia (1%); mydriasis, vertigo, dysarthria (0.1% to 1%); EEG abnormality, abnormal neurological exam, impaired attention, sciatica, aphasia (< 0.1%).

Neuropsychiatric (see Precautions): Mania/hypomania, increased libido, hallucinations, decreased sexual function, depression (1%); memory impairment, depersonalization, psychosis, dysphoria, mood instability, paranoia, formal thought disorder, frigidity (0.1% to 1%); suicidal ideation (< 0.1%).

Oral: Stomatitis (1%); toothache, bruxism, gum irritation, oral edema (0.1% to 1%); glossitis (< 0.1%).

Respiratory: Bronchitis, shortness of breath/dyspnea (0.1% to 1%); epistaxis, rate or rhythm disorder, pneumonia, pulmonary embolism (< 0.1%).

Special Senses: Visual disturbance (0.1% to 1%); diplopia (< 0.1%.)

Miscellaneous: Flu-like symptoms (1%); nonspecific pain (0.1% to 1%); body odor, surgically related pain, infection, medication reaction, musculoskeletal chest pain, overdose (< 0.1%).

Overdosage:

Thirteen overdoses occurred during clinical trials; 12 patients ingested 850 to 4200 mg and recovered without significant sequelae. Another patient who ingested 9000 mg bupropion and 300 mg tranylcypromine experienced a grand mal seizure and recovered without further sequelae.

Treatment: Hospitalize. If the patient is conscious, induce vomiting by syrup of ipecac, administer activated charcoal every 6 hours during the first 12 hours after ingestion and obtain baseline laboratory values; perform ECG and EEG monitoring for the next 48 hours. Provide adequate fluid intake. If the patient is stuporous, comatose, or convulsing, perform airway intubation prior to undertaking gastric lavage. Although there is little clinical experience, lavage is likely to be of benefit within the first 12 hours after ingestion since absorption of the drug may not yet be complete. Refer to General Management of Acute Overdosage.

Because diffusion of bupropion from tissue to plasma may be slow, dialysis may be of minimal benefit several hours after overdose. Treat seizures with IV benzodiazepines and other supportive measures.

(Continued on following page)

BUPROPION HCl (Cont.)

Patient Information:

Take in equally divided doses 3 or 4 times a day to minimize the risk of seizure.

May impair ability to perform tasks requiring judgment or motor and cognitive skills; patients should refrain from driving an automobile or operating complex, hazardous machinery until they are reasonably certain the drug does not adversely affect their performance.

Use and cessation of use of alcohol may alter the seizure threshold; therefore, minimize the consumption of alcohol and, if possible, avoid completely.

Administration and Dosage:

General: It is particularly important to administer bupropion in a manner most likely to minimize the risk of seizure (see Warnings). Do not exceed dose increases of 100 mg/day in a 3 day period. Gradual escalation of dosage is also important to minimize agitation, motor restlessness and insomnia often seen during the initial days of treatment. If necessary, these effects may be managed by temporary reduction of dose or the short-term administration of an intermediate to long acting sedative/hypnotic. A sedative/hypnotic is not usually required beyond the first week of treatment. Insomnia may also be minimized by avoiding bedtime doses. If distressing, untoward effects supervene, stop dose escalation.

No single dose of bupropion should exceed 150 mg. Administer 3 times daily, preferably with at least 6 hours between successive doses.

Adults: 300 mg/day, given 3 times daily. Begin dosing at 200 mg/day, given as 100 mg twice daily. Based on clinical response, this dose may be increased to 300 mg/day, given as 100 mg 3 times daily no sooner than 3 days after beginning therapy (see table below).

Bupropion Dosing Regimen					
Treatment Day	Total Daily Dose	Tablet Strength	Number of Tablets		
			Morning	Midday	Evening
1	200 mg	100 mg	1	0	1
4	300 mg	100 mg	1	1	1

Increasing the dosage above 300 mg/day: As with other antidepressants, the full antidepressant effect of bupropion may not be evident until 4 weeks of treatment or longer. An increase in dosage, up to a maximum of 450 mg/day, given in divided doses of not more than 150 mg each, may be considered for patients in whom no clinical improvement is noted after several weeks of treatment at 300 mg/day. Dosing above 300 mg/day may be accomplished using the 75 or 100 mg tablets. The 100 mg tablets must be administered 4 times daily with at least 4 hours between successive doses in order not to exceed the limit of 150 mg in a single dose. Discontinue in patients who do not demonstrate an adequate response after an appropriate period of 450 mg/day.

Maintenance: Use the lowest dose that maintains remission. Although it is not known how long the patient should remain on bupropion, acute episodes of depression generally require several months or longer of treatment. **C.I.***

				C.I.*
Rx	**Wellbutrin** (Burroughs Wellcome)	**Tablets:** 75 mg	(#Wellbutrin 75). Yellow-gold. Biconvex. In 100s.	23
		100 mg	(#Wellbutrin 100). Red. Biconvex. In 100s.	24

* Cost Index based on cost per 100 mg.

\# Product identification code.

Monoamine Oxidase Inhibitors

Actions:

Pharmacology: Monoamine oxidase is a complex enzyme system, widely distributed throughout the body, which is responsible for the metabolic decomposition of biogenic amines, thus terminating their activity. Drugs which inhibit this enzyme system (MAOIs) cause an increase in the concentration of endogenous epinephrine, norepinephrine and serotonin (5HT) in storage sites throughout the nervous system. The increase in the concentration of monoamines in the CNS is the basis for the antidepressant activity of these agents.

Tranylcypromine is a non-hydrazine MAOI. It has a rapid onset of activity of 10 days, rather than 3 to 4 weeks for the hydrazine derivatives (isocarboxazid and phenelzine).

Drugs that have MAOI activity cause a wide range of clinical effects and have the potential for serious interactions with other substances. Clinicians and patients should be fully aware of the potential hazards associated with their use.

Pharmacokinetics: Isocarboxazid, phenelzine and tranylcypromine are well absorbed orally. The clinical effects of isocarboxazid and phenelzine may continue for up to 2 weeks after discontinuation of therapy. When tranylcypromine is withdrawn, MAO activity is recovered in 3 to 5 days (possibly up to 10 days), although the drug is excreted in 24 hours.

Indications:

In general, the MAOIs appear to be indicated in patients with atypical (exogenous) depression, and in some patients unresponsive to other antidepressive therapy. They are rarely a drug of first choice.

Unlabeled uses: MAOIs have shown promise in the treatment of bulimia (having characteristics of atypical depression). Phenelzine (15 mg on alternate days to 90 mg/day) has been investigated in the treatment of cocaine addiction as a deterrent; careful supervision is required. MAOIs have also been used in the treatment of panic disorder with associated agoraphobia.

For indications of specific agents, see individual product listings.

Contraindications:

Hypersensitivity to these agents; pheochromocytoma; congestive heart failure; a history of liver disease or abnormal liver function tests; severe impairment of renal function; confirmed or suspected cerebrovascular defect; cardiovascular disease; hypertension; history of headache; in patients over 60 because of the possibility of existing cerebral sclerosis with damaged vessels.

Refer also to the Drug Interactions section.

Warnings:

Hypertensive crises: The most serious reactions involve changes in blood pressure; it is inadvisable to use these drugs in elderly or debilitated patients or in the presence of hypertension, cardiovascular or cerebrovascular disease. Not recommended in patients with frequent or severe headaches because headache during therapy may be the first symptom of a hypertensive reaction.

Hypertensive crises have sometimes been fatal. These crises usually occur within several hours after ingestion of a contraindicated substance and are characterized by some or all of the following symptoms: Occipital headache which may radiate frontally; palpitation; neck stiffness or soreness; nausea; vomiting; sweating (sometimes with fever or cold, clammy skin); dilated pupils; photophobia. Either tachycardia or bradycardia may be present, and can be associated with constricting chest pain. *Note:* Intracranial bleeding (sometimes fatal) has been reported in association with the paradoxical increase in blood pressure.

Monitor blood pressure frequently to detect evidence of any pressor response. Do not place full reliance on blood pressure readings, but observe patient frequently.

Discontinue therapy immediately if palpitations or frequent headaches occur. These signs may be prodromal of a hypertensive crisis.

Treatment: If a hypertensive crisis occurs, discontinue these drugs immediately and institute therapy to lower blood pressure. Do not use parenteral reserpine. Headaches tend to abate as blood pressure is lowered. Administer alpha-adrenergic blocking agents such as phentolamine 5 mg IV slowly to avoid producing an excessive hypotensive effect. The use of sublingual nifedipine 10 mg may be useful in treating hypertensive crisis. Manage fever by means of external cooling.

(Warnings continued on following page)

Warnings (Cont.):

Hypertensive crises (Cont.):

Warning to the patient – Warn all patients against eating foods with high tyramine or tryptophan content (see table) and for 2 weeks after discontinuing MAOIs. Any high protein food that is aged or undergoes breakdown by putrefaction process to improve flavor is suspect of being able to produce a hypertensive crisis in patients taking MAOIs. Also warn patients against drinking alcoholic beverages and against self-medication with certain proprietary agents such as cold, hay fever or weight reduction preparations containing sympathomimetic amines while undergoing therapy. Instruct patients not to consume excessive amounts of caffeine in any form and to report promptly the occurrence of headache or other unusual symptoms.

Tyramine-Containing Foods[1]		
	Cheese/Dairy Products	
American, processed Blue * Boursault Brick, natural Brie	* Camembert * Cheddar * Emmenthaler Gruyere Mozzarella Parmesan	Romano Roquefort Sour cream * Stilton Yogurt
	Meat/Fish	
Beef or chicken liver, other meats, fish (unrefrigerated, fermented) Meats prepared with tenderizer	* Fermented sausages (bologna, pepperoni, salami, summer sausage) Game meat	Caviar Dried fish (salted herring) * Herring, pickled, spoiled Shrimp paste
	Alcoholic Beverages (Undistilled)	
Beer and ale (imports, some nonalcoholic)	Red wine (especially Chianti)	Sherry
	Fruit/Vegetables	
Avocados (especially overripe) * Yeast extracts (Marmite, etc.)	Bananas Figs, canned (overripe) Raisins	Soy sauce Miso soup Bean curd
	Foods Containing Other Vasopressors	
Fava beans (overripe) – dopamine	Caffeine (eg, coffee, tea, colas) – caffeine	Chocolate – phenylethylamine Ginseng

[1] Tyramine contents are not predictable and may vary. The amounts of tyramine are estimated from low to very high.

* Contain high to very high amounts.

Suicidal risks: In patients who may be suicidal risks, no single form of treatment, such as MAOIs, electroconvulsive or other therapy should be relied upon as a sole therapeutic measure. Strict supervision and, preferably, hospitalization are advised.

Renal function impairment: Use isocarboxazid cautiously in these patients.

Carcinogenesis: **Phenelzine,** like other hydrazine derivatives, has induced pulmonary and vascular tumors in an uncontrolled lifetime study in mice.

Pregnancy: Safety for use during pregnancy has not been established. Use during pregnancy or in women of childbearing age only when clearly needed and when the potential benefits outweigh the potential hazards to the fetus.

Doses of **phenelzine** in pregnant mice, well exceeding the maximum recommended human dose, have caused a significant decrease in the number of viable offspring per mouse. The growth of dogs and rats has been retarded by doses exceeding the maximum human dose. **Tranylcypromine sulfate** passes through the placental barrier of animals into the fetus.

Lactation: Safety for use during lactation has not been established. **Tranylcypromine** is excreted in breast milk.

Children: Not recommended for patients $<$ 16 years of age.

(Continued on following page)

The discussion below applies to antipsychotics as a therapeutic class. Due to pharmacological similarities, consider all information when using these drugs. Reserpine, not discussed in this section, was used as an antipsychotic prior to the newer, more effective compounds.

Lithium, pimozide and clozapine are discussed separately (see individual monographs).

Actions:

Select Dosage and Pharmacologic Parameters of Antipsychotics

Incidence of Side Effects: +++ = High ++ = Moderate + = Low Antipsychotic Agent	Approx. Equiv Dose (mg)	Adult Daily Dosage Range (mg)	Sedation	Extrapyramidal Symptoms	Anticholinergic Effects	Orthostatic Hypotension	Therapeutic Plasma Concentration (ng/ml)
Phenothiazines: Aliphatic							
Chlorpromazine	100	30-800	+++	++	++	+++	30-500
Promazine	200	40-1200	++	++	+++	++	
Triflupromazine	25	60-150	+++	++	+++	++	
Phenothiazines: Piperidine							
Thioridazine	100	150-800	+++	+	+++	+++	
Mesoridazine	50	30-400	+++	+	+++	++	
Phenothiazines: Piperazine							
Acetophenazine	20	60-120	++	+++	+	+	
Perphenazine	10	12-64	+	+++	+	+	0.8-1.2
Prochlorperazine	15	15-150	++	+++	+	+	
Fluphenazine	2	0.5-40	+	+++	+	+	0.13-2.8
Trifluoperazine	5	2-40	+	+++	+	+	
Thioxanthenes							
Chlorprothixene	100	75-600	+++	++	++	++	
Thiothixene	4	8-30	+	+++	+	+	2-57
Butyrophenone							
Haloperidol	2	1-15	+	+++	+	+	5-20
Dihydroindolone							
Molindone	10	15-225	+	+++	+	+	
Dibenzoxazepine							
Loxapine	15	20-250	++	+++	+	++	
Dibenzodiazepine							
Clozapine	50	300-900	+++	+	+++	+++	
Diphenylbutylpiperidine							
Pimozide	0.3-0.5	1-10	++	+++	++	+	

Chemical classes of antipsychotics include phenothiazines, thioxanthenes, butyrophenones, dihydroindolones, dibenzoxazepines, dibenzodiazepines and diphenylbutylpiperidines. The phenothiazines are subdivided into three groups, based on side chain substitution at position 10 of the chemical structure: Aliphatic, piperidine and piperazine. Aliphatics cause more sedation, hypotension, dermatitis and convulsions and fewer extrapyramidal side effects (EPS). Piperazines cause more EPS and less sedation, hypotension and lens opacities. Piperidines cause more retinal toxicity, ejaculatory disturbances and ECG effects and the fewest EPS. Though chemically distinct, these agents share many pharmacological and clinical properties.

The exact mode of action is not fully understood. Antipsychotics block postsynaptic dopamine receptors in the basal ganglia, hypothalamus, limbic system, brain stem and medulla. Inhibition or alteration of dopamine release, an increased neuronal cell firing rate in the midbrain and an increased turnover rate of dopamine in the forebrain have been noted. These observations support the theory that antipsychotics interfere with dopamine, but do not prove that dopaminolytic activity is sufficient for antipsychotic efficacy. The phenothiazines appear to act at both D_1 and D_2 receptors, whereas haloperidol appears to act primarily at D_2 receptors.

(Actions continued on following page)

Actions (Cont.):

The phenothiazines are believed to depress various components of the reticular activating system which is involved in the control of basal metabolism and body temperature, wakefulness, vasomotor tone, emesis and hormonal balance. In addition, the drugs exert anticholinergic and alpha-adrenergic blocking effects.

The term "neuroleptic," used as a synonym for antipsychotic agent, refers to the effects of these agents that differ from the classical CNS depressants. They diminish conditional behavioral responses, selectively dampen neurophysiologic effects of peripheral stimuli on the forebrain and have limited ability to induce generalized sedation. These drugs cause a lack of initiative and interest in the environment, little display of emotion and limited affect; they also cause neurological (ie, EPS and parkinsonian) effects.

Pharmacokinetics:

Absorption – Oral absorption tends to be erratic and variable. Peak plasma levels are seen 2 to 4 hours following oral administration. Oral liquid formulations are most predictably absorbed. Conventional tablet dosage forms are preferred over controlled release forms which are usually more expensive and are not necessary due to long duration of effects of these agents. IM use provides 4 to 10 times more active drug than oral doses.

Distribution – These agents are widely distributed in tissues; CNS concentrations exceed those in the plasma. They are highly bound to plasma proteins (91% to 99%). Because these agents are highly lipophilic, the antipsychotic agents and their metabolites accumulate in the brain, lungs and other tissues with high blood supply. They are stored in these tissues and may be found in the urine for up to 6 months after the last dose.

Metabolism – Extensive biotransformation occurs in the liver. Numerous active metabolites, which persist for prolonged periods, have important side effects and contribute to the biological activity of the parent drug.

Excretion – One-half of the excretion of these agents occurs via the kidneys and the other half occurs through enterohepatic circulation. Elimination half-lives range from 10 to 20 hours. Less than 1% is excreted as unchanged drug.

Clinical pharmacology: There is little evidence of clinical differences in efficacy among these agents (except clozapine) when used in equitherapeutic dosages; however, a patient who fails to respond to one agent may respond to another and agents are not necessarily interchangeable. Clozapine is used for severely ill schizophrenic patients who fail to respond adequately to standard antipsychotic treatment.

The principal differences between antipsychotic agents are the type and severity of side effects which include: Sedation, extrapyramidal effects, anticholinergic effects and anti-adrenergic effects (orthostatic hypotension). Clozapine also differs in its effects on various dopamine mediated behaviors. Changing agents may minimize undesirable or intolerable side effects (refer to table). Coadministration of two or more antipsychotics does not improve clinical response and may increase the potential for adverse effects.

In chronic therapy, full clinical effects may not be achieved for 6 weeks or longer. Approximately 4 to 7 days are required to achieve steady-state plasma levels; therefore, do not make more than weekly dosage adjustments in chronic therapy.

Since plasma concentrations of antipsychotics are highly variable from patient to patient, plasma monitoring of these agents may not be useful for determining therapeutic response. Plus, therapeutic levels are only available for a small number of these agents. However, monitoring may help decrease the incidence of toxicity since plasma levels are relatively stable in each individual.

Indications:

Management of psychotic disorders.

Some of these agents are used as antiemetics (refer to Antiemetic/Antivertigo Agents).

Refer to individual product listings for approved indications.

Unlabeled uses: Chlorpromazine and haloperidol are effective in the treatment of phencyclidine (PCP) psychosis; coadministration of ascorbic acid with haloperidol may be more effective than haloperidol alone.

IV or IM chlorpromazine may be beneficial in the treatment of migraine headaches, and IV prochlorperazine may be effective in treating severe vascular or tension headaches.

Neuroleptics appear useful for the treatment of Tourette's syndrome; switching from one agent to another may occasionally be necessary. Haloperidol (approved for Tourette's) and nicotine polacrilex gum coadministration resulted in improvement of symptoms in two children. Further study is needed.

Neuroleptics are effective in control of acute agitation in the elderly; use lowest dose for shortest duration possible. May also be useful in treating some symptoms of dementia including agitation, hyperactivity, hallucinations, suspiciousness, hostility and uncooperativeness; however, they do not improve memory loss and may impair cognitive function.

Other potential uses include treatment of: Huntington's chorea (chlorpromazine, fluphenazine, haloperidol); hemiballismus (perphenazine, haloperidol); chorea associated with rheumatic fever or SLE, spasmodic torticollis and Meige's syndrome (haloperidol).

(Continued on following page)

Contraindications:

Comatose or severely depressed states; hypersensitivity (cross sensitivity between phenothiazines may occur); presence of large amounts of other CNS depressants; bone marrow depression; blood dyscrasias; circulatory collapse (thioxanthenes); subcortical brain damage; Parkinson's disease (haloperidol); liver damage; cerebral arteriosclerosis; coronary artery disease; severe hypotension or hypertension; pediatric surgery (prochlorperazine).

Warnings:

Tardive dyskinesia, a syndrome consisting of potentially irreversible, involuntary dyskinetic movements, may develop in patients treated with neuroleptic drugs. Although the prevalence of the syndrome appears highest among the elderly, especially women, it is impossible to rely upon prevalence estimates to predict, at the inception of neuroleptic treatment, which patients are likely to develop the syndrome. Whether neuroleptic drugs differ in their potential to cause tardive dyskinesia is unknown. Both the risk of developing the syndrome and the likelihood that it will become irreversible are increased as the duration of treatment and the total cumulative dose of drug administered increase. However, the syndrome can develop, although much less commonly, after relatively brief treatment periods at low doses. Anticholinergic agents may worsen these effects.

There is no known treatment for established cases of tardive dyskinesia, although the syndrome may remit, partially or completely, if neuroleptic treatment is withdrawn. Neuroleptic treatment itself, however, may suppress (or partially suppress) signs and symptoms of the syndrome, possibly masking the underlying disease process. The effect of symptomatic suppression on the long-term course of the syndrome is unknown.

Given these considerations, prescribe neuroleptics in a manner most likely to minimize the occurrence of tardive dyskinesia. In general, reserve chronic neuroleptic treatment for patients who suffer from a chronic illness that responds to neuroleptic drugs and for whom alternative, equally effective, but potentially less harmful treatments are not available or appropriate. In patients who require chronic treatment, use the smallest dose and the shortest duration of treatment producing a satisfactory clinical response. Periodically reassess the need for continued treatment.

If signs and symptoms of tardive dyskinesia appear, consider drug discontinuation. However, some patients may require treatment despite the presence of the syndrome.

Neuroleptic malignant syndrome (NMS) is a rare idiosyncratic combination of EPS, hyperthermia and autonomic disturbance. Onset may be hours to months after drug initiation, but once started, proceeds rapidly over 24 to 72 hours. It is most commonly associated with **haloperidol** and depot **fluphenazines**, but has occurred with **thiothixene** and **thioridazine** and may occur with other agents. NMS is potentially fatal, and requires intensive symptomatic treatment and immediate discontinuation of neuroleptic treatment. Treatment of choice is not yet established, but dantrolene may be beneficial (see individual monograph). Rechallenge with a neuroleptic may result in an 80% recurrence of NMS; however, some success has occurred by using a low-potency agent and gradually increasing the dose. See Adverse Reactions.

CNS effects: These agents may impair mental or physical abilities, especially during the first few days of therapy. Drowsiness may occur, particularly during the first or second week, after which it generally disappears. If troublesome, lower the dosage. Caution patients against activities requiring alertness (eg, operating vehicles or machinery). Use cautiously in depressed patients. When used to treat agitated states accompanying depression, caution is indicated (particularly if a suicidal tendency is recognized). When **haloperidol** is used for mania in cyclic disorders, a rapid mood swing to depression may occur.

Antiemetic effects: Those drugs that have an antiemetic effect can obscure signs of toxicity of other drugs, or mask symptoms of disease (eg, brain tumor, intestinal obstruction, Reye's syndrome). Because these drugs can suppress the cough reflex, aspiration of vomitus is possible.

Pulmonary: Cases of bronchopneumonia (some fatal) have followed the use of antipsychotic agents. Lethargy and decreased sensation of thirst due to central inhibition may lead to dehydration, hemoconcentration and reduced pulmonary ventilation. If the above signs appear, especially in the elderly, institute remedial therapy promptly.

Use with caution in respiratory impairment due to acute pulmonary infections or chronic respiratory disorders, such as severe asthma or emphysema. "Silent pneumonias" may develop in patients treated with phenothiazines.

Decreased serum cholesterol has occurred. **Chlorpromazine** may raise plasma cholesterol.

Cardiovascular: Use with caution in patients with cardiovascular disease or mitral insufficiency. Increased pulse rates occur in most patients. One result of therapy may be an increase in mental and physical activity. For example, a few patients with angina pectoris have complained of increased pain while taking **trifluoperazine**. Therefore, withdraw the drug from angina patients if an unfavorable response is noted.

Hypertension – Pulse rates have increased in most patients receiving antipsychotics. Rebound hypertension may occur in pheochromocytoma patients.

(Warnings continued on following page)

Warnings (Cont.):

Cardiovascular (Cont.):

Hypotension – Carefully watch patients who are undergoing surgery, and who are on large doses of phenothiazines, for hypotensive phenomena. It may be necessary to reduce amounts of anesthetics or CNS depressants. The hypotensive effects may occur after the first injection of the antipsychotic, occasionally after subsequent injections, and rarely after the first oral dose. Recovery is usually spontaneous and symptoms disappear within 0.5 to 2 hours. If hypotension occurs, place the patient in a recumbent position. Females appear to have a greater tendency to orthostatic hypotension. Patients with hypovolemia have increased sensitivity to the hypotensive effects of these agents. Volume replacement, when needed, should precede use of vasopressors. If a vasopressor is indicated, use phenylephrine or norepinephrine. Avoid administering epinephrine in drug-induced hypotension (see Drug Interactions).

Ophthalmic: Use with caution in patients with a history of glaucoma. The anticholinergic effects may precipitate angle closure in susceptible patients. During prolonged therapy, ocular changes may occur; these include particle deposition in the cornea and lens, progressing in more severe cases to star-shaped lenticular opacities.

Pigmentary retinopathy occurs most frequently in patients receiving **thioridazine** dosages > 1 g/day. Pigmentary retinopathy is characterized by diminution of visual acuity, brownish coloring of vision, impairment of night vision and pigment deposits on the fundus. Ophthalmological (slit lamp) evaluation is recommended. Discontinue use if retinal changes occur.

Seizure disorders: These drugs can lower the convulsive threshold and may precipitate seizures. Petit mal and grand mal seizures have occurred, particularly in patients with EEG abnormalities or a history of such disorders. Use cautiously in patients with a history of epilepsy and only when absolutely necessary. These drugs may be used concomitantly with anticonvulsants; maintain an adequate anticonvulsant dosage (see Adverse Reactions). In animals, **molindone** does not lower the seizure threshold to the degree noted with more sedating agents. However, convulsive seizures have occurred in humans.

Adynamic ileus occasionally occurs with phenothiazine therapy and, if severe, can result in complications and death.

Sudden death: Previous brain damage or seizures may be predisposing factors; avoid high doses in known seizure patients. Several patients have shown sudden flare-ups of psychotic behavior patterns shortly before death. In some cases, death was apparently due to cardiac arrest; in others, asphyxia was due to failure of the cough reflex. Autopsy findings usually reveal acute fulminating pneumonia or pneumonitis, aspiration of gastric contents or intramyocardial lesions. In some patients, cause could not be determined. Phenothiazine use in infants < 1 year may be a factor in sudden infant death syndrome (SIDS).

Hepatic effects: Jaundice usually occurs between the second and fourth weeks of treatment and is regarded as a hypersensitivity reaction. The clinical picture resembles infectious hepatitis with laboratory features of obstructive jaundice. It is usually reversible; however, chronic jaundice and biliary stasis have occurred. If fever with flu-like symptoms occurs, perform liver function tests. If tests are positive, discontinue treatment. Withhold exploratory laparotomy until extrahepatic obstruction is confirmed. Because of the possibility of liver damage, periodically monitor hepatic function. AST and ALT elevation has occurred with **loxapine**.

Hepatic function impairment: Use with caution in patients with impaired hepatic function. Patients with a history of hepatic encephalopathy due to cirrhosis have increased sensitivity to the CNS effects of antipsychotic drugs (ie, impaired cerebration and abnormal slowing of the EEG).

There is no conclusive evidence that preexisting liver disease makes patients more susceptible to jaundice. Alcoholics with cirrhosis have been successfully treated with chlorpromazine without complications. Nevertheless, use cautiously in patients with liver disease. Patients who have experienced jaundice with a phenothiazine should not, if possible, be reexposed.

Renal function impairment: Administer cautiously to those with diminished renal function. Monitor renal function in long-term therapy; lower the dose or discontinue if BUN becomes abnormal.

Carcinogenicity/prolactin stimulation: Neuroleptic drugs (except promazine) elevate prolactin levels which persist during chronic administration. Tissue culture experiments indicate that approximately ⅓ of human breast cancers are prolactin-dependent in vitro, a factor of potential importance if use of these drugs is contemplated in a patient with a previously detected breast cancer. Although disturbances such as galactorrhea, amenorrhea, gynecomastia and impotence have occurred, clinical significance of elevated serum prolactin levels is unknown for most patients. An increase in mammary neoplasms has occurred in rodents after chronic use of neuroleptics. Studies, however, have not shown an association between chronic use of these drugs and mammary tumorigenesis.

(Warnings continued on following page)

Overdosage (Cont.):

Treatment includes usual supportive measures. Refer to General Management of Acute Overdosage. Emetics are unlikely to be of value due to the antiemetic effects of these drugs, and induction of emesis may result in a dystonic reaction of the head or neck that could result in aspiration of vomitus. Extrapyramidal symptoms may be treated with antiparkinson drugs, barbiturates or diphenhydramine (see Adverse Reactions).

If hypotension occurs, initiate the standard measures for managing circulatory shock, including volume replacement. If a vasoconstrictor is desired, use norepinephrine or phenylephrine. Do not administer epinephrine (see Drug Interactions).

Phenytoin, 1 mg/kg IV, not to exceed 50 mg/min, with ECG control may be used for ventricular arrhythmias; may repeat every 5 minutes, up to 10 mg/kg.

Control convulsions or hyperactivity with pentobarbital or diazepam.

Limited experience indicates that these drugs are not dialyzable.

Sustained release formulations – Direct therapy at reversing the effects of ingested drug and supporting the patient for as long as overdosage symptoms remain. Saline cathartics are useful for hastening evacuation of pellets that have not already released medication.

Patient Information:

Because some patients exposed chronically to neuroleptics will develop tardive dyskinesia, inform all patients in whom chronic use is contemplated, if possible, about this risk. The decision to inform patients or their guardians must obviously take into account the clinical circumstances and the patient's competence to understand the information. See Warnings.

May cause drowsiness; use caution while driving or performing other tasks requiring alertness. Avoid alcohol and other CNS depressants due to possible additive effects and hypotension.

Liquid concentrates: Avoid contact with skin (contact dermatitis may occur). The liquid concentrates are light sensitive; keep in amber or opaque bottles, protect from light. These solutions are most conveniently used when diluted in fruit juices or other liquids. Use solutions immediately after dilution. See individual products for specific guidelines.

Phenothiazines:

Avoid prolonged exposure to sunlight or use sunscreens conscientiously; photosensitivity may occur.

May discolor the urine pink or reddish-brown.

If dizziness or fainting occurs, avoid sudden changes in posture and use caution when climbing stairs, etc (more common during first week of therapy).

Use caution in hot weather. These drugs may increase susceptibility to heat stroke.

Notify physician if sore throat, fever, skin rash, weakness, tremors, impaired vision or jaundice occurs.

Other agents: Notify physician if impaired vision, tremors, involuntary muscle twitching or jaundice occurs.

Administration:

Although divided daily dosages are recommended for initiation of therapy, once-daily dosing may be used during chronic therapy because of the long-acting effects of these agents. Administration at bedtime may be preferred to minimize the effects of sedation and orthostatic hypotension.

Individualize dosage. The milligram for milligram potency relationship among all dosage forms has not been precisely established. Increase dosage until symptoms are controlled. Increase dosage gradually in elderly, debilitated or emaciated patients. In continued therapy, gradually reduce dosage to the lowest effective maintenance level after symptoms have been controlled. Increase parenteral dosage only if hypotension has not occurred.

Elderly patients: Institute doses at ¼ to ⅓ that recommended for younger adults and increase more gradually.

Combative patients or those who have other serious manifestations of acute psychosis: Repeat parenteral administration every 1 to 4 hours until the desired effects are obtained or until cardiac arrhythmias or rhythm changes, hypotension or other disturbing side effects emerge.

Maintenance therapy can be administered as a single daily bedtime dose.

Oral liquid concentrates are light sensitive; dispense in amber or opaque bottles and protect from light. These solutions are most conveniently administered by dilution in fruit juices or other liquids. Administer these solutions immediately after dilution.

Bioequivalence:

Bioavailability differences between solid oral dosage forms and suppositories marketed by different manufacturers have been documented for various phenothiazines. Brand interchange is not recommended unless comparative bioavailability data which provide evidence of therapeutic equivalence are available.

(Products listed on following pages)

Complete prescribing information for these products begins on page 1323

Phenothiazine Derivatives

CHLORPROMAZINE HCl

Indications:

Management of manifestations of psychotic disorders; control of the manifestations of the manic type of manic depressive illness; relief of restlessness and apprehension prior to surgery; an adjunct in treatment of tetanus; treatment of acute intermittent porphyria.

Treatment of severe behavioral problems in children marked by combativeness or explosive hyperexcitable behavior (out of proportion to immediate provocations), and in the short-term treatment of hyperactive children who show excessive motor activity with accompanying conduct disorders consisting of some or all of the following symptoms: Impulsivity, difficulty sustaining attention, aggressivity, mood lability and poor frustration tolerance.

Also indicated for the control of nausea and vomiting and relief of intractable hiccoughs (see Antiemetic/Antivertigo Agents).

Unlabeled uses: Treatment of phencyclidine (PCP) psychosis; treatment of migraine headaches (IV or IM).

Administration and Dosage – Adults:

Concentrate: Add desired dosage to ≥ 60 ml of diluent just prior to administration. Suggested vehicles are tomato or fruit juice, milk, simple syrup, orange syrup, carbonated beverages, coffee, tea or water. Semisolid foods (eg, soups, puddings) may also be used.

Sustained release capsules: Do not crush or chew. Swallow whole.

Injection: Do not inject SC. Inject IM slowly, deep into upper outer quadrant of buttock. Because of possible hypotensive effects, reserve for bedfast patients or for acute ambulatory cases, and keep patient recumbent for at least ½ hour after injection. If irritation is a problem, dilute injection with saline or 2% procaine; do not mix with other agents in the syringe. Avoid injecting undiluted into vein. Use the IV route only for severe hiccoughs, surgery and tetanus.

Because of the possibility of contact dermatitis, avoid getting solution on hands or clothing.

Outpatients: For prompt control of severe symptoms 25 mg IM; if necessary, repeat in 1 hour. Give subsequent oral doses of 25 to 50 mg 3 times daily.

The usual initial oral dose is 10 mg 3 or 4 times daily or 25 mg 2 or 3 times daily. For more serious cases, give 25 mg 3 times/day. After 1 or 2 days, increase daily dosage by 20 to 50 mg semiweekly, until patient becomes calm and cooperative. Maximum improvement may not be seen for weeks or even months. Continue optimum dosage for 2 weeks, then gradually reduce to maintenance level; 200 mg per day is not unusual. Some patients require higher dosages (eg, 800 mg per day is not uncommon in discharged mental patients).

Surgery:

Preoperative – 25 to 50 mg orally 2 to 3 hours before surgery or 12.5 to 25 mg IM 1 to 2 hours before surgery.

Intraoperative (to control acute nausea and vomiting) –

IM: 12.5 mg. Repeat in ½ hour if necessary and if no hypotension occurs.

IV: 2 mg per fractional injection at 2 minute intervals. Do not exceed 25 mg (dilute to 1 mg/ml with saline).

Acute intermittent porphyria: 25 to 50 mg orally or 25 mg IM 3 or 4 times daily until patient can take oral therapy.

Tetanus: 25 to 50 mg IM 3 or 4 times daily, usually with barbiturates. For IV use, 25 to 50 mg diluted to at least 1 mg/ml and administered at a rate of 1 mg/minute.

Psychiatry, hospitalized patients (acutely manic or disturbed):

IM – 25 mg initially. If necessary, give an additional 25 to 50 mg injection in 1 hour. Increase gradually over several days (up to 400 mg every 4 to 6 hours in severe cases) until patient is controlled. Patient usually becomes quiet and cooperative within 24 to 48 hours. Substitute oral dosage and increase until the patient is calm; 500 mg/day is usually sufficient. While gradual increases to 2000 mg or more/day may be necessary, little therapeutic gain is achieved by exceeding 1000 mg/day for extended periods.

Psychiatry, hospitalized patients (less acutely disturbed):

Oral – 25 mg 3 times daily. Increase gradually until effective dose is reached, usually 400 mg/day.

(Administration and Dosage continued on following page)

CHLORPROMAZINE HCl (Cont.)

Administration and Dosage – Children:

Chlorpromazine should generally not be used in children < 6 months old except where potentially lifesaving. It should not be used in conditions for which specific children's dosages have not been established.

Psychiatric outpatients:

Oral – 0.5 mg/kg (0.25 mg/lb) every 4 to 6 hours, as needed.
Rectal – 1 mg/kg (0.5 mg/lb) every 6 to 8 hours, as needed.
IM – 0.5 mg/kg (0.25 mg/lb) every 6 to 8 hours, as needed.

Surgery:

Preoperative – 0.5 mg/kg (0.25 mg/lb) orally 2 to 3 hours before operation or 0.5 mg/kg (0.25 mg/lb) IM 1 to 2 hours before operation.

Intraoperative (administer only to control acute nausea and vomiting) –

IM: 0.25 mg/kg (0.125 mg/lb); repeat in ½ hour if needed, and if no hypotension occurs.

IV: 1 mg per fractional injection at 2 minute intervals; do not exceed IM dosage. Always dilute to 1 mg/ml with saline.

Psychiatry: Hospitalized patients –

Oral: Start with low doses and increase gradually. In severe behavior disorders or psychotic conditions, 50 to 100 mg daily, or in older children, 200 mg or more daily may be necessary. There is little evidence that improvement in severely disturbed mentally retarded patients is enhanced by doses > 500 mg/day.

IM: Up to 5 years – Do not exceed 40 mg/day. *5 to 12 years old* – Do not exceed 75 mg/day, except in unmanageable cases.

Tetanus (IM or IV): 0.5 mg/kg (0.25 mg/lb) every 6 to 8 hours. When given IV, dilute to at least 1 mg/ml and administer at a rate of 1 mg per 2 minutes. In children up to 23 kg (50 lbs), do not exceed 40 mg daily; 23 to 45 kg (50 to 100 lbs), do not exceed 75 mg/day, except in severe cases.

Concentrate: Slight yellowing will not alter potency. Discard if markedly discolored.

Admixture compatibility: A mixture of chlorpromazine, hydroxyzine and meperidine in the same glass or plastic syringe is stable for 1 year when stored at refrigeration (4°C; 39°F) or room temperature (25°C; 77°F). The combination was unstable at higher temperatures.

A precipitate or discoloration may occur when chlorpromazine is admixed with morphine, meperidine or other products preserved with cresols.

	Product	Form	Description	C.I.*
Rx	**Chlorpromazine HCl** (Various, eg, Balan, Geneva, Goldline, Lannett, Major, Moore, Parmed, Purepac, Rugby, Schein)	**Tablets:** 10 mg	In 100s, 1000s and UD 100s.	73+
Rx	**Thorazine** (SKF)		(SKF T73). Orange. In 100s, 1000s and UD 100s.	596
Rx	**Chlorpromazine HCl** (Various, eg, Balan, Geneva, Goldline, Lederle, Major, Moore, Parmed, Purepac, Rugby, Schein)	**Tablets:** 25 mg	In 100s, 1000s and UD 100s.	28+
Rx	**Thorazine** (SKF)		(SKF T74). Orange. In 100s, 1000s and UD 100s.	323
Rx	**Chlorpromazine HCl** (Various, eg, Balan, Geneva, Goldline, Lederle, Major, Moore, Parmed, Purepac, Rugby, Schein)	**Tablets:** 50 mg	In 100s, 1000s and UD 100s.	19+
Rx	**Thorazine** (SKF)		(SKF T76). Orange. In 100s, 1000s and UD 100s.	201

* Cost Index based on cost per 50 mg.

(Continued on following page)

Phenothiazine Derivatives (Cont.)

CHLORPROMAZINE HCl (Cont.)

	Product	Form/Strength	Description	C.I.*
Rx	**Chlorpromazine HCl** (Various, eg, Balan, Geneva, Goldline, Lederle, Major, Moore, Parmed, Purepac, Rugby, Schein)	**Tablets:** 100 mg	In 100s, 1000s and UD 100s.	12+
Rx	**Thorazine** (SKF)		(SKF T77). Orange. In 100s, 1000s and UD 100s.	130
Rx	**Chlorpromazine HCl** (Various, eg, Balan, Geneva, Goldline, Lederle, Major, Moore, Parmed, Purepac, Rugby, Schein)	**Tablets:** 200 mg	In 100s, 1000s and UD 100s.	10+
Rx	**Thorazine** (SKF)		(SKF T79). Orange. In 100s, 1000s and UD 100s.	83
Rx	**Thorazine Spansules** (SKF)	**Capsules, sustained release:** 30 mg	(SKF T63). Orange/natural. In 50s, 500s and UD 100s.	530
		75 mg	(SKF T64). Orange/natural. In 50s, 500s and UD 100s.	285
		150 mg	(SKF T66). Orange/natural. In 50s, 500s and UD 100s.	192
		200 mg	(SKF T67). Orange/natural. In 50s, 500s and UD 100s.	161
		300 mg	(SKF T69). In 50s and UD 100s.	121
Rx	**Chlorpromazine HCl** (Geneva)	**Syrup:** 10 mg per 5 ml	Wintergreen flavor. In 120 ml.	1156
Rx	**Thorazine** (SKF)		Sucrose. Orange-custard flavor. In 120 ml.	1469
Rx	**Chlorpromazine HCl** (Various, eg, Balan, Geneva, Harber, Moore, PBI, RID, Raway, Roxane, Warner Chilcott)	**Concentrate:** 30 mg per ml	In 120 ml.	23+
Rx	**Thorazine** (SKF)		In 120 ml	145
Rx	**Chlorpromazine HCl** (Various, eg, Balan, Geneva, Harber, Lederle, Moore, PBI, Raway, Roxane, Schein, Warner Chilcott)	**Concentrate:** 100 mg per ml	In 60 and 240 ml.	14+
Rx	**Thorazine** (SKF)		Saccharin. Custard flavor. In 240 ml.	120
Rx	**Thorazine** (SKF)	**Suppositories (as base):** 25 mg	(T70). In 12s.	1904
		100 mg	(T71). In 12s.	603
Rx	**Chlorpromazine HCl** (Various, eg, Balan, Elkins-Sinn, Geneva, Goldline, Lannett, Major, Moore, Parmed, Rugby, Schein)	**Injection:** 25 mg per ml	In 1 & 2 ml amps and 10 ml vials.	209+
Rx	**Ormazine** (Hauck)		In 10 ml vials.[1]	411
Rx	**Thorazine** (SKF)		In 1 and 2 ml amps[2] and 10 ml vials.[3]	3035

* Cost Index based on cost per 50 mg.
[1] With sodium metabisulfite, sodium sulfite and 2% benzyl alcohol.
[2] With sodium bisulfite and sodium sulfite.
[3] With sodium bisulfite, sodium sulfite and 2% benzyl alcohol.

Complete prescribing information for these products begins on page 1323

Phenothiazine Derivatives (Cont.)

PROMAZINE HCl

Indications:

Management of the manifestations of psychotic disorders.

Administration and Dosage:

Reserve parenteral administration for bedfast patients, although acute states in ambulatory patients may also be treated by IM injection, provided proper precautions are taken to eliminate the possibility of postural hypotension.

Injection IM is preferred. Give IM injections deep into large muscle masses (eg, gluteal region).

IV administration is not recommended. Do not give intra-arterially.

Adults: Dosage for acute or chronic mental disease varies with the severity of condition.

In the management of severely agitated patients, administer initial doses of 50 to 150 mg IM, depending on the degree of excitation. In general, these doses are sufficient, but if the desired calming effect is not apparent within 30 minutes, may give additional doses up to a total of 300 mg. Once control is obtained, administer orally. The oral or IM dose is 10 to 200 mg at 4 to 6 hour intervals. In less severe disturbances, adjust dosage downward. Maintenance dosage may range from 10 to 200 mg given at 4 to 6 hour intervals.

The degree of CNS depression induced by promazine has not been great; however, in the acutely inebriated patient the initial dose should not exceed 50 mg, to avoid potentiation of the depressant effect of alcohol.

Do not exceed a total daily dose of 1000 mg, since higher doses have not yielded greater results.

Children (> 12 years of age): In acute episodes of chronic psychotic disease, 10 to 25 mg may be given every 4 to 6 hours.

	Product	Dosage form	Description	C.I.*
Rx	**Sparine** (Wyeth-Ayerst)	**Tablets:** 25 mg	(Wyeth 29). Yellow. In 50s.	301
		50 mg	(Wyeth 28). Orange. In 50s.	183
		100 mg	(Wyeth 200). Pink. In 50s.	121
Rx	**Promazine HCl** (Various, eg, General Injectables, Schein)	**Injection:** 25 mg per ml	In 10 ml vials.	156+
Rx	**Promazine HCl** (Various, eg, Balan, Baxter, General Injectables, Pasadena, Rugby, Schein, Steris, Veratex, Vita-Rx)	**Injection:** 50 mg per ml	In 10 ml vials.	105+
Rx	**Prozine-50** (Hauck)		In 10 ml vials.	347
Rx	**Sparine** (Wyeth-Ayerst)		In 2 and 10 ml vials and 1 ml Tubex.[1]	1208

TRIFLUPROMAZINE HCl

Indications:

Management of manifestations of psychotic disorders (excluding psychotic depressive reactions).

Also indicated for the control of severe nausea and vomiting (see Antiemetic/Antivertigo Agents).

Administration and Dosage:

Psychotic disorders: 60 mg IM, up to a maximum of 150 mg/day.

Children – The recommended IM dosage range is 0.2 to 0.25 mg/kg (0.1 to 0.125 mg/lb), up to a maximum total dose of 10 mg/day. Do not administer to children < 2½ years of age.

	Product	Dosage form	Description	C.I.*
Rx	**Vesprin** (Princeton)	**Injection:** 10 mg per ml	In 10 ml vials.[2]	1887
		20 mg per ml	In 1 ml vials.[2]	2583

* Cost Index based on cost per 50 mg promazine HCl or 10 mg triflupromazine HCl.

[1] With EDTA and sodium metabisulfite.

[2] With 1.5% benzyl alcohol.

Complete prescribing information for these products begins on page 1323

Phenothiazine Derivatives (Cont.)

THIORIDAZINE HCl

Indications:

Management of manifestations of psychotic disorders and short-term treatment of moderate to marked depression with variable degrees of anxiety in adults.

Treatment of multiple symptoms such as agitation, anxiety, depressed mood, tension, sleep disturbances and fears in the geriatric patient.

Treatment of severe behavioral problems in children marked by combativeness or explosive hyperexcitable behavior (out of proportion to immediate provocations), and in the short-term treatment of hyperactive children who show excessive motor activity with accompanying conduct disorders consisting of some or all of the following symptoms: Impulsivity, difficulty sustaining attention, aggressivity, mood lability and poor frustration tolerance.

Administration and Dosage:

Psychotic manifestations: Usual initial dose is 50 to 100 mg 3 times daily; increase gradually to a maximum of 800 mg/day, if necessary, to control symptoms; then reduce gradually to the minimum maintenance dose. Total daily dosage ranges from 200 to 800 mg divided into 2 to 4 doses.

Short-term treatment of moderate to marked depression with variable degrees of anxiety, and treatment of multiple symptoms such as agitation, anxiety, depressed mood, tension, sleep disturbances and fears in geriatric patients: Usual initial dose is 25 mg 3 times daily. Dosage ranges from 10 mg 2 to 4 times daily in milder cases, to 50 mg 3 or 4 times daily for more severely disturbed patients. Total daily dosage ranges from 20 to 200 mg.

Children: Not recommended for children < 2 years of age. For children aged 2 to 12, the dosage ranges from 0.5 mg to a maximum of 3 mg/kg/day.

Moderate disorders – 10 mg 2 or 3 times daily is the usual starting dose.

Hospitalized, severely disturbed or psychotic children – 25 mg 2 or 3 times daily.

Concentrate may be administered in distilled or acidified tap water or suitable juices. **C.I.***

	Product	Form	Description	C.I.
Rx	**Thioridazine HCl** (Various, eg, Balan, Geneva, Goldline, Lederle, Major, Moore, Roxane, Rugby, Schein, Warner Chilcott)	**Tablets:** 10 mg	In 100s, 500s, 1000s and UD 100s.	101+
Rx	**Mellaril** (Sandoz)		(78-2). Chartreuse. In 100s, 1000s & UD 100s.	495
Rx	**Thioridazine HCl** (Various, eg, Balan, Bioline, Bolar, Dixon-Shane, Geneva, Goldline, Major, Moore, Parmed, Schein)	**Tablets:** 15 mg	In 100s, 500s, 1000s and UD 100s.	80+
Rx	**Mellaril** (Sandoz)		(78-8). Pink. In 100s, 1000s & UD 100s.	390
Rx	**Thioridazine HCl** (Various, eg, Balan, Geneva, Goldline, Lederle, Major, Moore, Roxane, Rugby, Schein, Warner Chilcott)	**Tablets:** 25 mg	In 100s, 500s, 1000s and UD 100s.	63+
Rx	**Mellaril** (Sandoz)		(Mellaril 25). Tan. In 100s, 1000s & UD 100s.	279
Rx	**Thioridazine HCl** (Various, eg, Balan, Geneva, Goldline, Lederle, Major, Moore, Roxane, Rugby, Schein, Warner Chilcott)	**Tablets:** 50 mg	In 100s, 500s, 1000s and UD 100s.	41+
Rx	**Mellaril** (Sandoz)		(Mellaril 50). White. In 100s, 1000s & UD 100s.	170

* Cost Index based on cost per 50 mg.

(Continued on following page)

Phenothiazine Derivatives (Cont.)

THIORIDAZINE HCl (Cont.)

	Product	Form/Strength	Description/Packaging	C.I.*
Rx	**Thioridazine HCl** (Various, eg, Balan, Geneva, Goldline, Lederle, Major, Moore, Roxane, Rugby, Schein, Warner Chilcott)	**Tablets:** 100 mg	In 100s, 500s, 1000s and UD 100s.	63+
Rx	**Mellaril** (Sandoz)		(Mellaril 100). Green. In 100s, 1000s and UD 100s.	100
Rx	**Thioridazine HCl** (Various, eg, Balan, Barr, Bioline, Bolar, Geneva, Goldline, Major, Parmed, Rugby, Schein)	**Tablets:** 150 mg	In 100s, 500s, 1000s and UD 100s.	36+
Rx	**Mellaril** (Sandoz)		(Mellaril 150). Yellow. In 100s & 1000s.	88
Rx	**Thioridazine HCl** (Various, eg, Balan, Bioline, Geneva, Goldline, Major, Moore, Parmed, Purepac, Rugby, Schein)	**Tablets:** 200 mg	In 100s, 500s, 1000s and UD 100s.	41+
Rx	**Mellaril** (Sandoz)		(Mellaril 200). Pink. In 100s, 1000s and UD 100s.	75
Rx	**Thioridazine HCl** (Various, eg, Balan, Geneva, Goldline, Harber, Major, Moore, PBI, Rugby, Schein, Warner Chilcott)	**Concentrate:** 30 mg per ml	In 120 ml.	83+
Rx	**Thioridazine HCl Intensol** (Roxane)		In 120 ml w/dropper.	70
Rx	**Thioridazine HCl** (Various, eg, Balan, Geneva, Harber, Major, Moore, PBI, Rugby, Schein, Warner Chilcott, Xactdose)	**Concentrate:** 100 mg per ml	In 120 ml and 3.4 ml (UD 100s).	110+
Rx	**Thioridazine HCl Intensol** (Roxane)		In 120 ml w/dropper.	51
Rx	**Mellaril** (Sandoz)	**Concentrate:** 30 mg per ml	3% alcohol. In 118 ml w/dropper.	133
		100 mg per ml	4.2% alcohol. In 118 ml w/dropper.	210
Rx	**Mellaril-S** (Sandoz)	**Suspension:** 25 mg per 5 ml	Buttermint flavor. In pt.	316
		100 mg per 5 ml	Buttermint flavor. In pt.	163

* Cost Index based on cost per 50 mg.

Complete prescribing information for these products begins on page 1323

Phenothiazine Derivatives (Cont.)

MESORIDAZINE

Indications:

Schizophrenia: Reduces the severity of emotional withdrawal, conceptual disorganization, anxiety, tension, hallucinatory behavior, suspiciousness and blunted affect.

Behavioral problems in mental deficiency and chronic brain syndrome: Reduces hyperactivity and uncooperativeness associated with mental deficiency and chronic brain syndrome.

Alcoholism (acute and chronic): Ameliorates anxiety, tension, depression, nausea and vomiting in acute and chronic alcoholics without producing hepatic dysfunction or hindering the functional recovery of the impaired liver.

Psychoneurotic manifestations: Reduces the symptoms of anxiety and tension and prevalent symptoms often associated with neurotic components of many disorders. It also benefits personality disorders in general.

Administration and Dosage:

Mesoridazine Dosage Guidelines

Disease state	Initial oral dose	Optimum total dosage range (mg/day)
Schizophrenia	50 mg tid	100-400
Behavior problems in mental deficiency and chronic brain syndrome	25 mg tid	75-300
Alcoholism	25 mg bid	50-200
Psychoneurotic manifestations	10 mg tid	30-150

IM administration: For most patients, 25 mg initially. May repeat dose in 30 to 60 minutes, if necessary. The usual optimum dosage range is 25 to 200 mg/day.

Concentrate may be diluted just prior to administration with distilled water, acidified tap water, orange or grape juice. Do not prepare and store bulk dilutions.

	Product	Formulation	Package	C.I.*
Rx	**Serentil** (Boehringer Ingelheim)	**Tablets:** Mesoridazine (as besylate). 10 mg	In 100s.	449
		25 mg	In 100s.	240
		50 mg	In 100s.	136
		100 mg	In 100s.	83
sf		**Concentrate:** Mesoridazine (as besylate). 25 mg per ml	0.61% alcohol. In 118 ml w/dropper.	134
		Injection: Mesoridazine (as besylate). 25 mg per ml	In 1 ml amps.[1]	1445

* Cost Index based on cost per 25 mg. *sf* – Sugar free. [1] With EDTA.

TRIFLUOPERAZINE HCl

Indications:

Management of manifestations of psychotic disorders; short-term treatment of nonpsychotic anxiety (not the drug of choice in most patients).

Administration and Dosage:

Individualize dosage. Increase dosage more gradually in debilitated or emaciated patients. When maximum response is achieved, reduce dosage gradually to a maintenance level. Patients may be controlled with once or twice daily administration.

Psychotic disorders: 2 to 5 mg orally twice daily. (Start small or emaciated patients on the lower dosage.) Most patients will show optimum response with 15 or 20 mg/day, although a few may require ≥ 40 mg/day. Optimum therapeutic dosage levels should be reached within 2 or 3 weeks.

IM (for prompt control of severe symptoms): 1 to 2 mg by deep injection every 4 to 6 hours, as needed. More than 6 mg/24 hours is rarely necessary.

Only in very exceptional cases should IM dosage exceed 10 mg/24 hours. Do not give injections at less than 4 hour intervals because of a possible cumulative effect. Equivalent oral dosage may be substituted once symptoms are controlled.

Children: Adjust dosage to the weight of the child and severity of symptoms. These dosages are for children, aged 6 to 12, who are hospitalized or under close supervision.

Oral – Initial dose is 1 mg once or twice daily. While it is usually not necessary to exceed 15 mg/day, older children with severe symptoms may require higher doses.

IM – There has been little experience in children. However, if it is necessary to achieve rapid control of severe symptoms, administer 1 mg once or twice a day.

(Administration and Dosage continued on following page)

Complete prescribing information for these products begins on page 1323

Phenothiazine Derivatives (Cont.)

TRIFLUOPERAZINE HCl (Cont.)

Administration and Dosage (Cont.):

Elderly patients: Usually, lower dosages are sufficient. The elderly appear more susceptible to hypotension and neuromuscular reactions; observe closely and increase dosage gradually.

Treatment of nonpsychotic anxiety: 1 or 2 mg twice daily. Do not administer > 6 mg per day or for > 12 weeks.

Concentrate: For institutional use only. Use in severe neuropsychiatric conditions when oral medication is preferred and other oral forms are impractical. Add dose to 60 ml or more of diluent just prior to administration. Vehicles suggested for dilution are: Tomato or fruit juice, milk, simple syrup, orange syrup, carbonated beverages, coffee, tea or water. Semisolid foods (soup, puddings, etc) may also be used.

				C.I.*
Rx	**Trifluoperazine** (Various, eg, Balan, Geneva, Goldline, Major, Moore, Parmed, Rugby, Schein, Warner-C, Zenith)	**Tablets:** 1 mg	In 100s, 500s, 1000s & UD 100s.	53+
Rx	**Stelazine** (SKF)		(SKF S03). Blue. Film coated. In 100s, 1000s and UD 100s.	357
Rx	**Trifluoperazine** (Various, eg, Balan, Geneva, Goldline, Major, Moore, Parmed, Rugby, Schein, Warner-C, Zenith)	**Tablets:** 2 mg	In 100s, 500s, 1000s and UD 100s and 1000s.	36+
Rx	**Stelazine** (SKF)		(SKF S04). Blue. Film coated. In 100s, 1000s and UD 100s.	263
Rx	**Trifluoperazine** (Various, eg, Balan, Geneva, Goldline, Major, Moore, Parmed, Rugby, Schein, Warner-C, Zenith)	**Tablets:** 5 mg	In 100s, 500s, 1000s and UD 100s.	16+
Rx	**Stelazine** (SKF)		(#SKF S06). Blue. Film coated. In 100s, 1000s and UD 100s.	132
Rx	**Trifluoperazine** (Various, eg, Balan, Geneva, Goldline, Major, Moore, Parmed, Rugby, Schein, Warner-C, Zenith)	**Tablets:** 10 mg	In 100s, 500s, 1000s & UD 100s.	10+
Rx	**Stelazine** (SKF)		(SKF S07). Blue. Film coated. In 100s, 1000s and UD 100s.	100
Rx	**Trifluoperazine** (Various, eg, Geneva, Harber, Moore, PBI, Raway, UDL, Warner-C)	**Concentrate:** 10 mg per ml	In 60 ml.	31+
Rx	**Stelazine** (SKF)		Sucrose. Banana-vanilla flavor. In 60 ml w/dropper.[1]	103
Rx	**Trifluoperazine** (Quad)	**Injection:** 2 mg/ml	In 10 ml vials.	1233
Rx	**Stelazine** (SKF)		In 10 ml vials.[2]	1425

* Cost Index based on cost per 2 mg.

[1] With sodium bisulfite.

[2] With sodium saccharin and 0.75% benzyl alcohol.

Complete prescribing information for these products begins on page 1323

Phenothiazine Derivatives (Cont.)

PERPHENAZINE

Indications:

Management of manifestations of psychotic disorders.

IV only: To control severe nausea and vomiting and intractable hiccoughs (see Antiemetic/Antivertigo Agents).

Administration and Dosage:

Oral: Moderately disturbed nonhospitalized patients – 4 to 8 mg 3 times/day; reduce as soon as possible to minimum effective dosage.

Hospitalized patients – 8 to 16 mg 2 to 4 times/day; avoid dosages > 64 mg/day.

IM: Use when rapid effect and prompt control are required or when oral administration is not feasible. Administer by deep IM injection to a seated or recumbent patient; observe patient for a short period after administration. Therapeutic effect usually occurs in 10 minutes and is maximal in 1 to 2 hours. The average duration of effect is 6 hours, occasionally, 12 to 24 hours.

Initial dose – 5 mg every 6 hours. The total daily dosage should not exceed 15 mg in ambulatory patients or 30 mg in hospitalized patients. Initiate oral therapy as soon as possible, generally within 24 hours. However, patients have been maintained on parenteral therapy for several months. Use equal or higher dosage when the patient is transferred to oral therapy after receiving the injection.

Psychotic conditions – While 5 mg IM has a definite tranquilizing effect, it may be necessary to use 10 mg to initiate therapy in severely agitated states. Most patients are controlled and oral therapy can be instituted within a maximum of 24 to 48 hours. Acute conditions (hysteria, panic reaction) often respond well to a single dose, whereas in chronic conditions, several injections may be required.

Children: Pediatric dosage has not been established. Children > 12 years of age may receive the lowest limit of the adult dosage.

Elderly or debilitated: Administer one-third to one-half the adult dose.

Concentrate: Dilute only with water, saline, homogenized milk, carbonated orange drink and pineapple, apricot, prune, orange, tomato and grapefruit juices. Do NOT mix with beverages containing caffeine (coffee, cola), tannics (tea) or pectinates (apple juice), since physical incompatibility may result. Use approximately 60 ml diluent for each 16 mg (5 ml) concentrate. Store concentrate between 2°C and 30°C (36° and 86°F).

	Product	Form	Description	C.I.*
Rx	**Perphenazine** (Various, eg, Balan, Bioline, Geneva, Goldline, Lemmon, Major, Moore, Rugby, URL, Zenith)	**Tablets:** 2 mg	In 100s and 500s.	268
Rx	**Trilafon** (Schering)		(Schering ADH or 705). Gray. Sugar coated. In 100s and 500s.	400
Rx	**Perphenazine** (Various, eg, Balan, Bioline, Geneva, Goldline, Lemmon, Major, Moore, Rugby, URL, Zenith)	**Tablets:** 4 mg	In 100s and 500s.	183
Rx	**Trilafon** (Schering)		(Schering ADK or 940). Gray. Sugar coated. In 100s and 500s.	274
Rx	**Perphenazine** (Various, eg, Balan, Bioline, Geneva, Goldline, Lemmon, Major, Moore, Rugby, URL, Zenith)	**Tablets:** 8 mg	In 100s, 250s and 500s.	109
Rx	**Trilafon** (Schering)		(Schering ADJ or 313). Gray. Sugar coated. In 100s and 500s.	166
Rx	**Perphenazine** (Various, eg, Balan, Bioline, Geneva, Goldline, Lemmon, Major, Moore, Rugby, URL, Zenith)	**Tablets:** 16 mg	In 100s and 500s.	75
Rx	**Trilafon** (Schering)		(Schering ADM or 077). Gray. Sugar coated. In 100s and 500s.	112
Rx	**Trilafon** (Schering)	**Concentrate:** 16 mg/5 ml	Alcohol. Sorbitol. In 118 ml w/dropper.	121
		Injection: 5 mg/ml	In 1 ml amps.[1]	1356

* Cost Index based on cost per 4 mg perphenazine.

[1] With sodium bisulfite.

Complete prescribing information for these products begins on page 1323

Phenothiazine Derivatives (Cont.)

ACETOPHENAZINE MALEATE

Indications: Management of manifestations of psychotic disorders.

Administration and Dosage:

20 mg 3 times daily. In patients who have difficulty sleeping, take the last tablet 1 hour before bedtime. Total dosage range is 40 to 80 mg/day.

Hospitalized patients: Optimum dosage is 80 to 120 mg/day in divided doses. Certain hospitalized patients with severe schizophrenia have received doses as high as 400 to 600 mg/day.

				C.I.*
Rx	**Tindal** (Schering)	**Tablets:** 20 mg	(BBA or 968). Salmon. Sugar coated. In 100s.	172

* Cost Index based on cost per 20 mg acetophenazine.

PROCHLORPERAZINE

Indications:

Management of manifestations of psychotic disorders. Short-term treatment of generalized nonpsychotic anxiety; however, prochlorperazine is not the drug of choice for this indication.

To control severe nausea and vomiting (see Antiemetic/Antivertigo Agents).

Administration and Dosage – Adults:

Administration SC is not advisable because of local irritation.

Individualize dosage. Begin with the lowest recommended dosage.

Elderly: Lower doses are sufficient for most elderly patients. Since they appear more susceptible to hypotension and neuromuscular reactions, observe patients closely. Monitor response and adjust dosage accordingly; increase dosage gradually.

Nonpsychotic anxiety:

Oral – 5 mg 3 or 4 times daily; 15 mg (sustained release) on arising, or 10 mg (sustained release) every 12 hours. Do not administer > 20 mg/day or for > 12 weeks.

Psychiatry: Although response ordinarily is seen within 1 to 2 days, longer treatment is usually required before maximal improvement is observed.

Oral – In mild conditions, give 5 or 10 mg 3 or 4 times daily. In moderate to severe conditions, for hospitalized or adequately supervised patients, give 10 mg 3 or 4 times daily. Increase dosage gradually until symptoms are controlled or side effects become bothersome. When dosage is increased by small increments every 2 or 3 days, side effects either do not occur or are easily controlled. Some patients respond to 50 to 75 mg/day. In more severe disturbances, optimum dosage is 100 to 150 mg/day.

IM – For immediate control of severely disturbed adults, inject an initial dose of 10 to 20 mg deeply into the upper outer quadrant of the buttock. Many patients respond shortly after the first injection. If necessary, repeat every 2 to 4 hours (or in resistant cases, every hour) to gain control. More than 3 or 4 doses are seldom necessary. After control is achieved, switch patient to the oral drug at the same dosage level or higher. If prolonged parenteral therapy is needed, give 10 to 20 mg every 4 to 6 hours.

Administration and Dosage – Children:

Do not use in children < 20 lbs (9.1 kg) or < 2 years of age. Do not use in pediatric surgery. Children seem more prone to develop extrapyramidal reactions, even on moderate doses. Use the lowest effective dose. Occasionally, the patient may react to the drug with signs of restlessness and excitement; if this occurs, do not administer additional doses. Use with caution in children with acute illnesses or dehydration. Do not use in conditions for which children's dosages are not established.

Oral or rectal: Children 2 to 12 years – 2.5 mg 2 or 3 times daily. Do not give > 10 mg on first day. Increase dosage according to patient response. *Children 2 to 5 years* – Do not exceed 20 mg total daily dose. *Children 6 to 12 years* – Do not exceed 25 mg total daily dose.

IM: Children < 12 years – 0.03 mg/kg (0.06 mg/lb) by deep IM injection. After control is achieved, usually after 1 dose, switch to oral form at same dosage level or higher.

Compatibility: Do not mix prochlorperazine injection with other agents in the syringe. Do not dilute with any diluent containing parabens as a preservative.

(Products listed on following page)

Phenothiazine Derivatives (Cont.)

PROCHLORPERAZINE (Cont.)			C.I.*
Rx **Prochlorperazine** (Various, eg, Balan, Bioline, Bolar, Geneva, Goldline, Major, Moore, Parmed, Rugby, Schein)	**Tablets (as maleate):** 5 mg	In 30s, 100s, 1000s and UD 100s.	38+
Rx **Compazine** (SKF)		Sucrose. (SKF C66). Yellow-green. In 100s, 1000s and UD 100s.	209
Rx **Prochlorperazine** (Various, eg, Balan, Bioline, Bolar, Geneva, Goldline, Major, Moore, Parmed, Rugby, Schein)	**Tablets (as maleate):** 10 mg	In 30s, 100s, 1000s and UD 100s.	24+
Rx **Compazine** (SKF)		Sucrose. (SKF C67). Yellow-green. In 100s, 1000s and UD 100s.	157
Rx **Prochlorperazine** (Various, eg, Balan, Bolar, Geneva, Gen-King, Harber, Major, Moore, Parmed, Raway, Rugby)	**Tablets (as maleate):** 25 mg	In 100s, 1000s and UD 100s.	12+
Rx **Compazine** (SKF)		Sucrose. (SKF C69). Yellow-green. In 100s and 1000s.	79
Rx **Compazine** (SKF)	**Spansules (sustained release capsules as maleate):** 10 mg	Benzyl alcohol, sucrose. (SKF C44). Black/natural. In 50s, 500s & UD 100s.	191
	15 mg	Benzyl alcohol, sucrose. (SKF C46). Black/natural. In 50s, 500s & UD 100s.	196
	30 mg	Benzyl alcohol, sucrose. (SKF C47). Black/natural. In 50s, 500s & UD 100s.	115
Rx **Compazine** (SKF)	**Suppositories:** 2.5 mg	In 12s.	1496
	5 mg	In 12s.	833
	25 mg	In 12s.	206
Rx **Compazine** (SKF)	**Syrup (as edisylate):** 5 mg per 5 ml	Sucrose. Fruit flavor. In 120 ml.	284
Rx **Prochlorperazine** (Various, eg, Dixon-Shane, Elkins-Sinn, Goldline, Rugby, Schein, Squibb Marsam)	**Injection (as edisylate):** 5 mg per ml	In 2 ml amps and 10 ml vials.	420+
Rx **Prochlorperazine** (Wyeth-Ayerst)		In 1 and 2 ml Tubex.[1]	1500
Rx **Compazine** (SKF)		In 2 ml amps[2], 2 ml syringes[1] and 2 and 10 ml vials.[1]	1228

* Cost Index based on cost per 5 mg.

[1] With sodium saccharin and benzyl alcohol.

[2] With sodium sulfite and sodium bisulfite.

Complete prescribing information for these products begins on page 1323

Phenothiazine Derivatives (Cont.)

FLUPHENAZINE HCl

Indications:

Management of manifestations of psychotic disorders.

Administration and Dosage:

Individualize dosage. The oral dose is approximately 2 to 3 times the parenteral dose. Institute treatment with a low initial dosage; increase as necessary. Therapeutic effect is often achieved with doses < 20 mg/day. However, daily doses up to 40 mg may be needed. Acutely ill patients may respond to lower doses and may require a rapid dosage increase. Elderly, debilitated and adolescent patients may respond to low dosages. Outpatients should receive smaller doses than hospitalized patients.

Administration IM is useful when patients are unable or unwilling to take oral therapy. When symptoms are controlled, oral maintenance therapy can be instituted, often with single daily doses. Continued treatment, by the oral route if possible, is needed to achieve maximum therapeutic benefits; further dosage adjustments may be necessary.

Oral: Adults – Initially 0.5 to 10 mg/day in divided doses administered at 6 to 8 hour intervals. In general, a daily dose in excess of 3 mg is rarely necessary. Use doses in excess of 20 mg with caution. When symptoms are controlled, reduce dosage gradually to daily maintenance doses of 1 to 5 mg, often given as a single daily dose.

Geriatric patients – Starting dose is 1 to 2.5 mg/day, adjusted according to response.

IM: The average starting dose is 1.25 mg IM. The initial total daily dosage may range from 2.5 to 10 mg, divided and given at 6 to 8 hour intervals. In general, the parenteral dose is approximately ⅓ to ½ the oral dose. Institute treatment with a low initial dosage and increase, if necessary, until desired clinical effects are achieved. Use dosages exceeding 10 mg/day IM with caution.

For psychotic patients stabilized on a fixed daily dosage of fluphenazine HCl tablets or liquid, conversion from oral therapy to the long-acting injectable fluphenazine decanoate may be indicated.

Concentrate: Suitable for administration only with the following diluents: Water, saline, *Seven-Up,* homogenized milk, carbonated orange beverage, and pineapple, apricot, prune, orange, *V-8,* tomato and grapefruit juices. Do NOT mix with beverages containing caffeine (coffee, cola), tannics (tea) or pectinates (apple juice), since physical incompatibility may result.

Storage: Store concentrate between 2° and 30°C (36° and 86°F). Avoid freezing.

	Product	Form	Packaging	C.I.*
Rx	**Fluphenazine HCl** (Various, eg, Balan, Bioline, Geneva, Goldline, Major, Moore, Rugby, Schein, URL, Warner Chilcott)	**Tablets:** 1 mg	In 50s, 100s, 500s, 1000s and UD 100s.	152+
Rx	**Prolixin** (Princeton)		(863). In 50s, 100s, 500s and UD 100s.	317
Rx	**Fluphenazine HCl** (Various, eg, Balan, Bioline, Geneva, Goldline, Major, Moore, Rugby, Schein, URL, Warner Chilcott)	**Tablets:** 2.5 mg	In 50s, 100s, 500s and UD 100s.	87+
Rx	**Permitil** (Schering)		(WDR or 442). Orange, scored. Oval. In 100s.	136
Rx	**Prolixin** (Princeton)		Tartrazine. (864). In 50s, 100s, 500s and UD 100s.	180
Rx	**Fluphenazine HCl** (Various, eg, Balan, Bioline, Geneva, Goldline, Major, Moore, Rugby, Schein, URL, Warner Chilcott)	**Tablets:** 5 mg	In 50s, 100s, 500s and UD 100s.	56+
Rx	**Permitil** (Schering)		(WFF or 550). Purple-pink, scored. Oval. In 100s.	91
Rx	**Prolixin)** (Princeton)		Tartrazine. (877). In 50s, 100s and UD 100s.	118

* Cost Index based on cost per 1 mg.

(Products continued on following page)

Complete prescribing information for these products begins on page 1323

Phenothiazine Derivatives (Cont.)

	FLUPHENAZINE HCl (Cont.)			**C.I.***
Rx	**Fluphenazine HCl** (Various, eg, Balan, Bioline, Geneva, Goldline, Major, Moore, Rugby, Schein, URL, Warner Chilcott)	**Tablets:** 10 mg	In 50s, 100s, 500s and UD 100s.	36+
Rx	**Permitil** (Schering)		(WFG or 316). Red, scored. Oval. In 1000s.	54
Rx	**Prolixin** (Princeton)		Tartrazine. (956). In 50s, 100s, 500s and UD 100s.	75
Rx	**Prolixin** (Princeton)	**Elixir:** 2.5 mg per 5 ml	14% alcohol, sucrose. In 60 ml w/dropper, 473 ml.	230
Rx	**Permitil** (Schering)	**Concentrate:** 5 mg per ml	1% alcohol. In 118 ml w/ dropper.	75
Rx	**Prolixin** (Princeton)		14% alcohol. In 120 ml w/ dropper.	75
Rx	**Fluphenazine HCl** (Quad)	**Injection:** 2.5 mg per ml	In 10 ml vials.	525
Rx	**Prolixin** (Princeton)		In 10 ml vials.[1]	857

FLUPHENAZINE ENANTHATE AND DECANOATE

Actions:

The esterification of fluphenazine markedly prolongs the duration of effects without unduly attenuating its beneficial action.

Selected Fluphenazine Pharmacokinetic Parameters					
Fluphenazine Ester	Peak Plasma Level (days)	Half-life (days)		Onset of Action (days)	Duration (weeks)
		Single-dose	Multiple-dose		
Enanthate	2 to 3	3.5 to 4		1 to 3	1 to 3
Decanoate	1 to 2	6.8 to 9.6	14.3	1 to 3	≥4

Indications: Management of patients requiring prolonged parenteral neuroleptic therapy (eg, chronic schizophrenics).

Administration and Dosage:

Administer IM or SC. Initiate with 12.5 to 25 mg. Determine subsequent injections and dosage interval in accordance with patient response. Do not exceed 100 mg. If doses > 50 mg are needed, increase succeeding doses cautiously in 12.5 mg increments.

In one study, significantly more injection site leakage occurred after IM administration compared to SC use; consider this possibility with nonresponders to IM therapy.

Initially, treat patients who have never taken phenothiazines with a shorter-acting form of the drug before administering the enanthate or decanoate. This helps to determine the response to fluphenazine and to establish appropriate dosage. The equivalent dosage of fluphenazine HCl to the longer-acting forms is not known; exercise caution when switching from shorter-acting forms to the enanthate.

No precise formula can be given to convert to use of fluphenazine decanoate. However, in a controlled multicenter study, 20 mg fluphenazine HCl daily was equivalent to 25 mg decanoate every 3 weeks. This represents an approximate conversion ratio of 0.5 ml (12.5 mg) decanoate every 3 weeks for every 10 mg fluphenazine HCl daily.

Severely agitated patients: Treat initially with a rapid-acting phenothiazine such as fluphenazine HCl injection. When acute symptoms have subsided, administer 25 mg of the enanthate or decanoate; adjust subsequent dosage as necessary.

"Poor risk" patients (those with known hypersensitivity to phenothiazines or with disorders that predispose to undue reactions): Initiate therapy cautiously with oral or parenteral fluphenazine HCl. When an appropriate dosage is established, administer an equivalent dose of fluphenazine enanthate or decanoate.

				C.I.*
Rx	**Prolixin Enanthate** (Princeton)	**Injection:** 25 mg per ml[2]	In 5 ml vials.	232
Rx	**Fluphenazine Decanoate** (Quad)	**Injection:** 25 mg per ml[2]	In 5 ml vials.	131
Rx	**Prolixin Decanoate** (Princeton)		In 5 ml vials and 1 ml Unimatic syringes.	218

* Cost Index based on cost per 1 mg.

[1] With methyl and propyl parabens.

[2] In sesame oil with benzyl alcohol.

Complete prescribing information for these products begins on page 1323

Thioxanthene Derivatives

Indications:

Management of manifestations of psychotic disorders.

CHLORPROTHIXENE

Administration and Dosage:

Safety and efficacy not established for oral administration in children < 6 years of age or for parenteral use in those < 12 years of age.

Oral: Adults – Initially, 25 to 50 mg 3 or 4 times daily; increase as needed. Dosages exceeding 600 mg daily are rarely required. For elderly or debilitated patients, initiate lower doses of 10 to 25 mg 3 or 4 times daily.

Children (> 6 years) – 10 to 25 mg 3 or 4 times daily.

IM: Adults and children > 12 years – 25 to 50 mg IM up to 3 or 4 times daily. Postural hypotension may occur, but recovery is usually spontaneous; inject with the patient seated or recumbent. Institute oral medication as soon as feasible. Gradually give oral and parenteral doses alternately on the same day, then oral doses only. Individualize dosage.

Concentrate: Administer undiluted or in milk, water, fruit juice, coffee or carbonated beverages.

				C.I.*
Rx	**Taractan** (Roche)	**Tablets:** 10 mg[1]	(Taractan 10). In 100s.	837
		25 mg[1]	(Taractan 25). In 100s and 500s.	461
		50 mg[1]	(Taractan 50). In 100s and 500s.	274
		100 mg[1]	(Taractan 100). In 100s and 500s.	173
		Concentrate: 100 mg (as lactate and HCl) per 5 ml	Sorbitol, sucrose. Fruit flavor. In 480 ml.	152
		Injection: 12.5 mg (as HCl) per ml	In 2 ml amps.[2]	4020

* Cost Index based on cost per 50 mg.

[1] Contains tartrazine.

[2] With methyl and propyl parabens.

Complete prescribing information for these products begins on page 1323

Thioxanthene Derivatives (Cont.)

THIOTHIXENE

Administration and Dosage:

Not recommended in children < 12 years of age.

Oral: Mild conditions – Initially 2 mg 3 times daily. If indicated, an increase to 15 mg/day is often effective. *Severe conditions* – Initially 5 mg twice daily. The optimal dose is 20 to 30 mg/day. If indicated, an increase to 60 mg/day is often effective. Exceeding 60 mg/day rarely increases the beneficial response.

IM: 4 mg 2 to 4 times daily. Most patients are controlled on 16 to 20 mg/day (maximum 30 mg/day). Used for more rapid control and treatment of acute behavior and when oral administration is impractical. Institute oral medication as soon as feasible. May need to adjust dosage when changing from IM to oral forms.

Preparation and storage – Reconstitute powder for injection with 2.2 ml Sterile Water for Injection; may then store at room temperature for 48 hours before discarding. The IM solution is stable for 12 months at room temperature.

	Product	Form	Packaging	C.I.*
Rx	**Thiothixene** (Various, eg, Balan, Bioline, Danbury, Geneva, Goldline, Major, Moore, Parmed, Rugby, Schein)	**Capsules:** 1 mg	In 100s, 500s, 1000s and UD 100s.	125+
Rx	**Navane** (Roerig)		(Navane Roerig 571). In 100s and UD 100s.	288
Rx	**Thiothixene** (Various, eg, Balan, Bioline, Danbury, Geneva, Goldline, Major, Moore, Parmed, Rugby, Schein)	**Capsules:** 2 mg	In 100s, 500s, 1000s and UD 100s.	81+
Rx	**Navane** (Roerig)		(Navane Roerig 572). In 100s, 1000s and UD 100s.	158
Rx	**Thiothixene** (Various, eg, Balan, Bioline, Danbury, Geneva, Goldline, Major, Moore, Parmed, Rugby)	**Capsules:** 5 mg	In 100s, 500s, 1000s and UD 100s.	43+
Rx	**Navane** (Roerig)		(Navane Roerig 573). In 100s, 1000s and UD 100s.	99
Rx	**Thiothixene** (Various, eg, Balan, Bioline, Danbury, Geneva, Goldline, Major, Moore, Parmed, Rugby, Schein)	**Capsules:** 10 mg	In 100s, 500s, 1000s and UD 100s.	31+
Rx	**Navane** (Roerig)		(Navane Roerig 574). In 100s, 1000s and UD 100s.	68
Rx	**Thiothixene** (Various, eg, Balan, Bioline, Dixon-Shane, Geneva, Goldline, Major, Moore, Parmed, Rugby, Schein)	**Capsules:** 20 mg	In 100s, 500s and 1000s.	33+
Rx	**Navane** (Roerig)		(Navane Roerig 577). In 100s, 500s and UD 100s.	40
Rx	**Thiothixene** (Various, eg, Barre-National, Bioline, Goldline, Lemmon, Major, Rugby, Schein, Warner-C)	**Concentrate:** 5 mg (as HCl) per ml	In 30 and 120 ml.	56
Rx	**Navane** (Roerig)		7% alcohol, sorbitol. Fruit flavor. In 30 and 120 ml w/dropper.	83
Rx	**Navane** (Roerig)	**IM Solution:** 2 mg (as HCl) per ml	In 2 ml vials.[1]	130
		Powder for Injection: 5 mg (as HCl) per ml when reconstituted	In 2 ml vials.[2]	79

* Cost Index based on cost per 2 mg.
[1] With 5% dextrose, 0.9% benzyl alcohol, 0.02% propyl gallate.
[2] With 59.6 mg mannitol per ml.

Complete prescribing information for these products begins on page 1323

Dibenzoxazepine

LOXAPINE

Actions:

Loxapine is chemically distinct from the thioxanthenes, butyrophenones and phenothiazines. No clear advantages over other antipsychotic agents are established.

Pharmacokinetics: Loxapine is metabolized extensively and is excreted within the first 24 hours. Metabolites are excreted in the urine as conjugates and in the feces unconjugated. Signs of sedation are usually seen within 20 to 30 minutes after administration, are most pronounced within 1.5 to 3 hours and last approximately 12 hours.

Indications:

Management of the manifestations of psychotic disorders.

Administration and Dosage:

Oral: Individualize dosage. Administer in divided doses, 2 to 4 times daily.

Initial dosage – 10 mg twice daily. In severely disturbed patients, up to 50 mg/day may be desirable. Increase dosage fairly rapidly over the first 7 to 10 days until psychotic symptoms are controlled. The usual range is 60 to 100 mg/day. Dosage > 250 mg/day is not recommended.

Maintenance therapy – Reduce dosage to the lowest level compatible with control of symptoms; usual range is 20 to 60 mg/day.

Mix the concentrate with orange or grapefruit juice shortly before administration.

IM: For prompt symptomatic control in the acutely agitated patient and in patients whose symptoms render oral medication temporarily impractical.

Administer IM (not IV) in 12.5 to 50 mg doses at intervals of 4 to 6 hours or longer. Many patients respond satisfactorily to twice daily dosage. Individualize dosage. Once control is achieved, institute oral medication, usually within 5 days.

	Product	Form/Strength	Description	C.I.*
Rx	**Loxapine Succinate** (Various, eg, Bristol-Myers Squibb, Geneva Marsam, Goldline, Major, Moore, Parmed, Schein, Warner Chilcott)	**Capsules:** 5 mg	In 100s.	NA
		10 mg	In 100s.	NA
		25 mg	In 100s.	NA
		50 mg	In 100s.	NA
Rx	**Loxitane** (Lederle)	**Capsules (as succinate):** 5 mg	(Lederle L1 5 mg). Green. In 100s and UD 100s.	564
		10 mg	(Lederle L2 10 mg). Green and yellow. In 100s, 1000s and UD 100s.	365
		25 mg	(Lederle L3 25 mg). Two-tone green. In 100s, 1000s and UD 100s.	220
		50 mg	(Lederle L4 50 mg). Green and blue. In 100s, 1000s and UD 100s.	147
Rx	**Loxitane C** (Lederle)	**Concentrate (as HCl):** 25 mg per ml	In 120 ml with dropper.	266
Rx	**Loxitane IM** (Lederle)	**Injection (as HCl):** 50 mg per ml	In 1 ml amps and 10 ml vials.[1]	655

* Cost Index based on cost per 10 mg.

[1] With 5% polysorbate 80 and 70% propylene glycol.

CLOZAPINE

Actions:

Pharmacology: Clozapine, a tricyclic dibenzodiazepine derivative, is classified as an "atypical" antipsychotic drug because its profile of binding to dopamine receptors and its effects on various dopamine mediated behaviors differ from those exhibited by more typical antipsychotic drug products. In particular, although clozapine does interfere with the binding of dopamine at both D-1 and D-2 receptors, it does not induce catalepsy nor inhibit apomorphine-induced stereotypy. This evidence, consistent with the view that clozapine is preferentially more active at limbic than at striatal dopamine receptors, may explain clozapine's relative freedom from extrapyramidal side effects. Clozapine also acts as an antagonist at adrenergic, cholinergic, histaminergic and serotonergic receptors. In contrast to more typical antipsychotic drugs, clozapine therapy produces little or no prolactin elevation.

As is true of more typical antipsychotic drugs, clozapine increases delta and theta activity and slows dominant alpha frequencies of the EEG. Enhanced synchronization occurs, and sharp wave activity and spike and wave complexes may also develop. Patients rarely may report intensification of dream activity. REM sleep was increased to 85% of the total sleep time. In these patients, the onset of REM sleep occurred almost immediately after falling asleep.

Pharmacokinetics: Absorption/Distribution – Clozapine tablets (25 and 100 mg) are equally bioavailable relative to a clozapine solution. Following a dosage of 100 mg twice daily, the average steady-state peak plasma concentration was 319 ng/ml (range: 102 to 771 ng/ml), occurring at an average of 2.5 hours (range: 1 to 6 hours) after dosing. The average minimum concentration at steady state was 122 ng/ml (range: 41 to 343 ng/ml) after 100 mg twice daily dosing. Food does not appear to affect the systemic bioavailability of clozapine; thus clozapine may be administered with or without food.

Clozapine is approximately 95% bound to serum proteins. The interaction between clozapine and other highly protein-bound drugs has not been fully evaluated but may be important (see Drug Interactions).

Metabolism/Excretion – Clozapine is almost completely metabolized prior to excretion and only trace amounts of unchanged drug are detected in the urine and feces. Approximately 50% of the administered dose is excreted in the urine and 30% in the feces as demethylated, hydroxylated and N-oxide derivatives. The desmethyl metabolite has only limited activity, while the hydroxylated and N-oxide derivatives are inactive.

The mean elimination half-life of clozapine after a single 75 mg dose was 8 hours (range: 4 to 12 hours), compared to a mean elimination half-life of 12 hours (range: 4 to 66 hours) after achieving steady state with 100 mg twice daily dosing. In comparisons of single and multiple dose administration of clozapine, the elimination half-life increased significantly after multiple dosing relative to that after single dose administration, suggesting concentration dependent pharmacokinetics. However, at steady state, linearly dose-proportional changes with respect to area under the curve, peak and minimum clozapine plasma concentrations were observed after administration of 37.5, 75 and 150 mg twice daily.

Indications:

Management of severely ill schizophrenic patients who fail to respond adequately to standard antipsychotic drug treatment.

Contraindications:

Myeloproliferative disorders; history of clozapine-induced agranulocytosis or severe granulocytopenia; simultaneous administration with other agents having a well-known potential to suppress bone marrow function; severe CNS depression or comatose states from any cause.

(Continued on following page)

CLOZAPINE (Cont.)

Warnings:

Because of the significant risk of agranulocytosis, a potentially life-threatening adverse event (see below), reserve clozapine for use in the treatment of severely ill schizophrenic patients who fail to show an acceptable response to adequate courses of standard antipsychotic drug treatment, either because of insufficient effectiveness or the inability to achieve an effective dose due to intolerable adverse effects from those drugs. Consequently, before initiating treatment with clozapine, it is strongly recommended that a patient be given at least two trials, each with a different standard antipsychotic drug product, at an adequate dose and for an adequate duration. Patients who are being treated with clozapine must have a baseline white blood cell (WBC) and differential count before initiation of treatment, and a WBC count every week throughout treatment and for 4 weeks after the discontinuation of clozapine.

Agranulocytosis, defined as a granulocyte count of < 500/mm³, occurs in association with clozapine use at a cumulative incidence at 1 year of approximately 1.3%, based on 15 cases out of 1743 patients exposed to clozapine during clinical testing. All of these cases occurred when the need for close monitoring of WBC counts was already recognized. This reaction could prove fatal if not detected early and therapy interrupted. While no fatalities have been associated with these agranulocytosis cases, and all cases have recovered fully, the sample is too small to reliably estimate the case fatality rate. Of the 112 cases of agranulocytosis reported worldwide in association with clozapine use as of December 31, 1986, 35% were fatal. However, few of these deaths occurred since 1977, when knowledge of clozapine-induced agranulocytosis became more widespread, and close monitoring of WBC counts more widely practiced.

Patients must have a blood sample drawn for a WBC count before initiation of treatment with clozapine, and must have subsequent WBC counts done at least weekly for the duration of therapy, as well as for 4 weeks thereafter. The distribution of clozapine is contingent upon performance of the required blood tests.

Clozapine Therapy Guidelines Based on WBC and Granulocyte Count

WBC Count (mm³)	Granulocyte Count (mm³)	Guidelines
< 3500, or history of myeloproliferative disorder, or previous clozapine-induced agranulocytosis or granulocytopenia		Do not initiate treatment.
< 3500, or > 3500 with a substantial drop from baseline, following initiation of treatment		Repeat WBC and differential counts. Symptoms of infection: Lethargy, weakness, fever, sore throat.
3000 to 3500 on subsequent counts	> 1500	Perform twice weekly WBC and differential counts.
< 3000	< 1500	Interrupt therapy, monitor for flu-like symptoms or other symptoms of infection. May resume therapy if no signs of infection develop, WBC count > 3000 and granulocyte count > 1500. However, continue twice weekly WBC and differential counts until WBC returns to 3500.
< 2000	< 1000	Consider bone marrow aspiration to ascertain granulopoietic status. If granulopoiesis is deficient, consider protective isolation. If infection develops, perform cultures and institute antibiotics. Do *not* rechallenge with clozapine since agranulocytosis may develop with a shorter latency.

(Warnings continued on following page)

CLOZAPINE (Cont.)

Warnings (Cont):

Except for evidence of significant bone marrow suppression during initial clozapine therapy, there are no established risk factors for the development of agranulocytosis. However, a disproportionate number of the US cases of agranulocytosis occurred in patients of Jewish background compared to the overall proportion of such patients exposed during clozapine's domestic development. Most of the US cases occurred with 4 to 10 weeks of exposure, but neither dose nor duration is a reliable predictor. No patient characteristics have been clearly linked to the development of agranulocytosis in association with clozapine use, but agranulocytosis associated with other antipsychotic drugs has been reported to occur with a greater frequency in women, the elderly and in patients who are cachectic or have serious underlying medical illness; such patients may also be at particular risk with clozapine.

To reduce the risk of agranulocytosis developing undetected, clozapine will be dispensed only within the clozapine Patient Management System.

Seizure occurs in association with clozapine use at a cumulative incidence at 1 year of approximately 5%, based on 61 of 1743 patients exposed to clozapine during its clinical testing (ie, a crude rate of 3.5%). Dose appears to be an important predictor of seizure, with a greater likelihood of seizure at the higher clozapine doses used.

Use caution when administering clozapine to patients with a history of seizures or other predisposing factors. Advise patients not to engage in any activity where sudden loss of consciousness could cause serious risk to themselves or others, (eg, the operation of complex machinery, driving an an automobile, swimming, climbing).

Cardiovascular disease: Use clozapine with caution; carefully observe the recommendation for gradual titration of dose.

Orthostatic hypotension can occur, especially during initial titration in association with rapid dose escalation, and may represent a continuing risk in some patients.

Tachycardia, which may be sustained, has also been observed in approximately 25% of patients, with patients having an average increase in pulse rate of 10 to 15 bpm. The sustained tachycardia is not simply a reflex response to hypotension, and is present in all positions monitored.

Either tachycardia or hypotension may pose a serious risk for an individual with compromised cardiovascular function.

ECG Changes: A minority of patients experience ECG repolarization changes similar to those seen with other antipsychotic drugs, including S-T segment depression and flattening or inversion of T waves, which all normalize after discontinuation of clozapine. The clinical significance is unclear. However, several patients have experienced significant cardiac events, including ischemic changes, myocardial infarction, nonfatal arrhythmias and sudden unexplained death. Causality assessment was difficult in many of these cases because of serious preexisting cardiac disease and plausible alternative causes. Rare instances of sudden, unexplained death have been reported in psychiatric patients, with or without associated antipsychotic drug treatment, and the relationship of these events to antipsychotic drug use is unknown.

Neuroleptic Malignant Syndrome (NMS), a potentially fatal symptom complex has occurred in association with antipsychotic drugs. Clinical manifestations of NMS are hyperpyrexia, muscle rigidity, altered mental status and evidence of autonomic instability (irregular pulse or blood pressure, tachycardia, diaphoresis and cardiac dysrhythmias).

Management of NMS should include 1) immediate discontinuation of antipsychotic drugs and other drugs not essential to concurrent therapy, 2) intensive symptomatic treatment and medical monitoring, and 3) treatment of any concomitant serious medical problems for which specific treatments are available. There is no general agreement about specific pharmacological treatment regimens for uncomplicated NMS.

If a patient requires antipsychotic drug treatment after recovery from NMS, the potential reintroduction of drug therapy should be carefully considered. The patient should be carefully monitored, since recurrences of NMS have been reported.

No cases of NMS have been attributed to clozapine alone. However, there have been several reported cases of NMS in patients treated concomitantly with lithium or other CNS-active agents.

(Warnings continued on following page)

CLOZAPINE (Cont.)

Warnings (Cont.)

Tardive dyskinesia, a syndrome consisting of potentially irreversible, involuntary, dyskinetic movements may develop in patients treated with antipsychotic drugs. Although the prevalence of the syndrome appears to be highest among the elderly, especially elderly women, it is impossible to predict which patients are likely to develop the syndrome. There have been no confirmed cases of tardive dyskinesia developing in association with clozapine use. Nevertheless, it cannot yet be concluded, without more extended experience, that clozapine is incapable of inducing this syndrome. Prescribe clozapine in a manner that is most likely to minimize the occurrence of tardive dyskinesia. If signs and symptoms of tardive dyskinesia appear in a patient on clozapine, consider drug discontinuation. However, some patients may require treatment with clozapine despite the presence of the syndrome.

Both the risk of developing the syndrome and the likelihood that it will become irreversible are believed to increase as the duration of treatment and the total cumulative dose of antipsychotic drugs administered to the patient increase. However, the syndrome can develop, although much less commonly, after relatively brief treatment periods at low doses. There is no known treatment, although the syndrome may remit, partially or completely, if antipsychotic drug treatment is withdrawn. Antipsychotic drug treatment itself, however, may suppress (or partially suppress) the signs and symptoms of the syndrome and thereby may possibly mask the underlying process. The effect that symptom suppression has upon the long-term course of the syndrome is unknown.

Pregnancy: Category B – There are no adequate or well controlled studies in pregnant women. Use during pregnancy only if clearly needed.

Lactation: Animal studies suggest that clozapine may be excreted in breast milk and have an effect on the nursing infant. Therefore, women on clozapine should not nurse.

Children: Safety and efficacy in children < 16 years old have not been established.

Precautions:

Fever: Patients may experience transient temperature elevations > 100.4°F (38°C), with the peak incidence within the first 3 weeks of treatment. While this fever is generally benign and self-limiting, it may necessitate discontinuing patients from treatment. On occasion, there may be an associated increase or decrease in WBC count. Carefully evaluate patients with fever to rule out the possibility of an underlying infectious process or the development of agranulocytosis. In the presence of high fever, the possibility of NMS must be considered (see Warnings).

Anticholinergic effects of clozapine are very potent; exercise great care in using this drug in the presence of prostatic enlargement or narrow angle glaucoma.

Interference with cognitive and motor performance: Because of initial sedation, clozapine may impair mental or physical abilities, especially during the first few days of therapy. Carefully adhere to the recommendations for gradual dose escalation, and caution patients about activities requiring alertness.

Concomitant illness: Clinical experience is limited. Nevertheless, caution is advisable in using clozapine in patients with hepatic, renal or cardiac disease.

Drug Interactions:

Anticholinergics: The anticholinergic effects may be potentiated by clozapine.

Antihypertensives: The hypotensive effects may be potentiated by clozapine.

CNS drugs: Given the primary CNS effects of clozapine, caution is advised in using it concomitantly with other CNS-active drugs.

Agents that suppress bone marrow function: Mechanism of clozapine in agranulocytosis is unknown; nonetheless, consider the possibility that causative factors may interact synergistically to increase the risk or severity of bone marrow suppression. Do not use with other agents that suppress bone marrow function.

Protein binding: Because clozapine is highly bound to serum protein, the administration of clozapine to a patient taking another drug which is highly bound to protein (eg, warfarin, digoxin) may cause an increase in plasma concentrations of these drugs, potentially resulting in adverse effects. Conversely, adverse effects may result from displacement of protein-bound clozapine by other highly bound drugs.

Adverse Reactions:

Of 1080 patients who received clozapine in premarketing clinical trials, 16% discontinued treatment due to an adverse event which included:

CNS – Drowsiness/sedation; seizures; dizziness/syncope.
Cardiovascular – Tachycardia; hypotension; ECG changes.
GI – Nausea/vomiting.
Hematologic – Leukopenia/granulocytopenia/agranulocytosis.
Miscellaneous – Fever.

(Adverse Reactions continued on following page)

CLOZAPINE (Cont.)

Adverse Reactions (Cont.):

The following table lists adverse events that occurred at a frequency of ≥ 1% among patients who participated in clinical trials.

Clozapine Adverse Reactions (n = 842)			
Adverse Reaction (%)		Adverse Reaction (%)	
CNS		*Cardiovascular*	
Drowsiness/sedation	39	Tachycardia	25
Dizziness/vertigo	19	Hypotension	9
Headache	7	Hypertension	4
Tremor	6	Chest pain/angina	1
Syncope	6	ECG change/cardiac abnormality	1
Disturbed sleep/ nightmares	4	*GI*	
Restlessness	4	Constipation	14
Hypokinesia/akinesia	4	Nausea	5
Agitation	4	Abdominal discomfort/ heartburn	4
Seizures (convulsions)	3	Nausea/vomiting	3
Rigidity	3	Diarrhea	2
Akathisia	3	Liver test abnormality	1
Confusion	3	Anorexia	1
Fatigue	2	*GU*	
Insomnia	2	Urinary abnormalities	2
Hyperkinesia	1	Incontinence	1
Weakness	1	Abnormal ejaculation	1
Lethargy	1	Urinary urgency/frequency	1
Ataxia	1	Urinary retention	1
Slurred speech	1	*Respiratory*	
Depression	1	Throat discomfort	1
Epileptiform movements/ Myoclonic jerks	1	Dyspnea, shortness of breath	1
Anxiety	1	Nasal congestion	1
Autonomic Nervous System		*Hemic/Lymphatic*	
Salivation	31	Leukopenia/decreased WBC/neutropenia	3
Sweating	6	Agranulocytosis	1
Dry mouth	6	Eosinophilia	1
Visual disturbances	5	*Miscellaneous*	
Musculoskeletal		Fever	5
Muscle weakness	1	Weight gain	4
Pain (back, neck, legs)	1	Rash	2
Muscle spasm	1	Tongue numb/sore	1
Muscle pain, ache	1		

Overdosage:

Symptoms: Most common – Altered states of consciousness, including drowsiness, delirium and coma; tachycardia; hypotension; respiratory depression; hypersalivation. Seizures have occurred in a minority of reported cases. Fatal overdoses have been reported with clozapine, generally at doses > 2.5 g. There have also been reports of patients recovering from overdoses well in excess of 4 g.

Treatment: Establish and maintain an airway; ensure adequate oxygenation and ventilation. Activated charcoal, which may be used with sorbitol, may be as or more effective than emesis or lavage. Monitoring cardiac and vital signs is recommended along with general symptomatic and supportive measures. Continue additional surveillance for several days because of the risk of delayed effects. Avoid epinephrine and derivatives when treating hypotension, and quinidine and procainamide when treating cardiac arrhythmia. Refer to General Management of Acute Overdosage.

Forced diuresis, dialysis, hemoperfusion and exchange transfusion are unlikely to be of benefit.

(Continued on following page)

CLOZAPINE (Cont.)

Patient Information:

Warn patients about the significant risk of developing agranulocytosis. Inform them that weekly blood tests are required to monitor for the occurrence of agranulocytosis, and that clozapine tablets will be made available only through a special program designed to ensure the required blood monitoring. Advise patients to report immediately the appearance of lethargy, weakness, fever, sore throat, malaise, mucous membrane ulceration or other possible signs of infection. Pay particular attention to any "flu-like" complaints or other symptoms that might suggest infection.

Inform patients of the significant risk of seizure during clozapine treatment, and advise them to avoid driving and any other potentially hazardous activity while taking clozapine.

Advise patients of the risk of orthostatic hypotension, especially during the period of initial dose titration.

Patients should notify their physician if they are taking, or plan to take, any prescription or over-the-counter drugs or alcohol.

Patients should notify their physician if they become pregnant or intend to become pregnant during therapy.

Patients should not breast feed an infant if they are taking clozapine.

Administration and Dosage:

Initial: 25 mg once or twice daily, and then continued with daily dosage increments of 25 to 50 mg/day, if well tolerated, to achieve a target dose of 300 to 450 mg/day by the end of 2 weeks. Make subsequent dosage increments no more than once or twice weekly, in increments not to exceed 100 mg. Cautious titration and a divided dosage schedule are necessary to minimize the risks of hypotension, seizure and sedation.

In a multicenter study, patients were titrated during the first 2 weeks up to a maximum dose of 500 mg/day, on a 3 times daily basis, and were then dosed in a total daily dose range of 100 to 900 mg/day, on a 3 times daily basis thereafter, with clinical response and adverse effects as guides to correct dosing.

Dose adjustment: Continue daily dosing on a divided basis to an effective and tolerable dose level. While many patients may respond adequately at doses between 300 to 600 mg/day, it may be necessary to raise the dose to the 600 to 900 mg/day range. Do not exceed 900 mg/day. The mean and median clozapine doses are approximately 600 mg/day.

Because of the possibility of increased adverse reactions at higher doses, particularly seizures, give patients adequate time to respond to a given dose level before escalation to a higher dose.

Because of the significant risk of agranulocytosis and seizure, events which both present a continuing risk over time, avoid the extended treatment of patients failing to show an acceptable level of clinical response.

Maintenance: Continue clozapine at the lowest level needed to maintain remission. Periodically reassess patients to determine the need for maintenance treatment.

Discontinuation: In the event of planned termination of clozapine therapy, gradual reduction in dose is recommended over a 1 to 2 week period. However, should a patient's medical condition require abrupt discontinuation (eg, leukopenia), carefully observe the patient for the recurrence of psychotic symptoms.

Reinitiation of treatment: Follow the original dosage build-up guidelines. However, certain additional precautions seem prudent. Reexposure of a patient might enhance the risk of an untoward event's occurrence and increase its severity. Patients discontinued for WBC counts < 2000 per mm^3 or a granulocyte count < 1000 per mm^3 must *not* be restarted on clozapine. (See Warnings.)

Clozapine is available only through the *Clozaril* Patient Management System, a program that combines WBC testing, patient monitoring, pharmacy, and drug distribution services, all linked to compliance with required safety monitoring. Do not dispense more than a 1 week supply.

Rx	**Clozaril** (Sandoz)	**Tablets:** 25 mg 100 mg	(#Clozaril 25 or 100). Yellow. In UD 100s. Also in total daily dose packages, each containing 1 week's worth of medication and containing various combinations of 25 and 100 mg tablets; in 150, 200, 250, 300, 400, 500 and 600 mg/day.

\# Product identification code.

Diphenylbutylpiperidine

PIMOZIDE

Actions:

Pharmacology: Pimozide is a neuroleptic which blocks CNS dopaminergic receptors. It has no effect on norepinephrine receptors. Its ability to suppress motor and phonic tics in Tourette's Disorder is thought to be a function of its dopaminergic blocking activity.

Pharmacokinetics: More than 50% of a dose of pimozide is absorbed after oral administration. Peak serum levels occur 6 to 8 hours (range 4 to 12 hours) after dosing. There are few correlations between plasma levels and clinical findings. Pimozide is extensively metabolized in the liver; mean elimination half-life in schizophrenic patients is approximately 55 hours. Two major metabolites with undetermined neuroleptic activity have been identified. The major route of elimination is via the kidney; 38% to 45% of the dose is recovered in the urine, mostly as metabolites.

Indications:

For the suppression of severely compromising motor and phonic tics in patients with Tourette's Disorder who have failed to respond satisfactorily to standard treatment.

Contraindications:

Treatment of simple tics or tics other than those associated with Tourette's Disorder.

Drug-induced motor and phonic tics (eg, pemoline, methylphenidate, amphetamines) until it is determined whether the tics are caused by the drugs or Tourette's Disorder.

Patients with congenital long QT syndrome or history of cardiac arrhythmias.

Administration with other drugs that prolong the QT interval.

Severe toxic CNS depression or comatose states from any cause.

Hypersensitivity to pimozide. It is not known whether cross-sensitivity exists among antipsychotics. Use pimozide with caution in patients hypersensitive to other antipsychotics.

Warnings:

Persistent tardive dyskinesia may appear on long-term therapy or after drug therapy has been discontinued. The risk appears to be greater in elderly patients on high-dose therapy, especially females. The symptoms are persistent, and in some patients appear irreversible. The risk of developing tardive dyskinesia and the likelihood that it will become irreversible are believed to increase as treatment duration and total cumulative dose increase. However, the syndrome can develop after relatively brief treatment periods at low doses. The syndrome is characterized by rhythmical involuntary movements of tongue, face, mouth or jaw (eg, protrusion of tongue, puffing of cheeks, puckering of mouth, chewing movements), sometimes accompanied by involuntary movements of extremities. Fine vermicular movement of the tongue may be an early sign of the syndrome; if the medication is stopped at this time, the syndrome may not develop. There is no known treatment for established cases of tardive dyskinesia, although the syndrome may remit, partially or completely, if antipsychotics are withdrawn. However, antipsychotic drugs may suppress (or partially suppress) signs and symptoms of the syndrome, possibly masking the underlying process. The effect of symptomatic suppression on the long-term course of the syndrome is unknown.

Given these considerations, administer antipsychotics with caution to minimize occurrence of tardive dyskinesia. Reserve chronic antipsychotic treatment for patients who suffer from a chronic illness that is known to respond to antipsychotic drugs, and for whom alternative, equieffective, but potentially less harmful treatments are **not** available or appropriate. In patients requiring chronic treatment, use the smallest dose and the shortest duration of treatment producing a satisfactory clinical response.

Prolongation of QT interval: Sudden death has occurred in conditions other than Tourette's Disorder in patients receiving dosages of ≈ 1 mg/kg. Sudden, unexpected deaths and grand mal seizure have occurred at doses above 20 mg/day. One possible mechanism is prolongation of the QT interval predisposing patients to ventricular arrhythmias. Perform an ECG before treatment is initiated and periodically thereafter, especially during dose adjustment. If the QT interval is prolonged beyond a limit of 0.47 seconds (children) or 0.52 seconds (adults), or more than 25% above the patient's original baseline, stop further dose increase and consider a lower dose.

Tumorigenicity: Pimozide may be tumorigenic. In mice, pimozide produced a dose-related increase in pituitary and mammary tumors. The significance is not known. Consider this effect, especially in young patients and when chronic use is anticipated.

(Warnings continued on following page)

LITHIUM (Cont.)

Drug Interactions:

Lithium Drug Interactions			
Precipitant Drug	Object Drug*		Description
Acetazolamide	Lithium	↓	Increased renal excretion of lithium
Carbamazepine	Lithium	↑	Increased neurotoxic effects despite therapeutic serum levels and normal dosage range
Fluoxetine	Lithium	↑	Increased lithium serum levels; mechanism unknown
Haloperidol	Lithium	↑	Increased neurotoxic effects despite therapeutic serum levels and normal dosage range
Loop diuretics	Lithium	↑	Increased lithium serum levels; mechanism unknown
Methyldopa	Lithium	↑	Increased neurotoxic effects with or without increased lithium serum levels
NSAIDS	Lithium	↑	Decreased renal clearance of lithium possibly due to inhibition of renal prostaglandin synthesis
Osmotic diuretics (urea)	Lithium	↓	Increased renal excretion of lithium
Theophyllines	Lithium	↓	Increased renal excretion of lithium
Thiazide diuretics	Lithium	↑	Increased lithium serum levels due to decreased renal lithium clearance
Urinary alkalinizers	Lithium	↓	Enhanced renal lithium clearance
Verapamil	Lithium	↔	Both a reduction in lithium levels and lithium toxicity have occurred
Lithium	Iodide salts	↑	Synergistic action to more readily produce hypothyroidism
Lithium	Neuromuscular blocking agents	↑	Neuromuscular blocking effects may be increased; profound and severe respiratory depression may occur
Lithium	Phenothiazines	↔	Neurotoxicity, decreased phenothiazine concentrations or increased lithium concentrations may occur
Lithium	Sympathomimetics	↓	The pressor sensitivity of the sympathomimetic may be decreased.
Lithium	Tricyclic antidepressants	↑	Pharmacologic effects of the tricyclic may be increased

*↑ = Object drug increased ↓ = Object drug decreased ↔ = Undetermined effect

Adverse Reactions:

Adverse reactions are seldom encountered at serum lithium levels < 1.5 mEq/L, except in the occasional patient sensitive to lithium. Mild to moderate toxic reactions may occur at levels from 1.5 to 2.5 mEq/L, and moderate to severe reactions may be seen at levels from 2 to 2.5 mEq/L, depending upon individual response. See Overdosage.

Fine hand tremor, polyuria and mild thirst may occur during initial therapy for the acute manic phase, and may persist throughout treatment. Transient and mild nausea and general discomfort may also appear during the first few days of administration. These side effects are an inconvenience rather than a disabling condition, and usually subside with continued treatment or a temporary reduction or cessation of dosage. If persistent, a cessation of dosage is indicated.

Reactions related to serum levels by organ system (see also Overdosage):

Cardiovascular – Arrhythmia; hypotension; peripheral circulatory collapse; bradycardia; sinus node dysfunction with severe bradycardia (which may result in syncope).

ECG changes – Reversible flattening, isoelectricity or inversion of T-waves.

(Adverse Reactions continued on following page)

LITHIUM (Cont.)

Adverse Reactions (Cont.):

Reactions related to serum levels by organ system (Cont.):

Neuromuscular – Tremor; muscle hyperirritability (fasciculations, twitching, clonic movements); ataxia; choreo-athetotic movements; hyperactive deep tendon reflexes.

CNS – Blackout spells; epileptiform seizures; slurred speech; dizziness; vertigo; incontinence of urine or feces; somnolence; psychomotor retardation; restlessness; confusion; stupor; coma; acute dystonia; downbeat nystagmus; blurred vision; startled response; hypertonicity; slowed intellectual functioning; hallucinations; poor memory; tongue movements; tics; tinnitus; cog wheel rigidity.

Neurological – Pseudotumor cerebri (increased intracranial pressure and papilledema) has been reported. If undetected, this condition may result in enlargement of the blind spot, constriction of visual fields and eventual blindness due to optic atrophy. Discontinue lithium, if clinically possible, if this syndrome occurs.

GI – Anorexia; nausea; vomiting; diarrhea; dry mouth; gastritis; salivary gland swelling; abdominal pain; excessive salivation; flatulence; indigestion.

GU – Albuminuria; oliguria; polyuria; glycosuria; decreased creatinine clearance; symptoms of nephrogenic diabetes.

Dermatologic – Drying and thinning of hair; anesthesia of skin; chronic folliculitis; xerosis cutis; alopecia; exacerbation of psoriasis; acne; angioedema.

Thyroid – Euthyroid goiter or hypothyroidism (including myxedema) accompanied by lower T_3 and T_4. Iodine 131 uptake may be elevated. (See Precautions.) Paradoxically, rare cases of hyperthyroidism have occurred.

EEG changes – Diffuse slowing; widening of frequency spectrum; potentiation; disorganization of background rhythm.

Miscellaneous – Fatigue; lethargy; sleepiness; dehydration; weight loss; transient scotomata; impotence/sexual dysfunction; dysgeusia/taste distortion; tightness in chest; hypercalcemia; hyperparathyroidism; salty taste; thirst; swollen lips; swollen, painful joints; fever; polyarthralgia; dental caries.

Reactions unrelated to dosage:

Transient EEG and ECG changes; leukocytosis; headache; diffuse nontoxic goiter with or without hypothyroidism; transient hyperglycemia; generalized pruritis with or without rash; cutaneous ulcers; albuminuria; worsening of organic brain syndromes; excessive weight gain; edematous swelling of ankles or wrists; thirst or polyuria, sometimes resembling diabetes insipidus; metallic taste.

The development of painful discoloration of fingers and toes and coldness of the extremities within 1 day of the starting of treatment of lithium has occurred. The mechanism through which these symptoms (resembling Raynaud's Syndrome) developed is not known. Recovery followed discontinuance.

Overdosage:

Symptoms:

Lithium toxicity – Toxic lithium levels are close to therapeutic. The likelihood of toxicity increases with increasing serum lithium levels. Serum lithium levels > 1.5 mEq/L carry a greater risk than lower levels. Do not permit levels to exceed 2 mEq/L during the acute treatment phase. Discontinue the drug if early toxic symptoms occur.

Lithium levels < 2 mEq/L: Diarrhea; vomiting; nausea; drowsiness; muscular weakness; lack of coordination. May be early signs of toxicity.

Lithium levels 2 to 3 mEq/L: Giddiness; ataxia; blurred vision; tinnitus; vertigo; increasing confusion; slurred speech; blackouts; fasciculations; myoclonic twitching or movement of entire limbs; choreoathetoid movements; urinary or fecal incontinence; agitation or manic-like behavior; hyperreflexia; hypertonia; dysarthria.

Lithium levels > 3 mEq/L may produce a complex clinical picture involving multiple organs and organ systems including: Seizures (generalized and focal); arrhythmias; hypotension; peripheral vascular collapse; stupor; muscle group twitching; spasticity; coma.

Treatment: Early symptoms of toxicity can usually be treated by dosage reduction or cessation and resumption of the treatment at a lower dose after 24 to 48 hours. In severe cases, first eliminate the ion from the patient. Treatment is essentially the same as that used in barbiturate toxicity: Gastric lavage; correction of fluid and electrolyte imbalance including the use of normal saline; regulation of kidney function. Charcoal is of no value. Urea, mannitol and aminophylline all produce significant increases in lithium excretion. Infection prophylaxis, chest x-rays, preservation of respiration and monitoring of thyroid status are essential. Hemodialysis effectively and rapidly lowers serum lithium levels in the severely toxic patient (generally, levels > 3.5 to 4 mEq/L); however, in some circumstances it may be indicated for patients with lower lithium levels. Refer to General Management of Acute Overdosage.

(Continued on following page)

LITHIUM (Cont.)

Patient Information:

Take immediately after meals or with food or milk to avoid stomach upset.

Stop the medication and contact the physician if signs of overdose or toxicity occur, such as diarrhea, vomiting, unsteady walking, tremor, drowsiness or muscle weakness.

May cause drowsiness. Use caution while driving or performing other tasks requiring alertness.

Drink 8 to 12 glasses of water or other liquid every day while taking this medication. Maintain a regular diet (including salt). Contact physician if fever or diarrhea develops.

Administration and Dosage:

Individualize dosage according to both serum levels and clinical response.

Serum lithium levels: Draw blood samples immediately prior to the next dose (8 to 12 hours after the previous dose) when lithium concentrations are relatively stable. Do not rely on serum levels alone.

Acute mania: Optimal patient response is usually established and maintained with 600 mg 3 times daily or 900 mg twice daily for the slow release form. Such doses normally produce an effective serum lithium level ranging between 1 and 1.5 mEq/L.

Determine serum levels twice weekly during the acute phase, and until the serum level and clinical condition of the patient have been stabilized.

Long-term use: The desirable serum levels are 0.6 to 1.2 mEq/L. Dosage will vary, but 300 mg 3-4 times/day will usually maintain this level. Monitor serum levels in uncomplicated cases on maintenance therapy during remission every 2 to 3 months.

	Product	Form	Description	C.I.*
Rx	**Lithium Carbonate** (Roxane)	**Capsules:** 150 mg lithium carbonate (4.06 mEq lithium)	(54 213). White. In 100s, 1000s and UD 100s.	47
Rx	**Lithium Carbonate** (Various, eg, Dixon-Shane, Geneva, Goldline, Major, Moore, Roxane, Rugby, Schein, URL)	**Capsules:** 300 mg lithium carbonate (8.12 mEq lithium)	In 100s, 1000s and UD 100s.	21+
Rx	**Eskalith** (SKF)		(Eskalith SKF). Yellow and gray. In 100s and 500s.	50
Rx	**Lithonate** (Solvay Pharm.)		(RR 7512). Peach. In 100s, 1000s, UD 100s.	32
Rx	**Lithium Carbonate** (Roxane)	**Capsules:** 600 mg lithium carbonate (16.24 mEq lithium)	(54 702). White and flesh. In 100s, 1000s and UD 100s.	20
Rx	**Lithium Carbonate** (Various, eg, Harber, International Labs, R.I.D. Inc., Roxane)	**Tablets:** 300 mg lithium carbonate (8.12 mEq lithium)	In 100s, 1000s and UD 100s.	19+
Rx	**Eskalith** (SK-Beecham)		(SKF J09). Gray, scored. In 100s.	50
Rx	**Lithane** (Miles Pharm.)		Tartrazine. (Miles 951). Green, scored. In 100s.	56
Rx	**Lithotabs** (Solvay Pharm.)		(RR 7516). White, scored. Film coated. In 100s, 1000s & UD 100s.	32
Rx	**Lithobid** (Ciba)	**Tablets, slow release:** 300 mg lithium carbonate (8.12 mEq lithium)	(Ciba 65). Peach. Film coated. In 100s, 1000s and UD 100s.	65
Rx	**Eskalith CR** (SK-Beecham)	**Tablets, controlled release:** 450 mg lithium carbonate (12.18 mEq lithium)	(SKF J10). Buff, scored. In 100s.	71
Rx	**Lithium Citrate** (Various, eg, Geneva, Major, PBI, Raway, Roxane, Schein, Xactdose)	**Syrup:** 8 mEq lithium (as citrate equivalent to 300 mg lithium carbonate) per 5 ml	In 480 and 500 ml and UD 5 and 10 ml.	43+
Rx *sf*	**Cibalith-S** (Ciba)		0.3% alcohol, saccharin, sorbitol. Raspberry flavor. In 480 ml.	99

* Cost Index based on cost per 300 mg lithium carbonate. *sf* – Sugar free.

METHYLPHENIDATE HCl

Actions:

A mild cortical stimulant with CNS actions similar to the amphetamines. The exact mechanism of action is not fully understood.

Pharmacokinetics: Rapidly and well absorbed from the GI tract, methylphenidate achieves peak blood levels in 1 to 3 hours. Plasma half-life ranges from 1 to 3 hours, but pharmacologic effects persist up to 4 to 6 hours. About 80% of a dose is metabolized to ritalinic acid and excreted in urine. Sustained release tablets are more slowly but as extensively absorbed as regular tablets. Relative bioavailability compared to the regular tablet was 105% in children and 101% in adults. The time to peak rate in children was 4.7 hours. In children, an average of 67% of a dose was excreted vs 86% in adults.

Indications:

Attention deficit disorders: As part of a total treatment program in children with a behavioral syndrome characterized by moderate to severe distractibility, short attention span, hyperactivity, emotional lability and impulsivity.

Stimulants are not for the child who exhibits symptoms secondary to environmental factors or primary psychiatric disorders, including psychosis. When symptoms are associated with acute stress reactions, methylphenidate is usually not indicated.

Narcolepsy.

Unlabeled Uses: Some success has been reported in the treatment of depression in elderly, cancer and post-stroke patients.

Contraindications:

Marked anxiety, tension and agitation, since the drug may aggravate these symptoms; hypersensitivity to methylphenidate; glaucoma.

Patients with motor tics or with a family history or diagnosis of Tourette's syndrome.

Warnings:

Do not use for severe depression of either exogenous or endogenous origin. Do not use for the prevention or treatment of normal fatigue states.

Seizure disorders: Methylphenidate may lower the seizure threshold in patients with history of seizures, with prior EEG abnormalities in absence of seizures and, very rarely, in the absence of history of seizures and no prior EEG evidence of seizures. Safe concomitant use with anticonvulsants has not been established. If seizures occur, discontinue the drug.

Hypertension: Use cautiously; monitor blood pressure in all patients, especially those with hypertension.

Drug dependence: Give cautiously to emotionally unstable patients, such as those with a history of drug dependence or alcoholism, because such patients may increase dosage on their own initiative.

Chronic abuse can lead to marked tolerance, psychic dependence and abnormal behavior. Frank psychotic episodes can occur, especially with parenteral abuse. Carefully supervise drug withdrawal, since severe depression as well as the effects of chronic overactivity can be unmasked. Long-term follow-up may be required.

Visual disturbances have been encountered rarely. Difficulties with accommodation and blurring of vision have been reported.

Pregnancy: Use in women of childbearing age only when clearly needed and when potential benefits outweigh potential hazards to the fetus. In the small numbers of patients reported who received methylphenidate during their pregnancy, no evidence of increased malformation rate was found.

Lactation: Because the amount of methylphenidate excretion into breast milk is not known, safety for use in the nursing mother has not been established.

Children: Do not use in children under 6 years, since safety and efficacy have not been established. In psychotic children, the drug may exacerbate symptoms of behavior disturbance and thought disorder. Precipitation of Tourette's syndrome has been reported following the initiation of methylphenidate therapy.

Safety and efficacy of long-term use in children are not established. Although a causal relationship has not been established, suppression of growth (ie, weight gain or height) has been reported with long-term use of stimulants in children. Carefully monitor patients on long-term therapy.

(Continued on following page)

METHYLPHENIDATE HCl (Cont.)

Precautions:

Patients with an element of agitation may react adversely; discontinue therapy if necessary.

Perform periodic CBC, differential and platelet counts during prolonged therapy.

Drug treatment is not indicated in all cases of this behavioral syndrome; consider only in light of the complete history and evaluation of the child. The decision to prescribe methylphenidate should depend on the physician's assessment of the chronicity and severity of the child's symptoms and their appropriateness for his or her age. Prescription should not depend solely on the presence of one or more of the behavioral characteristics.

When symptoms are associated with acute stress reactions, treatment with methylphenidate is usually not indicated.

Drug Interactions:

Guanethidine: Antihypertensive effect of guanethidine may be decreased by concurrent methylphenidate. This interaction may be dose-dependent. Avoid this combination when possible.

Monoamine oxidase (MAO) inhibitors: Pharmacologic effects of methylphenidate may be increased by concurrent use of these agents. Headache, GI symptoms and hypertension may occur. The effects may occur up to several weeks after discontinuation of the MAO inhibitors. If hypertension occurs, administer phentolamine.

Adverse Reactions:

Most common: Nervousness and insomnia, usually controlled by reducing dosage and omitting the drug in the afternoon or evening.

Hypersensitivity: Skin rash; urticaria; fever; arthralgia; exfoliative dermatitis; erythema multiforme with necrotizing vasculitis; thrombocytopenic purpura.

CNS: Dizziness; headache; dyskinesia; drowsiness; Tourette's syndrome (rare); toxic psychosis.

Cardiovascular: Blood pressure and pulse changes, increased and decreased; tachycardia; angina; cardiac arrhythmias; palpitations.

GI: Anorexia; nausea; abdominal pain; weight loss during prolonged therapy.

Other (causal relationship not established): Leukopenia; anemia; scalp hair loss.

Children: Loss of appetite, abdominal pain, weight loss during prolonged therapy, insomnia and tachycardia may occur more frequently; however, any of the other adverse reactions listed above may also occur.

Patient Information:

Take last daily dose early in the evening (prior to 6 pm) to avoid insomnia. Although it is often recommended that methylphenidate be taken 30 to 45 minutes before meals, there is evidence that suggests meals do not significantly affect the pharmacokinetics or therapeutic effects of methylphenidate and it may therefore be taken without regard to meals.

May mask symptoms of fatigue, impair physical coordination or produce dizziness or drowsiness. Use caution while driving or performing other tasks requiring alertness.

Notify physician of nervousness, insomnia, palpitations, vomiting, fever or skin rash.

Do not crush or chew timed release medication.

Overdosage:

Symptoms result principally from CNS overstimulation and excessive sympathomimetic effects and include: Vomiting; agitation; tremors; hyperreflexia; muscle twitching; convulsions (may be followed by coma); euphoria; confusion; hallucinations; delirium; sweating; flushing; headache; hyperpyrexia; tachycardia; palpitations; cardiac arrhythmias; hypertension; mydriasis; dry mucous membranes.

Treatment consists of supportive measures. Protect the patient against self-injury and against external stimuli that would aggravate overstimulation. If signs and symptoms are not too severe and the patient is conscious, evacuate gastric contents by emesis or gastric lavage. In severe intoxication, use a carefully titrated dosage of a short-acting barbiturate before gastric lavage. Maintain adequate circulation and respiratory exchange; external cooling procedures may be required for hyperpyrexia. Efficacy of peritoneal dialysis or extracorporeal hemodialysis has not been established.

(Continued on following page)

METHYLPHENIDATE HCl (Cont.)

Administration and Dosage:

Adults: Individualize dosage. Administer in divided doses 2 or 3 times daily, preferably 30 to 45 minutes before meals. Average dose is 20 to 30 mg/day. Dosage ranges from 10 to 15 mg/day up to 40 to 60 mg/day. In patients who are unable to sleep if medication is taken late in the day, take the last dose before 6 pm.

All patients – Timed release tablets have a duration of approximately 8 hours and may be used in place of regular tablets when the 8 hour dosage of the timed release tablets corresponds to the titrated 8 hour dosage of the regular tablets. Timed release tablets must be swallowed whole, never crushed or chewed.

Children (6 years and over): Start with small doses (eg, 5 mg before breakfast and lunch) with gradual increments of 5 to 10 mg weekly. Daily dosage above 60 mg is not recommended. If improvement is not observed after dosage adjustment over 1 month, discontinue use. If paradoxical aggravation of symptoms or other adverse effects occurs, reduce dosage or discontinue the drug.

Discontinue periodically to assess condition. Improvement may be sustained when the drug is either temporarily or permanently discontinued. Drug treatment should not be indefinite and usually may be discontinued after puberty.

	Product	Form/Strength	Description	C.I*
c-II	**Methylphenidate HCl** (Various, eg, Bioline, Goldline, Major, Parmed, Purepac, Qualitest, Regal, Rugby, Schein, Towne Paulsen)	**Tablets:** 5 mg	In 100s and 1000s.	3+
		10 mg	In 100s and 1000s.	2+
		20 mg	In 100s and 1000s.	1+
c-II	**Ritalin** (Ciba)	**Tablets:** 5 mg	(#Ciba 7). Yellow. In 100s, 500s and 1000s.	11
		10 mg	(#Ciba 3). Green, scored. In 100s, 500s and 1000s.	8
		20 mg	(#Ciba 34). Yellow, scored. In 100s and 1000s.	6
c-II	**Ritalin-SR** (Ciba)	**Tablets, sustained release:** 20 mg	Dye free. (#Ciba 16). White. In 100s.	9

* Cost Index based on cost per 5 mg.

Product identification code.

PEMOLINE

Actions:

Pharmacology: Pemoline is a CNS stimulant. Although structurally dissimilar from the amphetamines and methylphenidate, it has pharmacologic activity similar to that of other stimulants but with minimal sympathomimetic effects. Although the exact mechanism of action is unknown, pemoline may act through dopaminergic mechanisms.

Pharmacokinetics: Pemoline is rapidly absorbed from the GI tract. Approximately 50% is protein bound. Peak serum levels occur within 2 to 4 hours after ingestion of a single dose. The serum half-life is approximately 12 hours; however, in two studies of 35 children 5 to 12 years of age, the mean half-life ranged from 7 to 8.6 hours. Steady state is reached in approximately 2 to 3 days. Pemoline is metabolized by the liver and is primarily excreted by the kidneys. Approximately 50% is excreted unchanged and only minor fractions are present as metabolites. The drug is widely distributed throughout body tissues, including the brain.

Pemoline has a gradual onset of action. Using the recommended schedule of dosage titration, significant clinical benefit may not be evident until the third or fourth week of drug administration.

Indications:

Attention deficit disorder: As part of a total treatment program in children with a behavioral syndrome characterized by moderate to severe distractibility, short attention span, hyperactivity, emotional lability and impulsivity.

Unlabeled Uses: Pemoline 50 to 200 mg/day in two divided doses has been used in the treatment of narcolepsy and excessive daytime sleepiness.

Contraindications:

Known hypersensitivity or idiosyncrasy to pemoline; hepatic insufficiency.

Warnings:

Renal insufficiency: Administer with caution to patients with significantly impaired renal function.

Pregnancy: Category B. There are no adequate and well controlled studies in pregnant women. Use pemoline during pregnancy only if clearly needed. Studies in rats have shown an increased incidence of stillbirths and cannibalization when pemoline was administered at a dose of 37.5 mg/kg/day. Postnatal survival was reduced at doses of 18.75 and 37.5 mg/kg/day.

Lactation: It is not known whether pemoline is excreted in breast milk. Exercise caution when administering pemoline to a nursing woman.

Children: Safety and efficacy in children under 6 years of age have not been established.

In psychotic children, administration may exacerbate symptoms of behavior disturbance and thought disorder. CNS stimulants, including pemoline, can precipitate motor and phonic tics and Tourette's syndrome. Therefore, clinical evaluation for tics and Tourette's syndrome in children and their families should precede use of stimulants.

Chronic administration may be associated with growth inhibition; therefore, monitor growth during treatment. Long-term effects in children have not been well established.

Treatment is not indicated in all cases of attention deficit disorder with hyperactivity; consider therapy only in light of complete history and evaluation of the child. The decision to prescribe pemoline should depend on the physician's assessment of the chronicity and severity of the child's symptoms and their appropriateness for his or her age. Prescription should not depend solely on the presence of one or more of the behavioral characteristics.

Precautions:

Hepatic effects: Perform liver function tests prior to and periodically during therapy. Discontinue use if abnormalities are revealed and confirmed by follow-up tests (see Adverse Reactions).

Drug dependence: The pharmacologic similarity of pemoline to other psychostimulants with known dependence liability suggests that psychological or physical dependence might occur. There have been isolated reports of transient psychotic symptoms occurring in adults following the long-term misuse of excessive oral doses. Give with caution to emotionally unstable patients who may increase the dosage on their own initiative.

(Continued on following page)

PEMOLINE

Adverse Reactions:

Mild adverse reactions appearing early in treatment often remit with continuing therapy.

If adverse reactions are significant or protracted, reduce dosage or discontinue drug.

Most frequent: Insomnia usually occurs early in therapy prior to optimum therapeutic response; it is often transient or responds to dosage reduction.

CNS: Dyskinetic movements of tongue, lips, face and extremities; Tourette's syndrome; abnormal oculomotor function (eg, nystagmus and oculogyric crisis); convulsive seizures; increased irritability; mild depression; dizziness; headache; drowsiness; hallucinations.

GI: Anorexia with weight loss may occur during the first weeks of therapy. In the majority of cases it is transient; weight gain usually resumes within 3 to 6 months. Stomachache; nausea.

GU: A case of elevated acid phosphatase in association with prostatic enlargement occurred in a 63-year-old male who received pemoline for sleepiness. The acid phosphatase normalized with discontinuation of pemoline and was again elevated with rechallenge.

Hepatic: Hepatic dysfunction including elevated liver enzymes, hepatitis and jaundice has occurred. Elevated liver enzymes are not rare and appear reversible upon drug discontinuance. Most patients with elevated liver enzymes were asymptomatic. Although no causal relationship has been established, two hepatic-related fatalities occurred in patients taking pemoline.

Other: Skin rashes; growth suppression with long-term use of stimulants in children; aplastic anemia (rare).

Overdosage:

Symptoms of acute overdosage result principally from CNS overstimulation and excessive sympathomimetic effects and include: Vomiting; agitation; tremors; hyperreflexia; muscle twitching; convulsions (may be followed by coma); euphoria; confusion; hallucinations; delirium; sweating; flushing; headache; hyperpyrexia; tachycardia; hypertension; mydriasis.

Other – Overactivity, irregular respiration, increased salivation, intermittent tongue protrusion, generalized hyperreflexia and severe choreoathetosis with rhabdomyolysis have occurred.

Treatment consists of appropriate supportive measures. Protect the patient against self-injury and external stimuli that would aggravate overstimulation already present. If symptoms are not too severe and the patient is conscious, gastric contents may be evacuated. Chlorpromazine is reported useful in decreasing CNS stimulation and sympathomimetic effects.

Efficacy of peritoneal dialysis or extracorporeal hemodialysis for pemoline overdosage is not established.

Patient Information:

Take daily dose in the morning.

If dizziness occurs, use caution when performing tasks requiring alertness.

Notify physician if insomnia occurs and continues.

Administration and Dosage:

Administer as a single dose each morning. Recommended starting dose is 37.5 mg/day. Gradually increase at 1 week intervals using increments of 18.75 mg until desired response is obtained. Mean effective doses range from 56.25 to 75 mg/day. Maximum recommended dose is 112.5 mg/day.

Clinical improvement is gradual; significant benefit may not be evident until week 3 or 4 of administration.

Interrupt drug administration occasionally to determine if there is a recurrence of behavioral symptoms sufficient to require continued therapy.

				C.I.*
c-iv	**Cylert** (Abbott)	**Tablets:** 18.75 mg	(#TH). White, scored. In 100s.	30
		37.5 mg	(#TI). Orange, scored. In 100s.	24
		75 mg	(#TJ). Tan, scored. In 100s.	21
		Chewable Tablets: 37.5 mg	(#TK). Orange, scored. In 100s.	26

AMPHETAMINES

Amphetamine, dextroamphetamine and methamphetamine are also indicated for attention deficit disorders in children, as part of a total treatment program.

For complete prescribing information on the amphetamines for this and other uses, consult the general amphetamine monograph.

* Cost Index based on cost per 37.5 mg.

Product identification code.

Psychotherapeutic Combinations

MEPROBAMATE AND BENACTYZINE HCl

Actions:

In the following combination:

MEPROBAMATE is used for its antianxiety effect. (For complete prescribing information refer to the general Antianxiety Agent monograph.)

BENACTYZINE HCl is a mild antidepressant and anticholinergic agent which in animals reduces the autonomic response to emotion-provoking stress.

Indications:

"Possibly effective" in the management of depression, both acute (reactive) and chronic. Useful in the less severe depressions and where the depression is accompanied by anxiety, insomnia, agitation or rumination. Also useful for managing depression and associated anxiety accompanying or related to organic illnesses. Final classification of this indication requires further investigation.

Contraindications:

Acute intermittent porphyria; glaucoma; allergic or idiosyncratic reactions to meprobamate, benactyzine or related compounds.

Precautions:

Tartrazine sensitivity: This product contains tartrazine, which may cause an allergic-type reaction (including bronchial asthma) in susceptible individuals. Although the incidence of sensitivity is low, it is frequently seen in patients who also have aspirin hypersensitivity.

Adverse Reactions:

Nausea, dry mouth and other GI symptoms; syncope; severe nervousness and loss of power of concentration (one case each).

The following side effects, which have occurred after administration of the components alone, have either occurred or might occur when the combination is taken.

Benactyzine hydrochloride (particularly in high dosage): Dizziness; thought-blocking; depersonalization; aggravation of anxiety; disturbance of sleep patterns; a subjective feeling of muscle relaxation; blurred vision; dry mouth; failure of visual accommodation; gastric distress; allergic response; ataxia; euphoria.

Meprobamate: CNS – Drowsiness; ataxia; dizziness; slurred speech; headache, vertigo; weakness; paresthesias; impairment of visual accommodation; euphoria; overstimulation; paradoxical excitement; fast EEG activity.

GI – Nausea; vomiting; diarrhea.

Cardiovascular – Palpitations; tachycardia; arrhythmias; transient ECG changes; syncope; hypotensive crises (including one fatal case).

Allergic or idiosyncratic – Reactions are usually seen within the period of the first to fourth dose in patients having had no previous contact with the drug. Milder reactions are characterized by an itchy, urticarial, or erythematous maculopapular rash which may be generalized or confined to the groin. Other reactions have included: Leukopenia; acute nonthrombocytopenic purpura; petechiae; ecchymoses; eosinophilia; peripheral edema; adenopathy; fever; fixed drug eruption with cross reaction to carisoprodol.

More severe hypersensitivity reactions, rarely reported, include: Hyperpyrexia; chills; angioneurotic edema; bronchospasm; oliguria; anuria; anaphylaxis; erythema multiforme; exfoliative dermatitis; stomatitis; proctitis; Stevens-Johnson syndrome; bullous dermatitis, including one fatal case following administration of meprobamate in combination with prednisolone.

Treatment – In case of allergic or idiosyncratic reactions to meprobamate, discontinue the drug and initiate appropriate symptomatic therapy, which may include epinephrine, antihistamines, and in severe cases corticosteroids. In evaluating possible allergic reactions, also consider allergy to excipients.

Hematologic – Agranulocytosis and aplastic anemia (rarely fatal, no causal relationship established); thrombocytopenic purpura (rare).

Other – Exacerbation of porphyric symptoms.

Administration and Dosage:

Adults: One tablet 3 or 4 times daily. May gradually increase to a maximum of 6 tablets daily. Gradually reduce dosage to maintenance level when relief is achieved. Doses above 6 tablets daily are not recommended, although higher doses have been used to control depression and in chronic psychotic patients.

Children: Not intended for use in children.

				C.I.*
c-IV	**Deprol** (Wallace)	**Tablets:** 400 mg meprobamate and 1 mg benactyzine HCl	Tartrazine. Light pink, scored. In 100s and 500s.	32

* Cost Index based on cost per 200 mg. # Product identification code.

Psychotherapeutic Combinations

CHLORDIAZEPOXIDE AND AMITRIPTYLINE

Consider the prescribing information for chlordiazepoxide in the Antianxiety Agents monograph and amitriptyline in the Antidepressants monograph.

Indications:

Treatment of moderate to severe depression associated with moderate to severe anxiety. The therapeutic response to this combination has occurred earlier and with fewer treatment failures than when either ingredient is used alone. Symptoms likely to respond in the first week of treatment include: Insomnia; feelings of guilt or worthlessness; agitation; psychic and somatic anxiety; suicidal ideation; anorexia.

Contraindications:

Hypersensitivity to either benzodiazepines or tricyclic antidepressants; concomitant monoamine oxidase inhibitors (MAOIs; see Drug Interactions); during the acute recovery phase following myocardial infarction.

Drug Interactions:

MAOIs: Hyperpyretic crises, severe convulsions and deaths have occurred in patients receiving a tricyclic antidepressant and an MAOI simultaneously. When it is desired to replace an MAOI with this combination, allow a minimum of 14 days to elapse after the former is discontinued. Cautiously initiate this combination with a gradual increase in dosage until optimum response is achieved.

Patient Information:

May cause drowsiness or dizziness; use caution while driving or performing other tasks requiring alertness.

Avoid alcohol and other CNS depressants.

Consult a physician before either increasing the dose or abruptly discontinuing the drug.

Administration and Dosage:

Initially, administer 10 mg chlordiazepoxide with 25 mg amitriptyline 3 or 4 times daily in divided doses; increase to 6 times daily, as required. Some patients respond to smaller doses and can be maintained on 2 tablets daily.

After a satisfactory response is obtained, reduce dosage to smallest amount needed. The larger portion of the total daily dose may be taken at bedtime. In some patients, a single dose at bedtime may be sufficient. In general, lower dosages are recommended for elderly patients.

	Product	Form	Packaging	C.I.*
c-iv	**Chlordiazepoxide and Amitriptyline** (Various, eg, Bioline, Geneva, Goldline, Lederle, Lemmon, Major, Moore, Par, Rugby, Schein)	**Tablets:** 5 mg chlordiazepoxide and 12.5 mg amitriptyline	In 100s and 500s.	9+
c-iv	**Chlordiazepoxide and Amitriptyline** (Various, eg, Bioline, Geneva, Goldline, Lederle, Lemmon, Major, Moore, Par, Rugby, Schein)	**Tablets:** 10 mg chlordiazepoxide and 25 mg amitriptyline	In 100s and 500s.	6+
c-iv	**Limbitrol DS 10-25** (Roche)		(#Limbitrol DS). White. Film coated. In 100s, 500s, unit-of-use 50s and UD 100s.	14

* Cost Index based on cost per 5 mg.
# Product identification code.

Psychotherapeutic Combinations (Cont.)

PERPHENAZINE AND AMITRIPTYLINE HCl

Consider the prescribing information for perphenazine in the Antipsychotic Agents monograph and amitriptyline in the Antidepressants monograph.

Indications:

Treatment of moderate to severe anxiety or agitation and depressed mood; patients with depression in whom anxiety or agitation are moderate or severe; patients with anxiety and depression associated with chronic physical disease; patients in whom depression and anxiety cannot be clearly differentiated; schizophrenic patients who have associated symptoms of depression.

Many patients presenting symptoms such as agitation, anxiety, insomnia, psychomotor retardation, functional somatic complaints, tiredness, loss of interest and anorexia have responded well to this combination.

Patient Information:

May cause drowsiness or dizziness, and response to alcohol and other CNS depressants may be enhanced. Use caution while driving or performing other tasks requiring alertness.

Administration and Dosage:

Initially, 2 to 4 mg perphenazine with 10 to 50 mg amitriptyline, 3 or 4 times daily. After a satisfactory response is noted, reduce to smallest amount necessary to obtain relief. Not recommended for use in children.

	Product & Distributor	Perphenazine (mg)	Amitriptyline (mg)	How Supplied	C.I.*
Rx	**Perphenazine/Amitriptyline Tablets** (Various, eg, Bolar, Geneva, Goldline, Lemmon, Par, Rugby, Schein, Zenith)	2	10	In 21s, 100s, 500s and 1000s.	4+
Rx	**Etrafon 2-10 Tablets** (Schering)			(#Schering ANA or 287). Yellow. In 100s, 500s and UD 100s.	21
Rx	**Triavil 2-10 Tablets** (MSD)			(#MSD 914). Blue. Film coated. In 100s, 500s and UD 100s.	22
Rx	**Perphenazine/Amitriptyline Tablets** (Various, eg, Bolar, Geneva, Goldline, Lemmon, Par, Rugby, Schein, Zenith)	2	25	In 100s, 500s and 1000s.	5+
Rx	**Etrafon Tablets** (Schering)			(#Schering ANC or 598). Pink. Sugar coated. In 100s, 500s and UD 100s.	27
Rx	**Triavil 2-25 Tablets** (MSD)			(#MSD 921). Orange. Film coated. In 100s, 500s and UD 100s.	28
Rx	**Perphenazine/Amitriptyline Tablets** (Various, eg, Bolar, Geneva, Goldline, Lemmon, Par, Rugby, Schein, Zenith)	4	10	In 100s, 250s, 500s and 1000s.	2+
Rx	**Etrafon-A Tablets** (Schering)			(#Schering ANB or 119). Orange. In 100s, 500s and UD 100s.	12
Rx	**Triavil 4-10 Tablets** (MSD)			(#MSD 934). Salmon. Film coated. In 100s, 500s and UD 100s.	12
Rx	**Perphenazine/Amitriptyline Tablets** (Various, eg, Bolar, Geneva, Goldline, Lemmon, Par, Rugby, Schein, Zenith)	4	25	In 100s, 500s, 800s and 1000s.	3+
Rx	**Etrafon-Forte Tablets** (Schering)			(#Schering ANE or 720). Red. Sugar coated. In 100s, 500s and UD 100s.	14
Rx	**Triavil 4-25 Tablets** (MSD)			(#MSD 946). Yellow. Film coated. In 100s, 500s and UD 100s.	15
Rx	**Perphenazine/Amitriptyline Tablets** (Various, eg, Bolar, Geneva, Goldline, Lemmon, Par, Rugby, Schein, Zenith)	4	50	In 100s and 250s.	5+
Rx	**Triavil 4-50 Tablets** (MSD)			(#MSD 517). Orange. Film coated. In 60s, 100s and UD 100s.	25

* Cost Index based on cost per 2 mg perphenazine. # Product identification code.

ERGOLOID MESYLATES (Dihydrogenated Ergot Alkaloids, Dihydroergotoxine)

Actions:

Ergoloid mesylates contain equal proportions of dihydroergocornine mesylate, dihydroergocristine mesylate and dihydroergocryptine mesylate.

Pharmacology: The mechanism by which ergoloid mesylates produce mental effects is unknown. There is no conclusive evidence they directly affect cerebral arteriosclerosis or cerebrovascular insufficiency. Formerly, it was believed this drug caused cerebral vasodilation by alpha-adrenergic blockade; recent evidence suggests it may act primarily to increase brain metabolism, possibly increasing cerebral blood flow. It does not possess the vasoconstrictor properties of the natural ergot alkaloids.

Pharmacokinetics: Ergoloid mesylates are rapidly absorbed from the GI tract; peak plasma concentrations are achieved within 0.6 to 3 hours. The drug undergoes rapid first-pass biotransformation in the liver. Systemic bioavailability is approximately 6% to 25%. The liquid capsule has a 12% greater bioavailability than the oral tablet. The mean half-life of unchanged ergoloid in plasma is about 2.6 to 5.1 hours.

Clinical Pharmacology: In efficacy studies, modest but statistically significant changes were observed at the end of 12 weeks in the following parameters: Mental alertness, confusion, recent memory, orientation, emotional lability, self-care, depression, anxiety/fears, cooperation, sociability, appetite, dizziness, fatigue, bothersomeness and an overall impression of clinical status.

Indications:

Age-related mental capacity decline: Individuals over 60 years of age who manifest signs and symptoms of an idiopathic decline in mental capacity (ie, cognitive and interpersonal skills, mood, self-care, apparent motivation). Patients who respond suffer from some process related to aging or have some underlying dementing condition (ie, primary progressive dementia; Alzheimer's dementia; senile onset; multi-infarct dementia).

Contraindications:

Hypersensitivity to ergoloid mesylates.

Acute or chronic psychosis, regardless of etiology.

Precautions:

Before prescribing ergoloid mesylates, exclude the possibility that the patient's signs and symptoms arise from a potentially reversible and treatable condition. Exclude delirium and dementiform illness secondary to systemic disease, primary neurological disease or primary disturbance of mood.

Periodically reassess the diagnosis and the benefit of current therapy to the patient.

Do not chew or crush sublingual tablets.

Adverse Reactions:

Sublingual irritation; transient nausea; GI disturbances.

Patient Information:

May cause transient nausea and GI disturbances.

Allow sublingual tablets to completely dissolve under tongue.

Administration and Dosage:

The usual starting dose is 1 mg 3 times daily. Alleviation of symptoms is usually gradual; results may not be observed for 3 to 4 weeks. Doses up to 4.5 to 12 mg/day have been used. Up to 6 months of treatment may be necessary to determine efficacy, using doses of at least 6 mg/day.

(Products listed on following page)

ERGOLOID MESYLATES (Dihydrogenated Ergot Alkaloids; Dihydroergotoxine) (Cont.)

	Product	Form	Description	C.I.*
Rx	**Ergoloid Mesylates** (Various, eg, Bioline, Bolar, Dixon-Shane, Geneva, Goldline, Lederle, Major, Moore, Parmed, Qualitest)	**Tablets, sublingual:** 0.5 mg	In 100s, 500s, 1000s and UD 100s.	3+
Rx	**Gerimal** (Rugby)		(Rugby 3859). White. In 100s, 500s and 1000s.	6
Rx	**Hydergine** (Sandoz)		(S Hydergine 0.5). White. In 100s and 1000s.	28
Rx	**Ergoloid Mesylates** (Various, eg, Cenci, Martec, R.I.D.)	**Tablets, oral:** 0.5 mg	In 100s and 1000s.	3+
Rx	**Ergoloid Mesylates** (Various, eg, Bioline, Bolar, Dixon-Shane, Geneva, Goldline, Major, Moore, Parmed, Qualitest, Zenith)	**Tablets, sublingual:** 1 mg	In 100s, 500s, 1000s and UD 100s.	2+
Rx	**Gerimal** (Rugby)		(Rugby 3857). White. In 100s, 500s and 1000s.	5
Rx	**Hydergine** (Sandoz)		(Hydergine 78-77). White. In 100s and 1000s.	27
Rx	**Niloric** (Ascher)		(415). White. In 100s.	11
Rx	**Ergoloid Mesylates** (Various, eg, Bioline, Bolar, Dixon-Shane, Geneva, Goldline, Lederle, Major, Moore, Parmed, Qualitest)	**Tablets, oral:** 1 mg	In 60s, 100s, 500s, 1000s and UD 32s, 100s and 1000s.	4+
Rx	**Gerimal** (Rugby)		(Rugby 3856). White. In 100s, 500s and 1000s.	6
Rx	**Hydergine** (Sandoz)		(S Hydergine 1). White. In 100s, 500s and UD 100s and 500s.	15
Rx	**Hydergine LC** (Sandoz)	**Capsules, liquid:** 1 mg	(S Hydergine LC 1 mg). Off-white. In 100s, 500s and UD 100s and 500s.	18
Rx	**Hydergine** (Sandoz)	**Liquid:** 1 mg per ml	30% alcohol. In 100 ml with dropper.	18

* Cost Index based on cost per mg.

The following is a general discussion of nonbarbiturate sedative/hypnotics.

To facilitate comparison, the products are divided into two groups: The miscellaneous nonbarbiturates and the benzodiazepines. Although sedative doses can be given, these agents are primarily intended to be hypnotics (agents that produce drowsiness and facilitate sleep). Agents intended primarily for sedation or tranquilization are discussed in other parts of this chapter.

In the table below, some pharmacokinetic properties of the nonbarbiturate sedative/hypnotics are compared. Do not use this table to predict exact duration of effect, but use as a guide in drug selection.

Nonbarbiturate Sedative/Hypnotics Pharmacokinetic Parameters

Drug	Adult Oral Dose		Onset (min)	Duration of Action (hrs)	Half-Life (hrs)	Protein Binding (%)	Urinary Excretion % unchanged
	Hypnotic	Sedative					
Miscellaneous Nonbarbiturates							
Acetylcarbromal		250-500 mg bid or tid					
Chloral Hydrate	0.5-1 g	250 mg tid pc	30		7-10[1]	35-41	
Ethchlorvynol	500 mg	100-200 mg bid or tid	15-60	5	10-20[2]		40[3]
Ethinamate	0.5-1 g		20	4	2.5		small
Glutethimide	250-500 mg		30	4-8	10-12	50	<2
Methyprylon	200-400 mg	50-100 mg up to qid	45	5-8	3-6	60	<1
Paraldehyde	10-30 ml	5-10 ml	10-15	8-12	3.4-9.8		small
Propiomazine		10-20 mg					
Benzodiazepines							
Flurazepam	15-30 mg	na	17	7-8	50-100[4]	97	<1[4]
Quazepam	15 mg	na			25-41	>95	trace
Temazepam	15-30 mg	na			10-17	98	1.5
Triazolam	0.125-0.5 mg	na			1.5-5.5	90	2

na – Not applicable.

[1] Trichloroethanol, the principal metabolite.

[2] In acute use, half-life of the distribution phase (1 to 3 hours) is more appropriate.

[3] Free and conjugated forms of the major metabolite, secondary alcohol of ethchlorvynol.

[4] Active metabolite, desalkyflurazepam.

PARALDEHYDE

Actions:

Pharmacology: Paraldehyde, a polymer of acetaldehyde, is a colorless, bitter tasting liquid with a strong, unpleasant odor; it produces nonspecific, reversible depression of the CNS. With usual therapeutic doses, paraldehyde has little effect on respiration and blood pressure; large doses may cause respiratory depression and hypotension. It has generally been replaced by safer and more effective agents.

Pharmacokinetics: Absorption/Distribution – The drug is rapidly absorbed after oral administration. Peak serum concentrations are attained 30 to 60 minutes following oral use. Paraldehyde acts rapidly, producing sleep within 10 to 15 minutes after a therapeutic dose; sleep lasts about 8 to 12 hours.

Metabolism/Excretion – Plasma half-life ranges from 3.4 to 9.8 hours. Approximately 70% to 80% of the drug is metabolized in the liver, 11% to 28% is exhaled unchanged via the lungs and a negligible amount is excreted in the urine. In hepatic disease, elimination rate is decreased and more drug is excreted through the lungs.

Indications:

Sedative and hypnotic. Also used to quiet the patient and to produce sleep in delirium tremens and in other psychiatric states characterized by excitement.

Contraindications:

Bronchopulmonary disease (excretion of the drug by the lungs).

Hepatic insufficiency (metabolized by the liver).

Gastroenteritis; especially if ulceration is present.

Warnings:

Hepatic function impairment: Patients with liver dysfunction may be more susceptible to effects of paraldehyde.

Mucous membrane irritation: Paraldehyde is irritating to mucous membranes and must be well diluted. Esophagitis, hemorrhagic gastritis and proctitis have occurred.

Pregnancy: Category C. Paraldehyde crosses the placenta and appears in the fetal circulation. It is not known whether the drug can cause fetal harm. Use during pregnancy only if potential benefits outweigh potential hazards to the fetus.

Labor: Use during labor may cause respiratory depression in the neonate.

Lactation: Problems in the nursing infant have not been documented; however, consider the risk-benefit.

Children: Safety and efficacy for use in children have not been established.

Precautions:

Strong, unpleasant breath: Although medically insignificant, paraldehyde has a strong odor that is imparted to the exhaled air for as long as 24 hours after ingestion. The patient is often unaware of the odor.

May be habit forming; avoid sudden withdrawal after chronic use.

Drug Interactions:

CNS depressants (eg, **barbiturates, narcotics**) will have additive effects when given with paraldehyde.

Disulfiram inhibits acetaldehyde dehydrogenase. Avoid concomitant use.

Adverse Reactions:

Prolonged use may result in addiction resembling alcoholism. Withdrawal may produce delirium tremens and vivid hallucinations. Several cases of metabolic acidosis have occurred in association with paraldehyde addiction, although the etiology is uncertain. Prolonged use may produce yellowing of eyes or skin (hepatitis).

Miscellaneous: Strong, unpleasant breath may occur (see Precautions).

(Continued on following page)

PARALDEHYDE (Cont.)

Overdosage:

Symptoms: Death has occurred following 25 ml orally or 12 ml rectally. The hallmark of toxicity is metabolic acidosis; treat with IV sodium bicarbonate or sodium lactate. Clinical features are: Unconsciousness; coma; rapid, labored respirations; pulmonary hemorrhage; edema; irritation of the throat, stomach and rectum (enema); nausea; vomiting; esophagitis; hemorrhagic gastritis; hepatitis; renal damage; agitation; pseudoketosis; hyperacetaldehydemia; right heart dilation.

Treatment: Intensive support therapy is paramount. Support respiratory function, treat acidosis and protect the liver. Gastric lavage is inappropriate since the drug is rapidly absorbed after administration. Hemodialysis or peritoneal dialysis may be required to treat acidosis and to support renal function.

Patient Information:

May cause GI upset; take with food or mix with milk or iced fruit juice to improve taste.

Avoid alcohol and other sedatives while taking this drug.

May cause drowsiness; use caution while driving or performing tasks requiring alertness.

Do not use paraldehyde in any plastic container; do not dispense with a plastic spoon or syringe.

Discard any unused paraldehyde after opening bottle.

Do not use if liquid has a brownish color or a strong vinegar odor.

Administration and Dosage:

Hypnosis:

Adults – Oral: 4 to 8 ml in milk or iced fruit juice to mask the taste and odor. *Delirium tremens:* 10 to 35 ml may be necessary.

Rectal: Dissolve in oil as a retention enema. Mix 10 to 20 ml with 1 or 2 parts of olive oil or isotonic sodium chloride solution to avoid rectal irritation.

Children – 0.3 ml/kg orally or rectally.

Sedation:

Adults – 5 to 10 ml orally or rectally.

Children – 0.15 ml/kg orally or rectally

Stability and storage: Upon exposure to light and air, paraldehyde decomposes to acetaldehyde and oxidizes to acetic acid. Do not use if liquid has a brownish color or sharp odor of acetic acid. Keep away from heat, open flame or sparks. Paraldehyde solidifies at approximately 12°C (54°F) and must be liquefied before use. Do not store in direct sunlight or expose to temperatures above 25°C (77°F). Keep product covered in box until use. Discard unused portion. Do not use paraldehyde from a container that has been opened for longer than 24 hours.

				C.I.*
c-IV	**Paral** (Forest)	**Liquid (Oral, Rectal)**	In 30 ml.	197
c-IV	**Paraldehyde** (Various, eg, J.T. Baker, Spectrum)	**Liquid (Oral, Rectal):** 1 g per ml	In 30 ml.	350+

* Cost Index based on cost per 4 ml oral or rectal.

Piperidine Derivatives

GLUTETHIMIDE

Actions:

Pharmacology: Produces CNS depression similar to the barbiturates. Glutethimide exhibits pronounced anticholinergic activity, which is manifested by mydriasis, inhibition of salivary secretions and decreased intestinal motility. It suppresses REM sleep and is associated with REM rebound. It has generally been replaced by safer and more effective agents.

Pharmacokinetics:

Absorption/Distribution – It is erratically absorbed from the GI tract. Following single oral doses of 500 mg, the peak plasma concentration occurs from 1 to 6 hours after administration. The average plasma half-life is 10 to 12 hours. About 50% of the drug is bound to plasma proteins. Glutethimide stimulates hepatic microsomal enzymes.

Metabolism/Excretion – Glutethimide is a racemate; both isomers are hydroxylated and then conjugated with glucuronic acid. The glucuronides pass into the enterohepatic circulation and are excreted in the urine (< 2% unchanged).

Indications:

For short-term relief of insomnia (3 to 7 days). Not indicated for chronic administration. Should insomnia persist, a drug free interval of 1 or more weeks should elapse before retreatment is considered. Attempt to find alternative nondrug therapy in chronic insomnia.

Contraindications:

Hypersensitivity to glutethimide; porphyria.

Warnings:

Physical and psychological dependence occur; carefully evaluate patients before prescribing glutethimide. Ordinarily, an amount adequate for 1 week is sufficient, then reevaluate the patient. Withdrawal symptoms include nausea, abdominal discomfort, tremors, convulsions and delirium. In the presence of dependence, reduce dosage gradually.

Pregnancy: Category C. It is not known whether glutethimide can cause fetal harm or can affect reproduction capacity. Give to a pregnant woman only if clearly needed. Newborn infants of mothers dependent on glutethimide may exhibit withdrawal symptoms.

Lactation: Because of the potential for serious adverse reactions in nursing infants, decide whether to discontinue nursing or to discontinue the drug, taking into account the importance of the drug to the mother.

Children: Safety and efficacy have not been established. Use is not recommended.

Precautions:

Potentially hazardous tasks: May produce drowsiness; observe caution while driving or performing other tasks requiring alertness.

Drug Interactions:

Alcohol and **CNS depressants** (eg, **barbiturates, narcotics**): Additive CNS effects may occur when used concomitantly with glutethimide.

Anticoagulants, oral: Glutethimide induces hepatic microsomal enzymes, resulting in increased metabolism of the anticoagulant and possibly a decreased anticoagulant response.

Charcoal may prevent the GI absorption of glutethimide. Depending on the clinical situation, this will reduce the toxicity or effectiveness of glutethimide.

Adverse Reactions:

Clinical studies revealed the following effects: Skin rash (8.6%); nausea (2.7%); hangover (1.1%); drowsiness (1%). When a generalized skin rash occurs, withdraw the drug. The rash usually clears spontaneously, a few days after withdrawal.

The following occurred in < 1% of patients: Vertigo; headache; depression; dizziness; ataxia; confusion; edema; indigestion; lightheadedness; nocturnal diaphoresis; vomiting; dry mouth; euphoria; impaired memory; slurred speech; tinnitus.

Rare: Paradoxical excitation; blurred vision; acute hypersensitivity; porphyria; blood dyscrasia such as thrombocytopenic purpura, aplastic anemia and leukopenia.

(Continued on following page)

GLUTETHIMIDE (Cont.)

Overdosage:

Acute overdosage: The lethal dose ranges from 10 to 20 g; patients have died from 5 g and other patients have recovered from single doses as high as 35 g. A single oral dose of 5 g usually produces severe intoxication. A plasma level of 3 mg/dl is indicative of severe poisoning. A lower level does not preclude the possibility of severe poisoning because of sequestration of the drug in body fat depots and in the GI tract. Serial plasma level determinations are mandatory for proper patient evaluation.

Symptoms are dose-dependent and indistinguishable from barbiturate intoxication. The degree of CNS depression often fluctuates, possibly due to irregular absorption of the drug or accumulation of an active toxic metabolite. Symptoms include: CNS depression, including coma (profound and prolonged in severe intoxication); hypothermia, which may be followed by fever; depressed or lost deep tendon reflexes; depression or absence of corneal and pupillary reflexes; dilation of pupils; depressed or absent response to painful stimuli; inadequate ventilation (even with relatively normal respiratory rate), sometimes with cyanosis; sudden apnea, especially with manipulation such as gastric lavage or endotracheal intubation; diminished or absent peristalsis. Severe hypotension unresponsive to volume expansion, tonic muscular spasms, twitching and convulsions may occur.

Treatment – Cardiopulmonary supportive measures should include: Maintenance of a patent airway with assisted ventilation; monitoring of vital signs and level of consciousness; continuous ECG to detect arrhythmias; maintenance of blood pressure with plasma volume expanders and, if essential, pressor drugs.

Gastric lavage: Induce vomiting only if the patient is fully conscious. Institute gastric lavage in all cases, regardless of elapsed time since ingestion. Lavage with a 1:1 mixture of castor oil and water. Leave 50 ml of castor oil in the stomach as a cathartic. Delay absorption by giving activated charcoal in water. Follow up as soon as possible with production of emesis or gastric lavage.

Intestinal lavage is used to remove unabsorbed drug (100 to 250 ml of 20% to 40% sorbitol or mannitol).

Urinary output: If coma is prolonged, monitor and maintain urine output while preventing overhydration which might contribute to pulmonary or cerebral edema.

Dialysis/hemoperfusion: Consider in Grade III or Grade IV coma, when renal shutdown or impaired renal function are manifest, and in life-threatening situations complicated by pulmonary edema, heart failure, circulatory collapse, significant liver disease, major metabolic disturbance or uremia.

Use of pure food grade soybean oil as the dialysate enhances removal of glutethimide by hemodialysis. While aqueous hemodialysis is less effective for glutethimide than for readily water-soluble compounds, glutethimide blood levels may decline more rapidly with hemodialysis, and the duration of coma may be shortened; efficacy of the procedure, however, is controversial. Peritoneal dialysis is of minimal value.

Charcoal hemoperfusion has been simpler and more effective than hemodialysis. Similarly, a microcapsule artificial kidney has been developed using activated charcoal granules. Resin hemoperfusion with an Amberlite XAD-2 column has shown exceptionally high clearance capabilities in glutethimide intoxication and has been clinically superior to hemodialysis.

Lipid storage: Glutethimide is highly lipid soluble; it rapidly accumulates in lipoid tissue. As the drug is removed from the bloodstream by any technique, it is gradually released from fat storage back into the bloodstream. Even after substantial quantities of the drug have been extracted, this blood-level rebound can cause coma to persist or recur. Continue drug extraction techniques for at least 2 hours after the patient regains consciousness.

(Overdosage continued on following page)

GLUTETHIMIDE (Cont.)

Overdosage (Cont.):

Chronic overdosage:

Symptoms – Impairment of memory and ability to concentrate; impaired gait; ataxia; tremors; hyporeflexia; slurring of speech. Abrupt discontinuation after chronic overdosage frequently causes withdrawal reactions including: Nervousness; anxiety; grand mal seizures; abdominal cramping; chills; numbness of extremities; dysphagia.

Treatment – Gradual, stepwise reduction of dosage over a period of days or weeks. If withdrawal reactions occur, readminister glutethimide, or substitute pentobarbital and subsequently withdraw gradually.

Patient Information:

May decrease alertness or physical ability. Use caution when driving or performing tasks requiring alertness.

Avoid alcohol and other CNS depressants.

Administration and Dosage:

Individualize dosage. Not recommended for children.

Adults: Usual adult dose is 250 to 500 mg at bedtime.

For elderly or debilitated patients, initial daily dosage should not exceed 500 mg at bedtime, to avoid oversedation.

				C.I.*
c-II	**Glutethimide** (Halsey)	**Tablets:** 250 mg	(HD 564). White, scored. In 100s.	113
c-II	**Glutethimide** (Various, eg, Balan, Bioline, Dixon-Shane, Geneva, Goldline, Halsey, Parmed, Purepac, Rugby, Schein)	**Tablets:** 500 mg	In 100s and 1000s.	11+

* Cost Index based on cost per 250 mg.

METHYPRYLON

Actions:

Pharmacology: Methyprylon increases the threshold of the arousal centers in the brain stem and produces CNS depression similar to the barbiturates. It suppresses REM sleep and is associated with REM rebound following discontinuation of therapy. Methyprylon stimulates the hepatic microsomal enzyme system. It has generally been replaced by safer and more effective agents.

Pharmacokinetics: Absorption/Distribution – The drug is rapidly absorbed following oral administration and is ≈ 60% bound to plasma proteins. Mean plasma concentrations in six subjects following a single 650 mg dose peaked in 1 to 2 hours at 5.7 to 10 mcg/ml. Concentrations declined to 3.3 to 7.9 mcg/ml at 4 hours. Therapeutic blood concentrations are approximately 1 mg/dl. Concentrations > 30 mg/L cause unconsciousness in the acutely poisoned patient.

Metabolism/Excretion – Following a 400 mg dose, < 1% was recovered in the urine as intact drug and ≈ 23% as identified metabolites in 72 hours. The drug is metabolized by two pathways: Dehydrogenation with subsequent oxidation to form the alcohol and corresponding acid, and oxidation to form 6-oxymethyprylon. The plasma half-life is 4 hours; it is prolonged in acute intoxication.

Onset/Duration – When taken at bedtime, it usually induces sleep within 45 minutes and provides sleep for 5 to 8 hours.

Indications:

As a hypnotic, it is effective for at least 7 consecutive nights. Prolonged administration is generally not recommended.

Contraindications:

Hypersensitivity to methyprylon.

Warnings:

Physical and psychological dependence have occurred. Withdrawal symptoms resemble those associated with withdrawal of barbiturates; treat in a similar fashion (see Barbiturate group monograph). Exercise caution in individuals known to be addiction prone or those whose history suggests they may increase the dosage on their own initiative. Limit repeated prescriptions without adequate medical supervision.

Hepatic or renal function impairment: Observe the usual precautions in the presence of hepatic or renal disorders.

Pregnancy: Category B. At a dose of 50 mg/kg/day, methyprylon caused an increased incidence of resorptions in the rabbit. There are no adequate and well controlled studies in pregnant women. Use only when clearly needed and when the potential benefits outweigh the potential hazards to the fetus.

Lactation: It is not known whether this drug is excreted in breast milk. Use caution when administering to a nursing mother.

Children: Safety and efficacy in children < 12 years old have not been established.

Precautions:

Total daily intake should not exceed 400 mg; greater amounts do not increase hypnotic benefits.

Potentially hazardous tasks: Observe caution while driving or performing other tasks requiring alertness.

Monitoring: If used repeatedly or over prolonged periods, perform periodic blood counts.

Acute intermittent porphyria: May exacerbate porphyria; use with caution in susceptible patients.

Hepatic effects: Methyprylon stimulates the hepatic microsomal enzyme system.

Drug Interactions:

Alcohol or other **CNS depressants** (eg, **barbiturates, narcotics**): Additive CNS depressant effects may occur when used concomitantly.

(Continued on following page)

METHYPRYLON (Cont.)

Adverse Reactions:

CNS: Convulsions; hallucinations; ataxia; EEG changes; pyrexia; morning drowsiness; headache; dizziness; vertigo.

Psychiatric: Acute brain syndrome and confusion (particularly in the elderly); paradoxical excitation; anxiety; depression; nightmares; dreaming.

Hematologic: Aplastic anemia; thrombocytopenic purpura; neutropenia.

Cardiovascular: Hypotension; syncope.

Ophthalmic: Diplopia; blurred vision.

GI: Esophagitis; vomiting; nausea; diarrhea; constipation.

Dermatologic: Pruritus; rash.

Miscellaneous: Hangover effect; generalized allergic reactions.

Overdosage:

Symptoms: Somnolence, confusion, coma, shock, constricted pupils, respiratory depression, hypotension, tachycardia, edema and hepatic dysfunction. Blood concentrations associated with serious toxic symptoms range from 3 to 6 mg/dl. Concentrations that have caused fatalities range from 5.3 to 114 mg/dl. A fatality occurred after ingestion of 6 g of the drug.

Treatment: Monitor respiration, pulse and blood pressure. Employ general supportive measures, along with immediate gastric lavage with precautions to prevent pulmonary aspiration. Administer appropriate IV fluids and maintain an adequate airway. Combat hypotension with norepinephrine, metaraminol or other accepted antihypotensive measures. Refer to General Management of Acute Overdosage.

Hemodialysis – Hemodialysis is of value, especially in those cases where supportive measures are failing and adequate urinary output cannot be maintained.

CNS stimulation/convulsions – Excitation and convulsions have followed methyprylon overdosage during the recovery phase. Barbiturates may be used with great caution.

Patient Information:

May cause drowsiness or dizziness. Use caution while driving or performing other tasks requiring alertness. Avoid alcohol and other CNS depressants.

Do not exceed prescribed dosage.

May be habit forming. Do not discontinue the drug abruptly.

Total daily intake should not exceed 400 mg. Greater amounts do not increase the sleep-inducing benefits.

Administration and Dosage:

Individualize dosage.

Adults: Usual dosage is 200 to 400 mg before bedtime.

Children (> 12 years of age): Effective dosage varies greatly. Initiate treatment with 50 mg at bedtime and increase to 200 mg, if required.

				C.I.*
c-III	**Noludar** (Roche)	**Capsules:** 300 mg	(Noludar 300 Roche). Amethyst/white. In 100s and 500s.	95
		Tablets: 200 mg	(Noludar 200 Roche). White, scored. In 100s.	118

* Cost Index based on cost per 200 mg.

Tertiary Acetylenic Alcohols

ETHCHLORVYNOL

Actions:

Pharmacology: Ethchlorvynol has sedative-hypnotic, anticonvulsant and muscle relaxant properties. It produces EEG patterns similar to those produced by barbiturates. It has generally been replaced by safer and more effective agents.

Pharmacokinetics: Absorption/Distribution – Ethchlorvynol is rapidly absorbed from the GI tract with peak plasma concentrations occurring within 2 hours after a single oral fasting dose. Maximum blood concentrations occur in 1 to 1.5 hours; approximately 90% of the drug is destroyed in the liver. There is extensive tissue concentration, particularly in adipose tissue.

Metabolism/Excretion – Within 24 hours, 33% of a single 500 mg dose is excreted in the urine, mostly as metabolites. The free and conjugated forms of the major metabolite, the secondary alcohol of ethchlorvynol, in the urine accounts for about 40% of the dose. The parent compound and its metabolites undergo extensive enterohepatic recirculation. The plasma half-life of the parent compound is 10 to 20 hours.

Onset/Duration – The usual hypnotic dose induces sleep within 15 to 60 minutes. The duration of effect is about 5 hours.

Indications:

Short-term hypnotic therapy for periods up to 1 week in the management of insomnia. If retreatment becomes necessary after drug free intervals of 1 or more weeks, undertake only upon further evaluation of the patient.

Unlabeled use: A sedative dose for ethchlorvynol is 100 to 200 mg 2 or 3 times daily.

Contraindications:

Hypersensitivity to ethchlorvynol; porphyria.

Warnings:

Psychological and physical dependence: Administer with caution to mentally depressed patients, with or without suicidal tendencies, and to those who have a psychological potential for drug dependence. Prescribe the least amount of drug that is practical. Prolonged use may result in tolerance and psychological and physical dependence.

Intoxication symptoms have been reported with the prolonged use of doses as low as 1 g/day. Signs and symptoms may include incoordination, tremors, ataxia, confusion, slurred speech, hyperreflexia, diplopia and generalized muscle weakness. Toxic amblyopia, scotoma, nystagmus and peripheral neuropathy have also occurred; these symptoms are usually reversible.

Withdrawal symptoms similar to those seen during barbiturate and alcohol withdrawal follow abrupt discontinuance after prolonged use. Symptoms can appear as late as 9 days after sudden drug withdrawal and may include: Convulsions; delirium; schizoid reaction; perceptual distortions; memory loss; ataxia; insomnia; slurring of speech; unusual anxiety; irritability; agitation; tremors; anorexia; nausea; vomiting; weakness; dizziness; sweating; muscle twitching; weight loss.

Withdrawal management – Readminister drug to approximately the same level of intoxication that existed before the abrupt discontinuance. Phenobarbital may be substituted for ethchlorvynol. Make a gradual, stepwise reduction of dosage over a period of days or weeks. In addition, a phenothiazine may be used for patients who exhibit psychotic symptoms during withdrawal. Hospitalize or closely observe the patient and give general supportive care as indicated.

Hepatic or renal function impairment: Use caution when treating patients with impaired hepatic or renal function.

Elderly or debilitated patients should receive the smallest effective dose.

Pregnancy: Category C. The drug is associated with a high percentage of stillbirths and a low survival rate of progeny in rats given 40 mg/kg/day. Ethchlorvynol crosses the placental barrier. Not recommended for use during the first and second trimesters of pregnancy. Use during the third trimester of pregnancy may produce CNS depression and transient withdrawal symptoms in the newborn (eg, episodic jitteriness, hyperactivity, restlessness, irritability disturbed sleep, hunger). Use during pregnancy only if the potential benefit justifies the potential risk to the fetus.

Lactation: It is not known whether this drug is excreted in breast milk. Because of the potential for serious adverse reactions in the infant, decide whether to discontinue nursing or to discontinue the drug, taking into account the importance of the drug to the mother.

Children: Safety and efficacy are not been determined; use is not recommended.

Precautions:

Potentially hazardous tasks: May cause dizziness; observe caution while driving or performing other tasks requiring alertness.

(Precautions continued on following page)

ETHCHLORVYNOL (Cont.)

Precautions (Cont.):

CNS effects: Patients who exhibit unpredictable behavior or paradoxical restlessness or excitement in response to barbiturates or alcohol may react in this manner to ethchlorvynol. Do not use for the management of insomnia in the presence of pain, unless insomnia persists after pain is controlled with analgesics.

Tartrazine sensitivity: Some of these products contain tartrazine, which may cause allergic-type reactions (including bronchial asthma) in susceptible individuals. Although the incidence of tartrazine sensitivity in the general population is low, it is frequently seen in patients who also have aspirin hypersensitivity.

Drug Interactions:

Alcohol or other **CNS depressants** (eg, **barbiturates, narcotics**): Exaggerated depressant effects will occur when used concomitantly with ethchlorvynol.

Anticoagulants, oral: Ethchlorvynol may decrease the hypoprothrombinemic effect of the anti-coagulant. Dosage adjustment may be required at initiation and discontinuation of therapy. Alternatively, consider the use of a benzodiazepine in place of ethchlorvynol.

Adverse Reactions:

Reactions within each category are given in decreasing order of severity.

GI: Vomiting; gastric upset; nausea; aftertaste.

CNS: Dizziness; facial numbness. Transient giddiness and ataxia have occurred when absorption of the drug is especially rapid.

Hematologic: Thrombocytopenia; fatal immune thrombocytopenia (one case).

Hypersensitivity: Cholestatic jaundice; urticaria; rash.

Miscellaneous: Blurred vision; hypotension; mild "hangover."

Idiosyncratic (occasional): Syncope without marked hypotension; mild stimulation; marked excitement; hysteria; prolonged hypnosis; profound muscular weakness.

Overdosage:

Symptoms: Acute intoxication is characterized by prolonged deep coma, severe respiratory depression, hypothermia, hypotension and relative bradycardia. Nystagmus and pancytopenia have been reported. Death has occurred following ingestion of 6 g; however, patients have survived overdoses of 50 g and more with intensive care. Fatal blood concentrations range from 20 to 50 mcg/ml. Because large amounts are taken up by adipose tissue, the blood concentration is an unreliable parameter.

Treatment: Perform immediate gastric evacuation. In the unconscious patient, precede gastric lavage by tracheal intubation with a cuffed tube. Supportive care is essential. Place emphasis on pulmonary care and monitoring of blood gases. Hemoperfusion using the Amberlite column technique (XAD-4 resin) has been the most effective method of managing acute overdose. Hemodialysis and peritoneal dialysis (aqueous and oil dialysates) are of some value. Hemoperfusion with charcoal has been effective. Forced diuresis with maintenance of a high urinary output is also of value. Refer to General Management of Acute Overdosage.

Patient Information:

May cause drowsiness, dizziness or blurred vision; observe caution while driving or performing other tasks requiring alertness.

Avoid alcohol and other CNS depressants. Do not exceed prescribed dosage.

Symptoms of giddiness, ataxia or GI upset may be reduced if drug is taken with food.

Administration and Dosage:

Hypnotic: Usual adult dose is 500 mg at bedtime; 750 mg may be required for patients whose response to 500 mg is inadequate, or for patients being changed from barbiturates or nonbarbiturate hypnotics. Give the smallest effective dose to elderly or debilitated patients. Do not prescribe for > 1 week.

Severe insomnia: Up to 1000 mg may be given as a single bedtime dose.

Supplemental dose in insomnia characterized by untimely awakening during early morning hours. Administer 200 mg to reinstitute sleep in patients who awaken after the original bedtime dose of 500 or 750 mg.

				C.I.*
c-IV	**Placidyl** (Abbott)	**Capsules:** 200 mg	Red. In 100s.	667
		500 mg	Red. In 100s, 500s and Abbo-Pac 100s.	329
		750 mg[1]	(KN). Green. In 100s and Abbo-Pac 100s.	242

* Cost Index based on cost per 500 mg.

[1] Contains tartrazine.

PROPIOMAZINE HCl

Actions:

Pharmacology: Propiomazine is a phenothiazine compound with sedative, antiemetic and antihistaminic properties. It is a potent premedicant, with a short duration of action.

Pharmacokinetics: Following IM administration, peak serum concentrations are reached in 1 to 3 hours; mean bioavailability is 60%. Mean elimination half-lives reported in five healthy volunteers after IV and IM doses of 20 mg each were 7.7 ± 3.9 hours and 10.8 ± 1.9 hours, respectively.

Indications:

Sedative: Relief of restlessness and apprehension, preoperatively or during surgery.

Analgesic adjunct: Relief of restlessness and apprehension during labor.

Contraindications:

Intra-arterial injection: Arterial or arteriolar spasm with resultant local impairment of circulation may occur.

Warnings:

Pregnancy: Safety for use during the first trimester of pregnancy has not been established.

Precautions:

Neuroleptic malignant syndrome (NMS), a potentially fatal symptom complex, has occurred in association with antipsychotic drugs, which may include propiomazine. See Antipsychotic agents for a more complete discussion.

Thrombophlebitis: Inject IV only into vessels previously undamaged by multiple injections or trauma. Do not allow extravasation, since chemical irritation may be severe.

Potentially hazardous tasks: May produce drowsiness or dizziness; observe caution while driving or performing other tasks requiring alertness.

Drug Interactions:

CNS depressants: Propiomazine enhances the CNS effects. Eliminate or reduce the dose of **barbiturates** by at least ½ in the presence of propiomazine. Reduce the doses of **meperidine, morphine** and other **analgesic depressants** by ¼ to ½.

Adverse Reactions:

Autonomic reactions are rare. Dry mouth may occur, but this is usually desirable in patients undergoing anesthesia.

Cardiovascular: Moderate elevation in blood pressure (desirable in many cases) and hypotension (rare). Tachycardia has also occurred.

Norepinephrine appears to be most suitable if a vasopressor must be administered to patients receiving propiomazine. The pressor response to epinephrine is usually reduced and may even be reversed in the presence of propiomazine.

Neuroleptic malignant syndrome has occurred (see Warnings).

Administration and Dosage:

Adults: Administer IV or IM.

Preoperative medication – 20 mg propiomazine with 50 mg meperidine. Although 20 mg propiomazine is sufficient for most patients, some will require as much as 40 mg for adequate sedation. Belladonna alkaloids may be added as required.

Sedation during surgery with local, nerve block or spinal anesthesia – 10 to 20 mg.

Obstetrics – 20 mg will provide sedation and relieve apprehension in the early stages of labor. Some patients may require up to 40 mg. When labor is definitely established, administer 20 to 40 mg of propiomazine with 25 to 75 mg of meperidine (average dose, 50 mg). Amnesic agents may be administered as required. If the average doses of propiomazine and meperidine are used, it is seldom necessary to repeat the medication during normal labor. Additional doses may be repeated at 3 hour intervals. Neither prolongation of labor nor significant maternal or fetal depression has been observed.

Children: Use as a sedative the night before surgery and for preanesthetic and postoperative medication. In children under 27 kg (60 lb), calculate dosage on the basis of 0.55 to 1.1 mg/kg (0.25 to 0.5 mg/lb). The higher dosage recommendation should be necessary only in the extremely nervous, excitable child.

Satisfactory results were obtained with the following dosage schedule:

Propiomazine HCl Pediatric Dosage

Age (yrs)	Single Dosage
2 to 4	10 mg
4 to 6	15 mg
6 to 12	25 mg

Stability: Do not use if solution is cloudy or contains a precipitate.

				C.I.*
Rx	**Largon** (Wyeth-Ayerst)	**Injection:** 20 mg per ml	In 1 ml amps.	1675

* Cost Index based on cost per 20 mg.

Adverse Reactions (Cont.):

Estazolam: Other adverse reactions reported only for estazolam include the following:

CNS – Somnolence (42%); asthenia (11%); hypokinesia (8%); hangover (3%); abnormal thinking (2%); anxiety (1%); agitation, amnesia, apathy, emotional lability, hostility, seizure, sleep disorder, stupor, twitch (0.1% to 1%); ataxia, decreased libido, decreased reflexes, neuritis (< 0.1%).

GI – Dyspepsia (2%); decreased/increased appetite, flatulence, gastritis (0.1% to 1%); enterocolitis, melena, mouth ulceration (< 0.1%).

Cardiovascular – Arrhythmia, syncope (< 0.1%).

Dermatologic – Urticaria (0.1% to 1%); acne, dry skin, photosensitivity (< 0.1%).

Respiratory – Cold symptoms (3%); pharyngitis (1%); asthma, cough, dyspnea, rhinitis, sinusitis (0.1% to 1%); epistaxis, hyperventilation, laryngitis (< 0.1%).

Special senses – Ear pain, eye irritation/pain/swelling, photophobia (0.1% to 1%); decreased hearing, diplopia, nystagmus, scotomata (< 0.1%).

GU – Frequent urination, menstrual cramps, urinary hesitancy/urgency, vaginal discharge/itching (0.1% to 1%); hematuria, nocturia, oliguria, penile discharge, urinary incontinence (< 0.1%).

Miscellaneous – Lower extremity/back/abdominal pain (1% to 3%); stiffness (1%); allergic reaction, chills, fever, neck/upper extremity pain, thirst, arthritis, muscle spasm, myalgia (0.1% to 1%); edema, jaw pain, swollen breast, thyroid nodule, purpura, swollen lymph nodes, agranulocytosis, increased AST, weight gain/loss, arthralgia (< 0.1%).

Overdosage:

Symptoms: Somnolence; confusion with reduced or absent reflexes; respiratory depression; apnea; hypotension; impaired coordination; slurred speech; seizures; ultimately, coma. Death has occurred with overdoses of benzodiazepines alone and with alcohol.

Treatment: If excitation occurs, do not use barbiturates. Consider the possibility that multiple agents may have been ingested. Monitor respiration, pulse and blood pressure. Employ general supportive measures. Administer IV fluids and maintain an adequate airway. Perform gastric lavage. Refer to General Management of Acute Overdosage. Hemodialysis and forced diuresis are of little value.

Use of IV pressor agents may be necessary to treat hypotension. Administer IV fluids to encourage diuresis.

Patient Information:

Avoid alcohol and other CNS depressants. Do not exceed prescribed dosage.

Do not discontinue medication abruptly after prolonged therapy.

Advise patients that they may experience disturbed nocturnal sleep for the first or second night after discontinuing the drug.

May cause drowsiness or dizziness; observe caution while driving or performing other tasks requiring alertness.

Inform your physician if you are planning to become pregnant, if you are pregnant, or if you become pregnant while taking this medicine.

Triazolam: Advise patients not to take triazolam in circumstances where a full night's sleep and clearance of the drug from the body are not possible before they would again need to be active and functional.

ESTAZOLAM

Administration and Dosage:

Adults: 1 mg at bedtime; however, some patients may need a 2 mg dose.

Elderly: If healthy, 1 mg at bedtime; initiate increases with particular care.

Debilitated or small elderly patients: Consider a starting dose of 0.5 mg, although this is only marginally effective in the overall elderly population.

				C.I.*
c-IV	**ProSom** (Abbott)	**Tablets:** 1 mg	Lactose. White, scored. In 100s and UD 100s.	8.1
		2 mg	Lactose. Coral, scored. In 100s and UD 100s.	4.6

* Cost Index based on cost per 1 mg estazolam.

Benzodiazepine Compounds (Cont.)

FLURAZEPAM HCl

Administration and Dosage: Individualize dosage.

Adults: 30 mg before bedtime. In some patients, 15 mg may suffice.

Elderly or debilitated: Initiate with 15 mg until individual response is determined.

	Product	Form/Strength	Description	C.I.*
c-iv	**Flurazepam** (Various, eg, Goldline, Major, Moore, PBI, Rugby, Schein, Warner-C)	**Capsules:** 15 mg	In 100s and 500s.	3.1+
c-iv	**Dalmane** (Roche)		Orange and ivory. In 100s, 500s, Reverse number pack 100s and UD 100s.	5.4
c-iv	**Flurazepam** (Various, eg, Goldline, Major, Moore, PBI, Rugby, Schein, Warner-C)	**Capsules:** 30 mg	In 100s and 500s.	2.1+
c-iv	**Dalmane** (Roche)		Red and ivory. In 100s, 500s, Reverse number pack 100s and UD 100s.	5.9

TEMAZEPAM

Administration and Dosage: *Adults:* Individualize dosage. Give 15 to 30 mg before bedtime.

Elderly or debilitated: Initiate with 15 mg until individual response is determined.

	Product	Form/Strength	Description	C.I.*
c-iv	**Temazepam** (Various, eg, Goldline, Lederle, Major, Moore, PBI, Rugby, Warner Chilcott)	**Capsules:** 15 mg	In 100s, 500s and UD 100s.	1.7+
c-iv	**Restoril** (Sandoz)		(Restoril 15 mg). Maroon and pink. In 100s, 500s, Control Pak 25s and Sando Pak 100s.	13
c-iv	**Temazepam** (Various, eg, Goldline, Major, Moore, PBI, Rugby, Warner Chilcott)	**Capsules:** 30 mg	In 100s, 500s and UD 100s.	1+
c-iv	**Restoril** (Sandoz)		(Restoril 30 mg). Maroon and blue. In 100s, 500s, Control Pak 25s & Sando Pak 100s.	7.1

TRIAZOLAM

Administration and Dosage: *Adults:* 0.125 to 0.5 mg before bedtime.

Elderly or debilitated: 0.125 to 0.25 mg. Initiate with 0.125 mg until individual response is determined.

	Product	Form/Strength	Description	C.I.*
c-iv	**Halcion** (Upjohn)	**Tablets:** 0.125 mg	(0.125 Halcion 10). White. In 100s, 500s, UD 100s and Visipak 100s.	27
		0.25 mg	(0.25 Halcion 17). Blue, scored. In 100s, 500s, UD 100s and Visipak 100s.	15

QUAZEPAM

Administration and Dosage: *Adults:* Initiate at 15 mg until individual responses are determined; may reduce to 7.5 mg in some patients.

Elderly or debilitated: Attempt to reduce nightly dosage after the first one or two nights of therapy.

	Product	Form/Strength	Description	C.I.*
c-iv	**Doral** (Wallace)	**Tablets:** 7.5 mg	(7.5 Doral). Capsule shaped, light orange with white speckles. In 100s, 500s and UD 100s.	11
		15 mg	(15 Doral). Capsule shaped, light orange with white speckles. In 100s, 500s and UD 100s.	6.1

* Cost Index based on cost per 30 mg flurazepam or temazepam, 0.5 mg triazolam or 15 mg quazepam.

For a complete listing of diphenhydramine HCl products, refer to pages 970 to 971.
For a complete listing of pyrilamine maleate products, refer to page 972.

Actions: These products contain antihistamines which act on the CNS, producing prominent sedative effects. For complete monograph information on the antihistamines, refer to p. 964.

Indications: Aid in the relief of insomnia.

Traditionally, products containing analgesics have been used for relief of insomnia due to minor pain.

Contraindications:

Asthma, glaucoma or prostate gland enlargement, except under a physician's advice.

Warnings:

Hazardous tasks: May cause drowsiness; observe caution while driving or performing other tasks requiring alertness.

Prolonged insomnia: Not for use over 2 weeks. If insomnia persists for more than 2 weeks, consult a physician; it may be a symptom of a serious underlying illness.

Usage in Pregnancy and Lactation: Consult a physician before using these products. **Doxylamine** should not be taken by pregnant or nursing women.

Usage in Children: Do not use in children less than 12 years of age.

Drug Interactions: Alcohol or other **CNS depressants:** Use with caution due to additive effects.

Adverse Reactions: Occasional anticholinergic effects may occur with doxylamine.

Overdosage: Antihistamine overdosage reactions may vary from CNS depression to stimulation. See page 968 for a more complete description of reactions.

Administration and Dosage:

Administer 25 mg doxylamine or 50 mg diphenhydramine before bedtime. Give 50 mg pyrilamine maleate at bedtime; do not exceed 100 mg in 24 hours.

	Product	Formulation	Description	C.I.*
otc	**Doxysom Nighttime Sleep-Aid** (Quantum)	**Tablets:** 25 mg doxylamine succinate	In 8s.	56
otc	**Unisom Nighttime Sleep-Aid** (Leeming)		Blue, scored. In 8s, 16s, 32s and 48s.	62
otc	**Nervine Nighttime Sleep-Aid** (Miles Labs)	**Tablets:** 25 mg diphenhydramine HCl	White. In 12s, 30s and 50s.	58
otc	**Nytol** (Block)		In 16s, 32s and 72s.	37
otc	**Sleep-Eze 3** (Whitehall)		(S). Yellow. In 12s, 26s and 52s.	57
otc	**Sominex 2** (Beecham)		In 16s, 32s and 72s.	38
otc	**Sominex Caplets** (SK-Beecham)	**Tablets:** 50 mg diphenhydramine HCl	In 8s.	NA
otc	**Sominex 2 Pain Relief** (Beecham Products)	**Tablets:** 25 mg diphenhydramine HCl & 500 mg acetaminophen	(PR 2). White and blue. In 16s, 32s and 72s.	47
otc	**Extra Strength Tylenol PM Caplets & Tablets** (McNeil-CPC)	**Tablets:** 25 mg diphenhydramine & 500 mg acetaminophen	(Tylenol PM). In 24s & 50s.	NA
otc	**Bufferin AF Nite Time** (B-M Squibb)	**Tablets:** 38 mg diphenhydramine citrate, simethicone, 500 mg acetaminophen	Light blue, capsule shape. In 24s and 50s.	NA
otc	**Compoz Nighttime Sleep Aid** (Med-Tech)	**Tablets:** 50 mg diphenhydramine HCl	In 12s.	55
otc	**Dormarex 2** (Republic)		In 16s and 32s.	61
otc	**Maximum Strength Nytol** (Block)		Lactose. In 8s.	73
otc	**Twilite Caplets** (Pfeiffer)		In 20s.	31
otc	**Dormin** (Randob)	**Capsules:** 25 mg diphenhydramine HCl	Lactose, mineral oil. In 72s.	NA
otc	**Dormarex** (Republic)	**Capsules:** 25 mg pyrilamine maleate	In 20s, 40s and 100s.	30
otc	**Sleepinal** (Thompson)	**Capsules:** 50 mg diphenhydramine HCl	Lactose. In 16s.	NA
otc	**Quiet World** (Whitehall)	**Tablets:** 25 mg pyrilamine maleate, 162 mg acetaminophen and 227 mg aspirin	(Q). Blue. In 12s and 30s.	69

* Cost Index based on cost per capsule or tablet.

The following general discussion of the barbiturates refers to their use as sedative-hypnotic agents and as anticonvulsants. In addition, barbiturates are discussed under General Anesthetics, Barbiturates (see page 1414).

Actions:

Pharmacology: Barbiturates can produce all levels of CNS mood alteration from excitation to mild sedation, hypnosis and deep coma. In sufficiently high therapeutic doses, barbiturates induce anesthesia. Overdosage can produce death.

These agents depress the sensory cortex, decrease motor activity, alter cerebellar function and produce drowsiness, sedation and hypnosis. Barbiturates appear to act at the level of the thalamus where they inhibit ascending conduction in the reticular formation, thereby interfering with impulse transmission to the cortex.

Barbiturates have little analgesic action at subanesthetic doses and may increase the reaction to painful stimuli. All barbiturates exhibit anticonvulsant activity in anesthetic doses. However, only phenobarbital, mephobarbital and metharbital are effective as oral anticonvulsants in subhypnotic doses.

Barbiturates are respiratory depressants; the degree of respiratory depression is dose-dependent. With hypnotic doses, respiratory depression is similar to that which occurs during physiologic sleep.

Pharmacokinetics:

Absorption – Barbiturates are absorbed in varying degrees following oral, rectal or parenteral administration. The salts are more rapidly absorbed than the acids. The rate of absorption is increased if the sodium salt is ingested as a dilute solution or taken on an empty stomach.

Onset of action for oral or rectal administration varies from 20 to 60 minutes. For IM administration, onset is slightly faster. Following IV administration, onset ranges from almost immediate for pentobarbital sodium to 5 minutes for phenobarbital sodium. Maximal CNS depression may not occur for 15 minutes or more after IV administration of phenobarbital sodium.

Duration of action varies and is related to dose and to the rate at which the barbiturates are redistributed throughout the body. In the table below, the barbiturates are classified according to their duration of action. Do not use this classification to predict the exact duration of effect, but use as a guide in drug selection.

	Barbiturate	Half-life (hrs)[1]		Oral Dosage Range (mg)		Onset (minutes)	Duration (hours)
		Range	Mean	Sedative[2]	Hypnotic		
Long-Acting	Phenobarbital	53-118	79	30-120	100-320	≥ 60	10-12
	Mephobarbital	11-67	34	90-400	—		
	Metharbital	—	—	†	†		
Intermediate	Amobarbital	16-40	25	30-480	65-200	45-60	6-8
	Aprobarbital	14-34	24	120	40-160		
	Butabarbital	66-140	100	45-120	50-100		
	Talbutal	—	15	60-180	120		
Short-Acting	Secobarbital	15-40	28	—	100	10-15	3-4
	Pentobarbital	15-50	††	40-120	100		

[1] Data are inadequate on the half-life of metharbital and talbutal.
[2] Total daily dose; administered in 2 to 4 divided doses.
† Indicated only as an anticonvulsant.
†† May follow dose-dependent kinetics. Mean t½ is 50 hrs for 50 mg and 22 hrs for 100 mg.

(Actions continued on following page)

Actions (Cont.)

Pharmacokinetics (Cont.):

Distribution – Barbiturates are weak acids which are rapidly distributed to all tissues and fluids with high concentrations in the brain, liver and kidneys. Lipid solubility of the barbiturates is the dominant factor in their distribution. The more lipid soluble the barbiturate, the more rapidly it penetrates body tissue. Barbiturates are bound to plasma and tissue proteins; the degree of binding increases directly as a function of lipid solubility.

Phenobarbital has the lowest lipid solubility, plasma binding and brain protein binding, the longest delay in onset of activity and the longest duration of action. Secobarbital has the highest lipid solubility, plasma protein binding and brain protein binding, the shortest delay in onset of activity and the shortest duration of action. Butabarbital is an intermediate-acting barbiturate.

Elimination - Barbiturates are metabolized primarily by the hepatic microsomal enzyme system, and the metabolic products are excreted in the urine, and less commonly, in the feces. Approximately 25% to 50% of a dose of aprobarbital or phenobarbital is eliminated unchanged in the urine, whereas the amount of other barbiturates excreted unchanged in the urine is negligible. The excretion of unmetabolized barbiturate is one feature that distinguishes the long-acting agents. The inactive metabolites of the barbiturates are excreted as conjugates of glucuronic acid.

Clinical Pharmacology: Barbiturate-induced sleep reduces the amount of time spent in the rapid eye movement (REM) phase of sleep or dreaming stage. Also, Stages III and IV sleep are decreased. Following abrupt cessation of barbiturates used regularly, patients may experience markedly increased dreaming, nightmares or insomnia.

Secobarbital and pentobarbital lose most of their effectiveness for inducing and maintaining sleep by the end of 2 weeks of continued drug administration, even with the use of multiple doses. Other barbiturates might also be expected to lose their effectiveness for inducing and maintaining sleep after about 2 weeks. However, definitions of tolerance vary and these two barbiturates have been given for weeks to months for chronic sedation with little tolerance developing. The short, intermediate and, to a lesser degree, long-acting barbiturates have been widely prescribed for treating insomnia. Although the clinical literature abounds with claims that the short-acting agents are superior for producing sleep, while the intermediate-acting compounds are more effective in maintaining sleep, controlled studies have failed to demonstrate these differential effects.

Indications:

Sedation: Although traditionally used as nonspecific CNS depressants for daytime sedation, the barbiturates have generally been replaced by the benzodiazepines.

Hypnosis: For the short-term treatment of insomnia, since barbiturates appear to lose their effectiveness in sleep induction and maintenance after 2 weeks. If insomnia persists, drug free intervals of 1 or more weeks should elapse before retreatment. Seek alternative nondrug therapy for chronic insomnia.

Preanesthesia: As preoperative medication to help allay anxiety and facilitate induction of anesthesia.

Long-term anticonvulsant therapy (**phenobarbital, mephobarbital** and **metharbital**): For the treatment of generalized tonic-clonic and cortical focal seizures; and, in the emergency control of certain acute convulsive episodes, eg, those associated with status epilepticus, eclampsia, meningitis, tetanus and toxic reactions to strychnine or local anesthetics.

Pentobarbital sodium is also used as an anticonvulsant, in anesthetic doses, for emergency control of the acute convulsive episodes listed above.

Rectal administration: Barbiturates are absorbed from the colon and are used occasionally in infants for prolonged convulsive states, or when oral or parenteral administration may be undesirable. If the rectal form is not available, the soluble sodium salt may be incorporated in a retention enema.

Contraindications:

Barbiturate sensitivity; in patients with a history of manifest or latent porphyria or marked impairment of liver function. Large doses are contraindicated in nephritic patients and in patients with severe respiratory distress and respiratory disease where dyspnea, obstruction or cor pulmonale is present.

Do not administer to persons with previous addiction to the sedative/hypnotic group; ordinary doses may be ineffective and may contribute to further addiction.

Do not administer barbiturates in the presence of acute or chronic pain.

Parenteral secobarbital is contraindicated in obstetrical delivery.

(Continued on following page)

Warnings:

Habit forming: Tolerance or psychological and physical dependence may occur with continued use. (See Drug Abuse and Dependence.) Administer with caution, if at all, to patients who are mentally depressed, have suicidal tendencies or a history of drug abuse.

IV administration: Too rapid administration may cause respiratory depression, apnea, laryngospasm or vasodilation with fall in blood pressure. Parenteral solutions of barbiturates are highly alkaline. Therefore, use extreme care to avoid perivascular extravasation or intra-arterial injection. Extravascular injection may cause local tissue damage with subsequent necrosis; consequences of intra-arterial injection may vary from transient pain to gangrene of the limb. Any complaint of pain in the limb warrants stopping the injection.

Phenobarbital sodium may be administered IM or IV as an anticonvulsant for emergency use. When administered IV, it may require 15 or more minutes before reaching peak concentrations in the brain. Therefore, injecting phenobarbital sodium until the convulsions stop may cause the brain level to exceed that required to control the convulsions and may lead to severe barbiturate-induced depression.

Acute or chronic pain: Exercise caution when administering to patients with acute or chronic pain, because paradoxical excitement could be induced or important symptoms could be masked. However, the use of barbiturates as sedatives in postoperative surgery and as adjuncts to cancer chemotherapy is well established.

Use in impaired renal function: Barbiturates that are excreted either partially or completely unchanged in the urine (ie, phenobarbital, mephobarbital, aprobarbital and talbutal) are contraindicated in patients with impaired renal function.

Use in seizure disorders: Status epilepticus may result from abrupt discontinuation, even when administered in regular daily doses in the treatment of epilepsy.

Effects on vitamin D: Barbiturates may increase vitamin D requirements, possibly by increasing the metabolism of vitamin D via enzyme induction. Rickets and osteomalacia have been reported rarely following prolonged usage of barbiturates.

Use in elderly or debilitated patients: May produce marked excitement, depression and confusion. In some persons, barbiturates repeatedly produce excitement rather than depression.

Use in impaired hepatic function: Administer with caution and initially in reduced doses. Do not use in patients showing premonitory signs of hepatic coma.

Usage in Pregnancy: Category D. Barbiturates can cause fetal damage when administered to a pregnant woman. Studies suggest a connection between maternal consumption of barbiturates and a higher incidence of fetal abnormalities. If this drug is used during pregnancy, or if the patient becomes pregnant while taking this drug, apprise her of the potential hazards to the fetus.

Barbiturates readily cross the placental barrier and are distributed throughout fetal tissues. Fetal blood levels approach maternal blood levels following parenteral use.

Withdrawal symptoms occur in infants born to mothers who receive barbiturates throughout the last trimester of pregnancy. Reports include the acute withdrawal syndrome of seizures and hyperirritability from birth to a delayed onset of up to 14 days.

Anticonvulsant use – Because of the strong possibility of precipitating status epilepticus with attendant hypoxia and risk to both mother and unborn child, do not discontinue anticonvulsants when used to prevent major seizures. However, consider discontinuing anticonvulsants prior to and during pregnancy when the nature, frequency and severity of the seizures do not pose a serious threat to the patient. It is not known whether even minor seizures constitute some risk to the embryo or fetus.

Maternal ingestion of anticonvulsants, particularly barbiturates, may be associated with a neonatal coagulation defect that may cause bleeding usually within 24 hours of birth. The defect is characterized by decreased levels of vitamin K-dependent clotting factors, and prolongation of prothrombin time, partial thromboplastin time or both. Give prophylactic vitamin K to the mother 1 month prior to, and during, delivery and to the infant, IV, immediately after birth.

Labor and delivery: Hypnotic doses do not appear to significantly impair uterine activity during labor. Full anesthetic doses decrease the force and frequency of uterine contractions. Administration to the mother during labor may result in respiratory depression in the newborn; premature infants are particularly susceptible. If barbiturates are used during labor and delivery, have resuscitation equipment available.

A delayed interest in breast-feeding and a depressed response to auditory and visual stimuli have been noted in neonates. Long-term effects are unknown.

Usage in Lactation: Exercise caution when administering to the nursing mother, since small amounts are excreted in breast milk. Drowsiness in the nursing infant has been reported.

Usage in Children: Barbiturates may produce irritability, excitability, inappropriate tearfulness and aggression in children. Hyperkinetic states may also be induced or aggravated and are primarily related to a specific drug sensitivity.

(Continued on following page)

Precautions:

General: Reactions may occur in the presence of fever, hyperthyroidism, diabetes mellitus and severe anemia. Use with extreme caution in cases of debility, severely impaired liver function, pulmonary or cardiac disease, status asthmaticus, shock or uremia.

Use **mephobarbital** with caution in patients with myasthenia gravis and myxedema.

Laboratory evaluations: During prolonged therapy, perform periodic laboratory evaluation of organ systems, including hematopoietic, renal and hepatic systems.

Hypoadrenal function: Systemic effects of exogenous hydrocortisone and endogenous hydrocortisone (cortisol) may be diminished by barbiturates (see Drug Interactions). Therefore, administer with caution to patients with borderline hypoadrenal function, regardless of whether it is of pituitary or of primary adrenal origin.

Tartrazine sensitivity: Some of these products contain tartrazine, which may cause allergic-type reactions (including bronchial asthma) in susceptible individuals. Although the incidence of tartrazine sensitivity in the general population is low, it is frequently seen in patients who also have aspirin hypersensitivity. Specific products containing tartrazine are identified in the product listings.

Drug Interactions:

Most reports of clinically significant drug interactions occurring with the barbiturates have involved phenobarbital.

Agents which may increase the effects of barbiturates:

CNS depressants, including other sedatives, hypnotics, anesthetics, antihistamines, tranquilizers, phenothiazines or alcohol may produce additive depressant effects.

Valproic acid appears to decrease barbiturate metabolism. Monitor barbiturate blood levels and adjust dosage accordingly. The half-life of valproic acid may be decreased.

Chloramphenicol may inhibit phenobarbital metabolism. Barbiturates may enhance chloramphenicol metabolism.

Monoamine oxidase inhibitors (MAOIs) prolong the effects of barbiturates, probably because metabolism of the barbiturate is inhibited.

Barbiturates decrease the effects of the following drugs:

Oral anticoagulants (eg, warfarin) - Barbiturates can induce hepatic microsomal enzymes, resulting in increased metabolism and decreased anticoagulant response. Patients stabilized on anticoagulants may require dosage adjustments if barbiturates are added to or withdrawn from their regimen.

Digitoxin and **tricyclic antidepressants** - Barbiturates may increase metabolism by hepatic microsomal enzyme induction.

Corticosteroids - Barbiturates may enhance metabolism through the induction of hepatic microsomal enzymes. Patients stabilized on steroids may require dosage adjustments if barbiturates are added to or withdrawn from their regimen.

Doxycycline - Phenobarbital shortens the half-life for 2 weeks after barbiturate therapy is discontinued, probably through the induction of hepatic microsomal enzymes. If they are administered concurrently, monitor clinical response to doxycycline.

Oral contraceptives and estrogens - Decreased contraceptive effect and estrogen effect by induction of microsomal enzymes. Menstrual irregularities (spotting, breakthrough bleeding) or pregnancy may occur. An alternate form of birth control is suggested.

Acetaminophen - Effects may be decreased due to barbiturate-induced hepatic enzyme induction. Risk of increased hepatotoxicity may exist.

Beta-adrenergic blockers: Possible decreased β-blocker effect, especially with concomitant use of β-blockers metabolized by the liver (metoprolol and propranolol) with pentobarbital or phenobarbital.

Quinidine: Concurrent administration of phenobarbital may induce hepatic enzymes and significantly reduce the serum half-life of quinidine.

Rifampin induces hepatic microsomal enzymes and may decrease the effectiveness of barbiturates, especially phenobarbital.

Theophylline - Phenobarbital (and possibly pentobarbital and secobarbital) enhances xanthine metabolism and decreases theophylline effects. Monitor theophylline levels.

Metronidazole - Barbiturates may decrease the antimicrobial effectiveness of metronidazole when administered concurrently.

Phenmetrazine - The weight-reducing effects are decreased by amobarbital. The effect of barbiturates on other anorexiants is not known.

Miscellaneous drug interactions:

Phenytoin - The effect of barbiturates on metabolism is unpredictable; monitor phenytoin and barbiturate blood levels frequently if these drugs are given concurrently.

Griseofulvin - Phenobarbital appears to interfere with the absorption of oral griseofulvin, thus decreasing its blood level; however, the effect on therapeutic response has not been established. Avoid concomitant administration of these drugs.

Furosemide - Concomitant use may produce or aggravate orthostatic hypotension.

(Continued on following page)

Adverse Reactions:

The following adverse reactions and their incidence were compiled from observations of thousands of hospitalized patients. Because such patients may be less aware of certain milder adverse effects of barbiturates, the incidence of these reactions may be somewhat higher in fully ambulatory patients.

CNS: Somnolence is most common. Agitation, confusion, hyperkinesia, ataxia, vertigo, CNS depression, nightmares, lethargy, residual sedation (hangover effect), paradoxical excitement, nervousness, psychiatric disturbance, hallucinations, insomnia, anxiety, dizziness, thinking abnormality; delirium and stupor with excessive amounts.

Headache and fever with chronic phenobarbital use.

Respiratory: Hypoventilation, apnea, respiratory depression, laryngospasm, bronchospasm and circulatory collapse.

Cardiovascular: Bradycardia, hypotension, syncope.

GI: Nausea, vomiting, constipation, diarrhea and epigastric pain.

Liver damage with chronic phenobarbital use.

Hypersensitivity: Skin rashes, angioneurotic edema, serum sickness, morbilliform rash and urticaria are most likely in patients with asthma. Exfoliative dermatitis and Stevens-Johnson syndrome are rare reactions that may prove fatal.

Local reactions: Inadvertent intra-arterial injection may produce arterial spasm with resultant thrombosis and gangrene of an extremity. Reactions range from transient pain to severe tissue necrosis and neurological deficit. Injection SC may produce tissue necrosis, pain, tenderness and redness. Injection into or near peripheral nerves may result in permanent neurological deficit. Thrombophlebitis after IV use and pain at IM injection site have been reported.

Hematologic: Megaloblastic anemia following chronic phenobarbital use. Blood dyscrasias (eg, agranulocytosis, thrombocytopenia) are extremely rare. Patients should be encouraged to report symptoms of sore throat, easy bruising, nosebleed or petechiae.

Other: Rarely, barbiturates may produce a pain syndrome suggestive of myalgic, neuralgic or arthritic pain. Rickets and osteomalacia are rare following prolonged use.

Overdosage:

The toxic dose of barbiturates varies considerably. In general, an oral dose of 1 g produces serious poisoning in an adult. Death commonly occurs after 2 to 10 g of ingested barbiturate.

Symptoms: Acute barbiturate overdosage is manifested by CNS and respiratory depression which may progress to Cheyne-Stokes respiration, areflexia, constriction of the pupils to a slight degree (though in severe poisoning they may show paralytic dilation), oliguria, tachycardia, hypotension, lowered body temperature and coma. Typical shock syndrome (apnea, circulatory collapse, respiratory arrest and death) may occur.

In extreme overdose, all electrical activity in the brain may cease, in which case a "flat" EEG normally equated with clinical death cannot be accepted. This effect is fully reversible unless hypoxic damage occurs. Consider the possibility of barbiturate intoxication even in situations that appear to involve trauma.

Complications such as pneumonia, pulmonary edema, cardiac arrhythmias, congestive heart failure and renal failure may occur. Uremia may increase CNS sensitivity to barbiturates if renal function is impaired. Differential diagnosis should include hypoglycemia, head trauma, cerebrovascular accidents, convulsive states and diabetic coma.

Treatment is mainly supportive. Maintain an adequate airway, with assisted respiration and oxygen administration, as necessary. Monitor vital signs and fluid balance. Refer to General Management of Acute Overdosage on p. 2895

If the patient is conscious and has not lost the gag reflex, emesis may be induced with ipecac. Take care to prevent pulmonary aspiration of vomitus. After completion of vomiting, administer 30 g activated charcoal in a glass of water. Nasogastric administration of multiple doses of activated charcoal has been successful in accelerating the elimination of phenobarbital from the body. If emesis is contraindicated, perform gastric lavage with a cuffed endotracheal tube in place with the patient in the face down position. Activated charcoal may be left in the emptied stomach and a saline cathartic administered.

Administer fluid and other standard treatments for shock, if needed. If renal function is normal, forced diuresis may aid in the elimination of the barbiturate. Alkalinization of the urine increases renal excretion of some barbiturates, especially phenobarbital, aprobarbital and mephobarbital (which is metabolized to phenobarbital).

Hemodialysis may be used in severe barbiturate intoxication or if the patient is anuric or in shock. Patient should be rolled from side to side every 30 minutes.

(Continued on following page)

Complete prescribing information for these products begins on page 1398

Intermediate-Acting

AMOBARBITAL AND AMOBARBITAL SODIUM

Indications:

Oral: For sedation and relief of anxiety (at minimum doses); for hypnotic effects; as preanesthetic medication; for control of convulsive disorders.

Parenteral: For the management of catatonic and negativistic reactions, manic reactions and epileptiform seizures. It is also useful in narcoanalysis and narcotherapy and as a diagnostic aid in schizophrenia. Also indicated IV or IM for the control of convulsive seizures such as may be due to chorea, eclampsia, meningitis, tetanus, procaine or cocaine reactions, or poisoning from such drugs as strychnine or picrotoxin.

Administration and Dosage:

Individualize dosage.

Daytime sedation: The adult dosage range may be from 15 to 120 mg, 2 to 4 times per day. However, the usual adult dosage for daytime sedation is 30 to 50 mg, 2 or 3 times per day.

Hypnotic: The usual adult dose is 100 to 200 mg. On occasion, a larger dose may be necessary to produce the desired degree of hypnosis.

Insomnia: 65 to 200 mg (as sodium) at bedtime.

Preanesthetic sedation: 200 mg (as sodium) 1 or 2 hours before surgery.

Labor: Initial dose is 200 to 400 mg (as sodium); additional quantities of 200 to 400 mg may be given at 1 to 3 hour intervals for a total dose of not more than 1 g.

IM: The maximum IM dose should not exceed 500 mg. No greater volume than 5 ml, irrespective of drug concentration, should be injected IM at any one site. The average IM dose ranges from 65 to 500 mg. Solutions of 20% may be used so that a small volume can contain a large dose. Inject deeply into a large muscle, such as the gluteus maximus. Superficial IM or SC injections may be painful and may produce sterile abscesses or sloughs.

IV: Do not exceed the rate of 1 ml/minute. When the 10% solution is used, faster rates of administration may precipitate serious respiratory depression. Because of their higher metabolic rate, children tolerate comparatively larger doses. Ordinarily, 65 to 500 mg may be given to a child 6 to 12 years of age. The final dosage is determined to a great extent by the patient's reaction to the slow administration of the drug.

Preparation of solution: Add Sterile Water for Injection to the vial and rotate to facilitate solution of the powder. Do not shake the vial.

Stability: Do not use a solution which is not absolutely clear after 5 minutes. Amobarbital sodium hydrolyzes in solution or upon exposure to air. No more than 30 minutes should elapse from the time the vial is opened until contents are injected.

	Product	Form	Description	C.I.*
c-II	**Amytal Sodium Pulvules** (Lilly)	**Capsules:** 65 mg	(#Lilly F23). Blue. In 100s and 500s.	36
c-II	**Amobarbital Sodium** (Lannett)	**Capsules:** 200 mg	In 100s, 500s and 1000s.	5
c-II	**Amytal Sodium Pulvules** (Lilly)		(#Lilly F33). Blue. In 100s.	27
c-II	**Amobarbital Sodium** (Lannett)	**Powder**	In 15 and 30 g.	N/A
c-II	**Amytal** (Lilly)	**Tablets:** 30 mg	(#Lilly T56). Yellow, scored. In 100s.	24
		50 mg	(#Lilly T37). Orange, scored. In 100s.	16
		100 mg	(#Lilly T32). Pink, scored. In 100s.	13
c-II	**Amytal Sodium** (Lilly)	**Powder for Injection**	In 250 mg vials.	690
			In 500 mg vials.	510

* Cost Index based on cost per 30 mg oral amobarbital, 65 mg oral amobarbital sodium or 100 mg parenteral amobarbital sodium.

Product identification code.

Complete prescribing information for these products begins on page 1398

Intermediate-Acting (Cont.)

APROBARBITAL

Indications:

For short-term sedation and sleep induction.

Administration and Dosage:

Sedative: 40 mg, 3 times per day.

Mild insomnia: 40 to 80 mg before retiring.

Pronounced insomnia: 80 to 160 mg before retiring.

	Product	Form	Description	C.I.*
c-III	**Alurate** (Roche)	**Elixir:** 40 mg per 5 ml	20% alcohol. Contains saccharin and sorbitol. In pt.	74

BUTABARBITAL SODIUM

Indications:

For use as a sedative or hypnotic. Barbiturates appear to lose their effectiveness for sleep induction and maintenance after 2 weeks.

Administration and Dosage:

Adults: Daytime sedation – 15 to 30 mg, 3 or 4 times daily.

Bedtime hypnotic – 50 to 100 mg.

Preoperative sedation – 50 to 100 mg, 60 to 90 minutes before surgery.

Children: Preoperative sedation – 2 to 6 mg/kg; maximum 100 mg.

Daytime sedation – 7.5 to 30 mg, depending on age, weight and sedation desired.

Hypnotic – Dosage based on age and weight.

	Product	Form	Description	C.I.*
c-III	**Butabarbital Sodium** (Various)	**Tablets:** 15 mg	In 1000s.	2+
c-III	**Barbased** (Major)		In 1000s.	5
c-III	**Butisol Sodium** (Wallace)		Lavender, scored. In 100s and 1000s.	47
c-III	**Buticaps** (Wallace)	**Capsules:** 15 mg	Lavender and white. In 100s.	65
c-III	**Butabarbital Sodium** (Various)	**Tablets:** 30 mg	In 100s and 1000s.	1+
c-III	**Barbased** (Major)		In 1000s.	3
c-III	**Butatran** (Hauck)		In 100s and 1000s.	15
c-III	**Butisol Sodium** (Wallace)		Contains tartrazine. Green, scored. In 100s and 1000s.	31
c-III	**Sarisol No. 2** (Halsey)		Contains tartrazine. In 100s and 1000s.	2
c-III	**Buticaps** (Wallace)	**Capsules:** 30 mg	Contains tartrazine. Green and white. In 100s.	37
c-III	**Butisol Sodium** (Wallace)	**Tablets:** 50 mg	Contains tartrazine. Orange, scored. In 100s.	24
c-III	**Butabarbital Sodium** (Lannett)	**Tablets:** 100 mg	In 100s and 1000s.	1
c-III	**Butisol Sodium** (Wallace)		Pink, scored. In 100s.	15
c-III	**Butabarbital Sodium** (Various)	**Elixir:** 30 mg per 5 ml	In pt and gal.	4+
c-III	**Barbased** (Major)		7% alcohol. In 480 ml.	9
c-III	**Butisol Sodium** (Wallace)		7% alcohol. Contains tartrazine and saccharin. In pt and gal.	46
c-III	**Butalan** (Lannett)	**Elixir:** 33.3 mg per 5 ml	7% alcohol. In pt and gal.	3

TALBUTAL

Indications:

As a hypnotic for the short-term treatment of insomnia. Barbiturates appear to lose their effectiveness for sleep induction and maintenance after 2 weeks.

Administration and Dosage:

Adults: 120 mg 15 to 30 minutes before retiring.

	Product	Form	Description	C.I.*
c-III	**Lotusate** (Winthrop-Breon)	**Tablets:** 120 mg	Purple. In 100s.	66

* Cost Index based on cost per 40 mg aprobarbital, 15 mg butabarbital or 120 mg talbutal.

Complete prescribing information for these products begins on page 1398

Short-Acting

SECOBARBITAL AND SECOBARBITAL SODIUM

Indications:

Oral: For use as a hypnotic; for short-term treatment of insomnia and as a preanesthetic agent. Prolonged administration is not recommended, since it is not effective for a period of more than 14 days.

Rectal: For intermittent use as a sedative or hypnotic whenever rectal administration is indicated.

Parenteral: For intermittent use as a sedative, hypnotic or preanesthetic.

Also indicated in anesthetic doses for the emergency control of certain acute convulsive conditions associated with tetanus.

Administration and Dosage:

Oral: Adults – Preoperative sedation: 200 to 300 mg, 1 to 2 hours before surgery.
Bedtime hypnotic: 100 mg.

Oral: Children – Preoperative sedation: 2 to 6 mg/kg (max. 100 mg).

Rectal: Injectable solution – For rectal administration of the solution to children prior to ear, nose and throat procedures, the solution is usually diluted with lukewarm tap water to a concentration of 1% to 1.5%. It is administered after a cleansing enema. Children weighing less than 40 kg (88 pounds) may receive 5 mg/kg (2.3 mg per lb). Investigators recommend larger children receive only 4 mg/kg (1.8 mg/lb). Atropine may be administered for its drying effect on respiratory tract secretions. After rectal administration, hypnosis follows within 15 to 20 minutes. Children should be attended during this period.

Parenteral: Adjust dosage on basis of age, weight and patient's condition. Elderly or debilitated patients may be unusually sensitive to barbiturates and may require significant dosage reduction.

IM – Inject deeply into a large muscle mass. Inject no more than 250 mg (5 ml) into any one site because of possible tissue irritation.

IV – Restrict IV use to conditions in which other routes are not feasible, including patient unconsciousness (as in cerebral hemorrhage, eclampsia or status epilepticus) or because of resistance (as in delirium) or because prompt action is imperative.

Bedtime hypnotic: Usual adult dose is 100 to 200 mg IM.

Anesthetic procedures: To provide basal hypnosis for general, spinal or regional anesthesia or to facilitate intubation procedures, secobarbital is usually given IV at a rate not to exceed 50 mg per 15 second period. Discontinue administration as soon as the desired degree of hypnosis is attained. Total dosage in excess of 250 mg is not recommended. If hypnosis is inadequate after 250 mg, add a small quantity of meperidine. When employed as an adjunct to spinal or regional anesthesia, minimum quantities (50 to 100 mg) are required.

For children, the IM dose is 4 to 5 mg/kg.

Dentistry: As a sedative for apprehensive patients, the usual dose for adults or children is 2.2 mg/kg (1 mg/lb), maximum 100 mg. Intramuscular, rather than IV, administration is recommended 10 to 15 minutes before the procedure is started. Sedative effects persist for 3 to 4 hours. For light sedation, 1.1 to 1.6 mg/kg (0.5 to 0.75 mg/lb) will suffice.

In patients who are to receive nerve blocks, 100 to 150 mg may be given IV. With this dosage range and this route, the patient will awaken in 15 minutes and can be discharged in the company of another person after 30 minutes. If nitrous oxide is used, administer secobarbital as above (see Anesthetic Procedures).

Convulsions in tetanus: An initial dose of 5.5 mg/kg (2.5 mg/lb) may be used. Repeat every 3 or 4 hours, as needed. The rate of IV injections should not exceed 50 mg per 15 second period.

Stability and storage: Refrigerate; protect from light. Do not use if solution is discolored or contains a precipitate.

(Products listed on following page)

Short-Acting (Cont.)

SECOBARBITAL AND SECOBARBITAL SODIUM (Cont.)			C.I.*
c-II **Secobarbital Sodium** (Lannett)	**Capsules:** 50 mg	Orange. In 500s and 1000s.	12
c-II **Seconal Sodium Pulvules** (Lilly)		(#Lilly F42). Orange. In 100s.	78
c-II **Secobarbital Sodium** (Various)	**Capsules:** 100 mg	In 100s, 500s and 1000s.	7+
c-II **Seconal Sodium Pulvules** (Lilly)		(#Lilly F40). Orange. In 100s, 500s, 1000s and UD 100s.	56
c-II **Secobarbital Sodium** (Goldline)	**Tablets:** 100 mg	In 100s.	180
c-II **Seconal Sodium** (Lilly)	**Rectal Injection:** 50 mg per ml	In 20 ml vials.[1]	75
c-II **Secobarbital Sodium** (Wyeth)	**Injection:** 50 mg per ml	In 1 and 2 ml Tubex.[1]	395
c-II **Seconal Sodium** (Lilly)		In 20 ml vials.[1]	125

* Cost Index based on cost per 100 mg oral, 30 mg rectal or 50 mg parenteral secobarbital.
# Product identification code.
[1] With 50% polyethylene glycol and 0.25% phenol.

Complete prescribing information for these products begins on page 1398

Short-Acting (Cont.)

PENTOBARBITAL AND PENTOBARBITAL SODIUM

Indications:

Oral: Sedative or hypnotic for the short-term treatment of insomnia, since it appears to lose its effectiveness for sleep induction and maintenance after 2 weeks; may be used as preanesthetic medication.

Rectal: For sedation when oral or parenteral administration may be undesirable.

As a hypnotic, for the short-term treatment of insomnia, since the suppositories appear to lose their effectiveness for sleep induction and sleep maintenance after 2 weeks.

Parenteral: As a sedative. It may be used as a preanesthetic medication.

As a hypnotic for the short-term treatment of insomnia. Barbiturates appear to lose effectiveness for sleep induction and maintenance after 2 weeks.

Also for use as an anticonvulsant, in anesthetic doses, for the emergency control of certain acute convulsive episodes, (eg, those associated with status epilepticus, eclampsia, meningitis, tetanus and toxic reactions to strychnine or local anesthetics).

Administration and Dosage:

Oral: Adults – Daytime sedation: 20 mg, 3 or 4 times per day.

Hypnotic: 100 mg at bedtime.

Oral: Children – Preoperative sedation: 2 to 6 mg/kg/day (max. 100 mg), depending on age, weight and degree of sedation desired.

Hypnotic: Base dosage on age and weight.

Rectal: Do not divide suppositories.

Adults – 120 to 200 mg.

Children – 12 to 14 years (80 to 110 lbs) – 60 or 120 mg.

Children – 5 to 12 years (40 to 80 lbs) – 60 mg.

Children – 1 to 4 years (20 to 40 lbs) – 30 or 60 mg.

Children – 2 months to 1 year (10 to 20 lbs) – 30 mg.

Parenteral: Pentobarbital solutions are highly alkaline. Therefore, exercise extreme care to avoid perivascular extravasation or intra-arterial injection.

IV – Restrict IV use to conditions in which other routes are not feasible, including patient unconsciousness (as in cerebral hemorrhage, eclampsia or status epilepticus), because of resistance (as in delirium), or because prompt action is imperative. Slow IV injection is essential; carefully observe patients during administration. The rate of IV injection should not exceed 50 mg/min. No average IV dose can be relied upon to produce similar effects in different patients. The possibility of overdose and respiratory depression is remote when the drug is injected slowly in fractional doses. The clinical response is the basis for dosage determination, although the patient's weight and age may influence the total amount of the drug required. Watch the physical signs closely to accurately obtain and maintain the desired degree of sedation.

Initially administer 100 mg in the 70 kg adult. Reduce dosage proportionally for pediatric or debilitated patients. At least 1 minute is necessary to determine the full effect. If needed, additional small increments of the drug may be given to a total of 200 to 500 mg for normal adults.

In convulsive states, keep dosages to a minimum to avoid compounding the depression which may follow convulsions. Inject slowly with regard to the time required for the drug to penetrate the blood-brain barrier.

IM – Inject deeply into a large muscle mass. Do not exceed a volume of 5 ml at any one site because of possible tissue irritation.

Calculate dosage on basis of age, weight and the patient's condition. The usual adult dosage is 150 to 200 mg; children's dosage frequently ranges from 25 to 80 mg or 2 to 6 mg/kg as a single IM injection, not to exceed 100 mg.

Stability – Do not use if solution is discolored or contains a precipitate.

(Products listed on following page)

Short-Acting (Cont.)

PENTOBARBITAL AND PENTOBARBITAL SODIUM (Cont.)				C.I.*
c-II	**Pentobarbital Sodium** (Lannett)	**Capsules:** 50 mg	In 500s and 1000s.	9
c-II	**Nembutal Sodium** (Abbott)		(#CF). Orange and clear. In 100s, 500s and 1000s.	96
c-II	**Pentobarbital Sodium** (Various)	**Capsules:** 100 mg	In 25s, 100s, 500s and 1000s.	7+
c-II	**Nembutal Sodium** (Abbott)		Contains tartrazine. (#CH). Yellow. In 100s, 500s, 1000s, UD 100s and Display Pack 20 x 25 (500).	71
c-II	**Nembutal** (Abbott)	**Elixir:** 18.2 mg pentobarbital (equiv. to 20 mg pentobarbital sodium) per 5 ml	18% alcohol. In pt and gal.	457
c-III	**Nembutal Sodium** (Abbott)	**Suppositories:** 30 mg	In 12s.	476
		60 mg	In 12s.	250
		120 mg	In 12s.	153
		200 mg	In 12s.	113
c-II	**Pentobarbital Sodium** (Elkins-Sinn)	**Injection:** 50 mg per ml	In 2 ml Dosette vials.	240
c-II	**Pentobarbital Sodium** (Wyeth)		In 1 and 2 ml Tubex.[1]	635
c-II	**Nembutal Sodium Solution** (Abbott)		In 20 and 50 ml vials.[1]	172

* Cost Index based on cost per 100 mg oral or parenteral or 30 mg rectal pentobarbital.
# Product identification code.
[1] With propylene glycol and 10% alcohol.

Oral Combinations

Combined barbiturate products are promoted to provide a more balanced effect through the combination of those with differing rates of action and dissipation.

Consider the information given for Barbiturates on page 1398 when using these products.

			C.I.*
c-II	**Tuinal 50 mg Pulvules** (Lilly)	**Capsules:** 25 mg amobarbital sodium and 25 mg secobarbital sodium. (#Lilly F64). Blue and orange. In 100s.	50
c-II	**Tuinal 100 mg Pulvules** (Lilly)	**Capsules:** 50 mg amobarbital sodium and 50 mg secobarbital sodium. (#Lilly F65). Blue and orange. In 100s, 1000s and UD 100s and 1000s.	70
c-II	**Tuinal 200 mg Pulvules** (Lilly)	**Capsules:** 100 mg amobarbital sodium and 100 mg secobarbital sodium. (#Lilly F66). Blue and orange. In 100s, 1000s and UD 100s.	94
c-II	**Tri-Barbs** (Lannett)	**Capsules:** 32 mg phenobarbital, 32 mg butabarbital sodium and 32 mg secobarbital sodium. In 1000s.	15
c-II	**S.B.P.** (Lemmon)	**Tablets:** 15 mg phenobarbital, 30 mg butabarbital sodium and 50 mg secobarbital sodium. (#Lemmon 86/86). White, scored. In 1000s.	18

* Cost Index based on cost per capsule or tablet.
# Product identification code.

Barbiturates

Actions:

Pharmacology: The ultrashort-acting barbiturates, thiopental, thiamylal and methohexital, depress the CNS to produce hypnosis and anesthesia without analgesia. Methohexital does not possess muscle relaxant properties. These drugs are frequently used to provide hypnosis during balanced anesthesia with other agents for muscle relaxation and analgesia.

Pharmacokinetics: The rapid onset and brief duration of action of these drugs is a function of their high lipid solubility. They quickly cross the blood-brain barrier, but are rapidly redistributed from the brain to other body tissues, first to highly perfused visceral organs (liver, kidneys, heart) and muscle, and later to fatty tissues.

Administered IV as the sodium salts, these agents produce anesthesia within 1 minute. Recovery after a small dose is rapid, with somnolence and retrograde amnesia. Muscle relaxation occurs at the onset of anesthesia. The duration of anesthetic activity following a single IV dose is 20 to 30 minutes for thiopental and thiamylal and somewhat shorter for methohexital. Thiopental is readily absorbed by the rectal route when administered as a suspension; onset of action usually occurs within 8 to 10 minutes. Thiopental IV produces hypnosis within 30 to 40 seconds following administration. Repeated doses or continuous infusion of these agents causes accumulation. Slow release of the drug from lipoidal storage sites results in prolonged anesthesia, somnolence and respiratory and circulatory depression. The plasma half-life is 3 to 8 hours.

Indications:

Induction of anesthesia; supplementation of other anesthetic agents; IV anesthesia for short surgical procedures with minimal painful stimuli; induction of a hypnotic state.

Thiopental sodium for IV use is indicated for control of convulsive states, in neurosurgical patients with increased intracranial pressure if adequate ventilation is provided and for narcoanalysis and narcosynthesis in psychiatric disorders.

Thiopental sodium rectal suspension is used when preanesthetic sedation or basal narcosis by the rectal route is desired. It may be employed as the sole agent in selected brief, minor procedures where muscular relaxation and analgesia are not required.

Contraindications:

Absolute: Latent or manifest porphyria; known hypersensitivity to barbiturates; absence of suitable veins for IV administration; status asthmaticus (**thiopental**).

Relative: Severe cardiovascular disease; hypotension or shock; conditions in which hypnotic effects may be prolonged or potentiated (excessive premedication, Addison's disease, hepatic or renal dysfunction, myxedema, increased blood urea and severe anemia); increased intracranial pressure; asthma; myasthenia gravis.

If barbiturates are used in conditions involving relative contraindications, reduce dosage and administer slowly.

Do not use the rectal suspension in patients who are to undergo rectal surgery, or in the presence of inflammatory, ulcerative, bleeding or neoplastic lesions of the lower bowel.

Warnings:

Usage in status asthmaticus: Use **methohexital** and **thiamylal** with extreme caution in patients with status asthmaticus.

May be habit forming. Repeated or continuous infusion may cause cumulative effects resulting in prolonged somnolence and respiratory and circulatory depression. Resuscitative and endotracheal intubation equipment, oxygen and drugs should be immediately available. Maintain patency of the airway at all times.

Usage in Pregnancy: Category C. Safety for use during pregnancy has not been established. Use only when clearly needed and when the potential benefits outweigh the unknown potential hazards to the fetus.

Thiopental readily crosses the placental barrier.

Usage in Lactation: Small amounts of **thiopental** may appear in breast milk following administration of large doses.

Precautions:

Respiratory depression, apnea or hypotension may occur due to individual variations in tolerance or to the physical status of the patient. Exercise caution in debilitated patients, or those with impaired function of respiratory, circulatory, renal, hepatic or endocrine systems.

Extravascular injection may cause pain, swelling, ulceration and necrosis. Intra-arterial injection is dangerous and may produce gangrene of an extremity.

If evacuation of the instilled rectal dose occurs, assess the effects of any retained portion before administering a repeat dose.

(Continued on following page)

KETAMINE HCl

Warning:

Emergence reactions occur in approximately 12% of patients. The incidence is least in young (15 years of age or less) and elderly (over 65 years of age) patients. Reactions are also less frequent when the drug is given IM.

Psychological manifestations – Severity varies between pleasant dream-like states, vivid imagery, hallucinations and emergence delirium sometimes accompanied by confusion, excitement and irrational behavior. The duration is ordinarily a few hours; however, recurrences have been seen up to 24 hours postoperatively. No residual psychological effects are known.

The incidence may be reduced by using lower dosages with IV diazepam. These reactions may be reduced if verbal, tactile and visual patient stimulation is minimized during recovery. This does not preclude monitoring vital signs.

Management – To terminate a severe emergence reaction, a small hypnotic dose of a short-acting or ultrashort-acting barbiturate may be required.

When used on an outpatient basis, do not release patient until recovery from anesthesia is complete. Patients should be accompanied by an adult.

Actions:

Pharmacology: Ketamine is a rapid-acting general anesthetic producing an anesthetic state characterized by profound analgesia, normal pharyngeal-laryngeal reflexes, normal or slightly enhanced skeletal muscle tone, cardiovascular and respiratory stimulation, and occasionally, a transient and minimal respiratory depression. A patent airway is maintained partly by virtue of unimpaired pharyngeal and laryngeal reflexes.

Pharmacokinetics: Following IV administration, the ketamine concentration has an initial slope (α-phase) lasting about 45 minutes with a half-life of 10 to 15 minutes, corresponding to the anesthetic effect. The anesthetic action is terminated by redistribution from the CNS and by hepatic biotransformation. The major metabolite is about ⅓ as active as ketamine. The β-phase half-life of ketamine is 2.5 hours.

Elevation of blood pressure begins shortly after injection, reaches a maximum in minutes and returns to preanesthetic values within 15 minutes. The systolic and diastolic blood pressure peaks from 10% to 50% above preanesthetic levels.

An IV dose of 2 mg/kg (1 mg/lb) usually produces surgical anesthesia within 30 seconds after injection, lasting 5 to 10 minutes. Additional increments can be administered IV or IM to maintain anesthesia without significant cumulative effects.

Intramuscular doses of 9 to 13 mg/kg (4 to 6 mg/lb) usually produce surgical anesthesia within 3 to 4 minutes, and last approximately 12 to 25 minutes.

Indications:

Sole anesthetic agent for diagnostic and surgical procedures that do not require skeletal muscle relaxation. Ketamine is best suited for short procedures, but it can be used with additional doses for longer procedures.

For the induction of anesthesia prior to the administration of other general anesthetics.

Also used to supplement low-potency agents, such as nitrous oxide.

Contraindications:

Patients in whom a significant elevation of blood pressure would be a serious hazard.

Psychiatric disorders (schizophrenic or acute psychoses); hypersensitivity.

Warnings:

Cardiac effects: Monitor cardiac function continuously during the procedure in patients with hypertension or cardiac decompensation.

Emergence reactions and postoperative confusional states: See Warning Box.

Usage in Pregnancy: Ketamine crosses the placenta. Safety for use during pregnancy, including obstetrics, has not been established; use is not recommended.

Precautions:

In surgery or diagnostic procedures of the pharynx, larynx or bronchial tree: Because pharyngeal and laryngeal reflexes are usually active, do not administer ketamine alone. Muscle relaxants, with proper attention to respiration, may be required.

In surgical procedures involving visceral pain pathways, supplement with an agent which obtunds visceral pain.

Chronic alcoholic and the acutely alcohol intoxicated patient: Use with caution.

Cerebrospinal fluid pressure increase has been reported following administration.

Hazardous tasks: Warn patients not to drive, operate hazardous machinery or engage in hazardous activities for 24 hours or more after anesthesia.

(Continued on following page)

KETAMINE HCl (Cont.)

Drug Interactions:

Barbiturates or **narcotics:** Prolonged recovery time may occur if used with ketamine.

Halothane: Cardiac output, blood pressure and pulse rate may be decreased. Halothane blocks the cardiovascular stimulatory effects of ketamine. Closely monitor cardiac function if ketamine and halothane are used together.

Tubocurarine and **nondepolarizing muscle relaxants:** Ketamine may increase the neuromuscular effects resulting in prolonged respiratory depression.

Thyroid hormones: Concurrent use may produce hypertension and tachycardia.

Adverse Reactions:

Cardiovascular: Elevated blood pressure and pulse rate (frequent); hypotension; bradycardia; arrhythmia.

Respiration: Although respiration is frequently stimulated, severe depression of respiration or apnea may occur following rapid IV administration of high doses. Laryngospasm and other forms of airway obstruction have occurred.

Ophthalmic: Diplopia; nystagmus; slight elevation in intraocular pressure.

Psychological: (See Warning Box).

Neurological: Enhanced skeletal muscle tone manifested by tonic and clonic movements, sometimes resembling seizures.

GI: Anorexia; nausea; vomiting, hypersalivation.

General: Local pain and exanthema at the injection site (infrequent); transient erythema or morbilliform rash.

Overdosage:

Respiratory depression may occur with overdosage or too rapid a rate of administration; employ supportive ventilation. Mechanical support of respiration is preferred to administration of analeptics.

Administration and Dosage:

Individualize dosage.

Induction:

IV route – Initial dose ranges from 1 to 4.5 mg/kg (0.5 to 2 mg/lb). The average amount to produce 5 to 10 minutes of surgical anesthesia is 2 mg/kg (1 mg/lb).

Alternatively, in adults, 1 to 2 mg/kg administered at a rate of 0.5 mg/kg/min may be used for induction of anesthesia. In addition, diazepam in 2 to 5 mg doses (total: 15 mg IV or less), administered in a separate syringe over 60 seconds, may be used. This may reduce the incidence of psychological manifestations during emergence.

Administer slowly (over a period of 60 seconds). More rapid administration may result in respiratory depression and enhanced pressor response.

Note: *Do not* inject the 100 mg/ml concentration IV without proper dilution. Dilute the drug with an equal volume of Sterile Water for Injection, Normal Saline or 5% Dextrose in Water.

IM route – Initial dose ranges from 6.5 to 13 mg/kg (3 to 6 mg/lb). A dose of 10 mg/kg (5 mg/lb) will usually produce 12 to 25 minutes of surgical anesthesia.

Maintenance: Increments of one-half to the full induction dose may be repeated as needed for maintenance of anesthesia. The larger the total dose administered, the longer the time to complete recovery.

Adults induced with ketamine augmented with IV diazepam may be maintained on ketamine given by slow microdrip infusion at 0.1 to 0.5 mg/minute, augmented with 2 to 5 mg IV diazepam, given as needed. Often, 20 mg or less of IV diazepam total for combined induction and maintenance will suffice. The incidence of psychological manifestations during emergence may be reduced.

Dilution – To prepare a dilute solution containing 1 mg per ml, transfer 10 ml (50 mg per ml vial) or 5 ml (100 mg per ml vial) to 500 ml of 5% Dextrose Injection or Sodium Chloride (0.9%) Injection and mix well.

Vials of 10 mg/ml are not recommended for dilution.

If fluid restriction is required, add ketamine to a 250 ml infusion, as described above, to provide a 2 mg/ml concentration.

Compatibility: Barbiturates and ketamine are incompatible (precipitate); do not inject from the same syringe. Do not mix ketamine and diazepam in syringe or infusion flask.

Ketamine is clinically compatible with the commonly used general and local anesthetic agents when an adequate respiratory exchange is maintained.

Rx	**Ketalar** (Parke-Davis)	**Injection:** Ketamine base supplied as the HCl:	
		10 mg per ml	In 20, 25 and 50 ml vials.[1]
		50 mg per ml	In 10 ml vials.[1]
		100 mg per ml	In 5 ml vials.[1]

[1] With benzethonium chloride.

ETOMIDATE

Actions:

Etomidate, a nonbarbiturate hypnotic without analgesic activity, has fewer cardiovascular and respiratory depressant effects than thiopental sodium. Up to 0.6 mg/kg administered to patients with severe cardiovascular disease has little or no effect on myocardial metabolism, cardiac output, peripheral circulation or pulmonary circulation. The hemodynamic effects are qualitatively similar to those of thiopental sodium.

Etomidate lowers cerebral blood flow and cerebral oxygen consumption about as much as ketamine, methohexital or thiopental. Etomidate will usually lower intracranial pressure slightly and lower intraocular pressure moderately. Changes in EEG are similar to those produced by ultrashort-acting barbiturates. Reduced cortisol plasma levels have been reported with induction doses of 0.3 mg/kg and persisted for 6 to 8 hours.

Pharmacokinetics: Injection IV produces hypnosis rapidly, usually within one minute. Duration is usually 3 to 5 minutes and dissipation of effect following a single dose is a function of redistribution. The immediate recovery period will usually be shortened in adults by administration of approximately 0.1 mg of IV fentanyl, 1 or 2 minutes before induction of anesthesia, probably because less etomidate is generally required. Plasma levels required to induce anesthesia are about 2 mcg/ml, but hypnosis is maintained with concentrations $\geq$ 0.23 mcg/ml. Protein binding, primarily to albumin, is 76%.

Etomidate is rapidly metabolized in the liver. Plasma levels of unchanged drug decrease rapidly up to 30 minutes following injection and thereafter more slowly with a half-life of about 75 minutes. Approximately 75% of the dose is excreted in the urine as an inactive metabolite, 10% in bile and 13% in feces.

Indications:

Induction of general anesthesia.

Supplementation of subpotent anesthetic agents, such as nitrous oxide in oxygen, during maintenance of anesthesia for short operative procedures.

Unlabeled Use: Etomidate has been used for prolonged sedation of critically ill patients or ventilator-dependent patients; however, this use has been associated with increased risks, including acute adrenal insufficiency.

Contraindications:

Hypersensitivity to etomidate.

Warnings:

Although no changes in vital signs or increased mortality have been reported with etomidate-induced reduced plasma cortisol levels, consider exogenous corticosteroid replacement in patients undergoing severe stress.

Usage in Pregnancy: Category C. Etomidate has embryocidal effects in rats when given in doses 1 and 4 times the human dose. Reproductive studies have shown decreased survival in small animals. It has caused maternal toxicity with deaths in rats and rabbits at approximately 15 times the human dose. Use only when clearly needed and when the potential benefits outweigh the unknown potential hazards to the fetus.

Usage in Lactation: It is not known whether etomidate is excreted in breast milk. Use caution when administering to a nursing mother.

Usage in Children: Safety and efficacy for use in children less than 10 years of age have not been established. Use is not recommended.

Adverse Reactions:

Most frequent: Transient skeletal muscle movements (32%) classified as myoclonic in the majority of cases (74%); transient venous pain (20%); tonic movements (10%); eye movements (9%); averting movements (7%).

Respiratory: Hyperventilation; hypoventilation; apnea of short duration (5 to 90 seconds with spontaneous recovery); laryngospasm; hiccoughs; snoring.

Cardiovascular: Hypertension; hypotension; tachycardia; bradycardia; other arrhythmias.

GI: Postoperative nausea or vomiting following induction of anesthesia.

Administration and Dosage:

For IV use only. Individualize dosage.

Induction of anesthesia: Adults and children over 10 years, 0.2 to 0.6 mg/kg. The usual dose is 0.3 mg/kg, injected over 30 to 60 seconds.

Concomitant anesthesia: Smaller increments of etomidate may be administered to adults during short operative procedures to supplement subpotent anesthetic agents.

Premedication: Etomidate is compatible with commonly used preanesthetic medication.

Storage: Protect from freezing and extreme heat.

Rx	**Amidate** (Abbott)	**Injection:** 2 mg per ml[1]	In 10 and 20 ml amps and 20 ml Abboject.

[1] With propylene glycol.

Benzodiazepine compounds used as antianxiety agents appear on page 1255

MIDAZOLAM HCl

Warning:

Midazolam IV has been associated with respiratory depression and respiratory arrest, especially when used for conscious sedation. In some cases, where this was not recognized promptly and treated effectively, death or hypoxic encephalopathy resulted. Use midazolam IV only in hospital or ambulatory care settings, including physicians' offices, that provide for continuous monitoring of respiratory and cardiac function. Assure immediate availability of resuscitative drugs and equipment and personnel trained in their use. (See Warnings.)

The initial IV dose for conscious sedation may be as little as 1 mg, but should not exceed 2.5 mg in a normal healthy adult. Lower doses are necessary for older (over 60 years) or debilitated patients and in patients receiving concomitant narcotics or other CNS depressants. Never give the initial dose and all subsequent doses as a bolus; administer over at least 2 minutes and allow additional 2 or more minutes to fully evaluate sedative effect. Use of 1 mg/ml formulation or dilution of 1 mg/ml or 5 mg/ml formulation is recommended to facilitate slower injection. See Administration and Dosage for complete dosing information.

Actions:

Pharmacology: Midazolam is a short-acting benzodiazepine CNS depressant.

In patients without intracranial lesions, induction is associated with a moderate decrease in cerebrospinal fluid pressure, similar to thiopental. Preliminary data in intracranial surgical patients with normal intracranial pressure but decreased compliance show comparable elevations of intracranial pressure with midazolam and with thiopental during intubation.

May moderately lower intraocular pressure in patients without eye disease.

Induction doses depress the ventilatory response to carbon dioxide stimulation for 15 minutes or more beyond the duration of ventilatory depression following administration of thiopental. Impairment of ventilatory response is more marked in patients with chronic obstructive pulmonary disease (COPD). Sedation with IV midazolam does not adversely affect the mechanics of respiration; total lung capacity and peak expiratory flow decrease significantly, but static compliance and maximum expiratory flow at 50% of awake total lung capacity (V_{max}) increase.

Induction is associated with a slight to moderate decrease in mean arterial pressure, cardiac output, stroke volume and systemic vascular resistance. Slow heart rates (less than 65/minute), particularly in patients taking propranolol for angina, tend to rise slightly; faster heart rates (eg, 85/minute) tend to slow slightly.

Pharmacokinetics: Absorption/Distribution – The mean absolute bioavailability following IM use is > 90%. The mean time of maximum plasma concentrations following IM dosing occurs within 45 minutes. Peak concentrations of midazolam as well as 1-hydroxymethyl midazolam after IM administration are about one-half of those achieved after equivalent IV doses. Clinical effects do not directly correlate with blood concentrations.

Midazolam is approximately 97% plasma protein bound. It crosses the placenta and enters fetal circulation.

Metabolism/Excretion – Midazolam IV has an elimination half-life of 1.2 to 12.3 hours, a large volume of distribution (0.95 to 6.6 L/kg) and a plasma clearance of 0.15 to 0.77 L/hr/kg; less than 0.03% of the dose is excreted in the urine intact. It is rapidly metabolized to 1-hydroxymethyl midazolam, which is conjugated, with subsequent urinary excretion (45% to 57%). The metabolite elimination half-life is similar to that of the parent compound. The concentration of midazolam is 10-fold to 30-fold greater than that of 1-hydroxymethyl midazolam after single IV administration.

A small group of patients with congestive heart failure (CHF), appeared to have a twofold to threefold increase in the elimination half-life and volume of distribution; however, total body clearance appeared unchanged. There was no apparent change in the pharmacokinetics (IV) in patients with hepatic dysfunction. There was a 1.5-fold to 2-fold increase in elimination half-life, total body clearance and volume of distribution in patients with chronic renal failure.

Onset/Duration – Onset of sedation (IM) was 15 min.; peak sedation, 30 to 60 min.

Sedation after IV injection was achieved within 3 to 5 minutes. In the endoscopy studies, 71% of patients had no recall of introduction of the endoscope; 82% of patients had no recall of withdrawal of the endoscope.

When given IV, induction of anesthesia occurs in ≈1.5 minutes when narcotic premedication has been administered and in 2 to 2.5 minutes without narcotic or with sedative premedication. Some memory impairment was noted in 90% of the patients.

Midazolam does not delay awakening from general anesthesia, which usually occurs within 2 hours but may take up to 6 hours.

(Continued on following page)

PROPOFOL (Cont.)

Actions (Cont.):

The pharmacokinetics of propofol do not appear to be altered by gender, chronic hepatic cirrhosis or chronic renal failure. With increasing age, the clearance of propofol decreases from a mean of 1.8 ± 0.4 L/min in young (18 to 35 years) patients to 1.4 ± 0.4 L/min in elderly (65 to 80 years) patients. When given by an infusion for up to 2 hours, the pharmacokinetics of propofol appear to be independent of dose (0.05 to 0.15 mg/kg/min) and similar to IV bolus pharmacokinetics. The steady-state propofol blood concentrations are proportional to the rate of administration.

Indications:

Induction or maintenance of anesthesia as part of a balanced anesthetic technique for inpatient and outpatient surgery.

Contraindications:

When general anesthesia is contraindicated; hypersensitivity to propofol or its components.

Warnings:

Only persons trained in the administration of general anesthesia should administer propofol. Facilities for maintenance of a patent airway, artificial ventilation, and oxygen enrichment and circulatory resuscitation must be immediately available.

Do not coadminister through the same IV catheter with blood or plasma because compatibility has not been established. In vitro, aggregates of the globular component of the emulsion vehicle have occurred with blood/plasma/serum from humans and animals. The clinical significance is not known.

Neurosurgical Anesthesia: Propofol decreases cerebral blood flow, cerebral metabolic oxygen consumption and intracranial pressure, and increases cerebrovascular resistance. Propofol does not seem to affect cerebrovascular reactivity to changes in arterial carbon dioxide tension. Despite these findings, propofol is not recommended for use at this time in patients with increased intracranial pressure or impaired cerebral circulation because it may cause substantial decreases in mean arterial pressure, and consequently, substantial decreases in cerebral perfusion pressure. Further studies are needed to substantiate what happens to intracranial pressure following propofol when decreases in mean arterial and cerebral perfusion pressures are prevented by appropriate measures.

Pregnancy: Category B – Propofol causes maternal deaths in rats and rabbits and decreased pup survival during the lactating period in animals treated with 15 mg/kg/day (or 6 times the recommended human induction dose). The pharmacological activity (anesthesia) of the drug on the mother is probably responsible for the adverse effects seen in the offspring. There are, however, no adequate and well controlled studies in pregnant women. Use during pregnancy only if clearly needed.

Labor and Delivery: Not recommended for obstetrics, including cesarean section deliveries, because there are insufficient data to support its safety to the fetus.

Lactation: Not recommended for use in nursing mothers because propofol is excreted in breast milk and the effects of oral absorption of small amounts of propofol are not known.

Children: Not recommended for use in pediatric patients because safety and efficacy have not been established.

Precautions:

Use a lower induction dose and a slower maintenance rate of administration in elderly, debilitated or patients with circulatory disorders, and those rated ASA III or IV (see Administration and Dosage). Continuously monitor patients for early signs of significant hypotension or bradycardia. Treatment may include increasing the rate of IV fluid, elevation of lower extremities, use of pressor agents or administration of atropine. Apnea often occurs during induction and may persist for > 60 seconds. Ventilatory support may be required. Because propofol is an emulsion, use caution in patients with lipid metabolism disorders (eg, primary hyperlipoproteinemia, diabetic hyperlipemia, pancreatitis).

Since propofol is never used alone, an adequate period of evaluation of the awakened patient is indicated to ensure satisfactory recovery from general anesthesia prior to discharge of the patient from the recovery room or to home.

Transient local pain may occur during IV injection, which may be reduced by prior injection of IV lidocaine (1 ml of a 1% solution). Venous sequelae (phlebitis or thrombosis) have occurred rarely (< 1%). In two well controlled clinical studies using dedicated IV catheters, no instances of venous sequelae were reported up to 14 days following induction. Pain can be minimized if the larger veins of the forearm or antecubital fossa are used. Accidental clinical extravasation and intentional injection into SC or perivascular tissues of animals caused minimal tissue reaction. Intra-arterial injection in animals did not induce local tissue effects. One accidental intra-arterial injection has been reported in a patient, and other than pain, there were no major sequelae.

(Precautions continued on following page)

PROPOFOL (Cont.)

Precautions (Cont.):

Perioperative myoclonia, rarely including opisthotonus, has occurred in a temporal relationship in cases in which propofol has been administered.

Rarely, a clinical syndrome which may include bronchospasm and erythema accompanied by hypotension has occurred shortly after the administration of propofol, although the use of other drugs in most instances makes the relationship to propofol unclear.

Drug Interactions:

CNS depressants (eg, hypnotics/sedatives, inhalational anesthetics, narcotics) can increase the CNS depression induced by propofol. Morphine premedication with nitrous oxide decreases the necessary propofol maintenance infusion rate and therapeutic blood concentrations when compared to nonnarcotic (lorazepam) premedication. In addition, the induction dose requirements of propofol may be reduced in patients with IM or IV premedication, particularly with narcotics alone or in combination with sedatives. These agents may increase the anesthetic effects of propofol and may also result in more pronounced decreases in systolic, diastolic and mean arterial pressures and cardiac output.

Adverse Reactions:

The following estimates of adverse events for propofol are derived from reports of 1573 patients. These studies were conducted using a variety of premedicants, varying lengths of surgical procedures and various other anesthetic agents. Most adverse events were mild and transient.

Incidence > 1%:

Body as a whole: Fever (1% to 3%).

Cardiovascular: Hypotension (3% to 10%; see also Pharmacology); bradycardia, hypertension (1% to 3%).

CNS: Movement (3% to 10%); headache, dizziness, twitching, bucking/jerking/thrashing, clonic/myoclonic movement (1% to 3%).

Digestive: Nausea (≥ 10%); vomiting (3% to 10%); abdominal cramping (1% to 3%).

Injection site: Burning/stinging, pain (≥ 10%); tingling/numbness, coldness (1% to 3%).

Respiratory: Cough, hiccough, apnea (1% to 3%; see also Pharmacology).

Skin: Flushing (1% to 3%).

Incidence < 1%:

Body as a whole: Pain in extremities; chest pain; neck stiffness; trunk pain.

Cardiovascular: Tachycardia; premature ventricular and atrial contractions; syncope; abnormal ECG; ST segment depression.

CNS: Shivering; somnolence; hypertonia/dystonia; paresthesia; tremor; abnormal dreams; agitation; confusion; delirium; euphoria; fatigue; moaning; rigidity.

Digestive: Hypersalivation; dry mouth; swallowing.

Injection site: Discomfort; phlebitis; hives/itching; redness/discoloration.

Musculoskeletal: Myalgia.

Respiratory: Upper airway obstruction; bronchospasm; dyspnea; wheezing; hypoventilation; burning in throat; sneezing; tachypnea; hyperventilation; hypoxia.

Skin and appendages: Rash; urticaria.

Special senses: Amblyopia; diplopia; eye pain; taste perversion; tinnitus.

Urogenital: Urine retention; green urine.

Causal relationship unknown:

Cardiovascular: Arrhythmia; bigeminy; edema; ventricular fibrillation; heart block; myocardial ischemia.

CNS: Anxiety; emotional lability; depression; hysteria; insomnia; generalized and localized seizures; opisthotonus.

Respiratory: Laryngospasm.

Skin and appendages: Diaphoresis; pruritus; conjunctival hyperemia.

Special senses: Ear pain; nystagmus.

Miscellaneous: Abnormal urine; diarrhea; laryngospasm.

(Continued on following page)

PROPOFOL (Cont.)

Overdosage:

If accidental overdosage occurs discontinue propofol immediately. Overdosage is likely to cause cardiorespiratory depression. Treat respiratory depression by artificial ventilation with oxygen. Cardiovascular depression may require raising the patient's legs, increasing the flow rate of IV fluids and administering pressor agents or anticholinergic agents. Refer to General Management of Acute Overdosage on p. 2895

Administration and Dosage:

Induction: Individualize dosage and titrate to desired effect according to patient's age and clinical status. Most adults < 55 years of age and classified ASA I and II are likely to need 2 to 2.5 mg/kg of propofol for induction when unpremedicated or when premedicated with oral benzodiazepines or IM narcotics. For induction, titrate (≈ 40 mg every 10 sec) against the response of the patient until clinical signs show the onset of anesthesia.

It is important to be familiar and experienced with the IV use of propofol before treating elderly, debilitated, hypovolemic patients or those in ASA Physical Status Classes III or IV. These patients may be more sensitive to the effects of propofol; therefore, decrease the dosage in these patients by approximately 50% (20 mg every 10 seconds) according to their conditions and responses (see Precautions and Dosage Guide).

Additionally, as with most anesthetic agents, the effects of propofol may be increased in patients who have received IV sedative or narcotic premedications shortly prior to induction.

Maintenance: Anesthesia can be maintained by administering propofol by infusion or intermittent IV bolus injection. The patient's clinical response will determine the infusion rate or the amount and frequency of incremental injections.

When administering propofol by infusion, it is recommended that drop counters, syringe pumps or volumetric pumps be used to provide controlled infusion rates.

Continous infusion: Propofol 0.1 to 0.2 mg/kg/min administered in a variable rate infusion with 60% to 70% nitrous oxide and oxygen provides anesthesia for patients undergoing general surgery. Maintenance by infusion of propofol should immediately follow the induction dose in order to provide satisfactory or continuous anesthesia during the induction phase. During this initial period following the induction injection higher rates of infusion are generally required (0.15 to 0.2 mg/kg/min) for the first 10 to 15 minutes. Subsequently decrease infusion rates by 30% to 50% during the first half-hour of maintenance. Changes in vital signs (increases in pulse rate, blood pressure, sweating or tearing) that indicate a response to surgical stimulation or lightening of anesthesia may be controlled by the administration of propofol 25 mg (2.5 ml) or 50 mg (5 ml) incremental boluses or by increasing the infusion rate. If vital sign changes are not controlled after a 5 minute period initiate other means such as a narcotic, barbiturate, vasodilator or inhalation agent therapy to control these responses.

For minor surgical procedures (ie, body surface) 60% to 70% nitrous oxide can be combined with a variable rate propofol infusion to provide satisfactory anesthesia. With more stimulating surgical procedures (ie, intra-abdominal), consider supplementation with analgesic agents to provide a satisfactory anesthetic and recovery profile.

Always titrate infusion rates downward in the absence of clinical signs of light anesthesia until a mild response to surgical stimulation is obtained in order to avoid administration of propofol at rates higher than are clinically necessary. Generally, achieve rates of 0.05 to 0.1 mg/kg/min during maintenance in order to optimize recovery times.

Intermittent bolus: Increments of propofol 25 mg (2.5 ml) or 50 mg (5 ml) may be administered with nitrous oxide in patients undergoing general surgery. Administer the incremental boluses when changes in vital signs indicate a response to surgical stimulation or light anesthesia.

Propofol Dosage Guide

Indication	Dosage and Administration
Induction	Individualize dosage. *Adults:* Likely to require 2 to 2.5 mg/kg (approximately 40 mg every 10 seconds until induction onset). *Elderly, debilitated, hypovolemic or ASA III or IV patients:* Likely to require 1 to 1.5 mg/kg (approximately 20 mg every 10 seconds until induction onset).
Maintenance Infusion	*Variable rate infusion:* Titrated to the desired clinical effect. *Adults:* Generally 0.1 to 0.2 mg/kg/min (6 to 12 mg/kg/h). *Elderly, debilitated, hypovolemic or ASA III or IV patients:* Generally 0.05 to 0.1 mg/kg/min (3 to 6 mg/kg/h).
Intermittent Bolus	Increments of 25 mg to 50 mg, as needed.

(Administration and Dosage continued on following page)

PROPOFOL (Cont.)

Administration and Dosage (Cont.):

Concomitant therapy: Propofol has been used with a variety of agents commonly used in anesthesia such as atropine, scopolamine, glycopyrrolate, diazepam, depolarizing and nondepolarizing muscle relaxants and narcotic analgesics, as well as with inhalational and regional anesthetic agents. (See also Drug Interactions.)

Admixture compatibility and stability: Propofol should not be mixed with other therapeutic agents prior to administration.

Dilution prior to administration: Only dilute with 5% Dextrose Injection, USP and do not dilute to a concentration < 2 mg/ml because it is an emulsion. In diluted form it is more stable when in contact with glass than with plastic (95% potency after 2 hours of running infusion in plastic).

Administration into a running IV catheter: Compatibility of propofol with the coadministration of blood/serum/plasma has not been established. (See Warnings.) Propofol is compatible with the following IV fluids when administered into a running IV catheter: 5% Dextrose Injection, USP; Lactated Ringers Injection, USP; Lactated Ringers and 5% Dextrose Injection; 5% Dextrose and 0.45% Sodium Chloride Injection, USP; 5% Dextrose and 0.2% Sodium Chloride Injection, USP.

Storage/Stability: Do not use if there is evidence of separation of the phases of the emulsion.

Discard any unused portions of propofol or solutions containing propofol at the end of the surgical procedure.

Store below 22°C (72° F). Do not store below 4°C (40° F). Refrigeration is not recommended. Protect from light. Shake well before use.

Rx	**Diprivan** (ICI)	**Injection:** 10 mg/ml	In 20 ml amps.[1]

[1] With 100 mg/ml soybean oil, 22.5 mg/ml glycerol and 12 mg/ml egg lecithin.

DROPERIDOL

Actions:

Pharmacology: Droperidol, a butyrophenone derivative, produces marked tranquilization, sedation and an antiemetic effect. It also produces mild alpha-adrenergic blockade, peripheral vascular dilatation and reduction of the pressor effect of epinephrine, resulting in hypotension and decreased peripheral vascular resistance. It may decrease pulmonary arterial pressure (particularly if it is abnormally high). It may reduce the incidence of epinephrine-induced arrhythmias, but it does not prevent other cardiac arrhythmias.

Pharmacokinetics: The onset of action occurs in 3 to 10 minutes following IV or IM administration. The full effect may not be apparent for 30 minutes. The duration of the sedative and tranquilizing effect is generally 2 to 4 hours. Alteration of consciousness may persist as long as 12 hours. Droperidol is metabolized in the liver and is excreted in the urine and feces. Approximately 1% is excreted unchanged in the urine. Terminal half-life averages 2.2 hours.

Indications:

To produce tranquilization and reduce the incidence of nausea and vomiting in surgical and diagnostic procedures.

Premedication, induction and as an adjunct in the maintenance of general and regional anesthesia.

Neuroleptanalgesia, in which droperidol is given concurrently with a narcotic analgesic (eg, fentanyl), to aid in producing tranquility and decreasing anxiety and pain.

Unlabeled use: Droperidol has been used as an IV antiemetic in cancer chemotherapy.

Contraindications:

Hypersensitivity to droperidol.

Warnings:

Concomitant narcotic analgesic therapy: If administered with a narcotic analgesic such as fentanyl, be familiar with the special properties of each drug, particularly the widely differing durations of action. In addition, when such a combination is used, resuscitative equipment and a narcotic antagonist should be readily available to manage apnea.

Hepatic and renal function impairment: Administer with caution because of the importance of these organs in the metabolism and excretion of drugs.

Elderly, debilitated and other poor risk patients: Reduce the initial dose of droperidol. Consider the effect of the initial dose in determining incremental doses.

Pregnancy: Category C. There are no adequate and well controlled studies in pregnant women. Use only when clearly needed or when the potential benefit justifies the potential risk to the fetus. Droperidol administered IV has caused a slight increase in newborn rat mortality at 4.4 times the upper human dose. Following IM administration, increased mortality of the offspring at 1.8 times the upper human dose is attributed to CNS depression in the dams. Droperidol has not been teratogenic in animals.

Labor and delivery: Droperidol has been used to promote analgesia for cesarean section patients without respiratory effects in the neonate. Placental transfer is slow. The drug has been used as a continuous IV infusion for hyperemesis gravidarum during the 2nd and 3rd trimesters without apparent fetal harm.

Lactation: It is not known whether droperidol is excreted in breast milk. Exercise caution when administering to a nursing mother.

Children: Safety and efficacy for use in children $<$ 2 years of age have not been established.

Precautions:

Hypotension: If hypotension occurs, consider the possibility of hypovolemia and manage with appropriate parenteral fluid therapy. Reposition patient to improve venous return to the heart when operative conditions permit. In spinal and peridural anesthesia, tilting the patient into a head down position may result in a higher level of anesthesia than desired, and impair venous return to the heart. Exercise care in moving and positioning patients because of the possibility of orthostatic hypotension. If volume expansion with fluids plus other countermeasures do not correct the hypotension, use pressor agents other than epinephrine. Epinephrine may paradoxically decrease the blood pressure in patients treated with droperidol due to the α-adrenergic blocking action of droperidol. Droperidol may also decrease pulmonary arterial pressure.

EEG: When the EEG is used for postoperative monitoring, the EEG pattern may slowly return to normal.

(Continued on following page)

DROPERIDOL (Cont.)

Drug Interactions:

Anesthesia: Certain forms of conduction anesthesia (eg, spinal anesthesia and some peridural anesthetics) can cause peripheral vasodilatation and hypotension because of sympathetic blockade. Droperidol can also alter circulation through other mechanisms.

CNS depressants (eg, **antidepressants, barbiturates)** have additive or potentiating CNS effects with droperidol; thus, the dose of droperidol required will be less than usual. Likewise, following the administration of droperidol, reduce the dose of other CNS depressant drugs.

Adverse Reactions:

Most common: Postoperative drowsiness. Mild to moderate hypotension and occasionally tachycardia usually subside without treatment. If hypotension is severe or persists, consider hypovolemia and manage with appropriate parenteral therapy.

Extrapyramidal symptoms (dystonia, akathisia and oculogyric crisis) occur in about 1% of patients. Restlessness, hyperactivity and anxiety which can be the result of inadequate dosage or a part of the symptom complex of akathisia may occur. When these occur, they can usually be controlled with antiparkinson agents.

Respiratory depression: When droperidol is used with a narcotic analgesic such as fentanyl, respiratory depression, apnea and muscular rigidity can occur; if these remain untreated, respiratory arrest could occur.

Elevated blood pressure, with or without preexisting hypertension, has occurred following use of droperidol combined with fentanyl or other parenteral analgesics. This may be due to unexplained alterations in sympathetic activity following large doses; it is also frequently attributed to anesthetic or surgical stimulation during light anesthesia.

Other: Dizziness; chills or shivering; laryngospasm; bronchospasm; postoperative hallucinatory episodes (sometimes associated with transient mental depression).

Overdosage:

Symptoms: Extension of pharmacologic actions (eg, sedation, hypotension).

Treatment: In the presence of hypoventilation or apnea, administer oxygen and assist or control respiration as indicated. Maintain a patent airway. Observe the patient for 24 hours; maintain body warmth and fluid intake. If hypotension occurs and is severe or persists, consider hypovolemia and manage with parenteral fluid therapy. Refer to General Management of Acute Overdosage.

Administration and Dosage:

Individualize dosage. Monitor vital signs routinely.

Adults: Premedication – 2.5 to 10 mg IM 30 to 60 minutes preoperatively.

Adjunct to general anesthesia – Induction: 2.5 mg/9 to 11 kg (20 to 25 lb) usually IV with an analgesic or general anesthetic. Smaller doses may be adequate. Titrate total amount. *Maintenance:* 1.25 to 2.5 mg (usually IV).

If fentanyl plus droperidol *(Innovar)* injection is administered with droperidol, consider the amount of droperidol in the injection when calculating the recommended dose.

Use without a general anesthetic in diagnostic procedures – 2.5 to 10 mg IM 30 to 60 minutes before the procedure. Additional 1.25 to 2.5 mg amounts may be administered (usually IV). When droperidol is used in procedures such as bronchoscopy, appropriate topical anesthesia is still necessary.

Adjunct to regional anesthesia – 2.5 to 5 mg IM or slowly IV.

Children (2 to 12 years) – For premedication or induction of anesthesia, reduced dose as low as 1 to 1.5 mg/9 to 11 kg (20 to 25 lb) is recommended.

Stability: Stable in 5% Dextrose Injection, 0.9% Sodium Chloride Injection and Lactated Ringers' Injection for 7 to 10 days in glass bottles and for 7 days in polyvinyl chloride bags (only for the 5% Dextrose Injection and 0.9% Sodium Chloride Injection) all at a concentration of 20 mcg/ml (1 mg/50 ml).

Admixtures: Droperidol in a concentration of 2.5 mg/ml is physically compatible for at least 15 minutes with the following admixed in a syringe: Atropine sulfate, butorphanol tartrate, chlorpromazine HCl, diphenhydramine HCl, fentanyl citrate, glycopyrrolate, hydroxyzine HCl, meperidine HCl, morphine sulfate, perphenazine, promazine HCl, promethazine HCl, scopolamine HBr. Precipitation occurs if mixed with barbiturates.

				C.I.*
Rx	**Droperidol** (Various, eg, American Regent Labs, Astra, DuPont, Lyphomed, Quad, Solopak, VHA Supply)	**Injection:** 2.5 mg per ml	In 2, 5 and 10 ml vials.	475+
Rx	**Inapsine** (Janssen Pharm.)		In 1, 2 & 5 ml amps & 10 ml vials.[1]	612

* Cost Index based on cost per 2.5 mg.

[1] With methyl and propyl parabens.

FENTANYL CITRATE AND DROPERIDOL

Actions:

A combination containing a narcotic analgesic, fentanyl, and a neuroleptic (major tranquilizer), droperidol (see individual monographs). The combined effect, sometimes referred to as neuroleptanalgesia, is characterized by general quiescence, reduced motor activity and profound analgesia; complete loss of consciousness usually does not occur from use of this combination alone.

Indications:

To produce tranquilization and analgesia for surgical and diagnostic procedures. It may be used as an anesthetic premedication, for the induction of anesthesia and as an adjunct in the maintenance of general and regional anesthesia.

Dosage:

Varies depending upon application and patient. Consult package literature.

c-II	**Fentanyl Citrate and Droperidol** (Astra)	**Injection:** 0.05 mg fentanyl (as citrate) and 2.5 mg droperidol per ml	In 2 and 5 ml amps and vials.
c-II	**Innovar** (Janssen Pharmaceutica)	**Injection:** 0.05 mg fentanyl (as citrate) and 2.5 mg droperidol per ml	In 2 and 5 ml amps.

ATROPINE SULFATE AND MEPERIDINE HCl

Actions:

A combination containing a belladonna alkaloid, atropine, and a synthetic narcotic analgesic, meperidine (see individual monographs).

Indications:

For preoperative sedation and antisecretory effect.

Dosage:

Administer the appropriate dose, IM, 30 to 90 minutes prior to beginning anesthesia.

c-II	**Atropine and Demerol** (Winthrop Pharm.)	**Injection:** 0.4 mg atropine sulfate and 50 mg meperidine HCl per ml[1]	In 1 ml fill in 2 ml Carpuject.
		0.4 mg atropine sulfate and 75 mg meperidine HCl per ml[1]	In 1 ml fill in 2 ml Carpuject.

ATROPINE SULFATE AND MORPHINE SULFATE

Actions:

A combination containing a belladonna alkaloid, atropine, and a narcotic analgesic, morphine (see individual monographs).

Indications:

For preoperative sedation and antisecretory effect.

Dosage:

Give 0.25 to 2 ml SC, IM or IV, as condition demands.

c-II	**Morphine and Atropine Sulfates** (Beecham Labs)	**Injection:** 0.4 mg atropine sulfate and 16 mg morphine sulfate per ml[2]	In 30 ml vials.

[1] With 1.5 mg sodium metabisulfite and 5 mg phenol.
[2] With 0.5% chlorobutanol.

Gases

The information on General Anesthetic Gases is not intended to supply complete information on actions, uses, cautions and contraindications. Recommended uses and product availability are given. Consult detailed literature before using. These agents should be administered only by those with appropriate training and experience.

NITROUS OXIDE (N_2O)

The most commonly used anesthetic gas, nitrous oxide is a weak anesthetic usually used in combination with other anesthetics. It does not cause skeletal muscle relaxation. The chief danger in the use of nitrous oxide is hypoxia; at least 20% oxygen should be used. An increased risk of renal and hepatic diseases and peripheral neuropathy have been reported in dental personnel who work in areas where nitrous oxide is used.

The gas can diffuse into air-containing cavities faster than nitrogen can leave, causing potentially dangerous pressure accumulation (eg, middle ear abnormalities, bowel obstruction, pneumothorax). Nitrous oxide also oxidizes and inactivates vitamin B_{12}, thus affecting some enzymes. This action may be linked to observations of adversely affected hematological, immune, neurological and reproductive systems.

In high concentrations, nitrous oxide may cause vomiting, respiratory depression and death. A primary advantage of nitrous oxide is that it is nonexplosive.

Abuse and dependence have been documented, with speculation that interaction with the endogenous opioid system may be involved.

Malignant hyperthermia may be triggered by most of the potent, fat-soluble, inhalational anesthetics and by many skeletal muscle relaxants, especially when used concurrently. Monitor the patient closely; dantrolene (page 1531) has been used as prophylaxis and treatment.

Supplied in blue cylinders.

CYCLOPROPANE

An anesthetic gas with a rapid onset of action. May be used for analgesia and induction and maintenance of anesthesia. Produces skeletal muscle relaxation in full anesthetic doses. Administer in a closed system with oxygen. Disadvantages include difficulty in detection of planes of anesthesia, occasional laryngospasm and cardiac arrhythmias. Postanesthetic nausea, vomiting and headache are frequent.

Malignant hyperthermia may be triggered by most of the potent, fat-soluble, inhalational anesthetics and by many skeletal muscle relaxants, especially when used concurrently. Monitor the patient closely; dantrolene (page 1531) has been used as prophylaxis and treatment.

Caution: Cyclopropane/oxygen mixtures are EXPLOSIVE. Due to this undesirable property, cyclopropane is rarely used.

Supplied in orange cylinders.

ETHYLENE

An anesthetic gas with rapid onset and recovery. Provides adequate analgesia but has poor muscle relaxation properties. Must be administered in high (80%) concentrations with oxygen (20%). Advantages include minimal bronchospasm and laryngospasm and minimal postanesthetic vomiting. Ethylene is nontoxic; hypoxia is the primary complication.

*Caution:*Ethylene/oxygen mixtures are flammable and EXPLOSIVE. Due to this undesirable property, ethylene is rarely used.

Supplied in red cylinders.

Anticonvulsants: Indications and Pharmacokinetics

	Drug	Labeled indications	Protein binding (%)	Metabolism/ Excretion	t½ (hrs)	Therapeutic serum levels (mcg/ml)
Barbiturates	Phenobarbital[1] (PB)	Status epilepticus Epilepsy, all forms Tonic-clonic	40-60	Liver; 25% eliminated unchanged in urine	53-140	15-40
Hydantoins	Phenytoin	Tonic-clonic Psychomotor	≈ 90	Liver; renal excretion. < 5% excreted unchanged	Dose-dependent[2]	5-20
	Mephenytoin	Tonic-clonic Psychomotor Focal Jacksonian	nd	Liver	95 (active metabolite)	nd
	Ethotoin	Tonic-clonic Psychomotor	nd	Liver; renal excretion of metabolites	3-9[3]	15-50
Succinimides	Ethosuximide	Absence	0	Liver; 25% excreted unchanged in urine	30 (children 7-9 yrs) 40-60 (adults)	40-100
	Methsuximide	Absence	nd	Liver; < 1% excreted unchanged in urine	< 2 (40, active metabolite)	nd
	Phensuximide	Absence	nd	Urine, bile	8 (active metabolite)	nd
Oxazolidinediones	Paramethadione	Absence	nd	Demethylated to active metabolite; excreted in urine	nd	nd
	Trimethadione	Absence	0	Demethylated to dimethadione; 3% excreted unchanged	6-13 days (dimethadione)	≥ 700 (dimethadione)
Benzodiazepines	Clonazepam	Absence Myoclonic Akinetic	50-85	5 metabolites identified; urine is major route of excretion	18-60	20-80 ng/ml
	Clorazepate	Partial[4]	97	Hydrolyzed in stomach to desmethyldiazepam (active); metabolized in liver and renally excreted	30-100	nd
	Diazepam	Status epilepticus[4] Epilepsy, all forms[4]	97-99	Liver, active metabolites	20-50	nd
Miscellaneous	Primidone	Tonic-clonic Psychomotor Focal	20-25	Metabolized to PB and PEMA, both active	5-15 (primidone) 10-18 (PEMA) 53-140 (PB)	5-12 (primidone) 15-40 (PB)
	Valproic acid	Absence	80-94	Liver; excreted in urine	5-20	50-150
	Carbamazepine	Tonic-clonic Mixed Psychomotor	≈ 75	Liver to active 10, 11-epoxide. 72% excreted in urine, 28% in feces	18-54 (initial) 10-20[5] ≈ 6 (10, 11-epoxide)	4-12
	Phenacemide	Severe mixed psychomotor	nd	Liver	nd	nd

[1] Other barbiturates are also used as anticonvulsants. See Sedatives/Hypnotics section.
[2] Exhibits dose-dependent, nonlinear pharmacokinetics.
[3] Below 8 mcg/ml; > 8 mcg/ml, t½ not defined due to dose-dependent, nonlinear pharmacokinetics.
[4] Recommended for adjunctive use.
[5] Undergoes autoinduction. Half-life after repeated doses.

Actions:

Pharmacology: The primary site of action of the hydantoins appears to be the motor cortex, where the spread of seizure activity is inhibited. Possibly by promoting sodium efflux from neurons, hydantoins tend to stabilize the threshold against hyperexcitability caused by excessive stimulation or environmental changes capable of reducing membrane sodium gradient. This includes the reduction of post-tetanic potentiation at synapses. Loss of posttetanic potentiation prevents cortical seizure foci from detonating adjacent cortical areas. Hydantoins reduce the maximal activity of brain stem centers responsible for the tonic phase of grand mal seizures.

Phenytoin is available as phenytoin acid (chewable tablets, suspension) or phenytoin sodium (capsules, injection); phenytoin sodium contains 92% phenytoin.

Pharmacokinetics: Absorption/Distribution – Phenytoin is slowly absorbed from the small intestine. Rate and extent of absorption varies and is dependent on the product formulation. Bioavailability may differ among products of different manufacturers. Oral phenytoin sodium extended reaches peak plasma levels in 12 hours; phenytoin sodium prompt peaks within 1.5 to 3 hours. Administration IM results in precipitation of phenytoin at the injection site, resulting in slow and erratic absorption, which may continue for up to 5 days or more; 50% to 75% of an IM dose is absorbed within 24 hours. Plasma levels vary and are significantly lower than those achieved with an equal oral dose. Plasma protein binding is 87% to 93% and is lower in uremic patients and neonates. Volume of distribution averages 0.6 L/kg.

The therapeutic plasma concentration for phenytoin is 10 to 20 mcg/ml, although many patients achieve complete seizure control at lower serum concentrations. At plasma concentrations > 20 mcg/ml, far-lateral nystagmus may occur and at concentrations > 30 and 40 mcg/ml, ataxia and gross mental changes are usually seen.

Metabolism/Excretion – Phenytoin is metabolized in the liver to inactive hydroxylated metabolites and excreted in the urine by tubular secretion. The metabolism of phenytoin is capacity-limited and shows saturability. The major metabolite is 5-(p-hydroxyphenyl)-5-phenylhydantoin (p-HPPH); 1% to 5% is excreted unchanged. Because the elimination of p-HPPH glucuronide is rate-limited by its formation from phenytoin, measurement of the metabolite in urine can be used to assess the rate of phenytoin metabolism, patient compliance or bioavailability. Elimination is exponential (first-order) at plasma concentrations < 10 mcg/ml, and plasma half-life ranges from 6 to 24 hours. Dose-dependent elimination is apparent at higher concentrations, and half-life increases; values of 20 to 60 hours may be found at therapeutic levels. A genetically determined limitation in ability to metabolize phenytoin has been noted. Good correlation is generally observed between total concentration of phenytoin in plasma and therapeutic effects. Serum level monitoring is essential.

Ethotoin is fairly rapidly absorbed. The drug exhibits saturable metabolism with respect to the formation of N-deethyl and p-hydroxyl-ethotoin, the major metabolites. The drug is apparently biotransformed by the liver. Where plasma concentrations are below about 8 mcg/ml, the elimination half-life of ethotoin is in the range of 3 to 9 hours. Experience suggests that therapeutic plasma concentrations fall in the range of 15 to 50 mcg/ml.

Indications:

Control of grand mal and psychomotor seizures.

Phenytoin: Prevention and treatment of seizures occurring during or following neurosurgery.

Parenteral: For the control of status epilepticus of the grand mal type.

Mephenytoin: For patients refractory to less toxic anticonvulsants; focal and Jacksonian seizures.

Unlabeled uses: Phenytoin is useful as an antiarrhythmic agent, particularly in cardiac glycoside-induced arrhythmias. (Oral loading dose = 14 mg/kg; oral maintenance = 200 to 400 mg/day. IV loading dose = 50 mg every 5 minutes to total dose of 1 g; IV maintenance dose = 200 to 400 mg/day.) Pharmacokinetic, electrophysiologic and ECG effects of phenytoin are summarized in the Antiarrhythmic Agents monograph.

Phenytoin has been used as an alternative to magnesium sulfate for severe preeclampsia (15 mg/kg IV, given as 10 mg/kg initially and 5 mg/kg 2 hours later).

Phenytoin has been used in the treatment of trigeminal neuralgia (tic douloureux), recessive dystrophic epidermolysis bullosa and junctional epidermolysis bullosa.

Contraindications:

Hypersensitivity to hydantoins.

Ethotoin: Hepatic abnormalities or hematologic disorders.

Phenytoin: Because of its effect on ventricular automaticity, do not use phenytoin in sinus bradycardia, sino-atrial block, second and third degree AV block or in patients with Adams-Stokes syndrome.

(Continued on following page)

Hydantoins (Cont.)

Warnings:

Abrupt withdrawal of hydantoins in epileptic patients may precipitate status epilepticus. Reduce dosage, discontinue or substitute other anticonvulsant medication gradually.

Other seizures: Hydantoins are not indicated in seizures due to hypoglycemia or other metabolic causes. Perform appropriate diagnostic procedures.

Mephenytoin: Use only if safer anticonvulsants have failed after an adequate trial.

Phenytoin: Use with caution in hypotension and severe myocardial insufficiency.

Hepatic effects: Impairment – Biotransformation of hydantoins occurs in the liver; elderly patients or those with impaired liver function or severe illness may show early signs of toxicity. Discontinue drug if hepatic dysfunction occurs.

Induced abnormalities – Phenytoin-induced hepatitis is one of the more commonly reported hypersensitivity syndromes.

Pregnancy: Refer to information for use during pregnancy in the Anticonvulsant introduction. If megaloblastic anemia occurs during gestation, consider folic acid therapy.

Lactation: These drugs are excreted in breast milk. Because of the potential for serious adverse reactions in nursing infants, decide whether to discontinue nursing or to discontinue the drug.

Precautions:

Hematologic effects: Perform blood counts and urinalyses when therapy is begun and at monthly intervals for several months thereafter. Blood dyscrasias have occurred. Avoid use in combination with other drugs known to adversely affect the hematopoietic system. Be alert for general malaise, sore throat, fever, mucous membrane bleeding, glandular swelling, petechiae, epistaxis, easy bruising, cutaneous reactions and other symptoms indicative of blood dyscrasias. Signs of marked depression of the blood count indicate the need for drug withdrawal.

Some evidence suggests that hydantoins may interfere with folic acid metabolism, precipitating megaloblastic anemia.

Dermatologic effects: Discontinue these drugs if a skin rash appears. If the rash is exfoliative, purpuric or bullous, do not resume use of these drugs. If the rash is milder (measles-like or scarlatiniform), resume therapy after the rash has completely disappeared. If the rash recurs upon reinstitution of therapy, further medication is contraindicated.

Lymph node hyperplasia has been associated with hydantoins, and may represent a hypersensitivity reaction. Rarely, this may progress to frank malignant lymphoma. If lymph node enlargement occurs, attempt to substitute another anticonvulsant drug or drug combination.

Differentiate lymphadenopathy from other lymph gland pathology. Lymphadenopathy which simulates Hodgkin's disease has been observed. If a lymphoma-like syndrome develops, withdraw the drug and observe the patient closely for regression of signs and symptoms before resuming treatment.

Monoclonal gammopathy and multiple myeloma have occurred during prolonged **phenytoin** therapy.

Hypersensitivity: In the event of an allergic or hypersensitivity reaction, rapid substitution of alternative therapy may be necessary. Alternative therapy should be an anticonvulsant not belonging to the hydantoin chemical class. Phenytoin hypersensitivity reactions are not typical; they may present as one of many different syndromes (eg, lymphoma, hepatitis, Stevens-Johnson syndrome) and may include such symptoms as fever, rash, arthralgias or lymphadenopathy.

Hyperglycemia, resulting from the drug's inhibitory effect on insulin release, has occurred. Hydantoins may also raise blood sugar levels in hyperglycemic persons.

Cardiovascular: Death from cardiac arrest has occurred after too-rapid IV administration, sometimes preceded by marked QRS widening. Observe the patient closely when the drug is administered IV when possible SA node depression exists. Administer cautiously in the presence of advanced AV block. Do not exceed an IV infusion rate of 50 mg/minute.

Grand mal and petit mal seizures: Drugs that control grand mal seizures are not effective for petit mal seizures. Therefore, if both conditions are present, combined drug therapy is needed.

Slow metabolism: A small percentage of individuals treated with hydantoins metabolize the drug slowly. Slow metabolism may be due to limited enzyme availability and lack of induction. It appears to be genetically determined. Metabolism of phenytoin is dose-dependent.

Osteomalacia has been associated with phenytoin therapy.

Acute intermittent porphyria: Administer hydantoins cautiously to patients with acute intermittent porphyria.

(Continued on following page)

Drug Interactions:

The following drug interactions have occurred with the use of phenytoin; however, they may occur when using any of the hydantoins.

Increased pharmacologic effects of hydantoins may occur when the following drugs are administered concurrently. Mechanisms of these interactions may include:

Hydantoin Drug Interactions: Increased Hydantoin Effects			
Inhibit metabolism		Displace anticonvulsant	Unknown
Allopurinol Amiodarone Benzodiazepines Chloramphenicol Cimetidine Disulfiram Ethanol (acute ingestion) Fluconazole Isoniazid	Metronidazole Miconazole Omeprazole Phenacemide Phenylbutazone Succinimides Sulfonamides Trimethoprim Valproic acid[2]	Salicylates[1] Tricyclic antidepressants Valproic acid[2]	Chlorpheniramine Ibuprofen Phenothiazines

[1] **Salicylates** displace phenytoin from its plasma protein binding sites in a dose-dependent manner; no significant change occurs in the free phenytoin concentration.

[2] **Valproic acid** affects phenytoin disposition in different ways. Displacement of phenytoin from plasma proteins increases the free fraction and decreases total phenytoin levels; the concentration of unbound phenytoin is not significantly altered. Increased levels may result from inhibition of phenytoin metabolism. Conversely, phenytoin increases metabolism of valproic acid.

Decreased pharmacologic effects of hydantoins may occur when the following drugs are administered concurrently. Mechanisms of these interactions may include:

Hydantoin Drug Interactions: Decreased Hydantoin Effects		
Increase metabolism	Decrease absorption	Unknown
Barbiturates[3] Carbamazepine[4] Diazoxide Ethanol (chronic ingestion) Rifampin Theophylline	Antacids Charcoal Sucralfate	Antineoplastics Folic acid[5] Influenza virus vaccine[6] Loxapine Nitrofurantoin Pyridoxine

[3] **Barbiturates** effect on phenytoin is variable and unpredictable. Addition of phenytoin generally increases phenobarbital serum concentrations. Individual monitoring is needed, especially when starting or stopping either drug.

[4] **Carbamazepine's** effect on phenytoin is variable. Carbamazepine serum levels may also be decreased.

[5] See also Drug/Food interactions.

[6] **Influenza virus vaccine** may increase, decrease, or have no effect on total serum phenytoin concentrations.

Phenytoin may decrease the pharmacologic effects of the following drugs:

Hydantoin Drug Interactions: Decreased Effects of Other Drugs		
Increased metabolism by phenytoin		Other
Acetaminophen[7] Amiodarone Carbamazepine Cardiac glycosides Corticosteroids Dicumarol Disopyramide Doxycycline Estrogens	Haloperidol Methadone Metyrapone[8] Mexiletine Oral contraceptives Quinidine Theophylline Valproic acid	Cyclosporine Dopamine Furosemide Levodopa Levonorgestrel Mebendazole Nondepolarizing muscle relaxants Phenothiazines Sulfonylureas

[7] **Acetaminophen:** Although the therapeutic effects of acetaminophen may be reduced by concomitant phenytoin use, the potential hepatotoxicity of acetaminophen may be increased, especially with chronic phenytoin administration.

[8] See also Drug/Lab test interactions.

(Drug Interactions continued on following page)

Drug Interactions (Cont.):

Clonazepam: Plasma levels of clonazepam or phenytoin may be decreased with concomitant use, or phenytoin toxicity may occur.

Corticosteroid use may mask systemic manifestations of phenytoin hypersensitivity reactions.

Dopamine: Five critically ill patients requiring dopamine to maintain blood pressure developed severe hypotension when IV phenytoin was administered.

Lithium toxicity may be increased by coadministration of phenytoin. Marked neurologic symptoms were reported despite normal serum levels of lithium.

Meperidine's analgesic effectiveness may be decreased, while the toxic effects could be increased by phenytoin. The hepatic metabolism of meperidine is increased, but the formation of normeperidine, a potentially toxic metabolite, is increased.

Primidone's pharmacologic effects may be increased by phenytoin administration; toxicity has occurred. The metabolic conversion of primidone to phenobarbital and phenylethylmalonamide (PEMA) may also be increased. Monitor serum concentrations of primidone and primidone metabolites following alterations in hydantoin therapy.

Warfarin may be displaced by phenytoin; in one report, a patient died of bleeding complications.

Drug/Food interactions: Several case reports and single-dose studies suggest that enteral nutritional therapy may decrease phenytoin concentrations; however, this has not been substantiated. Monitor phenytoin concentrations. Consider giving phenytoin 2 hours before and after the enteral feeding, or stopping the enteral therapy for 2 hours before and after phenytoin administration.

Long-term phenytoin therapy may result in folate deficiency, possibly progressing to megaloblastic anemia (rare).

Drug/Lab test interactions: Phenytoin may interfere with the **metyrapone** and the 1 mg **dexamethasone** tests. Discontinuing hydantoins prior to metyrapone testing would be ideal, but not practical; consider doubling the oral metyrapone dose.

Adverse Reactions:

CNS (most common): Nystagmus; ataxia; dysarthria; slurred speech; mental confusion; dizziness; insomnia; transient nervousness; motor twitchings; diplopia; fatigue; irritability; drowsiness; depression; numbness; tremor; headache. These side effects may disappear by reducing dosage. Psychotic disturbances and increased seizures have occurred, but a definite causal relationship is uncertain. Choreoathetosis following IV phenytoin infusion has occurred.

Cardiovascular: Phenytoin IV – Cardiovascular collapse; CNS depression; hypotension (when the drug is administered rapidly IV). Rate of administration is very important; do not exceed 50 mg/minute. Severe cardiotoxic reactions and fatalities have occurred with atrial and ventricular conduction depression and ventricular fibrillation, most commonly in elderly or gravely ill patients.

GI: Nausea; vomiting; diarrhea; constipation. Administration of the drug with or immediately after meals may help prevent GI discomfort.

Gingival hyperplasia occurs frequently with **phenytoin;** incidence may be reduced by good oral hygiene, including gum massage, frequent brushing and appropriate dental care.

Hepatic: Toxic hepatitis and liver damage may occur and rarely can be fatal. Hypersensitivity reactions with hepatic involvement include hepatocellular degeneration and fatal hepatocellular necrosis. Hepatitis, jaundice and nephrosis have been reported, but a definite cause and effect relationship has not been established. See Warnings.

Dermatologic manifestations sometimes accompanied by fever have included scarlatiniform, morbilliform, maculopapular, urticarial and nonspecific rashes; a morbilliform rash is the most common. Rashes are more frequent in children and young adults. Serious forms which may be fatal include bullous, exfoliative or purpuric dermatitis, lupus erythematosus syndrome, Stevens-Johnson syndrome and toxic epidermal necrolysis. Hirsutism and alopecia have occurred.

(Adverse Reactions continued on following page)

Adverse Reactions (Cont.):

Hematopoietic complications, some fatal, include thrombocytopenia, leukopenia, granulocytopenia, agranulocytosis and pancytopenia. Macrocytosis and megaloblastic anemia usually respond to folic acid therapy. Eosinophilia; monocytosis; leukocytosis; simple anemia; hemolytic anemia; aplastic anemia.

Connective tissue system: Coarsening of the facial features; enlargement of the lips; Peyronie's disease.

Miscellaneous: Polyarthropathy; hyperglycemia; weight gain; chest pain; edema; IgA depression; fever; photophobia; conjunctivitis; gynecomastia; periarteritis nodosa; pulmonary fibrosis; soft tissue injury at the injection site with and without extravasation of IV phenytoin; lymph node hyperplasia (see Precautions).

Lab test abnormalities: Phenytoin may decrease serum thyroxine and free thyroxine concentrations. Although these decreases are generally not associated with clinical hypothyroidism, some patients may develop goiter or hypothyroidism.

Overdosage:

Symptoms: The lethal dose in adults is estimated to be 2 to 5 g. Initial symptoms are nystagmus, ataxia and dysarthria; the patient may then become comatose and hypotensive, with pupils unresponsive. At plasma concentrations > 20 mcg/ml, far-lateral nystagmus may occur and at concentrations > 30 mcg/ml, ataxia is usually seen. Significantly diminished mental capacity occurs at levels > 40 mcg/ml. Death is due to respiratory and circulatory depression.

Treatment is nonspecific; there is no known antidote. Refer to General Management of Acute Overdosage. Consider hemodialysis, since phenytoin is not completely bound to plasma proteins. Total exchange transfusion has been utilized in the treatment of severe intoxication in children.

Patient Information:

Take medication with food to reduce GI upset.

Phenytoin suspension must be thoroughly shaken immediately prior to use.

Do not discontinue medication abruptly or change dosage, except on advice of physician.

Maintain good oral hygiene (regular brushing and flossing) while taking phenytoin. Inform dentist of medication usage.

Patients should carry identification (Medic Alert) indicating medication usage and epilepsy.

May cause drowsiness, dizziness or blurred vision; alcohol may intensify these effects. Observe caution while driving or performing other tasks requiring alertness, coordination or physical dexterity. Notify physician if drowsiness, slurred speech or impaired coordination (ataxia) occurs.

Do not use capsules which are discolored.

Diabetic patients: Monitor urine sugar regularly and report any abnormalities to physician.

Notify physician if any of the following occurs: Skin rash; severe nausea or vomiting; swollen glands; bleeding, swollen or tender gums; yellowish discoloration of the skin or eyes; joint pain; unexplained fever; sore throat; unusual bleeding or bruising; persistent headache; malaise; any indication of an infection or bleeding tendency; pregnancy.

(Products listed on following pages)

Complete prescribing information for these products begins on page 1439.

PHENYTOIN SODIUM, PARENTERAL

Administration and Dosage:

Phenytoin sodium contains 92% phenytoin.

IV administration: The addition of phenytoin solution to an IV infusion is not recommended due to lack of solubility and resultant precipitation.

Inject parenteral phenytoin slowly and directly into a large vein through a large-gauge needle or IV catheter.

Do not exceed an IV infusion rate of 50 mg/minute in adults or 1 to 3 mg/kg/minute in neonates. There is a relatively small margin between full therapeutic effect and minimally toxic doses. Monitor ECG and blood pressure continuously. In status epilepticus, the IV route is preferred because of the delay in absorption with IM administration.

Follow each IV injection with an injection of sterile saline through the same needle or IV catheter to avoid local venous irritation due to alkalinity of the solution. Avoid continuous infusion.

Soft tissue irritation and injury, with and without extravasation of IV phenytoin, have occurred at the injection site.

Although not recommended, some studies indicate that an IV infusion of phenytoin may be feasible if proper precautions are observed, such as a suitable vehicle (eg, Sodium Chloride 0.9% or Lactated Ringer's injection), appropriate concentration, preparing the infusion shortly before administration and using an inline filter.

IM administration: Avoid the IM route due to erratic absorption of phenytoin and pain and muscle damage at the injection site. When IM administration is required for a patient previously stabilized orally, compensating dosage adjustments are necessary to maintain therapeutic plasma levels; an IM dose 50% greater than the oral dose is necessary. When returned to oral administration, reduce the dose by 50% of the original oral dose for 1 week to prevent excessive plasma levels due to sustained release from IM tissue sites. Determine serum drug levels when possible drug interactions are suspected.

If the patient requires > 1 week of IM therapy, consider alternative routes (eg, gastric intubation), using oral preparations. For periods < 1 week, the patient shifted back from IM administration should receive ½ the original oral dose for the same period of time the patient received IM therapy. Monitor plasma levels.

Status epilepticus: In adults, administer loading dose of 10 to 15 mg/kg slowly. Follow by maintenance doses of 100 mg orally or IV every 6 to 8 hours. For neonates and children, oral absorption of phenytoin is unreliable; IV loading dose is 15 to 20 mg/kg in divided doses of 5 to 10 mg/kg. If administration does not terminate the seizure, consider the use of other anticonvulsants, IV barbiturates, general anesthesia or other measures.

Neurosurgery (prophylactic dosage): 100 to 200 mg IM at approximately 4 hour intervals during surgery and the postoperative period.

Storage of solution: The solution is suitable for use as long as it remains free of haziness and precipitate. Upon refrigeration or freezing, a precipitate might form; this will dissolve again after the solution is allowed to stand at room temperature. The solution is still suitable for use. Use only a clear solution. A faint yellow color may develop, but has no effect on the potency of the solution.

	Product	Form	Packaging	C.I.*
Rx	**Phenytoin Sodium** (Elkins-Sinn)	**Injection:** 50 mg per ml (46 mg phenytoin)[1]	In 2 and 5 ml Dosette amps, 2 ml Dosette vials and 5 ml vials.	805
Rx	**Phenytoin Sodium** (Lyphomed)		In 2 and 5 ml single dose vials.	NA
Rx	**Phenytoin Sodium** (Smith & Nephew SoloPak)		In 2 and 5 ml single dose vials and 2 ml fill in 3 ml and 5 ml Ky-Pod syringes.	800
Rx	**Dilantin** (Parke-Davis)		In 2 and 5 ml amps, 2 ml Steri-Dose disp. syringes, 2 and 5 ml Steri-Vials, and UD 5 ml amps.	600

* Cost Index based on cost per 100 mg.

[1] With propylene glycol and alcohol.

Complete prescribing information for these products begins on page 1439 .

Hydantoins (Cont.)

PHENYTOIN and PHENYTOIN SODIUM, ORAL

Administration and Dosage:

Phenytoin sodium contains 92% phenytoin.

Individualize dosage. Determine serum levels for optimal dosage adjustments; the clinically effective serum level is usually in the range of 10 to 20 mcg/ml.

Monitor serum concentrations and exercise care when switching a patient from the sodium salt to the free acid form or vice versa. The free acid form of phenytoin is used in the *Dilantin Infatabs* and the *Dilantin-30 Pediatric* and *Dilantin-125* suspensions, as opposed to the sodium salt in the other products. Because there is an ≈ 8% increase in drug content with the free acid form, dosage adjustment and serum monitoring may be necessary.

Loading dose: Some authorities have advocated use of an oral loading dose of phenytoin in adults who require rapid steady-state serum levels and where IV administration is not desirable. Reserve this dosing regimen for patients in a clinic or hospital setting where phenytoin serum levels can be monitored. Patients with a history of renal or liver disease should not receive the oral loading regimen.

Initially, 1 g of phenytoin capsules is divided into 3 doses (400 mg, 300 mg, 300 mg) and administered at intervals of 2 hours. Normal maintenance dosage is then instituted 24 hours after the loading dose, with frequent serum level determinations.

Adults who have received no previous treatment may be started on 100 mg (125 mg suspension) 3 times daily; individualize dosage. Satisfactory maintenance dosage - 300 to 400 mg/day. An increase to 600 mg/day (625 mg/day suspension) may be necessary.

Pediatric: Initially, 5 mg/kg/day in 2 or 3 equally divided doses with subsequent dosage individualized to a maximum of 300 mg/day. Daily maintenance dosage - 4 to 8 mg/kg. Children over 6 years may require the minimum adult dose (300 mg/day).

Single daily dosage: In adults, if seizure control is established with divided doses of three 100 mg extended phenytoin sodium capsules daily, once-a-day dosage with 300 mg may be considered. Once-a-day dosage offers convenience to the patient or to nursing personnel for institutionalized patients; it may improve compliance and it is intended to be used only for patients requiring this amount of drug daily. Caution patients not to miss a dose. Only extended phenytoin sodium capsules are recommended once-a-day.

Bioavailability: Because of potential bioavailability differences between products, brand interchange is not recommended. Dosage adjustments may be required when switching from the extended to the prompt products.

PHENYTOIN

Not for once-a-day dosing.

	Product	Form	Description	C.I.*
Rx	**Dilantin Infatab** (Parke-Davis)	**Tablets, chewable:** 50 mg	(P-D 007). Saccharin, sucrose. Yellow, scored. Triangular. In 100s and UD 100s.	95
Rx	**Dilantin-30 Pediatric** (Parke-Davis)	**Oral Suspension:** 30 mg per 5 ml	≤ 0.6% alcohol. Banana-orange-vanilla flavor. In 240 ml and UD 5 ml.	355
Rx	**Dilantin-125** (Parke-Davis)	**Oral Suspension:** 125 mg per 5 ml	≤ 0.6% alcohol. Orange-vanilla flavor. In 240 ml and 5 ml UD.	110

PHENYTOIN SODIUM, PROMPT

Not for once-a-day dosing.

Dissolution rate: Not < 85% in 30 minutes.

	Product	Form	Description	C.I.*
Rx	**Diphenylan Sodium** (Lannett)	**Capsules:** 30 mg (27.6 mg phenytoin)	In 500s and 1000s.	25
Rx	**Phenytoin Sodium** (Various, eg, Dixon-Shane, Genetco, IDE, Major, Parmed, Rugby, Zenith)	**Capsules:** 100 mg (92 mg phenytoin)	In 100s, 1000s and UD 100s.	30+
Rx	**Diphenylan Sodium** (Lannett)		In 500s and 1000s.	NA

* Cost Index based on cost per 100 mg.

Oxazolidinediones

> **Warning:** Because of their potential to produce fetal malformations and serious side effects, use these agents only when other less toxic drugs have been found ineffective in controlling petit mal seizures.

Actions:

Pharmacology: Unlike the hydantoins and the anticonvulsant barbiturates, neither drug modifies the maximal seizure pattern in humans receiving electroconvulsive therapy. These agents have a sedative effect which may increase to ataxia with excessive doses.

Pharmacokinetics: Readily absorbed from the GI tract. The oxazolidinediones are demethylated by liver microsomes to an active metabolite, dimethadione, which is slowly excreted by the kidneys. About 3% of a daily trimethadione dose is recovered in urine as unchanged drug. Almost no unmetabolized paramethadione is excreted. Trimethadione has a plasma half-life of 16 to 24 hours, whereas that of dimethadione is 6 to 13 days. While no definite therapeutic trimethadione levels have been determined, patients with petit mal attacks are usually controlled by serum dimethadione levels ≥ 700 mcg/ml.

Indications:

For the control of absence (petit mal) seizures refractory to treatment with other drugs.

Contraindications:

Hypersensitivity to oxazolidinediones.

Warnings:

Side effects: May cause serious side effects. Strict medical supervision of the patient is mandatory, especially during the initial year of therapy.

Pregnancy: Category D. Refer to information for use during pregnancy in the Anticonvulsant introduction.

Lactation: It is not known whether these drugs are excreted in breast milk. Decide whether to discontinue nursing or to discontinue the drug, taking into account the importance of the drug to the mother.

Precautions:

Lupus: Manifestations of systemic lupus erythematosus have been associated with the use of the oxazolidinediones. Lymphadenopathies simulating malignant lymphoma have also occurred. Lupus-like manifestations or lymph node enlargement are indications for drug withdrawal. Signs and symptoms may disappear after discontinuation of therapy, and specific treatment may be unnecessary.

Withdrawal: Abrupt discontinuation of paramethadione or trimethadione may precipitate absence (petit mal) status. Withdraw gradually unless serious adverse effects dictate otherwise. If this occurs, another anticonvulsant may be substituted.

Dermatologic effects: Withdraw these agents promptly if skin rash appears, because of the possibility of exfoliative dermatitis or severe erythema multiforme. Even a minor acneiform or morbilliform rash should be allowed to clear completely before treatment is resumed; reinstitute therapy cautiously.

Hepatic effects: Perform liver function tests prior to initiating therapy and at monthly intervals thereafter. Hepatitis has been associated rarely with the use of oxazolidinediones. Jaundice or other signs of liver dysfunction are an indication for withdrawal of the drug. These agents should ordinarily not be used in patients with severe hepatic impairment.

Renal effects: Perform urinalysis prior to therapy and at monthly intervals. Fatal nephrosis has occurred. If persistent or increasing proteinuria, or any other significant renal abnormality occurs, withdraw the drug. Oxazolidinediones should ordinarily not be used in patients with severe renal dysfunction.

Ophthalmic effects: Hemeralopia has occurred with the use of these agents; this appears to be an effect on the neural layers of the retina, and usually can be reversed by a reduction in dosage. Scotomata are an indication for withdrawal of the drug. Use caution when treating patients who have diseases of the retina or optic nerve.

Hematologic effects: Perform a complete blood count prior to initiating therapy and monthly thereafter. If a marked depression of the blood count occurs, withdraw the drug. If no abnormality appears within 12 months, the interval between blood counts may be extended. A moderate degree of neutropenia, with or without a corresponding drop in the leukocyte count, is not uncommon. Therapy need not be withdrawn unless the neutrophil count is ≤ 2500; more frequent blood examinations should be done when the count is < 3000. Leukopenia, eosinophilia, thrombocytopenia, pancytopenia, agranulocytosis, hypoplastic anemia and fatal aplastic anemia have also occurred.

These agents are not ordinarily used in patients with severe blood dyscrasias.

CNS effects: May produce drowsiness or blurred vision. Observe caution while driving or performing other tasks requiring alertness, coordination or physical dexterity.

(Precautions continued on following page)

Oxazolidinediones (Cont.)

Precautions (Cont.):

Myasthenia gravis-like syndrome has been associated with the chronic use of the oxazolidinediones. If symptoms suggest this condition, withdraw the drug.

Porphyria: Use trimethadione with caution in patients with acute intermittent porphyria.

Tartrazine sensitivity: Paramethadione 300 mg capsules contain tartrazine, which may cause allergic-type reactions (including bronchial asthma) in susceptible individuals. Although the incidence of tartrazine sensitivity in the general population is low, it is frequently seen in patients who also have aspirin hypersensitivity.

Photosensitivity: Photosensitization may occur; therefore, caution patients to take protective measures (ie, sunscreens, protective clothing) against exposure to ultraviolet light or sunlight until tolerance is determined.

Adverse Reactions:

Renal: Fatal nephrosis; proteinuria.

Hematologic: Fatal aplastic anemia; hypoplastic anemia; pancytopenia; agranulocytosis; leukopenia; neutropenia; thrombocytopenia; eosinophilia; retinal and petechial hemorrhages; vaginal bleeding; epistaxis; bleeding gums.

Dermatologic: Acneiform or morbilliform skin rash that may progress to severe forms of erythema multiforme or to exfoliative dermatitis; hair loss.

CNS: Myasthenia gravis-like syndrome (see Precautions); precipitation of tonic-clonic (grand mal) seizures; vertigo; personality changes; increased irritability; drowsiness; headache; paresthesias; fatigue; malaise; insomnia; diplopia; hemeralopia; photophobia. Drowsiness usually subsides with continued therapy; if it persists, a reduction in dosage is indicated.

GI: Vomiting; abdominal pain; gastric distress; nausea; anorexia; weight loss; hiccoughs.

Other: Hepatitis (rare); lupus erythematosus and lymphadenopathies simulating malignant lymphoma; pruritus associated with lymphadenopathy and hepatosplenomegaly in hypersensitive individuals; changes in blood pressure.

Overdosage:

Symptoms: Nausea; drowsiness; dizziness; ataxia; visual disturbances. Coma may follow massive overdosage.

Treatment: Gastric evacuation by induced emesis, lavage or both, should be done immediately. General supportive care, including frequent monitoring of the vital signs is required. Refer to General Management of Acute Overdosage. Alkalinization of urine has increased the renal excretion of the active metabolite of both drugs. Monitor blood counts and hepatic and renal function following recovery.

Patient Information:

If GI upset occurs, may be taken with food.

Photosensitivity may occur. Avoid exposure to ultraviolet light or sunlight. Use sunscreen and protective clothing until tolerance is determined.

Do not discontinue medication abruptly or change dosage except on advice of physician.

Patients should carry identification (Medic Alert) indicating medication usage and epilepsy.

Medication may cause sensitivity to bright light.

May cause drowsiness or blurred vision; patients should observe caution while driving or performing other tasks requiring alertness, coordination or physical dexterity.

Notify physician if any of the following should occur: Visual disturbances, excessive drowsiness or dizziness, sore throat, fever, skin rash, pregnancy, malaise, easy bruising, petechiae or epistaxis, or others that may be indicative of an infection or bleeding tendency.

Administration and Dosage:

Adults: 900 mg to 2.4 g/day in 3 or 4 equally divided doses (300 to 600 mg 3 or 4 times daily). Initially, give 900 mg daily; increase this by 300 mg at weekly intervals until therapeutic results are seen or until toxic symptoms appear. Adjust maintenance dosage to the minimum required to maintain control.

Children: 300 to 900 mg/day in 3 or 4 equally divided doses.

PARAMETHADIONE				C.I.*
Rx	**Paradione** (Abbott)	**Capsules:** 150 mg	Orange. In 100s.	770
		300 mg	Tartrazine. Green. In 100s.	695
TRIMETHADIONE				
Rx	**Tridione** (Abbott)	**Dulcets (Tablets, chewable):** 150 mg	Sucrose. White. In 100s.	680
		Capsules: 300 mg	White. In 100s.	385
		Solution: 40 mg per ml	Sucrose. In pt.	425

* Cost Index based on cost per 900 mg.

For complete prescribing information, refer to the Benzodiazepine monograph in the Antianxiety Agents section.

Benzodiazepines

CLONAZEPAM

Indications:

Used alone or as adjunctive treatment of the Lennox-Gastaut syndrome (petit mal variant), akinetic and myoclonic seizures. It may be useful in patients with absence (petit mal) seizures who have failed to respond to succinimides.

Up to 30% of patients have shown a loss of anticonvulsant activity, often within 3 months of administration; dosage adjustment may reestablish efficacy.

Unlabeled uses:

Periodic leg movements during sleep (0.5 to 2 mg/night).
Parkinsonian (hypokinetic) dysarthria (0.25 to 0.5 mg/day).
Acute manic episodes of bipolar affective disorder (0.75 to 16 mg/day).
Multifocal tic disorders (1.5 to 12 mg/day).
Adjunct in the treatment of schizophrenia (0.5 to 2 mg/day).
Neuralgias (deafferentation pain syndromes; 2 to 4 mg/day).

Administration and Dosage:

Adults: Initial dose should not exceed 1.5 mg/day in 3 divided doses. Increase in increments of 0.5 to 1 mg every 3 days until seizures are adequately controlled or until side effects preclude any further increase. Individualize maintenance dosage. Maximum recommended dosage is 20 mg/day.

Infants and children (up to 10 years or 30 kg): To minimize drowsiness, the initial dose should be between 0.01 to 0.03 mg/kg/day, not to exceed 0.05 mg/kg/day, given in 2 or 3 divided doses. Increase dosage by not more than 0.25 to 0.5 mg every third day until a daily maintenance dose of 0.1 to 0.2 mg/kg has been reached, unless seizures are controlled or side effects preclude further increase. When possible, divide the daily dose into 3 equal doses. If doses are not equally divided, give the largest dose at bedtime.

Therapeutic serum concentrations of clonazepam are 20 to 80 ng/ml.

Multiple anticonvulsant use may result in an increase of depressant effects. Consider this before adding clonazepam to an existing anticonvulsant regimen.

				C.I.*
c-IV	**Klonopin** (Roche)	**Tablets:** 0.5 mg	Orange, scored. In Rx Pak 100s and *Tel-E-Dose* 100s.	230
		1 mg	Blue, scored. In Rx Pak 100s and *Tel-E-Dose* 100s.	130
		2 mg	White, scored. In Rx Pak 100s and *Tel-E-Dose* 100s.	90

* Cost Index based on cost per 0.5 mg clonazepam or 7.5 mg clorazepate.

For complete prescribing information, refer to the benzodiazepine monograph in the Antianxiety Agents section.

Benzodiazepines (Cont.)

CLORAZEPATE DIPOTASSIUM

Indications:

As adjunctive therapy in the management of partial seizures.

Symptomatic relief of anxiety and for the symptomatic relief of acute alcohol withdrawal (see monograph in the Antianxiety Agents section).

Administration and Dosage:

To minimize drowsiness, do not exceed recommended initial dosages and increments.

Adults and children (> 12 years): The maximum initial dose is 7.5 mg 3 times daily. Increase dosage by no more than 7.5 mg every week and do not exceed 90 mg/day.

Children (9 to 12 years): The maximum initial dose is 7.5 mg 2 times daily. Increase dosage by no more than 7.5 mg every week and do not exceed 60 mg/day. Not recommended in patients < 9 years of age.

	Product	Dosage form	Description	C.I.*
c-iv	**Clorazepate** (Various, eg, American Therapeutics, Geneva Marsam, Lederle, Martec, Moore, PBI, Rugby, URL)	**Capsules:** 3.75 mg	In 100s, 500s and 1000s.	120+
c-iv	**Clorazepate** (Various, eg, American Therapeutics, Geneva Marsam, Lederle, Martec, Moore, PBI, Rugby, URL)	**Capsules:** 7.5 mg	In 100s, 500s and 1000s.	85+
c-iv	**Clorazepate** (Various, eg, American Therapeutics, Geneva Marsam, Lederle, Martec, Moore, PBI, Rugby, URL)	**Capsules:** 15 mg	In 100s, 500s and 1000s.	5+
c-iv	**Clorazepate** (Various, eg, Geneva Marsam, Goldline, Lederle, Major, Moore, Mylan, Parmed, Rugby, Schein, Warner Chilcott)	**Tablets:** 3.75 mg	In 100s, 500s and UD 1000s.	90+
c-iv	**Gen-Xene** (Alra)		(Alra GX). Gray, scored. In 30s, 100s, 500s and UD 100s.	210
c-iv	**Tranxene** (Abbott)		(TL). Blue, scored. Six sided. In 100s, 500s and Abbo-pac 100s.	600
c-iv	**Clorazepate** (Various, eg, Geneva Marsam, Goldline, Lederle, Major, Moore, Mylan, Parmed, Rugby, Schein, Warner Chilcott)	**Tablets:** 7.5 mg	In 100s and 500s.	60+
c-iv	**Gen-Xene** (Alra)		(Alra GT). Yellow, scored. In 30s, 100s, 500s and UD 100s.	135
c-iv	**Tranxene** (Abbott)		(TM). Peach, scored. Six sided. In 100s, 500s and Abbo-pac 100s.	375
c-iv	**Tranxene-SD Half Strength** (Abbott)	**Tablets:** 11.25 mg	Lactose. Blue. In 100s.	485
c-iv	**Clorazepate** (Various, eg, Geneva Marsam, Goldline, Lederle, Major, Moore, Mylan, Parmed, Rugby, Schein, Warner Chilcott)	**Tablets:** 15 mg	In 100s and 500s.	35+
c-iv	**Gen-Xene** (Alra)		(Alra GN). Green, scored. In 30s, 100s, 500s and UD 100s.	100
c-iv	**Tranxene** (Abbott)		(TN). Lavender, scored. Six sided. In 100s, 500s and Abbo-pac 100s.	255
c-iv	**Tranxene-SD** (Abbott)	**Tablets:** 22.5 mg	Lactose. Tan. In 100s.	340

* Cost Index based on cost per 7.5 mg clorazepate.

For complete prescribing information, refer to the Benzodiazepine monograph in the Antianxiety Agents section.

Benzodiazepines (Cont.)

DIAZEPAM

Indications:

Oral: May be used adjunctively in convulsive disorders; it is not proven useful as sole therapy. When used as an adjunct in convulsive disorders, the possibility of an increase in frequency or severity of grand mal seizures may require an increase in the dosage of standard anticonvulsant medication. Abrupt diazepam withdrawal in such cases may also be associated with a temporary increase in frequency or severity of seizures.

Parenteral: Adjunct in status epilepticus and severe recurrent convulsive seizures.

Diazepam is also used as a muscle relaxant (see individual monograph in the Skeletal Muscle Relaxants section), as an antianxiety agent and in acute alcohol withdrawal (see group monograph in Antianxiety Agents section).

Administration and Dosage:

Individualize dosage. Some patients may require higher doses than those given below. In such cases, increase dosage cautiously to avoid adverse effects. Use lower doses and slowly increase the dose in elderly or debilitated patients and when other sedative drugs are administered.

Oral (tablets, oral solution and Intensol):

Adults – 2 to 10 mg 2 to 4 times daily.

Geriatric or debilitated patients – 2 to 2.5 mg once or twice daily initially. Limit dosage to the smallest effective amount to preclude the development of ataxia or oversedation.

Children – Not for use in children < 6 months. Give 1 to 2.5 mg 3 or 4 times daily initially; increase gradually as needed and tolerated.

Oral, sustained release:

Adults – 15 to 30 mg once daily.

Intensol preparation: Mix with liquid or semi-solid food such as water, juices, soda or soda-like beverages, applesauce and puddings. Consume the entire amount immediately. Do not store.

Parenteral: Although seizures may be brought under control promptly, a significant proportion of patients experience a return to seizure activity due to the short-lived effect of IV diazepam. Be prepared to readminister. Not recommended for maintenance; once seizures are controlled, administer agents indicated for long-term seizure control.

Tonic status epilepticus has been precipitated in patients treated with IV diazepam for petit mal status or petit mal variant status.

Use extreme care in administering IV diazepam to the elderly, to very ill patients and to those with limited pulmonary reserve; apnea or cardiac arrest may occur.

To reduce possibility of venous thrombosis, phlebitis, swelling, local irritation and rarely, vascular impairment: Inject slowly IV (at least 1 min for each 5 mg); do not use small veins (eg, dorsum of hand or wrist); avoid intra-arterial use and extravasation.

Do not mix or dilute with other solutions or drugs in syringe or infusion flask. If it is not feasible to administer directly IV, it may be injected slowly through the infusion tubing as close as possible to the vein insertion. Diazepam interacts with plastic containers and administration sets, significantly decreasing availability of drug delivered.

The IV route is preferred in the convulsing patient. However, if IV administration is impossible, the IM route may be used. Inject deeply. Administration IM results in low or erratic plasma levels.

Adults – 5 to 10 mg initially. May be repeated at 10 to 15 minute intervals up to a maximum dose of 30 mg, if necessary. Therapy may be repeated in 2 to 4 hours; however, residual active metabolites may persist. Exercise extreme caution in individuals with chronic lung disease or unstable cardiovascular status.

Children ≥ 5 years – 1 mg every 2 to 5 minutes up to a maximum of 10 mg. Repeat in 2 to 4 hours if necessary. EEG monitoring of the seizure may be helpful.

Infants > 30 days of age and children < 5 years – 0.2 to 0.5 mg slowly every 2 to 5 minutes up to a maximum of 5 mg.

Safety and efficacy of parenteral diazepam has not been established in the neonate (≤ 30 days of age). Prolonged CNS depression has been observed in neonates, apparently due to inability to biotransform diazepam into inactive metabolites. In pediatric use, give slowly over a 3 minute period at a dosage not to exceed 0.25 mg/kg. After an interval of 15 to 30 minutes, the initial dosage can be repeated. If relief of symptoms is not obtained after a third administration, other therapy is recommended. Have facilities for respiratory assistance readily available.

(Products listed on following page)

Benzodiazepines (Cont.)

DIAZEPAM (Cont.)

	Product	Form	Description	C.I.*
c-IV	**Diazepam** (Various, eg, Barr, Dixon-Shane, Major, Mylan, Parmed, Schein, Zenith)	**Tablets:** 2 mg	In 100s, 500s, 1000s and 2500s.	15+
c-IV	**Valium** (Roche)		(Roche 2 Valium). White, scored. Round with cut out V. In 100s, 500s and Tel-E-Dose 100s.	165
c-IV	**Diazepam** (Various, eg, Barr, Dixon-Shane, Major, Mylan, Parmed, Schein, Zenith)	**Tablets:** 5 mg	In 100s, 500s, 1000s and 2500s.	6+
c-IV	**Valium** (Roche)		(Roche 5 Valium). Yellow, scored. Round with cut out V. In 100s, 500s and Tel-E-Dose 100s.	102
c-IV	**Diazepam** (Various, eg, Barr, Dixon-Shane, Major, Mylan, Parmed, Schein, Zenith)	**Tablets:** 10 mg	In 100s, 500s, 1000s and 2500s.	3+
c-IV	**Valium** (Roche)		(Roche 10 Valium). Blue, scored. Round with cut out V. In 100s, 500s and Tel-E-Dose 100s.	87
c-IV	**Valrelease** (Roche)	**Capsules, sustained release:** 15 mg	(Roche Valrelease 15). Yellow and blue. In 100s and Rx pak 30s.	82
c-IV	**Diazepam** (Roxane)	**Intensol:** 5 mg per ml	In 30 ml w/dropper.	80
c-IV *sf*	**Diazepam** (Roxane)	**Oral Solution:** 5 mg per 5 ml	Wintergreen-spice flavor. In 500 ml and UD 5 and 10 ml.	NA
c-IV	**Diazepam** (Schein)	**Injection:** 5 mg per ml	In 2 ml amps, 1, 2, 5 and 10 ml vials and 1 and 2 ml syringes.	265
c-IV	**Valium** (Roche)		In 2 ml ampuls, 10 ml vials & 2 ml Tel-E-Ject disp. syringes[1].	315

* Cost Index based on cost per 2 mg.

sf – Sugar free.

[1] In 40% propylene glycol and 10% ethyl alcohol with 5% sodium benzoate, benzoic acid and 1.5% benzyl alcohol.

CARBAMAZEPINE

Warning:

Aplastic anemia and agranulocytosis have been reported in association with carbamazepine therapy. The risk of developing these reactions is 5 to 8 times greater than in the general population. However, the overall risk of these reactions in the untreated general population is low, approximately six and two patients per one million per year for agranulocytosis and aplastic anemia, respectively. Although reports of transient or persistent decreased platelet or white blood cell counts are not uncommon in association with the use of carbamazepine, data are not available to estimate accurately their incidence or outcome. However, the vast majority of the cases of leukopenia have not progressed to the more serious conditions of aplastic anemia or agranulocytosis. Because of the very low incidence of agranulocytosis and aplastic anemia, the vast majority of minor hematologic changes observed in monitoring of patients on carbamazepine are unlikely to signal the occurrence of either abnormality. Nonetheless, obtain complete pretreatment hematological testing as a baseline. If a patient in the course of treatment exhibits low or decreased white blood cell or platelet counts, monitor the patient closely. Consider discontinuation of the drug if any evidence of significant bone marrow depression develops.

Actions:

Pharmacology: Carbamazepine is an iminostilbene derivative chemically related to the tricyclic antidepressants. It is chemically unrelated to other anticonvulsants or agents used to control the pain of trigeminal neuralgia. Its mechanism of action is unknown. It appears to act by reducing polysynaptic responses and blocking the post-tetanic potentiation.

Pharmacokinetics:

Absorption/Distribution – Carbamazepine is adequately absorbed, with peak serum levels achieved 4 to 5 hours following administration. Both the suspension and tablet deliver equivalent amounts of drug to the systemic circulation; however, the suspension is absorbed somewhat faster than the tablet. Following a twice-daily dosage regimen, the suspension has higher peak levels and lower trough levels than those obtained from the tablet formulation for the same dosage regimen. However, the suspension given three times daily affords steady-state plasma levels comparable to the tablets given twice daily when administered at the same total daily dose in mg. Plasma levels are variable and may range from 0.5 to 25 mcg/ml, with no apparent relationship to the daily intake of the drug. Usual adult therapeutic levels are between 4 and 12 mcg/ml. Carbamazepine is 76% bound to plasma proteins. The CSF/serum ratio is 0.22, similar to 22% unbound carbamazepine in serum. Transplacental passage of carbamazepine is rapid (30 to 60 minutes); the drug accumulates in fetal tissues, with higher levels found in liver and kidney than in brain and lungs.

Metabolism/Excretion – Carbamazepine is metabolized in the liver to the 10,11-epoxide, which also has anticonvulsant activity. It may induce its own metabolism. Initial half-life ranges from 25 to 65 hours, and decreases to 12 to 17 hours with repeated doses. The half-life of the metabolite is somewhat shorter than the parent drug.

After administration, 72% of a dose is found in urine and 28% in feces. Urinary products are composed largely of hydroxylated and conjugated metabolites, with only 3% unchanged carbamazepine.

Indications:

Epilepsy: Partial seizures with complex symptoms (psychomotor, temporal lobe). Patients with these seizures appear to show greatest improvement. Generalized tonic-clonic seizures (grand mal); mixed seizure patterns or other partial or generalized seizures.

Reserve carbamazepine for patients who have not responded satisfactorily to other agents such as phenytoin, phenobarbital or primidone, whose seizures are difficult to control or patients experiencing marked side effects (eg, excessive sedation).

Trigeminal neuralgia: Treatment of pain associated with true trigeminal neuralgia. Beneficial results have also been reported in glossopharyngeal neuralgia.

Unlabeled uses: Neurogenic diabetes insipidus.

Certain psychiatric disorders, including bipolar disorders, schizoaffective illness, resistant schizophrenia and dyscontrol syndrome associated with limbic system dysfunction.

Management of alcohol withdrawal.

Restless legs syndrome (100 to 300 mg at bedtime).

(Continued on following page)

CARBAMAZEPINE (Cont.)

Contraindications:

History of bone marrow depression; hypersensitivity to carbamazepine and tricyclic antidepressants; concomitant use of monoamine oxidase (MAO) inhibitors. Discontinue MAO inhibitors for a minimum of 14 days before carbamazepine administration.

Warnings:

This drug is not a simple analgesic. Do not use for the relief of minor aches or pains.

Hematologic: Patients with a history of adverse hematologic reaction to any drug may be particularly at risk.

Glaucoma: Carbamazepine has shown mild anticholinergic activity; therefore, use with caution in patients with increased intraocular pressure.

CNS effects: Because of the drug's relationship to other tricyclic compounds, the possibility of activating latent psychosis, or confusion or agitation in elderly patients may occur.

Carcinogenesis: Carbamazepine administered to rats for 2 years at doses of 25 to 250 mg/kg/day resulted in a dose-related increase in the incidence of hepatocellular tumors in females and benign interstitial cell adenomas in the testes of males. The significance of these findings to humans is unknown.

Pregnancy: Category C. Adverse effects have been observed in animal studies.

Use only when clearly needed and when the potential benefits outweigh the unknown potential hazards to the fetus. For information on use during pregnancy, refer to the Anticonvulsants group monograph.

Lactation: Concentration of carbamazepine in milk is approximately 60% of the maternal plasma concentration. Because of the potential for serious adverse reactions, decide whether to discontinue nursing or to discontinue the drug, taking into account the importance of the drug to the mother.

Children: Safety and efficacy for use in children below the age of 6 years have not been established.

Precautions:

Absence seizures (petit mal) do not appear to be controlled by carbamazepine. Use with caution in patients with a mixed seizure disorder that includes atypical absence seizures since carbamazepine has been associated with increased frequency of generalized convulsions in these patients.

Potentially hazardous tasks: May produce drowsiness, dizziness or blurred vision; patients should observe caution while driving or performing other tasks requiring alertness.

Special risk patients: Prescribe carbamazepine only after benefit-to-risk appraisal in patients with a history of: Cardiac, hepatic or renal damage; adverse hematologic reaction to other drugs; interrupted courses of therapy with the drug.

Laboratory tests: Perform baseline liver function tests and periodic evaluations. Discontinue drug immediately if liver dysfunction occurs. Obtain baseline and periodic eye examinations (slit lamp, funduscopy and tonometry), urinalysis and BUN determinations.

The monitoring of blood levels may be particularly useful in cases of dramatic increase in seizure frequency, for verification of compliance and in determining the cause of toxicity when more than one medication is being used.

Obtain complete pretreatment hematological testing as a baseline. Repeat these tests at monthly intervals during the first 2 months and thereafter obtain yearly or every other year CBC, white cell differential and platelet count.

(Continued on following page)

CARBAMAZEPINE (Cont.)

Drug Interactions:

The following agents may inhibit the hepatic metabolism of carbamazepine; resultant elevated carbamazepine levels may result in toxicity (eg, nausea, vomiting, somnolence, nystagmus, ataxia and other cerebellar symptoms):

Cimetidine	**Nicotinamide**
Danazol	**Propoxyphene**
Diltiazem	**Troleandomycin**
Erythromycin	**Verapamil**
Isoniazid[1]	

[1] Conversely, carbamazepine may increase the risk of isoniazid-induced hepatotoxicity.

Acetaminophen: Carbamazepine may increase the metabolism of acetaminophen, increasing the risk of acetaminophen-induced hepatotoxicity or decreasing its analgesic/antipyretic effectiveness.

Anticoagulants, oral: Carbamazepine may increase the metabolism of these agents due to induction of hepatic microsomal enzyme induction. Hypoprothrombinemic effect of the anticoagulants may be decreased.

Barbiturates, primidone: The concurrent administration of these agents may lower serum levels of carbamazepine. No loss of seizure control has been reported with the addition of phenobarbital, since the anticonvulsant action is probably additive with carbamazepine. In addition, studies indicate that the active metabolite of primidone (phenobarbital) may be increased by carbamazepine.

Charcoal may decrease the GI absorption of carbamazepine. See Overdosage.

Doxycycline half-life may be reduced when coadministered with carbamazepine.

Haloperidol serum levels and therapeutic efficacy may be decreased by carbamazepine.

Hydantoins: Both increased and decreased hydantoin plasma levels as well as decreased carbamazepine plasma levels have occurred during coadministration.

Lithium: Increased CNS toxicity may occur during concomitant carbamazepine therapy.

Nondepolarizing muscle relaxants: Carbamazepine may cause resistance to, or reversal of, the neuromuscular blocking effects of these agents.

Posterior pituitary hormones: Carbamazepine, which potentiates ADH, may potentiate the antidiuretic effects of **vasopressin, lypressin** or **desmopressin.**

Succinimides: Plasma levels of these agents may be reduced by carbamazepine due to induction of hepatic microsomal enzymes, although there may be no loss of seizure control since the anticonvulsant action is probably additive.

Theophylline: During coadministration, pharmacologic effects of both drugs may be decreased.

Valproic acid plasma levels may be decreased by carbamazepine. However, valproic acid may prolong carbamazepine's half-life, decrease its protein binding and increase the plasma ratio of carbamazepine 10,11-epoxide/carbamazepine. Clinical effects are difficult to predict.

Drug/Lab Test Interactions: **Thyroid function tests** show decreased values with carbamazepine. Thyroid function alterations have occurred in combination with other anticonvulsants.

Adverse Reactions:

If adverse reactions are so severe that the drug must be discontinued, abrupt discontinuation in a responsive epileptic patient may lead to seizures or even status epilepticus.

Most frequent: Dizziness; drowsiness; unsteadiness; nausea; vomiting. To minimize such reactions, initiate therapy at low doses.

Hematopoietic: Aplastic anemia; leukopenia; agranulocytosis; eosinophilia; leukocytosis; thrombocytopenia; pancytopenia; bone marrow depression. (See Warning Box).

Hepatic: Abnormal liver function tests; cholestatic and hepatocellular jaundice; hepatitis.

GU: Urinary frequency; acute urinary retention; oliguria with hypertension; renal failure; azotemia; impotence; albuminuria; glycosuria; elevated BUN; microscopic deposits in urine.

CNS: Dizziness; drowsiness; disturbances of coordination; confusion; headache; fatigue; blurred vision; visual hallucinations; speech disturbances; abnormal involuntary movements; peripheral neuritis and paresthesias; depression with agitation; talkativeness; tinnitus; hyperacusis; behavioral changes in children; paralysis and other symptoms of cerebral arterial insufficiency.

(Adverse Reactions continued on following page)

CARBAMAZEPINE (Cont.)

Adverse Reactions (Cont.):

Pulmonary hypersensitivity characterized by fever, dyspnea, pneumonitis or pneumonia; pulmonary eosinophilia and asthma occurred in one patient.

Dermatologic: Pruritic and erythematous rashes; urticaria; Stevens-Johnson syndrome; photosensitivity reactions; alterations in pigmentation; exfoliative dermatitis; alopecia; diaphoresis; erythema multiforme and nodosum; purpura; aggravation of disseminated lupus erythematosus and toxic epidermal necrolysis (Lyell's syndrome). Discontinuation of therapy may be necessary.

GI: Nausea; vomiting; gastric distress; abdominal pain; diarrhea; constipation; anorexia; dryness of mouth or pharynx; glossitis and stomatitis.

Cardiovascular: Congestive heart failure; aggravation of hypertension; hypotension; syncope and collapse; edema; primary thrombophlebitis; recurrence of thrombophlebitis; aggravation of coronary artery disease; arrhythmias and AV block; adenopathy or lymphadenopathy. Some cardiovascular complications have resulted in fatalities.

Ophthalmologic: Transient diplopia and oculomotor disturbances; nystagmus; scattered, punctate cortical lens opacities; conjunctivitis.

Musculoskeletal: Aching joints and muscles; leg cramps.

Metabolic: Fever and chills; inappropriate antidiuretic hormone secretion syndrome (SIADH).

Overdosage:

Toxic doses: Lowest known lethal dose – *Adults,* $>$ 60 g (39-year-old man). Highest known doses survived – *Adults,* 30 g (31-year-old woman); *children,* 10 g (6-year-old boy); *small children,* 5 g (3-year-old girl).

Symptoms and signs first appear after 1 to 3 hours. Neuromuscular disturbances are the most prominent. Cardiovascular disorders are generally mild, and severe cardiac complications occur only when very high doses ($>$ 60 g) have been ingested.

Respiration – Irregular breathing; respiratory depression.

Cardiovascular – Tachycardia; hypotension or hypertension; shock; conduction disorders.

CNS – Impaired consciousness ranging to deep coma; convulsions, especially in small children; motor restlessness; muscular twitching; tremor; athetoid movements; opisthotonos; ataxia; drowsiness; dizziness; mydriasis; nystagmus; adiadochokinesia; ballism; psychomotor disturbances; dysmetria; initial hyperreflexia followed by hyporeflexia; EEG may show dysrhythmias.

GI/GU – Nausea; vomiting; anuria or oliguria; urinary retention.

Laboratory findings: Isolated instances of overdosage have included leukocytosis, reduced leukocyte count, glycosuria and acetonuria.

Treatment: The prognosis in cases of severe poisoning is dependent upon prompt elimination of the drug. Even when more than 4 hours have elapsed following ingestion of the drug, irrigate the stomach repeatedly, especially if the patient has also consumed alcohol. There is no specific antidote. Refer to General Management of Acute Overdosage. Charcoal administration is effective in increasing the total body clearance of carbamazepine. The recommended dosage is 50 to 100 g initially followed by a rate of $\geq$ 12.5 g/hour, preferably via a nasogastric tube; continue until the patient is symptom free.

Dialysis is indicated only in severe poisoning associated with renal failure. Replacement transfusion is indicated in severe poisoning in small children.

In treating convulsions, diazepam or barbiturates may aggravate respiratory depression (especially in children), hypotension and coma. Do not use barbiturates if MAO inhibitors have also been taken by the patient either in overdosage or in recent therapy (within 1 week).

Monitor respiration, ECG, blood pressure, body temperature, pupillary reflexes and kidney and bladder function for several days.

Treatment of blood count abnormalities – If evidence of significant bone marrow depression develops: Discontinue drug; perform daily CBC, platelet and reticulocyte counts; perform bone marrow aspiration and trephine biopsy immediately and repeat with sufficient frequency to monitor recovery. Fully developed aplastic anemia requires intensive monitoring and therapy; specialized consultation should be sought.

Special periodic studies might be helpful as follows: White cell and platelet antibodies; ^{59}Fe – ferrokinetic studies; peripheral blood cell typing; cytogenetic studies on marrow and peripheral blood; bone marrow culture studies for colony-forming units; hemoglobin electrophoresis for A_2 and F hemoglobin; serum folic acid; B_{12} levels.

(Continued on following page)

MAGNESIUM SULFATE (Cont.)

Overdosage:

Symptoms: Sharp drop in blood pressure and respiratory paralysis. ECG changes reported include increased PR interval, increased QRS complex and prolonged QT interval. Heart block and asystole may occur.

An approximate correlation of magnesium toxicity versus serum level is presented in the table.

Serum level (mEq/L)	Effect
1.5 to 3	Normal serum concentration
4 to 7	"Therapeutic" level for preeclampsia/eclampsia/convulsions
7 to 10	Loss of deep tendon reflexes, hypotension, narcosis
12 to 15	Respiratory paralysis
> 15	Cardiac conduction affected[1]
> 25	Cardiac arrest

[1] PR interval lengthening, QRS widening, prolonged QT interval dysrhythmias.

Treatment: Provide artificial ventilation until a calcium salt can be injected IV to antagonize the effects of magnesium. A dose of 5 to 10 mEq calcium will usually reverse the respiratory depression and heart block. Peritoneal dialysis or hemodialysis is also effective.

Administration and Dosage:

Individualize dosage. Monitor the patient's clinical status to avoid toxicity. Discontinue as soon as the desired effect is obtained. When repeated doses are given, test knee jerk reflexes before each dose; if they are absent, do not give magnesium. Administration beyond the point of suppression of knee jerks may cause respiratory center failure and thus necessitate artificial respiration or IV calcium.

IM: 1 to 5 g of a 25 to 50% solution 6 times a day as necessary.

IV: 1 to 4 g of a 10 to 20% solution; not exceeding 1.5 ml/minute of a 10% solution.

IV infusion: 4 g in 250 ml of 5% Dextrose, not exceeding 3 ml/minute.

Pediatric: IM - 20 to 40 mg/kg in a 20% solution; repeat as necessary.

			C.I.*
Rx	**Magnesium Sulfate** (Various)	**Injection:** 10%. (0.8 mEq/ml). In 10 and 20 ml amps and 20 ml vials.	14+
		50%. (4 mEq/ml). In 2 and 10 ml amps, 5, 10, 30 and 50 ml vials and 5 and 10 ml disp. syringes.	20+
Rx	**Magnesium Sulfate** (Abbott)	**Injection:** 12.5%. (1 mEq/ml). In 8 ml vials.	89+
Rx	**Magnesium Sulfate Concentrated** (American McGaw)	**Injection:** 25% (2 mEq/ml). In 150 ml vials.	38

* Cost Index based on cost per ml.

This is an abbreviated monograph. For complete prescribing information, see page 558 .

Miscellaneous (Cont.)

ACETAZOLAMIDE

Actions:

Pharmacology: Acetazolamide has been used as an adjuvant in the treatment of certain CNS dysfunctions (eg, epilepsy). Inhibition of carbonic anhydrase in this area appears to retard abnormal, paroxysmal, excessive discharge from CNS neurons. The mechanism of this anticonvulsant action is not fully understood. Beneficial effects may be related to direct inhibition of carbonic anhydrase, or due to acidosis produced by therapy.

Pharmacokinetics: Acetazolamide is absorbed from the GI tract; it is distributed in body tissues, including the CNS, and is excreted unchanged in the urine.

Indications:

Centrencephalic epilepsies (petit mal, unlocalized seizures). The best results have been in petit mal seizures in children. Good results, however, have been seen in both children and adults with other seizure disorders.

Edema due to congestive heart failure and drug-induced edema; glaucoma (see p. 558).

For the prevention or amelioration of symptoms of acute mountain sickness in climbers attempting rapid ascent and in those who are susceptible to acute mountain sickness despite gradual ascent.

Contraindications:

Known allergy or hypersensitivity to sulfonamides. Depressed sodium or potassium serum levels; in marked kidney and liver disease or dysfunction; suprarenal gland failure; hyperchloremic acidosis.

The sustained release dosage form is not recommended for use as an anticonvulsant.

Administration and Dosage:

Epilepsy: 8 to 30 mg/kg/day in divided doses. Optimum range is 375 to 1000 mg daily.

Concomitant anticonvulsant therapy: When given in combination with other anticonvulsants, the starting dose is 250 mg/day. Increase to levels as indicated above.

Replacement therapy: The change from other medication to acetazolamide should be gradual.

Acute mountain sickness: 500 to 1000 mg/day in divided doses of tablets or sustained release capsules. In circumstances of rapid ascent, such as in rescue or military operations, the higher dose (1000 mg) is recommended. If possible, initiate dosage 24 to 48 hours before ascent, and continue for 48 hours while at high altitude, or longer as needed to control symptoms.

Parenteral: Direct IV administration is preferred because IM administration is painful, due to the alkaline pH of the solution.

Preparation and storage of parenteral solution: Reconstitute each 500 mg vial with at least 5 ml Sterile Water for Injection. Reconstituted solutions retain potency for 1 week if refrigerated; however, since this product contains no preservative, use within 24 hours of reconstitution.

	Product	Form	Description	C.I.*
Rx	**Diamox** (Lederle)	**Tablets:** 125 mg	(#LL D1/Diamox 125). White, scored. In 100s.	144
Rx	**Acetazolamide** (Various)	**Tablets:** 250 mg	In 100s, 1000s and UD 100s.	20+
Rx	**AK-Zol** (Akorn)		White, scored. In 100s and 1000s.	44
Rx	**Dazamide** (Major)		In 100s, 250s, 1000s and UD 100s.	39
Rx	**Diamox** (Lederle)		(#LL D2/Diamox 250). White, scored. In 100s, 1000s and UD 100s.	105
Rx	**Storzolamide** (Storz)		(#S19 Storz). White, scored in quarters. In 100s.	N/A
Rx	**Diamox** (Lederle)	**Injection:** 500 mg per vial	In 500 mg vials.	3613

* Cost Index based on cost per 250 mg.

Product identification code.

Actions:

Pharmacology: Curare preparations block nerve impulses to skeletal muscles at the myoneural junction. This is a nondepolarizing (competitive) neuromuscular blockade. **Metocurine iodide** may not produce the autonomic ganglionic blockade seen with other nondepolarizing muscle relaxants. Metocurine iodide reaches the neuromuscular junction more rapidly than does tubocurarine and is approximately twice as potent.

Repeated doses may have a cumulative effect. The duration of action and degree of muscle relaxation are altered by dehydration, body temperature changes, hypocalcemia, excess magnesium, acid-base imbalance or by some carcinomas. Since these drugs are excreted by the kidneys, severe renal disease, conditions associated with poor renal perfusion (shock states) or hypotension may result in a more prolonged action.

Coadministered general anesthetics, certain antibiotics, abnormal states (eg, acidosis), electrolyte imbalance and neuromuscular disease may potentiate activity of these drugs.

Curare preparations do not affect consciousness or cerebration, and do not relieve pain.

Pharmacokinetics: Following IV infusion, onset of flaccid paralysis occurs within a few minutes. Maximum relaxation occurs within a mean time of $\approx$ 6 minutes following IV use. Maximal effects persist for 35 to 60 minutes and effective muscle paralysis may persist for 25 to 90 minutes. Complete recovery may require several hours.

Tubocurarine – Approximately 50% is bound in plasma. First phase half-life is < 5 minutes, second phase half-life ranges from 7 to 40 minutes. Third phase half-life is 2 ± 1.1 hours; approximately 30% to 43% is excreted unchanged in the urine. Tubocurarine is also excreted to a lesser extent (up to 11%) in the bile. Approximately 1% undergoes hepatic metabolism (N-demethylation); the metabolite is excreted in bile.

Metocurine – Half-life is 3.6 hours with approximately 50% of the drug excreted unchanged in the urine and approximately 35% bound to plasma globulins.

Indications:

Adjunct to anesthesia to induce skeletal muscle relaxation; to reduce the intensity of muscle contractions in pharmacologically or electrically induced convulsions; to facilitate management of patients undergoing mechanical ventilation.

Tubocurarine is used as a diagnostic agent for myasthenia gravis when the results of tests with neostigmine or edrophonium are inconclusive.

Contraindications:

Allergic reaction or hypersensitivity to these drugs.

Tubocurarine: Patients in whom histamine release is a definite hazard.

Metocurine iodide: Patients sensitive to it or to its iodide content.

Warnings:

Respiratory effects: These drugs may cause respiratory depression and should be used only by those experienced in artificial respiration and administration of oxygen under positive pressure. Facilities for these procedures (including intubation of the trachea and availability of antagonistic agents for reversing nondepolarizing block) should be immediately available. Prolonged apnea may result from overdosage.

Rapid IV injection may produce histamine release with resultant decreased respiratory capacity due to bronchospasm and paralysis of the respiratory muscles. Hypotension may occur due to ganglionic blockade, or it may be a complication of positive pressure respiration. Histamine release with **metocurine** occurs less frequently and is related to dosage and rapidity of administration; cardiovascular effects (eg, changes in the pulse rate, hypotension) are less than those with equipotent doses of tubocurarine and gallamine.

Myasthenia gravis: Use with extreme caution in patients with known myasthenia gravis since prolonged respiratory paralysis may occur. A peripheral nerve stimulator may be valuable in assessing the effects of administration.

Elderly: Dosage requirements and recovery times may be increased.

(Warnings continued on following page)

Nondepolarizing Neuromuscular Blockers (Cont.)

Curare Preparations (Cont.)

Warnings (Cont.):

Pregnancy: Category C. Safety for use during pregnancy has not been established. There are no adequate and well controlled studies in pregnant women. Use in women of childbearing potential, especially during early pregnancy, only when clearly needed and when the potential benefits outweigh the potential hazards to the fetus.

Metocurine passes the placental barrier; 6 minutes following IV injection in the mother, fetal plasma concentration is ≈ one-tenth the maternal level.

Tubocurarine in prolonged doses (used in management of tetanus in a patient during early pregnancy), may be associated with fetal contractures. Following a total dose of ≈ 1.3 g tubocurarine chloride injected IV and IM over 10 days to a 10 to 12 week pregnant woman suffering from severe generalized tetanus, the infant was born at term with joint contractures. The condition was attributed to immobilization of the fetus at the time of joint formation.

Placental transfer and fetal distribution of tubocurarine has been reported. When given during delivery, blood levels in the newborn are directly related to maternal dose and time interval between injection and delivery. Although most infants do not grossly manifest drug effect following delivery, myoneural block has been reported in the newborn following repeated doses of tubocurarine to the mother (245 mg total) for prolonged management of eclampsia.

Lactation: It is not known whether these drugs are excreted in breast milk. Exercise caution when administering to a nursing woman.

Children: Metocurine is twice as potent as tubocurarine in children, but the recovery rate is the same. There may be a slight increase in heart rate, but no change in blood pressure or ECG. Doses calculated on the basis of body weight or body surface area may be applicable.

Premature infants and neonates may be more sensitive to these drugs. Infants and children exhibit the same widely variable responses as do adults.

Doses based on body weight appear to be suitable for children (as for adults) whereas doses based on body surface area are more accurate for premature infants and neonates. Incremental doses of 0.25 mg may constitute a useful practical titration to obtain satisfactory conditions in infants and neonates.

Reduce dosage in event of prematurity, acidosis, hypothermia or halothane use.

Precautions:

Concomitant conditions: Use with caution in patients with respiratory depression or with impaired cardiovascular, renal, hepatic, pulmonary or endocrine function. Hypotension can follow rapid injection or the administration of large doses. The action of the drug may be altered by electrolyte imbalance (hypokalemia potentiates the paralysis), body temperature, some carcinomas, dehydration and renal disease.

Histamine release: Use with caution in patients in whom a sudden increase of histamine release is a definite hazard.

Drug accumulation: Tubocurarine accumulates and may be present for several hours after the effects are not clinically apparent. Keep this in mind should a patient require successive doses or a second anesthesia after having previously received this drug.

Sulfite sensitivity: Some of these products may contain sulfites which may cause allergic-type reactions (eg, hives, itching, wheezing, anaphylaxis) in certain susceptible persons. Although the overall prevalence of sulfite sensitivity in the general population is probably low, it is seen more frequently in asthmatics or in atopic nonasthmatic persons. Specific products containing sulfites are identified in the product listings.

(Continued on following page)

MIVACURIUM CHLORIDE (Cont.)

Actions (Cont.):

Pharmacodynamics (Cont.):

Interpatient variability in duration of action occurs. However, analysis of data from 224 diverse patients in clinical studies indicated that approximately 90% of the patients had clinically effective durations of block within 8 minutes of the median duration predicted from the dose-response data. Variations in plasma cholinesterase activity were not associated with clinically significant effects or duration. The variability in duration, however, was greater in patients with plasma cholinesterase activity at or slightly below the lower limit of the normal range.

A dose of 0.15 mg/kg (2 x ED_{95}) administered during the induction of anesthesia produced generally good-to-excellent conditions for tracheal intubation in 2.5 minutes. Doses of 0.2 and 0.25 mg/kg (3 and 3.5 x ED_{95}) yielded similar conditions in 2 minutes.

Repeated administration of maintenance doses or continuous infusion for up to 2.5 hours is not associated with development of tachyphylaxis or cumulative neuromuscular blocking effects in ASA Physical Status I-II patients. Spontaneous recovery of neuromuscular function after infusion is independent of the duration of infusion and comparable to recovery reported for single doses.

The neuromuscular block produced by the stereoisomers in mivacurium is readily antagonized by anticholinesterase agents. The more profound the neuromuscular block at the time of reversal, the longer the time and the greater the dose of anticholinesterase agent required for recovery of neuromuscular function.

Children – In children 2 to 12 years, mivacurium has a higher ED_{95} (0.1 mg/kg), faster onset, and shorter duration of action than in adults. The mean time for spontaneous recovery of the twitch response from 25% to 75% of control amplitude is about 5 minutes (n = 4) following an initial dose of 0.2 mg/kg. Recovery following reversal is faster in children than in adults.

Hemodynamics: Administration of doses up to and including 0.15 mg/kg (2 x ED_{95}) over 5 to 15 seconds to ASA Physical Status I-II patients during opioid/nitrous oxide/oxygen anesthesia is associated with minimal change in mean arterial blood pressure (MAP) or heart rate.

Higher doses of $\geq$ 0.2 mg/kg ($\geq$ 3 x ED_{95}) may be associated with transient decreases in MAP and increases in heart rate in some patients. These decreases in MAP are usually maximal within 1 to 3 minutes following the dose, typically resolved without treatment in an additional 1 to 3 minutes, and are usually associated with increases in plasma histamine concentration. Decreases in MAP can be minimized by administering mivacurium over 30 or 60 seconds.

Analysis of 426 patients in clinical studies receiving initial doses $\leq$ 0.3 mg/kg (2 times the recommended intubating dose) during anesthesia showed that high initial doses and a rapid rate of injection contributed to a greater probability of experiencing a decrease of $\geq$ 30% in MAP after administration. Obese patients also had a greater probability of experiencing a decrease of $\geq$ 30% in MAP when dosed on the basis of actual body weight, thereby receiving a larger dose than if dosed on the basis of ideal body weight.

Children experience minimal changes in MAP or heart rate after doses $\leq$ 0.2 mg/kg over 5 to 15 seconds, but higher doses ($\geq$ 0.25 mg/kg) may be associated with transient decreases in MAP.

Pharmacokinetics: The following table describes the results from a study of 9 adult patients receiving an infusion of mivacurium at 5 mcg/kg/min for 60 minutes followed by 10 mcg/kg/min for 60 minutes. Mivacurium is a mixture of isomers which do not interconvert in vivo. The two more potent isomers, *cis-trans* (36% of the mixture) and *trans-trans* (57% of the mixture), have very high clearances that exceed cardiac output reflecting the extensive metabolism by plasma cholinesterase. The volume of distribution is relatively small, reflecting limited tissue distribution secondary to the polarity and large molecular weight of mivacurium. The combination of high metabolic clearance and low distribution volume results in the short elimination half-life of approximately 2 minutes for the two active isomers. The pharmacokinetics of the *cis-trans* and *trans-trans* isomers are dose-proportional. The *cis-cis* isomer (6% of the mixture) has approximately one-tenth the neuromuscular blocking potency of the *trans-trans* and *cis-trans* isomers in cats and data suggest that it produces minimal (< 5%) neuromuscular block during a 2 hour infusion.

(Actions continued on following page)

MIVACURIUM CHLORIDE (Cont.)

Actions (Cont.):

Pharmacokinetics (Cont.)

Stereoisomer Pharmacokinetic Parameters of Mivacurium in ASA Physical Status I-II Adult Patients (n = 9)[1]			
Parameter	*trans-trans* isomer	*cis-trans* isomer	*cis-cis* isomer
Elimination half-life (min)	2.3 (1.4-3.6)	2.1 (0.8-4.8)	55 (32-102)
Volume of distribution (L/kg)	0.15 (0.06-0.24)	0.27 (0.08-0.56)	0.31 (0.18-0.46)
Plasma clearance (ml/min/kg)	53 (32-105)	99 (52-230)	4.2 (2.4-5.4)

[1] Values shown are mean (range).

Metabolism/Excretion – Enzymatic hydrolysis by plasma cholinesterase is the primary mechanism for inactivation of mivacurium and yields a quaternary alcohol and a quaternary monoester metabolite. Renal and biliary excretion of unchanged mivacurium are minor elimination pathways; urine and bile are important elimination pathways for the two metabolites. Each metabolite is unlikely to produce clinically significant neuromuscular, autonomic or cardiovascular effects.

Special populations – Preliminary evidence indicates that reduced clearance of one or more isomers is responsible for the longer duration of action of mivacurium seen in patients with end-stage kidney or liver disease. The data did not provide a pharmacokinetic explanation for the 15% to 20% longer duration of block seen in the elderly.

Indications:

As an adjunct to general anesthesia, to facilitate tracheal intubation and to provide skeletal muscle relaxation during surgery or mechanical ventilation.

Contraindications:

Allergic hypersensitivity to mivacurium or other benzylisoquinolinium agents, as manifested by reactions such as urticaria, severe respiratory distress or hypotension; use of multi-dose vials in patients with allergy to benzyl alcohol.

Warnings:

Administration: Administer in carefully adjusted dosage by or under the supervision of experienced clinicians who are familiar with the drug's actions and the possible complications of its use. The drug should not be administered unless personnel and facilities for resuscitation and life support (tracheal intubation, artificial ventilation, oxygen therapy), and an antagonist of mivacurium are immediately available. Use a peripheral nerve stimulator to measure neuromuscular function during administration in order to monitor drug effect.

Conscious patients: Mivacurium has no known effect on consciousness, pain threshold, or cerebration. To avoid distress to the patient, neuromuscular block should not be induced before unconsciousness.

Renal function impairment: The clinically effective duration of action of 0.15 mg/kg mivacurium was about 1.5 times longer in patients with end-stage kidney disease, presumably due to reduced clearance of one or more isomers.

Hepatic function impairment: The clinically effective duration of action of 0.15 mg/kg mivacurium was 3 times longer in patients with end-stage liver disease than in healthy patients and is likely related to the markedly decreased plasma cholinesterase activity (30% of healthy patient values) which could decrease the clearance of one or more isomers.

Elderly: Mivacurium was safely administered during clinical trials to 64 elderly patients ($\geq$ 65 years of age), including 31 patients with significant cardiovascular disease. The duration of neuromuscular block may be slightly longer in elderly patients than in young adult patients.

Pregnancy: Category C. There are no adequate and well controlled studies in pregnant women. Use during pregnancy only if the potential benefit justifies the potential risk to the fetus.

Lactation: It is not known whether mivacurium or any of the stereoisomers are excreted in breast milk. Exercise caution following administration to a nursing woman.

Children: Mivacurium has not been studied in children $<$ 2 years of age (see Administration and Dosage for use in children 2 to 12 years of age). In children 2 to 12 years of age, mivacurium has a faster onset, a shorter duration, and recovery following reversal is faster compared to adults (see Pharmacodynamics).

(Continued on following page)

MIVACURIUM CHLORIDE (Cont.)

Precautions:

Histamine release: Although mivacurium is not a potent histamine releaser, the possibility of substantial histamine release must be considered. Release of histamine is related to the dose and speed of injection.

Exercise caution in administering mivacurium to patients with clinically significant cardiovascular disease and patients with any history suggesting a greater sensitivity to the release of histamine or related mediators (eg, asthma). In such patients, use an initial dose of ≤ 0.15 mg/kg, administered over 60 seconds; maintain adequate hydration and carefully monitor hemodynamic status.

Obese patients may be more likely to experience clinically significant transient decreases in MAP than non-obese patients when the dose is based on actual rather than ideal body weight. Determine the initial dose using the patient's ideal body weight.

Bradycardia: Recommended doses have no clinically significant effects on heart rate; therefore, mivacurium will not counteract the bradycardia produced by many anesthetic agents or by vagal stimulation.

Neuromuscular diseases: Neuromuscular blocking agents may have a profound effect in patients with neuromuscular diseases (eg, myasthenia gravis and the myasthenic syndrome). In these and other conditions in which prolonged neuromuscular block is a possibility (eg, carcinomatosis), the use of a peripheral nerve stimulator and a dose of ≤ 0.015 to 0.02 mg/kg is recommended.

Burn patients: Mivacurium has not been studied, but resistance to nondepolarizing neuromuscular blocking agents may develop in patients with burns depending upon the time elapsed since the injury and the size of the burn. Patients with burns may have reduced plasma cholinesterase activity which may offset this resistance.

Acid-base or serum electrolyte abnormalities may potentiate or antagonize the action of neuromuscular blocking agents; their action may be enhanced by magnesium salts administered for the management of toxemia of pregnancy.

Reduced plasma cholinesterase activity: Mivacurium is metabolized by plasma cholinesterase. Prolonged neuromuscular block following administration of mivacurium must be considered in patients with reduced plasma cholinesterase (pseudocholinesterase) activity. Plasma cholinesterase activity may be diminished in the presence of genetic abnormalities of plasma cholinesterase (eg, patients heterozygous or homozygous for the atypical plasma cholinesterase gene), pregnancy, liver or kidney disease, malignant tumors, infections, burns, anemia, decompensated heart disease, peptic ulcer or myxedema. Plasma cholinesterase activity may also be diminished by chronic administration of oral contraceptives, glucocorticoids, or certain MAO inhibitors and by irreversible inhibitors of plasma cholinesterase (eg, organophosphate insecticides, echothiophate, certain antineoplastic drugs).

Mivacurium has been used safely in patients heterozygous for the atypical plasma cholinesterase gene. At doses of 0.1 to 0.2 mg/kg, the clinically effective duration of action was 8 to 11 minutes longer in patients heterozygous for the atypical gene than in genotypically normal patients.

As with succinylcholine, patients homozygous for the atypical plasma cholinesterase gene (1 in 2500 patients) are extremely sensitive to the neuromuscular blocking effect of mivacurium. In three such adult patients, a small dose of 0.03 mg/kg (approximately the ED_{10-20} in genotypically normal patients) produced complete neuromuscular block for 26 to 128 minutes. Once spontaneous recovery had begun, neuromuscular block in these patients was antagonized with conventional doses of neostigmine. One adult patient, who was homozygous for the atypical plasma cholinesterase gene, received a dose of 0.18 mg/kg and exhibited complete neuromuscular block for about 4 hours. The patient was extubated after 8 hours; reversal was not attempted. Use with great caution, if at all, in patients known to be or suspected of being homozygous for the atypical plasma cholinesterase gene.

Drug Interactions:

Mivacurium can be expected to interact similarly to other nondepolarizing neuromuscular blockers. Refer to the Nondepolarizing Neuromuscular Blockers – Curare Preparations monograph.

(Continued on following page)

MIVACURIUM CHLORIDE (Cont.)

Adverse Reactions:

Prolonged neuromuscular block was reported in 3 of 2074 patients. The most common adverse experience was transient, dose-dependent cutaneous flushing about the face, neck or chest, most frequently after the initial dose in about 20% of adult patients who received 0.15 mg/kg over 5 to 15 seconds. Flushing typically began within 1 to 2 minutes after the dose and lasted for 3 to 5 minutes. Of 60 patients who experienced flushing after 0.15 mg/kg, one patient also experienced mild hypotension that was not treated, and one patient experienced moderate wheezing that was successfully treated.

Cardiovascular: Flushing (15%); tachycardia, bradycardia, cardiac arrhythmia, phlebitis (< 1%).

Hypotension: 1% to 2% of healthy adults given ≥ 0.2 mg/kg over 5 to 15 seconds and 2% to 4% of cardiac surgery patients given ≥ 0.2 mg/kg over 60 seconds were treated for decreases in blood pressure associated with the administration of mivacurium.

Respiratory: Bronchospasm, wheezing, hypoxemia (< 1%).

Dermatologic: Rash, urticaria, erythema, injection site reaction (< 1%).

Other: Prolonged drug effect, dizziness, muscle spasms (< 1%).

Overdosage:

Overdosage with neuromuscular blocking agents may result in neuromuscular block beyond the time needed for surgery and anesthesia. The primary treatment is maintenance of a patent airway and controlled ventilation until recovery of normal neuromuscular function is assured. Once evidence of recovery from neuromuscular block is observed, further recovery may be facilitated by administration of an anticholinesterase agent (eg, neostigmine, edrophonium) in conjunction with an appropriate anticholinergic agent. Overdosage may increase the risk of hemodynamic side effects, especially decreases in blood pressure. If needed, cardiovascular support may be provided by proper positioning of the patient, fluid administration, or vasopressor agent administration.

Antagonism of neuromuscular block: Antagonists (such as neostigmine) should not be administered when complete neuromuscular block is evident or suspected. Use a peripheral nerve stimulator to evaluate recovery and antagonism of neuromuscular block. Administration of 0.03 to 0.064 mg/kg neostigmine or 0.5 mg/kg edrophonium at ≈ 10% recovery from neuromuscular block produced 95% recovery of the muscle twitch response and a T_4/T_1 ratio ≥ 75% in about 10 minutes. The times from 25% recovery of the muscle twitch response to T_4/T_1 ratio ≥ 75% following these doses of antagonists averaged about 7 to 9 minutes. In comparison, average times for spontaneous recovery from 25% to T_4/T_1 ≥ 75% were 12 to 13 minutes. Evaluate patients administered antagonists for adequate clinical evidence of antagonism (eg, 5 second head lift and grip strength). Ventilation must be supported until no longer required.

Antagonism may be delayed in the presence of debilitation, carcinomatosis, and the concomitant use of certain broad spectrum antibiotics, anesthetic agents and other drugs which enhance neuromuscular block or cause respiratory depression. Management is the same as that of prolonged neuromuscular block.

Administration and Dosage:

Approved by the FDA on January 22, 1992.

Administer IV only. Individualize doses. Factors that may warrant dosage adjustment include but may not be limited to: The presence of significant kidney, liver or cardiovascular disease, obesity (patients weighing ≥ 30% more than ideal body weight for height), asthma, reduction in plasma cholinesterase activity and the presence of inhalational anesthetic agents. The use of a peripheral nerve stimulator will permit the most advantageous use of mivacurium, minimize the possibility of overdosage or underdosage, and assist in the evaluation of recovery.

Renal or hepatic impairment: 0.15 mg/kg for facilitation of tracheal intubation. However, the clinically effective duration of block produced by this dose is about 1.5 times longer in patients with end-stage kidney disease and about 3 times longer in patients with end-stage liver disease. Decrease infusion rates by as much as 50% in these patients depending on the degree of renal or hepatic impairment.

(Administration and Dosage continued on following page)

GALLAMINE TRIETHIODIDE (Cont.)

Management of Prolonged Neuromuscular Blockade:

The same antagonists that effectively dissipate the action of d-tubocurarine will also interrupt the action of gallamine by inhibiting the enzymatic hydrolysis of acetylcholine so that it accumulates and displaces the gallamine. The antagonists are merely adjuncts to adequate ventilation until the patient has resumed respiratory control.

Neostigmine (p. 2716 is an effective antidote, but it is advisable to administer atropine before or with neostigmine to counteract neostigmine's muscarinic action. Neostigmine has a prolonged action which may be cumulative; use with caution.

Another antidote is edrophonium chloride (p. 2717 given IV in 10 mg doses and repeated when necessary. Occasionally, bradycardia follows edrophonium use; it may be treated with atropine. Observe the patient since the effect may be transitory.

Use antidotes cautiously in asthmatic patients who may be sensitive to their action and who may have bronchoconstriction or excessive secretions upon administration; administer atropine if these reactions occur.

Overdosage may be aggravated by antidotes; treat by adequate artificial ventilation and systemic support. Refer to General Management of Acute Overdosage.

Administration and Dosage:

For IV use only.

Initial dose: Individualize dosage. Preferably administer as soon as the patient is unconscious and before attempting intubation. The theoretical initial dose is about 1 mg/kg, which produces a 50% reduction in respiratory minute volume. A 50% increase in the dose (1.5 mg/kg) will produce a 75% decrease in respiratory minute volume. Never inject more than 100 mg at any one time, regardless of the weight of the patient.

Weight appears to be the most important factor in determining dosage; also consider muscularity, age, sex and pathologic conditions. Use particular caution for patients weighing < 11 pounds (5 kg).

Repeat doses: For prolonged procedures, reinject the drug after 30 to 40 minutes or less, using 0.5 to 1 mg/kg. Gallamine may accumulate.

Compatibility: Can be mixed with barbiturates without altering either component, but it is preferable to inject each drug separately to control their effects. May be used with atropine, scopolamine or other premedications. May be effectively employed with all commonly used anesthetic agents. The solution has a pH of 6.5 to 7.5.

Do not mix gallamine with anesthetic agents as a precipitate will form. Do not administer any gallamine solution with a visible precipitate.

				C.I.*
Rx	**Flaxedil** (Davis + Geck)	**Injection:** 20 mg per ml	In 10 ml vials.[1]	447

* Cost Index based on cost per 20 mg.

[1] With 2.5 mg sodium metabisulfite and 0.13 mg EDTA per ml.

PANCURONIUM BROMIDE

Actions:

Pharmacology: Pancuronium, a nondepolarizing neuromuscular blocking agent, possesses all of the characteristic pharmacological actions on the myoneural junction. It is approximately 5 times as potent as d-tubocurarine chloride and approximately ⅓ less potent than vecuronium.

Pancuronium has little effect on the circulatory system, except for a moderate rise in heart rate, mean arterial pressure and cardiac output. Histamine release rarely occurs.

Pharmacokinetics: The ED_{95} (dose required to produce 95% suppression of the muscle twitch response) is approximately 0.05 mg/kg under balanced anesthesia and 0.03 mg/kg under halothane anesthesia. These doses produce effective skeletal muscle relaxation (as judged by time from maximum effect to 25% recovery of control twitch height) for approximately 22 minutes. Recovery to 90% of control twitch height usually occurs in approximately 65 minutes. Supplemental incremental doses following the initial dose slightly increase the magnitude of blockade and significantly increase the duration of blockade.

The elimination half-life of pancuronium ranges between 89 to 161 minutes. Approximately 40% of the total dose of pancuronium has been recovered in urine as unchanged pancuronium and its metabolites while approximately 11% has been recovered in bile. As much as 25% of an injected dose may be recovered as 3-hydroxy metabolite, which is half as potent a blocking agent as pancuronium.

Pancuronium exhibits strong binding to gamma globulin, and moderate binding to albumin. Approximately 87% is bound to plasma protein.

Patients with renal failure – The elimination half-life is doubled and the plasma clearance is reduced by approximately 50%.

Indications:

Adjunct to anesthesia to induce skeletal muscle relaxation; to facilitate the management of patients undergoing mechanical ventilation; to facilitate tracheal intubation.

Contraindications:

Hypersensitivity to pancuronium.

Warnings:

Administer in carefully adjusted dosage only by, or under the supervision of, experienced clinicians. Do not administer unless reversal agents and facilities for intubation, artificial respiration and oxygen therapy are immediately available. Be prepared to assist or control respiration.

Use in myasthenia gravis: In patients with myasthenia gravis or the myasthenic (Eaton-Lambert) syndrome, small doses of pancuronium may have profound effects. In such patients, a peripheral nerve stimulator and use of a small test dose may be of value in monitoring the response to administration of muscle relaxants.

Usage in Pregnancy: Category C. Safety for use during pregnancy has not been established. Do not use during early pregnancy, unless the potential benefits outweigh the unknown potential hazards to the fetus.

May be used in cesarean section, but reversal of pancuronium may be unsatisfactory in patients receiving magnesium sulfate for preeclampsia, because magnesium salts enhance neuromuscular blockade. Dosage should usually be reduced. Interval between use of pancuronium and delivery should be reasonably short to avoid clinically significant placental transfer.

Usage in Children: The prolonged use in neonates undergoing mechanical ventilation has been associated in rare cases with severe skeletal muscle weakness that may be first noted during attempts to wean such patients from the ventilator; these patients usually receive other drugs such as antibiotics which may enhance neuromuscular blockade. Microscopic changes consistent with disuse atrophy have been noted at autopsy. Although a cause-and-effect relationship has not been established, the benefit-to-risk ratio must be considered when there is a need for neuromuscular blockade to facilitate long term mechanical ventilation of neonates.

Rare cases of unexplained, clinically significant methemoglobinemia have been reported in premature neonates undergoing emergency anesthesia and surgery which included combined use of pancuronium, fentanyl and atropine. A direct cause-and-effect relationship has not been established.

(Continued on following page)

PANCURONIUM BROMIDE (Cont.)

Precautions:

Use of a peripheral nerve stimulator will usually be of value for monitoring of neuromuscular blocking effect, avoiding overdosage and assisting in evaluation of recovery.

Although it has been used successfully in preexisting pulmonary, hepatic or renal disease, exercise caution in these situations, especially in renal disease, since a major portion is excreted unchanged in the urine.

Altered circulation time: Conditions associated with slower circulation time (cardiovascular disease, old age and edematous states resulting in increased volume of distribution) may contribute to a delay in onset time; therefore dosage should not be increased.

Hepatic or biliary tract disease: The doubled elimination half-life and reduced plasma clearance determined in patients with hepatic or biliary tract disease, as well as limited data showing that recovery time is prolonged an average of 65% in patients with biliary tract obstruction, suggests that prolongation of neuromuscular blockade may occur. At the same time, these conditions are characterized by an approximately 50% increase in volume of distribution of pancuronium, suggesting that the total initial dose to achieve adequate relaxation may in some cases be high. The possibility of slower onset, higher total dosage and prolongation of neuromuscular blockade must be taken into consideration when pancuronium is used in these patients.

Severe obesity or neuromuscular disease: Patients with severe obesity or neuromuscular disease may pose airway or ventilatory problems requiring special care before, during and after the use of neuromuscular blocking agents such as pancuronium.

Pancuronium has no known effect on consciousness, the pain threshold or cerebration. Administration should be accompanied by adequate anesthesia.

Electrolyte imbalance and diseases which lead to electrolyte imbalance, such as adrenal cortical insufficiency, alter neuromuscular blockade. Depending on the nature of the imbalance, either enhancement or inhibition may be expected.

Drug Interactions:

Antibiotics: Parenteral/intraperitoneal administration of high doses of certain antibiotics may produce neuromuscular block on their own. The following have been associated with various degrees of paralysis: **Aminoglycosides; tetracyclines; bacitracin; polymyxin B; clindamycin; lincomycin; colistin;** and **sodium colistimethate.** If these agents are used preoperatively or in conjunction with pancuronium during surgery, unexpected prolongation of neuromuscular block should be considered a possibility.

Azathioprine may cause a reversal of the neuromuscular blocking effects of pancuronium.

Inhalation anesthetics (eg, halothane, enflurane, isoflurane): Use of these drugs with pancuronium will enhance neuromuscular blockade. Potentiation is most prominent with use of **enflurane** and **isoflurane.**

Patients receiving chronic **tricyclic antidepressant** therapy who are anesthetized with **halothane** should have pancuronium administered with caution because severe ventricular arrhythmias may result from the combination. The severity of the arrhythmias appear in part related to the dose of pancuronium.

Magnesium sulfate: When administered for the management of toxemia of pregnancy, may enhance neuromuscular blockade of pancuronium.

Other neuromuscular blocking agents: The combination of pancuronium and either **metocurine** or **tubocurarine** appears to be synergistic; however, the duration of blockade is not prolonged.

Quinidine injected during recovery from use of other muscle relaxants suggests that recurrent paralysis may occur. Also consider this possibility for pancuronium bromide injection. **Quinine** may increase the action of pancuronium.

Succinylcholine: Prior administration, such as that used for endotracheal intubation, enhances the relaxant effect of pancuronium and its duration of action. If succinylcholine is used before pancuronium, delay administration of pancuronium until the effects of succinylcholine begin to subside.

If a small dose of pancuronium is given at least 3 minutes prior to the administration of succinylcholine in order to reduce the incidence and intensity of succinylcholine-induced fasiculations, this dose may induce a degree of neuromuscular block sufficient to cause respiratory depression in some patients.

Theophyllines: Possible resistance to, or reversal of, the effects of pancuronium. Cardiac arrhythmias might also occur.

(Continued on following page)

PANCURONIUM BROMIDE (Cont.)

Adverse Reactions:

Neuromuscular: The most frequent reactions are an extension of pharmacological actions beyond the time period needed for surgery and anesthesia. This varies from skeletal muscle weakness to profound and prolonged skeletal muscle relaxation, resulting in respiratory insufficiency or apnea. Inadequate reversal of the neuromuscular blockade by anticholinesterases has also been observed. Manage adverse reactions by manual or mechanical ventilation until there is adequate recovery.

Cardiovascular: See discussion in Pharmacology.

GI: Salivation during very light anesthesia, especially with no anticholinergic premedication.

Dermatologic: Transient rash (occasional).

Hypersensitivity reactions (rare) characterized by bronchospasm, flushing, redness, hypotension, tachycardia and other reactions possibly mediated by histamine release.

Management of Prolonged Neuromuscular Blockade:

Residual neuromuscular blockade beyond the time period needed for surgery and anesthesia may occur, manifested by skeletal muscle weakness, decreased respiratory reserve, low tidal volume or apnea. A peripheral nerve stimulator may be used to assess the degree of residual neuromuscular blockade. The primary treatment is manual or mechanical ventilation and maintenance of a patent airway until complete recovery of normal respiration is assured.

Pyridostigmine bromide, neostigmine or edrophonium, in conjunction with atropine or glycopyrrolate, will usually antagonize the action of pancuronium. Judge satisfactory reversal by adequacy of skeletal muscle tone and respiration. Failure of prompt reversal (within 30 minutes) may occur in the presence of extreme debilitation and carcinomatosis and with concomitant use of certain broad spectrum antibiotics or anesthetic agents and adjuncts which enhance neuromuscular blockade or cause respiratory depression of their own. Under such circumstances, the management is the same as that of prolonged neuromuscular blockade; support ventilation by artificial means until the patient has resumed respiratory control.

Administration and Dosage:

For IV use only.

Administer only by, or under the supervision of, clinicians experienced in the use of these drugs. Individualize dosage.

Concomitant therapy: Since potent inhalation agents or prior administration of succinylcholine enhance the intensity and duration of blockade of pancuronium, consider these factors when determining initial and incremental dosage.

Adults: Initial IV dosage is 0.04 to 0.1 mg/kg. Later, use incremental doses starting at 0.01 mg/kg. These increments slightly increase the magnitude of the blockade and significantly increase the duration of blockade because a significant number of myoneural junctions are still blocked when there is clinical need for more drug.

Skeletal muscle relaxation for endotracheal intubation – Bolus dose of 0.06 to 0.1 mg/kg. Conditions satisfactory for intubation usually occur in 2 to 3 min.

Cesarean section – The dosage to provide relaxation for intubation and operation and the dosage to provide relaxation following use of succinylcholine for intubation (see Drug Interactions) are the same as for general surgical procedures.

Children: With the exception of neonates, dosage requirements are the same as for adults. Neonates are especially sensitive to nondepolarizing neuromuscular blockers during the first month of life. Give a test dose of 0.02 mg/kg to assess responsiveness.

Compatibility/Stability: Pancuronium is compatible in solution with 0.9% sodium chloride, 5% dextrose, 5% dextrose and sodium chloride and Lactated Ringer's injections. Mixed with these solutions in glass or plastic containers, pancuronium will remain stable for 48 hours with no alteration in potency or pH.

Storage: Refrigerate at 2° to 8°C (36° to 46°F) to maintain potency for 2 years. If stored at 18° to 22°C (65°to 72°F), potency is maintained for 6 months.

				C.I.*
Rx	**Pancuronium Bromide** (Various, eg, Astra, Elkins-Sinn, Quad)	**Injection:** 1 mg per ml	In 10 ml vials.	1263+
Rx	**Pavulon** (Organon)		In 10 ml vials.[1]	1346
Rx	**Pancuronium Bromide** (Various, eg, Astra, Elkins-Sinn, Quad)	**Injection:** 2 mg per ml	In 2 & 5 ml vials, amps and syringes.	1391+
Rx	**Pavulon** (Organon)		In 2 and 5 ml amps.[1]	1440

* Cost Index based on cost per 2 mg.

[1] With benzyl alcohol.

ATRACURIUM BESYLATE

Actions:

Pharmacology: Atracurium, a nondepolarizing skeletal muscle relaxant, antagonizes the neurotransmitter action of acetylcholine by binding competitively with cholinergic receptor sites on the motor end-plate.

Atracurium is a less potent histamine releaser than d-tubocurarine or metocurine. Histamine release is minimal with initial doses up to 0.5 mg/kg, and hemodynamic changes are minimal within the recommended dose range. A moderate histamine release and significant fall in blood pressure have occurred following 0.6 mg/kg. The effects were generally short-lived and manageable.

Pharmacokinetics are essentially linear within the range of 0.3 to 0.6 mg/kg.

Onset, Peak and Duration of Action – The time to onset of paralysis decreases and the duration of maximum effect increases with increasing doses. The duration of neuromuscular blockade is approximately one-third to one-half that of d-tubocurarine, metocurine and pancuronium at initially equipotent doses.

The ED_{95} (dose required to produce 95% suppression of the muscle twitch response with balanced anesthesia) has averaged 0.23 mg/kg (0.11 to 0.26 mg/kg). An initial dose of 0.4 to 0.5 mg/kg generally produces maximum neuromuscular blockade within 3 to 5 minutes of injection. Recovery from neuromuscular blockade (under balanced anesthesia) begins approximately 20 to 35 minutes after injection; recovery to 25% of control is achieved approximately 35 to 45 minutes after injection, and recovery is usually 95% complete approximately 60 to 70 minutes after injection.

Repeated administration of maintenance doses has no cumulative effect on the duration of neuromuscular blockade if recovery is allowed to begin prior to repeat dosing. After the initial dose, the first maintenance dose (0.08 to 0.1 mg/kg) is generally required within 20 to 45 minutes, and subsequent doses are required at approximately 15 to 25 minute intervals.

Recovery proceeds more rapidly than recovery from d-tubocurarine, metocurine and pancuronium. Regardless of dose, the time from start of recovery to complete (95%) recovery is approximately 30 minutes under balanced anesthesia and approximately 40 minutes under halothane, enflurane or isoflurane anesthesia. Repeated doses have no cumulative effect on recovery rate.

Excretion – The elimination half-life is approximately 20 minutes. The duration of neuromuscular blockade does not correlate with plasma pseudocholinesterase levels and is not altered by the absence of renal function. Atracurium is inactivated in plasma via two nonoxidative pathways. Some placental transfer occurs.

Indications:

As an adjunct to general anesthesia to facilitate endotracheal intubation and to relax skeletal muscle during surgery or mechanical ventilation.

Contraindications:

Hypersensitivity to atracurium besylate.

Warnings:

Atracurium should be used only by those skilled in airway management and respiratory support. Equipment and personnel must be immediately available for endotracheal intubation and support of ventilation, including use of positive pressure oxygen. Have anticholinesterase reversal agents immediately available.

Do not give by IM administration.

Atracurium has no known effect on consciousness, pain threshold or cerebration. Use only with adequate anesthesia.

Usage in Pregnancy: Category C. Atracurium was potentially teratogenic in rabbits in doses up to ≈ half the human dose. There are no adequate and well controlled studies in pregnant women. Use during pregnancy only if the potential benefits outweigh the potential hazards to the fetus.

(Warnings continued on following page)

ATRACURIUM BESYLATE (Cont.)

Warnings (Cont.):

Usage in Labor and Delivery: Atracurium (0.3 mg/kg) has been administered to 26 pregnant women during delivery by cesarean section. No harmful effects occurred in any of the newborn infants, although small amounts crossed the placental barrier. Consider the possibility of respiratory depression in the newborn.

It is not known whether muscle relaxants given during vaginal delivery have immediate or delayed adverse effects on the fetus or increase the likelihood that resuscitation of the newborn will be necessary. The possibility of forceps delivery may increase.

Usage in Lactation: It is not known whether this drug is excreted in breast milk. Safety for use in the nursing mother has not been established.

Usage in Children: Safety and efficacy for children < 1 month old are not established.

Precautions:

Histamine release: Exercise special caution, especially when substantial histamine release would be hazardous (eg, patients with clinically significant cardiovascular disease, severe anaphylactoid reactions or asthma). The recommended initial dose is lower (0.3 to 0.4 mg/kg); administer slowly or in divided doses over 1 minute.

Bradycardia during anesthesia may be more common with atracurium than with other muscle relaxants since atracurium has no clinically significant effects on heart rate in the recommended dosage range. It will not counteract bradycardia or vagal stimulation.

Usage in neuromuscular diseases in which potentiation of nondepolarizing agents has been noted (ie, myasthenia gravis, Eaton-Lambert syndrome) may cause profound effects. The use of a peripheral nerve stimulator is especially important for assessing neuromuscular blockade in these patients. Take similar precautions in patients with severe electrolyte disorders or carcinomatosis.

Usage in bronchial asthma: Safety has not been established in these patients.

Drug Interactions:

Diuretics: The neuromuscular blocking effects of atracurium may be increased by **thiazide diuretics.** Hypokalemia enhances the neuromuscular blockade, possibly by hyperpolarizing the end plate membrane, increasing resistance to depolarization.

Enflurane, isoflurane and **halothane;** certain antibiotics, especially the **aminoglycosides, polypeptide antibiotics** (bacitracin, capreomycin, colistimethate, polymyxin B), **clindamycin** and **lincomycin; lithium; verapamil; trimethaphan; procainamide;** and **quinidine** may enhance the neuromuscular blocking action of atracurium. Neuromuscular blockade was prolonged 20% by halothane and 35% by enflurane and isoflurane.

Magnesium sulfate: In patients on magnesium sulfate, reversal of neuromuscular blockade may be unsatisfactory; lower atracurium dose as indicated. However, in one patient, reversal of neuromuscular blockade was not affected by magnesium sulfate.

Other muscle relaxants: If administered during the same procedure, consider the possibility of a synergistic or antagonist effect.

Phenytoin and **theophylline** may cause resistance to, or reversal of, the neuromuscular blocking action of atracurium.

Succinylcholine does not enhance duration, but quickens onset and may increase depth of atracurium-induced neuromuscular blockade. Do not give atracurium until patient recovers from succinylcholine-induced neuromuscular blockade.

Loop diuretics have been reported to both increase and decrease the neuromuscular blocking effects of nondepolarizing muscle relaxants.

Adverse Reactions:

Observed in clinical practice: In ≈ 3 million patients in the US and United Kingdom, spontaneously reported adverse reactions were uncommon (≈ 0.01% to 0.02%). The following are among those reported most frequently, but data are insufficient to estimate incidence.

General: Allergic reactions (anaphylactic or anaphylactoid responses), rarely severe.
Musculoskeletal: Inadequate block, prolonged block.
Cardiovascular: Hypotension, vasodilatation (flushing), tachycardia, bradycardia.
Respiratory: Dyspnea, bronchospasm, laryngospasm.
Integumentary: Rash, urticaria, reaction at injection site.

Controlled clinical studies: Most adverse reactions suggest histamine release. In studies of 875 patients, atracurium was discontinued in only one patient (who required treatment for bronchial secretions), and six other patients required treatment (wheezing in one, hypotension in five). Of the five patients who required treatment for hypotension, three had a history of significant cardiovascular disease. The overall incidence rate for clinically important adverse reactions was 7/875 (0.8%).

(Adverse Reactions continued on following page)

ATRACURIUM BESYLATE (Cont.)

Adverse Reactions (Cont.):

	Initial Dose (mg/kg)			
Adverse Reaction	0-0.3 (n = 485)	0.31-0.5[1] (n = 366)	≥ 0.6 (n = 24)	Total (n = 875)
Skin Flush	1%	8.7%	29.2%	5%
Erythema	0.6%	0.5%	0%	0.6%
Itching	0.4%	0%	0%	0.2%
Wheezing/Bronchial Secretions	0.2%	0.3%	0%	0.2%
Hives	0.2%	0%	0%	0.1%
Vital Sign Change[2] (≥ 30%)	(n = 365)	(n = 144)	(n = 21)	(n = 530)
Mean Arterial Pressure				
Increase	1.9%	2.8%	0%	2.1%
Decrease	1.1%	2.1%	14.3%	1.9%
Heart Rate				
Increase	1.6%	2.8%	4.8%	2.1%
Decrease	0.8%	0%	0%	0.6%

[1] Recommended range for most patients. [2] Clinical trials w/530 patients without cardiovascular disease.

Overdosage:

Minimize possibility of overdosage by monitoring muscle twitch response to peripheral nerve stimulation. Expect excessive doses to produce enhanced pharmacological effects. Overdosage may increase risk of histamine release and cardiovascular effects, especially hypotension. Provide cardiovascular support when necessary. Assure airway and ventilation. A longer duration of neuromuscular blockade may occur. To facilitate recovery, use an anticholinesterase reversing agent (eg, neostigmine, edrophonium, pyridostigmine) in conjunction with an anticholinergic agent such as atropine or glycopyrrolate.

Three pediatric patients (3 weeks, 4 and 5 months of age) unintentionally received doses of 0.8 mg/kg to 1 mg/kg of atracurium. The time to 25% recovery (50 to 55 minutes) following these doses, which were 5 to 6 times the ED_{95} dose, was moderately longer than the corresponding time observed following doses 2 to 2.5 times the atracurium ED_{95} dose in infants (22 to 36 min). Cardiovascular changes were minimal.

A 17-year-old patient unintentionally received an initial dose of 1.3 mg/kg atracurium. The time from injection to 25% recovery (83 minutes) was ≈ twice that observed following maximum recommended doses in adults (35 to 45 minutes). The patient experienced moderate hemodynamic changes (13% increase in mean arterial pressure and 27% increase in heart rate) persisting for 40 minutes, but not requiring treatment.

Reversal of neuromuscular blockade can be achieved with an anticholinesterase agent such as neostigmine, edrophonium or pyridostigmine, in conjunction with an anticholinergic agent such as atropine or glycopyrrolate. Reversal can usually be attempted approximately 20 to 35 minutes after an initial dose or 10 to 30 minutes after a maintenance dose. Complete reversal is usually attained within 8 to 10 minutes. Rare instances of breathing difficulties have been reported following attempted pharmacologic antagonism of atracurium-induced neuromuscular blockade. The tendency for residual neuromuscular block is increased if reversal is attempted at deep levels of blockade or if inadequate doses of reversal agents are used.

Administration and Dosage:

To avoid patient distress, do not administer before unconsciousness has been induced.

Administer IV. IM use may result in tissue irritation.

Using a peripheral nerve stimulator to monitor muscle twitch suppression and recovery permits the best use of atracurium and minimizes overdosage.

Neuromuscular blocking effect is potentiated by enflurane or isoflurane and, to a lesser extent, by halothane. Consider reducing initial atracurium dose or infusion rate in patients on inhalation anesthesia. Reduce dose by ≈ ⅓ in the presence of steady-state enflurane or isoflurane anesthesia; consider smaller reductions with concurrent halothane.

Bolus doses for intubation and maintenance of neuromuscular blockade: Initial adult dose – 0.4 to 0.5 mg/kg (1.7 to 2.2 times the ED_{95}) IV bolus injection. Expect good or excellent conditions for nonemergency intubation in 2 to 2.5 minutes in most patients; maximum neuromuscular blockade is achieved ≈ 3 to 5 minutes after injection.

Maintaining neuromuscular blockade during prolonged surgical procedures – 0.08 to 0.1 mg/kg. The first maintenance dose will generally be required 20 to 45 minutes after the initial injection. Give maintenance doses at regular intervals, every 15 to 25 minutes under balanced anesthesia, slightly longer under isoflurane or enflurane. Higher doses (up to 0.2 mg/kg) permit maintenance dosing at longer intervals.

(Administration and Dosage continued on following page)

ATRACURIUM BESYLATE (Cont.)

Administration and Dosage (Cont.):

Bolus doses for intubation and maintenance of neuromuscular blockade (Cont.):

Significant cardiovascular disease and history (eg, severe anaphylactoid reactions or asthma) *suggesting a greater risk of histamine release* – Initially, 0.3 to 0.4 mg/kg given slowly or in divided doses over 1 minute.

Neuromuscular disease, severe electrolyte disorders or carcinomatosis: Consider dosage reductions in which potentiation of neuromuscular blockade or difficulties with reversal have been demonstrated. There has been no clinical experience in these patients, and no specific dosage adjustments. No dosage adjustments are required for patients with *renal diseases.*

Following use of succinylcholine for intubation under balanced anesthesia – Initially, 0.3 to 0.4 mg/kg. Further reductions may be desirable with the use of potent inhalation anesthetics. Permit the patient to recover from the effects of succinylcholine prior to atracurium administration. Data are insufficient to recommend specific initial doses following administration of succinylcholine in infants and children.

Pediatrics – No dosage adjustments are required for patients 2 years of age or older. An initial dose of 0.3 to 0.4 mg/kg is recommended for infants (1 month to 2 years of age) under halothane anesthesia. More frequent maintenance doses may be required.

Use by infusion: After administration of an initial bolus dose of 0.3 to 0.5 mg/kg, give a diluted solution by continuous infusion to adults and children aged 2 or more years for maintenance of neuromuscular blockade during extended surgical procedures. Long-term IV infusion to support mechanical ventilation in the intensive care unit has not been studied sufficiently to support dosage recommendations. Individualize infusion. Accurate dosing is best achieved using a precision infusion device.

Initiate infusion only after early evidence of spontaneous recovery from the bolus dose. An initial infusion rate of 9 to 10 mcg/kg/min may be required to rapidly counteract the spontaneous recovery of neuromuscular function. Thereafter, a rate of 5 to 9 mcg/kg/min (range 2 to 15 mcg/kg/min) should maintain continuous neuromuscular blockade in the range of 89% to 99% in most pediatric and adult patients under balanced anesthesia.

In patients undergoing cardiopulmonary bypass with induced hypothermia, the rate of infusion required to maintain adequate surgical relaxation during hypothermia (25° to 28°C) is approximately half the rate required during normothermia.

Infusion solutions may be prepared by admixing atracurium with an appropriate diluent: 5% Dextrose Injection, 0.9% Sodium Chloride Injection or 5% Dextrose and 0.9% Sodium Chloride Injection. Spontaneous degradation has been demonstrated to occur more rapidly in Lactated Ringer's solution than in 0.9% Sodium Chloride solution. Therefore, do not use Lactated Ringer's Injection. The amount of infusion solutions required per minute will depend upon the concentration and dose desired (see table). Use infusion solutions within 24 hours of preparation. Discard unused solutions. Solutions containing 0.2 or 0.5 mg/ml in the above diluents may be stored either under refrigeration or at room temperature for 24 hours without significant loss of potency.

Atracurium Infusion Rates
Concentrations for 0.2 and 0.5 mg/ml

Drug Delivery Rate (mcg/kg/min)	Infusion Delivery Rate (ml/kg/min)	
	0.2 mg/ml†	0.5 mg/ml††
5	0.025	0.01
6	0.03	0.012
7	0.035	0.014
8	0.04	0.016
9	0.045	0.018
10	0.05	0.02

† 2 ml of 1% (10 mg/ml) added to 98 ml diluent.
†† 5 ml of 1% (10 mg/ml) added to 95 ml diluent.

Stability: Atracurium has an acid pH; do not mix with alkaline solutions (eg, barbiturates) in the same syringe or administer simultaneously during IV infusion through the same needle. The drug may be inactivated and precipitated.

Storage: Atracurium loses potency at the rate of 6% per year under refrigeration (5° C). Rate of loss in potency increases to approximately 5% per month at 25°C (77°F). Refrigerate at 2° to 8°C (36° to 46°F) to preserve potency. Do not freeze. **C.I.***

Rx	**Tracrium** (Burroughs Wellcome)	**Injection:** 10 mg per ml[1]	In 5 ml amps and 10 ml vials.[2]	1532

* Cost Index based on cost per 10 mg. [1] With benzenesulfonic acid. [2] With 0.9% benzyl alcohol.

PIPECURONIUM BROMIDE (Cont.)

Actions (Cont.):

Pharmacokinetics (Cont.):

In animals, pipecuronium is eliminated primarily by the kidneys (> 75% of drug recovered in the urine, primarily as the unchanged drug). The 3-deacetyl, 17-deacetyl, and 3,17-dideacetyl derivatives have been identified in urine; these metabolites account for approximately 20% of the administered dose. The 3-deacetyl derivative is the only metabolite with substantial neuromuscular blocking activity, manifesting approximately 40% to 50% of the activity of the parent drug.

Only the 3-deacetyl metabolite has been detected in the urine of humans undergoing coronary artery bypass surgery. Following 200 mcg/kg, 56% of the administered dose was recovered in the urine, of which 41% was unchanged drug, and the remaining 15% was the 3-deacetyl metabolite. No metabolites were found in the plasma.

Hemodynamics: Clinically significant bradycardia, hypotension and hypertension have occurred in approximately 3% of 592 patients. The most common observations, comparing vital signs immediately prior to initial dosage with pipecuronium and 2 minutes after injection, are a slight decrease in heart rate, systolic and diastolic blood pressure.

In patients undergoing surgery for coronary artery bypass grafting using 100 and 200 mcg/kg during induction of anesthesia with a narcotic or etomidate/narcotic combination, respectively, hemodynamic effects were small and included reductions in mean systolic and mean arterial pressures (10% to 14%), ventricular stroke-work index (8% to 25%) and cardiac output (20%).

Indications:

As an adjunct to general anesthesia, to provide skeletal muscle relaxation during surgery. Pipecuronium can also be used to provide skeletal muscle relaxation for endotracheal intubation. It is only recommended for procedures anticipated to last ≥ 90 minutes.

Warnings:

Monitoring: Administer pipecuronium in carefully adjusted dosage by or under the supervision of experienced clinicians familiar with the drug's actions and the possible complications of its use. Do not administer unless facilities for intubation, artificial respiration, oxygen therapy and an antagonist are within immediate reach. Clinicians administering long-acting neuromuscular blocking agents should employ a peripheral nerve stimulator to monitor drug response, need for additional relaxant, and adequacy of spontaneous recovery or antagonism.

Myasthenia gravis or myasthenic (Eaton-Lambert) syndrome: Small doses of nondepolarizing neuromuscular blocking agents may have profound effects. Shorter acting muscle relaxants may be more suitable for these patients.

Pipecuronium is not recommended for use in patients requiring prolonged mechanical ventilation in the ICU or prior to or following other nondepolarizing neuromuscular blocking agents.

Renal failure: In a limited number of patients (n = 20) undergoing renal transplant surgery, the mean clinical duration (injection to 25% recovery) of 103 minutes was not judged prolonged following a dose of 70 mg/kg; however, there was wide individual variation (30 to 267 minutes). Because it is primarily excreted by the kidney, and because some shorter acting drugs (vecuronium and atracurium) have a more predictable duration of action in patients with renal dysfunction, use with extra caution in patients with renal failure (see Administration and Dosage).

Pregnancy: Category C. An embryotoxic effect (secondary to maternal toxicity) was observed in rats at the highest dose administered (50 mcg/kg) as demonstrated by an increase in earlier fetal resorptions. There are no adequate and well controlled studies in pregnant women. Use during pregnancy only if the potential benefit justifies the potential risk to the fetus.

Obstetrics (cesarean section): There are insufficient data on placental transfer of pipecuronium and possible related effect(s) upon the neonate following cesarean section delivery. In addition, the duration of action of pipecuronium exceeds the duration of operative obstetrics (cesarean section). Therefore pipecuronium is not recommended for use in patients undergoing C-section.

Children: Infants (3 months to 1 year) under balanced anesthesia or halothane anesthesia, manifest similar dose response to pipecuronium as do adults on a mcg/kg basis. Children (1 to 14 years) under balanced anesthesia or halothane anesthesia, may be less sensitive than adults. There are no data on either onset time or clinical duration of larger doses in infants or children. There are no data on maintenance dosing in infants and children.

(Continued on following page)

PIPECURONIUM BROMIDE (Cont.)

Precautions:

Bradycardia: Since pipecuronium has little or no effect on the heart rate, the drug will not counteract the bradycardia produced by many opioid anesthetic agents or vagal stimulation. Consequently, bradycardia during anesthesia may be more common with pipecuronium than when muscle relaxants (eg, pancuronium), which exert vagolytic action are employed.

Increased volume of distribution: Conditions associated with an increased volume of distribution (eg, slower circulation time in cardiovascular disease, old age, edematous states) may be associated with a delay in onset time. Because higher doses may produce a longer duration of action, the initial dosage should not usually be increased to enhance onset time; allow more time for the drug to achieve maximum effect.

Obesity: The most common patient condition associated with prolonged clinical duration was obesity, defined as ≥ 30% over ideal body weight. Clinical study subjects were dosed on the basis of actual body weight, which may have contributed to the higher incidence of prolonged duration. Base dose on ideal body weight for height in obese patients (see Administration and Dosage).

Fluid/Electrolyte imbalance: Experience with other drugs has suggested that acute (eg, diarrhea) or chronic (eg, adrenocortical insufficiency) electrolyte imbalance may alter neuromuscular blockade. Since electrolyte imbalance and acid-base imbalance are usually mixed, either enhancement or inhibition may occur.

Drug Interactions:

Anesthetics, inhalational: Use of volatile inhalation anesthetics enhances the activity of other neuromuscular blocking agents on the order of enflurane > isoflurane > halothane. Since the neuromuscular blocking agents are routinely administered before or shortly after the administration of the inhalation anesthetic, minimal effects are generally observed on onset time and peak effect. In routine use of neuromuscular blocking agents, only clinical duration is generally affected (prolonged). Use of isoflurane has resulted in an increase in mean clinical duration of 12%. In 25 patients first anesthetized with enflurane for ≥ 5 minutes, the mean clinical duration was increased by 50%. Therefore, anticipate a prolonged clinical duration following initial or maintenance doses and prolonged recovery from the neuromuscular blocking effect of pipecuronium.

Antibiotics: Parenteral/intraperitoneal administration of high doses of certain antibiotics may intensify or produce neuromuscular block on their own.

The following antibiotics have been associated with various degrees of paralysis: Aminoglycosides; tetracyclines; bacitracin; polymyxin B; colistin; sodium colistimethate. If these antibiotics are used in conjunction with pipecuronium during surgery, consider prolongation of neuromuscular block a possibility.

Magnesium salts, administered for the management of toxemia of pregnancy, may enhance neuromuscular blockade.

Quinidine: Experience concerning injection of quinidine during recovery from use of other muscle relaxants suggests that recurrent paralysis may occur. This possibility must also be considered for pipecuronium.

Succinylcholine: Pipecuronium can be administered following recovery from succinylcholine when the latter is used to facilitate endotracheal intubation. The use of pipecuronium before succinylcholine, in order to attenuate some of the side effects of succinylcholine is not recommended. See Pharmacology.

(Continued on following page)

PIPECURONIUM BROMIDE (Cont.)

Adverse Reactions:

The most frequent side effect of nondepolarizing blocking agents is an extension of the drug's pharmacological action beyond the time period needed for surgery and anesthesia. Clinical signs may vary from skeletal muscle weakness to skeletal muscle paralysis resulting in respiratory insufficiency or apnea. This may be due to the drug's effect or inadequate antagonism.

The following listings are based on US clinical studies involving nearly 600 patients, using a variety of premedications, varying lengths of surgical procedures and various anesthetic agents.

Cardiovascular: Hypotension (2.5%); bradycardia (1.4%); hypertension, myocardial ischemia, cerebrovascular accident, thrombosis, atrial fibrillation, ventricular extrasystole (< 1%).

Metabolic/Nutritional: Hypoglycemia, hyperkalemia, increased creatinine (< 1%).

Musculoskeletal: Muscle atrophy, difficult intubation (< 1%).

CNS: Hypesthesia, CNS depression (< 1%).

Respiratory: Dyspnea, respiratory depression, laryngismus, atelectasis (< 1%).

Skin/Appendages: Rash, urticaria (< 1%).

GU: Anuria (< 1%).

Overdosage:

Support ventilation by artificial means until no longer required. Intensified monitoring of vital organ function is required for the period of paralysis and during an extended period postrecovery.

Antagonism of neuromuscular blockade: Antagonists (such as neostigmine) should not be administered prior to the demonstration of some spontaneous recovery from neuromuscular blockade. The use of a nerve stimulator to document recovery and antagonism of neuromuscular blockade is recommended.

Evaluate patients for adequate clinical evidence of antagonism (eg, 5 second head lift, adequate phonation, ventilation and upper airway maintenance). As with other neuromuscular blocking agents, physicians should be alert to the possibility that the action of the drugs used to antagonize neuromuscular blockade may wear off before plasma levels of pipecuronium have declined sufficiently.

Antagonism may be delayed in the presence of debilitation, carcinomatosis, and concomitant use of certain broad-spectrum antibiotics, or anesthetic agents and other drugs that enhance neuromuscular blockade or separately cause respiratory depression. Management is the same as that of prolonged neuromuscular blockade.

Edrophonium doses of 0.5 mg/kg are not as effective as neostigmine doses of 0.04 mg/kg in antagonizing pipecuronium-induced neuromuscular block, and is often inadequate. Therefore, the use of edrophonium 0.5 mg/kg is not recommended to antagonize pipecuronium-induced neuromuscular blockade. The use of greater (1 mg/kg) doses of edrophonium or of pyridostigmine has not been investigated.

Administration and Dosage:

For IV use only. Administer by or under the supervision of experienced clinicians familiar with the use of neuromuscular blocking agents. Individualize dosage.

The dosage information that follows serves as an initial guide to clinicians familiar with other neuromuscular blocking agents to acquire experience with pipecuronium. The monitoring of twitch response is recommended to evaluate recovery from pipecuronium and decrease the hazards of overdosage if additional doses are administered.

Clinicians administering long-acting neuromuscular blocking agents such as pipecuronium should employ a peripheral nerve stimulator to monitor drug response, need for additional relaxant and adequacy of spontaneous recovery or antagonism.

(Administration and Dosage continued on following page)

PIPECURONIUM BROMIDE (Cont.)

Administration and Dosage (Cont.):

Individualize dosage: Pipecuronium, like other long-acting neuromuscular blocking agents, displays a great deal of variability in the clinical duration of its effect. With experience, anesthesiologists will determine when and how to modify dosage on individual patients based on clinical factors like age, sex, weight/degree of obesity, renal, hepatic or other diseases, much as they do with pancuronium. The following table is to assist those physicians who wish to adjust dosage based on ideal body weight and renal function.

For small patients with decreased renal function, the initial dose is < 70 to 85 mcg/kg, ie, less than two times the average ED_{95} dose, which is generally the recommended intubating dose for neuromuscular blocking agents. Use extra care during intubation of any patient in whom, in order to decrease the possibility of prolonged clinical duration, < 70 mcg/kg is used for intubation. Dosing in accordance with the following table may reduce the variability in clinical duration to bring approximately 20% more patients to within ± 30 minutes of the duration predicted by the dose adjusted by ideal body weight and calculated creatinine clearance.

Calculated Dose of Pipecuronium (mg)[1]

Creatinine clearance (ml/min)[3]	Ideal body weight (kg)[2]						Dose in mcg/kg
	50	60	70	80	90	100	
≤ 40	2.5[4]	3[4]	3.5[4]	4[4]	4.5[4]	5[4]	50[4]
60	2.5[4]	3[4]	3.8	4.9	6.2	7.7	55
80	2.6	3.7	5	6.5	8.3	10[5]	70
100							85
≥ 100	3.2	4.6	6.3	8.2	9	10[5]	100[5]

[1] Based on ideal body weight (IBW) in kg and estimated creatinine clearance; mg = ml if 10 mg vial is reconstituted with 10 ml.

[2] IBW (kg): Men = (106 + [6 lbs/inch in height > 5 ft])/2.2
Women = (100 + [5 lbs/inch in height > 5 ft])/2.2
Use actual body weight in the calculation if it is less than IBW.

[3] Estimated Ccr = $\frac{(140 - \text{age in years}) \times \text{IBW (kg)}}{72 \times \text{serum creatinine (mg/dl)}} \times 0.85$ (for females only)

[4] Minimum calculated dose for intubation; anticipate prolonged clinical blockade.

[5] Maximum calculated dose for intubation; anticipate use of maintenance doses.

Endotracheal intubation: The recommended initial dose under balanced anesthesia, halothane, isoflurane, or enflurane anesthesia in patients with normal renal function who were not obese is 0.07 to 0.085 mg/kg (70 to 85 mcg/kg). Good to excellent intubating conditions are generally provided within 2.5 to 3 minutes. Maximum blockade, usually > 95%, is achieved in approximately 5 minutes. Doses in this range provide approximately 1 to 2 hours of clinical relaxation under balanced anesthesia (range, 47 to 124 minutes). Under halothane, isoflurane and enflurane anesthesia, expect extension of the period of clinical relaxation.

For obese patients (≥ 30% above ideal body weight for height) it is particularly important to consider dosage adjustment according to ideal body weight.

Use following succinylcholine: If succinylcholine is used to facilitate endotracheal intubation, pipecuronium may be administered after recovery from succinylcholine paralysis. In patients with normal renal function who are not obese, starting doses of 0.05 mg/kg (50 mcg/kg) of pipecuronium are recommended and will provide approximately 45 minutes of clinical relaxation. In nonobese patients with normal renal function, higher pipecuronium doses of 0.07 to 0.085 mg/kg (70 to 85 mcg/kg), if administered after recovery from succinylcholine, are associated with approximately the same clinical duration as pipecuronium without prior succinylcholine administration.

Maintenance dosing: Maintenance doses of 0.01 to 0.015 mg/kg (10 to 15 mcg/kg) administered at 25% recovery of control T_1, provide approximately 50 minutes (range, 17 to 175 minutes) clinical duration under balanced anesthesia. Consider a lower dose in patients receiving inhalation anesthetics. In all cases, guide dosing based on the clinical duration following initial dose or prior maintenance dose and do not administer until signs of neuromuscular function are evident.

(Administration and Dosage continued on following page)

PIPECURONIUM BROMIDE (Cont.)

Administration and Dosage (Cont.):

Children: Infants (3 months to 1 year) under balanced anesthesia or halothane anesthesia manifest similar dose response to pipecuronium as do adults on a mcg/kg basis. Children (1 to 14 years) under balanced anesthesia or halothane anesthesia may be less sensitive than adults. The clinical duration of doses averaging 0.04 mg/kg (40 mcg/kg) in infants, and 0.57 mg/kg (57 mcg/kg) in children, ranged from 10 to 44 minutes, and from 18 to 52 minutes, respectively. These doses were approximately 1.2 times ED_{95}.

IV compatibility: Pipecuronium can be reconstituted using the following IV solutions: 0.9% NaCl solution; 5% Dextrose in Saline; 5% Dextrose in Water; Lactated Ringer's; Sterile Water for Injection; Bacteriostatic Water for Injection.

Pipecuronium is not recommended for dilution into or administration from large volume IV solutions.

Storage/Stability: Store at 2° to 30°C (35° to 86°F). Protect from light.

When reconstituted with Bacteriostatic Water for Injection, USP: Contains benzyl alcohol, which is not intended for use in newborns. Use within 5 days. May be stored at room temperature or refrigerated.

When reconstituted with Sterile Water for Injection or other compatible IV solutions: Refrigerate vial. Use within 24 hours. Single use only. Discard unused portion.

Rx	**Arduan** (Organon)	**Powder for Injection (lyophilized):**[1] 10 mg	In 10 ml vials.

[1] Freeze-dried cake with 380 mg mannitol.

DOXACURIUM CHLORIDE

Actions:

Pharmacology: Doxacurium was approved by the FDA in March 1991. Doxacurium chloride is a long-acting, nondepolarizing skeletal muscle relaxant for IV administration. It binds competitively to cholinergic receptors on the motor end-plate to antagonize the action of acetylcholine, resulting in a block of neuromuscular transmission. This action is antagonized by acetylcholinesterase inhibitors, such as neostigmine.

Doxacurium is ≈ 2.5 to 3 times more potent than pancuronium and 10 to 12 times more potent than metocurine. Doxacurium in doses of 1.5 to 2 x ED_{95} has a clinical duration of action similar to that of equipotent doses of pancuronium and metocurine. The average ED_{95} (dose required to produce 95% suppression of the adductor pollicis muscle twitch response to ulnar nerve stimulation) is 0.025 mg/kg (range, 0.02 to 0.033) in adults receiving balanced anesthesia.

The onset and clinically effective duration (time from injection to 25% recovery) of doxacurium administered alone or after succinylcholine during stable balanced anesthesia are shown in the following table:

Pharmacodynamic Dose Response to Doxacurium During Balanced Anesthesia[1]			
	Initial doxacurium dose (mg/kg)		
Parameter	0.025[2] (n = 34)	0.05 (n = 27)	0.08 (n = 9)
Time to maximum block (min)	9.3 (5.4-16)	5.2 (2.5-13)	3.5 (2.4-5)
Clinical duration (min) (time to 25% recovery)	55 (9-145)	100 (39-232)	160 (110-338)

[1] Values shown are means (range).
[2] Doxacurium administered after 10% to 100% recovery from an intubating dose of succinylcholine.

Initial doses of 0.05 mg/kg (2 x ED_{95}) and 0.08 mg/kg (3 x ED_{95}) administered during the induction of thiopental-narcotic anesthesia produce good-to-excellent conditions for tracheal intubation in 5 and 4 minutes (which are before maximum block), respectively.

The clinical duration of neuromuscular block associated with doxacurium shows considerable interpatient variability. Approximately two-thirds of the patients had clinical durations within 30 minutes of the duration predicted by dose (based on mg/kg actual body weight). Patients ≥ 60 years old are approximately twice as likely to experience prolonged clinical duration (30 minutes longer than predicted) than patients < 60 years old; thus, use care in older patients when prolonged recovery is undesirable (see Warnings). In addition, obese patients (≥ 30% more than ideal body weight for height) were almost twice as likely to experience prolonged clinical duration than non-obese patients; therefore, base dosing on ideal body weight (IBW) for obese patients.

The mean time for spontaneous T_1 recovery from 25% to 50% of control following initial doses of doxacurium is ≈ 26 minutes (range, 7 to 104) during balanced anesthesia. The mean time for spontaneous T_1 recovery from 25% to 75% is 54 minutes (range, 14 to 184).

Most patients required pharmacologic reversal prior to full spontaneous recovery from neuromuscular block. As with other long-acting neuromuscular blocking agents, doxacurium may be associated with prolonged times to full spontaneous recovery. Following an initial dose of 0.025 mg/kg, some patients may require as long as 4 hours to exhibit full spontaneous recovery.

Cumulative neuromuscular blocking effects are not associated with repeated administration of maintenance doses of doxacurium at 25% T_1 recovery. As with initial doses, however, the duration of action following maintenance doses may vary considerably among patients.

The doxacurium ED_{95} for children 2 to 12 years of age receiving halothane anesthesia is approximately 0.03 mg/kg. Children require higher doses on a mg/kg basis than adults to achieve comparable levels of block. The onset, time and duration of block are shorter in children than adults. During halothane anesthesia, doses of 0.03 and 0.05 mg/kg produce maximum block in ≈ 7 and 4 minutes, respectively. The duration of clinically effective block is ≈ 30 minutes after an initial dose of 0.03 mg/kg and ≈ 45 minutes after 0.05 mg/kg. Doxacurium has not been studied in children below the age of 2 years.

(Actions continued on following page)

DOXACURIUM CHLORIDE (Cont.)

Actions (Cont.):

Pharmacology (Cont.):

The neuromuscular block produced by doxacurium may be antagonized by anticholinesterase agents. The more profound the neuromuscular block at reversal, the longer the time and the greater the dose of anticholinesterase required for recovery of neuromuscular function.

Hemodynamics: In healthy adult patients, children (2 to 12 years of age) and patients with serious cardiovascular disease undergoing coronary artery bypass grafting, cardiac valvular repair or vascular repair, doxacurium produced no dose-related effects on mean arterial blood pressure or heart rate.

Doses of 0.03 to 0.08 mg/kg (1.2 to 3 x ED_{95}) were not associated with dose-dependent changes in mean plasma histamine concentration. Adverse experiences typically associated with histamine release (eg, bronchospasm, hypotension, tachycardia, cutaneous flushing, urticaria) are very rare following the administration of doxacurium (see Adverse Reactions).

Pharmacokinetics: The pharmacokinetics appear linear. The pharmacokinetics are similar in healthy young adult and elderly patients; although some healthy elderly patients tend to be more sensitive to the neuromuscular blocking effects. The time to maximum block is longer in elderly patients than in young adult patients (11.2 vs 7.7 minutes at 0.025 mg/kg). In addition, the clinically effective durations of block are more variable and tend to be longer in healthy elderly patients.

A longer half life can be expected in patients with end-stage kidney disease; in addition, these patients may be more sensitive to the neuromuscular blocking effects of doxacurium. The time to maximum block was slightly longer and the clinically effective duration of block was prolonged in patients with end-stage kidney disease.

Sensitivity to the neuromuscular blocking effects of doxacurium was highly variable in patients undergoing liver transplantation. Three of 7 patients developed ≤ 50% block, indicating that a reduced sensitivity to doxacurium may occur in such patients. In those patients who developed > 50% neuromuscular block, the time to maximum block and the clinically effective duration tended to be longer than in healthy young adult patients.

Pharmacokinetic and Pharmacodynamic Parameters of Doxacurium[1]

Parameter	Healthy young adult patients (22 to 49 yrs)				Kidney transplant patients	Liver transplant patients	Healthy elderly patients (67 to 72 yrs)
	Dose (mg/kg)				Dose (mg/kg)	Dose (mg/kg)	Dose (mg/kg)
	0.015 (n = 9)	0.025 (n = 8)	0.05 (n = 8)	0.08 (n = 8)	0.015 (n = 8)	0.015 (n = 7)	0.025 (n = 8)
Elimination half-life (min)	99 (48-193)	86 (25-171)	123 (61-163)	98 (47-163)	221 (84-592)	115 (69-148)	96 (50-114)
Volume of distribution at steady state (L/kg)	0.22 (0.11-0.43)	0.15 (0.1-0.21)	0.24 (0.13-0.3)	0.22 (0.16-0.33)	0.27 (0.17-0.55)	0.29 (0.17-0.35)	0.22 (0.14-0.4)
Plasma clearance (ml/min/kg)	2.66 (1.35-6.66)	2.22 (1.02-3.95)	2.62 (1.21-5.7)	2.53 (1.88-3.38)	1.23 (0.48-2.4)	2.3 (1.96-3.05)	2.47 (1.58-3.6)
Maximum block (%)	86 (59-100)	97 (88-100)	100	100	98 (95-100)	70 (0-100)	96 (90-100)
Clinically effective duration of block[2] (min)	36 (19-80)	68 (35-90)	91 (47-132)	177 (74-268)	80 (29-133)	52 (20-91)	97 (36-179)

[1] Values shown are means (range).
[2] Time from injection to 25% recovery of the control twitch height.

(Actions continued on following page)

DOXACURIUM CHLORIDE (Cont.)

Actions (Cont.):

Pharmacokinetics (Cont.):

Consecutively administered maintenance doses of 0.005 mg/kg, each given at 25% T_1 recovery following the preceding dose, do not result in a progressive increase in the plasma concentration of doxacurium or a progressive increase in the depth or duration of block produced by each dose. Plasma protein binding is approximately 30%.

Doxacurium is not metabolized; the major elimination pathway is excretion of unchanged drug in urine and bile. In studies of healthy adult patients, 24% to 38% of an administered dose was recovered as parent drug in urine over 6 to 12 hours after dosing. High bile concentrations (relative to plasma) have been found 35 to 90 minutes after administration. The overall extent of biliary excretion is unknown.

Indications:

Adjunct to general anesthesia, to provide skeletal muscle relaxation during surgery.

Provide skeletal muscle relaxation for endotracheal intubation.

Contraindications:

Hypersensitivity to the drug.

Warnings:

Clinical supervision: Administer in carefully adjusted dosage by or under the supervision of experienced clinicians who are familiar with the drug's actions and the possible complications of its use. Do not administer unless facilities for intubation, artificial respiration, oxygen therapy, and an antagonist are immediately available. Employ a peripheral nerve stimulator to monitor drug response, need for additional relaxants and adequacy of spontaneous recovery or antagonism.

Doxacurium has no known effect on consciousness, pain threshold or cerebration; to avoid patient distress, do not induce neuromuscular blockade before unconsciousness.

Benzyl alcohol: Doxacurium injection contains benzyl alcohol. In newborn infants, benzyl alcohol has been associated with an increased incidence of neurological and other complications which are sometimes fatal.

Elderly: In elderly patients the onset of maximum block is slower and the duration of neuromuscular block is more variable and, in some cases, longer than in young adult patients.

Pregnancy: Category C. There are no adequate or well controlled studies in pregnant women. Use during pregnancy only if the potential benefit justifies the potential risk to the fetus. Since the duration of action of doxacurium exceeds the usual duration of operative obstetrics (cesarean section), doxacurium is not recommended for use in patients undergoing C-section.

Lactation: It is not known whether doxacurium is excreted in breast milk. Exercise caution following administration to a nursing woman.

Children: Doxacurium has not been studied in children $<$ 2 years of age. See Actions and Administration and Dosage for clinical experience and recommendations for use in children 2 to 12 years of age.

Precautions:

Neuromuscular diseases: Neuromuscular blocking agents may have a profound effect in patients with neuromuscular diseases (eg, myasthenia gravis and the myasthenic syndrome). In these and other conditions in which prolonged neuromuscular block is a possibility (eg, carcinomatosis), use a peripheral nerve stimulator and a small test dose of doxacurium to assess the level of neuromuscular block and to monitor dosage requirements. Shorter acting muscle relaxants may be more suitable.

Resistance to nondepolarizing neuromuscular blocking agents may develop in patients with burns depending upon the time elapsed since the injury and the size of the burn.

Acid-base or serum electrolyte abnormalities may potentiate or antagonize the action of neuromuscular blocking agents. Their action may be enhanced by magnesium salts administered for the management eclampsia or preeclampsia.

(Precautions continued on following page)

SUCCINYLCHOLINE CHLORIDE (Cont.)

Warnings:

Malignant hyperthermia: The abrupt onset of malignant hyperthermia, a rare hypermetabolic process of skeletal muscle, may be triggered by succinylcholine. Early premonitory signs include: Muscle rigidity, particularly involving jaw muscles; tachycardia and tachypnea unresponsive to increased depth of anesthesia; evidence of increased oxygen requirement and carbon dioxide production (change in color of the CO_2 absorber); rising temperature; and metabolic acidosis. Considerations important to the management of this problem are: Early recognition of premonitory signs; immediate discontinuation of anesthesia and succinylcholine (either agent may induce the syndrome); and implementation of supportive measures including administration of oxygen and sodium bicarbonate, lowering body temperature, restoration of fluid and electrolyte balance, maintenance of adequate urinary output and administration of IV dantrolene (see p. 1531). Establish a standard protocol to implement when the syndrome becomes apparent.

Use succinylcholine only when facilities for endotracheal intubation, artificial respiration and oxygen administration are instantly available. Be prepared to assist or control respiration.

Usage in Pregnancy: Category C. Safety for use during pregnancy has not been established. It is not known whether the drug can cause fetal harm when administered to a pregnant woman or can affect reproduction capacity. Use in pregnant women only when clearly needed and when the potential benefits outweigh the potential hazards.

Pseudocholinesterase levels are decreased by approximately 24% during pregnancy and for several days postpartum. Therefore, pregnant patients may be expected to show greater sensitivity (prolonged apnea) to succinylcholine than nonpregnant patients.

Usage in Labor and Delivery: Succinylcholine is commonly used to provide muscle relaxation during cesarean section. While small amounts cross the placenta, the amount that enters fetal circulation after a single dose of 1 mg/kg to the mother will not endanger the fetus. However, since the amount of drug that crosses the placenta depends on the concentration gradient between the maternal and fetal circulations, residual neuromuscular blockade (apnea and flaccidity) may occur in the neonate after repeated high doses to the mother or in the presence of atypical pseudocholinesterase in the mother.

The drug may be used during obstetrical anesthesia in patients with normal plasma cholinesterase activity. It is not known whether depolarizing muscle relaxants prolong the duration of labor, increase the possibility of obstetric intervention, or have immediate or delayed adverse effects on the fetus or the later growth, development or functional maturation of the child.

Usage in Lactation: It is not known whether this drug is excreted in human milk. Exercise caution when succinylcholine is administered to a woman currently nursing or one who anticipates nursing following delivery.

Precautions:

Use with caution in cardiovascular, hepatic, pulmonary, metabolic or renal disorders.

Administer with great caution to patients with severe burns, electrolyte imbalance, hyperkalemia, those receiving quinidine and those who are digitalized or recovering from severe trauma, as serious cardiac arrhythmias or cardiac arrest may result. Observe caution in patients with preexisting hyperkalemia or those who are paraplegic, who have suffered spinal cord injury or have degenerative or dystrophic neuromuscular disease, since such patients tend to become severely hyperkalemic when succinylcholine is given.

The action of succinylcholine may be altered in patients with myasthenia gravis, renal failure, disturbed electrolyte balance (prolonged blockade in patients with hypokalemia or hypocalcemia), hepatic disorders, and cardiovascular and pulmonary disorders.

Myoglobinemia/myoglobinuria have been associated with single or repeated IV and IM injections, especially in children. Inject small doses of nondepolarizing agents such as tubocurarine before injecting succinylcholine to reduce severity of muscle fasciculations and to decrease the incidence of myoglobinuria.

(Precautions continued on following page)

SUCCINYLCHOLINE CHLORIDE (Cont.)

Precautions (Cont.):

Low plasma pseudocholinesterase may be associated with a prolonged paralysis of respiration following succinylcholine. Low levels are often found in patients with severe liver disease or cirrhosis, anemia, malnutrition, dehydration, burns, cancer, collagen diseases, myxedema, abnormal body temperatures, pregnancy, exposure to neurotoxic insecticides; those receiving antimalarial drugs, anticancer drugs, irradiation, MAO inhibitors, oral contraceptives, pancuronium, chlorpromazine, echothiophate iodide or neostigmine; or those with a recessive hereditary trait. Administer minimal doses with extreme care to such patients. If low plasma pseudocholinesterase activity is suspected, administer a test dose of 5 to 10 mg or produce relaxation by the cautious administration of a 0.1% IV drip.

Respiratory depression or prolonged apnea may occur if given in amounts greater than recommended. Generally, single doses of 0.4 mg/kg or less given to adults, or infusions of 2.5 mg/minute do not cause complete or prolonged respiratory paralysis; however, transient apnea usually occurs at the time of maximal effect. Spontaneous respiration generally returns in a few seconds, or at most, in 3 or 4 minutes. Until then, initiate and continue controlled respiration with oxygen.

Nondepolarizing blockade: During repeated or prolonged administration of succinylcholine, the characteristic Phase I block may convert to a Phase II block. Prolonged respiratory depression or apnea may be observed in patients manifesting this transition. The transition from Phase I to Phase II block was reported in 7 of 7 patients studied under halothane anesthesia after an accumulated dose of 2 to 4 mg/kg succinylcholine (administered in repeated, divided doses). The onset of Phase II block coincided with the onset of tachyphylaxis and prolongation of spontaneous recovery. In another study, using balanced anesthesia (N_2O/O_2/narcotic-thiopental) and succinylcholine infusion, the transition was less abrupt, with great variability in the dose required to produce Phase II block. Of 32 patients studied, 24 developed Phase II block. Tachyphylaxis was not associated with the transition and 50% of the patients who developed Phase II block experienced prolonged recovery.

When Phase II block is suspected, base the decision to reverse the block with an anticholinesterase drug upon a positive diagnosis using a peripheral nerve stimulator, since an anticholinesterase agent will potentiate a succinylcholine-induced Phase I block. Phase II block is indicated by fade of responses to successive stimuli (preferably "train of four"). Accompany anticholinesterase drugs to reverse Phase II block by appropriate doses of atropine to prevent cardiac arrhythmias. After adequate reversal of Phase II block with an anticholinesterase agent, observe the patient for at least 1 hour for signs of return of muscle relaxation. Do not attempt reversal unless: (1) A peripheral nerve stimulator is used to determine the presence of Phase II block, and (2) spontaneous recovery of muscle twitch has occurred for at least 20 minutes and has reached a plateau with further recovery proceeding slowly; this delay ensures complete hydrolysis of succinylcholine by pseudocholinesterase prior to administration of the anticholinesterase agent.

Concurrent use of a depolarizing and a nondepolarizing (competitive) muscle relaxant is not recommended since a prolonged mixed block may occur. In this instance, determine the dominant feature of the block by the use of a nerve stimulator and treat accordingly.

Use in eye surgery: Succinylcholine causes a slight, transient increase in intraocular pressure immediately after its injection and during the fasciculation phase; slight increases may persist after onset of complete paralysis. Do not use the drug when open eye injury is present and use with caution, if at all, during intraocular surgery and in patients with glaucoma.

Use in patients with fractures or muscle spasm requires caution since the muscle fasciculations may cause additional trauma.

Reduce muscle fasciculations and hyperkalemia by administering a small dose of a nondepolarizing relaxant prior to succinylcholine. If other relaxants are to be used during the procedure, consider the possibility of a synergistic or antagonistic effect.

Succinylcholine may increase intragastric pressure, which could result in regurgitation and possible aspiration of stomach contents.

(Continued on following page)

SUCCINYLCHOLINE CHLORIDE (Cont.)

Drug Interactions:

Diazepam may reduce the duration of neuromuscular blockade produced by succinylcholine.

Phenelzine, promazine, oxytocin, certain **nonpenicillin antibiotics, quinidine, beta-adrenergic blocking agents, procainamide, lidocaine, trimethaphan, lithium carbonate, furosemide, magnesium sulfate, quinine, chloroquine, acetylcholine, anticholinesterases, procaine-type local anesthetics** and **isoflurane**: All of these drugs may enhance the neuromuscular blocking action of succinylcholine.

Amphotericin B and **thiazide diuretics** may increase effects of succinylcholine secondary to induced electrolyte imbalance. Patients with hypocalcemia and hypokalemia usually require reduced succinylcholine doses.

Nondepolarizing muscle relaxants: Consider the possibility of a synergistic or antagonistic effect with succinylcholine.

Cyclophosphamide (decreases plasma pseudocholinesterase) or **IV procaine** (competes for the enzyme) may prolong the effect of succinylcholine.

Digitalis glycosides: Succinylcholine may cause a sudden extrusion of potassium from muscle cells, possibly causing arrhythmias in **digitalized** patients. Toxicity (cardiac arrhythmias) of both drugs may be increased.

Inhalation anesthetics (eg, cyclopropane, diethyl ether, halothane and nitrous oxide): Coadministration with succinylcholine may increase incidence of bradycardia, arrhythmias, sinus arrest and apnea, as well as the occurrence of malignant hyperthermia in susceptible individuals.

Narcotic analgesics may increase the incidence of bradycardia and sinus arrest.

Adverse Reactions:

As with other neuromuscular blockers, the potential for releasing histamine is present following succinylcholine use. Serious histamine-mediated flushing, hypotension and bronchoconstriction are, however, uncommon in normal clinical usage.

Adverse reactions consist primarily of an extension of the drug's pharmacological actions. Profound and prolonged muscle relaxation may occur, resulting in respiratory depression to the point of apnea. Hypersensitivity and anaphylactic reactions have been reported rarely. The following reactions have been reported:

Cardiovascular: Bradycardia (frequently noted after a second IV injection of a 2% solution in children); tachycardia; hypertension; hypotension; cardiac arrest; arrhythmias.

Respiratory: Respiratory depression or apnea.

Miscellaneous: Malignant hyperthermia (see Warnings); increased intraocular pressure; muscle fasciculation; postoperative muscle pain; excessive salivation; hyperkalemia; rash; myoglobinemia; myoglobinuria.

(Continued on following page)

SUCCINYLCHOLINE CHLORIDE (Cont.)

Administration and Dosage:

Individualize dosage. Usually administered IV; may be given IM to infants, older children or adults when a suitable vein is inaccessible. Give a dose of up to 2.5 mg/kg; give no more than 150 mg total dose. An initial test dose of 0.1 mg/kg may determine patient sensitivity and recovery time.

To avoid patient distress, administer after unconsciousness has been induced.

Short surgical procedures: The average dose required to induce muscle relaxation of short duration is 0.6 mg/kg IV given over 10 to 30 seconds. The optimum dose varies among individuals and may range from 0.3 to 1.1 mg/kg.

Following an injection of an effective dose of succinylcholine, relaxation sufficient for endotracheal intubation generally occurs in approximately 1 minute. More succinylcholine should be given at appropriate intervals if relaxation is not complete.

Long surgical procedures: Dosage depends on duration of procedure. Average rate for an adult ranges between 2.5 and 4.3 mg/minute. Solutions containing from 0.1% to 0.2% (1 to 2 mg/ml) are commonly used for continuous IV drip. The more dilute solution is probably preferable for ease of control of the rate of administration and, hence, of relaxation. Give this 1 mg/ml IV drip solution at 0.5 to 10 mg/minute to obtain required amount of relaxation. The 0.2% solution may be useful when it is desirable to avoid overburdening circulation with a large volume of fluid.

Prolonged muscular relaxation may be achieved with intermittent IV injections. Give an initial dose of 0.3 to 1.1 mg/kg then give 0.04 to 0.07 mg/kg at appropriate intervals to maintain the required degree of relaxation.

Children:

IV – For infants and small children, 2 mg/kg; for older children and adolescents, 1 mg/kg. IV bolus use may result in profound bradycardia or, rarely, asystole. As in adults, the incidence of bradycardia is higher after a second dose. Reduce occurrence of bradyarrhythmias by pretreatment with atropine.

IM – In the absence of a suitable vein for IV administration, a dose of 3 to 4 mg/kg (not exceeding a total dose of 150 mg) is suggested.

Preparation of solution: Use only freshly prepared solutions. Succinylcholine is incompatible with alkaline solutions and will precipitate if mixed or administered simultaneously. Discard unused solutions within 24 hours. Inject separately; do not mix in the same syringe or administer simultaneously through the same needle with solutions of short-acting barbiturates, such as sodium thiopental or other drugs with an alkaline pH.

Storage: Refrigerate at 2° to 8°C (35° to 46°F). Multi-dose vials are stable for up to 14 days at room temperature without significant loss of potency.

Powder for infusion does not require refrigeration.

	Product	Form	Packaging	C.I.*
Rx	**Anectine** (Burroughs Wellcome)	**Injection:** 20 mg per ml	In 10 ml vials[1].	121
Rx	**Quelicin** (Abbott)		In 10 ml vials.[2]	495
Rx	**Sucostrin** (Apothecon)		In 10 ml vials.[2]	208
Rx	**Quelicin** (Abbott)	**Injection:** 50 mg per ml	In 10 ml amps.	68
Rx	**Quelicin** (Abbott)	**Injection:** 100 mg per ml	In 10 ml vials and 10 ml in 20 ml vials and 5 ml in 10 ml vials.	53
Rx	**Sucostrin** (Apothecon)		In 10 ml vials.[2]	118
Rx	**Succinylcholine Chloride Min-i-Mix** (I.M.S.)	**Powder for Injection:** 100 mg per vial	In UD 5 ml vial with diluent and Min-i-Mix injector.	612
Rx	**Anectine Flo-Pack** (Burroughs Wellcome)	**Powder for Infusion:** 500 mg or		41
		1 g per vial		35

* Cost Index based on cost per 20 mg.

[1] With methylparaben.

[2] With methyl and propyl parabens.

CYCLOBENZAPRINE HCl

Actions:

Pharmacology: Cyclobenzaprine, structurally related to the tricyclic antidepressants (TCAs), relieves skeletal muscle spasm of local origin without interfering with muscle function. It is ineffective in muscle spasm due to CNS disease. In animals, the drug reduces or abolishes muscle hyperactivity, does not act at the neuromuscular junction or directly on skeletal muscle, and acts primarily within the CNS at the brain stem as opposed to spinal cord levels; however, its action on the latter may contribute to its overall skeletal muscle relaxant activity. The net effect is a reduction of tonic somatic motor activity, influencing both gamma and alpha motor systems.

Animal studies also showed a similarity between the effects of cyclobenzaprine and TCAs, including reserpine antagonism, norepinephrine potentiation, potent peripheral and central anticholinergic effects and sedation. In animals, cyclobenzaprine caused a slight to moderate increase in heart rate.

Pharmacokinetics: Cyclobenzaprine is well absorbed after oral administration, but there is a large intersubject variation in plasma levels. Peak plasma levels are reached in 4 to 6 hours. The onset of action occurs in 1 hour with a duration of 12 to 24 hours. It is highly bound to plasma proteins, is extensively metabolized primarily to glucuronide-like conjugates and is excreted primarily via the kidneys. Elimination half-life is 1 to 3 days.

Clinical Pharmacology: Cyclobenzaprine significantly improves the signs and symptoms of skeletal muscle spasm as compared with placebo. Clinical responses include improvement in muscle spasm as determined by palpation, reduction in local pain and tenderness, increased range of motion and less restriction in activities of daily living. Clinical improvement was observed as early as the first day of therapy. In controlled trials comparing cyclobenzaprine, diazepam and placebo, cyclobenzaprine demonstrated comparable or greater improvement in muscle spasm when compared with diazepam. Side effects were comparable (cyclobenzaprine – drowsiness, dry mouth; diazepam – drowsiness, dizziness).

No studies have been performed to indicate whether cyclobenzaprine enhances the clinical effect of aspirin or other analgesics, or whether analgesics enhance the clinical effect of cyclobenzaprine in acute musculoskeletal conditions.

Indications:

Adjunct to rest and physical therapy for relief of muscle spasm associated with acute painful musculoskeletal conditions.

Cyclobenzaprine is not effective in the treatment of spasticity associated with cerebral or spinal cord disease, or in children with cerebral palsy.

Contraindications:

Hypersensitivity to cyclobenzaprine; concomitant use of monoamine oxidase (MAO) inhibitors or within 14 days after their discontinuation; acute recovery phase of myocardial infarction (MI) and in patients with arrhythmias, heart block or conduction disturbances, or congestive heart failure (CHF); hyperthyroidism.

Warnings:

Use only for short periods (up to 2 or 3 weeks); effectiveness for more prolonged use is not proven. Muscle spasm associated with acute, painful musculoskeletal conditions is generally of short duration; specific therapy for longer periods is seldom warranted.

Cyclobenzaprine is closely related to the TCAs. In short-term studies for indications other than muscle spasm associated with acute musculoskeletal conditions, and usually at doses somewhat greater than those recommended, some of the more serious CNS reactions noted with the TCAs have occurred. Because of pharmacologic similarities to tricyclic drugs, consider certain withdrawal symptoms with cyclobenzaprine, although they have not been reported. Abrupt cessation of treatment after prolonged administration may produce nausea, headache and malaise; these do not indicate addiction.

Usage in Pregnancy: Category B. Use only when clearly needed and when the potential benefits outweigh the unknown potential hazards to the fetus.

Usage in Lactation: It is not known whether cyclobenzaprine is excreted in milk. Some of the TCAs are excreted in breast milk. Exercise caution when administering cyclobenzaprine to a nursing woman.

Usage in Children: Safety and efficacy in children under 15 have not been established.

(Continued on following page)

CYCLOBENZAPRINE HCl (Cont.)

Precautions:

Hazardous tasks: May impair mental or physical abilities required for performance of hazardous tasks; patients should observe caution while driving or performing other tasks requiring alertness.

Because of its anticholinergic action, use with caution in patients with a history of urinary retention, angle-closure glaucoma and increased intraocular pressure.

Drug Interactions:

Alcohol, barbiturates and other **CNS depressants:** Effects may be enhanced by cyclobenzaprine.

Anticholinergics: Because of cyclobenzaprine's anticholinergic action, use with caution in patients receiving these agents.

MAO inhibitors: Hyperpyretic crisis, severe convulsions and deaths have occurred in patients receiving TCAs and MAO inhibitors. Cyclobenzaprine may interact similarly.

Because of similarities to the TCAs, consider all interactions listed with TCAs (p. 1291).

Adverse Reactions:

Most frequent: Drowsiness (39%); dry mouth (27%); dizziness (11%).

Less frequent (1% to 3%): Fatigue; tiredness; asthenia; nausea; constipation; dyspepsia; unpleasant taste; blurred vision; headache; nervousness; confusion.

The following have been noted in < 1% of patients:

Cardiovascular – Tachycardia; syncope; arrhythmias; vasodilatation; palpitations; hypotension.

CNS – Ataxia; vertigo; dysarthria; paresthesia; tremors; hypertonia; malaise; tinnitus.

Psychiatric – Disorientation; insomnia; depressed mood; abnormal sensations; anxiety; agitation; abnormal thinking and dreaming; hallucinations; excitement.

GI – Vomiting; anorexia; diarrhea; GI pain; gastritis; thirst; flatulence; ageusia.

GU – Urinary frequency or retention.

Hepatic – Abnormal liver function and rare reports of hepatitis, jaundice and cholestasis.

Integumentary – Sweating; skin rash; urticaria.

Musculoskeletal – Muscle twitching; local weakness.

Miscellaneous – Edema of face and tongue.

Causal relationship unknown:

Body as a Whole – Chest pain; edema.

Cardiovascular – Hypertension; myocardial infarction; heart block; stroke.

Digestive – Paralytic ileus; tongue discoloration; stomatitis; parotid swelling.

Endocrine – Inappropriate ADH syndrome.

Hematic and Lymphatic – Purpura; bone marrow depression; leukopenia; eosinophilia; thrombocytopenia.

Metabolic, Nutritional and Immune – Elevation and lowering of blood sugar levels; weight gain or loss.

Musculoskeletal – Myalgia.

Nervous System and Psychiatric – Decreased or increased libido; abnormal gait; delusions; peripheral neuropathy; Bell's palsy; alteration in EEG patterns; extrapyramidal symptoms.

Respiratory – Dyspnea.

Skin – Pruritus; photosensitization; alopecia.

Urogenital – Impaired urination; dilatation of urinary tract; impotence; testicular swelling; gynecomastia; breast enlargement; galactorrhea.

Because of the similarities to TCAs, consider all reactions listed in the Adverse Reaction section on TCAs (p. 1292).

(Continued on following page)

CYCLOBENZAPRINE HCl (Cont.)

Overdosage:

Symptoms: High doses may cause temporary confusion, disturbed concentration, transient visual hallucinations, agitation, hyperactive reflexes, muscle rigidity, vomiting or hyperpyrexia, in addition to the effects listed under adverse reactions. Overdosage may cause drowsiness, hypothermia, tachycardia and other cardiac arrhythmias such as bundle branch block, ECG evidence of impaired conduction and CHF, dilated pupils, convulsions, severe hypotension, stupor and coma. Paradoxical diaphoresis has been reported.

Treatment includes usual supportive measures. Refer to General Management of Acute Overdosage on p. vi. Closely monitor patients with ECG abnormalities.

Physostigmine, 1 to 3 mg IV, has been used to reverse anticholinergic effects. However, profound bradycardia and asystole may occur as a result (see p. 711). The role of physostigmine is not clear; avoid its use if other therapeutic agents are successful in reversing cardiac dysrhythmias.

Dialysis is probably of no value because of low plasma concentrations of the drug.

Patient Information:

May cause drowsiness, dizziness or blurred vision. Patients should observe caution while driving or performing other tasks requiring alertness.

Avoid alcohol and other CNS depressants.

May cause dry mouth.

Administration and Dosage:

Give 10 mg 3 times daily (range 20 to 40 mg daily in divided doses). Do not exceed 60 mg/day. Do not use longer than 2 or 3 weeks.

	Product	Form	Description	C.I.*
Rx	**Cyclobenzaprine HCl** (Various, eg, Danbury, Goldline, Major, Moore, Parmed, Rugby, Schein, Schiapparelli Searle	**Tablets:** 10 mg	In 100s and UD 100s.	
Rx	**Flexeril** (MSD)		(MSD 931). Yellow, film coated. In 100s, unit-of-use 30s and UD 100s.	342

* Cost Index based on cost per 10 mg.

METAXALONE

Actions:

Pharmacology: The mechanism of action of metaxalone has not been established, but it may be due to general CNS depression. The drug has no direct action on the contractile mechanism of striated muscle, the motor endplate or the nerve fiber. Metaxalone does not directly relax tense skeletal muscles.

Pharmacokinetics: Onset of action is 1 hour and duration of action is 4 to 6 hours. Peak plasma levels of approximately 300 mcg/ml occur 2 hours after administration of 800 mg metaxalone. The half-life is 2 to 3 hours; metabolites are excreted in the urine.

Indications:

As an adjunct to rest, physical therapy and other measures for the relief of discomfort associated with acute, painful musculoskeletal conditions.

Contraindications:

Hypersensitivity to metaxalone; known tendency to drug-induced hemolytic or other anemias; significantly impaired renal or hepatic function.

Warnings:

Usage in Pregnancy: Human experience has not revealed evidence of fetal injury, but the possibility of infrequent or subtle damage to the human fetus cannot be excluded. Do not use during pregnancy, especially during early pregnancy, or in women who may become pregnant, unless the potential benefits outweigh the potential hazards to the fetus.

Usage in Lactation: It is not known whether this drug is excreted in breast milk. Safety for use in the nursing mother has not been established.

Usage in Children: Safety and efficacy for use in children 12 years and under have not been established.

Precautions:

Usage in impaired hepatic function: Administer with great care to patients with preexisting liver damage and perform serial liver function studies as required. Elevations in cephalin flocculation tests without concurrent changes in other liver function parameters have been noted.

Drug Interactions:

Drug/Lab Tests: **False-positive Benedict's tests**, due to an unknown reducing substance, have been noted. A glucose-specific test will differentiate findings.

Adverse Reactions:

GI: Nausea, vomiting, GI upset.

CNS: Drowsiness, dizziness, headache, nervousness, irritability.

Other: Hypersensitivity reaction (light rash with or without pruritus), leukopenia, hemolytic anemia, jaundice.

Overdosage:

Employ gastric lavage and supportive therapy as indicated. No documented case of major toxicity has been reported. Refer to General Management of Acute Overdosage on p. 2895

Patient Information:

May cause drowsiness or dizziness. Patients should observe caution while driving or performing other tasks requiring alertness.

Avoid alcohol and other CNS depressants.

Notify physician if skin rash or yellowish discoloration of the skin or eyes occurs.

Administration and Dosage:

Adults and children (over 12 years): 800 mg 3 to 4 times daily.

				C.I.*
Rx	**Skelaxin** (Carnrick)	**Tablets:** 400 mg	(#C 8662). Pale rose, scored. In 100s.	167

* Cost Index based on cost per 800 mg.

Product identification code.

The following is an abbreviated monograph. For complete prescribing information see p. 1255

Centrally Acting (Cont.)

DIAZEPAM

Actions:

Diazepam is a benzodiazepine derivative. In animals, it acts on the thalamus and hypothalamus, inducing calming effects. Diazepam, unlike chlorpromazine and reserpine, has no demonstrable peripheral autonomic blocking action, nor does it produce extrapyramidal side effects; however, animals treated with diazepam do have a transient ataxia at higher doses.

Major muscle relaxant actions occur in two proposed sites: At the spinal level resulting in enhancement of GABA-mediated presynaptic inhibition, and at supraspinal sites, probably in the brain stem reticular formation.

Indications:

An adjunct for the relief of skeletal muscle spasm due to reflex spasm to local pathology (such as inflammation of the muscles or joints, or secondary to trauma); spasticity caused by upper motor neuron disorders (eg, cerebral palsy and paraplegia); athetosis; stiff-man syndrome. Injectable diazepam may also be used as an adjunct in tetanus.

Also used as an antianxiety agent (see p. 1264 and an anticonvulsant (see p. 1455).

Administration and Dosage:

Oral: Individualize dosage for maximum beneficial effect.

Adults – 2 to 10 mg 3 or 4 times daily.

Geriatric or debilitated patients – 2 to 2.5 mg 1 or 2 times daily initially, increasing as needed and tolerated.

Children – 1 to 2.5 mg 3 or 4 times daily initially, increasing as needed and tolerated (not for use in children under 6 months of age).

Intensol – Dosages are same as those listed above. Mix with liquid or semi-solid food such as water, juices, soda or soda-like beverages, applesauce and puddings. Stir in gently. Consume the entire mixture immediately. Do not store for future use.

Sustained release – 15 to 30 mg once daily.

Parenteral: Use lower doses (2 to 5 mg) and slow dosage increases for elderly or debilitated patients and when other sedatives are given. When acute symptoms are controlled with the injectable form, administer oral therapy if further treatment is required.

Neonates (30 days or less) – Safety and efficacy have not been established. Prolonged CNS depression has been observed in neonates, apparently due to inability to biotransform diazepam into inactive metabolites.

Children – Give slowly over 3 minutes in a dosage not to exceed 0.25 mg/kg. After a 15 to 30 minute interval, the initial dosage can be safely repeated. If relief is not obtained after a third administration, begin adjunctive therapy appropriate to the condition being treated.

IM – Inject deeply into the muscle.

IV – Inject slowly, taking at least 1 minute for each 5 mg (1 ml). Do not use small veins (ie, dorsum of hand or wrist). Avoid intra-arterial administration or extravasation. Do not mix or dilute with other solutions or drugs.

Adults: 5 to 10 mg, IM or IV initially, then 5 to 10 mg in 3 to 4 hours, if necessary. For tetanus, larger doses may be required.

Children: For tetanus in infants over 30 days of age, 1 to 2 mg IM or IV slowly; repeat every 3 to 4 hours as necessary. In children 5 years or older, 5 to 10 mg. Repeat every 3 to 4 hours if necessary to control tetanus spasms. Have respiratory assistance available.

(Products on following page)

DIAZEPAM (Cont.)

	Product	Form	Description	C.I.
c-IV	**Diazepam** (Various)	**Tablets:** 2 mg	In 30s, 56s, 100s, 500s, 1000s and UD 32s and 100s.	9+
c-IV	**Q-Pam** (Quantum)		(#2 Quantum 181). White, scored. In 100s, 500s and 1000s.	8
c-IV	**Valium** (Roche)		(#Roche 2 Valium). White, scored. In 100s, 500s and Rx pak 500s.	103
c-IV	**Vazepam** (Major)		In 100s, 500s and 1000s.	22
c-IV	**Diazepam** (Various)	**Tablets:** 5 mg	In 15s, 30s, 56s, 60s, 100s, 500s, 1000s and UD 32s and 100s.	5+
c-IV	**Q-Pam** (Quantum)		(#5 Quantum 182). Yellow, scored. In 100s, 500s and 1000s.	4
c-IV	**Valium** (Roche)		(#Roche 5 Valium). Yellow, scored. In 60s, 90s, 100s, 120s, 500s and Rx pak 500s.	64
c-IV	**Vazepam** (Major)		In 100s, 500s and 1000s.	13
c-IV	**Diazepam** (Various)	**Tablets:** 10 mg	In 15s, 30s, 56s, 100s, 500s, 1000s and UD 100s.	3+
c-IV	**Q-Pam** (Quantum)		(#10 Quantum 183). Blue, scored. In 100s, 500s, 1000s.	3
c-IV	**Valium** (Roche)		(#Roche 10 Valium). Blue, scored. In 60s, 90s, 100s, 120s, 500s and Rx pak 500s.	54
c-IV	**Vazepam** (Major)		In 100s, 500s and 1000s.	9
c-IV	**Valrelease** (Roche)	**Capsules, sustained release:** 15 mg	(#Roche 15 Valrelease). Yellow and blue. In 100s and Rx pak 30s.	62
c-IV	**Diazepam** (Roxane)	**Oral Solution:** 5 mg/5 ml	Wintergreen-spice flavor. In 500 ml and UD 5 and 10 ml.	42
c-IV	**Diazepam Intensol** (Roxane)	**Concentrated Oral Solution:** 5 mg/ml	In 30 ml with calibrated dropper.	75
c-IV	**Diazepam** (Various)	**Injection:** 5 mg/ml	In 2 ml amps, 1, 2, 5 and 10 ml vials and 1 and 2 ml syringe.	120+
c-IV	**Valium** (Roche)		In 2 ml amps,[1] 10 ml vials[1] and 2 ml disp. syringe.[1]	270
c-IV	**Vazepam** (Major)		In 10 ml vials.	221
c-IV	**Zetran** (Hauck)		In 10 ml vials.[1]	220

* Cost Index based on cost per 2 mg. # Product identification code.

[1] With 40% propylene glycol, 10% ethyl alcohol, 5% sodium benzoate and 1.5% benzyl alcohol.

BACLOFEN

Actions:

Pharmacology: The precise mechanism of action is not known. Baclofen can inhibit both monosynaptic and polysynaptic reflexes at the spinal level, possibly by hyperpolarization of afferent terminals, although actions at supraspinal sites may also contribute to its clinical effect. Although it is an analog of the inhibitory neurotransmitter gamma-aminobutyric acid (GABA), there is no conclusive evidence that actions on GABA systems produce clinical effects. In animal studies, it has been a CNS depressant as indicated by sedation with tolerance, somnolence, ataxia, and respiratory and cardiovascular depression.

Pharmacokinetics: Baclofen is rapidly and extensively absorbed. Absorption may be dose-dependent, being reduced with increasing doses. Peak serum levels are reached in approximately 2 hours; half-life is 3 to 4 hours. It is excreted primarily by the kidney in unchanged form with intersubject variation in absorption or elimination.

Indications:

For the alleviation of signs and symptoms of spasticity resulting from multiple sclerosis, particularly for the relief of flexor spasms and concomitant pain, clonus and muscular rigidity. Patients should have reversible spasticity so that treatment will aid in restoring residual function.

May be of some value in patients with spinal cord injuries and other spinal cord diseases.

Unlabeled Uses: Baclofen has been used to treat trigeminal neuralgia (tic douloureux).

It has also been used (40 mg/day), in combination with neuroleptics, to treat tardive dyskinesia.

Contraindications:

Hypersensitivity to baclofen.

Not indicated in the treatment of skeletal muscle spasm resulting from rheumatic disorders. Since efficacy in stroke, cerebral palsy and Parkinson's disease has not been established, it is not recommended for these conditions.

Warnings:

Abrupt drug withdrawal: Hallucinations and seizures have occurred on abrupt withdrawal. An isolated case of manic psychosis has been reported. Therefore, except in cases of serious adverse reactions, reduce the dose slowly when the drug is discontinued.

Use in impaired renal function: Because baclofen is primarily excreted unchanged through the kidneys, give with caution to patients with impaired renal function. Dosage reduction may be necessary.

Stroke: Baclofen has not significantly benefited patients with stroke; they also have poor drug tolerance.

Usage in Pregnancy: Developmental and skeletal abnormalities have been demonstrated in fetuses of several animal species who received 7 to 34 times the maximum recommended human dose of baclofen; other species failed to show defects. There are no studies in pregnant women. Use only when clearly needed and when the potential benefits outweigh the potential hazards to the fetus.

Usage in Lactation: It is not known whether this drug is excreted in human milk.

Usage in Children: Safety for use in children under 12 years of age has not been established. Baclofen is not recommended for use in children

Precautions:

Potentially hazardous tasks: Because of the possibility of sedation, patients should observe caution while driving or performing other tasks requiring alertness.

Usage in epilepsy: Monitor the clinical state and EEG at regular intervals, since deterioration in seizure control and EEG changes have been reported occasionally in patients taking this drug.

Use with caution where spasticity is utilized to sustain upright posture and balance in locomotion, or whenever spasticity is utilized to obtain increased function.

Ovarian cysts have been found by palpation in about 4% of multiple sclerosis patients treated with baclofen for up to 1 year. In most cases, these cysts disappeared spontaneously while patients continued to receive the drug. Ovarian cysts are estimated to occur spontaneously in approximately 1% to 5% of the normal female population.

Drug Interactions:

Alcohol and other **CNS depressants**: The CNS effects of baclofen may be additive.

(Continued on following page)

BACLOFEN (Cont.)

Adverse Reactions:

CNS: Transient drowsiness (10% to 63%); dizziness, weakness (5% to 15%); fatigue (2% to 4%); confusion (1% to 11%); headache (4% to 8%); insomnia (2% to 7%). Rarely, euphoria, excitement, depression, hallucinations, paresthesia, muscle pain, tinnitus, slurred speech, coordination disorder, tremor, rigidity, dystonia, ataxia, blurred vision, nystagmus, strabismus, miosis, mydriasis, diplopia, dysarthria, seizures.

Cardiovascular: Hypotension (< 9%). Rare instances of dyspnea, palpitations, chest pain, syncope.

GI: Nausea (4% to 12%); constipation (2% to 6%). Rarely, dry mouth, anorexia, taste disorder, abdominal pain, vomiting, diarrhea, positive test for occult blood in stool.

GU: Urinary frequency (2% to 6%). Rarely, enuresis, urinary retention, dysuria, impotence, inability to ejaculate, nocturia, hematuria.

Miscellaneous: Rash; pruritus; ankle edema; excessive perspiration; weight gain; nasal congestion.

Abnormal laboratory tests: Increased SGOT; elevated alkaline phosphatase; elevation of blood sugar.

Overdosage:

Symptoms: Vomiting, muscular hypotonia, muscle twitching, drowsiness, accommodation disorders, coma, respiratory depression and seizures.

Treatment: In the alert patient, empty the stomach promptly by induced emesis followed by lavage. In the obtunded patient, secure the airway with a cuffed endotracheal tube before beginning lavage (do not induce emesis). Maintain adequate respiratory exchange; do not use respiratory stimulants. Atropine has been used to improve ventilation, heart rate, blood pressure and core body temperature.

Patient Information:

May cause drowsiness, dizziness and fatigue. Patients should observe caution while driving or performing other tasks requiring alertness.

Avoid alcohol and other CNS depressants.

Do not discontinue therapy except on advice of physician. Abrupt withdrawal may result in hallucinations.

May cause frequent urge to urinate or painful urination, constipation, nausea, headache, insomnia or confusion. Notify physician if these effects persist.

Administration and Dosage:

Individualize dosage. Start at a low dosage and increase gradually until the optimum effect is achieved (usually 40 to 80 mg daily).

The following dosage schedule is suggested: 5 mg 3 times daily for 3 days; 10 mg 3 times daily for 3 days; 15 mg 3 times daily for 3 days; 20 mg 3 times daily for 3 days. Thereafter, additional increases may be necessary, but the total daily dose should not exceed 80 mg daily (20 mg 4 times daily).

The lowest effective dose is recommended. If benefits are not evident after a reasonable trial period, withdraw the drug slowly.

				C.I.*
Rx	**Baclofen** (Various, eg, Bristol-Myers Squibb, Geneva, Goldline, Major, Moore, Rugby, Schein, Vitarine, Warner Chilcott, Zenith)	**Tablets:** 10 mg	In 100s, 250s and UD 100s.	150+
Rx	**Lioresal** (Geigy)		(Geigy 23). White, scored. In 100s and UD 100s.	164
Rx	**Baclofen** (Various, eg, Bristol-Myers Squibb, Geneva, Goldline, Major, Moore, Rugby, Schein, Vitarine, Warner Chilcott, Zenith)	**Tablets:** 20 mg	In 100s, 250s and UD 100s.	130+
Rx	**Lioresal** (Geigy)		(Geigy 33). White, scored. In 100s and UD 100s.	146

* Cost Index based on cost per 10 mg.

DANTROLENE SODIUM (Cont.)

Patient Information (Cont.):

Notify physician if skin rash, itching, bloody or black tarry stools or yellowish discoloration of the skin or eyes occurs.

Dantrolene IV may decrease the grip strength and increase weakness of leg muscles, especially walking down stairs.

Exercise caution at meals on the day of administration because difficulty swallowing and choking has been reported.

Administration and Dosage:

Chronic spasticity: Prior to administration, consider the potential response to treatment. Decreased spasticity sufficient to allow a daily function not otherwise attainable should be the therapeutic goal. Establish a therapeutic goal (regain and maintain a specific function such as therapeutic exercise program, utilization of braces, transfer maneuvers, etc) before beginning therapy. Increase dosage until the maximum performance compatible with the dysfunction due to underlying disease is achieved. No further increase in dosage is then indicated.

Titrate and individualize dosage. In view of the potential for liver damage in long-term use, discontinue therapy if benefits are not evident within 45 days.

Adults – Begin with 25 mg once daily; increase to 25 mg, 2 to 4 times daily; then by increments of 25 mg up to as high as 100 mg, 2 to 4 times daily if necessary. As most patients will respond to 400 mg/day or less, higher doses are rarely needed. (See Warning Box.) Maintain each dosage level for 4 to 7 days to determine response. Adjust dosage to achieve maximal benefit without adverse effects.

Children – Use a similar approach. Start with 0.5 mg/kg twice daily; increase to 0.5 mg/kg, 3 or 4 times daily; then by increments of 0.5 mg/kg, up to 3 mg/kg, 2 to 4 times daily if necessary. Do not exceed doses higher than 100 mg 4 times daily.

Malignant hyperthermia:

Preoperative prophylaxis – Dantrolene may be given orally or IV to patients judged susceptible to malignant hyperthermia as part of the overall patient management to prevent or attenuate development of clinical and laboratory signs of MH.

Oral: Give 4 to 8 mg/kg/day orally in 3 or 4 divided doses for 1 or 2 days prior to surgery, with last dose given ≈ 3 to 4 hours before scheduled surgery with a minimum of water. This dosage will usually be associated with skeletal muscle weakness and sedation (sleepiness or drowsiness) or excessive GI irritation (nausea or vomiting); adjust within the recommended dosage range to avoid incapacitation or excessive GI irritation.

IV: 2.5 mg/kg ≈ 1¼ hours before anesthesia and infused over ≈ 1 hour. Additional dantrolene IV may be indicated during anesthesia and surgery by malignant hyperthermia signs or prolonged surgery. Individualize additional doses.

Treatment – As soon as the malignant hyperthermia reaction is recognized, discontinue all anesthetic agents. Use of 100% oxygen is recommended. Administer dantrolene by continuous rapid IV push beginning at a minimum dose of 1 mg/kg, and continuing until symptoms subside or a maximum cumulative dose of 10 mg/kg has been reached. If the physiologic and metabolic abnormalities reappear, repeat the regimen. Note: Administration should be continuous until symptoms subside. The effective dose to reverse the crisis depends upon the degree of susceptibility to malignant hyperthermia, the amount and time of exposure to the triggering agent and the time elapsed between onset of the crisis and initiation of treatment.

Children: Dose is the same as for adults.

Post-crisis follow-up – Following a malignant hyperthermia crisis, give 4 to 8 mg/kg/day orally, in 4 divided doses for 1 to 3 days to prevent recurrence. IV dantrolene may be used when oral administration is not practical. The IV dose must be individualized, starting with 1 mg/kg or more as the clinical situation dictates.

Preparation of solution: Add 60 ml of Sterile Water for Injection, USP (without a bacteriostatic agent) to each vial, and shake until solution is clear. Protect from direct light and use within 6 hours after reconstitution. Store reconstituted solutions at controlled room temperature (59°F to 86°F or 15°C to 30°C). Avoid prolonged exposure to light.

				C.I.*
Rx	**Dantrium** (Procter & Gamble Pharm.)	**Capsules:** 25 mg	Orange and light brown. In 100s, 500s and UD 100s.	106
		50 mg	Orange and dark brown. In 100s.	73
		100 mg	Orange and light brown. In 100s and UD 100s.	43
Rx	**Dantrium Intravenous** (Procter & Gamble Pharm.)	**Powder for Injection:** 20 mg/vial. Concentration following reconstitution is approximately 0.32 mg/ml. In 70 ml vials.[1]		24,000

* Cost Index based on cost per 25 mg.

[1] With 3 g mannitol per vial.

Uses:

The methocarbamol and aspirin combinations and the carisoprodol and aspirin (with or without codeine) combinations are indicated as adjuncts to rest, physical therapy and other measures for relief of discomfort associated with acute, painful musculoskeletal conditions. The other combinations are classified as *"probably effective"* for this indication. Components of these combinations include:

MUSCLE RELAXANTS: Methocarbamol (p.1523; Chlorzoxazone (p. 1518); Carisoprodol (p. 1515); Orphenadrine Citrate (p. 1525).

ANALGESICS: Acetaminophen (p.1147); Aspirin (p.1153); Codeine (p.1098).

CAFFEINE (p1078), used as a CNS stimulant, also has minor analgesic activity.

	Product	Composition	Supply	C.I.*
Rx	**Methocarbamol w/ASA** (Various)	**Tablets:** 400 mg methocarbamol and 325 mg aspirin *Dose:* 2 tablets 4 times daily	In 15s, 30s, 40s, 100s, 500s and 1000s.	107+
Rx	**Robaxisal** (Robins)		(AHR Robaxisal). Pink and white. In 100s, 500s and Dis-Co 100s.	503
Rx	**Carisoprodol Compound** (Various)	**Tablets:** 200 mg carisoprodol and 325 mg aspirin *Dose:* 1 or 2 tablets 4 times daily	In 15s, 30s, 40s, 100s, 500s and 1000s.	183+
Rx	**Sodol Compound** (Major)		In 100s and 500s.	279
Rx	**Soma Compound** (Wallace)		(Wallace-2103). White and orange. In 100s, 500s and UD 500s.	477
c-III	**Soma Compound w/Codeine** (Wallace)	**Tablets:** 200 mg carisoprodol, 325 mg aspirin and 16 mg codeine phosphate *Dose:* 1 or 2 tablets 4 times daily	(Wallace-2403). White and yellow. In 100s.[1]	646
Rx	**Chlorzoxazone w/APAP** (Various)	**Tablets:** 250 mg chlorzoxazone and 300 mg acetaminophen *Dose:* 2 tablets 4 times daily	In 20s, 28s, 30s, 40s, 60s, 100s, 500s, 1000s and UD 32s, 100s and 200s.	26+
Rx	**Chlorofon-F** (Rugby)		In 100s and 1000s.	36
Rx	**Flexaphen** (Trimen)	**Capsules:** 250 mg chlorzoxazone and 300 mg acetaminophen *Dose:* 2 capsules 4 times daily	Tan. In 100s.	130
Rx	**Miflex** (Misemer)		In 100s.	175
Rx	**Mus-Lax** (Jones Medical)		Red. In 100s.	200
Rx	**Lobac** (Seatrace)	**Capsules:** 200 mg salicylamide, 20 mg phenyltoloxamine and 300 mg acetaminophen *Dose:* 2 capsules 4 times daily	Eggshell. In 100s.	NA
Rx	**Orphengesic** (Various)	**Tablets:** 25 mg orphenadrine citrate, 385 mg aspirin and 30 mg caffeine *Dose:* 1 or 2 tablets 3 or 4 times daily	In 100s and 500s.	338+
Rx	**Norgesic** (Riker)		(Riker Norgesic). Green, white and yellow. In 100s, 500s and UD 100s.	440
Rx	**Orphengesic Forte** (Various)	**Tablets:** 50 mg orphenadrine citrate, 770 mg aspirin and 60 mg caffeine *Dose:* ½ or 1 tablet 3 or 4 times daily	In 100s and 500s.	240+
Rx	**Norgesic Forte** (Riker)		(Riker Norgesic Forte). Green, white and yellow, scored. In 100s, 500s and UD 100s.	307

*Cost Index based on cost per 1.5 g methocarbamol, 350 mg carisoprodol, 500 mg chlorzoxazone or 50 mg orphenadrine citrate.

[1] With sodium metabisulfite.

Parkinson's Disease:

Parkinsonism is a neurological disease with a variety of origins characterized by tremor, rigidity, akinesia, and disorders of posture and equilibrium. The onset is slow and progressive with symptoms advancing over months to years.

Although the biochemical basis of parkinsonism is complex, the primary defect appears to be an imbalance of neurotransmitters (ie, a relative excess of acetylcholine and a deficiency/absence of dopamine in the basal ganglia). Other central neurotransmitters may have some modifying influence on these primary substances. This defect may be part of a more generalized, structural and enzymatic defect.

Currently, therapy for Parkinson's disease is palliative, as there is no cure for this disease. The goal of therapy is to provide maximum relief from the symptoms and to attempt to maintain the independence and mobility of the patient.

Drug therapy of Parkinson's disease is aimed at correcting or modifying these neurotransmitter defects by inhibiting the effects of acetylcholine or enhancing the effects of dopamine.

Anticholinergic agents – Centrally-acting anticholinergics tend to diminish the characteristic tremor. Patients with minimal involvement who are functioning relatively well may not require medication. However, as the disease progresses, the anticholinergics may be considered.

Dopaminergic agents – Dopamine deficiency appears to be the central feature of the pathogenesis of parkinsonism. **Levodopa**, the immediate precursor of dopamine, directly increases dopamine content in the brain; it is currently the most effective treatment for parkinsonism. Other drugs are available that also affect the dopamine content of the brain: **Bromocriptine** and **pergolide** directly stimulate dopamine receptors. Pergolide is 10 to 1000 times more potent than bromocriptine on a milligram per milligram basis; **amantadine** may increase dopamine at the receptor either by releasing intact striatal dopamine stores or by blocking neuronal dopamine reuptake; **selegiline** increases dopaminergic activity through inhibition of monoamine oxidase type B, however, other mechanisms may exist such as interference of dopamine reuptake at the synapse.

Levodopa is used for symptomatic patients with moderate disabilities; therapy is usually initiated with a combination of levodopa and carbidopa (a dopa decarboxylase inhibitor that prevents peripheral metabolism of levodopa). Unfortunately, the response to levodopa gradually diminishes after 2 to 5 years in most patients, at which time the dopaminergic agonists, bromocriptine or pergolide, selegiline or amantadine may be added to the drug regimen. Amantadine may also be used in patients with minimal involvement when the patients cannot tolerate an anticholinergic drug.

The table below summarizes the drug therapy available for parkinsonism:

Drug Therapy for Parkinsonism

	Indications					
Drugs	Post-encephalitic	Arterio-sclerotic	Idiopathic	Drug/chemical induced	Adjunct to Levodopa/Carbidopa	Usual daily dose range (mg)
Anticholinergics						
Procyclidine	✓	✓	✓	✓		7.5-20
Trihexyphenidyl	✓	✓	✓	✓	✓	1-15
Benztropine	✓	✓	✓	✓		0.5-6
Biperiden	✓	✓	✓	✓		2-8
Ethopropazine	✓	✓	✓	✓		50-600
Diphenhydramine	✓	✓	✓	✓		10-400
Dopaminergic Agents						
Levodopa	✓	✓	✓	✓[1]		500-8000
Carbidopa/levodopa	✓		✓	✓[1]		10/100-200/2000
Amantadine	✓	✓	✓	✓		200-400
Bromocriptine	✓		✓			2.5-100
Pergolide					✓	1-5
Selegiline					✓	10

[1] Not effective in drug-induced extrapyramidal symptoms.

(Continued on following page)

Anticholinergics

Actions:

Pharmacology: The anticholinergic agents, although generally less effective than levodopa, are useful in the treatment of all forms of parkinsonism: Postencephalitic, arteriosclerotic, idiopathic and drug-induced extrapyramidal symptoms. They reduce the incidence and severity of akinesia, rigidity and tremor by about 20%; secondary symptoms such as drooling are also reduced. In addition to suppressing central cholinergic activity, these agents may also inhibit the reuptake and storage of dopamine at central dopamine receptors, thereby prolonging the action of dopamine.

The naturally occurring belladonna alkaloids (atropine, scopolamine, hyoscyamine) are active anticholinergic agents; however, they have largely been replaced by synthetic agents (eg, benztropine, trihexyphenidyl) with a more selective CNS activity. Peripheral anticholinergic side effects (eg, urinary retention, tachycardia, constipation) frequently limit the size of dosages utilized.

Antihistamines (eg, diphenhydramine) with central anticholinergic effects are also used; they may have a lower incidence of peripheral side effects than the belladonna alkaloids or synthetic derivatives. These agents are generally better tolerated by elderly patients. Some antihistamines provide mild antiparkinson effects, and are useful for initiating therapy in patients with minimal symptoms. Because of their sedative effects, the antihistamines may be useful in certain patients with insomnia.

Ethopropazine is a phenothiazine with prominent anticholinergic effects. It is less effective than the synthetic anticholinergic agents.

In spite of their limited efficacy, the anticholinergic drugs are useful in mild cases of Parkinson's disease where the risks and demands of levodopa therapy are not warranted.

Pharmacokinetics: Little pharmacokinetic data are available for these agents. The following table lists some of the available parameters.

Various Antiparkinson Anticholinergic Pharmacokinetic Parameters				
Anticholinergic	Time to peak concentration (hrs)	Peak concentration (mcg/L)	Half-life (hrs)	Oral bioavailability (%)
Benztropine[1]				
Biperiden	1-1.5	4-5	18.4-24.3	29
Diphenhydramine	2-4	65-90	4-15	50-72
Ethopropazine[1]				
Procyclidine	1.1-2	80	11.5-12.6	52-97
Trihexyphenidyl	1-1.3	87.2	5.6-10.2	≈ 100

[1] No data available.

Indications:

Adjunctive therapy in all forms of parkinsonism (postencephalitic, arteriosclerotic and idiopathic) and in the control of drug-induced extrapyramidal disorders. Refer to individual drug monographs for specific indications of individual agents.

Contraindications:

Hypersensitivity to any component; glaucoma, particularly angle-closure glaucoma (simple type glaucomas do not appear to be adversely affected); pyloric or duodenal obstruction; stenosing peptic ulcers; prostatic hypertrophy or bladder neck obstructions; achalasia (megaesophagus); myasthenia gravis; megacolon.

Benztropine: Children < 3 years of age; use with caution in older children.

Warnings:

Ophthalmic: Incipient narrow-angle glaucoma may be precipitated by these drugs. Perform gonioscopy and closely monitor intraocular pressures at regular intervals.

Elderly: Geriatric patients, particularly > 60 years of age, frequently develop increased sensitivity to anticholinergic drugs and require strict dosage regulation. Occasionally, mental confusion and disorientation may occur; agitation, hallucinations and psychotic-like symptoms may develop.

Pregnancy: Category C. Safety for use during pregnancy has not been established. Use only when clearly needed and when the potential benefits outweigh the potential hazards to the fetus.

Lactation: Safety for use in the nursing mother has not been established. An inhibitory effect on lactation may occur. Although infants are particularly sensitive to anticholinergic agents, no adverse effects have been reported in nursing infants whose mothers were taking atropine.

Children: Safety and efficacy for use in children have not been established.

(Continued on following page)

Complete prescribing information for these products begins on page 1537.

Anticholinergics (Cont.)

BENZTROPINE MESYLATE

Indications:

For use as an adjunct in the therapy of all forms of parkinsonism. May also be used in the control of extrapyramidal disorders (except tardive dyskinesia) due to neuroleptic drugs (eg, phenothiazines).

Dosage:

Injection is useful for psychotic patients with acute dystonic reactions or other reactions which make oral medication difficult or impossible, or when a more rapid response is desired.

Since there is no significant difference in onset of action after IV or IM injection, there is usually no need to use the IV route. Improvement is sometimes noticeable a few minutes after injection. In emergency situations, when the condition of the patient is alarming, 1 to 2 ml will normally provide quick relief. If the parkinsonian effect begins to return, repeat the dose.

Dosage titration: Because of cumulative action, initiate therapy with a low dose, increase in increments of 0.5 mg gradually at 5 or 6 day intervals to the smallest amount necessary for optimal relief. Maximum daily dose is 6 mg.

Generally, older patients and thin patients cannot tolerate large doses.

Dosage intervals: Some patients experience greatest relief by taking the entire dose at bedtime; others react more favorably to divided doses, 2 to 4 times a day. The drug's long duration of action makes it particularly suitable for bedtime medication; its effects may last throughout the night, enabling patients to turn in bed during the night more easily, and to rise in the morning.

Parkinsonism: 1 to 2 mg/day, with a range of 0.5 to 6 mg/day, orally or parenterally.

Idiopathic parkinsonism – Start with 0.5 to 1 mg at bedtime; 4 to 6 mg per day may be required.

Postencephalitic parkinsonism – 2 mg per day in one or more doses. In highly sensitive patients, begin therapy with 0.5 mg at bedtime; increase as necessary.

Concomitant therapy: If other antiparkinson agents are to be reduced or discontinued, do so gradually. Many patients obtain greatest relief with combination therapy.

Drug-induced extrapyramidal disorders: Administer 1 to 4 mg once or twice daily.

Acute dystonic reactions – 1 to 2 ml IM or IV usually relieves the condition quickly. After that, 1 to 2 ml orally 2 times daily usually prevents recurrence.

Extrapyramidal disorders which develop soon after initiating treatment with neuroleptic drugs are likely to be transient. A dosage of 1 to 2 mg orally 2 or 3 times a day usually provides relief within 1 or 2 days. After 1 or 2 weeks, withdraw drug to determine its continued need. If such disorders recur, reinstitute benztropine.

Certain drug-induced extrapyramidal disorders which develop slowly may not respond to benztropine.

	Product	Form	Description	C.I.*
Rx	**Benztropine Mesylate** (Various, eg, Dixon-Shane, Geneva Marsam, Harber, Moore, Par, Parmed, Rugby, Schein)	**Tablets:** 0.5 mg	In 100s and UD 100s.	33+
Rx	**Cogentin** (MSD)		(MSD 21). White, scored. In 100s.	9
Rx	**Benztropine Mesylate** (Various, eg, Geneva Marsam, Goldline, Lederle, Moore, Purepac, Rugby, Schein, Vangard)	**Tablets:** 1 mg	In 100s, 1000s and UD 100s.	34+
Rx	**Cogentin** (MSD)		(MSD 635). White, scored. Oval. In 100s and UD 100s.	3
Rx	**Benztropine Mesylate** (Various, eg, Geneva Marsam, Goldline, Lederle, Moore, Purepac, Rugby, Schein, Vangard)	**Tablets:** 2 mg	In 100s, 1000s and UD 100s.	45+
Rx	**Cogentin** (MSD)		(MSD 60). White, scored. In 100s, 1000s and UD 100s.	3
Rx	**Cogentin** (MSD)	**Injection:** 1 mg/ml	In 2 ml amps.	167

* Cost Index based on cost per 1 mg.

Complete prescribing information for these products begins on page 1537.

Anticholinergics (Cont.)

BIPERIDEN

Indications:

Adjunct in the therapy of all forms of parkinsonism (postencephalitic, arteriosclerotic and idiopathic). Useful in the control of extrapyramidal disorders secondary to neuroleptic drug therapy (eg, phenothiazines).

Dosage:

Parkinsonism: 2 mg 3 or 4 times daily, orally. Individualize dosage with dosing titrated to a maximum of 16 mg/24 hours.

Drug-induced extrapyramidal disorders: Oral – 2 mg 1 to 3 times daily.

Parenteral – 2 mg IM or IV. Repeat every half-hour until symptoms are resolved, but do not give more than 4 consecutive doses per 24 hours.

				C.I.*
Rx	**Akineton** (Knoll)	**Tablets:** 2 mg (as HCl)	(11). White, scored. In 100s and 1000s.	86
		Injection: 5 mg/ml (as lactate)	In 1 ml amps.	514

ETHOPROPAZINE HCl

A phenothiazine derivative.

Indications:

Effective as an adjunct in the therapy of all forms of parkinsonism (postencephalitic, idiopathic and arteriosclerotic). Although chemically a phenothiazine derivative, it is distinct from other drugs of its class. Ethopropazine is useful in the control of extrapyramidal disorders due to CNS drugs such as reserpine and phenothiazines.

Dosage:

Initially: 50 mg once or twice daily; increase gradually, if necessary.

Mild to moderate symptoms: 100 to 400 mg daily.

Severe cases: Gradually increase to 500 or 600 mg or more daily.

				C.I.*
Rx	**Parsidol** (Parke-Davis)	**Tablets:** 10 mg	White. In 100s.	4
		50 mg	White, scored. In 100s.	3

DIPHENHYDRAMINE

For complete prescribing information and product availability, see Antihistamines group monograph.

Indications:

For parkinsonism and drug-induced extrapyramidal reactions in the elderly unable to tolerate more potent agents; mild cases of parkinsonism (including drug-induced) in other age groups; in other cases of parkinsonism (including drug-induced) in combination with centrally-acting anticholinergic agents.

Dosage:

Oral:

Adults – 25 to 50 mg 3 to 4 times daily.

Children > 20 lbs (9 kg) – 12.5 to 25 mg 3 or 4 times daily or 5 mg/kg/day. Do not exceed 300 mg/day or 150 mg/m²/day.

Parenteral: Administer IV or deeply IM.

Adults – 10 to 50 mg; 100 mg if required. Maximum daily dosage is 400 mg.

Children – 5 mg/kg/day or 150 mg/m²/day, divided into 4 doses. Maximum daily dosage is 300 mg.

* Cost Index based on cost per 2 mg biperiden or 50 mg ethopropazine.

LEVODOPA

> In order to reduce the high incidence of adverse reactions, individualize therapy and gradually increase dosage to the desired therapeutic level.

Actions:

Pharmacology: The symptoms of Parkinson's disease are related to depletion of striatal dopamine. Dopamine does not cross the blood-brain barrier; however, levodopa, the metabolic precursor of dopamine, does cross the blood-brain barrier. It is decarboxylated into dopamine in the basal ganglia and in the periphery. Hence, blood dopamine is markedly increased, accounting for many of levodopa's pharmacologic and adverse effects.

Pharmacokinetics: Absorption/Distribution – Levodopa is absorbed from the small bowel; peak plasma levels occur in 0.5 to 2 hours, and may be delayed in the presence of food. The rate of absorption is dependent upon the rate of gastric emptying, pH of gastric juice, and the length of time the drug is exposed to degradative enzymes of gastric mucosa and intestinal flora.

Metabolism/Elimination – The drug is extensively metabolized (> 95%) in the periphery and by the liver; < 1% of unchanged drug penetrates the CNS. Plasma half-life ranges from 1 to 3 hours. It is excreted primarily in the urine. The major urinary metabolites of levodopa appear to be dihydroxyphenylacetic acid (DOPAC) and homovanillic acid (HVA). In 24 hour urine samples, HVA accounts for 13% to 42% of the ingested dose of levodopa.

Indications:

Treatment of idiopathic, postencephalitic and symptomatic parkinsonism which may follow injury to the nervous system by carbon monoxide and manganese intoxication, and in elderly patients with parkinsonism associated with cerebral arteriosclerosis.

Concomitant therapy: Levodopa is often used in combination with carbidopa, which inhibits decarboxylation of levodopa and makes more levodopa available for transport to the brain (see Levodopa/Carbidopa monograph).

Selegiline and pergolide are each used as adjuncts in the management of parkinsonian patients being treated with levodopa/carbidopa; the dose of the levodopa/carbidopa may be decreased with concomitant therapy (see individual monographs).

Unlabeled uses: Levodopa has been used with some benefit to relieve herpes zoster (shingles) pain and restless legs syndrome.

Contraindications:

Hypersensitivity to the drug; narrow-angle glaucoma; patients on MAOI therapy (does not apply to MAOI-type B agents such as selegiline). Discontinue MAOIs 2 weeks prior to initiating levodopa therapy.

Because levodopa may activate a malignant melanoma, do not use in patients with suspicious, undiagnosed skin lesions or history of melanoma.

Warnings:

Concomitant conditions: Administer cautiously to patients with severe cardiovascular or pulmonary disease, bronchial asthma, occlusive cerebrovascular disease, renal, hepatic or endocrine disease, affective disorders, major psychoses and cardiac arrhythmias. Periodically evaluate hepatic, hematopoietic, cardiovascular and renal functions during extended therapy in all patients.

Myocardial infarction: Administer cautiously to patients with a history of myocardial infarction who have residual atrial, nodal or ventricular arrhythmias. Use in a facility with a coronary or intensive care unit.

Upper GI hemorrhage may occur in those patients with a history of peptic ulcer.

Psychiatric patients: Observe all patients for the development of depression with suicidal tendencies. Treat psychotic patients with caution.

Pregnancy: Safety for use during pregnancy has not been established. Use only when clearly needed and when potential benefits outweigh potential hazards to the fetus. At dosages in excess of 200 mg/kg/day, levodopa has an adverse effect in rodents on fetal and postnatal growth and viability.

Lactation: Do not use in nursing mothers.

Children: Safety for use in children < 12 years has not been established.

Precautions:

Wide-angle glaucoma: Patients with chronic wide-angle glaucoma may be treated cautiously with levodopa, if the intraocular pressure is well controlled and the patient is carefully monitored for changes in intraocular pressure during therapy.

(Precautions continued on following page)

LEVODOPA (Cont.)

Precautions (Cont.):

"On-off" phenomenon: Some patients who initially respond to levodopa therapy may develop the "on-off" phenomenon, a condition where patients suddenly oscillate between improved clinical status and loss of therapeutic effect (abrupt onset of akinesia). This effect may occur within minutes or hours and is associated with long-term levodopa treatment. Approximately 15% to 40% of patients develop this phenomenon after 2 to 3 years of treatment; this frequency increases after 5 years. In other patients, a deteriorating response to levodopa occurs ("wearing-off" effect).

Suggestions to alleviate these conditions include keeping the dose low, reserving the drug for severe cases, or the use of a "drug holiday" which includes complete withdrawal of levodopa for a period of time (5 to 14 days) followed by a slow reintroduction of the drug at a lower dose. A protein-restricted diet and adjunctive therapy (eg, pergolide, selegiline), allowing for a decreased levodopa dose, may also be beneficial. Further study is needed.

Tartrazine sensitivity: Some of these products contain tartrazine, which may cause allergic-type reactions (including bronchial asthma) in certain susceptible individuals. Although the overall incidence of tartrazine sensitivity is low, it is frequently seen in patients who also have aspirin hypersensitivity. Specific products containing tartrazine are identified in the product listings.

Drug Interactions:

Levodopa Drug Interactions			
Precipitant drug	Object drug*		Description
Antacids	Levodopa	⬆	Levodopa bioavailability may be increased, possibly increasing its efficacy.
Anticholinergics	Levodopa	⬇	Increased gastric deactivation and decreased intestinal absorption of levodopa may occur.
Benzodiazepines	Levodopa	⬇	Levodopa's therapeutic value may be attenuated.
Hydantoins	Levodopa	⬇	Levodopa's effectiveness may be reduced.
Methionine	Levodopa	⬇	Levodopa's effectiveness may be reduced.
Metoclopramide	Levodopa	⬌	Levodopa's bioavailability may be increased; levodopa may decrease the effects of metoclopramide on gastric emptying and lower esophageal pressure.
MAO inhibitors	Levodopa	⬆	Hypertensive reactions occur with levodopa and MAOI coadministration. Avoid concurrent use. The MAO-type B inhibitor selegiline is used with levodopa and is not associated with such a reaction.
Papaverine	Levodopa	⬇	Levodopa's effectiveness may be reduced.
Pyridoxine	Levodopa	⬇	Levodopa's effectiveness is reduced.
Tricyclic antidepressants	Levodopa	⬇	Delayed absorption and decreased bioavailability of levodopa may occur. Hypertensive episodes have occurred.

* ⬆ = Object drug increased ⬇ = Object drug decreased ⬌ = Undetermined effect

Drug/Food interactions: In six of nine patients, meals reduced the peak plasma concentrations of levodopa by 29%; the peak was delayed by 34 minutes. A protein-restricted diet may also help minimize the "fluctuations" (decreased response to levodopa at the end of each day or at various times of day) that occur in some patients.

Drug/Lab test interactions: The **Coombs test** has occasionally become positive during extended therapy. Elevations of **uric acid** have occurred with the colorimetric method, but not with the uricase method.

Adverse Reactions:

Frequent: Adventitious movements, such as choreiform or dystonic movements (10% to 90%); anorexia (50%); nausea and vomiting (80%) with or without abdominal pain and distress; dry mouth; dysphagia; dysgeusia (4.5% to 22%); sialorrhea; ataxia; increased hand tremor; headache; dizziness; numbness; weakness and faintness; bruxism; confusion; insomnia; nightmares; hallucinations and delusions; agitation and anxiety; malaise; fatigue; euphoria.

(Adverse Reactions continued on following page)

LEVODOPA AND CARBIDOPA (Cont.)

Administration and Dosage (Cont.):

Patients currently treated with conventional carbidopa/levodopa preparations: Substitute dosage with *Sinemet CR* at an amount that provides ≈ 10% more levodopa per day, although this may need to be increased to a dosage that provides up to 30% more levodopa per day. Use intervals of 4 to 8 hours while awake.

Guidelines for Initial Conversion from *Sinemet* to *Sinemet CR*	
Sinemet Total daily levodopa dose (mg)	*Sinemet CR* Suggested dosage regimen
300 to 400	1 tablet twice daily
500 to 600	1½ tablets twice daily or 1 tablet 3 times daily
700 to 800	Total of 4 tablets in ≥ 3 divided doses (eg, 1½ tablets am, 1½ tablets early pm, 1 tablet later pm)
900 to 1000	Total of 5 tablets in ≥ 3 divided doses (eg, 2 tablets am, 2 tablets early pm, 1 tablet later pm)

Combination therapy: Other antiparkinson drugs can be given concurrently; dosage adjustment may be necessary.

Sinemet (25/100 or 10/100) can be added to the dosage regimen of *Sinemet CR* in selected patients with advanced disease who need additional levodopa.

				C.I.*
Rx	**Sinemet-10/100** (DuPont Pharm)	**Tablets:** 10 mg carbidopa and 100 mg levodopa	(647). Dark blue, scored. Oval. In 100s and UD 100s.	332
Rx	**Sinemet-25/100** (DuPont Pharm)	**Tablets:** 25 mg carbidopa and 100 mg levodopa	(650). Yellow, scored. Oval. In 100s and UD 100s.	504
Rx	**Sinemet-25/250** (DuPont Pharm)	**Tablets:** 25 mg carbidopa and 250 mg levodopa	(654). Light blue, scored. Oval. In 100s and UD 100s.	217
Rx	**Sinemet CR** (DuPont Pharm)	**Tablets, sustained release:** 50 mg carbidopa and 200 mg levodopa	(521). Peach, scored. Oval, biconvex. In 100s and UD 100s.	NA

Amantadine is also used as an antiviral agent. For information regarding this use and for full prescribing information, refer to page 1958

AMANTADINE HCl

Actions:

The exact mechanism of action is unknown, but amantadine is thought to release dopamine from intact dopaminergic terminals that remain in the substantia nigra of parkinson patients. Dopamine release may also occur from other central sites.

Amantadine is less effective than levodopa in the treatment of Parkinson's disease, but slightly more effective than anticholinergic agents. Although anticholinergic-type side effects have been noted with amantadine when used in patients with drug-induced extrapyramidal reactions, there is a lower incidence of these side effects than with anticholinergic antiparkinson drugs.

Indications:

Parkinson's disease/syndrome and drug-induced extrapyramidal reactions: Idiopathic Parkinson's disease (paralysis agitans); postencephalitic parkinsonism; arteriosclerotic parkinsonism; drug-induced extrapyramidal reactions; symptomatic parkinsonism following injury to the nervous system by carbon monoxide intoxication.

Administration and Dosage:

Parkinson's disease: 100 mg twice/day when used alone. Onset of action is usually within 48 hrs. Initial dose is 100 mg/day for patients with serious associated medical illnesses or those who are receiving high doses of other antiparkinson drugs. After one to several weeks at 100 mg once/day, increase to 100 mg twice/day, if necessary. Patients whose responses are not optimal at 200 mg/day may occasionally benefit from an increase up to 400 mg/day in divided doses; supervise closely. Patients initially benefiting from amantadine often experience decreased effectiveness after a few months. Benefit may be regained by increasing to 300 mg/day, or by temporary discontinuation for several weeks. Other antiparkinson drugs may be necessary.

Concomitant therapy – Some patients who do not respond to anticholinergic antiparkinson drugs may respond to amantadine. When each is used with marginal benefit, concomitant use may produce additional benefit.

When amantadine and levodopa are initiated concurrently, the patient can exhibit rapid therapeutic benefits. Maintain the dose at 100 mg daily or twice a day, while levodopa is gradually increased to optimal benefit. When amantadine is added to optimal, well tolerated doses of levodopa, additional benefit may result; this includes minimizing the fluctuations in improvement which sometimes occur on levodopa alone. Patients who require a reduction in their usual dose of levodopa because of side effects may regain lost benefit with addition of amantadine.

Dosage in renal impairment: The following table, designed to yield steady-state plasma concentrations of 0.7 to 1 mcg/ml, is a guide for dosage in renal impairment:

Suggested Guidelines for Amantadine in Patients with Impaired Renal Function

Creatinine Clearance *(ml/min/1.73 m²)*	Estimated Half-Life *(hours)*	Suggested Maintenance Regimen*
100	11	100 mg twice a day or 200 mg daily
80	14	100 mg twice a day
60	19	200 mg alternated with 100 mg daily
50	23	100 mg daily
40	29	100 mg daily
30	40	200 mg twice weekly
20	66	100 mg three times weekly
10	178	200 mg alternated with 100 mg every 7 days
Three times weekly chronic hemodialysis	199	200 mg alternated with 100 mg every 7 days

* Loading dose on first day of 200 mg.
Reproduced with permission from Horadam VW, Sharp JG, Smilack JD, et al. Pharmacokinetics of amantadine HCl in subjects with normal and impaired renal function. *Ann Intern Med* 1981;94 (Part 1):454-58.

Drug-induced extrapyramidal reactions: 100 mg twice a day. Patients with suboptimal responses may occasionally benefit from 300 mg daily in divided doses.

	Product	Form	Packaging	C.I.*
Rx	**Amantadine HCl** (Various)	**Capsules:** 100 mg	In 100s, 250s, 500s and UD 100s.	119+
Rx	**Symadine** (Solvay Pharm.)		(RR 4140). Red. In 100s.	150
Rx	**Symmetrel** (DuPont)		(Symmetrel/DuPont). Red. In 100s, 500s and UD 100s.	189
Rx	**Symmetrel** (DuPont)	**Syrup:** 50 mg/5 ml	In pt.	338

* Cost Index based on cost per 100 mg.

Bromocriptine is also used in the treatment of amenorrhea/galactorrhea, female infertility, acromegaly and prevention of physiological lactation. Refer to page 2778 for full prescribing information.

BROMOCRIPTINE MESYLATE

Actions:

Pharmacology: Experiments in rodents suggest a direct action of bromocriptine on striatal dopamine receptors.

Clinical Pharmacology (Parkinson's disease): Bromocriptine produces its therapeutic effect by directly stimulating the dopamine receptors in the corpus striatum.

As adjunctive treatment to levodopa (alone or with a peripheral decarboxylase inhibitor), bromocriptine therapy may provide additional therapeutic benefits in those patients who are currently maintained on optimal dosages of levodopa, those who are beginning to develop tolerance to levodopa therapy, and those who are experiencing levodopa "end of dose failure." Bromocriptine may permit reducing the maintenance dose of levodopa and thus, may ameliorate the occurrence or severity of adverse reactions associated with long-term levodopa therapy such as abnormal involuntary movements (eg, dyskinesias) and the marked swings in motor function ("on-off" phenomenon). Continued efficacy of bromocriptine during treatment of more than 2 years has not been established.

Data are insufficient to evaluate benefit from treating newly diagnosed Parkinson's disease with bromocriptine. Studies show more adverse reactions (notably nausea, hallucinations, confusion and hypotension) in bromocriptine-treated patients than in levodopa/carbidopa-treated patients. Patients unresponsive to levodopa are poor candidates for bromocriptine therapy.

Indications:

Parkinson's disease: In the treatment of idiopathic or postencephalitic Parkinson's disease.

Administration and Dosage:

Parkinson's disease: Initiate treatment at a low dosage and individualize; increase the daily dosage slowly until a maximum therapeutic response is achieved. If possible, maintain the dosage of levodopa during this introductory period.

One-half of a 2.5 mg tablet twice daily with meals. Assess dosage titrations every 2 weeks to ensure that the lowest dosage producing an optimal therapeutic response is not exceeded. If necessary, increase the dosage every 2 to 4 weeks by 2.5 mg/day with meals. If it is necessary to reduce the dose because of adverse reactions, reduce dose gradually in 2.5 mg increments.

The safety of bromocriptine has not been demonstrated in dosages exceeding 100 mg per day.

			C.I.*
Rx	**Parlodel** (Sandoz)	**Tablets:** 2.5 mg (as mesylate). (#Parlodel 2½). White, scored. In 30s.	309
		Capsules: 5 mg (as mesylate). (#Parlodel 5 mg/S). Caramel and white. In 30s and 100s.	280

* Cost Index based on cost per 2.5 mg.

Product identification code.

SELEGILINE HCl (L-Deprenyl)

Actions:

Pharmacology: Selegiline hydrochloride is a levorotatory acetylenic derivative of phenethylamine. The mechanism of action in the adjunctive treatment of Parkinson's disease is not fully understood. Inhibition of monoamine oxidase (MAO) type B activity is of primary importance; selegiline may act through other mechanisms to increase dopaminergic activity.

Selegiline is an irreversible inhibitor of MAO by acting as a 'suicide' substrate for the enzyme; ie, it is converted by MAO to an active moiety that combines irreversibly with the active site or the enzyme's essential FAD cofactor. Because selegiline has greater affinity for type B than for type A active sites, it can serve as a selective inhibitor of MAO type B at the recommended dose.

MAOs are widely distributed throughout the body; their concentration is especially high in liver, kidney, stomach, intestinal wall and brain. MAOs are currently subclassified into two types, A and B, which differ in their substrate specificity and tissue distribution in humans. Intestinal MAO is predominantly type A, while most of that in the brain is type B. In CNS neurons, MAO plays an important role in the catabolism of catecholamines (dopamine, norepinephrine and epinephrine) and serotonin. MAOs are also important in the catabolism of various exogenous amines found in a variety of food and drugs. MAO in the GI tract and liver (primarily type A) provides vital protection from exogenous amines (eg, tyramine) that have the capacity, if absorbed intact, to cause a hypertensive crisis.

Selegiline may have pharmacological effects unrelated to MAO type B inhibition. There is some evidence that it may increase dopaminergic activity by other mechanisms, including interfering with dopamine reuptake at the synapse. Effects resulting from selegiline administration may also be mediated through its metabolites. Two of its three principal metabolites, amphetamine and methamphetamine, have pharmacological actions of their own; they interfere with neuronal uptake and enhance release of several neurotransmitters (eg, norepinephrine, dopamine, serotonin). However, the extent to which these metabolites contribute to the effects of selegiline are unknown.

Pharmacokinetics: Absorption/Distribution – Selegiline is rapidly absorbed; approximately 73% of a dose is absorbed and the maximum plasma concentration occurs 0.5 to 2 hours following administration. Following the oral administration of a single dose of 10 mg to 12 healthy subjects, serum levels of intact selegiline were below the limit of detection (less than 10 ng/ml).

Metabolism/Excretion – The drug is rapidly metabolized. Three metabolites, N-desmethyldeprenyl (the major metabolite; mean half-life 2 hours), amphetamine (mean half-life 17.7 hours), and methamphetamine (mean half-life 20.5 hours), were found in serum and urine. Over 48 hours, 45% of the dose administered appeared in the urine as these 3 metabolites. Unchanged selegiline is not detected in the urine.

The rate of MAO B regeneration following discontinuation of treatment has not been quantitated. It is this rate, dependent upon de novo protein synthesis, that seems likely to determine how fast normal MAO B activity can be restored.

Clinical Trials: Selegiline's benefit in Parkinson's disease has only been documented as an adjunct to levodopa/carbidopa. Its effectiveness as a sole treatment is unknown but attempts to treat Parkinson's disease with nonselective MAO inhibitor monotherapy have been unsuccessful. Selegiline was significantly superior to placebo on all three principal outcome measures used: Change from baseline in daily levodopa/carbidopa dose; the amount of 'off' time; patient self-rating of treatment success (eg, measures of reduced end of dose akinesia, decreased tremor and sialorrhea, improved speech and dressing ability and improved overall disability as assessed by walking and comparison to previous state). Attempts to treat Parkinsonian patients with combinations of levodopa and currently marketed nonselective MAO inhibitors were abandoned because of multiple side effects including hypertension, increase in involuntary movement and toxic delirium.

Indications:

Adjunct in the management of Parkinsonian patients being treated with levodopa/carbidopa who exhibit deterioration in the quality of their response to this therapy.

Contraindications:

Hypersensitivity to the drug.

(Continued on following page)

Complete prescribing information for these products begins on page 1564.

ALUMINUM HYDROXIDE GEL

Administration and Dosage: 500 to 1800 mg, 3 to 6 times daily, between meals and at bedtime.

Children: For hyperphosphatemia – 50 to 150 mg/kg/24 hr in divided doses every 4 to 6 hours; titrate to normal serum phosphorus.

	Product	Form	Description	Sodium[1] (mg)	ANC[1] (mEq)	C.I.*
otc	**Alu-Cap** (Riker)	**Capsules:** 475 mg	Red/green. In 100s.			186
otc	**Dialume** (Armour)	**Capsules:** 500 mg	In 100s and 500s.	<1.2	10	256
otc	**Amphojel** (Wyeth-Ayerst)	**Tablets:** 300 mg	(119). In 100s.	1.8	8	75
		600 mg	(13). In 100s.	2.9	16	118
		Suspension: 320 mg per 5 ml	Saccharin and sorbitol. Plain or peppermint. In 360 ml.	<2.3	10	104
otc	**Aluminum Hydroxide** (Rugby)	**Tablets:** 600 mg	In 100s and UD 100s.			42
otc	**Alu-Tab** (Riker)		Green, film coated. In 250s.			170
otc	**Aluminum Hydroxide** (Roxane)	**Tablets:** Aluminum hydroxide equivalent to 608 mg dried aluminum hydroxide gel	In 100s and UD 100s.			77
otc	**Aluminum Hydroxide Gel** (Various)	**Suspension:** 320 mg per 5 ml	In 180 and 360 ml, pt, gal & UD 15 and 30 ml (100s).			34+
otc	**Aluminum Hydroxide Gel** (Various)	**Suspension:** 600 mg per 5 ml	In 180, 360 and 500 ml and UD 20 and 30 ml (100s).			64+
otc *sf*	**Concentrated Aluminum Hydroxide** (Roxane)	**Suspension:** 675 mg per 5 ml	In 20, 30, 180 and 500 ml.	1-2.5		94
otc	**Alternagel** (J & J-Merck)	**Liquid:** 600 mg/5 ml[2]	In 30, 150 and 360 ml.	<2.5	16	148

ALUMINUM PHOSPHATE GEL

Indications:

To reduce fecal excretion of phosphates.

This product is no longer labeled for use as an antacid.

Administration and Dosage:

15 to 30 ml undiluted every 2 hrs between meals and at bedtime.

	Product	Form	Description	Sodium[1] (mg)	ANC[1] (mEq)	C.I.*
otc *sf*	**Phosphaljel** (Wyeth-Ayerst)	**Suspension:** 233 mg (12.5 mg sodium) per 5 ml	In 360 ml.	7	na	101

DIHYDROXYALUMINUM SODIUM CARBONATE

Administration and Dosage:

Chew 1 or 2 tablets as required.

	Product	Form	Description	Sodium[1] (mg)	ANC[1] (mEq)	C.I.*
otc	**Rolaids Antacid** (Warner-Lambert Consumer)	**Tablets, chewable:** 334 mg	In rolls of 12s, 36s, 75s and 150s.	53	7.5	77

* Cost Index based on cost per capsule, tablet or 5 ml.

sf- Sugar free.

na – not applicable

[1] Acid neutralizing capacity and sodium content per capsule, tablet or 5 ml.

[2] With simethicone.

Complete prescribing information for these products begins on page 1564.

ALUMINUM CARBONATE GEL, BASIC

Indications: In addition to its use as an antacid, it is also used for hyperphosphatemia.

Administration and Dosage: *Antacid:* 2 capsules or tablets or 10 ml of regular suspension (in water or fruit juice) as often as every 2 hours, up to 12 times daily.

Hyperphosphatemia: Administer 3 to 4 times per day with meals.
Caps or Tabs – Take 2. *Suspension* – Take 2.5 tsp. (12 ml).

	Product	Form	Description	Sodium[1] (mg)	ANC[1] (mEq)	C.I.*
otc	**Basaljel** (Wyeth-Ayerst)	**Capsules:** Equivalent to 608 mg dried aluminum hydroxide gel or 500 mg aluminum hydroxide	(Wyeth 472). In 100s and 500s.	2.8	12	183
		Swallow Tablets: Equiv. to 608 mg dried aluminum hydroxide gel or 500 mg aluminum hydroxide	(Wyeth 473). Scored. In 100s.	2.8	13	156
		Suspension: Equiv. to 400 mg aluminum hydroxide per 5 ml[2]	Saccharin, sorbitol. In 360 ml.	2.9	12	115

MAGNESIA (Magnesium Hydroxide)

Administration and Dosage:

Adults and children over 12: Antacid dose is 5 to 15 ml liquid or 650 mg to 1.3 g tablets 4 times daily.
Laxative dose – See product listing in Laxative monograph.

	Product	Form	Description	Sodium[1] (mg)	ANC[1] (mEq)	C.I.*
otc	**Milk of Magnesia** (Various)	**Tablets:** 325 mg	In 250s and 1000s.			25+
		Liquid: 390 mg/5 ml	In 120, 360, 720 ml; pt, qt, gal; UD 10, 15, 20, 30, 100, 180, 400 ml.	0.12	14	26+
		Suspension	Pt, qt, gal, UD 15, 30 ml.			23+
otc	**Concentrated Phillips' Milk of Magnesia** (Phillips)	**Liquid:** 800 mg/5 ml	Sorbitol, sugar. Strawberry and orange vanilla creme flavors. In 240 ml.			NA

MAGNESIUM OXIDE

Administration and Dosage:

Capsules: 140 mg taken with water or milk 3 to 4 times daily.
Tablets: 400 to 840 mg/day.

	Product	Form	Description	Sodium[1] (mg)	ANC[1] (mEq)	C.I.*
otc	**Uro-Mag** (Blaine)	**Capsules:** 140 mg	Clear. In 100s, 1000s.			144
otc	**Mag-Ox 400** (Blaine)	**Tablets:** 400 mg	In 100s and 1000s.			150
otc	**Maox** (Kenneth M)	**Tablets:** 420 mg	Tartrazine. In 250s, 1000s.		21	84

MAGALDRATE (Hydroxymagnesium Aluminate)

Magaldrate is a chemical entity of aluminum and magnesium hydroxides (not a physical mixture). Also known as hydroxymagnesium aluminate, it contains the equivalent of 29% to 40% magnesium oxide and 18% to 26% aluminum oxide.

Administration and Dosage:

480 to 1080 mg between meals and at bedtime.

	Product	Form	Description	Sodium[1] (mg)	ANC[1] (mEq)	C.I.*
otc	**Lowsium** (Rugby)	**Tablets, chewable:** 480 mg	20 mg simethicone. In 60s.	<0.5		51
		Suspension: 540 mg per 5 ml	In 360 ml.			53
otc	**Riopan** (Whitehall)	**Swallow Tablets:** 480 mg	(Riopan). White. In 60s and 100s.	<0.1	13.5	73
		Tablets, chewable: 480 mg	Sorbitol. (Riopan). White. In 60s, 100s.	<0.1	13.5	84
		Suspension: 540 mg per 5 ml	Menthol. Saccharin. In 355 ml.	<0.1	15	94
otc	**Riopan Extra Strength** (Whitehall)	**Liquid:** 1080 mg per 5 ml.	In 176 ml and 355 ml.	<0.3	30	129

* Cost Index based on cost per capsule, tablet or 5 ml.
[1] Acid neutralizing capacity and sodium content per capsule, tablet or 5 ml.
[2] With simethicone.

Complete prescribing information for these products begins on page 1564.

CALCIUM CARBONATE

Contains 40% calcium; 20 mEq calcium/g.

Administration and Dosage:
0.5 to 1.5 g, as needed.

	Product	Form	Description	Sodium[1] (mg)	ANC[1] (mEq)	C.I.*
otc	**Amitone** (SK-Beecham)	**Tablets, chewable:** 350 mg	(Amitone). Peppermint flavor. White. In 100s.	<2	7	57
otc *sf*	**Mallamint** (Hauck)	**Tablets, chewable:** 420 mg	Mint flavor. In 100s.	<0.1		50
otc	**Calcium Carbonate** (Various)	**Tablets:** 500 mg	In 100s, 120s and UD 100s.			75+
otc	**Chooz** (Plough)	**Tablets, chewable:** 500 mg	Mint flavor. In 16s.	<1		136
otc	**Dicarbosil** (SK-Beecham)		Peppermint flavor. White. In rolls of 12.	<2	10	65
otc	**Equilet** (Mission Pharm.)		Neutral, scored. In 100s.	0.3		50
otc	**Tums** (SK-Beecham)		(Tums). Wintergreen, peppermint or fruit flavors. In rolls of 12 and bottles of 75 and 150.	≤2	10	49
otc	**Rolaids Calcium Rich** (Warner-Lambert)	**Tablets, chewable:** 550 mg	Cherry or assorted fruit flavors. In rolls of 12 and bottles of 75s and 150s.	<0.4	11	52
otc	**Calcium Carbonate** (Various)	**Tablets:** 650 mg	In 60s, 72s, 90s, 100s and 1000s.			48+
otc	**Tums E-X Extra Strength** (SK-Beecham)	**Tablets, chewable:** 750 mg	(Tums). Wintergreen or fruit flavors. In 12s, 48s and 96s.	≤2	15	77
otc	**Alka-Mints** (Miles Labs)	**Tablets, chewable:** 850 mg	Sorbitol. (#Alka-Mints). Spearmint flavor. In 30s.	<0.5	16	107
otc	**Calcium Carbonate** (Roxane)	**Tablets:** 1250 mg	Film coated. In 60s, 100s and UD 100s.			130
otc	**Calcium Carbonate** (Roxane)	**Suspension:** 500 mg per 5 ml	In 500 ml and UD 5 ml.			130
otc	**Tums Extra Strength** (SK-Beecham)	**Liquid:** 1000 mg per 5 ml	Sorbitol. Peppermint flavor. In 360 ml.	<5		73

SODIUM BICARBONATE (Contains 27% sodium.)

Administration and Dosage:
0.3 to 2 g, 1 to 4 times daily.

	Product	Form	Description	Sodium[1] (mg)	ANC[1] (mEq)	C.I.*
otc	**Sodium Bicarbonate** (Various)	**Tablets:** 325 mg	In 100s, 200s and 1000s.			15+
otc	**Soda Mint** (Various)		In 100s and 1000s.			22+
otc	**Bell/ans** (C.S. Dent)	**Tablets:** 520 mg	Ginger/wintergreen flavor. In 30s and 60s.	144		58
otc	**Sodium Bicarbonate** (Various)	**Tablets:** 650 mg	In 100s and 1000s.			15+
otc	**Sparkles** (Lafayette)	**Granules, effervescent:** 2 g sodium bicarbonate, 1.5 g citric acid simethicone per 4 g packet	In UD 50s.			NA

* Cost Index based on cost per tablet or 5 ml. *sf* – Sugar free.
[1] Acid-neutralizing capacity and sodium content per tablet or 5 ml.

ANTACID COMBINATIONS

Refer to the general discussion of these products beginning on page 1564.

Capsules and Tablets

Content given in mg per tablet or wafer.

	Product & Distributor	Aluminum Hydroxide	Magnesium Hydroxide	Calcium Carbonate	Other Content	Sodium[1] (mg)	ANC[2] (mEq)	How Supplied	C.I.*
otc	**WinGel Tablets** (Winthrop Pharm.)	180	160		Saccharin	< 2.5	12.3	Chewable. In 50s and 100s.	83
otc	**Maalox Tablets** (Rorer)	200	200		Saccharin, sorbitol	0.7	9.7	(#Maalox). Chewable. In 100s.	72
otc	**Rulox #1 Tablets** (Rugby)							Chewable. Mint flavor. In 100s and 1000s.	35
otc	**Extra Strength Maalox Tablets** (Rorer)	400	400		Saccharin, sorbitol	1.4	23.4	(#ES Maalox). Chewable. In 24s, 50s and 100s.	94
otc	**Rulox #2 Tablets** (Rugby)				Sorbitol			Chewable. Mint flavor. In 100s and 1000s.	47
otc	**Maalox TC Tablets** (Rorer)	600	300		Sorbitol	0.5	28	(#Maalox TC). Chewable. Peppermint-lemon-creme flavor. In 48s.	229
otc	**Magnatril Tablets** (Lannett)	260	130		455 mg magnesium trisilicate			Chewable. In 50s and 100s.	52
otc	**Bicalma Tablets** (Ferndale)			250	300 mg magnesium trisilicate			Chewable. In 100s and 1000s.	44

* Cost Index based on cost per tablet or wafer.
# Product identification code.
[1] 23 mg = 1 mEq sodium.
[2] Acid Neutralizing Capacity per tablet.

(Continued on following page)

ANTACID COMBINATIONS (Cont.)

Refer to the general discussion of these products beginning in the Antacids monograph.

Liquids

Content given in mg per 5 ml.

	Product & Distributor	Aluminum Hydroxide	Magnesium Hydroxide	Calcium Carbonate	Other Content	Sodium[1] (mg)	ANC[2] (mEq)	How Supplied	C.I.*
otc *sf*	**Nephrox Suspension** (Fleming)	320			10% mineral oil	3.3	9	Watermelon flavor. In pt and gal.	63
otc	**Magnatril Suspension** (Lannett)	150		80	400 mg magnesium trisilicate			In 360 ml.	72
otc	**Kolantyl Gel** (Lakeside Pharm.)	150	150		0.2% alcohol, saccharin, sorbitol	<5	10.5	In 360 ml.	134
otc	**WinGel Liquid** (Winthrop Pharm.)	180	160		Saccharin, sorbitol		≥ 10	In 180 and 360 ml.	127
otc	**Alamag Suspension** (Goldline)	225	200					Mint flavor. In 360 ml.	52
otc	**Alumid Suspension** (Vangard)							In 360 ml.	49
otc	**Maalox Suspension** (Rorer)				Saccharin, sorbitol	≈ 1.4	13.3	In 150, 360 and 780 ml and UD 30 ml.	126
otc	**Mintox Suspension** (Major)				25 mg simethicone			Mint flavor. In 360 and 780 ml and gal.	47
otc	**Rulox Suspension** (Rugby)					0.82	12	In 360 and 780 ml and gal.	50

* Cost Index based on cost per 5 ml.
sf- Sugar free.

[1] 23 mg = 1 mEq sodium.
[2] Acid Neutralizing Capacity per 5 ml.

(Continued on following page)

ANTACID COMBINATIONS (Cont.)

Refer to the general discussion of these products beginning in the Antacids monograph.

Liquids (Cont.)

Content given in mg per 5 ml.

	Product & Distributor	Aluminum Hydroxide	Magnesium Hydroxide	Calcium Carbonate	Other Content	Sodium[1] (mg)	ANC[2] (mEq)	How Supplied	C.I.*
otc	**Aludrox Suspension** (Wyeth-Ayerst)	307	103		Simethicone, saccharin, sorbitol	2.3		In 360 ml.	104
otc sf	**Extra Strength Maalox Plus** (Rorer)	500	450		40 mg simethicone, saccharin, sorbitol	1.2	29	In 150 and 355 ml.	28
otc	**Maalox TC Susp.** (Rorer)	600	300		Sorbitol	0.8	27.2	Peppermint flavor. In UD 30 ml (100s).	203
otc	**Kudrox Double Strength Liquid** (Schwartz Pharma Kremers Urban)	565	180			≤15	25	In 360 ml.	203
otc	**Camalox Suspension** (Rorer)	225	200	250	Saccharin, sorbitol	1.2	18.5	Vanilla-mint flavor. In 360 ml.	249
otc	**Algenic Alka Liquid** (Rugby)	31.7			412 mg magnesium carbonate, sodium alginate, EDTA, saccharin, sorbitol			In 355 ml.	86
otc	**Gaviscon Liquid** (Marion Merrell Dow)				137.3 mg magnesium carbonate, sodium alginate, EDTA, saccharin, sorbitol	13		In 177 and 355 ml.	188
otc sf	**Marblen Suspension** (Fleming)			520	400 mg magnesium carbonate	3	18	Peach/apricot flavor or unflavored. In pt and gal.	58
otc sf	**Titralac Plus Liquid** (3M Personal Care)			500	20 mg simethicone	0.0005	11	In 360 ml.	93
otc	**Tums Liquid Extra Strength w/Simethicone** (Norcliff-T)			1000	30 mg simethicone, sorbitol	<5		In 360 ml.	15
otc	**Tums Extra Strength Liquid** (Norcliff Thayer)			1000	Sorbitol	<5		Peppermint flavor. In 360 ml.	15

* Cost Index based on cost per 5 ml. *sf*- Sugar free. [1] 23 mg = 1 mEq sodium. [2] Acid Neutralizing Capacity per 5 ml. [3] As dried gel.

(Continued on following page)

ANTACID COMBINATIONS (Cont.)

Refer to the general discussion of these products beginning in the Antacids monograph.

Liquids (Cont.)

Content given in mg per 5 ml.

	Product & Distributor	Aluminum Hydroxide	Magnesium Hydroxide	Other Content	Sodium[1] (mg)	ANC[2] (mEq)	How Supplied	C.I.*
otc	**Almacone Liquid** (Rugby)	200	200	20 mg simethicone			In 360 ml and gal.	47
otc	**Alumid Plus Liquid** (Vangard)				1.38		In 360 ml.	65
otc	**Anta Gel Liquid** (Halsey)						In 360 ml.	35
otc	**Di-Gel Liquid** (Plough)			20 mg simethicone, saccharin, sorbitol	<5		Mint and lemon-orange flavors. In 180 and 360 ml.	97
otc	**Improved Alma-Mag Liquid** (Rugby)			25 mg simethicone			In 360 ml.	52
otc	**Gelusil Liquid** (Parke-Davis)			25 mg simethicone, saccharin, sorbitol	0.7	12	Spearmint and peppermint flavors. In 360 ml.	105
otc	**Mi-Acid Liquid** (Major)			20 mg simethicone			In 360 ml and gal.	54
otc	**Mygel Suspension** (Geneva Generics)						In 360 ml.	58
otc	**Mylanta Liquid** (J & J-Merck)			20 mg simethicone, sorbitol	0.68	12.7	In 150, 360, 720 ml and UD 30 ml.	115
otc	**Simaal Gel** (Schein)			20 mg simethicone, saccharin, sorbitol			In 360 ml and gal.	72
otc	**Mintox Plus Liquid** (Major)	225	200	25 mg simethicone			Lemon flavor. In 360 ml.	74
otc	**Silain-Gel** (Robins)	282	285	25 mg simethicone	4.4	15	Lemon-orange flavor. In 360 ml.	97
otc	**Gelusil-M Liquid** (Parke-Davis)	300	200	25 mg simethicone, saccharin, sorbitol	1.2	15	Spearmint flavor. In 360 ml.	132

* Cost Index based on cost per 5 ml. [1] 23 mg = 1 mEq sodium. [2] Acid Neutralizing Capacity per 5 ml.

(Continued on following page)

Refer to the general discussion of these products beginning on page 1564 .

Liquids (Cont.)

Content given in mg per 5 ml.

	Product & Distributor	Aluminum Hydroxide	Magnesium Hydroxide	Other Content	Sodium[1] (mg)	ANC[2] (mEq)	How Supplied	C.I.*
otc	**Maalox HRF** (RP-Rorer)	280		350 mg magnesium carbonate per 10 ml, saccharin, tartrazine, sorbitol			Mint flavor. In 355 ml.	NA
otc	**Anta Gel-II Liquid** (Halsey)	400	400	30 mg simethicone	9		In 360 ml.	46
otc	**Gelusil-II Liquid** (Parke-Davis)			30 mg simethicone, saccharin, sorbitol	1.3	24	Lemon-mint flavor. In 360 ml.	161
otc	**Mygel II Suspension** (Geneva Generics)			30 mg simethicone	1.3		In 360 ml.	68
otc	**Simaal 2 Gel** (Schein)						In 360 ml.	75
otc	**Almacone II Suspension** (Rugby)			40 mg simethicone, saccharin, sorbitol			In 360 ml and gal.	59
otc	**Mylanta-II Liquid** (J & J-Merck)			40 mg simethicone, sorbitol	1.14	25.4	In 15, 360 and 720 ml and UD 30 ml (100s).	101
otc	**Extra Strength Maalox Plus Liquid** (Rorer)	500	450	40 mg simethicone, saccharin, sorbitol	0.65	29	Lemon swiss creme flavor. In 360 ml.	100
otc	**Losotron Plus Liquid** (Dixon-Shane)	†		540 mg magaldrate, 20 mg simethicone			In 360 ml.	62+
otc	**Lowsium Plus Suspension** (Rugby)						In 360 ml.	83
otc	**Riopan Plus Suspension** (Whitehall)			540 mg magaldrate, 20 mg simethicone, saccharin, sorbitol	< 0.1	15	In 180 and 355 ml and UD 30 ml (100s).	184
otc	**Riopan Plus 2 Suspension** (Whitehall)	†		1080 mg magaldrate and 30 mg simethicone, saccharin, sorbitol	≤ 0.3	30	Saccharin and sorbitol. In 176 and 355 ml.	184

* Cost Index based on cost per 5 ml.

† See Other Content Column.

[1] 23 mg = 1 mEq sodium.

[2] Acid Neutralizing Capacity per 5 ml.

ANTACID COMBINATIONS (Cont.)

Refer to the general discussion of these products beginning on page 1564 .

Powders and Effervescent Tablets

	Product	Content	Other	C.I.*
otc *sf*	**Citrocarbonate** (Upjohn)	**Effervescent Granules:** 780 mg sodium bicarbonate, 1820 mg sodium citrate and 700.6 mg sodium per 3.9 g dose	In 120 and 240 g.	215
otc	**Bromo Seltzer** (Warner-Lambert)	**Effervescent Granules:** 2781 mg sodium bicarbonate, 325 mg acetaminophen, 2224 mg citric acid (when dissolved forms 2848 mg sodium citrate) and 0.761 g sodium per dosage measure	In 78.75, 127.5 and 270 g.	106
Rx	**Sparkles** (Lafayette)	**Effervescent Granules:** 2 g sodium bicarbonate, 1.5 g citric acid and simethicone per 4 g packet	In UD 50s.	NA
otc	**Alka-Seltzer Advanced Formula** (Miles Inc)	**Effervescent Tablets:** 465 mg sodium bicarbonate, 280 mg calcium carbonate, 325 mg acetaminophen, 900 mg citric acid, 300 mg potassium bicarbonate	4.2 mg phenylalanine. Aspartame, saccharin, lactose and sorbitol. In 36s.	NA
otc	**Alka-Seltzer** (Miles Inc)	**Effervescent Tablets:** 958 mg sodium bicarbonate, 832 mg citric acid, 312 mg potassium bicarbonate and 311 mg sodium. 10.6 mEq acid neutralizing capacity per dry tablet	In 20s and 36s.	141
otc	**Flavored Alka-Seltzer** (Miles Inc)	**Effervescent Tablets:** 1710 mg sodium bicarbonate, 1220 mg citric acid, 325 mg aspirin and 506 mg sodium	Saccharin. In 12s, 24s and 36s.	230
otc	**Alka-Seltzer w/Aspirin** (Miles Inc)	**Effervescent Tablets:** 1916 mg sodium bicarbonate, 1000 mg citric acid, 325 mg aspirin and 567 mg sodium. 17.2 mEq acid neutralizing capacity	In 8s, 12s, 24s, 26s and 36s.	150
otc	**Extra Strength Alka-Seltzer** (Miles Inc)	**Effervescent Tablets:** 1985 mg sodium bicarbonate (heat treated), 1000 mg citric acid, 500 mg aspirin and 588 mg sodium	In 12s, 24s, 36s and 72s.	138
otc	**Bisodol** (Whitehall)	**Powder:** 716 mg sodium bicarbonate, 528 mg magnesium carbonate and 196 mg sodium per 5 ml	Mint flavor. In 90 and 150 g.	315
otc *sf*	**ENO** (Beecham Products)	**Powder:** 1620 mg sodium tartrate, 1172 mg sodium citrate and 819 mg sodium per 5 ml	In 105 and 210 g.	160

* Cost Index based on cost per single dose, packet or tablet.
sf – Sugar free.

SUCRALFATE

Actions:

Pharmacology: Sucralfate, a basic aluminum salt of sulfated sucrose, is a polysaccharide with antipeptic activity. In the acidic medium of gastric juice, the aluminum ion splits off, leaving a highly polar anion which is essentially nonabsorbable. It exerts a local rather than systemic action. Sucralfate forms an ulcer-adherent complex with proteinaceous exudate. The ulcer-adherent complex covers the ulcer site and protects it against acid, pepsin and bile salts. Sucralfate has minimal acid neutralizing capacity.

Sucralfate aids in ulcer healing by forming the protective layer at the ulcer site, providing a barrier to hydrogen ion diffusion, inhibiting pepsin's action 32% and adsorbing bile salts. The acid neutralizing effects do not contribute to antiulcer effects.

Pharmacokinetics: Sucralfate is minimally absorbed (3% to 5%) from the GI tract. Approximately 90% is excreted in the stool. The small amounts of the sulfated disaccharide absorbed are excreted primarily in the urine.

Clinical studies: Acute duodenal ulcer – In two multicenter placebo controlled trials, endoscopic evaluation at 2 and 4 weeks demonstrated statistically significant sucralfate-placebo differences at 4 weeks but not at 2 weeks. At 4 weeks, the overall ulcer healing rate for sucralfate and placebo ranged from 75% to 92% and 58% to 64%, respectively.

Maintenance therapy – In two double-blind randomized placebo controlled trials, endoscopic evaluation at 4, 6 and 12 months revealed the following results:

Duodenal Ulcer Recurrence Rate with Sucralfate (%)						
	Months of therapy					
Drug	1[1]	2[1]	3[1]	4[1]	6[2]	12[2]
Sucralfate	20	30	38	42	19	27
Placebo	33	46	55	63	54	65

[1] Sucralfate (n = 122); placebo (n = 117). "As needed" antacids not permitted.
[2] Sucralfate (n = 48); placebo (n = 46). "As needed" antacids permitted.

Indications:

Short-term treatment (up to 8 weeks) of duodenal ulcer.

Maintenance therapy for duodenal ulcer patients at reduced dosage after healing of acute ulcers.

Unlabeled uses: Sucralfate has been used in the following conditions: Accelerating healing of gastric ulcers; long-term treatment of gastric ulcers; treatment of reflux and peptic esophagitis; treatment of NSAID- and aspirin-induced GI symptoms and mucosal damage; prevention of stress ulcers and GI bleeding in critically ill patients. Since increased gastric pH may be implicated in causing nosocomial infections in critically ill patients, sucralfate may offer an advantage over antacids and histamine H_2 antagonists in stress ulcer prophylaxis.

Sucralfate in suspension has also been used in treatment of oral and esophageal ulcers due to radiation, chemotherapy and sclerotherapy.

Warnings:

Chronic renal failure/dialysis: During sucralfate administration, small amounts of aluminum are absorbed from the GI tract. Concomitant use with other aluminum-containing products (eg, antacids) may increase the total body burden of aluminum. Patients with normal renal function receiving these agents concomitantly adequately excrete aluminum in the urine. However, patients with chronic renal failure or receiving dialysis have impaired excretion of absorbed aluminum, and aluminum does not cross dialysis membranes. Aluminum accumulation and toxicity (eg, aluminum osteodystrophy, osteomalacia, encephalopathy) have occurred. Use with caution in these patients.

Pregnancy: Category B. There are no adequate and well controlled studies in pregnant women. Use this drug during pregnancy only if clearly needed.

Lactation: It is not known whether this drug is excreted in breast milk. Exercise caution when sucralfate is administered to a nursing mother.

Children: Safety and efficacy in children have not been established.

Precautions:

Duodenal ulcer is a chronic recurrent disease. While short-term treatment can completely heal the ulcer, do not expect a successful course to alter post-healing frequency or severity of duodenal ulceration.

(Continued on following page)

SUCRALFATE (Cont.)

Drug Interactions:

Antacids, aluminum-containing: The total body burden of aluminum may be increased with sucralfate coadministration. See Warnings.

Phenytoin plasma levels may be reduced by concurrent sucralfate, possibly with a suboptimal response. Adjust the phenytoin dose if necessary.

Warfarin: A decrease in the hypoprothrombinemic effect of warfarin with sucralfate coadministration has been described in two reports. However, no interaction was detected in two other studies.

In addition, some studies have shown that simultaneous sucralfate administration in healthy volunteers reduced the bioavailability of single doses of the following drugs: Cimetidine; ciprofloxacin; digoxin; norfloxacin; phenytoin; ranitidine; tetracycline; theophylline. The mechanism appears to be due to binding of sucralfate to the concomitant drug in the GI tract. Administering the agent 2 hours before sucralfate eliminated the interaction.

Adverse Reactions:

Adverse reactions in clinical trials were minor and rarely led to drug discontinuation. In over 2,700 patients, adverse effects occurred in 129 (4.7%).

Constipation was the most frequent complaint (2%). Other adverse effects ($<$ 0.5%) include: Diarrhea; nausea; vomiting; gastric discomfort; indigestion; flatulence; dry mouth; rash; pruritus; back pain; headache; dizziness; sleepiness; vertigo.

Overdosage:

Risks associated with overdosage appear minimal.

Patient Information:

Take on an empty stomach at least 1 hour before meals and at bedtime.

Do not take antacids ½ hour before or after taking sucralfate.

Administration and Dosage:

Active duodenal ulcer: Adults – 1 g 4 times a day on an empty stomach (1 hour before meals and at bedtime).

Take antacids as needed for pain relief, but not within ½ hour before or after sucralfate.

While healing with sucralfate may occur within the first 2 weeks, continue treatment for 4 to 8 weeks unless healing is demonstrated by x-ray or endoscopic examination.

Maintenance therapy: Adults – 1 g twice daily.

Rx	**Carafate** (Marion Merrell Dow)	**Tablets:** 1 g	(Carafate 1712). Pink, scored. In 100s, 500s and UD 100s.

Anticholinergic agents are also known as antimuscarinic drugs. In addition to the Gastrointestinal Anticholinergics/Antispasmodics discussed below, related drugs include:

Anticholinergic Antiparkinson Agents
Cycloplegic Mydriatics
Urinary Antispasmodics

See specific monographs.

Gastrointestinal anticholinergic agents are used primarily to decrease motility (smooth muscle tone) in the GI, biliary and urinary tracts and for their antisecretory effects. Antispasmodic agents are related compounds that decrease GI motility by acting on smooth muscle.

Gastrointestinal Anticholinergic/Antispasmodic Dosage		
	Adult Dosage	
Drug	Oral	Parenteral
Anticholinergics		
Atropine	0.4-0.6 mg	0.4-0.6 mg
Scopolamine		0.32-0.65 mg
L-hyoscyamine	0.125-0.25 mg tid-qid (0.375 to 0.7 mg q 12 hrs – sustained release)	0.25-0.5 mg q 4 h
L-alkaloids of belladonna	0.25-0.5 mg tid	
Belladonna alkaloids	0.18-0.3 mg tid-qid	
Quaternary Anticholinergics		
Methscopolamine bromide	2.5 mg ac; 2.5-5 mg hs	
Anisotropine MBr	50 mg tid	
Clidinium bromide	2.5-5 mg tid-qid	
Glycopyrrolate	1-2 mg bid-tid	0.1-0.2 mg tid-qid
Hexocyclium	25 mg qid	
Isopropamide iodide	5-10 mg q 12 hrs	
Mepenzolate bromide	25-50 mg qid	
Methantheline bromide	50-100 mg q 4-6 hrs	
Propantheline bromide	7.5-15 mg tid; 30 mg hs	
Tridihexethyl chloride	25-50 mg tid-qid	
Antispasmodics		
Dicyclomine HCl	20-40 mg qid	20 mg qid
Oxyphencyclimine HCl	10 mg bid	

Actions:

Pharmacology: These agents inhibit the muscarinic actions of acetylcholine at postganglionic parasympathetic neuroeffector sites including smooth muscle, secretory glands and CNS sites. Large doses may block nicotinic receptors at the autonomic ganglia and at the neuromuscular junction.

Specific anticholinergic responses are dose-related. Small doses inhibit salivary and bronchial secretions and sweating; moderate doses dilate the pupil, inhibit accommodation and increase the heart rate (vagolytic effect); larger doses will decrease motility of the GI and urinary tracts; very large doses will inhibit gastric acid secretion.

Belladonna alkaloids are rapidly absorbed following oral administration. They readily cross the blood-brain barrier, and exert their effects on the CNS. The major difference between these agents is that atropine at usual therapeutic doses is a stimulant, whereas scopolamine is a CNS depressant. Undesirable peripheral and central effects occur when given in doses sufficient to control GI motility and gastric acid secretion.

Atropine has a half-life of about 2.5 hours; 94% of a dose is eliminated through the urine in 24 hours.

(Actions continued on following page)

Actions (Cont.):

Quaternary anticholinergics: Synthetic or semisynthetic derivatives structurally related to the belladonna alkaloids, they are poorly and unreliably absorbed orally. Since they do not cross the blood-brain barrier, CNS effects are negligible. They are also less likely to affect the pupil or ciliary muscle of the eye. The duration of action is more prolonged than the alkaloids. In addition, these agents may cause some degree of ganglionic blockade; neuromuscular blockade may occur at toxic doses.

Antispasmodics: The tertiary ammonium compounds have little or no antimuscarinic activity, and therefore, no significant effect on gastric acid secretion. They exhibit a nonspecific direct relaxant effect on smooth muscle.

Indications:

The general uses for these agents are listed below. Refer to the individual product listings for specific indications.

Peptic ulcer: Adjunctive therapy for peptic ulcer. These agents suppress gastric acid secretion. There is no conclusive evidence they aid in the healing of a peptic ulcer, decrease the rate of recurrence or prevent complications. Anticholinergics are used much less frequently in modern ulcer management.

Other GI conditions: Functional GI disorders (diarrhea, pylorospasm, hypermotility, neurogenic colon), irritable bowel syndrome (spastic colon, mucous colitis), acute enterocolitis, ulcerative colitis, diverticulitis, mild dysenteries, pancreatitis, splenic flexure syndrome and infant colic.

Biliary tract: For spastic disorders of the biliary tract. Given in conjunction with a narcotic analgesic.

Urogenital tract: Uninhibited hypertonic neurogenic bladder.

Bradycardia: Atropine is used in the suppression of vagally-mediated bradycardias.

Preoperative medication: Atropine, scopolamine, hyoscyamine and glycopyrrolate are used as preanesthetic medication to control bronchial, nasal, pharyngeal and salivary secretions; and to block cardiac vagal inhibitory reflexes during induction of anesthesia and intubation. Scopolamine is used for preanesthetic sedation and for obstetric amnesia.

Antidotes for poisoning by cholinergic drugs: Atropine is used for poisoning by organophosphorous insecticides, chemical warfare nerve gases and as an antidote for mushroom poisoning due to muscarine in certain species such as *Amanita muscaria* (see Pralidoxime Chloride).

Miscellaneous Uses: Calming delirium; motion sickness (scopolamine), see Antiemetic/Antivertigo Agents monograph; parkinsonism, see Antiparkinson Agents monograph.

Unlabeled Uses: Bronchial asthma: Atropine and related agents are effective in some patients with cholinergic-mediated bronchospasm. Use in patients with chronic lung disease is not generally recommended due to the effect of these agents on bronchial secretions (ie, reduced bronchial secretions resulting in decreased fluidity and thickening of the residual secretion).

Glycopyrrolate may be effective in the treatment of bronchial asthma; doses of 1 mg (nebulization) and 1.3 mg (solution) have been used.

Contraindications:

Hypersensitivity to anticholinergic drugs. Patients hypersensitive to belladonna or to barbiturates may be hypersensitive to **scopolamine.**

Ocular: Narrow-angle glaucoma; adhesions (synechiae) between the iris and lens.

Cardiovascular: Tachycardia; unstable cardiovascular status in acute hemorrhage; myocardial ischemia.

GI: Obstructive disease (eg, achalasia, pyloroduodenal stenosis or pyloric obstruction, cardiospasm); paralytic ileus; intestinal atony of the elderly or debilitated patient; severe ulcerative colitis; toxic megacolon complicating ulcerative colitis; hepatic disease.

GU: Obstructive uropathy (eg, bladder neck obstruction due to prostatic hypertrophy); renal disease.

Musculoskeletal: Myasthenia gravis.

Atropine is contraindicated in asthma patients.

Dicyclomine: Infants $<$ 6 months of age (see Warnings).

Warnings:

Heat prostration can occur with anticholinergic drug use (fever and heat stroke due to decreased sweating) in the presence of a high environmental temperature.

Diarrhea may be an early symptom of incomplete intestinal obstruction, especially in patients with ileostomy or colostomy. Treatment of diarrhea with these drugs is inappropriate and possibly harmful.

Parkinsonism: Vomiting, malaise, sweating and salivation may occur in patients with parkinsonism upon sudden withdrawal of large doses of **scopolamine.**

(Warnings continued on following page)

Warnings (Cont.):

Anticholinergic psychosis has been reported in sensitive individuals given anticholinergic drugs. CNS signs and symptoms include confusion, disorientation, short-term memory loss, hallucinations, dysarthria, ataxia, coma, euphoria, decreased anxiety, fatigue, insomnia, agitation and mannerisms, and inappropriate affect. These CNS signs and symptoms usually resolve within 12 to 24 hours after discontinuation of the drug.

Gastric ulcer may produce a delay in gastric emptying time and may complicate therapy (antral stasis).

Elderly: Elderly patients may react with excitement, agitation, drowsiness and other untoward manifestations to even small doses of anticholinergic drugs.

Pregnancy: Category B (glycopyrrolate, parenteral); *Category C* (hyoscyamine, atropine, scopolamine, isopropamide, propantheline, methantheline). Hyoscyamine crosses the placental barrier; atropine and scopolamine cross the placenta rapidly after IV injection. Effects on the fetus depend on maturity of its parasympathetic nervous system. In the neonate, scopolamine may cause respiratory depression and may contribute to neonatal hemorrhage due to reduction in Vitamin K-dependent clotting factors.

Safety for use during pregnancy has not been established. Use only when clearly needed and when the potential benefits outweigh the potential hazards to the fetus.

Labor and Delivery: Scopolamine does not affect uterine contractions during labor or increase duration of labor. It crosses the placenta but has not been reported to affect the fetus adversely.

Lactation: Hyoscyamine is excreted in breast milk; other anticholinergics (especially atropine) may be excreted in milk, causing infant toxicity, and may reduce milk production. Documentation is lacking or conflicting. Generally, do not use in nursing women.

Children: Safety and efficacy are not established. Hyoscyamine has been used in infant colic. **Isopropamide** is not recommended in children under 12. Safety and efficacy of **glycopyrrolate** in children under 12 are not established for peptic ulcer.

There are reports of infants in the first 3 months of life, administered **dicyclomine** syrup, who experienced respiratory distress, seizures, syncope, asphyxia, pulse rate fluctuations, muscular hypotonia and coma. These symptoms occurred within minutes of ingestion and lasted 20 to 30 minutes; this suggests that they were a consequence of local irritation or aspiration rather than a pharmacologic effect. A few deaths have been reported in infants $\leq$ 3 months of age. Two of these were associated with excessively high dicyclomine blood levels. Dicyclomine is contraindicated in infants $<$ 6 months old.

Precautions:

Potentially hazardous tasks: May produce drowsiness, dizziness or blurred vision; patients should observe caution while driving or performing other tasks requiring alertness.

Use with caution in:

Ocular – Glaucoma; light irides. If there is mydriasis and photophobia, wear dark glasses. Use caution in the elderly because of increased incidence of glaucoma.

GI – Hepatic disease; early evidence of ileus, as in peritonitis; ulcerative colitis (large doses may suppress intestinal motility and precipitate or aggravate toxic megacolon); hiatal hernia associated with reflux esophagitis (anticholinergics may aggravate it).

GU – Renal disease; prostatic hypertrophy. Patients with prostatism can have dysuria and may require catheterization.

Cardiovascular – Coronary heart disease; congestive heart failure; cardiac arrhythmias; tachycardia; hypertension.

Pulmonary – Debilitated patients with chronic lung disease; reduction in bronchial secretions can lead to inspissation and formation of bronchial plugs. Use cautiously in patients with asthma or allergies.

Miscellaneous: Autonomic neuropathy; hyperthyroidism.

In the presence of pain or severe anxiety, scopolamine is usually given with analgesic or sedative agents to avoid behavioral disturbances. Risk of hyperpyrexia is increased in patients with fever. In elderly patients, confusional states are more common.

Special risk patients: Use cautiously in infants, small children, blondes, and persons with Down's syndrome, brain damage or spastic paralysis.

Sulfite sensitivity: Some of these products contain sulfites that may cause allergic-type reactions including anaphylactic symptoms and life-threatening asthmatic episodes in certain susceptible persons. Although the overall prevalence of sulfite sensitivity in the general population is probably low, it is seen more frequently in asthmatic or atopic nonasthmatic persons.

Tartrazine sensitivity: Some of these products contain tartrazine, which may cause allergic-type reactions (including bronchial asthma) in certain susceptible persons. Although the overall incidence of tartrazine sensitivity in the general population is low, it is often seen in patients who have aspirin hypersensitivity. Specific products containing tartrazine are identified in the product listings.

(Continued on following page)

Drug Interactions:

Amantadine: Coadministration of anticholinergics may result in an increase in anticholinergic side effects. Consider decreasing the anticholinergic dose.

Atenolol: The pharmacologic effects may be increased by concurrent anticholinergic administration. Metoprolol and propranolol were not affected in two studies.

Digoxin: Pharmacologic effects may be increased by anticholinergic coadministration. This interaction may be product specific, ie, slow dissolving digoxin tablets interact whereas digoxin capsules and elixir are not affected. However, since USP standards require a minimum dissolution rate, tablets available in the US are not likely to be affected.

Phenothiazines: The antipsychotic effectiveness may be decreased by anticholinergic coadministration. Anticholinergic side effects may also be increased by concurrent therapy. Adjust the phenothiazine dose as necessary.

Tricyclic antidepressants: Coadministration with anticholinergics may result in increased anticholinergic side effects (eg, dry mouth, constipation, urinary retention) due to an additive effect. Using a tricyclic antidepressant with less anticholinergic activity may be beneficial.

Drug/Lab Test Interaction: The iodine in **isopropamide iodide** may alter **thyroid function tests** and will suppress I^{131} uptake. Substitute a thyroid function test unaffected by exogenous iodides.

Adverse Reactions:

GI: Xerostomia; altered taste perception; nausea; vomiting; dysphagia; heartburn; constipation; bloated feeling; paralytic ileus.

GU: Urinary hesitancy and retention; impotence.

Ocular: Blurred vision; mydriasis; photophobia; cycloplegia; increased intraocular pressure; dilated pupils.

Cardiovascular: Palpitations; bradycardia (following low doses of atropine); tachycardia (after higher doses).

CNS: Headache; flushing; nervousness; drowsiness; weakness; dizziness; confusion; insomnia; fever (especially in children); mental confusion or excitement especially in elderly patients with even small doses. Large doses may produce CNS stimulation (restlessness, tremor). In the presence of pain, **scopolamine** may produce excitement, restlessness, hallucinations or delirium. Parenteral **dicyclomine** may cause temporary lightheadedness.

Dermatologic/Hypersensitivity: Severe allergic reactions including anaphylaxis, urticaria and other dermal manifestations. Local irritation may occur with parenteral **dicyclomine**.

Other: Suppression of lactation; nasal congestion; decreased sweating.

Overdosage:

Symptoms:

GI – Dry mouth; thirst; vomiting; nausea; abdominal distention; difficulty swallowing.

CNS – Theoretically, a curare-like action may occur (ie, neuromuscular blockade leading to muscular weakness and paralysis); CNS stimulation; delirium; drowsiness; restlessness; anxiety; stupor; fever; disorientation; dizziness; headache; seizures; hallucinations; ataxia; convulsions; coma; psychotic behavior; other signs of an acute organic psychosis.

Cardiovascular – Circulatory failure; rapid pulse and respiration; vasodilation; tachycardia with weak pulse; hypertension; hypotension; respiratory depression; palpitations.

GU – Urinary urgency with difficulty in micturition.

Ocular – Blurred vision; photophobia; dilated pupils.

Miscellaneous – Leukocytosis; flushed hot dry skin; rash; respiratory failure.

Children, especially those with mongolism, spastic paralysis or brain damage, are more sensitive than adults to toxic effects.

Treatment: Induce emesis or perform gastric lavage, then administer activated charcoal slurry, and supportive and symptomatic therapy, as indicated. See also General Management of Acute Overdosage on p. 2895

Physostigmine by slow IV injection of 0.2 to 4 mg has been used to reverse anticholinergic effects. Since physostigmine is rapidly metabolized, the patient may relapse into coma after 1 to 2 hours; repeat doses as necessary to a total of 6 mg (2 mg in children). However, profound bradycardia, asystole and seizures may occur (see Antidotes monograph). The role of physostigmine is not clear; avoid it if other therapeutic agents successfully reverse cardiac dysrhythmias.

Neostigmine methylsulfate 0.25 to 2.5 mg IV, repeated as needed, may be given.

Diazepam, short-acting barbiturates, IV sodium thiopental (2% solution) or chloral hydrate (100 to 200 ml of a 2% solution) by rectal infusion may control excitement. Hyoscyamine is dialyzable, but hemodialysis is ineffective for atropine poisoning. Treat hyperpyrexia with physical cooling measures.

In the event of progression of the curare-like effect to paralysis of the respiratory muscles, artificial respiration should be instituted and maintained until effective respiratory action returns.

(Continued on following page)

Complete prescribing information for these products begins on page 1582

Belladonna Alkaloids

Patient Information:

Usually taken 30 to 60 minutes before a meal.

May cause drowsiness, dizziness or blurred vision; patients should observe caution while driving or performing other tasks requiring alertness.

Notify physician if skin rash, flushing or eye pain occurs.

May cause dry mouth, difficulty in urination, constipation or increased sensitivity to light; notify physician if these effects persist or become severe.

L-HYOSCYAMINE SULFATE

Indications:

GI: To aid in the control of gastric secretion, visceral spasm, hypermotility in spastic colitis, spastic bladder, pylorospasm and associated abdominal cramps. May be used to relieve symptoms in functional intestinal disorders (eg, mild dysenteries and diverticulitis), infant colic, biliary and renal colic. As adjunctive therapy in peptic ulcer; irritable bowel syndrome (irritable colon, spastic colon, mucus colitis, acute enterocolitis and functional GI disorders); neurogenic bowel disturbances including the splenic flexure syndrome and neurogenic colon; to reduce pain and hypersecretion in pancreatitis.

Respiratory tract: As a "drying agent" in the relief of symptoms of acute rhinitis.

CNS: In parkinsonism to reduce rigidity and tremors and to control associated sialorrhea and hyperhidrosis. May be used for poisoning by anticholinesterase agents.

GU: Cystitis; renal colic.

Cardiovascular: Use in certain cases of partial heart block associated with vagal activity.

Parenteral: Reduces duodenal motility to facilitate the diagnostic radiologic procedure, hypotonic duodenography. May also improve radiologic visibility of the kidneys.

Preoperative medication: Parenteral hyoscyamine is indicated as a pre-operative antimuscarinic to reduce salivary, tracheobronchial, and pharyngeal secretions; to reduce the volume and acidity of gastric secretions, and to block cardiac vagal inhibitory reflexes during induction of anesthesia and intubation. Hyoscyamine protects against the peripheral muscarinic effects such as bradycardia and excessive secretions produced by halogenated hydrocarbons and cholinergic agents such as physostigmine, neostigmine, and pyridostigmine given to reverse the actions of curariform agents.

Administration and Dosage:

Oral: Adults – 0.125 to 0.25 mg, 3 or 4 times/day orally or sublingually; or 0.375 to 0.75 mg in sustained release form every 12 hours.

Children – Individualize dosage according to weight.

Parenteral: 0.25 to 0.5 mg SC, IM or IV, 2 to 4 times daily, as needed.

	Product	Form	Description	C.I.*
Rx	**Anaspaz** (Ascher)	**Tablets:** 0.125 mg	(225/295). In 100s, 500s.	226
Rx	**Gastrosed** (Hauck)		In 100s.	NA
Rx	**Levsin** (Schwarz Pharma Kremers Urban)		(K-U 531). White, scored. In 100s and 500s.	320
Rx	**Neoquess** (Forest)		In 1000s.	42
Rx	**Cystospaz** (Webcon)	**Tablets:** 0.15 mg	(W 2225). Blue. In 100s.	415
Rx	**Levsin/SL** (Schwarz Pharma Kremers Urban)	**Tablets, sublingual:** 0.125 mg	(Schwarz 532). Blue-green, scored. Octagonal. Peppermint flavor. In 100s & 500s.	NA
Rx	**Cystospaz-M** (Webcon)	**Capsules, timed release:** 0.375 mg	(W 2260). Blue. In 100s.	250
Rx	**Levsinex Timecaps** (Schwarz Pharma Kremers Urban)		(Kremers Urban 537). Brown/clear. In 100s & 500s.	254
Rx	**Gastrosed** (Hauck)	**Solution:** 0.125 mg/ml	Alcohol free. In 5 ml bottle.	NA
Rx	**Levsin Drops** (Schwarz Pharma Kremers Urban)		5% alcohol. Sorbitol. Orange flavor. In 15 ml w/dropper.	1131
Rx	**Levsin** (Schwarz Pharma Kremers Urban)	**Elixir:** 0.125 mg/5 ml	20% alcohol. Sorbitol. Orange flavor. In pt.	450
Rx	**Gastrosed** (Hauck)	**Drops:** 0.125 mg/ml hyoscyamine sulfate	Alcohol free. In 5 ml dropper bottle.	NA
Rx	**Levsin** (Schwarz Pharma Kremers Urban)	**Injection:** 0.5 mg/ml	In 1 ml amps and 10 ml[1] vials.	933

* Cost Index based on cost per 0.125 mg.

[1] With 1.5% benzyl alcohol and 0.1% sodium metabisulfite.

Complete prescribing information for these products begins on page 1582

ATROPINE SULFATE

For information on atropine sulfate inhalation and ophthalmic preparations, refer to individual monographs.

Indications:

Antisialogogue for preanesthetic medication to prevent or reduce secretions of the respiratory tract.

Treatment of parkinsonism. Rigidity and tremor are relieved by the apparently selective depressant action.

Restore cardiac rate and arterial pressure during anesthesia when vagal stimulation produced by intra-abdominal surgical traction causes a sudden decrease in pulse rate and cardiac action.

Lessen the degree of atrioventricular heart block when increased vagal tone is a major factor in the conduction defect as in some cases due to digitalis.

Overcome severe bradycardia and syncope due to a hyperactive carotid sinus reflex.

Antidote (with external cardiac massage) for cardiovascular collapse from the injudicious use of a choline ester (cholinergic) drug, pilocarpine, physostigmine or isofluorophate.

Relieve pylorospasm, hypertonicity of the small intestine and hypermotility of the colon.

Relax the spasm of biliary and ureteral colic and bronchial spasm.

Relaxation of the upper GI tract and colon during hypertonic radiography.

Diminish the tone of the detrusor muscle of the urinary bladder in the treatment of urinary tract disorders.

Control the crying and laughing episodes in patients with brain lesions.

In cases of closed head injuries which cause acetylcholine to be released or to be present in cerebrospinal fluid, which in turn causes abnormal EEG patterns, stupor and neurological signs.

Relieve hypertonicity of the uterine muscle.

Management of peptic ulcer.

Control rhinorrhea of acute rhinitis or hay fever.

Poisoning: Treatment of anticholinesterase poisoning from organophosphorus insecticides; as an antidote for mushroom poisoning due to muscarine, in certain species such as *Amanita muscaria*.

Administration and Dosage:

Adults: 0.4 to 0.6 mg.

Children:

Atropine Dosage Recommendations in Children

Weight		Dose
lb	kg	mg
7 to 16	3.2 to 7.3	0.1
16 to 24	7.3 to 10.9	0.15
24 to 40	10.9 to 18.1	0.2
40 to 65	18.1 to 29.5	0.3
65 to 90	29.5 to 40.8	0.4
> 90	40.8	0.4 to 0.6

Hypotonic radiography: 1 mg IM.

Surgery: Give SC, IM or IV. The average adult dose is 0.5 mg (range 0.4 to 0.6 mg). As an antisialogogue, it is usually injected IM prior to induction of anesthesia. In children, it has been suggested to use a dose of 0.01 mg/kg to a maximum of 0.4 mg, repeated every 4 to 6 hours as needed. A recommended infant dose is 0.04 mg/kg (infants < 5 kg) or 0.03 mg/kg (infants > 5 kg), repeated every 4 to 6 hours as needed. During surgery, the drug is given IV when reduction in pulse rate and cessation of cardiac action are due to increased vagal activity. However, if the anesthetic is cyclopropane, use doses less than 0.4 mg and give slowly to avoid production of ventricular arrhythmia. Usual doses reduce severe bradycardia and syncope associated with hyperactive carotid sinus reflex.

(Administration and Dosage continued on following page)

Complete prescribing information for these products begins on page 1582

Belladonna Alkaloids (Cont.)

ATROPINE SULFATE (Cont.)

Administration and Dosage (Cont.)

Bradyarrhythmias: The usual IV adult dosage ranges from 0.4 to 1 mg every 1 to 2 hours as needed; larger doses, up to a maximum of 2 mg, may be required. In children, IV dosage ranges from 0.01 to 0.03 mg/kg. Atropine is also a specific antidote for cardiovascular collapse resulting from injudicious administration of choline ester. When cardiac arrest has occurred, external cardiac massage or other method of resuscitation is required to distribute the drug after IV injection.

Poisoning: In anticholinesterase poisoning from exposure to insecticides, give large doses of at least 2 to 3 mg parenterally and repeat until signs of atropine intoxication appear. In the "rapid" type of mushroom poisoning, give in doses sufficient to control parasympathomimetic signs before coma and cardiovascular collapse supervene.

	Product	Form/Strength	Supplied	C.I.*
Rx	**Atropine Sulfate** (Abbott)	**Injection:** 0.05 mg/ml	In 5 ml Abboject syringes.	22144
Rx	**Atropine Sulfate** (Abbott)	**Injection:** 0.1 mg/ml	In 5 and 10 ml Abboject syringes.	7160
Rx	**Atropine Sulfate** (Various, eg, American Regent, Burroughs Wellcome, Elkins-Sinn, Lilly, Loch, LyphoMed, Moore, Rugby, Schein, Vortech)	**Injection:** 0.3 mg/ml	In 1 and 30 ml vials.	827+
		0.4 mg/ml	In 1 ml amps and 1, 20 and 30 ml vials.	780+
		0.5 mg/ml	In 1 and 30 ml vials and 5 ml syringes.	170+
		0.8 mg/ml	In 0.5 and 1 ml amps and 0.5 ml syringes.	283+
		1 mg/ml	In 1 ml amps & vials and 10 ml syringes.	219+
Rx	**Atropine Sulfate** (Lilly)	**Tablets:** 0.4 mg	In 100s.	67
		Tablets, soluble: 0.4 mg	In 100s.	57
		0.6 mg	In 100s.	39

SCOPOLAMINE HBr (Hyoscine HBr)

Indications:

Preanesthetic sedation and obstetric amnesia in conjunction with analgesics; also used for calming delirium.

Motion sickness (see Antiemetic/Antivertigo Agents monograph).

Administration and Dosage:

Give SC or IM; may give IV after dilution with Sterile Water for Injection.

Adults: 0.32 to 0.65 mg.

Children: 0.006 mg/kg (0.003 mg/lb). Maximum dosage, 0.3 mg.

	Product	Form/Strength	Supplied	C.I.*
Rx	**Scopolamine HBr** (Various, eg, Loch, LyphoMed)	**Injection:** 0.3 mg/ml	In 1 ml vials.	1440+
Rx	**Scopolamine HBr** (Various, eg, Burroughs Wellcome, LyphoMed)	**Injection:** 0.4 mg/ml	In 0.5 ml amps and 1 ml vials.	561+
Rx	**Scopolamine HBr** (Burroughs Wellcome)	**Injection:** 0.86 mg/ml	In 0.5 ml amps.[1]	2102
Rx	**Scopolamine HBr** (Various, eg, Loch, LyphoMed)	**Injection:** 1 mg/ml	In 1 ml vials.	208+

LEVOROTATORY ALKALOIDS OF BELLADONNA

Indications:

GI: Spasm; peptic ulcer; pylorospasm; spastic colitis; intestinal and biliary colic.

GU: Dysmenorrhea; renal colic; enuresis; nocturia.

Respiratory tract: Hypersecretion; bronchial asthma.

CNS: Vagal inhibition; parkinsonism (postencephalitic); motion sickness.

Administration and Dosage:

Oral: Adults – 0.25 to 0.5 mg, 3 times daily.

Children (over 6 years) – 0.125 to 0.25 mg, 3 times daily.

	Product	Form/Strength	Supplied	C.I.*
Rx	**Bellafoline** (Sandoz)	**Tablets:** 0.25 mg	(#Sandoz 78/30). White, scored. In 100s.	556

* Cost Index based on cost per 0.4 mg atropine sulfate or scopolamine HBr or 0.25 mg levorotatory alkaloids.

\# Product identification code.

[1] With alcohol and mannitol.

Complete prescribing information for these products begins on page 1582

Belladonna Alkaloids (Cont.)

BELLADONNA

Belladonna, a crude botanical preparation, contains the anticholinergic alkaloids hyoscyamine (which racemizes to atropine on extraction), scopolamine (hyoscine) and other minor alkaloids. Belladonna leaf contains approximately 0.35% alkaloids. Pharmaceutical preparations of belladonna include *belladonna tincture,* which contains 27 to 33 mg alkaloids/100 ml.

Indications:

GI: As adjunctive therapy in the treatment of peptic ulcer, functional digestive disorders (including spastic, mucous and ulcerative colitis), diarrhea, diverticulitis, pancreatitis.

GU: Dysmenorrhea, nocturnal enuresis.

CNS: Parkinsonism (idiopathic and postencephalitic). Large doses may provide some symptomatic relief; tremor, rigidity, sialorrhea and oculogyric crises are reduced; posture, gait and speech are improved.

Other: Motion sickness; nausea and vomiting of pregnancy.

Administration and Dosage:

Belladonna Tincture: Adults - 0.6 to 1 ml, 3 to 4 times daily.
Children - 0.03 ml/kg (0.8 ml/m²) 3 times daily.

				C.I.*
Rx	**Belladonna Tincture** (Various, eg, Lannett, Life, Lilly, Rugby, Texas Drug)	**Liquid:** 27 to 33 mg belladonna alkaloids/100 ml	65% to 70% alcohol. In 120 ml, pt and gal.	27+

Quaternary Anticholinergics

METHSCOPOLAMINE BROMIDE

Indications:

Adjunctive therapy in the treatment of peptic ulcer.

Administration and Dosage:

2.5 mg 30 minutes before meals and 2.5 to 5 mg at bedtime.

				C.I.*
Rx	**Pamine** (Upjohn)	**Tablets:** 2.5 mg	White. In 100s and 500s.	380

ANISOTROPINE METHYLBROMIDE

Indications:

Adjunctive therapy in the treatment of peptic ulcer.

Administration and Dosage:

50 mg 3 times daily.

				C.I.*
Rx	**Anisotropine Methylbromide** (Various, eg, Balan, Rugby)	**Tablets:** 50 mg	In 100s.	198+
Rx	**Valpin 50** (DuPont)		Beige, scored. In 100s.	436

CLIDINIUM BROMIDE

Indications:

Adjunctive therapy in the treatment of peptic ulcer.

Administration and Dosage:

Adults: 2.5 to 5 mg, 3 or 4 times daily before meals and at bedtime.
Geriatric or debilitated patients: 2.5 mg, 3 times daily before meals.

				C.I.*
Rx	**Quarzan** (Roche)	**Capsules:** 2.5 mg	(#Quarzan 2.5 Roche). Green and red. In 100s.	248
		5 mg	(#Quarzan 5.0 Roche). Green and gray. In 100s.	169

* Cost Index based on cost per ml tincture belladonna, 2.5 mg methscopolamine, 50 mg anisotropine or 2.5 mg clidinium.
# Product identification code.

Complete prescribing information for these products begins on page 1582

Quaternary Anticholinergics (Cont.)

GLYCOPYRROLATE

Indications:

Oral: Adjunctive therapy in the treatment of peptic ulcer.

Parenteral: Used preoperatively to reduce salivary, tracheobronchial and pharyngeal secretions; to reduce the volume and free acidity of gastric secretions; to block cardiac vagal inhibitory reflexes during induction of anesthesia and intubation. May be used intraoperatively to counteract drug-induced or vagal traction reflexes with the associated arrhythmias. Glycopyrrolate protects against the peripheral muscarinic effects (eg, bradycardia and excessive secretions) of cholinergic agents such as neostigmine and pyridostigmine given to reverse the neuromuscular blockade due to nondepolarizing muscle relaxants.

Administration and Dosage:

Not recommended for children under age 12 for the management of peptic ulcer.

Oral: 1 mg 3 times daily or 2 mg 2 to 3 times daily.

Maintenance – 1 mg 2 times daily.

Parenteral: Peptic ulcer – 0.1 to 0.2 mg IM or IV, 3 or 4 times daily.

Preanesthetic medication – 0.002 mg/lb (0.004 mg/kg) IM, 30 minutes to 1 hour prior to anesthesia. Children less than 2 years of age may require up to 0.004 mg/lb. Children under 12, give 0.002 to 0.004 mg/lb IM.

Intraoperative medication – Adults, 0.1 mg IV. Repeat as needed at 2 to 3 minute intervals. Children, give 0.002 mg/lb (0.004 mg/kg) IV, not to exceed 0.1 mg in a single dose; may be repeated at 2 to 3 minute intervals.

Reversal of neuromuscular blockade – Adults and children, 0.2 mg for each 1 mg neostigmine or 5 mg pyridostigmine. Administer IV simultaneously.

				C.I.*
Rx	**Robinul** (Robins)	**Tablets:** 1 mg	(AHR 7824). White, scored. In 100s and 500s.	184
Rx	**Robinul Forte** (Robins)	**Tablets:** 2 mg	(AHR 2/7840). White, scored. In 100s.	147
Rx	**Glycopyrrolate** (Various, eg, American Regent, LyphoMed, Quad, Schein, Texas Drug, VHA)	**Injection:** 0.2 mg per ml	In 1, 2, 5 and 20 ml vials.	4000+
Rx	**Robinul** (Robins)		In 1, 2, 5 and 20 ml vials.[1]	6400

HEXOCYCLIUM METHYLSULFATE

Indications:

Adjunctive therapy in the treatment of peptic ulcer.

Administration and Dosage:

Adults: 25 mg 4 times daily before meals and at bedtime.

Children: Not for use in children.

				C.I.*
Rx	**Tral Filmtabs** (Abbott)	**Tablets:** 25 mg	Tartrazine. Film coated. In 100s.	389

ISOPROPAMIDE IODIDE

Indications:

Adjunctive therapy in the treatment of peptic ulcer.

Administration and Dosage:

Adults: 5 mg every 12 hours; 10 mg twice daily or more may be required.

Children: Not for use in children less than 12 years old.

				C.I.*
Rx	**Darbid** (SKF)	**Tablets:** 5 mg	(SKF D62). Pink. In 50s.	410

* Cost Index based on cost per 1 mg glycopyrrolate, 25 mg hexocyclium or 5 mg isopropamide.

[1] With 0.9% benzyl alcohol.

Complete prescribing information for these products begins on page 1582

Quaternary Anticholinergics (Cont.)

MEPENZOLATE BROMIDE

Indications:

Adjunctive therapy in the treatment of peptic ulcer.

Administration and Dosage:

Adults: 25 to 50 mg 4 times daily with meals and at bedtime.

Children: Safety and efficacy have not been established.

	Product	Form	Description	C.I.*
Rx	**Cantil** (Merrell Dow)	**Tablets:** 25 mg	Tartrazine. (Merrell 37). Yellow. In 100s.	845

METHANTHELINE BROMIDE

Indications:

Adjunctive therapy in the treatment of peptic ulcer.

Treatment of an uninhibited hypertonic neurogenic bladder.

Administration and Dosage:

Adults: 50 to 100 mg every 6 hours.

Pediatric: Newborns – 12.5 mg 2 times daily, then 12.5 mg 3 times daily. *Infants* (1 to 12 months) –12.5 mg 4 times daily, increased to 25 mg 4 times daily. *Children* (over 1 year) – 12.5 to 50 mg 4 times daily.

	Product	Form	Description	C.I.*
Rx	**Banthine** (Schiapparelli Searle)	**Tablets:** 50 mg	(Searle 1501). Peach, scored. In 100s.	448

PROPANTHELINE BROMIDE

Indications:

As adjunctive therapy in the treatment of peptic ulcer.

Unlabeled Uses: Has been used for its antisecretory and antispasmodic effects.

Administration and Dosage:

Adults: 15 mg 30 minutes before meals and 30 mg at bedtime. For patients with mild manifestations, geriatric patients or those of small stature, take 7.5 mg, 3 times daily.

Children: Peptic ulcer – Safety and efficacy have not been established.

Antisecretory – 1.5 mg/kg/day divided 3 to 4 times daily.

Antispasmodic – 2 to 3 mg/kg/day divided every 4 to 6 hours and at bedtime.

	Product	Form	Description	C.I.*
Rx	**Pro-Banthine** (Schiapparelli Searle)	**Tablets:** 7.5 mg	(Searle 611). White. Sugar coated. In 100s.	1080
Rx	**Propantheline Bromide** (Various, eg, Balan, Bioline, Goldline, Harber, Major, Moore, Par, Richlyn, Roxane, Rugby)	**Tablets:** 15 mg	In 100s, 500s, 1000s and UD 100s.	34+
Rx	**Pro-Banthine** (Schiapparelli Searle)		(Searle 601). Peach. Sugar coated. In 100s, 500s and UD 100s.	823

TRIDIHEXETHYL CHLORIDE

Indications:

Adjunctive therapy in peptic ulcer treatment.

Administration and Dosage:

25 to 50 mg 3 or 4 times daily before meals and at bedtime. Bedtime dose: 50 mg.

	Product	Form	Description	C.I.*
Rx	**Pathilon** (Lederle)	**Tablets:** 25 mg	(LL/P4). Pink. Film coated. In 100s.	1152

* Cost Index based on cost per 25 mg mepenzolate, 50 mg methantheline, 10 mg oxyphenonium, 15 mg propantheline or 25 mg tridihexethyl.

Complete prescribing information for these products begins on page 1582

Antispasmodics

DICYCLOMINE HCl

Indications:

Treatment of functional bowel/irritable bowel syndrome (irritable colon, spastic colon, mucous colitis).

Administration and Dosage:

Oral: Adults – The only oral dose shown to be effective is 160 mg/day in 4 equally divided doses. However, because of side effects, begin with 80 mg/day (in 4 equally divided doses). Increase dose to 160 mg/day unless side effects limit dosage.

Parenteral: IM only. Not for IV use.

Adults – 80 mg/day in 4 divided doses.

	Product	Form	Description	C.I.*
Rx	**Dicyclomine HCl** (Various, eg, Bioline, Bolar, Geneva, Goldline, Lannett, Lederle, Major, Rugby, Schein, Vangard)	**Capsules:** 10 mg	In 30s, 100s, 120s, 1000s and UD 100s.	36+
Rx	**Bemote** (Everett)		In 100s.	180
Rx	**Bentyl** (Lakeside Pharm.)		(#Merrell 120/Bentyl or Bentyl 10). In 100s, 500s and UD 100s.	300
Rx	**Byclomine** (Major)		In 100s, 250s, 1000s & UD 100s.	81
Rx	**Di-Spaz** (Vortech)		In 1000s.	57
Rx	**Dicyclomine HCl** (Various, eg, Bioline, Bolar, Geneva, Goldline, Lannett, Lederle, Major, Rugby, Schein, Vangard)	**Tablets:** 20 mg	In 15s, 20s, 30s, 100s, 120s, 250s, 1000s and UD 100s.	19+
Rx	**Bemote** (Everett)		In 100s.	100
Rx	**Bentyl** (Lakeside Pharm.)		(#Merrell 123 or Bentyl 20). In 100s, 500s, 1000s and UD 100s.	214
Rx	**Byclomine** (Major)		In 100s, 250s, 1000s & UD 100s.	25
Rx	**Dicyclomine HCl** (Various, eg, Moore, Richie)	**Capsules:** 20 mg	In 100s and 1000s.	17+
Rx	**Dicyclomine HCl** (Various, eg, Balan, Bioline, Dixon-Shane, Gen-King, Goldline, Harber, Moore, Qualitest, Rugby, Schein)	**Syrup:** 10 mg/5 ml	In 118 ml, pt and gal.	73+
Rx	**Bentyl** (Lakeside Pharm.)		Saccharin. In pt.	349
Rx	**Dicyclomine HCl** (Various, eg, Baxter, Bioline, Goldline, Major, Moore, Richie, Rugby, Schein, Steris, Veratex)	**Injection:** 10 mg/ml	In 2 and 10 ml vials.	728+
Rx	**Antispas** (Keene)		In 10 ml vials.[1]	1372
Rx	**Bentyl** (Lakeside Pharm.)		In 2 ml amps and 10 ml vials[1].	4942
Rx	**Dibent** (Hauck)		In 10 ml vials.[1]	4888
Rx	**Dilomine** (Kay Drug)		In 10 ml vials.[1]	850
Rx	**Di-Spaz** (Vortech)		In 10 ml vials.[1]	790
Rx	**Neoquess** (Forest)		In 10 ml vials.[1]	1750
Rx	**Or-Tyl** (Ortega)		In 10 ml vials.[1]	800
Rx	**Spasmoject** (Mayrand)		In 10 ml vials.[1]	1800

OXYPHENCYCLIMINE HCl

Indications:

Adjunctive therapy in the treatment of peptic ulcer.

Administration and Dosage:

Adults: 5 to 10 mg, 2 or 3 times daily, preferably in the morning and at bedtime. Some respond to 5 mg, 2 times daily, while some may require a higher dosage 3 times daily.

Children: Not for use in children less than 12 years of age.

	Product	Form	Description	C.I.*
Rx	**Daricon** (Beecham Labs)	**Tablets:** 10 mg	White, scored. In 60s and 500s.	597

* Cost Index based on cost per 10 mg dicyclomine or 10 mg oxyphencyclimine.

\# Product identification code.

[1] With chlorobutanol.

GASTROINTESTINAL ANTICHOLINERGIC COMBINATIONS

Refer to the general discussion of these products on page 1582

Combination anticholinergic preparations may include the following components:
SEDATIVES and ANTIANXIETY AGENTS. See: Barbiturates, Prochlorperazine, Hydroxyzine, Meprobamate, Chlordiazepoxide.
ERGOTAMINE TARTRATE provides inhibition of the sympathetic nervous system.
ANTIHISTAMINES may be included for antihistaminic effects, sedative or anticholinergic side effects.
KAOLIN is used for its adsorbent properties.

Capsules and Tablets

Content given per tablet.

		Anticholinergic (mg)						
	Product and Distributor	Atropine Sulfate	Scopolamine HBr	Hyoscyamine HBr or SO_4	Sedative	Daily Dose (Tablets)	How Supplied	C.I.*
Rx	**Barbidonna No. 2 Tablets** (Wallace)	0.025	0.0074	0.1286	32 mg phenobarbital	3	(#Wallace 311). Brown, scored. In 100s.	456
Rx	**Barbidonna Tablets** (Wallace)	0.025	0.0074	0.1286	16 mg phenobarbital	3 to 6	(#Wallace 301). White, scored. In 100s and 500s.	406
Rx	**Kinesed Tablets** (Stuart)	0.12	0.007	0.12	16 mg phenobarbital	3 to 8	Chewable. Saccharin. (#Stuart 220). Scored. Fruit flavor. In 100s.	240
Rx	**Donphen Tablets** (Lemmon)	0.02	0.006	0.1	15 mg phenobarbital	3 to 8	Saccharin. (#Lemmon 93/205). Pink, scored. In 100s and 1000s.	79
Rx	**Donnatal No. 2 Tablets** (Robins)	0.0194	0.0065	0.1037	32.4 mg phenobarbital	3 to 6	(#R). Green, scored. In 100s and 1000s.	148
Rx	**Spasmophen Tablets** (Lannett)	0.0194	0.0065	0.1037	15 mg phenobarbital	3 to 8	In 1000s.	14

* Cost Index based on cost per tablet.
# Product identification code.

(Continued on following page)

GASTROINTESTINAL ANTICHOLINERGIC COMBINATIONS (Cont.)

Refer to the general discussion of these products on page 1593.

Capsules and Tablets (Cont.)

Content given per capsule or tablet.

	Product and Distributor	Anticholinergic (mg) Atropine Sulfate	Scopolamine HBr	Hyoscyamine HBr or SO_4	Sedative	Daily Dose (Caps or Tabs)	How Supplied	C.I.*
Rx	**Belladonna Alkaloids w/Phenobarbital Tablets** (Various, eg, Harber, Purepac, Qualitest, Redi-Med, Regal, Rondex, Rugby, Scripts)	0.0194	0.0065	0.1037	16.2 mg phenobarbital	3 to 8	In 20s, 30s, 50s, 100s and 1000s.	43+
Rx	**Donnapine Tablets** (Major)						In 100s, 1000s and UD 100s.	38
Rx	**Donnatal Capsules and Tablets** (Robins)						**Capsules:** (#AHR 4207). Green and white. In 100s and 1000s.	145
							Tablets: (#R 4250). White, scored. In 100s, 1000s and Dis-Co Pack 100s.	121
Rx	**Hyosophen Tablets** (Rugby)						In 1000s.	14
Rx	**Malatal Tablets** (Hauck)						In 1000s.	24
Rx	**Relaxadon Tablets** (Geneva Generics)						White. In 1000s.	15
Rx	**Spaslin Tablets** (Blaine)						White, scored. In 100s and 1000s.	50
Rx	**Spasmolin Capsules and Tablets** (Various, eg, Richlyn, Spencer-Mead, Texas Drug)						**Capsules:** In 100s and 1000s.	34+
							Tablets: In 100s and 1000s.	14+
Rx	**Susano Tablets** (Halsey)						In 1000s.	14

* Cost Index based on cost per capsule or tablet.
# Product identification code.

(Continued on following page)

GASTROINTESTINAL ANTICHOLINERGIC COMBINATIONS (Cont.)

Refer to the general discussion of these products on page 1593.

Liquids (Cont.)

Content given per 5 ml liquid or 1 ml drops.

	Product and Distributor	Anticholinergic	Sedative	Other Content	Daily Dose	How Supplied	C.I.*
Rx	**Butibel Elixir** (Wallace)	15 mg belladonna extract	15 mg butabarbital sodium	7% alcohol	20 to 40 ml	Tartrazine, saccharin. In pt.	570
Rx *sf*	**Antrocol Elixir** (Poythress)	0.195 mg atropine sulfate	16 mg phenobarbital	20% alcohol	Children: 0.5 ml per 15 lbs every 4 to 6 hours	Citrus flavor. In 30 ml and pt.	436
Rx	**Levsin w/Phenobarbital Elixir** (Schwarz Pharma Kremers Urban)	0.125 mg hyoscyamine sulfate	15 mg phenobarbital	20% alcohol	15 to 40 ml	Raspberry flavor. In pt.	571
Rx	**Levsin-PB Drops** (Schwarz Pharma Kremers Urban)	0.125 mg hyoscyamine sulfate per ml	15 mg phenobarbital per ml	5% alcohol	1 to 2 ml. Children: 0.5 to 1 ml	Cherry flavor. In 15 ml.	1473

* Cost Index based on cost per 5 ml liquid or 1 ml drops.
sf – Sugar free.

Actions:

Pharmacology: Histamine H_2 antagonists are reversible competitive blockers of histamine at the H_2 receptors, particularly those in the gastric parietal cells. The H_2 antagonists are highly selective, do not affect the H_1 receptors, and are not anticholinergic agents. Potent inhibitors of all phases of gastric acid secretion, they inhibit secretions caused by histamine, muscarinic agonists and gastrin. They also inhibit fasting and nocturnal secretions, and secretions stimulated by food, insulin, caffeine, pentagastrin and betazole. In addition, the volume and the hydrogen ion concentration of gastric juice are reduced. Cimetidine, ranitidine and famotidine have no effect on gastric emptying, and cimetidine and famotidine have no effect on lower esophageal sphincter pressure. Ranitidine, nizatidine and famotidine have little or no effect on fasting or postprandial serum gastrin. Ranitidine is 5 to 12 times more potent and famotidine is 30 to 60 times more potent than cimetidine on a molar basis in controlling gastric acid hypersecretion, although there is no indication the greater potency offers any advantage.

The histamine H_2 antagonists are effective in alleviating symptoms and in preventing complications of peptic ulcer disease. The drugs have similar adverse reaction profiles. Cimetidine appears to have the greatest degree of antiandrogenic (eg, gynecomastia, impotence) and CNS (eg, mental confusion). Cimetidine inhibits the cytochrome P-450 oxidase system that affects other drugs (eg, warfarin, theophylline). Ranitidine also affects the microsomal enzyme system, but its influence on elimination of other drugs is not significant. Famotidine and nizatidine do not affect the cytochrome P-450 enzyme system.

Treatment failures have been documented with all of the H_2 antagonists. Since all of the drugs act to inhibit gastric acid secretion, it is doubtful ulcers "resistant" to one drug will heal with another.

Ranitidine: Basal, nocturnal and betazole-stimulated secretion are most sensitive to inhibition by ranitidine, responding almost completely to doses of 100 mg or less. Ranitidine does not affect pepsin secretion or pentagastrin-stimulated intrinsic factor secretion. Other pharmacological actions include an increase in gastric nitrate-reducing organisms; small, transient dose-related increases in serum prolactin after IV bolus injections of 100 mg or more and possible impairment of vasopressin release. No effect on prolactin levels has been noted with recommended oral or IV doses.

Famotidine: Both the acid concentration and volume of gastric secretion are suppressed while changes in pepsin secretion are proportional to volume output. Exocrine pancreatic function is not affected. After oral use, the onset of antisecretory effect occurred within 1 hour; the maximum effect was dose-dependent, occurring within 1 to 3 hours. Duration of secretion inhibition by doses of 20 and 40 mg was 10 and 12 hours, respectively.

After IV administration, the maximum effect was achieved within 30 minutes. Single IV doses of 10 and 20 mg inhibited nocturnal secretion for 10 and 12 hours, respectively.

There is no cumulative effect with repeated doses. The nocturnal intragastric pH was raised by evening doses of 20 and 40 mg to mean values of 5 and 6.4, respectively. When famotidine was given after breakfast, the basal daytime interdigestive pH at 3 and 8 hours after 20 or 40 mg was raised to about 5.

Nizatidine's effect on gastric acid secretion is presented in the following table:

Effect of Oral Nizatidine on Gastric Acid Secretion

Method	Time After Dose (hrs)	% Inhibition of Gastric Acid Output by Dose (mg)				
		20-50	75	100	150	300
Basal	Up to 8	45-57	–	72	–	–
Nocturnal	Up to 10	57	–	73	–	90
Betazole	Up to 3	–	93	–	100	99
Pentagastrin	Up to 6	–	25	–	64	67
Meal	Up to 4	41	64	–	98	97
Caffeine	Up to 3	–	73	–	85	96

Total pepsin output was reduced in proportion to the reduced volume of gastric secretions. Oral administration of 75 to 300 mg nizatidine increased betazole-stimulated secretion of intrinsic factor. There was no effect on hormone levels, including androgens.

(Actions continued on following page)

Actions (Cont.):

Clinical Pharmacology:

Cimetidine – Antisecretory activity: Nocturnal – Cimetidine 800 mg at bedtime reduces mean hourly hydrogen ion (H +) activity by greater than 85% over an 8 hour period in duodenal ulcer patients, with no effect on daytime acid secretion. The 1600 mg bedtime dose produces 100% inhibition of mean hourly H + activity over an 8 hour period in ulcer patients, but also reduces H + activity by 35% for an additional 5 hours into the following morning. Both the 400 mg twice daily and 300 mg 4 times daily doses decrease nocturnal acid secretion in a dose-related manner, 47% to 83% over a 6 to 8 hour period and 54% over a 9 hour period, respectively.

During the first hour after a standard meal, 300 mg inhibited gastric acid secretion in ulcer patients by at least 50% and during the subsequent 2 hours by at least 75%. The effect of a 300 mg breakfast dose continued for at least 4 hours, with partial suppression of the rise in gastric acid secretion following lunch in duodenal ulcer patients.

Total pepsin output is also reduced as a result of the decrease in volume of gastric juice. Cimetidine 300 mg inhibited the rise in intrinsic factor concentration produced by betazole, but some intrinsic factor was secreted at all times.

Ranitidine – Duodenal ulcer: Ranitidine 200 to 300 mg/day has been compared to placebo in numerous studies of 4 weeks duration with healing rates (verified endoscopically) of 60% to 100% and 16% to 52%, respectively.

Maintenance therapy in duodenal ulcer: In two multicenter, double-blind controlled studies, the number of duodenal ulcers observed was significantly less in patients treated with ranitidine than in patients treated with placebo over a 12 month period. Prevalence was 20% for ranitidine and 44% for placebo after 4 months and 35% for ranitidine and 59% for placebo after 12 months.

Gastric ulcer: In a multicenter, double-blind controlled study, 19% of ranitidine patients and 12% of placebo patients showed healing by week 2 of therapy. Healing rates by week 6 were 68% vs 51% for ranitidine and placebo, respectively.

Pathological hypersecretory conditions (eg, Zollinger-Ellison syndrome, systemic mastocytosis): Ulcer healing occurred in 8 of 19 (42%) patients who used ranitidine and were intractable to previous therapy.

Gastroesophageal reflux disease (GERD): In two multicenter, double-blind, placebo controlled 6 week trials, ranitidine was more effective than placebo for relief of symptoms associated with GERD. Ranitidine-treated patients consumed significantly less antacid than did placebo-treated patients. In one trial, ranitidine significantly reduced the frequency of heartburn attacks and severity of heartburn pain within 1 to 2 weeks after starting therapy. Improvement was maintained throughout the 6 week trial, extending through both the day and night.

Famotidine – Gastric ulcer: In an international multicenter trial, famotidine at a dose of 40 mg at bedtime was more effective than placebo in healing gastric ulcers. At 4, 6 and 8 weeks, healing rates versus placebo were 47% vs 31%, 65% vs 46% and 80% vs 54%, respectively.

Nizatidine – Duodenal ulcer: In several studies, nizatidine 50 to 300 mg/day was more effective than placebo in healing duodenal ulcers. At 4 and 8 weeks, healing rates versus placebo were 50% to 76% vs 28.5% to 39% and 77% to 82% vs 49% to 50%, respectively.

Comparative Studies:

DUODENAL ULCER HEALING RATES – COMPARISONS*				
Drug	Dose (mg/day)	Healing Rate 4 week	Healing Rate 8 week	Side Effect Incidence
Cimetidine	1000	60% to 84%	82% to 95%	4% to 5%
Famotidine	40	67% to 77%		
Nizatidine	300	73% to 81%		
Ranitidine	300	63% to 77%		

*Combined results. Studies did not compare all drugs simultaneously

In the treatment of gastric ulcers, healing rates after 6 weeks of therapy with ranitidine 150 mg twice daily or cimetidine 300 mg 4 times daily were 65% to 70%; after 8 weeks of treatment, the rates increased to 75% to 85%.

Studies evaluating an evening meal or bedtime dose of ranitidine 150 mg or cimetidine 400 mg for maintenance therapy for duodenal ulcers indicated that the relapse rate was lower in patients receiving ranitidine. However, these doses are not equipotent in reducing gastric acid secretion. A one year multicenter study indicated nizatidine 150 mg at night is similar in efficacy to ranitidine in preventing ulcer recurrence.

(Actions continued on following page)

Actions (Cont.):

Pharmacokinetics:

Pharmacokinetic Properties of Histamine H_2 Antagonists									
H_2 Receptor Antagonist	Bioavailability (%)	Time to Peak Plasma Concentration (hrs)	Peak Plasma Concentration[1] (mcg/ml)	Half-life (hrs)	Protein Binding (%)	Volume of Distribution (L/kg)	Elimination (%) Urine, Unchanged Oral	Elimination (%) Urine, Unchanged IV	Elimination (%) Metabolized
Cimetidine	60-70	0.75-1.5	0.7-3.2 (300 mg dose) (3.5-7.5 IV)	≈ 2[2]	13-25	0.8-1.2	48	75	30-40
Ranitidine	50-60 (90-100 IM)	1-3 (0.25 IM)	0.44-0.55 (0.58 IM)	2-3[3]	15	1.2-1.9	30-35	68-79	< 10
Famotidine	40-45	1-3	0.076-0.1 (40 mg dose)	2.5-3.5[3]	15-20	1.1-1.4	25-30	65-70	30-35
Nizatidine	> 90	0.5-3	0.7-1.8/ 1.4-3.6 (150/300 mg dose)	1-2[3]	≈ 35	0.8-1.5	60	na	< 18

[1] Dose dependent na = not applicable
[2] Increased in renal and hepatic impairment and in the elderly
[3] Increased in renal impairment

Additional pharmacokinetic information for these agents is discussed individually.

Cimetidine: Absorption may be decreased by antacids, but is unaffected by food. Both oral and parenteral administration provide comparable serum levels. Plasma concentrations of 0.5 to 1 mcg/ml are required to suppress basal or gastric acid secretion; however, plasma concentrations of cimetidine have not correlated with duodenal ulcer healing. Blood concentrations remain above those required to provide 80% inhibition of basal gastric acid secretion for 4 to 5 hours following a 300 mg dose. Cimetidine is widely distributed. Following oral administration, about 30% to 40% is metabolized in the liver, the sulfoxide being the major metabolite. Cimetidine is not significantly removed by hemodialysis or peritoneal dialysis.

Ranitidine: Absorption of oral ranitidine is not significantly impaired by the administration of food. Coadministration of antacids may reduce its absorption. Hepatic metabolism results in three metabolites. Maintenance of serum concentration necessary to inhibit 50% of stimulated gastric acid secretion (36 to 94 ng/ml) is 12 hours orally and 6 to 8 hours IV. Blood levels, however, bear no consistent relationship to dose or degree of acid inhibition.

Famotidine: Plasma levels after multiple doses of famotidine are similar to those after single doses. Famotidine is eliminated by renal (65% to 70%) and metabolic (30% to 35%) routes. The only metabolite identified is the S-oxide.

Nizatidine: A concentration of 1000 mcg/L is equivalent to 3 μmol/L; a dose of 300 mg is equivalent to 905 μmoles. Plasma concentrations 12 hours after administration are less than 10 mcg/L. Plasma clearance is 40 to 60 L/hour. Because of the short half-life and rapid clearance, drug accumulation would not be expected in individuals with normal renal function who take either 300 mg at bedtime or 150 mg twice daily. Nizatidine exhibits dose proportionality over the recommended dose range.

Antacids consisting of aluminum and magnesium hydroxides with simethicone decrease nizatidine absorption by about 10%. With food, AUC and maximum concentration increase by ≈ 10%.

In humans, less than 7% of an oral dose is metabolized as N2-monodesmethylnizatidine, an H_2-receptor antagonist. Other likely metabolites are the N2-oxide (less than 5% of the dose) and the S-oxide (less than 6% of the dose). More than 90% of an oral dose of nizatidine is excreted in the urine within 12 hours. Renal clearance is about 500 ml/min, which indicates excretion by active tubular secretion. Less than 6% of an administered dose is eliminated in the feces.

(Continued on following page)

Adverse Reactions (Cont.):

Famotidine (causal relationship not established): Anorexia; dry mouth; musculoskeletal pain; paresthesias; grand mal seizure (one report); acne; dry skin; flushing; tinnitus; taste disorder; fever; asthenia; palpitations; orbital edema; conjunctival injection.

Nizatidine: Sweating (1%); asymptomatic ventricular tachycardia; hyperuricemia unassociated with gout or nephrolithiasis; eosinophilia; fever.

Laboratory test abnormalities: Small increases in serum creatinine and elevated ALT levels (at least twice pretreatment levels) occurred with **ranitidine**. Small possibly dose-related increases in plasma creatinine and serum transaminase occurred with **cimetidine**; these are not common and do not signify deteriorating renal function. Elevated AST, ALT and alkaline phosphatase levels occur with **nizatidine** (see Precautions).

Overdosage:

Symptoms: There is no experience with deliberate overdosage. Toxic doses in animals are associated with rapid respiration or respiratory failure, tachycardia, muscular tremors, vomiting, restlessness, pallor of mucous membranes or redness of mouth and ears, hypotension, collapse and cholinergic-type effects including lacrimation, salivation, emesis, miosis and diarrhea.

Reported ingestions of up to 20 g **cimetidine** have been associated with transient adverse effects similar to those encountered in normal clinical experience. Two deaths have occurred in adults who were reported to ingest $>$ 40 g on a single occasion.

Famotidine doses of up to 640 mg/day have been given to patients with pathological hypersecretory conditions with no serious adverse effects.

Treatment: Symptomatic and supportive. Remove unabsorbed material from the GI tract, monitor the patient and employ supportive therapy. Refer to General Management of Acute Overdosage.

With **nizatidine**, renal dialysis for 4 to 6 hours increased plasma clearance by approximately 84%.

Physostigmine has been reported to arouse obtunded patients with evidence of **cimetidine**-induced CNS toxicity; data are insufficient to recommend this use.

Patient Information:

Inform physician or pharmacist of any concomitant drug therapy, especially when taking **cimetidine**.

Stagger doses of antacids and **cimetidine** or **rantidine**.

These agents may be taken without regard to meals.

(Products listed on following pages)

Refer to the general discussion of these agents on page 1600

CIMETIDINE

Cimetidine was approved by the FDA in 1977.

Indications:

Duodenal ulcer: Short-term treatment and maintenance therapy.

Benign gastric ulcer: Short-term treatment.

Gastroesophageal reflux disease (GERD), erosive.

Pathological hypersecretory conditions.

Prevention of upper GI bleeding in critically ill patients.

Administration and Dosage:

Duodenal ulcer: Short-term treatment of active duodenal ulcer – 800 mg at bedtime. Alternate regimens are 300 mg 4 times a day with meals and at bedtime, or 400 mg twice a day. Give antacids as needed for pain relief. While healing often occurs during the first few weeks, continue treatment for 4 to 6 weeks unless healing is demonstrated by endoscopy.

Maintenance therapy – 400 mg at bedtime.

Active benign gastric ulcer: For short-term treatment, 800 mg at bedtime or 300 mg 4 times a day with meals and at bedtime. The preferred regimen is 800 mg at bedtime based on convenience and lowered potential for drug interaction. There is no information concerning usefulness of treatment periods longer than 8 weeks.

Erosive gastroesophageal reflux disease (GERD): Adults – 1600 mg daily in divided doses (800 mg twice daily or 400 mg 4 times a day) for 12 weeks. Use beyond 12 weeks has not been established.

The doses and regimen for parenteral administration in patients with GERD have not been established.

Pathological hypersecretory conditions: 300 mg 4 times a day with meals and at bedtime. If necessary, give 300 mg doses more often. Individualize dosage. Do not exceed 2400 mg/day; continue as long as clinically indicated.

Prevention of upper GI bleeding: Continuous IV infusion of 50 mg/hour. Patients with creatinine clearance < 30 ml/min should receive half the recommended dose. Treatment beyond 7 days has not been studied.

Severely impaired renal function: Accumulation may occur. Use the lowest dose; 300 mg every 12 hours orally or IV has been recommended. According to the patient's condition, dosage frequency may be increased to every 8 hours or even further with caution. Whether hemodialysis reduces the level of circulating cimetidine is controversial. Give the dose at the end of hemodialysis. When liver impairment is also present, further dosage reductions may be necessary.

Parenteral: For hospitalized patients with pathological hypersecretory conditions or intractable ulcers, or patients unable to take oral medication. The usual dose is 300 mg IM or IV every 6 to 8 hours. If it is necessary to increase dosage, do so by more frequent administration of a 300 mg dose, not to exceed 2400 mg/day.

IM – Administer undiluted.

IV – Dilute in 0.9% Sodium Chloride Injection or other compatible IV solution to a total volume of 20 ml; inject over not less than 2 minutes.

Intermittent IV infusion – Dilute 300 mg in at least 50 ml of 5% Dextrose Injection or other compatible IV solution; infuse over 15 to 20 minutes.

Continuous IV infusion: 37.5 mg/hour (900 mg/day). For patients requiring a more rapid elevation of gastric pH, continuous infusion may be preceded by a 150 mg loading dose administered by IV infusion as described above. Dilute 900 mg cimetidine injection in a compatible IV fluid (see Stability) for a constant rate infusion over a 24 hour period.

Note: Cimetidine may be diluted in 100 to 1000 ml; however, a volumetric pump is recommended if the volume for 24 hour infusion is < 250 ml.

Plastic containers – Do not add drugs to the solution in these containers or introduce any additives.

Stability – Stable for 48 hours at room temperature when added to commonly used IV solutions (eg, 0.9% Sodium Chloride Injection, 5% or 10% Dextrose Injection, Lactated Ringer's Solution, 5% Sodium Bicarbonate Injection) or when added to a total parenteral nutrition admixture containing amino acids, dextrose, fat emulsion, electrolytes and vitamins.

Premixed, single-dose: Avoid exposure of the premixed product to excessive heat. The product should be stored at controlled room temperature (15° to 30°C; 59° to 86°F). Brief exposure up to 40°C does not adversely affect the premixed product.

(Administration and Dosage continued on following page)

Refer to the general discussion of these agents on page 1600

CIMETIDINE (Cont.)

Administration and Dosage (Cont.):

Parenteral (Cont.):

Incompatibility – Incompatible with aminophylline and barbiturates in IV solutions. Incompatible in the same syringe with pentobarbital sodium and a pentobarbital sodium/atropine sulfate combination. In one study, cimetidine and aminophylline were chemically stable and physically compatible for 48 hours at room temperature when admixed in 5% Dextrose in Water.

				C.I.*
Rx	**Tagamet** (SK-Beecham)	**Tablets:** 200 mg	(Tagamet 200 SKF). Light green. Film coated. In 100s.	1.7
		300 mg	(Tagamet 300 SKF). Light green. Film coated. In 100s and UD 100s.	1.2
		400 mg	(Tagamet 400 SKF). Light green. Capsule shaped. Film coated. In 60s and UD 100s.	1.5
		800 mg	(Tagamet 800 SKF). Light green. Oval. Film coated. In 30s and UD 100s.	1.5
		Liquid: 300 mg (as HCl) per 5 ml	2.8% alcohol. Saccharin, sorbitol. Mint-peach flavor. In 240 ml and UD 5 ml (10s).	2.8
		Injection: 300 mg (as HCl) per 2 ml[1] aqueous solution	In single-dose vials, disp. syringes and *ADD-Vantage* vials and 8 ml multiple-dose vials.	4.6
		300 mg (as HCl) in 50 ml 0.9% sodium chloride	In single-dose containers.	10

* Cost Index based on cost per 1200 mg cimetidine. [1] With phenol.

RANITIDINE

Indications:

Duodenal ulcer: Short-term treatment and maintenance therapy.

Benign gastric ulcer: Short-term treatment.

Pathological hypersecretory conditions.

Gastroesophageal reflux disease (GERD).

Erosive esophagitis.

Administration and Dosage:

Approved by the FDA in June 1983.

Duodenal ulcer: Short-term treatment of active duodenal ulcer – 150 mg orally twice daily. An alternate dosage of 300 mg once daily at bedtime can be used for patients in whom dosing convenience is important; 100 mg twice daily is as effective as the 150 mg dose. Smaller doses are equally effective in inhibiting gastric acid secretion.

Maintenance therapy – 150 mg at bedtime.

Pathological hypersecretory conditions: 150 mg orally twice a day. More frequent doses may be necessary. Individualize dosage and continue as long as indicated. Doses up to 6 g/day have been used.

Benign gastric ulcer (oral doseforms only) and GERD: 150 mg twice daily.

Erosive esophagitis: 150 mg 4 times daily.

Renal impairment (Ccr $<$ 50 ml/min): 150 mg orally every 24 hours or 50 mg parenterally every 18 to 24 hours. The frequency of dosing may be increased to every 12 hours or further with caution. Hemodialysis reduces the level of circulating ranitidine. Adjust dosage timing so that a scheduled dose coincides with the end of hemodialysis.

Parenteral: Do not exceed recommended rates of administration.

IM – 50 mg (2 ml) every 6 to 8 hours. (No dilution necessary.)

IV injection – 50 mg (2 ml) every 6 to 8 hours. Dilute 50 mg in 0.9% Sodium Chloride or other compatible IV solution to a total volume of 20 ml; inject over $\geq$ 5 min.

Intermittent IV infusion – 50 mg (2 ml) every 6 to 8 hours. Dilute 50 mg in 100 ml 5% Dextrose Injection or other compatible IV solution, or use 100 ml of 0.5 mg/ml premixed solution and infuse over 15 to 20 minutes; do not exceed 400 mg/day.

Premixed injection – Requires no dilution and should be infused over 15 to 20 minutes. Administer by slow IV drip infusion only. Do not introduce additives into the solution. If used with a primary IV fluid system, discontinue primary solution during premixed infusion. Do not use equipment containing aluminum that might contact the drug solution.

(Administration and Dosage continued on following page)

Refer to the general discussion of these agents on page 1600

RANITIDINE (Cont.)

Administration and Dosage (Cont.):

Parenteral (Cont.):

Continuous IV infusion: Add ranitidine injection to 5% Dextrose Injection or other compatible IV solution (see Stability). Deliver at a rate of 6.25 mg/hr (eg, 150 mg [6 ml] ranitidine injection in 250 ml of 5% Dextrose Injection at 10.7 ml/hr).

For Zollinger-Ellison patients, dilute ranitidine injection in 5% Dextrose Injection or other compatible IV solution (see Stability) to a concentration no greater than 2.5 mg/ml. Start the infusion at a rate of 1 mg/kg/hr. If after 4 hours either a measured gastric acid output is > 10 mEq/hr or the patient becomes symptomatic, adjust the dose upwards in 0.5 mg/kg/hr increments and remeasure the acid output. Doses up to 2.5 mg/kg/hr and infusion rates as high as 220 mg/hr have been used.

Storage/Stability – Stable for 48 hours at room temperature when added to or diluted with most commonly used IV solutions (eg, 0.9% Sodium Chloride Injection, 5% or 10% Dextrose Injection, Lactated Ringer's Solution, 5% Sodium Bicarbonate Injection).

Studies have shown ranitidine is stable in minibags with 5% Dextrose or 0.9% Sodium Chloride when frozen (–30°C; –22°F) for 30 days in concentrations of 0.5, 1 and 2 mg/ml and for 100 days at a concentration of 2 mg/ml or refrigerated (4°C; 39°F) for 10 days in a concentration of 1 mg/ml. Concentrations of 83 to 250 mcg/ml in standard TPN solutions decreased by < 10% when stored at room temperature for < 48 hours. TPN solutions with 4.25% and 2.125% crystalline amino acids and 50 and 100 mcg/ml concentrations of ranitidine were stable 24 hours at room temperature.

Syrup: Store between 4° and 25° C (39° and 77°F). Dispense in tight, light-resistant containers.

				C.I.*
Rx	**Zantac** (Glaxo and Roche)	**Tablets:** 150 mg (as HCl)	(Zantac 150 Glaxo). Peach. Film-coated. Five sided. In 60s, 100s and UD 100s.	1.1
		300 mg (as HCl)	(Zantac 300 Glaxo). Yellow. Film coated. Capsule shape. In 30s and UD 100s.	1
		Syrup: 15 mg (as HCl) per ml	7.5% alcohol, saccharin, sorbitol, parabens. Peppermint flavor. In pt.	NA
		Injection: 0.5 mg (as HCl) per ml	Preservative free. In 100 ml single-dose plastic containers.[1]	6.8
		25 mg (as HCl) per ml	In 2, 10 and 40 ml vials and 2 ml syringes.[2]	8.4

NIZATIDINE

Indications:

Duodenal ulcer: Short-term treatment and maintenance therapy.

Administration and Dosage:

Approved by the FDA in April 1988.

Active duodenal ulcer: 300 mg once daily at bedtime. An alternative dosage regimen is 150 mg twice daily.

Maintenance of healed duodenal ulcer: 150 mg once daily at bedtime.

Moderate to severe renal insufficiency:

Nizatidine Dosage in Renal Insufficiency		
	Dosage	
Creatinine clearance	Active duodenal ulcer	Maintenance therapy
20 to 50 ml/min	150 mg/day	150 mg every other day
< 20 ml/min	150 mg every other day	150 mg every 3 days

Extemporaneous liquid preparation: When a typical 150 or 300 mg dose was mixed in various commercial juices (eg, *Gatorade,* apple juice, *Ocean Spray*), nizatidine solutions were stable for at least 48 hours under refrigeration and at room temperature (except in *V8* and *Cran-Grape* juices, which had 10% loss of nizatidine potency at room temperature).

				C.I.*
Rx	**Axid Pulvules** (Lilly)	**Capsules:** 150 mg	Two-tone yellow. In 60s.	1.8
		300 mg	Yellow and peach. In 30s and UD 30s.	1.6

* Cost Index based on cost per 300 mg ranitidine tablet or 150 mg injection, or 300 mg nizatidine.

[1] Premixed in 0.45% sodium chloride.

[2] With phenol.

FAMOTIDINE

Famotidine was approved by the FDA in October 1986.

Indications:

Duodenal ulcer: Short-term treatment and maintenance therapy.

Benign gastric ulcer: Short-term treatment.

Pathological hypersecretory conditions.

Gastroesophageal reflux disease (GERD): Short-term treatment. Also for esophagitis due to GERD, including erosive or ulcerative disease (short-term treatment).

Administration and Dosage:

Duodenal ulcer: Acute therapy – 40 mg once a day at bedtime. Most patients heal in 4 weeks; there is rarely reason to use the drug at full dosage for > 6 to 8 weeks. A regimen of 20 mg twice a day is also effective.

Maintenance therapy – 20 mg once a day at bedtime.

Benign gastric ulcer: Acute therapy – 40 mg orally once a day at bedtime.

Pathological hypersecretory conditions: Individualize dosage. The adult starting dose is 20 mg every 6 hours; some patients may require a higher starting dose. Continue as long as clinically indicated. Doses up to 160 mg every 6 hours have been administered to some patients with severe Zollinger-Ellison syndrome.

GERD: 20 mg twice daily for up to 6 weeks. For esophagitis including erosions and ulcerations and accompanying symptoms due to GERD, 20 or 40 mg twice daily for up to 12 weeks.

Concomitant use of antacids: Antacids may be given concomitantly if needed.

Severe renal insufficiency: Ccr < 10 ml/min – The elimination half-life may exceed 20 hours, reaching ≈ 24 hours in anuric patients. Although no relationship of adverse effects to high plasma levels has been established, to avoid excess accumulation of the drug, the dose may be reduced to 20 mg at bedtime or the dosing interval may be prolonged to 36 to 48 hours, as indicated.

Parenteral:

IV administration – In some hospitalized patients with pathological hypersecretory conditions or intractable ulcers, or in patients who are unable to take oral medication, administer famotidine IV 20 mg every 12 hours. The doses and regimen for GERD have not been established.

Preparation of IV solutions – Dilute 2 ml famotidine IV (solution containing 10 mg/ml) with 0.9% Sodium Chloride Injection or other compatible IV solution to a total volume of either 5 or 10 ml and inject over not less than 2 minutes.

Preparation of IV infusion solutions – Famotidine IV may also be administered as an infusion, 2 ml diluted with 100 ml of 5% Dextrose or other compatible solution, and infused over 15 to 30 minutes.

Stability – Solution is stable for 48 hours at room temperature when added to or diluted with most commonly used IV solutions (eg, Water for Injection, 0.9% Sodium Chloride Injection, 5% or 10% Dextrose Injection, Lactated Ringer's Injection, 5% Sodium Bicarbonate Injection). Famotidine, 20 to 50 mg/L, is also stable when mixed with various total parenteral nutrition solutions: 24 hours at 4°C, then 24 hours at 20° to 22°C in a mixture of dextrose, amino acids and fat emulsion; up to 72 hours at room temperature in dextrose, amino acids, electrolytes, vitamins, minerals and fat emulsion; 35 days under refrigeration in dextrose, amino acids, electrolytes and trace elements.

Storage: Do not store powder > 40°C (104°F). After reconstitution of powder, store oral suspension < 30°C (86°F). Do not freeze. Discard unused suspension after 30 days.

Store IV at 2° to 8°C (36° to 46°F). When mixed with dextrose or sodium chloride in polyvinyl chloride minibags, famotidine is stable for 14 days at 4°C (39°F), or when frozen for 28 days and subsequently refrigerated for 14 days. Also, when stored at –20°C (–4°F) in polypropylene syringes, famotidine is stable for 3 weeks in dextrose and for 8 weeks in sodium chloride.

				C.I.*
Rx	**Pepcid** (MSD)	**Tablets:** 20 mg	(MSD 963). Beige. Film coated. In unit-of-use 30s, 90s, 100s and UD 100s.	1.2
		40 mg	(MSD 964). Lt. brownish-orange. Film coated. In unit-of-use 30s, 90s, 100s & UD 100s.	1.1
Rx	**Pepcid** (MSD)	**Powder for Oral Suspension:** 40 mg per 5 ml when reconstituted	Cherry-banana-mint flavor. In bottles of 400 mg.	3.1
Rx	**Pepcid IV** (MSD)	**Injection:** 10 mg per ml	Mannitol. In 2 ml single-dose vials[1] & 4 ml multi-dose vials.[2]	5.4

* Cost Index based on cost per 40 mg famotidine.

[1] Preservative free. [2] With 0.9% benzyl alcohol.

MISOPROSTOL

Warning:

Misoprostol is contraindicated because of its abortifacient property in pregnant women. Advise patients of the abortifacient property and warn them not to give the drug to others. Do not use in women of childbearing potential unless the patient requires nonsteroidal anti-inflammatory drugs (NSAIDs) and is at high risk of complications from gastric ulcers associated with use of NSAIDs, or is at high risk of developing gastric ulceration. In such patients, misoprostol may be prescribed if the patient:

- Is capable of complying with effective contraceptive measures;
- Has received both oral and written warnings of the hazards of misoprostol, the risk of possible contraception failure and the danger to other women of childbearing potential should the drug be taken by mistake;
- Has had a negative *serum* pregnancy test within 2 weeks prior to beginning therapy;
- Will begin therapy only on second or third day of next normal menstrual period.

Actions:

Misoprostol was approved by the FDA in 1988.

Pharmacology: Misoprostol, a synthetic prostaglandin E_1 analog, has both antisecretory (inhibiting gastric acid secretion) and (in animals) mucosal protective properties. NSAIDs inhibit prostaglandin synthesis; a deficiency of prostaglandins within the gastric mucosa may lead to diminishing bicarbonate and mucous secretion and may contribute to the mucosal damage caused by these agents. Misoprostol can increase bicarbonate and mucus production.

Prostaglandin receptor binding is saturable, reversible and stereospecific. The sites have a high affinity for misoprostol, for its acid metabolite, and for other E type prostaglandins, but not for F or I prostaglandins and unrelated compounds, such as histamine or cimetidine. It is likely that these specific receptors allow misoprostol taken with food to be effective topically, despite the lower serum concentrations attained.

Misoprostol produces a moderate decrease in pepsin concentration during basal conditions, but not during histamine stimulation. It has no significant effect on fasting or postprandial gastrin nor on intrinsic factor output.

Effects on gastric acid secretion: Misoprostol over the range of 50 to 200 mcg inhibits basal and nocturnal gastric acid secretion, and acid secretion in response to a variety of stimuli, including meals, histamine, pentagastrin and coffee. Activity is apparent 30 minutes after oral administration and persists for at least 3 hours. Only the 200 mcg dose had substantial effects on nocturnal secretion or on histamine and meal-stimulated secretion.

Uterine effects: Misoprostol produces uterine contractions that may endanger pregnancy (see Warnings). In studies in women undergoing elective termination of pregnancy during the first trimester, misoprostol caused partial or complete expulsion of the uterine contents in 11% of the subjects and increased uterine bleeding in 41%.

Pharmacokinetics: Misoprostol is extensively absorbed, and undergoes rapid deesterification to its free acid, which is responsible for its clinical activity and, unlike the parent compound, is detectable in plasma. In healthy volunteers, misoprostol is rapidly absorbed after oral administration with a time to reach peak concentration of misoprostol acid of 12 ± 3 minutes and a terminal half-life of 20 to 40 minutes.

Mean plasma levels after single doses show a linear relationship with doses over the range of 200 to 400 mcg. No accumulation was noted in multiple-dose studies; plasma steady state was achieved within 2 days. After oral administration of radiolabeled misoprostol, $\approx$ 80% of detected radioactivity appears in urine.

Misoprostol does not affect the hepatic mixed function oxidase (cytochrome P-450) enzyme system in animals. The serum protein binding of misoprostol acid is $<$ 90% and is concentration-independent in the therapeutic range.

(Actions continued on following page)

MISOPROSTOL (Cont.)

Actions (Cont.):

Clinical pharmacology: A series of small short-term (about 1 week) placebo controlled studies in healthy human volunteers using misoprostol 200 mcg 4 times a day with tolmetin and naproxen or 100 and 200 mcg 4 times a day with ibuprofen showed reduction of the rate of significant endoscopic injury from about 70% to 75% on placebo to 10% to 30% on misoprostol. Doses of 25 to 200 mcg 4 times a day reduced aspirin-induced mucosal injury and bleeding.

Two 12 week randomized, double-blind trials in osteoarthritic patients who had GI symptoms but no ulcer on endoscopy while taking an NSAID compared the ability of 100 or 200 mcg of misoprostol or placebo to prevent gastric ulcer formation. Patients were equally divided between ibuprofen, piroxicam and naproxen and continued this treatment throughout the 12 weeks. The 200 mcg dose caused a marked, statistically significant reduction in gastric ulcers in both studies. The 100 mcg dose was somewhat less effective, with a significant result in only one of the studies.

In another clinical trial, 239 patients receiving aspirin 650 to 1300 mg 4 times a day for rheumatoid arthritis and who had endoscopic evidence of duodenal or gastric inflammation were randomized to misoprostol 200 mcg 4 times a day or placebo for 8 weeks while continuing to receive aspirin. Misoprostol did not interfere with the efficacy of aspirin in these patients with rheumatoid arthritis.

Indications:

Prevention of NSAID- (including aspirin) induced gastric ulcers in patients at high risk of complications from a gastric ulcer, eg, the elderly and patients with concomitant debilitating disease, as well as patients at high risk of developing gastric ulceration, such as patients with a history of ulcer. Take misoprostol for the duration of NSAID therapy.

Unlabeled uses: In doses of at least 400 mcg/day, misoprostol appears effective in treating duodenal ulcers, and may be useful in treating duodenal ulcers unresponsive to histamine H_2 antagonists; however, it does not prevent duodenal ulcers in patients on NSAIDs (see Warnings).

In one study, misoprostol 200 mcg 4 times daily for 12 weeks (concurrently with cyclosporine and prednisone) reduced the incidence of acute graft rejection in renal transplant recipients by improving renal function.

Contraindications:

History of allergy to prostaglandins; pregnancy (see Warnings).

Warnings:

Renal function impairment: Pharmacokinetic studies in patients with varying degrees of renal impairment showed an approximate doubling of half-life, maximum concentration and area under the curve (AUC), but no clear correlation between degree of impairment and AUC was shown. No routine dosage adjustment is recommended, but dosage may need to be reduced if usual dose is not tolerated.

Duodenal ulcers: Misoprostol does not prevent duodenal ulcers in patients on NSAIDs. It had no effect, compared to placebo, on GI pain or discomfort associated with NSAIDs.

Fertility impairment: Misoprostol, when administered to breeding male and female rats at doses 6.25 times to 625 times the maximum recommended human therapeutic dose, produced dose related pre- and post-implantation losses and a significant decrease in the number of live pups born at the highest dose. These findings suggest the possibility of a general adverse effect on fertility in males and females.

Elderly: In subjects $>$ 64 years of age, the AUC for misoprostol acid is increased; however, no routine dosage adjustment is recommended. Reduce the dose if the usual dose is not tolerated.

Pregnancy: Category X. Misoprostol may cause miscarriage. Uterine contractions, uterine bleeding and expulsion of the products of conception occur. Miscarriages caused by misoprostol may be incomplete. In studies in women undergoing elective termination of pregnancy during the first trimester, misoprostol caused partial or complete expulsion of the products of conception in 11% of subjects and increased uterine bleeding in 41%. If a woman is or becomes pregnant while taking this drug, discontinue the drug and apprise the patient of potential hazards to the fetus.

Lactation: It is unlikely that misoprostol is excreted in breast milk, since it is rapidly metabolized. However, it is not known if the active metabolite (misoprostol acid) is excreted in breast milk. Therefore, do not administer to nursing mothers because the potential excretion of misoprostol acid could cause significant diarrhea in nursing infants.

Children: Safety and efficacy in children $<$ 18 years of age have not been established.

(Continued on following page)

MISOPROSTOL (Cont.)

Precautions:

Women of childbearing potential: Advise women of childbearing potential that they must not be pregnant when misoprostol therapy is initiated, and that they must use an effective contraception method while taking misoprostol. See Warnings.

Diarrhea (13% to 40%) is dose-related and usually develops early in the course of therapy (after 13 days), usually is self-limiting (often resolving after 8 days), but sometimes requires discontinuation of misoprostol (2% of the patients). The incidence of diarrhea can be minimized by administering after meals and at bedtime, and by avoiding coadministration of misoprostol with magnesium-containing antacids.

Drug Interactions:

Antacids reduce the total availability of misoprostol acid but this does not appear clinically important.

Drug/Food interaction: Maximum plasma concentrations of misoprostol acid are diminished when taken with food.

Adverse Reactions:

GI: Diarrhea (13% to 40%); abdominal pain (7% to 20%); nausea (3.2%); flatulence (2.9%); dyspepsia (2%); vomiting (1.3%); constipation (1.1%).

Gynecological: Spotting (0.7%); cramps (0.6%); hypermenorrhea (0.5%); menstrual disorder (0.3%); dysmenorrhea (0.1%). Postmenopausal vaginal bleeding may be related to misoprostol administration. If it occurs, perform diagnostic workup to rule out gynecological pathology.

Other: Headache (2.4%).

Overdosage:

Symptoms: The toxic dose in humans has not been determined. Cumulative total daily doses of 1600 mcg have been tolerated with only symptoms of GI discomfort. In animals, the acute toxic effects are diarrhea, GI lesions, focal cardiac, hepatic and renal tubular necrosis, testicular atrophy, respiratory difficulties and CNS depression. Clinical signs that may indicate an overdose are sedation, tremor, convulsions, dyspnea, abdominal pain, diarrhea, fever, palpitations, hypotension or bradycardia.

Treatment: Treat with supportive therapy; refer to Management of Acute Overdosage.

It is not known if misoprostol acid is dialyzable. However, because misoprostol is metabolized like a fatty acid, it is unlikely that dialysis would be appropriate treatment for overdosage.

Patient Information:

Misoprostol can cause miscarriage, often associated with potentially dangerous bleeding. This may result in hospitalization, surgery, infertility or death. Do not take misoprostol if pregnant and do not become pregnant while taking this medication. If pregnancy occurs during misoprostol therapy, discontinue the drug and contact physician immediately.

Take misoprostol only according to the directions given by the physician.

Do not give misoprostol to anyone else.

Administration and Dosage:

Adults: 200 mcg 4 times daily with food. If this dose cannot be tolerated, 100 mcg can be used. Take misoprostol for the duration of NSAID therapy as prescribed. Take with meals, the last dose of the day taken at bedtime.

Renal impairment: Dosage adjustment is not routinely needed, but dosage can be reduced if the 200 mcg dose is not tolerated.

Rx	**Cytotec** (Searle)	**Tablets:** 100 mcg	(Searle 1451). White. In UD 100s and unit-of-use 60s and 120s.
		200 mcg	(Searle 1461). White, scored. Hexagonal. In UD 100s and unit-of-use 60s and 100s.

OMEPRAZOLE

Actions:

Pharmacology: Omeprazole belongs to a new class of antisecretory compounds, the substituted benzimidazoles, that do not exhibit anticholinergic or H_2 histamine antagonistic properties, but that suppress gastric acid secretion by specific inhibition of the H^+/K^+ ATPase enzyme system at the secretory surface of the gastric parietal cell. Because this enzyme system is the 'acid (proton) pump' within the gastric mucosa, omeprazole has been characterized as a gastric acid pump inhibitor; it blocks the final step of acid production. This effect is dose-related and inhibits both basal and stimulated acid secretion irrespective of the stimulus. In animals, after rapid disappearance from plasma, omeprazole is found within the gastric mucosa for a day or more.

Antisecretory activity – Onset after oral administration of omeprazole occurs within 1 hour, and is maximum within 2 hours. Inhibition of secretion is about 50% of maximum at 24 hours and the duration of inhibition lasts up to 72 hours. The antisecretory effect thus lasts far longer than would be expected from the very short (< 1 hour) plasma half-life, apparently due to prolonged binding to the parietal H^+/K^+ ATPase enzyme. When the drug is discontinued, secretory activity returns over 3 to 5 days. The inhibitory effect of omeprazole on acid secretion increases with repeated once-daily dosing, plateauing after 4 days.

Results from numerous studies on the antisecretory effect of multiple doses of 20 and 40 mg omeprazole in healthy volunteers and patients are shown below. The "max" value represents determinations at a time of maximum effect (2 to 6 hours after dosing), while "min" values are those 24 hours after the last omeprazole dose.

Mean Antisecretory Effects of Omeprazole After Multiple Daily Dosing

Parameter	Omeprazole 20 mg		Omeprazole 40 mg	
	Max	Min	Max	Min
% Decrease in basal acid output	78*	58-80	94*	80-93
% Decrease in peak acid output	79*	50-59	88*	62-68
% Decrease in 24 hr intragastric acidity		80-97		92-94

* Single studies.

Single daily oral doses of omeprazole 10 to 40 mg have produced 100% inhibition of 24 hour intragastric acidity in some patients.

Serum gastrin effects – In studies involving > 200 patients, serum gastrin levels increased during the first 1 to 2 weeks of once-daily therapeutic omeprazole doses in parallel with inhibition of acid secretion. No further increase in serum gastrin occurred with continued treatment. In comparison with histamine H_2-receptor antagonists, the median increases produced by 20 mg omeprazole were higher (1.3- to 3.6-fold vs 1.1- to 1.8-fold increase). Gastrin values returned to pretreatment levels, usually within 1 to 2 weeks after discontinuation of therapy.

Other effects – No effect on gastric emptying was demonstrated after a single 90 mg dose. In healthy subjects, a single IV dose (0.35 mg/kg) had no effect on intrinsic factor secretion. No dose-dependent effect has been observed on basal or stimulated pepsin output. However, when intragastric pH is maintained at ≥ 4, basal pepsin output is low, and pepsin activity is decreased.

As seen with other agents that elevate intragastric pH, omeprazole administered for 14 days in healthy subjects produced a significant increase in the intragastric concentrations of viable bacteria. The pattern of the bacterial species was unchanged from that commonly found in saliva. All changes resolved within 3 days of stopping treatment.

(Actions continued on following page)

OMEPRAZOLE (Cont.)

Actions (Cont.):

Clinical studies:

Active duodenal ulcer: In a multicenter, double-blind, placebo controlled study of 147 patients with endoscopically documented duodenal ulcer, the percentage of patients healed (per protocol) at 2 and 4 weeks was significantly higher with omeprazole 20 mg once a day than with placebo. Complete daytime and nighttime pain relief occurred significantly faster in patients treated with omeprazole 20 mg than in patients treated with placebo. At the end of the study, significantly more patients who had received omeprazole had complete relief of daytime and nighttime pain.

In a multicenter, double-blind study of 293 patients with endoscopically documented duodenal ulcer, the percentage of patients healed (per protocol) at 4 weeks was significantly higher with omeprazole 20 mg once a day than with ranitidine 150 mg twice a day. Healing occurred significantly faster in patients treated with omeprazole than in those treated with ranitidine 150 mg twice daily.

In a foreign multinational, randomized, double-blind study of 105 patients with endoscopically documented duodenal ulcer, 20 and 40 mg omeprazole were compared to 150 mg ranitidine twice daily at 2, 4 and 8 weeks. At 2 and 4 weeks, both doses of omeprazole were statistically superior (per protocol) to ranitidine, but 40 mg was not superior to 20 mg omeprazole, and at 8 weeks there was no significant difference between any of the active drugs:

Omeprazole Treatment of Active Duodenal Ulcer

	% of patients healed						
Week	Omeprazole 20 mg (n = 99)	Placebo (n = 48)	Omeprazole 20 mg (n = 145)	Ranitidine 150 mg bid (n = 148)	Omeprazole 20 mg (n = 34)	Omeprazole 40 mg (n = 36)	Ranitidine 150 mg bid (n = 35)
2	41[1]	13	42	34	83[1]	83[1]	53
4	75[1]	27	82[1]	63	97[1]	100[1]	82
8	—	—	—	—	100	100	94

[1] $p \leq 0.01$

Gastroesophageal reflux disease (GERD) – In a US multicenter double-blind placebo controlled study of 20 or 40 mg omeprazole in patients with symptomatic esophagitis and endoscopically diagnosed erosive esophagitis of grade 2 or above, the percentage healing rates (per protocol) were as follows:

GERD Healing Rates with Omeprazole (%)

Week	20 mg (n = 83)	40 mg (n = 87)	Placebo (n = 43)
4	39	45	7
8	74	75	14

In comparisons with histamine H_2-receptor antagonists in patients with erosive esophagitis, grade 2 or above, a 20 mg dose of omeprazole was significantly more effective than the active controls. Complete daytime and nighttime heartburn relief occurred significantly faster in patients treated with omeprazole than in those taking placebo or histamine H_2-receptor antagonists.

Pathological hypersecretory conditions – In studies of patients with pathological hypersecretory conditions, such as Zollinger-Ellison (ZE) syndrome with or without multiple endocrine adenomas, omeprazole significantly inhibited gastric acid secretion and controlled associated symptoms of diarrhea, anorexia and pain; 20 mg every other day to 360 mg per day maintained basal acid secretion < 10 mEq/hr in patients without prior gastric surgery, and < 5 mEq/hr in patients with prior gastric surgery.

Omeprazole was well tolerated for > 5 years in some patients. In most ZE patients, serum gastrin levels were not modified. However, in some patients serum gastrin increased. At least 2 patients with ZE syndrome on long-term treatment developed gastric carcinoids. This finding was believed to be a manifestation of the underlying condition, rather than the result of omeprazole administration.

(Actions continued on following page)

OMEPRAZOLE (Cont.)

Actions (Cont.)

Pharmacokinetics: Absorption/Distribution – Omeprazole contains an enteric coated granule formulation (because omeprazole is acid-labile). Absorption is rapid, with peak plasma levels occurring within 0.5 to 3.5 hours. Peak plasma concentrations of omeprazole and AUC are approximately proportional to doses up to 40 mg, but because of a saturable first-pass effect a greater than linear response in peak plasma concentration and AUC occurs with doses > 40 mg. Absolute bioavailability is about 30% to 40% at doses of 20 to 40 mg, due to presystemic metabolism. Plasma half-life is 0.5 to 1 hour, and total body clearance is 500 to 600 ml/min. Protein binding is approximately 95%. The bioavailability of omeprazole increases slightly upon repeated administration.

Metabolism/Excretion – Little unchanged drug is excreted in urine. The majority of the dose (about 77%) is eliminated in urine as at least six metabolites. Two are hydroxyomeprazole and the corresponding carboxylic acid. The remainder of the dose was recoverable in feces. This implies a significant biliary excretion of the metabolites of omeprazole. Three metabolites have been identified in plasma – the sulfide and sulfone derivatives and hydroxyomeprazole. These metabolites have very little or no antisecretory activity.

In patients with chronic hepatic disease, the bioavailability increased to approximately 100%, reflecting decreased first-pass effect; plasma half-life increased to nearly 3 hours. Plasma clearance averaged 70 ml/min, compared to 500 to 600 ml/min in healthy subjects.

In patients with chronic renal impairment (creatinine clearance, 10 to 62 ml/min/1.73 m^2), the disposition of omeprazole was very similar to that in healthy volunteers, with a slight increase in bioavailability. Because urinary excretion is a primary route of excretion of omeprazole metabolites, their elimination slowed in proportion to the decreased creatinine clearance.

Elderly: The elimination rate of omeprazole was somewhat decreased and bioavailability was increased. Omeprazole was 76% bioavailable with a 40 mg oral dose in elderly volunteers vs 58% in young volunteers. Nearly 70% of the dose was recovered in urine as metabolites; no unchanged drug was detected. The plasma clearance of omeprazole was 250 ml/min and its plasma half-life averaged 1 hour.

Indications:

Active duodenal ulcer: Short-term treatment of active duodenal ulcer. Most patients heal within 4 weeks, although some may require an additional 4 weeks.

Omeprazole should not be used as maintenance therapy for treatment of patients with duodenal ulcer disease.

Gastroesophageal reflux disease (GERD):

Severe erosive esophagitis – Short-term treatment (4 to 8 weeks) of severe erosive esophagitis (grade 2 or above), diagnosed by endoscopy.

Poorly responsive symptomatic GERD – Short-term treatment (4 to 8 weeks) of symptomatic GERD (esophagitis) poorly responsive to customary medical treatment, usually including histamine H_2-receptor antagonists.

The efficacy of omeprazole used for > 8 weeks has not been established. In the rare patient not responding to 8 weeks of treatment, an additional 4 weeks of treatment may help. If there is recurrence of severe or symptomatic GERD poorly responsive to customary medical treatment, additional 4 to 8 week courses of omeprazole may be considered. Do not use as maintenance therapy (see boxed Warning).

Pathological hypersecretory conditions (eg, Zollinger-Ellison syndrome, multiple endocrine adenomas and systemic mastocytosis): Long-term treatment.

Unlabeled uses: Omeprazole appears to be effective in the treatment of gastric ulcers at doses of 20 to 40 mg/day. It is similar in efficacy to the H_2-receptor antagonists and possibly more effective (40 mg/day) in the treatment of resistant gastric ulcers. It is also useful in healing gastric ulcers in patients receiving NSAIDs.

Contraindications:

Hypersensitivity to any component of the formulation.

(Continued on following page)

OMEPRAZOLE (Cont.)

Warnings:

> In long-term (2 year) studies in rats, omeprazole produced a dose-related increase in gastric carcinoid tumors (see Carcinogenesis). While endoscopic evaluations and histologic examinations of biopsy specimens from human stomachs have not detected a risk from short-term exposure to omeprazole, further human data on the effect of sustained hypochlorhydria and hypergastrinemia are needed to rule out the possibility of increased risk for development of tumors in humans receiving long-term omeprazole therapy. Prescribe only for the conditions, dosage and duration described (see Indications and Administration and Dosage).

Carcinogenesis: In two 24 month carcinogenicity studies in rats, omeprazole at daily doses approximately 4 to 352 times the human dose, produced gastric enterochromaffin-like (ECL) cell carcinoids in a dose-related manner in both male and female rats; the incidence was markedly higher in female rats, which had higher blood levels of omeprazole. In addition, ECL cell hyperplasia was present in all treated groups of both sexes. In one study, female rats were treated with 35 times the human dose for 1 year, then followed for an additional year without the drug. No carcinoids were seen in these rats. An increased incidence of treatment-related ECL cell hyperplasia was observed at the end of 1 year (94% treated vs 10% controls). By the second year the difference between treated and control rats was much smaller (46% vs 26%). An unusual primary malignant tumor in the stomach was seen in one rat (2%).

Elderly: Bioavailability may be increased. See Pharmacokinetics.

Pregnancy: Category C. In rabbits, omeprazole 17 to 172 times the human dose produced dose-related increases in embryo-lethality, fetal resorptions and pregnancy disruptions. In rats, dose-related embryo/fetal toxicity and postnatal developmental toxicity were observed in offspring resulting from parents treated with 35 to 345 times the human dose. There are no adequate or well controlled studies in pregnant women. Use during pregnancy only if the potential benefit justifies the potential risk to the fetus.

Lactation: It is not known whether omeprazole is excreted in breast milk. In rats, omeprazole administration during late gestation and lactation at doses of 35 to 345 times the human dose resulted in decreased weight gain in pups. Decide whether to discontinue nursing or to discontinue the drug, taking into account the importance of the drug to the mother.

Children: Safety and efficacy in children have not been established.

Precautions:

Gastric malignancy: Symptomatic response to therapy with omeprazole does not preclude gastric malignancy.

Drug Interactions:

Omeprazole Drug Interactions			
Precipitant drug	Object drug *		Description
Omeprazole	Diazepam	↑	Omeprazole produced a 130% increase in the half-life of diazepam, probably due to inhibition of oxidative metabolism. Plasma concentrations were also increased and total clearance of diazepam was decreased. Clinical significance was not determined.
Omeprazole	Phenytoin	↑	Omeprazole reduced the plasma clearance of phenytoin by 15% and increased its half-life by 27%, probably due to inhibition of oxidative metabolism. Clinical significance was not determined.
Omeprazole	Warfarin	↑	Omeprazole may prolong the elimination of warfarin via inhibition of oxidative metabolism.

* ↑ = Object drug increased.

There may be interactions with other drugs also metabolized via the cytochrome P-450 system, although in healthy subjects no interaction with theophylline or propranolol has been found. Because of its profound and long-lasting inhibition of gastric acid secretion, omeprazole may interfere with absorption of drugs where gastric pH is a determinant of their bioavailability (eg, ketoconazole, ampicillin esters, iron salts). In clinical trials, antacids were used concomitantly with omeprazole.

(Continued on following page)

OMEPRAZOLE (Cont.)

Adverse Reactions:

Omeprazole is generally well tolerated. In clinical trials of 3096 patients (including duodenal ulcer, Zollinger-Ellison syndrome and resistant ulcer patients), the following adverse experiences occurred in ≥ 1% of patients.

Selected Omeprazole Adverse Reactions (%)					
	Causal relationship				
	Assessed			Not Assessed	
Adverse reaction	Omeprazole (n = 465)	Placebo (n = 64)	Ranitidine (n = 195)	Omeprazole (n = 2631)	Placebo (n = 120)
Headache	6.9	6.3	7.7	2.9	2.5
Diarrhea	3	3.1	2.1	3.7	2.5
Abdominal pain	2.4	3.1	2.1	5.2	3.3
Nausea	2.2	3.1	4.1	4	6.7
URI	1.9	1.6	2.6		
Vomiting	1.5	4.7	1.5	3.2	10
Dizziness	1.5	0	2.6		
Rash	1.5	0	0		
Constipation	1.1	0	0	1.5	0.8
Asthenia	1.1	1.6	1.5	1.3	0.8
Cough	1.1	0	1.5		
Back pain	1.1	0	0.5		
Flatulence				2.7	5.8
Acid regurgitation				1.9	3.3

Adverse reactions occurring in < 1% of patients (relationship to omeprazole unclear).

Body as a whole: Fever; pain; fatigue; malaise; abdominal swelling.

Cardiovascular: Chest pain/angina; tachycardia; bradycardia; palpitation; peripheral edema.

GI: Hepatitis; elevated AST, ALT, γ-glutamyl transpeptidase, alkaline phosphatase and bilirubin (jaundice); anorexia; irritable colon; fecal discoloration; esophageal candidiasis; mucosal atrophy of the tongue; dry mouth.

Metabolic/Nutritional: Hypoglycemia; weight gain.

Musculoskeletal: Muscle cramps; myalgia; joint pain; leg pain.

CNS: Dizziness; vertigo; insomnia; nervousness; apathy; somnolence; anxiety disorders; paresthesia; dream abnormalities; hemifacial dysesthesia.

Respiratory: Epistaxis; pharyngeal pain.

Skin: Skin inflammation; urticaria; pruritus; alopecia; dry skin; hyperhidrosis.

Special senses: Tinnitus; taste perversion.

GU: Urinary tract infection; microscopic pyuria; urinary frequency; elevated serum creatinine; proteinuria; hematuria; glycosuria; testicular pain.

Hematologic: Agranulocytosis occurred in a 65-year-old diabetic male on several drugs in addition to omeprazole; the relationship of the agranulocytosis to omeprazole is uncertain. Pancytopenia; thrombocytopenia; neutropenia; anemia; leukocytosis.

Elderly: The incidence of clinical adverse experiences in patients > 65 years of age was similar to that in patients ≤ 65 years of age.

(Continued on following page)

OMEPRAZOLE (Cont.)

Overdosage:

Symptoms: Lethal doses of omeprazole after single oral administration are about 1500 mg/kg in mice and > 4000 mg/kg in rats, and about 100 mg/kg in mice and > 40 mg/kg in rats given single IV injections. Animals given these doses showed sedation, ptosis, convulsions, increased depth of respiration, and decreased activity, body temperature and respiratory rate. There is no experience to date with deliberate overdosage. Dosages of up to 360 mg/day have been well tolerated.

Treatment: Omeprazole is extensively protein bound and is, therefore, not readily dialyzable. Treatment should be symptomatic and supportive. Refer to General Management of Acute Overdosage.

Patient Information:

Take before eating.

Swallow capsule whole; do not open, chew or crush.

Administration and Dosage:

Active duodenal ulcer: Adults – 20 mg daily for 4 to 8 weeks (see Indications).

Severe erosive esophagitis or poorly responsive gastroesophageal reflux disease (GERD): Adults – 20 mg daily for 4 to 8 weeks (see Indications).

Pathological hypersecretory conditions: Individualize dosage. Initial adult dose is 60 mg once a day. Doses up to 120 mg 3 times/day have been administered. Administer daily dosages > 80 mg in divided doses. Some patients with Zollinger-Ellison syndrome have been treated continuously for > 5 years.

No dosage adjustment is necessary for patients with renal impairment, hepatic dysfunction or for the elderly.

Take before eating. In the clinical trials, antacids were used concomitantly with omeprazole.

Rx	**Prilosec** (MSD)	**Capsules, sustained release:** 20 mg	(MSD 742). Amethyst. In 30s and UD 100s.

SIMETHICONE

Actions:

The defoaming action relieves flatulence by dispersing and preventing the formation of mucus-surrounded gas pockets in the GI tract. It acts in the stomach and intestines to change the surface tension of gas bubbles, enabling them to coalesce; thus, gas is freed and eliminated more easily by belching or passing flatus.

Indications:

For relief of the painful symptoms of excess gas in the digestive tract. Used as an adjunct in the treatment of many conditions in which gas retention may be a problem, such as: Postoperative gaseous distention, air swallowing, functional dyspepsia, peptic ulcer, spastic or irritable colon, or diverticulosis.

Administration and Dosage:

Capsules: 125 mg, 4 times daily after each meal and at bedtime.

Tablets: 40 to 125 mg, 4 times daily after each meal and at bedtime. Chew thoroughly.

Drops: Take after meals and at bedtime. Shake well before using.

	Product	Form	Description	C.I.*
otc	**Simethicone** (Various)	**Drops:** 40 mg per 0.6 ml	In 30 ml w/calibrated oral syringe.	NA
otc	**Flatulex** (Dayton)		In 30 ml w/calibrated dropper.	NA
otc	**Mylicon** (J & J-Merck)		In 30 ml dropper bottle.	128
otc	**Phazyme** (Reed & C)		Saccharin. In 30 ml w/dropper.	NA
otc	**Mylanta Gas** (J & J-Merck)	**Tablets, chewable:** 40 mg	(Stuart 450). White, scored. In 100s, 500s and UD 100s.	68
otc	**Gax-X** (Sandoz)	**Tablets, chewable:** 80 mg	(Gas-X). White, scored. In 12s, 30s.	37
otc	**Mylanta Gas** (J & J-Merck)		(Stuart 858). Pink, scored. In 12s, 48s, 100s and UD 100s.	34
otc	**Extra Strength Gas-X** (Sandoz)	**Tablets, chewable:** 125 mg	(Gas-X). Yellow, scored. In 18s.	31
otc	**Maximum Strength Mylanta Gas** (J & J-Merck)		Sorbitol. White, scored. In 12s and 60s.	NA
otc	**Phazyme** (Reed & Carnrick)	**Tablets:** 60 mg	Enteric coated inner core. In 50s, 100s and 1000s.	68
otc	**Phazyme 95** (Reed & Carnrick)	**Tablets:** 95 mg	Enteric coated inner core. In 50s, 100s, 500s and Consumer Pak 10s.	43
otc	**Phazyme 125** (Reed & C)	**Capsules:** 125 mg	Red. In 50s.	44

CHARCOAL

Actions: Charcoal is an adsorbent (detoxicant). It reduces the volume of intestinal gas and allays related discomfort.

Indications: For relief of intestinal gas, diarrhea and GI distress associated with ingestion. Also for the prevention of nonspecific pruritus associated with kidney dialysis treatment and intestinal motility studies. For use as an antidote in poisonings, see p. 2523.

Warnings: Evidence indicates that high dosage or prolonged use does not cause side effects or harm the patient's nutritional state.

Usage in Children: Do not use in children less than 3 years of age.

Drug Interactions: Activated charcoal can adsorb drugs while they are in the GI tract. Therefore, take charcoal 2 hours before, or 1 or more hours after other oral medication.

Administration and Dosage: Usual adult dosage is 520 mg to 975 mg after meals or at first sign of discomfort. Repeat as needed, up to 4.16 g daily.

	Product	Form	Description	C.I.*
otc	**Charcoal** (Paddock)	**Tablets:** 325 mg	In 1000s.	19
otc	**Charcocaps** (Requa)	**Capsules:** 260 mg	In 36s.	76

CHARCOAL AND SIMETHICONE

Actions: Charcoal reduces the volume of gas. Simethicone dispenses and prevents the formation of gas, and allows for its elimination.

Indications: For the relief of gas and the syumptoms associated with it.

Administration and Dosage: 1 tablet 3 times daily and at bedtime.

	Product	Form	Description	C.I.*
otc	**Charcoal Plus** (Kramer)	**Tablets:** 200 mg activated charcoal and 40 mg simethicone	In 120s.	NA
otc	**Flatulex** (Dayton)	**Tablets:** 250 mg activated charcoal and 80 mg simethicone	In 100s.	NA

* Cost Index based on cost per minimum daily dose.

METOCLOPRAMIDE

Actions:

Pharmacology: Metoclopramide stimulates motility of the upper GI tract without stimulating gastric, biliary or pancreatic secretions. Its mode of action is unclear, but it appears to sensitize tissues to the action of acetylcholine. The effect on motility does not depend on intact vagal innervation, but it can be abolished by anticholinergic drugs.

Metoclopramide increases the tone and amplitude of gastric (especially antral) contractions, relaxes the pyloric sphincter and the duodenal bulb, and increases peristalsis of the duodenum and jejunum, resulting in accelerated gastric emptying and intestinal transit. It has little, if any, effect on colon or gallbladder motility. It produces dose-related increases in lower esophageal sphincter pressure (LESP). Effects on LESP begin at about 5 mg and increase through 20 mg. The increase in LESP from a 5 mg dose lasts about 45 minutes and that of 20 mg lasts between 2 and 3 hours. Increased rate of stomach emptying has been observed with single oral doses of 10 mg.

Like the phenothiazines and related dopamine antagonists, metoclopramide produces sedation and, rarely, may produce extrapyramidal reactions. The drug inhibits the central and peripheral effects of apomorphine, induces release of prolactin and transiently increases circulating aldosterone levels.

Pharmacokinetics: Onset of action is 1 to 3 minutes following an IV dose, 10 to 15 minutes following IM administration, and 30 to 60 minutes following an oral dose. Effects persist for 1 to 2 hours.

Absorption/Distribution - Metoclopramide is well absorbed after oral administration, but is subject to significant first-pass metabolism, with total bioavailability about 50% to 70%. When the drug is taken on an empty stomach, absorption is rapid, with peak concentrations observed in 1 hour. It is weakly protein bound (13% to 22%) and rapidly distributed to most tissues.

Metabolism/Excretion - Metoclopramide is primarily excreted in the urine (80% in 24 hours) either unchanged (up to 25%) or conjugated to sulfate or glucuronide in the bile. Half-life is approximately 3 to 6 hours. Impaired renal function prolongs the half-life (up to 24 hours); estimated adjustments reduce doses by one-half. Dialysis effectively removes the drug.

Indications:

Diabetic gastroparesis: Relief of symptoms associated with acute and recurrent diabetic gastroparesis (diabetic gastric stasis). Usual manifestations of delayed gastric emptying (ie, nausea, vomiting, heartburn, persistent fullness after meals and anorexia) respond within different time intervals. Significant relief of nausea occurs early and improves over 3 weeks. Relief of vomiting and anorexia may precede the relief of abdominal fullness by 1 week or more.

Symptomatic gastroesophageal reflux: As short-term (4 to 12 weeks) therapy for adults with symptomatic documented gastroesophageal reflux who fail to respond to conventional therapy.

Parenteral: For prevention of nausea and vomiting associated with emetogenic cancer chemotherapy.

Single doses may facilitate small bowel intubation when the tube does not pass the pylorus with conventional maneuvers.

Stimulates gastric emptying and intestinal transit of barium in cases where delayed emptying interferes with radiological examination of the stomach or small intestine.

Unlabeled Uses: Used to improve lactation. Doses of 30 to 45 mg/day have increased milk secretion, possibly by elevating serum prolactin levels. (See Warnings).

Studies have indicated some potential value of metoclopramide in the following conditions: Nausea and vomiting of a variety of etiologies (uncontrolled studies report 80% to 90% efficacy), including emesis during pregnancy and labor; gastric ulcer and anorexia nervosa (due to GI stimulation). It has also been used to improve patient response to ergotamine, analgesics and sedatives in migraine, perhaps by enhancing absorption of the other medications.

Contraindications:

When stimulation of GI motility might be dangerous (eg, in the presence of GI hemorrhage, mechanical obstruction or perforation).

In pheochromocytoma, as the drug may cause a hypertensive crisis, probably due to release of catecholamines from the tumor. Control such crises with phentolamine.

In patients with known sensitivity or intolerance to metoclopramide.

In epileptics or in patients receiving drugs likely to cause extrapyramidal reactions, the frequency and severity of seizures or extrapyramidal reactions may be increased.

(Continued on following page)

METOCLOPRAMIDE (Cont.)

Warnings:

Extrapyramidal symptoms occur in 0.2% to 1% of patients. They occur more frequently in children and young adults and at the higher doses used in prophylaxis of vomiting due to cancer chemotherapy. Treat with 50 mg diphenhydramine IM. Symptoms include involuntary movements of limbs and facial grimacing; torticollis, oculogyric crisis, rhythmic protrusion of tongue, bulbar type of speech, trismus or dystonic reactions resembling tetanus. Rare persistent dyskinesias have been reported.

Depression may be related to metoclopramide administration.

Usage in Pregnancy: Category B. Studies in animals at 12 to 250 times the human dose have revealed no evidence of impaired fertility or significant fetal harm. However, the drug does cross the human placental barrier to the fetus. There are no well controlled studies in pregnant women. Use only when clearly needed and when the potential benefits outweigh the unknown potential hazards to the fetus.

Usage in Lactation: Metoclopramide readily enters into breast milk and may concentrate at about twice the plasma level at 2 hours postdose. Exercise caution when administering to a nursing mother.

Usage in Children: Methemoglobinemia has been reported in premature and full term neonates given metoclopramide IM, 1 to 2 mg/kg/day for 3 or more days; this was not reported at 0.5 mg/kg/day. Reverse methemoglobinemia by IV administration of methylene blue.

Precautions:

Hypoglycemia: Gastroparesis (gastric stasis) may be responsible for poor diabetic control. Exogenously administered insulins may act before food has left the stomach, leading to hypoglycemia.

Potentially hazardous tasks: May cause drowsiness; observe caution while driving or performing other tasks requiring alertness.

Carcinogenesis: Elevated prolactin levels persist during chronic administration. Approximately one-third of human breast cancers are prolactin-dependent in vitro; use caution if metoclopramide is contemplated in a patient with previously detected breast cancer. Although galactorrhea, amenorrhea, gynecomastia and impotence have been reported with prolactin-elevating drugs, the clinical significance of elevated serum prolactin levels is unknown. An increase in mammary neoplasms has been found in rodents after chronic administration of prolactin-stimulating neuroleptic drugs; however, studies have not shown an association and evidence is not conclusive.

Drug Interactions:

Anticholinergic drugs and **narcotic analgesics:** Metoclopramide effects on GI motility are antagonized by these drugs.

Alcohol, sedatives, hypnotics, narcotics or **tranquilizers:** Additive sedative effects may occur.

Absorption of drugs from the stomach may be diminished (eg, **digoxin, cimetidine**) by metoclopramide, whereas absorption of drugs from the small bowel may be accelerated (eg, **acetaminophen, tetracycline, levodopa, ethanol**). Although metoclopramide increases ethanol absorption, other factors may account for synergistic sedation.

Insulin: Metoclopramide influences the delivery of food to the intestines and the rate of absorption; therefore, dosage or timing of insulin may require adjustment.

Phenothiazine, butyrophenone and **thioxanthine drugs:** Concomitant use with metoclopramide may potentiate extrapyramidal effects.

Adverse Reactions:

Approximately 20% to 30% of patients experience side effects that are usually mild, transient and reversible upon drug withdrawal. High doses of 2 mg/kg for control of cisplatin-induced vomiting have produced CNS and GI side effects with an incidence of 81% and 43%, respectively.

CNS (12% to 24%): Restlessness, drowsiness, fatigue, lassitude ($\approx$ 10%); extrapyramidal reactions (1% to 9%) and parkinsonism-like reactions; akathisia (1% to 8%); dizziness (3%); anxiety, dystonia, insomnia, headache; myoclonus; rarely, depression and persistent dyskinesia.

GI (2% to 9%): Nausea; diarrhea.

Cardiovascular: Transient hypertension. A single instance of supraventricular tachycardia following IM administration has been reported.

Miscellaneous: Elevated serum prolactin levels may cause galactorrhea, reversible amenorrhea, nipple tenderness and gynecomastia in males.

(Continued on following page)

METOCLOPRAMIDE (Cont.)

Overdosage:

Symptoms: Drowsiness, disorientation and extrapyramidal reactions which are self-limiting and usually disappear within 24 hours. Muscle hypertonia, irritability and agitation are common.

Treatment: Anticholinergic or antiparkinson drugs or antihistamines with anticholinergic properties may help control extrapyramidal reactions. Hemodialysis appears ineffective in removing metoclopramide. See also General Management of Acute Overdosage on p. 2895

Patient Information:

May produce drowsiness and dizziness; observe caution while driving or performing other tasks requiring alertness.

Notify physician if involuntary movement of eyes, face or limbs occurs.

Take medication 30 minutes before each meal.

Administration and Dosage:

Relief of symptoms associated with diabetic gastroparesis: 10 mg orally, 30 minutes before each meal and at bedtime for 2 to 8 weeks.

Determine initial route of administration by the severity of symptoms. With only the earliest manifestations of diabetic gastric stasis, initiate oral administration. If symptoms are severe, begin with parenteral therapy. Administer 10 mg IV over 1 to 2 minutes. Parenteral administration up to 10 days may be required before symptoms subside, then oral administration may be instituted. Reinstitute therapy at the earliest manifestation.

Rectal administration: For outpatient treatment when oral dosing is not possible, suppositories containing 25 mg metoclopramide have been extemporaneously compounded (5 pulverized oral tablets in polyethylene glycol). Administer 1 suppository 30 to 60 minutes before each meal and at bedtime.[1]

Symptomatic gastroesophageal reflux: 10 to 15 mg orally up to 4 times daily 30 minutes before each meal and at bedtime. If symptoms occur only intermittently or at specific times of the day, single doses up to 20 mg prior to the provoking situation may be preferred rather than continuous treatment. Guide therapy directed at esophageal lesions by endoscopy. Therapy longer than 12 weeks has not been evaluated and cannot be recommended.

Prevention of chemotherapy-induced emesis: For doses in excess of 10 mg, dilute injection in 50 ml of a parenteral solution (Dextrose 5% in Water, Sodium Chloride Injection, Dextrose 5% in 0.45% Sodium Chloride, Ringer's Injection or Lactated Ringer's Injection). Infuse slowly IV over not less than 15 minutes, 30 minutes before beginning cancer chemotherapy; repeat every 2 hours for 2 doses, then every 3 hours for 3 doses.

The initial 2 doses should be 2 mg/kg if highly emetogenic drugs such as cisplatin or dacarbazine are used alone or in combination. For less emetogenic regimens, 1 mg/kg/dose may be adequate.

If extrapyramidal symptoms occur, administer 50 mg diphenhydramine IM.

Direct IV injection: Inject slowly IV over 1 to 2 minutes. A transient but intense feeling of anxiety and restlessness, followed by drowsiness, may occur with rapid administration.

Facilitation of small bowel intubation - If the tube has not passed the pylorus with conventional maneuvers in 10 minutes, administer a single dose slowly IV over 1 to 2 minutes.

The recommended single dose is -

Adults: 10 mg (2 ml).

Children (6 to 14 years): 2.5 to 5 mg (0.5 to 1 ml).

Children (under 6 years): 0.1 mg/kg.

Radiological examinations - In patients where delayed gastric emptying interferes with radiological examination of the stomach or small intestine, a single dose may be administered slowly IV over 1 to 2 minutes.

(Administration and Dosage continued on following page)

[1] *Arch Intern Med* 1986;146:2278-79.

METOCLOPRAMIDE (Cont.)

Administration and Dosage (Cont.):

Admixture and Compatibilities:

Physically and chemically compatible up to 48 hours – Cimetidine; mannitol; potassium acetate; potassium chloride; potassium phosphate.

Physcially compatible up to 48 hours – Ascorbic acid; benztropine; cytarabine; dexamethasone sodium phosphate; diphenhydramine; doxorubicin; heparin sodium; hydrocortisone sodium phosphate; lidocaine; magnesium sulfate; vitamine B complex with ascorbic acid.

Incompatible – Cephalothin; chloramphenicol; sodium bicarbonate.

	Product	Form	Description	C.I.*
Rx	**Metoclopramide HCl** (Various, eg, Goldline, Invamed, Major)	**Tablets:** 5 mg metoclopramide HCl (as monohydrochloride monohydrate)	In 100s, 500s and 1000s.	NA
Rx	**Reglan** (Robins)		Lactose. (Reglan 5 AHR). Green. Elliptical. In 100s and *Dis-Co* UD 100s.	30
Rx	**Metoclopramide** (Various, eg, Geneva, Goldline, Invamed, Major, Martec, Parmed, Rugby, Schein, Warner Chilcott)	**Tablets:** 10 mg (as monohydrochloride monohydrate)	In 100s, 500s, 1000s, 2500s and UD 100s.	12+
Rx	**Maxolon** (SK-Beecham)		Lactose. (BMP 192). Blue, scored. In 100s.	20
Rx	**Reglan** (Robins)		(Reglan AHR 10). Pink, scored. Capsule shape. In 100s, 500s and *Dis-Co* UD 100s.	50
Rx	**Metoclopramide HCl** (Various, eg, Goldline, Major, Roxane, Rugby, Warner Chilcott)	**Syrup:** 5 mg/5 ml (as monohydrochloride monohydrate)	In pt and UD 10 ml.	62+
Rx *sf*	**Reglan** (Robins)		Parabens, sorbitol. In pt and *Dis-Co* UD 10 ml (100s).	77
Rx	**Metoclopramide HCl** (Various, eg, DuPont, Smith + Nephew Solopak)	**Injection:** 5 mg/ml (as monohydrochloride monohydrate)	In 2, 10, 20 and 30 ml vials and 2 ml amps.	292
Rx	**Octamide PFS** (Adria)		Preservative free. In 2, 10 and 30 ml single-dose vials.	NA
Rx	**Reglan** (Robins)		Preservative free. In 2 and 10 ml amps and 2, 10 and 30 ml vials.	380

* Cost Index based on cost per 10 mg.

sf – Sugar free.

DEXPANTHENOL (Dextro-Pantothenyl Alcohol)

Actions:

Dexpanthenol is the alcohol analog of D-pantothenic acid. Pantothenic acid is a precursor of coenzyme A, which is a cofactor for enzyme-catalyzed reactions involving transfer of acetyl groups. The final step in acetylcholine synthesis is the choline acetylase transfer of an acetyl group from acetylcoenzyme A to choline. Acetylcholine, the neurohumoral transmitter in the parasympathetic system, maintains normal intestinal functions. Decreased acetylcholine content results in decreased peristalsis and in extreme cases, adynamic ileus. Dexpanthenol's mechanism of action is unknown.

Choline, in addition to being the precursor for acetylcholine, is essential for normal transport of fat, as a constituent of the phospholipid lecithin and as an intermediary methyl donor. Choline has the same pharmacological actions as acetylcholine, but is less active; single oral 10 g doses produce no obvious pharmacodynamic response.

Indications:

Prophylactic use immediately after major abdominal surgery to minimize paralytic ileus. Intestinal atony causing abdominal distention; postoperative or postpartum retention of flatus; postoperative delay in resumption of intestinal motility; paralytic ileus.

Contraindications:

Hemophilia; ileus due to mechanical obstruction.

Warnings:

Usage in Pregnancy and Lactation: Category C. Safety for use during pregnancy and lactation has not been established. Use only when clearly needed and when the potential benefits outweigh the unknown potential hazards to the fetus or nursing infant.

Usage in Children: Safety and efficacy for use in children have not been established.

Precautions:

Hypersensitivity: If signs of a hypersensitivity reaction appear, discontinue drug. Refer to Management of Acute Hypersensitivity Reactions.

Mechanical obstruction: If ileus is secondary to mechanical obstruction, direct primary attention to the obstruction. Management of adynamic ileus includes: Correction of any fluid and electrolyte imbalance (especially hypokalemia), anemia and hypoproteinemia; treatment of infection; avoidance of drugs which decrease GI motility; and GI tract decompression by nasogastric suction or by use of a long intestinal tube.

Drug Interactions:

Antibiotics or **narcotics:** Allergic reactions have occurred rarely during concomitant use of dexpanthenol.

Succinylcholine: Temporary respiratory difficulty occurred following dexpanthenol administration 5 minutes after succinylcholine was discontinued. Its effects appeared to have been prolonged. Do not administer within 1 hour of succinylcholine.

Adverse Reactions:

Itching; tingling; dyspnea; red patches of skin; generalized dermatitis; urticaria; slight drop in blood pressure; intestinal colic (½ hour after administration); vomiting; diarrhea (10 days postsurgery); agitation in an elderly patient. Causal relationship is uncertain.

Administration and Dosage:

Prevention of postoperative adynamic ileus: 250 or 500 mg IM. Repeat in 2 hours, followed by doses every 6 hours, or until danger of adynamic ileus has passed.

Treatment of adynamic ileus: 500 mg IM. Repeat in 2 hours, followed by doses every 6 hours, as needed.

IV administration: Not for direct IV administration. The 500 mg dose has been mixed with IV bulk solutions such as glucose or Lactated Ringer's and infused slowly IV.

				C.I.*
Rx	**Dexpanthenol** (Various)	**Injection:** 250 mg per ml	In 10 and 30 ml vials.	33+
Rx	**Ilopan** (Adria)		In 2 ml amps and 2 ml disp. syringes.	353

DEXPANTHENOL WITH CHOLINE BITARTRATE

Indications:

May help relieve gas retention associated with splenic flexure syndrome, cholecystitis, gastritis, gastric hyperacidity, irritable colon, regional ileitis, postantibiotic and postoperative gas retention or during laxative withdrawal.

Administration and Dosage:

Take 2 to 3 tablets, 3 times daily.

			C.I.*
Rx	**Ilopan-Choline** (Adria)	**Tablets:** 50 mg dexpanthenol and 25 mg choline bitartrate. (#Adria 231). White. In 100s and 500s.	228

* Cost Index based on cost per 250 mg dexpanthenol.

Product identification code.

Actions:

Pharmacology: Pancreatin and pancrelipase hydrolyze fats to glycerol and fatty acids, change protein into proteoses and derived substances, and convert starch into dextrins and sugars. Administration reduces the fat and nitrogen content in the stool. These agents exert their primary effects in the duodenum and upper jejunum. Pancreatic enzymes are normally secreted in great excess. There is a tenfold reserve for exocrine pancreatic enzyme secretion. Generally, steatorrhea and malabsorption occur only after a $\geq$ 90% reduction in secretion of lipase and proteolytic enzymes. It has been estimated that $\approx$ 8000 units of lipase per hour should be delivered into the duodenum postprandially. Even if all the enzymes taken orally reached the proximal intestine in active form, ingestion of 24,000 units of lipase (8000 units per hour) for 3 postprandial hours would be required. If one could deliver sufficient pancreatic enzymes to the small intestine, malabsorption could be corrected. It is rarely possible to achieve complete relief of steatorrhea although major improvement in fat absorption can be achieved in most patients.

There are many factors which may influence the ability to deliver pancreatic enzymes to the duodenum including asynchrony of gastric emptying of food and enzyme, sensitivity of pancreatic enzymes to permanent inactivation by gastric acid and pepsin secreted in response to the meal, and acidic precipitation of bile acids.

Pancreatic lipase is irreversibly inactivated at pH $\leq$ 4. An enteric coating may prevent destruction or inactivation by gastric pepsin and acid pH, but may inhibit enzyme delivery to the duodenum. Cimetidine or antacids may increase the amount of pancreatin in the duodenum by decreasing its destruction by the gastric acid.

Pancreatic Extract Activity

Enzyme concentrate	Source	Minimal USP standards (USP units/mg)		
		Lipase	Protease	Amylase
Pancrelipase	Porcine	24	100	100
Pancreatin	Bovine, porcine or vegetable	2	25	25

Indications:

Enzyme replacement therapy in patients with deficient exocrine pancreatic secretions, cystic fibrosis, chronic pancreatitis, postpancreatectomy, ductal obstructions caused by cancer of the pancreas or common bile duct, pancreatic insufficiency and for steatorrhea of malabsorption syndrome and postgastrectomy (Billroth II and Total) or, post-GI surgery (eg, Billroth II gastroenterostomy).

Presumptive test for pancreatic function, especially in pancreatic insufficiency due to chronic pancreatitis.

Contraindications:

Hypersensitivity to pork protein or enzymes; acute pancreatitis; acute exacerbations of chronic pancreatic diseases.

Warnings:

Replacement therapy: Pancreatic exocrine replacement therapy should not delay or supplant treatment of the primary disorder.

Pregnancy: Category C. It is not known whether the drug can cause fetal harm when administered to a pregnant woman or can affect reproduction capacity. Give to a pregnant woman only if clearly needed. The enteric coating component, diethyl phthalate, has been teratogenic in rats with high intraperitoneal dosing.

Lactation: It is not known whether pancreatin is excreted in breast milk. Exercise caution when administering to a nursing mother.

Precautions:

Excessive doses may cause nausea, abdominal cramps or diarrhea. Extremely high doses have been associated with hyperuricosuria and hyperuricemia.

Pork sensitivity: Use pork products with caution in patients sensitive to pork. Discontinue use if symptoms of sensitivity appear and initiate symptomatic and supportive treatment if necessary. Individuals previously sensitized to trypsin, pancreatin or pancrelipase may have allergic reactions.

Irritation of skin/mucous membranes: Do not spill powder on hands since it may irritate skin. The dust of finely powdered concentrates irritates the nasal mucosa and the respiratory tract. Inhalation of airborne powder can precipitate an asthma attack. Asthma can also occur in patients sensitized to pancreatic enzyme concentrates.

(Continued on following page)

Drug Interactions:

Antacids: Calcium carbonate or magnesium hydroxide may negate the beneficial effect of the enzymes.

Iron: The serum iron response to oral iron may be decreased by concomitant pancreatic extracts.

Adverse Reactions:

The most frequently reported adverse reactions are GI in nature. Less frequently, allergic-type reactions have also been observed. Perianal irritation may occur with pancreatin and rarely, inflammation with large doses.

Overdosage:

Overdosage may cause diarrhea or transient intestinal upset.

Patient Information:

Take before or with meals.

Do not inhale powder dosage form or powder from capsules since it may irritate skin or mucous membranes.

To protect enteric coating, do not crush or chew the microspheres/tablets in the enteric coated capsule formulations. Microsphere contact with foods having a pH > 5.5 can dissolve the enteric shell.

Do not change brands without consulting with the physician or pharmacist.

Administration:

Microspheres/Microtablets: To protect enteric coating, do not crush or chew the microspheres or microtablets. Where swallowing of capsules is difficult, they may be opened and shaken onto a small quantity of soft non-hot food (eg, applesauce, gelatin), which does not require chewing. Swallow immediately without chewing as the proteolytic action may cause irritation of the mucosa. Follow with a glass of juice or water to ensure complete swallowing of the microspheres/microtablets. Contact of the microspheres/microtablets with foods having a pH > 5.5 can dissolve the protective enteric shell. Use any mixture of food or liquid with the microspheres/microtablets immediately; do not store.

Brand interchange: These products are not bioequivalent. Therefore, do not substitute one brand for another without first consulting the physician.

PANCRELIPASE

Dosage:

Adjust dosage according to the severity of the exocrine pancreatic enzyme deficiency. Estimate dosage by assessing which dose minimizes steatorrhea and maintains good nutritional status. The assessment of the end points in children is aided by charting growth curves.

Capsules and tablets:

Children – < 6 months old, dosage not established.

6 months to 1 year, 2000 units lipase per meal.

1 to 6 years, 4000 to 8000 units lipase with each meal and 4000 units with snacks.

7 to 12 years, 4000 to 12,000 units lipase (or more if necessary) with each meal and with snacks.

Adults – 4000 to 48,000 units lipase with each meal and with snacks.

In patients with pancreatectomy or obstruction of pancreatic ducts, administer 8000 to 16,000 units lipase at 2 hour intervals or as directed by physician *(Viokase).* In severe deficiencies, the dose may be increased to 64,000 to 88,000 units lipase with meals or the frequency of administration may increase to hourly intervals if nausea, cramps or diarrhea do not occur.

Powder (in cystic fibrosis): 0.7 g with meals.

(Products listed on following page)

Refer to the general discussion of these products on page 1627

PANCRELIPASE (Cont.)

Content given per capsule, tablet or 0.7 g powder.

	Product and Distributor	Lipase (units)	Protease (units)	Amylase (units)	Other Content	How Supplied	C.I.*
Rx	**Pancrease MT 4 Capsules** (McNeil)	4,000	12,000	12,000	Parabens	Enteric coated micro-tablets. (McNeil Pancrease MT 4). Yellow/clear. In 100s.	2.7
Rx	**Pancrease Capsules** (McNeil)	4,000	25,000	20,000	Sugar	Dye free. Enteric coated microspheres. (McNeil Pancrease). White. In 100s and 250s.	2.1
Rx	**Pancrelipase Capsules** (Geneva)	4,000	25,000	20,000		Enteric coated pellets. White. In 100s and 250s.	2.1
Rx	**Protilase Capsules** (Rugby)					Enteric coated spheres. In 100s and 500s.	3.4
Rx	**Cotazym-S Capsules** (Organon)	5,000	20,000	20,000		Enteric coated spheres. (Organon 388). Clear. In 100s and 500s.	2.5
Rx	**Cotazym Capsules** (Organon)	8,000	30,000	30,000	25 mg calcium carbonate	(Organon 381). In 100s & 500s.	NA
Rx	**Ku-Zyme HP Capsules** (Schwarz Pharma Kremers-Urban)	8,000	30,000	30,000	Lactose	(Kremers Urban 525). White. In 100s.	2.1
Rx	**Viokase Tablets** (Robins)					(Viokase/AHR 9111). Tan. In 100s and 500s.	1.7
Rx	**Pancrease MT 10 Capsules** (McNeil)	10,000	30,000	30,000	Parabens	Enteric coated micro-tablets. (McNeil Pancrease MT 10). Pink/clear. In 100s.	6.7
Rx	**Ilozyme Tablets** (Adria)	11,000	≥ 30,000	≥ 30,000		(200). Buff. In 250s.	3.4
Rx	**Zymase Capsules** (Organon)	12,000	24,000	24,000		Enteric coated spheres. In 100s.	6.5
Rx	**Ultrase MT12 Capsules** (Scandipharm)	12,000	39,000	39,000		(Ultrase MT12). White/yellow. In 100s.	4.5
Rx	**Pancrease MT 16 Capsules** (McNeil)	16,000	48,000	48,000	Parabens	Enteric coated micro-tablets. (McNeil Pancrease MT 16). Salmon/clear. In 100s.	11
Rx	**Viokase Powder** (Robins)	16,800	70,000	70,000	Lactose	In 113.5 and 227 g.	6.4
Rx	**Ultrase MT20 Capsules** (Scandipharm)	20,000	65,000	65,000		(Ultrase MT20). Gray/yellow. In 100s.	7.3
Rx	**Ultrase MT24 Capsules** (Scandipharm)	24,000	78,000	78,000		(Ultrase MT24). Gray/orange. In 100s.	8.7

* Cost Index based on cost per capsule, tablet or 0.7 g of powder.

PANCREATIN

Dosage:

Take 1 to 2 with meals or snacks. Adjust according to individual requirements for control of steatorrhea.

Content given per tablet or capsule.

	Product and Distributor	Pancreatin (mg)	Lipase (units)	Protease (units)	Amylase (units)	How Supplied	C.I.*
otc	**Dizymes Tablets** (Recsei)	250	6,750	41,250	43,750	Enteric coated. In 100s and 500s.	1
Rx	**Entozyme Tablets** (Robins)	300	600	7,500	7,500	Sucrose. (AHR 5050). White. In 100s.	NA
Rx	**Donnazyme Tablets** (Robins)	500	1,000	12,500	12,500	Parabens, sucrose. Green. In 100s.	NA
otc sf	**Pancrezyme 4X Tablets** (Vitaline)	2,400	12,000	60,000	60,000	In 90s	NA
otc sf	**4X Pancreatin 600 mg Tablets** (Vitaline)					In 90s.	1.1
otc sf	**Hi-Vegi-Lip Tablets** (Freeda)	2,400	4,800	60,000	60,000	In 100s and 250s.	NA
otc sf	**8X Pancreatin 900 mg Tablets** (Vitaline)	7,200	22,500	180,000	180,000	In 60s.	2
Rx	**Creon Capsules** (Solvay)	Strength not known	8,000	13,000	30,000	Enteric coated microspheres. Brown/clear. In 100s and 250s.	3.5

GASTRIC ACIDIFIERS

Actions:

Gastric acidifiers counterbalance a deficiency of hydrochloric acid in the gastric juice and destroy or inhibit growth of putrefactive microorganisms in ingested food. A deficiency of hydrochloric acid is often associated with pernicious anemia, allergies, gastric carcinoma and congenital achlorhydria.

Contraindications:

Gastric hyperacidity or peptic ulcer.

GLUTAMIC ACID HCl

340 mg contains approximately 1.8 mEq hydrochloric acid.

Dose:

1 to 3 capsules 3 times daily before meals.

	Product	Strength	How Supplied	C.I.*
otc	**Glutamic Acid HCl** (Various)	**Capsules:** 340 mg	In 100s.	NA

* Cost Index based on cost per capsule or tablet.

sf – Sugar free.

DEHYDROCHOLIC ACID

Actions:

Pharmacology: Dehydrocholic acid is an oxidation product of cholic acid (a natural bile acid). At recommended dosage levels, dehydrocholic acid exerts laxative and hydrocholeretic (increased volume and water content of bile) actions. The mechanisms of action are unknown. Unlike the natural bile acids and their conjugates, dehydrocholic acid does not readily form micelles (small aggregates of bile acids, fats and phospholipids necessary for normal fat absorption).

Indications:

Temporary relief of constipation.

Adjunctive therapy of biliary stasis, without complete mechanical obstruction of the common or hepatic bile ducts, where hydrocholeresis is desired.

Contraindications:

Significant cholelithiasis; presence of jaundice; marked hepatic insufficiency; complete obstruction of the common or hepatic bile ducts or of the GI or GU tracts; hypersensitivity to bile acids or their conjugates; use as a diuretic or adjunct.

Warnings:

Rectal bleeding or failure to have a bowel movement after use as a laxative may indicate a serious condition. Discontinue use and consult a physician.

Duration: Do not use as a laxative for > 1 week unless directed otherwise.

GI effects: Do not use as a laxative if abdominal pain, nausea or vomiting are present unless directed otherwise.

Elderly: Use with caution. If promotion of true bile flow is desired, use a cholagogue.

Children: No data supporting a recommended pediatric dose are available. Therefore, do not use in children < 12 years of age.

Adverse Reactions:

Hypersensitivity (pruritus, dermatitis).

Administration and Dosage:

250 to 500 mg 3 times daily after meals. Thereafter, titrate dosage to individual patient's needs. Do not exceed 1.5 g in 24 hours.

When used as a laxative, a bowel movement is generally produced in 6 to 12 hours.

				C.I.*
Rx	**Dehydrocholic Acid** (Various, eg, Goldline)	**Tablets:** 250 mg	In 100s.	87+
otc	**Cholan-HMB** (Fisons)		Lactose. Dye free. (Cholan HMB). In 100s.	333
otc	**Decholin** (Miles Pharm.)		Lactose. In 100s.	420

* Cost Index based on cost per 250 mg.

These products are used in the symptomatic treatment of various digestive dysfunctions, to supplement deficiencies of natural digestive enzymes and for a variety of vague GI disorders. Treat specific deficiency states with the deficient substance rather than with a mixture of components.

Components of these combinations include:

DIGESTIVE ENZYMES

Pepsin and papain aid in protein digestion.

Pancreatic enzymes (see individual monograph) aid in the intestinal digestion of starch, fat and protein.

Cellulase aids in dietary cellulose digestion.

DEHYDROCHOLIC ACID (see individual monograph) and *DESOXYCHOLIC ACID* increase secretion of bile and aid in digestion of fats.

ANTICHOLINERGICS relieve spasm and reduce hypermotility (see GI Anticholinergic/Antispasmodic monograph).

BARBITURATES (see individual monograph) and *PHENYLTOLOXAMINE CITRATE*, an antihistamine, are used for their sedative effects.

Dosage:

Capsules and tablets: Take 1 to 3 with or after meals (see individual dosing instructions).

				C.I.*
Rx	**Arco-Lase Plus** (Arco)	**Tablets:** 30 mg amylase, 6 mg protease, 25 mg lipase, 2 mg cellulase, 0.1 mg hyoscyamine sulfate, 0.02 mg atropine sulfate, 7.5 mg phenobarbital	In 50s.	148
Rx	**Bilezyme** (Geriatric Pharm.)	**Tablets:** 30 mg amylase, 6 mg protease, 200 mg dehydrocholic acid, 50 mg desoxycholic acid	In 42s, 100s and 500s.	NA
Rx	**Digestozyme** (Various, eg, Major)	**Tablets:** 300 mg pancreatin, 250 mg pepsin, 25 mg dehydrocholic acid	In 50s, 100s and 1000s.	71+
otc	**Gustase** (Geriatric Pharm.)	**Tablets:** 30 mg amylase, 6 mg protease, 2 mg cellulase	In 42s, 100s and 500s.	NA
Rx	**Gustase Plus** (Geriatric Pharm.)	**Tablets:** 30 mg amylase, 6 mg protease, 2 mg cellulase, 2.5 mg homatropine MBr, 8 mg phenobarbital	In 42s, 100s and 500s.	NA
Rx	**Kutrase** (Schwarz Pharma Kremers Urban)	**Capsules:** 30 mg amylase, 6 mg protease, 75 mg lipase, 2 mg cellulase, 0.0625 mg hyoscyamine sulfate, 15 mg phenyltoloxamine citrate	Lactose. (Kremers Urban 475). Green and white. In 100s.	422
Rx	**Ku-Zyme** (Schwarz Pharma Kremers Urban)	**Capsules:** 30 mg amylase, 6 mg protease, 75 mg lipase, 2 mg cellulase	Lactose. (Kremers Urban 522). Yellow and white. In 100s.	333
otc	**Arco-Lase** (Arco)	**Tablets, chewable:** 30 mg amylase, 6 mg protease, 25 mg lipase, 2 mg cellulase	Mint flavor. In 50s.	148
otc	**Enzyme** (Nature's Bounty)	**Tablets, chewable:** 30 mg amylase, 6 mg protease, 2 mg cellulase, 25 mg lipase	In 100s.	NA
otc	**Papaya Enzyme** (Nature's Bounty)	**Tablets, chewable:** 60 mg papain (from papaya leaves) and 60 mg amylase	In 100s.	NA

* Cost Index based on cost per capsule or tablet.

CHENODIOL (Chenodeoxycholic Acid)

Because of potential hepatotoxicity and poor response rates in some subgroups of chenodiol-treated patients, this agent is not appropriate treatment for many patients with gallstones. Reserve chenodiol for carefully selected patients and monitor for liver function alterations. (See Warnings.)

Actions:

Pharmacology: Chenodiol is a naturally occurring human bile acid. It suppresses hepatic synthesis of both cholesterol and cholic acid, gradually replacing cholic acid and its metabolite, deoxycholic acid, in an expanded bile acid pool. These actions contribute to biliary cholesterol desaturation and gradual dissolution of radiolucent cholesterol gallstones. Chenodiol has no effect on radiopaque (calcified) gallstones or on radiolucent bile pigment stones.

Pharmacokinetics:

Absorption/Distribution – Chenodiol is well absorbed from the small intestine. It is conjugated by the liver and secreted in bile. Owing to 60% to 80% first-pass hepatic clearance, the body pool of chenodiol resides mainly in the enterohepatic circulation; serum and urinary bile acid levels are not significantly affected.

Metabolism/Excretion – At steady-state, an amount of chenodiol approximating the daily dose escapes to the colon and is converted by bacterial action to lithocholic acid. About 80% of the lithocholate is excreted in the feces; the remainder is absorbed and converted in the liver to poorly absorbed conjugates. There is only a minor increase in biliary lithocholate, while fecal bile acids are increased threefold to fourfold.

Clinical Pharmacology:

General clinical results - In the National Cooperative Gallstone Study (NCGS) involving 305 patients in each treatment group, placebo and chenodiol dosages of 375 mg and 750 mg/day showed that stone dissolution rates achieved with chenodiol treatment are higher in subgroups having certain pretreatment characteristics. The studies and results are summarized in the table.

Criteria	NCGS[1]			Uncontrolled Trials 13-16 mg/kg/day
	Placebo	375 mg/day	750 mg/day	
Overall results				
Complete dissolution rate in 24 months				
Overall	0.8%	5.2%	13.5%	28%-38%
Small (< 15 mm diameter) radiolucent stones			20%	42%-60%
Floatable Stones[2]				
Complete dissolution rate				
Small stones				70%
Biliary pain	47%		27%	
Cholecystectomy rate	19%		1.5%	
Nonfloatable Stones				
Complete dissolution rate				
Large stones				11%
Small stones				35%
Overall				27%
Cholecystectomy rate	4%		8%	

[1] National Cooperative Gallstone Study (NCGS), 305 patients/group, 916 patients total.
[2] In the NCSG, 17.8% of patients had floatable stones.

Even higher dissolution rates have been observed in patients with small floatable stones. For unknown reasons, some obese patients and occasional normal weight patients fail to achieve bile desaturation even with doses up to 19 mg/kg/day.

Although dissolution is generally higher with increased dosage of chenodiol, doses that are too low are associated with increased cholecystectomy rates.

(Actions continued on following page)

CHENODIOL (Chenodeoxycholic Acid) (Cont.)

Actions (Cont.):

Clinical Pharmacology (Cont.):

Other radiographic and laboratory features – Pigment stones and partially calcified radiolucent stones do not respond to chenodiol. As stone size, number and volume increase, the probability of dissolution within 24 months decreases.

Patient selection/evaluation of surgical risk – Surgery offers the advantage of immediate and permanent stone removal, but carries a fairly high risk in some patients. About 5% of cholecystectomized patients have residual symptoms or retain common duct stones.

Women in good health, or having only moderate systemic disease, under 49 years of age have the lowest surgical mortality rate (0.054%); men in all categories have a rate twice that of women; common duct exploration quadruples the rates in all categories; the rates rise with each decade of life and increase tenfold or more in all categories with severe or extreme systemic disease.

Stones have recurred within 5 years in about 50% of patients following complete confirmed dissolutions. Although retreatment with chenodiol has proven successful in dissolving newly formed stones, the long-term consequences of repeated courses in terms of liver toxicity, neoplasia and elevated cholesterol levels are not known.

The patient most likely to respond to chenodiol therapy is a thin woman with serum cholesterol $\geq$ 227 mg/dl having a small number of small floatable, radiolucent (cholesterol) gallstones, and able to tolerate the higher recommended doses for 24 months.

Indications:

For patients with radiolucent stones in well-opacifying gallbladders, in whom elective surgery would be undertaken except for the presence of increased surgical risk due to systemic disease or age. The likelihood of successful dissolution is far greater if the stones are floatable or small.

Contraindications:

Known hepatocyte dysfunction or bile ductal abnormalities such as intrahepatic cholestasis, primary biliary cirrhosis or sclerosing cholangitis; a gallbladder confirmed as nonvisualizing after two consecutive single doses of dye; radiopaque or radiolucent bile pigment stones; or gallstone complications or compelling reasons for gallbladder surgery including unremitting acute cholecystitis, cholangitis, biliary obstruction, gallstone pancreatitis or biliary GI fistula.

Usage in Pregnancy: Category X. Chenodiol may cause fetal harm when administered to a pregnant woman. Serious hepatic, renal and adrenal lesions occurred in fetuses of Rhesus monkeys given 4 to 6 times the maximum recommended human dose (MRHD). Hepatic lesions also occurred in neonatal baboons whose mothers had received 1 to 2 times the MRHD during pregnancy. Fetal malformations were not observed. No human data are available at this time. Chenodiol is contraindicated in women who are or who may become pregnant. If this drug is used during pregnancy, or if the patient becomes pregnant while taking this drug, apprise her of the potential hazard to the fetus.

Warnings:

Hepatic effects: Chenodiol is unequivocally hepatotoxic in many animal species, including sub-human primates at doses close to the human dose. Although the theoretical cause is the metabolite, lithocholic acid, an established hepatotoxin, and man has an efficient mechanism for sulfating and eliminating this substance, there is some evidence that the demonstrated hepatotoxicity is partly due to chenodiol *per se.*

Humans can form sulfate conjugates of lithocholic acid. Variation in this capacity has not been well established; patients who develop chenodiol-induced serum aminotransferase elevations may be poor sulfators of lithocholic acid.

Safe use of chenodiol depends upon selection of patients without preexisting liver disease and upon monitoring of serum aminotransferase levels. Aminotransferase elevations over 3 times the upper limit of normal have required discontinuation of chenodiol in 2% to 3% of patients. Although clinical and biopsy studies have not shown fulminant lesions, an occasional patient may develop serious hepatic disease.

Three patients with biochemical and histologic pictures of chronic active hepatitis while on chenodiol, 375 or 750 mg/day, have been reported. The biochemical abnormalities returned spontaneously to normal in two of the patients within 13 and 17 months, and after 17 months of prednisone in the third. The causal relationship could not be determined. Another patient was terminated from therapy because of elevated aminotransferase levels and a liver biopsy showing active drug hepatitis.

One patient with sclerosing cholangitis, biliary cirrhosis and a history of jaundice died during chenodiol treatment for hepatic duct stones. A contribution of chenodiol to the fatal outcome could not be ruled out.

(Warnings continued on following page)

CHENODIOL (Chenodeoxycholic Acid) (Cont.)

Warnings (Cont.):

Colon cancer: The possibility that chenodiol therapy might contribute to colon cancer in otherwise susceptible individuals cannot be ruled out.

Usage in Pregnancy: Category X. See Contraindications.

Usage in Lactation: Safety for use in the nursing mother has not been established.

Usage in Children: Safety and efficacy for use in children have not been established.

Precautions:

Carcinogenesis, mutagenesis and impairment of fertility: Chenodiol given in long-term studies at oral doses 40 to 65 times the maximum recommended human dose induced benign and malignant liver cell tumors in female rats and cholangiomata in female rats and male mice. The dietary administration of lithocholic acid to chickens is reported to cause hepatic adenomatous hyperplasia.

Drug Interactions:

Bile acid sequestering agents, such as cholestyramine and colestipol, may interfere with the action of chenodiol by reducing its absorption.

Aluminum-based antacids have been shown to adsorb bile acids in vitro, and may interfere with chenodiol in the same manner as the sequestering agents.

Estrogens, oral contraceptives, clofibrate and perhaps other lipid-lowering drugs increase biliary cholesterol secretion and the incidence of cholesterol gallstones; as a result, these drugs may counteract the effectiveness of chenodiol.

Adverse Reactions:

Hepatobiliary: Dose-related serum aminotransferase (mainly SGPT) elevations, usually not accompanied by rises in alkaline phosphatase or bilirubin, occurred in 20% to 50% of patients treated with the recommended dose of chenodiol. Most elevations were minor (1½ to 3 times the upper limit of laboratory normal) and transient, returning to the normal range within 6 months, despite continued administration. In 2% to 3% of patients, SGPT levels rose to over 3 times the upper limit of laboratory normal, recurred on rechallenge with the drug, and required chenodiol discontinuation. Enzyme levels returned to normal following withdrawal of chenodiol.

Morphologic studies before and after 9 and 24 months of chenodiol treatment show that 63% of patients had evidence of intrahepatic cholestasis prior to treatment. Almost all pretreatment patients had electron microscopic abnormalities. By the ninth treatment month, reexamination showed an 89% incidence of signs of intrahepatic cholestasis.

Increased cholecystectomy rates: NCGS patients with a history of biliary pain prior to treatment had higher cholecystectomy rates during the study if assigned to low dosage chenodiol (375 mg/day) than if assigned to either placebo or high dosage chenodiol (750 mg/day). (Refer to the table on p. 1633)

GI: Dose-related diarrhea (30% to 50%) may occur at any time during treatment, but most commonly at treatment initiation. Usually, the diarrhea is mild and transient. Dose reduction has been required in 10% to 15% of patients; about half of these may require a permanent dose reduction. Antidiarrheal agents are useful in some patients. Discontinuation of chenodiol is expected in approximately 3% of patients.

Less frequent GI side effects include cramps, nausea, vomiting, flatulence, dyspepsia (4% to 9% in one study); biliary pain (10% to 30%); heartburn, constipation, anorexia, epigastric distress and nonspecific abdominal pain.

Serum lipids: Serum total cholesterol and low density lipoprotein (LDL) cholesterol may rise 10% or more during administration of chenodiol; no change has been seen in the high density lipoprotein (HDL) fraction; average decreases of 14% in serum triglyceride levels have been reported.

Hematologic: Decreases in white cell count, never below 3000, have been noted in a few patients; the drug was continued in all patients without incident.

(Continued on following page)

CHENODIOL (Chenodeoxycholic Acid) (Cont.)

Overdosage:

Accidental or intentional overdoses have not been reported. One patient tolerated 4 g/day (58 mg/kg/day) for 6 months without incident.

Patient Information:

Counsel patients on the importance of periodic visits for liver function tests and oral cholecystograms (or ultrasonograms) for monitoring stone dissolution.

Patients should see a physician immediately if any symptoms of gallstone complications occur (ie, nonspecific abdominal pain; severe, sudden right upper quadrant pain radiating to shoulder; nausea; vomiting).

Instruct patients on compliance with the dosage regimen.

Temporary dose reduction may relieve diarrhea; patients should consult physician.

Administration and Dosage:

The recommended dose range is 13 to 16 mg/kg/day in 2 divided doses, morning and night, starting with 250 mg twice daily the first 2 weeks and increasing by 250 mg/day each week thereafter until the recommended or maximum tolerated dose is reached. If diarrhea occurs, it can usually be controlled by temporary dosage adjustment until symptoms abate, after which the previous dose is usually tolerated. Dosage less than 10 mg/kg is usually ineffective and may be associated with *increased* risk of cholecystectomy.

Weight/Dosage Guide			
Body Weight		Recommended Dose Range	
lb	kg	Tablets/Day	mg/kg
100-130	45-58	3	17-13
131-165	59-75	4	17-13
166-200	76-90	5	16-14
201-235	91-107	6	16-14
236-275	108-125	7	16-14

Lab test monitoring: Monitor *serum aminotransferase levels* monthly for the first 3 months and every 3 months thereafter during administration. Under NCGS guidelines, if a minor, usually transient elevation (1½ to 3 times the upper limit of normal) persisted longer than 3 to 6 months, chenodiol was discontinued and resumed only after the aminotransferase level returned to normal; however, the safety of allowing minor elevations to persist over such an interval is not established. Elevations over 3 times the upper limit of normal require immediate discontinuation, and usually recur on challenge.

Monitor *serum cholesterol* at 6 month intervals. Discontinue chenodiol if cholesterol rises above the acceptable age-adjusted limit for a given patient.

Oral cholecystograms or ultrasonograms are recommended at 6 to 9 month intervals. Confirm complete dissolutions after 1 to 3 months of continued administration. Most patients who achieve complete dissolution will show partial (or complete) dissolution at the first on-treatment test. If partial dissolution is not seen by 9 to 12 months, the likelihood of success of continued treatment is greatly reduced; discontinue chenodiol if there is no response by 18 months.

Use beyond 24 months is not established.

Stone recurrence can be expected within 5 years in 50% of cases. After confirmed dissolution, stop treatment. Monitor serial cholecystograms or ultrasonograms for recurrence. A prophylactic dose is not established. Reduced doses cannot be recommended; stones have recurred on 500 mg/day. Low cholesterol or carbohydrate diets and dietary bran reportedly reduce biliary cholesterol; maintenance of reduced weight is recommended to forestall stone recurrence.

Rx	**Chenix** (Solvay Pharm.)	**Tablets:** 250 mg. (#Rowell 7720). White. Film coated. In 100s.

Product identification code.

URSODIOL (Ursodeoxycholic acid)

Gallbladder stone dissolution with ursodiol treatment requires months of therapy. Complete dissolution does not occur in all patients and recurrence of stones within 5 years has been observed in up to 50% of patients who do dissolve their stones on bile acid therapy. Carefully select patients for therapy with ursodiol, and consider alternative therapies.

Actions:

Pharmacology: Ursodiol, an agent intended for dissolution of radiolucent gallstones, is a naturally-occurring bile acid found in small quantities in normal human bile and in larger quantities in the biles of certain species of bears. Ursodiol suppresses hepatic synthesis and secretion of cholesterol, and also inhibits intestinal absorption of cholesterol. It has little inhibitory effect on synthesis and secretion into bile of endogenous bile acids, and does not appear to affect phospholipid secretion into bile.

With repeated dosing, bile ursodeoxycholic acid concentrations reach steady state in about 3 weeks. Although insoluble in aqueous media, cholesterol can be solubilized in at least two ways in the presence of dihydroxy bile acids. In addition to solubilizing cholesterol in micelles, ursodiol acts by an apparently unique mechanism to cause dispersion of cholesterol as liquid crystals in aqueous media. Thus, even though administration of high doses (eg, 15 to 18 mg/kg/day) does not result in a concentration of ursodiol higher than 60% of the total bile acid pool, ursodiol-rich bile solubilizes cholesterol. The overall effect of ursodiol is to increase the concentration level at which saturation of cholesterol occurs. The various actions of ursodiol combine to change the bile of patients with gallstones from cholesterol-precipitating to cholesterol-solubilizing.

After ursodiol dosing is stopped, its concentration in bile falls exponentially, declining to about 5% to 10% of its steady-state level in about 1 week.

Pharmacokinetics: About 90% of a therapeutic dose of ursodiol is absorbed in the small bowel after oral administration. After absorption, ursodiol enters the portal vein and undergoes extraction from portal blood by the liver (ie, "first pass" effect) where it is conjugated with either glycine or taurine and is then secreted into the hepatic bile ducts. Ursodiol in bile is concentrated in the gallbladder and expelled into the duodenum in gallbladder bile via the cystic and common ducts by gallbladder contractions provoked by physiologic responses to eating.

Small quantities of ursodiol appear in the systemic circulation and very small amounts are excreted into urine. A small portion of orally administered drug undergoes bacterial degradation with each cycle of enterohepatic circulation. Ursodiol can be both oxidized and reduced, yielding either 7-keto-lithocholic acid or lithocholic acid, respectively. Free ursodiol, 7-keto-lithocholic acid and lithocholic acid are relatively insoluble in aqueous media and larger proportions of these compounds are excreted via the feces. Reabsorbed free ursodiol is reconjugated by the liver. Eighty percent of lithocholic acid formed in the small bowel is excreted in the feces, but the 20% that is absorbed is sulfated in the liver to relatively insoluble lithocholyl conjugates which are excreted into bile and lost in feces. Absorbed 7-keto-lithocholic acid is stereospecifically reduced in the liver to chenodiol.

Clinical Pharmacology: Based on clinical trials in 868 patients with radiolucent gallstones treated for 6 to 78 months with ursodiol doses ranging from about 5 to 20 mg/kg/day, a dose of about 8 to 10 mg/kg/day appeared to be best. Complete stone dissolution occurs in about 30% of unselected patients with uncalcified gallstones < 20 mm in maximal diameter treated for up to 2 years. Patients with calcified gallstones prior to treatment, or patients who develop stone calcification or gallbladder nonvisualization on treatment, and patients with stones larger than 20 mm in maximal diameter rarely dissolve their stones. The chance of gallstone dissolution is increased up to 50% in patients with floating or floatable stones (ie, those with high cholesterol content), and is inversely related to stone size for those < 20 mm in maximal diameter. Complete dissolution was observed in 81% of patients with stones up to 5 mm in diameter. Age, sex, weight, degree of obesity and serum cholesterol level are not related to the chance of stone dissolution with ursodiol.

Partial stone dissolution occurring within 6 months of beginning therapy with ursodiol appears to be associated with a > 70% chance of eventual complete stone dissolution with further treatment; partial dissolution observed within 1 year of starting therapy indicates a 40% probability of complete dissolution.

(Actions continued on following page)

URSODIOL (Ursodeoxycholic acid) (Cont.)

Actions (Cont.):

Clinical Pharmacology (Cont.): Stone recurrence after dissolution with ursodiol therapy was seen within 2 years in 30% of patients. Of 16 patients whose stones had previously dissolved with chenodiol but later recurred, 11 had complete dissolution with ursodiol. Stone recurrence occurs in up to 50% of patients within 5 years of complete stone dissolution with ursodiol therapy. Obtain serial ultrasonographic examinations to monitor for recurrence of stones; establish radiolucency of the stones before instituting another course of ursodiol. A prophylactic dose of ursodiol has not been established.

Alternative therapies: Watchful waiting has the advantage that no therapy may ever be required. For patients with silent or minimally symptomatic stones, the rate of development of moderate to severe symptoms or gallstone complications is between 2% and 6% per year; 7% to 27% in 5 years. Presumably the rate is higher for patients already having symptoms.

Surgery (cholecystectomy) offers the advantage of immediate and permanent stone removal, but carries a high risk in some patients. About 5% of cholecystectomized patients have residual symptoms of retained common duct stones. The spectrum of surgical risk varies as a function of age and the presence of disease other than cholelithiasis.

Indications:

Dissolution of gallstones in patients with radiolucent, noncalcified, gallbladder stones < 20 mm in greatest diameter in whom elective cholecystectomy would be undertaken except for the presence of increased surgical risk due to systemic disease, advanced age, idiosyncratic reaction to general anesthesia, or for those patients who refuse surgery. Safety of use of ursodiol beyond 24 months is not established.

Contraindications:

Ursodiol will not dissolve calcified cholesterol stones, radiopaque stones or radiolucent bile pigment stones. Hence, patients with such stones are not candidates for ursodiol.

Patients with compelling reasons for cholecystectomy including unremitting acute cholecystitis, cholangitis, biliary obstruction, gallstone pancreatitis or biliary-gastrointestinal fistula are not candidates for ursodiol therapy.

Allergy to bile acids.

Chronic liver disease.

Warnings:

A nonfunctioning (ie, nonvisualizing) gallbladder by oral cholecystogram prior to the initiation of therapy is not a contraindication to ursodiol therapy. However, gallbladder nonvisualization developing during ursodiol treatment predicts failure of complete stone dissolution and therapy should be discontinued.

Carcinogenesis, Mutagenesis, Impairment of Fertility: Bile acids might be involved in the pathogenesis of human colon cancer in patients who have undergone a cholecystectomy, but direct evidence is lacking.

Usage in Pregnancy: Category B. There have been no adequate and well controlled studies of the use of ursodiol in pregnant women, but inadvertent exposure of four women to therapeutic doses of the drug in the first trimester of pregnancy during the ursodiol trials led to no evidence of effects on the fetus or newborn baby. The possibility that ursodiol can cause fetal harm cannot be ruled out; hence, the drug is not recommended during pregnancy.

Usage in Lactation: It is not known whether ursodiol is excreted in breast milk. Exercise caution when ursodiol is administered to a nursing mother.

Usage in Children: Safety and efficacy for use of ursodiol in children have not been established.

(Continued on following page)

URSODIOL (Ursodeoxycholic acid) (Cont.)

Precautions:

Ursodiol therapy has not been associated with liver damage. Lithocholic acid, a naturally occurring bile acid and metabolite of ursodiol, is known to be a liver-toxic metabolite. This bile acid is formed in the gut from ursodiol less efficiently and in smaller amounts than that seen from chenodiol. Lithocholic acid is detoxified in the liver by sulfation and although man appears to be an efficient sulfater, it is possible that some patients may have a congenital or acquired deficiency in sulfation, thereby predisposing them to lithocholate-induced liver damage. Therefore, measure SGOT and SGPT at the initiation of therapy, after 1 and 3 months of therapy, and every 6 months thereafter.

Patients with significant abnormalities in liver tests at any point should be monitored frequently; evaluate carefully for worsening gallstone disease which, in the controlled clinical trials, has been the only identified cause of significant liver test abnormality. Discontinue therapy with ursodiol if increased levels persist.

Estrogens, oral contraceptives and **clofibrate** (and perhaps other lipid-lowering drugs) increase hepatic cholesterol secretion, and encourage cholesterol gallstone formation and hence may counteract the effectiveness of ursodiol.

Drug Interactions:

Aluminum-based antacids adsorb bile acids in vitro and interfere with the action of ursodiol by reducing its absorption.

Cholestyramine and **colestipol** may interfere with the action of urosdiol by reducing its absorption.

Adverse Reactions:

Gastrointestinal: Doses of 8 to 10 mg/kg/day rarely cause diarrhea (< 1%). Nausea, vomiting, dyspepsia, metallic taste, abdominal pain, biliary pain, cholecystitis, constipation, stomatitis and flatulence have also occurred.

Dermatological: One patient with preexisting psoriasis apparently developed exacerbation of itching which remitted on withdrawal of the drug. Pruritis, rash, urticaria, dry skin, sweating and hair thinning have also occurred.

Other: Headache; fatigue; anxiety; depression; sleep disorder; arthralgia; myalgia; back pain; cough; rhinitis.

Overdosage:

The most likely manifestation of severe overdose with ursodiol would probably be diarrhea; treat symptomatically. Treatment includes usual supportive measures. Refer to General Management of Acute Overdosage on p. 2895

Administration and Dosage:

Radiolucent gallbladder stones: 8 to 10 mg/kg/day given in 2 or 3 divided doses.

Obtain ultrasound images of the gallbladder at 6 month intervals for the first year of ursodiol therapy to monitor gallstone response. If gallstones appear to have dissolved, continue therapy and confirm dissolution on a repeat ultrasound within 1 to 3 months. Most patients who eventually achieve complete stone dissolution will show partial or complete dissolution at the first on-treatment reevaluation. If partial stone dissolution is not seen by 12 months, the likelihood of success is greatly reduced.

Storage: Do not store above 86°F (30°C).

Rx	**Actigall** (Ciba)	**Capsules:** 300 mg	In 100s.

MONOCTANOIN

Actions:

Monoctanoin is a semisynthetic esterified glycerol intended for cholesterol stone dissolution via perfusion of the common bile duct. The mixed mono-di-glyceride has the following approximate composition: Glyceryl-1-mono-octanoate (80% to 85%); glyceryl-1-mono-decanoate and glyceryl-1-2-di-octanoate (10% to 15%); and free glycerol (maximum 2.5%).

Monoctanoin is readily hydrolyzed by pancreatic and other digestive lipases. The liberated fatty acids are excreted or absorbed and metabolized in a normal fashion.

Treatment results in complete stone dissolution about one-third of the time and in reduction in stone size in approximately one-third of patients. When reduced in size, these stones may pass spontaneously or may be more susceptible to simple physical extraction. Complete dissolution is much more likely (almost 50%) when there is a single stone than when there are multiple stones (about 20%). Complete dissolution is uncommon in diabetic patients (about 10%).

Indications:

A solubilizing agent for cholesterol (radiolucent) gallstones retained in the biliary tract following cholecystectomy, via perfusion of the common bile duct, when other means of removing cholesterol stones retained in the common bile duct have failed or cannot be undertaken.

Contraindications:

Impaired hepatic function, significant biliary tract infection or a history of recent duodenal ulcer or jejunitis; porto-systemic shunting, such that there is saturation of the hepatic uptake and metabolism of material absorbed from the gut lumen; acute pancreatitis, or any active life-threatening problems that would be complicated by perfusion into the biliary tract.

Warnings:

Intended for biliary tract perfusion only; not for parenteral use. Monoctanoin is irritating to the GI and biliary tracts. The irritation seems closely related to perfusion pressure and rate of administration; monitor both closely. Such irritation is reversible and disappears 2 to 7 days after therapy. (See Adverse Reactions.) Ascending cholangitis has occurred, possibly related to obstruction in the common bile duct. If fever, anorexia, chills, leukocytosis, severe right upper quadrant abdominal pain or jaundice occurs, discontinue treatment.

Biopsies from the gastric antrum, duodenum and bile ducts have shown diffuse erythema in the antral and duodenal mucosa. Ulceration or irritation of the common bile duct mucosa has also been observed on endoscopic examination. Duodenal erosion, inflammatory cell infiltration and localized inflammation have occurred. Multiple duodenal ulcerations adjacent to the infusion catheter were observed in one patient. No mucosal abnormalities were seen 1 month after therapy was discontinued.

Usage in Pregnancy: Category C. It is not known whether monoctanoin can cause fetal harm when administered to a pregnant woman or can affect reproduction capacity. Use only when clearly needed and when the potential benefits outweigh the potential hazards to the fetus.

Usage in Lactation: It is not known whether monoctanoin is excreted in breast milk. Exercise caution when administering to a nursing woman.

Usage in Children: Safety and efficacy for use in children have not been established.

Precautions:

Impaired hepatic function: Perform routine liver function tests since patients with impaired function may experience metabolic acidosis during drug perfusion.

(Continued on following page)

MONOCTANOIN (Cont.)

Adverse Reactions:

The incidences of adverse reactions are based on 326 patients. Overall, 251 (77%) of the patients had side effects; 134 (41%) had multiple side effects. Most of these were mild GI symptoms. Some were tolerated; some abated with reduced perfusion rate and discontinuation during meals. Side effects and other events caused discontinuation in 41 (12.5%).

Although a causal relationship has not been established with monoctanoin therapy, four deaths have occurred that are attributed to cholangitis, gallbladder perforation and biliary peritonitis, pulmonary embolism, and pancreatitis, respectively.

GI: Abdominal pain/discomfort (50.3%); nausea (32%); vomiting (20%); diarrhea (19%); loose stool (1.5%); anorexia (3%); indigestion (1.2%); increased serum amylase (0.6%); burning, increased fistula drainage, bile shock (0.3%). Irritation of the duodenal mucosa during perfusion has been observed by endoscopy. This was reversible and disappeared 2 to 7 days after therapy was completed.

Hematologic: Leukopenia (0.3%).

Other: Fever (6.3%); pruritus, fatigue/lethargy (0.9%); intolerance (0.6%); chills, depression, diaphoresis, headache, hypokalemia, allergic reaction (0.3%). One patient developed lupus erythematosus, which abated when the drug was discontinued.

Administration and Dosage:

The value of monoctanoin therapy should be determined. Gallstones must be radiolucent and readily accessible to the perfusate. If recently removed stones are available, analyze them for composition or incubate in monoctanoin at body temperature with stirring. If analysis shows the stone to be other than cholesterol or if no dissolution is observed after 72 hours of incubation, do not institute or discontinue therapy.

Do not administer IV or IM. Perfuse into the biliary tract either directly via catheter inserted through the T-tube or a catheter inserted through the mature sinus tract through a nasobiliary tube placed endoscopically. The gravity feed method is recommended if a positive pressure infusion pump is not available. The tip of the catheter must be placed as close to the stone(s) as possible (preferably within 1 cm) to insure stone contact and complete bathing. Monoctanoin is effective only when in direct contact with the stone.

Sterile Water for Injection must be added to each 120 ml vial to reduce the viscosity and enhance the bathing of the stone(s). This dilution reduces the viscosity by nearly 50%. The benefits of therapy will be maximized if the drug is maintained at 37°C (98.6°F) to obtain optimal levels of cholesterol solubility and further reduce viscosity. Maintain this procedure during perfusion.

Continuously perfuse on a 24 hour basis at a rate of 3 to 5 ml/hr. Continuous perfusion usually requires 2 to 10 days for elimination or size reduction of stones. Average duration is 5 days. If, after 10 days, cholangiography shows neither elimination nor reduction in size or density of stones, perform endoscopy to determine advisability of additional perfusion based on friability, softness or reduction of stone density.

If abdominal pain, nausea, diarrhea or emesis occurs and is not tolerated, stop perfusion for 1 hour, aspirate duct, then restart; if symptoms persist, stop perfusion for 1 hour, aspirate duct, then restart at a reduced rate of 3 ml/hr; if symptoms still persist, temporarily discontinue perfusion during mealtimes.

Storage: When stored at temperatures below 59°F, the drug may form a semisolid. Warming will reliquify. Store at room temperature 15°-30°C (59°-86°F).

Rx	**Moctanin** (Ethitek)	**Infusion:**	In 120 ml bottles. Ready for use with disposable bottle hangers.

Laxatives promote bowel evacuation. Nonprescription laxatives are frequently misused due to lack of understanding of normal bowel function. Restrict self-medication to short-term therapy of constipation; chronic use of laxatives (particularly stimulants) may lead to dependence. Prior to institution of laxative use, consider living habits affecting bowel function including disease state and drug history. Rational therapy and prevention of constipation includes: Adequate fluid intake (4 to 6 glasses [8 oz] of water daily), proper dietary habits including sufficient bulk or roughage, responding to the urge to defecate and daily exercise.

Actions:

Pharmacologic Actions of Laxatives

	Laxatives	Onset of action (hrs)	Site of action	Mechanism of action	Comments
Saline	Magnesium sulfate Magnesium hydroxide Magnesium citrate Sodium phosphate	0.5-3	Small & large intestine	Attract/retain water in intestinal lumen increasing intraluminal pressure; cholecystokinin release	May alter fluid and electrolyte balance. Sulfate salts are considered the most potent.
	Sod. phosphate/ biphosphate enema	0.03-0.25	Colon		
Irritant/Stimulant	Cascara Senna Phenolphthalein Bisacodyl Tablets Casanthranol	6-10	Colon	Direct action on intestinal mucosa; stimulate myenteric plexus; alters water and electrolyte secretion	Bile must be present for phenolphthalein to produce its effects. May prefer castor oil when more complete evacuation is required.
	Bisacodyl suppository	0.25-1			
	Castor oil	2-6	Small intestine		Castor oil is converted to ricinoleic acid (active component) in the gut.
Bulk-Producing	Methylcellulose Psyllium Polycarbophil	12-24 (up to 72)	Small & large intestine	Holds water in stool; mechanical distention; malt soup extract reduces fecal pH	Safest and most physiological.
Lubricant	Mineral oil	6-8	Colon	Retards colonic absorption of fecal water; softens stool	May decrease absorption of fat soluble vitamins.
Surfactants	Docusate	24-72	Small & large intestine	Detergent activity; facilitates admixture of fat & water to soften stool	Beneficial when feces are hard or dry, or in anorectal conditions where passage of a firm stool is painful.
Miscellaneous	Glycerin suppository	0.25-0.5	Colon	Local irritation; hyperosmotic action	Sodium stearate in preparation causes the local irritation.
	Lactulose	24-48	Colon	Delivers osmotically active molecules to colon	Also indicated in portal-systemic encephalopathy.

Indications:

Short-term treatment of constipation; certain stimulant, lubricant and saline laxatives are used to evacuate the colon for rectal and bowel examinations. Lubricant laxatives or fecal softeners are useful prophylactically in patients who should not strain during defecation (ie, following anorectal surgery, myocardial infarction). Psyllium is also useful in patients with irritable bowel syndrome, diverticular disease, spastic colon and hemorrhoids. Polycarbophil is indicated for constipation or diarrhea associated with conditions such as irritable bowel syndrome and diverticulosis; it is also for acute non-specific diarrhea. Mineral oil enema is indicated for relief of fecal impaction.

Unlabeled uses: Psyllium appears to be useful in the reduction of cholesterol levels as an adjunct to a dietary program. In two studies of 101 patients with mild to moderate hypercholesterolemia, 3.4 g psyllium 3 times a day for 8 weeks resulted in a mean reduction in cholesterol of approximately 5% to 15% and an 8% to 20% reduction in LDL.

(Continued on following page)

Contraindications:

Hypersensitivity to any ingredient; nausea, vomiting or other symptoms of appendicitis; acute surgical abdomen; fecal impaction (except mineral oil enema); intestinal obstruction; undiagnosed abdominal pain.

Do not use **bisacodyl tannex** in patients with ulcerative lesions of the colon or in children < 10 years old.

Do not give **docusate sodium** if mineral oil is being given.

Warnings:

Fluid and electrolyte balance: Excessive laxative use may lead to significant fluid and electrolyte imbalance. Monitor patients periodically.

Preparations containing sodium should not be used by individuals on a sodium restricted diet or in the presence of edema, congestive heart failure or hypertension.

Megacolon, imperforate anus or CHF: Do not use sodium phosphate and sodium biphosphate in these patients; hypernatremic dehydration may occur.

Abuse/Dependency: Chronic use of laxatives, particularly stimulants, may lead to laxative dependency, which in turn may result in fluid and electrolyte imbalances, steatorrhea, osteomalacia and vitamin and mineral deficiencies. Also known as laxative abuse syndrome (LAS), it is difficult to diagnose. It is often seen in women with depression, personality disorders or anorexia nervosa. Many agents can be detected in urine or stool samples; however, it is important to follow up negative test results if LAS is suspected since patients may be intermittent abusers or change laxative products frequently.

Cathartic colon, a poorly functioning colon, results from the chronic abuse of stimulant cathartics. Pathologic presentation resembles ulcerative colitis.

Melanosis coli is a darkened pigmentation of the colonic mucosa resulting from chronic use of anthraquinone derivatives. It resolves within 5 to 11 months of drug discontinuation.

Bisacodyl tannex: Use with caution when multiple enemas are administered. Tannic acid is hepatotoxic if absorbed in sufficient quantity. Deaths have occurred from hepatic damage due to tannic acid used in barium enema examination.

Lipid pneumonitis may result from oral ingestion and aspiration of mineral oil, especially when patient reclines. The young, elderly, debilitated and dysphagic are at greatest risk.

Renal function impairment: Up to 20% of the magnesium in magnesium salts may be absorbed. Do not use products containing phosphate, sodium, magnesium or potassium salts in the presence of renal dysfunction. Use sodium phosphate and sodium biphosphate with caution in these patients; hyperphosphatemia, hypernatremia, acidosis and hypocalcemia may occur.

Pregnancy: (*Category C* – Docusate sodium, cascara sagrada, mineral oil, senna) Do not use castor oil during pregnancy; its irritant effect may induce premature labor. Mineral oil may decrease absorption of fat-soluble vitamins. Improper use of saline cathartics can lead to dangerous electrolyte imbalance. If needed, limit use to bulk forming or surfactant laxatives.

Lactation: Cascara sagrada is excreted in breast milk. There may be an increased incidence of diarrhea in the nursing infant. It is not known whether docusate sodium or lactulose are excreted in breast milk.

Children: Physical manipulation of a glycerin suppository in infants often initiates defecation; hence, adverse effects are minimal. Do not administer enemas to children < 2 years of age. Do not use bisacodyl tannex in children < 10 years of age.

An 11-month-old infant died following an overdose of a sodium phosphate enema. A 6-week-old infant developed magnesium poisoning following 16 doses of $\approx$ 1.7 ml over 48 hours of a magnesium hydroxide mixture (550 mg/10 ml) for constipation.

Precautions:

Rectal bleeding or failure to respond to therapy may indicate a serious condition which may require further medical attention.

Phenolphthalein may cause a skin hypersensitivity characterized by a fixed drug eruption. Discontinue the drug if this occurs.

Discoloration of acid urine to yellow-brown may occur with cascara sagrada or senna. Pink-red, red-violet or red-brown discoloration of alkaline urine may occur with phenolphthalein, cascara sagrada or senna.

Impaction or obstruction may be caused by bulk-forming agents if temporarily arrested in their passage through the alimentary canal (eg, patients with esophageal strictures). Use in patients with intestinal ulcerations, stenosis or disabling adhesions may be hazardous.

Tartrazine sensitivity: Some of these products contain tartrazine, which may cause allergic-type reactions (including bronchial asthma) in susceptible individuals. Although the incidence of tartrazine sensitivity in the general population is low, it is frequently seen in patients who also have aspirin hypersensitivity. Specific products containing tartrazine are identified in the product listings.

(Continued on following page)

Drug Interactions:

Mineral oil: Surfactants (ie, docusate) may facilitate absorption, thus increasing the toxicity of mineral oil.

Milk or **antacids:** Concomitant administration of **bisacodyl** tablets may cause the enteric coating to dissolve, resulting in gastric lining irritation or dyspepsia.

Lipid soluble vitamins (vitamins **A, D, E** and **K**)**:** Absorption may decrease during prolonged administration with **mineral oil.**

Tetracycline: Laxatives containing aluminum, calcium or magnesium (ie, polycarbophil) impair absorption of tetracycline, due to release of free calcium.

Adverse Reactions:

Excessive bowel activity (griping, diarrhea, nausea, vomiting); perianal irritation; weakness; dizziness; fainting; palpitations; sweating; bloating; flatulence.

Abdominal cramps have occurred.

Esophageal, gastric, small intestinal and rectal obstruction due to the accumulation of mucilaginous components of bulk laxatives have occurred.

Large doses of mineral oil may cause anal seepage, resulting in itching (pruritis ani), irritation, hemorrhoids and perianal discomfort.

Bisacodyl suppositories may cause proctitis and inflammation. Not recommended for long-term use.

Patient Information:

Direct attention to proper dietary fiber intake, adequate fluids and regular exercise.

Do not use in the presence of abdominal pain, nausea or vomiting.

Laxative use is only a temporary measure; do not use longer than 1 week. When regularity returns, discontinue use. Prolonged, frequent or excessive use may result in dependence or electrolyte imbalance.

Notify physician if unrelieved constipation, rectal bleeding or symptoms of electrolyte imbalance (eg, muscle cramps or pain, weakness, dizziness) occurs.

Pink-red, red-violet or red-brown discoloration of alkaline urine may occur with cascara sagrada, phenolphthalein or senna.

Yellow-brown discoloration of acid urine may occur with cascara sagrada or senna.

Refrigerate magnesium citrate solutions to retain potency and palatability.

Take with a full glass of water or juice.

Mineral oil: Preferably administered on an empty stomach.

Bisacodyl tablets: Swallow whole; do not take within 1 hour of antacids or milk.

(Products listed on following pages)

Saline Laxatives

	Product	Form/Dose	Supplied	C.I.*
otc	**Epsom Salt** (Various, eg, Dixon-Shane, Humco, Purepac)	**Granules:** Magnesium sulfate. ≃ 40 mEq magnesium/5 g *Dose:* Adults – 10 to 15 g in glass of water. Children – 5 to 10 g in glass of water.	In 150 and 240 g and 1 and 4 lb.	21+
otc	**Milk of Magnesia - Concentrated** (Various, eg, Roxane, Vangard)	**Liquid:** Magnesium hydroxide *Dose:* 10 to 20 ml.	Lemon flavor. In 100, 400 and 480 ml and UD 10, 15 and 20 ml.	220+
otc	**Phillips' Milk of Magnesia, Concentrated** (Glenbrook)	**Liquid:** Magnesium hydroxide. *Dose:* 15 to 30 ml.	Sorbitol, sugar. Strawberry and orange vanilla creme flavors. In 240 ml.	150
otc	**Milk of Magnesia** (Various, eg, Apothecon, Geneva Marsam, Goldline, Major, Moore, Purepac, Roxane, Rugby, Schein, URL)	**Liquid:** Magnesium hydroxide. 7% to 8.5% aqueous suspension; ≃ 80 mEq magnesium per 30 ml *Dose:* Adults – 30 to 60 ml/day, taken with liquid. Children ≥ 2 years – 5 to 30 ml, depending on age.	In 180, 360, 480, 720 and 960 ml, and UD 15 and 30 ml.	80+
otc	**Phillips' Milk of Magnesia** (Glenbrook)		Mint and regular flavors. In 120, 360 and 780 ml.	280
otc	**Citrate of Magnesia** (Dixon-Shane)	**Solution:** Magnesium citrate *Dose:* Adults – 1 glassful (approx. 240 ml) as needed. Children – ½ the adult dose; repeat if necessary.	In 300 ml.	1344
otc	**Citro-Nesia** (Century)		In 296 ml.	1000
otc *sf*	**Fleet Phospho-soda** (Fleet)	**Solution:** 18 g sodium phosphate and 48 g sodium biphosphate per 100 ml (96.4 mEq sodium per 20 ml) *Dose:* Adults – 20 to 30 ml mixed with ½ glass cool water. Children – 5 to 15 ml.	Regular and ginger-lemon flavors. In 45, 90 and 237 ml.	140
otc *sf*	**Sodium Phosphates** (Roxane)		Lemon flavor. In UD 30 ml.	450

Irritant or Stimulant Laxatives

CASCARA SAGRADA

	Product	Form/Dose	Supplied	C.I.*
otc	**Cascara Sagrada** (Various, eg, Dixon-Shane, Rugby)	**Tablets:** 325 mg *Dose:* 1 tablet at bedtime.	In 100s and 1000s.	30+
otc	**Cascara Sagrada Aromatic Fluid Extract** (Various, eg, Major, Purepac, Rugby)	**Liquid:** ≈ 18% alcohol *Dose:* 5 ml.	In 120 ml and pt.	80+

CALCIUM SALTS OF SENNOSIDES A & B (The laxative principle of senna)

	Product	Form/Dose	Supplied	C.I.*
otc	**Ex-Lax Gentle Nature** (Sandoz)	**Tablets:** 20 mg *Dose:* Adults – 1 to 2 tablets with water at bedtime. Children (≥ 6 years) – 1 tablet/day	In 16s.	148

* Cost Index based on cost per minimum adult dose.
sf – Sugar free.

Complete prescribing information for these products begins on page 1642

Irritant or Stimulant Laxatives (Cont.)

PHENOLPHTHALEIN

Yellow phenolphthalein is 2 to 3 times more potent than white phenolphthalein.

Dose: 60 to 194 mg, preferably at bedtime.

	Product	Form	Description	C.I.*
otc	**Alophen Pills No. 973** (Parke-Davis)	**Tablets:** 60 mg phenolphthalein	Sucrose, sugar. In 100s.	10
otc	**Ex-Lax Unflavored** (Sandoz Consumer)	**Tablets:** 90 mg yellow phenolphthalein	Sucrose. In 8s, 30s and 60s.	10
otc	**Lax Pills** (G&W)		In 30s and 60s.	100
otc	**Laxative Pills** (Rugby)		Sugar coated. In 30s.	NA
otc	**Espotabs** (Combe)	**Tablets:** 97.2 mg yellow phenolphthalein	Lactose, sucrose. In 12s, 30s and 60s.	20
otc	**Feen-a-mint** (Schering-Plough)		In 20s.	50
otc	**Modane** (Adria)	**Tablets:** 130 mg phenolphthalein	Lactose, sucrose. (A 513). Red. Sugar coated. In 10s, 30s and 100s.	40
otc	**Prulet** (Mission)	**Tablets:** 60 mg white phenolphthalein	Green, scored. Lemon-lime flavor. In 12s and 40s.	50
otc	**Feen-a-mint Chocolated** (Schering-Plough)	**Tablets, chewable:** 65 mg yellow phenolphthalein	Sugar. Chocolate mint flavor. In 4s, 18s and 36s.	NA
otc	**Ex-Lax Chocolated** (Sandoz Consumer)	**Tablets, chewable:** 90 mg yellow phenolphthalein	Sugar. In 6s, 18s, 48s and 72s.	20
otc	**Evac-U-Gen** (Walker)	**Tablets, chewable:** 97.2 mg yellow phenolphthalein	Corn syrup, lactose, saccharin, sugar. In 35s and 100s.	10
otc	**Feen-a-mint** (Schering-Plough)		Sugar, methylsalicylate. Scored. Square shape. Mint flavor. In 20s.	50
otc	**Medilax** (Mission)	**Tablets, chewable:** 120 mg phenolphthalein	Aspartame, 1.5 mg phenylalanine. Citrus flavor. In 24s.	NA
otc	**Phenolax** (Upjohn)	**Wafers:** 64.8 mg phenolphthalein	Tartrazine, glucose, sucrose. (Phenolax). In 100s.	20
otc	**Evac-U-Lax Tablets** (Hauck)	**Wafers, chewable:** 80 mg phenolphthalein	In 1000s.	1
otc	**Feen-a-mint** (Schering-Plough)	**Gum:** 97.2 mg yellow phenolphthalein	Sugar. Peppermint flavor. In 5s, 16s and 40s.	30

SENNA

	Product	Form	Description	C.I.*
otc	**Senexon** (Rugby)	**Tablets:** 187 mg senna concentrate *Dose:* Adults – 2 tablets at bedtime (up to 8/day). Children > 60 lbs (27 kg) – 1 tablet at bedtime (up to 4/day).	Sucrose. In 100s and 1000s.	70
otc	**Senolax** (Schein)	**Tablets:** 187 mg senna concentrate *Dose:* Adults – 2 tablets (up to 8/day) Children (6 to 12 years) – 1 tablet (up to 4/day)	In 100s and 1000s.	35

* Cost Index based on cost per minimum adult dose, 30 mg or 10 ml pediatric dose.

(Continued on following page)

Complete prescribing information for these products begins on page 1642

Irritant or Stimulant Laxatives (Cont.)

SENNA (Cont.)

	Product (Manufacturer)	Formulation / Dose	How Supplied	C.I.*
otc	**Senokot** (Purdue Frederick)	**Tablets:** 187 mg standardized senna concentrate	Lactose. In 20s, 50s, 100s, 1000s and UD 100s.	200
		Granules: 326 mg standardized senna concentrate per tsp	Sucrose. In 60, 170 & 340 g.	9
		Suppositories: 652 mg standardized senna concentrate *Dose:* Adults – 2 tablets (up to 8/day), 1 tsp granules (up to 4 tsp/day) or 1 suppository at bedtime (repeat in 2 hrs if necessary). Children (6 to < 12 years) – 1 tablet (up to 4/day), > 60 lbs (27 kg) – ½ tsp granules (up to 2 tsp/day) or ½ suppository at bedtime.	In 6s.	1400
		Syrup: 218 mg/5 ml standardized senna extract *Dose:* Adults – 10 to 15 ml at bedtime (up to 30 ml/day). Children (5 to 15 years) – 5 to 10 ml at bedtime (up to 20 ml/day). Children (1 to 5 years) – 2.5 to 5 ml at bedtime (up to 10 ml/day). Children (1 month to 1 year) – 1.25 to 2.5 ml at bedtime (up to 5 ml/day).	7% alcohol. In 60 and 240 ml.	470
otc	**Senna-Gen** (Goldline)	**Tablets:** 217 mg senna concentrate *Dose:* Adults – 2 tablets at bedtime (up to 8/day). Children > 60 lbs (27 kg) – 1 tablet at bedtime (up to 4/day).	Brown. In 100s and 1000s.	60
otc	**Senokotxtra** (Purdue Fredrick)	**Tablets:** 374 mg senna concentrate *Dose:* Adults – 1 tablet at bedtime (up to 4/day)	In 12s.	NA
otc	**Black-Draught** (Chattem)	**Tablets:** 600 mg senna equivalent	Sucrose. In 30s.	920
		Granules: 1.65 g senna equivalent per ½ tsp *Dose:* Adults – 2 tablets at bedtime (up to 3/day) or ¼ to ½ level tsp granules with water.	Tartrazine, sucrose. In 22.5 g.	240
otc	**Gentlax** (Blair)	**Granules:** 326 mg standardized senna concentrate per tsp *Dose:* Adults – 1 tsp once/day (up to 4 tsp/day). Children 6 to < 12 years – ½ tsp once/day (up to 2 tsp/day).	Malt extract, sucrose. In 180 g.	360
otc	**Dr. Caldwell Senna Laxative** (Gebauer)	**Liquid:** 33.3 mg/ml senna concentrate *Dose:* Adults – 15 to 30 ml with or after meals or at bedtime. Children (6 to 15 years) – 10 to 15 ml at bedtime. Children (2 to 5 years) – 5 to 10 ml at bedtime.	4.9% alcohol, salicylic acid, sucrose. In 150 and 360 ml.	249
otc	**Fletcher's Castoria** (Mentholatum)	**Liquid:** 33.3 mg/ml senna concentrate *Dose:* Children (6 to 15 years) – 10 to 15 ml. Children (2 to 5 years) – 5 to 10 ml.	3.5% alcohol, sucrose. In 75 and 150 ml.	260

* Cost Index based on cost per minimum adult dose or per 10 ml pediatric dose.

Complete prescribing information for these products begins on page 1642

Irritant or Stimulant Laxatives (Cont.)

CASTOR OIL

	Product	Description	C.I.*
otc	**Castor Oil** (Various, eg, Apothecon, Dixon-Shane, Purepac)	**Liquid:** In 60 and 120 ml and pt. *Dose:* Adults – 15 to 60 ml. Children (6 to 12 years) – 5 to 15 ml.	450+
otc	**Neoloid** (Lederle)	**Emulsion:** 36.4% castor oil with emulsifying agents. Saccharin. Peppermint flavor. In 118 ml. *Dose:* Adults – 30 to 60 ml. Children – 7.5 to 30 ml. Infants – 2.5 to 7.5 ml.	680
otc	**Alphamul** (Lannett)	**Emulsion:** 60% castor oil with emulsifying and flavoring agents. In 90 ml and gal. *Dose:* Adults – 15 to 45 ml. Children – 5 to 15 ml. Infants – 1.25 to 5 ml.	130
otc	**Fleet Flavored Castor Oil** (Fleet)	**Emulsion:** 67% castor oil with emulsifying agents. In 45 and 90 ml. *Dose:* Adults – 45 ml. Children (2 to 12 years) – 15 ml. Children (< 2 years) – 5 ml.	20
otc	**Purge** (Fleming)	**Liquid:** 95% castor oil. Lemon flavor. In 30 and 60 ml. *Dose:* Adults – 30 to 60 ml. Children – 7.5 to 30 ml. Infants – 2.5 to 7.5 ml.	1130
otc *sf*	**Emulsoil** (Paddock)	**Emulsion:** 95% castor oil with emulsifying agents. In 63 ml. *Dose:* Adults – 15 to 60 ml mixed with ½ to 1 glass liquid. Children – 5 to 10 ml mixed with ½ to 1 glass liquid.	390

BISACODYL

Dose:

Tablets: Swallow whole; do not chew. Do not take within 1 hour of antacids or milk.

Adults – 10 to 15 mg. Up to 30 mg has been used for preparation of lower GI tract for special procedures.

Children (> 6 years) – 5 to 10 mg (0.3 mg/kg) at bedtime or before breakfast.

Suppositories:

Adults and children (> 2 years) – 10 mg to induce bowel movement.

Children (< 2 years) – 5 mg.

	Product	Form	Description	C.I.*
otc	**Bisacodyl** (Various, eg, Dixon-Shane, Geneva Marsam, Major, Moore, Parmed, Purepac, URL)	**Tablets, enteric coated:** 5 mg	In 25s, 100s, 250s, 1000s and UD 100s.	30+
otc	**Dulcagen** (Goldline)		Yellow. In 100s and 1000s.	54
otc	**Dulcolax** (Boehringer Ingelheim)		Lactose, sucrose. (BI-12). Yellow. In 24s, 100s, 1000s and UD 100s.	160
otc	**Fleet Laxative** (Fleet)		In 24s and 100s.	30
otc	**Bisacodyl Uniserts** (Upsher-Smith)	**Suppositories, pediatric:** 5 mg	In 12s.	210
otc	**Bisacodyl** (Various, eg, Dixon-Shane, Geneva Marsam, Major, Moore, Purepac, URL)	**Suppositories:** 10 mg	In 8s, 12s, 100s and 1000s.	60+
otc	**Bisco-Lax** (Raway)		In UD 12s, 50s, 100s, 500s and 1000s.	NA
otc	**Dulcagen** (Goldline)		In 100s and 500s.	165
otc	**Dulcolax** (Boehringer Ingelheim)		In 2s, 4s, 8s, 50s and 500s.	30
otc	**Fleet Laxative** (Fleet)		In 4s, 50s and 100s.	80

* Cost Index based on cost per minimum adult dose of castor oil or 5 mg bisacodyl.

sf – Sugar free.

Complete prescribing information for these products begins on page 1634.

Bulk-Producing Laxatives

Take with a full glass of water; encourage additional fluid intake.

				C.I.*
otc	**Citrucel** (Marion Merrell Dow)	**Powder:** 2 g methylcellulose per heaping tbsp *Dose:* Adults and children ≥ 12 – 1 heaping tbsp (19 g) in 8 oz cold water, 1 to 3 times daily. Children (6 to < 12) – 1 level tbsp in 4 oz cold water, 1 to 3 times daily.	Sucrose. Regular and orange flavor. In 480 and 900 g.	30
otc sf	**Citrucel Sugar Free** (Marion Merrell-Dow)	**Powder:** 2 g methylcellulose, 52 mg phenylalanine *Dose:* Adults and children ≥ 12 – 1 heaping tbsp (10.2 g) in 8 oz cold water, up to 3 times daily. Children 6 to 12 – 1 level tbsp in 4 oz cold water, up to 3 times daily.	Aspartame. In 479 g.	NA
otc	**Unifiber** (Dow B. Hickam)	**Powder:** 3 g powdered cellulose per tbsp. < 4 calories per serving. *Dose:* 1 to 2 tbsp (4 to 8 g) once or twice/day into liquid.	Corn syrup solids, xanthan gum. In 454 g.	NA
otc	**Maltsupex** (Wallace)	**Tablets:** 750 mg nondiastatic barley malt extract. *Dose:* Adults – 4 tablets, 4 times daily (with meals and at bedtime) with liquid.	In 100s.	890
otc	**Maltsupex** (Wallace)	**Powder:** 16 g nondiastatic barley malt extract per heaping tbsp	In 240 and 480 g.	890
		Liquid: 16 g per tbsp *Dose:* Adults – 2 heaping tbsp twice daily for 3 or 4 days, then 1 to 2 tbsp at bedtime. Drink 8 oz of liquid with each dose. Children: 1 or 2 heaping tbsp once or twice daily. Infants (> 1 month): ½ to 2 tbsp in day's total formula or, in breastfed infants, 1 to 2 tsp in 2 to 4 oz water or juice once or twice daily.	In 240 and 480 ml.	870

* Cost Index based on cost per minimum single adult dose of bulk-producing laxatives.
sf – Sugar free.

POLYCARBOPHIL

Actions:

Calcium polycarbophil is a hydrophilic agent. As a *bulk laxative,* it retains free water within the intestinal lumen, and indirectly opposes dehydrating forces of the bowel, promoting well-formed stools. In *diarrhea,* when the intestinal mucosa is incapable of absorbing water at normal rates, calcium polycarbophil absorbs free fecal water, forming a gel and producing formed stools. Thus, in both diarrhea and constipation, it works by restoring a more normal moisture level and providing bulk.

Indications:

Treatment of constipation or diarrhea associated with conditions such as irritable bowel syndrome and diverticulosis; acute nonspecific diarrhea.

Adverse Reactions:

Abdominal fullness is noted occasionally. Smaller doses given more frequently but spaced evenly throughout the day may provide relief.

Administration and Dosage:

Individualize dosage.

Adults: 1 g 1 to 4 times daily or as needed. Do not exceed 6 g in 24 hours.

Children (6 to < 12 years): 500 mg 1 to 3 times daily or as needed. Do not exceed 3 g in 24 hours.

Children (3 to < 6 years): 500 mg 2 times daily or as needed. Do not exceed 1.5 g in 24 hours.

For severe diarrhea, repeat dose every half hour; do not exceed maximum daily dosage.
When using as a laxative, drink 8 fl. oz water or other liquid with each dose.

(Continued on following page)

Complete prescribing information for these products begins on page 1642

Bulk-Producing Laxatives (Cont.)

	POLYCARBOPHIL (Cont.)			**C.I.***
otc	**FiberCon** (Lederle)	**Tablets:** 500 mg (as calcium). Sodium free	(LL F66). Film coated. In 36s, 60s and 90s.	240
otc	**Equalactin** (Numark)	**Tablets, chewable:** 500 mg (as calcium)	Sorbitol. In 16s and 36s.	NA
otc	**Mitrolan** (Robins)	**Tablets, chewable:** 500 mg (as calcium). < 0.02 mEq (0.46 mg) sodium per tablet	(AHR 1535). Sucrose. In 36s and 100s.	180
otc	**Fiber-Lax** (Rugby)	**Tablets:** 625 mg calcium polycarbophil (equivalent to 500 mg polycarbophil)	In 60s.	NA
otc	**Fiberall** (Ciba Consumer)	**Tablets, chewable:** 1250 mg calcium carbophil (equivalent to 1000 mg polycarbophil)	Dextrose. Scored. Lemon flavor. In 18s.	NA

	PSYLLIUM			**C.I.***
otc *sf*	**Fiberall Natural Flavor** (Ciba Consumer)	**Powder:** 3.4 g psyllium hydrophilic mucilloid, wheat bran, < 10 mg sodium, < 60 mg potassium and < 6 calories per dose *Dose:* 1 rounded tsp (5 to 5.9 g) in 8 oz cool water or juice, 1 to 3 times daily.	In 284 and 426 g.	90
otc *sf*	**Fiberall Orange Flavor** (Ciba Consumer)		Saccharin. In 284 and 426 g.	110
otc *sf*	**Hydrocil Instant** (Solvay Pharm.)	**Powder:** 3.5 g psyllium hydrophilic mucilloid per dose *Dose:* 1 packet or level scoopful (3.7 g) in liquid, morning & evening	In 250 g and UD 3.7 g packets (30s & 500s).	110
otc *sf*	**Konsyl** (Lafayette)	**Powder:** 100% psyllium. Sodium free *Dose:* 1 packet or rounded tsp (6 g) in liquid, 1 to 3 times daily.	In 300 and 450 g and UD 6 g packets (25s).	150
otc	**Metamucil** (Procter & Gamble)	**Powder:** ≈ 3.4 g psyllium hydrophilic mucilloid, 3.5 g carbohydrates, < 10 mg sodium, 31 mg potassium & 14 calories per dose *Dose:* 1 rounded tsp (7 g) in liquid, 1 to 3 times a day.	Dextrose. In 210, 420, 630 and 960 g and 30 and 100 UD single-dose packs (100s).	120
otc	**Metamucil, Orange Flavor** (Procter & Gamble)	**Powder:** ≈ 3.4 g psyllium hydrophilic mucilloid, 7.1 g carbohydrate (sucrose), < 10 mg sodium, 31 mg potassium and 30 calories per dose *Dose:* 1 rounded tbsp (11 g) in liquid, 1 to 3 times a day.	In 210, 420, 630 and 960 g and UD 30s.	190
otc *sf*	**Metamucil, Sugar Free** (Procter & Gamble)	**Powder:** ≈ 3.4 g psyllium hydrophilic mucilloid, 0.3 g carbohydrates, < 10 mg sodium, 31 mg potassium and 1 calorie per dose *Dose:* 1 rounded tsp (3.7 g) in liquid, 1 to 3 times a day.	Aspartame, 6 mg phenylalanine. In 111, 222, 333 and 507 g and UD single-dose packs (100s).	120
otc	**Alramucil** (Alra)	**Powder, effervescent:** 3.6 g psyllium hydrophilic mucilloid, citric acid, potassium bicarbonate, sodium bicarbonate *Dose:* 1 packet dissolved into 8 oz water, 1 to 3 times daily.	Sucrose, saccharin. Regular or orange flavor. In 30s.	NA
otc	**Metamucil** (Procter & Gamble)	**Wafers:** ≈ 1.7 g psyllium mucilloid, 18 g carbohydrate, 18 mg sodium, 4.5 g fat, 96 calories per dose	Sugar, fructose, molasses, sucrose. In 24s.	NA

* Cost Index based on cost per minimum single adult dose of bulk-producing laxatives.
sf – Sugar free.

(Continued on following page)

Complete prescribing information for these products begins on page 1642

Bulk-Producing Laxatives (Cont.)

PSYLLIUM (Cont.)

	Product	Description	Notes	C.I.*
otc *sf*	**Metamucil, Sugar Free, Orange Flavor** (Procter & Gamble)	**Powder:** ≈ 3.4 mg psyllium hydrophilic mucilloid, 1.4 mg carbohydrate, < 10 mg sodium, 31 mg potassium and 5 calories per dose. *Dose:* 1 rounded tsp (5.2 g) in liquid 1 to 3 times a day.	Aspartame, 30 mg phenylalanine per dose. In 141, 261, 387 and 621 g.	100
otc	**Natural Vegetable** (Various, eg, Dixon-Shane, Geneva Marsam, Moore, Schein)	**Powder:** 3.4 g psyllium hydrophilic mucilloid with dextrose, < 10 mg sodium and 14 calories per dose *Dose:* 1 rounded tsp (7 g) in liquid, 1 to 3 times daily.	In 210, 420 and 630 g.	NA
otc	**Reguloid, Orange** (Rugby)	**Powder:** 3.4 g psyllium mucilloid & 70% sucrose/rounded tbsp *Dose:* Adults – 1 rounded tbsp, 2 to 3 times daily. Children – ½ adult dose	Orange flavor. In 420 and 630 g.	100
otc *sf*	**Reguloid, Sugar Free Orange** (Rugby)	**Powder:** ≈ 3.4 g psyllium hydrophilic mucilloid, < 0.01 g sodium and ≈ 5 calories per rounded tsp *Dose:* Adults – 1 rounded tsp (5.2 g) in 8 oz liquid 1 to 3 times/day. Children (6 to 12) – ½ adult dose in 8 oz liquid 1 to 3 times/day.	Aspartame, 30 mg phenylalanine per dose. In 246 and 387 g.	70
otc *sf*	**Reguloid, Sugar Free Regular** (Rugby)	**Powder:** ≈ 3.4 g psyllium hydrophilic mucilloid, < 0.01 g sodium and ≈ 1 calorie per 3.7 g dose *Dose:* Adults – 1 rounded tsp (3.7 g) in 8 oz liquid, 1 to 3 times/day. Children (6 to 12) – ½ adult dose in 8 oz liquid 1 to 3 times a day.	Aspartame, 6 mg phenylalanine per dose. In 222 and 333 g.	70
otc	**Serutan** (Menley & James)	**Powder:** 3.4 g psyllium (< 0.1 g sodium) per heaping tsp *Dose:* 1 heaping tsp in 240 ml water, 1 to 3 times daily, preferably with meals.	Dextrose (regular flavor). In regular and fruit flavors. In 210, 420 and 630 g.	120
otc	**Syllact** (Wallace)	**Powder:** 3.3 g psyllium seed husks and ≈ 14 calories per rounded tsp *Dose:* 1 rounded tsp in 8 oz liquid, 1 to 3 times daily. Children ≥ 6 – ½ adult dose in 8 oz liquid	Dextrose, saccharin. Fruit flavor. In 300 g.	200
otc *sf*	**Konsyl-D** (Lafayette)	**Powder:** 3.4 g psyllium hydrophilic mucilloid, 14 calories per rounded tsp *Dose:* Adults – 1 tsp (6.5 g) in 8 oz liquid 1 to 3 times per day. Children – ½ adult dose	Dextrose. In 325 & 500 g & UD 6.5 g (25s).	120
otc	**Modane Bulk** (Adria)	**Powder:** 50% psyllium hydrophilic mucilloid and 50% dextrose per dose *Dose:* Adults – 1 rounded tsp in 8 oz liquid, 1 to 3 times a day. Children (6-13) – ½ adult dose in 8 oz liquid	2 mg sodium, 37 mg potassium and 14 calories per tsp. In 396 g.	120
otc	**Reguloid, Natural** (Rugby)		14 calories per tsp. Sodium free. In 420 and 630 g.	60
otc	**V-Lax** (Century)		In 120 and 480 g.	80

* Cost Index based on cost per minimum single adult dose of bulk-producing laxatives.
sf – Sugar free.

(Continued on following page)

Complete prescribing information for these products begins on page 1642

Bulk-Producing Laxatives (Cont.)

PSYLLIUM (Cont.)				C.I.*
otc	**Effer-syllium** (J & J-Merck)	**Effervescent Powder:** 3 g psyllium hydrocolloid per 7 g packet or rounded tsp (< 5 mg sodium/rounded tsp) *Dose:* Adults – 1 rounded tsp or packet in water, 1 to 3 times/day. Children ≥ 6 – 1 level tsp or ½ packet in ½ glass of water at bedtime.	Saccharin, sucrose. Lemon-lime flavor. In 270 and 480 g and single dose packets (24s).	150
otc *sf*	**Metamucil Lemon-Lime Flavor** (Procter & Gamble)	**Effervescent Powder:** ≈ 3.4 g psyllium hydrophilic mucilloid, sodium and potassium bicarbonate, < 10 mg sodium, calcium carbonate, 290 mg potassium and 1 calorie per dose *Dose:* 1 packet in 8 oz water 1 to 3 times daily.	Aspartame, 30 mg phenylalanine per dose. In single dose packets (30s and 100s).	250
otc *sf*	**Metamucil Orange Flavor** (Procter & Gamble)	**Effervescent Powder:** ≈ 3.4 g psyllium hydrophilic mucilloid, sodium and potassium bicarbonate, 310 mg potassium, < 10 mg sodium and 1 calorie per dose *Dose:* 1 packet in 8 oz water, 1 to 3 times a day.	Aspartame, 30 mg phenylalanine per dose. In single dose packets (30s).	250
otc	**Perdiem Fiber** (Rhone-Poulenc Rorer)	**Granules:** 4.03 g psyllium, 1.8 mg sodium, 36.1 mg potassium and 4 calories/rounded tsp (6 g) *Dose: Adults* – 1 to 2 rounded tsp with 8 oz liquid, once or twice daily. Do not chew. Children (7 to 11) – 1 rounded tsp with 8 oz liquid once or twice daily	Sucrose. Dye free. Mint flavor. In 100 and 250 g.	220
otc	**Serutan** (Menley & James)	**Granules:** 2.5 g psyllium and < 0.03 g sodium per heaping tsp *Dose:* Adults – 1 to 3 heaping tsp on cereal or other food, 1 to 3 times daily. Children (6 to 12) – ½ adult dose with 8 oz liquid.	Saccharin, sugar. In 180 and 540 g.	190
otc	**Siblin** (Warner-Lambert Consumer)	**Granules:** 2.5 g blond psyllium seed coatings per rounded tsp *Dose:* Adults – 1 rounded tsp up to 12 times daily in liquid. Children (6 to 12) – ½ rounded tsp up to 12 times daily.	Sugar. In 480 g.	170
otc	**Fiberall** (Ciba Consumer)	**Wafers:** 3.4 g psyllium hydrophilic mucilloid, 0.03 g sodium and 78 calories per wafer. With wheat bran and oats. *Dose:* Adults – 1 or 2 wafers with 8 oz liquid, 1 to 3 times a day. Children (6 to 12) – ½ adult dosage.	Corn syrup, molasses, sugar. Oatmeal raisin and fruit & nut flavors. In 14s.	209

* Cost Index based on cost per minimum single adult dose of bulk-producing laxatives.
sf – Sugar free.

Complete prescribing information for these products begins on page 1642

Emollient Laxatives

MINERAL OIL

Dose: *Adults* – 5-45 ml. *Children* – 5-20 ml. Although usual directions are to give at bedtime, caution is advised because of lipid pneumonitis (see Laxative monograph).

	Product	Form	Packaging	C.I.*
otc	**Mineral Oil** (Various, eg, Apothecon, Barre, Century, Dixon-Shane, Lannett, Paddock, Pharm Assoc., Purepac, Roxane, UDL)	**Liquid:** Heavy mineral oil	In 30 and 180 ml, pt, qt and gal.	69+
otc	**Neo-Cultol** (Fisons)	**Jelly:** Refined mineral oil	Sugar. Chocolate flavor. In 180 ml.	680
otc	**Milkinol** (Schwarz Pharma Kremers-Urban)	**Emulsion:** Mineral oil with an emulsifier	In 355 ml.	250
otc sf	**Agoral Plain** (Warner-Lambert)	**Emulsion:** 1.4 g mineral oil per 5 ml with agar, tragacanth, egg albumin, acacia and glycerin	In 480 ml.	160
otc sf	**Kondremul Plain** (Fisons)	**Emulsion:** Mineral oil	Irish moss, acacia, glycerin. Maple walnut flavor. In 480 ml.	170

Fecal Softeners

DOCUSATE SODIUM (Dioctyl Sodium Sulfosuccinate; DSS)

Administration and Dosage:

Increase the daily fluid intake by drinking a glass of water with each dose.

Adults and older children: 50 to 500 mg.
Children (6 to 12): 40 to 120 mg.
Children (3 to 6): 20 to 60 mg.
Children (< 3): 10 to 40 mg.

Give higher doses for initial therapy; individualize dosage.

Liquid: Give in milk, fruit juice or infant formula to mask taste. In enemas, add 50 to 100 mg (5 to 10 ml liquid) to a retention or flushing enema.

	Product	Form	Packaging	C.I.*
otc	**Regutol** (Schering-Plough)	**Tablets:** 100 mg	Lactose, sugar. In UD 30s, 60s and 90s.	153
otc	**Docusate Sodium** (Roxane)	**Capsules:** 50 mg	In 100s and UD 100s.	20
otc	**Colace** (Mead Johnson)		In 30s, 60s, 250s, 1000s and UD 100s.	220
otc	**Docusate Sodium** (Various, eg, Geneva Marsam, Lederle, Major, Purepac, Rugby, Schein, URL)	**Capsules:** 100 mg	In 100s, 1000s and UD 100s.	20+
otc	**Colace** (Mead Johnson)		In 30s, 60s, 250s, 1000s and UD 100s.	140
otc	**Disonate** (Lannett)		Amber. In 100s, 500s, 1000s.	20
otc	**DOK** (Major)		In 1000s.	30
otc	**DOS Softgel** (Goldline)		Red-orange. Oval. In 60s, 100s and 1000s.	50
otc	**D-S-S** (Warner Chilcott)		(WC 247). In 100s, 1000s and UD 100s.	30
otc	**Modane Soft** (Adria)		Sorbitol. In UD 30s.	150
otc	**Pro-Sof** (Vangard)		In 30s, 60s, 90s, 100s, 1000s and UD 100s and Metripak 640s.	60
otc	**Regulax SS** (Republic)		In 100s.	NA

* Cost Index based on cost per 15 ml mineral oil or 100 mg DSS.
sf – Sugar free.

(Continued on following page)

Complete prescribing information for these products begins on page 1642

Fecal Softeners (Cont.)

DOCUSATE SODIUM (Dioctyl Sodium Sulfosuccinate; DSS) (Cont.)				C.I.*
otc	**Disonate** (Lannett)	**Capsules:** 240 mg	Amber. In 100s, 500s and 1000s.	41
otc	**Doxinate** (Hoechst-Roussel)		Sorbitol. Yellow. In 100s.	84
otc	**Docusate Sodium** (Various, eg, Geneva Marsam, Goldline, Major, Purepac, Rugby, Schein, URL, Vitarine)	**Capsules:** 250 mg	In 100s and 1000s.	17+
otc	**Dioeze** (Century)		In 100s and 1000s.	13
otc	**DOK** (Major)		In 100s and 1000s.	NA
otc	**DOS Softgels** (Goldline)		Red-orange. In 30s, 100s and 500s.	17
otc	**Pro-Sof** (Vangard)		In UD 100s.	NA
otc	**Regulax SS** (Republic)		In 100s.	NA
otc	**Correctol Extra Gentle** (Schering-Plough)	**Capsules, soft gel:** 100 mg	Rose. In 30s.	NA
otc	**Docusate Sodium** (Roxane)	**Syrup:** 50 mg per 15 ml	Saccharin, sucrose. In UD 15 and 30 ml (100s).	369
otc	**Docusate Sodium** (Various, eg, Geneva Marsam, Lederle, Major, PBI, Schein)	**Syrup:** 60 mg per 15 ml	In pt and gal.	177+
otc	**Diocto** (Various, eg, Dixon-Shane, Goldline, Moore, PBI, Rugby, URL)		In pt and gal.	208+
otc	**Colace** (Mead Johnson)		≤ 1% alcohol, menthol, sucrose. In 240 & 480 ml.	533
otc	**Disonate** (Lannett)		In 240 ml, pt and gal.	156
otc	**DOK** (Major)		In pt and gal.	177
otc	**Pro-Sof** (Vangard)		In pt.	NA
otc	**Diocto** (Various, eg, Dixon-Shane, Goldline, Moore, Rugby)	**Liquid:** 150 mg per 15 ml	In pt and gal.	NA
otc	**Colace** (Mead Johnson)		With calibrated dropper. In 30 and 480 ml.	1010
otc	**Disonate** (Lannett)		In pt.	245
otc	**DOK** (Major)		In pt.	266
otc	**Doxinate** (Hoechst-Roussel)	**Solution:** 50 mg per ml	5% alcohol. In 60 ml and gal.	490

* Cost Index based on cost per 100 mg.

Complete prescribing information for these products begins on page 1642

Fecal Softeners (Cont.)

DOCUSATE CALCIUM (Dioctyl Calcium Sulfosuccinate)

Administration and Dosage:

Adults: 240 mg daily until bowel movements are normal.

Children (≥ 6 years) and adults with minimal needs: 50 to 150 mg daily.

				C.I.*
otc	**Surfak Liquigels** (Hoechst-Roussel)	**Capsules:** 50 mg	≤ 1.3% alcohol, sorbitol. Orange. In 30s and 100s.	510
otc	**Docusate Calcium** (Various, eg, Dixon-Shane, Geneva Marsam, Major, Parmed, Rugby, Schein)	**Capsules:** 240 mg	In 100s, 250s, 500s, 1000s and UD 100s.	60+
otc	**DC Softgels** (Goldline)		Red, oblong. In 100s and 500s.	90+
otc	**Pro-Cal-Sof** (Vangard)		In 1000s, UD 100s, Metripak 640s.	100
otc	**Sulfalax Calcium** (Major)		In 500s.	230
otc	**Surfak Liquigels** (Hoechst-Roussel)		≤ 3% alcohol, sorbitol. Red. In 7s, 30s, 100s, 500s and UD 100s.	140

DOCUSATE POTASSIUM (Dioctyl Potassium Sulfosuccinate)

Administration and Dosage:

Adults: 100 to 300 mg daily until bowel movements are normal.

Children (≥ 6 years): 100 mg at bedtime.

				C.I.*
otc	**Dialose** (J & J-Merck)	**Tablets:** 100 mg	Lactose. (Dialose.) Pink. In 36s.	420
otc	**Diocto-K** (Rugby)		Pink. In 100s.	100
otc	**Kasof** (J & J-Merck)	**Capsules:** 240 mg	Sorbitol. Brown. In 30s and 60s.	100

Hyperosmolar Agents

GLYCERIN

Administration and Dosage:

Suppositories: Insert one suppository high in the rectum and retain 15 minutes; it need not melt to produce laxative action.

Rectal liquid: With gentle, steady pressure, insert stem with tip pointing towards navel. Squeeze unit until nearly all the liquid is expelled, then remove. A small amount of liquid will remain in unit.

				C.I.*
otc	**Glycerin, USP** (Various, eg, Dixon-Shane, Goldline, Major, Moore, Purepac, Rugby, Schein, URL)	**Suppositories:** Glycerin and sodium stearate	**Adults:** In 10s, 12s, 25s, 50s and 100s. **Pediatric:** In 10s, 12s and 25s.	50+ 50+
otc	**Sani-Supp** (G & W Labs)		**Adults:** In 10s, 25s and 50s. **Pediatric:** In 10s and 25s.	50+ 50+
otc	**Fleet Babylax** (Fleet)	**Liquid:** 4 ml per applicator	In 6 applicators.	460+

* Cost Index based on cost per 240 mg docusate calcium or docusate potassium or per glycerin suppository or applicator.

Complete prescribing information for these products begins on page 1642

	Enemas			C.I.*
otc	**Fleet** (Fleet)	**Disposable Enema:** 7 g sodium phosphate and 19 g sodium biphosphate per 118 ml delivered dose (4.4 g sodium per dose) *Dose:* Adults – 118 ml. Children (≥ 2 years) – ½ the adult dose.	In squeeze bottles. **Pediatric:** In 67.5 ml. **Adult:** In 133 ml.	 780 840
otc	**Fleet Bisacodyl** (Fleet)	**Disposable Enema:** 10 mg bisacodyl per 30 ml delivered dose *Dose:* Adults – 30 ml.	In 37 ml squeeze bottles.	1570
otc	**Fleet Bisacodyl Prep** (Fleet)	**Enema:** 10 mg bisacodyl in 10 ml aqueous suspension per packet *Dose:* Cleansing enema – 1 packet in 1.5 L water. Barium enema – 1 packet into barium suspension.	In 36 packets.	1180
otc	**Fleet Mineral Oil** (Fleet)	**Disposable Enema:** Mineral oil *Dose:* Adults – 118 ml. Children (> 2 years) – ½ adult dose.	In 133 ml plastic squeeze bottles.	940
otc	**Therevac-SB** (Jones Medical)	**Disposable Enema:** 283 mg docusate sodium in a base of soft soap, PEG 400 and glycerin per 3.9 g capsule *Dose:* 3.9 g.	In 30 disposable capsules per bottle.	1090
otc	**Therevac-Plus** (Jones Medical)	**Disposable Enema:** 283 mg docusate sodium and 20 mg benzocaine in a base of soft soap, PEG 400 and glycerin per 3.9 g capsule *Dose:* 3.9 g.	In 50 disposable capsules per bottle.	1090

BISACODYL TANNEX

Administration and Dosage:

Cleansing enema: 2.5 g (1 packet) in 1 L warm water.

Barium enema: 2.5 or 5 g in 1 L barium suspension.

Total dosage for one colonic examination should not exceed 7.5 g. Do not give > 10 g within a 72 hour period.

Do not administer to children < 10 years of age.

				C.I.*
Rx	**Clysodrast** (Rhone-Poulenc Rorer)	**Powder:** 1.5 mg bisacodyl and 2.5 g tannic acid per packet	In 25s and 50s.	1640

	CO_2 Releasing Suppositories			C.I.*
otc	**Ceo-Two** (Beutlich)	**Suppositories:** Sodium bicarbonate and potassium bitartrate in a water soluble polyethylene glycol base Before inserting, moisten suppository with warm water.	In 10s.	3430

* Cost Index based on cost per single enema unit, powder packet or suppository.

LACTULOSE

Actions:

Pharmacology: Lactulose, a synthetic disaccharide analog of lactose containing galactose and fructose, decreases blood ammonia concentrations and reduces the degree of portal-systemic encephalopathy.

The human GI tissue does not have an enzyme capable of hydrolysis of this disaccharide; as a result, oral doses pass to the colon virtually unchanged. After reaching the colon, lactulose is metabolized by bacteria *(Lactobacillus, Bacteroides, Escherichia coli* and *Streptococcus faecalis)* resulting in the formation of low molecular weight acids (lactic acid, formic acid, acetic acid) and carbon dioxide. These products produce an increased osmotic pressure and slightly acidify the colonic contents, resulting in an increase in stool water content and stool softening. Since the colonic contents are more acidic than the blood, ammonia can migrate from the blood into the colon. The acid colonic contents convert NH_3 to the ammonium ion $[NH_4]^+$, trapping it and preventing its absorption. The laxative action of the lactulose metabolites then expels the trapped ammonium ion from the colon.

Lactulose may also interfere with glutamine-dependent non-bacterial ammonia production in the intestinal wall.

Pharmacokinetics: Lactulose is poorly absorbed. When given orally, only small amounts reach the blood. Urinary excretion is $\leq$ 3% and is essentially complete within 24 hours. Lactulose does not exert its effect until it reaches the colon. Transit time through the colon may be slow; therefore, 24 to 48 hours may be required to produce a normal bowel movement.

Indications:

Chronulac, Constilac, Duphalac: Treatment of constipation.

Cephulac, Cholac, Enulose: Prevention and treatment of portal-systemic encephalopathy, including the stages of hepatic pre-coma and coma. Lactulose reduces blood ammonia levels by 25% to 50%; this generally parallels improved mental state and EEG patterns.

Clinical response has been observed in about 75% of patients. An increase in protein tolerance is also frequent. In chronic portal-systemic encephalopathy, lactulose has been given for > 2 years in controlled studies.

Contraindications:

Patients who require a low galactose diet.

Warnings:

Electrocautery procedures: A theoretical hazard may exist for patients being treated with lactulose who may undergo electrocautery procedures during proctoscopy or colonoscopy. Accumulation of H_2 gas in significant concentration in the presence of an electrical spark may result in an explosion. Although this complication has not been reported with lactulose, patients should have a thorough bowel cleansing with a nonfermentable solution. Insufflation of CO_2 as an additional safeguard may be pursued, but is considered a redundant measure.

Pregnancy: Category B. The safety of lactulose during pregnancy and its effect on the fetus or the mother have not been evaluated in humans. Use only when clearly needed and when the potential benefits outweigh the potential hazards to the mother and fetus.

Lactation: It is not known whether lactulose is excreted in breast milk. Exercise caution when administering lactulose to a nursing mother.

Children: Safety and efficacy for use in children have not been established. Infants receiving lactulose may develop hyponatremia and dehydration.

Precautions:

Diabetics: Lactulose syrup contains galactose (< 2.2 g/15 ml) and lactose (< 1.2 g/15 ml). Use with caution in these individuals.

Concomitant laxative use: Do not use other laxatives, especially during the initial phase of therapy for portal-systemic encephalopathy; the resulting loose stools may falsely suggest adequate lactulose dosage.

Monitoring: In the overall management of portal-systemic encephalopathy, there is serious underlying liver disease with complications such as electrolyte disturbance (eg, hypokalemia and hypernatremia) which may require other specific therapy. Elderly, debilitated patients who receive lactulose for > 6 months should have serum electrolytes (potassium, chloride) and carbon dioxide measured periodically.

Drug Interactions:

Neomycin and other anti-infectives: Reports conflict about concomitant use of lactulose syrup. The elimination of certain colonic bacteria may interfere with the desired degradation of lactulose and prevent the acidification of colonic contents. Monitor the patient if concomitant oral anti-infectives are given.

Antacids: Nonabsorbable antacids given concurrently with lactulose may inhibit the desired lactulose-induced drop in colonic pH.

(Continued on following page)

LACTULOSE (Cont.)

Adverse Reactions:

Gaseous distention with flatulence or belching and abdominal discomfort, such as cramping (20%). Excessive dosage can lead to diarrhea. Nausea and vomiting have occurred.

Overdosage:

There have been no reports of accidental overdose. It is expected that diarrhea and abdominal cramps would be the major symptoms. Discontinue the medication.

Patient Information:

May be mixed with fruit juice, water or milk to increase palatability.

May cause belching, flatulence or abdominal cramps; notify physician if these effects become bothersome or if diarrhea occurs.

Do not take other laxatives while on lactulose therapy.

In the event that an unusual diarrheal condition occurs, contact your physician.

Administration and Dosage:

Chronulac, Constilac, Duphalac: Treatment of constipation – 15 to 30 ml (10 to 20 g lactulose) daily, increased to 60 ml/day, if necessary.

Cephulac, Cholac, Enulose: Prevention and treatment of portal-systemic encephalopathy.

Oral – Adults: 30 to 45 ml, 3 or 4 times daily. Adjust dosage every day or two to produce 2 or 3 soft stools daily. Hourly doses of 30 to 45 ml may be used to induce rapid laxation in the initial phase of therapy. When the laxative effect has been achieved, reduce dosage to recommended daily dose. Improvement may occur within 24 hours, but may not begin before 48 hours or later. Continuous long-term therapy is indicated to lessen severity and prevent recurrence of portal-systemic encephalopathy.

Children: There is little information on use in children and adolescents. The goal is to produce 2 or 3 soft stools daily. Recommended initial daily oral dose in infants is 2.5 to 10 ml in divided doses. For older children and adolescents, the total daily dose is 40 to 90 ml. If the initial dose causes diarrhea, reduce immediately. If diarrhea persists, discontinue use.

Rectal – Administer to adults during impending coma or coma stage of portal-systemic encephalopathy when the danger of aspiration exists or when endoscopic or intubation procedures interfere with oral administration. The goal of treatment is reversal of the coma stage so the patient can take oral medication. Reversal of coma may occur within 2 hours of the first enema. Start recommended oral doses before enema is stopped entirely.

Lactulose may be given as a retention enema via a rectal balloon catheter. Do not use cleansing enemas containing soap suds or other alkaline agents.

Mix 300 ml lactulose with 700 ml water or physiologic saline and retain for 30 to 60 minutes. The enema may be repeated every 4 to 6 hours. If the enema is inadvertently evacuated too promptly, it may be repeated immediately.

May be more palatable when mixed with fruit juice, water or milk.

Storage: Store below 86°F (30°C); do not freeze.

	Product	Form	Packaging	C.I.*
Rx	**Cephulac** (Marion Merrell Dow)	**Syrup:** 10 g lactulose per 15 ml. (<2.2 g galactose, <1.2 g lactose and ≤ 1.2 g of other sugars).	In 480 ml, 1.9 L and UD 30 ml.	956
Rx	**Cholac** (Alra)		In 240, 480 and 960 ml, 1.9 L, gal and UD 30 ml.	906
Rx	**Chronulac** (Marion Merrell Dow)		In 240 and 960 ml and UD 30 ml.	854
Rx	**Constilac** (Alra)		In 240, 480 and 960 ml, 1.9 L, gal and UD 30 ml.	560
Rx	**Constulose** (Barre-National)		In 237, 473 and 946 ml and 1.89 L.	559
Rx	**Duphalac** (Solvay Pharm.)		In 240, 480 and 960 ml and UD 30 ml.	664
Rx	**Enulose** (Barre-National)		In pt and 1.89 L.	696+
Rx	**Lactulose** (Various, eg, Moore, Schiapparelli Searle)		In 240 and 960 ml and UD 30 ml.	670+

* Cost Index based on cost per 15 ml.

Refer to the general discussion of these products beginning on page 1642

In addition to the laxatives listed on the previous pages, these combinations include:
DEHYDROCHOLIC ACID, used as a choleretic (see p. 1630
CASANTHRANOL is a stimulant laxative.

Dose: 1 or 2 at bedtime with a full glass of water.

Capsules and Tablets

		Docusate (mg)	Senna Concentrate (mg)	Phenolphthalein (mg)	Casanthranol (mg)	Other Content and How Supplied	C.I.*
otc	**Gentlax S Tablets** (Blair)	50[1]	8.6[2]			Lactose. In 60s.	170
otc	**Senokot-S Tablets** (Purdue Frederick)	50[1]	187			Lactose. In 30s, 60s, 1000s and UD 100s.	220
otc	**Doxidan Capsules** (Upjohn)	60[3]		65		Sorbitol. Maroon. In 10s, 30s, 100s, 1000s and UD 100s.	120
otc	**Docucal-P Softgels (Capsules)** (Parmed)					In 100s and 1000s.	43
otc	**Ex-Lax, Extra Gentle Pills (Tablets)** (Sandoz Consumer)	75[1]		65		Sucose. Pink. In 24s.	100
otc	**Phillips' LaxCaps (Capsules)** (Glenbrook)	83[1]		90		Sorbitol. In 8s and 24s.	100
otc	**Colax Tablets** (Rugby)	100[1]		65		In 30s.	50
otc	**Correctol Tablets** (Schering Plough)					Sugar. In 15s, 30s, 60s and 90s.	80
otc	**Disolan Capsules** (Lannett)					Blue and yellow. In 100s, 500s and 1000s.	40
otc	**Feen-a-mint Pills (Tablets)** (Schering Plough)					Sugar. In 15s, 30s and 60s.	80
otc	**Femilax Tablets** (G & W Labs)					In 30s, 60s and 90s.	40
otc	**Modane Plus Tablets** (Adria)					Sucrose. In 10s, 30s and 100s.	180
otc	**Unilax Capsules** (B.F. Ascher)	230[1]		130		Sorbitol. In 15s and 60s.	120

* Cost Index based on cost per capsule or tablet.
[1] As sodium.
[2] As sennosides.
[3] As calcium.

(Continued on following page)

Refer to the general discussion of these products beginning on page 1661.

Capsules and Tablets (Cont.)

		Docusate (mg)	Senna Concentrate (mg)	Phenolphthalein (mg)	Casanthranol (mg)	Other Content and How Supplied	C.I.*
otc	**Docusate w/ Casanthranol Caps** (Various, eg, Geneva Marsam, Major, Schein)	100[1]			30	In 100s, 1000s and UD 100s.	30+
otc	**Disanthrol Capsules** (Lannett)					In 100s and 1000s.	40
otc	**D-S-S plus Capsules** (Warner-Chilcott)					Maroon. In 100s, 1000s and UD 100s.	30
otc	**Genasoft Plus Softgels (Capsules)** (Goldline)					Maroon. In 60s.	60
otc	**Peri-Colace Capsules** (Mead Johnson)					Maroon. In 30s, 60s, 250s, 1000s and UD 100s.	170
otc	**Peri-Dos Softgels (Capsules)** (Goldline)					Maroon. In 100s and 1000s.	40
otc	**Pro-Sof Plus Capsules** (Vangard)					In 100s, 1000s and UD 32s and 100s.	60
otc	**Regulace Capsules** (Republic)					In 100s.	NA
otc	**Docusate Potassium w/ Casanthranol Capsules** (Various, eg, UDL, URL)	100[2]			30	In 100s, 1000s and UD 100s.	NA
otc	**Dialose Plus Capsules** (J & J-Merck)					Lactose. (Dialose Plus). Yellow. In 36s, 100s, 500s and UD 100s.	200
otc	**Diocto-K Plus Capsules** (Rugby)					Sorbitol. Yellow. In 100s and 1000s.	50
otc	**Dioctolose Plus Capsules** (Goldline)					Yellow. In 100s and 1000s.	80
otc	**DSMC Plus Capsules** (Geneva Marsam)					Yellow. In 100s.	60

* Cost Index based on cost per capsule.
[1] As sodium.
[2] As potassium.

(Continued on following page)

Refer to the general discussion of these products beginning on page 1661 .

Capsules and Tablets (Cont.)

		Docusate (mg)	Senna Concentrate (mg)	Phenolphthalein (mg)	Casanthranol (mg)	Cascara Sagrada (mg)	Sodium Carboxymethylcellulose (mg)	Other Content and How Supplied	C.I.*
otc	**Disoplex Capsules** (Lannett)	100[1]					400	Pink. In 100s, 500s and 1000s.	20
otc	**Disolan Forte Capsules** (Lannett)	100[1]			30		400	Yellow. In 100s, 500s and 1000s.	40
otc *sf*	**Herbal Laxative Tablets** (Nature's Bounty)		125[2]			20[3]		5 mg buckthorn bark PDR. In 100s.	NA
otc	**Caroid Laxative Tablets** (Mentholatum)			32.4		50[4]		In 20s, 50s and 100s.	70
otc	**Nature's Remedy Tablets** (SK Beecham Consumer)					150		100 mg aloe, lactose. In 12s, 30s and 60s.	150

* Cost Index based on cost per capsule or tablet.
[1] As sodium.
[2] As senna leaves.
[3] As cascara sagada bark.
[4] As extract.

Refer to the general discussion of these products beginning on page 1642

Liquids

Dose: Usual adult dose is 5 to 45 ml with a full glass of water at bedtime.

	Product	Content	Notes	C.I.*
otc	**Diocto C** (Various, eg, Barre National, Dixon-Shane, Moore, Rugby, URL)	**Syrup:** 60 mg docusate sodium and 30 mg casanthranol per 15 ml	In 240 ml, pt and gal.	140+
otc	**Docusate Sodium w/Casanthranol** (Various, eg, Geneva Marsam, Major, Schein)		In pt and gal.	130+
otc	**Peri-Colace** (Mead Johnson)		10% alcohol. Sorbitol, sucrose. In 240 and 480 ml.	320
otc sf	**Liqui-Doss** (Ferndale)	**Emulsion:** Mineral oil in an emulsifying base	Alcohol free. In pt.	150
otc sf	**Kondremul w/Phenolphthalein** (Fisons)	**Emulsion:** 55% mineral oil and 150 mg phenolphthalein per 15 ml with Irish Moss	In pt.	190
otc sf	**Agoral** (Warner-Lambert)	**Emulsion:** 4.2 g mineral oil and 0.2 g phenolphthalein per 15 ml with agar, tragacanth, egg albumin, acacia, glycerin and saccharin	Plain, marshmallow and raspberry flavors. In 480 ml.	160
otc	**Haley's M-O** (Glenbrook)	**Liquid:** 900 mg magnesium hydroxide and 3.75 ml mineral oil per 15 ml	Saccharin. Regular or flavored. In 120, 360 and 780 ml.	110
otc	**Black-Draught** (Chattem)	**Syrup:** 90 mg per 15 ml casanthranol with senna extract, fluid rhubarb aromatic, methyl salicylate and menthol	5% alcohol. Tartrazine, sugar. In 150 ml.	200

Powders and Granules

Dose: Usual adult dose is 1 or 2 rounded tsp, 1 to 3 times daily, with a full glass of water.

	Product	Content	Notes	C.I.*
otc	**Syllamalt** (Wallace)	**Powder:** 4 g malt soup extract, 3 g psyllium seed husks and 13 calories/rounded tsp	In 300 g.	1130
otc	**Perdiem** (Rhone-Poulenc Rorer)	**Granules:** 3.25 g psyllium, 0.74 g senna, 1.8 mg sodium, 35.5 mg potassium and 4 calories per rounded teaspoonful (6 g)	Dye free. Sucrose. In 100 and 250 g.	550

* Cost Index based on cost per 15 ml or tsp powder or granules.

sf – Sugar free.

DIFENOXIN HCl WITH ATROPINE SULFATE

Actions:

Difenoxin is an antidiarrheal agent chemically related to meperidine. Atropine sulfate is present to discourage deliberate overdosage.

Pharmacology: Animal studies have shown that difenoxin manifests its antidiarrheal effect by slowing intestinal motility. The mechanism of action is by a local effect on the gastrointestinal wall.

Difenoxin is the principal active metabolite of diphenoxylate and is effective at one-fifth the dosage of diphenoxylate.

Pharmacokinetics: Difenoxin is rapidly and extensively absorbed orally. Mean peak plasma levels of 160 ng/ml occur within 40 to 60 minutes in most patients following a 2 mg dose. Plasma levels decline to less than 10% of their peak values within 24 hours and to less than 1% of their peak values within 72 hours. This decline parallels the appearance of difenoxin and its metabolites in the urine. Difenoxin is metabolized to an inactive hydroxylated metabolite. Both the drug and its metabolites are excreted, mainly as conjugates, in urine and feces.

Indications:

Adjunctive therapy in management of acute nonspecific diarrhea and acute exacerbations of chronic functional diarrhea.

Contraindications:

Diarrhea associated with organisms that penetrate the intestinal mucosa (eg, toxigenic *E coli, Salmonella* sp, *Shigella*) and pseudomembranous colitis associated with broad-spectrum antibiotics. Antiperistaltic agents may prolong or worsen diarrhea.

Children under 2 years of age because of the decreased margin of safety of drugs in this class in younger age groups.

Hypersensitivity to difenoxin, atropine or any of the inactive ingredients; jaundice.

Warnings:

Difenoxin HCl with atropine sulfate is *not* innocuous; strictly adhere to dosage recommendations. It is not recommended for children under 2 years of age. Overdosage may result in severe respiratory depression and coma, possibly leading to permanent brain damage or death (see Overdosage).

Fluid and electrolyte balance: The use of this drug does not preclude the administration of appropriate fluid and electrolyte therapy. Dehydration, particularly in children, may further influence the variability of response and may predispose to delayed difenoxin intoxication. Drug-induced inhibition of peristalsis may result in fluid retention in the colon, and this may further aggravate dehydration and electrolyte imbalance. If severe dehydration or electrolyte imbalance is manifested, withhold the drug until appropriate corrective therapy has been initiated.

Ulcerative colitis: Agents which inhibit intestinal motility or delay intestinal transit time have induced toxic megacolon. Consequently, carefully observe patients with acute ulcerative colitis. Discontinue promptly if abdominal distention occurs or if other untoward symptoms develop.

Liver and kidney disease: Use with extreme caution in patients with advanced hepatorenal disease and in all patients with abnormal liver function tests since hepatic coma may be precipitated.

Atropine: A subtherapeutic dose of atropine has been added to difenoxin to discourage deliberate overdosage. A recommended dose is not likely to cause prominent anticholinergic side effects, but avoid in patients in whom anticholinergic drugs are contraindicated. Observe the warnings and precautions for use of anticholinergic agents. In children, signs of atropinism may occur even with recommended doses, particularly in patients with Down's Syndrome.

Pregnancy: Category C. Reproduction studies in rats and rabbits with doses up to 75 times the human therapeutic dose demonstrated no evidence of teratogenesis. Pregnant rats receiving oral doses 20 times the maximum human dose had an increase in delivery time as well as a significant increase in the percent of stillbirths. Neonatal survival in rats was also reduced with most deaths occurring within 4 days of delivery. There are no well controlled studies in pregnant women. Use during pregnancy only if the potential benefit justifies the potential risk to the fetus.

Lactation: Because of the potential for serious adverse reactions in nursing infants, decide whether to discontinue nursing or to discontinue the drug, taking into account the importance of the drug to the mother.

Children: Contraindicated in children under 2 years of age. Safety and efficacy in children below the age of 12 have not been established. See Overdosage section for information on hazards from accidental poisoning in children.

(Continued on following page)

DIFENOXIN HCl WITH ATROPINE SULFATE (Cont.)

Drug Interactions:

Monoamine oxidase (MAO) inhibitors: Since the chemical structure of difenoxin is similar to meperidine, concurrent use with MAO inhibitors may, in theory, precipitate a hypertensive crisis.

Barbiturates, tranquilizers, narcotics and **alcohol** may be potentiated by coadministration of difenoxin. Closely monitor patients.

Adverse Reactions:

Anticholinergic: In view of the small amount of atropine present (0.025 mg/tablet), effects such as dryness of the skin and mucous membranes, flushing, hyperthermia, tachycardia and urinary retention are very unlikely to occur, except perhaps in children.

Many adverse effects reported during clinical investigation are difficult to distinguish from symptoms of diarrheal syndrome. However, the following events have occurred:

GI: Nausea (7%), vomiting, dry mouth (3%); epigastric distress, constipation (≤ 1%).

CNS: Dizziness, lightheadedness (5%); drowsiness (4%); headache (2.5%); tiredness, nervousness, insomnia, confusion (< 1%).

Ophthalmic: Burning eyes, blurred vision (infrequent).

Overdosage:

Symptoms: Initial signs may include dryness of the skin and mucous membranes, flushing, hyperthermia and tachycardia followed by lethargy or coma, hypotonic reflexes, nystagmus, pinpoint pupils and respiratory depression.

Treatment: Gastric lavage, establishment of a patent airway and, possibly, mechanically assisted respiration are advised. Refer to General Management of Acute Overdosage.

Naloxone may be used in the treatment of respiratory depression. When administered IV, the onset is generally apparent within 2 minutes. Naloxone may also be administered SC or IM providing a slightly less rapid onset but a more prolonged effect.

Since the duration of action of difenoxin is longer than that of naloxone, improvement of respiration following administration may be followed by recurrent respiratory depression. Continuous observation is necessary until the effect of difenoxin on respiration (which may persist for many hours) has passed. Supplemental IM naloxone doses may be used to produce a longer lasting effect. Treat all possible overdosages as serious; observe for at least 48 hours, preferably under continuous hospital care.

Although signs of overdosage and respiratory depression may not be evident soon after ingestion of difenoxin, respiratory depression may occur 12 to 30 hours later.

Drug Abuse/Dependence:

Addiction to (dependence on) difenoxin is theoretically possible at high dosage. Therefore, do not exceed recommended dosage. Because of the structural and pharmacological similarities of difenoxin to drugs with definite addiction potential, administer with caution to patients receiving addicting drugs, to addiction-prone individuals, or to those whose histories suggest they may increase the dosage on their own initiative.

Patient Information:

Adhere strictly to recommended dosage schedules. Keep out of reach of children since accidental overdosage may result in severe, even fatal, respiratory depression.

Drowsiness or dizziness may occur. Exercise caution in activities requiring mental alertness, coordination or physical dexterity, eg, driving or operating dangerous machinery.

Administration and Dosage:

Adults: Recommended starting dose: 2 tablets, then 1 tablet after each loose stool; 1 tablet every 3 to 4 hours as needed. The total dosage during any 24 hour treatment period should not exceed 8 tablets. For diarrhea in which clinical improvement is not observed in 48 hours, continued administration is not recommended. For acute diarrhea and acute exacerbations of functional diarrhea, treatment beyond 48 hours is usually not necessary.

Children: Studies in children < 12 years old are inadequate to evaluate safety and efficacy. Contraindicated in children < 2 years old.

				C.I.*
c-iv	**Motofen** (Carnrick)	**Tablets:** 1 mg difenoxin (as HCl) and 0.025 mg atropine sulfate	Dye free. (C 8674). White, scored. Five-sided. In 50s and 100s.	598

*Cost Index based on cost per tablet.

DIPHENOXYLATE HCl WITH ATROPINE SULFATE

Actions:

Pharmacology: Diphenoxylate, a constipating meperidine congener, lacks analgesic activity. High doses (40 to 60 mg) cause opioid activity, including euphoria, suppression of morphine abstinence syndrome and physical dependence after chronic use.

Pharmacokinetics: The bioavailability of the tablet compared with the liquid is ≈ 90%. Diphenoxylate is rapidly and extensively metabolized to diphenoxylic acid (difenoxine), which is biologically active and the major metabolite. Elimination half-life of diphenoxine is ≈ 12 to 14 hours. An average of 14% of the drug and its metabolites are excreted over 4 days in urine, 49% in feces. Urinary excretion of unmetabolized drug is < 1%; difenoxine plus its glucuronide conjugate constitutes ≈ 6%.

Indications:

Adjunctive therapy in the management of diarrhea.

Contraindications:

Children < 2 years old due to greater variability of response; hypersensitivity to diphenoxylate or atropine; obstructive jaundice; diarrhea associated with pseudomembranous enterocolitis or enterotoxin-producing bacteria (see Warnings).

Warnings:

Diarrhea: Diphenoxylate may prolong or aggravate diarrhea associated with organisms that penetrate the intestinal mucosa (ie, toxigenic *Escherichia coli, Salmonella, Shigella*) or in pseudomembranous enterocolitis associated with broad-spectrum antibiotic therapy. Do not use diphenoxylate in these conditions. In some patients with acute ulcerative colitis, diphenoxylate may induce toxic megacolon. Discontinue therapy promptly if abdominal distention or other untoward symptoms develop.

Hepatic function impairment: Use with extreme caution in patients with advanced hepatorenal disease or abnormal liver function; hepatic coma may be precipitated.

Fluid/electrolyte balance: Dehydration, particularly in younger children, may influence variability of response and may predispose to delayed diphenoxylate intoxication. Inhibition of peristalsis may result in fluid retention in the intestine, which may further aggravate dehydration and electrolyte imbalance. If severe dehydration or electrolyte imbalance occurs, withhold the drug until initiating corrective therapy.

Pregnancy: Category C. There are no adequate and well controlled studies in pregnant women. Use in women of childbearing potential only when clearly needed and when the potential benefits outweigh the potential hazards to the fetus.

Lactation: Exercise caution when administering to a nursing mother. Diphenoxylic acid may be excreted in breast milk and atropine is excreted in breast milk.

Children: Use with caution; signs of atropinism may occur with recommended doses, particularly in Down's syndrome patients. Use with caution in young children due to variable response. Not recommended in children < 2 years old.

Precautions:

Drug dependence: In recommended doses, diphenoxylate has not produced addiction and is devoid of morphine-like subjective effects. At high doses, it exhibits codeine-like subjective effects; therefore, addiction to diphenoxylate is possible. A subtherapeutic dose of atropine has been added to discourage deliberate abuse.

Hazardous tasks: May cause drowsiness or dizziness; observe caution while driving or performing other tasks requiring alertness, coordination or physical dexterity.

Drug Interactions:

Monoamine oxidase inhibitors: Since the chemical structure of diphenoxylate is similar to meperidine, concurrent use may precipitate hypertensive crises.

Barbiturates, tranquilizers and **alcohol**: Diphenoxylate may potentiate the depressant action. Closely observe the patient when these medications are used concomitantly.

Adverse Reactions:

Allergic: Pruritus; swelling of gums; angioneurotic edema; urticaria; anaphylaxis.

CNS: Dizziness; drowsiness; sedation; headache; malaise; lethargy; restlessness; euphoria; depression; numbness of extremities; confusion.

GI: Anorexia; nausea; vomiting; abdominal discomfort; paralytic ileus; toxic megacolon; pancreatitis.

Atropine effects: Dry skin and mucous membranes, flushing, hyperthermia, tachycardia, urinary retention, especially in children.

Overdosage:

Symptoms: Initial signs include dry skin and mucous membranes, mydriasis, restlessness, flushing, hyperthermia and tachycardia followed by lethargy or coma, hypotonic reflexes, nystagmus and pinpoint pupils. Severe, even fatal, respiratory depression may result. Although signs of overdosage and respiratory depression may not be evident soon after ingestion, respiratory depression may occur 12 to 30 hours later.

(Overdosage continued on following page)

DIPHENOXYLATE HCl WITH ATROPINE SULFATE (Cont.)

Overdosage (Cont.):

Treatment includes usual supportive measures. Refer to General Management of Acute Overdosage. Gastric lavage, induction of emesis, establishment of a patent airway, and, possibly, mechanically assisted respiration are advised. Use naloxone for respiratory depression (see individual monograph). Diphenoxylate's duration of action is longer than that of naloxone; improved respiration after administration may be followed by recurrent respiratory depression. Consequently, continuous observation for at least 48 hours is necessary until diphenoxylate's effect on respiration has passed. Activated charcoal may significantly decrease bioavailability of diphenoxylate. In non-comatose patients, 100 g activated charcoal slurry can be given immediately after induction of vomiting or gastric lavage.

Patient Information:

Do not exceed prescribed dosage. Avoid alcohol and other CNS depressants.

May cause drowsiness or dizziness; use caution while driving or performing other tasks requiring alertness, coordination or physical dexterity.

May cause dry mouth.

Notify physician if diarrhea persists or if fever, palpitations or abnormal distention occur.

Administration and Dosage:

Adults: Individualize dosage. Initial dose is 5 mg 4 times a day.

Children: See Warnings. In children 2 to 12 years of age, use liquid form only. The recommended initial dosage is 0.3 to 0.4 mg/kg daily, in 4 divided doses.

Diphenoxylate w/Atropine Pediatric Dosage

Age (years)	Approximate weight		Dosage (ml) (4 times daily)
	kg	lb	
2	11-14	24-31	1.5-3
3	12-16	26-35	2-3
4	14-20	31-44	2-4
5	16-23	35-51	2.5-4.5
6-8	17-32	38-71	2.5-5
9-12	23-55	51-121	3.5-5

This pediatric schedule is the best approximation of an average dose recommendation which may be adjusted downwards according to the overall nutritional status and degree of dehydration encountered in the sick child.

Reduce dosage as soon as initial control of symptoms is achieved. Maintenance dosage may be as low as ¼ of the initial daily dosage. Do not exceed recommended dosage. Clinical improvement of acute diarrhea is usually observed within 48 hours. If clinical improvement of chronic diarrhea is not seen within 10 days after a maximum daily dose of 20 mg, symptoms are unlikely to be controlled by further use.

	Product	Form	Packaging	C.I.*
c-v	**Diphenoxylate HCl w/ Atropine Sulfate** (Various, eg, Barr, Major, Mylan, Purepac, Rugby, Schein)	**Tablets:** 2.5 mg diphenoxylate HCl and 0.025 mg atropine sulfate	In 100s, 500s, 1000s, 2500s and UD 100s.	1+
c-v	**Lofene** (Lannett)		In 100s, 500s and 1000s.	1+
c-v	**Logen** (Goldline)		White. In 100s, 500s & 1000s.	1+
c-v	**Lomodix** (Dixon-Shane)		In 1000s.	1
c-v	**Lomotil** (Searle)		Sorbitol, sucrose. (Searle 61). White. In 100s, 500s, 1000s, 2500s and UD 100s.	6.6
c-v	**Lonox** (Geneva Marsam)		White. In 100s, 500s, 1000s & UD 100s.	1
c-v	**Low-Quel** (Halsey)		White. In 100s and 1000s.	1
c-v	**Diphenoxylate HCl w/ Atropine Sulfate** (Various, eg, Goldline, Major, Roxane, Rugby)	**Liquid:** 2.5 mg diphenoxylate HCl and 0.025 mg atropine sulfate per 5 ml	In 60 ml, UD 4 and 10 ml.	15+
c-v	**Lomanate** (Various, eg, Barre-National, Qualitest)		In 60 ml.	NA
c-v	**Lomotil** (Searle)		15% alcohol. Sorbitol. Cherry flavor. In 60 ml w/dropper.	16

* Cost Index based on cost per 2.5 mg diphenoxylate.

LOPERAMIDE HCl

Actions:

Pharmacology: Loperamide slows intestinal motility and affects water and electrolyte movement through the bowel. It inhibits peristalsis by a direct effect on the circular and longitudinal muscles of the intestinal wall. It reduces daily fecal volume, increases viscosity and bulk density and diminishes the loss of fluid and electrolytes. Tolerance to the antidiarrheal effect has not been observed.

In morphine-dependent monkeys, loperamide at higher than recommended doses prevented signs of morphine withdrawal. However, in humans, opiate-like effects have not been demonstrated after > 2 years of therapeutic use of loperamide.

Pharmacokinetics:

Absorption/Distribution – Loperamide is 40% absorbed after oral administration and does not penetrate well into the brain. Peak plasma levels occur approximately 5 hours after capsule administration, 2.5 hours after liquid administration and are similar for both formulations.

Metabolism/Excretion – The apparent elimination half-life is 10.8 hours (range, 9.1 to 14.4 hours). Of a 4 mg oral dose, 25% is excreted unchanged in the feces, and 1.3% is excreted in the urine as free drug and glucuronic acid conjugate within 3 days.

Indications:

Control and symptomatic relief of acute nonspecific diarrhea and of chronic diarrhea associated with inflammatory bowel disease.

For reducing the volume of discharge from ileostomies.

Unlabeled use: In one study, the combination of loperamide (4 mg loading dose, 2 mg after each loose stool) plus trimethoprim-sulfamethoxazole for 3 days resulted in more rapid relief from traveler's diarrhea than either agent alone.

Contraindications:

Hypersensitivity to the drug and in patients who must avoid constipation.

OTC use: Bloody diarrhea; body temperature > 101°F.

Warnings:

Diarrhea: Do not use loperamide in acute diarrhea associated with organisms that penetrate the intestinal mucosa (enteroinvasive *Escherichia coli, Salmonella* and *Shigella*) or in pseudomembranous colitis associated with broad-spectrum antibiotics.

Acute ulcerative colitis: In some patients with acute ulcerative colitis, agents which inhibit intestinal motility or delay intestinal transit time may induce toxic megacolon. Discontinue therapy promptly if abdominal distention occurs or if other untoward symptoms develop in patients with acute ulcerative colitis.

Fluid/electrolyte depletion may occur in patients who have diarrhea. The use of loperamide does not preclude administration of appropriate fluid and electrolyte therapy.

Pregnancy: Category B. There are no adequate and well controlled studies in pregnant women. Safety for use during pregnancy has not been established. Use only when clearly needed and when the potential benefits outweigh the potential hazards to the fetus.

Lactation: It is not known whether loperamide is excreted in breast milk. Safety for use in the nursing mother has not been established.

Children: Not recommended for use in children < 2 years old. Use loperamide with special caution in young children because of the greater variability of response in this age group. Dehydration may further influence the variability of response. A loperamide dosage has not been established for children in the treatment of chronic diarrhea.

Precautions:

Acute diarrhea: If clinical improvement is not observed in 48 hours, discontinue use.

Hepatic dysfunction: Monitor patients with hepatic dysfunction closely for signs of CNS toxicity because of the apparent large first-pass biotransformation.

Abuse and dependence: Physical dependence in humans has not been observed.

Adverse Reactions:

Adverse experiences are generally minor and self-limiting. They are more commonly observed during the treatment of chronic diarrhea.

Abdominal pain, distention or discomfort; constipation; dry mouth; nausea; vomiting; tiredness; drowsiness or dizziness; hypersensitivity reactions (including skin rash).

Overdosage:

Symptoms: Constipation, CNS depression and GI irritation. In clinical trials, nausea and vomiting occurred in an adult who took 60 mg within 24 hours. Ingestion of up to 60 mg loperamide in a single dose caused no significant adverse effects in healthy subjects. A 15-month-old, 8 kg child developed opioid toxicity (eg, pale skin, increased pulse rate, respiratory depression) following a single 1 g dose of loperamide.

(Overdosage continued on following page)

LOPERAMIDE HCl (Cont.)

Overdosage (Cont.):

Treatment: Activated charcoal administered promptly after loperamide ingestion can reduce the amount of drug absorbed into systemic circulation by up to ninefold. If vomiting has occurred spontaneously, administer a slurry of 100 g activated charcoal orally as soon as fluids can be retained. If vomiting has not occurred, perform gastric lavage, followed by 100 g activated charcoal through the gastric tube.

Monitor for signs of CNS depression for at least 24 hours; if CNS depression is observed, administer naloxone. Children may be more sensitive to CNS effects than adults. If responsive to naloxone, monitor vital signs for recurrence of symptoms for at least 24 hours after the last dose of naloxone. In view of the prolonged action of loperamide and the short duration (1 to 3 hours) of naloxone (see individual monograph), monitor the patient closely and repeat naloxone as indicated.

Since relatively little drug is excreted in the urine, forced diuresis is not expected to be effective for overdosage.

Patient Information:

Do not exceed prescribed dosage.

May cause drowsiness or dizziness; patients should observe caution while driving or performing other tasks requiring alertness, coordination or physical dexterity.

May cause dry mouth.

Notify physician if diarrhea does not stop after a few days or if abdominal pain or distention or fever occurs.

Administration and Dosage:

Acute diarrhea (Imodium capsules; Rx): Adults – Initial dosage is 4 mg followed by 2 mg after each unformed stool. Do not exceed 16 mg/day. Clinical improvement is usually observed within 48 hours.

Children – First day dosage schedule:

Loperamide Pediatric Dosage (First Day Schedule)			
Age (years)	Weight (kg)	Doseform	Amount
2-5	13-20	liquid	1 mg tid
6-8	20-30	liquid or capsule	2 mg bid
8-12	> 30	liquid or capsule	2 mg tid

This pediatric schedule is the best approximation of an average dose recommendation which may be adjusted downwards according to the overall nutritional status and degree of dehydration encountered in the sick child.

Subsequent doses: Administer 1 mg/10 kg only after a loose stool. Total daily dosage should not exceed recommended dosages for the first day.

Acute diarrhea (Imodium A-D tablets and liquid; otc): Adults – 4 mg after first loose bowel movement followed by 2 mg after each subsequent loose bowel movement but no more than 8 mg/day for no more than 2 days.

Children – 9 to 11 years old (60 to 95 lbs), 2 mg after first loose bowel movement followed by 1 mg after each subsequent loose bowel movement but no more than 6 mg/day for no more than 2 days; *6 to 8 years old* (48 to 59 lbs), 1 mg after first loose bowel movement followed by 1 mg after each subsequent loose bowel movement but no more than 4 mg/day for no more than 2 days; < *6 years old* (up to 47 lbs), consult physician (not intended for use in children < 6 years old.

Chronic diarrhea: Adults – Initial dosage is 4 mg followed by 2 mg after each unformed stool until diarrhea is controlled; then, individualize dosage. When optimal daily dosage (average, 4 to 8 mg) has been established, administer as a single dose or in divided doses.

If clinical improvement is not observed after treatment with 16 mg/day for at least 10 days, symptoms are unlikely to be controlled by further use. Continue administration if diarrhea cannot be adequately controlled with diet or specific treatment.

Children – Dose has not been established.

				C.I.*
otc	**Imodium A-D Caplets** (McNeil-CPC)	**Tablets:** 2 mg	Lactose. In 6s and 12s.	NA
Rx	**Imodium** (Janssen)	**Capsules:** 2 mg	Lactose. (Janssen Imodium). Two-tone green. In 100s, 500s and UD 100s.	1187
Rx	**Loperamide** (Various, eg, Mylan, Novopharm)	**Capsules:** 2 mg	In 100s, 500s and 1000s.	NA
otc	**Imodium A-D** (McNeil-CPC)	**Liquid:** 1 mg per 5 ml	5.25% alcohol. Cherry/licorice flavor. In 60, 90 and 120 ml.	2850

* Cost Index based on cost per 4 mg.

BISMUTH SUBSALICYLATE (BSS)

Actions:

Pharmacology: Bismuth subsalicylate (BSS) appears to have antisecretory and antimicrobial effects in vitro and may have some anti-inflammatory effects. The salicylate moiety provides the antisecretory effect, while the bismuth moiety may exert direct antimicrobial effects against bacterial and viral enteropathogens.

Pharmacokinetics: BSS undergoes chemical dissociation in the GI tract. Two BSS tablets yield 204 mg salicylate; the 30 ml suspension yields 258 mg salicylate. Following ingestion, salicylate is absorbed, with > 90% recovered in the urine; plasma levels are similar to levels achieved after a comparable dose of aspirin. Absorption of bismuth is negligible.

Indications:

For indigestion without causing constipation; nausea; control of diarrhea, including traveler's diarrhea, within 24 hours. Also relieves abdominal cramps.

Unlabeled uses: Bismuth subsalicylate has also been used in the prevention of traveler's diarrhea (enterotoxigenic *Escherichia coli*), in doses of 2.1 g/day (2 tablets 4 times daily, before meals and at bedtime) for up to 3 weeks during brief periods of high risk. The suspension has also been used (4.2 g/day). BSS has been effective in up to 65% of patients.

BSS has also been used for chronic infantile diarrhea (2.5 ml every 4 hours for children 2 to 24 months old; 5 ml for those 24 to 48 months old; 10 ml for those 48 to 70 months old) and for symptoms associated with Norwalk virus-induced gastroenteritis.

Precautions:

Impaction may occur in infants and debilitated patients.

Radiologic examinations: May interfere with radiologic examinations of GI tract. Bismuth is radiopaque.

Drug Interactions:

Aspirin: BSS contains salicylate. If taken with aspirin and ringing of the ears occurs, discontinue use. If taking medicines for anticoagulation, diabetes or gout, consult a physician.

Tetracycline: Bismuth may decrease GI absorption and bioavailability of tetracyclines, reducing their antimicrobial effectiveness.

Patient Information:

Shake liquid well before using. Chew tablets or allow to dissolve in mouth.

Stool may temporarily appear gray-black.

If diarrhea is accompanied by high fever or continues for > 2 days, consult physician.

Administration and Dosage:

Adults: 2 tablets or 30 ml.

Children: 9 to 12 years – 1 tablet or 15 ml.
6 to 9 years – ⅔ tablet or 10 ml.
3 to 6 years – ⅓ tablet or 5 ml.
< 3 years – Consult physician.

Repeat above dosage every 30 minutes to 1 hour, as needed, up to 8 doses in 24 hours.

	Product	Form	Description	C.I.*
otc sf	**Pepto-Bismol** (Procter & Gamble)	**Tablets, chewable:** 262 mg	< 2 mg sodium/tablet. Saccharin, mannitol. (Pepto-Bismol). Pink. Original and cherry flavors. In 30s and 42s (cherry flavor). In 24s and 42s (original flavor).	360
otc	**Bismatrol** (Major)		Saccharin. In 240 ml.	4
otc sf	**Pepto-Bismol** (Procter & Gamble)	**Liquid:** 262 mg/15 ml	5 mg sodium/15 ml. Saccharin. In 120, 240, 360 & 480 ml.	970
otc	**Pink Bismuth** (Various, eg, Dixon-Shane, Goldline, Schein)		In 240 ml.	6.4+
otc	**Bismatrol Extra Strength** (Major)	**Liquid:** 524 mg/15 ml	In 240 ml.	4.7
otc sf	**Pepto-Bismol Maximum Strength** (Procter & Gamble)		< 5 mg sodium/15 ml. Saccharin. In 120, 240 and 360 ml.	1930

* Cost Index based on cost per minimum single adult dose. *sf* – Sugar free.

ANTIDIARRHEAL COMBINATION PRODUCTS

LACTOBACILLUS

A viable culture of the naturally occurring metabolic products produced by *Lactobacillus acidophilus* and *L bulgaricus.*

Uses:

As a dietary supplement.

Treatment of uncomplicated diarrhea, including that due to antibiotic therapy.

Treatment of acute fever blisters (cold sores).

The FDA has determined that these ingredients are not generally recognized as safe and effective as antidiarrheal drug products.

Contraindications:

Allergy to milk or sensitivity to lactose.

Precautions:

Unless directed by physician, do not use for > 2 days or in the presence of high fever or in children < 3 years old.

	Product	Description	Supply	C.I.*
otc	**Bacid** (Fisons)	**Capsules:** Cultured strain of not less than 500 million viable *L acidophilus* with carboxymethylcellulose sodium. *Dose:* 2 capsules 2 to 4 times/day	In 50s and 100s. Must be refrigerated.	9
otc	**Lactinex** (HW & D)	Mixed culture of *L acidophilus* and *L bulgaricus* **Granules:** 1 packet added to or taken with cereal, food, milk, fruit juice or water 3 or 4 times daily.	In 1 g packets (12s). Must be refrigerated.	101
		Tablets, chewable: 4 tablets, 3 or 4 times daily. May follow each dose with a small amount of milk, fruit juice or water.	In 50s.	71
otc *sf*	**More-Dophilus** (Freeda)	**Powder:** 4 billion units of acidophilus-carrot derivative per g *Dose:* 1 tsp daily with liquid.	In 120 g. Store at room temperature.	20

* Cost Index based on cost per minimum single adult dose. *sf* – Sugar free.

These products are used for the symptomatic treatment of diarrhea by reducing intestinal motility or adsorbing fluid.

Warnings:

Do not use antiperistaltic agents for diarrhea associated with pseudomembranous enterocolitis or in diarrhea caused by toxigenic bacteria.

Do not use these preparations for > 2 days, in the presence of high fever or in infants and children < 3 years of age, except under a physician's direction.

Salicylate absorption may occur from bismuth subsalicylate; therefore, observe caution in patients with bleeding disorders or salicylate sensitivity and in children.

The use of the ingredients in combination in the following products as nonspecific antidiarrheal agents has, to a large extent, been empiric. Adequate controlled clinical studies demonstrating the efficacy of these antidiarrheal combinations are lacking. The FDA has determined that the following ingredients are not generally recognized as safe and effective and are misbranded when present in *otc* antidiarrheal preparations: Aluminum hydroxide, atropine sulfate, calcium carbonate, carboxymethylcellulose, glycine, homatropine methylbromide, hyoscyamine sulfate, *Lactobacillus acidophilus* and *bulgaricus*, opium (powdered and tincture), paregoric, phenyl salicylate, scopolamine hydrobromide and zinc phenolsulfonate.

OPIUM (tincture, powder or paregoric) is used to reduce intestinal motility and to relieve tenesmus and pain associated with diarrhea. See Narcotic Agonist Analgesics monograph.

BELLADONNA ALKALOIDS and *HOMATROPINE METHYLBROMIDE* are used to control hypermotility and hypersecretion in the gastrointestinal tract. See GI Anticholinergics/Antispasmodics monograph.

ACTIVATED ATTAPULGITE, KAOLIN and *PECTIN* are used for their adsorbent actions.

BISMUTH SALTS have antacid and adsorbent properties.

	Opiate-Containing			C.I.*
c-v	**Parepectolin** (Rhone-Poulenc Rorer)	**Liquid:** 15 mg opium (3.7 ml paregoric), 5.5 g kaolin and 162 mg pectin/30 ml *Dose:* 15 or 30 ml after each loose bowel movement up to 120 ml in 12 hours.	0.69% alcohol. Saccharin. In 120 and 240 ml.	502
c-v	**Kapectolin w/Paregoric** (Various, eg, Barre-National, Major)		0.69% alcohol. In 120 and 473 ml.	370+
c-v	**Kapectolin PG** (Various, eg, Barre-National, Dixon-Shane, Goldline, URL)	**Liquid:** 24 mg powdered opium, 6 g kaolin, 142.8 mg pectin, 0.1037 mg hyoscyamine sulfate, 0.0194 mg atropine sulfate and 0.0065 mg scopolamine HBr per 30 ml with 5% alcohol *Dose:* 30 ml; then 15 ml every 3 hours.	In 120 and 180 ml, pt and gal.	172+
c-v	**Donnagel-PG** (Robins)		Corn syrup. Banana flavor. In 180 and 480 ml.	443
c-v	**Donnapectolin-PG** (Major)		Sucrose. In 240 ml and pt.	500

* Cost Index based on cost per minimum single adult dose.

(Continued on following page)

Refer to the general discussion of these products on page 1673

Opiate Free

	Product	Description	Packaging	C.I.*
otc	**Kao-Spen** (Century)	**Suspension:** 5.2 g kaolin and 260 mg pectin per 30 ml *Dose:* 60 to 120 ml after each bowel movement.	Peppermint flavor. In 120 ml, pt and gal.	6.4
otc	**Kaolin w/Pectin** (Various, eg, Barre-National, Hauck, Interstate, Major, Pharm Assoc., Roxane)	**Suspension:** 5.85 g kaolin and 130 mg pectin per 30 ml *Dose:* 60 to 120 ml after each bowel movement. *Children –* *3 to 6 years* – 15 to 30 ml/dose. *6 to 12 years* – 30 to 60 ml/dose.	In 120, 180, 240 & 360 ml, pt, gal & UD 15 and 30 ml.	NA
otc	**Kapectolin** (Various, eg, Barre-National, Goldline, Major, Moore, URL)		In 120 and 240 ml, pt and gal.	15+
otc	**Kaopectate Advanced Formula** (Upjohn)	**Concentrated liquid:** 600 mg attapulgite per 15 ml *Dose: Adults* – 30 ml after each bowel movement up to 7 times/day. *Children –* *6 to 12 years* – 15 ml/dose *3 to < 6 years* – 7.5 ml/dose	Alcohol free. Sucrose. Vanilla flavor. In 240, 360 and 480 ml. Peppermint flavor. In 240 and 360 ml.	5.8
otc	**Parepectolin** (Rhone-Poulenc Rorer)		Sucrose. In 240 ml.	NA
otc	**K-Pek** (Rugby)	**Suspension:** 600 mg attapulgite/15 ml *Dose: Adults* – 30 ml after each bowel movement up to 7 times a day. *Children –* *6 to < 12 years* – 15 ml/dose *3 to < 6 years* – 7.5 ml/dose	Sucrose. Regular flavor. In 237 ml, pt and gal. Peppermint flavor. In 237 ml.	3.8
otc	**K-C** (Century)	**Suspension:** 5.2 g kaolin, 260 mg pectin and 260 mg bismuth subcarbonate per 30 ml *Dose:* 10 to 20 ml every 6 hours.	Peppermint flavor. In 120 ml, pt and gal.	1
otc	**Kaodene Non-Narcotic** (Pfeiffer)	**Liquid:** 3.9 g kaolin, 194.4 mg pectin per 30 ml, with sodium carboxymethylcellulose and bismuth subsalicylate. *Dose: Adults* – 45 ml 1 to 3 times daily or after each loose stool. *Children –* *6 to 12 years* – ½ adult dose *3 to 6 years* – ⅓ adult dose	Sucrose. Alcohol free. In 120 ml.	20
otc	**Devrom** (Parthenon)	**Tablets, chewable:** 200 mg bismuth subgallate *Dose:* 1 or 2 tabs 3 times/day w/meals.	In 100s.	1
otc	**Children's Kaopectate** (Upjohn)	**Tablets, chewable:** 300 mg attapulgite *Dose: Adults* – 4 tabs after each bowel movement. *Children –* *6 to < 12 years* – 2/dose *3 to < 6 years* – 1/dose	Sucrose, dextrose. Cherry flavor. In 16s.	13
		Liquid: 600 mg attapulgite per 15 ml *Dose: Adults* – 30 ml after each bowel movement up to 7 times a day. *Children –* *6 to < 12 years* – 15 ml/dose *3 to < 6 years* – 7.5 ml/dose	Sucrose. In 180 ml.	NA

* Cost Index based on cost per minimum single dose.

(Continued on following page)

Refer to the general discussion of these products on page 1673

		Opiate Free (Cont.)		C.I.*
otc	**Donnagel** (Robins)	**Liquid:** 600 mg attapulgite per 15 ml *Dose: Adults* – 30 ml after each bowel movement up to 7 times/day. *Children –* *6 to 11 years* – 15 ml/dose *3 to 5 years* – 7.5 ml/dose	1.4% alcohol, saccharin, sorbitol. In 120 and 240 ml.	NA
otc sf	**Donnagel** (Robins)	**Tablets, chewable:** 600 mg attapulgite *Dose: Adults* – 2 tabs after each bowel movement up to 7 times/day. *Children –* 6 to 11 years – 1/dose 3 to 5 years – ½/dose	Saccharin, sorbitol. (AHR Donnagel). Green with darker green specks. Mint flavor. In 18s.	NA
otc	**Rheaban Maximum Strength** (Pfizer)	**Tablets:** 750 mg activated attapulgite, pectin *Dose: Adults* – 2 after each bowel movement. *Children – 6 to 12 years* – 1/dose	Sucrose. In 12s.	8.6
otc	**Diar•Aid** (Thompson Medical)	**Tablets:** 750 mg activated attapulgite and 150 mg pectin *Dose:* 2 to 4 initially, then 2 after each bowel movement.	In 12s and 24s.	5.2
otc	**Diasorb** (Columbia)	**Tablets:** 750 mg activated attapulgite *Dose: Adults* – 4 tablets initially; then after each bowel movement up to 3 doses/day. *Children –* *6 to 12 years* – 2/dose *3 to 6 years* – 1/dose	Sorbitol. In 24s.	17
otc sf	**Diasorb** (Columbia)	**Liquid:** 750 mg activated attapulgite per 5 ml *Dose: Adults* – 20 ml initially; then after each bowel movement up to 3 doses per day. *Children –* *6 to 12 years* – 10 ml/dose *3 to 6 years* – 5 ml/dose	Sorbitol, saccharin. Cola flavor. In 120 ml.	17
otc	**Kaopectate Maximum Strength Caplets** (Upjohn)	**Tablets:** 750 mg attapulgite, pectin *Dose: Adults* – 2 after each bowel movement up to 12/day. *Children – 6 to 12 years* – 1/dose	Sucrose. In 12s and 20s.	7.8

* Cost Index based on cost per minimum single dose.

MESALAMINE (5-aminosalicylic acid, 5-ASA)

Actions:

Pharmacology: Sulfasalazine is split by bacterial action in the colon into sulfapyridine (SP) and mesalamine (5-ASA). It is thought that the mesalamine component is therapeutically active in ulcerative colitis. The usual oral dose of sulfasalazine for active ulcerative colitis in adults is 2 to 4 g per day in divided doses. Four grams of sulfasalazine provide 1.6 g of free mesalamine to the colon. Each suspension enema delivers up to 4 g mesalamine to the left side of the colon; each suppository delivers 500 mg to the rectum.

The mechanism of action of mesalamine (and sulfasalazine) is unknown, but appears to be topical rather than systemic. Mucosal production of arachidonic acid (AA) metabolites, both through cyclooxygenase pathways (ie, prostanoids) and through lipoxygenase pathways (ie, leukotrienes [LTs] and hydroxyeicosatetraenoic acids [HETEs]) is increased in patients with chronic inflammatory bowel disease, and it is possible that mesalamine diminishes inflammation by blocking cyclooxygenase and inhibiting prostaglandin (PG) production in the colon.

Pharmacokinetics: Absorption/Distribution – Rectal: Mesalamine administered rectally as a suspension enema is poorly absorbed from the colon and is excreted principally in the feces during subsequent bowel movements. The extent of absorption is dependent upon the retention time of the drug product, and there is considerable individual variation. At steady state, approximately 10% to 30% of the daily 4 g dose can be recovered in cumulative 24 hour urine collections. Other than the kidneys, the organ distribution and other bioavailability characteristics of absorbed mesalamine are not known. The compound undergoes acetylation, but whether this process takes place at colonic or systemic sites has not been elucidated.

Oral: Mesalamine tablets are coated with an acrylic-based resin that delays release of mesalamine until it reaches the terminal ileum and beyond. Approximately 28% is absorbed after oral ingestion, leaving the remainder available for topical action and excretion in the feces. Absorption is similar with or without food. Mesalamine from oral mesalamine tablets appears to be more extensively absorbed than that released from sulfasalazine. Maximum plasma levels of mesalamine and N-acetyl-5-ASA following multiple doses are about 1.5 to 2 times higher than those following an equivalent dose of sulfasalazine; combined parent drug and metabolite area under the concentration-time curves and urine drug dose recoveries are also about 1.3 to 1.5 times higher. The time to reach maximum plasma concentration for mesalamine and its metabolite is usually delayed (due to the delayed release formulation) and ranges from 4 to 12 hours.

Metabolism/Excretion – Rectal: Whatever the metabolic site, most absorbed mesalamine is excreted in urine as the N-acetyl-5-ASA metabolite. Patients demonstrated plasma levels of 2 mcg/ml 10 to 12 hours after administration; about two-thirds of this was the N-acetyl metabolite. While the elimination half-life of mesalamine is short (0.5 to 1.5 hr), the acetylated metabolite exhibits a half-life of 5 to 10 hours. In addition, steady-state plasma levels demonstrated a lack of accumulation of either free or metabolized drug during repeated daily administrations.

Oral: Following oral administration, the absorbed mesalamine is rapidly acetylated in the gut mucosal wall and by the liver. It is excreted mainly by the kidney as N-acetyl-5-ASA. The half-lives of elimination for mesalamine and the metabolite are usually about 12 hours, but are variable ranging from 2 to 15 hours. There is large intersubject variability in plasma concentrations of mesalamine and N-acetyl-5-ASA and in their elimination half-lives following administration of the tablets.

Indications:

Treatment of active mild to moderate distal ulcerative colitis, proctosigmoiditis or proctitis.

Contraindications:

Hypersensitivity to mesalamine, salicylates or any component of the formulation.

(Continued on following page)

MESALAMINE (Cont.)

Warnings:

Intolerance/Colitis exacerbation: Mesalamine has been implicated in the production of an acute intolerance syndrome or exacerbation of colitis ($\approx$ 3% of patients) characterized by cramping, acute abdominal pain and bloody diarrhea, and occasionally fever, headache, malaise, pruritus, conjunctivitis and rash. Symptoms usually abate when mesalamine is discontinued. Re-evaluate the patient's history of sulfasalazine intolerance, if any. If a rechallenge is performed to validate the hypersensitivity, do it under close supervision and only if clearly needed, giving consideration to reduced dosage. One patient previously sensitive to sulfasalazine was rechallenged with 400 mg oral mesalamine; within 8 hours she experienced headache, fever, intensive abdominal colic, profuse diarrhea and was readmitted as an emergency. She responded poorly to steroid therapy; 2 weeks later, a pancolectomy was required.

Hypersensitivity: In a clinical trial, most patients who were hypersensitive to sulfasalazine were able to take mesalamine enemas without evidence of any allergic reaction. Nevertheless, exercise caution when mesalamine is initially used in patients known to be allergic to sulfasalazine. Instruct these patients to discontinue therapy if signs of rash or fever become apparent.

Pancolitis: While using mesalamine some patients have developed pancolitis. However, extension of upper disease boundary or flare-ups occurred less often in mesalamine patients than in placebo patients.

Renal function impairment: Renal impairment, including minimal change nephropathy, and acute and chronic interstitial nephritis, has occurred. In animals, the kidney is the principal target organ for toxicity; at doses $\approx$ 15 to 20 times the recommended human dose, mesalamine causes renal papillary necrosis. Exercise caution when using mesalamine in patients with renal dysfunction or history of renal disease. Evaluate renal function of all patients prior to therapy and periodically during therapy.

Pregnancy: Category B. There are no adequate and well controlled studies in pregnant women. Use during pregnancy only if clearly needed.

Lactation: Low concentrations of mesalamine and higher concentrations of N-acetyl-5-ASA have been detected in breast milk. Clinical significance has not been determined. However, exercise caution when administering to a nursing woman.

Children: Safety and efficacy for use in children have not been established.

Precautions:

Pericarditis has occurred rarely with mesalamine-containing products including sulfasalazine. Cases of pericarditis have also occurred as manifestations of inflammatory bowel disease. In cases reported with mesalamine rectal suspension, there have been positive rechallenges. In one of these cases, however, a second rechallenge with sulfasalazine was negative throughout a 2 month follow-up. Investigate chest pain or dyspnea in mesalamine-treated patients with this in mind. Discontinuation of the drug may be warranted in some patients, but rechallenge can be performed under careful clinical observation.

Pyloric stenosis patients may have prolonged gastric retention of mesalamine tablets which could delay release of mesalamine in the colon.

Sulfite sensitivity: May cause allergic-type reactions (eg, hives, itching, wheezing, anaphylaxis) in certain susceptible persons. Although the overall prevalence of sulfite sensitivity in the general population is probably low, it is seen more frequently in asthmatics or in atopic nonasthmatic persons.

Epinephrine is the preferred treatment for serious allergic or emergency situations even though epinephrine injection contains sodium or potassium metabisulfite. The alternatives to using epinephrine in a life-threatening situation may not be satisfactory. The presence of a sulfite(s) in epinephrine injection should not deter the administration of the drug for treatment of serious allergic or other emergency situations.

(Continued on folowing page)

MESALAMINE (Cont.)

Adverse Reactions:

Mesalamine is usually well tolerated. Most adverse effects have been mild and transient.

Mesalamine Adverse Reactions (%)

Adverse reaction	Mesalamine			
	Oral (n = 152)	Suppository (n = 168)	Suspension (n = 815)	Placebo[1] (n = 301)
GI				
Abdominal pain/cramps/ discomfort	18	3	8.1	9.3
Bloating			1.5	1.6
Colitis exacerbation[2]	3	1.2		0
Constipation	5		< 1	2.3
Diarrhea	7	3	2.1	6
Dyspepsia	6			1
Eructation	16			13
Flatulence/Gas	3	3.6	6.1	5.6
Hemorrhoids			1.3	0
Nausea	13	1.2	5.8	10.3
Pain on insertion of enema	na	na	1.3	< 1
Rectal pain/soreness/ burning		1.8	1.2	0
Vomiting	5			2
CNS				
Asthenia	7	1.2	< 1	7
Chills	3			2
Dizziness	8	3	1.8	4
Fever	7	1.2	3.2	2.3
Headache	35	6.5	6.5	18.9
Insomnia	✓		< 1	2.3
Malaise/Fatigue/Weakness	1-2		3.4	6.2
Sweating	3			1
Respiratory				
Cold/Sore throat		1.8	2.3	5.2
Cough increased	1-2			0
Pharyngitis	11			9
Rhinitis	5			5
Dermatologic				
Acne	1-2	1.2		0
Itching			1.2	< 1
Pruritus	3			0
Rash/Spots	6	1.2	2.8	2.3
Musculoskeletal				
Arthralgia	5			3
Arthritis	1-2			0
Back pain	7		1.3	2.3
Hypertonia	5			4
Leg/Joint pain	✓		2.1	< 1
Myalgia	3			1
Miscellaneous				
Chest pain	3			2
Conjunctivitis	1-2			0
Dysmenorrhea	3			3
Edema	3	1.2	< 1	4.6
Flu syndrome	3		5.3	1.4
Hair loss[3]	✓		< 1	0
Pain	14			8
UTI/Urinary burning	✓		< 1	3.1

✓ = Occurred, no incidence reported. na = Not applicable

[1] Data pooled from oral and rectal studies.

[2] See Warnings.

[3] Mild hair loss characterized by "more hair in the comb." There are at least six additional cases in the literature of mild hair loss with mesalamine or sulfasalazine. Retreatment is not always associated with repeated hair loss.

(Adverse Reactions continued on following page)

MESALAMINE (Cont.)

Adverse Reactions (Cont.):

Other adverse reactions have occurred with oral mesalamine.

Cardiovascular: Pericarditis (see Precautions); myocarditis; vasodilation; migraine.

CNS: Anxiety; depression; somnolence; emotional lability; hyperesthesia; vertigo; nervousness; confusion; paresthesia; tremor; peripheral neuropathy; transverse myelitis; Guillain-Barre syndrome.

GI: Anorexia; pancreatitis (also for rectal mesalamine); gastroenteritis; gastritis; increased appetite; cholecystitis; dry mouth; oral ulcers; perforated peptic ulcer; bloody diarrhea; tenesmus.

GU: Interstitial nephritis, nephropathy (see Warnings); dysuria; urinary urgency; hematuria; epididymitis; menorrhagia.

Hematologic: Agranulocytosis; thrombocytopenia; eosinophilia; leukopenia; anemia; lymphadenopathy.

Respiratory/Pulmonary: Sinusitis; interstitial pneumonitis; asthma exacerbation.

Dermatologic: Psoriasis; pyoderma gangrenosum; dry skin; erythema nodosum; urticaria.

Special senses: Ear/Eye pain; taste perversion; blurred vision; tinnitus.

Other: Neck pain; abdominal enlargement; facial edema; gout.

Lab test abnormalities: Elevated AST, ALT, alkaline phosphatase, serum creatinine and BUN.

Hepatitis occurs rarely. More commonly, asymptomatic elevations of liver enzymes have occurred which usually resolve during continued use or with discontinuation of the drug.

Overdosage:

One case of overdosage has been reported. A 3-year-old male ingested 2 g of mesalamine tablets. He was treated with ipecac and charcoal, and no adverse events occurred. Oral doses in mice and rats of ≈ 5000 mg/kg cause significant lethality.

Patient Information:

Oral: Swallow tablets whole; do not break the outer coating, which is designed to remain intact to protect the active ingredient. In 2% to 3% of patients, intact or partially intact tablets are found in the stool. If this occurs repeatedly, notify the physician.

Suppository: Remove the foil wrapper. Avoid excessive handling of the suppository which is designed to melt at body temperature. Insert completely into rectum with gentle pressure, pointed end first.

Suspension: Patient instructions are included with the product. Shake well. Remove protective sheath from applicator tip, and gently insert applicator tip into the rectum.

Administration and Dosage:

Oral: 800 mg 3 times daily for a total dose of 2.4 g/day for 6 weeks.

Suppository: One suppository (500 mg) 2 times daily. Retain the suppository in the rectum for 1 to 3 hours or more if possible to achieve maximum benefit. While the effect may be seen within 3 to 21 days, the usual course of therapy is 3 to 6 weeks depending on symptoms and sigmoidoscopic findings. Studies have not assessed if the suppositories will modify relapse rates after the 6 week short-term treatment.

Suspension: The usual dosage of mesalamine suspension enema in 60 ml units is one rectal instillation (4 g) once a day, preferably at bedtime, and retained for ≈ 8 hours. While the effect may be seen within 3 to 21 days, the usual course of therapy is 3 to 6 weeks depending on symptoms and sigmoidoscopic findings. Studies have not assessed if suspension enema will modify relapse rates after the 6 week short-term treatment.

Shake the bottle well to make sure the suspension is homogenous. Remove the protective sheath from the applicator tip. Holding the bottle at the neck will not cause any of the medication to be discharged. The position most often used is to lie on the left side (to facilitate migration into the sigmoid colon), with the lower leg extended and the upper right leg flexed forward for balance. An alternative is the knee-chest position. Gently insert the applicator tip in the rectum pointing toward the umbilicus. A steady squeezing of the bottle will discharge most of the preparation. Patient instructions are included with every 7 units.

C.I.*

Rx	**Asacol** (Procter & Gamble Pharm.)	**Tablets, delayed release:** 400 mg	Lactose. (Asacol NE). Red-brown. Capsule shape. In 100s.
Rx	**Rowasa** (Solvay)	**Suppositories:** 500 mg	Light tan. Bullet shape. In 12s and 24s.
Rx	**Rowasa** (Solvay)	**Rectal Suspension:** 4 g per 60 ml[1]	In units of 7 disposable bottles.

[1] With potassium metabisulfite.

OLSALAZINE SODIUM

Actions:

Pharmacology: Olsalazine sodium is a sodium salt of a salicylate compound that is effectively bioconverted to 5-aminosalicylic acid (mesalamine; 5-ASA), which has anti-inflammatory activity in ulcerative colitis. Approximately 98% to 99% of an oral dose will reach the colon where each molecule is rapidly converted into two molecules of 5-ASA by colonic bacteria and the low prevailing redox potential found in this environment. More than 0.9 g mesalamine would usually be made available in the colon from 1 g olsalazine. The liberated 5-ASA is absorbed slowly, resulting in very high local concentrations in the colon.

The mechanism of action of mesalamine is unknown, but appears to be topical rather than systemic. It is possible that mesalamine diminishes colonic inflammation by blocking cyclooxygenase and inhibiting colon prostaglandin production in the bowel mucosa.

In rats the kidney is the major target organ of olsalazine toxicity. At an oral daily dose of ≥ 400 mg/kg, olsalazine treatment produced nephritis and tubular necrosis in a 4 week study, interstitial nephritis and tubular calcinosis in a 6 month study and renal fibrosis, mineralization and transitional cell hyperplasia in a 1 year study.

Pharmacokinetics: After oral administration approximately 2.4% of a single 1 g oral dose is absorbed. Maximum serum concentrations appear after approximately 1 hour, and are low (eg, 1.6 to 6.2 mcmol/L) even after a 1 g single dose. Olsalazine has a very short serum half-life of ≈ 0.9 hours and is > 99% bound to plasma proteins. The urinary recovery is < 1%. Total recovery of oral olsalazine ranges from 90% to 97%.

Approximately 0.1% of an oral dose is metabolized in the liver to olsalazine-O-sulfate (olsalazine-S), which has a half-life of 7 days and accumulates to steady state within 2 to 3 weeks. Patients on daily doses of 1 g olsalazine for 2 to 4 years show a stable plasma concentration of olsalazine-S (3.3 to 12.4 mcmol/L). Olsalazine-S is > 99% bound to plasma proteins. Its long half-life is mainly due to slow dissociation from the protein binding site. Less than 1% of olsalazine and olsalazine-S appears undissociated in plasma.

Serum concentrations of 5-ASA are detected after 4 to 8 hours. The peak levels of 5-ASA after an oral dose of 1 g olsalazine are low (0 to 4.3 mcmol/L). Of the total urinary 5-ASA, > 90% is in the form of N-acetyl-5-ASA (Ac-5-ASA).

Ac-5-ASA is acetylated (deactivated) in at least two sites, the colonic epithelium and the liver. Ac-5-ASA is found in the serum, with peak values of 1.7 to 8.7 mcmol/L after a single 1 g dose. In the urine, approximately 20% of total 5-ASA is found almost exclusively as Ac-5-ASA. The remaining 5-ASA is partially acetylated and is excreted in the feces. After dosing, the concentration of 5-ASA in the colon has been calculated to be 18 to 49 mmol/L. No accumulation of 5-ASA or Ac-5-ASA in plasma has been detected. 5-ASA and Ac-5-ASA are 74% and 81% bound to plasma proteins, respectively.

Clinical studies: In one controlled study, ulcerative colitis patients in remission were randomized to olsalazine 500 mg twice a day or placebo, and relapse rates for a 6 month period of time were compared. For the 52 patients randomized to olsalazine, 12 relapses occurred, while for the 49 placebo patients, 22 relapses occurred. This difference in relapse rates was significant.

In a second controlled study, 164 ulcerative colitis patients in remission were randomized to olsalazine 500 mg twice a day or sulfasalazine 1 g twice a day and relapse rates were compared after 6 months. The relapse rate for olsalazine was 19.5% while that for sulfasalazine was 12.2%; the difference was not significant.

Indications:

Maintenance of remission of ulcerative colitis in patients intolerant of sulfasalazine.

Contraindications:

Hypersensitivity to salicylates.

Warnings:

Carcinogenesis: In animals, olsalazine was tested at daily doses of 200 to 2000 mg/kg/day (approximately 10 to 100 times the human maintenance dose). Urinary bladder transitional cell carcinomas were found in three male rats (6%); liver hemangiosarcomata were found in two male mice (4%).

Pregnancy: Category C. Olsalazine produces fetal developmental toxicity ie, reduced fetal weights, retarded ossifications and immaturity of visceral organs when given during organogenesis to pregnant rats in doses 5 to 20 times the human dose (100 to 400 mg/kg). There are no adequate and well controlled studies in pregnant women. Use during pregnancy only if the potential benefit justifies the potential risk to the fetus.

Lactation: Oral administration of olsalazine to lactating rats in doses 5 to 20 times the human dose produced growth retardation in their pups. It is not known whether this drug is excreted in human breast milk. Exercise caution when olsalazine is administered to a nursing woman.

Children: Safety and efficacy in children have not been established.

(Continued on following page)

OLSALAZINE SODIUM (Cont.)

Precautions:

Diarrhea: Approximately 17%, resulting in treatment withdrawal in 6%; appears to be dose-related, although it may be difficult to distinguish from underlying disease symptoms.

Exacerbation of the symptoms of colitis thought to have been caused by mesalamine or sulfasalazine has been noted.

Renal abnormalities were not reported in clinical trials with olsalazine; however, the possibility of renal tubular damage due to absorbed mesalamine or its n-acetylated metabolite must be kept in mind, particularly for patients with pre-existing renal disease. In these patients, monitor urinalysis, BUN and creatinine determination.

Adverse Reactions:

Overall, 10.4% of patients discontinued olsalazine because of an adverse experience compared with 6.7% of placebo patients.

Olsalazine Adverse Reactions

Adverse Reactions	Olsalazine (n = 441)	Placebo (n = 208)	Adverse Reactions	Olsalazine (n = 441)	Placebo (n = 208)
CNS			*Miscellaneous*		
Headache	5%	4.8%	Arthralgia	4%	2.9%
Fatigue/Drowsiness/Lethargy	1.8%	2.9%	Upper respiratory infection	1.5%	—
Depression	1.5%	—	*Withdrawal from therapy* (No. patients)		
Vertigo/Dizziness	1%	—			
Insomnia	—	2.4%			
GI			Diarrhea	26	10
Diarrhea	11.1%	6.7%	Nausea	3	2
Pain/Cramps	10.1%	7.2%	Abdominal pain	5	0
Nausea	5%	3.9%	Rash/Itching	5	0
Dyspepsia	4%	4.3%	Headache	3	0
Bloating	1.5%	1.4%	Heartburn	2	0
Anorexia	1.3%	1.9%	Rectal bleeding	1	0
Vomiting	1%	—	Insomnia	1	0
Stomatitis	1%	—	Dizziness	1	0
Blood in stool	—	3.4%	Anorexia	1	0
Skin			Lightheadedness	1	0
Rash	2.3%	1.4%	Depression	1	0
Itching	1.3%	—	Miscellaneous	4	3

A causal relationship to the drug has not been demonstrated for the following.

GI: Pancreatitis; rectal bleeding; flare in symptoms; rectal discomfort; epigastric discomfort; flatulence; granulomatous hepatitis and nonspecific, reactive hepatitis. A patient developed mild cholestatic hepatitis with sulfasalazine and when changed to olsalazine 2 weeks later. Withdrawal of olsalazine led to complete recovery.

Neurologic: Paresthesia; tremors; mood swings; irritability; fever; chills.

Dermatologic: Erythema nodosum; photosensitivity; erythema; hot flashes; alopecia.

Musculoskeletal: Muscle cramps.

Cardiovascular/Pulmonary: Pericarditis; second degree heart block; hypertension; orthostatic hypotension; peripheral edema; chest pains; tachycardia; palpitations; bronchospasm; shortness of breath.

GU: Urinary frequency; dysuria; hematuria; proteinuria; impotence; menorrhagia.

Hematologic: Leukopenia; neutropenia; lymphopenia; eosinophilia; thrombocytopenia; anemia; reticulocytosis.

Laboratory: Elevated ALT or AST.

Special senses: Dry mouth; dry eyes; watery eyes; blurred vision.

Overdosage:

Symptoms of acute toxicity were decreased motor activity and diarrhea in all species tested and, in addition, vomiting in dogs.

Patient Information:

Take with food. Take in evenly divided doses.

Approximately 17% of subjects in clinical studies developed diarrhea some time during therapy. Contact your physician if diarrhea occurs.

Administration and Dosage:

1 g per day in 2 divided doses.

Rx	**Dipentum** (Pharmacia)	**Capsules:** 250 mg	(Dipentum 250 mg). Beige. In 100s and 500s.

chapter 8

anti-infectives

ANTIBIOTICS

ANTIFUNGALS

SULFONAMIDES, 1900

ANTIMALARIAL PREPARATIONS

ANTITUBERCULOUS DRUGS, 1924

AMEBICIDES

ANTIVIRAL AGENTS

MISCELLANEOUS ANTI-INFECTIVES

LEPROSTATICS

ANTHELMINTICS, 2025

URINARY ANTI-INFECTIVES

GENITOURINARY IRRIGANTS, 2050

CDC ANTI-INFECTIVE AGENTS, 2057

Actions:

The penicillins are bactericidal antibiotics that include natural and semisynthetic derivatives. All of these agents contain the 6-β-aminopenicillanic acid nucleus and have a similar mechanism of action. All of the penicillins share cross-allergenicity. The significant differences among agents include: Resistance to gastric acid inactivation; resistance to inactivation by penicillinase; spectrum of antimicrobial activity. In addition to the prototype penicillin G, this class includes an acid stable penicillin G derivative (penicillin V), penicillinase-resistant penicillins, the aminopenicillins and the extended spectrum derivatives. Bacampicillin is hydrolyzed in vivo to ampicillin; amoxicillin is closely related to ampicillin. Several of these penicillins are also available in combination with agents that inactivate β-lactamase enzymes (eg, clavulanic acid, sulbactam), thereby extending the antibiotic spectrum to include many bacteria normally resistant to it and to other β-lactam antibiotics (see Pharmacokinetics). The available combinations include: Ampicillin/sulbactam sodium; amoxicillin/potassium clavulanate; ticarcillin/potassium clavulanate.

Penicillins

	Routes of administration	Penicillinase-resistant	Acid stable	% Protein bound	May be taken with meals
Natural Penicillins					
Penicillin G	IM-IV-Oral	no	no	60	no
Penicillin V	Oral	no	yes	80	yes
Penicillinase-Resistant					
Cloxacillin	Oral	yes	yes	95	no
Dicloxacillin	Oral	yes	yes	98	no
Methicillin	IM-IV	yes	†	40	†
Nafcillin	IM-IV-Oral	yes	yes	87 to 90	no
Oxacillin	IM-IV-Oral	yes	yes	94	no
Aminopenicillins					
Amoxicillin	Oral	no	yes	20	yes
Amoxicillin/potassium clavulanate	Oral	yes	yes	20/30	yes
Ampicillin	IM-IV-Oral	no	yes	20	no
Ampicillin/sulbactam	IM-IV	yes	†	28/38	†
Bacampicillin	Oral	no	yes	20	yes[1]
Extended Spectrum					
Carbenicillin	Oral	no	yes	50	no
Mezlocillin	IM-IV	no	†	16 to 42	†
Piperacillin	IM-IV	no	†	16	†
Ticarcillin	IM-IV	no	†	45	†
Ticarcillin/potassium clavulanate	IV	yes	†	45/9	†

† Available only for IM or IV use. [1]Tablets only; not the suspension.

Mechanism: Penicillins inhibit the biosynthesis of cell wall mucopeptide. They are bactericidal against sensitive organisms when adequate concentrations are reached, and they are most effective during the stage of active multiplication. Inadequate concentrations may produce only bacteriostatic effects.

(Actions continued on following page)

Actions (Cont.)

Pharmacokinetics:

Absorption – Oral preparations of penicillin G are slightly affected by normal gastric acidity (pH 2 to 3.5); however, a pH < 2 may partially or totally inactivate it. Oral penicillin G is absorbed (about 30%) chiefly in the duodenum. Since gastric acidity, stomach emptying time and other factors affecting absorption may vary considerably, serum levels may be reduced to nontherapeutic levels in certain individuals. Penicillin V is preferred for oral therapy since it achieves blood levels 2 to 5 times higher than the same dose of penicillin G and shows less individual variation. Methicillin is the only acid labile penicillinase-resistant penicillin, and is only used parenterally. Nafcillin's oral absorption is inferior to oxacillin, cloxacillin and dicloxacillin. Ampicillin and carbenicillin indanyl have good GI absorption, but amoxicillin and bacampicillin are more completely absorbed.

Absorption of most penicillins is affected by food; these medications are best taken on an empty stomach, 1 hour before or 2 hours after meals. Penicillin V may be given with meals; however blood levels may be slightly higher when given on an empty stomach. Amoxicillin, bacampicillin tablets and amoxicillin/potassium clavulanate may be given without regard to meals.

Peak serum levels occur approximately 1 hour after oral use. After a 500 mg oral dose, peak serum concentrations for oxacillin, cloxacillin and dicloxacillin range from 5 to 7, 7.5 to 14.4 and 10 to 17 mcg/ml, respectively. One hour after a 1 g oral nafcillin dose, average serum concentration was 1.19 mcg/ml (range, 0 to 3.12). IM injections of 1 g nafcillin, 560 mg oxacillin and 1 g methicillin produced peak serum levels in 0.5 to 1 hour of 7.61, 15 and 17 mcg/ml, respectively.

Parenteral penicillin G (sodium and potassium) gives rapid and high but transient blood levels; derivatives provide prolonged penicillin blood levels with IM use. Procaine penicillin G, an equimolecular suspension of procaine and penicillin G, must be given IM; it dissolves slowly at the injection site and plateaus in about 4 hours; levels decline gradually over 15 to 20 hours. Benzathine penicillin G IM is absorbed very slowly from the injection site and is hydrolyzed to penicillin G; hence, serum levels are much lower but more prolonged, sustaining serum levels for up to 4 weeks.

Distribution – Penicillins are bound to plasma proteins, primarily albumin, in varying degrees (see table in Pharmacology section). They diffuse readily into most body tissues and fluids, including kidneys, liver, lungs, heart, skin, synovial fluid, intestines, bile, peritoneal fluid, bronchial and wound secretions, bone, prostate, pericardial and ascitic fluids, spleen and other tissues. Penetration into cerebrospinal fluid (CSF), the brain and the eye occurs only with inflammation. CSF levels usually do not exceed 5% of penicillin G's peak serum concentration. Penicillins cross the placenta and appear in amniotic fluid and cord serum.

Excretion – Penicillins are excreted largely unchanged in the urine by glomerular filtration and active tubular secretion. Nonrenal elimination includes hepatic inactivation and excretion in bile; this is only a minor route for all penicillins except nafcillin and oxacillin. Excretion by renal tubular secretion can be delayed by coadministration of probenecid. Excretion is delayed in neonates and infants. Elimination half-life of most penicillins is short (≤ 1.5 hr). Impaired renal function prolongs the serum half-life of penicillins eliminated primarily by renal excretion. The half-life is not greatly affected for nafcillin, oxacillin, cloxacillin and dicloxacillin due to increased biotransformation and biliary excretion. Because piperacillin is excreted by biliary and renal routes, it can be used safely in appropriate dosage in patients with severe renal impairment and in the treatment of hepato-biliary infections.

β-lactamase inhibitors (clavulanic acid and sulbactam) have weak antimicrobial activity, but irreversibly inactivate bacterial β-lactamase enzymes. Used with β-lactam antibiotics, they protect antibiotics from inactivation by β-lactamase-producing organisms.

Clavulanic acid, used in combination with amoxicillin and ticarcillin, inhibits plasmid-mediated β-lactamases (eg, *Hemophilus influenzae, Neisseria gonorrheae, E coli,* salmonella, shigella, staphylococci) and chromosomal-mediated β-lactamases (eg, *Klebsiella, Bacteroides fragilis* and *Legionella*). It does not inhibit β-lactamases produced by *Enterobacter, Serratia, Morganella, Citrobacter, Pseudomonas* or *Acinetobacter* species.

Clavulanic acid is well absorbed orally and widely distributed to many body tissues. Half-life is approximately 1 hour; 35% to 45% is excreted unchanged in the urine during the first 6 hours after administration. Probenecid does not alter renal excretion of clavulanic acid.

Sulbactam, another β-lactamase inhibitor, extends the bacterial spectrum of ampicillin to include such β-lactamase-producing organisms as *S aureus, H influenzae, B fragilis* and most strains of *E coli.*

(Actions continued on following page)

Actions (Cont.):

Microbiology: The following table indicates the organisms that are generally susceptible to the penicillins in vitro:

Organisms Generally Susceptible to Penicillins

	Organisms	Natural penicillins		Penicillinase-resistant					Aminopenicillins					Extended spectrum				
	✓ = generally susceptible	Penicillin G	Penicillin V	Cloxacillin	Dicloxacillin	Methicillin	Nafcillin	Oxacillin	Amoxicillin	Ampicillin	Bacampicillin	Amoxicillin/potassium clavulanate	Ampicillin/sulbactam	Carbenicillin	Mezlocillin	Piperacillin	Ticarcillin	Ticarcillin/potassium clavulanate
Gram-positive	Staphylococci	✓[1]	✓[1]	✓	✓	✓	✓	✓	✓[1]	✓[1]	✓[1]	✓	✓	✓[1]		✓[1]	✓[1]	✓
	Staphylococcus aureus	✓[1]	✓[1]	✓	✓	✓	✓	✓				✓	✓	✓[1]	✓[1]	✓[1]	✓[1]	✓
	Streptococci	✓	✓			✓				✓			✓					
	Streptococcus pneumoniae	✓	✓	✓	✓	✓	✓	✓	✓	✓	✓	✓	✓	✓	✓	✓	✓	✓
	Beta-hemolytic streptococci	✓	✓				✓		✓	✓	✓	✓	✓	✓	✓	✓	✓	✓
	Streptococcus faecalis	✓	✓						✓	✓	✓	✓	✓	✓	✓	✓	✓	✓
	Streptococcus viridans	✓	✓				✓		✓	✓		✓	✓			✓		✓
	Corynebacterium diphtheriae	✓	✓															
	Bacillus anthracis	✓	✓							✓			✓					
	Listeria monocytogenes	✓	✓							✓			✓					
Gram-negative	Escherichia coli	✓							✓	✓	✓	✓	✓	✓	✓	✓	✓	✓
	Hemophilus influenzae								✓	✓	✓	✓	✓	✓	✓	✓[2]	✓	✓
	Klebsiella sp											✓	✓		✓	✓		✓
	Neisseria gonorrhoeae	✓[1]	✓						✓	✓	✓	✓	✓	✓	✓	✓	✓	✓
	Neisseria meningitidis	✓								✓		✓	✓			✓	✓	✓
	Proteus mirabilis	✓							✓	✓	✓	✓	✓	✓	✓	✓	✓	✓
	Salmonella sp	✓								✓			✓	✓	✓	✓	✓	✓
	Shigella sp	✓								✓			✓		✓	✓		
	Morganella morganii												✓	✓	✓	✓	✓	✓
	Proteus vulgaris												✓	✓	✓	✓	✓	✓
	Providencia sp																	
	Providencia rettgeri												✓	✓	✓	✓	✓	✓
	Providencia stuartii												✓		✓			✓
	Enterobacter sp	✓										✓	✓	✓	✓	✓	✓	✓
	Citrobacter sp													✓	✓	✓	✓	✓
	Pseudomonas aeruginosa													✓	✓	✓	✓	✓
	Serratia sp													✓	✓	✓	✓	✓
	Acinetobacter sp												✓		✓	✓		✓
	Streptobacillus moniliformis	✓	✓															
	Moraxella (Branhamella) catarrhalis											✓	✓			✓		✓
Anaerobic	Clostridium sp	✓	✓						✓	✓		✓	✓	✓	✓	✓	✓	✓
	Peptococcus sp	✓	✓						✓	✓		✓	✓	✓	✓	✓	✓	✓
	Peptostreptococcus sp	✓	✓						✓			✓	✓	✓	✓	✓	✓	✓
	Bacteroides sp	✓[3]											✓	✓	✓	✓	✓	✓
	Fusobacterium sp	✓											✓	✓	✓	✓	✓	✓
	Eubacterium sp	✓													✓	✓	✓	✓
	Treponema pallidum	✓	✓															
	Actinomyces bovis	✓	✓													✓		
	Veillonella sp														✓	✓		✓

[1] Non-penicillinase-producing.
[2] Non-beta-lactamase-producing.
[3] B fragilis is resistant.

(Continued on following page)

Indications:

Oral: Penicillins are generally indicated in the treatment of mild to moderately severe infections due to penicillin-sensitive microorganisms.

Penicillin V is preferred over penicillin G for oral administration due to better absorption.

Penicillinase-resistant penicillins: The percentage of staphylococcal isolates resistant to penicillin G outside the hospital is increasing, approximating the high percentage found in the hospital. Therefore, use a penicillinase-resistant penicillin as initial therapy for any suspected staphylococcal infection until culture and sensitivity results are known.

When treatment is initiated before definitive culture and sensitivity results are known, consider that these agents are only effective in the treatment of infections caused by pneumococci, group A beta-hemolytic streptococci and penicillin G-resistant and penicillin G-sensitive staphylococci.

Parenteral: In patients with severe infection, or when there is nausea, vomiting, gastric dilatation, cardiospasm or intestinal hypermotility. Parenteral aqueous penicillin G (eg, potassium, sodium) is the dosage form of choice in severe infections caused by penicillin-sensitive microorganisms when rapid and high penicillin serum levels are required.

For specific labeled indications, refer to individual drug monographs.

Contraindications:

History of hypersensitivity to penicillins, cephalosporins or imipenem.

Do not treat severe pneumonia, empyema, bacteremia, pericarditis, meningitis and purulent or septic arthritis with an oral penicillin during the acute stage.

Warnings:

Hypersensitivity (estimated incidence, 1% to 10%): Serious and occasionally fatal immediate hypersensitivity reactions have occurred. The incidence of anaphylactic shock is between 0.015% and 0.04%. Anaphylactic shock resulting in death has occurred in approximately 0.002% of the patients treated. Although anaphylaxis is more frequent following parenteral therapy, it may occur with oral use. Accelerated reactions (including urticaria and laryngeal edema) and delayed reactions (serum sickness-like reactions) may also occur. These reactions are likely to be immediate and severe in penicillin-sensitive individuals with a history of atopic conditions (see Adverse Reactions).

Hypersensitivity myocarditis is not dose-dependent and may occur at any time during treatment. The initial reaction involves rash, fever and eosinophilia. The second stage reflects cardiac involvement: Sinus tachycardia, ST-T changes, slight increase in cardiac enzymes (creatine phosphokinase) and cardiomegaly.

A urticarial rash, not representing a true penicillin allergy, occasionally occurs with **ampicillin** (9%). This reaction is more frequent in patients on allopurinol (14% to 22.4%), patients with lymphatic leukemia (90%) and in those with infectious mononucleosis (43% to 100%). Typically, the rash appears 7 to 10 days after the start of oral ampicillin therapy and remains for a few days to a week after drug discontinuance. In most cases, the rash is maculopapular, pruritic and generalized.

Before therapy, inquire about previous hypersensitivity reactions to penicillins, cephalosporins and other allergens. Skin testing with benzylpenicilloyl-polylysine may be used to evaluate penicillin hypersensitivity (see individual monograph in In Vivo Diagnostic Aids section).

Desensitization – Patients who have a positive skin test to one of the penicillin determinants can be desensitized, which is a relatively safe procedure. This is recommended in those instances when penicillin must be administered (eg, neurosyphilis, congenital syphilis or syphilis in pregnancy) where no proven alternatives exist. This procedure can be done orally, IV or SC; however, oral is thought to be safest and easiest. Various protocols are described for desensitization, but each protocol utilizes the same principles, which involve the administration of gradually increasing doses of penicillin, increasing each dose every 15 to 20 minutes. For example, one oral protocol using penicillin V uses 14 total doses, each dose given 15 minutes apart. The units per dose are doubled at each interval (eg, 100, 200, 400, 800) for a total cumulative dose of 1.3 million units over 4 hours. Following desensitization, maintain patients on penicillin for the duration of therapy.

Cross-allergenicity with cephalosporins – Individuals with a history of penicillin hypersensitivity have experienced severe reactions when treated with a cephalosporin. The incidence of cross-allergenicity between penicillins and cephalosporins is estimated to range from 5% to 16%; however, it is possible the incidence is much lower, possibly 3% to 7%.

Urticaria, other skin rashes and serum sickness-like reactions may be controlled by antihistamines and, if necessary, corticosteroids. Discontinue use unless the condition being treated is life-threatening and amenable only to penicillin therapy. Serious anaphylactoid reactions require emergency measures. See Management of Acute Hypersensitivity Reactions.

(Warnings continued on following page)

Warnings (Cont.):

Bleeding abnormalities: **Ticarcillin, mezlocillin or piperacillin** may induce hemorrhagic manifestations associated with abnormalities of coagulation tests (eg, bleeding time, prothrombin time, platelet aggregation). Upon withdrawal of the drug, bleeding should cease and coagulation abnormalities revert to normal. Observe patients with renal impairment, in whom excretion of these drugs is delayed, for prolonged bleeding manifestations.

Cystic fibrosis patients have a higher incidence of side effects (eg, fever, rash) when treated with extended spectrum penicillins (eg, piperacillin, carbenicillin). This may be due to the higher IgE, IgG and eosinophil levels in this population.

Pregnancy: Category B. There are no adequate or well controlled studies in pregnant women. Penicillins cross the placenta. Use during pregnancy only if clearly needed.

Labor and delivery: Oral aminopenicillins are poorly absorbed during labor. It is not known whether use has immediate or delayed adverse effects on the fetus, or alters normal labor.

Lactation: Penicillins are excreted in breast milk in low concentrations; use may cause diarrhea, candidiasis or allergic response in the nursing infant.

Children: Safety and efficacy of carbenicillin, piperacillin and the β-lactamase inhibitor/penicillin combinations have not been established in infants and children < 12 years old. Penicillins are excreted largely unchanged by the kidney. Because of incompletely developed renal function in infants, the rate of elimination will be slow. Penicillinase-resistant penicillins (especially methicillin) may not be completely excreted, with abnormally high blood levels resulting. Oral aminopenicillins are not absorbed as well in neonates as in adults. Use caution in administering to newborns and evaluate organ system function frequently. Frequent blood levels are advisable, with dosage adjustments when necessary. Monitor all newborns closely for clinical and laboratory evidence of toxic or adverse effects.

Precautions:

Streptococcal infections: Therapy must be sufficient to eliminate the organism (a minimum of 10 days); otherwise, sequelae (eg, endocarditis, rheumatic fever) may occur. Take cultures following treatment to confirm that streptococci have been eradicated.

Sexually transmitted diseases: When treating gonococcal infections in which primary and secondary syphilis are suspected, perform proper diagnostic procedures, including darkfield examinations and monthly serological tests for at least 4 months. All cases of penicillin-treated syphilis should receive clinical and serological examinations every 6 months for 2 to 3 years.

Renal function impairment: Since carbenicillin is primarily excreted by the kidney, patients with severe renal impairment (creatinine clearance, < 10 ml/min) will not achieve the therapeutic urine levels of carbenecillin.

In patients with creatinine clearance 10 to 20 ml/min, it may be necessary to adjust dosage to prevent accumulation of the drug.

Monitoring: Perform bacteriologic studies to determine causative organisms and their susceptibility so that appropriate therapy is administered.

Obtain blood cultures, white blood cell and differential cell counts prior to initiation of therapy and at least weekly during therapy with penicillinase-resistant penicillins. Measure AST and ALT during therapy to monitor for liver function abnormalities.

Perform periodic urinalysis, BUN and creatinine determinations during therapy with penicillinase-resistant penicillins, and consider dosage alterations if these values become elevated. If renal impairment is known or suspected, reduce the total dosage and monitor blood levels to avoid possible neurotoxic reactions.

Monitoring is particularly important in newborns and other infants, and when high dosages are used.

Superinfection: Use of antibiotics (especially prolonged or repeated therapy) may result in bacterial or fungal overgrowth of nonsusceptible organisms. Such overgrowth may lead to a secondary infection. Take appropriate measures if superinfection occurs.

Indwelling IV catheters encourage superinfections.

Resistance: The number of strains of staphylococci resistant to penicillinase-resistant penicillins has been increasing; widespread use of penicillinase-resistant penicillins may result in an increasing number of resistant staphylococcal strains. Interpret resistance to any penicillinase-resistant penicillin as evidence of clinical resistance to all. Cross-resistance with cephalosporin derivatives also occurs frequently.

Pseudomembranous colitis has occurred with the use of broad spectrum antibiotics due to overgrowth of clostridia; therefore, it is important to consider its diagnosis in patients who develop diarrhea in association with antibiotic use. Mild cases may respond to drug discontinuation alone. Manage moderate-to-severe cases with fluid, electrolyte and protein supplementation. If it is not relieved by drug withdrawal or when it is severe, oral vancomycin is the treatment of choice.

(Precautions continued on following page)

Precautions (Cont.):

Procaine sensitivity: If sensitivity to the procaine in **penicillin G procaine** is suspected, inject 0.1 ml of a 1% to 2% procaine solution intradermally. Development of erythema, wheal, flare or eruption indicates procaine sensitivity; treat by the usual methods. Do not use procaine penicillin preparations.

Tartrazine sensitivity: Some of these products contain tartrazine, which may cause allergic-type reactions (including bronchial asthma) in susceptible individuals. Although the incidence of tartrazine sensitivity in the general population is low, it is frequently seen in patients who also have aspirin hypersensitivity. Specific products containing tartrazine are identified in the product listings.

Sulfite sensitivity: Some of these products contain sodium formaldehyde sulfoxylate, a sulfite that may cause allergic-type reactions including anaphylactic symptoms and life-threatening or less severe asthmatic episodes in certain susceptible people. The overall prevalence of sulfite sensitivity in the general population is unknown and probably low. Sulfite sensitivity is seen more frequently in asthmatic than in nonasthmatic people.

Parenteral administration: Inadvertent intravascular administration, including direct intra-arterial injection or injection immediately adjacent to arteries, has resulted in severe neurovascular damage, including transverse myelitis with permanent paralysis, gangrene requiring amputation of digits and more proximal portions of extremities, and necrosis and sloughing at and surrounding the injection site. Such severe effects have occurred following injections into the buttock, thigh and deltoid areas. Other serious complications include immediate pallor, mottling or cyanosis of the extremity, both distal and proximal to the injection site, followed by bleb formation; severe edema requiring anterior or posterior compartment fasciotomy in the lower extremity. These severe effects have most often occurred in infants and small children. Promptly consult specialist if any evidence of compromise of the blood supply occurs at, proximal to or distal to the site of injection.

Quadriceps femoris fibrosis and atrophy have occurred following repeated IM injections of penicillin preparations into the anterolateral thigh.

Take particular care with IV administration because of the possibility of thrombophlebitis. Higher than recommended IV doses of most of the penicillins may cause neuromuscular excitability or convulsions.

Avoid SC and fat layer injections; pain and induration may occur. If these occur, apply an ice pack.

Electrolyte imbalance: Administer **aqueous penicillin G** IV in high doses (▷ 10 million units) slowly because of electrolyte imbalance from either the potassium or sodium content. When sodium restriction is necessary (eg, cardiac patients), make periodic electrolyte determinations and monitor cardiac status.

Patients given continuous IV therapy with **potassium penicillin G** in high dosage (▷ 10 million units daily) may suffer severe or even fatal potassium poisoning, particularly if renal insufficiency is present. Hyperreflexia, convulsions, coma, cardiac arrhythmias and cardiac arrest may be indicative of this syndrome. High dosage of **sodium salts of penicillins** may result in or aggravate CHF due to high sodium intake. Individuals with liver disease or those receiving cytotoxic therapy or diuretics rarely demonstrated a decrease in serum potassium concentrations with high doses of **piperacillin.**

Sodium penicillin G contains 2 mEq sodium per million units, **potassium penicillin G** contains 1.7 mEq potassium and 0.3 mEq sodium per million units. The sodium content of other IV penicillin derivatives is listed below:

Sodium Content of IV Penicillins

Penicillin	Maximum daily dose (g)	Sodium content (mEq/g)[1]	Sodium (mEq/day)[1,2]
Ampicillin sodium	12	2.9	34.8
Methicillin sodium	12	3	36
Mezlocillin sodium	24	1.85	44.4
Nafcillin sodium	9	2.9	26
Oxacillin sodium	12	2.5	30
Piperacillin sodium	24	1.85	44.4
Ticarcillin disodium	24	4.7 to 5	112.8 to 120

[1] 1 mEq sodium equals 23 mg. [2] Based on maximum daily dose.

Hypokalemia has occurred in a few patients receiving **mezlocillin, ticarcillin** and **piperacillin**. It may also occur in patients with low potassium reserves and in patients receiving cytotoxic therapy or diuretics. Monitor serum potassium and supplement when necessary.

(Continued on following page)

Drug Interactions:

Penicillin Drug Interactions			
Precipitant drug	Object drug*		Description
Penicillins, parenteral	Aminoglycosides, parenteral	↔	Although these agents are often used together to achieve a synergistic action, certain penicillins may inactivate certain aminoglycosides in vitro. Do not mix in the same IV solution. Also, oral neomycin may reduce the serum concentrations of oral penicillin.
Penicillins, parenteral	Anticoagulants	↑	Large IV doses of penicillins can increase bleeding risks of anticoagulants by prolonging bleeding time. Conversely, nafcillin has been associated with warfarin resistance.
Penicillins, oral	Beta blockers	↔	Ampicillin may reduce the bioavailability of atenolol. Case reports indicated that beta blockers may potentiate anaphylactic reactions of penicillin.
Penicillins	Contraceptives, oral	↓	The efficacy of oral contraceptives may be reduced. Although infrequently reported, the use of an additional form of contraception during penicillin therapy is advisable.
Penicilllins, parenteral	Heparin	↑	An increased risk of bleeding may occur, possibly due to additive effects.
Allopurinol	Ampicillin	↑	The rate of ampicillin-induced skin rash appears much higher when coadministered with allopurinol than with either drug by itself (see Warnings).
Chloramphenicol	Penicillins	↔	Synergistic effects may develop, but antagonism has been reported in animal studies.
Erythromycin	Penicillins	↔	In vitro tests and clinical studies have demonstrated both antagonism and synergism with coadministration.
Tetracyclines	Penicillins	↓	The bacteriostatic action of tetracycline derivatives may impair the bactericidal effects of penicillins.

* ↑ = Object drug increased ↓ = Object drug decreased ↔ = Undetermined effect

Drug/Food interaction: Absorption of most penicillins is affected by food; these medications are best taken on an empty stomach, 1 hour before or 2 hours after meals. Penicillin V may be given with meals; however, blood levels may be slightly higher when taken on an empty stomach. Amoxicillin, amoxicillin/potassium clavulanate and bacampicillin tablets may be given without regard to meals; absorption of bacampicillin suspension is affected by food.

Drug/Lab test interactions: False-positive **urine glucose** reactions may occur with penicillin therapy if Clinitest, Benedict's Solution or Fehling's Solution are used. It is recommended that enzymatic glucose oxidase tests (such as *Clinistix* or *Tes-Tape*) be used. Positive **Coombs' tests** have occurred. Positive direct antiglobulin tests (DAT) have been reported after large IV doses of **piperacillin**; **clavulanic acid** has also been reported to cause a positive DAT. High urine concentrations of some penicillins may produce false-positive protein reactions (pseudoproteinuria) with the following methods: Sulfosalicylic acid and boiling test, acetic acid test, biuret reaction and nitric acid test. The bromphenol blue *(Multi-Stix)* reagent strip test has been reported to be reliable.

(Continued on following page)

Adverse Reactions:

Hypersensitivity: Adverse reactions (estimated incidence, 1% to 10%) are more likely to occur in individuals with previously demonstrated hypersensitivity. In penicillin-sensitive individuals with a history of allergy, asthma or hay fever, the reactions may be immediate and severe. (See Warnings).

Allergic symptoms include urticaria, angioneurotic edema, laryngospasm, bronchospasm, hypotension, vascular collapse; death; maculopapular to exfoliative dermatitis; vesicular eruptions; erythema multiforme (rarely, Stevens-Johnson syndrome); reactions resembling serum sickness (chills, fever, edema, arthralgia, arthritis, malaise); laryngeal edema; skin rashes; prostration.

GI (usually with oral use): Glossitis; stomatitis; gastritis; sore mouth or tongue; dry mouth; furry tongue; black "hairy" tongue; abnormal taste sensation; nausea; vomiting; abdominal pain or cramp; epigastric distress; diarrhea or bloody diarrhea; rectal bleeding; flatulence; enterocolitis; pseudomembranous colitis (see Precautions). Incidence of symptoms, particularly diarrhea, is less with amoxicillin and bacampicillin than with ampicillin.

Hematopoietic and lymphatic systems: Anemia; hemolytic anemia; thrombocytopenia; thrombocytopenic purpura; eosinophilia; leukopenia; granulocytopenia; neutropenia; bone marrow depression; agranulocytosis; a reduction of hemoglobin or hematocrit; prolongation of bleeding and prothrombin time; decrease in WBC and lymphocyte counts; increase in lymphocytes, monocytes, basophils and platelets. These reactions are usually reversible on discontinuation of therapy, and are believed to be hypersensitivity phenomena. A slight thrombocytosis occurred in $< 1\%$ of patients treated with amoxicillin and clavulanate potassium.

Bleeding abnormalities: Hemorrhagic manifestations associated with abnormalities of coagulation tests such as clotting and prothrombin time have occurred (see Warnings).

Renal: Interstitial nephritis (eg, oliguria, proteinuria, hematuria, hyaline casts, pyuria) and nephropathy are infrequent and usually associated with high doses of parenteral penicillins (most frequently **methicillin**); this has also occurred with all of the penicillins. Such reactions are hypersensitivity responses and are usually associated with fever, skin rash and eosinophilia. Methicillin-induced nephropathy does not appear to be dose-related and is generally reversible upon prompt discontinuation of the drug. Elevations of creatinine or BUN may occur.

CNS: Penicillins have caused neurotoxicity (manifested as lethargy, neuromuscular irritability, hallucinations, convulsions and seizures) when given in large IV doses especially in patients with renal failure. Mental disturbances including anxiety, confusion, agitation, depression, hallucinations, weakness, seizures, combativeness and expressed "fear of impending death" have been reported in individuals following single dose therapy for gonorrhea with **penicillin G procaine**, which may have been a reaction to procaine. Reactions have been transient, lasting from 15 to 30 minutes. Dizziness, fatigue, insomnia, reversible hyperactivity and prolonged muscle relaxation have occurred.

Local reactions: Pain (accompanied by induration) at the site of injection; ecchymosis; deep vein thrombosis; hematomas. Vein irritation and phlebitis can occur, particularly when undiluted solution is injected directly into the vein. Tissue necrosis due to extravasated **nafcillin** has been successfully modified with hyaluronidase.

Miscellaneous: Vaginitis; anorexia; hyperthermia, itchy eyes, transient hepatitis and cholestatic jaundice (rare); sciatic neuritis caused by IM injection of penicillin. The Jarisch-Herxheimer reaction has been reported in the treatment of syphilis.

Laboratory test abnormalities: Elevations of AST, ALT, bilirubin and LDH have been noted in patients receiving semisynthetic penicillins (particularly **oxacillin** and **cloxacillin**); such reactions are more common in infants. Elevations of serum alkaline phosphatase and hypernatremia, and reduction in serum potassium, albumin, total proteins and uric acid may occur. Evidence indicates glutamic oxaloacetic transaminase (GOT) is released at the site of IM injection of **ampicillin**. Increased amounts of this enzyme in the blood do not necessarily indicate liver involvement.

(Continued on following page)

Overdosage:

Penicillin overdosage can result in neuromuscular hyperexcitability or convulsive seizures. Dose-related toxicity may arise with the use of massive doses of IV penicillins (40 to 100 million units/day), particularly in patients with severe renal impairment. Manifestations may include agitation, confusion, asterixis, hallucinations, stupor, coma, multifocal myoclonus, seizures and encephalopathy. Hyperkalemia is also possible.

In case of overdosage, discontinue penicillin, treat symptomatically and institute supportive measures as required. Refer to General Management of Acute Overdosage. If necessary, hemodialysis may be used to reduce blood levels of penicillin, although the degree of effectiveness of this procedure is questionable. The metabolic by-products of carbenicillin indanyl sodium, indanyl sulfate and glucuronide, as well as free carbenicillin, are dialyzable. In renal function impairment, aminopenicillins can be removed by hemodialysis, but not peritoneal dialysis. The molecular weight, degree of protein binding and pharmacokinetic profile of sulbactam and clavulanic acid suggest these compounds may also be removed by hemodialysis.

Patient Information:

Complete full course of therapy.

Take on an empty stomach 1 hour before or 2 hours after meals. Absorption of penicillin V, amoxicillin, bacampicillin tablets and amoxicillin/potassium clavulanate is not significantly affected by food.

Take each oral dose with a full glass of water, not fruit juice or carbonated beverage (cloxacillin, penicillin G).

Take at even intervals, preferably around the clock.

Notify physician if skin rash, itching, hives, severe diarrhea, shortness of breath, wheezing, black tongue, sore thoat, nausea, vomiting, fever, swollen joints or any unusual bleeding or bruising occurs.

Discard any liquid forms of penicillin after 7 days if stored at room temperature or after 14 days if refrigerated.

Administration:

Therapy may be initiated prior to obtaining results of bacteriologic studies when there is reason to believe the causative organisms may be susceptible. Once results are known, adjust therapy.

Dosage for any individual patient must take into consideration the severity of infection, the susceptibility of the organisms causing the infection and the status of the patient's host defense mechanism. Duration of therapy depends on the severity of the infection.

Continue treatment of all infections for a minimum of 48 to 72 hours beyond the time that the patient becomes asymptomatic or evidence of bacterial eradication has been obtained, unless single dose therapy is employed. A minimum of 10 days treatment is recommended for any infection caused by group A beta-hemolytic streptococci to prevent the occurrence of acute rheumatic fever or acute glomerulonephritis.

Patients with a history of rheumatic fever and receiving continuous prophylaxis may harbor increased numbers of penicillin-resistant organisms.

(Products listed on following pages)

Complete prescribing information for these products begins on page 1686

Natural Penicillins

PENICILLIN G (AQUEOUS), PARENTERAL

Dosage:

Children: 100,000 to 250,000 units/kg/day in divided doses every 4 hours.

Infants (over 7 days and > 2000 g): 100,000 units/kg/day in divided doses every 6 hours (meningitis – 200,000 units).

Over 7 days and < 2000 g: 75,000 units/kg/day in divided doses every 8 hours (meningitis – 150,000 units).

Under 7 days and > 2000 g: 50,000 units/kg/day in divided doses every 8 hours (meningitis – 150,000 units).

Under 7 days and < 2000 g: 50,000 units/kg/day in divided doses every 12 hours (meningitis – 100,000 units).

Streptococci in groups A, C, G, H, L and M are very sensitive to penicillin G. Some group D organisms are sensitive to the high serum levels obtained with aqueous penicillin G.

Parenteral Penicillin G Use and Dosages	
Organisms/Infections	Dosage
Labeled uses:	
Meningococcal meningitis	1 to 2 million units IM every 2 hours; or 20 to 30 million units/day continuous IV drip for 14 days or until afebrile for 7 days; or 200,000 to 300,000 units/kg/day every 2 to 4 hours divided doses for a total of 24 doses.
Actinomycosis For cervicofacial cases	1 to 6 million units/day
For thoracic and abdominal disease	12 to 20 million units/day IV for 6 weeks. May be followed by oral penicillin V, 500 mg 4 times daily for 2 to 3 months
Clostridial infections	20 million units/day as adjunct to antitoxin
Fusospirochetal infections: Severe infections of oropharynx, lower respiratory tract and genital area	5 to 10 million units/day
Rat-bite fever (Spirillum minus, Streptobacillus moniliformis), Haverhill fever	12 to 20 million units/day for 3 to 4 weeks
Listeria infections (Listeria monocytogenes):	
Meningitis (adults)	15 to 20 million units/day for 2 weeks
Endocarditis (adults)	15 to 20 million units/day for 4 weeks
Pasteurella infections (Pasteurella multocida): Bacteremia and meningitis	4 to 6 million units/day for 2 weeks
Erysipeloid (Erysipelothrix rhusiopathiae): Endocarditis	12 to 20 million units/day for 4 to 6 weeks
Gram-negative bacillary bacteremia (Escherichia coli, Enterobacter aerogenes, Alcaligenes faecalis, Salmonella, Shigella, Proteus mirabilis)	≥ 20 million units/day
Diphtheria: Adjunct to antitoxin to prevent carrier state	2 to 3 million units/day in divided doses for 10 to 12 days
Anthrax: (*B anthracis* is often resistant)	Minimum 5 million units/day; 12 to 20 million units/day have been used
Pneumococcal infections (S pneumoniae):	
Empyema	5 to 24 million units/day in divided doses every 4 to 6 hours
Meningitis	20 to 24 million units/day for 14 days
Suppurative arthritis, osteomyelitis, mastoiditis, endocarditis, peritonitis, pericarditis	12 to 20 million units/day for ≥ 2 to 4 weeks

(Continued on following page)

PENICILLIN G (AQUEOUS), PARENTERAL (Cont.)

Dosage (Cont.):

Parenteral Penicillin G Uses and Dosages (Cont.)	
Organisms/Infections	Dosage
Syphilis:[1]	
Neurosyphilis	12 to 24 million units/day IV (2 to 4 million units every 4 hours) for 10 to 14 days. Many recommend benzathine penicillin G 2.4 million units IM weekly for 3 weeks following the completion of this regimen.
Congenital syphilis: Symptomatic or asymptomatic infants	*Newborns:* 50,000 units/kg/day IV every 8 to 12 hours for 10 to 14 days. If > 1 day of therapy is missed, restart the entire course. *Infants* (after newborn period): 50,000 units/kg every 4 to 6 hours for 10 to 14 days.
Gonococcal infections:[1] Infants with disseminated gonococcal infection or gonococcal ophthalmia (hospitalization recommended)	If the gonococcal isolate is proven to be susceptible to penicillin: 100,000 units/kg/day in 2 equal doses (4 equal doses per day for infants > 1 week old). Increase the dose to 150,000 units/kg/day for meningitis.
Unlabeled uses:	
Lyme disease (Borrelia burgdorferi):	
Erythema chronicum migrans	Use oral penicillin V
Neurologic complications (eg, meningitis, encephalitis)	200,000 to 300,000 units/kg/day (up to 20 million units) IV for 10 to 14 days
Carditis	200,000 to 300,000 units/kg/day (up to 20 million units) IV for 10 days with cardiac monitoring and a temporary pacemaker for complete heart block
Arthritis	200,000 to 300,000 units/kg/day (up to 20 million units) IV for 10 to 20 days

[1] CDC 1989 Sexually Transmitted Diseases Treatment Guidelines. *Morbidity and Mortality Weekly Report* 1989 Sept. 1;38 (No. S-8):1-43.

Since alpha-hemolytic streptococci resistant to penicillin may be found when patients are receiving continuous oral penicillin for secondary prevention of rheumatic fever, prophylactic agents other than penicillin may be prescribed in addition to their continuous rheumatic fever prophylactic regimen.

(Continued on following page)

PENICILLIN G (AQUEOUS), PARENTERAL (Cont.)

Administration:

Penicillin G potassium contains 1.7 mEq potassium and 0.3 mEq sodium per million units; Penicillin G sodium contains 2 mEq sodium per million units.

Give recommended daily dosage IM or by continuous IV infusion.

Administer 10 or 20 million units by IV infusion only.

IM: Keep total volume of injection small. The IM route is the preferred route of administration. Solutions containing up to 100,000 units/ml may be used with a minimum of discomfort. Use greater concentrations as required.

Continuous IV infusion: When larger doses are required, administer aqueous solutions by means of continuous IV infusion. Determine volume and rate of fluid administration required by the patient in a 24 hour period. Add appropriate daily dosage to this fluid.

Intrapleural or other local infusion: If fluid is aspirated, give infusion in a volume equal to ¼ or ½ the amount of fluid aspirated; otherwise, prepare as for the IM injection.

Intrathecal use: Must be highly individualized. Use only with full consideration of the possible irritating effects of penicillin when used by this route. The preferred route of therapy in bacterial meningitis is IV, supplemented by IM injection. It has been suggested that intrathecal use has no place in therapy.

Preparation of solutions: Depending on the route of administration, use Sterile Water for Injection, Isotonic Sodium Chloride Injection or Dextrose Injection. Penicillins are rapidly inactivated in the presence of carbohydrate solutions at alkaline pH.

Stability/Storage: The dry powder is stable and does not require refrigeration. Sterile solutions may be kept in the refrigerator for 1 week without loss of potency. Solutions prepared for IV infusion are stable at room temperature for at least 24 hours.

Premixed, frozen solution: Thaw frozen container at room temperature (25°C; 77°F) or in a refrigerator (5°C; 41°F). Do not force thaw by immersion in water baths or by microwave irradiation.

The thawed solution is stable for 24 hours at room temperature or for 14 days under refrigeration. Do not refreeze thawed antibiotics.

	Product	Form/Strength	Package	C.I.*
Rx	**Penicillin G Potassium** (Baxter)	**Injection, premixed, frozen:** 1,000,000 units	In 50 ml	105
		2,000,000 units	In 50 ml	54
		3,000,000 units	In 50 ml	38
Rx	**Penicillin G Potassium** (Apothecon)	**Powder for Injection:** 1,000,000 units	In vials	12
Rx	**Pfizerpen** (Roerig)		In vials	16
Rx	**Penicillin G Potassium** (Apothecon)	**Powder for Injection:** 5,000,000 units	In vials.	37
Rx	**Pfizerpen** (Roerig)		In vials.	42
Rx	**Penicillin G Potassium** (Apothecon)	**Powder for Injection:** 10,000,000 units	In vials.	62
Rx	**Penicillin G Potassium** (Apothecon)	**Powder for Injection:** 20,000,000 units per vial	In vials.	101
Rx	**Pfizerpen** (Roerig)		In vials.	122
Rx	**Penicillin G Sodium** (Apothecon)	**Powder for Injection:** 5,000,000 units per vial		62

* Cost Index based on cost per 800,000 units.

Complete prescribing information for these products begins on page 1686

Natural Penicillins (Cont.)

PENICILLIN G POTASSIUM, ORAL

Administration and Dosage:

250 mg = 400,000 units.

Administer at least 1 hour before or 2 hours after meals.

Streptococci in groups A, C, G, H, L and M are very sensitive to penicillin G. Other groups, including group D (enterococci), are resistant.

Penicillin V is the preferred agent for oral therapy.

Children (< 12 years): 25,000 to 90,000 units/kg/day in 3 to 6 divided doses. 40,000 to 80,000 units/kg/day divided every 6 hours has been suggested.

Oral Penicillin G Uses and Dosages

Organisms/Infections	Dosage
Streptococcal infections of the upper respiratory tract (ie, otitis media, scarlet fever and mild erysipelas): Mild infections	200,000 to 250,000 units every 6 to 8 hours for 10 days.
Moderately severe infections	400,000 to 500,000 units every 8 hours for 10 days or 800,000 units every 12 hours.
Pneumococcal infections: Mild to moderately severe infections of the respiratory tract (eg, otitis media)	400,000 to 500,000 units every 6 hours until afebrile for at least 2 days.
Staphylococcal infections: Mild infections of skin and skin structures	200,000 to 500,000 units every 6 to 8 hours until infection is cured.
Fusospirochetosis (Vincent's gingivitis and pharyngitis) of the oropharynx: Mild to moderately severe infections	400,000 to 500,000 units every 6 to 8 hours. Obtain necessary dental care in infections involving the gum tissue.
Prevention of recurrent rheumatic fever and/or chorea	200,000 to 250,000 units twice daily on a continuing basis.

	Product	Form	Description	C.I.*
Rx	**Penicillin G Potassium** (Various, eg, Purepac, Rugby, URL)	**Tablets:** 200,000 units	In 100s and 1000s.	2+
Rx	**Penicillin G Potassium** (Various, eg, Dixon-Shane Geneva Marsam, Goldline, Major, Rugby, URL)	**Tablets:** 250,000 units	In 100s and 1000s.	1+
Rx	**Penicillin G Potassium** (Various, eg, Dixon-Shane, Geneva Marsam, Goldline, Major, Moore, Mylan, Rugby, Schein, URL, Warner Chilcott)	**Tablets:** 400,000 units	In 100s and 1000s.	1.4+
Rx	**Pentids '400'** (Apothecon)		Lactose. (165). White, scored. Oval. In 100s.	3
Rx	**Penicillin G Potassium** (Rugby)	**Tablets:** 500,000 units	In 100s.	NA
Rx	**Pentids '800'** (Apothecon)	**Tablets:** 800,000 units	Tartrazine, lactose. (168). Yellow, scored. Oval. In 100s.	2.2
Rx	**Pentids '400' for Syrup** (Apothecon)	**Powder for Oral Solution:** 400,000 units per 5 ml when reconstituted	Tartrazine, saccharin. Fruit flavor. In 100 and 200 ml.	5.9

* Cost Index based on cost per 800,000 units.

Complete prescribing information for these products begins on page 1686

PENICILLIN G PROCAINE, AQUEOUS (APPG)

Indications:

A long-acting parenteral penicillin indicated in the treatment of moderately severe infections due to penicillin G-sensitive microorganisms sensitive to low and persistent serum levels achievable with this dosage form. When high sustained serum levels are required, use aqueous penicillin G, either IM or IV.

Administration and Dosage:

Administer by deep IM injection into the upper, outer quadrant of the buttock. In infants and small children, the midlateral aspect of the thigh may be preferable. When doses are repeated, rotate the injection site.

Streptococci in groups A, C, G, H, L and M are very sensitive to penicillin G. Other groups, including group D (enterococci), are resistant. Use aqueous penicillin for streptococcal infections with bacteremia.

An increasing number of strains of staphylococci are resistant to penicillin G, emphasizing the need for culture and sensitivity studies.

Gonorrhea: Some isolates of *Neisseria gonorrhoeae* have decreased susceptibility to penicillin, but penicillin in large doses remains the drug of choice for these strains. Strains producing penicillinase, however, are resistant to penicillin G and another drug should be used.

Retreatment – The CDC recommends follow-up cultures 3 to 7 days after treatment is completed.[1] In the male, a gram-stained smear is adequate if positive; otherwise, obtain a culture specimen from the anterior urethra. In the female, obtain culture specimens from both the endocervical and anal canal sites. Retreatment in the male is indicated if urethral discharge persists for ≥ 3 days following initial therapy and the smear or culture remains positive. If gonorrhea persists after a nonspectinomycin treatment regimen, treat with **spectinomycin** 2 g IM or **ceftriaxone** 250 mg IM.[1]

Perform a serologic test for syphilis at the time of diagnosis. If patients with gonorrhea have concurrent syphilis, give additional treatment appropriate to the stage of syphilis.

Adults and children: 600,000 to 1.2 million units/day IM in one or two doses (up to a maximum of 4.8 million units/day) for 10 days to 2 weeks.

Newborns: 50,000 units/kg IM once daily. Avoid use in these patients since sterile abscesses and procaine toxicity are of much greater concern than in older children.

Severe pneumonia, empyema, bacteremia, pericarditis, meningitis, peritonitis and purulent or septic arthritis of pneumococcal etiology are better treated with aqueous penicillin G during the acute stage.

Penicillin G Procaine Uses and Dosages	
Organisms/Infections	Dosage
Pneumococcal infections: Moderately severe uncomplicated pneumonia and middle ear and paranasal sinus infections	600,000 to 1.2 million units/day
Streptococcal infections (group A): Moderately severe to severe tonsillitis, erysipelas, scarlet fever, upper respiratory tract (ie, otitis media) and skin and skin structure infections	600,000 to 1.2 million units/day for a minimum of 10 days
Bacterial endocarditis – Only in extremely sensitive infections *(S viridans, S bovis)*	1.2 million units 4 times daily for 2 to 4 weeks plus streptomycin 500 mg twice daily for the first 2 weeks
Staphylococcal infections: Moderately severe to severe infections of the skin and skin structure	600,000 to 1.2 million units/day
Diphtheria: Adjunctive therapy with antitoxin	300,000 to 600,000 units/day
Carrier state	300,000 units/day for 10 days
Anthrax: Cutaneous	600,000 to 1.2 million units/day
Vincent's gingivitis and pharyngitis (fusospirochetosis):	600,000 to 1.2 million units/day. Obtain necessary dental care in infections involving gum tissue.
Erysipeloid:	600,000 to 1.2 million units/day
Rat-bite fever (Streptobacillus moniliformis and Spirillum minus):	600,000 to 1.2 million units/day

[1] CDC 1989 Sexually Transmitted Diseases Treatment Guidelines. *Morbidity and Mortality Weekly Report* 1989 Sept 1;38(No. S-8):1-43.

(Continued on following page)

Natural Penicillins (Cont.)

PENICILLIN G PROCAINE, AQUEOUS (APPG)(Cont.)

Administration and Dosage (Cont.):

Penicillin G Procaine Uses and Dosages	
Organisms/Infections	Dosage
Gonorrheal infections (uncomplicated):	4.8 million units divided into at least two doses at one visit; 1 g oral probenecid is given 30 minutes before the injections. Obtain follow-up cultures from the original site(s) of infection 7 to 14 days after therapy. In women, it is also desirable to obtain culture test-of-cure from both the endocervical and anal canals. Note: Treat gonorrheal endocarditis intensively with aqueous penicillin G
Syphilis: Primary, secondary and latent with a negative spinal fluid (adults and children > 12 years of age):	600,000 units daily for 8 days; total 4.8 million units
Neurosyphilis[1] (as an alternative to the recommended regimen of penicillin G aqueous)	2 to 4 million units/day plus probenecid 500 mg orally 4 times daily, both for 10 to 14 days; many recommend benzathine penicillin G 2.4 million units weekly for 3 doses following the completion of this regimen.
Congenital syphilis:[1] Symptomatic and asymptomatic infants	50,000 units/kg/day (administered once IM) for 10 to 14 days
Yaws, Bejel and Pinta:	Treat same as syphilis in corresponding stage of disease

Storage: Refrigerate (stable for 24 months); avoid freezing.

	Product	Form	Package	C.I.*
Rx	**Crysticillin 300 A.S.** (Apothecon)	**Injection:** 300,000 units per ml	In 10 ml vials.[2]	46
Rx	**Pfizerpen-AS** (Roerig)		In 10 ml vials.[3]	42
Rx	**Crysticillin 600 A.S.** (Apothecon)	**Injection:** 500,000 units per ml (600,000 units/1.2 ml)	In 12 ml vials.[4]	45
Rx	**Wycillin** (Wyeth-Ayerst)	**Injection:** 600,000 units per unit dose	In 1 ml Tubex.[5]	207
Rx	**Wycillin** (Wyeth-Ayerst)	**Injection:** 1,200,000 units per unit dose	In 2 ml Tubex.[5]	172
Rx	**Wycillin** (Wyeth-Ayerst)	**Injection:** 2,400,000 units per unit dose	In 4 ml disp. syringe.[5]	183
Rx	**Wycillin Injection & Probenecid Tablets** (Wyeth-Ayerst)	**Combination Package:** Two 4 ml disposable syringes containing 2,400,000 units penicillin G procaine each[5] and two 500 mg probenecid tablets.		NA

* Cost Index based on cost per 800,000 units.

[1] CDC 1989 Sexually Transmitted Diseases Treatment Guidelines. *Morbidity and Mortality Weekly Report* 1989 Sept 1;38 (No. S-8):1-43.

[2] With parabens, lecithin, povidone and sodium formaldehyde sulfoxylate.

[3] With parabens, sorbitol, polyvinylpyrrolidone and lecithin.

[4] With parabens, phenol, povidone, lecithin and sodium formaldehyde sulfoxylate.

[5] With parabens, lecithin and povidone.

Complete prescribing information for these products begins on page 1686

PENICILLIN G BENZATHINE, PARENTERAL

Administration and Dosage:

Administer by deep IM injection in the upper outer quadrant of the buttock. In infants and small children, the midlateral aspect of the thigh may be preferable. Do not inject benzathine penicillin into the gluteal region of children < 2 years of age. When doses are repeated, rotate the injection site.

Adults: 1.2 million units in one dose.

Children (> 27 kg): 900,000 to 1.2 million units in one dose.

Children and infants (< 27 kg): 300,000 to 600,000 units in one dose.

Neonates: 50,000 units/kg in one dose.

Parenteral Penicillin G Benzathine Uses and Dosages

Organisms/Infections	Dosage
Streptococcal (group A): Prevention of recurrent rheumatic fever.	1.2 million units every 4 weeks
Syphilis:[1]	
Early syphilis – Primary, secondary or latent syphilis of < 1 year's duration.	2.4 million units IM in single dose
Syphilis of > 1 year's duration, gummas and cardiovascular syphilis – Latent, cardiovascular or late benign syphilis.	2.4 million units once weekly for 3 weeks
Neurosyphilis	Aqueous penicillin G, 12 to 24 million units/day IV (2 to 4 million units every 4 hours) for 10 to 14 days. Many recommend benzathine penicillin G, 2.4 million units IM weekly for 3 doses following completion of this regimen. or Aqueous procaine penicillin G, 2.4 million units/day IM *plus* probenecid 500 mg orally 4 times daily, both for 10 to 14 days. Many recommend benzathine penicillin G, 2.4 million units IM weekly for 3 doses following completion of this regimen.
Syphilis in pregnancy	Dosage schedule appropriate for stage of syphilis recommended for nonpregnant patients.
Congenital syphilis – Older children with definite acquired syphilis and a normal neurologic examination	50,000 units/kg IM, up to the adult dose of 2.4 million units
Yaws, Bejel and Pinta	1.2 million units in a single dose
Erysipeloid (Erysipelothrix rhusiopathiae): Uncomplicated infection	1.2 million units in a single dose

Storage: Refrigerate (stable for 24 months); avoid freezing.

				C.I.*
Rx	**Bicillin L-A** (Wyeth-Ayerst)	**Injection:** 300,000 units per ml	In 10 ml vials.[2]	288
		600,000 units/dose	In 1 ml Tubex.[2]	625
		1,200,000 units/dose	In 2 ml Tubex.[2]	614
		2,400,000 units/dose	In 4 ml syringe.[2]	657
Rx	**Permapen** (Roerig)	**Injection:** 1,200,000 units per dose	In 2 ml Isoject.[3]	390

* Cost Index based on cost per 800,000 units.

[1] CDC 1989 Sexually Transmitted Diseases Treatment Guidelines. *Morbidity and Mortality Weekly Report* 1989 Sept 1;38(No. S-8):1-43.

[2] With lecithin, povidone, methyl and propyl parabens.

[3] With lecithin, methyl and propyl parabens.

Complete prescribing information for these products begins on page 1686

PENICILLIN G BENZATHINE AND PROCAINE COMBINED

Indications:

Treatment of moderately severe infections due to microorganisms that are susceptible to the serum levels of penicillin G achievable with this dosage form. Guide therapy by bacteriological studies and clinical response. When high, sustained serum levels are required, use IV or IM aqueous penicillin G (potassium or sodium). This drug should not be used in the treatment of venereal diseases, including syphilis and gonorrhea, or yaws, bejel and pinta. The following infections will usually respond to adequate doses of this drug:

Streptococcal infections: Moderately severe to severe infections of the upper respiratory tract, skin and soft tissue infections, scarlet fever and erysipelas.

Pneumococcal infections: Moderately severe pneumonia and otitis media.

Administration and Dosage:

Administer by deep IM injection in the upper outer quadrant of the buttock. In infants and small children, the midlateral aspect of the thigh may be preferable. When doses are repeated, rotate the injection site.

Streptococcal infections: Streptococci in groups A, C, G, H, L and M are very sensitive to penicillin G. Other groups, including group D (enterococci), are resistant. Penicillin G sodium or potassium is recommended for streptococcal infections with bacteremia.

Treatment with the recommended dosage is usually given in a single session using multiple IM sites when indicated. An alternative dosage schedule may be used, giving half the total dose on day 1 and half on day 3. This will also ensure adequate serum levels over a 10 day period; however, use only when the patient's cooperation can be assured.

Adults and children (> 60 lbs; 27 kg) – 2.4 million units.
Children (30 to 60 lbs; 14 to 27 kg) – 900,000 to 1.2 million units.
Infants and children (< 30 lbs; 14 kg) – 600,000 units.

Pneumococcal infections (except pneumococcal meningitis):

Children: 600,000 units. *Adults:* 1.2 million units. Repeat every 2 or 3 days until the patient has been afebrile for 48 hours. Severe pneumonia, empyema, bacteremia, pericarditis, meningitis, peritonitis and arthritis of pneumococcal etiology are better treated with aqueous penicillin G during the acute stage.

Storage: Refrigerate.

				C.I.*
Rx	**Bicillin C-R** (Wyeth-Ayerst)	**Injection:** 300,000 units/ml (150,000 units each penicillin G benzathine and penicillin G procaine)	In 10 ml vials.[1]	208
		600,000 units/dose (300,000 units each penicillin G benzathine and penicillin G procaine)	In 1 ml Tubex.[1]	NA
		1,200,000 units/dose	In 2 ml Tubex.[1]	360
		2,400,000 units/dose	In 4 ml syringe.[1]	385
Rx	**Bicillin C-R 900/300** (Wyeth-Ayerst)	**Injection:** 900,000 units penicillin G benzathine and 300,000 units penicillin G procaine per dose	In 2 ml Tubex.[1]	374

* Cost Index based on cost per 800,000 units.
[1] With parabens, lecithin and povidone.

Complete prescribing information for these products begins on page 1686

Natural Penicillins (Cont.)

PENICILLIN V (Phenoxymethyl Penicillin)

Administration and Dosage:

250 mg = 400,000 units.

Each g of penicillin V potassium contains 2.6 mmol (2.6 mEq) potassium.

Severe pneumonia, empyema, bacteremia, pericarditis, meningitis and arthritis should not be treated with oral penicillin V during the acute stage.

Streptococci in groups A, C, G, H, L and M are very sensitive to penicillin. Other groups, including group D (enterococci), are resistant.

An increasing number of strains of staphylococci are resistant to penicillin G (and V), emphasizing the need for culture and susceptibility studies.

Adults: 125 to 500 mg 4 times a day; in renal impairment (creatinine clearance, ≤ 10 ml/min) – Do not exceed 250 mg every 6 hours.

Children: 25 to 50 mg/kg/day in divided doses every 6 to 8 hours.

Penicillin V Uses and Dosages

Organisms/Infections	Dosage
Labeled uses:	
Streptococcal infections: Infections of the upper respiratory tract, including scarlet fever and mild erysipelas	125 to 250 mg every 6 to 8 hours for 10 days for mild to moderately severe infections
Pharyngitis in children	250 mg 2 times daily for 10 days
Otitis media and sinusitis	250 to 500 mg every 6 hours for 2 weeks
Prevention of bacterial endocarditis[1] in patients with rheumatic, congenital or other acquired valvular heart disease undergoing dental procedures or upper respiratory tract surgical procedures	Amoxicillin is the recommended agent; however, the choice of penicillin V is rational and acceptable (see amoxicillin monograph for dosage)
Pneumococcal infections: Mild to moderately severe respiratory tract infections including otitis media	250 to 500 mg every 6 hours until afebrile at least 2 days
Staphylococcal infections: Mild infections of skin and soft tissue	250 to 500 mg every 6 to 8 hours
Fusospirochetosis (Vincent's infection) of the oropharynx: Mild to moderately severe infections	250 to 500 mg every 6 to 8 hours
Unlabeled uses:	
Prophylactic treatment of children with sickle cell anemia (to reduce the incidence of *S pneumoniae* septicemia)	125 mg 2 times daily
Anaerobic infections: Mild to moderate infections	250 mg 4 times daily
Lyme disease (Borrelia burgdorferi):	
Erythema chronicum migrans:	
Pregnant or lactating women, tetracycline treatment failures	250 to 500 mg 4 times a day for 10 to 20 days
Children < 2 years of age	50 mg/kg/day (up to 2 g/day) in 4 divided doses for 10 to 20 days
Neurologic complications (eg, meningitis, encephalitis), carditis, arthritis	Use penicillin G IV

[1] American Heart Association Statement. *JAMA* 1990;264:2919-2922.

Storage/Stability: Reconstituted oral suspension is stable for 24 to 48 hours at room temperature (not exceeding 25°C; 77°F.)

Complete prescribing information for these products begins on page 1686

Natural Penicillins (Cont.)

PENICILLIN V POTASSIUM

See Administration and Dosage information on page 1703.

				C.I.*
Rx	**V-Cillin K** (Lilly)	**Tablets:** 125 mg	Lactose. In 100s.	6
Rx	**Penicillin VK** (Various, eg, Dixon-Shane, Major, Mylan, Parmed, Rugby, URL, Warner Chilcott)	**Tablets:** 250 mg	In 100s and 1000s.	1.3+
Rx	**Beepen-VK** (SK-Beecham)		Lactose. In 1000s.	1.8
Rx	**Betapen-VK** (Apothecon)		Lactose. Film coated. In 100s and 1000s.	1.8
Rx	**Ledercillin VK** (Lederle)		Lactose. (L10 LL). White, scored. In 100s, 1000s and unit-of-issue 480s.	2.9
Rx	**Pen-V** (Goldline)		White. Oval or round. In 100s and 1000s.	1.4
Rx	**Pen•Vee K** (Wyeth-Ayerst)		Lactose. (Wyeth 59). White, scored. In 100s, 500s and UD 100s.	3
Rx	**Robicillin VK** (Robins)		In 100s and 1000s.	1.1
Rx	**V-Cillin K** (Lilly)		Lactose. In 100s and 500s.	5
Rx	**Veetids '250'** (Apothecon)		Lactose. Film coated. In 100s and 1000s.	NA
Rx	**Penicillin VK** (Various, eg, Dixon-Shane, Geneva Marsam, Major, Mylan, Parmed, Rugby, URL, Warner Chilcott)	**Tablets:** 500 mg	In 100s, 500s, 1000s and UD 100s.	1+
Rx	**Beepen-VK** (SK-Beecham)		Lactose. In 500s.	1.8
Rx	**Betapen-VK** (Apothecon)		Lactose. Film coated. In 100s and 500s.	1.6
Rx	**Ledercillin VK** (Lederle)		(L9 LL). White, scored. In 100s and 500s.	2.6
Rx	**Pen-V** (Goldline)		White. Oval or round. In 100s and 1000s.	1.3
Rx	**Pen•Vee K** (Wyeth-Ayerst)		(Wyeth 390). White, scored. In 100s, 500s and UD 100s.	2.8
Rx	**Robicillin VK** (Robins)		In 100s and 500s.	1.1
Rx	**V-Cillin K** (Lilly)		Lactose. In 100s and 500s.	4.8
Rx	**Veetids '500'** (Apothecon)		Lactose. Film coated. In 100s and 1000s.	2

* Cost Index based on cost per 500 mg.

(Continued on following page)

Natural Penicillins (Cont.)

PENICILLIN V POTASSIUM (Cont.)

See Administration and Dosage information on page 1703.

	Product	Form	Description	C.I.*
Rx	**Penicillin VK** (Various, eg, Major, Rugby, URL, Warner Chilcott)	**Powder for Oral Solution:** 125 mg per 5 ml when reconstituted	In 100 and 200 ml.	3.5+
Rx	**Beepen-VK** (SK-Beecham)		Saccharin, sucrose. In 100 and 200 ml.	5.9
Rx	**Betapen-VK** (Apothecon)		DL-menthol, saccharin, sucrose. In 100 and 200 ml.	5.3
Rx	**Pen•Vee K** (Wyeth-Ayerst)		Saccharin, sucrose. In 100 and 200 ml.	4.4
Rx	**V-Cillin K** (Lilly)		Saccharin, sucrose. In 100, 150 and 200 ml.	7.6
Rx	**Veetids '125'** (Apothecon)		DL-menthol, saccharin, sucrose. In 100 and 200 ml.	3.5
Rx	**Penicillin VK** (Various, eg, Rugby, URL, Warner Chilcott)	**Powder for Oral Solution:** 250 mg per 5 ml when reconstituted	In 100 and 200 ml.	2.4+
Rx	**Beepen-VK** (SK-Beecham)		Saccharin, sucrose. In 100 and 200 ml.	3.9
Rx	**Betapen-VK** (Apothecon)		DL-menthol, saccharin, sucrose. In 100 and 200 ml.	3.6
Rx	**Ledercillin VK** (Lederle)		Saccharin, sugar. Cherry flavor. In 100, 150 and 200 ml.	3.8
Rx	**Pen•Vee K** (Wyeth-Ayerst)		Saccharin, sucrose. In 100, 150 and 200 ml.	3.3
Rx	**V-Cillin K** (Lilly)		Saccharin, sucrose. In 100, 150 and 200 ml.	5.1
Rx	**Veetids '250'** (Apothecon)		DL-menthol, saccharin, sucrose. In 100 and 200 ml.	2.3

* Cost Index based on cost per 500 mg.

Complete prescribing information for these products begins on page 1686

Penicillinase-Resistant Penicillins

METHICILLIN SODIUM

Indications:

Treatment of infections due to penicillinase-producing staphylococci. May be used to initiate therapy when a staphylococcal infection is suspected. (See Indications in the group monograph concerning use of penicillinase-resistant penicillins.)

Oral penicillinase-resistant penicillins should not be used as initial therapy. Oral therapy may be used as follow-up therapy as soon as the clinical condition warrants.

Administration and Dosage:

IM: Take care to avoid sciatic nerve injury.

IV: Take care due to possibility of thrombophlebitis, especially in the elderly.

Treatment of osteomyelitis and endocarditis may require a longer term of intensive therapy.

Adults: 4 to 12 g/day in divided doses every 4 to 6 hours; in severe renal impairment (creatinine clearance ≤ 10 ml/min) do not exceed 2 g every 12 hours.

Children: 100 to 300 mg/kg/day in divided doses every 4 to 6 hours.

Infants: Over 7 days and > 2000 g – 100 mg/kg/day in divided doses every 6 hours; for meningitis – 200 mg/kg/day.

Over 7 days and < 2000 g – 75 mg/kg/day in divided doses every 8 hours; for meningitis – 150 mg/kg/day.

Under 7 days and > 2000 g – 75 mg/kg/day in divided doses every 8 hours; for meningitis – 150 mg/kg/day.

Under 7 days and < 2000 g – 50 mg/kg/day in divided doses every 12 hours; for meningitis – 100 mg/kg/day.

Preparation of solutions: Reconstitute with Sterile Water for Injection or Sodium Chloride Injection. If another agent is used in conjunction with methicillin therapy, do not physically mix with methicillin, but administer separately.

IM – Dilute as indicated in the table below. Each reconstituted ml contains approximately 500 mg methicillin.

Methicillin IM Administration Dilution	
Vial size	Minimum amount of diluent
1 g	1.5 ml
4 g	5.7 ml
6 g	8.6 ml

IV administration – Dilute each ml of reconstituted solution with 25 ml Sodium Chloride Injection.

Reconstitute piggyback units according to manufacturer's product label.

Compatible IV solutions: The drug will lose < 10% activity at room temperature (21°C; 70°F) during an 8 hour period when given in the solutions listed below. Dilute methicillin for IV infusion only in these solutions: 5% Dextrose in Normal Saline; 10% D-Fructose in Water or in Normal Saline; Lactated Potassic Saline Injection; 5% Plasma Hydrolysate in Water; 10% Invert Sugar in Normal Saline††; 10% Invert Sugar plus 0.3% Potassium Chloride in Water; *Travert* 10% Electrolyte #1, #2 or #3.

††At a concentration of 2 mg/ml, methicillin is stable for only 4 hours. Concentrations between 10 and 30 mg/ml are stable for 8 hours.

				C.I.*
Rx	**Staphcillin** (Apothecon)	**Powder for Injection:** (Contains 3 mEq sodium/g) 1 g	In vials and piggyback vials.	40
		4 g	In vials.	37
		6 g	In vials.	37
		10 g	In bulk vials.	39

* Cost Index based on cost per 500 mg.

Complete prescribing information for these products begins on page 1686

Penicillinase-Resistant Penicillins (Cont.)

NAFCILLIN SODIUM

Indications:

The treatment of infections due to penicillinase-producing staphylococci. They may be used to initiate therapy in any patient in whom a staphylococcal infection is suspected. (See Indications in the group monograph for use of penicillinase-resistant penicillins.)

Administration and Dosage:

Use parenteral therapy initially in severe infections. Very severe infections may require very high doses. Change to oral therapy as condition warrants.

Parenteral: IV – 3 to 6 g per 24 hours. Use this route for short-term therapy (24 to 48 hours) because of occasional occurrence of thrombophlebitis, particularly in the elderly.

IM – Adults: 500 mg every 4 to 6 hours.

Infants and children: 25 mg/kg twice daily.

Neonates: 10 mg/kg twice daily. Other suggested doses include: Weight < 2000 g – 50 mg/kg/day divided every 12 hours (age < 7 days) or 75 mg/kg/day divided every 8 hours (age > 7 days).

Weight > 2000 g – 50 mg/kg/day divided every 8 hours (age < 7 days) or 75 mg/kg/day divided every 6 hours (age > 7 days).

Oral: Serum levels of nafcillin after oral administration are low and unpredictable.

Adults – 250 to 500 mg every 4 to 6 hours for mild to moderate infections. In severe infections – 1 g every 4 to 6 hours.

Children – Staph infections: 50 mg/kg/day in 4 divided doses. For neonates, 10 mg/kg 3 to 4 times daily. If inadequate, change to parenteral nafcillin sodium.

Scarlet fever and pneumonia: 25 mg/kg/day in 4 divided doses.

Streptococcal pharyngitis: 250 mg, 3 times daily for 10 days. (Penicillin V is the drug of choice for streptococcal infections.)

Preparation of solutions:

IV – Dilute in 15 to 30 ml Sterile Water for Injection or Sodium Chloride for Injection; inject over 5 to 10 min. or longer. Stability studies show that nafcillin sodium at concentrations of 2 to 40 mg/ml loses < 10% activity at 21°C (70°F) for 24 hours or at 4°C (40°F) for 96 hours in the following IV solutions: Isotonic sodium chloride; Sterile Water for Injection; 5% Dextrose in Water; 5% Dextrose in 0.4% Sodium Chloride Solution; Ringer's Solution; M/6 Sodium Lactate Solution. Discard unused portions of IV solution after time period stated. Use only those solutions listed above for IV infusion. Concentration of the antibiotic should be within the range of 2 to 40 mg/ml.

IM – Reconstitute with Sterile Water for Injection or Sodium Chloride Injection. Administer clear solution immediately by deep intragluteal injection. After reconstitution, refrigerate (2° to 8°C; 36 to 46°F) and use within 7 days or keep at room temperature (25°C; 77°F) and use within 3 days or keep frozen (– 20°C; – 4°F) for up to 3 months.

(Products listed on following page)

Complete prescribing information for these products begins on page 1686

Penicillinase-Resistant Penicillins (Cont.)

NAFCILLIN SODIUM (Cont.):				C.I.*
Rx	**Unipen** (Wyeth-Ayerst)	**Tablets:** 500 mg	(Wyeth 464). White, scored. Film coated. Capsule shape. In 50s.	13
Rx	**Unipen** (Wyeth-Ayerst)	**Capsules:** 250 mg	(Wyeth 57). Green and yellow. In 100s.	15
Rx	**Nafcillin Sodium** (Geneva Marsam)	**Powder for Injection:** 500 mg[1]	In vials.	30
Rx	**Nafcil** (Apothecon)		In vials.	48+
Rx	**Nallpen** (SK-Beecham)		In vials.	22
Rx	**Unipen** (Wyeth-Ayerst)		In vials.	33
Rx	**Nafcillin Sodium** (Geneva Marsam)	**Powder for Injection:** 1 g[1]	In vials, piggyback and *ADD-Vantage* vials.	28
Rx	**Nafcil** (Apothecon)		In vials, piggyback vials and *ADD-Vantage* vials.	45
Rx	**Nallpen** (SK-Beecham)		In vials, piggyback and *ADD-Vantage* vials.	17
Rx	**Unipen** (Wyeth-Ayerst)		In vials, piggyback and *ADD-Vantage* vials.	39
Rx	**Nafcillin Sodium** (Geneva Marsam)	**Powder for Injection:** 2 g[1]	In vials, piggyback and *ADD-Vantage* vials.	27
Rx	**Nafcil** (Apothecon)		In vials, piggyback and *ADD-Vantage* vials.	44
Rx	**Nallpen** (SK-Beecham)		In vials, piggyback and *ADD-Vantage* vials.	17
Rx	**Unipen** (Wyeth-Ayerst)		In vials, piggyback and *ADD-Vantage* vials.	36
Rx	**Nafcillin Sodium** (Geneva Marsam)	**Powder for Injection:** 10 g[1]	In bulk package.	27
Rx	**Nafcil** (Apothecon)		In bulk package.	44
Rx	**Nallpen** (SK-Beecham)		In bulk package.	14
Rx	**Unipen** (Wyeth-Ayerst)		In bulk package.	32

* Cost Index based on cost per 500 mg. [1] Contains 2.9 mEq sodium/gram.

Complete prescribing information for these products begins on page 1686

OXACILLIN SODIUM

Indications:

Treatment of infections due to penicillinase-producing staphylococci. May be used to initiate therapy when a staphylococcal infection is suspected. (See Indications in the group monograph concerning use of penicillinase-resistant penicillins.)

Administration and Dosage:

Oral: Mild to moderate infections of the skin, soft tissue or upper respiratory tract –

Adults and children (> 20 kg): 500 mg every 4 to 6 hours for a minimum of 5 days.

Children (< 20 kg): 50 mg/kg/day in divided doses every 6 hrs for at least 5 days.

In serious or life-threatening infections, such as staphylococcal septicemia or other deep-seated severe infection – Following initial parenteral treatment, oral oxacillin may be given for follow-up therapy. Continue therapy 1 to 2 weeks after the patient is afebrile and cultures are sterile. Treatment of osteomyelitis may require several months of intensive therapy.

Adults – 1 g every 4 to 6 hours.

Children – ≥ 100 mg/kg/day in equally divided doses every 4 to 6 hours.

Parenteral: Consider for patients who are unable to take oral form. Oral use is most appropriate as prolonged follow-up therapy after successful initial parenteral use.

Mild to moderate upper respiratory and localized skin and soft tissue infections –

Adults and children (≥ 40 kg) – 250 to 500 mg every 4 to 6 hours.

Children (< 40 kg) – 50 mg/kg/day in equally divided doses every 6 hours.

Absorption and excretion data indicate that 25 mg/kg/day in prematures and neonates provided adequate therapeutic levels.

Severe infections (lower respiratory tract or disseminated infections) –

Adults and children (≥ 40 kg) – ≥ 1 g every 4 to 6 hours.

Children (< 40 kg) – ≥ 100 mg/kg/day in equally divided doses every 4 to 6 hrs.

Very severe infections may require very high doses and prolonged therapy. Maximum daily dose for adults is 12 g/day and for children 100 to 300 mg/kg/day.

Other suggested doses for children and neonates include:

Children – 50 to 100 mg/kg/day divided every 6 hours.

Neonates – Weight < 2000 g – 50 mg/kg/day divided every 12 hours (age < 7 days) or 100 mg/kg/day divided every 8 hours (age > 7 days).

Weight > 2000 g: 75 mg/kg/day divided every 8 hours (age < 7 days) or 150 mg/kg/day divided every 6 hours (age > 7 days).

Preparation of solutions: Reconstitute vials only with Sterile Water for Injection or Sodium Chloride (normal saline) Injection in the appropriate volume.

IM – Reconstitute to a dilution of 250 mg/1.5 ml. Discard unused solution after 3 days at room temperature (21°C; 70°F) or 7 days under refrigeration (4°C; 40°F).

Direct IV – Reconstitute with Sterile Water for Injection or Sodium Chloride Injection. Administer slowly over approximately 10 minutes to avoid vein irritation.

Continuous IV – Prior to diluting with IV solution, reconstitute as directed.

IV solutions: Use only the solutions listed below for IV infusions. At concentrations from 0.5 to 40 mg/ml, these dilutions are stable at least 6 hours at room temperature: 5% Dextrose in Normal Saline; 10% D-Fructose in Water or Normal Saline; Lactated Potassic Saline Injections; 10% Invert Sugar in Normal Saline; 10% Invert Sugar plus 0.3% Potassium Chloride in Water; *Travert* 10% Electrolyte #1, #2 or #3.

	Product	Form	Description	Cost Index*
Rx	**Oxacillin Sodium** (Various, eg, Dixon-Shane, Geneva Marsam, Major, Rugby, Schein)	**Capsules:** 250 mg	In 100s.	7.4+
Rx	**Bactocill** (SK-Beecham)		Lactose. (BMP 143). In 100s.	8.9
Rx	**Prostaphlin** (Apothecon)		In 48s, 100s and UD 100s.	25
Rx	**Oxacillin Sodium** (Various, eg, Geneva Marsam, Major, Rugby, Schein)	**Capsules:** 500 mg	In 100s.	6.9+
Rx	**Bactocill** (SK-Beecham)		Lactose. (BMP 144). In 100s.	8.4
Rx	**Prostaphlin** (Apothecon)		In 48s, 100s and UD 100s.	14
Rx	**Prostaphlin** (Apothecon)	**Powder for Oral Solution:** 250 mg/5 ml when reconstituted	Saccharin, sucrose. In 100 ml.	16

* Cost Index based on cost per 500 mg.

(Continued on following page)

Complete prescribing information for these products begins on page 1686

Penicillinase-Resistant Penicillins (Cont.)

OXACILLIN SODIUM (Cont.)				C.I.*
Rx	**Oxacillin Sodium**[1] (Apothecon)	**Powder for Injection:** 250 mg	In vials.	NA
Rx	**Bactocill**[2] (SK-Beecham)		In vials.	80
Rx	**Oxacillin Sodium**[1] (Apothecon)	**Powder for Injection:** 500 mg	In vials.	NA
Rx	**Bactocill**[2] (SK-Beecham)		In vials.	21
Rx	**Prostaphlin** (Apothecon)		In vials.	63
Rx	**Oxacillin Sodium**[1] (Apothecon)	**Powder for Injection:** 1 g	In vials and piggyback vials.	NA
Rx	**Bactocill**[2] (SK-Beecham)		In vials, piggyback and *Add-Vantage* vials.	16
Rx	**Prostaphlin** (Apothecon)		In vials and piggyback vials.	61
Rx	**Oxacillin Sodium**[1] (Apothecon)	**Powder for Injection:** 2 g	In vials and piggyback vials.	NA
Rx	**Bactocill**[2] (SK-Beecham)		In vials, piggyback and *Add-Vantage* vials.	13
Rx	**Prostaphlin** (Apothecon)		In vials and piggyback vials.	59
Rx	**Oxacillin Sodium**[1] (Apothecon)	**Powder for Injection:** 4 g	In vials.	NA
Rx	**Bactocill**[2] (SK-Beecham)		In bulk vials.	12
Rx	**Prostaphlin** (Apothecon)		In vials.	56
Rx	**Oxacillin Sodium**[1] (Apothecon)	**Powder for Injection:** 10 g	In bulk vials.	NA
Rx	**Bactocill**[2] (SK-Beecham)		In bulk vials.	12
Rx	**Prostaphlin** (Apothecon)		In bulk vials.	59

* Cost Index based on cost per 500 mg.
[1] Contains 2.5 mEq sodium/g.
[2] Contains 3.1 mEq sodium/g.

DICLOXACILLIN SODIUM

Indications:

Treatment of infections due to penicillinase-producing staphylococci. May be used to initiate therapy when a staphylococcal infection is suspected. (See Indications in the group monograph concerning use of penicillinase-resistant penicillins.)

Administration and Dosage:

For mild to moderate upper respiratory and localized skin and soft tissue infections:

Adults and children (> 40 kg) – 125 mg every 6 hours.

Children (< 40 kg) – 12.5 mg/kg/day in equal doses every 6 hours.

For more severe infections, such as lower respiratory tract or disseminated infections:

Adults and children (> 40 kg) – 250 mg every 6 hours.

Children (< 40 kg) – 25 mg/kg/day in equally divided doses every 6 hours.

Another suggested dosage for children is 12 to 25 mg/kg/day divided every 6 hours. Use in the newborn is not recommended.

Storage/Stability: When the reconstituted oral solution is stored in polypropylene oral syringes for unit dose purposes, it is stable for 7 days (ambient conditions), 10 days (refrigerated) and 21 days (frozen). The manufacturer states a 14 day stability when reconstituted and refrigerated in its original container.

(Products listed on following page)

Complete prescribing information for these products begins on page 1686

Penicillinase-Resistant Penicillins (Cont.)

DICLOXACILLIN SODIUM (Cont.)				C.I.*
Rx	**Dynapen** (Apothecon)	**Capsules:** 125 mg	Lactose. In 24s and 100s.	28
Rx	**Dicloxacillin Sodium** (Various, eg, Apothecon, Dixon-Shane, Geneva Marsam, Lederle, Goldline, Major, Moore, Rugby, URL, Warner Chilcott)	**Capsules:** 250 mg	In 100s.	7.8+
Rx	**Dycill** (SK-Beecham)		Lactose. In 100s.	13
Rx	**Dynapen** (Apothecon)		Lactose. In 24s, 100s and UD 100s.	25
Rx	**Pathocil** (Wyeth-Ayerst)		Lactose. Purple and white. (Wyeth 360). In 100s.	13
Rx	**Dicloxacillin Sodium** (Various, eg, Apothecon, Dixon-Shane, Geneva Marsam, Goldline, Lederle, Major, Moore, Rugby, URL, Warner Chilcott)	**Capsules:** 500 mg	In 40s and 100s.	6.9+
Rx	**Dycill** (SK-Beecham)		In 100s.	11
Rx	**Dynapen** (Apothecon)		Lactose. In 50s.	23
Rx	**Pathocil** (Wyeth-Ayerst)		Lactose. Purple and white. (Wyeth 593). In 50s.	12
Rx	**Dynapen** (Apothecon)	**Powder for Oral Suspension:** 62.5 mg/5 ml reconstituted[1]	In 80, 100 and 200 ml.	46
Rx	**Pathocil** (Wyeth-Ayerst)		In 100 ml.	29

CLOXACILLIN SODIUM

Indications:

Treatment of infections due to penicillinase-producing staphylococci. May be used to initiate therapy when a staphylococcal infection is suspected. (See Indications in the group monograph concerning use of penicillinase-resistant penicillins.)

Administration and Dosage:

Mild to moderate upper respiratory and localized skin and soft tissue infections:

Adults and children (> 20 kg) – 250 mg every 6 hours.

Children (< 20 kg) – 50 mg/kg/day in equally divided doses every 6 hours.

Severe infections (lower respiratory tract or disseminated infections):

Adults and children (> 20 kg) – ≥ 500 mg every 6 hours.

Children (< 20 kg) – ≥ 100 mg/kg/day in equal doses every 6 hours.

Another suggested dosage for infants and children is 50 to 100 mg/kg/day, up to a maximum of 4 g/day, divided every 6 hours.

				C.I.*
Rx	**Cloxacillin Sodium** (Various, eg, Biocraft, Dixon-Shane, Geneva Marsam, Major, Rugby, Schein, Warner Chilcott)	**Capsules:** 250 mg	In 100s.	6.5+
Rx	**Cloxapen** (SK-Beecham)		In 100s.	11
Rx	**Tegopen** (Apothecon)		In 100s.	20
Rx	**Cloxacillin Sodium** (Various, eg, Biocraft, Dixon-Shane, Geneva Marsam, Major, Rugby, Schein, Warner Chilcott)	**Capsules:** 500 mg	In 100s.	6.1+
Rx	**Cloxapen** (SK-Beecham)		In 100s.	11
Rx	**Tegopen** (Apothecon)		In 100s.	20
Rx	**Cloxacillin Sodium** (Various, eg, Biocraft, Major, Rugby, Warner Chilcott)	**Powder for Oral Solution:** 125 mg per 5 ml when reconstituted	In 100 and 200 ml.	8.6+
Rx	**Tegopen** (Apothecon)		In 100 and 200 ml.[1]	29

* Cost Index based on cost per 500 mg. [1] With saccharin and sucrose.

Complete prescribing information for these products begins on page 1686

Aminopenicillins

AMPICILLIN

Indications:

Treatment of infections caused by susceptible strains of *Shigella, Salmonella* (including *S typhosa*), *Escherichia coli, Hemophilus influenzae, Proteus mirabilis, Neisseria gonorrhoeae* and enterococci. It is also effective in the treatment of meningitis due to *N meningitidis* and in infections caused by susceptible gram-positive organisms: Penicillin G-sensitive staphylococci, streptococci and pneumococci.

Ampicillin Uses and Dosages	
Organisms/Infections	Dosage
Labeled uses: *Respiratory tract and soft tissue infections:*	*Parenteral:* Patients ≥ 40 kg – 250 to 500 mg every 6 hours; < 40 kg – 25 to 50 mg/kg/day in divided doses at 6 to 8 hour intervals. *Oral:* Patients ≥ 20 kg – 250 mg every 6 hours; < 20 kg – 50 mg/kg/day in divided doses at 6 to 8 hour intervals.
Bacterial meningitis: H influenzae, S pneumoniae or *N meningitidis*	8 to 14 g/day (100 to 200 mg/kg/day for children) in divided doses every 3 to 4 hours. Initial treatment is usually by IV drip, followed by frequent (every 3 to 4 hour) IM injections.
Septicemia:	*Parenteral:* 150 to 200 mg/kg/day. Administer IV at least 3 days, then continue IM every 3 to 4 hours.
Gonococcal infections:[1] Disseminated gonococcal infection (hospitalization recommended)	When the infecting organism is proven to be penicillin-sensitive, parenteral treatment may be switched to ampicillin 1 g every 6 hours (or equivalent).
Rape victims (prophylaxis of infection): Alternative regimen for pregnant women or when tetracycline is contraindicated.	3.5 g orally with 1 g probenecid.
Prevention of bacterial endocarditis:[2] For dental, oral or upper respiratory tract procedures in patients at high risk: Alternate regimen.	1 to 2 g (50 mg/kg for children) plus gentamicin 1.5 mg/kg (2 mg/kg for children) not to exceed 80 mg, both IM or IV one-half hour prior to procedure, followed by 1.5 g amoxicillin (25 mg/kg for children) 6 hours after initial dose or repeat parenteral dose 8 hours after initial dose.
For GU or GI procedures: Standard regimen.	2 g (50 mg/kg for children) IM or IV plus gentamicin 1.5 mg/kg (not to exceed 80 mg) IM or IV (2 mg/kg for children) one-half hour prior to procedure, followed by 1.5 g amoxicillin (25 mg/kg for children) 6 hours after initial dose; or repeat parenteral dose 8 hours after initial dose.
Unlabeled use: Prophylaxis in cesarean section in certain high risk patients	Single IV dose, administered immediately after cord clamping.

[1] CDC 1989 Sexually Transmitted Diseases Treatment Guidelines. *Morbidity and Mortality Weekly Report* 1989 Sept. 1;38(No.S-8):1-43

[2] American Heart Association Statement. *JAMA* 1990;264:2919-2922

Administration and Dosage:

Reserve parenteral form (IM or IV) for moderately severe and severe infections and for patients unable to take oral medication. Change to oral therapy as soon as appropriate.

Renal impairment: Increase dosing interval to 12 hours in severe renal impairment (creatinine clearance ≤ 10 ml/min).

In the treatment of chronic urinary tract and intestinal infections, frequent bacteriologic and clinical appraisal is necessary. Higher doses should be used for persistent or severe infections. In persistent infections, therapy may be required for several weeks. It may be necessary to continue clinical or bacteriologic follow-up for several months after cessation of therapy.

In the treatment of complications of gonorrheal urethritis, such as prostatitis and epididymitis, prolonged and intensive therapy is recommended. Cases of gonorrhea with a suspected primary lesion of syphilis should have dark-field examinations before receiving treatment. In all other cases where concomitant syphilis is suspected, perform monthly serologic tests for a minimum of 4 months.

(Administration and Dosage continued on following page)

Aminopenicillins (Cont.)

AMPICILLIN (Cont.)

Administration and Dosage (Cont.):

Adults: 1 to 12 g daily in divided doses every 4 to 6 hours.

Children: 50 to 200 mg/kg/day in divided doses every 4 to 6 hours.

Infants (over 7 days and > 2000 g) – 100 mg/kg/day in divided doses every 6 hours (meningitis 200 mg/kg/day).

Over 7 days and < 2000 g – 75 mg/kg/day in divided doses every 8 hours (meningitis 150 mg/kg/day).

Under 7 days and > 2000 g – 75 mg/kg/day in divided doses every 8 hours (meningitis 150 mg/kg/day).

Under 7 days and < 2000 g – 50 mg/kg/day in divided doses every 12 hours (meningitis 100 mg/kg/day).

Preparation of solutions: Use only freshly prepared solutions. Administer IM and IV injections within 1 hour after preparation since the potency may decrease significantly after this period. Reconstitute with Sterile or Bacteriostatic Water for Injection (piggyback vials may be reconstituted with Sodium Chloride Injection).

Direct IV administration – Administer slowly over at least 10 to 15 minutes. Caution: More rapid administration may result in convulsive seizures.

IV drip (standard vials) – Dilute as above for direct IV use prior to further dilution with compatible IV solutions.

IV drip (piggyback vials) – After reconstitution, administer alone or further dilute with suitable IV solutions. To assure compatibility and stability of ampicillin solutions for IV use, use only the solutions specified below:

IV Solutions Compatible with Ampicillin

IV solution	Concentrations up to (mg/ml)	Stability (hours)
0.9% Sodium Chloride	30	8
5% Dextrose in Water	2	4
5% Dextrose in Water	10-20	2
5% Dextrose in 0.45% Sodium Chloride Solution	2	4
10% Invert Sugar in Water	2	4
M/6 Sodium Lactate Solution	30	8
Lactated Ringer's Solution	30	8
Sterile Water for Injection	30	8

Stability studies on ampicillin sodium in various IV solutions indicate that the drug will lose < 10% activity at room temperature (21°C; 70°F) for the time periods and concentrations stated.

Oral: Reconstituted oral solution is stable for 7 days at room temperature (not exceeding 25°C; 77°F).

AMPICILLIN WITH PROBENECID

Indications: Treatment of uncomplicated infections (urethral, endocervical or rectal) caused by *Neisseria gonorrhoeae* in adults.

Administration and Dosage:

Administer 3.5 g ampicillin and 1 g probenecid as a single dose.

	Product	Form	Packaging	C.I.*
Rx	**Polycillin-PRB** (Apothecon)	**Powder For Oral Suspension:** 3.5 g ampicillin (as trihydrate) & 1 g probenecid per bottle	In single-dose bottles.	26
Rx	**Probampacin** (Various, eg, Goldline, Schein)		In single-dose bottles.	64+

* Cost Index based on cost per 500 mg ampicillin.

Aminopenicillins (Cont.)

AMPICILLIN SODIUM, PARENTERAL (Contains 3 mEq sodium/g.)
See Administration and Dosage information beginning on page 1712

	Product	Form	Packaging	C.I.*
Rx	**Ampicillin Sodium** (Various, eg, Apothecon, Elkins-Sinn, Geneva Marsam)	**Powder for Injection:** 125 mg	In vials.	NA
Rx	**Omnipen-N** (Wyeth-Ayerst)		In vials and *ADD-Vantage* vials.	95
Rx	**Polycillin-N** (Apothecon)		In vials.	109
Rx	**Ampicillin Sodium** (Various, eg, Apothecon, Elkins-Sinn, Geneva Marsam)	**Powder for Injection:** 250 mg	In vials.	NA
Rx	**Omnipen-N** (Wyeth-Ayerst)		In vials and *ADD-Vantage* vials.	56
Rx	**Polycillin-N** (Apothecon)		In vials.	64
Rx	**Totacillin-N** (SK-Beecham)		In vials.	21
Rx	**Ampicillin Sodium** (Various, eg, Apothecon, Elkins-Sinn, Geneva Marsam, Lilly)	**Powder for Injection:** 500 mg	In vials and piggyback vials.	26+
Rx	**Omnipen-N** (Wyeth-Ayerst)		In vials, piggyback and *ADD-Vantage* vials.	41
Rx	**Polycillin-N** (Apothecon)		In vials	42
Rx	**Totacillin-N** (SK-Beecham)		In vials and piggyback vials.	14
Rx	**Ampicillin Sodium** (Various, eg, Apothecon, Elkins-Sinn, Geneva Marsam)	**Powder for Injection:** 1 g	In vials and piggyback vials.	17+
Rx	**Omnipen-N** (Wyeth-Ayerst)		In vials, piggyback and *ADD-Vantage* vials.	23
Rx	**Polycillin-N** (Apothecon)		In vials and piggyback vials.	27
Rx	**Totacillin-N** (SK-Beecham)		In vials, piggyback and *ADD-Vantage* vials.	9.8
Rx	**Ampicillin Sodium** (Various, eg, Apothecon, Elkins-Sinn, Geneva Marsam)	**Powder for Injection:** 2 g	In vials and piggyback vials.	15+
Rx	**Omnipen-N** (Wyeth-Ayerst)		In vials, piggyback and *ADD-Vantage* vials.	22
Rx	**Polycillin-N** (Apothecon)		In vials and piggyback vials.	24
Rx	**Totacillin-N** (SK-Beecham)		In vials, piggyback and *ADD-Vantage* vials.	7.9
Rx	**Ampicillin Sodium** (Various, eg, Apothecon, Elkins-Sinn, Geneva Marsam)	**Powder for Injection:** 10 g bulk	In vials.	NA
Rx	**Omnipen-N** (Wyeth-Ayerst)		In vials.	23
Rx	**Polycillin-N** (Apothecon)		In vials.	26
Rx	**Totacillin-N** (SK-Beecham)		In vials.	8.5

* Cost Index based on cost per 500 mg.

(Continued on following page)

Aminopenicillins (Cont.)

AMPICILLIN, ORAL

See Administration and Dosage information beginning on page 1712

	Product	Form	Description	C.I.*
Rx	**Ampicillin** (Various, eg, Dixon-Shane, Geneva Marsam, Major, Mylan, Parke-Davis, Parmed, Rugby, Schein, URL, Warner Chilcott)	**Capsules:** 250 mg (as trihydrate)	In 28s, 40s, 100s, 500s, 1000s and UD 100s.	11+
Rx	**Polycillin** (Apothecon)		In 100s, 500s, 1000s and UD 100s.	4.1
Rx	**Principen** (Apothecon)		(Squibb 971). Red/gray. In 100s, 500s and UD 100s.	2.4
Rx	**Totacillin** (SK-Beecham)		In 500s.	3
Rx	**Omnipen** (Wyeth-Ayerst)	**Capsules:** 250 mg (anhydrous)	Lactose. (Wyeth 53). Violet and pink. In 500s.	3
Rx	**Ampicillin** (Various, eg, Biocraft, Dixon-Shane, Geneva Marsam, Mylan, Parmed, Rugby, Schein, URL)	**Capsules:** 500 mg (as trihydrate)	In 21s, 28s, 40s, 100s, 500s, 1000s and UD 100s.	1.5+
Rx	**D-Amp** (Dunhall)		In 100s.	NA
Rx	**Polycillin** (Apothecon)		In 100s, 500s and UD 100s.	3.6
Rx	**Principen** (Apothecon)		(Squibb 974). Red/gray. In 100s, 500s and UD 100s.	1.8
Rx	**Totacillin** (SK-Beecham)		In 500s.	15
Rx	**Omnipen** (Wyeth-Ayerst)	**Capsules:** 500 mg (anhydrous)	Lactose. (Wyeth 309). Violet and pink. In 100s and 500s.	33
Rx	**Polycillin Pediatric Drops** (Apothecon)	**Powder for Oral Suspension:** 100 mg per ml (as trihydrate) when reconstituted	Sucrose. In 20 ml.	14
Rx	**Ampicillin** (Various, eg, Biocraft, Dixon-Shane, Mylan, Schein, URL, Warner-C)	**Powder for Oral Suspension:** 125 mg per 5 ml (as trihydrate) when reconstituted	In 80, 100, 150 and 200 ml.	5.1+
Rx	**Omnipen** (Wyeth-Ayerst)		Sucrose. In 100, 150 and 200 ml.	5.4
Rx	**Polycillin** (Apothecon)		Sucrose. In 100, 150 and 200 ml and UD 5 ml (25s).	7.9
Rx	**Principen** (Apothecon)		Sucrose. In 100, 150 and 200 ml and UD 5 ml.	4.6
Rx	**Totacillin** (SK-Beecham)		Sucrose. In 100 and 200 ml.	6
Rx	**Ampicillin** (Various, eg, Biocraft, Dixon-Shane, Major, Mylan, Rugby, Schein, URL, Warner Chilcott)	**Powder for Oral Suspension:** 250 mg per 5 ml (as trihydrate) when reconstituted	Sucrose. In 80, 100, 150 and 200 ml.	3.5+
Rx	**Omnipen** (Wyeth-Ayerst)		Sucrose. In 100, 150 and 200 ml.	4
Rx	**Polycillin** (Apothecon)		Sucrose. In 100, 150 and 200 ml and UD 5 ml (25s).	5.4
Rx	**Principen** (Apothecon)		Sucrose. In 100, 150 and 200 ml and UD 5 ml.	3.5
Rx	**Totacillin** (SK-Beecham)		Sucrose. In 100 and 200 ml.	4.4
Rx	**Polycillin** (Apothecon)	**Powder for Oral Suspension:** 500 mg per 5 ml (as trihydrate) when reconstituted	Sucrose. In 100 ml and UD 5 ml (25s).	4.6

* Cost Index based on cost per 500 mg ampicillin.

Complete prescribing information for these products begins on page 1686

AMPICILLIN SODIUM AND SULBACTAM SODIUM

Actions:

Pharmacokinetics: Peak serum concentrations of ampicillin and sulbactam are attained immediately following a 15 minute IV infusion. Ampicillin serum levels are similar to those produced by the administration of equivalent amounts of ampicillin alone. Peak ampicillin serum levels ranging from 109 to 150 mcg/ml are attained after administration of 2000 mg ampicillin plus 1000 mg sulbactam and 40 to 71 mcg/ml after administration of 1000 mg ampicillin plus 500 mg sulbactam. The corresponding mean peak serum levels for sulbactam range from 48 to 88 mcg/ml and 21 to 40 mcg/ml, respectively. After an IM injection of 1000 mg ampicillin plus 500 mg sulbactam, peak ampicillin serum levels ranging from 8 to 37 mcg/ml and peak sulbactam serum levels ranging from 6 to 24 mcg/ml are attained. The mean serum half-life of both drugs is ≈ 1 hour in healthy volunteers.

Approximately 75% to 85% of both ampicillin and sulbactam is excreted unchanged in the urine during the first 8 hours after administration to individuals with normal renal function. Higher and more prolonged serum levels can be achieved with the coadministration of probenecid. Ampicillin is ≈ 28% reversibly bound to human serum protein and sulbactam is ≈ 38% reversibly bound.

Microbiology: A wide range of β-lactamases found in microorganisms resistant to penicillins and cephalosporins are irreversibly inhibited by sulbactam. Although sulbactam alone possesses little useful antibacterial activity except against the Neisseriaceae, sulbactam restores ampicillin activity against β-lactamase producing strains. Sulbactam has good inhibitory activity against the clinically important plasmid mediated β-lactamases most frequently responsible for transferred drug resistance. Sulbactam has no effect on the activity of ampicillin against ampicillin-susceptible strains.

The presence of sulbactam in the formulation effectively extends the antibiotic spectrum of ampicillin to include many bacteria normally resistant to it and to other β-lactam antibiotics. Thus, this combination possesses the properties of a broad-spectrum antibiotic and a β-lactamase inhibitor.

Indications:

For the treatment of infections due to susceptible strains of the microorganisms in the conditions listed below.

Skin and skin structure infections caused by β-lactamase producing strains of *Staphylococcus aureus, Escherichia coli,* Klebsiella* sp* (including *K pneumoniae**), *Proteus mirabilis,* Bacteroides fragilis,* Enterobacter* sp* and *Acinetobacter calcoaceticus.**

Intra-abdominal infections caused by β-lactamase producing strains of *E coli, Klebsiella* sp (including *K pneumoniae**), *Bacteroides* (including *B fragilis*) and *Enterobacter* sp.*

Gynecological infections caused by β-lactamase producing strains of *E coli** and *Bacteroides* sp* (including *B fragilis**).

While this combination is indicated only for the conditions listed above, infections caused by ampicillin-susceptible organisms are also amenable to treatment due to the ampicillin content. Therefore, mixed infections caused by ampicillin-susceptible organisms and β-lactamase producing organisms susceptible to this combination should not require the addition of another antibiotic.

Adverse Reactions:

Local: Pain at IM injection site (16%); pain at IV injection site, thrombophlebitis (3%).

Systemic: Most frequent – Diarrhea (3%); rash (< 2%). In < 1% of patients: Itching; nausea; vomiting; candidiasis; fatigue; malaise; headache; chest pain; flatulence; abdominal distension; glossitis; urine retention; dysuria; edema; facial swelling; erythema; chills; tightness in throat; substernal pain; epistaxis; mucosal bleeding.

Laboratory changes: Increased AST, ALT, alkaline phosphatase and LDH. Decreased hemoglobin, hematocrit, RBC, WBC, neutrophils, lymphocytes, platelets and increased lymphocytes, monocytes, basophils, eosinophils and platelets; decreased serum albumin and total proteins; increased BUN and creatinine; presence of RBCs and hyaline casts in urine.

Overdosage:

Neurological adverse reactions, including convulsions, may occur with the attainment of high CSF levels of β-lactams. Ampicillin may be removed from circulation by hemodialysis. The molecular weight, degree of protein binding and pharmacokinetic profile of sulbactam suggest that this compound may also be removed by hemodialysis.

*Efficacy for this organism in this organ system was studied in fewer than 10 infections.

(Continued on following page)

Aminopenicillins (Cont.)

AMPICILLIN SODIUM AND SULBACTAM SODIUM (Cont.)

Administration and Dosage:

May be administered by either the IV or the IM routes. The recommended adult dosage is 1.5 g (1 g ampicillin plus 0.5 g sulbactam) to 3 g (2 g ampicillin plus 1 g sulbactam) every 6 hours. Do not exceed 4 g/day sulbactam.

Renal function impairment: The elimination kinetics of ampicillin and sulbactam are similarly affected; hence, the ratio of one to the other will remain constant whatever the renal function. In patients with renal impairment, give as follows:

Ampicillin/Sulbactam Dosage Guide For Patients With Renal Impairment		
Ccr (ml/min/1.73m^2)	Half-life (hours)	Recommended dosage
≥ 30	1	1.5-3 g q 6-8 h
15-29	5	1.5-3 g q 12 h
5-14	9	1.5-3 g q 24 h

Children: Safety and efficacy in children < 12 years old have not been established.

Dissolution: Reconstitute powder for IV and IM use with any of the compatible diluents described below. Allow solutions to stand after dissolution so that any foaming will dissipate. This permits visual inspection for complete solubilization.

Preparation for IV use: 1.5 and 3 g bottles – Reconstitute powder in piggyback units to the desired concentrations using any of the following diluents. Discard unused solutions after indicated time periods:

Preparation of Ampicillin/Sulbactam for IV Use		
Diluent	Maximum concentration (mg/ml)	Stability
Sterile Water for Injection	45 (30/15) 45 (30/15) 30 (20/10)	8 hrs @ 25°C 48 hrs @ 4°C 72 hrs @ 4°C
0.9% Sodium Chloride Injection	45 (30/15) 45 (30/15) 30 (20/10)	8 hrs @ 25°C 48 hrs @ 4°C 72 hrs @ 4°C
5% Dextrose Injection	30 (20/10) 30 (20/10) 3 (2/1)	2 hrs @ 25°C 4 hrs @ 4°C 4 hrs @ 25°C
Lactated Ringer's Injection	45 (30/15) 45 (30/15)	8 hrs @ 25°C 24 hrs @ 4°C
M/6 Sodium Lactate Injection	45 (30/15) 45 (30/15)	8 hrs @ 25°C 8 hrs @ 4°C
5% Dextrose in 0.45% Saline	3 (2/1) 15 (10/5)	4 hrs @ 25°C 4 hrs @ 4°C
10% Invert Sugar	3 (2/1) 30 (20/10)	4 hrs @ 25°C 3 hrs @ 4°C

If piggyback bottles are unavailable, use standard vials of sterile powder. Initially, reconstitute with Sterile Water for Injection to yield solutions of 375 mg/ml (250 mg ampicillin/125 mg sulbactam). Then immediately dilute an appropriate volume with a suitable diluent to yield solutions of 3 to 45 mg/ml (2 to 30 mg ampicillin/1 to 15 mg sulbactam per ml). Give by slow injection over at least 10 to 15 minutes or infuse in greater dilutions with 50 to 100 ml of a compatible diluent over 15 to 30 minutes.

Preparation for IM injection: Reconstitute with Sterile Water for Injection or 0.5% or 2% Lidocaine HCl Injection. Consult the following table for recommended volumes needed to obtain 375 mg/ml solutions (250 mg ampicillin/125 mg sulbactam/ml). *Use only freshly prepared solutions; give within 1 hour after preparation.*

Preparation of Ampicillin/Sulbactam for IM Use		
Vial size	Diluent to be added	Withdrawal volume
1.5 g	3.2 ml	4 ml
3 g	6.4 ml	8 ml

Stability and storage: Store at ≤ 30°C (86°F) prior to reconstitution. When concomitant aminoglycosides are indicated, reconstitute and administer this product and aminoglycosides separately; aminopenicillins inactivate aminoglycosides in vitro.

				C.I.*
Rx	**Unasyn** (Roerig)	**Powder for Injection:** 1.5 g (1 g ampicillin sodium/ 0.5 g sulbactam sodium)	In vials, bottles and *Add-Vantage* vials.	61
		3 g (2 g ampicillin sodium/1 g sulbactam sodium)	In vials and bottles.	58

* Cost Index based on cost per 1.5 g.

Complete prescribing information for these products begins on page 1686

Aminopenicillins (Cont.)

BACAMPICILLIN HCl

Bacampicillin is hydrolyzed to ampicillin during absorption from the GI tract. Because bacampicillin is more completely absorbed than ampicillin, it is administered in lower total daily dosages, and sustains effective serum levels when given every 12 hours.

Indications:

Upper and lower respiratory tract infections (including acute exacerbations of chronic bronchitis) due to streptococci (β-hemolytic streptococci, *S pyogenes*), pneumococci (*S pneumoniae*), nonpenicillinase-producing staphylococci and *Hemophilus influenzae*.

Urinary tract infections due to *Escherichia coli, Proteus mirabilis* and *S faecalis* (enterococci).

Skin and skin structure infections due to streptococci and susceptible staphylococci.

Gonorrhea (acute uncomplicated urogenital infections) due to *Neisseria gonorrhoeae*.

Administration and Dosage:

Tablets may be given without regard to meals; administer suspension to fasting patients.

Upper respiratory tract infections (including otitis media) due to streptococci, pneumococci, nonpenicillinase-producing staphylococci and *H influenzae; urinary tract* infections due to *E coli, P mirabilis* and *S faecalis; skin and skin structure* infections due to streptococci and susceptible staphylococci:

Adults (≥ 25 kg) – 400 mg every 12 hours.
Children – 25 mg/kg/day in equally divided doses at 12 hour intervals.

Severe infections or those caused by less susceptible organisms:

Adults (≥ 25 kg) – 800 mg every 12 hours.
Children – 50 mg/kg/day in equally divided doses at 12 hour intervals.

Lower respiratory tract infections due to streptococci, pneumococci, nonpenicillinase-producing staphylococci and *H influenzae:*

Adults (≥ 25 kg) – 800 mg every 12 hours.
Children – 50 mg/kg/day in equally divided doses at 12 hour intervals.

Gonorrhea: The usual adult dosage (males and females) is 1.6 g bacampicillin plus 1 g probenecid as a single oral dose. No pediatric dosage has been established.

Larger doses may be needed for persistent or severe infections.

				C.I.*
Rx	**Spectrobid** (Roerig)	**Tablets:** 400 mg (chemically equivalent to 280 mg ampicillin)	Lactose. White. Film coated. Oblong. In 100s.	13
		Powder for Oral Suspension: 125 mg per 5 ml reconstituted suspension (chemically equivalent to 87.5 mg ampicillin)	Saccharin, sugar. In 70 ml.	2.2

* Cost Index based on cost per 200 mg ampicillin equivalent.

Complete prescribing information for these products begins on page 1686

Aminopenicillins (Cont.)

AMOXICILLIN

The spectrum of amoxicillin is essentially identical to ampicillin, except that ampicillin is more effective against *Shigella* sp. Amoxicillin has the advantage of more complete absorption than ampicillin, a 3 times a day regimen for most infections and less diarrhea than ampicillin.

Indications:

Infections due to susceptible strains of the following organisms: Gram-negative – *Hemophilus influenzae, E coli, P mirabilis* and *N gonorrhoeae*. Gram-positive – Streptococci (including *S faecalis*), *S pneumoniae* and nonpenicillinase-producing staphylococci.

Administration and Dosage:

Larger doses may be required for persistent or severe infections.

The children's dose is intended for individuals whose weight will not cause the calculated dosage to be greater than that recommended for adults; the children's dose should not exceed the maximum adult dose.

Amoxicillin Uses and Dosages

Organisms/Infections	Dosage
Infections of the ear, nose and throat due to streptococci, pneumococci, nonpenicillinase-producing staphylococci and *H influenzae* *Infections of the GU tract* due to *E coli, P mirabilis* and *S faecalis* *Infections of the skin and soft tissues* due to streptococci, susceptible staphylococci and *E coli*	*Adults and children* (> *20 kg)* – 250 to 500 mg every 8 hours. *Children* – 20 to 40 mg/kg/day in divided doses every 8 hours.
Infections of the lower respiratory tract due to streptococci, pneumococci, nonpenicillinase-producing staphylococci and *H influenzae*	*Adults and children (*> *20 kg)* – 500 mg q 8 h. *Children* – 40 mg/kg/day in divided doses q 8 h.
Gonococcal infections: Uncomplicated urethral, endocervical or rectal infection (alternative regimen)[1]	*Adults* – If infection was acquired from a source proven not to have penicillin-resistant gonorrhea, a penicillin such as amoxicillin 3 g plus 1 g probenecid *followed by* doxycycline may be used.
Prevention of bacterial endocarditis:[2]	
For dental, oral or upper respiratory tract procedures in patients at risk	
Standard regimen:	3 g 1 hour before procedure, then 1.5 g 6 hours after initial dose
Alternate regimen:	1 to 2 g (50 mg/kg for children) ampicillin plus 1.5 mg/kg gentamicin (2 mg/kg for children) not to exceed 80 mg, both IM or IV one-half hour prior to procedure, followed by 1.5 g amoxicillin (25 mg/kg for children) 6 hours after initial dose or, repeat parenteral dose 8 hours after initial dose.
For GU or GI procedures	
Standard regimen:	2 g ampicillin (50 mg/kg for children) plus 1.5 mg/kg gentamicin (2 mg/kg for children) not to exceed 80 mg, both IM or IV one-half hour prior to procedure, followed by 1.5 g amoxicillin (25 mg/kg for children)
Alternate low-risk patient regimen:	3 g 1 hour before procedure, then 1.5 g 6 hours after initial dose
Unlabeled use:	
Chlamydia trachomatis in pregnancy	As an alternative to erythromycin; 500 mg 3 times a day for 7 days.

[1] CDC 1989 Sexually Transmitted Diseases Treatment Guidelines. *Morbidity and Mortality Weekly Report* 1989 Sept 1;38 (No S-8):1-43.

[2] American Heart Association Statement. *JAMA* 1990;264:2919-2922.

Storage/stability: Reconstituted oral suspension stable for 7 days at room temperature (not exceeding 25°C; 77°F).

(Continued on following page)

Aminopenicillins (Cont.)

AMOXICILLIN (Cont.)				C.I.*
Rx	**Amoxil** (SK Beecham)	**Tablets, chewable:** 125 mg (as trihydrate)	Saccharin, sucrose. In 60s.	35
		250 mg (as trihydrate)	Saccharin, sucrose. In 100s.	30
Rx	**Amoxicillin** (Various, eg, Geneva Marsam, Goldline, Lemmon, Major, Mylan, Parmed, Rugby, Schein, URL, Warner Chilcott)	**Capsules:** 250 mg (as trihydrate)	In 50s, 100s, 500s and UD 1000s.	13+
Rx	**Amoxil** (SK Beecham)		In 100s, 500s and UD 100s.	32
Rx	**Biomox** (Inter. Ethical Labs[1])		In 100s.	NA
Rx	**Polymox** (Apothecon)		In 100s, 500s and UD 100s.	49
Rx	**Trimox 250** (Apothecon)		In 100s, 500s and UD 100s.	35
Rx	**Wymox** (Wyeth-Ayerst)		(Wyeth 559). Gray and green. In 100s & 500s.	42
Rx	**Amoxicillin** (Various, eg, Dixon-Shane, Geneva Marsam, Goldline, Lemmon, Major, Mylan, Parmed, Rugby, URL, Warner-C)	**Capsules:** 500 mg (as trihydrate)	In 50s, 100s, 500s and UD 100s.	13+
Rx	**Amoxil** (SK Beecham)		In 100s, 500s and UD 100s.	30
Rx	**Biomox** (Inter. Ethical Labs[1])		In 100s.	NA
Rx	**Polymox** (Apothecon)		In 50s, 100s, 500s, UD 100s.	481
Rx	**Trimox 500** (Apothecon)		In 50s, 500s and UD 100s.	33
Rx	**Wymox** (Wyeth-Ayerst)		(Wyeth 560). Gray and green. In 50s & 500s.	40
Rx	**Amoxil Pediatric Drops** (SK Beecham)	**Powder for Oral Suspension:** 50 mg per ml (as trihydrate) when reconstituted	Sucrose. In 15 and 30 ml.	87
Rx	**Polymox Drops** (Apothecon)		Sucrose. In 15 ml.	177
Rx	**Amoxicillin** (Various, eg, Dixon-Shane, Geneva Marsam, Major, Mylan, Parmed, Rugby, URL, Warner Chilcott)	**Powder for Oral Suspension:** 125 mg per 5 ml (as trihydrate) when reconstituted	In 80, 100, 150 and 200 ml.	24+
Rx	**Amoxil** (SK Beecham)		Sucrose. In 80, 100 & 150 ml and UD 5 ml.	45
Rx	**Polymox** (Apothecon)		Sucrose. In 80, 100 & 150 ml and UD 5 ml.	105
Rx	**Trimox 125** (Apothecon)		Sucrose. In 80, 100, 150 ml and UD 5 ml.	50
Rx	**Wymox** (Wyeth-Ayerst)		Sucrose. In 100 and 150 ml.	61
Rx	**Amoxicillin** (Various, eg, Dixon-Shane, Geneva Marsam, Major, Mylan, Parmed, Rugby, Schein, URL, Warner Chilcott)	**Powder for Oral Suspension:** 250 mg per 5 ml (as trihydrate) when reconstituted	In 80, 100, 150 and 200 ml.	19+
Rx	**Amoxil** (SK Beecham)		Sucrose. In 80, 100 & 150 ml and UD 5 ml.	39
Rx	**Biomox** (Inter. Ethical Labs[1])		In 100 and 150 ml.	NA
Rx	**Polymox** (Apothecon)		Sucrose. In 80, 100 & 150 ml and UD 5 ml.	69
Rx	**Trimox 250** (Apothecon)		Sucrose. In 80, 100, 150 ml and UD 5 ml.	43
Rx	**Wymox** (Wyeth-Ayerst)		Sucrose. In 80, 100 & 150 ml.	52

* Cost Index based on cost per 375 mg.

[1] International Ethical Laboratories, Rio Piedras, Puerto Rico 00921 (809) 765-3510.

Complete prescribing information for these products begins on page 1686

AMOXICILLIN AND POTASSIUM CLAVULANATE

Actions:

Pharmacology: Amoxicillin has a spectrum of bacterial activity essentially identical to ampicillin, except that ampicillin is more effective against *Shigella* sp. Amoxicillin is more completely absorbed from the GI tract than ampicillin. Clavulanic acid is a β-lactam structurally related to the penicillins that inactivates β-lactamase enzymes commonly found in microorganisms resistant to penicillin. The combination of amoxicillin/clavulanic acid extends the antibiotic spectrum of amoxicillin to include bacteria normally resistant to amoxicillin and other β-lactam antibiotics (see Microbiology table in the group monograph).

Indications:

Lower respiratory infections caused by β-lactamase-producing strains of *Hemophilus influenzae.*

Otitis media and *sinusitis* caused by β-lactamase-producing strains of *H influenzae* and *Moraxella (Branhamella) catarrhalis.*

Skin and skin structure infections caused by β-lactamase-producing strains of *Staphylococcus aureus, Escherichia coli* and *Klebsiella* species.

Urinary tract infections caused by β-lactamase producing strains of *E coli, Klebsiella* sp and *Enterobacter* sp.

While amoxicillin/potassium clavulanate is indicated only for the conditions listed above, infections caused by ampicillin susceptible organisms are also amenable to this drug due to its amoxicillin content. Therefore, mixed infections caused by ampicillin susceptible organisms and β-lactamase-producing organisms susceptible to amoxicillin/potassium clavulanate should not require an additional antibiotic. Therapy may be instituted prior to obtaining the results from bacteriologic studies when there is reason to believe the infection may involve any of the β-lactamase-producing organisms listed above. Once the results are known, adjust therapy.

Administration and Dosage: May be administered without regard to meals.

Since both the '250' and '500' tablets contain the same amount of clavulanic acid (125 mg as potassium salt), two '250' tablets are not equivalent to one '500' tablet.

Usual dose: Children's dose is based on amoxicillin content.

Adults – One '250' tablet every 8 hours.

Children (< 40 kg) – 20 mg/kg/day, in divided doses every 8 hours.

Severe infections and respiratory tract infections:

Adults – One '500' tablet every 8 hours.

Children (< 40 kg) – 40 mg/kg/day, in divided doses every 8 hours.

Otitis media, sinusitis and lower respiratory infections:

Children (< 40 kg) – 40 mg/kg/day, in divided doses every 8 hours.

Chancroid (Hemophilus ducreyi infection)[1]: One '500' tablet 3 times daily for 7 days as an alternative to erythromycin or ceftriaxone (not evaluated in the U.S.).

Disseminated gonococcal infection[1]*:* Following appropriate parenteral therapy with ceftriaxone, ceftizoxime or cefotaxime, reliable patients with uncomplicated disease may be discharged from the hospital 24 to 48 hours after all symptoms resolve and may complete the therapy (for a total of 1 week of antibiotic therapy) with an oral regimen of one '500' tablet 3 times a day.

Storage: Refrigerate reconstituted suspension and discard after 10 days.

[1] CDC 1989 Sexually Transmitted Diseases Treatment Guidelines. *Morbidity and Mortality Weekly Report* 1989 Sept 1;38(No.S-8):1-43.

(Products listed on following page)

Complete prescribing information for these products begins on page 1686

Aminopenicillins (Cont.)

AMOXICILLIN AND POTASSIUM CLAVULANATE (Cont.)				C.I.*
Rx	**Augmentin** (SK-Beecham)	**'250' Tablets:** 250 mg amoxicillin (as trihydrate) and 125 mg clavulanic acid[1]	0.63 mEq potassium/tablet. (Augmentin 250/125). White. Oval. Film coated. In 30s & UD 100s.	32
		'500' Tablets: 500 mg amoxicillin (as trihydrate) and 125 mg clavulanic acid[1]	0.63 mEq potassium/tablet. (Augmentin 500/125). White. Oval. Film coated. In 30s & UD 100s.	26
		'125' Tablets, chewable: 125 mg amoxicillin (as trihydrate) and 31.25 mg clavulanic acid[1]	0.16 mEq potassium/tablet. Saccharin. (BMP 189). Yellow, mottled. In 30s.	33
		'250' Tablets, chewable: 250 mg amoxicillin (as trihydrate) and 62.5 mg clavulanic acid[1]	0.32 mEq potassium/tablet. Saccharin. (BMP 190). Yellow, mottled. In 30s.	32
		'125' Powder for Oral Suspension: 125 mg amoxicillin and 31.25 mg clavulanic acid[1] per 5 ml.	0.16 mEq potassium/5 ml. Saccharin. Banana flavor. In 75 and 150 ml.	34
		'250' Powder for Oral Suspension: 250 mg amoxicillin and 62.5 mg clavulanic acid[1] per 5 ml	0.32 mEq potassium/5 ml. Saccharin. Orange flavor. In 75 and 150 ml.	32

* Cost Index based on cost per 500 mg ampicillin equivalent.

[1] As the potassium salt.

Complete prescribing information for these products begins on page 1686

Extended Spectrum Penicillins (Cont.)

TICARCILLIN DISODIUM

Indications:

For the treatment of the following infections: Bacterial septicemia, skin and soft tissue infections, acute and chronic respiratory tract infections caused by susceptible strains of *Pseudomonas aeruginosa, Proteus* species (both indole-positive and indole-negative), and *Escherichia coli*. Although clinical improvement has been shown, bacteriological cures cannot be expected in patients with chronic respiratory disease or cystic fibrosis.

Genitourinary tract infections (complicated and uncomplicated) due to susceptible strains of *P aeruginosa, Proteus* species (both indole-positive and indole-negative), *E coli, Enterobacter* and *Streptococcus faecalis* (enterococcus).

Infections due to susceptible *anaerobic bacteria:* Bacterial septicemia; lower respiratory tract infections such as empyema, anaerobic pneumonitis and lung abscess; intra-abdominal infections such as peritonitis and intra-abdominal abscess (typically resulting from anaerobic organisms resident in the normal GI tract); infections of the female pelvis and genital tract such as endometritis, pelvic inflammatory disease, pelvic abscess and salpingitis; skin and soft tissue infections.

Although ticarcillin is primarily indicated in gram-negative infections, consider its in vitro activity against gram-positive organisms in infections caused by both gram-negative and gram-positive organisms.

Based on the in vitro synergism between ticarcillin and gentamicin or tobramycin against certain strains of *P aeruginosa,* combined therapy has been successful using full therapeutic dosages.

Dosage:

Use IV therapy in higher doses in serious urinary tract and systemic infections. Intramuscular injections should not exceed 2 g/injection.

Seriously ill patients should receive higher doses. Ticarcillin is useful in infections in which protective mechanisms are impaired, such as acute leukemia, and during therapy with immunosuppressive or oncolytic drugs.

Ticarcillin Uses and Dosages

Organisms/Infections	Dosage
Bacterial septicemia, respiratory tract infections, skin and soft tissue infections, intra-abdominal infections and infections of the female pelvis and genital tract	*Adults:* 200 to 300 mg/kg/day by IV infusion in divided doses every 3, 4 or 6 hours (3 g every 3, 4 or 6 hours), depending on weight of patient and severity of infection.
	Children (< 40 kg): 200 to 300 mg/kg/day by IV infusion in divided doses every 4 or 6 hours.[1]
Urinary tract infections: Complicated infections.	150 to 200 mg/kg/day IV infusion in divided doses every 4 or 6 hours. Usual dose for average adult (70 kg) is 3 g 4 times daily.
Uncomplicated infections.	*Adults:* 1 g IM or direct IV every 6 hours.
	Children (< 40 kg): 50 to 100 mg/kg/day IM or direct IV in divided doses every 6 or 8 hours.
Neonates: Severe infections (sepsis) due to susceptible strains of *Pseudomonas* species, *Proteus* species and *E coli.*	Give IM or by 10 to 20 minute IV infusions.
< 2 kg –	< *7 days* – 75 mg/kg/12 hr (150 mg/kg/day). > *7 days* – 75 mg/kg/8 hr (225 mg/kg/day).
> 2 kg –	< *7 days* – 75 mg/kg/8 hr (225 mg/kg/day). > *7 days* – 100 mg/kg/8 hr (300 mg/kg/day).
Dosage in renal insufficiency:[2]	Initial loading dose of 3 g IV followed by IV doses based on creatinine clearance and type of dialysis.
Creatinine clearance (ml/min) –	
> 60	3 g every 4 hours.
30 to 60	2 g every 4 hours.
10 to 30	2 g every 8 hours.
< 10	2 g every 12 hours or 1 g IM every 6 hours.
< 10 with hepatic dysfunction	2 g every 24 hours or 1 g IM every 12 hours.
Patients on peritoneal dialysis	3 g every 12 hours.
Patients on hemodialysis	2 g every 12 hours supplemented with 3 g after each dialysis.

[1] Daily dose for children should not exceed adult dosage.

[2] Half-life in patients with renal failure is approximately 13 hours.

(Dosage continued on following page)

TICARCILLIN DISODIUM (Cont.)

Dosage (Cont.):

Use the following formula to calculate creatinine clearance from serum creatinine value:

$$\text{Males: } \frac{\text{Weight (kg)} \times (140 - \text{Age})}{72 \times \text{serum creatinine (mg/dl)}} = \text{Ccr}$$

Females: 0.85 × above value

Children weighing > 40 kg should receive adult dose. In children under 40 kg, data are insufficient to recommend an optimum dose.

Administration:

IM: Reconstitute each g ticarcillin with 2 ml Sterile Water for Injection, Sodium Chloride Injection or 1% lidocaine HCl solution (without epinephrine) to obtain 1 g ticarcillin per 2.6 ml solution and use promptly.

Inject well into a relatively large muscle, using usual techniques and precautions.

IV: Reconstitute each g of ticarcillin with 4 ml of desired IV solution. Each 1 ml of the resulting solution will have an approximate average concentration of 200 mg. When dissolved, dilute further to desired volume. When injecting solution directly, administer as slowly as possible to avoid vein irritation.

For IV infusions, administer by continuous or intermittent IV drip. Administer intermittent infusion over a 30 minute to 2 hour period in 6 equally divided doses.

Reconstitute 3 g piggyback vials with a minimum of 30 ml of desired IV solution. A dilution of ≈ 1 g/20 ml or more will reduce the incidence of vein irritation.

Stability and Storage of Ticarcillin IV Solutions			
		Stability (loss of potency < 10%)	
Concentration	Compatible diluents	Controlled room temperature	Refrigeration
10 mg/ml & 50 mg/ml	Sodium Chloride Injection[1]	72 hours	14 days
	Dextrose Injection 5%[1]	72 hours	14 days
	Lactated Ringer's Injection[1]	48 hours	14 days

IV infusion: Use a 50 ml or 100 ml *ADD-Vantage* container of either Sodium Chloride Injection or 5% Dextrose in Water. The resulting concentration of the 3 g dose reconstituted in 50 ml diluent is ≈ 60 mg/ml. The resulting concentration of the 3 g dose reconstituted in 100 ml diluent is ≈ 30 mg/ml. Administer by continuous or intermittent IV drip. Give intermittent infusion over 30 minutes to 2 hours in equally divided doses. To avoid vein irritation, administer as slowly as possible.

The IV solutions, Sodium Chloride Injection and 5% Dextrose in Water, in concentrations of ≈ 30 or ≈ 60 mg/ml are stable for 72 hours when stored at room temperature (21° to 24°C; 70° to 75°F).

Incompatibilities: Do NOT mix ticarcillin together with gentamicin, amikacin or tobramycin in the same IV solution, due to the gradual inactivation of gentamicin, amikacin or tobramycin under these circumstances. The therapeutic effect of these drugs remains unimpaired when administered separately. **C.I.***

Rx				
Rx	**Ticar** (SK-Beecham)	**Powder for Injection:** (Contains 5.2 mEq sodium/g)		
		1 g (as disodium)	In vials.	15
		3 g (as disodium)	In vials, piggyback and *ADD-Vantage* vials.	15
		6 g (as disodium)	In vials.	15
		20 g (as disodium)	In bulk vials.	14
		30 g (as disodium	In bulk vials.	14

* Cost Index based on cost per 500 mg.

[1] These solutions remain stable up to 100 mg/ml concentration. After reconstitution, they can be frozen (approximately -18°C; 0°F) and stored for up to 30 days without loss of potency. The stabilities of the thawed solutions are identical to the unfrozen ones listed above.

Complete prescribing information for these products begins on page 1686

TICARCILLIN AND CLAVULANATE POTASSIUM

Actions:

Pharmacology: The formulation of ticarcillin with clavulanic acid protects ticarcillin from degradation by β-lactamase enzymes (see group monograph).

Indications:

Treatment of infections caused by susceptible strains of the designated organisms in the conditions listed below:

Septicemia including bacteremia, caused by β-lactamase-producing strains of *Klebsiella* sp*, *Escherichia coli**, *Staphylococcus aureus** and *Pseudomonas aeruginosa** (and other *Pseudomonas* species*).

Lower respiratory infections caused by β-lactamase-producing strains of *S aureus, Hemophilus influenzae** and *Klebsiella* sp.*

Bone and joint infections caused by β-lactamase-producing strains of *S aureus.*

Skin and skin structure infections caused by β-lactamase-producing strains of *S aureus, Klebsiella* sp* and *E coli.**

Urinary tract infections (complicated and uncomplicated) caused by β-lactamase-producing strains of *E coli, Klebsiella* sp, *P aeruginosa** (and other *Pseudomonas* species*), *Citrobacter* sp*, *Enterobacter cloacae**, *Serratia marcescens** and *S aureus.**

Gynecologic infections: Endometritis caused by β-lactamase producing strains of *B melaninogenicus**, *Enterobacter* sp. (including *E cloacae**), *E coli, Klebsiella pneumoniae**, *S aureus* and *Staphylococcus epidermidis*.

While this combination is indicated only for the conditions listed above, infections caused by ticarcillin-susceptible organisms are also amenable to this combination treatment due to its ticarcillin content.

Treatment of mixed infections and for presumptive therapy prior to the identification of the causative organisms.

Based on the in vitro synergism between this drug and aminoglycosides against certain strains of *P aeruginosa,* combined therapy has been successful, especially in patients with impaired host defenses. Use both drugs in full therapeutic doses. As soon as results of culture and susceptibility tests become available, adjust antimicrobial therapy.

Administration and Dosage:

Administer by IV infusion over 30 minutes.

Generally, continue treatment for at least 2 days after signs and symptoms of infection have disappeared. The usual duration is 10 to 14 days; however, in difficult and complicated infections, more prolonged therapy may be required.

Frequent bacteriologic and clinical appraisal is necessary during therapy of chronic urinary tract infections and may be required for several months after therapy has been completed; persistent infections may require treatment for several weeks; do not use doses smaller than those indicated.

In certain infections involving abscess formation, perform appropriate surgical drainage in conjunction with antimicrobial therapy.

When administering in combination with another antimicrobial (eg, an aminoglycoside), administer each drug separately.

Ticarcillin/Clavulanate Potassium Uses and Dosages

Infection	Dosage
Systemic and urinary tract infections:	
Adults (≥ 60 kg)	3.1 g[1] every 4 to 6 hours
(≤ 60 kg)[2]	200 to 300 mg/kg/day (based on ticarcillin content) given in divided doses every 4 to 6 hours
Gynecologic infections:	
Adults (≥ 60 kg)	
moderate infections	200 mg/kg/day in divided doses every 6 hours
severe infections	300 mg/kg/day in divided doses every 4 hours

* Efficacy for this organism in this organ system was studied in < 10 infections.
[1] 3 g ticarcillin plus 100 mg clavulanic acid.
[2] Dosage in children < 12 years of age is not established.

(Administration and Dosage continued on following page)

Extended Spectrum Penicillins (Cont.)

TICARCILLIN AND CLAVULANATE POTASSIUM (Cont.)

Administration and Dosage (Cont.):

Dosage of Ticarcillin/Clavulanate Potassium in Renal Insufficiency[1]	
Initial loading dose is 3.1 g[2]. Follow with doses based on creatinine clearance and type of dialysis.	
Creatinine clearance (ml/min)	*Dosage*
> 60	3.1 g[2] every 4 hours
30 to 60	2 g every 4 hours
10 to 30	2 g every 8 hours
< 10	2 g every 12 hours
< 10 with hepatic dysfunction	2 g every 24 hours
Patients on peritoneal dialysis	3.1 g[2] every 12 hours
Patients on hemodialysis	2 g every 12 hours supplemented with 3.1 g[2] after each dialysis

[1] Half-life of ticarcillin in patients with renal failure is ≈ 13 hours.
[2] 3 g ticarcillin plus 100 mg clavulanic acid.

Use the following formula to calculate creatinine clearance from serum creatinine values:

$$\text{Males: } \frac{\text{Weight (kg)} \times (140 - \text{age})}{72 \times \text{serum creatinine (mg/dl)}} = \text{Ccr} \qquad \text{Females: } 0.85 \times \text{Ccr for males}$$

IV: Reconstitute by shaking with ≈ 13 ml of Sterile Water for Injection or NaCl Injection. The resulting ticarcillin concentration is ≈ 200 mg/ml and 6.7 mg/ml clavulanic acid for the 3.1 g dose. Conversely, each 5 ml of the 3.1 g dose reconstituted with ≈ 13 ml of diluent will contain ≈ 1 g ticarcillin and 33 mg clavulanic acid.

Further dilute the solution with Sodium Chloride Injection, 5% Dextrose Injection or Lactated Ringer's Injection to a concentration between 10 to 100 mg/ml. Administer over 30 minutes by direct infusion or through a Y-type IV infusion set already in place. If this method or the "piggyback" method is used, temporarily discontinue administering any other solutions during the infusion of ticarcillin and clavulanate potassium.

The concentrated stock solution (200 mg/ml) is stable for up to 6 hours at room temperature (21° to 23°C; 70° to 75°F) or up to 72 hours under refrigeration (4°C; 40°F); if further diluted to a concentration between 10 mg/ml and 100 mg/ml with any of the recommended diluents, the following stability periods apply:

Stability and Storage for IV Solutions of Ticarcillin/Clavulanate Potassium				
		Stability		
Concentration	Compatible diluents	Controlled room temp.	Refrigeration	Frozen
10 mg/ml to 100 mg/ml	Sodium Chloride Injection	24 hours	7 days	30 days
	5% Dextrose Injection	24 hours	3 days	7 days
	Lactated Ringer's Injection	24 hours	7 days	30 days

Unused solutions must be discarded after the time period stated above. Use all thawed solutions within 8 hours. Do not refreeze thawed solutions.

Premixed, frozen solutions: Store at ≤ –20°C (–4°F). Thaw at room temperature 22°C (72°F) or in a refrigerator 4°C (40°F). Do not force thaw by immersion in water baths or by microwave irradiation. Thawed solution is stable for 7 days if stored under refrigeration or for 24 hours at room temperature. Do not refreeze.

Incompatibility: Incompatible with sodium bicarbonate.

				C.I.*
Rx	**Timentin** (SK-Beecham Labs)	**Powder for Injection:** Contains 4.75 mEq sodium/g. 3 g ticarcillin (as disodium) and 0.1 g clavulanic acid	In 3.1 g vials, piggyback bottles, *ADD-Vantage* vials and 31 g pharmacy bulk packages.[1]	24
		Solution: Contains 18.7 mEq sodium/100 ml 3 g ticarcillin (as disodium) and 0.1 g clavulanic acid.	In 100 ml premixed, frozen vials.	NA

* Cost Index based on cost per 500 mg.
[1] Pharmacy bulk package contains 30 g ticarcillin (as disodium) and 1 g clavulanic acid.

Complete prescribing information for these products begins on page 1686

MEZLOCILLIN SODIUM

Indications:

Lower respiratory tract infections: Including pneumonia and lung abscess caused by *Hemophilus influenzae, Klebsiella* sp including *K pneumoniae, Proteus mirabilis, Pseudomonas* sp including *P aeruginosa, E coli* and *Bacteroides* sp including *B fragilis.*

Intra-abdominal infections: Including acute cholecystitis, cholangitis, peritonitis, hepatic abscess and intra-abdominal abscess caused by susceptible *E coli, P mirabilis, Klebsiella* sp, *Pseudomonas* sp, *Streptococcus faecalis* (enterococcus), *Bacteroides* sp, *Peptococcus* sp and *Peptostreptococcus* sp.

Urinary tract infections: Caused by susceptible *E coli; P mirabilis;* the indole-positive *Proteus* sp, *Morganella morganii; Klebsiella* sp; *Enterobacter* sp; *Serratia* sp; *Pseudomonas* sp; *S faecalis* (enterococcus).

Uncomplicated gonorrhea due to susceptible *Neisseria gonorrhoeae.*

Gynecological infections: Including endometritis, pelvic cellulitis and pelvic inflammatory disease associated with susceptible *N gonorrhoeae, Peptococcus* sp, *Peptostreptococcus* sp, *Bacteroides* sp, *E coli, P mirabilis, Klebsiella* sp and *Enterobacter* sp.

Skin and skin structure infections: Caused by susceptible *S faecalis* (enterococcus); *E coli; P mirabilis;* the indole-positive *Proteus* sp, *P vulgaris* and *Providencia rettgeri; Klebsiella* sp; *Enterobacter* sp; *Pseudomonas* sp; *Peptococcus* sp; *Bacteroides* sp.

Septicemia: Including bacteremia caused by susceptible *E coli, Klebsiella* sp, *Enterobacter* sp, *Pseudomonas* sp, *Bacteroides* sp and *Peptococcus* sp.

Streptococcal infections: Caused by *Streptococcus* sp including group A beta-hemolytic *Streptococcus* and *S pneumoniae;* however, such infections are ordinarily treated with more narrow spectrum penicillins. Mezlocillin's broad spectrum of activity makes it useful for treating mixed infections caused by susceptible strains of both gram-negative and gram-positive aerobic or anaerobic bacteria. It is not effective, however, against infections caused by penicillinase-producing *Staphylococcus aureus.*

Severe infections: In certain severe infections when the causative organisms are unknown, administer in conjunction with an aminoglycoside or a cephalosporin antibiotic as initial therapy. When results of culture and susceptibility tests become available, adjust antimicrobial therapy if indicated.

Pseudomonas infections: Mezlocillin is effective in combination with an aminoglycoside for the treatment of life-threatening infections caused by *P aeruginosa.* For the treatment of febrile episodes in immunosuppressed patients with granulocytopenia, combine with an aminoglycoside or a cephalosporin.

Prophylaxis: Perioperative administration may reduce the incidence of infection in patients undergoing surgical procedures that are classified as contaminated or potentially contaminated (eg, vaginal hysterectomy, colorectal surgery). Effective use depends on time of administration. To achieve effective tissue levels, give ½ to 1½ hours before surgery.

In patients undergoing Caesarean section, intraoperative (after clamping the umbilical cord) and postoperative use may reduce the incidence of postoperative infections.

For patients undergoing colorectal surgery, preoperative bowel preparation by mechanical cleansing as well as with a non-absorbable antibiotic (eg, neomycin) is recommended.

Dosage:

Administer IV for serious infections. IM doses should not exceed 2 g/injection. Individualize dosage.

Adults: The recommended adult dosage for serious infections is 200 to 300 mg/kg/day given in 4 to 6 divided doses. The usual dose is 3 g given every 4 hours (18 g/day) or 4 g given every 6 hours (16 g/day).

Infants and children: Limited data are available on the safety and effectiveness in the treatment of infants and children with serious infection.

Mezlocillin Dosage Guidelines for Neonates

Body weight (g)	Age	
	≤ 7 Days	> 7 Days
≤ 2000	75 mg/kg every 12 hours (150 mg/kg/day)	75 mg/kg every 8 hours (225 mg/kg/day)
> 2000	75 mg/kg every 12 hours (150 mg/kg/day)	75 mg/kg every 6 hours (300 mg/kg/day)

For infants > 1 month of age and children < 12 years, administer 50 mg/kg every 4 hours (300 mg/kg/day); infuse IV over 30 minutes or administer by IM injection.

(Dosage continued on following page)

MEZLOCILLIN SODIUM (Cont.)

Dosage (Cont.):

Renal function impairment: The rate of elimination of mezlocillin is dose-dependent and related to the degree of renal function impairment. After an IV dose of 3 g, the serum half-life is approximately 1 hour in patients with creatinine clearances > 60 ml/min, 1.3 hours in those with clearances of 30 to 59 ml/min, 1.6 hours in those with clearances of 10 to 29 ml/min, and approximately 3.6 hours in patients with clearances of < 10 ml/min. Dosage adjustments are not required in patients with mild impairment of renal function.

Renal failure and hepatic insufficiency – Measurement of serum levels of mezlocillin will provide additional guidance for adjusting dosage; however, this may not be practical.

Mezlocillin Uses and Dosages

Organisms/Infections	Dosage
Urinary infection: Uncomplicated with normal renal function (creatinine clearance ≥ 30 ml/min).	100 to 125 mg/kg/day (6 to 8 g/day); 1.5 to 2 g every 6 hours IV or IM.
Uncomplicated with renal impairment	1.5 g every 8 hours
Complicated with normal renal function	150 to 200 mg/kg/day (12 g/day); 3 g every 6 hours IV.
Complicated with renal impairment – Creatinine clearance	
10 to 30 ml/min	1.5 g every 6 hours.
< 10 ml/min	1.5 g every 8 hours.
Lower respiratory tract infection, intra-abdominal infection, gynecological infection, skin and skin structure infections, septicemia:	225 to 300 mg/kg/day (16 to 18 g/day); 4 g every 6 hours or 3 g every 4 hours IV.
Serious systemic infection with renal impairment – Creatinine clearance	
10 to 30 ml/min	3 g every 8 hours.
< 10 ml/min	2 g every 8 hours.
Serious systemic infection undergoing hemodialysis for renal failure	3 to 4 g after each dialysis; then every 12 hours.
peritoneal dialysis	3 g every 2 hours
Life-threatening infections:	Up to 350 mg/kg/day; 4 g every 4 hours (24 g/day maximum).
In patients with renal impairment – Creatinine clearance	
10 to 30 ml/min	3 g every 6 hours.
< 10 ml/min	2 g every 6 hours.
Acute, uncomplicated gonococcal urethritis:	1 to 2 g IV or IM; plus 1 g probenecid at time of dosing or up to ½ hour before.
Prophylaxis:	
To prevent postoperative infection in contaminated or potentially contaminated surgery	4 g IV, ½ to 1½ hr prior to start of surgery; 4 g IV, 6 and 12 hours later.
Caesarean section patients –	First dose: 4 g IV when umbilical cord is clamped; Second dose: 4 g IV, 4 hrs after first dose; Third dose: 4 g IV, 8 hrs after first dose.

(Continued on following page)

MEZLOCILLIN SODIUM (Cont.)

Administration:

IV administration: Administer IV by intermittent infusion or by direct IV injection. In combination with another antimicrobial, such as an aminoglycoside, give each drug separately in accordance with the recommended dosage and routes of administration for each drug.

Infusion – Reconstitute each g of mezlocillin by vigorous shaking with at least 9 to 10 ml of Sterile Water for Injection, 5% Dextrose Injection or 0.9% Sodium Chloride Injection. Further dilute to desired volume (50 to 100 ml) with an appropriate IV solution. The solution may then be administered over a period of 30 minutes by direct infusion or through a Y-type IV infusion set. If this method or the piggyback method of administration is used, temporarily discontinue the administration of any other solutions during the infusion.

Injection – The reconstituted solution may be injected directly into a vein or into IV tubing; when so administered, give the injection slowly over a period of 3 to 5 minutes. To minimize venous irritation, the concentration of drug should not exceed 10%.

IM administration: Reconstitute each g of mezlocillin by vigorous shaking with 3 to 4 ml of Sterile Water for Injection or with 3 to 4 ml of 0.5% or 1% lidocaine HCl solution (without epinephrine). Do not exceed 2 g/injection.

Inject well within the body of a relatively large muscle, such as the upper outer quadrant of the buttock (ie, gluteus maximus); aspirate to avoid unintentional injection into a blood vessel. Slow injection (12 to 15 seconds) will minimize the discomfort of IM administration.

Stability and Storage of Mezlocillin IV Solutions

Concentration	Compatible diluents	Stability (loss of potency < 10%): Controlled room temperature	Refrigeration
10 mg/ml & 100 mg/ml	Sterile Water for Injection[1]	48 hours	7 days
	0.9% Sodium Chloride Injection[1]	48 hours	7 days
	5% Dextrose Injection[1]	48 hours	7 days
	5% Dextrose in 0.225% Sodium Chloride Injection	72 hours	7 days
	Lactated Ringer's Injection	24 hours	7 days
	5% Dextrose in Electrolyte #75 Injection	72 hours	7 days
	5% Dextrose in 0.45% Sodium Chloride Injection[2]	48 hours	48 hours
	Ringer's Injection	24 hours	24 hours
	10% Dextrose Injection	24 hours	24 hours
	5% Fructose Injection	24 hours	24 hours
Up to 250 mg/ml	Sterile Water for Injection	24 hours	
	0.9% Sodium Chloride Injection	24 hours	
	0.5% and 1% Lidocaine HCl Solution (without epinephrine)	24 hours	

[1] These solutions are stable for up to 28 days when frozen at −12°C (10°F).
[2] This solution is stable from 10 mg/ml to 50 mg/ml refrigerated.

If precipitation occurs under refrigeration, warm product to 37°C (98.6°F) for 20 minutes in a water bath and shake well.

Store vials and infusion bottles at or below 30°C (86°F). Product may darken slightly depending on storage conditions, but potency is not affected. **C.I.***

				C.I.
Rx	**Mezlin** (Miles Pharm.)	**Powder for Injection:** Contains 1.85 mEq sodium/g		
		1 g mezlocillin (as sodium)	In vials.	35
		2 g mezlocillin (as sodium)	In vials and infusion bottles.	28
		3 g mezlocillin (as sodium)	In vials and infusion bottles and *ADD-Vantage* vials.	23
		4 g mezlocillin (as sodium)	In vials, infusion bottles and *ADD-Vantage* vials.	21
		20 g mezlocillin (as sodium)	In pharmacy bulk packages.	20

* Cost Index based on cost per 500 mg.

Complete prescribing information for these products begins on page 1686

PIPERACILLIN SODIUM

Indications:

Treatment of mixed infections and presumptive therapy prior to the identification of the causative organisms. Also, it may be used as single drug therapy in some situations where two antibiotics are normally used.

Intra-abdominal infections (including hepatobiliary and surgical infections): Caused by *Escherichia coli; Pseudomonas aeruginosa;* enterococci; *Clostridium* sp; anaerobic cocci; *Bacteroides* sp, including *B fragilis.*

Urinary tract infections (UTIs): Caused by *E coli, Klebsiella* sp, *P aeruginosa, Proteus* sp, including *P mirabilis* and enterococci.

Gynecologic infections (including endometritis, pelvic inflammatory disease, pelvic cellulitis): Caused by *Bacteroides* sp, including *B fragilis;* anaerobic cocci; *Neisseria gonorrhoeae;* enterococci (*Streptococcus faecalis*).

Septicemia (including bacteremia): Caused by *E coli, Klebsiella* sp, *Enterobacter* sp, *Serratia* sp, *P mirabilis, S pneumoniae,* enterococci, *P aeruginosa, Bacteroides* sp and anaerobic cocci.

Lower respiratory tract infections: Caused by *E coli, Klebsiella* sp, *Enterobacter* sp, *P aeruginosa, Serratia* sp, *Hemophilus influenzae, Bacteroides* sp and anaerobic cocci. Although improvement has been noted in cystic fibrosis patients, long-term bacterial eradication may not be achieved.

Skin and skin structure infections: Caused by *E coli; Klebsiella* sp; *Serratia* sp; *Acinetobacter* sp; *Enterobacter* sp; *P aeruginosa;* indole-positive *Proteus* sp; *P mirabilis; Bacteroides* sp, including *B fragilis;* anaerobic cocci; enterococci.

Bone and joint infections: Caused by *P aeruginosa,* enterococci, *Bacteroides* sp and anaerobic cocci.

Gonococcal infections: Treatment of uncomplicated gonococcal urethritis.

Streptococcal infections: Infections caused by streptococcus species including group A β-hemolytic *Streptococcus* and *S pneumoniae;* however, these infections are ordinarily treated with more narrow spectrum penicillins.

Prophylaxis: For prophylactic use in surgery including intra-abdominal (GI and biliary) procedures, vaginal and abdominal hysterectomy and cesarean section. Effective prophylaxis depends on the time of administration; give ½ to 1 hour before the operation so that effective levels can be achieved in the wound prior to the procedure.

Stop the prophylactic use of piperacillin within 24 hours. Continuing administration of any antibiotic increases the possibility of adverse reactions, but in the majority of surgical procedures does not reduce the incidence of subsequent infections. If there are signs of infection, obtain specimens for culture so that appropriate therapy can begin.

Administration and Dosage:

Administer IM or IV. For serious infections, give 3 to 4 g every 4 to 6 hours as a 20 to 30 minute IV infusion. Maximum daily dose is 24 g/day, although higher doses have been used. Limit IM injections to 2 g/site.

Hemodialysis: Maximum dose is 6 g/day (2 g every 8 hours). Hemodialysis removes 30% to 50% of piperacillin in 4 hours; administer an additional 1 g after each dialysis.

Renal failure and hepatic insufficiency: Measure serum levels to provide additional guidance for adjusting dosage; however, this may not be practical.

Infants and children < 12 years of age: Dosages have not been established; however, the following dosages have been suggested:

Neonates – 100 mg/kg/dose every 12 hours.

Children – Cystic fibrosis, 350 to 500 mg/kg/day divided every 4 to 6 hours.

Other conditions, 200 to 300 mg/kg/day, up to a maximum of 24 g/day divided every 4 to 6 hours.

Concomitant therapy with aminoglycosides has been used successfully, especially in patients with impaired host defenses. Use both drugs in full therapeutic doses.

(Administration and Dosage continued on following page)

Extended Spectrum Penicillins (Cont.)

PIPERACILLIN SODIUM (Cont.)

Administration and Dosage (Cont.):

Piperacillin Uses and Dosages	
Organisms/Infections	Dosage
Serious infections (septicemia, nosocomial pneumonia, intra-abdominal infections, aerobic and anaerobic gynecologic infections and skin and soft tissue infections):	12 to 18 g/day IV (200 to 300 mg/kg/day) in divided doses every 4 to 6 hours.
Renal impairment –	
Creatinine clearance 20 to 40 ml/min	12 g/day; 4 g every 8 hours.
< 20 ml/min	8 g/day; 4 g every 12 hours.
Urinary tract infections: Complicated (normal renal function)	8 to 16 g/day IV (125 to 200 mg/kg/day) in divided doses every 6 to 8 hours.
Renal impairment	
Creatinine clearance 20 to 40 ml/min	9 g/day; 3 g every 8 hours.
< 20 ml/min	6 g/day; 3 g every 12 hours.
Uncomplicated UTI and most community-acquired pneumonia (normal renal function)	6 to 8 g/day IM or IV (100 to 125 mg/kg/day) in divided doses every 6 to 12 hours.
Uncomplicated UTI with renal impairment – Creatinine clearance < 20 ml/min	6 g/day; 3 g every 12 hours.
Uncomplicated gonorrhea infections:	2 g IM in a single dose accompanied by 1 g probenecid ½ hour prior to injection.
Prophylaxis: Intra-abdominal surgery	2 g IV just prior to surgery; 2 g during surgery; 2 g every 6 hours post-op for no more than 24 hours.
Vaginal hysterectomy	2 g IV just prior to surgery; 2 g 6 hours after initial dose; 2 g 12 hours after first dose.
Cesarean section	2 g IV after cord is clamped; 2 g 4 hours after initial dose; 2 g 8 hours after first dose.
Abdominal hysterectomy	2 g IV just prior to surgery; 2 g on return to recovery room; 2 g after 6 hours.

Diluents for Reconstitution of Piperacillin	
Sterile Water for Injection	Bacteriostatic* Sodium Chloride Injection
Bacteriostatic* Water for Injection	Dextrose 5% in Water
Sodium Chloride Injection	Dextrose 5% and 0.9% Sodium Chloride
	**Lidocaine HCl 0.5% to 1% (w/o epinephrine)

* Either parabens or benzyl alcohol.
**For IM use only. Lidocaine is contraindicated in patients with a known history of hypersensitivity to local anesthetics of the amide type.

IV Solutions	IV Admixtures	ADD-Vantage vials
Dextrose 5% in Water	Normal Saline [+ KCl 40 mEq]	Dextrose 5% in Water
0.9% Sodium Chloride	5% Dextrose in Water [+ KCl 40 mEq]	0.9% Sodium Chloride
Dextrose 5% and 0.9% Sodium Chloride	5% Dextrose/Normal Saline [+ KCl 40 mEq]	
Lactated Ringer's Injection	Ringer's Injection [+ KCl 40 mEq]	
Dextran 6% in 0.9% Sodium Chloride	Lactated Ringer's Injection [+ KCl 40 mEq]	

IV administration:

Reconstitution directions – Reconstitute each g piperacillin with at least 5 ml of a suitable diluent (except Lidocaine HCl 0.5% to 1% without epinephrine) listed above. Shake well until dissolved. Reconstituted solution may be further diluted to the desired volume (eg, 50 or 100 ml) in the above listed IV solutions and admixtures.

Reconstitution directions for bulk vial – Reconstitute the 40 g vial with 172 ml of a suitable diluent (except Lidocaine HCl 0.5% to 1% without epinephrine) listed above to achieve a concentration of 1 g per 5 ml.

Directions for administration:

Intermittent IV infusion – Infuse diluted solution over a period of about 30 minutes. During infusion it is desirable to discontinue the primary IV solution.

IV injection (bolus) – Reconstituted solution should be injected slowly over a 3 to 5 minute period to help avoid vein irritation.

(Administration and Dosage continued on following page)

Extended Spectrum Penicillins (Cont.)

PIPERACILLIN SODIUM (Cont.)

Administration and Dosage (Cont.):

IM administration:

Reconstitution directions – Reconstitute each g of piperacillin with 2 ml of a suitable diluent listed in the previous table to achieve a concentration of 1 g per 2.5 ml. Shake well until dissolved.

Directions for administration: When indicated by clinical and bacteriological findings, IM administration of 6 to 8 g daily, in divided doses, may be used for initiation of therapy. In addition, consider IM administration of the drug for maintenance therapy after clinical and bacteriologic improvement has been obtained with IV piperacillin sodium treatment. Administration IM should not exceed 2 g per injection at any one site. The preferred site is the upper outer quadrant of the buttock (ie, gluteus maximus). Use the deltoid area only if well developed, and then only with caution to avoid radial nerve injury. Injections IM should not be made into the lower or mid-third of the upper arm.

Stability following reconstitution: Stable in both glass and plastic containers when reconstituted with recommended diluents and when diluted with the IV solutions and IV admixtures indicated above.

Extensive stability studies have demonstrated chemical stability (potency, pH and clarity) through 24 hours at room temperature, up to 1 week refrigerated, and up to 1 month frozen (–10° to –20°C;14 to –4°F). (*Note:* The 40 g bulk vial should not be frozen after reconstitution.) Appropriate consideration of aseptic technique and individual hospital policy, however, may recommend discarding unused portions after storage for 48 hours under refrigeration and recommend discarding after 24 hours storage at room temperature. **C.I.***

Rx	**Pipracil** (Lederle)	**Powder for injection:** Contains 1.85 mEq (42.5 mg) sodium/g		
		2 g	In vials, infusion bottles and *ADD-Vantage* vials.	26
		3 g	In vials, infusion bottles and *ADD-Vantage* vials.	24
		4 g	In vials, infusion bottles and *ADD-Vantage* vials.	23
		40 g	In pharmacy bulk vials.	21

CARBENICILLIN INDANYL SODIUM

Indications:

Treatment of acute and chronic infections of the upper and lower urinary tract and in asymptomatic bacteriuria due to susceptible strains of: *Escherichia coli, Proteus mirabilis, Morganella morganii, Providencia rettgeri, P vulgaris, Pseudomonas, Enterobacter* and enterococci. Also indicated in the treatment of prostatitis due to susceptible strains of: *E coli,* enterococcus *(S faecalis), P mirabilis* and *Enterobacter* species.

Administration and Dosage:

Urinary tract infections:

E coli, Proteus species and *Enterobacter* – 382 to 764 mg, 4 times daily.

Pseudomonas and enterococci – 764 mg, 4 times daily.

Prostatitis due to E coli, P mirabilis, Enterobacter and enterococcus *(S faecalis):* 764 mg, 4 times daily. **C.I.***

Rx	**Geocillin** (Roerig)	**Tablets, film coated:** 382 mg carbenicillin (118 mg indanyl sodium ester)	Yellow. Capsule shape. In 100s and UD 100s.	23

* Cost Index based on cost per 500 mg.

Actions:

Pharmacology: Structurally and pharmacologically related to penicillins. Cefoxitin and cefotetan (cephamycins), moxalactam (a β-lactam) and loracarbef (a carbacephem) are included due to their similarity.

Cephalosporins and related compounds are divided into first, second and third generation agents (see table). Within each group, differentiation is primarily by pharmacokinetics; groups are divided by antibacterial spectrum. In general, progression from first to third generation reveals broadening gram-negative spectrum, loss of efficacy against gram-positive organisms, greater efficacy against resistant organisms and increased cost.

Mechanism – Cephalosporins inhibit mucopeptide synthesis in the bacterial cell wall, making it defective and osmotically unstable. The drugs are usually bactericidal, depending on organism susceptibility, dose, tissue concentrations and the rate at which organisms are multiplying. They are more effective against rapidly growing organisms forming cell walls.

Pharmacokinetics:

Pharmacokinetic Parameters of Cephalosporins

	Drug	Routes	Half-Life			Protein bound (%)	Recovered unchanged in urine (%)	Peak serum level 1 g IV dose (mcg/ml)	Sodium (mEq/g)
			Normal renal function (minutes)	ESRD[1] (hours)	Hemo-dialysis (hours)				
First	Cephalexin	Oral	50-80	19-22	4-6	10	>90	—	—
	Cefadroxil	Oral	78-96	20-25	3-4	20	>90	—	—
	Cephradine	Oral/IM-IV	48-80	8-15	—	8-17	>90	86	6[2]
	Cephalothin	IM-IV	30-50	3-15	3	70	68-70	30	2.8
	Cephapirin	IM-IV	24-36	1.8-4	1.8	54	68-70	73	2.4
	Cefazolin	IM-IV	90-120	3-7	9-14	80-86	80-96	185-189	2-2.1
Second	Cefaclor	Oral	35-54	2-3	1.6-2.1	25	60-85	—	—
	Cefamandole	IM-IV	30-60	8-11	7	70	65-85	139	3.3
	Cefoxitin	IM-IV	40-60	20	4	73	85-99	64-110	2.3
	Cefuroxime	Oral/IM-IV	80	16-22[3]	3.5	33-50	66-100	100[4]	2.4[3]
	Cefonicid	IM-IV	270	11	—	98	95-99	221.3	3.7
	Ceforanide	IM-IV	156-180	19	5	80	78-95	125	0
	Cefmetazole	IV	72	—	—	65	85	—	2
	Cefotetan	IM-IV	180-276	13-35	5	88-90	51-81	158	3.5
	Cefprozil	Oral	78	5.2-5.9	decreased	36	60	—	—
	Loracarbef	Oral	60	32	4	25	>90	—	—
Third	Cefoperazone	IM-IV	102-156	1.3-2.9	2	82-93	20-30	73-153	1.5
	Moxalactam	IM-IV	114-150	19-30	2-5	57	60-90	94-101	3.8
	Cefotaxime	IM-IV	60	3-11	2.5	30-40	20-36	42-102	2.2
	Ceftizoxime	IM-IV	84-114	25-30	6	30	80	60-87	2.6
	Ceftriaxone	IM-IV	348-522	15.7	14.7	85-95	33-67	151	3.6
	Ceftazidime	IM-IV	114-120	14-30	—	<10-17	80-90	69-90	2.3
	Cefixime	Oral	180-240	11.5	—	65	50	—	—

[1] ESRD = End stage renal disease (Ccr < 10 ml/min/1.73 m^2). [2] Also available in sodium free form.
[3] Injection only. [4] Following 1.5 g IV dose.

Absorption – Cephalexin, cephradine, cefaclor, cefixime, cefprozil, cefadroxil and loracarbef are well absorbed from the GI tract; absorption may be delayed by food, except cefadroxil and cefprozil, but the amount absorbed is not affected. Peak plasma levels of loracarbef (capsules) are decreased by food and occur later. The absorption of oral cefuroxime is increased when given with food.

Distribution – Cephalosporins are widely distributed to most tissues and fluids. First and second generation agents do not readily enter cerebrospinal fluid (CSF), except cefuroxime, even when meninges are inflamed. Third generation compounds (little data for cefixime) and cefuroxime readily diffuse into the CSF of patients with inflamed meninges. However, CSF levels of cefoperazone are relatively low. Therapeutic levels are reached in bone after usual doses of most agents. Cefazolin penetrates into acutely inflamed bone at higher concentrations than into normal bone.

High concentrations of ceftriaxone, cefamandole and cefoperazone are attained in bile. Therapeutic levels of ceftizoxime, ceforanide, cefuroxime, cefotetan, ceftazidime, cefoxitin and cefonicid are attained in bile. Bile levels of cefazolin can reach or exceed serum levels by up to 5 times in patients without obstructive biliary disease.

(Actions continued on following page)

Actions (Cont.):

Pharmacokinetics (Cont.):

Metabolism/Excretion – Cefuroxime axetil is metabolized to free cefuroxime plus acetaldehyde and acetic acid. Cephalothin and cephapirin are metabolized to less active compounds; however, desacetylcephapirin contributes to the drug's antibacterial activity. Desacetylcefotaxime, a major metabolite of cefotaxime, contributes to cefotaxime's bactericidal activity. The metabolite increases the spectrum to include anaerobes, specifically *Bacteroides* sp; the synergy with the parent drug appears to extend the dosing interval to 8 to 12 hours due to the prolonged half-life of the metabolite. Most cephalosporins and their metabolites are primarily excreted renally. Cefoperazone is excreted mainly in the bile; peak serum concentrations and serum half-lives are unchanged, even in patients with severe renal insufficiency. In hepatic dysfunction, serum half-life and urinary excretion are increased.

Microbiology:

Organisms Generally Susceptible to Cephalosporins																	
Organisms		First Generation						Second Generation									
✓ = generally susceptible ‡ = demonstrated in vitro activity		Cephalexin	Cefadroxil	Cephradine	Cephalothin	Cephapirin	Cefazolin	Cefaclor	Cefamandole	Cefoxitin	Cefuroxime	Cefonicid	Ceforanide	Cefmetazole	Cefotetan	Cefprozil	Loracarbef
Gram-positive	Staphylococci[1]	✓[2]	✓	✓	✓	✓	✓	✓[2]	✓	✓	✓	✓[2]	✓[2]	✓	✓	✓	✓
	Streptococci, beta-hemolytic	✓	✓	✓	✓	✓	✓	✓	✓	✓	✓	✓	✓	✓	✓	✓	✓
	Streptococcus pneumoniae	✓	✓	✓	✓	✓	✓	✓	✓	✓	✓	✓	✓	✓	✓	✓	✓
Gram-negative	Acinetobacter sp																
	Citrobacter sp										✓[2]	‡	✓	‡	‡	‡	‡
	Enterobacter sp						✓[2]		✓		✓[2]	‡	✓	‡	✓		
	Escherichia coli	✓	✓	✓	✓	✓	✓	✓	✓	✓	✓	✓	✓	✓	✓	‡	✓
	Hemophilus influenzae	✓		✓	✓	✓	✓	✓[3]	✓[3]	✓[3]	✓[3]	✓[3]	✓[3]	✓[3]	✓[3]	✓[3]	✓[3]
	Hemophilus parainfluenzae										‡		‡				‡
	Klebsiella sp	✓	✓	✓	✓	✓	✓	✓	✓	✓	✓	✓	✓	✓	✓	‡	‡
	Moraxella (Branhamella) catarrhalis	‡						✓			‡			‡		✓	✓[3]
	Morganella morganii (Proteus morganii)								✓	✓	✓[2]	✓		✓	✓		
	Neisseria gonorrhoeae							‡		✓	✓	‡	✓	‡	✓	‡	‡
	Neisseria meningitidis										✓				‡		
	Proteus mirabilis	✓	✓	✓	✓	✓	✓	✓	✓	✓	✓	✓	✓	✓	✓	‡	‡
	Proteus vulgaris								✓[2]	✓		✓		✓	✓		
	Providencia sp									✓	✓		✓	✓	✓		
	Providencia rettgeri								✓	✓	✓	✓	✓	‡	✓		
	Pseudomonas aeruginosa																
	Salmonella sp				✓						✓			‡	‡	‡	‡
	Salmonella typhi												✓		‡		
	Serratia sp														‡		
	Shigella sp				✓						✓			‡	‡	‡	‡
Anaerobes	Bacteroides sp							✓	✓	✓	✓		✓[2]	✓	✓[2]	‡	
	Bacteroides fragilis									✓				✓	✓		
	Clostridium sp								✓	✓	✓	‡		✓	✓	‡	‡
	Clostridium difficile															‡	
	Eubacterium sp																
	Fusobacterium sp								✓		✓	‡	✓	✓	✓	‡	‡
	Peptococcus sp							‡	✓	✓	✓	‡	✓	‡	✓		‡
	Peptostreptococcus sp							‡	✓	✓	✓	‡	✓	‡	✓	‡	‡

[1] Coagulase-positive, coagulase-negative and penicillinase-producing.

[2] Some strains are resistant.

[3] Including some β-lactamase-producing strains.

(Actions continued on following page)

Actions (Cont.):

Microbiology (Cont.):

β-lactamase resistance – First generation cephalosporins are generally inactivated by β-lactamase-producing organisms. Newer agents are distinguished by an increasing resistance to β-lactamase inactivation. Ceforanide, cefonicid and cefixime have a high degree of stability to some β-lactamases. Cefoxitin, cefuroxime, ceftriaxone, cefotaxime, ceftizoxime, cefotetan and moxalactam have a high degree of stability in the presence of both penicillinases and cephalosporinases produced by gram-negative and gram-positive bacteria. Cefoperazone and ceftazidime are also highly stable in the presence of β-lactamases produced by most gram-negative pathogens, and are active against organisms that are resistant to other β-lactam antibiotics because of β-lactamase production.

Organisms Generally Susceptible to Cephalosporins

Third Generation							Organisms	
Cefoperazone	Moxalactam	Cefotaxime	Ceftizoxime	Ceftriaxone	Ceftazidime	Cefixime	✓ = generally susceptible ‡ = demonstrated in vitro activity	
✓	✓	✓[3]	✓	✓	✓		Staphylococci[1]	Gram-positive
✓	✓	✓	✓	✓	✓	✓	Streptococci, beta-hemolytic	Gram-positive
✓	✓	✓	✓	✓	✓	✓	Streptococcus pneumoniae	Gram-positive
✓[2]		✓	✓	‡	‡		Acinetobacter sp	Gram-negative
✓		✓	‡	‡	✓	‡	Citrobacter sp	Gram-negative
✓	✓	✓	✓	✓	✓		Enterobacter sp	Gram-negative
✓	✓	✓	✓	✓	✓	✓	Escherichia coli	Gram-negative
✓[3]	✓[3]	✓[3]	✓[3]	✓[3]	✓[3]	✓[3]	Hemophilus influenzae	Gram-negative
		✓		✓	‡	‡[3]	Hemophilus parainfluenzae	Gram-negative
✓	✓	✓	✓	✓	✓	‡	Klebsiella sp	Gram-negative
			‡		✓	✓[3]	Moraxella catarrhalis (Branhamella catarrhalis)	Gram-negative
✓	✓	✓	✓	✓	‡		Morganella morganii (Proteus morganii)	Gram-negative
✓[3]	‡	✓	✓	✓	‡	‡[3]	Neisseria gonorrhoeae	Gram-negative
‡	‡	✓	‡	✓	✓		Neisseria meningitidis	Gram-negative
✓	✓	✓	✓	✓	✓	✓	Proteus mirabilis	Gram-negative
✓	✓	✓	✓	✓	✓	‡	Proteus vulgaris	Gram-negative
	‡	‡	‡	‡	‡	‡	Providencia sp	Gram-negative
✓	✓	✓	✓	‡	‡	‡	Providencia rettgeri	Gram-negative
✓	✓[2]	✓[2]	✓[2]	✓[2]	✓		Pseudomonas aeruginosa	Gram-negative
‡	‡	‡	‡	‡	‡	‡	Salmonella sp	Gram-negative
	‡	‡		‡			Salmonella typhi	Gram-negative
✓	✓	✓	✓	✓	✓	‡	Serratia sp	Gram-negative
‡	‡	‡	‡	‡	‡	‡	Shigella sp	Gram-negative
✓	✓	✓	‡	✓			Bacteroides sp	Anaerobes
✓	✓	✓	✓	‡			Bacteroides fragilis	Anaerobes
✓	✓	✓	‡	‡	‡		Clostridium sp	Anaerobes
‡							Clostridium difficile	Anaerobes
‡	✓		‡				Eubacterium sp	Anaerobes
‡	✓	✓	‡	‡			Fusobacterium sp	Anaerobes
✓	✓	✓	✓	‡	‡		Peptococcus sp	Anaerobes
✓	✓	✓	✓	‡	‡		Peptostreptococcus sp	Anaerobes

[1] Coagulase-positive, coagulase-negative and penicillinase-producing.
[2] Some strains are resistant.
[3] Including some β-lactamase-producing strains.

(Continued on following page)

Indications:

Perform culture and sensitivity tests.

Some of these agents are indicated for preoperative, intraoperative and postoperative prophylaxis to reduce the incidence of infection in patients undergoing surgical procedures that are classified as contaminated or potentially contaminated (eg, GI surgery, cesarean section, vaginal hysterectomy or cholecystectomy in high-risk patients).

For specific approved indications, refer to individual drug monographs.

Contraindications:

Hypersensitivity to cephalosporins or related antibiotics (see Warnings).

Warnings:

Coagulation abnormalities: **Moxalactam** (with which most experience is reported), **cefamandole** and **cefoperazone** can interfere with hemostasis through three different mechanisms: Hypoprothrombinemia with or without bleeding (due to destruction of vitamin K-producing intestinal bacteria; or a molecular attachment common to these three drugs, a methyltetrazolethiol side chain that prevents activation of prothrombin), platelet dysfunction and very rarely, immune-mediated thrombocytopenia. A total of 2.5% of clinical trial patients treated for 4 or more days with moxalactam experienced bleeding which was usually serious. At least 13 deaths occurred. Alterations in prothrombin times (PT) have occurred rarely in patients treated with **ceftriaxone. Cefotetan** also contains the methyltetrazolethiol side chain, but bleeding has not yet been a problem. However, several case reports have noted hypoprothrombinemia.

Bleeding associated with *hypoprothrombinemia* can be prevented with vitamin K. Give patients who receive moxalactam 10 mg of vitamin K/week prophylactically. The inhibition of *platelet function,* which may be accompanied by a prolonged bleeding time, is dose-dependent and can generally be avoided by limiting dosage to 4 g/day. Monitor the bleeding time in patients with normal renal function who receive more than 4 g of moxalactam/day for more than 3 days. Reduce dosage in all patients with significantly impaired renal function, and monitor bleeding times. If the bleeding time becomes unduly prolonged, discontinue these agents.

If bleeding occurs and if the PT is prolonged, give vitamin K. Administration of fresh frozen plasma, packed red cells and platelet concentrates may be indicated. Discontinue moxalactam if bleeding is due to platelet dysfunction; use cefamandole, cefoperazone, ceftriaxone and cefotetan with caution.

Bleeding during therapy may also be related to complications of underlying diseases (eg, sepsis, malignancy, renal and hepatic dysfunction) or may result from the combined effects of underlying diseases and drug therapy. When bleeding occurs, rule out disseminated intravascular coagulation (DIC) since DIC is more likely to occur in patients with sepsis, malignancy or hepatic disease.

Predisposing factors to cephalosporin bleeding abnormalities include hepatic and renal dysfunction, thrombocytopenia and the concomitant use of "high dose" heparin (more than 20,000 units/day), oral anticoagulants or other drugs that affect hemostasis (eg, aspirin). Elderly, malnourished or debilitated patients are more likely to experience bleeding abnormalities than other patients.

Hypersensitivity: Reactions range in severity from mild to life-threatening. Before therapy is instituted, inquire about previous hypersensitivity reactions to cephalosporins and penicillins. If a hypersensitivity reaction occurs, discontinue the drug and institute appropriate therapy. See also Management of Acute Hypersensitivity Reactions.

Cross-allergenicity with penicillin – Administer cephalosporins cautiously to penicillin-sensitive patients. There is evidence of partial cross-allergenicity between penicillins and cephalosporins; they cannot be assumed to be an absolutely safe alternative to penicillin in the penicillin-allergic patient. The estimated incidence of cross-sensitivity is 5% to 16%; however, it is possible the incidence is much lower, possibly 3% to 7%.

Serum sickness-like reactions (erythema multiforme or skin rashes accompanied by polyarthritis, arthralgia and, frequently, fever) have been reported; these reactions usually occurred following a second course of therapy. Signs and symptoms occur after a few days of therapy and resolve a few days after drug discontinuation with no serious sequelae. Antihistamines and corticosteroids may be of benefit in managing symptoms.

(Warnings continued on following page)

Warnings (Cont.):

Pseudomembranous colitis occurs with the use of cephalosporins (and other broad spectrum antibiotics); therefore, consider its diagnosis in patients who develop diarrhea with antibiotic use. Colitis may range in severity from mild to life-threatening. Treatment alters normal flora of the colon and may permit overgrowth of *Clostridia* species. A toxin produced by *C difficile* is a primary cause of antibiotic-associated colitis. Cholestyramine and colestipol resins bind the toxin in vitro.

Mild cases of colitis may respond to drug discontinuation alone. Manage moderate to severe cases by sigmoidoscopy, bacteriologic studies and with fluid, electrolyte and protein supplementation, as indicated. When the colitis is not relieved by drug discontinuation, or when it is severe, oral vancomycin or metronidazole (see individual monographs) is the treatment of choice. Rule out other causes of colitis.

Prescribe broad spectrum antibiotics with caution in individuals with a history of GI disease, especially colitis.

Renal function impairment: Cephalosporins may be nephrotoxic; use with caution in the presence of markedly impaired renal function (creatinine clearance rate of < 50 ml/min/1.73 m^2). In the elderly and in patients with known or suspected renal impairment, monitor carefully prior to and during therapy.

Reduce total daily antibiotic dosage in patients with transient or persistent reduction of urinary output due to renal insufficiency; high and prolonged serum concentrations can occur in such patients from usual doses. See individual product monographs for information on dosage adjustments in patients with impaired renal function.

Hepatic function impairment: **Cefoperazone** is extensively excreted in bile. Serum half-life increases twofold to fourfold in patients with hepatic disease or biliary obstruction. If higher dosages are used (> 4 g), monitor serum concentrations.

Pregnancy: Category B (*Category C* – Moxalactam). Safety for use during pregnancy has not been established. Use only when potential benefits outweigh potential hazards to the fetus. Cephalosporins appear safe to use in pregnant patients, although relatively few controlled studies exist. Few case reports are available for the newer agents.

These agents cross the placenta; peak umbilical cord concentrations for the various agents range from 3 to 29 mcg/ml following doses of 0.5 to 2 g. These data yielded a maternal:fetal serum ratio range of 0.16 to 1. Drug levels in cord blood after administration of **cefazolin** are approximately ¼ to ⅓ maternal drug levels. **Cefotetan** reaches therapeutic levels in cord blood.

In addition, the pharmacokinetic parameters of these drugs appear to change in the pregnant woman; tendencies are toward shorter half-lives, lower serum levels, larger volumes of distribution and increased clearance.

Lactation: Most of these agents are excreted in breast milk in small quantities. Levels range from 0.16 to 4 mcg/ml, or a breast milk:maternal serum ratio of 0.01 to 0.5 following doses of 0.5 to 2 g. However, consider the following problems for the nursing infant: Modification/alteration of bowel flora; pharmacological effects; interference with the interpretation of culture results if a fever/infection workup is needed.

Infants and Children: When using cephalosporins in infants, consider the relative benefit to risk. In neonates, accumulation of cephalosporin antibiotics (with resulting prolongation of drug half-life) has occurred.

In children ≥ 3 months of age, higher doses of **cefoxitin** have been associated with an increased incidence of eosinophilia and elevated AST.

In children ≥ 6 months of age, treatment with **ceftizoxime** has been associated with transient elevated levels of eosinophils, AST, ALT and CPK.

Safety and efficacy in children < 1 month (**cefaclor, cefamandole, cefazolin** and **parenteral cephradine**), < 3 months (**cefuroxime**), < 6 months (**cefixime**), < 9 months (**oral cephradine**) and < 1 year (**ceforanide**) have not been established.

Safety and efficacy for use of **cefoperazone** and **cefotetan** in children have not been established.

Precautions:

Superinfection: Use of antibiotics (especially prolonged or repeated therapy) may result in bacterial or fungal overgrowth of nonsusceptible organisms. Such overgrowth may lead to a secondary infection. Take appropriate measures if superinfection occurs.

Parenteral use: Inject preparations for IM administration deep into the musculature; properly dilute preparations for IV injection and administer over an appropriate time interval. See individual product monographs. Prolonged or high dosage IV use may be associated with thrombophlebitis; use small IV needles, larger veins and alternate infusion sites.

Gonorrhea: In the treatment of gonorrhea, all patients should have a serologic test for syphilis. Patients with incubating syphilis (seronegative without clinical signs of syphilis) are likely to be cured by the regimens used for gonorrhea.

(Continued on following page)

Drug Interactions:

Alcohol, ethyl: Alcoholic beverages consumed concurrently with or up to 72 hours after cefamandole, cefoperazone, moxalactam or cefotetan may produce acute alcohol intolerance (disulfiram-like reaction). These four antibiotics possess a methyltetrazolethiol side chain that may inhibit aldehyde dehydrogenase. The reaction begins within 30 minutes after alcohol ingestion and may subside 30 minutes to several hours afterwards; the reaction may occur up to 3 days after the last dose of the antibiotic.

Aminoglycosides: Nephrotoxicity of the aminoglycosides may be potentiated by the coadministration of some cephalosporins, specifically cephalothin. No interaction has occurred between tobramycin and ceftazidime or cefotaxime. Monitor renal function closely.

Anticoagulants, oral: Hypoprothrombinemic effects of anticoagulants may be increased by cephalosporins with the methyltetrazolethiol side chain (cefamandole, cefoperazone, cefotetan, moxalactam). Bleeding complications may occur. See Warnings. Although a causal relationship has not been clearly established, bleeding disorders have occurred with some of the other cephalosporins; therefore, the risk of bleeding episodes might be increased in anticoagulated patients. The concurrent use of heparin may also theoretically increase the risk of bleeding.

Bacteriostatic agents (eg, chloramphenicol) may interfere with the bactericidal action of cephalosporins, particularly in acute infections where organisms are proliferating rapidly; avoid concurrent administration with bacteriostatic agents.

Polypeptide antibiotics (eg, colistimethate): The nephrotoxic effects of colistimethate may be increased by cephalothin. Monitor renal function.

Probenecid administered concurrently with cephalosporins may increase and prolong plasma levels by competitively inhibiting renal tubular secretion. This interaction is most significant for those cephalosporins eliminated primarily by tubular secretion.

Drug/Lab Test Interactions: A false-positive reaction for **urine glucose** may occur with Benedict's solution, Fehling's solution or with *Clinitest* tablets, but not with enzyme-based tests such as *Clinistix* and *Tes-Tape*. **Moxalactam** does not interfere with *Clinitest*. There may be a false-positive test for **proteinuria** with acid and denaturization-precipitation tests.

Cephradine may cause false-positive reactions in urinary protein tests that use sulfosalicylic acid.

Cefuroxime may cause a false-negative reaction in the ferricyanide test for **blood glucose**.

A false-positive direct **Coombs' test** has occurred in some patients receiving cephalosporins, particularly those with azotemia, in hematologic studies, in transfusion crossmatching procedures when **antiglobulin tests** are performed on the minor side or in Coombs' testing of newborns of mothers receiving cephalosporins before parturition. This reaction is nonimmunological.

Cephalosporins may falsely elevate **urinary 17-ketosteroid** values.

High concentrations of **cephalothin** or **cefoxitin** (> 100 mcg/ml) may interfere with measurement of **creatinine levels** by the Jaffe reaction and produce false results. Serum samples from cefoxitin-treated patients should not be analyzed for creatinine if obtained within 2 hours of drug administration. **Cefotetan** may also affect these measurements.

Adverse Reactions:

Most common: GI disturbances and hypersensitivity phenomena. The latter are more likely to occur in individuals who have previously demonstrated hypersensitivity and in those with a history of allergy, asthma, hay fever or urticaria.

Hypersensitivity (see Warnings): Most common reactions appear as urticaria, pruritis or morbilliform eruptions. Other reactions: Drug fever; eosinophilia; maculopapular rash; joint pain; chest tightness; myalgia; angioedema; edema; erythema; erythema multiforme; itching; rash; exfoliative dermatitis; numbness; chills; Stevens-Johnson syndrome; toxic epidermal necrolysis (rare); severe bronchospasm (oral cefuroxime, one case).

Serum sickness-like reactions: See Warnings.

GI: Nausea, vomiting; diarrhea; anorexia; dysgeusia; dysuria; glossitis; abdominal pain; flatulence; heartburn; stomach cramps; gallbladder sludge; cholestasis; dyspepsia. Colitis, including pseudomembranous colitis, can appear during or after treatment (see Warnings). Adverse GI effects may occur after parenteral administration of some cephalosporins.

(Adverse Reactions continued on following page)

Adverse Reactions (Cont.):

Hematologic: Eosinophilia; transient neutropenia; lymphocytosis; leukocytosis; leukopenia; thrombocythemia; thrombocytopenia; agranulocytosis; granulocytopenia; hemolytic anemia; bone marrow depression; pancytopenia; decreased platelet function; bleeding in association with hypoprothrombinemia; anemia; aplastic anemia; hemorrhage; transient thrombocytosis. Lymphocytosis, lymphopenia, monocytosis, basophilia, jaundice, glycosuria, bronchospasm, palpitations and epistaxis occurred rarely with **ceftriaxone**. Neutropenia due to an immunologic reaction and characterized by rapid destruction of peripheral neutrophils may require drug discontinuation. Transient fluctuations in leukocyte count with **cefaclor,** predominantly lymphocytosis, occurred in infants and young children. Slight decreases in neutrophil count and decreased hemoglobin or hematocrit, disturbances in vitamin K-dependent clotting function (increased PT), increased platelets and increased bleeding have occurred (see Warnings).

Hepatic: Elevated AST, ALT, GGTP, total bilirubin, alkaline phosphatase, LDH; hepatomegaly; hepatitis. One case of significantly elevated liver enzymes accompanied by clinical signs and symptoms of hepatitis has occurred with **cefoperazone**. Values tend to return to normal after the end of therapy. Cholestatic jaundice has occurred with **cefaclor, cephalexin** and **cefamandole**.

Renal: Transitory elevations in BUN with and without elevated serum creatinine (frequency increases in patients > 50 years old and in children < 3); pyuria; dysuria; reversible interstitial nephritis; hematuria; toxic nephropathy; acute renal failure (rare). **Cefamandole** may cause decreased creatinine clearance in patients with prior renal impairment. Casts in the urine have been noted with **ceftriaxone**.

CNS: Headache; dizziness; lethargy; fatigue; paresthesia; confusion; diaphoresis; flushing; generalized tonic-clonic seizures, mild hemiparesis and extreme confusion following large doses of **cefazolin** in renal failure.

Local: Administration IM commonly results in pain, induration, temperature elevation and tenderness. Sterile abscesses have occurred following accidental SC injection. Administration IV or IM has produced local swelling, inflammation, burning, cellulitis, paresthesia, phlebitis and thrombophlebitis.

Miscellaneous: Hypotension, fever, dyspnea and interstitial pneumonitis. Candidal overgrowth consisting of oral candidiasis, vaginitis, genital moniliasis, vaginal discharge and genito-anal pruritus has been reported. Elevated CPK following IM injection of **ceforanide** has occurred. Reversible hyperactivity, nervousness, insomnia, confusion, hypertonia, dizziness and somnolence (causal relationship unknown).

Overdosage:

Parenteral cephalosporins: Inappropriately large doses may cause seizures, particularly in renal impairment. Reduce dosage when renal function is impaired. If seizures occur, promptly discontinue the drug; administer anticonvulsant therapy if clinically indicated and consider hemodialysis in cases of overwhelming overdosage.

Administration:

Duration of therapy: Continue administration for a minimum of 48 to 72 hours after fever abates or after evidence of bacterial eradication has been obtained. A minimum of 10 days of treatment is recommended for infections caused by group A β-hemolytic streptococci to guard against the risk of rheumatic fever or glomerulonephritis.

Perioperative prophylaxis: Discontinue prophylactic administration within 24 hours after the surgical procedure. In surgery where infection may be particularly devastating (eg, open heart surgery and prosthetic arthroplasty), prophylactic administration may be continued for 3 to 5 days following the completion of surgery. If there are signs of infection, obtain cultures and perform sensitivity tests so that appropriate therapy may be instituted.

Patient Information (oral preparations):

Complete full course of therapy.

May cause GI upset; may take with food or milk.

Notify your physician or pharmacist if you have experienced allergic reactions to the cephalosporins, penicillins or their relatives.

Notify physician of nausea, vomiting or diarrhea, especially if the diarrhea is severe or contains blood, mucus or pus.

Notify physician if breast-feeding; cephalosporins enter breast milk.

A false-positive reaction for urine glucose may occur with the nonspecific urine tests. Use an enzyme-based test.

Diabetic patients receiving cephradine – Notify physician before changing diet or dosage of diabetes medication.

(Continued on following page)

Complete prescribing information for these products begins on page 1733

CEFACLOR

Indications:

Lower respiratory tract infections, including pneumonia caused by *S pneumoniae, H influenzae* and *S pyogenes* (group A β-hemolytic streptococci).

Upper respiratory tract infections, including pharyngitis and tonsillitis caused by *S pyogenes* (group A β-hemolytic streptococci).

Otitis media caused by *S pneumoniae, H influenzae,* staphylococci and *S pyogenes* (group A β-hemolytic streptococci).

Skin and skin structure infections caused by *S aureus* and *S pyogenes* (group A β-hemolytic streptococci).

Urinary tract infections including pyelonephritis and cystitis caused by *E coli, P mirabilis, Klebsiella* species and coagulase-negative staphylococci.

Unlabeled Uses: A single 2 g dose may be effective for acute uncomplicated UTI in select populations.

Administration and Dosage:

Adults: Usual dosage is 250 mg every 8 hours. In severe infections or those caused by less susceptible organisms, dosage may be doubled.

Children: Give 20 mg/kg/day in divided doses, every 8 hours. In more serious infections, otitis media and infections caused by less susceptible organisms, administer 40 mg/kg/day, with a maximum dosage of 1 g/day.

Twice daily treatment option: For otitis media and pharyngitis, the total daily dosage may be divided and administered every 12 hours.

Refrigerate suspension after reconstitution; discard after 14 days. **C.I.***

Rx	**Ceclor** (Lilly)	**Pulvules (Capsules):** 250 mg	(#Lilly 3061 Ceclor 250 mg). White and purple. In 15s, 100s and UD 100s.	56
		500 mg	(#Lilly 3062). Gray and purple. In 15s, 100s and UD 100s.	55
		Powder for Oral Suspension: 125 mg per 5 ml	Strawberry flavor. In 75 and 150 ml.	54
		187 mg per 5 ml	Strawberry flavor. In 50 and 100 ml.	53
		250 mg per 5 ml	Strawberry flavor. In 75 and 150 ml.	50
		375 mg per 5 ml	Strawberry flavor. In 50 and 100 ml.	48

CEPHALEXIN

Indications: *Respiratory tract infections* due to *S pneumoniae* and group A β-hemolytic streptococci.

Otitis media caused by *S pneumoniae, H influenzae,* staphylococci, streptococci and *M catarrhalis* (monohydrate only).

Skin and skin structure infections caused by staphylococci or streptococci.

Bone infections caused by staphylococci or *Proteus mirabilis*.

GU infections, including acute prostatitis, caused by *E coli, P mirabilis* and *Klebsiella* sp.

Administration and Dosage:

Adults: 1 to 4 g/day in divided doses. Usual dose – 250 mg every 6 hours. Streptococcal pharyngitis, skin and skin structure infections, uncomplicated cystitis in patients > 15 years – 500 mg every 12 hours. May need larger doses for more severe infections or less susceptible organisms. If dose is > 4 g/day, use parenteral drugs.

Children (monohydrate): 25 to 50 mg/kg/day in divided doses. For streptococcal pharyngitis in patients > 1 year and for skin and skin structure infections, divide total daily dose and give every 12 hours. In severe infections, double the dose. *Otitis media* – 75 to 100 mg/kg/day in 4 divided doses. *β-hemolytic streptococcal infections* – Continue treatment for at least 10 days.

HCl monohydrate – Safety and efficacy not established for use in children.

* Cost Index based on cost per 100 mg.
\# Product identification code.

(Products listed on following page)

CEPHALEXIN MONOHYDRATE

				C.I.*
Rx	**Cephalexin** (Various, eg, Geneva, Goldline, Lederle, Lemmon, Lyphomed, Major, Rugby, Schein, Squibb-Mark, Zenith)	**Capsules:** 250 mg	In 20s, 28s, 30s, 40s, 100s, 500s, 1000s and UD 100s.	7+
Rx	**Cefanex** (Apothecon)		In 100s.	NA
Rx	**Keflex** (Dista)		(402). White and dark green. In 20s, 100s and UD 100s.	36
Rx	**Cephalexin** (Various, eg, Geneva, Goldline, Lederle, Lemmon, Lyphomed, Major, Rugby, Schein, Squibb-Mark, Zenith)	**Capsules:** 500 mg	In 14s, 20s, 28s, 30s, 40s, 100s, 250s, 500s, 1000s and UD 100s and 500s.	7+
Rx	**Biocef** (Inter. Ethical Labs)		In 100s.	NA
Rx	**Cefanex** (Apothecon)		In 100s.	NA
Rx	**Keflex** (Dista)		(403). Two-tone green. In 20s, 100s and UD 100s.	35
Rx	**Cephalexin** (Various, eg, Balan, Barr, Best, Goldline, Harber, Major, Moore, Parmed, Schein, Warner Chilcott)	**Tablets:** 250 mg	Capsule shaped. In 100s and 500s.	13+
Rx	**Keflet** (Dista)		(4202). Light blue-green. In 100s.	36
Rx	**Cephalexin** (Various, eg, Balan, Barr, Best, Goldline, Harber, Major, Moore, Parmed, Schein, Warner-Chilcott)	**Tablets:** 500 mg	Capsule shaped. In 100s and 500s.	13+
Rx	**Keflet** (Dista)		(4203). Dark green. In 100s.	35
Rx	**Cephalexin** (Major)	**Tablets:** 1 g	In 24s.	21
Rx	**Keflet** (Dista)		(1896). Dark green. In 24s and UD 100s.	32
Rx	**Cephalexin** (Various, eg, Best, Geneva, Goldline, Lederle, Lemmon, Lyphomed, Major, Rugby, Schein, Squibb-Mark)	**Oral Suspension:**[1] 125 mg/5 ml	In 100 and 200 ml.	17+
Rx	**Biocef** (Inter. Ethical Labs)		In 100 ml.	NA
Rx	**Keflex** (Dista)		In 60, 100, 200 and UD 5 ml.	35
Rx	**Cephalexin** (Various, eg, Best, Geneva, Goldline, Lederle, Lemmon, Lyphomed, Major, Rugby, Schein, Squibb-Mark)	**Oral Suspension:**[1] 250 mg/5 ml	In 100 and 200 ml.	12+
Rx	**Biocef** (Inter. Ethical Labs)		In 100 ml.	NA
Rx	**Keflex** (Dista)		In 100, 200 and UD 5 ml.	33
Rx	**Keflex** (Dista)	**Pediatric Oral Suspension:**[1] 100 mg/ml (5 mg/drop)	In 10 ml, with dropper calibrated at 25 and 50 mg.	38

CEPHALEXIN HCl MONOHYDRATE

Cephalexin HCl monohydrate does not require conversion in the stomach before absorption.

				C.I.*
Rx	**Keftab** (Dista)	**Tablets:** 250 mg	(4142). Light green. In 100s.	30
		500 mg	(4143). Dark green. In 100s.	29

* Cost Index based on cost per 100 mg.

[1] Refrigerate reconstituted suspension; discard after 14 days.

Complete prescribing information for these products begins on page 1733

CEFADROXIL

Indications:

Urinary tract infections caused by *Escherichia coli, Proteus mirabilis* and *Klebsiella* species.

Skin and skin structure infections caused by staphylococci or streptococci.

Pharyngitis and tonsillitis caused by group A β-hemolytic streptococci.

Administration and Dosage:

Can be given without regard to meals. Shake suspension well before using.

Urinary tract infections: For uncomplicated lower urinary tract infection (ie, cystitis), the usual dosage is 1 or 2 g/day in single or 2 divided doses. For all other urinary tract infections, the usual dosage is 2 g/day in 2 divided doses.

Skin and skin structure infections: 1 g/day in single or 2 divided doses.

Pharyngitis and tonsillitis: Group A β-hemolytic streptococci – 1 g/day in single or 2 divided doses for 10 days.

Children: Urinary tract infections, skin and skin structure infections – 30 mg/kg/day in divided doses every 12 hours. *Pharyngitis, tonsillitis* – 30 mg/kg/day in single or 2 divided doses. For β-hemolytic streptococcal infections, continue treatment for at least 10 days.

Renal impairment: Adjust dosage according to creatinine clearance rates to prevent drug accumulation. *Initial adult dose* – 1 g; the maintenance dose (based on creatinine clearance rate, ml/min/1.73 m^2) is 500 mg at the intervals below:

Cefadroxil Dosage in Renal Impairment	
Creatinine Clearance (ml/min)	Dosage Interval (hours)
0-10	36
10-25	24
25-50	12
>50	No adjustment

	Product	Form	Package	C.I.*
Rx	**Cefadroxil** (Various, eg, Best, Bioline, Geneva, Goldline, Lemmon, Major, Rugby, Schein, Warner-Chilcott, Zenith)	**Capsules:** 500 mg[1]	In 50s and 100s.	32+
Rx	**Duricef** (Mead Johnson)		In 20s, 50s, 100s and UD 100s.	42
Rx	**Ultracef** (Bristol Labs)		In 50s, 100s and UD 100s.	45
Rx	**Cefadroxil** (Various, eg, Bioline, Goldline, Lemmon, Zenith)	**Tablets:** 1 g[1]	In 24s and 100s.	35+
Rx	**Duricef** (Mead Johnson)		In 24s, 50s, 100s and UD 100s.	40
Rx	**Ultracef** (Bristol Labs)		In UD 100s.	35
Rx	**Cefadroxil** (Various, eg, Biocraft, Bioline, Goldline, Major)	**Oral Suspension:**[2] 125 mg/5 ml	In 50 and 100 ml.	65+
Rx	**Duricef** (Mead Johnson)		Orange-pineapple flavor. In 50 and 100 ml.	67
Rx	**Ultracef** (Bristol Labs)		In 50 and 100 ml.	70
Rx	**Cefadroxil** (Various, eg, Biocraft, Bioline, Goldline, Major)	**Oral Suspension:**[2] 250 mg/5 ml	In 50 and 100 ml.	58+
Rx	**Duricef** (Mead Johnson)		Orange-pineapple flavor. In 50 and 100 ml.	63
Rx	**Ultracef** (Bristol Labs)		In 50 and 100 ml.	65
Rx	**Cefadroxil** (Various, eg, Biocraft, Goldline, Major)	**Oral Suspension:**[2] 500 mg/5 ml	In 100 ml.	39+
Rx	**Duricef** (Mead Johnson)		Orange-pineapple flavor. In 50 and 100 ml.	44

* Cost Index based on cost per 100 mg.

\# Product identification code.

[1] As monohydrate.

[2] Refrigerate reconstituted suspension; discard after 14 days.

Complete prescribing information for these products begins on page 1733

CEPHRADINE

Indications:

Oral:

Respiratory tract infections (eg, tonsillitis, pharyngitis and lobar pneumonia) caused by group A β-hemolytic streptococci and *Streptococcus pneumoniae.*

Otitis media caused by group A β-hemolytic streptococci, *S pneumoniae, Hemophilus influenzae* and staphylococci.

Skin and skin structure infections caused by staphylococci (penicillinase/nonpenicillinase-producing) and β-hemolytic streptococci.

Urinary tract infections, including prostatitis, caused by Escherichia coli, Proteus mirabilis and *Klebsiella* species.

Cephradine may be used in the treatment of some enterococcal *(S faecalis)* infections confined to the urinary tract. The high concentrations of cephradine achieved in the urinary tract will be effective against many strains of enterococci for which disc susceptibility studies indicate relative resistance. Ampicillin is the drug of choice for enterococcal urinary tract *(S faecalis)* infections.

Parenteral:

Respiratory tract infections due to *S pneumoniae, Klebsiella* sp, *H influenzae, S aureus* (penicillinase/nonpenicillinase-producing) and group A β-hemolytic streptococci.

Urinary tract infections due to *E coli, P mirabilis* and *Klebsiella* sp.

Skin and skin structure infections due to *S aureus* (penicillinase/nonpenicillinase-producing) and group A β-hemolytic streptococci.

Bone infections due to *S aureus* (penicillinase/nonpenicillinase-producing).

Septicemia due to *S pneumoniae, S aureus* (penicillinase/nonpenicillinase-producing), *P mirabilis* and *E coli.*

Perioperative prophylaxis administration (preoperatively, intraoperatively and postoperatively) may reduce the incidence of certain postoperative infections in patients undergoing surgical procedures (eg, vaginal hysterectomy) that are classified as contaminated or potentially contaminated.

In cesarean section, intraoperative (after clamping the umbilical cord) and postoperative use may reduce the incidence of certain postoperative infections.

Effective perioperative use depends on time of administration. Give 30 to 90 minutes before surgery, which is sufficient time to achieve effective tissue levels.

Dosage:

Oral: May be given without regard to meals.

Adults – Skin, skin structures and respiratory tract infections (other than lobar pneumonia): Usual dose is 250 mg every 6 hours or 500 mg every 12 hours.

For lobar pneumonia: 500 mg every 6 hours or 1 g every 12 hours.

For uncomplicated urinary tract infections: The usual dose is 500 mg every 12 hours. In more serious infections and prostatitis, 500 mg every 6 hours or 1 g every 12 hours. Severe or chronic infections may require larger doses (up to 1 g every 6 hours).

Children – No adequate information is available on the efficacy of twice a day regimens in children less than 9 months of age. For children over 9 months, the usual dose is 25 to 50 mg/kg/day, in equally divided doses every 6 or 12 hours. For otitis media due to *H influenzae*, 75 to 100 mg/kg/day in equally divided doses every 6 or 12 hours is recommended; do not exceed 4 g/day.

All patients, regardless of age and weight – Larger doses (up to 1 g 4 times/day) may be given for severe or chronic infections.

Parenteral: Parenteral therapy may be followed by oral. To minimize pain and induration, inject IM deep into a large muscle mass.

Adults – Daily dose is 2 to 4 g in equally divided doses 4 times/day, IM or IV. In bone infections, the usual dosage is 1 g IV, 4 times/day. A dose of 500 mg, 4 times/day is adequate in uncomplicated pneumonia, skin and skin structure infections and most urinary tract infections. In severe infections, dose may be increased by giving every 4 hours or by increasing dose up to a maximum of 8 g/day.

Perioperative prophylaxis: Recommended doses are 1 g IV or IM administered 30 to 90 minutes prior to start of surgery, followed by 1 g every 4 to 6 hours after the first dose for 1 or 2 doses, or for up to 24 hours postoperatively.

Cesarean section: Give 1 g IV as soon as the umbilical cord is clamped. Give the second and third doses as 1 g IM or IV at 6 and 12 hours after the first dose.

(Dosage continued on following page)

CEPHRADINE (Cont.)

Dosage (Cont.):

Parenteral (Cont.): Infants and children – 50 to 100 mg/kg/day in 4 equally divided doses; determine by age, weight and infection severity. Weigh benefits of use in infants < 1 yr against risks. In neonates, accumulation of other cephalosporins (with resultant half-life prolongation) may occur. Do not exceed adult dose.

Pediatric Dosage of Cephradine

Weight		50 mg/kg/day		100 mg/kg/day	
lbs	kg	Approx. single dose (mg q 6 h)	Volume needed @ 208 mg/ml	Approx. single dose (mg q 6 h)	Volume needed @ 227 mg/ml
10	4.5	56	0.27 ml	112	0.5 ml
20	9.1	114	0.55 ml	227	1 ml
30	13.6	170	0.82 ml	340	1.5 ml
40	18.2	227	1.1 ml	455	2 ml
50	22.7	284	1.4 ml	567	2.5 ml

Renal impairment dosage: Patients not on dialysis – Use the following initial dosage schedule as a guideline based on creatinine clearance. Further modification in the dosage schedule may be required because of individual variations in absorption.

Cephradine Dosage in Renal Impairment

Ccr (ml/min)	Dose (mg)	Time Interval (hours)
> 20	500	6
5 to 20	250	6
< 5	250	12

Patients on chronic, intermittent hemodialysis – 250 mg initially; repeat at 12 hours and after 36 to 48 hours. Children may require dosage modification proportional to their weight and severity of infection.

Administration:

IM: Add Sterile Water for Injection or Bacteriostatic Water for Injection.

IV: A 3 mcg/ml serum concentration can be maintained for each mg of cephradine/kg of body weight per hour of infusion.

Direct IV – Add 5 ml of diluent to the 250 or 500 mg vials, 10 ml to the 1 g vial or 20 ml to the 2 g bottle. Inject slowly over 3 to 5 minutes or give through tubing.

Diluents for direct IV injection are: Sterile Water for Injection; 5% Dextrose Injection; Sodium Chloride Injection.

Continuous or intermittent IV infusion – Add 10 or 20 ml of Sterile Water for Injection or a suitable infusion fluid to the 1 g vial or 2 g bottles, respectively, to prepare solution. Withdraw entire contents; transfer to an IV infusion container.

2 g IV bottle: Reconstitute with 40 ml; infuse directly.

Infusion solutions include: 5% and 10% Dextrose Injection; Sodium Chloride Injection; M/6 Sodium Lactate; Dextrose and Sodium Chloride Injection; 10% Invert Sugar in Water; *Normosol-R; Ionosol B* with 5% Dextrose. Use Sterile Water for Injection at a concentration of 30 to 50 mg/ml.

Stability and Storage: Use IM or direct IV solutions within 2 hours at room temperature. Solutions refrigerated at 5°C (41°F) retain potency for 24 hours. The IV infusion solutions retain potency for 10 hours at room temperature or 48 hours at 5°C (41°F); infusion solutions in Sterile Water for Injection, frozen immediately after reconstitution, are stable for 6 weeks at –20°C (–4°F). For prolonged infusions, replace the infusion every 10 hours with fresh solution. Protect from concentrated light or direct sunlight.

Oral Suspension – Do not store above 86°F prior to reconstitution. After reconsitution, suspensions retain their potency for 7 days at room temperature and 14 days if refrigerated.

Admixture Incompatibility: Do not mix cephradine with other antibiotics. Do not use with Lactated Ringer's Injection.

(Products listed on following page)

CEPHRADINE (Cont.)

				C.I.*
Rx	**Cephradine** (Various, eg, Baxter, Biocraft, Geneva, Lederle, Lemmon, Major, Parmed, Rugby, Schein, Zenith)	**Capsules:** 250 mg	In 24s, 100s, 500s and UD 100s.	18+
Rx	**Velosef** (Apothecon)		(Squibb 113). In 24s, 100s and UD 100s.	31
Rx	**Cephradine** (Various, eg, Baxter, Biocraft, Geneva, Lederle, Lemmon, Major, Parmed, Rugby, Schein, Zenith)	**Capsules:** 500 mg	In 24s, 100s, 500s and UD 100s.	18+
Rx	**Velosef** (Apothecon)		(Squibb 114). In 24s, 100s and UD 100s.	30
Rx	**Cephradine** (Various, eg, Barr, Biocraft, Major, Parmed, Schein)	**Oral Suspension:** 125 mg/5 ml when reconstituted	In 100 ml.	26+
Rx	**Velosef** (Apothecon)		Fruit flavor. In 100, 200 and UD 5 ml.	34
Rx	**Cephradine** (Various, eg, Barr, Biocraft, Major, Parmed, Schein)	**Oral Suspension:** 250 mg/5 ml when reconstituted	In 100 ml.	23+
Rx	**Velosef** (Apothecon)		Fruit flavor. In 100, 200 and UD 5 ml.	33
Rx	**Velosef** (Apothecon)	**Powder for Injection:**[1] 250 mg	In vials.	467
		500 mg	In vials.	413
		1 g	In vials.	389
		2 g	In 100 ml infusion bottles.	386

* Cost Index based on cost per 100 mg oral, 500 mg parenteral.
[1] Contains 6 mEq (136 mg) sodium per g.

LORACARBEF

Indications:

Lower respiratory tract:

Secondary bacterial infection of acute bronchitis and *acute bacterial exacerbations of chronic bronchitis* caused by *S pneumoniae, H influenzae* (including β-lactamase-producing strains) or *M catarrhalis* (including β-lactamase-producing strains).

Pneumonia caused by *S pneumoniae* or *H influenzae* (non-β-lactamase-producing strains only).

Upper respiratory tract:

Otitis media caused by *S pneumoniae, H influenzae* (including β-lactamase-producing strains), *M catarrhalis* (including β-lactamase-producing strains) or *S pyogenes*.

Acute maxillary sinusitis caused by *S pneumoniae, H influenzae* (non-β-lactamase-producing strains only) or *M catarrhalis* (including β-lactamase-producing strains).

In a patient population with significant numbers of β-lactamase-producing organisms, loracarbef's clinical cure and bacteriological eradication rates were somewhat less than those observed with a product containing a β-lactamase inhibitor. Take into account loracarbef's decreased potential for toxicity compared to products containing β-lactamase inhibitors along with the susceptibility patterns of the common microbes.

Pharyngitis and tonsillitis caused by *S pyogenes*. The usual drug of choice in the treatment and prevention of streptococcal infections, including the prophylaxis of rheumatic fever, is IM penicillin. Loracarbef is generally effective in the eradication of *S pyogenes* from the nasopharynx; however, data establishing the efficacy of loracarbef in the subsequent prevention of rheumatic fever are not available at present.

Skin and skin structure:

Uncomplicated skin and skin structure infections caused by *S aureus* (including penicillinase-producing strains) or *S pyogenes*. Surgically drain abscesses as clinically indicated.

Urinary tract:

Uncomplicated UTIs (cystitis) caused by *E coli* or *S saprophyticus*†.

In considering the use of loracarbef in the treatment of cystitis, weigh its lower bacterial eradication rates and lower potential for toxicity against the increased eradication rates and increased potential for toxicity demonstrated by some other classes.

Uncomplicated pyelonephritis caused by *E coli*.

† Efficacy for this organism in this organ system was studied in fewer than 10 infections.

(Continued on following page)

LORACARBEF (Cont.)

Administration and Dosage:

Approved by the FDA on December 31, 1991.

Administer at least 1 hour before or 2 hours after a meal.

Dosage/Duration of Loracarbef		
Population/Infection	Dosage (mg)	Duration (days)
Adults ≥ 13 years of age		
Lower respiratory tract		
Secondary bacterial infection of acute bronchitis	200-400 q 12 h	7
Acute bacterial exacerbation of chronic bronchitis	400 q 12 h	7
Pneumonia	400 q 12 h	14
Upper respiratory tract		
Pharyngitis/Tonsillitis	200 q 12 h	10[1]
Sinusitis	400 q 12 h	10
Skin and skin structure		
Uncomplicated	200 q 12 h	7
Urinary tract		
Uncomplicated cystitis	200 q 24 h	7
Uncomplicated pyelonephritis	400 q 12 h	14
Infants and children (6 months to 12 years)		
Upper respiratory tract		
Acute otitis media[2]	30 mg/kg/day in divided doses q 12 h	10
Pharyngitis/Tonsillitis	15 mg/kg/day in divided doses q 12 h	10[1]
Skin and skin structure		
Impetigo	15 mg/kg/day in divided doses q 12 h	7

[1] In the treatment of infections due to *S pyogenes,* administer for at least 10 days.

[2] Use the suspension; it is more rapidly absorbed than the capsules, resulting in higher peak plasma concentrations when administered at the same dose.

Loracarbef Pediatric Suspension Dosage									
Weight		Daily dose 15 mg/kg/day				Daily dose 30 mg/kg/day			
		100 mg/5 ml twice daily		200 mg/5 ml twice daily		100 mg/5 ml twice daily		200 mg/5 ml twice daily	
lb	kg	ml	tsp	ml	tsp	ml	tsp	ml	tsp
15	7	2.6	0.5	—	—	5.2	1	2.6	0.5
29	13	4.9	1	2.5	0.5	9.8	2	4.9	1
44	20	7.5	1.5	3.8	0.75	—	—	7.5	1.5
57	26	9.8	2	4.9	1	—	—	9.8	2

Renal function impairment: Use the usual dose and schedule in patients with creatinine clearance (Ccr) levels of ≥ 50 ml/min. Patients with Ccr between 10 and 49 ml/min may be given half of the recommended dose at the usual dosage interval. Patients with Ccr levels < 10 ml/min may be treated with the recommended dose given every 3 to 5 days; patients on hemodialysis should receive another dose following dialysis.

When only the serum creatinine is available, the following formula may be used to convert this value into Ccr. The equation assumes the patient's renal function is stable.

$$\text{Males: } \frac{\text{Weight (kg)} \times (140 - \text{age})}{72 \times \text{serum creatinine (mg/dl)}} = \text{Ccr} \qquad \text{Females: } 0.85 \times \text{male value}$$

Reconstitution of oral suspension: Add 30 or 60 ml water in 2 portions to the dry mixture in the 50 or 100 ml bottle, respectively.

Storage/Stability: After mixing, the suspension may be kept at room temperature, 15° to 30°C (59° to 86°F), for 14 days without significant loss of potency. Keep tightly closed. Discard unused portion after 14 days.

Rx	**Lorabid** (Lilly)	**Pulvules (capsules):** 200 mg	(3170). Blue/gray. In 30s.
		Powder for suspension: 100 mg/5 ml	Parabens. Strawberry bubble gum flavor. In 100 ml.

Complete prescribing information for these products begins on page 1733

CEFPROZIL

Indications:

Pharyngitis/tonsillitis caused by *Streptococcus pyogenes.*

Note: The usual drug of choice in the treatment and prevention of streptococcal infections, including the prophylaxis of rheumatic fever, is penicillin given by the IM route. Cefprozil is generally effective in the eradication of *S pyogenes* from the nasopharynx; however, substantial data establishing the efficacy of cefprozil in the subsequent prevention of rheumatic fever are not available at present.

Otitis media caused by *S pneumoniae, Hemophilus influenzae* and *Moraxella (Branhamella) catarrhalis.*

Note: In the treatment of otitis media due to beta-lactamase producing organisms, cefprozil had bacteriologic eradication rates somewhat lower than those observed with a product containing a specific beta-lactamase inhibitor. In considering the use of cefprozil, balance lower overall eradication rates against the susceptibility patterns of the common microbes in a given geographic area and the increased potential for toxicity with products containing beta-lactamase inhibitors.

Secondary bacterial infection of acute bronchitis and acute bacterial exacerbation of chronic bronchitis caused by *S pneumoniae, H influenzae* (beta-lactamase positive and negative strains), and *Moraxella catarrhalis.*

Uncomplicated skin and skin structure infections caused by *Staphylococcus aureus* (including penicillinase-producing strains) and *S pyogenes.* Abscesses usually require surgical drainage.

Administration and Dosage:

Approved by the FDA in December 1991.

Cefprozil is administered orally.

Dosage and Duration of Ceprozil		
Population/Infection	Dosage (mg)	Duration (days)
Adults (≥ 13 years of age)		
Upper respiratory tract		
Pharyngitis/Tonsillitis	500 q 24 h	10*
Lower respiratory tract		
Secondary bacterial infection of acute bronchitis and acute bacterial exacerbation of chronic bronchitis	500 q 12 h	10
Skin and skin structure		
Uncomplicated skin and skin structure infections	250 q 12 h or 500 q 24 h or 500 q 12 h	10
Infants and children (6 months to 12 years)		
Otitis media	15 mg/kg q 12 h	10

* In the treatment of infections due to *Streptococcus pyogenes,* administer for at least 10 days.

Renal function impairment: Cefprozil may be administered to patients with impaired renal function. Use the following dosage schedule.

Cefprozil Dosage in Renal Impairment		
Creatinine clearance (ml/min)	Dosage (mg)	Dosing interval
30 to 120	standard	standard
0 to 30*	50% of standard	standard

* Cefprozil is in part removed by hemodialysis; therefore, administer cefprozil after the completion of hemodialysis.

Storage/Stability: Suspension – After reconstitution, store in a refrigerator and discard unused portion after 14 days.

Rx	**Cefzil** (Bristol Labs)	**Tablets:** 250 mg (as anhydrous)	(BMS 7720 250). Light orange. Film coated. In 100s and UD 100s.
		500 mg (as anhydrous)	(BMS 7721 500). White. Film coated. In 100s and UD 100s.
Rx	**Cefzil** (Bristol Labs)	**Powder for suspension:** 125 mg/5 ml (as anhydrous)[1]	Bubble gum flavor. In 50 and 100 ml.
		250 mg/5 ml (as anhydrous)[1]	Bubble gum flavor. In 50 and 100 ml.

[1] With aspartame (28 mg/5 ml phenylalanine) and sucrose.

Complete prescribing information for these products begins on page 1733

CEPHALOTHIN SODIUM

Indications:

Respiratory tract infections caused by *Streptococcus pneumoniae,* staphylococci (penicillinase/nonpenicillinase-producing), group A β-hemolytic streptococci, *Klebsiella* species and *Hemophilus influenzae.*

Skin and soft tissue infections, including peritonitis, caused by staphylococci (penicillinase/nonpenicillinase-producing), group A β-hemolytic streptococci, *Escherichia coli, Proteus mirabilis* and *Klebsiella* species.

Genitourinary tract infections caused by *E coli, P mirabilis* and *Klebsiella* species.

Septicemia, including endocarditis, caused by *S pneumoniae,* staphylococci (penicillinase/nonpenicillinase-producing), group A β-hemolytic streptococci, *S viridans, E coli, P mirabilis* and *Klebsiella* species.

Gastrointestinal infections caused by *Salmonella* and *Shigella* species.

Meningitis caused by *S pneumoniae,* group A β-hemolytic streptococci and staphylococci (penicillinase/nonpenicillinase-producing).

Because only low drug levels are found in the cerebrospinal fluid, the drug is not reliable in treatment of meningitis and cannot be recommended for that purpose. However, the drug has been effective in a number of cases of meningitis, and may be considered for unusual circumstances in which other more reliable antibiotics cannot be used.

Bone and joint infections caused by staphylococci (penicillinase/nonpenicillinase-producing).

Perioperative prophylaxis to reduce the incidence of certain postoperative infections in patients undergoing contaminated or potentially contaminated surgical procedures (eg, vaginal hysterectomy). Perioperative use also may be effective in surgical patients in whom infection at the operative site would present a serious risk (eg, open heart surgery, prosthetic arthroplasty).

Dosage:

Adults: 500 mg to 1 g every 4 to 6 hours.

Uncomplicated pneumonia, furunculosis with cellulitis, most urinary tract infections – 500 mg every 6 hours.

Severe infections – Increase the dose to 1 g or administer 500 mg every 4 hours.

Life-threatening infections – Up to 2 g every 4 hours.

Normal renal function (bacteremia, septicemia or other severe or life-threatening infections): The IV dosage is 4 to 12 g daily. In conditions such as septicemia, 6 to 8 g per day may be administered IV for several days at the beginning of therapy; reduce the dosage gradually.

Infants and children: The dosage is proportionately less according to age, weight and severity of infection. Daily administration of 100 mg/kg (80 to 160 mg/kg or 40 to 80 mg/lb) in divided doses is effective for most infections susceptible to cephalothin.

Perioperative prophylaxis:

Preoperative – 1 to 2 g administered IV ½ to 1 hour prior to initial incision.

Intraoperative – 1 to 2 g during surgery, administered according to the duration of surgery.

Postoperative – 1 to 2 g every 6 hours; discontinue within 24 hours after surgery. If there are signs of infection, obtain specimens for culture and sensitivity testing and institute appropriate therapy.

Children – 20 to 30 mg/kg given at the times designated above.

Renal function impairment: Give an IV loading dose of 1 to 2 g. Determine the continued dosage schedule by degree of renal impairment, severity of infection and susceptibility of the causative organism. Base maximum doses on the following recommendations:

Cephalothin Dosage in Renal Impairment		
Renal function	Creatinine clearance (ml/min)	Maximum adult dosage (maintenance)
Mild impairment	50 - 80	2 g every 6 hours
Moderate impairment	25 - 50	1.5 g every 6 hours
Severe impairment	10 - 25	1 g every 6 hours
Marked impairment	2 - 10	0.5 g every 6 hours
Essentially no function	< 2	0.5 g every 8 hours

(Continued on following page)

CEPHALOTHIN SODIUM (Cont.)

Administration:

Administer IV or by deep IM injection. The IV route may be preferable in bacteremia, septicemia or other severe or life-threatening infections.

IM: Administer deeply IM into a large muscle mass (eg, the gluteus or lateral aspect of the thigh) to minimize pain and induration.

Intermittent IV administration: Slowly inject a solution of 1 g in 10 ml diluent directly into the vein over 3 to 5 minutes, or give through IV tubing.

Intermittent infusion with Y-type administration set: Can be accomplished while bulk IV solutions are infused. However, during infusion, discontinue the other solutions.

Continuous IV infusion: 1 or 2 g of cephalothin, diluted and mixed with at least 10 ml of Sterile Water for Injection, may be added to an IV container of one of the following IV solutions: Acetated Ringer's Injection; 5% Dextrose Injection; 5% Dextrose in Lactated Ringer's Injection; *Ionosol B* in D5-W; *Isolyte M* with 5% Dextrose; Lactated Ringer's Injection; *Normosol-M* in D5-W; *Plasma-Lyte Injection; Plasma-Lyte-M* in 5% Dextrose; Ringer's Injection; 0.9% Sodium Chloride Injection.

Intraperitoneal: Cephalothin has been added to peritoneal dialysis fluid in concentrations up to 6 mg/100 ml and instilled into the peritoneal cavity throughout an entire dialysis (16 to 30 hours); 44% was absorbed. Serum levels of 10 mcg/ml were reported; accumulation and untoward local or systemic reactions were not evident.

Intraperitoneal administration of 0.1% to 4% cephalothin solutions in saline has been used to treat peritonitis or contaminated peritoneal cavities. (The total daily dosage should take into account the amount given by the intraperitoneal route.)

Preparation of solution: For IM use, reconstitute each gram with 4 ml Sterile Water for Injection. If the vial contents do not completely dissolve, add an additional small amount of diluent (0.2 to 0.4 ml) and warm the contents slightly.

Stability and storage: Concentrated solutions will darken, especially at room temperature; slight discoloration is permissible.

Room temperature – Give solutions for IM injection within 12 hours after reconstitution. Start IV infusions within 12 hours and complete within 24 hours. For prolonged infusion, replace with a freshly prepared solution at least every 24 hours.

Refrigeration – The solution is stable for 96 hours after reconstitution. Redissolve solutions which precipitate by warming to room temperature and constantly agitating.

Freezing – Solutions in Sterile Water for Injection, 5% Dextrose Injection or 0.9% Sodium Chloride Injection frozen immediately after reconstitution in the original container are stable for 12 weeks when stored at −20°C (−4°F). If warmed, avoid heating after thawing is complete; do not refreeze.

				C.I.*
Rx	**Cephalothin Sodium** (Baxter)	**Injection:**[1] 1 g in 5% Dextrose	Premixed, frozen. In 50 ml single dose *Viaflex Plus* containers.	399
		2 g in 5% Dextrose	Premixed, frozen. In 50 ml single dose *Viaflex Plus* containers.	264
Rx	**Cephalothin Sodium** (Various, eg, Lyphomed, Pasadena)	**Powder for Injection:**[2] 1 g	In 10 ml vials and 100 ml piggyback vials.	137+
Rx	**Keflin, Neutral** (Lilly)		In 10 and 100 ml vials and Faspak.	144
Rx	**Cephalothin Sodium** (Lyphomed)	**Powder for Injection:**[2] 2 g	In 20 ml vials and 100 ml piggyback vials.	137
Rx	**Keflin, Neutral** (Lilly)		In 20 and 100 ml vials and Faspak.	144
Rx	**Keflin, Neutral** (Lilly)	**Powder for Injection:**[2] 20 g	In 200 ml vials.	144

* Cost Index based on cost per 500 mg.

[1] Contains 2.4 mEq sodium/g

[2] Contains 2.8 mEq sodium/g

Complete prescribing information for these products begins on page 1733

CEPHAPIRIN SODIUM

Indications:

Respiratory tract infections caused by *Streptococcus pneumoniae, Staphylococcus aureus* (penicillinase/nonpenicillinase-producing), *Klebsiella* sp, *Hemophilus influenzae* and group A β-hemolytic streptococci.

Skin and skin structure infections caused by *S aureus* (penicillinase/nonpenicillinase-producing), *S epidermidis* (methicillin-susceptible strains), *Escherichia coli, Proteus mirabilis, Klebsiella* sp and group A β-hemolytic streptococci.

Urinary tract infections caused by *S aureus* (penicillinase/nonpenicillinase-producing), *E coli, P mirabilis* and *Klebsiella* species.

Septicemia caused by *S aureus* (penicillinase/nonpenicillinase-producing), *S viridans, E coli, Klebsiella* sp and group A β-hemolytic streptococci.

Endocarditis caused by *S viridans* and *S aureus* (penicillinase/nonpenicillinase-producing).

Osteomyelitis caused by *S aureus* (penicillinase/nonpenicillinase-producing), *Klebsiella* sp, *P mirabilis* and group A β-hemolytic streptococci.

Perioperative prophylaxis: Preoperative and postoperative administration may reduce the incidence of certain postoperative infections in patients undergoing contaminated or potentially contaminated surgical procedures (eg, vaginal hysterectomy).

Perioperative use may also be effective in surgical patients in whom infection at the operative site would present a serious risk (eg, open heart surgery and prosthetic arthroplasty).

Dosage:

Adults: 500 mg to 1 g every 4 to 6 hours IM or IV. The lower dose is adequate for certain infections, such as skin and skin structure and most urinary tract infections; the higher dose is recommended for more serious infections.

Serious or life-threatening infections - Up to 12 g daily. Use the IV route when high doses are indicated.

Renal function impairment – Depending upon the causative organism and the severity of infection, patients with reduced renal function (moderately severe oliguria or serum creatinine > 5 mg/100 ml) may be treated adequately with a lower dose, 7.5 to 15 mg/kg every 12 hours. Patients who are to be dialyzed should receive the same dose just prior to dialysis and every 12 hours thereafter.

Perioperative prophylaxis – 1 to 2 g IM or IV administered ½ to 1 hour prior to the start of surgery; 1 to 2 g during surgery (administration modified depending on the duration of the operation); 1 to 2 g IV or IM every 6 hours for 24 hours postoperatively.

Give the preoperative dose just prior to surgery (½ to 1 hour) so that adequate antibiotic levels are present in the serum and tissues at initial surgical incision. Administer cephapirin, if necessary, at appropriate intervals during surgery to provide sufficient levels of the antibiotic at the anticipated moments of greatest exposure to infective organisms.

In surgery in which the occurrence of infection may be particularly devastating (eg, open heart surgery and prosthetic arthroplasty), prophylactic administration may be continued for 3 to 5 days following surgery.

Children: Dosage is in accordance with age, weight and severity of infection. Recommended total daily dose is 40 to 80 mg/kg (20 to 40 mg/lb) administered in 4 equally divided doses.

Infants: Cephapirin has not been extensively studied in infants; therefore, in the treatment of children < 3 months of age, consider the relative benefit to risk.

Administration:

IM: Reconstitute the 500 mg and 1 g vials with 1 or 2 ml of Sterile Water for Injection or Bacteriostatic Water for Injection, respectively. Each 1.2 ml contains 500 mg of cephapirin. Inject deep in the muscle mass.

(Administration continued on following page)

CEPHAPIRIN SODIUM (Cont.)

Administration (Cont.):

IV: Patients with bacteremia, septicemia or other severe or life-threatening infections may be poor risks because of resistance-lowering conditions such as malnutrition, trauma, surgery, diabetes, heart failure and malignancy. The IV route may be preferable in these patients particularly if shock is present or impending.

Intermittent IV injection – Dilute the 500 mg or 1 or 2 g vial with 10 ml or more diluent and give slowly over 3 to 5 minutes, or administer with IV infusions.

Piggyback vials contain labeled quantities of cephapirin for IV use. Diluent and volume are specified on the label.

Intermittent IV infusion with Y-tube – Can be accomplished while bulk IV solutions are being infused. However, during infusion, discontinue the other solution. When Y-tube arrangement is used, dilute 4 g vial with 40 ml Bacteriostatic Water for Injection, Dextrose Injection or Sodium Chloride Injection.

Pharmacy bulk package – Add 67 ml of Sodium Chloride Injection or Dextrose Injection. The resulting solution contains 250 mg cephapirin activity per ml. Reconstituted solutions are stable for 24 hours at room temperature or 10 days under refrigeration.

Stability:

Stability of Cephapirin in Various Diluents

Diluent	Approximate Concentration (mg/ml)	Stability Time	
		25°C	4°C
Water for Injection	50 to 400	12 hrs	10 days
Bacteriostatic Water for Injection	250 to 400	48 hrs	10 days
Normal Saline	20 to 100	24 hrs	10 days
5% Dextrose in Water	20 to 100	24 hrs	10 days

Solutions can be frozen immediately after reconstitution and stored at –15°C (5°F) for 60 days before use. After thawing at room temperature (25°C; 77°F), solutions are stable for at least 12 hours at room temperature or 10 days under refrigeration (4°C; 39°F).

Compatibility with infusion solutions: Stable and compatible for 24 hours at room temperature at concentrations between 2 and 30 mg/ml in the following solutions: Sodium Chloride Injection; 5% Sodium Chloride in Water; 5%, 10% and 20% Dextrose in Water; Sodium Lactate Injection; 10% Invert Sugar in Normal Saline or Water; 5% Dextrose + 0.2% or 0.45% Sodium Chloride Injection; 5% Dextrose in Normal Saline; Lactated Ringer's Injection; Lactated Ringer's with 5% Dextrose; Ringer's Injection; Sterile Water for Injection; 5% Dextrose in Ringer's Injection; *Normosol R; Normosol R* in 5% Dextrose Injection; *Ionosol D-CM; Ionosol G* in 10% Dextrose Injection.

Cephapirin 4 mg/ml is stable and compatible for 10 days under refrigeration (4°C; 39°F) or 14 days in the frozen state (–15°C; 5°F) followed by 24 hours at room temperature (25°C; 77°F) in all solutions listed above.

				C.I.*
Rx	**Cephapirin Sodium** (Lyphomed)	**Powder for Injection:**[1] 500 mg	In 10 ml vials.	229
Rx	**Cefadyl** (Apothecon)		In vials.	229
Rx	**Cephapirin Sodium** (Lyphomed)	**Powder for Injection:**[1] 1 g	In 10 and 100 ml vials.	188
Rx	**Cefadyl** (Apothecon)		In vials and piggyback vials.	188
Rx	**Cephapirin Sodium** (Various, eg, Lyphomed, VHA Supply)	**Powder for Injection:**[1] 2 g	In 20 and 100 ml vials.	145+
Rx	**Cefadyl** (Apothecon)		In vials and piggyback vials.	186
Rx	**Cephapirin Sodium** (Lyphomed)	**Powder for Injection:**[1] 4 g	In 100 ml vials.	191
Rx	**Cefadyl** (Apothecon)		In piggyback vials.	187
Rx	**Cephapirin Sodium** (Lyphomed)	**Powder for Injection:**[1] 20 g	In 100 ml vials.	186
Rx	**Cefadyl** (Apothecon)		In bulk packages.	180

* Cost Index based on cost per 500 mg.

[1] Contains 2.36 mEq sodium per g.

Complete prescribing information for these products begins on page 1733

CEFAZOLIN SODIUM

Indications:

Respiratory tract infections due to *Streptococcus pneumoniae, Klebsiella* species, *Hemophilus influenzae, Staphylococcus aureus* (penicillinase/nonpenicillinase-producing) and group A β-hemolytic streptococci.

Genitourinary tract infections due to *Escherichia coli, Proteus mirabilis, Klebsiella* species and some strains of *Enterobacter* and enterococci.

Skin and skin structure infections due to *S aureus* (penicillinase/nonpenicillinase-producing) and group A β-hemolytic streptococci and other strains of streptococci.

Biliary tract infections due to *E coli,* various strains of streptococci, *P mirabilis, Klebsiella* species and *S aureus.*

Bone and joint infections due to *S aureus.*

Septicemia due to *S pneumoniae, S aureus* (penicillinase/nonpenicillinase-producing), *P mirabilis, E coli* and *Klebsiella* species.

Endocarditis due to *S aureus* (penicillinase/nonpenicillinase-producing) and group A β-hemolytic streptococci.

Perioperative prophylaxis may reduce the incidence of certain postoperative infections in patients undergoing contaminated or potentially contaminated surgical procedures (eg, vaginal hysterectomy and cholecystectomy in high risk patients such as those over 70 years of age, with acute cholecystitis, obstructive jaundice or common duct bile stones).

May also be effective in surgical patients in whom infection at the operative site would present a serious risk (eg, open heart surgery and prosthetic arthroplasty).

Dosage:

Total daily dosages are the same for IV and IM administration.

Mild infections caused by susceptible gram-positive cocci: 250 to 500 mg every 8 hours.

Moderate to severe infections: 500 mg to 1 g every 6 to 8 hours.

Pneumococcal pneumonia: 500 mg every 12 hours.

Severe, life-threatening infections (eg, endocarditis, septicemia): 1 to 1.5 g every 6 hours. Rarely, 12 g per day have been used.

Acute uncomplicated urinary tract infections: 1 g every 12 hours.

Perioperative prophylaxis:

Preoperative – 1 g IV or IM, ½ to 1 hour prior to surgery.

Intraoperative (2 hours or more) – 0.5 to 1 g IV or IM during surgery at appropriate intervals.

Postoperative – 0.5 to 1 g IV or IM every 6 to 8 hours for 24 hours after surgery. Prophylactic administration may be continued for 3 to 5 days, especially where the occurrence of infection may be particularly devastating (eg, open heart surgery, prosthetic arthroplasty).

Renal function impairment: All reduced dosage recommendations apply after an initial loading dose appropriate to the severity of the infection.

Cefazolin Dosage in Renal Impairment

Serum Creatinine (mg%)	Ccr (ml/min)	Dose: Mild to Moderate Infection (mg)	Dose: Moderate to Severe Infection (mg)	Dosage Interval (hrs)
≤ 1.5	≥ 55	250 to 500	500 to 1000	6-8
1.6-3	35-54	250 to 500	500 to 1000	≥ 8
3.1-4.5	11-34	125 to 250	250 to 500	12
≥ 4.6	≤10	125 to 250	250 to 500	18-24

(Dosage continued on following page)

CEFAZOLIN SODIUM (Cont.)

Dosage (Cont.):

Children: Mild to moderately severe infections – A total daily dosage of 25 to 50 mg/kg (approximately 10 to 20 mg/lb) in 3 or 4 equal doses. *Severe infections* – Total daily dosage may be increased to 100 mg/kg (45 mg/lb).

Pediatric Dosage of Cefazolin[1]

Weight		25 mg/kg/day				50 mg/kg/day			
		Approx. single dose		Volume needed @ 125 mg/ml		Approx. single dose		Volume needed @ 225 mg/ml	
lbs	kg	mg q 8 h	mg q 6 h	mg q 8 h	mg q 6 h	mg q 8 h	mg q 6 h	mg q 8 h	mg q 6 h
10	4.5	40	30	0.35 ml	0.25 ml	75	55	0.35 ml	0.25 ml
20	9.1	75	55	0.6 ml	0.45 ml	150	110	0.7 ml	0.5 ml
30	13.6	115	85	0.9 ml	0.7 ml	225	170	1 ml	0.75 ml
40	18.2	150	115	1.2 ml	0.9 ml	300	225	1.35 ml	1 ml
50	22.7	190	140	1.5 ml	1.1 ml	375	285	1.7 ml	1.25 ml

[1] Infants (premature and < 1 month): Safety not established; use is not recommended.

Renal function impairment – Recommendations apply after an initial loading dose.

Ccr 40 to 70 ml/min, 60% of normal daily dose every 12 hrs; Ccr 20 to 40 ml/min, 25% of normal daily dose every 12 hrs; Ccr 5 to 20 ml/min, 10% of normal daily dose every 24 hrs.

Administration:

IM administration: Inject into a large muscle mass. Pain on injection is infrequent.

Intermittent IV infusion: Administer in a volume control set or in a separate, secondary IV container. Reconstituted 500 mg or 1 g may be diluted in 50 to 100 ml of: 0.9% NaCl Injection; 5% or 10% Dextrose Injection; 5% Dextrose in Lactated Ringer's Injection; 5% Dextrose and 0.2%, 0.45% or 0.9% NaCl; Lactated Ringer's Injection; 5% or 10% Invert Sugar in Sterile Water for Injection; 5% Sodium Bicarbonate (*Ancef*); Ringer's Injection; *Normosol-M* in D5-W; *Ionosol B* w/Dextrose 5%; *Plasma-Lyte* with 5% Dextrose.

Direct IV injection: Dilute reconstituted 500 mg or 1 g cefazolin in minimum of 10 ml Sterile Water for Injection. Inject slowly into vein or through IV fluid tubing over 3 to 5 minutes.

Preparation of solution: IM – Reconstitute with Sterile Water, Bacteriostatic Water or 0.9% Sodium Chloride Injections. Shake well until dissolved. *IV* – Dilute as required.

Stability and storage: Reconstituted cefazolin is stable for 24 hours at room temperature, 96 hours refrigerated (5°C; 41°F). Solutions in Sterile Water for Injection, 5% Dextrose Injection or 0.9% Sodium Chloride Injection frozen immediately after reconstitution in original container are stable up to 12 weeks when stored at –20°C (–4°F). If warmed, avoid heating after thawing is complete; do not refreeze. Thaw premixed frozen solution at room temperature. Do not introduce additives. After thawing, it is stable 48 hours at room temperature and 10 days refrigerated. Do not refreeze.

	Product	Form/Strength	Description	C.I.*
Rx	**Cefazolin Sodium** (Apothecon)	**Powder for Injection:** 250 mg	In vials.	NA
		500 mg	In vials and piggyback vials.	NA
		1 g	In vials and piggyback vials.	NA
		5 g	In pharmacy bulk packages.	NA
		10 g	In pharmacy bulk packages.	NA
		20 g	In pharmacy bulk packages.	NA
Rx	**Ancef** (SKF)	**Powder for Injection:**[1] 250 mg	In vials.	266
		500 mg	In vials and piggyback vials.	141
		1 g	In vials and piggyback vials.	141
		5 g	In bulk vials.	141
		10 g	In bulk vials.	141
Rx	**Ancef** (SKF)	**Injection:**[1] 500 mg in 5% Dextrose in Water	Premixed, frozen. In 50 ml plastic containers.	373
		1 g in 5% Dextrose in Water	Premixed, frozen. In 50 ml plastic containers.	253
Rx	**Kefzol** (Lilly)	**Powder for Injection:**[1] 250 mg	In vials.	550
		500 mg	In vials.	328
		1 g	In vials.	328
		10 g	In 100 ml bulk vials.	328
		20 g	In 100 ml bulk vials.	328

* Cost Index based on cost per 500 mg. [1] Contains 2 mEq sodium/g.

(Products continued on following page)

CEFAZOLIN SODIUM (Cont.)

				C.I.*
Rx	**Kefzol** (Lilly)	**Injection:**[1] 500 mg	In 10 ml Redi-vials, Faspacks and *ADD-Vantage* vials.	76
		1 g	In 10 ml Redi-vials, Faspacks and *ADD-Vantage* vials.	352
Rx	**Zolicef** (Apothecon)	**Powder for Injection:**[1] 500 mg	In 10 ml vials.	235
		1 g	In 10 ml vials.	223

* Cost Index based on cost per 500 mg.

[1] Contains 2.1 mEq sodium/g.

CEFMETAZOLE SODIUM

Indications:

Urinary tract infections (complicated or uncomplicated) caused by *E coli.*

Lower respiratory tract infections: Pneumonia and bronchitis caused by *S pneumoniae, S aureus* (penicillinase- and non-penicillinase-producing strains), *E coli, H influenzae* (non-penicillinase-producing strains).

Skin and structure infections: S aureus (penicillinase- and non-penicillinase-producing strains), *S epidermidis, S pyogenes, S agalactiae, E coli, P mirabilis, P vulgaris*, M morganii*, P stuartii*, K pneumoniae, K oxytoca*, B fragilis* and *B melaninogenicus.**

Intra-abdominal infections: E coli, K pneumoniae, K oxytoca*, B fragilis, C perfringens.**

Prophylaxis: Preoperative administration may reduce the incidence of certain postoperative infections in patients who undergo cesarean section, abdominal or vaginal hysterectomy, cholecystectomy (high-risk patients) and colorectal surgery.

Administration and Dosage:

Adults: General guidelines – 2 g IV every 6 to 12 hours for 5 to 14 days.

Prophylaxis:

Cefmetazole Dosing Regimen for Prophylaxis	
Surgery	Dosing Regimen
Vaginal hysterectomy	2 g single dose 30 to 90 minutes before surgery or 1 g doses 30 to 90 minutes before surgery and repeated 8 and 16 hours later
Abdominal hysterectomy	1 g doses 30 to 90 minutes before surgery and repeated 8 and 16 hours later
Cesarean section	2 g single dose after clamping cord or 1 g doses after clamping cord; repeated at 8 and 16 hours
Colorectal surgery	2 g single dose 30 to 90 minutes before surgery or 2 g doses 30 to 90 minutes before surgery and repeated 8 and 16 hours later
Cholecystectomy (high risk)	1 g doses 30 to 90 minutes before surgery and repeated 8 and 16 hours later

Renal function impairment:

Cefmetazole Dosage Guidelines in Renal Function Impairment			
Renal Function	Creatinine Clearance (ml/min/1.73 m²)	Dose (g)	Frequency (hrs)
Mild impairment	50-90	1 to 2	q 12
Moderate impairment	30-49	1 to 2	q 16
Severe impairment	10-29	1 to 2	q 24
Essentially no function	< 10	1 to 2	q 48[1]

[1] Administered after hemodialysis.

Reconstitution: Reconstitute with Sterile Water for Injection, Bacteriostatic Water for Injection or 0.9% Sodium Chloride Injection.

Stability and storage: Following reconstitution, cefmetazole maintains satisfactory potency for 24 hours at room temperature (25°C; 77°F) , for 7 days under refrigeration (8°C; 46°F) and for 6 weeks in the frozen state (≤ -20°C; -4°F).

Primary solutions may be further diluted to concentrations of 1 to 20 mg/ml in 0.9% Sodium Chloride Injection, 5% Dextrose Injection or Lactated Ringer's Injection and maintain potency for 24 hours at room temperature (25°C; 77°F), for 7 days under refrigeration (8°C; 46°F) and for 6 weeks in the frozen state (≤-20°C; -4°F).

Do not refreeze thawed solutions. Discard any unused solutions or frozen material.

Rx	**Zefazone** (Upjohn)	**Powder for Injection:** 1 g	In vials.
		2 g	In vials.

* Efficacy of this organism in this organ system was studied in fewer than 10 infections.

Complete prescribing information for these products begins on page 1733

CEFAMANDOLE NAFATE

Indications:

Lower respiratory infections, including pneumonia caused by *Streptococcus pneumoniae, Hemophilus influenzae, Klebsiella* species, *Staphylococcus aureus* (penicillinase/nonpenicillinase-producing), β-hemolytic streptococci and *Proteus mirabilis*.

Urinary tract infections caused by *Escherichia coli, Proteus* species (both indole-negative and positive), *Enterobacter* species, *Klebsiella* species, group D streptococci (*Note:* Most enterococci, eg, *S faecalis*, are resistant) and *S epidermidis*.

Peritonitis caused by *E coli* and *Enterobacter* species.

Septicemia caused by *E coli, S aureus* (penicillinase/nonpenicillinase-producing), *S pneumoniae, S pyogenes* (group A β-hemolytic streptococci), *H influenzae* and *Klebsiella* species.

Skin and skin structure infections caused by *S aureus* (penicillinase/nonpenicillinase-producing), *S pyogenes* (group A β-hemolytic streptococci), *H influenzae, E coli, Enterobacter* species and *P mirabilis*.

Bone and joint infections caused by *S aureus* (penicillinase/nonpenicillinase-producing).

Mixed infections: Nongonococcal pelvic inflammatory disease in females, lower respiratory and skin infections. Cefamandole has been successful in infections in which several organisms were isolated. Most *Bacteroides fragilis* strains are resistant in vitro; however, infections caused by susceptible strains have been treated successfully.

Concomitant aminoglycoside therapy: In confirmed or suspected gram-positive or gram-negative sepsis or in patients with other serious infections in which the causative organism has not been identified, cefamandole may be used concomitantly with an aminoglycoside. Monitor renal function carefully, especially with higher dosages.

Perioperative prophylaxis may reduce the incidence of certain postoperative infections in patients undergoing surgical procedures that are classified as contaminated or potentially contaminated (eg, GI surgery, cesarean section, vaginal hysterectomy or cholecystectomy in high risk patients such as those with acute cholecystitis, obstructive jaundice or common bile duct stones).

In major surgery in which the risk of postoperative infection is low but serious (cardiovascular surgery, neurosurgery or prosthetic arthroplasty), cefamandole may effectively prevent such infections.

Discontinue use after 24 hours; however, in prosthetic arthroplasty, continue for 72 hours. If signs of infection occur, obtain culture specimens for identification of the causative organism so that appropriate antibiotic therapy may be instituted.

Dosage:

Administer IV or by deep IM injection into a large muscle mass to minimize pain.

Adults: Usual dosage range is 500 mg to 1 g every 4 to 8 hours; 500 mg every 6 hours is adequate in uncomplicated pneumonia and skin structure infections. In uncomplicated urinary tract infections, 500 mg every 8 hours; in more serious urinary tract infections, the dose may be increased to 1 g every 8 hours. In severe infections, administer 1 g at 4 to 6 hour intervals. In life-threatening infections or infections due to less susceptible organisms, up to 2 g every 4 hours may be needed.

Infants and children: 50 to 100 mg/kg/day in equally divided doses every 4 to 8 hours is effective for most infections susceptible to cefamandole. This may be increased to 150 mg/kg/day (not to exceed the maximum adult dose) for severe infections.

Perioperative prophylaxis:

Adults - 1 or 2 g IM or IV, ½ to 1 hour prior to the surgical incision, followed by 1 or 2 g every 6 hours for 24 to 48 hours.

Children (3 months of age and older) - 50 to 100 mg/kg/day in equally divided doses by the routes and schedule designated above.

In patients undergoing prosthetic arthroplasty, administer up to 72 hours.

In patients undergoing cesarean section, administer the initial dose just prior to surgery or immediately after the cord has been clamped.

Renal function impairment: Reduce dosages and monitor the serum levels. After an initial dose of 1 to 2 g (depending on the severity of infection), follow maintenance dosage in table. Determine further dosage by degree of renal impairment, severity of infection and susceptibility of the causative organism.

When only serum creatinine is available, use the following formula to obtain creatinine clearance. The serum creatinine should represent steady-state renal function.

$$\text{Males: } \frac{\text{Weight (kg)} \times (140 - \text{age})}{72 \times \text{serum creatinine (mg/dl)}} = \text{Ccr}$$

Females: 0.85 x above value

(Dosage continued on following page)

CEFAMANDOLE NAFATE (Cont.)

Dosage (Cont.):

Maintenance Cefamandole Dosage Guide for Patients with Renal Impairment			
Renal Function	Creatinine Clearance (ml/min/1.73 m²)	Life-threatening Infections (Maximum Dosage)	Less Severe Infections
Normal Impairment	>80	2 g q 4 h	1-2 g q 6 h
Mild Impairment	50-80	1.5 g q 4 h or 2 g q 6 h	0.75-1.5 g q 6 h
Moderate Impairment	25-50	1.5 g q 6 h or 2 g q 8 h	0.75-1.5 g q 8 h
Severe Impairment	10-25	1 g q 6 h or 1.25 g q 8 h	0.5-1 g q 8 h
Marked Impairment	2-10	0.67 g q 8 h or 1 g q 12 h	0.5-0.75 g q 12 h
None	<2	0.5 g q 8 h or 0.75 g q 12 h	0.25-0.5 g q 12 h

Administration:

IM: Dilute each gram with 3 ml of one of the following diluents: Sterile Water for Injection; Bacteriostatic Water for Injection; 0.9% Sodium Chloride Injection; Bacteriostatic Sodium Chloride Injection. Shake well until dissolved.

IV: The IV route may be preferable for bacterial septicemia, localized parenchymal abscesses (ie, intra-abdominal abscess), peritonitis or other severe or life-threatening infections when patients may be poor risks because of lowered resistance. In patients with normal renal function, the IV dosage is 3 to 12 g daily. In conditions such as bacterial septicemia, give 6 to 12 g/day IV initially for several days, and gradually reduce.

Concomitant aminoglycoside therapy – If combination therapy with cefamandole and an aminoglycoside is indicated, administer each of these antibiotics in different sites. Do not mix an aminoglycoside with cefamandole in the same IV fluid container.

Intermittent IV – Reconstitute each gram with 10 ml of Sterile Water for Injection, 5% Dextrose Injection or 0.9% Sodium Chloride Injection. Slowly inject into the vein over 3 to 5 minutes, or through IV fluid containing: 0.9% Sodium Chloride Injection; 5% Dextrose Injection; 5% or 10% Dextrose and 0.2%, 0.45% or 0.9% Sodium Chloride Injection; Sodium Lactate Injection (M/6).

Intermittent IV infusion with a Y-type administration set or volume control set can also be accomplished while any of the mentioned IV fluids are being infused. However, during infusion, discontinue the other solution. When a Y-tube arrangement is used, add 100 ml of the appropriate diluent to the 1 or 2 g piggyback (100 ml) vial. If Sterile Water for Injection is used as the diluent, reconstitute with approximately 20 ml/g to avoid a hypotonic solution.

Continuous IV infusion – Dilute each gram with 10 ml of Sterile Water for Injection. An appropriate quantity of the resulting solution may be added to an IV container of one of the fluids listed under *Intermittent IV* administration.

Stability: Room temperature – Reconstituted cefamandole is stable for 24 hours at room temperature (25°C; 77°F). During storage, carbon dioxide develops inside the vial after reconstitution. This pressure may be dissipated prior to withdrawal of the vial contents, or it may be used to aid withdrawal if the vial is inverted over the syringe needle and the contents are allowed to flow into the syringe.

Refrigeration – The solution is stable for 96 hours when refrigerated (5°C; 41°F).

Freezing – Solutions in Sterile Water for Injection, 5% Dextrose Injection or 0.9% Sodium Chloride Injection that are frozen immediately after reconstitution in the original container are stable for 6 months when stored at -20°C (-4°F). If the product is warmed (to a maximum of 37°C; 99°F), avoid heating after thawing is complete; do not refreeze.

				C.I.*
Rx	**Mandol** (Lilly)	**Powder for Injection:**[1] 500 mg	In 10 ml vials.	416
		1 g	In 10 and 100 ml vials, *ADD-Vantage* vials and Faspacks.	416
		2 g	In 20 and 100 ml vials, *ADD-Vantage* vials and Faspacks.	416
		10 g	In 100 ml vials.	416

* Cost Index based on cost per 500 mg.

[1] Contains 3.3 mEq sodium/g.

Complete prescribing information for these products begins on page 1733

CEFOXITIN SODIUM

Indications:

Cefoxitin and cephalothin were comparable for management of infections caused by susceptible gram-positive cocci and gram-negative rods. Many infections caused by gram-negative bacteria resistant to some cephalosporins and penicillins respond to cefoxitin.

Lower respiratory tract infections (pneumonia and lung abscess) caused by *Streptococcus pneumoniae*, other streptococci (excluding enterococci, eg, *S faecalis*), *Staphylococcus aureus* (penicillinase/nonpenicillinase-producing), *Escherichia coli*, *Klebsiella* species, *Hemophilus influenzae* and *Bacteroides* species.

Urinary tract infections caused by *E coli, Klebsiella* species, *Proteus mirabilis*, indole-positive *Proteus* (ie, *Morganella morganii* and *P vulgaris*) and *Providencia* species (including P rettgeri). Uncomplicated gonorrhea due to *Neisseria gonorrhoeae* (penicillinase/nonpenicillinase-producing).

Intra-abdominal infections (peritonitis and intra-abdominal abscess), caused by *E coli, Klebsiella* species, *Bacteroides* species including *B fragilis* and *Clostridium* species.

Gynecological infections (endometritis, pelvic cellulitis and pelvic inflammatory disease) caused by *E coli, N gonorrhoeae* (penicillinase/nonpenicillinase-producing), *Bacteroides* species including the *B fragilis* group, *Clostridium* species, *Peptococcus* species, *Peptostreptococcus* species and group B streptococci.

Septicemia caused by *S pneumoniae, S aureus* (penicillinase/nonpenicillinase-producing), *E coli, Klebsiella* species and *Bacteroides* species including *B fragilis*.

Bone and joint infections caused by *S aureus* (penicillinase/nonpenicillinase-producing).

Skin and skin structure infections caused by *S aureus* (penicillinase/nonpenicillinase-producing), *S epidermidis*, streptococci (excluding enterococci, eg, *S faecalis*), *E coli, P mirabilis, Klebsiella* species, *Bacteroides* species including the *B fragilis* group, *Clostridium* species, *Peptococcus* species and *Peptostreptococcus* species.

Perioperative prophylaxis may reduce the incidence of certain postoperative infections following surgical procedures (eg, vaginal hysterectomy, GI surgery, transurethral prostatectomy) that are classified as contaminated or potentially contaminated and in patients in whom infection at the operative site would present a serious risk (eg, prosthetic arthroplasty). In cesarean section, intraoperative (after clamping the umbilical cord) and postoperative use may reduce the incidence of postoperative infections.

Give cefoxitin 30 to 60 minutes before the operation, to achieve effective levels in the wound during the procedure. Prophylactic administration should usually be stopped within 24 hours.

Dosage:

Adult dosage range is 1 to 2 g every 6 to 8 hours. Determine dosage and route of administration by susceptibility of the causative organisms, severity of infection and the patient's condition (see table for dosage guidelines). Maintain antibiotic therapy for group A β-hemolytic streptococcal infections for at least 10 days to guard against the risk of rheumatic fever or glomerulonephritis.

Cefoxitin Dosage Guidelines		
Type of Infection	Daily Dosage	Frequency and Route
Uncomplicated (pneumonia, urinary tract, cutaneous)†	3 to 4 g	1 g every 6 to 8 hours IV or IM
Moderately severe or severe	6 to 8 g	1 g every 4 hours or 2 g every 6 to 8 hours IV
Infections commonly requiring higher dosage (eg, gas gangrene)	12 g	2 g every 4 hours or 3 g every 6 hours IV

† Including patients in whom bacteremia is absent or unlikely.

Uncomplicated gonorrhea: 2 g IM with 1 g oral probenecid given concurrently or up to 30 minutes before cefoxitin.

Prophylactic use, surgery: Administer 2 g IV or IM 30 to 60 minutes prior to surgery followed by 2 g every 6 hours after the first dose for no more than 24 hours (continued for 72 hours after prosthetic arthroplasty).

Prophylactic use, cesarean section: Administer 2 g IV as soon as the umbilical cord is clamped. If a three dose regimen is used, give the second and third 2 g dose IV, 4 and 8 hours after the first dose.

Prophylactic use, transurethral prostatectomy: Administer 1 g prior to surgery; 1 g every 8 hours for up to 5 days.

(Dosage continued on following page)

CEFOXITIN SODIUM (Cont.)

Dosage (Cont.):

Renal function impairment: Adults - Initial loading dose is 1 to 2 g. Maintenance doses:

Maintenance Cefoxitin Dosage in Renal Impairment			
Renal Function	Ccr (ml/min/1.73 m²)	Dose (g)	Frequency (hrs)
Mild impairment	30-50	1-2	8-12
Moderate impairment	10-29	1-2	12-24
Severe impairment	5-9	0.5-1	12-24
Essentially no function	<5	0.5-1	24-48

When only serum creatinine level is available, use the following formula to obtain creatinine clearance. Serum creatinine should represent steady-state renal function.

$$\text{Males:} \quad \frac{\text{Weight (kg)} \times (140 - \text{age})}{72 \times \text{serum creatinine (mg/dl)}} = \text{Ccr}$$

Females: 0.85 x above value

Hemodialysis - Administer a loading dose of 1 to 2 g after each hemodialysis. Give the maintenance dose as indicated in the table above.

Infants and Children ≥ 3 months: 80 to 160 mg/kg/day divided every 4 to 6 hours. Use higher dosages for more severe or serious infections. Do not exceed 12 g/day.

Prophylactic use (≥ 3 months) – 30 to 40 mg/kg/dose every 6 hours.

Renal function impairment – Modify consistently with the recommendations for adults.

CDC recommended treatment schedules for gonorrhea and acute pelvic inflammatory disease (PID):[1,2]

Disseminated gonococcal infection - 1 g cefoxitin IV, 4 times/day for at least 7 days for disseminated infections caused by PPNG.

Gonococcal ophthalmia in adults - For PPNG, use 1 g cefoxitin IV, 4 times/day.

Acute PID - For hospitalized patients, give 100 mg doxycycline, IV, twice/day plus 2 g cefoxitin, IV, 4 times/day. Continue drugs IV for at least 4 days and at least 48 hours after patient improves. Continue 100 mg oral doxycycline, twice/day after discharge to complete 10 to 14 days of therapy. For outpatients, give 2 g cefoxitin IM with 1 g oral probenecid, followed by 100 mg oral doxycycline, twice/day for 10 to 14 days.

Administration: *Preparation of solution:*

Preparation of Cefoxitin Solution			
Package Size	Diluent to Add (ml)	≈ Withdrawable Volume (ml)	≈ Concentration (mg/ml)
1 g vial (IM)	2	2.5	400
2 g vial (IM)	4	5	400
1 g vial (IV)	10	10.5	95
2 g vial (IV)	10 or 20	11.1 or 21	180 or 95
1 g infusion bottle (IV)	50 or 100	50 or 100	20 or 10
2 g infusion bottle (IV)	50 or 100	50 or 100	40 or 20
10 g bulk (IV)	43 or 93	49 or 98.5	200 or 100

IV use – Reconstitute 1 g with at least 10 ml of Sterile Water for Injection, and 2 g with 10 to 20 ml. May reconstitute 10 g vial with 43 or 93 ml Sterile Water for Injection or any solutions listed under IV Compatibility and Stability. Benzyl alcohol as a preservative has caused toxicity in neonates. This has not occurred in infants > 3 months of age, but they may also be at risk. Do not use diluents with benzyl alcohol in infants.

IM use – Reconstitute each gram with 2 ml of Sterile Water for Injection or 2 ml of 0.5% lidocaine HCl solution (without epinephrine) to minimize IM injection discomfort.

Administration of solution:

IV administration is preferable for patients with bacteremia, bacterial septicemia or other severe or life-threatening infections, or for patients who are poor risks because of lowered resistance from debilitating conditions (malnutrition, trauma, surgery, diabetes, heart failure, malignancy), particularly if shock is present or impending.

Intermittent IV administration: 1 or 2 g in 10 ml of Sterile Water for Injection over 3 to 5 minutes; may also give over longer periods through an existing system. Temporarily discontinue administration of any other solutions at the same site.

Continuous IV infusion: For higher doses, add solution to an IV container of 5% Dextrose Injection, 0.9% Sodium Chloride Injection, 5% Dextrose and 0.9% Sodium Chloride Injection or 5% Dextrose Injection with 0.02% Sodium Bicarbonate Solution.

[1] Morbidity and Mortality Weekly Report 1985 (Oct 18); 34 (Suppl 4S);75S-108S.
[2] Morbidity and Mortality Weekly Report 1987 (Sep 11); 36 (Suppl 5S);1S-18S.

(Administration continued on following page)

CEFOXITIN SODIUM (Cont.)

Administration (Cont.):

Storage: Store dry powder below 30°C (86°F). Avoid exposure to temperatures above 50°C (122°F). The dry material, as well as solutions, darkens depending on storage conditions; product potency, however, is not adversely affected.

Premixed frozen: Maintains satisfactory potency after thawing for 24 hours at room temperature and 5 days if stored under refrigeration (2° to 8°C; 35.6° to 46.4°F). Discard any unused thawed solutions. Do not refreeze.

Admixture incompatibility: Do not add solutions of cefoxitin to aminoglycoside solutions because of potential interaction; administer separately to the same patient.

Compatibility/Stability: After time periods indicated in table, discard unused solution.

Stability/Storage for Diluents of Cefoxitin

Diluent	24 hrs at Room Temp.	Refrigeration		Freezer	
		48 hours	1 week	26 weeks	30 weeks
Sterile Water for Injection	✓[1,2,3,4]	✓[2]	✓[1,3,4]		✓[1,3]
Bacteriostatic Water for Injection	✓[1,3]		✓[1,3]		✓[1,3]
0.9% Sodium Chloride Injection	✓[1,4,5]	✓[4,5]	✓[1]	✓[5]	✓[1]
5% Dextrose Injection	✓[1,4,6]	✓[6]	✓[1,4]	✓[6]	✓[1]
10% Dextrose Injection	✓[4]		✓[4]		
Lactated Ringer's	✓[4,6]	✓[6]	✓[4]	✓[6]	
5% Dextrose in Lactated Ringer's	✓[4]		✓[4]		
Neut (4% Sodium Bicarbonate)	✓[4]		✓[4]		
Normosol-M in D5-W	✓[4]		✓[4]		
Ionosol B with 5% Dextrose	✓[4]		✓[4]		
10% Mannitol	✓[4]		✓[4]		
5% Dextrose and 0.9% NaCl	✓[4]	✓[4]			
5% Dextrose with 0.02% Sodium Bicarbonate Solution	✓[4]	✓[4]			
5% Dextrose with 0.2% or 0.45% Saline Solution	✓[4]	✓[4]			
Ringer's Injection	✓[4]	✓[4]			
5% or 10% Invert Sugar in Water	✓[4]	✓[4]			
10% Invert Sugar in Saline	✓[4]	✓[4]			
5% Sodium Bicarbonate Injection	✓[4]	✓[4]			
M/6 Sodium Lactate Solution	✓[4]	✓[4]			
Polyonic M56 in 5% Dextrose	✓[4]	✓[4]			
2.5% and 5% Mannitol	✓[4]	✓[4]			
Isolyte E	✓[4]	✓[4]			
Isolyte E with 5% Dextrose	✓[4]	✓[4]			
0.5% or 1% Lidocaine without Epinephrine	✓[3]		✓[3]		✓[3]

[1] When reconstituted to 1 g/10 ml. [2] After reconstitution and subsequent storage in plastic syringes.
[3] After reconstitution for IM use. [4] After reconstitution and further dilution in 50 to 1000 ml.
[5] After storage in IV bags, plastic tubing, drip chambers, volume control devices of IV infusion sets.
[6] After storage in IV bags.

				C.I.*
Rx	**Mefoxin** (MSD)	**Powder for Injection:**[1] 1 g	In vials, infusion bottles and *ADD-Vantage* vials.	426
		2 g	In vials, infusion bottles and *ADD-Vantage* vials.	425
		10 g	In bulk bottles.	425
		Injection: 1 g in 5% Dextrose in Water	Premixed, frozen. In 50 ml plastic containers.	545
		2 g in 5% Dextrose in Water	Premixed, frozen. In 50 ml plastic containers.	484

* Cost Index based on cost per 500 mg.
[1] Contains 2.3 mEq sodium/g.

Complete prescribing information for these products begins on page 1733

CEFUROXIME

Indications:

Oral (axetil): Pharyngitis and tonsillitis caused by *S pyogenes* (group A β-hemolytic streptococci). Penicillin is the usual drug of choice in treatment and prevention of streptococcal infections, including prophylaxis of rheumatic fever. Cefuroxime axetil generally eradicates streptococci from the oropharynx. Not for prophylaxis of subsequent rheumatic fever.

Otitis media caused by *S pneumoniae, H influenzae* (ampicillin-susceptible and -resistant), *M catarrhalis* (ampicillin-susceptible strains) and *S pyogenes* (group A β-hemolytic streptococci).

Lower respiratory tract infections (bronchitis) caused by *S pneumoniae, H influenzae* (ampicillin-susceptible strains), *H parainfluenzae* (ampicillin-susceptible strains).

Urinary tract infections caused by *E coli* and *K pneumoniae* in the absence of urological complications.

Skin and skin structure infections caused by *S aureus* and *S pyogenes* (group A β-hemolytic streptococci).

Uncomplicated gonorrhea (urethral and endocervical) caused by nonpenicillinase-producing strains of *N gonorrhoeae.*

Parenteral: Lower respiratory infections, including pneumonia caused by *S pneumoniae, H influenzae* (including ampicillin-resistant), *Klebsiella* sp, *S aureus* (penicillinase/nonpenicillinase-producing), *S pyogenes, E coli.*

Urinary tract infections caused by *E coli* and *Klebsiella* sp.

Skin and skin structure infections caused by *S aureus* (penicillinase/nonpenicillinase-producing), *S pyogenes, E coli, Klebsiella* sp and *Enterobacter* sp.

Septicemia caused by *S aureus* (penicillinase/nonpenicillinase-producing), *S pneumoniae, E coli, H influenzae* (including ampicillin-resistant strains) and *Klebsiella* sp.

Meningitis caused by *S pneumoniae, H influenzae* (including ampicillin-resistant strains), *N meningitidis* and *S aureus* (penicillinase/nonpenicillinase-producing).

Gonorrhea – Uncomplicated and disseminated gonococcal infections due to *N gonorrhoeae* (penicillinase/nonpenicillinase-producing) in both males and females.

Bone and joint infections caused by *S aureus* (penicillinase/nonpenicillinase-producing).

Mixed infections – Clinical microbiological studies in skin and skin structure infections frequently reveal the growth of susceptible strains of both aerobic and anaerobic organisms. Cefuroxime has been used successfully in these mixed infections in which several organisms have been isolated. In certain cases of confirmed or suspected gram-positive or gram-negative sepsis, or in patients with other serious infections in which the causative organism has not been identified, the drug may be used concomitantly with an aminoglycoside. The recommended doses of both antibiotics may be given, depending on the severity of the infection and on the patient's condition.

Preoperative prophylaxis may reduce incidence of certain postoperative infections in patients undergoing surgical procedures (eg, vaginal hysterectomy) classified as clean-contaminated or potentially contaminated. Stop prophylaxis within 24 hours. Preoperative use is effective during open heart surgery when operative site infections present a serious risk. For these patients, continue therapy at least 48 hours after procedure ends. If infection is present, obtain culture specimens; institute appropriate therapy.

Dosage:

Oral: Adults and children $\geq$ *12 yrs* – 250 mg twice daily. For severe infections or infections caused by less susceptible organisms, increase to 500 mg twice daily.

Uncomplicated urinary tract infections: 125 mg twice daily. Dosage may be increased to 250 mg twice daily for some patients.

Uncomplicated gonorrhea (urethral and endocervical): A single 1 g dose.

Infants and children $<$ *12 yrs* – Usual dosage is 125 mg twice daily.

Otitis media: 125 mg twice a day for children $<$ 2 yrs and 250 mg twice daily for children $\geq$ 2 yrs.

Cefuroxime axetil administered as a crushed tablet has a strong, persistent bitter taste. Consider alternative therapy for children who cannot swallow tablets. In infections due to *S pyogenes,* administer therapeutic dosage for at least 10 days.

Absorption of cefuroxime axetil is enhanced when administered with food.

(Dosage continued on following page)

CEFUROXIME (Cont.)

Dosage (Cont.):

Parenteral: Adults – 750 mg to 1.5 g IM or IV every 8 hours, usually for 5 to 10 days.

Cefuroxime Dosage Guidelines		
Type of Infection	Daily Dosage (g)	Frequency
Uncomplicated urinary tract, skin and skin structure, disseminated gonococcal, uncomplicated pneumonia	2.25	750 mg every 8 hours
Severe or complicated	4.5	1.5 g every 8 hours
Bone and joint	4.5	1.5 g every 8 hours
Life-threatening or due to less susceptible organisms	6	1.5 g every 6 hours
Bacterial meningitis	9	≤ 3 g every 8 hours
Uncomplicated gonococcal	1.5 g IM†	Single dose

† Administered at 2 different sites together with 1 g oral probenecid.

Preoperative prophylaxis – For clean-contaminated or potentially contaminated surgical procedures, administer 1.5 g IV prior to surgery (≈ ½ to 1 hour before). Thereafter, give 750 mg IV or IM every 8 hours when the procedure is prolonged.

For preventive use during open heart surgery, give 1.5 g IV at the induction of anesthesia and every 12 hours thereafter for a total of 6 g.

Renal function impairment – Reduce dosage.

Cefuroxime Dosage in Renal Impairment	
Dosage in Adults with Reduced Function	
Creatinine Clearance (ml/min)	Dose and Frequency
> 20	750 mg to 1.5 g every 8 hours
10-20	750 mg every 12 hours
< 10	750 mg every 24 hours††

†† Since cefuroxime is dialyzable, give patients on hemodialysis a further dose at the end of the dialysis.

When only serum creatinine is available, refer to the formula on p. ix.

Infants and children (over 3 months) – 50 to 100 mg/kg/day in equally divided doses every 6 to 8 hours. Use 100 mg/kg/day (not to exceed the maximum adult dose) for more severe or serious infections.

Bone and joint infections – 150 mg/kg/day (not to exceed maximum adult dose) in equally divided doses every 8 hours. In clinical trials, oral antibiotics were administered to children following the completion of parenteral therapy.

Bacterial meningitis – Initially, 200 to 240 mg/kg/day IV in divided doses every 6 to 8 hours.

In children with renal insufficiency, modify dosage frequency per adult guidelines.

CDC recommended treatment schedules for acute pelvic inflammatory disease:[1]

Cefuroxime 150 mg/kg/day IV plus erythromycin 40 mg/kg/day IV in 4 doses or sulfisoxazole 100 mg/kg/day IV in 4 doses or tetracycline (children > 7 years of age) 30 mg/kg/day IV in 3 doses. Continue for at least 4 days and at least 2 days after marked improvement occurs. Continue the non-cephalosporin agents orally for at least 14 days.

Administration:

Parenteral: IV administration – May be preferable for patients with bacterial septicemia or other severe or life-threatening infections, or for patients who may be poor risks because of lowered resistance, particularly if shock is present or impending.

Direct intermittent IV: Slowly inject solution into a vein over 3 to 5 minutes or give it through the tubing by which the patient receives other IV solutions.

Intermittent IV infusion with a Y-type administration set: Dose through the tubing by which the patient is receiving other IV solutions. However, during infusion, temporarily discontinue administration of other solutions at the same site.

Continuous IV infusion: A solution may be added to an IV bottle containing one of the following fluids: 0.9% Sodium Chloride Injection; 5% or 10% Dextrose Injection; 5% Dextrose and 0.45% or 0.9% Sodium Chloride Injection; M/6 Sodium Lactate Injection.

Premixed, frozen solution: For either continuous or intermittent IV infusion.

[1] Morbidity and Mortality Weekly Report 1985; 34 (Supp 4S):75S-108S.

(Administration continued on following page)

CEFUROXIME (Cont.)

Administration (Cont.):

Parenteral (Cont.):

IM administration – Give by deep IM injection into a large muscle mass. Prior to IM injection, aspiration is necessary to avoid injection into a blood vessel.

Preparation of Cefuroxime Solution and Suspension						
	Kefurox			Zinacef		
Strength	Diluent to Add (ml)	Volume to be Withdrawn (ml)	Approximate Concentration (mg/ml)	Diluent to Add (ml)	Volume to be Withdrawn (ml)	Approximate Concentration (mg/ml)
750 mg vial	3.6 (IM)	3.6[1]	200	3 (IM)	Total[1]	220
750 mg vial	9 (IV)	8	100	8 (IV)	Total	90
1.5 g vial	14 (IV)	Total	100	16 (IV)	Total	90
750 mg Infusion Pack	50 (IV)	—	15	100 (IV)	—	7.5
750 mg Infusion Pack	100 (IV)	—	7.5			
1.5 g Infusion Pack	50 (IV)	—	30	100 (IV)	—	15
1.5 g Infusion Pack	100 (IV)	—	15			
750 mg bottle	50 (IV)	—	15			
750 mg bottle	100 (IV)	—	7.5			
1.5 g bottle	50 (IV)	—	30			
1.5 g bottle	100 (IV)	—	15			
750 mg ADD-Vantage	50 (IV)	—	15			
750 mg ADD-Vantage	100 (IV)	—	7.5			
1.5 g ADD-Vantage	50 (IV)	—	30			
1.5 g ADD-Vantage	100 (IV)	—	15			
7.5 g Pharmacy Bulk Package				77 (IV)	Amount needed[2]	95

[1] Cefuroxime sodium is a suspension at IM concentrations.
[2] 8 ml of solution contains 750 mg cefuroxime; 16 ml of solution contains 1.5 g cefuroxime.

Use Sterile Water for Injection, 5% Dextrose in Water, 0.9% Sodium Chloride or any solution listed under the IV portion of the Compatibility/Stability section. If Sterile Water for Injection is used, reconstitute with ≈ 20 ml/g to avoid a hypotonic solution.

Compatibility/Stability – Discard unused solutions after the specified time periods.

IV: When the 750 mg, 1.5 g and 7.5 g Pharmacy Bulk vials are reconstituted as directed with Sterile Water for Injection, the solutions for IV administration maintain potency for 24 hours at room temperature and for 48 hours (750 mg and 1.5 g vials) and for 7 days (Pharmacy Bulk Vial) when refrigerated at 5°C (41°F). More dilute solutions such as 750 mg or 1.5 g plus 50 to 100 ml Sterile Water for Injection, 5% Dextrose Injection or 0.9% Sodium Chloride Injection maintain potency for 24 hours at room temperature and for 7 days refrigerated.

These solutions may be further diluted to concentrations between 1 and 30 mg/ml in the following solutions, and will lose not more than 10% activity for 24 hours at room temperature or for at least 7 days under refrigeration: 0.9% Sodium Chloride Injection; M/6 Sodium Lactate Injection; Ringer's Injection; Lactated Ringer's Injection; 5% Dextrose and 0.225%, 0.45% or 0.9% Sodium Chloride Injection; 5% or 10% Dextrose Injection; 10% Invert Sugar in Water for Injection.

The following are compatible for 24 hours at room temperature when admixed in IV infusion: Heparin (10 and 50 units/ml) in 0.9% Sodium Chloride Injection and Potassium Chloride (10 and 40 mEq/L) in 0.9% Sodium Chloride Injection.

Sodium bicarbonate injection is not recommended for dilution.

Premixed, frozen solution – Thaw at room temperature or under refrigeration. Do not force thaw by immersion in water bath or by microwave irradiation. Components of the solution may precipitate in the frozen state and will dissolve upon reaching room temperature with little or no agitation. Potency is not affected. Mix after solution has reached room temperature. Do not add supplementary medication. The thawed solution is stable for 21 days under refrigeration (5°C; 41°F) or for 24 hours at room temperature (25°C; 77°F). Do not refreeze. The maximum frozen stability of premixed Zinacef is 12 months from the day of manufacturing when stored at −20°C.

(Administration continued on following page)

CEFUROXIME (Cont.)

Administration (Cont.):

Parenteral (Cont.):

Compatibility/Stability (Cont.):

IM: When reconstituted with Sterile Water for Injection, suspensions for IM injection maintain satisfactory potency for 24 hours at room temperature and for 48 hours when refrigerated at 5°C (41°F).

Frozen, reconstituted: Zinacef – Reconstitute 750 mg or 1.5 or 7.5 g vial as directed for IV administration. Immediately withdraw total contents of 750 mg or 1.5 g vial or 8 or 16 ml from the 7.5 g bulk vial and add to a *Viaflex Mini-bag* containing 50 or 100 ml of 0.9% Sodium Chloride Injection or 5% Dextrose Injection and freeze. Frozen solutions are stable for 6 months when stored at –20°C (–4°F). Thaw frozen solutions at room temperature. Do not refreeze. Do not force thaw by immersion in water bath, or by microwave irradiation. Thawed solutions may be stored for 24 hours at room temperature or 7 days in refrigerator.

Incompatibility – Do not add cefuroxime to aminoglycoside solutions. However, each may be administered separately to the same patient.

Storage: Parenteral – Store cefuroxime in the dry state between 15° and 30°C (59° and 86°F) and protect from light. Powder, solutions and suspensions tend to darken, depending on storage conditions, without adversely affecting the product's potency.

Premixed, frozen – Do not store above –20°C (–4°F).

Patient Information:

Pediatric cefuroxime axetil is only available in tablet form. Children who cannot swallow the tablet whole may have the tablet crushed and mixed with food (eg, applesauce, ice cream) or beverages (eg, orange or grape juice, chocolate milk). However, *the crushed tablet has a strong, persistent, bitter taste*. Discontinuance of therapy due to taste or problems of administration occurred in 13% of children (range, 2% to 28%). Ascertain, preferably while still in physician's office, that the child can ingest cefuroxime axetil reliably. If not, consider alternative therapy.

	Product	Form	Description	C.I.*
Rx	**Ceftin** (Allen & Hanburys)	**Tablets:** (as axetil) 125 mg	(#Glaxo 395). White. Capsule shaped. In 20s, 60s and UD 100s.	220
		250 mg	(#Glaxo 387). Light blue. Capsule shaped. In 20s, 60s and UD 100s.	209
		500 mg	(#Glaxo 394). Dark blue. Capsule shaped. In 20s, 60s and UD 50s.	205
Rx	**Kefurox** (Lilly)	**Powder for Injection:** 750 mg (as sodium). 2.4 mEq sodium/g	In 10 and 100 ml vials, Faspak and *ADD-Vantage* vials.	451
Rx	**Zinacef** (Glaxo)		In vials and infusion pack.	474
Rx	**Kefurox** (Lilly)	**Powder for Injection:** 1.5 g (as sodium). 2.4 mEq sodium/g	In 20 and 100 ml vials, Faspak and *ADD-Vantage* vials.	465
Rx	**Zinacef** (Glaxo)		In vials and infusion pack.	460
Rx	**Zinacef** (Glaxo)	**Powder for Injection:** 7.5 g (as sodium) per vial. 2.4 mEq sodium/g	In Pharmacy Bulk Package.	440
Rx	**Kefurox** (Lilly)		In Pharmacy Bulk Package.	439
Rx	**Zinacef** (Glaxo)	**Injection:** 750 mg (as sodium). 2.4 mEq sodium/g	Premixed, frozen. In 50 ml.	451
		1.5 g (as sodium). 2.4 mEq sodium/g	Premixed, frozen. In 50 ml.	449

* Cost Index based on cost per 250 mg cefuroxime axetil or 500 mg cefuroxime sodium.

Complete prescribing information for these products begins on page 1733

CEFONICID SODIUM

Indications:

Lower respiratory tract infections due to *Streptococcus pneumoniae; Klebsiella pneumoniae**; *Escherichia coli;* and *Hemophilus influenzae* (ampicillin-resistant and ampicillin-sensitive).

Urinary tract infections due to *E coli; Proteus* sp (which may include the organisms now called *Proteus vulgaris**, *Providencia rettgeri* and *Morganella morganii*); and *K pneumoniae.**

Skin and skin structure infections due to *Staphylococcus aureus* and *S epidermidis; S pyogenes* (group A *Streptococcus*) and *S agalactiae* (group B *Streptococcus*).

Septicemia due to *S pneumoniae* and *E coli.**

Bone and joint infections due to *S aureus.*

Preoperative prophylaxis: A single 1 g dose administered before surgery may reduce the incidence of postoperative infections in patients undergoing surgical procedures classified as contaminated or potentially contaminated (eg, colorectal surgery, vaginal hysterectomy or cholecystectomy in high risk patients), or in patients in whom infection at the operative site would present a serious risk (eg, prosthetic arthroplasty, open heart surgery). Although cefonicid is as effective as cefazolin in preventing infection following coronary artery bypass surgery, no placebo controlled trials have evaluated any cephalosporin antibiotic in preventing infections following coronary artery bypass surgery or prosthetic heart valve replacement.

In cesarean section, the use of cefonicid (after the umbilical cord has been clamped) may reduce the incidence of certain postoperative infections.

Dosage:

Adults: Usual dose is 1 g/24 hours, IV or by deep IM injection. Doses > 1 g/day are rarely necessary; however, up to 2 g/day have been well tolerated.

General Cefonicid Dosage Guidelines (IM or IV)		
Type of Infection	Daily Dosage (g)	Frequency
Uncomplicated urinary tract	0.5	once every 24 hours
Mild to moderate	1	once every 24 hours
Severe or life-threatening	2[1]	once every 24 hours
Surgical prophylaxis	1	1 hr preoperatively

[1] When administering 2 g IM doses once daily, divide dose in half and give each half in different large muscle masses.

Preoperative prophylaxis: Administer 1 g, 1 hour prior to appropriate surgical procedures, to provide protection from most infections due to susceptible organisms for approximately 24 hours after administration. Intraoperative and postoperative administration is not necessary. Daily doses may be administered for 2 additional days in patients undergoing prosthetic arthroplasty or open heart surgery.

In cesarean section, administer only after the umbilical cord has been clamped.

Renal function impairment requires modification of dosage. Following an initial loading dosage of 7.5 mg/kg, IM or IV, follow the maintenance schedule below. Individualize further dosing.

Cefonicid Dosage in Adults with Reduced Renal Function		
Creatinine Clearance (ml/min/1.73 m²)	Mild to Moderate Infections	Severe Infections
60-79	10 mg/kg q 24 h	25 mg/kg q 24 h
40-59	8 mg/kg q 24 h	20 mg/kg q 24 h
20-39	4 mg/kg q 24 h	15 mg/kg q 24 h
10-19	4 mg/kg q 48 h	15 mg/kg q 48 h
5-9	4 mg/kg q 3 to 5 days	15 mg/kg q 3 to 5 days
< 5	3 mg/kg q 3 to 5 days	4 mg/kg q 3 to 5 days

Note: It is not necessary to administer additional dosage following dialysis.

Administration:

IM injection: Inject well within the body of a relatively large muscle and aspirate. When administering 2 g IM doses once daily, divide the dose in half and give in different large muscle masses.

(Administration continued on following page)

Complete prescribing information for these products begins on page 1733

CEFONICID SODIUM (Cont.)

Administration (Cont.):

IV administration:

Direct (bolus) injection – Administer reconstituted solution slowly over 3 to 5 minutes, directly or through tubing for patients receiving parenteral fluids (see list below).

Infusion – Dilute reconstituted cefonicid in 50 to 100 ml of one of the following solutions: 0.9% Sodium Chloride Injection; 5% or 10% Dextrose Injection; 5% Dextrose and 0.2%, 0.45% or 0.9% Sodium Chloride Injection; Ringer's Injection; Lactated Ringer's Injection; 5% Dextrose and Lactated Ringer's Injection; 10% Invert Sugar in Sterile Water for Injection; 5% Dextrose and 0.15% Potassium Chloride Injection; Sodium Lactate Injection.

Preparation of solution:

Single dose vials – Reconstitute with Sterile Water for Injection according to the following table. Shake well.

Pharmacy bulk vials – Reconstitute with Sterile Water for Injection, Bacteriostatic Water for Injection or Sodium Chloride Injection according to the following table:

Preparation of Cefonicid Solution			
Vial size	Diluent to add (ml)	≈ Available volume (ml)	≈ Average concentration
500 mg	2	2.2	220 mg/ml
1 g	2.5	3.1	325 mg/ml
10 g	25 45	31 51	333 mg/ml 200 mg/ml

For IV infusion, dilute reconstituted solution in 50 to 100 ml of the parenteral fluids listed under IV administration.

Piggyback vials – Reconstitute with 50 to 100 ml Sodium Chloride Injection or other IV solution listed under IV administration. Give with primary IV fluids as a single dose.

Stability: After reconstitution or dilution, all of these solutions are stable for 24 hours at room temperature or 72 hours if refrigerated (5°C; 41°F).

A solution of 1 g cefonicid in 18 ml Sterile Water for Injection is isotonic.

				C.I.*
Rx	**Monocid** (SmithKline Beecham)	**Powder for Injection:** Contains 3.7 mEq sodium/g		
		500 mg	In vials.	960
		1 g	In vials and piggyback vials.	998
		10 g	In pharmacy bulk vials.	957

* Cost Index based on cost per 500 mg.

CEFTRIAXONE SODIUM

Indications:

Lower respiratory tract infections caused by *Streptococcus pneumoniae, Streptococcus* species (excluding enterococci), *Staphylococcus aureus, Hemophilus influenzae, H parainfluenzae, Klebsiella* species (including *K pneumoniae), Escherichia coli, E aerogenes, Proteus mirabilis* and *Serratia marcescens.*

Skin and skin structure infections caused by *S aureus, S epidermidis, Streptococcus* species (excluding enterococci), *Enterobacter cloacae, Klebsiella* species (including *K pneumoniae*), *P mirabilis* and *Pseudomonas aeruginosa.*

Urinary tract infections (complicated and uncomplicated) caused by *E coli, P mirabilis, P vulgaris, Morganella morganii* and *Klebsiella* species (including *K pneumoniae*).

Uncomplicated gonorrhea (cervical/urethral and rectal) caused by *Neisseria gonorrhoeae,* including both penicillinase/nonpenicillinase-producing strains (considered treatment of choice) and pharyngeal gonorrhea caused by nonpenicillinase producing strains of *N gonorrhoeae*.

Pelvic inflammatory disease caused by *N gonorrhoeae.*

Bacterial septicemia caused by *S aureus, S pneumoniae, E coli, H influenzae* and *K pneumoniae.*

Bone and joint infections caused by *S aureus, S pneumoniae, Streptococcus* species (excluding enterococci), *E coli, P mirabilis, K pneumoniae* and *Enterobacter* species.

Intra-abdominal infections caused by *E coli* and *K pneumoniae.*

Meningitis caused by *H influenzae, N meningitidis* and *S pneumoniae.* Has been used successfully in a limited number of cases of meningitis and shunt infections caused by *S epidermidis* and *E coli.*

(Indications continued on following page)

CEFTRIAXONE SODIUM (Cont.)

Indications (Cont.):

Prophylaxis: The use of a single preoperative dose may reduce the incidence of postoperative infections in patients undergoing surgical procedures classified as contaminated or potentially contaminated (eg, vaginal or abdominal hysterectomy) and in surgical patients for whom infection at the operative site would present serious risk (eg, coronary artery bypass surgery). Ceftriaxone is as effective as cefazolin in preventing infection following coronary artery bypass surgery.

Unlabeled use: Ceftriaxone 2 to 4 g daily IV for 10 to 14 days is effective in treating neurologic complications, arthritis and carditis associated with Lyme disease in patients refractory to penicillin G.

Dosage:

Administer IV or IM. Continue therapy for at least 2 days after signs and symptoms of infection have disappeared. Usual duration is 4 to 14 days; in complicated infections, longer therapy may be required. For *S pyogenes,* continue therapy for at least 10 days.

Adults: Usual daily dose is 1 to 2 g once a day (or in equally divided doses twice a day) depending on type and severity of infection. Do not exceed a total daily dose of 4 g.

Uncomplicated gonococcal infections – Give a single IM dose of 250 mg.

Surgical prophylaxis – Give a single 1 g dose ½ to 2 hours before surgery.

Children: To treat serious infections other than meningitis, administer 50 to 75 mg/kg/day (not to exceed 2 g) in divided doses every 12 hours.

Meningitis – Administer 100 mg/kg/day (not to exceed 4 g) in divided doses every 12 hours, with or without a loading dose of 75 mg/kg.

Skin and skin structure infections – Give 50 to 75 mg/kg once daily (or in equally divided doses twice daily), not to exceed 2 g.

Renal and hepatic impairment: No dosage adjustment is necessary; however, monitor blood levels.

CDC recommended treatment schedules for chancroid, gonorrhea and acute pelvic inflammatory disease (PID):†

Chancroid (Hemophilus ducreyi infection) – 250 mg IM as a single dose.

Gonococcal infections –

Uncomplicated urethral/endocervical/rectal: 250 mg IM once plus doxycycline.
Pharyngeal: 250 mg IM once.
Pregnancy: 250 mg IM once plus erythromycin.
Disseminated: 1 g IM or IV every 24 hours.
Meningitis/Endocarditis: 1 to 2 g IV every 12 hours.
Ophthalmia (adults and children > 20 kg): 1 g IM once.
Children (< 45 kg): 125 mg IM once.
Infants: 25 to 50 mg/kg/day IV or IM in a single daily dose. If born to mothers with gonococcal infection, 50 mg/kg IV or IM once, not to exceed 125 mg.

Acute PID (ambulatory) – 250 mg IM plus doxycycline or tetracycline.

Administration:

Reconstitution of Ceftriaxone			
	Vial/Bottle dosage size	Amount of diluent to add (ml)	Resultant concentration (mg/ml)
IM[1]	250 mg	0.9	250
	500 mg	1.8	250
	1 g	3.6	250
	2 g	7.2	250
IV[2]	250 mg	2.4	100
	500 mg	4.8	100
	1 g	9.6	100
	2 g	19.2	100
Piggy-back[3]	1 g	10	
	2 g	20	

[1] If required, use more dilute solutions. Inject well within the body of a large muscle.
[2] Administer by intermittent infusion. Concentrations between 10 and 40 mg/ml are recommended; however, lower concentrations may be used.
[3] After reconstitution, further dilute to 50 or 100 ml with appropriate IV diluent.

10 g bulk container – This dosage size is not for direct administration. Reconstitute with 95 ml of an appropriate IV diluent. Before parenteral administration, withdraw the required amount, then further dilute to the desired concentration.

† CDC 1989 Sexually Transmitted Diseases Treatment Guidelines. *Morbidity and Mortality Weekly Report* 1989 Sept 1; 38 (No. S-8):1-43.

(Administration continued on following page)

CEFTRIAXONE SODIUM (Cont.)

Administration (Cont.):

Compatibility, Stability and Storage: Do not physically mix with other antimicrobial drugs because of possible incompatibility. Protect from light. After reconstitution, protection from normal light is not necessary.

IM – Solutions remain stable (loss of potency less than 10%) for the following time periods:

Stability/Storage of Ceftriaxone (IM)			
Diluent	Concentration mg/ml	Storage	
		Room Temp (25°C)	Refrigerated (4°C)
Sterile Water for Injection	100 250	3 days 24 hours	10 days 3 days
0.9% Sodium Chloride Solution	100 250	3 days 24 hours	10 days 3 days
5% Dextrose Solution	100 250	3 days 24 hours	10 days 3 days
Bacteriostatic Water and 0.9% Benzyl Alcohol	100 250	24 hours 24 hours	10 days 3 days
1% Lidocaine Solution (without epinephrine)	100 250	24 hours 24 hours	10 days 3 days

IV – At concentrations of 10, 20 and 40 mg/ml, solutions stored in glass or PVC containers and IV solutions at concentrations of 100 mg/ml in the IV piggyback glass containers remain stable (loss of potency less than 10%) for the following time periods:

Stability/Storage of Ceftriaxone (IV)		
Diluent	Storage	
	Room Temp (25°C)	Refrigerated (4°C)
Sterile Water	3 days	10 days
0.9% Sodium Chloride Solution	3 days	10 days
5% or 10% Dextrose Solution	3 days	10 days
5% Dextrose and 0.9% Sodium Chloride Solution†	3 days	Incompatible
5% Dextrose and 0.45% Sodium Chloride Solution	3 days	Incompatible

† Data available for 10 to 40 mg/ml concentrations in this diluent in PVC containers only.

The following IV solutions are stable at room temperature (25°C; 77°F) for 24 hours at concentrations between 10 mg/ml and 40 mg/ml: Sodium Lactate (PVC container), 10% Invert Sugar (glass container), 5% Sodium Bicarbonate (glass container), *Freamine III* (glass container), *Normosol-M* in 5% Dextrose (glass and PVC containers), *Ionosol-B* in 5% Dextrose (glass container), 5% or 10% Mannitol (glass container).

Solutions reconstituted with 5% Dextrose or 0.9% Sodium Chloride solution at concentrations between 10 mg/ml and 40 mg/ml, and then frozen (–20°C; –4°F) in PVC or polyolefin containers, remain stable for 26 weeks. Thaw frozen solutions at room temperature before use. After thawing, discard unused portions. Do not refreeze.

				C.I.*
Rx	**Rocephin** (Roche)	**Powder for Injection:**[1] 250 mg	In vials.	1848
		500 mg	In vials.	1590
		1 g	In vials, piggyback vials and *ADD-Vantage* vials.	1434
		2 g	In vials, piggyback vials and *ADD-Vantage* vials.	1425
		10 g	In bulk containers.	1398
		Injection:[1] 1 g	Premixed, frozen. In 50 ml plastic containers.	1634
		2 g	Premixed, frozen. In 50 ml plastic containers.	1434

* Cost Index based on cost per 500 mg.

[1] Contains 3.6 mEq sodium/g.

Complete prescribing information for these products begins on page 1733

CEFORANIDE

Indications:

Lower respiratory tract infections caused by *Staphylococcus aureus* (penicillinase/nonpenicillinase-producing strains), *Streptococcus pneumoniae, Klebsiella pneumoniae* and *Hemophilus influenzae* (including β-lactamase producing strains).

Urinary tract infections caused by *Escherichia coli, Proteus mirabilis* and *K pneumoniae*.

Skin and skin structure infections caused by *S aureus* (penicillinase/nonpenicillinase-producing strains), *S epidermidis*, group A and group B streptococci, *E coli, P mirabilis* and *K pneumoniae*.

Septicemia caused by *S aureus* (penicillinase/nonpenicillinase-producing strains), *S pneumoniae* and *E coli*.

Bone and joint infections caused by *S aureus* (penicillinase/nonpenicillinase-producing strains).

Endocarditis caused by *S aureus* (penicillinase/nonpenicillinase-producing strains).

Perioperative prophylaxis may reduce the incidence of certain postoperative infections in patients undergoing surgical procedures classified as contaminated or potentially contaminated (eg, vaginal hysterectomy). Administer 1 hour before the operation. Discontinue prophylactic administration, usually not required after the surgical procedure ends, within 24 hours. In most surgical procedures, continuing prophylactic administration does not reduce incidence of subsequent infections but will increase possibility of adverse reactions and development of bacterial resistance.

Perioperative use may also be effective in patients in whom infections at the operative site would present a serious risk (eg, during prosthetic arthroplasty and open heart surgery). Although ceforanide is as effective as cephalothin for preventing infections following coronary artery bypass surgery, no placebo controlled trials have evaluated any cephalosporin for preventing infection following either coronary artery bypass surgery or prosthetic heart valve replacement. In these procedures, prophylactic administration may be continued for 2 days, administered every 12 hours following completion of surgery. If there are signs of infection, obtain culture specimens for the identification of the causative organism so that appropriate therapy may be instituted.

Administration and Dosage:

Adults: The usual dosage range is 0.5 to 1 g every 12 hours IM or IV.

Children: Administer 20 to 40 mg/kg/day in equally divided doses every 12 hours.

Perioperative prophylaxis in contaminated or potentially contaminated surgery: Administer 0.5 to 1 g IM or IV, 1 hour prior to the start of surgery.

In surgery in which infection may be particularly devastating (eg, prosthetic arthroplasty and open heart surgery), prophylactic administration may be continued for 2 days following completion of surgery.

Renal function impairment: Determine dosage by the degree of renal impairment, the severity of infection, the susceptibility of the causative organism and monitoring.

Ceforanide Dosage in Renal Impairment

Creatinine Clearance (ml/min/1.73 m²)	Dosage Interval (hours)
≥ 60	12
20-59	24
5-19	48
< 5	48 to 72*

* Monitoring of plasma ceforanide concentrations is recommended.

If only serum creatinine is available, creatinine clearance may be calculated from the following formula when renal function and serum creatinine levels are at steady state:

Males: $$\frac{\text{Weight (kg)} \times (140 - \text{age})}{72 \times \text{serum creatinine (mg/dl)}} = \text{Ccr}$$

Females: 0.85 x above value

IV administration may be preferable for patients with bacterial septicemia, or other severe or life-threatening infections. These patients may be poor risks because of lowered resistance resulting from such debilitating conditions as malnutrition, trauma, surgery, diabetes, heart failure or malignancy, particularly if shock is present or impending.

IV infusion – Dilute the contents of the 500 mg vial in 5 ml or more of the specified diluent; dilute the 1 g vial in ≥ 10 ml of the specified diluent. Administer slowly by direct IV administration over 3 to 5 minutes or give with IV infusion over 30 minutes.

(Administration and Dosage continued on following page)

CEFORANIDE (Cont.)

Administration and Dosage (Cont.):

IM: Reconstitute 500 mg and 1 g vials with 1.7 and 3.2 ml, respectively, of Bacteriostatic Water for Injection, 0.9% Sodium Chloride Injection, Sterile Water for Injection or Bacteriostatic Sodium Chloride Injection. Each ml contains 250 mg.

Compatibility/Stability:

IM – The 500 mg and 1 g vials, when reconstituted with 1.7 ml and 3.2 ml, respectively, of the solutions listed above, are stable for 48 hours at room temperature (25°C; 77°F), 14 days if refrigerated (4°C; 39°F) and 90 days if frozen (–15°C; 5°F). After thawing, the solution is stable for 48 hours at room temperature.

IV – At concentrations up to 10 mg/ml, ceforanide is stable and compatible for 48 hours at room temperature (25°C: 77°F), for 14 days under refrigeration (4°C; 39°F) and 90 days in the frozen state (–15°C; 5°F) followed by 48 hours at 25°C (77°F) when thawed, in the following infusion solutions: Sterile Water for Injection; 0.9% Sodium Chloride Injection; 5% Dextrose in Water; 5% Dextrose and 0.45% Sodium Chloride Injection; 5% Dextrose and 0.2% Sodium Chloride Injection; Lactated Ringer's Injection; 5% Dextrose in Lactated Ringer's Injection; 10% Dextrose in Water.

Reconstitute piggyback containers with ≥ 10 ml of the appropriate diluent as specified on container label. Following reconstitution, solutions are stable for 48 hours at room temperature, 14 days when refrigerated at 4°C and 90 days when frozen. **C.I.***

Rx	**Precef** (ICN)	**Powder for Injection:** 500 mg	In vials and StrapKap piggyback vials.	755
		1 g	In vials and StrapKap piggyback vials.	653

CEFIXIME

Indications:

Uncomplicated urinary tract infections caused by *E coli* and *P mirabilis*.

Otitis media caused by *H influenzae* (beta-lactamase positive and negative strains), *Moraxella catarrhalis* and *S pyogenes*.

Pharyngitis and tonsillitis caused by *S pyogenes*.

Acute bronchitis and acute exacerbations of chronic bronchitis caused by *S pneumoniae* and *H influenzae* (beta-lactamase positive and negative strains).

Administration and Dosage:

Adults: 400 mg/day as a single 400 mg tablet or as 200 mg every 12 hours.

Children: 8 mg/kg/day suspension as a single daily dose or as 4 mg/kg every 12 hours. Treat children > 50 kg or > 12 years of age with the recommended adult dose.

Pediatric Dosage of Cefixime

Weight		Dose/Day		
lb	kg	mg	tsp of suspension	ml
13	6	46	0.5	2.4
27.5	12.5	100	1	5
42	19	152	1.5	7.6
55	25	200	2	10
77	35	280	3	14

Treat otitis media with the suspension. In clinical studies, the suspension resulted in higher peak blood levels than the tablet administered at the same dosage.

For *S pyogenes* infections, administer cefixime for at least 10 days.

Renal function impairment:

Cefixime Dosage in Renal Impairment

Creatinine Clearance (ml/min)	Dosage
> 60	Standard
21-60 or renal hemodialysis	75% of standard
≤ 20 or continuous ambulatory peritoneal dialysis	50% of standard

C.I.*

Rx	**Suprax** (Lederle)	**Tablets:** 200 mg	(#Suprax 200 LL). White, scored. Film coated. In 100s.	487
		400 mg	(#Suprax 400 LL). White, scored. Film coated. In 50s and 100s.	414
		Powder for Oral Suspension: 100 mg/5 ml	Strawberry flavor. In 50 and 100 ml.	754

* Cost Index based on cost per 500 mg ceforanide or 400 mg cefixime. # Product identification code.

Complete prescribing information for these products begins on page 1733

CEFOPERAZONE SODIUM

Indications:

Respiratory tract infections caused by *Streptococcus pneumoniae, Hemophilus influenzae, Staphylococcus aureus* (penicillinase/nonpenicillinase-producing), *S pyogenes** (group A β-hemolytic streptococci), *Pseudomonas aeruginosa, Klebsiella pneumoniae, Escherichia coli, Proteus mirabilis* and *Enterobacter* sp.

Peritonitis and other intra-abdominal infections caused by *E coli, P aeruginosa**, enterococci, anaerobic gram-negative bacilli (including *Bacteroides fragilis*).

Bacterial septicemia caused by *S pneumoniae, S agalactiae*, S aureus,* enterococci, *P aeruginosa*, E coli, Klebsiella* sp*, *Proteus* sp* (indole-positive and indole-negative), *Clostridium* sp* and anaerobic gram-positive cocci.*

Skin and skin structure infections caused by *S aureus* (penicillinase/nonpenicillinase-producing), *S pyogenes**, and *P aeruginosa* and enterococci.

Pelvic inflammatory disease, endometritis and other infections of the female genital tract caused by *N gonorrhoeae, S epidermidis*, S agalactiae, E coli, Clostridium* sp*, enterococci, *Bacteroides* sp (including *B fragilis*) and anaerobic gram-positive cocci.

Urinary tract infections caused by enterococci*, *E coli* and *P aeruginosa*.

Dosage:

Administer IM or IV.

Usual adult dose is 2 to 4 g/day administered in equally divided doses every 12 hours.

In severe infections or infections caused by less sensitive organisms, the total daily dose or frequency may be increased. Patients have been successfully treated with a total daily dosage of 6 to 12 g divided into 2, 3 or 4 administrations ranging from 1.5 to 4 g/dose. A total daily dose of 16 g by constant infusion has been given without complications. Steady-state serum concentrations were approximately 150 mcg/ml.

Hepatic disease or biliary obstruction: Cefoperazone is extensively excreted in bile. The serum half-life is increased twofold to fourfold in patients with hepatic disease or biliary obstruction. In general, total daily dosage above 4 g should not be necessary. If higher dosages are used, monitor serum concentrations.

Renal function impairment: Because renal excretion is not the main route of elimination, patients with renal failure require no adjustment in dosage when usual doses are administered. When high doses are used, monitor serum drug concentrations.

Hemodialysis: The half-life is reduced slightly during hemodialysis. Thus, schedule dosing to follow a dialysis period. In patients with both hepatic dysfunction and significant renal disease, do not exceed 1 to 2 g daily without monitoring serum concentration.

Administration:

IV administration: Vials – In general, concentrations of between 2 and 50 mg/ml are recommended. Vials of sterile powder may be initially reconstituted with a minimum of 2.8 ml diluent per g of cefoperazone. Use any compatible diluent listed appropriate for IV administration. Reconstitute, using 5 ml of compatible diluent per g of cefoperazone. Withdraw the entire quantity for further dilution and administer via an IV administration system using one of the following methods:

Piggyback units: Intermittent infusion – Further dilute reconstituted cefoperazone in 20 to 40 ml of diluent per g and administer over 15 to 30 minutes.

Continuous infusion – After dilution to a final concentration of between 2 and 25 mg per ml, use cefoperazone for continuous infusion.

IM administration: Any suitable diluent listed may be used to prepare solutions for IM injection. Where concentrations ≥ 250 mg/ml are to be administered, prepare solutions using 0.5% Lidocaine HCl Injection.

After reconstitution, the following volumes and concentrations will be obtained:

Volume and Concentration Following Reconstitution of Cefoperazone			
Package Size	Concentration (mg/ml)	Diluent to Add (ml)	Withdrawable Volume (ml)
1 g vial	333 250	2.6 3.8	3 4
2 g vial	333 250	5.0 7.2	6 8

* Efficacy of this organism in this organ system was studied in fewer than 10 infections.

(Administration continued on following page)

CEFOPERAZONE SODIUM (Cont.)

Administration (Cont.):

Preparation of solution: Reconstitute powder for IV or IM use with any compatible solution for infusion mentioned below. After reconstitution, allow any foaming to dissipate to permit visual inspection for complete solubilization. Vigorous prolonged agitation may be needed to solubilize cefoperazone in higher concentrations (> 333 mg/ml). Maximum solubility of cefoperazone is ≈ 475 mg/ml of compatible diluent.

IV use – Reconstitute with 5% Dextrose Injection; 5% Dextrose and Lactated Ringer's Injection; 5% Dextrose and 0.2% or 0.9% Sodium Chloride Injection; 10% Dextrose Injection; Lactated Ringer's Injection; 0.9% Sodium Chloride Injection; *Normosol M* and 5% Dextrose Injection; *Normosol R*.

IM use – Reconstitute with Bacteriostatic Water for Injection (benzyl alcohol or parabens); 0.5% Lidocaine HCl Injection; Sterile Water for Injection.

Do not use preparations containing benzyl alcohol in neonates.

Compatibility, Stability and Storage: The following parenteral diluents and approximate concentrations of cefoperazone provide stable solutions under the following conditions for the indicated time periods. (After indicated time periods, discard unused portions.)

Compatibility, Stability and Storage of Cefoperazone

Diluent	24 hours Room Temperature (15°C to 25°C)	5 days Refrigeration (2°C to 8°C)	Freezer: 3 weeks (–20°C to –10°C)	Freezer: 5 weeks (–20°C to –10°C)	Approximate Concentration (mg/ml)
Bacteriostatic Water for Injection (benzyl alcohol or parabens)	✓	✓			300
5% Dextrose Injection	✓	✓	✓[1]		2-50
5% Dextrose & Lactated Ringer's Injection	✓				2-50
5% Dextrose & 0.2% or 0.9% Sodium Chloride Injection	✓	✓	✓[2]		2-50
10% Dextrose Injection	✓				2-50
Lactated Ringer's Injection	✓	✓			2
0.5% Lidocaine HCl Injection	✓	✓			300
0.9% Sodium Chloride Injection	✓	✓		✓[3]	2-300
Normosol M and 5% Dextrose Injection	✓	✓			2-50
Normosol R	✓	✓			2-50
Sterile Water for Injection	✓	✓		✓	300

[1] The 50 mg/ml injection only. [2] The 2 mg/ml injection only. [3] The 300 mg/ml injection only.

Thaw frozen samples at room temperature before use. After thawing, discard unused portions. Do not refreeze.

Sterile powder: Prior to reconstitution, protect sterile powder from light and store at or below 25°C (77°F). After reconstitution, protection from light is not necessary.

Frozen solution: Do not store above –20°C (–4°F). After thawing, solution is stable for 10 days at 5°C (41°F) and for 48 hours at room temperature. Do not refreeze.

Admixture incompatibility: Do not mix cefoperazone directly with an aminoglycoside. If concomitant therapy is necessary, use sequential intermittent IV infusion provided that separate secondary IV tubing is used and the primary IV tubing is irrigated between doses. Administer cefoperazone prior to the aminoglycoside.

				C.I.*
Rx	**Cefobid** (Roerig)	**Powder for Injection:**[1] 1 g	In vials and Piggyback units.	564
		2 g	In vials and Piggyback units.	564
		Injection:[1] 1 g	Premixed, frozen. In 50 ml plastic containers.[2]	590
		2 g	Premixed, frozen. In 50 ml plastic containers.[3]	532

* Cost Index based on cost per 500 mg.
[1] Contains 1.5 mEq sodium/g.
[2] With 2.3 g dextrose hydrous.
[3] With 1.8 g dextrose hydrous.

Complete prescribing information for these products begins on page 1733

MOXALACTAM DISODIUM

Indications:

Lower respiratory infections, including pneumonia, caused by *Streptococcus pneumoniae, Hemophilus influenzae* (including β-lactamase producing strains), *Klebsiella* sp, *Enterobacter* sp, *Staphylococcus aureus* (penicillinase/nonpenicillinase-producing), *Escherichia coli* and *Proteus mirabilis.*

Urinary tract infections caused by *E coli, Klebsiella* sp, *Enterobacter* sp, *Proteus* sp (indole-positive and indole-negative) and *Serratia* sp.

Intra-abdominal infections (eg, peritonitis, endometritis and pelvic cellulitis) caused by *E coli; Peptostreptococcus* sp; *Bacteroides* sp, including *B fragilis,* mixed aerobic and anaerobic organisms, such as *K pneumoniae, S agalactiae* (group B streptococci), *P mirabilis, Enterobacter* sp, *Pseudomonas aeruginosa, Peptococcus, Clostridium* sp, *Fusobacterium* sp and *Eubacterium* sp.

Bacterial septicemia caused by *S aureus, E coli, S pneumoniae, Klebsiella* sp, *Serratia* sp, *Pseudomonas* sp and *B fragilis.*

CNS infections (eg, meningitis and ventriculitis) caused by *E coli* and *Klebsiella* sp. Has been used successfully in the treatment of a limited number of patients with meningitis and ventriculitis caused by other Enterobacteriaceae and *H influenzae.*

Skin and skin structure infections caused by *S aureus* (penicillinase/nonpenicillinase-producing), *S pyogenes* (group A β-hemolytic streptococci), *E coli* and *Serratia* sp. Mixed aerobic and anaerobic organisms, such as *Proteus* sp, *Klebsiella* sp, *Enterobacter* sp, *Peptococcus, Peptostreptococcus, Bacteroides* sp and *Clostridium* sp.

Bone and joint infections caused by *S aureus* (penicillinase/nonpenicillinase-producing), *P aeruginosa* and *Serratia* sp.

Pseudomonas infections: Because many strains of *Pseudomonas* sp are moderately susceptible to moxalactam, higher dosage is recommended (see Administration and Dosage). Moxalactam has been used successfully in the treatment of some patients with serious lower respiratory tract infections caused by *P aeruginosa* and *Serratia* sp. Higher dosage is recommended; institute other therapy if response is not prompt.

Concomitant aminoglycoside therapy: In certain cases of confirmed or suspected gram-positive or gram-negative sepsis, or in patients with other serious infections in which the causative organism has not been identified, moxalactam may be used concomitantly with an aminoglycoside. The dosage of both antibiotics depends on the severity of the infection and the patient's condition. Monitor renal function, especially if higher dosages of the aminoglycosides are administered or if therapy is prolonged, because of the potential nephrotoxicity and ototoxicity of aminoglycoside antibiotics. Some β-lactam antibiotics also have a certain degree of nephrotoxicity. Although not noted when moxalactam was given alone, it is possible that nephrotoxicity may be potentiated if it is used concomitantly with an aminoglycoside.

Dosage:

Adults: The usual dose is 2 to 4 g/day administered in divided doses every 8 to 12 hours for 5 to 10 days or up to 14 days. Most mild to moderate infections can be expected to respond to a dosage of 500 mg to 2 g every 12 hours. Individual IM doses of 2 g or more at one site are not recommended.

Mild skin and skin structure infections and uncomplicated pneumonia – 500 mg every 8 hours.

Mild, uncomplicated urinary tract infections – 250 mg every 12 hours.

Urinary tract infections (persistent) – 500 mg every 12 hours.

Serious urinary tract infections – Dosage frequency may be increased to every 8 hours.

Life-threatening infections or infections due to less susceptible organisms (eg, *P aeruginosa*) – Doses up to 4 g every 8 hours (ie, 12 g/day) may be needed.

Give prophylactic vitamin K, 10 mg/week, to patients receiving moxalactam.

Neonates, infants and children:

Neonates (0 to 1 week of age) – 50 mg/kg every 12 hours.

Neonates (1 to 4 weeks of age) – 50 mg/kg every 8 hours.

Infants – 50 mg/kg every 6 hours.

Children – 50 mg/kg every 6 or 8 hours.

This may be increased to 200 mg/kg/day (not to exceed the maximum adult dose) for serious infections. In pediatric gram-negative meningitis, an initial loading dose of 100 mg/kg is recommended prior to using the above dosage schedule.

(Dosage continued on following page)

MOXALACTAM DISODIUM (Cont.)

Dosage (Cont.):

Renal function impairment: Reduce dose and monitor serum levels. After an initial dose of 1 to 2 g (depending on the severity of the infection), a maintenance dosage schedule is determined by the degree of renal impairment, the severity of infection and the susceptibility of the causative organism.

When only serum creatinine is available, use the following formula to convert this value into creatinine clearance. The serum creatinine should represent steady-state renal function.

$$\text{Males:} \quad \frac{\text{Weight (kg)} \times (140 - \text{age})}{72 \times \text{serum creatinine (mg/dl)}} = \text{Ccr}$$

Females: 0.85 x above value

Moxalactam Dosage in Renal Impairment

Renal Function Impairment	Creatinine Clearance (ml/min/1.73 m^2)	Life-Threatening Infections (Maximum Dosage)	Less Severe Infections
Normal	> 80	4 g every 8 hours	0.5-2 g every 8-12 hours
Mild	50-80	3 g every 8 hours	0.5-1 g every 8 hours
Moderate	25-50	2 g every 8 hours or 3 g every 12 hours	0.25-1 g every 12 hours
Severe	2-25	1 g every 8 hours or 1.25 g every 12 hours	0.25-0.5 g every 8 hours
None	< 2	1 g every 24 hours	0.25-0.5 g every 12 hours

The serum half-life of moxalactam during hemodialysis has ranged from 2 to 5 hours. Repeat maintenance doses following regular hemodialysis.

Administration:

Give IV or by deep IM injection into a large muscle mass (ie, gluteus maximus or lateral part of the thigh).

IM: Dilute each g with 3 ml of: Sterile Water; Bacteriostatic Water; 0.9% Sodium Chloride; Bacteriostatic Sodium Chloride; 0.5% or 1% Lidocaine HCl. Shake well until dissolved.

IV: The IV route may be preferable for patients with bacterial septicemia, localized parenchymal abscesses (such as intra-abdominal abscess), peritonitis, meningitis or other severe or life-threatening infections.

Direct IV administration – Add 10 ml of Sterile Water for Injection, 5% Dextrose Injection or 0.9% Sodium Chloride Injection/gram of moxalactam. Slowly inject directly into the vein over 3 to 5 minutes, or through the tubing of an administration set while the patient is also receiving one of the following IV fluids: 0.9% Sodium Chloride; 5% or 10% Dextrose; 6% *Gentran* 75 injection and 10% *Travert;* 5% Dextrose and 0.2%, 0.45% or 0.9% Sodium Chloride; 5% Dextrose and 0.15% Potassium Chloride; 10% Fructose; 5% Dextrose and 0.2% Sodium Bicarbonate Injection; 5% *Osmitrol* in Water; Sodium Lactate (M/6); *Normosol-M* in D5-W; *Ionosol B* in 5% Dextrose; *Plasma-Lyte-M* in 5% Dextrose; Ringer's Injection; Acetated Ringer's Injection; Lactated Ringer's Injection; Lactated Ringer's in 5% Dextrose. Avoid IV solutions containing alcohol.

Intermittent IV infusion with a Y-type administration set or volume control set can also be accomplished while any of the above mentioned IV fluids are being infused. However, during infusion, discontinue the other solution. If Sterile Water for Injection is the diluent, reconstitute with approximately 20 ml/g to avoid a hypotonic solution.

Continuous IV infusion – Dilute each gram with 10 ml of Sterile Water for Injection. An appropriate quantity of the resulting solution may be added to an IV bottle containing one of the compatible fluids listed above.

Storage: Reconstituted moxalactam is stable for 96 hours if refrigerated (5°C) and for 24 hours at room temperature. Dry powder should be stored below 26°C (78°F). **C.I.***

Rx	**Moxam** (Lilly)	**Powder for Injection:** Contains 3.8 mEq sodium/g		
		1 g per vial	In 10 ml vials.[1]	610
		2 g per vial	In 20 ml vials.[1]	610
		10 g per vial	In 100 ml vials.[1]	610

* Cost Index based on cost per 500 mg.

[1] With 150 mg mannitol per gram.

Complete prescribing information for these products begins on page 1733

CEFOTAXIME SODIUM

Indications:

Lower respiratory tract infections, including pneumonia, caused by *Streptococcus pneumoniae, S pyogenes** (group A streptococci) and other streptococci (excluding enterococci, eg, *S faecalis*), *Staphylococcus aureus* (penicillinase/nonpenicillinase-producing), *Escherichia coli, Klebsiella* sp, *Hemophilus influenzae* (including ampicillin-resistant strains), *H parainfluenzae, Proteus mirabilis, Serratia marcescens** and *Enterobacter* sp, indole-positive *Proteus* and *Pseudomonas* sp.

Urinary tract infections caused by *Enterococcus* sp, *S epidermidis, S aureus** (penicillinase/nonpenicillinase-producing), *Citrobacter* species, *Enterobacter* species, *E coli, Klebsiella* species, *P mirabilis, P vulgaris*, P inconstans* group B, *Morganella morganii*, Providencia rettgeri*, S marcescens* and *Pseudomonas* sp. Also, uncomplicated gonorrhea caused by *Neisseria gonorrhoeae,* including penicillinase-producing strains.

Gynecological infections, including pelvic inflammatory disease, endometritis and pelvic cellulitis caused by *S epidermidis,* streptococci, *Enterococcus, Enterobacter* sp*, *Klebsiella* sp*, *E coli, P mirabilis, Bacteroides* species (including *B fragilis*)*, *Clostridium* species and anaerobic cocci (including *Peptostreptococcus* and *Peptococcus*).

Bacteremia/septicemia caused by *E coli, Klebsiella* sp, *S marcescens, S aureus* and streptococci.

Skin and skin structure infections caused by *S aureus* (penicillinase/nonpenicillinase-producing), *S epidermidis, S pyogenes* (group A streptococci) and other streptococci, *Enterococcus, Acinetobacter* sp*, *Citrobacter* sp, *E coli, Enterobacter, Klebsiella* sp, *P mirabilis, M morganii, P rettgeri*, P vulgaris*, Pseudomonas* sp, *S marcescens, Bacteroides* sp and anaerobic cocci (including *Peptostreptococcus** and *Peptococcus*).

Intra-abdominal infections including peritonitis caused by streptococci*, *E coli, Klebsiella* sp, *Bacteroides* sp and anaerobic cocci (including *Peptostreptococcus** and *Peptococcus*, P mirabilis** and *Clostridium* sp).

Bone or joint infections caused by *S aureus* (penicillinase/nonpenicillinase-producing strains), streptococci, *Pseudomonas* sp and *P mirabilis.**

CNS infections (eg, meningitis and ventriculitis) caused by *N meningitidis, H influenzae, S pneumoniae, K pneumoniae** and *E coli.**

Although many strains of enterococci (eg, *S faecalis*) and *Pseudomonas* species are resistant to cefotaxime in vitro, it has been used successfully in treating patients with infections caused by susceptible organisms.

Perioperative prophylaxis may reduce the incidence of certain postoperative infections in patients undergoing surgical procedures (eg, abdominal or vaginal hysterectomy, GI and GU surgery) that are classified as contaminated or potentially contaminated. Effective perioperative use depends on the time of administration. For patients undergoing GI surgery, preoperative bowel preparation by mechanical cleansing as well as with a nonabsorbable antibiotic (eg, neomycin) is recommended.

Cesarean section – Intraoperative (after clamping the umbilical cord) and postoperative use may reduce the incidence of certain postoperative infections.

If there are signs of infection, obtain specimens for identification of the causative organism so that appropriate therapy may be instituted.

Concomitant aminoglycoside therapy: In certain cases of confirmed or suspected gram-positive or gram-negative sepsis, or other serious infections in which the causative organism has not been identified, cefotaxime may be used concomitantly with an aminoglycoside. The dosage recommended for both antibiotics may be given, and dosage depends on the severity of the infection and the patient's condition. Monitor renal function, especially if higher dosages of the aminoglycosides are used or if therapy is prolonged, because of the potential nephrotoxicity and ototoxicity of aminoglycoside antibiotics. Some β-lactam antibiotics also have a certain degree of nephrotoxicity. Although not noted when cefotaxime was given alone, nephrotoxicity may be potentiated if it is used concomitantly with an aminoglycoside.

* Efficacy for this organism in this organ system has been studied in fewer than 10 infections.

(Continued on following page)

CEFOTAXIME SODIUM (Cont.)

Dosage:

Adults: Administer IV or IM. The maximum daily dosage should not exceed 12 g. Determine dosage and route of administration by susceptibility of the causative organisms, severity of the infection and the patient's condition (see table for dosage guidelines).

Cefotaxime Dosage Guidelines for Adults		
Type of Infection	Daily Dosage (g)	Frequency and Route
Gonorrhea	1	1 g IM (single dose)
Uncomplicated infections	2	1 g every 12 hours IM or IV
Moderate to severe	3 to 6	1 to 2 g every 8 hours IM or IV
Infections commonly needing higher dosage (eg, septicemia)	6 to 8	2 g every 6 to 8 hours IV
Life-threatening infections	up to 12	2 g every 4 hours IV

Perioperative prophylaxis: 1 g IV or IM, 30 to 90 minutes prior to surgery.

Cesarean section: Administer the first 1 g dose IV as soon as the umbilical cord is clamped. Administer the second and third doses as 1 g IV or IM at 6 and 12 hour intervals after the first dose.

Pediatric: It is not necessary to differentiate between premature and normal gestational age infants. The following dosage recommendations may serve as a guide:

Cefotaxime Dosage Guidelines in Pediatrics			
Age	Weight (kg)	Dosage Schedule	Route
0 to 1 week	—	50 mg/kg every 12 hours	IV
1 to 4 weeks	—	50 mg/kg every 8 hours	IV
1 month to 12 years	< 50†	50 to 180 mg/kg/day in 4 to 6 divided doses‡	IV or IM

† For children $\geq$ 50 kg, use adult dosage.

‡ Use higher doses for more severe or serious infections including meningitis.

Renal function impairment: Determine dosage by degree of renal impairment, severity of infection and susceptibility of the causative organism. In patients with estimated creatinine clearances of less than 20 ml/min/1.73m^2, reduce dosage by one-half.

When only serum creatinine is available, the following formula may be used to convert this value into creatinine clearance. The serum creatinine should represent steady-state renal function.

$$\text{Males:} \quad \frac{\text{Weight (kg)} \times (140 - \text{age})}{72 \times \text{serum creatinine (mg/dl)}} = \text{Ccr}$$

Females: 0.85 x above value

CDC recommended treatment schedules for gonorrhea:[1]

Disseminated gonococcal infection – Give 500 mg cefotaxime IV 4 times per day for at least 7 days.

Gonococcal ophthalmia in adults – For penicillinase-producing Neisseria gonorrhoeae (PPNG), give 500 mg, IV, 4 times per day.

Administration:

IV administration: The IV route is preferable for patients with bacteremia, bacterial septicemia, peritonitis, meningitis, or other severe or life-threatening infections, or for patients who may be poor risks because of lowered resistance resulting from such debilitating conditions as malnutrition, trauma, surgery, diabetes, heart failure or malignancy, particularly if shock is present or impending.

Intermittent IV – 1 or 2 g in 10 ml of Sterile Water for Injection over 3 to 5 minutes; may also be given over a longer period of time through the tubing system by which the patient may be receiving other IV solutions. However, temporarily discontinue administration of other solutions at the same site.

Continuous IV infusion – May add to IV bottles containing solutions discussed below.

IM administration: Inject well within the body of a relatively large muscle (ie, gluteus maximus). Divide doses of 2 g and administer in different IM sites.

[1] Morbidity and Mortality Weekly Report 1985 (Oct 18); 34 (Supp 4S):76S-108S.

(Administration continued on following page)

CEFOTAXIME SODIUM (Cont.)

Administration (Cont.):

Preparation of Solution: Use the following table as a guide for reconstitution:

Volume and Concentration Following Reconstitution of Cefotaxime			
Package Size	Diluent to Add (ml)	≈ Withdrawable Volume (ml)	≈ Concentration (mg/ml)
1 g vial 2 g vial	3 (IM) 5 (IM)	3.4 6	300 330
1 g vial 2 g vial	10 (IV) 10 (IV)	10.4 11	95 180
1 g infusion 2 g infusion	50-100 50-100	50-100 50-100	10-20 20-40
10 g bottle 10 g bottle	47 97	52 102	200 100

Shake to dissolve. Solutions range in color from light yellow to amber, depending on concentration, diluent used, and length and condition of storage. A solution of 1 g cefotaxime in 14 ml of Sterile Water for Injection is isotonic.

IV – Reconstitute with at least 10 ml of Sterile Water for Injection. Infusion bottles may be reconstituted with 50 or 100 ml of 0.9% Sodium Chloride Injection or 5% Dextrose Injection.

IM – Reconstitute with Sterile Water or Bacteriostatic Water for Injection.

Compatibility, Stability and Storage: Solutions reconstituted as described above maintain potency for 24 hours at room temperature (≤ 22°C; 72°F), for 10 days under refrigeration (≤ 5°C; 41°F) and for at least 13 weeks frozen. After reconstitution and subsequent storage in disposable glass or plastic syringes, cefotaxime is stable for 24 hours at room temperature, 5 days under refrigeration and 13 weeks frozen.

Reconstituted solutions may be further diluted up to 50 to 1000 ml with the following solutions and will maintain potency for 24 hours at room temperature and at least 5 days under refrigeration: 0.9% Sodium Chloride; 5% or 10% Dextrose; 5% Dextrose and 0.2%, 0.45% or 0.9% Sodium Chloride; Lactated Ringer's Solution; Sodium Lactate Injection (M/6); 10% Invert Sugar.

IV bags: Solutions of cefotaxime in 0.9% Sodium Chloride Injection and 5% Dextrose Injection in IV bags are stable for 24 hours at room temperature, 5 days under refrigeration and 13 weeks frozen.

Thaw frozen samples at room temperature before use; do not heat. After the periods mentioned above, discard any unused solutions or frozen material. Do not refreeze.

Cefotaxime solutions exhibit maximum stability in the pH 5 to 7 range. Do not use with diluents having a pH above 7.5 (eg, Sodium Bicarbonate Injection).

Admixtures: Do not admix with aminoglycoside solutions. If cefotaxime and aminoglycosides are to be administered to the same patient, administer separately.

Storage: Powder – Store cefotaxime in the dry state below 30°C (86°F). The dry material, as well as the solutions, tends to darken depending on storage conditions; protect from elevated temperatures and excessive light.

Frozen solutions – Thawed solutions are stable for 24 hours at room temperature (≤ 22°C; 72°F) or for 10 days under refrigeration (≤ 5°C; 41°F).

				C.I.*
Rx	**Claforan** (Hoechst-Roussel)	**Powder for Injection:**[1] 1 g	In vials, packages of 10s, 25s, 50s. Infusion bottles in 10s. *ADD-Vantage* system vials in 25s.	540
		2 g	In vials, packages of 10s, 25s, 50s. Infusion bottles in 10s. *ADD-Vantage* system vials in 25s.	500
		10 g	In bulk vials.	472
		Injection:[1] 1 g	Premixed, frozen. In 50 ml, package of 24s.	639
		2 g	Premixed, frozen. In 50 ml, package of 24s.	537

* Cost Index based on cost per 500 mg.

[1] Contains 2.2 mEq sodium/g.

Complete prescribing information for these products begins on page 1733

CEFTIZOXIME SODIUM

Indications:

Lower respiratory tract infections caused by *Streptococcus* sp including *S pneumoniae*, but excluding enterococci, *Klebsiella* sp, *Proteus mirabilis, Escherichia coli, Hemophilus influenzae* (including ampicillin-resistant strains), *Staphylococcus aureus* (penicillinase/nonpenicillinase-producing), *Serratia* sp, *Enterobacter* sp and *Bacteroides* sp.

Urinary tract infections caused by *S aureus* (penicillinase/nonpenicillinase-producing), *E coli, Pseudomonas* sp including *P aeruginosa, P mirabilis, P vulgaris, Providencia rettgeri, Morganella morganii, Klebsiella* sp, *Serratia* sp including *S marcescens and Enterobacter* sp.

Gonorrhea: Uncomplicated cervical and urethral gonorrhea caused by *Neisseria gonorrhoeae*.

Intra-abdominal infections caused by *E coli, S epidermidis, Streptococcus* sp (excluding enterococci), *Enterobacter* sp, *Klebsiella* sp, *Bacteroides* sp including *B fragilis* and anaerobic cocci, including *Peptococcus* sp and *Peptostreptococcus* sp.

Septicemia caused by *Streptococcus* sp including *S pneumoniae*, but excluding enterococci, *S aureus* (penicillinase/nonpenicillinase-producing), *E coli, Bacteroides* sp including *B fragilis, Klebsiella* sp and *Serratia* sp.

Skin and skin structure infections caused by *S aureus* (penicillinase/nonpenicillinase-producing), *S epidermidis, E coli, Klebsiella* sp, *Streptococcus* sp including *S pyogenes* (group A β-hemolytic), but excluding enterococci, *P mirabilis, Serratia* sp, *Enterobacter* sp, *Bacteroides* sp including *B fragilis* and anaerobic cocci, including *Peptococcus* sp and *Peptostreptococcus* sp.

Bone and joint infections caused by *S aureus* (penicillinase/nonpenicillinase-producing), *Streptococcus* sp (excluding enterococci), *P mirabilis, Bacteroides* sp and anaerobic cocci, including *Peptococcus* sp and *Peptostreptococcus* sp.

Meningitis caused by *H influenzae*. Used to treat limited cases of meningitis caused by *S pneumoniae*.

Dosage:

Adults: Usual dosage is 1 or 2 g every 8 to 12 hours. Individualize dosage.

Ceftizoxime Dosage Guidelines in Adults		
Type of Infection	Daily Dose (grams)	Frequency and Route
Uncomplicated urinary tract	1	500 mg every 12 hours IM or IV
Other sites	2-3	1 g every 8 to 12 hours IM or IV
Severe or refractory	3-6	1 g every 8 hours IM or IV 2 g every 8 to 12 hours IM* or IV
Life-threatening†	9-12	3 to 4 g every 8 hours IV

* Divide 2 g IM doses and give in different large muscle masses.
† Dosages up to 2 g every 4 hours have been given.

Urinary tract infections: Because of the serious nature of urinary tract infections due to *P aeruginosa* and because many strains of *Pseudomonas* species are only moderately susceptible to ceftizoxime, higher dosage is recommended. Institute other therapy if the response is not prompt.

Gonorrhea, uncomplicated: A single 1 g IM injection is the usual dose.

Life-threatening infections: The IV route may be preferable for patients with bacterial septicemia, localized parenchymal abscesses (such as intra-abdominal abscess), peritonitis or other severe or life-threatening infections.

In those patients with normal renal function, the IV dosage is 2 to 12 g daily. In conditions such as bacterial septicemia, 6 to 12 g/day IV may be given initially for several days, and the dosage gradually reduced according to clinical response and laboratory findings.

Pediatric:

Children (≥ 6 months) – 50 mg/kg every 6 to 8 hours. Dosage may be increased to 200 mg/kg/day. Do not exceed the maximum adult dose for serious infection.

Renal function impairment requires modification of dosage. Following an initial loading dose of 500 mg to 1 g, IM or IV, use the maintenance dosing schedule in the following table. Determine further dosing by therapeutic monitoring, severity of the infection and susceptibility of the causative organisms.

(Dosage continued on following page)

CEFTIZOXIME SODIUM (Cont.)

Dosage (Cont.):

Renal function impairment (Cont.):

When only serum creatinine is available, calculate creatinine clearance from the formula below. The serum creatinine should represent steady-state renal function.

Males: $$\frac{\text{Weight (kg)} \times (140 - \text{age})}{72 \times \text{serum creatinine (mg/dl)}} = \text{Ccr}$$

Females: 0.85 x above value

Hemodialysis – No additional supplemental dosing is required following hemodialysis; give the dose (according to the table below) at the end of dialysis.

Ceftizoxime Dosage in Adults with Renal Impairment			
Renal Function	Creatinine Clearance (ml/min)	Less Severe Infections	Life-threatening Infections
Mild impairment	50-79	500 mg q 8 h	0.75-1.5 g q 8 h
Moderate to severe impairment	5-49	250-500 mg q 12 h	0.5-1 g q 12 h
Dialysis patients	0-4	500 mg q 48 h or 250 mg q 24 h	0.5-1 g q 48 h or 0.5 g q 24 h

Administration:

IV administration: Direct (bolus) injection, slowly over 3 to 5 minutes, directly or through tubing for patients receiving parenteral fluids (see list below). For intermittent or continuous infusion, dilute reconstituted ceftizoxime in 50 to 100 ml of one of the following solutions: Sodium Chloride Injection; 5% or 10% Dextrose Injection; 5% Dextrose and 0.9%, 0.45% or 0.2% Sodium Chloride Injection; Ringer's Injection; Lactated Ringer's Injection; Invert Sugar 10% in Sterile Water for Injection; 5% Sodium Bicarbonate in Sterile Water for Injection; 5% Dextrose in Lactated Ringer's Injection (only when reconstituted with 4% Sodium Bicarbonate Injection).

Preparation of solution: Reconstitute with Sterile Water for Injection. Shake well.

Volume and Concentration Following Reconstitution of Ceftizoxime			
Package Size	Diluent to Add (ml)	≈ Available Volume (ml)	≈ Concentration (mg/ml)
1 g vial	3 (IM)	3.7	270
2 g vial†	6 (IM)	7.4	270
1 g vial	10 (IV)	10.7	95
2 g vial	20 (IV)	21.4	95
10 g vial	30 (Bulk vial)	37	1g/3.5 ml
	45 (Bulk vial)	51	1 g/5 ml

† Divide 2 g IM doses and give in different large muscle masses.

Piggyback vials – Reconstitute with 50 to 100 ml of any IV solution listed above. Shake well. Administer as a single dose with primary IV fluids.

A solution of 1 g ceftizoxime in 13 ml Sterile Water for Injection is isotonic.

Frozen injection: Thaw container at room temperature. Do not introduce additives into the solution.

Storage: After reconstitution or dilution in the IV fluids above, these solutions are stable for 24 hours at room temperature and for 96 hours if refrigerated (5°C; 41°F).

After thawing the frozen injection, the solution is stable for 24 hours at room temperature or for 10 days if refrigerated. Do not refreeze.

				C.I.*
Rx	**Cefizox** (SKF)	**Powder for Injection:**[1] 1 g (as sodium)	In 28 ml vials and 100 ml piggyback vials.	559
		2 g (as sodium)	In 28 ml vials and 100 ml piggyback vials.	518
		10 g (as sodium)	In pharmacy bulk vials.	512
		Injection: In 5% Dextrose in Water[1] 1 g (as sodium)	Frozen, premixed. In 50 ml single dose plastic containers.	647
		2 g (as sodium)	Frozen, premixed. In 50 ml single dose plastic containers.	549

* Cost Index based on cost per 500 mg.

[1] Contains 2.6 mEq sodium/g.

Complete prescribing information for these products begins on page 1733

CEFOTETAN DISODIUM

Indications:

Urinary tract infections caused by *Escherichia coli, Klebsiella* sp (including *K pneumoniae)* and *Proteus* sp (including *P vulgaris, P mirabilis, Providencia rettgeri* and *Morganella morganii*).

Lower respiratory tract infections caused by *Streptococcus pneumoniae, Staphylococcus aureus* (penicillinase/nonpenicillinase-producing), *Hemophilus influenzae* (including ampicillin-resistant strains), *Klebsiella* sp (including *K pneumoniae*) and *E coli.*

Skin and skin structure infections caused by *S aureus* (penicillinase/nonpenicillinase-producing), *S epidermidis, S pyogenes, Streptococcus* sp (excluding enterococci) and *E coli.*

Gynecologic infections caused by *S aureus** (including penicillinase/nonpenicillinase-producing), *S epidermidis, Streptococcus* sp (excluding enterococci), *E coli, P mirabilis, Neisseria gonorrhoeae, Bacteroides* sp (excluding *B distasonis, B ovatus, B thetaiotaomicron*), *Fusobacterium* sp* and gram-positive anaerobic cocci (including *Peptococcus* and *Peptostreptococcus* sp*).

Intra-abdominal infections caused by *E coli, Klebsiella* sp (including *K pneumoniae**), *Streptococcus* sp (excluding enterococci) and *Bacteroides* sp (excluding *B distasonis, B ovatus, B thetaiotaomicron).*

Bone and joint infections caused by *S aureus.**

Concomitant antibiotic therapy: If cefotetan and an aminoglycoside are used concomitantly, carefully monitor renal function, especially if higher dosages of the aminoglycoside are to be administered or if therapy is prolonged, because of the potential nephrotoxicity and ototoxicity of aminoglycosides. Although to date, nephrotoxicity has not been noted when cefotetan was given alone, it is possible that nephrotoxicity may be potentiated if used concomitantly with an aminoglycoside.

Perioperative prophylaxis: Preoperative administration of cefotetan may reduce incidence of certain postoperative infections in patients undergoing surgical procedures classified as clean contaminated or potentially contaminated (eg, cesarean section, abdominal or vaginal hysterectomy, transurethral surgery, GI and biliary tract surgery).

If there are signs and symptoms of infection, obtain specimens for identification of the causative organism so that appropriate therapeutic measures may be initiated.

Dosage:

Adults: The usual dosage is 1 or 2 g IV or IM every 12 hours for 5 to 10 days. Determine proper dosage and route of administration by the condition of the patient, severity of the infection and susceptibility of the causative organism.

General Cefotetan Dosage Guidelines		
Type of Infection	Daily Dose	Frequency and Route
Urinary Tract	1 to 4 g	500 mg every 12 hours IV or IM 1 or 2 g every 24 hours IV or IM 1 or 2 g every 12 hours IV or IM
Other Sites	2 to 4 g	1 or 2 g every 12 hours IV or IM
Severe	4 g	2 g every 12 hours IV
Life-threatening	6 g†	3 g every 12 hours IV

† Maximum daily dosage should not exceed 6 g.

Prophylaxis: To prevent postoperative infection in clean contaminated or potentially contaminated surgery in adults, give a single 1 or 2 g IV dose 30 to 60 minutes prior to surgery. In patients undergoing cesarean section, give the dose as soon as the umbilical cord is clamped.

Renal function impairment: Reduce the dosage schedule using the following guidelines:

Cefotetan Dosage in Renal Impairment		
Ccr (ml/min)	Dose	Frequency
> 30	Usual Recommended Dose††	Every 12 hours
10-30	Usual Recommended Dose††	Every 24 hours
< 10	Usual Recommended Dose††	Every 48 hours

†† Dose determined by the type and severity of infection, and susceptibility of the causative organism.

* Efficacy for this organism in this organ system was studied in fewer than ten infections.

(Dosage continued on following page)

CEFOTETAN DISODIUM (Cont.)

Dosage (Cont.):

Renal Function Impairment (Cont.):

Alternatively, the dosing interval may remain constant at 12 hour intervals, but reduce dose by one-half for patients with a creatinine clearance of 10 to 30 ml/min, and by one-quarter for patients with a creatinine clearance of less than 10 ml/min.

When only serum creatinine is available, use the following formula to estimate creatinine clearance. Serum creatinine level should represent steady-state renal function.

$$\text{Males:} \quad \frac{\text{Weight (kg)} \times (140 - \text{age})}{72 \times \text{serum creatinine (mg/dl)}} = \text{Ccr}$$

Females: 0.85 x above value

Dialysis: Cefotetan is dialyzable; for patients undergoing intermittent hemodialysis, give one-quarter of the usual recommended dose every 24 hours on days between dialysis and one-half the usual recommended dose on the day of dialysis.

Administration:

IV: The IV route is preferable for patients with bacteremia, bacterial septicemia or other severe or life-threatening infections, or for patients who may be poor risks because of lowered resistance resulting from such debilitating conditions as malnutrition, trauma, surgery, diabetes, heart failure or malignancy, particularly if shock is present or impending.

Intermittent IV administration – Inject a solution containing 1 or 2 g in Sterile Water for Injection over 3 to 5 minutes. Using an infusion system, the solution may be given over a longer period through the tubing system by which the patient may be receiving other IV solutions. Butterfly or scalp vein-type needles are preferred. However, during infusion of cefotetan, temporarily discontinue the administration of other solutions at the same site.

IM: As with all IM preparations, inject well within the body of a relatively large muscle such as the upper outer quadrant of the buttock (ie, gluteus maximus).

Preparation of Solution:

For IV use – Reconstitute with Sterile Water for Injection.

For IM use – Reconstitute with Sterile Water for Injection, Bacteriostatic Water for Injection, Normal Saline USP or 0.5% or 1% Lidocaine HCl.

Volume and Concentration Following Reconstitution of Cefotetan			
Vial Size (g)	Amount of Diluent to Add (ml)	≈ Withdrawable Volume (ml)	≈ Average Concentration (mg/ml)
IV			
1	10	10.5	95
2	10-20	11-21	182-195
IM			
1	2	2.5	400
2	3	4	500

Infusion bottles (100 ml) may be reconstituted with 50 to 100 ml of 5% Dextrose Solution or 0.9% Sodium Chloride Solution.

Compatibility and Stability: Reconstituted as described above, cefotetan maintains potency for 24 hours at room temperature (25°C; 77°F), for 96 hours refrigerated (5°C; 40°F) and for at least 1 week frozen. After reconstitution and subsequent storage in disposable glass or plastic syringes, cefotetan is stable for 24 hours at room temperature and 96 hours refrigerated.

Thaw frozen samples at room temperature before use. After the periods mentioned above, discard any unused solutions or frozen materials. Do not refreeze.

Admixtures – Do not admix with solutions containing aminoglycosides. If cefotetan and aminoglycosides are to be administered to the same patient, they must be administered separately and not as a mixed injection.

Storage – Do not store vials above 22°C (72°F); protect from light. **C.I.***

Rx	**Cefotan** (Stuart)	**Powder for Injection:** Contains 3.5 mEq sodium/g		
		1 g	In 10 and 100 ml vials.	526
		2 g	In 20 and 100 ml vials.	516
		10 g	In 100ml vials	558

* Cost Index based on cost per 500 mg.

Complete prescribing information for these products begins on page 1733

CEFTAZIDIME

Indications:

Lower respiratory tract infections, including pneumonia, caused by *Pseudomonas aeruginosa* and other *Pseudomonas* species; *Hemophilus influenzae*, including ampicillin-resistant strains; *Klebsiella* species; *Enterobacter* species; *Proteus mirabilis; Escherichia coli; Serratia* species; *Citrobacter* species; *Staphylococcus pneumoniae; S aureus* (methicillin-susceptible strains).

Skin and skin structure infections, caused by *P aeruginosa; Klebsiella* species; *E coli; Proteus* species, including *P mirabilis* and indole-positive *Proteus; Enterobacter* species; *Serratia* species; *S aureus* (methicillin-susceptible strains); *S pyogenes* (group A β-hemolytic streptococci).

Urinary tract infections, both complicated and uncomplicated, caused by *P aeruginosa; Enterobacter* species; *Proteus* species, including *P mirabilis* and indole-positive *Proteus; Klebsiella* species; *E coli.*

Bacterial septicemia, caused by *P aeruginosa; Klebsiella* species; *H influenzae; E coli; Serratia* species; *S pneumoniae; S aureus* (methicillin-susceptible strains).

Bone and joint infections, caused by *P aeruginosa; Klebsiella* species; *Enterobacter* species; *S aureus* (methicillin-susceptible strains).

Gynecological infections, including endometritis, pelvic cellulitis and other infections of the female genital tract, caused by *E coli.*

Intra-abdominal infections, including peritonitis caused by *E coli; Klebsiella* species; *S aureus* (methicillin-susceptible strains); polymicrobial infections caused by aerobic and anaerobic organisms and *Bacteroides* species (many strains of *B fragilis* are resistant).

CNS infections, including meningitis caused by *H influenzae* and *Neisseria meningitidis.* Ceftazidime has also been used successfully in a limited number of cases of meningitis due to *P aeruginosa* and *S pneumoniae.*

Concomitant antibiotic therapy: Ceftazidime may be used concomitantly with other antibiotics (eg, aminoglycosides, vancomycin and clindamycin) in severe and life-threatening infections and in the immunocompromised patient. Dose depends on the severity of the infection and the patient's condition.

Dosage:

Determine dosage and route by the susceptibility of the causative organisms, severity of infection and patient's condition and renal function.

Ceftazidime Dosage Guidelines

Patient/Infection site	Dose	Frequency
Adults Usual recommended dose	1 g IV or IM	q 8-12 h
Uncomplicated urinary tract infections	250 mg IV or IM	q 12 h
Complicated urinary tract infections	500 mg IV or IM	q 8-12 h
Uncomplicated pneumonia; mild skin and skin structure infections	500 mg to 1 g IV or IM	q 8 h
Bone and joint infections	2 g IV	q 12 h
Serious gynecological and intra-abdominal infections	2 g IV	q 8 h
Meningitis		
Very severe life-threatening infections, especially in immunocompromised patients		
Pseudomonal lung infections in cystic fibrosis patients w/normal renal function†	30 to 50 mg/kg IV to a max 6 g/day	q 8 h
Neonates (0 to 4 weeks)	30 mg/kg IV	q 12 h
Infants and children (1 month to 12 years)	30 to 50 mg/kg IV to a max 6 g/day††	q 8 h

† Although clinical improvement has been shown, bacteriological cures cannot be expected in patients with chronic respiratory disease and cystic fibrosis.

†† Reserve the higher dose for immunocompromised children or children with cystic fibrosis or meningitis.

(Dosage continued on following page)

CEFTAZIDIME (Cont.)

Dosage (Cont.):

Hepatic function impairment: No dosage adjustment is required.

Renal function impairment: Ceftazidime is excreted by the kidneys, almost exclusively by glomerular filtration. In patients with impaired renal function (GFR < 50 ml/min), reduce dosage to compensate for slower excretion. In patients with suspected renal insufficiency, give an initial loading dose of 1 g. Estimate GFR to determine the appropriate maintenance dose.

Ceftazidime Dosage in Renal Impairment

Creatinine clearance (ml/min)	Recommended unit dose of ceftazidime	Frequency of dosing
31-50	1 g	q 12 h
16-30	1 g	q 24 h
6-15	500 mg	q 24 h
≤ 5	500 mg	q 48 h

When only serum creatinine is available, use the following formula to estimate creatinine clearance. Serum creatinine should represent steady-state renal function.

$$\text{Males:} \quad \frac{\text{Weight (kg)} \times (140 - \text{age})}{72 \times \text{serum creatinine (mg/dl)}} = \text{Ccr}$$

Females: 0.85 x above value

In patients with severe infections who would normally receive 6 g ceftazidime daily were it not for renal insufficiency, the unit dose given in the table above may be increased by 50% or the dosing frequency increased appropriately. Determine further dosing by therapeutic monitoring, severity of the infection and susceptibility of the causative organism.

In children, as for adults, adjust creatinine clearance for body surface area or lean body mass and reduce the dosing frequency in cases of renal insufficiency.

Dialysis: Give a 1 g loading dose, followed by 1 g after each hemodialysis period.

Ceftazidime can also be used in patients undergoing intraperitoneal dialysis (IPD) and continuous ambulatory peritoneal dialysis (CAPD). Give a loading dose of 1 g, followed by 500 mg every 24 hours. In addition to IV use, ceftazidime can be incorporated in the dialysis fluid at a concentration of 250 mg per 2 L of dialysis fluid.

Administration:

Preparation of Ceftazidime Solutions

Package size	Diluent to add (ml)	≈ Available volume (ml)	≈ Ceftazidime concentration (mg/ml)
IM			
500 mg vial	1.5	1.8	280
1 g vial	3	3.6	280
IV			
500 mg vial	5	5.3	100
1 g vial	5 or 10	5.6 or 10.6	180 or 100
2 g vial	10	2-11.5	170-180
Infusion pack			
1 g vial	50 or 100†	50 or 100	20 or 10
2 g vial	50 or 100†	50 or 100	40 or 20
Bulk package			
6 g vial	26	30	200

† *Note:* Addition should be in two stages (see *IV infusion*).

Inject IV or deeply IM into a large muscle mass such as the upper outer quadrant of the gluteus maximus or lateral part of the thigh.

IM: Reconstitute with one of the following diluents: Sterile or Bacteriostatic Water for Injection or 0.5% or 1% Lidocaine HCl Injection. Refer to the Preparation of Ceftazidime Solutions table.

IV: This route is preferable for patients with bacterial septicemia, bacterial meningitis, peritonitis or other severe or life-threatening infections, or for patients who may be poor risks because of lowered resistance resulting from malnutrition, trauma, surgery, diabetes, heart failure or malignancy, particularly if shock is present or impending.

(Administration continued on following page)

CEFTAZIDIME (Cont.)

Administration (Cont.):

Direct intermittent IV administration – Reconstitute ceftazidime as directed in the table with Sterile Water for Injection. Slowly inject directly into the vein over a period of 3 to 5 minutes or give through the tubing of an administration set while the patient is also receiving one of the compatible IV fluids.

IV infusion – Reconstitute the 1 or 2 g infusion pack with 100 ml Sterile Water for Injection or one of the compatible IV fluids. Alternatively, reconstitute the 500 mg, 1 or 2 g vial and add an appropriate quantity of the resulting solution to an IV container with one of the compatible IV fluids.

Intermittent IV infusion (Y-type) can be accomplished with compatible solutions. However, during infusion of ceftazidime solution, discontinue other solution.

Compatibility and stability:

IM – When reconstituted as directed with Sterile or Bacteriostatic Water for Injection or 0.5% or 1% Lidocaine HCl Injection, the solution maintains potency for 18 to 24 hours at room temperature or for 7 to 10 days if refrigerated. Solutions in Sterile Water for Injection, frozen immediately after reconstitution in the original container, are stable for 3 months at –20°C (–4°F). Once thawed, do not refreeze. Thawed solutions may be stored for 8 to 24 hours at room temperature or 4 days in a refrigerator.

IV – When reconstituted as directed with Sterile Water for Injection, the solution maintains potency for 18 to 24 hours at room temperature or for 7 to 10 days under refrigeration. Solutions in Sterile Water for Injection in the original container or in 0.9% Sodium Chloride or 5% Dextrose Injection in PVC small volume containers, frozen immediately after reconstitution, are stable for 3 months at –20°C (–4°F). For larger volumes, when it is necessary to warm the frozen product (to a maximum of 40°C; 104°F), avoid heating after thawing is complete. Once thawed, do not refreeze. Store thawed solutions for 8 to 24 hrs at room temp. or for 4 days in a refrigerator.

Ceftazidime is compatible with the more common IV infusion fluids. Solutions at concentrations between 1 mg/ml and 40 mg/ml in the following infusion fluids may be stored for up to 18 to 24 hours at room temperature or 7 to 10 days if refrigerated: 0.9% Sodium Chloride; M/6 Sodium Lactate; Ringer's; Lactated Ringer's; 5% or 10% Dextrose; 5% Dextrose and 0.225%, 0.45% or 0.9% Sodium Chloride; 10% Invert Sugar in Water; *Normosol M* in 5% Dextrose.

Ceftazidime is less stable in Sodium Bicarbonate Injection than in other IV fluids. It is not recommended as a diluent. Solutions in 5% Dextrose and 0.9% Sodium Chloride Injection are stable for at least 6 hours at room temperature in plastic tubing, drip chambers and volume control devices of common IV infusion sets.

Ceftazidime at a concentration of 4 mg/ml is compatible for 18 to 24 hours at room temperature or 7 to 10 days under refrigeration in 0.9% Sodium Chloride Injection or 5% Dextrose Injection when admixed with: Cefuroxime 3 mg/ml; heparin 10 or 50 units/ml; or potassium chloride 10 or 40 mEq/L.

Admixtures: Do not add aminoglycoside antibiotics to ceftazidime. If aminoglycoside cotherapy is indicated, give separately.

	Product	Dosage form	Package	C.I.*
Rx	**Ceptaz** (Glaxo)	**Powder for Injection:**[1] 340 mg/g	In 500 mg, 1 g and 2 g vials, 1 and 2 g infusions and 10 g.	NA
Rx	**Fortaz** (Glaxo)	**Powder for Injection:**[2] 500 mg	In vials.	711
Rx	**Tazidime** (Lilly)		In 10 ml vials.	711
Rx	**Fortaz** (Glaxo)	**Powder for Injection:**[2] 1 g	In vials and infusion packs.	711
Rx	**Tazicef** (SK-Beecham)		In vials and Piggyback vials.	697
Rx	**Tazidime** (Lilly)		In 20 and 100 ml vials, *Faspak* and *ADD-Vantage* vials.	665
Rx	**Fortaz** (Glaxo)	**Powder for Injection:**[2] 2 g	In vials and infusion packs.	711
Rx	**Tazicef** (SK-Beecham)		In vials and Piggyback vials.	697
Rx	**Tazidime** (Lilly)		In 50 and 100 ml vials, *Faspak* and *ADD-Vantage* vials.	711
Rx	**Fortaz** (Glaxo)	**Powder for Injection:**[2] 6 g	In bulk package.	690
Rx	**Tazicef** (SK-Beecham)		In bulk package.	676
Rx	**Tazidime** (Lilly)		In 100 ml vial.	690
Rx	**Ceptaz** (Glaxo)	**Powder for Injection:** 500 mg	In 1 and 2 g vials, 1 and 2 g infusions and 10 g.	NA
Rx	**Fortaz** (Glaxo)	**Injection:** 1 g	Premixed, frozen. In 50 ml.[3]	706
		2 g	Premixed, frozen. In 50 ml.[4]	649

* Cost Index based on cost per 500 mg.
[1] As pentahydrate with L-arginine.
[2] Contains 2.3 mEq sodium/g.
[3] With 2.2 g dextrose hydrous.
[4] With 1.6 g dextrose hydrous.

IMIPENEM-CILASTATIN

Actions:

Pharmacology: This product is a formulation of imipenem, a thienamycin antibiotic, and cilastatin sodium, the inhibitor of the renal dipeptidase, dehydropeptidase-1. Dehydropeptidase-1 is responsible for the extensive metabolism of imipenem when it is administered alone. Cilastatin, by inhibiting this dipeptidase, prevents the metabolism of imipenem, thereby increasing urinary recovery and decreasing possible renal toxicity.

Pharmacokinetics: Absorption/Distribution (IV) – IV infusion over 20 minutes results in peak plasma levels of imipenem antimicrobial activity that range from 14 to 24 mcg/ml for the 250 mg dose, from 21 to 58 mcg/ml for the 500 mg dose and from 41 to 83 mcg/ml for the 1 g dose. Plasma levels declined to ≤ 1 mcg/ml in 4 to 6 hours. Peak plasma levels of cilastatin following a 20 minute IV infusion range from 15 to 25 mcg/ml for the 250 mg dose, from 31 to 49 mcg/ml for the 500 mg dose and from 56 to 88 mcg/ml for the 1 g dose.

The plasma half-life of each component is approximately 1 hour. Urine concentrations of imipenem in excess of 10 mcg/ml can be maintained for up to 8 hours at the 500 mg dose.

After a 1 g dose, the following average levels (mcg/ml or mcg/g) of imipenem were measured (usually 1 hour post-dose except where indicated) in the following tissues and fluids: Peritoneal 23.9 (2 hours); pleural 22; interstitial 16.4; fallopian tubes 13.6; endometrium 11.1; lung 5.6; bile 5.3 (2.25 hours); myometrium 5; skin 4.4; fascia 4.4; vitreous humor 3.4 (3.5 hours); aqueous humor 2.99 (2 hours); CSF (inflamed) 2.6 (2 hours); bone 2.6; sputum 2.1; CSF (uninflamed) 1 (4 hours).

Absorption/Distribution (IM) – Following IM administration of 500 or 750 mg doses, peak plasma levels of imipenem antimicrobial activity occur within 2 hours and average 10 and 12 mcg/ml, respectively. For cilastatin, peak plasma levels average 24 and 33 mcg/ml, respectively, and occur within 1 hour. When compared to IV administration, imipenem is approximately 75% bioavailable following IM administration while cilastatin is approximately 95% bioavailable. The absorption of imipenem from the IM injection site continues for 6 to 8 hours while that for cilastatin is essentially complete within 4 hours. This prolonged absorption of imipenem following IM use results in an effective plasma half-life of approximately 2 to 3 hours and plasma levels which remain above 2 mcg/ml for at least 6 or 8 hours following a 500 or 750 mg dose, respectively. This plasma profile for imipenem permits IM administration of every 12 hours with no accumulation of cilastatin and only slight accumulation of imipenem.

A comparison of plasma levels of imipenem after a single IV or IM dose of 500 or 750 mg is as follows:

Plasma Concentrations of Imipenem, IV vs IM (mcg/ml)

Time	500 mg dose		750 mg dose	
	IV	IM	IV	IM
25 min	45.1	6	57	6.7
1 hr	21.6	9.4	28.1	10
2 hr	10	9.9	12	11.4
4 hr	2.6	5.6	3.4	7.3
6 hr	0.6	2.5	1.1	3.8
12 hr	ND	0.5	ND	0.8

ND – Not detectable (< 0.3 mcg/ml)

Imipenem urine levels remain above 10 mcg/ml for the 12 hour dosing interval following the IM administration of 500 or 750 mg doses. Total urinary excretion of imipenem averages 50% while that for cilastatin averages 75% following either IM dose.

In a clinical study in which a 500 mg dose of the IM formulation was administered to healthy subjects, the average peak level of imipenem in interstitial fluid (skin blister fluid) was approximately 5 mcg/ml within 3.5 hours after administration.

Metabolism/Excretion – Imipenem, when administered alone, is metabolized in the kidneys by dehydropeptidase-1 resulting in relatively low levels in urine. Cilastatin, an inhibitor of this enzyme, prevents renal metabolism of imipenem. The protein binding of imipenem is approximately 20% and that of cilastatin is approximately 40%.

Approximately 70% of administered imipenem and cilastatin is recovered in urine within 10 hours of administration.

(Actions continued on following page)

IMIPENEM-CILASTATIN

Actions (Cont.):

Microbiology: The bactericidal activity of imipenem results from the inhibition of cell wall synthesis, related to binding to penicillin binding proteins (PBP) 2 and 1B. It has in vitro activity against a wide range of gram-positive and gram-negative organisms.

Imipenem has a high degree of stability in the presence of β-lactamases. It is a potent inhibitor of β-lactamases from certain gram-negative bacteria resistant to most β-lactam antibiotics, eg, *Pseudomonas aeruginosa, Serratia* sp and *Enterobacter* sp.

In vitro, imipenem is active against most strains of clinical isolates of the following microorganisms:

Gram-positive aerobes: Staphylococcus aureus including penicillinase-producing strains. (Note: Methicillin-resistant staphylococci are resistant.)

Group D streptococcus including *Enterococcus faecalis* (formerly *S faecalis).* (Note: Inactive in vitro against *Enterococcus faecium* [formerly *S faecium*].) *Streptococcus pneumoniae; S pyogenes* (Group A streptococcus); *S viridans* group.

Gram-negative aerobes: Acinetobacter sp, including *A calcoaceticus; Citrobacter* sp; *Enterobacter cloacae; Escherichia coli; Hemophilus influenzae; Klebsiella pneumoniae; P aeruginosa.* (Note: Inactive in vitro against *Xanthomonas (Pseudomonas) maltophilia* and *P cepacia.*)

Gram-positive anaerobes: Peptostreptococcus sp.

Gram-negative anaerobes: Bacteroides sp, including *B distasonis, B intermedius* (formerly *B melaninogenicus intermedius*), *B fragilis* and *B thetaiotaomicron; and Fusobacterium* sp.

Imipenem is active in vitro against the following microorganisms; however, the clinical significance of these data is unknown.

Gram-positive aerobes: Listeria monocytogenes; Nocardia sp; *Staphylococcus epidermidis* including penicillinase-producing strains. (Note: Methicillin-resistant staphylococci are resistant.)

S agalactiae (Group B streptococcus); Group C and G streptococcus.

Gram-negative aerobes: Achromobacter sp; *Aeromonas hydrophilia; Alcaligenes* sp; *Bordetella bronchiseptica; Campylobacter* sp; *Enterobacter* sp; *Gardnerella vaginalis; H parainfluenzae; Hafnia* sp, including *Hafnia alvei; Klebsiella* sp, including *K oxytoca; Moraxella* sp; *Morganella morganii; Neisseria gonorrhoeae* (including penicillinase-producing strains); *Pasteurella multocida; Plesiomonas shigelloides; Proteus mirabilis; P vulgaris; Providencia rettgeri; P stuartii; Salmonella* sp; *Serratia* sp, including *S marcescens* and *S proteamaculans* (formerly *S liquefaciens*); *Shigella* sp; *Yersinia* sp, including *Y enterocolitica* and *Y pseudotuberculosis.*

Gram-positive anaerobes: Actinomyces sp; *Clostridia* sp, including *C perfringens; Eubacterium* sp; *Peptococcus niger; Propionibacterium* sp, including *P acnes.*

Gram-negative anaerobes: Bacteroides bivius; B disiens; B ovatus; B vulgatus; Porphyromonas asaccharolytica (formerly *B asaccharolyticus*); *Veillonella* sp.

In vitro tests show imipenem to act synergistically with aminoglycoside antibiotics against some isolates of *P aeruginosa.*

Indications:

IV: Treatment of serious infections caused by susceptible strains of the designated microorganisms in the diseases listed below:

Lower respiratory tract infections – *S aureus* (penicillinase-producing), *E coli, Klebsiella* sp, *Enterobacter* sp, *H influenzae, H parainfluenzae**, *Acinetobacter* sp, *S marcescens.*

Urinary tract infections (complicated and uncomplicated) – *S aureus* (penicillinase-producing)*, group D streptococci (enterococci), *E coli, Klebsiella* sp, *Enterobacter* sp, *P vulgaris**, *P rettgeri**, *M morganii**, *P aeruginosa.*

Intra-abdominal infections – *S aureus* (penicillinase-producing)*, *S epidermidis,* group D streptococci (enterococci), *E coli, Klebsiella* sp, *Enterobacter* sp, *Proteus* sp (indole-positive and indole-negative), *M morganii**, *P aeruginosa, Citrobacter* sp, *Clostridium* sp, gram-positive anaerobes including *Peptococcus* sp, *Peptostreptococcus* sp, *Eubacterium* sp, *Propionibacterium* sp*, *Bifidobacterium* sp, *Bacteroides* sp including *B fragilis, Fusobacterium* sp.

Gynecologic infections – *S aureus* (penicillinase-producing)*, *S epidermidis,* group B streptococci, group D streptococci (enterococci), *E coli, Klebsiella* sp*, *Proteus* sp (indole-positive and indole-negative), *Enterobacter* sp*, gram-positive anaerobes including *Peptococcus* sp*, *Peptostreptococcus* sp, *Propionibacterium* sp*, *Bifidobacterium* sp*, *Bacteroides* sp, *B fragilis**, *Gardnerella vaginalis.*

Bacterial septicemia – *S aureus* (penicillinase-producing), group D streptococci (enterococci), *E coli, Klebsiella* sp, *P aeruginosa, Serratia* sp*, *Enterobacter* sp, *Bacteroides* sp, *B fragilis.**

*Efficacy for this organism in this organ system was demonstrated in less than ten infections.

(Indications continued on following page)

IMIPENEM-CILASTATIN (Cont.)

Indications (Cont.):

IV (Cont.):

Bone and joint infections – *S aureus* (penicillinase-producing), *S epidermidis,* group D streptococci (enterococci), *Enterobacter* sp, *P aeruginosa.*

Skin and skin structure infections – *S aureus* (penicillinase-producing), *S epidermidis,* group D streptococci (enterococci), *E coli, Klebsiella* sp, *Enterobacter* sp, *P vulgaris, P rettgeri**, *M morganii, P aeruginosa, Serratia* sp, *Citrobacter* sp, *Acinetobacter* sp, gram-positive anaerobes including *Peptococcus* sp and *Peptostreptococcus* sp, *Bacteroides* sp including *B fragilis, Fusobacterium* sp*.

Endocarditis – *S aureus* (penicillinase-producing).

Polymicrobic infections, including those in which *S pneumoniae* (pneumonia, septicemia), group A β-hemolytic streptococcus (skin and skin structure) or nonpenicillinase-producing *S aureus* is one of the causative organisms. However, these monobacterial infections are usually treated with narrower spectrum antibiotics, ie, penicillin G.

Although clinical improvement has been observed in patients with cystic fibrosis, chronic pulmonary disease and lower respiratory tract infections caused by *P aeruginosa,* bacterial eradication may not be achieved.

IM: Treatment of serious infections of mild to moderate severity for which IM therapy is appropriate. Not intended for severe or life-threatening infections, including bacterial sepsis or endocarditis, or in instances of major physiological impairments (eg, shock).

Lower respiratory tract infections, including pneumonia and bronchitis as an exacerbation of COPD, caused by *S pneumoniae* and *H influenzae.*

Intra-abdominal infections, including acute gangrenous or perforated appendicitis and appendicitis with peritonitis, caused by Group D streptococcus including *Enterococcus faecalis**; *S viridans* group*; *E coli; K pneumoniae**; *P aeruginosa**; *Bacteroides* sp including *B fragilis, B distasonis**, *B intermedius** and *B thetaiotaomicron**; *Fusobacterium* sp; *Peptostreptococcus* sp*.

Skin and skin structure infections, including abscesses, cellulitis, infected skin ulcers and wound infections caused by *S aureus* (including penicillinase-producing strains); *Streptococcus pyogenes**, Group D streptococcus including *Enterococcus faecalis; Acinetobacter sp** including *A calcoaceticus**; *Citrobacter* sp*; *E coli; Enterobacter cloacae; K pneumoniae**; *P aeruginosa**; *Bacteroides* sp* including *B fragilis**.

Gynecologic infections, including postpartum endomyometritis, caused by Group D streptococcus including *Enterococcus faecalis**; *E coli; K pneumoniae**; *B intermedius**; *Peptostreptococcus* sp*.

As with other β-lactam antibiotics, some strains of *P aeruginosa* may develop resistance fairly rapidly; periodically perform clinically appropriate susceptibility testing.

Infections resistant to other antibiotics (eg, cephalosporins, penicillins, aminoglycosides) have responded to treatment with imipenem.

Contraindications:

Hypersensitivity to any component of this product.

IM: Hypersensitivity to local anesthetics of the amide type and in patients with severe shock or heart block due to the use of lidocaine HCl diluent.

Warnings:

Hypersensitivity and cross-resistance: Serious and occasionally fatal hypersensitivity (anaphylactic) reactions have occurred in patients receiving therapy with β-lactams. They are more apt to occur in persons with a history of sensitivity to multiple allergens. Patients with a history of penicillin hypersensitivity have experienced severe reactions when treated with another β-lactam. If a reaction occurs, discontinue the drug. Serious reactions may require emergency measures. See Management of Acute Hypersensitivity Reactions.

Pseudomembranous colitis has been reported with virtually all antibiotics. Consider its diagnosis in patients developing diarrhea while on antibiotics. Severity ranges from mild to life-threatening. Mild cases may respond to drug discontinuation. More severe cases may require sigmoidoscopy, appropriate bacteriological studies, fluid, electrolyte and protein supplementation and a drug such as oral vancomycin, as indicated. Isolating the patient may be advisable. Consider other causes of colitis.

Pregnancy: Category C. There are no adequate and well controlled studies in pregnant women. Use only when potential benefits outweigh potential hazards to the fetus.

Lactation: It is not known whether this drug is excreted in breast milk. Exercise caution when administering to a nursing woman.

Children: Safety and efficacy for use in children $<$ 12 years of age have not been established.

*Efficacy for this organism in this organ system was demonstrated in less than ten infections.

(Continued on following page)

IMIPENEM-CILASTATIN (Cont.)

Precautions:

CNS adverse experiences (eg, myoclonic activity, confusional states, seizures) have been reported with the IV formulation, especially when recommended dosages were exceeded. They are most common in patients with CNS disorders (eg, brain lesions, history of seizures) who also have compromised renal function and rare when no underlying CNS disorder exists. Closely adhere to recommended dosage schedules, especially in patients with known factors that predispose to convulsive activity. Continue anticonvulsants in patients with a known seizure disorder. If focal tremors, myoclonus or seizures occur, neurologically evaluate patient and institute anticonvulsants. Re-examine the dosage and determine whether to decrease dosage or discontinue the drug. If these effects occur with the IM formulation, discontinue the drug.

Monitoring: While imipenem has the characteristic low toxicity of the β-lactam group of antibiotics, periodically assess organ system function during prolonged therapy.

Superinfection: Use of antibiotics (especially prolonged or repeated therapy) may result in bacterial or fungal overgrowth of nonsusceptible organisms. Such overgrowth may lead to a secondary infection. Take appropriate measures if superinfection occurs.

Drug Interactions:

Ganciclovir: Generalized seizures have occurred in patients receiving concomitant imipenem-cilastatin IV. Do not use concomitantly unless potential benefits outweigh the risks.

Probenecid and concurrent imipenem-cilastatin results in only minimal increases in imipenem plasma levels and half-life; therefore, it is not recommended that probenecid be given concurrently.

Adverse Reactions:

IV: Local – Phlebitis/thrombophlebitis (3.1%); pain at the injection site (0.7%); erythema at the injection site (0.4%); vein induration (0.2%); infused vein infection (0.1%).

GI – Nausea (2%); diarrhea (1.8%); vomiting (1.5%); pseudomembranous colitis, hemorrhagic colitis, hepatitis, gastroenteritis, abdominal pain, glossitis, tongue papillar hypertrophy, heartburn, pharyngeal pain, increased salivation (< 0.2%).

CNS – Fever (0.5%); seizures (0.4%); dizziness (0.3%); somnolence (0.2%); encephalopathy, tremor, confusion, myoclonus, paresthesia, vertigo, headache, psychic disturbances (< 0.2%).

Respiratory – Chest discomfort, dyspnea, hyperventilation (< 0.2%).

Cardiovascular – Hypotension (0.4%); palpitations, tachycardia (< 0.2%).

Dermatologic – Rash (0.9%); pruritus (0.3%); urticaria (0.2%); erythema multiforme, toxic epidermal necrolysis, facial edema, flushing, cyanosis, skin texture changes, candidiasis, pruritus vulvae (< 0.2%).

Other – Transient hearing loss in patients with impaired hearing, tinnitus, polyarthralgia, taste perversion, asthenia/weakness, thoracic spine pain, thrombocytopenia, leukopenia, oliguria/anuria, polyuria, acute renal failure, hyperhidrosis (< 0.2%).

Altered laboratory findings –

Hepatic: Increased AST, ALT, alkaline phosphatase, bilirubin and LDH.

Hemic: Increased eosinophils, monocytes, lymphocytes, basophils; decreased neutrophils (including agranulocytosis [< 0.2%]), hemoglobin, hematocrit; increased/decreased WBCs and platelets; positive Coombs' test; abnormal prothrombin time.

Electrolytes: Decreased serum sodium; increased potassium and chloride.

Renal: Increased BUN and creatinine.

Urinalysis: Presence of protein, RBCs, WBCs, casts, bilirubin or urobilinogen in the urine.

IM: Local – Pain at the injection site.

Systemic – Nausea, diarrhea (0.6%); vomiting (0.3%); rash (0.4%).

Altered laboratory findings – *Hemic:* Decreased hemoglobin and hematocrit; eosinophilia; increased/decreased WBCs and platelets; decreased erythrocytes; increased prothrombin time.

Hepatic: Increased AST, ALT, alkaline phosphatase and bilirubin.

Renal: Increased BUN and creatinine.

Urinalysis: Presence of RBCs, WBCs, casts and bacteria in the urine.

Overdosage:

In the case of overdosage, discontinue the drug. Treat symptomatically and institute supportive measures as required. Refer to General Management of Acute Overdosage. Imipenem-cilastatin is hemodialyzable; however, usefulness of this procedure in the overdosage setting is questionable.

(Continued on following page)

IMIPENEM-CILASTATIN (Cont.)

Administration and Dosage:

Dosage recommendations represent the quantity of imipenem to be administered. An equivalent amount of cilastatin is also present in the solution.

Base the initial dosage on the type or severity of infection and administer in equally divided doses. Base subsequent dosing on severity of illness, degree of susceptibility of the pathogen(s), weight and creatinine clearance.

IV: Give each 250 or 500 mg dose by IV infusion over 20 to 30 minutes. Infuse each 1 g dose over 40 to 60 minutes. In patients who develop nausea, slow the infusion rate.

Due to high antimicrobial activity, do not exceed 50 mg/kg/day or 4 g/day, whichever is lower. There is no evidence that higher doses provide greater efficacy.

Imipenem-Cilastatin IV Dosing Schedule for Adults with Normal Renal Function		
Type or severity of infection	Fully susceptible organisms including gram-positive and gram-negative aerobes and anaerobes	Moderately susceptible organisms, primarily some strains of *P aeruginosa*
Mild	250 mg q 6 h	500 mg q 6 h
Moderate	500 mg q 8 h - 500 mg q 6 h	500 mg q 6 h - 1 g q 8 h
Severe, life-threatening	500 mg q 6 h	1 g q 8 h - 1 g q 6 h
Uncomplicated UTI	250 mg q 6 h	250 mg q 6 h
Complicated UTI	500 mg q 6 h	500 mg q 6 h

IM:

Imipenem-Cilastatin IM Dosage Guidelines		
Type/Location of infection	Severity	Dosage regimen
Lower respiratory tract Skin and skin structure Gynecologic	Mild/Moderate	500 or 750 mg q 12 h depending on the severity of infection
Intra-abdominal	Mild/Moderate	750 mg q 12 h

Total daily IM dosages > 1500 mg/day are not recommended.

The duration of therapy depends upon the type and severity of the infection. Generally, continue for at least 2 days after the signs and symptoms of infection have resolved. Safety and efficacy of treatment beyond 14 days have not been established.

Administer by deep IM injection into a large muscle mass (such as the gluteal muscles or lateral part of the thigh) with a 21 gauge 2" needle. Aspiration is necessary to avoid inadvertent injection into a blood vessel.

Renal function impairment: Patients with creatinine clearance (Ccr) of ≤ 70 ml/min/1.73 m^2 require dosage adjustment (see table below). Base doses on 70 kg body weight.

Serum creatinine alone may not be a sufficiently accurate measure of renal function. Ccr may be estimated from the following equation:

Males: $$\frac{\text{Weight (kg)} \times (140 - \text{age})}{72 \times \text{serum creatinine (mg/dl)}} = \text{Ccr}$$

Females: 0.85 x above value

<table>
<tr><th colspan="4">Imipenem-Cilastatin IV Dosage in Renal Impairment</th></tr>
<tr><th>Ccr (ml/min/ 1.73 m²)</th><th>Renal function impairment</th><th>Fully susceptible organisms including gram-positive and gram-negative aerobes and anaerobes</th><th>Moderately susceptible organisms, primarily some strains of P aeruginosa</th></tr>
<tr><td>31-70</td><td>Mild</td><td>500 mg q 8 h</td><td>500 mg q 6 h</td></tr>
<tr><td>21-30</td><td>Moderate</td><td>500 mg q 12 h</td><td>500 mg q 8 h</td></tr>
<tr><td>6-20</td><td>Severe to marked</td><td rowspan="2">250 mg q 12 h</td><td rowspan="2">500 mg q 12 h</td></tr>
<tr><td>0-5[1]</td><td>None, but on hemodialysis</td></tr>
</table>

[1] Do not administer imipenem-cilastatin unless hemodialysis is instituted within 48 hours.

(Administration and Dosage continued on following page)

IMIPENEM-CILASTATIN (Cont.)

Administration and Dosage (Cont.):

Hemodialysis: Imipenem-cilastatin is cleared by hemodialysis. The patient should receive imipenem-cilastatin after hemodialysis and at 12 hour intervals timed from the end of that dialysis session. For patients on hemodialysis, imipenem-cilastatin is recommended only when the benefits outweigh the potential risk of seizures. There is inadequate information to recommend usage for patients undergoing peritoneal dialysis. Carefully monitor dialysis patients, especially those with CNS diseases.

Preparation of solution: IV – Restore contents of the infusion bottles with 100 ml of diluent (see Compatibility/Stability). Shake until a clear solution is obtained. Contents of the vials must be suspended and transferred to 100 ml of an appropriate infusion solution. Add approximately 10 ml from the infusion solution (see Compatibility/Stability) to the vial. Shake well and transfer the resulting suspension to the infusion solution container. Caution: The suspension is not for direct infusion.

Repeat with an additional 10 ml of infusion solution to ensure complete transfer of vial contents to the infusion solution. Agitate the resulting mixture until clear.

IM – Prepare with 1% lidocaine HCl solution (without epinephrine). Prepare the 500 mg vial with 2 ml and the 750 mg vial with 3 ml lidocaine HCl. Agitate to form a suspension, then withdraw and inject the entire contents of vial IM. Note: The IM formulation is not for IV use.

Compatibility/Stability: Before reconstitution – Store powder below 30°C (86°F).

Reconstituted IV solutions: Solutions range from colorless to yellow. Variations of color within this range do not affect product potency.

Imipenem-cilastatin in infusion bottles and vials, reconstituted as directed with the following diluents, maintains satisfactory potency for 4 hours at room temperature and for 24 hours when refrigerated (5°C; 41°F). Note exception below. Do not freeze solutions.

- 0.9% Sodium Chloride Injection (stable in 0.9% Sodium Chloride Injection for 10 hours at room temperature and 48 hours refrigerated)
- 5% or 10% Dextrose Injection
- 5% Dextrose Injection with 0.02% sodium bicarbonate solution
- 5% Dextrose and 0.9% Sodium Chloride Injection
- 5% Dextrose Injection with 0.225% or 0.45% saline solution
- *Normosol-M* in D5-W
- 5% Dextrose Injection with 0.15% potassium chloride solution
- Mannitol 2.5%, 5% and 10%

Reconstituted IM suspensions: Suspensions are white to light tan in color. Variations of color within this range do not affect the potency of the product.

Use this suspension within 1 hour after preparation.

Admixture incompatibility: Do not mix with or physically add to other antibiotics. However, it may be administered concomitantly with other antibiotics, such as aminoglycosides.

				C.I.*
Rx	**Primaxin I.V.** (MSD)	**Powder for Injection:** Contains 3.2 mEq sodium per g.		
		250 mg imipenem equivalent and 250 mg cilastatin equivalent	In vials, infusion bottles and *ADD-Vantage* vials.	1024
		500 mg imipenem equivalent and 500 mg cilastatin equivalent	In vials, infusion bottles and *ADD-Vantage* vials.	962
Rx	**Primaxin I.M.** (MSD)	**Powder for Injection:** 500 mg imipenem equivalent and 500 mg cilastatin equivalent. Contains 1.4 mEq sodium	In vials.	NA
		750 mg imipenem equivalent and 750 mg cilastatin equivalent Contains 2.1 mEq sodium	In vials.	NA

* Cost Index based on cost per 250 mg imipenem equivalent.

AZTREONAM

Actions:

Pharmacology: Aztreonam, a synthetic bactericidal antibiotic, is the first of a new class of antibiotics identified as monobactams. The monobactams have a monocyclic β-lactam nucleus and are structurally different from other β-lactams (eg, penicillins, cephalosporins, cephamycins). Aztreonam has a wide spectrum of activity against gram-negative aerobic pathogens.

Pharmacokinetics: Absorption/Distribution – Single 30 minute IV infusions of 500 mg, 1 and 2 g doses in healthy subjects produced peak serum levels of 54, 90 and 204 mcg/ml, respectively, immediately after administration; at 8 hours, serum levels were 1, 3 and 6 mcg/ml, respectively.

Following single IM injections of 500 mg and 1 g, maximum serum concentrations occur at about 1 hour. After identical single IV or IM doses, the serum concentrations of aztreonam are comparable at 1 hour (1.5 hours from start of IV infusion) with similar slopes of serum concentrations thereafter.

The serum half-life averaged 1.7 hours (range, 1.5 to 2) in subjects with normal renal function, independent of the dose and route. In healthy subjects, based on a 70 kg person, the serum clearance was 91 ml/min and renal clearance was 56 ml/min; the apparent mean volume of distribution at steady state averaged 12.6 L, approximately equivalent to extracellular fluid volume.

The average elimination half-life appears slightly longer in healthy elderly males.

In patients with impaired renal function, the serum half-life is prolonged. Serum half-life is slightly prolonged in patients with hepatic impairment since the liver is a minor pathway of excretion.

The concentration in breast milk at 2 hours after a single 1 g IV dose (6 patients) was 0.2 mcg/ml; in amniotic fluid at 6 to 8 hours after a single 1 g IV dose (5 patients), it was 2 mcg/ml. The concentration in peritoneal fluid obtained 1 to 6 hours after multiple 2 g IV doses ranged between 12 and 90 mcg/ml in 7 of 8 patients studied.

Aztreonam, given IV, rapidly reaches therapeutic concentrations in peritoneal dialysis fluid; conversely, given intraperitoneally in dialysis fluid, it rapidly produces therapeutic serum levels.

Metabolism/Excretion – After IM injection of single 500 mg and 1 g doses, urinary levels were approximately 500 and 1200 mcg/ml, respectively, within the first 2 hours, declining to 180 and 470 mcg/ml in the 6 to 8 hour specimens. In healthy subjects, aztreonam is excreted in the urine about equally by active tubular secretion and glomerular filtration. Approximately 60% to 70% of an IV or IM dose was recovered in the urine by 8 hours; recovery was complete by 12 hours. About 12% of a single IV dose was recovered in the feces.

Administration IV or IM of a single 500 mg or 1 g dose every 8 hours for 7 days to healthy subjects produced no apparent accumulation; serum protein binding averaged 56% and was independent of dose. An average of about 6% of a 1 g IM dose was excreted as an inactive open β-lactam ring hydrolysis product (serum half-life approximately 26 hours).

Microbiology: Aztreonam exhibits potent and specific activity in vitro against a wide spectrum of gram-negative aerobic pathogens including *Pseudomonas aeruginosa*. The bactericidal action results from the inhibition of bacterial cell wall synthesis due to a high affinity of aztreonam for penicillin binding protein 3 (PBP3). Aztreonam does not induce β-lactamase activity, and its molecular structure confers a high degree of resistance to hydrolysis by β-lactamases; it is therefore usually active against gram-negative aerobic organisms. Aztreonam maintains its antimicrobial activity over a pH of 6 to 8. Aztreonam is effective in clinical infections against most strains of the following organisms: *Escherichia coli; Enterobacter* sp; *Klebsiella pneumoniae* and *K oxytoca; Proteus mirabilis; P aeruginosa; Serratia marcescens; Hemophilus influenzae,* including ampicillin-resistant and other penicillinase-producing strains; *Citrobacter* sp.

While in vitro studies have demonstrated susceptibility to aztreonam in most of these strains, clinical efficacy for infections other than those included in the indications section has not been documented: *Neisseria gonorrhoeae* (including penicillinase-producing strains); *P vulgaris; Morganella morganii* (formerly *Proteus morganii*); *Providencia* species, including *P stuartii* and *P rettgeri; Pseudomonas* sp; *Shigella* sp; *Pasteurella multocida; Yersinia enterocolitica; Aeromonas hydrophila; N meningitidis*.

Aztreonam and aminoglycosides are synergistic in vitro against most strains of *P aeruginosa*, many strains of Enterobacteriaceae, and other gram-negative aerobic bacilli.

Aztreonam has little effect on the anaerobic intestinal microflora in in vitro studies. *Clostridium difficile* and its cytotoxin were not found in animal models following administration of aztreonam.

(Continued on following page)

AZTREONAM (Cont.)

Indications:

For the treatment of the following infections caused by susceptible gram-negative microorganisms:

Urinary tract infections (complicated and uncomplicated), including pyelonephritis and cystitis (initial and recurrent) caused by *E coli, K pneumoniae, P mirabilis, P aeruginosa, E cloacae, K oxytoca, Citrobacter* sp and *S marcescens*.

Lower respiratory tract infections, including pneumonia and bronchitis caused by *E coli, K pneumoniae, P aeruginosa, H influenzae, P mirabilis, Enterobacter* sp and *S marcescens*.

Septicemia caused by *E coli, K pneumoniae, P aeruginosa, P mirabilis, S marcescens* and *Enterobacter* sp.

Skin and skin structure infections, including those associated with postoperative wounds, ulcers and burns caused by *E coli, P mirabilis, S marcescens, Enterobacter* sp, *P aeruginosa, K pneumoniae* and *Citrobacter* sp.

Intra-abdominal infections, including peritonitis caused by *E coli, Klebsiella* sp including *K pneumoniae, Enterobacter* sp including *E cloacae, P aeruginosa, Citrobacter* sp including *C freundii* and *Serratia* sp including *S marcescens*.

Gynecologic infections, including endometritis and pelvic cellulitis caused by *E coli, K pneumoniae, Enterobacter* sp including *E cloacae* and *P mirabilis*.

For adjunctive therapy to surgery to manage infections caused by susceptible organisms.

Concurrent initial therapy with other antimicrobials and aztreonam is recommended before the causative organism(s) are known in seriously ill patients who are also at risk of having an infection due to gram-positive aerobic pathogens. If anaerobic organisms are also suspected, initiate therapy concurrently with aztreonam.

Contraindications:

Allergy to aztreonam.

Warnings:

Acute hypersensitivity reaction: Make careful inquiry for a history of hypersensitivity reactions. Monitor patients who have had immediate hypersensitivity reactions (eg, anaphylactic or urticarial) to penicillins or cephalosporins. If an allergic reaction to aztreonam occurs, discontinue the drug and institute supportive treatment. Refer to Management of Acute Hypersensitivity Reactions

Usage in Pregnancy: Category B. Aztreonam crosses the placenta and enters fetal circulation. There are no adequate and well controlled studies in pregnant women. Use during pregnancy only if clearly needed.

Usage in Lactation: Aztreonam is excreted in breast milk in concentrations that are less than 1% of maternal serum. Consider temporary discontinuation of nursing.

Usage in Children: Safety and efficacy for use in infants and children have not been established.

Precautions:

Impaired renal or hepatic function: Appropriate monitoring is recommended.

If an **aminoglycoside** is used concurrently with aztreonam, especially if high dosages of the former are used or if therapy is prolonged, monitor renal function because of the potential nephrotoxicity and ototoxicity of aminoglycoside antibiotics.

Superinfection: Use of antibiotics (especially prolonged or repeated therapy) may result in bacterial (including gram-positive *S aureus* and *S faecalis*) or fungal overgrowth of nonsusceptible organisms. Such overgrowth may lead to a secondary infection. Take appropriate measures if superinfection occurs.

Drug Interactions:

Probenecid or **furosemide:** Concomitant administration causes clinically insignificant increases in aztreonam serum levels.

Antibiotics (eg, cefoxitin, imipenem) may induce high levels of β-lactamase in vitro in some gram-negative aerobes such as *Enterobacter* and *Pseudomonas* species, resulting in antagonism to many β-lactam antibiotics including aztreonam. These in vitro findings suggest that such β-lactamase-inducing antibiotics not be used concurrently with aztreonam.

(Continued on following page)

AZTREONAM (Cont.)

Adverse Reactions:

Local reactions such as phlebitis/thrombophlebitis following IV administration (1.9%); discomfort/swelling at the injection site following IM administration (2.4%).

Systemic reactions (1% to 1.3%) include diarrhea, nausea, vomiting and rash. Reactions occurring at an incidence < 1% are listed below.

Hypersensitivity: Anaphylaxis.

Hematologic: Pancytopenia, neutropenia, thrombocytopenia, anemia, leukocytosis, thrombocytosis.

GI: Abdominal cramps; *C difficile*-associated diarrhea or GI bleeding (rare).

Dermatologic: Purpura, erythema multiforme, urticaria, exfoliative dermatitis, petechiae, pruritus, diaphoresis.

Cardiovascular: Hypotension, transient ECG changes (ventricular bigeminy and PVC).

Hepatic: Hepatitis, jaundice.

CNS: Seizure, confusion, headache, vertigo, paresthesia, insomnia, dizziness.

Special senses: Tinnitus, diplopia, mouth ulcer, altered taste, numb tongue, sneezing and nasal congestion, halitosis.

Other: Vaginal candidiasis, vaginitis, breast tenderness, weakness, muscular aches, fever, malaise. One patient experienced flushing, chest pain and dyspnea.

Laboratory: Elevations of AST (SGOT), ALT (SGPT) and alkaline phosphatase; increases in prothrombin and partial thromboplastin times, eosinophilia, positive Coombs test; increases in serum creatinine.

Overdosage:

If necessary, clear aztreonam from the serum by hemodialysis or peritoneal dialysis.

Dosage:

Give IM or IV. Individualize dosage.

DOSAGE GUIDE (Adults)		
Type of infection	**Dose†**	**Frequency (hours)**
Urinary tract infection	500 mg or 1 g	8 or 12
Moderately severe systemic infections	1 or 2 g	8 or 12
Severe systemic or life-threatening infections	2 g	6 or 8

† Maximum recommended dose is 8 g per day.

The IV route is recommended for patients requiring single doses greater than 1 g or those with bacterial septicemia, localized parenchymal abscess (eg, intra-abdominal abscess), peritonitis or other severe systemic or life-threatening infections. For infections due to *P aeruginosa,* a dosage of 2 g every 6 or 8 hours is recommended, at least upon initiation of therapy.

Duration of therapy depends on the severity of infection. Generally, continue aztreonam for at least 48 hours after the patient becomes asymptomatic or evidence of bacterial eradication has been obtained. Persistent infections may require treatment for several weeks. Do not use doses smaller than those indicated.

Impaired renal function: Prolonged aztreonam serum levels may occur in patients with transient or persistent renal insufficiency. Therefore, reduce dosage by one-half in patients with estimated creatinine clearances between 10 and 30 ml/min/1.73 m² after an initial loading dose of 1 g or 2 g.

When only the serum creatinine concentration is available, the following formula may be used to approximate creatinine clearance (Ccr). The serum creatinine should represent steady-state renal function.

$$\text{Males:} \quad \frac{\text{Weight (kg)} \times (140 - \text{age})}{72 \times \text{serum creatinine (mg/100 ml)}} = \text{Ccr}$$

Females: 0.85 x above value

In patients with severe renal failure (creatinine clearance < 10 ml/min/1.73 m²), such as those supported by hemodialysis, give 500 mg, 1 g or 2 g initially. The maintenance dose should be one-fourth of the usual initial dose given at the usual fixed interval of 6, 8 or 12 hours. For serious or life-threatening infections, in addition to the maintenance doses, give one-eighth of the initial dose after each hemodialysis session.

Dosage in the elderly: Renal status is a major determinant of dosage in the elderly. Serum creatinine may not be an accurate determinant of renal status. Therefore, obtain estimates of creatinine clearance and make appropriate dosage modifications.

(Continued on following page)

AZTREONAM (Cont.)

Administration:

IV: Bolus injection may be used to initiate therapy. Slowly inject directly into a vein, or into the tubing of a suitable administration set, over 3 to 5 minutes.

Infusion – With any intermittent infusion of aztreonam and another drug not pharmaceutically compatible, flush the common delivery tube before and after delivery of aztreonam with an infusion solution compatible with both drug solutions. Do not deliver the drugs simultaneously. Complete the infusion within 20 to 60 minutes. With a Y-type administration set, give careful attention to the calculated volume of aztreonam solution required so that the entire dose will be infused. If a volume control administration set is used to deliver an initial dilution of aztreonam during administration, the final aztreonam dilution should provide a concentration not > 2% w/v.

IM: Inject deeply into a large muscle mass (ie, upper outer quadrant of gluteus maximus or lateral thigh). Aztreonam is well tolerated; do not admix with local anesthetics.

Preparation of solutions: After adding diluent to container, shake **immediately** and **vigorously.** Constituted solutions are not for multiple-dose use; discard unused solution.

Constituted aztreonam yields a colorless to light straw yellow solution which may develop a slight pink tint on standing (potency is not affected).

IV solutions – For bolus injection: Constitute the contents of the 15 ml vial with 6 to 10 ml Sterile Water for Injection.

For infusion: Constitute the contents of the 100 ml bottle to a final concentration not > 2% w/v (at least 50 ml of any infusion solution listed below per g aztreonam). Most solutions may be frozen in the original container immediately after constitution.

If the contents of a 15 ml vial are to be transferred to an infusion solution, initially constitute each g of aztreonam with at least 3 ml Sterile Water for Injection. Further dilute with one of the following IV infusion solutions:

Sodium Chloride Injection, 0.9%
Ringer's or Lactated Ringer's Injection
Dextrose Injection, 5% or 10%
Dextrose and Sodium Chloride Injection, (5%:0.9%), (5%:0.45%) or (5%:0.2%)
Sodium Lactate Injection (M/6 Sodium Lactate)
Ionosol B and 5% Dextrose
Isolyte E or Isolyte E with 5% Dextrose
Isolyte M with 5% Dextrose
Normosol R
Normosol R and 5% Dextrose
Normosol M and 5% Dextrose
Mannitol Injection, 5% or 10%
Lactated Ringer's and 5% Dextrose Injection
Plasma-Lyte M and 5% Dextrose
10% Travert Injection
10% Travert and Electrolyte No. 2 Injection

IM Solutions – Constitute a 15 ml vial with at least 3 ml of diluent per g aztreonam. The following diluents may be used: Sterile Water for Injection; Bacteriostatic Water for Injection (with benzyl alcohol or methyl and propyl parabens); Sodium Chloride Injection, 0.9%; Bacteriostatic Sodium Chloride Injection (with benzyl alcohol or parabens).

Stability of IV and IM solutions: Use solutions for IV infusion at concentrations not > 2% w/v within 48 hours following constitution if kept at controlled room temperature (59° to 86°F/15° to 30°C) or within 7 days if refrigerated (36° to 46°F/2° to 8°C).

Frozen aztreonam infusion solutions, except for solutions prepared with Mannitol Injection 10% or Lactated Ringer's and 5% Dextrose Injection which have not been tested, may be stored for up to 3 months at −4°F/−20°C. Use frozen solutions that have been thawed and maintained at controlled room temperature or by overnight refrigeration within 24 or 72 hours, respectively, after removal from the freezer. Do not refreeze solutions.

Solutions at concentrations exceeding 2% w/v, except those prepared with Sterile Water for Injection or Sodium Chloride Injection, should be used promptly after preparation. The two excepted solutions must be used within 48 hours if stored at controlled room temperature or within 7 days if refrigerated.

Admixtures with other antibiotics: IV infusion solutions of aztreonam prepared with Sodium Chloride Injection 0.9% or Dextrose Injection 5%, to which clindamycin phosphate, gentamicin sulfate, tobramycin sulfate or cefazolin sodium have been added at clinical concentrations, are stable for 48 hours at room temperature or 7 days refrigerated. Ampicillin sodium admixtures with aztreonam in Sodium Chloride Injection 0.9% are stable for 24 hours at room temperature and 48 hours under refrigeration; stability in Dextrose Injection 5% is 2 hours at room temperature and 8 hours refrigerated. Aztreonam-cloxacillin sodium and aztreonam-vancomycin HCl admixtures are stable in *Dianeal 137* (peritoneal dialysis solution) with 4.25% Dextrose for 24 hours at room temperature.

Incompatible with aztreonam: Nafcillin sodium, cephradine and metronidazole. Other admixtures are not recommended, since compatibility data are not available.

Rx	**Azactam** (Squibb)	**Powder for Injection:** 500 mg.[1]	In 15 ml vials and 100 ml infusion bottles.
		1 g.[1]	In 15 ml vials and 100 ml infusion bottles.
		2 g.[1]	In 15 ml vials and 100 ml infusion bottles.

[1] With ≈ 780 mg L-arginine per g aztreonam.

CHLORAMPHENICOL

Warning:

Serious and fatal blood dyscrasias (aplastic anemia, hypoplastic anemia, thrombocytopenia and granulocytopenia) occur after chloramphenicol administration. There have been reports of aplastic anemia, which later terminated in leukemia. Blood dyscrasias have occurred after both short-term and prolonged therapy. Chloramphenicol must not be used when less potentially dangerous agents are effective. *It must not be used to treat trivial infections (ie, influenza, colds, throat infections), infections other than indicated, or as prophylaxis for bacterial infections.*

It is essential that adequate blood studies be performed during treatment. While blood studies may detect early peripheral blood changes, such as leukopenia, reticulocytopenia or granulocytopenia before they become irreversible, such studies cannot be relied upon to detect bone marrow depression prior to development of aplastic anemia. To facilitate appropriate studies and observation, patients should be hospitalized.

Actions:

Microbiology: Chloramphenicol binds to the 50 S ribosomal subunits of bacteria and interferes with or inhibits protein synthesis. In vitro, chloramphenicol exerts mainly a bacteriostatic effect on a wide range of gram-negative and gram-positive bacteria, and is active in vitro against rickettsiae, the lymphogranuloma-psittacosis group and *Vibrio cholerae.* It is particularly active against *Salmonella typhi* and *Hemophilus influenzae.*

Pharmacokinetics:

Absorption – Chloramphenicol base is absorbed rapidly from the intestinal tract and is 75% to 90% bioavailable. In adults, at doses of 1 g every 6 hours for 8 doses, the average peak serum level was 11.2 mcg/ml 1 hour after the first dose, and 18.4 mcg/ml after the fifth 1 g dose. Mean serum levels ranged from 8 to 14 mcg/ml over the 48 hour period.

The inactive prodrug, chloramphenicol palmitate, is rapidly hydrolyzed to active chloramphenicol base. Bioavailability is approximately 80% for the palmitate ester. The bioavailability of the IV succinate is approximately 70%. Hydrolysis of the succinate is probably by esterases of the liver, kidney and lungs. Approximately 30% is eliminated in the urine as unhydrolyzed ester.

Distribution – The therapeutic range for total serum chloramphenicol concentration is peak, 10 to 20 mcg/ml; trough, 5 to 10 mcg/ml. The drug is approximately 60% bound to plasma proteins. Because of the significantly greater concentration of free drug in the serum of premature infants, the therapeutic range for total serum concentration of chloramphenicol may be lower.

Chloramphenicol diffuses rapidly, but its distribution is not uniform. Highest concentrations are found in liver and kidney, and lowest concentrations are found in brain and cerebrospinal fluid (CSF). However, chloramphenicol enters the CSF, even in the absence of meningeal inflammation, appearing in concentrations 45% to 99% of those found in the blood. Measurable levels are also detected in pleural and ascitic fluids, saliva, milk and in the aqueous and vitreous humors. Transport across the placental barrier occurs with somewhat lower concentrations in the cord blood of newborns than in maternal blood.

Metabolism/Elimination – Total urinary excretion of chloramphenicol ranges from 68% to 99% over 3 days. From 5% to 15% is excreted as free chloramphenicol; the remainder consists of inactive metabolites via the liver, principally the glucuronide. Since the glucuronide is excreted rapidly, most chloramphenicol detected in the blood is in the active free form. Small amounts of active drug are found in bile and feces.

The elimination half-life of chloramphenicol is approximately 4 hours, and correlates well with serum bilirubin concentration. Protein binding and clearance are decreased in patients with severe liver dysfunction, leading to potentially toxic serum concentrations of free drug.

(Continued on following page)

CHLORAMPHENICOL (Cont.)

Indications:

Serious infections for which less potentially dangerous drugs are ineffective or contraindicated. If presumptive therapy is initiated, perform in vitro sensitivity tests concurrently, so that the drug may be discontinued if less potentially dangerous agents are indicated.

Acute infections caused by *S typhi.* Chloramphenicol is a drug of choice. (In treatment of typhoid fever, some authorities recommend that chloramphenicol be used at therapeutic levels for 8 to 10 days after the patient becomes afebrile, to lessen the possibility of relapse.) It is not recommended for the routine treatment of the typhoid "carrier state."

Serious infections caused by susceptible strains of *Salmonella* species; *H influenzae,* specifically, meningeal infections; rickettsiae; lymphogranuloma-psittacosis group; various gram-negative bacteria causing bacteremia, meningitis or other serious gram-negative infections; infections involving anaerobic organisms, when *Bacteroides fragilis* is suspected; other susceptible organisms which have been demonstrated to be resistant to all other appropriate antimicrobial agents.

Cystic fibrosis regimens.

Contraindications:

History of hypersensitivity to, or toxicity from, chloramphenicol.

Chloramphenicol must not be used to treat trivial infections (ie, colds, influenza, throat infections), infections other than indicated or as prophylaxis for bacterial infections.

Warnings:

Usage in Pregnancy: There are no studies to establish the safety of this drug in pregnancy. Since it readily crosses the placental barrier, cautious use is particularly important during pregnancy at term or during labor because of potential toxic effects on the fetus (gray syndrome).

Usage in Lactation: Chloramphenicol appears in breast milk with a milk:plasma ratio of 0.5. Use with caution, if at all, during lactation, because of the possibility of toxic effects on the nursing infant.

Usage in Infants: Use with caution and in reduced dosages in premature and full-term infants to avoid gray syndrome toxicity. (See Adverse Reactions.) Monitor drug serum levels carefully during therapy of the newborn.

Precautions:

Hematology: Evaluate baseline and periodic blood studies approximately every 2 days during therapy. Discontinue the drug upon appearance of reticulocytopenia, leukopenia, thrombocytopenia, anemia or any other findings attributable to chloramphenicol. *Such studies do not exclude the possible later appearance of the irreversible type of bone marrow depression.* Avoid concurrent therapy with other drugs that may cause bone marrow depression.

Avoid repeated courses if at all possible. Do not continue treatment longer than required to produce a cure.

Usage in impaired hepatic or renal function: Excessive blood levels may result from the use of the recommended dose in patients with impaired liver or kidney function, including that due to immature metabolic processes in the infant. Adjust dosage accordingly or, preferably, determine the blood concentration at appropriate intervals.

Acute intermittent porphyria or glucose-6-phosphate dehydrogenase deficiency: Use with caution in patients with these conditions.

Superinfection: Use of antibiotics (especially prolonged or repeated therapy) may result in bacterial or fungal overgrowth of nonsusceptible organisms. Such overgrowth may lead to a secondary infection. Take appropriate measures if superinfection occurs.

(Continued on following page)

CHLORAMPHENICOL (Cont.)

Drug Interactions:

Dicumarol, phenytoin, phenobarbital, tolbutamide, chlorpropamide and **cyclophosphamide:** Chloramphenicol inhibits the metabolism of these drugs. Half-life may be prolonged and pharmacologic effects enhanced when chloramphenicol is administered concomitantly. Because cyclophosphamide's activity may be mediated through active metabolites, its therapeutic value may theoretically be reduced.

Acetaminophen: Data conflict; however, elevated serum levels of chloramphenicol may occur during concomitant administration The pharmacologic effects of chloramphenicol may be increased; hence, the dosage may need to be decreased.

Iron salts and **vitamin B_{12}:** The hematologic response may be decreased when given concomitantly with chloramphenicol.

Penicillin and concurrent chloramphenicol may decrease penicillin's effect and increase the half-life of chloramphenicol. Conversely, the combination has been beneficial.

Rifampin: Concomitant administration may reduce serum chloramphenicol levels, presumably through hepatic enzyme induction.

Adverse Reactions:

Blood dyscrasias: The most serious adverse effect is bone marrow depression. Serious and fatal blood dyscrasias (aplastic anemia, hypoplastic anemia, thrombocytopenia and granulocytopenia) occur. An irreversible type of marrow depression leading to aplastic anemia with a high rate of mortality is characterized by appearance of bone marrow aplasia or hypoplasia weeks or months after therapy. Peripherally, pancytopenia is most often observed, but only one or two of the three major cell types (erythrocytes, leukocytes and platelets) may be depressed. This complication appears unrelated to administration route. One estimate based on 149 cases stated the route was oral in 83%, parenteral in 14% and rectal in 3%. Several cases of aplastic anemia have been associated with chloramphenicol ophthalmic ointment.

A dose-related reversible type of bone marrow depression may occur and is associated with sustained serum levels at peak ≥ 25 mcg/ml; trough ≥ 10 mcg/ml. This type of marrow depression is characterized by vacuolization of the erythroid cells, a decrease in red cell iron uptake, an increase in circulating serum iron with saturation of iron-binding globulin (usually within 6 to 10 days) and reduction of reticulocytes (usually within 5 to 7 days) and leukopenia; it responds promptly to withdrawal of the drug.

Aplastic anemia is estimated to occur in 1:40,000 cases (range 1:19,000 to 1:200,000). There have been reports of aplastic anemia attributed to the drug which later terminated in leukemia.

Hemoglobinuria – Paroxysmal nocturnal hemoglobinuria has been reported.

GI: Nausea; vomiting; glossitis; stomatitis; diarrhea; enterocolitis (low incidence).

CNS: Headache; mild depression; mental confusion; delirium. Optic and peripheral neuritis have been reported, usually following long-term therapy; if this occurs, promptly withdraw the drug.

Hypersensitivity: Fever; macular and vesicular rashes; angioedema; urticaria; anaphylaxis. Herxheimer reactions have occurred during therapy for typhoid fever.

Gray syndrome: Toxic reactions including fatalities (approximately 40%) have occurred in the premature infant and newborn; the signs and symptoms associated with these reactions have been referred to as the "gray syndrome". The following summarizes the clinical and laboratory studies:

- In most cases, therapy was instituted within the first 48 hours of life.
- Symptoms first appeared after 3 to 4 days of treatment with high doses.
- Symptoms appeared in the following order: Abdominal distension with or without emesis; progressive pallid cyanosis; vasomotor collapse, frequently accompanied by irregular respiration; death within a few hours of onset. Other initial symptoms may include refusal to suck, loose green stools, flaccidity, ashen color, decrease in temperature and refractory lactic acidosis. Death occurs in approximately 40% of the patients within 2 days of initial symptoms.
- Progression of symptoms was accelerated with higher doses.
- Serum level studies revealed unusually high drug concentrations (≥ 40 mcg/ml after repeated doses) with doses in excess of 25 mg/kg/day in newborns.
- Termination of therapy upon early evidence of associated symptoms frequently reversed the process with complete recovery.
- Preexisting liver dysfunction may be a significant risk factor.

Patient Information:

Preferably taken on an empty stomach at least 1 hour before or 2 hours after meals. Take with food if GI upset occurs.

Take at evenly spaced intervals (every 6 hours) around the clock.

Notify physician if fever, sore throat, tiredness or unusual bleeding or bruising occurs.

(Continued on following page)

CHLORAMPHENICOL (Cont.)

Administration and Dosage:

Therapeutic concentrations generally should be maintained as follows: Peak 10 to 20 mcg/ml; trough 5 to 10 mcg/ml.

Monitoring serum levels is important because of the variability of chloramphenicol's pharmacokinetics. Monitor serum concentrations weekly; monitor more often in patients with hepatic dysfunction, in therapy longer than 2 weeks or with potentially interacting drugs (see Drug Interactions).

Adults: 50 mg/kg/day in divided doses every 6 hours for typhoid fever and rickettsial infections. Exceptional infections (ie, meningitis or brain abscess) due to moderately resistant organisms may require dosage up to 100 mg/kg/day to achieve blood levels inhibiting the pathogen; decrease high doses as soon as possible.

Impaired hepatic or renal function reduces the ability to metabolize and excrete the drug. Impaired metabolic processes require that doses be adjusted based on drug concentration in the blood. *In adults,* an initial loading dose of 1 g followed by 500 mg every 6 hours has been recommended in impaired hepatic function.

Children: 50 to 75 mg/kg/day in divided doses every 6 hours has been recommended for most indications. For meningitis, 50 to 100 mg/kg/day in divided doses every 6 hours has been recommended.

Newborns (See Gray syndrome under Adverse Reactions): 25 mg/kg/day in 4 doses every 6 hours usually produces and maintains adequate concentrations in blood and tissues. Increased dosage demanded by severe infections should be given only to maintain the blood concentration within an effective range. After the first 2 weeks of life, full-term infants ordinarily may receive up to 50 mg/kg/day in 4 doses every 6 hours.

Neonates (< 2 kg) – 25 mg/kg once daily.

Neonates from birth to 7 days (> 2 kg) – 25 mg/kg once daily.

Neonates over 7 days (> 2 kg) – 50 mg/kg/day in divided doses every 12 hours.

These dosage recommendations are extremely important because blood concentration in all premature and full-term infants under 2 weeks of age differs from that of other infants due to variations in the maturity of the metabolic functions of the liver and kidneys. When these functions are immature (or seriously impaired in adults), the drug is found in high concentrations which tend to increase with succeeding doses.

Infants and children with immature metabolic processes: 25 mg/kg/day usually produces therapeutic concentrations. In this group particularly, carefully monitor the concentration of drug in the blood.

IV administration: Chloramphenicol sodium succinate is intended for IV use only; it is ineffective when given IM. It must be hydrolyzed to its active form, and there is a lag in achieving adequate blood levels following infusion. Administer IV as a 10% solution injected over at least 1 minute. Prepare by adding 10 ml of an aqueous diluent (eg, Water for Injection or 5% Dextrose Injection). Substitute oral dosage as soon as feasible.

	Product	Dosage form	Notes	C.I.*
Rx	**Chloramphenicol** (Qualitest)	**Capsules:** 250 mg	In 100s.	1
Rx	**Chloromycetin Kapseals** (Parke-Davis)		Lactose. (P-D 379). In 100s.	2.6
Rx	**Chloromycetin Palmitate** (Parke-Davis)	**Oral Suspension:** 150 mg (as palmitate) per 5 ml	Alcohol, sucrose, 0.5% sodium benzoate. Custard flavor. In 60 ml.	4.8
Rx	**Chloramphenicol Sodium Succinate** (Lyphomed)	**Powder for Injection:** 100 mg/ml (as sodium succinate) when reconstituted	In 1 g in 15 ml vials.	3.4
Rx	**Chloromycetin Sodium Succinate** (Parke-Davis)		In 1 g vials.	2.8

* Cost Index based on cost per 100 mg.

[1] Each g contains 2.25 mEq sodium.

Actions:

Pharmacology: The fluoroquinolones are synthetic, broad-spectrum antibacterial agents related to the other quinolones, nalidixic acid and cinoxacin. These agents contain a 6-fluoro and 7-piperazine substituent which greatly enhances their antimicrobial efficacy when compared to nalidixic acid. The fluorine molecule provides increased potency against gram-negative organisms and broadens the spectrum to include gram-positive organisms; the piperazine moiety is responsible for antipseudomonal activity. These agents are bactericidal; they interfere with the enzyme DNA gyrase needed for the synthesis of bacterial DNA.

Pharmacokinetics:

Pharmacokinetics of Fluoroquinolones							
Fluoroquinolone	Bio-availability (%)	Max urine concentration (mcg/ml) (dose)	Mean peak plasma concentration (mcg/ml) (dose)	Area under curve (AUC) (mcg • hr/ml) (dose)	Protein binding (%)	t½ (hr)	Urine recovery unchanged (%)
Ciprofloxacin Oral	70-80	160-700 (500 mg)	1.2 (250 mg) 2.4 (500 mg) 4.3 (750 mg) 5.4 (1000 mg)	4.8 (250 mg) 11.6 (500 mg) 20.2 (750 mg) 30.8 (1000 mg)	20-40	4	40-50
IV		> 200 (200 mg) > 400 (400 mg)	4.3 (400 mg)	4.8 (200 mg) 11.6 (400 mg)	20-40	5-6	50-70
Enoxacin	90	nd	0.83 (200 mg) 2 (400 mg)	16 (400 mg)	40	3-6	> 40
Lomefloxacin	95-98	> 300 (400 mg)	4.2 (400 mg)	5.6 (100 mg) 10.9 (200 mg) 26.1 (400 mg)	10	8	65
Norfloxacin	30-40	200-500 (400 mg)	0.8 (200 mg) 1.5 (400 mg)	5.4 (400 mg)	10-15	3-4.5	26-32
Ofloxacin Oral	≈ 98	220 (200 mg)	1.5 (200 mg) 2.4 (300 mg) 2.9 (400 mg)	14.1 (200 mg) 21.2 (300 mg) 31.4 (400 mg)	32	5-7	70-80
IV		nd	2.7 (200 mg) 4 (400 mg)	43.5 (400 mg)	32	5-10	nd

nd = no data. [1] Dose-dependent trend toward increased AUC as doses increase > 600 mg.

Norfloxacin – Absorption/Distribution: Absorption is rapid. Food may decrease absorption. Steady-state concentrations of norfloxacin will be attained within 2 days of dosing. Urinary concentrations of ≥ 200 mcg/ml are attained 2 to 3 hours after a single 400 mg dose. Mean urinary concentrations of norfloxacin remain above 30 mcg/ml for at least 12 hours following a 400 mg dose. Norfloxacin is least soluble at urinary pH of 7.5 with greater solubility occurring at pHs above and below this value.

Metabolism/Excretion: Norfloxacin is eliminated through metabolism, biliary excretion and renal excretion. Renal excretion occurs by both glomerular filtration and tubular secretion, as evidenced by the high rate of renal clearance (≈ 275 ml/min). Within 24 hours of administration, 5% to 8% of the dose is recovered in the urine as six less active metabolites. Fecal recovery accounts for another 30%. In healthy elderly volunteers (65 to 75 years of age), norfloxacin is eliminated more slowly because of decreased renal function. Drug absorption appears unaffected. Disposition of norfloxacin in patients with creatinine clearance (Ccr) rates > 30 ml/min/1.73 m^2 is similar to that in healthy volunteers. In patients with Ccr rates ≤ 30 ml/min/1.73 m^2, the renal elimination decreases so that the effective serum half-life is 6.5 hours; dosage alteration is necessary. See Administration and Dosage.

Enoxacin – Absorption/Distribution: Peak plasma concentrations are achieved in 1 to 3 hours. Effect of food on absorption has not been studied. In elderly patients, mean peak plasma concentrations are 50% higher than in young adults. Enoxacin diffuses into cervix, fallopian tube and myometrium at levels ≈ 1 to 2 times those achieved in plasma, and into kidney and prostate at levels ≈ 2 to 4 times plasma levels.

Metabolism/Excretion: Five metabolites have been identified in the urine and account for 15% to 20% of a dose. Some isozymes of the cytochrome P-450 hepatic microsomal enzyme system are inhibited by enoxacin, resulting in significant drug interactions with some agents (see Drug Interactions). Clearance is reduced in renal impairment; dosage adjustment is necessary (see Administration and Dosage).

(Actions continued on following page)

Actions (Cont.):

Pharmacokinetics (Cont.):

Ciprofloxacin – Absorption/Distribution: Ciprofloxacin is rapidly and well absorbed from the GI tract after oral administration with no substantial loss by first-pass metabolism. When given concomitantly with food, there is a delay in the absorption of the drug, resulting in peak concentrations that are closer to 2 hours after dosing rather than 1 hour. The overall absorption, however, is not substantially affected. Maximum serum concentrations are attained 1 to 2 hours after oral dosing. Mean concentrations 12 hours after dosing with 250, 500 or 750 mg are 0.1, 0.2 and 0.4 mcg/ml, respectively. Following 60 minute IV infusions of 200 and 400 mg, mean maximum serum concentrations achieved were 2.1 and 4.6 mcg/ml, respectively; concentrations at 12 hours were 0.1 and 0.2 mcg/ml, respectively. Ciprofloxacin is widely distributed throughout the body. Tissue concentrations often exceed serum concentrations in both men and women, particularly in genital tissue. The drug diffuses into the cerebrospinal fluid (CSF); however, CSF concentrations are generally only about 10% of peak serum concentrations.

Metabolism/Excretion: Four metabolites have been identified in urine which, together, account for approximately 15% of an oral dose. The metabolites have antimicrobial activity, but are less active than unchanged ciprofloxacin. After IV administration, three metabolites have been identified in urine which account for ≈ 10% of the IV dose. After a 250 mg oral dose, urine concentrations usually exceed 200 mcg/ml during the first 2 hours and are ≈ 30 mcg/ml at 8 to 12 hours after dosing. Following a 200 or 400 mg IV dose, urine concentrations usually exceed 200 and 400 mcg/ml, respectively, during the first 2 hours and are generally > 15 and > 30 mcg/ml, respectively, at 8 to 12 hours after dosing. Urinary ciprofloxacin excretion is virtually complete within 24 hours after dosing. Renal clearance is ≈ 300 ml/min; active tubular secretion plays a significant role. Although bile concentrations are several fold higher than serum after oral dosing, only a small amount is recovered from the bile. Approximately 20% to 35% of an oral dose is recovered from feces within 5 days after dosing. In patients with reduced renal function, the half-life is slightly prolonged; dosage adjustments may be required. See Administration and Dosage.

Ofloxacin – Absorption/Distribution: Maximum serum concentrations are achieved 1 to 2 hours after an oral dose. The amount absorbed increases proportionately with the dose. The effect of food on absorption has not been studied. Elimination is biphasic; half-lives are approximately 4 to 5 hours and 20 to 25 hours, although accumulation at steady state can be estimated using a half-life of 9 hours. Steady-state concentrations are achieved after four doses and are ≈ 50% higher than concentrations after single doses. Ofloxacin is widely distributed to body tissues and fluids.

Metabolism/Excretion: Ofloxacin has a pyridobenzoxazine ring that appears to decrease the extent of parent compound metabolism; < 5% of a dose is recovered in the urine as the desmethyl or N-oxide metabolites. Elimination is mainly by renal excretion; 4% to 8% is excreted in the feces. In healthy elderly volunteers with normal renal function, the apparent half-life is 6 to 8 hours (compared to ≈ 5 hours in younger adults); however, absorption is unaffected by age. Clearance is reduced in patients with renal function impairment (Ccr ≤ 50 ml/min); dosage adjustment is necessary. See Administration and Dosage.

Lomefloxacin – Absorption/Distribution: Absorption is rapid. Following coadministration with food, rate of absorption is delayed (time to reach maximum plasma concentration delayed by 41%, maximum concentration decreased by 18%) and the extent of absorption (AUC) is decreased by 12%. At 24 hours post-dose, single doses of 200 or 400 mg result in mean plasma levels of 0.1 and 0.24 mcg/ml, respectively. Steady-state concentrations are achieved within 48 hours of initiating once-daily dosing. The mean urine concentration exceeds 35 mcg/ml for at least 24 hours after dosing. Urine pH appears to affect the solubility of lomefloxacin, with solubilities ranging from 3.03 to 7.8 mg/ml at pH of 8.12 to 5.2, respectively.

Metabolism/Excretion: Mean renal clearance is 145 ml/min in subjects with normal renal function, which may indicate tubular secretion. Approximately 9% of a dose is recovered in the urine as the glucuronide metabolite; four other metabolites have been identified and account for < 0.5% of the dose. Approximately 10% of a dose is recovered unchanged in the feces. In healthy elderly volunteers, plasma clearance was reduced by ≈ 25% and the AUC was increased by ≈ 33%, which may be due to decreased renal function in this population. In patients with Ccr between 10 and 40 ml/min/1.73 m^2, the mean AUC after a single dose increased 335% over the AUC in patients with Ccr > 80 ml/min/1.73 m^2, and mean half-life increased to 21 hours. In patients with Ccr < 10 ml/min/1.73 m^2, AUC increased 700% and half-life increased to 45 hours. Adjustment of dosage is necessary. See Administration and Dosage.

(Actions continued on following page)

Actions (Cont.):

Microbiology:

Table I: Organisms Generally Susceptible to Fluoroquinolones In Vitro

	Organism	Ciprofloxacin	Enoxacin	Lomefloxacin	Norfloxacin	Ofloxacin
Gram-negative	Acinetobacter sp	✓			✓	✓
	Aeromonas sp	✓	✓[1]	✓[1]	✓	✓[1]
	Alcaligenes sp				✓	
	Brucella melitensis	✓				
	Campylobacter sp	✓			✓	✓[1]
	Citrobacter sp	✓	✓[1]	✓[1]	✓[1]	✓[1]
	Edwardsiella tarda	✓			✓	
	Enterobacter sp	✓	✓[1]	✓	✓[1]	✓[1]
	Escherichia coli	✓	✓	✓	✓	✓
	Flavobacterium sp				✓	
	Hafnia alvei			✓	✓	
	Hemophilus ducreyi	✓	✓			
	Hemophilus influenzae	✓		✓	✓	✓
	Hemophilus parainfluenzae	✓		✓	✓	✓
	Klebsiella pneumoniae	✓	✓	✓	✓	✓
	Klebsiella sp	✓	✓[1]	✓	✓[1]	✓[1]
	Legionella sp	✓		✓	✓	✓
	Listeria monocytogenes	✓				
	Moraxella (Branhamella) catarrhalis	✓		✓	✓	✓
	Morganella morganii	✓	✓	✓	✓	✓
	Neisseria gonorrhoeae	✓	✓		✓	✓
	Neisseria meningitidis	✓			✓	✓
	Pasteurella multocida	✓				
	Plesiomonas shigelloides					✓
	Proteus mirabilis	✓	✓	✓	✓	✓
	Proteus vulgaris	✓	✓	✓	✓	✓
	Providencia alcalifaciens		✓	✓	✓	
	Providencia rettgeri	✓		✓	✓	✓
	Providencia stuartii	✓	✓		✓	✓
	Pseudomonas aeruginosa	✓	✓	✓	✓	✓
	Pseudomonas fluorescens					✓
	Salmonella sp	✓			✓	✓
	Serratia sp	✓	✓[1]	✓	✓[1]	✓[1]
	Shigella sp	✓			✓	✓
	Vibrio sp	✓			✓[1]	✓[1]
	Xanthomonas (Pseudomonas) maltophilia					✓
	Yersinia enterocolitica	✓			✓	✓
Gram-positive	Staphylococcus aureus	✓[2]		✓[2]	✓[2]	✓[2]
	coagulase-negative sp	✓				
	epidermidis	✓	✓	✓[2]	✓	✓[2]
	hemolyticus	✓			✓	
	saprophyticus	✓	✓	✓	✓	✓
	Streptococci group D				✓	
	agalactiae				✓	✓
	faecalis	✓			✓	✓
	pneumoniae	✓				✓
	pyogenes	✓				✓
	Bacillus cereus				✓	

[1] May be species-dependent.

[2] Including methicillin-susceptible and methicillin-resistant strains.

(Actions continued on following page)

Actions (Cont.):

Microbiology (Cont.):

These agents have in vitro activity against a wide range of gram-negative and gram-positive organisms. Ciprofloxacin, lomefloxacin and norfloxacin are generally inactive against anaerobic bacteria. Refer to Table I for a listing of organisms generally susceptible to fluoroquinolones in vitro.

Ciprofloxacin – Most strains of streptococci are only moderately susceptible as are *Mycobacterium tuberculosis, M fortuitum* and *Chlamydia trachomatis. Mycoplasma pneumoniae, M hominis* and *Ureaplasma urealyticum* are susceptible in vitro. Some strains of *Pseudomonas aeruginosa* may develop resistance fairly rapidly.

Ciprofloxacin does not cross-react with other antimicrobial agents such as beta-lactams or aminoglycosides; however, additive activity may result when it is combined with beta-lactams, aminoglycosides, clindamycin or metronidazole.

Norfloxacin – U urealyticum is susceptible in vitro. Resistance to norfloxacin due to spontaneous mutation in vitro is rare (< 1%). Development of resistance is greatest in the following: *Pseudomonas aeruginosa; Klebsiella pneumoniae; Acinetobacter* sp; enterococci. Norfloxacin is not generally active against obligate anaerobes.

Ofloxacin – The following organisms are susceptible in vitro:

Anaerobes – Bacteroides fragilis and *B intermedius; Clostridium perfringens* and *C welchii; Gardnerella vaginalis; Peptococcus niger; Peptostreptococcus* sp.

Other – Chlamydia pneumoniae; C trachomatis (also active in vivo); *M tuberculosis; Mycoplasma pneumoniae; U urealyticum.*

Many strains of other streptococcal sp, enterococcus sp and anaerobes are resistant. It is not active against *Treponema pallidum.* Although cross-resistance has been observed between ofloxacin and other fluoroquinolones, some organisms resistant to other quinolones may be susceptible to ofloxacin.

Lomefloxacin – Most group A, B, D and G streptococci, *S pneumoniae, Pseudomonas cepacia, U urealyticum, Mycoplasma hominis* and anaerobic bacteria are resistant.

Cross-resistance has occurred between lomefloxacin and other quinolone-class antimicrobial agents, but not between lomefloxacin and other antimicrobials, such as aminoglycosides, penicillins, tetracyclines, cephalosporins or sulfonamides. Lomefloxacin is active in vitro against some strains of cephalosporin- and aminoglycoside-resistant gram-negative bacteria.

Indications:

For specific approved indications, refer to individual drug monographs.

Unlabeled uses: Ciprofloxacin 750 mg twice daily appears effective in patients with cystic fibrosis who have pulmonary exacerbations associated with susceptible microorganisms. However, restrict use to patients > 14 years of age. Also, long-term therapy is inadvisable due to emergence of resistant organisms. It may also be useful in the treatment of malignant external otitis (750 mg twice daily) and for tuberculosis in combination with rifampin and other antituberculosis agents. It has been used as part of a multi-drug regimen (1500 mg/day divided every 12 hours) for the treatment of *Mycobacterium avium* complex infection, a common infection in AIDS patients.

Fluoroquinolones may also be useful in the following conditions (some agents are specifically indicated for these conditions; refer to drug monographs): Bronchitis; pneumonia (including Legionella and Mycoplasma); prostatitis; osteomyelitis (selected types); prophylaxis in urological surgery; traveler's diarrhea; gonorrheal cervicitis or urethritis; pelvic inflammatory disease; sinusitis; otitis media; septic arthritis; bacterial meningitis; bacteremia (pseudomonal or staphylococcal); endocarditis. Further study is needed.

Contraindications:

Hypersensitivity to fluoroquinolones or the quinolone group of antibacterial agents (cinoxacin and nalidixic acid).

Warnings:

Convulsions, increased intracranial pressure and toxic psychosis have occurred. CNS stimulation may also occur, which may lead to tremor, restlessness, lightheadedness, confusion and hallucinations. Use with caution in patients with known or suspected CNS disorders, (eg, severe cerebral arteriosclerosis, epilepsy) or other factors which predispose to seizures. If these reactions occur, stop the drug and institute appropriate measures.

Syphilis: **Ofloxacin** and **enoxacin** are not effective for syphilis. High doses of antimicrobial agents for short periods of time to treat gonorrhea may mask or delay symptoms of incubating syphilis. All patients should have a serologic test for syphilis at the time of gonorrhea diagnosis. Patients treated with ofloxacin and enoxacin should have a follow-up serologic test after 3 months.

Renal function impairment: Alteration in dosage regimen is necessary. See Administration and Dosage.

(Warnings continued on following page)

Warnings (Cont.):

Chronic bronchitis due to S pneumoniae: **Lomefloxacin** is not indicated for the empiric treatment of acute bacterial exacerbation of chronic bronchitis when it is probable that *S pneumoniae* is a causative pathogen since it exhibits in vitro resistance to lomefloxacin. Use only if sputum gram stain demonstrates an adequate quality of specimen and there is a predominance of gram-negative and not gram-positive organisms.

Hypersensitivity reactions, serious and occasionally fatal, have occurred in patients receiving quinolone therapy, some following the first dose. Some reactions were accompanied by cardiovascular collapse, loss of consciousness, tingling, pharyngeal or facial edema, dyspnea, urticaria and itching. If an allergic reaction occurs, discontinue the drug. Refer to Management of Acute Hypersensitivity Reactions.

Pseudomembranous colitis has been reported with nearly all antibacterial agents, including fluoroquinolones, and may range from mild to life-threatening in severity. Therefore, it is important to consider this diagnosis in patients who present with diarrhea subsequent to the administration of antibacterial agents. After the diagnosis of pseudomembranous colitis has been established, initiate therapeutic measures. Mild cases of pseudomembranous colitis usually respond to discontinuation of drug alone. In moderate to severe cases, consider management with fluid and electrolytes, protein supplementation, and treatment with an antibacterial drug clinically effective against *C difficile* colitis.

Fertility impairment: Decreased spermatogenesis and subsequent decreased fertility occurred in animals given **enoxacin** doses that produced plasma levels 3 times higher than those in humans at the recommended therapeutic dosage.

Elderly: **Norfloxacin** is eliminated more slowly because of decreased renal function; absorption appears unaffected. The apparent half-life of **ofloxacin** is 6 to 8 hours, compared to ≈ 5 hours in younger adults; absorption is unaffected. **Lomefloxacin** plasma clearance was reduced by ≈ 25% and the AUC was increased by ≈ 33% in the elderly, which may be due to decreased renal function in this population. **Enoxacin** plasma concentrations are 50% higher in the elderly than in young adults.

Pregnancy: Category C. Do not use in pregnant women. There are no adequate and well controlled studies in pregnant women. Use during pregnancy only if the potential benefit justifies the potential risk to the fetus.

Norfloxacin produces embryonic loss in monkeys when given in doses 10 times the maximum human dose.

Ciprofloxacin and **norfloxacin** caused lameness in immature dogs due to permanent cartilage lesions, and caused arthropathy in immature animals.

Ofloxacin in doses equivalent to 10 to 50 times the maximum therapeutic dose were fetotoxic (ie, decreased fetal body weight, increased fetal mortality) in rats and rabbits, and minor skeletal variations occurred in rats; it also caused arthropathy in immature animals.

Lomefloxacin increased the incidence of fetal loss in monkeys at approximately 3 to 6 times the recommended human dose. In rabbits, maternal toxicity and associated fetotoxicity, decreased placental weight and variations of the coccygeal vertebrae occurred at doses 2 times the recommended human dose.

Enoxacin caused dose-related maternal toxicity (eg, venous irritation, weight loss) and fetal toxicity (increased post-implantation loss and stunted fetuses) following IV doses of 10 to 50 mg/kg. At 50 mg/kg, the incidence of fetal malformations was significantly increased in the presence of overt maternal and fetal toxicity.

Lactation: **Norfloxacin** was not detected in breast milk following the administration of 200 mg to nursing mothers; however, this was a low dose. **Ciprofloxacin** is excreted in breast milk; however, the amount ingested by the infant appears to be low. **Ofloxacin** as a single 200 mg dose resulted in breast milk concentrations in nursing females that were similar to those found in plasma. It is not known whether **lomefloxacin** or **enoxacin** are excreted in breast milk. Because of the potential for serious adverse reactions in nursing infants, decide whether to discontinue nursing or to discontinue the drug, taking into account the importance of the drug to the mother.

Children: Do not use in children. Safety and efficacy of **lomefloxacin, enoxacin** and **ofloxacin** in children < 18 years of age have not been established. **Ciprofloxacin, enoxacin, lomefloxacin** and **ofloxacin** cause arthropathy and osteochondrosis in immature animals. Administration of **norfloxacin** and **ciprofloxacin** caused lameness in immature dogs due to permanent cartilage lesions.

Precautions:

Superinfection: Use of antibiotics (especially prolonged or repeated therapy) may result in bacterial or fungal overgrowth of nonsusceptible organisms. Such overgrowth may lead to a secondary infection. Take appropriate measures if superinfection occurs.

Ophthalmologic abnormalities, including cataracts and multiple punctate lenticular opacities, have occurred during therapy with some quinolones. With multiple dose therapy, ophthalmic tissue levels of the quinolones were significantly higher than plasma levels. A causal relationship has not been established.

(Precautions continued on following page)

Precautions (Cont.):

Crystalluria: Needle shaped crystals were found in the urine of some volunteers who received either placebo or 800 or 1600 mg norfloxacin. While crystalluria is not expected to occur under usual conditions with 400 mg twice daily, do not exceed the daily recommended dosage. Crystalluria related to ciprofloxacin has occurred only rarely in man because human urine is usually acidic. The patient should drink sufficient fluids to ensure proper hydration and adequate urinary output. Avoid alkalinity of the urine and do not exceed the recommended daily dose.

Phototoxicity reactions, moderate to severe, have occurred in patients who are exposed to direct sunlight while receiving some drugs in this class. Avoid excessive sunlight. Discontinue therapy if phototoxicity occurs.

Monitoring: Periodic assessment of organ system functions, including renal, hepatic and hematopoietic is advisable during prolonged therapy.

Drug Interactions:

Fluoroquinolone Drug Interactions

Precipitant drug	Object drug*		Description
Antacids (aluminum/ magnesium hydroxide) Iron salts Sucralfate Zinc salts	Fluoroquinolones	↓	Interference of GI absorption of the fluoroquinolones, resulting in decreased serum levels. Avoid simultaneous use; administer antacids 2 to 4 hours before or after the fluoroquinolone.
Antineoplastic agents	Fluoroquinolones	↓	Fluoroquinolone serum levels may be decreased.
Azlocillin	Ciprofloxacin	↑	The clearance of ciprofloxacin is decreased, possibly increasing its pharmacologic effects. This combination may be beneficial for some serious gram-negative infections, although it is not known if toxicity also increases.
Bismuth subsalicylate	Enoxacin	↓	Enoxacin bioavailability is decreased when bismuth subsalicylate is given with or 60 minutes after enoxacin. Avoid concurrent use.
Cimetidine	Fluoroquinolones	↑	Cimetidine may interfere with the elimination of the fluoroquinolones.
Nitrofurantoin	Norfloxacin	↓	Antibacterial effect of norfloxacin in the urinary tract may be antagonized.
Probenecid	Fluoroquinolones	↑	Ciprofloxacin renal clearance is reduced 50%, and its serum concentration is increased 50%; diminished norfloxacin and lomefloxacin urinary excretion has also occurred.
Ciprofloxacin Enoxacin	Caffeine	↑	Total body clearance of caffeine is reduced, possibly resulting in increased pharmacologic effects. Ofloxacin and lomefloxacin do not appear to affect caffeine. Enoxacin trough plasma levels were also 20% higher.
Enoxacin	Digoxin	↑	Digoxin serum levels may be increased. Monitor digoxin levels.
Fluoroquinolones	Anticoagulants	↑	The effects of the anticoagulant may be increased. Monitor prothrombin time.
Fluoroquinolones	Cyclosporine	↑	Nephrotoxic effects may be increased. Closely monitor renal function. Conflicting data exist.
Fluoroquinolones	Theophylline	↑	Decreased clearance and increased plasma levels and toxicity of theophylline has occurred with concurrent ciprofloxacin and enoxacin. Data conflict with norfloxacin and ofloxacin; some studies report no interaction, others suggest increased theophylline levels. Lomefloxacin does not appear to alter theophylline levels. Monitor theophylline levels.

* ↑ = Object drug increased. ↓ = Object drug decreased.

Drug/Food interactions: Food may decrease the absorption of **norfloxacin.** Food delays the absorption of **ciprofloxacin,** resulting in peak concentrations that are closer to 2 hours after dosing rather than 1 hour; however, overall absorption is not substantially affected. Dairy products such as milk and yogurt reduce the absorption of ciprofloxacin; avoid concurrent use. The bioavailability of ciprofloxacin may also be decreased by enteral feedings. Food delays the rate of absorption of **lomefloxacin** (time to reach maximum plasma concentration delayed by 41%, maximum concentration decreased by 18%) and decreases the extent of absorption (AUC) by 12%.

(Continued on following page)

Adverse Reactions:

Fluoroquinolone Adverse Reactions (%)						
	Adverse reactions	Ciprofloxacin[1]	Enoxacin	Lomefloxacin	Norfloxacin	Ofloxacin[1]
GI	Nausea	5.2	2-9	3.7	2.8	3-10
	Abdominal pain/discomfort	1.7	≤2	<1	0.3-1	1-3
	Diarrhea	2.3	1-2	1.4	✓	1-4
	Vomiting	2	6-9	<1	✓	1-3
	Dry/painful mouth	<1	<1	<1	✓	1-3
	Dyspepsia/Heartburn	✓	1	<1	0.3-1	<1
	Constipation	✓	<1	<1	0.3-1	<1
	Flatulence	✓	<1	<1	0.3-1	1-3
	Pseudomembranous colitis[2]	✓	✓	✓	✓	✓
CNS	Headache	1.2	≤2	3.2	2.7	1-9
	Dizziness	<1	≤3	2.3	1.8	1-5
	Fatigue/Lethargy/Malaise	<1	<1	<1	0.3-1	1-3
	Somnolence/Drowsiness	<1	<1	<1	0.3-1	1-3
	Depression	<1	<1	<1	0.3-1	<1
	Insomnia	<1	1	<1	0.3-1	3-7
	Seizures/Convulsions[2]	<1	<1	<1	rare	✓
	Confusion	✓	<1	<1	✓	
	Psychotic reactions	<1			✓	
	Paresthesia	<1	<1	<1	✓	<1
	Hallucinations	<1				<1
Dermatologic	Photosensitivity[2]	<1	<1	2.4	✓	✓
	Rash	1.1	≤1	<1	0.3-1	1-3
	Pruritus		1	<1	✓	1-3
	Toxic epidermal necrolysis	✓	<1		✓	
	Stevens-Johnson syndrome	✓	<1		✓	
	Exfoliative dermatitis	✓			✓	
	Hypersensitivity[2]	<1		✓	✓	✓
Other	Visual disturbances	<1	<1	<1	✓	1-3
	Hearing loss	<1			✓	<1
	Vaginitis	<1	<1	<1		1-3
	Hypertension	<1		<1		<1
	Palpitations	<1	<1			<1
	Syncope	<1	<1	<1		<1
	Chills	<1	<1	<1		<1
	Edema	<1	<1	<1		<1
	Fever		<1		✓	1-3
Abnormal laboratory values	↑ ALT/↑ AST	1.9/1.7	<1	≤0.4	1.8/1.8	≥1/0
	↑ Alkaline phosphatase	0.8	<1	0.1	1.4	
	↑ LDH	0.4			✓	
	↑ Bilirubin	0.3	<1	0.1		
	Eosinophilia	0.6	<1	≤0.1	1.8	≥1
	Leukopenia	0.4	<1	≤0.1	1.2	
	↑ or ↓ Platelets	0.1	<1	≤1	✓	
	Pancytopenia	0.1				
	↑ ESR/Lymphocytopenia			0.1		≥1
	Neutropenia				1.2	
	↑ Serum creatinine	1.1			✓	
	↑ BUN	0.9		0.1	✓	
	Crystalluria/Cylinduria/Candiduria	✓			✓	
	Hematuria	✓				≥1
	Glucosuria/Pyuria					≥1
	Proteinuria/Albuminuria	✓	<1	≤0.1		≥1
	↑ γ-glutamyltransferase	<0.1		≤0.1		
	↑ Serum amylase	<0.1				
	↑ Uric acid	<0.1				
	↑ or ↓ Blood glucose	<0.1		≤0.1		≥1
	↓ Hemoglobin/hematocrit	<0.1	<1	≤0.1	✓	
	↑ or ↓ Potassium	<0.1	<1	0.1		
	Anemia	<0.1		≤0.1		
	Bleeding/↑ PT	<0.1		≤0.1		
	↑ Monocytes	<0.1		0.3		
	Leukocytosis	<0.1	<1			≥1
	↑ Triglycerides/cholesterol	✓				

✓ = Adverse reaction observed, incidence not reported.

[1] Includes data for oral and IV formulations.
[2] See Warnings or Precautions.

(Adverse Reactions continued on following page)

Adverse Reactions (Cont.):

Other adverse reactions listed only for the individual agents:

Ciprofloxacin:

Renal/GU (< 1%) – Acidosis; interstitial nephritis; nephritis; renal failure; polyuria; urinary retention; urethral bleeding. Also, vaginal candidiasis, renal calculi.

Cardiovascular (< 1%) – Angina pectoris; atrial flutter; cardiopulmonary arrest; cerebral thrombosis; myocardial infarction; ventricular ectopy. Also, postural hypotension.

Respiratory (< 1%) – Bronchospasm; dyspnea; epistaxis; hemoptysis; hiccoughs; laryngeal/pulmonary edema; pulmonary embolism.

Special senses (< 1%) – Bad taste in mouth; eye pain; tinnitus. Also, nystagmus.

Miscellaneous – Restlessness (1.1%); oral/cutaneous candidiasis, intestinal perforation, GI bleeding, nightmares, irritability, tremor, ataxia, anorexia, urticaria, flushing, hyperpigmentation, erythema nodosum (< 1%); hepatic necrosis; exacerbation of myasthenia gravis; dysphasia; agranulocytosis; cholestatic jaundice.

Norfloxacin:

Miscellaneous – Erythema; myoclonus (rare); erythema multiforme; hepatitis; pancreatitis; stomatitis; arthralgia.

Ofloxacin:

Renal/GU – Vaginal discharge, genital pruritus (1% to 3%); burning/irritation/pain of female genitalia, dysmenorrhea, menorrhagia, metrorrhagia, urinary frequency/pain (< 1%).

Cardiovascular – Chest pain (1% to 3%); vasodilation (< 1%).

Respiratory – Cough, rhinorrhea (< 1%).

Special senses – Dysgeusia (1% to 3%); photophobia (< 1%).

CNS – Sleep disorders, nervousness (1% to 3%); anxiety, cognitive change, dream abnormality, euphoria, vertigo (< 1%).

Miscellaneous – Decreased appetite (1% to 3%); arthralgia, asthenia, diaphoresis, myalgia, thirst, vasculitis, weight loss (< 1%).

Lomefloxacin:

Renal/GU (< 1%) – Dysuria; hematuria; strangury; micturition disorder; anuria; leukorrhea; intermenstrual bleeding; perineal pain; vaginal moniliasis; orchitis; epididymitis.

Cardiovascular (< 1%) – Hypotension; tachycardia; bradycardia; arrhythmia; extrasystoles; cyanosis; cardiac failure; angina pectoris; myocardial infarction; pulmonary embolism; cerebrovascular disorder; cardiomyopathy; phlebitis.

Respiratory (< 1%) – Dyspnea; respiratory infection; epistaxis; respiratory disorder; bronchospasm; cough; increased sputum; stridor.

CNS (< 1%) – Coma; hyperkinesia; tremor; vertigo; nervousness; anorexia; anxiety; agitation; increased appetite; depersonalization; paroniria.

GI (< 1%) – GI inflammation/bleeding; dysphagia; tongue discoloration; bad taste in mouth.

Special senses (< 1%) – Earache; tinnitus; conjunctivitis; eye pain.

Dermatologic (< 1%) – Urticaria; eczema; skin exfoliation; skin disorder.

Miscellaneous – Flushing, increased sweating, back/chest pain, asthenia, facial edema, influenza-like symptoms, decreased heat tolerance, purpura, lymphadenopathy, increased fibrinolysis, thirst, gout, hypoglycemia, leg cramps, arthralgia, myalgia (< 1%); abnormalities of urine specific gravity or serum electrolytes (≤ 0.1%).

Enoxacin:

GI (< 1%) – Anorexia; bloody stools; gastritis; stomatitis.

CNS (≤ 1%) – Nervousness; anxiety; tremor; agitation; myoclonus; depersonalization; hypertonia.

Dermatologic (< 1%) – Urticaria; hyperhidrosis; mycotic infection; erythema multiforme.

Special senses – Vertigo (3%); unusual taste (1%); tinnitus, conjunctivitis (< 1%).

Respiratory (< 1%) – Dyspnea; cough; epistaxis.

GU (< 1%) – Vaginal moniliasis; urinary incontinence; renal failure.

Miscellaneous (< 1%) – Asthenia; back/chest pain; myalgia; arthralgia; tachycardia; vasodilation; purpura.

Overdosage:

Symptoms: One patient developed oliguric acute renal failure following ingestion of 21 g of **ciprofloxacin** (serum concentration 12 mcg/ml). The patient responded to prednisone therapy.

Treatment: For acute overdosage, empty the stomach by inducing vomiting or by gastric lavage. Observe patient carefully and give symptomatic and supportive treatment. Maintain adequate hydration. Refer to General Management of Acute Overdosage.

Hemodialysis or peritoneal dialysis may aid in the removal of **ciprofloxacin** from the body, particularly if renal function is compromised. **Ofloxacin, enoxacin, norfloxacin** and **lomefloxacin** are not efficiently removed by hemodialysis or peritoneal dialysis.

(Continued on following page)

Patient Information:

Drink fluids liberally.

Do not take antacids containing magnesium or aluminum or products containing iron or zinc simultaneously or within 4 hours before or 2 hours after dosing.

May cause dizziness or lightheadedness; observe caution while driving or performing other tasks requiring alertness, coordination or physical dexterity. CNS stimulation may occur (eg, tremor, restlessness, confusion); use with caution in patients predisposed to seizures or with other CNS disorders.

Take **norfloxacin** and **enoxacin** 1 hour before or 2 hours after meals. Do not take **ofloxacin** with food. **Ciprofloxacin** and **lomefloxacin** can be taken without regard to meals; however, the preferred time of ciprofloxacin dosing is 2 hours after a meal.

Hypersensitivity reactions may occur, even following the first dose; discontinue the drug at the first sign of skin rash or other allergic reaction.

Avoid excessive sunlight/artificial ultraviolet light; discontinue drug if phototoxicity occurs.

CIPROFLOXACIN

Indications:

For the treatment of infections caused by susceptible strains of the designated microorganisms in the conditions listed below:

Lower respiratory infections caused by *E coli, K pneumoniae, Enterobacter cloacae, P mirabilis, P aeruginosa, Hemophilus influenzae, parainfluenzae* and *pneumoniae*.

Skin and skin structure infections caused by *E coli, K pneumoniae, E cloacae, P mirabilis, P vulgaris, Providencia stuartii, Morganella morganii, Citrobacter freundii, S pyogenes, P aeruginosa* and *S aureus* (penicillinase- and nonpenicillinase-producing strains) and *epidermidis*.

Bone/joint infections caused by *E cloacae, Serratia marcescens* and *P aeruginosa*.

Urinary tract infections caused by *E coli, K pneumoniae, E cloacae, S marcescens, P mirabilis, Providencia rettgeri, M morganii, C diversus, C freundii, P aeruginosa, S epidermidis* and *S faecalis*.

Infectious diarrhea caused by *E coli* (enterotoxigenic strains), *Campylobacter jejuni, Shigella flexneri** and *Shigella sonnei** when antibacterial therapy is indicated.

Administration and Dosage:

Approved by the FDA in 1987.

Ciprofloxacin Dosage Guidelines				
Location of infection	Type or severity	Unit dose	Frequency	Daily dose
Urinary tract	Mild/Moderate	250 mg (200 mg IV)	q 12 h	500 mg (400 mg IV)
	Severe/Complicated	500 mg (400 mg IV)	q 12 h	1000 mg (800 mg IV)
Respiratory tract Bone and joint Skin & skin structure	Mild/Moderate	500 mg (400 mg IV)	q 12 h	1000 mg (800 mg IV)
	Severe/Complicated	750 mg	q 12 h	1500 mg
Infectious diarrhea	Mild/Moderate/Severe	500 mg	q 12 h	1000 mg

The duration of treatment depends upon the severity of infection. Generally, continue ciprofloxacin for at least 2 days after the signs and symptoms of infection have disappeared. The usual duration is 7 to 14 days; however, for severe and complicated infections, more prolonged therapy may be required. Bone and joint infections may require treatment for 4 to 6 weeks or longer. Infectious diarrhea may be treated for 5 to 7 days.

Renal function impairment: The following table provides dosage guidelines; however, monitoring of serum drug levels provides the most reliable basis for dosage adjustment:

Ciprofloxacin Dosage in Impaired Renal Function	
Creatinine clearance (ml/min)	Dose
> 50 (oral); ≥ 30 (IV)	See usual dosage
30-50	250-500 mg q 12 h
5-29	250-500 mg q 18 h (oral); 200-400 mg q 18-24 h (IV)
Hemodialysis or peritoneal dialysis	250-500 mg q 24 h (after dialysis)

When only the serum creatinine concentration is known, this formula may be used to estimate Ccr. Serum creatinine should represent a steady state of renal function.

$$\text{Males: } \frac{\text{Weight (kg)} \times (140 - \text{age})}{72 \times \text{serum creatinine (mg/dl)}} = \text{Ccr} \qquad \text{Females: } 0.85 \times \text{male value}$$

* Efficacy for this organism in this organ system was studied in fewer than ten infections.

(Administration and Dosage continued on following page)

Refer to the general discussion of these agents on page 1798.

CIPROFLOXACIN (Cont.)

Administration and Dosage (Cont.):

Renal function impairment (cont.):

In patients with severe infections and severe renal impairment, a unit dose of 750 mg may be administered orally at the intervals noted in the table; however, carefully monitor patients and measure serum ciprofloxacin concentration periodically. Avoid peak concentrations (1 to 2 hours after dosing) > 5 mcg/ml. For patients with changing renal function or with renal impairment and hepatic insufficiency, measurement of serum levels will provide additional guidance for adjusting dosage.

IV: Administer by IV infusion over 60 minutes. Slow infusion of a dilute solution into a large vein will minimize patient discomfort and reduce the risk of venous irritation.

Vials (injection concentrate) – Dilute before use with a suitable IV solution to a final concentration of 1 to 2 mg/ml (see Compatibility/Stability). If a Y-type IV infusion set or a piggyback method is used, temporarily discontinue the administration of any other solutions during the ciprofloxacin infusion.

Compatibility/Stability – Stable up to 14 days at refrigerated or room temperature (5° to 25°C; 41° to 77°F) when diluted with 0.9% NaCl Injection, USP or 5% Dextrose Injection, USP. Protect from freezing.

				C.I.*
Rx	**Cipro** (Miles Pharm.)	**Tablets:** 250 mg	(Miles 512). Film coated. In 50s and UD 100s.	1.7
		500 mg	(Miles 513). Film coated. In 50s and UD 100s.	1
		750 mg	(Miles 514). Film coated. In 50s and UD 100s.	1.2
Rx	**Cipro I.V.** (Miles Pharm.)	**Injection:** 200 mg	With lactic acid. In 20 ml vials (1%) and 100 ml in 5% Dextrose or 0.9% NaCl flexible containers (0.2%).	NA
		400 mg	With lactic acid. In 40 ml vials (1%) and 200 ml in 5% Dextrose flexible containers (0.2%).	NA

NORFLOXACIN

Indications:

For the treatment of adults with the following infections caused by susceptible strains of the designated microorganisms in the conditions listed below:

Urinary tract infections – *Uncomplicated* (including cystitis) caused by *Enterococcus faecalis, E coli, K pneumoniae, P mirabilis, P aeruginosa, S epidermidis, S saprophyticus, C freundii*†, *Enterobacter aerogenes*†, *Enterobacter cloacae*†, *P vulgaris*†, *S aureus*† or *S agalactiae*†; *complicated* caused by *Enterococcus faecalis, E coli, K pneumoniae, P mirabilis, P aeruginosa* or *Serratia marcescens*†.

Sexually transmitted diseases – *Uncomplicated urethral and cervical gonorrhea* caused by *N gonorrhoeae.*

Administration and Dosage:

Approved by the FDA in 1986.

Take 1 hr before or 2 hrs after meals with glass of water. Patients should be well hydrated.

Recommended Norfloxacin Dosage					
Infection	Description	Dose	Frequency	Duration	Daily dose
Urinary tract infections (UTI)	Uncomplicated (cystitis) due to *E coli, K pneumoniae* or *P mirabilis*	400 mg	q 12 h	3 days	800 mg
	Uncomplicated due to other organisms	400 mg	q 12 h	7-10 days	800 mg
	Complicated	400 mg	q 12 h	10-21 days	800 mg
Sexually transmitted diseases	Uncomplicated gonorrhea	800 mg	single dose	1 day	800 mg

Renal function impairment: In patients with a Ccr rate ≤ 30 ml/min/1.73 m², administer 400 mg once daily for the duration given above.

When only the serum creatinine is known, the following formula may be used to estimate Ccr. The serum creatinine should represent a steady state of renal function.

$$\text{Males: } \frac{\text{Weight (kg)} \times (140 - \text{age})}{72 \times \text{serum creatinine (mg/dl)}} = \text{Ccr} \qquad \text{Females: } 0.85 \times \text{male value}$$

Elderly: Dose based on normal or impaired renal function.

				C.I.*
Rx	**Noroxin** (MSD)	**Tablets:** 400 mg	(MSD 705 Noroxin). Dark pink. Film coated. In 100s and UD 20s and 100s.	1.5

* Cost Index based on cost per adult daily dose of 500 mg ciprofloxacin or 800 mg norfloxacin.

† Efficacy for this organism in this organ system was studied in fewer than 10 infections.

Refer to the general discussion of these agents on page 1798.

OFLOXACIN

Indications:

For the treatment of adults with the following infections caused by susceptible strains of the designated microorganisms. Use IV administration when this route is advantageous to the patient (eg, patient cannot tolerate an oral dosage form).

In the absence of vomiting or other factors interfering with the absorption of orally administered drug, patients receive essentially the same systemic antimicrobial therapy after equivalent doses of ofloxacin administered by either the oral or the IV route. Therefore, the IV formulation does not provide a higher degree of efficacy or more potent antimicrobial activity than an equivalent dose of the oral formulation.

Lower respiratory tract infections – Acute bacterial exacerbations of chronic bronchitis or community-acquired pneumonia due to *H influenzae* or *S pneumoniae*.

Sexually transmitted diseases (see Warnings) – Acute, uncomplicated urethral and cervical gonorrhea due to *N gonorrhoeae;* nongonococcal urethritis and cervicitis due to *Chlamydia trachomatis;* mixed infections of urethra and cervix due to both organisms.

Skin and skin structure infections (uncomplicated) due to *S aureus, S pyogenes* or *P mirabilis*†.

Urinary tract infections – Uncomplicated cystitis due to *Citrobacter diversus, Enterobacter aerogenes, E coli, K pneumoniae, P mirabilis* or *P aeruginosa;* complicated UTIs due to *E coli, K pneumoniae, P mirabilis, Citrobacter diversus*† or *P aeruginosa*†.

Prostatitis due to *E coli*.

Administration and Dosage:

Approved by the FDA in 1990.

Usual daily dose is 200 to 400 mg every 12 hours as described in the following table:

Ofloxacin Dosage Guidelines (Oral and IV)					
Infection	Description	Unit dose	Frequency	Duration	Daily dose
Lower respiratory tract	Exacerbation of chronic bronchitis	400 mg	q 12 h	10 days	800 mg
	Pneumonia	400 mg	q 12 h	10 days	800 mg
Sexually transmitted diseases	Acute, uncomplicated gonorrhea	400 mg	single dose	1 day	400 mg
	Cervicitis/urethritis due to *C trachomatis*	300 mg	q 12 h	7 days	600 mg
	Cervicitis/urethritis due to *C trachomatis* and *N gonorrhoeae*	300 mg	q 12 h	7 days	600 mg
Skin and skin structure	Mild to moderate	400 mg	q 12 h	10 days	800 mg
Urinary tract	Cystitis due to *E coli* or *K pneumoniae*	200 mg	q 12 h	3 days	400 mg
	Cystitis due to other organisms	200 mg	q 12 h	7 days	400 mg
	Complicated UTIs	200 mg	q 12 h	10 days	400 mg
Prostatitis		300 mg	q 12 h	6 weeks[1]	600 mg

[1] Because there are no safety data presently available to support the use of the IV formulation for > 10 days, switch to oral therapy or other appropriate therapy after 10 days.

IV: Administer by IV infusion only. Do not give IM, intrathecally, intraperitoneally or SC. Avoid rapid or bolus IV infusion; administer slowly over a period of not less than 60 min.

Single-use vials – Must be diluted prior to use (see Compatible IV solutions). The resulting concentration is 4 mg/ml. Prepare the desired dosage as follows:

Preparation of Ofloxacin Dosage From Single-Use Vials				
Desired strength (mg)	Volume to withdraw (ml)		Volume of diluent	Infusion time (min)
	From 10 ml vial	From 20 ml vial		
200	5	10	qs 50 ml	60
300	7.5	15	qs 75 ml	60
400	10	20	qs 100 ml	60

† Efficacy for this organism in this organ system was studied in fewer than 10 infections.

Compatible IV solutions: 0.9% Sodium Chloride; 5% Dextrose; 5% Dextrose/0.9% Sodium Chloride; 5% Dextrose in Lactated Ringer's; 5% Sodium Bicarbonate; *Plasma-Lyte* 56 in 5% Dextrose; 5% Dextrose, 0.45% Sodium Chloride and 0.15% Potassium Chloride; Sodium Lactate (M/6); Water for Injection.

(Administration and Dosage continued on following page)

Refer to the general discussion of these agents on page 1798 .

OFLOXACIN (Cont.)

Administration and Dosage (Cont.):

IV (Cont.):

Premixed bottles/flexible containers – No further dilution is necessary; already premixed in 5% Dextrose.

Storage/Stability – Preservative free; discard unused portions. Store premixed flexible containers at ≤ 25°C (77°F). Brief exposure up to 40°C (104°F) does not adversely affect the product. Avoid excessive heat and protect from freezing and light.

Renal function impairment: Adjust dosage in patients with a Ccr value of ≤ 50 ml/min. After a normal initial dose, adjust the dosing interval as follows: Ccr 10-50 ml/min, use a 24 hour interval and do not adjust dosage; Ccr < 10 ml/min, use a 24 hour interval and one-half the recommended dosage.

When only the serum creatinine is known, the following formula may be used to estimate Ccr. Serum creatinine should represent a steady state of renal function.

$$\text{Males: } \frac{\text{Weight (kg)} \times (140 - \text{age})}{72 \times \text{serum creatinine (mg/dl)}} = \text{Ccr} \qquad \text{Females: } 0.85 \times \text{male value}$$

				C.I.*
Rx	Floxin (Ortho)	Tablets: 200 mg	(Floxin 200). Pale gold. Film coated. In 50s and UD 100s.	2
		300 mg	(Floxin 300). Pale gold. Film coated. In 50s and UD 100s.	1.6
		400 mg	(Floxin 400). Pale gold. Film coated. In 50s and UD 100s.	1.3
		Injection: 200 mg[1]	In 50 ml single-use premixed flexible containers in 5% dextrose.	NA
		400 mg[1]	In 10 and 20 ml single-use vials in Water for Injection, and 100 ml single-use premixed bottles or flexible containers in 5% dextrose.	NA

ENOXACIN

Indications:

For the treatment of adults (≥ 18 years of age) with infections caused by susceptible strains of the designated microorganisms in the conditions listed below:

Sexually transmitted diseases – Uncomplicated urethral or cervical gonorrhea due to *Neisseria gonorrhoeae.*

Urinary tract infections – Uncomplicated (cystitis) due to *Escherichia coli, Staphylococcus epidermidis*† or *S saprophyticus*†; complicated due to *E coli, Klebsiella pneumoniae, Proteus mirabilis, Pseudomonas aeruginosa, S epidermidis* or *Enterobacter cloacae*†.

Administration and Dosage:

Approved by the FDA on December 31, 1991.

Take at least 1 hour before or 2 hours after a meal.

Enoxacin Dosage Guidelines

Infection	Description	Dose	Frequency	Duration	Daily dose
Urinary tract infections	Uncomplicated (cystitis)	200 mg	q 12 h	7 days	400 mg
	Complicated	400 mg	q 12 h	14 days	800 mg
Sexually transmitted diseases	Uncomplicated gonorrhea	400 mg	single dose	1 day	400 mg

Renal function impairment: Adjust dosage in patients with a creatinine clearance (Ccr) ≤ 30 ml/min/1.73 m^2. After a normal initial dose, use a 12 hour interval and one-half the recommended dose.

When only the serum creatinine is known, the following formula may be used to estimate Ccr. Serum creatinine should represent a steady state of renal function.

$$\text{Males: } \frac{\text{Weight (kg)} \times (140 - \text{age})}{72 \times \text{serum creatinine (mg/dl)}} = \text{Ccr} \qquad \text{Females: } 0.85 \times \text{male value}$$

Elderly: Dosage adjustment is not necessary with normal renal function; however, adjust according to previous guidelines in patients with compromised renal function.

Rx	Penetrex (Rhone-Poulenc Rorer)	Tablets: 200 mg	(5100). Light blue. Film coated. In 50s.
		400 mg	(5140). Dark blue. Film coated. In 50s.

† Efficacy for this organism in this organ system was studied in fewer than 10 infections.
* Cost Index based on cost per daily dose of 400 mg.
[1] Preservative free.

Refer to the general discussion of these agents on page 1798 .

LOMEFLOXACIN HCl

Indications:

For the treatment of adults with mild to moderate infections caused by susceptible strains of the designated microorganisms in the conditions listed below:

Lower respiratory tract infections – Acute bacterial exacerbation of chronic bronchitis caused by *H influenzae* or *Moraxella (Branhamella) catarrhalis**. *Note:* Lomefloxacin is not indicated for the empiric treatment of acute bacterial exacerbation of chronic bronchitis when it is probable that *S pneumoniae* is a causative pathogen (see Warnings).

Urinary tract infections – Uncomplicated (cystitis) caused by *E coli, K pneumoniae, P mirabilis* or *S saprophyticus; complicated* caused by *E coli, K pneumoniae, P mirabilis, P aeruginosa, C diversus** or *Enterobacter cloacae**.

Prophylaxis – Preoperatively to reduce the incidence of urinary tract infections in the early postoperative period (3 to 5 days postsurgery) in patients undergoing transurethral procedures. Efficacy in decreasing the incidence of other infections in the early postoperative period has not been established. Do not use in minor urologic procedures for which prophylaxis is not indicated (eg, simple cystoscopy, retrograde pyelography).

Administration and Dosage:

Approved by the FDA on February 21, 1992.

Lomefloxacin may be taken without regard to meals (see Clinical Pharmacology).

Recommended Daily Dose of Lomefloxacin					
Body system	Infection	Dose	Frequency	Duration	Daily dose
Lower respiratory tract	Acute bacterial exacerbation of chronic bronchitis	400 mg	once daily	10 days	400 mg
Urinary tract	Cystitis	400 mg	once daily	10 days	400 mg
	Complicated urinary tract infections	400 mg	once daily	14 days	400 mg

Elderly: No dosage adjustment is needed for elderly patients with normal renal function (Ccr $\geq$ 40 ml/min/1.73 m²).

Renal function impairment: Lomefloxacin is primarily eliminated by renal excretion. Modification of dosage is recommended in patients with renal dysfunction. In patients with a Ccr $>$ 10 but $<$ 40 ml/min/1.73 m², the recommended dosage is an initial loading dose of 400 mg followed by daily maintenance doses of 200 mg once daily for the duration of treatment. It is suggested that serial determinations of lomefloxacin levels be performed to determine any necessary alteration in the appropriate next dosing interval.

If only the serum creatinine is known, the following formula may be used to estimate Ccr.

$$\text{Males:} \quad \frac{\text{Weight (kg)} \times (140 - \text{age})}{72 \times \text{serum creatinine (mg/dl)}} = \text{Ccr}$$

Females: 0.85 x above value

Dialysis patients: Hemodialysis removes only a negligible amount of lomefloxacin (3% in 4 hours). Hemodialysis patients should receive an initial loading dose of 400 mg followed by maintenance doses of 200 mg once daily for the duration of treatment.

Cirrhosis: Cirrhosis does not reduce the non-renal clearance of lomefloxacin. Base the need for a dosage reduction in this population on the degree of renal function and plasma concentrations.

Prophylaxis: A single dose of 400 mg 2 to 6 hours prior to surgery when oral preoperative prophylaxis for transurethral surgical procedures is considered appropriate.

Rx	**Maxaquin** (Searle)	**Tablets:** 400 mg	Lactose. (Maxaquin 400). White, scored. Film coated. Oval. In 20s and UD 100s.

* Efficacy for this organism in this organ system was studied in fewer than 10 infections.

Actions:

Pharmacokinetics: Absorption/Distribution – Tetracyclines are adequately but incompletely absorbed in children and adults in the fasting state. The percentage of an oral dose absorbed is highest for doxycycline and minocycline, and intermediate for oxytetracycline, methacycline, demeclocycline and tetracycline. Achlorhydria has no effect on absorption. Food decreases absorption of tetracyclines, except doxycycline and minocycline; take these two agents with food.

Doxycycline and minocycline are highly lipid soluble, and readily penetrate into the cerebrospinal fluid (CSF), brain, eye and prostate. In addition, minocycline displays good penetration of saliva, making it useful in eliminating meningococci from asymptomatic carriers. Tetracycline and demeclocycline are intermediate in terms of lipid solubility, whereas oxytetracycline is the least lipid soluble. Oxytetracycline diffuses readily through the placenta into fetal circulation, into pleural fluid and under some circumstances into the CSF.

Metabolism/Excretion – *Hemodialysis* removes 20% to 30% of tetracycline, but has little effect on doxycycline or minocycline. *Peritoneal dialysis* has no effect on any of the tetracyclines.

The tetracyclines are concentrated by the liver in the bile and excreted in the urine and feces, largely unchanged; therefore, make appropriate dosage adjustments in patients with impaired renal function. Conventional tetracyclines are contraindicated in anuria. Doxycycline and minocycline are excreted largely by nonrenal routes; their serum half-lives do not significantly increase in renal impairment. Doxycycline is secreted in an inactive form into the intestinal lumen and eliminated with feces; hence, its half-life is largely independent of renal or hepatic function. Minocycline is metabolized, and its half-life is prolonged in oliguria.

Tetracycline Pharmacokinetic Variables and Dosage Regimens

Tetracyclines	Serum Protein Binding (%)	Normal Serum Half-Life (hrs)	% Excreted Unchanged in Urine	Usual Oral Adult Maintenance Dosage	Lipid Solubility
Tetracycline	65	6 to 12	60	250 mg q 6 h or 500 mg q 6 to 12 h	Intermediate
Demeclocycline	65 to 91	12 to 16	39	150 mg q 6 h or 300 mg q 12 h	Intermediate
Doxycycline	80 to 95	15 to 25	30 to 42	50 mg q 12 h or 100 mg q 24 h	High
Methacycline	80 to 90	14 to 16	50 to 60	150 mg q 6 h or 300 mg q 12 h	
Minocycline	70 to 80	11 to 18	6 to 12	100 mg q 12 h	High
Oxytetracycline	20 to 40	6 to 12	70	250 to 500 mg q 6 h	Low

Microbiology: The tetracyclines are bacteriostatic. They exert their antimicrobial effect by inhibition of protein synthesis. Tetracyclines are active against a wide range of gram-negative and gram-positive organisms (see Indications). The tetracyclines have similar antimicrobial spectra, and cross-resistance is common.

Indications:

Infections caused by the following microorganisms: Rickettsiae (Rocky Mountain spotted fever, typhus fever and the typhus group, Q fever, rickettsialpox and tick fevers); *Mycoplasma pneumoniae* (PPLO, Eaton agent); agents of psittacosis and ornithosis; agents of lymphogranuloma venereum and granuloma inguinale; the spirochetal agent of relapsing fever *(Borrelia recurrentis)*.

Infections caused by the following gram-negative microorganisms: *Hemophilus ducreyi* (chancroid); *Yersinia pestis* and *Francisella tularensis* (formerly *Pasteurella pestis* and *P tularensis*); *Bartonella bacilliformis; Bacteroides* sp; *Campylobacter fetus* (formerly *Vibrio fetus*); *V cholerae* (formerly *V comma*); *Brucella* sp (in conjunction with streptomycin).

Infections caused by the following microorganisms, when bacteriologic testing indicates appropriate susceptibility to the drug:

Gram-negative: Escherichia coli; Enterobacter aerogenes (formerly *Aerobacter aerogenes); Shigella* sp; *Acinetobacter calcoaceticus* (formerly *Mima* and *Herellea* sp); *H influenzae* (respiratory infections); *Klebsiella* sp (respiratory and urinary infections).

Gram-positive: Streptococcus sp including *S pneumoniae.* Up to 44% of strains of *S pyogenes* and 74% of *S faecalis* are resistant to tetracyclines. Therefore, do not use tetracyclines unless the organism has been demonstrated to be sensitive.

For upper respiratory infections due to group A β-hemolytic streptococci, including prophylaxis of rheumatic fever, penicillin is the usual drug of choice.

Staphylococcus aureus, skin and soft tissue infections. Tetracyclines are not the drugs of choice in the treatment of any type of staphylococcal infection.

(Indications continued on following page)

Indications (Cont.):

Treatment of trachoma, although the infectious agent is not always eliminated, as judged by immunofluorescence.

When penicillin is contraindicated, tetracyclines are alternative drugs in the treatment of infections due to: *Neisseria gonorrhoeae; Treponema pallidum* and *T pertenue* (syphilis and yaws); *Listeria monocytogenes; Clostridium* species; *Bacillus anthracis; Fusobacterium fusiforme* (Vincent's infection); *Actinomyces* species; *N meningitidis* (IV only).

Acute intestinal amebiasis: Tetracyclines may be a useful adjunct to amebicides.

Oral tetracyclines: Adults – Treatment of uncomplicated urethral, endocervical or rectal infections caused by *Chlamydia trachomatis.*

Severe acne (where it may be useful as adjunctive therapy).

Inclusion conjunctivitis (which may be treated with oral tetracyclines or with a combination of oral and topical agents).

Doxycycline, oral: Treatment of uncomplicated gonococcal infections in adults (except for anorectal infections in men); gonococcal arthritis-dermatitis syndrome; acute epididymo-orchitis caused by *N gonorrhoeae* and *C trachomatis;* nongonococcal urethritis caused by *C trachomatis* and *Ureaplasma urealyticum.*

Minocycline, oral: Treatment of asymptomatic carriers of *N meningitidis* to eliminate meningococci from the nasopharynx. In order to preserve the usefulness of minocycline in this indication, perform diagnostic laboratory procedures, including serotyping and susceptibility testing, to establish the carrier state and the correct treatment. Reserve the drug for situations in which the risk of meningococcal meningitis is high. *Not* indicated for the treatment of meningococcal infection.

Oral minocycline has been used successfully in *Mycobacterium marinum* infections.

Minocycline is also indicated for the treatment of uncomplicated urethral, endocervical or rectal infections in adults caused by *U urealyticum;* uncomplicated gonococcal urethritis in men due to *N gonorrhoeae.*

Methacycline: Mycoplasma pneumonia; nongonococcal urethritis caused by *C trachomatis;* early Lyme disease.

Unlabeled Uses: **Demeclocycline** has been used successfully in the treatment of chronic hyponatremia associated with the syndrome of inappropriate antidiuretic hormone (SIADH) secretion. Experience with this therapy is limited.

Doxycycline has been used to prevent "Traveler's Diarrhea" commonly caused by enterotoxigenic *E coli.*

Minocycline has been used as an alternative to sulfonamides in nocardiosis.

Tetracycline instilled through a chest tube is employed as a pleural sclerosing agent in malignant pleural effusions. Tetracycline plus gentamicin is recommended for *V vulnificus* infections caused by wound infection after trauma or by ingestion of contaminated seafood.

Tetracycline suspension has been used as a mouthwash in the treatment of nonspecific mouth ulcerations, aphthous ulcers and canker sores. Dosages have ranged from 5 to 10 ml of 125 mg/ml 3 times/day for 5 to 7 days.

Lyme disease (the etiologic agent is a spirochete, *Borrelia burgdorferi*): Oral **tetracycline** 250 mg daily for 10 days is the drug of choice for stage I disease (skin rash: erythema chronicum migrans) in adults; **doxycycline** has also been recommended for early disease. Both agents have been recommended for stage II disease (mild cardiac and neurologic illness), and they are being evaluated for treatment of stage III disease (arthritis). However, the efficacy of tetracycline at the recommended dose for early Lyme disease has been questioned.

Refer to individual product listings for CDC recommendations for treatment of sexually transmitted diseases.

Contraindications:

Hypersensitivity to any of the tetracyclines.

Warnings:

Renal function impairment: If renal impairment exists, even usual doses may lead to excessive systemic accumulation of the tetracyclines (with the exception of doxycycline and minocycline) and possible liver toxicity. Use lower than usual doses; if therapy is prolonged, drug serum level determinations may be advisable.

The hazard of liver toxicity is of particular importance in parenteral administration to pregnant or postpartum patients with pyelonephritis.

The antianabolic action of the tetracyclines may cause an increase in BUN. In patients with significantly impaired renal function, higher serum levels of tetracycline may lead to azotemia, hyperphosphatemia and acidosis. This does not occur with doxycycline.

(Warnings continued on following page)

Warnings (Cont.):

Photosensitivity: Photosensitivity manifested by an exaggerated sunburn reaction has been observed in some individuals taking tetracyclines. Advise patients who are apt to be exposed to direct sunlight or ultraviolet light that this reaction can occur with tetracycline drugs, and discontinue treatment at the first evidence of skin erythema.

In patients taking **demeclocycline**, exaggerated sunburn reactions are characterized by severe burns of exposed surfaces, resulting from direct exposure to sunlight during therapy with moderate or large doses. Phototoxic reactions are most frequent with demeclocycline, and occur less frequently with the other tetracyclines; minocycline is least likely to cause phototoxic reactions.

Parenteral therapy: Reserve parenteral use for situations in which oral therapy is not indicated. Institute oral therapy as soon as possible. If IV therapy is given over prolonged periods of time, thrombophlebitis may result. Administration IM produces lower blood levels than oral administration in recommended dosages. If high blood levels are needed rapidly, administer IV.

Hepatic effects: Doses in excess of 2 g/day IV can be extremely dangerous. In the presence of renal dysfunction, and particularly in pregnancy, IV tetracycline in daily doses exceeding 2 g has been associated with death secondary to liver failure. When the need for intensive treatment outweighs its potential dangers (especially during pregnancy or in individuals with known or suspected renal and liver impairment), monitor renal and liver function tests. Serum tetracycline concentrations should not exceed 15 mcg/ml. Do not prescribe other potentially hepatotoxic drugs concomitantly.

Nephrogenic diabetes insipidus: Administration of **demeclocycline** has resulted in appearance of the diabetes insipidus syndrome (polyuria, polydipsia and weakness) in some patients on long-term therapy. The syndrome has been shown to be nephrogenic, dose-dependent and reversible on discontinuation of therapy.

Hazardous Tasks: Lightheadedness, dizziness or vertigo may occur with **minocycline.** Patients should observe caution while driving or performing other tasks requiring alertness. These symptoms may disappear during therapy and always disappear rapidly when the drug is discontinued.

Pregnancy: Category D (doxycycline; methacycline). (See Warnings about use during tooth development.) Tetracyclines should not be used during pregnancy. They readily cross the placenta; concentrations of oxytetracycline in cord blood are ≈ 50% of those of the mother. Tetracyclines are found in fetal tissues and can have toxic effects on the developing fetus (retardation of skeletal development). Evidence of embryotoxicity has also been noted in animals treated early in pregnancy.

Lactation: Tetracyclines are excreted in breast milk. A dosage of 2 g/day for 3 days has achieved a milk:plasma ratio of 0.6 to 0.8. Because of the potential for serious adverse reactions decide whether to discontinue nursing or discontinue the drug.

Children: Tetracyclines should not generally be used in children under 8 years of age, unless other drugs are not likely to be effective, or are contraindicated.

Teeth – The use of tetracyclines during the period of tooth development (from the last half of pregnancy through the eighth year of life) may cause permanent discoloration (yellow-gray-brown) of deciduous and permanent teeth. This adverse reaction is more common during long-term use of the drugs, but has been observed following repeated short-term courses. Enamel hypoplasia has also been reported. Doxycycline and oxytetracycline may be less likely to affect teeth.

Bone – Tetracycline forms a stable calcium complex in any bone-forming tissue. A decrease in the fibula growth rate has been observed in premature infants given oral tetracycline in doses of 25 mg/kg every 6 hours. This reaction was reversible when the drug was discontinued.

Precautions:

Pseudotumor cerebri (benign intracranial hypertension) in adults has been associated with tetracycline use. Usual clinical manifestations are headache and blurred vision. Bulging fontanels have been associated with tetracycline use in infants. While both conditions and related symptoms usually resolve soon after tetracycline discontinuation, the possibility for permanent sequelae exists.

Superinfection: Use of antibiotics (especially prolonged or repeated therapy) may result in bacterial or fungal overgrowth of nonsusceptible organisms. Such overgrowth may lead to a secondary infection. Take appropriate measures if superinfection occurs. Superinfection of the bowel by staphylococci may be life-threatening.

Laboratory tests: In sexually transmitted diseases when coexistent syphilis is suspected, perform darkfield examination before treatment is started and repeat the blood serology monthly for at least 4 months.

In long-term therapy, perform periodic laboratory evaluation of organ systems, including hematopoietic, renal and hepatic studies.

(Precautions continued on following page)

Precautions (Cont.):

Outdated products: Under no circumstances should outdated tetracyclines be administered; the degradation products of tetracyclines are highly nephrotoxic and have, on occasion, produced a Fanconi-like syndrome.

Sulfite sensitivity: Some of these products contain sulfites that may cause allergic-type reactions (including anaphylactic symptoms and life-threatening or less severe asthmatic episodes) in certain susceptible people. The overall prevalence of sulfite sensitivity in the general population is unknown and probably low. It is seen more frequently in asthmatic or atopic nonasthmatic people. Specific products containing sulfites are identified in the product listings.

Drug Interactions:

Antacids containing **aluminum, calcium, zinc or magnesium** and **bismuth salts** and other **divalent** and **trivalent cations** impair absorption of tetracyclines due to formation of a poorly soluble chelate, possibly decreasing the antimicrobial efficacy. Administer tetracyclines at least 2 hours before or after these agents.

Anticoagulants, oral: Tetracyclines may alter normal hemostasis; therefore these agents may increase the hypoprothrombinemic effects of concurrent anticoagulants. Monitor prothrombin activity.

Barbiturates, carbamazepine and **hydantoins** may increase the rate of metabolism, and therefore, decrease the half-life and serum levels of doxycycline. Antimicrobial effectiveness may be decreased.

Cimetidine may decrease the GI absorption of tetracyclines due to a pH-dependent inhibition of dissolution; antimicrobial effectiveness may be decreased.

Digoxin: Tetracyclines may increase the serum levels of **digoxin** in a small portion (< 10%) of patients; this could lead to digoxin toxicity. These effects may last for months after tetracycline administration is discontinued.

Insulin: Tetracyclines may reduce insulin requirements. Controlled studies are needed. Monitor blood glucose.

Iron salts, oral may decrease the GI absorption of tetracyclines due to formation of poorly soluble chelate; antimicrobial effectiveness may be decreased. Give iron salts in non-enteric coated, non-sustained release form at least 3 hours before or 2 hours after tetracyclines.

Lithium: Tetracycline may increase or decrease lithium levels. Monitor serum lithium levels.

Methoxyflurane and tetracycline coadministration may increase the nephrotoxic effects of both drugs. Avoid this combination.

Oral contraceptives: Coadministration of tetracyclines may decrease the pharmacologic effects of oral contraceptives; breakthrough bleeding or pregnancy may occur.

Penicillins: Bacteriostatic drugs (eg, tetracycline) may interfere with the bactericidal action of penicillins; avoid concomitant administration.

Sodium bicarbonate may impair the GI absorption of tetracyclines; this may depend on differences in tetracycline product formulations. Alkalinization of the urine may also alter urinary tetracycline excretion.

Drug/Food Interactions: Food and some dairy products interfere with absorption of tetracyclines. Administer oral tetracycline 1 hour before or 2 hours after meals. Doxycycline has a low affinity for calcium binding. Gastrointestinal absorption of minocycline and doxycycline is not significantly affected by food or dairy products.

Drug/Lab Test Interactions: Following a course of therapy, persistence for several days in both urine and blood of bacteriosuppressive levels of **demeclocycline** may interfere with culture studies. These levels should not be considered therapeutic.

Adverse Reactions:

GI: Oral and parenteral – Anorexia; nausea; vomiting; diarrhea; epigastric distress; bulky loose stools; stomatitis; sore throat; glossitis; hoarseness; black hairy tongue; dysphagia; enterocolitis; inflammatory lesions (with monilial overgrowth) in the anogenital region, including proctitis and pruritis ani.

Oral: Esophageal ulcers, most commonly in patients with an esophageal obstructive element or hiatal hernia. Having the patient remain standing for at least 90 seconds after medication ingestion and taking the medication with a full glass of water at least 1 hour before going to bed may minimize this problem.

Dermatologic: Maculopapular and erythematous rashes; exfoliative dermatitis (uncommon). Photosensitivity (See Warnings). Onycholysis and discoloration of the nails (rare). Onycholysis has been reported to occur in up to 25% of patients experiencing phototoxic reactions to tetracyclines. This may also occur without phototoxicity. Blue-gray pigmentation of the skin and mucous membranes has been reported, primarily with **minocycline**.

Stevens-Johnson syndrome (rare) has occurred with **minocycline**.

Renal: Rise in BUN (dose-related). (See Warnings).

(Adverse Reactions continued on following page)

Adverse Reactions (Cont.):

Hepatic: Fatty liver; hepatotoxicity (rare); increases in liver enzymes; hepatitis (rare). Hepatic cholestasis (rare), is usually associated with high dosage levels. (See Warnings).

CNS: Lightheadedness, dizziness or vertigo has been reported with **minocycline**; (see Warnings). Transient myopathy has been reported.

Hypersensitivity: Urticaria; angioneurotic edema; anaphylaxis; anaphylactoid purpura; pericarditis; exacerbation of systemic lupus erythematosus; polyarthralgia; serum sickness-like reactions, such as fever, rash and arthralgia; pulmonary infiltrates with eosinophilia.

Hematologic: Hemolytic anemia; thrombocytopenia; thrombocytopenic purpura; neutropenia; eosinophilia.

Miscellaneous: Pseudotumor cerebri (adults) and bulging fontanels (infants). (See Warnings.) Nephrogenic diabetes insipidus has been reported with **demeclocycline**. (See Warnings.) When given over prolonged periods, tetracyclines have been reported to produce brown-black microscopic discoloration of thyroid glands. No abnormalities of thyroid function studies are known to occur. Drug deposition in the eye may produce abnormal pigmentation of the conjunctiva. Tooth discoloration in adults is rare.

Local: Irritation may occur with IM administration.

Patient Information:

Take on an empty stomach, at least 1 hour before or 2 hours after meals (**doxycycline** and **minocycline** may be taken with food or milk). Take with a full glass of water (240 ml).

Avoid simultaneous dairy products (milk, cheese), antacids, laxatives or iron-containing products. If an antacid must be taken, take at least 2 hours before or after tetracycline.

Avoid prolonged exposure to sunlight or sunlamps; may cause photosensitivity (especially **demeclocycline**).

Administration:

Avoid rapid IV administration. Thrombophlebitis may result from prolonged IV therapy.

Continue therapy for at least 24 to 48 hours after symptoms and fever have subsided. Treat all infections due to group A β-hemolytic streptococci for at least 10 days.

TETRACYCLINE HCl

Administration and Dosage:

Oral: Adults – Usual dose: 1 to 2 g/day in 2 or 4 equal doses.

Mild to moderate infections: 500 mg, 2 times/day or 250 mg, 4 times/day.

Severe infections: 500 mg, 4 times/day.

Children (over 8 years of age) – Daily dose is 10 to 20 mg/lb (25 to 50 mg/kg) in 4 equal doses.

Brucellosis – 500 mg, 4 times/day for 3 weeks, accompanied by 1 g streptomycin IM twice/day the first week, and once daily the second week.

Syphilis – 30 to 40 g in equally divided doses over 10 to 15 days. Perform close follow-up and laboratory tests.

Gonorrhea – 1.5 g initially, then 500 mg every 6 hours, to a total of 9 g.

Gonorrhea in patients sensitive to penicillin – Initially, 1.5 g; follow with 500 mg every 6 hours for 4 days to a total of 9 g.

Uncomplicated urethral, endocervical or rectal infections caused by Chlamydia trachomatis – 500 mg, 4 times/day for at least 7 days.

Severe acne (long-term therapy) – Initially, 1 g/day in divided doses. For maintenance, give 125 to 500 mg/day.

CDC recommended treatment schedules for sexually transmitted diseases:[1]

Chlamydia trachomatis - Uncomplicated urethral, endocervical or rectal infections in adults: 500 mg, 4 times/day for 7 days.

Gonococcal infections - Uncomplicated urethral, endocervical or rectal infections in adults: 3 g amoxicillin, 3.5 g oral ampicillin, 4.8 million units IM aqueous procaine penicillin G or 250 mg IM ceftriaxone. Each (except ceftriaxone) should be accompanied by 1 g oral probenecid. Follow with 500 mg tetracycline, 4 times/day for 7 days.

In adults allergic to penicillins, cephalosporins or probenecid: 500 mg, 4 times/day for 7 days.

In PPNG-endemic and -hyperendemic areas: 250 mg IM ceftriaxone plus 100 mg oral doxycycline twice daily for 7 days or 500 mg oral tetracycline 4 times a day for 7 days. If tetracyclines are contraindicated or not tolerated, follow the single-dose regimen with erythromycin.

Penicillinase-producing Neisseria gonorrhoeae – 2 g IM spectinomycin or 250 mg IM ceftriaxone. Follow with 500 mg tetracycline, 4 times/day for 7 days.

Children (> 8 years) allergic to penicillins or cephalosporins: 40 mg/kg/day in 4 divided doses for 5 days.

Disseminated gonococcal infections in patients allergic to penicillins or cephalosporins – 500 mg, 4 times/day for at least 7 days.

[1] MMWR 1985 (Oct 18); 34 (Suppl 4S):75S-108S and 1987 (Sep 11); 36 (Suppl 5S):1S-18S.

(Administration and Dosage continued on following page)

TETRACYCLINE HCl (Cont.)

Administration and Dosage (Cont.):

Lymphogranuloma venereum - Genital, inguinal or anorectal: 500 mg, 4 times/day for at least 2 weeks.

Nongonococcal urethritis – 500 mg, 4 times/day for 7 days.

Acute pelvic inflammatory disease - Ambulatory treatment: 2 g IM cefoxitin, 3 g amoxicillin, 3.5 g oral ampicillin, 4.8 million units IM aqueous procaine penicillin G at 2 sites or 250 mg IM ceftriaxone. Each (except for ceftriaxone) should be accompanied by 1 g oral probenecid. Follow with 500 mg tetracycline, 4 times/day. (However, doxycycline is preferred.)

Children over 7 years of age: 150 mg/kg/day IV cefuroxime or 100 mg/kg/day IV ceftriaxone followed by 30 mg/kg/day IV tetracycline in 3 doses, continued for at least 4 days. Thereafter, continue tetracycline orally to complete at least 14 days of therapy.

Syphilis (penicillin-allergic patients) - Early: 500 mg, 4 times/day for 15 days. *More than 1 year's duration:* 500 mg, 4 times/day for 30 days.

Sexually transmitted epididymo-orchitis – 3 g oral amoxicillin, 3.5 g oral ampicillin, 4.8 million units IM aqueous procaine penicillin G at 2 sites (each with 1 g oral probenecid), 2 g IM spectinomycin or 250 mg IM ceftriaxone followed by 500 mg tetracycline, 4 times/day for 10 days.

Urethral syndrome in women – 500 mg, 4 times/day for 7 days.

Rape victims - Prophylaxis: 500 mg, 4 times/day for 7 days.

Parenteral:

IM – Inject deeply into a large muscle mass such as the gluteal region. Inadvertent injection into the subcutaneous or fat layers may cause pain and induration.

Adults: The usual daily dose is 250 mg once every 24 hours or 300 mg in divided doses at 8 to 12 hour intervals.

Children (over 8 years of age): 15 to 25 mg/kg, up to a maximum of 250 mg per single daily injection. Dosage may be divided and given at 8 to 12 hour intervals.

Preparation and storage of solution (IM) – Add 2 ml Sterile Water for Injection or Sodium Chloride Injection to the 100 or 250 mg vial. Store resulting solution at room temperature; do not use after 24 hours.

IV – Adults: 250 to 500 mg every 12 hours; do not exceed 500 mg every 6 hours.

Children (over 8 years of age): 12 mg/kg/day, divided into 2 doses; from 10 to 20 mg/kg/day may be given, depending on the severity of the infection.

Preparation of solution (IV): Initially, reconstitute 250 and 500 mg vials by adding 5 or 10 ml, respectively, of Sterile Water for Injection; further dilute, prior to administration, to at least 100 ml (up to 1000 ml) with any of the following: Ringer's Injection; Sodium Chloride Injection; 5% Dextrose Injection; 5% Dextrose and Sodium Chloride Injection; Lactated Ringer's Injection; 5% Protein Hydrolysate Injection Low Sodium with 5% Dextrose or with 10% Invert Sugar.

Avoid use of solutions containing calcium, unless necessary. These tend to form precipitates (especially in neutral to alkaline solution). However, Ringer's Injection and Lactated Ringer's Injection can be used with caution since the calcium ion content in these diluents does not normally precipitate tetracycline in an acid medium.

Storage: The initial reconstituted solutions are stable at room temperature for 12 hours without significant loss of potency. Administer the final dilution immediately.

				C.I.*
Rx	**Tetracycline HCl Syrup** (Various, eg, Balan, Bioline, Geneva, Gen-King, Goldline, Harber, Major, Moore, Rugby, Schein)	**Oral Suspension:** 125 mg/5 ml	In 60 and 480 ml.	11+
Rx	**Achromycin V** (Lederle)		Cherry flavor. In 473 ml.	139
Rx	**Sumycin Syrup** (Apothecon)		Fruit flavor. In 473 ml.	44
Rx	**Tetralan Syrup** (Lannett)		Cherry flavor. In 480 ml.	21
Rx	**Tetracycline HCl** (Richlyn)	**Capsules:** 100 mg	In 1000s.	9

(Continued on following page)

Complete prescribing information for these products begins on page 1811

TETRACYCLINE HCl (Cont.)

	Product	Form	Description	C.I.*
Rx	**Tetracycline** (Various, eg, Bioline, Geneva, Goldline, Major, Moore, Rugby, Wyeth-Ayerst, Zenith)	**Capsules:** 250 mg	In 20s, 28s, 30s, 40s, 60s, 100s, 500s, 1000s and UD 32s and 100s.	4+
Rx	**Achromycin V** (Lederle)		(Lederle A3 250 mg). Blue/ yellow. In 100s, 1000s, UD 100s, unit-of-issue 120s, 240s, 336s, 480s, 1200s.	14
Rx	**Ala-Tet** (Del-Ray)		In 100s and 1000s.	18
Rx	**Nor-Tet** (Vortech)		(H214). In 100s and 1000s.	15
Rx	**Panmycin** (Upjohn)		Tartrazine. Grey and yellow. In 100s and 1000s.	18
Rx	**Robitet Robicaps** (Robins)		Pink/brown. In 100s, 1000s.	8
Rx	**Sumycin '250'** (Apothecon)		In 100s, 1000s and UD 100s.	11
Rx	**Teline** (Hauck)		In 100s and 1000s.	10
Rx	**Tetracap** (Circle)		In 100s.	8
Rx	**Tetracyn** (Pfizer)		Black/white. In 100s, 1000s.	NA
Rx	**Tetralan "250"** (Lannett)		White/orange. In 100s, 1000s.	6
Rx	**Tetram** (Dunhall)		In 100s.	16
Rx	**Tetracycline** (Dr.'s Pharm.)	**Tablets:** 250 mg	In 30s and 60s.	11
Rx	**Sumycin '250'** (Apothecon)		In 100s and 1000s.	11
Rx	**Tetracycline HCl** (Various, eg, Bioline, Geneva, Goldline, Major, Moore, Rugby, Wyeth-Ayerst, Zenith)	**Capsules:** 500 mg	In 20s, 28s, 40s, 50s, 100s, 500s, 1000s and UD 100s.	4+
Rx	**Achromycin V** (Lederle)		(Lederle A5 500 mg). Blue and yellow. In 100s, 1000s, UD 100s, unit-of-issue 240s.	13
Rx	**Ala-Tet** (Del-Ray)		In 100s and 1000s.	NA
Rx	**Nor-Tet** (Vortech)		(H203). In 100s and 1000s.	9
Rx	**Robitet Robicaps** (Robins)		Cream/brown. In 100s, 500s.	7
Rx	**Sumycin '500'** (Apothecon)		In 100s, 500s and UD 100s.	11
Rx	**Teline-500** (Hauck)		In 100s.	9
Rx	**Tetracyn 500** (Pfizer)		Black/blue. In 100s.	NA
Rx	**Tetralan-500** (Lannett)		Black/yellow. In 100s, 1000s.	7
Rx	**Tetracycline** (Dr.'s Pharm.)	**Tablets:** 500 mg	In 30s and 60s.	6
Rx	**Sumycin '500'** (Apothecon)		In 100s and 500s.	11
Rx	**Achromycin IM** (Lederle)	**Powder for IM Injection:** 100 or 250 mg	In vials.[1]	2434
Rx	**Achromycin IV** (Lederle)	**Powder for IV Injection:** 250 or 500 mg	In vials.	2434

DEMECLOCYCLINE HCl

Caution: May cause photosensitivity (see group monograph).

Administration and Dosage:

Adults: Daily dose – 4 divided doses of 150 mg each or 2 divided doses of 300 mg each.

Children (over 8 years of age): Usual daily dose – 3 to 6 mg/lb (6 to 12 mg/kg), depending upon the severity of the disease, divided into 2 or 4 doses.

Gonorrhea patients sensitive to penicillin: Initially, 600 mg; follow with 300 mg every 12 hours for 4 days to a total of 3 g.

	Product	Form	Description	C.I.*
Rx	**Declomycin** (Lederle)	**Capsules:** 150 mg	(LL D9). Two-tone coral. In 100s.	409
		Tablets: 150 mg	(LL D11). Red, film coated. Convex, round. In 100s.	409
		300 mg	(LL D12). Red, film coated. Convex, round. In 48s.	372

* Cost Index based on cost per 500 mg.

[1] With 40 mg procaine HCl per vial.

Complete prescribing information for these products begins on page 1811

DOXYCYCLINE

Administration and Dosage:

Oral:

The therapeutic antibacterial serum activity will usually persist for 24 hours.

Adults – Usual dose: 200 mg on the first day of treatment (100 mg every 12 hours); follow with a maintenance dose of 100 mg/day. The maintenance dose may be administered as a single dose or as 50 mg every 12 hours. *More severe infections (particularly chronic urinary tract infections):* 100 mg every 12 hours.

Children (over 8 years of age) – 100 pounds or less (< 45 kg): 2 mg/lb (4.4 mg/kg) divided into 2 doses on the first day of treatment; follow with 1 mg/lb (2.2 mg/kg) given as a single daily dose or divided into 2 doses on subsequent days. *More severe infections* - Up to 2 mg/lb (4.4 mg/kg) may be used. For children over 100 pounds (45 kg), use the usual adult dose.

Acute gonococcal infection - 200 mg immediately, then 100 mg at bedtime on the first day. Follow by 100 mg 2 times/day for 3 days.

Single visit dose: Immediately give 300 mg; follow with 300 mg in 1 hour, which may be administered with food, milk or carbonated beverage.

Primary and secondary syphilis - 300 mg/day in divided doses for at least 10 days.

Uncomplicated urethral, endocervical or rectal infections in adults caused by Chlamydia trachomatis - 100 mg twice daily for at least 7 days.

Unlabeled Use - Doxycycline has been used to prevent "Traveler's Diarrhea" commonly caused by enterotoxigenic *Escherichia coli*. In limited trials, this prophylactic (100 mg/day) therapy appears to be superior to placebo.

Endometritis, salpingitis, parametritis or peritonitis: Give 100 mg doxycycline IV, twice daily and 2 g cefoxitin IV, 4 times/day. Continue IV administration for at least 4 days and for at least 48 hours after patient improves. Then continue oral doxycycline (100 mg), twice daily to complete 10 to 14 days total therapy.

Parenteral:

Do not inject IM or SC. The duration of IV infusion may vary with the dose (100 to 200 mg per day), but is usually 1 to 4 hours. A recommended minimum infusion time for 100 mg of a 0.5 mg/ml solution is 1 hour. Continue therapy for at least 24 to 48 hours after symptoms and fever have subsided. Therapeutic antibacterial serum activity usually persists for 24 hours following recommended dosage.

Renal impairment - Doxycycline at recommended doses does not lead to excessive accumulation in patients with renal impairment.

Adults - The usual dosage is 200 mg IV on the first day of treatment, administered in 1 or 2 infusions. Subsequent daily dosage is 100 to 200 mg, depending upon the severity of infection, with 200 mg administered in 1 or 2 infusions.

Primary and secondary syphilis: 300 mg daily for at least 10 days.

Children (over 8 years) - ≤ 100 pounds (45 kg), give 2 mg/lb (4.4 mg/kg) on the first day of treatment, in 1 or 2 infusions. Subsequent daily dosage is 1 to 2 mg/lb (2.2 to 4.4 mg/kg) given as 1 or 2 infusions, depending on the severity of the infection. For children > 100 pounds (45 kg), use the usual adult dose.

Children (< 8 years): Safety of IV use has not been established (see Warnings, p. 341b).

Preparation of solution: To prepare a solution containing 10 mg/ml, reconstitute the contents of the vial with 10 ml (for the 100 mg/vial) or 20 ml (for the 200 mg/vial) of Sterile Water for Injection or any of the IV infusion solutions listed below. Dilute the 100 mg vial further with 100 to 1000 ml (or 200 to 2000 ml for the 200 mg vial) of the following IV solutions: Sodium Chloride Injection; 5% Dextrose Injection; Ringer's Injection; 10% Invert Sugar in Water; Lactated Ringer's Injection; 5% Dextrose in Lactated Ringer's; *Normosol-M* in D5-W; *Normosol-R* in D5-W; *Plasma-Lyte 56* in 5% Dextrose; *Plasma-Lyte 148* in 5% Dextrose. This will result in the recommended concentrations of 0.1 to 1 mg/ml.

Storage: When diluted with Lactated Ringer's Injection or 5% Dextrose in Lactated Ringer's, complete infusion of the solution (0.1 to 1 mg/ml) within 6 hours after reconstitution to assure stability. Use solutions within this time period or discard.

When diluted with the remaining solutions listed above, doxycycline may be stored up to 72 hours prior to infusion, if refrigerated and protected from light. Complete infusion within 12 hours to ensure stability; discard remaining solution.

Stability: Solutions at concentrations of 10 mg/ml in Sterile Water for Injection, when frozen immediately after reconstitution, are stable for 8 weeks when stored at –20°C. If product is warmed, avoid heating after thawing is complete. Do not refreeze.

(Administration and Dosage continued on following page)

DOXYCYCLINE (Cont.)

Administration and Dosage (Cont.):

CDC recommended treatment schedules for sexually transmitted diseases:[1]

Chlamydia trachomatis – Uncomplicated urethral, endocervical or rectal infections in adults: 100 mg, 2 times/day for 7 days.

Gonococcal infections – Uncomplicated urethral, endocervical or rectal infections in adults: 3 g oral amoxicillin, 3.5 g oral ampicillin, 4.8 million units IM aqueous procaine penicillin G or 250 mg IM ceftriaxone. Each (except for ceftriaxone) should be accompanied by 1 g oral probenecid. Follow with 100 mg doxycycline, twice daily for 7 days.

In adults allergic to penicillins, cephalosporins or probenecid: 100 mg, twice daily for 7 days.

In PPNG-endemic and -hyperendemic areas: 250 mg IM ceftriaxone plus 100 mg oral doxycycline twice daily for 7 days or 500 mg oral tetracycline 4 times a day for 7 days. If tetracyclines are contraindicated or not tolerated, follow the single-dose regimen with erythromycin.

Penicillinase-producing Neisseria gonorrhoeae - 2 g IM spectinomycin or 250 mg IM ceftriaxone. Follow with 100 mg doxycycline, twice daily for 7 days.

Disseminated gonococcal infections in patients allergic to penicillins or cephalosporins - 100 mg, twice daily for at least 7 days.

Lymphogranuloma venereum - Genital, inguinal or anorectal: 100 mg, twice daily for at least 2 weeks.

Nongonococcal urethritis - 100 mg, twice daily for 7 days.

Acute pelvic inflammatory disease – Ambulatory treatment: 250 mg single IM dose of ceftriaxone plus 100 mg oral doxycycline twice daily for 10 to 14 days. Other effective third generation cephalosporins may be substituted in the appropriate doses for ceftriaxone.

Inpatient treatment – 100 mg IV doxycycline twice daily, plus 2 g IV cefoxitin 4 times a day. Continue drugs IV for at least 4 days and at least 48 hours after patient improves. Then continue doxycycline 100 mg orally twice daily to complete 10 to 14 days of total therapy.

Sexually transmitted epididymo-orchitis - 3 g oral amoxicillin, 3.5 g oral ampicillin, 4.8 million units IM aqueous procaine penicillin G at 2 sites (each with 1 g oral probenecid), 2 g IM spectinomycin or 250 mg IM ceftriaxone followed by 100 mg doxycycline, twice daily for 10 days.

Urethral syndrome in women - 100 mg, twice daily for 7 days.

Rape victims – Prophylaxis: 100 mg, twice daily for 7 days.

	Product	Form	Packaging	C.I.*
Rx	**Doxycycline** (Various, eg, Geneva, Goldline, Lederle, Lemmon, Squibb-Mark, Warner-Chilcott, Zenith)	**Capsules:** 50 mg (as hyclate)	In 50s, 60s, 100s, 500s and UD 50s and 100s.	7+
Rx	**Doxychel Hyclate** (Rachelle)		In 50s and 500s.	6
Rx	**Vibramycin** (Pfizer)		(094). In 50s and UD 100s.	126
Rx	**Doxychel Hyclate** (Rachelle)	**Tablets:** 50 mg (as hyclate)	In 50s and 500s.	6
Rx	**Doxycycline** (Various, eg, Geneva, Goldline, Lederle, Lemmon, Squibb-Mark, Warner-Chilcott, Zenith)	**Capsules:** 100 mg (as hyclate)	In 10s, 11s, 14s, 20s, 40s, 50s, 100s, 200s, 500s and UD 100s.	5+
Rx	**Doxy Caps** (Edwards)		In 50s.	20
Rx	**Doxychel Hyclate** (Rachelle)		In 50s, 500s and UD 100s.	3
Rx	**Vibramycin** (Pfizer)		(095). In 50s, 500s and UD 100s.	113
Rx	**Monodox** (Oclassen)	**Capsules:** 100 mg (as monohydrate)	(Monodox 100 M 259). Yellow/brown. In 50s.	NA
Rx	**Doryx** (Parke-Davis)	**Capsules, coated pellets:** 100 mg (as hyclate)	(Doryx). Yellow and blue. In 50s.	74

* Cost Index based on cost per 50 mg.

[1] Morbidity and Mortality Weekly Report 1985 (Oct 18); 34 (Suppl 4S):75S-108S and 1987 (Sep 11); 36 (Suppl 5S):1S-18S.

(Continued on following page)

Complete prescribing information for these products begins on page 1811

DOXYCYCLINE (Cont.)

				C.I.*
Rx	**Doxycycline** (Various, eg, Geneva, Goldline, Lederle, Lemmon, Major, Purepac, Rugby, Squibb-Mark, Warner-Chilcott, Zenith)	**Tablets:** 100 mg (as hyclate)	In 20s, 28s, 30s, 32s, 50s, 200s, 500s and UD 100s.	5+
Rx	**Bio-Tab** (Inter. Ethical Labs.)		Film coated. In 50s, 100s and 500s.	NA
Rx	**Doxychel Hyclate** (Rachelle)		In 50s and 500s.	3
Rx	**Vibra-Tabs** (Pfizer)		(099). Film coated. In 50s, 500s and UD 100s.	113
Rx	**Vibramycin** (Pfizer)	**Powder for Oral Suspension:** 25 mg (as monohydrate) per 5 ml when reconstituted	Raspberry flavor. In 60 ml.	115
Rx	**Vibramycin** (Pfizer)	**Syrup:** 50 mg (as calcium) per 5 ml	Raspberry-apple flavor. In 30 and 473 ml.	115
Rx	**Doxycycline** (Various, eg, DuPont Crit Care, Elkins-Sinn, Loch, Lyphomed, Quad)	**Powder for Injection:** 100 mg (as hyclate)	In vials.	100+
Rx	**Doxy 100** (Lyphomed)		In vials.	840
Rx	**Doxychel Hyclate** (Rachelle)		In vials.	400
Rx	**Vibramycin IV** (Pfizer)		In vials.	1023
Rx	**Doxycycline** (Various, eg, DuPont Crit Care, Elkins-Sinn, Loch, Lyphomed)	**Powder for Injection:** 200 mg (as hyclate)	In vials.	150+
Rx	**Doxy 200** (Lyphomed)		In vials.	842
Rx	**Doxychel Hyclate** (Rachelle)		In vials.	375
Rx	**Vibramycin IV** (Roerig)		In vials.	1007

* Cost Index based on cost per 50 mg doxycycline or 300 mg methacycline.

Complete prescribing information for these products begins on page 1811

MINOCYCLINE

Administration and Dosage:

Oral:

Usual dosage – Adults: 200 mg initially, followed by 100 mg every 12 hours. If more frequent doses are preferred, give 100 or 200 mg initially; follow with 50 mg, 4 times/day.

Children (over 8 years of age): Initially, 4 mg/kg; follow with 2 mg/kg every 12 hours.

Syphilis – Administer usual dose over a period of 10 to 15 days. Close follow-up, including laboratory tests, is recommended.

Uncomplicated urethral, endocervical or rectal infections in adults caused by Chlamydia trachomatis or Ureaplasma urealyticum – 100 mg, 2 times/day for at least 7 days.

Uncomplicated gonococcal urethritis in men – 100 mg, 2 times/day for 5 days.

Gonorrhea patients sensitive to penicillin –200 mg initially, followed by 100 mg every 12 hours for a minimum of 4 days, with post-therapy cultures within 2 to 3 days.

Meningococcal carrier state –100 mg every 12 hours for 5 days.

Mycobacterium marinum infections – Although optimal doses are not established, 100 mg twice daily for 6 to 8 weeks has been successful in a limited number of cases.

Parenteral:

Adults – 200 mg followed by 100 mg every 12 hours; do not exceed 400 mg in 24 hours.

Children (over 8 years of age) – Usual pediatric dose is 4 mg/kg, followed by 2 mg/kg every 12 hours.

Preparation of solution: Initially dissolve the drug and then further dilute to 500 to 1000 ml with either Sodium Chloride Injection, Dextrose Injection, Dextrose and Sodium Chloride Injection, Ringer's Injection or Lactated Ringer's Injection, but not in other solutions containing calcium (a precipitate may form).

Storage: The prepared solution is stable at room temperature for 24 hours without significant loss of potency. Discard unused portions after that period. Administer the final dilution immediately.

				C.I.*
Rx	**Minocycline HCl** (Warner Chilcott)	**Capsules:** 50 mg	(WC 815). Olive/brown. In 100s.	NA
		100 mg	(WC 816). White/olive. In 50s.	NA
Rx	**Minocin** (Lederle)	**Capsules, pellet filled:** 50 mg (as HCl)	(Lederle M45 50 mg). Yellow and green. In 100s.	NA
		100 mg (as HCl)	(Lederle M46 100 mg). Green. In 50s.	NA
		Oral Suspension: 50 mg (as HCl) per 5 ml	5% alcohol. Custard flavor. In 60 ml.	184
Rx	**Minocin IV** (Lederle)	**Powder for Injection:** 100 mg	In vials.	1702

* Cost Index based on cost per 100 mg.

Complete prescribing information for these products begins on page 1811

OXYTETRACYCLINE

Administration and Dosage:

Oral: See Tetracycline HCl.

Parenteral:

Adults – The usual daily dose is 250 mg administered once every 24 hours or 300 mg given in divided doses at 8 to 12 hour intervals.

Children (over 8 years of age) – 15 to 25 mg/kg, up to a maximum of 250 mg per single daily injection. Dosage may be divided and given at 8 to 12 hour intervals.

	Product	Form	Packaging	**C.I.***
Rx	**Oxytetracycline HCl** (Various, eg, Balan, Bioline, Dixon-Shane, Geneva, Goldline, Major, Moore, Parmed, Rugby, Schein)	**Capsules:** 250 mg (as HCl)	In 100s and 1000s.	6+
Rx	**E.P. Mycin** (Edwards)		In 100s.	30
Rx	**Terramycin** (Pfizer)		(#Terramycin Pfizer 073). Yellow. In 100s and 500s.	100
Rx	**Uri-Tet** (American Urologicals)		In 100s.	51
Rx	**Terramycin IM** (Various, eg, Roerig, Texas Drug)	**Injection:** 50 mg per ml with 2% lidocaine	In 2 ml amps and 10 ml vials.	904
Rx	**Terramycin IM** (Roerig)	**Injection:** 125 mg per ml with 2% lidocaine	In 2 ml amps.	1294

* Cost Index based on cost per 500 mg oxytetracycline oral or IM.

Product identification code.

MACROLIDES

This macrolide discussion briefly summarizes the Actions of the group. Specific information for the individual agents follows.

Actions:

Pharmacology: Macrolide antibiotics, which include azithromycin, clarithromycin, erythromycin and troleandomycin, reversibly bind to the P site of the 50S ribosomal subunit of susceptible organisms and inhibit RNA-dependent protein synthesis by stimulating the dissociation of peptidyl t-RNA from ribosomes. They may be bacteriostatic or bactericidal, depending on such factors as drug concentration.

Rearrangement of erythromycin's 9-oxime derivative, followed by reduction and N-methylation, yields the ring-expanded derivative azithromycin, an azalide. Alkylation of the hydroxyl group at C-6 yields clarithromycin. The classical erythromycins A, B, C and D and oleandomycin are 14-membered macrolides; azithromycin is a 15-membered-ring macrolide.

Despite their differing structures, macrolides are characterized by similar antibacterial spectrum, mechanisms of action and resistance, but relatively different pharmacokinetics (see Pharmacokinetic table).

Macrolides are weak bases; their activity increases in alkaline pH. Macrolides enter pleural fluid, ascitic fluid, middle-ear exudates and sputum. When meninges are inflamed, macrolides may enter the CSF.

Erythromycin base, the active form, is marketed in acid-resistant enteric coated form to retard gastric inactivation. Converting the base to its acid-stable salt (stearate), ester (ethyl succinate and propionate) or salt of an ester (estolate) also improves oral bioavailability. For IV injection, a relatively water-soluble salt, lactobionate, is available.

Macrolides are used for respiratory, genital, GI tract and skin and soft tissue infections, especially when beta-lactam antibiotics or tetracyclines are contraindicated.

Microbiology:

Organisms Generally Susceptible to Macrolides In Vitro

	Organisms (✓ = generally susceptible)	Azithromycin	Clarithromycin	Erythromycin	Troleandomycin[1]
Gram-positive aerobes	*Staphylococcus aureus*	✓	✓	✓	
	Streptococcus pyogenes	✓	✓	✓	✓
	Streptococcus pneumoniae	✓	✓	✓	✓
	Streptococcus agalactiae	✓	✓	✓	
	Streptococcus sp	✓	✓		
	Streptococcus viridans	✓	✓	✓	
	Listeria monocytogenes		✓	✓	
	Corynebacterium diphtheriae			✓	
	Corynebacterium minutissimum			✓	
Gram-negative aerobes	*Hemophilus influenzae*	✓	✓	†	
	Hemophilus ducreyi	✓			
	Moraxella catarrhalis	✓	✓	✓	
	Bordetella pertussis	✓	✓	✓	
	Legionella pneumophila	✓	✓	✓	
	Campylobacter jejuni	✓	✓		
	Neisseria gonorrhoeae		✓	✓	
	Pasteurella multocida		✓		
Anaerobes	*Bacteroides bivius*	✓			
	Bacteroides melaninogenicus		✓		
	Clostridium perfringens	✓	✓		
	Propionibacterium acnes		✓		
	Peptococcus niger		✓		
	Peptostreptococcus sp	✓			
Other	*Borrelia burgdorferi*	✓			
	Chlamydia trachomatis	✓	✓	✓	
	Mycobacterium kansasii		✓		
	Mycoplasma pneumoniae	✓	✓	✓	
	Treponema pallidum	✓		✓	
	Ureaplasma urealyticum	✓		✓	
	Entamoeba histolytica			✓	

† Many strains resistant to erythromycin alone; may be susceptible to erythromycin plus a sulfonamide.

[1] Data is limited for troleandomycin.

(Continued on following page)

MACROLIDES (Cont.)

Actions (Cont.):

Microbiology (Cont.):

The in vitro spectrum of erythromycin covers primarily gram-positive microorganisms and gram-negative cocci.

Azithromycin is less active than erythromycin against most *Staphylococcus* and *Streptococcus* sp, but it is more potent against other organisms, including many gram-negative bacteria considered resistant to erythromycin. Azithromycin may expand the therapeutic range traditionally assigned to macrolides.

Clarithromycin exhibits the same spectrum of in vitro activity as erythromycin, but appears to have significantly increased potency against those organisms.

Troleandomycin, an acetylated ester of oleandomycin, is less active than erythromycin and offers no advantage. It can also cause hepatotoxicity.

Pharmacokinetics (refer to table): Azithromycin has an extended half-life and high tissue penetration. Without a loading dose, minimum plasma concentrations take 5 to 7 days to reach steady state. It is rapidly absorbed and widely distributed throughout the body. It is also rapidly distributed into tissues and reaches high concentrations within cells; therefore, significantly higher concentrations are achieved in tissues compared to plasma or serum. The prolonged half-life appears to be due to uptake and subsequent release of drug from tissues.

Clarithromycin is rapidly absorbed, reaching peak concentrations in serum 2 hours after dosing, regardless of dose size.

Various Pharmacokinetic Parameters of Macrolides								
Macrolide	Protein binding (%)	Metabolism	Elimination	Bioavailability (%)	Effect of food	Cmax (mcg/ml)	Tmax (hr)	Half-life (hr)
Azithromycin	50 (0.02 mg/L) 7 (1 mg/L)		4.5% excreted unchanged in urine; primarily excreted unchanged in bile	≈ 40	Food decreases absorption, Cmax and AUC by ≈ 50%; take on empty stomach	0.4	2-3	68[1]
Clarithromycin		Metabolized to active metabolite (14-OH clarithromycin)	Primarily renal; rate approximates normal GFR	≈ 50	Food delays onset of absorption and formation of metabolite; does not affect extent of bioavailability. Take without regard to meals	1-3	1.7	3-7
Erythromycin	70-74	Hepatic; demethylation	<5% (oral) and 12% to 15% (IV) excreted unchanged in urine; significant quantity excreted in bile		Base or stearate: Preferably take on an empty stomach. Estolate, ethylsuccinate, delayed release base: Take without regard to meals			1.4
Troleandomycin			20% excreted in urine; significant quantity excreted in bile		Take on an empty stomach	2	2	

Cmax = Maximum concentration; Tmax = Time to reach maximum concentration.

[1] Average terminal half-life.

CLARITHROMYCIN

Actions:

Clarithromycin was approved by the FDA in October 1991.

Pharmacology: Clarithromycin is a semi-synthetic macrolide antibiotic. It exerts its antibacterial action by binding to the 50S ribosomal subunit of susceptible organisms and inhibiting protein synthesis.

Pharmacokinetics: Clarithromycin is rapidly absorbed from the GI tract after oral administration. The absolute bioavailability of 250 mg tablets was approximately 50%. Food slightly delays both the onset of absorption and the formation of the antimicrobially active metabolite, 14-OH clarithromycin, but does not affect the extent of the bioavailability. Therefore, clarithromycin may be given without regard to meals.

In fasting healthy human subjects, peak serum concentrations were attained within 2 hours after oral dosing. Steady-state peak serum clarithromycin concentrations were attained in 2 to 3 days and were approximately 1 mcg/ml with a 250 mg dose every 12 hours and 2 to 3 mcg/ml with a 500 mg dose every 12 hours. The elimination half-life was about 3 to 4 hours with 250 mg every 12 hours but increased to 5 to 7 hours with 500 mg every 12 hours. With a 250 mg dose every 12 hours, the principal metabolite, 14-OH clarithromycin, attains a peak steady-state concentration of about 0.6 mcg/ml and has an elimination half-life of 5 to 6 hours. With a 500 mg dose every 12 hours, the peak steady-state concentrations of 14-OH clarithromycin are slightly higher (up to 1 mcg/ml), and its elimination half-life is about 7 hours. With either dose, the steady-state concentration of this metabolite is generally attained within 2 to 3 days.

After a 250 mg dose every 12 hours, approximately 20% of the dose is excreted in the urine as the unchanged parent drug. After a 500 mg dose every 12 hours, the urinary excretion of clarithromycin is somewhat greater, approximately 30%. The renal clearance of clarithromycin is, however, relatively independent of the dose size and approximates the normal glomerular filtration rate. The major metabolite found in urine is 14-OH clarithromycin which accounts for an additional 10% to 15% of the dose with either 250 or 500 mg every 12 hours.

The steady-state concentrations of clarithromycin in subjects with impaired hepatic function did not differ from those in healthy subjects; however, the 14-OH clarithromycin concentrations were lower in the hepatically impaired subjects. The decreased formation of 14-OH clarithromycin was at least partially offset by an increase in renal clearance of clarithromycin in subjects with impaired hepatic function when compared to healthy subjects. The pharmacokinetics of clarithromycin were also altered in subjects with impaired renal function. (See Warnings.)

Clarithromycin and the 14-OH clarithromycin metabolite distribute readily into body tissues and fluids. No data are available on CSF penetration. Because of high intracellular concentrations, tissue concentrations are higher than serum concentrations.

Microbiology: Clarithromycin is active in vitro against a variety of aerobic and anaerobic gram-positive and gram-negative organisms. Refer to the table in the Macrolide introduction.

Additionally, the 14-OH clarithromycin metabolite has clinically significant antimicrobial activity. Against *Hemophilus influenzae,* 14-OH clarithromycin is twice as active as the parent compound.

Beta-lactamase production should have no effect on clarithromycin activity.

Indications:

For the treatment of mild to moderate infections caused by susceptible strains of the designated microorganisms in the conditions listed below:

Upper respiratory tract infections – Pharyngitis/Tonsillitis due to *Streptococcus pyogenes*. Acute maxillary sinusitis due to *S pneumoniae.*

Lower respiratory tract infections – Acute bacterial exacerbation of chronic bronchitis due to *Hemophilus influenzae, Moraxella catarrhalis* or *S pneumoniae.* Pneumonia due to *Mycoplasma pneumoniae* or *S pneumoniae.*

Uncomplicated skin and skin structure infections due to *Staphylococcus aureus* or *S pyogenes.* Abscesses usually require surgical drainage.

Contraindications:

Hypersensitivity to clarithromycin, erythromycin, or any of the macrolide antibiotics.

(Continued on following page)

CLARITHROMYCIN (Cont.)

Warnings:

Pseudomembranous colitis has occurred with nearly all antibacterial agents, including macrolides, and may range in severity from mild to life-threatening. Therefore, it is important to consider this diagnosis in patients who present with diarrhea subsequent to the administration of antibacterial agents.

Treatment with antibacterial agents alters the normal flora of the colon and may permit overgrowth of clostridia. Studies indicate that a toxin produced by *Clostridium difficile* is a primary cause of "antibiotic-associated colitis."

After the diagnosis of pseudomembranous colitis has been established, initiate therapeutic measures. Mild cases of pseudomembranous colitis usually respond to discontinuation of the drug alone. In moderate to severe cases, give consideration to management with fluids and electrolytes, protein supplementation and treatment with an antibacterial drug effective against *C difficile*.

Hepatic/renal function impairment: Clarithromycin is principally excreted via the liver and kidney and may be administered without dosage adjustment to patients with hepatic impairment and normal renal function. However, in the presence of severe renal impairment with or without coexisting hepatic impairment, decreased dosage or prolonged dosing intervals may be appropriate.

Elderly: In a steady-state study in which healthy elderly subjects (ages 65 to 81 years old) were given 500 mg every 12 hours, the maximum concentrations of clarithromycin and 14-OH clarithromycin were increased. The AUC was also increased. These changes in pharmacokinetics parallel known age-related decreases in renal function. In clinical trials, elderly patients did not have an increased incidence of adverse events when compared to younger patients. Consider dosage adjustment in elderly patients with severe renal impairment.

Pregnancy: Category C. Clarithromycin has demonstrated adverse effects on pregnancy outcome or embryo-fetal development in monkeys, rats, mice and rabbits at doses that produced plasma levels 2 to 17 times the serum levels achieved in humans treated at the maximum recommended human doses. There are no adequate and well controlled studies in pregnant women. Clarithromycin should not be used in pregnant women except in clinical circumstances where no alternative therapy is appropriate. If pregnancy occurs while taking this drug, apprise the patient of the potential hazard to the fetus.

Lactation: Clarithromycin is excreted in the milk of lactating animals, and other drugs of this class are excreted in human breast milk. It is not known whether clarithromycin is excreted in human breast milk. Exercise caution when clarithromycin is administered to a nursing woman.

Children: Safety and efficacy in children < 12 years of age have not been established.

Drug Interactions:

Carbamazepine: Single-dose administration of clarithromycin resulted in increased concentrations of carbamazepine. Consider blood level monitoring of carbamazepine.

Theophylline: Concurrent use may be associated with an increase of serum theophylline concentrations. Consider monitoring serum theophylline concentrations in patients receiving high doses of theophylline or with baseline concentrations in the upper therapeutic range. In two studies, theophylline steady-state levels of C_{max}, C_{min} and the AUC increased about 20%.

Also consider all drug interactions listed with erythromycin (see individual monograph).

Drug/Food interaction: Food delays both the onset of clarithromycin absorption and the formation of 14-OH clarithromycin (the active metabolite) but does not affect the extent of bioavailability. Clarithromycin may be given without regard to meals.

Adverse Reactions:

The majority of side effects observed in clinical trials were of a mild and transient nature. Fewer than 3% of patients discontinued therapy because of drug-related side effects.

The most frequently reported adverse events were: Diarrhea, nausea, abnormal taste (3%); dyspepsia, abdominal pain/discomfort, headache (2%). Most of these events were described as mild or moderate in severity; only 1% were described as severe.

In studies of pneumonia comparing clarithromycin to erythromycin base or erythromycin stearate, there were fewer adverse events involving the digestive system in clarithromycin-treated patients (13%) compared to erythromycin-treated patients (13% vs 32%). Of erythromycin-treated patients, 20% discontinued therapy due to adverse events compared to 4% of clarithromycin-treated patients.

Patient Information:

Clarithromycin may be given without regard to meals.

(Continued on following page)

CLARITHROMYCIN (Cont.)

Administration and Dosage:

Clarithromycin may be given with or without meals.

Clarithromycin Dosage Guidelines		
Infection	Dosage (every 12 hr)	Normal duration (days)
Pharyngitis/Tonsillitis	250 mg	10
Acute maxillary sinusitis	500 mg	14
Lower respiratory tract	250-500 mg	7 to 14
Acute exacerbation of chronic bronchitis due to:		
S pneumoniae	250 mg	7 to 14
M catarrhalis	250 mg	7 to 14
H influenzae	500 mg	7 to 14
Pneumonia due to:		
S pneumoniae	250 mg	7 to 14
M pneumoniae	250 mg	7 to 14
Uncomplicated skin and skin structure	250 mg	7 to 14

Clarithromycin may be administered without dosage adjustment in the presence of hepatic impairment if there is normal renal function. However, in the presence of severe renal impairment with or without coexisting hepatic impairment, decreased doses or prolongation of dosing intervals may be appropriate.

Rx	**Biaxin Filmtabs** (Abbott)	**Tablets:** 250 mg clarithromycin	Yellow. Film coated. Oval. In 60s.
		500 mg clarithromycin	Yellow. Film coated. Oval. In 60s.

AZITHROMYCIN

Actions:

Azithromycin was approved by the FDA in November 1991.

Pharmacology: Azithromycin is an azalide antibiotic, a subclass of the macrolides. Azithromycin is derived from erythromycin; however, it differs chemically from erythromycin in that a methyl-substituted nitrogen atom is incorporated into the lactone ring. Azithromycin acts by binding to the 50S ribosomal subunit of susceptible organisms and thus interfering with microbial protein synthesis. Nucleic acid synthesis is not affected.

Pharmacokinetics: Following oral administration, azithromycin is rapidly absorbed and widely distributed throughout the body. Rapid distribution into tissues and high concentration within cells result in significantly higher azithromycin concentrations in tissues than in plasma or serum.

The pharmacokinetic parameters of azithromycin in plasma after a 500 mg loading dose on day 1 followed by 250 mg every day on days 2 through 5 in healthy young adults (ages 18 to 40 years old) are listed in the following table.

Azithromycin Pharmacokinetics (n = 12)		
Parameter (mean)	Day 1	Day 5
C_{max} (mcg/ml)	0.41	0.24
T_{max} (hr)	2.5	3.2
AUC 0-24 (mcg • hr/ml)	2.6	2.1
C_{min} (mcg/ml)	0.05	0.05
Urinary excretion (% dose)	4.5	6.5

Plasma azithromycin concentrations declined in a polyphasic pattern resulting in an average terminal half-life of 68 hours. On the recommended dosing regimen, C_{min} and C_{max} remained essentially unchanged from day 2 through day 5 of therapy. However, without a loading dose, C_{min} levels required 5 to 7 days to reach steady state.

The pharmacokinetic parameters of azithromycin in elderly men were similar to those in young adults; however, in elderly women, although higher peak concentrations (increased by 30% to 50%) were observed, no significant accumulation occurred.

The high values for apparent steady-state volume of distribution (31.1 L/kg) and plasma clearance (630 ml/min) suggest that the prolonged half-life is due to extensive uptake and subsequent release of drug from tissues. Selected tissue (or fluid) to plasma/serum concentration ratios are shown in the following table:

Azithromycin Concentrations Following Recommended Clinical Dosage Regimen				
Tissue or fluid	Time after dose (hr)	Tissue or fluid concentration (mcg/g or mcg/ml)[1]	Plasma or serum level (mcg/ml)	Tissue (fluid): Plasma (serum) ratio[1]
Skin	72-96	0.4	0.012	35
Lung	72-96	4	0.012	> 100
Sputum	2-4	1	0.64	2
Sputum	10-12	2.9	0.1	30
Tonsil	9-16	4.5	0.03	> 100
Tonsil	180	0.9	0.006	> 100
Cervix	19	2.8	0.04	70

[1] High tissue concentrations should not be interpreted to be quantitatively related to clinical efficacy. The antimicrobial activity of azithromycin is pH related. Azithromycin is concentrated in cell lysosomes which have a low intraorganelle pH, at which the drug's activity is reduced. However, the extensive distribution of drug to tissues may be relevant to clinical activity.

Only very low concentrations were noted in CSF (< 0.01 mcg/ml) in the presence of non-inflamed meninges.

The serum protein binding of azithromycin is variable, decreasing from 51% at 0.02 mcg/ml to 7% at 2 mcg/ml.

Biliary excretion of azithromycin, predominantly as unchanged drug, is a major route of elimination. Over the course of a week, approximately 6% of the administered dose appears as unchanged drug in urine. Food decreases the absorption of azithromycin, reducing the C_{max} by 52% and the AUC by 43%. Azithromycin concentrates in phagocytes and fibroblasts; concentration in phagocytes may contribute to drug distribution to inflamed tissues.

Microbiology: Azithromycin is active against a variety of organisms. Refer to the table in the Macrolides introduction.

(Continued on following page)

AZITHROMYCIN (Cont.)

Indications:

For the treatment of individuals ≥ 16 years of age with mild to moderate infections caused by susceptible strains of the designated microorganisms in the specific conditions listed below:

Lower respiratory tract: Acute bacterial exacerbations of chronic obstructive pulmonary disease due to *Hemophilus influenzae, Moraxella catarrhalis* or *Streptococcus pneumoniae.* Community-acquired pneumonia of mild severity due to *S pneumoniae* or *H influenzae* in patients appropriate for outpatient oral therapy (see Warnings).

Upper respiratory tract: Streptococcal pharyngitis/tonsillitis – As an alternative to first-line therapy of acute pharyngitis/tonsillitis due to *S pyogenes* in individuals who cannot use first-line therapy.

Note: Penicillin is the usual drug of choice in the treatment of *S pyogenes* infections and the prophylaxis of rheumatic fever. Azithromycin is often effective in the eradication of susceptible strains of *S pyogenes* from the nasopharynx. Because some strains are resistant to azithromycin, perform susceptibility tests when patients are treated with azithromycin.

Skin/Skin structure: Uncomplicated skin and skin structure infections due to *Staphylococcus aureus, S pyogenes* or *S agalactiae*. Abscesses usually require surgical drainage.

Sexually transmitted diseases: Non-gonococcal urethritis and cervicitis due to *Chlamydia trachomatis*.

Contraindications:

Hypersensitivity to azithromycin, erythromycin or any macrolide antibiotic.

Warnings:

Pneumonia: Azithromycin is only safe and effective in the treatment of community-acquired pneumonia of mild severity due to *S pneumoniae* and *H influenzae* in patients appropriate for outpatient oral therapy. Do not use in patients with pneumonia who are judged to be inappropriate for outpatient oral therapy because of moderate to severe illness or risk factors such as any of the following: Nosocomially acquired infections; known or suspected bacteremia; conditions requiring hospitalization; significant underlying health problems that may compromise the patients' ability to respond to their illness (including immunodeficiency or functional asplenia); elderly or debilitated patients.

Gonorrhea or syphilis: Azithromycin at the recommended dose should not be relied upon to treat gonorrhea or syphilis. Antimicrobial agents used in high doses for short periods of time to treat non-gonococcal urethritis may mask or delay the symptoms of incubating gonorrhea or syphilis. All patients with sexually transmitted urethritis or cervicitis should have a serologic test for syphilis and appropriate cultures for gonorrhea performed at the time of diagnosis. Initiate appropriate antimicrobial therapy and follow-up tests for these diseases if infection is confirmed.

Pseudomembranous colitis has been reported with nearly all antibacterial agents and may range in severity from mild to life-threatening. Therefore, it is important to consider this diagnosis in patients who present with diarrhea subsequent to the administration of antibacterial agents.

Treatment with antibacterial agents alters the normal flora of the colon and may permit overgrowth of clostridia. Studies indicate that a toxin produced by *Clostridium difficile* is a primary cause of "antibiotic-associated colitis."

After the diagnosis of pseudomembranous colitis has been established, initiate therapeutic measures. Mild cases of pseudomembranous colitis usually respond to discontinuation of the drug alone. In moderate to severe cases, give consideration to management with fluids and electrolytes, protein supplementation and treatment with an antibacterial drug effective against *C difficile* colitis.

Hepatic/Renal function impairment: Because azithromycin is principally eliminated via the liver, exercise caution when azithromycin is administered to patients with impaired hepatic function. There are no data regarding azithromycin usage in patients with renal impairment; thus, exercise caution when prescribing azithromycin in these patients.

Cardiac effects: Ventricular arrhythmias, including ventricular tachycardia and torsade de pointes, in individuals with prolonged QT intervals have not been reported in clinical trials with azithromycin; however, it has occurred with macrolide products.

Elderly: Pharmacokinetic parameters in older volunteers (65 to 85 years old) were similar to those in younger volunteers (18 to 40 years old) for the 5 day therapeutic regimen. Dosage adjustment does not appear to be necessary for older patients with normal renal and hepatic function receiving treatment with this dosage regimen.

Pregnancy: Category B. There are no adequate and well controlled studies in pregnant women. Use during pregnancy only if clearly needed.

(Warnings continued on following page)

AZITHROMYCIN (Cont.)

Warnings (Cont.):

Lactation: It is not known whether azithromycin is excreted in breast milk. Exercise caution when administering to a nursing woman.

Children: Safety and efficacy in children < 16 years old have not been established.

Drug Interactions:

Aluminum- and magnesium-containing antacids reduce the peak serum levels but not the extent of azithromycin absorption.

Theophylline: Azithromycin did not affect the plasma levels or pharmacokinetics of theophylline administered as a single IV dose. The effect of azithromycin on the plasma levels or pharmacokinetics of theophylline administered in multiple doses resulting in therapeutic steady-state levels of theophylline is not known. However, concurrent use of macrolides and theophylline has been associated with increases in serum concentrations of theophylline. Therefore, until further data are available, carefully monitor plasma theophylline levels in patients receiving azithromycin and theophylline concomitantly.

Warfarin: Azithromycin did not affect the prothrombin time response to a single dose of warfarin. However, concurrent use of macrolides and warfarin has been associated with increased anticoagulant effects. Carefully monitor prothrombin time in all patients treated with azithromycin and warfarin concomitantly.

Also consider all drug interactions listed with erythromycin (see individual monograph).

Drug/Food interaction: Food decreases the absorption of azithromycin, reducing the maximum concentration by 52% and bioavailability by 43%. Take 1 hour before or 2 hours after a meal.

Adverse Reactions:

Most side effects are mild to moderate in severity and are reversible upon discontinuation of the drug. Approximately 0.7% of the patients from the multiple-dose clinical trials discontinued therapy because of treatment-related side effects. Most of the side effects leading to discontinuation were related to the GI tract (eg, nausea, vomiting, diarrhea, abdominal pain). Rare, but potentially serious side effects, were angioedema (1 case) and cholestatic jaundice (1 case).

Multiple-dose regimen: Overall, the most common side effects in patients receiving the multiple-dose regimen were related to the GI system with diarrhea/loose stools (5%), nausea and abdominal pain (3%) being the most frequently reported. The following adverse reactions occurred in ≤ 1% of patients:

Cardiovascular – Palpitations; chest pain.
GI – Dyspepsia; flatulence; vomiting; melena; cholestatic jaundice.
GU – Monilia; vaginitis; nephritis.
CNS – Dizziness; headache; vertigo; somnolence; fatigue.
Allergic – Rash; photosensitivity; angioedema.

Single 1 g dose regimen: The most common side effects in patients receiving a 1 g single dose were related to the GI system and were more frequently reported than in patients receiving the multiple-dose regimen. Side effects that occurred with a frequency of ≥ 1% included: Diarrhea/loose stools (7%); nausea (5%); vomiting, vaginitis (2%).

Lab test abnormalities: Elevated serum creatine phosphokinase, potassium, ALT, GGT and AST (1% to 2%); leukopenia, neutropenia, decreased platelet count and elevated serum alkaline phosphatase, bilirubin, BUN, creatinine, blood glucose, LDH and phosphate (≤ 1%). When follow-up was provided, changes in laboratory tests appeared to be reversible. In multiple-dose clinical trials involving > 3000 patients, three patients discontinued therapy because of treatment-related liver enzyme abnormalities and one because of a renal function abnormality.

Patient Information:

Caution patients to take this medication at least 1 hour prior to a meal or at least 2 hours after a meal. This medication should not be taken with food.

Caution patients not to take aluminum- and magnesium-containing antacids and azithromycin simultaneously.

Administration and Dosage:

Approved by the FDA in November 1991.

Administer at least 1 hour before or 2 hours after a meal.

Mild to moderate acute bacterial exacerbations of chronic obstructive pulmonary disease, pneumonia, pharyngitis/tonsillitis (as second-line therapy), and uncomplicated skin and skin structure infections (≥ 16 years of age): 500 mg as a single dose on the first day followed by 250 mg once daily on days 2 through 5 for a total dose of 1.5 g.

Non-gonococcal urethritis and cervicitis due to C trachomatis: Give a single 1 g dose.

Rx	**Zithromax** (Pfizer)	**Capsules:** 250 mg azithromycin (as dihydrate)	Lactose. (Pfizer 305). Red. In 50s and UD 100s.

ERYTHROMYCIN

Actions:

Pharmacology: Erythromycin is a macrolide antibiotic which may be bactericidal or bacteriostatic. Erythromycin binds to the 50 S ribosomal subunits of susceptible bacteria and suppresses protein synthesis without affecting nucleic acid synthesis.

The strength of erythromycin products is expressed as erythromycin base equivalents. Because of differences in absorption and biotransformation, varying quantities of each erythromycin salt form are required to produce the same free erythromycin serum levels. For example, expressed in base equivalents, 400 mg erythromycin ethylsuccinate produces the same free erythromycin serum levels as 250 mg of erythromycin base, stearate or estolate.

Microbiology: Erythromycin is usually active against the following organisms in vitro: *Gram positive – Staphylococcus aureus* (resistant organisms may emerge during treatment); *Streptococcus pyogenes* (group A beta-hemolytic streptococci); alpha-hemolytic streptococci (viridans group); *S pneumonia; Corynebacterium diphtheriae; C minutissimum.*

Gram-negative – Moraxella catarrhalis; Neisseria gonorrhoeae; Legionella pneumophila; Bordetella pertussis.

Mycoplasma – Mycoplasma pneumoniae; Ureaplasma urealyticum.

Other – Chlamydia trachomatis; Entamoeba histolytica; Treponema pallidum; Listeria monocytogenes.

Hemophilus influenzae: Many strains are resistant to erythromycin alone but are susceptible to erythromycin and sulfonamides together.

Pharmacokinetics: Absorption – Erythromycin base is acid labile and is usually formulated in enteric coated or film coated forms for oral administration. Acid stable salts and esters (estolate, ethylsuccinate, stearate) are well absorbed. Generally, administer the base and stearate preparations in the fasting state or immediately before meals. Absorption of the estolate and ethylsuccinate preparations and the base in a delayed release dosage form is unaffected or enhanced by food.

Distribution – Erythromycin is approximately 70% bound to plasma proteins. It diffuses into most body fluids, including prostatic fluid, where it reaches concentrations approximately 40% of those in plasma. Low concentrations are normally achieved in the spinal fluid, but passage of the drug across the blood-brain barrier increases in meningitis. Erythromycin crosses the placental barrier and is excreted in breast milk.

Metabolism/Elimination – In normal hepatic function, the drug is concentrated in the liver and excreted via the bile. Erythromycin's plasma half-life is approximately 1.4 hours in patients with normal renal function; it is prolonged to 4.8 to 5.8 hours in anuria. From 12% to 15% of IV erythromycin is excreted in active form in the urine. After oral administration, < 5% is recovered in the urine. Erythromycin is not dialyzable.

Alkalinization of the urine (pH 8.5) increases the gram-negative antibacterial activity of erythromycin; several investigators have suggested coadministration of urinary alkalinizing agents (eg, sodium bicarbonate) and erythromycin for urinary tract infections.

Indications:

Indicated for treatment of infections caused by susceptible strains of the designated microorganisms in the diseases listed below:

Upper respiratory tract infections of mild to moderate severity caused by: *Streptococcus pyogenes* (group A beta-hemolytic streptococci); *S pneumoniae; H influenzae* (with concomitant sulfonamides).

Lower respiratory tract infections of mild to moderate severity caused by: *S pyogenes* (group A beta-hemolytic streptococci); *S pneumoniae.*

Respiratory tract infections due to *Mycoplasma pneumoniae*

Skin and skin structure infections of mild to moderate severity caused by: *S pyogenes; Staphylococcus aureus* (resistant staphylococci may emerge during treatment).

Pertussis (whooping cough) caused by *Bordetella pertussis.* Effective in eliminating the organism from the nasopharynx of infected patients. May be helpful in the prophylaxis of pertussis in exposed susceptible individuals.

Diphtheria – As an adjunct to antitoxin in infections due to *Corynebacterium diphtheriae,* to prevent establishment of carriers and to eradicate the organism in carriers.

Erythrasma – Treatment of infections due to *C minutissimum.*

Intestinal amebiasis caused by *Entamoeba histolytica* (oral erythromycin only). Extraenteric amebiasis requires treatment with other agents.

Pelvic inflammatory disease (PID), acute caused by *Neisseria gonorrhoeae*: Erythromycin lactobionate IV followed by oral erythromycin as an alternative to penicillin in patients with a history of penicillin sensitivity.

Conjunctivitis of the newborn, pneumonia of infancy, urogenital infections during pregnancy caused by *Chlamydia trachomatis.*

(Indications continued on following page)

ERYTHROMYCIN (Cont.)

Indications (Cont.):

Uncomplicated urethral, endocervical or rectal infections in adults due to *C trachomatis* when tetracyclines are contraindicated or not tolerated.

Nongonococcal urethritis caused by *Ureaplasma urealyticum* when tetracyclines are contraindicated or not tolerated.

Primary syphilis caused by *Treponema pallidum*: Erythromycin (oral only) as an alternative to penicillin in penicillin-allergic patients.

Legionnaire's disease caused by *Legionella pneumophila*. Although no controlled clinical efficacy studies have been conducted, in vitro and limited preliminary clinical data suggest effectiveness.

Rheumatic fever: Prevention of initial or recurrent attacks as an alternative in patients who are allergic to penicillins or sulfonamides

Bacterial endocarditis (due to alpha-hemolytic streptococci, Viridans group): Prevention as an alternative in patients allergic to penicillins.

Listeria monocytogenes infections.

Unlabeled uses:

Neisseria gonorrhoeae – Uncomplicated urethral, endocervical or rectal infection and in penicillinase-producing *N gonorrhoeae* (PPNG); in pregnancy.

Treponema pallidum – Early syphilis (primary, secondary or early latent syphilis of < 1 year duration).

Campylobacter jejuni – Erythromycin has been used successfully in prolonged diarrhea associated with campylobacter enteritis.

Lymphogranuloma venereum – Genital, inguinal or anorectal.

Hemophilus ducreyi (chancroid) – Treat until ulcers or lymph nodes are healed.

Prior to elective colorectal surgery, to reduce wound complications, the combination of erythromycin base and oral neomycin is a popular preoperative combination.

Other unlabeled uses, as an alternative to penicillins, include: Anthrax; Vincent's gingivitis; erysipeloid; tetanus; actinomycosis; *Nocardia* infections (with a sulfonamide); *Eikenella corrodens* infections; *Borrelia* infections (including early Lyme disease).

Contraindications:

Hypersensitivity to erythromycin.

Erythromycin estolate: Preexisting liver disease.

Warnings:

Hepatic function impairment: Erythromycin is principally excreted by the liver. Exercise caution in administering to patients with impaired hepatic function. There have been reports of hepatic dysfunction with or without jaundice.

Hepatotoxicity: Erythromycin administration has been associated with the infrequent occurrence of cholestatic hepatitis. This effect is most common with erythromycin estolate; however, it has also occurred with other erythromycin salts. Laboratory findings include abnormal hepatic function, peripheral eosinophilia and leukocytosis. Symptoms may include malaise, nausea, vomiting, abdominal cramps and fever. Jaundice may or may not be present. In some instances, severe abdominal pain may simulate the pain of biliary colic, pancreatitis, perforated ulcer or an acute abdominal surgical problem. In other instances, clinical symptoms and results of liver function tests have resembled findings in extrahepatic obstructive jaundice. Although initial symptoms have developed after a few days of treatment, they generally have followed 1 or 2 weeks of continuous therapy. Symptoms reappear promptly, usually within 48 hours after the drug is readministered to sensitive patients. The syndrome seems to result from a form of sensitization, occurs chiefly in adults, and is reversible when medication is discontinued.

Pseudomembranous colitis has occurred with virtually all broad-spectrum antibiotics (including macrolides, semi-synthetic penicillins and cephalosporins). Therefore, consider its diagnosis in patients who develop diarrhea in association with antibiotic use. Broad-spectrum antibiotics alter the normal flora of the colon; this may permit overgrowth of *Clostridia.* A toxin produced by *Clostridium difficile* is a primary cause of antibiotic-associated colitis. Such colitis may range in severity from mild to life-threatening.

Mild cases usually respond to discontinuation. Management of moderate to severe cases should include sigmoidoscopy, bacteriologic studies and fluid, electrolyte and protein supplementation. When colitis does not improve after discontinuation, or when it is severe, oral vancomycin or metronidazole is the drug of choice; rule out other causes.

Hypersensitivity reactions: Serious allergic reactions, including anaphylaxis, have occurred. Refer to Management of Acute Hypersensitivity Reactions.

(Warnings continued on following page)

ERYTHROMYCIN (Cont.)

Warnings (Cont.):

Pregnancy: Category B. Safety for use during pregnancy has not been established. Erythromycin crosses the placental barrier but fetal levels are low (5% to 20% of maternal concentrations). There are no adequate and well controlled studies in pregnant women. Use only when clearly needed. **Erythromycin estolate** abnormally elevated liver function tests in 10% of pregnant patients.

Lactation: Erythromycin is excreted in breast milk, and may concentrate (observed milk:plasma ratio of 0.5 to 3). Although no infant adverse effects are reported, potential problems for the nursing infant include modification of bowel flora, pharmacological effects and interference with fever work-ups. Erythromycin is considered compatible with breastfeeding by the American Academy of Pediatrics.

Precautions:

Superinfection: Use of antibiotics (especially prolonged or repeated therapy) may result in bacterial or fungal overgrowth of nonsusceptible organisms. Take appropriate measures if superinfection occurs.

Drug Interactions:

Erythromycin Drug Interactions			
Precipitant drug	Object drug*		Description
Erythromycin	Alfentanil	↑	The alfentanil clearance may be decreased and its elimination half-life increased.
Erythromycin	Anticoagulants	↑	The anticoagulant effect is increased; hemorrhage has occurred.
Erythromycin	Bromocriptine	↑	Serum bromocriptine levels may be increased, resulting in an increase in pharmacologic and toxic effects.
Erythromycin	Carbamazepine	↑	Carbamazepine toxicity sufficient to require hospitalization or resuscitative measures may result.
Erythromycin	Cyclosporine	↑	Increased cyclosporine concentrations with renal toxicity may occur.
Erythromycin	Digoxin	↑	Increased serum digoxin levels may occur in a small population of patients (≈ 10%); toxic effects may occur.
Erythromycin	Disopyramide	↑	Increased disopyramide plasma levels may occur. Arrhythmias and increased QTc intervals have occurred.
Erythromycin	Ergot alkaloids	↑	Acute ergotism manifested as peripheral ischemia has occurred.
Erythromycin	Lincosamides	↓	Under some conditions, coadministration may be antagonistic.
Erythromycin	Methylprednisolone	↑	Methylprednisolone clearance may be decreased.
Erythromycin	Penicillins	↔	Both antagonism and synergism have occurred with coadministration.
Erythromycin	Theophyllines	↔	Increased theophylline serum levels with toxicity are possible. Decreased erythromycin levels may also occur.
Erythromycin	Triazolam	↑	Triazolam bioavailability may be increased, resulting in increased CNS depression.

* ↑ = Object drug increased ↓ = Object drug decreased ↔ = Undetermined effect

Drug/Food interaction: Antimicrobial effectiveness of erythromycin stearate and certain formulations of erythromycin base may be reduced. Take at least 2 hours before or after a meal. Erythromycin estolate and ethylsuccinate and the base in a delayed release form may be administered without regard to meals.

(Continued on following page)

ERYTHROMYCIN (Cont.)

Adverse Reactions:

Allergic reactions: Serious allergic reactions, including anaphylaxis, have occurred. Mild allergic reactions include rashes with or without pruritus, urticaria, bullous fixed eruptions and eczema. See Warnings.

Parenteral administration: Venous irritation and phlebitis have occurred, but the risk of such reactions may be reduced if the infusion is given slowly, in dilute solution, by continuous IV infusion or intermittent infusion over 20 to 60 minutes.

GI: The most frequent dose-related side effects following oral use include abdominal cramping and discomfort, anorexia, nausea, vomiting and diarrhea. Pseudomembranous colitis associated with erythromycin therapy has occurred (see Warnings). Several cases of nausea and vomiting following IV erythromycin lactobionate have occurred.

Ototoxicity: There have been isolated reports of reversible hearing loss occurring chiefly in patients with renal or hepatic insufficiency, in the elderly ($>$ 50 years old) and in those receiving high doses ($>$ 4 g/day). In rare instances involving IV use, the ototoxic effect has been irreversible.

Hepatotoxicity: Hepatotoxicity is most commonly associated with **erythromycin estolate** (see Warnings).

Cardiovascular: Rarely, production of ventricular arrhythmias, including ventricular tachycardia and torsade de pointes in individuals with prolonged QT intervals.

Overdosage:

Symptoms may include nausea, vomiting, epigastric distress and diarrhea. The severity of the epigastric distress and diarrhea are dose-related. Reversible mild acute pancreatitis has occurred. Hearing loss, with or without tinnitus and vertigo, may occur, especially in patients with renal or hepatic insufficiency.

Treatment includes usual supportive measures. Refer to General Management of Acute Overdosage. Induce prompt elimination of unabsorbed drug. However, unless 5 times the normal single dose has been ingested, GI decontamination should not be necessary. An accidental ingestion of erythromycin should not be predicted to have minimal toxicity unless there is a good approximation of how much was ingested and unless only a single medication was involved. Control allergic reactions with conventional therapy as indicated. Hemodialysis and peritoneal dialysis are not particularly effective.

Patient Information:

Preferably taken on an empty stomach (at least 1 hour before or 2 hours after meals); if GI upset occurs, may be taken with food. Erythromycin estolate, ethylsuccinate and certain brands of erythromycin base enteric coated tablets may be taken without regard to meals; consult the current package literature.

Complete full course of therapy; take until finished.

Take each dose with an adequate amount of water (180 to 240 ml).

Take at evenly spaced intervals during the day, preferably around the clock.

Notify physician if nausea, vomiting, diarrhea or stomach cramps, severe abdominal pain, yellow discoloration of the skin or eyes, darkened urine, pale stools or unusual tiredness occurs.

(Products listed on following pages)

Complete prescribing information for these products begins on page 1831

ERYTHROMYCIN, IV

Administration and Dosage:

Erythromycin IV is indicated when oral use is impossible, or when severity of the infection requires immediate high serum levels. Replace IV therapy with oral as soon as possible.

Continuous infusion is preferable, but intermittent infusion in 20 to 60 minute periods at intervals of ≤ 6 hours is also effective. Due to irritative properties of erythromycin, IV push is unacceptable.

Severe infections: 15 to 20 mg/kg/day. Up to 4 g/day in very severe infections.

Preparation of solution: Vials – Prepare the initial solution by adding 10 ml Sterile Water for Injection, USP to the 500 mg vial or 20 ml Sterile Water for Injection, USP to the 1 g vial. Use only Sterile Water for Injection, USP as other diluents may cause precipitation during reconstitution. Do not use diluents containing preservatives or inorganic salts. Note: When the product is reconstituted as directed above, the resulting solution contains an effective microbial preservative. After reconstitution, each ml contains 50 mg erythromycin activity.

Add the initial dilution to one of the following diluents before administration to give a concentration of 1 g/L (1 mg/ml) erythromycin activity for continuous infusion or 1 to 5 mg/ml for intermittent infusion: 0.9% Sodium Chloride Injection, USP; Lactated Ringer's Injection, USP; *Normosol-R*.

The following solutions may also be used providing they are first buffered with 4% sodium bicarbonate or *Neut* by adding 1 ml of the 4% Sodium Bicarbonate Injection or *Neut* per 100 ml of solution: 5% Dextrose Injection, USP; 5% Dextrose and Lactated Ringer's Injection; 5% Dextrose and 0.9% Sodium Chloride Injection.

Piggyback vial – Add 100 ml 0.9% Sodium Chloride Injection, USP or Lactated Ringer's Injection, USP or *Normosol-R* to the dispensing vial. Immediately after adding diluent, shake the product to aid dissolution. Lack of immediate agitation will greatly increase time required for complete dissolution. May also be reconstituted using 100 ml of the following solutions to which 1 ml of 4% Sodium Bicarbonate Injection or *Neut* has first been added: 5% Dextrose Injection, USP; 5% Dextrose and Lactated Ringer's Injection; 5% Dextrose and 0.9% Sodium Chloride Injection, USP; *Normosol-M* and 5% Dextrose Injection; *Normosol-R* and 5% Dextrose Injection.

The 4% sodium bicarbonate injection or *Neut* must be added to these solutions so that their pH is in the optimum range for erythromycin lactobionate stability. Acidic solutions of erythromycin lactobionate are unstable and lose their potency rapidly. A pH of at least 5.5 is desirable for the final diluted solution of erythromycin lactobionate.

Storage/Stability: The *initial* solution is stable for 2 weeks if refrigerated or for 24 hours at room temperature. Completely administer the final diluted solution within 8 hours in order to assure proper potency since it is not suitable for storage.

Use the solution in the piggyback vial within 8 hours if stored at room temperature and 24 hours if stored in the refrigerator. If the solution is to be frozen, freeze at –10° to –20° C (14° to –4°F) within 4 hours of preparation. Frozen solution may be stored for 30 days. Thaw the frozen solution in the refrigerator and use within 8 hours after thawing is completed. Thawed solution must not be refrozen.

			C.I.*
Rx	**Erythromycin Lactobionate** (Various, eg, Abbott, Elkins-Sinn, Lederle, Lyphomed)	**Powder for Injection:** 500 mg (as lactobionate) per vial or piggyback vial.	27+
		1 g (as lactobionate) per vial.	25+

* Cost Index based on cost per 500 mg.

Complete prescribing information for these products begins on page 1831

ERYTHROMYCIN, ORAL

Administration and Dosage:

Dosages and product strengths are expressed as erythromycin base equivalents. Because of differences in absorption and biotransformation, varying quantities of each salt form are required to produce the same free erythromycin serum levels. For example, expressed in base equivalents, 400 mg erythromycin ethylsuccinate produces the same free erythromycin serum levels as 250 mg of erythromycin base, stearate or estolate.

Optimal serum levels of erythromycin are reached when erythromycin base or stearate is taken in the fasting state or immediately before meals. Erythromycin ethylsuccinate, estolate and enteric coated erythromycin may be administered without regard to meals.

Usual dosage:

Adults – 250 mg (or 400 mg ethylsuccinate) every 6 hours, or 500 mg every 12 hours, or 333 mg every 8 hours. May increase up to $\geq$ 4 g/day, according to severity of infection. If twice-a-day dosage is desired, the recommended dose is 500 mg every 12 hours. Twice-a-day dosing is not recommended when doses $>$ 1 g daily are administered.

Children – 30 to 50 mg/kg/day (15 to 25 mg/lb/day) in divided doses. Proper dosage is determined by age, weight and severity of infection. For more severe infections, dosage may be doubled.

Erythromycin Uses and Dosages

Indication (Organism)	Dosage (Stated as erythromycin base)
Labeled uses:	
Upper respiratory tract infections of mild to moderate severity	
Streptococcus pyogenes (group A beta-hemolytic streptococcus)	250 to 500 mg 4 times a day or 20 to 50 mg/kg/day in divided doses for 10 days.
S pneumoniae	250 to 500 mg every 6 hours.
Hemophilus influenzae (used concomitantly with a sulfonamide)	Erythromycin ethylsuccinate: 50 mg/kg/day. Sulfisoxazole: 150 mg/kg/day. Combination given for 10 days.
Lower respiratory tract infections of mild to moderate severity	
S pyogenes	250 to 500 mg 4 times a day or 20 to 50 mg/kg/day in divided doses for 10 days.
S pneumoniae	250 to 500 mg every 6 hours.
Respiratory tract infections	
Mycoplasma pneumoniae (Eaton agent, PPLO)	500 mg every 6 hours for 5 to 10 days. Treat severe infections for up to 3 weeks.
Skin and skin structure infections of mild to moderate severity	
S pyogenes	250 to 500 mg 4 times a day or 20 to 50 mg/kg/day in divided doses for 10 days.
Staphylococcus aureus (resistant organisms may emerge)	250 mg every 6 hours or 500 mg every 12 hours, maximum 4 g/day.
Pertussis (whooping cough) *Bordetella pertussis:* Effective in eliminating the organism from the nasopharynx of infected patients. May be helpful in prophylaxis of pertussis in exposed individuals.	40 to 50 mg/kg/day in divided doses for 5 to 14 days, or 500 mg 4 times a day for 10 days.
Diphtheria *Corynebacterium diphtheriae:* Adjunct to antitoxin to prevent establishment of carriers and to eradicate the organism in carriers.	500 mg every 6 hours for 10 days.
Erythrasma *C minutissimum*	250 mg 3 times daily for 21 days
Intestinal amebiasis *Entamoeba histolytica:* Oral erythromycin only.	*Adults:* 250 mg 4 times daily for 10 to 14 days. *Children:* 30 to 50 mg/kg/day in divided doses for 10 to 14 days.

(Administration and Dosage continued on following page)

ERYTHROMYCIN, ORAL (Cont.)

Administration and Dosage (Cont.):

Indication (Organism)	Dosage (Stated as erythromycin base)
Pelvic inflammatory disease (PID), acute *Neisseria gonorrhoeae:* Erythromycin lactobionate IV followed by oral erythromycin.[1]	500 mg IV every 6 hours for 3 days, then 250 mg orally every 6 hours for 7 days. An alternative regimen for ambulatory management of PID is 500 mg orally 4 times a day for 10 to 14 days.[2]
Conjunctivitis of the newborn, pneumonia of infancy, urogenital infections during pregnancy *Chlamydia trachomatis*	50 mg/kg/day in 4 divided doses for 14 days (conjunctivitis) or 21 days (pneumonia); 500 mg 4 times daily for 7 days or 250 mg 4 times daily for 14 days (urogenital infections).
Urethral, endocervical or rectal infections, uncomplicated *C trachomatis*[1]	500 mg 4 times daily for 7 days or 250 mg 4 times daily for 14 days.[2]
Nongonococcal urethritis *Ureaplasma urealyticum*[1]	500 mg 4 times daily for at least 7 days.
Primary syphilis *Treponema pallidum:* (Oral only)[1]	20 g in divided doses over a period of 10 days.
Legionnaire's disease *Legionella pneumophila:* No controlled clinical efficacy studies have been conducted, but data suggest effectiveness	1 to 4 g daily in divided doses or 500 mg to 1 g 4 times daily for 21 days.
Rheumatic fever *S pyogenes* (group A beta-hemolytic streptococci): Prevention of initial or recurrent attacks.[1]	250 mg 2 times daily.
Bacterial endocarditis *Alpha-hemolytic streptococcus* (viridans)[1]	*Adults:* 1 g 2 hours prior to procedure, then 500 mg 6 hours after initial dose.[3] *Children:* 20 mg/kg 2 hours prior to procedure, then 10 mg/kg 6 hours after initial dose.[3]
Listeria monocytogenes	*Adults:* 250 mg every 6 hours or 500 mg every 12 hours, maximum 4 g/day.
Unlabeled uses: *Campylobacter jejuni*: Has been successful in severe or prolonged diarrhea associated with *Campylobacter enteritis* or enterocolitis.[2]	500 mg 4 times a day for 7 days.
Lymphogranuloma venereum: Genital, inguinal or anorectal.[2]	500 mg 4 times a day for 21 days.
Hemophilus ducreyi (chancroid): Treat until ulcers or lymph nodes are healed.[2]	500 mg 4 times a day for 7 days.
Neisseria gonorrhoeae: Uncomplicated urethral, endocervical or rectal infections and in penicillinase-producing *N gonorrhoeae* (PPNG)[2] In pregnancy[2]	500 mg 4 times a day for 7 days **or** spectinomycin 2 g IM followed by erythromycin regimen. 500 mg 4 times a day for 7 days.
Treponema pallidum: Early syphilis (primary, secondary or latent syphilis of < 1 year duration)	500 mg 4 times a day for 14 days.
Prior to elective colorectal surgery, to reduce wound complications	Combination of erythromycin base and neomycin is a popular preoperative preparation.
Clostridium tetani: Tetanus[1]	500 mg every 6 hours for 10 days.

[1] Use as alternative drug in penicillin or tetracycline hypersensitivity or when penicillin or tetracycline are contraindicated or not tolerated.

[2] CDC 1989 Sexually Transmitted Diseases Treatment Guidelines. *Morbidity and Mortality Weekly Report* 1989 Sept 1;38(No. S-8):1-43.

[3] American Heart Association statement. *JAMA* 1990;264:2919-2922.

Refer to the general discussion of these products on page 1831

ERYTHROMYCIN BASE

	Product	Form	Description	C.I.*
Rx	**E-Mycin** (Boots)	**Tablets, enteric coated:** 250 mg	Orange. In 40s, 100s, 500s and UD 100s.	1
Rx	**Ery-Tab** (Abbott)		Delayed release. Pink. In 30s, 40s, 100s, 500s and UD 100s.	3.5
Rx	**Robimycin Robitabs** (Robins)		Lactose. Green. In 100s and 500s.	1.4
Rx	**E-Base Caplets and Tablets** (Barr)	**Tablets, enteric coated:** 333 mg	Delayed release. (E-Base/333 barr). White. In 100s, 500s and 1000s.	NA
Rx	**E-Mycin** (Boots)		White. In 30s, 100s, 500s and UD 100s.	1.9
Rx	**Ery-Tab** (Abbott)		Delayed release. White. In 30s, 100s, 500s and UD 100s.	3.8
Rx	**PCE Dispertab** (Abbott)	**Tablets with polymer coated particles:** 333 mg	Lactose. (PCE). White with pink speckles. Oval. In 60s and 500s.	5.6
Rx	**Erythromycin** (Various, eg, Boots, Parmed)	**Tablets, delayed release:** 333 mg	In 100s.	NA
Rx	**E-Base** (Barr)	**Tablets, enteric coated:** 500 mg	(E-Base/500 mg barr). White. Capsule shape. In 100s, 500s.	NA
Rx	**Ery-Tab** (Abbott)		Delayed release. Pink. In 100s and UD 100s.	2.6
Rx	**PCE Dispertab** (Abbott)	**Tablets with polymer coated particles:** 500 mg	(EK). White. Oval. In 100s.	NA
Rx	**Erythromycin Filmtabs** (Abbott)	**Tablets, film coated:** 250 mg	Pink. In 100s, 500s and UD 100s.	1.8
Rx	**Erythromycin Filmtabs** (Abbott)	**Tablets, film coated:** 500 mg	Pink. In 100s.	1.7
Rx	**Eryc** (Parke-Davis)	**Capsules, delayed release, enteric coated pellets:** 250 mg	(P-D 696). Clear and orange. In 40s, 100s, 500s and UD 100s.	3.3
Rx	**Erythromycin Base** (Various, eg, Abbott, Parmed)	**Capsules, delayed release:** 250 mg	In 100s and 500s.	1.6+

ERYTHROMYCIN ESTOLATE

	Product	Form	Description	C.I.*
Rx	**Ilosone** (Dista)	**Tablets:** 500 mg (as estolate)	White, scored. Capsule shape. In 50s.	5.8
Rx	**Erythromycin Estolate** (Various, eg, Barr, Geneva, Major, Parmed, Rugby, Schein, URL)	**Capsules:** 250 mg (as estolate)	In 100s.	2.5+
Rx	**Ilosone Pulvules** (Dista)		Ivory and red. In 100s and UD 100s.	6.1
Rx	**Erythromycin Estolate** (Various, eg, Dixon-Shane)	**Suspension:** 125 mg (as estolate) per 5 ml	In 480 ml.	4.3+
Rx	**Ilosone** (Dista)		Sucrose. Orange flavor. In 480 ml.	10.5
Rx	**Erythromycin Estolate** (Various, eg, Dixon-Shane)	**Suspension:** 250 mg (as estolate) per 5 ml	In 480 ml.	3.6+
Rx	**Ilosone** (Dista)		Sucrose. Cherry flavor. In 100 & 480 ml.	9.5

* Cost Index based on cost per 500 mg erythromycin.

Refer to the general discussion of these products on page 1831

ERYTHROMYCIN STEARATE

	Product	Form	Packaging	C.I.*
Rx	**Erythromycin Stearate** (Various, eg, Barr, Geneva, Major, Mylan, Rugby, Schein, Warner Chilcott, Zenith)	**Tablets, film coated:** 250 mg (as stearate)	In 100s, 500s and 1000s.	1.3+
Rx	**Eramycin** (Wesley)		In 100s and 500s.	NA
Rx	**Erythrocin Stearate** (Abbott)		In 20s, 40s, 100s, 500s and UD 100s.	NA
Rx	**Wyamycin S** (Wyeth-Ayerst)		(Wyeth 576). Yellow. In 500s.	1.5
Rx	**Erythromycin Stearate** (Various, eg, Geneva, Lederle, Major, Moore, Mylan, Purepac, Rugby, URL, Warner-C, Zenith)	**Tablets, film coated:** 500 mg (as stearate)	In 100s, 500s and UD 100s.	1.2+
Rx	**Erythrocin Stearate** (Abbott)		In 20s and 100s.	1.6
Rx	**Wyamycin S** (Wyeth-Ayerst)		(Wyeth 578). Yellow. Elliptical. In 100s.	1.3

ERYTHROMYCIN ETHYLSUCCINATE

Expressed in base equivalents, 400 mg erythromycin ethylsuccinate produces the same free erythromycin serum levels as 250 mg of erythromycin base, stearate or estolate.

	Product	Form	Packaging	C.I.*
Rx	**EryPed** (Abbott)	**Tablets, chewable:** 200 mg (as ethylsuccinate)	Sugar. Fruit flavor. Scored. In 40s.	9.7
Rx	**Erythromycin Ethylsuccinate** (Various, eg, Abbott, Barr, Geneva, Lederle, Major, Moore, Parmed, Rugby, Schein)	**Tablets:** 400 mg (as ethylsuccinate)	In 100s and 500s.	2.1+
Rx	**E.E.S. 400** (Various, eg, Abbott, Dixon-Shane)		Film coated. In 100s, 500s and UD 100s.	2.9
Rx	**Erythromycin Ethylsuccinate** (Various, eg, Barr, Lederle, Major, Purepac, Rugby, Schein, URL, Warner Chilcott)	**Suspension:** 200 mg (as ethylsuccinate) per 5 ml	In 100, 200 and 480 ml.	5.6+
Rx	**E.E.S. 200** (Various, eg, Abbott, Dixon-Shane)		In 100 and 480 ml.	5.4
Rx	**EryPed 200** (Abbott)		Sucrose. Fruit flavor. In 100 and 200 ml and UD 5 ml.	NA
Rx	**Erythromycin Ethylsuccinate** (Various, eg, Lederle, Major, Schein, Warner Chilcott)	**Suspension:** 400 mg (as ethylsuccinate) per 5 ml	In 480 ml.	3.4+
Rx	**E.E.S. 400** (Various, eg, Abbott, Dixon-Shane)		In 100 and 480 ml.	4.7
Rx	**EryPed 400** (Abbott)		Sucrose. Banana flavor. In 60, 100, 200 and UD 5 ml (100s).	NA
Rx	**EryPed Drops** (Abbott)	**Suspension:** 100 mg (as ethylsuccinate)/2.5 ml	Sucrose. Fruit flavor. In 50 ml.	NA
Rx	**E.E.S. Granules** (Abbott)	**Powder for Oral Suspension:** 200 mg (as ethylsuccinate)/5 ml when reconstituted	Sucrose. Cherry flavor. In 100 and 200 ml.	7.8
Rx	**EryPed** (Abbott)	**Granules for Oral Suspension:** 400 mg (as ethylsuccinate)/5 ml when reconstituted	In 60, 100 and 200 ml.	3.7

* Cost Index based on cost per 500 mg erythromycin (800 mg ethylsuccinate).

TROLEANDOMYCIN (Triacetyloleandomycin)

Actions:

Troleandomycin is a synthetically derived acetylated ester of the macrolide oleandomycin.

Pharmacokinetics: Peak serum levels of 2 mcg/ml are attained 2 hours following a 500 mg dose. Serum levels are still detected 12 hours later; 20% of the drug is recovered in the urine. Significant quantities are also excreted in bile.

Indications:

Streptococcus pneumoniae: Pneumococcal pneumonia due to susceptible strains.

Streptococcus pyogenes: Group A β-hemolytic streptococcal infections of the upper respiratory tract. Troleandomycin is generally effective in the eradication of streptococci from the nasopharynx. However, substantial data establishing efficacy in the subsequent prevention of rheumatic fever are not available.

Contraindications:

Hypersensitivity to troleandomycin.

Warnings:

Hepatic effects: Troleandomycin has been associated with an allergic cholestatic hepatitis. Some patients receiving troleandomycin for > 2 weeks or in repeated courses have developed jaundice accompanied by right upper quadrant pain, fever, nausea, vomiting, eosinophilia and leukocytosis. The changes have been reversible on discontinuance of the drug. Readministration reproduces hepatotoxicity, often within 24 to 48 hours. Monitor liver function tests and discontinue the drug if abnormalities develop.

Hepatic function impairment: Troleandomycin is principally excreted by the liver. Exercise caution in administering to patients with impaired hepatic function.

Pregnancy: Safety for use during pregnancy has not been established.

Precautions:

Superinfection: Use of antibiotics (especially prolonged or repeated therapy) may result in bacterial or fungal overgrowth of nonsusceptible organisms. Such overgrowth may lead to a secondary infection. Take appropriate measures if superinfection occurs.

Drug Interactions:

Troleandomycin Drug Interactions			
Precipitant drug	Object drug *		Description
Troleandomycin	Carbamazepine	↑	Carbamazepine toxicity sufficient to require resuscitative measures may result.
Troleandomycin	Contraceptives, oral	↑	Concurrent use may result in an increased risk of intrahepatic cholestasis due to decreased metabolism and accumulation of the contraceptive.
Troleandomycin	Ergot alkaloids	↑	Acute ergotism manifested as peripheral ischemia has occurred.
Troleandomycin	Methylprednisolone	↑	The clearance of methylprednisolone is greatly reduced. This has been used as a therapeutic advantage to reduce the dose.
Troleandomycin	Theophyllines	↑	Increased theophylline serum levels with toxicity may occur.
Troleandomycin	Triazolam	↑	Triazolam bioavailability may be increased, resulting in increased CNS depression.

* ↑ = Object drug increased

Adverse Reactions:

Most frequent: Abdominal cramping and discomfort (dose-related). *Infrequent:* Nausea; vomiting; diarrhea.

Allergic: Serious – Anaphylaxis. *Mild* – Urticaria and other skin rashes.

Patient Information:

Take at evenly spaced intervals during the day, preferably around the clock. Complete full course of therapy; take until gone.

Administration and Dosage:

Continue therapy for 10 days when used for streptococcal infection.

Adults: 250 to 500 mg, 4 times a day.

Children: 125 to 250 mg (6.6 to 11 mg/kg) every 6 hours.

				C.I.*
Rx	**Tao** (Roerig)	**Capsules:** 250 mg oleandomycin (as troleandomycin)	Lactose. (Roerig 159). In 100s.	95

* Cost Index based on cost per 500 mg.

SPECTINOMYCIN

Actions:

Pharmacology: Spectinomycin, structurally different from related aminoglycosides, inhibits protein synthesis in the bacterial cell. Site of action is the 30S ribosomal subunit.

Microbiology: Active in vitro against most strains of *Neisseria gonorrhoeae,* studies show no cross-resistance between spectinomycin and penicillin.

Pharmacokinetics: Rapidly absorbed after IM injection. A single 2 g injection produces average peak serum concentrations of 100 mcg/ml at 1 hour; a single 4 g injection, 160 mcg/ml at 2 hours. Eight hours following a 2 or 4 g injection, concentrations in plasma are 15 and 31 mcg/ml, respectively. The majority of the drug is excreted in the urine in the biologically active form.

Indications:

Acute gonorrheal urethritis and proctitis in the male and acute gonorrheal cervicitis and proctitis in the female due to susceptible strains of *N gonorrhoeae.* Treat men and women with known recent exposure to gonorrhea as those with gonorrhea.

Contraindications:

Hypersensitivity to spectinomycin.

Warnings:

Syphilis: Not effective in the treatment of syphilis. Antibiotics used to treat gonorrhea may mask or delay the symptoms of incubating syphilis. All patients with gonorrhea should have a serologic test for syphilis at time of diagnosis and a follow-up test after 3 months.

Pharyngeal infections: Not effective in pharyngeal infections due to *N gonorrhoeae.*

Pregnancy: Safety for use during pregnancy has not been established.

Infants and Children: Safety for use has not been established.

Precautions:

The diluent provided with this product contains benzyl alcohol which has been associated with a fatal gasping syndrome in infants.

Monitoring: Monitor clinical effectiveness to detect resistance by *N gonorrhoeae.*

Hypersensitivity: A few cases of anaphylaxis or anaphylactoid reactions have been reported. Have epinephrine immediately available. Refer to Management of Acute Hypersensitivity Reactions.

Adverse Reactions:

Single dose trials: Soreness at the injection site; urticaria; dizziness; nausea; chills; fever; insomnia.

Multiple dose studies: Decrease in hemoglobin, hematocrit and creatinine clearance; elevation of alkaline phosphatase, BUN and ALT.

In single and multiple dose studies in healthy volunteers, a reduction in urine output was noted; however, renal toxicity has not been demonstrated.

Administration and Dosage:

For IM use only. Shake vials vigorously immediately after adding diluent and before withdrawing dose. Inject 5 ml (2 g) IM deep into the upper outer quadrant of the gluteus. Also recommended for patients being treated after failure of previous antibiotic therapy. In geographic areas where antibiotic resistance is prevalent, initial treatment with 4 g (10 ml) IM is preferred, and may be divided between 2 gluteal injection sites.

CDC recommended treatment schedules for gonorrhea[1]:

Uncomplicated urethral, endocervical or rectal gonococcal infections, alternative regimen – For patients who cannot take ceftriaxone, the preferred alternative is spectinomycin 2 g IM as a single dose followed by doxycycline.

Children weighing $\geq$ 45 kg (100 lbs) should receive adult regimens. Children weighing $<$ 45 kg (100 lbs) with uncomplicated vulvovaginitis, cervicitis, urethritis, pharyngitis or proctitis and who cannot tolerate ceftriaxone may be treated with 40 mg/kg IM once.

Gonococcal infections in pregnancy – Treat pregnant women allergic to β-lactams with 2 g IM followed by erythromycin.

Disseminated gonococcal infection – Treat patients allergic to β-lactams with 2 g IM every 12 hours.

Stability: Use reconstituted suspension within 24 hours.

				C.I.*
Rx	**Trobicin** (Upjohn)	**Powder for Injection:** 400 mg spectinomycin (as HCl) per ml when reconstituted	In 2 g vial with 3.2 ml diluent.[2]	1049
			In 4 g vial with 6.2 ml diluent.[2]	994

* Cost Index based on cost per 2 g.

[1] CDC 1989 Sexually Transmitted Diseases Treatment Guidelines. *Morbidity and Mortality Weekly Report* 1989 Sept 1;38 (No. S-8):1-43.

[2] Bacteriostatic water for injection with 0.9% benzyl alcohol.

VANCOMYCIN

Actions:

Pharmacology: Vancomycin is a tricyclic glycopeptide antibiotic which interferes with bacterial cell wall synthesis in multiplying microorganisms. It also exerts a smaller effect on inhibition of RNA synthesis and bacterial cytoplasmic membranes.

Microbiology: At clinically achievable concentrations, vancomycin is active only against gram-positive bacteria. In vitro, at concentrations of 0.5 to 5 mcg/ml, it is active against many strains of streptococci, staphylococci, *Clostridium difficile, Corynebacterium, Listeria monocytogenes* and other gram-positive bacteria. A few *S aureus* strains require 10 to 20 mcg/ml for inhibition. It is bacteriostatic against enterococci.

No cross-resistance between vancomycin and any other antibiotic has been reported.

Pharmacokinetics: Absorption/Distribution – Systemic absorption of oral vancomycin is generally poor, although clinically significant serum concentrations have been reported in patients with active *C difficile*-induced colitis. In patients with normal renal function, 500 mg IV produces peak concentrations of 33 mcg/ml 5 minutes after infusion, 7 mcg/ml after 1 hour and 3 mcg/ml after 6 hours. A 1 g dose produces peak levels of 48 mcg/ml at 5 minutes, and trough levels of 2 mcg/ml after 12 hours. *Oral* doses of 2 g/day produce stool concentrations of vancomycin between 900 to 9000 mcg/g; serum concentrations are less than 1 mcg/ml.

Vancomycin IV penetrates inflamed meninges at levels about 15% of those found in serum; approximate mean, 2.5 mcg/ml in adults and 3.1 mcg/ml in infants. In the presence of inflammation, it also penetrates into pleural fluid, pericardial fluid, ascitic fluid, synovial fluid and bile (≈ 15%). It is 50% to 60% bound to serum albumin.

Metabolism/Excretion – Systemic vancomycin is eliminated in its active form in the urine (80% to 90%) through glomerular filtration. Urine concentrations of 90 to 300 mcg/ml are achieved 1 hour after a 500 mg IV dose. Creatinine clearance is linearly associated with vancomycin clearance. Elimination half-life is 4 to 8 hours in adults and 2 to 3 hours in children. Accumulation occurs in renal failure. Serum half-life in anuric patients is approximately 7.5 days. In anephric patients, the drug is slowly eliminated by unknown routes and mechanisms. Vancomycin is not significantly removed by hemodialysis or continuous ambulatory peritoneal dialysis.

Indications:

Parenteral: Potentially life-threatening infections not treatable with other effective, less toxic antimicrobials, including the penicillins and cephalosporins.

Severe staphylococcal infections (including methicillin-resistant staphylococci) in patients who cannot receive or who have failed to respond to penicillins and cephalosporins, or who have infections with resistant staphylococci. Infections may include endocarditis, osteomyelitis, pneumonia, septicemia and skin and skin structure infections.

Concomitant Use: Vancomycin has been effective alone or in combination with an aminoglycoside for endocarditis caused by *Streptococcus viridans* or *S bovis.* It is only effective in combination with an aminoglycoside for endocarditis caused by enterococci (eg, *S faecalis*).

Vancomycin has been effective for diphtheroid endocarditis, and has been used successfully with rifampin, an aminoglycoside or both in early onset prosthetic valve endocarditis caused by *S epidermidis* or diphtheroids.

Although no controlled clinical efficacy studies have been conducted, IV vancomycin has been suggested for prophylaxis against bacterial endocarditis in penicillin-allergic patients who have congenital heart disease or rheumatic or other acquired or valvular heart disease when these patients undergo dental procedures or surgical procedures of the upper respiratory tract.

Oral: Staphylococcal enterocolitis and antibiotic-associated pseudomembranous colitis produced by *C difficile.* Parenteral administration may be used concomitantly.

Contraindications: Known hypersensitivity to vancomycin.

Warnings:

Usage in renal impairment: Because of its nephrotoxicity, use carefully in renal insufficiency. The risk of toxicity may be appreciably increased by high serum concentrations or prolonged therapy. Factors that may increase the risk of nephrotoxicity include use in elderly and neonatal patients and concomitant use with other nephrotoxic drugs.

Ototoxicity: Avoid use in patients with previous hearing loss. If used, regulate dosage by periodic determination of drug serum levels; serum concentrations of 60 to 80 mcg/ml are associated with toxicity. Tinnitus and high-tone hearing loss may precede deafness. The elderly are more susceptible to auditory damage. Deafness may progress despite cessation of treatment. Vertigo, dizziness and tinnitus (rarely) have also been reported.

Hypotension: Rapid bolus administration may produce a sudden drop in blood pressure and, rarely, cardiac arrest. To avoid hypotension, administer in a dilute solution over 60 minutes and frequently monitor blood pressure and heart rate.

(Warnings continued on following page)

VANCOMYCIN (Cont.)

Warnings (Cont.):

Usage in Pregnancy – Category C: Animal reproduction studies have not been conducted. It is not known if vancomycin causes fetal harm when administered to a pregnant woman. Give only if the potential benefit justifies the potential risk to the fetus.

Usage in Lactation: Safety for use in the nursing mother has not been established. It is not known whether the drug is excreted in breast milk.

Usage in premature and full term neonates: Use with caution. Renal function is not completely developed in neonates.

Precautions:

Monitoring: Perform serial tests of auditory function and serum levels in patients with borderline renal function and in individuals over the age of 60. Perform periodic hematologic studies, urinalyses and liver and renal function tests in all patients.

For IV administration only: Injection IM causes tissue irritation and necrosis. Pain and thrombophlebitis, occasionally severe, may occur and are minimized by administering the drug slowly as a dilute solution (2.5 to 5 g/L) and by rotating injection sites.

Redneck or Red Man syndrome is characterized by a sudden and profound fall in blood pressure with or without a maculopapular rash over the face, neck, upper chest and extremities. The reaction appears to be at least partially mediated through a histaminergic response.

The reaction is usually stimulated by a too rapid IV infusion (dose given over a few minutes), but it has been reported rarely, when given as recommended (up to a 2 hour administration). This is not an allergic-type reaction. The onset may occur anytime within a few minutes of starting an IV infusion, to a short time after infusion completion. The rash generally resolves some hours after termination of administration.

Monitor blood pressure throughout the infusion; if treatment is necessary, fluids, antihistamines or corticosteroids may be beneficial.

Superinfection: Use of antibiotics (especially prolonged or repeated therapy) may result in bacterial or fungal overgrowth. Such overgrowth may lead to a secondary infection. Take appropriate measures if superinfection occurs.

Drug Interactions:

Concurrent or sequential use of other neurotoxic or nephrotoxic antibiotics (ie, **colistin, streptomycin, neomycin, kanamycin, tobramycin, gentamicin, amikacin, amphotericin B, bacitracin, cisplatin, paromomycin, polymyxin B**) requires careful monitoring.

Adverse Reactions:

Nausea, urticaria, macular rashes, chills, eosinophilia, anaphylactoid reactions; reversible neutropenia and drug fever (rare); ototoxicity and nephrotoxicity (see Warnings).

Concomitant use of vancomycin and **anesthetic agents** has been associated with erythema and histamine-like flushing in children.

Parenteral: Thrombocytopenia, phlebitis, hypotension, wheezing, dyspnea, pruritus. Increased serum creatinine or BUN concentrations in patients given vancomycin IV have been reported.

Redneck or Red Man syndrome – See Precautions.

Patient Information:

Complete full course of therapy; do not discontinue therapy without notifying physician.

Dosage:

Oral: Adults – 500 mg every 6 hours or 1 g every 12 hours.

Pseudomembranous colitis produced by C difficile – 500 mg to 2 g/day given in 3 or 4 divided doses for 7 to 10 days.

Children – 40 mg/kg/day in 4 divided doses. Do not exceed 2 g/day.

Neonates: (See Precautions). 10 mg/kg/day in divided doses.

Parenteral: Administer each dose over at least 60 minutes.

Adults – 500 mg IV every 6 hours or 1 g every 12 hours.

Children – 40 mg/kg/day in divided doses, added to fluids.

Infants and Neonates – Initial dose of 15 mg/kg, followed by 10 mg/kg every 12 hours for neonates in the first week of life up to the age of 1 month and every 8 hours thereafter.

For prevention of bacterial endocarditis in penicillin-allergic patients undergoing dental procedures or upper respiratory tract surgery or instrumentation:

Adults and Children (> 27 kg) – 1 g IV slowly over 1 hour beginning 1 hour prior to procedure. For patients considered to be at higher risk, may repeat in 8 to 12 hours.

Children (< 27 kg) – 20 mg/kg IV slowly over 1 hour beginning 1 hour prior to procedure. For patients considered to be at higher risk, may repeat in 8 to 12 hours.

(Dosage continued on following page)

VANCOMYCIN (Cont.)

Dosage (Cont.):

For prevention of bacterial endocarditis in penicillin-allergic patients undergoing GI or GU surgery and instrumentation[1]:

Adults and Children (> 27 kg) – 1 g IV slowly over 1 hour and 1.5 mg/kg gentamicin IM or IV concurrently 1 hour prior to the procedure. For patients considered to be at higher risk, may repeat in 8 to 12 hours.

Children (< 27 kg) – 20 mg/kg IV slowly over 1 hour and 2 mg/kg gentamicin IM or IV concurrently 1 hour prior to the procedure. For patients considered to be at higher risk, may repeat in 8 to 12 hours.

Dosage guidelines in renal failure: Adjust dosage; check serum levels regularly. In the elderly, dosage reduction may be necessary due to decreasing renal function.

For most patients, dosage may be calculated by using the following table.

Dosage in Impaired Renal Function	
Ccr (ml/min)	Dose (mg/24 hr)
100	1545
90	1390
80	1235
70	1080
60	925
50	770
40	620
30	465
20	310
10	155

The table is not valid for functionally anephric patients on dialysis. For such patients, give a loading dose of 15 mg/kg to achieve therapeutic serum levels promptly and a maintenance dose of 1.9 mg/kg/24 hr.

When only serum creatinine is available, use the formula below to calculate est. creatinine clearance. Serum creatinine should represent a steady state of renal function.

Males: $\frac{\text{Weight (kg)} \times (140 - \text{age})}{72 \times \text{serum creatinine}}$

Females: $0.85 \times$ above value

Administration:

Preparation of oral solution: Add 115 ml distilled water to the 10 g container. Each 6 ml of solution provides ≈ 500 mg vancomycin. Alternatively, dilute the contents of one 500 mg vial for injection in 30 ml water for oral or nasogastric tube administration.

Preparation of parenteral solution: Reconstitute by adding 10 ml Sterile Water for Injection to the 500 mg vial or 20 ml to the 1 g vial. Further dilution is required.

Intermittent infusion is the preferred administration method.

Dilute reconstituted solutions containing 500 mg or 1 g vancomycin with at least 100 or 200 ml respectively of diluent. Give the diluted dose IV over at least 60 minutes.

Compatible diluents: 5% Dextrose Injection, 5% Dextrose Injection and 0.9% NaCl, Lactated Ringer's Injection, Lactated Ringer's and 5% Dextrose Injection, *Normosol-M* and 5% Dextrose, 0.9% NaCl Injection, *Isolyte E,* Acetated Ringer's Injection.

Stability and storage: **Oral** and **parenteral** solutions are stable for 14 days if refrigerated after initial reconstitution. After further dilution, the parenteral solution is stable for 24 hours at room temperature.

			C.I.*
Rx	**Vancomycin HCl** (Various)	**Powder for Injection (Lyophilized):** 500 mg/vial. In 10s.	1400+
		1000 mg per vial. In 20 ml flip-top vials. In 5s.	1500+
Rx	**Lyphocin** (Lyphomed)	**Powder for Injection (Lyophilized):** 500 mg (as HCl) per vial. In 10 ml flip-top vials.	2046
Rx	**Vancocin** (Lilly)	**Pulvules:** 125 mg. (#3125). Blue and brown. In UD 20s.	1890
		250 mg. (#3126). Blue and gray. In UD 20s.	1890
		Powder for Oral Solution: 1 and 10 g (as HCl) in screw cap container.	1710
		Powder for Injection: 500 mg (as HCl) per 10 ml vial.	2047
Rx	**Vancoled** (Lederle)	**Powder for Injection:** 500 mg (as HCl) per vial.	1645
Rx	**Vancor IV** (Adria)	**Powder for Injection:** 500 mg (as HCl) or 1 g (as HCl) per vial.	1500

* Cost Index based on cost per 500 mg. # Product identification code.

[1] Committee on Rheumatic Fever and Bacterial Endocarditis, American Heart Association. "Prevention of Bacterial Endocarditis", *Circulation* 1984;70:1123A-1127A.

CLINDAMYCIN AND LINCOMYCIN

Warning:

These agents can cause severe and possibly fatal colitis, characterized by severe persistent diarrhea, severe abdominal cramps and possibly, the passage of blood and mucus. Endoscopic examination may reveal pseudomembranous colitis. A toxin(s) produced by *Clostridia* is a primary cause of antibiotic-associated colitis.

When significant diarrhea occurs, discontinue the drug or, if necessary, continue only with close observation of the patient. Large bowel endoscopy is recommended.

Mild cases of colitis and diarrhea may respond to drug discontinuation. Promptly manage moderate to severe cases with fluid, electrolyte and protein supplementation as indicated. Systemic corticoids and corticoid retention enemas may help relieve the colitis. Also consider other causes of colitis such as previous sensitivities to drugs or other allergens.

Antiperistaltic agents such as opiates and diphenoxylate with atropine may prolong or aggravate the condition. Diarrhea, colitis and pseudomembranous colitis can begin up to several weeks following cessation of therapy.

Vancomycin is effective in the treatment of antibiotic-associated pseudomembranous colitis produced by *C difficile.* (See page 1842 for complete prescribing information.)

Reserve for serious infections where less toxic antimicrobial agents are inappropriate (see Indications). Do not use in patients with nonbacterial infections (ie, most upper respiratory tract infections).

Actions:

Lincomycin and clindamycin (7-deoxy, 7-chloro derivative of lincomycin), known collectively as lincosamides, bind exclusively to the 50 S subunit of bacterial ribosomes and suppress protein synthesis.

Since bacterial resistance to these agents has been demonstrated, perform susceptibility testing. Cross-resistance has been demonstrated between these two agents.

Clindamycin is the preferred drug of the two because it is better absorbed, more potent and less toxic.

Microbiology: The following table indicates (✓) organisms generally susceptible in vitro:

	Microorganism	Lincosamides	
		Lincomycin	Clindamycin
Gram-positive	Staphylococcus aureus	✓	✓
	S albus	✓	
	S epidermidis[1]	✓	✓
	S pyogenes	✓	✓
	Streptococcus pneumoniae	✓	✓
	β-hemolytic streptococci	✓	✓
	S viridans	✓	✓
	Corynebacterium diphtheriae	✓	✓
	Nocardia asteroides	✓	✓
Anaerobes	Bacteroides species	✓	✓[2]
	Fusobacterium		✓
	Propionibacterium (same as C acnes)	✓	✓
	Eubacterium	✓	✓
	Actinomyces species	✓	✓
	Peptococcus	✓	✓
	Peptostreptococcus	✓	✓
	Microaerophilic streptococci		✓
	Clostridium perfringens	✓	✓
	C tetani	✓	✓
	Veillonella		✓

[1] Penicillinase and nonpenicillinase.
[2] Including B fragilis and B melaninogenicus.

(Actions continued on following page)

CLINDAMYCIN AND LINCOMYCIN (Cont.)

Actions (Cont.):

Pharmacokinetics: Administration with food markedly impairs lincomycin (but not clindamycin) oral absorption. Both agents achieve significant tissue penetration; lincomycin may reach a cerebrospinal fluid (CSF) concentration 40% of serum levels with inflamed meninges, but neither agent crosses well into the CSF with normal meninges.

Lincomycin levels above the MIC for most gram-positive organisms are maintained with oral doses of 500 mg for 6 to 8 hours and for 14 hours after a 600 mg IV infusion. Following a 600 mg IM dose, detectable levels persist for 24 hours.

Clindamycin serum levels exceed MIC for most indicated organisms for at least 6 hrs after recommended doses. Levels can be maintained above the in vitro MIC for most indicated organisms by giving clindamycin phosphate every 8 to 12 hrs to adults, every 6 to 8 hrs to children or by continuous IV infusion. Equilibrium is reached by dose 3.

Hemodialysis and *peritoneal dialysis* do not remove either agent from the blood.

The following table summarizes selected pharmacokinetic data:

Lincosamides			Bioavailability (%)	Mean Peak Serum Level[1] (mcg/ml)	Time to Peak Serum Level (hours)	Protein Binding (%)	Half-Life (hours)			Elimination (%)		
							Normal	Anephric	Liver Disease	Hepatic	Unchanged in Urine (range)	Feces
Clindamycin	HCl & Palmitate[2]	Oral	23-38	4	0.75	60-95	2.4-3	3.5-5	7-14	85	10-15	3.6
	Phosphate[2]	IM		4.9	1-3							
		IV		14.7	0							
Lincomycin		Oral	30	2.6	2-4	70-72	4-6.4	10	11.8	50-70	4 (1-31)	40
		IM		9.5	0.5						17.3 (2-25)	
		IV		19	0						13.8 (5-30)	

[1] Clindamycin 300 mg; lincomycin, oral 500 mg, IM/IV 600 mg.

[2] Clindamycin palmitate and phosphate are rapidly hydrolyzed to the clindamycin base.

Indications:

For the treatment of serious infections due to susceptible strains of streptococci, pneumococci and staphylococci. Reserve use for penicillin-allergic patients or when penicillin is inappropriate. Because of the risk of colitis (see Warning Box), consider the nature of the infection and the suitability of less toxic alternatives (eg, erythromycin).

Refer to individual monographs for complete information.

Contraindications:

Hypersensitivity to one of these agents is a contraindication to use of both agents.

Do not use in the treatment of minor bacterial or viral infections.

Warnings:

Colitis: Studies indicate a toxin(s) produced by *Clostridia* is one primary cause of antibiotic-associated colitis (see Warning Box).

Sensitivity: Use with caution in patients with a history of asthma or significant allergies. If hypersensitivity occurs, discontinue the drug and institute emergency treatment. Have epinephrine 1:1000 immediately available. Refer to Management of Acute Hypersensitivity Reactions on p. viii.

Usage in meningitis: Since **clindamycin** does not diffuse adequately into cerebrospinal fluid, do not use in the treatment of meningitis.

Usage in Pregnancy: Safety for use in pregnancy has not been established. Clindamycin and lincomycin cross the placenta in amounts approximately 50% and 25% of maternal serum levels, respectively. No reports of congenital defects are known.

Usage in Lactation: **Clindamycin** appears in breast milk in ranges of 0.7 to 3.8 mcg/ml following doses of 300 mg orally to 600 mg IV, every 6 hours. **Lincomycin** appears in breast milk in ranges of 0.5 to 2.4 mcg/ml. Breast-feeding is probably best discontinued when taking these agents to avoid potential problems in the infant.

Usage in Newborns and Infants: When **clindamycin** is administered to newborns and infants, monitor organ system functions. Each ml of clindamycin and lincomycin contains 9.45 mg benzyl alcohol. **Lincomycin** is not indicated for use in the newborn.

(Continued on following page)

CLINDAMYCIN AND LINCOMYCIN (Cont.)

Precautions:

Usage in the elderly: Older patients with associated severe illness may not tolerate diarrhea well; carefully monitor these patients for changes in bowel frequency. Cautiously prescribe to those with GI disease, particularly colitis.

Usage in renal and hepatic disease: Cautiously give **clindamycin** to patients with severe renal or hepatic disease accompanied by severe metabolic aberrations; monitor serum clindamycin levels during high dose therapy.

Since adequate data are not available for using **lincomycin** in preexisting liver disease, it is not recommended unless special clinical circumstances so indicate.

Prolonged therapy dictates performing liver and kidney function tests and blood counts.

Do NOT inject IV undiluted as a bolus; infuse over at least 10 to 60 minutes as directed in Administration and Dosage.

Superinfection: Use of antibiotics (especially prolonged or repeated therapy) may result in bacterial or fungal overgrowth of nonsusceptible organisms, particularly yeasts. Such overgrowth may lead to a secondary infection. Take appropriate measures if superinfection occurs.

When preexisting monilial infections require **lincomycin** therapy, give concomitant antimonilial treatment.

Tartrazine sensitivity: Cleocin Capsules contain tartrazine, which may cause allergic-type reactions (including bronchial asthma) in susceptible individuals. Although the incidence of tartrazine sensitivity in the general population is low, it is frequently seen in patients who also have aspirin hypersensitivity. See the product listings.

Drug Interactions:

Neuromuscular blocking agents: Clindamycin and lincomycin have neuromuscular blocking properties that may enhance the action of other similar agents. Use with caution in patients receiving such agents.

Kaolin: Simultaneous administration reduces GI absorption of lincomycin.

Antagonism has been seen between **clindamycin** and **erythromycin** in vitro.

Adverse Reactions:

GI: Nausea; vomiting; diarrhea (clindamycin 3.4% to 30%); pseudomembranous colitis (clindamycin 0.01% to 10%; 3 to 4 times more frequent with oral administration).

Hematopoietic: Neutropenia (sometimes transient); leukopenia; agranulocytosis; thrombocytopenia.

Hypersensitivity: Skin rashes, urticaria, erythema multiforme, some cases resembling Stevens-Johnson syndrome (rare); anaphylaxis.

Hepatic: Jaundice; liver function test abnormalities (serum transaminase elevations).

Renal: Rare dysfunction has been evidenced by azotemia, oliguria and proteinuria (no direct causal relationship established).

Cardiovascular: Hypotension and cardiopulmonary arrest following too rapid IV administration (rare).

Local reactions: Pain following injection. Induration and sterile abscess have occurred after IM injection and thrombophlebitis after IV infusion with clindamycin. Give deep IM injections and avoid prolonged use of IV catheters.

Clindamycin:

GI – Abdominal pain; esophagitis; anorexia.

Hematopoietic – Eosinophilia.

Hypersensitivity – Maculopapular rash; generalized mild to moderate morbilliform-like rash (3% to 5%, most frequent).

Musculoskeletal – Polyarthritis (rare).

Lincomycin:

GI – Glossitis; stomatitis; pruritus ani.

Hematopoietic – Aplastic anemia and pancytopenia (rare).

Hypersensitivity – Angioneurotic edema; serum sickness.

Skin and mucous membranes – Vaginitis; exfoliative, vesiculobullous dermatitis (rare).

Special senses – Tinnitus; vertigo.

Patient Information:

May cause diarrhea; notify physician if this occurs.

Take each dose with a full glass of water. Complete full course of therapy.

Lincomycin: Take on an empty stomach at least 1 hour before or 2 hours after meals.

(Products listed on following page)

Complete prescribing information begins on page 1845

LINCOMYCIN

Indications:

Effective in the treatment of some streptococcal and staphylococcal infections resistant to other antibiotics. Administer concomitantly with other antimicrobial agents when indicated.

Dosage:

Oral: Take at least 1 to 2 hours before or after eating to ensure optimum absorption of lincomycin.

Adults – Serious infections: 500 mg every 8 hours. *More severe infections:* 500 mg or more every 6 hours. With B-hemolytic streptococcal infections, continue treatment for at least 10 days to diminish the likelihood of subsequent rheumatic fever or glomerulonephritis.

Children over 1 month of age – Serious infections: 30 mg/kg/day (15 mg/lb/day) divided into 3 or 4 equal doses. *More severe infections:* 60 mg/kg/day (30 mg/lb/day) divided into 3 or 4 equal doses.

IM: IM administration is well tolerated.

Adults – Serious infections: 600 mg every 24 hours.*More severe infections:* 600 mg every 12 hours or more often.

Children over 1 month of age – Serious infections: 10 mg/kg (5 mg/lb) every 24 hours. *More severe infections:* 10 mg/kg (5 mg/lb) every 12 hours or more often.

IV: Dilute to 1 g/100 ml and infuse over 1 hour. Severe cardiopulmonary reactions have occurred when given at greater than the recommended concentration and rate. Intravenous administration in 250 to 500 ml of 5% Dextrose in Water or normal saline produced no local irritation or phlebitis.

Adults – Determine dose by the severity of the infection. *Serious infections:* 600 mg to 1 g every 8 to 12 hours. *Severe to life-threatening situations:* Doses of 8 g/day have been given.

The *maximum recommended dose* is 8 g/day.

Children over 1 month of age – Infuse 10 to 20 mg/kg/day (5 to 10 mg/lb/day), (depending on severity of infection), in divided doses as described above for adults.

Subconjunctival injection: 75 mg/0.25 ml injected subconjunctivally results in ocular fluid levels of antibiotic (lasting for at least 5 hours) with MICs sufficient for most susceptible pathogens.

Impaired renal function: When required, an appropriate dose is 25% to 30% of that recommended for patients with normal renal function.

Administration:

For IV use, dilute 1 g in a minimum of 100 ml solution.

Physical compatibilities:

The compatible and incompatible determinations are physical observations only, not chemical determinations. Adequate clinical evaluation of the safety and efficacy of these combinations has not been performed. **Compatible** for 24 hours at room temperature unless otherwise indicated in:

Infusion solutions:
5% and 10% Dextrose in Water
5% and 10% Dextrose in Saline
Ringer's Solution
Sodium Lactate ⅙ Molar
Travert 10% – Electrolyte No. 1
Dextran in 6% Saline

Vitamins in infusion solutions:
B-Complex
B-Complex with Ascorbic Acid

Antibiotics in infusion solutions:
Penicillin G Sodium (satisfactory for 4 hours)
Cephalothin
Tetracycline HCl
Colistimethate (satisfactory for 4 hours)
Ampicillin
Methicillin
Chloramphenicol
Polymyxin B Sulfate

Incompatibilities: Lincomycin is incompatible with novobiocin, kanamycin and phenytoin sodium.

			C.I.*
Rx	**Lincocin** (Upjohn)	**Capsules:** 500 mg (as HCl). In 24s and 100s.	15
		Capsules, pediatric: 250 mg (as HCl). In 24s.	16
		Injection: 300 mg (as HCl)/ml. In 2 and 10 ml vials[1] and 2 ml U-ject[1].	61
Rx	**Lincorex** (Roman)	**Injection:** 300 mg (as HCl) and 9.45 mg benzyl alcohol per ml. In 10 ml vials.	NA

* Cost Index based on cost per 100 mg.
[1] With 0.9% benzyl alcohol.

Complete prescribing information begins on page 1845

CLINDAMYCIN

Indications:

Anaerobes: Serious respiratory tract infections such as empyema, anaerobic pneumonitis and lung abscess; serious skin and soft tissue infections; septicemia, intra-abdominal infections such as peritonitis and intra-abdominal abscess (typically resulting from anaerobic organisms resident in the normal GI tract); infections of the female pelvis and genital tract such as endometritis, nongonococcal tubo-ovarian abscess, pelvic cellulitis and postsurgical vaginal cuff infection.

Streptococci and Staphylococci: Serious respiratory tract infections; serious skin and soft tissue infections.

Pneumococci: Serious respiratory tract infections.

In addition, **injectable clindamycin** is indicated in infections caused by:

Streptococci: Septicemia.

Staphylococci: Septicemia; acute hematogenous osteomyelitis.

Adjunctive therapy: In the surgical treatment of chronic bone and joint infections due to susceptible organisms.

Dosage:

In the treatment of anaerobic infections, use parenteral clindamycin initially. This may be followed by oral therapy.

In cases of β-hemolytic streptococcal infections, continue treatment for at least 10 days.

Oral: Take with a full glass of water or with food to avoid esophageal irritation.

Adults – *Serious infections:* 150 to 300 mg every 6 hours. *More severe infections:* 300 to 450 mg every 6 hours.

Children –

Clindamycin HCl – *Serious infections:* 8 to 16 mg/kg/day divided into 3 or 4 equal doses. *More severe infections:* 16 to 20 mg/kg/day divided into 3 or 4 equal doses.

Clindamycin palmitate HCl – *Serious infections:* 8 to 12 mg/kg/day divided into 3 or 4 equal doses. *Severe infections:* 13 to 25 mg/kg/day divided into 3 or 4 equal doses. In children weighing 10 kg or less, administer 37.5 mg 3 times daily as the minimum dose.

Topical: See Clindamycin, Topical p. 2305.

Parenteral:

Adults – *Serious infections* due to aerobic gram-positive cocci and the more sensitive anaerobes: 600 to 1200 mg/day in 2 to 4 equal doses. *More severe infections,* particularly those due to *B fragilis, Peptococcus* species or *Clostridium* species other than *C perfringens:* 1.2 to 2.7 g/day in 2 to 4 equal doses. For more serious infections, these doses may have to be increased. In *life-threatening situations* due to aerobes or anaerobes, doses of 4.8 g/day have been given IV to adults.

CDC Recommendation *for Acute Pelvic Inflammatory Disease*[1]: 600 mg IV, 4 times a day plus gentamicin 2 mg/kg IV, followed by 1.5 mg/kg, 3 times a day. Continue IV for 4 days and at least 48 hours after patient improves. To complete the 10 to 14 day treatment regimen, continue clindamycin 450 mg orally, 4 times a day.

Alternatively, administer in the form of a single rapid infusion of the first dose, followed by continuous IV infusion, as follows:

To maintain serum clindamycin levels	Rapid infusion rate	Maintenance infusion rate
Above 4 mcg/ml	10 mg/min for 30 min	0.75 mg/min
Above 5 mcg/ml	15 mg/min for 30 min	1.00 mg/min
Above 6 mcg/ml	20 mg/min for 30 min	1.25 mg/min

Children (over 1 month of age) –*Serious infections:* 15 to 25 mg/kg/day (350 mg/m²/day) in 3 or 4 equal doses. *More severe infections:* 25 to 40 mg/kg/day (450 mg/m²/day) in 3 or 4 equal doses.

[1] Morbidity and Mortality Weekly Report 1985(Oct 18);34(Supp 4S):75S-108S.

(Continued on following page)

CLINDAMYCIN (Cont.)

Administration:

Dilution and Infusion Rates: Single IM injections of greater than 600 mg are not recommended. Dilute clindamycin phosphate prior to IV administration to a concentration of not more than 12 mg/ml. Infusion rates are as follows:

Dose (mg)	Diluent (ml)	Time (min)
300	50	10
600	50	20
900	100	30
1200	100	40

Do not administer more than 1200 mg in a single 1 hour infusion.

Compatibility in IV solutions:

Compatible at room temperature for 24 hours		Incompatible
IV solutions containing: sodium chloride glucose potassium	vitamin B complex cephalothin kanamycin gentamicin penicillin carbenicillin	ampicillin phenytoin sodium barbiturates aminophylline magnesium sulfate calcium salts†

† Certain admixtures or concentrations.

Reconstitution – Add 75 ml water to 100 ml bottle of palmitate in 2 portions; shake.

Storage and Stability – Store unreconstituted palmitate product at room temperature 15° to 30°C (59° to 86°F). Do **NOT** refrigerate the reconstituted solution; it may thicken and be difficult to pour when chilled. The solution is stable for 2 weeks at room temperature.

Clindamycin phosphate is stable in 0.9% Sodium Chloride Injection, 5% Dextrose Injection and Lactated Ringer's Solution, in both glass and polyvinyl chloride containers, at concentrations of 6, 9 and 12 mg/ml for 8 weeks frozen (–10°C), 32 days refrigerated (4°C) and 16 days at room temperature (25°C).

	Product	Description	C.I.*
Rx	**Clindamycin HCl** (Various, eg, Biocraft, Vitarine)	**Capsules:** 75 mg (as HCl). In 16s, 100s, 500s and 1000s.	15
		150 mg (as HCl). In 16s, 100s, 500s and 1000s.	20
Rx	**Cleocin HCl** (Upjohn)	**Capsules:** 75 mg (as HCl). Contains tartrazine. (#Cleocin 75 mg Upjohn 331). Lavender. In 100s.	30
		150 mg (as HCl). Contains tartrazine. (#Cleocin 150 mg). Lavender and maroon. In 16s, 100s and UD 100s.	27
		300 mg (as HCl). In 16s, 100s and UD 100s.	16
Rx	**Cleocin Pediatric** (Upjohn)	**Granules, flavored:** 75 mg (as palmitate HCl)/5 ml when reconstituted. In 100 ml bottles.	35
Rx	**Clindamycin Phosphate** (Various, eg, Abbott, Bioline, Elkins-Sinn, Goldline, Lederle, Lemmon, Lyphomed, Squibb-Marsam)	**Injection:** 150 mg (as phosphate) per ml. In 2 and 4 ml amps and 2, 4, 6 and 60 ml vials.	100+
Rx	**Cleocin Phosphate** (Upjohn)	**Injection:** 300 mg (as phosphate)/2 ml vial.[1]	134
		600 mg (as phosphate)/4 ml vial.[1]	121
		900 mg (as phosphate)/6 ml vial.[1]	108

* Cost Index based on cost per 50 mg.

Product identification code.

[1] With benzyl alcohol and EDTA.

The aminoglycosides are bactericidal antibiotics. Used primarily in the treatment of gram-negative infections caused by *Pseudomonas* sp, *Escherichia coli, Proteus* sp, *Klebsiella* sp and *Enterobacter* sp.

Actions:

Pharmacology: Aminoglycosides irreversibly bind to the 30S subunit of bacterial ribosomes, blocking the recognition step in protein synthesis and causing misreading of the genetic code. The ribosomes separate from messenger RNA; cell death ensues.

Pharmacokinetics: Absorption – Absorption from the GI tract is poor. Therefore, treat systemic infections parenterally. Aminoglycosides are occasionally used orally for enteric infections (see Aminoglycosides Oral, page 1868 Absorption from IM injection is rapid, with peak blood levels achieved within 1 hour after injection.

Distribution – Aminoglycosides are widely distributed in extracellular fluids; peak serum concentrations may be lower than usual in patients whose extracellular fluid volume is expanded (eg, patients with edema or ascites). These drugs cross the placental barrier. Measurable concentrations are found in unobstructed bile, synovial fluid, renal lymph, sputum, bronchial secretions and pleural fluid. Aminoglycosides exhibit low protein binding with the exception of streptomycin. They do NOT achieve significant levels in the cerebrospinal fluid (CSF) in normal patients. Although penetration is enhanced in the presence of inflamed meninges, only low levels are achieved. When intrathecal gentamicin is given with systemic gentamicin, CSF levels are substantially increased, depending on location of injection. Peak CSF concentrations following intralumbar administration generally occur at 1 to 6 hours after injection.

Newborn infants, postpartum females and patients with fever, liver disease and ascites, spinal cord injury and cystic fibrosis may have an enlarged apparent volume of distribution. Obesity will artificially contract the apparent volume of distribution because adipose tissue contains less water than lean body mass of equal weight.

Excretion is by glomerular filtration, largely as unchanged drug; thus, high urine levels are attained. Probenecid does not affect renal tubular transport. The serum half-lives of all the agents are between 2 to 3 hours in patients with normal renal function. Approximately 53% to 98% of a single IV dose is excreted in the urine in 24 hours. However, when renal function is impaired, significant accumulation and subsequent toxicity may occur rapidly if dosage is not adjusted. The serum half-life is longer in young infants, as the immature renal system is unable to excrete these drugs rapidly; during the first days of life, the half-life may exceed 5 to 6 hours. Prolonged half-life may also be noted in the elderly. In severely burned patients, the half-life may be significantly decreased and result in serum concentrations lower than anticipated. Febrile and anemic states may be associated with a shorter serum half-life; dosage adjustment is usually not necessary. Aminoglycosides are removed by hemodialysis (4 to 6 hours removes approximately 50%) and peritoneal dialysis (range-removal of 23% in 8 hours to only 4% in 22 hours).

Serum levels – Because of the narrow range between therapeutic and toxic serum levels, careful attention to dosage calculations is essential, especially in patients with renal impairment, geriatric and female patients, those requiring high peak serum levels, patients on prolonged (> 10 days) therapy, patients with unstable renal function or those undergoing dialysis, those with abnormal extracellular fluid volume, or those with prior exposure to ototoxic or nephrotoxic drugs. Monitor drug serum levels. Peak serum levels indicate achievement of therapeutic serum levels. Trough serum level determinations (just prior to the next dose) best indicate drug accumulation. Serum levels should be obtained within 48 hours of the start of therapy and every 3 to 4 days assuming stable renal function; also, levels are indicated when the dose is changed or in changing renal function. The following table summarizes various pharmacokinetic parameters:

	Half-life (hrs)		Therapeutic Serum Levels	Toxic Serum Levels (mcg/ml)		Dose (mg/kg/day)
Aminoglycoside	Normal	ESRD	(mcg/ml)	Peak[1]	Trough[2]	Normal Ccr
Neomycin	2-3	—	5-10	—	—	15
Streptomycin	2-2.5	100	25	> 50	—	15-25
Kanamycin	2-3	24-60	8-16	> 30	> 5	15
Gentamicin	2	24-60	4-8	> 12	> 2	3-5
Tobramycin	2-2.5	24-60	4-8	> 12	> 2	3-5
Amikacin	2-3	24-60	8-16	> 35	> 5	15
Netilmicin	2-3	40	0.5-10	> 16	> 4	3-6.5

[1] Measured 1 hour after IM administration.
[2] Measured immediately prior to next dose.

(Actions continued on following page)

Actions (Cont.):

Microbiology:

The bactericidal activity of aminoglycosides is through inhibition of bacterial protein synthesis. One-way cross resistance is frequently noted. Three mechanisms for the development of bacterial resistance to aminoglycosides have been identified: Alteration of the drug target site (the bacterial ribosome); reduction or elimination of transport of the drug into the bacterial cell; inactivation of the drug by enzymatic modification (most significant). Bactericidal serum levels are usually 2 to 4 times greater than bacteriostatic levels. These agents are more active in an alkaline medium. Therefore, alkalinization of the urine with bicarbonate may be beneficial in the therapy of urinary tract infections.

Perform culture and sensitivity testing to determine appropriate antimicrobial therapy. Treat susceptible organisms with agents less toxic than aminoglycosides, especially if renal function is compromised. Resistance to aminoglycosides develops slowly, except with streptomycin. Development of streptomycin resistance may be a single step process and may occur rapidly. Anaerobic bacteria, including *Bacteroides fragilis, Clostridia* and anaerobic cocci are resistant to the aminoglycosides.

The following table indicates (✓) the organisms which are generally susceptible to aminoglycosides:

	Microorganisms	Neomycin	Streptomycin	Kanamycin	Gentamicin	Tobramycin	Amikacin	Netilmicin
Gram-positive	Mycobacterium tuberculosis		✓[1]					
	Staphylococcus species				✓[2]	✓	✓[2]	✓[2]
	Staphylococcus aureus			✓[2]		✓		
	Staphylococcus epidermidis			✓				
	Streptococcus species		✓[1]					
	Streptococcus faecalis		✓[1]	✓[1]	✓[1]	✓[1]		✓[1]
Gram-negative	Acinetobacter species			✓			✓	✓
	Citrobacter species				✓	✓	✓	✓
	Enterobacter species				✓	✓	✓	✓
	Enterobacter aerogenes	✓	✓	✓				
	Escherichia coli	✓	✓	✓	✓	✓	✓	✓
	Hemophilus influenzae		✓[1]	✓				
	Hemophilus ducreyi		✓					
	Klebsiella species	✓	✓[1]	✓	✓	✓	✓	✓
	Morganella morganii					✓		
	Neisseria species							✓
	Neisseria gonorrhoeae			✓				
	Proteus species	✓	✓	✓[3]	✓[3]	✓[3]	✓[3]	✓
	Proteus mirabilis					✓		✓
	Proteus vulgaris	✓				✓		
	Providencia species					✓	✓	
	Providencia rettgeri					✓	✓	
	Pseudomonas aeruginosa	✓			✓[1]	✓	✓	✓
	Salmonella species			✓	✓			✓
	Serratia species			✓	✓	✓	✓	✓
	Shigella species			✓	✓			✓
	Yersinia pestis (Pasteurella pestis)		✓					

1 Usually used concomitantly with other anti-infective agents.
2 Penicillinase-producing and nonpenicillinase-producing.
3 Indole-positive and indole-negative.

(Continued on following page)

Indications:

The indications for specific agents are listed in individual drug monographs on the following pages. Reserve these drugs for treatment of infections caused by organisms not sensitive to less toxic agents.

Contraindications:

In patients who have shown previous reactions to these agents. With the exception of the use of streptomycin in tuberculosis, these agents are generally NOT indicated in long-term therapy because of the ototoxic and nephrotoxic hazards of extended administration.

Warnings:

The aminoglycosides are associated with significant nephrotoxicity or ototoxicity. These agents are excreted primarily by glomerular filtration; thus, the serum half-life will be prolonged and significant accumulation will occur in patients with impaired renal function. Toxicity may develop even with conventional doses, particularly in patients with prerenal azotemia or impaired renal function.

Closely observe all patients treated with aminoglycosides. Monitoring of renal and eighth cranial nerve function at the onset of therapy is essential for patients with known or suspected renal impairment and also in those whose renal function is initially normal, but who develop signs of renal dysfunction. Evidence of renal impairment or ototoxicity requires discontinuation of the drug or appropriate dosage adjustments. When feasible, monitor drug serum concentrations. Avoid concomitant use with other ototoxic, neurotoxic or nephrotoxic drugs. Other factors which may increase the risk of toxicity are dehydration and advanced age.

Ototoxicity, both auditory (cochlear) and vestibular, can occur with any of these agents. The incidence of ototoxicity is directly proportional to the duration (> 10 days) and amount of drug administered. The risk is greater in patients with renal impairment and with preexisting hearing loss. High frequency deafness usually occurs first and can be detected by audiometric testing. When feasible, obtain serial audiograms. There may be no clinical symptoms to warn of developing cochlear damage. Tinnitus or vertigo may occur, and are evidence of vestibular injury and impending bilateral irreversible deafness. The onset of deafness may occur several weeks after the drug has been discontinued and may progress to a complete hearing loss. Vestibular toxicity is more predominant with gentamicin and streptomycin; auditory toxicity is more common with kanamycin, amikacin, netilmicin and neomycin. Tobramycin affects both functions equally. The relative ototoxicity of these agents is: Neomycin > Streptomycin = Kanamycin > Amikacin = Gentamicin = Tobramycin > Netilmicin. Kanamycin and streptomycin appear in this relative comparison based on high dose therapy and antituberculosis therapy, respectively.

Renal toxicity may be characterized by decreased creatinine clearance, cells or casts in the urine, decreased urine specific gravity, oliguria, proteinuria or evidence of nitrogen retention (increasing BUN, nonprotein nitrogen or creatinine). Renal tubular damage is usually reversible. The relative nephrotoxicity of these agents is estimated to be: Neomycin > Kanamycin = Amikacin = Gentamicin = Netilmicin > Tobramycin > Streptomycin.

Neuromuscular blockade: Aminoglycosides may aggravate muscle weakness because of a potential curare-like effect on the neuromuscular function. Use with caution in patients with neuromuscular disorders, (ie, myasthenia gravis, parkinsonism, infant botulism).

Neuromuscular blockade resulting in respiratory paralysis has occurred with aminoglycosides, especially if given with or soon after anesthesia or muscle relaxants. This effect is pronounced with neomycin and streptomycin, but is also seen with kanamycin in humans, and with amikacin, gentamicin, tobramycin and netilmicin in animals.

Use caution in newborns of mothers receiving magnesium sulfate; these hypermagnesemic infants may experience respiratory arrest after receiving aminoglycosides.

Usage in Pregnancy and Lactation: Category D (tobramycin, netilmicin). Aminoglycosides can cause fetal harm when given to pregnant women. These agents cross the placenta. Fetal serum levels may reach 15% to 50% of maternal levels. There are reports of total irreversible bilateral congenital deafness in children whose mothers received **streptomycin** during pregnancy. Serious side effects to the fetus or newborn have not been reported with other aminoglycosides, but the potential for harm exists. Use only when clearly needed and when the potential benefits outweigh the unknown hazards.

Small amounts of **streptomycin** and **netilmicin** are excreted in breast milk.

Usage in Children: Use with caution in premature infants and neonates because of their renal immaturity and the resulting prolongation of serum half-life of these drugs. **Neomycin** is not recommended for use in infants or children.

A syndrome of apparent CNS depression, characterized by stupor and flaccidity to coma and deep respiratory depression, has been reported in very young infants given **streptomycin** in doses greater than those recommended. Do not exceed recommended doses in infants.

(Continued on following page)

Precautions:

Intrathecal gentamicin: A patient with multiple sclerosis for 7 years was treated with intralumbar gentamicin; disseminated microscopic lesions of the brainstem were reported at autopsy. Tissue rarefaction and marked swelling of axis cylinders with occasional calcification, loss of oligodendroglia and astroglia and a poor inflammatory response were seen.

Cross-allergenicity among the aminoglycosides has been demonstrated.

Assess renal function prior to and periodically during therapy. If signs of renal irritation appear (ie, casts, white or red cells, albumin), increase hydration. Reduce dosage if other evidence of renal dysfunction occurs (decreased creatinine clearance or urine specific gravity, increased BUN or creatinine or oliguria). These usually disappear when therapy is complete. If azotemia or a progressive decrease in urine output occurs, stop treatment.

Hydration: These drugs reach high concentrations in the renal system; keep patients well hydrated to prevent chemical irritation of tubules. Well hydrated patients with normal renal function have low risk of nephrotoxic reactions if maximum dosage is not exceeded.

Streptomycin, given to patients with preexisting renal insufficiency, calls for extreme caution. In severely uremic patients, a single dose may produce high blood levels for several days and the cumulative effect may produce ototoxic sequelae. Alkalinize the urine to minimize or prevent renal irritation.

Usage in the elderly - Elderly patients may have reduced renal function that is not evident in the results of routine screening tests, such as BUN or serum creatinine. A creatinine clearance determination may be more useful. Monitoring of renal function during treatment is particularly important in such patients.

Laboratory Tests: In the treatment of sexually transmitted disease, if concomitant syphilis is suspected, perform a darkfield examination before treatment is started. Perform monthly serologic tests for at least 4 months.

Superinfection: Use of antibiotics (especially prolonged or repeated therapy) may result in bacterial or fungal overgrowth of nonsusceptible organisms. Such overgrowth may lead to a secondary infection. Take appropriate measures if superinfection occurs.

Irrigation: Neurotoxic and nephrotoxic antibiotics may be absorbed after local irrigation or application. In some cases, aminoglycosides (ie, neomycin) are absorbed from wounds and granulating surfaces similar to IM injection. Consider potential toxicity of topical use.

Drug Interactions:

Concurrent or sequential administration with other ototoxic, neurotoxic or nephrotoxic agents may increase the potential for adverse effects. Avoid concurrent use with **other aminoglycosides** or with **amphotericin B, bacitracin, cisplatin, cephalothin** (and potentially other cephalosporins), **vancomycin, methoxyflurane** or with **potent diuretics** (ethacrynic acid, furosemide, bumetanide or mannitol). Some diuretics themselves cause ototoxicity, and IV administered diuretics enhance aminoglycoside toxicity by altering antibiotic concentrations in serum and tissue.

Anesthetics, nondepolarizing neuromuscular blocking drugs (eg, tubocurarine, gallamine, metocurine iodide or pancuronium) or **succinylcholine** or in patients receiving massive transfusions of **citrate-anticoagulated blood:** Consider risk of neuromuscular blockade and respiratory paralysis when aminoglycosides are given concomitantly or sequentially. If blockade occurs, calcium salts or neostigmine may reverse the phenomenon.

Beta-lactam antibiotics (penicillins and cephalosporins) may inactivate aminoglycosides when admixed or coadministered. Ticarcillin and carbenicillin are the worst β-lactam offenders; tobramycin and gentamicin are more susceptible than netilmicin or amikacin. This is most likely to occur: When the agents are mixed in the same container; during the aminoglycoside assay procedure (see Drug/Lab Tests); and in poor renal function.

These penicillins have also decreased aminoglycoside serum levels (see Overdosage).

Inactivation of **tobramycin** has not occurred in patients with normal renal function if given the drugs by separate routes. **Kanamycin** and **methicillin** inactivate each other in vitro, but this has not been seen in patients who receive them by different routes.

Synergism: In vitro studies indicate that aminoglycosides combined with **penicillins** or **cephalosporins** act synergistically against some strains of gram-negative organisms and enterococci *(Streptococcus faecalis).* Aminoglycosides may exhibit a synergistic effect when combined with **carbenicillin** or **ticarcillin** for *Pseudomonas* infections. Tests for antibiotic synergy are necessary. Because of reported in vivo inactivation of aminoglycosides by these penicillins, adjust dose and spacing appropriately.

Drug/Lab Tests: Aminoglycoside serum levels - Guard against in vitro inactivation of aminoglycosides by β-lactam antibiotics in patients on combination therapy: 1) Place sample on ice immediately after drawing the specimen; test immediately. If testing is delayed, freeze serum as soon as possible. 2) Draw the aminoglycoside level when the β-lactam antibiotic is at its trough level. 3) Inactivation can still occur when the specimen is frozen (eg, kanamycin and ampicillin). If samples are to be frozen for a long period of time, inactivate the penicillin with penicillinase prior to freezing.

(Continued on following page)

Adverse Reactions:

Nephrotoxic: Proteinuria; hematuria and granular casts; azotemia; oliguria; rising BUN, non-protein nitrogen and serum creatinine. See Warnings and Drug Interactions.

Hepatic: Increased serum transaminases (SGOT, SGPT), serum LDH and bilirubin; hepatomegaly; hepatic necrosis.

Hematologic: Increased and decreased reticulocyte count; immature circulating white blood cells; leukemoid reaction; transient agranulocytosis; leukopenia; leukocytosis; thrombocytopenia; eosinophilia; pancytopenia; anemia; hemolytic anemia.

Ototoxic: Tinnitus, roaring in the ears, dizziness, vertigo, vestibular paralysis (gentamicin), and partial reversible to irreversible deafness have been reported, usually associated with higher than recommended dosage. See Warnings and Drug Interactions.

CNS: Confusion; disorientation; depression; lethargy; respiratory depression; nystagmus; visual disturbances; amblyopia; headache; fever; pseudotumor cerebri; acute organic brain syndrome; delirium (tobramycin).

Hypersensitivity: Purpura; rash; urticaria; angioneurotic edema; itching; exfoliative dermatitis; generalized burning; alopecia; anaphylactoid reactions; laryngeal edema; drug fever.

Neurotoxic: Numbness; skin tingling; circumoral or peripheral paresthesia; tremor; muscle twitching; convulsions; muscular weakness; neuromuscular blockade (acute muscular paralysis and apnea). Hypomagnesemia may occur in more than ⅓ of patients; patients whose oral diet is restricted or who are eating poorly are at high risk.

Gastrointestinal: Nausea; vomiting; anorexia; weight loss; hypersalivation; stomatitis.

Other: Pulmonary fibrosis; myocarditis (streptomycin); palpitations; splenomegaly; arthralgia; hypotension; hypertension; hyperkalemia; decreased serum calcium, magnesium, sodium and potassium; serum sickness (streptomycin); toxic epidermal necrolysis (streptomycin and neomycin).

Local: Local irritation or pain may follow IM injections. Rare subcutaneous atrophy or fat necrosis; a few cases of severe pain, induration and hematomas following **netilmicin** injection; arachnoiditis or burning at the injection site after intrathecal **gentamicin.**

Overdosage:

In the event of overdosage or toxic reaction, peritoneal dialysis or hemodialysis will aid in removal from the blood. Hemodialysis is preferable because it is more efficient in reducing serum levels. Complexation with ticarcillin or carbenicillin (12 to 20 g/day) appears as effective as continuous hemodialysis in lowering excessive aminoglycoside serum concentrations. In newborns, consider exchange transfusions. See the table below:

Range of half-lives (hours)[1]			
Aminoglycoside	Interdialysis	Hemodialysis	Peritoneal dialysis
Kanamycin	40-96	5	12
Gentamicin	21-59	6-11	5-29
Tobramycin	27-70	3-10	10-37
Amikacin	28-87	4-7	18-29
Netilmicin	24-52	5	

[1] Patient renal function creatinine clearance ≤ 5 ml/min.

Complete prescribing information for these products begins on page 1851
SPECIAL NOTE: See WARNING BOX on page 1853 concerning aminoglycoside toxicity.

STREPTOMYCIN SULFATE

Indications:

Mycobacterium tuberculosis: All forms when the infecting organisms are susceptible. Use only in combination with other antituberculous drugs.

Nontuberculous infections: Use only in serious infections caused by organisms shown by in vitro sensitivity studies to be susceptible, and when less potentially hazardous therapeutic agents are ineffective or contraindicated. Organisms usually sensitive include: *Yersinia pestis* (plague); *Francisella tularensis* (tularemia); *Brucella;* Donovanosis (granuloma inguinale); *Hemophilus ducreyi* (chancroid); *H influenzae* (with another agent); *Klebsiella pneumoniae* (with another agent); *Escherichia coli, Proteus* sp, *Enterobacter aerogenes, K pneumoniae* and *Streptococcus faecalis* in urinary tract infections; *S viridans,* gram-negative bacilli (in bacteremia, with another agent).

Administration and Dosage:

Administer IM only.

Tuberculosis: Therapy includes 1 g daily streptomycin and one or more additional antituberculars (isoniazid, ethambutol or rifampin). In pediatric patients, administer 20 to 40 mg/kg/24 hr and in patients with a creatinine clearance < 50 ml/min administer 500 mg twice weekly. Give elderly patients smaller doses in accordance with age, renal function and eighth nerve function. Ultimately, reduce dosage to 1 g, 2 or 3 times weekly. Terminate therapy when toxic symptoms appear, toxicity is feared, organisms become resistant or full therapeutic effect has been obtained. The total treatment period is a minimum of 1 year.

Tularemia: 1 to 2 g daily in divided doses for 7 to 10 days, or until the patient is afebrile for 5 to 7 days.

Plague: 2 to 4 g daily in divided doses until patient is afebrile for 3 days.

Bacterial endocarditis due to penicillin-sensitive alpha and non-hemolytic streptococci (sensitive to 0.1 mcg/ml or less of penicillin), use streptomycin for 2 weeks concomitantly with penicillin: 1 g twice daily for 1 week and 0.5 g twice daily for the second week. If patient is over 60, give 0.5 g twice daily for the entire 2 week period.

Enterococcal endocarditis: Give 1 g twice daily for 2 weeks and 0.5 g twice daily for 4 weeks in combination with penicillin.

For use with other agents to which infecting organism is also sensitive: (Streptomycin is a secondary choice.) Gram-negative bacillary bacteremia, meningitis and pneumonia; brucellosis; granuloma inguinale; chancroid; UTI.

Severe fulminating infections, 2 to 4 g/day IM (children – 20 to 40 mg/kg/day or 8 to 20 mg/lb/day) in divided doses every 6 to 12 hours; less severe infections and highly susceptible organisms, 1 to 2 g daily.

				C.I.*
Rx	**Streptomycin Sulfate** (Pharma-Tek)	**Injection:** 400 mg per ml	In 12.5 ml (5 g) vials.	20+
Rx	**Streptomycin Sulfate** (Lilly)	**Powder for Injection**	In 1 & 5 g for reconstitution.	40
Rx	**Streptomycin Sulfate** (Roerig)		In 1 & 5 g for reconstitution.	44

* Cost Index based on cost per 500 mg.

Complete prescribing information for these products begins on page 1851
SPECIAL NOTE: See WARNING BOX on page 1853 concerning aminoglycoside toxicity.

KANAMYCIN SULFATE

Warning:
Elderly patients with preexisting tinnitus or vertigo or known subclinical deafness, those having received prior ototoxic drugs, and patients receiving a total dose of > 15 g kanamycin sulfate should be carefully observed for signs of eighth nerve damage. Loss of hearing may occur, even with normal renal function.

Indications:

Consider initial therapy for one or more of the following: *Escherichia coli, Proteus* sp (both indole-positive and indole-negative), *Enterobacter aerogenes, Klebsiella pneumoniae, Serratia marcescens* and *Acinetobacter.* May be used as initial therapy with a penicillin or cephalosporin before obtaining results of susceptibility testing. Not the drug of choice for staphylococcal infections; may be indicated for initial therapy of severe infections where the strain is thought to be susceptible in patients allergic to other antibiotics, or in mixed staphylococcal/gram-negative infections.

Not indicated in long-term therapy (eg, tuberculosis) because of the toxic hazard associated with extended administration.

Administration and Dosage: Do not exceed a total of 1.5 g/day by any route.

IM: Inject deeply into the upper outer quadrant of the gluteal muscle. For adults or children, 7.5 mg/kg every 12 hours (15 mg/kg/day). If continuously high blood levels are desired, give the daily dose of 15 mg/kg in equally divided doses every 6 or 8 hours. Usual treatment duration is 7 to 10 days. Doses of 7.5 mg/kg give mean peak levels of 22 mcg/ml. At 8 hours after a 7.5 mg/kg dose, mean serum levels are 3.2 mcg/ml.

Uncomplicated infections should respond in 24 to 48 hours. If a clinical response does not occur within 3 to 5 days, stop therapy and reevaluate. Failure may be due to resistance of the organism or the presence of septic foci requiring surgical drainage.

IV: Do not admix with other antibacterial agents; administer separately.

Adults – Give slowly. Prepare by adding contents of 500 mg vial to 100 to 200 ml sterile diluent (Normal saline or 5% Dextrose in Water) or the contents of a 1 g vial to 200 to 400 ml of sterile diluent. Give over 30 to 60 min. Divide daily dose into 2 to 3 equal doses.

Children – Use sufficient diluent to infuse the drug over 30 to 60 minutes.

Dosing in renal failure: Follow therapy by appropriate serum assays. If not feasible, reduce frequency of administration. Calculate the dosage interval with the following formula: Serum creatinine (mg/100 ml) × 9 = dosage interval (in hours).

Intraperitoneal (following exploration for peritonitis or after peritoneal contamination due to fecal spill during surgery): 500 mg diluted in 20 ml sterile distilled water instilled through a catheter into the wound. If possible, postpone instillation until patient has recovered from anesthesia and muscle relaxants. Absorption after intraperitoneal instillation is equal to IM administration. After a single instillation of 250 or 500 mg, peak serum concentrations of 24 mcg/ml and 13.5 mcg/ml respectively, have been seen.

Aerosol treatment: 250 mg, 2 to 4 times a day. Withdraw 250 mg (1 ml) from 500 mg vial, dilute with 3 ml normal saline and nebulize.

Other routes: Concentrations of 0.25% have been used as irrigating solutions in abscess cavities, pleural space, peritoneal and ventricular cavities.

Stability: Darkening of vials during shelf life does not indicate loss of potency.

	Product	Form	Package	C.I.*
Rx	**Kanamycin Sulfate** (Various)	**Injection**: 500 mg	In 2 ml vials.	275+
Rx	**Kantrex** (Apothecon)		In 2 ml vials[1] & 2 ml disp. syringes.[1]	1077
Rx	**Klebcil** (Beecham Labs)		In 2 ml vials[1] & 2 ml disp. syringes.[1]	770
Rx	**Kanamycin Sulfate** (Various)	**Injection**: 1 g	In 3 ml vials.	248+
Rx	**Kantrex** (Apothecon)		In 3 ml vials.[1]	1068
Rx	**Klebcil** (Beecham Labs)		In 3 ml vials.[1]	760
Rx	**Kanamycin Sulfate** (Various)	**Pediatric Injection**: 75 mg	In 2 ml vials.	1033+
Rx	**Kantrex** (Apothecon)		In 2 ml vials.[1]	3193
Rx	**Klebcil** (Beecham Labs)		In 2 ml vials.[1]	2367

* Cost Index based on cost per 500 mg.

[1] With sodium bisulfite.

Complete prescribing information for these products begins on page 1851
SPECIAL NOTE: See Warning Box on page 1853 concerning aminoglycoside toxicity.

GENTAMICIN

Indications:

Treatment of serious infections caused by susceptible strains of *Pseudomonas aeruginosa, Proteus* sp (indole-positive and indole-negative), *Escherichia coli, Klebsiella-Enterobacter-Serratia* sp, *Citrobacter* sp and *Staphylococcus* sp (coagulase-positive and coagulase-negative).

Effective in neonatal sepsis; septicemia; serious infections of the CNS (meningitis), urinary tract, respiratory tract, GI tract (including peritonitis), skin, bone and soft tissue (including burns).

Not indicated in uncomplicated initial episodes of urinary tract infections, unless causative organisms are susceptible to these antibiotics and are not susceptible to antibiotics with less potential for toxicity. Perform bacterial cultures.

Gram-negative infections: Consider as initial therapy in suspected or confirmed gram-negative infections; institute therapy before obtaining results of susceptibility testing, but continue therapy based on susceptibility test results, infection severity and the concepts in the Warning Box on page 1853.

Unknown causative organisms: In serious infections, administer gentamicin as initial therapy in conjunction with a penicillin or cephalosporin before obtaining results of susceptibility tests. Following identification of the organism and its susceptibility, continue appropriate antibiotic therapy.

Combination therapy: Effective in combination with carbenicillin for the treatment of life-threatening infections caused by *P aeruginosa.* Also effective when combined with a penicillin for treatment of endocarditis caused by group D streptococci. In the neonate with suspected sepsis or staphylococcal pneumonia, penicillin is usually indicated concomitantly with gentamicin.

Staphylococcal infections: While not the antibiotic of first choice, consider gentamicin when penicillins or other less toxic drugs are contraindicated, when bacterial susceptibility tests and clinical judgment indicate its use and in mixed infections caused by susceptible strains of staphylococci and gram-negative organisms.

Intrathecal administration is indicated as adjunctive therapy to systemic gentamicin sulfate in the treatment of serious CNS infections (meningitis, ventriculitis) caused by susceptible *Pseudomonas* sp. Perform bacteriologic tests to determine that the causative organisms are susceptible to gentamicin.

Unlabeled Use: An alternative regimen for *pelvic inflammatory disease* is gentamicin 2 mg/kg IV followed by 1.5 mg/kg 3 times daily (normal renal function) plus clindamycin 600 mg IV 4 times daily. Continue for at least 4 days and at least 48 hours after patient improves; then continue clindamycin 450 mg orally 4 times daily for 10 to 14 days total therapy.

Administration and Dosage:

Monitoring: Because of the potential for toxicity, serum level monitoring is recommended when the drug is used in patients with impaired renal function, when doses in excess of 3 mg/kg/day are used, or when the drug is used in any patient in whom altered pharmacokinetics are suspected (ie, patients with extensive burns).

Generally, the peak concentration (at 30 to 60 minutes after IM injection or immediately after a slow IV infusion) is expected to be in the range of 4 to 6 mcg/ml. When monitoring peak concentrations, avoid prolonged levels above 12 mcg/ml. When monitoring trough concentrations (just prior to the next dose), avoid levels above 2 mcg/ml. When determining the adequacy of a serum level for a particular patient, consider susceptibility of the causative organism, infection severity and the status of the patient's host-defense mechanisms.

Dosage: May be given IM or IV. For patients with serious infections and normal renal function, give 3 mg/kg/day in 3 equal doses every 8 hours. For patients with life-threatening infections, administer up to 5 mg/kg/day in 3 or 4 equal doses. Reduce dosage to 3 mg/kg/day as soon as clinically indicated. *Obese patients* – Base dosage on an estimate of lean body mass.

Children – 6 to 7.5 mg/kg/day (2 to 2.5 mg/kg every 8 hours).

Infants and neonates – 7.5 mg/kg/day (2.5 mg/kg every 8 hours).

Premature or full term neonates (1 week of age or less) – 5 mg/kg/day (2.5 mg/kg every 12 hours). A regimen of either 2.5 mg/kg every 18 hours or 3 mg/kg every 24 hours may also provide satisfactory peak and trough levels in preterm infants less than 32 weeks gestational age.

(Administration and Dosage continued on following page)

GENTAMICIN (Cont.)

Administration and Dosage (Cont.):

Duration of therapy is usually 7 to 10 days. In difficult and complicated infections, a longer course of therapy may be necessary. In such cases, monitor renal, auditory and vestibular function, since toxicity is more apt to occur with treatment extended beyond 10 days. Reduce dosage if clinically indicated.

For prevention of bacterial endocarditis in dental/respiratory tract procedures: Special regimen for maximal protection (eg, patients with prosthetic valves) – Ampicillin 1 to 2 g IM or IV plus gentamicin 1.5 mg/kg IM or IV, ½ hour before procedure; follow by 1 g oral penicillin V, 6 hours after initial dose. Alternatively, the parenteral regimen may be repeated once, 8 hours after the initial dose.

For prevention of bacterial endocarditis in GI or GU tract surgery or instrumentation[1]*:* Give 2 g ampicillin IM or IV, plus 1.5 mg/kg gentamicin (not to exceed 80 mg) IM or IV. Administer ½ to 1 hour prior to procedure; give 1 additional dose in 8 hours. Pediatric doses are: 30,000 units/kg aqueous penicillin G or 50 mg/kg ampicillin; 2 mg/kg gentamicin. Pediatric doses should not exceed the recommended single dose or 24 hour dose for adults.

Penicillin allergic patients, vancomycin 1 g slowly IV over 1 hour may be substituted for ampicillin; the combination may be repeated in 8 to 12 hours.

Usage in impaired renal function: Adjust dosage; whenever possible, monitor serum concentrations of gentamicin. One method of dosage adjustment is to increase the interval between the doses administered.

Rule of eights – The serum creatinine concentration roughly correlates with the serum half-life of gentamicin. Creatinine clearance is better, but still roughly correlated with serum aminoglycoside levels. Approximate the interval between doses (in hours) by multiplying the serum creatinine level (mg/100 ml) by 8. For example, a patient weighing 60 kg with a serum creatinine level of 2 mg/100 ml could be given 60 mg (1 mg/kg) every 16 hours (2 x 8).

In patients with serious systemic infections and renal impairment, administer the antibiotic more frequently, but in reduced dosage. Measure serum concentrations of gentamicin so that appropriate levels result. Peak and trough concentrations, measured intermittently during therapy, will provide optimal guidance for adjusting dosage.

After the usual initial dose, a rough guide for determining reduced dosage at 8 hour intervals is to divide the normally recommended dose by the serum creatinine level. For example, after an initial dose of 60 mg (1 mg/kg), a patient weighing 60 kg with a serum creatinine level of 2 mg/100 ml could be given 30 mg every 8 hours (60 ÷ 2).

The status of renal function may change over the course of the infectious process. Deteriorating renal function may require a greater reduction in dosage than that specified in the above guidelines for patients with stable renal impairment. The above dosage schedules are not rigid recommendations, but are provided as rough guides to dosage when the measurement of gentamicin serum levels is not feasible.

Several predictive methods and published nomograms have been compared, none of which performed as well as individualized pharmacokinetic dosing with serum levels.

Hemodialysis – The amount of gentamicin removed from the blood may vary depending upon several factors, including the dialysis method used. An 8 hour hemodialysis may reduce serum concentrations of gentamicin by approximately 50%. The recommended dosage at the end of each dialysis period is 1 to 1.7 mg/kg, depending upon the severity of infection. In children, administer a dose of 2 to 2.5 mg/kg.

IV: The dose for IV and IM administration is identical; Administration IV is useful for treating patients with septicemia or those in shock. It may also be the preferred route for some patients with CHF, hematologic disorders, severe burns or reduced muscle mass. A 1 to 2 mg/kg loading dose is infused over 30 to 60 minutes, followed by a maintenance dose.

For intermittent IV administration in adults, dilute a single dose in 50 to 200 ml sterile isotonic saline or in a sterile solution of 5% Dextrose in Water. In infants and children, the volume of diluent should be less. Infuse over a period of ½ to 2 hours. Do not physically premix gentamicin with other drugs; administer separately in accordance with route and dosage schedule.

[1] Prevention of bacterial endocarditis. American Heart Association guidelines. *Circulation* 1984;70:1123A-1127A.

(Administration and Dosage continued on following page)

GENTAMICIN (Cont.)

Administration and Dosage (Cont.):

Intrathecal: Administer only the 2 mg/ml intrathecal preparation without preservatives.

Dosage will vary depending upon factors such as age and weight of the patient, site of injection, degree of obstruction to CSF flow and the amount of CSF estimated to be present. In general, the recommended dose for infants and children 3 months of age and older is 1 to 2 mg once a day. For adults, administer 4 to 8 mg once a day.

Continue administration as long as sensitive organisms are demonstrated in the CSF. Since the intralumbar or intraventricular dose is administered immediately after specimens are taken for laboratory study, continue treatment for at least 1 day after negative results have been obtained from CSF cultures or stained smears.

The suggested method for administering the intrathecal injection into the lumbar area is as follows: Perform the lumbar puncture and remove a specimen of the spinal fluid for laboratory tests, then insert syringe containing injection into the hub of the spinal needle. Allow a quantity of CSF (approximately 10% of the estimated total CSF volume) to flow into the syringe and mix with the gentamicin. Inject the resultant solution over a period of 3 to 5 minutes with the bevel of the needle directed upward.

If the CSF is grossly purulent, or if it is unobtainable, dilute gentamicin with sterile normal saline before injection.

May also be administered directly into the subdural space or directly into the ventricles, including administration by use of an implanted reservoir.

	Product	Strength	Package	C.I.*
Rx	**Gentamicin Sulfate IV Piggyback** (I.M.S.)	**Injection:** 100 mg per dose (as sulfate)	In 100 ml piggyback unit.	418
Rx	**Gentamicin Sulfate** (Elkins-Sinn)	**Injection:** 80 mg per dose (as sulfate)	In 2 ml Dosette.[1]	164
Rx	**Gentamicin Sulfate IV Piggyback** (I.M.S.)		In 80 ml piggyback unit.	491
Rx	**Garamycin IV Piggyback** (Schering)		In 80 ml piggyback unit.	419
Rx	**Gentamicin Sulfate** (Elkins-Sinn)	**Injection:** 60 mg per dose (as sulfate)	In 1.5 ml Dosette.[1]	192
Rx	**Gentamicin Sulfate IV Piggyback** (I.M.S.)		In 60 ml piggyback unit.	625
Rx	**Garamycin IV Piggyback** (Schering)		In 60 ml piggyback unit.	455
Rx	**Gentamicin Sulfate** (Elkins-Sinn)	**Injection:** 40 mg per ml (as sulfate)	In 2 and 20 ml vials.	100
Rx	**Gentamicin Sulfate** (Various)		In 2, 10 and 20 ml vials.	175+
Rx	**Garamycin** (Schering)		In 2 and 20 ml vials[1] and 1.5 and 2 ml disp. syringes.[1]	382
Rx	**Jenamicin** (Hauck)		In 2 ml vials.[1]	275
Rx	**Pediatric Gentamicin Sulfate** (Elkins-Sinn)	**Injection:** 10 mg per ml (as sulfate)	In 2 ml vials.[1]	272
Rx	**Garamycin Pediatric** (Schering)		In 2 ml vials.[1]	832
Rx	**Garamycin Intrathecal** (Schering)	**Injection:** 2 mg per ml (as sulfate)	In 2 ml amps.	4700

* Cost Index based on cost per 80 mg.

[1] With methyl and propyl parabens, EDTA and sodium bisulfite.

Information beginning on page 1851 must be considered when using these products.
SPECIAL NOTE: See WARNING BOX on page 1853 concerning aminoglycoside toxicity.

TOBRAMYCIN SULFATE

Indications:

Treatment of serious infections caused by susceptible strains of *Pseudomonas aeruginosa, Escherichia coli, Proteus* sp (indole-positive and indole-negative), *Providencia* sp, *Klebsiella-Enterobacter-Serratia* group, *Citrobacter* sp and staphylococci, including *S aureus* (coagulase-positive and coagulase-negative).

Septicemia in the neonate, child and adult caused by *P aeruginosa, E coli* and *Klebsiella* sp.

Lower respiratory tract infections caused by *P aeruginosa, Klebsiella* sp, *Enterobacter* sp, *Serratia* sp, *E coli* and *S aureus* (penicillinase and nonpenicillinase producing strains).

Serious CNS infections (meningitis) caused by susceptible organisms.

Intra-abdominal infections, including peritonitis, caused by *E coli, Klebsiella* sp and *Enterobacter* sp.

Skin, bone and skin structure infections caused by *P aeruginosa, Proteus* sp, *E coli, Klebsiella* sp, *Enterobacter* sp and *S aureus.*

Complicated and recurrent urinary tract infections caused by P aeruginosa, Proteus sp (indole-positive and indole-negative), *E coli, Klebsiella* sp, *Enterobacter* sp, *Serratia* sp, *S aureus, Providencia* sp and *Citrobacter* sp. Not indicated in uncomplicated initial episodes of UTIs unless the organisms are not susceptible to less toxic antibiotics.

Tobramycin may be considered in serious staphylococcal infections when penicillin or other potentially less toxic drugs are contraindicated and when bacterial susceptibility testing and clinical judgment indicate its use.

In patients in whom serious life-threatening gram-negative infection is suspected, including those in whom concurrent therapy with a penicillin or cephalosporin and an aminoglycoside may be indicated, initiate treatment with tobramycin before the results of susceptibility studies are obtained. Base the decision to continue therapy on susceptibility study results, infection severity and the concepts discussed in the Warning Box on page 1853 .

Administration and Dosage:

Use the patient's ideal body weight for dosage calculation. For obese patients, calculate appropriate dosage by using patient's estimated lean body weight plus 40% of the excess as the basic weight on which to figure mg/kg. Following 1 mg/kg IM, maximum serum concentrations reach about 4 mcg/ml, and measurable levels persist for as long as 8 hours. Serum concentrations of the drug given by IV infusion over 1 hour are similar to those obtained by IM use.

The usual duration of treatment is 7 to 10 days. A longer course of therapy may be necessary in difficult and complicated infections. In such cases, monitor renal, auditory and vestibular functions; toxicity can occur when treatment is extended > 10 days.

Monitor serum concentrations when feasible; avoid prolonged concentrations > 12 mcg/ml. Examine urine for decreased specific gravity and for increased excretion of protein, cells and casts.

Adults with serious infections: Administer 3 mg/kg/day in 3 equal doses every 8 hours.
Life-threatening infections – Administer up to 5 mg/kg/day in 3 or 4 equal doses. Reduce dosage to 3 mg/kg/day as soon as clinically indicated. To prevent increased toxicity due to excessive blood levels, do not exceed 5 mg/kg/day, unless serum levels are monitored.

Children: Administer 6 to 7.5 mg/kg/day in 3 or 4 equally divided doses (2 to 2.5 mg/kg every 8 hours or 1.5 to 1.9 mg/kg every 6 hours).

Prematures or full-term neonates (1 week of age or less): Administer up to 4 mg/kg/day in 2 equal doses every 12 hours. Preliminary data suggest that 2.5 mg/kg every 18 hours or 3 mg/kg every 24 hours may achieve safe and effective peak and trough serum concentrations in newborn infants weighing less than 1 kg at birth.

(Administration and Dosage continued on following page)

TOBRAMYCIN SULFATE (Cont.)

Administration and Dosage (Cont.):

Dosage in impaired renal function: Whenever possible, determine serum tobramycin concentrations.

Following a loading dose of 1 mg/kg, adjust subsequent dosage, either with reduced doses administered at 8 hour intervals or with normal doses given at prolonged intervals. Both of these methods are suggested as guides when serum levels of tobramycin cannot be measured directly. They are based on either creatinine clearance (preferred) or serum creatinine, because these values correlate with the half-life of tobramycin. The dosage schedules derived from either method should be used with careful clinical and laboratory observations of the patient; modify as necessary. These calculation methods may be misleading in patients who have undergone severe wasting and in the elderly. Do not use either method when dialysis is performed.

Reduced dosage at 8 hour intervals – When the creatinine clearance rate is 70 ml or less per minute, or when the serum creatinine value is known, determine the amount of the reduced dose by multiplying the normal dose by the percent of normal dose from the accompanying nomogram.

REDUCED DOSAGE NOMOGRAM†

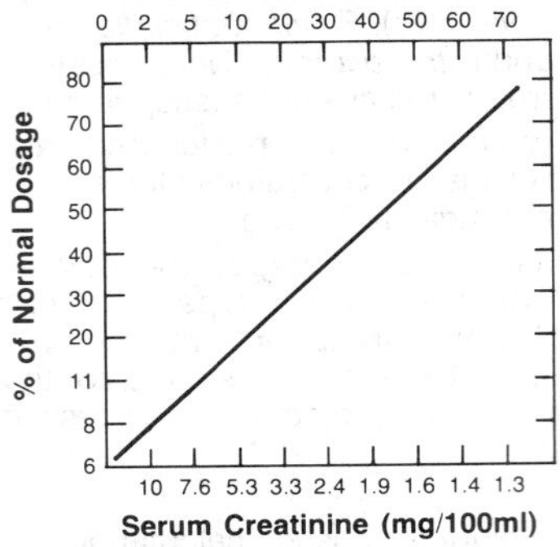

†Scales have been adjusted to facilitate dosage calculations.

An alternate guide for determining reduced dosage at 8 hour intervals (for patients whose steady-state serum creatinine values are known) is to divide the normally recommended dose by the patient's serum creatinine.

Normal dosage at prolonged intervals – If the creatinine clearance rate is not available and the patient's condition is stable, determine a dosage frequency (in hours) for the normal dosage by multiplying the patient's serum creatinine by 6.

Several predictive methods and published nomograms have been compared for gentamicin, none of which performed as well as individualized pharmacokinetic dosing with serum levels. This would probably also be true for tobramycin.

Hemodialysis removes approximately 50% of a dose in 6 hours. In anephric patients maintained by regular dialysis, the usual dose of 1.5 to 2 mg/kg given after every dialysis usually maintains therapeutic, nontoxic serum levels. In patients receiving intermittent peritoneal dialysis, patients dialyzed twice weekly should receive a 1.5 to 2 mg/kg loading dose followed by 1 mg/kg every 3 days. Where dialysis occurs every 2 days, a 1.5 mg/kg loading dose is given after the first dialysis and 0.75 mg/kg after each subsequent dialysis.

IV administration: The IV dose is the same as the IM. The usual volume of diluent (0.9% Sodium Chloride Injection or 5% Dextrose Injection) for adult doses is 50 to 100 ml. For children, the volume of diluent should be proportionately less than for adults. Infuse the diluted solution over a period of 20 to 60 minutes. Infusion periods of less than 20 minutes are not recommended, because peak serum levels may exceed 12 mcg/ml.

Do not physically premix with other drugs. Administer separately according to the recommended dose and route.

			C.I.*
Rx	**Tobramycin Sulfate** (Apothecon)	**Injection:** 40 mg/ml. In 1.5 and 2 ml disposable syringes and 2 ml vials.	NA
		Pediatric Injection: 10 mg/ml. In 2 ml vials.	NA
Rx	**Nebcin** (Lilly)	**Injection:** 80 mg/2 ml. In 2 ml Hyporets and 2 ml vials.[1]	633
		60 mg/1.5 ml. In 1.5 ml Hyporets.[1]	755
		Powder for Injection: 40 mg/ml after reconstitution. In 1.2 g vials.	573
		30 mg/ml after reconstitution. In 1.2 g vials.	573
		Pediatric Injection: 20 mg/2 ml. In 2 ml vials.[1]	1144

* Cost Index based on cost per 80 mg.

[1] With phenol, EDTA and sodium bisulfite.

Information beginning on page 1851 must be considered when using these products.
SPECIAL NOTE: See WARNING BOX on page 1853 concerning aminoglycoside toxicity.

AMIKACIN SULFATE

Indications:

Organisms: Short-term treatment of serious infections due to susceptible strains of gram-negative bacteria, including *Pseudomonas* sp, *Escherichia coli, Proteus* sp (indole-positive and indole-negative), *Providencia* sp, *Klebsiella-Enterobacter-Serratia* sp and *Acinetobacter (Mima-Herellea)* sp.

Infections: Effective in bacteremia and septicemia (including neonatal sepsis); in serious infections of the respiratory tract, bones and joints, CNS (including meningitis) and skin and soft tissue; in intra-abdominal infections (including peritonitis); and in burns and postoperative infections (including postvascular surgery). Also effective in serious complicated and recurrent urinary tract infections (UTIs) due to these organisms. Not indicated in uncomplicated initial episodes of UTIs unless the causative organisms are not susceptible to antibiotics having less toxicity.

Suspected gram-negative infections: Consider amikacin as initial therapy in suspected gram-negative infections, and institute therapy before obtaining the results of susceptibility testing. It is effective in infections caused by gentamicin or tobramycin resistant strains of gram-negative organisms, particularly *Proteus rettgeri, Providencia stuartii, Serratia marcescens* and *Pseudomonas aeruginosa.* Continue therapy based on susceptibility test results, infection severity, patient response and the concepts discussed in the Warning Box on page 1853 .

Staphylococcal infections: Consider as initial therapy under certain conditions in the treatment of known or suspected staphylococcal disease, such as: Severe infections where the causative organism may be either a gram-negative bacterium or a staphylococcus; infections due to susceptible strains of staphylococci in patients allergic to other antibiotics; and in mixed staphylococcal/gram-negative infections.

Neonatal sepsis when other aminoglycosides cannot be used. In severe infections, concomitant therapy with a penicillin-type drug may be indicated because of the possibility of infections due to gram-positive organisms, such as streptococci or pneumococci.

Unlabeled Use: Intrathecal/intraventricular administration has been suggested at 8 mg/24 hours.

Administration and Dosage:

Monitor the patient's renal status. Evidence of impairment in renal, vestibular or auditory function requires drug discontinuation or dosage adjustment. Examine urine for increased protein excretion, the presence of cells and casts and decreased specific gravity. Monitor serum concentrations and avoid prolonged peak concentrations above 35 mcg/ml. In normal adult volunteers, average peak serum concentrations of about 12, 16 and 21 mcg/ml are obtained 1 hour after IM administration of 250 mg (3.7 mg/ kg), 375 mg (5 mg/kg) and 500 mg (7.5 mg/kg) single doses, respectively. At 10 hours, serum levels are about 0.3 mcg/ml, 1.2 mcg/ml and 2.1 mcg/ml, respectively.

Use the patient's ideal body weight for dosage calculation. Administer IM or IV.

Adults, children and older infants: Administer 15 mg/kg/day divided into 2 or 3 equal doses at equally divided intervals. Treatment of heavier patients should not exceed 1.5 g/day. In UTIs, use 250 mg twice daily.

Neonates – A loading dose of 10 mg/kg is recommended, followed by 7.5 mg/kg every 12 hours. Preliminary IM studies in newborns of different weights (<1.5 kg, 1.5 to 2 kg, >2 kg) at a dose of 7.5 mg/kg revealed that, like other aminoglycosides, serum half-life values were correlated inversely with postnatal age and renal clearances of amikacin. Lower dosages may be safer during the first 2 weeks of life.

The usual duration of treatment is 7 to 10 days. Do not exceed 15 mg/kg/day. If treatment beyond 10 days is considered, monitor renal and auditory functions daily. Uncomplicated infections due to sensitive organisms should respond in 24 to 48 hours. If definite clinical response does not occur within 3 to 5 days, stop therapy and reevaluate. Failure of the infection to respond may be due to resistance of the organism or to the presence of septic foci requiring surgical drainage.

(Administration and Dosage continued on following page)

AMIKACIN SULFATE (Cont.)

Administration and Dosage (Cont.):

Usage in impaired renal function: Whenever possible, monitor serum concentrations. Adjust doses in patients with impaired renal function by administering normal doses at prolonged intervals or by administering reduced doses at a fixed interval. Both methods are based on the patient's creatinine clearance (preferred) or serum creatinine values, since these have been found to correlate with aminoglycoside half-lives. Use these dosage schedules in conjunction with clinical and laboratory observations of the patient, and modify, as necessary. These methods of dosage calculation may be misleading in patients who have undergone severe wasting, and in the elderly. Neither method should be used when dialysis is being performed.

Normal dosage at prolonged intervals – If the creatinine clearance rate is not available and the patient's condition is stable, calculate a dosage interval (in hours) for the normal dose by multiplying the patient's serum creatinine by 9.

Reduced dosage at fixed time intervals – Measure serum concentrations to assure accurate administration and to avoid concentrations above 35 mcg/ml. Initiate therapy by administering a normal dose, 7.5 mg/kg, as a loading dose.

To determine maintenance doses administered every 12 hours, reduce the loading dose in proportion to the reduction in the patient's creatinine clearance rate (Ccr):

$$\text{Maintenance Dose Every 12 Hours} = \frac{\text{observed Ccr (ml/min)}}{\text{normal Ccr (ml/min)}} \times \text{calculated loading dose (mg)}$$

An alternate rough guide for determining reduced dosage at 12 hour intervals (for patients whose steady-state serum creatinine values are known) is to divide the normally recommended dose by the patient's serum creatinine.

Several predictive methods and published nomograms have been compared for gentamicin, none of which performed as well as individualized pharmacokinetic dosing with serum levels. This would probably also be true for amikacin.

Dialysis: Approximately half the normal mg/kg dose can be given after hemodialysis; in peritoneal dialysis, a parenteral dose of 7.5 mg/kg is given, and then amikacin is instilled in peritoneal dialysate at a concentration desired in serum.

IV administration: Dose is identical to IM dose.

Normal adults – Single doses of 500 mg (7.5 mg/kg), administered as an infusion over a period of 30 minutes, produced a mean peak serum concentration of 38 mcg/ml at the end of the infusion, and levels of 24 mcg/ml, 18 mcg/ml and 0.75 mcg/ml at 30 minutes, 1 hour and 10 hours postinfusion, respectively. Repeated infusions of 7.5 mg/kg every 12 hours were well tolerated and caused no drug accumulation.

Preparation of solution – Prepare the solution for IV use by adding the contents of a 500 mg vial to 100 or 200 ml of sterile diluent. Administer the solution to adults over 30 to 60 minutes. Do not exceed 15 mg/kg/day, and divide into either 2 or 3 equal doses at equal intervals.

Infants – In pediatric patients, the amount of fluid used will depend on the amount ordered for the patient. It should be a sufficient amount to infuse the amikacin over 30 to 60 minutes. Infants should receive a 1 to 2 hour infusion.

Stability in IV fluids: Amikacin is stable for 24 hours at room temperature, at concentrations of 0.25 and 5 mg/ml in the following solutions: 5% Dextrose Injection; 5% Dextrose and 0.2% Sodium Chloride Injection; 5% Dextrose and 0.45% Sodium Chloride Injection; 0.9% Sodium Chloride Injection; Lactated Ringer's Injection; *Normosol M* in 5% Dextrose Injection (or *Plasma-Lyte 56* Injection in 5% Dextrose in Water); *Normosol R* in 5% Dextrose Injection (or *Plasma-Lyte 148* Injection in 5% Dextrose in Water). Do not physically premix amikacin with other drugs; administer separately according to recommended dose and route.

			C.I.*
Rx	**Amikacin Sulfate** (Elkins-Sinn)	**Injection:** 250 mg/ml.[2] In 4 ml and 2 ml *Dosette* vials.	NA
Rx	**Amikin** (Bristol Labs)	**Injection:** 100 mg per 2 ml vial.[1]	3729
		500 mg per 2 ml vial.[1]	1252
		500 mg per 2 ml disp. syringe.	1306
		1 g per 4 ml vial.[1]	1228

* Cost Index based on cost per 300 mg.

[1] With sodium bisulfite and sulfuric acid.

[2] With 6.6 mg sodium metabisulfite per ml.

Information beginning on page 1851 must be considered when using these products.
SPECIAL NOTE: See WARNING BOX on page 1853 concerning aminoglycoside toxicity.

NETILMICIN SULFATE

Indications:

For the short-term treatment of patients with serious or life-threatening bacterial infections caused by susceptible strains of the following organisms:

Complicated urinary tract infections caused by *Escherichia coli, Klebsiella pneumoniae, Pseudomonas aeruginosa, Enterobacter* sp, *Proteus mirabilis, Proteus* sp (indole-positive), *Serratia* and *Citrobacter* sp and *Staphylococcus aureus.*

Septicemia caused by *E coli, K pneumoniae, P aeruginosa, Enterobacter* sp, *Serratia* sp and *P mirabilis.*

Skin and skin structure infections caused by *E coli, K pneumoniae, P aeruginosa, Enterobacter* sp, *Serratia* sp, *P mirabilis, Proteus* sp (indole-positive) and *S aureus* (penicillinase and nonpenicillinase-producing strains).

Intraabdominal infections including peritonitis and intraabdominal abscess caused by *E coli, K pneumoniae, P aeruginosa, Enterobacter* sp, *P mirabilis, Proteus* sp (indole-positive), and *S aureus* (penicillinase and nonpenicillinase- producing strains).

Lower respiratory tract infections caused by *E coli, K pneumoniae, P aeruginosa, Enterobacter* sp, *Serratia* sp, *P mirabilis, Proteus* sp (indole-positive) and *S aureus* (penicillinase and nonpenicillinase-producing strains).

Consider netilmicin as initial therapy in suspected or confirmed gram-negative infections; institute therapy before obtaining results of susceptibility testing. Continue therapy based on the susceptibility test results, infection severity and the concepts contained in the Warning Box on page 1853 .

While not the antibiotic class of first choice, consider netilmicin for the treatment of serious staphylococcal infections when penicillins or other less potentially toxic drugs are contraindicated and when bacterial susceptibility tests and clinical judgment indicate their use. It may also be considered in mixed infections caused by susceptible strains of staphylococci and gram-negative organisms.

Netilmicin is indicated for those infections for which potentially less toxic antimicrobial agents are ineffective or contraindicated. It is not indicated in the treatment of uncomplicated initial episodes of urinary tract infection unless the causative organisms are resistant to antimicrobial agents having less potential toxicity.

In serious infections when the causative organisms are unknown, netilmicin may be administered as initial therapy in conjunction with a penicillin-type or cephalosporin-type drug before obtaining results of susceptibility testing. In neonates with suspected sepsis, a penicillin-type drug is also usually indicated as concomitant therapy with netilmicin. If anaerobic organisms are suspected, also give other suitable antimicrobial therapy. Following identification of the organism and its susceptibility, continue appropriate antibiotic therapy.

Has been used effectively in combination with carbenicillin or ticarcillin for the treatment of life-threatening infections caused by *P aeruginosa*.

Has been effective in the treatment of serious infections caused by some organisms resistant to other aminoglycosides.

Administration and Dosage:

Administer IM or IV. The recommended dosage for both methods is identical.

Obtain patient's pretreatment body weight for calculation of correct dosage. Base the dosage in obese patients on an estimate of the lean body mass.

Estimate status of renal function by measurement of the serum creatinine concentration or calculation of the endogenous creatinine clearance rate. The BUN level is much less reliable for this purpose. Periodically reassess renal function during therapy.

Burn patients: In patients with extensive body surface burns, altered pharmacokinetics may result in reduced serum concentrations. Measurement of netilmicin serum concentrations is particularly important as a basis for dosage adjustment.

Duration of treatment: Limit the duration of treatment to short-term whenever feasible. The usual duration of treatment is 7 to 14 days. In complicated infections, a longer course of therapy may be necessary. Although prolonged courses of netilmicin therapy have been well tolerated, it is particularly important to monitor patients carefully for changes in renal, auditory and vestibular functions. Adjust dosage if clinically indicated.

(Administration and Dosage continued on following page)

NETILMICIN SULFATE (Cont.)

Administration and Dosage (Cont.):

Measure serum concentrations periodically during therapy, both peak and trough, to determine the safety and efficacy of the administered dosage.

Peak serum concentrations range from 4 to 12 mcg/ml. Adjust dosage to attain the desired peak and trough concentrations and to avoid prolonged peak serum concentrations above 16 mcg/ml. When monitoring trough concentrations (just prior to the next dose), adjust dosage to avoid levels above 4 mcg/ml. Generally, desirable peak and trough concentrations range from 6 to 10 and 0.5 to 2 mcg/ml, respectively.

To determine the adequacy of a serum level, consider the susceptibility of the causative organism, the severity of the infection and the status of the patient's host-defense mechanisms.

The following dosage recommendations are intended as guides for initial therapy, or for when the measurement of netilmicin serum levels during therapy is not feasible.

Patients with normal renal function:

Adults – Complicated UTIs: 1.5 to 2 mg/kg every 12 hours (3 to 4 mg/kg/day).

Serious systemic infections: 1.3 to 2.2 mg/kg every 8 hours or 2 to 3.25 mg/kg every 12 hours (4 to 6.5 mg/kg/day).

Infants and children (6 weeks through 12 years) – Administer 1.8 to 2.7 mg/kg every 8 hours or 2.7 to 4 mg/kg every 12 hours (5.5 to 8 mg/kg/day).

Neonates (less than 6 weeks) – Administer 2 to 3.25 mg/kg every 12 hours (4 to 6.5 mg/kg/day).

Patients with impaired renal function: Individualize dosage. Dosage adjustment based upon serum drug concentrations during treatment is the most accurate.

If netilmicin serum concentrations are not available and renal function is stable, serum creatinine and creatinine clearance values are the most reliable, readily available indicators of the degree of renal impairment to guide dosage adjustment.

Deteriorating renal function may require a greater reduction in dosage than that specified in the guidelines given below for patients with stable renal impairment.

The initial or loading dose is the same as that for a patient with normal renal function. Three suggested methods to adjust the total daily dosage for the degree of renal impairment are:

1) Divide the suggested dosage value for patients with normal renal function by the serum creatinine level to obtain the adjusted size of each dose.

2) Determine the adjusted daily dose of netilmicin by multiplying the dose for patients with normal renal function by:

$$\frac{\text{Patient's Ccr}}{\text{Normal Ccr}}$$

3) Alternatively, use the following graph to obtain the percentage of the dose selected; it should be administered at 8 hour intervals:

REDUCED DOSAGE NOMOGRAM

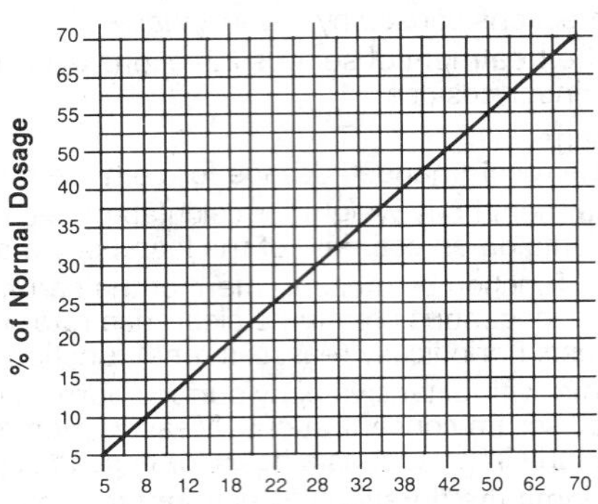

(Administration and Dosage continued on following page)

NETILMICIN SULFATE (Cont.)

Administration and Dosage (Cont.):

Patients with impaired renal function (Cont.):

Creatinine clearance can be estimated from serum creatinine levels by the following formula:

Males: $$\frac{\text{Weight (kg)} \times (140 - \text{age})}{72 \times \text{serum creatinine (mg/100 ml)}} = \text{Ccr}$$

Females: 0.85 x above value

The adjusted total daily dose may be administered as one dose at 24 hour intervals, or as 2 or 3 equally divided doses at 12 hour or 8 hour intervals, respectively. Generally, each individual dose should not exceed 3.25 mg/kg.

Hemodialysis – In adults with renal failure who are undergoing hemodialysis, the amount of netilmicin removed from the blood may vary, depending upon the dialysis equipment and methods used. In adults, a dose of 2 mg/kg at the end of each dialysis period is recommended until the results of tests measuring serum levels become available. Adjust dosage appropriately based on these tests.

Alternate dosing method (normal or impaired renal function): An alternate method of determining dosage regimen (dose and dosing interval) applicable to all ages and all states of renal function is to employ pharmacokinetic parameters derived from measurements of serum concentrations. This is probably the most reliable and accurate method.

IV administration: In adults, a single dose may be diluted in 50 to 200 ml of one of the parenteral solutions listed below. In infants and children, the volume of diluent should be less, according to the fluid requirements of the patient. The solution may be infused over a period of ½ to 2 hours.

Compatible solutions: Tested at concentrations of 2.1 to 3 mg/ml, netilmicin is stable in the following large volume parenteral solutions for up to 72 hours when stored in glass containers, both when refrigerated and at room temperature. Do not use after this time period. Sterile Water for Injection; 0.9% Sodium Chloride Injection alone or with 5% Dextrose; 5% or 10% Dextrose Injection in Water or 5% Dextrose with Electrolyte #48 or #75; Ringer's and Lactated Ringer's, and Lactated Ringer's with 5% Dextrose Injection; *10% Travert with Electrolyte #2* or *#3 Injection; Isolyte E, M* or *P* with 5% Dextrose Injection; 10% Dextran 40 or 6% Dextran 75 in 5% Dextrose Injection; *Plasma-Lyte 56* or *148* Injection with 5% Dextrose; *Plasma-Lyte M* Injection with 5% Dextrose; *Ionosol B* in D5-W; *Normosol-R; Plasma-Lyte 148* Injection (approx. pH 7.4); 10% Fructose Injection; Electrolyte #3 with 10% Invert Sugar Injection; *Normosol-M* or *R* in D5-W; *Isolyte H* or *S* with 5% Dextrose; *Isolyte S; Plasma-Lyte 148* Injection in Water; *Normosol-R* pH 7.4.

Storage: Store between 2° and 30°C (36° and 86°F). Protect from freezing.

			C.I.*
Rx	**Netromycin** (Schering)	**Injection:** 100 mg/ml. In 1.5 ml vials.[1]	534
		Pediatric Injection: 25 mg/ml. In 2 ml vials.[2]	560
		Neonatal Injection: 10 mg/ml. In 2 ml amps.[3]	2925

* Cost Index based on cost per 100 mg.

[1] With benzyl alcohol, EDTA, sodium metabisulfite and sodium sulfite.

[2] With methyl and propyl parabens, EDTA, sodium metabisulfite and sodium sulfite.

[3] With sodium metabisulfite and sodium sulfite.

Actions:

Oral aminoglycosides are not significantly absorbed; therefore use only for suppression of GI bacterial flora. The small absorbed fraction is rapidly excreted with normal kidney function. The unabsorbed drug is eliminated unchanged in the feces. Rarely, systemic toxicity may result from unintended absorption. Growth of most intestinal bacteria is rapidly suppressed, persisting for 48 to 72 hours. Nonpathogenic yeasts and occasionally resistant strains of *Enterobacter aerogenes* replace the intestinal bacteria. For complete information on the pharmacology of the aminoglycosides, refer to page 1851

Contraindications:

In the presence of intestinal obstruction; hypersensitivity to aminoglycosides.

Warnings:

Although negligible amounts are absorbed through intact mucosa, consider the possibility of increased absorption from ulcerated or denuded areas. In patients with renal dysfunction, this could lead to accumulation and toxicity.

Because of reported cases of deafness and potential nephrotoxic effects, closely observe patients. Perform urine and blood examinations and audiometric tests prior to and during extended therapy, especially in those with hepatic or renal disease. If renal insufficiency develops, reduce dosage or discontinue the drug.

Usage in Pregnancy: Safety for use during pregnancy has not been established. Use only when clearly needed and when the potential benefits outweigh the potential hazards.

Precautions:

Superinfection: Use of antibiotics (especially prolonged or repeated therapy) may result in bacterial or fungal overgrowth of nonsusceptible organisms. Such overgrowth may lead to a secondary infection. Take appropriate measures if superinfection occurs.

Drug Interactions:

Penicillin V potassium: Avoid concomitant use of oral neomycin, since malabsorption of penicillin V potassium has been reported.

Digitalis: Decreased therapeutic effect due to inhibition of absorption may occur with concurrent neomycin. Spacing doses of the two drugs may not circumvent the interaction. However, a small portion of the population ($<$ 10%) metabolizes digoxin in the GI tract; neomycin may increase digoxin serum levels in these patients. Addition or withdrawal of oral neomycin in patients stabilized on digoxin may result in fluctuations of serum digoxin concentration.

Oral anticoagulants: Oral aminoglycosides may increase the effects by causing malabsorption of vitamin K. It may be necessary to reduce the anticoagulant dose.

Methotrexate: Neomycin and paromomycin may decrease the oral absorption whereas kanamycin may have the opposite effect. The mechanism is unclear, but may relate to the known ability of these drugs to produce malabsorption.

Potent diuretics: Avoid concurrent use of aminoglycosides with such diuretics as ethacrynic acid, furosemide, bumetanide, urea and mannitol (particularly when the diuretics are given IV). They may cause cumulative adverse effects on the kidney and auditory nerve.

Other ototoxic or **nephrotoxic antimicrobial drugs:** Use caution with concurrent use.

Adverse Reactions:

Nausea, vomiting and diarrhea are most common. The "malabsorption syndrome" characterized by increased fecal fat, decreased serum carotene and fall in xylose absorption has been reported with prolonged therapy. *Clostridium difficile* associated colitis has been reported following neomycin therapy. Nephrotoxicity and ototoxicity have been reported following prolonged and high dosage therapy in hepatic coma.

Patient Information:

Complete full course of therapy; take until gone. May cause nausea, vomiting or diarrhea. Notify physician if ringing in the ears, hearing impairment or dizziness occurs.

KANAMYCIN SULFATE

Indications:

Suppression of intestinal bacteria: For short-term adjunctive therapy.

Hepatic coma: Prolonged administration is effective adjunctive therapy by reduction of the ammonia-forming bacteria in the intestinal tract. The subsequent reduction in blood ammonia has resulted in neurologic improvement.

Administration and Dosage:

Suppression of intestinal bacteria: As an adjunct to mechanical cleansing of the large bowel - 1 g every hour for 4 hours, followed by 1 g every 6 hours for 36 to 72 hours.

Hepatic coma: 8 to 12 g per day in divided doses.

			C.I.*
Rx	**Kantrex** (Apothecon)	**Capsules:** 500 mg (as sulfate). (Bristol 3506). In 20s & 100s.	180

* Cost Index based on cost per 500 mg.

Refer to the general discussion of these products on page 1868

NEOMYCIN SULFATE

Indications:

Preoperative suppression of intestinal bacteria for short or long-term adjunctive therapy.

Hepatic coma: Prolonged administration has been effective adjunctive therapy in hepatic coma by reduction of the ammonia-forming bacteria in the intestinal tract. The subsequent reduction in blood ammonia has resulted in neurologic improvement.

Unlabeled Use: Many studies have documented the lipid-lowering efficacy of neomycin. Administered alone, it reduced LDL cholesterol levels by 24%. Combined with niacin, it reduced LDL cholesterol level to below the 90th percentile in 92% of patients.

Administration and Dosage:

Preoperative prophylaxis for elective colorectal surgery: Give 3 doses of 1 g neomycin with 3 doses of 1 g erythromycin base enteric coated tablets on the third day of a 3 day regimen to prepare the patient for GI surgery. In this regimen, give bisacodyl orally on day 1. On day 2, give 30 mg of a 50% magnesium sulfate solution at 3 equally spaced intervals and 2 or more evening enemas until no solid feces are returned. On day 3, give 2 oral neomycin and erythromycin doses in the early afternoon 1 hour apart and give dose 3 at bedtime. Evacuate the rectum the next day, 1½ hours before surgery.

Below is a recommended bowel preparation regimen. Proposed surgery time is 8 am.

	Day 3	Day 2	Day 1
Diet	Minimum residue or clear liquid	Minimum residue or clear liquid	Clear liquid
Bisacodyl, one oral capsule	6 pm (−62 hrs)		
Magnesium sulfate, 30 ml of a 50% solution orally		10 am (−46 hrs). Repeat at 2 pm (−42 hrs) and 6 pm (−38 hrs).	10 am (−22 hrs). Repeat at 2 pm (−18 hrs).
Enema		7 pm (−37 hrs) & 8 pm (−36 hrs). Repeat hourly until no solid feces return with last enema.	None
Supplemental IV Fluids			As needed
Neomycin and Erythromycin tablets, 1 g each, orally			1 pm (−19 hrs). Repeat at 2 pm (−18 hrs) and 11 pm (−9 hrs).

On day of surgery the patient should evacuate the rectum at 6:30 am (−1½ hrs) for an 8 am procedure.

Hepatic coma (as an adjunct); the following regimen has been used: Withdraw protein from diet. Avoid diuretics. Use supportive therapy, including transfusions, as needed.

Neomycin sulfate orally in doses of 4 to 12 g/day in divided doses. In children, 50 to 100 mg/kg/day in divided doses. Continue treatment over a period of 5 to 6 days; during this time, return protein to the diet incrementally. Chronic hepatic insufficiency may require up to 4 g/day over an indefinite period.

			C.I.*
Rx	**Neomycin Sulfate** (Various)	**Tablets:** 500 mg. In 20s, 100s, 500s and UD 100s.	9+
Rx	**Mycifradin Sulfate** (Upjohn)	**Tablets:** 500 mg. (#Upjohn 521). In 100s and 500s.	47
		Oral Solution: 125 mg per 5 ml. In 480 ml.	78

PAROMOMYCIN SULFATE

Indications:

Intestinal amebiasis (acute and chronic): Note: Paromomycin is not effective in extraintestinal amebiasis. (See also p. 1945)

Hepatic coma: As adjunctive therapy.

Unlabeled Uses: Has been recommended for other parasitic infections – *Dientamoeba fragilis* (25 to 30 mg/kg/day in 3 doses for 7 days); *Diphyllobothrium latum, Taenia saginata, T solium, Dipylidium caninum* (adults: 1 g every 15 min for 4 doses, pediatric: 11 mg/kg every 15 min for 4 doses); *Hymenolepis nana* (45 mg/kg/day for 5 to 7 days).

Administration and Dosage:

Intestinal amebiasis: Adults and children - Usual dose is 25 to 35 mg/kg/day, in 3 doses with meals for 5 to 10 days.

Management of hepatic coma: Adults - Usual dose is 4 g/day in divided doses given at regular intervals for 5 to 6 days.

			C.I.*
Rx	**Humatin** (Parke-Davis)	**Capsules:** 250 mg paromomycin (as sulfate). (#P-D 529). Yellow and brown. In 16s.	87

* Cost Index based on cost per 500 mg neomycin or 250 mg paromomycin.

Product identification code.

COLISTIN SULFATE (POLYMYXIN E)

Actions:

Has in vitro bactericidal activity against most gram-negative enteric pathogens, especially enteropathogenic *Escherichia coli* and *Shigella* sp, but not *Proteus* sp. In infants and children, it has effectively controlled acute infections of the intestinal tract due to these pathogens. Susceptible strains of *E coli* and *Shigella* sp in vitro or in vivo rarely develop resistance. Cross-resistance to polymyxin B sulfate does exist, but cross-resistance to broad spectrum antibiotics has not been encountered.

When administered orally, colistin sulfate is not significantly absorbed into the systemic circulation.

Indications:

Diarrhea in infants and children, caused by susceptible strains of enteropathogenic *E coli.*

Gastroenteritis due to *Shigella* organisms. Clinical response may vary due to the absence of tissue levels in the bowel wall.

Contraindications:

Hypersensitivity to colistin sulfate.

Warnings:

Although colistin sulfate is not absorbed systemically in measurable amounts, it is assumed that slight absorption may occur. Therefore, a potential for renal toxicity exists in the presence of azotemia or if dosages above those recommended are used.

Superinfection: Use of antibiotics (especially prolonged or repeated therapy) may result in bacterial or fungal overgrowth of nonsusceptible organisms (ie, *Proteus*). Such overgrowth may lead to secondary infection. Take appropriate measures if superinfection occurs.

Precautions:

Assess renal function prior to initiation of therapy.

Adverse Reactions:

No adverse reactions or side effects have been reported within the recommended dosage range.

Administration and Dosage:

Usual dose is 5 to 15 mg/kg/day given in 3 divided doses. Higher doses may be necessary.

Preparation and storage: Reconstitute with 37 ml distilled water. Slowly add one-half of the diluent, replace the cap and shake well. Add remaining diluent and repeat shaking. When reconstituted, it is stable for 2 weeks when kept below 15°C (59°F).

			C.I.*
Rx	**Coly-Mycin S** (Parke-Davis)	**Powder for Oral Suspension:** 25 mg colistin (as sulfate) per 5 ml when reconstituted. Chocolate flavor. In 300 mg bottles.	368

* Cost Index based on cost per 100 mg.

COLISTIMETHATE SODIUM

Actions:

Microbiology: Has bactericidal activity against the following gram-negative bacilli: *Enterobacter aerogenes, Escherichia coli, Klebsiella pneumoniae* and *Pseudomonas aeruginosa.*

Pharmacokinetics: Administer either IV or IM. Higher initial blood levels are obtained following IV administration. Blood levels peak at over 5 mcg/ml between 1 and 2 hours after IM administration. Serum half-life is 2 to 3 hours.

Average urine levels range from about 270 mcg/ml at 2 hours to about 15 mcg/ml at 8 hours after IV administration and from about 200 to 25 mcg/ml during a similar period following IM administration.

Indications:

For the treatment of acute or chronic infections due to sensitive strains of certain gram-negative bacilli. Particularly indicated when the infection is caused by sensitive strains of *P aeruginosa.* Has proven clinically effective in treatment of infections due to the following gram-negative organisms: *E aerogenes, E coli, K pneumoniae* and *P aeruginosa.* Pending results of bacteriologic cultures and sensitivity tests, colistimethate may be used to initiate therapy in serious infections that are suspected to be due to gram-negative organisms.

Contraindications:

History of sensitivity to colistimethate sodium.

Not indicated for infections due to *Proteus* or *Neisseria* species.

Warnings:

Do not exceed 5 mg/kg/day in patients with normal renal function.

Neurologic effects may occur transiently. These include circumoral paresthesias or numbness, tingling or formication of the extremities, generalized pruritus, vertigo, dizziness and slurring of speech. Warn patients not to drive vehicles or use hazardous machinery while on therapy. Dosage reduction may alleviate symptoms. Therapy need not be discontinued, but observe such patients carefully. Overdosage can result in renal insufficiency, muscle weakness and apnea.

Usage in Pregnancy: Colistimethate sodium is transferred across the placental barrier, and blood levels of about 1 mcg/ml are obtained in the fetus following IV administration to the mother. Safety for use during pregnancy has not been established. Use only when clearly needed and when the potential benefits outweigh the unknown potential hazards.

Precautions:

Renal function impairment: Since colistimethate is eliminated mainly by renal excretion, use with caution when the possibility of impaired renal function exists. Consider the decline in renal function with advanced age.

When actual renal impairment is present, use colistimethate with extreme caution; reduce the dosage in proportion to the extent of the impairment. Administration of amounts in excess of renal excretory capacity will lead to high serum levels. This can result in further impairment of renal function, initiating a cycle which, if not recognized, can lead to acute renal insufficiency, renal shutdown and further concentration of the antibiotic to toxic levels in the body. Interference with nerve transmission at neuromuscular junctions may occur and result in muscle weakness and apnea.

Signs indicating the development of impaired renal function are diminishing urine output and rising BUN or serum creatinine. If present, discontinue therapy immediately. If a life-threatening situation exists, reinstate therapy at a lower dosage after blood levels have fallen.

If apnea occurs, treat with assisted respiration, oxygen and calcium chloride injections.

Drug Interactions:

Aminoglycosides and **cephalothin:** Avoid concurrent use with other **nephrotoxic** drugs. These toxic effects will be additive.

Anesthetics, neuromuscular blocking agents or **other drugs with neuromuscular blocking activity** (ie, aminoglycosides): Neuromuscular blockade and muscular paralysis may occur; this effect is additive when administered concomitantly. Avoid concurrent use of colistimethate sodium and these agents.

(Continued on following page)

COLISTIMETHATE SODIUM (Cont.)

Adverse Reactions:

Respiratory arrest has been reported following IM administration. Impaired renal function increases the possibility of apnea and neuromuscular blockade, generally because of failure to follow recommended guidelines, overdosage, failure to reduce dose commensurate with degree of renal impairment or concomitant use of other antibiotics or drugs with neuromuscular blocking potential.

Renal: A decrease in urine output or increase in BUN or serum creatinine can be signs of nephrotoxicity, which is probably a dose-dependent effect. These manifestations are reversible following discontinuation. Increases of BUN have been reported at dose levels of 1.6 to 5 mg/kg/day. Values returned to normal following cessation.

Miscellaneous: Paresthesia, tingling of the extremities or the tongue and generalized itching or urticaria have been reported by patients who received IV or IM injections. In addition, drug fever, GI upset, vertigo and slurring of speech have been reported. The subjective symptoms reported by the adult may not be manifest in infants or young children, thus requiring close attention to renal function.

Administration and Dosage:

For IM or IV use.

Adults and children: 2.5 to 5 mg/kg/day in 2 to 4 divided doses for patients with normal renal function, depending upon the severity of the infection. Reduce the daily dose in the presence of any renal impairment.

Suggested Modification of Dosage Schedules for Adults with Impaired Renal Function

RENAL FUNCTION			DOSAGE			
Degree of Impairment	Plasma Creatinine (mg/100 ml)	Urea Clearance % (of normal)	Dose (mg)	Frequency (times per day)	Total daily dose (mg)	Approx. daily dose (mg/kg)
Normal	0.7 - 1.2	80 - 100	100 - 150	4 to 2	300	5
Mild	1.3 - 1.5	40 - 70	75 - 115	2	150 - 230	2.5 - 3.8
Moderate	1.6 - 2.5	25 - 40	66 - 150	2 or 1	133 - 150	2.5
Severe	2.6 - 4	10 - 25	100 - 150	q 36 h	100	1.5

Note: Suggested unit dose is 2.5 to 5 mg/kg; increase time interval between injections in presence of impaired renal function.

IV administration:

Direct intermittent administration – Inject one-half the total daily dose over a period of 3 to 5 minutes every 12 hours.

Continuous infusion – Slowly inject one-half the daily dose over 3 to 5 minutes. Add the remaining half of the total daily dose of colistimethate to one of the following: 0.9% Sodium Chloride; 5% Dextrose in Water; 5% Dextrose with 0.9% Sodium Chloride; 5% Dextrose with 0.45% Sodium Chloride; 5% Dextrose with 0.225% Sodium Chloride; Lactated Ringer's solution or 10% invert sugar solution. Swirl gently to avoid frothing. Data are insufficient to recommend use with other drugs or other infusion solutions.

Administer by slow IV infusion starting 1 to 2 hours after the initial dose at a rate of 5 to 6 mg/hr in the presence of normal renal function. In the presence of impaired renal function, reduce infusion rate. Choice of IV solution and volume to be employed are dictated by requirements of fluid and electrolyte management.

Stability: Freshly prepare any infusion solution containing colistimethate and use for no longer than 24 hours.

			C.I.*
Rx	**Coly-Mycin M** (Parke-Davis)	**Powder for Injection:** 150 mg colistin (as colistimethate sodium) per vial for reconstitution.	959

* Cost Index based on cost per 100 mg.

POLYMYXIN B SULFATE, PARENTERAL

> **Warning:** When this drug is given intramuscularly or intrathecally, administer only to hospitalized patients to provide constant physician supervision.
>
> Carefully determine renal function; patients with renal damage and nitrogen retention should have reduced dosage. Patients with nephrotoxicity due to polymyxin B sulfate usually show proteinuria, cellular casts and azotemia. Diminishing urine output and a rising BUN are indications to discontinue therapy.
>
> Neurotoxic reactions may be manifested by irritability, weakness, drowsiness, ataxia, perioral paresthesia, numbness of the extremities and blurring of vision. These are usually associated with high serum levels found in patients with impaired renal function or nephrotoxicity. Avoid concurrent or sequential use of other nephrotoxic and neurotoxic drugs, particularly bacitracin, kanamycin, streptomycin, paromomycin, colistin, tobramycin, neomycin, gentamicin and amikacin.
>
> The drug's neurotoxicity can result in respiratory paralysis from neuromuscular blockade, especially when the drug is given soon after anesthesia or muscle relaxants.

Actions:

Polymyxin is bactericidal against almost all gram-negative bacilli except the *Proteus* group; it increases the permeability of bacterial cell membranes. All gram-positive bacteria, fungi and gram-negative cocci, *Neisseria gonorrhoeae* and *N meningitidis,* are resistant.

Pharmacokinetics: Polymyxin B sulfate is not absorbed from the normal GI tract. Since the drug loses 50% of its activity in the presence of serum, active blood levels are low. Repeated injections may give a cumulative effect. Levels tend to be higher in infants and children. Tissue diffusion is poor, and the drug does not pass the blood-brain barrier into the cerebrospinal fluid (CSF). The drug is excreted slowly by the kidneys. In therapeutic dosage, it causes some nephrotoxicity with slight tubule damage.

Indications:

Acute infections caused by susceptible strains of *Pseudomonas aeruginosa.* It may be used topically and subconjunctively in the treatment of infections of the eye caused by susceptible strains of *P aeruginosa.*

It may be indicated (when less toxic drugs are ineffective or contraindicated) in serious infections caused by susceptible strains of the following organisms: *Hemophilus influenzae* (meningeal infections); *Escherichia coli* (urinary tract infections); *Enterobacter aerogenes* (bacteremia); *Klebsiella pneumoniae* (bacteremia).

Note: In meningeal infections, administer polymyxin B sulfate only intrathecally.

Contraindications:

History of hypersensitivity reactions to the polymyxins.

Warnings:

Usage in Pregnancy: Safety for use during pregnancy has not been established.

Precautions:

Determine baseline renal function prior to therapy. Frequently monitor renal function and drug blood levels during therapy. The use of doses higher than those recommended is dangerous and potentially fatal. In doses of 3 mg/kg/day (30,000 U), polymyxin B may cause nephrotoxicity in patients with normal renal function, but lower doses may cause renal damage in patients with preexisting renal impairment.

Superinfection: Use of antibiotics (especially prolonged or repeated therapy) may result in bacterial or fungal overgrowth of nonsusceptible organisms. Such overgrowth may lead to a secondary infection. Take appropriate measures if superinfection occurs.

Drug Interactions:

Aminoglycosides and other **nephrotoxic** drugs: Avoid concurrent use; these toxic effects will be additive.

Anesthetics, neuromuscular blocking agents or **other drugs with neuromuscular blocking activity** (ie, aminoglycosides): Neuromuscular blockade and muscular paralysis may occur; this effect is additive when administered concomitantly. Avoid concurrent use.

(Continued on following page)

POLYMYXIN B SULFATE, PARENTERAL (Cont.)

Adverse Reactions:

Nephrotoxic: Proteinuria, casts, azotemia, rising blood levels without increase in dosage.

Neurotoxic: Facial flushing; dizziness progressing to ataxia; drowsiness; peripheral paresthesias, circumoral and stocking-glove; apnea due to concurrent use of curariform muscle relaxants, other neurotoxic drugs or inadvertent overdosage.

Meningeal irritation with intrathecal administration, eg, fever, headache, stiff neck and increased cell count and protein in cerebrospinal fluid (CSF).

Other: Occasionally reported – Drug fever, urticarial rash; severe pain at IM injection sites; thrombophlebitis at IV injection sites.

Administration and Dosage:

Intravenous: Dissolve 500,000 units polymyxin B sulfate in 300 to 500 ml of 5% Dextrose in Water for continuous IV drip.

Adults and children – 15,000 to 25,000 units/kg/day in individuals with normal renal function. Reduce this amount from 15,000 units/kg downward for individuals with renal impairment. Infusions may be given every 12 hours; however, the total daily dose must not exceed 25,000 units/kg/day.

Infants – Infants with normal renal function may receive up to 40,000 units/kg/day.

Intramuscular: Not recommended routinely because of severe pain at injection sites, particularly in infants and children. Dissolve 500,000 units polymyxin B sulfate in 2 ml sterile distilled water (Water for Injection, USP) or sterile physiologic saline (Sodium Chloride Injection) or 1% procaine HCl solution.

Adults and children – 25,000 to 30,000 units/kg/day. Reduce dosage in the presence of renal impairment. Dosage may be divided and given at either 4 or 6 hour intervals.

Infants with normal renal function may receive up to 40,000 units/kg/day.

Note: Doses as high as 45,000 units/kg/day have been used in limited clinical studies in treating premature and newborn infants for sepsis caused by *Pseudomonas aeruginosa.*

Intrathecal: A treatment of choice for *P aeruginosa* meningitis. Dissolve 500,000 units polymyxin B sulfate in 10 ml sterile physiologic saline for a concentration of 50,000 units/ml.

Adults and children over 2 years of age – Dosage is 50,000 units once daily intrathecally for 3 to 4 days, then 50,000 units once every other day for at least 2 weeks after cultures of the CSF are negative and glucose content has returned to normal.

Children less than 2 years of age – 20,000 units once daily, intrathecally for 3 to 4 days or 25,000 units once every other day. Continue with a dose of 25,000 units once every other day for at least 2 weeks after cultures of the CSF are negative and glucose content has returned to normal.

Storage of solution: Refrigerate and discard any unused portion after 72 hours.

			C.I.*
Rx	**Polymyxin B Sulfate** (Roerig)	**Injection:** 500,000 units per 20 ml vial.	1056
Rx	**Aerosporin** (Burroughs Wellcome)	**Powder for Injection:** 500,000 units per vial.	1840

* Cost Index based on cost per 1,000,000 units.

BACITRACIN, INTRAMUSCULAR

Warning:

Nephrotoxicity: Parenteral (IM) bacitracin may cause renal failure due to tubular and glomerular necrosis. Restrict its use to infants with staphylococcal pneumonia and empyema when due to organisms shown to be susceptible to bacitracin. Use only where adequate laboratory facilities are available and when constant supervision of the patient is possible.

Carefully determine renal function prior to therapy, and daily during therapy. Do not exceed the recommended daily dose, and maintain fluid intake and urinary output at proper levels to avoid renal toxicity. If renal toxicity occurs, discontinue the drug.

Actions:

Bacitracin exerts pronounced antibacterial action in vitro against a variety of gram-positive and a few gram-negative organisms. However, among systemic diseases, only staphylococcal infections qualify for consideration of bacitracin therapy. Bacitracin is assayed against a standard, and its activity is expressed in units, 1 mg having a potency of not less than 50 units.

Susceptibility plate testing: If the Kirby-Bauer method of disk susceptibility is used, a 10 unit bacitracin disk should give a zone of over 13 mm when tested against a bacitracin-susceptible strain of *Staphylococcus aureus*.

Pharmacokinetics: Absorption of bacitracin following IM injection is rapid and complete. A dose of 200 or 300 units/kg every 6 hours gives serum levels of 0.2 to 2 mcg/ml in individuals with normal renal function. It is widely distributed in all body organs and is demonstrable in ascitic and pleural fluids. It is excreted slowly by glomerular filtration.

Indications:

Limit use of IM bacitracin to the treatment of infants with pneumonia and empyema caused by staphylococci shown to be sensitive to the drug (see Warning Box).

Unlabeled Use: Bacitracin administered orally has been used successfully in the treatment of antibiotic-associated colitis.

Contraindications:

Previous hypersensitivity or toxic reaction to bacitracin.

Precautions:

See Warning Box.

Maintain adequate fluid intake orally, or if necessary, parenterally.

Superinfection: Use of antibiotics (especially prolonged or repeated therapy) may result in bacterial or fungal overgrowth of nonsusceptible organisms. Such overgrowth may lead to a secondary infection. Take appropriate measures if superinfection occurs.

Drug Interactions:

Aminoglycosides and other **nephrotoxic** drugs: Avoid concurrent use; these toxic effects will be additive.

Anesthetics, neuromuscular blocking agents or **other drugs with neuromuscular blocking activity** (ie, aminoglycosides): Neuromuscular blockade and muscular paralysis may occur; this effect is additive when administered concomitantly. Avoid concurrent use with bacitracin IM.

Adverse Reactions:

Proteinuria; casts; azotemia; rising blood levels without increase in dosage; nausea and vomiting; pain at injection site; skin rashes.

Administration and Dosage:

For IM use only.

Infants under 2.5 kg: 900 units/kg/24 hours, in 2 or 3 divided doses.

Infants over 2.5 kg: 1000 units/kg/24 hours, in 2 or 3 divided doses.

Preparation of solutions: Dissolve in Sodium Chloride Injection containing 2% procaine HCl. The concentration of the antibiotic in the solution should not be less than 5000 units/ml nor more than 10,000 units/ml.

Do not use diluents containing parabens to reconstitute bacitracin; cloudy solutions and precipitate formation have occurred. Reconstitution of the 50,000 unit vial with 9.8 ml of diluent and the 10,000 unit vial with 2 ml of diluent will result in a concentration of 5000 units/ml.

Storage: Refrigerate the unreconstituted product at 2° to 8°C (36° to 46°F). Solutions are stable for 1 week when refrigerated at 2° to 8°C (36° to 46°F).

			C.I.*
Rx	**Bacitracin USP** (Upjohn)	**Powder for Injection:** 10,000 unit vials.	310
		50,000 unit vials.	1702
Rx	**Bacitracin Sterile** (Roerig)	**Injection:** 50,000 unit vials.	1790

* Cost Index based on cost per 10,000 units.

NOVOBIOCIN

Warning: Use only for serious infections where less toxic drugs are ineffective or contraindicated because of: (1) High frequency of adverse reactions, principally urticaria and maculopapular dermatitis. Hepatic dysfunction and blood dyscrasias are less frequent. (2) Rapid and frequent emergence of resistant strains, especially staphylococci.

Actions:

Novobiocin, primarily bacteriostatic, inhibits protein and nucleic acid synthesis and interferes with bacterial cell wall synthesis. In vitro, it is active against *Staphylococcus aureus* and some *Proteus vulgaris* strains. In vitro, *S aureus* rapidly develops resistance.

Pharmacokinetics: Novobiocin is well absorbed from the GI tract. Peak serum levels, which occur in about 2 hours, are higher when taken in the fasting state. The drug is highly bound to serum proteins (>90%) and diffusion into body fluids is poor. Small amounts may penetrate into the cerebrospinal fluid if the meninges are inflamed. Excretion is primarily via the bile and feces; 3% is excreted in the urine.

Indications:

Serious infections due to susceptible *S aureus* when other effective antibiotics are contraindicated. May be useful in the few urinary tract infections caused by *Proteus* sp sensitive to novobiocin but resistant to other therapy.

Contraindications: Known sensitivity to novobiocin.

Warnings:

Usage in Pregnancy: Category C. It is not known whether novobiocin causes fetal harm when administered to a pregnant woman. Use only when clearly needed.

Usage in Lactation: Safety and efficacy for use in the nursing mother have not been established. Novobiocin reaches low levels in milk (0.34 to 0.54 mg/100 ml); kernicterus may develop in the neonate. Effects on the neonate may include modification of bowel flora, direct effects and interference of cultures for fever evaluation.

Usage in Infants: Affects bilirubin metabolism; avoid use in newborns and prematures.

Precautions:

Novobiocin possesses a high index of sensitization. If allergic reactions develop during treatment and are not readily controlled by the usual measures, discontinue use.

Routinely perform hepatic and hematologic studies. Discontinue use if liver dysfunction develops and if hematologic studies show evidence of leukopenia or blood dyscrasias.

Superinfection: Use of antibiotics (especially prolonged or repeated therapy) may result in bacterial or fungal overgrowth of nonsusceptible organisms. Such overgrowth may lead to a secondary infection. Take appropriate measures if superinfection occurs.

Drug Interactions:

Drug/Lab: Novobiocin may cause "pseudojaundice" (yellow skin and plasma). This may interfere with **serum bilirubin** and **icterus index determinations**.

The drug may interfere with the hepatic uptake or biliary excretion of **sulfobromophthalein** in the bromsulphalein test.

Adverse Reactions:

Hypersensitivity: Reactions consist of skin eruptions, including urticarial, erythematous, maculopapular or scarlatiniform rash (10% to 15% of patients receiving therapy for 1 week or longer develop a rash). Erythema multiforme has occurred, but is rare.

Hematopoietic: Blood dyscrasias including leukopenia, eosinophilia (with or without fever), anemia, pancytopenia, agranulocytosis and thrombocytopenia have occurred.

Hepatic dysfunction: Jaundice, elevation of unconjugated bilirubin, impaired bromsulphalein excretion. Yellow discoloration of plasma, skin and sclerae may occur due to lipochrome pigment metabolite; normal serum bilirubin distinguishes this from jaundice.

Miscellaneous: Nausea and vomiting; loose stools and diarrhea (fairly common but usually doesn't necessitate discontinuing therapy); intestinal hemorrhage; alopecia.

Patient Information:

Complete full course of therapy. Notify physician of skin rash or hives; yellowish discoloration of skin or eyes; fever, sore throat; or unusual bleeding or bruising.

Administration and Dosage:

Adults: 250 mg every 6 hours or 500 mg every 12 hours. Continue for at least 48 hours after temperature has returned to normal and evidence of infection has disappeared. In severe or unusually resistant infections, give 0.5 g every 6 hours or 1 g every 12 hours.

Children: 15 mg/kg/day for moderate acute infections; up to 30 to 45 mg/kg/day for severe infections. Give in divided doses every 6 to 12 hours.

			C.I.*
Rx	**Albamycin** (Upjohn)	**Capsules:** 250 mg novobiocin (as sodium). (#Upjohn 101). White and maroon. In 100s.	112

* Cost Index based on cost per 250 mg. # Product identification code.

METRONIDAZOLE

> **Warning:**
> Metronidazole has been shown to be carcinogenic in rodents. Avoid unnecessary use.

Actions:

Pharmacology:

Metronidazole, a nitroimidazole, is active against various anaerobic bacteria and protozoa. Its mode of action is not well understood. It appears to enter the target cell, where its nitro group is reduced. Unstable intermediate compounds are formed which bind to DNA and inhibit synthesis, causing cell death.

Microbiology: Metronidazole is active in vitro against most obligate anaerobes, but does not appear to possess activity against facultative anaerobes or obligate aerobes. Against susceptible organisms, it is generally bactericidal at concentrations equal to or slightly higher than the minimal inhibitory concentrations (MICs). Metronidazole is active against anaerobic gram-negative bacilli, including *Bacteroides* sp, (eg, *B fragilis, B distasonis, B ovatus, B thetaiotaomicron, B vulgatus*); *Fusobacterium* sp; anaerobic gram-positive bacilli, including: *Clostridium* sp and susceptible strains of *Eubacterium*; anaerobic gram-positive cocci, including *Peptococcus* sp and *Peptostreptococcus* sp; anaerobic protozoa, including *Trichomonas vaginalis, Entamoeba histolytica, Giardia lamblia* and *Balantidium coli.*

Perform bacteriologic studies to determine the causative organisms and their susceptibility; however, therapy may be started while awaiting these results.

Pharmacokinetics:

Absorption – Metronidazole is well absorbed after oral administration (similar to IV values). It is absorbed about one-half and one-fifth as well via rectal and vaginal administration, respectively. Peak serum levels occur at about 1 hour, 4 hours and 8 to 24 hours, respectively. Oral bioavailability is not affected by food, but peak serum levels will be delayed to about 2 hours.

Distribution – Metronidazole has a large apparent volume of distribution. It diffuses well into all tissues, achieving therapeutic levels in bone, pelvic tissues, bile, saliva, seminal fluid, breast milk, placenta, abscesses (including hepatic abscesses), empyema fluid, middle ear fluid and cerebrospinal fluid (approximately 50% of serum concentration in patients with normal meninges, approximates serum concentration in patients with inflamed meninges). Less than 20% of the circulating drug is bound to plasma proteins. Plasma concentrations are proportional (linear) to the administered dose, both IV and oral. A dosage regimen of 15 mg/kg loading dose, followed by 7.5 mg/kg every 6 hours, produces peak steady-state plasma concentrations averaging 25 mcg/ml, with trough concentrations averaging 18 mcg/ml. Multiple dosing results in some drug accumulation.

Metabolism – Metronidazole is the major component appearing in the plasma, along with lesser quantities of the 2-hydroxymethyl metabolite and an acidic metabolite. The metabolites that appear in the urine result primarily from side-chain oxidation and glucuronide conjugation, with unchanged metronidazole accounting for approximately 20% of the total. Both the parent compound and the 2-hydroxymethyl metabolite possess in vitro bactericidal activity against most strains of anaerobic bacteria.

Elimination – The major route of elimination of metronidazole and its metabolites is via the urine (60% to 80% of the dose); fecal excretion accounts for 6% to 15% of the dose. Renal clearance is approximately 10 ml/min/1.73 m^2.

Metronidazole has an elimination half-life range in healthy humans of 6.2 to 10 hours. The hydroxy-metabolite has a half-life of $\approx$ 15 hours. In patients with creatinine clearances $>$ 10 ml/min, the accumulation of metronidazole or its metabolites is unlikely to produce toxicity. Patients with creatinine clearances $<$ 10 ml/min (not receiving dialysis) will accumulate both metabolites. Metronidazole and its two major metabolites are extensively removed by hemodialysis. Mean dialysis clearance values for parent compound and metabolites range from 60 to 125 ml/min, depending on the membrane used. Metronidazole is also removed by peritoneal dialysis. Plasma clearance is decreased in patients with decreased liver function.

Pharmacokinetic parameters are not significantly altered in patients with serious anaerobic infections or during pregnancy. However, neonates have a slower elimination of metronidazole; dosage adjustment may be necessary.

(Continued on following page)

METRONIDAZOLE (Cont.)

Indications:

Anaerobic infections: The treatment of serious infections caused by susceptible anaerobic bacteria. Effective in *Bacteroides fragilis* infections resistant to clindamycin, chloramphenicol and penicillin.

Intraabdominal infections (peritonitis, intraabdominal abscess and liver abscess), caused by *Bacteroides* sp (*B fragilis, B distasonis, B ovatus, B thetaiotaomicron, B vulgatus*); Clostridium sp, *Eubacterium* sp, *Peptostreptococcus* sp, *Peptococcus* sp.

Skin and skin structure infections, caused by *Bacteroides* sp including the *B fragilis* group, *Clostridium* sp, *Peptococcus* sp, *Peptostreptococcus* sp and *Fusobacterium* sp.

Gynecologic infections (endometritis, endomyometritis, tubo-ovarian abscess and postsurgical vaginal cuff infection), caused by *Bacteroides* sp including the *B fragilis* group, *Clostridium* sp, *Peptococcus* sp and *Peptostreptococcus* sp.

Bacterial septicemia caused by *Bacteroides* sp including the *B fragilis* group and *Clostridium* sp.

Bone and joint infections caused by *Bacteroides* sp including the *B fragilis* group, as adjunctive therapy.

CNS infections (meningitis and brain abscess), *lower respiratory tract infections* (pneumonia, empyema and lung abscess) and *endocarditis* caused by *Bacteroides* sp including the *B fragilis* group.

Also indicated orally for amebiasis and trichomoniasis (see page1947).

Prophylaxis: Preoperative, intraoperative and postoperative IV metronidazole may reduce the incidence of postoperative infection in patients undergoing elective colorectal surgery which is classified as contaminated or potentially contaminated.

Discontinue within 12 hours after surgery. If there are signs of infection, obtain specimens for cultures to identify the causative organisms.

Unlabeled Uses: Metronidazole has shown efficacy, alone and in combination, as prophylaxis in reducing infection rates in gynecologic and abdominal surgery.

Hepatic encephalopathy: Metronidazole has compared favorably to neomycin.

Radiosensitizers, rendering resistant tumors more susceptible to radiation therapy. Results have not been convincing; more data are needed.

Crohn's disease: Metronidazole has been successful, with particular improvement of perineal manifestations.

Antibiotic-associated pseudomembranous colitis: Metronidazole is as effective as vancomycin (1 to 2 g/day for 7 to 10 days).

The **CDC** has recommended the use of oral metronidazole for bacterial vaginosis (500 mg, twice daily for 7 days) and for giardiasis (alternative to quinacrine; 250 mg, 3 times daily for 7 days).

Contraindications:

Hypersensitivity to metronidazole or other nitroimidazole derivatives.

Contraindicated in the first trimester of pregnancy in patients with trichomoniasis. (See Warnings.)

Warnings:

Neurologic effects: Seizures (associated with high cumulative doses) and peripheral neuropathy (characterized by numbness or paresthesia of an extremity) have been reported. Peripheral neuropathy occurs rarely when metronidazole is used in low doses for short durations. Carefully monitor patients receiving high doses for long periods (eg, Crohn's disease). In some cases, neuropathy is not reversible. Appearance of abnormal neurologic signs demands prompt evaluation of the benefit/risk ratio of the continuation of therapy. Administer metronidazole with caution to patients with CNS diseases.

Sodium retention may result from solutions containing sodium ions. Carefully give metronidazole to patients on corticosteroids or to patients predisposed to edema.

Usage in impaired hepatic function: Patients with severe hepatic disease metabolize metronidazole slowly. Accumulation of the drug and its metabolites may occur. Cautiously administer doses below those usually recommended.

Usage in Pregnancy: Metronidazole crosses the placenta and enters fetal circulation rapidly. Animal studies at doses up to 5 times the human dose have revealed no evidence of impaired fertility or harm to the fetus. There are no adequate and well controlled studies in pregnant women. Use during pregnancy only if clearly needed.

Restrict metronidazole for trichomoniasis in the second and third trimesters to those in whom local palliative treatment has been inadequate to control symptoms.

Usage in Lactation: Safety for use in the nursing mother has not been established. Metronidazole is secreted in breast milk in concentrations similar to those found in plasma. Its half-life in breast milk is about 9 to 10 hours. A nursing mother should express and discard any breast milk produced while on the drug and resume nursing 24 to 48 hours after the drug is discontinued.

(Warnings continued on following page)

METRONIDAZOLE (Cont.)

Warnings (Cont.):

Usage in Children: Safety and efficacy in children have not been established, except for the treatment of amebiasis. Newborns demonstrate a diminished capacity to eliminate metronidazole. The elimination half-life is inversely related to gestational age. In infants whose gestational ages were between 28 and 40 weeks, the corresponding elimination half-lives ranged from 109 to 22.5 hours.

Precautions:

Candidiasis, known or previously unrecognized, may present more prominent symptoms during therapy and requires treatment with a candicidal agent.

Hematologic effects: Metronidazole is a nitroimidazole; use with care in patients with evidence or history of blood dyscrasia. Mild leukopenia has been seen during administration; however, no persistent hematologic abnormalities attributable to the drug have been observed. Perform total and differential leukocyte counts before and after therapy.

Carcinogenesis and mutagenesis: Metronidazole has shown evidence of carcinogenic activity with chronic oral administration in rodents. In several long-term studies in rats, there was an increase in the incidence of neoplasms, particularly mammary and hepatic tumors, among female rats. Two lifetime tumorigenicity studies in hamsters were negative. Also, metronidazole has shown mutagenic activity in a number of in vitro assay systems, but studies in mammals failed to demonstrate a potential for genetic damage.

Amebic liver abscess: Metronidazole does not obviate the need for aspiration of pus.

Drug Interactions:

Warfarin and other coumarin anticoagulants: Metronidazole potentiates the anticoagulant effect, resulting in a prolongation of prothrombin time.

Alcoholic beverages: Do not consume during metronidazole therapy and for at least 1 day afterward because abdominal cramps, nausea, vomiting, headache and flushing may occur.

Disulfiram: Concurrent use may result in an acute psychotic reaction or confusional state caused by the combined toxicity.

Phenobarbital and phenytoin: The antimicrobial effectiveness of metronidazole may be decreased when administered concurrently probably due to increased metronidazole metabolism. A higher dose of the anti-infective may be required.

Cimetidine may inhibit the metabolism of metronidazole and may increase the likelihood of dose-dependent metronidazole adverse effects.

Drug/Lab tests: The drug may interfere with chemical analyses for AST, SGOT, ALT, SGPT, LDH, triglycerides and hexokinase glucose. Zero values may occur.

Adverse Reactions:

CNS: Most serious – Seizures and peripheral neuropathy, the latter characterized mainly by numbness or paresthesia of an extremity.

Less serious – Dizziness; vertigo; incoordination; ataxia; confusion; irritability; depression; weakness; insomnia; headache; syncope.

Toxic encephalopathy has been associated with high dose or prolonged dosing; controversy exists as to whether it is concentration-related.

GI: Most common – Nausea, sometimes accompanied by headache, anorexia and occasionally, vomiting; diarrhea; epigastric distress; abdominal cramping; constipation; proctitis; sharp, unpleasant metallic taste; a modification of the taste of alcoholic beverages; furry tongue, glossitis, stomatitis (these may be associated with a sudden overgrowth of *Candida*). Paradoxically, metronidazole has been implicated in causing pseudomembranous colitis.

Hematologic: Reversible neutropenia (leukopenia).

Renal/GU: Dysuria; cystitis; polyuria; incontinence; sense of pelvic pressure. Darkened urine (deep red-brown color) has been reported. The pigment appears to be a metabolite of metronidazole and it seems to have no clinical significance. Proliferation of *Candida* in the vagina; dyspareunia; decreased libido.

Cardiac: Flattening of the T-wave may be seen in electrocardiographic tracings.

Hypersensitivity: Urticaria; erythematous rash; flushing; nasal congestion; dryness of the mouth (or vagina or vulva); fever.

Local reactions: Thrombophlebitis after IV infusion can be minimized or eliminated by avoiding prolonged use of indwelling IV catheters.

Other: Fleeting joint pains, sometimes resembling "serum sickness". One case of metronidazole-induced pancreatitis, confirmed with rechallenge, has been reported.

(Continued on following page)

METRONIDAZOLE (Cont.)

Overdosage: Single oral doses, up to 15 g, have been reported in suicide attempts and accidental overdoses.

Symptoms – Nausea, vomiting and ataxia. Neurotoxic effects (seizures and peripheral neuropathy) have been reported after 5 to 7 days of 6 to 10.4 g every other day.

Treatment – No specific antidote for metronidazole overdose. Treatment consists of usual supportive measures. Refer to General Management of Acute Overdosage on p. 2895

Patient Information:

May cause GI upset; take with food. Avoid alcoholic beverages.

Complete full course of therapy; take until gone. May cause darkening of urine.

An unpleasant metallic taste may be noticeable.

During treatment for trichomoniasis, the patient should refrain from sexual intercourse, or the partner should wear a condom to avoid reinfection.

Administration and Dosage:

Anaerobic bacterial infections: In the treatment of most serious anaerobic infections, metronidazole is usually administered IV initially.

Loading dose – 15 mg/kg infused over 1 hour (≈ 1 g for a 70 kg adult).

Maintenance dose – 7.5 mg/kg infused over 1 hour every 6 hours (≈ 500 mg for a 70 kg adult). Administer the first maintenance dose 6 hours following the initial loading dose. Do not exceed a maximum of 4 g in 24 hours.

The usual duration of therapy is 7 to 10 days; however, infections of the bone and joints, lower respiratory tract and endocardium may require longer treatment.

Administer by slow IV, continuous or intermittent drip infusion only. Do not use syringes with aluminum needles or hubs. If used with a primary IV fluid system, discontinue the primary solution during infusion. Do not give by direct IV bolus injection because of the low pH (0.5 to 2) of the reconstituted product. The drug must be further diluted and neutralized for infusion. Do not introduce additives into the solution.

Following IV therapy, use oral metronidazole when conditions warrant. The usual adult oral dosage is 7.5 mg/kg every 6 hours.

Prophylaxis: To prevent postoperative infection in contaminated or potentially contaminated colorectal surgery, the recommended adult dosage is 15 mg/kg infused over 30 to 60 minutes and completed ≈ 1 hour before surgery, followed by 7.5 mg/kg infused over 30 to 60 minutes at 6 and 12 hours after the initial dose.

Complete administration of the initial preoperative dose ≈ 1 hour before surgery so that adequate drug levels are present in the serum and tissues at the time of initial incision, and administer, if necessary, at 6 hour intervals to maintain effective drug levels. Limit prophylactic use to the day of surgery only, following the above guidelines.

Amebiasis: Acute intestinal amebiasis (acute amebic dysentery) – 750 mg, 3 times daily for 5 to 10 days. The **CDC** recommends it be combined with iodoquinol (650 mg orally 3 times daily for 20 days).

Amebic liver abscess – 500 or 750 mg, 3 times daily for 5 to 10 days.

Children – 35 to 50 mg/kg/24 hours, in 3 divided doses, for 10 days.

Trichomoniasis: 1 day treatment – 2 g either as a single dose or in 2 divided doses of 1 g each given in the same day. *7 day course of treatment* – 250 mg, 3 times daily for 7 consecutive days.

Cure rates may be higher after a 7 day course than after a 1 day treatment. Individualize dosage. Single dose treatment can assure compliance, especially if administered under supervision, in patients who will not continue the 7 day regimen. A 7 day treatment may minimize reinfection of the female long enough to treat sexual contacts. Some patients may tolerate one course of therapy better than the other.

Do not treat pregnant patients during the first trimester. In the second or third trimester, when local palliative treatment has failed to control symptoms, do not use the 1 day course of therapy. It causes higher serum levels to reach the fetal circulation.

When repeat courses of the drug are required, allow 4 to 6 weeks between courses and reconfirm the presence of the trichomonad by appropriate laboratory measures. Perform total and differential leukocyte counts before and after retreatment.

The **CDC** recommends sex partners of women with trichomoniasis be treated with a 2 g single dose or 250 mg metronidazole twice daily for 7 days.

Infants with symptomatic trichomoniasis or with persistent urogenital trichomonal colonization beyond the fourth week of life can be treated with metronidazole 10 to 30 mg/kg/day for 5 to 8 days. *Children* with trichomonal infection should be treated with metronidazole 15 mg/kg by mouth daily divided into 3 doses for 7 to 10 days.

Hepatic disease patients metabolize metronidazole slowly; accumulation of metronidazole and its metabolites occurs. Therefore, reduce doses below those usually recommended. Monitor plasma metronidazole levels and observe for toxicity.

(Administration and Dosage continued on following page)

METRONIDAZOLE (Cont.)

Administration and Dosage (Cont.):

Renal disease: Do not specifically reduce the dose in anuric patients, since accumulated metabolites may be rapidly removed by dialysis.

Preparation of parenteral solution: NOTE: Order of mixing is important. (1) Reconstitution; (2) Dilution in IV solution; (3) pH neutralization with sodium bicarbonate injection.

Do not use aluminum-containing equipment with lyophilized metronidazole IV. The solution will interact, turning an orange/rust color, although drug potency is not affected. This interaction does not occur with the neutralized or ready-to-use product.

Reconstitution – Add 4.4 ml of one of the following diluents to the vial and mix thoroughly: Sterile Water for Injection; Bacteriostatic Water for Injection; 0.9% Sodium Chloride Injection; or Bacteriostatic 0.9% Sodium Chloride Injection. The resultant volume is 5 ml with an approximate concentration of 100 mg/ml.

The pH of the reconstituted product will be between 0.5 to 2; the solution is clear, and pale yellow to yellow-green in color. Do not use if cloudy or precipitated.

Dilution in IV solutions – Add the properly reconstituted product to a glass or plastic IV container. Do not exceed a concentration of 8 mg/ml. Use any of the following: 0.9% Sodium Chloride Injection; 5% Dextrose Injection; Lactated Ringer's Injection.

Neutralization for IV infusion – Prior to administration, neutralize the IV solution containing metronidazole with approximately 5 mEq sodium bicarbonate injection for each 500 mg used. Mix thoroughly. The pH of the neutralized IV solution will be approximately 6 to 7. Carbon dioxide gas will be generated with neutralization. It may be necessary to relieve gas pressure within the container.

When the contents of one vial (500 mg) are diluted and neutralized to 100 ml, the resultant concentration is 5 mg/ml. Do not exceed an 8 mg/ml concentration in the neutralized IV solution; neutralization will decrease aqueous solubility and precipitation may occur. *Do not refrigerate neutralized solutions;* precipitation may occur.

Ready-to-use: Do not use plastic containers in series connections; it could result in air embolism due to residual air (approximately 15 ml) being drawn from the primary container before administration of the fluid from the secondary container is complete.

Storage and stability: Reconstituted *Flagyl IV* is stable for 96 hours when stored below 30°C (86°F) in room light. Use diluted and neutralized IV solutions within 24 hours. Store ready-to-use solution at 15° to 30°C (59° to 86°F); protect from light.

	Product	Form	Description	C.I.*
Rx	**Metronidazole** (Various)	**Tablets:** 250 mg	In 50s, 100s, 500s, 1000s, UD 100s.	15+
Rx	**Femazole** (Major)		In 100s, 250s and 500s.	40
Rx	**Flagyl** (Searle)		(Searle 1831/Flagyl 250). Blue. In 50s, 100s, 250s, 500s, UD 100s.	149
Rx	**Metizol** (Glenwood)		(PP-551). White. In 100s.	39
Rx	**Metric 21** (Fielding)		In 100s.	NA
Rx	**Metryl** (Lemmon)		(Metryl 93). In 100s, 250s, 500s.	48
Rx	**Protostat** (Ortho)		(Ortho 1570). White. In 100s.	117
Rx	**Satric** (Savage)		(3681). White. In 100s and 250s.	94
Rx	**Metronidazole** (Various)	**Tablets:** 500 mg	In 50s, 100s, 500s, 1000s, UD 100s.	12+
Rx	**Femazole** (Major)		In 50s and 100s.	26
Rx	**Flagyl** (Searle)		(Flagyl 500). Blue. Film coated. In 100s, 500s and UD 100s.	136
Rx	**Metryl** (Lemmon)		(Metryl 500/93-93). White, scored. In 100s and 500s.	44
Rx	**Protostat** (Ortho)		(Ortho 1571). White. In 50s.	102
Rx	**Satric** (Savage)		(3688). White. In 60s.	89
Rx	**Flagyl I.V.** (Schiapparelli Searle)	**Powder for Injection:** 500 mg (as HCl) per vial.[1]		1163
Rx	**Metronidazole** (Abbott)	**Injection, ready-to-use:** 500 mg per 100 ml	In 100 ml vials.	1659
Rx	**Metronidazole Redi-Infusion** (Elkins-Sinn)		In 100 ml vials.[2]	750
Rx	**Flagyl I.V. RTU** (Schiapparelli Searle)		In 100 ml single dose vials[2] and 100 ml *Viaflex* containers.[2]	138
Rx	**Metro I.V.** (Kendall-McGaw)		In 100 ml vials[3] and 100 ml plastic containers.[3]	1573
Rx	**Metryl I.V.** (Lemmon)		In 100 ml vials.[2]	437

* Cost Index based on cost per 500 mg.

[1] With 415 mg mannitol. [2] 14 mEq sodium per vial. [3] 13.5 mEq sodium per vial.

FLUCYTOSINE (5-FC; 5-Fluorocytosine)

Warning: Use with extreme caution in patients with renal impairment. Close monitoring of hematologic, renal and hepatic status of all patients is essential.

Actions:

Pharmacology: Flucytosine has in vitro and in vivo activity against *Candida* and *Cryptococcus*, but the exact mode is not known. It is rarely used alone; generally it is used in combination with amphotericin B (see Drug Interactions).

Pharmacokinetics: Absorption/Distribution – Flucytosine is well absorbed after oral administration; peak serum levels are reached within 2 hours. The drug is well distributed into the aqueous humor, joints, peritoneal fluid and other body fluids and tissues; CSF concentrations are about 65% to 90% of serum levels. Plasma protein binding is minimal. Toxicity occurs at blood levels > 100 mcg/ml.

Metabolism/Excretion – ≈ 80% to 90% of a dose is excreted unchanged in urine by glomerular filtration; < 10% is found unchanged in the feces. Serum half-life is 2 to 5 hours in patients with normal renal function; half-life increases significantly in renal failure. The drug is easily removed by hemodialysis or peritoneal dialysis.

Indications:

Treatment of serious infections caused by susceptible strains of *Candida* or *Cryptococcus*.

Candida: Septicemia, endocarditis and urinary tract infections have been effectively treated. Trials in pulmonary infections have been limited.

Cryptococcus: Meningitis and pulmonary infections. Good responses in septicemias and urinary tract infections have occurred.

Unlabeled use: Flucytosine has been used for the treatment of chromomycosis.

Contraindications:

Hypersensitivity to flucytosine.

Warnings:

Bone marrow depression: Give with extreme caution to patients with bone marrow depression. Patients may be more prone to bone marrow depression if they have a hematologic disease, are being treated with radiation or marrow-suppressant drugs, or have a history of treatment with such drugs or radiation. Frequently monitor hepatic function and the hematopoietic system during therapy.

Renal function impairment: Give with extreme caution; drug accumulation may occur. Monitor blood levels to determine the adequacy of renal excretion in such patients. Adjust dosage or dosing interval to maintain blood levels at < 100 mcg/ml.

Pregnancy: Category C. Flucytosine is teratogenic in the rat and mouse at doses of 40 mg/kg/day; teratogenicity is apparently species-related. There are no adequate and well controlled studies in pregnant women. Use during pregnancy only if the potential benefit justifies the potential risk to the fetus.

Lactation: It is not known whether this drug is excreted in breast milk. Because of the potential for serious adverse reactions in nursing infants from flucytosine, decide whether to discontinue nursing or to discontinue the drug, taking into account the importance of the drug to the mother.

Children: Safety and efficacy in children have not been established.

Precautions:

Before therapy is instituted, determine hematologic, renal status and electrolytes. Monitor hepatic function at frequent intervals during therapy.

Drug Interactions:

Amphotericin B may increase the therapeutic action and toxicity of flucytosine.

Cytosine may inactivate the antifungal activity of flucytosine.

Drug/Lab test interactions: Flucytosine interferes with creatinine value determinations with the dry-slide enzymatic method (Kodak Ektachem analyzer). Use Jaffe method.

Adverse Reactions:

Respiratory: Respiratory arrest; chest pain; dyspnea.

Dermatologic: Rash; pruritus; urticaria; photosensitivity.

GI: Nausea; emesis; abdominal pain; diarrhea; anorexia; dry mouth; duodenal ulcer; GI hemorrhage; hepatic dysfunction; jaundice; ulcerative colitis; bilirubin elevation; elevation of hepatic enzymes.

Genitourinary: Azotemia; creatinine and BUN elevation; crystalluria; renal failure.

Hematologic: Anemia; agranulocytosis; aplastic anemia; eosinophilia; leukopenia; pancytopenia; thrombocytopenia.

CNS: Ataxia; hearing loss; headache; paresthesia; parkinsonism; peripheral neuropathy; pyrexia; vertigo; sedation; confusion; hallucinations; psychosis.

Miscellaneous: Cardiac arrest; fatigue; hypoglycemia; hypokalemia; weakness.

(Continued on following page)

FLUCYTOSINE (5-FC; 5-Fluorocytosine) (Cont.)

Overdosage:

Symptoms: There is no experience with intentional overdosage. It is reasonable to expect that overdosage may produce pronounced manifestations of the known clinical adverse reactions. Prolonged serum concentration in excess of 100 mcg/ml may be associated with an increased incidence of toxicity, especially GI (diarrhea, nausea, vomiting), hematologic (leukopenia, thrombocytopenia) and hepatic (hepatitis).

Treatment: In the management of overdosage, prompt gastric lavage or the use of an emetic is recommended. Maintain adequate fluid intake by the IV route if necessary, since flucytosine is excreted unchanged via the renal tract. Monitor hematologic parameters frequently; monitor liver and kidney function carefully. Should any abnormalities appear in any of these parameters, institute appropriate therapeutic measures. Refer also to General Management of Acute Overdosage. Since hemodialysis has been shown to rapidly reduce serum concentrations in anuric patients, consider this method in the management of overdosage.

Patient Information:

May cause GI upset (nausea, vomiting). Reduce or avoid by taking capsules a few at a time over a 15 minute period. Notify physician if effects become intolerable.

Administration and Dosage:

The usual dosage is 50 to 150 mg/kg/day in divided doses at 6 hour intervals. To reduce or avoid nausea or vomiting, take capsules a few at a time over 15 minutes. If BUN or serum creatinine is elevated, or if there are other signs of renal impairment, the initial dose should be at the lower level (see Warnings).

				C.I.*
Rx	**Ancobon** (Roche)	**Capsules:** 250 mg	(Ancobon Roche 250). Green and gray. In 100s.	9
		500 mg	(Ancobon Roche 500). White and gray. In 100s.	9

NYSTATIN, ORAL

Actions:

Pharmacology: A polyene antibiotic with antifungal activity. Nystatin probably acts by binding to sterols in the cell membrane of the fungus, with a resultant change in membrane permeability allowing leakage of intracellular components.

Pharmacokinetics: Following oral administration, nystatin is sparingly absorbed, with no detectable blood levels when given in the recommended doses. Most of the unabsorbed nystatin is passed unchanged in the stool. The antibiotic exhibits no appreciable activity against bacteria or trichomonads.

Indications:

Treatment of intestinal candidiasis.

For information on nystatin oral suspension and troches for the treatment of oral candidiasis, refer to the monograph in the Mouth and Throat Products section.

Contraindications:

Hypersensitivity to nystatin.

Warnings:

Pregnancy: No adverse effects or complications have been attributed to nystatin in infants born to women treated with nystatin.

Adverse Reactions:

Nystatin is virtually nontoxic and nonsensitizing and is well tolerated by all age groups including debilitated infants, even on prolonged administration. Large oral doses have occasionally produced diarrhea, GI distress, nausea and vomiting.

Patient Information:

Continue therapy for at least 2 days after symptoms have disappeared.

Administration and Dosage:

500,000 to 1,000,000 units 3 times daily. Continue treatment for at least 48 hours after clinical cure to prevent relapse.

				C.I.*
Rx	**Nystatin** (Various, eg, Major, Rugby)	**Tablets:** 500,000 units	In 15s, 30s, 100s, 500s and 1000s.	2+
Rx	**Mycostatin** (Apothecon)		Lactose. (580). Film coated. In 100s and Unimatic 100s.	4
Rx	**Nilstat** (Lederle)		(LL N5). Pink. Convex. Film coated. In 100s and UD 100s.	4

* Cost Index based on cost per 500 mg flucytosine or 500,000 units nystatin.

For information on vaginal and topical miconazole, refer to individual monographs.

MICONAZOLE

Actions:

Pharmacology: Miconazole, an imidazole derivative, exerts a fungicidal effect by altering the permeability of the fungal cell membrane. Its mechanism of action may also involve an alteration of RNA and DNA metabolism or an intracellular accumulation of peroxides toxic to the fungal cell.

Pharmacokinetics: Absorption/Distribution – Recommended doses of miconazole produce serum concentrations which exceed in vitro minimum inhibitory concentration (MIC) values for the fungal species noted in the microbiology section. Doses > 9 mg/kg produce peak blood levels > 1 mcg/ml in most cases. Intrathecal administration of a 20 mg dose produces CSF concentrations > 1 mcg/ml for 24 hours; CSF levels following IV administration are undetectable. Penetration of the drug into inflamed joints, the vitreous body of the eye and the peritoneal cavity is good; penetration into sputum and saliva is poor. Greater than 90% is bound to serum protein.

Metabolism/Excretion – Miconazole is rapidly metabolized in the liver. About 14% to 22% of the administered dose is excreted in the urine, mainly as inactive metabolites. The terminal elimination half-life is 20 to 25 hours. The pharmacokinetic profile is unaltered in patients with renal insufficiency, including those on hemodialysis.

Microbiology: The in vitro antifungal activity is broad. Clinical efficacy has been demonstrated against the following: *Coccidioides immitis; Candida albicans; Cryptococcus neoformans; Pseudoallescheria boydii (Petriellidium boydii, Allescheria boydii); Paracoccidioides brasiliensis.*

Indications:

Treatment of the following severe systemic fungal infections: Coccidioidomycosis, candidiasis, cryptococcosis, pseudoallescheriosis (petriellidiosis, allescheriosis), paracoccidioidomycosis and for the treatment of chronic mucocutaneous candidiasis.

In the treatment of fungal meningitis or *Candida* urinary bladder infections, IV infusion alone is inadequate. It must be supplemented with intrathecal administration or bladder irrigation. Follow appropriate diagnostic procedures and determine MICs.

Use only to treat severe systemic fungal disease.

Contraindications:

Hypersensitivity to miconazole.

Warnings:

Cardiac effects: Cardiorespiratory arrest or anaphylaxis has occurred, possibly due to excessively rapid administration in some cases. Rapid injection of undiluted miconazole may produce transient tachycardia or arrhythmia.

Pregnancy: Category C. There are no adequate and well controlled studies in pregnant women. Give to a pregnant woman only if clearly needed.

Children: Safety for use in children < 1 year of age has not been extensively studied; however, there are reports of 21 neonates who received 3 to 50 mg/kg/day with no unanticipated adverse reactions. Seven of 11 evaluable children recovered or improved.

Precautions:

Give by IV infusion. Start treatment under stringent conditions of hospitalization. Subsequently, it may be given to suitable patients under ambulatory conditions with close clinical monitoring. Give an initial dose of 200 mg with the physician in attendance. Monitor hemoglobin, hematocrit, electrolytes and lipids. Since *Pseudoallescheria* is difficult to distinguish histologically from species of *Aspergillus,* grow cultures.

Systemic fungal mycoses may be complications of chronic underlying conditions which, in themselves, may require appropriate measures.

Drugs containing cremophor-type vehicles (eg, PEG 40, castor oil) cause electrophoretic abnormalities of the lipoprotein. These effects are reversible upon discontinuation of treatment, but are usually not an indication that treatment should be discontinued.

Drug Interactions:

Amphotericin B: Limited data indicate that miconazole and amphotericin B are antagonistic both in vitro and in vivo. The antifungal activity of the two drugs when used in combination is less than that of either drug used alone.

Anticoagulants, oral: An enhanced anticoagulant effect has occurred; carefully titrate the anticoagulant effect since reductions of the anticoagulant doses may be indicated.

Phenytoin levels were increased in a single patient receiving miconazole, which resulted in toxicity.

Due to structural similarity with ketoconazole, consider the possibility of similar drug interactions occurring with miconazole (see ketoconazole monograph).

(Continued on following page)

MICONAZOLE (Cont.)

Adverse Reactions:

Integumentary: Phlebitis at infusion site (29%); pruritus (21%); rash (9%). If pruritus and skin rashes are severe, discontinuation of treatment may be necessary.

GI: Nausea (18%); vomiting (7%); diarrhea; anorexia. Nausea and vomiting can be lessened with antihistaminic or antiemetic drugs given prior to infusion, or by reducing the dose, slowing the rate of infusion or avoiding administration at mealtime.

Hematologic: Transient decreases in hematocrit have been observed following infusion. Thrombocytopenia, aggregation of erythrocytes or rouleau formation on blood smears has occurred.

Miscellaneous: Fever and chills (10%), drowsiness, flushes, transient decreases in serum sodium, anaphylaxis. Hyperlipemia has occurred and is reported to be due to the vehicle, *Cremophor EL* (PEG 40, castor oil).

Dosage:

Adults: The following daily doses are recommended:

Recommended Miconazole Daily Doses

Organism	Total daily dosage range[1] (mg)	Duration of therapy (weeks)
Coccidioidomycosis	1800 to 3600	3 to > 20
Cryptococcosis	1200 to 2400	3 to > 12
Pseudoallescheriosis	600 to 3000	5 to > 20
Candidiasis	600 to 1800	1 to > 20
Paracoccidioidomycosis	200 to 1200	2 to > 16

[1] May be divided over 3 infusions.

Repeated courses may be necessitated by relapse or reinfection.

Children: < *1 year old* – 15 to 30 mg/kg/day. *1 to 12 years old* – 20 to 40 mg/kg/day. Do not exceed 15 mg/kg/dose.

Administration:

IV: For doses ≤ 2400 mg/day, dilute in at least 200 ml of fluid per amp. The diluent of choice is 0.9% Sodium Chloride Injection or, alternatively, 5% Dextrose Injection. Infuse at a rate of approximately 2 hours/amp. For doses > 2400 mg/day, adjust infusion rate and diluent according to patient tolerability.

Continue treatment until clinical and laboratory tests no longer indicate presence of active fungal infection. Inadequate treatment periods may yield poor response and lead to early recurrence of clinical symptoms. Dosing intervals, sites and duration of treatment vary and depend on the causative organism.

Intrathecal: Administer undiluted solution by various intrathecal routes (20 mg per dose) as an adjunct to IV treatment in fungal meningitis. Succeeding intrathecal injections may be alternated between lumbar, cervical and cisternal punctures every 3 to 7 days.

Bladder instillation: 200 mg diluted solution for *Candida* of the urinary bladder.

				C.I.*
Rx	**Monistat i.v.** (Janssen)	**Injection:** 10 mg per ml	In 20 ml amps.[2]	166

* Cost Index based on cost per 200 mg.

[2] With PEG 40, castor oil and parabens.

For information on topical ketoconazole, refer to the individual monograph in the Topical Anti-infectives section.

KETOCONAZOLE

Warning:
Ketoconazole has been associated with hepatic toxicity, including some fatalities. Closely monitor patients and inform them of the risk. See Warnings.

Actions:

Pharmacology: Ketoconazole, an imidazole broad-spectrum antifungal agent, impairs the synthesis of ergosterol, the main sterol of fungal cell membranes, allowing increased permeability and leakage of cellular components.

Pharmacokinetics: Absorption/Distribution – Bioavailability depends on an acidic pH for dissolution and absorption (see Precautions). Peak plasma levels of 1.6 to 6.9 mcg/ml occur 1 to 2 hours after a 200 mg oral dose taken with a meal. Administration with food may decrease absorption. In vitro, plasma protein binding is about 95% to 99%, mainly to albumin. At recommended doses, cerebrospinal fluid penetration is negligible. Detectable concentrations are achieved in urine, saliva, sebum and cerumen.

Metabolism/Excretion – The drug undergoes extensive hepatic metabolism to inactive metabolites. Plasma elimination is biphasic; half-life is 2 hours during the first 10 hours, 8 hours thereafter. The major excretory route is enterohepatic. From 85% to 90% is excreted in bile and feces, 10% to 15% in urine, 2% to 4% unchanged.

Renal failure does not alter ketoconazole dosing requirements; the drug does not appear to be dialyzable.

Microbiology: Active against clinical infections with *Blastomyces dermatitidis, Candida* sp, *Coccidioides immitis, Histoplasma capsulatum, Paracoccidioides brasiliensis, Phialophora* sp, *Trichophyton* sp, *Epidermophyton* sp and *Microsporum* sp. In animals, activity has been demonstrated against *Malassezia furfur* and *Cryptococcus neoformans*.

Indications:

Treatment of the following systemic fungal infections: Candidiasis, chronic mucocutaneous candidiasis, oral thrush, candiduria, blastomycosis, coccidioidomycosis, histoplasmosis, chromomycosis and paracoccidioidomycosis.

Treatment of severe recalcitrant cutaneous dermatophyte infections not responding to topical therapy or oral griseofulvin or in patients unable to take griseofulvin.

Unlabeled uses: Ketoconazole has been used successfully in the treatment of onychomycosis (caused by *Trichophyton* and *Candida* sp); pityriasis versicolor (Tinea versicolor); tinea pedis, corporis and cruris (200 to 400 mg/day); tinea capitis (3.3 to 6.6 mg/kg/day); and vaginal candidiasis.

High dose (800 to 1200 mg/day) ketoconazole has shown some success in treating CNS fungal infections.

Ketoconazole in doses of 400 mg every 8 hours has been used in the treatment of advanced prostate cancer (see Warnings).

Ketoconazole 800 to 1200 mg/day has been used to effectively treat Cushing's syndrome due to its ability to inhibit adrenal steroidogenesis.

Contraindications:

Hypersensitivity to ketoconazole. Do not use for the treatment of fungal meningitis because it penetrates poorly into the CSF (see Unlabeled uses).

Warnings:

Hepatotoxicity, primarily of the hepatocellular type, has been associated with ketoconazole including rare fatalities. The incidence has been about 1:10,000 exposed patients, but this probably represents under-reporting. The median duration of therapy in patients who developed symptomatic hepatotoxicity was about 28 days, although the range extended to as low as 3 days. The hepatic injury is usually reversible upon discontinuation of treatment. Several cases of hepatitis have occurred in children.

Prompt recognition of liver injury is essential. Measure liver function (eg, AST, ALT, alkaline phosphatase, bilirubin) before starting treatment and frequently during treatment. Monitor patients receiving ketoconazole concurrently with other potentially hepatotoxic drugs, particularly those patients requiring prolonged therapy or those with a history of liver disease.

Transient minor elevations in liver enzymes have occurred. Discontinue ketoconazole if these persist or worsen, or are accompanied by symptoms of possible liver injury.

Prostatic cancer: In clinical trials involving 350 patients with metastatic prostatic cancer, 11 deaths were reported within 2 weeks of starting high dose ketoconazole (1200 mg/day). It is not known whether death was related to therapy. High ketoconazole doses are known to suppress adrenal corticosteroid secretion.

(Warnings continued on following page)

KETOCONAZOLE (Cont.)

Warnings (Cont.):

Hypersensitivity: Anaphylaxis occurs rarely after the first dose. Hypersensitivity reactions, including urticaria, have been reported. Have epinephrine 1:1000 immediately available. Refer to Management of Acute Hypersensitivity Reactions.

Pregnancy: Category C. Teratogenic effects (syndactylia and oligodactylia), embryotoxic effects and dystocia have been seen in animals at doses in excess of the maximum human dose. There are no adequate and well controlled studies in pregnant women. Use only if the potential benefit justifies the potential risk to the fetus.

Lactation: Ketoconazole is probably excreted in breast milk; mothers who are under treatment should not nurse.

Children: Safety for use in children < 2 years of age has not been established. Do not use in pediatric patients unless the potential benefits outweigh the risks.

Precautions:

Hormone levels: Ketoconazole lowers serum testosterone. Testosterone levels are impaired with doses of 800 mg/day and abolished by 1600 mg/day. Once therapy has been discontinued, levels return to baseline values. It also decreases ACTH-induced corticosteroid serum levels at similar high doses. Closely follow the recommended dose of 200 to 400 mg/day.

Gastric acidity: Ketoconazole requires acidity for dissolution and absorption. If antacids, anticholinergics or H_2 blockers are needed, give at least 2 hours after administration. In achlorhydria, dissolve each tablet in 4 ml aqueous solution of 0.2 N HCl. Use a glass or plastic straw to avoid contact with the teeth. Follow with a glass of water.

Drug Interactions:

Ketoconazole Drug Interactions			
Precipitant Drug	Object Drug*		Description
Antacids	Ketoconazole	↓	Increased gastric pH may inhibit ketoconazole absorption. Consider giving antacids ≥ 2 hrs after ketoconazole.
Histamine H_2 antagonists	Ketoconazole	↓	Increased gastric pH may inhibit ketoconazole absorption.
Isoniazid	Ketoconazole	↓	Bioavailability of ketoconazole may be decreased.
Rifampin	Ketoconazole	↓	Decreased serum levels of either drug may occur. Avoid concurrent use if possible.
Ketoconazole	Anticoagulants, oral	↑	The anticoagulant response may be enhanced.
Ketoconazole	Corticosteroids	↑	Corticosteroid bioavailability may be increased and clearance may be decreased, possibly resulting in toxicity.
Ketoconazole	Cyclosporine	↑	Increased cyclosporine concentrations may occur, possibly resulting in toxicity. Since the effect on cyclosporine levels is consistent and predictable, this interaction has been used beneficially to decrease cyclosporine dosage in some patients.
Ketoconazole	Theophyllines	↓	Theophylline serum levels may be decreased.

* ↑ = Object drug increased. ↓ = Object drug decreased.

Adverse Reactions:

Most reactions are mild, transient and rarely require discontinuation. The rare occurrences of hepatic dysfunction require special attention.

GI: Nausea/vomiting (3% to 10%); abdominal pain (1.2%); diarrhea (< 1%); hepatotoxicity.

CNS: Headache, dizziness, somnolence, photophobia (< 1%).

Neuropsychiatric: Suicidal tendencies, severe depression (rare).

Other: Pruritus (1.5%), fever, chills, impotence, gynecomastia, thrombocytopenia, leukopenia, hemolytic anemia, bulging fontanelles (< 1%). Hypersensitivity including urticaria (see Warnings). Oligospermia at dosages above those approved but not at dosages up to 400 mg/day; sperm counts were obtained infrequently at these dosages.

(Continued on following page)

KETOCONAZOLE (Cont.)

Overdosage:

Institute supportive measures, including gastric lavage with sodium bicarbonate. Refer to General Management of Acute Overdosage.

Patient Information:

Do not take with antacids; if antacids are required, delay administration by 2 hours.

Take with food to alleviate GI disturbance.

May produce headache, dizziness and drowsiness; observe caution while driving or performing other tasks requiring alertness.

Notify physician of any signs or symptoms suggesting liver dysfunction (eg, unusual fatigue, anorexia, nausea, vomiting, jaundice, dark urine, pale stools), or if abdominal pain, fever or diarrhea become pronounced.

Administration and Dosage:

Prior to starting therapy, determine laboratory and clinical documentation of infection. Continue therapy until tests indicate that active fungal infection has subsided.

Adults: Initially, 200 mg once daily. In very serious infections, or if clinical response is insufficient, increase dose to 400 mg once daily.

Children: (> 2 years) – 3.3 to 6.6 mg/kg/day as a single daily dose.
(< 2 years) – Daily dosage has not been established.

Inadequate treatment periods may yield poor response and lead to early recurrence of clinical symptoms. Minimum treatment for candidiasis is 1 or 2 weeks and for the other indicated systemic mycoses, 6 months. Chronic mucocutaneous candidiasis usually requires maintenance therapy.

Minimum treatment of recalcitrant dermatophyte infections is 4 weeks in cases involving glabrous skin. Palmar and plantar infections may respond more slowly. Apparent cures may subsequently recur after discontinuation of therapy in some cases.

				C.I.*
Rx	**Nizoral** (Janssen)	**Tablets:** 200 mg	(Janssen/Nizoral). White, scored. In 100s and UD 100s.	14

* Cost Index based on cost per 200 mg.

For information on topical amphotericin B, refer to individual monograph in the Topical Anti-infectives section.

AMPHOTERICIN B

Warning: Use primarily for treatment of patients with progressive and potentially fatal fungal infections. Do not use to treat the common clinically inapparent forms of fungal disease which show only positive skin or serologic tests.

Actions:

Pharmacology: Amphotericin B is fungistatic or fungicidal, depending on the concentration obtained in body fluids and on the susceptibility of the fungus. It probably acts by binding to sterols in the fungal cell membrane with a resultant change in membrane permeability, allowing leakage of a variety of small molecules. Mammalian cell membranes also contain sterols, and the damage to human cells (toxicity) and fungal cells (antibiotic effect) may share common mechanisms.

Pharmacokinetics:

Absorption/Distribution – An initial IV infusion of 1 to 5 mg/day, gradually increased to 0.4 to 0.6 mg/kg/day, produces peak plasma concentrations of approximately 0.5 to 2 mcg/ml. Amphotericin B is highly protein bound (> 90%) and is poorly dialyzable. Penetration of the drug into inflamed pleural cavities and joints is good; penetration is poor into the parotid gland, bronchial secretions, cerebrospinal fluid, aqueous humor, brain, pancreas, muscle and bone.

Metabolism/Excretion – Metabolic pathways of amphotericin B are not known. It has a relatively short initial serum half-life of 24 hours, followed by a second elimination phase with a half-life of about 15 days. The drug is very slowly excreted by the kidneys with 2% to 5% as the biologically active form. After treatment is discontinued, amphotericin B can be detected in the urine for at least 7 weeks. The cumulative urinary output over 7 days amounts to approximately 40% of the drug infused. Dosage alteration is not required in patients with renal dysfunction.

Children – Based on studies in a small number of premature infants and children, the pharmacokinetics for amphotericin B differ from those seen in adults, and also vary with the age of the child. Therefore, consider these differences when determining a dosing regimen and individualize doses based on therapeutic drug monitoring.

Microbiology: Amphotericin B, a polyene antibiotic, is active in vitro against many species of fungi. *Histoplasma capsulatum, Coccidioides immitis, Candida* sp, *Blastomyces dermatitidis, Rhodotorula* sp, *Cryptococcus neoformans, Sporothrix schenckii, Mucor mucedo* and *Aspergillus fumigatus* are inhibited by concentrations ranging from 0.03 to 1 mcg/ml in vitro. It has no effect on bacteria, rickettsiae and viruses.

Indications:

Specifically intended to treat cryptococcosis (torulosis); North American blastomycosis; the disseminated forms of moniliasis, coccidioidomycosis and histoplasmosis; mucormycosis (phycomycosis) caused by species of the genera *Mucor, Rhizopus, Absidia, Entomophthora* and *Basidiobolus;* sporotrichosis *(S schenckii)*; aspergillosis *(A fumigatus)*.

May be helpful in the treatment of American mucocutaneous leishmaniasis, but it is not the drug of choice in primary therapy.

For patients with progressive, potentially fatal infections. Do not use to treat common inapparent forms of fungal disease which show only positive skin or serologic tests.

Contraindications:

Hypersensitivity to amphotericin B, unless the condition requiring treatment is life-threatening and amenable only to amphotericin B therapy.

Warnings:

Fatal fungal diseases: Amphotericin B is frequently the only effective treatment for potentially fatal fungal diseases. Balance its possible lifesaving effect against its dangerous side effects.

Nephrotoxicity: Renal damage, the most important toxic effect, is a limiting factor for the use of amphotericin B. Renal dysfunction usually improves upon interruption of therapy, dose reduction or increased dosing interval; however, some permanent impairment often occurs, especially in patients receiving large doses (> 5 g). Decreased glomerular filtration rate and renal blood flow, increased serum creatinine and renal tubular dysfunction are prominent. Sodium loading may be effective in reducing nephrotoxicity of amphotericin B in sodium-depleted patients, but this may be a problem in patients with cardiac or hepatic disease.

Pregnancy: Category B. Systemic fungal infections have been successfully treated in pregnant women with amphotericin B without obvious effects to the fetus, but the number of cases reported has been small. Adequate and well controlled studies have not been conducted; therefore, use during pregnancy only if clearly needed.

(Warnings continued on following page)

AMPHOTERICIN B (Cont.)

Warnings (Cont.):

Lactation: It is not known whether amphotericin B is excreted in breast milk. However, consider discontinuing nursing and eliminating IV amphotericin B.

Children: Safety and efficacy in children have not been established. Systemic fungal infections have been successfully treated in children without reports of unusual side effects. Limit administration to the least amount compatible with an effective therapeutic regimen.

Precautions:

Prolonged therapy is usually necessary. Unpleasant reactions are common and some are potentially dangerous. Use only in hospitalized patients or in those under close medical observation. Reserve use for those patients in whom a diagnosis of the progressive, potentially fatal forms of susceptible mycotic infections has been firmly established, preferably by positive culture or histologic study.

Monitoring: Perform BUN and serum creatinine or endogenous creatinine clearance tests at least weekly during therapy. If BUN exceeds 40 mg/dl or if serum creatinine exceeds 3 mg/dl, discontinue the drug or reduce dosage until renal function improves. Weekly hemograms, serum potassium and magnesium determinations are also advisable. Low serum magnesium levels have been noted during treatment. Discontinue therapy if liver function test results are abnormal (elevated alkaline phosphatase and bilirubin).

Therapy interruption: Whenever medication is interrupted for > 7 days, resume therapy with the lowest dosage level; increase gradually.

Pulmonary reactions characterized by acute dyspnea, hypoxemia and interstitial infiltrates have been observed in neutropenic patients receiving amphotericin B and leukocyte transfusions. Although pulmonary toxicity has occurred in association with either agent used alone, it was more frequent when amphotericin B was given after or during initiation of leukocyte transfusions. Administer amphotericin B cautiously in patients receiving leukocyte transfusions and separate the infusion as far as possible from the time of a leukocyte transfusion.

Drug Interactions:

Corticosteroids should not be administered concomitantly, due to the possibility of hypokalemia, unless they are necessary to control drug reactions.

Cyclosporine: Nephrotoxic effects of cyclosporine appear to be increased. Consider alternative immunosuppressive therapy. Also, use great caution when administering amphotericin B with other nephrotoxic agents (eg, aminoglycosides) due to a possible synergistic effect.

Because of its hypokalemic effect, amphotericin B may potentiate the effects of the **digitalis glycosides** and **neuromuscular blocking agents**; however, a drug interaction has not been documented.

Adverse Reactions:

Most patients will exhibit some intolerance, often at less than full therapeutic dosage. Severe reactions may be lessened by giving aspirin, antipyretics (eg, acetaminophen), antihistamines and antiemetics before the infusion and by maintaining sodium balance. Administration on alternate days may decrease anorexia and phlebitis. Small doses of IV adrenal corticosteroids given just prior to or during the infusion may decrease febrile reactions. Keep the dosage and duration of such corticosteroid therapy to a minimum. In three patients, dantrolene was a successful adjunctive agent for the prophylaxis (50 mg oral) and treatment (50 mg IV) of amphotericin B-induced rigors. Adding a small amount of heparin to the infusion (500 to 2000 units), rapid infusion rate, removal of needle after infusion, rotation of infusion sites, administration through a large central vein or distal veins and using a pediatric scalp-vein needle may lessen the incidence of thrombophlebitis. Extravasation may cause chemical irritation.

Most frequent:

General toxic reactions – Fever (sometimes with shaking chills); headache; anorexia; malaise; generalized pain, including muscle and joint pains.

Renal – Hypokalemia; azotemia; hyposthenuria; nephrocalcinosis; renal tubular acidosis (supplemental alkali medication may decrease complications).

GI – Nausea; vomiting; dyspepsia; diarrhea; cramping; epigastric pain.

Hematologic – Normochromic, normocytic anemia.

Local – Venous pain at the injection site with phlebitis and thrombophlebitis.

Miscellaneous – Weight loss.

(Adverse Reactions continued on following page)

AMPHOTERICIN B (Cont.)

Adverse Reactions (Cont.):

Less frequent (or rare):

Cardiovascular – Arrhythmias; ventricular fibrillation; cardiac arrest; hypertension; hypotension.

Hematologic – Coagulation defects; thrombocytopenia; leukopenia; agranulocytosis; eosinophilia; leukocytosis.

CNS – Peripheral neuropathy; convulsions; other neurologic symptoms.

Special senses – Hearing loss; tinnitus; transient vertigo; blurred vision; diplopia.

GI – Melena or hemorrhagic gastroenteritis; acute liver failure.

Renal – Anuria; oliguria; permanent damage is often related to a large total dose (> 5 g).

Dermatologic – Maculopapular rash; pruritus (without rash).

Miscellaneous – Anaphylactoid reactions; flushing; dyspnea.

Administration and Dosage:

Test dose: Infuse 1 mg slowly to determine patient tolerance. Increase dosage gradually.

Administer by slow IV infusion over 6 hours at a concentration of 0.1 mg/ml.

Individualize dosage. Therapy is usually instituted with a daily dose of 0.25 mg/kg and gradually increased as tolerance permits. Data are insufficient to define total dosage requirements and duration of treatment necessary for eradication of mycoses such as phycomycosis. Optimal dose is unknown. Total daily dosage may range up to 1 mg/kg; alternate day dosages range up to 1.5 mg/kg. Several months of therapy are usually necessary; a shorter period of therapy may be inadequate and lead to relapse.

Do not exceed a total daily dose of 1.5 mg/kg.

Sporotrichosis: Usual dose per injection is 20 mg. Therapy has ranged up to 9 months.

Aspergillosis has been treated for up to 11 months with a total dose of up to 3.6 g.

Rhinocerebral phycomycosis, a fulminating disease, generally occurs in association with diabetic ketoacidosis. Diabetic control must be instituted before successful treatment with amphotericin B can be accomplished. Pulmonary phycomycosis, which is more common in association with hematologic malignancies, is often an incidental finding at autopsy. A cumulative dose of at least 3 g amphotericin B is recommended. Although a total dose of 3 to 4 g will infrequently cause permanent renal impairment, it is a reasonable minimum where there is clinical evidence of deep tissue invasion. Rhinocerebral phycomycosis usually follows a rapidly fatal course; therapy must be more aggressive than that for more indolent mycoses.

Unlabeled administration: Because of amphotericin's poor CNS penetration, fungal meningitis may require intrathecal or intraventricular administration. Doses range from 0.1 mg initially, increased gradually up to 0.5 mg every 48 to 72 hours.

Bladder irrigations have been used for the treatment of candidal cystitis with minimal toxicity. It has been administered in concentrations ranging from 5 to 15 mg/dl, instilled periodically or continuously for 5 to 10 days.

IV infusion of 45 minutes to 2 hours has been successful without resulting in hypotension and other local side effects.

Preparation of solutions: For initial concentration of 5 mg/ml, rapidly inject 10 ml Sterile Water for Injection without a bacteriostatic agent directly into the lyophilized cake, using a sterile needle (minimum diameter: 20 gauge). Shake the vial immediately until the colloidal solution is clear. The infusion solution, providing 0.1 mg/ml, is then obtained by further dilution (1:50) with 5% Dextrose Injection of pH above 4.2.

Caution – Strictly observe aseptic technique in all handling, since no preservative or bacteriostatic agent is present. Do not reconstitute with saline solutions. Use of any other diluent or presence of a bacteriostatic agent in the diluent may cause precipitation. Do not use if there is any evidence of precipitation or foreign matter.

An in-line membrane filter may be used for IV infusion. To assure passage of the antibiotic colloidal dispersion, the filter's mean pore diameter should be ≥ 1 micron.

The manufacturer recommends that the solution be protected from light during administration. Although solutions of amphotericin B are light sensitive, loss of drug activity is reported to be negligible when solutions are exposed to light for 8 hours. Therefore, it is probably not necessary to cover infusion containers if administered within 8 hours of reconstitution.

Storage: Refrigerate vials; protect against exposure to light. The concentrate (after reconstitution) may be stored in the dark at room temperature for 24 hours, or under refrigeration for 1 week with minimal loss of potency and clarity. Discard any unused material. Use solutions prepared for IV infusions promptly after preparation.

	Product	Form	C.I.*
Rx	**Amphotericin B** (Lyphomed)	**Injection:** 50 mg per vial.[1]	1.2
Rx	**Fungizone Intravenous** (Squibb)	Sterile lyophilized cake (may partially reduce to powder following manufacture).	1

* Cost Index based on cost per 50 mg.

[1] With 41 mg sodium desoxycholate.

GRISEOFULVIN

Actions:

Pharmacology: Griseofulvin, an antibiotic derived from a species of *Penicillium*, is deposited in the keratin precursor cells, which are gradually exfoliated and replaced by noninfected tissue; it has a greater affinity for diseased tissue. The drug is tightly bound to the new keratin, which becomes highly resistant to fungal invasions.

Pharmacokinetics: The peak serum level found in fasting adults given 0.5 g griseofulvin microsize occurs at about 4 hours and ranges between 0.5 to 2 mcg/ml. Some individuals are consistently "poor absorbers" and tend to attain lower blood levels at all times. The serum level may be increased by giving the drug with a meal with a high fat content. GI absorption varies considerably among individuals, due to insolubility of the drug in aqueous media of the upper GI tract. The efficiency of GI absorption of the ultramicrocrystalline formulation is approximately 1.5 times that of conventional microsized griseofulvin. This factor permits the oral intake of two-thirds as much ultramicrocrystalline griseofulvin as the microsized form; but there is no evidence that this confers any significant clinical differences in regard to safety and efficacy.

Microbiology: Fungistatic with in vitro activity against species of *Microsporum, Epidermophyton* and *Trichophyton.* It has no effect on bacteria or other fungi.

Indications:

Treatment of ringworm infections of the skin, hair and nails, namely: Tinea corporis, tinea pedis, tinea cruris, tinea barbae, tinea capitis, tinea unguium (onychomycosis) when caused by one or more of the following genera of fungi: *Trichophyton rubrum; T tonsurans; T mentagrophytes; T interdigitalis; T verrucosum; T megnini; T gallinae; T crateriform; T sulphureum; T schoenleini; Microsporum audouini; M canis; M gypseum; Epidermophyton floccosum.*

Note: Prior to therapy, identify the types of fungi responsible for the infection. Use of this drug is not justified in minor or trivial infections which will respond to topical agents alone.

Griseofulvin is NOT effective in bacterial infections; candidiasis (moniliasis); histoplasmosis; actinomycosis; sporotrichosis; chromoblastomycosis; coccidioidomycosis; North American blastomycosis; cryptococcosis (torulosis); tinea versicolor; nocardiosis.

Contraindications:

Hypersensitivity to griseofulvin; porphyria; hepatocellular failure.

Warnings:

Prophylaxis: Safety and efficacy for prophylaxis of fungal infections have not been established.

Hypersensitivity reactions (eg, skin rashes, urticaria, angioneurotic edema) may occur and necessitate withdrawal of therapy. Institute appropriate counter measures; see Management of Acute Hypersensitivity Reactions.

Carcinogenesis: Chronic feeding of griseofulvin to mice, at levels ranging from 0.5% to 2.5% of the diet, resulted in the development of liver tumors. Smaller particle sizes resulted in an enhanced effect. Thyroid tumors developed in male rats receiving griseofulvin at levels of 2%, 1% and 0.2% of the diet.

In subacute toxicity studies, griseofulvin produced hepatocellular necrosis in mice, but not in other species. Griseofulvin produced disturbances in porphyrin metabolism, a colchicine-like effect on mitosis and cocarcinogenicity with methylcholanthrene in cutaneous tumor induction in laboratory animals.

Pregnancy: Category C. Griseofulvin was embryotoxic and teratogenic in rats. Rare cases of conjoined twins have been reported in patients taking griseofulvin during the first trimester of pregnancy. Do not give to pregnant women or women contemplating pregnancy.

Precautions:

Prolonged therapy: Closely observe patients on prolonged therapy. Periodically monitor renal, hepatic and hematopoietic function.

Penicillin cross-sensitivity is possible since griseofulvin is derived from species of *Penicillium;* however, known penicillin-sensitive patients have been treated without difficulty.

Lupus erythematosus, lupus-like syndromes or exacerbation of lupus erythematosus have occurred in patients receiving griseofulvin.

Photosensitivity may occur; therefore, caution patients to take protective measures (ie, sunscreens, protective clothing) against exposure to ultraviolet light or sunlight.

Photosensitivity reactions may aggravate lupus erythematosus.

(Continued on following page)

GRISEOFULVIN (Cont.)

Drug Interactions:

Anticoagulants: Griseofulvin may decrease the hypoprothrombinemic activity of warfarin; patients may require anticoagulant dosage adjustment.

Barbiturates may depress griseofulvin serum levels; concomitant administration may require a dosage adjustment of the antifungal agent.

Contraceptives, oral: Loss of contraceptive effectiveness may occur during griseofulvin coadministration, possibly leading to breakthrough bleeding, amenorrhea or unintended pregnancy.

Adverse Reactions:

Most common: Hypersensitivity reactions, such as skin rashes, urticaria, and rarely, angioneurotic edema may occur. See Warnings.

Occasional: Oral thrush; nausea; vomiting; epigastric distress; diarrhea; headache; fatigue; dizziness; insomnia; mental confusion; impairment of performance of routine activities.

Rare: Griseofulvin interferes with porphyrin metabolism. Proteinuria; leukopenia; hepatic toxicity; GI bleeding; menstrual irregularities; paresthesias of the hands and feet after extended therapy. Discontinue administration if granulocytopenia occurs. When rare, serious reactions occur with griseofulvin, they are usually associated with high dosages, long periods of therapy or both.

Patient Information:

Beneficial effects may not be noticeable for some time; continue taking medication for entire course of therapy.

Photosensitivity reactions may occur; avoid prolonged exposure to sunlight or sunlamps.

Notify physician if fever, sore throat or skin rash occurs.

Oral suspension: Store at room temperature in a light resistant container.

Administration and Dosage:

Accurate diagnosis of the infecting organism is essential.

Duration of therapy: Continue medication until the infecting organism is completely eradicated, as indicated by appropriate clinical or laboratory examination. Representative treatment periods are: Tinea capitis, 4 to 6 weeks; tinea corporis, 2 to 4 weeks; tinea pedis, 4 to 8 weeks; tinea unguium (depending on rate of growth) – fingernails, at least 4 months, toenails, at least 6 months.

Hygiene: Observe good hygiene to control sources of infection or reinfection. Concomitant use of appropriate topical agents is usually required, particularly in treatment of tinea pedis. In some forms of athlete's foot, yeasts and bacteria may be involved, as well as fungi. Griseofulvin will not eradicate the bacterial or monilial infection.

Adults: Tinea corporis, tinea cruris and tinea capitis – A single or divided daily dose of 500 mg microsize (330 to 375 mg ultramicrosize) will give a satisfactory response in most patients.

Tinea pedis and tinea unguium – 0.75 to 1 g microsize (660 to 750 mg ultramicrosize) per day in divided doses.

Children: Approximately 11 mg microsize/kg/day (5 mg/lb/day) or 7.3 mg ultramicrosize/kg/day (3.3 mg/lb/day) is an effective dose for most children. The following dosage schedule is suggested:

Griseofulvin Dosage for Children Based on Weight

Weight		Daily dose (mg)	
lb	kg	microsize	ultramicrosize
30 to 50	13.6 to 23	125 to 250	82.5 to 165
> 50	> 23	250 to 500	165 to 330

Clinical experience indicates that a single daily dose is effective in children with tinea capitis.

Children (≤ 2 years of age): Dosage not established.

(Products listed on following page)

GRISEOFULVIN MICROSIZE

	Product	Dosage form	Description	C.I.*
Rx	**Fulvicin U/F** (Schering)	**Tablets:** 250 mg	(Schering AUF or 948). White, scored. In 60s and 250s.	7
Rx	**Grifulvin V** (Ortho Derm)		(Ortho 211). White, scored. In 100s.	6
Rx	**Fulvicin U/F** (Schering)	**Tablets:** 500 mg	(Schering AUG or 496). White, scored. In 60s and 250s.	6
Rx	**Grifulvin V** (Ortho Derm)		(Ortho 214). White, scored. In 100s and 500s.	5
Rx	**Grisactin 500** (Wyeth-Ayerst)		(Grisactin 500444). Scored. In 60s.	4
Rx	**Grisactin** (Wyeth-Ayerst)	**Capsules:** 125 mg	(Grisactin 125442). In 100s.	5
Rx	**Grisactin** (Wyeth-Ayerst)	**Capsules:** 250 mg	(Grisactin 250443). In 100s and 500s.	5
Rx	**Grifulvin V** (Ortho Derm)	**Oral Suspension:** 125 mg/5 ml	0.2% alcohol, saccharin, sucrose. In 120 ml.	18

GRISEOFULVIN ULTRAMICROSIZE

The efficiency of GI absorption of griseofulvin ultramicrosize is approximately 1.5 times that of conventional microsized griseofulvin. This factor permits the oral intake of two-thirds as much ultramicrosize as the microsize form, but there is no evidence that this confers any significant clinical difference in regard to safety and efficacy.

	Product	Dosage form	Description	C.I.*
Rx	**Fulvicin P/G** (Schering)	**Tablets:** 125 mg	(Schering 228). White, scored. In 100s.	5
Rx	**Grisactin Ultra** (Wyeth-Ayerst)		(Grisactin Ultra 125). White. Square. In 100s.	4
Rx	**Gris-PEG** (Herbert)		(Gris-PEG 125). White, scored. Elliptical. Film coated. In 100s and 500s.	5
Rx	**Fulvicin P/G** (Schering)	**Tablets:** 165 mg	(Fulvicin P/G 654). Off-white, scored. Oval. In 100s.	6
Rx	**Fulvicin P/G** (Schering)	**Tablets:** 250 mg	(Schering 507). White, scored. In 100s.	5
Rx	**Grisactin Ultra** (Wyeth-Ayerst)		(Grisactin Ultra 250). White. Square. In 100s.	4
Rx	**Gris-PEG** (Herbert)		(Gris-PEG 250). White, scored. Capsule shape. Film coated. In 100s, 250s, 500s.	5
Rx	**Fulvicin P/G** (Schering)	**Tablets:** 330 mg	(Fulvicin P/G 352). Off-white, scored. Oval. In 100s.	5
Rx	**Grisactin Ultra** (Wyeth-Ayerst)		(Grisactin Ultra 330). White, scored. Oval. In 100s.	4

* Cost Index based on cost per 500 mg griseofulvin microsize or 330 mg ultramicrosize.

FLUCONAZOLE

Actions:

Pharmacology: Fluconazole, a synthetic broad spectrum bis-triazole antifungal agent, is a highly selective inhibitor of fungal cytochrome P-450 and sterol C-14 alpha-demethylation. Mammalian cell demethylation is much less sensitive to fluconazole inhibition. The subsequent loss of normal sterols correlates with the accumulation of 14 alpha-methyl sterols in fungi and may be responsible for the fungistatic activity of fluconazole.

In healthy volunteers, fluconazole administration (doses ranging from 200 mg to 400 mg once daily for up to 14 days) was associated with small and inconsistent effects on testosterone concentrations, endogenous corticosteroid concentrations and the ACTH-stimulated cortisol response.

Pharmacokinetics: Absorption/Distribution – The pharmacokinetic properties of fluconazole are similar following administration by the IV or oral routes. In healthy volunteers, the bioavailability of oral fluconazole is > 90% compared with IV administration.

Peak plasma concentration (C_{max}) in fasted healthy volunteers occur between 1 and 2 hours with a terminal plasma elimination half-life of ≈ 30 hours (range, 20 to 50 hours) after oral administration. A single oral 400 mg dose leads to a mean C_{max} of 6.72 mcg/ml (range, 4.12 to 8.08 mcg/ml); after single oral doses of 50 to 400 mg, plasma concentrations and AUC are dose proportional.

Steady-state concentrations are reached within 5 to 10 days following oral doses of 50 to 400 mg given once daily. Administration of a loading dose (day 1) of twice the usual daily dose results in plasma concentrations close to steady state by day 2. The apparent volume of distribution approximates that of total body water. Plasma protein binding is low (11% to 12%). Following either single- or multiple-oral doses for up to 14 days, fluconazole penetrates into all body fluids studied (see table). In healthy volunteers, saliva concentrations were equal to or slightly greater than plasma concentrations regardless of dose, route or duration of dosing. In patients with bronchiectasis, sputum concentrations following a single 150 mg oral dose were equal to plasma concentrations at both 4 and 24 hours post dose. In patients with fungal meningitis, concentrations in the CSF are ≈ 80% of the corresponding plasma concentrations.

Tissue/Fluid Concentration of Fluconazole

Tissue or Fluid	Concentration*
Cerebrospinal fluid†	0.5-0.9
Saliva	1
Sputum	1
Blister fluid	1
Urine	10
Normal skin	10
Nails	1
Blister skin	2

* Relative to plasma concentrations in subjects with normal renal function.
† Independent of degree of meningeal inflammation.

Metabolism/Excretion – In healthy volunteers, fluconazole is cleared primarily by renal excretion, with ≈ 80% of the administered dose appearing in the urine unchanged, about 11% as metabolites. The pharmacokinetics of fluconazole are markedly affected by reduction in renal function. There is an inverse relationship between the elimination half-life and creatinine clearance. The dose of fluconazole may need to be reduced in patients with impaired renal function (see Administration and Dosage). A 3 hour hemodialysis session decreases plasma concentrations by ≈ 50%.

Microbiology: Fluconazole exhibits in vitro activity against *Cryptococcus neoformans* and *Candida sp.* Fungistatic activity has also been demonstrated in normal and immunocompromised animal models for systemic and intracranial fungal infections due to *C neoformans* and for systemic infections due to *C albicans.* Development of resistance to fluconazole has not been studied.

In common with other azole antifungal agents, most fungi show a higher apparent sensitivity to fluconazole in vivo than in vitro. Activity has been demonstrated against fungal infections caused by *Aspergillus flavus* and *A fumigatus* in mice. Fluconazole is active in animal models of endemic mycoses, including one model of *Blastomyces dermatidis* pulmonary infections, one model of *Coccidioides immitis* intracranial infections and several models of *Histoplasma capsulatum* pulmonary infection.

Coadministration of fluconazole and amphotericin B in infected normal and immunosuppressed mice showed the following results: A small additive antifungal effect in systemic infection with *C albicans,* no interaction in intracranial infection with *C neoformans,* and antagonism of the two drugs in systemic infection with *A fumigatus.*

(Continued on following page)

FLUCONAZOLE (Cont.)

Indications:

Oropharyngeal and esophageal candidiasis.

Also effective for the treatment of serious systemic candidal infections, including urinary tract infection, peritonitis and pneumonia.

Cryptococcal meningitis: Obtain specimens for fungal culture and other relevant laboratory studies (serology, histopathology) prior to therapy to isolate and identify causative organisms. Therapy may be instituted before the results are known; however, once these results become available, adjust anti-infective therapy accordingly.

Contraindications:

Hypersensitivity to fluconazole or to any excipients in the product. There is no information regarding cross hypersensitivity between fluconazole and other azole antifungal agents; use with caution in patients with hypersensitivity to other azoles.

Warnings:

Liver function test abnormalities: Monitor patients who develop abnormal liver function tests during fluconazole therapy for the development of more severe hepatic injury. Although serious hepatic reactions have been rare and the causal association with fluconazole uncertain, if clinical signs and symptoms consistent with liver disease develop that may be attributable to fluconazole, discontinue the drug. (See Adverse Reactions.)

Rashes: Closely monitor immunocompromised patients who develop rashes during treatment with fluconazole and discontinue the drug if lesions progress. (See Adverse Reactions.)

Carcinogenesis and impairment of fertility: Male rats treated with 5 and 10 mg/kg/day had an increased incidence of hepatocellular adenomas.

Fluconazole did not affect the fertility of male or female rats treated orally with daily doses of 5, 10 or 20 mg/kg or with parenteral doses of 5, 25 or 75 mg/kg, although the onset of parturition was slightly delayed at 20 mg/kg oral administration. In an IV perinatal study in rats at 5, 20 and 40 mg/kg, dystocia and prolongation of parturition were observed in a few dams at 20 mg/kg (approximately 5 to 15 times the recommended human dose) and 40 mg/kg, but not at 5 mg/kg. The effects on parturition in rats are consistent with the species-specific, estrogen-lowering property produced by high doses of fluconazole. Such a hormone change has not been observed in women treated with fluconazole. (See Pharmacology.)

Pregnancy: Category C. Fluconazole was administered orally to pregnant rabbits during organogenesis in two studies, at 5, 10 and 20 mg/kg and at 5, 25 and 75 mg/kg respectively. Maternal weight gain was impaired at all dose levels and abortions occurred at 75 mg/kg (approximately 20 to 60 times the recommended human dose); no adverse fetal effects were detected. In several studies in which pregnant rats were treated orally with fluconazole during organogenesis, maternal weight gain was impaired and placental weights were increased at 25 mg/kg. There were no fetal effects at 5 or 10 mg/kg; increases in fetal anatomical variants (eg, supernumerary ribs, renal pelvis dilation) and delays in ossification were observed at 25 and 50 mg/kg and higher doses. At doses ranging from 80 mg/kg (approximately 20 to 60 times the recommended human dose) to 320 mg/kg, embryolethality in rats was increased and fetal abnormalities included wavy ribs, cleft palate and abnormal cranio-facial ossification. These effects are consistent with the inhibition of estrogen synthesis in rats and may be a result of known effects of lowered estrogen on pregnancy, organogenesis and parturition.

There are no adequate and well controlled studies in pregnant women. Use in pregnancy only if the potential benefit justifies the possible risk to the fetus.

Lactation: It is not known whether fluconazole is excreted in breast milk. Exercise caution when fluconazole is administered to a nursing woman.

Children: Efficacy has not been established in children. A small number of patients from age 3 to 13 years have been treated safely with fluconazole using doses of 3 to 6 mg/kg daily.

(Continued on following page)

FLUCONAZOLE (Cont.)

Drug Interactions:

Cimetidine: Single dose administration of fluconazole (100 mg) with cimetidine (400 mg) resulted in a 4% to 32% reduction in AUC and a 20% to 40% reduction in C_{max} of fluconazole.

Cyclosporine: Stable bone marrow transplant patients receiving twice daily doses of cyclosporine and fluconazole (100 mg) as a single oral dose for 14 days demonstrated slight increases in cyclosporine C_{max}, C_{min} and AUC values which did not achieve statistical significance. There have been several literature reports associating concomitant administration of high doses of fluconazole with an increase in cyclosporine plasma concentrations in renal transplant patients with or without renal function. Carefully monitor cyclosporine concentrations.

Hydrochlorothiazide: Concomitant oral administration of 100 mg fluconazole and 50 mg hydrochlorothiazide for 10 days in healthy volunteers resulted in an increase of 41% in C_{max} and an increase of 43% in AUC of fluconazole, compared to fluconazole given alone. Overall, the plasma concentrations of fluconazole were approximately 1 to 2 mcg/ml higher. These changes are attributable to a mean net reduction of approximately 20% in the renal clearance of fluconazole.

Oral contraceptives: Single and multiple 50 mg oral doses of fluconazole were administered to healthy women taking oral contraceptives. The AUC for ethinyl estradiol was decreased by 16%, but no changes were observed in levonorgestrel pharmacokinetics.

Phenytoin: Coadministration of oral fluconazole (200 mg) and phenytoin at steady state resulted in an average increase of 75% of phenytoin AUC values in healthy volunteers. Carefully monitor phenytoin concentrations.

Rifampin: Administration of a single oral dose of fluconzaole after chronic rifampin administration resulted in a 25% decrease in AUC and a 20% shorter half-life of fluconazole in healthy volunteers. Consider increasing the fluconazole dose.

Sulfonylureas: In three studies, fluconazole administration resulted in significant increases in C_{max} and AUC of **tolbutamide, glyburide** and **glipizide**. Several subjects experienced symptoms consistent with hypoglycemia. In the glyburide study, several volunteers required oral glucose treatment. Monitor blood glucose and adjust the sulfonylurea dose as necessary.

Warfarin: A single dose of warfarin (15 mg) given to healthy volunteers following 14 days of orally administered fluconazole (200 mg) resulted in a 12% increase in the prothrombin time (PT) response (area under the prothrombin time-time curve). One of 13 subjects experienced a twofold increase in his PT response. Carefully monitor PT.

Adverse Reactions:

In $>$ 4000 patients treated with fluconazole in clinical trials $\geq$ 7 days, 16% experienced adverse events. Treatment was discontinued in 1.5% of patients due to adverse clinical events and in 1.3% of patients due to laboratory test abnormalities.

In combined clinical trials and foreign marketing experience prior to U.S. marketing, patients with serious underlying disease (predominantly AIDS or malignancy) rarely have developed serious hepatic reactions or exfoliative skin disorders during treatment with fluconazole (see Warnings). Two of these hepatic reactions and one exfoliative skin disorder (Stevens-Johnson syndrome) were associated with a fatal outcome. Because many confounding factors were present, the causal association of these reactions with fluconazole therapy is uncertain.

Clinical adverse events were reported more frequently in HIV infected patients (21%) than in non-HIV infected patients (13%); however, the patterns in both patients were similar. The proportions of patients discontinuing therapy due to clinical adverse events were similar in the two groups (1.5%).

The following adverse events occurred at an incidence of $\geq$ 1% in 4048 patients receiving fluconazole for $\geq$ 7 days in clinical trials: Nausea (3.7%); headache (1.9%); skin rash (1.8%); vomiting (1.7%); abdominal pain (1.7%); diarrhea (1.5%).

(Adverse Reactions continued on following page)

FLUCONAZOLE (Cont.)

Adverse Reactions (Cont.):

Laboratory test abnormalities: In two comparative trials a statistically significant increase was observed in median AST levels from a baseline value of 30 to 41 IU/L in one trial and 34 to 66 IU/L in the other. The overall rate of serum transaminase elevations of more than 8 times the upper limit of normal was approximately 1% in fluconazole-treated patients in clinical trials. These elevations occurred in patients with severe underlying disease, predominantly AIDS or malignancies, most of whom were receiving multiple concomitant medications, including many known to be hepatotoxic. The incidence of abnormally elevated serum transaminases was greater in patients taking fluconazole concomitantly with one or more of the following medications: Rifampin, phenytoin, isoniazid, valproic acid or oral sulfonylurea hypoglycemic agents.

Overdosage:

Symptoms: In mice and rats receiving very high doses of fluconazole, clinical effects, included decreased motility and respiration, ptosis, lacrimation, salivation, urinary incontinence, loss of righting reflex and cyanosis; death was sometimes preceded by clonic convulsions.

Treatment: In the event of overdose, institute symptomatic treatment (with supportive measures and gastric lavage if clinically indicated). Refer to General Management of Acute Overdosage.

Fluconazole is largely excreted in urine. A 3 hour hemodialysis session decreases plasma levels by approximately 50%.

Administration and Dosage:

Individualize dosage. Since oral absorption is rapid and almost complete, the daily dose of fluconazole is the same for oral and IV administration. Patients with AIDS and cryptococcal meningitis or recurrent oropharyngeal candidiasis usually require maintenance therapy to prevent relapse.

Oropharyngeal candidiasis: 200 mg on the first day, followed by 100 mg once daily. Clinical evidence of oropharyngeal candidiasis generally resolves within several days, but continue treatment for at least 2 weeks to decrease the likelihood of relapse.

Esophageal candidiasis: 200 mg on the first day, followed by 100 mg once daily. Doses up to 400 mg/day may be used, based on the patient's response. Treat patients with esophageal candidiasis for a minimum of 3 weeks and for at least 2 weeks following resolution of symptoms.

Systemic candidiasis: 400 mg on the first day, followed by 200 mg once daily. Treat these patients for a minimum of 4 weeks for at least 2 weeks following resolution of symptoms.

Cryptococcal meningitis: 400 mg on the first day, followed by 200 mg once daily. A dosage of 400 mg once daily may be used, based on the patient's response to therapy. The duration of treatment for initial therapy of cryptococcal meningitis is 10 to 12 weeks after the cerebrospinal fluid becomes culture negative. The dosage of fluconazole for suppression of relapse of cryptococcal meningitis in patients with AIDS is 200 mg once daily.

Renal function impairment: Fluconazole is cleared primarily by renal excretion as unchanged drug. In patients with impaired renal function, give an initial loading dose of 50 to 400 mg. After the loading dose, base the daily dose on the following table:

Fluconazole Dose in Impaired Renal Function

Creatinine Clearance (ml/min)	Percent of Recommended Dose
> 50	100%
21-50	50%
11-20	25%
Patients receiving regular hemodialysis	One recommended dose after each dialysis

These are suggested dose adjustments based on pharmacokinetics following administration of single doses. Further adjustment may be needed depending upon clinical condition.

(Administration and Dosage continued on following page)

FLUCONAZOLE (Cont.)

Administration and Dosage (Cont.):

When serum creatinine is the only measure of renal function available, use the following formula to estimate the creatinine clearance.

$$\text{Males: } \frac{\text{Weight (kg)} \times (140 - \text{age})}{72 \times \text{serum creatinine (mg/dl)}}$$

Females: 0.85 x above value

Fluconazole injection has been used safely for up to 14 days of IV therapy. Administer the IV infusion of fluconazole at a maximum rate of approximately 200 mg/hr, given as a continuous infusion.

Fluconazole injections are intended only for IV administration using sterile equipment.

Do not use if the solution is cloudy or precipitated or if the seal is not intact.

Directions for IV use: Do not remove unit from overwrap until ready for use. The overwrap is a moisture barrier. The inner bag maintains the sterility of the product. Do not use plastic containers in series connections; such use could result in air embolism due to residual air being drawn from the primary container before administration of the fluid from the secondary container is completed.

Tear overwrap down side at slit and remove solution container. Some opacity of the plastic due to moisture absorption during the sterilization process may be observed. This is normal and does not affect the solution quality or safety. The opacity will diminish gradually. After removing overwrap, check for minute leaks by squeezing inner bag firmly. If leaks are found, discard solution as sterility may be impaired.

IV admixture incompatibility: Do not add supplementary medication.

Rx	**Diflucan** (Roerig)	**Tablets:** 50 mg	(#Diflucan 50 Roerig). Pink. Trapezoid shape. In 30s.
		100 mg	(#Diflucan 100 Roerig). Pink. Trapezoid shape. In 30s and UD 100s.
		200 mg	(#Diflucan 200 Roerig). Pink. Trapezoid shape. In 30s and UD 100s.
		Injection: 200 mg/100 ml[1]	In 100 ml vials and Viaflex Plus containers.
		400 mg/200 ml[1]	In 200 ml vials and Viaflex Plus containers.

Product identification code.

[1] Contains 9 mg sodium chloride per ml.

In addition to the sulfonamides listed on the following pages, other preparations that contain sulfonamides include: Ophthalmic; vaginal; burn preparations (eg, mafenide, silver sulfadiazine). See individual monographs or sections.

Actions:

Pharmacology: Sulfonamides exert their bacteriostatic action by competitive antagonism of para-aminobenzoic acid (PABA), an essential component in folic acid synthesis. Microorganisms that require exogenous folic acid and do not synthesize folic acid are not susceptible to the action of sulfonamides.

Microbiology: Sulfonamides have a broad antibacterial spectrum which includes both gram-positive and gram-negative organisms.

Resistance develops in organisms which produce excessive amounts of PABA; resistance may also be due to destruction of the sulfonamide molecule. The increasing frequency of resistant organisms is a limitation to the usefulness of the sulfonamides alone, especially in the treatment of chronic and recurrent urinary tract infections. Cross-resistance between sulfonamides is common, once resistance develops. Minimize resistance by initiating treatment promptly with adequate doses and continue for a sufficient period. In vitro sensitivity tests are not always reliable; carefully coordinate the test with bacteriologic and clinical response.

Pharmacokinetics: Absorption/Distribution – The oral sulfonamides are readily absorbed from the GI tract. Approximately 70% to 100% of an oral dose is absorbed. These agents are distributed throughout all body tissues and readily enter the cerebrospinal fluid, pleura, synovial fluids, the eye, the placenta and the fetus. Sulfonamides are bound to plasma proteins in varying degrees. Wide interpatient variation in serum levels may result from identical doses. "Free" sulfonamide serum levels of 5 to 15 mg/dl may be therapeutically effective for most infections. Avoid levels > 20 mg/dl.

Metabolism – The duration of antibacterial activity depends on the rate of metabolism and renal excretion. Metabolism occurs in the liver by conjugation, acetylation and other metabolic pathways to inactive metabolites. Sulfonamide acetylation requires a coenzyme which is a pantothenic acid derivative; individuals who are pantothenic acid deficient or are slow acetylators have an increased risk of toxicity from sulfonamide accumulation.

Excretion – Renal excretion is mainly by glomerular filtration; tubular reabsorption occurs in varying degrees. Urinary solubility of these compounds is pH dependent. Some of the acetylated metabolites are less soluble and may contribute to crystalluria and renal complications. To prevent the possibility of crystalluria, alkalinization of the urine and adequate fluid intake are recommended when using the less soluble sulfonamides (eg, sulfadiazine, sulfamerazine). Small amounts are eliminated in the feces, and in bile, breast milk and other secretions.

(Continued on following page)

Indications:

Sulfonamide Indications							
Indications ✓ – Labeled × – Unlabeled	Multiple Sulfas	Sulfacytine	Sulfadiazine	Sulfamethizole	Sulfamethoxazole	Sulfasalazine	Sulfisoxazole
Chancroid	✓		✓		✓		✓
Colitis, ulcerative						✓	
Inclusion conjunctivitis	✓		✓		✓		✓
Malaria[1]	✓		✓		✓		✓
Meningitis, *H influenzae*[2]	✓		✓				✓
Meningitis, meningococcal[3]	✓		✓		✓		✓
Nocardiosis	✓		✓		✓		✓
Otitis media, acute[4]	✓		✓		✓		✓
Rheumatic fever			✓				
Toxoplasmosis[5]	✓		✓		✓		✓
Trachoma	✓		✓		✓		✓
Urinary tract infections[6] (pyelonephritis, cystitis)	✓	✓	✓	✓	✓		✓
Ankylosing spondylitis						×	
Colitis, collagenous						×	
Crohn's disease						×	
Otitis media, recurrent							×
Rheumatoid arthritis						×	

[1] As adjunctive therapy due to chloroquine-resistant strains of *P falciparum*.
[2] As adjunctive therapy with parenteral streptomycin.
[3] When the organism is susceptible and for prophylaxis when sulfonamide-sensitive group A strains prevail.
[4] Due to *H influenzae* when used with penicillin or erythromycin.
[5] As adjunctive therapy with pyrimethamine.
[6] In the absence of obstructive uropathy or foreign bodies, when caused by *E coli, Klebsiella-Enterobacter, S aureus, P mirabilis* and *P vulgaris*.

Contraindications:

Hypersensitivity to sulfonamides or chemically related drugs (eg, sulfonylureas, thiazide and loop diuretics, carbonic anhydrase inhibitors, sunscreens containing PABA, local anesthetics); pregnancy at term (see Warnings); lactation (see Warnings); infants $<$ 2 months of age (except in the treatment of congenital toxoplasmosis as adjunctive therapy with pyrimethamine); porphyria (see Warnings); hypersensitivity to salicylates; intestinal or urinary obstruction (**sulfasalazine**).

Warnings:

Group A beta-hemolytic streptococcal infections: Do not use for treatment of these infections. In an established infection, they will not eradicate the streptococcus and will not prevent sequelae, such as rheumatic fever and glomerulonephritis.

Severe reactions including deaths due to sulfonamides have been associated with hypersensitivity reactions, agranulocytosis, aplastic anemia, other blood dyscrasias and renal and hepatic damage. Irreversible neuromuscular and CNS changes and fibrosing alveolitis may occur. Sore throat, fever, pallor, purpura or jaundice may be early indications of serious blood disorders. Perform complete blood counts.

Porphyria: In patients with porphyria, these drugs have precipitated an acute attack.

Renal or hepatic function impairment: Use with caution. The frequency of renal complications is considerably lower in patients receiving the more soluble sulfonamides (sulfisoxazole and sulfamethizole). Obtain urinalysis with microscopic examinations and perform liver and kidney function tests during long-term treatment. Maintain adequate fluid intake to prevent crystalluria and stone formation.

Photosensitivity: Photosensitization (photoallergy or phototoxicity) may occur; therefore, caution patients to take protective measures (ie, sunscreens, protective clothing) against exposure to ultraviolet light or sunlight until tolerance is determined.

(Warnings continued on following page)

Warnings (Cont.):

Fertility impairment: Oligospermia and infertility have been described in men treated with **sulfasalazine.** Withdrawal of the drug appears to reverse these effects.

Pregnancy: Safety for use during pregnancy has not been established. Sulfonamides cross the placenta with fetal levels averaging 70% to 90% of maternal serum levels. Significant levels may persist in the neonate if these drugs are given near term and may produce jaundice, hemolytic anemia and kernicterus. Although most reports do not demonstrate congenital malformations, teratogenicity (eg, cleft palate, other bony abnormalities) has been observed in some animal species. Do not use during pregnancy at term.

Lactation: Sulfonamides are excreted in breast milk in low concentrations. Milk: plasma ratios for sulfonamides are as low as 0.06 (sulfisoxazole). According to the American Academy of Pediatrics, breast feeding and sulfonamide use are compatible since sulfonamide excretion into breast milk does not pose a significant risk to the healthy full-term neonate. However, do not nurse premature infants or those with hyperbilirubinemia or G-6-PD deficiency.

Children: Do not use in infants < 2 months of age (except in the treatment of congenital toxoplasmosis as adjunctive therapy with pyrimethamine). **Sulfacytine** is not recommended for use in children < 14 years. There are insufficient clinical data on prolonged or recurrent therapy with **sulfamethoxazole** in chronic renal diseases of children < 6 years.

Precautions:

Allergy or asthma: Give sulfonamides with caution to patients with severe allergy or bronchial asthma. If toxicity or hypersensitivity reactions occur, discontinue immediately.

Hemolytic anemia, frequently dose-related, may occur in G-6-PD deficient individuals.

Drug Interactions:

Sulfonamide Drug Interactions			
Precipitant Drug	Object Drug*		Description
Sulfonamides	Anticoagulants, oral	↑	Warfarin's anticoagulation action may be enhanced. Hemorrhage could occur
Sulfisoxazole	Barbiturate anesthetics	↑	The anesthetic effects of thiopental may be enhanced
Sulfonamides	Cyclosporine	↔	Cyclosporine concentrations are decreased, and the risk of nephrotoxicity may be increased
Sulfasalazine	Digoxin	↓	Digoxin's bioavailability may be decreased, possibly resulting in a reduced therapeutic effect
Sulfasalazine	Folic acid	↓	Signs of folate deficiency have occurred (eg, low serum folate, megaloblastic anemia, macrocytosis, reticulocytosis), but specific symptoms related to the deficiency have not been reported
Sulfonamides	Hydantoins	↑	Serum hydantoin levels may be increased
Sulfonamides	Methotrexate	↑	The risk of methotrexate-induced bone marrow suppression may be enhanced
Sulfonamides	Sulfonylureas	↑	Increased sulfonylurea half-lives and hypoglycemia have occurred

*↑ = Object drug increased ↓ = Object drug decreased ↔ = Undetermined effect.

Drug/Lab test interactions: Sulfonamides may produce false-positive **urinary glucose tests** when performed by Benedict's method. Sulfisoxazole may interfere with the **Urobilistix test** and may produce false-positive results with sulfosalicylic acid tests for urinary protein.

Adverse Reactions:

Hematologic: Agranulocytosis; aplastic anemia; thrombocytopenia; leukopenia; hemolytic anemia; purpura; hypoprothrombinemia; cyanosis; methemoglobinemia; megaloblastic (macrocytic) anemia; Heinz body anemia.

Hypersensitivity: Erythema multiforme of the Stevens-Johnson type; parapsoriasis varioliformis acuta (Mucha-Habermann syndrome); generalized skin eruptions; allergic myocarditis; epidermal necrolysis, with or without corneal damage; urticaria; serum sickness; pruritus; exfoliative dermatitis; anaphylactoid reactions; periorbital edema; conjunctival and scleral injection; photosensitization; arthralgia; allergic myocarditis; transient pulmonary changes with eosinophilia and decreased pulmonary function.

(Adverse Reactions continued on following page)

Adverse Reactions (Cont.):

GI: Nausea; emesis; abdominal pains; diarrhea; bloody diarrhea; anorexia; pancreatitis; stomatitis; impaired folic acid absorption; hepatitis; hepatocellular necrosis; pseudomembranous enterocolitis; glossitis.

CNS: Headache; peripheral neuropathy; mental depression; convulsions; ataxia; hallucinations; tinnitus; vertigo; insomnia; hearing loss; drowsiness; transient lesions of posterior spinal column; transverse myelitis; apathy.

Renal: Crystalluria; hematuria; proteinuria; elevated creatinine; nephrotic syndrome; toxic nephrosis with oliguria and anuria.

Miscellaneous: Drug fever; chills; pyrexia; alopecia; arthralgia; myalgia; pulmonary infiltrates; periarteritis nodosum; L.E. phenomenon.

The sulfonamides bear chemical similarities to some goitrogens, diuretics (acetazolamide and the thiazides) and oral hypoglycemic agents. Goiter production, diuresis and hypoglycemia have occurred rarely in patients receiving sulfonamides. Cross-sensitivity may exist with these agents (see Contraindications).

Sulfasalazine produces an orange-yellow color urine when the urine is alkaline. Similar discoloration of the skin has also occurred.

Overdosage:

Therapeutic doses of 2 to 5 g/day may produce toxicity or fatalities. The aniline radical is largely responsible for the effects on the blood or hematopoietic system.

Symptoms:

GI – Anorexia; colic; nausea; vomiting.

CNS – Dizziness; headache; drowsiness; unconsciousness.

Toxic fever – Precedes serious manifestations and may develop ≥ 1 day after the fever due to infection has subsided.

Serious manifestations – Acidosis; acute hemolytic anemia; agranulocytosis; sensitivity reactions; dermatitis (maculopapular); toxic neuritis; hepatic jaundice; death (occurring several days after first dose).

Treatment: Discontinue the drug immediately. Within 1 or 2 days after discontinuation, the less serious symptoms disappear; grave symptoms require 1 to 3 weeks for remission. Empty the stomach if large doses have been ingested. Alkalinize the urine to enhance solubility and excretion. Force fluids if kidney function is normal, up to 4 L/day, to increase excretion. If anuria is present, treat for renal failure. Catheterization of the ureters may be indicated for complete renal blockage by crystals. For agranulocytosis, give antibiotic therapy to combat infection, and blood or platelet transfusions for severe anemia or thrombocytopenia.

Patient Information:

Complete full course of therapy.

Take on an empty stomach with a full glass of water.

Avoid prolonged exposure to sunlight; photosensitivity may occur. If outside, wear protective clothing and apply sunscreen to exposed areas.

Notify physician if any of the following occurs: Blood in urine, rash, ringing in ears, difficulty in breathing, fever, sore throat or chills.

Sulfasalazine: Take with food if GI irritation occurs. May cause an orange-yellow discoloration of the urine or skin. May permanently stain soft contact lenses yellow.

Oral suspension: Shake well; refrigerate after opening. Discard unused portion after 14 days.

Administration and Dosage:

See individual products for specific guidelines based on indication.

CDC recommended treatment schedules for sexually transmitted diseases:[1]

Lymphogranuloma venereum: As an alternative regimen to doxycycline, sulfisoxazole 500 mg 4 times a day for 21 days or equivalent sulfonamide course.

Treatment of uncomplicated urethral, endocervical or rectal Chlamydia trachomatis infections: As an alternative regimen to doxycycline or tetracycline (or if erythromycin is not tolerated), sulfisoxazole 500 mg 4 times a day for 10 days or equivalent sulfonamide course.

[1] Morbidity and Mortality Weekly Report 1989 (Sept 1);38 (No. S-8):1-43.

(Products listed on following pages)

Complete prescribing information for these products begins on page 1900

SULFADIAZINE

Administration and Dosage:

Adults: Loading dose – 2 to 4 g. *Maintenance dose* – 4 to 8 g/day in 4 to 6 divided doses.

Children (> 2 months of age): Loading dose – 75 mg/kg (or 2 g/m²). *Maintenance dose* – 120 to 150 mg/kg/day (4 g/m²/day) in 4 to 6 divided doses. *Maximum dose* – 6 g/day.

Infants (< 2 months of age): Contraindicated, except as adjunctive therapy with pyrimethamine in the treatment of congenital toxoplasmosis. *Loading dose* – 75 to 100 mg/kg. *Maintenance dose* – 100 to 150 mg/kg/day in 4 divided doses.

Other recommended doses for toxoplasmosis (for 3 to 4 weeks) include – *Infants (< 2 months of age):* 25 mg/kg/dose 4 times daily; *children (> 2 months of age):* 25 to 50 mg/kg/dose 4 times daily.

Prevention of recurrent attacks of rheumatic fever (not recommended for initial treatment of streptococcal infections): Patients > 30 kg (> 66 lbs) – 1 g/day; patients < 30 kg (< 66 lbs) – 0.5 g/day.

				C.I.*
Rx	**Sulfadiazine** (Various, eg, Lannett)	**Tablets:** 500 mg	In 100s and 1000s.	1+

SULFACYTINE

Administration and Dosage:

Loading dose: 500 mg. *Maintenance dose:* 250 mg 4 times daily for 10 days.

Not recommended in children < 14 years of age.

				C.I.*
Rx	**Renoquid** (Glenwood)	**Tablets:** 250 mg	In 100s.	N/A

SULFISOXAZOLE

Administration and Dosage:

Loading dose: 2 to 4 g. *Maintenance dose:* 4 to 8 g/day in 4 to 6 divided doses. Although recommended, a loading dose is unnecessary because sulfisoxazole is rapidly absorbed and appears in high concentrations in the urine.

Children and infants (> 2 months) – Initial dose: 75 mg/kg. *Maintenance dose:* 120 to 150 mg/kg/day (4 g/m²/day) in 4 to 6 divided doses (maximum, 6 g/day).

				C.I.*
Rx	**Sulfisoxazole** (Various, eg, Balan, Geneva, Goldline, Major, Moore, Parmed, Rugby, Schein, URL, Zenith)	**Tablets:** 500 mg	In 100s, 1000s and UD 100s.	1.3+
Rx	**Gantrisin** (Roche)		(Roche Gantrisin). White, scored. In 100s, 500s and Tel-E-Dose 100s.	8
Rx	**Gantrisin** (Roche)	**Syrup:** 500 mg acetyl sulfisoxazole per 5 ml	0.9% alcohol. Chocolate flavor. In pt.	9.3
		Pediatric Suspension: 500 mg acetyl sulfisoxazole per 5 ml	0.3% alcohol, sucrose. Raspberry flavor. In 120 and 480 ml.	9.3

SULFAMETHOXAZOLE

Administration and Dosage:

Adults: Mild to moderate infections – 2 g initially; maintenance dose is 1 g morning and evening thereafter. *Severe infections* – 2 g initially, then 1 g 3 times daily.

Children and infants (> 2 months): Initially, 50 to 60 mg/kg; maintenance dose is 25 to 30 mg/kg morning and evening. Do not exceed 75 mg/kg/day.

Another recommended dose is 50 to 60 mg/kg/day divided every 12 hours, not to exceed 3 g/24 hours.

				C.I.*
Rx	**Sulfamethoxazole** (Various, eg, Balan, Bioline, Bolar, Geneva, Parmed, Rugby, URL)	**Tablets:** 500 mg	In 100s and 1000s.	2.3+
Rx	**Gantanol** (Roche)		(Roche Gantanol). Green, scored. In 100s and Tel-E-Dose 100s.	11
Rx	**Urobak** (Shionogi)		Scored. In 100s, 1000s.	2.3
Rx	**Gantanol** (Roche)	**Oral Suspension:** 500 mg per 5 ml	Saccharin, sorbitol, sucrose, EDTA. Cherry flavor. In pt.	18

* Cost Index based on cost per 500 mg.

Complete prescribing information for these products begins on page 1900

SULFAMETHIZOLE

Administration and Dosage:

Adults: 0.5 to 1 g 3 or 4 times daily.

Children and infants (> 2 months): 30 to 45 mg/kg/day in 4 divided doses. **C.I.***

	Product	Form	Description	C.I.*
Rx	**Thiosulfil Forte** (W-A)	**Tablets:** 500 mg	White, scored. Oval. In 100s.	13

MULTIPLE SULFONAMIDES (Trisulfapyrimidines)

Provides therapeutic effect of total sulfonamide content; reduces chance of precipitation in kidneys and crystalluria, as solubility of each sulfonamide is independent of others.

Administration and Dosage:

Adults: 2 to 4 g initially, then 2 to 4 g daily in 3 to 6 divided doses.

Children or infants (> 2 months): 75 mg/kg initially, then 120 to 150 mg/kg/day (4 g/m^2/day) in 4 to 6 divided doses. Do not exceed 6 g daily.

Recommended doses for toxoplasmosis (with pyrimethamine) for 3 to 4 wks: *Infants* – 100 mg/kg/day divided 4 times; *children* – 25 to 50 mg/kg 4 times/day. **C.I.***

	Product	Form	Description	C.I.*
Rx	**Triple Sulfa No. 2** (Rugby)	**Tablets:** 167 mg each of sulfadiazine, sulfamerazine and sulfamethazine	In 100s and 1000s.	1.5+

SULFASALAZINE

About one-third of an oral dose of sulfasalazine is absorbed from the small intestine. The remaining two-thirds passes to the colon where it is split into 5-aminosalicylic acid (5-ASA) and sulfapyridine. Most of the sylfapyridine thus liberated is absorbed, whereas only about one-third of the 5-ASA is absorbed, the remainder being excreted in the feces.

Administration and Dosage: Individualize dosage. Administer in evenly divided doses over each 24 hour period; intervals between nighttime doses should not exceed 8 hours. Administer after meals. Doses of ≥ 4 g/day tend to increase adverse reactions.

GI intolerance (eg, anorexia, nausea, vomiting) after the first few doses is probably due to mucosal irritation and may be alleviated by distributing the total daily dose more evenly or by giving enteric coated tablets. If such symptoms occur after the first few days of treatment, they are probably due to increased serum levels of total sulfapyridine and may be alleviated by halving the dose and subsequently increasing it gradually over several days. If symptoms continue, stop the drug for 5 to 7 days, then reinstitute at a lower daily dose.

It is often necessary to continue medication, even when clinical symptoms, including diarrhea, have been controlled. When endoscopic examination confirms satisfactory improvement, reduce dosage to maintenance level. If diarrhea recurs, increase dosage to previously effective levels.

Desensitization regimens: Upon reinstituting sulfasalazine, various regimens comprise a total daily dose of 50 to 250 mg which, every 4 to 7 days thereafter, is doubled until the desired therapeutic level is achieved. Administration of small doses is achieved most easily with the oral suspension. If sensitivity symptoms recur, discontinue the drug. Do not attempt desensitization in patients who have a history of agranulocytosis or who have had anaphylactoid reactions to sulfasalazine.

Initial therapy: Adults – 3 to 4 g/day in evenly divided doses; however, initial doses of 1 to 2 g/day may lessen adverse GI effects. Doses of ≥ 4 g/day increase the risk of toxicity.

Children (≥ 2 years old) – 40 to 60 mg/kg/24 hours in 4 to 6 divided doses.

Maintenance therapy: Adults – 2 g/day (500 mg 4 times daily).

Children – 20 to 30 mg/kg/day, in 4 divided doses, maximum 2 g/day. **C.I.***

	Product	Form	Description	C.I.*
Rx	**Sulfasalazine** (Various, eg, Balan, Geneva, Goldline, Lederle, Major, Parmed, Rugby, Schein, URL)	**Tablets:** 500 mg	In 100s, 250s, 500s, 1000s and UD 100s.	3+
Rx	**Azulfidine** (Pharmacia)		(101). Gold, scored. In 100s, 500s and UD 100s & 1000s.	4.3
Rx	**Sulfasalazine** (Various, eg, Bolar, Dixon-Shane, Genetco, Major, Moore, Parmed, Quali-test, Rugby, URL)	**Tablets, enteric coated:** 500 mg	In 100s, 500s and 1000s.	5+
Rx	**Azulfidine EN-tabs** (Pharmacia)		(102). Gold, elliptical. In 100s and 500s.	6
Rx	**Azulfidine** (Pharmacia)	**Oral Suspension:** 250 mg per 5 ml	In pt.	12

* Cost Index based on cost per 500 mg.

QUININE SULFATE

Actions:

Pharmacology: Quinine, a cinchona alkaloid, acts primarily as a blood schizonticide. Quinine's antimalarial action is unclear. It was once believed to be due to the intercalation of the quinoline moiety into the DNA of the parasite, thereby reducing the effectiveness of DNA to act as a template, as well as depression of the oxygen uptake and carbohydrate metabolism of plasmodia. Recently it is thought that pH elevation in intracellular organelles of the parasites by quinine plays a role in the mechanism.

Quinine has a skeletal muscle relaxant effect, increasing the refractory period by direct action on the muscle fiber, decreasing the excitability of the motor end-plate by a curariform action, and affecting the distribution of calcium within the muscle fiber. It also has analgesic, antipyretic and oxytocic effects. An optical isomer of quinidine, quinine has cardiovascular effects similar to quinidine.

Pharmacokinetics:

Absorption – Quinine is readily absorbed orally, mainly from the upper small intestine. Absorption is almost complete, even in patients with marked diarrhea. Peak plasma concentrations occur within 1 to 3 hours after a single oral dose. Chronic administration of 1 g/day produces an average plasma concentration of 7 mcg/ml.

Tinnitus and hearing impairment rarely occur at plasma concentrations of $<$ 10 mcg/ml. However, an occasional patient may have some evidence of cinchonism such as tinnitus from use of one or two tablets daily (see Warnings).

Distribution – Quinine is approximately 70% to 85% protein bound. The concentration of the alkaloid in cerebrospinal fluid is only 2% to 7% of that in the plasma. However, it can cross the placenta and readily reach fetal tissues.

Metabolism/Excretion – The cinchona alkaloids are primarily metabolized in the liver; $<$ 5% is excreted unaltered in the urine. There is no accumulation in the body upon continued administration. Half-life is 4 to 5 hours. After termination of therapy, the plasma level falls rapidly and only a negligible concentration is detectable after 24 hours.

The metabolites are excreted in the urine, many as hydroxy derivatives; small amounts also appear in the feces, gastric juice, bile and saliva. Renal excretion of quinine is twice as rapid when the urine is acidic as when it is alkaline; greater tubular reabsorption of the alkaloidal base occurs in an alkaline medium.

The pharmacokinetics of quinine are affected by malarial infection, with volume of distribution and systemic clearance decreasing. Also, protein binding increases (to $>$ 90%) in patients with cerebral malaria, in pregnant patients and in children.

Indications:

Chloroquine-resistant falciparum malaria: Either alone, with pyrimethamine and a sulfonamide or with a tetracycline. It is also considered alternative therapy for chloroquine-sensitive strains of *P falciparum, P malariae, P ovale* and *P vivax*. Mefloquine and clindamycin may also be used with quinine depending on where the malaria was acquired (eg, Southeast Asia, Bangladesh, East Africa).

Quinine dihydrochloride, a parenteral preparation available only from the CDC, may also be used (see CDC Anti-infective Agents).

Nocturnal recumbency leg cramps, prevention and treatment.

Contraindications:

Hypersensitivity to quinine; glucose-6-phosphate dehydrogenase (G-6-PD) deficiency; optic neuritis; tinnitus; history of blackwater fever and thrombocytopenic purpura (associated with previous quinine ingestion); pregnancy (see Warnings).

Warnings:

Cinchonism: Repeated doses or overdosage of quinine may precipitate cinchonism. The mildest symptoms include tinnitus, headache, nausea and slightly disturbed vision, which usually subside rapidly upon discontinuation of the drug. When quinine is continued or after large single doses, symptoms also involve the GI tract, the nervous and cardiovascular systems and the skin.

Tinnitus and impaired hearing may occur at plasma quinine concentrations $>$ 10 mcg/ml, a level not normally attained with quinine 260 to 520 mg/day. In a hypersensitive patient, as little as 300 mg may produce tinnitus.

Hemolysis (with the potential for hemolytic anemia) has been associated with a G-6-PD deficiency in patients taking quinine. Stop therapy immediately if hemolysis appears.

Cardiac disease: Use with caution in patients with cardiac arrhythmias; quinine has quinidine-like activity. In patients with atrial fibrillation, quinine use requires the same precautions as those for quinidine (see Drug Interactions). May cause cardiotoxicity.

(Warnings continued on following page)

QUININE SULFATE (Cont.)

Warnings (Cont.):

Hypersensitivity: Discontinue quinine if there is any evidence of hypersensitivity. Cutaneous flushing, pruritus, skin rashes, fever, gastric distress, dyspnea, ringing in the ears and visual impairment may occur, particularly with only small doses of quinine. Extreme flushing of the skin accompanied by intense, generalized pruritus is most common. Hemoglobinuria and asthma are idiosyncratic. Refer to Management of Acute Hypersensitivity Reactions.

Pregnancy: Category X. Quinine has an oxytocic action that appears to occur only with doses that are higher than those recommended. It also crosses the placenta. Congenital malformations have occurred primarily with large doses (up to 30 g) for attempted abortion. In about 50%, the malformation was deafness related to auditory nerve hypoplasia. Other abnormalities were limb anomalies, visceral defects and visual changes.

Lactation: Quinine is excreted in breast milk in small amounts. Although no adverse effects have been reported in the nursing infant, rule out patients at risk for G-6-PD deficiency before breastfeeding.

Drug Interactions:

Antacids, aluminum-containing may delay or decrease absorption of concurrent quinine.

Anticoagulants, oral: Quinine may depress the hepatic enzyme system that synthesizes the vitamin K dependent clotting factors and thus may enhance the action of warfarin and other oral anticoagulants.

Cimetidine may reduce quinine's oral clearance and increase its elimination half-life.

Digoxin serum concentrations may be increased by concurrent quinine.

Mefloquine: Do not use concurrently with quinine. If these agents are to be used in the initial treatment of severe malaria, delay mefloquine administration at least 12 hours after the last dose of quinine. ECG abnormalities or cardiac arrest may occur. The risk of convulsions may also be increased with coadministration.

Neuromuscular blocking agents (depolarizing and nondepolarizing): The neuromuscular blockade of these agents may be potentiated by quinine, and may result in respiratory difficulties.

Urinary alkalinizers (eg, acetazolamide and sodium bicarbonate) administered concurrently with quinine may increase quinine blood levels with potential for toxicity.

Drug/Lab test interactions: Elevated values for urinary **17 ketogenic steroids** may occur with the Zimmerman method.

Adverse Reactions:

Cinchonism (see Warnings) may occur at therapeutic doses.

Hematologic: Acute hemolysis; hemolytic anemia; thrombocytopenic purpura; agranulocytosis; hypoprothrombinemia.

Ophthalmic: Visual disturbances including – Disturbed color vision and perception; photophobia; blurred vision with scotomata; night blindness; amblyopia; diplopia; diminished visual fields; mydriasis; optic atrophy.

CNS: Tinnitus; deafness; vertigo; headache; fever; apprehension; restlessness; confusion; syncope; excitement; delirium; hypothermia; convulsions.

GI: Nausea; vomiting; epigastric pain; hepatitis.

Hypersensitivity: Cutaneous rashes (urticarial, papular, scarlatinal); pruritus; flushing; sweating; facial edema; asthmatic symptoms. See Warnings.

Cardiovascular: Anginal symptoms.

Overdosage:

Symptoms: The more common signs and symptoms of overdosage are tinnitus, dizziness, skin rash and GI disturbance (intestinal cramping). With higher doses, cardiovascular and CNS effects may occur, including headache, fever, vomiting, apprehension, confusion and convulsions. Other effects are listed in the Adverse Reactions section.

Fatalities with quinine have occurred from single oral doses of 2 to 8 g; a single fatality reported with a dose of 1.5 g may reflect an idiosyncratic effect. Several cases of blindness following large overdoses of quinine, with partial recovery of vision in each instance, have been reported.

(Overdosage continued on following page)

QUININE SULFATE (Cont.)

Overdosage (Cont.):

Treatment: Employ gastric lavage or induce emesis. Support blood pressure and maintain renal function; provide mechanical ventilation if needed. Use sedatives, oxygen and other supportive measures as necessary. Maintain fluid and electrolyte balance with IV fluids. Refer also to General Management of Acute Overdosage.

Urinary acidification will promote renal excretion of quinine. In the presence of hemoglobinuria, however, acidification of the urine may augment renal blockade. Quinine should be readily dialyzable by hemodialysis or hemoperfusion.

Angioedema or asthma may require epinephrine, corticosteroids and antihistamines.

In the acute phase of toxic amaurosis caused by quinine, IV vasodilators may have a salutory effect. Stellate block has also been used effectively for quinine-associated blindness. Residual visual impairment occasionally yields to vasodilators.

Patient Information:

Take with food or after meals to minimize GI irritation.

Medication may cause diarrhea, nausea, stomach cramps or pain, vomiting or ringing in the ears; notify physician if these become pronounced.

May produce blurred vision, vertigo, restlessness, confusion or dizziness; patients should observe caution while driving or performing other tasks requiring alertness.

Stop the drug if there is any evidence of allergy such as flushing, itching, rash, fever, stomach pain, difficult breathing, ringing in the ears and vision problems.

Administration and Dosage:

Chloroquine-resistant malaria:

Adults – 650 mg every 8 hours for 5 to 7 days.

Children – 25 mg/kg/day in divided doses every 8 hours for 5 to 7 days.

Chloroquine-sensitive malaria:

Adults – 600 mg every 8 hours for 5 to 7 days.

Children – 10 mg/kg every 8 hours for 5 to 7 days.

Nocturnal leg cramps: 260 to 300 mg at bedtime; if needed, may be taken after the evening meal and at bedtime.

	Product	Dosage form	Description/Packaging	C.I.*
otc sf	**M-KYA**[1] (Nature's Bounty)	**Capsules:** 64.8 mg[2]	In 50s.	6.3
otc	**Q-vel Soft Caplets**[1] (Ciba Consumer)		In 16s, 30s, 50s and 100s.	N/A
otc	**Formula Q**[1] (Major)	**Capsules:** 65 mg[3]	In 50s.	1.5
otc	**Legatrin**[1] (Columbia)	**Tablets:** 162.5 mg[4]	(480). Brick red. Oblong. In blister pack 30s and 50s.	3.6
otc	**Quinine Sulfate**[1] (Various, eg, Balan, Geneva, Major, Moore, Parmed, Purepac, R.I.D., Westward, Zenith)	**Capsules:** 200 mg	In 100s, 1000s and UD 100s.	1.4+
Rx[5]	**Quinine Sulfate**[1] (Various, eg, Balan, Baxter, Bolar, Moore, Parmed, Rugby, Schein, UDL, URL, Zenith)	**Tablets:** 260 mg	In 100s, 250s, 500s, 1000s and UD 100s.	1.1+
Rx	**Quinamm**[1] (Marion Merrell Dow)		Sucrose. (Merrell 547). White. In 100s.	7.1
Rx	**Quiphile**[1] (Geneva)		White. In 100s.	1.6
otc	**Quinine Sulfate**[1] (Major)	**Capsules:** 300 mg	In 100s, 500s and UD 100s.	1+
otc	**Quinine Sulfate**[6] (Various, eg, Balan, Geneva, Goldline, Lederle, Moore, Parmed, Purepac, Rugby, Schein, Zenith)	**Capsules:** 325 mg	In 100s, 500s, 1000s and UD 100s.	1+

* Cost Index based on cost per 325 mg.

sf – Sugar free.

[1] Product indicated only for treatment of nocturnal leg cramps.

[2] With 400 IU vitamin E (as dl-alpha tocopheryl acetate) and lecithin.

[3] With 400 IU vitamin E (as dl-alpha tocopheryl acetate).

[4] With calcium phosphate dibasic.

[5] Also available *otc* depending on distributor discretion.

[6] Indicated for nocturnal leg cramps, malaria, or both depending on specific distributor.

MEFLOQUINE HCl

Actions:

Pharmacology: Mefloquine is an antimalarial agent which acts as a blood schizonticide. Its exact mechanism of action is not known, but may act by raising intravesicular pH in parasite acid vesicles. It is a structural analog of quinine.

Pharmacokinetics: Studies of mefloquine in healthy male subjects showed that a significant lagtime occurred after drug administration, and the terminal elimination half-life varied widely (13 to 24 days) with a mean of about 3 weeks. Mefloquine is a mixture of enantiomeric molecules whose rates of release, absorption, transport, action, degradation and elimination may differ.

Additional studies showed slightly greater concentrations of drug for longer periods of time. The absorption half-life was 0.36 to 2 hours, and the terminal elimination half-life was 15 to 33 days. The primary metabolite was identified, and its concentrations were found to surpass the concentrations of mefloquine. In multiple-dose studies, the mean metabolite to mefloquine ratio measured at steady state was found to range between 2.3 and 8.6

The total clearance of the drug, which is essentially all hepatic, is ≈ 30 ml/min. The volume of distribution, ≈ 20 L/kg, indicates extensive distribution. The drug is highly bound (98%) to plasma proteins and concentrated in blood erythrocytes, the target cells in malaria, at a relatively constant erythrocyte-to-plasma concentration ratio of ≈ 2.

Indications:

Treatment of acute malaria infections: Treatment of mild to moderate acute malaria caused by mefloquine-susceptible strains of *Plasmodium falciparum* (both chloroquine-susceptible and resistant strains) or by *P vivax*. There are insufficient clinical data to document the effect of mefloquine in malaria caused by *P ovale* or *P malariae*.

Prevention of malaria: Prophylaxis of *P falciparum* and *P vivax* malaria infections, including prophylaxis of chloroquine-resistant strains of *P falciparum*. The use of mefloquine alone is recommended by the CDC for travel to areas of risk where chloroquine-resistant *P falciparum* exists.

Contraindications:

Hypersensitivity to mefloquine or related compounds.

Warnings:

In case of life-threatening, serious or overwhelming malaria infections due to *P falciparum*, treat patients with an IV antimalarial drug. Following completion of IV treatment, mefloquine may be given orally to complete the course of therapy.

Pregnancy: Category C. Mefloquine is teratogenic in rats and mice at a dose of 100 mg/kg/day. In rabbits, 160 mg/kg/day was embryotoxic and teratogenic, and 80 mg/kg/day was teratogenic but not embryotoxic. There are no adequate and well controlled studies in pregnant women. Use during pregnancy only if potential benefit justifies potential risk to the fetus. Warn women of childbearing potential traveling to areas where malaria is endemic against becoming pregnant and to take reliable contraceptive measures for 2 months after the last dose.

Lactation: Based on a study in a few subjects, low concentrations (3% to 4%) of mefloquine were excreted in breast milk following a dose equivalent to 250 mg of the free base. Exercise caution when mefloquine is administered to a nursing woman.

Children: Safety and efficacy in children have not been established. Two studies of mefloquine in children living in endemic areas for *P falciparum* were conducted. All children in these studies had at least a low level of parasitemia and 18% to 40% had significant parasitemia with or without mild malaria symptoms. When given a single 20 to 30 mg/kg dose, all children with fever became afebrile, and 92% of those with significant parasitemia had a satisfactory response to treatment. Nausea and vomiting occurred in ≈ 10% and 20%, respectively, and dizziness was seen in ≈ 40% of children.

Precautions:

Potentially hazardous tasks: Exercise caution while driving or operating hazardous machinery, as dizziness, a disturbed sense of balance or neuropsychiatric reactions have occurred during the use of mefloquine. During prophylactic use, if signs of unexplained anxiety, depression, restlessness or confusion are noticed, these may be considered prodromal to a more serious event. In these cases, the drug must be discontinued.

Monitoring: This drug has not been administered for > 1 year. If the drug is to be administered for a prolonged period, perform periodic evaluations including liver function tests.

Ocular lesions were observed in rats fed mefloquine daily for 2 years. All surviving rats given 30 mg/kg/day had ocular lesions in both eyes characterized by retinal degeneration, opacity of the lens and retinal edema. Similar but less severe lesions were observed in 80% of female and 22% of male rats fed 12.5 mg/kg/day for 2 years. At doses of 5 mg/kg/day, only corneal lesions were observed (9% of rats studied). Periodic ophthalmic examinations are recommended.

(Continued on following page)

MEFLOQUINE HCl (Cont.)

Drug Interactions:

Beta-adrenergic blockers: ECG abnormalities or cardiac arrest may occur with concurrent mefloquine. There is one report of cardiopulmonary arrest with full recovery in a patient taking propranolol.

Chloroquine: The risk of convulsions may be increased with concomitant mefloquine.

Quinine or quinidine: Do not use concurrently with mefloquine. If these agents are to be used in the initial treatment of severe malaria, delay mefloquine administration at least 12 hours after the last dose of quinine or quinidine. ECG abnormalities or cardiac arrest may occur. Although no cardiovascular action of mefloquine, a myocardial depressant, has been observed during clinical trials, parenteral studies in animals show that it possesses 20% of the antifibrillatory action of quinidine and produces 50% of the increase in the PR interval reported with quinine. The risk of convulsions may also be increased with concurrent mefloquine and quinine.

Valproic acid and concurrent mefloquine resulted in loss of seizure control and lower than expected valproic acid blood levels. Therefore, monitor valproic acid blood levels and adjust the dosage as necessary.

Adverse Reactions:

At the doses used for treatment of acute malaria infections, the symptoms possibly attributable to drug administration cannot be distinguished from those symptoms usually attributable to the disease itself.

Prophylaxis of malaria: Vomiting (3%); dizziness, syncope, extrasystoles ($<$ 1%); encephalopathy of unknown etiology (relationship to drug administration not established).

Treatment of malaria: The most frequently observed adverse reactions included: Dizziness; myalgia; nausea; fever; headache; vomiting; chills; diarrhea; skin rash; abdominal pain; fatigue; loss of appetite; tinnitus. Side effects occurring in $<$ 1% included: Bradycardia; hair loss; emotional problems; pruritus; asthenia; transient emotional disturbances; telogen effluvium (loss of resting hair); seizures.

Postmarketing surveillance: Vertigo; visual disturbances; CNS disturbances (eg, psychotic manifestations, hallucinations, confusion, anxiety, depression, convulsions).

Laboratory test abnormalities: Decreased hematocrit; transient elevation of transaminases; leukopenia; thrombocytopenia. These alterations were observed in patients with acute malaria who received treatment doses of the drug and were attributed to the disease itself. During prophylactic administration of mefloquine to indigenous populations in malaria-endemic areas, the following occasional alterations in laboratory values were observed: Transient elevation of transaminases; leukocytosis; thrombocytopenia.

Overdosage:

Induce vomiting and see a physician immediately because of the potential cardiotoxic effect. Treat vomiting or diarrhea with standard fluid therapy. Refer to General Management of Acute Overdosage.

Administration and Dosage:

Treatment of mild to moderate malaria in adults caused by P vivax or mefloquine-susceptible strains of P falciparum: Five tablets (1250 mg) mefloquine as a single dose. Do not take on an empty stomach. Administer with at least 240 ml (8 oz) of water.

Patients with acute *P vivax* malaria treated with mefloquine are at high risk of relapse because mefloquine does not eliminate exoerythrocytic (hepatic phase) parasites. To avoid relapse after initial treatment of the acute infection with mefloquine, subsequently treat with an 8-aminoquinolone (eg, primaquine).

Malaria prophylaxis: Adult – 250 mg once weekly for 4 weeks, then 250 mg every other week. The CDC recommends a single dose taken weekly starting 1 week before travel, continued weekly during travel and for 4 weeks after leaving such areas.[1]

Children – The CDC has recommended the following pediatric doses to be taken weekly, starting 1 week before travel, continued weekly during travel and for 4 weeks after leaving such areas: 15 to 19 kg, ¼ tab; 20 to 30 kg, ½ tab; 31 to 45 kg, ¾ tab; $>$ 45 kg, 1 tab.[1]

Initiate prophylactic drug administration 1 week prior to departure to an endemic area. It is suggested that the same day of the week be used each time the drug is administered. To avoid development of malaria after return from an endemic area, continue prophylaxis for 4 additional weeks. For prolonged stays in an endemic area this may be achieved by continuing the recommended dosage schedule, once weekly for 4 weeks, then once every other week, until the traveler has taken 3 doses following return to a malaria-free area. Do not take on an empty stomach. Administer with at least 240 ml (8 oz) of water.

C.I.*

Rx	**Lariam** (Roche)	**Tablets:** 250 mg mefloquine HCl	(Lariam 250 Roche). White, scored. In UD 25s.	56

* Cost Index based on cost per 250 mg.

[1] Morbidity and Mortality Weekly Report 1990 (March 9);39 (RR-3):1-10 and 1990 (Sept. 14);39:630.

QUINACRINE HCl

Actions:

Pharmacology: Quinacrine couples with and fixes DNA so that it is unable to replicate or serve for the transcription of RNA. Protein synthesis is thus decreased through ribosomal destruction.

Microbiology: Exerts both suppressive and therapeutic action in malaria. It destroys erythrocytic asexual forms (trophozoites) of vivax, falciparum and quartan malaria, and sexual forms (gametocytes) of vivax and quartan malaria. It is ineffective against falciparum gametocytes and sporozoites of all forms of malaria.

Pharmacokinetics: Oral administration produces maximum plasma levels in 1 to 3 hours and is widely distributed to tissues. Excretion is slow and the drug tends to accumulate; thus, quinacrine persists in the body for long periods of time. The metabolic fate is unknown. Biological half-life is about 5 days. The main route of excretion is the urine (11%); small amounts of unchanged drug are excreted in feces, sweat, milk, saliva and bile.

Indications:

Malaria: Occasionally used for malaria treatment and suppression, although the use of this drug for malaria has generally become obsolete and replaced by other therapies.

Giardiasis and cestodiasis treatment (see quinacrine monograph in Anthelmintic section).

Unlabeled uses: Quinacrine has been used intrapleurally in the prevention of recurrence of pneumothorax in patients at high risk of recurrence (eg, cystic fibrosis).

Contraindications:

Concomitant use with primaquine; see Drug Interactions.

Warnings:

Psoriasis or porphyria: Use in patients with psoriasis or porphyria may precipitate a severe attack or exacerbate the condition. Do not use in these conditions unless the benefit to the patient outweighs the possible hazard.

Resistant strains of *Plasmodium falciparum* have developed in recent years to synthetic antimalarial compounds (including quinacrine). Treat resistant strain of parasites with quinine or other specific forms of therapy.

Hepatic function impairment: Since the drug is known to concentrate in the liver, use with caution in patients with hepatic disease or alcoholism or in conjunction with known hepatotoxic drugs.

Elderly or debilitated: Quinacrine occasionally causes a transitory psychosis; therefore, use with special caution in patients > 60 years of age or in those with a history of psychosis.

Pregnancy: Use only when clearly needed and when the potential benefits outweigh the potential hazards to the fetus.

Precautions:

Hematologic effects: Periodically perform complete blood cell counts if patients are given prolonged therapy. If any severe blood disorder appears which is not attributable to the disease under treatment, discontinue use. Administer cautiously to patients with glucose-6-phosphate dehydrogenase (G-6-PD) deficiency.

Ophthalmologic effects: Instruct patients receiving prolonged therapy to promptly report any visual disturbances and to receive periodic complete ophthalmologic examinations.

Drug Interactions:

Primaquine toxicity is increased by quinacrine; concomitant use is contraindicated.

Adverse Reactions:

Temporarily imparts a yellow color to the urine and skin (but does not cause jaundice).

Frequent: Mild and transient headache; dizziness; GI complaints (eg, diarrhea, anorexia, nausea, abdominal cramps).

Infrequent, reversible: Pleomorphic skin eruptions; neuropsychiatric disturbances (eg, nervousness, vertigo, irritability, emotional change, nightmares, transient psychosis).

Rarely: Vomiting. Episodes of convulsions and transient toxic psychosis have been observed after doses of only 50 to 100 mg 3 times daily for a few days.

Prolonged therapy: Aplastic anemia; hepatitis; lichen planus-like eruptions.

Dermatologic: Exfoliative dermatitis; contact dermatitis.

Ophthalmic: Reversible corneal edema or deposits, manifested by visual halos, focusing difficulty and blurred vision, have occurred in patients during long-term suppressive therapy for malaria.

Retinopathy has occurred rarely in patients who received relatively high doses for prolonged periods. It has not been reported as a result of use in malaria suppression or in the short-term treatment of parasitic diseases.

(Continued on following page)

QUINACRINE HCl (Cont.)

Overdosage:

Symptoms: Extremely large doses may prove fatal. Toxic effects include CNS excitation with restlessness, insomnia, psychic stimulation and convulsions; GI disorders (nausea, vomiting, abdominal cramps, diarrhea); vascular collapse with hypotension, shock, cardiac arrhythmias or arrest; yellow pigmentation of the skin.

Treatment is symptomatic; evacuate the stomach by emesis or gastric lavage. Control seizures before attempting gastric lavage. If seizure is due to cerebral stimulation, cautiously administer an ultrashort-acting barbiturate. Correct anoxia-induced convulsions by administration of oxygen, mechanical ventilation or, in shock with hypotension, by vasopressor therapy. Because of the importance of supporting respiration, tracheal intubation or tracheostomy may be advisable.

Closely observe a patient who survives the acute phase and is asymptomatic for at least 6 hours. Fluids may be forced; urinary acidification helps promote urinary excretion of quinacrine.

Patient Information:

Take after meals with a full glass of water, tea or fruit juice.

May impart a yellow color to skin or urine.

Promptly report any visual disturbances to physician.

Administration and Dosage:

Treatment:

Adults and children > 8 years old – 200 mg with 1 g sodium bicarbonate every 6 hours for 5 doses; then 100 mg 3 times daily for 6 days (total dosage, 2.8 g in 7 days).

Children (4 to 8 years old) – 200 mg 3 times daily the first day; then 100 mg every 12 hours for 6 days.

Children (1 to 4 years old) – 100 mg 3 times daily the first day; then 100 mg once daily for 6 days.

Suppression: Maintain therapy for 1 to 3 months.

Adults – 100 mg daily.

Children – 50 mg daily.

				C.I.*
Rx	**Atabrine HCl** (Winthrop)	**Tablets:** 100 mg	In 100s.	33

* Cost Index based on cost per 100 mg.

The following is an abbreviated monograph. For complete prescribing information refer to the Tetracyclines monograph.

DOXYCYCLINE

CDC recommendations for use of doxycycline in malaria:[1]

Doxycycline alone taken daily is an alternative regimen for malaria prophylaxis for short-term travelers who are intolerant of mefloquine or for whom the drug is contraindicated. Doxycycline prophylaxis can begin 1 to 2 days before travel to malarious areas and continued daily during travel in the malarious area and for 4 weeks after the traveler leaves the area.

Caution patients that the drug may cause photosensitivity. Do not use during pregnancy or in children < 8 years of age.

Administration and Dosage:[1]

Adults: 100 mg once daily.

Children (> 8 years of age): 2 mg/kg/day up to adult dose of 100 mg/day.

For complete listing of available products, see Doxycycline monograph in the Tetracyclines section.

[1] Morbidity and Mortality Weekly Report 1990 (March 9);39 (RR-3):1-10.

4-Aminoquinoline Compounds

Actions:

Pharmacology: Although the exact mechanism of action of chloroquine is not known, several mechanisms have been suggested. The drug concentrates within parasite acid vesicles and raises the internal pH. The "non-weak base effect" results in inhibition of the parasite growth at extracellular chloroquine concentrations; this effect may occur due to an active chloroquine-concentrating mechanism in the acid vesicles of the parasite. Another mechanism may involve aggregates of ferriprotoporphyrin IX, which are released by parasitized erythrocytes during hemoglobin degradation and serve as chloroquine receptors, thus causing membrane damage with lysis of parasites or erythrocytes. Chloroquine may also influence hemoglobin digestion by the parasite or interfere with parasite/nucleoprotein synthesis.

Pharmacokinetics: Absorbed readily from the GI tract, peak plasma levels are reached in 1 to 6 hours. Plasma protein binding is 55%. The drug concentrates in the liver, spleen, kidney, heart and brain and is strongly bound in melanin-containing cells such as those in the eyes and skin. Chloroquine is eliminated very slowly and may persist in tissues for a prolonged period. Up to 70% of a dose may be excreted unchanged in the urine and up to 25% as a metabolite. Renal excretion is enhanced by urinary acidification.

Microbiology: Highly active against the erythrocytic forms of *Plasmodium vivax* and *malariae* and most strains of *P falciparum* (but not the gametocytes of *P falciparum*). It provides suppression without prevention of the infection.

These drugs do not prevent relapses or infection of vivax or malariae malaria; they are not effective against exoerythrocytic forms of the parasite. Highly effective as suppressive agents in vivax or malariae malaria, in terminating acute attacks and significantly lengthening the interval between treatment and relapse. In patients with falciparum malaria, they abolish the acute attack and completely cure the infection, unless due to a resistant strain. Hydroxychloroquine is not effective against chloroquine-resistant strains of *P falciparum.*

Indications:

Prophylaxis and treatment of acute attacks of malaria due to *P vivax, P malariae, P ovale* and susceptible strains of *P falciparum.* Chloroquine phosphate is the drug of choice in this situation. Chloroquine HCl is used when oral therapy is not feasible. For radical cure of vivax and malariae malaria, concomitant primaquine therapy is required.

Unlabeled use: Chloroquine has been used to suppress rheumatoid arthritis and in the treatment of systemic and discoid lupus erythematosus, scleroderma, pemphigus, lichen planus, polymyositis, sarcoidosis and porphyria cutanea tarda.

For other uses, refer to individual product monographs.

Contraindications:

Retinal or visual field changes; hypersensitivity. Consider an exception in acute malarial attacks caused by *Plasmodia* strains susceptible only to 4-aminoquinoline compounds.

Hydroxychloroquine is not for long-term therapy in children.

Warnings:

Resistance: Certain strains of *P falciparum* are resistant to 4-aminoquinoline compounds; normally adequate doses fail to prevent or cure clinical malaria or parasitemia. Treatment with quinine or other specific forms of therapy is advised for such an infection.

Retinopathy: Irreversible retinal damage has been observed with long-term or high dosages. Retinopathy has been reported to be dose-related.

When prolonged therapy is contemplated, perform baseline and periodic ophthalmologic examinations (including visual acuity, expert slit-lamp, funduscopic and visual field tests). If there is any past or present indication of abnormality in the visual acuity, visual field or retinal macular areas (pigmentary changes, loss of foveal reflex) or any visual symptoms (light flashes and streaks) not explainable by difficulties of accommodation or corneal opacities, discontinue therapy immediately and observe for possible progression. Retinal changes and visual disturbances may progress even after cessation of therapy.

Muscular weakness: Question and examine patients periodically; test knee and ankle reflexes to detect muscular weakness. If weakness occurs, discontinue therapy.

Psoriasis or porphyria: Use of these drugs may exacerbate these conditions. Do not use in these conditions unless the benefit to the patient outweighs the possible hazard.

Pregnancy: Use only when clearly needed and when potential benefits outweigh potential hazards to the fetus. In mice, IV chloroquine rapidly crosses the placenta, accumulates in melanin structures of fetal eyes and remains in ocular tissue 5 months after elimination from the rest of the body.

Lactation: Safety for use has not been established; these agents are excreted in breast milk. A nursing infant may consume ≈ 0.55% of a 300 mg maternal dose over 24 hours. One study determined the milk:blood ratio of the nursing mother to be 0.358.

(Warnings continued on following page)

4-Aminoquinoline Compounds (Cont.)

Warnings (Cont.):

Children: Children are especially sensitive to the 4-aminoquinoline compounds. Fatalities following accidental ingestion of relatively small doses and sudden deaths from parenteral chloroquine have been recorded. Do not exceed a single dose of 5 mg base/kg of chloroquine HCl in infants or children.

Precautions:

Hepatic function impairment: Since these drugs concentrate in the liver, use with caution in patients with hepatic disease or alcoholism or in conjunction with hepatotoxic drugs.

Monitoring: Perform periodic CBCs during prolonged therapy. If any severe blood disorder not attributable to the disease appears, consider discontinuing therapy. Measure glucose-6-phosphate dehydrogenase (G-6-PD) in susceptible individuals prior to initiating therapy. Although probably safe when given in normal therapeutic doses, these compounds may induce hemolysis in G-6-PD deficient individuals in the presence of infection or stressful conditions. An acute drop in hematocrit, hemoglobin and red blood cell count may occur.

Drug Interactions:

Cimetidine may reduce the oral clearance rate and metabolism of chloroquine.

Kaolin or **magnesium trisilicate:** GI absorption of chloroquine may be decreased by concomitant administration of these agents.

Adverse Reactions:

Cardiovascular: Hypotension; ECG changes (particularly inversion or depression of the T-wave, widening of QRS complex).

CNS: Mild, transient headache; psychic stimulation; psychotic episodes or convulsions (rare).

GI: Anorexia; nausea; vomiting; diarrhea; abdominal cramps.

Otologic: A few cases of a nerve-type deafness have occurred after prolonged high doses. Tinnitus and reduced hearing occurred in a patient with preexistent auditory damage after administration of 500 mg once a week for a few months.

Ophthalmic: Irreversible retinal damage in patients receiving long-term or high-dosage 4-aminoquinoline therapy; visual disturbances (blurring of vision and difficulty of focusing or accommodation); nyctalopia; scotomatous vision with field defects of paracentral, pericentral ring types and typically temporal scotomas, eg, difficulty in reading with words tending to disappear, seeing half an object, misty vision and fog before the eyes.

Other: Agranulocytosis; pruritus; neuropathy, blood dyscrasias, lichen planus-like eruptions, skin and mucosal pigmentary changes, pleomorphic skin eruptions (prolonged therapy).

Overdosage:

Symptoms may occur within 30 minutes in overdosage (or rarely with lower doses in hypersensitive patients) and consist of headache, drowsiness, visual disturbances, cardiovascular collapse and convulsions followed by sudden and early respiratory and cardiac arrest. Respiratory depression, cardiovascular collapse, shock, convulsions and death have occurred with overdose of parenteral **chloroquine HCl,** especially in infants and children. The ECG may reveal atrial standstill, nodal rhythm, prolonged intraventricular conduction and bradycardia progressing to ventricular fibrillation or arrest. In a retrospective study it was determined that ingestion of $>$ 5 g of chloroquine was an accurate predictor of fatal outcome in adults, although the amount may be as low as 2 g (250 mg in children).

Treatment is symptomatic; the stomach must be immediately evacuated by emesis or gastric lavage. After lavage, activated charcoal (a dose not less than five times estimated dose ingested) may inhibit further absorption if given within 30 minutes of ingestion.

Control convulsions before attempting gastric lavage. If due to cerebral stimulation, cautious administration of a short-acting anticonvulsant may be tried. Treat anoxia-induced convulsions by oxygen, mechanical ventilation or, in shock with hypotension, by vasopressor therapy. Tracheal intubation or tracheostomy may be necessary. Peritoneal dialysis and exchange transfusions have been suggested.

For at least 6 hours, closely observe an asymptomatic patient who survives the acute phase. Force fluids and acidify the urine to help promote excretion.

In one study, 10 of 11 patients who ingested $>$ 5 g of chloroquine survived after treatment with diazepam and epinephrine for several days along with mechanical ventilation. The use of diazepam has also been successful in other reports.

Patient Information:

May cause GI upset; take with food. Complete full course of therapy.

Report any visual disturbances or difficulty in hearing or ringing in the ears to physician.

Keep out of reach of children; overdosage is especially dangerous in children.

Medication may cause diarrhea, loss of appetite, nausea, stomach pain or vomiting, muscle weakness or rash. Notify physician if these become pronounced or bothersome.

(Products listed on following pages)

Refer to the general discussion of these products beginning on page 1913

4-Aminoquinoline Compounds (Cont.)

CHLOROQUINE PHOSPHATE

Chloroquine phosphate 500 mg is equivalent to 300 mg chloroquine base and 400 mg hydroxychloroquine sulfate.

Indications:

Prophylaxis and treatment of acute attacks of malaria due to *P vivax, P malariae, P ovale* and susceptible strains of *P falciparum.*

Also used for treatment of extraintestinal amebiasis (see Amebicides section).

Administration and Dosage:

Children's doses, expressed in mg/kg, should not exceed the recommended adult dose.

Suppression: Adults – 300 mg (base) weekly, on the same day each week. Begin 1 to 2 weeks prior to exposure; continue for 4 weeks after leaving endemic area.

If suppressive therapy is not begun prior to exposure, double the initial loading dose (adults – 600 mg base; children – 10 mg base/kg) and give in 2 divided doses, 6 hours apart.

Children – Administer 5 mg base/kg weekly, up to a maximum adult dose of 300 mg base.[1]

Children's Chloroquine Dose Based on Age	
Age (years)	Chloroquine base equivalent
< 1	37.5 mg
1 to 3	75 mg
4 to 6	100 mg
7 to 10	150 mg
11 to 16	225 mg

CDC recommended schedule for chloroquine as an alternative to mefloquine:[1] Travelers to areas of risk where chloroquine-resistant *P falciparum* is endemic and for whom mefloquine is contraindicated may elect to use an alternative regimen. Chloroquine alone taken weekly is recommended for travelers who cannot use mefloquine or doxycycline, especially pregnant women and children < 15 kg. In addition, give these travelers a single treatment dose of sulfadoxine/pyrimethamine (see individual monograph) to keep during travel and to take promptly in the event of a febrile illness during their travel when professional medical care is not readily available. Continue weekly chloroquine prophylaxis after presumptive treatment with sulfadoxine/pyrimethamine.

Acute attack:

Chloroquine Phosphate Dose in Acute Malarial Attack			
		Dosage (in mg of base)	
Dose	Time	Adults	Children
Initial dose	Day 1	600 mg	10 mg/kg
2nd dose	6 hours later	300 mg	5 mg/kg
3rd dose	Day 2	300 mg	5 mg/kg
4th dose	Day 3	300 mg	5 mg/kg

	Product	Dosage form	Packaging	C.I.*
Rx	**Chloroquine Phosphate** (Various, eg, Balan, Danbury, Geneva, Goldline, Major, Moore, Rugby, Schein, URL, West-Ward)	**Tablets:** 250 mg	In 100s, 250s, 1000s and UD 100s.	1+
Rx	**Aralen Phosphate** (Winthrop)	**Tablets:** 500 mg (equiv. to 300 mg base)	Pink. Sugar coated. In 25s.	26

* Cost Index based on cost per 500 mg.

[1] Morbidity and Mortality Weekly Report 1990 (March 9);39 (RR-3):1-10.

Refer to the general discussion of these products beginning on page 1913

4-Aminoquinoline Compounds (Cont.)

CHLOROQUINE HCl

Chloroquine HCl 50 mg is equivalent to 40 mg chloroquine base.

Indications:

Treatment of malaria when oral therapy is not feasible.

Also used for treatment of extraintestinal amebiasis (see Amebicides section).

Administration and Dosage:

Adults: 160 to 200 mg base (4 to 5 ml) IM initially; repeat in 6 hours if necessary. Do not exceed 800 mg (base) total dose in the first 24 hours. Begin oral dosage as soon as possible and continue for 3 days until approximately 1.5 g base has been administered.

Other suggested dosages include 2.5 mg base/kg every 4 hours or 3.5 mg/kg every 6 hours; repeat if necessary, maximum 25 mg/kg/day.

Children: Infants and children are extremely susceptible to overdosage. Severe reactions and deaths have occurred. The recommended single dose is 5 mg base/kg; repeat in 6 hours. Do not exceed 10 mg base/kg/24 hours.

				C.I.*
Rx	**Aralen HCl** (Winthrop)	**Injection:** 50 mg (equiv. to 40 mg chloroquine base) per ml	In 5 ml amps.	201

HYDROXYCHLOROQUINE SULFATE

Hydroxychloroquine sulfate 200 mg is equivalent to 155 mg hydroxychloroquine base and 250 mg chloroquine phosphate.

Indications:

Prophylaxis and treatment of acute attacks of malaria due to *P vivax, P malariae, P ovale* and susceptible strains of *P falciparum.*

Also used for the treatment of discoid and systemic lupus erythematosus and rheumatoid arthritis (see monograph in Antirheumatic Agents section).

Administration and Dosage:

Children's doses, expressed in mg/kg, should not exceed the recommended adult dose.

Suppression: Adults – 310 mg base weekly on the same day each week. Begin 1 to 2 weeks prior to exposure; continue for 4 weeks after leaving endemic area.

If suppressive therapy is not begun prior to exposure, double the initial loading dose (adults – 620 mg base; children – 10 mg base/kg) and give in 2 doses, 6 hours apart.

Children – Administer 5 mg base/kg weekly, up to a maximum adult dose.

Children's Hydroxychloroquine Dose Based on Age

Age (years)	Hydroxychloroquine base equivalent
< 1	37.5 mg
1 to 3	75 mg
4 to 6	100 mg
7 to 10	150 mg
11 to 16	225 mg

Acute attack:

Hydroxychloroquine Dose in Acute Malarial Attack

		Dosage (in mg of base)	
Dose	Time	Adults	Children
Initial dose	Day 1	620 mg	10 mg/kg
2nd dose	6 hours later	310 mg	5 mg/kg
3rd dose	Day 2	310 mg	5 mg/kg
4th dose	Day 3	310 mg	5 mg/kg

An alternative method, using a single dose of 620 mg base, has also proved effective.

				C.I.*
Rx	**Plaquenil Sulfate** (Winthrop)	**Tablets:** 200 mg (equiv. to 155 mg base)	In 100s.	19

* Cost Index based on cost per 500 mg chloroquine HCl or 400 mg hydroxychloroquine sulfate.

8-Aminoquinoline Compound

PRIMAQUINE PHOSPHATE

Primaquine phosphate 26.3 mg is equivalent to 15 mg primaquine base.

Actions:

An 8-aminoquinoline, primaquine is structurally similar to the 4-aminoquinolines but possesses markedly different antimalarial activities.

Pharmacology: Primaquine may disrupt the parasite's mitochondria and bind to native DNA. The resulting structural changes create a major disruption in the metabolic process. The gametocyte and exoerythrocyte forms are inhibited. Some gametocytes are destroyed while others are rendered incapable of undergoing maturation division in the mosquito gut. By eliminating tissue (exoerythrocyte) infection, primaquine prevents development of blood (erythrocytic) forms responsible for relapses in vivax malaria.

Pharmacokinetics: After oral administration, peak plasma concentrations of primaquine are reached in 1 to 3 hours. Primaquine, as compared to other antimalarials, is found in relatively low concentrations in the tissues. Highest concentrations are in the liver, lungs, brain, heart and skeletal muscle.

Primaquine is rapidly metabolized to a carboxylic acid derivative and then to further metabolites which have varying degrees of activity; elimination half-life is around 4 hours. Approximately 1% is excreted unchanged in the urine.

Microbiology: Active against *Plasmodium vivax, P ovale* and the gametocytial forms of *P falciparum.*

Indications:

Recommended only for the radical cure of vivax malaria, the prevention of relapse in vivax malaria or following the termination of chloroquine phosphate suppressive therapy in an area where vivax malaria is endemic.

Contraindications:

Concomitant administration of quinacrine and primaquine (see Drug Interactions); the acutely ill suffering from systemic disease manifested by tendency to granulocytopenia (eg, rheumatoid arthritis and lupus erythematosus); concurrent administration of other potentially hemolytic drugs or bone marrow depressants.

Warnings:

Hemolytic reactions (moderate to severe) may occur in the following groups of people while receiving primaquine: Glucose-6-phosphate dehydrogenase (G-6-PD) deficient patients; individuals with idiosyncratic reactions (manifested by hemolytic anemia, methemoglobinemia or leukopenia); or individuals with nicotinamide adenine dinucleotide (NADH) methemoglobin reductase deficiency. Discontinue if marked darkening of the urine or sudden decrease in hemoglobin concentration or leukocyte count occurs.

Pregnancy: Safety for use during pregnancy has not been established. Use only when clearly needed and when potential benefits outweigh potential hazards to the fetus.

Precautions:

Anemia, methemoglobinemia and leukopenia have occurred following large doses; do not exceed recommended dose. Perform routine blood examinations (particularly blood cell counts and hemoglobin determinations) during therapy.

Drug Interactions:

Quinacrine may potentiate the toxicity of antimalarial compounds which are structurally related to primaquine. Do not administer primaquine to patients who have recently received quinacrine.

Adverse Reactions:

GI: Nausea; vomiting; epigastric distress; abdominal cramps.

Hematologic: Leukopenia; hemolytic anemia in G-6-PD deficient individuals; methemoglobinemia in NADH methemoglobin reductase deficient individuals.

Overdosage:

Symptoms: Abdominal cramps; vomiting; burning, epigastric distress; CNS and cardiovascular disturbances; cyanosis; methemoglobinemia; moderate leukocytosis or leukopenia; anemia. The most striking symptoms are granulocytopenia and acute hemolytic anemia in sensitive persons. Acute hemolysis occurs, but patients recover completely if the dosage is discontinued.

Treatment is symptomatic.

(Continued on following page)

8-Aminoquinoline Compound (Cont.)

PRIMAQUINE PHOSPHATE (Cont.)

Patient Information:

Complete full course of therapy.

If GI upset occurs, may be taken with food. If stomach upset (nausea, vomiting or stomach pain) continues, notify physician.

Notify physician if a darkening of the urine occurs.

Administration and Dosage:

Patients suffering from an attack of vivax malaria or having parasitized red blood cells should receive a course of chloroquine phosphate which quickly destroys the erythrocytic parasites and terminates the paroxysm. Administer primaquine concurrently to eradicate the exoerythrocytic parasites in a dosage of 15 mg (base) daily for 14 days.

CDC recommended treatment schedule[1]:

Begin therapy during the last 2 weeks of, or following a course of, suppression with chloroquine or a comparable drug.

Adults – 26.3 mg (15 mg base) daily for 14 days.

Children – 0.5 mg/kg/day (0.3 mg base/kg/day; maximum 15 mg base/dose) for 14 days.

C.I.*

			C.I.*
Rx	**Primaquine Phosphate**[2] (Winthrop)	**Tablets:** 26.3 mg (equivalent to 15 mg base). Lactose, sucrose. In 100s.	4.5

CHLOROQUINE PHOSPHATE WITH PRIMAQUINE PHOSPHATE

Consider the prescribing information for chloroquine phosphate and for primaquine phosphate when using this product.

Indications:

Prophylaxis of malaria, regardless of species, in all areas where the disease is endemic.

Administration and Dosage:

Adults: Start at least 1 day before entering the endemic area. Take 1 tablet weekly on the same day each week. Continue for 8 weeks after leaving the endemic area.

Children: The following dosage (based on body weight) is suggested:

Chloroquine Phosphate/Primaquine Phosphate Dosage for Children Based on Body Weight

Weight		Chloroquine base (mg)	Primaquine base (mg)	Dose† (ml)
(lb)	(kg)			
10-15	4.5-6.8	20	3	2.5
16-25	7.3-11.4	40	6	5
26-35	11.8-15.9	60	9	7.5
36-45	16.4-20.5	80	12	10
46-55	20.9-25	100	15	12.5
56-100	25.4-45.4	150	22.5	½ tab.
100+	>45.4	300	45	1 tab.

† Dose based on liquid containing approx. 40 mg of chloroquine base and 6 mg primaquine base per 5 ml, prepared from chloroquine phosphate with primaquine phosphate tablets (1 crushed tablet suspended in 40 ml liquid. Chocolate syrup may be used to prepare a suspension). Shake well before using.

			C.I.*
Rx	**Aralen Phosphate With Primaquine Phosphate** (Winthrop)	**Tablets:** 500 mg chloroquine phosphate (300 mg base) and 79 mg primaquine phosphate (45 mg base). Lactose. In 100s.	32

* Cost Index based on cost per 26.3 mg or tablet.

[1] Morbidity and Mortality Weekly Report 1990 (March 9);39(No. RR-3):1-10.

[2] Production temporarily discontinued; expected to be commercially available again in mid-1991. In the meantime, CDC has acquired a supply in sufficient quantity for treatment of nonmilitary cases of *P vivax* and *P ovale* infections. Because of the limited supply, CDC is unable to provide the drug for persons who wish to use it as part of a chemoprophylactic regimen. For further information, call 404-639-3670.

For information on the sulfadoxine and pyrimethamine combination, see individual monograph.

Folic Acid Antagonists

PYRIMETHAMINE

Actions:

Pharmacology: Pyrimethamine is a folic acid antagonist; its therapeutic action is based on differential requirement between host and parasite for nucleic acid precursors involved in growth as it selectively inhibits plasmodial dihydrofolate reductase. Pyrimethamine inhibits the enzyme dihydrofolate reductase which catalyzes the reduction of dihydrofolate to tetrahydrofolate. This activity is highly selective against plasmodia and *Toxoplasma gondii.* It does not destroy gametocytes, but arrests sporogony in the mosquito. Pyrimethamine possesses blood schizonticidal, and some tissue schizonticidal activity may be slower than that of 4-amino-quinoline compounds.

Pharmacokinetics: Pyrimethamine is well absorbed after oral administration. Peak plasma concentrations occur in 2 to 6 hours. It has a plasma half-life of about 4 days and suppressive concentrations are maintained for approximately 2 weeks. It is approximately 87% bound to plasma proteins. Pyrimethamine is hepatically metabolized. Several metabolites appear in the urine, but metabolic disposition is not well characterized.

Indications:

Chemoprophylaxis of malaria due to susceptible strains of plasmodia. Fast-acting schizonticides (chloroquine or quinine) are preferable for treatment of acute attacks. However, concurrent pyrimethamine will initiate transmission control and suppressive cure.

Toxoplasmosis: Use with a sulfonamide; synergism exists with this combination.

Contraindications:

Hypersensitivity to the drug; documented megaloblastic anemia due to folate deficiency.

Warnings:

Folic acid deficiency: The dosage required for treatment of toxoplasmosis is 10 to 20 times the recommended antimalarial dosage and approaches the toxic level. If signs of folate deficiency develop, reduce dosage or discontinue drug according to patient response. Folinic acid (leucovorin) may be given in a dosage of 5 to 15 mg/day (orally, IM or IV) until normal hematopoiesis is restored. Use with caution in patients with possible folate deficiency (eg, malabsorption syndrome, alcoholism, pregnancy).

Carcinogenesis/Mutagenesis/Impairment of fertility: Pyrimethamine produces a significant increase in the number of lung tumors per mouse when given intraperitoneally at high doses (0.025 g/kg). There have been two reports of cancer associated with pyrimethamine: A 51-year-old female who developed chronic granulocytic leukemia after taking the drug for 2 years for toxoplasmosis; a 56-year-old patient who developed reticulum cell sarcoma after 14 months of pyrimethamine for toxoplasmosis.

In vivo, chromosomes analyzed from the bone marrow of rats dosed with pyrimethamine showed an increased number of structural and numerical aberrations.

The fertility index of rats treated with pyrimethamine is lowered only when the higher dosage is used, suggesting a possible toxic effect upon the whole organism or the conceptuses.

Hypersensitivity reactions, occasionally severe, can occur at any dose, particularly when pyrimethamine is coadministered with a sulfonamide. Refer to Management of Acute Hypersensitivity Reactions.

Renal or hepatic function impairment: Use with caution.

Pregnancy: Category C. Large doses may produce teratogenic effects in animals. Use pyrimethamine for confirmed acute toxoplasmosis only after weighing the possibility of teratogenic effects against the possible risks of permanent damage to the fetus from the infection. Coadministration of folinic acid is recommended.

Lactation: Pyrimethamine is excreted in breast milk with a milk:plasma ratio of 0.2 to 0.43. Milk samples obtained from lactating mothers after pyrimethamine treatment had measurable concentrations of the drug with peak concentration at 6 hours postadministration. It is estimated that after a single 75 mg dose of oral pyrimethamine, approximately 3 to 4 mg of the drug would be passed on to the feeding child over a 48 hour period. Safety for use has not been established. Because of the potential for serious adverse reactions in nursing infants from pyrimethamine, decide whether to discontinue nursing or discontinue the drug, taking into account the importance of the drug to the mother.

Precautions:

Do not exceed the recommended dosage for malaria suppression. For toxoplasmosis, perform semiweekly blood counts, including platelet counts. In patients with convulsive disorders, use a lower initial dose (for toxoplasmosis) to avoid potential CNS toxicity.

G-6-PD: May precipitate hemolytic anemia in patients with glucose-6-phosphate dehydrogenase deficiency, generally in the presence of other stressful events.

(Continued on following page)

PYRIMETHAMINE (Cont.)

Drug Interactions:

Antifolic drugs (eg, **methotrexate, sulfonamides, TMP-SMZ**) and concurrent pyrimethamine may increase the risk of bone marrow suppression. Discontinue pyrimethamine if signs of folate deficiency develop (see Warnings).

Adverse Reactions:

GI: Anorexia, vomiting (large doses); atrophic glossitis. Vomiting may be minimized by giving with meals; it usually disappears promptly upon reduction of dosage.

Hematologic: Megaloblastic anemia, leukopenia, thrombocytopenia, pancytopenia, hematuria (large doses). Hematologic effects, however, may also occur at low doses.

Rare: Insomnia; diarrhea; headache; lightheadedness; dryness of the mouth or throat; fever; malaise; dermatitis; abnormal skin pigmentation; depression; seizures; pulmonary eosinophilia; hyperphenylalaninemia.

Other: Cardiac rhythm disorders (large doses).

Overdosage:

Symptoms: Acute intoxication may involve GI symptoms or CNS stimulation including convulsions. Initial symptoms are usually GI and may include abdominal pain, nausea, and severe and repeated vomiting possibly including hematemesis. CNS toxicity may be manifest by initial excitability, generalized and prolonged convulsions which may be followed by respiratory depression, circulatory collapse and death within a few hours. Neurological symptoms appear rapidly (30 min to 2 hours after drug ingestion), suggesting that in gross overdosage pyrimethamine has a direct toxic effect on the CNS.

The fatal dose is variable; the smallest reported fatal single dose is 250 to 300 mg. There are reports of children who have recovered after taking 375 to 625 mg.

Treatment: There is no specific antidote. Gastric lavage is effective if carried out very soon after drug ingestion. A parenteral barbiturate may be indicated to control convulsions. Folinic acid (leucovorin) may also be given to counteract effects on the hematopoietic system. Treatment includes usual supportive measures. Refer to General Management of Acute Overdosage.

Patient Information:

May cause anorexia or vomiting; take with food or meals.

At first appearance of a skin rash, discontinue the drug and seek medical attention.

Notify physician if sore throat, pallor, purpura or glossitis occurs.

Blood counts at scheduled intervals are essential in patients receiving high dosage and should not be delayed or missed.

Administration and Dosage:

Chemoprophylaxis of malaria:

Adults and children (> 10 years old) – 25 mg once weekly.

Children (4 to 10 years old) – 12.5 mg once weekly.

Infants and children (< 4 years old) – 6.25 mg once weekly.

Extend regimens to include suppressive cure through any characteristic periods of early recrudescence and late relapse for at least 6 to 10 weeks in each case.

Treatment of acute attacks: Recommended in areas where only susceptible plasmodia exist. Not recommended alone in treatment of acute attacks of malaria in nonimmune persons. Fast-acting schizonticides (chloroquine or quinine) are indicated for treatment of acute attacks. However, concomitant pyrimethamine, 25 mg daily for 2 days, will initiate transmission control and suppressive cure.

If pyrimethamine must be used alone in semi-immune persons for acute attack: *Adults and children (> 10 years old)* – 50 mg daily for 2 days. *Children (4 to 10 years old)* – 25 mg daily for 2 days.

Follow clinical cure by the once weekly chemoprophylactic regimen described above.

Toxoplasmosis: At the high dosage, there is marked variation in tolerance. Young patients may tolerate higher doses than older patients.

Adults – Initially, 50 to 75 mg daily with 1 to 4 g of a sulfapyrimidine. Continue for 1 to 3 weeks, depending on response and tolerance. Dosage for each drug may then be reduced by one-half and continued for an additional 4 or 5 weeks.

Pediatric dosage is 1 mg/kg/day divided into 2 equal daily doses; after 2 to 4 days, reduce to one-half and continue for approximately 1 month. Usual pediatric sulfonamide dosage is used in conjunction with pyrimethamine.

Another recommended dosage is a loading dose of 2 mg/kg/day for 3 days, then a maintenance dose of 1 mg/kg/day or divided twice daily for 4 weeks; maximum 25 mg/day.

				C.I.*
Rx	**Daraprim** (Burroughs Wellcome)	**Tablets:** 25 mg	(Daraprim A3A). White, scored. In 100s.	68

* Cost Index based on cost per 50 mg.

SULFADOXINE AND PYRIMETHAMINE

Warning:
Fatalities associated with sulfadoxine/pyrimethamine have occurred due to severe reactions, including Stevens-Johnson syndrome and toxic epidermal necrolysis. Discontinue prophylaxis if skin rash appears, if the count of any formed blood elements is reduced significantly, or if active bacterial or fungal infections occur.

Actions:

Pharmacology: Sulfadoxine/pyrimethamine is an antimalarial agent which acts by reciprocal potentiation of its components, achieved by a sequential blockade of two enzymes involved in the biosynthesis of folinic acid within the parasites. The bacteriostatic action of sulfonamides occurs through competitive antagonism of para-aminobenzoic acid, an essential component in folic acid synthesis. Pyrimethamine inhibits the enzyme dihydrofolate reductase, which catalyzes the reduction of dihydrofolate to tetrahydrofolate and is important to cellular biosynthesis of purines, pyrimidines and some amino acids.

Pharmacokinetics: Both sulfadoxine and pyrimethamine are orally absorbed and excreted mainly by the kidneys. Following a single tablet, sulfadoxine peak plasma concentrations of 51 to 76 mcg/ml are achieved in 2.5 to 6 hours and pyrimethamine peak plasma concentrations of 0.13 to 0.4 mcg/ml are achieved in 1.5 to 8 hours. Elimination half-life of sulfadoxine ranges from 100 to 231 hours (mean, 169 hours); that of pyrimethamine ranges from 54 to 148 hours (mean, 111 hours).

Indications:

Treatment of Plasmodium falciparum malaria in patients in whom chloroquine resistance is suspected. Chloroquine remains the drug of choice for travelers to malarious areas.

Prophylaxis of malaria is indicated for travelers to areas where chloroquine-resistant *P falciparum* malaria is endemic. However, resistant strains may be encountered. Regardless of the prophylactic regimen used, it is still possible to contract malaria.

Unlabeled use: Sulfadoxine/pyrimethamine has been used as a prophylactic agent for the prevention of *Pneumocystis carinii* pneumonia in patients with AIDS, usually as a second-line agent.

Contraindications:

Hypersensitivity to pyrimethamine or sulfonamides; patients with documented megaloblastic anemia due to folate deficiency; infants $<$ 2 months of age; pregnancy at term and during the nursing period (see Warnings); prophylactic (repeated) use in patients with severe renal insufficiency, marked liver parenchymal damage or blood dyscrasias.

Warnings:

Deaths associated with sulfonamide administration, although rare, have occurred due to severe reactions, including fulminant hepatic necrosis, agranulocytosis, aplastic anemia and other blood dyscrasias. The prophylactic regimen has caused leukopenia, generally mild and reversible, during treatment $\geq$ 2 months. See Warning Box.

Renal or hepatic function impairment: Use cautiously. Prophylactic use is contraindicated in patients with severe renal insufficiency or marked liver parenchymal damage.

Mutagenesis: Pyrimethamine was found to be mutagenic in laboratory animals and also in human bone marrow following 3 or 4 consecutive daily doses totaling 200 to 300 mg. Testicular changes have been observed in rats treated with 105 mg/kg/day of the combination of sulfadoxine and pyrimethamine and with 15 mg/kg/day of pyrimethamine alone.

Pregnancy: Category C. Sulfadoxine/pyrimethamine is teratogenic in rats when given in weekly doses approximately 12 times the weekly human prophylactic dose. There are no adequate and well controlled studies in pregnant women. However, due to the teratogenic effects shown in animals and because sulfadoxine/pyrimethamine may interfere with folic acid metabolism, use during pregnancy only if the potential benefits outweigh the potential risk to the fetus.

Contraindicated in pregnancy at term; sulfonamides cross the placenta and may cause kernicterus.

Lactation: Both drugs appear in breast milk. Sulfonamides are excreted in breast milk and may cause kernicterus. Discontinue nursing during this period.

Children: Do not give to infants $<$ 2 months of age because of inadequate development of the glucuronide-forming enzyme system.

(Continued on following page)

SULFADOXINE AND PYRIMETHAMINE (Cont.)

Precautions:

Administer cautiously to patients with possible folate deficiency, severe allergy or bronchial asthma. During therapy, perform urinalysis with microscopic examination and renal function tests in patients with impaired renal function. Hemolysis may occur in glucose-6-phosphate dehydrogenase deficient individuals.

Folic acid deficiency: If signs of folic acid deficiency develop, discontinue the drug. Administer folinic acid (leucovorin) in doses of 5 to 15 mg IM daily, for ≥ 3 days, for depressed platelet or white blood cell counts when recovery is too slow.

Monitoring: Perform periodic blood counts and analyze urine for crystalluria during prolonged prophylaxis.

Drug Interactions:

Antifolic drugs (eg, **methotrexate, sulfonamides, TMP-SMZ**): Do not use while the patient is receiving sulfadoxine/pyrimethamine for antimalarial prophylaxis.

Adverse Reactions:

Major reactions to sulfonamides and to pyrimethamine are listed, even though they may not have been reported with this combination.

There have been reports which may indicate an increase in incidence and severity of adverse effects when **chloroquine** is used with sulfadoxine/pyrimethamine as compared to the use of the sulfadoxine/pyrimethamine combination alone.

Hematologic: Agranulocytosis; aplastic, megaloblastic or hemolytic anemia; thrombocytopenia; leukopenia; eosinophilia; purpura; hypoprothrombinemia; methemoglobinemia.

GI: Glossitis; stomatitis; nausea; emesis; abdominal pains; hepatitis; hepatocellular necrosis; diarrhea; pancreatitis.

CNS: Headache; peripheral neuritis; mental depression; convulsions; ataxia; hallucinations; tinnitus; vertigo; insomnia; apathy; fatigue; muscle weakness; nervousness.

Hypersensitivity: Erythema multiforme (Stevens-Johnson syndrome); generalized skin eruptions; toxic epidermal necrolysis; urticaria; serum sickness; pruritus; exfoliative dermatitis; anaphylactoid reactions; periorbital edema; conjunctival and scleral injection; photosensitization; arthralgia; allergic myocarditis.

Miscellaneous: Drug fever; chills; toxic nephrosis with oliguria and anuria; periarteritis nodosa and LE phenomenon; pulmonary infiltrates.

The sulfonamides bear certain chemical similarities to some goitrogens, diuretics (acetazolamide and the thiazides) and oral hypoglycemic agents. Diuresis and hypoglycemia have occurred rarely in patients receiving sulfonamides. Cross-sensitivity may exist with these agents.

Overdosage:

Symptoms: Anorexia, vomiting and CNS stimulation (including convulsions), followed by megaloblastic anemia, leukopenia, thrombocytopenia, glossitis and crystalluria.

Treatment: In acute intoxication, emesis and gastric lavage followed by purges may be beneficial. Treatment includes usual supportive measures. Refer to General Management of Acute Overdosage. Adequately hydrate the patient to prevent renal damage. Monitor the renal and hematopoietic systems for at least 1 month after an overdose. A parenteral barbiturate is indicated for convulsions. For depressed platelet or white blood cell counts, administer leucovorin 5 to 15 mg IM daily for ≥ 3 days.

Patient Information:

Maintain adequate fluid intake to prevent crystalluria and stone formation.

Notify physician if any of the following occurs: Sore throat, fever, pallor, purpura, jaundice, glossitis, arthralgia, cough or shortness of breath. These symptoms may be early indications of serious disorders which require prophylactic treatment to be stopped and medical treatment to be sought.

At the first appearance of skin rash, discontinue the drug and seek medical attention immediately.

Regardless of the prophylactic regimen used, it is still possible to contract malaria. Seek medical attention immediately in the event of a febrile illness. Malaria can be effectively treated early in the course of the disease, but delays before instituting appropriate therapy can have serious or fatal consequences.

Take contraceptive measures to avoid pregnancy during therapy.

Avoid breastfeeding during therapy.

(Continued on following page)

Folic Acid Antagonists (Cont.)

SULFADOXINE AND PYRIMETHAMINE (Cont.)

Administration and Dosage:

Manufacturer's Recommended Dosage for Sulfadoxine/Pyrimethamine			
		Malaria prophylaxis[2]	
Age	Acute malarial attack[1]	Once weekly	Once every 2 weeks
Adults	2 to 3 tablets	1 tablet	2 tablets
9 to 14 years	2 tablets	¾ tablet	1½ tablets
4 to 8 years	1 tablet	½ tablet	1 tablet
< 4 years	½ tablet	¼ tablet	½ tablet

[1] Single dose used in sequence with quinine or alone.

[2] Take the first dose 1 or 2 days before departure to an endemic area; continue administration during the stay and for 4 to 6 weeks after return.

CDC recommendations for use of sulfadoxine/pyrimethamine in malaria:[1]

Travelers to areas of risk where drug-resistant *P falciparum* is endemic and for whom mefloquine is contraindicated may elect to use an alternative regimen. Chloroquine alone taken weekly is recommended for travelers who cannot use mefloquine or doxycycline, especially pregnant women and children < 15 kg. In addition, give these travelers (except those with histories of sulfonamide or pyrimethamine intolerance) a single treatment dose of sulfadoxine/pyrimethamine (see table above) to keep during travel and to take promptly in the event of a febrile illness during their travel when professional medical care is not readily available. Emphasize to travelers that such self-treatment of a possible malarial infection is only a temporary measure and that professional medical follow-up care as soon as possible is imperative. Continue weekly chloroquine prophylaxis after presumptive treatment with sulfadoxine/pyrimethamine.

Presumptive Treatment of Malaria with Sulfadoxine/Pyrimethamine Acquired in Areas with CRPF		
	Presumptive Treatment	
Drug	Adult dose	Pediatric dose
Sulfadoxine/pyrimethamine	3 tablets (1500 mg sulfadoxine/ 75 mg pyrimethamine) orally, as a single dose	5-10 kg: ½ tab 11-20 kg: 1 tab 21-30 kg: 1½ tabs 31-45 kg: 2 tabs > 45 kg: 3 tabs

				C.I.*
Rx	**Fansidar** (Roche)	**Tablets:** 500 mg sulfadoxine and 25 mg pyrimethamine	(Fansidar). Scored. In UD Tel-E-Dose 25s.	31

* Cost Index based on cost per tablet.

[1] Morbidity and Mortality Weekly Report 1990 (March 9);39(RR-3):1-10.

Antituberculous drugs are categorized as primary and retreatment agents, indicating their approximate place and usefulness in treatment of tuberculosis. The foundation of treatment should include the primary agents, most of which are bactericidal (ie, destructive to mycobacteria) and are necessary for sterilization of the tuberculous lesions.

The retreatment agents are generally less effective or more toxic than the primary group. A number of these agents are bacteriostatic (ie, inhibit the growth or multiplication of mycobacteria). They are indicated for use in combination with the primary drugs for partial or complete drug-resistant organisms or to treat extrapulmonary tuberculosis.

Antituberculosis Drugs

Drugs	Activity	Route	Pediatric Daily Dose (mg/kg)	Adult Daily Dose (mg/kg/day)	Usual Adult Daily Dose	Max. Daily Dose (Children & Adults)	Toxicity
Primary Agents							
Isoniazid[1]	Bactericidal	oral	10-20 (20-40 twice weekly)	5-10 once daily (15 mg/kg twice weekly)	300 mg	300 mg (900 mg twice wkly)	Hepatic Neurologic
Rifampin	Bactericidal	oral	10-20 (10-20 twice weekly)	10 once daily (10 mg/kg twice weekly)	600 mg	600 mg	Hepatic Hematologic
Ethambutol[2]	Bacteriostatic	oral	15-25 (50 twice weekly)	15-25 once daily (50 twice weekly)	800-1600 mg	2.5 g	Optic neuritis
Pyrazinamide[2]	Bactericidal	oral	15-30 (50-70 twice weekly)	15-30 once daily (50-70 twice weekly)	1-2 g	2 g	Hepatic Hyperuricemia
Streptomycin[2]	Bactericidal	IM	20-40 (25-30 twice weekly)	7-15 once daily (25-30 twice weekly)	0.75-1 g	1 g (750 mg > 60 yrs)	Eighth nerve Renal
Retreatment Agents							
P-aminosalicylic acid	Bacteriostatic	oral	150-200	200, 4 equal doses 6-hourly	12-16 g	12 g	GI intolerance
Ethionamide	Bacteriostatic	oral	15-20	7-15, 4 equal doses 6-hourly	0.75-1 g	1 g	GI intolerance Hepatic
Cycloserine	Bacteriostatic	oral	10-20	10-15, 4 equal doses 6-hourly	0.75-1 g	1 g	Psychoses Seizures
Capreomycin	Bactericidal	IM	15	15 once daily	1 g	1 g	Eighth nerve Renal
Kanamycin	Bactericidal	IM	7.5-15	15 once daily	0.5-1 g	1 g	Eighth nerve Renal

Adapted from Hoeprich PD, Jordan MC. *Infectious Diseases,* ed. 4. Philadelphia: J.B. Lippincott Co., 1989.
[1] Always include in retreatment regimen if susceptibility remains. [2] May use as primary or retreatment.

The most generally effective and widely used regimen for pulmonary tuberculosis is the combination of the primary agents, isoniazid 300 mg and rifampin 600 mg, both given in single daily doses. Sputum conversion (ie, failure of growth of *M tuberculosis* in cultures) occurs within 1 month in the majority of patients and within 3 months in > 95% of previously untreated cases with drug susceptible organisms. The major disadvantage of the isoniazid/rifampin combination is that as many as 20% to 30% of patients will develop laboratory evidence of impaired hepatic function; most will have no symptoms and liver function returns to normal despite continuation of drug administration. It is estimated that < 5% of patients develop symptoms (anorexia, nausea, vomiting), jaundice and progressive deterioration of liver function; if symptoms occur, discontinue isoniazid/rifampin immediately and substitute another regimen temporarily or permanently.

Treatment regimens of isoniazid-streptomycin-ethambutol (initial therapy) followed by isoniazid-ethambutol have typically been continued for 18 to 24 months. Regimens of isoniazid-rifampin for 12 months, or isoniazid-rifampin for 20 weeks, followed by isoniazid-ethambutol for 12 months following sputum conversion, have proven to be highly effective.

Other regimens recommended include: (a) Isoniazid (5 mg/kg/day, up to 500 mg in adults or 10 to 20 mg/kg/day, up to 300 mg in children) and ethambutol, 15 mg/kg/day for 18 to 24 months – a third drug may be used for the initial 2 to 3 months; (b) after sputum conversion an 18 month, twice weekly regimen of isoniazid, 15 mg/kg/dose and streptomycin, 25 mg/kg/dose *or* isoniazid and ethambutol, 50 mg/kg/dose.

(Continued on following page)

Short-course regimen: The American Thoracic Society and the Tuberculosis Control Division of the Centers for Disease Control have recommended a 9 month regimen of isoniazid-rifampin as an acceptable alternative for adults with previously untreated, drug susceptible, uncomplicated pulmonary tuberculosis. In some circumstances after 2 weeks to 2 months of daily therapy, treatment may be continued with twice weekly supervised doses of isoniazid (15 mg/kg) and rifampin (600 mg). Add ethambutol if isoniazid resistance is suspected. Patients with extrapulmonary tuberculosis, those who have received previous therapy for tuberculosis and those following irregular or inconsistent regimens because of toxicity are not candidates for short-course chemotherapy.

A more recent regimen is isoniazid, rifampin and pyrazinamide daily for 2 months followed by isoniazid-rifampin daily (or twice weekly with an increased isoniazid dose) for 4 months. If isoniazid resistance is suspected, add ethambutol during the initial phase. Continuing pyrazinamide for > 2 months does not appear to improve the outcome. Substituting ethambutol or streptomycin for pyrazinamide appears to decrease efficacy of the therapy.

Although good results with regimens < 6 months have been reported, relapse rates are unacceptably high. Rifampin and isoniazid are essential components of any regimen < 9 or 12 months for at least the first 2 months.

In Southeast Asia and Central and South America, primary drug resistance is common. Therefore, patients should be given ethambutol in addition to isoniazid-rifampin until susceptibility tests are completed.

Retreatment regimens generally consist of two or three agents that were not previously used. Always include isoniazid in the retreatment regimen if susceptibility remains; occasionally isoniazid is recommended when in vitro resistance is determined since the degree of resistance may vary. Treat patients resistant to isoniazid with rifampin 600 mg/day combined with ethambutol and streptomycin; pyrazinamide may also be used in place of ethambutol. If the patient is resistant to streptomycin, capreomycin (preferred) or kanamycin are recommended. Ethionamide, p-aminosalicylic acid and cycloserine are rarely required. Continuous therapy for 18 to 24 months is generally required; delete the most toxic agents during treatment if possible.

HIV: Treat patients with HIV infection who develop tuberculosis with the standard antituberculous drug regimen. The recommended regimen is the short-course 9 month regimen (see above). However, the treatment period may need to be longer. Preventive therapy with isoniazid may also be considered (see Chemoprophylaxis). Again, the treatment period may need to be extended.

Pregnancy: Tuberculosis in pregnancy should be treated, but presents a therapeutic dilemma. The best therapeutic choices with the least danger to the fetus appear to be combinations of isoniazid, ethambutol and rifampin.

Resistance to antituberculosis drugs is not uncommon although relatively low in North American and European-born patients. In the US, approximately 7% are resistant to one or more drugs and 3% to 5% are resistant to isoniazid. Primary resistance to rifampin is low.

Chemoprophylaxis: The administration of isoniazid for 1 year in a single daily dose of 300 mg for adults and 10 to 14 mg/kg (not to exceed 300 mg/day) for children prevents active pulmonary tuberculosis. Isoniazid diminishes the mycobacterial population of roentgenographically detectable, quiescent pulmonary lesions or of pulmonary foci which are radiologically inapparent. The United States Public Health Service has demonstrated a significant reduction of morbidity in treated subjects. Chemoprophylaxis not only reduces the risk of active disease in those treated, but also prevents the spread of disease to uninfected persons. Evidence suggests that 6 month therapy may be comparable. Therapy for < 6 months is of little value and therapy for > 1 year provides no additional benefit.

Additionally, an international, multiclinic study of > 27,000 patients with fibrotic chest lesions, revealed that patients taking prophylactic isoniazid for 24 to 52 weeks had a reduction in tuberculosis development of 65% to 93% with minimal side effects.

However, wide-spread prophylactic treatment is still questioned because of the isoniaizid-induced hepatitis risk. The following priorities have been recommended and are widely accepted in identifying candidates for chemoprophylaxis. (1) Household members and other close associates of persons with recently diagnosed tuberculosis. (2) Tuberculin reactors with chest roentgenograms demonstrating nonprogressive, healed or quiescent lesions, and in whom there are neither positive bacteriologic findings nor a history of adequate chemotherapy. (3) Persons whose tuberculin reaction has become positive within the last 2 years. (4) Tuberculin reactors at increased risk of developing tuberculous disease (ie, prolonged adrenocorticosteroid therapy, immunosuppressive therapy, diabetes mellitus, silicosis, leukemia, Hodgkin's disease, post-gastrectomy). (5) Regardless of age, persons with AIDS, ARC or HIV-seropositivity who are skin test positive, or who have a negative skin test but a history of prior significant reaction to PPD. (6) Any positive tuberculin reactor > 35 years and particularly children < 7 years.

Isoniazid prophylaxis is indicated during pregnancy by some for recent tuberculin converters and in any tuberculin reactor with inactive disease. Therapy for nearly all other pregnant candidates should probably be withheld during pregnancy until the postpartum period.

(Products listed on following pages)

Refer to the general discussion of these agents beginning on page 1924

ISONIAZID (Isonicotinic acid hydrazide; INH)

Warning:

Severe and sometimes fatal hepatitis associated with isoniazid therapy may occur or develop even after many months of treatment. The risk of developing hepatitis is age-related. Approximate case rates by age are 0 per 1000 for persons $<$ 20 years of age, 3 per 1000 for persons 20 to 34, 12 per 1000 for persons 35 to 49, 23 per 1000 for persons 50 to 64, and 8 per 1000 for persons $>$ 65 years of age.

The risk of hepatitis is increased with daily consumption of alcohol. Precise data to provide a fatality rate for isoniazid-related hepatitis are not available; however, in a study of 13,838 persons taking isoniazid, there were eight deaths among 174 cases of hepatitis.

Carefully monitor and interview patients at monthly intervals. Serum transaminase concentration becomes elevated in about 10% to 20% of patients, usually during the first few months of therapy but can occur at any time. Enzyme levels generally return to normal despite continuance of the drug, but in some cases, progressive liver dysfunction occurs. Instruct patients to report immediately any of the prodromal symptoms of hepatitis, such as fatigue, weakness, malaise, anorexia, nausea or vomiting. If these symptoms appear, or if signs suggestive of hepatic damage are detected, discontinue isoniazid promptly since continued use of the drug in such cases may cause a more severe form of liver damage.

Reinstitute isoniazid after symptoms and laboratory abnormalities have become normal. Restart the drug in very small doses; gradually increase doses and withdraw immediately if there is any indication of recurrent liver involvement.

Defer preventive treatment in persons with acute hepatic diseases.

Actions:

Isoniazid (INH) acts against actively growing tubercle bacilli. It is bactericidal and interferes with lipid and nucleic acid biosynthesis in the growing organism.

Pyridoxine (vitamin B_6) deficiency is sometimes observed in adults taking high doses of INH, and is probably due to the drug's competition with pyridoxal phosphate for the enzyme apotryptophanase.

Pharmacokinetics:

Absorption – INH is rapidly and completely absorbed orally and parenterally and produces peak blood levels within 1 to 2 hours; these decline to $\leq$ 50% within 6 hours. However, the rate and extent of absorption is decreased by food.

Distribution – INH readily diffuses into all body fluids including cerebrospinal (90% serum concentrations), pleural and ascitic, tissues, organs, and excreta (saliva, sputum, feces). It also passes through the placental barrier and into breast milk in concentrations comparable to those in plasma.

Metabolism – The half-life of INH is widely variable and dependent on acetylator status. Isoniazid is primarily acetylated by the liver; this process is genetically controlled. Liver disease can prolong the clearance of isoniazid. Fast acetylators metabolize the drug about 5 to 6 times faster than slow acetylators. Several minor metabolites have been identified, one or more of which may be "reactive" (monoacetylhydrazine is suspected), and responsible for liver damage. Approximately 50% of Blacks and Caucasians are "slow acetylators" and the rest are "rapid acetylators"; the majority of Eskimos and Orientals are "rapid acetylators". The rate of acetylation does not significantly alter the effectiveness of INH. However, slow acetylation may lead to higher blood levels of the drug, and thus to an increase in toxic reactions. Rapid acetylators may be more likely to develop hepatitis, since hepatotoxicity is caused by the acetylated metabolite of INH; however, this remains controversial.

Excretion – Approximately 50% to 70% of a dose of isoniazid is excreted as unchanged drug and metabolites by the kidneys in 24 hours. Elimination is largely independent of renal function.

Indications:

Used for all forms of tuberculosis in which organisms are susceptible.

Also recommended as preventive therapy (chemoprophylaxis) for specific situations (see the Antituberculous Drugs Introduction).

IM administration is intended for use whenever oral administration is not possible.

Unlabeled uses: Isoniazid (300 to 400 mg/day, increased over 2 weeks to 20 mg/kg/day) may be beneficial in improving severe tremor in patients with multiple sclerosis.

(Continued on following page)

ISONIAZID (Isonicotinic acid hydrazide; INH) (Cont.)

Contraindications:

Patients with previous isoniazid-associated hepatic injury or other severe adverse reactions to isoniazid, (eg, drug fever, chills, arthritis; acute liver disease of any etiology).

Warnings:

Hypersensitivity: Stop all drugs and evaluate at the first sign of a hypersensitivity reaction. If isoniazid must be reinstituted, give only after symptoms have cleared. Restart the drug in very small and gradually increasing doses and withdraw immediately if there is any indication of recurrent hypersensitivity reaction. Refer to Management of Acute Hypersensitivity Reactions.

Hepatic and renal function impairment: Monitor patients with active chronic liver disease or severe renal dysfunction.

Carcinogenesis: Isoniazid induces pulmonary tumors in a number of strains of mice.

Pregnancy: Isoniazid exerts an embryocidal effect in both rats and rabbits, but no isoniazid-related congenital anomalies have been found in reproduction studies in mammalian species (mice, rats and rabbits). Prescribe during pregnancy only when therapeutically necessary. Weigh the benefit of preventive therapy against a possible risk to the fetus. Start preventive treatment generally after delivery because of the increased risk of tuberculosis for new mothers.

Refer to the Antituberculous Drugs Introduction for treatment regimens suggested during pregnancy.

Lactation: Since isoniazid appears in breast milk, observe breastfed infants of isoniazid-treated mothers for any evidence of adverse effects.

Precautions:

Periodic ophthalmologic examinations during isoniazid therapy are recommended even when visual symptoms do not occur.

Pyridoxine administration is recommended in individuals likely to develop peripheral neuropathies secondary to INH therapy (see Adverse Reactions). Prophylactic doses of 6 to 50 mg of pyridoxine daily have been recommended.

Drug Interactions:

Alcohol ingestion on a daily basis may be associated with a higher incidence of isoniazid-related hepatitis.

Aluminum salts may reduce the oral absorption of isoniazid, thereby decreasing its serum levels. Administer isoniazid 1 to 2 hours before aluminum salts.

Anticoagulants, oral: Anticoagulant activity may be enhanced by concurrent isoniazid.

Benzodiazepines: Isoniazid may inhibit the metabolic clearance of benzodiazepines that undergo oxidative metabolism (eg, diazepam, triazolam), possibly increasing the activity of the benzodiazepine.

Carbamazepine toxicity or isoniazid hepatotoxicity may result from concurrent use. Monitor carbamazepine concentrations and liver function.

Cycloserine in combination with isoniazid may result in increased cycloserine CNS side effects, most notably dizziness.

Disulfiram and isoniazid coadministration may result in acute behavioral and coordination changes.

Enflurane: In rapid acetylators of isoniazid, high output renal failure may occur due to nephrotoxic concentrations of inorganic fluoride. Isoniazid may produce high concentrations of hydrazine which then facilitates defluorination of enflurane. Monitor renal function in patients receiving these agents concurrently.

Halothane: Hepatotoxicity and hepatic encephalopathy have occurred when rifampin and isoniazid were given after halothane anesthesia.

Hydantoins: Serum hydantoin levels may be increased by isoniazid due to inhibition of hepatic microsomal enzymes. An increase in the pharmacologic or toxic effects of the hydantoins may occur. This may be most significant in slow acetylators of isoniazid.

Ketoconazole serum concentrations may be decreased by isoniazid, possibly resulting in antifungal treatment resistance.

Meperidine coadministration may result in a hypotensive episode or CNS depression.

Rifampin and isoniazid coadministration may result in a higher rate of hepatotoxicity than with either agent alone. If alterations in liver function tests occur, consider discontinuation of one or both agents.

Drug/Food interactions: Since isoniazid has some monoamine oxidase inhibitor activity, an interaction may occur with tyramine-containing foods (see Monoamine Oxidase Inhibitors group monograph). Diamine oxidase may also be inhibited, causing exaggerated responses (eg, headache, palpitations, sweating, hypotension, flushing, diarrhea, itching) to foods containing histamine (eg, tuna, sauerkraut juice, yeast extract).

(Continued on following page)

ISONIAZID (Isonicotinic acid hydrazide; INH) (Cont.)

Adverse Reactions:

Toxic effects are usually encountered with higher doses of isoniazid; the most frequent are those affecting the nervous system and the liver.

CNS: Peripheral neuropathy, the most common toxic effect, is characterized by symmetrical numbness and tingling of the extremities. The incidence correlates closely with the dose of isoniazid, ie, ≈ 2%, 10% to 20% and 44% of patients may develop pyridoxine deficiency-induced peripheral neuropathy while taking 3 to 5 mg/kg/day, 10 mg/kg/day and 16 to 24 mg/kg/day, respectively. Patients predisposed to this condition include the malnourished, slow isoniazid acetylators, pregnant women, elderly, diabetics and patients with chronic liver disease, including alcoholics. Some advocate pyridoxine (B_6) prophylaxis for all patients, others advocate prophylaxis only for those predisposed. Recommended prophylactic doses range from 6 to 50 mg daily, but the lower doses of 6 to 25 mg appear more common. Treatment of established neuropathy requires 50 to 200 mg pyridoxine daily.

Other neurotoxic effects uncommon with conventional doses: Convulsions; toxic encephalopathy; optic neuritis and atrophy; memory impairment; toxic psychosis.

GI: Nausea; vomiting; epigastric distress.

Hepatic: Elevated serum transaminase levels (AST, ALT); bilirubinemia; bilirubinuria; jaundice; occasionally, severe and sometimes fatal hepatitis. The common prodromal symptoms are anorexia, nausea, vomiting, fatigue, malaise and weakness. Mild and transient elevation of serum transaminase levels occurs in 10% to 20% of patients taking isoniazid. This abnormality usually appears in the first 4 to 6 months of treatment, but can develop at any time during therapy. Enzyme levels return to normal in most instances, and there is no need to discontinue medication. Occasionally, progressive liver damage with accompanying symptoms may occur. In such cases, discontinue the drug immediately. The frequency of progressive liver damage increases with age. It is rare in individuals < 20 years, but is seen in as many as 2.3% of those patients > 50 years old.

Concurrent ethanol use may increase the risk of hepatitis. In addition, it is more commonly believed that rapid acetylators are at greater risk; however, the same has been shown for slow acetylators.

Hematologic: Agranulocytosis; hemolytic, sideroblastic or aplastic anemia; thrombocytopenia; eosinophilia.

Hypersensitivity: Fever; skin eruptions (morbilliform, maculopapular, purpuric or exfoliative); lymphadenopathy; vasculitis (see Warnings).

Metabolic/Endocrine: Pyridoxine deficiency; pellagra; hyperglycemia; metabolic acidosis; gynecomastia. Isoniazid may cause hypocalcemia and hypophosphatemia due to alterations of vitamin D metabolism.

Miscellaneous: Rheumatic syndrome and systemic lupus erythematosus-like syndrome. Local irritation has been observed at the site of IM injection.

Overdosage:

Symptoms occur within 30 minutes to 3 hours. Nausea, vomiting, dizziness, slurring of speech, blurring of vision and visual hallucinations (including bright colors and strange designs) are among the early manifestations. With marked overdosage, respiratory distress and CNS depression, progressing rapidly from stupor to profound coma, are to be expected along with severe, intractable seizures. Ingestion of 80 to 150 mg/kg usually results in severe seizures and a high likelihood of fatality. Severe metabolic acidosis, acetonuria and hyperglycemia are typical laboratory findings.

Treatment: INH overdosage can be fatal, but good response has been reported in most patients adequately treated within the first few hours after drug ingestion.

Secure the airway and establish adequate respiratory exchange. Gastric lavage is advised within the first 2 to 3 hours, but do not attempt it until convulsions are under control. To control convulsions, administer a short-acting IV barbiturate or diazepam, followed by pyridoxine IV (usually 1 mg per 1 mg of isoniazid ingested). Pyridoxine can be toxic, but doses of 70 to 357 mg/kg have been administered without incident.

Obtain blood samples for immediate determination of gases, electrolytes, BUN, glucose, etc; type and crossmatch blood in preparation for possible hemodialysis.

Rapid control of metabolic acidosis is fundamental to management. Give sodium bicarbonate IV immediately and repeat as needed, adjusting subsequent dosage on the basis of laboratory findings (ie, serum sodium, pH).

Start forced osmotic diuresis early and continue for some hours after clinical improvement has been noted to hasten renal clearance of the drug and help prevent relapse. Monitor fluid intake and output.

Hemodialysis is advised for severe cases. If this is not available, peritoneal dialysis can be used concomitantly with forced diuresis. In addition, protect against hypoxia, hypotension, aspiration pneumonitis, etc.

(Continued on following page)

ISONIAZID (Isonicotinic acid hydrazide; INH) (Cont.)

Patient Information:

Take on an empty stomach, at least 1 hour before or 2 hours after meals; it may be taken with food to decrease GI upset.

Take medication as directed. Do not discontinue therapy except on advice of physician.

Patients should minimize daily alcohol consumption while on INH therapy due to the increased risk of hepatitis.

Avoid certain foods (ie, fish-skipjack, tuna, and perhaps tyramine-containing products) (see Monoamine Oxidase Inhibitor group monograph).

Notify physician if weakness, fatigue, loss of appetite, nausea and vomiting, yellowing of skin or eyes, darkening of urine, or numbness or tingling in hands and feet occurs.

Administration and Dosage:

Treatment of tuberculosis: Use in conjunction with other effective antituberculosis agents. If the bacilli become resistant, therapy must be changed to agents to which the bacilli are susceptible.

Adults – 5 mg/kg/day (up to 300 mg total) in a single dose.

Infants and children – 10 to 20 mg/kg/day (300 mg total) in a single dose, depending on the severity of infection.

Preventive treatment:

Adults – 300 mg/day in a single dose.

Infants and children – 10 mg/kg/day (up to 300 mg total) in a single dose.

Continuous administration of isoniazid for a sufficient period is an essential part of the regimen, because relapse rates are higher if chemotherapy is stopped prematurely. In the treatment of tuberculosis, resistant organisms may multiply and the emergence of resistant organisms may necessitate a change in the regimen.

Concomitant administration of 6 to 50 mg/day pyridoxine is recommended in the malnourished and in those predisposed to neuropathy (eg, alcoholics and diabetics). See Adverse Reactions.

				C.I.*
Rx	**Laniazid** (Lannett)	**Tablets:** 50 mg	Scored. In 100s and 500s.	3
Rx	**Isoniazid** (Various, eg, Barr, Baxter, Geneva, Halsey, Lilly, Major, Moore, Qualitest, Rugby, Schein)	**Tablets:** 100 mg	In 100s, 1000s and UD 100s.	4+
Rx	**Laniazid** (Lannett)		Scored. In 100s, 500s and 1000s.	4
Rx	**Isoniazid** (Various, eg, Barr, Baxter, Geneva, Goldline, Halsey, Lilly, Major, Moore, Rugby, Schein)	**Tablets:** 300 mg	In 30s, 100s, 1000s & UD 100s.	2+
Rx	**Laniazid C.T.** (Lannett)		White, scored. Convex. In 100s and 1000s.	NA
Rx	**Isoniazid** (Carolina Medical)	**Syrup:** 50 mg per 5 ml	Sorbitol. Orange flavor. In pt.	15
Rx	**Laniazid** (Lannett)		Sorbitol. Raspberry flavor. In pt.	NA
Rx	**Isoniazid** (Quad)	**Injection:** 100 mg per ml	In 10 ml vials.	540
Rx	**Nydrazid** (Apothecon)		In 10 ml vials.[1]	410

ISONIAZID COMBINATIONS

ISONIAZID acts against actively growing tubercle bacilli. See individual monograph.

PYRIDOXINE is included as a supplement due to the increased need for pyridoxine induced by isoniazid treatment. See individual monograph.

RIFAMPIN is used as an adjunct to isoniazid in the treatment of tuberculosis. See individual monograph.

				C.I.*
Rx	**Rifamate** (Merrell Dow)	**Capsules:** 150 mg isoniazid and 300 mg rifampin	Red. In 60s.	282
Rx	**Rimactane/INH Dual Pack** (Ciba)	**Pack:** Thirty 300 mg isoniazid tablets and sixty 300 mg rifampin capsules	In 30 day supplies.	261

* Cost Index based on cost per 300 mg isoniazid.

[1] With 0.25% chlorobutanol.

Refer to the general discussion of these agents beginning on page 1924

RIFAMPIN

Actions:

Pharmacology: Rifampin inhibits DNA-dependent RNA polymerase activity in susceptible cells. Specifically, it interacts with bacterial RNA polymerase, but does not inhibit the mammalian enzyme. Cross-resistance has only been shown with other rifamycins.

Pharmacokinetics:

Oral –

Absorption/Distribution: Rifampin, 600 mg administered orally, is almost completely absorbed and achieves mean peak plasma levels within 1 to 4 hours. The peak level averages 7 mcg/ml but may vary from 4 to 32 mcg/ml. In children, mean peak serum levels range from 3.5 to 15 mcg/ml. Food interferes with absorption. It is 80% protein bound but very lipid soluble; it penetrates and concentrates in many body tissues, including the cerebrospinal fluid, which is increased with meningitis (12% to 25% of serum concentrations).

Metabolism: Rifampin is metabolized in the liver by deacetylation; the metabolite is still active against *Mycobacterium tuberculosis*. About 40% is excreted in bile and undergoes enterohepatic circulation; however, the deacetylated metabolite is poorly absorbed. The half-life is approximately 3 hours after a 600 mg oral dose, up to 5.1 hours after a 900 mg oral dose. With repeated administration, the half-life decreases and averages approximately 2 to 3 hours. In children, the half-life is 2.9 hours following a dose of 10 mg/kg.

Excretion: 6% to 30% of rifampin is excreted in the urine; 30% to 60% in the deacetylated form, approximately 50% unchanged. Dosage adjustment is not necessary in renal failure, but is with hepatic dysfunction. Neither peritoneal dialysis nor hemodialysis removes significant amounts of rifampin from the plasma.

IV –

Following administration of a 300 or 600 mg IV dose in 12 volunteers, mean peak plasma concentrations were 9 and 17 mcg/ml, respectively. The average plasma concentrations remained detectable for 8 and 12 hours, respectively. The elimination of the larger dose was not as rapid. After repeated once daily infusions of 600 mg in five patients for 7 days, concentrations decreased from 5.8 mcg/ml 8 hours after the infusion on day 1 to 2.6 mcg/ml 8 hours after the infusion on day 7.

In children, the mean peak serum concentration was 26 mcg/ml following a 300 mg/m^2 infusion, 11.7 to 41.5 mcg/ml 1 to 4 days after initiation of therapy, and 13.6 to 37.4 mcg/ml 5 to 14 days after initiation of therapy. The half-life was 1.17 to 3.24 hours.

Microbiology: Rifampin has initial in vitro activity against the following organisms; however, clinical efficacy has not been established: *M leprae; Hemophilus influenzae; Staphylococcus aureus; S epidermidis.* Both penicillinase- and non-penicillinase- producing strains and β-lactam resistant staphylococci (MRSA) are initially susceptible in vitro.

Indications:

Tuberculosis: Oral – Treatment of all forms of tuberculosis in conjunction with at least one other antituberculous drug. Frequently used regimens include: Isoniazid and rifampin; ethambutol and rifampin; isoniazid, ethambutol and rifampin; isoniazid, pyrazinamide and rifampin.

IV – Initial treatment and retreatment of tuberculosis when the drug cannot be taken by mouth.

Neisseria meningitidis carriers: Treatment of asymptomatic carriers of *N meningitidis* to eliminate meningococci from the nasopharynx. Not indicated for treatment of meningococcal infection.

To avoid indiscriminate use, perform diagnostic laboratory procedures, including serotyping and susceptibility testing. Reserve the drug for situations in which the risk of meningococcal meningitis is high. Since rapid emergence of resistance can occur, perform culture and susceptibility tests in the event of persistent positive cultures.

Unlabeled uses: Rifampin has a broad antibacterial spectrum. Some uses showing promise with a reasonable amount of human data include: Infections caused by *Staphylococcus aureus* and *S epidermidis* (eg, endocarditis, osteomyelitis, prostatitis), usually in combination with other effective drugs; gram-negative bacteremia in infancy; Legionella (*Legionella pneumophilia*) when not responsive to erythromycin; leprosy (in combination with dapsone); prophylaxis of meningitis due to *Hemophilus influenzae*.

Contraindications:

Hypersensitivity to any rifamycin.

(Continued on following page)

RIFAMPIN (Cont.)

Warnings:

Hepatotoxicity: There have been fatalities associated with jaundice in patients with liver disease or patients receiving rifampin concomitantly with other hepatotoxic agents. Since an increased risk may exist for individuals with liver disease, weigh benefits against risk of further liver damage. Carefully monitor liver function, especially AST and ALT, prior to therapy and then every 2 to 4 weeks during therapy. Withdraw rifampin if signs of hepatocellular damage occur.

Hyperbilirubinemia, resulting from competition between rifampin and bilirubin for excretory pathways of the liver at the cell level, can occur in the early days of treatment. An isolated report showing a moderate rise in bilirubin or transaminase level is not in itself an indication to interrupt treatment. Make the decision based on repeat tests and the patient's clinical condition.

Porphyria: Isolated reports have associated porphyria exacerbation with rifampin administration.

Meningococci resistance: The possibility of rapid emergence of resistant meningococci restricts use to short-term treatment of asymptomatic carrier state. Not for treatment of meningococcal disease.

Hypersensitivity reactions have occurred during intermittent therapy or when treatment was resumed following accidental or intentional interruption and were reversible with rifampin discontinuation and appropriate therapy. Refer to General Management of Acute Hypersensitivity Reactions. See Adverse Reactions.

Hepatic function impairment: Dosage adjustment is necessary.

Carcinogenesis: A few cases of accelerated growth of lung carcinoma have occurred in man, but a causal relationship has not been established. An increase in the incidence of hepatomas in female mice (of a strain known to be particularly susceptible to the spontaneous development of hepatomas) was observed when rifampin was administered in doses 2 to 10 times the average daily human dose for 60 weeks. Rifampin possesses immunosuppressive potential in animals and humans. Antitumor activity in vitro has also occurred.

Pregnancy: Category C. The effect of rifampin (alone or in combination with other antituberculous drugs) on the human fetus is not known. Rifampin crosses the placental barrier and appears in cord blood. It is teratogenic in rodents given oral doses of 15 to 25 times the human dose. An increase in congenital malformations, primarily spina bifida and cleft palate, has occurred in the offspring of rodents given oral doses of 150 to 250 mg/kg/day. Imperfect osteogenesis and embryotoxicity occurred in rabbits given doses up to 20 times the usual human daily dose. When administered during the last few weeks of pregnancy, rifampin can cause postnatal hemorrhages in the mother and infant for which treatment with vitamin K may be indicated. Carefully weigh possible teratogenic potential in women capable of bearing children against benefits of therapy (see also Antituberculous Drugs introduction).

Carefully observe neonates of rifampin-treated mothers for any adverse effects.

Lactation: Rifampin is excreted in breast milk with a milk/plasma ratio of 0.2 to 0.6. Decide whether to discontinue nursing or discontinue the drug, taking into account the importance of the drug to the mother.

Precautions:

Intermittent therapy may be used if the patient cannot or will not self-administer drugs on a daily basis. Closely monitor patients on intermittent therapy for compliance, and caution against intentional or accidental interruption of prescribed therapy because of increased risk of serious adverse reactions.

Urine, feces, saliva, sputum, sweat and tears may be colored red-orange. Soft contact lenses may be permanently stained. Advise patients of these possibilities. Rifampin may impart a yellow color to cerebrospinal fluid.

IV: For IV infusion only. Must not be administered by IM or SC route. Avoid extravasation during injection; local irritation and inflammation due to extravascular infiltration of the infusion have been observed. If these occur, discontinue and restart at another site.

Monitoring: Obtain a complete blood count prior to instituting therapy and periodically throughout the course of therapy. Because of a possible transient rise in transaminase and bilirubin values, obtain blood for baseline clinical chemistries before rifampin dosing.

Thrombocytopenia has occurred, primarily with high dose intermittent therapy, but has also been noted after resumption of interrupted treatment. It rarely occurs during well supervised daily therapy. This effect is reversible if the drug is discontinued as soon as purpura occurs. Cerebral hemorrhage and fatalities have occurred when rifampin administration has continued or resumed after the appearance of purpura.

(Continued on following page)

RIFAMPIN (Cont.)

Drug Interactions:

Rifampin is known to induce the hepatic microsomal enzymes that metabolize various drugs listed in the table below. The therapeutic effects of these drugs may be decreased.

Rifampin Drug Interactions Due to Hepatic Microsomal Enzyme Induction		
Acetaminophen	Corticosteroids	Mexiletine
Anticoagulants, oral	Cyclosporine	Quinidine
Barbiturates	Digitoxin	Sulfones
Benzodiazepines[1]	Disopyramide	Sulfonylureas
Beta-blockers	Estrogens	Theophyllines[2]
Chloramphenicol	Hydantoins	Tocainide
Clofibrate	Methadone	Verapamil
Contraceptives, oral		

[1] Benzodiazepines metabolized by oxidation.
[2] Dyphylline probably does not interact.

Digoxin serum concentrations may be decreased by rifampin.

Enalapril: A significant increase in blood pressure occurred in a patient receiving enalapril and rifampin concurrently.

Halothane: Hepatotoxicity and hepatic encephalopathy have occurred when rifampin and isoniazid were given after halothane anesthesia.

Isoniazid and rifampin coadministration may result in a higher rate of hepatotoxicity than with either agent alone. If alterations in liver function tests occur, consider discontinuation of one or both agents.

Ketoconazole: Treatment failure of either ketoconazole or rifampin may occur.

Drug/Lab test interactions: Therapeutic levels of rifampin inhibit standard assays for serum **folate** and **vitamin B_{12}**. Consider alternative methods when determining folate and vitamin B_{12} concentrations in the presence of rifampin.

Transient abnormalities in liver function tests (eg, elevation in serum bilirubin, abnormal bromsulphalein [BSP] excretion, alkaline phosphatase and serum transaminases), and reduced biliary excretion of contrast media used for visualization of the gallbladder have also been observed. Therefore, perform these tests before the morning dose of rifampin.

Drug/Food interaction: Food interferes with the absorption of rifampin, possibly resulting in decreased peak plasma concentrations. Take on an empty stomach.

Adverse Reactions:

High doses of rifampin (> 600 mg) given once or twice weekly have resulted in a high incidence of adverse reactions including: The "flu-like" syndrome (eg, fever, chills, malaise); hematopoietic reactions (eg, leukopenia, thrombocytopenia, acute hemolytic anemia); cutaneous, GI and hepatic reactions; shortness of breath; shock; renal failure. Recent studies indicate that regimens using twice-weekly doses of rifampin 600 mg plus isoniazid 15 mg/kg are much better tolerated.

GI (1% to 2%): Heartburn; epigastric distress; anorexia; nausea; vomiting; gas; cramps; diarrhea; sore mouth and tongue; pseudomembranous colitis; pancreatitis.

Hepatic: Asymptomatic elevations of liver enzymes (up to 14%) and hepatitis (< 1%). Hepatitis or shock-like syndrome with hepatic involvement (rare); abnormal liver function tests; transient abnormalities in liver function tests (elevations in serum bilirubin, BSP, alkaline phosphatase, serum transaminases). Perform BSP test prior to the morning dose of rifampin to avoid false-positive results.

Dermatologic: Rash (1% to 5%); pruritus; urticaria; pemphigoid reaction; flushing.

CNS: Headache; drowsiness; fatigue; dizziness; inability to concentrate; mental confusion; generalized numbness; behavioral changes; myopathy (rare).

Hematologic: Eosinophilia; transient leukopenia; hemolytic anemia; decreased hemoglobin; hemolysis; thrombocytopenia (see Precautions).

Musculoskeletal: Ataxia; muscular weakness; pain in extremities; osteomalacia; myopathy.

Ophthalmologic: Visual disturbances; exudative conjunctivitis.

Renal: Hemoglobinuria; hematuria; renal insufficiency; acute renal failure. These are considered hypersensitivity reactions (see Warnings).

Miscellaneous: Menstrual disturbances; fever; elevations in BUN and elevated serum uric acid; possible immunosuppression; isolated reports of abnormal growth of lung tumors; reduced 25-hydroxycholecalciferol levels; edema of face and extremities; shortness of breath; wheezing; decrease in blood pressure; shock.

(Continued on following page)

RIFAMPIN (Cont.)

Overdosage:

Signs and symptoms: Nausea, vomiting and increasing lethargy will probably occur within a short time after ingestion; unconsciousness may occur with severe hepatic involvement. Brownish-red or orange discoloration of the skin, urine, sweat, saliva, tears and feces is proportional to amount ingested. Liver enlargement, possibly with tenderness, can develop within a few hours after severe overdosage, and jaundice may develop rapidly. Hepatic involvement may be more marked in patients with prior impairment of hepatic function. Other physical findings remain essentially normal.

Direct and total bilirubin levels may increase rapidly with severe overdosage; hepatic enzyme levels may be affected, especially with prior impairment of hepatic function. A direct effect on the hematopoietic system, electrolyte levels or acid-base balance is unlikely.

Non-fatal overdoses with as high as 12 g of rifampin have been reported. One case of fatal overdose occurred in a 26-year-old man after self-administering 60 g.

Treatment: Nausea and vomiting are likely to be present. Gastric lavage is probably preferable to induction of emesis. Activated charcoal slurry instilled into the stomach following evacuation of gastric contents can help absorb any remaining drug in the GI tract. Antiemetic medication may be required to control severe nausea or vomiting.

Forced diuresis (with measured intake and output) will promote excretion of the drug. Bile drainage may be indicated in the presence of serious impairment of hepatic function lasting more than 24 to 48 hours; extracorporeal hemodialysis may be required. In patients with previously adequate hepatic function, reversal of liver enlargement and impaired hepatic excretory function probably will be noted within 72 hours, with rapid return toward normal thereafter.

Patient Information:

Take on an empty stomach, at least 1 hour before or 2 hours after meals.

Take medication on a regular basis; avoid missing doses. Do not discontinue therapy except on advice of physician.

Medication may cause a reddish-orange discoloration of urine, stools, saliva, tears, sweat and sputum. This is to be expected and is not harmful. May also permanently discolor soft contact lenses.

Notify physician if flu-like symptoms (fever, chills, muscle and bone pain, headache), excessive tiredness or weakness, anorexia, nausea and vomiting, sore throat, unusual bleeding or bruising, yellowish discoloration of the skin or eyes, skin rash or itching occurs.

Administration and Dosage:

Oral:

Administer once daily, either 1 hour before or 2 hours after meals.

Data is not available to determine dosage for children $<$ 5 years of age. For pediatric and adult patients in whom capsule swallowing is difficult or when lower doses are needed, a rifampin suspension can be prepared (see Preparation of Extemporaneous Oral Suspension).

Oral and IV: Tuberculosis: Adults – 600 mg once daily. *Children* – 10 to 20 mg/kg, not to exceed 600 mg/day.

Use rifampin in conjunction with at least one other antituberculous agent. In general, continue therapy until bacterial conversion and maximal improvement have occurred.

In general, continue therapy for tuberculosis for 6 to 9 months or until at least 6 months have elapsed from conversion of sputum to culture negativity. In patients who cannot be relied upon for compliance, intermittent therapy with 600 mg/day 2 or 3 times per week under close supervision may be prescribed and substituted for the daily regimen after 1 to 2 months of an initial daily phase of therapy.

The 6 month regimen ordinarily consists of an initial 2 month phase of rifampin, isoniazid and pyrazinamide and, if clinically indicated, streptomycin or ethambutol, followed by 4 months of rifampin and isoniazid.

The 9 month regimen ordinarily consists of rifampin and isoniazid, usually supplemented during the initial phase by pyrazinamide, streptomycin or ethambutol.

Either of the above regimens is recommended as standard therapy.

Meningococcal carriers: Administer once daily for 4 consecutive days in the following doses: *Adults* – 600 mg. *Children* – 10 to 20 mg/kg, not to exceed 600 mg/day.

The following dosage has also been recommended: *Adults* – 600 mg every 12 hours for 2 days; *children* ($\geq$ 1 month of age) – 10 mg/kg every 12 hours for 2 days; *children* ($<$ 1 month of age) – 5 mg/kg every 12 hours for 2 days.

(Administration and Dosage continued on following page)

RIFAMPIN (Cont.)

Administration and Dosage (Cont.):

Preparation/Stability of solution for IV infusion: Reconstitute the lyophilized powder by transferring 10 ml of Sterile Water for Injection to a vial containing 600 mg of rifampin for injection. Swirl vial gently to completely dissolve the antibiotic. The resultant solution contains rifampin 60 mg/ml and is stable at room temperature for 24 hours. Withdraw a volume equivalent to the amount of rifampin calculated to be administered and add to 500 ml of infusion medium. Mix well and infuse at a rate allowing for complete infusion in 3 hours. In some cases, the amount of rifampin calculated to be administered may be added to 100 ml of infusion medium and infused in 30 minutes. The 500 and 100 ml dilutions are also stable at room temperature for 24 hours.

Dextrose 5% for injection is the recommended infusion medium. Sterile Saline may be used when dextrose is contraindicated, but the stability of rifampin is slightly reduced. Other solutions are not recommended.

Preparation of extemporaneous oral suspension (according to Merrell Dow Pharmaceuticals): Preparation of suspension (to contain rifampin 10 mg/ml) – 1) Empty the contents of four rifampin 300 mg (or eight rifampin 150 mg) capsules into a 4 oz amber glass bottle. 2) Add 20 ml of simple syrup (Syrup, NF). Shake vigorously. 3) Add 100 ml of simple syrup. Shake again.

Storage – The suspension is stable for 4 weeks when stored at room temperature (25°C ± 3°C) or in refrigerator (2° to 8°C; 36° to 46°F).

				C.I.*
Rx	**Rifadin** (Marion Merrell Dow)	**Capsules:** 150 mg	(Rifadin 150). Maroon and scarlet. In 30s.	2.1
Rx	**Rifadin** (Marion Merrell Dow)	**Capsules:** 300 mg	(Rifadin 300). Maroon and scarlet. In 30s, 60s and 100s.	1.6
Rx	**Rimactane** (Ciba)		(Ciba 154). Scarlet and caramel. In 30s, 60s and 100s.	1
Rx	**Rifadin** (Marion Merrell Dow)	**Powder for Injection:** 600 mg	In vials.	26

* Cost Index based on cost per 600 mg.

Refer to the general discussion of these agents beginning on page 1935

ETHAMBUTOL HCl

Actions:

Pharmacology: Ethambutol diffuses into actively growing mycobacterium cells such as tubercle bacilli. It inhibits the synthesis of one or more metabolites, thus causing impairment of cell metabolism, arrest of multiplication, and cell death. No cross-resistance with other agents has been demonstrated.

Pharmacokinetics:

Absorption/Distribution – Ethambutol absorption is not influenced by food. Following a single oral dose of 15 to 25 mg/kg, ethambutol attains a peak of 2 to 5 mcg/ml in serum 2 to 4 hours after administration. Serum levels are similar after prolonged dosing. The serum level is undetectable 24 hours after the last dose except in some patients with abnormal renal function. Cerebrospinal fluid concentrations may attain 10% to 50% of simultaneous serum concentrations in the presence of meningeal inflammation.

Metabolism – During the 24 hours following oral administration, about 20% of ethambutol is metabolized by the liver.

Excretion – Approximately 50% of unchanged drug is excreted in the urine, 8% to 15% as metabolites and 20% to 25% unchanged in the feces. Marked accumulation may occur with renal insufficiency.

Microbiology: Ethambutol is effective against strains of *Mycobacterium tuberculosis,* but does not seem to be active against fungi, viruses or other bacteria. *M tuberculosis* strains previously unexposed to ethambutol have been uniformly sensitive to concentrations of $\leq$ 8 mcg/ml, depending on the nature of the culture media. When used alone for treatment of tuberculosis, tubercle bacilli from these patients have developed resistance by in vitro susceptibility tests; the development of resistance has been unpredictable and appears to occur in a stepwise manner. Ethambutol has reduced the incidence of mycobacterial resistance to isoniazid when used concurrently.

Indications:

Pulmonary tuberculosis: Use in conjunction with at least one other antituberculous drug.

In patients who have received previous therapy, mycobacterial resistance to other drugs used in initial therapy is frequent. In retreatment patients, combine ethambutol with at least one of the second-line drugs not previously administered to the patient, and to which bacterial susceptibility has been indicated.

Contraindications:

Hypersensitivity to ethambutol; known optic neuritis, unless clinical judgment determines that it may be used.

Warnings:

Renal function impairment: Patients with decreased renal function require reduced dosage (as determined by serum levels) since this drug is excreted by the kidneys.

Pregnancy: The effects of combinations of ethambutol with other antituberculous drugs on the fetus are not known. Administration to pregnant patients has produced no detectable effect upon the fetus; use only when clearly needed and when the potential benefits outweigh the potential hazards to the fetus.

In fetuses born of mice treated with high doses of ethambutol during pregnancy, a low incidence of cleft palate, exencephaly and abnormality of the vertebral column were observed. Minor abnormalities of the cervical vertebra were seen in the newborn of rats treated with high doses of ethambutol during pregnancy. Rabbits receiving high doses during pregnancy gave birth to two fetuses with monophthalmia, one with a shortened right forearm accompanied by bilateral wrist-joint contracture and one with hare lip and cleft palate.

Children: Not recommended for use in children $<$ 13 years.

Precautions:

Monitoring: Perform periodic assessment of renal, hepatic and hematopoietic systems during long-term therapy.

(Precautions continued on following page)

ETHAMBUTOL HCl (Cont.)

Precautions (Cont.):

Visual effects: This drug may have adverse effects on vision. The effects are generally reversible when the drug is discontinued promptly. In rare cases, recovery may be delayed for up to 1 year or more, and the effect may possibly be irreversible. Patients have then received the drug again without recurrence of loss of visual acuity. Acuity changes may be unilateral or bilateral; therefore, each eye must be tested separately and both eyes tested together. Perform testing before beginning therapy and periodically during drug administration (monthly when a patient is receiving > 15 mg/kg/day). Use Snellen eye charts for testing of visual acuity. Physical examination should include ophthalmoscopy, finger perimetry and testing of color discrimination.

In patients with visual defects such as cataracts, recurrent inflammatory conditions of the eye, optic neuritis, and diabetic retinopathy, the evaluation of changes in visual acuity is more difficult; the variations in vision may be due to the underlying disease conditions. In such patients, consider the relationship between benefits expected and possible visual deterioration, since evaluation of visual changes is difficult.

Advise patients to report promptly any change in visual acuity. Changes in color perception are probably the first signs of toxicity. These changes can be detected with the use of hue charts. If evaluation confirms visual change and fails to reveal other causes, discontinue drug and reevaluate patient at frequent intervals. Consider progressive decreases in visual acuity during therapy to be due to the drug.

Patients developing visual abnormality during treatment may show subjective visual symptoms before, or simultaneously with, the demonstration of decreases in visual acuity; periodically question all patients receiving ethambutol about blurred vision and other subjective eye symptoms.

Drug Interactions:

Aluminum salts may delay and reduce the absorption of ethambutol. Separate their administration by several hours.

Adverse Reactions:

Ophthalmic: May produce decreases in visual acuity, which appear to be due to optic neuritis and to be related to dose and duration of treatment. See Precautions.

Allergic: Anaphylactoid reactions; dermatitis; pruritus.

GI: Anorexia; nausea; vomiting; GI upset; abdominal pain.

CNS: Fever; malaise; headache; dizziness; mental confusion; disorientation; possible hallucinations. Numbness and tingling of the extremities due to peripheral neuritis have occurred infrequently.

Metabolic: Elevated serum uric acid levels; precipitation of acute gout; transient impairment of liver function as indicated by abnormal liver function.

Miscellaneous: Toxic epidermal necrolysis; thrombocytopenia; joint pain.

Patient Information:

May cause stomach upset; take with food.

Notify physician if changes in vision (eg, blurring, red-green color blindness) or skin rash occurs.

Administration and Dosage:

Do not use ethambutol alone. Administer once every 24 hours only. Absorption is not significantly altered by administration with food. Continue therapy until bacteriological conversion has become permanent and maximal clinical improvement has occurred.

Initial treatment: In patients who have not received previous antituberculous therapy, administer 15 mg/kg (7 mg/lb) as a single oral dose once every 24 hours. Isoniazid has been administered concurrently in a single, daily oral dose.

Retreatment: In patients who have received previous antituberculous therapy, administer 25 mg/kg (11 mg/lb) as a single oral dose once every 24 hours. Concurrently administer at least one other antituberculous drug to which the organisms have been demonstrated to be susceptible by in vitro tests. Suitable drugs usually include those not previously used in the treatment of the patient. After 60 days of administration, decrease the dose to 15 mg/kg and administer as a single oral dose once every 24 hours.

During the period when a patient is receiving a daily dose of 25 mg/kg, monthly eye examinations are advised (see Precautions).

Children: Not recommended for use in children < 13 years old.

				C.I.*
Rx	**Myambutol** (Lederle)	**Tablets:** 100 mg	(LL M6). White, coated. Convex. In 100s.	9.5
		400 mg	(LL M7). White, scored. Film coated. In 1000s, UD 100s and unit-of-use 100s.	2.2

* Cost Index based on cost per 1 gram.

Refer to the general discussion of these agents beginning on page 1924

PYRAZINAMIDE

Actions:

Pharmacology: Pyrazinamide is an analog of nicotinamide and is bacteriostatic against *Mycobacterium tuberculosis.* Little is known of its mechanism.

Pharmacokinetics:

Absorption/Distribution – Pyrazinamide is well absorbed from the GI tract; it reaches peak plasma concentrations after an oral dose in 2 hours and is widely distributed throughout the body, including cerebrospinal fluid (100% of serum concentrations in normal and inflamed meninges).

Metabolism/Excretion – The drug is primarily metabolized by the liver; the metabolites and about 3% to 4% of unchanged drug is excreted in the urine. There may be some concentration in the bile.

Indications:

Recommended for any form of active tuberculosis when treatment with primary drugs has failed. Give pyrazinamide only with other effective antituberculous agents.

New information indicates that pyrazinamide is considered a primary agent and is used with other primary agents in certain situations. Refer to the Antituberculous Drugs introduction for details.

Contraindications:

Hypersensitivity to the drug; severe hepatic damage.

Warnings:

Discontinue pyrazinamide and do not resume therapy if signs of hepatocellular damage or hyperuricemia accompanied by an acute gouty arthritis become manifest.

Children: Safety for use in children has not been established. Because of its potential toxicity, avoid use in children unless crucial to therapy.

Precautions:

Pretreatment examinations should include in vitro susceptibility tests of recent cultures of *M tuberculosis* as measured against pyrazinamide and the usual primary drugs; however, there is no reliable in vitro test for pyrazinamide resistance.

Monitoring: Use only when close observation of the patient is possible and when laboratory facilities are available for performing frequent, reliable liver function tests and blood uric acid determinations. Perform liver function tests (especially AST, ALT determinations) prior to and every 2 to 4 weeks during therapy.

Gout or diabetes mellitus: Use pyrazinamide with caution in patients with a history of gout or diabetes mellitus, as management may be more difficult.

Porphyria: Use with caution in patients with acute intermittent porphyria.

Adverse Reactions:

Hepatotoxicity: The principal untoward effect is a hepatic reaction. This varies from a symptomless abnormality of hepatic cell function, detectable only by laboratory tests, through a mild syndrome of fever, anorexia, malaise, liver tenderness, hepatomegaly, and splenomegaly, to more serious reactions such as clinical jaundice and rare cases of progressive fulminating acute yellow atrophy and death. The incidence of hepatotoxicity ranges from 2% to 20%, generally the higher doses (50 mg/kg) will result in a higher incidence.

GI: Nausea; vomiting; diarrhea.

Miscellaneous: Active gout; sideroblastic anemia and adverse effects on the blood clotting mechanism or vascular integrity; urticaria; pruritis; rashes; photosensitivity.

Patient Information:

Take as directed; do not stop taking this drug before consulting a physician.

Notify physician if fever, loss of appetite, malaise, nausea and vomiting, darkened urine, yellowish discoloration of the skin and eyes, or symptoms of acute gouty arthritis (severe pain in the great toe, instep, ankle, heel, knee or wrist) occurs.

Administration and Dosage:

Administer with at least one other effective antituberculous drug. Average adult dose is 20 to 35 mg/kg/day in 3 or 4 divided doses. Do not exceed 3 g/day. A dose of 15 to 30 mg/kg/day has also been suggested.

				C.I.*
Rx	**Pyrazinamide** (Lederle)	**Tablets:** 500 mg	(LL P36). White, scored. Convex. In 100s and 500s.	1.8

* Cost Index based on cost per 1.5 g.

AMINOSALICYLATE SODIUM (Para-Aminosalicylate Sodium)

Aminosalicylate sodium is the sodium salt of para-aminosalicylic acid (PAS). It contains 73% aminosalicylic acid equivalent and 10.9% sodium (54.5 mg sodium/500 mg tablet).

Actions:

Aminosalicylate sodium is bacteriostatic against *Mycobacterium tuberculosis.* It inhibits the onset of bacterial resistance to streptomycin and isoniazid.

Pharmacokinetics:

Absorption/Distribution – PAS is readily absorbed from the GI tract; the sodium salt is absorbed more rapidly than the free acid. It is widely distributed, concentrates in pleural and caseous tissue, but achieves low cerebrospinal fluid concentration.

Metabolism – The half-life of PAS is about 1 hour. It is metabolized in the liver; $>$ 50% is acetylated.

Excretion – Over 80% is excreted through the kidneys as metabolites and free acid. Excretion is retarded in the presence of renal dysfunction.

Indications:

Treatment of tuberculosis in combination with other antituberculous drugs when due to susceptible strains of tubercle bacilli.

Unlabeled uses: PAS has been shown to have serum lipid-lowering activity.

Contraindications:

Severe hypersensitivity to aminosalicylate sodium and its congeners.

Warnings:

Hypersensitivity: Stop all medication if symptoms of hypersensitivity develop. Refer to General Management of Acute Hypersensitivity Reactions. After the symptoms have abated, restart medications one at a time, in very small but gradually increasing doses, to determine if the symptoms were drug-induced and, if so, which medication was responsible. Oral hyposensitization can only occasionally be accomplished. See Adverse Reactions.

Hepatic or renal function impairment: Use with caution.

Precautions:

Gastric ulcer: Use cautiously in patients with gastric ulcer.

Crystalluria may be prevented by maintaining the urine at a neutral or alkaline pH.

Tablet deterioration: Aminosalicylate sodium deteriorates rapidly in contact with water, heat and sunlight. A brownish or purplish color of powder or tablets, especially of a solution made with them, is indicative of such deterioration. If deterioration is evident, discard the drug.

Use with caution in patients with known or impending congestive heart failure and in other situations in which excess sodium is potentially harmful.

Drug Interactions:

Digoxin: Oral absorption of digoxin may be reduced with a subsequent reduction in serum levels by PAS. Digoxin doses need to be increased.

Vitamin B_{12} (oral) deficiency may be induced due to PAS interference of its GI absorption; parenteral vitamin B_{12} may be required.

Adverse Reactions:

Most common: GI – Nausea; vomiting; diarrhea; abdominal pain.

Less common: Hypersensitivity – Fever; skin eruptions of various types; infectious mononucleosis-like syndrome; leukopenia; agranulocytosis; thrombocytopenia; hemolytic anemia; jaundice; hepatitis; encephalopathy; Loffler's syndrome; vasculitis. See Warnings.

Endocrine – Goiter with or without myxedema.

Patient Information:

Take as directed. Do not stop taking before consulting your doctor.

May cause stomach upset. Take with food or meals.

Do not use products that are brown or purple in color. Aminosalicylate will not work if it becomes wet or is left in extreme heat or direct sunlight. Therefore, do not store in the kitchen or bathroom cabinet.

Notify your doctor if fever, sore throat, unusual bleeding or bruising, or skin rash occurs.

Administration and Dosage:

Administer aminosalicylate sodium with other antituberculous drugs.

Adults: 14 to 16 g/day in 2 to 3 divided doses.

Children: 275 to 420 mg/kg/day in 3 to 4 divided doses daily.

				C.I.*
Rx	**Sodium P.A.S.** (Lannett)	**Tablets:** 0.5 g	In 100s, 500s and 1000s.	43

* Cost Index based on cost per 10 g.

Refer to the general discussion of these agents beginning on page 1924

ETHIONAMIDE

Actions:

Bacteriostatic against *Mycobacterium tuberculosis.*

Pharmacokinetics: Oral administration of ethionamide yields peak plasma concentrations in 3 hours. It is widely and rapidly distributed, including into the cerebrospinal fluid. The drug is metabolized in the liver and $<$ 1% is excreted in the urine unchanged.

Indications:

Recommended for any form of active tuberculosis when treatment with first-line drugs (isoniazid, rifampin) has failed. Use only with other effective antituberculous agents.

Contraindications:

Severe hypersensitivity to ethionamide; severe hepatic damage.

Warnings:

Pregnancy: Teratogenic effects have been demonstrated in small animals receiving doses in excess of those recommended in humans. Use during pregnancy only when clearly needed and when the potential benefits outweigh the potential hazards to the fetus.

Children: Optimum dosage for children has not been established. This does not preclude use of the drug when crucial to therapy.

Precautions:

Pretreatment examinations should include in vitro susceptibility tests of recent cultures of *M tuberculosis* from the patient as measured against ethionamide and the usual first-line antituberculous drugs.

Monitoring: Make determinations of serum transaminase (AST, ALT) prior to and every 2 to 4 weeks during therapy.

Diabetes mellitus: Management of the diabetes may be more difficult and hepatitis occurs more frequently.

Adverse Reactions:

GI: Anorexia, nausea and vomiting are most common (50% unable to tolerate doses $>$ 500 mg); diarrhea; metallic taste; hepatitis (5%); jaundice; stomatitis.

Neurotoxicity: Depression, drowsiness and asthenia (common); convulsions; peripheral neuritis and neuropathy; olfactory disturbances; blurred vision; diplopia; optic neuritis; dizziness; headache; restlessness; tremors; psychosis.

Miscellaneous: Postural hypotension; skin rash; acne; alopecia; thrombocytopenia; pellagra-like syndrome; gynecomastia; impotence; menorrhagia; increased difficulty managing diabetes mellitus.

Patient Information:

May cause stomach upset, loss of appetite, metallic taste or salivation. Notify physician if these effects persist or are severe. Taking with food may help reduce GI upset.

Administration and Dosage:

Administer with at least 1 other effective antituberculous drug.

Average adult dose: 0.5 to 1 g/day in divided doses.

Children: A dose of 15 to 20 mg/kg/day (maximum 1 g) has been recommended.

Concomitant administration of pyridoxine is recommended.

				C.I.*
Rx	**Trecator-SC** (Wyeth-Ayerst)	**Tablets:** 250 mg	(#Wyeth 4130). Orange. Sugar coated. In 100s.	246

* Cost Index based on cost per 500 mg.

\# Product identification code.

Refer to the general discussion of these agents beginning on page 1924

CYCLOSERINE

Actions:

Pharmacology: Inhibits cell wall synthesis in susceptible strains of gram-positive and gram-negative bacteria and in *Mycobacterium tuberculosis.* Cycloserine, a structural analogue of D-alanine, antagonizes D-alanine's role in bacterial cell wall synthesis.

Pharmacokinetics:

Absorption/Distribution – When given orally, cycloserine is rapidly absorbed, reaching peak plasma concentrations in 3 to 8 hours. It is widely distributed throughout body fluids and tissues; cerebrospinal fluid levels are similar to plasma.

Metabolism/Excretion – Approximately 35% of the drug is metabolized; 50% of a parenteral dose is excreted unchanged in the urine in the first 12 hours. About 65% of the drug is recoverable in 72 hours. Renal insufficiency will lead to toxic accumulation; it may be removed by dialysis.

Indications:

For the treatment of active pulmonary and extrapulmonary tuberculosis (including renal disease) when organisms are susceptible, after failure of adequate treatment with the primary medications. Administer in conjunction with other effective chemotherapy.

May be effective in the treatment of acute urinary tract infections caused by susceptible strains of gram-positive and gram-negative bacteria, especially *Enterobacter* sp and *Escherichia coli*. It is usually less effective than other antimicrobial agents in the treatment of urinary tract infections caused by bacteria other than mycobacteria. Consider using only when the more conventional therapy has failed and when the organism has demonstrated sensitivity.

Contraindications:

Hypersensitivity to cycloserine; epilepsy; depression, severe anxiety or psychosis; severe renal insufficiency; excessive concurrent use of alcohol.

Warnings:

CNS toxicity: Discontinue the drug or reduce dosage if patient develops allergic dermatitis or symptoms of CNS toxicity, such as convulsions, psychosis, somnolence, depression, confusion, hyperreflexia, headache, tremor, vertigo, paresis or dysarthria. The risk of convulsions is increased in chronic alcoholics.

Toxicity is closely related to excessive blood levels (> 30 mcg/ml), which are due to high dosage or inadequate renal clearance. The therapeutic index in tuberculosis is small.

Monitor patients by hematologic, renal excretion, blood level and liver function studies.

Renal function impairment: Patients will accumulate cycloserine and may develop toxicity if the dosage regimen is not modified. Patients with severe impairment should not receive the drug.

Pregnancy: Category C. It is not known whether this drug can cause fetal harm when administered to a pregnant woman or can affect reproduction capacity. Use only if clearly needed.

Lactation: Because of the potential for serious adverse reactions in nursing infants, decide whether to discontinue nursing or to discontinue the drug, taking into account the importance of the drug to the mother.

Children: Safety and dosage not established for pediatric use.

Precautions:

Obtain cultures and determine susceptibility before treatment.

Determine blood levels weekly for patients having reduced renal function, for individuals receiving > 500 mg/day, and for those with symptoms of toxicity. Adjust dosage to maintain blood level < 30 mcg/ml.

Anticonvulsant drugs or sedatives may be effective in controlling symptoms of CNS toxicity, such as convulsions, anxiety and tremor. Closely observe patients receiving > 500 mg/day for such symptoms. Pyridoxine may prevent CNS toxicity, but its efficacy has not been proven.

Anemia: Administration has been associated in a few cases with vitamin B_{12} or folic acid deficiency, megaloblastic anemia and sideroblastic anemia. If evidence of anemia develops, institute appropriate studies and therapy.

Drug Interactions:

Alcohol and cycloserine are incompatible; alcohol increases the possibility and risk of epileptic episodes.

Isoniazid in combination with cycloserine may result in increased cycloserine CNS side effects, most notably dizziness.

(Continued on following page)

CYCLOSERINE (Cont.)

Adverse Reactions:

CNS (related to dosages > 500 mg/day): Convulsions; drowsiness and somnolence; headache; tremor; dysarthria; vertigo; confusion and disorientation with loss of memory; psychoses, possibly with suicidal tendencies, character changes, hyperirritability, aggression; paresis; hyperreflexia; paresthesias; major and minor (localized) clonic seizures; coma.

Cardiovascular: Sudden development of congestive heart failure has been reported.

Allergic (not related to dosage): Skin rash.

Miscellaneous: Elevated transaminase, especially in patients with liver disease.

Overdosage:

Symptoms: Acute toxicity can occur if > 1 g is ingested; chronic toxicity is dose-related and can occur if > 500 mg/day is administered. Toxic effects may include CNS depression with accompanying drowsiness, mental confusion, headache, vertigo, hyperirritability, paresthesias, dysarthrias and psychosis. Paresis, convulsions and coma may occur after larger doses.

Management includes supportive therapy. Charcoal may be more effective than emesis or lavage; consider charcoal instead of or in addition to gastric emptying. Hemodialysis removes the drug from the bloodstream; reserve for patients with life-threatening toxicity. Pyridoxine 200 to 300 mg/day may treat the neurotoxic effects. Refer also to General Managment of Acute Overdosage.

Patient Information:

May cause drowsiness. Observe caution when driving or performing other tasks requiring alertness. Avoid excessive alcohol consumption.

Notify physician if skin rash, mental confusion, dizziness, headache or tremors occur.

Administration and Dosage:

Administer 500 mg to 1 g daily in divided doses monitored by blood levels. The usual initial dosage is 250 mg twice daily at 12 hour intervals for the first 2 weeks. Do not exceed 1 g/day.

Pyridoxine 200 to 300 mg/day may prevent the neurotoxic effects.

Children: A dose of 10 to 20 mg/kg/day (maximum 0.75 to 1 g) has been recommended.

				C.I.*
Rx	**Seromycin Pulvules** (Lilly)	**Capsules:** 250 mg	In 40s.	157

STREPTOMYCIN SULFATE

The following is an abbreviated monograph for streptomycin sulfate. For complete prescribing information, see individual monograph in Aminoglycosides, Parenteral section.

Indications:

Recommended in the treatment of all forms of *Mycobacterium tuberculosis* when the infecting organisms are susceptible. Use only in combination with other antituberculous drugs.

For nontuberculous infection indications, see individual monograph in Aminoglycosides, Parenteral section.

Administration and Dosage:

Administer by the IM route only.

Combined therapy for adults: 1 g streptomycin and an appropriate dosage of additional antitubercular drugs (usually isoniazid, ethambutol or rifampin). Elderly patients should have a smaller daily dose of streptomycin in accordance with age, renal function and eighth nerve function.

Discontinue the streptomycin or reduce dosage to 1 g 2 to 3 times weekly. Therapy with streptomycin may be terminated when toxic symptoms appear, impending toxicity is feared, organisms have become resistant, or full therapeutic effect has been obtained. The total period of treatment for tuberculosis is a minimum of 1 year; however, indications for terminating streptomycin therapy may occur at any time.

Children: A dose of 20 to 40 mg/kg/day (maximum 0.75 to 1 g) has been recommended.

As with other aminoglycosides, reduce dosage in patients with impaired renal function.

For a complete listing of streptomycin sulfate products, refer to individual monograph in Aminoglycosides, Parenteral section.

* Cost Index based on cost per 500 mg cycloserine.

Product identification code.

Refer to the general discussion of these agents beginning on page 1924

CAPREOMYCIN

Warning:

The use of capreomycin in patients with renal insufficiency or preexisting auditory impairment must be undertaken with great caution, and weigh the risk of additional eighth nerve impairment or renal injury against benefits to be derived from therapy.

Since other parenteral antituberculous agents (eg, streptomycin) also have similar and sometimes irreversible toxic effects, particularly on eighth cranial nerve and renal function, simultaneous administration of these agents with capreomycin is not recommended. Use concurrent nonantituberculous drugs (eg, aminoglycoside antibiotics) having ototoxic or nephrotoxic potential only with great caution.

Actions:

A polypeptide antibiotic isolated from *Streptomyces capreolus.*

Microbiology: Active against human strains of *Mycobacterium tuberculosis.*

Cross-resistance – Varying degrees of cross-resistance between capreomycin and kanamycin and neomycin have occurred. No cross-resistance has been observed between capreomycin and isoniazid, aminosalicylate sodium, cycloserine, streptomycin, ethionamide or ethambutol.

Pharmacokinetics:

Distribution – Capreomycin sulfate is not absorbed in significant quantities from the GI tract and must be administered parenterally. Peak serum concentrations following IM administration of 1 g are achieved in 1 to 2 hours. Low serum concentrations are present at 24 hours. Doses of 1 g daily for ≥ 30 days produce no significant accumulation in subjects with normal renal function.

Excretion – Capreomycin is excreted essentially unaltered; 52% is excreted in the urine within 12 hours. Urine concentrations average 1680 mcg/ml during the 6 hours following a 1 g dose.

Indications:

Intended for use concomitantly with other antituberculous agents in pulmonary infections caused by capreomycin-susceptible strains of *M tuberculosis*, when the primary agents (eg, isoniazid, rifampin) have been ineffective or cannot be used because of toxicity or the presence of resistant tubercle bacilli.

Perform susceptibility studies to determine the presence of a capreomycin-susceptible strain of *M tuberculosis*.

Contraindications:

Hypersensitivity to capreomycin.

Warnings:

Renal function impairment: Dosage reduction is necessary. See Administration and Dosage.

Hypersensitivity has occurred when capreomycin and other antituberculous drugs were given concomitantly. Refer to General Management of Acute Hypersensitivity Reactions.

Pregnancy: Category C. Well controlled studies have not been performed in pregnant women. Use only if clearly needed and when potential benefits justify potential risks to the fetus. Safety for use during pregnancy has not been established.

Lactation: It is not known whether this drug is excreted in breast milk. Therefore, exercise caution when administering capreomycin to nursing mothers.

Children: Safety for use in infants and children has not been established.

Precautions:

Ototoxicity: Perform audiometric measurements and assessment of vestibular function prior to initiation of therapy and at regular intervals during treatment.

Nephrotoxicity: Perform regular tests of renal function throughout treatment, and reduce dose in patients with renal impairment. Renal injury with tubular necrosis, elevation of BUN or serum creatinine and abnormal sediment has been noted. Monitor renal function both before therapy is started and on a weekly basis during treatment. Slight elevation of the BUN or serum creatinine has been observed in a significant number of patients receiving prolonged therapy. The appearance of casts, red cells and white cells in the urine has been noted in a high percentage of these cases.

Elevation of the BUN > 30 mg/dl or any other evidence of decreasing renal function with or without a rise in BUN level should indicate careful evaluation of the patient; reduce the dosage or withdraw the drug. The clinical significance of abnormal urine sediment and slight elevation in the BUN (or serum creatinine) during long-term therapy has not been established.

Hypokalemia may occur during therapy; therefore, determine serum potassium levels frequently.

(Continued on following page)

CAPREOMYCIN (Cont.)

Drug Interactions:

Aminoglycosides and capreomycin coadministration may increase the risk of respiratory paralysis and renal dysfunction.

Nondepolarizing neuromuscular blocking agents: Neuromuscular blockade may be enhanced by concurrent capreomycin due to a synergistic effect on myoneural function.

Adverse Reactions:

Nephrotoxicity: In 36% of 722 patients treated with capreomycin, elevation of the BUN > 20 mg/dl has been observed. In many instances, there was also depression of PSP excretion and abnormal urine sediment. In 10% of this series, the BUN elevation exceeded 30 mg/dl.

Toxic nephritis was reported in one patient with tuberculosis and portal cirrhosis who was treated with capreomycin (1 g) and aminosalicylate sodium daily for 1 month. This patient developed renal insufficiency and oliguria and died. Autopsy showed subsiding acute tubular necrosis.

Electrolyte disturbances resembling Bartter's syndrome occurred in one patient.

Ototoxicity: Subclinical auditory loss was noted in approximately 11% of patients. This has been a 5 to 10 decibel loss in the 4,000 to 8,000 CPS range. Clinically apparent hearing loss occurred in 3% of 722 subjects. Some audiometric changes were reversible. Other cases with permanent loss were not progressive following withdrawal of capreomycin.

Tinnitus and vertigo have also occurred.

Hepatic: Serial tests of liver function have demonstrated a decrease in BSP excretion without change in AST or ALT in the presence of preexisting liver disease. Abnormal results in liver function tests have occurred in many persons receiving capreomycin in combination with other antituberculous agents which are also known to cause changes in hepatic function. The role of capreomycin is not clear; however, periodic determinations of liver function are recommended.

Blood: Leukocytosis and leukopenia have been observed. The majority of patients treated have had eosinophilia exceeding 5% while receiving daily injections of capreomycin. This subsided with reduction of the capreomycin dosage to 2 or 3 g weekly.

Rare cases of thrombocytopenia have occurred.

Hypersensitivity: Urticaria and maculopapular skin rashes, associated in some cases with febrile reactions. See Warnings.

Other: Pain and induration and excessive bleeding at the injection sites; sterile abscesses.

Overdosage:

Adverse reactions listed above may be seen in capreomycin overdose. Management includes supportive therapy. Refer to General Management of Acute Overdosage.

Hemodialysis may be useful in patients with significant renal disease.

(Continued on following page)

CAPREOMYCIN (Cont.)

Administration and Dosage:

Give by deep IM injection into a large muscle mass; superficial injections may be associated with increased pain and sterile abscesses. Always administer in combination with at least one other antituberculous agent to which the patient's strain of tubercle bacilli is susceptible.

Usual dose: 1 g daily (not to exceed 20 mg/kg/day) given IM for 60 to 120 days, followed by 1 g IM 2 or 3 times weekly.

Note: Maintain therapy for tuberculosis for 12 to 24 months. If facilities for administering injectable medication are not available, a change to oral therapy is indicated upon the patient's release from the hospital.

Children: A dose of 15 mg/kg/day (maximum 1 g) has been recommended.

Renal function impairment: Reduce the dosage based on creatinine clearance (Ccr) using the guidelines in the table. These dosages are designed to achieve a mean steady-state capreomycin level of 10 mg/L.

Capreomycin Dosage in Renal Function Impairment

Ccr (ml/min)	Capreomycin clearance (L/kg/h × 10^{-2})	Half-life (hours)	Dose[1] (mg/kg) for the following dosing intervals		
			24 hr	48 hr	72 hr
0	0.54	55.5	1.29	2.58	3.87
10	1.01	29.4	2.43	4.87	7.3
20	1.49	20.0	3.58	7.16	10.7
30	1.97	15.1	4.72	9.45	14.2
40	2.45	12.2	5.87	11.7	
50	2.92	10.2	7.01	14	
60	3.40	8.8	8.16		
80	4.35	6.8	10.4		
100	5.31	5.6	12.7		
110	5.78	5.2	13.9		

[1] Initial maintenance dose estimates are given for optional dosing intervals; longer dosing intervals are expected to provide greater peak and lower trough serum capreomycin levels than shorter dosing intervals.

Preparation of solution: Dissolve in 2 ml of 0.9% Sodium Chloride Injection or Sterile Water for Injection. Allow 2 to 3 minutes for complete dissolution. For administration of a 1 g dose, give the entire contents of the vial. For dosages < 1 g, the following dilution table may be used.

Preparation of Capreomycin Solution

Concentration† (Approx.)	Diluent added to 1 g vial	Volume of solution
350 mg/ml	2.15 ml	2.85 ml
300 mg/ml	2.63 ml	3.33 ml
250 mg/ml	3.3 ml	4 ml
200 mg/ml	4.3 ml	5 ml

† Stated in terms of mg of capreomycin activity.

Storage/Stability: The solution may acquire a pale straw color and darken with time, but this is not associated with loss of potency or the development of toxicity. After reconstitution, solutions may be stored for 48 hours at room temperature and up to 14 days under refrigeration.

			C.I.*
Rx	**Capastat Sulfate** (Lilly)	**Powder for Injection:** 1 g (as sulfate) per 10 ml vial.	2301

* Cost Index based on cost per 1 gram.

The agents listed in this group are recommended for the following disorders (see individual monographs):

Intestinal amebiasis:	*Extraintestinal amebiasis:*
Paromomycin	Metronidazole
Iodoquinol	Emetine HCl
Metronidazole	Chloroquine
Emetine HCl	

PAROMOMYCIN

Actions:

Paromomycin is an amebicidal and antibacterial aminoglycoside obtained from a strain of *Streptomyces rimosus,* and is active in intestinal amebiasis. Its in vitro and in vivo antibacterial activity closely parallels that of neomycin; complete cross-resistance exists between paromomycin, kanamycin and neomycin. Effective against enteric bacteria *Salmonella* and *Shigella.*

Gastrointestinal absorption of paromomycin is poor; almost 100% of the drug is recovered in the stool.

Indications:

Acute and chronic intestinal amebiasis.

Adjunctive therapy in the management of hepatic coma.

Not indicated in extraintestinal amebiasis because it is not absorbed.

Unlabeled uses: Has been recommended for other parasitic infections – *Dientamoeba fragilis* (25 to 30 mg/kg/day in 3 doses for 7 days); *Diphyllobothrium latum, Taenia saginata, T solium, Dipylidium caninum* (adults: 1 g every 15 min for 4 doses; pediatric: 11 mg/kg every 15 min for 4 doses); *Hymenolepis nana* (45 mg/kg/day for 5 to 7 days).

Contraindications:

Hypersensitivity reactions to paromomycin; intestinal obstruction.

Precautions:

Ototoxicity and renal damage: Inadvertent absorption through ulcerative bowel lesions may result in eighth cranial nerve damage and renal damage.

Superinfection: Use of antibiotics (especially prolonged or repeated therapy) may result in bacterial or fungal overgrowth of nonsusceptible organisms. Such overgrowth may lead to secondary infections. Take appropriate measures if superinfection occurs.

Drug Interactions:

Since paromomycin is an aminoglycoside, consider the interactions that may occur with the other oral aminoglycosides as potentially occurring with paromomycin as well (see Aminoglycosides, Oral section).

Adverse Reactions:

GI: Doses > 3 g daily have reportedly produced nausea, abdominal cramps and diarrhea.

Patient Information:

Complete full course of therapy.

May cause nausea, vomiting or diarrhea.

Notify physician if ringing in the ears, hearing impairment or dizziness occurs.

Administration and Dosage:

Intestinal amebiasis: Adults and children – 25 to 35 mg/kg/day in 3 divided doses with meals for 5 to 10 days.

Management of hepatic coma: Adults – 4 g daily in divided doses administered at regular intervals for 5 to 6 days.

				C.I.*
Rx	**Humatin** (Parke-Davis)	**Capsules:** 250 mg (as sulfate)	In 16s.	247

* Cost Index based on cost per 500 mg.

IODOQUINOL (Diiodohydroxyquin)

Actions:

Iodoquinol is effective against the trophozoites and cysts of *Entamoeba histolytica* located in the large intestine. Because it is poorly absorbed in the GI tract, the drug can reach high concentrations in the intestinal lumen, and produce its potent amebicidal effect precisely at the site of infection, without significant systemic absorption (approximately 8%). This is useful for the prevention of extraintestinal (liver, lung) complications of amebic dysentery. The drug is not effective in amebic hepatitis and amebic abscess of the liver.

Indications:

Treatment of intestinal amebiasis.

Not indicated for treatment of chronic diarrhea, particularly in children, because of potential association with optic atrophy and permanent loss of vision.

Contraindications:

Hypersensitivity to any 8-hydroxyquinoline (eg, iodoquinol, iodochlorhydroxyquin) or iodine-containing preparations; hepatic damage.

Warnings:

Optic neuritis, optic atrophy and peripheral neuropathy have occurred following prolonged high dosage therapy; avoid long-term therapy.

Pregnancy and lactation: Safety for use during pregnancy and in the nursing mother has not been established.

Precautions:

Use with caution in patients with thyroid disease.

Drug Interactions:

Drug/Lab test interactions: Protein bound iodine levels may be increased during treatment and interfere with the results of certain **thyroid** function tests. These effects may persist for as long as 6 months after discontinuance of therapy.

Adverse Reactions:

Dermatologic: Various forms of skin eruptions (acneiform, papular, pustular, bullae, vegetating or tuberous iododerma); urticaria; pruritus.

GI: Nausea; vomiting; abdominal cramps; diarrhea; pruritus ani.

Other: Fever; chills; headache; vertigo; enlargement of thyroid. Optic neuritis, optic atrophy and peripheral neuropathy have occurred in association with prolonged high dosage 8-hydroxyquinoline therapy.

Patient Information:

Complete full course of therapy.

May cause nausea, vomiting, diarrhea or GI upset.

Administration and Dosage:

Adults: 650 mg 3 times daily after meals for 20 days.

Children: 40 mg/kg daily (maximum 650 mg/dose) in 3 divided doses for 20 days. Do not exceed 1.95 g in 24 hours for 20 days.

				C.I.*
Rx	**Yodoxin** (Glenwood)	**Tablets:** 210 mg	In 100s and 1000s.	87
		650 mg	In 100s and 1000s.	35
		Powder	In 25 g.	60

* Cost Index based on cost per 650 mg.

METRONIDAZOLE

The following is an abbreviated monograph for metronidazole. Complete prescribing information begins on page 1877.

Warning: Metronidazole has been shown to be carcinogenic in rodents. Avoid unnecessary use.

Actions:

Microbiology: Metronidazole is a nitroimidazole that possesses direct trichomonacidal and amebicidal activity against *Trichomonas vaginalis* and *Entamoeba histolytica*. The in vitro minimal inhibitory concentration (MIC) for most strains of these organisms is ≤ 1 mcg/ml. Metronidazole's mechanism of antiprotozoal action is unknown.

Indications:

Amebiasis: Treatment of acute intestinal amebiasis (amebic dysentery) and amebic liver abscess. In amebic liver abscess, therapy does not obviate the need for aspiration or drainage of pus.

Trichomoniasis, symptomatic: Treatment in females and males when the presence of the trichomonad has been confirmed by appropriate laboratory procedures (wet smears or cultures).

Trichomoniasis, asymptomatic: Treatment of asymptomatic females with endocervicitis, cervicitis or cervical erosion. Since there is evidence that presence of the trichomonad can interfere with accurate assessment of abnormal cytological smears, perform additional smears after eradication of the parasite.

Treatment of asymptomatic partner: T vaginalis infection is a sexually transmitted disease. Therefore, in order to prevent reinfection, simultaneously treat asymptomatic sexual partners of treated patients if the organism has been found to be present. Since there can be difficulty in isolating the organism from the asymptomatic male carrier, negative smears and cultures cannot be relied upon. Women may become reinfected if the male partner is not treated. Therefore, it may be advisable to treat an asymptomatic male partner with a negative culture or when no culture has been attempted.

Anaerobic bacterial infections: Refer to page 1878.

Unlabeled uses: The CDC has recommended the use of oral metronidazole for *Gardnerella vaginalis* (500 mg twice daily for 7 days) and for giardiasis (alternative to quinacrine; 250 mg 3 times daily for 7 days).

Patient Information:

May cause GI upset; take with food.

Complete full course of therapy; take until gone.

Avoid alcoholic beverages.

May cause darkening of urine.

An unpleasant metallic taste may be noticeable.

During treatment for trichomoniasis, it is recommended that the patient refrain from sexual intercourse or the male partner wear a condom to avoid reinfection.

(Continued on following page)

METRONIDAZOLE (Cont.)

Administration and Dosage:

Amebiasis:

Acute intestinal amebiasis (acute amebic dysentery) - 750 mg 3 times daily for 5 to 10 days.

Amebic liver abscess – 500 or 750 mg 3 times daily for 5 to 10 days.

Children – 35 to 50 mg/kg/24 hours (maximum 750 mg/dose) in 3 divided doses for 10 days.

Trichomoniasis: 1 day treatment – 2 g given either as a single dose or in 2 divided doses of 1 g each given in the same day.

7 day course of treatment – Adults: 250 mg 3 times daily for 7 consecutive days; *children:* 5 mg/kg/dose 3 times daily for 7 days.

Cure rates, as determined by vaginal smears, signs and symptoms, may be higher after a 7 day course of treatment than after the 1 day treatment regimen. Individualize dosage. Single dose treatment can assure compliance, especially if administered under supervision, in those patients who cannot be relied upon to continue the 7 day regimen. A 7 day course of treatment may minimize reinfection of the female long enough to treat sexual contacts. Further, some patients may tolerate one course of therapy better than the other.

Do not treat pregnant patients during the first trimester. If treated during the second or third trimester in those whom local palliative treatment has been inadequate to control symptoms, do not use the 1 day course of therapy as it results in higher serum levels which reach the fetal circulation.

When repeat courses of the drug are required, 4 to 6 weeks should elapse between courses and reconfirm the presence of the trichomonad by appropriate laboratory measures. Perform total and differential leukocyte counts before and after retreatment.

Patients with severe hepatic disease metabolize metronidazole slowly, with resultant accumulation of metronidazole and its metabolites in the plasma. Accordingly, cautiously administer doses below those usually recommended. Monitor plasma metronidazole levels and toxicity.

Do not specifically reduce the dose of metronidazole in anuric patients since accumulated metabolites may be rapidly removed by dialysis.

				C.I.*
Rx	**Metronidazole** (Various, eg, Baxter, Geneva, Goldline, Lederle, Lemmon, Moore, Rugby, Schein, Squibb Mark, Zenith)	**Tablets:** 250 mg	In 8s, 21s, 28s, 50s, 100s, 250s, 500s, 1000s and UD 32s and 100s.	99+
Rx	**Flagyl** (Searle)		(Searle 1831 Flagyl 250). Blue. Film coated. In 50s, 100s, 250s, 1000s, 2500s and UD 100s.	310
Rx	**Metizol** (Glenwood)		In 100s.	56
Rx	**Metric 21** (Fielding)		In 100s.	NA
Rx	**Protostat** (Ortho)		(Ortho 1570). White, scored. Convex, capsule shape. In 100s.	222
Rx	**Metronidazole** (Various, eg, Baxter, Geneva, Goldline, Lederle, Lemmon, Moore, Rugby, Schein, Squibb Mark, Zenith)	**Tablets:** 500 mg	In 4s, 8s, 10s, 14s, 21s, 30s, 50s, 64s, 100s, 200s, 250s, 500s and UD 32s and 100s.	119+
Rx	**Flagyl** (Searle)		(Flagyl 500). Blue. Film coated. Oblong. In 50s, 100s, 500s and UD 100s.	235
Rx	**Protostat** (Ortho)		(Ortho 1571). White, scored. Convex, capsule shape. In 50s.	194

* Cost Index based on cost per 500 mg.

EMETINE HCl

Actions:

Emetine has a direct lethal action on *Entamoeba histolytica.*

Pharmacology: An alkaloid related to ipecac, emetine is an amebicide which acts primarily in the bowel wall and in the liver. Emetine inhibits polypeptide chain elongation, thereby blocking protein synthesis in parasitic and mammalian cells, but not in bacteria.

Pharmacokinetics: Emetine is a general protoplasmic poison which, because of its slow elimination following parenteral administration, tends to accumulate in the body. The drug is not administered orally because it produces nausea and vomiting. Subcutaneous and IM doses are concentrated primarily in the liver; appreciable levels are also attained in the kidney, spleen and lungs, and persist in these tissues for several months. Very little of the drug is excreted into the bowel after parenteral administration; however, it may continue to be eliminated in the urine for 40 to 60 days after administration since renal excretion is slow.

Clinical pharmacology: In comparative studies of emetine and chloroquine, emetine has demonstrated superior efficacy in amebic liver abscess. Combined therapy with emetine given for 10 days and chloroquine given for 3 weeks results in a satisfactory response with few relapses.

Indications:

Intestinal amebiasis: Useful in the symptomatic management of acute fulminating amebic dysentery or acute exacerbations of chronic amebic dysentery. It is not indicated in the treatment of mild symptoms or carriers. The effect is symptomatic; cure can be expected in only 10% to 15% of cases with the use of emetine alone. Give patients another effective antiamebic preparation simultaneously.

Extraintestinal amebiasis: Highly effective against amebae in tissues; it is of value in the treatment of amebic abscess and "amebic hepatitis" because of the high concentration of the drug in the liver.

In all cases of extraintestinal amebiasis, institute other amebicidal treatment simultaneously or as an immediate follow-up to guarantee that *E histolytica* has been eradicated from primary lesions in the intestine.

Other parasitic infections: Useful in certain cases of balantidiasis, fascioliasis and paragonimiasis.

Contraindications:

Patients with organic disease of the heart or kidney, except those with amebic abscess or hepatitis not controlled by chloroquine; patients who have received a course of emetine less than 6 weeks to 2 months previously; pregnancy and children (see Warnings); IV administration.

Warnings:

Medical Supervision: A potentially dangerous drug, emetine requires strict medical supervision including: Daily examinations, complete bed rest during and for several days after administration, pulse and blood pressure recorded 2 to 3 times daily, and an electrocardiogram (ECG) performed before initial administration, after the fifth dose, at the completion of therapy, and 1 week later.

Fatalities: No fatalities from a single dose have been reported; however, several have resulted from repeated doses, even when the total dose did not exceed the 600 mg upper limit for the drug. There is insufficient absorption from oral administration to cause systemic poisoning in humans.

The drug is very irritating and should not be allowed to come in contact with the cornea or with mucous membranes, especially of the conjunctiva.

Pregnancy. Category X. Emetine may cause fetal harm when administered to a pregnant woman and is contraindicated in women who are or who may become pregnant. If this drug is used during pregnancy or if the patient becomes pregnant while taking this drug, apprise her of the potential hazard to the fetus.

Lactation: Safety for use in the nursing mother has not been established.

Children: Use in children is contraindicated except in those with severe dysentery not controlled by other amebicides.

Elderly: Exercise caution in administering emetine to the aged or debilitated.

(Continued on following page)

EMETINE HCl (Cont.)

Precautions:

Discontinue emetine upon appearance of tachycardia, precipitous fall in blood pressure, neuromuscular symptoms, marked GI effects, or considerable weakness.

Some investigators consider the appearance of any ECG abnormalities an indication for immediate cessation of therapy (eg, widening of the QRS complex and prolongation of the PR interval). However, the significance of ECG changes rests upon the judgment of the clinician as to the severity and type of disease.

Adverse Reactions:

Toxic manifestations may occur at any dose level.

Local: Common reactions include aching, tenderness and muscle weakness in the area of the injection site. Eczematous, urticarial or purpuric lesions may also appear.

GI: Severe GI side effects are unusual; nausea and vomiting, in association with dizziness and headache, are more common.

Neuromuscular: Weakness; aching; tenderness; skeletal muscle stiffness. The weakness and muscle pain tend to persist until emetine is discontinued; they usually appear before more serious symptoms develop and serve as a guide for avoiding overdosage.

Cardiovascular: The most severe toxic effects are related to the cardiovascular system and include: Hypotension; tachycardia; precordial pain; dyspnea; ECG abnormalities; gallop rhythm; cardiac dilatation; congestive heart failure. Death has occurred.

In 45 patients undergoing emetine therapy, the most noteworthy change observed was inversion of the T-wave in the precordial leads; this change is the first to appear, the most consistent (100%), and the last to disappear. Second in importance is prolongation of the QT interval (in 90% of cases). The ECG patterns observed sometimes resemble those of myocardial infarction (eg, ST elevation, T-wave inversion and prolongation of the QT interval). ECG changes appear about 7 days after the drug is administered and are reversible. The average time required for complete return of the tracing to normal is over 6 weeks.

Overdosage:

Symptoms: Systemic toxicity will generally involve the cardiovascular, neuromuscular and GI systems and may occur from a single overdose or from a chronic accumulation of emetine that is the result of the drug's very slow (40 to 60 days) renal excretion. Degenerative changes in the heart, kidneys, liver, skeletal muscles and GI tract may result. Fatalities have been associated with chronic toxicity (see Adverse Reactions).

Centrally mediated toxicity may result in nausea, vomiting, diarrhea, dizziness and marked prostration. Other symptoms may include epigastric burning or pain; crampy abdominal pain; hyperperistalsis; blood, mucus or pus in stools; and, rarely, constipation.

The neuromuscular signs and symptoms of toxicity generally appear early following an overdose. These symptoms may include muscle ache, tenderness, stiffness, edema, fatigue and listlessness. Depression, peripheral neuropathies, paresthesias, paralysis and encephalitis have been reported with overdoses of emetine. The lethal dose is 10 to 25 mg/kg.

Treatment: Discontinue administration of the drug and begin supportive measures. Refer to General Management of Acute Overdosage. Syrup of ipecac is contraindicated because it contains emetine.

If PVCs require therapy, lidocaine or phenytoin is preferred. Quinidine, procainamide and other antiarrhythmic agents that prolong intraventricular conduction are contraindicated.

Forced diuresis, peritoneal dialysis, hemodialysis or charcoal hemoperfusion have not been established as beneficial.

Administration and Dosage:

Do NOT give IV. This route is dangerous and is contraindicated. Deep SC injection is usually preferred; may be given IM.

Maximum dosage: Do not exceed 65 mg/day or 10 days of therapy (650 mg total dosage). Do not repeat a course of therapy in less than 6 weeks. Some authorities recommend a dose of 1 mg/kg/day, not to exceed 65 mg. May be administered as a single 65 mg dose or 32 mg morning and evening.

Children: Use ONLY in severe dysentery not controlled by other amebicides.

Under 8 years – Do not exceed 10 mg/day.

Over 8 years – Do not exceed 20 mg/day.

1 mg/kg/day in 2 doses for no more than 5 days has also been suggested.

Acute fulminating amebic dysentery: Administer only long enough to control diarrheal or dysenteric symptoms; usually 3 to 5 days.

Amebic hepatitis or abscess: Administer for 10 days.

				C.I.*
Rx	**Emetine HCl** (Lilly)	**Injection:** 65 mg per ml	In 1 ml amps.	502

* Cost Index based on cost per 65 mg.

The following are abbreviated monographs for chloroquine phosphate and chloroquine HCl. For complete prescribing information, see 4-Aminoquinoline Compounds in the Antimalarial Preparations section.

CHLOROQUINE PHOSPHATE

Indications:

Treatment of extraintestinal amebiasis.

Administration and Dosage:

Adults: 1 g (600 mg base) daily for 2 days, followed by 500 mg (300 mg base) daily for at least 2 to 3 weeks. Treatment is usually combined with an effective intestinal amebicide.

				C.I.*
Rx	**Chloroquine Phosphate** (Various, eg, Balan, Bioline, Danbury, Geneva, Goldline, Major, Moore, Rugby, Schein, URL)	**Tablets:** 250 mg (equiv. to 150 mg base)	In 20s, 22s, 30s, 100s, 1000s and UD 100s.	21+
Rx	**Aralen Phosphate** (Winthrop)	**Tablets:** 500 mg (equiv. to 300 mg base)	In 25s.	529

CHLOROQUINE HCl

Indications:

Treatment of extraintestinal amebiasis when oral therapy is not feasible.

Administration and Dosage:

Adults: 4 to 5 ml (200 to 250 mg; 160 to 200 mg base) IM daily for 10 to 12 days. Substitute or resume oral administration as soon as possible.

				C.I.*
Rx	**Aralen HCl** (Winthrop)	**Injection:** 50 mg (equiv. to 40 mg base) per ml	In 5 ml amps.	832

* Cost Index based on cost per 1 g chloroquine phosphate or 200 mg chloroquine HCl.

ZIDOVUDINE (Azidothymidine; AZT; Compound S)

Warnings:

Zidovudine is often associated with hematologic toxicity including granulocytopenia and severe anemia requiring transfusions (see Warnings).

Zidovudine patients may continue to develop opportunistic infections (OI's) and other complications of the acquired immunodeficiency syndrome (AIDS) and AIDS-related complex (ARC) caused by the human immunodeficiency virus (HIV). Therefore, patients should be under close clinical observation by physicians experienced in the treatment of patients with diseases associated with HIV.

Actions:

Pharmacology: Zidovudine is a thymidine analog and an inhibitor of the in vitro replication of some retroviruses, including HIV (also known as HTLV III, LAV or ARV). Cellular thymidine kinase converts zidovudine into zidovudine monophosphate and finally to the triphosphate derivative by other cellular enzymes. Zidovudine triphosphate interferes with the HIV viral RNA-dependent DNA polymerase (reverse transcriptase) and thus, inhibits viral replication. Zidovudine triphosphate also inhibits cellular α-DNA polymerase, but at concentrations 100-fold higher than those required to inhibit reverse transcriptase. In vitro, zidovudine triphosphate is incorporated into growing chains of DNA by viral reverse transcriptase, and the DNA chain is terminated.

Pharmacokinetics: Absorption/Distribution – The following pharmacokinetic data was obtained in adults. Overall, the pharmacokinetics in pediatric patients > 3 months of age is similar to that in adults. After oral dosing, zidovudine is rapidly absorbed from the GI tract with peak serum concentrations occurring within 0.5 to 1.5 hours. The rate of absorption of the syrup is greater than that of the capsules. Dose-dependent kinetics were observed over the range of 2 mg/kg every 8 hours to 10 mg/kg every 4 hours. Zidovudine plasma protein binding is 34% to 38%.

Steady-state serum concentrations following chronic oral use of 250 mg every 4 hours (3 to 5.4 mg/kg) were determined in 21 patients. Mean steady-state predose and 1.5 hours postdose concentrations were 0.16 mcg/ml (range, 0 to 0.84 mcg/ml) and 0.62 mcg/ml (range, 0.05 to 1.46 mcg/ml), respectively.

Metabolism/Elimination – Zidovudine is rapidly metabolized in the liver to the inactive 3′-azido-3′-deoxy-5′-O-β-D-glucopyranuronosylthymidine (GAZT) which has an apparent elimination half-life of 1 hour (range, 0.61 to 1.73 hours). The mean zidovudine half-life was approximately 1 hour (range, 0.78 to 1.93 hours). Following oral administration, urinary recovery of zidovudine and GAZT was 14% and 74% of the dose, respectively, and the total urinary recovery averaged 90% (range, 63% to 95%). However, as a result of first-pass metabolism, the average oral capsule bioavailability is 65% (range, 52% to 75%).

Following IV dosing (1 to 5 mg/kg) total body clearance averaged 1900 ml/min/70 kg and the apparent volume of distribution was 1.6 L/kg. Renal clearance is estimated to be 400 ml/min/70 kg, indicating glomerular filtration and active tubular secretion by the kidneys. The zidovudine CSF/plasma concentration ratios measured at 2 to 4 hours following IV dosing of 2.5 and 5 mg/kg were 0.2 and 0.64, respectively.

Microbiology: Zidovudine has antiviral activity against some mammalian retroviruses in addition to HIV. No significant inhibitory activity was exhibited against a variety of other human and animal viruses, except against the Epstein-Barr virus (clinical significance not known). Many Enterobacteriaceae, including strains of *Shigella, Salmonella, Klebsiella, Enterobacter, Citrobacter* and *Escherichia coli* are inhibited in vitro by low concentrations of zidovudine (0.005 to 0.5 mcg/ml). The clinical significance is not known. Synergy of zidovudine with trimethoprim has been observed against some of these bacteria. Limited data suggest that bacterial resistance to zidovudine develops rapidly. Although *Giardia lamblia* is inhibited by 1.9 mcg/ml of zidovudine, no activity was observed against other protozoal pathogens.

Indications:

Oral: Adults – For the management of patients with HIV infection who have evidence of impaired immunity (CD4 cell count of ≤ 500/mm³) before therapy is begun.

Children – For HIV-infected children > 3 months of age who have HIV-related symptoms or who are asymptomatic with abnormal laboratory values indicating significant HIV-related immunosuppression.

IV: For the management of certain adult patients with symptomatic HIV infection (AIDS and advanced ARC) who have a history of cytologically confirmed *Pneumocystis carinii* pneumonia (PCP) or an absolute CD4 (T4 helper/inducer) lymphocyte count of < 200/mm³ in the peripheral blood before therapy is begun.

Contraindications:

Patients who have life-threatening allergic reactions to any of the components.

(Continued on following page)

ZIDOVUDINE (Azidothymidine; AZT; Compound S) (Cont.)

Warnings:

Zidovudine has been studied in controlled trials in significant numbers of asymptomatic and symptomatic HIV-infected patients, but only for limited periods of time. Therefore, the full safety and efficacy profile of zidovudine has not been completely defined, especially with prolonged use and in HIV-infected individuals who have less advanced disease.

Hematologic effects: Use with extreme caution in patients who have bone marrow compromise evidenced by granulocyte count < 1000/mm³ or hemoglobin < 9.5 g/dl. Anemia and granulocytopenia are the most significant adverse events observed. There have been reports of reversible pancytopenia.

Significant anemia most commonly occurred after 4 to 6 weeks of therapy and in many cases required dose adjustment, discontinuation of drug or blood transfusions. Frequent blood counts are strongly recommended for advanced HIV disease patients, less frequent for asymptomatic and early HIV disease depending on overall status. If anemia or granulocytopenia develops, dosage adjustments may be necessary.

Hypersensitivity: Sensitization reactions, including anaphylaxis in one patient, have occurred with zidovudine therapy. Patients experiencing a rash should undergo medical evaluation. Refer to Management of Acute Hypersensitivity Reactions.

Renal and hepatic function impairment: There are currently no data available concerning the use of zidovudine in patients with impaired renal or hepatic function; such patients may be at a greater risk of toxicity from zidovudine.

Carcinogenesis and mutagenesis: In mice, seven late-appearing (after 19 months) vaginal neoplasms (five non-metastasizing squamous cell carcinomas, one squamous cell papilloma, one squamous polyp) occurred in animals given the highest dose of zidovudine; one squamous cell papilloma occurred with the middle dose. In rats, two late-appearing (after 20 months) non-metastasizing vaginal squamous cell carcinomas occurred in animals given the highest dose.

Zidovudine was weakly mutagenic in the absence of metabolic activation only at the highest concentrations tested (4000 and 5000 mcg/ml) in mouse lymphoma cells. In the presence of metabolic activation the drug was weakly mutagenic at concentrations of 1000 mcg/ml and higher. In cultured human lymphocytes, zidovudine caused dose-related structural chromosomal abnormalities at concentrations ≥ 3 mcg/ml.

Pregnancy: Category C. It is not known whether zidovudine can cause fetal harm when administered to a pregnant woman or can affect reproductive capacity. Zidovudine should be given to a pregnant woman only if clearly needed.

Lactation: It is not known whether zidovudine is excreted in breast milk. Because of the potential for serious adverse reactions from zidovudine in nursing infants, mothers should discontinue nursing if they are receiving zidovudine.

Children: Insufficient clinical experience exists to recommend a dosing regimen in infants < 3 months of age. Zidovudine clearance may be reduced in children < 1 month old.

A positive test for HIV-antibody in children < 15 months of age may represent passively acquired maternal antibodies, rather than an active antibody response to infection in the infant. Thus, the presence of HIV-antibody in a child < 15 months of age must be interpreted with caution, especially in the asymptomatic infant. Pursue confirmatory tests such as serum P_{24} antigen or viral culture in such children.

Drug Interactions:

Dapsone, pentamidine, amphotericin B, flucytosine, vincristine, vinblastine, adriamycin, interferon: Coadministration of zidovudine with drugs that are nephrotoxic, cytotoxic or interfere with RBC/WBC number or function may increase the toxicity risk.

Probenecid may inhibit glucuronidation or reduce renal excretion of zidovudine. Avoid coadministration of zidovudine with other drugs metabolized by glucuronidation because the toxicity of either drug may be potentiated. In addition, other drugs (eg, **acetaminophen, aspirin** or **indomethacin**) may competitively inhibit glucuronidation. Zidovudine recipients who used acetaminophen had an increased incidence of granulocytopenia associated with the duration of acetaminophen use.

Experimental nucleoside analogs which are being evaluated in AIDS and ARC patients may affect RBC/WBC number or function and may increase the potential for hematologic toxicity of zidovudine. Some analogs affecting DNA replication antagonize the in vitro antiviral activity of zidovudine against HIV; avoid concomitant use.

Trimethoprim-sulfamethoxazole, pyrimethamine and **acyclovir** may be necessary for the management or prevention of opportunistic infections. In the controlled trial, increased toxicity was not detected with limited exposure to these drugs. However, there are two reports of neurotoxicity (one of profound lethargy and one of seizure) associated with concomitant use of zidovudine and acyclovir.

(Continued on following page)

ZIDOVUDINE (Azidothymidine; AZT; Compound S) (Cont.)

Adverse Reactions:

The most frequent adverse events and abnormal laboratory values reported in the placebo controlled clinical trial of oral zidovudine were granulocytopenia and anemia. The occurrence of hematologic toxicities was inversely related to CD4 (T4) lymphocyte number, hemoglobin and granulocyte count at study entry, and directly related to dose and duration of therapy. The anemia appeared to be the result of impaired erythrocyte maturation as evidenced by increasing macrocytosis (MCV) while on drug. Similar results occurred in children.

The 281 patients (144 zidovudine; 137 placebo) treated in this trial had serious underlying disease. Headache, nausea, insomnia and myalgia occurred at a significantly greater rate in zidovudine recipients.

Zidovudine Adverse Reactions (≥ 5% Advanced Adult HIV Patients) %

Adverse Reaction	Zidovudine (n = 144)	Placebo (n = 137)	Adverse Reaction	Zidovudine (n = 144)	Placebo (n = 137)
Body as a whole			*GI*		
Asthenia	19	18	Anorexia	11	8
Diaphoresis	5	4	Diarrhea	12	18
Fever	16	12	Dyspepsia	5	4
Headache	42	37	GI pain	20	19
Malaise	8	7	Nausea	46	18
			Vomiting	6	3
CNS			*Other*		
Dizziness	6	4	Dyspnea	5	3
Insomnia	5	1	Myalgia	8	2
Paresthesia	6	3	Rash	17	15
Somnolence	8	9	Taste perversion	5	8

Other reactions (< 5% of adults, advanced HIV); causal relationship not established.

Body as a whole: Body odor; chills; edema of the lip; flu syndrome; hyperalgesia; back pain; chest pain; lymphadenopathy.

Cardiovascular: Vasodilation.

GI: Constipation; dysphagia; edema of the tongue; eructation; flatulence; bleeding gums; rectal hemorrhage; mouth ulcer.

Musculoskeletal: Arthralgia; muscle spasm; tremor; twitch.

CNS: Anxiety; confusion; depression; emotional lability; nervousness; syncope; loss of mental acuity; vertigo.

Respiratory: Cough; epistaxis; pharyngitis; rhinitis; sinusitis; hoarseness.

Skin: Acne; pruritus; urticaria.

Special senses: Amblyopia; hearing loss; photophobia.

GU: Dysuria; polyuria; urinary frequency; urinary hesitancy.

Zidovudine Adverse Reactions (Early Symptomatic and Asymptomatic Adult HIV Patients) %

Adverse Reaction	Early Symptomatic HIV Disease		Asymptomatic HIV Infection		
	Zidovudine (n = 361)	Placebo (n = 352)	Zidovudine 500 mg (n = 453)	Zidovudine 1500 mg[1] (n = 457)	Placebo (n = 428)
Body as a whole					
Asthenia	69	62	8.6	10.1	5.8
Headache	—	—	62.5	58	52.6
Malaise	—	—	53.2	55.6	44.9
GI					
Anorexia	—	—	20.1	19.3	10.5
Constipation	—	—	6.4	8.1	3.5
Dyspepsia	6	1			
Nausea	61	41	51.4	57.3	29.9
Vomiting	25	13	17.2	16.4	9.8
CNS					
Dizziness	—	—	17.9	20.8	15.2

[1] Three times the currently recommended dose in asymptomatic patients.

Children (the adverse effects reported in adults may also occur in children):

Body as a whole – Fever (3.2%); phlebitis/bacteremia (1.6%); headache (1.6%).

GI – Vomiting (4.8%); abdominal pain (3.2%); nausea, diarrhea, weight loss (0.8%).

CNS – Decreased reflexes (5.6%); insomnia (2.4%); nervousness/irritability (1.6%); seizure (0.8%).

Cardiovascular – ECG abnormality (2.4%); left ventricular dilation, cardiomyopathy, S_3 gallop, CHF, generalized edema (0.8%).

GU – Hematuria/viral cystitis (0.8%).

(Continued on following page)

ZIDOVUDINE (Azidothymidine; AZT; Compound S) (Cont.)

Overdosage:

Cases of acute overdoses in both children and adults have occurred with doses up to 50 g; none were fatal. The only consistent finding was spontaneous or induced nausea and vomiting. Hematologic changes were transient and not severe. All patients recovered without permanent sequelae. Hemodialysis appears to have a negligible effect on zidovudine while elimination of its primary metabolite, GAZT, is enhanced.

Patient Information:

Zidovudine is not a cure for HIV infections, and patients may continue to acquire illnesses associated with AIDS or ARC, including opportunistic infections. Patients should seek medical care for any significant change in their health status.

The major toxicities of zidovudine are granulocytopenia or anemia that may require transfusions or dose modifications including possible discontinuation. It is extremely important to have blood counts followed closely while on therapy.

Warn patients about the use of other medications (eg, acetaminophen) that may exacerbate the toxicity of zidovudine.

Long-term effects of zidovudine are unknown at this time.

Zidovudine therapy has not been shown to reduce the risk of transmission of HIV to others through sexual contact or blood contamination.

Oral: Take exactly as prescribed; administration every 4 hours includes dosing around the clock, even though it may interrupt normal sleep (except asymptomatic patients which is every 4 hours while awake). Do not share medication and do not exceed the recommended dose.

Administration and Dosage:

Oral:

Adults –

Symptomatic HIV infection: Initial –200 mg (two 100 mg capsules or 4 teaspoonfuls [20 ml] syrup) every 4 hours around the clock. In a 70 kg patient, this dose corresponds to 2.9 mg/kg every 4 hours. After 1 month, dose may be reduced to 100 mg every 4 hours. The effectiveness of this lower dose in improving neurologic dysfunction associated with HIV disease, however, is unknown.

Asymptomatic HIV infection: 100 mg every 4 hours while awake (500 mg/day).

Children (3 months to 12 years) – The recommended starting dose is 180 mg/m^2 every 6 hours (720 mg/m^2/day, not to exceed 200 mg every 6 hours.

Monitor hematologic indices every 2 weeks to detect serious anemia or granulocytopenia. In patients with hematologic toxicity, reduction in hemoglobin may occur as early as 2 to 4 weeks, and granulocytopenia usually occurs after 6 to 8 weeks.

Dose adjustment: Significant anemia (hemoglobin of $<$ 7.5 g/dl or reduction of $>$ 25% of baseline) or significant granulocytopenia (granulocyte count of $<$ 750/mm^3 or reduction of $>$ 50% from baseline) may require a dose interruption until evidence of marrow recovery is observed. For less severe anemia or granulocytopenia, dose reduction may be adequate. In patients who develop significant anemia, dose modification does not necessarily eliminate the need for transfusion. If marrow recovery occurs following dose modification, gradual increases in dose may be appropriate depending on hematologic indices and patient tolerance.

Storage: Capsules/Syrup – Protect from light.

IV: 1 to 2 mg/kg infused over 1 hour at a constant rate; administer every 4 hours around the clock (6 times daily). Avoid rapid infusion or bolus injection. Do not give IM. Patients should receive the IV infusion only until oral therapy can be administered. The IV dosing regimen equivalent to the oral administration of 100 mg every 4 hours is approximately 1 mg/kg IV every 4 hours.

Preparation: Dilute prior to administration. Remove the calculated dose from the vial; add to 5% Dextrose Injection to achieve a concentration of $\leq$ 4 mg/ml.

IV admixture incompatibility: Admixture in biologic or colloidal fluids (eg, blood products, protein solutions) is not recommended.

Storage/Stability: After dilution, the solution is physically and chemically stable for 24 hours at room temperature and 48 hours if refrigerated at 2°C to 8°C (36°F to 46°F). As an additional precaution, administer the diluted solution within 8 hours if stored at 25°C (77°F) or 24 hours if refrigerated at 2°C to 8°C to minimize the potential administration of a microbially contaminated solution. Store undiluted vials at 15°C to 25°C (59°F to 77°F) and protect from light.

				C.I.*
Rx	**Retrovir** (Burroughs Wellcome)	**Capsules:** 100 mg	(Wellcome Y9C 100). White with blue band. In 100s.	515
		Syrup: 50 mg/5 ml	Strawberry flavor. In 240 ml.	412
		Injection: 10 mg/ml	In 20 ml single use vial.	2229

* Cost Index based on 200 mg zidovudine.

RIBAVIRIN

Warning:

Do not use for infants requiring assisted ventilation because precipitation of the drug in the respiratory equipment may interfere with safe and effective patient ventilation.

Deterioration of respiratory function has been associated with ribavirin use in infants, and in adults with chronic obstructive lung disease or asthma. Carefully monitor respiratory function during treatment. If ribavirin aerosol treatment produces sudden deterioration of respiratory function, stop treatment and reinstitute only with extreme caution and continuous monitoring.

Actions:

Pharmacology: Antiviral effects – Ribavirin has antiviral inhibitory activity in vitro against respiratory syncytial virus (RSV), influenza virus and herpes simplex virus. The mechanism of action is unknown.

Immunologic effects – Neutralizing antibody responses to RSV were decreased in ribavirin-treated infants compared to placebo-treated infants; clinical significance of this observation is unknown. In rats, ribavirin resulted in lymphoid atrophy of thymus, spleen and lymph nodes. Humoral immunity was reduced in guinea pigs and ferrets. Cellular immunity was also mildly depressed in animal studies.

Pharmacokinetics: Absorption – Ribavirin administered by aerosol is absorbed systemically. Four pediatric patients inhaling ribavirin aerosol by face mask for 2.5 hours each day for 3 days had plasma concentrations ranging from 0.44 to 1.55 μM (mean, 0.76 μM). The plasma half-life was 9.5 hours. Three pediatric patients inhaling ribavirin aerosol by face mask or mist tent for 20 hours/day for 5 days had plasma concentrations ranging from 1.5 to 14.3 μM (mean, 6.8 μM).

Distribution – The bioavailability of ribavirin aerosol is unknown and may depend on the mode of aerosol delivery. After aerosol treatment, peak plasma concentrations are less than the concentration that reduced RSV plaque formation in tissue culture by 85% to 98%. After aerosol treatment, respiratory tract secretions are likely to contain ribavirin in concentrations many times higher than those required to reduce plaque formation. However, RSV is an intracellular virus and serum concentrations may better reflect intracellular concentrations in the respiratory tract than respiratory secretion concentrations.

Accumulation of ribavirin or metabolites in the red blood cells has been noted, with plateauing in red cells in about 4 days. Accumulation gradually declines with an apparent half-life of 40 days. Accumulation following inhalation is not well defined.

Indications:

Treatment of carefully selected hospitalized infants and young children with severe lower respiratory tract infections due to RSV.

The vast majority of infants and children with RSV infection have no lower respiratory tract disease or have disease that is mild, self-limited and does not require hospitalization or antiviral treatment.

The presence of underlying conditions such as prematurity or cardiopulmonary disease may increase the severity of the infection and its risk to the patient. High risk infants and young children with such conditions may benefit from treatment.

Ribavirin aerosol treatment must be accompanied by, and does not replace, standard supportive respiratory and fluid management for infants and children with severe respiratory tract infection.

Unlabeled uses: Aerosol ribavirin has shown some success against influenza A and B.

Oral ribavirin (600 mg to 1800 mg/day for 10 to 14 days) has been variously effective against other viral diseases including acute and chronic hepatitis, herpes genitalis, measles and Lassa fever.

Contraindications:

Females who are, or who may become pregnant during exposure to the drug. Ribavirin may cause fetal harm and RSV infection is self-limited in this population. Although there are no pertinent human data, ribavirin has been found to be teratogenic (malformation of skull, palate, eye, jaw, skeleton and GI tract) or embryolethal in nearly all species in which it has been tested in dosages of 1 to 10 mg/kg.

Warnings:

Animal toxicology: Ribavirin administered by aerosol produced cardiac lesions in mice and rats after 30 and 36 mg/kg, respectively, for 4 weeks, and after oral administration in monkeys at 120 mg/kg and rats at 154 to 200 mg/kg, for 1 to 6 months. Ribavirin aerosol administered to developing ferrets at 60 mg/kg for 10 or 30 days resulted in inflammatory and possibly emphysematous changes in the lungs. Proliferative changes were seen at 131 mg/kg for 30 days. The significance of these findings to human administration is unknown.

(Warnings continued on following page)

RIBAVIRIN (Cont.)

Warnings (Cont.):

Carcinogenesis, mutagenesis, impairment of fertility: Ribavirin induces cell transformation in an in vitro mammalian system. However, in vivo carcinogenicity studies are incomplete. Results thus far suggest that chronic feeding of ribavirin to rats at doses of 16 to 60 mg/kg can induce benign mammary, pancreatic, pituitary and adrenal tumors.

Pregnancy: Category X. See Contraindications.

Lactation: Use of ribavirin aerosol in nursing mothers is not indicated because RSV infection is self-limited in this population. Ribavirin is toxic to lactating animals and their offspring. It is not known whether the drug is excreted in breast milk.

Precautions:

Patients with lower respiratory tract infection due to RSV require optimum monitoring and attention to respiratory and fluid status.

Ribavirin is mutagenic to mammalian cells in culture.

Ribavirin causes testicular lesions (tubular atrophy) in adult rats at oral dose levels as low as 16 mg/kg/day, but fertility of ribavirin-treated animals is unknown.

Adverse Reactions:

Several serious adverse events occurred in severely ill infants with life-threatening underlying diseases, many of whom required assisted ventilation. The role of ribavirin aerosol in these events is undetermined.

Pulmonary: Worsening of respiratory status; bacterial pneumonia; pneumothorax; apnea; ventilator dependence.

Some subjects requiring assisted ventilation have experienced serious difficulties, which may jeopardize adequate ventilation and gas exchange. Precipitation of drug within the ventilatory apparatus, including the endotracheal tube, has resulted in increased positive end expiratory pressure and increased positive inspiratory pressure. Accumulation of fluid in tubing ("rain out") has also been noted.

Pulmonary function significantly deteriorated during ribavirin aerosol treatment in all of six adults with chronic obstructive lung disease, and in four of six asthmatic adults. Dyspnea and chest soreness were also reported in the latter group. Minor abnormalities in pulmonary function were also seen in healthy adult volunteers.

Cardiovascular: Cardiac arrest; hypotension; digitalis toxicity.

Hematologic: Although anemia has not been reported with use of the aerosol, it occurs frequently with oral and IV ribavirin, and most infants treated with the aerosol have not been evaluated 1 to 2 weeks posttreatment when anemia is likely to occur. Reticulocytosis has been reported with aerosol use.

Miscellaneous: Rash; conjunctivitis.

Administration and Dosage:

For aerosol administration only.

Before use, read thoroughly the Viratek Small Particle Aerosol Generator (SPAG) Model SPAG-2 Operator's Manual for small particle aerosol generator operating instructions.

Treatment was effective when instituted within the first 3 days of RSV lower respiratory tract infection.

Treatment is carried out for 12 to 18 hours per day for at least 3, but no more than 7 days, and is part of a total treatment program. The aerosol is delivered to an infant oxygen hood from the SPAG-2 aerosol generator. Administration by face mask or oxygen tent may be necessary if a hood cannot be used. However, the volume of distribution and condensation area are larger in a tent, and efficacy of this method has been evaluated in only a few patients. Ribavirin aerosol is not to be administered with any other aerosol generating device or together with other aerosolized medications, and it is not to be used for patients requiring simultaneous assisted ventilation.

Solubilize drug with sterile USP water for injection or inhalation in the 100 ml vial. Transfer to the clean, sterilized 500 ml wide-mouth Erlenmeyer flask (SPAG-2 Reservoir) and further dilute to a final volume of 300 ml with sterile USP water for injection or inhalation. The final concentration should be 20 mg/ml.

Important: This water should not have any antimicrobial agent or other substance added. Discard solutions placed in the SPAG-2 unit at least every 24 hours and when the liquid level is low before adding newly reconstituted solution. Using the recommended drug concentration of 20 mg/ml ribavirin as the starting solution in the SPAG unit's drug reservoir, the average aerosol concentration for a 12 hour period is 190 mcg/L of air.

Storage: Store powder at 15° to 25°C (59° to 78°F). May store reconstituted solutions at room temperature for up to 24 hours.

Rx	Virazole (ICN)	**Powder for reconstitution for aerosol:** 6 g powder per 100 ml vial. Contains 20 mg per ml when reconstituted with 300 ml sterile water.

Amantadine is also used as an antiparkinson agent. For information regarding this use, refer to amantadine in the Antiparkinson Agents section.

AMANTADINE HCl

Actions:

Pharmacology: Amantadine's antiviral activity against influenza A virus is not completely understood. Its mode of action appears to be the prevention of the release of infectious viral nucleic acid into the host cell. It may also interfere with viral penetration into cells. The reaction appears to be virus specific (for influenza A) but not host specific. Amantadine does not appear to interfere with the immunogenicity of inactivated influenza A virus vaccine.

Amantadine is 70% to 90% effective in preventing illnesses caused by circulating strains of type A influenza viruses (it is not effective against type B influenza). When administered within 24 to 48 hours after onset of illness, amantadine reduces the duration of fever and other systemic symptoms with a more rapid return to routine daily activities and improvement in peripheral airway function.

Pharmacokinetics: Absorption/Distribution – After oral administration of a single dose of 100 mg, maximum blood levels are reached in approximately 4 hours, based on the mean time of the peak urinary excretion rate; the peak excretion rate is approximately 5 mg/hr; the mean half-life of the excretion rate approximates 15 hours.

Compared with otherwise healthy adult individuals, the clearance of amantadine is significantly reduced in adult patients with renal insufficiency. The elimination half-life increases two- to threefold when creatinine clearance is less than 40 ml/min/1.73 m^2 and averages 8 days in patients on chronic maintenance hemodialysis.

The renal clearance of amantadine is reduced and plasma levels are increased in otherwise healthy elderly patients age 65 years and older. The drug plasma levels in elderly patients receiving 100 mg daily have been reported to approximate those determined in younger adults taking 200 mg daily. Whether these changes are due to the normal decline in renal function or other age related factors is not known.

Metabolism/Excretion – Amantadine is readily absorbed, is not metabolized, and is excreted in the urine.

Indications:

Influenza A virus respiratory tract illness: Prevention or chemoprophylaxis of and treatment of respiratory tract illness caused by influenza A virus strains. Indicated especially for high risk patients because of underlying disease (eg, cardiovascular, pulmonary, metabolic, neuromuscular or immunodeficiency disease), close household or hospital ward contacts of index cases, immunocompromised patients and health care and community services personnel. Early immunization is the prophylaxis method of choice. When early immunization is contraindicated, not feasible or not available, amantadine can be used for chemoprophylaxis.

Amantadine prophylaxis recommendations:

1. Short-term prophylaxis during the course of a presumed influenza A outbreak (eg, in institutions for persons at high risk), particularly when the vaccine may be relatively ineffective.
2. Adjunct to late immunization of high risk individuals. It is not too late to immunize even when influenza A is known to be in the community. Since the development of a protective response following vaccination takes about 2 weeks, use amantadine in the interim.
3. To reduce disruption of medical care and to reduce spread of virus to high risk persons when influenza A virus outbreaks occur. Prophylaxis is desirable for those physicians, nurses and other personnel who have extensive contact with high risk patients but who failed to receive the recommended annual influenza vaccination before the onset of influenza A activity.
4. To supplement vaccination protection in those with impaired immune responses. Consider chemoprophylaxis for high risk patients who may have a poor response to influenza vaccine, eg, those with severe immunodeficiency.
5. As chemoprophylaxis throughout the influenza season for those few high risk individuals for whom influenza vaccine is contraindicated because of anaphylactic hypersensitivity to egg protein or prior severe reactions associated with influenza vaccination.

Parkinson's disease and drug-induced extrapyramidal reactions: See amantadine in the Antiparkinson Agents section.

Contraindications:

Hypersensitivity to amantadine.

(Continued on following page)

AMANTADINE HCl (Cont.)

Warnings:

Seizures: Closely observe patients with a history of epilepsy or other seizures for increased seizure activity. Dosage reduction is recommended (see Administration and Dosage).

Exercise care when administering to patients with liver disease, a history of recurrent eczematoid rash, or psychosis or severe psychoneurosis not controlled by chemotherapeutic agents.

Congestive heart failure (CHF): CHF or peripheral edema requires careful observation and dosage titration; patients have developed CHF while receiving amantadine.

Renal impairment: Reduce the dose in renal impairment. Amantadine is not metabolized and is mainly excreted in the urine; therefore, it accumulates in plasma and the body when renal function declines. See Administration and Dosage.

Elderly: Reduce dose in individuals 65 years of age and older.

Pregnancy: Category C. Amantadine in high doses is embryotoxic and teratogenic in animals. Cardiovascular malformation was reported in an infant exposed to amantadine during the first trimester. There are no adequate and well controlled studies of amantadine in pregnant women. Use only when clearly needed and when the potential benefits outweigh the potential hazards to the fetus.

Lactation: Amantadine is excreted in breast milk. Exercise caution when administering to a nursing woman.

Infants: Safety and efficacy for use in neonates and infants < 1 year of age have not been established.

Precautions:

May cause CNS effects or blurred vision; observe caution while driving or performing other tasks requiring alertness.

Do not discontinue abruptly; a few patients with Parkinson's disease experienced a parkinsonian crisis (ie, a sudden marked clinical deterioration) when this medication was stopped suddenly.

Drug Interactions:

Anticholinergic drugs: Reduce the dose of anticholinergic drugs or of amantadine if atropine-like effects appear when these drugs are used concurrently.

Hydrochlorothiazide plus triamterene: Decreased urinary excretion of amantadine with subsequent increased plasma concentrations occurred when hydrochlorothiazide plus triamterene was administered concurrently with amantadine.

Adverse Reactions:

Most frequent (5% to 10%): Nausea; dizziness; lightheadedness; insomnia.

Less frequent (1% to 5%): Depression; anxiety; irritability; hallucinations; confusion; anorexia; dry mouth; constipation; ataxia; livedo reticularis; peripheral edema; orthostatic hypotension; headache.

Infrequent (0.1% to 1%): CHF; psychosis; urinary retention; dyspnea; fatigue; skin rash; vomiting; weakness; slurred speech; visual disturbance.

Rare ($<$ 0.1%): Convulsions; leukopenia; neutropenia; eczematoid dermatitis; oculogyric episodes.

Overdosage:

Symptoms: Nausea, vomiting, anorexia and CNS effects (including hyperexcitability, tremors, ataxia, blurred vision, lethargy, depression, slurred speech and convulsions). Ventricular arrhythmias manifested by torsade de pointes and ventricular fibrillation were observed in a patient who ingested 2.5 g amantadine. Death has occurred from a major overdose.

Treatment: There is no specific antidote. *CNS toxicity* – IV physostigmine, 1 to 2 mg slowly administered every 1 to 2 hours in adults or 0.5 mg at 5 to 10 minute intervals up to a maximum of 2 mg/hour in children. *Acute overdosing* – Employ general supportive measures along with immediate gastric lavage or induction of emesis. Refer to General Management of Acute Overdosage. Force fluids; administer IV if necessary. Urinary acidification may increase elimination from the body. Monitor blood pressure, pulse, respiration, temperature, electrolytes, urine pH and urinary output. Observe the patient for hyperactivity and convulsions; administer sedatives and anticonvulsants if required. Give appropriate antiarrhythmic and vasopressor therapy when warranted.

Hemodialysis does not remove significant amounts of amantadine.

(Continued on following page)

AMANTADINE HCl (Cont.)

Patient Information:

May cause blurred vision; observe caution while driving or performing other tasks requiring alertness.

If dizziness or lightheadedness occurs, avoid sudden changes in posture; notify physician of this effect.

Notify physician if mood or mental changes, swelling of the extremities, difficult urination or shortness of breath occurs.

Administration and Dosage:

Influenza A virus illness:

Prophylaxis – Start in anticipation of contact or as soon as possible after exposure. Continue daily for at least 10 days following a known exposure. The infectious period extends from shortly before onset of symptoms to up to 1 week after. When vaccine is unavailable or contraindicated, administer for up to 90 days in case of possible repeated and unknown exposures. Because amantadine does not appear to suppress antibody response, it can be used in conjunction with inactivated influenza A virus vaccine until protective antibody responses develop; administer for 2 to 3 weeks after vaccine has been given.

Symptomatic management – Start as soon as possible after onset of symptoms and continue for 24 to 48 hours after symptoms disappear.

Adults – 200 mg daily as a single dose or 100 mg twice a day. Splitting the dose may reduce the frequency of CNS side effects.

Children (9 to 12 years) – 100 mg twice a day.

Children (1 to 9 years) – 2 to 4 mg/lb/day (4.4 to 8.8 mg/kg/day) given once daily or divided twice daily; not to exceed 150 mg per day.

The following table may serve as a guideline for dosage:

Amantadine Dosage by Patient Age and Renal Function

Renal function	Dosage[1]
No recognized renal disease	
1 to 9 yrs[2]	4.4 to 8.8 mg/kg/day once daily or divided twice daily, not to exceed 150 mg/day
10 to 64 yrs[3]	200 mg once daily or divided twice daily
≥ 65 yrs	100 mg once daily[4]
Renal function impairment Creatinine clearance: (ml/min/1.73m²)	
30 to 50	200 mg 1st day; 100 mg daily thereafter
15 to 29	200 mg 1st day; then 100 mg on alternate days
< 15	200 mg every 7 days
Hemodialysis patients	200 mg every 7 days

[1] For prophylaxis, take amantadine each day for the duration of influenza A activity in the community (generally 6 to 12 weeks). For therapy, institute amantadine as soon as possible after onset of symptoms and continue for 24 to 48 hours after symptoms disappear (generally 5 to 7 days).

[2] Use in children < 1 year of age has not been evaluated adequately. In one study, a dose of 6.6 mg/kg/day was well tolerated by children > 2 years of age.

[3] Reduce dosage to 100 mg/day for persons with an active seizure disorder, because they may be at increased risk of seizure frequency when given 200 mg/day.

[4] Recommended to minimize the risk of toxicity, because renal function normally declines with age, and side effects are more frequent in the elderly.

	Product	Form	Description	C.I.*
Rx	**Amantadine HCl** (Various, eg, Balan, Geneva, Goldline, Major, Parmed, Pharmaceutical Basics, Purepac, Rugby, Schein, Warner Chilcott)	**Capsules:** 100 mg	In 100s, 250s, 500s and UD 100s.	32+
Rx	**Symadine** (Reid-Rowell)		(RR 4140). Red. In 100s.	40
Rx	**Symmetrel** (DuPont)		Lecithin. (DuPont Symmetrel). Red. In 100s, 500s and UD 100s.	75
Rx	**Symmetrel** (DuPont)	**Syrup:** 50 mg per 5 ml	Sorbitol. Raspberry flavor. In 480 ml.	147

* Cost Index based on cost per 100 mg.

FOSCARNET SODIUM (Phosphonoformic acid)

Warning:

Renal impairment, the major toxicity of foscarnet, occurs to some degree in most patients. Consequently, continual assessment of a patient's risk and frequent monitoring of serum creatinine with dose adjustment for changes in renal function are imperative.

Foscarnet causes alterations in plasma minerals and electrolytes that have led to seizures. Monitor patients frequently for such changes and their potential sequelae.

Actions:

Pharmacology: Foscarnet is an organic analog of inorganic pyrophosphate that inhibits replication of all known herpesviruses in vitro including cytomegalovirus (CMV), herpes simplex virus types 1 and 2 (HSV-1, HSV-2), human herpesvirus 6 (HHV-6), Epstein-Barr virus (EBV) and varicella-zoster virus (VZV).

Foscarnet exerts its antiviral activity by a selective inhibition at the pyrophosphate binding site on virus-specific DNA polymerases and reverse transcriptases at concentrations that do not affect cellular DNA polymerases. Foscarnet does not require activation (phosphorylation) by thymidine kinase or other kinases, and therefore is active in vivo against HSV mutants deficient in thymidine kinase. CMV strains resistant to ganciclovir may be sensitive to foscarnet.

The quantitative relationship between the in vitro susceptibility of human CMV to foscarnet and clinical response to therapy has not been clearly established in man and virus sensitivity testing has not been standardized. If no clinical response to foscarnet is observed, test viral isolates for sensitivity to foscarnet; naturally resistant mutants may emerge under selective pressure both in vitro and in vivo. The latent state of any of the human herpesviruses is not known to be sensitive to foscarnet and viral reactivation of CMV occurs after foscarnet therapy is terminated.

Pharmacokinetics: Foscarnet is 14% to 17% bound to plasma protein at plasma drug concentrations of 1 to 1000 mcM. Plasma foscarnet concentrations in two studies are summarized in the following table:

Foscarnet Plasma Concentrations			
Mean dose (Infusion time)	Day of sampling	Mean plasma concentration (mcM)	
		C_{max} (range)	C_{min} (range)
57 ± 6 mg/kg q 8 hr (1 hour)	1	573 (213 to 1305)[1]	78 (< 33 to 139)[3]
47 ± 12 mg/kg q 8 hr (1 hour)	14 or 15	579 (246 to 922)[2]	110 (< 33 to 148)[4]
55 ± 6 mg/kg q 8 hr (2 hours)	3	445 (306 to 720)[1]	88 (< 33 to 162)[3]
57 ± 7 mg/kg q 8 hr (2 hours)	14 or 15	517 (348 to 789)[2]	105 (43 to 205)[4]

[1] Observed 0.9 to 2.4 hr after start of infusion.
[2] Observed 0.8 to 2.6 hr after start of infusion.
[3] Observed 4 to 8.1 hr after start of infusion.
[4] Observed 6.3 to 8.7 hr after start of infusion.

Mean plasma clearances were 130 ± 44 and 178 ± 48 ml/min in two studies in which foscarnet was given by intermittent infusion and 152 ± 59 and 214 ± 25 ml/min/1.73 m² in two studies using continuous infusion. Approximately 80% to 90% of IV foscarnet is excreted unchanged in the urine of patients with normal renal function. Both tubular secretion and glomerular filtration account for urinary elimination of foscarnet. In one study, plasma clearance was less than creatinine clearance (Ccr), suggesting that foscarnet may also undergo tubular reabsorption. In three studies, decreases in plasma clearance of foscarnet were proportional to decreases in Ccr.

Two studies in patients with initially normal renal function who were treated with intermittent infusions showed average drug plasma half-lives of about 3 hours determined on days 1 or 3 of therapy. This may be an underestimate of the effective half-life due to the limited observation period. Plasma half-life increases with the severity of renal impairment. Half-lives of 2 to 8 hours occurred in patients having estimated or measured 24 hour Ccr of 44 to 90 ml/min. Careful monitoring of renal function and dose adjustment is imperative (see Warnings and Administration and Dosage).

Following continuous foscarnet infusion for 72 hours in six HIV-positive patients, plasma half-lives of 0.45 ± 0.32 and 3.3 ± 1.3 hours were determined. A terminal half-life of 18 ± 2.8 hours was estimated from foscarnet urinary excretion over 48 hours after stopping infusion. When foscarnet was given as a continuous infusion to 13 patients with HIV infection for 8 to 21 days, plasma half-lives of 1.4 ± 0.6 and 6.8 ± 5 hours were determined. A terminal half-life of 87.5 ± 41.8 hours was estimated from foscarnet urinary excretion over 6 days after the last infusion; however, renal function at the time of discontinuing the infusion was not known.

(Actions continued on following page)

FOSCARNET SODIUM (Phosphonoformic acid) (Cont.)

Actions (Cont.):

Pharmacokinetics (Cont.):

Measurements of urinary excretion are required to detect the longer terminal half-life assumed to represent release of foscarnet from bone. In animal studies (mice), 40% of an IV dose is deposited in bone in young animals and 7% in adults. Evidence indicates that foscarnet accumulates in human bone; however, the extent to which this occurs has not been determined. Mean volumes of distribution at steady state range from 0.3 to 0.6 L/kg.

Variable penetration into cerebrospinal fluid (CSF) has been observed. Intermittent infusion of 50 mg/kg every 8 hours for 28 days in 9 patients produced CSF levels of 150 to 260 mcM 3 hours after the end of infusion or 39% to 103% of the plasma levels. In another 4 patients, CSF concentrations were 35% to 69% of the plasma drug level after a dose of 230 mg/kg/day by continuous infusion for 2 to 13 days. However, the CSF:plasma ratio was only 13% in one patient receiving a continuous infusion at a rate of 274 mg/kg/day. Disease-related defects in the blood-brain barrier may be responsible for the variations seen.

Clinical trials: In most clinical studies, treatment for CMV retinitis was begun with an induction dosage regimen of 60 mg/kg every 8 hours for the first 2 to 3 weeks, followed by a once-daily maintenance regimen at doses ranging from 60 to 120 mg/kg.

A prospective, randomized, masked, controlled clinical trial was conducted in 24 patients with acquired immunodeficiency syndrome (AIDS) and CMV retinitis. Patients received induction treatment of 60 mg/kg every 8 hours for 3 weeks, followed by maintenance treatment with 90 mg/kg/day until retinitis progression (appearance of a new lesion or advancement of the border of a posterior lesion > 750 microns in diameter). The 13 patients randomized to treatment with foscarnet had a significant delay in progression of CMV retinitis compared to untreated controls. Median times to retinitis progression from study entry were 93 days (range, 21 to > 364) and 22 days (range, 7 to 42), respectively.

In another prospective clinical trial of CMV retinitis in AIDS patients, 33 were treated with 2 to 3 weeks of foscarnet induction (60 mg/kg 3 times a day) and then randomized to two maintenance dose groups, 90 and 120 mg/kg/day. Median times from study entry to retinitis progression were 96 days (range, 14 to > 176) and 140 days (range, 16 to > 233), respectively. This difference was not statistically significant.

Indications:

Treatment of CMV retinitis in patients with AIDS.

Contraindications:

Hypersensitivity to foscarnet.

Warnings:

Renal function impairment: The major toxicity of foscarnet is renal impairment, which occurs to some degree in most patients. Approximately 33% of 189 patients with AIDS and CMV retinitis who received IV foscarnet in clinical studies developed significant impairment of renal function, manifested by a rise in serum creatinine concentration to ≥ 2 mg/dl. Therefore, use foscarnet with caution in all patients, especially those with a history of renal function impairment. Patients vary in their sensitivity to foscarnet-induced nephrotoxicity, and initial renal function may not be predictive of the potential for drug-induced renal impairment.

Renal impairment is most likely to become clinically evident as assessed by increasing serum creatinine during the second week of induction therapy at 60 mg/kg 3 times a day. Renal impairment, however, may occur at any time in any patient during treatment; therefore, monitor renal function carefully (see Monitoring).

Elevations in serum creatinine are usually, but not uniformly, reversible following discontinuation or dose adjustment. Recovery of renal function after foscarnet-induced impairment usually occurs within 1 week of drug discontinuation. However, of 35 patients who experienced grade II renal impairment (serum creatinine 2 to 3 times the upper limit of normal), two died with renal failure within 4 weeks of stopping foscarnet and three others died with renal insufficiency still present < 4 weeks after drug cessation.

Because of foscarnet's potential to cause renal impairment, dose adjustment for decreased baseline renal function and any change in renal function during treatment is necessary. In addition, it may be beneficial for adequate hydration to be established (eg, by inducing diuresis) prior to and during administration.

(Warnings continued on following page)

FOSCARNET SODIUM (Phosphonoformic acid) (Cont.)

Warnings (Cont.):

Mineral and electrolyte imbalances: Foscarnet has been associated with changes in serum electrolytes including hypocalcemia (15%), hypophosphatemia (8%) and hyperphosphatemia (6%), hypomagnesemia (15%) and hypokalemia (16%). Foscarnet is associated with a transient, dose-related decrease in ionized serum calcium, which may not be reflected in total serum calcium. This effect most likely is related to foscarnet's chelation of divalent metal ions such as calcium. Therefore, advise patients to report symptoms of low ionized calcium such as perioral tingling, numbness in the extremities and paresthesias. Be prepared to treat these as well as severe manifestations of electrolyte abnormalities, such as tetany and seizures. The rate of infusion may affect the transient decrease in ionized calcium; slowing the rate may decrease or prevent symptoms.

Transient changes in calcium or other electrolytes (including magnesium, potassium or phosphate) may also contribute to a patient's risk for cardiac disturbances and seizures (see Neurotoxicity and Seizures). Therefore, particular caution is advised in patients with altered calcium or other electrolyte levels before treatment, especially those with neurologic or cardiac abnormalities and those receiving other drugs known to influence minerals and electrolytes (see Monitoring and Drug Interactions).

Neurotoxicity and seizures: Foscarnet was associated with seizures in 18/189 (10%) of AIDS patients in five controlled studies. These patients were not taking foscarnet at the time of seizure. In most cases (15/18), the patients had an active CNS condition (eg, toxoplasmosis, HIV encephalopathy) or a history of CNS diseases. The rate of seizures did not increase with duration of treatment. Three cases were associated with overdoses of foscarnet (see Overdosage).

Statistically significant risk factors associated with seizures were low baseline absolute neutrophil count (ANC), impaired baseline renal function and low total serum calcium. Several cases of seizures were associated with death. However, occurrence of seizures did not always necessitate discontinuation of foscarnet. Ten of fifteen patients with seizures that occurred while receiving the drug continued or resumed foscarnet following treatment of their underlying disease, electrolyte disturbances or dose decreases. If factors predisposing a patient to seizures are present, carefully monitor electrolytes, including calcium and magnesium (see Monitoring).

Other CMV infections: Safety and efficacy have not been established for the treatment of other CMV infections (eg, pneumonitis, gastroenteritis); congenital or neonatal CMV disease; non-immunocompromised individuals.

Mutagenesis: Foscarnet showed genotoxic effects in an in vitro transformation assay at concentrations $>$0.5 mcg/ml and an increased frequency of chromosome aberrations in the sister chromatid exchange assay at 1000 mcg/ml. A high dose of foscarnet (3650 mg/kg) caused an increase in micronucleated polychromatic erythrocytes in mice at doses that produced exposures comparable to that anticipated clinically.

Elderly: Since these individuals frequently have reduced glomerular filtration, pay particular attention to assessing renal function before and during administration (see Administration and Dosage).

Pregnancy: Category C. Daily SC doses up to 75 mg/kg (one-eighth the maximal daily human exposure) administered to female rats prior to and during mating, during gestation and 21 days postpartum caused a slight increase ($<$ 5%) in the number of skeletal anomalies compared with the control group. Daily SC doses up to 75 mg/kg (one-third the maximal daily human exposure) administered to rabbits and 150 mg/kg administered to rats during gestation caused an increase in the frequency of skeletal anomalies/variations. These studies are inadequate to define the potential teratogenicity at levels to which women will be exposed. There are no adequate and well controlled studies in pregnant women. Use during pregnancy only if clearly needed.

Lactation: It is not known whether foscarnet is excreted in breast milk; however, in lactating rats administered 75 mg/kg, foscarnet was excreted in maternal milk at concentrations three times higher than peak maternal blood concentrations. Exercise caution if foscarnet is administered to a nursing woman.

Children: The safety and efficacy of foscarnet in children have not been studied. Foscarnet is deposited in teeth and bone, and deposition is greater in young and growing animals. Foscarnet adversely affects development of tooth enamel in mice and rats. The effects of this deposition on skeletal development have not been studied. Since deposition in human bone also occurs, it is likely that it does so to a greater degree in developing bone in children. Administer to children only after careful evaluation and only if the potential benefits for treatment outweigh the risks.

(Continued on following page)

FOSCARNET SODIUM (Phosphonoformic acid) (Cont.)

Precautions:

Diagnosis of CMV retinitis should be made by indirect ophthalmoscopy. Other conditions in the differential diagnosis of CMV retinitis include candidiasis, toxoplasmosis and other diseases producing a similar retinal pattern, any of which may produce a retinal appearance similar to CMV. For this reason it is essential that the diagnosis of CMV retinitis be established by an ophthalmologist familiar with the retinal presentation of these conditions. The diagnosis of CMV retinitis may be supported by culture of CMV from urine, blood, throat or other sites, but a negative CMV culture does not rule out CMV retinitis.

Toxicity/local irritation: In controlled clinical studies, the maximum single-dose administered was 120 mg/kg by IV infusion over 2 hours. It is likely that larger doses, or more rapid infusions, would result in increased toxicity. Take care to infuse solutions containing foscarnet only into veins with adequate blood flow to permit rapid dilution and distribution, and avoid local irritation (see Administration and Dosage). Local irritation and ulcerations of penile epithelium have occurred in male patients receiving foscarnet, possibly related to the presence of drug in urine. One case of vulvovaginal ulceration in a female has occurred. Adequate hydration with close attention to personal hygiene may minimize the occurrence of such events.

Anemia occurred in 33% of patients. This anemia was usually manageable with transfusions and required discontinuation of foscarnet in < 1% (1/189) of patients in the studies. Granulocytopenia occurred in 17% of patients; however, only 1% (2/189) were terminated from these studies because of neutropenia.

Monitoring: The majority of patients will experience some decrease in renal function due to foscarnet administration. Therefore it is recommended that Ccr, either measured or estimated using the modified Cockcroft and Gault equation based on serum creatinine, be determined at baseline, 2 to 3 times per week during induction therapy and at least once every 1 to 2 weeks during maintenance therapy, with foscarnet dose adjusted accordingly (see Dose Adjustment). More frequent monitoring may be required for some patients. It is also recommended that a 24 hour Ccr be determined at baseline and periodically thereafter to ensure correct dosing. Discontinue foscarnet if Ccr drops to < 0.4 ml/min/kg.

Due to foscarnet's propensity to chelate divalent metal ions and alter levels of serum electrolytes, closely monitor patients for such changes. It is recommended that a schedule similar to that recommended for serum creatinine (see above) be used to monitor serum calcium, magnesium, potassium and phosphorus. Particular caution is advised in patients with decreased total serum calcium or other electrolyte levels before treatment, as well as in patients with neurologic or cardiac abnormalities, and in patients receiving other drugs known to influence serum calcium levels. Correct any clinically significant metabolic changes. Also, patients who experience mild (eg, perioral numbness or paresthesias) or severe symptoms (eg, seizures) of electrolyte abnormalities should have serum electrolyte and mineral levels assessed as close in time to the event as possible.

Careful monitoring and appropriate management of electrolytes, calcium, magnesium and creatinine are of particular importance in patients with conditions that may predispose them to seizures (see Warnings).

Drug Interactions:

Nephrotoxic drugs: The elimination of foscarnet may be impaired by drugs that inhibit renal tubular secretion. Because of foscarnet's tendency to cause renal impairment, avoid the use of foscarnet in combination with potentially nephrotoxic drugs such as aminoglycosides, amphotericin B and IV pentamidine unless the potential benefits outweigh the risks to the patient.

Pentamidine: Concomitant treatment of four patients with foscarnet and IV pentamidine may have caused hypocalcemia; one patient died with severe hypocalcemia. Toxicity associated with concomitant use of aerosolized pentamidine has not been reported.

Zidovudine: Foscarnet was used concomitantly with zidovudine in approximately one-third of patients in the US studies. Although the combination was generally well tolerated, additive effects on anemia may have occurred. However, no evidence of increased myelosuppression was seen.

Foscarnet decreases serum levels of ionized calcium. Exercise particular caution when other drugs known to influence serum calcium levels are used concurrently.

(Continued on following page)

FOSCARNET SODIUM (Phosphonoformic acid) (Cont.)

Adverse Reactions:

The most frequently reported events were: Fever (65%); nausea (47%); anemia (33%); diarrhea (30%); abnormal renal function including acute renal failure, decreased Ccr and increased serum creatinine (27%); vomiting, headache (26%); seizure (10%) (see Warnings and Precautions).

Adverse events categorized as "severe" were: Death (14%); abnormal renal function (14%); marrow suppression (10%); anemia (9%); seizures (7%). Although death was specifically attributed to foscarnet in only one case, other complications of foscarnet (ie, renal impairment, electrolyte abnormalities, seizures) may have contributed to patient deaths (see Warnings and Precautions).

Body as a whole: Fever, fatigue, rigors, asthenia, malaise, pain, infection, sepsis, death (≥ 5%); back/chest pain, edema, influenza-like symptoms, bacterial/fungal infections, moniliasis, abscess (1% to 5%); hypothermia, leg edema, peripheral edema, syncope, ascites, substernal chest pain, abnormal crying, malignant hyperpyrexia, herpes simplex, viral infection, toxoplasmosis (< 1%).

Central and peripheral nervous system: Headache, paresthesia, dizziness, involuntary muscle contractions, hypoesthesia, neuropathy, seizures (including grand mal; see Warnings) (≥ 5%); tremor, ataxia, dementia, stupor, generalized spasms, sensory disturbances, meningitis, aphasia, abnormal coordination, leg cramps, EEG abnormalities (see Warnings) (1% to 5%); vertigo, coma, encephalopathy, abnormal gait, hyperesthesia, hypertonia, visual field defects, dyskinesia, extrapyramidal disorders, hemiparesis, hyperkinesia, vocal cord paralysis, paralysis, paraplegia, speech disorders, tetany, hyporeflexia, hyperreflexia, neuralgia, neuritis, peripheral neuropathy, cerebral edema, nystagmus (< 1%).

GI: Anorexia, nausea, diarrhea, vomiting, abdominal pain (≥ 5%); constipation, dysphagia, dyspepsia, rectal hemorrhage, dry mouth, melena, flatulence, ulcerative stomatitis, pancreatitis (1% to 5%); enteritis, enterocolitis, glossitis, proctitis, stomatitis, tenesmus, increased amylase, pseudomembranous colitis, gastroenteritis, oral leukoplakia, oral hemorrhage, rectal disorders, colitis, duodenal ulcer, hematemesis, paralytic ileus, esophageal ulceration, ulcerative proctitis, tongue ulceration (< 1%).

Hematologic: Anemia, granulocytopenia, leukopenia (see Precautions) (≥ 5%); thrombocytopenia, platelet abnormalities, thrombosis, WBC abnormalities, lymphadenopathy (1% to 5%); pulmonary embolism, coagulation disorders, decreased coagulation factors, epistaxis, decreased prothrombin, hypochromic anemia, pancytopenia, hemolysis, leukocytosis, cervical lymphadenopathy, lymphopenia (< 1%).

Metabolic/Nutritional: Mineral/electrolyte imbalances (see Warnings), including hypokalemia, hypocalcemia, hypomagnesemia, hypo- or hyperphosphatemia (≥ 5%); hyponatremia, decreased weight, increased alkaline phosphatase, LDH and BUN, acidosis, cachexia, thirst, hypercalcemia (1% to 5%); dehydration, glycosuria, increased creatine phosphokinase, diabetes mellitus, abnormal glucose tolerance, hypervolemia, hypochloremia, periorbital edema, hypoproteinemia (< 1%).

Psychiatric: Depression, confusion, anxiety (≥ 5%); insomnia, somnolence, nervousness, amnesia, agitation, aggressive reaction, hallucination (1% to 5%); impaired concentration, emotional lability, psychosis, suicide attempt, delirium, personality disorders, sleep disorders (< 1%).

Respiratory: Coughing, dyspnea (≥ 5%); pneumonia, sinusitis, pharyngitis, rhinitis, respiratory disorders or insufficiency, pulmonary infiltration, stridor, pneumothorax, hemoptysis, bronchospasm (1% to 5%); bronchitis, laryngitis, respiratory depression, abnormal chest x-ray, pleural effusion, pulmonary hemorrhage, pneumonitis (< 1%).

Dermatologic: Rash, increased sweating (≥ 5%); pruritus, skin ulceration, seborrhea, erythematous rash, maculopapular rash, skin discoloration, facial edema (1% to 5%); acne, alopecia, dermatitis, anal pruritus, genital pruritus, aggravated psoriasis, psoriaform rash, skin disorders, dry skin, urticaria, verruca (< 1%).

(Adverse Reactions continued on following page)

FOSCARNET SODIUM (Phosphonoformic acid) (Cont.)

Adverse Reactions (Cont.):

Urinary: Alterations in renal function, including serum creatinine, decreased Ccr and abnormal renal function (see Warnings) (≥ 5%); albuminuria, dysuria, polyuria, urethral disorder, urinary retention, urinary tract infections, acute renal failure, nocturia (1% to 5%); hematuria, glomerulonephritis, micturition disorders/frequency, toxic nephropathy, nephrosis, urinary incontinence, renal tubular disorders, pyelonephritis, urethral irritation, uremia (< 1%).

Special senses: Vision abnormalities (≥ 5%); taste perversions, eye abnormalities, eye pain, conjunctivitis (1% to 5%); diplopia, blindness, retinal detachment, mydriasis, photophobia, deafness, earache, tinnitus, otitis (< 1%).

Cardiovascular: Hypertension, palpitations, ECG abnormalities including sinus tachycardia, first degree AV block and non-specific ST-T segment changes, hypotension, flushing, cerebrovascular disorder (see Warnings) (1% to 5%); cardiomyopathy, cardiac failure/arrest, bradycardia, extrasystole, arrhythmias, atrial arrhythmias/fibrillation, phlebitis, superficial thrombophlebitis of arm, mesenteric vein thrombophlebitis (< 1%).

Application site: Injection site pain or inflammation (1% to 5%).

Hepatic/biliary: Abnormal A-G ratio, abnormal hepatic function, increased AST and ALT (1% to 5%); cholecystitis, cholelithiasis, hepatitis, cholestatic hepatitis, hepatosplenomegaly, jaundice (< 1%).

Musculoskeletal: Arthralgia, myalgia (1% to 5%); arthrosis, synovitis, torticollis (< 1%).

Neoplasms: Lymphoma-like disorder, sarcoma (1% to 5%); malignant lymphoma, skin hypertrophy (< 1%).

Endocrine: Antidiuretic hormone disorders, decreased gonadotropins, gynecomastia (< 1%).

Reproductive: Perineal pain in women, penile inflammation (< 1%).

Overdosage:

Symptoms: In controlled clinical trials, overdosage was reported in 10 patients. All 10 patients experienced adverse events and all except one made a complete recovery. One patient died after receiving a total daily dose of 12.5 g for 3 days instead of the intended 10.9 g. The patient suffered a grand mal seizure and became comatose. Three days later the patient died with the cause of death listed as respiratory/cardiac arrest. The other nine patients received doses ranging from 1.14 times to 8 times their recommended doses with an average of 4 times their recommended doses. Overall, three patients had seizures, three patients had renal function impairment, four patients had paresthesias either in limbs or periorally, and five patients had documented electrolyte disturbances primarily involving calcium and phosphate.

Treatment: There is no specific antidote. Hemodialysis and hydration may be of benefit in reducing drug plasma levels in patients who receive an overdosage, but these have not been evaluated in a clinical trial setting. Observe the patient for signs and symptoms of renal impairment and electrolyte imbalance. Institute medical treatment if clinically warranted. Refer to General Management of Acute Overdosage.

Patient Information:

Foscarnet is not a cure for CMV retinitis; patients may continue to experience progression of retinitis during or following treatment.

Regular ophthalmologic examinations are necessary. The major toxicities of foscarnet are renal impairment, electrolyte disturbances and seizures; dose modifications and possibly discontinuation may be required.

Close monitoring while on therapy is essential. Advise patients of the importance of perioral tingling, numbness in the extremities or paresthesias during or after infusion as possible symptoms of electrolyte abnormalities. Should such symptoms occur, stop the infusion, obtain appropriate laboratory samples for assessment of electrolyte concentrations and consult physician before resuming treatment. The rate of infusion must be no more than 1 mg/kg/min.

The potential for renal impairment may be minimized by accompanying administration with hydration adequate to establish and maintain diuresis during dosing.

(Continued on following page)

FOSCARNET SODIUM (Phosphonoformic acid) (Cont.)

Administration and Dosage:

Caution: Do not administer by rapid or bolus IV injection. Toxicity may be increased as a result of excessive plasma levels. Take care to avoid unintentional overdose by carefully controlling the rate of infusion. Therefore, an infusion pump must be used. In spite of the use of an infusion pump, overdoses have occurred.

Administer by controlled IV infusion, either by using a central venous line or by using a peripheral vein. The standard 24 mg/ml solution may be used without dilution when using a central venous catheter for infusion. When a peripheral vein catheter is used, dilute the 24 mg/ml solution to 12 mg/ml with 5% Dextrose in Water or with a normal saline solution prior to administration to avoid local irritation of peripheral veins. Since the dose is calculated on the basis of body weight, it may be desirable to remove and discard any unneeded quantity from the bottle before starting with the infusion to avoid overdosage. Use solutions thus prepared within 24 hours of first entry into a sealed bottle.

Do not exceed the recommended dosage, frequency or infusion rates. All doses must be individualized for patients' renal function.

Induction treatment: The recommended initial dose for patients with normal renal function is 60 mg/kg, adjusted for individual patients' renal function, given IV at a constant rate over a minimum of 1 hour every 8 hours for 2 to 3 weeks depending on clinical response. An infusion pump must be used to control the rate of infusion. Adequate hydration is recommended to establish diuresis, both prior to and during treatment to minimize renal toxicity (see Warnings), provided there are no clinical contraindications.

Maintenance treatment: 90 to 120 mg/kg/day (individualized for renal function) given as an IV infusion over 2 hours. Because the superiority of the 120 mg/kg/day has not been established in controlled trials, and given the likely relationship of higher plasma foscarnet levels to toxicity, it is recommended that most patients be started on maintenance treatment with a dose of 90 mg/kg/day. Escalation to 120 mg/kg/day may be considered should early reinduction be required because of retinitis progression. Some patients who show excellent tolerance to foscarnet may benefit from initiation of maintenance treatment at 120 mg/kg/day earlier in their treatment. An infusion pump must be used to control the rate of infusion with all doses. Again, hydration to establish diuresis both prior to and during treatment is recommended to minimize renal toxicity.

Patients who experience progression of retinitis while receiving maintenance therapy may be retreated with the induction and maintenance regimens given above.

Renal function abnormalities: Use with caution in patients with abnormal renal function because reduced plasma clearance of foscarnet will result in elevated plasma levels. In addition, foscarnet has the potential to further impair renal function (see Warnings). Foscarnet has not been specifically studied in patients with Ccr < 50 ml/min or serum creatinine > 2.8 mg/dl. Carefully monitor renal function at baseline and during induction and maintenance therapy with appropriate dose adjustments. If Ccr falls below the limits of the dosing nomograms (0.4 ml/min/kg) during therapy, discontinue foscarnet and monitor the patient daily until resolution of renal impairment is ensured.

(Administration and Dosage continued on following page)

FOSCARNET SODIUM (Phosphonoformic acid) (Cont.)

Administration and Dosage (Cont.):

Dose adjustment in renal impairment: Individualize foscarnet dosing according to the patient's renal function status. Refer to the table below for recommended doses and adjust the dose as indicated.

To use this dosing guide, actual 24 hour Ccr (ml/min) must be divided by body weight (kg) or the estimated Ccr in ml/min/kg can be calculated from serum creatinine (mg/dl) using the following formula (modified Cockcroft and Gault equation).

$$\text{Males: } \frac{140 - \text{age}}{\text{serum creatinine} \times 72} = \text{Ccr}$$

Females: 0.85 x above value

Foscarnet Dosing Guide Based on Ccr

Induction

Ccr (ml/min/kg)	Equivalent to 60 mg/kg dose every 8 hours
≥ 1.6	60
1.5	57
1.4	53
1.3	49
1.2	46
1.1	42
1	39
0.9	35
0.8	32
0.7	28
0.6	25
0.5	21
0.4	18

Maintenance

Ccr (ml/min/kg)	Equivalent to 90 mg/kg dose every 24 hours	Equivalent to 120 mg/kg dose every 24 hours
≥ 1.4	90	120
1.2-1.4	78	104
1-1.2	75	100
0.8-1	71	94
0.6-0.8	63	84
0.4-0.6	57	76

IV incompatibility: Other drugs and supplements can be administered to a patient receiving foscarnet. However, take care to ensure that foscarnet is only administered with normal saline or 5% Dextrose Solution and that no other drug or supplement is administered concurrently via the same catheter. Foscarnet is chemically incompatible with 30% dextrose, amphotericin B, and solutions containing calcium such as Ringer's Lactate and TPN. Physical incompatibility with other IV drugs includes: Acyclovir sodium, ganciclovir, trimetrexate, pentamidine, vancomycin, trimethoprim/sulfamethoxazole, diazepam, midazolam, digoxin, phenytoin, leucovorin and prochlorperazine. Because of foscarnet's chelating properties, a precipitate can potentially occur when divalent cations are administered concurrently in the same catheter.

Rx	**Foscavir** (Astra)	**Injection:** 24 mg/ml	In 250 and 500 ml bottles.

DIDANOSINE (ddI; dideoxyinosine)

Warning:

Didanosine is indicated for the treatment of adult and pediatric patients (> 6 months of age) with advanced HIV infection who are intolerant of zidovudine therapy or who have demonstrated significant clinical or immunologic deterioration during zidovudine therapy. This indication is based primarily on the results of non-randomized, phase I studies in which an increase in CD4 cell counts was observed for many patients during therapy. There are no results from controlled studies regarding the effect of didanosine therapy on the clinical progression of HIV infection, such as incidence of opportunistic infections and survival. Because zidovudine prolongs survival and decreases the incidence of opportunistic infections in patients with advanced HIV disease, consider zidovudine as initial therapy, unless contraindicated.

The major clinical toxicities of didanosine are pancreatitis and peripheral neuropathy.

Pancreatitis, which can be fatal, occurred in 9% of the phase I patients treated with didanosine at or below the recommended dose. Pancreatitis must be considered whenever a patient receiving didanosine develops abdominal pain, nausea, vomiting or elevated biochemical markers. Suspend use of didanosine until the diagnosis of pancreatitis is excluded (see Warnings).

Peripheral neuropathy occurred in 34% of phase I patients treated with didanosine at or below the recommended dose (see Warnings).

Patients receiving didanosine or any antiretroviral therapy may continue to develop opportunistic infections and other complications of HIV infection, and should remain under close clinical observation by physicians experienced in the treatment of patients with HIV-associated diseases.

Actions:

Didanosine was approved by the FDA in October 1991.

Pharmacology: Didanosine is a synthetic purine nucleoside analog of deoxyadenosine, active against the human immunodeficiency virus (HIV). The chemical name for didanosine is 2′,3′-dideoxyinosine; it is also called ddI. It inhibits in vitro replication of HIV (also known as HTLV III or LAV) in human primary cell cultures and in established cell lines. After didanosine enters the cell, it is converted by cellular enzymes to the active antiviral metabolite, dideoxyadenosine triphosphate (ddATP). The intracellular half-life of ddATP varies from 8 to 24 hours.

A common feature of dideoxynucleosides (the class of compounds to which didanosine belongs) is the lack of a free 3′-hydroxyl group. In nucleic acid replication, the 3′-hydroxyl of a naturally occurring nucleoside is the acceptor for covalent attachment of subsequent nucleoside 5′-monophosphates; its presence is therefore requisite for continued DNA chain extension. Because ddATP lacks a 3′-hydroxyl group, incorporation of ddATP into viral DNA leads to chain termination and, thus, inhibition of viral replication. In addition, ddATP further contributes to inhibition of viral replication through interference with the HIV-RNA dependent DNA polymerase (reverse transcriptase) by competing with the natural nucleoside triphosphate, dATP, for binding to the active site of the enzyme.

Microbiology: The relationship between in vitro susceptibility of HIV to didanosine and the inhibition of HIV replication in man or clinical response to therapy is not established.

Didanosine has in vitro antiviral activity in a variety of HIV-infected T cell and monocyte/macrophage cell cultures. The concentration of drug necessary to inhibit viral replication 50% ranges from 2.5 to 10 mcM (1 mcM = 0.2 mcg/ml) in T cells and from 0.01 to 0.1 mcM in monocyte/macrophage cell cultures.

The development of clinically significant didanosine resistance in patients with HIV infection receiving didanosine therapy has not been studied adequately and the frequency of didanosine-resistant isolates in the general population remains unknown.

Didanosine inhibits human hepatitis B virus replication in vitro; the clinical significance is unknown.

Pharmacokinetics: Didanosine is rapidly degraded at acidic pH. Therefore, all oral formulations contain buffering agents designed to increase gastric pH. When the tablets are administered, each adult and pediatric dose must consist of 2 tablets to achieve adequate acid-neutralizing capacity for maximal absorption. For pediatric patients < 1 year of age, only 1 tablet is necessary.

(Actions continued on following page)

DIDANOSINE (ddI; dideoxyinosine) (Cont.)

Actions (Cont.):

Pharmacokinetics (Cont.):

Bioequivalence of dosage formulations – A study of 18 asymptomatic, HIV seropositive patients comparing a 375 mg dose of powder for oral solution and buffered tablets indicated that didanosine is 20% to 25% more bioavailable from the tablet than the solution. A 375 mg dose of the buffered powder for oral solution produced similar plasma concentrations to a 300 mg (2 x 150 mg tablets) dose of the tablets. Mean peak plasma concentrations (C_{max}) were 1.6 ± 0.6 mcg/ml (range, 0.6 to 2.9) for the buffered solution and 1.6 ± 0.5 mcg/ml (range, 0.5 to 2.6) for the tablet. Mean area under the plasma concentration vs time curve (AUC) values were 3 ± 0.8 mcg • hr/ml (range, 1.6 to 5.1) for the buffered solution and 2.6 ± 0.7 mcg • hr/ml (range, 1.1 to 3.9) for the chewable tablet.

Effect of food on oral absorption – Administer all didanosine formulations on an empty stomach. The administration of didanosine tablets within 5 minutes of a meal results in a 50% decrease in mean C_{max} and AUC values.

Adults – The pharmacokinetics of didanosine were evaluated in 69 adult patients with AIDS or severe AIDS-Related Complex (ARC) after single and multiple IV and oral doses. Patients received a 60 minute IV infusion once or twice a day for 2 weeks, at total daily doses ranging from 0.8 to 33 mg/kg. Oral doses equivalent to twice the IV dose were administered for an additional 4 weeks. Plasma concentrations were obtained on the first day of dosing and at steady state after IV and oral dosing.

Absorption: Although there was significant variability between patients, the C_{max} and AUC values increased in proportion to dose over the range of doses administered. At doses of ≤ 7 mg/kg, the average absolute bioavailability was 33% ± 14% after a single dose and 37% ± 14% after 4 weeks of dosing. Pharmacokinetic parameters at steady state were not significantly different from values obtained after the initial IV or oral dose.

Distribution: The steady-state volume of distribution after IV administration averaged 54 L (range, 22 to 103). In a study of five adults, the concentration in the CSF 1 hour after infusion averaged 21% of the simultaneous plasma concentration.

Elimination: After oral administration, average elimination half-life was 1.6 hours (range, 0.52 to 4.64). Total body clearance averaged 800 ml/min (range, 412 to 1505). Renal clearance represented ≈ 50% of total body clearance (average 400 ml/min; range, 95 to 860) when didanosine was given either IV or orally. This indicates that active tubular secretion, in addition to glomerular filtration, is responsible for the renal elimination. Urinary recovery after a single dose was ≈ 55% (range, 27% to 98%), and 20% (range, 3% to 31%) of the dose after IV and oral administration, respectively. There was no evidence of accumulation after either IV or oral dosing.

Children – The pharmacokinetics of didanosine have been evaluated in two pediatric studies. In one study, 16 children and 4 adolescents received a single IV dose ranging from 40 to 90 mg/m² and multiple, twice daily oral doses of 80 to 180 mg/m² of didanosine. In another study, 48 pediatric patients received a single IV dose and then multiple, 3 times daily oral doses ranging from 20 to 180 mg/m².

Absorption: Although there was significant variability between patients, the C_{max} and AUC values increased in proportion to dose in both studies. These findings were similar to those in adult patients. The absolute bioavailability varied between patients in one study and averaged 32% ± 12% (range, 13% to 53%) and 42% ± 18% (range, 21% to 78%), after the first oral dose and at steady state, respectively. The other study also demonstrated significant variability in the oral absorption of didanosine with an average absolute bioavailability of 19% ± 17% (range, 2% to 89%). In one study, the average steady-state AUC was 1.4 ± 0.4, 1.6 ± 0.9 and 2.3 ± 0.9 mcg • hr/ml after the administration of oral doses of 80, 120, and 180 mg/m², respectively. The average corresponding steady-state C_{max} values were 0.8 ± 0.4, 1.4 ± 0.7, and 1.7 ± 0.9 mcg/ml, respectively.

Distribution: In one study, the volume of distribution after IV administration averaged 35.6 L/m² (range, 18.4 to 60.7). In this study, the concentration of didanosine ranged from 0.04 to 0.12 mcg/ml in CSF samples collected from seven patients at times ranging from 1.5 to 3.5 hr after a single IV or oral dose. These CSF concentrations corresponded to 12% to 85% (mean, 46%) of the concentration in a simultaneous plasma sample.

(Actions continued on following page)

DIDANOSINE (ddI; dideoxyinosine) (Cont.)

Actions (Cont.):

Pharmacokinetics (Cont.):

Children (Cont.):

Elimination: In one study, the elimination half-life following oral administration averaged 0.8 hours (range, 0.51 to 1.2). Total body clearance following IV administration averaged 532 ml/min/m² (range, 294 to 920). Mean renal clearance ranged from 190 to 319 ml/min/m² after the first oral dose and from 231 to 265 ml/min/m² at steady state. Urinary recovery averaged 17% (range, 5.4% to 30.4%) at steady state. There was no evidence of accumulation of didanosine after the administration of oral doses for an average of 26 days.

Metabolism: The metabolism of didanosine has not been evaluated in humans. When didanosine was administered to dogs as a single IV or oral dose, extensive metabolism occurred. The major metabolite identified in the urine, allantoin, represented ≈ 61% after oral administration. Three putative metabolites tentatively identified in the urine were hypoxanthine, xanthine and uric acid. Based on data from animal studies, it is presumed that the metabolism of didanosine in humans will occur by the same pathways responsible for elimination of endogenous purines.

The intracellular half-life of ddATP, the metabolite presumed to be responsible for the antiretroviral activity of didanosine, is 8 to 24 hours in vitro.

In vitro human plasma protein binding is $< 5\%$.

Clinical trials:

Adults – Median CD4 count at entry was 62 cells/mcl. Dosages ranged from 0.8 to 66 mg/kg/day, and were given using several schedules and by two routes of administration (IV and oral) for a median duration of 38 weeks (range, 0 to 99). The median average daily dose was 10.3 mg/kg. Analyses included the following:

a) Presence of a "response," where response was defined as i) the greater of a 50-cell or 50% increase over baseline CD4 cell count maintained for a minimum of any consecutive 4 weeks during therapy (50:50); ii) the greater of a 10 cell or 10% increase over baseline CD4 cell count maintained for a minimum of any consecutive 4 weeks during therapy (10:10).

b) Percent change from baseline in CD4 cell count at various time points on therapy.

c) Longitudinal changes during study weeks 0 to 12: Time weighted average of serial CD4 cell counts corrected for (normalized by) baseline CD4 cell count (NAUC). NAUCs that exceed a value of 1 indicate that the average CD4 level during therapy is increased over the baseline CD4 cell count.

d) Dose response analyses.

Results –

a) *Response:* i) 22% of patients receiving didanosine had a 50:50 response in CD4 counts vs 2% to 12% of the historical control patients; ii) 50% of patients receiving didanosine had a 10:10 response in CD4 counts vs 17% to 31% of the historical control patients.

b) *Percent change from baseline:* In patients receiving didanosine the increase from baseline CD4 cell counts was 29% at 4 weeks, 27% at 8 weeks and 14% at 12 weeks. In comparison, historical control groups had progressive declines in CD4 cell counts, ranging from 6% to 24% below baseline at week 8 and 5% to 27% at week 12.

c) *Longitudinal changes during study weeks 0 to 12:* 70% of patients receiving didanosine had NAUC values exceeding 1 vs 34% to 46% of the historical control patients. The mean NAUC in patients receiving didanosine was 1.38 vs 0.99 to 1.04 in historical control groups.

d) *Dose response:* Attempts to demonstrate a dose response among patients receiving didanosine were inconclusive.

Results from an ongoing study: An interim analysis of summary CD4 data was obtained from an ongoing, randomized, double-blind study comparing continued zidovudine therapy (comparison group) to didanosine therapy in patients previously treated with zidovudine. Preliminary results showed that the mean percent increase from baseline in CD4 cell counts after 12 weeks of didanosine therapy was 11% vs a decrease of 3.2% in the comparison group. Of patients taking didanosine, 55% had NAUCs exceeding 1 vs 39.7% of patients in the comparison group, while mean NAUCs were 1.14 and 0.97, respectively. The clinical significance of these differences is not known.

(Actions continued on following page)

DIDANOSINE (ddI; dideoxyinosine) (Cont.)

Actions (Cont.):

Clinical trials (Cont.):

Children: Patients received doses from 60 to 540 mg/m²/day. Based on an increased incidence of pancreatitis observed at the higher doses administered, all patients treated at doses > 360 mg/m²/day were dose reduced to this level or lower. Due to multiple dose adjustments, 77% of patients received average daily doses ≤ 300 mg/m²/day. Results were obtained from open-label studies without controls.

Activity of didanosine was based on the criteria previously described for the adult patients. Weight gain in children was also analyzed as either a 10% increase in weight (for smaller children) or a 2.5 kg increase (for children > 25 kg), also occurring at any time during therapy and maintained for at least 4 weeks.

The effect of didanosine on survival and the incidence of opportunistic infections in children could not be assessed in these studies, and data evaluating the impact of didanosine therapy on clinical parameters of HIV infection in children are not currently available. Therefore, consider zidovudine as initial therapy for the treatment of advanced HIV infection, unless contraindicated.

Thirty-seven percent of patients had a 10:10 response in CD4 counts, and 23% had a 50:50 response. The percent increase from baseline CD4 counts was 27% at 8 weeks. A weight response occurred in 39% of patients.

In general, hematologic parameters were stable during treatment with didanosine. In addition, improvement in platelet counts was seen in 3 of 6 patients with idiopathic thrombocytopenic purpura who entered the pediatric studies with this diagnosis. Some children exhibited improvements in detailed neuropsychometric tests. An increment in an individual's IQ score of 10% and a minimum of 8 points relative to baseline was considered a response. Improvement was seen in 12 of 43 evaluable patients with a baseline IQ < 115. In the absence of a control group, the contribution of drug to this increase is uncertain.

Indications:

For the treatment of adult and pediatric patients (> 6 months of age) with advanced HIV infection who are intolerant of zidovudine therapy or who have demonstrated significant clinical or immunologic deterioration during zidovudine therapy.

Because zidovudine prolongs survival and decreases the incidence of opportunistic infections in patients with advanced HIV disease, consider zidovudine as initial therapy for the treatment of advanced HIV infection, unless contraindicated.

Contraindications:

Hypersensitivity to any of the components of the formulations.

Warnings:

Peripheral neuropathy occurred in 34% of patients in phase I studies treated with didanosine doses at or below the currently recommended dose. Monitor patients for the development of a neuropathy that is usually characterized by distal numbness, tingling, or pain in the feet or hands.

The table below describes the incidence of neuropathy during therapy in the combined adult phase I studies.

Incidence of Neuropathy with Didanosine			
Parameter	All phase I (n = 170)	Phase I ≤ 12.5 mg/kg/day (n = 91)	Phase I > 12.5 mg/kg/day (n = 79)
Neuropathy	71 (42%)	31 (34%)	40 (51%)
Neuropathy requiring dose modification	38 (22%)	11 (12%)	27 (34%)

Among the 91 adult phase I patients who received an average oral daily dose similar to the recommended dose, 12% had neuropathy requiring dose modification. In the Expanded Access Program, where the median duration of exposure to didanosine was shorter than in the adult phase I studies, the incidence of neuropathy was 16%. Many patients tolerated a reduced dose of didanosine.

Neuropathy occurred more frequently in patients with a history of neuropathy or neurotoxic drug therapy. These patients may be at increased risk of neuropathy during didanosine therapy.

Neuropathy has been reported rarely in children treated with didanosine. However, because signs and symptoms of neuropathy are difficult to assess in children, physicians should be alerted to this possibility.

(Warnings continued on following page)

DIDANOSINE (ddI; dideoxyinosine) (Cont.)

Warnings (Cont.):

Pancreatitis occurred in 9% of patients in phase I studies treated with didanosine at or below the recommended dose. This condition can be fatal. Pancreatitis must be considered whenever a patient receiving didanosine develops abdominal pain, nausea, vomiting or elevated biochemical markers. Under these circumstances, suspend use of didanosine until the diagnosis of pancreatitis is excluded. When treatment with other drugs known to cause pancreatic toxicity is required (eg, IV pentamidine), consider suspension of didanosine. The incidence of pancreatitis and potential manifestations of pancreatitis in the adult phase I studies are described in the following table.

Incidence of Pancreatitis with Didanosine

Parameter	All phase I (n = 170)	Phase I ≤ 12.5 mg/kg/day (n = 91)	Phase I > 12.5 mg/kg/day (n = 79)
Pancreatitis	29 (17%)	8 (9%)	21 (27%)
Abdominal pain	14 (8%)	9 (10%)	5 (6%)
Increased amylase	26 (16%)	16 (18%)	12 (15%)
Abdominal pain and increased amylase	11 (6%)	6 (7%)	5 (6%)

In the Expanded Access Program for didanosine, where the median duration of exposure was shorter than in the phase I studies (5 months vs 8.5 months), lower incidences of pancreatitis (5%) and potential manifestations of pancreatitis (abdominal pain 5%, increased amylase 8%) were reported. For 27 patients treated with didanosine who had a history of pancreatitis, 8 (30%) developed pancreatitis. Fatal pancreatitis occurred in 27 of 7806 treated patients (0.35%).

Positive relationships have been found between risk of pancreatitis and steady-state plasma concentration of didanosine as well as with daily oral dose. Patients with renal impairment may be at greater risk for pancreatitis if treated without dose adjustment. Follow patients with a history of pancreatitis more closely, as well as those with other risk factors such as diagnosis of AIDS, CD4 cell counts < 100 cells/mcl, and risk factors for pancreatitis in general, such as alcohol consumption and elevated triglycerides.

In pediatric studies, pancreatitis occurred in 2 of 60 (3%) patients treated at entry doses < 300 mg/m²/day and in 5 of 38 (13%) of patients treated at higher doses. In pediatric patients with symptoms similar to those described above, suspend didanosine until the diagnosis of pancreatitis is excluded.

Liver failure of unknown etiology has occurred in < 0.2% of patients.

Retinal depigmentation: Four pediatric patients demonstrated retinal depigmentation at doses > 300 mg/m²/day. Two of the patients, treated at doses of 540 mg/m²/day, had progression of disease when treated with lower doses. One patient treated at lower doses has continued therapy without progression of disease. Children receiving didanosine should undergo dilated retinal examination every 6 months or if a change in vision occurs.

Myopathy: Evidence of a dose-limiting skeletal muscle toxicity has been observed in mice and rats (but not in dogs) following long-term (> 90 days) dosing with didanosine at doses that were approximately 1.2 to 12 times the estimated human exposure. Human myopathy has been associated with administration of other nucleoside analogs.

Renal function impairment: Patients with renal impairment (serum creatinine > 1.5 mg/dl or creatinine clearance < 60 ml/min) may be at greater risk of toxicity from didanosine due to decreased drug clearance; consider a dose reduction. The magnesium hydroxide content of each tablet (15.7 mEq) may present an excessive magnesium load to patients with significant renal impairment, particularly after prolonged dosing.

Hepatic function impairment: Patients with hepatic impairment may be at greater risk for toxicity due to altered metabolism; a dose reduction may be necessary.

Mutagenesis: In an in vitro cytogenic study, high concentrations of didanosine (≥ 500 mcg/ml) elevated the frequency of cells bearing chromosome aberrations. Another in vitro study revealed that didanosine produces chromosome aberrations at ≥ 500 mcg/ml after 48 hours of exposure. Similar chromosomal aberration effects were induced by the natural nucleoside of didanosine (2′-deoxyinosine), suggesting that these effects of didanosine were not due to a direct genotoxic interaction.

At significantly elevated doses in vitro, the genotoxic effects of didanosine are similar in magnitude to those seen with natural DNA nucleosides.

(Warnings continued on following page)

DIDANOSINE (ddI; dideoxyinosine) (Cont.)

Warnings (Cont.):

Pregnancy: Category B. At approximately 12 times the estimated human exposure, didanosine was slightly toxic to female rats and their pups during mid and late lactation. These rats showed reduced food intake and body weight gains but the physical and functional development of the offspring was not impaired and there were no major changes in the F2 generation. There are no adequate and well controlled studies in pregnant women. Use during pregnancy only if clearly needed.

Lactation: It is not known whether didanosine is excreted in breast milk. Because of the potential for serious adverse reactions from didanosine in nursing infants, instruct mothers to discontinue nursing when taking didanosine.

Children: See Indications, Warnings and Administration and Dosage.

Precautions:

Opportunistic infections: Patients receiving didanosine or any other antiretroviral therapy may continue to develop opportunistic infections and other complications of HIV infection and, therefore, should remain under close clinical observation by physicians experienced in the treatment of patients with associated HIV diseases.

Progression of HIV infection: At present there are no results from controlled studies regarding the effect of didanosine therapy on the clinical progression of HIV infection, such as incidence of opportunistic infections and survival.

Phenylketonuria: Didanosine tablets contain 22.5 mg phenylalanine (33.7 mg in the 150 mg tablet).

Sodium-restricted diets: Each buffered tablet contains 264.5 mg sodium. Each single-dose packet of buffered powder for oral solution contains 1380 mg sodium.

Hyperuricemia: Didanosine has been associated with asymptomatic hyperuricemia; consider suspending treatment if clinical measures aimed at reducing uric acid levels fail.

Diarrhea: Didanosine buffered powder for oral solution was associated with diarrhea in 34% of patients in the phase I adult studies. No data are available to demonstrate whether other formulations are associated with lower rates of diarrhea. However, if diarrhea develops in a patient receiving buffered powder for oral solution, consider a trial of chewable/dispersible buffered tablets.

Drug Interactions:

Administer drugs whose absorption can be affected by the level of acidity in the stomach (eg, ketoconazole, dapsone) at least 2 hours prior to dosing with didanosine.

Coadministration of didanosine with drugs that are known to cause peripheral neuropathy or pancreatitis may increase the risk of these toxicities. Closely observe patients who receive these drugs.

Tetracyclines: As with other products containing magnesium or aluminum antacid components, do not simultaneously administer didanosine tablets or pediatric powder for oral solution with a prescription antibiotic containing any form of tetracycline.

Fluoroquinolones: Plasma concentrations of some quinolone antibiotics are decreased when administered with antacids containing magnesium or aluminum. Therefore, doses of quinolone antibiotics should not be administered within 2 hours of taking didanosine tablets or pediatric powder for oral solution. Coadministration of antacids containing magnesium or aluminum with didanosine buffered tablets or pediatric powder for oral solution may potentiate adverse effects associated with the antacid components.

Drug/Food interaction: Ingestion of didanosine with food reduces the absorption of didanosine by as much as 50%. Therefore, administer didanosine on an empty stomach.

(Continued on following page)

DIDANOSINE (ddI; dideoxyinosine) (Cont.)

Adverse Reactions:

The major toxicities of didanosine are pancreatitis and peripheral neuropathy (see Warnings).

Didanosine Adverse Reactions (Adults)			
Adverse Reaction	Phase I ≤ 12.5 mg/kg/day (n = 91)	Phase I all patients (n = 170)	US expanded access (n = 7806)
Headache	36%	32%	5%
Diarrhea	34%	29%	18%
Peripheral neuropathy	34%	42%	16%
Asthenia	25%	24%	3%
Insomnia	25%	22%	2%
Nausea/Vomiting	25%	25%	8%
Rash/Pruritus	24%	25%	4%
Abdominal pain	21%	22%	5%
CNS depression	19%	16%	< 1%
Constipation	16%	13%	< 1%
Stomatitis	14%	11%	< 1%
Myalgia	13%	13%	1%
Arthritis	11%	11%	1%
Taste loss/perversion	10%	8%	< 1%
Pain	10%	16%	4%
Dry mouth	9%	8%	1%
Pancreatitis	9%	17%	5%
Alopecia	8%	7%	< 1%
Dizziness	7%	8%	1%

Body as a whole: Pneumonia, infection (2%); anorexia, weight loss, sepsis (1%); ascites, facial edema, enlarged abdomen, flu syndrome (< 1%).

Cardiovascular: Hypertension (1%); syncope, congestive heart failure, pericardial effusion, vasodilation, cardiomyopathy, palpitation (< 1%).

CNS: Seizure/convulsions (3%); confusion (2%); anxiety, nervousness, hypertonia, abnormal thinking (1%); dementia, agitation, ataxia, amnesia, speech disorder, cerebrovascular disorder (< 1%).

GI: Dyspepsia, GI disorder, liver abnormalities, flatulence (1%); GI hemorrhage, dysphagia, oral moniliasis, colitis, esophagitis, sialadenitis (< 1%).

Metabolic/nutritional: CPK increase, edema, hyperlipidemia (1%).

Respiratory: Cough (1%); dyspnea, pharyngitis, apnea, sinusitus, bronchitis, pleural effusion, rhinitis, pneumothorax (< 1%).

Skin: Sweating, herpes, acne (< 1%).

Special senses: Eye disorder, amblyopia, deafness (< 1%).

Other: Myopathy (1%); kidney failure, polyuria (< 1%).

In pediatric studies, pancreatitis occurred in 2 of 60 (3%) patients treated at entry doses < 300 mg/m²/day and in 5 of 38 (13%) patients treated at higher doses.

(Adverse Reactions continued on following page)

DIDANOSINE (ddI; dideoxyinosine) (Cont.)

Actions (Cont.):

Didanosine Adverse Reactions (Children)					
Adverse reaction	< 300 mg/ m^2/day (n = 60)	All patients (n = 98)	Adverse reaction	< 300 mg/ m^2/day (n = 60)	All patients (n = 98)
Body as whole			*CNS*		
Chills/Fever	82%	82%	Headache	58%	55%
Anorexia	52%	51%	Nervousness	33%	27%
Asthenia	42%	41%	Insomnia	10%	8%
Pain	27%	31%	Dizziness	5%	7%
Malaise	38%	29%	Poor coordination	8%	6%
Failure to thrive	13%	9%	Lethargy	7%	4%
Weight loss	10%	8%	Neurologic	2%	< 1%
Flu syndrome	7%	7%	Seizure	1%	< 1%
Change in appetite	10%	6%	*Respiratory*		
Alopecia	7%	5%	Cough	87%	85%
Dehydration	7%	5%	Rhinitis	48%	48%
Increased appetite	5%	0%	Dyspnea	27%	23%
GI			Asthma	28%	21%
Diarrhea	82%	81%	Rhinorrhea	20%	21%
Nausea/Vomiting	57%	58%	Epistaxis	13%	14%
Liver abnormalities	32%	38%	Pharyngitis	17%	14%
Abdominal pain	32%	35%	Hypoventilation	10%	8%
Stomatitis/Mouth sores	17%	16%	Sinusitis	8%	7%
			Rhonchi/Rales	8%	6%
Pancreatitis	3%	13%	Congestion	5%	3%
Constipation	10%	12%	Pneumonia	1%	< 1%
Oral thrush	13%	9%	*Skin and appendages*		
Melena	7%	7%	Rash/Pruritus	72%	70%
Dry mouth	7%	4%	Skin disorder	12%	13%
Lympho-Hematologic			Eczema	13%	12%
Ecchymosis	15%	15%	Sweating	8%	7%
Hemorrhage	10%	10%	Impetigo	5%	6%
Petechiae	3%	7%	Excoriation	7%	4%
Musculoskeletal			Erythema	5%	4%
Arthritis	12%	11%	*Special senses*		
Myalgia	12%	9%	Ear pain/otitis	13%	11%
Muscle atrophy	12%	8%	Photophobia	8%	5%
Decreased strength	3%	6%	Strabismus	8%	5%
Cardiovascular			Visual impairment	5%	5%
Vasodilation	22%	22%	*Other*		
Arrhythmia	10%	6%	Urinary frequency	5%	4%
			Diabetes mellitus	1%	< 1%
			Diabetes insipidus	1%	< 1%

Laboratory Test Abnormalities with Didanosine				
	Children		Adults	
Laboratory test (seriously abnormal level)	Normal baseline	Abnormal baseline	Normal baseline	Abnormal baseline
Leukopenia (< 2000/mcl)	3%	36%	5%	37%
Granulocytopenia (< 1000/mcl)	24%	62%	3%	56%
Thrombocytopenia (< 50,000/mcl)	2%	67%	1%	25%
Anemia (Hb < 8 g/dl)	4%	27%	5%	0
ALT (> 5 x ULN)	3%	25%	10%	12%
AST (> 5 x ULN)	0	36%	10%	12%
Alkaline phosphatase (> 5 x ULN)	0	0	4%	17%
Bilirubin (> 5 x ULN)	2%	0	3%	0
Uric acid (> 1.25 x ULN)	0	0	6%	50%
Amylase (≥ 5 x ULN)	0	0	3%	0

ULN = Upper limit of normal.

(Continued on following page)

DIDANOSINE (ddI; dideoxyinosine) (Cont.)

Overdosage:

There is no known antidote for overdosage. Experience in the phase I studies in which didanosine was initially administered at doses 10 times the currently recommended dose indicates that the complications of chronic overdosage would include pancreatitis, peripheral neuropathy, diarrhea, hyperuricemia or, possibly, hepatic dysfunction. It is not known whether didanosine is dialyzable by peritoneal or hemodialysis.

Administration and Dosage:

Dosage: Use a 12 hour dosing interval. Administer all formulations on an empty stomach.

Adults: Take 2 tablets at each dose so that adequate buffering is provided to prevent gastric acid degradation of didanosine. The recommended starting dose in adults is dependent on weight as outlined in the table below:

Adult Didanosine Dosing		
Patient weight (kg)	Tablets	Buffered powder
≥ 75	300 mg bid	375 mg bid
50-74	200 mg bid	250 mg bid
35-49	125 mg bid	167 mg bid

Children: To prevent gastric acid degradation, children > 1 year of age should receive a 2 tablet dose; children < 1 year should receive a 1 tablet dose. The recommended dose in children is dependent on body surface area as outlined in the table below. Doses equivalent to 100 to 300 mg/m²/day of the pediatric powder are being further evaluated in controlled clinical trials.

Pediatric Didanosine Dosing (based on 200 mg/m²/day average recommended dose)[1]			
		Pediatric powder (m²)	
Body surface area (m²)	Tablets	Dose	Vol/10 mg/ml admixture
1.1-1.4	100 mg bid	125 mg bid	12.5 ml bid
0.8-1	75 mg bid	94 mg bid	9.5 ml bid
0.5-0.7	50 mg bid	62 mg bid	6 ml bid
< 0.4	25 mg bid	31 mg bid	3 ml bid

[1] Based on didanosine pediatric powder.

Dose adjustment: If clinical signs suggest pancreatitis, suspend dose and carefully evaluate the possibility of pancreatitis. Resume dosing only after pancreatitis has been ruled out.

Many patients who have presented with symptoms of neuropathy will tolerate a reduced dose after resolution of these symptoms following drug discontinuation.

There are insufficient data to recommend dose adjustment in patients with impaired renal or hepatic function. Consider a dose reduction in patients with renal insufficiency or hepatic impairment.

(Administration and Dosage continued on following page)

DIDANOSINE (ddI; dideoxyinosine) (Cont.)

Administration and Dosage (Cont.):

Method of preparation:

Adults – Chewable/dispersible buffered tablets: Thoroughly chew tablets or manually crush or disperse 2 tablets in at least 1 ounce of water prior to consumption. To disperse tablets, add 2 tablets to at least 1 ounce of water. Stir until a uniform dispersion forms, and drink entire dispersion immediately.

Buffered powder for oral solution:

1. Open packet carefully and pour contents into approximately 4 ounces of water. Do not mix with fruit juice or other acid-containing liquid.
2. Stir until the powder completely dissolves (approximately 2 to 3 minutes).
3. Drink the entire solution immediately.

Children – Chewable/dispersible buffered tablets: Chew tablets or manually crush or disperse 1 or 2 tablets in water prior to consumption, as described for adults.

Pediatric powder for oral solution: Prior to dispensing, the pharmacist must constitute dry powder with Purified Water, USP, to an initial concentration of 20 mg/ml and immediately mix the resulting solution with antacid to a final concentration of 10 mg/ml as follows:

20 mg/ml initial solution – Reconstitute the product to 20 mg/ml by adding 100 or 200 ml Purified Water, USP, to the 2 or 4 g of powder, respectively, in the product bottle. Prepare final admixture as described below.

10 mg/ml final admixture – 1. Immediately mix one part of the 20 mg/ml initial solution with one part of either *Mylanta Double Strength Liquid* or *Maalox TC Suspension* for a final dispensing concentration of 10 mg/ml. For patient home use, dispense the admixture in flint-glass bottles with child-resistant closures. This admixture is stable for 30 days under refrigeration at 2° to 8°C (36° to 46°F).

2. Instruct the patient to shake the admixture thoroughly prior to use and to store the tightly closed container in the refrigerator at 2° to 8°C (36° to 46°F), up to 30 days.

Spill, leak and disposal procedure: Avoid generating dust during clean-up of powdered products; use wet mop or damp sponge. Clean surface with soap and water as necessary. Containerize larger spills.

Rx	**Videx** (Bristol-Myers Squibb)	**Tablets, buffered, chewable/dispersible:**[1]	
		25 mg	(Videx BL 25). White. Mint flavor. In 60s.
		50 mg	(Videx BL 50). White. Mint flavor. In 60s.
		100 mg	(Videx BL 100). White. Mint flavor. In 60s.
		150 mg	(Videx BL 150). White. Mint flavor. In 60s.
		Powder for Oral Solution, buffered:[2]	
		100 mg	In single-dose packets.
		167 mg	In single-dose packets.
		250 mg	In single-dose packets.
		375 mg	In single-dose packets.
		Powder for Oral Solution, pediatric:	
		2 g	In bottles.
		4 g	In bottles.

[1] Buffered with dihydroaluminum sodium carbonate, magnesium hydroxide and sodium citrate. With aspartame and sugar.

[2] Buffered with dibasic sodium phosphate, sodium citrate and citric acid. With sucrose.

VIDARABINE (Adenine Arabinoside; Ara-A)

Actions:

Pharmacology: Vidarabine is a purine nucleoside obtained from fermentation cultures of *streptomyces antibioticus* that possesses in vitro and in vivo antiviral activity against Herpes simplex virus (HSV) types 1 and 2.

The antiviral mechanism of action has not yet been established. Within cells, it is phosphorylated to a triphosphate form that is a relatively selective competitive inhibitor of DNA polymerase. Vidarabine may also incorporate into the viral DNA molecule at different positions and produce chain termination. The main metabolite, arabinosyl hypoxanthine (Ara-Hx) has approximately 1/10 the activity of vidarabine.

Pharmacokinetics:

Distribution – Following IV administration, vidarabine is rapidly deaminated to Ara-Hx, which is promptly distributed into tissues. Peak Ara-Hx and Ara-A plasma levels ranging from 3 to 6 mcg/ml and 0.2 to 0.4 mcg/ml, respectively, are attained after doses of 10 mg/kg. These levels reflect the rate of infusion and show no accumulation over time. Ara-Hx penetrates into the cerebrospinal fluid (CSF) to give a CSF:plasma ratio of approximately 1:3 to 1:2.

Metabolism/Excretion – The mean half-life of Ara-A is 1 hour and of Ara-Hx is 3.3 hours. Excretion is principally via the kidneys; 41% to 53% of the daily dose is recovered in the urine as Ara-Hx, with 1% to 3% appearing as the parent compound. In patients with impaired renal function, Ara-Hx may accumulate.

Indications:

Herpes simplex virus encephalitis: Vidarabine reduces mortality caused by HSV encephalitis from 70% to 28%. It does not alter morbidity and resulting serious neurological sequelae in the comatose patient.

Neonatal herpes simplex virus infections including disseminated infection with visceral involvement, encephalitis, and infections of the skin, eyes and mouth. Vidarabine reduces mortality in encephalitis and disseminated infection from 74% to 38%.

Herpes zoster in immunosuppressed patients: Vidarabine significantly reduced the severity of acute pain, new vesicle formation, time to pustulation and scabbing, cutaneous dissemination inside and outside the primary dermatome(s) and the overall frequency of visceral complications (uveitis or keratitis, hepatitis, encephalitis and peripheral neuropathy).

Contraindications:

Hypersensitivity to vidarabine.

Warnings:

There are no reports to indicate that vidarabine is effective in the management of encephalitis due to varicella-zoster or vaccinia viruses. It is not effective against infections caused by adenovirus or RNA viruses, bacteria or fungi. There are no data to support efficacy against cytomegalovirus, vaccinia virus or smallpox virus.

HSV encephalitis: Early diagnosis and treatment are essential. Studies which may support the suspected diagnosis include examination of CSF and localization of an intracerebral lesion by brain scan, EEG or computerized axial tomography (CAT). Brain biopsy is required to confirm the etiological diagnosis by means of viral isolation in cell cultures or by specific fluorescent antibody techniques.

Neonatal HSV infections: Following vidarabine therapy, the evidence of neurological abnormalities at 1 year of age was 44% in infants with localized CNS infection and 67% in infants with disseminated infection. Therefore, early diagnosis and treatment are essential to reduce both mortality and morbidity.

Renal function impairment: Patients may have a slower rate of renal excretion of Ara-Hx. Therefore, the dose may need to be adjusted.

Hepatic function impairment: Observe patients for possible adverse effects.

Carcinogenesis: In chronic studies conducted in mice and rats, there was a statistically significant increase in liver tumors among the vidarabine-treated female mice; some treated male mice developed kidney neoplasia. Intestinal, testicular and thyroid neoplasia occurred in rats.

Hepatic megalocytosis associated with vidarabine treatment has been found in short- and long-term rodent studies. It is not clear whether this represents a preneoplastic change.

Mutagenesis: In vitro, vidarabine can incorporate into mammalian DNA and induce mutation in mammalian cells. In vivo, vidarabine may be capable of producing mutagenic effects in male germ cells.

Vidarabine causes chromosome breaks and gaps when added to human leukocytes in vitro. While the significance is not fully understood, there is a correlation between the ability of various agents to produce such effects and their ability to produce inheritable genetic damage.

(Warnings continued on following page)

VIDARABINE (Adenine Arabinoside; Ara-A) (Cont.)

Warnings (Cont.)

Herpes zoster: To be effective, initiate vidarabine therapy as early as possible, within 72 hours after the appearance of vesicular lesions.

Pregnancy: Category C. Vidarabine is teratogenic in small animals and produces maternal toxicity. There are no adequate and well controlled studies in pregnant women. Use during pregnancy only if the potential benefit justifies the potential risk to the fetus.

Lactation: It is not known whether vidarabine is excreted in breast milk. Decide whether to discontinue nursing or to discontinue the drug, taking into account the importance of the drug to the mother.

Precautions:

Discontinue treatment in the patient with a brain biopsy negative for HSV in cell culture.

Fluid overload: Because vidarabine is relatively insoluble, its administration often requires a large fluid load. Exercise special care when administering to patients susceptible to fluid overloading or cerebral edema (ie, patients with CNS infections or impaired renal function).

Hematologic effects: Perform appropriate hematologic tests during administration since hemoglobin, hematocrit, white blood cells and platelets may be depressed during therapy.

Some degree of immunocompetence must be present to achieve clinical response.

Drug Interactions:

Allopurinol: Although clear evidence of adverse experience has not been reported, allopurinol may interfere with vidarabine metabolism. Exercise caution when administering these two drugs concomitantly.

Adverse Reactions:

GI: Anorexia, nausea, vomiting and diarrhea are all usually mild to moderate and seldom require termination of therapy. AST and total bilirubin may be elevated. Hematemesis has also occurred.

CNS: Tremor, dizziness, headache, hallucinations, confusion, psychosis and ataxia have occurred mostly in patients with impaired hepatic or renal function. Malaise and fatal metabolic encephalopathy have also occurred.

Hematologic: Decrease in reticulocyte count, hemoglobin or hematocrit, WBC count and platelet count.

Miscellaneous: Weight loss; pruritus; rash; pain at injection site.

Overdosage:

Acute massive overdose has occurred without any serious effects. Acute fluid overloading poses a greater threat to the patient than vidarabine due to its low solubility. Doses $>$ 20 mg/kg/day can produce bone marrow depression with thrombocytopenia and leukopenia. If overdose occurs, monitor hematologic, liver and renal functions.

Administration and Dosage:

For slow IV infusion only. Avoid rapid or bolus injection. Do not inject IM or SC because of low solubility and poor absorption. The contents of the vial must be diluted in an appropriate IV solution prior to administration. Slowly infuse the total daily dose over 12 to 24 hours.

Herpes simplex virus encephalitis: 15 mg/kg/day for 10 days.

Neonatal herpes simplex virus infections: 15 mg/kg/day for 10 days.

Herpes zoster: 10 mg/kg/day for 5 days.

Preparation: Solubility in IV fluids is limited. Each 1 mg requires 2.22 ml of IV fluid for complete solubilization. Therefore, each liter will solubilize a maximum of 450 mg of vidarabine. *Newborns* – Due to the small quantity required by the infant, add 1 ml to 9 ml of sterile normal saline or sterile water for injection to provide a suspension of 20 mg/ml.

Any appropriate IV solution is suitable for use as a diluent EXCEPT biologic or colloidal fluids (eg, blood products, protein solutions).

Prewarm the IV infusion fluid to 35° to 40°C (95° to 100°F) to facilitate solution of the drug following its transference. Depending on the dose, more than 1 L of IV fluid may be required. Thoroughly agitate the prepared admixture until completely clear. Final filtration with an in-line membrane filter ($\leq$ 0.45 micron pore size) is necessary.

Stability/Storage: Dilute just prior to administration and use within 48 hours. Do not refrigerate the dilution.

				C.I.*
Rx	**Vira-A** (Parke-Davis)	**Injection:** 200 mg/ml suspension vidarabine monohydrate (equiv. to 187.4 mg vidarabine)	In 5 ml vials.[1]	737

* Cost Index based on cost per 200 mg vidarabine monohydrate.

[1] With 0.1 mg benzethonium chloride per ml.

ACYCLOVIR (Acycloguanosine)

Actions:

Pharmacology: A synthetic acyclic purine nucleoside analog, acyclovir has in vitro inhibitory activity against Herpes simplex virus types 1 and 2 (HSV-1 and HSV-2), varicella zoster, Epstein-Barr and cytomegalovirus. Acyclovir is preferentially taken up and selectively converted to the active triphosphate form by HSV-infected cells. Acyclovir triphosphate interferes with HSV DNA polymerase and inhibits viral DNA replication. In vitro, acyclovir triphosphate can be incorporated into growing chains of DNA by viral DNA polymerase and, to a much smaller extent, by cellular DNA polymerase. When incorporation occurs, the DNA chain is terminated.

The relationship between in vitro susceptibility of HSV to antiviral drugs and clinical response has not been established.

Clinical pharmacology: Genital herpes (oral therapy) –

Initial episodes: Oral acyclovir reduced the duration of acute infection and lesion healing. Duration of pain and new lesion formation was decreased in some patients. The promptness of initiation of therapy or the patient's prior exposure to HSV may influence the degree of benefit from therapy.

Recurrent episodes: In patients with frequent recurrences (≥ 6 episodes per year), oral acyclovir given for 4 months to 3 years prevented or reduced the frequency or severity of recurrences in > 95% of patients. In a study of 283 patients who received 400 mg twice daily for 3 years, 45%, 52% and 63% of patients remained free of recurrences in the first, second and third years, respectively. Serial analysis of the 3 month recurrence rates for the 283 patients showed that 71% to 87% were recurrence-free in each quarter, indicating that the effects are consistent over time.

In general, do not use for suppression of recurrent disease in mildly affected patients. Immunocompromised patients with recurrent HSV can be treated with either intermittent or chronic suppressive therapy. Clinically significant resistance, although rare, is more likely to be seen with prolonged or repeated therapy in severely immunocompromised patients with active lesions.

Herpes zoster – In two studies of 270 patients with localized cutaneous zoster infection, acyclovir 800 mg 5 times daily for 7 to 10 days shortened the times to lesion scabbing, healing and complete cessation of pain, and reduced the duration of viral shedding, the duration of new lesion formation and the prevalence of localized zoster-associated neurologic symptoms (paresthesia, dysesthesia or hyperesthesia).

Chickenpox – In 110 patients (ages 5 to 16 years) who presented within 24 hours of the onset of a typical chickenpox rash, acyclovir 4 times daily for 5 to 7 days at doses of 10, 15, or 20 mg/kg orally depending on the age group reduced the maximum number of lesions (336 vs > 500; lesions beyond 500 were not counted). Acyclovir also shortened the mean time to 50% healing (7.1 vs 8.7 days), reduced the number of vesicular lesions by the second day of treatment (49 vs 113), and decreased the proportion of patients with fever (temperature > 38°C or 100°F) by the second day (19% vs 57%).

In two studies, 883 patients (ages 2 to 18 years) were enrolled within 24 hours of the onset of a typical chickenpox rash. In the larger study (n = 815, ages 2 to 12 years), acyclovir 20 mg/kg orally up to 800 mg 4 times daily for 5 days reduced the median maximum number of lesions (277 vs 386), reduced the median number of vesicular lesions by the second day of treatment (26 vs 40), and reduced the proportion of patients with moderate to severe itching by the third day of treatment (15% vs 34%). In addition, in both studies acyclovir also decreased the proportion of patients with fever (temperature > 38°C or 100°F), anorexia and lethargy by the second day of treatment, and decreased the mean number of residual lesions on day 28.

Pharmacokinetics: Absorption/Distribution – Proportionality between dose and plasma levels is seen after single doses or at steady state after multiple dosing. When acyclovir was administered to adults at 5 mg/kg (≈ 250 mg/m²) by 1 hour infusions every 8 hours, mean steady-state peak and trough concentrations were 9.8 mcg/ml (5.5 to 13.8 mcg/ml) and 0.7 mcg/ml (0.2 to 1 mcg/ml), respectively. Similar concentrations are achieved in children > 1 year old when doses of 250 mg/m² are given every 8 hours. Oral acyclovir is slowly and incompletely absorbed from the GI tract. Peak concentrations are reached in 1.5 to 2 hours; absorption is unaffected by food. Bioavailability is between 15% and 30% and decreases with increasing doses. Concentrations achieved in CSF are ≈ 50% of plasma values. Plasma protein binding is 9% to 33%. Acyclovir is widely distributed in tissues and body fluids, including brain, kidney, lung, liver, muscle, spleen, uterus, vaginal mucosa, vaginal secretions, CSF and herpetic vesicular fluid.

(Actions continued on following page)

ACYCLOVIR (Acycloguanosine) (Cont.)

Actions (Cont.):

Pharmacokinetics (Cont.):

Metabolism/Excretion – Renal excretion of unchanged drug by glomerular filtration and tubular secretion following IV use accounts for 62% to 91% of the dose. Mean renal excretion of unchanged drug following oral use is 14.4% (8.6% to 19.8%). The only major urinary metabolite is 9-carboxymethoxymethylguanine; this may account for up to 14% of the dose in patients with normal renal function. An insignificant amount is recovered in feces and expired CO_2; there is no evidence of tissue retention.

Half-life and total body clearance depend on renal function:

Acyclovir Half-Life and Total Body Clearance Based on Renal Function		
Creatinine clearance (ml/min/1.73 m²)	Half-life (hr)	Total body clearance (ml/min/1.73 m²)
> 80	2.5	327
50-80	3	248
15-50	3.5	190
0 (Anuric)	19.5	29

The half-life and total body clearance of acyclovir in pediatric patients > 1 year of age is similar to those in adults with normal renal function.

Indications:

Parenteral: Treatment of initial and recurrent mucosal and cutaneous HSV-1 and HSV-2 and varicella-zoster (shingles) infections in immunocompromised patients.

Herpes simplex encephalitis in patients > 6 months of age.

Severe initial clinical episodes of genital herpes in patients who are not immunocompromised.

Oral: Treatment of initial episodes and management of recurrent episodes of genital herpes in certain patients. Severity of the disease (and hence, patient selection) depends upon the immune status of the patient, frequency and duration of episodes and degree of cutaneous or systemic involvement.

Acute treatment of herpes zoster (shingles) and chickenpox (varicella).

Unlabeled uses: Other potential uses of oral or parenteral acyclovir include:

Unlabeled Uses of Acyclovir	
Cytomegalovirus and HSV infection following bone marrow or renal transplantation	Herpes simplex proctitis
Disseminated primary eczema herpeticum	Herpes simplex whitlow
Herpes simplex-associated erythema multiforme	Herpes zoster encephalitis
Herpes simplex labialis	Infectious mononucleosis
Herpes simplex ocular infections	Varicella pneumonia

Contraindications:

Hypersensitivity to acyclovir or any component of the formulation.

Warnings:

Testicular atrophy occurred in rats administered acyclovir intraperitoneally at 320 or 80 mg/kg/day for 1 and 6 months, respectively. Some recovery of sperm production was evident 30 days postdose.

Pregnancy: Category C. In a non-standard test in rats given 3 SC doses of 100 mg/kg (plasma levels of 63 and 125 times human levels), there was maternal toxicity and fetal abnormalities such as head and tail anomalies. There are no adequate and well controlled studies in pregnant women. Use during pregnancy only if the potential benefit outweighs the potential risk to the fetus. Potential uses in pregnancy would be for life-threatening infections such as disseminated maternal HSV infection and varicella pneumonia.

Lactation: Acyclovir concentrations in breast milk in women following oral administration have ranged from 0.6 to 4.1 times corresponding plasma levels. These concentrations would potentially expose the nursing infant to a dose of acyclovir up to 0.3 mg/kg/day. Exercise caution when administering to a nursing woman.

Children: Safety and efficacy of oral acyclovir in children < 2 years of age have not been established.

(Continued on following page)

ACYCLOVIR (Acycloguanosine) (Cont.)

Precautions:

Diagnosis: Proof of HSV infection rests on viral isolation and identification in tissue culture. Although the cutaneous vesicular lesions associated with HSV are often characteristic, other etiologic agents can cause similar lesions.

Genital herpes: Avoid sexual intercourse when visible lesions are present because of the risk of infecting intimate partners.

Herpes zoster infections: Adults ≥ 50 years of age tend to have more severe shingles, and acyclovir treatment showed more significant benefit for older patients. Treatment was begun within 72 hours of rash onset in these studies, and was more useful if started within the first 48 hours.

Chickenpox: Although chickenpox in otherwise healthy children is usually a self-limited disease of mild to moderate severity, adolescents and adults tend to have more severe disease. Treatment was initiated within 24 hours of the typical chickenpox rash in the controlled studies, and there is no information regarding the effects of treatment begun later in the disease course. It is unknown whether the treatment of chickenpox in childhood has any effect on long-term immunity. However, there is no evidence to indicate that acyclovir treatment of chickenpox would have any effect on either decreasing or increasing the incidence or severity of subsequent recurrences of herpes zoster (shingles) later in life. IV acyclovir is indicated for the treatment of varicella-zoster infections in immunocompromised patients.

Do not exceed the recommended dosage, frequency or length of treatment. Base dosage adjustments on estimated creatinine clearance.

Renal effects: Precipitation of acyclovir crystals in renal tubules can occur if the maximum solubility of free acyclovir (2.5 mg/ml at 37°C in water) is exceeded or if the drug is administered by bolus injection. Serum creatinine and blood urea nitrogen (BUN) rise and creatinine clearance decreases.

Bolus administration of the drug leads to a 10% incidence of renal dysfunction, while infusion of 5 mg/kg (250 mg/m²) over an hour was associated with a lower frequency (4.6%). Concomitant use of other nephrotoxic drugs, preexisting renal disease and dehydration make further renal impairment with acyclovir more likely. In most instances, alterations of renal function were transient and resolved spontaneously or with improvement of water and electrolyte balance, with drug dosage adjustments or with drug discontinuation. However, these changes may progress to acute renal failure.

Hydration: Accompany IV infusion by adequate hydration. Since maximum urine concentration occurs within the first 2 hours following infusion, establish sufficient urine flow during that period to prevent precipitation in renal tubules.

Encephalopathic changes: Approximately 1% of patients receiving acyclovir IV have manifested encephalopathic changes characterized by either lethargy, obtundation, tremors, confusion, hallucinations, agitation, seizures or coma. Use with caution in those patients who have underlying neurologic abnormalities; those with serious renal, hepatic or electrolyte abnormalities or significant hypoxia; and those who have manifested prior neurologic reactions to cytotoxic drugs.

Resistance: Exposure of HSV isolates to acyclovir in vitro can lead to the emergence of less sensitive viruses. In severely immunocompromised patients, prolonged or repeated courses of acyclovir may result in resistant viruses which may not fully respond to continued acyclovir therapy.

Drug Interactions:

Acyclovir Drug Interactions			
Precipitant drug	Object drug*		Description
Probenecid	Acyclovir	↑	Acyclovir bioavailability and terminal plasma half-life may be increased, and renal clearance may be decreased.
Zidovudine	Acyclovir	↑	Severe drowsiness and lethargy may occur.

* ↑ = Object drug increased.

(Continued on following page)

ACYCLOVIR (Acycloguanosine) (Cont.)

Adverse Reactions:

Parenteral:

Frequency ≥ *1%* – Inflammation or phlebitis at injection site (≈ 9%); transient elevations of serum creatinine or BUN (5% to 10%, the higher incidence usually occurring following rapid [< 10 minutes] IV infusion); nausea or vomiting (≈ 7%); itching, rash, hives (≈ 2%); elevation of transaminases (1% to 2%); encephalopathic changes characterized by either lethargy, obtundation, tremors, confusion, hallucinations, agitation, seizures or coma (≈ 1%; see Precautions).

Frequency < *1%* – Anemia; anuria; hematuria; hypotension; edema; anorexia; lightheadedness; thirst; headache; diaphoresis; fever; neutropenia; thrombocytopenia; abnormal urinalysis (characterized by an increase in formed elements in urine sediment); pain on urination; pulmonary edema with cardiac tamponade; abdominal pain; chest pain; thrombocytosis; leukocytosis; neutrophilia; ischemia of digits; hypokalemia; purpura fulminans; pressure on urination; hemoglobinemia; rigors.

Oral:

Oral Acyclovir Adverse Reactions (Treatment of Herpes Simplex)

Body system	Short-term administration	Long-term administration	Intermittent administration
GI	Nausea/vomiting (2.7%); diarrhea (0.3%)	Nausea (4.8%); diarrhea (2.4%)	Diarrhea (2.7%); nausea (2.4%)
CNS	Headache (0.6%); dizziness, fatigue (0.3%)	Headache (0.9% to 1.9%)	Headache (2.2%)
Dermatologic	Skin rash (0.3%)	Skin rash (1.3% to 1.7%)	Skin rash (1.5%)
Other	Anorexia, edema, inguinal adenopathy, leg pain, medication taste, sore throat (0.3%)	Asthenia (1.2%); paresthesia (0.8% to 1.2%)	

Oral Acyclovir Adverse Reactions (Treatment of Herpes Zoster and Chickenpox)

	Herpes zoster		Chickenpox	
Adverse Reaction	Acyclovir	Placebo	Acyclovir	Placebo
Malaise	11.5%	11.1%	—	—
Nausea	8%	11.5%	—	—
Headache	5.9%	11.1%	—	—
Vomiting	2.5%	2.5%	0.6%	—
Diarrhea	1.5%	0.3%	3.2%	2.2%
Constipation	0.9%	2.4%	—	—
Abdominal pain	—	—	0.6%	—
Rash	—	—	0.6%	—
Flatulence	—	—	0.4%	0.8%

Overdosage:

Symptoms: Precipitation of acyclovir in renal tubules may occur when the solubility (2.5 mg/ml) in the intratubular fluid is exceeded.

Parenteral – Overdosage has occurred with bolus injections, or inappropriately high doses, and in patients whose fluid and electrolyte balance was not properly monitored. Elevations in BUN, serum creatinine and subsequent renal failure resulted.

Oral – Doses as high as 800 mg 6 times daily for 5 days have been administered without acute untoward effects. This should not be construed as a recommended dosage for patients with more severe herpes.

Treatment: Acyclovir is dialyzable. A 6 hour hemodialysis results in a 60% decrease in plasma acyclovir concentration. Peritoneal dialysis appears less efficient in removing acyclovir from the blood. In the event of acute renal failure and anuria, the patient may benefit from hemodialysis until renal function is restored.

Patient Information

Avoid sexual intercourse when visible herpes lesions are present.

Oral acyclovir does not eliminate latent HSV virus and is not a cure.

Do not exceed recommended dosage; do not share medication with others.

Notify physician if frequency and severity of recurrences do not improve.

(Continued on following page)

ACYCLOVIR (Acycloguanosine) (Cont.)

Administration and Dosage:

Approved by the FDA in 1984.

Parenteral:

Avoid rapid or bolus IV, IM or SC injection. Initiate therapy as soon as possible following onset of signs and symptoms. For IV infusion only. Administer over at least 1 hour to prevent renal tubular damage.

IV Acyclovir Dosage/Management Guidelines		
Indication	Dosage	
	Adults	Children (< 12 years)
Mucosal and cutaneous HSV infections in immunocompromised patients	5 mg/kg infused at a constant rate over 1 hour every 8 hours (15 mg/kg/day) for 7 days[1]	250 mg/m² infused at a constant rate over 1 hour every 8 hours (750 mg/m²/day) for 7 days[1]
Varicella-zoster infections (shingles) in immunocompromised patients[2]	10 mg/kg infused at a constant rate over 1 hour every 8 hours for 7 days[3]	500 mg/m² infused at a constant rate over at least 1 hour every 8 hours for 7 days[3]
Herpes simplex encephalitis	10 mg/kg infused at a constant rate over at least 1 hour every 8 hours for 10 days	500 mg/m² infused at a constant rate over at least 1 hour every 8 hours for 10 days[4]

[1] For severe initial clinical episodes of herpes genitalis, use the same dose for 5 days.
[2] Base dosage for obese patients on ideal body weight (10 mg/kg).
[3] Do not exceed 500 mg/m² every 8 hours.
[4] > 6 months of age.

Renal function impairment, acute or chronic – Adjust the dosing interval as indicated below:

Parenteral Acyclovir Dosage in Renal Function Impairment		
Creatinine clearance (ml/min/1.73 m²)	Percent of recommended dose	Dosing interval (hours)
> 50	100%	8
25-50	100%	12
10-25	100%	24
0-10	50%	24

Hemodialysis – The mean plasma half-life of acyclovir during hemodialysis is approximately 5 hours; a 60% decrease in plasma concentrations follows a 6 hour dialysis period. Therefore, administer a dose after each dialysis.

Preparation of IV solution: Dissolve the contents of the 500 or 1000 mg vial in 10 or 20 ml Sterile Water for Injection, respectively, to yield a final concentration of 50 mg/ml acyclovir (pH ≈ 11). Do not use bacteriostatic water containing benzyl alcohol or parabens; it is incompatible and may cause precipitation.

Add the calculated dose to an appropriate IV solution at a volume selected for administration during each 1 hour infusion. Infusion concentrations of approximately 7 mg/ml or lower are recommended. In clinical studies, the average 70 kg adult received approximately 60 ml of fluid per dose. Higher concentrations (eg, 10 mg/ml) may produce phlebitis or inflammation at the injection site upon inadvertent extravasation. The addition of acyclovir to biologic or colloidal fluids (eg, blood products, protein solutions) is not recommended.

(Administration and Dosage continued on following page)

ACYCLOVIR (Acycloguanosine) (Cont.)

Administration and Dosage (Cont.):

Oral:

Herpes simplex –

Initial genital herpes: 200 mg every 4 hours 5 times daily for 10 days. In patients with extremely severe episodes in which prostration, CNS involvement, urinary retention or inability to take oral medication requires hospitalization and more aggressive management, initiate therapy with IV acyclovir (see above).

Chronic suppressive therapy for recurrent disease: 400 mg 2 times daily for up to 12 months, followed by reevaluation. Reevaluate the frequency and severity of the patient's HSV after 1 year of therapy to assess the need for continuation of therapy; frequency and severity of episodes of untreated genital herpes may change over time. Reevaluation usually requires a trial off acyclovir to assess the need for reinstitution of suppressive therapy. Some patients, such as those with very frequent or severe episodes before treatment, may warrant uninterrupted suppression for > 1 year.

Alternative regimens have included doses ranging from 200 mg 3 times daily to 200 mg 5 times daily.

Intermittent therapy: 200 mg every 4 hours 5 times daily for 5 days. Initiate therapy at the earliest sign or symptom (prodrome) of recurrence.

Herpes zoster, acute treatment – 800 mg every 4 hours 5 times daily for 7 to 10 days.

Chickenpox – 20 mg/kg (not to exceed 800 mg) 4 times daily for 5 days. Initiate at earliest sign or symptom.

Renal impairment, acute or chronic –

Oral Acyclovir Dosage in Renal Function Impairment			
Normal dosage regimen (5x daily)	Creatinine clearance (ml/min/1.73 m²)	Adjusted dosage regimen	
		Dose (mg)	Dosing interval
200 mg every 4 hours	> 10 0-10	200 200	Every 4 hours, 5x daily Every 12 hours
400 mg every 12 hours	> 10 0-10	400 200	Every 12 hours Every 12 hours
800 mg every 4 hours	> 25 10-25 0-10	800 800 800	Every 4 hours, 5x daily Every 8 hours Every 12 hours

Hemodialysis – For patients that require hemodialysis, adjust dosing schedule so that a dose is administered after each dialysis. No supplemental dose is necessary after peritoneal dialysis.

Stability/Storage: Use reconstituted solution within 12 hours. Once diluted for administration, use each dose within 24 hours. Refrigeration of reconstituted solutions may result in formation of a precipitate which redissolves at room temperature.

				C.I.*
Rx	**Zovirax** (Burroughs Wellcome)	**Tablets:** 800 mg	(Zovirax 800 mg). Blue. Oval. In 100s.	NA
		Capsules: 200 mg	(Wellcome Zovirax 200). Blue. In 100s and UD 100s.	184
		Suspension: 200 mg/5 ml	Banana flavor. In 473 ml.[1]	NA
		Powder for Injection: 500 mg/vial (as sodium)	In 10 ml vials.	4083
		1000 mg/vial (as sodium)	In 20 ml vials.	NA

* Cost Index based on cost per 500 mg.

[1] With 0.1% methylparaben, 0.02% propylparaben and sorbitol.

GANCICLOVIR SODIUM (DHPG)

Warning:

The clinical toxicity of ganciclovir includes granulocytopenia and thrombocytopenia. In animal studies, the drug was carcinogenic, teratogenic, and caused aspermatogenesis. Ganciclovir is indicated for use *only* in the treatment of cytomegalovirus (CMV) retinitis in immunocompromised patients and for the prevention of CMV disease in transplant patients at risk for CMV disease.

Actions:

Pharmacology: Ganciclovir sodium is an antiviral drug active against cytomegalovirus (CMV). It is a synthetic nucleoside analog of 2′-deoxyguanosine. Sensitive human viruses include CMV, herpes simplex virus-1 and -2 (HSV-1, HSV-2), Epstein-Barr virus and varicella zoster virus. Clinical studies have been limited to assessment of efficacy in patients with CMV infection.

Median effective inhibitory doses (ED_{50}) of ganciclovir for human CMV isolates tested in vitro in several cell lines ranged from 0.2 to 3 mcg/ml. The relationship between in vitro sensitivity of CMV to ganciclovir and clinical response has not been established. Ganciclovir inhibits mammalian cell proliferation in vitro at higher concentrations (10 to 60 mcg/ml) with bone marrow colony forming cells being the most sensitive ($ID_{50} \geq 10$ mcg/ml) of those cell types tested.

Upon entry into host cells, CMVs induce one or more cellular kinases that phosphorylate ganciclovir to its triphosphate. There is approximately a tenfold greater concentration of ganciclovir-triphosphate in CMV-infected cells than in uninfected cells, indicating a preferential phosphorylation of ganciclovir in virus-infected cells. In vitro, ganciclovir-triphosphate is catabolized slowly, with 60% to 70% of the original level remaining in the infected cells 18 hours after removal of ganciclovir from the extracellular medium. The antiviral activity of ganciclovir-triphosphate is believed to be the result of inhibition of viral DNA synthesis by two known modes: Competitive inhibition of viral DNA polymerases and direct incorporation into viral DNA, resulting in eventual termination of viral DNA elongation. The cellular DNA polymerase alpha is inhibited, but at a higher concentration than required for viral DNA polymerase.

Pharmacokinetics: Twenty-two immunocompromised patients with serious CMV disease and normal renal function received ganciclovir 5 mg/kg, each dose infused IV over 1 hour. The mean plasma level of ganciclovir at the end of the first 1 hour infusion (C_{max}) was 8.3 ± 4 mcg/ml and the plasma level 11 hours after the start of infusion (C_{min}) was 0.56 ± 0.66 mcg/ml. The plasma half-life was 2.9 ± 1.3 hours and the systemic clearance was 3.64 ± 1.86 ml/kg/min (approximately 250 ml/1.73 m^2/min). Dose-independent kinetics were demonstrated over the range of 1.6 to 5 mg/kg. Multiple-dose kinetics were measured in eight patients with normal renal function who received ganciclovir 5 mg/kg twice daily for 12 to 14 days. After the first dose and after multiple dosing, plasma levels at the end of infusion were 7.1 mcg/ml (3.1 to 14 mcg/ml) and 9.5 mcg/ml (2.7 to 24.2 mcg/ml), respectively. At 7 hours after infusion, plasma levels after the first dose were 0.85 mcg/ml (0.2 to 1.8 mcg/ml) and were 1.2 mcg/ml (0.6 to 1.8 mcg/ml) after multiple dosing.

Renal excretion of unchanged drug by glomerular filtration is the major route of elimination. In patients with normal renal function, more than 90% of the administered ganciclovir was recovered unmetabolized in the urine. In four patients with mild renal impairment (creatinine clearance [Ccr] 50 to 79 ml/min/1.73 m^2), the systemic clearance of ganciclovir was 128 ± 63 ml/min/1.73 m^2, and the plasma half-life was 4.6 ± 1.4 hours. In three patients with moderate renal impairment (Ccr 25 to 49 ml/min/1.73 m^2), the systemic clearance of ganciclovir was 57 ± 8 ml/min/1.73 m^2, and the plasma half-life was 4.4 ± 0.4 hours. In 3 patients with severe renal impairment (Ccr < 25 ml/min/1.73 m^2) the systemic clearance was 30 ± 13 ml/min/1.73 m^2, and the plasma half-life was 10.7 ± 5.7 hours. There was positive correlation between systemic clearance of ganciclovir and Ccr.

Data from four patients with severe renal impairment showed that hemodialysis reduced plasma drug levels by ≈ 50%. Binding of ganciclovir to plasma proteins is 1% to 2%. Drug interactions involving binding site displacement are not expected.

(Actions continued on following page)

GANCICLOVIR SODIUM (DHPG) (Cont.)

Actions (Cont.):

Pharmacokinetics (Cont.):

There is limited evidence to suggest that ganciclovir crosses the blood brain barrier. Cerebrospinal fluid (CSF) concentrations have been measured in three patients:

Ganciclovir CSF Concentrations				
Patient	CSF conc. (mcg/ml)	Plasma conc. (mcg/ml)	Hr after dose	CSF/Plasma ratio
1	0.62	0.92	5.67	0.67
	0.68	2.2	3.5	0.31
	0.51	1.96	2.75	0.26
2	0.5	2.05	0.25	0.24
3	0.31	0.44	5.5	0.7

Clinical trials: Immunocompromised patients – Of 314 immunocompromised patients enrolled in an open label study of the treatment of life- or sight-threatening CMV disease, 121 patients had a positive culture for CMV within 7 days prior to treatment.

Virologic Response to Ganciclovir Treatment			
Culture source	No. patients cultured	No. (%) patients responding	Median days to response
Urine	107	93 (87)	8
Blood	41	34 (83)	8
Throat	21	19 (90)	7
Semen	6	6 (100)	15

Transplant recipients – In 149 CMV seropositive heart allograft recipients and 72 CMV culture positive allogeneic bone marrow transplant recipients, ganciclovir prevented recrudescence of CMV shedding in the heart allograft patients and suppressed CMV shedding in the bone marrow allograft patients.

Patients with Positive CMV Cultures Following Ganciclovir				
	Heart allograft		Bone marrow allograft	
Time	Ganciclovir	Placebo	Ganciclovir	Placebo
Pre-Treatment	2% (1/67)	8% (5/64)	100% (37/37)	100% (35/35)
Week 2	3% (2/75)	16% (11/67)	6% (2/31)	68% (19/28)
Week 4	5% (3/66)	43% (28/66)	0% (0/24)	80% (16/20)

Emergence of viral resistance has occurred. The prevalence of resistant isolates is unknown, and some patients may be infected with strains of CMV resistant to ganciclovir. Therefore, consider the possibility of viral resistance in patients who show poor clinical response or experience persistent viral excretion during therapy.

Indications:

CMV retinitis: Treatment of immunocompromised patients, including those with acquired immunodeficiency syndrome (AIDS).

CMV disease: Prevention in transplant patients at risk for CMV disease.

Unlabeled uses: Ganciclovir may also be beneficial in some immunocompromised patients in the treatment of other CMV infections (eg, pneumonitis, gastroenteritis, hepatitis). See Warnings.

Contraindications:

Hypersensitivity to ganciclovir or acyclovir.

Warnings:

CMV disease: Safety and efficacy have not been established for congenital or neonatal CMV disease nor for the treatment of established CMV disease other than retinitis (eg, pneumonitis, colitis), nor for use in nonimmunocompromised individuals.

(Warnings continued on following page)

GANCICLOVIR SODIUM (DHPG) (Cont.)

Warnings (Cont.):

Diagnosis of CMV retinitis is ophthalmologic and should be made by indirect opthalmoscopy. Other conditions in the differential diagnosis of CMV retinitis include candidiasis, toxoplasmosis, histoplasmosis, retinal scars and cotton wool spots, any of which may produce a retinal appearance similar to CMV. The diagnosis may be supported by culture of CMV from urine, blood, throat, etc, but a negative CMV culture does not rule out CMV retinitis.

Hematologic: Granulocytopenia – Approximately 40% of 522 immunocompromised patients with serious CMV infections who received IV ganciclovir developed granulocytopenia (neutropenia, ie, neutrophil count < 1,000/mm³). Therefore, use with caution in patients with pre-existing cytopenias, or with a history of cytopenic reactions to other drugs, chemicals or irradiation. Granulocytopenia usually occurs during the first or second week of treatment, but may occur at any time during treatment. Cell counts usually begin to recover within 3 to 7 days of discontinuing the drug. Do not administer if the absolute neutrophil count is < 500/mm³ or the platelet count is < 25,000/mm³.

Thrombocytopenia (platelet count < 50,000/mm³) was observed in approximately 20% of the same 522 patients treated with ganciclovir. Patients with iatrogenic immunosuppression were more likely to develop thrombocytopenia than patients with AIDS (46% vs 14%).

Retinal detachment in CMV retinitis patients has occurred both before and after initiation of therapy. The relationship to therapy is unknown. Frequent ophthalmologic evaluations to monitor the status of retinitis and to detect any other retinal lesions is advised.

Renal toxicity: In heart allograft recipients, patients receiving ganciclovir had more elevation of serum creatinine to values exceeding > 2.5 mg/dl than patients receiving placebo (18% vs 4%, respectively). These increases in serum creatinine, up to 5.5 mg/dl in one patient, were transient and occurred primarily during the first week of treatment. In bone marrow allograft recipients, more ganciclovir-treated patients than untreated patients experienced serum creatinine values exceeding 1.5 mg/dl (70% vs 35%, respectively). These elevations in serum creatinine, up to 3.2 mg/dl in one patient, were transient and occurred intermittently throughout the 3 month study. Most patients in these studies received cyclosporine. Careful monitoring of renal function during therapy is essential, especially for those patients receiving concomitant agents that may cause nephrotoxicity.

Renal function impairment: Use with caution because the plasma half-life and peak plasma levels of ganciclovir will be increased due to reduced renal clearance (see Administration and Dosage).

Carcinogenesis, mutagenesis, impairment of fertility: In mice, daily oral doses of 1,000 mg/kg may have caused an increased incidence of tumors in the preputial gland of males, nonglandular mucosa of the stomach of males and females, and ovary, vagina and liver of females. A slightly increased incidence of tumors occurred in the preputial gland (males) and nonglandular mucosa (males and females) of the stomach in mice given 20 mg/kg/day. Consider ganciclovir a potential carcinogen in humans.

Ganciclovir caused point mutations and chromosomal damage in mammalian cells in vitro and in vivo. Because of the mutagenic potential of ganciclovir, advise women of childbearing potential to use effective contraception during treatment. Similarly, advise male patients to practice barrier contraception during and for at least 90 days following treatment with ganciclovir.

Ganciclovir caused decreased mating behavior, decreased fertility, and increased embryolethality in female mice at doses approximately equivalent to the recommended human dose. Animal data indicate that ganciclovir causes inhibition of spermatogenesis and subsequent infertility. These effects were reversible at lower doses and irreversible at higher doses. Although data in humans is lacking, IV ganciclovir at recommended doses probably causes temporary or permanent inhibition of spermatogenesis.

Elderly: Since elderly individuals frequently have reduced glomerular filtration, pay particular attention to assessing renal function before and during ganciclovir administration.

(Warnings continued on following page)

GANCICLOVIR SODIUM (DHPG) (Cont.)

Warnings (Cont.):

Pregnancy: Category C. Ganciclovir is teratogenic and embryotoxic in rabbits and embryotoxic in mice in doses approximately equivalent to the recommended human dose. The adverse effects observed in mice were maternal/fetal toxicity and embryolethality. In rabbits, the effects were: Fetal growth retardation, embryolethality, teratogenicity and maternal toxicity. Teratogenic changes included cleft palate, anophthalmia/microphthalmia, aplastic organs (kidneys and pancreas), hydrocephaly and brachygnathia.

Ganciclovir may be teratogenic or embryotoxic at the dose levels recommended for human use. There are no adequate and well controlled studies in pregnant women. Use during pregnancy only if the potential benefit justifies the potential risk to the fetus.

Lactation: It is not known if ganciclovir is excreted in breast milk. Daily IV doses of 90 mg/kg administered to female mice prior to mating, during gestation, and during lactation caused hypoplasia of the testes and seminal vesicles in the month-old male offspring, as well as pathologic changes in the nonglandular region of the stomach. Because of the potential for serious adverse reactions from ganciclovir in nursing infants, instruct mothers to discontinue nursing if they are receiving ganciclovir. Do not resume nursing until at least 72 hours after the last dose of ganciclovir.

Children: Safety and efficacy in children have not been established. The use of ganciclovir warrants extreme caution due to the probability of long-term carcinogenicity and reproductive toxicity. Administer to children only after careful evaluation and only if the potential benefits of treatment outweigh the risks.

There has been very limited clinical experience in treating CMV retinitis in patients < 12 years of age. Two children (ages 9 and 5 years) showed improvement or stabilization of retinitis for 23 and 9 months, respectively. These children received induction treatment with 2.5 mg/kg 3 times daily followed by maintenance therapy with 6 to 6.5 mg/kg once per day, 5 to 7 days per week. When retinitis progressed during once daily maintenance therapy, both children were treated with the 5 mg/kg twice daily regimen. Two other children (ages 2.5 and 4 years) who received similar induction regimens showed only partial or no response to treatment. A 6-year-old with T-cell dysfunction showed stabilization of retinitis for 3 months while receiving continuous infusions of ganciclovir at doses of 2 to 5 mg/kg/24 hours. Continuous infusion treatment was discontinued due to granulocytopenia.

Adverse events reported in 120 immunocompromised children with serious CMV infections receiving ganciclovir were similar to those reported in adults. Granulocytopenia (17%) and thrombocytopenia (10%) were most commonly reported.

Five bone marrow transplant children, ranging in age from 3 to 10 years, received 5 mg/kg twice daily for 7 days and then 5 mg/kg once daily until day 100 post-transplant. Results were similar to those observed in the ganciclovir once-daily-treated adult transplant recipients. Two of 6 placebo-treated pediatric patients developed CMV pneumonia vs zero of 5 ganciclovir-treated patients. Toxicity in the pediatric group was similar to that observed in the adult patients.

Precautions:

Large doses/rapid infusion: The maximum single dose administered was 6 mg/kg by IV infusion over 1 hour. Larger doses, or more rapid infusions, will probably result in increased toxicity.

Phlebitis/Pain at injection site: Initially reconstituted ganciclovir solutions have a high pH (pH 11). Despite further dilution in IV fluids, phlebitis or pain may occur at the site of IV infusion. Care must be taken to infuse solutions containing ganciclovir only into veins with adequate blood flow to permit rapid dilution and distribution.

Hydration: Administration of ganciclovir by IV infusion should be accompanied by adequate hydration, since ganciclovir is excreted by the kidneys and normal clearance depends on adequate renal function.

Monitoring: Perform neutrophil and platelet counts every 2 days during twice-daily dosing of ganciclovir and at least weekly thereafter. Monitor neutrophil counts daily in patients in whom ganciclovir or other nucleoside analogs have previously resulted in leukopenia, or in whom neutrophil counts are $< 1000/mm^3$ at the beginning of treatment. Because dosing must be modified in patients with renal impairment, monitor serum creatinine or Ccr at least once every 2 weeks.

(Continued on following page)

GANCICLOVIR SODIUM (DHPG) (Cont.)

Drug Interactions:

Ganciclovir Drug Interactions			
Precipitant drug	Object drug*		Description
Cytotoxic drugs	Ganciclovir	↑	Cytotoxic drugs that inhibit replication of rapidly dividing cell populations such as bone marrow, spermatogonia and germinal layers of skin and GI mucosa may have additive toxicity when administered concomitantly with ganciclovir. Therefore, consider the concomitant use of drugs such as dapsone, pentamidine, flucytosine, vincristine, vinblastine, adriamycin, amphotericin B, trimethoprim/sulfamethoxazole combinations or other nucleoside analogs only if potential benefits are judged to outweigh the risks.
Imipenem-cilastatin	Ganciclovir	↑	Generalized seizures occurred in seven patients who received ganciclovir and imipenem-cilastatin. Do not use these drugs concomitantly unless the potential benefits outweigh the risks.
Nephrotoxic drugs	Ganciclovir	↑	Increases in serum creatinine were observed following concurrent use of ganciclovir and either cyclosporine or amphotericin B (see Warnings).
Probenecid	Ganciclovir	↑	Probenecid and other drugs that inhibit renal tubular secretion or resorption may reduce renal clearance of ganciclovir.
Zidovudine	Ganciclovir	↑	Patients with AIDS may be receiving, or may have received, treatment with zidovudine. Because both zidovudine and ganciclovir can cause granulocytopenia, many patients will not tolerate combination therapy at full dosage strength.

* ↑ = Object drug increased

Adverse Reactions:

During clinical trials, ganciclovir was withdrawn or interrupted in approximately 32% of patients because of adverse reactions. In some instances, treatment was restarted and the reappearance of adverse reactions again necessitated withdrawal or interruption.

Hematologic: Granulocytopenia (absolute neutrophil count $< 1{,}000/mm^3$; 40%); thrombocytopenia (platelet count $< 50{,}000/mm^3$; 20%). In most cases, withdrawal of ganciclovir resulted in increased neutrophil or platelet counts. While granulocytopenia was generally reversible with discontinuation of treatment, some patients experienced irreversible neutropenia or died with severe bacteriological or fungal infections during neutropenic episodes.

Anemia (2%); eosinophilia (≤ 1%).

Cardiovascular: Arrhythmia, hypertension, hypotension (≤ 1%).

CNS: Headache (17%); confusion (6%); abnormal thoughts or dreams, ataxia, coma, dizziness, nervousness, paresthesia, psychosis, somnolence, tremor (≤ 1%).

GI: Nausea, vomiting, anorexia, diarrhea, hemorrhage, abdominal pain (≤ 1%).

Dermatologic: Rash (2%); alopecia, pruritus, urticaria (≤ 1%).

GU: Hematuria (≤ 1%); increased serum creatinine (see Warnings); increased BUN.

Injection site: Inflammation, pain, phlebitis (≤ 1%).

Miscellaneous: Sepsis (6%); fever (2%); chills, edema, infections, malaise, dyspnea (≤ 1%); retinal detachment (see Warnings).

Lab test abnormalities: Abnormal liver function values (2%); decrease in blood glucose (≤ 1%).

Overdosage:

Overdosage has been reported in 11 patients. In three of these patients, no adverse effects were observed. The doses received were: 7 doses of 11 mg/kg over a 3 day period, 9 mg/kg twice daily for 3 days, and 2 doses of 500 mg in a 21-month-old child.

(Overdosage continued on following page)

GANCICLOVIR SODIUM (DHPG) (Cont.)

Overdosage (Cont.):

Symptoms: Neutropenia in three patients: One had a history of bone marrow suppression prior to treatment and received ganciclovir 5 mg/kg twice daily for 14 days followed by 8 mg/kg given as single daily doses for 4 days, one patient received a single dose of 1675 mg (approximately 24 mg/kg), and a 60-year-old patient with preexisting neutropenia received a single 20 mg/kg dose. In all cases the neutropenia was reversible (17 days, 1 day and 9 days, respectively) following discontinuation of ganciclovir. Irreversible pancytopenia occurred in one 28-year-old AIDS patient with CMV colitis and abdominal pain who inadvertently received 3000 mg on each of 2 consecutive days. One patient with a history of renal insufficiency and hematuria developed worsening of the hematuria following a single 500 mg dose; the hematuria resolved in 2 days.

Treatment: Hemodialysis and hydration may be of benefit in reducing drug plasma levels. Data from four patients indicate that ganciclovir plasma levels are reduced approximately 50% following hemodialysis.

Patient Information:

Ganciclovir is not a cure for CMV retinitis, and immunocompromised patients may continue to experience progression of retinitis during or following treatment. Advise patients to have regular ophthalmologic examinations at a minimum of every 6 weeks while being treated.

The major toxicities of ganciclovir are granulocytopenia and thrombocytopenia. Dose modifications may be required, including possible discontinuation. Emphasize the importance of close monitoring of blood counts while on therapy.

Patients with AIDS may be receiving zidovudine. Treatment with zidovudine and ganciclovir will not be tolerated by many patients and may result in severe granulocytopenia.

Advise patients that ganciclovir has caused decreased sperm production in animals and may cause infertility in humans. Advise women of childbearing potential that ganciclovir causes birth defects in animals and should not be used during pregnancy; use effective contraception during ganciclovir treatment. Similarly, advise men to practice barrier contraception during and for at least 90 days following ganciclovir treatment.

Ganciclovir causes tumors in animals. Although there is no information from human studies, consider ganciclovir a potential carcinogen.

Transplant recipients: Counsel transplant recipients regarding the high frequency of impaired renal function, particularly in patients receiving concomitant administration of nephrotoxic agents such as cyclosporine and amphotericin B.

Administration and Dosage:

Approved by the FDA in 1989.

Administer IV; IM or SC injection of reconstituted ganciclovir may result in severe tissue irritation due to high pH (11). Do not administer ganciclovir by rapid or bolus IV injection. The toxicity of ganciclovir may be increased as a result of excessive plasma levels.

Do not exceed the recommended dosage, frequency or infusion rates.

CMV retinitis treatment:

Induction treatment – Initial dose in normal renal function is 5 mg/kg (given IV at a constant rate of 1 hour) every 12 hours for 14 to 21 days.

Maintenance treatment – Following induction, 5 mg/kg given as an IV infusion over 1 hour once per day 7 days each week, or 6 mg/kg once per day 5 days each week. Patients who experience progression of retinitis while receiving maintenance therapy may be re-treated with the twice-daily regimen.

Perform frequent hematologic monitoring throughout treatment. Do not administer if the neutrophil count falls below 500/mm³ or the platelet count falls below 25,000/mm³.

CMV disease prevention in transplant recipients: Initial dose in normal renal function is 5 mg/kg (given IV at a constant rate over 1 hour) every 12 hours for 7 to 14 days, followed by 5 mg/kg once per day on 7 days each week, or 6 mg/kg once per day on 5 days each week.

Duration is dependent on the duration and degree of immunosuppression. In controlled clinical trials in bone marrow allograft recipients, treatment was continued until day 100 to 120 post-transplantation. CMV disease occurred in several patients who discontinued treatment prematurely. In heart allograft recipients, the onset of newly diagnosed CMV disease occurred after treatment was stopped at day 28 post-transplant, suggesting that continued dosing may be necessary to prevent late occurrence of CMV disease in this patient population.

(Administration and Dosage continued on following page)

GANCICLOVIR SODIUM (DHPG) (Cont.)

Administration and Dosage (Cont.):

Renal function impairment:

Ganciclovir Dose in Renal Impairment		
Ccr (ml/min/1.73 m^2)	Ganciclovir dose (mg/kg)	Dosing interval (hours)
≥ 80	5	12
50-79	2.5	12
25-49	2.5	24
< 25	1.25	24

Ccr can be related to serum creatinine by the following formula:

Males: $$\frac{\text{Weight (kg)} \times (140 - \text{age})}{72 \times \text{serum creatinine (mg/dl)}} \times 1.73/\text{body surface } [m^2]$$

Females: 0.85 x above value

The optimal maintenance dose for patients with renal impairment is not known. Physicians may elect to reduce the dose to 50% of the induction dose and monitor the patient for disease progression.

Hemodialysis: Only limited data are available on ganciclovir elimination in patients undergoing hemodialysis. Do not exceed 1.25 mg/kg/24 hours. On days when hemodialysis is performed, administer shortly after the completion of the hemodialysis session, since hemodialysis reduces plasma levels by ≈ 50%. Monitor neutrophil and platelet counts daily.

Monitoring: Due to the frequency of granulocytopenia and thrombocytopenia in patients receiving ganciclovir (see Adverse Reactions), perform neutrophil and platelet counts every 2 days during twice-daily dosing and at least weekly thereafter. In patients in whom ganciclovir or other nucleoside analogs have previously resulted in leukopenia, or in whom neutrophil counts are < 1000/mm³ at the beginning of treatment, monitor neutrophil counts daily. Because dosing must be modified in renal impairment, monitor serum creatinine or Ccr at least once every 2 weeks.

Dose reduction: Perform frequent white blood cell counts. Severe neutropenia (ANC < 500/mm³) or severe thrombocytopenia (platelets < 25,000/mm³) requires a dose interruption until evidence of marrow recovery is observed (ANC ≥ 750/mm³).

Method of preparation: Each 10 ml vial contains ganciclovir sodium equivalent to 500 mg of the free base form of ganciclovir and 46 mg of sodium. Prepare the contents of the vial for administration in the following manner:

Reconstituted solution –

1. Reconstitute lyophilized ganciclovir by injecting 10 ml of Sterile Water for Injection into the vial. *Do not* use bacteriostatic water for injection containing parabens. It is incompatible with ganciclovir sterile powder and may cause precipitation.
2. Shake the vial to dissolve the drug.
3. If particulate matter or discoloration is observed, discard the vial.
4. Reconstituted solution in the vial is stable at room temperature for 12 hours. *Do not refrigerate.*

Infusion solution – Based on patient weight, remove the appropriate calculated dose volume from the vial (ganciclovir concentration 50 mg/ml) and add to an acceptable (see below) infusion fluid (typically 100 ml) for delivery over 1 hour. Infusion concentrations > 10 mg/ml are not recommended. The following infusion fluids are chemically and physically compatible with ganciclovir: 0.9% Sodium Chloride, 5% Dextrose, Ringer's Injection and Lactated Ringer's Injection.

Storage: Because nonbacteriostatic infusion fluid must be used with ganciclovir, the infusion solution must be used within 24 hours of dilution to reduce the risk of bacterial contamination. Refrigerate the infusion solution. Freezing is not recommended.

Disposal: Because ganciclovir is a nucleoside analog, consider procedures for proper handling and disposal of unused solution. (See Handling of Cytotoxic Agents in the Antineoplastics introduction.)

Rx	**Cytovene** (Syntex)	**Powder for Injection, lyophilized:** 500 mg/vial ganciclovir (as sodium)	In 10 ml vials.

ZALCITABINE (Dideoxycytidine; ddC)

Warning:

Zalcitabine in combination with zidovudine is indicated for the treatment of adult patients with advanced HIV infection (CD4 cell count $\leq 300/mm^3$) who have demonstrated significant clinical or immunologic deterioration. This indication is based on limited data from two small studies in which zidovudine-naive patients with a CD4 cell count $\leq 300/mm^3$ who were treated with zalcitabine plus zidovudine had a greater CD4 response than patients treated with zidovudine alone. Neither study included a concurrent control group taking the currently recommended zidovudine dose of 100 mg every 4 hours, and these studies were not designed to measure the clinical efficacy of the combination. No data are available on the combined use of zalcitabine and zidovudine in patients who have previously received zidovudine monotherapy, although controlled studies are ongoing. Results are also unavailable from controlled studies evaluating the effect of combined use on the clinical progression of HIV infection (such as survival or the incidence of opportunistic infections).

Because zidovudine prolongs survival and decreases the incidence of opportunistic infections in patients with advanced HIV disease, consider zidovudine as initial therapy for adult patients with HIV infection who have evidence of impaired immunity (CD4 cell counts of $\leq 500/mm^3$).

The major clinical toxicities of zalcitabine are peripheral neuropathy and, much less frequently, pancreatitis. Moderate or severe peripheral neuropathy, which for some patients was clinically disabling, occurred in 17% to 31% of patients treated with zalcitabine monotherapy. It is unknown whether the risk of peripheral neuropathy is increased with combination therapy vs monotherapy. There are no data regarding the use of zalcitabine in patients with preexisting peripheral neuropathy since these patients were excluded from clinical trials; therefore, use with extreme caution in these patients. The occurrence of peripheral neuropathy in patients treated with zalcitabine was greater in patients with more advanced HIV disease (see Warnings).

Documented fatal pancreatitis has been observed with the administration of zalcitabine alone or in combination with zidovudine. Suspend the use of both agents immediately in patients who develop any symptoms suggestive of pancreatitis until this diagnosis is excluded. Overall, pancreatitis is an uncommon complication of zalcitabine monotherapy, occurring in $< 1\%$ of patients.

Toxicities previously associated with zidovudine monotherapy are likely to occur in patients treated with combined therapy. Refer to the zidovudine product information before using combination therapy.

Actions:

Pharmacology: Zalcitabine, active against the human immunodeficiency virus (HIV), is a synthetic pyrimidine nucleoside analog of the naturally occurring nucleoside 2'-deoxycytidine in which the 3'-hydroxyl group is replaced by hydrogen. Within cells, zalcitabine is converted to the active metabolite, dideoxycytidine 5'-triphosphate (ddCTP), by cellular enzymes. ddCTP serves as an alternative substrate to deoxycytidine triphosphate (dCTP) for HIV-reverse transcriptase and inhibits the in vitro replication of HIV-1 by inhibition of viral DNA synthesis. Because ddCTP lacks the 3-hydroxyl group required for DNA chain elongation, its incorporation into a growing DNA chain leads to premature chain termination. ddCTP serves as a competitive inhibitor of the natural substrate dCTP for the active site of the viral reverse transcriptase, and thus further inhibits viral DNA synthesis. The active metabolite, ddCTP, also has a high affinity for cellular mitochondrial DNA polymerase gamma and appears to be incorporated into the DNA of cells in culture. However, DNA chain termination with cellular DNA polymerases has not been demonstrated. The half-life of ddCTP in established cell lines and in human peripheral blood mononuclear cells in culture is in the range of 2.6 to 10 hours.

(Actions continued on following page)

ZALCITABINE (Dideoxycytidine; ddC) (Cont.)

Actions (Cont.):

Microbiology: The anti-HIV activity of zalcitabine was determined in a variety of human T-cell lines infected with different strains of HIV. The in vitro anti-HIV activity of zalcitabine varied greatly depending on the time between virus infection and zalcitabine treatment of cell cultures, the ratio of the number of infectious virus particles to the number of cells, the kind of assay and the cell type used. In vitro, the concentration of zalcitabine required to inhibit HIV-1 replication by 50% (ID_{50}) was generally in the range of 30 to 500 nM (1 nM = 0.21 ng/ml). In these cell lines, > 95% inhibition of viral replication was achieved with 100 to 1000 nM zalcitabine. Comparative studies of the antiviral activity of zalcitabine against HIV-1 and HIV-2 in vitro revealed no significant difference in sensitivity between the two viruses when activity was determined by measuring viral cytopathic effect. The relationship of the in vitro inhibition of HIV by zalcitabine to the inhibition of HIV replication in infected people, or the clinical response to therapy, has not been established.

In vitro combination studies have demonstrated that zalcitabine and zidovudine have an additive or synergistic antiviral effect, depending on the cell line used, without increased cytotoxicity over that observed for either agent alone. Combination therapy of zalcitabine plus zidovudine does not appear to prevent the emergence of zidovudine-resistant isolates. However, studies with zidovudine-resistant virus isolates indicate zidovudine-resistant strains remain sensitive to zalcitabine.

Pharmacokinetics: Adults – Absorption/Distribution: Following oral administration to HIV-infected patients, the mean absolute bioavailability of zalcitabine was > 80%. The absorption rate of a 1.5 mg oral dose was reduced when administered with food. This resulted in a 39% decrease in mean maximum plasma concentrations (C_{max}) from 25.2 to 15.5 ng/ml, and a twofold increase in time to achieve C_{max} from a mean of 0.8 hours under fasting conditions to 1.6 hours when the drug was given with food. The extent of absorption was decreased by 14% (from 72 to 62 ng • hr/ml).

The steady-state volume of distribution following IV administration of a 1.5 mg dose averaged 0.534 L/kg. Cerebrospinal fluid obtained from 9 patients at 2 to 3.5 hours following 0.06 or 0.09 mg/kg IV infusion showed measurable concentrations of zalcitabine. The CSF:plasma concentration ratio ranged from 9% to 37% (mean, 20%), demonstrating penetration of the drug through the blood-brain barrier.

Metabolism/Elimination: Zalcitabine is phosphorylated intracellularly to zalcitabine triphosphate, the active substrate for HIV-reverse transcriptase. Concentrations of zalcitabine triphosphate are too low for quantitation. Metabolism has not been fully evaluated. Zalcitabine does not appear to undergo a significant degree of metabolism by the liver. Renal excretion appears to be the primary route of elimination, and accounted for approximately 70% of an orally administered dose within 24 hours after dosing. The mean elimination half-life is 2 hours and generally ranges from 1 to 3 hours. Total body clearance following an IV dose averages 285 ml/min. Less than 10% of a dose appears in the feces.

In patients with impaired kidney function, prolonged elimination of zalcitabine may be expected. Results from 7 patients with renal impairment (estimated Ccr < 55 ml/min) indicate that the half-life was prolonged (up to 8.5 hours) in these patients compared to those with normal renal function. C_{max} was higher in some patients after a single dose. In patients with normal renal function, the pharmacokinetics of zalcitabine were not altered during three times daily multiple dosing. Accumulation of drug in plasma during this regimen was negligible. The drug was < 4% bound to plasma proteins, indicating that drug interactions involving binding-site displacement are unlikely (see Drug Interactions).

Children – Limited pharmacokinetic data have been reported for five HIV-positive children using doses of 0.03 and 0.04 mg/kg administered orally every 6 hours. The mean bioavailability of zalcitabine in this study was 54% and mean apparent systemic clearance was 150 ml/min/m^2.

Clinical trials: The combined use of zalcitabine and zidovudine is based on limited data from two small studies. The first was a Phase 1/2, open-label, dose-ranging study that evaluated several dose combinations of zalcitabine and zidovudine. The second study was a randomized Phase 2 study designed to evaluate the virologic and immunologic effects of the combined administration of two nucleoside analogs (zidovudine combined with either zalcitabine or didanosine).

(Actions continued on following page)

ZALCITABINE (Dideoxycytidine; ddC) (Cont.)

Actions (Cont.):

Clinical trials (Cont.):

Analysis of CD4 cell counts in combination trials – The activity of combination zalcitabine and zidovudine was assessed using CD4 cell counts as a marker of biologic activity. In controlled trials, zidovudine monotherapy was associated with clinical benefit (improved survival and decreased incidence of opportunistic infection) and transient increases in CD4 cell counts. Evidence of efficacy of zalcitabine in combination with zidovudine is based only on improvements in CD4 cell counts. Analyses included the following:

1. Mean change from baseline in CD4 cell counts at various times during therapy.
2. Longitudinal changes during study: Time weighted average of serial CD4 cell counts adjusted (normalized) for baseline CD4 cell counts (NAUC). NAUC = Cumulative AUC of CD4 cell count up to time t/baseline CD4 count x t. NAUCs that exceed a value of 1 indicate that the average CD4 level during therapy is increased over the baseline CD4 cell count.
3. Presence of a "response" where response was defined as one of the following: a) The greater of either a 75-cell or 75% increase over baseline CD4 cell count maintained for a minimum of two consecutive visits at least 21 days apart (75:75 response) or b) the greater of either a 50-cell or 50% increase over baseline CD4 cell count maintained for a minimum of two consecutive visits at least 21 days apart (50:50 response).

Response Analyses to Zalcitabine/Zidovudine (ZDV) Combinations

Response	Zalcitabine + ZDV vs ZDV alone		No prior ZDV	Zalcitabine + ZDV
	Zalcitabine 0.75 mg q8h + ZDV 200 mg q8h	ZDV 200 mg q8h	ZDV[1] 200 mg q4h	Four pooled combination arms[2]
Mean peak increase in CD4	+94 cells/mm³ (week 8)	+53 cells/mm³ (week 12)	+57 cells/mm³ (week 4)	+97 cells/mm³ (week 4)
Week 12				
NAUC > 1	84%	72%	87%	97%
Median NAUC	1.4	1.2	1.5	2.37
25:25	—	—	47%	82%
50:50	—	—	29%	70%
75:75	—	—	13%	46%
Week 24				
NAUC > 1	89%	68%	81%	97%
Median NAUC	1.5	1.3	1.39	2.1
25:25	51%	43%	54%	85%
50:50	38%	21%	34%	70%
75:75	31%	9%	18%	49%

[1] Reduced to 100 mg every 4 hours ZDV when dose was approved.

[2] The pooled concomitant regimens of zalcitabine + ZDV included:
Zalcitabine 0.005 mg/kg every 8 hours + ZDV 100 mg every 8 hours.
Zalcitabine 0.005 mg/kg every 8 hours + ZDV 200 mg every 8 hours.
Zalcitabine 0.01 mg/kg every 8 hours + ZDV 100 mg every 8 hours.
Zalcitabine 0.01 mg/kg every 8 hours + ZDV 200 mg every 8 hours.

Additional monotherapy and combination studies – Zalcitabine was studied in two controlled comparative trials of patients with AIDS or advanced ARC (CD4 cell count ≤ 200/mm³) and in a randomized, dose-comparison, expanded-access safety study in patients with advanced HIV disease who were intolerant to zidovudine or who showed evidence of clinical progression while on zidovudine therapy.

Zalcitabine monotherapy in adults with AIDS or advanced ARC and ≤ 3 months of prior zidovudine therapy: This study was terminated on the basis of 1 year survival results that showed a significant difference in survival favoring zidovudine, with 59 deaths in the zalcitabine group vs 33 deaths with zidovudine. One hundred and thirty patients (41%) in the zalcitabine group and 95 patients (30%) in the zidovudine group progressed to a critical event at the time of the 1 year analysis (eg, death or first occurrence of an AIDS-defining opportunistic infection, neoplasm or condition).

Zalcitabine monotherapy in adults with AIDS or advanced ARC and ≥ 48 weeks of prior zidovudine therapy: At the time of this analysis, there were 10 (17%) deaths in the zalcitabine-treatment group and 13 (25%) deaths in the zidovudine group. Nineteen (33%) patients in the zalcitabine group and 17 (33%) in the zidovudine group progressed to a critical event (ie, death or first occurrence of an AIDS-defining opportunistic infection, neoplasm or condition). Due to the small number of patients enrolled in this study, definitive conclusions cannot be reached.

(Actions continued on following page)

ZALCITABINE (Dideoxycytidine; ddC) (Cont.)

Actions (Cont.):

Clinical trials (Cont.):

Additional monotherapy and combination studies (Cont.) –

Expanded-access safety study of zalcitabine therapy in adult patients with advanced HIV disease who are intolerant to zidovudine or had failed zidovudine therapy: An interim analysis was performed for 3479 patients, 1757 in the zalcitabine 0.375 mg every 8 hours and 1722 in the zalcitabine 0.75 mg every 8 hours groups, with a median duration of treatment of 16 weeks (range, 0.1 to 61). No statistically significant difference in survival was found for the deaths reported at the interim analysis. Subsequently, in survival data on 3920 patients there was a total of 556 deaths (296 in the low-dose group and 260 in the high-dose group).

Alternating trials: Alternating regimens of zalcitabine and zidovudine were studied in two open-label, controlled, multi-arm, dose-ranging trials. One trial evaluated regimens of zalcitabine and zidovudine alternating weekly and alternating monthly. Regimens were also included with zidovudine alternating weekly with no therapy, zidovudine alternating weekly with no therapy and continuous zidovudine therapy. All patients were zidovudine-naive. In one trial, 3 of the 4 alternating regimens had improvements in CD4 cell counts that were higher and sustained above baseline longer than the continuous zidovudine-monotherapy control arm. The occurrence of toxicity in some of the alternating arms was higher than that seen in the monotherapy studies of zalcitabine.

Indications:

Combination therapy with zidovudine in advanced HIV infection: For the treatment of adult patients with advanced HIV infection (CD4 cell count $\leq$ 300/mm^3) who have demonstrated significant clinical or immunologic deterioration.

This indication is based on limited data from two small studies in which zidovudine-naive patients with a CD4 cell count $\leq$ 300/mm^3 who were treated with zalcitabine plus zidovudine had a greater CD4 response than patients treated with zidovudine alone (see Warning box). Because zidovudine prolongs survival and decreases the incidence of opportunistic infections in patients with advanced HIV disease, consider zidovudine monotherapy as initial therapy for adult patients with HIV infection who have evidence of impaired immunity (CD4 cell counts $\leq$ 500/mm^3).

Contraindications:

Hypersensitivity to zalcitabine or any components of the product.

Warnings:

Peripheral neuropathy: The major clinical toxicity of zalcitabine is peripheral neuropathy, which occurred in 17% to 31% of subjects. By comparison, neuropathy occurred in 0% to 12% of zidovudine-treated patients. Data are very limited on the occurrence of peripheral neuropathy with the combined use of zalcitabine and zidovudine.

Zalcitabine-related peripheral neuropathy is a sensorimotor neuropathy characterized initially by numbness and burning dysesthesia involving the distal extremities. These symptoms may be followed by sharp shooting pains or severe continuous burning pain if the drug is not withdrawn. The neuropathy may progress to severe pain requiring narcotic analgesics and is potentially irreversible, especially if zalcitabine is not stopped promptly. In some patients, symptoms of neuropathy may initially progress despite discontinuation of zalcitabine. With prompt discontinuation, the neuropathy is usually slowly reversible.

There are no data regarding the use of zalcitabine in patients with preexisting peripheral neuropathy since these patients were excluded from clinical trials; therefore, use with extreme caution in patients with low CD4 cell counts ($<$ 50/mm^3) for whom the risk of developing peripheral neuropathy while on therapy is greater. Careful monitoring is strongly recommended for these individuals. Avoid zalcitabine in individuals with moderate or severe peripheral neuropathy, as evidenced by symptoms accompanied by objective findings.

Promptly discontinue the drug when moderate discomfort from numbness, tingling, burning or pain of the extremities progresses, or any related symptoms occur that are accompanied by an objective finding. In a large ongoing clinical trial, peripheral neuropathy requiring zalcitabine interruption is defined as moderate discomfort of the lower extremities (requiring non-narcotic analgesics) that is bilateral and persists for $\geq$ 3 days, or mild symptoms accompanied by the loss of a previously present Achilles reflex. If symptoms resolve to mild intensity, rechallenge with half-dosage is permitted. Peripheral neuropathy requiring permanent discontinuation of zalcitabine has been defined in clinical trials as any severe discomfort of the extremities requiring narcotic analgesics or moderate discomfort progressing for $\geq$ 1 week.

(Warnings continued on following page)

ZALCITABINE (Dideoxycytidine; ddC) (Cont.)

Warnings (Cont.):

Pancreatitis: Documented fatal pancreatitis has occurred with the administration of zalcitabine alone or in combination with zidovudine. Pancreatitis is an uncommon complication of zalcitabine monotherapy, occurring in < 1% of patients. The occurrence of asymptomatic elevated serum amylase of any etiology while on zalcitabine monotherapy was also < 1%. Of 633 patients treated with zalcitabine in the expanded-access safety study who had a history of prior pancreatitis or increased amylase, 10 (1.6%) developed pancreatitis and an additional 10 developed asymptomatic elevated serum amylase.

Exercise caution when administering zalcitabine to any patient with a history of pancreatitis or known risk factor for the development of pancreatitis. To date, one patient died of fulminant pancreatitis possibly related to zalcitabine or zidovudine. Another patient who received concomitant IV pentamidine and zalcitabine died of fulminant pancreatitis possibly related to the concomitant use of zalcitabine and IV pentamidine.

Follow patients with a history of pancreatitis or a history of elevated serum amylase more closely while on zalcitabine therapy. The significance of an asymptomatic increase in serum amylase levels in HIV-infected patients prior to starting zalcitabine or while on zalcitabine is unclear. Interrupt treatment in patients with a rising serum amylase level associated with dysglycemia, rising triglyceride level, decreasing serum calcium or other parameters or symptoms (eg, nausea, vomiting, abdominal pain) suggestive of impending pancreatitis, until a clinical diagnosis is reached. Also interrupt treatment if another drug known to cause pancreatitis (eg, IV pentamidine) is required (see Drug Interactions). Restart zalcitabine only after pancreatitis has been ruled out. If clinical pancreatitis develops during zalcitabine administration, permanently discontinue the drug.

Esophageal ulcers: Infrequent cases of esophageal ulcers have been attributed to zalcitabine therapy. Consider interruption of therapy in patients who develop esophageal ulcers that do not respond to specific treatment for opportunistic pathogens in order to assess a possible relationship to zalcitabine.

Cardiomyopathy/Congestive heart failure (CHF) has occurred with the use of nucleoside antiretroviral agents in AIDS patients; infrequent cases have occurred in patients receiving zalcitabine. In one case, the exacerbation of preexisting cardiomyopathy was possibly related to zalcitabine. Approach treatment with caution in patients with baseline cardiomyopathy or history of CHF.

Anaphylactoid reaction: There has been one report of an anaphylactoid reaction occurring in a patient receiving both zalcitabine and zidovudine in an alternating regimen. In addition, there have been several reports of urticaria without other signs of anaphylaxis.

Combination therapy: Because severe adverse effects may be attributable to either the zalcitabine or the zidovudine components of combination therapy, or to their combination, consult the complete product information for zidovudine before initiation of combination therapy or reinstitution of monotherapy with zidovudine following an adverse reaction.

Renal function impairment: Patients with renal impairment (estimated Ccr < 55 ml/min) may be at a greater risk of toxicity due to decreased drug clearance. Consider dosage reduction (see Administration and Dosage).

Hepatic function impairment: The use of zalcitabine may be associated with exacerbation of hepatic dysfunction, especially in individuals with preexisting liver disease or with a history of ethanol abuse. Of 85 patients in the expanded-access safety study with a prior history of liver function test (LFT) elevation before starting zalcitabine 10 (12%) developed increases in LFTs > 5 times the upper limit of normal while on zalcitabine. Closely monitor such patients. Consider dose reduction or interruption of drug therapy if necessary. Zidovudine use has also been associated with increases in liver function tests.

(Warnings continued on following page)

ZALCITABINE (Dideoxycytidine; ddC) (Cont.)

Warnings (Cont.):

Mutagenesis: Human peripheral blood lymphocytes were exposed to zalcitabine, and at ≥ 1.5 mcg/ml, dose-related increases in chromosomal aberrations were seen. Oral doses of zalcitabine at 2500 and 4500 mg/kg were clastogenic in the mouse micronucleus assay.

Pregnancy: Category C. Zalcitabine is teratogenic in mice and rats. Increased embryolethality was observed and average fetal body weight was significantly decreased in mice and rats. There are no adequate and well controlled studies in pregnant women. Use during pregnancy only if the potential benefit justifies the potential risk to the fetus. Fertile women should not receive zalcitabine unless they are using an effective contraceptive during therapy.

Lactation: It is not known whether zalcitabine is excreted in breast milk. Decide whether to discontinue nursing or to discontinue the drug, taking into account the importance of the drug to the mother. It is currently recommended practice in the US that HIV-infected women do not breastfeed infants regardless of the use of antiretroviral agents.

Children: Safety and efficacy of zalcitabine in combination with zidovudine or as monotherapy in HIV-infected children < 13 years of age has not been established.

Precautions:

HIV infection complications: Patients receiving zalcitabine or any other antiretroviral therapy may continue to develop opportunistic infections and other complications of HIV infection, and therefore should remain under close clinical observation by healthcare personnel experienced in the treatment of patients with HIV-associated diseases.

Monitoring: Perform complete blood counts and clinical chemistry tests prior to initiating combination therapy with zalcitabine and zidovudine and at appropriate intervals thereafter. Perform baseline testing on serum amylase and triglyceride levels in individuals with a prior history of pancreatitis, increased amylase, those on parenteral nutrition or with a history of ethanol abuse.

Drug Interactions:

Drugs that have the potential to cause peripheral neuropathy: Avoid concomitant use where possible. Drugs which have been associated with peripheral neuropathy include: Chloramphenicol; cisplatin; dapsone; disulfiram; ethionamide; glutethimide; gold; hydralazine; iodoquinol; isoniazid; metronidazole; nitrofurantoin; phenytoin; ribavirin; vincristine. Concomitant use of zalcitabine with didanosine is not recommended.

Drugs such as amphotericin, foscarnet and aminoglycosides may increase the risk of developing peripheral neuropathy or other zalcitabine-associated toxicities by interfering with the renal clearance of zalcitabine (and thereby raising systemic exposure). Patients who require the use of one of these drugs with zalcitabine and zidovudine should have frequent clinical and laboratory monitoring with dosage adjustment for any significant change in renal function.

Drugs that have the potential to cause pancreatitis: Interrupt treatment when the use of a drug that has the potential to cause pancreatitis is required. One death due to fulminant pancreatitis possibly related to zalcitabine and IV pentamidine was reported. If IV pentamidine is required to treat *Pneumocystis carinii* pneumonia, interrupt treatment with zalcitabine (see Warnings).

Drug/Food interaction: The absorption rate of a 1.5 mg dose is reduced when administered with food resulting in a 39% decrease in mean C_{max} and a twofold increase in time to achieve C_{max}. The extent of absorption is decreased by 14%.

(Continued on following page)

ZALCITABINE (Dideoxycytidine; ddC) (Cont.)

Adverse Reactions:

The following data on adverse reactions are based primarily on the administration of zalcitabine at the recommended dose, as a single agent, to patients with AIDS or advanced ARC (CD4 cell count ≤ 200/mm³).

Zalcitabine Adverse Reactions (%)

	≤ 3 months prior ZDV		≥ 12 months prior ZDV		No prior ZDV	ZDV intolerant or failure	
Adverse reaction	Zalcitabine 0.75 mg q8h (n = 320)	ZDV 200 mg q4h (n = 318)	Zalcitabine 0.75 mg q8h (n = 59)	ZDV 100 mg q4h (n = 52)	Zalcitabine & ZDV Combination trial (n = 47)	Zalcitabine 0.375 mg q8h (n = 1757)	Zalcitabine 0.75 mg q8h (n = 1722)
GI							
Oral ulcers	7.8-13.4	3.1-6.3	15.3-16.9	1.9	4.3-27.7	—	—
Nausea	2.8-7.2	8.2-19.5	1.7-3.4	0	8.5-36.2	0.8-1.5	0.9-1.5
Dysphagia	3.1-3.4	0	1.7	0	—	—	—
Anorexia	1.9-3.1	2.5-6	0	0	6.4-12.8	< 1	< 1
Abdominal pain	0.9-2.8	1.6-2.5	3.4-5.1	0	8.5-21.3	0.9-1.3	0.6-1.2
Vomiting	0.9-2.2	3.5-5	1.7	0	2.1-14.9	< 1	< 1
Constipation	< 1	—	—	—	2.1-6.4	< 1	< 1
Ulcerative stomatitis	—	—	—	—	—	0.6-1.4	1.7-2.6
Aphthous stomatitis	—	—	—	—	—	0.6-1.1	1.3-2.2
Diarrhea	2.5	—	—	—	10.6-14.9	0.4-0.9	0.6-1
Dermatologic							
Rash (including erythematous, maculopapular and follicular)	4.1-7.8	3.1-5.3	0	0	≤ 14.9	0.6-1.2	0.6-1.4
Pruritus	2.8-4.7	2.2-5.3	0	0	4.3-14.9	< 1	< 1
Night sweats	< 1	—	—	—	2.1-6.4	—	—
Central/Peripheral nervous system							
Headache	5-8.8	6.6-12.6	0	0	8.5-38.3	0.2-0.7	0.7-1.2
Dizziness	1.3-3.1	1.3-2.8	0	0	—	< 1	< 1
Musculoskeletal							
Myalgia	2.2-5.3	3.1-6.3	1.7	1.9	2.1-14.9	< 1	< 1
Arthralgia	1.9	—	—	—	2.1-8.5	< 1	< 1
Pain, feet	< 1	—	—	—	—	0.3-0.9	1.2-2.1
Other							
Fatigue	3.8-7.8	8.5-12.3	1.7-3.4	3.8	8.5-34	< 1	< 1
Pharyngitis	1.9-2.2	0	3.4-5.1	0	2.1-8.5	< 1	< 1
Fever	< 1	—	—	—	2.1-14.9	< 1	< 1
Rigors	—	—	—	—	2.1-8.5	—	—
Chest pain	1.6	—	—	—	2.1-6.4	< 1	< 1
Weight decrease	1.9	—	—	—	4.3-6.4	< 1	< 1

Other adverse reactions that occurred in the expanded access study (zalcitabine 0.375 or 0.75 mg every 8 hours in patients with zidovudine intolerance or failure) are listed below.

Body as a whole: Pain, malaise, asthenia, generalized edema (< 1%).

Cardiovascular: Hypertension, palpitation, syncope, atrial fibrillation, tachycardia, heart racing (< 1%).

GI: Dry mouth, esophageal ulcers (1.6%); dyspepsia, glossitis (1.3%); rectal hemorrhage, hemorrhoids, enlarged abdomen, gum disorders, increased amylase, flatulence, anorexia, stomatitis, tongue ulceration, dysphagia, eructation, gastritis, GI hemorrhage, pancreatitis (see Warnings), left quadrant pain, salivary gland enlargement, jaundice, esophageal pain, esophagitis, rectal ulcers (< 1%).

Endocrine: Diabetes mellitus, hyperglycemia, hypocalcemia, impotence, hot flushes (< 1%).

Hematologic: Epistaxis (< 1%).

Hepatic: Abnormal hepatic function, hepatitis, jaundice, hepatocellular damage (< 1%).

Musculoskeletal: Arm pain, arthritis, arthropathy, cold feet, leg cramps, myositis, shoulder pain, wrist pain, cold extremities (< 1%).

(Adverse Reactions continued on following page)

ZALCITABINE (Dideoxycytidine; ddC) (Cont.)

Adverse Reactions (Cont.):

CNS: Seizures, ataxia, abnormal coordination, Bell's palsy, dysphonia, hyperkinesia, hypokinesia, migraine, neuralgia, neuritis, stupor, tremor, vertigo, hypertonia, hand tremor, twitching (< 1%).

Psychiatric: Confusion, impaired concentration (1.3%), insomnia, agitation, depersonalization, hallucination, emotional lability, nervousness, anxiety, depression, euphoria, manic reaction, dementia, amnesia, somnolence, abnormal thinking/crying (< 1%).

Respiratory: Coughing, dyspnea, flu-like symptoms, cyanosis (< 1%).

Skin: Dermatitis (1.3%); skin lesions, acne, alopecia, bullous eruptions, follicular rash, flushing, increased sweating, urticaria, erythematous papules (< 1%).

Special senses: Abnormal vision, ear blockage, parosmia, loss of taste, taste perversion, burning/itching eyes, deafness, xerophthalmia, eye pain/abnormality, tinnitus (< 1%).

Urinary: Gout, toxic nephropathy, polyuria, renal calculus, acute renal failure, hyperuricemia, micturition frequency, abnormal renal function, renal cyst (< 1%).

Zalcitabine Laboratory Test Abnormalities

	Monotherapy				Combination therapy		
	≤ 3 Months Prior ZDV (n = 635)		≥ 12 Months Prior ZDV (n = 111)		No prior ZDV (n= 47)	ZDV-intolerant or failure (n = 3479)	
						Zalcitabine	
Lab test abnormality	Zalcitabine 0.75 mg q 8 h (n = 320)	ZDV 200 mg q 4 h (n = 315)	Zalcitabine 0.75 mg q 8 h (n = 59)	ZDV 100 mg q 4 h (n = 52)	Pooled concomitant regimens	0.375 mg q 8 h (n = 1757)	0.75 mg q 8 h (n = 1722)
Anemia (< 7.5 g/dl)	5	14.3	5.1	7.7	8.5	3.5	4.1
Leukopenia (< 1500/mm³)	9.4	12.1	11.9	15.4	2.1	8.8	10.2
Neutropenia (< 750/mm³)	8.8	19.7	5.1	11.5	8.5	9.3	9.5
Eosinophilia (> 1000 or 25%)	5.8	2.3	5.2	0	4.3	2	2.8
Thrombocytopenia (< 50,000/mm³)	4.4	2.9	0	5.8	4.3	3.2	2.3
ALT (> 250 U/L)	10	8.6	8.5	7.7	8.5	2.7	3.3
AST (> 250 U/L)	5.6	5.1	6.8	5.8	4.3	2.4	2.6
Alkaline Phosphatase (> 625 U/L)	3.1	3.2	0	9.6	2.1	2.8	2.3

Overdosage:

In a study in which zalcitabine was administered at doses 25 times (0.25 mg/kg every 8 hours) the currently recommended dose, one patient discontinued zalcitabine after 1.5 weeks of treatment subsequent to the development of a rash and fever.

In the early Phase 1 studies, all patients receiving zalcitabine at approximately six times the current total daily recommended dose experienced peripheral neuropathy by week 10; 80% who received approximately two times the current total daily recommended dose experienced peripheral neuropathy by week 12. There is little experience with acute zalcitabine overdosage and the sequelae are unknown. There is no known antidote for zalcitabine overdosage. It is not known whether zalcitabine is dialyzable by peritoneal dialysis or hemodialysis.

Patient Information:

Zalcitabine is not a cure for HIV infection; patients may continue to develop illnesses associated with advanced HIV infection including opportunistic infections, and zalcitabine does not reduce the incidence or frequency of such illnesses. Since it is frequently difficult to determine whether symptoms are a result of drug effect or underlying disease manifestation, encourage patients to report all changes in their condition to their physician. The use of zalcitabine or other antiretroviral drugs do not preclude the ongoing need to maintain practices designed to prevent transmission of HIV.

Instruct patients that the major toxicity of zalcitabine is peripheral neuropathy. Pancreatitis is another serious and potentially life-threatening toxicity that has been reported in < 1% of patients treated with zalcitabine monotherapy. Advise patients of the early symptoms of both of these conditions and instruct them to promptly report these symptoms to their physician. Since the development of peripheral neuropathy appears to be dose-related, advise patients to follow the prescribed dose. Inform patients that the long-term effects of zalcitabine in combination with zidovudine are presently unknown.

Women of childbearing age should use effective contraception while using zalcitabine.

(Continued on following page)

ZALCITABINE (Dideoxycytidine; ddC) (Cont.)

Administration and Dosage:

Approved by the FDA on June 19, 1992.

Combination therapy with zidovudine in advanced HIV infection: 0.75 mg administered concomitantly with 200 mg zidovudine every 8 hours (2.25 mg zalcitabine total daily dose and 600 mg zidovudine total daily dose). Dose reduction not necessary for patient weights down to 30 kg.

Monitoring: Perform periodic complete blood counts and clinical chemistry tests. Monitor serum amylase levels in those individuals who have a history of elevated amylase, pancreatitis, ethanol abuse, who are on parenteral nutrition or who are otherwise at high risk of pancreatitis. Carefully monitor for signs or symptoms suggestive of peripheral neuropathy, particularly in individuals with a low CD4 cell count or who are at a greater risk of developing peripheral neuropathy while on therapy (see Warnings).

Dose adjustment: Combination therapy – For recipients of combination therapy with zalcitabine and zidovudine, base dose adjustments for either drug on the known toxicity profile of the individual drugs. For toxicities more likely to be associated with zalcitabine (eg, peripheral neuropathy, severe oral ulcers), interrupt or reduce the dose (see Warnings and Precautions). For patients experiencing toxicities more likely to be associated with zidovudine (eg, anemia, granulocytopenia), interrupt zidovudine or reduce the dose first. For any interruption of zalcitabine and especially if zalcitabine is permanently discontinued, adjust the zidovudine dosage schedule from 200 mg every 8 hours to 100 mg as recommended in the complete product information for zidovudine. For severe toxicities or toxicities in which the causative drug is unclear or those persisting after dose interruption or reduction of one drug, interrupt or reduce the dose of the other drug. Since zalcitabine is not indicated for use as monotherapy, consider alternative antiretroviral therapy for patients who are unable to tolerate zidovudine as part of a combination regimen.

Peripheral neuropathy – Patients developing moderate discomfort with signs or symptoms of peripheral neuropathy (eg, numbness, tingling, hypesthesias, burning or shooting pains of the lower or upper extremities, loss of vibratory sense or ankle reflex) should stop zalcitabine, especially when these symptoms are bilateral and progress for $>$ 72 hours. Zalcitabine-associated peripheral neuropathy may continue to worsen despite interruption of therapy. Reintroduce the drug at 50% dose (0.375 mg every 8 hours) only if all findings related to peripheral neuropathy have improved to mild symptoms. Permanently discontinue the drug when patients experience severe discomfort related to peripheral neuropathy or moderate discomfort progressing for $\geq$ 1 week. If other moderate to severe clinical adverse reactions or laboratory abnormalities (eg, increased liver function tests) occur, then interrupt both zalcitabine and zidovudine until the adverse reaction abates. Carefully reintroduce either zidovudine monotherapy or combination therapy at lower doses if appropriate. If adverse reactions recur at the reduced dose, discontinue therapy.

Hematologic toxicities – In patients with poor bone marrow reserve, particularly those patients with advanced symptomatic HIV disease, frequent monitoring of hematologic indices is recommended to detect serious anemia or granulocytopenia (see Warnings). Significant toxicities, such as anemia (hemoglobin $<$ 7.5 g/dl or reduction $>$ 25% of baseline) or granulocytopenia (granulocyte count $<$ 750/mm^3 or reduction of $>$ 50% from baseline), may require a treatment interruption of zalcitabine and zidovudine until evidence of marrow recovery is observed. For less severe anemia or granulocytopenia, a reduction in the zidovudine daily dose may be adequate. In patients who experience hematologic toxicity, reduction in hemoglobin may occur as early as 2 to 4 weeks after initiation of therapy and granulocytopenia usually occurs after 6 to 8 weeks of therapy. In patients who develop significant anemia, dose modification does not necessarily eliminate the need for transfusion. If marrow recovery occurs following dose modification, gradual increases in dose may be appropriate depending on hematologic indices and patient intolerance.

Renal function impairment – Consider dosage reduction as follows: Estimated Ccr 10 to 40 ml/min, reduce the dose to 0.75 mg every 12 hours; estimated Ccr $<$ 10 ml/min, reduce the dose to 0.75 mg every 24 hours.

Rx	**Hivid** (Roche)	**Tablets:** 0.375 mg	Lactose. (Hivid 0.375 Roche). Beige, oval. Film coated. In 100s.
		0.75 mg	Lactose. (Hivid 0.750 Roche). Gray, oval. Film coated. In 100s.

TRIMETHOPRIM (TMP)

Actions:

Pharmacology: Trimethoprim blocks the production of tetrahydrofolic acid from dihydrofolic acid by binding to and reversibly inhibiting the enzyme dihydrofolate reductase. This binding is much stronger for the bacterial enzyme than for the corresponding mammalian enzyme. Bacterial biosynthesis of nucleic acids and proteins is blocked by trimethoprim's interference with the normal bacterial metabolism of folinic acid.

Microbiology: In vitro, the spectrum of antibacterial activity includes common urinary tract pathogens except *Pseudomonas aeruginosa.*

Using the dilution method for determining the minimum inhibitory concentrations (MIC), the MIC for susceptible organisms is ≤ 8 mcg/ml. Resistant species have an MIC of ≥ 16 mcg/ml.

Representative Trimethoprim MICs For Susceptible Organisms	
Bacteria	Trimethoprim MIC (mcg/ml)
Escherichia coli	0.05-1.5
Proteus mirabilis	0.5-1.5
Klebsiella pneumoniae	0.5-5
Enterobacter species	0.5-5
Staphylococcus species (coagulase-negative)	0.15-5

Normal vaginal and fecal flora are the source of most pathogens causing urinary tract infections (UTIs). Concentrations in vaginal secretions are consistently greater (1.6 fold) than those in serum. Sufficient trimethoprim is excreted in the feces to markedly reduce or eliminate susceptible organisms. Dominant fecal organisms (non-*Enterobacteriaceae, Bacteroides* and *Lactobacillus* species), are generally not susceptible.

Trimethoprim acts synergistically with sulfonamides, blocking sequential steps in the biosynthesis of folic acid. See trimethoprim-sulfamethoxazole monograph.

Pharmacokinetics:

Absorption/Distribution – Oral trimethoprim is rapidly absorbed. Mean peak serum levels of approximately 1 mcg/ml occur 1 to 4 hours after a single 100 mg dose. Approximately 44% is serum protein bound. Urine concentrations are considerably higher than blood concentrations. After a single oral dose of 100 mg, urine levels ranged from 30 to 160 mcg/ml during the 0 to 4 hour period and declined to approximately 18 to 91 mcg/ml during the 8 to 24 hour period.

Metabolism/Excretion – Trimethoprim is metabolized less than 20%. The half-life is 8 to 10 hours. Elimination is delayed in patients with renal function impairment and half-life is prolonged. Excretion is chiefly by the kidneys through glomerular filtration and tubular secretion. After oral administration, 50% to 60% is excreted in the urine within 24 hours; ≈ 80% is unmetabolized, and ≈ 4% is detectable in feces.

Indications:

For the treatment of initial uncomplicated UTIs due to susceptible strains including: *E coli, P mirabilis, K pneumoniae, Enterobacter* species, and coagulase-negative *Staphylococcus* species, including *S saprophyticus.*

Perform culture and susceptibility tests. May initiate therapy prior to obtaining test results.

Contraindications:

Hypersensitivity to trimethoprim; megaloblastic anemia due to folate deficiency.

Warnings:

Hematologic effects: Trimethoprim rarely interferes with hematopoiesis, especially in large doses or for prolonged periods. Sore throat, fever, pallor, or purpura may be early indications of serious blood disorders; obtain complete blood counts. Discontinue drug if a significant reduction in the count of any formed blood element is found.

Pregnancy: Category C. Teratogenic in small animals at 40 times the human dose; increased fetal loss occurred with 6 times the human therapeutic dose.

Trimethoprim crosses the placenta, producing similar levels in fetal and maternal serum and in amniotic fluid. In a report of 186 pregnancies in which the mother received either placebo or trimethoprim/sulfamethoxazole, the incidence of congenital abnormalities was 4.5% (3 of 66) for placebo and 3.3% (4 of 120) for the drug combination. There were no abnormalities in 10 children exposed during the first trimester or in 35 children exposed to trimethoprim/sulfamethoxazole at conception or shortly after.

Trimethoprim may interfere with folic acid metabolism; use only when potential benefits outweigh potential hazards to the fetus.

(Warnings continued on following page)

TRIMETHOPRIM (TMP) (Cont.)

Warnings (Cont.):

Renal or hepatic impairment: Use with caution.

Lactation: Following 160 mg twice daily for 5 days, milk concentrations ranged from 1.2 to 2.4 mcg/ml; observed milk:plasma ratios were 1.25. Because it may interfere with folic acid metabolism, use caution when administering to nursing women.

Children: Safety for use in infants < 2 months has not been established. The efficacy for use in children < 12 has not been established.

Precautions:

Folate deficiency: Use with caution. Folates may be administered concomitantly without interfering with antibacterial action.

Drug Interactions:

Phenytoin's pharmacologic effects may be increased by coadministration of trimethoprim, apparently due to inhibition of hepatic metabolism.

Adverse Reactions:

Dermatologic: Rash (3% to 7%); pruritus; exfoliative dermatitis. In high-dose studies, an increased incidence of mild to moderate maculopapular, morbilliform and pruritic rashes occurred 7 to 14 days after therapy began.

GI: Epigastric distress; nausea; vomiting; glossitis.

Hematologic: Thrombocytopenia; leukopenia; neutropenia; megaloblastic anemia; methemoglobinemia.

Miscellaneous: Fever; elevation of serum transaminase and bilirubin; increased BUN and serum creatinine levels.

Overdosage:

Acute:

Symptoms – After ingestion of ≥ 1 g, nausea, vomiting, dizziness, headaches, mental depression, confusion, and bone marrow depression may occur (see Chronic Overdosage).

Treatment – Gastric lavage and general supportive measures. Urine acidification increases renal elimination. Peritoneal dialysis is not effective and hemodialysis is only moderately effective.

Chronic:

Symptoms – Use at high doses or for extended periods may cause bone marrow depression manifested as thrombocytopenia, leukopenia or megaloblastic anemia.

Treatment – Discontinue use and give leucovorin, 3 to 6 mg IM daily for 3 days, or as required to restore normal hematopoiesis. Alternatively, 5 to 15 mg daily of oral leucovorin has been recommended.

Patient Information:

Take for full course of therapy until medication is gone.

Administration and Dosage:

Adults: 100 mg every 12 hours or 200 mg every 24 hours for 10 days.

Renal impairment: If creatinine clearance is 15 to 30 ml/min, give 50 mg every 12 hours. If it is < 15 ml/min, use is not recommended.

Children (< 12): Effectiveness has not been established.

Storage: Protect the 200 mg tablet from light.

				C.I.*
Rx	**Trimethoprim** (Various, eg, Biocraft, Major, Moore, Parmed, Rugby, Schein)	**Tablets:** 100 mg	In 14s, 30s, 100s and UD 100s.	14+
Rx	**Proloprim** (Burroughs Wellcome)		(Proloprim 09A). White, scored. In 100s.	66
Rx	**Trimpex** (Roche)		(Trimpex 100 Roche). White, scored. In 100s and Tel-E-Dose 100s.	68
Rx	**Trimethoprim** (Various, eg, Biocraft, Moore, Rugby,)	**Tablets:** 200 mg	In 100s.	9
Rx	**Proloprim** (Burroughs Wellcome)		(Proloprim 200). Yellow, scored. In 100s.	132

* Cost Index based on cost per 100 mg.

TRIMETHOPRIM AND SULFAMETHOXAZOLE (Co-Trimoxazole; TMP-SMZ)

See also individual monographs for trimethoprim and sulfonamides.

Actions:

Pharmacology: Sulfamethoxazole (SMZ) inhibits bacterial synthesis of dihydrofolic acid by competing with para-aminobenzoic acid. Trimethoprim (TMP) blocks the production of tetrahydrofolic acid by inhibiting the enzyme dihydrofolate reductase. Thus, this combination blocks two consecutive steps in the bacterial biosynthesis of essential nucleic acids and proteins. In vitro, bacterial resistance develops more slowly with this combination than with either drug alone.

Pharmacokinetics: Absorption/Distribution – Rapidly and completely absorbed following oral administration. Peak plasma levels occur in 1 to 4 hours following oral administration and 1 to 1.5 hours after IV infusion. The 1:5 ratio of TMP to SMZ achieves an approximate 1:20 ratio of peak serum concentrations. Detectable amounts of TMP–SMZ are present in the blood 24 hours after administration. During 3 days of administration of 160 mg TMP/800 mg SMZ twice daily, the mean steady-state plasma TMP concentration was 1.72 mcg/ml. The steady-state mean plasma levels of free and total SMZ were 57.4 mcg/ml and 68 mcg/ml, respectively. Approximately 44% of TMP and 70% of SMZ are protein bound. Both distribute to sputum, vaginal fluid and middle ear fluid, pass the placental barrier and are excreted in breast milk; TMP also distributes to bronchial secretion. Two to three times the serum concentration of TMP is achieved in prostatic fluid. Therapeutic concentrations are achieved in vaginal secretions, cerebrospinal fluid, pulmonary tissue, pleural effusion, bile and aqueous humor. It is also detectable in breast milk, amniotic fluid and fetal serum. Following oral administration, the half-lives of TMP (8 to 11 hours) and SMZ (10 to 12 hours) are similar. Following IV administration, the mean plasma half-life was 11.3 ± 0.7 hours for TMP and 12.8 ± 1.8 hours for SMZ. Patients with severely impaired renal function exhibit an increase in the half-lives of both components, requiring dosage regimen adjustment.

Metabolism/Excretion – TMP is metabolized to a relatively small extent; SMZ undergoes biotransformation to inactive compounds. The metabolism of SMZ occurs predominantly by N_4-acetylation, although the glucuronide conjugate has been identified. The principal metabolites of TMP are the 1- and 3-oxides and the 3′- and 4′-hydroxy derivatives. The free forms are the therapeutically active forms.

Excretion is chiefly by the kidneys through both glomerular filtration and tubular secretion. Urine concentrations are considerably higher than serum concentrations. Concurrent administration does not affect the excretion pattern of either drug. The average percentage of the dose recovered in urine from 0 to 72 hours after a single oral dose is 84.5% for total sulfonamide and 66.8% for free TMP. Of the total sulfonamide, 30% is excreted as free SMZ, with the remaining as N_4-acetylated metabolite.

Microbiology: The antibacterial activity of TMP–SMZ includes the common urinary tract pathogens except *Pseudomonas aeruginosa.* The following are usually susceptible: *Escherichia coli, Klebsiella* and *Enterobacter* species, *Morganella morganii, Proteus mirabilis* and indole-positive *Proteus* species including *P vulgaris.* The following pathogens isolated from middle ear exudate and bronchial secretions are usually susceptible: *Hemophilus influenzae* (including ampicillin-resistant strains), *Streptococcus pneumoniae, Shigella flexneri* and *S sonnei.*

Indications:

Oral and parenteral: Urinary tract infections (UTIs) due to susceptible strains of *E coli, Klebsiella* and *Enterobacter* species, *M morganii, P mirabilis* and *P vulgaris* – Treat initial uncomplicated UTIs with a single antibacterial agent. Parenteral therapy is indicated in severe or complicated infections when oral therapy is not feasible.

Shigellosis enteritis caused by susceptible strains of *S flexneri* and *S sonnei.*

Pneumocystis carinii pneumonitis in children and adults.

Oral: Acute otitis media in children due to susceptible strains of *H influenzae* or *S pneumoniae.* There are limited data on the safety of repeated use in children < 2 years of age. Not indicated for prophylactic use or prolonged administration.

Acute exacerbations of chronic bronchitis in adults due to susceptible strains of *H influenzae* and *S pneumoniae.*

Travelers' diarrhea in adults due to susceptible strains of enterotoxigenic *E coli.*

(Indications continued on following page)

TRIMETHOPRIM AND SULFAMETHOXAZOLE (Co-Trimoxazole; TMP-SMZ) (Cont.)

Indications (Cont.):

Unlabeled uses: Treatment of cholera and salmonella-type infections and nocardiosis.

TMP 40 mg and SMZ 200 mg daily at bedtime, a minimum of three times weekly or postcoitally has been used to prevent recurrent UTIs in females.

Low-dose TMP–SMZ has been studied in the prophylaxis of neutropenic patients with *Pneumocystis carinii* infections or leukemia patients to reduce the incidence of gram-negative rod bacteremia.

Prophylaxis with TMP-SMZ (320/1600 mg per day) appears beneficial in reducing the incidence of bacterial infection (especially of the urinary tract and blood) following renal transplantation, and may provide protection against *P carinii* pneumonia.

Treatment of prostatitis: Acute bacterial – 160 mg TMP/800 mg SMZ twice daily until patient is afebrile 48 hours; less intensive treatment may be continued up to 30 days. Chronic bacterial – 160 mg TMP/800 mg SMZ twice daily for 4 to 6 weeks; regimens up to 12 weeks have been used.

Contraindications:

Hypersensitivity to trimethoprim or sulfonamides; megaloblastic anemia due to folate deficiency; during pregnancy at term and during lactation (see Warnings); infants < 2 months of age.

Warnings:

Streptococcal pharyngitis: Do not use to treat streptococcal pharyngitis. Patients with group A β-hemolytic streptococcal tonsillopharyngitis have a greater incidence of bacteriologic failure with this combination than with penicillin.

Hematologic effects: Sulfonamide-associated deaths, although rare, have occurred from hypersensitivity of the respiratory tract, Stevens-Johnson syndrome, toxic epidermal necrolysis, fulminant hepatic necrosis, agranulocytosis, aplastic anemia and other blood dyscrasias. Both TMP and SMZ can interfere with hematopoiesis. In elderly patients receiving diuretics (primarily thiazides), an increased incidence of thrombocytopenia with purpura occurred. Discontinue the drug at the first appearance of skin rash or any sign of adverse reaction. Rash, sore throat, fever, arthralgia, cough, shortness of breath, pallor, purpura or jaundice may be early indications of serious reactions. Obtain complete blood counts frequently. If significant reduction in the count of any formed blood element is noted, discontinue therapy.

IV use at high doses or for extended periods of time may cause bone marrow depression manifested as thrombocytopenia, leukopenia or megaloblastic anemia. If signs of bone marrow depression occur, administer leucovorin as required to restore normal hematopoiesis. Oral leucovorin, 5 to 15 mg daily has been recommended.

Pneumocystis carinii pneumonitis in patients with Acquired Immunodeficiency Syndrome (AIDS): Because of their unique immune dysfunction, AIDS patients may not tolerate or respond to TMP–SMZ. The incidence of side effects, particularly rash, fever and leukopenia, in these patients is greatly increased compared with non-AIDS patients.

Renal and hepatic function impairment: Use with caution. Maintain adequate fluid intake to prevent crystalluria and stone formation. Perform urinalyses and renal function tests during therapy, particularly in impaired renal function. Fatal renal failure has occurred.

Elderly: There may be an increased risk of severe adverse reactions, particularly when complicating conditions exist (eg, impaired kidney or liver function, concomitant use of other drugs). Severe skin reactions, generalized bone marrow suppression or a decrease in platelets (with or without purpura) are the most frequently reported severe adverse reactions. In those concurrently receiving certain diuretics, primarily thiazides, an increased incidence of thrombocytopenia with purpura has occurred. Make appropriate dosage adjustments for impaired kidney function.

Pregnancy: Category C. Do not use at term. Sulfonamides readily cross the placenta. Fetal levels average 70% to 90% of maternal levels. Toxicities observed in the neonate include jaundice, hemolytic anemia and kernicterus. Trimethoprim crosses the placenta, producing similar levels in fetal and maternal serum. There are no large, well controlled studies; however, in one study of 186 pregnancies where the mother received either placebo or oral TMP–SMZ, the incidence of congenital abnormalities was 4.5% (3 of 66) in those who received placebo and 3.3% (4 of 120) in those receiving TMP–SMZ. There were no abnormalities in 10 children whose mothers received the drug during the first trimester or in 35 children whose mothers had taken the drug at conception or shortly thereafter.

Because TMP-SMZ may interfere with folic acid metabolism, use during pregnancy only if the potential benefits outweigh the potential hazards to the fetus.

Lactation: TMP–SMZ is not recommended in the nursing period because sulfonamides are excreted in breast milk and may cause kernicterus. Premature infants and infants with hyperbilirubinemia or G-6-PD deficiency are also at risk for adverse effects.

Children: Not recommended for infants < 2 months old. See Indications.

(Continued on following page)

TRIMETHOPRIM AND SULFAMETHOXAZOLE (Co-Trimoxazole; TMP-SMZ) (Cont.)

Precautions:

Use with caution in patients with possible folate deficiency (eg, elderly patients, chronic alcoholics, anticonvulsant therapy, malabsorption syndrome, patients in malnutrition states), severe allergy or bronchial asthma. In G-6-PD deficient individuals, hemolysis may occur; it is frequently dose-related.

Extravascular infiltration: If local irritation and inflammation due to extravascular infiltration of the infusion occurs, discontinue the infusion and restart at another site.

Sulfite sensitivity: Sulfites may cause allergic-type reactions (eg, hives, itching, wheezing, anaphylaxis) in susceptible persons. Although the prevalence of sulfite sensitivity in the general population is probably low, it is more frequent in asthmatics or atopic nonasthmatic persons. Products containing sulfites are identified in the product listings.

Superinfection: Use of antibiotics (especially prolonged or repeated therapy) may result in bacterial or fungal overgrowth of nonsusceptible organisms. Such overgrowth may lead to a secondary infection. Take appropriate measures if superinfection occurs.

Drug Interactions:

Cyclosporine: A decrease in the therapeutic effect of cyclosporine and an increased risk of nephrotoxicity have occurred during concurrent administration of trimethoprim.

Methotrexate: Sulfonamides can displace methotrexate from plasma protein binding sites, thus increasing free methotrexate concentrations. The bone marrow depressant effects of methotrexate may be potentiated.

Phenytoin's hepatic clearance may be decreased (27%) and the half-life prolonged (39%).

Sulfonylureas: The hypoglycemic response to these agents may be increased due to displacement from protein binding sites or an inhibition of hepatic metabolism.

Thiazide diuretics: In elderly patients, concomitant use has caused an increased incidence of thrombocytopenia with purpura.

Warfarin: TMP–SMZ may prolong the prothrombin time of patients receiving warfarin. Monitor coagulation tests and adjust dosage as required.

Drug/Lab test interactions: Trimethoprim can interfere with a serum methotrexate assay as determined by the competitive binding protein technique (CBPA) when a bacterial dihydrofolate reductase is used as the binding protein. No interference occurs if methotrexate is measured by a radioimmunoassay.

TMP-SMZ may interfere with the Jaffe alkaline picrate reaction assay for creatinine, resulting in overestimations of about 10% in the range of normal values.

Adverse Reactions:

Most common: GI disturbances (nausea, vomiting, anorexia); allergic skin reactions (eg, rash, urticaria).

Hematologic: Agranulocytosis; aplastic, hemolytic or megaloblastic anemia; thrombocytopenia; leukopenia; neutropenia; hypoprothrombinemia; eosinophilia; methemoglobinemia.

Allergic: Erythema multiforme; Stevens-Johnson syndrome; generalized skin eruptions; rash; toxic epidermal necrolysis; urticaria; serum sickness; pruritus; exfoliative dermatitis; anaphylactoid reactions; conjunctival and scleral injection; photosensitization; allergic myocarditis; angioedema; drug fever; chills; Henoch-Schoenlein purpura; systemic lupus erythematosus; generalized allergic reactions; periarteritis nodosa.

GI: Glossitis; anorexia; stomatitis; nausea; emesis; abdominal pain; diarrhea; pseudomembranous enterocolitis; hepatitis (including cholestatic jaundice and hepatic necrosis); pancreatitis; elevation of serum transaminase and bilirubin. Tablets taken without food or water have lodged in the esophagus and produced esophageal ulcers.

CNS: Headache; mental depression; convulsions; ataxia; hallucinations; tinnitus; vertigo; insomnia; apathy; fatigue; weakness; nervousness; aseptic meningitis; peripheral neuritis.

GU: Renal failure; interstitial nephritis; BUN and serum creatinine elevation; toxic nephrosis with oliguria and anuria; crystalluria.

Musculoskeletal: Arthralgia; myalgia.

Respiratory: Pulmonary infiltrates; cough; shortness of breath.

Other: The sulfonamides are chemically similar to some goitrogens, diuretics (acetazolamide and the thiazides) and oral hypoglycemic agents. Goiter production, diuresis and hypoglycemia occur rarely in patients receiving sulfonamides. Cross-sensitivity may exist with these agents.

Parenteral therapy: Infrequent – Local reaction, pain and slight irritation on IV administration. Thrombophlebitis has occurred rarely.

(Continued on following page)

TRIMETHOPRIM AND SULFAMETHOXAZOLE (Co-trimoxazole; TMP-SMZ) (Cont.)

Overdosage:

Symptoms: Signs and symptoms observed with either TMP or SMZ alone include: Anorexia; colic; nausea; vomiting; dizziness; headache; drowsiness; unconsciousness; pyrexia; hematuria; crystalluria; depression; confusion; blood dyscrasias and jaundice (late manifestations). High doses or use for extended periods may cause bone marrow depression manifested as thrombocytopenia, leukopenia or megaloblastic anemia. Give leucovorin; 5 to 15 mg/day has been recommended.

Treatment: Treatment includes usual supportive measures. Refer to General Management of Acute Overdosage. Perform gastric lavage or emesis, force oral fluids and administer IV fluids if urine output is low and renal function is normal. Acidifying urine will increase renal elimination of TMP. Monitor patient with blood counts and appropriate blood chemistries, including electrolytes. If significant blood dyscrasia or jaundice occurs, institute specific therapy for these complications. Peritoneal dialysis is not effective and hemodialysis is only moderately effective in eliminating TMP and SMZ.

Patient Information:

Complete full course of therapy. Take each oral dose with a full glass of water.

Maintain adequate fluid intake.

Notify physician of skin rash, sore throat, fever or unusual bruising or bleeding.

Administration and Dosage:

Administration and Dosage of TMP-SMZ

Organisms/Infections	Dosage
Urinary tract infections, shigellosis and acute otitis media:	
Adults	160 mg TMP/800 mg SMZ every 12 hours for 10 to 14 days (5 days for shigellosis).
Children (≥ 2 months of age)	8 mg/kg TMP/40 mg/kg SMZ per day given in 2 divided doses every 12 hours for 10 days (5 days for shigellosis).
Guideline for proper dosage:	Dose every 12 hours:
Weight in kg	Teaspoonfuls / Tablets
10	1 (5 ml) / —
20	2 (10 ml) / 1
30	3 (15 ml) / 1½
40	4 (20 ml) / 2 (or 1 double strength tablet)
Patients with impaired renal function	Recommended dosage regimen:
Ccr (ml/min):	
> 30	Usual regimen.
15-30	½ usual regimen.
< 15	Not recommended.
IV: Adults and children > 2 months with normal renal function for severe UTIs and shigellosis.	8 to 10 mg/kg/day (based on TMP) in 2 to 4 divided doses every 6, 8 or 12 hours for up to 14 days for severe UTIs and 5 days for shigellosis.
Traveler's diarrhea in adults:	160 mg TMP/800 mg SMZ every 12 hrs for 5 days.
Acute exacerbations of chronic bronchitis in adults:	160 mg TMP/800 mg SMZ every 12 hrs for 14 days.
Pneumocystis carinii pneumonitis:	20 mg/kg TMP/100 mg/kg SMZ per day in divided doses every 6 hours for 14 days.
Guideline for proper dosage in children	Dose every 6 hours:
Weight in kg	Teaspoonfuls / Tablets
8	1 (5 ml) / —
16	2 (10 ml) / 1
24	3 (15 ml) / 1½
32	4 (20 ml) / 2 (or 1 double strength tablet)
IV for adults and children > 2 months:	15 to 20 mg/kg/day (based on TMP) in 3 or 4 divided doses every 6 to 8 hours for up to 14 days.
Chancroid (Hemophilus ducreyi infection): Alternative treatment regimen.[1]	160 mg TMP/800 mg SMZ orally twice daily for 7 days.

[1] CDC recommendations: Morbidity and Mortality Weekly Report 1989;38 (S-8):1-43.

(Administration and Dosage continued on following page)

TRIMETHOPRIM AND SULFAMETHOXAZOLE (Co-Trimoxazole; TMP-SMZ) (Cont.)

Administration and Dosage (Cont.):

IV: Administer over 60 to 90 minutes. Avoid rapid infusion or bolus injection. Do not give IM. When administered by an infusion device, thoroughly flush all lines used to remove any residual TMP-SMZ.

Preparation of solution – Infusion must be diluted; add the contents of each 5 ml amp to 125 ml of 5% Dextrose in Water. Do not mix with other drugs or solutions. Use within 6 hours. When fluid restriction is desirable, add each 5 ml amp to 75 ml of 5% Dextrose in Water. Mix solution just prior to use and administer within 2 hours. If solution is cloudy or precipitates after mixing, discard and prepare fresh solution.

Storage: Store infusion at room temperature (15° to 30°C; 59° to 86°F). Do not refrigerate.

	Product	Form	Description	C.I.*
Rx	**Trimethoprim and Sulfamethoxazole** (Various, eg, Balan, Bioline, Geneva, Goldline, Lederle, Lemmon, Major, Moore, Rugby, Schein)	**Tablets:** 80 mg trimethoprim and 400 mg sulfamethoxazole	In 100s and 500s.	2.2+
Rx	**Bactrim** (Roche)		(Bactrim Roche). Green, scored. Capsule shape. In 40s, 100s and UD 100s.	10.5
Rx	**Cotrim** (Lemmon)		White, scored. In 100s, 500s and UD 100s.	3.8
Rx	**Septra** (Burroughs Wellcome)		(Septra Y2B). Pink, scored. In 100s, 500s and UD 100s.	9.6
Rx	**Uroplus SS** (Shionogi)		(S/T SS 510). White, scored. In 100s, 500s and UD 100s.	2.6
Rx	**Trimethoprim and Sulfamethoxazole DS** (Various, eg, Goldline, Lederle, Lemmon, Major, Moore, Parmed, Purepac, Rugby, Schein, URL)	**Tablets, Double Strength:** 160 mg trimethoprim and 800 mg sulfamethoxazole	In 20s, 100s and 500s.	1+
Rx	**Bactrim DS** (Roche)		(Bactrim-DS Roche). White, scored. Capsule shape. In 20s, 100s, 250s, 500s and UD 100s.	8.7
Rx	**Cotrim D.S.** (Lemmon)		White, scored. Oval. In 100s, 500s and UD 100s.	3
Rx	**Septra DS** (Burroughs Wellcome)		(Septra DS O2C). Pink, scored. Oval. In 20s, 100s, 250s and UD 100s.	7.9
Rx	**Sulfatrim DS** (Schein)		In 100s.	1.2+
Rx	**Uroplus DS** (Shionogi)		(S/T DS 511). White, scored. In 20s, 100s, 500s, UD 100s.	1.7

* Cost Index based on cost per 160 mg trimethoprim with 800 mg sulfamethoxazole.

(Continued on following page)

TRIMETHOPRIM AND SULFAMETHOXAZOLE (Co-Trimoxazole; TMP-SMZ) (Cont.) C.I.*

	Product	Formulation	How supplied	C.I.*
Rx	**Trimethoprim and Sulfamethoxazole** (Various, eg, Balan, Bioline, Geneva, Lederle, Major, Moore, Purepac, Rugby, Schein, URL)	**Oral Suspension:** 40 mg trimethoprim and 200 mg sulfamethoxazole per 5 ml	In 150, 200 and 480 ml.	4.6+
Rx	**Bactrim** (Roche)		Regular: Fruit-licorice flavor. In 480 ml.[1]	7.3
			Pediatric: Cherry flavor. In 100 and 480 ml.[1]	7.3
Rx	**Cotrim Pediatric** (Lemmon)		Cherry flavor. In 480 ml.	2.7
Rx	**Septra** (Burroughs Wellcome)		Cherry flavor in 20, 100, 150, 200 and 473 ml.[2] Grape flavor in 473 ml.	5.9
Rx	**Sulfatrim** (Various, eg, Goldline, Schein, URL)		In 480 ml.	2+
Rx	**Trimethoprim and Sulfamethoxazole** (DuPont)	**Infusion:** 80 mg trimethoprim and 400 mg sulfamethoxazole per 5 ml	In 5, 10 and 30 ml vials.	61
Rx	**Bactrim I.V.** (Roche)		In 5 ml amps and 5, 10, 30 and 50 ml vials.[3]	14
Rx	**Cotrim IV** (Lemmon)		In 5, 10 and 30 ml vials.	27
Rx	**Septra IV** (Burroughs Wellcome)		In 5 ml amps, 5, 10, 20 and 50 ml vials and 5 and 10 ml Add-Vantage vials.	59
Rx	**Sulfamethoprim** (Quad)		In 5, 10, 30 and 50 ml vials.	100

* Cost Index based on cost per 160 mg trimethoprim with 800 mg sulfamethoxazole.

[1] With 0.3% alcohol, saccharin, sorbitol, sucrose, EDTA.

[2] With 0.26% alcohol, saccharin and sorbitol.

[3] With 40% propylene glycol, 10% ethyl alcohol, 0.3% diethanolamine, 0.1% sodium metabisulfite and 1% benzyl alcohol.

ERYTHROMYCIN ETHYLSUCCINATE AND SULFISOXAZOLE

For complete information on each of the components refer to Erythromycin and sulfisoxazole individual monographs.

Indications:

Children: Acute otitis media caused by susceptible strains of *Hemophilus influenzae.*

Administration and Dosage:

Do not administer to infants < 2 months old; systemic sulfonamides are contraindicated in this age group.

Acute otitis media: 50 mg/kg/day erythromycin and 150 mg/kg/day (to a maximum of 6 g/day), sulfisoxazole. Give in equally divided doses 4 times daily for 10 days. Administer without regard to meals. The following dosage schedule is recommended:

Erythromycin/Sulfisoxazole Dosage Based on Weight		
Weight		
kg	lb	Dose (every 6 hours)
<8	<18	Adjust dosage by body weight
8	18	2.5 ml
16	35	5 ml
24	53	7.5 ml
>45	>100	10 ml

	Product	Description	Package	C.I.*
Rx	**Erythromycin and Sulfisoxasole** (Various, eg, Barr, Geneva Marsam, Goldline, Harber, Lederle, Major, Moore, Rugby, Schein, URL	**Granules for Oral Suspension:** Erythromycin ethylsuccinate (equivalent to 200 mg erythromycin activity) and sulfisoxazole acetyl (equivalent to 600 mg sulfisoxazole) per 5 ml when reconstituted	In 100, 150 and 200 ml.	1+
Rx	**Eryzole** (Alra)		Sucrose. Strawberry flavor. In 100, 150 and 200 ml.	40
Rx	**Pediazole** (Ross)		Sucrose. Strawberry-banana flavor. In 100, 150, 200 and 250 ml.	1.4

* Cost Index based on cost per 200 mg erythromycin with 600 mg sulfisoxazole.

FURAZOLIDONE

Actions:

Pharmacology: Furazolidone exerts bactericidal activity via interference with several bacterial enzyme systems, minimizing the development of resistant organisms. It neither significantly alters the normal bowel flora nor results in fungal overgrowth.

Microbiology: Its broad antibacterial spectrum covers the majority of GI tract pathogens, including *Escherichia coli,* staphylococci, *Salmonella, Shigella* and *Proteus* species, *Aerobacter aerogenes, Vibrio cholerae* and *Giardia lamblia.*

Pharmacokinetics: There are limited data in humans. Previously it was thought that very little drug was absorbed following oral administration. However, recent data indicate significant absorption. It is rapidly and extensively metabolized, possibly in the intestine. Colored metabolites are excreted in the urine.

Indications:

Specific and symptomatic treatment of bacterial or protozoal diarrhea and enteritis caused by susceptible organisms.

Unlabeled uses: Furazolidone 7.5 mg/kg plus oral rehydration therapy for 5 days was more effective than oral rehydration therapy alone in the treatment of acute infantile diarrhea (when fecal leukocytes were present) in children 3 to 73 months of age.

Furazolidone appears effective in the treatment of typhoid fever in adults (800 mg/day for 14 days) and for the treatment of giardiasis in children (67 to 266 mg/day for 10 days).

Furazolidone may also be useful in treating traveler's diarrhea, cholera and bacteremic salmonellosis.

Contraindications:

Do not administer to infants < 1 month of age.

Prior sensitivity to furazolidone.

Warnings:

Pregnancy: Category C. Safety for use during pregnancy has not been established. Use only when clearly needed and when the potential benefits outweigh the potential hazards to the fetus. Theoretically, furazolidone could produce hemolytic anemia in a glucose-6-phosphate dehydrogenase (G-6-PD) deficient neonate if given at term.

Lactation: Safety for use in the nursing mother has not been established. Drug concentration in breast milk has not been determined.

Precautions:

Orthostatic hypotension and hypoglycemia may occur.

Hemolysis may occur in G-6-PD deficient individuals.

Hypertensive crisis: When considering the administration of larger than recommended doses, or for > 5 days, consider the possibility of hypertensive crises.

Monoamine oxidase (MAO) inhibition: Furazolidone inhibits the enzyme MAO. Doses of 400 mg/day for 5 days increased tyramine and amphetamine sensitivity two- to threefold. See Drug Interactions. Use caution if administering with other MAOIs.

(Continued on following page)

FURAZOLIDONE (Cont.)

Drug Interactions:

Furazolidone Drug Interactions			
Precipitant Drug	Object Drug*		Description
Furazolidone	Alcohol	↑	A disulfiram-like reaction (eg, facial flushing, light-headedness, weakness, lacrimation) has occurred. See Adverse Reactions.
Furazolidone	Anorexiants	↑	Increased sensitivity to the pressor response of the anorexiants due to MAO inhibition.
Furazolidone	Levodopa	↑	Both the efficacy and adverse effects of levodopa may be increased, specifically hypertensive crisis. This may occur for several weeks after stopping furazolidone.
Furazolidone	Meperidine	↑	Effects are difficult to characterize, but may include agitation, seizures, diaphoresis, fever and progress to coma and apnea.
Furazolidone	Sympathomimetics (indirect and mixed)	↑	Increased pressor sensitivity to the indirect- and mixed-acting sympathomimetics due to MAO inhibition. Direct-acting agents are not affected.
Furazolidone	Tricyclic antidepessants	↑	Variable effects, including hypertension, hyperpyrexia, seizures, tachycardia; acute psychosis has occurred.

* ↑ = Object drug increased.

Drug/Food interactions: Patients taking furazolidone may experience marked elevation of blood pressure, hypertensive crisis or hemorrhagic strokes if foods high in amine content are consumed concurrently or after therapy. For a list of foods, see the MAOI group monograph.

Adverse Reactions:

Allergic: Hypotension; urticaria; fever; arthralgia; vesicular morbilliform rash. These reactions subsided following withdrawal of the drug.

GI: Colitis; proctitis; anal pruritus; staphylococcic enteritis. Nausea or emesis occurs occasionally and may be minimized or eliminated by reducing or withdrawing the drug.

CNS: Headache; malaise.

Disulfiram-like reaction: Rarely, individuals have exhibited a disulfiram-like reaction to alcohol characterized by flushing, fever, dyspnea, and in some instances, chest tightness. All symptoms disappeared within 24 hours with no lasting ill effects. During 9 years of clinical use, 43 cases have been reported (14 under experimental conditions with doses in excess of those recommended). Three experienced hypotension necessitating active therapy. Norepinephrine may be used for hypotensive episodes, since it is not potentiated by furazolidone. Avoid indirectly acting pressor agents. Avoid ingestion of alcohol in any form during therapy and for 4 days thereafter.

Hematologic: May cause mild reversible intravascular hemolysis in G-6-PD deficient patients. Observe patients closely; discontinue the drug if there is any indication of hemolysis.

Do not administer to infants $<$ 1 month of age because of possible hemolytic anemia due to immature enzyme systems (glutathione instability).

Other: Renal or hepatic toxicity have not been significant with furazolidone.

(Continued on following page)

FURAZOLIDONE (Cont.)

Patient Information:

Avoid ingestion of alcohol during and within 4 days after furazolidone therapy (a disulfiram-like reaction may occur; see Adverse Reactions).

Avoid foods containing tyramine, especially if therapy extends beyond 5 days (see Drug Interactions).

Avoid over-the-counter or prescription medications containing sympathomimetic drugs (eg, cold and hay fever remedies, anorexiants).

Medication may color the urine brown.

May cause nausea, vomiting or headache. Notify physician if these symptoms become severe.

Administration and Dosage:

Dosage is based on an average dose of 5 mg/kg/day given in 4 equally divided doses. Do not exceed 8.8 mg/kg/day due to the possibility of nausea and emesis. If these are severe, reduce dosage.

Adults: 100 mg 4 times daily.

Children: (≥ 5 years of age) – 25 to 50 mg 4 times daily (tablet or liquid).
(1 to 4 years) – 17 to 25 mg 4 times daily (liquid).
(1 month to 1 year) – 8 to 17 mg 4 times daily (liquid).

If satisfactory clinical response is not obtained within 7 days, the pathogen is refractory to furazolidone; discontinue the drug. Adjunctive therapy with other antibacterial agents or bismuth salts is not contraindicated.

				C.I.*
Rx	**Furoxone** (Procter & Gamble Pharm.)	**Tablets:** 100 mg	Sucrose. (Eaton 072). Green, scored. In 20s and 100s.	2.4
		Liquid: 50 mg per 15 ml	Saccharin. In 60 and 473 ml.	5.6

* Cost Index based on cost per 100 mg.

PENTAMIDINE ISETHIONATE

Actions:

Pharmacology: Pentamidine isethionate, an aromatic diamidine antiprotozoal agent, has activity against *Pneumocystis carinii.* The mode of action is not fully understood. In vitro studies indicate that the drug interferes with nuclear metabolism and inhibits the synthesis of DNA, RNA, phospholipids and protein synthesis.

Pharmacokinetics: Absorption/Distribution – Pentamidine is well absorbed after IM administration. It is detectable in the blood briefly, due to extensive tissue binding.

The mean concentrations of pentamidine determined 18 to 24 hours after inhalation therapy were 23.2 ng/ml in bronchoalveolar lavage fluid and 705 ng/ml in sediment after administration of a 300 mg single dose via the Respirgard® II nebulizer. The mean concentrations of pentamidine determined 18 to 24 hours after a 4 mg/kg IV dose were 2.6 ng/ml in bronchoalveolar lavage fluid and 9.3 ng/ml in sediment. In the patients who received aerosolized pentamidine, the peak plasma levels of pentamidine were at or below the lower limit of detection of the assay (2.3 ng/ml).

Metabolism/Excretion – Approximately ⅓ of the dose is excreted unchanged by the kidneys in the first 6 hours; however, small amounts are found in the urine up to 6 to 8 weeks following administration. Pentamidine may accumulate in renal failure. Following a single 2 hour IV infusion of 4 mg/kg of pentamidine the mean maximum plasma concentration, half-life and clearance were 612 ± 371 ng/ml, 6.4 ± 1.3 hr and 248 ± 91 L/hr respectively.

Plasma concentrations after aerosol administration are substantially lower than those observed after a comparable IV dose. The extent of pentamidine accumulation and distribution following chronic inhalation therapy are not known.

Indications:

Injection: Treatment of *Pneumocystis carinii* pneumonia (PCP).

Inhalation: Prevention of PCP in high-risk, HIV-infected patients defined by one or both of the following criteria:

1) a history of one or more episodes of PCP
2) a peripheral CD4+ (T4 helper/inducer) lymphocyte count ≤ 200 cu mm.

Unlabeled uses: Pentamidine has been used in the treatment of trypanosomiasis and visceral leishmaniasis.

Contraindications:

Injection: Once the diagnosis of PCP has been established, there are no absolute contraindications to the use of pentamidine.

Inhalation: Patients with a history of an anaphylactic reaction to inhaled or parenteral pentamidine isethionate.

Warnings:

Development of acute PCP still exists in patients receiving pentamidine prophylaxis. Therefore, any patient with symptoms suggestive of the presence of a pulmonary infection, including but not limited to dyspnea, fever or cough, should receive a thorough medical evaluation and appropriate diagnostic tests for possible acute PCP and for other opportunistic and non-opportunistic pathogens. The use of pentamidine may alter the clinical and radiographic features of PCP and could result in an atypical presentation, including but not limited to mild diseases or focal infection.

Prior to initiating pentamidine prophylaxis, evaluate symptomatic patients to exclude the presence of PCP. The recommended dose of pentamidine for the prevention of PCP is insufficient to treat acute PCP.

Fatalities due to severe hypotension, hypoglycemia and cardiac arrhythmias have been reported, both by the IM and IV routes. Severe hypotension may result after a single dose. Limit administration of the drug to patients in whom *P carinii* has been demonstrated. Closely monitor patients for serious adverse reactions.

Pregnancy: Category C. Safety and efficacy for use during pregnancy have not been established. Use only when clearly needed and when the potential benefits outweigh the unknown potential hazards to the fetus.

Lactation: It is not known whether pentamidine is excreted in breast milk. Because of the potential for serious adverse reactions in nursing infants decide whether to discontinue nursing or to discontinue the drug, taking into account the importance of the drug to the mother.

Children: Inhalation Solution – Safety and efficacy have not been established.

(Continued on following page)

PENTAMIDINE ISETHIONATE (Cont.)

Precautions:

Use with caution in patients with hypertension, hypotension, hypoglycemia, hyperglycemia, hypocalcemia, leukopenia, thrombocytopenia, anemia, hepatic or renal dysfunction, ventricular tachycardia, pancreatitis, Stevens-Johnson syndrome.

Hypotension: Patients may develop sudden, severe hypotension after a single dose, whether given IV or IM. Therefore, patients receiving the drug should be supine; monitor blood pressure closely during drug administration and several times thereafter until the blood pressure is stable. Have equipment for emergency resuscitation readily available. If pentamidine is administered IV, infuse over 60 minutes.

Hypoglycemia: Pentamidine-induced hypoglycemia has been associated with pancreatic islet cell necrosis and inappropriately high plasma insulin concentrations. Hyperglycemia and diabetes mellitus, with or without preceding hypoglycemia, have also occurred, sometimes several months after therapy. Therefore, monitor blood glucose levels daily during therapy and several times thereafter.

Pulmonary: Inhalation of pentamidine isethionate may induce bronchospasm or cough particularly in patients who have a history of smoking or asthma. In clinical trials, cough and bronchospasm were the most frequently reported adverse experiences associated with pentamidine administration (38% and 15%, respectively of patients receiving the 300 mg dose); however less than 1% of the doses were interrupted or terminated due to these effects. For the majority of patients, cough and bronchospasm were controlled by administration of an aerosolized bronchodilator (only 1% of patients withdrew from the study due to treatment-associated cough or bronchospasm). In patients who experience bronchospasm or cough, administration of an inhaled bronchodilator prior to giving each pentamidine dose may minimize recurrence of the symptoms.

Extrapulmonary infection with *P carinii* has been reported infrequently with inhalation use. Most have been reported in patients who have a history of PCP. Consider the presence of extrapulmonary pneumocystosis when evaluating patients with unexplained signs and symptoms.

Laboratory tests to perform before, during and after therapy:

1. Daily BUN, serum creatinine and blood glucose.
2. Complete blood count and platelet counts.
3. Liver function test, including bilirubin, alkaline phosphatase, AST and ALT.
4. Serum calcium.
5. ECG at regular intervals.

Adverse Reactions:

Injection: 244 of 424 (57.5%) patients treated with pentamidine injection developed some adverse reaction. Most of the patients had acquired immunodeficiency syndrome (AIDS). In the following, "severe" refers to life-threatening reactions or reactions that required immediate corrective measures and led to discontinuation of pentamidine.

Severe: Leukopenia (< 1000/cu mm) 2.8%; hypoglycemia (< 25 mg/dl) 2.4%; thrombocytopenia (< 20,000/cu mm) 1.7%; hypotension (< 60 mm Hg systolic) 0.9%; acute renal failure (serum creatinine > 6 mg/dl) 0.5%; hypocalcemia (0.2%); Stevens-Johnson syndrome and ventricular tachycardia (0.2%); fatalities due to severe hypotension, hypoglycemia and cardiac arrhythmias.

Moderate: Elevated serum creatinine (2.4 to 6 mg/dl) 23.1%; sterile abscess, pain or induration at the IM injection site (11.1%); elevated liver function tests (8.7%); leukopenia (7.5%); nausea, anorexia (5.9%); hypotension (4%); fever, hypoglycemia (3.5%); rash (3.3%); bad taste in mouth, confusion/hallucinations (1.7%); anemia (1.2%); neuralgia, thrombocytopenia (0.9%); hyperkalemia, phlebitis (0.7%); dizziness without hypotension (0.5%).

Each of the following was reported in one patient: Abnormal ST segment of ECG, bronchospasm, diarrhea, hypocalcemia and hyperglycemia.

(Adverse Reactions continued on following page)

PENTAMIDINE ISETHIONATE (Cont.)

Adverse Reactions (Cont.):

Aerosol: Most Frequent – Fatigue, metallic taste, shortness of breath, decreased appetite (53% to 72%); dizziness, rash, cough (31% to 47%); nausea, pharyngitis, chest pain/congestion, night sweats, chills, vomiting, bronchospasm (10% to 23%).

Less frequent – Pneumothorax, diarrhea, headache, anemia (generally associated with zidovudine use), myalgia, abdominal pain, edema (1% to 5%).

Causal relationship unknown (≤ 1%):

Cardiovascular: Tachycardia; hypotension; hypertension; palpitations; syncope; cerebrovascular accident; vasodilation; vasculitis.

Metabolic: Hypoglycemia; hyperglycemia; hypocalcemia.

GI: Gingivitis; dyspepsia; oral ulcer/abscess; gastritis; gastric ulcer; hypersalivation; dry mouth; splenomegaly; melena; hematochezia; esophagitis; colitis; pancreatitis.

Hematologic: Pancytopenia; neutropenia; eosinophilia; thrombocytopenia.

Hepatic: Hepatitis; hepatomegaly; hepatic dysfunction.

Renal: Renal failure; flank pain; nephritis.

Neurological: Tremors; confusion; anxiety; memory loss; seizure; neuropathy; paresthesia; insomnia; hypesthesia; drowsiness; emotional lability; vertigo; paranoia; neuralgia; hallucination; depression; unsteady gait.

Respiratory: Rhinitis; laryngitis; laryngospasm; hyperventilation; hemoptysis; gagging; eosinophilic or interstitial pneumonitis; pleuritis; cyanosis; tachypnea; rales.

Dermatologic: Pruritis; erythema; dry skin; desquamation; urticaria.

Special Senses: Eye discomfort; conjunctivitis; blurred vision; blepharitis; loss of taste and smell.

Miscellaneous: Incontinence; miscarriage; arthralgia; allergic reactions; extrapulmonary pneumocystosis.

Administration and Dosage:

Injection: Adults and Children – 4 mg/kg once a day for 14 days administered deep IM or IV only. The benefits and risks of therapy for more than 14 days are not well defined. Dosage in renal failure should be patient-specific. If necessary, reduce dosage, use a longer infusion time or extend the dosing interval.

Preparation of Solution:

IM – Dissolve the contents of 1 vial in 3 ml of Sterile Water for Injection.

IV – Dissolve the contents of 1 vial in 3 to 5 ml of Sterile Water for Injection or 5% Dextrose Injection. Further dilute the calculated dose in 50 to 250 ml of 5% Dextrose solution.

Infuse the diluted IV solution over 60 minutes.

Aerosol: Prevention of PCP – 300 mg once every 4 weeks administered via the Respirgard® II nebulizer by Marquest.

Deliver the dose until the nebulizer chamber is empty (approximately 30 to 45 minutes). The flow rate should be 5 to 7 L/min from a 40 to 50 pounds per square inch (PSI) air or oxygen source. Alternatively, a 40 to 50 PSI air compressor can be used with flow limited by setting the flowmeter at 5 to 7 L/min or by setting the pressure at 22 to 25 PSI. Do not use low pressure (less than 20 PSI) compressors.

Reconstitution: The contents of one vial must be dissolved in 6 ml Sterile Water for Injection, USP. It is important to use *only* sterile water; saline solution will cause the drug to precipitate. Place the entire reconstituted contents of the vial into the Respirgard® II nebulizer reservoir for administration. Do not mix the pentamidine solution with any other drugs.

Stability and storage: Injection – IV solutions of 1 and 2.5 mg/ml prepared in 5% Dextrose Injection are stable at room temperature for up to 48 hours. Store dry product between 15° to 30° C (59° to 86°F). Protect from light. Discard unused portion.

Aerosol: Use freshly prepared solutions. After reconstitution with sterile water, the solution is stable for 48 hours in the original vial at room temperature if protected from light. Store dry product at controlled room temperature 15° to 30° C (59° to 86° F).

Rx	**Pentam 300** (Lyphomed)	**Injection**: 300 mg per vial	In single dose vials.
Rx	**NebuPent** (Lyphomed)	**Aerosol**: 300 mg	In single dose vials.

EFLORNITHINE HCl (DFMO)

Actions:

Pharmacology: Eflornithine is an antiprotozoal agent for IV injection. Its activity has been attributed to inhibition of the enzyme ornithine decarboxylase. Eflornithine differs from other currently available antiprotozoal drugs in both structure and mode of action. It is a specific, enzyme-activated, irreversible inhibitor of ornithine decarboxylase. In all mammalian and many non-mammalian cells, decarboxylation of ornithine by ornithine decarboxylase is an obligatory step in the biosynthesis of polyamines such as putrescine, spermidine and spermine, which are ubiquitous in living cells and thought to play important roles in cell division and differentiation.

Pharmacokinetics: Following IV administration to humans, approximately 80% of the administered dose is excreted unchanged in the urine within 24 hours, and the terminal plasma elimination half-life is approximately 3 hours. Eflornithine's excretion through the kidney approximates that of creatinine clearance. Therefore, in patients with impaired renal function, dose adjustments are necessary to compensate for the slower excretion of the drug.

Eflornithine does not bind significantly to human plasma proteins. It crosses the blood-brain barrier and produces cerebrospinal fluid:blood ratios between 0.13 and 0.51 (studies in 5 patients).

Microbiology: In tissue culture, eflornithine inhibits growth of *Trypanosoma brucei brucei.* This effect is reversed by the addition of polyamine putrescine to the culture medium.

Eflornithine is active in treatment of African trypanosomal infections in various animal models, including *Trypanosoma brucei gambiense* infection in a monkey model.

Indications:

Treatment of meningoencephalitic stage of *Trypanosoma brucei gambiense* infection (sleeping sickness). Extended follow-up of patients is required to assure adequate further therapy should relapse occur (see Precautions).

Warnings:

Concentrate: Must be diluted before use.

Hematologic effects: Myelosuppression – The safe and effective use of eflornithine demands thorough knowledge of the natural history of trypanosomiasis due to *T brucei gambiense* and of the condition of the patient. The most frequent, serious, toxic effect of eflornithine is myelosuppression, which may be unavoidable if successful treatment is to be completed. Base decisions to modify dosage or to interrupt or cease treatment upon the response to treatment, the severity of the observed adverse event(s) and the availability of support facilities.

Anemia (hemoglobin < 10 g/dl, a decrease of ≥ 2 g/dl hemoglobin during treatment of hematocrit $< 35\%$, or a decrease of $> 5\%$ in hematocrit during treatment) occurred in about 55% of monitored patients, but was generally found to be reversible upon stopping treatment. Many of these patients were chronically anemic prior to the start of therapy.

Leukopenia ($\leq 4{,}000$ WBC/mm^3) occurred in about 37% of the patients monitored. The minimum value usually occurred within 8 days of the start of therapy, and the condition usually resolved after discontinuation of therapy.

Thrombocytopenia ($< 100{,}000$ platelets/mm^3) developed in approximately 14% of the patients in clinical trials. In these patients, thrombocytopenia was reversible with interruption of or after completion of eflornithine therapy.

Seizures: Eflornithine has been temporally associated with seizures, an adverse event that can also be caused by the underlying disease. Seizures occurred in approximately 8% of patients treated with IV eflornithine in clinical trials. The etiology of the seizures (intrinsic meningoencephalitis or drug or combination) has not been determined. Be aware of the potential for seizure activity.

Occasional hearing impairment has occurred. When feasible, it is recommended that serial audiograms be obtained.

Relapse: Due to limited data on the risk of relapse after eflornithine therapy for Stage II *gambiense* trypanosomiasis, physicians are advised to follow their patients for at least 24 months to assure further therapy should relapses occur.

Renal function impairment: Since approximately 80% of the IV dose is eliminated unchanged in the urine, exercise caution in patients with renal impairment.

(Warnings continued on following page)

Antiprotozoals (Cont.)

EFLORNITHINE HCl (DFMO) (Cont.)

Warnings (Cont.)

Fertility impairment: Decreased spermatogenetic effects in rats and rabbits were observed at doses equivalent to one-half the recommended human dose and in mice at approximately twice the human dose.

Pregnancy: Category C. Eflornithine is contragestational in rats, rabbits and mice when given, respectively, in doses 0.5, 0.5 and 2 times the human dose. There are no adequate and well controlled studies in pregnant women. Use during pregnancy only if the potential benefit justifies the potential risk to the fetus. In postnatal studies, retarded development occurred in rat pups on doses slightly higher than the human dose.

Lactation: It is not known whether this drug is excreted in breast milk. Because of the potential for serious adverse reactions in nursing infants from eflornithine, decide whether to discontinue nursing or to discontinue the drug, taking into account the importance of the drug to the mother.

Children: Safety and efficacy in children have not been established.

Precautions:

Monitoring: Perform complete blood counts, including platelet counts, before treatment, twice weekly during therapy, and weekly after completion of therapy until hematologic values return to baseline levels.

Adverse Reactions:

Most frequent: Anemia (55%), leukopenia (37%), thrombocytopenia (14%), see Warnings; diarrhea (9%); seizures (8%), see Warnings; hearing impairment (5%), see Warnings; vomiting (5%); alopecia (3%); abdominal pain, anorexia, headache, asthenia, facial edema, eosinophilia (2%); dizziness (1%).

Four percent of patients died during therapy or shortly after completion of treatment. It could not be established whether these deaths were caused by underlying disease or the use of eflornithine.

Overdosage:

In mice and rats given intraperitoneal doses of 3 g/kg, moderate CNS depression was observed after 2 to 4 hours. Convulsions were observed in 3 out of 10 rats, and 2 of them died within 3 hours following receipt of the drug.

Administration and Dosage:

Trypanosoma brucei gambiense (sleeping sickness): 100 mg/kg/dose (46 mg/lb/dose) administered every 6 hours by IV infusion for 14 days. Administer infusion over a minimum of 45 consecutive minutes. Other drugs should not be administered intravenously during the infusion of eflornithine.

Renal function impairment: In patients with impaired renal function, dose adjustments are necessary to compensate for the slower excretion of the drug. When only serum creatinine is available, the following formula (Cockcroft's equation) may be used to estimate creatinine clearance. The serum creatinine should represent a steady state of renal function:

$$\text{Males:} \quad \frac{\text{Weight (kg)} \times (140 - \text{age})}{72 \times \text{serum creatinine (mg/dl)}} = \text{Ccr}$$

Females: 0.85 x above value

Preparation for IV administration: Eflornithine concentrate is hypertonic and must be diluted with Sterile Water for Injection, USP, before infusion.

Solutions within 10% of plasma tonicity can be produced using 1 part eflornithine concentrate to 4 parts Sterile Water for Injection, USP, by volume as described below.

Using strict aseptic technique, withdraw the entire contents of each 100 ml vial. Inject 25 ml into each of four IV diluent bags, each of which contains 100 ml of Sterile Water, USP. The eflornithine concentration following dilution will be 40 mg/ml (5000 mg of eflornithine in 125 ml total volume).

Storage/Stability: The diluted drug must be used within 24 hours of preparation. Store bags containing diluted eflornithine at 4°C (39°F) to minimize the risk of microbial proliferation. Store undiluted vial at room temperature, preferably below 30°C (86°F). Protect from freezing and light.

Rx	**Ornidyl** (Marion Merrell Dow)	**Injection Concentrate:** 200 mg/ml (as monohydrate)	In 100 ml vials.

DAPSONE (DDS)

Actions:

Pharmacology: Dapsone (4,4-diaminodiphenylsulphone; DDS), a sulfone, is bactericidal as well as bacteriostatic against *Mycobacterium leprae.* The mechanism of action in dermatitis herpetiformis has not been established.

Pharmacokinetics: Absorption/Distribution - Dapsone is rapidly and nearly completely absorbed from the GI tract; peak plasma concentrations are reached in 4 to 8 hours. Daily administration of 200 mg for at least 8 days is necessary to achieve a plateau level of 0.1 to 7 mcg/ml (average 2.3). Approximately 70% to 90% of dapsone is plasma protein bound. Its main metabolite is monoacetyl dapsone (MADDS) which is 99% protein bound. Enterohepatic circulation accounts for appreciable tissue levels of dapsone 3 weeks after therapy is discontinued.

Metabolism/Excretion - Dapsone is acetylated in the liver, and the degree of acetylation is genetically determined. The plasma half-life ranges from 10 to 50 hours (average 28 hours). Repeat tests in the same individual show the clearance rate to be constant. Daily administration (50 to 100 mg) in leprosy patients will provide blood levels in excess of the usual minimum inhibitory concentration even for patients with a short dapsone half-life.

About 70% to 85% is excreted in urine as conjugates and unidentified metabolites. Excretion of the drug is slow and a constant blood level can be maintained with the usual dosage.

Indications:

All forms of leprosy (Hansen's disease) except for cases of proven dapsone resistance; dermatitis herpetiformis.

Unlabeled Uses: Treatment of relapsing polychondritis and prophylaxis of malaria.

Contraindications:

Hypersensitivity to dapsone or its derivatives.

Warnings:

Deaths associated with dapsone administration have been reported from agranulocytosis, aplastic anemia and other blood dyscrasias. Sore throat, fever, pallor, purpura or jaundice may occur.

Perform blood counts weekly for the first month, monthly for 6 months and semiannually thereafter. If a significant reduction in leukocytes, platelets or hematopoiesis occurs, discontinue dapsone; follow the patient intensively.

Anemia: Treat prior to initiation of therapy and monitor hemoglobin. Hemolysis and methemoglobin may be poorly tolerated by patients with severe cardiopulmonary disease.

Hypersensitivity: Cutaneous reactions (especially bullous), include exfoliative dermatitis, toxic erythema, erythema multiforme, toxic epidermal necrolysis, morbilliform and scarlatiniform reactions, urticaria and erythema nodosum. These are some of the most serious and rare complications of dapsone therapy. They are directly due to drug sensitization. If new or toxic dermatologic reactions occur, promptly discontinue sulfone therapy and institute appropriate therapy.

Sulfone syndrome is an unusual and potentially fatal hypersensitivity reaction. It consists of fever, malaise, hepatitis with hepatic necrosis, exfoliative dermatitis, lymphadenopathy, methemoglobinemia and hemolytic anemia.

Leprosy reactional states, including cutaneous, are not hypersensitivity reactions to dapsone and do not require discontinuation (see Precautions).

Usage in Pregnancy: Category C. Extensive, but uncontrolled, experience and two published surveys in pregnant women have not shown that dapsone increases the risk of fetal abnormalities if administered during all trimesters. Because of the lack of controlled studies, use during pregnancy only if necessary.

In general, for leprosy, the United States Public Health Service (USPHS) at Carville, Louisiana recommends maintenance of dapsone. Dapsone has been important for the management of some pregnant dermatitis herpetiformis patients. It is generally not considered to have an effect on the later growth, development and functional maturation of the child.

Usage in Lactation: Dapsone is excreted in breast milk in substantial amounts. Hemolytic reactions can occur in neonates. Because of the potential for tumorigenicity shown in animal studies, discontinue nursing or discontinue the drug.

(Continued on following page)

DAPSONE (DDS) (Cont.)

Precautions:

Hemolysis and Heinz body formation may be exaggerated in individuals with glucose-6-phosphate dehydrogenase (G-6-PD) deficiency, or methemoglobin reductase deficiency, or hemoglobin M. This reaction is frequently dose-related. Give dapsone with caution to these patients or if the patient is exposed to other agents or conditions such as infection or diabetic ketosis capable of producing hemolysis.

Toxic hepatitis and cholestatic jaundice have been reported early in therapy. Hyperbilirubinemia may occur more often in G-6-PD deficient patients. When feasible, baseline and subsequent monitoring of liver function is recommended. If abnormal, discontinue dapsone until the source of the abnormality is established.

Leprosy reactional states are abrupt changes in clinical activity occurring in leprosy with any effective treatment and are classified into two groups.

Type 1 (reversal reaction; downgrading) may occur in borderline or tuberculoid leprosy patients often soon after chemotherapy is started, and is presumed to result from a reduction in the antigenic load. The patient has an enhanced delayed hypersensitivity response to residual infection leading to swelling ("reversal") of existing skin and nerve lesions. If severe, or if neuritis is present, use large doses of steroids and hospitalize the patient. In general, continue antileprosy treatment and therapy to suppress the reaction, using measures such as analgesics, steroids or surgical decompression of swollen nerve trunks. Contact USPHS[1] for advice in management.

Type 2 (Erythema nodosum leprosum, ENL, lepromatous lepra reaction) occurs mainly in lepromatous patients and small numbers of borderline patients. Approximately 50% of treated patients show this reaction in the first year. The principal clinical features are fever and tender erythematous skin nodules sometimes associated with malaise, neuritis, orchitis, proteinuria, joint swelling, iritis, epistaxis or depression. Skin lesions can become pustular or ulcerate. Histologically, there is a vasculitis with an intense polymorphonuclear infiltrate. Elevated circulating immune complexes are considered the mechanism of the reaction. If severe, hospitalize patients. In general, antileprosy treatment is continued. Analgesics, steroids and other agents (ie, thalidomide or clofazimine) available from USPHS[1] are used to suppress the reaction.

Carcinogenicity: Dapsone has been found carcinogenic (sarcomagenic) in small animals.

Drug Interactions:

Rifampin lowers dapsone levels seven to tenfold by accelerating plasma clearance.

Folic acid antagonists such as pyrimethamine may increase the likelihood of hematologic reactions. Weekly concomitant use has caused granulocytosis during the second and third months of therapy.

Para-aminobenzoic acid may antagonize the effect of dapsone by interfering with the primary mechanism of action.

Activated charcoal may decrease the GI absorption and enterohepatic recycling of dapsone.

Probenecid reduces urinary excretion of dapsone, increasing plasma concentrations.

Adverse Reactions:

Hematologic: Dose-related hemolysis is the most common adverse effect, including hemolytic anemia (in patients with or without G-6-PD deficiency). Hemolysis develops in almost every individual treated with 200 to 300 mg dapsone per day. Doses of 100 mg or less in normal healthy individuals and 50 mg or less in healthy individuals with G-6-PD deficiency do not cause hemolysis. Almost all patients demonstrate the interrelated changes of a loss of 1 to 2 g hemoglobin, an increase in the reticulocytes (2% to 12%), a shortened red cell life span and a rise in methemoglobin. G-6-PD deficient patients have greater responses.

Hypoalbuminemia without proteinuria has occurred.

Dermatologic: Drug-induced lupus erythematosus; phototoxicity.

CNS: Peripheral neuropathy is an unusual complication in nonleprosy patients. Motor loss is predominant. If muscle weakness appears, withdraw dapsone. Recovery on withdrawal is usually substantially complete. The mechanism of recovery is reportedly by axonal regeneration. In leprosy, this complication may be difficult to distinguish from a leprosy reactional state.

Other CNS reactions include - Headache; psychosis; insomnia; vertigo; paresthesia.

GI: Nausea; vomiting; abdominal pain; anorexia.

Renal: Proteinuria; the nephrotic syndrome; renal papillary necrosis.

Other: Blurred vision; tinnitus; fever; male infertility; tachycardia; an infectious mononucleosis-like syndrome.

[1] National Hansen's Disease Center; Carville, LA 70721: (504) 642-7771.

(Continued on following page)

DAPSONE (DDS) (Cont.)

Overdosage:

Symptoms: Nausea, vomiting and hyperexcitability can appear a few minutes up to 24 hours after ingestion of an overdose. Methemoglobin-induced depression, convulsions and severe cyanosis require prompt treatment. Headache, hemolysis and permanent retinal damage have occurred.

Treatment: Empty the stomach by aspiration and lavage. In normal and methemoglobin reductase deficient patients, methylene blue, 1 to 2 mg/kg, given slowly IV is the treatment of choice. The effect is complete in 30 minutes, but may have to be repeated if methemoglobin reaccumulates. For nonemergencies, if treatment is needed, methylene blue may be given orally in doses of 3 to 5 mg/kg every 4 to 6 hours. Methylene blue reduction depends on G-6-PD; do not give to fully expressed G-6-PD deficient patients. Hemolysis may be treated by blood transfusions to replace damaged cells. Other supportive measures include oxygen and IV fluids to maintain renal flow.

Use of activated charcoal in intoxicated patients increased the rate of elimination by 3 to 5 times. The half-life of dapsone and MADDS was reduced by 50%.

Administration and Dosage:

Dermatitis herpetiformis: Individualize dosage. Start with 50 mg daily in adults and correspondingly smaller doses in children. If full control is not achieved within the range of 50 to 300 mg daily, higher doses may be tried. Reduce dosage to a minimum maintenance level as soon as possible. In responsive patients, there is a prompt reduction in pruritus followed by clearance of skin lesions. There is no effect on the GI component of the disease.

Dapsone levels are influenced by acetylation rates. Patients with high acetylation rates or who are receiving treatment affecting acetylation may require a dosage adjustment.

Maintenance dosage often may be reduced or eliminated on a strict gluten free diet.

Leprosy: To reduce a secondary dapsone resistance, the WHO Expert Committee on Leprosy recommends therapy be commenced and maintained at full dosage without interruption.

Recommended dosage: The schedule amounts to 50 to 100 mg daily in adults, with correspondingly smaller doses for children.

In bacteriologically negative tuberculoid and indeterminate type leprosy: An adult dosage of 100 mg daily with 6 months of rifampin 600 mg/day is recommended. After all signs of clinical activity are controlled, continue dapsone therapy a minimum of 3 years for tuberculoid and indeterminate patients.

In lepromatous and borderline patients: Administer dapsone therapy in full dosage (100 mg/day) for many years, perhaps for life. The WHO Committee recommends administration for *at least* 10 years after the patient is bacteriologically negative. More than 5 years of continuous therapy is required to render most patients with lepromatous leprosy bacteriologically negative.

Suspect secondary dapsone resistance whenever a lepromatous or borderline lepromatous patient receiving dapsone treatment relapses clinically and bacteriologically. If such cases show no response to regular and supervised dapsone therapy within 3 to 6 months, consider dapsone resistance confirmed clinically. Determination of drug sensitivity after prior arrangement is available without charge from USPHS[1]. Treat patients with proven dapsone resistance with other drugs.

			C.I.*
Rx	**Dapsone** (Jacobus)	**Tablets:** 25 mg. (#Jacobus 102). White, scored. In 100s.	33
		100 mg. (#Jacobus 101). White, scored. In 100s.	9

* Cost Index based on cost per 50 mg.

Product identification code.

[1] National Hansen's Disease Center; Carville, LA 70721: (504) 642-7771.

CLOFAZIMINE

Actions:

Pharmacology: Clofazimine exerts a slow bactericidal effect on *Mycobacterium leprae* (Hansen's bacillus). It inhibits mycobacterial growth and binds preferentially to mycobacterial DNA. The drug also exerts anti-inflammatory properties in controlling erythema nodosum leprosum reactions. Precise mechanism of action is unknown.

Microbiology: Measurement of the minimum inhibitory concentration (MIC) of clofazimine against leprosy bacilli in vitro is not yet feasible. Although bacterial killing may begin shortly after starting the drug, it cannot be measured in patient biopsy tissues until approximately 50 days after therapy starts.

Clofazimine does not show cross-resistance with dapsone or rifampin. Rarely are microorganisms other than mycobacteria inhibited by the drug.

Pharmacokinetics: Absorption/Distribution - Absorption rate ranges from 45% to 62% after oral administration. Average serum concentrations in patients treated with 100 mg and 300 mg daily were 0.7 mcg and 1 mcg per ml, respectively.

Clofazimine is highly lipophilic and is deposited predominantly in fatty tissue and in the reticuloendothelial system. It is taken up by macrophages.

Metabolism/Elimination - After ingestion of a single 300 mg dose, elimination of unchanged drug and its metabolites in urine in 24 hours was negligible. Clofazimine is retained in the human body for a long time. The half-life after repeated doses is estimated to be at least 70 days. Part of the drug recovered from the feces may represent excretion via bile. A small amount is also eliminated in sputum, sebum and sweat.

Indications:

Treatment of lepromatous leprosy, including dapsone-resistant lepromatous leprosy and lepromatous leprosy complicated by erythema nodosum leprosum.

Combination drug therapy has been recommended for initial treatment of multibacillary leprosy to prevent the development of drug resistance.

Contraindications: None known.

Warnings:

GI effects: Severe abdominal symptoms have necessitated exploratory laparotomies in patients receiving clofazimine. Rare reports have included splenic infarction, bowel obstruction and GI bleeding. Death has been reported following severe abdominal symptoms. Autopsies have revealed crystalline deposits of clofazimine in the intestinal mucosa, liver, gallbladder, bile, spleen, adrenals, subcutaneous fat, mesenteric lymph nodes, muscles, bone and skin.

Use with caution in patients who have GI problems such as abdominal pain and diarrhea. Give dosages of more than 100 mg daily for as short a period as possible and only under close medical supervision. If a patient complains of colicky or burning pain in the abdomen, nausea, vomiting or diarrhea, reduce the dose and, if necessary, increase the interval between doses or discontinue the drug.

Usage in Pregnancy: Category C. Clofazimine crosses the human placenta. The infant skin was deeply pigmented at birth. No evidence of teratogenicity was found in these infants. There are no adequate and well controlled studies in pregnant women. Use during pregnancy only if clearly needed and when the potential benefits outweigh the unknown potential hazards to the fetus.

Clofazimine was not teratogenic in laboratory animals at dose levels equivalent to 8 to 25 times the human daily dose. However, there was evidence of fetotoxicity in the mouse at 12 to 25 times the human dose. Skin and fatty tissue of offspring became discolored ≈ 3 days after birth; this was attributed to the presence of the drug in maternal milk.

Usage in Lactation: Clofazimine is excreted in beast milk. Do not administer to a nursing woman unless clearly indicated.

Usage in Children: Safety and efficacy in children have not been established. Several cases of children treated with clofazimine have been reported in the literature.

Drug Interactions:

Dapsone: Preliminary data which suggest that dapsone may inhibit the anti-inflammatory activity of clofazimine have not been confirmed. If leprosy-associated inflammatory reactions develop in patients being treated with dapsone and clofazimine, it is still advisable to continue treatment with both drugs.

(Continued on following page)

CLOFAZIMINE (Cont.)

Precautions:

Skin discoloration due to the drug may result in depression. Two suicides have been reported in patients receiving clofazimine. For skin dryness and ichthyosis, apply oil to the skin.

Adverse Reactions:

In general, clofazimine is well tolerated when administered in dosages no greater than 100 mg daily. The most consistent adverse reactions are usually dose-related and reversible when the drug is discontinued.

Skin: Pigmentation (pink to brownish black) in 75% to 100% of patients within a few weeks of treatment; ichthyosis and dryness (8% to 28%); rash and pruritus (1% to 5%). Less than 1% of patients reported phototoxicity, erythroderma, acneiform eruptions and monilial cheilosis.

GI: Abdominal/epigastric pain, diarrhea, nausea, vomiting, GI intolerance (40% to 50%). Less than 1% of patients reported bowel obstruction and GI bleeding (see Warnings), anorexia, constipation, weight loss, hepatitis, jaundice, eosinophilic enteritis and enlarged liver.

Ocular: Conjunctival and corneal pigmentation due to clofazimine crystal deposits; dryness; burning; itching; irritation.

Other: Discolored urine, feces, sputum or sweat; elevated blood sugar or ESR. Less than 1% of patients reported splenic infarction (see Warnings), thromboembolism, anemia, cystitis, bone pain, edema, fever, lymphadenopathy, vascular pain and diminished vision.

CNS (< 1%): Dizziness, drowsiness, fatigue, headache, giddiness, neuralgia, taste disorder.

Psychiatric (< 1%): Depression secondary to skin discoloration; two suicides have occurred.

Laboratory (< 1%): Elevated albumin, serum bilirubin and AST; eosinophilia; hypokalemia.

Overdosage:

No specific data are available. In case of overdose, empty the stomach by inducing vomiting or by gastric lavage. Treatment includes usual supportive measures. Refer to General Management of Acute Overdosage.

Patient Information:

Take with meals.

Warn patients that clofazimine may discolor the skin from red to brownish black, as well as discoloring the conjunctivae, lacrimal fluid, sweat, sputum, urine and feces. Skin discoloration, although reversible, may take several months or years to disappear after the conclusion of therapy.

Administration and Dosage:

Take with meals.

Clofazimine should be used preferably in combination with one or more other antileprosy agents to prevent the emergence of drug resistance.[1]

Dapsone-resistant leprosy: Give 100 mg clofazimine/day in combination with one or more other antileprosy drugs for 3 years, followed by monotherapy with 100 mg clofazimine/day. Clinical improvement usually can be detected between the first and third months of treatment and is usually clearly evident by the sixth month.

Dapsone-sensitive multibacillary leprosy: Combination therapy with two other antileprosy drugs is recommended. Give the triple-drug regimen for at least 2 years and continue, if possible, until negative skin smears are obtained. At this time, monotherapy with an appropriate antileprosy drug can be instituted.

Erythema nodosum leprosum: Treatment depends on the severity of symptoms. In general, continue basic antileprosy treatment; if nerve injury or skin ulceration is threatened, give corticosteroids. Where prolonged corticosteroid therapy becomes necessary, clofazimine at dosages of 100 to 200 mg daily for up to 3 months may be useful in eliminating or reducing corticosteroid requirements. Dosages above 200 mg daily are not recommended; taper dosage to 100 mg daily as quickly as possible after the reactive episode is controlled. Keep patient under medical surveillance.

Storage: Store below 86°F; protect from moisture.

				C.I.*
Rx	Lamprene (Geigy)	Capsules: 50 mg	Brown. In 100s.	30
		100 mg	(Geigy GM). Brown. In 100s.	27

* Cost Index based on cost per 100 mg

[1] For information about combination drug regimens, contact the USPHS Gillis W. Long Hansen's Disease Center, Carville, LA (504-642-7771).

The following table lists the major parasitic infections, causative organisms and drugs of choice for treatment. For investigational antiparasitic agents available from the Centers for Disease Control, refer to page2057.

Major Parasite Infections

	Infection (common name)	Organism	Drug(s) of Choice
Intestinal Nematodes	Ascariasis[1] (Roundworm)	*Ascaris lumbricoides*	Mebendazole or Pyrantel pamoate
	Uncinariasis (hookworm)	*Ancylostoma duodenale* *Necator americanus*	Mebendazole or Pyrantel pamoate[2]
	Strongyloidiasis (Threadworm)	*Strongyloides stercoralis*	Thiabendazole
	Trichuriasis (Whipworm)	*Trichuris trichiura*	Mebendazole
	Enterobiasis[3] (Pinworm)	*Enterobius vermicularis*	Pyrantel pamoate or Mebendazole
	Capillariasis	*Capillaria philippinensis*	Mebendazole or Thiabendazole
Tissue Nematodes	Trichinosis	*Trichinella spiralis*	Steroids for severe symptoms plus Thiabendazole or Mebendazole[2]
	Cutaneous larva migrans (creeping eruption)	*Ancylostoma braziliense and others*	Thiabendazole
	Onchocerciasis (River blindness)	*Onchocerca volvulus*	Suramin[4]
	Dracontiasis (guinea worm)	*Dracunculus medinensis*	Metronidazole or Thiabendazole
	Angiostrongyliasis (rat lungworm)	*Angiostrongylus cantonensis*	Thiabendazole or Mebendazole
Cestodes	Taeniasis (Beef tapeworm)	*Taenia saginata*	Niclosamide or Praziquantel[2]
	(Pork tapeworm)	*Taenia solium*	Niclosamide or Praziquantel[2]
	Diphyllobothriasis (Fish tapeworm)	*Diphyllobothrium latum*	Niclosamide or Praziquantel[2]
	Dog tapeworm	*Dipylidium caninum*	Niclosamide or Praziquantel[2]
	Hymenolepiasis (Dwarf tapeworm)	*Hymenolepis nana*	Praziquantel[2] or Niclosamide
Trematodes	Schistosomiasis	*Schistosoma mansoni*	Fraziquantel or Oxamniquine
		Schistosoma japonicum	Praziquantel
		Schistosoma haematobium	Praziquantel
		Schistosoma mekongi	Praziquantel
	Hermaphroditic Flukes		
	Fasciolopsiasis (Intestinal fluke)	*Fasciolopsis buski*	Praziquantel or Niclosamide
		Heterophyes heterophyes *Metagonimus yokogawai*	Praziquantel
	Clonorchiasis (Chinese liver fluke)	*Clonorchis sinensis*	Praziquantel
	Fascioliasis (Sheep liver fluke)	*Fasciola hepatica*	Praziquantel or Bithionol[4]
	Opisthorchiasis (Liver fluke)	*Opisthorchis viverrini*	Praziquantel
	Paragonimiasis (Lung fluke)	*Paragonimus westermani*	Praziquantel or Bithionol[4] (alternate)

[1] The following drugs are also indicated in Ascariasis: Piperazine, diethylcarbamazine and thiabendazole.
[2] Unlabeled use.
[3] The following drugs are also indicated in Enterobiasis: Piperazine, pyrvinium pamoate & thiabendazole.
[4] Available from the CDC (see page 444).

Refer to the general discussion of these products on page 2025

MEBENDAZOLE

Actions:

Pharmacology: Mebendazole inhibits the formation of the worms' microtubules and irreversibly blocks glucose uptake by the susceptible helminths, thereby depleting endogenous glycogen stored within the parasite which is required for survival and reproduction of the helminth. Mebendazole does not affect blood glucose concentrations in the host.

Microbiology: Active against *Trichuris trichiura* (whipworm), *Enterobius vermicularis* (pinworm), *Ascaris lumbricoides* (roundworm), *Ancylostoma duodenale* (common hookworm) and *Necator americanus* (American hookworm). Parasite immobilization and death are slow, and complete clearance from the GI tract may take up to 3 days after treatment. Efficacy varies as a function of such factors as preexisting diarrhea and GI transit time, degree of infection and helminth strains.

Pharmacokinetics: Mebendazole is poorly absorbed (5% to 10%) after oral administration. Peak plasma levels are reached in 2 to 4 hours. Following administration of 100 mg of mebendazole twice daily for 3 consecutive days, plasma levels of mebendazole and its primary metabolite did not exceed 0.03 mcg/ml and 0.09 mcg/ml, respectively. Approximately 2% of the drug is excreted in the urine during the first 24 to 48 hours. Most of the dose is excreted in the feces as unchanged drug or primary metabolites.

Indications:

For the treatment of *Trichuris trichiura* (whipworm), *Enterobius vermicularis* (pinworm), *Ascaris lumbricoides* (roundworm), *Ancylostoma duodenale* (common hookworm) or *Necator americanus* (American hookworm), in single or mixed infections.

Contraindications:

Hypersensitivity to mebendazole.

Warnings:

There is no evidence that mebendazole is effective for hydatid disease.

Pregnancy: Category C. Mebendazole was embryotoxic and teratogenic in pregnant rats at single oral doses as low as 10 mg/kg. This drug is not recommended for use in pregnant women. Based on a limited number of women, the incidence of spontaneous abortion, malformation and teratogenesis did not exceed that in the general population. During pregnancy, especially during the first trimester, use mebendazole only if the potential benefit justifies the potential risk to the fetus.

Lactation: Safety for use in the nursing mother has not been established.

Children: Safety and efficacy for use in children $<$ 2 years of age have not been established; consider the relative benefit/risk.

Drug Interactions:

Carbamazepine and **hydantoins** may reduce the plasma levels of concomitant mebendazole, possibly decreasing its therapeutic effect.

Adverse Reactions:

Transient abdominal pain and diarrhea have occurred in cases of massive infection and expulsion of worms.

Fever, a possible response to drug-induced tissue necrosis, has occurred.

Two patients receiving high doses of mebendazole for echinococcosis developed a severe but reversible neutropenia apparently due to marrow suppression.

Patient Information:

Chew or crush tablet and mix with food.

Parasite death may be slow. Removal from digestive tract may take up to 3 days after treatment. Effectiveness depends on factors such as degree of infection or resistance of parasite to treatment, presence of diarrhea and how quickly things pass through the digestive system. Laxative therapy and fasting are not necessary.

If not cured in 3 weeks, a second treatment is recommended.

Pinworm infections are easily spread to others. If one family member has a pinworm infection, treat all family members in close contact with the patient. This decreases the chance of spreading the infection.

Strict hygiene is essential to prevent reinfection. Disinfect toilet facilities daily. Change and launder undergarments, bed linens, towels and nightclothes daily.

(Continued on following page)

MEBENDAZOLE (Cont.)

Overdosage:

GI complaints lasting up to a few hours may occur. Induce vomiting and purging. Refer to General Management of Acute Overdosage.

Administration and Dosage:

The same dosage schedule applies to children and adults.

Tablets may be chewed, swallowed or crushed and mixed with food. No special procedures, such as fasting or purging, are required.

If the patient is not cured 3 weeks after treatment, a second treatment course is advised.

Trichuriasis, ascariasis and hookworm infection: One tablet morning and evening on 3 consecutive days. In one study, treatment with a single 500 mg dose was effective against *Ascaris lumbricoides.*

Enterobiasis: A single tablet given once.

				C.I.*
Rx	**Vermox** (Janssen)	**Tablets, chewable:** 100 mg	In 36s.	470

* Cost Index based on cost per 100 mg.

DIETHYLCARBAMAZINE CITRATE

Actions:

Diethylcarbamazine does not resemble other antiparasitic compounds. It is a synthetic organic compound which is highly specific for several common parasites and does not contain any toxic metallic elements.

The drug is effective against the following organisms: *Wuchereria bancrofti, Onchocerca volvulus, Loa loa* and *Ascaris lumbricoides.*

Diethylcarbamazine has demonstrated a low order of toxicity in animals.

Indications:

Treatment of Bancroft's filariasis, onchocerciasis, ascariasis, tropical eosinophilia, loiasis.

Precautions:

Administer carefully to avoid or to control allergic or other untoward reactions.

Adverse Reactions:

Wuchereria bancrofti: Mild reactions are transient but fairly frequent. Headache, lassitude, weakness or general malaise are most common. Nausea, vomiting and skin rash occasionally occur. These effects are not considered serious and do not usually require discontinuation of therapy. However, it may be necessary to stop therapy when severe allergic phenomena appear in conjunction with skin rash. It has not yet been determined what proportion or type of reactions result from the death of parasites rather than from the influence of the drug.

Onchocerciasis: Facial edema and pruritus, especially of the eyes, are often encountered. Severe reactions may develop after a single dose when intense infestations are treated. In such cases, only 1 dose should be given on the first day, 2 doses the second day and 3 daily thereafter for 30 days. If very severe reactions occur, discontinue the drug and start antihistamine therapy. After 1 or 2 days, therapy may be resumed, but if severe allergic phenomena again supervene, use the drug only with extreme caution.

Ascariasis: Giddiness, nausea, vomiting and malaise may occur more frequently following treatment of ascariasis in children who are malnourished or who suffer from various debilitating diseases.

Administration and Dosage:

Bancroft's filariasis, onchocerciasis and loiasis: Usual dose is 2 mg/kg 3 times a day immediately following meals. When the disease is in the acute stage, continue treatment for 3 to 4 weeks. Recurrences have been more frequent with smaller doses. When, as a public health measure, it is desirable to treat large numbers of patients known to harbor microfilariae, use the same dosage schedule for 3 to 5 days. Laboratory tests in randomly selected patients are helpful in assessing efficacy of therapy.

Ascariasis: Outpatients – 13 mg/kg, given once a day for 7 days, should reduce the number of worms by 85% to 100%. No pretreatment fasting or post-treatment purging is required. Expulsion of ascarids usually begins 1 or 2 days after therapy initiation.

Children – Give 6 to 10 mg/kg 3 times daily for 7 to 10 days. In particularly obstinate cases, an additional course consisting of 10 mg/kg 3 times daily is indicated.

Topical eosinophilia: 13 mg/kg/day for 4 to 7 days.

Rx	**Hetrazan**[1] (Lederle)	**Tablets:** 50 mg	In 100s.

[1] Hetrazan is available without charge from Lederle Labs. For more information, physicians should contact: David H. Wu, MD, Professional Medical Services, Lederle Labs, Middletown Road, Pearl River, NY 10965, 914/732-5000.

Refer to the general discussion of these products on page 2025

PYRANTEL

Actions:

Pharmacology: Pyrantel is a depolarizing neuromuscular blocking agent, resulting in spastic paralysis of the worm. It also inhibits cholinesterases. It is active against *Enterobius vermicularis* (pinworm) and *Ascaris lumbricoides* (roundworm); it is also effective against hookworm.

Pharmacokinetics: Pyrantel is poorly absorbed from the GI tract. Plasma levels of unchanged drug are low. Greater than 50% is excreted in feces as unchanged drug; $\leq$ 7% of the dose is found in the urine as parent drug and metabolites.

Indications:

Treatment of ascariasis (roundworm infection) and enterobiasis (pinworm infection).

Contraindications:

Hepatic disease; pregnancy (see Warnings).

Warnings:

Pregnancy: Do not use during pregnancy unless otherwise directed by a physician.

Children: Safety and efficacy for use in children $<$ 2 years have not been established.

Drug Interactions:

Piperazine: In ascariasis, pyrantel and piperazine are mutually antagonistic; concomitant use, therefore, is unwise.

Theophylline serum levels increased in a pediatric patient following pyrantel pamoate administration. Further study is needed.

Adverse Reactions:

GI and hepatic (most frequent): Anorexia; nausea; vomiting; abdominal cramps; diarrhea.

CNS: Headache; dizziness; drowsiness; insomnia.

Skin: Rash.

Patient Information:

A single dose is required. The dose is based on body weight.

May be taken with food, milk, juice, or on an empty stomach anytime during the day. Be certain to take entire dose.

Using a laxative after taking the drug to facilitate removal of the parasites is not necessary.

Pinworm infections are easily spread to others. If one family member has a pinworm infection, treat all family members in close contact with the patient. This decreases the chance of spreading the infection.

Strict hygiene is essential to prevent reinfection. Disinfect toilet facilities daily. Change and launder undergarments, bed linens, towels and nightclothes daily.

A package insert is available for patients containing the following information: Symptoms of pinworm infestations; how to find and identify the pinworm; pinworm life cycle; how it is spread from person to person.

Administration and Dosage:

A single dose of 11 mg/kg (5 mg/lb). This corresponds to a simplified dosage regimen of 1 ml/10 lb. Maximum total dose is 1 g.

May be administered without regard to ingestion of food or time of day. Purging is not necessary. May be taken with milk or fruit juices.

				C.I.*
otc	**Pin-Rid** (Apothecary)	**Capsules, soft gel:** 180 mg pyrantel (as pamoate)	In 24s.	NA
otc	**Antiminth** (Pfizer Labs)	**Oral Suspension:** 50 mg pyrantel (as pamoate) per ml	Sorbitol. Caramel-currant flavor. In 60 ml.	946
otc	**Pin-Rid** (Apothecary)	**Liquid:** 144 mg pyrantel (as pamoate) per ml	Sucrose, saccharin. Cherry flavor. In 30 ml.	NA
otc	**Pin-X** (Effcon)	**Liquid:** 50 mg pyrantel (as pamoate) per ml	Sorbitol. Carmel flavor. In 30 ml.	NA
otc	**Reese's Pinworm** (Reese)		In 30 ml.	513

* Cost Index based on cost per 750 mg.

Refer to the general discussion of these products on page 2025

THIABENDAZOLE

Actions:

Microbiology: Thiabendazole is vermicidal or vermifugal against *Enterobius vermicularis* (pinworm); *Ascaris lumbricoides* (roundworm); *Strongyloides stercoralis* (threadworm); *Necator americanus* and *Ancylostoma duodenale* (hookworm); *Trichuris trichiura* (whipworm); *Ancylostoma braziliense* (dog and cat hookworm); and *Toxocara canis* and *Toxocara cati* (ascarids).

Thiabendazole's effect on larvae of *Trichinella spiralis* that have migrated to muscle is questionable. It suppresses egg or larval production and may inhibit the subsequent development of those eggs or larvae which are passed in the feces. While the exact mechanism is unknown, the drug inhibits the helminth-specific enzyme fumarate reductase. The anthelmintic activity against *Trichuris trichiura* (whipworm) is least predictable.

Pharmacokinetics: Thiabendazole is rapidly absorbed and peak plasma concentrations occur within 1 to 2 hours. It is metabolized almost completely and appears in the urine as conjugates. In 48 hours, about 5% of the administered dose is recovered from the feces and about 90% from the urine. Most is excreted within the first 24 hours.

Indications:

For the treatment of strongyloidiasis (threadworm infection), cutaneous larva migrans (creeping eruption) and visceral larva migrans.

Although not indicated as primary therapy, when enterobiasis (pinworm) occurs with any of the conditions listed above, additional therapy is not required for most patients. Use thiabendazole only in the following infestations when more specific therapy is not available or cannot be used or when further therapy with a second agent is desirable: Uncinariasis (hookworm: *Necator americanus* and *Ancylostoma duodenale*); Trichuriasis (whipworm); Ascariasis (large roundworm).

Also indicated for alleviating symptoms of trichinosis during the invasive phase.

Contraindications:

Hypersensitivity to thiabendazole.

Warnings:

Hypersensitivity: If hypersensitivity reactions occur, discontinue the drug immediately. Erythema multiforme has been associated with therapy; in severe cases (ie, Stevens-Johnson syndrome), fatalities have occurred. Refer to Management of Acute Hypersensitivity Reactions.

CNS effects: Because CNS side effects may occur, avoid activities requiring mental alertness.

Pregnancy: Category C. There are no adequate and well controlled studies in pregnant women. Use during pregnancy only if potential benefit outweighs risk to the fetus.

Lactation: It is not known whether this drug is excreted in breast milk. Because of the potential for serious adverse reactions in nursing infants, decide whether to discontinue nursing or to discontinue the drug taking into account the importance of the drug to the mother.

Children: Safety and efficacy for use in children weighing < 13.6 kg (30 lbs) has not been established.

Precautions:

Supportive therapy is indicated for anemic, dehydrated or malnourished patients prior to initiation of therapy. Monitor patients with hepatic or renal dysfunction carefully.

Some patients may excrete a metabolite that imparts an odor to urine similar to that occurring after ingestion of asparagus.

Thiabendazole is not suitable for the treatment of mixed infections with ascaris because it may cause these worms to migrate. Use only in patients in whom susceptible worm infestation has been diagnosed; do not use prophylactically.

Laboratory test abnormalities: Rarely, a transient rise in cephalin flocculation and AST has occurred in patients receiving thiabendazole.

Drug Interactions:

Xanthines: Thiabendazole may compete with these agents for sites of metabolism in the liver, thus elevating the serum levels of the xanthine to potentially toxic levels. Monitor xanthine serum levels and reduce the dose if necessary.

(Continued on following page)

THIABENDAZOLE (Cont.)

Adverse Reactions:

CNS: Dizziness; weariness; drowsiness; giddiness; headache; numbness; hyperirritability; convulsions; collapse.

GI: Anorexia; nausea; vomiting; diarrhea; epigastric distress; jaundice; cholestasis; parenchymal liver damage.

GU: Hematuria; enuresis; malodor of the urine; crystalluria.

Hypersensitivity: Pruritus; fever; facial flush; chills; conjunctival injection ("red eye"); angioedema; anaphylaxis; skin rashes (including perianal); erythema multiforme (including Stevens-Johnson syndrome); lymphadenopathy. See Warnings.

Special senses: Tinnitus; abnormal sensation in eyes; xanthopsia (objects appear yellow); blurring of vision; drying of mucous membranes (eg, mouth, eyes).

Miscellaneous: Appearance of live Ascaris in the mouth and nose; hypotension; transient leukopenia.

Overdosage:

Symptoms: Possible transient disturbances of vision and psychic alterations.

Treatment: There is no specific antidote. Use symptomatic and supportive measures. Induce emesis or carefully perform gastric lavage. Refer to General Management of Acute Overdosage.

Patient Information:

May cause stomach upset. Take with food.

Chewable tablets – Chew thoroughly before swallowing.

Cleansing enemas are not needed after drug therapy.

Duration of therapy varies from 1 to 4 days depending upon the condition being treated.

Pinworm infections are easily spread to others. If one family member has a pinworm infection, treat all family members in close contact with the patient. This decreases the chance of spreading the infection.

Repeat therapy in 7 days to prevent reinfection.

Strict hygiene is essential to prevent reinfection. Disinfect toilet facilities daily. Change and launder undergarments, bed linens, towels and nightclothes daily.

May produce drowsiness or dizziness. Use caution when driving or performing other tasks requiring alertness.

Administration and Dosage:

< 150 lbs (68 kg): 10 mg/lb/dose (22 mg/kg/dose).

≥ 150 lbs: 1.5 g/dose.

The usual dosage schedule for all conditions is 2 doses per day. Maximum daily dose is 3 g after meals if possible.

Dietary restriction, complementary medications and cleansing enemas are not needed.

Thiabendazole Dosage Regimen for Each Indication

Indication	Regimen	Comments
Strongyloidiasis† Ascariasis† Uncinariasis† Trichuriasis†	2 doses/day for 2 successive days	May also use single dose of 20 mg/lb (44 mg/kg) but with higher incidence of side effects.
Cutaneous larva migrans (creeping eruption)	2 doses/day for 2 successive days	If active lesions are still present 2 days after end of therapy, a second course is recommended.
Trichinosis†	2 doses/day for 2 to 4 successive days. Individualize dosage	Optimal dosage has not been established.
Visceral larva migrans	2 doses/day for 7 successive days	Safety and efficacy data on the 7 day treatment are limited.

† Clinical experience with thiabendazole in children weighing < 13.6 kg (30 lbs) is limited.

				C.I.*
Rx	**Mintezol** (MSD)	**Tablets, chewable:** 500 mg	Saccharin. (MSD 907). White, scored. Orange flavor. In 36s.	674
		Oral Suspension: 500 mg/5 ml	In 120 ml.	291

* Cost Index based on cost per 3 g.

Refer to the general discussion of these products on page 2025

PIPERAZINE

Actions:

Pharmacology: Piperazine blocks the response of Ascaris muscle to acetylcholine, causing flaccid paralysis of the worm. The paralyzed Ascaris are dislodged and expelled via peristalsis. Piperazine affects all stages of the parasite in the gut, but has little effect on larvae in the tissues.

Pharmacokinetics: Although excretion is variable, piperazine is readily absorbed from the GI tract. Approximately 25% is metabolized. It is excreted in urine essentially unchanged within 24 hours.

Indications:

Treatment of enterobiasis (pinworm infection) and ascariasis (roundworm infection).

Contraindications:

Renal or hepatic function impairment; convulsive disorders; hypersensitivity to piperazine.

Warnings:

Because of potential neurotoxicity, especially in children, avoid prolonged, repeated or excessive treatment.

Pregnancy: Safety for use during pregnancy has not been established.

Lactation: Safety for use in the nursing mother has not been established. The drug is probably excreted in breast milk. The potential for neuromuscular blockade exists. Women who are breastfeeding should not take the drug.

Precautions:

Piperazine is best taken on an empty stomach. The surface contact between drug and parasite is diminished in the presence of food.

If CNS, significant GI or hypersensitivity reactions occur, discontinue the drug.

Use caution in patients with severe malnutrition or anemia.

Adverse Reactions:

GI: Nausea; vomiting; abdominal cramps; diarrhea.

CNS: Headache; vertigo; ataxia; tremors; chorea; muscular weakness; hyporeflexia; paresthesia; seizures; EEG abnormalities; sense of detachment; memory defect.

Ocular: Cataracts; blurred vision; nystagmus; paralytic strabismus.

Hypersensitivity: Urticaria; erythema multiforme; purpura; fever; arthralgia; eczematous skin reactions; lacrimation; rhinorrhea; productive cough; bronchospasm.

Patient Information:

Take on an empty stomach (at least 1 hour before or 2 hours after a meal).

If symptoms such as headache, vertigo, lack of coordination, muscle weakness, seizures, confusion, dizziness, nausea, vomiting, diarrhea, rash or difficult breathing occurs, contact physician.

Pinworm infections are easily spread to others. If one family member has a pinworm infection, all family members in close contact with the patient should be treated. This decreases the chance of spreading the infection. In severe infections, repeat treatment 1 week after the first course of therapy.

Strict hygiene is essential to prevent reinfection. Disinfect toilet facilities daily. Change and launder undergarments, bed linens, towels and nightclothes daily.

The dose for treating pinworms and roundworms is based on body weight.

Administration and Dosage:

All doses are given in terms of hexahydrate equivalent.

Ascariasis (roundworm infection):

Adults – Single daily dose of 3.5 g for 2 consecutive days.

Children – Single daily dose of 75 mg/kg for 2 consecutive days; maximum daily dose is 3.5 g.

Enterobiasis (pinworm infection): Adults and children – Single daily dose of 65 mg/kg; maximum daily dose is 2.5 g for 7 consecutive days.

Severe infections - Repeat treatment course after a 1 week interval.

				C.I.*
Rx	**Piperazine** (Various, eg, Richlyn, Schein)	**Tablets:** Piperazine citrate equivalent to 250 mg piperazine hexahydrate	In 100s and 1000s.	24+
Rx	**Piperazine** (Various, eg, Balan, Lannett)	**Syrup:** Piperazine citrate equiv. to 500 mg piperazine hexahydrate/5 ml	In pt and gal.	27+

* Cost Index based on cost per 3.5 g.

Refer to the general discussion of these products on page 2025

Quinacrine is also used in the treatment and suppression of malaria. For information regarding this use and full prescribing information, refer to monograph in Antimalarial section.

QUINACRINE HCl

Actions:

Quinacrine eradicates certain intestinal cestodes: *Taenia saginata* (beef tapeworm), *T solium* (pork tapeworm), *Hymenolepis nana* (dwarf tapeworm) and probably *Diphyllobothrium latum* (fish tapeworm); it also eliminates *Giardia lamblia* from the intestinal tract.

Indications:

For the treatment of giardiasis and cestodiasis.

Unlabeled use: Quinacrine in total doses of 100 to 1500 mg has been used as a sclerosing agent for pleural effusions.

Contraindications:

Pregnancy (see Warnings).

Warnings:

Hepatic function impairment: Since quinacrine concentrates in the liver, use with caution in patients with hepatic disease or alcoholism or in conjunction with known hepatotoxic drugs.

Elderly or patients with history of psychosis: Quinacrine can cause transitory psychosis; use with caution in patients > 60 years of age or those with a history of psychosis.

Pregnancy: Postpone treatment of pregnant women with cestodiasis or giardiasis until after delivery because quinacrine crosses the placenta. Cestodiasis and giardiasis are generally not life-threatening.

Patient Information:

May impart a yellow color to skin or urine.

Promptly report any visual disturbances.

Administration and Dosage:

Dwarf tapeworm:

Adults – The night before medication, give 1 tablespoonful sodium sulfate dissolved in water. On day 1, take 900 mg on an empty stomach in 3 portions 20 minutes apart, with sodium sulfate purge 1½ hours later. On the following 3 days, take 100 mg 3 times daily.

Children – Give ½ tablespoonful sodium sulfate on the night before medication.

Quinacrine Dosage for Dwarf Tapeworm in Children		
Age (years)	Initial dose (mg)	Maintenance therapy
4 to 8	200	100 mg after breakfast for 3 days
8 to 10	300	100 mg 2 times daily for 3 days
11 to 14	400	100 mg 3 times daily for 3 days

Tapeworm (beef, pork and fish): Preliminary bland, semisolid, nonfat diet or milk diet on the day before medication, with fasting following the evening meal. Administer a saline purge or purge and cleansing enema before treatment if desired. Saline purge 1 to 2 hours later. The expelled worm is stained yellow, facilitating identification of scolex.

Adults – 4 doses of 200 mg (800 mg) 10 minutes apart. Give sodium bicarbonate 600 mg with each dose to reduce nausea and vomiting.

Children – Administer in 3 to 4 divided doses 10 minutes apart. Give 300 mg sodium bicarbonate with each dose if desired.

(5 to 10 yrs): 400 mg total dose.
(11 to 14 yrs): 600 mg total dose.

Giardiasis:

Adults – 100 mg, 3 times daily, for 5 to 7 days.

Children – 7 mg/kg/day given in 3 divided doses (maximum, 300 mg/day) after meals for 5 days. Examine stool 2 weeks later and give a repeat course if indicated. The bitter taste of the pulverized tablets may be disguised in jam or honey.

				C.I.*
Rx	**Atabrine HCl** (Winthrop Pharm)	**Tablets:** 100 mg	In 100s.	91

* Cost Index based on cost per 300 mg.

Refer to the general discussion of these products on page 2025

NICLOSAMIDE

Actions:

Niclosamide inhibits oxidative phosphorylation in the mitochondria of cestodes. The scolex and proximal segments are killed on contact with the drug. The scolex of the tapeworm, loosened from the gut wall, may be digested in the intestine, and thus may not be identified in the feces even after extensive purging.

Indications:

Treatment of *Taenia saginata* (beef tapeworm), *Diphyllobothrium latum* (fish tapeworm) and *Hymenolepis nana* (dwarf tapeworm).

Contraindications:

Hypersensitivity to niclosamide or any of its components.

Warnings:

Pregnancy: Category B. Safety for use during pregnancy has not been established. Use only when clearly needed and when the potential benefits outweigh the potential hazards to the fetus.

Lactation: Safety for use in the nursing mother has not been established.

Children: Safety and efficacy for use in children < 2 years old have not been established.

Precautions:

Niclosamide affects the cestodes of the intestine only. It is without effect in cysticercosis.

Adverse Reactions:

GI: Nausea/vomiting (4.1%); abdominal discomfort, loss of appetite (3.4%); diarrhea (1.6%); constipation; rectal bleeding; oral irritation; bad taste in mouth.

CNS: Drowsiness, dizziness, headache (1.4%); weakness.

Dermatologic: Skin rash, including pruritus ani (0.3%); alopecia. Two cases of urticaria reported may have been related to tapeworm breakdown products.

Miscellaneous: Fever; sweating; palpitations; edema of an arm; backache; irritability. There was one report of a transient rise in AST in an IV narcotic addict. All side effects were mild or moderate and transitory, and did not necessitate discontinuing treatment.

Overdosage:

In the event of overdose, give a fast-acting laxative and enema. Do not induce vomiting.

Patient Information:

Chew tablets, then swallow with a small amount of water.

May cause GI upset; take with food after a light meal (eg, breakfast).

Use a mild laxative, if necessary, to relieve constipation.

Administration and Dosage:

Chew thoroughly, then swallow tablets with a little water. For young children, crush the tablets to a fine powder and mix with a small amount of water to form a paste. No special dietary restrictions are necessary. Take after a light meal (eg, breakfast). Constipated patients may need a mild laxative.

T saginata and D latum (beef and fish tapeworm):

Adults – 4 tablets (2 g) as a single dose.
Children 11 to 34 kg (25 to 75 lbs) – 2 tablets (1 g) as a single dose.
Children > 34 kg (75 lbs) – 3 tablets (1.5 g) as a single dose.

Hymenolepis nana (dwarf tapeworm):

Observe strict personal and environmental hygiene to avoid autoinfection.
Adults – 4 tablets (2 g) as a single daily dose for 7 days.
Children 11 to 34 kg (25 to 75 lbs) – 2 tablets (1 g) on the first day, then one tablet (0.5 g) daily for the next 6 days.
Children > 34 kg (75 lbs) – 3 tablets (1.5 g) on the first day, then 2 tablets (1 g) daily for next 6 days.

Follow-up: Niclosamide renders the tapeworm vulnerable to destruction during its passage through the gut; thus, it is not always possible to identify the scolex in stools. The sooner the tapeworm is passed and examined after treatment, the better the chance to identify the scolex. Segments or ova of beef or fish tapeworm may be present in the stool for up to 3 days after therapy. Persistent *T saginata* or *D latum* segments or ova on the 7th day of post-therapy indicate failure. Give a second course of treatment at that time. A patient is not cured unless the stool is negative for a minimum of 3 months. **C.I.***

Rx	**Niclocide** (Miles Inc.)	**Tablets, chewable:** 500 mg	(Miles 721). Yellow, scored. Vanilla flavor. In 4s.	1310

* Cost Index based on cost per 2 g.

Refer to the general discussion of these products on page 2025

OXAMNIQUINE

Actions:

Microbiology: Male schistosomes are more susceptible than female, but after treatment with oxamniquine, the residual female schistosomes cease to lay eggs, thus losing the parasitological aspect of their pathological significance.

Pharmacokinetics: Oxamniquine is well absorbed; plasma concentrations reach a peak at 1 to 1.5 hours after oral administration of therapeutic doses, with a plasma half-life of 1 to 2.5 hours. It is extensively metabolized to inactive acidic metabolites which are largely excreted in the urine.

Indications:

All stages of *Schistosoma mansoni* infection, including acute and chronic phase with hepatosplenic involvement.

Unlabeled use: Concurrent low dose administration of oxamniquine plus praziquantel has been used successfully as a single dose treatment of neurocysticercosis.

Warnings:

Convulsions: Epileptiform convulsions have occurred rarely within the first few hours after ingestion, most often in patients with a previous seizure history. Use with care in such individuals and keep under medical supervision with facilities available to treat a convulsion. EEG abnormalities have also developed in patients with normal pretreatment recordings.

Pregnancy: Category C. Oxamniquine was embryocidal in rabbits and mice when given in doses 10 times the human dose. There are no adequate and well controlled studies in pregnant women. Use only when clearly needed and when the potential benefits outweigh the potential hazards to the fetus.

Lactation: It is not known whether this drug is excreted in breast milk. Exercise caution when administering to a nursing mother.

Adverse Reactions:

Generally well tolerated. Tolerance improves when doses are given after food.

CNS: Transitory dizziness/drowsiness (33%); headache; epileptiform convulsions (rare), see Warnings; EEG abnormalities.

GI: Nausea; vomiting; abdominal pain; anorexia.

Other: Urticaria.

Minor and transient abnormalities observed after treatment (not drug-related, and of no clinical significance): Mild to moderate liver enzyme elevations, but no evidence of hepatotoxicity, even in patients with severe hepatosplenic involvement.

Patient Information:

Take with food to improve tolerance.

Administration and Dosage:

Adults: 12 to 15 mg/kg as a single oral dose in patients with Western Hemisphere strains of *S mansoni.* Recommended dosage according to weight is as follows:

Recommended Oxamniquine Adult Dosage	
Weight (kg)	Dose (mg)
30 to 40	500
41 to 60	750
61 to 80	1000
81 to 100	1250

Children (< 30 kg): 20 mg/kg given in 2 divided doses of 10 mg/kg with 2 to 8 hours between doses.

				C.I.*
Rx	**Vansil** (Pfizer Labs)	**Capsules:** 250 mg.	Green and yellow. In 24s.	1495

* Cost Index based on cost per 1 g.

Refer to the general discussion of these products on page 2025

PRAZIQUANTEL

Actions:

Praziquantel increases cell membrane permeability in susceptible worms, resulting in a loss of intracellular calcium, massive contractions and paralysis of their musculature. The drug further results in vacuolization and disintegration of the schistosome tegument. This effect is followed by attachment of phagocytes to the parasite and death.

Pharmacokinetics: Praziquantel is rapidly absorbed (80%), reaching maximal serum concentration in 1 to 3 hours. Cerebrospinal fluid levels are ≈ 14% to 20% the total amount of drug in plasma. The drug undergoes a significant first-pass biotransformation; elimination half-life of the parent drug is 0.8 to 1.5 hours and the metabolites, 4 to 5 hours. Metabolites are excreted primarily in urine and have little or no activity.

Indications:

For infections due to: *Schistosoma mekongi, S japonicum, S mansoni* and *S hematobium*; infections due to liver flukes, *Clonorchis sinensis/Opisthorchis viverrini* (approval of this indication was based on studies in which the two species were not differentiated).

Unlabeled uses: Praziquantel demonstrates promise for the treatment of neurocysticercosis. Further study is needed. It may also be beneficial in the treatment of other tissue flukes (eg, opisthorchis, felineus, *Paragonimus westermani* and other species, *Fasciola hepatica*), intestinal flukes (eg, *Heterophyes heterophyes, Fascilopsis buski*) and intestinal cestodes (eg, *Diphyllobothrium latum, Taenia saginata* and *solium, Dipylidium caninum, Hymenolepsis nana*).

Concurrent low dose administration of oxamniquine plus praziquantel has been used successfully as a single dose treatment of schistosomiasis.

Contraindications:

Previous hypersensitivity to praziquantel.

Since parasite destruction within the eyes may cause irreparable lesions, do not treat ocular cysticercosis with praziquantel.

Warnings:

Pregnancy: Category B. An increase in the abortion rate was found in rats at three times the single human therapeutic dose. There are no adequate and well controlled studies in pregnant women. Use this drug during pregnancy only if clearly needed.

Lactation: Praziquantel appeared in the milk of nursing women at a concentration of about 25% that of maternal serum. Do not nurse on the day of treatment and during the subsequent 72 hours.

Children: Safety in children $<$ 4 years of age has not been established.

Precautions:

Potentially hazardous tasks: May produce drowsiness; observe caution while driving or performing other tasks requiring alertness on the day of praziquantel treatment and the following day.

Minimal increases in liver enzymes have occurred in some patients.

When schistosomiasis or fluke infection is found to be associated with cerebral cysticercosis, hospitalize the patient for the duration of treatment.

Adverse Reactions:

Praziquantel is well tolerated. Side effects are usually mild and transient and do not need treatment, but may be more frequent or serious in patients with a heavy worm burden.

In order of severity: Malaise; headache; dizziness; abdominal discomfort (with or without nausea); rising temperature; rarely, urticaria. Such symptoms can, however, also result from the infection itself. In patients with liver impairment caused by the infection, no adverse effects occurred that necessitated restriction in use.

Overdosage:

In the event of overdose, give a fast-acting laxative.

Patient Information:

Take with liquids during meals. Do not chew tablets.

May cause dizziness or drowsiness; observe caution while driving or performing other tasks requiring alertness.

Administration and Dosage:

Schistosomiasis: Administer 3 doses of 20 mg/kg as a 1 day treatment. The interval between the doses should not be $<$ 4 and not $>$ 6 hours.

Clonorchiasis and opisthorchiasis: Administer 3 doses of 25 mg/kg as a 1 day treatment.

Swallow the tablets unchewed with some liquid during meals. Keeping the tablets in the mouth may reveal a bitter taste which can produce gagging or vomiting. **C.I.***

Rx	**Biltricide** (Miles Inc.)	**Tablets:** 600 mg	White, tri-scored. Film coated. In 6s.	1215

* Cost Index based on cost per 600 mg.

Urinary tract antiseptics are effective in inhibiting bacterial proliferation in the urinary tract. Concentrated in the renal tubules, these drugs may be used to treat urinary tract infections. They do not achieve significant serum or tissue levels and are therefore not useful in systemic or localized infections in other tissues. The urinary tract antiseptics are commonly used for treatment and prevention of urinary tract infections.

Other anti-infective agents with more general utility are considered primary agents for the treatment of acute urinary tract infections (UTIs). These include:

Ampicillin, p. 1712
Cephalosporins, p. 1733
Aminoglycosides, parenteral, p. 1851
Sulfonamides, p. 1900
Trimethoprim, p. 1987
Trimethoprim/Sulfamethoxazole, p. 2003
Norfloxacin, p. 1807

METHYLENE BLUE

Actions:

Methylene blue is a dye that is a weak germicide and is used as a mild genitourinary antiseptic. It is primarily bacteriostatic.

Pharmacology: This compound has an oxidation-reduction action and a tissue staining property. In high concentrations, methylene blue converts the ferrous iron of reduced hemoglobin to the ferric form; as a result, methemoglobin is produced. This action is the basis for the antidotal action of methylene blue in cyanide poisoning (p. 2697). In contrast, low concentrations of methylene blue are capable of hastening the conversion of methemoglobin to hemoglobin. Oral absorption is reported to be 53% to 97% (74% average).

Indications:

A mild genitourinary antiseptic for cystitis and urethritis.

For treatment of idiopathic and drug-induced methemoglobinemia and as an antidote for cyanide poisoning.

May be useful in the management of patients with oxalate urinary tract calculi.

Contraindications:

Renal insufficiency; patients allergic to methylene blue.

Precautions:

Methylene blue may induce hemolysis in glucose-6-phosphate dehydrogenase (G-6-PD) deficient patients.

Continued administration may cause a marked anemia due to accelerated destruction of erythrocytes. Therefore, perform frequent hemoglobin checks.

Cyanosis and cardiovascular abnormalities have accompanied treatment in humans.

Adverse Reactions:

Turns the urine and sometimes the stool blue-green. May cause bladder irritation, and in some cases, nausea, vomiting and diarrhea. Large doses may cause fever.

Patient Information:

Take after meals with a glass of water.

May discolor the urine or stool blue-green.

Administration and Dosage:

Take 55 to 130 mg, 3 times daily after meals with a full glass of water.

				C.I.*
Rx	**Methylene Blue** (Kenneth Manne)	**Tablets:** 55 mg	In 100s and 1000s.	8
Rx	**Urolene Blue** (Star)	**Tablets:** 65 mg	In 100s and 1000s.	22

* Cost Index based on cost per minimum daily dose.

NALIDIXIC ACID

Actions:

Pharmacology: Nalidixic acid appears to interfere with DNA polymerization.

Microbiology: Nalidixic acid is bactericidal and has marked antibacterial activity over the urinary pH against gram-negative bacteria (ie, *Proteus mirabilis, Morganella morganii, P vulgaris, Providencia rettgeri, Escherichia coli, Enterobacter* and *Klebsiella* species). *Pseudomonas* strains are generally resistant. Conventional chromosomal resistance to full dosage emerges in approximately 2% to 14% of patients during treatment; however, bacterial resistance has not been transferable via R plasmid-mediated factor.

Pharmacokinetics: Absorption/Distribution – Nalidixic acid is well absorbed (96%) from the GI tract; peak serum levels of 20 to 50 mcg/ml (67% nalidixic acid, 33% hydroxynalidixic acid) are attained 1 to 2 hours after an oral 1 g dose. The drug concentrates in renal tissue and seminal fluid; it does not penetrate prostatic tissue.

Metabolism/Elimination – Hepatic metabolism to hydroxynalidixic acid (16 times more active than nalidixic acid) and inactive conjugates is followed by rapid renal excretion. Protein binding is approximately 93% for nalidixic acid and 63% for hydroxynalidixic acid. Approximately 2% to 3% of nalidixic acid and 13% of hydroxynalidixic acid appear in the urine. Plasma half-life in normal renal function is 1 to 2.5 hours; half-life in urine is about 6 hours. Although renal failure does not significantly affect renal clearance of nalidixic acid, it does decrease the elimination rate of hydroxynalidixic acid. Approximately 4% of nalidixic acid is excreted in the feces.

Indications:

Urinary tract infections caused by susceptible gram-negative microorganisms, including the majority of *Proteus* strains, *Klebsiella* and *Enterobacter* species and *E coli*.

Contraindications: Hypersensitivity to nalidixic acid; history of convulsive disorders.

Warnings:

CNS: Brief convulsions, increased intracranial pressure and toxic psychosis (rare) usually occur from overdosage or with predisposing factors, such as epilepsy, cerebral vascular insufficiency, parkinsonism, mental instability or cerebral arteriosclerosis. They usually completely and rapidly disappear upon drug discontinuation. If these reactions occur, discontinue use and institute therapeutic measures. If CNS symptoms do not disappear within 48 hours, perform diagnostic procedures even if risky to the patient. In infants and children receiving therapeutic doses, intracranial hypertension, increased intracranial pressure with bulging anterior fontanelle, papilledema and headache have occasionally occurred. A few cases of sixth cranial nerve palsy were reported. Signs and symptoms usually disappear rapidly with no sequelae upon discontinuation.

Hematologic: Nalidixic acid has been reported to induce clinically significant hemolysis in patients with glucose-6-phosphate dehydrogenase deficiency (G-6-PD).

Usage in Pregnancy: Safe use during the first trimester has not been established. The drug has been used during the last two trimesters without apparent ill effects on mother or child. Traces of nalidixic acid were found in blood and urine of an infant whose mother had received the drug during the last trimester. No drug-linked congenital defects have been reported. One author has cautioned against use in the third trimester because of possible hydrocephalus, but this has not been corroborated.

Usage in Lactation: Data are scant; reported milk:plasma ratios are 0.08 to 0.13. Milk levels of 4 mcg/ml have been noted. Although the amounts are small, hemolytic anemia has been reported in one infant whose mother received 1 g nalidixic acid, 4 times/day.

Usage in Children: Nalidixic acid and related drugs can produce erosions of the cartilage in weight-bearing joints and other signs of arthropathy in several species of immature animals. No joint lesions have been reported in humans, but exercise care when prescribing for prepubertal children.

Precautions:

Perform periodic blood counts and renal and liver function tests if treatment is continued for more than 2 weeks.

Use with caution in liver disease, epilepsy or severe cerebral arteriosclerosis patients.

Use in renal failure: Therapeutic concentrations in the urine, without increased toxicity due to drug accumulation in the blood, have occurred in patients on full dosage with creatinine clearances as low as 2 to 8 ml/min. However, exercise caution.

Resistance: If bacterial resistance emerges, it is usually within 48 hours, permitting rapid change to another drug. If clinical response is unsatisfactory or if relapse occurs, repeat cultures and sensitivity tests. Underdosage ($<$ 4 g/day for adults) may predispose to resistance. Cross-resistance between nalidixic acid and **cinoxacin** has occurred.

Photosensitivity: Photosensitization (photoallergy or phototoxicity) may occur; therefore, caution patients to take protective measures against exposure to ultraviolet light or sunlight (ie, sunscreens, protective clothing) until tolerance is determined.

(Continued on following page)

NALIDIXIC ACID (Cont.)

Drug Interactions:

Oral anticoagulants (warfarin or dicumarol): Nalidixic acid may enhance the effects by displacing significant amounts of these drugs from serum albumin binding sites.

Drug/Lab Tests: Urinary metabolites of nalidixic acid liberate glucuronic acid and produce false-positive **urinary glucose** results when Benedict's or Fehling's solutions or Clinitest reagent tablets are used. Avoid this problem by using Clinistix or Tes-Tape.

Urinary 17-keto and ketogenic steroids may be falsely elevated due to an interaction between nalidixic acid and the m-dinitrobenzene used in the assay. In such cases, use the Porter-Silber method.

Adverse Reactions:

CNS: Drowsiness, weakness, headache, dizziness and vertigo. Toxic psychosis or brief convulsions are rare. Intracranial hypertension, increased intracranial pressure, sixth cranial nerve palsy in children and infants (see Warnings).

Visual: Reversible subjective visual disturbances occur infrequently (generally with each dose during the first few days of treatment) and include overbrightness of lights, change in color perception, focusing difficulty, decrease in visual acuity and double vision. They usually disappear promptly with reduced dosage or drug discontinuation.

GI: Abdominal pain, nausea, vomiting and diarrhea.

Allergic: Rash, pruritus, urticaria, angioedema, eosinophilia, arthralgia with joint stiffness and swelling, and rarely, anaphylactoid reaction.

Photosensitivity reactions (eg, erythema and pruritic, painful bullae on exposed skin surfaces) may be initiated with as little as 15 minutes exposure, usually resolve completely 2 to 8 weeks after discontinuation, but may persist up to 1 year. However, bullae may continue to appear with successive exposures to sunlight or with mild skin trauma for up to 3 months after discontinuation.

Hematologic: Rarely, thrombocytopenia, leukopenia or hemolytic anemia, sometimes associated with G-6-PD deficiency or acute immune mechanism.

Other: Rarely, cholestatic jaundice, cholestasis, paresthesia or metabolic acidosis.

Overdosage:

Symptoms: Toxic psychosis, convulsions, increased intracranial pressure, hyperglycemia, metabolic acidosis, vomiting, nausea and lethargy may occur in patients taking more than the recommended dosage.

Treatment: Reactions are short lived (2 to 3 hours) because the drug is rapidly excreted. If overdosage is noted early, gastric lavage is indicated. If absorption has occurred, increase fluid administration and have supportive measures available. Anticonvulsants may be indicated in severe cases.

Patient Information:

May cause GI upset; take with food.

May produce drowsiness, dizziness or blurred vision; observe caution while driving or performing other tasks requiring alertness.

Avoid prolonged exposure to sunlight; photosensitivity may occur.

Administration and Dosage:

Underdosage during initial treatment may predispose to emergence of bacterial resistance.

Adults: Initial therapy – 1 g, 4 times/day (total dose 4 g/day) for 1 or 2 weeks. *Prolonged therapy* – May be reduced to 2 g/day after the initial treatment period.

Children: Do not administer to infants younger than 3 months. *Children 12 years of age and under: Total daily dosage for initial therapy* – 25 mg/lb/day (55 mg/kg/day) in 4 equally divided doses. *Prolonged therapy* – May be reduced to 15 mg/lb/day (33 mg/kg/day).

				C.I.*
Rx	**NegGram Caplets** (Winthrop-Breon)	**Tablets:** 250 mg	(#W N21). Scored. In 56s.	616
		500 mg	(#W N22). Scored. In 56s, 500s, 1000s and UD 100s.	510
		1 g	(#W N23). Scored. In 100s and UD 100s.	384
Rx	**NegGram** (Winthrop-Breon)	**Suspension:** 250 mg per 5 ml	Saccharin and sorbitol. Raspberry flavor. In pt.	925

* Cost Index based on cost per adult daily dose (4 g). # Product identification code.

CINOXACIN

Actions:

Pharmacology: Cinoxacin, a synthetic organic acid chemically related to nalidixic acid, inhibits DNA replication. The drug is active within the range of urinary pH.

Microbiology: Cinoxacin has in vitro activity against a wide variety of aerobic gram-negative bacilli, particularly strains of Enterobacteriaceae. It is active against most strains of the following organisms: *Escherichia coli, Klebsiella* sp, *Enterobacter* sp (including *E aerogenes, E cloacae* and *E hafniae*), *Proteus mirabilis* and *P vulgaris.*

Cinoxacin is NOT active against *Pseudomonas,* enterococci or staphylococci. Cross-resistance with **nalidixic acid** has been demonstrated. Bacterial resistance to cinoxacin has been reported in less than 4% of patients treated with recommended doses; bacterial resistance to cinoxacin has not been shown to be transferable via R-factor (plasmids).

Susceptibility tests - Quantitative methods give the most precise estimates of susceptibility. Reports giving results of the standardized test using the 100 mcg cinoxacin disc should be used.

Pharmacokinetics: Absorption/Distribution - Cinoxacin is rapidly and completely absorbed after oral administration. Mean peak plasma concentrations of 15 mcg/ml occur ≈ 2 hours after a single 500 mg dose and detectable levels persist 10 to 12 hours. Food decreases peak serum concentrations by about 30%, although the total extent of absorption is not altered. Cinoxacin concentrates in renal tissue; prostatic levels achieve a 30% to 60% concentration versus plasma (approximately 2.3 mcg/g). It is 60% to 80% protein bound.

Metabolism/Elimination - Peak urine concentrations of 300 to 400 mcg/ml (up to 700 mcg/ml) occur within 2 to 4 hours; urine concentrations usually exceed the MIC (ie, 10 to 30 mcg/ml) for at least 12 hours after a dose. The mean serum half-life is 1 to 1.5 hours with normal renal function; renal failure increases half-life (up to 16 hours in end-stage renal failure). Oral cinoxacin is 97% excreted in the urine within 24 hours. Approximately 60% to 65% of cinoxacin is excreted unchanged; 30% to 40% as inactive hepatic metabolites. Cinoxacin is removed by hemodialysis, the extent is unknown.

Indications:

Treatment of initial and recurrent urinary tract infections in adults caused by the following susceptible microorganisms: *E coli, P mirabilis, P vulgaris, K pneumoniae, Klebsiella* sp and *Enterobacter* sp.

Contraindications:

Hypersensitivity to cinoxacin.

Warnings:

Usage in Pregnancy: Category B. Reproduction studies have been performed in animals at doses up to 10 times the daily human dose and revealed no evidence of impaired fertility or harm to the fetus. There are, however, no adequate and well controlled studies in pregnant women. Since cinoxacin causes arthropathy in immature animals (see Usage in Children below), its use during pregnancy is not recommended.

Usage in Lactation: It is not known whether cinoxacin is excreted in human milk. Because other drugs in this class are excreted in human milk and because of the potential for serious adverse reactions in nursing infants, discontinue nursing or discontinue the drug, taking into account the importance of the drug to the mother.

Usage in Children: Use in prepubertal children is not recommended. Cinoxacin and nalidixic acid have produced erosions of the cartilage in weight-bearing joints and other signs of arthropathy in immature animals of various species.

Precautions:

Renal failure: Since cinoxacin is primarily eliminated by the kidney, decrease dosage in patients with reduced renal function. In patients with creatinine clearance < 30 ml/min, cinoxacin serum half-life may increase threefold. Administration is not recommended for anuric patients.

Hepatic disease: Use with caution in patients with a history of hepatic disease.

Drug Interactions:

Probenecid pretreatment will block tubule secretion of cinoxacin, and thus, will reduce the elimination rate, increase half-life, decrease urine concentrations by 20% and double serum concentrations.

Acidification and **alkalinization** of the urine will double and halve cinoxacin's half-life, respectively. However, it does not appear clinically significant.

(Continued on following page)

CINOXACIN (Cont.)

Adverse Reactions:

The overall incidence of adverse reactions is approximately 4%.

GI/GU: Most common (< 3%) – Nausea.

Less frequent (< 1%) – Anorexia; vomiting; abdominal cramps; diarrhea; perineal burning; distorted taste sensation.

CNS: Most frequent (1% to 2%) – Headache; dizziness.

Less frequent (< 1%) – Insomnia; confusion; drowsiness; tingling sensation; photophobia; blurred vision; tinnitus.

Hypersensitivity (< 3%): Rash; urticaria; pruritus; edema; angioedema; eosinophilia; anaphylactoid reactions (rare); toxic epidermal necrolysis (very rare).

Hematologic (rare): Thrombocytopenia.

Laboratory tests: Laboratory values reported to be abnormally elevated were, in order of frequency – BUN, AST, ALT, serum creatinine and alkaline phosphatase (each ≤ 1%). Reduction in hematocrit/hemoglobin has also been reported.

Although not observed in patients treated with cinoxacin, the following reversible side effects have been reported for other drugs in the same pharmacologically active and chemically related class: Constipation; sore gums; metallic taste; restlessness; nervousness; weakness; disorientation; agitation; acute anxiety; toxic psychosis; convulsions (rare); swelling of the extremities; joint stiffness; change in color perception; difficulty in focusing; decrease in visual acuity; double vision; erythema and bullae; palpitations.

Patient Information:

May cause dizziness; observe caution while driving or performing other tasks requiring alertness.

Eyes may be more sensitive to light than normal.

Administration and Dosage:

The usual adult dosage is 1 g/day, in 2 or 4 divided doses for 7 to 14 days. Although susceptible organisms may be eradicated within a few days after therapy has begun, the full treatment course is recommended.

Impaired renal function: A reduced dosage must be employed. After an initial dose of 500 mg, use the following maintenance dosage schedule:

Cinoxacin Maintenance Dosage Guide for Renal Impairment		
Creatinine Clearance (ml/min/1.73 m²)	Renal Function	Dosage
> 80	Normal	500 mg bid
80-50	Mild Impairment	250 mg tid
50-20	Moderate Impairment	250 mg bid
< 20	Marked Impairment	250 mg daily

Administration of cinoxacin to anuric patients is not recommended.

When only serum creatinine is available, use the following formula to convert this value into creatinine clearance. The serum creatinine should represent a steady-state of renal function.

Males: $$\frac{\text{Weight (kg)} \times (140 - \text{age})}{72 \times \text{serum creatinine (mg/100 ml)}} = \text{Ccr}$$

Females: 0.85 x above value

				C.I.*
Rx	**Cinobac Pulvules** (Dista)	**Capsules:** 250 mg	(3055). Orange and green. In 40s.	399
otc	**Cinoxacin** (Biocraft)		(Biocraft 163). Blue/yellow. In 40s and 100s.	NA
Rx	**Cinobac Pulvules** (Dista)	**Capsules:** 500 mg	(Dista 3056 Cinobac 500 mg). Orange and green. In 50s.	397
otc	**Cinoxacin** (Biocraft)		(Biocraft 164). Blue/yellow. In 50s and 100s.	NA

* Cost Index based on cost per adult daily dose (1 g).

NITROFURANTOIN

Actions:

Pharmacology: A synthetic nitrofuran that is bacteriostatic in low concentrations (5 to 10 mcg/ml) and bactericidal in higher concentrations. Nitrofurantoin may inhibit acetyl-coenzyme A, interfering with bacterial carbohydrate metabolism. It may also disrupt bacterial cell wall formation.

Microbiology: The MIC in urine for most susceptible organisms is ≤ 25 mcg/ml. Resistant species generally have an MIC of ≥ 100 mcg/ml. Most gram-negative bacilli and gram-positive cocci associated with urinary tract infections are susceptible, including: *Escherichia coli, Klebsiella* and *Enterobacter* sp, enterococci (eg, *Streptococcus faecalis*), *Staphylococcus aureus* and *S saprophyticus.* Some strains of *Enterobacter* and *Klebsiella* sp are resistant. Most strains of *Proteus, Serratia* and *Acinetobacter* species are resistant. It has no activity against *Pseudomonas* sp. Usually, sensitive organisms develop only a limited resistance clinically.

Pharmacokinetics: Absorption/Distribution – Nitrofurantoin is well absorbed from the GI tract after oral administration. The macrocrystalline form is absorbed more slowly due to slower dissolution and causes less GI distress. Bioavailability of micro- and macrocrystalline forms is enhanced by concomitant ingestion of food. Therapeutic serum and tissue concentrations are not achieved after usual oral doses, except in the urinary tract. Protein binding is about 60%.

Metabolism/Elimination – Approximately 50% to 70% of the drug is rapidly metabolized by body tissues. The plasma half-life is about 20 minutes in normal individuals and increases to 60 minutes in the anephric patient. In patients with impaired renal function, nitrofurantoin accumulates in the serum. Renal excretion is via glomerular filtration and tubular secretion. About 30% to 50% of a dose is excreted unchanged in the urine. Usual doses produce urinary levels of 50 to 250 mcg/ml in patients with normal renal function. If creatinine clearance is < 40 ml/min, antibacterial concentrations attained in the urine are inadequate, and the subsequent elevated blood levels increase the danger of toxicity. Antibacterial activity is greater in an acidic urine. Acid urine enhances tubular reabsorption of nitrofurantoin, enhancing antibacterial activity in the renal tissues and lowering urinary concentrations. However, do not alkalinize urine to increase urinary concentration of nitrofurantoin, because the antimicrobial activity is decreased at higher pH.

Indications:

Treatment of urinary tract infections due to susceptible strains of *E coli,* enterococci, *S aureus* (not for treatment of associated renal cortical or perinephric abscesses) and certain strains of *Klebsiella, Enterobacter* and *Proteus* species.

Contraindications:

Renal function impairment (creatinine clearance < 40 ml/minute), anuria or oliguria. Treatment is much less effective and carries an increased risk of toxicity because of impaired excretion of the drug.

Hypersensitivity to nitrofurantoin.

Pregnant patients at term and in infants under 1 month of age: Possibility of hemolytic anemia due to immature enzyme systems (glutathione instability).

Warnings:

Pulmonary reactions:

Acute – May occur within hours and up to 3 weeks after nitrofurantoin therapy is initiated. Manifested by sudden onset of dyspnea, chest pain, cough, fever and chills. Chest x-rays show alveolar infiltrates or effusions; elevated sedimentation rate and eosinophilia are also present. Resolution of clinical and radiological abnormalities occurs within 24 to 48 hours after discontinuation. Rechallenge is dangerous and will produce similar symptoms.

Subacute/chronic – Associated with prolonged therapy. These reactions are characterized by insidious development of dyspnea, nonproductive cough and malaise after 1 to 6 months or more of therapy. Pulmonary function tests demonstrate a restrictive pattern. Radiographs show an interstitial pneumonitis. Usually, symptoms regress with discontinuation of the drug over weeks to months. Pulmonary function may be permanently impaired, even after cessation of nitrofurantoin. Respiratory failure and death have been reported.

Hemolysis: Hemolytic anemia of the primaquine sensitivity type has been induced by nitrofurantoin. The hemolysis appears to be linked to a glucose-6-phosphate dehydrogenase (G-6-PD) deficiency in the red blood cells of affected patients. At any sign of hemolysis, discontinue the drug. Hemolysis ceases when the drug is withdrawn.

(Warnings continued on following page)

NITROFURANTOIN (Cont.)

Warnings (Cont.):

Hepatitis, including chronic active hepatitis, has been observed rarely. Fatalities have been reported. The mechanism appears to be of an idiosyncratic hypersensitivity type.

The onset of chronic active hepatitis may be insidious. Periodically monitor patients receiving long-term therapy for changes in liver function. If hepatitis occurs, withdraw the drug and take appropriate measures.

Usage in Pregnancy: Safety for use during pregnancy has not been established. Use in women of childbearing potential only when clearly needed and when the potential benefits outweigh the unknown potential hazards to the fetus. Do not give to pregnant patients with G-6-PD deficiency because of the risk of hemolysis in the mother and fetus, although fetal hemolysis has not been documented. Contraindicated in pregnant women at term.

Usage in Lactation: Minimal concentrations of nitrofurantoin (taken in recommended doses) are found in breast milk. Concentrations of 0.3 to 0.5 mcg/ml were reported in two women who received 100 mg nitrofurantoin every 6 hours for 1 day followed by 200 mg the next morning. However, infants with G-6-PD deficiency may be adversely affected. Safety for use in the nursing mother has not been established.

Contraindicated in infants less than 1 month of age.

Precautions:

Peripheral neuropathy may occur and may become severe or irreversible. Fatalities have been reported. Predisposing conditions such as renal impairment, anemia, diabetes, electrolyte imbalance, vitamin B deficiency and debilitating disease may enhance such occurrences.

Superinfection: Use of antibiotics (especially prolonged or repeated therapy) may result in bacterial or fungal overgrowth of nonsusceptible organisms. Such overgrowth may lead to a secondary infection. *Pseudomonas* is the organism most commonly implicated in superinfections. Take appropriate measures if superinfection occurs.

Monitoring: Obtain specimens for culture and susceptibility testing prior to and during drug administration.

Drug Interactions:

Anticholinergic drugs and **food** increase nitrofurantoin bioavailability by delaying gastric emptying and increasing absorption.

Probenecid: Administration of high doses of probenecid with nitrofurantoin decreases renal clearance and increases serum levels of nitrofurantoin. The result could be increased toxic effects.

Magnesium trisilicate may delay or decrease the absorption of nitrofurantoin.

Drug/Lab Tests: Serum glucose may be decreased; bilirubin and alkaline phosphatase may be elevated. Urinary creatinine elevation and a false-positive urine glucose determination using Benedict's reagent (cupric sulfate solution) may also occur.

Adverse Reactions:

GI: Most frequent – Anorexia, nausea, emesis.

Less frequent – Abdominal pain, diarrhea, parotitis, pancreatitis. Hepatitis (rare).

Hepatotoxicity is not dose-related and jaundice is not invariable. Although hepatotoxicity usually reverses upon drug discontinuation, permanent liver dysfunction and death have been reported. Chronic active hepatitis and cholestatic jaundice have also been reported.

Pulmonary sensitivity reactions (acute, subacute or chronic) are documented with outcomes ranging from complete resolution to death. See Warnings.

Dermatologic: Exfoliative dermatitis and erythema multiforme (including Stevens-Johnson syndrome) have been reported rarely; maculopapular, erythematous or eczematous eruption; pruritus; urticaria; angioedema.

Other sensitivity reactions: Anaphylaxis; asthmatic attack in patients with history of asthma; drug fever; arthralgia; sialadenitis.

Hematologic: Hemolytic anemia due to G-6-PD deficiency (see Warnings); granulocytopenia; agranulocytosis; leukopenia; thrombocytopenia; eosinophilia; megaloblastic anemia. Return of the blood picture to normal has followed cessation of therapy. Aplastic anemia (rare).

Neurological: Peripheral neuropathy (see Precautions); headache; dizziness; nystagmus; drowsiness.

Miscellaneous: Transient alopecia; superinfections in GU tract by resistant organisms; muscular aches.

(Continued on following page)

NITROFURANTOIN (Cont.)

Patient Information:

Complete full course of therapy; do not discontinue without notifying physician.

May cause GI upset; take with food or milk.

May cause brown discoloration of the urine.

Notify physician if fever, chills, cough, chest pain, difficult breathing, skin rash, numbness or tingling of the fingers or toes, or intolerable GI upset occurs.

Administration and Dosage:

Oral: Give with food or milk to minimize gastric upset. Continue for at least 1 week and for at least 3 days after sterile urine is obtained. Continued infection indicates need for reevaluation.

Adults – 50 to 100 mg, 4 times/day with meals and at bedtime (5 to 7 mg/kg/24 hrs; not to exceed 400 mg). For long-term suppressive therapy, reduce dosage (50 to 100 mg at bedtime).

Children – 5 to 7 mg/kg/24 hrs given in 4 divided doses. For long-term suppressive therapy, doses as low as 1 mg/kg/24 hrs, given in single or in 2 divided doses, may be adequate. (Contraindicated in children less than 1 month of age.) **C.I.***

	Product	Form	Description	C.I.
Rx	**Nitrofurantoin** (Various)	**Tablets:** 50 mg	In 100s, 500s, 1000s, UD 100s.	3+
Rx	**Furadantin** (Proctor & Gamble Pharm.)		(Eaton 036). Yellow, scored. In 100s, 500s and UD 100s.	119
Rx	**Furalan** (Lannett)		Scored. In 100s, 500s, 1000s.	11
Rx	**Furan** (American Urologicals)		(2075). Yellow, scored. In 100s and 1000s.	93
Rx	**Furanite** (Major)		In 100s.	15
Rx	**Nitrofurantoin** (Various)	**Capsules:** 50 mg	In 28s, 40s, 100s, 500s, 1000s and UD 100s.	40+
Rx	**Nitrofan** (Major)		In 100s and 500s.	65
Rx	**Nitrofurantoin** (Various)	**Tablets:** 100 mg	In 100s and 1000s.	2+
Rx	**Furadantin** (Procter & Gamble Pharm.)		(Eaton 037). Yellow, scored. In 100s, 500s and UD 100s.	120
Rx	**Furalan** (Lannett)		Scored. In 100s, 500s, 1000s.	10
Rx	**Furan** (American Urologicals)		(2076). Yellow, scored. In 100s and 1000s.	77
Rx	**Furanite** (Major)		In 100s.	9
Rx	**Nitrofurantoin** (Various)	**Capsules:** 100 mg	In 100s, 500s, 1000s, UD 100s.	29+
Rx	**Nitrofan** (Major)		In 100s and 500s.	49
Rx	**Furadantin** (Procter & Gamble Pharm.)	**Oral Suspension:** 25 mg per 5 ml	Saccharin, sorbitol. In 60 and 470 ml.	272

NITROFURANTOIN MACROCRYSTALS

The large crystal size improves GI tolerance. **C.I.***

	Product	Form	Description	C.I.
Rx	**Macrodantin** (Procter & Gamble Pharm.)	**Capsules:** 25 mg	(Macrodantin 25 mg/ 0149-0007). White. In 100s.	328
		50 mg	(Macrodantin 50 mg/ 0149-0008). Yellow/white. In 100s, 500s, 1000s, UD 100s.	185
		100 mg	(Macrodantin 100 mg/ 0149-0009). Yellow. In 100s, 500s, 1000s, UD 100s.	183
Rx	**Macrodantin MACPAC** (Procter & Gamble Pharm.)	**Capsules:** 50 mg	(Macrodantin 50 mg/0149-0008). Yellow/white. In box of 7 Daycard blisters, 4 capsules each.	185
		100 mg	(Macrodantin 100 mg/0149-0009). Yellow. In box of 7 Daycard blisters, 4 capsules each.	183
Rx	**Macrobid** (Procter & Gamble Pharm.)	**Capsules:** 100 mg	Sugar, lactose. Black and yellow. In 100s.	NA
		250 mg	Blue/yellow. In 40s and 100s.	NA
		500 mg	Blue/yellow. In 50s and 100s.	NA

* Cost Index based on cost per average daily adult dose (200 mg).

Methenamine and Methenamine Salts

Actions:

Pharmacology: In acid urine, methenamine is hydrolyzed to ammonia and formaldehyde, which is bactericidal. Methenamine does not liberate formaldehyde in the serum. The acid salts (mandelate and hippurate) help maintain a low urine pH.

Microbiology: The nonspecific antibacterial action of formaldehyde is effective against gram-positive and gram-negative organisms and fungi. *Escherichia coli,* enterococci and staphylococci are usually susceptible. *Enterobacter aerogenes* and *Proteus vulgaris* are generally resistant. Urea-splitting organisms (eg, *Proteus, Pseudomonas*) may be resistant since they raise the pH of the urine inhibiting the release of formaldehyde. An effective urine concentration of formaldehyde must persist for a minimum of 2 hours.

Methenamine is effective clinically against most common urinary tract pathogens. It has demonstrable antibacterial activity in vitro against *E coli, Micrococcus pyogenes, E aerogenes, P aeruginosa* and *P vulgaris* at pH 5 to 6.8. The minimal inhibitory concentrations are significantly lower in more acidic media; therefore, efficacy can be increased by urine acidification.

Methenamine is particularly suited for therapy of chronic infections, since bacteria and fungi do not develop resistance to formaldehyde.

Pharmacokinetics: Absorption – Methenamine and its acid salts are readily absorbed following oral administration; 10% to 30% of the drug will be hydrolyzed by the gastric juices unless it is protected by an enteric coating.

Metabolism/Elimination – Approximately 10% to 25% of methenamine is metabolized in the liver and has a half-life of 3 to 6 hours. Generation of formaldehyde depends upon urinary pH, the concentration of methenamine and the duration that the urine is retained in the bladder. Peak concentrations of formaldehyde occur at a urine pH of 5.5 or less and are seen approximately 2 hours after a dose of methenamine hippurate and 3 to 8 hours after a dose of methenamine mandelate. A urinary formaldehyde concentration of greater than 25 mcg/ml is necessary for antimicrobial activity. Steady-state urinary formaldehyde concentrations are achieved in 2 to 3 days. Formaldehyde levels range from 1 to 85 mcg/ml, and decrease with increasing pH, urinary volume or flow rate.

In some instances, supplementary urine acidification may be desirable, especially in infections caused by urea-splitting organisms. Ingestion of acidifying agents (ie, mandelic acid, hippuric acid, ammonium chloride, monobasic sodium phosphate) or acid-producing foods (ie, cranberries, plums, prunes) aid in maintaining an acid urine; however, effects may be negligible. Ammonium chloride 8 to 12 g/day, methionine 8 to 15 g/day and cranberry juice 1200 to 4000 ml/day, have all been recommended, but with marginal results. There is no reliable oral urinary acidifier at present. Monitor urine pH.

Excretion occurs via glomerular filtration and tubular secretion. Approximately 75% to $>$ 90% of the methenamine moiety is excreted in the urine within 24 hours. The influence of renal dysfunction on the pharmacology of methenamine is unknown.

In clinical studies, symptomatic relief was usually reported within 24 to 72 hours followed by culture reversal in the majority of patients monitored.

Indications:

Suppression or elimination of bacteriuria associated with pyelonephritis, cystitis and other chronic urinary tract infections. Also for infected residual urine, sometimes accompanying neurologic diseases.

Contraindications:

In renal insufficiency and severe dehydration.

In severe hepatic insufficiency because it facilitates ammonia production in the intestine.

Do not use alone for acute infections with parenchymal involvement causing systemic symptoms.

Hypersensitivity to the drug.

Warnings:

Usage in Pregnancy: Category C. Safe use of methenamine in early pregnancy has not been established. Safety in the last trimester is suggested, but not proven. Methenamine passes into the fetus, but there is no evidence that methenamine salts cause fetal abnormalities, based on several nonrigid studies. It is not known whether the drug can cause fetal harm when administered to a pregnant woman or can affect reproduction capacity. Give to pregnant women only if clearly needed.

Usage in Lactation: Methenamine passes into breast milk, levels are about equivalent to maternal serum and peak in 1 hour. One estimate revealed an infant would receive about 0.15 to 0.4 mg methenamine/feeding. No adverse effects on the nursing infant have been reported.

(Continued on following page)

Methenamine and Methenamine Salts (Cont.)

Precautions:

Large doses (8 g daily for 3 to 4 weeks) have caused bladder irritation, painful and frequent micturition, proteinuria and gross hematuria. Dysuria can be controlled by reducing the dosage and acidification.

Acid urine pH should be maintained, especially when treating infections due to urea-splitting organisms such as *Proteus* and strains of *Pseudomonas.* When acidification is contraindicated or unattainable (as with some urea-splitting bacteria) the drug is not recommended.

Serum transaminases have elevated mildly during treatment in a few instances and returned to normal while patients were still receiving methenamine hippurate. Perform liver function studies periodically on patients receiving methenamine hippurate, especially those with liver dysfunction.

Methenamine mandelate oral suspensions have a vegetable oil base; administer with caution to elderly, debilitated or otherwise susceptible patients to avoid inducing lipid pneumonia.

Gout: Methenamine salts may cause precipitation of urate crystals in the urine.

Tartrazine sensitivity: Some of these products contain tartrazine, which may cause allergic-type reactions (including bronchial asthma) in certain susceptible individuals. Although the overall incidence of tartrazine sensitivity in the general population is low, it is frequently seen in patients who also have aspirin hypersensitivity. Specific products containing tartrazine are identified in the product listings.

Drug Interactions:

Sulfonamides: Avoid concurrent use; the sulfonamide may precipitate.

Sodium bicarbonate and **acetazolamide** can decrease the effectiveness of methenamine by alkalinizing the urine and inhibiting the conversion of methenamine to formaldehyde.

Drug/Lab Tests: Methenamine may interfere with laboratory urine determinations of **17-hydroxycorticosteroids, catecholamines** and **vanillylmandelic acid** (false increases); and **5-hydroxyindoleacetic acid** (false decrease).

Methenamine taken during pregnancy can interfere with laboratory tests of **urine estriol** (resulting in unmeasurably low values) when an acid hydrolysis procedure is used. This is due to the presence in the urine of methenamine or formaldehyde. Use enzymatic hydrolysis in place of acid hydrolysis.

Adverse Reactions:

Overall incidence: Approximately 1% to 7%.

GI: Nausea; vomiting; cramps; diarrhea; stomatitis; anorexia.

GU (large doses): Bladder irritation; dysuria; proteinuria; hematuria; frequency; urgency; crystalluria.

Dermatologic: Pruritus (rare); urticaria; erythematous eruptions; rashes.

Miscellaneous: Rare – Headache; dyspnea; lipoid pneumonitis; generalized edema.

Patient Information:

Take with food to minimize GI upset.

Drink sufficient fluids to ensure adequate urine flow.

Avoid excessive intake of alkalinizing foods (citrus fruits and milk products) or medication (bicarbonate, acetazolamide).

Complete full course of therapy; take until gone.

Notify physician if skin rash, painful urination or intolerable GI upset occurs.

(Products listed on following page)

Complete prescribing information for these products begins on page 2044

Methenamine and Methenamine Salts (Cont.)

METHENAMINE HIPPURATE

Administration and Dosage:

Adults and children over 12 years: 1 g twice daily.
Children (6 to 12 years): 0.5 to 1 g twice daily.

	Product	Form	Description	C.I.*
Rx	**Hiprex** (Merrell Dow)	**Tablets:** 1 g	Tartrazine, saccharin. (#Merrell 277). Yellow, scored. In 100s.	235
Rx	**Urex** (Riker)		Saccharin. (#Riker Urex). White, scored. In 100s and 500s.	269

METHENAMINE MANDELATE

Administration and Dosage:

Adults: 1 g, 4 times daily, after meals and at bedtime.
Children (6 to 12 years): 0.5 g, 4 times daily.
Children (less than 6 years): 0.25 g/30 lb (14 kg), 4 times daily.

	Product	Form	Description	C.I.*
Rx	**Methenamine Mandelate** (Various)	**Tablets:** 0.5 g	In 100s, 500s 1000s and UD 100s and 1000s.	23+
Rx	**Mandelamine** (Parke-Davis)		(#P-D 166). Brown. Film coated. In 100s, 1000s and UD 100s.	140
Rx	**Methenamine Mandelate** (Various)	**Tablets, enteric coated:** 0.5 g	In 1000s.	27+
Rx	**Mandameth** (Major)		Brown. In 100s and 250s.	45
Rx	**Methenamine Mandelate** (Various)	**Tablets:** 1 g	In 100s, 500s and 1000s.	19+
Rx	**Mandelamine** (Parke-Davis)		(#P-D 167). Purple. Film coated. In 100s, 1000s and UD 100s.	112
Rx	**Methenamine Mandelate** (Various)	**Tablets, enteric coated:** 1 g	In 100s, 1000s and UD 100s.	22+
Rx	**Mandameth** (Major)		In 100s and 250s.	33
Rx	**Mandelamine** (Parke-Davis)	**Oral Suspension:** 0.25 g per 5 ml	Coconut flavor. In 480 ml.[1]	549
Rx	**Methenamine Mandelate** (Various)	**Suspension Forte:** 0.5 g per 5 ml	In 480 ml.	147+
Rx	**Mandelamine** (Parke-Davis)		Cherry flavor. In 240 and 480 ml.[1]	422
Rx	**Mandelamine** (Parke-Davis)	**Granules:** 1 g packets	Orange flavor. In 56s.	286

* Cost Index based on cost per daily adult dose (4 g).
\# Product identification code.
[1] In a vegetable oil base.

The following anti-infective agents are used in these combinations:

TETRACYCLINE and *OXYTETRACYCLINE,* see p. 1811

SULFONAMIDES, see p. 1900

METHENAMINE and *METHENAMINE SALTS,* see p. 2044

METHYLENE BLUE, see p. 2036

Additional ingredients include:

PHENAZOPYRIDINE HCl, used as a urinary analgesic, see p. 2733

SALICYLAMIDE (see p. 1162 *SODIUM SALICYLATE* (see p. 1161 and *PHENYL SALICYLATE,* used as analgesics.

BELLADONNA ALKALOIDS, used as urinary antispasmodics, see p. 1586

SODIUM BIPHOSPHATE (SODIUM ACID PHOSPHATE), POTASSIUM ACID PHOSPHATE and BENZOIC ACID, used to acidify the urine.

Usual adult doses are listed, unless otherwise specified. Take doses with a full glass of water.

	Sulfonamide Combinations			C.I.*
Rx	**Urobiotic-250** (Roerig)	**Capsules:** 250 mg oxytetracycline (as HCl), 250 mg sulfamethizole and 50 mg phenazopyridine HCl. *Dose:* 1 capsule, 4 times daily.	(#Pfizer 092). Yellow and green. In 50s and UD 100s.	436
Rx	**Thiosulfil-A** (Ayerst)	**Tablets:** 250 mg sulfamethizole and 50 mg phenazopyridine HCl. *Dose:* 2 to 4 tablets, 3 or 4 times daily.	(#Ayerst 784). In 100s.	154
Rx	**Thiosulfil-A Forte** (Ayerst)	**Tablets:** 500 mg sulfamethizole and 50 mg phenazopyridine HCl. *Dose:* 2 tablets, 3 or 4 times daily.	(#Ayerst 783). Yellow. In 100s.	224
Rx	**Azo Gantanol** (Roche)	**Tablets:** 500 mg sulfamethoxazole and 100 mg phenazopyridine HCl. *Dose:* 4 tablets initially, then 2 tablets morning and evening for up to 2 days. Continue treatment beyond 2 days with sulfamethoxazole only.	(#Roche Azo Gantanol). Red. Film coated. In 100s and 500s.	218
Rx	**Azo-Sulfisoxazole** (Various)	**Tablets:** 500 mg sulfisoxazole and 50 mg phenazopyridine HCl. *Dose:* 4 to 6 tablets initially, then 2 tablets 4 times daily, up to 2 days. Continue treatment beyond 2 days with sulfisoxazole only.	In 100s and 1000s.	27+
Rx	**Azo Gantrisin** (Roche)		(#Roche Azo Gantrisin). Red. Film coated. In 100s and 500s.	92
Rx	**Suldiazo** (Kay Pharm.)		Red. Film coated. In 1000s.	23
Rx	**Thiosulfil Duo-Pak** (Ayerst)	*This package contains two products:* **Tablets:** Thiosulfil-A-Forte (500 mg sulfamethizole and 50 mg phenazopyridine HCl).	Yellow. In 16s.	
		Tablets: Thiosulfil Forte (500 mg sulfamethizole). *Dose:* Initial – 2 yellow tablets, 3 or 4 times per day for 2 days. Continue with 2 white tablets, 4 times/day for 5 days.	White. In 40s.	222

* Cost Index based on cost per minimum adult daily dose.

Product identification code.

Refer to the general statement concerning these products on page 2047

	Methenamine Combinations			C.I.*
Rx	**Prosed/DS** (Star)	**Tablets:** 81.6 mg methanemine, 36.2 mg phenyl salicylate.	Sugar. Deep blue. Sugar coated. In 100s and 1000s.	NA
Rx	**Urogesic Blue** (Edwards)	**Tablets:** 81.6 mg methenamine, 40.8 mg sodium biphosphate, 32.2 mg phenyl salicylate.	Sucrose. Purple. Sugar coated. In 100s.	NA
Rx	**Uro-Phosphate** (Poythress)	**Tablets:** 300 mg methenamine and 500 mg sodium biphosphate. *Dose:* 1 or 2 tablets at 4 to 6 hour intervals.	(WmP 9531). White. In 100s and 1000s.	55
Rx	**Uroqid-Acid** (Beach)	**Tablets:** 350 mg methenamine mandelate and 200 mg sodium acid phosphate. *Dose:* Initial – 3 tablets, 4 times daily. Maintenance – 1 or 2 tablets 4 times daily.	(Beach 1112). Yellow. Sugar coated. In 100s and 500s.	59
Rx	**Uroqid-Acid No. 2** (Beach)	**Tablets:** 500 mg methenamine mandelate and 500 mg sodium acid phosphate. *Dose:* Initial – 2 tablets, 4 times daily. Maintenance – 2 to 4 tablets daily, in divided doses.	(Beach 1114). Yellow, scored. Film coated. In 100s and 500s.	36
Rx	**Thiacide** (Beach)	**Tablets:** 500 mg methenamine mandelate and 250 mg potassium acid phosphate. *Dose:* 1 tablet every 2 to 4 hours; do not exceed 8 tablets in 24 hours.	Tartrazine. Sodium free. (Beach 1115). Green, scored. Film coated. In 100s.	29
Rx	**Urisedamine** (Webcon)	**Tablets:** 500 mg methenamine mandelate and 0.15 mg l-hyoscyamine. *Dose:* 2 tablets, 4 times daily.	(W 2210). Blue. In 100s.	270
Rx	**Trac Tabs 2X** (Hyrex)	**Tablets:** 120 mg methenamine, 30 mg phenyl salicylate, 0.06 mg atropine sulfate, 0.03 mg hyoscyamine sulfate, 7.5 mg benzoic acid and 6 mg methylene blue. *Dose:* 1 or 2 tablets, 4 times daily.	(HY-408). Blue. Sugar coated. In 100s and 1000s.	68
Rx	**U-Eze** (T.E. Williams)	**Tablets:** 81.6 mg methenamine, 40.8 mg sodium biphosphate, 36.2 mg phenyl salicylate, 10.8 mg methylene blue and 0.12 mg hyoscyamine (as sulfate). *Dose:* 1 tablet, 4 times daily.	In 100s.	79

* Cost Index based on cost per minimum adult dose.

(Continued on following page)

Refer to the general statement concerning these products on page 2047

Methenamine Combinations (Cont.)

	Product (Manufacturer)	Composition / Dose	How Supplied	C.I.*
Rx	**Atrosept** (Geneva Generics)	**Tablets:** 40.8 mg methenamine, 18.1 mg phenyl salicylate, 0.03 mg atropine sulfate, 0.03 mg hyoscyamine, 4.5 mg benzoic acid and 5.4 mg methylene blue. *Dose:* Adults – 2 tablets, 4 times daily. Children (≥ 6 years) – Reduce dosage in proportion to age and weight.	In 100s and 1000s.	75
Rx	**Dolsed** (American Urologicals)		(#Dolsed). Blue. Sugar coated. In 100s and 1000s.	157
Rx	**Hexalol** (Central)		(#93/845). Purple. Sugar coated. In 100s.	91
Rx	**Prosed** (Star)		In 100s and 1000s.	126
Rx	**UAA** (Econo Med)		(#UAA). Blue. Sugar coated. In 100s and 1000s.	75
Rx	**Uridon Modified** (Rugby)		Blue. Sugar coated. In 100s and 1000s.	22
Rx	**Urinary Antiseptic No. 2** (Various)		In 100s, 1000s and UD 100s.	41+
Rx	**Urised** (Webcon)		(#W 2183). Purple. Sugar coated. In 100s, 500s and 1000s.	229
Rx	**Uritab** (Vortech)		In 100s.	61
Rx	**Uritin** (Various)		In 1000s.	19+
Rx	**Uro-Ves** (Mallard)		Blue. In 1000s.	30
Rx	**Mandex** (Vale)	**Tablets, enteric coated:** 250 mg methenamine mandelate, 120 mg salicylamide and 5 mg extract belladonna. *Dose:* Adults – Initially, 4 tablets, 4 times daily. Maintenance – 1 tablet, 3 times daily. Children (> 5) – 1 tablet, 3 times daily. Children (< 5) – 1 tablet, 2 times daily.	Red. In 100s, 500s and 1000s.	81
otc	**Cystex** (CooperVision)	**Tablets:** 162 mg methenamine, 65 mg salicylamide, 97 mg sodium salicylate and 32 mg benzoic acid. *Dose:* Adults and children > 16 – 2 tablets, 4 times daily with meals and at bedtime.	In 40s and 100s.	91

* Cost Index based on cost per minimum adult daily dose.
# Product identification code.

NEOMYCIN AND POLYMYXIN B IRRIGANT

Actions:

Polymyxin B sulfate is bactericidal to most gram-negative bacilli, particularly against *Pseudomonas* infections. Neomycin sulfate is bactericidal against a wide range of gram-negative organisms including *Proteus vulgaris,* and gram-positive organisms. When used topically, these drugs are rarely irritating.

Indications:

Continuous irrigant or rinse for short-term use (up to 10 days) in the urinary bladder of abacteriuric patients to help prevent bacteriuria and gram-negative rod bacteremia associated with the use of indwelling catheters.

Contraindications:

Hypersensitivity to any component.

Precautions:

Safety and efficacy have not been established for use in patients with recent lower urinary tract surgery.

Superinfection: Use of antibiotics (especially prolonged or repeated therapy) may result in bacterial or fungal overgrowth of nonsusceptible organisms. Such overgrowth may lead to a secondary infection. Take appropriate measures if superinfection occurs.

Neomycin toxicity: Neomycin is nephrotoxic and ototoxic, particularly when given parenterally in higher than recommended doses. Cases of nephrotoxicity or ototoxicity have been reported following its topical use for extensive burns and wound irrigation. Although the possibility of these reactions is remote with use of the minimal amount in bladder irrigations, such reactions may occur if irrigations are continued beyond the recommended maximum of 10 days; observe caution.

Adverse Reactions:

The prevalence of neomycin hypersensitivity has increased; however, topical application to mucous membranes rarely results in local or systemic reactions.

Administration and Dosage:

Not for injection.

For use with catheter systems permitting continuous irrigation of the urinary bladder: Add 1 ml irrigant to 1 L isotonic saline solution. Connect the container to the inflow lumen of the three-way catheter. Connect the outflow lumen via a sterile disposable plastic tube to a disposable plastic collection bag.

Adjust flow rate to 1 L/24 hours. If the patient's urine output exceeds 2 L/day, increase flow rate to 2 L/24 hours.

The rinse of the bladder must be continuous. Do not interrupt the inflow or rinse solution for more than a few minutes.

Rx	**Neosporin G.U. Irrigant** (Burroughs Wellcome)	**Solution:** 40 mg neomycin (as sulfate) and 200,000 units polymyxin B sulfate per ml	In 1 ml amps and 20 ml vials.[1]

[1] With methylparaben.

CITRIC ACID, GLUCONO-DELTA-LACTONE AND MAGNESIUM CARBONATE IRRIGANT (Hemiacidrin)

Actions:

The action of hemiacidrin on susceptible apatite calculi results from an exchange of magnesium from the irrigating solution for the insoluble calcium contained in the stone matrix or calcification. The magnesium salts thereby formed are soluble in the gluconocitrate irrigating solution resulting in the dissolution of the calculus. Struvite calculi are composed mainly of magnesium ammonium phosphates which are solubilized by hemiacidrin due to its acidic pH.

Hemiacidrin is not effective for dissolution of calcium oxalate, uric acid or cysteine stones.

Indications:

Solution: For use as local irrigation for the dissolution of renal calculi composed of apatite (a calcium carbonate-phosphate compound) or struvite (magnesium ammonium phosphates) in patients who are not candidates for surgical removal of the calculi.

As adjunctive therapy to dissolve residual apatite or struvite calculi and fragments after surgery or to achieve partial dissolution of renal calculi to facilitate surgical removal.

For dissolution of bladder calculi of the struvite or apatite variety by local intermittent irrigation through a urethral catheter or cystostomy catheter as an alternative or adjunct to surgical procedures.

For use as an intermittent irrigating solution to prevent or minimize encrustations of indwelling urinary tract catheters.

Powder for solution: For use in preparing solutions for irrigating indwelling urethral catheters and the urinary bladder, to dissolve or prevent formation of calcifications.

Unlabeled use: Hemiacidrin has been used as a renal pelvis irrigation, with meticulous attention to intrapelvic pressure and urosepsis.

Contraindications:

Solution: Urinary tract infections (see Warnings); presence of demonstrable urinary tract extravasation.

Powder for solution: Biliary calculi; therapy or preventive therapy above the ureteral-vesical junction, therefore contraindicated for use with ureteral catheters, nephrostomy or pyelostomy tubes or renal lavage for dissolving calculi.

Warnings:

Urinary tract infection: Stop the hemiacidrin immediately if the patient develops fever, urinary tract infection, signs and symptoms consistent with urinary tract infection, or persistent flank pain or if hypermagnesemia or elevated serum creatinine develops.

Urea-splitting bacteria reside within struvite and apatite stones which therefore serve as a source of infection. Dissolution therapy with hemiacidrin in the presence of an infected urinary tract may lead to sepsis and death. Obtain urine specimens for culture prior to initiating chemolytic therapy of the renal pelvis. Institute appropriate antibiotic therapy to treat any infection detected. A sterile urine must be present prior to initiating therapy. An infected stone can serve as a continual source for infection; therefore, continue antibiotic therapy throughout the course of dissolution therapy.

Severe hypermagnesemia has occurred. Use caution when irrigating the renal pelvis of patients with impaired renal function. Observe patients for early signs and symptoms of hypermagnesemia including nausea, lethargy, confusion and hypotension. Severe hypermagnesemia may result in hyporeflexia, dyspnea, apnea, coma, cardiac arrest and subsequent death. Monitor serum magnesium levels and evaluate deep tendon reflexes. Treatment of hypermagnesemia should include discontinuation of hemiacidrin followed by therapy with IV calcium gluconate, fluids and diuresis in severe cases.

Not indicated for dissolution of calcium oxalate, uric acid or cysteine calculi.

Pregnancy: Category C. It is not known whether hemiacidrin can cause fetal harm when administered to a pregnant woman or can affect reproduction capacity. Give to a pregnant woman only if clearly needed.

Lactation: Magnesium is known to be excreted into breast milk. However, it is not known whether hemiacidrin is excreted in breast milk. Exercise caution when hemiacidrin is administered to a nursing woman.

Precautions:

Vesicoureteral reflux frequently occurs in patients with indwelling urethral or cystostomy catheters. Cystogram prior to initiation of hemiacidrin is essential for such patients. If reflux is demonstrated, all precautions recommended for renal pelvis irrigation must be taken.

(Precautions continued on following page)

CITRIC ACID, GLUCONO-DELTA-LACTONE AND MAGNESIUM CARBONATE IRRIGANT (Hemiacidrin) (Cont.)

Precautions (Cont.):

Catheter care: Hospitalization is prolonged for days to weeks when chemolytic therapy is used in lieu of, or following, surgery. Reserve this therapy for selected patients. Care must be taken during chemolysis of renal calculi with hemiacidrin to maintain the patency of the irrigating catheter. Calculus fragments and debris may obstruct the outflow catheter. Continued irrigation under those circumstances leads to increased intrapelvic pressure with a danger of tissue damage or absorption of the irrigating solution. Catheter outflow blockage may be prevented by flushing the catheter with saline and repositioning of the catheter. Frequent monitoring of the system should be performed by a nurse, an aide or any person with sufficient skills to be able to detect any problems with the patency of the catheter. At the first sign of obstruction, discontinue the irrigation and disconnect the system.

Intrapelvic pressures must be maintained at or below 25 cm of water. The preferred method of pressure control is the insertion of an open Y connection pop-off valve into the infusion line allowing immediate decompression if pressure exceeds 25 cm of water. An alternative method has been proposed to direct or stop the flow of the irrigating solution to prevent increased intrapelvic pressure: Placement of a pinch clamp on the inflow line which can be used by the patient or nurse to stop the irrigation at the first sign of flank pain. However, extreme caution must be taken when relying on cooperation of the patient. Patients may not be sufficiently alert to detect signs and symptoms of outflow obstruction. This is especially true in elderly patients, sedated patients or those with severe neurological dysfunction with varying degrees of sensory loss or motor paralysis.

Monitoring: Throughout the course of therapy, monitor patients to ensure safety. Obtain serum creatinine phosphate and magnesium every few days. Collect urine specimens for culture and antibacterial sensitivity every 3 days or less and at the first sign of fever. Stop the irrigation if any culture exhibits growth and initiate appropriate antibacterial therapy. The irrigation may be started again after a course of antibacterial therapy upon demonstration of a sterile urine. Struvite calculi frequently contain bacteria within the stone; therefore, continue antibacterial therapy throughout the course of dissolution therapy. Hypermagnesemia or an elevated serum creatinine level are indications to halt the irrigation until they return to pre-irrigation levels. Evidence of severe urothelial edema on X-ray is also an indication for temporarily halting the irrigation until the complication resolves.

Drug Interactions:

Magnesium-containing medications: Concurrent use may contribute to production of hypermagnesemia and is not recommended.

Adverse Reactions:

Solution: The most common adverse reaction in selected case series is transient flank pain which occurs in most patients. Additional reactions include: Urothelial ulceration or edema (13%); fever (20% but up to 40% in some case series); urinary tract infection, back pain, dysuria, transient hematuria, nausea, hypermagnesemia, hyperphosphatemia, elevated serum creatinine, candidiasis, bladder irritability (1% to 10%); septicemia, ileus, vomiting, thrombophlebitis (< 1%). Death from sepsis has occurred.

Powder for solution: Occasional temporary pain or burning sensation from this procedure; discontinue use if this occurs.

Administration and Dosage:

Solution:

Renal calculi – It is essential that patients be free from urinary tract infections prior to initiating chemolytic therapy. A nephrostomy tube is placed at surgery or percutaneously to permit lavage of the calculi. A single catheter may be sufficient if the calculus is not obstructing the ureter or ureteropelvic junction. In patients with an obstructed ureter, a retrograde catheter can be placed through the ureter to the renal pelvis via a cystoscope. This second catheter is used to irrigate the calculus while the percutaneous nephrostomy tube is used for drainage. Pressure measurements are made under fluoroscopy to assure that 2 to 3 ml/min can be infused without causing pain, pyelovenous or pyelotubular backflow or manometric evidence of elevated pressure within the collecting system.

For postoperative patients, irrigation should not be started before the fourth or fifth postoperative day. Irrigation of the renal pelvis is begun with sterile saline only after a sterile urine has been demonstrated. The saline is infused at a rate of 60 ml/hr initially, and the rate is increased until pain or an elevated pressure (25 cm H_2O) appears, or until a maximum flow rate of 120 ml/hr is achieved. Inspect the site of insertion for leakage. If leakage occurs, the irrigation is discontinued temporarily to allow for complete healing around the nephrostomy tube.

(Administration and Dosage continued on following page)

CITRIC ACID, GLUCONO-DELTA-LACTONE AND MAGNESIUM CARBONATE IRRIGANT (Hemiacidrin) (Cont.)

Administration and Dosage (Cont.)

Solution: Renal calculi (Cont.):

If no leakage or flank pain occurs, irrigation is then started with hemiacidrin with a flow rate equal to the maximum rate achieved with the saline solution. Place a clamp on the inflow tube and patients and nursing personnel should be instructed to stop the irrigating solution whenever pain develops. Nursing personnel who are responsible for performing the irrigation must be instructed concerning the location of the nephrostomy tube(s) and the direction of flow of the irrigating solution to ensure against misconnection of the inflowing and egress tubes. Perform nephrostomograms periodically to assure proper placement of the catheter tip and to assess efficacy. If stones fail to change size after several days of adequate irrigation, discontinue the procedure.

Upon demonstration of complete dissolution of the calculus, the inflow tube is clamped and left in place for a few days to ensure that no obstruction exists, after which time the nephrostomy tube is removed.

Bladder calculi – Chemolysis of bladder calculi is used as an alternative to cystoscopic or surgical removal of the stones in patients who refuse surgery or cystoscopic removal or in whom these procedures constitute an unwarranted risk. Following appropriate studies to evaluate possible vesicoureteral reflux, 30 ml of hemiacidrin is instilled through a urinary catheter into the bladder and the catheter is clamped for 30 to 60 minutes. The clamp is then released and the bladder is drained. This is repeated 4 to 6 times a day. A continuous drip through a 3 way Foley catheter is an alternative means of dissolving bladder stones. In the presence of bladder spasm and associated high pressure reflux, all precautions required for irrigation of the renal pelvis must be observed.

Indwelling urinary tract catheter encrustation – Periodic instillation of hemiacidrin is indicated to minimize or prevent encrustation of indwelling catheters which frequently results in plugging of the catheter and discomfort to the patient. This is accomplished by instilling 30 ml of the solution through the catheter and then clamping the catheter for 10 minutes, after which the clamp is removed to allow drainage of the bladder. This process is repeated 3 times a day.

Powder for solution:

Irrigating indwelling catheters – Administer as a 10% solution (sterile) in distilled water. Irrigation is carried out with 30 to 60 ml 2 to 3 times daily by means of a rubber syringe.

Preparation of the solution: Always add powder to the water; do not add water to the powder when preparing solutions.

Dissolve the contents of one 300 g bottle in 3000 ml of sterile distilled water, or any smaller quantity of powder in the proportionately smaller amount of water. Since powder may be reactive upon addition to water, add slowly to the water, with constant agitation, in a container larger than that which the amount of solution actually requires. Do not stopper or cap the container during preparation. Thoroughly mix the solution for as long as possible (up to 15 to 20 minutes). This can be achieved through the use of a mechanical mixer where available. Solutions often vary in color from almost colorless to a definite clear yellow solution.

After thorough mixing, filter the solution through a coarse filter to remove any undissolved matter. Alternatively, if desired, the solution may be allowed to stand and decant. (A 10% solution was filtered after 24 hours and the residue dried at 105°C for 8 hours, then weighed. The weight of the residue equalled 0.008% of the solution.)

The residue which may be noted on a filter consists primarily of the insolubles present in the original magnesium hydroxycarbonate, which has about 0.03% to 0.05% acid insolubles in the form of a small amount of silica (or calcium, as the silicate) and iron oxides which remain undissolved when the solution is prepared. It may be yellow or even brown or black in color.

Storage (solution): Minimize exposure of hemiacidrin to heat or cold. Store at controlled room temperature (15° to 30°C; 59° to 86°F). Avoid excessive heat or cold (keep from freezing). Brief exposure to temperatures of up to 40°C (104°F) or temperatures down to 5°C (41°F) does not adversely affect the product.

Rx	**Renacidin** (Guardian)	**Powder for Solution:** 156 to 171 g citric acid (anhydrous) and 21 to 30 g d-gluconic acid (as the lactone) with 75 to 87 g purified magnesium hydroxycarbonate, 9 to 15 g magnesium acid citrate, 2 to 6 g calcium (as carbonate) and 17 to 21 g water (combined and free) per 300 g bottle	In 150 or 300 g.
		Solution: 6.602 g citric acid (anhydrous), 0.198 g glucono-delta-lactone, 3.177 g magnesium carbonate and 0.023 g benzoic acid per 100 ml	In 500 ml.

Hexitol Irrigants

Actions:

Hexitol irrigants are nonelectrolytic and nonhemolytic urologic irrigation solutions. The amount of solution absorbed intravascularly during transurethral prostatic surgery is variable and depends primarily on the extent and duration of the surgery. Mannitol is confined to the extracellular space, only slightly metabolized, rapidly excreted in the urine and is, therefore, an effective osmotic diuretic. The sorbitol-containing products will be metabolized to carbon dioxide (70%) and dextrose (30%) or excreted by the kidneys.

Indications:

In transurethral prostatic resection or other transurethral surgical procedures.

Contraindications:

Anuria; injection.

Warnings:

Use with caution in patients with significant cardiopulmonary or renal dysfunction (see Precautions).

Systemic effects: Irrigating fluids used during transurethral prostatectomy may enter the systemic circulation in relatively large volumes. Therefore, the irrigation solution must be considered as a systemic drug. The osmotic diuresis it may produce can significantly alter cardiopulmonary and renal dynamics.

Diabetes mellitus: Hyperglycemia from metabolism of sorbitol may occur in patients with diabetes mellitus.

Sorbitol solution: Use with caution in patients unable to metabolize sorbitol rapidly enough to avoid the development of hyperosmolar states.

Precautions:

Cardiovascular effects: Carefully evalute the cardiovascular status of the patient, particularly one with cardiac disease, before and during transurethral prostatic resection when mannitol solution is used as an irrigant. The quantity of fluid absorbed into the systemic circulation may cause expansion of the extracellular fluid, leading to fulminating congestive heart failure.

Fluid and electrolyte balance: Systemic absorption of the solutions may cause a shift of sodium free intracellular fluid into the extracellular compartment, lowering serum sodium concentration and aggravating any preexisting hyponatremia.

A significant diuresis resulting from the irrigating solution may obscure and intensify inadequate hydration or hypovolemia. Excessive loss of water and electrolytes may lead to hypernatremia.

Adverse Reactions:

Since significant systemic absorption occurs, the potential for systemic effects must be considered. The following effects have been noted from *intravenous infusion:*

Fluid and electrolyte disturbances – Acidosis; electrolyte loss; marked diuresis; urinary retention; edema; dry mouth; thirst; dehydration.

Cardiovascular/pulmonary disorders – Pulmonary congestion; hypotension; tachycardia; angina-like pains; thrombophlebitis.

Miscellaneous – Blurred vision; convulsions; nausea; vomiting; rhinitis; chills; vertigo; backache; urticaria; diarrhea.

Additional reactions associated with sorbitol solution include slight increases in postoperative serum glucose and inhibition of intestinal absorption of vitamin B_{12}.

Administration and Dosage:

Do not use unless solution is clear and seal unbroken. Use as required for irrigation.

Storage: Promptly use the contents of opened containers; discard unused portions of the solution. Do not warm above 66°C (150°F). Protect from freezing and avoid storage above 40°C (104°F).

MANNITOL			
Rx	**Resectisol** (Kendall McGaw)	**Solution:** 5 g per 100 ml in distilled water (275 mOsm/L)	In 2000 ml.
SORBITOL			
Rx	Kendall McGaw	**Solution:** 3.3% (183 mOsm/L)	In 2000 ml.
Rx	Travenol	**Solution:** 3% (165 mOsm/L)	In 1500 and 3000 ml.
MANNITOL AND SORBITOL			
Rx	**Sorbitol-Mannitol** (Abbott)	**Solution:** 0.54 g mannitol and 2.7 g sorbitol per 100 ml (178 mOsm/L)	In 1500 and 3000 ml.

SUBY'S SOLUTION G

Indications:

To dissolve phosphatic calculi or incrustations in the bladder and urethra; to irrigate the bladder and urethra with an acidic solution.

Contraindications:

Do not use in presence of fulminating bladder infections, bleeding, ulcerations or other open wounds.

Not for injection into body tissue.

Not for irrigation during transurethral surgical procedures.

These solutions are conductive; do not use in the presence of electrical instrumentation.

Warning:

For use in irrigation of the lower urinary tract only.

Not recommended for dissolving phosphate calculi in the renal pelvis because of the risk of creating back pressure that may reactivate an existing pyelonephritis.

Do not use solution to replace other indicated measures including correction of underlying metabolic disorders, surgical intervention and treatment of infection.

Usage in Pregnancy: Category C. It is not known whether this irrigation solution can cause fetal harm when given to a pregnant woman or can affect reproduction capacity. Administer to a pregnant woman only if clearly needed.

Precautions:

Avoid reflux of the solution up the ureters into the renal pelvis. Repeated or continuous use may cause bleeding. Solution is irritating to urethra; after each treatment, irrigate with sterile saline or water.

Four cases of sudden death were reported during lavage therapy with a similarly acting solution. The autopsy indicated that calcium phosphate sludge resulting from dissolving stone is a severe irritant to the renal pelvis and is probably absorbed to some degree as evidenced by a terminal serum phosphorus of three times the normal level in one case. Disintegration of calculi into phosphate sludge by acids might form a variety of toxic compounds in small quantities. Since pyelonephritis accompanies renal calculus disease in many cases, pyelorenal backflow of chemicals may aggravate the infectious process causing progression to a severe toxemia.

Adverse Reactions:

Discomfort or pain due to bladder irritation during irrigation. In the presence of undetected mucosal lesions, irrigation may initiate bleeding from the bladder.

Administration and Dosage:

Not for IV, SC or IM injection.

Administer 1 to 3 liters daily by intermittent irrigation or by tidal instillation and drainage to allow continuous irrigation of the bladder for periods of several hours. Intermittent irrigation of the bladder (after the manner of intermittent peritoneal dialysis) may be preferred to promote more prolonged contact of the irrigation with bladder stones; tidal (continuous in and out flow) irrigation may be less efficient and require larger amounts of irrigation fluid.

Use contents of opened container promptly to minimize the possibility of bacterial growth or pyrogen formation. Do not use solution unless clear and seal is intact. Discard unused portion.

Rx	Abbott	**Solution:** 3.24 g citric acid (monohydrate), 0.43 g sodium carbonate (anhydrous) and 0.38 g magnesium oxide (anhydrous) per 100 ml	In 1000 ml.
Rx	Travenol		In 1000 ml.

ACETIC ACID FOR IRRIGATION

Indications:

For bladder irrigation.

Rx	Abbott	**Solution:** 0.25%	In 250 and 1000 ml.
Rx	Baxter		In 1000 ml.
Rx	Kendall McGaw		In 500 and 1000 ml.

GLYCINE (AMINOACETIC ACID) FOR IRRIGATION

Indications:

For urological irrigation.

Rx	Abbott	**Solution:** 1.5%	In 1500 and 3000 ml.
Rx	Baxter		In 3000 and 5000 ml.
Rx	Kendall McGaw		In 2000 and 4000 ml.

SODIUM CHLORIDE FOR IRRIGATION

Indications:

For use as an irrigating solution.

Rx	Abbott	**Solution (Isotonic):** 0.9%	In 250, 500, 1000, 1500 and 2000 ml.
Rx	Baxter		In 150, 250, 500, 1000 and 1500 ml.
Rx	Kendall McGaw		In 500, 1000, 2000 and 4000 ml.
Rx	Abbott	**Solution (Hypotonic):** 0.45%	In 500, 1000 and 1500 ml.
Rx	Baxter		In 1000 ml.

STERILE WATER FOR IRRIGATION

Indications:

For use as an irrigating solution.

Rx	Abbott		In 250, 500 and 1000 ml.
Rx	Baxter		In 1000 ml.
Rx	Kendall McGaw		In 500, 1000, 2000 and 4000 ml.

In addition to the commercially available anti-infective agents, the Centers for Disease Control (CDC) can supply several investigational agents upon request. These agents may be requested from the Drug Service, Division of Host Factors, Center for Infectious Disease, by calling 404-639-3670, 8:00 a.m. to 4:30 p.m. EST Monday through Friday; for emergencies (evenings, weekends or holidays), call 404-639-2888.

The following drugs are available:

Generic	Trade Name	Disease/Infestation	Organism
Bithionol	Lorothidol Bitin	Paragonimiasis Fascioliasis	*Paragonimus westermani* *Fasciola hepatica*
Dehydroemetine	Mebadin	Amebiasis Amebic dysentery	*Entamoeba histolytica*
Diloxanide furoate	Furamide	Amebiasis, asymptomatic cyst passers	*Entamoeba histolytica*
Melarsoprol (Mel B)	Arsobal	Trypanosomiasis (African sleeping sickness)	*Trypanosoma gambiense* *Trypanosoma rhodesiense*
Nifurtimox	Lampit (Bayer 2502)	Chagas' disease (megaesophagus, megacolon)	*Trypanosoma cruzi*
Sodium antimony gluconate or sodium stibogluconate	Pentostam	Leishmaniasis (kala azar, espundia ulcer, oriental sore)	*Leishmania brasiliensis* *Leishmania mexicana* *Leishmania donovani* *Leishmania tropica*
Suramin	Fourneau 309 Bayer 205 Germanin Moranyl Belganyl Naphuride Antrypol Naganol	Trypanosomiasis Onchocerciasis	*Trypanosoma gambiense* *Trypanosoma rhodesiense* *Onchocerca volvulus*
Quinine dihydrochloride (parenteral)		Pernicious malaria	*Plasmodium falciparum*
Rifabutin	Ansamycin LM 427	Mycobacterial disease Acquired Immune Deficiency Syndrome (AIDS)	*Mycobacterium avium*

chapter 9

biologicals

Standard immune globulins contain approximately 16.5% gamma globulin. Immune globulin IV contains 5% immune globulins. These products are obtained, purified and standardized from human serum or plasma. They are obtained from pooled plasma either of donors from the general population or of hyperimmunized donors (for immune globulins for specific diseases).

The following general information applies to all immune sera. For specific information on individual agents, refer to specific monographs:

Immune Globulin, Intramuscular
Immune Globulin, Intravenous
Hepatitis B Immune Globulin
Tetanus Immune Globulin
Varicella-Zoster Immune Globulin
Rh_O (D) Immune Globulin
Lymphocyte Immune Globulin

Indications:

To provide passive immunization to one or more infectious diseases. Protection derived will be of rapid onset, but of short duration (1 to 3 months). See individual monographs for specific indications.

Contraindications:

Allergic response to gamma globulin or anti-immunoglobulin A (IgA) antibodies.

Allergic response to thimerosal.

Persons with isolated immunoglobulin A (IgA) deficiency. Such persons have the potential for developing antibodies to IgA and could have anaphylactic reactions to subsequent administration of blood products that contain IgA.

Immune Globulin, intramuscular should not be administered to patients who have severe thrombocytopenia or any coagulation disorder that would contraindicate IM use.

Warnings:

Do not give these products IV (except immune globulin IV). IV injections can cause a precipitous fall in blood pressure and a picture similar to anaphylaxis. Administer IM.

Hypersensitivity reactions: Give with caution to patients with prior systemic allergic reactions following administration of human immunoglobulin preparations. Hypersensitivity reactions occur rarely; the incidence may be increased in patients receiving large IM doses or in patients receiving repeated injections of immune globulin. Epinephrine should be available for treatment of acute allergic symptoms. Refer to Management of Acute Hypersensitivity Reactions

Anaphylactic reactions (rare) may occur following the injection of human immune globulin preparations. Anaphylaxis is more likely to occur if immune globulin is given IV; therefore, except for immune globulin IV, these products must only be administered IM. In highly allergic individuals, repeated injections may lead to anaphylactic shock.

Usage in Pregnancy: Category C. No studies have been conducted in pregnant patients. Clinical experience suggests no adverse effects on the fetus per se; however, it is not known whether these agents can cause fetal harm.

Usage in Lactation: Safety for use in the nursing mother has not been established. It is not known whether immune globulin is excreted in breast milk.

Precautions:

Skin testing should not be performed. Intradermal injection of concentrated gamma globulin causes a localized area of inflammation which can be misinterpreted as a positive allergic reaction. It is actually localized chemical tissue irritation. Misinterpretation can cause necessary medication to be withheld from a patient not actually allergic to this material. True allergic responses to human gamma globulin given in the prescribed IM manner are extremely rare.

Admixture incompatibilities: Do not admix with other medications.

Drug Interactions:

Live virus vaccines: Do not administer within 3 months of immune globulin administration because antibodies in the globulin preparation may interfere with the immune response to the vaccination. It may be necessary to revaccinate persons who received immune globulin shortly after live virus vaccination.

Adverse Reactions:

Local: Tenderness, pain, muscle stiffness at the injection site; may persist for several hours.

Systemic: Urticaria; angioedema. Less frequently reported reactions include: Emesis; chills; fever; myalgia; lethargy; chest tightness; nausea. Isolated cases of angioneurotic edema and nephrotic syndrome have occurred.

(Products listed on following pages)

Complete prescribing information for these products begins on page 2062.

IMMUNE GLOBULIN INTRAVENOUS (IGIV)

Intravenous immune globulin (IGIV) provides immediate antibody levels, whereas IM administration involves a 2 to 5 day delay before adequate serum levels are attained. The half-life is approximately 3 weeks.

IGIV can cause a precipitous fall in blood pressure and the clinical picture of anaphylaxis, even when the patient is not known to be sensitive to immune globulin preparations. These reactions appear to be related to the infusion rate. Closely follow the infusion rates given under Administration and Dosage. Monitor vital signs continuously and observe for any symptoms throughout the infusion. Have epinephrine available.

Mechanism of action in idiopathic thrombocytopenic purpura (ITP) is not determined.

Indications:

Immunodeficiency syndrome: For the maintenance treatment of patients who are unable to produce sufficient amounts of IgG antibodies. IGIV may be preferred to IM immunoglobulin, especially in patients who require an immediate increase in intravascular immunoglobulin levels, in patients with a small muscle mass, and in patients with bleeding tendencies in whom IM injections are contraindicated. It may be used in disease states such as congenital agammaglobulinemia (eg, x-linked agammaglobulinemia), common variable hypogammaglobulinemia, x-linked immunodeficiency with hyper IgM and combined immunodeficiency.

Idiopathic thrombocytopenic purpura (Gamimune N, Gammagard, Sandoglobulin and *Venoglobulin-I only):* Some children and adults with ITP have shown an increase (albeit temporary) in platelet counts upon administration of IGIV. Therefore, consider administration in situations that require a rapid, temporary rise in the platelet count (eg, prior to surgery or to control excessive bleeding). Not all patients will respond. Even in those patients who do respond, this treatment should not be considered curative.

B-cell chronic lymphocytic leukemia (CLL) (Gammagard only): Prevention of bacterial infections in patients with hypogammaglobulinemia or recurrent bacterial infections associated with B-cell CLL. In one study, bacterial infections were significantly reduced in 41 patients receiving *Gammagard* compared to 40 patients receiving placebo. The placebo group had twice as many bacterial infections.

Administration and Dosage:

Administer IV only.

IGIV is well tolerated and less likely to produce side effects if infused at indicated rates.

Sandoglobulin: Usual dosage in immunodeficiency syndrome – 200 mg/kg administered once a month by IV infusion. If clinical response or the level of IgG achieved is insufficient (minimum serum level of 300 mg/dl), increase dose to 300 mg/kg or repeat the infusion more frequently.

Rate of administration – Give the first infusion to previously untreated agammaglobulinemic or hypogammaglobulinemic patients as a 3% immunoglobulin solution. Start with a flow rate of 0.5 to 1 ml/min. After 15 to 30 minutes, further increase the infusion rate to 1.5 to 2.5 ml/min. Administer subsequent infusions at a rate of 2 to 2.5 ml/min.

If high doses must be administered repeatedly after the first dose, a 6% solution may be used; the initial infusion rate should be 1 to 1.5 ml/min, increased after 15 to 30 minutes to a maximum of 2.5 ml/min.

Idiopathic thrombocytopenic purpura – 400 mg/kg for 2 to 5 consecutive days.

Reconstitution – 3% solution: Invert bottles so that solvent flows into IV bottle.

6% solution: For 1 g vial, use 16.5 ml diluent; for 3 g vial, use 50 ml diluent; for 6 g vial, use 100 ml diluent.

Proceed with infusion only if solution is clear and at approximately body temperature.

Gammagard: Initial dosage in immunodeficiency syndrome – 200 to 400 mg/kg. Monthly doses of at least 100 mg/kg are recommended.

B-Cell CLL – 400 mg/kg every 3 to 4 weeks.

Idiopathic thrombocytopenic purpura – 1000 mg/kg. Need for additional doses can be determined by clinical response and platelet count. Give up to 3 doses on alternate days if required.

Rate of administration – Initially 0.5 ml/kg/hr. If rate causes the patient no distress, it may be gradually increased, not to exceed 4 ml/kg/hr.

Gammar-IV: Usual dosage in immunodeficiency syndrome – 100 to 200 mg/kg every 3 to 4 weeks. An initial loading dose of at least 200 mg/kg at more frequent intervals, proceeding to 100 to 200 mg/kg at 3 week intervals once a therapeutic plasma level has been established can be used. Individualize treatment.

Rate of administration – 0.01 ml/kg/min, increasing to 0.02 ml/kg/min after 15 to 30 min. Most patients tolerate a gradual increase to 0.03 to 0.06 ml/kg/min. If adverse reactions develop, slowing the infusion rate will usually eliminate the reaction.

(Administration and Dosage continued on following page)

IMMUNE GLOBULIN INTRAVENOUS (IGIV) (Cont.)

Administration and Dosage (Cont.):

Venoglobulin-I: Initial dosage in immunodeficiency syndrome – 200 mg/kg, administered monthly. If clinical response or the level of IgG achieved is insufficient, increase to 300 to 400 mg/kg monthly or repeat infusion more frequently than once a month.

Rate of administration – Infuse at a rate of 0.01 to 0.02 ml/kg/min for the first 30 minutes. If rate causes the patient no distress, it may be increased to 0.04 ml/kg/min. If tolerated, subsequent infusions to the same patient may be at the higher rate.

Idiopathic thrombocytopenic purpura – Induction: 500 mg/kg/day for 2 to 7 consecutive days.

Acute: Patients who respond to induction therapy by manifesting a platelet count of 30,000 to 50,000/mm³ may be discontinued after 2 to 7 daily doses.

Maintenance: If platelet count falls to < 30,000/mm³ or the patient manifests clinically significant bleeding, 500 to 2000 mg/kg may be given as a single infusion every 2 weeks or less as needed to maintain the platelet count above 30,000/mm³ in children and 20,000/mm³ in adults.

Gamimune N: Usual dosage in immunodeficiency syndrome – 100 to 200 mg/kg (2 to 4 ml/kg) administered once a month by IV infusion. May dilute in 5% dextrose. If clinical response or the level of IgG achieved is insufficient, increase to 400 mg/kg (8 ml/kg) or repeat the infusion more frequently than once a month.

Rate of administration – 0.01 to 0.02 ml/kg/min for 30 minutes by itself. If the patient does not experience any discomfort, the rate may be increased to a maximum of 0.08 ml/kg/min. If side effects occur, reduce the rate or interrupt the infusion until symptoms subside; resume at a rate tolerable by the patient.

Idiopathic thrombocytopenic purpura – 400 mg/kg for 5 consecutive days.

Iveegam: Usual dosage in immunodeficiency syndrome – 200 mg/kg per month. If desired clinical results are not obtained, the dosage may be increased up to fourfold or intervals shortened. Doses up to 800 mg/kg per month have been tolerated.

Rate of administration – 1 ml/min up to a maximum of 2 ml/min for the 5% solution. The drug may be further diluted with 5% dextrose or saline; with gradually increasing dosage levels and protein concentrations (up to 5% protein) adverse reactions were not observed.

Storage: Sandoglobulin and Gammagard – Store at room temperature not exceeding 25°C (77°F). Discard partially used vials.

Gamimune N and Iveegam – Store at 2° to 8°C (35° to 46°F). Do not freeze. Do not use a solution that has been frozen. Discard partially used vials.

Venoglobulin-I – Store at a temperature below 30°C (86°F).

Gammar-IV – Store at temperatures not exceeding 30°C (86°F). Avoid freezing. Discard any unused solution.

Rx	**Gamimune N** (Cutter Biological)	**Injection**: 5% (in 10% maltose)	In 10, 50 and 100 ml single-dose vials.
Rx	**Gammagard** (Hyland)	**Powder for Injection (lyophilized)**: 50 mg protein per ml containing at least 90% gamma globulin when reconstituted	In 0.5, 2.5, 5 and 10 g single-dose vials.
Rx	**Gammar-IV** (Armour)	**Powder for Injection (lyophilized)**	In 120 ml single-dose vial with Sterile Water for Injection as diluent.
Rx	**Iveegam** (Immuno)	**Powder for Injection (freeze-dried, lyophilized)**	In 500 mg and 1 g vials with 10 and 20 ml Sterile Water for Injection as diluent, respectively, and 2.5 and 5 g infusion bottles with 50 and 100 ml Sterile Water for Injection as diluent, respectively.
Rx	**Sandoglobulin** (American Red Cross, Sandoz)	**Powder for Injection (lyophilized)**	1, 3 and 6 g vials with 33, 100 and 200 ml 0.9% NaCl injection as diluent, respectively.
Rx	**Venoglobulin-I** (Alpha Therapeutic)	**Powder for Injection (lyophilized)**	In 2.5 or 5 g individual vial or in reconstitution kit containing Sterile Water for Injection, USP (50 ml and 100 ml, respectively).[1]

[1] Preservative free.

Complete prescribing information for these products begins on page 2062.

CYTOMEGALOVIRUS IMMUNE GLOBULIN INTRAVENOUS, HUMAN (CMV-IGIV)

Actions:

Pharmacology: This product contains IgG antibodies representative of the large number of healthy persons who contributed to the plasma pools from which the product was derived. The globulin contains a relatively high concentration of antibodies directed against cytomegalovirus (CMV). In persons who may be exposed to CMV, this product can raise the relevant antibodies to levels sufficient to attenuate or reduce the incidence of serious CMV disease. In two separate clinical trials, CMV-IGIV provided effective prophylaxis in renal transplant recipients at risk for primary CMV disease. In the first randomized trial, the incidence of virologically confirmed CMV-associated syndromes was reduced from 60% in controls (n = 35) to 21% in recipients of CMV immune globulin (n = 24); marked leukopenia was reduced from 37% in controls to 4% in globulin recipients. Fungal or parasitic superinfections were not seen in globulin recipients but occurred in 20% of controls. Serious CMV disease was reduced from 46% to 13%. There was a concomitant but statistically significant reduction in the incidence of CMV pneumonia (17% of controls as compared with 4% of globulin recipients). There was no effect on rates of viral isolation or seroconversion although the rate of viremia was less in CMV-IGIV recipients. In a subsequent non-randomized trial in renal transplant recipients (n = 36), the incidence of virologically confirmed CMV-associated syndrome was reduced to 36% in the globulin recipients. The rates of CMV-associated pneumonia, CMV-associated hepatitis and concomitant fungal and parasitic superinfection were similar to those in the first trial.

Indications:

For the attenuation of primary CMV disease associated with kidney transplantation. Specifically, the product is indicated for kidney transplant recipients who are seronegative for CMV and who receive a kidney from a CMV seropositive donor. In a population of seronegative recipients of seropositive kidneys, approximately 75% of the untreated recipients would be expected to develop CMV disease. Clinical studies have shown a 50% reduction in primary CMV disease in renal transplant patients given CMV-IGIV.

Administration and Dosage:

The maximum recommended total dosage per infusion is 150 mg/kg, administered according to the following schedule:

Dosage Schedule for CMV-IGIV	
Time of infusion	Dosage (mg/kg)
Within 72 hours of transplant	150
2 weeks post transplant	100
4 weeks post transplant	100
6 weeks post transplant	100
8 weeks post transplant	100
12 weeks post transplant	50
16 weeks post transplant	50

Preparation for administration: Reconstitute the lyophilized powder with 50 ml of Sterile Water for Injection, USP. Do not shake the vials; avoid foaming. A double-ended transfer needle or large syringe is suitable for adding the water for reconstitution. When using a double-ended transfer needle, insert one end first into the vial of water. The lyophilized powder is supplied in an evacuated vial so the water will transfer by suction. After the water is transferred into the evacuated vial, release the residual vacuum to hasten the dissolving process. Rotate the container gently to wet all the undissolved powder. Allow a 30 minute interval for dissolving the powder. Infuse the solution only if it is colorless, free of particulate matter and not turbid.

Infusion: Begin infusion within 6 hours after reconstitution and complete within 12 hours of reconstitution. Monitor vital signs pre-infusion, mid-way and post-infusion as well as before any rate increase. Administer through an IV line using a constant infusion pump. Pre-dilution of CMV-IGIV before infusion is not recommended. Administer through a separate IV line. If this is not possible, it may be "piggybacked" into a pre-existing line if that line contains either Sodium Chloride Injection, USP, or one of the following dextrose solutions (with or without NaCl added): 2.5%, 5%, 10% or 20% Dextrose in Water. If a pre-existing line must be used, do not dilute the CMV-IGIV more than 1:2 with any of the above solutions. Admixtures of CMV-IGIV with any other solutions have not been evaluated. Filters are not necessary for the administration of CMV-IGIV.

(Administration and Dosage continued on following page)

Complete prescribing information for these products begins on page 2062 .

CYTOMEGALOVIRUS IMMUNE GLOBULIN INTRAVENOUS, HUMAN (CMV-IGIV) (Cont.)

Administration and Dosage (Cont.):

Initial dose: Administer IV at 15 mg/kg/hr. If no untoward reactions occur after 30 minutes, the rate may be increased to 30 mg/kg/hr; if no untoward reactions occur after a subsequent 30 minutes, the infusion may be increased to 60 mg/kg/hr (volume not to exceed 75 ml/hour). Do not exceed this rate of administration. Monitor the patient closely during and after each rate change.

Subsequent doses: Administer at 15 mg/kg/hr for 15 minutes. If no untoward reactions occur, increase to 30 mg/kg/hr for 15 minutes and then increase to a maximum rate of 60 mg/kg/hr (volume not to exceed 75 ml/hr). Do not exceed this rate of administration. Monitor the patient closely during each rate change.

Potential adverse reactions are: Flushing; chills; muscle cramps; back pain; fever; nausea; vomiting; wheezing; drop in blood pressure. Minor adverse reactions have been infusion rate related. If the patient develops a minor side effect (eg, nausea, back pain, flushing), slow the rate or temporarily interrupt the infusion. If anaphylaxis or drop in blood pressure occurs, discontinue infusion and use an antidote such as diphenhydramine and epinephrine.

To prevent the transmission of hepatitis viruses or other infectious agents from one person to another, use sterile disposable syringes and needles. The syringes and needles should not be reused.

Storage: Store between 2° to 8°C (36° to 46°F). Use reconstituted CMV-IGIV within 6 hours. CMV-IGIV should not be stored in the reconstituted state.

Rx	**CytoGam** (Connaught)	**Powder for Injection (lyophilized):** 2500 mg ± 250 mg[2]	In single-dose vial with 50 ml Sterile Water for Injection, USP, as diluent.

[1] With 5% sucrose and 1% albumin (human).

Complete prescribing information for these products begins on page 2062.

IMMUNE GLOBULIN INTRAMUSCULAR (IG; Gamma Globulin; ISG)

Indications:

Hepatitis A: The prophylactic value of IG is greatest when given before or soon after exposure to hepatitis A. Not indicated in persons with clinical manifestations of hepatitis A or in those exposed more than 2 weeks previously.

Measles (Rubeola): For the prevention or modification of measles in susceptible contacts (one who has not been vaccinated and has not had measles previously) exposed less than 6 days previously. May be especially indicated for susceptible household contacts of measles patients, particularly those under 1 year of age, for whom the risk of complications is highest. Do not give with measles vaccine. If a child older than 12 months has received IG, give measles vaccine about 3 months later, when the measles antibody titer will have disappeared.

If a susceptible child exposed to measles is immunocompromised, administer IG immediately. Children who are immunocompromised should not receive measles vaccine or any other live viral vaccine.

Immunoglobulin deficiency: IG therapy may prevent serious infection if circulating IgG levels of ≈ 200 mg/dl plasma are maintained. However, it may not prevent chronic infections of external secretory tissues such as the respiratory and GI tracts.

Prophylactic therapy, especially against infections due to encapsulated bacteria, is often effective in Bruton-type, sex-linked congenital agammaglobulinemia, agammaglobulinemia associated with thymoma and acquired agammaglobulinemia.

Varicella: Passive immunization against varicella in immunosuppressed patients is best accomplished with varicella zoster immune globulin. If unavailable, IG may be used.

Rubella: The routine use of IG for rubella prophylaxis in early pregnancy is of dubious value and cannot be justified. Some studies suggest that the use of IG in exposed susceptible women can lessen the likelihood of infection and fetal damage. See Administration and Dosage below.

Administration and Dosage:

For IM injection only.

Hepatitis A: A dose of 0.02 ml/kg (0.01 ml/lb) is recommended for household and institutional hepatitis A case contacts. The following doses are recommended for persons who plan to travel in areas where hepatitis A is common:

IG Dose for Common Hepatitis A Areas	
Length of Stay	Dose (ml/kg)
< 3 months	0.02
Prolonged (> 3 months)	0.06 (repeat every 4 to 6 months)

Measles (Rubeola): To prevent or modify measles in a susceptible person exposed less than 6 days previously, give 0.11 ml/lb (0.25 ml/kg). If a susceptible child who is also immunocompromised is exposed to measles, give 0.5 ml/kg (15 ml maximum) immediately.

Immunoglobulin deficiency: The usual dosage consists of an initial dose of 1.3 ml/kg followed in 3 or 4 weeks by 0.66 ml/kg (at least 100 mg/kg) to be given every 3 to 4 weeks. Some patients may require more frequent injections.

Varicella: Give 0.6 to 1.2 ml/kg promptly, if zoster immune globulin is unavailable.

Rubella: Some studies suggest that the use of IG in exposed susceptible women can lessen the likelihood of infection and fetal damage; therefore, a dose of 0.55 ml/kg within 72 hours of exposure has been recommended and may benefit those women who do not consider a therapeutic abortion.

Storage: Store between 2° to 8°C (35° to 46°F). Do not freeze.

			C.I.*
Rx	**Gamastan** (Cutter Biological)	In 2 and 10 ml vials.[1]	1
Rx	**Gammar** (Armour)	In 2 and 10 ml vials.[1]	1.5

* Cost Index based on cost per ml.

[1] Dissolved in 0.3 M glycine with thimerosal.

Complete prescribing information for these products begins on page 2062.

HEPATITIS B IMMUNE GLOBULIN (HBIG)

A sterile solution of immunoglobulin (10% to 18% protein) containing a high titer of antibody to hepatitis B surface antigen (HB_SAg).

Indications:

Postexposure prophylaxis following either parenteral exposure (eg, accidental "needle-stick"), direct mucous membrane contact (eg, accidental splash) or oral ingestion (eg, pipetting accident) involving HB_SAg-positive materials such as blood, plasma or serum.

Prophylaxis of infants born to HB_SAg-positive mothers: Such infants are at risk of being infected with hepatitis B virus and becoming chronic carriers. The risk is especially great if the mother is HB_eAg-positive. The carrier state can be prevented in about 75% of such infections in newborns given HBIG immediately after birth and in the early months of life; 98% are prevented in newborns when HBIG is administered at birth and again at 3 months of age, then active immunization with hepatitis B vaccine is begun.

Individuals at increased risk of infection with hepatitis B virus may be candidates for active vaccination with hepatitis B vaccine. Administration of HBIG either preceding or concomitant with the commencement of active immunization with hepatitis B vaccine does not interfere with the active immune response to the vaccine, and provides for more rapid achievement of protective levels of hepatitis B antibody than when the vaccine alone is administered. Rapid achievement of protective levels of antibody to hepatitis B virus may be desirable in certain clinical situations as in cases of accidental inoculations with contaminated medical instruments.

Administration and Dosage:

Give injections IM, preferably in the gluteal or deltoid region.

Postexposure prophylaxis: The recommended dose is 0.06 ml/kg; the usual adult dose is 3 to 5 ml. Administer the appropriate dose as soon after exposure as possible (preferably within 7 days) and repeat 28 to 30 days after exposure.

Prophylaxis of infants born to HB_SAG-positive mothers: The recommended dose for at-risk newborns is 0.5 ml IM into the anterolateral thigh, as soon after birth as possible, preferably within 12 hours.

Prevention of carrier state: A similar or higher rate of prevention of the carrier state may be achieved in at-risk infants by administering HBIG 0.5 ml IM as soon after birth as possible, preferably no later than 24 hours and repeated at 3 months of age. At this time, an active vaccination program with hepatitis B vaccine is begun.

Individuals at increased risk: HBIG may be administered at the same time (but at a different site), or up to 1 month preceding hepatitis B vaccination without impairing the active immune response from hepatitis B vaccination.

Storage: Store at 2° to 8°C (35° to 46°F). Do not freeze.

Hepatitis B Virus Postexposure Recommendations†

Exposure	Hepatitis B Immune Globulin		Vaccine	
	Dose (IM)	Recommended Timing	Dose (IM)	Recommended Timing
Perinatal	0.5 ml	Within 12 hrs of birth	0.5 ml	Within 12 hrs of birth;[1] repeat at 1 and 6 months
Percutaneous[2]	0.06 ml/kg	Single dose within 24 hours	1 ml[3]	Within 7 days; repeat at 1 and 6 months
Sexual	0.06 ml/kg	Single dose within 14 days of sexual contact[4]	1 ml[5]	Within 7 days; repeat at 1 and 6 months

	Product	Packaging	C.I.*
Rx	**H-BIG** (Abbott)	In 4 and 5 ml vials.[6]	1
Rx	**Hep-B-Gammagee** (MSD)	In 5 ml vials.[6]	1.6
Rx	**HyperHep** (Cutter Biological)	In 1 and 5 ml vials[7] and 0.5 ml prefilled syringe.	1

* Cost Index based on cost per ml.

† Morbidity and Mortality Weekly Report 1985;34:313-35 and 1988;37:341-46.

1 First dose can be given the same time as the HBIG dose, but at a different site.

2 Needlestick, ocular or mucosal exposure.

3 < 10 years old, give 0.5 ml.

4 In heterosexuals, if vaccine is not given, give a second dose of HBIG and a course of the vaccine if the index patient remains HB_SAg-positive for 3 months after detection.

5 Vaccine recommended for homosexual men and for regular sexual contacts of HBV carriers. Vaccine optional in initial treatment of heterosexual contacts of persons with acute HBV.

6 Dissolved in 0.3 M glycine with 1:10,000 thimerosal.

7 Dissolved in 0.21 to 0.32 M glycine with 80 to 120 mcg/ml thimerosal.

Complete prescribing information for these products begins on page 2062 .

TETANUS IMMUNE GLOBULIN

Indications:

For passive immunization against tetanus. Passive immunization is indicated for any person with a wound that might be contaminated with tetanus spores (ie, a wound other than a clean, minor wound), when the following conditions exist: The history of active immunization with tetanus toxoid is unknown or uncertain. A history of having received "tetanus shots" is not sufficient unless it can be confirmed that prior "shots" were tetanus toxoid and not tetanus antitoxin or TIG; or that the person has received either less than two prior doses of tetanus toxoid or two prior doses of tetanus toxoid, but a delay of 24 hours or more has occurred between the time of injury and initiation of tetanus prophylaxis.

If given at the time of injury, it will not interfere with the primary immune response to tetanus toxoid given at the same time at a different site, should it be necessary to begin a series of active immunization.

Tetanus antibodies of homologous origin have a half-life of 3.5 to 4.5 weeks.

Administration and Dosage:

Good medical care is essential in the prevention of tetanus in fresh wounds. Thorough cleansing and removal of all foreign and necrotic material from the injury is important.

Administer IM. Do NOT inject IV.

Prophylaxis: Adults – 250 units. *Children* – In small children, the dose may be calculated by the body weight (4 units/kg). However, it may be advisable to administer the entire contents of the vial or syringe (250 units) regardless of the child's size, since theoretically the same amount of toxin will be produced in his body by the infecting tetanus organisms as in an adult.

Therapy: Several studies suggest the value of human tetanus antitoxin in the actual treatment of active tetanus using single doses of 3000 to 6000 units in combination with other accepted clinical procedures.

The table below is a guide to active and passive tetanus immunization at the time of wound cleansing or debridement. It presumes a reliable knowledge of the patient's immunization history.

Guide to Tetanus Prophylaxis in Wound Management

History of Tetanus Immunization (Doses)	Clean, Minor Wounds		All Other Wounds	
	Tetanus Toxoid	Tetanus Immune Globulin	Tetanus Toxoid	Tetanus Immune Globulin
Uncertain	Yes	No	Yes	Yes
0 to 1	Yes	No	Yes	Yes
2	Yes	No	Yes	No[1]
3 or more	No[2]	No	No[3]	No

Storage: Store between 2° and 8°C (35° and 46°F). Do not freeze.

			C.I.*
Rx	**Hyper-Tet** (Cutter Biological)	In 250 unit vial[4] and 250 unit disp. syringe.[4]	63

* Cost Index based on cost per single dose (250 units).

[1] Unless wound is more than 24 hours old.

[2] Unless more than 10 years since last dose.

[3] Unless more than 5 years since last dose.

[4] Dissolved in 0.21 to 0.32 M glycine with 80 to 120 mcg thimerosal.

Complete prescribing information for these products begins on page 2062 .

VARICELLA-ZOSTER IMMUNE GLOBULIN (HUMAN) (VZIG)

Actions:

Varicella-Zoster Immune Globulin (Human) is the globulin fraction of human plasma, primarily immunoglobulin G (IgG) found in routine screening of normal volunteer blood donors. When absorbed into the circulation, the antibodies persist for 1 month or longer and are sufficient to mitigate or prevent varicella infection. It significantly reduces mortality and morbidity from varicella among immunodeficient children.

Indications:

Passive immunization of susceptible immunodeficient individuals after significant exposure to varicella (see criteria below). Most effective if begun within 96 hrs of exposure. There is no evidence VZIG modifies established Varicella-Zoster infections.

VZIG supplies are limited; restrict administration to those meeting the following criteria:

1. One of the following underlying illnesses or conditions:
   a. Neoplastic disease (eg, leukemia or lymphoma)
   b. Congenital or acquired immunodeficiency
   c. Immunosuppressive therapy with steroids, antimetabolites or other immunosuppressive treatment regimens.
   d. Newborn of mother who had onset of chickenpox within 5 days before delivery or within 48 hours after delivery
   e. Premature ($\geq$ 28 weeks' gestation) whose mother has no history of chickenpox
   f. Premature ($<$ 28 weeks' gestation or $\leq$ 1000 g VZIG) regardless of maternal history
2. One of the following types of exposure to chickenpox or zoster patient(s):
   a. Continuous household contact
   b. Playmate contact ($>$1 hour play indoors)
   c. Hospital contact (in same 2 to 4 bed room or adjacent beds in a large ward or prolonged face-to-face contact with an infectious staff member or patient)
3. Susceptible to varicella zoster.
4. Age of $<$ 15 years; administer to immunocompromised adolescents and adults and to other older patients on an *individual* basis.
5. If VZIG can be administered within 96 hours after exposure, but preferably sooner.

Not for prophylactic use in immunodeficient patients with history of varicella, unless patient's immunosuppression is associated with bone marrow transplantation.

Not recommended for nonimmunodeficient patients, including pregnant women, because the severity of chickenpox is much less than in immunosuppressed patients.

Administration and Dosage:

For maximum benefit, administer as soon as possible after presumed exposure, as late as 96 hours after exposure. High risk susceptible patients who are exposed again more than 3 weeks after a prior dose of VZIG should receive another full dose.

Do not inject IV. Administer by deep IM injection in the gluteal muscle, or in another large muscle mass. Inject 125 units per 10 kg (22 lbs), up to a maximum dose of 625 units (5 vials). The minimum dose is 125 units; do not give fractional doses.

VZIG Dose Based on Weight			
Weight of Patient		Dose	
Kilograms	Pounds	Units	Number of Vials
0 to 10	0 to 22	125	1
10.1 to 20	22.1 to 44	250	2
20.1 to 30	44.1 to 66	375	3
30.1 to 40	66.1 to 88	500	4
$>$40	$>$88	625	5

Administer the entire contents of each vial. For patients $\leq$ 10 kg, administer 1.25 ml at a single site. For patients $>$ 10 kg, give no more than 2.5 ml at a single site. Each vial of varicella-zoster virus antibody contains 125 units in a volume of 2.5 ml or less.

The dosage regimen is effective in modifying the severity of chickenpox, and reducing the frequency of death, pneumonia and encephalitis to $<$ 25% expected without treatment.

Storage: Store at 2° to 8°C (35° to 46°F).

Rx	**Varicella-Zoster Immune Globulin (Human)** (American Red Cross, Northeast Region)[1]	**Injection:** A sterile 10% to 18% solution of the globulin fraction of human plasma, primarily IgG, in single dose vials[2] containing 125 units of varicella-zoster virus antibody in 2.5 ml or less.

[1] Within Mass., VZIG is distributed by the Mass. Public Health Biologic Laboratories. Outside Mass., distribution is arranged by the American Red Cross Blood Services – Northeast Region through other regional distribution centers. VZIG is distributed free of charge to Mass. residents.

[2] In 0.3 M glycine as a stabilizer and 1:10,000 thimerosal.

Complete prescribing information for these products begins on page 2062 .

RHO (D) IMMUNE GLOBULIN

Actions:

Effectively suppresses the immune response of nonsensitized Rh_O (D) negative individuals who receive Rh_O (D) positive blood as the result of a fetomaternal hemorrhage, as a consequence of abdominal trauma, amniocentesis, abortion or full-term delivery, or a transfusion accident.

Each vial of Rh_O (D) completely suppresses immunity to 15 ml of Rh-positive packed red blood cells (≈ 30 ml whole blood). One vial contains approximately 300 mcg immunoglobulin.

Indications:

Full Term Delivery: To prevent sensitization to the Rh_O (D) factor and to prevent hemolytic disease of the newborn (Erythroblastosis fetalis) in a subsequent pregnancy. It effectively suppresses the immune response of nonsensitized Rh-negative mothers after delivery of an Rh-positive infant.

Criteria for an Rh-incompatible pregnancy requiring administration are:

1. The mother must be Rh_O (D) negative.
2. Mother not previously sensitized to Rh_O (D) factor.
3. The infant must be Rh_O (D) positive and direct antiglobulin negative.

Incomplete Pregnancy: Administer to all nonsensitized Rh-negative women after spontaneous or induced abortions, ruptured tubal pregnancies, amniocentesis and other abdominal trauma, or any occurrence of transplacental hemorrhage, unless the blood type of the fetus or the father has been determined to be Rh_O (D) negative.

For antepartum prophylaxis.

Note: In a case of abortion or ectopic pregnancy when Rh typing of the fetus is not possible, assume the fetus to be Rh_O (D) positive and consider the patient a candidate for administration of Rh_O (D) immune globulin. If the father can be determined to be Rh_O (D) negative, Rh_O (D) immune globulin need not be given.

Transfusions: To prevent Rh_O (D) sensitization in Rh_O (D) negative patients accidentally transfused with Rh_O (D) positive blood (which may include massive platelet transfusion).

Unlabeled Uses: Although controversial, some physicians advocate administration prior to *external version* attempts for breech presentations (due to induced fetal-maternal hemorrhage) and following *tubal ligation* after delivery of a Rh_O (D) positive infant (to prevent problems should the sterilization fail or subsequent tubal reanastomoses occur).

Administration and Dosage:

Do not give IV.

Do not give Rh_O (D) immune globulin to: The postpartum infant; to a Rh_O (D) positive individual; or to a Rh_O (D) negative individual previously sensitized to the Rh_O (D) antigen.

Note: Although there is no need to administer Rh_O (D) immune globulin to a woman who is already sensitized to the Rh factor, there is no more risk than when it is given to a woman who is not sensitized. When in doubt, administer Rh_O (D) immune globulin.

Administer within 72 hours after Rh incompatible delivery, miscarriage, abortion or transfusion.

Preadministration Laboratory Procedure: Immediately postpartum, determine the infant's blood type (ABO, Rh_O (D)) and perform a direct antiglobulin test using umbilical cord, venous or capillary blood.

Confirm that the mother is RH_O (D) negative.

(Administration and Dosage continued on following page)

RH$_O$ (D) IMMUNE GLOBULIN (Cont.)

Administration and Dosage (Cont.):

Obstetrical usage: One vial prevents maternal sensitization to the Rh factor if the fetal packed red blood cell volume, that entered the mother's blood due to fetomaternal hemorrhage, is less than 15 ml (30 ml of whole blood). When the fetomaternal hemorrhage exceeds this, administer more than one vial.

Postpartum prophylaxis – Administer one vial IM, preferably within 72 hours of delivery. If an unusually large fetomaternal hemorrhage is suspected, determine the number of vials required as described below.

Antepartum prophylaxis – Inject one vial (approximately 300 mcg) IM at 26 to 28 weeks gestation and one vial within 72 hours after an Rh-incompatible delivery to prevent Rh isoimmunization during pregnancy.

To determine number of vials required, determine volume of packed fetal red blood cells by approved laboratory assay. The volume of fetomaternal hemorrhage divided by 2 gives volume of packed fetal red blood cells in maternal blood. Determine number of vials to be administered by dividing volume (ml) of packed red blood cells by 15.

Following amniocentesis, miscarriage, abortion or ectopic pregnancy at or beyond 13 weeks' gestation: One vial IM.

Transfusion accidents: The number of vials to be administered depends on the volume of packed red cells or whole blood transfused. Multiply the volume (in ml) of Rh-positive whole blood administered by the hematocrit of the donor unit. This value equals the volume of packed red blood cells transfused. Divide the volume (in ml) of packed red blood cells by 15 to obtain the number of vials to be administered. If the dosage calculation results in a fraction, administer the next whole number of vials.

One vial dose: Withdraw and inject IM the entire contents of the vial.

Two or more vial dose: Using 5 or 10 ml syringes, withdraw the contents from the vials to be administered at one time and inject IM. The contents of the total number of vials may be injected as a divided dose at different injection sites at the same time, or the total dosage may be divided and injected at intervals (provided the total dosage is injected within 72 hours postpartum or after a transfusion accident).

Storage: Store at 2° to 8°C (35° to 46°F). Do not freeze.

			C.I.*
Rx	**Gamulin Rh** (Armour)	Each package contains one single dose vial of Rh$_O$ (D) Immune Globulin[1], patient ID card, directions for use and a patient information brochure.	1219
Rx	**HypRho-D** (Cutter Biological)	Each package contains one single dose vial or prefilled syringe of Rh$_O$ (D) Immune Globulin[2], directions for use and a patient ID card.	702
Rx	**Rhesonativ** (KabiVitrum)	Each package contains one vial of Human Immunoglobulin anti-Rh$_O$ (D) 0.2 g, glycine 70 mg and a 2 ml vial of diluent (water for injection).	753
Rx	**RhoGAM** (Ortho Diagnostics)	Each package contains one single dose vial or prefilled syringe of Rh$_O$ (D) Immune Globulin[3], a package insert, control form and patient ID card.	900

RH$_O$ (D) IMMUNE GLOBULIN MICRO-DOSE

One vial will suppress the immune response to 2.5 ml of Rh$_O$ (D) positive packed red blood cells. One vial contains approximately 50 mcg immunoglobulin.

This dose is indicated for the prevention of isoimmunization in Rh negative women following spontaneous or induced abortion or termination of ectopic pregnancy up to and including 12 weeks gestation, unless the father is Rh negative. At or beyond 13 weeks gestation, administer RH$_O$ (D) Immune Globulin.

Give one vial IM as soon as possible after termination of pregnancy.

Storage: Store at 2° to 8°C (35° to 46°F). Do not freeze.

			C.I.*
Rx	**HypRho-D Mini-Dose** (Cutter Biological)	Each package contains a single dose syringe of Rh$_O$ (D) Immune Globulin micro-dose[2], package insert, patient ID cards.	150
Rx	**MICRhoGAM** (Ortho Diagnostics)	Each package contains a single dose syringe of Rh$_O$ (D) Immune Globulin micro-dose,[4] package insert, injection control form and patient ID card.	500
Rx	**Mini-Gamulin Rh** (Armour)	Each package contains a single dose vial of Rh$_O$ (D) Immune Globulin micro-dose,[1] package insert, injection control form and patient ID card	320

* Cost Index based on cost per single dose.
[1] Dissolved in 0.3 M glycine with 0.01% thimerosal.
[2] Dissolved in 0.21 to 0.32 M glycine with 80 to 120 mcg thimerosal.
[3] Dissolved in 15 mg glycine per ml with 0.01% thimerosal.
[4] Dissolved in 15 mg glycine per ml with 0.003% thimerosal.

LYMPHOCYTE IMMUNE GLOBULIN, ANTI-THYMOCYTE GLOBULIN (EQUINE)

Warning:

Only physicians experienced in immunosuppressive therapy and management of renal transplant patients should use this product.

Patients receiving this drug should be managed in facilities equipped and staffed with adequate laboratory and supportive medical resources.

Actions:

Lymphocyte Immune Globulin, Anti-Thymocyte Globulin (Equine), is a lymphocyte-selective immunosuppressant. It reduces the number of circulating, thymus-dependent lymphocytes that form rosettes with sheep erythrocytes. This antilymphocytic effect is believed to reflect an alteration of the function of the T-lymphocytes, which are responsible, in part, for cell mediated immunity and are involved in humoral immunity. It also contains low concentrations of antibodies against other formed elements of the blood. In rhesus and cynomolgus monkeys, this drug reduces lymphocytes in the thymus-dependent areas of the spleen and lymph nodes. It also decreases the circulating sheep-erythrocyte-rosetting lymphocytes that can be detected, but ordinarily does not cause severe lymphopenia.

In general, when administered with other immunosuppressive therapy, such as antimetabolites and corticosteroids, the patient's own antibody response to horse gamma globulin is minimal. When administered with other immunosuppressive therapy and measured as horse IgG, it had a serum half-life of 5.7 ± 3 days.

Precise methods of determining potency have not been established, thus activity may potentially vary from lot to lot.

Indications:

Management of allograft rejection in renal transplant patients. When administered with conventional therapy at the time of rejection, it increases the frequency of resolution of the acute rejection episode.

Administered as an adjunct to other immunosuppressive therapy to delay the onset of the first rejection episode. Data have not consistently demonstrated improvement in functional graft survival associated with therapy to delay the onset of the first rejection episode.

Contraindications:

Do not administer to a patient who has had a severe systemic reaction during prior administration of the drug or any other equine gamma globulin preparation.

Warnings:

Discontinue treatment if any of the following occurs: Anaphylaxis; severe and unremitting thrombocytopenia; or severe and unremitting leukopenia.

Usage in Pregnancy and Lactation: Category C. Safety for use during pregnancy has not been established. Use only when clearly needed and when the potential benefits outweigh the unknown potential hazards to the fetus.

Usage in Children: Experience with children has been limited. The drug has been administered safely to a small number of pediatric renal allograft recipients at dosage levels comparable to those used in adults on a mg per kg basis.

Precautions:

Skin testing: Test patients with an intradermal injection of 0.1 ml of a 1:1000 dilution (5 mcg horse IgG) in normal saline and a saline control. If this causes a wheal or erythema greater than 10 mm or both with or without pseudopod formation and itching or a marked local swelling, be particularly cautious during infusion. A systemic reaction such as a generalized rash, tachycardia, dyspnea, hypotension or anaphylaxis precludes any additional administration of the drug. The predictive value of this test is not proven; allergic reactions can occur in patients whose skin test is negative.

Because this agent is ordinarily given with corticosteroids and antimetabolites, monitor patients carefully for signs of leukopenia, thrombocytopenia or concurrent infection. If infection occurs, institute adjunctive therapy promptly. On the basis of the clinical circumstances, decide whether therapy will continue.

Safety and efficacy have not been demonstrated in renal transplant patients not receiving concomitant immunosuppressive therapy.

When the dose of corticosteroids and other immunosuppressants is being reduced, some previously masked reactions to the drug may appear; observe patients carefully during therapy.

(Continued on following page)

LYMPHOCYTE IMMUNE GLOBULIN, ANTI-THYMOCYTE GLOBULIN (EQUINE) (Cont.)

Adverse Reactions:

In controlled trials, investigators frequently reported the following adverse reactions: Fever in 1 of 3 patients; chills in 1 of 7; leukopenia in 1 of 7; thrombocytopenia in 1 of 9; and dermatological reactions, such as rash, pruritus, urticaria, wheal and flare, in 1 of 8.

The following were reported in 1% to 5% of patients: Arthralgia, chest or back pain or both, clotted A/V fistula, diarrhea, dyspnea, headache, hypotension, nausea, vomiting, night sweats, pain at the infusion site, peripheral thrombophlebitis and stomatitis.

Reactions reported in $< 1\%$ of patients were anaphylaxis, dizziness, weakness or faintness, edema, herpes simplex reactivation, hiccoughs or epigastric pain, hyperglycemia, hypertension, iliac vein obstruction, laryngospasm, localized infection, lymphadenopathy, malaise, myalgia, paresthesia, possible serum sickness, pulmonary edema, renal artery thrombosis, seizures, systemic infection, tachycardia, toxic epidermal necrosis and wound dehiscence.

Management of adverse reactions:

Anaphylaxis: Uncommon but serious, it may occur at any time during therapy. Stop infusion immediately; administer 0.3 ml aqueous epinephrine 1:1000 IM. Administer steroids, assist respiration and provide other resuscitative measures. Do not resume therapy. Respiratory distress or hypotension may indicate anaphylaxis. **Pain in chest, flank or back** may indicate anaphylaxis or hemolysis. Stop infusion; treat appropriately.

Hemolysis: Clinically significant hemolysis is rare. Treatment may include transfusion of erythrocytes; if necessary, administer IV mannitol, furosemide, sodium bicarbonate and fluids. Severe and unremitting hemolysis may require discontinuation of therapy.

Thrombocytopenia is usually transient; platelet counts generally return to adequate levels without discontinuing therapy and without transfusions.

Chills and fever occur frequently. This drug may release endogenous leukocyte pyrogens. Prophylactic or therapeutic administration of antihistamines or corticosteroids generally controls this reaction.

Chemical phlebitis can be caused by infusion through peripheral veins. Avoid by administering the solution into a high-flow vein.

Itching and erythema probably result from the drug's effect on blood elements. Antihistamines control the symptoms.

Administration and Dosage:

Adults: 10 to 30 mg/kg/day.

Children: 5 to 25 mg/kg/day.

The drug has been used to delay the onset of the first rejection episode and at the time of the first rejection episode. Most patients who received it for the treatment of acute rejection had not received it at the time of transplantation. Usually, it is used concomitantly with azathioprine and corticosteroids. Exercise caution during repeat courses of therapy; carefully observe patients for signs of allergic reactions.

Delaying the onset of renal allograft rejection: Give a fixed dose of 15 mg/kg/day for 14 days, then every other day for 14 days, for a total of 21 doses in 28 days. Administer the first dose within 24 hours before or after the transplant.

Treatment of allograft rejection: The first dose can be delayed until the diagnosis of the first rejection episode. The recommended dose is 10 to 15 mg/kg/day for 14 days. Additional alternate day therapy up to a total of 21 doses can be given.

Infusion instructions: Dilute in saline solution before IV infusion. Invert the IV saline bottle so undiluted drug does not contact the air inside. Add the total daily dose to a sterile 0.45% or 0.9% saline solution. Ideally, concentration should not exceed 1 mg per ml.

Adding the drug to dextrose solutions is not recommended, as low salt concentrations can cause precipitation. Highly acidic infusion solutions can also contribute to physical instability over time.

During clinical trials, most investigators infused into a vascular shunt, arterial venous fistula or a high-flow central vein through an in-line filter with a pore size of 0.2 to 1 micron to prevent inadvertent administration of any insoluble material that may develop in the product during storage. Using high-flow veins will minimize the occurrence of phlebitis and thrombosis.

Do not infuse a dose in less than 4 hours.

Always keep a tray containing epinephrine, antihistamines, corticosteroids, syringes and an airway at the patient's bedside while this agent is being administered. Observe the patient continuously for possible allergic reactions throughout the infusion.

Storage: Refrigerate at 2° to 8°C (35° to 46°F). Do not freeze. Do not keep in diluted form for more than 12 hours (including actual infusion time). Refrigerate diluted solution if prepared prior to time of infusion. Even if refrigerated, total time in dilution should not exceed 12 hours.

Rx	**Atgam** (Upjohn)	**Injection:** 50 mg per ml. In 5 ml amps.[1]

[1] In 0.3 M glycine with 0.01% thimerosal.

Antitoxins and antivenins are used for passive immunization. Antitoxins are antibodies which combine with the toxins and neutralize them. Most antitoxins for human use are derived from horse serum (antivenins, diphtheria, etc). However, there is a tetanus immune globulin of human origin. The following general information applies to antitoxins and antivenins. For specific indications and dosage guidelines, refer to individual product listings.

Warnings:

Hypersensitivity: In the parenteral administration of any biological product, observe every precaution to prevent or arrest allergic or other untoward reactions. A careful history should review possible sensitivity to the type of protein being injected. Administer animal serums with caution even in individuals with a negative sensitivity test.

Have epinephrine injection (1:1000) available while performing sensitivity tests or administering antitoxin. Refer to Management of Acute Hypersensitivity Reactions, 2897.

Precautions:

History and Sensitivity Testing: Before administration of any product prepared from animal serum, make a complete record of previous injections of "serum" of any type and any previous allergic manifestations of the patient. Test for sensitivity to animal serum. Do the scratch test or "eye" sensitivity test before proceeding to the intradermal tests. These tests should be performed by skilled personnel familiar with management of acute anaphylaxis. Fatalities have resulted from intradermal testing. Positive tests indicate probable sensitivity. A negative skin or conjunctival sensitivity test is usually reliable, but does not completely rule out systemic sensitivity. *The following is a general procedure for sensitivity testing. Manufacturers' recommendations may vary. Consult package literature prior to use of a specific product.*

Scratch test – Make a ¼" skin scratch through a drop of 1:100 dilution in normal saline. To serve as a control, make a similar scratch through a drop of normal saline on a different but comparable skin site. After 20 minutes, compare the sites. A positive sensitivity test consists of an urticarial wheal, with or without pseudopods, surrounded by a halo of erythema. A negative or minimal reaction, with no wheal or pseudopods, occurs at the control site.

Conjunctival test ("eye" test) – Instill into the conjunctival sac one drop of a 1:10 saline dilution. A drop of normal saline placed in the opposite conjunctival sac provides a control. A positive reaction consists of itching, burning, redness and lacrimation appearing within 10 to 30 minutes; these symptoms can be relieved by instilling a drop of epinephrine solution. The control eye should remain normal. If both eyes remain normal, the conjunctival test is negative.

Intradermal test – In patients with a negative allergy history and negative scratch or eye test, inject with 0.02 to 0.1 ml of 1:100 saline diluted serum; refer to manufacturers' recommendations for specific instructions. In patients with a history or allergy, especially to animal serums, inject with 1:1000 saline diluted serum. Inject a separate but comparable skin site intracutaneously with normal saline to serve as a control. After 10 to 30 minutes, compare the injection sites. A positive sensitivity test consists of an urticarial wheal, with or without pseudopods, surrounded by a halo of erythema. A negative or minimal reaction, with no wheal or pseudopods, occurs at the control site.

Desensitization: In the event of a positive sensitivity test or a doubtful reaction, perform careful desensitization of the patient. Serial injections of diluted antitoxin or antivenin may be made at 15 minute intervals, provided no reaction occurs. If a reaction occurs after an injection, wait an hour and then repeat the last dose which failed to cause a reaction.

Antihistamines: Concomitant use may interfere with sensitivity tests.

Adverse Reactions:

Systemic: Acute anaphylaxis is characterized by sudden onset of urticaria, respiratory distress and vascular collapse, and serum sickness (usually appearing 7 to 12 days after administration). Symptoms of lymphadenopathy, polyarthritis, arthralgias, skin rash and fever, etc, may develop. Anaphylaxis is largely related to the amount of serum administered, patient hypersensitivity and history of previous serum injection. The incidence of serum sickness with modern enzyme-treated serum is about 5% to 10%. This occurs more frequently after the largest dose.

Local: Pain or erythema and urticaria without constitutional disturbance may occur 7 to 10 days after administration and may last for about 2 days.

(Products listed on following pages)

Complete prescribing information for these products begins on page 2075

DIPHTHERIA ANTITOXIN

A sterile solution of purified antitoxic substances obtained from the blood of horses immunized against diphtheria toxin.

Indications:

For prevention or treatment of diphtheria; neutralizes the toxins produced by *Corynebacterium diphtheriae*.

Administration and Dosage:

Administer IM or by slow IV infusion. Warm antitoxin to 32° to 34°C (90° to 95°F).

Therapeutic regimen: Any person with clinical symptoms of diphtheria should receive diphtheria antitoxin immediately without waiting for bacteriologic confirmation. Continue treatment until all local and general symptoms are controlled, or until some other etiologic agent has been identified.

1. Perform sensitivity tests.
2. Immediately give all of the required antitoxin IM or IV. Each hour's delay increases dosage requirement and decreases beneficial effects.
3. Suggested ranges: Pharyngeal or laryngeal disease of 48 hours duration - 20,000 to 40,000 units; nasopharyngeal lesions - 40,000 to 60,000 units; extensive disease of 3 or more days duration or any patient with brawny swelling of the neck - 80,000 to 120,000 units.
4. Give children the same dose as adults.
5. Start appropriate antimicrobial agents in full therapeutic dosage.

Prophylactic regimen: Give all asymptomatic, unimmunized contacts of patients with diphtheria prompt prophylaxis with antimicrobial therapy with cultures before and after treatment. Immunize with diphtheria toxoid and continue surveillance for 7 days.

Close contacts not under surveillance should receive appropriate antimicrobial therapy and immunization with diphtheria toxoid and diphtheria antitoxin.

1. Perform sensitivity tests.
2. If sensitivity test is negative, give 10,000 units IM. Dose depends upon length of time since exposure, extent of exposure and medical condition of the individual.
3. If sensitivity test is positive, proceed with desensitization schedule.

Storage: Store between 2° to 8°C (35° to 46°F). Do not freeze.

Rx	**Diphtheria Antitoxin** (Squibb/Connaught)	**Injection:** Not less than 500 units/ml	In 20,000 units per vial.[1]
Rx	**Diphtheria Antitoxin** (Sclavo)	**Injection:** Not less than 500 units/ml	In 10,000 units and 20,000 units per vial.[2]

TETANUS ANTITOXIN

Solution of refined and concentrated proteins, chiefly globulins, containing antitoxic antibodies obtained from the blood of horses immunized against tetanus toxin.

Tetanus Immune Globulin is preferred for the prevention and treatment of tetanus. Use Tetanus Antitoxin only when Tetanus Immune Globulin is not available.

Indications:

For prevention of tetanus when Tetanus Immune Globulin is not available and for treatment of tetanus. Give prophylactic doses to those individuals who have had less than two previous injections of tetanus toxoid and if the wound is untended for more than 24 hours.

The concomitant administration of tetanus antitoxin and tetanus toxoid adsorbed is indicated for those persons who must receive an immediate injection of tetanus antitoxin and for whom it is desirable to begin the process of active immunization. Complete the active immunization with tetanus toxoid adsorbed (and diphtheria toxoid adsorbed, if indicated) in accordance with ACIP guidelines.

Administration and Dosage:

Perform equine serum sensitivity tests.

Prophylaxis: 1500 to 5000 units IM or SC according to body weight (1500 units up to 65 pounds [29.5 kg] and 3000 to 5000 units over this weight). Protection from tetanus antitoxin lasts about 15 days or even less in individuals who have already received an injection of horse serum.

Treatment: A single dose of about 50,000 to 100,000 units. Preferably, give at least part of the dose IV; give the remainder IM. Institute antitoxin treatment as soon as possible.

Storage: Store between 2° to 8°C (35° to 46°F). Do not freeze.

Rx	**Tetanus Antitoxin** (Sclavo)	**Injection:** Not less than 400 units/ml	In 1,500 unit and 20,000 unit vials.[2]

[1] With 0.4% tricresol.

[2] With 0.3% m-cresol.

Complete prescribing information for these products begins on page 2075

ANTIVENIN (CROTALIDAE) POLYVALENT

Concentrated serum globulins from horses immunized with the following venoms: *Crotalus adamanteus* (eastern diamond rattlesnake), *C atrox* (western diamond rattlesnake), *C durissus terrificus* (tropical rattlesnake, Cascabel) and *Bothrops atrox* (Fer-de-lance).

The location of antivenins for rare species and names and telephone numbers of experts on venomous bites can be obtained at any hour from the Arizona Poison Control Center (602-626-6016).

Indications:

To neutralize the toxic effects of venoms of crotalids (pit vipers) native to North, Central and South America, including rattlesnakes (*Crotalus, Sistrurus*); copperhead and cottonmouth moccasins (*Agkistrodon*), including *A halys* of Korea and Japan; the Fer-de-lance and other species of *Bothrops*; the tropical rattler (*C durissus* and similar species); the Cantil (*A bilineatus*); and bushmaster (*Lachesis mutus*) of South and Central America.

Pit Viper Bites and Envenomation:

Symptoms, signs and severity of snake venom poisoning depend on many factors, including species, age and size of the snake; number and location of bite(s); depth of venom deposit; condition of the snake's fangs and venom glands; length of time the snake "hangs on"; age, general health and size of the victim; timing, type and efficacy of first aid treatment rendered to remove venom. In any snake bite, the actual amount of venom introduced is unknown. The type of clothing or leg-footwear through which the snake's fangs pass may affect the amount of venom delivered. Although most North American pit vipers tend to bite and introduce venom superficially, their fangs may get hung up in subcutaneous tissues during the biting act and penetrate deeper tissues during the attempt to release the bitten part. In some bites, fangs may penetrate into muscle. In such cases, the usual local superficial manifestations of envenomation may not appear early in the course of poisoning. In bites by some species, systemic evidence of envenomation may be present in the absence of significant local manifestations. It may be difficult to determine the severity of envenomation during the first several hours after a pit viper bite; estimates of severity may need to be revised as poisoning progresses. Not all pit viper bites result in envenomation. In approximately 20% of rattlesnake bites, the snake may not inject any venom. Local and systemic signs and symptoms of envenomation include the following:

Local: Fang punctures – Swelling: Edema, usually seen around the bite area within 5 minutes, may progress rapidly and involve the entire extremity within an hour.

Ecchymosis and skin discoloration often appear in the bite area within a few hours. Vesicles may form in a few hours and are usually present at 24 hours. Hemorrhagic blebs and petechiae are common. Necrosis may develop, necessitating amputation.

Pain frequently begins shortly after the bite by most pit vipers. Pain may be absent after bites by Mojave rattlers.

Systemic: Weakness; faintness; nausea; sweating; numbness or tingling around the mouth, tongue, scalp, fingers, toes, bite area; muscle fasciculations; hypotension; prolonged bleeding and clotting times; hemoconcentration followed by decrease in erythrocytes; thrombocytopenia; hematuria; proteinuria; vomiting, including hematemesis; melena; hemoptysis; epistaxis.

In fatal poisoning, cause of death is frequently associated with destruction of erythrocytes and changes in capillary permeability, especially of the pulmonary vascular system, leading to pulmonary edema; hemoconcentration usually occurs early, probably as a result of plasma loss secondary to vascular permeability; hemoglobin may fall, and bleeding may occur throughout the body as early as 6 hours after the bite. Renal involvement is uncommon. Mojave rattler venom may cause neuromuscular changes leading to respiratory failure.

(Continued on following page)

ANTIVENIN (CROTALIDAE) POLYVALENT (Cont.)

Supportive Care:

Treat suspected envenomation as a medical emergency. Until careful observation provides clear evidence that envenomation has not occurred or is minimal, follow these procedures: Monitor vital signs frequently. Draw blood as soon as possible for baseline lab studies, including type and cross-match, CBC, hematocrit, platelet count, prothrombin time, clot retraction, bleeding and coagulation times, BUN, electrolytes and bilirubin. During the first 4 or 5 days after a severe envenomation, perform hemoglobin, hematocrit and platelet counts several times a day. Obtain urine samples at frequent intervals, with special attention to microscopic examination for presence of erythrocytes. Chart fluid intake and urine output. To monitor progression of edema, measure the circumference of the bitten extremity, every 15 to 30 minutes, just proximal to the bite and at one or more additional points, each several inches closer to the trunk.

Have available for immediate use: Oxygen and resuscitation equipment including airway, tourniquet, epinephrine, parenteral antihistamines and corticosteroids. Start IV infusions: Use one line for supportive therapy, if needed and the other line for administration of the antivenin and electrolytes.

Treat shock following envenomation like the shock resulting from hypovolemia of any cause, including administration of blood products or plasma expanders, as indicated.

Administration:

Test for sensitivity to horse serum (see introduction to this section). Whenever a product containing horse serum is administered, there is a possibility of a severe immediate reaction. Constant observation for untoward reactions is mandatory. Should any systemic reaction occur, discontinue use and initiate appropriate treatment. See also Management of Acute Hypersensitivity Reactions.

IV route is preferred. If shock is present, IV use is mandatory. Administer within 4 hours of bite; it is less effective when given after 8 hours, and may be of questionable value after 12 hours. However, in severe poisonings, administer antivenin even if 24 hours have elapsed since time of bite. Maximum blood levels of antivenin may not be obtained for 8 or more hours following IM administration.

Reconstituting dried antivenin: Withdraw diluent and inject into the vial of antivenin. Gentle agitation will hasten complete dissolution of the lyophilized drug.

For IV infusion, prepare a 1:1 to 1:10 dilution of reconstituted drug in Sodium Chloride Injection or 5% Dextrose Injection. Gently swirl to avoid foaming. Infuse initial 5 to 10 ml over 3 to 5 minutes, while observing patient; if no immediate systemic reactions appear, continue infusion with delivery at the maximum safe rate for IV fluid administration. To determine dilution, type of electrolyte solution and delivery rate, consider the patient's age, weight and cardiac status; severity of envenomation; estimated total amount of parenteral fluids needed; and interval between bite and therapy initiation.

Dosage:

Give entire initial dose as soon as possible based on the best estimate of the severity of envenomation. The following doses are recommended:

No envenomation – No local or systemic manifestations. None.

Minimal envenomation – Local swelling and other local changes; no systemic manifestations; normal laboratory findings. 20 to 40 ml (2 to 4 vials).

Moderate envenomation – Swelling progresses beyond the site of bite; one or more systemic manifestations; abnormal laboratory findings (eg, fall in hematocrit or platelets). 50 to 90 ml (5 to 9 vials).

Severe envenomation – Marked local response, severe systemic manifestations and significant alteration in laboratory findings. 100 to 150 ml or more ($\geq$ 10 to 15 vials).

Base the need for additional antivenin on clinical response to initial dose and continuing assessment of severity of poisoning. If swelling progresses, if systemic symptoms increase in severity, or if new manifestations appear, administer an additional 10 to 50 ml (1 to 5 vials) IV.

Children: Envenomation by large snakes in children or small adults requires larger doses of antivenin. The amount administered to a child is *not* based on weight.

IM: Administer into large muscle mass, preferably the gluteal area, taking care to avoid nerve trunks. Never inject into a finger or toe.

Rx	**Antivenin (Crotalidae) Polyvalent** (Wyeth)	**Injection: Combination Package** – 1 vial of lyophilized serum[1], 1 vial of 10 ml Bacteriostatic Water for Injection, USP[2], and one 1 ml vial of normal horse serum[3] (diluted 1:10) as sensitivity testing material.

[1] With 0.25% phenol and 0.005% thimerosal.
[2] With 0.001% phenylmercuric nitrate.
[3] With 0.35% phenol and 0.005% thimerosal.

Complete prescribing information for these products begins on page 2075

ANTIVENIN (MICRURUS FULVIUS) (North American Coral Snake Antivenin)

Refined, concentrated, lyophilized preparation of serum globulins from healthy horses immunized with eastern coral snake *(Micrurus fulvius fulvius)* venom.

Indications:

Two genera of coral snakes are found in the United States – *Micrurus* (including the eastern and Texas varieties) and *Micruroides* (the Sonoran or Arizona variety), found only in southeastern Arizona and southwestern New Mexico. This antivenin will neutralize the venom of *M fulvius fulvius* (eastern coral snake) and *M fulvius tenere* (Texas coral snake) but will NOT neutralize the venom of *M euryxanthus* (Arizona or Sonoran coral snake).

Envenomation:

Coral snake venom is chiefly paralytic (neurotoxic), and usually causes only minimal to moderate tissue reaction and pain at the bite area. Coral snakebites, like bites by crotalids, are not always followed by envenomation. However, severe and even fatal envenomation from a coral snakebite may be present without significant local tissue reaction.

Symptoms of envenomation usually begin 1 to 7 hours after the bite, but may be delayed for as long as 18 hours. If envenomation occurs, symptoms and signs may progress rapidly and precipitously. Paralysis has been observed 2½ hours post-bite and appears to be of a bulbar type, involving cranial motor nerves. Death from respiratory paralysis has occurred within 4 hours of the bite.

Systemic signs and symptoms may include euphoria, lethargy, weakness, nausea, vomiting, excessive salivation, ptosis of the eyelids, dyspnea, abnormal reflexes, seizures and motor weakness or paralysis, including complete respiratory paralysis.

Local signs and symptoms may include scratch marks or fang puncture wounds, no edema to moderate edema, erythema, pain at the bite area and paresthesia in the bitten extremity.

Administration and Dosage:

Supportive therapy: Appropriate tetanus prophylaxis is indicated. Morphine or other narcotics that depress respiration are contraindicated. Use sedatives with extreme caution.

Test for sensitivity to horse serum (see p.2075). Whenever a product containing horse serum is administered, there is a possibility of a severe immediate reaction. Have appropriate therapeutic agents available (not corticosteroids). See also Management of Acute Hypersensitivity Reactions

If practical, immobilize victim immediately and completely. If complete immobilization is not practical, splint bitten extremity to limit spread of venom.

If symptoms or signs of envenomation occur or are already present at the time the patient is first seen, give antivenin promptly IV. With vigorous treatment and careful observation, patients with complete respiratory paralysis have recovered.

Hemoglobinuria has occurred in animals. Therefore, continuous bladder drainage with careful attention to urinary output and blood electrolyte balance is recommended.

Reconstituting dried antivenin: Withdraw diluent and inject into the vial of antivenin. Gentle agitation will hasten complete dissolution of the lyophilized drug.

Start an IV drip of 250 to 500 ml of Sodium Chloride Injection, USP. If the patient is not dangerously hypersensitive to horse serum (and depending on the nature and severity of envenomation), administer 3 to 5 vials (30 to 50 ml) by slow IV injection directly into tubing or by adding to the reservoir bottle of the IV drip. Inject the first 1 or 2 ml over 3 to 5 minutes, carefully observing the patient for evidence of allergic reaction. If no signs or symptoms of anaphylaxis appear, continue injection. Rate of delivery is regulated by severity of envenomation and tolerance of antivenin. Until 30 to 50 ml of antivenin has been given, administer at the maximum safe rate for IV fluids based on body weight and general condition of the patient. Response may be rapid and dramatic. Observe patient carefully and administer additional antivenin IV as required.

Some patients may require 10 or more vials to neutralize the venom dose.

Rx	**Antivenin (Micrurus fulvius)** (Wyeth)	**Injection: Combination Package** – One vial antivenin[1] and one vial diluent (10 ml Bacteriostatic Water for Injection)[2].

[1] With 0.25% phenol and 0.005% thimerosal.

[2] With 1:100,000 phenylmercuric nitrate.

Complete prescribing information for these products begins on page 2075

BLACK WIDOW SPIDER SPECIES ANTIVENIN (Latrodectus Mactans)

Prepared from blood serum of horses immunized against black widow spider venom.

Indications:

Used to treat patients with symptoms of black widow spider bites *(Latrodectus mactans)*. Early use is emphasized for prompt relief.

Warnings:

Usage in Pregnancy: (Category C). Animal reproduction studies have not been conducted. It is also not known whether the antivenin can cause fetal harm when administered to a pregnant woman or can affect reproduction capacity. Give to a pregnant woman only if clearly needed and when potential benefits outweigh potential hazards to the fetus.

Usage in Lactation: It is not known whether this drug is excreted in breast milk. Use caution when administering to a nursing woman.

Usage in Children: Controlled studies have not been conducted. However, there have been virtually no adverse effects in children receiving this product.

Envenomation:

Symptoms: Local muscular cramps begin from 15 minutes to several hours after bite, usually producing sharp pain similar to that caused by needle puncture. The exact sequence of symptoms depends on location of the bite. Venom acts on the myoneural junctions or nerve endings, causing ascending motor paralysis or destruction of peripheral nerve endings. Muscles most frequently affected first are thigh, shoulder and back. Later, pain becomes more severe, spreading to the abdomen, and weakness and tremor usually develop. Abdominal muscles assume a board-like rigidity, but tenderness is slight. Respiration is thoracic; patient is restless and anxious. Feeble pulse, cold, clammy skin, labored breathing and speech, light stupor and delirium may occur. Convulsions may also occur, particularly in small children. Temperature may be normal or slightly elevated. Urinary retention, shock, cyanosis, nausea, vomiting, insomnia and cold sweats have been reported. The syndrome following the bite of the black widow spider may be confused with any medical or surgical condition with acute abdominal symptoms.

The symptoms of black widow spider bite increase in severity for several hours, perhaps a day, and then very slowly become less severe, gradually passing off in 2 or 3 days, except in fatal cases. Residual symptoms such as general weakness, tingling, nervousness and transient muscle spasm may persist for weeks or months after recovery from the acute stage.

Supportive therapy is indicated by the condition of the patient. If possible, hospitalize patient. Additional treatment consists of prolonged warm baths and IV injection of 10 ml of calcium gluconate 10%, repeated as necessary to control muscle pain. Morphine may be required to control pain. Barbiturates may be used for extreme restlessness. However, because venom can cause respiratory paralysis, consider this when using morphine or a barbiturate. Corticosteroids have been used with varying degrees of success. Local treatment of the bite is of no value; nothing is gained by applying a tourniquet or attempting to remove venom by incision and suction.

In otherwise healthy individuals between the ages of 16 and 60, the use of antivenin may be deferred and treatment with muscle relaxants may be considered.

Administration and Dosage:

Test for sensitivity to horse serum (see p. 2075

Adults and children: Inject one vial (2.5 ml) of antivenin IM, preferably in the region of the anterolateral thigh so that a tourniquet may be applied in the event of a systemic reaction. Symptoms usually subside in 1 to 3 hours. Although one dose is usually adequate, a second dose may be necessary.

May also be given IV in 10 to 50 ml of saline over 15 minutes. This is the preferred route in severe cases, when the patient is under 12 years of age, or in shock. One vial is usually adequate.

Rx	**Antivenin (Latrodectus mactans)** (MSD)	**Powder for Injection:** 6000 antivenin units per vial[1]. Supplied with a 2.5 ml vial of Sterile Water for Injection and a 1 ml vial[1] of normal horse serum (1:10 dilution) for sensitivity testing.

[1] With 1:10,000 thimerosal.

Although rabies rarely affects humans in the United States, every year approximately 25,000 persons receive rabies prophylaxis. Appropriate management depends on the interpretation of the risk of infection and the efficacy and risk of prophylactic treatment. There are two types of immunizing products: Vaccines and globulins. Use both types of products concurrently for rabies postexposure prophylaxis.

Vaccines induce an active immune response that requires about 7 to 10 days to develop, but persists for as long as a year or more.

Human Diploid Cell Rabies Vaccine (HDCV) (see p. 2084 An inactivated virus vaccine prepared from fixed rabies virus grown in human diploid cell culture.

Rabies Vaccine, Adsorbed (RVA): A cell culture-derived vaccine prepared from the Kissling strain of rabies virus adapted to a diploid cell line of the fetal rhesus lung. Currently, RVA is available only to residents of Michigan; however, out-of-state distribution is being planned. For further information, contact the biologics Products Program, Michigan Department of Public Health (517-335-8050), which developed, and now produces and distributes RVA.

RVA differs from HDCV in several aspects: A different virus strain, cell line and concentration process are used in making RVA, and it is liquid rather than lyophilized. Also, approximately 6% of patients receiving HDCV develop an "immune complex-like" reaction, apparently due to the presence of a small amount of human serum albumin. Since this is not a component of the medium used to grow the rabies virus for RVA, this reaction should be less likely to occur. However, an allergic reaction to RVA has occurred in < 1% of patients. Other adverse reactions to RVA appear similar to HDCV. RVA should be used IM and should not be given intradermally. Administration and dosage is the same as for HDCV.

Globulins provide rapid passive immune protection that persists for a short time (half-life of about 21 days).

Rabies Immune Globulin, Human (RIG) (see p. 2086 Antirabies gamma globulin, concentrated from plasma of hyperimmunized human donors.

Antirabies Serum, Equine (ARS) (see p. 2087): A refined, concentrated serum obtained from hyperimmunized horses.

RIG and ARS are both effective; however, ARS causes serum sickness in over 40% of adult recipients, while RIG rarely causes adverse reactions. RIG is preferred over ARS because the latter has a higher risk of adverse reactions.

Rationale of Treatment:

Individually evaluate each possible rabies exposure. Consult local or state public health officials if questions arise about the need for prophylaxis. Consider the following factors before specific treatment is initiated:

Species of biting animal: Carnivorous animals (especially skunks, foxes, coyotes, raccoons, dogs and cats) and bats are more likely to be infective than other animals. Unless the animal is tested and shown not rabid, post-exposure prophylaxis should be initiated upon bite or non-bite exposure to these animals. If treatment has been initiated and subsequent testing shows the exposing animal is not rabid, treatment can be discontinued.

Since the likelihood that a domestic dog or cat is infected with rabies varies from region to region, the need for post-exposure prophylaxis also varies. Bites of rabbits, hares, squirrels, chipmunks, rats, mice, hamsters, guinea pigs, gerbils and other rodents seldom call for specific rabies prophylaxis.

Circumstances of biting incident: An unprovoked attack is more likely to mean that the animal is rabid. Bites inflicted during attempts to feed or handle an apparently healthy animal should generally be regarded as provoked.

Type of exposure: Rabies is transmitted by introducing the virus into open cuts or wounds in skin via mucous membranes. The likelihood of rabies infection varies with the nature and extent of the exposure.

Bite – Any penetration of the skin by teeth.

Nonbite – Scratches, abrasions, open wounds or mucous membranes contaminated with saliva or other potentially infectious material, such as brain tissue from a rabid animal. There have been two instances of airborne rabies acquired in laboratories and two probable airborne rabies cases acquired in one bat-infested cave.

Casual contact with a rabid animal, such as petting it (without a bite or nonbite exposure), is not an indication for prophylaxis.

The only documented cases of rabies due to human-to-human transmission occurred in four patients who received corneal transplants from persons who died of rabies undiagnosed at the time of death.

(Continued on following page)

Preexposure Prophylaxis:

Preexposure immunization does not eliminate the need for prompt postexposure prophylaxis following an exposure; it only reduces the postexposure regimen.

Consider preexposure immunization for persons in high risk groups: Veterinarians, animal handlers, certain laboratory workers, and persons, especially children, living in places where rabies is a constant threat. Also consider others whose vocational or avocational pursuits bring them into contact with potentially rabid dogs, cats, foxes, skunks or bats. Preexposure immunization of immunosuppressed persons is not recommended.

Preexposure immunization consists of 3 doses of HDCV, 1 ml/dose, IM (ie, deltoid area), one each on days 0, 7 and 21 or 28. The intradermal dose is 0.1 ml in the deltoid area of either arm on days 0, 7 and 28. Administration of routine booster doses of vaccine depends on exposure risk category as noted below.

Criteria for Preexposure Immunization			
Risk category	**Nature of risk**	**Typical populations**	**Preexposure regimen**
Continuous	Virus present continuously, often in high concentrations. Aerosol, mucous membrane, bite or nonbite exposure possible. Specific exposures may go unrecognized.	Rabies research lab workers.[1] Rabies biologics production workers.	Primary preexposure immunization course. Serology every 6 months. Booster immunization when antibody titer falls below acceptable level.[2]
Frequent	Exposure usually episodic, with source recognized or unrecognized. Aerosol, mucous membrane, bite or nonbite exposure.	Rabies diagnostic lab workers,[1] spelunkers, veterinarians and animal control and wildlife workers in rabies epizootic areas.	Primary preexposure immunization course. Booster immunization or serology every 2 years.[2]
Infrequent (greater than population-at-large)	Exposure nearly always episodic with source recognized. Mucous membrane, bite or nonbite exposure.	Veterinarians and animal control wildlife workers in areas of low rabies endemicity. Travelers to foreign rabies epizootic areas. Veterinary students.	Primary preexposure immunization course. No routine booster immunization or serology.
Rare (population-at-large)	Exposure always episodic, mucous membrane or bite with source recognized.	US population-at-large, including individuals in rabies epizootic areas.	No preexposure immunization.

[1] Judgment of relative risk and extra monitoring of immunization status of laboratory workers is the responsibility of the laboratory supervisor (see US Department of Health and Human Services' *Biosafety in Microbiological and Biomedical Laboratories,* 1984).

[2] Preexposure booster immunization consists of one dose of HDCV, 1 ml/dose, IM or 0.1 ml ID. Acceptable antibody level is 1:5 titer (complete inhibition in RFFIT at 1:5 dilution). Boost if titer falls below 1:5.

Postexposure Prophylaxis – Local wound treatment:

Immediate and thorough washing of all bite wounds and scratches with soap and water is perhaps the most effective means of preventing rabies. Give tetanus prophylaxis and control bacterial infection as indicated.

(Continued on following page)

Postexposure Prophylaxis - Immunization:

Postexposure antirabies immunization should always include both passive immunization (preferably RIG) and vaccine, with one exception: Persons previously immunized with HDCV in recommended preexposure or postexposure regimens or with other types of vaccines and who have a documented adequate rabies antibody titer should receive only vaccine. The globulin/vaccine combination is recommended for both bite and nonbite exposures, regardless of the interval between exposure and treatment.

Postexposure rabies treatment: Use the following recommendations below as a guide in conjunction with knowledge of the circumstances of the situation. Consult public health officials with questions about the need for rabies prophylaxis.

Animal Species	Condition of Animal at Time of Attack	Treatment of Exposed Person:[1]
Domestic: Dog and cat	Healthy & available for 10 days of observation	None, unless animal develops rabies[2]
	Rabid/suspected rabid	RIG[3] and HDCV[4]
	Unknown (escaped)	Consult public health officials. If treatment is indicated, give RIG[3] and HDCV[4]
Wild: Skunk, bat, fox, coyote, raccoon, bobcat & other carnivores	Regard as rabid unless proven negative by laboratory test[5]	RIG[3] and HDCV[4]
Other: Livestock, rodents, rabbits and hares	Consider individually – Bites of squirrels, hamsters, guinea pigs, gerbils, chipmunks, rats, mice, other rodents, rabbits and hares almost never call for antirabies prophylaxis.	

[1] If treatment is indicated, administer both RIG and HDCV as soon as possible, regardless of the interval from exposure.

[2] Begin treatment with RIG and HDCV at first sign of rabies in biting domestic animals during the usual holding period of 10 days. Kill the symptomatic animal immediately and test.

[3] If RIG is not available, use ARS. Do not exceed the recommended dosage.

[4] Discontinue vaccine if fluorescent antibody tests of animal are negative.

[5] Kill animal and test as soon as possible. Holding for observation is not recommended.

Postexposure immunization:

Persons not previously immunized	RIG, 20 IU/kg, one-half infiltrated at bite site (if possible), remainder IM; 5 doses of HDCV, 1 ml/dose, IM, one each on days 0, 3, 7, 14 and 28.
Persons previously immunized†	2 doses of HDCV, 1 ml/dose, IM, one each on days 0 and 3.

† Preexposure immunization with HDCV; prior postexposure prophylaxis with HDCV; or persons previously immunized with any other type of rabies vaccine and a documented history of positive antibody response to the prior vaccination.

Passive immunization: Administer RIG (ARS if RIG is not available) only once, at the beginning of antirabies therapy. If not given when vaccination was begun, RIG can be given up to the eighth day after the first dose of vaccine. After that, RIG is not indicated, since an antibody response is presumed to have occurred. The recommended RIG dose is 20 IU/kg, ≈ 9 IU/lb (ARS – 40 IU/kg, ≈ 18 IU/lb). Thoroughly infiltrate up to half the dose of RIG around the wound and administer the rest IM. Because RIG may partially suppress active production of antibody, do not exceed the recommended dose.

Active immunization: Administer HDCV in conjunction with RIG on Day 0. Give five 1 ml doses of HDCV IM. Administer the first dose as soon as possible after the exposure; give an additional dose on each of days 3, 7, 14 and 28 after the first dose (Day 0). WHO recommends a sixth dose at 90 days after the first dose. In unusual instances, as when the patient is known to be immunosuppressed, serologic testing is indicated.

Previously immunized persons: When an immunized person who was vaccinated by the recommended regimen with HDCV or who had previously demonstrated rabies antibody is exposed to rabies, that person should receive two doses of HDCV 1 ml/dose, IM, one immediately and one 3 days later. If the person's immune status is not known, postexposure antirabies treatment may be necessary. If antibody can be demonstrated in a serum sample collected before vaccine is given, treatment can be discontinued after at least two doses of HDCV.

(Continued on following page)

Refer to the general discussion of rabies prophylaxis on page 2081

RABIES VACCINE, HUMAN DIPLOID CELL CULTURES (HDCV)

Actions:

Preexposure immunization: High titer antibody responses of HDCV have been demonstrated. Seroconversion was often obtained with only one dose. With two doses 1 month apart, 100% of recipients developed specific antibody.

Postexposure immunization efficacy was proven in conjunction with antirabies serum. Persons severely bitten by rabid dogs and wolves received the vaccine within hours of, and up to 14 days after, the bites. All individuals were fully protected against rabies.

Indications:

Preexposure rabies immunization for persons in high risk groups.

Postexposure antirabies immunization in conjunction with local treatment and immune globulin.

Contraindications:

Postexposure treatment: None known.

Preexposure treatment: Developing febrile illness.

Warnings:

Report any serious reactions immediately to the State Health Department or the Viral Disease Division, Centers for Infectious Diseases, CDC, (404) 329-3095 during working hours, or (404) 329-2888 at other times.

Guillain-Barre syndrome: Two cases of acute polyradiculoneuropathy (Guillain-Barre syndrome) that resolved within 12 weeks, and a focal subacute CNS disorder temporally associated with HDCV have been reported.

Recently, a significant increase has been noted in "immune complex-like" reactions (6%) in persons receiving booster doses of HDCV. The illness, characterized by onset at 2 to 21 days postbooster, presents with a generalized urticaria and may also include arthralgia, arthritis, angioedema, nausea, vomiting, fever and malaise. In no case were the illnesses life-threatening. This reaction occurred much less frequently in persons receiving primary immunization.

Usage in Pregnancy: Category C. Animal studies have not been conducted with HDCV. It is also not known whether the product can cause fetal harm when administered to a pregnant woman or can affect reproductive capacity. Rabies Vaccine should be given to a pregnant woman only if clearly needed. Pregnancy is not a contraindication to postexposure therapy. There have been no fetal abnormalities associated with rabies vaccination. If there is substantial risk of rabies exposure, preexposure prophylaxis may also be indicated during pregnancy.

Usage in Children: Although specific intradermal studies in children have not been conducted, vaccine given IM (1 ml) has been safe. There are no known specific hazards expected from intradermal use of the vaccine in children.

Precautions:

Hypersensitivity: Antihistamines may be given. Have epinephrine available to counteract anaphylactic reactions. Refer to Management of Acute Hypersensitivity Reactions on p. viii.

While the concentration of antibiotics in each dose of vaccine is extremely small, persons with known hypersensitivity to any of these agents could manifest an allergic reaction.

Drug Interactions:

Corticosteroids and **immunosuppressive agents** may interfere with the development of active immunity and predispose the patient to developing rabies. Do not administer during postexposure therapy unless essential. If rabies postexposure therapy is administered to these persons, test serum for rabies antibody to ensure that an adequate response has developed.

Antimalarial drugs such as chloroquine are associated with a reduction in the antibody response to Rabies Vaccine administered intradermally. Although antimalarial agents are not solely responsible for the reduced antibody response, persons on antimalarial drugs should receive Rabies Vaccine (3 doses/1 ml each) by the IM route until more definitive data are available.

Adverse Reactions:

Local (25%): Swelling; erythema; itching; pain; local discomfort.

Systemic (20%): Nausea; headache; abdominal pain; muscle aches; dizziness; malaise; neuroparalytic reactions (see Warnings).

Mild local or systemic reactions can be treated with anti-inflammatory or antipyretic agents (eg, aspirin and antihistamines).

(Continued on following page)

RABIES VACCINE, HUMAN DIPLOID CELL CULTURES (HDCV) (Cont.)

Administration and Dosage:

For IM injection; administer into the deltoid region or upper, outer quadrant of the buttock.

Preexposure dosage:

Primary vaccination – In the US, the Immunization Practices Advisory Committee (ACIP) recommends 3 IM injections of 1 ml each, on days 0, 7 and 21 or 28.

Booster dose – Persons working with live rabies virus in research laboratories and in vaccine production facilities should have rabies antibody titers checked every 6 months and boosters given as needed to maintain an adequate titer. Persons with continuing risk of exposure should receive booster doses or have serum tested for rabies antibody every 2 years; if the titer is inadequate, administer a booster dose.

Postexposure dosage: The ACIP recommends a 5 dose regimen. Five 1 ml doses are given IM on each of days 0, 3, 7, 14 and 28 in conjunction with RIG on day 0. The WHO currently recommends a sixth dose 90 days after the first dose.

Previously immunized persons – Give 2 doses (1 ml each), 1 immediately and 1 3 days later. Do not give RIG in these cases. If the immune status of a previously immunized person is not known, full primary postexposure antirabies treatment (RIG plus 5 days of HDCV) may be necessary. In such cases, if antibody can be demonstrated in a serum sample before vaccine is given, treatment can be discontinued after at least 2 doses of HDCV.

Antibody testing: Routine antibody testing is not recommended. Serologic testing is recommended for persons with diminished immune responses.

Preparation and storage of suspension: Reconstitute the vaccine in its vial with the 1 ml of diluent supplied in the disposable syringe, using the longer of the 2 needles. Gently stir the contents until completely dissolved and withdraw the dissolved vaccine into the syringe by setting the vial in an upright position on the table. Remove the reconstitution needle and replace it with the smaller needle for administration.

Stability: Refrigerate dried vaccine at 2° to 8°C (36° to 46°F). Do not freeze.

Rx	**Imovax Rabies Vaccine** (Merieux Institute)	**Injection:** Freeze-dried suspension of Wistar rabies virus strain PM-1503-3M grown in human diploid cell cultures. (Inactivated whole virus). Contains 2.5 IU rabies antigen per ml. In single dose vial[1] with disposable needle and syringe containing diluent and disposable needle for administration.

RABIES VACCINES, HUMAN DIPLOID CELL CULTURES (For Intradermal Use)

This product is for pre-exposure use only by the intradermal route.

Administration and Dosage:

Primary Vaccination: Based on studies in Europe and the US, the ACIP recommends three 0.1 ml injections; one injection on day 0, one on day 7 and one either on day 21 or 28. The ACIP cites studies in which more than 1500 persons received 0.1 ml of vaccine intradermally as the 2 or 3 dose pre-exposure vaccination. All subjects developed antibody as shown by the rapid fluorescent focus inhibition test (RFFIT). Routine serologic testing to confirm a satisfactory antibody response is not necessary according to the ACIP.

Booster Dose: Persons working with live rabies virus in laboratories and vaccine production facilities should have rabies antibody titers checked every 6 months and boosters given as needed to maintain an adequate titer. Give boosters or test serum every 2 years in laboratory workers (such as those doing rabies diagnostic tests), spelunkers, veterinarians and animal control and wildlife officers in areas where rabies is epizootic. If the titer is inadequate, give a booster dose. Veterinarians and those working in areas of low rabies endemicity do not require routine doses of HDCV after primary pre-exposure immunization. Persons who have had "immune complex-like" hypersensitivity reactions should not receive further HDCV doses unless they are exposed or are likely to be exposed to rabies virus and have unsatisfactory antibody titers.

Rx	**Imovax Rabies I.D. Vaccine** (Merieux Institute)	**Injection:** Freeze-dried suspension of Wistar rabies virus strain PM-1503-3M grown in human diploid cell cultures. Contains 0.25 IU rabies antigen per intradermal dose. In single dose syringe with 1 vial diluent.[2]

[1] With < 100 mg human albumin, < 150 mcg neomycin sulfate and 20 mcg phenol red indicator.
[2] With < 15 mg human albumin, < 22 mcg neomycin sulfate and 3 mcg phenol red indicator/dose.

Refer to the general discussion of rabies prophylaxis on page 2081

RABIES IMMUNE GLOBULIN, HUMAN (RIG)

Actions:

Provides passive protection when given immediately to individuals exposed to rabies virus. Studies of RIG with the first of five doses of human diploid cell vaccine (HDCV) confirmed that passive immunization with RIG provides maximum circulating antibody with minimum interference of active immunization by HDCV.

After initiation of the vaccine series, it takes approximately 1 week to develop immunity to rabies; therefore, the value of immediate passive immunization with rabies antibody cannot be overemphasized.

Indications:

For passive protection against rabies when administered to persons suspected of exposure to rabies, particularly to severe exposure, with one exception: Persons previously immunized with Rabies Vaccine and who have confirmed adequate rabies antibody titers should receive only vaccine. Inject RIG as promptly as possible after exposure.

Contraindications:

Do not administer in repeated doses once vaccine treatment has been initiated. Repeating the dose may interfere with maximum active immunity expected from the vaccine.

Precautions:

Use with caution in individuals who are allergic to human immunoglobulin or thimerosal.

Warnings:

Usage in Pregnancy: Category C. Safety for use during pregnancy has not been established. Use only when clearly needed and when the potential benefits outweigh the potential hazards to the fetus.

Drug Interations:

Measles, mumps, polio or rubella live vaccines: Other antibodies in the RIG preparation may interfere with the response to these live vaccines. Immunization with live vaccines should not be administered within 3 months after RIG administration.

Adverse Reactions:

Local tenderness, muscle soreness or stiffness at the injection site and low grade fever may occur. Sensitization to repeated injections of human globulin has occurred occasionally in immunoglobulin-deficient patients.

There have been a few isolated occurrences of angioedema, urticara nephrotic syndrome and anaphylactic shock after injection. See also Management of Acute Hypersensitivity Reactions on p. viii.

Administration and Dosage:

For IM administration only; do not administer IV. Use in conjunction with HDCV. Inject a single dose of 20 IU/kg (0.133 ml/kg) or 9 IU/lb (0.06 ml/lb) at the time of the first vaccine dose. It may be given up to the eighth day after the first dose of vaccine is given. Use up to one-half the dose to infiltrate the wound area, if the nature and location of the wound site permits. Administer remaining dose IM at a different site, and in a different extremity from the vaccine.

Storage: Refrigerate between 2° to 8°C (35° to 46°F). Do not freeze.

Rx	**Hyperab** (Cutter)	**Injection:** 150 IU per ml	In 2 ml pediatric vial[1] and 10 ml adult vial[1].
Rx	**Imogam** (Merieux)		In 2 ml pediatric vial[1] and 10 ml adult vial[1].

[1] In 0.3 M glycine with 1:10,000 thimerosal.

Refer to the general discussion of rabies prophylaxis on page 2081

ANTIRABIES SERUM, EQUINE ORIGIN (ARS)

Because of a significantly lower incidence of adverse reactions, Rabies Immune Globulin, Human (see page 2086 is preferred over Antirabies Serum Equine.

Actions:

Refined and concentrated antiserum for passive immunity against rabies. Obtained from horses hyperimmunized by repeated injections of fixed rabies virus. Delays virus propagation, thus allowing more time for rabies vaccine to induce antibodies to the virus.

Indications:

For the prevention of rabies in patients who have received severe bites from rabid animals or animals suspected of being rabid. Give in conjunction with HDCV. When ARS is indicated, regardless of the interval between exposure and treatment.

Contraindications:

Use with extreme caution in patients with a history of allergic symptoms or hypersensitivity to horse serum.

Warnings:

Sensitivity testing: Perform a sensitivity test to horse proteins in all patients; take a careful history of asthma, angioneurotic edema or other allergies, including sensitivity to horse serum.

Skin test - Inject intracutaneously 0.1 ml of a 1:100 saline dilution of ARS (0.05 ml of a 1:1000 dilution for persons with a history of allergy), followed by observation for 10 to 30 minutes. A positive reaction consists of urticarial wheal, with or without pseudopods, surrounded by a halo of erythema.

Conjunctival test - Use whenever there may be danger of a severe systemic reaction to the intradermal test. Instill 0.1 ml of 1:10 normal saline dilution of ARS into the lower conjunctival sac. Dilated vessels, edema, itching and lacrimation within 10 to 30 minutes indicate a positive reaction. Wash the eye with epinephrine (1:1000) and normal saline to provide local relief.

Desensitization: In the event of a positive sensitivity test, "desensitization" may be undertaken with extreme caution. Have epinephrine available in the event that an acute anaphylactic reaction develops. See also Management of Acute Hypersensitivity Reactions

Administer small amounts of serum diluted with normal saline at 15 minute intervals, with a gradual increase in the amount used if the injections are tolerated. The following schedule has been recommended:

1. 0.05 ml of 1:20 dilution SC
2. 0.1 ml of 1:10 dilution SC
3. 0.3 ml of 1:10 dilution SC
4. 0.1 ml undiluted serum SC
5. 0.2 ml undiluted serum SC
6. 0.5 ml undiluted serum IM
7. Inject remaining therapeutic dose IM.

Adverse Reactions:

Serum sickness; local pain, erythema and urticaria.

Administration and Dosage:

Administer in a single dose of 1000 IU/55 lbs. (39.6 IU/Kg). Infiltrate up to 50% of the dose around the wound when feasible. Given in conjunction with HDCV.

Rx	**Antirabies Serum** (Sclavo)	**Injection:** 125 IU per ml	In 1000 unit vials.[1]

[1] With 0.3% m-Cresol.

In contrast to the immune serums and antitoxins, which contain exogenous antibodies to provide passive immunity, the Agents for Active Immunization include specific antigens which induce the endogenous production of antibodies. Agents which induce active immunity include vaccines and toxoids.

Vaccines contain whole, either killed or attenuated live, microorganisms capable of inducing antibody formation, but which are not pathogenic. Toxoids are detoxified by-products derived from organisms which induce disease primarily through the elaboration of exotoxins. Although toxoids are not toxic, they are antigenic, and therefore, stimulate specific antibody production. Active immunization induced through inoculation with vaccines and toxoids provides prolonged immunity, whereas passive immunization with immune sera or antitoxins is of short duration.

The table below indicates the recommended immunization schedule for infants and children. Routine smallpox immunization is no longer recommended in the U.S., as the risk of untoward reactions now exceeds the risk of the disease.

Recommended Immunization Schedules[1]

	2 months	4 months	6 months	15 months	18 months	4-6 years
Diphtheria Toxoid[2,3]	✓	✓	✓	✓[4]		✓
Tetanus Toxoid[2,3]	✓	✓	✓	✓[4]		✓
Pertussis Vaccine[2]	✓	✓	✓	✓[4]		✓
Trivalent Oral Polio Vaccine	✓	✓	✓[5]	✓[4]		✓
Measles Vaccine[6]				✓		
Rubella Vaccine[6]				✓		
Mumps Vaccine[6]				✓		
Hemophilus b Polysaccharide Vaccine[7]					✓	

[1] Adapted from MMWR 1986;35(37);577-79. Refer to this source for recommended immunization schedules of infants and children (up to the seventh birthday) and persons over 7 years old, not immunized according to the above schedule.

[2] Usually given as diphtheria and tetanus toxoids combined with pertussis vaccine absorbed (DTP).

[3] Tetanus and diphtheria toxoid boosters. Give at 10 year intervals to maintain immunity.

[4] Acceptable alternative is to administer at 18 months.

[5] OPV is optional. May be given in areas with increased risk of polio virus exposure.

[6] May be given as combined measles, mumps and rubella (MMR) live vaccine in a single dose.

[7] May give at 18 to 23 months for children who are at increased risk of disease (eg, attend a day-care center).

Concomitant vaccination: When Measles, Mumps and Rubella Virus Vaccine, Live, is given simultaneously with trivalent oral poliovirus vaccine, and DTP antibody responses can be expected to be comparable to those which follow administration of the vaccines at different times.

Immunization for other diseases is recommended for persons with a risk of exposure. Specific immunization requirements and recommendations for international travel can be obtained from the Superintendent of Documents, U.S. Government Printing Office, Washington, DC, 20402, in the publication "Health Information for International Travel".

Hypersensitivity to vaccine components: Vaccine antigens produced in systems containing allergenic substances, (ie, embryonated chicken eggs) may cause hypersensitivity reactions including anaphylaxis (ie, yellow fever vaccine). Such vaccines should not be given to persons with known hypersensitivity to components of the substrates. Contrarily, influenza vaccine antigens (whole or split), although prepared in embryonated eggs, are highly purified and only rarely are associated with hypersensitivity reactions.

Live virus vaccines prepared by growing viruses in cell cultures are essentially devoid of allergenic substances. On very rare occasions, hypersensitivity reactions to measles vaccine have been reported in persons with anaphylactic hypersensitivity to eggs. Measles vaccine, however, can be given safely to egg-allergic individuals provided the allergies are not manifested by anaphylactic symptoms. The same precautions apply to mumps vaccine.

Some vaccines contain preservatives (eg, thimerosal, a mercurial) or trace amounts of antibiotics (eg, neomycin) to which patients may be hypersensitive.

(Continued on following page)

Altered immunocompetence: Virus replication after administration of live, attenuated virus vaccines may be enhanced in persons with immune deficiency diseases, and in those with suppressed capability for immune response (ie, leukemia, lymphoma, generalized malignancy or therapy with corticosteroids, alkylating agents, antimetabolites or radiation). Do not give live, attenuated virus vaccines to such patients. Do not give live, attenuated virus vaccines to a member of a household in which there is a family history of congenital or hereditary immunodeficiency until the immune competence of the recipient is known.

Children with symptomatic HTLV-III/LAV infection (human T-lymphotropic virus type III/lymphadenopathy-associated virus): Do not give children and young adults who are immunosuppressed in association with AIDS or other clinical manifestations of HTLV-III/LAV infection live-virus and live-bacterial vaccines (MMR, BCG, OPV). After exposure to measles or varicella, these patients may receive passive immunization with immune globulin or varicella-zoster immune globulin.

Immunization with DTP, inactivated poliovaccine (IPV), and Hemophilus influenzae type b vaccines is recommended, although immunization may be less effective than it would be for immunocompetent children. Annual immunization with inactivated influenza vaccine for children over 6 months and one time administration of pneumococcal vaccine for children over 2 years is recommended.

Children with previously diagnosed asymptomatic HTLV-III/LAV infection have received live-virus vaccines without adverse reactions. However, observe for possible adverse reactions and for occurrence of vaccine-preventable diseases since immunization may be less effective than for uninfected persons.

Available data also suggest OPV may be administered without adverse reaction. However, it may be prudent to use IPV routinely to immunize asymptomatic children with HTLV-III/LAV infection. DTP and Hemophilus influenzae type b vaccines may be given in accordance with Immunization Practices Advisory Committee (ACIP) recommendations.

Severe febrile illnesses: Immunization of persons with severe febrile illnesses should generally be deferred until they have recovered.

Vaccination during pregnancy: On the grounds of a theoretical risk to the developing fetus, live, attenuated virus vaccines are not generally given to pregnant women or to those likely to become pregnant within 3 months after receiving vaccine(s). With some of these vaccines, particularly rubella, measles and mumps, pregnancy is a contraindication. When vaccine is to be given during pregnancy, waiting until the second or third trimester to minimize any concern over teratogenicity is a reasonable precaution. However, there has been no evidence of congenital rubella syndrome in infants born to susceptible mothers who received rubella vaccine during pregnancy.

Measles, mumps, rubella or oral polio vaccines may be administered with safety to children of pregnant women. Experience to date has not revealed any risks of poliovaccine virus to the fetus.

There is no convincing evidence of risk to the fetus from immunization of pregnant women using inactivated virus vaccines, bacterial vaccines or toxoids. Tetanus and diphtheria toxoid (Td) should be given to inadequately immunized pregnant women because it affords protection against neonatal tetanus.

Adverse events following immunization: Modern vaccines are extremely safe and effective, but not completely so. Adverse events following immunization have been reported with all vaccines. These range from frequent, minor, local reactions to extremely rare, severe, systemic illness such as paralysis associated with oral polio vaccine.

BCG VACCINE

Actions:

Pharmacology: BCG vaccine for intravesical or percutaneous use is an attenuated, live culture preparation of the Bacillus of Calmette and Guerin (BCG) strain of *Mycobacterium bovis.* The Tice strain was developed at the University of Illinois from a strain originated at the Pasteur Institute.

Immunization with BCG vaccine lowers the risk of serious complications of primary tuberculosis in children. Estimates of efficacy from observational studies in areas where vaccination is performed at birth show that the incidence of tuberculous meningitis and miliary tuberculosis is 52% to 100% lower and that the incidence of pulmonary tuberculosis is 2% to 80% lower in vaccinated children $<$15 years of age than in unvaccinated controls. However, estimates of vaccine efficacy may be distorted because of the following: Vaccination was not allocated randomly in observational studies; there were differences in BCG strains, methods and routes of administration; there were differences in the characteristics of the populations and environments in which the vaccines have been studied.

Indications:

Exposed tuberculin skin test-negative infants and children: BCG vaccination is recommended for infants and children with risk of intimate and prolonged exposure to persistently untreated or ineffectively treated patients with infectious pulmonary tuberculosis and who cannot be removed from the source of exposure and cannot be placed on long-term preventive therapy, or who are continuously exposed to persons with tuberculosis who have bacilli resistant to isoniazid and rifampin.

Groups with an excessive rate of new infections: BCG vaccination is also recommended for tuberculin-negative infants and children in groups in which the rate of new infections exceeds 1% per year and for whom the usual surveillance and treatment programs have been attempted but are not operationally feasible. These groups include persons without regular access to health care, those for whom usual health care is culturally or socially unacceptable, or groups who have demonstrated an inability to effectively use existing accessible care.

The US Immunization Practices Advisory Committee (ACIP) no longer recommends the use of BCG vaccination for health care workers at risk of repeated exposure to tuberculosis but recommends that these individuals be under tuberculin skin testing surveillance and receive isoniazid prophylaxis in case of tuberculin skin test conversion.

For international travelers, the CDC recommends that BCG vaccination be considered only for travelers with insignificant reaction to tuberculin skin test who will be in a high-risk environment for prolonged periods of time without access to tuberculin skin test surveillance.

Tice BCG vaccine is also indicated for carcinoma in situ of the bladder. See individual monograph in the Antineoplastics section.

Contraindications:

Persons with impaired immune responses, whether they be congenital, disease-produced, drug- or therapy-induced (ie, cytotoxic drugs and radiation used in cancer therapy). The concurrent use of steroids requires caution because of the possibility of the vaccine establishing a systemic infection; if necessary, the infection can be treated with antituberculous drugs.

Warnings:

Route of administration: Do not inject IV, SC or intradermally. Use percutaneous administration with the multiple puncture disc (see Administration and Dosage).

Immune deficiency syndromes: Do not use in infants, children or adults with severe immune deficiency syndromes. Administer with caution to persons in groups at high risk for HIV infection. Children with a family history of immune deficiency disease should not be vaccinated. If they are, consult an infectious disease specialist and administer antituberculous therapy if clinically indicated.

Pregnancy: Category C. It is not known whether BCG vaccine can cause fetal harm when administered to a pregnant woman or can affect reproduction capacity. Give to a pregnant woman only if clearly needed.

Lactation: It is not known whether BCG vaccine is excreted in breast milk. Because of the potential for serious adverse reactions in nursing infants from BCG vaccine, decide whether to discontinue nursing or not to vaccinate, taking into account the importance of tuberculosis vaccination to the mother.

Children: Take precautions with respect to infants vaccinated with BCG and exposed to persons with active tuberculosis. See Administration and Dosage.

(Continued on following page)

BCG VACCINE (Cont.):

Precautions:

Aseptic technique: Tice BCG contains live bacteria; use with aseptic technique. Handle and dispose of all equipment, supplies, and receptacles in contact with BCG vaccine as biohazardous.

Allergic reactions: Assess the possibility of allergic reactions.

Normal reaction: The intensity and duration of the local reaction depends on the depth of penetration of the multiple-puncture disc and individual variations in patients' tissue reactions. The initial skin lesions usually appear within 10 to 14 days and consist of small red papules at the site. The papules reach maximum diameter (about 3 mm) after 4 to 6 weeks, after which they may scale and then slowly subside.

Six months later, there is usually no visible sign of the vaccination, but on occasion a faintly discernible pattern of the disc points may be visible. On people whose skin tends to keloid formation, there may be slightly more visible evidence of the vaccination.

Vaccination is recommended only for those who are tuberculin negative to a recent skin test with 5 tuberculin units (5TU). Otherwise, vaccination of persons highly sensitive to mycobacterial antigens can result in hypersensitivity reactions including fever, anorexia, myalgia and neuralgia, which last a few days.

After vaccination, it is usually not possible to clearly distinguish between a tuberculin reaction caused by persistent postvaccination sensitivity and one caused by a virulent suprainfection. Caution is advised in attributing a positive skin test to BCG vaccination. Further investigate a sharp rise in the tuberculin reaction since the latest test (except in the immediate postvaccination period).

Lymphadenopathy: Occasionally, lymphadenopathy of the regional lymph node, which spontaneously resolves itself, is seen in young children. Only rarely does the node create a fistula followed by a short period of drainage. The usual treatment is to maintain cleanliness of the drainage site and allow the lesion to heal spontaneously without medical intervention.

Drug Interactions:

Antimicrobial or immunosuppressive agents may interfere with the development of the immune response; use only under medical supervision.

Adverse Reactions:

Lymphadenopathy (see Precautions); osteomyelitis (≈ 1 per 1,000,000 vaccinees); lupoid reactions; disseminated BCG infection and death are very rare (≈ 1 per 5,000,000 vaccinees) and occur almost exclusively in children with impaired immune responses.

Overdosage:

Accidental overdosages, if treated immediately with antituberculous drugs, have not led to complications. If the vaccination response is allowed to progress it can still be treated successfully with antituberculous drugs but complications can include regional adenitis, lupus vulgaris, subcutaneous cold abscesses, ocular lesions and others.

Patient Information:

Keep the vaccination site clean until the local reaction has disappeared.

Administration and Dosage:

Preparation: Add 1 ml Sterile Water for Injection, USP, to one amp of vaccine. Draw the mixture into a syringe and expel it back into the ampule three times to ensure thorough mixing.

Treatment and schedule: The vaccine is administered after fully explaining the risks and benefits to the vaccinee, parent or guardian. After the vaccine is prepared, the immunizing dose of 0.2 to 0.3 ml is dropped on the cleansed surface of the skin, and the vaccine is administered percutaneously utilizing a sterile multiple-puncture disc. After vaccination, the vaccine should flow into the wounds and dry. No dressing is required; however, it is recommended that the site be kept dry for 24 hours. Advise the patient that the vaccine contains live organisms. Although the vaccine will not survive in a dry state, infection of others is possible.

Repeat vaccination for those who remain tuberculin-negative to 5TU of tuberculin after 2 to 3 months.

Children: In infants < 1 month old, reduce the dosage of vaccine by one half by using 2 ml of Sterile Water when reconstituting. If a vaccinated infant remains tuberculin negative to 5TU on skin testing, and if indications for vaccination persist, the infant should receive a full dose after 1 year of age.

Storage/Stability: Refrigerate the intact amp at 2° to 8°C (36° to 46°F). Protect from light. Do not use after the expiration date printed on the label.

Keep reconstituted vaccine refrigerated, protect from exposure to light, and use within 2 hours.

Rx	**TICE BCG** (Organon)	**Powder for Injection, lyophilized:** Tice strain[1] (1 to 8 x 10^8 CFU equivalent to approximately 50 mg)	In 2 ml amps.[2]

[1] Developed at the University of Illinois. [2] Preservative free.

MIXED RESPIRATORY VACCINE

Actions:

Pharmacology: Mixed respiratory vaccine (MRV) is prepared from many strains of bacterial organisms commonly found in respiratory tract infections. Many of these strains are isolated in the preparation of autogenous vaccines for patients subject to respiratory infections.

These organisms consist of two general classes of streptococci (a variety of *viridans* and non-hemolytic types). Staphylococci is a mixture of several *aureus* strains. Four types of pneumococci are in this product. The other organisms in the vaccine are *Moraxella (Branhamella) catarrhalis, Klebsiella pneumoniae* (Friedlanders bacillus) and *Hemophilus influenzae.*

The mechanism of MRV is not known. Antigens injected into the skin are processed locally or in satellite lymph nodes by macrophages or lymphocytes. Subsequently this may lead to production of blocking antibody to specific antigens or activation of suppressor cells or helper cells that alter the immunologic status of the patient.

The antigens are metabolized in the macrophages of the immune system. It is not known how much of the antigenic material in bacterial vaccines passes through the immune barriers to be excreted or detoxified by other organs.

Clinical trials: Very few controlled studies have evaluated the effectiveness of MRV or delineated the kinds of illness likely to respond to MRV. Infectious asthma, chronic bronchitis, rhino-bronchitis and secretory otitis were conditions treated, but exact criteria for these diagnoses were generally vague. Criteria for judging severity of symptoms were generally subjective, but the same criteria were applied to both treated and control patients.

To various degrees, these studies indicated that patients given bacterial vaccines did better over the period of study and in some cases did less well later, after vaccines were discontinued. Many reports on the effectiveness of MRV have come from pediatric practices. The youngest patient reported is 3 years old.

Many diseases such as rhinitis, infectious asthma, chronic sinusitis, nasal polyposis and chronic, serous otitis are of unknown etiology. Bacterial or viral infections play a prominent role in these disorders. These disorders may respond transiently or incompletely to appropriate antibiotic, surgical, antihistamine and anti-inflammatory treatment. Bacterial vaccines have been used in the hopes of favorably altering the course of the chronic inflammatory process. There are numerous uncontrolled testimonial reports that indicate the benefits of mixed respiratory vaccines for a variety of common chronic disorders, including those listed above.

Indications:

Based on a review by the Panel on the safety, effectiveness and labeling of bacterial vaccines and bacterial antigens that have "No U.S. Standard of Potency" and other information, the Food and Drug Administration has directed that further investigation be conducted before this product is determined to be fully effective for the labeled indications.

Contraindications:

Rheumatoid arthritis; lupus erythematosus; other connective tissue disease; hypersensitivity to any component of the product (see Warnings). Occasionally a patient will develop excessively large, delayed local reactions after injection, and rarely, vague malaise or myalgia. Drastically reduce subsequent doses or discontinue.

Warnings:

Hypersensitivity: Systemic reactions are very rare. If any do occur, treat like other allergenic reactions using epinephrine and antihistamines. Delayed hypersensitivity to bacterial products is common, and if severe, may limit the dose that can be administered. If delayed skin reactions are accompanied by any systemic symptoms, stop administration. Refer also to Management of Acute Hypersensitivity Reactions.

Pregnancy: Category C. It is not known whether MRV can cause fetal harm when administered to a pregnant woman or can affect reproduction capacity. Give to a pregnant woman only if clearly needed.

Lactation: It is not known whether bacterial products appear in breast milk.

(Continued on following page)

MIXED RESPIRATORY VACCINE (Cont.)

Adverse Reactions:

Immediate systemic reactions are rare. When suspicion has arisen, other antigens were given that were known to be associated with immediate hypersensitivity. Delayed, local reactions are frequent but are no cause for alarm unless accompanied by fever, malaise or myalgia.

Administration and Dosage:

Inject SC. Do not inject IV. Always agitate the suspension to ensure uniform distribution while withdrawing the dose from the vial.

Initial dose: An initial prophylactic dose of 0.05 ml SC is recommended. Increase doses by 0.05 to 0.1 ml at 4 to 7 day intervals until a maximum dose of 0.5 to 1 ml has been reached. In acute conditions, give an initial dose of 0.02 ml and administer increments of 0.02 to 0.05 ml at 3 to 5 day intervals. Patient sensitivity varies and for some, doses may be increased faster; for others, more slowly. Do not administer another dose until all local reactions resulting from the previous dose have disappeared.

Dosage increments: When doses are being advanced, the time interval can be every 3 to 4 days with the lower concentration and 5 to 7 days with the more concentrated vaccine. Local reaction and generalized symptoms determine the final maintenance dose.

Maintenance dose: Generally, give 0.5 ml at weekly or alternate week intervals. The hyposensitizing dose for children is the same as for adults. The maximum volume of antigen tolerated without undue pain and swelling may be less for the smaller patient.

Increasingly large delayed reactions may occur after administering maintenance doses for many months. Further administration of vaccine, even at smaller doses, may continue to increase the reaction. Stop vaccine immediately. A rest period of 2 to 6 months may allow the delayed hypersensitivity to subside, and injections may be resumed at a lower dose if still needed. Individualize dosage. Smaller increments in doses may be necessary for extremely sensitive patients.

General reactions such as fatigue, drowsiness or a definite aggravation of allergic symptoms require a reduction in the size of the subsequent doses or further dilution of the vaccine. Severe systemic reactions mandate a decrease of at least 50% in the next dose, followed by cautious increases.

Storage: Store at 2° to 8°C (36° to 46°F).

Rx	**MRV** (Hollister-Stier, Miles)	**Injection:** 2000 million organisms per ml from:		In 20 ml vials with 0.4% phenol and dextrose.
		Staphylococcus aureus	1200 million	
		Streptococcus (viridans and *non-hemolytic)*	200 million	
		Streptococcus pneumoniae	150 million	
		Moraxella (Branhamella) catarrhalis	150 million	
		Klebsiella pneumoniae	150 million	
		Hemophilus influenzae	150 million	

STAPHAGE LYSATE (SPL)

Actions:

Pharmacology: Bacterial antigen made from *Staphylococcus,* staphage lysate (SPL) is a bacteriologically sterile staphylococcal vaccine containing components of *S aureus,* bacteriophage and culture medium ingredients.

In experimental conditions, *S aureus* or its cellular components may induce cell-mediated immunity. In uncontrolled studies in humans, favorable results have been reported using SPL for a variety of staphylococcal diseases, as well as for herpesvirus and aphthous ulcers (essentially treatment failures with other therapeutic modalities).

In vitro, SPL has stimulated lymphoproliferative responses in both T- and B-cell subpopulations present in peripheral and cord blood of healthy human subjects.

These findings appear to support the interpretation that SPL in staphylococcal-hypersensitive subjects acts as an immunopotentiator of nonspecific cell-mediated immunity.

Indications:

Treatment of either staphylococcal infections or polymicrobial infections with a staphylococcal component.

Based on a review by the Panel on Bacterial Vaccines and Bacterial Antigens with no US Standard of Potency and other information, the Food and Drug Administration has directed that further investigation be conducted before this product is determined fully effective for the labeled indication(s).

(Continued on following page)

STAPHAGE LYSATE (SPL) (Cont.)

Contraindications:

Intranasal use during an acute asthmatic episode.

Warnings:

Hypersensitivity: In common with all antigens employed to stimulate the production of antibodies that are protective in the event of subsequent disease, SPL presents the remote potential of host sensitization to staphylococcal or bovine protein. Anaphylaxis has never been observed in > 10 million doses, but consider this possibility and be prepared with emergency resuscitation equipment and medications. Refer to Management of Acute Hypersensitivity Reactions.

Allergies: Exercise caution when administering SPL intranasally to patients with known allergies (see Administration and Dosage).

Pregnancy: Category B. There are no adequate and well controlled studies in pregnant women. Use during pregnancy only if clearly needed and if the potential benefits outweigh the potential hazards to the fetus.

Lactation: It is not known whether SPL is excreted in breast milk. Exercise caution when administering to a nursing mother.

Children: Safety and effectiveness in children have not been established.

Precautions:

Preservative free: SPL does not contain a preservative; it must be handled aseptically. Do not use if it becomes cloudy or turbid.

Amps: Use 1 ml amps for SC injection and intranasal aerosol inhalation only. When a parenteral dose of SPL is withdrawn from the amp, use the remainder immediately or discard.

Vials: Use the 10 ml vial for intranasal (aerosol or drop instillation), oral or topical administration only; do not use for SC injection.

Adverse Reactions:

SPL may cause general vaccine-type reactions (eg, malaise, fever, chills). Excessive reactions may be lessened by dose reduction.

Reactions at the site of injection (redness, itching or swelling) may occur in 2 to 3 hours and may last up to 3 days, steadily decreasing. These reactions indicate a normal response to SPL and, if excessive, may be lessened by dose reduction.

Patient Information:

SPL may cause vaccine-type or injection site reactions and, if excessive, these reactions may be lessened by dose reduction.

Administration and Dosage:

Routes of administration: SPL is administered by several routes including: SC injection; intranasal aerosol inhalation or nasal drop instillation; oral; topical; irrigation; combinations of these routes. The severity of the infection and the response of the patient are the guiding factors in determining the proper dosage regimen.

Skin testing: It is highly recommended that all new patients first be skin-tested with 0.025 to 0.05 ml intracutaneously to assess their relative sensitivity to SPL. Based on relative sensitivity to skin test, the initial dose of SPL is small, followed by incremental increases at prescribed intervals (according to urgency and tolerance), to a maximum dose. The dose is continued until improvement is certain, then the interval may be lengthened gradually to the longest interval that maintains adequate clinical control.

Tolerance: The limit of tolerance is the maximum quantity that can be given to a patient without producing signs of a general vaccine-type reaction (see Adverse Reactions).

Chronic, recurrent, refractory or deep-seated infections: Cautiously increase the frequency or the dose to achieve the desired therapeutic response.

Children usually should receive about one-half the adult dose. Infants are best treated with nasal drop instillation, sprays or topical application.

Acute infections: Initial dose – 0.05 to 0.2 ml, followed by incremental increases (according to urgency and tolerance) of 0.1 to 0.2 ml at 1 to 2 day intervals, to a maximum dose of up to 0.5 ml.

Subacute and chronic infections: Initial dose – 0.05 to 0.1 ml, followed by incremental increases (according to urgency and tolerance) of 0.1 to 0.2 ml at 2 to 4 day intervals, to a maximum dose of 0.2 to 0.5 ml.

(Administration and Dosage continued on following page)

STAPHAGE LYSATE (SPL) (Cont.)

Administation and Dosage (Cont.):

SC administration: Administer in the deltoid region. Following the initial injection, subsequent injections are given in alternate arms, avoiding a previous site.

If an undue amount of local redness, itching or swelling ensues, await a partial subsidence of the reactions, proceed with one-half the previous dose and make incremental increases at longer intervals.

Following an SC injection, the unused contents of the 1 ml amp may be given orally, topically or intranasally to reinforce the SC dose.

Intranasal aerosol inhalation: SPL is rapidly absorbed through the anterior nares, the main reservoir of pathogenic staphylococci. The importance of intranasal aerosol inhalation is stressed because of the high absorptive characteristics of the nasal mucosa. When using this route, some patients may experience transient general vaccine-type reactions. If excessive, reactions may be lessened by dose reduction.

Intranasal aerosol inhalation allows direct access to the sinuses, throat and bronchi; when this route is combined with SC injection, better clinical results may be obtained.

A nebulizer with nasal tips is used, attached by rubber tubing having a hand-controlled air valve to an air supply (a DeVilbiss Air Compressor). Clean the nebulizer after each use according to the manufacturer's directions.

A measured dose of SPL is placed in the nebulizer, adding sufficient sterile preservative free water or isotonic saline to a total volume of 1 ml for efficient atomization. Nebulization is achieved by closing the air valve during inspiration, holding the breath a few seconds, and exhaling through the mouth, avoiding hyperventilation.

Patients without allergies – Initial dose: 0.1 ml, followed by incremental increases (according to urgency and tolerance) of up to 0.2 ml at 1 to 3 days, to a maximum dose of 0.5 to 1 ml.

Patients with known allergies – Exercise caution when administering SPL by this route to patients with allergies such as bronchial asthma, pulmonary fibrosis, emphysema, bronchiectasis, hay fever and multiple allergies.

It is highly recommended that these patients first be skin-tested with 0.025 to 0.05 ml intracutaneously to assess their relative sensitivity to SPL. Based on relative sensitivity to the skin test, the initial dose varies from 0.05 to 0.1 ml, followed by incremental increases (according to urgency and tolerance) of 0.05 to 0.1 ml at weekly intervals, to a maximum dose of 0.25 to 0.5 ml. These doses can be increased cautiously at shorter intervals if the patient tolerates SPL well.

For faster immunologic response, SPL may be given concomitantly by SC injection or orally without aftereffects.

Nasal drop instillation: If intranasal aerosol inhalation equipment is not available, administer SPL by nasal drop instillation, particularly to patients with upper respiratory symptoms. Administer by this route either alone or concomitantly with other routes.

Before using SPL by nasal drop instillation, review all information under *Intranasal aerosol inhalation.*

When using this route, withdraw appropriate dose with sterile tuberculin syringe and needle, remove the needle, and use the syringe as a dropper. Divide the dose equally between each nostril and keep in contact with the nasal mucosa for a minimum of 2 minutes to achieve adequate absorption.

Oral: The specific therapy of staphylococcal enterocolitis should include an oral dose of 1 to 2 ml, in water, 1 to 3 times a day as long as necessary to maintain adequate clinical control.

For systemic action, SPL by SC injection or intranasally will reinforce the oral dose.

Topical application: Concomitantly with other routes of administration, SPL in the form of sprays, drops, packs or irrigations may be used to treat accessible lesions of the skin and mucous membranes, including eye and ear infections, burns, sinus tracts and ulcers. The usual dose varies from 0.25 to 2 ml, as often as indicated to maintain adequate clinical control.

Storage/Stability: Store at 2° to 8°C (35° to 46°F). Do not freeze. Do not use if cloudy or turbid. Preservative free; handle aseptically.

Rx	**SPL-Serologic Types I and III** (Delmont Labs)	**Solution:** per ml 120 to 180 million *Staphylococcus aureus colony forming units* and 100 to 1000 million *Staphylococcus bacteriophage plaque forming units*	In 1 ml amps[1] and 10 ml vials.[2]

[1] Preservative free. For SC injection and intranasal aerosol inhalation only.

[2] Preservative free. For intranasal aerosol inhalation or nose drops, oral administration or topical application only.

MENINGOCOCCAL POLYSACCHARIDE VACCINE

Actions:

Pharmacology: Meningitis can be caused by a variety of microorganisms including several sero-groups of meningococci. This vaccine will not stimulate protection against infections caused by organisms other than *Neisseria meningitidis* Groups A, C, Y and W-135. The presence of human serum bactericidal antibodies to meningococcal antigens is strongly correlated with immunity to meningococcal disease; meningococcal polysaccharides induce the formation of such antibodies in humans.

Clinical trials: In one study, group A polysaccharide vaccine was 100% effective in preventing systemic disease caused by group A organisms occurring ≥ 2 weeks after immunization. Another study using group C polysaccharide vaccine was at least 87% effective in preventing disease caused by group C organisms. With A and C combined, there was at least a fourfold increase in bactericidal antibodies in 95% of subjects in a separate study. Another study using groups A, C, Y and W-135 showed at least a fourfold increase in antibodies in > 90% of subjects. In children (ages 2 to 12), the following seroconversion rates were obtained following the vaccine: Group A – 72% to 99%; Group C – 58% to 99%; Group Y – 90% to 97%; Group W-135 – 82% to 89%.

Indications:

Persons ≥ 2 years of age at risk in epidemic or highly endemic areas.

Consider vaccination for:

Household or institutional contacts of meningococcal disease as an adjunct to appropriate antibiotic chemoprophylaxis.

Medical and laboratory personnel at risk of exposure to meningococcal disease.

Travelers planning to visit countries having epidemic meningococcal disease.

Terminal complement component deficiency patients.

Anatomic or functional asplenia patients.

Routine vaccination is not recommended in the US for the following reasons: (1) Meningococcal disease is infrequent (≈ 3000 cases per year); (2) no vaccine exists for serogroup B, which accounts for ≈ 50% of cases in the US; and (3) vaccine is not efficacious against group C disease in children < 2 years of age, which account for 28% of the group C cases in the US.

Contraindications:

Acute illness; pregnancy (see Warnings).

Warnings:

Immunosuppressive therapy: The expected immune response may not be obtained if the vaccine is used in persons receiving immunosuppressive therapy.

Hypersensitivity: Have epinephrine 1:1000 available to control anaphylactic reactions. Refer to Management of Acute Hypersensitivity Reactions.

Pregnancy: Category C. Effects on the human fetus and on reproduction capacity are unknown. Do not administer to a pregnant woman unless clearly required.

Children: Not recommended in children < 2 years of age.

Adverse Reactions:

Systemic: Headache (1.2% to 4.1%); malaise (≤ 2.6%); fever (0.4% to 3.1%); chills (≤ 1.7%).

Local: Tenderness (24.2% to 29.1%); pain (17.5% to 25.1%); erythema (0.8% to 31.7%); induration (4.8% to 8.3%).

Administration and Dosage:

Inject SC. Avoid injecting intradermally or IV since clinical studies have not established safety and efficacy. The immunizing dose is one SC injection of 0.5 ml.

Preparation of solution: Reconstitute the vaccine using the diluent supplied. Shake until dissolved.

Storage/Stability: Store freeze-dried vaccine and reconstituted vaccine between 2° to 8°C (35° to 46°F). Discard remainder of vaccine within 5 days after reconstitution.

Rx	**Menomune-A/C/Y/W-135** (Connaught Labs)	**Powder for Injection:** When reconstituted, each 0.5 ml contains 50 mcg "isolated product" from each of groups A, C, Y and W-135.	Freeze-dried. In single dose vials with diluent.[1]

[1] With lactose (2.5 to 5 mg per dose) and 1:10,000 thimerosal.

CHOLERA VACCINE

Actions:

Pharmacology: Cholera vaccine is a sterile suspension of equal parts of phenol-inactivated Ogawa and Inaba serotypes of killed *Vibrio cholerae (V comma)* in buffered sodium chloride injection. The vaccine contains 8 units of each serotype antigen (Ogawa and Inaba) per ml.

Cholera vaccine is used for active immunization against cholera. In field studies carried out in endemic cholera areas, cholera vaccines were approximately 50% effective in reducing incidence of disease and for only 3 to 6 months. Use of cholera vaccine does not prevent transmission of infection.

Indications:

Active immunization against cholera is indicated only for individuals traveling to or residing in countries where cholera is endemic or epidemic.

The risk of cholera to most US travelers is so low that vaccination is of dubious benefit. The World Health Organization no longer recommends cholera vaccination for travel to or from cholera-infected areas; however, some countries affected or threatened by cholera may require evidence of vaccination as a condition of entry. The traveler's best protection against cholera is to avoid food and water that might be contaminated.

Contraindications:

Presence of any acute illness; history of severe systemic reaction or allergic response following a prior dose of cholera vaccine.

Warnings:

Route of administration: Do not inject IV. Inject IM, SC or intradermally. Do not administer IM to persons with thrombocytopenia or any coagulation disorder that would contraindicate IM injection.

Hypersensitivity: Before the injection of any biological, take all precautions known for prevention of allergic or other side effects, including a review of the patient's history regarding possible sensitivity, and a knowledge of the recent literature pertaining to the use of the biological concerned. Have epinephrine 1:1000 available for immediate use when this product is injected. Refer to Management of Acute Hypersensitivity Reactions.

Pregnancy: Category C. It is not known whether cholera vaccine can cause fetal harm when administered to a pregnant woman or can affect reproductive capacity. However, as with other inactivated bacterial vaccines, its use is not contraindicated during pregnancy unless the intended recipient has manifested significant systemic or allergic reaction following administration of prior doses. Individualize use of cholera vaccine during pregnancy to reflect actual need.

Precautions:

Hepatitis B: Use a separate, sterilized syringe and needle for each patient to prevent transmission of hepatitis B virus and other infectious agents from one person to another.

Aspirate: Before delivering the dose IM or SC, aspirate to help avoid inadvertent injection into a blood vessel.

Drug Interactions:

Yellow fever vaccine: Some data suggest that administration of cholera and yellow fever vaccines within 3 weeks of each other may result in decreased levels of antibody response to both vaccines as compared with administration at longer intervals. However, there is no evidence that protection to either disease is diminished following simultaneous administration. When feasible, administer cholera and yellow fever vaccines at a minimal interval of 3 weeks, unless time constraints preclude this. If the vaccines cannot be administered at least 3 weeks apart, give simultaneously.

Adverse Reactions:

Local reactions manifested by erythema, induration, pain and tenderness at the site of injection occur in most recipients, and such local reactions may persist for a few days.

Recipients frequently develop malaise, headache and mild-to-moderate temperature elevations which may persist for 1 to 2 days.

(Continued on following page)

CHOLERA VACCINE (Cont.)

Patient Information:

The traveler's best protection against cholera is to avoid food and water that may be contaminated.

Administration and Dosage:

Administer intradermally, SC or IM. The intracutaneous (intradermal) route is satisfactory for persons ≥ 5 years of age, but higher levels of antibody may be achieved in children < 5 years old by the SC and IM routes.

The primary immunizing course consists of 2 doses, 1 week to 1 month or more apart. The primary immunizing series does not need to be repeated for booster doses to be effective.

Primary and Booster Immunizations for Cholera Vaccine				
	Route and Age			
	Intradermal[1]	SC or IM		
Dose number	≥ 5 years	6 mos-4 years	5-10 years	> 10 years
1 & 2[2]	0.2 ml	0.2 ml	0.3 ml	0.5 ml
Boosters[3]	0.2 ml	0.2 ml	0.3 ml	0.5 ml

[1] Higher levels of antibody may be achieved in children < 5 years old by the SC or IM routes.
[2] Primary immunization requires 2 doses given at intervals of 1 week to 1 month (or more).
[3] Give booster every 6 months where cholera is epidemic or endemic.

Storage: Refrigerate between 2° to 8°C (35° to 46°F). Do not freeze.

Rx	**Cholera Vaccine** (Wyeth-Ayerst)	**Injection:** Suspension of killed *Vibrio cholerae* (Inaba and Ogawa types), 8 units of each serotype per ml	In 1.5 and 20 ml vials.[4]

[4] With 0.5% phenol.

PLAGUE VACCINE

Actions:

Pharmacology: Prepared from *Yersinia pestis* organisms grown in artificial media and inactivated with formaldehyde. Plague vaccine is used to promote active immunity to plague in individuals considered at high risk of infection. Inactivated bacilli present in plague vaccine promote the production of plague antibody; plague antibody neutralizes the bacilli so that the incidence and severity of infection are reduced.

Indications:

Persons at particularly high risk of exposure to plague. High risk areas include rural mountains or upland areas of South America, Asia and Africa. Routine vaccination is not necessary for persons residing in plague-enzootic areas (such as those in the western US) nor for travelers in countries where cases have been reported, particularly if travel is limited to urban areas. Vaccination is recommended in the following situations:

1. Following natural disaster or at times when regular sanitary practices are interrupted.
2. Laboratory and field personnel working with *Y pestis* organisms resistant to antimicrobics.
3. Persons engaged in aerosol experiments with *Y pestis.*
4. Persons engaged in field operations in plague-enzootic areas where prevention of exposure is not possible (such as some disaster areas).

Consider selective plague vaccination for:

1. Laboratory personnel regularly working with *Y pestis* or plague-infected rodents.
2. Workers (eg, Peace Corps volunteers, agricultural advisors) who reside in plague-enzootic or plague-epidemic rural areas where avoidance of rodents and fleas is impossible.
3. Persons whose vocation brings them into regular contact with wild rodents or rabbits in plague-enzootic areas.

Use of plague vaccine greatly increases the chances of recovery in those vaccinated individuals who may develop the insect-borne (bubonic) form of the infection. The degree of protection afforded against the pneumonic form is unknown; give adequate daily doses of a suitable antibiotic over 6 days to vaccinated persons exposed to the pneumonic form.

Contraindications:

Hypersensitivity to any of the product constituents; previous severe local or systemic reactions to plague vaccine injections; severe thrombocytopenia or any coagulation disorder that would contraindicate IM injections.

Warnings:

Severe febrile illness: Defer immunization until patients have recovered to avoid superimposing adverse effects of the vaccine on the underlying illness or to avoid mistakenly concluding that a manifestation of the underlying illness resulted from vaccination. Consult public health officials regarding the need for prophylaxis in these individuals. Do not postpone administration of plague vaccine to individuals with minor illnesses (eg, mild upper respiratory infections).

Hypersensitivity: Have epinephrine 1:1000 available to control immediate anaphylactic reactions. Refer to Management of Acute Hypersensitivity Reactions.

Pregnancy: Category C. It is not known whether plague vaccine can cause fetal harm when administered to a pregnant woman or can affect reproduction capacity. Give the vaccine to a pregnant woman only if clearly needed.

Children: Although clinical studies have not been conducted in children, the Immunization Practices Advisory Committee (ACIP) recommends the immunization of children who are at risk.

Precautions:

Concurrent vaccines: When practical, do not give plague vaccine on the same occasion as typhoid or cholera vaccines to avoid the possibility of accentuated side effects.

Repeated injections of plague vaccine may result in increasing reactivity of body tissues; therefore, the incidence and severity of reactions increases with the number of injections received.

(Continued on following page)

PLAGUE VACCINE (Cont.)

Adverse Reactions:

Adverse reactions are usually mild following primary immunization with plague vaccine and may occur more frequently and with more severity following repeated doses. The increased frequency and severity of adverse reactions following repeated doses appear to depend on the number of doses received, the method by which the doses are administered and the reactivity of the individual.

Local effects: Erythema and induration at the site of injection (≈ 10%, may occur more frequently following repeated injections); most local reactions subside within 2 days. Tenderness; edema; sterile abscesses (rare).

Systemic effects: Malaise, headache, lymphadenopathy, fever (≈ 10%; may occur more frequently following repeated doses); arthralgia; myalgia; leukocytosis; nausea; vomiting. Adverse systemic effects usually persist for only a few days. Sensitivity reactions, manifested by anaphylactic shock, tachycardia, urticaria, asthma or hypotension have occurred rarely.

Administration and Dosage:

Administer IM, preferably into the deltoid muscle. It may be used with the jet injector gun. Shake well before use.

Primary immunization: Administer a series of 2 to 3 IM injections, preferably in the deltoid. The series of 2 injections will produce adequate protection in the vast majority of persons who have never received the vaccine. Generally, plague antibody titers are increased by a third injection. Some patients not responding to the first 2 injections may produce an adequate response folowing the third injection.

Booster doses: Administer at 6 month intervals to individuals remaining in a known plague area. Approach the small dose as the total number of such injections increases. Booster doses at intervals > 6 months (eg, 1 to 2 years) may be appropriate for persons who have received ≥ 3 booster doses at 6 month intervals. In persons who have a history of serious reactions to the vaccine, determine passive hemagglutination titers in order to determine frequency of booster doses.

Recommended Doses of Plague Vaccine

Dose number	Age (years)			
	< 1	1-4	5-10	> 10
1	0.2 ml	0.4 ml	0.6 ml	1 ml
2 & 3[1]	0.04 ml	0.08 ml	0.12 ml	0.2 ml
Boosters[2]	0.02-0.04 ml	0.04-0.08 ml	0.06-0.12 ml	0.1-0.2 ml

[1] Give second dose 1 to 3 months after the first dose. Give third dose 3 to 6 months after the second dose.

[2] Give single booster doses at 6 month intervals.

CDC recommended vaccination schedules:[3]

Primary immunization – Administer all injections IM.

The primary series consists of 3 doses of vaccine. The first dose, 1 ml, is followed by the second dose, 0.2 ml, 4 weeks later. The third dose, 0.2 ml, is administered 5 months after the second dose.

Children (≤ 10 years old): The primary series is also 3 doses of vaccine, but the doses are less. The intervals between injections are the same as for adults.

Booster doses – When needed because of continuing exposure, give 2 booster doses, each 0.1 to 0.2 ml, at ≈ 6 month intervals. Thereafter, booster doses at 1 to 2 year intervals should provide good protection.

Storage: Store at 2° to 8°C (35° to 46°F). Do not freeze.

Rx	**Plague Vaccine** (Cutter, Miles)	**Injection:** 1.8 to 2.2 x 10^9 killed plague bacilli per ml	In 20 ml vials.[4]

[3] Morbidity and Mortality Weekly Report 1991 Nov 15;49(RR-12):41-2.

[4] With 0.5% phenol, 0.019% formaldehyde and trace amounts of beef heart extract, yeast extract, agar, and peptones and peptides of soya and casein.

TYPHOID VACCINE

Actions:

Typhoid vaccine is estimated to be > 70% effective in preventing typhoid fever, depending partly on the degree of exposure.

Oral: Typhoid vaccine live oral Ty21a is a live attenuated vaccine for oral administration. The vaccine contains the attenuated strain *Salmonella typhi* Ty21a. The vaccine strain is grown under controlled conditions and lyophilized. The lyophilized bacteria are filled into gelatin capsules which are coated with an organic solution to render them resistant to dissolution in stomach acid.

Parenteral: Typhoid vaccine for SC or intradermal use is a saline suspension containing not more than 1000 million *S typhi* (Ty-2 strain) organisms per ml. The vaccine strain is grown on veal infusion agar, the bacteria are washed off the medium, suspended in buffered sodium chloride injection and killed by a combination of phenol and heat.

Pharmacology: S typhi is the etiological agent of typhoid fever, an acute, febrile enteric disease. This vaccine will not afford protection against species of *Salmonella* other than *S typhi* or other bacteria that cause enteric disease.

There are approximately 500 cases of typhoid fever per year diagnosed in the US. In 62% of these patients (statistics from 1977 to 1979) the disease was acquired outside of the US while in 38% of the patients the disease was acquired within the US. Of the disease acquired in the US, 23% of the cases were associated with typhoid carriers, 24% were due to food outbreaks, 23% were associated with the ingestion of contaminated food or water, 6% due to household contact with an infected person and 4% following exposure to *S typhi* in a laboratory setting.

Virulent strains of *S typhi* upon ingestion are able to pass through the stomach acid barrier, colonize the intestinal tract, penetrate the lumen and enter the lymphatic system and blood stream, thereby causing disease.

The ability of *S typhi* to cause disease and to induce a protective immune response is dependent upon the bacteria possessing a complete lipopolysaccharide. The *S typhi* Ty21a vaccine strain is restricted in its ability to produce complete lipopolysaccharide. However, a sufficient quantity of complete lipopolysaccharide is synthesized to evoke a protective immune response.

At present, the precise mechanism(s) by which the oral vaccine confers protection against typhoid fever is unknown. However, it is known that immunization of adult subjects can elicit a humoral anti-*S typhi* LPS antibody response.

Clinical trials: Results from clinical studies indicate that adults and children > 6 years of age may be protected against typhoid fever following the oral ingestion of 4 doses of the vaccine. Immunization (ingestion of all 4 doses) should be completed at least 1 week prior to potential exposure to *S typhi*.

Parenterally administered typhoid vaccine is effective at reducing the incidence of disease in endemic areas. However, immunization with such vaccines is frequently accompanied by adverse reactions such as pain or swelling at the injection site, fever, malaise and headache. See Adverse Reactions.

Indications:

Parenteral: For active immunization against typhoid fever.

Oral: For immunization of adults and children > 6 years of age against disease caused by *S typhi*.

Routine immunization against typhoid fever is not recommended in the US. Selective immunization against typhoid fever is recommended under the following circumstances: 1) Expected intimate exposure to a household contact with typhoid fever, 2) travelers to areas of the world with a risk of exposure to typhoid fever, and 3) workers in microbiology laboratories with expected frequent contact with *S typhi*.

Although at one time typhoid immunization was suggested for persons attending rural summer camps or for residents of areas where flooding or other natural disasters have occurred, there are no data to support continuation of such practices.

Contraindications:

Hypersensitivity to any component of the vaccine or the enteric-coated capsule.

Safety of the vaccine has not been demonstrated in persons deficient in their ability to mount a humoral or cell-mediated immune response due to either a congenital or acquired immunodeficient state including treatment with immunosuppressive or antimitotic drugs. The vaccine should not be administered to these persons regardless of benefits.

Postpone administration in the presence of acute respiratory infection, acute febrile illness, acute GI illness, other active infection, or persistent diarrhea or vomiting.

(Continued on following page)

TYPHOID VACCINE

Warnings:

Pregnancy: Category C. It is not known whether typhoid vaccine can cause fetal harm when administered to pregnant women or can affect reproduction capacity. Give to a pregnant woman only if clearly needed.

Lactation: There are no data to warrant the use of the product in nursing mothers. It is not known if the vaccine is excreted in breast milk.

Children: Safety and efficacy have not been established for the oral vaccine in children $<$ 6 years of age and is therefore not recommended for use in this age group.

Precautions:

Not all recipients of typhoid vaccine will be fully protected against typhoid fever. Travelers should take all necessary precautions to avoid contact or ingestion of potentially contaminated food or water sources.

Oral typhoid vaccine will not afford protection against enteric microorganisms other than *S typhi.* An optimal booster dose has not yet been established. However, it is recommended that a booster dose consisting of 4 vaccine capsules taken on alternate days be given every 4 years under conditions of repeated or continued exposure to typhoid fever (see Administration and Dosage section).

Use a sterile syringe and needle for each patient to prevent transmission of hepatitis B virus and other infectious agents from one person to another.

Drug Interactions:

Sulfonamides and other **antibiotics:** The vaccine should not be administered to individuals receiving sulfonamides and antibiotics since these agents may be active against the vaccine strain and prevent a sufficient degree of multiplication to occur in order to induce a protective immune response.

Adverse Reactions:

Oral: Objectively monitored side effects did not occur at a statistically higher frequency in the vaccinated group as compared to a placebo group. Post-marketing surveillance outside of the US has found that side effects are infrequent, transient, and resolve of their own accord. Reported adverse reactions include: Nausea; abdominal cramps; vomiting; skin rash or urticaria on the trunk or extremities.

Parenteral: Most recipients of typhoid vaccine experience some degree of local and systemic response, usually beginning within 24 hours of administration and persisting for 1 or 2 days. Local reactions are usually manifested by erythema, induration, and tenderness and should be expected in all those injected intracutaneously.

Systemic manifestations may include: Malaise; headache; myalgia; elevated temperature.

Overdosage:

Oral: Five to eight doses of oral vaccine were administered to 155 healthy adult males. This dosage was, at a minimum, five-fold higher than the currently recommended dose. No significant reactions (eg, vomiting, acute abdominal distress, fever) were observed. At the recommended dosage, the *S typhi* Ty21a vaccine strain is not excreted in the feces. However, clinical studies in volunteers have shown that overdosing can increase the possibility of shedding the *S typhi* Ty21a vaccine strain in the feces.

Patient Information:

Oral: It is essential that all 4 doses of vaccine be taken at the prescribed alternate day interval to obtain a maximal protective immune response.

Vaccine potency is dependent upon storage under refrigeration (2°C to 8°C; 36°F to 46°F). Store the vaccine under refrigeration at all times. It is essential to replace unused vaccine in the refrigerator between doses.

Swallow the vaccine capsule approximately 1 hour before a meal with a cold or lukewarm drink, not to exceed body temperature (37°C; 98.6°F). Do not chew the vaccine capsule; swallow as soon as possible.

(Continued on following page)

TYPHOID VACCINE (Cont.)

Administration and Dosage:

Oral:

Primary immunization – One capsule on alternate days (eg, days 1, 3, 5 and 7), taken approximately 1 hour before a meal with a cold or lukewarm drink, not to exceed body temperature (37°C; 98.6°F). The vaccine capsule should not be chewed; swallow as soon after placing in the mouth as possible. A complete immunization schedule is the ingestion of 4 vaccine capsules as described above. Unless a complete immunization schedule is followed, an optimum immune response may not be achieved. Not all recipients will be fully protected against typhoid fever. Travelers should take all necessary precautions to avoid contact or ingestion of potentially contaminated food or water.

Booster dose: The optimum booster schedule has not been determined. Efficacy persists for at least 5 years. Further, there is no experience with oral vaccine as a booster in persons previously immunized with parenteral typhoid vaccine. Despite these limitations it is recommended that booster dose consisting of four vaccine capsules taken on alternate days be given every 5 years under conditions of repeated or continued exposure to typhoid fever.

Storage: The oral vaccine is not stable when exposed to ambient temperatures. Ship and store between 2°C and 8°C (36°F to 46°F). Each package of vaccine shows an expiration date. This expiration date is valid only if the product has been maintained at these temperatures.

Parenteral:

Primary immunization –

Adults and children (> 10 years old): Two doses of 0.5 ml each, administered SC at an interval of ≥ 4 weeks.

Children (< 10 years old): Two doses of 0.25 ml each, administered SC at an interval of ≥ 4 weeks.

In instances where there is insufficient time for two doses administered at the specified intervals, three doses of the appropriate volume may be given at weekly intervals.

Booster doses –

Adults and children (> 10 years old): 0.5 ml, administered SC, or 0.1 ml, injected intracutaneously (intradermally).

Children (6 months to 10 years old): 0.25 ml, administered SC, or 0.1 ml, intracutaneously (intradermally).

Under conditions of continued or repeated exposure, give a booster dose at least every 3 years. In instances where an interval of > 3 years has elapsed since primary immunization or the last booster dose, a single booster dose is considered sufficient; it is not necessary to repeat the primary immunizing series.

Rx	**Typhoid Vaccine** (Wyeth-Ayerst)	**Injection:** Suspension of killed Ty-2 strain of *S typhi* organisms. Provides 8 units/ml	In 5, 10 and 20 ml vials.[1]
Rx	**Vivotif Berna Vaccine** (Berna)	**Capsules, enteric coated:** 2 to 6 x 10^9 colony-forming units of viable *S typhi* Ty21a and 5 to 50 x 10^9 bacterial cells of non-viable *S typhi* Ty21a[2]	In a single foil blister containing 4 doses in a single package.

[1] With 0.5% phenol.

[2] With 26 to 130 mg sucrose, 1 to 5 mg ascorbic acid, 1.4 to 7 mg amino acid mixture, 100 to 180 mg lactose and 3.6 to 4.4 mg magnesium stearate.

PNEUMOCOCCAL VACCINE, POLYVALENT

Actions:

The 23-valent vaccine affords protection against the 23 most prevalent or invasive pneumococcal types, accounting for at least 90% of pneumococcal blood isolates and at least 85% of all pneumococcal isolates from sites which are generally sterile.

Because the polysaccharide capsules are immunogenic, they stimulate antipneumococcal antibody production and prevent pneumococcal disease. The vaccine will provide protection only against the capsular types of pneumococci contained in the vaccine.

Indications:

For immunization against pneumococcal pneumonia and bacteremia caused by the types of pneumococci included in the vaccine.

Adults:[1]

Immunocompetent adults who are at increased risk of pneumococcal disease or its complications because of chronic illnesses (eg, cardiovascular or pulmonary disease, diabetes mellitus, alcoholism, cirrhosis, or CSF leaks) or adults ≥ 65 years old.

Immunocompromised adults at increased risk of pneumococcal disease or its complications (eg, persons with splenic dysfunction or anatomic asplenia, Hodgkin's disease, lymphoma, multiple myeloma, chronic renal failure, nephrotic syndrome, or conditions such as organ transplantation associated with immunosuppression).

Asymptomatic or symptomatic HIV infection.

Children:[1]

Children ≥ 2 years old with chronic illnesses specifically associated with increased risk of pneumococcal disease or its complications (eg, anatomic or functional asplenia [including sickle cell disease], nephrotic syndrome, CSF leaks and conditions associated with immunosuppression).

Children ≥ 2 years old with asymptomatic or symptomatic HIV infection.

Prevention of pneumococcal otitis media in children ≥ 2 years old who are at risk of developing middle ear infections.

Note: The CDC states that recurrent upper respiratory diseases, including otitis media and sinusitis, are *not* considered indications for vaccine use in children.

Special groups: Persons living in special environments or social settings with an identified increased risk of pneumococcal disease or its complications (eg, certain native American populations).[1] Persons > 2 years old, as follows: (1) Closed groups (ie, residential schools, nursing homes, other institutions); (2) groups epidemiologically at risk in the community when there is a generalized outbreak due to a single pneumococcal type included in the vaccine; (3) patients at high risk of influenza complications, particularly pneumonia.

Contraindications:

Hypersensitivity to any component of the vaccine; previous immunization with any polyvalent pneumococcal vaccine. (See Adverse Reactions.)

Immunosuppressive therapy: Do not attempt immunization of patients < 10 days prior to or during treatment with immunosuppressive drugs or irradiation.

Hodgkin's disease patients immunized < 7 to 10 days prior to immunosuppressive therapy have postimmunization antibody levels below preimmunization levels.

These patients who have received extensive chemotherapy or nodal irradiation have an impaired antibody response to a 12-valent vaccine. Because, in some intensively treated patients, use of that vaccine depressed preexisting levels of antibody to some pneumococcal types, the 23-valent vaccine is not recommended for these patients.

Infections: Defer administration in the presence of acute respiratory or other active infections, except when withholding the agent entails even greater risk.

Warnings:

Hypersensitivity: Epinephrine 1:1000 must be available to control immediate allergic reactions. Refer to Management of Acute Hypersensitivity Reactions.

Limited effectiveness: The vaccine may not be effective in preventing infection resulting from basilar skull fracture or from external communication with CSF, or in patients with altered humoral immune responses due to agammaglobulinemia, multiple myeloma, lymphoproliferative diseases or immunosuppressive drugs. The vaccine may be less effective in splenectomized patients.

When elective splenectomy is considered, give pneumococcal vaccine at least 2 weeks before the operation, if possible. Similarly, when immunosuppressive therapy is planned, as in candidates for organ transplants, the interval between vaccination and initiation of immunosuppressive therapy should be as long as possible.

Although vaccine failures have occurred in some of these groups, especially those who are immunocompromised, vaccination is still recommended for such persons because they are at high risk of developing severe disease.

[1] *Morbidity and Mortality Weekly Report* 1989 (February 10);38(5):64-76.

(Warnings continued on following page)

PNEUMOCOCCAL VACCINE, POLYVALENT (Cont.)

Warnings (Cont.):

Pregnancy: Category C. Safety for use during pregnancy has not been established. Use only when clearly needed and when the potential benefits outweigh the potential hazards to the fetus. Ideally, vaccinate women at high risk before pregnancy.

Lactation: It is not known whether this drug is excreted in breast milk. Exercise caution when administering to a nursing woman.

Children: Not recommended for children < 2 years of age since they do not respond satisfactorily to the capsular types of the vaccine that are most often the cause of pneumococcal disease in this age group.

Certain groups at very high risk for pneumococcal disease (eg, sickle cell disease, nephrotic syndrome) may have lower peak levels of antibody response or more rapid rates of decline in antibody levels than do healthy adults. However, insufficient data are available to permit formulation of guidelines for reimmunization of high risk children.

Precautions:

History of pneumococcal pneumonia or other pneumococcal infection: Patients may have high levels of pre-existing pneumococcal antibodies which may result in increased reactions to this vaccine. These reactions are mostly local, but are occasionally systemic. Exercise caution if such patients are considered for vaccination.

Cardiac/pulmonary disease: Exercise caution when administering to individuals with severely compromised cardiac or pulmonary function in whom a systemic reaction would pose a significant risk.

Revaccination: Do not give a repeat (booster) injection of pneumococcal vaccine to previously vaccinated subjects. Arthus reactions and systemic reactions have been common among adults given second doses. Revaccination may result in more frequent and severe local reactions at the injection site, especially in persons who have retained high antibody titers. Such adverse reactions have occurred with booster doses given after long intervals from the initial vaccination. There is also evidence that booster doses do not result in increased antibody titers.

Without more information, persons who received the 14-valent pneumococcal vaccine should not be routinely revaccinated with the 23-valent vaccine, as increased coverage is modest and duration of protection is not well defined. However, strongly consider revaccination with the 23-valent vaccine for persons who received the 14-valent vaccine if they are at highest risk of fatal pneumococcal infection (eg, asplenic patients). Also consider revaccination for adults at highest risk who received the 23-valent vaccine ≥ 6 years before and for those shown to have rapid decline in pneumococcal antibody levels (eg, patients with nephrotic syndrome, renal failure, or transplant recipients). Consider revaccination after 3 to 5 years for children with nephrotic syndrome, asplenia, or sickle cell anemia who would be ≤ 10 years old at revaccination.

Antibiotic prophylaxis: In patients who require antibiotic prophylaxis against pneumococcal infection, do not discontinue prophylaxis after vaccination.

Concomitant use of influenza virus vaccine with this vaccine gives satisfactory antibody response without an increase in adverse reactions.

Adverse Reactions:

Local: Erythema, induration and soreness at the injection site (≈ 72%), usually of < 48 hours duration, occur within 2 to 3 days after vaccination.

Systemic: Low grade fever (< 37.7°C; 100°F) and mild myalgia occur occasionally, usually within 24 hours following vaccination. However, acute febrile reactions (> 38.8°C; 102°F), rash and arthralgia have occurred rarely.

Patients with otherwise stabilized idiopathic thrombocytopenic purpura have experienced a relapse, occurring 2 to 14 days after vaccination, and lasting up to 2 weeks.

Reactions of greater severity, duration or extent are unusual.

Neurological disorders such as paresthesias and acute radiculoneuropathy, including Guillain-Barré syndrome, have occurred rarely in temporal association with administration of pneumococcal vaccine. No cause and effect relationship has been established.

Anaphylactoid reactions have been rare (about 5 cases per million doses).

Administration and Dosage:

Give one 0.5 ml dose. Do not inject IV. Avoid intradermal administration. Administer SC or IM (preferably in the deltoid muscle or lateral mid-thigh).

Preparation and storage: Refrigerate at 2° to 8°C (36° to 46°F). Use the vaccine directly as supplied. No dilution or reconstitution is necessary. At room temperature, *Pnu-Imune 23* is stable for several days (temperature not exceeding 25°C; 77°F) and *Pneumovax 23* is stable for 1 month (temperature 15°C to 30°C; 59°F to 86°F).

Rx	**Pneumovax 23** (MSD)	**Injection:** 25 mcg each of 23 polysaccharide isolates per 0.5 ml dose	In 1 and 5 dose vials.[1]
Rx	**Pnu-Imune 23** (Lederle)		In 5 dose vials[2] and Lederject disp. syringes.[2]

[1] With 0.25% phenol. [2] With 0.01% thimerosal.

HEMOPHILUS b CONJUGATE VACCINE

Hemophilus influenzae type b (Hemophilus b; Hib) is a leading cause of serious systemic bacterial disease in the US. Most cases of *H influenzae* meningitis among children are caused by capsular strains of type b. In addition to bacterial meningitis, Hemophilus b is responsible for other invasive diseases, including epiglottitis, sepsis, septic arthritis, osteomyelitis, pericarditis and pneumonia.

Approximately 17% of all cases of Hib occur in infants < 6 months of age, 47% by 1 year of age and the remaining 53% over the next 4 years. Peak incidence occurs between 6 to 11 months of age. Incidence rates of Hib disease are increased in high-risk groups, such as daycare attendees, household contacts of cases, Caucasians who lack the G2m (n or 23) immunoglobulin allotype, Native Americans, blacks, individuals of lower socioeconomic status and patients with asplenia, sickle cell disease and antibody deficiency syndromes.

Actions:

The principal virulence factor is the capsular polysaccharide purified from *Hemophilus influenzae* type b, strain Eag, and is a polymer of ribose, ribitol and phosphate.

Diphtheria toxoid-conjugate and protein-conjugate are prepared from the purified capsular polysaccharide covalently bound to diphtheria toxoid (D) and diphtheria CRM_{197} protein, respectively. The meningococcal protein conjugate is prepared from the purified capsular polysaccharide covalently bound to an outer membrane complex (OMPC) of the B11 strain of *Neisseria meningitidis* serogroup B.

An antibody concentration of ≥ 0.15 mcg/ml is correlated with protection; in 3 week post-vaccination serum, antibody levels ≥ 1 mcg/ml were correlated with long-term protection.

The development of stable humoral immunity requires recognition of foreign material by at least two separate sets of lymphocytes: The B-lymphocytes, which are precursors of antibody-forming cells, and the T-lymphocytes, which can modulate B-cell function. Some antigens (ie, polysaccharides) stimulate B-cells directly to produce antibody (T-independent). Responses to many other antigens are augmented by helper T-lymphocytes (T-dependent). Hib conjugate vaccines use a new technology, covalent bonding of the capsular polysaccharide of *Hemophilus influenzae* type b to either diphtheria toxoid, diphtheria CRM_{197} protein or to an OMPC of *Neisseria meningitidis*, to produce an antigen which is postulated to convert the T-independent antigen into a T-dependent antigen. The protein carries both its own antigenic determinants and those of the covalently bound polysaccharide. Therefore, the polysaccharide is postulated to be presented as a T-dependent antigen resulting in both an enhanced antibody response and an immunologic memory.

Immunogenicity Studies of Conjugate Vaccines by Age

Parameter	*HibTITER*			*PedvaxHIB*				*ProHIBiT*	
	1-6 mos.[1] (n = 423)	7-14 mos.[2] (n = 432)	15-23 mos. (n = 377)	2-14 mos.[2] (n = 365)	15-17 mos. (n = 59)	18-23 mos. (n = 59)	24-71 mos. (n = 52)	15-17 mos. (n = 43)	18-23 mos. (n = 180)
% subjects responding with ≥ 1 mcg/ml	99.2	≈100	97.6	88-92	83	97	92	53	73
Geometric mean titer of PRP antibody (mcg/ml)	22.4	27.9-32.7	11.4	4.6-6	3.1	7.4	10.6	1.2	3.1

[1] Following 3 doses. [2] Following 2 doses.

Following immunization of 16- to 24-month-old children with a single dose of conjugate, 89% (109/123) had antibody levels ≥ 0.15 mcg/ml 12 months post-immunization, compared to 93% 1 month post-vaccination.

(Continued on following page)

HEMOPHILUS b CONJUGATE VACCINE (Cont.)

Indications:

For the routine immunization of children 2 months to 5 years of age *(HibTITER)*, 2 to 71 months of age *(PedvaxHIB)* and 18 months to 5 years of age *(ProHIBiT)* against invasive diseases caused by *H influenzae* type b. The duration of protection and need for booster doses have not yet been determined.

Administration may be considered for children as young as 15 months of age *(ProHIBiT)* when it is expected that the child will not return at 18 months for Hemophilus b immunization. However, the percentage of children at 15 months of age responding with > 1 mcg/ml may not be as high as in children ≥ 18 months of age (see table).

The Immunization Practices Advisory Committee (ACIP) recommends that all children receive one of the conjugate vaccines licensed for infant use beginning routinely at 2 months of age. The vaccine series may be initiated as early as age 6 weeks.

Children < 24 months of age who have had invasive Hib disease should still receive the vaccine, since many children of that age fail to develop adequate immunity following natural disease. The vaccine can be initiated (or continued) at the time of hospital discharge.

Chemoprophylaxis of household or daycare classroom contacts of children with Hib disease should be directed at both vaccinated and unvaccinated contacts because immune individuals may asymptomatically carry and transmit the organism.

Conjugate vaccines may be given simultaneously with diphtheria and tetanus toxoids and pertussis vaccine adsorbed (DPT); combined measles, mumps and rubella vaccine (MMR); oral poliovirus vaccine (OPV); or inactivated poliovirus vaccine (IPV).

Hemophilus b conjugate vaccines will not protect children against *H influenzae* other than type b or other microorganisms that cause meningitis or septic disease.

Contraindications:

Hypersensitivity to diphtheria toxoid or any component of the vaccine, including thimerosal.

Warnings:

The expected immune response may not be attained in persons deficient in producing antibody, whether due to genetic defect or to immunosuppressive therapy.

Any febrile illness or active infection is reason for delaying vaccine.

Pregnancy: Category C. It is not known whether these vaccines can cause fetal harm or affect reproduction capacity; they are NOT recommended for use in pregnant patients.

Children: ProHIBiT is not recommended for use in children < 15 months of age. *HibTITER* and *PedvaxHIB* are not recommended in children < 2 months of age; however, the ACIP states that the vaccine series may be initiated as early as age 6 weeks.

Precautions:

Hypersensitivity: Have epinephrine 1:1000 available for immediate use if an anaphylactoid reaction occurs. Refer to Management of Acute Hypersensitivity Reactions.

Hemophilus b disease may occur in the week after vaccination, prior to the onset of the protective effects of the vaccine.

Although some immune response to the diphtheria toxoid component of the conjugate vaccine may occur, it does not substitute for routine diphtheria immunization.

Drug Interactions:

Drug/Lab test interactions: Sensitive tests (eg, Latex Agglutination Kits) may detect PRP derived from the vaccine in urine of some vaccinees for up to 7 days following vaccination with *PedvaxHIB*.

Adverse Reactions:

Hemophilus b Vaccines Adverse Reactions		
Adverse reaction	< 24 hrs	> 24 hrs
Fever (> 38.3°C or 101°F)	1.1% to 3.8%[1]	1.5% to 2.1%
Erythema	1% to 3.3%	0.4% to 2.5%
Induration	1.5%	1% to 1.9%
Tenderness	3.7%	4.6%
Diarrhea/Vomiting	nd	< 1.2%
Crying	nd	< 1.2%

nd = no data reported [1] Higher in older children.

Other (causal relationship not established): Rash; hives; convulsions; early onset Hemophilus b disease; Guillain-Barré syndrome; irritability; sleepiness, respiratory infection/symptoms; ear infection/otitis media; thrombocytopenia (one case).

(Continued on following page)

HEMOPHILUS b CONJUGATE VACCINE (Cont.)

Administration and Dosage:

Administer IM doses in the outer aspect area of the vastus lateralis (mid-thigh) or deltoid. Do not inject IV.

Data are not available regarding the interchangeability of hemophilus b conjugate vaccines with regard to safety, immunogenicity or efficacy. Ideally, use the same conjugate vaccine throughout the entire vaccination series. However, situations will arise in which the vaccine provider does not know which vaccine was previously used. Under these circumstances, it is prudent for vaccine providers to ensure that, at a minimum, an infant 2 to 6 months of age receives a primary series of three doses of conjugate vaccine.

HibTITER: 2 to 6 months old – Three separate IM injections of 0.5 ml given at approximately 2 month intervals.

7 to 11 months old (previously unvaccinated) – Two separate IM injections of 0.5 ml given approximately 2 months apart.

12 to 14 months old (previously unvaccinated) – One IM injection.

All vaccinated children receive a single booster dose at ≥ 15 months of age, but not < 2 months after the previous dose. Previously unvaccinated children 15 to 60 months of age receive a single 0.5 ml IM injection in the mid-thigh or deltoid muscle.

PedvaxHIB: 2 to 14 months old – Two separate IM injections of 0.5 ml given at 2 months of age and 2 months later (or as soon as possible thereafter). When the primary two dose regimen is completed before 12 months of age, a 0.5 ml booster dose is required at 12 months of age but not earlier than 2 months after the second dose.

≥ 15 months old (previously unvaccinated) – Administer a single 0.5 ml IM injection.

Reconstitution – Use only the aluminum hydroxide diluent supplied.

ProHIBiT: 15 months to 5 years old – Administer a single 0.5 ml IM injection.

Vaccination Schedule for Hemophilus b Conjugate Vaccines

	HibTITER		*PedvaxHIB*		*ProHIBiT*	
Age at first dose (mos)	Primary series	Booster	Primary series	Booster	Primary series	Booster
2-6	3 doses, 2 months apart	15 mos.[1]	2 doses, 2 months apart	12 mos.[1]		
7-11	2 doses, 2 months apart	15 mos.[1]	2 doses, 2 months apart	15 mos.[1]		
12-14	1 dose	15 mos.[1]	1 dose	15 mos.[1]		
15-59	1 dose	—	1 dose	—	1 dose	—

[1] At least 2 months after previous dose.

Storage: HibTITER and *ProHIBiT* – Store at 2° to 8°C (36° to 46°F). Do not freeze.

PedvaxHIB – Before reconstitution, store at 2° to 8°C (36° to 46°F); store reconstituted vaccine at the same temperature and discard if not used within 24 hours. Do not freeze the reconstituted vaccine or the aluminum hydroxide diluent.

Rx	**HibTITER** (Lederle/Praxis Biologicals)	**Injection:** 10 mcg capsular oligosaccharide and ≈ 25 mcg diphtheria CRM_{197} protein per 0.5 ml dose.	In 1, 5 and 10 dose vials.[1]
Rx	**PedvaxHIB** (MSD)	**Powder for Injection:** 15 mcg purified capsular polysaccharide and 250 mcg *Neisseria meningitidis* OMPC per dose when reconstituted[2]	In single-dose vials with vial of aluminum hydroxide diluent.
Rx	**ProHIBiT** (Connaught)	**Injection:** 25 mcg purified capsular polysaccharide and 18 mcg conjugated diphtheria toxoid protein per 0.5 ml dose[3]	In 1, 5 and 10 dose vials.

[1] Multidose vials contain thimerosal 1:10,000.

[2] In 0.9% sodium chloride with 2 mg lactose and thimerosal 1:20,000.

[3] Dissolved in sodium phosphate buffered isotonic sodium chloride solution.

For information on recommended immunization schedules, refer to p. 2088

MEASLES (RUBEOLA) VIRUS VACCINE, LIVE, ATTENUATED

Actions:

Produces a modified measles infection in susceptible individuals. The vaccine is highly immunogenic and generally well tolerated. A single injection induces measles hemagglutination-inhibiting antibodies in 97% or more of susceptible persons. Vaccine-induced antibody levels persist for at least 8 years without substantial decline.

Indications:

Measles vaccine given immediately after exposure to natural measles may provide some protection. If given a few days before exposure, it provides substantial protection.

Children (≥ 15 months): Active immunization against measles (rubeola). A booster is not needed.

Strongly recommended for: Children living in schools, orphanages and similar institutions; malnourished children; those with inactive or active tuberculosis under treatment; those with chronic diseases such as cystic fibrosis, heart disease, asthma and other chronic pulmonary diseases.

Infants (< 15 months): May not respond to the vaccine due to the circulation of residual measles antibody of maternal origin; the younger the infant, the lower the likelihood of seroconversion. In populations for whom immunization programs are logistically difficult, and in population groups in which natural measles infection may occur in a significant proportion of infants before 15 months of age, it may be desirable to give the vaccine at an earlier age. Weigh the advantage of early protection against the chance for failure of response. Revaccinate infants after they reach 15 months of age.

Revaccination: Children vaccinated before 12 months of age (particularly if vaccine was administered with immune serum globulin [ISG] or measles immune globulin) should be revaccinated at about 15 months of age for optimal protection. There is no reason to routinely revaccinate children originally vaccinated when 12 months of age or older.

Despite the risk of local reactions (see Adverse Reactions), children who have previously been given inactivated vaccine alone or followed by live vaccine within 3 months, should be revaccinated with live vaccine to avoid the severe atypical form of natural measles that may occur.

Adults: Ordinarily, adults need not be immunized, since most are immune to measles. However, vaccination may be advisable for high school and college persons in epidemic situations and for adults in isolated communities where measles is not endemic.

Use with other live virus vaccines: Serologic evidence shows that when measles, mumps and rubella virus vaccine, live, containing the HPV-77 rubella strain, is given simultaneously with TOPV, expect antibody responses comparable to those which follow administration of the vaccines at different times. Therefore, when measles vaccine is given simultaneously with either monovalent or TOPV rubella virus vaccine, live or mumps virus vaccine, live, expect antibody responses comparable to those which follow administration of the vaccines at different times.

Contraindications:

Anaphylactic hypersensitivity to neomycin.

Infections: Defer administration in the presence of acute respiratory or other active infections or in active untreated tuberculosis.

Immune deficiency conditions: Patients receiving therapy with ACTH, corticosteroids (does not apply to patients receiving corticosteroids as replacement therapy, eg, for Addison's disease), irradiation, alkylating agents or antimetabolites; individuals with blood dyscrasias, leukemia, lymphomas or other malignant neoplasms affecting the bone marrow or lymphatic systems; primary immunodeficiency states, including cellular immune deficiencies, hypogammaglobulinemic and dysgammaglobulinemic states.

Note: If immediate protection against measles is required for persons in whom the vaccine is contraindicated, passive immunization with ISG is recommended. (See page 2063)

Warnings:

Do not give ISG concurrently with measles vaccination.

Usage in Pregnancy: Effects on fetal development are unknown; do not give to pregnant women. Avoid pregnancy for 3 months following vaccination.

Contracting natural measles during pregnancy enhances fetal risk. Increased rates of spontaneous abortion, stillbirth, congenital defects and prematurity have occurred. There are no adequate studies of measles virus vaccine in pregnancy. However, it is assumed that the vaccine strain of virus is also capable of inducing adverse fetal effects for up to 3 months following vaccination.

Advisory committees recommend vaccination of postpubertal females presumed to be susceptible to measles and not known to be pregnant. If measles exposure occurs during pregnancy, consider providing temporary passive immunity with ISG.

(Continued on following page)

MEASLES (RUBEOLA) VIRUS VACCINE, LIVE, ATTENUATED (Cont.)

Warnings (Cont.):

Usage in Children: Use caution in administering to children with a history of febrile convulsions, cerebral injury or other conditions in which stress due to fever should be avoided. Fever may occur following vaccination.

Precautions:

Hypersensitivity to eggs, chicken or chicken feathers: This vaccine is essentially devoid of potentially allergenic substances derived from host tissues (chick embryo). However, because it is propagated in cell cultures of chick embryo, there is a risk of hypersensitivity reactions in patients allergic to eggs, chicken or chicken feathers. When children with these known allergies were given a similarly prepared vaccine in a clinical study, none experienced related allergic reactions.

Have epinephrine 1:1000 available to control immediate allergic reactions. See also Management of Acute Hypersensitivity Reactions on p. 2897

Concomitant immunization: Do not give within one month of immunization with other live virus vaccines, with the exception of monovalent or trivalent polio vaccine, rubella vaccine or mumps vaccine, which may be administered simultaneously.

Defer vaccination for at least 3 months following blood or plasma transfusions, or administration of ISG.

Tuberculin skin test: Measles vaccine may temporarily depress tuberculin skin sensitivity. Administer the test before or simultaneously with the vaccine. Children under treatment for tuberculosis have not experienced exacerbation of the disease when immunized with measles vaccine.

Adverse Reactions:

Occasional: Moderate fever of 38.3° to 39.4°C (103°F) may occur during the month after vaccination. Generally, fever, rash, or both appear between the 5th and 12th days. Rash is usually minimal without generalized distribution.

Less common: High fever (over 39.4°C).

CNS: Children developing fever may rarely exhibit febrile convulsions. Significant CNS reactions (eg, encephalitis and encephalopathy) occurring within 30 days after vaccination have been associated with approximately one per every million vaccine doses. The risk following measles vaccine administration remains far less than that for encephalitis and encephalopathy with natural measles (1 per 1000 reported cases).

Isolated reports of ocular palsies and Guillain-Barre syndrome have occurred after immunization with vaccines containing live attenuated measles virus. The ocular palsies occurred approximately 3 to 24 days following vaccination. A causal relationship has not been established.

Subacute sclerosing panencephalitis (SSPE) has occurred in children who did not have a history of natural measles but received measles vaccine. The association of SSPE cases to measles vaccination is about one case per million doses, far less than that associated with natural measles, 5 to 10 cases per million.

Local: Because of the slightly acidic pH of the vaccine, patients may experience burning or stinging of short duration at injection site. Allergic reactions such as wheal and flare at the injection site or urticaria (rare) have been reported. Marked swelling, redness and vesiculation at the injection site have occurred in children previously vaccinated with killed measles.

Hematologic: Thrombocytopenia and purpura (extremely rare).

Administration and Dosage:

Inject the total volume of reconstituted vaccine SC, into the outer aspect of the upper arm. Do not inject IV. The dosage is the same for all patients. Each dose contains not less than 1000 $TCID_{50}$ (tissue culture infectious doses) of measles virus vaccine.

Use a sterile syringe free of preservatives, antiseptics and detergents for each injection, as these substances may inactivate the live virus vaccine. A 25-gauge, ⅝" needle is recommended.

Preparation and Storage: Store at 2° to 8°C (35° to 46°F). Protect from light. Use only the diluent supplied and reconstitute just before using. Store reconstituted vaccine in a dark place at 2° to 8°C. Discard if not used within 8 hours.

Rx	**Attenuvax** (MSD)	**Injection:** A more attenuated line of measles virus derived from Enders' attenuated Edmonston strain grown in cell cultures of chick embryo. In 1 and 10 dose vials[1].

[1] With 25 mcg neomycin.

For information on recommended immunization schedules, refer to p. 2088

RUBELLA VIRUS VACCINE, LIVE

Actions:

Antibody levels after immunization have persisted for at least 6 years without substantial decline. Expect more than 90% of vaccinees to have protection against both clinical rubella and asymptomatic viremia for at least 15 years. Vaccine-induced protection is expected to be life-long; therefore, vaccination is presumptive evidence of immunity.

Although vaccine-induced titers are generally lower than those stimulated by rubella infection, vaccine-induced immunity usually protects against both clinical illness and viremia after natural exposure.

Indications:

Persons can be considered immune to rubella only if they have documentation of:

1. Laboratory evidence of rubella immunity or
2. Adequate immunization with rubella vaccine on or after the first birthday.

The clinical diagnosis of rubella should not be considered in assessing immune status.

Children (12 months of age to puberty): For immunization against rubella. It is not recommended for infants less than one year old because persisting maternal antibodies may interfere with seroconversion. Children in kindergarten and the first grades of elementary school deserve priority for vaccination because often they are epidemiologically the major source of virus dissemination in the community.

When rubella vaccine is part of a combination that includes measles antigen, give the combination to children at 15 months of age or older to maximize measles seroconversion. Vaccinate promptly older children who have not received rubella vaccine.

Adolescent and adult males: Vaccination may be useful in preventing or controlling outbreaks of rubella in circumscribed population groups.

Nonpregnant adolescent and adult females: Vaccinating susceptible postpubertal females protects against subsequently acquiring rubella infection during pregnancy, which prevents infection of the fetus and consequent congenital rubella injury.

Subjects should not become pregnant within 3 months following vaccination. If a pregnant woman is inadvertently vaccinated or if she becomes pregnant within 3 months of vaccination, counsel her on the possible risks to the fetus.

Determine rubella susceptibility by serologic testing prior to immunization. If immune, as evidenced by a specific rubella antibody titer of 1:8 or greater (hemagglutination inhibition test), vaccination is unnecessary. Congenital malformations occur in up to 7% of all live births. Their chance appearance after vaccination could lead to misinterpretation of the cause, particularly if the prior rubella-immune status of vaccinees is unknown.

Pregnant women not known to be immune should be prenatally screened; vaccinate rubella-susceptible women in the immediate postpartum period.

Leukemia patients in remission whose chemotherapy has been terminated for at least 3 months may receive rubella vaccine. The exact interval after discontinuing immunosuppression that coincides with the ability to respond to individual vaccines is not known, but varies from 3 months to 1 year.

Protect persons without rubella immunity who travel abroad against rubella, since rubella is endemic and even epidemic, in many countries. No immunization or record of immunization is required for entry into the United States.

Revaccination: There is no reason to revaccinate children originally vaccinated when 12 months of age or older; however, revaccinate children vaccinated when younger than 12 months of age.

Previously unimmunized children of susceptible pregnant women should receive live attenuated rubella vaccine.

(Continued on following page)

RUBELLA VIRUS VACCINE, LIVE (Cont.)

Contraindications:

Hypersensitivity to neomycin. A history of dermatitis to neomycin is not a contraindication.

Infections: Defer administration in the presence of acute respiratory or other active infections. However, susceptible children with mild illnesses such as upper respiratory infection may be vaccinated.

Immune deficiency conditions: Patients receiving therapy with ACTH, corticosteroids (does not apply to patients receiving corticosteroids as replacement therapy, eg, for Addison's disease), irradiation, alkylating agents or antimetabolites; individuals with blood dyscrasias, leukemia, lymphomas or other malignant neoplasms affecting the bone marrow or lymphatic systems; primary immunodeficiency states, including cellular immune deficiencies, hypogammaglobulinemic and dysgammaglobulinemic states.

Short-term (less than 2 weeks) corticosteroid therapy, topical steroid therapy and intra-articular, bursal or tendon injection with corticosteroids should not be immunosuppressive and do not necessarily contraindicate live virus vaccine administration.

Pregnancy: Do not give to pregnant females. It is not known to what extent infection of the fetus with attenuated virus might occur following vaccination, or whether damage to the fetus could result. Avoid pregnancy for 3 months following vaccination.

The CDC has followed to term 214 known rubella-susceptible pregnant females who had been vaccinated with live vaccine within 3 months before or 3 months after conception. None of the 216 babies had malformations compatible with congenital rubella infection.

Maximum estimated theoretical risk of serious malformations attributable to rubella vaccine is 3%. The observed risk is zero. This risk is far less than the 20% or greater risk of congenital rubella syndrome associated with maternal infection during the first trimester of pregnancy.

Precautions:

Have epinephrine 1:1000 available to control immediate allergic reactions. See also Management of Acute Hypersensitivity Reactions

Inform postpubertal females of the frequent occurrence of self-limited arthralgia and possible arthritis beginning 2 to 4 weeks after vaccination.

Concomitant immunization: Do not give less than one month before or after immunization with other live virus vaccines, with the exception of monovalent or trivalent live poliovirus vaccine, live attenuated measles virus vaccine or live mumps virus vaccine, which may be administered simultaneously.

Postexposure vaccination: There is no evidence that giving live rubella virus vaccine after exposure will prevent illness or that vaccinating an individual incubating rubella or a child exposed to natural rubella is harmful. Consequently, vaccination is recommended unless otherwise contraindicated.

Blood transfusions/ISG: Defer vaccination for at least 3 months following blood or plasma transfusions or administration of human immune serum globulin (ISG). In addition, administer vaccine 2 weeks before receipt of ISG because passively acquired antibodies might interfere with response to the vaccine. Although studies have shown that rubella virus vaccine may be given in the immediate postpartum period to nonimmune women who have received anti-Rho (D) immune globulin (human) without interfering with vaccine effectiveness, perform 6 to 8 week postvaccination serologic testing on those who have received the globulin or blood products to assure seroconversion. Obtaining laboratory evidence of seroconversion in other vaccinees is not necessary.

Tuberculin skin test: Live attenuated rubella virus vaccine may temporarily depress tuberculin skin sensitivity. Administer a tuberculin test either before or simultaneously with rubella virus vaccine.

(Continued on following page)

RUBELLA VIRUS VACCINE, LIVE (Cont.)

Adverse Reactions:

Evaluate and report in detail all adverse effects following vaccination through local and state health officials to CDC and to the manufacturer.

Reactions are usually mild and transient; hypersensitivity reactions are very rare. Because the vaccine is slightly acidic, patients may experience burning or stinging of short duration at the injection site. Only susceptible vaccinees have reported side effects. There is no evidence of increased risk of these reactions for persons who are already immune when vaccinated. Symptoms similar to those seen following natural rubella may occur. These include regional lymphadenopathy, urticaria, rash, malaise, sore throat, fever, headache, polyneuritis, and occasionally, temporary arthralgia that is infrequently associated with inflammation. Local pain, induration and erythema may occur at the injection site. Moderate fever (38° to 39.4°C) occurs occasionally and high fever (> 39.4°C) occurs less commonly.

Arthritis/Arthralgia: Up to 40% of vaccinees in large-scale field trials have had joint pain, usually of the small peripheral joints, but frank arthritis has been reported for fewer than 2%. While up to 3% of susceptible childen have reported arthralgia, arthritis has rarely been reported. By contrast, up to 10% to 15% of susceptible female vaccinees have reported arthritis-like signs and symptoms. Transient peripheral neuritic complaints, such as paresthesias and pain in the arms and legs, are rare.

When joint symptoms or nonjoint-associated pain and paresthesias occur, they generally begin 3 to 25 days (mean 8 to 14 days) after immunization, persist for 1 to 11 days (mean 2 to 4 days) and rarely recur. Occasional reports of persistent or recurrent joint signs and symptoms probably represent a rare phenomenon. No joint destruction has been reported.

CNS effects: Encephalitis and other CNS reactions (rare). A causal relationship has not been established.

Hematologic: Decreases in platelet counts; thrombocytopenic purpura is a theoretical hazard.

Administration and Dosage:

Each dose contains not less than 1000 $TCID_{50}$ (tissue culture infectious doses) of rubella.

Inject total volume of reconstituted vaccine SC, into the outer aspect of the upper arm. Do not inject IV or administer intranasally.

Preparation and Storage: Prior to and after reconstitution, store at 2° to 8°C (35° to 46°F) and protect from light. To reconstitute, use only the diluent supplied. Use as soon as possible after reconstitution. Discard reconstituted vaccine if not used within 8 hours.

Ship vaccine at 10°C (50°F) or colder; it may be shipped on dry ice.

Rx	**Meruvax II** (MSD)	**Injection:** The Wistar Institute RA 27/3 strain of rubella virus, adapted to and propagated in human diploid cell (WI-38) culture. In single dose vials[1] in 1s and 10s.

[1] With 25 mcg neomycin.

For information on recommended immunization schedules, refer to p. 2088

MUMPS VIRUS VACCINE, LIVE

Do not use for delayed hypersensitivity (anergy) skin testing. Use Mumps Skin Test Antigen, a killed viral product (p. 2151).

Actions:

A single dose of this vaccine induced an effective antibody response in approximately 97% of susceptible children and 93% of susceptible adults. There are no reports of transmission of mumps from vaccinees to susceptible contacts.

Adequate antibody levels, with continuing protection of vaccinated children exposed to mumps, have persisted for 10 years without substantial decline.

The vaccine will not offer protection when given after exposure to natural mumps.

Indications:

Immunization against mumps in children 12 months of age or older and adults.

Revaccination: There is no reason to routinely revaccinate children originally vaccinated when 12 months of age or older.

Contraindications:

Not recommended for infants less than one year old because they may retain maternal mumps neutralizing antibodies which may interfere with the immune response.

Hypersensitivity to neomycin. A history of dermatitis to neomycin is not a contraindication.

Immune deficiency conditions: Individuals with blood dyscrasias, leukemia, lymphomas or other malignant neoplasms affecting the bone marrow or lymphatic systems; patients receiving therapy with ACTH, corticosteroids (does not apply to patients receiving corticosteroids as replacement therapy, eg, for Addison's disease), irradiation, alkylating agents or antimetabolites; primary immunodeficiency states, including cellular immune deficiencies, hypogammaglobulinemic and dysgammaglobulinemic states.

Infections: Defer administration in the presence of active infections.

Pregnancy: Do not give to pregnant women; the possible effects on fetal development are unknown. When vaccinating postpubertal women, rule out pregnancy and eliminate the possibility of pregnancy occurring in the 3 months following vaccination.

Precautions:

Hypersensitivity: Have epinephrine 1:1000 available to control immediate allergic reactions. See also Management of Acute Hypersensitivity Reactions

Allergies: This vaccine is essentially devoid of potentially allergenic substances derived from host tissues (chick embryo). However, since it is propagated in cell cultures of chick embryo, there is a potential risk of a hypersensitivity reaction in patients hypersensitive to eggs, chicken or chicken feathers. Widespread use has resulted in only rare reports of minor allergic reactions attributed to allergens of this kind.

Concomitant immunization: Do not give less than one month before or after immunization with other live virus vaccines, with the exception of live attenuated measles virus vaccine, live rubella virus vaccine or live oral monovalent or trivalent poliovirus vaccine, which may be administered simultaneously.

Defer vaccination for at least 3 months following blood or plasma transfusions, or administration of human immune serum globulin.

Tuberculin skin test: Live mumps virus vaccine may temporarily depress tuberculin skin sensitivity. Therefore, if a tuberculin test is to be done, administer either before or simultaneously with mumps vaccine.

Adverse Reactions:

Occasionally, mild fever. Fever above 39.4°C (103°F) is uncommon. Rarely, parotitis and orchitis. In most instances, prior exposure to natural mumps was established.

Purpura and allergic reactions such as wheal and flare at the injection site or urticaria (extremely rare).

CNS: Febrile seizures, unilateral nerve deafness and encephalitis have occurred rarely within 30 days of vaccination.

Administration and Dosage:

Each dose contains not less than 5000 $TCID_{50}$ of mumps virus vaccine.

Inject total volume of reconstituted vaccine SC, into the outer aspect of the upper arm. Do not inject IV. Use a sterile syringe free of preservatives, antiseptics and detergents. A 25-gauge ⅝" needle is recommended.

Preparation and storage: Prior to and after reconstitution, store at 2° to 8°C (35° to 46°F). Protect from light. To reconstitute, use only the diluent supplied and use as soon as possible after reconstitution. Discard within 8 hours.

Rx	**Mumpsvax** (MSD)	**Injection:** Prepared from the Jeryl Lynn (B Level) strain grown in cell cultures of chick embryo. In single dose vials[1] with vials of diluent.

[1] With 25 mcg neomycin.

For information on recommended immunization schedules, refer to p. 2088

RUBELLA AND MUMPS VIRUS VACCINE, LIVE

Consider the prescribing information for rubella virus vaccine (p. 2111 and for mumps virus vaccine (p.2114) when using this product.

Indications:

Children (12 months or older) and adults: Simultaneous immunization against rubella and mumps.

Infants (< 12 months of age): Not recommended. Infants may retain maternal rubella and mumps neutralizing antibodies which may interfere with the immune response.

Revaccination: There is no reason to routinely revaccinate children originally vaccinated when 12 months of age or older; however, children vaccinated when younger than 12 months of age should be revaccinated. Evaluate each case.

Administration and Dosage:

Inject the total volume of reconstituted vaccine SC, preferably into the outer aspect of the upper arm. Do not inject IV.

Each dose contains not less than 1000 $TCID_{50}$ (tissue culture infectious doses) of live rubella virus vaccine and 5000 $TCID_{50}$ of live mumps virus vaccine.

Preparation and storage: Prior to and after reconstitution, store at 2° to 8°C (35° to 46°F) and protect from light. To reconstitute, use only the diluent supplied. Use as soon as possible after reconstitution. Discard within 8 hours.

Rx	**Biavax II** (MSD)	**Injection:** Mixture of 2 viruses: (1) The Wistar RA 27/3 strain of rubella virus, propagated in human diploid cell (WI-38) culture; (2) The Jeryl Lynn (B Level) mumps strain grown in cell cultures of chick embryo. In single dose vials[1] with diluent.

MEASLES (RUBEOLA) AND RUBELLA VIRUS VACCINE, LIVE

Consider the prescribing information for measles (rubeola) virus vaccine (p.2109) and for rubella virus vaccine (p.2111) when using this product.

Indications:

Children (15 months or older) and adults: Simultaneous immunization against measles and rubella.

Infants (< 15 months of age) may fail to respond to one or both components of the vaccine due to residual measles or rubella antibody of maternal origin in the circulation; the younger the infant, the lower the likelihood of seroconversion.

In geographically isolated or other relatively inaccessible populations for whom immunization programs are logistically difficult, and in population groups in which natural measles infection may occur in a significant proportion of infants before 15 months of age, it may be desirable to give the vaccine to infants at an earlier age. Weigh the advantage of early protection against the chance for failure of response; revaccinate these infants after they reach 15 months of age.

Revaccination: There is no reason to routinely revaccinate children originally vaccinated when 12 months of age or older; however, children vaccinated when younger than 12 months of age should be revaccinated. Evaluate each case.

Administration and Dosage:

Each dose contains not less than 1000 $TCID_{50}$ (tissue culture infectious doses) of live attenuated measles virus vaccine and 1000 $TCID_{50}$ of live rubella virus vaccine.

Inject the total volume of reconstituted vaccine SC, preferably into the outer aspect of the upper arm. Do not inject IV.

Preparation and storage: Prior to and after reconstitution, store at 2° to 8°C (35° to 46°F). Protect from light. To reconstitute, use only the diluent supplied and use as soon as possible after reconstitution. Discard if not used within 8 hours.

Rx	**M-R-Vax II** (MSD)	**Injection:** Mixture of 2 viruses: (1) A more attenuated line of measles virus derived from Enders' attenuated Edmonston strain grown in cell cultures of chick embryo; (2) The Wistar RA 27/3 strain of rubella virus, propagated in human diploid cell (WI-38) culture. In single dose vials[1] with vial of diluent.

[1] With 25 mcg neomycin.

For information on recommended immunization schedules, refer to p. 2088

MEASLES, MUMPS AND RUBELLA VIRUS VACCINE, LIVE

Consider the prescribing information for measles virus vaccine (p.2109), mumps virus vaccine (p.2114) and rubella virus vaccine (p.2111) when using this product.

Indications:

Children (15 months or older) and adults: Simultaneous immunization against measles, mumps and rubella.

Infants (< 15 months of age): May fail to respond to one or all three components of the vaccine due to presence in the circulation of residual measles, mumps or rubella antibody of maternal origin; the younger the infant, the lower the likelihood of seroconversion.

In geographically isolated or other relatively inaccessible populations for whom immunization programs are logistically difficult, and in population groups in which natural measles infection may occur in a significant proportion of infants before 15 months of age, it may be desirable to give the vaccine to infants at an earlier age. Weigh the advantage of early protection against the chance for failure of response; revaccinate these infants after they reach 15 months of age.

Revaccination: There is no reason to routinely revaccinate children originally vaccinated when 12 months of age or older; however, children vaccinated when younger than 12 months of age should be revaccinated. Evaluate each case.

Administration and Dosage:

Each dose contains not less than 1000 $TCID_{50}$ (tissue culture infectious doses) of live attenuated measles virus vaccine; 5000 $TCID_{50}$ of live mumps virus vaccine; and 1000 $TCID_{50}$ of live rubella virus vaccine.

Inject the total volume of reconstituted vaccine SC, into the outer aspect of the upper arm. Do not inject IV.

Preparation and storage: Prior to and after reconstitution, store at 2° to 8°C (35° to 46°F) and protect from light. To reconstitute, use only the diluent supplied. Use as soon as possible after reconstitution. Discard within 8 hours.

Rx	**M-M-R II** (MSD)	**Injection:** Mixture of 3 viruses: (1) A more attenuated line of measles virus derived from Enders' attenuated Edmonston strain grown in cell cultures of chick embryo; (2) The Jeryl Lynn (B Level) mumps strain grown in cell cultures of chick embryo; (3) The Wistar RA 27/3 strain of rubella virus grown in human diploid cell (WI-38) culture. In single dose vials[1] with diluent.

[1] With 25 mcg neomycin.

For information on recommended immunization schedules, refer to p. 2088

POLIOVIRUS VACCINE, LIVE, ORAL, TRIVALENT (TOPV; Sabin)

Actions:

Attenuated, live virus vaccine produces an active immunity by simulating the natural infection without producing symptoms of the disease. To accomplish this with live poliovirus vaccine, the virus must multiply in the intestinal tract. A primary series of this vaccine is designed to produce an antibody response to poliovirus Types 1, 2 and 3 comparable to the immunity induced by the natural disease.

When used for primary immunization, type specific neutralizing antibodies will be induced in 90% or more of susceptible individuals.

Indications:

Prevention of poliomyelitis caused by Poliovirus Types 1, 2 and 3.

Infants from 6 to 12 weeks of age, all unimmunized children and adolescents through age 18 for routine prophylaxis.

Trivalent oral poliovirus vaccine (TOPV) and inactivated poliovirus vaccine (IPV) both prevent poliomyelitis. TOPV is the vaccine of choice for primary immunization of children in the United States because: It induces intestinal immunity; is simple to administer; is well accepted by patients; results in immunization of some contacts of vaccinated persons; has essentially eliminated disease associated with wild poliovirus in this country.

History of clinical poliomyelitis or prior vaccination with IPV in otherwise healthy individuals does not preclude the administration of TOPV when otherwise indicated.

Measles and rubella vaccines or combinations (measles-mumps-rubella vaccine) given simultaneously with TOPV produce adequate antibody response.

Adults: Routine poliomyelitis immunization for adults residing in the continental United States is not necessary because of extreme unlikelihood of exposure. However, primary immunization with IPV is recommended whenever feasible for unimmunized adults with increased risk of exposure, as by travel to or contact with epidemic or endemic areas, and for those employed in hospitals, medical laboratories, clinics or sanitation facilities. If less than 4 weeks are available before protection is needed, a single dose of TOPV is recommended, with IPV given later if the person remains at increased risk.

Contraindications:

Postpone or avoid the vaccine in the presence of persistent vomiting or diarrhea and in patients with any advanced debilitated condition.

Allergy to streptomycin or neomycin.

Infections: Defer administration in the presence of any acute illness.

Immune deficiency conditions: Do not administer in immune deficiency diseases such as combined immunodeficiency, hypogammaglobulinemia and agammaglobulinemia; also withhold the vaccine from siblings of a child known to have an immunodeficiency syndrome. Do not administer in altered immune states such as those occurring in thymic abnormalities, leukemia, lymphoma, or generalized malignancy or by lowered resistance from therapy with corticosteroids, alkylating drugs, antimetabolites, or radiation. Persons with altered immune status should avoid close household-type contact with recipients of the vaccine for at least 6 to 8 weeks. IPV is preferred for immunizing all persons in this setting.

Warnings:

Usage in Pregnancy: Safety for use during pregnancy has not been established. Use only when clearly needed and when the potential benefits outweigh the unknown hazards to the fetus. However, if immediate protection against poliomyelitis is needed, TOPV is recommended.

Precautions:

Other viruses (including poliovirus and other enterovirus) may interfere with the desired response to this vaccine, since their presence in the intestinal tract may interfere with the replication of the attenuated strains of poliovirus in the vaccine.

Do not administer TOPV shortly after Immune Serum Globulin (ISG) unless unavoidable, for example, with unexpected travel to or contact with epidemic areas or endemic areas. If TOPV is given with or shortly after ISG, the dose probably should be repeated after 3 months, if immunization is still indicated.

The vaccine will not modify or prevent cases of existing or incubating poliomyelitis.

(Continued on following page)

POLIOVIRUS VACCINE, LIVE, ORAL, TRIVALENT (TOPV; Sabin) (Cont.)

Adverse Reactions:

Vaccine-associated paralysis: Paralytic disease following ingestion of live poliovirus vaccines has been reported in individuals receiving the vaccine, and in persons who were in close contact with vaccinees. Most authorities believe that a causal relationship exists.

The Centers for Disease Control (CDC) reports that during the years 1969 through 1980 approximately 290 million doses of TOPV were distributed in the United States. In the same 12 years, 25 "vaccine-associated" and 55 "contact vaccine-associated" paralytic cases were reported. Twelve other "vaccine-associated" cases have been reported in persons (recipients or contacts) with immune deficiency conditions.

The risk of vaccine-associated paralysis is extremely small for vaccinees, susceptible family members and other close personal contacts; however, advise the vaccinee's parent, guardian or other responsible person of this possibility. When attenuated vaccine strains are introduced into a household with adults who have never been vaccinated or whose immune status cannot be determined, minimize risk by giving them 3 doses of IPV a month apart before the children receive TOPV.

Administration and Dosage:

Do not administer parenterally. Administer directly or mix with distilled water, tap water free of chlorine, simple syrup, USP, or milk. Alternatively, it may be adsorbed on any one of a number of foods such as bread, cake or cube sugar.

Community programs: TOPV has been recommended for epidemic control. Within an epidemic area, provide TOPV for all persons over 6 weeks of age who have not been completely immunized or whose immunization status is unknown, with the exceptions noted under immunodeficiency.

Dose: Each single dose consists of 0.5 ml.

Initial administration (primary series):

Infants – The primary series is 3 doses. The Immunization Practices Advisory Committee (Public Health Service) recommends that the series be started at 6 to 12 weeks of age, commonly with the first DTP inoculation. Give the second dose not less than 6 and preferably 8 weeks later. Administer the third dose 8 to 12 months after the second dose.

The American Academy of Pediatrics recommends that the vaccine be administered at 2 months, 4 months, and at approximately 18 months of age. An optional dose may be given at 6 months in areas where poliomyelitis is endemic.

Administration to the newborn (under 6 weeks) is not generally recommended because of the varying persistence of maternal antibodies. However, in certain tropical endemic areas, where poliomyelitis has been increasing in recent years, the physician may wish to administer TOPV to the infant at birth, and complete the basic course during the first 6 months of life. If immunizing the infant at birth, wait until the child is 3 days old; abstain from breast-feeding for 2 to 3 hours before and after TOPV to permit establishment of the vaccine viruses in the gut.

Older children and adolescents (through age 18) - Administer 2 doses not less than 6 and preferably 8 weeks apart and the third dose 6 to 12 months later.

Adults – See Indications and Adverse Reactions. When given to unimmunized adults, the dosage is as indicated for children and adolescents.

Booster doses:

School entrance – When entering elementary school, all children who have completed the primary series should receive a single follow-up dose of TOPV. All others should complete the primary series.

The Public Health Service Advisory Committee does not recommend routine booster doses of vaccine beyond that given when entering school.

Increased risk – If an individual who has completed a primary series is subjected to a substantially increased risk by virtue of contact, travel or occupation, a single dose of TOPV has been suggested.

Storage: Store vaccine at a temperature which will maintain ice continuously in a solid state. This vaccine may remain fluid at temperatures above – 14°C (+ 7°F) because of its sorbitol content. If frozen, thaw the vaccine prior to use. An unopened container of vaccine that has been frozen and then is thawed may be carried through a maximum of 10 freeze-thaw cycles, provided the temperature does not exceed 8°C (46°F) during the periods of thaw, and provided the total cumulative duration of thaw does not exceed 24 hours. If the 24 hour period is exceeded, use the vaccine within 30 days, during which time it must be stored at 2° to 8°C (35° to 46°F).

Rx	**Orimune** (Lederle)	**Oral Vaccine:** Mixture of 3 viruses (Types 1, 2 and 3) propagated in monkey kidney tissue culture. In 0.5 ml single dose Dispettes.[1] In 10s and 50s.

[1] Each dose contains sorbitol and less than 25 mcg each of streptomycin and neomycin.

POLIOVIRUS VACCINE, INACTIVATED (IPV)

Actions:

Pharmacology: Poliovirus vaccine, inactivated (IPV) is a sterile suspension of three types of poliovirus: Type 1 (Mahoney), Type 2 (MEF-1), and Type 3 (Saukett). The viruses are grown in cultures of VERO cells, a continuous line of monkey kidney cells *(IPOL)* or in human diploid cell cultures *(Poliovax)*, both by the microcarrier technique. This culture technique and improvements in purification, concentration and standardization of poliovirus antigen have resulted in a more potent and more consistently immunogenic vaccine than the poliovirus vaccine inactivated which was available in the US prior to 1988. These new methods allow for the production of vaccine that induces antibody responses in most children after administering fewer doses than with vaccine available prior to 1988. Studies in developed and developing countries with similar inactivated poliovirus vaccine produced by the same technology have shown that a direct relationship exists between the antigenic content of the vaccine, the frequency of seroconversion, and resulting antibody titer. Since the *Poliovax* vaccine will be available mainly as a backup to *IPOL*, this monograph will refer to prescribing information for *IPOL;* however, the prescribing information for *Poliovax* closely follows that of *IPOL*.

Clinical trials: Of 120 infants who received two doses of IPV at 2 and 4 months of age, detectable serum neutralizing antibody was induced after two doses of vaccine in 98.3% (Type 1), 100% (Type 2) and 97.5% (Type 3) of the children. In 83 children receiving three doses at 2, 4 and 12 months of age, detectable serum neutralizing antibodies were detected in 97.6% (Type 1) and 100% (Types 2 and 3) of the children. Paralytic polio has not been reported in association with administration of IPV.

Indications:

For active immunization of infants, children and adults for preventing poliomyelitis. Recommendations on the use of live and inactivated poliovirus vaccines are described in the ACIP Recommendations and the 1988 American Academy of Pediatrics Red Book.

Infants, children and adolescents: General recommendations – It is recommended that all infants, unimmunized children and adolescents not previously immunized be vaccinated routinely against paralytic poliomyelitis. IPV should be offered to individuals who have refused poliovirus vaccine live oral trivalent (OPV) or in whom OPV is contraindicated. Adequately inform parents of the risks and benefits of both inactivated and oral polio vaccines so that they can make an informed choice.

OPV should not be used in households with immunodeficient individuals because OPV is excreted in the stool by healthy vaccinees and can infect an immunocompromised household member, which may result in paralytic disease. In a household with an immunocompromised member, use only IPV for all those requiring poliovirus immunization.

Children incompletely immunized – Children of all ages should have their immunization status reviewed and be considered for supplemental immunization as follows for adults. Time intervals between doses longer than those recommended for routine primary immunization do not necessitate additional doses as long as a final total of four doses is reached (see Administration and Dosage).

Previous clinical poliomyelitis (usually due to only a single poliovirus type) or incomplete immunization with OPV are not contraindications to completing the primary series of immunization with IPV.

Adults: General recommendations – Routine primary poliovirus vaccination of adults (generally those ≥ 18 years of age) residing in the US is not recommended. Adults who have increased risk of exposure to either vaccine or wild poliovirus and have not been adequately immunized should receive polio vaccination in accordance with the schedule given in the Administration and Dosage section.

The following categories of adults run an increased risk of exposure to wild polioviruses:

1. Travelers to regions or countries where poliomyelitis is endemic or epidemic;
2. Health care workers in close contact with patients who may be excreting polioviruses;
3. Laboratory workers handling specimens that may contain polioviruses;
4. Members of communities or specific population groups with disease caused by wild polioviruses;
5. Incompletely vaccinated or unvaccinated adults in a household with (or other close contacts of) children given OPV provided that immunization of the child can be assured and not unduly delayed. Inform adult of the small OPV related risk to the contact.

(Indications continued on following page)

POLIOVIRUS VACCINE, INACTIVATED (IPV) (Cont.)

Indications (Cont.):

Immunodeficiency and altered immune status: Patients with recognized immunodeficiency are at a greater risk of developing paralysis when exposed to live poliovirus than persons with a normal immune system. Under no circumstances should OPV be used in such patients or introduced into a household where such a patient resides.

Use IPV in all patients with immunodeficiency diseases and members of such patients' households when vaccination of such persons is indicated. This includes patients with asymptomatic HIV infection, AIDS or AIDS-related complex, severe combined immunodeficiency, hypogammaglobulinemia or aggammaglobulinemia; altered immune states due to diseases such as leukemia, lymphoma or generalized malignancy; or an immune system compromised by treatment with corticosteroids, alkylating drugs, antimetabolites or radiation. Patients with an altered immune state may develop a protective response against paralytic poliomyelitis after IPV administration.

Contraindications:

Hypersensitivity to any component of the vaccine, including neomycin, streptomycin and polymyxin B (see Warnings).

Defer vaccination of persons with any acute, febrile illness until after recovery; however, minor illnesses such as mild upper respiratory infection, are not in themselves reasons for postponing vaccine administration.

Warnings:

Hypersensitivity reactions: Neomycin, streptomycin, and polymyxin B are used in producing this vaccine. Although purification procedures eliminate measurable amounts of these substances, traces may be present and allergic reactions may occur in persons sensitive to these substances. If anaphylaxis or anaphylactic shock occurs within 24 hours of administration of a dose, no further doses should be given. Epinephrine HCl (1:1000) and other appropriate agents should be available to control immediate allergic reactions. Refer to Management of Acute Hypersensitivity Reactions.

Pregnancy: Category C. It is not known whether IPV can cause fetal harm when administered to a pregnant woman or can affect reproduction capacity. Give to a pregnant woman only if clearly needed.

Children: Safety and efficacy of IPV have been shown in children > 6 weeks of age (see Administration and Dosage).

Precautions:

Patient review: Before injection of the vaccine, the physician should carefully review the recommendations for product use and the patient's medical history including possible hypersensitivities and side effects that may have occurred following previous doses of the vaccine.

HIV infection: Concerns have been raised that stimulation of the immune system of a patient with HIV infection by immunization with inactivated vaccines might cause deterioration in immunologic function. However, such effects have not been noted thus far among children with AIDS or among immunosuppressed individuals after immunizations with inactivated vaccines. The potential benefits of immunization of these children outweigh the undocumented risk of such adverse events.

Adverse Reactions:

In earlier studies with the vaccine grown in primary monkey kidney cells, transient local reactions at the site of injection have been observed. Erythema, induration and pain occurred in 3.2%, 1% and 13%, respectively, of vaccinees within 48 hours post-vaccination. Temperatures ≥ 39°C (≥ 102°F) were reported in up to 38% of vaccinees. Other symptoms noted included sleepiness, fussiness, crying, decreased appetite and spitting up of feedings. Because IPV was given in a different site but concurrently with Diphtheria and Tetanus Toxoids and Pertussis Vaccine Adsorbed (DTP), systemic reactions could not be attributed to a specific vaccine. However, these systemic reactions were comparable in frequency and severity to that reported for DTP given without IPV.

In another study using IPV in the US, there were no significant local or systemic reactions following injection of the vaccine. There were 7% (6/86), 12% (8/65) and 4% (2/45) of children with temperatures > 100.6°F, following the first, second and third doses, respectively. Most of the children received DTP at the same time as IPV and therefore it was not possible to attribute reactions to a particular vaccine; however, such reactions were not significantly different than when DTP is given alone.

(Adverse Reactions continued on following page)

POLIOVIRUS VACCINE, INACTIVATED (IPV) (Cont.)

Adverse Reactions (Cont.):

Although no causal relationship between IPV and Guillain-Barré Syndrome (GBS) has been established, GBS has been temporally related to administration of another IPV.

Note: The National Childhood Vaccine Injury Act of 1986 requires the keeping of certain records and the reporting of certain events occurring after the administration of vaccine, including the occurrence of any contraindicating reaction. Poliovirus vaccines are listed vaccines covered by this Act and health care providers should ensure that they comply with the terms thereof.

Administration and Dosage:

Administer SC; do not administer IV. In infants and small children, the mid-lateral aspect of the thigh is the preferred site. In adults, administer the vaccine in the deltoid area.

Take care to avoid administering the injection into or near blood vessels and nerves. After aspiration, if blood or any suspicious discoloration appears in the syringe, do not inject; discard contents and repeat procedures using a new dose of vaccine administered at a different site.

Children: Primary immunization – A primary series of IPV consists of three 0.5 ml doses administered SC. The interval between the first two doses should be at least 4 weeks, but preferably 8 weeks. The first two doses are usually administered with DTP immunization and are given at 2 and 4 months of age. The third dose should follow at least 6 months but preferably 12 months after the second dose. It may be desirable to administer this dose with MMR and other vaccines, but at a different site, in children 15 to 18 months of age. Give all children who received a primary series of IPV, or a combination of IPV and OPV, a booster dose of OPV or IPV before entering school, unless the first dose of the primary series was administered on or after the fourth birthday. The need to routinely administer additional doses is unknown at this time.

A final total of four doses is necessary to complete a series of primary and booster doses. Children and adolescents with a previously incomplete series of IPV should receive sufficient additional doses to reach this number.

Adults: Unvaccinated adults – For unvaccinated adults at increased risk of exposure to poliovirus, a primary series of IPV is recommended. While the responses of adults to primary series have not been studied, the recommended schedule for adults is two doses given at a 1 to 2 month interval and a third dose given 6 to 12 months later. If $<$ 3 months but $>$ 2 months are available before protection is needed, give 3 doses at least 1 month apart. Likewise, if only 1 or 2 months are available, give 2 doses of IPV at least 1 month apart. If $<$ 1 month is available, a single dose of either OPV or IPV is recommended.

Incompletely vaccinated adults – Adults who are at an increased risk of exposure to poliovirus and who have had at least one dose of OPV, $<$ 3 doses of conventional IPV or a combination of conventional IPV or OPV totalling $<$ 3 doses should receive at least 1 dose of OPV or IPV. Give additional doses to complete a primary series if time permits.

Completely vaccinated adults – Adults who are at an increased risk of exposure to poliovirus and who have previously completed a primary series with one or a combination of polio vaccines can be given a dose of either OPV or IPV.

Storage: The vaccine is stable if stored in the refrigerator between 2° and 8°C (35° and 46°F). The vaccine must not be frozen.

Rx	**IPOL** (Connaught)	**Injection:** Suspension of 3 types of poliovirus (Types 1, 2 and 3) grown in monkey kidney cell cultures	In 0.5 ml single-dose syringe with integrated needle.[1]
Rx	**Poliovax** (Connaught)	**Injection:** Mixture of 3 viruses (Types 1, 2 and 3) grown in human diploid cell cultures	In 0.5 ml single-dose amps.[2]

[1] Each dose contains 0.5% 2-phenoxyethanol, a maximum of 0.02% formaldehyde and not more than 200 ng streptomycin, 25 ng polymyxin B and 5 ng neomycin.

[2] With 27 ppm formaldehyde, 0.5% 2-phenoxyethanol and 0.5% albumin (human).

INFLUENZA VIRUS VACCINE

Actions:

Inoculation of antigens prepared from inactivated influenza virus stimulates the production of specific antibodies. Protection is afforded only against those strains from which the vaccine is prepared or against closely related strains.

An updated type A (H1N1) antigen will be a component of the influenza virus vaccines that will be used during the 1992-1993 influenza season, as well as the same A (H3N2) and B components that were used in the 1991-1992 vaccine. The antigens recommended by the FDA Vaccine Advisory Panel include A/Texas/36/91 (H1N1), A/Beijing/353/89 (H3N2) and B/Panama/45/90. Therefore, these strains will be included in the influenza virus vaccine for use during the 1992-1993 season. Remaining 1991-1992 vaccines should not be used for the 1992-1993 season. The vaccine is available as a "whole-virus," "split-virus" (subvirion) or "purified surface antigen" preparation. Having received a vaccination for the 1991-1992 flu season does not preclude the need to be revaccinated for the 1992-1993 season to provide optimal protection.

Indications:

For the production of immunity to influenza virus containing antigens related to those in the vaccine. Influenza vaccine is strongly recommended for any person ≥ 6 months of age who, because of age or underlying medical condition, is at increased risk for complications of influenza. Healthcare workers and others (including household members) in close contact with high-risk persons should also be vaccinated. In addition, influenza vaccine may be given to any person who wishes to reduce the chance of becoming infected with influenza. Guidelines for use of the vaccine in specific groups follow.

Groups at increased risk of influenza-related complications:

1. Persons ≥ 65 years of age.
2. Residents of nursing homes and other chronic-care facilities housing persons of any age with chronic medical conditions.
3. Adults and children with chronic disorders of the pulmonary or cardiovascular systems, including children with asthma.
4. Adults and children who have required regular medical follow-up or hospitalization during the preceding year because of chronic metabolic diseases (including diabetes mellitus), renal dysfunction, hemoglobinopathies or immunosuppression (including immunosuppression caused by medications).
5. Children and teenagers (6 months to 18 years of age) who are receiving long-term aspirin therapy and, therefore, may be at risk of developing Reye's syndrome after influenza.

Groups that can transmit influenza to high-risk persons: Persons who are clinically or subclinically infected and who attend or live with high-risk persons can transmit influenza virus to them. Some high-risk persons (eg, elderly, transplant recipients, persons with AIDS) can have low antibody responses to influenza vaccine. Efforts to protect these high-risk persons against influenza may be improved by reducing the chances of exposure to influenza from their care providers. Therefore, the following groups should be vaccinated:

1. Physicians, nurses and other personnel in both hospital and outpatient-care settings who have contact with high-risk persons in all age groups, including infants.
2. Employees of nursing homes and chronic-care facilities who have contact with patients or residents.
3. Providers of home care to high-risk persons (eg, visiting nurses, volunteer workers).
4. Household members (including children) of high-risk persons.

General population: Any individual wishing to reduce their chances of acquiring an influenza infection. Persons who provide essential community service (eg, police, fire department employees) and students or other persons in institutional settings may be considered for vaccination programs to minimize potential disruption of routine activities during outbreaks.

Persons infected with human immunodeficiency virus (HIV): Little information exists regarding the frequency and severity of influenza illness in HIV-infected persons, but recent reports suggest that symptoms may be prolonged and the risk of complications increased for this high-risk group. Because influenza may result in serious illness and complications, vaccination is a prudent precaution and will result in protective antibody levels in many recipients. However, the antibody response to vaccine may be low in persons with advanced HIV-related illnesses; a booster dose of vaccine has not improved the immune response for these individuals.

(Indications continued on following page)

INFLUENZA VIRUS VACCINE (Cont.)

Indications (Cont.):

Foreign travelers: The risk of exposure to influenza during foreign travel varies, depending on season and destination. In the tropics, influenza can occur throughout the year; in the southern hemisphere, the season of greatest activity is April through September. Because of the short incubation period for influenza, exposure to the virus during travel can result in clinical illness that also begins while traveling, an inconvenience or potential danger, especially for persons at increased risk for complications. Persons preparing to travel to the tropics at any time of year or to the southern hemisphere during April through September should review their influenza vaccination histories. If they were not vaccinated the previous fall/winter, they should consider influenza vaccination before travel. Persons in the high-risk categories should be especially encouraged to receive the most currently available vaccine. High-risk persons given the previous season's vaccine before travel should be revaccinated in the fall/winter with current vaccine.

Pregnancy: See Warnings.

Contraindications:

The use of products prepared from the embryonic fluid of chicken eggs is contraindicated in persons with a history of allergy to eggs or egg products. The vaccine is also contraindicated in individuals hypersensitive to any component of the vaccine.

In persons suspected of having an allergic condition, precede immunization procedures by a scratch test or an intradermal injection (0.05 to 0.1 ml) of vaccine diluted 1:100 in sterile saline to determine possible sensitivity to the minute residual egg protein that may be present in the vaccine. A positive skin reaction contraindicates immunization with the vaccine. See Warnings.

Defer immunization in the presence of acute respiratory disease or other active infection or acute febrile illness (see Warnings).

Warnings:

Hypersensitivity reactions: Have epinephrine 1:1000 immediately available. Refer to Management of Acute Hypersensitivity Reactions.

Immunosuppressed patients may experience a lower than expected antigenic response, although in one study, appropriate antibody responses occurred in patients with HIV who received trivalent influenza vaccine. Amantadine may be given to supplement the protection afforded by vaccination in high-risk patients.

Pregnancy: Category C. Pregnancy has not been demonstrated to be a risk factor for severe influenza infection, except in the largest pandemics of 1918-1919 and 1957-1958. However, vaccinate pregnant women with medical conditions that increase the risk of complications from influenza since influenza vaccine is considered safe for pregnant women without a specific severe egg allergy. To minimize any concern over the theoretical possibility of teratogenicity, give vaccine after the first trimester. However, it may be undesirable to delay vaccinating a pregnant woman who has a high-risk condition and will still be in the first trimester of pregnancy when influenza activity usually begins.

Precautions:

Concurrent vaccination: Because children are accessible when pediatric vaccines are administered, it may be desirable to administer influenza vaccine simultaneously with routine pediatric vaccine, but in a different site. Studies have not been done, but no diminution of immunogenicity or enhancement of adverse reactions is expected.

Pneumococcal vaccine and influenza vaccine can be given at the same time at different sites without increasing side effects. Note: Influenza vaccine is given annually; pneumococcal vaccine should be given only once.

High-risk children may receive influenza vaccine at the same time as measles-mumps-rubella, Hemophilus b, pneumococcal and oral polio vaccines, at different sites. Influenza vaccine should not be given within 3 days of vaccination with pertussis vaccine.

Febrile reaction: Because of the possibility of a febrile reaction following immunization, weigh the value of immunizing patients with a history of febrile convulsions. Persons with acute febrile illnesses usually should not be vaccinated until their temporary symptoms have abated. The likelihood of febrile convulsions is greater in children 6 months through 35 months of age. Minor illnesses with or without fever should not contraindicate the use of influenza vaccine, particularly among children with a mild upper respiratory tract infection or allergic rhinitis.

Sero-conversion: Vaccination may not result in sero-conversion in all individuals.

(Precautions continued on following page)

INFLUENZA VIRUS VACCINE (Cont.)

Precautions (Cont.):

Guillain-Barre syndrome (GBS), characterized by ascending paralysis, is usually self-limited and reversible. Although most persons recover without residual weakness, approximately 5% of cases are fatal. Before 1976, no association of GBS with influenza vaccination was recognized. However, that year, GBS appeared among persons who had received A/New Jersey/76 swine influenza vaccine. For the 10 weeks following vaccination, the risk was approximately ten cases of GBS for every million persons vaccinated – an incidence five to six times higher than that in unvaccinated persons. No significant excess risk of GBS was found for recipients of influenza vaccine during the influenza seasons 1978-1979 to 1980-1981. Subsequent vaccines have not been associated with an increased frequency of GBS. Nonetheless, advise persons who receive influenza vaccine of the possible risk as compared with the risk of influenza and its complications.

Other neurologic disorders, including encephalopathies, have been temporally associated with influenza vaccination.

Sulfite sensitivity: Sulfites may cause allergic-type reactions (eg, hives, itching, wheezing, anaphylaxis) in certain susceptible persons. Although the overall prevalence of sulfite sensitivity in the general population is probably low, it is seen more frequently in asthmatics or in atopic nonasthmatic persons. Although not detectable in the final product by current assay procedures, the manufacturing process for some formulations utilizes sodium bisulfite.

Drug Interactions:

Influenza Virus Vaccine Drug Interactions			
Precipitant drug	Object drug*		Description
Influenza virus vaccine	Phenytoin	↔	Although influenza vaccination reportedly inhibits the clearance of these agents, further studies have consistently failed to show any adverse effects of influenza vaccination among patients taking these drugs.
	Theophylline	↑	
	Warfarin	↑	

* ↑ = Object drug increased ↔ = Undetermined effect.

Adverse Reactions:

Side effects of influenza vaccine are generally inconsequential in adults and occur at low frequency. Severe reactions are uncommon in adults and disabling effects are exceedingly rare.

Local: Most frequent – Soreness at injection site for up to 1 or 2 days occurs in less than one-third of vaccinees.

Systemic: Two types: (1) Fever, malaise, myalgia and other symptoms of toxicity, although infrequent, occur more often in children and others who have had no exposure to the vaccine influenza virus antigen. These reactions, which begin 6 to 12 hours after vaccination and persist 1 to 2 days, are attributed to the influenza antigens (even though they are inactivated) and constitute most of the systemic side effects. (2) Immediate, presumably allergic, responses such as flare and wheal or various respiratory symptoms are extremely rare. They probably result from sensitivity to some vaccine component, most likely residual egg protein (see Contraindications).

Administration and Dosage:

Do not inject IV. Give injections IM, preferably in the deltoid muscle for adults and older children; for infants and young children, the preferred site is the anterolateral aspect of the thigh.

Vaccination schedules: Organized vaccination campaigns where high-risk persons are routinely accessible, such as in chronic-care facilities or worksites, may be optimally undertaken in November. Vaccination is desirable in September or October (1) if warranted by regional experience of earlier than normal epidemic activity (eg, in Alaska); or (2) for other persons recommended for vaccination who receive medical check-ups or treatment during September or October and who may not be seen again until after November. In addition, make arrangements to assure vaccination of hospitalized high-risk adults and children who are discharged between September and the time influenza activity begins to decline in their community; give vaccine as part of the discharge procedure.

Children < 9 years of age who have not been previously vaccinated require two doses of vaccine with at least 1 month between doses. Schedule programs for childhood influenza vaccination so the second dose can be given before December. Vaccine can be given to both children and adults up to and even after influenza virus activity is documented in a region, although temporary chemoprophylaxis may be indicated when influenza outbreaks are occurring.

(Administration and Dosage continued on following page)

INFLUENZA VIRUS VACCINE (Cont.)

Administration and Dosage (Cont.):

Vaccination schedules (cont.):

Influenza Vaccine Dosage Recommendations by Age Group			
Age	Product type†	Dosage (ml)	Number of Doses
≥ 12 years	whole-virus, split-virus or purified surface antigen	0.5	1
9-12 years	split-virus or purified surface antigen only	0.5	1
3-8 years	split-virus or purified surface antigen only	0.5	1 or 2††
6-35 months	split-virus or purified surface antigen only	0.25	1 or 2††

† Because of the lower potential for causing febrile reactions, use only split (subvirion) or purified surface antigen vaccine in children. Immunogenicity and side effects of split, whole and purified surface antigen virus vaccine are similar in adults when used as recommended.

†† ≥ 4 weeks between doses; both doses are recommended for maximum protection. However, if the individual received at least 1 dose of the 1978-1979 or later influenza vaccine, 1 dose is sufficient.

The only drug currently available for the specific prophylaxis and therapy of influenza virus infections is amantadine HCl (see individual monograph). Since it may not prevent actual infection, persons who take the drug may still develop immune responses that will protect them when exposed to antigenically-related viruses.

While amantadine chemoprophylaxis is effective against influenza A, it confers no protection against influenza B, and patient compliance could be a problem for continuous administration throughout epidemic periods, which generally last 6 to 12 weeks. *Under most circumstances do not use in lieu of vaccination.*

Consider amantadine for therapeutic use, particularly for persons in the high-risk groups if they develop an illness compatible with influenza during a period of known or suspected influenza A activity in the community.

Storage: Store between 2° to 8°C (36° to 46°F). Freezing destroys potency.

Rx	**Influenza Virus Vaccine, Trivalent, Types A & B** (Wyeth-Ayerst)	**Injection (Split-Virus):** 15 mcg A/Texas/36/91 (H1N1), 15 mcg A/Beijing/353/89 (H3N2) and 15 mcg B/Panama/45/90 hemagglutinin antigens per 0.5 ml	In 5 ml vials and 0.5 ml Tubex.
Rx	**Fluogen** (Parke-Davis)		In 5 ml Steri-Vials[1,2] and 0.5 ml Steri-Dose disp. syringes.[1,2]
Rx	**Fluzone** (Connaught)		In 5 ml vials[1] and 0.5 ml syringes.[1]
Rx	**Fluzone** (Connaught)	**Injection (Whole-Virus):** 15 mcg A/Texas/36/91 (H1N1), 15 mcg A/Beijing/353/89 (H3N2) and 15 mcg B/Panama/45/90 hemagglutinin antigens per 0.5 ml[1]	In 5 ml vials.
Rx	**Flu-Imune** (Lederle)	**Injection (Purified Surface Antigen):** 15 mcg A/Texas/36/91 (H1N1), 15 mcg A/Beijing/353/89 (H3N2) and 15 mcg B/Panama/45/90 hemagglutinin antigens per 0.5 ml[1]	In 5 ml vials.

[1] With 0.01% thimerosal.

[2] With sodium bisulfite.

YELLOW FEVER VACCINE

This vaccine is a live, attenuated virus preparation.

Indications:

For active immunization of all travelers 6 months of age or older planning a trip to countries which require a certificate of vaccination against yellow fever. Recommended for persons living in areas where yellow fever infection occurs. Do not vaccinate children under 6 months of age unless they live in or are traveling to a high risk area.

Immunity develops by the tenth day and the World Health Organization (WHO) requires revaccination every 10 years to maintain travelers' vaccination certificates. United States vaccination certificates are valid for 10 years, beginning 10 days after initial vaccination or revaccination.

Vaccinate laboratory personnel who might be exposed to virulent yellow fever virus.

Contraindications:

Sensitivity to egg or chick embryo protein.

Do not vaccinate pregnant women and children under 6 months of age, except in high risk areas.

Warnings:

Yellow fever vaccine virus infection might be potentiated by severe underlying diseases, such as leukemia, lymphoma or generalized malignancy; immunosuppressed patients, such as from therapy with steroids, alkylating drugs, antimetabolites, cytotoxic agents or radiation; or gamma globulin deficiency. Evaluate administration in such conditions individually.

Pregnancy: Category C. Safety for use during pregnancy has not been established. Use only when clearly needed and when the potential benefits outweigh the potential hazards to the fetus.

Precautions:

Hypersensitivity: Yellow fever vaccine is produced in chick embryos; do not administer to individuals hypersensitive to egg or chicken protein. Perform intradermal skin tests with the vaccine and sterile normal saline as a control on all such individuals. Inject 0.02 to 0.03 ml into the volar surface of the forearm. This should raise a noticeable intradermal wheal at each test site.

A positive sensitivity test consists of an urticarial wheal, with or without pseudopods, surrounded by an area of erythema and no response to the control. A positive reaction contraindicates vaccine administration. Have epinephrine 1:1000 and a tourniquet available while performing the sensitivity test.

An intracutaneous dose of 0.02 ml administered for hypersensitivity testing may induce immunity. However, in such individuals, the presence of specific protective antibodies must be confirmed through evaluation of serum obtained approximately 4 weeks after skin testing. Contact the state or public health laboratory for assistance.

Immediate hypersensitivity reactions characterized by rash, urticaria or asthma are very rare ($< 1/1,000,000$) and occur principally in persons with histories of egg allergy. Have epinephrine 1:1000 available. Refer to Management of Acute Hypersensitivity Reactions.

Concurrent vaccine administration: Administer Yellow Fever Vaccine at least 1 month apart from other live virus vaccines. However, administration of the most widely used live virus vaccines has not impaired antibody response or increased adverse reactions.

Defer vaccination with Yellow Fever Vaccine for 8 weeks following blood or plasma transfusion or administration of human immune globulin.

Adverse Reactions:

Frequent: Fever or malaise, usually appearing 7 to 14 days after administration (10%); treatment is symptomatic. Myalgia and headache (2% to 5%). Fewer than 0.2% curtail regular activities.

Rare: Encephalitis has developed in very young infants; only two cases have been reported in the US. One death has been reported.

Anaphylaxis may occur, even in individuals with no history of hypersensitivity to any vaccine component (see Precautions).

(Continued on following page)

YELLOW FEVER VACCINE (Cont.)

Administration and Dosage:

Adults and children: Administer a single immunizing dose of 0.5 ml SC.

Preparation of solution for needle injection: Reconstitute the vaccine using only the diluent supplied. The vaccine is slightly opalescent and light orange after reconstitution. Draw the volume of the diluent, shown on the diluent label, into a suitable size syringe and inject into the vial containing the vaccine. Slowly add diluent to vaccine, let set for 1 to 2 minutes and then carefully swirl mixture until suspension is uniform. Avoid vigorous shaking as it tends to cause foaming of the suspension. Use vaccine within 60 minutes of reconstitution.

Storage: Yellow Fever Vaccine is shipped in a container with dry ice; do not use vaccine unless shipping case contains some dry ice on arrival. Maintain vaccine continuously at a temperature between 0° to 5°C (32° to 41°F).

Stability: The following information is provided for areas of the world where an adequate cold chain is a problem and inadvertent exposure to abnormal temperatures has occurred.

Temperature (°C)	Test	Number of Lots Tested	Computed Half-Life (Days)
35°-37°	Mouse Assay	3	14
35°-37°	Vero Cell Assay	3	13.9
45°-47°	Mouse Assay	3	3.3
45°-47°	Vero Cell Assay	3	4.5

Sterilize and discard all unused rehydrated vaccine and containers after 1 hour.

Rx	**YF-Vax**[1] (Connaught)	**Injection:** Not less than 5.04 Log_{10} Plaque Forming Units (PFU) per 0.5 ml dose when reconstituted. Prepared by culturing the 17D strain virus in living chick embryo.[2] In 1 and 5 dose vials with diluent.

[1] Supplied only to designated Yellow Fever Vaccination Centers authorized to issue certificates of Yellow Fever Vaccination.

[2] With gelatin and sorbitol.

HEPATITIS B VACCINE

Actions:

Hepatitis B vaccine, plasma-derived *(Heptavax-B)*, consists of biochemically and biophysically inactivated human hepatitis B surface antigen (HBsAg) particles, obtained by plasmapheresis from plasma of screened healthy chronic HBsAG carriers. The recombinant vaccines *(Recombivax HB, Engerix-B)* are derived from HBsAg produced in yeast cells.

Clinical Pharmacology: Hepatitis B vaccine induces protective anti-HBs in most individuals receiving the recommended three dose regimen. Responsiveness is age-dependent; children respond more vigorously than adults. Immunocompromised and immunosuppressed persons do not respond as well as healthy individuals. Antibody titers $\geq$ 10 mIU/ml against HBsAg are recognized as conferring protection against hepatitis B. Seroconversion is defined as antibody titers $\geq$ 1 mIU/ml. Duration of protective effect is unknown. Anti-HBs levels may fall below 10 sample ratio units (protective level) over 3 to 4 years. Periodically determine anti-HBs level.

Hepatitis B vaccine was 80% to 95% effective in preventing acute hepatitis B, asymptomatic infection and antigenemia. Immunity (defined by predetermined serum titers of antibody which prevented hepatitis B infection) was obtained in 87% of vaccinated subjects after two doses; however, a third dose was needed in 96% of the population.

Follow-up data from clinical trials provide no evidence to suggest transmission of Acquired Immune Deficiency Syndrome (AIDS) by this vaccine. *Recombivax HB* and *Engerix-B* are prepared from recombinant yeast cultures and are free of association with human blood or blood products.

The recombinant vaccines, injected into the deltoid, induced protective antibody levels in 93% to 99% of healthy adults, adolescents, children and neonates who received the recommended regimen; in adults $\geq$ 40 years of age, the protective level is lower (88% to 89%). Studies with the plasma-derived vaccine show that a lower response rate (81%) may occur if the vaccine is administered as a buttock injection.

Revaccination (booster doses)[1]*:* The following recommendations from the Immunization Practices Advisory Committee of the Centers for Disease Control for booster doses are based on studies using the plasma-derived vaccine.

Adults and children with normal immune status: The antibody response to properly administered vaccine is excellent, and protection lasts for at least 5 years. Booster doses are not routinely recommended, nor is routine serologic testing to assess antibody levels in vaccine recipients necessary during this period.

Hemodialysis patients: The vaccine-induced protection is less complete and may persist only as long as antibody levels remain above 10 mIU/ml. Assess the need for booster doses by semiannual antibody testing; give booster doses when antibody levels are $<$ 10 mIU/ml.

Vaccinated persons who experience percutaneous or needle exposure to HBsAg positive blood: Serologic testing to assess immune status is recommended unless testing within the previous 12 months has indicated adequate antibody levels. If inadequate levels exist, treatment with HBIG or a booster dose of vaccine is indicated.

Nonrepsonders: Revaccination of persons who do not respond to the primary series produces adequate antibody in only one-third when the primary vaccination has been given in the deltoid. Therefore, revaccination of nonresponders to deltoid injection is not recommended. For persons who did not respond to a primary vaccine series given in the buttock, two small studies suggest that revaccination in the arm induces adequate antibody in over 75%. Strongly consider revaccination for such persons.

Postexposure prophylaxis: Hepatitis B Immune Globulin (HBIG), administered with hepatitis B vaccine at separate sites, does not interfere with induction of protective antibodies against hepatitis B virus.

Interchangeability with hepatitis B vaccines: It is possible to interchange the use of recombinant and plasma-derived vaccines, since in vitro and in vivo studies indicate the antibody produced in response to each type of vaccine is comparable. (However, see Contraindications.) Also, *Engerix-B* can be used to complete a vaccination course initiated with *Recombivax HB*.

[1] Morbidity and Mortality Weekly Report 1987 (June 19);36:353-366.

(Continued on following page)

HEPATITIS B VACCINE (Cont.)

Indications:

For immunization against infection caused by all known subtypes of hepatitis B virus.

Vaccination is recommended in persons of all ages, especially in those at increased risk of infection with hepatitis B virus.

Health care personnel: Dentists; oral surgeons, physicians; surgeons; nurses; paramedical personnel and custodial staff who may be exposed via blood or patient specimens; dental hygienists and nurses; blood bank and plasma fractionation workers; laboratory personnel handling blood, its products and patient specimens; dental, medical and nursing students.

Selected patients and patient contacts: Patients and staff in hemodialysis units and hematology/oncology units; patients requiring frequent or large volume blood transfusions or clotting factor concentrates (eg, persons with hemophilia, thalassemia); residents and staff of institutions for the mentally handicapped; classroom contacts of deinstitutionalized mentally handicapped persons who have persistent hepatitis B antigenemia and who show aggressive behavior; household and other intimate contacts of persons with persistent hepatitis B antigenemia.

Infants born to HBsAg-positive mothers: Immune globulin and hepatitis B vaccine are relatively effective in infants born to HBsAg-positive, HBeAg-positive mothers, following accidental percutaneous or permucosal exposure to HBsAg-positive blood or sexual exposure to HBsAg-positive persons.

Populations with high incidence of the disease: Alaskan Eskimos; Indochinese refugees; Haitian refugees.

Persons at increased risk due to their sexual practices (ie, persons who repeatedly contract sexually transmitted diseases; homosexually active males; prostitutes; persons with multiple sexual partners).

Others: Military personnel identified as being at increased risk; morticians and embalmers; prisoners; users of illicit injectable drugs; police and fire department personnel who render first aid or medical assistance.

Contraindications:

Hypersensitivity to yeast or any component of the vaccines.

Warnings:

Acute hypersensitivity reaction: Have epinephrine 1:1000 immediately available. Refer to Management of Acute Hypersensitivity Reactions on p. 2897

Immunosuppressed patients may require larger vaccine doses and may not respond as well as healthy individuals. Refer to Administration and Dosage.

Unrecognized hepatitis B infection may be present at the time the vaccine is given, and the vaccine may not prevent hepatitis B in such patients because of the long incubation period.

Pregnancy: Category C. Safety for use during pregnancy has not been established. Use only when clearly needed and when the potential benefits outweigh potential hazards to the fetus.

Lactation: Safety for use in the nursing mother has not been established.

Children: Hepatitis B vaccine is well tolerated and highly immunogenic in infants and children of all ages. Newborns also respond well; maternally transferred antibodies do not interfere with the active immune response to the vaccine.

Precautions:

Infection: Serious active infection is reason to delay use of hepatitis B vaccine, except when withholding the vaccine entails a greater risk.

Cautiously administer to individuals with severely compromised cardiopulmonary status or when a febrile or systemic reaction could be a significant risk.

Adverse Reactions:

Local: Injection site soreness (≈ 50% with plasma-derived vaccine); erythema; swelling; warmth; induration; pain; tenderness; pruritus; ecchymosis; nodule formation.

GI: Nausea; vomiting; abdominal pain/cramps; dyspepsia; diminished appetite; anorexia; diarrhea; abnormal liver function tests.

CNS: Headache; lightheadedness; vertigo; dizziness; paresthesia; insomnia; disturbed sleep; somnolence; irritability; agitation; migraine; syncope; paresis; neuropathy including hypoesthesia, Guillain-Barré syndrome and Bell's palsy; transverse myelitis.

Respiratory: Pharyngitis; upper respiratory infection; rhinitis; influenza-like symptoms; cough; bronchospasm.

Musculoskeletal: Arthralgia; myalgia; back, neck and shoulder pain; neck stiffness.

Dermatologic: Pruritus; rash (nonspecified); angioedema; urticaria; petechiae; erythema; eczema; purpura; herpes zoster.

(Adverse Reactions continued on following page)

HEPATITIS B VACCINE (Cont.)

Adverse Reactions (Cont.):

Body as a Whole: Fatigue/weakness; fever (≥ 100°F); malaise; sweating; achiness; sensation of warmth; chills; flushing; irritability; tingling.

Other: Lymphadenopathy; earache; hypotension; dysuria; tachycardia/palpitations; thrombocytopenia; conjunctivitis; keratitis; visual disturbances.

In addition, the following were reported with the plasma-derived vaccine *(Heptavax-B)*:

Hypersensitivity – Symptoms of immediate hypersensitivity (urticaria, angioedema, pruritus) are rare within the first few hours after vaccination. A hypersensitivity syndrome of delayed onset has occurred rarely, days to weeks after vaccination. This has included arthritis (usually transient), fever and dermatologic reactions (urticaria, erythema multiforme or ecchymoses).

CNS – Optic neuritis; myelitis, including transverse myelitis; herpes zoster.

Other – Tinnitus; visual disturbances; thrombocytopenia.

Administration and Dosage:

For IM use. The deltoid muscle is the preferred site in adults. Injections given in the buttocks frequently are given into fatty tissue instead of into muscle and have resulted in a lower seroconversion rate than expected. The anterolateral thigh is the recommended site in infants and young children. May be given SC to persons at risk of hemorrhage following IM injection (eg, hemophiliacs). The immune responses and clinical reactions following IM and SC use are comparable. However, an increased incidence of local reactions, including subcutaneous nodules, may occur.

Immunization Regimen of 3 IM Hepatitis B Vaccine Doses

Age Group	Initial			1 month			6 months		
	Recombivax HB	Heptavax-B	Engerix-B	Recombivax HB	Heptavax-B	Engerix-B	Recombivax HB	Heptavax-B	Engerix-B
Birth[1] through 10 years	0.25 ml	0.5 ml	0.5 ml	0.25 ml	0.5 ml	0.5 ml	0.25 ml	0.5 ml	0.5 ml
11 to 19 years	0.5 ml	1 ml	1 ml	0.5 ml	1 ml	1 ml	0.5 ml	1 ml	1 ml
≥ 20 years	1 ml	1 ml	1 ml	1 ml	1 ml	1 ml	1 ml	1 ml	1 ml
Dialysis or Immunocompromised Patients		2 ml[2]	2 ml[2]		2 ml[2]	2 ml[3]		2 ml[2]	2 ml[2]

[1] Infants born of HBsAg negative mothers. [2] Two 1 ml doses given at different sites.
[3] Two 1 ml doses given at different sites, plus an additional dose at 2 months.

Alternate schedule (Engerix-B): Designed for certain populations (eg, neonates born of hepatitis B infected mothers, others who have or might have been recently exposed to the virus, certain travelers to high-risk areas).

Alternate Dosing Schedule for Engerix-B

Age Group	Initial	1 month	2 months	12 months
Birth-10 yrs	0.5 ml	0.5 ml	0.5 ml	0.5 ml[1]
Children > 10 yrs and Adults	1 ml	1 ml	1 ml	1 ml[1]

[1] Recommended for infants born of infected mothers and for others for whom prolonged maintenance of protective titers is desired.

Revaccination (booster): See Clinical Pharmacology.

Engerix-B: Children ≤ 10 years of age – 10 mcg. *Adults and children ≥ 10 years of age* – 20 mcg. *Hemodialysis patients* – Assess need by semiannual antibody testing. Give 40 mcg (two 20 mcg doses) when antibody levels decline below 10 mIU/ml.

(Administration and Dosage continued on following page)

HEPATITIS B VACCINE (Cont.)

Administration and Dosage (Cont.):

Dosage for infants born of HBsAg-positive mothers (Heptavax-B): Infants born to HBsAg-positive mothers are at high risk of becoming chronic carriers of hepatitis B virus and of developing the chronic sequelae of hepatitis B virus infection. Administration of three 0.5 ml doses of HBIG starting at birth are 75% effective in preventing establishment of the chronic carrier state in these infants during the first year of life. Protection can be transient. Administration of one 0.5 ml dose of HBIG at birth and three 20 mcg (1 ml) doses of *Heptavax-B*, the first dose given within 1 week after birth, were 85% to 93% effective in preventing establishment of the chronic carrier state in infants born to HBsAg and HBeAg-positive mothers. Preliminary data from studies using one 0.5 ml dose of HBIG and three 10 mcg (0.5 ml) doses of *Heptavax-B* in the same type of population indicate that this lower dose is equally effective.

Test for HBsAg and anti-HBs at 12 to 15 months. If HBsAg is not detectable and anti-HBs is present, the child is protected.

Recommended Dosage for Infants Born to HBsAg Positive Mothers				
Treatment	Birth	Within 7 days	1 month	6 months
Heptavax-B (Pediatric formulation 10 mcg/0.5 ml)		0.5 ml*	0.5 ml	0.5 ml
Recombivax HB (Pediatric dose 5 mcg/0.5 ml)		0.5 ml*	0.5 ml	0.5 ml
Hepatitis B Immune Globulin	0.5 ml	—	—	—

* The first dose may be given at birth at the same time as HBIG, but give in the opposite anterolateral thigh. This may better ensure vaccine absorption.

Known or presumed exposure to HBsAg: The following guidelines are recommended for persons who have been exposed to hepatitis B virus through (1) percutaneous (needlestick), ocular, mucous membrane exposure to blood known or presumed to contain HBsAg, (2) human bites by known or presumed HBsAg carriers that penetrate the skin or (3) following sexual contact with known or presumed HBsAg carriers. Give HBIG (0.06 ml/kg) IM as soon as possible after exposure, preferably within 24 hours. Give hepatitis B vaccine IM at a separate site within 7 days of exposure, and give second and third doses 1 and 6 months, respectively, after the first dose.

Recombivax HB dialysis formulation is intended only for adult predialysis/dialysis patients.

Dosage: Recommended vaccination schedule is as follows: 1 ml initially, than 1 ml at 1 and 6 months.

Revaccination: A booster dose may be considered if the anti-HBs level is < 10 mIU/ml 1 to 2 months after the third dose.

Preparation: After thorough agitation, the vaccine is a slightly opaque, white suspension. Use as supplied; no dilution or reconstitution is necessary.

Storage: Store unopened and opened vials at 2°C to 8°C (35.6°F to 46.4°F). Do not freeze; freezing destroys potency.

Rx	**Heptavax-B** (MSD)	**Injection:** 20 mcg hepatitis B surface antigen per ml[1]	In 3 ml vials.
		Pediatric Injection: 10 mcg hepatitis B surface antigen per 0.5 ml[1]	In 0.5 ml vials.
Rx	**Recombivax HB** (MSD)	**Injection:** 10 mcg hepatitis B surface antigen per ml[2]	In 1 and 3 ml vials.
		Dialysis Formulation: 40 mcg hepatitis B surface antigen per ml[1]	In 1 ml vials.
Rx	**Engerix-B** (SK-Beecham)	**Injection:** 20 mcg hepatitis B surface antigen per ml	In single-dose vials.
		Pediatric Injection: 10 mcg hepatitis B surface antigen per 0.5 ml	In single-dose vials.

[1] Formulated in an alum adjuvant with 1:20,000 thimerosal.

[2] With 1:20,000 thimerosal.

TETANUS TOXOID

Actions:

In these preparations, the toxin produced by virulent tetanus bacilli has been modified by treatment with formaldehyde to lose its toxicity, while still retaining its antigenic ability, and thus can induce active immunity.

Adsorbed toxoids are superior to fluid toxoids in the production of antibody titers and in the duration of protection achieved.

Indications:

For active immunization against tetanus in adults and children. Tetanus Toxoid, Fluid, may be used, although Tetanus Toxoid, Adsorbed, is preferred for all basic immunizing and recall doses. Individuals with known sensitivity to horse serum and those with asthma or other allergies should maintain this immunity with tetanus toxoid and avoid the potential complications of equine tetanus antitoxin treatment, which still may be used in certain areas of the world. Tetanus immunization is recommended for all persons, particularly military personnel, farm and utility workers, those working with horses, firemen and all individuals whose occupation renders them liable to even minor lacerations and abrasions.

Tetanus Toxoid, Adsorbed is usually administered to patients at the time of injury, for recall, and can be used at all ages for establishing primary immunization and for booster injections.

Routine prophylaxis is now usually accomplished between infancy (2 months) and childhood (6 years) by Diphtheria and Tetanus Toxoids and Pertussis Vaccine, Adsorbed (DTP), or Diphtheria and Tetanus Toxoids, Adsorbed (pediatric). Tetanus and Diphtheria Toxoids, Adsorbed, for adult use (Td) is recommended to protect individuals over 6 years of age.

Contraindications:

Prior systemic allergic reaction to tetanus toxoid.

An acute respiratory infection or other active infection is reason for deferring routine primary immunizing or recall (booster) doses, but not emergency wound recall (booster) doses. Prolonging the interval between primary immunizing doses for 6 months or longer does not interfere with final immunity. Count any dose of tetanus toxoid an individual has received, even a decade earlier, as an immunizing injection.

Defer elective immunization for patients > 6 months during a poliomyelitis outbreak.

The occurrence of any type of neurological signs or symptoms after administration absolutely contraindicates further use.

Warnings:

Under no circumstances should tetanus toxoid be used to treat actual tetanus infections, nor should it be used for immediate prophylaxis of unimmunized individuals. Employ tetanus antitoxin, preferably Tetanus Immune Globulin (Human), in all such cases.

Allergic reactions: Take every precaution to prevent and arrest allergic and other untoward reactions. A careful history should review possible sensitivity to the type of protein to be injected. Epinephrine 1:1000 and other appropriate agents should be readily available to combat unexpected allergic reactions. Refer to Management of Acute Hypersensitivity Reactions.

Pregnancy: Tetanus toxoid has been administered to pregnant women in an effort to prevent neonatal tetanus in newborns considered to be at high risk. There are, however, inconclusive data on the safety of tetanus toxoid so used. Generally, avoid unnecessary drugs and biologics in pregnant women, especially in the first trimester.

Children: Cautiously inject infants or children with cerebral damage, neurological disorders or a history of febrile convulsions to test their tolerance. If a CNS reaction (eg, convulsions) occurs in infants, defer completion of immunization schedule until at least 1 year of age.

Precautions:

Concomitant immunosuppressive therapy: Avoid or postpone tetanus toxoid in persons receiving immunosuppressive therapy. The use of toxoids in such cases or in hypogammaglobulinemia or agammaglobulinemia is unlikely to initiate adequate antibody response.

Inject only healthy individuals.

Avoid injecting vaccine into a blood vessel.

(Continued on following page)

TETANUS TOXOID (Cont.)

Drug Interactions:

Therapeutic doses of **chloramphenicol** may interfere with the response to tetanus toxoid. Avoid concomitant administration of this antibiotic.

Adverse Reactions:

There is an increased incidence of local and systemic reactions to booster doses when given to previously immunized persons over 25 years of age. Severe systemic reactions are extremely rare. Over the past several years, reports have described extensive local reactions which, in some instances, were accompanied by mild to moderate systemic responses. A typical reaction of this type is manifested by a delayed onset of erythema, boggy edema and induration surrounding the site. Pain and tenderness may be present. Edema, occasionally extensive, is frequently accompanied by itching. Axillary lymphadenopathy has also been reported.

Local: A small area of erythema, local redness and induration surrounding the injection site may persist for a few days. A nodule may be palpable for a few weeks.

The majority of the extensive delayed local responses have occurred in adults following booster doses and in children who have received several doses of tetanus toxoid in the past. Local reactions have been reported following use of both fluid and adsorbed tetanus toxoids.

Arthus-type hypersensitivity reactions, characterized by severe local reactions (generally starting 2 to 8 hours after injection) may occur, particularly in those who have received multiple prior boosters. Although their cause is unknown, hypersensitivity to the toxin or bacillary protein of the tetanus organism itself may be a possibility in some; in others, interreaction between the injected antigen and high levels of preexisting tetanus antibody (antitoxin) from prior booster doses seems the most likely cause of the Arthus-type response.

Systemic: Low grade fever, chills, malaise, generalized aches and pains, flushing, generalized urticaria or pruritus, tachycardia and hypotension.

Neurologic – Paralysis of the radial nerve, paralysis of the recurrent nerve, cochlear lesions, brachial plexus neuropathies, difficulty in swallowing, accommodation paresis and EEG disturbances have been reported. In the differential diagnosis of polyradiculoneuropathies following administration of tetanus toxoid, consider it a possible etiology.

Postvaccinal neurologic disorders have been reported following the injection of almost all biological products; consider the possibility of their occurrence.

Administration and Dosage:

Tetanus Toxoid, Adsorbed: Administer IM, preferably into the deltoid or midlateral thigh muscles. In infants, the vastus lateralis (mid-thigh laterally) is the preferred site.

Tetanus Toxoid, Fluid: Administer IM or SC in the vastus lateralis or deltoid. Inject at sites not previously used for a vaccine or toxoid.

Depending on the manufacturer, each 0.5 ml dose of tetanus toxoid, fluid contains 4 or 5 Lf units of tetanus toxoid and each 0.5 ml dose of tetanus toxoid, adsorbed contains 5 or 10 Lf units of tetanus toxoid.

Primary immunization for adults and children:

Administration	Tetanus Toxoid	
	Adsorbed	Fluid
Dose (Route)	0.5 ml (IM)	0.5 ml (IM or SC)
Number of injections	2	3
Interval (weeks)	4 to 8	4 to 8
Additional dose	Give a third dose of 0.5 ml approximately 6 to 12 months after second injection	Give a fourth dose of 0.5 ml approximately 6 to 12 months after third injection
Booster dose	0.5 ml every 10 years	0.5 ml every 10 years

Tetanus prophylaxis in wound management: Determine proper procedure for protection, with special consideration of the wound, as well as the proper program for prophylaxis.

1. If primary immunization administered or booster dose administered less than 10 years prior to injury and simple clean wound or less than 5 years prior to all other wounds – No tetanus prophylaxis required.
2. If primary immunization administered or most recent booster dose administered more than 10 years prior to injury and simple clean wound or more than 5 years prior to all other wounds – Give 0.5 ml Tetanus Toxoid, Adsorbed IM.
3. Patient incompletely immunized or history of immunization uncertain – Give 0.5 ml of Tetanus Toxoid Adsorbed IM and complete primary immunization.
4. Patient not immunized – Initiate primary immunization.

(Administration and Dosage continued on following page)

TETANUS TOXOID (Cont.)

Administration and Dosage (Cont.):

Tetanus prophylaxis in wound management (Cont.):

Concurrent diphtheria immunization – Tetanus and Diphtheria Toxoids, Adsorbed (Td) is preferred for active tetanus immunization in patients ≥ 7 years old. This enhances diphtheria protection since a large portion of adults are susceptible. For children < 7 years old, use Diphtheria, Pertussis and Tetanus Toxoids, Adsorbed (pediatric) (DPT) or DT, if pertussis immunization is contraindicated, instead of Td or tetanus toxoid alone.

Alternate recommendations: The Committee on Infectious Diseases of the American Academy of Pediatrics and the CDC recommend the following:

IMMUNIZATION STATUS	
Type of Wound†	**Immunization Treatment**
Unimmunized, Uncertain or Incomplete (one or two doses of toxoid)	
Low risk wound	One dose of Td or DT followed by completion of immunization; booster every 10 years thereafter
Tetanus-prone wound and Wound neglected > 24 hr	One dose of Td or DT plus 250 to 500 U TIG followed by completion of immunization. Note: Use separate syringe and sites for TIG and toxoid
Full Primary Immunization with Booster Dose Within 10 Years of Wound	
Low risk wound	No toxoid necessary
Tetanus-prone wound	If more than 5 years since last dose, one dose of Td If less than 5 years, no toxoid necessary
Wound neglected > 24 hr	One dose of Td plus 250 to 500 U TIG
Full Primary Immunization with No Booster Doses or Last Booster Dose > 10 Years	
Low risk wound	One dose of Td
Tetanus-prone wound	One dose of Td
Wound neglected > 24 hr	One dose of Td plus 250 to 500 U TIG

†"Tetanus-prone" refers to wounds which yield anaerobic conditions or which were incurred in circumstances with probability of exposure to tetanus spores (eg, severe necrotizing machinery injuries, puncture wounds, wounds heavily contaminated with excreta). All others are considered low risk from the standpoint of tetanus. Neglected wounds are at greater risk. The decision to use concomitant passive prophylaxis with Tetanus Antitoxin depends on medical judgment, but is rarely indicated over TIG.

	TETANUS TOXOID, FLUID		**C.I.***
Rx	**Antigens Int.**	**Injection:** 4 Lf units tetanus per 0.5 ml dose. In 7.5 ml vials.[1]	83
Rx	**Lederle**	**Injection:** 5 Lf units tetanus per 0.5 ml dose. In 0.5 ml disp. syringe[1] and 7.5 ml vials.[1]	103
Rx	**Squibb/Connaught**	**Injection:** 4 Lf units tetanus per 0.5 ml dose. In 7.5 ml vials.[1]	83
Rx	**Wyeth**	**Injection:** 5 Lf units tetanus per 0.5 ml dose. In 0.5 ml Tubex[1] and 7.5 ml vials.[1]	89
	TETANUS TOXOID, ADSORBED		
Rx	**Lederle**	**Injection:** 5 Lf units tetanus per 0.5 ml dose. In 0.5 ml disp. syringe[2] and 5 ml vials.[2]	154
Rx	**Sclavo**	**Injection:** 10 Lf units tetanus per 0.5 ml dose. In 5 ml vials.[3]	109
Rx	**Squibb/Connaught**	**Injection:** 5 Lf units tetanus per 0.5 ml dose. In 5 ml vials.[4]	125
Rx	**Wyeth**	**Injection:** 5 Lf units tetanus per 0.5 ml dose. In 0.5 ml Tubex[2] and 5 ml vials.[2]	134
	TETANUS TOXOID, PLAIN		
Rx	**Sclavo**	**Injection:** 20 to 30 Lf units per 0.5 ml dose. In 0.5 and 7.5 ml vials.[5]	NA

* Cost Index based on cost per 0.5 ml.
[1] With thimerosal.
[2] With aluminum phosphate and thimerosal.
[3] With aluminum hydroxide and thimerosal.
[4] With aluminum potassium sulfate and thimerosal.
[5] With ≤ 0.02% residual free formaldehyde and 0.01% thimerosal.

Refer to general discussion of agents for active immunization on page 2088

DIPHTHERIA AND TETANUS TOXOIDS, COMBINED (Td)

Actions:

The diphtheria and tetanus toxins are inactivated by formaldehyde. The triple antigen combination (Diphtheria and Tetanus Toxoids and Pertussis Vaccine) is the agent of choice for routine immunization of children < 6 years of age; diphtheria and tetanus toxoids may be used when pertussis vaccine is contraindicated or used separately.

Tetanus: Adequate immunization with tetanus toxoid provides effective and durable protection against tetanus. Prior active immunization eliminates the need for passive therapy at the time of injury in most instances.

Diphtheria: Although the incidence of diphtheria has declined due to the high level of appropriate immunization among children, localized outbreaks occur. Most diphtheria cases occur in unimmunized or inadequately immunized individuals. Immunization does not eliminate carriage of *Corynebacterium diphtheriae* in the pharynx or nose or on the skin.

Recall Injection After Injury: If an injury occurs more than 5 years after the primary course of immunization or after a booster dose, give an exposure recall injection or emergency booster dose of Tetanus and Diphtheria Toxoids Adsorbed, Tetanus Toxoid Adsorbed or Tetanus Toxoid. This provides adequate protection in the majority of previously immunized patients. Antitoxin is not needed prophylactically for injured individuals who have been actively immunized unless the wounds are not treated promptly, are extensive, are severely contaminated or cannot be adequately debrided. If tetanus toxoid and TIG are given concurrently, use separate syringes. Adsorbed Td or tetanus toxoid is preferred over fluid toxoid for coadministration with TIG.

Indications:

Diphtheria and Tetanus Toxoids, Adsorbed (Pediatric) (DT): Active immunization against diphtheria and tetanus in infants and children through 6 years of age.

Tetanus and Diphtheria Toxoids, Adsorbed (Adult) (Td): Active immunization of adults and children 7 years of age and older against diphtheria and tetanus.

Contraindications:

Prior anaphylactic, allergic or systemic reactions.

Patients receiving immunosuppressive agents (corticosteroids, antimetabolites, alkylating compounds or irradiation) and in those with a recent injection of immune globulin or an immunodeficiency disorder, may not respond optimally to active immunization. When possible, interrupt treatment when immunization is contemplated with an injury.

In case of any acute respiratory infection or other active infection, defer routine immunizing or booster doses, but not emergency booster doses. A minor illness not associated with fever, such as a mild upper respiratory infection, need not preclude vaccination.

Defer elective immunization during an outbreak of poliomyelitis.

Warnings:

Do not use for treatment of actual tetanus or diphtheria infections.

Usage in Pregnancy: Tetanus toxoid has been administered to pregnant women to prevent neonatal tetanus in newborns at high risk. However, data regarding safety are inconclusive. There are no data on the safety of diphtheria toxoid in pregnancy; therefore, the combined product is not recommended for use in pregnant women.

Precautions:

Hypersensitivity: Have epinephrine 1:1000 immediately available. Refer to Management of Acute Hypersensitivity Reactions on p. 2897

History of CNS damage or convulsions: Postpone primary immunization until the second year of life; the use of single, rather than combined, antigens is preferred.

Adverse Reactions:

Although both components may evoke local and systemic allergic responses, the tetanus toxoid component may be the more common cause.

Systemic: Fretfulness (23%); drowsiness (15%); anorexia (7%); vomiting (3%); persistent crying (1%); transient fever ($> 38°C$ [100°F] in children is unusual); malaise; generalized aches and pains; flushing; generalized urticaria or pruritus; rash; tachycardia and hypotension may occur, especially in persons who received many booster injections. Itching of edematous area is frequent, and the area may resemble a giant "hive." Edema is occasionally extensive, shoulder to elbow or shoulder to wrist. Axillary lymphadenopathy has occurred.

Serious postvaccinal neurologic disorders are uncommon. Paralysis of the radial nerve, paralysis of the recurrent nerve, cochlear lesion, brachial plexus neuropathies, and a case of dysphagia, accommodation paresis and EEG disturbances have been reported following tetanus toxoid administration. In the differential diagnosis of polyradiculoneuropathies, consider tetanus toxoid a possible etiology.

(Adverse Reactions continued on following page)

DIPHTHERIA AND TETANUS TOXOIDS, COMBINED (Td) (Cont.)

Adverse Reactions (Cont.):

Local: Mild to moderate pain, tenderness, swelling and redness (8% to 10%); edema; erythema; induration surrounding the injection site for a few days. Persistent nodules and sterile abscesses may occur. A nodule may be palpable at injection site for a few weeks.

Severe local reactions (generally starting 2 to 8 hours after an injection) have been reported from tetanus toxoids prepared by different manufacturers. Hypersensitivity to the toxin or bacillary protein is a possible cause. Interreaction between the injected antigen and high levels of preexisting tetanus antibody (antitoxin) from prior booster doses seems the most likely cause of the Arthus-type response.

Administration and Dosage:

Interruption of the recommended schedule with a delay between doses does not interfere with the final immunity achieved, nor does it necessitate starting the series over again, regardless of the length of time elapsed between doses.

Shake vial well before withdrawing each dose.

Do not inject intracutaneously or SC. Ensure that injection does not enter a blood vessel. For adults, give IM in the vastus lateralis (mid-thigh laterally), gluteus or deltoid. For infants, the vastus lateralis is preferred. Avoid injection in the deltoid area in infants; also avoid the gluteus maximus due to the potential for sciatic nerve damage. During primary immunization, do not inject the same site more than once.

Pediatric, Adsorbed Toxoids: Recommended for children up to the 7th birthday, ideally beginning when the infant is 6 weeks to 2 months old. Start immunization at once if diphtheria is present in the community.

Infants (6 weeks through 1 year) – Give three 0.5 ml doses IM at least 4 weeks apart. Give a reinforcing dose 6 to 12 months after the third injection.

Children (1 year through 6 years) – Give two 0.5 ml doses IM at least 4 weeks apart. Give a reinforcing dose 6 to 12 months after the second injection. If the final immunizing dose is given after the 7th birthday, use the *adult* preparation.

Booster immunization (4 to 6 years of age) – 0.5 ml IM. Those who receive all 4 primary immunizing doses before the 4th birthday, should receive a single dose of DT. The booster dose is not necessary if the 4th dose in the primary series was given after the 4th birthday. Thereafter, give routine booster doses with the adult preparation at 10 year intervals.

Adult, Adsorbed Toxoids (7 years of age or older): 2 primary doses of 0.5 ml each, given at an interval of 4 to 6 weeks, followed by a third (reinforcing) 0.5 ml dose 6 to 12 months later; basic immunization is not complete until the third dose is given. Give a 0.5 ml routine recall (booster) dose every 10 years to maintain immunity.

Wound management: For tetanus prophylaxis in wound management, refer to page 2134

Storage: Store between 2° to 8°C (35° to 46°F). Do not freeze.

DIPHTHERIA AND TETANUS TOXOIDS, ADSORBED (FOR PEDIATRIC USE)

For use only in patients 6 years of age or younger.

				C.I.*
Rx	**Lederle**	**Injection:** 12.5 Lf units diphtheria and 5 Lf units tetanus per 0.5 ml dose	In 5 ml vials.[1]	172
Rx	**Sclavo**	**Injection:** 15 Lf units diphtheria and 10 Lf units tetanus per 0.5 ml dose	In 5 ml vials.[2]	139
Rx	**Connaught**	**Injection:** 6.6 Lf units diphtheria and 5 Lf units tetanus per 0.5 ml dose	In 5 ml vials.[3]	167
Rx	**Wyeth**	**Injection:** 10 Lf units diphtheria and 5 Lf units tetanus per 0.5 ml dose	In 5 ml vials[4] and 0.5 ml Tubex.[4]	185

DIPHTHERIA AND TETANUS TOXOIDS, ADSORBED (FOR ADULT USE)

Contains ≤ 2 Lf units of diphtheria toxoid per 0.5 ml.

Rx	**Lederle**	**Injection:** 2 Lf units diphtheria and 5 Lf units tetanus per 0.5 ml dose	In 0.5 ml disp. syringe[5] & 5 ml vials.[5]	172
Rx	**Sclavo**	**Injection:** 2 Lf units diphtheria and 10 Lf units tetanus per 0.5 ml dose	In 5 ml vials.[2]	148
Rx	**Connaught**	**Injection:** 2 Lf units diphtheria and 5 Lf units tetanus per 0.5 ml dose	In 5 ml vials.[3]	163
Rx	**Wyeth**	**Injection:** 1.5 Lf units diphtheria and 5 Lf units tetanus per 0.5 ml dose	In 5 ml vials[4] and 0.5 ml Tubex.[4]	185

* Cost Index based on cost per 0.5 ml dose.
[1] With aluminum phosphate, glycine, thimerosal.
[2] With aluminum hydroxide, thimerosal.
[3] In saline w/aluminum potassium sulfate, thimerosal.
[4] With aluminum phosphate, thimerosal.
[5] In saline w/aluminum phosphate, glycine, thimerosal.

Refer to general discussion of agents for active immunization on page 2088

DIPHTHERIA AND TETANUS TOXOIDS AND PERTUSSIS VACCINE, ADSORBED (DTP)

Actions:

These preparations combine diphtheria and tetanus toxins (detoxified by formaldehyde) with pertussis vaccine.

Pharmacology: Adequate immunization with diphtheria toxoid is thought to confer protection for at least 10 years. It significantly reduces both the risk of developing diphtheria and the severity of clinical illness. It does not, however, eliminate carriage of *Corynebacterium diphtheriae* in the pharynx or on the skin. A serum level $\geq$ 0.01 toxin neutralization units/ml is generally protective.

Tetanus toxoid is highly effective, with a failure rate in fully immunized persons of less than 4 per 100 million. Protective levels of serum antitoxin ($\geq$ 0.01 toxin neutralization units/ml) are achieved which persist for at least 10 years after full immunization.

Indications:

For active immunization of infants and children through 6 years of age (between 2 months and the 7th birthday) against diphtheria, tetanus and pertussis. Recommended for both primary immunization and routine recall. Start immunization at once if whooping cough or diphtheria is present in the community.

Contraindications:

Not recommended for use in adults or in children over 7 years of age.

Defer immunization during any acute illness or if any neurological signs or symptoms, including one or more seizures (see Warnings), occur following administration of these products.

Occurrence of any of the following after administration contraindicates further use of this product: Fever > 39°C (102°F), convulsions with or without accompanying fever, alterations of consciousness, focal neurologic signs, thrombocytopenia, screaming episodes, shock, collapse, somnolence, encephalopathy.

The presence of an evolving or changing neurologic disorder.

Anaphylactoid or allergic reactions, immunosuppressive therapy, recent gammaglobulin, plasma or blood transfusions, immunodeficiency disorders, leukemia, lymphoma or generalized malignancy.

Immunosuppressive therapy including irradiation, corticosteroids, antimetabolites, alkylating agents and cytotoxic agents, may result in aberrant responses to active immunization. Defer administration in such individuals.

Defer elective immunization of patients > 6 months old during a poliomyelitis outbreak.

Warnings:

Do not use DTP for treatment of actual tetanus, diphtheria or whooping cough infections.

History of convulsions: Although contraindicated by the manufacturers, the Immunization Practices Advisory Committee (ACIP) has reviewed the risks and benefits of pertussis vaccine for infants and children with a family history of convulsions. Based on this review, the ACIP believes that a family history of convulsions should not be a contraindication to DTP vaccination. Also, the Committee believes that antipyretic use with DTP vaccination may be reasonable in children with personal or family histories of convulsions.

Precautions:

When an infant or child returns for the next dose in the series, question the parent concerning occurrence of any symptoms or signs of adverse reactions after the previous dose. If such are reported, further doses of DTP are contraindicated; complete active immunization against diphtheria and tetanus with Diphtheria and Tetanus Toxoids, Adsorbed (Pediatric) (see p. 2136

Hypersensitivity: Review the patient's history regarding possible sensitivity. Have epinephrine 1:1000 immediately available. Refer to Management of Acute Hypersensitivity Reactions on p. 2897

(Continued on following page)

DIPHTHERIA AND TETANUS TOXOIDS AND PERTUSSIS VACCINE, ADSORBED (DTP) (Cont.)

Adverse Reactions:

Local: Erythema and induration with or without tenderness (common). Pain (51%), swelling (41%) and redness (37%). Local reactions are usually self-limited and require no therapy. A nodule may be palpable at the injection site for a few weeks. Abscess may form at the injection site.

Systemic: Mild to moderate temperature elevations, accompanied by malaise, chills and irritability. Other systemic reactions include fretfulness (53%), drowsiness (32%), anorexia (21%), vomiting (6%) and persistent crying (3%).

Rarely, serious and occasionally fatal adverse reactions have followed administration of pertussis vaccine-containing preparations. They almost always appear within 24 to 48 hours after injection, but may occur after as long as 7 days. Should such reactions occur, further immunization against pertussis is contraindicated. Reactions reported are: High fever of 40.5°C (105°F); collapse with rapid recovery; collapse followed by prolonged prostration; a transient shock-like episode; excessive screaming (persistent crying or screaming for 3 or more hours duration); somnolence; isolated convulsions with or without fever; encephalopathy with changes in the level of consciousness, focal neurological signs and convulsions, with or without permanent neurological or mental deficit (rare but may be fatal or result in permanent CNS damage); thrombocytopenic purpura; hemolytic anemia. Pertussis vaccine has been associated with a greater proportion of adverse reactions than many other childhood immunizations.

Neurological complications following tetanus toxoid administration, such as paralysis of the radial nerve, paralysis of the recurrent nerve, cochlear lesion, brachial plexus neuropathies, and a case with dysphagia, accommodation paresis and EEG disturbances, have been reported. In the differential diagnosis of polyradiculoneuropathies following administration, consider tetanus toxoid a possible etiology.

Sudden infant death syndrome (SIDS) has been reported following administration of DTP. The significance of these reports is unclear. Consider that the three primary immunizing doses are usually administered to infants between the age of 2 and 6 months and that approximately 85% of SIDS cases occur between 1 and 6 months of age, with peak incidence at 2 to 4 months.

Administration and Dosage:

Interruption of the recommended schedule with a delay between doses does not interfere with the final immunity achieved, nor does it necessitate starting the series over again, regardless of the length of time elapsed between doses.

Inject IM. The midlateral muscle of the thigh is preferred for infants. Do not inject the same muscle site more than once during the course of basic immunization.

Primary immunization: For children 2 months through 6 years (ideally beginning at age 2 to 3 months or at the 6 week check-up) administer 0.5 ml IM on 3 occasions at 4 to 8 week intervals with a reinforcing dose administered 1 year after the 3rd injection.

Booster doses: Administer 0.5 ml IM when the child is 4 to 6 years of age (preferably prior to entering kindergarten or elementary school). However, if the 4th dose of the basic immunization series was administered after the 4th birthday, a recall (booster) of DTP prior to school entry is not necessary.

For booster doses thereafter, use the recommended dose of Diphtheria and Tetanus Toxoids, Adsorbed (For Adult Use) every 10 years. Do not immunize persons 7 years of age and older with Pertussis Vaccine.

Storage: Store between 2° to 8°C (35° to 46°F). Do not freeze.

				C.I.*
Rx	**Acel-Immune** (Lederle)	**Injection**: 7.5 Lf units diphtheria, 5 Lf units tetanus and 300 hemagglutinating units of acellular pertussis[2]	In 5 ml vials.	NA
Rx	**Tri-Immunol** (Lederle)	**Injection**: 12.5 Lf units diphtheria, 5 Lf units tetanus and 4 protective units pertussis per 0.5 ml dose	In 7.5 ml vials.[1]	665

* Cost Index based on cost per 0.5 ml dose.

[1] In saline solution with aluminum phosphate, glycine and thimerosal.

[2] Also contains aluminum, formaldehyde and thimerosal.

Actions:

Allergenic extracts are derived individually from various biological sources containing antigens which possess immunologic activity. They are categorized based on the method of standardization and dosage form, including: 1) Immunogenically standardized, 2) weight-to-volume standardized, 3) protein nitrogen unit standardized and 4) alum-precipitated.

The mechanism of action is not completely defined. Specific Immunoglobulin G (IgG) appears in the serum following injection of allergenic extracts. IgG competes with specific IgE for a specific antigen. Bound to receptors on mast cell membranes, IgE produces an allergenic reaction by releasing histamine and other agents upon coupling with an antigen. Serum IgE levels decrease over time. Decreased leukocyte sensitivity to allergens and increased numbers of T-suppressor cells for IgE-producing plasma cells are also noted. The histamine release response of circulating basophils to a specific allergen may be reduced in some patients by hyposensitization.

Onset/Duration: Relief of symptoms is dose-related. It is rarely achieved before maintenance dosage levels are reached, which often takes 4 to 6 months, sometimes 12 months. Serum IgG levels remain elevated for weeks to months following injection and vary markedly between individuals.

Indications:

Diagnosis of specific allergies.

Relief of allergic symptoms (hay fever, rhinitis, etc) due to specifically identified materials by means of a graduated schedule of doses.

Contraindications:

As initial therapy when an allergen can be environmentally avoided.

Frequent large local reactions or systemic reactions are relative contraindications for continued immunotherapy.

Foodstuff allergen extracts are diagnostic tools; efficacy for hyposensitization immunotherapy has not been demonstrated.

Warnings:

Cross-sensitivity: Cross-immunoreactivity has been documented within botanical genus groups, especially among grasses. Exercise caution in prescribing since the additive effects could precipitate an allergic reaction. Markedly increased exposure to allergens in the environment may have an additive effect when coupled with an allergen extract injection. Dosage reduction may be necessary.

Anaphylactic reactions may occur with an overdose or in extremely sensitive individuals. Administer allergen extracts only where emergency facilities are *immediately* available. Refer to Management of Acute Hypersensitivity Reactions on p. 2897

Usage in Pregnancy: Category C. Controlled studies of hyposensitization with allergen extracts thoughout pregnancy failed to demonstrate any fetal or maternal risk. Because histamine can produce uterine contraction, avoid any reaction which releases significant amounts of histamine, whether from natural allergen exposure or from hyposensitization overdose. IgG crosses the placenta, especially in the third trimester. Administer during pregnancy only if clearly needed and with caution. Although pregnancy is not an indication to stop allergen extract therapy in women receiving maintenance doses without side effects, some allergists empirically decrease the maintenance dose by 50% throughout gestation.

Usage in Lactation: Minimal amounts of IgG are excreted in breast milk. No problems in humans have been documented. Rather, various nutritional, immunologic and other advantages of breast-feeding have been described, especially in children of atopic mothers.

Usage in Children: Dosage for children is generally the same as for adults. The larger dosage volumes may produce relatively greater discomfort. To achieve the total dose required, the volume of the dose may be distributed among several injection sites.

(Continued on following page)

Precautions:

Mixed allergens are not to be used for skin testing. In the case of a negative reaction, a mixture fails to indicate whether one of the individual components at the full labeled concentration is capable of evoking a positive reaction. If the patient responds positively, there is no indication which component of the mixture produced the antigenic response. Treatment with nonreactive allergens can lead to sensitization and induction of IgE production.

Do not combine allergens to which the patient is extremely sensitive with allergens for which only a nominal sensitivity is shown. Administer separately to individualize and better control dosage.

Delay the start of immunotherapy until after any period of symptoms from seasonal environmental exposure. Typical allergic symptoms may follow shortly after an injection, particularly when the sum of the antigen load from the environment and from the injection exceed the patient's antigen tolerance.

While routine immunizations may theoretically exacerbate autoimmune diseases, studies have failed to demonstrate this. Give hyposensitization cautiously to patients with autoimmune diseases and only if the risk from exposure exceeds the risk of exacerbating the underlying condition.

Drug Interactions:

Drug/lab tests: **H_1 histamine antagonists** (as well as possibly **H_2 antagonists** and **tricyclic antidepressants**) may produce a false-negative reaction to cutaneous diagnostic testing with allergen extracts unless a 72 hour period of antihistamine abstinence is observed.

Adverse Reactions:

Most serious reactions begin within 30 minutes of an injection. Observe patients for at least 30 minutes after every injection, even once they have achieved maintenance therapy.

Local: Erythema and swelling at the injection site are common, but not significant unless they persist longer than 24 hours or exceed the diameter of a nickel (about 2 cm).

Systemic: Fainting, pallor, bradycardia, hypotension, angioedema, wheezing, cough, conjunctivitis, rhinitis, generalized urticaria.

Patient Information:

Comply with full course of therapy. For the medication to work, it must be taken regularly and in the proper dosage. Medication will not cure allergies, but it will help control them.

Notify physician of increased environmental exposure to natural allergens; a dosage reduction may be required.

Missed dose: Depending on the amount of time elapsed, dosage reduction may be required. Do *not* double the dose to make up for the missed dose. More frequent injections may be necessary to return to maintenance doses.

Notify physician if erythema, swelling or generalized urticaria persists.

Notify physician immediately if fainting, wheezing, hypotension or bradycardia occurs.

Administration and Dosage:

Begin immunotherapy with very small doses; increase progressively until maintenance levels are reached. Dosages vary depending on the type of standardization used. Individualize dosage.

Do not inject IV. SC injection is preferable because it is less painful, allows better delineation of reaction size and slows the absorption rate, thus lowering the likelihood of an anaphylactic reaction. Although IM administration is acceptable, it is more painful and more difficult to assess the local reaction.

Do not combine allergens to which the patient is extremely sensitive with allergens for which only a nominal sensitivity is shown. Distinct treatment schedules for each formula are frequently employed. (See Precautions.)

Children: Dosage is the same as for adults; divide doses among several injection sites.

Diagnostic Testing: Perform puncture (prick) or intradermal testing with appropriate dilutions, employing positive and negative controls. Consult manufacturer's literature for each allergen. Do not conduct diagnostic testing with alum-precipitated allergen extracts.

Therapeutic dosing: Typical doses are given SC every 3 to 14 days (or 7 to 14 days with alum-precipitated allergen extracts). Progress to the maximum tolerated dose or a weekly maintenance dose. Consult manufacturer's literature for each allergen.

Admixtures: Limit combinations of allergens so that each allergen will be present at a therapeutic concentration. Do not combine allergens of different standardization types. Stability varies with diluent, storage condition and concentration. Stability will be shortest in the low concentration ranges.

Storage: Store between 2° and 8°C (35° to 46°F).

(Products listed on following page)

Rx	**Stinging Insect Antigen No. 108** (Barry)	Combined antigens of bumblebee, honeybee, wasp, hornet and yellow jacket. In three 5 ml vials, serially diluted. Refills available.
Rx	**Insect Antigens** (Hollister-Stier)	Antigens available: Bee, wasp, hornet, yellow jacket and fire ant. Insect antigen extract for hyposensitization and diagnosis available in appropriate dilutions in 5 ml vial plus 4.5 ml buffered saline with phenol.
Rx	**Pharmalgen** (Pharmacia)	For diagnosis and hyposensitization of allergic reactions to insect stings. 6 vials of freeze-dried venom/venom protein - one each of honeybee, yellow jacket, yellow hornet, white-faced hornet, mixed vespid and wasp. Each vial contains 100 mcg.
Rx	**Venomil** (Hollister-Stier)	For diagnosis and hyposensitization of allergic reactions to insect stings. Contains freeze-dried venom of honey bee, yellow jacket, yellow hornet, white-faced hornet, wasp and mixed vespid. In 1, 2 and 10 ml vials of powder for reconstitution.
Rx	**Albay** (Hollister-Stier)	For diagnosis and hyposensitization of allergic reactions to insect stings. 500 mcg freeze-dried venom (honeybee) and venom protein (yellow jacket, yellow hornet, white-faced hornet, wasp and mixed vespid). In 10 ml vials.
Rx	**Allergenic Extracts** (Barry)	Several hundred fluid allergens available from the following categories: Pollens, foods, dusts, epidermals, insects, fungi (molds and smuts), stinging insects, yeasts and others. **"50 Plus" Diagnostic Test Set:** Perennial and seasonal allergens for each of 5 botanical zones. **"60 Plus" Diagnostic Test Set:** Complete food allergen test set. **Regionalized Pollen Test Set:** For each of 5 botanical zones. **Immunorex:** Prescription allergy treatment sets; individualized 4 vial sets prepared from physician's instructions based on patient's skin test reactions and history. Refills available.
Rx	**Allergenic Extracts** (Berkeley Biologicals)	Antigens available: Pollen, protein/fungus, food and insect tests. Therapeutic extracts supplied in either buffered saline diluents or buffered diluents containing 50% glycerin. In multidose vials of 2, 5, 10, 20, 30 and 50 ml.
Rx	**Allergenic Extracts** (Greer Laboratories)	Several hundred allergens available from the following categories: Pollen, insect, mold, epidermals and food. Available in various size vials.
Rx	**Allergenic Extracts** (Hollister-Stier)	For hyposensitization. Extracts include epidermals, regular process molds, miscellaneous inhalants and insects. In 5 or 10 ml vials of 4 graduated dilutions.
Rx	**Allpyral** (Hollister-Stier)	Alum-precipitated allergenic extracts. Pollens, molds, epidermals, house dust and other inhalants and stinging insects. Available in various size vials.

Tuberculin Tests

Actions:

Tuberculin testing products contain soluble growth products derived from the tubercle bacillus. When administered intradermally, a hypersensitivity reaction, manifesting as induration and erythema, appears in sensitive individuals. A positive reaction indicates that the patient has had, at some time, a tuberculous infection, but may indicate previous BCG vaccination. A positive test does not indicate an active infection, but indicates that further evaluation is needed.

Two agents are used for tuberculin testing: Old tuberculin (OT) is a culture filtrate standardized to a uniform potency; Purified Protein Derivative (PPD) is a more refined preparation, and is recommended by the National Tuberculosis and Respiratory Disease Association.

Indications:

Skin test as an aid in the diagnosis of tuberculosis.

Routine tuberculin testing is recommended at 12 months of age and every 1 to 2 years thereafter, preferably before measles vaccination. The frequency of repeated tuberculin tests depends on the risk of exposure and the prevalence of tuberculosis in the population group. Also indicated for high risk groups such as hospital personnel and institutionalized individuals.

Warnings:

Repeated testing of the uninfected individual does not sensitize to tuberculin, but may have a "booster" effect in persons with low degrees of homologous or heterologous mycobacterial antigens or may even cause an apparent development of sensitivity in some cases.

Tuberculin positive reactors: Do not administer to known tuberculin-positive reactors because of the severity of reactions (eg, vesiculation, ulceration or necrosis) that may occur at the test site.

SC injection should be avoided. If this occurs, a general febrile reaction or acute inflammation around old tuberculous lesions may occur in sensitive individuals.

Usage in Pregnancy: Category C. It is not known whether the tuberculin test can cause fetal harm when administered to a pregnant woman or can affect reproduction capacity. Administer to a pregnant woman only if clearly needed.

During pregnancy, known positive reactors may demonstrate a negative response to a tine test.

Usage in Children: A child who has been exposed to a tuberculous adult must not be judged free of infection until there is a negative tuberculin reaction at least 10 weeks after ending contact with the tuberculous person.

Precautions:

Do not apply on acneiform skin, hairy areas or areas without adequate subcutaneous tissue.

Hypersensitivity reactions: Have epinephrine immediately available. See also Management of Acute Hypersensitivity Reactions on page viii.

Usage in active tuberculosis: Perform tuberculin testing with caution in persons with active tuberculosis. However, activation of quiescent lesions is rare.

Altered reactivity: Reactivity to tuberculin may be depressed or suppressed for as long as 4 weeks by viral infections, live virus vaccines (ie, measles, smallpox, polio, rubella and mumps), severe febrile illness, sarcoidosis or malignancy, overwhelming miliary or pulmonary tuberculosis, administration of corticosteroids or immunosuppressive drugs, old age and malnutrition. When of diagnostic importance, accept a negative test as proof that hypersensitivity is absent only after normal reactivity to nonspecific irritants has been demonstrated. In most patients who are very sick with tuberculosis, the previously negative tuberculin test becomes positive after a few weeks of treatment.

A positive reaction does not necessarily signify active disease. Perform further diagnostic procedures such as chest x-ray and bacteriologic examinations of sputa before making a diagnosis of tuberculosis.

Adverse Reactions:

In highly sensitive individuals, strong positive reactions including vesiculation, ulceration or necrosis may occur at the test site. Cold packs or topical steroids may provide symptomatic relief. Minimal bleeding at puncture site occurs infrequently and does not affect test interpretation. Strongly positive reactions may result in scarring at the test site.

(Products listed on following pages)

Tuberculin Tests (Cont.)

Complete prescribing information for these products begins on page 2142

TUBERCULIN PURIFIED PROTEIN DERIVATIVE (Mantoux; PPD)

Aqueous solutions of a purified protein fraction isolated from culture filtrates of human type strains of *Mycobacterium tuberculosis*.

Administration and Dosage:

Intradermal (Mantoux) test: For the initial test, use 5 tuberculin units (TU). The 1 TU dose is used for individuals suspected of being highly sensitized, since larger initial doses may result in severe skin reactions. Use the 250 TU test dose exclusively for the testing of individuals who fail to react to a previous injection of either 1 or 5 TU. *Never* use it for the initial injection.

Test method: The preferred test site is the flexor or dorsal surface of the forearm about 4 inches below the elbow. Inject intradermally with a disposable syringe using a 26- or 27-gauge x ½ inch needle.

If the intradermal injection is performed properly, a definite white bleb will rise at the needle point, about 6 to 10 mm (⅜") in diameter. This will disappear within minutes. No dressing is required.

If injected SC (ie, no bleb will form), or if a significant part of the dose leaks from the injection site, repeat the test immediately at least 5 cm (2") removed from the first site.

Interpretation: Read 48 to 72 hours after administration. Consider only induration in interpretation. Measure the diameter of induration transversely to the long axis of the forearm and record in millimeters. Disregard erythema of less than 10 mm. If the area of erythema is greater than 10 mm and induration is absent, the injection may have been too deep; retesting is indicated. Interpret reactions as follows:

Positive - Palpable induration measuring 10 mm or more. This indicates hypersensitivity to tuberculoprotein; interpret as positive for past or present infection.

Inconclusive - Induration of 5 to 9 mm. Retest using a different injection site. In the case of known contacts, interpret an induration measuring 5 mm or even smaller as positive. Rule out cross-reaction from other mycobacterial infection.

Negative - Induration of less than 5 mm. This indicates a lack of hypersensitivity to tuberculoprotein; tuberculous infection is highly unlikely.

Retesting: An individual who does not show a positive reaction to 1 or 5 TU on the first test may be retested with 5 TU, and if negative, with 250 TU. If a second test is employed, repeat on the other forearm.

An individual who does not positively react to 5 TU is considered tuberculin negative although the test may be positive to 250 TU. If negative to 250 TU, this individual is nonreactive.

			C.I.*
Rx	**Aplisol** (Parke-Davis)	5 TU per 0.1 ml.[1] In 1 ml (10 test) and 5 ml (50 test) vials.	10
Rx	**Tubersol** (Squibb/Connaught)	1 TU per 0.1 ml.[2] In 1 ml (10 test) vials.	12
		5 TU per 0.1 ml.[2] In 1 ml (10 test) and 5 ml (50 test) vials.	8
		250 TU per 0.1 ml.[2] In 1 ml (10 test) vials.	17

* Cost Index based on cost per one test.

[1] With potassium and sodium phosphates, 0.35% phenol and polysorbate 80.

[2] In isotonic phosphate buffer saline with 0.28% phenol and polysorbate 80.

Complete prescribing information for these products begins on page 2142

TUBERCULIN PPD MULTIPLE PUNCTURE DEVICE

A single use, multiple puncture type device for determining tuberculin sensitivity. Each unit consists of a cylindrical plastic holder bearing four stainless steel tines coated with tuberculin PPD. The units give reactions equivalent to 5 tuberculin units (TU) of PPD-S administered intradermally in the Mantoux test.

Regard all multiple puncture type devices as screening tools; employ appropriate diagnostic procedures for retesting "doubtful" reactors.

Administration and Dosage:

Test method: The volar surface of the upper one-third of the forearm, over a muscle belly, is preferred. Avoid hairy areas and areas without adequate subcutaneous tissue.

Grasp the patient's forearm firmly to stretch the skin taut at the site and to prevent any jerking motion of the arm that could cause scratching with the tines. Apply the unit firmly and without twisting to the test area for approximately 1 second. Exert sufficient pressure to assure that all 4 tines have penetrated the skin of the test area and a circular depression is visible.

Interpretation: Read tests at 48 to 72 hours. Vesiculation or the extent of induration are the determining factors; erythema without induration is of no significance. Determine the size of the induration in millimeters by inspection, measuring and palpation with gentle finger stroking. Measure the diameter of the largest single reaction around one of the puncture sites. With pronounced reactions, the areas of induration around the puncture sites may coalesce.

Positive reaction - If vesiculation is present, the test is positive; manage the patient as if classified positive to the Mantoux Test. The test may be interpreted as positive if induration is greater than 2 mm, but consider further diagnostic procedures.

Negative reaction - Induration less than 2 mm. There is no need for retesting unless the person is a contact of a patient with tuberculosis or there is clinical evidence suggestive of the disease.

			C.I.*
Rx	**Aplitest** (Parke-Davis)	In 25 test packages.[1]	13
Rx	**Sclavo Test-PPD** (Sclavo)	In 20 and 250 test packages.	13
Rx	**Tine Test PPD** (Lederle)	In 25 and 100 test packages.[2]	15

* Cost Index based on cost per one test.

[1] With potassium and sodium phosphate buffers and 0.5% phenol.

[2] With 7% acacia, 30% dextrose and 5% glycerol.

Tuberculin Tests (Cont.)

Complete prescribing information for these products begins on page 2142

OLD TUBERCULIN, MULTIPLE PUNCTURE DEVICES

Tuberculin, Old, Tine Test units give reactions equivalent to or more potent than 5 TU of standard old tuberculin administered intradermally in the Mantoux test. However, regard all multiple puncture-type devices as screening tools and use other appropriate diagnostic procedures such as the Mantoux test for retesting reactors.

Administration and Dosage:

Test method: The volar surface of the upper one-third of the forearm, over a muscle belly, is preferred. Avoid hairy areas and areas without adequate subcutaneous tissue.

Grasp the patient's forearm firmly, since the sharp momentary sting may cause a jerk of the arm, resulting in scratching. Stretch the skin of the forearm tightly and apply the disc with the other hand. Hold at least 1 second. Release tension grip on forearm. Withdraw tine unit. Exert sufficient pressure so that the 4 puncture sites and circular depression of the skin from the plastic base are visible.

Interpretation: Read tests at 48 to 72 hours following administration. Vesiculation or the extent of induration are the determining factors; erythema without induration is not significant. Determine the size of the induration in millimeters by inspection, measuring and palpation with gentle finger stroking. Measure the diameter of the largest single reaction around one of the puncture sites. With pronounced reactions, the areas of induration around the puncture sites may coalesce.

Positive reaction - If vesiculation is present, the test is positive. The management of the patient is the same as that for one classified as positive to the Mantoux test. If induration is 2 mm or greater, the test may be interpreted as positive, but consider further diagnostic procedures.

Negative reaction - Induration less than 2 mm. There is no need to retest unless the person is a contact of a patient with tuberculosis or clinical evidence suggests the disease.

			C.I.*
Rx	**Tuberculin, Old Mono-Vacc Test** (Merieux)	5 TU activity per test. In boxes of 25 tests.	16
Rx	**Tuberculin, Old, Tine Test** (Lederle)	5 TU activity per test. Solution of Old Tuberculin containing 7% acacia[1] and 8.5% lactose. Individual test units in sets of 25, 100 and 250.	15

* Cost Index based on cost per one test.

[1] Although clinical allergy to acacia is very rare, use this product with caution in patients with known allergy to this component.

DIPHTHERIA TOXIN

Indications:

To determine serologic immunity to diphtheria.

Warnings:

Hypersensitivity: Have epinephrine available for treatment of an anaphylactic reaction. See also Management of Acute Hypersensitivity Reactions on page viii.

Usage in Pregnancy: Category C. Animal reproduction studies have not been conducted. It is also not known whether it can cause fetal harm when administered to a pregnant woman or can affect reproduction capacity. Administer only if clearly needed.

Adverse Reactions:

Small areas of erythema at injection sites are normal. Some very sensitive individuals may have larger areas of redness at both the toxin and control injection sites.

Administration and Dosage:

Test method: Cleanse the skin of the flexor surface of both forearms. On the left arm inject 0.1 ml of the control into the epidermal layers of the skin with a 26- or 27-gauge ½ inch needle.

On the right arm inject 0.1 ml of the toxin intradermally. Do not guess at the amount from the size of the bleb produced by the injection. If the point of the needle has been properly inserted, the injection should produce a small, slightly raised bleb which moves with the skin and disappears in about 30 minutes. The test is not reliable if the injection is made under the skin. The injection causes little or no pain, it is not followed by constitutional symptoms and the injection site requires no subsequent care.

Observe the results of the test on the fourth or fifth day; earlier observations may confuse the reaction to toxin with that due to hypersensitivity.

Interpretation:

Positive reaction - A circumscribed area of redness and slight infiltration which measures 1 cm or more in diameter appearing in 24 to 36 hours on the right arm. It develops gradually, reaches its greatest intensity on or about the 4th or 5th day, then fades, leaving a faint brownish pigmented spot which eventually disappears. There is no reaction on the control arm. A positive test signifies that the individual possesses little or no antitoxin in the blood and is probably susceptible to diphtheria.

Combined reaction - Reactions appear at both injection sites but the reaction at the site of the toxin injection is larger at the end of 4 days and persists longer than that at the control site. A positive-combined test indicates possible susceptibility to diphtheria, and a sensitivity to the diphtheria bacillus proteins; use caution in administration of diphtheria toxoid.

Pseudo reaction - This reaction differs from the true positive test by the appearance of a reaction at the control site, and from a positive-combined test by the fact that reactions developing at both injection sites run a similar course, reach a maximum of intensity on the third day and then fade. Individuals showing this reaction are hypersensitive to the diphtheria bacillus protein and may have measurable amounts of antitoxin in their blood.

Negative reaction - There may be a slight mark incident to the needle puncture or a very small area of reddening at either or both injection sites. This negative reaction almost invariably indicates a circulating serum antitoxin titer of not less than 0.005 units per ml.

Storage: Store at 2° to 8°C (35° to 46°F). Discard all vial contents remaining after the day's use.

Rx	**Diphtheria Toxin for Schick Test** (Mass. Pub. Health Biological Labs.)	1 vial of toxin[1] and 1 vial of Control[1] (0.008 Lf per dose) with 50 doses of 0.1 ml each

[1] In diluent containing 1:30,000 thimerosal and 0.4% Normal Serum Albumin (Human).

COCCIDIOIDIN

Indications:

An intradermal skin test to aid in the diagnosis of coccidioidomycosis, and in the differential diagnosis of this disease from histoplasmosis, sarcoidosis and other mycotic and bacterial infections.

Contraindications:

Hypersensitivity to thimerosal; patients with erythema nodosum.

Warnings:

Usage in Pregnancy: Animal reproductive studies have not been conducted. It is not known whether coccidioidin can cause fetal harm when administered to a pregnant woman or can affect reproductive capacity. Administer to a pregnant woman only if clearly needed.

Usage in Children: Coccidioidin has been used routinely in children. No special problems of safety or specific hazards have been found in children including those under 5 years of age.

Adverse Reactions:

Systemic: Patients with great sensitivity may rarely develop a systemic reaction consisting of fever or erythema nodosum. There are no reports that skin testing can cause a recrudescence of the disease.

Hypersensitivity - Because of the possibility of an immediate systemic allergic reaction, observe the patient for 15 minutes after the injection. Have epinephrine available in case an acute hypersensitivity reaction occurs. See also Management of Acute Hypersensitivity Reactions on page viii.

Local: An occasional patient may develop an immediate local wheal reaction. Occasionally, large local reactions may lead to vesiculation, local tissue necrosis and scar formation.

Administration and Dosage:

Test method: Inject 0.1 ml of a 1:100 dilution intradermally on the flexor surface of the forearm.

Perform the 1:10 dilution skin test on persons nonreactive to the 1:100 dilution.

Interpretation: Consider the following points in interpretation: (1) A positive reaction may cause a transitory rise in titer of complement fixation antibody to histoplasma antigens, but not to coccidioidin. (2) Coccidioidin may elicit skin test cross-reactions in individuals infected with *Histoplasma, Blastomyces* and possibly other fungi. (3) Coccidioidin may boost level of skin sensitivity to coccidioidin in already sensitive individuals. (4) The skin test may be negative in severe forms of disease (anergy) or when prolonged periods of time have passed since infection.

Positive reaction - Induration of 5 mm or more. Erythema without induration is considered negative. Read tests both at 24 and 48 hours because some reactions may fade after 36 hours. A positive test reaction indicates present or past infection with *Coccidioides immitis*.

Negative reaction - A negative test means the individual has not been sensitized to coccidioidin or has lost sensitivity.

Storage: Store at 2° to 8°C (35° to 46°F).

Rx	**Spherulin** (Berkeley Biologicals)	1:10 dilution. In 0.5 ml vials.[1] 1:100 dilution. In 1 ml vials.[1]

[1] With 1:10,000 thimerosal.

HISTOPLASMIN

Histoplasmin skin test is seldom used since it may increase the complement fixation titer, which is the preferred method used to diagnose an active infection. Definitive diagnosis requires demonstration of the organism by culture or histology.

Indications:

An aid in diagnosing histoplasmosis, in detecting delayed hypersensitivity to *Histoplasma capsulatum* and in differentiating possible histoplasmosis from coccidioidomycosis, sarcoidosis and other mycotic or bacterial infections, and in interpreting x-rays showing pulmonary infiltration and calcification.

May also be useful in epidemiological studies of persons with exposure to histoplasmosis and other infectious disease.

Precautions:

Local reactions: Greater than recommended doses may produce severe erythema and induration followed by necrosis and ulceration that may last for several weeks.

Hypersensitivity reactions: Have epinephrine immediately available in case an anaphylactoid or acute hypersensitivity reaction occurs. See also Management of Acute Hypersensitivity Reactions

Laboratory tests: If serological studies are indicated, draw the blood sample prior to administering the skin test or within 48 to 96 hours following the skin test injection. After this time period, a rise in titer associated with a positive skin test may occur.

Adverse Reactions:

Local: In highly sensitive individuals, vesiculation, ulceration or necrosis may occur at the test site and may result in scarring. Cold packs or topical steroids may provide symptomatic relief of the associated pain, pruritus and discomfort.

Hypersensitivity: Urticaria, angioedema, shortness of breath and excessive perspiration.

Administration and Dosage:

Inject intradermally only.

Test method: Inject 0.1 ml intradermally into the flexor surface of the forearm. Use a tuberculin syringe and a 26-gauge x ⅜ inch or 27-gauge x ½ inch needle. If correctly injected, a small bleb will rise over the needle point. Read reactions 48 to 72 hours after injection. The usual delayed skin test reaction appears in 24 hours and reaches a maximum in 48 to 72 hours.

Interpretation: Describe and measure the reaction in terms of millimeters of induration and degree of reaction (from slight induration to vesiculation and necrosis). A reaction of 5 mm or greater induration is positive. In case of doubt and if clinically indicated, repeat the test only after obtaining serum for antibody titer.

Positive reaction - May indicate a past infection or a mild, subacute or chronic infection with *H capsulatum* or immunologically-related organisms, such as *Blastomyces* or *Coccidioides* species. It may also denote improvement in cases of serious illness of symptomatic histoplasmosis that previously may have been histoplasmin-negative.

Differential diagnosis - Histoplasmin is of little value in diagnosing acute fulminating infections because a negative reaction usually occurs. In mild infections, repeatedly negative reactions may suggest the exclusion of *Histoplasma* as the causative agent. Employ the tuberculin test in conjunction with histoplasmin to exclude the possibility of tuberculosis. The histoplasmin skin test sometimes causes elevation of serum antibody titers to histoplasmin.

To distinguish lesions associated with histoplasmin sensitivity from other causes, consider: (1) Skin sensitivity to histoplasmin but not tuberculin; (2) lesions must persist for 2 months (to exclude transient pneumonic lesions); and (3) laboratory and clinical examinations to exclude tuberculosis, Boeck's sarcoid, sarcoidosis, Hodgkin's disease, etc. These criteria may help interpret roentgenographic findings.

Storage: Store at 2° to 8°C (35° to 46°F).

Rx	**Histoplasmin, Diluted** (Parke-Davis)	Standardized sterile filtrate from cultures of *Histoplasma capsulatum.*	Each vial[1] contains ten 0.1 ml doses.
Rx	**Histolyn-CYL** (Berkeley Biologicals)		Each 1.3 ml vial[1] contains ten 0.1 ml doses.

[1] With phenol and polysorbate 80.

CANDIDA AND TRICHOPHYTON EXTRACTS

Indications:

Trichophytin injections will regularly and specifically hyposensitize the skin to *Trichophyton*. Ringworm of the hands and feet is most often due to *Trichophyton* or *Candida albicans*. Extracts of these fungi are used for the desensitizing treatment of mycotic skin infections caused by these organisms.

Unlabeled uses: As components of a battery of skin tests to screen for cell-mediated immunity (anergy).

Warnings:

Markedly sensitive patients may develop a local reaction; large cold packs will lessen discomfort.

Some patients have exhibited extraordinarily severe local and focal reactions to the test solution of 1:30. Retest such patients with a more dilute solution (1:30,000 to 1:3,000, etc). These results may indicate treatment initiation with a further dilution (1:10 or 1:100) of the weakest treatment mixture employed.

Occasionally, areas of epidermophytosis or "ID" reaction will become more inflamed a few hours after extract injection, indicating that allergy is present and probably controllable. However, greatly reduce dosage.

Observe caution in this treatment. Sometimes small quantities suffice and satisfactory desensitization can be achieved without significant reactions at the injection site. If the patient develops increasing local immediate or delayed reactions after the injection, stop injections for 14 days and then restart, using 0.1 ml of a 1:100 dilution of previous concentration.

Usage in Pregnancy: Studies indicate no increased risk to the fetus or to the mother who is treated cautiously with immunotherapy during a normal pregnancy. Because histamines may contract uterine muscle, avoid any allergic reaction that would release significant amounts of histamine, either from allergen exposure or hyposensitization overdose.

Precautions:

Hypersensitivity: Observe patients for 15 minutes after each treatment and instruct them to return to the office promptly if symptoms of an allergic reaction or shock occur. *If anaphylactic reaction* occurs, have epinephrine available. See also Management of Acute Hypersensitivity Reactions on p. viii.

Adverse Reactions:

Systemic: Mild exaggeration of the patient's allergic symptoms to hives or to anaphylactic reactions, shock or even death from anaphylaxis.

Local: Wheal or swelling at the injection site occurs frequently and is not a cause for alarm; if persistent, the dosage may need adjustment. Expect a mild burning immediately after injection; this subsides in 10 to 20 seconds. Prolonged pain or pain radiating up the arm indicates the injection has been given IM.

(Continued on following page)

CANDIDA AND TRICHOPHYTON EXTRACTS (Cont.)

Administration and Dosage:

Do not administer IV. Shallow SC or intradermal injection is recommended.

Use a sterile tuberculin syringe with a needle at least ⅝" long and graduated in 0.01 ml units to measure each dose.

Diagnosis: A positive trichophytin specific reaction must occur with a concentration no stronger than 1:30, given intradermally. A specific oidiomycin reaction must be positive in a concentration no stronger than 1:100. Inject 0.1 ml of the diluted extract intradermally into the volar forearm; observe sites 24 to 48 hours later. The reaction is of the tuberculin "delayed" type.

A delayed reaction consisting of erythema and induration 5 mm or greater is a positive reaction.

If the reaction area for either type extract is from 5 to 20 mm, use the test strength dilution to start treatment. If the reaction area is greater than 20 mm, further dilute the extracts; a dilution of 1:100 for trichophytin and 1:500 for oidiomycin is recommended.

Treatment: Judge hypersensitization by the diminution or disappearance of the skin reactivity. To constantly observe changes in skin reactivity, apply treatment by intracutaneous injections of 0.1 ml of the selected mixture at 5 to 7 day intervals. Shallow SC injection is a less painful alternate method.

When this treatment has produced a diminution in the sensitivity, the area of cutaneous reaction (24 to 72 hours after injection) will be lessened.

As the skin reaction diminishes, increase the dosage by 0.1 ml in each of 2 sites, then in 3 sites and so on, until the injections no longer cause any reaction and the dermatomycosis has disappeared.

In some cases it is advisable to carry the hyposensitization further and employ stronger extracts when the patient no longer reacts to trichophytin 1:30 or oidiomycin 1:100.

Prepare further dilutions by using prefilled 4.5 ml vials of albumin saline, normal saline or buffered saline.

Dilution schedule: 1:30 dilution - Add 0.5 ml of undiluted extract to a 4.5 ml diluent vial, which will result in a 1:10 dilution. Remove with sterile syringe 2.5 ml from a second 4.5 ml diluent vial and discard. To the remaining 2 ml of diluent, add 1 ml of the 1:10 dilution. This will provide 3 ml of 1:30 extract.

1:100 dilution - Prepare 1:10 dilution by adding 0.5 ml of undiluted extract to 4.5 ml diluent vial; mix and add 0.5 ml of 1:10 dilution to second 4.5 ml of diluent vial, which will provide 5 ml of 1:100 dilution.

1:500 dilution - Remove 0.5 ml from a 4.5 diluent vial and add 1 ml of the 1:100 dilution.

1:1000, 1:10,000, etc - Prepare dilutions by adding 0.5 ml of 1:100 to 4.5 ml diluent; 0.5 ml 1:1000 to 4.5 ml diluent, etc.

Storage: Store at 2° to 8°C (35° to 46°F).

Rx	**Dermatophytin (Trichophytin)** (Hollister-Stier)	Prepared from the filtrates of mixtures of 21 day maltose broth cultures of Trichophyton mentagrophytes, *T rubrum* (purpureum) and *T tonsurans.* In 5 ml vials (undiluted extract) and 5 ml (diluted 1:30) vials.
Rx	**Dermatophytin "O" (Oidiomycin)** (Hollister-Stier)	Prepared from the filtrate of a 21 day maltose broth culture of *Candida* (Monilia) *albicans.* In 5 ml vials (undiluted extract) and 5 ml (diluted 1:100) vials.

MUMPS SKIN TEST ANTIGEN

Indications:

Based on a report by the Panel on Review of Skin Test Antigens and other information, the Food and Drug Administration has directed that further investigation be conducted before this product is determined to be fully effective for labeled indications.

Used to assess immunocompetency. Since most of the population (except the very young) have had contact or infection with mumps virus, they usually demonstrate a delayed cutaneous hypersensitivity to mumps skin test antigen if the immune system is intact.

Contraindications:

Because the antigen is prepared from virus cultivated in chicken embryo, persons sensitive to avian protein may have a severe reaction following administration. Therefore, do not test those sensitive to chicken, eggs or feathers.

Hypersensitivity to thimerosal.

Precautions:

Hypersensitivity reactions: Treatment facilities should be readily available. See also Management of Acute Hypersensitivity Reactions

Neurologic effects: Encephalopathies and peripheral nervous system lesions have followed the administration of almost all biologicals, although this has not been reported after the injection of mumps skin test antigen.

Administration and Dosage:

Must be given intradermally. If it is injected SC, no reaction or an unreliable reaction may occur.

Test method: Inject 0.1 ml intradermally on the inner surface of the forearm after suitable preparation of the skin. Examine the reaction in 24 to 48 hours.

Interpretation:

Positive reaction – An area of erythema 1.5 cm or more in diameter, with or without induration, indicates sensitivity.

Negative reaction – If the test has been given correctly, probably indicates either anergy or nonsensitivity.

Pseudopositive reactions may develop in persons sensitive to egg protein.

Storage: Store between 2° and 8°C (35° to 46°F).

Rx	**MSTA** (Connaught)	**Antigen:** Suspension of killed mumps virus. 40 complement-fixing units per ml. In 1 ml vials[1] (10 tests).

[1] With 0.012 M glycine, < 1:8,000 formaldehyde solution and 1:10,000 thimerosal.

SKIN TEST ANTIGENS, MULTIPLE

The skin test for multiple antigens consists of a disposable applicator with eight sterile heads preloaded with the following seven delayed hypersensitivity skin test antigens and glycerin negative control for percutaneous administration: Tetanus Toxoid Antigen, Diphtheria Toxoid Antigen, Streptococcus Antigen, Old Tuberculin, Candida Antigen, Trichophyton Antigen and Proteus Antigen. The delayed cutaneous responses associated with this test appear to be typical cellular hypersensitivity reactions.

Indications:

For detection of anergy (nonresponsiveness to antigens) by means of delayed hypersensitivity skin testing.

Contraindications:

Do not apply on acneiform, infected or inflamed skin. Although severe systemic reactions are rare to diphtheria and tetanus antigens, persons known to have a history of systemic reactions should be tested only after the test heads containing these antigens have been removed.

Warnings:

Hypersensitivity: Epinephrine should be available. See also Management of Acute Hypersensitivity Reactions.

Pregnancy: Category C. Animal reproduction studies have not been conducted. It is not known whether skin test antigens can cause fetal harm when administered to a pregnant woman or can affect reproduction capacity. Give to a pregnant woman only if clearly needed. Pregnancy may result in a decreased level of sensitivity to the test antigens.

Children: Skin testing is recommended only for subjects $\geq$ 17 years. Safety and efficacy in children below this age have not been established.

Precautions:

Reactivity to delayed hypersensitivity skin test antigens may decrease or disappear temporarily as a result of: Febrile illness; measles and other viral infections; live virus vaccination including measles, mumps, rubella and poliomyelitis vaccines.

Loss of reactivity may occur in patients undergoing treatment with drugs or procedures that suppress immunity such as: Corticosteroids, chemotherapeutic agents, antilymphocyte globulin and irradiation.

Administration and Dosage:

Remove skin test antigens from refrigeration approximately 1 hour before use.

Select only test sites that permit sufficient surface area and subcutaneous tissue to allow adequate penetration of all points on all 8 test heads. Preferred sites are the volar surfaces of the arms and the back; skin of the posterior thighs may be used. If several tests are planned, alternate forearms. Avoid hairy areas when possible because reaction interpretation will be more difficult.

Interpretation: Read test sites at both 24 and 48 hours, if possible, and use the largest reaction recorded from the 2 readings at each test site. If 2 readings are not possible, a single 48 hour reading is recommended.

A positive reaction from any of the 7 antigens is induration of $\geq$ 2 mm, providing there is no induration at the negative control site.

Periodic testing can determine if anergy persists or if skin reactivity has returned. If periodic testing is done more frequently than every 2 months, rotate the test sites so that retesting is not conducted at the same site sooner than 2 months. Refer to the manufacturer's scoring system for instruction.

Storage: Store at 2° to 8°C (35° to 46°F).

Rx	**Multitest CMI** (Merieux)	In single use, preloaded applicators.

PEGADEMASE BOVINE

Actions:

Pharmacology: Pegademase bovine is a modified enzyme used for enzyme replacement therapy for the treatment of severe combined immunodeficiency disease (SCID) associated with a deficiency of adenosine deaminase. The drug will not benefit patients with immunodeficiency due to other causes. It is a conjugate of numerous strands of monomethoxypolyethylene glycol (PEG), covalently attached to the enzyme adenosine deaminase (ADA). ADA, used in the manufacture of pegademase bovine, is derived from bovine intestine.

Pegademase bovine provides specific replacement of the deficient enzyme. In the absence of the enzyme ADA, the purine substrates adenosine, 2'-deoxyadenosine and their metabolites are toxic to lymphocytes. The direct action of pegademase bovine is the correction of these metabolic abnormalities. Improvement in immune function and diminished frequency of opportunistic infections only occurs after metabolic abnormalities are corrected. There is a lag between the correction of the metabolic abnormalities and improved immune function. This period of time is variable, from a few weeks to as long as 6 months. In contrast to the natural history of combined immunodeficiency disease due to ADA deficiency, a trend toward diminished frequency of opportunistic infections and fewer complications of infections has occurred in patients receiving pegademase bovine.

SCID associated with a deficiency of ADA is a rare, inherited, and often fatal disease. In the absence of the ADA enzyme, the purine substrates adenosine and 2'-deoxyadenosine accumulate, causing metabolic abnormalities that are directly toxic to lymphocytes.

The immune deficiency can be cured by bone marrow transplantation. When a suitable bone marrow donor is unavailable or when bone marrow transplantation fails, nonselective replacement of the ADA enzyme has been provided by periodic irradiated red blood cell transfusions. However, transmission of viral infections and iron overload are serious risks, and relatively few ADA-deficient patients have benefited from chronic transfusion therapy.

In patients with ADA deficiency, rigorous adherence to a schedule of pegademase bovine administration can eliminate the toxic metabolites of ADA deficiency and result in improved immune function. Treatment must be carefully monitored by measurement of the level of ADA activity in plasma. Monitoring of the level of deoxyadenosine triphosphate (dATP) in erythrocytes is also helpful in determining that the dose is adequate.

Pharmacokinetics: The pharmacokinetics and biochemical effects have been studied in six children ranging in age from 6 weeks to 12 years with SCID associated with ADA deficiency. After IM injection, peak plasma levels of ADA activity were reached within 2 to 3 days. The plasma elimination half-life of ADA was variable, even for the same child. The range was 3 to > 6 days. Following weekly injections of 15 U/kg, the average trough level of ADA activity in plasma was between 20 and 25 mcmol/hr/ml.

The changes in red blood cell deoxyadenosine nucleotide (ie, dATP) and S-adenosylhomocysteine hydrolase (SAHase) have been evaluated. In patients with ADA deficiency, inadequate elimination of 2'-deoxyadenosine caused a marked elevation in dATP and a decrease in SAHase level in red blood cells. Prior to treatment with pegademase bovine, the levels of dATP in the red blood cells ranged from 0.056 to 0.899 mcmol/ml of erythrocytes. After 2 months of maintenance treatment, the levels decreased to 0.007 to 0.015 mcmol/ml. The normal value of dATP is below 0.001 mcmol/ml. In the same period of time, the levels of SAHase increased from the pretreatment range of 0.09 to 0.22 nmol/hr/mg protein to a range of 2.37 to 5.16 nmol/hr/mg protein. The normal value for SAHase is 4.18 ± 1.9 nmol/hr/mg protein.

Indications:

For enzyme replacement therapy for ADA deficiency in patients with severe combined immunodeficiency disease who are not suitable candidates for or who have failed bone marrow transplantation. Pegademase bovine is recommended for use in infants from birth or in children of any age at the time of diagnosis. It is not intended as a replacement for HLA identical bone marrow transplant therapy, and it is also not intended to replace continued close medical supervision and the initiation of appropriate diagnostic tests and therapy (eg, antibiotics, nutrition, oxygen, gammaglobulin) as indicated for intercurrent illnesses.

Contraindications:

There is no evidence to support the safety and efficacy of pegademase bovine as preparatory or support therapy for bone marrow transplantation. Since the drug is administered by IM injection, use with caution in patients with thrombocytopenia and do not use if thrombocytopenia is severe.

(Continued on following page)

PEGADEMASE BOVINE (Cont.)

Warnings:

Product potency testing prior to distribution may not assure the initial and continuing potency of each new lot of pegademase bovine. Report any laboratory or clinical indication of a decrease in potency *immediately* by telephone to Enzon (201-668-1800).

Pregnancy: Category C. It is not known whether pegademase bovine can cause fetal harm when administered to a pregnant woman or can affect reproduction capacity. Give to a pregnant woman only if clearly needed.

Lactation: It is not known whether pegademase bovine is excreted in breast milk. Exercise caution when administering to a nursing woman.

Precautions:

Immunodeficiency: Maintain appropriate care to protect immune-deficient patients until improvement in immune function has been documented. The degree of immune function improvement may vary from patient to patient and, therefore, each patient will require appropriate care consistent with immunologic status.

Laboratory test monitoring: Monitor the treatment of SCID associated with ADA deficiency with pegademase bovine by measuring plasma ADA activity and red blood cell dATP levels.

Determine plasma ADA activity and red cell dATP prior to treatment. Once treatment has been initiated, a desirable range of plasma ADA activity (trough level before maintenance injection) should be 15 to 35 mcmol/hr/ml. This minimum trough level will ensure that plasma ADA activity from injection to injection is maintained above the level of total erythrocyte ADA activity in the blood of normal individuals.

Determine plasma ADA activity (pre-injection) every 1 to 2 weeks during the first 8 to 12 weeks of treatment in order to establish an effective dose. After 2 months of maintenance treatment, red cell dATP levels should decrease to a range of $\leq$ 0.005 to 0.015 mcmol/ml. The normal value of dATP is below 0.001 mcmol/ml. Once the level of dATP has fallen adequately, measure 2 to 4 times during the remainder of the first year and 2 to 3 times a year thereafter, assuming no interruption in therapy.

Between 3 and 9 months, determine plasma ADA twice a month, then monthly until after 18 to 24 months of treatment. In patients who have successfully been maintained on therapy for 2 years, continue to have plasma ADA measured every 2 to 4 months and red cell dATP measured twice yearly. More frequent monitoring would be necessary if therapy were interrupted or if an enhanced rate of clearance of plasma ADA activity develops.

Once effective ADA plasma levels have been established, should a patient's plasma ADA activity level fall below 10 mcmol/hr/ml (which cannot be attributed to improper dosing, sample handling or antibody development) then all patients receiving this lot of pegademase bovine will be required to have a blood sample for plasma ADA determination taken prior to their next injection. The index patient will require retesting for determination of plasma ADA activity prior to their next injection. If this value, as well as the value from one of the other patients from a different site, is $<$ 10 mcmol/hr/ml, then the lot in use will be recalled and replaced with a new clinical lot by Enzon.

Immune function, including the ability to produce antibodies, generally improves after 2 to 6 months of therapy, and matures over a longer period. Compared with the natural history of combined immunodeficiency disease due to ADA deficiency, a trend toward diminished frequency of opportunistic infections and fewer complications of infections has occurred in patients receiving pegademase bovine. However, the lag between the correction of the metabolic abnormalities and improved immune function with a trend toward diminished frequency of infections and complications of infection is variable, and has ranged from a few weeks to $\approx$ 6 months. Improvement in the general clinical status of the patient may be gradual (as evidenced by improvement in various clinical parameters) but should be apparent by the end of the first year of therapy.

A decline in immune function, with increased risk of opportunistic infections and complications of infection, will result from failure to maintain adequate levels of plasma ADA activity (whether due to the development of antibody, improper calculation of dosage, interruption of treatment or to improper storage with subsequent loss of activity). If a persistent decline in plasma ADA activity occurs, monitor immune function and clinical status closely and take precautions to minimize the risk of infection. If antibody to ADA or pegademase bovine is found to be the cause of a persistent fall in plasma ADA activity, then adjustment in the dosage and other measures may be taken to induce tolerance and restore adequate ADA activity.

(Precautions continued on following page)

PEGADEMASE BOVINE (Cont.)

Precautions (Cont.):

Antibody to pegademase bovine may develop in patients and may result in more rapid clearance of the drug. Suspect antibody to pegademase bovine if a persistent fall in pre-injection level of plasma ADA to $<$ 10 mcmol/hr/ml occurs. If other causes for a decline in plasma ADA levels can be ruled out (eg, improper storage of vials [freezing or prolonged storage at temperatures $>$ 4°C], or improper handling of plasma samples [eg, repeated freezing and thawing during transport to laboratory]), then perform a specific assay for antibody to ADA and pegademase bovine (ELISA, enzyme inhibition).

One of 12 patients showed an enhanced rate of clearance of plasma ADA activity after 5 months of therapy at 15 U/kg/week. Enhanced clearance was correlated with the appearance of an antibody that directly inhibited both unmodified ADA and pegademase bovine. Subsequently, the patient was treated with twice weekly IM injections at an increased dose of 20 U/kg, or a total weekly dose of 40 U/kg. No adverse effects were observed at the higher dose and effective levels of plasma ADA were restored. After 4 months, the patient returned to a weekly dosage schedule of 20 U/kg and effective plasma levels have been maintained.

Drug Interactions:

Vidarabine is a substrate for ADA and **2'-deoxycoformycin** is a potent inhibitor of ADA. Thus, the activities of these drugs and pegademase bovine could be substantially altered if they are used in combination with one another.

Adverse Reactions:

Clinical experience with pegademase bovine is limited. The following adverse reactions have occurred: Headache (one patient) and pain at the injection site (two patients).

Overdosage:

An intraperitoneal dose of 50,000 U/kg of pegademase bovine in mice resulted in weight loss up to 9%.

Administration and Dosage:

Before prescribing pegademase bovine, the physician should be thoroughly familiar with the details of this prescribing information. For further information concerning the essential monitoring of therapy, contact Enzon, Inc., 40 Cragwood Road, South Plainfield, NJ 07080 (201-668-1800).

Pegademase bovine is recommended for use in infants from birth or in children of any age at the time of diagnosis.

Administer every 7 days as an IM injection. Individualize the dosage. *First dose:* 10 U/kg; *second dose:* 15 U/kg; *third dose:* 20 U/kg; *usual maintenance dose:* 20 U/kg/week. Further increases of 5 U/kg/week may be necessary, but a maximum single dose of 30 U/kg should not be exceeded.

Plasma levels of ADA more than twice the upper limit of 35 mcmol/hr/ml have occurred on occasion in several patients, and have been maintained for several weeks in one patient who received twice weekly injections (20 U/kg per dose). No adverse effects have been observed at these higher levels; there is no evidence that maintaining pre-injection plasma ADA $>$ 35 mcmol/hr/ml produces any additional clinical benefits.

Dose proportionality has not been established; closely monitor patients when the dosage is increased. Pegademase bovine is not recommended for IV administration.

Establish the optimal dosage and schedule of administration for each patient based on monitoring of plasma ADA activity levels (trough levels before maintenance injection), biochemical markers of ADA deficiency (primarily red cell dATP content). Since improvement in immune function follows correction of metabolic abnormalities, maintenance dosage in individual patients should be aimed at achieving the following biochemical goals: 1) Maintain plasma ADA activity (trough levels before maintenance injection) in the range of 15 to 35 mcmol/hr/ml (assayed at 37°C); and 2) decline in erythrocyte dATP to $\leq$ 0.005 to 0.015 mcmol/ml packed erythrocytes, or $\leq$ 1% of the total erythrocyte adenine nucleotide (ATP + dATP) content, with a normal ATP level, as measured in a pre-injection sample. In addition, continued monitoring of immune function and clinical status is essential in any patient with a primary immunodeficiency disease and should be continued in patients being treated with pegademase bovine.

Admixture incompatibility: Pegademase bovine should not be diluted nor mixed with any other drug prior to administration.

Storage: Refrigerate. Store between 2°C and 8°C (36°F and 46°F). Do not freeze. Pegademase bovine should not be stored at room temperature. This product should not be used if there are any indications that it may have been frozen.

Rx	**Adagen** (Enzon)	**Injection:** 250 units[1]/ml[2]	In 1.5 ml vials.

[1] One unit of activity is defined as the amount of ADA that converts 1 mcM of adenosine to inosine per minute at 25°C and pH 7.3.

[2] With 1.2 mg monobasic sodium phosphate, 5.58 mg dibasic sodium phosphate, 8.5 mg sodium chloride and water for injection.

In addition to the commercially available products, the Centers for Disease Control in Atlanta, GA can supply various rare immunobiological products for use in certain emergency situations or for special immunization needs. These biological products are available through the CDC Drug Service, Division of Immunologic, Oncologic, and Hematologic Diseases, Center for Infectious Diseases, Centers for Disease Control in Atlanta, Georgia. For further information, call 404-639-3356, Monday through Friday, 8 am to 4:30 pm, or refer to the numbers listed below. After working hours, on weekends and holidays, call 404-639-2888 (emergency requests only).

The following products are available:

	Telephone Number
Antitoxins Botulism Equine trivalent Antitoxin (ABE) – Licensed Diphtheria Equine Antitoxin – Licensed	404-639-3356 404-639-1867
Immune Serum Globulins Western Equine Encephalitis (WEE) Immune Globulin – IND* Vaccinia Immune Globulin (VIG) (Human) – Licensed	404-639-3356
Vaccines (for high laboratory risk immunization, nonemergency) Botulinum Toxoid, pentavalent (ABCDE) - IND* Japanese Encephalitis Vaccine – IND* Smallpox Vaccine	404-639-3356

* Investigational New Drug.

INTERFERON GAMMA-1B

Actions:

Pharmacology: Interferon gamma-1b, a biologic response modifier, is a single-chain polypeptide containing 140 amino acids. Production of interferon gamma is achieved by fermentation of a genetically engineered *Escherichia coli* bacterium containing the DNA which encodes for the human protein.

Interferons are a family of functionally related, species-specific proteins synthesized by eukaryotic cells in response to viruses and a variety of natural and synthetic stimuli. The most striking differences between interferon gamma and other classes of interferon concern the immunomodulatory properties of this molecule. While gamma, alpha and beta interferons share certain properties, interferon gamma has potent phagocyte-activating effects not seen with other interferon preparations, including generation of toxic oxygen metabolites within phagocytes, which are capable of mediating the killing of microorganisms such as *Staphylococcus aureus, Toxoplasma gondii, Leishmania donovani, Listeria monocytogenes*, and *Mycobacterium avium intracellulare*.

Clinical studies in patients using interferon gamma have revealed a broad range of biological activities including the enhancement of the oxidative metabolism of tissue macrophages, enhancement of antibody-dependent cellular cytotoxicity and natural killer cell activity. Additionally, effects of Fc receptor expression on monocytes and major histocompatibility antigen expression have been noted.

To the extent that interferon gamma is produced by antigen-stimulated T lymphocytes and regulates the activity of immune cells, it is appropriate to characterize interferon gamma as a lymphokine of the interleukin type. There is growing evidence that interferon gamma interacts functionally with other interleukin molecules such as interleukin-2, and that all of the interleukins form part of a complex, lymphokine regulatory network. For example, interferon gamma and interleukin-4 appear to reciprocally interact to regulate murine IgE levels; interferon gamma can suppress IgE levels and inhibit the production of collagen at the transcription level in human systems.

Pharmacokinetics: Following single-dose administration of 100 mcg/m², interferon gamma is rapidly cleared after IV use (1.4 L/minute) and slowly absorbed after IM or SC injection. After IM or SC injection, the apparent fraction of dose absorbed was > 89%. The mean elimination half-life after IV administration was 38 minutes. The mean elimination half-lives for IM and SC dosing were 2.9 and 5.9 hours, respectively. Peak plasma concentrations occurred approximately 4 hours (1.5 ng/ml) after IM dosing and 7 hours (0.6 ng/ml) after SC dosing. Multiple-dose SC pharmacokinetic studies were conducted in 38 healthy male subjects. There was no accumulation of drug after 12 consecutive daily injections of 100 mcg/m². Administration to nephrectomized mice and squirrel monkeys demonstrated a reduction in clearance of interferon gamma from blood; however, prior nephrectomy did not prevent elimination.

Clinical trials: A randomized, double-blind, placebo controlled study in patients (n = 128; 1 to 44 years of age) with chronic granulomatous disease (an inherited disorder characterized by deficient phagocyte oxidative metabolism) was performed to determine whether SC interferon gamma 3 times weekly could decrease the incidence of serious infectious episodes and improve existing infectious and inflammatory conditions. Most patients received prophylactic antibiotics. Serious infection was defined as a clinical event requiring hospitalization and the use of parenteral antibiotics. There was a 67% reduction in relative risk of serious infection in patients receiving interferon gamma (n = 63) compared to placebo (n = 65). Additional supportive evidence of treatment benefit included a twofold reduction in the number of primary serious infections in the interferon gamma group and the total number and rate of serious infections including recurrent events. Placebo patients required three times as many inpatient hospitalization days for treatment of clinical events compared to patients receiving interferon gamma. The beneficial effect of therapy was observed throughout the entire study, in which the mean duration of administration was 8.9 months per patient.

Indications:

For reducing the frequency and severity of serious infections associated with chronic granulomatous disease.

Contraindications:

Hypersensitivity to interferon gamma, *E coli* derived products or any component of the product.

Warnings:

Seizure disorders/compromised CNS function: Exercise caution in patients with these conditions. CNS adverse reactions including decreased mental status, gait disturbance and dizziness have been observed, particularly in patients receiving doses > 250 mcg/m²/day. Most of these abnormalities were mild and reversible within a few days upon dose reduction or discontinuation of therapy.

(Warnings continued on following page)

INTERFERON GAMMA-1B (Cont.)

Warnings (Cont.):

Cardiac disease: Use with caution in patients with pre-existing cardiac disease, including symptoms of ischemia, CHF or arrhythmia. No direct cardiotoxic effect has been demonstrated, but it is possible that acute and transient "flu-like" or constitutional symptoms such as fever and chills frequently associated with interferon gamma administration at doses of ≥ 250 mcg/m²/day may exacerbate pre-existing conditions.

Myelosuppression: Exercise caution in patients with myelosuppression. Reversible neutropenia and elevation of hepatic enzymes can be dose-limiting at doses > 250 mcg/m²/day. Thrombocytopenia and proteinuria have also occurred rarely.

Hypersensitivity: Acute serious hypersensitivity reactions have not been observed in patients receiving interferon gamma; however, if such an acute reaction develops, discontinue the drug immediately and institute appropriate medical therapy. Refer to Management of Acute Hypersensitivity Reactions. Transient cutaneous rashes have occurred in some patients following injection but have rarely necessitated treatment interruption.

Fertility impairment: Female monkeys treated with daily SC doses of 150 mcg/kg (approximately 100 times the human dose) exhibited irregular menstrual cycles or absence of cyclicity during treatment.

Pregnancy: Category C. Interferon gamma has shown an increased incidence of abortions in primates when given in doses approximately 100 times the human dose. There are no adequate and well controlled studies in pregnant women. Use during pregnancy only if the potential benefit justifies the potential risk to the fetus. In addition, studies evaluating recombinant murine interferon gamma in pregnant mice revealed increased incidences of uterine bleeding and abortifacient activity and decreased neonatal viability at maternally toxic doses. The clinical significance of this observation with recombinant murine interferon gamma tested in a homologous system is uncertain.

Lactation: It is not known whether interferon gamma is excreted in breast milk. Because of the potential for serious adverse reactions in nursing infants, decide whether to discontinue nursing or to discontinue the drug, depending on the importance of the drug to the mother.

Children: Safety and efficacy in children < 1 year of age has not been established.

Precautions:

Monitoring: In addition to tests normally required for monitoring patients with chronic granulomatous disease, the following laboratory tests are recommended for all patients prior to beginning therapy and at 3 month intervals during treatment: Hematologic tests including complete blood counts, differential and platelet counts; blood chemistries including renal and liver function tests; urinalysis.

Drug Interactions:

Myelosuppressive agents: Exercise caution when administering interferon gamma in combination with other potentially myelosuppressive agents (see Warnings).

Preclinical studies in rodents using species-specific interferon gamma have demonstrated a decrease in hepatic microsomal cytochrome P-450 concentrations. This could potentially lead to a depression of the hepatic metabolism of certain drugs that utilize this degradative pathway.

Adverse Reactions:

The following data on adverse reactions are based on the SC use of 50 mcg/m² interferon gamma 3 times weekly in 63 patients with chronic granulomatous disease.

Interferon Gamma-1B Adverse Reactions (%)					
Adverse reaction	Interferon gamma-1b (n = 63)	Placebo (n = 65)	Adverse reaction	Interferon gamma-1b (n = 63)	Placebo (n = 65)
Fever	52	28	Nausea	10	2
Headache	33	9	Abdominal pain[1]	8	3
Rash	17	6	Weight loss	6	6
Chills	14	0	Myalgia	6	0
Injection site erythema or tenderness	14	2	Anorexia	3	5
			Depression[1]	3	0
			Arthralgia	2	0
Fatigue	14	11	Back pain[1]	2	0
Diarrhea	14	12	Injection site pain	0	2
Vomiting	13	5			

[1] May have been related to underlying disease.

(Adverse Reactions continued on following page)

INTERFERON GAMMA-1B (Cont.)

Adverse Reactions (Cont.):

Interferon gamma has also been evaluated in additional disease states in studies in which patients have generally received higher doses (> 100 mcg/m²/day) administered by IM injection or IV infusion. All of the previously described adverse reactions which occurred in patients with chronic granulomatous disease have also been observed in patients receiving higher doses. Adverse reactions not observed in patients with chronic granulomatous disease receiving doses < 100 mcg/m²/day but seen rarely in patients receiving interferon gamma in other studies include:

Cardiovascular – Hypotension; syncope; tachyarrhythmia; heart block; heart failure; myocardial infarction.

CNS – Confusion; disorientation; gait disturbance; parkinsonian symptoms; seizure; hallucinations; transient ischemic attacks.

GI – Hepatic insufficiency; GI bleeding; pancreatitis.

Hematologic – Deep venous thrombosis; pulmonary embolism.

Pulmonary – Tachypnea; bronchospasm; interstitial pneumonitis.

Metabolic – Hyponatremia; hyperglycemia.

Other – Exacerbation of dermatomyositis; reversible renal insufficiency.

Patient Information:

Inform patients of the potential benefits and risks associated with treatment. If home use is determined to be desirable by the physician, give instructions on appropriate use, including a review of the contents of the Patient Information insert. This information is intended to aid in the safe and effective use of the medication; it is not a disclosure of all possible adverse or intended effects.

If home use is prescribed, supply the patients with a puncture resistant container for the disposal of used syringes and needles. Thoroughly instruct patients in the importance of proper disposal and caution against any reuse of needles and syringes. Dispose of the full container according to the directions provided by the physician.

The most common adverse experiences are "flu-like" or constitutional symptoms such as fever, headache, chills, myalgia or fatigue which may decrease in severity as treatment continues. Some of the "flu-like" symptoms may be minimized by bedtime administration. Acetaminophen may be used to prevent or partially alleviate the fever and headache.

Administration and Dosage:

Chronic granulomatous disease: 50 mcg/m² (1.5 million U/m²) for patients whose body surface area is > 0.5 m² and 1.5 mcg/kg/dose for patients whose body surface area is ≤ 0.5 m². Administer SC 3 times weekly (eg, Monday, Wednesday, Friday). The optimum sites of injection are the right and left deltoid and anterior thigh. Interferon gamma can be administered by a physician, nurse, family member or patient when trained in the administration of SC injections.

The formulation does not contain a preservative. A vial is suitable for a single dose only. Discard the unused portion of any vial.

Higher doses are not recommended. Safety and efficacy have not been established for interferon gamma given in doses greater or less than the recommended dose of 50 mcg/m². The minimum effective dose has not been established.

If severe reactions occur, modify the dosage (50% reduction) or discontinue therapy until the adverse reaction abates.

Interferon gamma may be administered using either sterilized glass or plastic disposable syringes.

Storage/Stability: Vials must be placed in a 2° to 8°C (36° to 46°F) refrigerator immediately upon receipt to ensure optimal retention of physical and biochemical integrity; do not freeze. Avoid excessive or vigorous agitation; do not shake. An unentered vial should not be left at room temperature for a total time exceeding 12 hours prior to use. Vials exceeding this time period should not be returned to the refrigerator; discard such vials.

Rx	**Actimmune** (Genentech)	**Injection:** 100 mcg (3 million U)	In single-dose vials.[1]

[1] With 20 mg mannitol, 0.36 mg sodium succinate, 0.05 mg polysorbate 20.

chapter 10

topical preparations

General Considerations in Topical Ophthalmic Drug Therapy:

Proper administration of a dosage form is essential to an optimal therapeutic response. In many instances, health professionals may be too casual when instructing patients on proper use of ophthalmic products. The technique used in administering such products often determines drug safety and efficacy.

- The normal eye can retain ≈ 10 mcl of fluid (adjusted for the effect of blinking). The average dropper delivers 25 to 50 mcl/drop. The value of more than one drop is questionable.
- Minimize systemic absorption of ophthalmic drops by compressing the lacrimal sac for 1 to 2 minutes following instillation of drops. This retards passage of drops via the nasolacrimal duct into areas of potential absorption such as nasal and pharyngeal mucosa.
- Because of rapid lacrimal drainage (16% per minute) and limited eye capacity, if multiple drop therapy is indicated, the best interval between drops is 5 minutes. This ensures that the first drop is not flushed away by the second or that the second drop is not diluted by the first.
- Topical anesthesia will increase the bioavailability of ophthalmic agents by decreasing the blink reflex and the production and turnover of tears.
- Factors that may increase absorption from ophthalmic dosage forms include lax eyelids of some patients, usually the elderly, which creates a greater reservoir for retention of drops, and hyperemic or diseased eyes.
- Use of eyecups is discouraged due to potential contamination and risk of spreading disease.
- Ophthalmic suspensions mix with tears less rapidly and remain in the cul-de-sac longer than solutions.
- Ophthalmic ointments maintain contact between the drug and ocular tissues by slowing the clearance rate to as little as 0.5% per minute. Ophthalmic ointments provide maximum contact between drug and external ocular tissues.
- Ophthalmic ointments may impede delivery of other ophthalmic drugs to the affected side by serving as a barrier to contact.
- Ointments may blur vision during the waking hours. Use with caution in conditions where visual clarity is critical (eg, operating motor equipment, reading).
- Monitor expiration dates closely. Do not use outdated medication.
- Ophthalmic solutions and ointments are frequently misused. Do not assume that patients know how to maximize safe and effective use of these agents. Appropriate patient education and counseling should accompany prescribing and dispensing of ophthalmics.

Topical application is the most common route of administration for ophthalmic drugs. Advantages of topical administration include convenience, simplicity, noninvasive nature and the ability of the patient to self-administer the medication. Because of blood and aqueous losses of drug, topical medications do not typically penetrate in useful concentrations to the posterior ocular structures and therefore are of no therapeutic benefit for diseases of the retina, optic nerve and other posterior segment structures.

Ingredients: The following inactive agents may be present in ophthalmic products:

PRESERVATIVES destroy or inhibit multiplication of microorganisms introduced into the product by accident.

benzalkonium chloride
benzethonium chloride
cetylpyridinium chloride
chlorobutanol
EDTA
mercurial preservatives (phenylmercuric nitrate, phenylmercuric acetate, thimerosal)
methyl and propylparabens
phenylethyl alcohol
sodium benzoate
sodium propionate
sorbic acid

VISCOSITY-INCREASING AGENTS slow drainage of the product from the eye, thus increasing retention time of the product. Increased bioavailability may result.

acetylated polyvinyl alcohol
carboxymethylcellulose sodium
dextran 70
gelatin
glycerin
hydroxyethylcellulose
hydroxypropyl methylcellulose
methylcellulose
polyethylene glycol 300
polysorbate 80
propylene glycol
polyvinyl alcohol 2%
polyvinylpyrrolidone
povidone

ANTIOXIDANTS:

EDTA
sodium bisulfite
sodium metabisulfite
sodium thiosulfate
thiourea

(Continued on following page)

Ingredients (Cont.):

WETTING AGENTS reduce surface tension, allowing the drug solution to spread over the eye.

polysorbate 20 and 80
poloxamer 282 (Pluronic L-92)
tyloxapol (Triton WR-1339)

BUFFERS: Ophthalmic products range from pH 6 to 8.

acetic acid
boric acid
hydrochloric acid
phosphoric acid
potassium bicarbonate
potassium borate and tetraborate
potassium carbonate
potassium citrate
potassium phosphates
sodium acetate
sodium bicarbonate
sodium biphosphate
sodium borate
sodium carbonate
sodium citrate
sodium hydroxide
sodium phosphate

TONICITY AGENTS help the ophthalmic product solutions to be isotonic with natural tears. Products in the sodium chloride equivalence range of 0.9% ± 0.2% are considered isotonic and will help prevent ocular pain and tissue damage. A range of 0.6% to 1.8% can usually be tolerated without damage.

buffers
dextran 40 and 70
dextrose
glycerin
potassium chloride
propylene glycol
sodium chloride

Medications:

Solutions and Suspensions: Most topical ocular preparations are commercially available as solutions or suspensions that are applied directly to the eye from the bottle, which serves as the eye dropper. Avoid touching the dropper tip to the eye because this can lead to contamination of the medication and may also cause ocular injury. Resuspend suspensions (notably, many ocular steroids) by shaking to provide an accurate dosage of drug.

Recommended Procedures for Administration of Solutions or Suspensions:

- Wash hands thoroughly before administration.
- Tilt head backward or lie down and gaze upward.
- Gently grasp lower eyelid below eyelashes and pull the eyelid away from the eye to form a pouch.
- Place dropper directly over eye. Avoid contact of the dropper with the eye, finger or any surface.
- Look upward just before applying a drop.
- After instilling the drop, look downward for several seconds.
- Release the lid slowly.
- Close eyes gently for 1 to 2 minutes. Closing the eyes tightly after instillation may expel medication from the cul-de-sac.
- Apply gentle pressure with fingers to the bridge of the nose (inside corner of eye). This retards drainage of solution from the intended area.
- Do not rub the eye. Minimize blinking.
- Do not rinse the dropper.
- Do not use eye drops that have changed color.
- If more than one type of ophthalmic drop is used, wait at least 5 minutes before administering the second agent.
- When the instillation of eye drops is difficult (eg, pediatric patients, adults with particularly strong blink reflex), the close-eye method may be used. This involves lying down, placing the prescribed number of drops on the eyelid in the inner corner of the eye, then opening eye so that drops will fall into the eye by gravity.

(Continued on following page)

Medications (Cont.):

Ointments: The primary purpose for an ophthalmic ointment vehicle is to prolong drug contact time with the external ocular surface. This is particularly useful for treating children, who may "cry out" topically applied solutions, and for medicating ocular injuries, such as corneal abrasions, when the eye is to be patched. Administer solutions before ointments. Ointments preclude entry of subsequent drops.

Recommended Procedures for Administration of Ointments:

- Wash hands thoroughly before administration.
- Holding the ointment tube in the hand for a few minutes will warm the ointment and facilitate flow.
- When opening the ointment tube for the first time, squeeze out and discard the first 0.25 inch of ointment as it may be too dry.
- Tilt head backward or lie down and gaze upward.
- Gently pull down the lower lid to form a pouch.
- Place 0.25 to 0.5 inch of ointment with a sweeping motion inside the lower lid by squeezing the tube gently.
- Close the eye for 1 to 2 minutes and roll the eyeball in all directions.
- Temporary blurring of vision may occur. Avoid activities requiring visual acuity until blurring clears.
- Remove excessive ointment around the eye or ointment tube tip with a tissue.
- If using more than one kind of ointment, wait about 10 minutes before applying the second drug.

Gels: Ophthalmic gels are similar in viscosity and clinical usage to ophthalmic ointments. Pilocarpine *(Pilopine HS)* is currently the only ophthalmic preparation available in gel form, and it is intended to serve as a "sustained release" pilocarpine, requiring only once-daily administration (at bedtime).

Sprays: Although not commercially available, some practitioners use mydriatics or cycloplegics, alone or in combination, administered as a spray to the eye to dilate the pupil or for cycloplegic examination. This is most often used for pediatric patients, and the solution is administered using a sterile perfume atomizer.

Lid Scrubs: Commercially available eyelid cleansers or antibiotic solutions or ointments can be applied directly to the lid margin for the treatment of blepharitis. This is best accomplished by applying the medication to the end of a cotton-tipped applicator and then scrubbing the eyelid margin several times daily.

Devices:

Contact Lenses: Soft contact lenses can absorb water-soluble drugs and release them to the eye over prolonged periods of time. This has the clinical advantage of promoting sustained release of solutions or suspensions that would otherwise be removed quickly from the external ocular tissues. Soft contact lenses as drug delivery devices are most often used in the management of dry eye disorders, but the technique is occasionally used for the treatment of ocular infections, including corneal ulcers.

Cotton Pledgets: Small pieces of cotton can be saturated with ophthalmic solutions and placed in the conjunctival sac. These devices allow a prolonged ocular contact time with solutions that are normally administered topically into the eye. The clinical use of pledgets is usually reserved for the administration of mydriatic solutions such as cocaine or phenylephrine. This drug delivery method promotes maximum mydriasis in an attempt to break posterior synechiae or to dilate sluggish pupils.

Filter Paper Strips: Sodium fluorescein and rose bengal dyes are commercially available as drug-impregnated filter paper strips. The strips help ensure sterility of sodium fluorescein which, when prepared in solution, can become easily contaminated with *Pseudomonas aeruginosa.* These dyes are used diagnostically to disclose corneal injuries, infections such as herpes simplex, and dry eye disorders.

Artificial Tear Inserts: A rod-shaped pellet of hydroxypropyl cellulose without preservative is commercially available *(Lacrisert).* It is inserted into the inferior conjunctival sac with a specially designed applicator. Following placement, the device absorbs fluid, swells, and then releases the nonmedicated polymer to the eye for up to 24 hours. The device is designed as a sustained release artificial tear for the treatment of dry eye disorders.

Membrane-Bound Inserts: A membrane controlled drug delivery system is commmercially available *(Ocusert)* that delivers a constant quantity of pilocarpine to the eye for up to 1 week. Placed onto the bulbar conjunctiva under the upper or lower eyelid, it is a useful substitute for pilocarpine drops or gel in glaucoma patients who cannot comply with more frequent drug instillation or in patients who have ocular or visual side effects from pilocarpine solutions.

Glaucoma is a condition of the eye in which an elevation of the intraocular pressure (IOP) leads to progressive cupping and atrophy of the optic nerve head, deterioration of the visual fields and ultimately to blindness. Primary open-angle glaucoma is the most common type of glaucoma. Angle-closure glaucoma and congenital glaucoma are treated primarily by surgical methods, although short-term drug therapy is used to decrease IOP prior to surgery.

Drugs used in the therapy of primary open-angle glaucoma include a variety of agents with different mechanisms of action. The therapeutic goal in treating glaucoma is reducing the elevated IOP, a major risk factor in the pathogenesis of glaucomatous visual field loss. The higher the level of IOP, the greater the likelihood of glaucomatous visual field loss and optic nerve damage. Reduction of IOP may be accomplished by: 1) Decreasing the rate of production of aqueous humor or 2) increasing the rate of outflow (drainage) of aqueous humor from the anterior chamber of the eye.

The five groups of agents used in therapy of primary open-angle glaucoma are listed in the table, which summarizes their mechanism of decreasing IOP, effects on pupil size and ciliary muscle, and duration of action.

AGENTS FOR GLAUCOMA

Drug	Strength	Duration (hrs)	Decrease Aqueous Production	Increase Aqueous Outflow	Effect on Pupil	Effect on Ciliary Muscle
Sympathomimetics						
Apraclonidine[1]	1%	3-5	NR	NR	NR	NR
Epinephrine	0.25%-2%	12	NR	++	mydriasis	NR
Dipivefrin	0.1%	12	NR	++	mydriasis	NR
Beta-Blockers						
Betaxolol	0.5%	12	+++	NR	NR	NR
Levobunolol	0.5%	12-24	+++	NR	NR	NR
Timolol	0.25%-0.5%	12-24	+++	+	NR	NR
Miotics, Direct-Acting						
Acetylcholine[2]	1%	10-20 min	NR	+++	miosis	accommodation
Carbachol[2]	0.75%-3%	8	NR	+++	miosis	accommodation
Pilocarpine	0.25%-10%	4-6	NR	+++	miosis	accommodation
Miotics, Cholinesterase Inhibitors						
Physostigmine	0.25%-0.5%	12-36	NR	+++	miosis	accommodation
Demecarium	0.125%-0.25%	days/wks	NR	+++	miosis	accommodation
Echothiophate	0.03%-0.25%	days/wks	NR	+++	miosis	accommodation
Isoflurophate	0.025%	days/wks	NR	+++	miosis	accommodation
Carbonic Anhydrase Inhibitors[3]						
Dichlorphenamide	50 mg	6-12	+++	NR	NR	NR
Acetazolamide	125-250 mg	8-12	+++	NR	NR	NR
Methazolamide	25-50 mg	10-18	+++	NR	NR	NR

+++ = significant activity ++ = moderate activity + = some activity NR = no activity reported

[1] Used only to decrease IOP in surgery. [2] Intraocular administration only for miosis during surgery.

[3] Systemic agents; for detailed information, see group monograph in Cardiovascular section.

Sympathomimetic agents have both α and β activity. They lower IOP mainly by increasing nonpressure-dependent uveal-scleral outflow. Epinephrine is used as an adjunct to miotic therapy; however, it is also used as primary therapy, especially in young patients who develop intolerable fluctuating myopia or in older patients with lens opacities. The combination of a miotic and epinephrine will have additive effects in lowering IOP and antagonistic effects on pupil size, thus overcoming the diminished vision caused by miosis because of its lower dose.

Dipivefrin HCl is a prodrug which is metabolized to epinephrine in vivo. The IOP-lowering effects are qualitatively and quantitatively similar to epinephrine; however, dipivefrin may be better tolerated and have a lower incidence of adverse effects because of its lower dose.

Beta-adrenergic blocking agents may be used alone or in conjunction with other agents. They may be more effective than either pilocarpine or epinephrine alone and have the advantage of not affecting either pupil size or accommodation. They lower IOP by decreasing the rate of aqueous production.

(Continued on following page)

Miotics, direct-acting were considered the first step in glaucoma therapy. They have now yielded to the β-blockers. They are useful adjunctive agents that are additive to either the β-blockers or the sympathomimetics. Dosage and frequency of administration must be individualized. Recent information indicates pilocarpine 2% and carbachol 1.5% every 12 hours provides maximum effect. Increasing the concentration and reducing dosage intervals may correct an inadequate response. Concentrations greater than pilocarpine 4% or carbachol 3% are occasionally required in patients with darkly pigmented irides.

Miotics, cholinesterase inhibitors include both reversible/short-acting (eg, physostigmine) and irreversible/long-acting (eg, echothiophate) agents which enhance the effects of endogenous acetylcholine by inactivation of the enzyme acetylcholinesterase. These agents are more potent and longer acting than the direct-acting cholinergic agents. Side effects and systemic toxicity are more common and of greater significance. These drugs are reserved for patients unresponsive to other agents. Using a direct-acting cholinergic and a cholinesterase inhibitor provides no improvement in response.

Carbonic anhydrase inhibitors are administered systemically. IOP is lowered by a direct action on the ciliary epithelium which decreases aqueous humor production. Carbonic anhydrase inhibitors are used as adjunctive therapy and do not replace topical therapy.

Hyperosmotic agents (mannitol, urea, glycerin and isosorbide) are administered systemically and are useful in lowering IOP in acute situations. These agents lower IOP by creating an osmotic gradient between the ocular fluids and plasma. They are not for chronic use.

(Products listed on following pages)

Refer to the general discussion of these products beginning on page 2167.

Sympathomimetics

EPINEPHRINE

Actions:

Sympathomimetic agents have a variety of effects on the eye, including pupil dilation, increased outflow of aqueous humor and vasoconstriction (α-adrenergic effects).

Systemic effects from ophthalmic instillation of these products are uncommon and minimal; however, systemic absorption may occur from drainage via the lacrimal drainage system into the nasal pharyngeal passages.

Epinephrine is available as the hydrochloride, borate and bitartrate salts. These preparations are therapeutically equal when given in equivalent doses of epinephrine base. A 2% solution of epinephrine bitartrate is the equivalent of a 1.1% solution of the hydrochloride or the borate. The borate salts may cause less local discomfort.

Epinephrine produces a significant decrease in IOP in approximately 70% of the population. The duration of decrease of IOP is 12 to 24 hours. It is additive with miotics, carbonic anhydrase inhibitors and somewhat with β-blockers.

Indications:

Management of open-angle (chronic simple) glaucoma; may be used in combination with miotics, β-adrenergic blocking agents or carbonic anhydrase inhibitors when indicated.

Contraindications:

Hypersensitivity to epinephrine; aphakia; patients with a narrow (occludable) angle who do not have glaucoma. Prior to peripheral iridectomy, epinephrine is contraindicated in patients in whom mydriatic action may precipitate angle closure.

Do not use if the nature of the glaucoma has not been clearly established.

Warnings:

Since pupil dilation may precipitate an acute attack of narrow-angle glaucoma, evaluate anterior chamber angle by gonioscopy prior to beginning therapy.

Do not use while wearing soft contact lenses; discoloration of lenses may occur.

Anesthesia: Discontinue use prior to general anesthesia with anesthetics which sensitize the myocardium to sympathomimetics (eg, cyclopropane or halothane).

Aphakic patients: Maculopathy with associated decrease in visual acuity may occur in the aphakic eye; if this occurs, promptly discontinue use.

Sulfite Sensitivity: Some of these products contain sulfites which may cause allergic-type reactions (eg, hives, itching, wheezing, anaphylaxis) in certain susceptible persons. Although the overall prevalence of sulfite sensitivity in the general population is probably low, it is seen more frequently in asthmatics or in atopic nonasthmatic persons. Specific products containing sulfites are identified in the product listings.

Elderly: Use with caution.

Pregnancy: Category C. Safety for use during pregnancy has not been established. Use only when clearly needed and when the potential benefits outweigh the potential hazards to the fetus.

Lactation: It is not known whether this drug is excreted in breast milk. Safety for use in the nursing mother has not been established.

Children: Safety and efficacy for use in children have not been established.

Precautions:

Epinephrine is relatively uncomfortable upon instillation. Discomfort lessens as concentration of epinephrine decreases. Not for injection.

Use with caution in the presence of: Hypertension; diabetes; hyperthyroidism; heart disease; cerebral arteriosclerosis; long-standing bronchial asthma.

Potentially hazardous tasks: Epinephrine may cause temporary blurred or unstable vision after instillation; observe caution while driving or operating machinery.

Drug Interactions:

Cyclopropane or **halothane:** Discontinue use prior to general anesthesia with anesthetics which sensitize the myocardium to sympathomimetics.

Chymotrypsin: Epinephrine 1:100 will inactivate chymotrypsin in approximately 1 hour.

Monoamine oxidase inhibitors (MAOIs): When administered simultaneously with, or up to 21 days after, administration of MAOIs, careful supervision and adjustment of dosages are required; exaggerated adrenergic effects may result.

Tricyclic antidepressants: The pressor response of adrenergic agents may also be potentiated by concurrent use of TCAs.

(Continued on following page)

Sympathomimetics (Cont.)

EPINEPHRINE (Cont.)

Adverse Reactions:

Local (up to 86%): Transitory stinging on initial instillation. Conjunctival hyperemia is a normal response. Headache or browache frequently occur, but usually diminish as treatment is continued. Also common are blurred vision, difficulty with night vision, photophobia and eye pain or ache. Conjunctival allergy occurs occasionally. Ocular irritation and pigmentary deposits in the conjunctiva, cornea or lids may occur after prolonged use. Reversible maculopathy with a central scotoma may result from use in aphakic patients.

Systemic effects: Palpitations; tachycardia; extrasystoles; cardiac arrhythmia; hypertension; faintness; trembling; sweating; pallor.

Patient Information:

Transitory stinging on initial instillation.

Headache or browache may occur on beginning therapy.

Patients should immediately report any decrease in visual acuity.

Refer to page 2164 for more complete information.

Administration and Dosage:

Instill 1 or 2 drops into affected eye(s) usually once or twice daily. Determine frequency of instillation by tonometry.

More frequent instillation than 1 drop twice daily does not usually elicit any further improvement in therapeutic response.

When used in conjunction with miotics, instill the miotic first.

Storage: Solutions are inherently unstable. Keep container tightly sealed. Protect solution from light and excessive heat; store in cool place. Discard if solution becomes brown or discolors, becomes cloudy or contains a precipitate.

				C.I.*
EPINEPHRINE (as HCl)				
Rx	**Epinephrine HCl** (Iolab)	**Solution:** 0.1%	In 1 ml Dropperettes.[1]	59
Rx	**Adrenalin Chloride** (Parke-Davis)		In 30 ml Steri-Vials.[1]	6
Rx	**Epifrin** (Allergan)	**Solution:** 0.25%	In 15 ml.[2]	24
Rx	**Epifrin** (Allergan)	**Solution:** 0.5%	In 15 ml.[2]	27
Rx	**Epinephrine HCl** (Various, eg, Iolab, Pharmafair, Raway)	**Solution:** 1%	In 1 ml.	19+
Rx	**Epifrin** (Allergan)		In 15 ml.[2]	29
Rx	**Glaucon** (Webcon)		In 10 ml.[2]	31
Rx	**Epinephrine HCl** (Various, eg, Pharmafair, Raway)	**Solution:** 2%	In 15 ml.[2]	20+
Rx	**Epifrin** (Allergan)		In 15 ml.[2]	33
Rx	**Glaucon** (Webcon)		In 10 ml.[2]	32
EPINEPHRINE (as Bitartrate)				
Rx	**Epitrate** (Wyeth-Ayerst)	**Solution:** 1% (as 2% bitartrate)	In 7.5 ml.[3]	42
EPINEPHRINE (as Borate)				
Rx	**Epinal** (Alcon)	**Solution:** 0.5%	In 7.5 ml.[4]	35
Rx	**Eppy/N ½%** (Sola/Barnes-Hind)		In 7.5 ml.[5]	27
Rx	**Epinal** (Alcon)	**Solution:** 1%	In 7.5 ml.[4]	37
Rx	**Eppy/N 1%** (Sola/Barnes-Hind)		In 7.5 ml.[5]	29
Rx	**Eppy/N 2%** (Sola/Barnes-Hind)	**Solution:** 2%	In 7.5 ml.[5]	30

* Cost Index based on cost per ml.

1 With 0.5% chlorobutanol and sodium bisulfite.

2 With benzalkonium chloride, sodium metabisulfite and EDTA.

3 With 0.6% chlorobutanol, polyoxypropylene-polyoxyethylenediol, sodium bisulfite and EDTA.

4 With 0.01% benzalkonium chloride, acetylcysteine, boric acid and sodium carbonate.

5 With 0.01% benzalkonium chloride, erythorbic acid, povidone and polyoxyl 40 stearate.

Refer to the general discussion of these products beginning on page 2167.

Sympathomimetics (Cont.)

DIPIVEFRIN HCl (Dipivalyl epinephrine)

Actions:

Pharmacology: Dipivefrin is a prodrug of epinephrine formed by the diesterification of epinephrine and pivalic acid, enhancing its lipophilic character and, as a consequence, its penetration into the anterior chamber. Penetration is ≈ 17 times that of epinephrine.

Dipivefrin HCl is converted to epinephrine within the eye by enzymatic hydrolysis. It appears to exert its action by enhancing outflow facility. Dipivefrin HCl delivers the same therapeutic effects as epinephrine with fewer local and systemic side effects than with conventional epinephrine therapy.

Pharmacokinetics: The onset of action with 1 drop occurs about 30 minutes after treatment, with maximum effect seen at about 1 hour.

Clinical Pharmacology: In patients with a history of epinephrine intolerance, only 3% of dipivefrin-treated patients exhibited intolerance, while 55% of those re-treated with epinephrine developed an intolerance.

Response to dipivefrin twice daily is less than that of 2% epinephrine twice daily and comparable to 2% pilocarpine 4 times daily. Patients using dipivefrin twice daily in studies of 76 to 146 days experienced mean IOP reductions ranging from 20% to 24%.

Dipivefrin does not produce miosis or accommodative spasm which cholinergic agents produce. The blurred vision and night blindness often associated with miotic agents do not occur with dipivefrin. In patients with cataracts the inability to see around lenticular opacities caused by constricted pupil is avoided.

Indications: Initial therapy or as an adjunct with other antiglaucoma agents for the control of IOP in chronic open-angle glaucoma.

Contraindications: Hypersensitivity to any component; narrow-angle glaucoma since any dilation of the pupil may predispose the patient to an attack of angle-closure glaucoma.

Warnings:

Sulfite Sensitivity: This product contains sulfites which may cause allergic-type reactions (eg, hives, itching, wheezing, anaphylaxis) in certain susceptible persons. Although the overall prevalence of sulfite sensitivity in the general population is probably low, it is seen more frequently in asthmatics or in atopic nonasthmatic persons.

Pregnancy: Category B. There are no adequate and well controlled studies in pregnant women. Safety for use in pregnancy is not established. Use only when clearly needed.

Lactation: It is not known whether this drug is excreted in breast milk. Use with caution.

Children: Safety and efficacy for use in children have not been established.

Adverse Reactions:

Cardiovascular: Tachycardia, arrhythmias and hypertension (reported with epinephrine).

Local: Conjunctival injection (6.5%); burning and stinging (6%). Infrequently, follicular conjunctivitis and allergic reactions occur. Epinephrine therapy can lead to adrenochrome deposits in the conjunctiva and cornea.

Dipivefrin 0.1% is less irritating than 1% epinephrine HCl or bitartrate. Only 1.8% of dipivefrin patients reported discomfort due to photophobia, glare or light sensitivity.

Aphakic patients: Macular edema occurs in up to 30% of aphakic patients treated with epinephrine. Discontinuation generally results in reversal of the maculopathy.

Patient Information:

Slight stinging or burning on initial instillation may occur.

Refer to page 2164 for complete information.

Administration and Dosage:

Initial glaucoma therapy: Instill 1 drop into the eye(s) every 12 hours. Not for injection.

Replacement therapy: When transferring patients to dipivefrin from antiglaucoma agents other than epinephrine, the first day continue the previous medication and add 1 drop of dipivefrin in affected eyes every 12 hours. The next day, discontinue the antiglaucoma agent and continue with dipivefrin. Monitor with tonometry.

In transferring patients from conventional epinephrine therapy, discontinue the epinephrine and institute the dipivefrin regimen.

Concomitant therapy: When patients receiving other antiglaucoma agents require additional therapy, add 1 drop of dipivefrin every 12 hours. For difficult to control patients, the addition of dipivefrin to other agents such as pilocarpine, carbachol, echothiophate iodide or acetazolamide is effective.

				C.I.*
Rx	**Propine** (Allergan)	**Solution:** 0.1%	In 5, 10 and 15 ml and 5 and 10 ml compliance cap bid.[1]	41

* Cost Index based on cost per ml.

[1] With 0.004% benzalkonium chloride, mannitol, sodium metabisulfite and EDTA.

APRACLONIDINE HYDROCHLORIDE

Actions:

Pharmacology: Apraclonidine HCl is a relatively selective α-adrenergic agonist that does not have significant membrane stabilizing (local anesthetic) activity. When instilled into the eyes, apraclonidine reduces intraocular pressure (IOP) and has minimal effect on cardiovascular parameters.

Optic nerve head damage and visual field loss may result from an acute elevation in IOP that can occur after argon laser surgical procedures. The higher the peak or spike of IOP, the greater the likelihood of visual field loss and optic nerve damage especially in patients with previously compromised optic nerves. The onset of action is usually within 1 hour and the maximum IOP reduction occurs 3 to 5 hours after application of a single dose. The mechanism of action of apraclonidine is not completely established, although its predominant action may be related to a reduction of aqueous formation.

Indications:

To control or prevent postsurgical elevations in IOP that occur in patients after argon laser trabeculoplasty or iridotomy.

Contraindications:

Hypersensitivity to any component of this medication or to **clonidine.**

Warnings:

Pregnancy: Category C. There are no adequate and well controlled studies in pregnant women. Use during pregnancy only when clearly needed and when the potential benefits outweigh the potential risks to the fetus.

Lactation: It is not known if topically applied apraclonidine is excreted in breast milk. Consider discontinuing nursing for the day on which apraclonidine is used.

Children: Safety and efficacy for use in children have not been established.

Precautions:

IOP reduction: Since apraclonidine is a potent depressor of IOP, closely monitor patients who develop exaggerated reductions in IOP.

Cardiovascular disease: Acute administration of two drops of apraclonidine has had minimal effect on heart rate or blood pressure; however, observe caution in treating patients with severe cardiovascular disease, including hypertension.

Vasovagal attack: Consider the possibility of a vasovagal attack occurring during laser surgery; use caution in patients with history of such episodes.

Corneal changes: Topical ocular administration of two drops of 0.5% and 1.5% apraclonidine to rabbits 3 times daily for 1 month resulted in sporadic and transient instances of minimal corneal cloudiness in the 1.5% group. No corneal changes were observed in 320 humans given at least one dose of 1% apraclonidine.

Adverse Reactions:

The following adverse effects were reported with the use of apraclonidine in laser surgery: Upper lid elevation (1.3%); conjunctival blanching (0.4%); mydriasis (0.4%).

The following adverse effects were observed in investigational studies with dosing once or twice daily for up to 28 days in nonlaser studies:

Ocular – Conjunctival blanching; upper lid elevation; mydriasis; burning; discomfort; foreign body sensation; dryness; itching; hypotony; blurred or dimmed vision; allergic response; conjunctival microhemorrhage.

GI – Abdominal pain; diarrhea; stomach discomfort; emesis.

Cardiovascular – Bradycardia; vasovagal attack; palpitations; orthostatic episode.

CNS – Insomnia; dream disturbances; irritability; decreased libido.

Other – Taste abnormalities; dry mouth; nasal burning or dryness; headache; head cold sensation; chest heaviness or burning; clammy or sweaty palms; body heat sensation; shortness of breath; increased pharyngeal secretion; extremity pain or numbness; fatigue; paresthesia; pruritus not associated with rash.

Administration and Dosage:

Instill 1 drop in scheduled operative eye 1 hour before initiating anterior segment laser surgery. Instill second drop into same eye immediately upon completion of surgery.

Storage: Store at room temperature. Protect from light.

Rx	**Iopidine** (Alcon)	**Solution:** 1% apraclonidine HCl and 0.01% benzalkonium chloride	In 0.25 ml dispenser.

Refer to the general discussion of these products beginning on page 2167.

Beta-Adrenergic Blocking Agents

Actions:

Pharmacology: Timolol, levobunolol, carteolol and metipranolol are noncardioselective (β_1 and β_2) β-blockers; betaxolol is a cardioselective (β_1) β-blocker. Topical β-blockers do not have significant membrane-stabilizing (local anesthetic) actions or intrinsic sympathomimetic activity. They reduce elevated and normal intraocular pressure (IOP), with or without glaucoma.

The exact mechanism of ocular antihypertensive action is not established, but it appears to be a reduction of aqueous production. However, some studies show a slight increase in outflow facility with timolol and metipranolol.

These agents reduce IOP with little or no effect on pupil size or accommodation. Blurred vision and night blindness often associated with miotics are not associated with these agents. In addition, in patients with cataracts, the inability to see around lenticular opacities when the pupil is constricted is avoided. These agents may be absorbed systemically (see Warnings).

Pharmacokinetics:

Pharmacokinetics of Ophthalmic β-Adrenergic Blocking Agents				
Drug	β-receptor selectivity	Onset (min)	Maximum effect (hr)	Duration (hr)
Carteolol	β_1 and β_2	nd	nd	12
Betaxolol	β_1	30	2	12
Levobunolol	β_1 and β_2	< 60	2 to 6	12 to 24
Metipranolol	β_1 and β_2	≤ 30	≈ 2	12 to 24
Timolol	β_1 and β_2	30	1 to 2	12 to 24

nd = No data

Clinical pharmacology: Timolol – In controlled studies of untreated IOP of ≥ 22 mm Hg, timolol 0.25% or 0.5% twice daily caused greater IOP reduction than 4% pilocarpine solution 4 times daily or 2% epinephrine HCl solution twice daily. In comparative studies, mean IOP reduction was 31% to 33% with timolol, 22% with pilocarpine and 28% with epinephrine.

In ocular hypertension, effects of timolol and acetazolamide are additive. Timolol, generally well tolerated, produces fewer and less severe side effects than pilocarpine or epinephrine. Timolol has been well tolerated in patients wearing conventional (PMMA) hard contact lenses.

Betaxolol ophthalmic was compared to ophthalmic timolol and placebo in patients with reactive airway disease. Betaxolol had no significant effect on pulmonary function as measured by Forced Expiratory Volume (FEV_1), Forced Vital Capacity (FVC) and FEV_1/VC. Also, action of isoproterenol was not inhibited. Timolol significantly decreased these pulmonary functions. No evidence of cardiovascular β-blockade during exercise was observed with betaxolol. Mean arterial blood pressure was not affected by any treatment; however, timolol significantly decreased mean heart rate. Betaxolol reduces mean IOP 25% from baseline. In controlled studies, the magnitude and duration of the ocular hypotensive effects of betaxolol and timolol were clinically equivalent.

Clinical observation of glaucoma patients treated with betaxolol solution for up to 3 years shows that the IOP-lowering effect is well maintained.

Betaxolol has been successfully used in glaucoma patients who have undergone laser trabeculoplasty and have needed long-term antihypertensive therapy. The drug is well tolerated in glaucoma patients with hard or soft contact lenses and in aphakic patients.

Levobunolol effectively reduced IOP in controlled clinical studies from 3 months to over 1 year when given topically twice daily; IOP was well maintained. The mean IOP decrease from baseline was between 6.8 and 9 mm Hg with 0.5% levobunolol.

Metipranolol reduced the average intraocular pressure approximately 20% to 26% in controlled studies of patients with IOP $>$ 24 mm Hg at baseline. Clinical studies in patients with glaucoma treated for up to 2 years indicate that an intraocular pressure lowering effect is maintained.

Carteolol produced a median percent IOP reduction of 22% to 25% when given twice daily in clinical trials ranging from 1.5 to 3 months.

Indications:

Lowering IOP in patients with chronic open-angle glaucoma.

For specific approved indications, refer to individual drug monographs.

(Continued on following page)

Contraindications:

Bronchial asthma, a history of bronchial asthma or severe chronic obstructive pulmonary disease; sinus bradycardia; second-degree and third-degree AV block; cardiac failure; cardiogenic shock; hypersensitivity to any component of the products.

Warnings:

Systemic absorption: These agents may be absorbed systemically. The same adverse reactions found with systemic β-blockers (see group monograph in Cardiovascular section) may occur with topical use. For example, severe respiratory reactions and cardiac reactions, including death due to bronchospasm in asthmatics, and rarely, death associated with cardiac failure, have been reported with topical β-blockers. Levobunolol and metipranolol may decrease heart rate and blood pressure, and betaxolol has had adverse effects on pulmonary and cardiovascular parameters. Detectable, perhaps significant serum timolol levels may be achieved in some patients. Exercise caution with all of these agents.

Cardiovascular: Timolol can decrease resting and maximal exercise heart rate even in normal subjects.

Cardiac failure – Sympathetic stimulation may be essential for circulation support in diminished myocardial contractility; its inhibition by β-receptor blockade may precipitate more severe failure.

In patients without history of cardiac failure, continued depression of myocardium with β-blockers may lead to cardiac failure. Discontinue at the first sign or symptom of cardiac failure.

Non-allergic bronchospasm patients, or patients with a history of chronic bronchitis, emphysema, etc, should receive β-blockers with caution; they may block bronchodilation produced by catecholamine stimulation of β_2-receptors.

Major surgery: Withdrawing β-blockers before major surgery is controversial. Beta-receptor blockade impairs the heart's ability to respond to β-adrenergically mediated reflex stimuli. This may augment the risk of general anesthesia. Some patients on β-blockers have had protracted severe hypotension during anesthesia. Difficulty restarting and maintaining heartbeat has been reported. In elective surgery, gradual withdrawal of β-blockers may be appropriate.

The effects of β-blocking agents may be reversed by β-agonists such as isoproterenol, dopamine, dobutamine or norepinephrine.

Diabetes mellitus: Administer with caution to patients subject to spontaneous hypoglycemia or to diabetic patients (especially labile diabetics). Beta-blocking agents may mask signs and symptoms of acute hypoglycemia.

Thyroid: Beta-adrenergic blocking agents may mask clinical signs of hyperthyroidism (eg, tachycardia). Manage patients suspected of developing thyrotoxicosis carefully to avoid abrupt withdrawal of β-blockers which might precipitate thyroid storm.

Cerebrovascular insufficiency: Because of potential effects of β-blockers on blood pressure and pulse, use with caution in patients with cerebrovascular insufficiency. If signs or symptoms suggesting reduced cerebral blood flow develop, consider alternative therapy.

Carcinogenesis: In mice receiving oral metipranolol doses of 5, 50 and 100 mg/kg/day, females receiving the low dose had an increased number of pulmonary adenomas.

Pregnancy: Category C. There are no adequate and well controlled studies in pregnant women. Use during pregnancy only if the potential benefits outweigh potential hazards to the fetus.

Carteolol – Increased resorptions and decreased fetal weights occurred in rabbits and rats at maternally toxic oral doses ≈ 1052 and 5264 times the maximum human dose, respectively. A dose-related increase in wavy ribs was noted in the developing rat fetus when pregnant rats received oral daily doses ≈ 212 times the maximum human dose.

Betaxolol – In oral studies with rats and rabbits, evidence of post-implantation loss was seen at dose levels above 12 mg/kg and 128 mg/kg, respectively. Betaxolol was not teratogenic, however, and there were no other adverse effects on reproduction at subtoxic dose levels.

Levobunolol – Fetotoxicity was observed in rabbits at doses 200 and 700 times the glaucoma dose.

Metipranolol – Increased fetal resorption, fetal death and delayed development occurred in rabbits receiving 50 mg/kg orally during organogenesis.

Timolol – Doses 1000 times the maximum recommended human oral dose were maternotoxic in mice and resulted in increased fetal resorptions. Increased fetal resorptions were seen in rabbits at 100 times the maximum recommended human oral dose.

(Warnings continued on following page)

Beta-Adrenergic Blocking Agents (Cont.)

Warnings (Cont.):

Lactation: It is not known whether betaxolol, levobunolol or metipranolol are excreted in breast milk. Systemic β-blockers and topical timolol maleate are excreted in milk. Carteolol is excreted in breast milk of animals. Exercise caution when administering to a nursing mother.

Because of the potential for serious adverse reactions from **timolol** in nursing infants, decide whether to discontinue nursing or discontinue the drug. Ophthalmic timolol that is absorbed appears to concentrate in breast milk approximately sixfold.

Children: Safety and efficacy for use in children have not been established.

Precautions:

Angle-closure glaucoma: The immediate objective is to reopen the angle, requiring constriction of the pupil with a miotic. These agents have little or no effect on the pupil. When they are used to reduce elevated IOP in angle-closure glaucoma, use with a miotic.

Muscle weakness: Beta-blockade may potentiate muscle weakness consistent with certain myasthenic symptoms (eg, diplopia, ptosis, generalized weakness). **Timolol** has increased muscle weakness in some patients with myasthenic symptoms.

Long-term therapy: Diminished responsiveness to **betaxolol** and **timolol** after prolonged therapy has been reported. However, in long-term studies (2 and 3 years), no significant differences in mean IOP were observed after initial stabilization.

Sulfite sensitivity: Some of these products contain sulfites which may cause allergic-type reactions (eg, hives, itching, wheezing, anaphylaxis) in certain susceptible persons. Although the overall prevalence of sulfite sensitivity in the general population is probably low, it is seen more frequently in asthmatics or in atopic nonasthmatic persons.

Drug Interactions:

Ophthalmic Beta Blocker Drug Interactions			
Precipitant drug	Object drug*		Description
Beta blockers, ophthalmic	Beta blockers, oral	↑	Use topical β-blockers with caution because of the potential for additive effects on systemic β-blockade.
Beta blockers, ophthalmic	Epinephrine, ophthalmic	↔	The use of epinephrine with topical β-blockers is controversial. Some reports indicate the initial effectiveness of the combination decreases over time. In one case verified by rechallenge, combined use of topical epinephrine and topical timolol appeared to result in hypertension resulting from unopposed α-adrenergic stimulation. However, this combination has been used to reduce IOP.
Beta blockers, ophthalmic	Quinidine	↑	One case of sinus bradycardia has been reported with the coadministration of ophthalmic timolol. The incidence was reaffirmed by a negative rechallenge with the β-blockers alone and positive rechallenge with the combination.
Beta blockers, ophthalmic	Verapamil	↑	Coadministration of ophthalmic timolol has caused bradycardia and asystole.

* ↑ = Object drug increased ↔ = Undetermined effect

Other drugs that may interact with the systemic β-adrenergic blocking agents may also interact with the ophthalmic agents. For further information refer to the β-blocker group monograph in the Cardiovascular section.

Adverse Reactions:

The following adverse reactions have occurred with ophthalmic use of the β_1 and β_2 (nonselective) adrenergic blocking agents:

Systemic:

CNS – Headache; depression.

Cardiovascular – Arrhythmia; syncope; heart block; cerebral vascular accident; cerebral ischemia; congestive heart failure; palpitation.

Digestive – Nausea.

Skin – Hypersensitivity, including localized and generalized rash.

Respiratory – Bronchospasm (predominantly in patients with preexisting bronchospastic disease); respiratory failure.

Endocrine – Masked symptoms of hypoglycemia in insulin-dependent diabetics (see Warnings).

Ophthalmic – Keratitis; blepharoptosis; visual disturbances including refractive changes (due to withdrawal of miotic therapy in some cases); diplopia; ptosis.

(Adverse Reactions continued on following page)

Beta-Adrenergic Blocking Agents (Cont.)

Adverse Reactions (Cont.)

The following adverse reactions have occurred with each individual agent:

Carteolol: Ophthalmic – Transient eye irritation, burning, tearing, conjunctival hyperemia, edema (≈25%); blurred/cloudy vision; photophobia; decreased night vision; ptosis; blepharoconjunctivitis; abnormal corneal staining; corneal sensitivity.

Systemic – Bradycardia; decreased blood pressure; arrhythmia; heart palpitation; dyspnea; asthenia; headache; dizziness; insomnia; sinusitis; taste perversion.

Betaxolol: Ophthalmic – Brief discomfort (> 25%); occasional tearing (5%). Rare: Decreased corneal sensitivity; erythema; itching; corneal punctate staining; keratitis; anisocoria; photophobia.

Systemic – Insomnia; depressive neurosis (rare).

Metipranolol: Ophthalmic – Transient local discomfort; conjunctivitis; eyelid dermatitis; blepharitis; blurred vision; tearing; browache; abnormal vision; photophobia; edema.

Systemic – Allergic reaction; headache; asthenia; hypertension; myocardial infarction; atrial fibrillation; angina; palpitation; bradycardia; nausea; rhinitis; dyspnea; epistaxis; bronchitis; coughing; dizziness; anxiety; depression; somnolence; nervousness; arthritis; myalgia; rash.

Levobunolol: Ophthalmic – Transient burning/stinging (25%); blepharoconjunctivitis (5%); iridocyclitis (rare); decreased corneal sensitivity.

Cardiovascular effects may resemble timolol.

CNS – Rare: Ataxia; dizziness; lethargy.

Dermatologic – Rare: Urticaria; pruritis.

Timolol: Ophthalmic – Ocular irritation including conjunctivitis; blepharitis; keratitis; blepharoptosis; decreased corneal sensitivity; visual disturbances including refractive changes (due, in some cases, to withdrawal of miotics); diplopia; ptosis.

CNS – Headache; dizziness; depression; fatigue; lethargy; hallucinations; confusion.

Cardiovascular – Bradycardia; arrhythmia; hypotension; syncope; heart block; cerebral vascular accident; cerebral ischemia; congestive heart failure; palpitation; cardiac arrest. These generally occur in the elderly or those with preexisting cardiovascular problems.

Respiratory – Bronchospasm (mainly in patients with preexisting bronchospastic disease); respiratory failure; dyspnea.

Other – Aggravation of myasthenia gravis; alopecia; nail pigmentary changes; nausea; hypersensitivity including localized and generalized rash; urticaria; asthenia; sexual dysfunction including impotence, decreased libido and decreased ejaculation; hyperkalemia; masked symptoms of hypoglycemia in insulin-dependent diabetics; diarrhea; paresthesia.

Causal relationship unknown – Hypertension; chest pain; dyspepsia; anorexia; dry mouth; behavioral changes including anxiety, disorientation, nervousness, somnolence and other psychic disturbance; aphakic cystoid macular edema; retroperitoneal fibrosis.

Systemic β-adrenergic blocker-associated reactions: Consider potential effects with ophthalmic use. See Warnings.

Overdosage:

If ocular overdosage occurs, flush eye(s) with water or normal saline. If accidentally ingested, efforts to decrease further absorption may be appropriate (gastric lavage).

The most common signs and symptoms of overdosage from systemic β-blockers are bradycardia, hypotension, bronchospasm and acute cardiac failure. If these occur, discontinue therapy and initiate appropriate supportive therapy. See group monograph in Cardiovascular section.

Patient Information:

Refer to page 2164 for more complete information.

Transient stinging/discomfort is relatively common with these agents. Notify physician if severe.

Administration:

Monitoring: The IOP-lowering response to betaxolol and timolol may require a few weeks to stabilize. Determine the IOP during the first month of treatment. Thereafter, determine IOP on an individual basis.

Because of diurnal IOP variations in individual patients, satisfactory response to twice a day therapy is best determined by measuring IOP at different times during the day. Intraocular pressures ≤ 22 mm Hg may not be optimal to control glaucoma in each patient; therefore, individualize therapy.

Concomitant therapy: If IOP is inadequately controlled with these agents, institute concomitant pilocarpine, other miotics, dipivefrin or systemic carbonic anhydrase inhibitors.

The use of epinephrine in combination with topical β-blockers is controversial. Some reports indicate the initial effectiveness of the combination decreases over time (see Drug Interactions).

(Products listed on following pages)

Beta-Adrenergic Blocking Agents (Cont.)

METIPRANOLOL HCl

Indications:

Treatment of ocular conditions in which lowering intraocular pressure is likely to be of therapeutic benefit, including patients with ocular hypertension and in patients with chronic open angle glaucoma.

Administration and Dosage:

Usual dose: One drop in the affected eye(s) twice a day. If the patient's IOP is not at a satisfactory level on this regimen, more frequent administration or a larger dose is not known to be of benefit. Concomitant therapy to lower IOP can be instituted. **C.I.***

Rx	**OptiPranolol** (Bausch & Lomb)	**Solution:** 0.3%	In 5 or 10 ml dropper bottles.[1]	1.3

CARTEOLOL HCl

Indications:

Treatment of chronic open-angle glaucoma and intraocular hypertension. It may be used alone or in combination with other intraocular pressure lowering drugs.

Administration and Dosage:

Usual dose: One drop in affected eye(s) twice daily. If the patient's IOP is not at a satisfactory level on this regimen, concomitant therapy can be instituted. **C.I.***

Rx	**Ocupress** (Otsuka America[2])	**Solution:** 1%	In 5 and 10 ml dropper bottles.[3]	86

LEVOBUNOLOL HCl

Indications:

Lowering IOP in chronic open-angle glaucoma or ocular hypertension.

Administration and Dosage:

Usual dose: 1 drop in the affected eye(s) once or twice a day. **C.I.***

Rx	**Betagan Liquifilm** (Allergan)	**Solution:** 0.25%	In 5 and 10 ml dropper bottles with B.I.D. *C Cap.*[4]	NA
		0.5%	In 2 ml dropper bottle[4] and 5, 10 and 15 ml dropper bottles with B.I.D. and Q.D. *C Cap.*[4]	2.2

* Cost Index based on cost per ml.

[1] With 0.004% benzalkonium chloride and EDTA.

[2] Otsuka America Pharmaceutical, Inc., 1201 Third Avenue, Suite 5300, Seattle, WA 98101; 206-682-5300.

[3] With 0.005% benzalkonium chloride.

[4] With 1.4% polyvinyl alcohol, 0.004% benzalkonium chloride, sodium metabisulfite and EDTA.

Complete prescribing information for these products begins on page 2172

Beta-Adrenergic Blocking Agents (Cont.)

BETAXOLOL HCl

Indications:

Treatment of ocular hypertension and chronic open-angle glaucoma. Betaxolol may be used alone or in combination with other antiglaucoma drugs.

Administration and Dosage:

Usual dose: One drop twice daily.

Replacement therapy (single agent): Continue the agent already used and add 1 drop of betaxolol twice daily. The following day, discontinue the previous agent and continue betaxolol. Monitor with tonometry.

Replacement therapy (multiple agents): When transferring from several concomitant antiglaucoma agents, individualize dosage. Adjust 1 agent at a time at intervals of not less than 1 week. One approach is to continue the agents being used and add 1 drop of betaxolol twice daily. The next day, discontinue one of the other agents. Decrease or discontinue the remaining antiglaucoma agents according to patient response.

				C.I.*
Rx	**Betoptic** (Alcon)	**Solution:** 5.6 mg (equiv. to 5 mg base) per ml (0.5%)	In 2.5, 5, 10 and 15 ml Drop-Tainer bottles.[1]	2.4
Rx	**Betoptic S** (Alcon)	**Suspension:** 2.8 mg (equiv. to 2.5 mg base) per ml (0.25%)	In 2.5, 5, 10 and 15 ml Drop-Tainer bottles.[1]	2.2

TIMOLOL MALEATE

Indications:

Effective in lowering IOP in patients with chronic open-angle glaucoma, aphakic patients with glaucoma, some patients with secondary glaucoma and patients with elevated IOP who require lowering of the ocular pressure.

In patients who respond inadequately to multiple antiglaucoma drug therapy, the addition of timolol may produce a further reduction of IOP.

Administration and Dosage:

Initial therapy: 1 drop of 0.25% twice a day. If clinical response is not adequate, change the dosage to 1 drop of 0.5% solution twice a day. If the IOP is maintained at satisfactory levels, change the dosage to 1 drop once a day.

Replacement therapy (single agent): When a patient is transferred from another topical ophthalmic β blocking agent, discontinue that agent after proper dosing on one day, and start treatment on the following day with 1 drop of 0.25% timolol. Increase the dose to 1 drop of 0.5% solution twice a day if clinical response is not adequate.

When changing from another antiglaucoma agent, other than a topical ophthalmic β-blocking agent, on the first day continue with the agent being used and add 1 drop of 0.25% timolol twice daily. The next day, discontinue the previously used agent completely and continue with timolol. If a higher dosage is required, substitute 1 drop of 0.5% twice daily.

Replacement therapy (multiple agents): When transferring from several concomitantly administered agents, individualize dosage. If any of the agents is an ophthalmic β-blocker, discontinue it before starting timolol. Adjust 1 agent at a time and at intervals of not less than 1 week. Continue the agents being used and add 1 drop of 0.25% twice a day. The next day, discontinue 1 of the other antiglaucoma agents. The remaining agents may be decreased or discontinued according to patient response. If a higher dosage is required, substitute 1 drop of 0.5% twice a day.

				C.I.*
Rx	**Timoptic** (MSD)	**Solution:** 0.25%	In 2.5, 5, 10 and 15 ml Ocumeter bottles.[2]	2.2
		0.5%	In 2.5, 5, 10 and 15 ml Ocumeter bottles.[2]	2.6
Rx	**Timoptic in Ocudose** (MSD)	**Solution:** 0.25%	Preservative free. In UD 60s.	1.3
		0.5%	Preservative free. In UD 60s.	1.5

* Cost Index based on cost per ml.

[1] With 0.01% benzalkonium chloride and EDTA.

[2] With 0.01% benzalkonium chloride.

Refer to the general discussion of these products beginning on page 2167

Miotics, Direct-Acting

Actions:

The direct-acting miotics are cholinergic agents which have effects on the muscarinic (parasympathomimetic) receptors in the eye. Pharmacologic effects include constriction of the pupil (miosis) and contraction of the ciliary muscle (accommodation).

In narrow-angle glaucoma, miosis may open the anterior chamber angle to improve the outflow of aqueous humor. In chronic open-angle glaucoma, the increase in outflow is independent of the miotic effect. Contraction of the ciliary muscle enhances the outflow of aqueous humor via indirect effects on the trabecular system. The exact mechanism of this action is not known.

Pilocarpine is most commonly used; carbachol is useful in patients experiencing irritation or who become refractory to pilocarpine. The pilocarpine therapeutic system *Ocusert* provides a continuous source of the medication, thus eliminating the need for frequent instillation of drops.

Pharmacokinetics:

Pharmacokinetics of the Direct-Acting Miotics			
Miotic	Onset of miosis (min)	Peak (hrs)	Duration (hrs)
Acetylcholine[1]	seconds	—	10-20 min
Carbachol	10-20	<4	8
Pilocarpine	10-30	2-4	4-8

[1] Intraocular administration.

Indications:

To decrease elevated intraocular pressure (IOP) in glaucoma.

Acetylcholine is used only for intraocular administration to induce miosis during surgery.

Unlabeled Use: **Pilocarpine,** 5 mg orally, has been used successfully to treat xerostomia (dry mouth) in patients with malfunctioning salivary glands.

Contraindications:

Hypersensitivity to any component of the products; where cholinergic effects are undesirable (eg, acute iritis, some forms of secondary glaucoma, acute inflammatory disease of the anterior chamber).

Warnings:

Use carbachol with caution in the presence of corneal abrasion to avoid excessive penetration; this can produce systemic toxicity.

Pregnancy and Lactation: Category C (**pilocarpine**). Safety for use during pregnancy and lactation has not been established. Use only when clearly needed and when the potential benefits outweigh the potential hazards to the fetus and nursing infant.

Children: Safety and efficacy for use in children have not been established.

Precautions:

Systemic reactions rarely occur during the treatment of chronic glaucoma, but in treating acute angle-closure glaucoma, consider the possibility of such reactions because of the relatively high dosage required over a short period of time.

Although systemic effects are uncommon at usual doses, caution is advised in patients with acute cardiac failure, bronchial asthma, peptic ulcer, hyperthyroidism, GI spasm, urinary tract obstruction and Parkinson's disease.

Retinal detachment has been caused by miotics in susceptible individuals, in individuals with preexisting retinal disease or in those who are predisposed to retinal tears. Fundus examination is advised for all patients prior to initiation of therapy.

Miosis usually causes difficulty in dark adaptation. Advise patients to use caution while night driving or performing hazardous tasks in poor illumination.

Use **pilocarpine** with caution in patients with narrow angles; it may produce acute angle closure.

(Continued on following page)

Miotics, Direct-Acting (Cont.)

Drug Interactions:

Flurbiprofen and **suprofen, ophthalmic**: Although clinical studies with acetylcholine chloride and animal studies with acetylcholine chloride or carbachol revealed no interference, and there is no known pharmacological basis for an interaction, there have been reports that both of these drugs have been ineffective when used in patients treated with flurbiprofen or suprofen.

Adverse Reactions:

Acetylcholine: Ophthalmic – Transient lenticular opacities.

Systemic – Bradycardia; hypotension; flushing; breathing difficulties; sweating.

Carbachol: Ophthalmic – Corneal clouding; persistent bullous keratopathy; postoperative iritis following cataract extraction with intraocular use. Retinal detachment; transient ciliary and conjunctival injection, ciliary spasm with resultant temporary decrease of visual acuity.

CNS – Headache.

Systemic – Salivation; GI cramps; vomiting; diarrhea; asthma; syncope; cardiac arrhythmia; flushing; sweating; epigastric distress; tightness in urinary bladder.

Pilocarpine: Approximately 80% of patients receiving pilocarpine may experience side effects.

Ophthalmic – Especially in younger patients who have recently started therapy: Burning; itching; smarting; blurring; ciliary spasm (not a contraindication to continued therapy unless the myopia is debilitating); conjunctival vascular congestion; induced myopia; sensitization of lids and conjunctiva; reduced visual acuity in poor illumination; lens changes (with chronic use); increased pupillary block; retinal detachments; vitreous hemorrhages.

The following reactions may occur at start of therapy, but rarely persist beyond a week or two: Conjunctival and ciliary congestion; ocular and periorbital pain; twitching lids; accommodative myopia; fixed iris leading to posterior synechiae; iris cysts at the pupillary border; allergic conjunctivitis; paradoxical rise in IOP due to pupillary block; lens opacities; superficial keratitis; subtle corneal granularity.

CNS – Browache; headache (especially in younger patients who have recently started therapy).

Systemic – Hypertension; tachycardia; bronchiolar spasm; pulmonary edema; salivation; sweating; nausea; vomiting; diarrhea; lacrimation and muscle tremors. Systemic reactions following ocular use are rare.

Pilocarpine Ocular Systems (Ocusert): Conjunctival irritation, including mild erythema with or without a slight increase in mucus secretion with first use. These symptoms tend to lessen or disappear after the first week of therapy. Occasionally, a sudden increase in pilocarpine effects has been reported during use due to rupture of the *Ocusert* device.

Although withdrawal of the peripheral iris from the anterior chamber angle by miosis may reduce the tendency for narrow-angle closure, miotics can occasionally precipitate angle closure by increasing resistance to aqueous flow from posterior to anterior chamber.

Irritation from pilocarpine has been infrequently encountered and may require cessation of therapy. True allergic reactions are uncommon, but require discontinuation of therapy.

Overdosage:

Should accidental overdosage in the eye(s) occur, flush with water or normal saline.

Treatment includes usual supportive measures. Refer to General Management of Acute Overdosage

If accidentally ingested, induce emesis or perform gastric lavage. Observe patients for signs of toxicity (ie, salivation, lacrimation, sweating, nausea, vomiting and diarrhea). If these occur, therapy with anticholinergics (atropine) may be necessary. Bronchial constriction may be a problem in asthmatic patients.

Patient Information:

May sting on instillation, especially first few doses.

May cause headache, browache, alteration of distance vision and decreased night vision.

Refer to page 477a for more complete information on administration and use.

(Products listed on following pages)

Complete prescribing information for these products begins on page 2179.

Miotics, Direct-Acting (Cont.)

ACETYLCHOLINE CHLORIDE, INTRAOCULAR

Indications:

To produce complete miosis in seconds, by irrigating the iris after delivery of the lens in cataract surgery. In penetrating keratoplasty, iridectomy and other anterior segment surgery where rapid, complete miosis may be required.

Administration and Dosage:

Instill the solution into the anterior chamber before or after securing one or more sutures. The pupil is rapidly constricted and the peripheral iris drawn away from the angle of the anterior chamber if there are no mechanical hindrances. Any anatomical hindrance to miosis may require surgery to permit the desired effect of the drug.

In cataract surgery, use only after delivery of the lens.

Solution: 0.5 to 2 ml produces satisfactory miosis. Solution need not be flushed from the chamber after miosis occurs. Since acetylcholine's action is of short duration (10 to 20 minutes), pilocarpine may be applied topically before dressing to maintain miosis.

Preparation of solution: Aqueous solutions of acetylcholine chloride are unstable. Prepare solution immediately before use. Discard any solution that has not been used.

Do not gas sterilize.

				C.I.*
Rx	**Miochol** (Iolab)	**Solution:** 1:100 acetylcholine chloride when reconstituted	In 2 ml dual chamber univial (lower chamber 20 mg lyophilized acetylcholine chloride and 60 mg mannitol; upper chamber 2 ml Sterile Water for Injection). Also available in system pak with 15 ml (2s) *Iocare* balanced salt solution.	305

CARBACHOL, INTRAOCULAR

Indications:

Miosis during surgery.

Administration and Dosage:

Gently instill no more than 0.5 ml into the anterior chamber before or after securing sutures. Miosis is usually maximal 2 to 5 minutes after application.

				C.I.*
Rx	**Miostat** (Alcon)	**Solution:** 0.01%	In 1.5 ml vials.	465

CARBACHOL, TOPICAL

Indications:

For lowering intraocular pressure in the treatment of glaucoma.

Administration and Dosage:

Instill 1 or 2 drops into eye(s) up to 4 times daily.

				C.I.*
Rx	**Isopto Carbachol** (Webcon)	**Solution:** 0.75%	In 15 and 30 ml.[1]	21
		1.5%	In 15 and 30 ml.[1]	22
		2.25%	In 15 ml.[1]	22
		3%	In 15 and 30 ml.[1]	23

* Cost Index based on cost per ml.

[1] With 0.005% benzalkonium chloride and 1% hydroxypropyl methylcellulose.

Complete prescribing information for these products begins on page 2179

Miotics, Direct-Acting (Cont.)

PILOCARPINE HCl

Indications:

Chronic simple glaucoma, especially open-angle glaucoma. Patients may be maintained on pilocarpine as long as intraocular pressure (IOP) is controlled and there is no deterioration in the visual fields.

Chronic angle-closure glaucoma, especially after iridectomy.

Acute (closed-angle) glaucoma: Alone, or in combination with other miotics, β-adrenergic blocking agents, epinephrine, carbonic anhydrase inhibitors or hyperosmotic agents to decrease IOP prior to surgery.

Miosis: Also indicated to counter the effect of cycloplegics and mydriatics.

Unlabeled uses: Pilocarpine 5 mg has been used orally to successfully treat xerostomia (dry mouth) in patients with malfunctioning salivary glands.

Administration and Dosage:

Initial: 1 or 2 drops up to 6 times daily. The frequency of instillation and the concentration are determined by patient response. The usual range is 0.5% to 4%. Concentrations > 4% are occasionally more effective, especially in patients with dark pigmented eyes, because pilocarpine is absorbed by melanin pigment; however, the incidence of adverse reactions is also increased.

				C.I.*
Rx	**Isopto Carpine** (Alcon)	**Solution:** 0.25%	In 15 ml.[1]	15
Rx	**Pilocarpine HCl** (Various, eg, Goldline, Moore, Parmed, Schein, Steris)	**Solution:** 0.5%	In 15 ml.	5+
Rx	**Isopto Carpine** (Alcon)		In 15 and 30 ml.[1]	15
Rx	**Pilocar** (Iolab)		In 15 ml[2] and twin-pack (2 × 15 ml).[2]	13
Rx	**Pilostat** (Bausch & Lomb)		In 15 ml.[3]	
Rx	**Pilocarpine HCl** (Various, eg, Alcon, Geneva, Goldline, Major, Moore, Parmed)	**Solution:** 1%	In 2 and 15 ml.	5+
Rx	**Adsorbocarpine** (Alcon)		In 15 ml.[4]	15
Rx	**Akarpine** (Akorn)		In 15 ml.[5]	9
Rx	**Isopto Carpine** (Alcon)		In 15 and 30 ml.[1]	15
Rx	**Pilocar** (Iolab)		In 15 ml[4], twin-pack (2 × 15 ml)[4] and 1 ml dropperettes.[4]	14
Rx	**Piloptic-1** (Optopics)		In 15 ml.[6]	12
Rx	**Pilostat** (Bausch & Lomb)		In 15 ml[3] and twin-pack (2 × 15 ml).	NA
Rx	**Pilocarpine HCl** (Various, eg, Alcon, Geneva, Goldline, Major, Moore, Parmed)	**Solution:** 2%	In 2 and 15 ml.	6+
Rx	**Adsorbocarpine** (Alcon)		In 15 ml.[4]	15
Rx	**Akarpine** (Akorn)		In 15 ml.[5]	9
Rx	**Isopto Carpine** (Alcon)		In 15 and 30 ml.[1]	15
Rx	**Pilocar** (Iolab)		In 15 ml[2], twin-pack (2 × 15 ml)[2] and 1 ml dropperettes.[2]	14
Rx	**Piloptic-2** (Optopics)		In 15 ml.[6]	12
Rx	**Pilostat** (Bausch & Lomb)		In 15 ml[3] and twin-pack (2 × 15 ml).	NA

* Cost Index based on cost per ml.

[1] With 0.5% hydroxypropyl methylcellulose and 0.01% benzalkonium chloride.

[2] With hydroxypropyl methylcellulose, benzalkonium chloride and EDTA.

[3] With 0.01% benzylkonium chloride.

[4] With 0.004% benzalkonium chloride, 0.1% EDTA, povidone and water soluble polymers.

[5] With hydroxyethylcellulose, 0.01% benzalkonium chloride and 0.01% EDTA.

[6] With polyvinyl alcohol, 0.02% benzalkonium chloride and 0.05% EDTA.

(Continued on following page)

Miotics, Direct-Acting (Cont.)

PILOCARPINE HCl (Cont.)

	Product	Form	Package	C.I.*
Rx	**Pilocarpine HCl** (Various, eg, Balan, Goldline, Major, Moore, Pharmafair)	**Solution:** 3%	In 15 ml.	8+
Rx	**Isopto Carpine** (Alcon)		In 15 and 30 ml.[1]	17
Rx	**Pilocar** (Iolab)		In 15 ml twin-pack.[2]	17
Rx	**Pilostat** (Bausch & Lomb)		In 15 ml.[3]	NA
Rx	**Pilocarpine HCl** (Various, eg, Alcon, Balan, Bioline, Geneva, Goldline, Major, Moore, Parmed, Pharmafair, URL)	**Solution:** 4%	In 2 and 15 ml.	7+
Rx	**Adsorbocarpine** (Alcon)		In 15 ml.[4]	17
Rx	**Akarpine** (Akorn)		In 15 ml.[5]	11
Rx	**I-Pilopine** (Americal)		In 15 ml.[5]	7
Rx	**Isopto Carpine** (Alcon)		In 15 and 30 ml.[1]	17
Rx	**Pilocar** (Iolab)		In 15 ml[6], twin-pack (2 x 15 ml)[6] and 1 ml dropperettes.[6]	15
Rx	**Pilostat** (Bausch & Lomb)		In 15 ml[3] and twin-pack 15 ml.	NA
Rx	**Pilocarpine HCl** (Various, eg, Pharmafair, Steris)	**Solution:** 5%	In 15 ml.	14+
Rx	**Isopto Carpine** (Alcon)		In 15 ml.[1]	18
Rx	**Pilocarpine HCl** (Various, eg, Balan, Dixon-Shane, Harber, Moore, Parmed, Pharmafair, Rugby, Schein, Steris)	**Solution:** 6%	In 15 ml.	5+
Rx	**Isopto Carpine** (Alcon)		In 15 and 30 ml.[1]	18
Rx	**Pilocar** (Iolab)		In 15 ml[6] and twin-pack (2 x 15 ml).[6]	17
Rx	**Pilostat** (Bausch & Lomb)		In 15 ml.[3]	NA
Rx	**Pilocarpine HCl** (Alcon)	**Solution:** 8%	In 2 ml.	56
Rx	**Isopto Carpine** (Alcon)		In 15 ml.[1]	22
Rx	**Isopto Carpine** (Alcon)	**Solution:** 10%	In 15 ml.[1]	19
Rx	**Pilopine HS** (Alcon)	**Gel:** 4%	In 5 g.[7]	79

PILOCARPINE NITRATE

Administration and Dosage:

Glaucoma: 1 to 2 drops 2 to 4 times daily; patient response may vary.

Emergency miosis: 1 to 2 drops of higher concentrations.

	Product	Form	Package	C.I.*
Rx	**Pilagan** (Allergan)	**Solution:** 1%	In 15 ml.[8]	16
		2%	In 15 ml.[8]	18
		4%	In 15 ml.[8]	19

* Cost Index based on cost per g or ml.

[1] With 0.5% hydroxypropyl methylcellulose and 0.01% benzalkonium chloride.

[2] With hydroxypropyl methylcellulose, benzalkonium chloride and EDTA.

[3] With 0.01% benzalkonium chloride.

[4] With 0.004% benzalkonium chloride, 0.1% EDTA, povidone and water soluble polymers.

[5] With hydroxyethylcellulose, 0.01% benzalkonium chloride and 0.01% EDTA.

[6] With hydroxypropyl methylcellulose, benzalkonium chloride and EDTA.

[7] With 0.008% benzalkonium chloride and EDTA.

[8] With 1.4% polyvinyl alcohol, 0.5% chlorobutanol, NaCl, citric acid, menthol, camphor, phenol and eucalyptol.

Refer to the general discussion of miotics on page 2179.

Miotics, Direct-Acting (Cont.)

PILOCARPINE OCULAR THERAPEUTIC SYSTEM

Actions:

An elliptical unit designed for continuous release of pilocarpine following placement in the cul-de-sac of the eye. Pilocarpine is released from the system as soon as it is placed in contact with the conjunctival surfaces.

Pharmacokinetics: Ocusert initially releases the drug at 3 times the rated value in the first hours and declines to the rated value in approximately 6 hours. A total of 0.3 to 0.7 mg pilocarpine is released during this initial 6 hour period (one drop of 2% pilocarpine ophthalmic solution contains 1 mg pilocarpine). During the remainder of the 7 day period, the release rate is within ± 20% of the rated value.

The ocular hypotensive effect is fully developed within 1½ to 2 hours after placement in the cul-de-sac. A satisfactory ocular hypotensive response is maintained around the clock. Because of the continuous release of the drug, adequate intraocular pressure (IOP) reduction is maintained with significantly lower doses than are required with conventional eye drops.

During the first several hours after insertion, induced myopia may occur. In contrast to the fluctuating and high levels of induced myopia typical of administration of pilocarpine drops, the amount of induced myopia with *Ocusert* decreases after the first several hours to a low baseline level (approximately 0.5 diopters or less), which persists for the therapeutic life of the system. Pilocarpine-induced miosis approximately parallels the induced myopia.

Indications:

Control of elevated IOP in pilocarpine responsive patients.

Concurrent therapy: Ocusert has been used concomitantly with various ophthalmic medications. Its release rate is not influenced by other ophthalmic preparations.

Administration and Dosage:

Damaged or deformed systems: Do not place or retain in the eye. Remove and replace systems believed to be associated with an unexpected increase in drug action.

Initiation of therapy: There is no direct correlation between the strength of *Ocusert* used and the strength of pilocarpine eyedrop solutions required to achieve a given level of pressure lowering. It has been estimated that *Ocusert* 20 mcg is roughly equal to 0.5% or 1% drops and 40 mcg is roughly equal to 2% or 3% drops. *Ocusert* reduces the amount of drug necessary to achieve adequate medical control; therefore, therapy may be started with the 20 mcg system, irrespective of the strength of pilocarpine solution the patient previously required. Because of the patient's age, family history and disease status or progression, however, therapy may be started with the 40 mcg system. The patient should return during the first week of therapy for evaluation of IOP, and as often thereafter as deemed necessary.

If pressure is satisfactorily reduced with the 20 mcg system, the patient should continue its use, replacing each unit every 7 days. If IOP reduction greater than that achieved by the 20 mcg system is needed, transfer the patient to the 40 mcg system. If necessary, an epinephrine ophthalmic solution, a β-blocker or a carbonic anhydrase inhibitor may be used concurrently.

Placement and removal of the system: The system is placed in the eye by the patient, according to patient instructions provided in the package. The instructions also describe procedures for removal of the system.

Since pilocarpine-induced myopia may occur during the first several hours of therapy (average of 1.4 diopters), place the system into the conjunctival cul-de-sac at bedtime. By morning, the induced myopia is at a stable level (about 0.5 diopters or less).

In those patients in whom retention of the system is a problem, superior cul-de-sac placement is often more desirable. The unit can be manipulated from the lower to the upper conjunctival cul-de-sac by gentle digital massage through the lid. If possible, move the unit before sleep to the upper conjunctival cul-de-sac for best retention. Should the unit slip out of the conjunctival cul-de-sac during sleep, its ocular hypotensive effect following loss continues for a period of time comparable to that following instillation of eyedrops.

Storage: Refrigerate at 2° to 8°C (36° to 46°F).

Rx	**Ocusert Pilo-20** (Alza)	**Ocular Therapeutic System:** Releases 20 mcg pilocarpine per hour for 1 week	In packages of 8 individual sterile systems.
Rx	**Ocusert Pilo-40** (Alza)	**Ocular Therapeutic System:** Releases 40 mcg pilocarpine per hour for 1 week	In packages of 8 individual sterile systems.

Refer to the general discussion of these products beginning on page 2167

Miotics, Cholinesterase Inhibitors

Actions:

Pharmacology: These agents inhibit the enzyme cholinesterase and thus enhance the effects of endogenous acetylcholine. In the eye, increase in cholinergic activity leads to intense miosis and contraction of the ciliary muscle (accommodation; myopia). Decrease in intraocular pressure (IOP) results primarily from increased facility of outflow of the aqueous humor.

Physostigmine and demecarium act principally on true cholinesterase, whereas isoflurophate and echothiophate depress both plasma and erythrocyte cholinesterase. Echothiophate is the most frequently used agent; demecarium is considered the most toxic of these agents; isoflurophate is available only in ointment form.

Combination therapy – A cholinesterase inhibitor with epinephrine, a β-blocker or a carbonic anhydrase inhibitor has additive effects. Concomitant use of a cholinesterase inhibitor and a direct-acting cholinergic agent offers no therapeutic advantage.

Pharmacokinetics: Physostigmine reversibly binds cholinesterase. Demecarium is also a reversible inhibitor, but has a prolonged action similar to the irreversible inhibitors. Echothiophate and isoflurophate irreversibly inactivate cholinesterase and have prolonged effects.

Pharmacokinetics of Cholinesterase-Inhibiting Miotics			
Miotic	Onset (minutes)	Peak (hours)	Duration
Physostigmine	10-30	—	12-48 hours
Demecarium	15-60	2-4	3-10 days[1]
Echothiophate	10-30	0.5	1-4 weeks
Isoflurophate	5-10	0.25-0.34	1-4 weeks

[1] Rarely 3 to 4 weeks.

Indications:

Demecarium, echothiophate and **isoflurophate:** Therapy of open-angle glaucoma; conditions obstructing aqueous outflow, eg, synechial formation, that are amenable to miotic therapy; following iridectomy; in accommodative esotropia (convergent strabismus).

Physostigmine is indicated only for reduction of IOP in primary glaucoma.

Echothiophate iodide may be used in subacute or chronic angle-closure glaucoma after iridectomy or where surgery is refused or contraindicated and in certain nonuveitic secondary types of glaucoma, especially glaucoma following cataract surgery.

In glaucoma, use cholinesterase inhibitors for patients who fail to respond to direct-acting cholinergics alone or in combination with epinephrine, a β-blocker or a carbonic anhydrase inhibitor.

Contraindications:

Active uveal inflammation or any inflammatory disease of the iris or ciliary body; most cases of angle-closure (narrow-angle) glaucoma (prior to iridectomy) or in patients with narrow angles, due to the possibility of producing pupillary block and increasing angle blockage; glaucoma associated with iridocyclitis; hypersensitivity to cholinesterase inhibitors.

Warnings:

Overdosage may produce systemic cholinergic and GI effects (see Adverse Reactions).

Pregnancy: Category C (**physostigmine**). Safety for use during pregnancy has not been established. Use only when clearly needed and when the potential benefits outweigh the potential hazards to the fetus.

Lactation: Exercise caution when administering **physostigmine** to nursing women.

Children: Safety and efficacy for use of **physostigmine** have not been established.

Precautions:

Ophthalmic ointments may retard corneal healing.

The miosis usually causes difficulty in dark adaptation. Use caution while driving at night or performing hazardous tasks in poor light.

Use in glaucoma only when shorter-acting miotics have proved inadequate, except in aphakic patients. Gonioscopy is recommended prior to use of medication.

Sulfite Sensitivity: Some of these products contain sulfites which may cause allergic-type reactions (eg, hives, itching, wheezing, anaphylaxis) in certain susceptible persons. Although the overall prevalence of sulfite sensitivity in the general population is probably low, it is seen more frequently in asthmatics or in atopic nonasthmatic persons.

(Precautions continued on following page)

Refer to the general discussion of these products beginning on page 2167

Miotics, Cholinesterase Inhibitors (Cont.)

Precautions (Cont.):

Concomitant ocular conditions: When an intraocular inflammatory process is present, breakdown of the blood-aqueous barrier from anticholinesterase therapy requires abstention from, or cautious use of, these drugs. Use with great caution, if at all, where there is a history of retinal detachment.

After long-term use, blood vessel dilation and resultant greater permeability increase possibility of hyphema during ophthalmic surgery. Discontinue at least 3 weeks before surgery.

Systemic effects: Repeated administration may cause depression of the concentration of cholinesterase in the serum and erythrocytes, with resultant systemic effects. Discontinue if salivation, urinary incontinence, diarrhea, profuse sweating, muscle weakness, respiratory difficulties, shock or cardiac irregularities occur.

Although systemic effects are infrequent, use digital compression of the nasolacrimal ducts for 1 to 2 minutes after instillation to minimize drainage into the nasal chamber.

Use caution in patients with marked vagotonia, bronchial asthma, spastic GI disturbances, peptic ulcer, pronounced bradycardia and hypotension, recent MI, epilepsy, parkinsonism and other disorders that may respond adversely to vagotonic effects.

Drug Interactions:

Carbamate or **organophosphate insecticides** and **pesticides:** Warn persons on cholinesterase inhibitors who are exposed to these substances (gardeners, organophosphate plant or warehouse workers, farmers, etc) of systemic effects possible from absorption through respiratory tract or skin. Advise respiratory masks, frequent washing and clothing changes.

Chymotrypsin: Activity is inhibited by isoflurophate.

Succinylcholine: Use extreme caution before or during general anesthesia to patients on cholinesterase inhibitors because of possible respiratory and cardiovascular collapse.

Systemic anticholinesterases for myasthenia gravis: Additive effects are possible; coadminister topical cholinesterase inhibitors cautiously, regardless of which therapy is added.

Adverse Reactions:

Ocular: Stinging; burning; lacrimation; eczematoid dermatitis; allergic follicular conjunctivitis; accommodative spasm; lid muscle twitching; conjunctival and ciliary redness; browache; headache; induced myopia with visual blurring.

Activation of latent iritis or uveitis may occur. Iris cysts may form, enlarge and obscure vision. Occurrence is more frequent in children. The iris cyst usually shrinks upon discontinuance of the miotic, or following reduction in strength of the drops or frequency of instillation. Rarely, the cyst may rupture or break free into the aqueous humor.

Retinal detachment and vitreous hemorrhage have been reported occasionally.

Prolonged use may cause conjunctival thickening and obstruction of nasolacrimal canals. Posterior synechiae to the lens may occur; dilation of the pupil once or twice yearly will prevent synechiae formation.

Lens opacities have been reported. Routine slit lamp examinations, including lens, should accompany prolonged use.

Paradoxical increase in IOP by pupillary block may follow instillation. Alleviate with pupil-dilating medication.

Systemic: Should systemic effects occur (ie, nausea, vomiting, abdominal cramps, diarrhea, urinary incontinence, salivation, difficulty in breathing, bradycardia or cardiac irregularities), parenteral administration of atropine sulfate is indicated (see Overdosage).

Overdosage:

If systemic effects occur, give parenteral atropine sulfate (IV if necessary; see GI Anticholinergics/Antispasmodics monograph). *Adults* – $\geq$ 0.4 to 0.6 mg. *Children* – organophosphate poisoning (similar compounds), 0.05 mg/kg IV initially, followed by maintenance with 0.02 to 0.05 mg/kg, titrated to signs of atropinization. Much larger atropine doses for anticholinesterase intoxication in adults have been used. Initially, 2 to 6 mg followed by 2 mg every hour or more often, as long as muscarinic effects continue. Consider the greater possibility of atropinization with large doses, particularly in sensitive individuals.

Pralidoxime chloride (see Antidotes) has been useful in treating systemic effects due to cholinesterase inhibitors. However, use in addition to, not as a substitute for, atropine.

A short-acting barbiturate is indicated for convulsions not relieved by atropine. Promptly treat marked weakness or paralysis of respiratory muscles by maintaining a clear airway and by artificial respiration.

Patient Information:

Local irritation and headache may occur at initiation of therapy.

Notify physician if abdominal cramps, diarrhea or excessive salivation occurs.

Refer to page 2164 for complete information.

(Products listed on following pages)

Complete prescribing information for these products begins on page 2185

Miotics, Cholinesterase Inhibitors (Cont.)

PHYSOSTIGMINE

A reversible cholinesterase inhibitor. Conjunctivitis occurs frequently with chronic use of physostigmine.

Administration and Dosage:

Solution: Instill 1 or 2 drops into the eye(s), up to 4 times/day.

Ointment: Apply small quantity to lower fornix, up to 3 times/day.

Storage: Store at 46° to 80°F. Do not use if solution becomes cloudy or dark brown.

				C.I.*
Rx	**Eserine Sulfate** (Various, eg, Harber, Iolab, Pharmaderm)	**Ointment:** 0.25% (as sulfate)	In 3.5 and 3.75 g.	10+
Rx	**Isopto Eserine** (Alcon)	**Solution:** 0.25% (as salicylate)	In 15 ml.[1]	22
Rx	**Eserine Salicylate** (Alcon)	**Solution:** 0.5% (as salicylate)	In 2 ml.	56
Rx	**Isopto Eserine** (Alcon)		In 15 ml[1]	24

DEMECARIUM BROMIDE

Administration and Dosage:

Because of the prolonged duration of action of demecarium, administration of the drug is required only twice daily; some patients may achieve adequate control with once daily or every other day administration. Because of the tendency to produce more severe adverse effects, including systemic reactions, use the lowest dose consistent with adequate control.

Closely observe the patient during the initial period. If the response is not adequate within the first 24 hours, consider other measures. Keep frequency of use to a minimum in all patients, especially children, to reduce chance of iris cyst development.

Glaucoma: For initial therapy, place 1 drop (children) or 1 or 2 drops (adults) into eye. A decrease in IOP should occur within a few hours. During this period, keep patient under supervision and perform tonometric examinations at least hourly for 3 or 4 hours to make sure no immediate rise in pressure occurs.

If necessary, increase dosage from 1 or 2 drops twice a week to 1 or 2 drops twice a day. The 0.125% strength used twice a day usually results in smooth control of the physiologic diurnal variation in IOP. This is probably the preferred dosage for most wide (open) angle glaucoma patients.

Accommodative esotropia: Essentially equal visual acuity of both eyes is a prerequisite to successful treatment.

Diagnosis – As a diagnostic aid to determine if an accommodative factor exists; especially useful preoperatively in young children and in patients with normal hypermetropic refractive errors. Instill 1 drop daily for 2 weeks, then 1 drop every 2 days for 2 to 3 weeks. If the eyes become straighter, an accommodative factor is demonstrated. This technique may supplement or complement standard testing with atropine and trial with glasses for the accommodative factor.

Therapy – In esotropia uncomplicated by amblyopia or anisometropia, instill not more than 1 drop at a time in both eyes every day for 2 to 3 weeks; too severe a degree of miosis may interfere with vision. Then reduce dosage to 1 drop every other day for 3 to 4 weeks and reevaluate the patient's status. Continue with a dosage of 1 drop every 2 days to 1 drop twice a week. (The latter dosage may be maintained for several months.) Evaluate the patient's condition every 4 to 12 weeks. If improvement continues, reduce to 1 drop once a week and eventually to a trial without medication. However, if, after 4 months, control of the condition still requires 1 drop every 2 days, discontinue therapy.

Demecarium bromide should not be used more often than directed. Caution is necessary to avoid overdosage.

Individualize dosage to obtain maximal therapeutic effect.

				C.I.*
Rx	**Humorsol** (MSD)	**Solution:** 0.125%	In 5 ml Ocumeter.[1]	61
		0.25%	In 5 ml Ocumeter.[1]	66

* Cost Index based on cost per g or ml.

[1] With 0.15% chlorobutanol, 0.5% hydroxypropyl methylcellulose and sodium bisulfite.

Complete prescribing information for these products begins on page 2185

Miotics, Cholinesterase Inhibitors (Cont.)

ECHOTHIOPHATE IODIDE

Administration and Dosage:

Because of the prolonged duration of action of the irreversible cholinesterase inhibitors, administration of the drug is required only twice daily; some patients may achieve adequate control with once daily or every other day administration. Because of the tendency to produce more severe adverse effects, including systemic reactions, use the lowest dose consistent with adequate control.

Tolerance may develop after prolonged use; a rest period restores response to the drug.

Glaucoma: Two doses per day are preferred to maintain as smooth a diurnal tension curve as possible, although 1 dose/day or every other day has been used with satisfactory results. It is unnecessary and undesirable to exceed a schedule of twice a day. Instill the daily dose or 1 of the 2 daily doses just before bedtime to avoid inconvenience due to miosis.

Early chronic simple glaucoma – Instill a 0.03% solution just before retiring and in the morning in cases not controlled with pilocarpine. Control during the night and early morning hours may then be obtained. Change therapy if IOP fails to remain at an acceptable level.

Advanced chronic simple glaucoma and glaucoma secondary to cataract surgery – Instill 0.03% solution twice daily, as above. When transferring a patient to echothiophate because of unsatisfactory control with other miotics, one of the higher strengths will usually be needed. In this case, a brief trial with 0.03% solution will be advantageous because higher strengths will then be more easily tolerated.

Concomitant therapy: May be used concomitantly with epinephrine, a β-blocker, a carbonic anhydrase inhibitor or all three.

Accommodative esotropia:

Diagnosis – Instill 1 drop of 0.125% solution once a day into both eyes at bedtime for 2 or 3 weeks. If the esotropia is accommodative, a favorable response may begin within a few hours.

Treatment – Use lowest concentration and frequency which gives satisfactory results. After initial period of treatment for diagnostic purposes, reduce schedule to 0.125% every other day or 0.06% every day. Dosages can often be gradually lowered as treatment progresses. The 0.03% strength has proven effective in some cases. The maximum recommended dose is 0.125% once a day, although more intensive therapy has been used for short periods.

Duration of treatment – In diagnosis, only a short period is required and little time will be lost in instituting other procedures if the esotropia proves to be unresponsive. In therapy, there is no definite limit if the drug is well tolerated. However, if the eyedrops, with or without eyeglasses, are gradually withdrawn after a year or two and deviation recurs, consider surgery.

				C.I.*
Rx	**Phospholine Iodide** (Wyeth-Ayerst)	**Powder for Reconstitution:**	1.5 mg to make 0.03%.	58
			3 mg to make 0.06%.	61
			6.25 mg to make 0.125%.	69
			12.5 mg to make 0.25%.	77
			With 5 ml diluent.[1]	

* Cost Index based on cost per ml.

[1] With potassium acetate, 0.55% chlorobutanol and 1.2% mannitol.

Complete prescribing information for these products begins on page 2185

Miotics, Cholinesterase Inhibitors (Cont.)

ISOFLUROPHATE

Isoflurophate hydrolyzes in the presence of water to form hydrofluoric acid. To prevent absorption of moisture and loss of potency, keep ointment tube tightly closed.

Administration and Dosage:

Because of the prolonged duration of action of the irreversible cholinesterase inhibitors, administration of the drug is required only twice daily; some patients may achieve adequate control with once daily or every other day administration. Because of the tendency to produce more severe adverse effects, including systemic reactions, use the lowest dose consistent with adequate control.

Whenever possible, apply before bedtime to lessen blurring of vision. Wash hands immediately after administration.

Caution is necessary to avoid overdosage. Keep frequency of use to a minimum in all patients, especially children, to reduce the chance of iris cyst development. If tolerance develops, use another miotic. Isoflurophate therapy may be resumed later.

Glaucoma: For initial therapy, place a 0.25 inch strip of ointment into the eye every 8 to 72 hours. A decrease in IOP should occur within a few hours. During this period, keep the patient under supervision and perform tonometric examinations at least hourly for 3 or 4 hours to be sure that no immediate rise in pressure occurs.

Accommodative esotropia: Essentially equal visual acuity of both eyes is a prerequisite to successful treatment.

Diagnosis - For initial evaluation, use isoflurophate as a diagnostic aid to determine if an accommodative factor exists. This is especially useful preoperatively in young children and in patients with normal hypermetropic refractive errors. Not more than a 0.25 inch strip of ointment is administered every night for 2 weeks. If the eyes become straighter, an accommodative factor is demonstrated. This technique may supplement or complement standard atropine testing and trial with glasses for the accommodative factor.

Therapy – In esotropia uncomplicated by amblyopia or anisometropia, use not more than a 0.25 inch strip at a time in both eyes every night for 2 weeks, as too severe a degree of miosis may interfere with vision. Dosage is then reduced from a 0.25 inch strip every other day to a 0.25 inch strip once a week for 2 months, after which reevaluate the patient's status. If benefit cannot be maintained with a dosage interval of at least 48 hours, discontinue therapy. Frequency of administration and duration of maintenance therapy depend on how long the eyes remain straight without medication. Gradually increase intervals between administration to the greatest length compatible with good results. Therapy may need to be continued indefinitely. Occasionally, however, the miotic may be needed only when the eyes begin to turn in. In a few instances, it has been possible to discontinue therapy entirely after several months.

				C.I.*
Rx	**Floropryl** (MSD)	**Ointment:** 0.025%	In a polyethylene mineral oil gel. In 3.5 g.	51

* Cost Index based on cost per g.

Also refer to the general discussion of these products beginning on page 2185

Combinations

PILOCARPINE AND EPINEPHRINE

PILOCARPINE lowers IOP by a direct cholinergic action that improves outflow facility on chronic administration (see Agents for Glaucoma: Miotics, Direct-Acting).

EPINEPHRINE reduces IOP by increasing outflow facility (see Agents for Glaucoma: Sympathomimetics).

The combination of pilocarpine and epinephrine provides additive effects in lowering IOP; opposing actions on the pupil may prevent marked miosis or mydriasis. These fixed combinations do not permit the flexibility necessary to adjust the dosage of each agent.

Administration and Dosage:

Instill 1 or 2 drops into the eye(s) 1 to 4 times daily. Determine concentration and frequency of instillation by severity of the glaucoma and response of patient.

	Product	Formulation	Size	C.I.*
Rx	**E-Pilo-1** (Iolab)	**Solution:** 1% pilocarpine HCl and 1% epinephrine bitartrate	In 10 ml.[1]	30
Rx	**P_1E_1** (Alcon)		In 15 ml.[2]	20
Rx	**E-Pilo-2** (Iolab)	**Solution:** 2% pilocarpine HCl and 1% epinephrine bitartrate	In 10 ml.[1]	31
Rx	**P_2E_1** (Alcon)		In 15 ml.[2]	21
Rx	**E-Pilo-3** (Iolab)	**Solution:** 3% pilocarpine HCl and 1% epinephrine bitartrate	In 10 ml.[1]	31
Rx	**P_3E_1** (Alcon)		In 15 ml.[2]	22
Rx	**E-Pilo-4** (Iolab)	**Solution:** 4% pilocarpine HCl and 1% epinephrine bitartrate	In 10 ml.[1]	33
Rx	**P_4E_1** (Alcon)		In 15 ml.[2]	22
Rx	**E-Pilo-6** (Iolab)	**Solution:** 6% pilocarpine HCl and 1% epinephrine bitartrate	In 10 ml.[1]	35
Rx	**P_6E_1** (Alcon)		In 15 ml.[2]	23

PILOCARPINE AND PHYSOSTIGMINE

PILOCARPINE lowers IOP by a direct cholinergic action that improves outflow facility on chronic administration (see Agents for Glaucoma: Miotics, Direct-Acting).

PHYSOSTIGMINE is a reversible inhibitor of cholinesterase and has indirect cholinergic effects (see Agents for Glaucoma: Miotics, Cholinesterase Inhibitors).

Combinations of pilocarpine and physostigmine have been used on the theory that improved response may be obtained. Studies indicate that no additive pressure lowering effects are achieved over either agent used alone. Such combinations are therefore not recommended.

Administration and Dosage:

Instill 1 or 2 drops into the eye(s) up to 4 times daily.

	Product	Formulation	Size	C.I.*
Rx	**Isopto P-ES** (Alcon)	**Solution:** 2% pilocarpine HCl and 0.25% physostigmine salicylate	In 15 ml.[3]	21

* Cost Index based on cost per ml.

[1] With benzalkonium chloride, EDTA, mannitol and sodium bisulfite.

[2] With 0.01% benzalkonium chloride, methylcellulose, EDTA, chlorobutanol, polyethylene glycol and sodium bisulfite.

[3] With 0.5% hydroxypropyl methylcellulose and 0.15% chlorobutanol.

DAPIPRAZOLE HCl

Actions:

Dapiprazole was approved by the FDA in December 1990.

Pharmacology: Dapiprazole is an ophthalmic alpha-adrenergic blocking agent. It acts through blocking the alpha-adrenergic receptors in smooth muscle. Dapiprazole produces miosis through an effect on the dilator muscle of the iris.

Dapiprazole does not have any significant activity on ciliary muscle contraction and, therefore, does not induce a significant change in the anterior chamber depth or the thickness of the lens.

Dapiprazole has demonstrated safe and rapid reversal of mydriasis produced by phenylephrine and, to a lesser degree, tropicamide. In patients with decreased accommodative amplitude due to treatment with tropicamide, the miotic effect of dapiprazole may partially increase the accommodative amplitude.

Eye color affects the rate of pupillary constriction. In individuals with brown irides, the rate of pupillary constriction may be slightly slower than in individuals with blue or green irides. Eye color does not appear to affect the final pupil size.

Dapiprazole does not significantly alter intraocular pressure in normotensive eyes or in eyes with elevated intraocular pressure.

Indications:

Treatment of iatrogenically induced mydriasis produced by adrenergic (phenylephrine) or parasympatholytic (tropicamide) agents.

Not indicated for the reduction of intraocular pressure or in the treatment of open angle glaucoma.

Contraindications:

When constriction is undesirable, such as acute iritis; hypersensitivity to any component of this preparation.

Warnings:

For topical ophthalmic use only. Not for injection.

Do not touch the dropper tip to lids or any surface as this may contaminate the solution. Do not use in the same patient more frequently than once a week.

Pregnancy: Category B. There are no adequate and well controlled studies in pregnant women. Use during pregnancy only if clearly needed.

Lactation: It is not known whether this drug is excreted in breast milk. Exercise caution when dapiprazole is administered to a nursing woman.

Children: Safety and efficacy has not been established.

Adverse Reactions:

The most frequent reaction was conjunctival injection, lasting 20 minutes in > 80% of patients. Burning on instillation occurred in approximately half of all patients. Reactions occurring in 10% to 40% of patients included: Ptosis; lid erythema; lid edema; chemosis; itching; punctate keratitis; corneal edema; browache; photophobia; headaches. Other reactions reported less frequently included dryness of eyes, tearing and blurring of vision.

Administration and Dosage:

Administer 2 drops followed 5 minutes later by an additional 2 drops applied topically to the conjunctiva of each eye after the ophthalmic examination to reverse the diagnostic mydriasis. Dapiprazole should not be used in the same patient more frequently than once per week.

Preparation: Tear off aluminum seals; remove and discard rubber plugs from both drug and diluent vials. Pour diluent into drug vial. Remove dropper assembly from its sterile wrapping and attach to the drug vial. Shake container for several minutes to ensure mixing.

Storage/stability: Once the eyedrops have been reconstituted they may be stored at room temperature (15° to 30°C; 59° to 86°F) for 21 days. Discard any solution that is not clear and colorless.

Rx	**Rēv-Eyes** (Storz/ Lederle)	**Powder, lyophilized:** 25 mg dapiprazole HCl[1] (0.5% solution when reconstituted)	In vial with 5 ml diluent and dropper.

[1] With 2% mannitol, 0.4% hydroxypropyl methylcellulose, 0.01% edetate sodium, sodium phosphate dibasic, sodium phosphate monobasic, water for injection and 0.01% benzalkonium chloride.

Actions:

The effects of sympathomimetic agents on the eye include: Pupil dilation, increase in outflow of aqueous humor and vasoconstriction (α-adrenergic effects); relaxation of the ciliary muscle and a decrease in the formation of aqueous humor (β-adrenergic effects).

The strong (alpha) vasoconstriction preparations (phenylephrine 2.5% and 10% and hydroxyamphetamine) are used to cause vasoconstriction and pupillary dilation for diagnostic eye examinations, during surgery and to prevent synechiae formation in uveitis. The intermediate strength solutions (epinephrine 0.5% to 2%) are used in the management of open-angle glaucoma (see p. 478b), and can be used alone or in combination with miotics, β-adrenergic blocking agents, hyperosmotic agents or carbonic anhydrase inhibitors. Weak solutions of sympathomimetics (phenylephrine 0.12%, naphazoline and tetrahydrozoline) are used as ophthalmic decongestants (vasoconstriction of conjunctival blood vessels) for symptomatic relief of minor eye irritations.

Ophthalmic Vasoconstrictors/Mydriatics			
Vasoconstrictor/ Mydriatic	Duration of action (hr)	Available concentration	Prescription status
Epinephrine	1 to 3	0.1%	*Rx*
Phenylephrine	0.5 to 1.5	0.8%	*otc*
		0.12%	*otc*
		2.5%	*Rx*
	5 to 7[1]	10%	*Rx*
Oxymetazoline	≤ 6	0.025%	*otc*
Hydroxyamphetamine	few hours	1%	*Rx*
Naphazoline	2 to 3	0.012%	*otc*
		0.02%	*otc*
		0.03%	*otc*
		0.05%	*otc*
		0.1%	*Rx*
Tetrahydrozoline	2 to 3	0.05%	*otc*

[1] For mydriasis with 5% to 10% solution.

Indications:

Refer to individual product listings for specific indications.

Contraindications:

Hypersensitivity to any of these agents; narrow-angle glaucoma or individuals with a narrow (occludable) angle that do not have glaucoma; prior to peripheral iridectomy, in eyes capable of angle closure because their mydriatic action may precipitate angle block.

Phenylephrine 10%: Patients with long-standing insulin-dependent diabetes; hypertensive patients receiving reserpine or guanethidine; advanced arteriosclerotic changes; aneurysms; idiopathic orthostatic hypotension; history of organic cardiac disease; infants, small children with low body weight; debilitated or elderly patients; patients with intraocular lens implants, due to the possibility of dislodging the lens.

Warnings:

Anesthetics: Discontinue prior to use of anesthetics which sensitize the myocardium to sympathomimetics (eg, cyclopropane or halothane).

Local anesthetics can increase absorption of topically applied drugs; exercise caution when applying prior to use of phenylephrine.

Pregnancy (Category C) and lactation: Safety for use during pregnancy and lactation has not been established. Use only if clearly needed and if the potential benefits outweigh the potential hazards to the fetus.

Precautions:

Use with caution in the presence of hypertension, diabetes, hyperthyroidism, heart disease, hypertensive cardiovascular disease, coronary artery disease, cerebral arteriosclerosis or long-standing bronchial asthma.

Narrow-angle glaucoma: Ordinarily, any mydriatic is contraindicated in patients with glaucoma. However, when temporary dilation of the pupil may free adhesions, or when vasoconstriction of the intrinsic vessels may lower intraocular tension, these advantages may temporarily outweigh the danger from coincident dilation of the pupil.

Corneal effects: If the corneal epithelium has been denuded or damaged, corneal clouding may occur if **phenylephrine 10%** is instilled. This may be especially serious following corneal epithelium removal during retinal detachment surgery or vitrectomy. The corneas of diabetic patients may manifest epithelial ulcerations as well as a slow rate of reepithelialization. Use of phenylephrine in such corneas may be especially hazardous.

(Precautions continued on following page)

Precautions (Cont.):

Corneal effects: If the corneal epithelium has been denuded or damaged, corneal clouding may occur if **phenylephrine 10%** is instilled. This may be especially serious following corneal epithelium removal during retinal detachment surgery or vitrectomy. The corneas of diabetic patients may manifest epithelial ulcerations as well as a slow rate of reepithelialization. Use of phenylephrine in such corneas may be especially hazardous.

Rebound congestion may occur with extended use of ophthalmic vasoconstrictors.

Sulfite sensitivity: Some of these products contain sulfites that may cause allergic-type reactions (eg, hives, itching, wheezing, anaphylaxis) in certain susceptible persons. Although the overall prevalence of sulfite sensitivity in the general population is probably low, it is seen more frequently in asthmatics or in atopic nonasthmatic persons. Specific products containing sulfites are identified in the product listings.

Systemic absorption: Exceeding recommended dosages of these agents or applying **phenylephrine** 2.5% to 10% solutions to the instrumented, traumatized, diseased or postsurgical eye or adnexa, or to patients with suppressed lacrimation, as during anesthesia, may result in the absorption of sufficient quantities to produce a systemic vasopressor response.

Epinephrine: Do not use while wearing soft contact lenses; lens discoloration may occur.

Potentially hazardous tasks: **Epinephrine** and **phenylephrine** may cause temporary blurred or unstable vision; observe caution while driving or performing other hazardous tasks.

Drug Interactions:

Anesthetics: Use anesthetics that sensitize the myocardium to sympathomimetics (eg, cyclopropane or halothane) cautiously. Local anesthetics can increase absorption of topical drugs; exercise caution when applying prior to use of phenylephrine.

β-adrenergic blocking agents: Systemic side effects may occur more readily in patients taking these drugs. A severe hypertensive episode and fatal intracranial hemorrhage, associated with ophthalmic phenylephrine 10%, was reported in one patient taking propranolol for hypertension.

MAOIs: When given with, or up to 21 days after MAOIs, exaggerated adrenergic effects may result. Supervise and adjust dosage carefully.

Adverse Reactions:

Ocular: Transitory stinging on initial instillation, blurring of vision. Rarely, maculopathy with a central scotoma results from use in aphakic patients; prompt reversal generally follows discontinuation.

Phenylephrine may cause rebound miosis and decreased mydriatic response to therapy in older persons.

Epinephrine has been reported to cause adrenochrome deposits in the conjunctiva and cornea after prolonged therapy. Eye pain or ache, conjunctival hyperemia, allergy and allergic lid reactions may occur. Pigmentary deposits in the lids, conjunctiva or cornea may occur after prolonged use.

Systemic effects (occasional):

Cardiovascular: Palpitation; tachycardia; collapse; extrasystoles; cardiac arrhythmia; hypertension; ventricular arrhythmias (ie, premature ventricular contractions); reflex bradycardia; coronary occlusion; pulmonary embolism; subarachnoid hemorrhage; myocardial infarction; stroke; death associated with cardiac reactions. Headache or browache may occur, but usually diminishes as treatment is continued.

Phenylephrine 10%: Significant elevation of blood pressure is rare but can occur after conjunctival instillation. Exercise caution with elderly patients and children of low body weight. Carefully monitor the blood pressure of these patients. (See Warnings and Contraindications.)

There have been rare reports of the development of serious cardiovascular reactions, including coronary artery spasm, ventricular arrhythmias and myocardial infarctions. These episodes, some fatal, have usually occurred in elderly patients with preexisting cardiovascular diseases.

Other: Occipital headache; blanching; tremor; trembling; sweating; faintness; pallor.

Patient Information:

Do not use beyond 72 hours without consulting a physician.

If severe eye pain, headache, vision changes, floating spots, acute eye redness or pain with light exposure occur, discontinue use and consult a physician.

Refer to page 477b for more complete information.

Potentially hazardous tasks: **Epinephrine** and **phenylephrine** may cause temporary blurred or unstable vision; observe caution while driving or performing other hazardous tasks.

(Products listed on following pages)

Complete prescribing information for these products begins on page 2191 .

PHENYLEPHRINE HCl

Indications:

10%: Decongestant and vasoconstrictor and for pupil dilation in uveitis (posterior synechiae), wide-angle glaucoma and surgery.

2.5%: Decongestant and vasoconstrictor and for pupil dilation in uveitis (posterior synechiae), open angle glaucoma in conjunction with miotics, refraction, ophthalmoscopic examination, diagnostic procedures and before intraocular surgery.

0.12%: A decongestant to provide temporary relief of minor eye irritations caused by hay fever, colds, dust, wind, sun, smog or hard contact lenses.

Administration and Dosage:

Vasoconstrictors and pupil dilation: Apply a drop of topical anesthetic. Follow in a few minutes by 1 drop of the 2.5% or 10% ophthalmic solution on the upper limbus. The anesthetic prevents stinging and consequent dilution of solution by lacrimation. It may be necessary to repeat the instillation after 1 hour, again preceded by the use of a topical anesthetic.

Uveitis and posterior synechiae: The formation of synechiae may be prevented by using the 2.5% or 10% ophthalmic solution and atropine to produce wide dilation of the pupil. However, the vasoconstrictor effect of phenylephrine HCl may be antagonistic to the increase of local blood flow in uveal infection.

To free recently formed posterior synechiae, instill 1 drop of the 2.5% or 10% ophthalmic solution to the upper surface of the cornea. Continue treatment the following day, if necessary. In the interim, apply hot compresses for 5 or 10 minutes, 3 times daily using 1 drop of 1% or 2% solution of atropine sulfate and before and after each series of compresses.

Glaucoma: Instill 1 drop of 10% solution on the upper surface of the cornea as often as necessary. The 2.5% solution, as well as the 10% solution, may be used in conjunction with miotics in patients with wide-angle glaucoma.

Surgery: When a short-acting mydriatic is needed for wide dilation of the pupil before intraocular surgery, the 2.5% or 10% solution may be instilled from 30 to 60 minutes before the operation.

Refraction: Prior to determination of refractive errors, the 2.5% solution may be used effectively with homatropine HBr or atropine sulfate.

Adults: Place 1 drop of the preferred cycloplegic in each eye; follow in 5 minutes with 1 drop phenylephrine 2.5% solution, and in 10 minutes with another drop of the cycloplegic. In 50 to 60 minutes, the eyes are ready for refraction.

Children: Place 1 drop of atropine sulfate 1% in each eye; follow in 10 to 15 minutes with 1 drop of phenylephrine 2.5% solution and in 5 to 10 minutes with a second drop of atropine sulfate 1%. In 1 to 2 hours, the eyes are ready for refraction.

For a "one application method", combine 2.5% phenylephrine solution with a cycloplegic to elicit synergistic action. The additive effect varies depending on the patient. Therefore, when using a "one application method", it may be desirable to increase the concentration of the cycloplegic.

Ophthalmoscopic examination: Place 1 drop of 2.5% phenylephrine solution in each eye. Sufficient mydriasis is produced in 15 to 30 minutes and lasts 1 to 3 hours.

Diagnostic procedures: Heavily pigmented irides may require larger doses in all the following procedures.

Provocative test for angle block in patients with glaucoma – The 2.5% solution may be used as a provocative test when latent increased IOP is suspected. Measure tension before application of phenylephrine and again after dilation. A 3 to 5 mm Hg rise in pressure suggests the presence of angle block in patients with glaucoma; however, failure to obtain such a rise does not preclude the presence of glaucoma from other causes.

Shadow test (retinoscopy) – When dilation of the pupil without cycloplegic action is desired, the 2.5% ophthalmic solution may be used alone.

Blanching test – Instill 1 to 2 drops of the 2.5% ophthalmic solution to the injected eye. After 5 minutes, examine for perilimbal blanching. If blanching occurs, the congestion is superficial and probably does not indicate iritis.

Minor eye irritations: Instill 1 or 2 drops of the 0.12% solution in eye(s) 2 to 4 times daily as needed.

Stability: Prolonged exposure to air or strong light may cause oxidation and discoloration. Do not use if solution is brown or contains a precipitate.

(Products listed on following page)

PHENYLEPHRINE HCl (Cont.)

	Product	Strength	How supplied	C.I.*
otc	**AK-Nefrin Ophthalmic** (Akorn)	**Solution:** 0.12%	In 15 ml.[1]	6
Rx	**Phenylephrine HCl** (IDE)		In 15 ml.	NA
otc	**Isopto Frin** (Alcon)		In 15 ml.[2]	15
Rx	**AK-Dilate** (Akorn)	**Solution:** 2.5%	In 2 and 15 ml.[3]	30
Rx	**I-Phrine 2.5%** (Americal)		In 2 and 15 ml.[3]	5
Rx	**2.5% Mydfrin Ophthalmic** (Alcon)		In 3 and 5 ml Drop-Tainers.[3]	38
Rx	**Neo-Synephrine 2.5% Ophthalmic** (Winthrop Pharm.)		In 15 ml.[4]	17
Rx	**Phenylephrine HCl** (Iolab)	**Solution:** 10%	In 1 ml Dropperettes.[5]	52
Rx	**AK-Dilate Ophthalmic** (Akorn)		In 2 and 5 ml.[3]	29
Rx	**I-Phrine 10%** (Americal)		In 2 and 5 ml.[3]	18
Rx	**Neo-Synephrine 10% Plain Ophthalmic** (Winthrop Pharm.)		In 5 ml.[6]	47
Rx	**Neo-Synephrine Viscous Ophthalmic** (Winthrop Pharm.)		In 5 ml.[7]	48

* Cost Index based on cost per ml.
[1] With 0.01% benzalkonium chloride, 0.5% hydroxyethylcellulose and EDTA.
[2] With 0.01% benzalkonium chloride and 0.5% hydroxypropyl methylcellulose.
[3] With 0.01% benzalkonium chloride, EDTA and sodium bisulfite.
[4] With 0.013% benzalkonium chloride.
[5] With 0.01% thimerosal and sodium bisulfite.
[6] With 0.01% benzalkonium chloride.
[7] With 0.01% benzalkonium chloride and methylcellulose.

Complete prescribing information for these products begins on page 2191

NAPHAZOLINE HCl

Indications: For use as a topical ocular vasoconstrictor.

To soothe, refresh, moisturize and remove redness due to minor eye irritation.

Administration and Dosage:
Instill 1 or 2 drops into the conjunctival sac of affected eye(s) every 3 to 4 hours.

	Product	Form	Size	C.I.*
otc	**Allerest Eye Drops** (Pharmacraft)	**Solution:** 0.012%	In 15 and 30 ml.[1]	7
otc	**Clear Eyes** (Ross)		In 15 and 30 ml.[2]	5
otc	**Degest 2** (Sola/Barnes-Hind)		In 15 ml.[3]	10
Rx	**Estivin II** (Alcon)		In 7.5 ml.[4]	15
otc	**Naphcon** (Alcon)		In 15 ml.[5]	15
otc	**VasoClear** (Iolab)	**Solution:** 0.02%	In 15 ml.[6]	11
Rx	**Naphazoline HCl** (Major)	**Solution:** 0.025%	In 15 ml.	8
otc	**Comfort Eye Drops** (Sola/B-H)	**Solution:** 0.03%	In 15 ml.[7]	5
Rx	**Naphazoline HCl** (Various)	**Solution:** 0.1%	In 15 and 480 ml.	2+
Rx	**AK-Con Ophthalmic** (Akorn)		In 15 ml.[8]	8
Rx	**Albalon Liquifilm** (Allergan)		In 15 ml.[9]	17
Rx	**I-Naphline** (Americal)		In 15 ml.[8]	4
Rx	**Nafazair** (Various, eg, Balan, Texas)		In 15 ml.	4+
Rx	**Naphcon Forte** (Alcon)		In 15 ml.[10]	17
Rx	**Opcon** (Bausch & Lomb)		In 15 ml.[11]	12
Rx	**Vasocon Regular** (Iolab)		In 15 ml.[12]	17

OXYMETAZOLINE HCl

Indications: For the relief of redness of the eye due to minor eye irritations.

Administration and Dosage: Instill 1 or 2 drops in the affected eye(s) every 6 hours.

	Product	Form	Size	C.I.*
otc	**OcuClear** (Schering)	**Solution:** 0.025%	In 15 and 30 ml.[11]	5
otc	**Visine L.R.** (Leeming)		In 15 and 30 ml.[13]	6

TETRAHYDROZOLINE HCl

Indications: For use as a topical ocular decongestant.

Administration and Dosage: Instill 1 or 2 drops into eye(s) 2 to 4 times a day.

	Product	Form	Size	C.I.*
otc	**Tetrahydrozoline HCl** (Various)	**Solution:** 0.05%	In 15 and 22.5 ml.	3+
otc	**Collyrium w/Tetrahydrozoline** (Wyeth-Ayerst)		In 15 ml.[12]	4
otc	**Eyesine** (Akorn)		In 15 ml.[14]	NA
otc	**Mallazine Drops** (Hauck)		In 15 ml.[15]	4
otc	**Murine Plus** (Ross)		In 15 and 30 ml.[1]	5
otc	**Optigene 3** (Pfeiffer)		In 15 ml.[16]	3
otc	**Soothe Eye Drops** (Alcon)		In 15 ml.[16]	11
otc	**Visine Extra** (Pfizer)		In 15 ml.[17]	NA
otc	**Visine Eye Drops** (Leeming)		In 15, 22.5, 30 ml.[1]	5

* Cost Index based on cost per ml.
[1] With 0.01% benzalkonium chloride and 0.1% EDTA.
[2] With 0.01% benzalkonium chloride, 0.1% EDTA and 0.2% glycerin.
[3] With 0.0067% benzalkonium chloride, 0.02% EDTA, hydroxyethylcellulose and povidone.
[4] With 0.01% benzalkonium chloride, 0.1% dextran 7, 0.3% hydroxypropyl methylcellulose and EDTA.
[5] With 0.01% benzalkonium chloride.
[6] With 0.01% benzalkonium chloride, polyvinyl alcohol, PEG-8000 and EDTA.
[7] With 0.005% benzalkonium chloride and 0.02% EDTA.
[8] With 0.01% benzalkonium chloride and 0.01% EDTA.
[9] With 0.004% benzalkonium chloride, EDTA and 1.4% polyvinyl alcohol.
[10] With 0.01% benzalkonium chloride, EDTA and hydroxypropyl methylcellulose.
[11] With 0.01% benzalkonium chloride and EDTA.
[12] With 0.01% benzalkonium chloride, 0.1% EDTA and 1% glycerin.
[13] With 0.01% benzalkonium chloride, 0.1% EDTA, sodium borate, boric acid, NaCl.
[14] With 0.1% benzalkonium chloride, EDTA, sodium borate, boric acid, NaCl.
[15] With sodium borate, boric acid, NaCl.
[16] With 0.004% benzalkonium chloride, 0.1% EDTA, povidone.
[17] With 0.013% benzalkonium Cl, boric acid, EDTA, sodium borate and 1% PEG-400.

In these combinations:

PHENYLEPHRINE HCl, NAPHAZOLINE HCl and *TETRAHYDROZOLINE* are used for their decongestant actions. See individual monographs for further information.

HYDROXYPROPYL METHYLCELLULOSE and *POLYVINYL ALCOHOL* are used to increase the viscosity of the solution, thereby increasing contact time.

ZINC SULFATE is used as an astringent and antiseptic.

ANTIPYRINE is a weak local anesthetic.

PHENIRAMINE MALEATE, PYRILAMINE MALEATE and *ANTAZOLINE* are antihistamines.

Warning: Topical antihistamines are potential sensitizers and may produce a local sensitivity reaction. Because they may produce angle closure, use with caution in persons with a narrow angle or a history of glaucoma.

Administration and Dosage:

Recommendations vary. Refer to manufacturer package insert for instructions.

		Dosage form	Decongestant	Antihistamine	Other		C.I.*
otc	**Optised** (Various, eg, Rugby, Vortech)	solution	phenylephrine HCl 0.12%		zinc sulfate 0.25%	In 15 ml.	5+
otc	**Phenylzin** (CooperVision)					In 15 ml.[1]	20
otc	**Zincfrin** (Alcon)					In 15 ml.[2]	15
otc	**Prefrin Liquifilm** (Allergan)	solution	phenylephrine HCl 0.12%		antipyrine 0.1%	In 20 ml.[3]	9
otc	**Relief** (Allergan)					In 0.3 and 1 ml.[4]	6
Rx	**Prefrin-A** (Allergan)	solution	phenylephrine HCl 0.12%	pyrilamine maleate 0.1%	antipyrine 0.1%	In 15 ml.[5]	14
Rx	**AK-Vernacon** (Akorn)	solution	phenylephrine HCl 0.125%	pheniramine maleate 0.5%		In 15 ml.[6]	10
otc	**Clear eyes ACR** (Ross)	solution	naphazoline HCl 0.012%		zinc sulfate 0.25%, glycerin 0.2%	In 15 and 30 ml.[13]	
otc	**VasoClear A** (Iolab)	solution	naphazoline HCl 0.02%		zinc sulfate 0.25%	In 15 ml.[7]	11
Rx	**AK-Con-A** (Akorn)	solution	naphazoline HCl 0.025%	pheniramine maleate 0.3%		In 15 ml.[8]	10
Rx	**Naphcon-A** (Alcon)					In 15 ml.[8]	17
Rx	**Opcon-A** (Bausch & Lomb)					In 15 ml.[9]	13
Rx	**Albalon-A Liquifilm** (Allergan)	solution	naphazoline HCl 0.05%	antazoline phosphate 0.5%		In 15 ml.[10]	17
Rx	**Antazoline-V** (Rugby)					In 5 and 15 ml dropper bottles.[11]	16
Rx	**Vasocon-A** (Iolab)					In 15 ml.[11]	18
otc	**Visine A.C.** (Leeming)	solution	tetrahydrozoline HCl 0.05%		zinc sulfate 0.25%	In 15 and 30 ml.[12]	5

* Cost Index based on cost per ml.

[1] With benzalkonium chloride, EDTA, hydroxypropyl methylcellulose and sodium bisulfite.

[2] With 0.01% benzalkonium chloride.

[3] With 0.004% benzalkonium chloride, 1.4% polyvinyl alcohol and EDTA.

[4] With 1.4% polyvinyl alcohol and EDTA.

[5] With benzalkonium chloride, EDTA and sodium bisulfite.

[6] With benzalkonium chloride, polyvinyl alcohol and EDTA.

[7] With 0.005% benzalkonium chloride, EDTA, 0.25% polyvinyl alcohol and PEG-8000.

[8] With 0.01% benzalkonium chloride and EDTA.

[9] With 0.01% benzalkonium chloride, EDTA and hydroxypropyl methylcellulose.

[10] With 0.004% benzalkonium chloride, EDTA, 1.4% polyvinyl alcohol and povidone.

[11] With 0.01% benzalkonium chloride, PEG-8000, polyvinyl alcohol and EDTA.

[12] With 0.01% benzalkonium chloride and 0.1% EDTA.

[13] With benzalkonium chloride, boric acid.

Actions:

These anticholinergic agents block the responses of the sphincter muscle of the iris and the muscle of the ciliary body to cholinergic stimulation, producing pupillary dilation (mydriasis) and paralysis of accommodation (cycloplegia).

Cycloplegic Mydriatics

Drug	Mydriasis		Cycloplegia		Solution Available (%)
	Peak (minutes)	Recovery (days)	Peak (minutes)	Recovery (days)	
Atropine	30-40	7-12	60-180	6-12	0.5-3
Homatropine	40-60	1-3	30-60	1-3	2-5
Scopolamine	20-30	3-7	30-60	3-7	0.25
Cyclopentolate	30-60	1	25-75	0.25-1	0.5-2
Tropicamide	20-40	0.25	20-35	0.25	0.5-1

Indications:

For cycloplegic refraction and for dilating the pupil in inflammatory conditions of the iris and uveal tract.

Contraindications:

Glaucoma or a tendency toward glaucoma (eg, narrow anterior chamber angle); hypersensitivity to belladonna alkaloids or any component of the products.

Atropine: In the elderly where undiagnosed glaucoma or excessive pressure in the eye may be present.

Warnings:

For topical ophthalmic use only.

Determine the intraocular tension and the depth of the angle of the anterior chamber before and during use to avoid glaucoma attacks.

Do not exceed recommended dosages.

Excessive use in children and in certain susceptible individuals may produce general toxic symptoms.

Pregnancy: Category C (atropine, homatropine). Safety for use during pregnancy has not been established. Use only if clearly needed and if the potential benefits outweigh the potential hazards to the fetus.

Lactation: **Atropine** and **homatropine** are absorbed systemically and are detectable, in very small amounts, in breast milk. Because of the potential for serious adverse reactions in nursing infants, decide whether to discontinue nursing or discontinue the drug, taking into account the importance of the drug to the mother.

Children: Do not use **atropine** or **homatropine** during the first 3 months of life, due to the possible association between the cycloplegia produced and development of amblyopia. Safety and efficacy for use in children have not been established. Use with extreme caution. Premature and small infants are especially prone to CNS and cardiopulmonary side effects from systemic absorption of **cyclopentolate**.

Precautions:

To avoid excessive systemic absorption, compress the lacrimal sac by digital pressure for 1 to 2 minutes after instillation.

Longer acting agents (atropine, scopolamine) may cause posterior synechiae to form when treating anterior segment inflammation, without moving the pupil.

Permanent mydriasis may occur in patients with keratocopus and Down's syndrome.

Acute Hypersensitivity Reaction: Have epinephrine 1:1000 immediately available. Refer to Management of Acute Hypersensitivity Reactions on p. viii. Discontinue use if signs of sensitivity develop.

Potentially hazardous tasks: May produce drowsiness, loss of neuromuscular coordination, blurred vision or sensitivity to light (due to dilated pupils); observe caution while driving or performing other tasks requiring alertness.

Sulfite Sensitivity: Some of these products contain sulfites which may cause allergic-type reactions (eg, hives, itching, wheezing, anaphylaxis) in certain susceptible persons. Although the overall prevalence of sulfite sensitivity in the general population is probably low, it is seen more frequently in asthmatics or in atopic nonasthmatic persons. Specific products containing sulfites are identified in the product listings.

Adverse Reactions:

Local: Increased intraocular pressure; transient stinging. Prolonged use may produce irritation (eg, allergic lid reactions, hyperemia, follicular conjunctivitis, vascular congestion, edema, exudate, photophobia, eczematoid dermatitis).

(Adverse Reactions continued on following page)

Adverse Reactions (Cont.:)

Systemic: Systemic **atropine** toxicity is manifested by: Flushing and dryness of the skin (a rash may be present in children); blurred vision; photophobia with or without corneal staining; dryness of the mouth and nose; anhidrosis; a rapid and irregular pulse; fever; abdominal distention in infants; bladder distention; dysarthric quality of speech; mental aberration (hallucinosis) with recovery frequently followed by retrograde amnesia; loss of neuromuscular coordination (ataxic gait). Severe reactions are manifested by hypotension with progressive respiratory depression. Coma, medullary paralysis and death have been reported in the very young.

Cardiac dysrhythmias (atrial fibrillation, supraventricular tachycardia) are reported in patients undergoing surgery for glaucoma.

Headache, parasympathetic stimulation, allergic reactions and somnolence may occur. Other toxic manifestations of anticholinergic drugs are vasodilation, urinary retention and diminished GI motility.

In addition, **cyclopentolate** and **tropicamide** have been associated with psychotic reactions and behavioral disturbances in children. CNS disturbances and cardiorespiratory collapse have occurred in children on **tropicamide**. Ataxia, incoherent speech, restlessness, hallucinations, hyperactivity, seizures, disorientation as to time and place, and failure to recognize people have occurred with **cyclopentolate**.

Overdosage:

When symptoms of atropine toxicity develop (see Adverse Reactions), administer parenteral physostigmine. In infants and children, keep body surface moist.

Patient Information:

May cause blurred vision and increased sensitivity to light.

If eye pain occurs, discontinue use and consult physician immediately.

Refer to page 2164 for more complete information on administration and use.

ATROPINE SULFATE

Indications:

A potent parasympatholytic for producing cycloplegia and mydriasis. Useful for cycloplegic refraction or pupil dilation in acute inflammatory conditions of iris and uveal tract.

Administration and Dosage:

Adults: For uveitis – Instill 1 to 2 drops into the eye(s) 4 times daily. *For refraction* – Instill 1 drop into the eye(s) twice daily for 1 or 2 days before examination.

Children: For uveitis – Instill 1 or 2 drops of 0.5% solution into eye(s) up to 3 times daily. *For refraction* – Instill 1 or 2 drops of 0.5% solution into the eye(s) twice daily for 1 to 3 days before examination and 1 hour before examination.

Individuals with heavily pigmented irides may require larger doses.

	Product	Form	Packaging	C.I.*
Rx	**Atropine Sulfate S.O.P.** (Allergan)	**Ointment:** 0.5%	In 3.5 g.[1]	39
Rx	**Atropine Sulfate Ophthalmic** (Various, eg, Akorn, Balan, Fougera, Harber, Lilly, Moore, Pharmaderm, Raway, Rugby, Schein)	**Ointment:** 1%	In 3.5 and 3.75 g.	9+
Rx	**Atropine Sulfate S.O.P.** (Allergan)		In 3.5 g.[1]	44
Rx	**Atropisol Ophthalmic** (Iolab)	**Solution:** 0.5%	In 1 ml.[2]	59
Rx	**Isopto Atropine** (Alcon)		In 5 ml.[3]	35
Rx	**Atropine Sulfate Ophthalmic** (Various, eg, Alcon, Allergan, Moore, Optopics, Raway, Rugby, Schein, Steris)	**Solution:** 1%	In 2 and 15 ml.	3+
Rx	**Atropine-Care Ophthalmic** (Akorn)		In 2, 5 and 15 ml.[3]	23
Rx	**Atropisol Ophthalmic** (Iolab)		In 1[2], 5[4] and 15[4] ml.	38
Rx	**Isopto Atropine** (Alcon)		In 5 and 15 ml.[3]	38
Rx	**I-Tropine** (Americal)		In 2, 5 and 15 ml.[5]	9
Rx	**Atropine Sulfate Ophthalmic** (Alcon)	**Solution:** 2%	In 2 ml.	53
Rx	**Atropisol** (Iolab)		In 1 ml.[2]	59
Rx	**Isopto Atropine Ophthalmic** (Alcon)	**Solution:** 3%	In 5 ml.[3]	46

* Cost Index based on cost per g or ml.

[1] With 0.5% chlorobutanol, white petrolatum, mineral oil and nonionic lanolin derivatives.

[2] With benzalkonium chloride.

[3] With 0.01% benzalkonium chloride and hydroxypropyl methylcellulose.

[4] With benzalkonium chloride and EDTA.

[5] With 0.01% benzalkonium chloride, 0.35% hydroxyethylcellulose, EDTA and sodium bisulfite.

Complete prescribing information for these products begins on page 2198 .

SCOPOLAMINE HBr (Hyoscine HBr)

Indications:

An anticholinergic agent for use in producing cycloplegia and mydriasis. For preoperative and postoperative states in the treatment of iridocyclitis.

Administration and Dosage:

For refraction: Instill 1 or 2 drops into the eye(s) 1 hour before refracting.

For uveitis: Instill 1 or 2 drops into the eye(s) up to 4 times daily.

				C.I.*
Rx	**Isopto Hyoscine** (Alcon)	**Solution:** 0.25%	In 5 and 15 ml.[1]	38

HOMATROPINE HBr

Indications:

A moderately long-acting mydriatic and cycloplegic for refraction, and in the treatment of inflammatory conditions of the uveal tract. For preoperative and postoperative states when mydriasis is required. As an optical aid in some cases of axial lens opacities.

Administration and Dosage:

For refraction: Instill 1 or 2 drops into the eye(s); repeat in 5 to 10 minutes if necessary.

For uveitis: Instill 1 or 2 drops into the eye(s) up to every 3 to 4 hours.

Individuals with heavily pigmented irides may require larger doses.

				C.I.*
Rx	**Homatropine HBr Ophthalmic** (Iolab)	**Solution:** 2%	In 1[2] and 5 ml.[3]	47
Rx	**Isopto Homatropine** (Alcon)		In 5 and 15 ml.[4]	38
Rx	**Homatropine HBr Ophthalmic** (Various, eg, Alcon, Iolab, Pharmafair)	**Solution:** 5%	In 1, 2 and 5 ml.	52+
Rx	**AK-Homatropine** (Akorn)		In 15 ml.[5]	9
Rx	**Homatrine** (Americal)		In 5 ml.[5]	53
Rx	**Isopto Homatropine** (Alcon)		In 5 and 15 ml.[6]	44

TROPICAMIDE

Indications:

For mydriasis and cycloplegia for diagnostic purposes. When a short-acting mydriatic is needed for some preoperative and postoperative states.

Administration and Dosage:

For refraction: Instill 1 or 2 drops of 1% solution into the eye(s); repeat in 5 minutes. If patient is not seen within 20 to 30 minutes, instill an additional drop to prolong mydriatic effect. For examination of fundus, instill 1 or 2 drops of 0.5% solution 15 or 20 minutes prior to examination.

Individuals with heavily pigmented irides may require larger doses.

				C.I.*
Rx	**Tropicamide** (Various, eg, Pharmafair, Raway, Schein)	**Solution:** 0.5%	In 2 and 15 ml.	8+
Rx	**Mydriacyl Ophthalmic** (Alcon)		In 15 ml.[7]	27
Rx	**Tropicacyl** (Akorn)		In 15 ml.[8]	17
Rx	**Tropicamide** (Various, eg, Harber, Pharmafair, Raway, Schein)	**Solution:** 1%	In 2 and 15 ml.	10+
Rx	**I-Picamide** (Americal)		In 2 and 15 ml.[7]	9
Rx	**Mydriacyl Ophthalmic** (Alcon)		In 3 and 15 ml.[7]	30
Rx	**Tropicacyl** (Akorn)		In 2 and 15 ml.[8]	19

* Cost Index based on cost per g or ml.

[1] With 0.01% benzalkonium chloride and 0.5% hydroxypropyl methylcellulose.

[2] With benzalkonium chloride.

[3] With benzalkonium chloride and EDTA.

[4] With 0.01% benzalkonium chloride, 0.5% hydroxypropyl methylcellulose and polysorbate 80.

[5] With 0.01% benzalkonium chloride, hydroxyethylcellulose and EDTA.

[6] With 0.005% benzethonium chloride and 0.5% hydroxypropyl methylcellulose.

[7] With 0.01% benzalkonium chloride and EDTA.

[8] With 0.1% benzalkonium chloride and EDTA.

Complete prescribing information for these products begins on page 2198 .

CYCLOPENTOLATE HCl

Indications:

For mydriasis and cycloplegia in diagnostic procedures.

Administration and Dosage:

Adults: Instill 1 drop of solution followed by a second drop in 5 to 10 minutes. Although complete recovery usually occurs in 24 hours, 1 or 2 drops of 1% or 2% pilocarpine reduces recovery time to 3 to 6 hours in most eyes.

Children: Pretreatment with cyclopentolate on the day before examination usually is not necessary. One drop of 0.5%, 1% or 2% solution is instilled into each eye, followed 5 minutes later by a second application of 0.5% or 1% solution, if necessary. For small infants, instill one drop of 0.5% solution into each eye. To minimize absorption, apply pressure over the nasolacrimal sac for 2 to 3 minutes. Observe patient closely for at least 30 minutes following instillation.

Individuals with heavily pigmented irides may require larger doses.

	Product	Form	Size	C.I.*
Rx	**AK-Pentolate** (Akorn)	**Solution:** 0.5%	In 15 ml.[1]	75
Rx	**Cyclogyl** (Alcon)		In 2, 5 and 15 ml.[1]	27
Rx	**Cyclopentolate** (Rugby)	**Solution:** 1%	In 2, 5 and 15 ml.[1]	9
Rx	**AK-Pentolate** (Akorn)		In 2 and 15 ml.[1]	19
Rx	**Cyclogyl** (Alcon)		In 2, 5 and 15 ml.[1]	30
Rx	**I-Pentolate** (Americal)		In 2 and 15 ml.[1]	8
Rx	**Cyclogyl** (Alcon)	**Solution:** 2%	In 2, 5 and 15 ml.[1]	35

MYDRIATRIC COMBINATIONS

In the combinations:

PHENYLEPHRINE HCl is used with *CYCLOPENTOLATE HCl* or *SCOPOLAMINE HBr* to induce mydriasis that is considerably greater than that of either drug alone. See individual monographs for complete prescribing information.

	Product	Description	C.I.*
Rx	**Cyclomydril Ophthalmic** (Alcon)	**Solution:** 0.2% cyclopentolate HCl and 1% phenylephrine HCl. In 2 and 5 ml.[2] **Indications:** For the production of mydriasis. **Dose:** Instill 1 drop into each eye every 5 to 10 minutes, not to exceed 3 times.	48
Rx	**Murocoll-2 Ophthalmic** (Bausch & Lomb)	**Drops:** 0.3% scopolamine HBr and 10% phenylephrine HCl. In 5 ml.[3] **Indications:** For mydriasis, cycloplegia and to break posterior synechiae in iritis. **Dose:** For mydriasis – 1 or 2 drops into eye(s); repeat in 5 minutes, if necessary. Postoperatively – 1 or 2 drops into eye(s), 3 or 4 times daily.	36
Rx	**Paremyd** (Allergan)	**Solution:** 1% hydroxyamphetamine hydrobromide, 0.25% tropicamide. In 5 and 15 ml.[4] **Indication:** For mydriasis.	NA

* Cost Index based on cost per ml.

[1] With benzalkonium chloride and EDTA.

[2] With 0.01% benzalkonium chloride and EDTA.

[3] With 0.01% benzalkonium chloride, sodium metabisulfite and EDTA.

[4] With 0.005% benzalkonium chloride and 0.015% EDTA.

Enzymes

CHYMOTRYPSIN

Actions:

Chymotrypsin is a proteolytic enzyme. The principal proteolytic effect is exerted by the splitting of peptide bonds of amino acids in the zonular fibers and ocular tissues.

Destruction of the equatorial pericapsular membrane of the lens occurs in 5 minutes. Zonular fibers are lysed within 10 to 15 minutes of application; complete lysis of the entire zonular membrane occurs in 30 minutes.

Indications:

For enzymatic zonulysis for intracapsular lens extraction.

Contraindications:

Significant anterior displacement of the lens iris diaphragm with impending vitreous loss; other conditions in which loss of vitreous is a significant problem (eg, intracapsular extraction of congenital cataracts); high vitreous pressure; gaping incisional wound; congenital cataracts; hypersensitivity to chymotrypsin or any component of the preparation; patients less than 20 years old because of probable lens-vitreous adhesion not responsive to alpha-chymotrypsin lysis.

Precautions:

Intraocular pressure (IOP): Chymotrypsin may produce an acute rise in IOP following surgery, especially in patients with poor facility of outflow.

Synechiae lysis: The enzyme will not lyse the synechiae that may exist between the lens and other eye structures.

Drug Interactions:

Epinephrine 1:100 will inactivate chymotrypsin in approximately 1 hour.

Isoflurophate and **chloramphenicol** inhibit chymotrypsin.

Adverse Reactions:

Transient increases in intraocular pressure; moderate uveitis; corneal edema; striation. Delayed healing of incisions has been reported, but not confirmed.

Administration and Dosage:

Instruments and syringes must be free of enzyme-inactivating alcohol and other chemicals. Excessive heat may alter chymotrypsin; do not autoclave the powder or reconstituted solution. Do not use solution if it is cloudy or contains a precipitate. Serum, blood, detergents, alkalies, acids and antiseptics (ie, alcohol) will inactivate chymotrypsin.

Potency: Chymotrypsin's potency is measured in Armour proteolytic activity (APA) units.

Reconstitution: Reconstitute immediately prior to use. The 750 unit vials may be reconstituted with 5 ml (150 units/ml) or 10 ml (75 units/ml) of the diluent provided. A solution of 150 units/ml is equivalent to a 1:5000 dilution; 75 units/ml is equivalent to a 1:10,000 dilution. The 300 unit vials reconstituted with 2 ml of diluent yields a 1:5000 dilution.

Procedure –

1) Dilate pupils with a suitable mydriatic. Use either local or general anesthesia.

2) Following incision, irrigate the posterior chamber (under the iris) with 0.25 to 2 ml chymotrypsin solution.

3) Wait 2 to 4 minutes, then irrigate with at least 2 ml of the unused portion of diluent or sodium chloride solution. If zonules are still intact, irrigate with additional chymotrypsin solution (0.5 to 2 ml). After 2 to 4 minutes, irrigate again with about 2 ml diluent or sodium chloride solution.

4) Following extraction, the pupils may be contracted with a suitable miotic.

			C.I.*
Rx	**Catarase 1:10,000** (Iolab)	**For Ophthalmic Solution:** 150 units with 2 ml sodium chloride diluent per dual chamber univial	718
Rx	**Catarase 1:5,000** (Iolab)	**For Ophthalmic Solution:** 300 units with 2 ml sodium chloride diluent per dual chamber univial	359
Rx	**Zolyse** (Alcon)	**For Ophthalmic Solution:** 750 units per vial. With 9 ml balanced salt solution diluent	160

* Cost Index based on cost per 150 units.

Nonsteroidal Anti-inflammatory Agents

Actions:

Flurbiprofen sodium 0.03%, suprofen 1% and diclofenac sodium 0.1% are topical nonsteroidal anti-inflammatory drugs (NSAIDs) available as solutions for ophthalmic use.

Pharmacology: Flurbiprofen and suprofen are phenylalkanoic acids and diclofenac is a phenylacetic acid; they have analgesic, antipyretic and anti-inflammatory activity. Their mechanism of action is believed to be through inhibition of the cyclo-oxygenase enzyme that is essential in the biosynthesis of prostaglandins.

In animals, prostaglandins are mediators of certain kinds of intraocular inflammation. Prostaglandins produce disruption of the blood-aqueous humor barrier, vasodilation, increased vascular permeability, leukocytosis and increased intraocular pressure (IOP). Diclofenac has no significant effect on IOP.

Prostaglandins also appear to play a role in the miotic response produced during ocular surgery by constricting the iris sphincter independently of cholinergic mechanisms. These agents inhibit the miosis induced during the course of cataract surgery.

Nonsteroidal Anti-Inflammatory Ophthalmic Agents

Ophthalmic NSAID	Trade name (manufacturer)	Solution concentration	Ophthalmic indication
Flurbiprofen	*Ocufen* (Allergan)	0.03%	Inhibition of intra-operative miosis
Suprofen	*Profenal* (Alcon)	1%	
Diclofenac	*Voltaren* (Ciba Vision Ophthalmics)	0.1%	Treatment of post-operative inflammation following cataract extraction

Indications:

Flurbiprofen, suprofen: For inhibition of intraoperative miosis.

Diclofenac: Treatment of postoperative inflammation following cataract extraction.

Unlabeled uses: Flurbiprofen – Topical treatment of cystoid macular edema, inflammation after cataract surgery and uveitis syndromes.

Contraindications:

Hypersensitivity to the drugs or any component of the products.

Flurbiprofen, suprofen: Epithelial herpes simplex keratitis (dendritic keratitis).

Diclofenac: Patients wearing soft contact lenses (see Precautions).

Warnings:

Cross-sensitivity: The potential for cross-sensitivity to acetylsalicylic acid and other NSAIDs exists. Therefore, use caution when treating individuals who have previously exhibited sensitivities to these drugs.

Systemic absorption occurs with drugs applied ocularly. Use with caution in surgical patients with known bleeding tendencies (see Precautions).

Pregnancy: Category C (flurbiprofen, suprofen); *Category B* (diclofenac). **Flurbiprofen** is embryocidal, delays parturition, prolongs gestation, reduces weight and slightly retards fetal growth in rats at daily oral doses of ≥ 0.4 mg/kg (approximately 185 times the human daily topical dose).

Oral doses of **suprofen** of up to 200 mg/kg/day in animals resulted in an increased incidence of fetal resorption associated with maternal toxicity. There was an increase in stillbirths and a decrease in postnatal survival in pregnant rats treated with ≥ 2.5 mg/kg/day.

Oral **diclofenac** in mice and rats crosses the placental barrier. In rats, maternally toxic doses were associated with dystocia, prolonged gestation, reduced fetal weights, growth and survival. Because of the known effects of prostaglandin-inhibiting drugs on the fetal cardiovascular system, avoid the use of ophthalmic diclofenac during late pregnancy.

There are no adequate and well controlled studies in pregnant women. Use during pregnancy only if the potential benefits outweigh the potential hazards to the fetus.

(Warnings continued on following page)

Warnings (Cont.):

Lactation: It is not known whether **flurbiprofen** is excreted in breast milk. Because of the potential for serious adverse reactions in nursing infants, decide whether to discontinue nursing or to discontinue the drug, taking into account the importance of the drug to the mother.

Suprofen is excreted in breast milk after a single oral dose. Based on measurements of plasma and milk levels in women taking oral suprofen, the milk concentration is about 1% of the plasma level. Because systemic absorption may occur from topical ocular administration, consider discontinuing nursing while on suprofen; its safety in human neonates has not been established.

Children: Safety and efficacy for use in children have not been established.

Precautions:

Wound healing may be delayed with the use of flurbiprofen.

Bleeding tendencies: Use with caution in surgical patients with known bleeding tendencies or who are on other medications that may prolong bleeding time. Some systemic absorption occurs with drugs applied ocularly, and NSAIDs increase bleeding time by interference with thrombocyte aggregation. NSAIDs applied ocularly may cause an increased bleeding tendency of ocular tissues in conjunction with surgery.

Contact lenses: Patients wearing hydrogel soft contact lenses who have used diclofenac concurrently have experienced ocular irritation manifested by redness and burning.

Drug Interactions:

Acetylcholine chloride and **carbachol:** Although clinical studies with acetylcholine chloride and animal studies with acetylcholine chloride or carbachol revealed no interference, and there is no known pharmacological basis for an interaction, both of these drugs have reportedly been ineffective when used in patients treated with flurbiprofen or suprofen.

Adverse Reactions:

Most frequent: Transient burning and stinging upon instillation (15% with diclofenac); other minor symptoms of ocular irritation.

Suprofen: Discomfort; itching; redness; allergy, iritis, pain, chemosis, photophobia, irritation, punctate epithelial staining ($< 0.5\%$).

Diclofenac: Keratitis (28%, although most cases occurred in cataract studies prior to drug therapy); elevated IOP (15%, although most cases occurred post surgery and prior to drug therapy); anterior chamber reaction; ocular allergy; nausea, vomiting (1%); viral infections ($\leq 1\%$).

Overdosage:

Overdosage will not ordinarily cause acute problems. If accidentally ingested, drink fluids to dilute.

FLURBIPROFEN SODIUM

Administration and Dosage:

Instill 1 drop approximately every ½ hour, beginning 2 hours before surgery (total of 4 drops).

				C.I.*
Rx	**Ocufen** (Allergan)	**Solution:** 0.03%	In 2.5, 5 and 10 ml dropper bottles.[1]	77

SUPROFEN

Administration and Dosage:

On the day of surgery, instill 2 drops into the conjunctival sac at 3, 2 and 1 hour prior to surgery. Two drops may be instilled into the conjunctival sac every 4 hours, while awake, the day preceding surgery.

Rx	**Profenal** (Alcon)	**Solution:** 1%	In 2.5 ml Drop-Tainers.[2]

DICLOFENAC SODIUM

Administration and Dosage:

Apply 1 drop to the affected eye 4 times daily beginning 24 hours after cataract surgery and continuing throughout the first 2 weeks of the postoperative period.

Rx	**Voltaren** (Ciba Vision Ophthalmics)	**Solution:** 0.1%	In 2.5 and 5 ml dropper bottles.[3]

* Cost index based on cost per ml.

[1] With 1.4% polyvinyl alcohol, 0.005% thimerosal and EDTA.

[2] With 0.005% thimerosal, 2% caffeine and EDTA.

[3] With 1 mg/ml EDTA, boric acid, polyoxyl 35 castor oil, 2 mg/ml sorbic acid and tromethamine.

Corticosteroids

Actions:

Topical corticosteroids exert an anti-inflammatory action. Aspects of the inflammatory process such as hyperemia, cellular infiltration, vascularization and fibroblastic proliferation are suppressed. Steroids cause inhibition of inflammatory response to inciting agents of mechanical, chemical or immunological nature. Topical corticosteroids are effective in acute inflammatory conditions of the conjunctiva, sclera, cornea, lids, iris, ciliary body and anterior segment of the globe; and in ocular allergic conditions. In the treatment of ocular disease, the route depends on the site and extent of the disorder.

The mechanism of the anti-inflammatory action is thought to be potentiation of epinephrine vasoconstriction, stabilization of lysosomal membranes, retardation of macrophage movement, prevention of kinin release, inhibition of lymphocyte and neutrophil function, inhibition of prostaglandin synthesis and, in prolonged use, decrease of antibody production.

By inhibiting fibroblastic proliferation, symblepharon formation in chemical and thermal burns may be prevented. Decreased scarring with clearer corneas following topical corticosteroid therapy is a result of inhibiting fibroblastic proliferation and vascularization.

Indications:

For treatment of steroid responsive inflammatory conditions of the palpebral and bulbar conjunctiva, lid, cornea and anterior segment of the globe, such as: Allergic conjunctivitis; nonspecific superficial keratitis; superficial punctate keratitis; herpes zoster keratitis; iritis; cyclitis; and selected infective conjunctivitis when the inherent hazard of steroid use is accepted to obtain a diminution in edema and inflammation. Also used for corneal injury from chemical, radiation or thermal burns or penetration of foreign bodies.

Use higher strengths for moderate to severe inflammations. In difficult cases of anterior segment eye disease, systemic therapy may be required. When deeper ocular structures are involved, use systemic therapy. May use to suppress graft reaction after keratoplasty.

Contraindications:

Acute superficial herpes simplex keratitis; fungal diseases of ocular structures; vaccinia, varicella and most other viral diseases of the cornea and conjunctiva; ocular tuberculosis; hypersensitivity; after uncomplicated removal of a superficial corneal foreign body.

Medrysone is not for use in iritis and uveitis; its efficacy has not been demonstrated.

Warnings:

Ocular damage: Prolonged use may result in glaucoma, elevated IOP, optic nerve damage, defects in visual acuity and fields of vision, posterior subcapsular cataract formation or secondary ocular infections from pathogens liberated from ocular tissues. Check IOP and lens frequently. In diseases causing thinning of cornea or sclera, perforation has occurred with topical steroids.

Mustard gas keratitis or Sjogren's keratoconjunctivitis: Topical steroids are not effective.

Infections: Acute, purulent, untreated eye infection may be masked or activity enhanced by steroids. Fungal infections of the cornea have been reported with long-term local steroid applications. Therefore, suspect fungal invasion in any persistent corneal ulceration where a steroid has been used, or is being used.

Stromal herpes simplex keratitis treatment with steroid medication requires great caution; frequent slit-lamp microscopy is mandatory. Numerous cases of herpes simplex keratitis have occurred after inappropriate use of these preparations.

Pregnancy: Category C. Safety of intensive or protracted use is not substantiated. Use only when clearly needed and when potential benefits outweigh potential hazards.

Lactation: It is not known whether topical steroids are excreted in breast milk. Exercise caution when administering to a nursing mother.

Children: Safety and efficacy have not been established in children.

Precautions:

Sulfite sensitivity: Some of these products contain sulfites which may cause allergic-type reactions (eg, hives, itching, wheezing, anaphylaxis) in certain susceptible persons. Although the overall prevalence of sulfite sensitivity in the general population is probably low, it is seen more frequently in asthmatics or in atopic nonasthmatic persons. Specific products containing sulfites are identified in the product listings.

Adverse Reactions:

Glaucoma with optic nerve damage, visual acuity and field defects; posterior subcapsular cataract formation; secondary ocular infection from pathogens, including herpes simplex liberated from ocular tissues; perforation of globe. Viral and fungal corneal infections may be exacerbated by steroids. Transient stinging or burning may occur on instillation. Rarely, filtering blebs have been reported with steroid use after cataract surgery.

Systemic side effects may occur with extensive use (see Adrenal Cortical Steroids group monograph).

(Continued on following page)

Corticosteroids (Cont.)

Patient Information:

Do not discontinue use without consulting physician.

May cause sensitivity to bright light; this may be minimized by wearing sunglasses. Notify physician if improvement is not seen after 7 to 8 days, if condition worsens, or if pain, itching or swelling of the eye occurs.

Refer to page 2165 for more complete information on administration and use.

Administration and Dosage:

Treatment duration varies with type of lesion and may extend from a few days to several weeks, depending on therapeutic response. Relapse may occur if therapy is reduced too rapidly; taper over several days. Relapses, more common in chronic active lesions than in self-limited conditions, usually respond to retreatment.

Solutions: Instill 1 or 2 drops into the conjunctival sac every hour during the day and every 2 hours during the night. When a favorable response is observed, reduce dosage to 1 drop every 4 hours. Later, 1 drop 3 or 4 times daily may suffice to control symptoms.

Ointments: Apply a thin coating in the lower conjunctival sac 3 or 4 times a day. When a favorable response is observed, reduce the number of daily applications to twice, and later to once a day as a maintenance dose if sufficient to control symptoms.

Ointments are particularly convenient when an eye pad is used and may be the preparation of choice when prolonged contact of drug with ocular tissues is needed.

Corticosteroid Drops

	Product	Formulation	How supplied	C.I.*
Rx	**Pred Mild Ophthalmic** (Allergan)	**Suspension:** 0.12% prednisolone acetate	In 5 and 10 ml dropper bottles.[1]	202
Rx	**Econopred Ophthalmic** (Alcon)	**Suspension:** 0.125% prednisolone acetate	In 5 and 10 ml Drop-Tainers.[2]	205
Rx	**Prednisolone Sodium Phosphate** (Various, eg, Harber, Pharmafair, Raway, Rugby)	**Solution:** 0.125% prednisolone sodium phosphate	In 5 and 15 ml.	47+
Rx	**AK-Pred Ophthalmic** (Akorn)		In 5 ml dropper bottles.[3]	127
Rx	**Inflamase Mild Ophthalmic** (Iolab)		In 5 and 10 ml dropper bottles.[4]	207
Rx	**Metreton Ophthalmic** (Schering)	**Solution:** 0.5% prednisolone phosphate (as sodium phosphate)	In 5 ml dropper bottles.[5]	265
Rx	**Prednisolone Acetate Ophthalmic** (Various, eg, Harber, Moore, Raway, Rugby, Schein)	**Suspension:** 1% prednisolone acetate	In 5, 10 and 15 ml.	63+
Rx	**Econopred Plus** (Alcon)		In 5 & 10 ml Drop-Tainers.[2]	214
Rx	**Pred Forte** (Allergan)		In 1, 5, 10 and 15 ml dropper bottles.[1]	217

* Cost Index based on cost per ml.

[1] With benzalkonium chloride, EDTA, polysorbate 80, hydroxypropyl methylcellulose, sodium bisulfite.

[2] With 0.01% benzalkonium chloride, EDTA, polysorbate 80 and hydroxypropyl methylcellulose.

[3] With 0.01% benzalkonium chloride, EDTA, hydroxyethylcellulose and sodium bisulfite.

[4] With benzalkonium chloride and EDTA.

[5] With benzalkonium chloride, EDTA, tyloxapol and phenylethyl alcohol.

(Continued on following page)

Complete prescribing information for these products begins on page 2205

Corticosteroid Drops (Cont.)

	Product	Formulation	How Supplied	C.I.*
Rx	**Prednisolone Sodium Phosphate** (Various, eg, Pharmafair, Rugby)	**Solution:** 1% prednisolone sodium phosphate	In 5 and 15 ml.	54+
Rx	**AK-Pred** (Akorn)		In 5 and 15 ml w/dropper.[1]	127
Rx	**Inflamase Forte Ophthalmic** (Iolab)		In 5 and 10 ml w/dropper.[2]	218
Rx	**AK-Dex Ophthalmic** (Akorn)	**Solution:** 0.1% dexamethasone phosphate (as sodium phosphate)	In 5 ml dropper bottles.[3]	135
Rx	**Baldex** (Bausch & Lomb)		In 5 ml dropper bottles.[4]	170
Rx	**Decadron Phosphate Ophthalmic** (MSD)		In 5 ml Ocumeter.[5]	279
Rx	**Dexotic** (Parnell)		In 5 ml w/dropper.[1]	100
Rx	**I-Methasone** (Akorn)		In 5 ml w/dropper.	50
Rx	**Dexamethasone Ophthalmic** (Various)	**Suspension:** 0.1% dexamethasone	In 5 ml.	NA
Rx	**Maxidex** (Alcon)		In 5 and 15 ml Drop-Tainers.[6]	268
Rx	**Fluor-Op** (Iolab)	**Suspension:** 0.1% fluorometholone	In 5, 10 and 15 ml bottles.[7]	134
Rx	**FML Liquifilm** (Allergan)		In 1, 5, 10 and 15 ml bottles.[7]	230
Rx	**Flarex** (Alcon)	**Suspension:** 0.1% fluorometholone, 0.01% benzalkonium chloride, EDTA	In 2.5 and 5 ml bottle w/ dropper.	NA
Rx	**FML Forte** (Allergan)	**Suspension:** 0.25% fluorometholone	In 2, 5, 10 and 15 ml dropper bottles.[8]	276
Rx	**HMS Liquifilm** (Allergan)	**Suspension:** 1% medrysone	In 5 and 10 ml dropper bottles.[9]	217

Corticosteroid Ointments

	Product	Formulation	How Supplied	C.I.*
Rx	**Dexamethasone Sodium Phosphate Ophthalmic** (Various)	**Ointment:** 0.05% dexamethasone phosphate (as sodium phosphate) in a white petrolatum and mineral oil base	In 3.75 g.	54+
Rx	**AK-Dex** (Akorn)		In 3.5 g.[10]	102
Rx	**Baldex** (Bausch & Lomb)		In 3.5 g.[10]	267
Rx	**Decadron Phosphate** (MSD)		In 3.5 g.	163
Rx	**Maxidex** (Alcon)		In 3.5 g.	465
Rx	**FML** (Allergan)	**Ointment:** 0.1% fluorometholone	In a white petrolatum and mineral oil base. In 3.5 g.[11]	351

Corticosteroid/Mydriatic Combination

Atropine is a cycloplegic mydriatic; it is combined with prednisolone when used for the treatment of anterior uveitis.

	Product	Formulation	How Supplied	C.I.*
Rx	**Mydrapred** (Alcon)	**Suspension:** 0.25% prednisolone acetate & 1% atropine sulfate	In 5 ml Drop-Tainers.[12]	250

* Cost Index based on cost per g or ml.

1 With 0.01% benzalkonium chloride, EDTA, polysorbate 80 and hydroxypropyl methylcellulose.

2 With 0.01% benzalkonium chloride, EDTA, hydroxyethylcellulose and sodium bisulfite.

3 With benzalkonium chloride and EDTA.

4 With benzalkonium chloride, EDTA, tyloxapol and phenylethyl alcohol.

5 With benzalkonium chloride, EDTA, polysorbate 80, polyvinyl alcohol and hydroxyethylcellulose.

6 With 0.01% benzalkonium chloride, EDTA, hydroxyethylcellulose, polysorbate 80, sodium bisulfite.

7 With 0.004% benzalkonium chloride, EDTA, polysorbate 80 and 1.4% polyvinyl alcohol.

8 With 0.005% benzalkonium chloride, EDTA, polysorbate 80 and 1.4% polyvinyl alcohol.

9 With 0.004% benzalkonium chloride, EDTA, 1.4% polyvinyl alcohol and hydroxypropyl methylcellulose.

10 With lanolin, parabens and polyethylene glycol 400.

11 With lanolin.

12 With 0.01% benzalkonium chloride.

Antiallergic

CROMOLYN SODIUM (Sodium Cromoglycate)

Actions:

Animal studies show that cromolyn sodium inhibits the degranulation of sensitized mast cells that occurs after exposure to specific antigens, thus inhibiting the release of histamine and SRS-A (slow-reacting substance of anaphylaxis) from the mast cell. It has no intrinsic vasoconstrictor, antihistaminic or anti-inflammatory activity.

Pharmacokinetics: Cromolyn sodium is poorly absorbed; approximately 0.03% of cromolyn is absorbed following administration to the eye. Systemically absorbed drug is excreted unchanged in the bile and urine.

Indications:

Treatment of allergic ocular disorders (vernal keratoconjunctivitis, vernal conjunctivitis, giant papillary conjunctivitis, vernal keratitis and allergic keratoconjunctivitis).

Contraindications:

Hypersensitivity to cromolyn or to any component of the product.

As with all ophthalmic preparations containing benzalkonium chloride, patients are advised not to wear soft contact lenses during cromolyn sodium treatment. Wear can be resumed within a few hours after discontinuation of the drug.

Warnings:

Pregnancy: Category B. There are no adequate and well controlled studies in pregnant women. Use during pregnancy only if clearly needed.

Lactation: It is not known whether this drug is excreted in breast milk. Exercise caution when administering to a nursing mother.

Children: Safety and efficacy in children < 4 years of age are not established.

Adverse Reactions:

Most frequent: Transient ocular stinging or burning upon instillation (13% to 77% of patients) that usually regresses with continued use.

Infrequent (unclear whether attributable to the drug): Conjunctival injection; watery, itchy and puffy eyes; dryness around eyes; eye irritation; styes.

Patient Information:

A transient stinging or burning sensation may occur after instillation.

Do not wear soft contact lenses during treatment. Lenses may be worn within a few hours after discontinuation of the drug.

Administer the drug at regular intervals.

Administration and Dosage:

Symptomatic response to therapy (decreased itching, tearing, redness and discharge) is usually evident within a few days, but treatment for up to 6 weeks is sometimes required. Effect of therapy depends upon administration at regular intervals. Continue therapy as long as needed to sustain improvement. Corticosteroids may be used concomitantly.

Adults and children: 1 to 2 drops in each eye 4 to 6 times per day at regular intervals. One drop contains approximately 1.6 mg cromolyn sodium.

Storage: Store below 30°C (86°F). Protect from direct sunlight. Discard any remaining contents after 4 weeks.

				C.I.*
Rx	**Opticrom 4%** (Fisons)	**Solution:** 40 mg per ml	In 10 ml dropper bottles.[1]	177

* Cost Index based on cost per ml.

[1] With 0.01% benzalkonium chloride and 0.1% EDTA.

Antibiotics

Indications:

Treatment of superficial ocular infections (eg, conjunctivitis, keratitis, keratoconjunctivitis, corneal ulcers, blepharitis, blepharoconjunctivitis, acute meibomianitis and dacryocystitis) due to strains of microorganisms susceptible to antibiotics.

Tetracycline HCl and erythromycin are also indicated for the prophylaxis of ophthalmia neonatorum due to *Neisseria gonorrhoeae* or *Chlamydia trachomatis*.

Use chloramphenicol only in those serious infections for which less potentially dangerous drugs are ineffective or contraindicated (see Warnings).

For a discussion of the microorganisms usually susceptible to these agents, refer to individual product monographs for the systemic preparations in the Anti-infectives chapter.

Organisms Generally Susceptible to Ophthalmic Antibiotics

							Quinolones		Aminoglycosides			Tetracyclines			Sulfonamides	
	Organism/Infection	Bacitracin	Gramicidin	Polymyxin B	Erythromycin	Chloramphenicol	Norfloxacin	Ciprofloxacin	Neomycin	Gentamicin	Tobramycin	Tetracycline	Chlortetracycline	Oxytetracycline	Sod. sulfacetamide	Sulfisoxazole
Gram-Positive	Staphylococcus sp		✓				✓	✓		✓	✓					
	S aureus	✓				✓	✓	✓	✓		✓	✓	✓			
	Streptococcus sp	✓	✓			✓		✓			✓	✓		✓		
	S pneumoniae	✓	✓			✓	✓	✓		✓	✓	✓	✓			
	S pyogenes							✓					✓		✓	
	β-hemolytic streptococci	✓				✓				✓	✓					
	Clostridia sp	✓														
	Diphtheria bacilli		✓													
Gram-Negative	Escherichia coli			✓		✓	✓	✓	✓	✓	✓	✓	✓	✓	✓	✓
	Hemophilus aegyptius (Koch-Weeks bacillus)						✓			✓	✓				✓	✓
	H ducreyi							✓					✓	✓		
	H influenzae			✓		✓	✓	✓	✓	✓	✓		✓	✓		
	Klebsiella sp					✓	✓		✓					✓		
	K pneumoniae						✓	✓		✓	✓		✓			
	Neisseria sp					✓			✓	✓	✓	✓				
	N gonorrhoeae	✓			✓‡		✓	✓		✓		✓‡	✓		✓	
	Proteus sp						✓	✓	✓	✓	✓					
	Acinetobacter calcoaceticus						✓	✓			✓					
	Enterobacter aerogenes			✓			✓	✓	✓	✓	✓			✓		
	Enterobacter sp					✓	✓		✓							
	Mima/Herellea sp													✓		
	Moraxella lacunata					✓				✓	✓					
	Chlamydia trachomatis				✓‡			✓				✓‡‡	✓‡‡	✓	✓**	✓**
	Pasteurella tularensis												✓	✓		
	Pseudomonas aeruginosa			✓		✓	✓	✓		✓	✓					
	Bartonella bacilliformis													✓		
	Bacteroides sp				✓							✓	✓	✓		
	Vibrio sp						✓							✓		
	Yersinia pestis												✓	✓		
	Brucella sp													✓*		
	Aeromonas hydrophilia						✓									
	Serratia marcescens						✓									

‡ For prophylaxis
‡‡ In conjunction with oral therapy
* In conjunction with streptomycin
** Adjunct in systemic sulfonamide therapy.

(Continued on following page)

Contraindications:

Hypersensitivity to any component of these products; epithelial herpes simplex keratitis (dendritic keratitis); vaccinia; varicella; mycobacterial infections of the eye; fungal diseases of the ocular structure; use after uncomplicated removal of a corneal foreign body.

Warnings:

Sensitization from the topical use of an antibiotic may contraindicate the drug's later systemic use in serious infections. For this reason, topical preparations containing antibiotics not ordinarily administered systemically are preferable.

Products with **neomycin sulfate** may cause cutaneous/conjunctival sensitization (10%).

Cross-sensitivity: Kanamycin, paromomycin, streptomycin, and possibly, gentamicin: Allergic cross-reactions may occur that could prevent future use of any or all of these antibiotics.

Ophthalmic ointments may retard corneal epithelial healing.

Hematologic: At least ten cases involving major adverse hematologic events (bone marrow hypoplasia, aplastic anemia and death) have occurred with ocular **chloramphenicol** after use for 1 to 23 months (prolonged or frequent intermittent use).

Hematopoietic toxicity has occurred occasionally with the systemic use of chloramphenicol and rarely with topical administration. It is generally a dose-related toxic effect on bone marrow, and is usually reversible on cessation of therapy.

Pregnancy: (Category B – tobramycin. Category C – gentamicin, ciprofloxacin, norfloxacin). Safety for use with tobramycin during pregnancy has not been established. Use only when clearly needed and when the potential benefits outweigh the potential hazards to the fetus.

Lactation: Because of the potential for adverse reactions in nursing infants from **norfloxacin** and **tobramycin,** decide whether to discontinue nursing or discontinue the drug, taking into account the importance of the drug to the mother. Exercise caution when administering **ciprofloxacin** to a nursing mother.

Children: **Tobramycin** is safe and effective in children. Safety and efficacy of **ciprofloxacin** in children < 12 years of age and **norfloxacin** in infants < 1 year of age have not been established.

Precautions:

Laboratory tests: Perform culture and susceptibility testing during treatment.

Superinfection: Use of antibiotics (especially prolonged or repeated therapy) may result in bacterial or fungal overgrowth of nonsusceptible organisms. Such overgrowth may lead to a secondary infection. Take appropriate measures if superinfection occurs.

Ophthalmic solutions are not for injection. Do not inject them subconjunctivally or directly introduce them into the anterior chamber of the eye.

Systemic antibiotics: In all except very superficial infections, supplement the topical use of antibiotics with appropriate systemic medication. Systemic aminoglycoside antibiotics require monitoring the total serum concentration (peak and trough).

Crystalline precipitate: A white crystalline precipitate located in the superficial portion of the corneal defect was observed in ≈ 17% of patients on **ciprofloxacin**. Onset was within 1 to 7 days after starting therapy. The precipitate resolved in most patients within 2 weeks, and did not preclude continued use nor adversely affect the clinical course or outcome.

Drug Interactions:

Chymotrypsin: Concomitant use with chloramphenicol will inhibit the enzyme.

Adverse Reactions:

Sensitivity reactions such as transient irritation, burning, stinging, itching, angioneurotic edema, urticaria, vesicular and maculopapular dermatitis have occurred in some patients.

Hematologic events (including aplastic anemia) have occurred with the use of **chloramphenicol** (see Warnings).

Dermatologic: Dermatitis and photosensitivity have occurred with **tetracycline HCl.**

Ophthalmic: Tobramycin – Localized ocular toxicity and hypersensitivity, lid itching, lid swelling, conjunctival erythema (< 3%). *Gentamicin* – mydriasis and conjunctival paresthesia. Similar reactions may occur with the topical use of other aminoglycoside antibiotics.

Ciprofloxacin – Lid margin crusting, crystals/scales, foreign body sensation, itching, conjunctival hyperemia, bad taste in mouth (< 10%); corneal staining, keratopathy/keratitis, allergic reactions, lid edema, tearing, photophobia, corneal infiltrates, nausea, decreased vision (< 1%).

Norfloxacin – Conjunctival hyperemia; chemosis; photophobia; bitter taste in mouth.

(Continued on following page)

Antibiotics (Cont.)

Overdosage:

Symptoms of **tobramycin** overdose include punctate keratitis, erythema, increased lacrimation, edema and lid itching. These may be similar to adverse reactions.

A topical overdose of **ciprofloxacin** may be flushed from the eyes with warm tap water.

Patient Information:

Tilt head back, place medication in conjunctival sac and close eyes. Apply light finger pressure on lacrimal sac for 1 minute following instillation.

May cause temporary blurring of vision or stinging following administration. Notify physician if stinging, burning or itching becomes pronounced or if redness, irritation, swelling, decreasing vision or pain persists or worsens.

Administration and Dosage:

For specific frequency and duration of dosage, refer to the individual package inserts. The following are general guidelines only.

Instill into the conjunctival sac of the affected eye(s).

Solutions: Acute infections – 1 to 2 drops every 15 to 30 minutes, initially, reducing the frequency of instillation gradually as infection is controlled.

Moderate infections – 1 to 2 drops 4 to 6 times daily or more often as needed.

Acute and chronic trachoma – Tetracycline suspension: 2 drops in each eye 4 times daily. Continue this treatment for 6 weeks. Concomitant oral tetracycline is helpful.

Ointments: Acute infections – 1.25 cm (0.5 inch) ribbon every 3 to 4 hours until improvement occurs; reduce treatment prior to discontinuation.

Mild to moderate infections – 1.25 cm (0.5 inch) ribbon 2 to 3 times daily.

Prophylaxis of neonatal gonococcal or chlamydial conjunctivitis – Ointments: 0.5 to 1 cm (0.2 to 0.4 inch) ribbon (erythromycin or tetracycline) into each conjunctival sac. Do not flush from eyes. Give to infants born by either cesarean section or vaginal route.

Do not initially prescribe more than 20 ml and do not refill without further evaluation.

Chloramphenicol

	Product	Formulation	Description	Cost*
Rx	**Chloramphenicol** (Various, eg, Bausch & Lomb, Goldline, Rugby)	**Ointment:** 10 mg chloramphenicol/g	In 3.5 g.	30+
Rx	**AK-Chlor** (Akorn)		In a white petrolatum base w/mineral oil and polysorbate 60. In 3.5 g.	173
Rx	**Chloromycetin Ophthalmic** (Parke-Davis)		In a liquid petrolatum and polyethylene base. In 3.5 g.	229
Rx	**Chloroptic S.O.P.** (Allergan)		In white petrolatum, mineral oil, polyoxyl 40 stearate, nonionic lanolin derivatives, PEG 300 and 0.5% chlorobutanol. In 3.5 g.	304
Rx	**Chloromycetin Ophthalmic** (Parke-Davis)	**Powder for solution:** 25 mg chloramphenicol/vial	Preservative free. For reconstitution to 0.16% to 0.5% solution. With 15 ml diluent.	70
Rx	**Chloramphenicol Ophthalmic** (Various, eg, Bausch & Lomb, Goldline, Moore, Rugby, Schein, Steris)	**Solution:** 5 mg chloramphenicol/ml[1]	In 7.5 and 15 ml.	37+
Rx	**AK-Chlor** (Akorn)		In 7.5 and 15 ml.	80
Rx	**Chloroptic** (Allergan)		In 2.5 and 7.5 ml.[2]	126
Rx	**Ophthochlor** (Parke-Davis)		Preservative free. In 15 ml dropper bottles.	51

* Cost Index based on cost per g or ml.

[1] Refrigerate until dispensed.

[2] With 0.5% chlorobutanol, PEG-300, polyoxyl 40 stearate.

(Continued on following page)

Antibiotics (Cont.)

	Product	Formulation	Packaging	C.I.*
		Polymyxin B Sulfate		
Rx	**Polymyxin B Sulfate Sterile Ophthalmic** (Pfizer)	**Powder for solution:** 500,000 units polymyxin B sulfate	For reconstitution with 20 to 50 ml diluent.	38
		Erythromycin		
Rx	**Erythromycin** (Various, eg, Fougera, Major, Moore, Parmed, Pharmaderm, Rugby, Schein, URL)	**Ointment:** 5 mg erythromycin/g	In 1, 3.5 and 3.75 g.	54+
Rx	**AK-Mycin** (Akorn)		With white petrolatum and mineral oil. In 3.5 g.	91
Rx	**Ilotycin** (Dista)		With white petrolatum, mineral oil & parabens. In 3.75 & UD 1 g.	126
		Gentamicin		**C.I.***
Rx	**Gentamicin** (Bausch & Lomb)	**Ointment:** 3 mg gentamicin per g	In 3.75 & 15 g.[1]	114
Rx	**Gent-AK** (Akorn)		In 3.5 g.[1]	173
Rx	**Gentacidin** (Iolab)		With mineral oil, white petrolatum. In 3.5 g.	196
Rx	**Gentrasul** (Bausch & Lomb)		In 3.5 g.[1]	188
Rx	**Gentamicin Ophthalmic** (Various, eg, Goldline, Moore, Parmed, Pharmafair, Rugby)	**Ointment:** 3 mg gentamicin (as sulfate)/g	In 3.5 g and UD 1 g.	138+
Rx	**Garamycin Ophthalmic** (Schering)		In a white petrolatum base w/parabens. In 3.5 g.	302
Rx	**Genoptic S.O.P. Ophthalmic** (Allergan)		In a white petrolatum base w/parabens. In 3.5 g.	300
Rx	**Gentamicin Ophthalmic** (Various, eg, Bausch & Lomb, Geneva Marsam, Goldline, Moore, Parmed, Pharmafair, Rugby, Schein)	**Solution:** 3 mg gentamicin/ml	In 2, 5 and 15 ml.	50+
Rx	**Garamycin** (Schering)		In 5 ml.[2]	226
Rx	**Genoptic Ophthalmic Liquifilm** (Allergan)		In 1 and 5 ml dropper bottles.[3]	205
Rx	**Gentacidin** (Iolab)		In 5 ml dropper bottles.[2]	134
Rx	**Gent-AK** (Akorn)		In 5 and 15 ml.[2]	60
Rx	**Gentrasul** (Bausch & Lomb)		In 5 and 15 ml dropper bottles.[5]	131
		Tobramycin		
Rx	**Tobrex** (Alcon)	**Ointment:** 3 mg tobramycin per g	In a white petrolatum base w/mineral oil, 0.5% chlorobutanol. In 3.5 g.	344
Rx	**Tobrex** (Alcon)	**Solution:** 3 mg tobramycin per ml	In 5 ml Drop-Tainers.[4]	241

* Cost Index based on cost per g or ml.
[1] With liquid lanolin, white petrolatum, mineral oil, parabens.
[2] With benzalkonium chloride.
[3] With benzalkonium chloride, 1.4% polyvinyl alcohol, EDTA.
[4] With 0.01% benzalkonium chloride and tyloxapol.
[5] With 0.01% benzalkonium chloride.

Antibiotics (Cont.)

Tetracycline

	Product	Form	Description	C.I.*
Rx	**Achromycin** (Lederle)	**Ointment:** 10 mg tetracycline HCl/g	In a lanolin-petrolatum base. In 3.5 g.	315
Rx	**Achromycin** (Lederle)	**Suspension:** 10 mg tetracycline/ml	With Plastibase 50W and light mineral oil. In 0.5, 1 and 4 ml.	470

Chlortetracycline

	Product	Form	Description	C.I.*
Rx	**Aureomycin Ophthalmic** (Lederle)	**Ointment:** 10 mg chlortetracycline HCl/g	In a lanolin-petrolatum base. In 3.5 g.	294

Bacitracin

	Product	Form	Description	C.I.*
Rx	**Bacitracin Ophthalmic** (Various, eg, Fougera, Goldline, Lilly, Major, Moore, Parmed, Pharmafair, Rugby)	**Ointment:** 500 units bacitracin/g	In 3.5 and 454 g and UD 1 g.	40+
Rx	**AK-Tracin** (Akorn)		Preservative free. In 3.5 g.	82

Ciprofloxacin

	Product	Form	Description	C.I.*
Rx	**Ciloxan** (Alcon)	**Solution:** 3.5 mg ciprofloxacin HCl/ml (equivalent to 3 mg base)	In 2.5 and 5 ml *Drop-Tainer* dispensers.[1]	

Norfloxacin

	Product	Form	Description	C.I.*
Rx	**Chibroxin** (MSD)	**Solution:** 3 mg/ml	In 5 ml dropper bottle.[2]	

[1] With 0.006% benzalkonium chloride, 4.6% mannitol and 0.05% EDTA.
[2] With 0.0025% benzalkonium chloride and EDTA.

Antibiotics (Cont.)

COMBINATION ANTIBIOTIC PRODUCTS

	Product and Distributor	Polymyxin B Sulfate (units/g or ml)	Neomycin Sulfate (mg/g or ml)	Bacitracin (units/g)	Other Antibiotics	How Supplied	C.I.*
Rx	**Neotal Ophthalmic Ointment** (Hauck)	5000	5	400		In a petrolatum and mineral oil base. In 3.75 g.	71
Rx	**Triple Antibiotic Ophthalmic Ointment** (Rugby)					In 3.75 g.	93
Rx	**Bacitracin Zinc-Neomycin Sulfate-Polymyxin B Sulfate Ointment** (Various, eg, Fougera, Parmed, Pharmaderm, Pharmafair, Rugby)	10,000	3.5	400		In white petrolatum and mineral oil. In 3.75 and 30 g.	45+
Rx	**AK-Spore Ointment** (Akorn)					In white petrolatum and mineral oil. In 3.75 g.	153
Rx	**Neosporin Ophthalmic Ointment** (Burroughs Wellcome)					In a white petrolatum base. In 3.75 g.	267
Rx	**Ocutricin Ointment** (Bausch & Lomb)					In white petrolatum and mineral oil. In 3.75 g.	268
Rx	**Neomycin Sulfate-Polymyxin B Sulfate-Gramicidin Solution** (Various, eg, Bioline, Goldline, Iolab, Pharmafair, Rugby, Steris)	10,000	1.75		0.025 mg/ml gramicidin	In 2 and 10 ml and UD 1 ml.	46+
Rx	**AK-Spore Solution** (Akorn)					In 2 and 10 ml dropper bottles.[2]	61
Rx	**Neocidin Solution** (Major)					In 10 ml.	56
Rx	**Neosporin Ophthalmic Solution** (Burroughs Wellcome)					In 10 ml Drop Dose.[2]	100
Rx	**Ocutricin Ophthalmic Solution** (Bausch & Lomb)					In 2 and 10 ml.[2]	94
Rx	**Statrol Ointment** (Alcon)	10,000	3.75			With parabens in a white petrolatum and lanolin base. In 3.75 g.	280
Rx	**Statrol Solution** (Alcon)	16,250	3.5			In 5 ml Drop-Tainers.[3]	197
Rx	**AK-Poly-Bac Ointment** (Akorn)	10,000		500[1]		Preservative free. In white petrolatum and mineral oil. In 3.5 g.	173
Rx	**Polysporin Ointment** (Burroughs Wellcome)					In a white petrolatum base. In 3.75 g.	267
Rx	**Terramycin w/Polymyxin B Ointment** (Roerig)	10,000			5 mg/g oxytetracycline HCl	In a white and liquid petrolatum base. In 3.75 g.	182
Rx	**Polytrim Ophthalmic Solution** (Allergan)	10,000			1 mg/ml trimethoprim	In 10 ml dropper bottle.	161

* Cost Index based on cost per g or ml.

[1] As zinc.

[2] With 0.001% thimerosal, 0.5% alcohol, propylene glycol, polyoxyethylene and polyoxypropylene.

[3] With 0.004% benzalkonium chloride and 0.5% hydroxypropyl methylcellulose.

OPHTHALMICS (Cont.)

Steroid and Antibiotic Drops

The information given for Steroid Preparations and for Antibiotic Preparations must be considered when using these combinations.
Administration and Dosage: Instill 1 or 2 drops into affected eye(s) every 3 or 4 hours.

	Product and Distributor	Steroid	Antibiotic	Other Content	How Supplied	C.I.*
Rx	**Chloromycetin Hydrocortisone Powder** (Parke-Davis)	0.5% hydrocortisone acetate† (2.5% as powder)	0.25% chloramphenicol† (1.25% as powder)	Cholesterol, methylcellulose and 0.01% benzethonium chloride	In 5 ml w/dropper.	305
Rx	**Neo-Cortef Suspension** (Upjohn)	0.5% hydrocortisone acetate	Neomycin sulfate equivalent to 0.35% neomycin base	Myristyl-gamma-picolinium chloride, polyethylene glycol 3350 and povidone	In 5 ml dropper bottles.	208
Rx	**AK-Spore H.C. Ophthalmic Suspension** (Akorn)	1% hydrocortisone	Neomycin sulfate equivalent to 0.35% neomycin base and 10,000 units polymyxin B sulfate/ml	0.01% benzalkonium Cl and sodium borate, mineral oil, propylene glycol, boric acid	In 5 and 7.5 ml.	NA
Rx	**Bacticort Suspension** (Rugby)			0.01% benzalkonium chloride, cetyl alcohol, glyceryl monostearate, mineral oil, polyoxyl 40 stearate, propylene glycol	In 7.5 ml plastic bottles.	134
Rx	**Triple-Gen Suspension** (Goldline)				In 7.5 ml plastic bottles.	98
Rx	**Cortisporin Suspension** (Burroughs Wellcome)			0.001% thimerosal, cetyl alcohol, glyceryl monostearate, polyoxyl 40 stearate, propylene glycol and mineral oil	In 7.5 ml w/dropper.	152
Rx	**Terra-Cortril Suspension** (Roerig)	1.5% hydrocortisone acetate	0.5% oxytetracycline (as HCl)	Mineral oil and aluminum tristearate	In 5 ml w/dropper.	325
Rx	**AK-Neo-Cort Suspension** (Akorn)	1.5% hydrocortisone acetate	Neomycin sulfate equivalent to 0.35% neomycin base	Polysorbate 80, carboxymethylcellulose, sodium metabisulfite and 0.5% chlorobutanol	In 5 ml dropper bottles.	143
Rx	**Cor-Oticin Suspension** (Americal)				In 5 ml dropper bottles.	49
Rx	**Ortho Drops Suspension** (Vortech)				In 5 ml dropper bottles.	124
Rx	**Poly-Pred Suspension** (Allergan)	0.5% prednisolone acetate	Neomycin sulfate equivalent to 0.35% neomycin base and 10,000 units polymyxin B sulfate/ml	1.4% polyvinyl alcohol, 0.001% thimerosal, polysorbate 80 and propylene glycol	In 5 and 10 ml dropper bottles.	256
Rx	**Pred-G Suspension** (Allergan)	1% prednisolone acetate	Gentamicin sulfate equivalent to 0.3% gentamicin base	Polyvinyl alcohol, benzalkonium chloride, EDTA, hydroxypropylmethylcellulose and polysorbate 80	In 5 and 10 ml dropper bottles.	321

* Cost Index based on cost per ml.　　† As a prepared solution.

(Continued on following page)

OPHTHALMICS (Cont.)

Steroid and Antibiotic Drops (Cont.)

	Product and Distributor	Steroid	Antibiotic	Other Content	How Supplied	C.I.*
Rx	**AK-Neo-Dex Solution** (Akorn)	0.1% dexamethasone phosphate (as sodium phosphate)	Neomycin sulfate equivalent to 0.35% neomycin base	Sodium citrate, creatinine base, EDTA, polysorbate 80, sodium bisulfite, sodium borate, 0.01% benzalkonium chloride	In 5 ml.	NA
Rx	**NeoDecadron Solution** (MSD)			Polysorbate 80, EDTA, 0.02% benzalkonium chloride and 0.1% sodium bisulfite	In 5 ml Ocumeter.	279
Rx	**TobraDex Suspension** (Alcon)	0.1% dexamethasone	0.3% tobramycin	0.001% thimerosal, 0.5% alcohol, propylene glycol, polyoxyethylene and polyoxypropylene	In 2.5 and 5 ml.	321
Rx	**AK-Trol Suspension** (Akorn)	0.1% dexamethasone	Neomycin sulfate equivalent to 0.35% neomycin base and 10,000 units polymyxin B sulfate/ml	Hydroxypropyl methylcellulose, polysorbate 20 and benzalkonium chloride	In 5 ml w/dropper.	143
Rx	**Dexacidin Suspension** (Iolab)				In 5 ml dropper bottles.	192
Rx	**Dexasporin Suspension** (Various, eg, Balan, Bioline, Dixon-Shane, Goldline, Moore, Pharmafair, Rugby, URL)				In 5 ml.	107+
Rx	**Infectrol Suspension** (Bausch & Lomb)				In 5 ml.	205
Rx	**Maxitrol Suspension** (Alcon)				In 5 ml Drop-Tainers.	286

* Cost Index based on cost per g or ml.

Steroid and Antibiotic Ointments

The information given for Steroid Preparations and for Antibiotic Preparations must be considered when using these combinations. See individual product monographs.

	Product and Distributor	Steroid	Antibiotic	Other Content	How Supplied	C.I.*
Rx	**Bacitracin Zinc-Neomycin Sulfate-Polymyxin B Sulfate-Hydrocortisone** (Various, eg, Major, Parmed)	1% hydrocortisone	Neomycin sulfate equivalent to 0.35% neomycin base, 400 units bacitracin zinc and 10,000 units polymyxin B sulfate/g	White petrolatum and mineral oil	In 3.75 g.	46
Rx	**Cortisporin** (B W)			White petrolatum	In 3.75 g	278
Rx	**Triple Antibiotic w/HC** (Various, eg, Bioline, Goldline, Harber, Rugby)			White petrolatum and mineral oil	In 3.5, 3.6 and 3.75 g.	61+
Rx	**Ophthocort** (Parke-Davis)	0.5% hydrocortisone acetate	1% chloramphenicol and 10,000 units polymyxin B (as sulfate)/g	Liquid petrolatum and polyethylene. Preservative free	In 3.75 g.	261
Rx	**Coracin** (Hauck)	1% hydrocortisone acetate	0.5% neomycin sulfate, 400 units bacitracin zinc and 10,000 units polymyxin B sulfate/g	White petrolatum and mineral oil	In 3.75 g.	95
Rx	**Pred-G** (Allergan)	0.6% prednisolone acetate	Gentamicin sulfate equivalent to 0.3% gentamicin base	0.5% chlorobutanol, white petrolatum, mineral oil, petrolatum and lanolin alcohol	In 3.5 g.	N/A
Rx	**NeoDecadron** (MSD)	0.05% dexamethasone phosphate (as sodium phosphate)	Neomycin sulfate equivalent to 0.35% neomycin base	White petrolatum and mineral oil	In 3.5 g.	163
Rx	**AK-Trol** (Akorn)	0.1% dexamethasone	Neomycin sulfate equivalent to 0.35% neomycin base and 10,000 units polymyxin B sulfate/g	White petrolatum, liquid lanolin, mineral oil, parabens	In 3.5 g.	168
Rx	**Dexacidin** (Iolab)			White petrolatum and mineral oil	In 3.5 g.	196
Rx	**Dexasporin** (Various, eg, Bioline, Goldline, Moore, Pharmafair)			White petrolatum, lanolin, mineral oil, parabens	In 3.5 & 3.75 g.	141+
Rx	**Infectrol** (Bausch & L)				In 3.5 g.	293
Rx	**Maxitrol** (Alcon)			White petrolatum, lanolin and parabens	In 3.5 g.	357
Rx	**TobraDex** (Alcon)	0.1% dexamethasone	0.3% tobramycin	0.5% chlorobutanol, mineral oil and white petrolatum	In 3.5 g.	N/A

* Cost Index based on cost per g or ml.

Sulfonamides

Actions:

Sulfonamides exert a bacteriostatic effect against a wide range of susceptible gram-positive and gram-negative microorganisms. Through competition with para-aminobenzoic acid (PABA), they restrict the synthesis of folic acid which bacteria require for growth. For complete information on sulfonamides, refer to the group monograph in the Anti-Infective section.

Indications:

Conjunctivitis, corneal ulcer and other superficial ocular infections due to susceptible microorganisms.

Adjunctive treatment in systemic sulfonamide therapy of trachoma.

Contraindications:

Hypersensitivity to sulfonamides or to any ingredients of the preparations.

Warnings:

A significant percentage of staphylococcal isolates are completely resistant to sulfonamides.

Severe sensitivity reactions (see Adverse Reactions) have been identified in individuals with no prior history of sulfonamide hypersensitivity.

Sensitization may occur when a sulfonamide is readministered, regardless of the route of administration. Cross sensitivity between different sulfonamides may occur. If signs of sensitivity or other untoward reactions occur, discontinue use of the preparation.

Pregnancy: (Category C – sulfacetamide sodium/phenylephrine HCl). Safety for use during pregnancy has not been established. Use only when clearly needed and when the potential benefits outweigh the potential hazards to the fetus.

Lactation: It is not known whether these drugs are excreted in breast milk. Safety for use in the nursing mother has not been established.

Children: Safety and efficacy for use in children have not been established.

Precautions:

Ophthalmic ointments may retard corneal epithelial healing.

Nonsusceptible organisms, including fungi, may proliferate with the use of sulfonamide preparations.

Use with caution in patients with severe dry eye.

PABA present in purulent exudates inactivates sulfonamides.

Sulfite sensitivity: May cause allergic-type reactions (eg, hives, itching, wheezing, anaphylaxis) in certain susceptible persons. Although the overall prevalence of sulfite sensitivity in the general population is probably low, it is seen more frequently in asthmatics or in atopic nonasthmatic persons. Specific products containing sulfites are identified in the product listings.

Drug Interactions:

Silver preparations are incompatible with these solutions.

Adverse Reactions:

Headache or browache; blurred vision; local irritation; reactive hyperemia; burning and transient stinging. Rarely, sensitization reactions to sulfacetamide sodium may occur. As with all sulfonamide preparations, severe sensitivity reactions include rare occurrences of Stevens-Johnson syndrome, exfoliative dermatitis, toxic epidermal necrolysis, photosensitivity, fever, skin rash, GI disturbance and bone marrow depression.

A single instance of local hypersensitivity was reported which progressed to a fatal syndrome resembling systemic lupus erythematosus.

Patient Information:

Do not discontinue use without consulting physician.

May cause sensitivity to bright light; this may be minimized by wearing sunglasses. Notify physician if improvement is not seen after 7 to 8 days, if condition worsens, or if pain, decreased vision, increased redness, itching or swelling of the eye occurs.

Refer to page 2164 for more complete information.

Administration and Dosage:

Solutions: Instill 1 to 3 drops into the lower conjunctival sac every 2 or 3 hours daily.

Ointments: Apply small amount in the lower conjunctival sac 1 to 4 times/day and at bedtime.

(Products listed on following page)

Refer to the general discussion of these products on page 2218

Sulfonamide Solutions

	Product	Formulation	How Supplied	C.I.*
Rx	**Sodium Sulfacetamide 10%** (Various, eg, Balan, Geneva, Goldline, Hauck, Major, Moore, Pharmafair, Rugby, Schein, URL)	**Ophthalmic Solution:** 10% sodium sulfacetamide	In 3.75 and 15 ml.	16+
Rx	**AK-Sulf** (Akorn)		In 2, 5 and 15 ml dropper bottles.[1]	26
Rx	**Bleph-10 Liquifilm** (Allergan)		In 2.5, 5 and 15 ml dropper bottles.[2]	82
Rx	**Ophthacet** (Vortech)		In 15 ml.[3]	36
Rx	**Sodium Sulamyd** (Schering)		In 5 and 15 ml dropper bottles.[4]	97
Rx	**SOSS-10** (Hauck)		In 15 ml.	23
Rx	**Sulf-10** (Iolab)		In 1 ml Dropperettes[5] and 15 ml dropper bottles.[6]	67
Rx	**Sulten-10** (Bausch & Lomb)		In 15 ml.[7]	38
Rx	**Sodium Sulfacetamide 15%** (Various, eg, Alcon, Moore, Raway, Rugby)	**Ophthalmic Solution:** 15% sodium sulfacetamide	In 2 and 15 ml.	22+
Rx	**AK-Sulf** (Akorn)		In 15 ml dropper bottles.[1]	43
Rx	**Isopto Cetamide** (Alcon)		In 5 and 15 ml Drop-Tainers.[8]	77
Rx	**Sulfair 15** (Pharmafair)		In 15 ml.[9]	20
Rx	**Sodium Sulfacetamide 30%** (Various, eg, Bioline, Geneva, Goldline, Major, Raway, Rugby, Schein, Steris)	**Ophthalmic Solution:** 30% sodium sulfacetamide	In 5 and 15 ml.	30+
Rx	**AK-Sulf Forte** (Akorn)		In 5 ml dropper bottles.[1]	114
Rx	**Sodium Sulamyd** (Schering)		In 15 ml dropper bottles.[10]	103
Rx	**Gantrisin** (Roche)	**Ophthalmic Solution:** 4% sulfisoxazole (as diolamine)	In 15 ml w/dropper.[11]	51

* Cost Index based on cost per ml.

[1] With hydroxyethylcellulose, 0.2% sodium thiosulfate, 0.2% chlorobutanol and parabens.

[2] With 1.4% polyvinyl alcohol, 0.005% thimerosal, polysorbate 80, sodium thiosulfate and EDTA.

[3] With 0.2% sodium thiosulfate, 0.2% chlorobutanol, poloxamer 188, EDTA, 0.1% sodium metabisulfite and parabens.

[4] With 0.5% methylcellulose, 0.31% sodium thiosulfate and parabens.

[5] With sodium thiosulfate and 0.005% thimerosal.

[6] With sodium thiosulfate, 0.01% thimerosal and hydroxypropyl methylcellulose.

[7] With 0.5% EDTA, sodium thiosulfate, propylene glycol, hydroxypropyl methylcellulose and parabens.

[8] With 0.3% sodium thiosulfate, 0.5% hydroxypropyl methylcellulose and parabens.

[9] With chlorobutanol, EDTA, sodium bisulfite and parabens.

[10] With 0.15% sodium thiosulfate and parabens.

[11] With 1:100,000 phenylmercuric nitrate.

Refer to the general discussion of these products on page 2218

Sulfonamide Ointments

	Product	Form	Supplied	C.I.*
Rx	**Sodium Sulfacetamide** (Various, eg, Fougera, Goldline, Harber, Major, Moore, Pharmafair, Raway, Rugby, Schein, URL)	**Ophthalmic Ointment:** 10% sodium sulfacetamide	In 3.5 and 3.75 g.	40+
Rx	**AK-Sulf** (Akorn)		In 3.5 g.[1]	89
Rx	**Bleph-10 S.O.P.** (Allergan)		In 3.5 g.[2]	271
Rx	**Cetamide** (Alcon)		In 3.5 g.[3]	281
Rx	**Sodium Sulamyd** (Schering)		In 3.5 g.[4]	341
Rx	**Gantrisin** (Roche)	**Ophthalmic Ointment:** 4% sulfisoxazole (as diolamine)	In 3.75 g.[5]	123

Sulfonamide Decongestant Combination

In this combination, phenylephrine HCl is used as an ophthalmic decongestant.

	Product	Form	Supplied	C.I.*
Rx	**Vasosulf** (Iolab)	**Ophthalmic Solution:** 15% sodium sulfacetamide and 0.125% phenylephrine HCl	In 5 and 15 ml dropper bottles.[6]	70

* Cost Index based on cost per g or ml.
[1] With parabens in a petrolatum base.
[2] With 0.0008% phenylmercuric acetate, white petrolatum, mineral oil, nonionic lanolin derivatives.
[3] With parabens in white petrolatum, mineral oil and liquid lanolin.
[4] With 0.025% benzalkonium chloride, sorbitan monolaurate and parabens in a petrolatum base.
[5] With 1:50,000 phenylmercuric nitrate, white petrolatum and mineral oil.
[6] With sodium thiosulfate, poloxamer 188 and parabens.

Steroid and Sulfonamide Combinations, Suspensions and Solutions

The information for steroid preparations and sulfonamide preparations must be considered when using these products. See individual monographs.

Administration and Dosage:

Solutions and Suspensions: Instill 1 to 3 drops into the conjunctival sac every 1 to 2 hours during the day and at bedtime until a favorable response is obtained.

Ointments: Apply a small amount in the conjunctival sac 3 or 4 times daily and once at bedtime.

	Product & Distributor	Steroid	Sulfonamide	Other Content	How Supplied	C.I.*
Rx	**AK-Cide Suspension** (Akorn)	0.5% prednisolone acetate	10% sodium sulfacetamide	Hydroxypropyl methylcellulose, polysorbate 80, sodium thiosulfate and 0.01% benzalkonium chloride	In 5 and 15 ml dropper bottles.	139
Rx	**Metimyd Suspension** (Schering)			0.5% phenylethyl alcohol, 0.025% benzalkonium chloride, sodium thiosulfate, EDTA and tyloxapol	In 5 ml dropper bottles.	406
Rx	**Ophtha P/S Ophthalmic Suspension** (Misemer)			Hydroxyethylcellulose, EDTA, polysorbate 80, sodium thiosulfate and 0.025% benzalkonium chloride	In 5 ml dropper bottles.	114
Rx	**Or-Toptic M Suspension** (Ortega)				In 5 ml dropper bottles.	157
Rx	**Predamide Suspension** (Americal)				In 5 and 15 ml dropper bottles.	36
Rx	**Predsulfair Suspension** (Pharmafair)			Hydroxypropyl methylcellulose, 0.5% polysorbate 80, sodium thiosulfate and 0.01% benzalkonium chloride	In 5 and 15 ml dropper bottles.	59
Rx	**Sulfamide Suspension** (Rugby)			Hydroxypropyl methylcellulose, polysorbate 80, sodium thiosulfate and 0.01% benzalkonium chloride	In 5 and 15 ml dropper bottles.	79
Rx	**Sulphrin Suspension** (Bausch & Lomb)			Hydroxypropyl methylcellulose, EDTA, polysorbate 80, sodium metabisulfite, propylene glycol, sodium thiosulfate and parabens	In 5 ml dropper bottles.	157

* Cost Index based on cost per ml.

(Continued on following page)

Steroid and Sulfonamide Combinations, Suspensions and Solutions (Cont.)

Refer to the general discussion of these products on page 497c.

	Product & Distributor	Steroid	Sulfonamide	Other Content	How Supplied	C.I.*
Rx	**Isopto Cetapred Suspension** (Alcon)	0.25% prednisolone acetate	10% sodium sulfacetamide	0.5% hydroxypropyl methylcellulose, EDTA, polysorbate 80, sodium thiosulfate, 0.025% benzalkonium chloride and parabens	In 5 and 15 ml Drop-Tainers.	125
Rx	**Blephamide Liquifilm Suspension** (Allergan)	0.2% prednisolone acetate	10% sodium sulfacetamide	EDTA, 1.4% polyvinyl alcohol, polysorbate 80, sodium thiosulfate and benzalkonium chloride	In 2.5, 5 and 10 ml dropper bottles.	156
Rx	**Sulpred** (Bausch & Lomb)			0.01% benzalkonium chloride	In 5 ml w/ applicator.	NA
Rx	**Optimyd Solution** (Schering)	0.5% prednisolone sodium phosphate	10% sodium sulfacetamide	EDTA, sodium thiosulfate, tyloxapol, 0.025% benzalkonium chloride and 0.5% phenylethyl alcohol	In 5 ml dropper bottles.	406
Rx	**Vasocidin Solution** (Iolab)	0.25% prednisolone sodium phosphate	10% sodium sulfacetamide	EDTA, 0.01% thimerosal and poloxamer 407	In 5 and 10 ml dropper bottles.	142
Rx	**FML-S Suspension** (Allergan)	0.1% fluorometholone	10% sodium sulfacetamide	EDTA, 1.4% polyvinyl alcohol, 0.006% benzalkonium chloride, polysorbate 80	In 5 and 10 ml dropper bottles.	N/A

Steroid and Sulfonamide Combinations, Ointments

	Product & Distributor	Steroid	Sulfonamide	Other Content	How Supplied	C.I.*
Rx	**AK-Cide** (Akorn)	0.5% prednisolone acetate	10% sodium sulfacetamide	Mineral oil, white petrolatum, lanolin and parabens	In 3.5 g.	179
Rx	**Predsulfair** (Pharmafair)				In 3.5 g.	60
Rx	**Metimyd** (Schering)			Mineral oil, white petrolatum and parabens	In 3.5 g.	509
Rx	**Vasocidin** (Iolab)			Mineral oil and white petrolatum	In 3.5 g.	286
Rx	**Cetapred** (Alcon)	0.25% prednisolone acetate	10% sodium sulfacetamide	Mineral oil, white petrolatum, liquid lanolin and parabens	In 3.5 g.	332
Rx	**Blephamide S.O.P.** (Allergan)	0.2% prednisolone acetate	10% sodium sulfacetamide	0.0008% phenylmercuric acetate, mineral oil, white petrolatum and nonionic lanolin derivatives	In 3.5 g.	304

* Cost Index based on cost per g or ml.

Antiseptic Preparations

YELLOW MERCURIC OXIDE

Indications:

Treatment of irritation and minor infections of the eyelids.

Warnings:

If irritation or rash develops or if condition persists, discontinue use and consult physician. Frequent or prolonged use may cause serious mercury poisoning.

Administration and Dosage:

Apply a small quantity to inner surface of lower eyelid once a day or as directed.

				C.I.*
otc	**Yellow Mercuric Oxide** (Various, eg, Balan, Harber, Lilly, Major, Moore, Rugby, Schein)	**Ointment:** 1%	In 3.5, 3.75 and 30 g.	39+
otc	**Yellow Mercuric Oxide** (Various, eg, Balan, Fougera, Harber, Lilly, Major, Moore, Rugby, Schein)	**Ointment:** 2%	In 3.5, 3.75 and 30 g.	39+

SILVER PROTEIN, MILD

Actions:

Instilled prior to eye surgery, it stains and coagulates mucus. It has antimicrobial action against gram-positive and gram-negative organisms.

Indications:

Preoperatively in eye surgery and in eye infections.

Contraindications:

Hypersensitivity to any of the components of this preparation.

Warnings:

Pregnancy: Category C. Safety for use during pregnancy has not been established. Use only when clearly needed and when the potential benefits outweigh the potential hazards to the fetus.

Lactation: It is not known whether this drug is excreted in breast milk. Safety for use in the nursing mother has not been established.

Children: Safety and efficacy for use in children have not been established.

Precautions:

Not for prolonged use. When used preoperatively, remove all stained material before entering the eye. This may reduce the incidence of postoperative infection.

Drug Interactions:

Sulfacetamide preparations are incompatible with silver preparations.

Adverse Reactions:

Uninterrupted or too frequent use over a long period may result in a permanent discoloration of the skin and conjunctiva (argyria).

Administration and Dosage:

Preoperatively: Instill 2 or 3 drops into eye(s); rinse out with sterile irrigating solution.

Infections: Instill 1 to 3 drops into eye(s) every 3 or 4 hours for several days.

				C.I.*
Rx	**Argyrol S.S. 20%** (Iolab)	**Solution:** 20%	With EDTA. In 1 ml Dropperettes.	251

* Cost Index based on cost per g or ml.

SILVER NITRATE

Actions:

Silver nitrate ophthalmic solution is an anti-infective. In weak solutions, it is used as a germicide and astringent to mucous membranes. The germicidal action is due to precipitation of bacterial proteins by liberated silver ions.

Indications:

Prevention of gonorrheal ophthalmia neonatorum.

Contraindications:

Hypersensitivity to any component of this preparation.

Warnings:

A 1% solution is considered optimal; however, it must be used with caution, since cauterization of the cornea and blindness may result, especially with repeated applications.

Silver nitrate is caustic and irritating to the skin and mucous membranes.

Precautions:

Handle solutions carefully since they tend to stain skin and utensils.

Drug Interactions:

Sulfacetamide preparations are incompatible with silver preparations.

Adverse Reactions:

A mild chemical conjunctivitis should result from a properly performed Credé prophylaxis using silver nitrate. A more severe chemical conjunctivitis occurs in 20% or less of cases.

Overdosage:

When ingested, silver nitrate is highly toxic to the GI tract and CNS. Swallowing can cause severe gastroenteritis that may be fatal. Sodium chloride may be used by gastric lavage to remove the chemical.

Administration and Dosage:

Immediately after birth, clean the child's eyelids with sterile absorbent cotton or gauze and sterile water. Use a separate pledget for each eye; wash unopened lids from the nose outward until free of blood, mucus or meconium. Next, separate the lids and instill 2 drops of 1% solution. Elevate lids away from the eyeball so that a lake of silver nitrate may lie for $\geq$ 30 seconds between them, contacting the entire conjunctival sac.

Irrigation of the eyes following instillation of silver nitrate is NOT recommended.

Storage: Keep ampules at controlled room temperature, 15° to 30°C (59° to 86°F). Do not freeze. Do not use when cold. Protect from light.

				C.I.*
Rx	**Silver Nitrate** (Lilly)	**Solution:** 1% with acetic acid and sodium acetate	In 100s (wax ampules).	83

* Cost Index based on cost per wax ampule.

Antifungal Agent

NATAMYCIN

Actions:

A tetraene polyene antibiotic derived from *Streptomyces natalensis.* It possesses in vitro activity against a variety of yeasts and filamentous fungi, including *Candida, Aspergillus, Cephalosporium, Fusarium* and *Penicillium.*

Pharmacology: Mechanism of action appears to be through binding of the molecule to the fungal cell membrane. The polyene sterol complex alters membrane permeability, depleting essential cellular constituents. Although activity against fungi is dose-related, natamycin is predominantly fungicidal. It is not effective in vitro against bacteria.

Pharmacokinetics: Topical administration appears to produce effective concentrations within the corneal stroma, but not in intraocular fluid. Absorption from the GI tract is very poor. Systemic absorption should not occur after topical administration.

Indications:

Fungal blepharitis, conjunctivitis and keratitis caused by susceptible organisms. Natamycin is the initial drug of choice in *Fusarium solani* keratitis.

Topical natamycin is inadequate as a single agent in fungal endophthalmitis.

Contraindications:

History of hypersensitivity to any component of the formulation.

Warnings:

Pregnancy: Safety for use during pregnancy has not been established. Use only when clearly needed and when potential benefits outweigh potential hazards to the fetus.

Precautions:

Failure of keratitis to improve following 7 to 10 days of administration suggests that the infection may be caused by a microorganism not susceptible to natamycin. Base continuation of therapy on clinical reevaluation and additional laboratory studies.

Adherence of the suspension to areas of epithelial ulceration or retention in the fornices occurs regularly. Should suspicion of drug toxicity occur, discontinue the drug.

Laboratory tests: Determine initial and sustained therapy of fungal keratitis by the clinical diagnosis (laboratory diagnosis by smear and culture of corneal scrapings) and by response to the drug. Whenever possible, determine the in vitro activity of natamycin against the responsible fungus. Monitor tolerance of natamycin at least twice weekly.

Adverse Reactions:

One case of conjunctival chemosis and hyperemia, thought to be allergic in nature, was reported.

Patient Information:

Refer to page 2164 for complete information.

Administration and Dosage:

Fungal keratitis: 1 drop instilled into the conjunctival sac at 1 or 2 hour intervals. The frequency of application can usually be reduced to 1 drop 6 to 8 times daily after the first 3 to 4 days. Generally, continue therapy for 14 to 21 days, or until there is resolution of active fungal keratitis. In many cases, it may help to reduce the dosage gradually at 4 to 7 day intervals to assure that the organism has been eliminated.

Fungal blepharitis and conjunctivitis: 4 to 6 daily applications may be sufficient.

Storage: May be stored at room temperature or in refrigerator 2° to 9°C (35° to 48°F). Do not freeze. Avoid exposure to light and excessive heat. Shake well before each use.

Rx	**Natacyn** (Alcon)	**Suspension:** 5%	In 15 ml.[1]

[1] With 0.02% benzalkonium chloride.

Antiviral Agents

The topical ophthalmic antiviral preparations idoxuridine, vidarabine and trifluridine appear to interfere with viral reproduction by altering DNA synthesis. They are effective treatment for herpes simplex infections of the conjunctiva and cornea.

Topical Ophthalmic Antiviral Preparations			
Generic Name	Trade Name (Manufacturer)	Preparations	Indications
Idoxuridine	*Herplex* (Allergan)	Solution 0.1%	Herpes simplex
	Stoxil (SKF)	Solution 0.1% Ointment 0.5%	
Vidarabine	*Vira-A* (Parke-Davis)	Ointment 3%	Herpes simplex types 1 and 2 Idoxuridine-resistant herpes
Trifluridine	*Viroptic* (Burroughs Wellcome)	Solution 1%	Herpes simplex types 1 and 2 Idoxuridine and vidarabine-resistant herpes

Viral infection, especially epidemic keratoconjunctivitis, is more often associated with a follicular conjunctivitis, a serous conjunctival discharge and preauricular lymphadenopathy. This exceptionally contagious organism is not susceptible to antibiotic therapy at this time. Pustular lesions of the nose and face, and spade-shaped fascicular keratitis in association with chronic blepharitis, suggesting acne rosacea, warrants a trial of systemic tetracycline or doxycycline as both an antibiotic and potentially anti-inflammatory regimen.

IDOXURIDINE (IDU)

Actions:

Idoxuridine (IDU) blocks reproduction of herpes simplex virus by altering normal DNA synthesis.

It irreversibly inhibits incorporation of thymidine into viral DNA. The production of faulty DNA results in a pseudostructure which cannot infect or destroy tissue.

Indications:

Treatment of herpes simplex keratitis. Epithelial infections (especially initial attacks), characterized by the presence of a dendritic figure, respond better than stromal infections. Recurrences are common. IDU will often control the infection, but will have no effect on accumulated scarring, vascularization or resultant progressive loss of vision.

Contraindications:

Hypersensitivity to IDU or any component of the formulation.

Since herpes infects and destroys nerves, a sterile trophic ulcer may result. A sterile trophic ulcer may not heal with continued IDU therapy. Discontinuation of therapy is often necessary to eliminate epithelial toxicity and allow healing.

Warnings:

Sensitization: IDU may be sensitizing; this is more common with dermal than with ocular use.

Carcinogenesis: Regard this cytotoxic drug as potentially carcinogenic, although data are inadequate for assessment. It can inhibit DNA synthesis or function, and is incorporated into the DNA of mammalian cells as well as into the genome of DNA viruses. IDU induces RNA tumor virus production from mouse cells and has caused in vitro cell transformation and induction of specific neoplasms (lymphatic leukemias and carcinomas) upon inoculation into syngeneic mice.

Pregnancy: IDU crosses the placental barrier and produces fetal malformations when administered topically to the eyes of pregnant rabbits in clinical doses and when administered by various routes in high doses to other rodents. Administer with caution in pregnancy or in women of childbearing potential.

Lactation: It is not known whether IDU is excreted in breast milk. Do not nurse while undergoing treatment; the drug and metabolites may be excreted in breast milk.

Precautions:

Resistance: Some strains of herpes simplex appear to be resistant. If there is no response in epithelial infections after 14 days of treatment, consider other forms of therapy.

Do not exceed the recommended frequency and duration of administration.

Recurrence may be seen if medication is not continued for 5 to 7 days after the epithelial lesion is apparently healed.

(Continued on following page)

IDOXURIDINE (IDU) (Cont.)

Drug Interactions:

Boric acid-containing solutions: Do not coadminister with IDU, since it may cause irritation in the presence of IDU.

Adverse Reactions:

Occasional irritation, pain, pruritus, inflammation or edema of the eyes or lids; allergic reactions; photophobia; corneal clouding; stippling; punctate defects in the corneal epithelium. (The punctate defects may be a manifestation of the infection, since healing usually takes place without interruption of therapy. These defects have been observed in untreated herpes simplex keratitis.) Follicular conjunctivitis, punctal occlusion and conjunctival scarring may be observed with prolonged use.

Squamous cell carcinoma has been reported at the site of topical treatment.

Overdosage:

Local: Overdosage due to frequent administration (see recommended dosage) is possible and may result in small defects ("pseudo-dendrites") on the epithelium of the cornea. Should such defects occur, discontinue therapy, either temporarily or permanently, as indicated after close observation of the progress of the infection.

Accidental ingestion: Animal data indicate that the minimum systemic dose that will produce toxic effects is many times greater than the quantity in a commercial bottle or tube. Also, metabolic breakdown and excretion take place very rapidly. Thus, no untoward consequences should be expected from accidental ingestion of even an entire bottle of the solution or tube of ointment; no treatment is indicated.

Patient Information:

May cause sensitivity to bright light; this may be minimized by wearing sunglasses. Notify physician if improvement is not seen after 7 to 8 days, if condition worsens, or if pain, decreased vision, itching or swelling of the eye occurs.

Refer to page 2164 for more complete information.

Administration and Dosage:

For optimal results, keep infected tissues saturated with IDU.

Examine patients at frequent intervals. In epithelial infections, improvement is usually seen within 7 to 8 days. If the patient continues to improve, continue therapy, usually not longer than 21 days.

Solution: Initially, place 1 drop into each infected eye every hour during the day and every 2 hours at night. Continue until definite improvement has taken place, as evidenced by loss of staining with fluorescein. Then reduce dosage to 1 drop every 2 hours during the day and every 4 hours at night. To minimize recurrences, continue therapy at this reduced dosage for 3 to 5 days after healing appears complete.

Alternate dosing schedule: Instill 1 drop every minute for 5 minutes. Repeat every 4 hours, night and day.

Ointment: 5 instillations daily, ≈ every 4 hours, with the last dose at bedtime. Place ointment inside the infected conjunctival sac. Continue for 3 to 5 days after healing appears complete.

Concomitant therapy: In the management of herpes simplex with stromal lesions, corneal edema or iritis, **topical corticosteroids** may be used with IDU. Use such combined therapy for as long as the condition warrants. It is important to continue IDU therapy a few days after the steroid has been withdrawn.

Antibiotics may be used with IDU to control secondary infections, and **atropine** preparations may be employed adjunctively as indicated.

Stability: Do not mix with other medications. Protect solution from light.

				C.I.*
Rx	**Herplex Liquifilm** (Allergan)	**Ophthalmic Solution:** 0.1%	In 15 ml dropper bottles.[1]	78
Rx	**Stoxil** (SKF)		In 15 ml w/dropper.[2]	111
Rx	**Stoxil** (SKF)	**Ophthalmic Ointment:** 0.5%	Petrolatum base. In 4 g.	346

* Cost Index based on cost per g or ml.

[1] With benzalkonium chloride, EDTA and 1.4% polyvinyl alcohol.

[2] Store under refrigeration. With 1:50,000 thimerosal.

VIDARABINE (Adenine Arabinoside; Ara-A)

Actions:

Pharmacology: The antiviral mechanism of action has not been established. Vidarabine appears to interfere with the early steps of viral DNA synthesis. It is rapidly deaminated to arabinosylhypoxanthine (Ara-Hx), the principal metabolite. Ara-Hx also possesses in vitro antiviral activity less than vidarabine's. In contrast to topical idoxuridine, vidarabine demonstrated less cellular toxicity in regenerating corneal epithelium of rabbits.

Pharmacokinetics: Absorption – Systemic absorption is not expected to occur following ocular administration and swallowing lacrimal secretions. In laboratory animals, vidarabine is rapidly deaminated in the GI tract to Ara-Hx.

Distribution – Because of its low solubility, trace amounts of both vidarabine and Ara-Hx can be detected in the aqueous humor only if there is an epithelial defect in the cornea. If the cornea is normal, only trace amounts of Ara-Hx can be recovered from the aqueous humor.

Microbiology: Vidarabine possesses in vitro and in vivo antiviral activity against herpes simplex types 1 and 2, varicella zoster and vaccinia viruses. Except for rhabdovirus and oncornavirus, it does not display antiviral activity against other RNA or DNA viruses, including adenovirus.

Indications:

For the treatment of acute keratoconjunctivitis and recurrent epithelial keratitis due to herpes simplex virus types 1 and 2. It is also effective in superficial keratitis caused by herpes simplex virus which has not responded to topical idoxuridine, or when toxic or hypersensitivity reactions to idoxuridine have occurred. Effectiveness against stromal keratitis and uveitis due to herpes simplex virus has not been established.

Vidarabine is not effective against RNA virus, adenoviral ocular infections, bacterial, fungal or chlamydial infections of the cornea, or nonviral trophic ulcers.

Contraindications:

Hypersensitivity to vidarabine; sterile trophic ulcers.

Warnings:

Corticosteroids alone are normally contraindicated in herpes simplex virus eye infections. If vidarabine is coadministered with topical corticosteroid therapy, consider corticosteroid-induced ocular side effects such as corticosteroid-induced glaucoma or cataract formation and progression of bacterial or viral infection.

Temporary visual haze may be produced with vidarabine.

Mutagenesis: In vitro, vidarabine can be incorporated into mammalian DNA and can induce mutation. Studies have not been conclusive; however, vidarabine may be capable of producing mutagenic effects in male germ cells.

Vidarabine has caused chromosome breaks and gaps when added to human leukocytes in vitro. While the significance is not fully understood, there is a well known correlation between the ability of various agents to produce such effects and their ability to produce heritable genetic damage.

Carcinogenesis: In mice, there was an increase in liver tumor incidence among the vidarabine-treated (IM) females; some male mice developed kidney neoplasia.

In rats, intestinal, testicular and thyroid neoplasia occurred with greater frequency among the vidarabine-treated animals.

Pregnancy: Category C. A 10% ointment applied to 10% of the body surface during organogenesis induced fetal abnormalities in rabbits. The possibility of embryonic or fetal damage in pregnant women is remote. The topical ophthalmic dose is small, and the drug is relatively insoluble. Its ocular penetration is very low. However, a safe dose for a human embryo or fetus has not been established. Therefore, use only if the potential benefit outweighs the potential risk to the fetus.

Lactation: It is not known whether vidarabine is excreted in breast milk. However, excretion of vidarabine in breast milk is unlikely because the drug is rapidly deaminated in the GI tract. However, it is still recommended that either nursing or the drug be discontinued, taking into account the importance of the drug to the mother.

Precautions:

Viral resistance to vidarabine has not been observed, although this possibility exists.

(Continued on following page)

VIDARABINE (Adenine Arabinoside; Ara-A) (Cont.)

Adverse Reactions:

Lacrimation; foreign body sensation; conjunctival injection; burning; irritation; superficial punctate keratitis; pain; photophobia; punctal occlusion; sensitivity.

The following have also been reported, but appear disease-related: Uveitis; stromal edema; secondary glaucoma; trophic defects; corneal vascularization; hyphema.

Overdosage:

The rapid deamination to Ara-Hx should preclude any difficulty. No untoward effects should result from ingestion of the entire contents of a tube. Overdosage by ocular instillation is unlikely because any excess is quickly expelled from the conjunctival sac.

Before use of another ointment, wait about 10 minutes. Instill ointments 10 minutes after eyedrops to allow for absorption.

Patient Information:

May cause sensitivity to bright light; this may be minimized by wearing sunglasses.

Do not discontinue use without consulting physician.

Notify physician if improvement is not seen after 7 days, if condition worsens, or if pain, decrease in vision, burning or irritation of the eye occurs.

Refer to page 2164 for more complete information.

Administration and Dosage:

Administer approximately 0.5 inch of ointment into the lower conjunctival sac 5 times daily at 3 hour intervals.

If there are no signs of improvement after 7 days, or if complete reepithelialization has not occurred in 21 days, consider other forms of therapy. Some severe cases may require longer treatment.

After reepithelialization has occurred, treat for an additional 7 days at a reduced dosage (such as twice daily) to prevent recurrence.

Concomitant therapy: Topical **antibiotics** (gentamicin, erythromycin, chloramphenicol) or topical **steroids** (prednisolone or dexamethasone) have been administered concurrently with vidarabine without an increase in adverse reactions, although their advantages and disadvantages must be considered (see Warnings).

				C.I.*
Rx	**Vira-A** (Parke-Davis)	**Ophthalmic Ointment:** 3% vidarabine monohydrate (equivalent to 2.8% vidarabine)	In a petrolatum base. In 3.5 g.	413

* Cost Index based on cost per g.

TRIFLURIDINE (Trifluorothymidine)

Actions:

Pharmacology: A fluorinated pyrimidine nucleoside with in vitro and in vivo activity against herpes simplex virus types 1 and 2, and vaccinia virus. Some strains of adenovirus are also inhibited in vitro. Trifluridine interferes with DNA synthesis in cultured mammalian cells. However, its antiviral mechanism of action is not completely known.

Pharmacokinetics: Absorption – Intraocular penetration occurs after topical instillation. Decreased corneal integrity or stromal or uveal inflammation may enhance the penetration into the aqueous humor. Systemic absorption following therapeutic dosing appears negligible.

Indications:

For the treatment of primary keratoconjunctivitis and recurrent epithelial keratitis due to herpes simplex virus types 1 and 2. Also effective in the treatment of epithelial keratitis that has not responded clinically to topical idoxuridine, or when ocular toxicity or hypersensitivity to idoxuridine has occurred. In a smaller number of patients resistant to topical vidarabine, trifluridine was also effective.

The clinical efficacy in the treatment of stromal keratitis and uveitis due to herpes simplex or ophthalmic infections caused by vaccinia virus and adenovirus, or in the prophylaxis of herpes simplex virus keratoconjunctivitis and epithelial keratitis has not been established by well controlled clinical trials.

Not effective against bacterial, fungal or chlamydial infections of the cornea or nonviral trophic lesions.

Contraindications:

Hypersensitivity reactions or chemical intolerance to trifluridine.

Warnings:

Do not exceed the recommended dosage or frequency of administration.

Mutagenesis: Has exerted mutagenic, DNA-damaging and cell-transforming activities in various standard in vitro test systems. Although the significance of these test results is not clear or fully understood, it is possible that mutagenic agents may cause genetic damage in humans.

Pregnancy: Based upon animal findings, it is unlikely that trifluridine would cause embryonic or fetal damage if given in the recommended ophthalmic dosage to pregnant women. A safe dose, however, has not been established for the human embryo or fetus. Safety for use during pregnancy has not been established. Use only when clearly needed and when the potential benefits outweigh the potential hazards to the fetus.

Lactation: It is unlikely that trifluridine is excreted in breast milk after ophthalmic instillation because of the relatively small dosage ($\leq$ 5 mg/day), its dilution in body fluids and its extremely short half-life ($\approx$ 12 minutes). However, do not prescribe for nursing mothers unless the potential benefits outweigh the potential risks.

Precautions:

Cross-sensitivity between idoxuridine and trifluridine appears rare, despite their structural relationship.

Mild local irritation of the conjunctiva and cornea may occur when instilled, but these effects are usually transient.

Viral resistance, although documented in vitro, has not been reported following multiple exposure to trifluridine; this possibility may exist.

(Continued on following page)

TRIFLURIDINE (Trifluorothymidine) (Cont.)

Adverse Reactions:

The most frequent adverse reactions reported are mild, transient burning or stinging upon instillation (4.6%) and palpebral edema (2.8%). Other adverse reactions in decreasing order of reported frequency were: Superficial punctate keratopathy; epithelial keratopathy; hypersensitivity reaction; stromal edema; irritation; keratitis sicca; hyperemia and increased intraocular pressure.

Overdosage:

Overdosage by ocular instillation is unlikely because any excess solution is quickly expelled from the conjunctival sac.

No untoward effects are likely to result from ingestion of the entire contents of a bottle. Single IV doses of 15 to 30 mg/kg/day in children and adults with neoplastic disease produce reversible bone marrow depression as the only potentially serious toxic effect and only after three to five courses of therapy.

Patient Information:

Do not discontinue use without consulting physician.

Transient stinging may occur upon instillation.

Notify physician if improvement is not seen after 7 days, if condition worsens or if irritation occurs.

Refer to page 2164 for more complete information.

Administration and Dosage:

Instill 1 drop onto the cornea of the affected eye every 2 hours while awake for a maximum daily dosage of 9 drops until the corneal ulcer has completely reepithelialized. Following reepithelialization, treat for an additional 7 days with 1 drop every 4 hours while awake for a minimum daily dosage of 5 drops.

If there are no signs of improvement after 7 days of therapy, or if complete reepithelialization has not occurred after 14 days of therapy, consider other forms of therapy. Avoid continuous administration for periods exceeding 21 days because of potential ocular toxicity.

Storage: Store at 2° to 8°C (36° to 46°F).

				C.I.*
Rx	**Viroptic** (Burroughs Wellcome)	**Ophthalmic Solution:** 1%	In 7.5 ml Drop-Dose.[1]	409

* Cost Index based on cost per ml.

[1] In aqueous solution with 0.001% thimerosal.

ARTIFICIAL TEAR SOLUTIONS

These products contain: Balanced amounts of salts to maintain ocular tonicity (0.9% NaCl equivalent); buffers to adjust pH; viscosity agents to prolong eye contact time; preservatives for sterility. See p. 2164 for a description and listing of these ingredients.

Indications:

These products offer tear-like lubrication for the relief of dry eyes and eye irritation associated with deficient tear production. Also used as ocular lubricants for artificial eyes. Some of these products can be used in conjunction with hard contact lenses.

Patient Information:

Wash hands thoroughly. Do not touch the tip of the container or dropper to any surface. Close container immediately after use.

If headache, eye pain, vision changes, continued redness or irritation occurs, or if condition worsens or persists for more than 3 days, discontinue use and consult a physician.

May cause mild stinging or temporary blurred vision.

Administration and Dosage:

Usually, 1 to 2 drops into eye(s) 3 or 4 times daily, as needed.

	Product	Ingredients	How supplied	C.I.*
otc	**Adsorbotear** (Alcon)	Hydroxyethylcellulose, 1.67% povidone, water soluble polymers, 0.004% thimerosal, 0.1% EDTA	In 15 ml with dropper.	35
otc	**Akwa Tears** (Akorn)	Polyvinyl alcohol, sodium chloride, 0.01% benzalkonium chloride, EDTA	In 2 and 15 ml.	20
otc	**Artificial Tears Solution** (Rugby)	1.4% polyvinyl alcohol, EDTA, chlorobutanol	In 15 ml.	13
otc	**Celluvisc** (Allergan)	1% carboxymethylcellulose sodium, calcium chloride, potassium chloride, sodium chloride, sodium lactate	In 0.3 ml single-use containers.	25
otc	**Dry Eye Therapy** (Bausch & Lomb)	0.3% glycerin, calcium chloride, magnesium chloride, NaCl, sodium citrate, sodium phosphate, zinc chloride	Preservative free. In 0.3 ml single-use container.	NA
otc	**HypoTears** (Iolab)	1% polyvinyl alcohol, PEG-8000, dextrose, benzalkonium chloride, EDTA	In 15 and 30 ml dropper bottles.	33
otc	**HypoTears PF** (Iolab)	1% polyvinyl alcohol, PEG-400, dextrose, EDTA	In 0.6 ml single-use containers.	33
otc	**I-Liqui Tears** (Americal)	0.5% hydroxyethylcellulose, 1% polyvinyl alcohol, 0.01% benzalkonium chloride, EDTA, sodium chloride	In 2 and 15 ml.	27
otc	**Isopto Alkaline** (Alcon)	1% hydroxypropyl methylcellulose, 0.01% benzalkonium chloride	In 15 ml.	49
otc	**Ultra Tears** (Alcon)		In 15 ml.	49
otc	**Isopto Plain** (Alcon)	0.5% hydroxypropyl methylcellulose, 0.01% benzalkonium chloride	In 15 ml.	35
otc	**Isopto Tears** (Alcon)		In 15 and 30 ml.	35
otc	**Just Tears** (Blairex)	Hydroxypropyl methylcellulose, 0.01% benzalkonium chloride, 0.025% EDTA, sodium chloride, boric acid	In 15 ml.	14
otc	**Lacril** (Allergan)	0.5% hydroxypropyl methylcellulose, gelatin A, 0.5% chlorobutanol, sodium chloride, polysorbate 80	In 15 ml dropper bottles.	41
otc	**Liquifilm Forte** (Allergan)	3% polyvinyl alcohol, 0.002% thimerosal, sodium chloride, EDTA	In 15 and 30 ml dropper bottles.	37
otc	**Liquifilm Tears** (Allergan)	1.4% polyvinyl alcohol, sodium chloride, 0.5% chlorobutanol	In 15 and 30 ml dropper bottles.	35
otc	**Moisture Drops** (Bausch & Lomb)	0.5% hydroxypropyl methylcellulose, 0.1% dextran 40, NaCl, potassium chloride, 0.01% benzalkonium chloride, EDTA, sodium borate, boric acid	In 15 and 30 ml.	16
otc	**Murine** (Ross)	1.4% polyvinyl alcohol, 0.6% povidone, benzalkonium chloride, dextrose, EDTA, potassium chloride, sodium bicarbonate, sodium chloride, sodium citrate, sodium phosphate	In 15 and 30 ml.	11

* Cost Index based on cost per ml.

(Continued on following page)

ARTIFICIAL TEAR SOLUTIONS (Cont.)

	Product	Contents	How supplied	C.I.*
otc	**Murocel** (Bausch & Lomb)	1% methylcellulose, propylene glycol, NaCl, boric acid, parabens	In 15 ml dropper bottles.	26
otc	**Muro Tears** (Bausch & Lomb)	Hydroxypropyl methylcellulose, dextran 40, 0.01% benzalkonium chloride, EDTA, sodium chloride, boric acid	In 15 ml dropper bottles.	23
otc	**Neo-Tears** (Sola/Barnes-Hind)	Polyvinyl alcohol, hydroxyethylcellulose, sodium chloride, PEG-300, ≤ 0.004% thimerosal, 0.02% EDTA	In 15 ml.	39
otc	**Refresh** (Allergan)	1.4% polyvinyl alcohol, sodium chloride, 0.6% povidone	Preservative free. In 0.3 ml UD 30s and 50s.	15
otc	**TearGard** (Medtech)	Hydroxyethylcellulose in a hypertonic base, 0.25% sorbic acid, 0.1% EDTA	In 15 ml.	23
otc	**Tearisol** (Iolab)	0.5% hydroxypropyl methylcellulose, benzalkonium chloride, EDTA, boric acid	In 15 ml with dropper.	39
otc	**Tears Naturale** (Alcon)	Hydroxypropyl methylcellulose, dextran 70, 0.01% benzalkonium chloride, 0.05% EDTA	In 15 and 30 ml Drop-Tainers.	33
otc	**Tears Naturale II** (Alcon)	0.1% dextran 70, 0.3% hydroxypropyl methylcellulose 2910, 0.001% polyquaternium-1, EDTA, potassium chloride, sodium chloride. May contain hydrochloric acid or sodium hydroxide	In 15 and 30 ml.	24
otc	**Tears Plus** (Allergan)	1.4% polyvinyl alcohol, sodium chloride, povidone, 0.5% chlorobutanol	In 15 and 30 ml dropper bottles.	33
otc	**Tears Renewed** (Akorn)	Dextran 70, sodium chloride, hydroxypropyl methylcellulose, 0.01% benzalkonium chloride, 0.05% EDTA	In 15 ml.	25

ARTIFICIAL TEAR INSERT

The hydroxypropyl cellulose insert acts to stabilize and thicken the precorneal tear film and prolong tear film breakup time.

Indications:

Moderate to severe dry eye syndromes including: Keratoconjunctivitis sicca; exposure keratitis; decreased corneal sensitivity; recurrent corneal erosions.

Contraindications:

Hypersensitivity to hydroxypropyl cellulose.

Adverse Reactions:

The following adverse reactions have been reported, but in most instances were mild and transient: Transient blurring of vision; ocular discomfort or irritation; matting or stickiness of eyelashes; photophobia; hypersensitivity; edema of the eyelids; hyperemia.

Patient Information:

May produce transient blurring of vision; exercise caution while operating hazardous machinery or driving a motor vehicle.

If improperly placed in the inferior cul-de-sac, corneal abrasion may result. The patient should practice insertion and removal of insert while in physician's office until proficiency is achieved.

Illustrated instructions are included in each package.

If symptoms worsen, remove insert and notify physician.

Administration:

One daily, inserted into the inferior cul-de-sac beneath the base of the torsus, not in apposition to the cornea. Individual patients may require twice daily use for optimal results.

	Product	Contents	How supplied	C.I.*
Rx	**Lacrisert** (MSD)	**Insert:** 5 mg hydroxypropyl cellulose ophthalmic insert	Preservative free. In 60s with applicator.	54

* Cost Index based on cost per ml or insert.

OCULAR LUBRICANTS

These products serve as lubricants and emollients.

Indications:

Protection and lubrication of the eye in: Exposure keratitis; decreased corneal sensitivity; recurrent corneal erosions; keratitis sicca, particularly for nighttime use; after removal of a foreign body; during and following surgery.

Contraindications:

Hypersensitivity to any component of the products.

Patient Information:

Do not touch tube tip to any surface since this may contaminate the ointment.

If eye pain, change in vision, continued redness or irritation occurs or if condition worsens or persists more than 72 hours, discontinue use and consult a physician.

Do not use with contact lenses.

Administration:

Instill small amount into the conjunctival cul-de-sac.

	Product	Composition	Supplied	C.I.*
otc	**Akwa Tears** (Akorn)	**Ointment:** White petrolatum, mineral oil and lanolin	Preservative free. In 3.5 g.	78
otc	**Artificial Tears** (Rugby)		In 3.75 g.	35
Rx	**Dey-Lube** (Dey)	**Ointment:** White petrolatum	Preservative free. In 0.5 g.	150
otc	**Duolube** (Bausch & Lomb)	**Ointment:** White petrolatum and mineral oil	Preservative free. In 3.5 g.	107
otc	**Duratears Naturale** (Alcon)	**Ointment:** White petrolatum, anhydrous liquid lanolin and mineral oil	In 3.5 g.	134
otc	**Hypotears** (Iolab)	**Ointment:** White petrolatum and light mineral oil	Preservative free. In 3.5 g.	128
otc	**Tears Renewed** (Akorn)		In 3.5 g.	NA
otc	**Lacri-Lube NP** (Allergan)	**Ointment:** 55.5% white petrolatum, 42.5% mineral oil and 2% petrolatum/lanolin alcohol	Preservative free. In 0.7 g.	172
otc	**Lacri-Lube S.O.P.** (Allergan)	**Ointment:** 55% white petrolatum, 42.5% mineral oil, 2% nonionic lanolin derivatives and 0.5% chlorobutanol	In 3.5 and 7 g and UD 0.7 g paks (24s).	138
otc	**Lipo-Tears** (Spectra)	**Drops:** Mineral oil and petrolatum	Preservative free. In 1 ml (30s).	28
otc	**Refresh PM** (Allergan)	**Ointment:** 55% white petrolatum, sodium chloride, 41.5% mineral oil and 2% petrolatum/lanolin alcohol	Preservative free. In 3.5 g.	139
otc	**Vit-A-Drops** (Vision Pharm.)	**Drops:** 5000 IU vitamin A, polysorbate 80, sodium chloride and 0.05% EDTA	In 15 ml.	43

* Cost Index based on cost per g or ml.

Ophthalmic Irrigation Solutions

Irrigating solutions are aqueous solutions used to cleanse and to maintain moisture of ocular tissue. Ideally these solutions are isotonic. The optimum pH is 7.4. A pH < 7 or > 8 has caused cellular stress and death when the tissues have been exposed for a prolonged period of time.

Intraocular Irrigating Solutions:
Used during ocular surgery to protect the lens and cornea in nondiabetic patients. Unlike physiological saline and lactated Ringer's solution, these balanced salt solutions provide the ions magnesium and calcium as cellular nutrients. These nutrients are required for intercellular and intracellular function during prolonged ocular surgery. In addition to magnesium and calcium, bicarbonate, glucose and glutathione are in these perfusion media *(BSS Plus)*. These components help to maintain a deturgesced or thin cornea by avoiding corneal swelling.

Extraocular Irrigating Solutions:
Sterile isotonic solutions for general ophthalmic use. Office uses include irrigating procedures following tonometry, gonioscopy, foreign body removal or use of fluorescein; they are also used to soothe and cleanse the eye, and in conjunction with hard contact lenses. Because these solutions have a short contact time with the eye, they do not need to provide nutrients to cells. Unlike intraocular irrigants, irrigants for extraocular use contain preservatives which prevent bacteriostatic contamination. However, the preservatives are exceedingly toxic to the corneal endothelium and intraocular use of extraocular irrigating fluids is contraindicated.

		Intraocular Irrigating Solutions		C.I.*
Rx	**BSS** (Various, eg, Abbott, Alcon, Balan, Kendall-McGaw, Pharmafair)	**Solution:** 0.64% sodium chloride, 0.075% potassium chloride, 0.03% magnesium chloride, 0.048% calcium chloride, 0.39% sodium acetate, 0.17% sodium citrate, and sodium hydroxide or hydrochloric acid	In 15, 30, 250, 300, 500 ml sterile vials.	33+
Rx	**BSS Plus** (Alcon)	**Solution:** Mix aseptically just prior to use. **Part I:** 480 ml containing 7.44 mg sodium chloride, 0.395 mg potassium chloride, 0.433 mg sodium phosphate, 2.19 mg sodium bicarbonate, and hydrochloric acid or sodium hydroxide/ml **Part II:** 20 ml containing 3.85 mg calcium chloride dihydrate, 5 mg magnesium chloride hexahydrate, 23 mg dextrose and 4.6 mg glutathione disulfide/ml	Preservative free. In **500 ml**.	12
		Solution: Mix aseptically just prior to use. **Part I:** 28.8 ml containing 7.44 mg sodium chloride, 0.395 mg potassium chloride, 0.433 mg sodium phosphate, 2.19 mg sodium bicarbonate, and hydrochloric acid or sodium hydroxide/ml **Part II:** 1.2 ml containing 3.85 mg calcium chloride dihydrate, 5 mg magnesium chloride hexahydrate, 23 mg dextrose and 4.6 mg glutathione disulfide/ml	Preservative free. In **30 ml**.	77

		Extraocular Irrigating Solutions		C.I.*
otc	**AK-Rinse** (Akorn)	**Solution:** 0.49% sodium chloride, 0.075% potassium chloride, 0.048% calcium chloride, 0.03% magnesium chloride, 0.39% sodium acetate and 0.17% sodium citrate with 0.013% benzalkonium chloride	In 30 and 118 ml.	8
otc	**Blinx** (Sola/Barnes-Hind)	**Solution:** Boric acid and sodium borate with 0.004% phenylmercuric acetate	In 30 and 120 ml.	10
otc	**Collyrium Eye Lotion** (Wyeth-Ayerst)	**Solution:** Boric acid and sodium borate with $\leq$ 0.002% thimerosal	In 180 ml with eyecup.	1

* Cost Index based on cost per ml.

(Continued on following page)

Ophthalmic Irrigation Solutions (Cont.)

Extraocular Irrigating Solutions (Cont.)

				C.I.*
otc	**Collyrium Fresh** (Wyeth-Ayerst)	**Solution:** 0.05% tetrahydrozoline, 1% glycerin, 0.01% benzalkonium chloride, 0.1% EDTA, boric acid, hydrochloric acid, sodium borate	In 15 ml.	15
otc	**Collyrium for Fresh Eyes** (Wyeth-Ayerst)	**Solution:** Neutral borate solution with boric acid, sodium borate, ≤ 0.002% thimerosal	In 177 ml.	2
otc	**Dacriose** (Iolab)	**Solution:** Sodium chloride, potassium chloride, sodium phosphate and sodium hydroxide with benzalkonium chloride and EDTA	In 15, 30 and 120 ml.	20
otc	**Eye-Stream** (Alcon)	**Solution:** 0.49% sodium chloride, 0.075% potassium chloride, 0.03% magnesium chloride, 0.048% calcium chloride, 0.39% sodium acetate and 0.17% sodium citrate with 0.013% benzalkonium chloride and sodium hydroxide or hydrochloric acid	In 30 and 120 ml.	14
otc	**Eye Wash** (Hauck)	**Solution:** 1.2% boric acid, 0.38% potassium chloride, 0.014% sodium carbonate anhydrous, 0.05% EDTA and 0.01% benzalkonium chloride	In 120 ml.	2
Rx	**Iocare** (Iolab)	**Solution:** 0.64% sodium chloride, 0.075% potassium chloride, 0.048% calcium chloride, 0.03% magnesium chloride, 0.39% sodium acetate and 0.17% sodium citrate	In 15 and 500 ml.	NA
otc	**I Rinse** (Americal)	**Solution:** 0.49% sodium chloride, 0.075% potassium chloride, 0.048% calcium chloride, 0.03% magnesium chloride, 0.39% sodium acetate, 0.17% sodium citrate and 0.013% benzalkonium chloride	In 30 and 120 ml.	5
Rx	**I-Sol** (Dey Labs)	**Solution:** 0.64% sodium chloride, 0.075% potassium chloride, 0.048% calcium chloride, 0.03% magnesium chloride, 0.39% sodium acetate, 0.17% sodium citrate and sodium hydroxide or hydrochloric acid	In 20 and 200 ml.	1
otc	**Lavoptik Eye Wash** (Lavoptik)	**Solution:** 0.49% sodium chloride, 0.4% sodium biphosphate and 0.45% sodium phosphate with 0.005% benzalkonium chloride	In 180 ml with eyecup.	1
otc	**Murine Regular Formula** (Ross)	**Solution:** Sodium chloride, potassium chloride, sodium phosphate and glycerin with 0.01% benzalkonium chloride and 0.05% EDTA	In 15 and 30 ml dropper bottles.	14
otc	**Ocu-Bath Eye Lotion** (Commerce Drug)	**Solution:** Sodium chloride, sodium propionate, sodium borate, boric acid, glycerin, rose and camphor water, extract of witch hazel, berberine bisulfate and benzalkonium chloride	In 120 ml with eyecup.	2
otc	**Ocu-Drop** (Commerce Drug)	**Solution:** 0.05% tetrahydrozoline HCl with sodium chloride, sodium borate, boric acid, 0.01% benzalkonium chloride and 0.1% EDTA	In 15 ml.	13
otc	**Star-Optic Eye Wash** (Stellar)	**Solution:** Sterile, isotonic, buffered solution containing sodium chloride, sodium phosphate mono- and dibasic, EDTA and benzalkonium chloride	In 120 ml dropper bottle with eye cup.	NA

* Cost Index based on cost per ml.

Hyperosmolar Preparations

Hypertonic (hyperosmolar) preparations reduce corneal edema by osmotic attraction of water through the semipermeable corneal epithelium.

SODIUM CHLORIDE, HYPERTONIC

Indications:

As adjunctive therapy in the reduction of corneal edema from various causes including bullous keratitis.

As a diagnostic aid in facilitating ophthalmoscopic examination in gonioscopy, funduscopy and biomicroscopy.

Contraindications: Hypersensitivity to any component.

Precautions:

Discontinue use if any of the following occur: Severe pain; headache; rapid change in vision (side and straight ahead); sudden appearance of floating spots; acute redness of eyes; pain on exposure to light; double vision.

Adverse Reactions: May cause temporary burning and irritation upon instillation.

Administration and Dosage:

Solution: Instill 1 or 2 drops in affected eye(s) every 3 or 4 hours, or as directed.

Ointment: Apply once a day or more often, as directed.

				C.I.*
otc	**Adsorbonac Ophthalmic** (Alcon)	**Solution:** 2% or 5% in povidone with water soluble polymers, 0.004% thimerosal and 0.1% EDTA	In 15 ml.	42
otc	**Muro-128 Ophthalmic** (Bausch & Lomb)	**Solution:** 2% or 5% with hydroxypropyl methylcellulose and parabens. 5% also contains propylene glycol, sodium borate and boric acid	2%: In 15 ml.	30
			5%: In 15 and 30 ml.	30
otc	**AK-NaCl** (Akorn)	**Ointment:** 5% with mineral oil, white petrolatum and anhydrous lanolin	In 3.5 g.	93
otc	**Muro-128 Ophthalmic** (Bausch & Lomb)		In 3.5 g.	114

GLYCERIN

Indications:

To clear an edematous cornea in order to facilitate ophthalmoscopic and gonioscopic examination in acute glaucoma, bullous keratitis and Fuchs' endothelial dystrophy.

Contraindications: Hypersensitivity to any component of the product.

Warnings:

Pregnancy: Category C. Safety for use during pregnancy has not been established. Use only when clearly needed and when the potential benefits outweigh the potential hazards to the fetus.

Lactation: It is not known whether glycerin is excreted in breast milk. Safety for use in the nursing mother has not been established.

Children: Safety and efficacy for use in children have not been established.

Precautions:

Because glycerin is an irritant and may cause pain, instill a local anesthetic before use.

Adverse Reactions: Some pain or irritation may occur upon instillation.

Administration and Dosage:

Instill 1 or 2 drops prior to examination. In gonioscopy of an edematous cornea, additional glycerin may be used as the lubricant.

				C.I.*
Rx	**Ophthalgan Ophthalmic** (Wyeth-Ayerst)	**Solution:** Glycerin with 0.55% chlorobutanol	In 7.5 ml.	117

GLUCOSE

Indications: Topical osmotherapy for reducing corneal edema.

Contraindications: Hypersensitivity to any component of the product.

Precautions: If irritation develops, discontinue use.

Administration and Dosage:

Depress lower lid with index finger while looking upward. Introduce a small amount of ointment behind depressed eyelid into conjunctival sac. Close and open eyes twice. Wipe off excess ointment. If eyelids are sticky, clean them before each application with a pledget of cotton and lukewarm boiled water. May be used 2 to 6 times daily.

				C.I.*
Rx	**Glucose-40 Ophthalmic** (Iolab)	**Ointment:** 40% in white petrolatum and anhydrous lanolin with parabens	In 3.75 g.	224

* Cost Index based on cost per ml or g.

Contact Lens Products

Inadequate cleaning can lead to lens discoloration and lens surface buildup of protein, lipids, minerals and other environmental contaminants, which can contribute to giant papillary conjunctivitis (GPC), superficial punctate keratitis (SPK) and corneal abrasion. Irregular contact lens disinfection can cause severe ocular infection.

Contact Lens Guidelines

- Proper contact lens care will increase success and decrease complications.
- Cleaning does not disinfect lenses.
- Disinfecting does not clean lenses.
- Wash and rinse hands thoroughly before handling contact lenses.
- Do not insert contact lenses if eyes are red or irritated.
- Do not wear contact lenses while sleeping unless they have been prescribed for extended wear.
- For soft lens care, use only products designed for soft lenses.
- For rigid lens care, use only products designed for rigid lenses.
- Do not change or substitute products from a different manufacturer without consulting a physician.
- Always follow label directions or the physician's recommendations.
- Do not store lenses in tap water.
- Never use saliva to wet contact lenses.
- Keep lens care products out of the reach of children.
- Do not instill topical medications while contact lenses are being worn unless directed by the physician.

Contact Lens Materials

Three types of contact lenses are manufactured: Hard, rigid gas permeable and soft.

Hard Contact Lenses: Hard contact lenses made from polymethylmethacrylate (PMMA) provide easy care, durability and excellent vision. However, PMMA does not transmit the oxygen needed for normal corneal integrity. Hard contact lenses have caused chronic corneal edema, corneal distortion, edematous corneal formations, spectacle blur, polymegathism and corneal abrasions. Because of these ocular complications, hard lenses are seldom the lens of choice for a new contact lens patient. Less than 1% of the contact lens population wear hard contact lenses.

Rigid Gas Permeable Lenses: Approximately 20% of contact lens patients wear rigid gas permeable (RGP) lenses. The major advantage of these lenses over hard lenses is that they are oxygen permeable. With this increased oxygen supply, the RGP patient does not have the severe physiological complications of the hard lens patient. Most doctors prescribe daily wear RGP lenses. Several new lens polymers with a high degree of oxygen permeability have been approved by the FDA for extended wear. RGP lenses provide the patient with good vision and easy care, but RGP lenses are not as durable as hard (PMMA) lenses. They are more susceptible to lens deposits and vulnerable to scratching and breaking.

Soft Contact Lenses: Soft contact lenses are made of hydroxyethylmethacrylate (HEMA), a plastic compound that had been used for making artificial blood vessels and organs. The first soft lens was marketed in the US in 1971. Today, most soft lenses manufactured from HEMA contain 30% to 50% water. In some, HEMA is combined with polyvinylpyrrolidone (PVP), which increases the hydration of methylmethacrylate (MMA). This enhances the firmness of the lens.

Daily wear soft contact lenses are designed to be worn all day (12 to 14 hours), but must be removed nightly to be cleaned and disinfected. Extended wear soft lenses can be worn for 24 hours or more. Some lenses are approved for up to 30 days of continuous wear, but most eye care practitioners recommend a maximum wearing period of 3 to 6 days. The lenses must then be removed overnight for cleaning and disinfection. The major advantage of extended wear lenses is convenience. Daily wear soft lenses provide the same level of comfort and vision as extended wear soft lenses; however, the popularity of extended wear soft lenses has decreased in the last few years due to the increased risk of infection.

Disposable Soft Lenses: These are extended wear soft lenses designed for maximum convenience. The concept is to totally eliminate lens cleaning and disinfection. The manufacturer recommends that the lenses be discarded after 1 or 2 weeks of continuous wear. Many doctors are concerned about patient compliance. Patients may be tempted to wear the disposable extended wear soft lens longer than recommended, increasing the risk of physiological complications. For example, if a patient wears these lenses on a daily wear basis in the presence of an upper respiratory infection, the patient may risk ocular infection in the absence of proper cleaning and disinfection.

(Continued on following page)

Contact Lens Care Products

Products for use with contact lenses possess the same general characteristics of all ophthalmic products; they are sterile, isotonic and free of particulate matter. Product formulations contain various components to achieve specific goals of contact lens care.

Although all contact lenses serve similar functions in correcting visual defects, there are distinct types of lens materials, each requiring unique lens care programs. In selecting appropriate accessory lens care solutions, it is essential to correctly identify the type of lens the patient is using.

Hard and Rigid Gas Permeable Lenses

Similar lens care is used for the hard and RGP lenses. Products include wetting/soaking/disinfection solutions, cleaning agents, lubricants and re-wetting solutions.

When a rigid contact lens is removed from the eye, it may be covered with lipids, proteins, eye makeup and other debris. After removal, immediately clean the lens with a *surfactant cleaner*. Improper cleaning can contribute to a lens surface buildup which can interfere with vision and potentially cause corneal irritation.

Soak rigid lenses overnight in a *wetting/soaking/disinfecting solution*. This solution has four major functions:

1. To enhance the lens surface wettability
2. To maintain the lens hydration similar to that achieved during daily wear
3. Lens disinfection
4. To act as a mechanical buffer between the lens and the cornea

It is not uncommon for a rigid lens patient to experience dryness after several hours of wear. This is especially true with RGP lens patients because of the hydrophobic nature of the lens material. *Re-wetting drops* can provide temporary relief by rinsing some debris off the lens surface and re-wetting the eye and the lens.

Many clinicians routinely recommend the weekly use of an enzyme (papain) cleaner with RGP lenses. This weekly cleaning process is very effective in removing protein deposits from the lens surface. A protein film on an RGP lens can decrease vision and cause GPC.

Soft Contact Lenses

Soft contact lens care systems are designed to clean, disinfect and re-wet the lenses. The first step is proper cleaning. Cleaning the lens gently in the palm of the hand with a *daily surfactant cleaner* will remove fresh lipids, oils and other environmental debris. Clean soft lenses thoroughly with a surfactant cleaner each time a lens is removed. After cleaning the lens, thoroughly rinse with a soft lens *rinsing/storage solution.* All rinsing/storage solutions contain 0.9% saline. Some are available with no preservatives in unit-dose vials or aerosol containers. Other saline solutions contain preservatives to decrease microorganism growth. Discourage use of saline made with salt tablets because of risk of contamination and infection (see Precautions).

Enzymatic cleaners are generally used weekly. They more effectively remove protein deposits than surfactant cleaners because they contain proteolytic enzymes (papain, pancreatin or subtilisin). Most enzymes are dissolved directly in saline, but a newer enzyme (subtilisin) tablet can be dissolved in a hydrogen peroxide disinfection solution.

Soft lens *disinfection* is the most important step in soft lens care. Disinfection is achieved by using a thermal (heat) or chemical (cold) system.

Thermal disinfection was the first system approved for soft lenses. A heat unit designed for soft lenses is used for 10 min at 80° C (176°F). This will kill most dangerous microorganisms. Recently *Acanthamoeba* keratitis has concerned many clinicians. Heat disinfection is the only procedure that will successfully kill *Acanthamoeba*; however, it cannot be used with all soft lenses. Also, continued use of heat can shorten soft lens life.

Chemical disinfection: The original chemical soft lens disinfection systems used thimerosal with either chlorhexidine or a quaternary ammonium compound. These systems had a high incidence of sensitivity reactions. Hydrogen peroxide disinfection systems have become the lens care system of choice for the majority of soft lens patients. Several systems require two steps to achieve disinfection and hydrogen peroxide neutralization; other systems combine disinfection and neutralization in one step. Hydrogen peroxide (3%) is very effective and can be used with all soft lens polymers, but these systems can be complex and expensive. Do not substitute generic peroxide solutions for solutions formulated for contact lenses. They may be contaminated with heavy metals, have different concentrations of hydrogen peroxide or use stabilizers that may discolor soft lenses.

(Continued on following page)

Contact Lens Products (Cont.)

Soft Contact Lenses (Cont.)

Soft lens re-wetting solutions permit the lubrication of the soft lens while it is on the eye. Most patients find these re-wetting drops minimally effective in reducing the symptoms of dryness. Maximum relief can be achieved by removing the lens, cleaning it with a daily surfactant cleaner and thoroughly rinsing it with a rinsing/storage saline solution.

Precautions:

Acanthamoeba keratitis: Soft contact lens wearers who use homemade saline solution are at risk of developing *Acanthamoeba* keratitis, a serious and painful corneal infection. This infection may cause blindness or impaired vision. Homemade saline solutions (nonsterile) may be used before and during the thermal disinfection phase but NOT after disinfection.

Drug interference with contact lens use: Many systemic and local medications have been associated with intolerance to or discoloration of contact lenses.

Drug Interference With Contact Lens Use		
Drug	**RGP[1]/Hard/Soft Lens**	**Action**
Anticholinergic	RGP, hard, soft	Tear volume decreased
Antihistamines, sympathomimetics	RGP, hard, soft	Tear volume decreased, blink rate decreased
Chlorthalidone	RGP, hard, soft	Causes lid or corneal edema
Clomiphene	RGP, hard, soft	Causes lid or corneal edema
Diuretics, Thiazide	RGP, hard, soft	Tear volume decreased
Dopamine	soft	Discoloration of contact lenses
Epinephrine, topical	soft	Lens absorbs the yellow dye
Fluorescein, topical	soft	Lens absorbs the yellow dye
Hypnotics, sedatives, muscle relaxants	RGP, hard, soft	Blink rate decreased
Iodine Groups	soft	Discoloration of contact lenses
Nitrofurantoin	soft	Discoloration of contact lenses
Oral contraceptives	RGP, hard, soft	Increased stickiness of mucus; corneal lid edema due to fluid retention properties of estrogens
Phenazopyridine	soft	Discoloration of contact lenses
Phenolphthaleins	soft	Discoloration of contact lenses
Phenylephrine	soft	Discoloration of contact lenses
Primidone	RGP, hard, soft	Causes lid or corneal edema
Rifampin	soft	Lens absorbs drug causing orange discoloration
Sulfasalazine	soft	Yellow staining
Tetracycline	soft	Discoloration of contact lenses
Tricyclic antidepressants	RGP, hard, soft	Tear volume decreased

[1] Rigid gas permeable.

Products are listed on the following pages and are grouped as follows:

Contact Lens Solutions	
Type of Lens	**Type of Solution**
Hard	Storage/Soaking Wetting Wetting/Soaking Cleaning/Soaking/Wetting Re-wetting Cleaning Cleaning/Soaking
Rigid Gas Permeable	Disinfecting/Wetting/Soaking Cleaning/Soaking Cleaning Cleaning/Disinfecting/Storage
Soft	Rinsing/Storage Surfactant Cleaning Enzymatic Cleaners Re-wetting Chemical Disinfection

(Products listed on following pages)

Contact Lens Products (Cont.)

Refer to the general discussion of these products on page 2238

Hard Contact Lens Products

Conventional hard lenses are made of a rigid hydrophobic polymer, polymethylmethacrylate (PMMA). For optimum comfort and to minimize problems, these lenses require care with separate wetting, cleaning and soaking solutions.

Storage/Soaking Solutions

Storage/soaking solutions serve to maintain the lens in a state of hydration, prevent growth of microbial contamination, and possibly remove debris from lens surface through chelation or solvation. Discard used soaking solutions and replace with fresh solution daily.

				C.I.*
otc	**Soakare** (Allergan)	**Solution:** 0.01% benzalkonium chloride and 0.25% EDTA	In 120 ml.	122
otc	**Soquette** (Sola/Barnes-Hind)	**Solution:** Polyvinyl alcohol with 0.01% benzalkonium chloride and 0.2% EDTA	In 120 ml.	124

Wetting Solutions

Wetting solutions contain surfactants to facilitate hydration of the hydrophobic hard lens surface. These solutions include methylcellulose and derivatives, polyvinyl alcohol, povidone, some newer polymers, preservatives and buffering agents. These agents increase solution viscosity and act as a physical cushioning agent between lens and cornea.

				C.I.*
otc	**Contique** (Alcon)	**Solution:** Hydroxypropyl methylcellulose, polyvinyl alcohol, 0.004% benzalkonium chloride, 0.025% EDTA	In 60 ml.	7
otc	**hy-Flow** (Wesley-Jessen)	**Solution:** Polyvinyl alcohol w/hydroxyethylcellulose, benzalkonium chloride, EDTA	In 60 ml.	8
otc	**Liquifilm Wetting** (Allergan)	**Solution:** Hydroxypropyl methylcellulose, NaCl, KCl, polyvinyl alcohol, 0.004% benzalkonium chloride, EDTA	In 20 and 60 ml.	7
otc	**Sereine** (Optikem)	**Solution:** Sterile, buffered solution with 0.1% EDTA and 0.01% benzalkonium chloride	In 60 ml.	5
otc	**Stay-Wet** (Sherman)	**Solution:** Polyvinyl alcohol, hydroxyethylcellulose, povidone, sodium chloride, potassium chloride, sodium carbonate, 0.01% benzalkonium chloride, 0.025% EDTA	In 30 ml.	19
otc	**Visalens Wetting** (Leeming)	**Solution:** Hydroxypropyl methylcellulose, NaCl, sodium hydroxide, polyvinyl alcohol, 0.01% benzalkonium chloride, 0.1% EDTA	In 60 and 120 ml.	5
otc	**Wetting** (Sola/Barnes-Hind)	**Solution:** Polyvinyl alcohol with 0.004% benzalkonium chloride and 0.02% EDTA	In 35 and 60 ml.	8

Wetting/Soaking Solutions

				C.I.*
otc	**Sereine** (Optikem)	**Solution:** Buffered, isotonic aqueous solution, 0.1% EDTA, 0.01% benzalkonium chloride	In 120 ml.	73
otc	**Soaclens** (Alcon)	**Solution:** Wetting agents, 0.004% thimerosal, 0.1% EDTA, buffering agents	In 120 ml.	111
otc	**SWS** (Ocular)	**Solution:** Polyvinyl alcohol, hydroxyethylcellulose, NaCl, KCl, 0.01% benzalkonium chloride and 0.025% EDTA	In 120 ml.	75
otc	**Wetting & Soaking** (Sola/Barnes-Hind)	**Solution:** Isotonic, buffered solution, 0.02% EDTA, 0.003% chlorhexidine gluconate, 0.002% thimerosal	In 120 ml.	122
otc	**Wet-N-Soak** (Allergan)	**Solution:** Isotonic, buffered solution of polyvinyl alcohol, 0.004% benzalkonium chloride, EDTA	In 120 and 180 ml.	119
otc	**Wet-N-Soak Plus** (Allergan)	**Solution:** Buffered, isotonic solution of polyvinyl alcohol, EDTA, 0.003% benzalkonium chloride	In 30 and 120 ml.	104

* Cost Index based on cost per 30 ml storage/soaking or wetting/soaking solutions, or 1 ml wetting solutions.

Refer to the general discussion of these products on page 2238

Hard Contact Lens Products (Cont.)

Cleaning/Soaking/Wetting Solutions

				C.I.*
otc	**Contactisol** (Ciba Vision)	**Solution:** Hydroxypropyl methylcellulose, boric acid, nonoxynol-15, 0.01% benzalkonium chloride and 0.01% EDTA	In 57 ml.	284
otc	**Lens-Mate** (Alcon)	**Solution:** Hydroxypropyl methylcellulose and polyvinyl alcohol with 0.01% benzalkonium chloride and 0.1% EDTA	In 59 ml.	194
otc	**Total** (Allergan)	**Solution:** Isotonic, buffered solution of polyvinyl alcohol, benzalkonium chloride and EDTA	In 60 and 120 ml.	220

Re-Wetting Solutions

Re-wetting solutions are intended for use directly in the eye in conjunction with a contact lens. These products improve wearing time by rehydrating the lens, which may become dry and contaminated during wear. The principle components of these solutions are wetting agents.

				C.I.*
otc	**Adapt** (Alcon)	**Solution:** Povidone and other water soluble polymers with 0.004% thimerosal and 0.1% EDTA	In 15 ml.	31
otc	**Blink-N-Clean** (Allergan)	**Solution:** Buffered solution with polyoxyl 40 stearate, PEG 300, 0.5% chlorobutanol	In 7.5 and 15 ml.	42
otc	**Clerz Drops** (Wesley-Jessen)	**Solution:** Hypertonic solution with hydroxyethylcellulose, sorbic acid, poloxamer 407, 0.1% EDTA and 0.001% thimerosal	In 25 ml.	17
otc	**Clerz 2** (Wesley-Jessen)	**Solution:** Isotonic solution with hydroxyethylcellulose, poloxamer 407, NaCl, KCl, sodium borate, boric acid, sorbic acid and EDTA	Thimerosal free. In 5 and 15 ml.	23
otc	**Lens Drops** (Ciba Vision)	**Solution:** Isotonic solution with NaCl, borate buffer, carbamide, poloxamer 407, 0.2% EDTA and 0.15% sorbic acid	In 15 ml.	19
otc	**Lens Fresh Drops** (Allergan)	**Solution:** Hydroxyethylcellulose, NaCl, sodium borate, boric acid, 0.1% sorbic acid and 0.2% EDTA	Thimerosal free. In 15 ml.	25
otc	**Lens Lubricant** (Bausch & Lomb)	**Solution:** Povidone and polyoxyethylene with 0.004% thimerosal and 0.1% EDTA	In 15 ml.	33
otc	**Lens-Wet** (Allergan)	**Solution:** Isotonic, buffered solution of polyvinyl alcohol, 0.002% thimerosal and 0.01% EDTA, dibasic sodium phosphate, monobasic sodium phosphate monohydrate and sodium chloride	In 15 ml.	27
otc	**Murine Sterile Lubricating and Rewetting Drops** (Ross)	**Solution:** Buffered, isotonic solution of hydroxyethylcellulose, NaCl, boric acid and sodium borate with 0.1% sorbic acid and 0.2% EDTA	Thimerosal free. In 15 ml.	22
otc	**Stay-Wet** (Sherman)	**Solution:** Polyvinyl alcohol, hydroxyethylcellulose, povidone, NaCl, KCl, sodium carbonate, 0.01% benzalkonium chloride, 0.025% EDTA	In 30 ml.	12

* Cost Index based on cost per 30 ml cleaning/soaking/wetting solutions, or 1 ml re-wetting solutions.

Refer to the general discussion of these products on page 2238

Hard Contact Lens Products (Cont.)

Cleaning Solutions and Gels

Cleaning solutions and gels contain surfactant cleaners to facilitate removal of oleaginous, proteinaceous and other types of debris from lens surface. To adequately clean, physically rub lens with solution or gel and rinse with water or sterile saline solution.

	Product	Composition	How Supplied	C.I.*
otc	**The Boston Cleaner** (Polymer Tech)	**Solution:** Anionic sulfate surfactant with friction-enhancing agents and NaCl	In 30 ml.	15
otc	**Concentrated Cleaner** (B & L)		In 30 ml.	12
otc	**Clens** (Alcon)	**Solution:** Cleaning agent with 0.02% benzalkonium chloride and 0.1% EDTA	In 60 ml.	10
otc	**LC-65** (Allergan)	**Solution:** Cleaning agent with 0.001% thimerosal and EDTA	In 15 and 60 ml.	22
otc	**Lensine Extra Strength** (Wesley-J)	**Solution:** Cleaning agent with 0.01% benzalkonium chloride and 0.1% EDTA	In 45 ml.	11
otc	**MiraFlow Extra Strength** (Ciba V)	**Solution:** 20% isopropyl alcohol, poloxamer 407 and amphoteric 10	Thimerosal free. In 25 ml.	14
otc	**Opti-Clean** (Alcon)	**Solution:** Polysorbate 21, polymeric cleaning beads, 0.004% thimerosal, 0.1% EDTA	In 12 and 20 ml.	26
otc	**Opti-Clean II** (Alcon)	**Solution:** Isotonic polymeric cleaning agent, hydroxyethylcellulose, polysorbate 21, 0.1% EDTA, 0.01% polyquaternium-1	Thimerosal free. In 12 and 20 ml.	26
otc	**Resolve/GP Daily Cleaner** (Allergan)	**Solution:** A surfactant with cocoamphocarboxyglycinate, sodium lauryl sulfate, hexylene glycol, alkyl ether sulfate	Preservative free. In 30 ml.	N/A
otc	**Sereine** (Optikem)	**Solution:** Surfactants and re-wetting agents, 0.1% EDTA, 0.01% benzalkonium chloride	In 60 ml.	5
otc	**SilaClean** (Professional Supplies)	**Solution:** Cleaning agent with benzalkonium chloride and EDTA	In 60 ml.	3
otc	**SLC** (Ocular)	**Solution:** Cleaning agent with 0.1% sorbic acid and 0.1% EDTA	In 30 ml.	10
otc	**Stay-Brite** (Sherman)	**Solution:** Cleaning agent with 0.25% EDTA and 0.01% benzalkonium chloride	In 30 ml pump spray.	10
otc	**Titan** (Sola/Barnes-Hind)	**Solution:** A surfactant with 2% EDTA and 0.02% benzalkonium chloride	In 30 and 60 ml.	16
otc	**Blairex Hard Lens Cleaner** (Blairex)	**Liquid:** Anionic detergent	In 60 ml.	NA
otc	**d-Film** (Wesley-Jessen)	**Gel:** Poloxamer 407 with 0.25% EDTA and 0.025% benzalkonium chloride	In 25 g.	21
otc	**Gel Clean** (Sola/Barnes-Hind)	**Gel:** Nonionic surfactant with 0.004% thimerosal	In 30 g.	20

Cleaning and Soaking Solutions

	Product	Composition	How Supplied	C.I.*
otc	**Boston Reconditioning Drops** (Polymer Tech)	**Solution:** Hydrophilic polyelectrolyte, polyvinyl alcohol, hydroxyethylcellulose with chlorhexidine gluconate and EDTA.	In 120 ml.	71
otc	**Clean-N-Soak** (Allergan)	**Solution:** Cleaning agent with 0.004% phenylmercuric nitrate	In 120 ml.	116
otc	**de•Stat** (Sherman)	**Solution:** Surfactant cleaner with 0.01% benzalkonium chloride and 0.25% EDTA	In 118 ml.	110
otc	**duo-Flow** (Wesley-Jessen)	**Solution:** Poloxamer 188 with 0.013% benzalkonium chloride and 0.25% EDTA	In 120 ml.	113
otc	**Sereine** (Optikem)	**Solution:** Sterile solution with 0.25% EDTA and 0.01% benzalkonium chloride	In 120 ml.	73
otc	**Visalens Soaking/Cleaning** (Leeming)	**Solution:** Cleaning agents with lauramide DEA, nonoxynol-15, poloxamer 188, NaCl, sodium borate, boric acid, 0.02% benzalkonium chloride and 0.1% EDTA	In 120 ml.	66

* Cost Index based on cost per ml or g cleaning solutions/gels or 30 ml cleaning/soaking solutions.

Refer to the general discussion of these products on page 2238

Rigid Gas Permeable Contact Lens Products

Gas Permeable Hard Lenses: Cellulose acetate butyrate (CAB) and silicon-containing polymers are used in gas (oxygen) permeable hard contact lenses. Lens care regimens include use of a surfactant cleaner and storage in a chemical disinfecting solution. Advise patients to follow the lens care protocol provided by the lens manufacturer. One advantage of the lenses is that they maintain the integrity and metabolism of the cornea, preventing complications. However, they are predisposed to dehydration and accumulating protein and lipid deposits.

Disinfecting/Wetting/Soaking Solutions

	Product	Composition	Supplied	C.I.*
otc	**Gas Permeable Wetting and Soaking** (Sola/Barnes-Hind)	**Solution:** Isotonic. With polyvinyl alcohol, 0.003% chlorhexidine gluconate, 0.002% thimerosal and 0.02% EDTA	In 35, 60 and 120 ml.	5
otc	**Stay-Wet 3** (Sherman)	**Solution:** Sodium and potassium chloride salts containing polyvinyl pyrrolidone, polyvinyl alcohol, hydroxyethyl cellulose, 0.02% sodium bisulfite, 0.1% pure benzyl alcohol, 0.05% sorbic acid, 0.1% trisodium edetate	In 30 ml.	NA
otc	**Wetting and Soaking Solution** (Bausch & Lomb)	**Solution:** Polyvinyl alcohol, hydroxyethyl cellulose with chlorhexidine gluconate and EDTA	In 120 ml.	3
otc	**Wet-N-Soak** (Allergan)	**Solution:** Isotonic, buffered. With polyvinyl alcohol, 0.004% benzalkonium chloride, EDTA	In 120 and 180 ml.	4
otc	**Wet-N-Soak Plus** (Allergan)	**Solution:** Buffered, isotonic. With polyvinyl alcohol, EDTA, 0.003% benzalkonium chloride	In 30 and 120 ml.	4

Cleaning/Soaking Solutions

	Product	Composition	Supplied	C.I.*
otc	**Boston Reconditioning Drops** (Polymer Tech)	**Solution:** Hydrophilic polyelectrolyte, polyvinyl alcohol, hydroxyethylcellulose, chlorhexidine gluconate, EDTA *For use with the Boston Lens*	In 120 ml.	2

Cleaning Solutions

	Product	Composition	Supplied	C.I.*
otc	**The Boston Cleaner** (Polymer Tech)	**Solution:** Anionic sulfate surfactant with friction-enhancing agents and NaCl	In 30 ml.	15
otc	**EasyClean/GP Daily Cleaner** (Allergan)	**Solution:** Cocoamphocarboxyglycinate, sodium lauryl sulfate, sodium chloride, sodium phosphate, hexylene glycol and EDTA	Preservative free. In 30 ml.	13
otc	**Gas Permeable Daily Cleaner** (Sola/Barnes-Hind)	**Solution:** Non-ionic cleaning agents with 0.004% thimerosal and 2% EDTA	In 30 ml.	14
otc	**LC-65 Daily Cleaner** (Allergan)	**Solution:** Cleaning agent with 0.001% thimerosal and EDTA	In 15 and 60 ml.	22
otc	**ProFree/GP Weekly Enzymatic Cleaner** (Allergan)	**Tablets:** Papain, sodium chloride, sodium carbonate, sodium borate and EDTA *To make a solution for soaking when diluted in distilled water*	In 24s.	24
otc	**Resolve/GP Daily Cleaner** (Allergan)	**Solution:** A surfactant with cocoamphocarboxyglycinate, sodium lauryl sulfate, hexylene glycol, alkyl ether sulfate	Preservative free. In 30 ml.	NA

Cleaning/Disinfecting/Storage Solutions

	Product	Composition	Supplied	C.I.*
otc	**de • Stat 3** (Sherman)	**Solution:** Octylphenoxypolyethoxyethanol, 0.1% benzyl alcohol, 0.5% trisodium edetate	In 30 and 118 ml.	4

* Cost Index based on cost per ml or tablet.

Refer to the general discussion of these products on page 2238

Soft (Hydrogel) Contact Lens Products

Soft (hydrogel) contact lenses are made of a hydrophilic polymer, hydroxyethylmethacrylate (HEMA). Hydrogel lenses must be maintained in a hydrated state in physiological saline to prevent them from becoming brittle. Hydrogel lenses will absorb many substances; therefore, use only solutions specifically formulated for hydrogel lenses. In addition, these lenses must be disinfected either by heating or by soaking in a chemical solution. *Heating a lens in solutions used for chemical disinfection may cause the lens to become opaque.*

Soft lens solutions are especially formulated to be compatible with, and to meet the particular needs of, soft (hydrogel) contact lenses. Of particular importance to soft lens care is the need for thorough cleaning to remove mucus deposits which coat and may discolor the lens, especially when subjected to asepticizing by heating.

Warning:
Do NOT use conventional (hard) lens solutions on soft contact lenses. Use caution in product selection. Not all products are intended for use in all types of soft lenses.

Rinsing/Storage Solutions

Use these solutions for rinsing and storage of hydrogel lenses in conjunction with heat disinfection. Prepared saline solutions for soft lenses are alkaline, which helps minimize mucus accumulation; they may contain chelating agents (EDTA) which prevent calcium deposits from forming. Thimerosal free preserved saline solutions may be used by patients sensitive to thimerosal or mercury-containing compounds. Preservative free solutions are for patients intolerant to preservatives. Salt tablets are available to make saline solution; however, these solutions are nonsterile and contain no preservatives; use only with heat disinfection methods.

	Preserved Saline Solutions			C.I.*
otc	**Allergan Hydrocare Preserved Saline** (Allergan)	**Solution:** Isotonic, buffered. With NaCl, sodium hexametaphosphate, sodium hydroxide, boric acid, sodium borate, 0.01% EDTA, 0.001% thimerosal	In 240 and 360 ml.	45
otc	**Boil n Soak** (Alcon)	**Solution:** Isotonic, buffered. With 0.7% sodium chloride, boric acid, sodium borate, 0.001% thimerosal, 0.1% EDTA	In 240 and 360 ml.	41
otc	**Lensrins** (Allergan)	**Solution:** Isotonic, buffered. With NaCl, monobasic monohydrate sodium phosphate, dibasic anhydrous sodium phosphate, sodium hydroxide or hydrochloric acid, 0.001% thimerosal, 0.1% EDTA	In 240 ml.	45
otc	**Opti-Soft** (Alcon)	**Solution:** Isotonic. With NaCl, borate buffer, 0.1% EDTA, 0.001% polyquaternium-1. For lenses with 45% or less water content	Thimerosal free. In 237 and 355 ml.	64
otc	**ReNu Saline** (Bausch & Lomb)	**Solution:** Isotonic, buffered. With NaCl, boric acid, 0.00003% polyaminopropyl biguanide, EDTA	In 237 and 355 ml.	24
otc	**Saline Solution, Sterile Preserved** (Bausch & Lomb)	**Solution:** Boric acid, sodium chloride, 0.001% thimerosal, EDTA	In 120, 240 and 360 ml.	77
otc	**Murine Preserved All-Purpose Saline Solution** (Ross)	**Solution:** Isotonic, buffered. With NaCl, 0.1% sorbic acid, 0.1% EDTA	Thimerosal free. In 60, 237 and 355 ml.	39
otc	**Sensitive Eyes Saline** (Bausch & Lomb)	**Solution:** Sodium chloride, borate buffer, 0.1% sorbic acid, EDTA	Thimerosal free. In 120, 240 and 360 ml.	77
otc	**Soft Mate Saline for Sensitive Eyes** (Sola/Barnes-Hind)	**Solution:** Isotonic. With NaCl, 0.13% potassium sorbate, 0.025% EDTA	In 120, 240 and 360 ml.	40
otc	**Allergan Sorbi-Care Saline** (Allergan)	**Solution:** Isotonic, buffered. With NaCl, sodium hexametaphosphate, sodium borate, boric acid, 0.1% sorbic acid	Thimerosal free. In 240 ml.	47
otc	**Sterile Saline** (Bausch & Lomb)	**Solution:** Sodium chloride, borate buffer, EDTA	Thimerosal free. In 60 ml.	54

* Cost Index based on cost per 30 ml.

Refer to the general discussion of these products on page 2238

Soft (Hydrogel) Contact Lens Products (Cont.)

Rinsing/Storage Solutions (Cont.)

Preservative Free Saline Solutions

	Product	Description	Packaging	C.I.*
otc	**Blairex Sterile Saline** (Blairex)	**Solution:** Isotonic. With 0.9% sodium chloride	In 240 ml aerosol.	33
otc	**Hypo-Clear** (Bausch & Lomb)		In 240 ml.	56
otc	**Lens Plus Preservative Free** (Allergan)		In 90, 240 and 360 ml aerosol.	44
otc	**Ciba Vision Saline** (Ciba Vision)	**Solution:** Buffered, isotonic. With NaCl, boric acid	In 90, 340 and 360 ml aerosol.	30
otc	**Hypo-Clear** (Bausch & Lomb)	**Solution:** Buffered, isotonic. With NaCl, EDTA	In 240 and 360 ml aerosol.	23
otc	**Purisol 4** (Amcon)	**Solution:** Buffered, isotonic. With NaCl, boric acid, sodium borate	In 236 ml.	35
otc	**Unisol** (Wesley-Jessen)	**Solution:** Buffered, isotonic. With sodium chloride, boric acid, sodium borate	In 15 ml.	46
otc	**Unisol 4** (Wesley-Jessen)		In 120 ml.	36
otc	**Soft Mate Saline Preservative-Free** (Sola/Barnes-Hind)	**Solution:** Sodium chloride w/borate buffer	In 15 ml.	83

Salt Tablets for Normal Saline

Reconstitute in container provided with Purified Water, USP. If pharmaceutical grade water is not available, use distilled water. These solutions are not sterile and are only for use with heat disinfection regimens. Not for use in the eye. See Precautions on p. 507.

	Product	Description	Packaging	C.I.*
otc	**Soft Rinse 135** (Professional Supplies)	**Tablets:** 135 mg	In 365s w/15 ml bottle.	2
otc	**Amcon 250** (Amcon)	**Tablets:** 250 mg	In 90s, 180s, 200s.	1
otc	**Easy Eyes** (Eaton Medicals)		In 90s, 180s w/ 27.7 ml bottle.	2
otc	**Marlin Salt System II** (Marlin)		In 200s w/ 27.7 ml bottle.	1
otc	**Soft Rinse 250** (Professional Supplies)		In 200s w/ 27.7 ml bottle.	1

Surfactant Cleaning Solutions

Cleaning solutions are used for daily prophylactic cleaning to prevent the accumulation of proteinaceous (mucus) deposits and to remove other debris.

	Product	Description	Packaging	C.I.*
otc	**Ciba Vision Cleaner** (Ciba Vision)	**Solution:** Cocoamphocarboxyglycinate, sodium lauryl sulfate, hexylene glycol with EDTA 0.2% and sorbic acid 0.1%	In 15 ml.	18
otc	**Daily Cleaner** (Bausch & Lomb)	**Solution:** Isotonic solution with NaCl, sodium phosphate, tyloxapol, hydroxyethylcellulose and polyvinyl alcohol and 0.2% EDTA	With thimerosal. In 45 ml.	7
otc	**Preflex Especially for Sensitive Eyes** (Alcon)		Thimerosal free. In 45 ml.	7
otc	**DURAcare** (Blairex)	**Solution:** Hypertonic w/salt buffers, detergents, 0.004% thimerosal, 0.1% EDTA	In 30 ml.	11
otc	**DURAcare II** (Blairex)	**Solution:** Hypertonic w/salt buffers, block copolymers of ethylene/propylene oxide, octyphenoxypolyethoxyethanol, lauryl sulfate salt of imidazole, sodium bisulfite 0.1%, sorbic acid 0.1%, trisodium EDTA	Thimerosal free. In 30 ml.	12

* Cost Index based on cost per 30 ml saline solution or prepared saline, or ml surfactant cleaning solution.

(Continued on following page)

Soft (Hydrogel) Contact Lens Products (Cont.)

Refer to the general discussion of these products on page 2238

Surfactant Cleaning Solutions (Cont.)

	Product	Description		C.I.*
otc	**LC-65** (Allergan)	**Solution:** Cleaning agent with 0.001% thimerosal and EDTA	In 15 and 60 ml.	22
otc	**Lens Clear** (Allergan)	**Solution:** Isotonic solution of cocoamphocarboxyglycinate, sodium lauryl sulfate, hexylene glycol, 0.1% sorbic acid and 0.2% EDTA	Thimerosal free. In 15 ml.	22
otc	**Lens Plus Daily Cleaner** (Allergan)	**Solution:** Buffered solution with cocoamphocarboxyglycinate, sodium lauryl sulfate, hexylene glycol, NaCl, sodium phosphate and EDTA	Preservative free. In 15 ml.	18
otc	**MiraFlow Extra Strength** (Ciba Vision)	**Solution:** 20% isopropyl alcohol, poloxamer 407 and amphoteric 10	Thimerosal free. In 25 ml.	13
otc	**Murine Contact Lens Cleaner** (Ross)	**Solution:** Buffered, isotonic solution containing poloxamine, borate buffers, NaCl, hydroxypropyl methylcellulose, 0.5% EDTA and 0.25% sorbic acid	Thimerosal free. In 15 and 30 ml.	11
otc	**Opti-Clean II** (Alcon)	**Solution:** Isotonic polymeric cleaning agent, hydroxyethylcellulose, polysorbate 21, 0.1% EDTA, 0.01% polyquaternium-1	Thimerosal free. In 12 and 20 ml.	12
otc	**Pliagel** (Wesley-Jessen)	**Solution:** NaCl, KCl, poloxamer 407, 0.25% sorbic acid and 0.5% EDTA	Thimerosal free. In 25 ml.	14
otc	**Sensitive Eyes Daily Cleaner** (Bausch & Lomb)	**Solution:** Isotonic solution, borate buffer, surfactant cleaner, NaCl, hydroxypropyl methylcellulose, 0.25% sorbic acid, 0.5% EDTA	Thimerosal free. In 30 ml.	10
otc	**Sensitive Eyes Saline/Cleaning Solution** (Bausch & Lomb)	**Solution:** Isotonic solution with borate buffer, NaCl, surfactant with sorbic acid and EDTA	In 240 ml.	1
otc	**Sof/Pro-Clean** (Sherman)	**Solution:** Buffered hypertonic solution with salt, detergents, 0.004% thimerosal and 0.1% EDTA	In 30 ml.	10
otc	**Sof/Pro-Clean (s.a.)** (Sherman)	**Solution:** Hypertonic solution of salt buffers, copolymers of ethylene and propylene oxide, octylphenoxypolyethoxyethanol, lauryl sulfate salt of imidazoline, 0.1% sodium bisulfite, 0.1% sorbic acid and 0.25% trisodium EDTA	Thimerosal free. In 30 ml.	12
otc	**Soft Mate Hands Off Daily Cleaner** (Sola/Barnes-Hind)	**Solution:** Isotonic solution with NaCl, octylphenoxy (oxyethylene) ethanol, hydroxyethylcellulose, 0.13% potassium sorbate and 0.2% EDTA. *For use with Hydra-Mat II cleaning system*	In 15 and 240 ml.	2
otc	**Soft Mate Protein Remover** (Sola/Barnes-Hind)	**Solution:** Sterile solution with alkyl carboxylic acid amine condensate, alkyl imidazoline dicarboxylate, polyoxyalkylene dimethylpolysiloxane, EDTA and borate buffers	Preservative free. In 8 ml bottles of 4s, 8s and 12s.	5
otc	**Soft Mate Daily Cleaning For Sensitive Eyes** (Sola/Barnes-Hind)	**Solution:** Isotonic solution with NaCl, octylphenoxy (oxyethylene) ethanol and hydroxyethylcellulose with 0.13% potassium sorbate and 0.2% EDTA	In 1 and 30 ml.	12

* Cost Index based on cost per ml.

Soft (Hydrogel) Contact Lens Products (Cont.)

Refer to the general discussion of these products on page 2238

Enzymatic Cleaners

Enzymatic cleaning is recommended once weekly to remove protein.

				C.I.*
otc	**Allergan Enzymatic** (Allergan)	**Tablets:** Papain, sodium chloride, sodium carbonate, sodium borate and EDTA. *To make solution for soaking when diluted in distilled water*	In 12s, 24s, 36s and 48s.	43
otc	**Extenzyme Protein Cleaner** (Allergan)		In 24s and 36s.	30
otc	**Opti-zyme Enzymatic Cleaner** (Alcon)	**Tablets:** Pork pancreatin. *For soaking when diluted in preserved saline solution*	In 4s, 8s, 24s, 36s and 56s.	44
otc	**ReNu Effervescent Enzymatic Cleaner** (Bausch & Lomb)	**Tablets:** Subtilisin, polyethylene glycol, sodium carbonate, sodium chloride and tartaric acid. *To make solution for soaking when diluted in preserved saline or sterile unpreserved saline solution*	In 10s and 20s.	31
otc	**ReNu Thermal Enzymatic Cleaner** (Bausch & Lomb)	**Tablets:** Subtilisin, sodium carbonate, sodium chloride and boric acid. *To make solution for heat disinfection directly in lens carrying case*	In 8s and 16s.	40
otc	**Soft Mate Enzyme Plus Cleaner** (Sola/Barnes-Hind)	**Tablets:** Subtilisin, poloxamer 338, povidone, citric acid, potassium bicarbonate, sodium carbonate and sodium benzoate. *To make solution for soaking when diluted in sterile saline*	In 4s.	NA
otc	**Ultrazyme Enzymatic Cleaner** (Allergan)	**Tablets:** Subtilisin A, effervescing, buffering and tableting agents. *For soaking, dilute in 3% hydrogen peroxide*	In 5s and 10s.	56

Re-Wetting Solutions

May be used directly in the eye to rehydrate and improve comfort of hydrogel lenses.

				C.I.*
otc	**Adapettes For Sensitive Eyes** (Alcon)	**Solution:** Isotonic. With povidone and other water-soluble polymers, 0.004% thimerosal and 0.1% EDTA	In 15 ml.	27
otc	**Clerz Drops** (Wesley-Jessen)	**Solution:** Hypertonic. With hydroxyethylcellulose, sodium borate, poloxamer 407, sorbic acid, 0.001% thimerosal, 0.1% EDTA	In 25 ml.	23
otc	**Clerz 2** (Wesley-Jessen)	**Solution:** Isotonic. With sodium chloride, potassium chloride, hydroxyethylcellulose, poloxamer 407, sodium borate, boric acid, sorbic acid and EDTA	Thimerosal free. In 5 and 15 ml.	23
otc	**Comfort Tears** (Sola/Barnes-Hind)	**Solution:** Isotonic w/hydroxyethylcellulose, 0.005% benzalkonium Cl and 0.02% EDTA	In 15 ml.	25
otc	**Lens Drops** (Ciba Vision)	**Solution:** Isotonic. With sodium chloride, borate buffer, carbamide, poloxamer 407, 0.2% EDTA, 0.15% sorbic acid	In 15 ml.	19
otc	**Lens Fresh** (Allergan)	**Solution:** Isotonic. With hydroxyethylcellulose, boric acid, sodium borate, sodium chloride, 0.1% sorbic acid, 0.2% EDTA	Thimerosal free. In 15 ml.	25
otc	**Lens Lubricant** (Bausch & Lomb)	**Solution:** Povidone and polyoxyethylene with 0.004% thimerosal and 0.1% EDTA	In 15 ml.	33
otc	**Lens Plus Rewetting Drops** (Allergan)	**Solution:** Isotonic solution with sodium chloride and boric acid	Thimerosal and preservative free. In 0.3 ml (30s).	38
otc	**Lens-Wet** (Allergan)	**Solution:** Buffered, isotonic. With polyvinyl alcohol, 0.002% thimerosal, 0.01% EDTA, dibasic and monobasic sodium phosphates, sodium chloride	In 15 ml.	27

* Cost Index based on cost per tablet or ml.

(Continued on following page)

Soft (Hydrogel) Contact Lens Products (Cont.)

Refer to the general discussion of these products on page 2238

Re-Wetting Solutions (Cont.)

	Product	Composition		C.I.*
otc	**Murine Sterile Lubricating and Rewetting Drops** (Ross)	**Solution:** Buffered, isotonic. With hydroxyethylcellulose, NaCl, boric acid, sodium borate, 0.1% sorbic acid, 0.2% EDTA	Thimerosal free. In 15 ml.	23
otc	**Opti-Tears** (Alcon)	**Solution:** Isotonic. With dextran, NaCl, potassium Cl, hydroxypropyl methylcellulose, 0.1% EDTA, 0.01% polyquaternium-1	Thimerosal free. In 15 ml.	25
otc	**Sensitive Eyes Drops** (Bausch & Lomb)	**Solution:** Isotonic. With a borate buffer system, 0.1% sorbic acid, EDTA	In 30 and 60 ml.	10
otc	**Soft Mate Comfort Drops** (Sola/Barnes-Hind)	**Solution:** Isotonic, buffered. With 0.004% thimerosal, 0.1% EDTA	In 15 ml dropper bottle.	25
otc	**Soft Mate Comfort Drops for Sensitive Eyes** (Sola/Barnes-Hind)	**Solution:** Borate buffered. With 0.13% potassium sorbate, 0.1% EDTA	In 15 ml dropper bottle.	29
otc	**Soft Mate Lens Drops** (Sola/Barnes-Hind)	**Solution:** Isotonic. With sodium chloride, 0.13% potassium sorbate, 0.025% EDTA	Thimerosal free. In 60 ml.	5
otc	**Sterile Lens Lubricant** (Blairex)	**Solution:** Isotonic. With borate buffer system, sodium chloride, hydroxypropyl methylcellulose, glycerin, 0.25% sorbic acid, 0.1% EDTA	Thimerosal free. In 15 ml.	19

Chemical Disinfection Systems

Chemical disinfection is an alternative to heat. Two-solution systems use separate disinfecting and rinsing solutions. One-solution systems use the same solution for rinsing and storage.

Warning: Lenses must not be disinfected by heating when using these solutions.

	Product	Composition		C.I.*
otc	**Allergan Hydrocare Cleaning and Disinfecting** (Allergan)	**Solution:** 0.013% tris (2-hydroxyethyl) tallow ammonium Cl; 0.002% thimerosal; bis (2-hydroxyethyl) tallow ammonium Cl; sodium bicarbonate; dibasic, monobasic & anhydrous sodium phosphate; hydrochloric acid; propylene glycol; polysorbate 80; special soluble polyhema	In 120, 240 and 360 ml.	49
otc	**Aosept** (Ciba Vision)	**Solution:** 3% hydrogen peroxide, 0.85% sodium chloride, sodium stannate, sodium nitrate and phosphate buffer	Thimerosal free. In 120, 237 & 355 ml.	125
otc	**Disinfecting Solution** (Bausch & Lomb)	**Solution:** NaCl, sodium borate, boric acid, 0.005% chlorhexidine gluconate, 0.1% EDTA, 0.001% thimerosal	In 237 and 355 ml.	62
otc	**Flex-Care** (Alcon)		In 120, 237, 355 ml.	51
otc	**Lens Plus Oxysept System** (Allergan)	**Disinfecting Solution:** 3% hydrogen peroxide with sodium stannate, sodium nitrate and phosphate buffer	Preservative free. In 240 ml.	39
		Rinse and Neutralizer: Isotonic, with NaCl, mono- and dibasic sodium phosphates, catalytic neutralizing agent, EDTA	In 15 ml. Includes lens case.	27
otc	**Lens Plus Oxysept 2 Neutralizing** (Allergan)	**Tablets:** Catalase with buffering agents. *Used to neutralize the Lens Plus Oxysept disinfecting solution*	In 12s (with Oxytab cup) and 36s.	N/A
otc	**Lensept** (Ciba Vision)	**Disinfecting Solution:** 3% micro-filtered hydrogen peroxide w/sodium stannate, sodium nitrate, phosphate buffers	In 237 and 355 ml.	38
		Rinse and Neutralizer: Buffered, isotonic. With NaCl, sodium borate decahydrate, boric acid, bovine catalase, sorbic acid, EDTA	In 237 ml. System includes lens cup and holder.	44

* Cost Index based on cost per ml re-wetting solution or per 30 ml chemical disinfection system.

(Continued on following page)

Soft (Hydrogel) Contact Lens Products (Cont.)

	Chemical Disinfection Systems (Cont.)			C.I.*
otc	**MiraSept System** (Wesley-Jessen)	**Disinfecting Solution:** 3% hydrogen peroxide with sodium stannate and sodium nitrate	Thimerosal free. In 30 and 120 ml.	113
		Rinsing and Neutralizing Solution: Isotonic solution, boric acid, sodium borate, sorbic acid, sodium pyruvate & EDTA	Thimerosal free. Includes lens case. In 20 ml.	413
otc	**Opti-Free** (Alcon)	**Solution:** Citrate buffer, NaCl, 0.05% EDTA, 0.001% polyquaternium-1	In 240 ml.	55
otc	**Pure Sept** (Ross)	**Disinfecting Solution:** Sterile hydrogen peroxide 3% solution, sodium stannate, sodium nitrate and phosphate buffers	Thimerosal free. In 237 ml.	46
		Murine Saline Solution: Buffered, isotonic solution with borate buffers, NaCl, 0.1% sorbic acid and 0.1% EDTA	In 60, 237 and 355 ml. Includes cups and lens holder.	39
otc	**Quik-Sept System** (Bausch & Lomb)	**Disinfecting Solution:** 3% hydrogen peroxide with sodium stannate, sodium nitrate and phosphate buffers	Thimerosal free. In 240 ml w/lens cup	46
		Sensitive Eyes Saline Solution: Isotonic NaCl w/borate buffer, 0.1% sorbic acid, EDTA	In 118, 237 and 355 ml.	77
		Sensitive Eyes Saline/Cleaning Solution: Isotonic solution of NaCl, borate buffer, surfactant, sorbic acid, EDTA	In 240 ml.	1
otc	**ReNu Multi-Action** (Bausch & Lomb)	**Disinfecting Solution:** Isotonic w/NaCl, sodium borate, boric acid, poloxamine, 0.00005% polyaminopropyl biguanide, EDTA. *For disinfection, rinsing, storage*	In 237 and 355 ml.	41
otc	**Soft Mate** (Sola/Barnes-Hind)	**Disinfecting Solution:** Sodium chloride, povidone, octylphenoxy (oxyethylene) ethanol, 0.1% EDTA and 0.005% chlorhexidine gluconate	Thimerosal free. In 240 and 360 ml.	52
otc	**Soft Mate Consept** (Sola/Barnes-Hind)	**Consept 1 Cleaning and Disinfecting Solution:** 3% hydrogen peroxide with polyoxyl 40 stearate, sodium stannate, sodium nitrate and phosphate buffer	Thimerosal free. In 240 ml	50
		Consept 2 Neutralizing and Rinsing Spray: Isotonic solution of 0.5% sodium thiosulfate, NaCl and borate buffers	In 240 ml. System includes lens case.	41

* Cost Index based on cost per 30 ml.

Local Anesthetics

Actions:

Pharmacology: Local anesthetics stabilize the neuronal membrane so that the neuron is less permeable to ions. This prevents the initiation and transmission of nerve impulses, thereby producing the local anesthetic action.

Studies indicate that they may limit sodium ion permeability by closing the pores through which the ions migrate in the lipid layer of the nerve cell membrane. This limitation prevents the fundamental change necessary for the generation of the action potential.

Pharmacokinetics: Tetracaine and proparacaine are approximately equally potent. They have a rapid onset of analgesia beginning within 15 to 20 seconds following instillation; the duration of action is 15 to 20 minutes.

Indications:

Corneal anesthesia of short duration (eg, tonometry, gonioscopy, removal of corneal foreign bodies and sutures); short corneal and conjunctival procedures; cataract surgery; conjunctival and corneal scraping for diagnostic purposes; paracentesis of the anterior chamber.

Contraindications:

Known hypersensitivity to similar drugs (ester-type local anesthetics), para-aminobenzoic acid or its derivatives or to any other ingredient in these preparations.

Prolonged use, especially for self-medication, is not recommended.

Warnings:

For topical ophthalmic use only. Prolonged use is not recommended; it may diminish duration of anesthesia, retard wound healing and cause corneal epithelial erosions. It may produce permanent corneal opacification with accompanying visual loss, severe keratitis, scarring or corneal perforation. If signs of sensitivity develop, discontinue use.

Systemic toxicity is rare with ophthalmic application of local anesthetics. It usually occurs as CNS stimulation followed by CNS and cardiovascular depression.

Pregnancy and Lactation: Pregnancy Category C. Safety for use during pregnancy and lactation has not been established. Use only when clearly needed and when potential benefits outweigh potential hazards to the fetus or nursing infant.

Children: Safety and efficacy of tetracaine have not been established.

Precautions:

Tolerance varies with the status of the patient; give debilitated, elderly or acutely ill patients reduced doses commensurate with their weight, age and physical status.

Use caution in patients with abnormal or reduced levels of plasma esterases.

Use cautiously and sparingly in patients with known allergies, cardiac disease or hyperthyroidism.

Protection of the eye from irritating chemicals, foreign bodies and rubbing during the period of anesthesia is important. Because the "blink" reflex is temporarily eliminated, cover eye with patch following these procedures.

Adverse Reactions:

Occasional temporary stinging, burning, lacrimation, photophobia, chemosis and conjunctival redness have been reported. Corneal epithelial erosions, retardation or prevention of healing of corneal erosions, severe keratitis, permanent corneal opacification and scarring have also been reported with prolonged use.

Proparacaine: Conjunctival congestion; softening and erosion of the corneal epithelium; diffuse stromal edema. Rarely, a severe, immediate, apparently hyperallergenic corneal reaction may occur with acute, intense and diffuse epithelial keratitis; a gray, ground glass appearance; sloughing of large areas of necrotic epithelium; corneal filaments; and sometimes, iritis.

Tetracaine: Transient stinging of the eye with use of concentrations $> 0.5\%$; systemic toxicity, usually manifest as CNS stimulation followed by CNS and cardiovascular depression.

(Continued on following page)

Local Anesthetics (Cont.)

Patient Information:

May retard wound healing; use sparingly and only as directed.

Avoid touching or rubbing the eye until the anesthesia has worn off because inadvertent damage may be done to the anesthetized cornea and conjunctiva.

Do not use if discolored; protect from light.

Refer to page 2164 for more complete information.

TETRACAINE

Administration and Dosage:

Solution: Instill 1 or 2 drops.

Ointment: Apply 0.5 to 1 inch to lower conjunctival fornix. Not for prolonged use.

	Product	Form	How Supplied	C.I.*
Rx	**Tetracaine** (Various, eg, Alcon, Iolab, Optopic, Pharmafair, Raway, Rugby, Schein)	**Solution:** 0.5% (as HCl)	In 1, 2 and 15 ml.	10+
Rx	**Pontocaine HCl** (Winthrop Pharm.)		In 15 ml Mono-drop and 59 ml.[1]	47
Rx	**Pontocaine Eye** (Winthrop Pharm.)	**Ointment:** 0.5% (as base)	In white petrolatum and light mineral oil. In 3.75 g.	144

PROPARACAINE HCl

Administration and Dosage:

Deep anesthesia: 1 drop every 5 to 10 minutes for 5 to 7 doses.

Removal of sutures: Instill 1 or 2 drops 2 or 3 minutes before removal of sutures.

Removal of foreign bodies: Instill 1 or 2 drops prior to operating.

Tonometry: Instill 1 or 2 drops immediately before measurement.

	Product	Form	How Supplied	C.I.*
Rx	**Proparacaine HCl** (Various, eg, Alcon, Iolab, Moore, Pharmafair, Raway, Rugby, Schein)	**Solution:** 0.5%	In 2 and 15 ml.	15+
Rx	**AK-Taine** (Akorn)		In 2 & 15 ml dropper bottles.[2]	30
Rx	**Alcaine** (Alcon)		In 15 ml Drop-Tainers.[3]	48
Rx	**I-Paracaine** (Americal)		In 15 ml.[3]	17
Rx	**Kainair** (Various, eg, Pharmafair, Texas Drug)		In 2 & 15 ml dropper bottles.[3]	24
Rx	**Ophthaine** (Apothecon)		In 15 ml dropper bottles.[2,4]	73
Rx	**Ophthetic** (Allergan)		In 15 ml dropper bottles.[3,4]	49

MISCELLANEOUS COMBINATIONS

Indications:

For procedures in which a topical ophthalmic anesthetic agent in conjunction with a disclosing agent is indicated: Corneal anesthesia of short duration (eg, tonometry, gonioscopy, removal of corneal foreign bodies); short corneal and conjunctival procedures.

Administration and Dosage:

Removal of foreign bodies, sutures and for tonometry: 1 to 2 drops (in single instillations) in each eye before operating.

Deep ophthalmic anesthesia: Proparacaine/fluorescein – 1 drop in each eye every 5 to 10 minutes for 5 to 7 doses. *Benoxinate/fluorescein* – Instill 2 drops into each eye at 90 second intervals for 3 instillations using the 0.4% benoxinate HCl solution.

	Product	Form	How Supplied	C.I.*
Rx	**Fluoracaine** (Akorn)	**Solution:** 0.5% proparacaine HCl and 0.25% fluorescein sodium	In 2 and 5 ml dropper bottles.[5]	135
Rx	**I-Parescein** (Americal)		In 5 ml.[4,5]	71
Rx	**Fluress** (Sola/Barnes-Hind)	**Solution:** 0.4% benoxinate HCl and 0.25% fluorescein sodium	In 5 ml[6] with dropper.	153

* Cost Index based on cost per ml or gram.
[1] With 0.4% chlorobutanol.
[2] With glycerin, chlorobutanol and benzalkonium Cl.
[3] With glycerin and benzalkonium Cl.
[4] Refrigerate.
[5] With glycerin, povidone and 0.01% thimerosal.
[6] With povidone and 1% chlorobutanol.

Diagnostic Products

In addition to the products listed below, the ophthalmic vasoconstrictors, cycloplegic mydriatics and topical local anesthetics are used in diagnostic procedures (see group monographs).

Vasoconstrictors/Mydriatics with α-sympathomimetic activity cause dilation of the pupil and are used to facilitate ophthalmoscopic examination and other diagnostic procedures.

Cycloplegic Mydriatics (anticholinergics) cause both a dilation of the pupil and paralysis of accommodation. These agents are used to facilitate refraction.

Local Anesthetics: Used to facilitate gonioscopy, tonometry and other procedures.

FLUORESCEIN SODIUM

Actions:

Sodium fluorescein, a yellow water-soluble dibasic acid xanthine dye, produces an intense green fluorescent color in alkaline (> pH 5) solution. Fluorescein demonstrates defects of corneal epithelium. It does not stain tissues, but is a useful indicator dye. Normal precorneal tear film will appear yellow or orange. The intact corneal epithelium resists fluorescein penetration and is not colored. Any break in the epithelial barrier permits rapid penetration. Whether resulting from trauma, infection or other causes, epithelial corneal defects appear bright green and are easily visualized. If epithelial loss is extensive, topical fluorescein penetrates into the aqueous and is readily visible biomicroscopically as a green flare.

Indications:

Topical: In fitting hard contact lenses; in applanation tonometry; diagnosis and detection of corneal stippling, abrasions, ulcerations, herpetic lesions, foreign bodies (not epithelialized), contact lens pressure points, wound leaks; making lacrimal drainage test; ascertaining postoperative sclerocorneal wound closure in delayed anterior chamber reformation.

Injection: Diagnostic aid in ophthalmic angiography, including examination of the fundus; evaluation of the iris vasculature; distinction between viable and nonviable tissue; observation of the aqueous flow; differential diagnosis of malignant and nonmalignant tumors; determination of circulation time and adequacy.

Unlabeled Use: Oral use as a diagnostic aid in detecting certain retinal vascular diseases.

Contraindications:

Hypersensitivity to fluorescein or any other component of the product. Do not use with hydrogel (soft) contact lenses; lenses may become discolored.

Warnings:

Exercise caution in administering to patients with a history of hypersensitivity, allergies or asthma. If signs of sensitivity develop, discontinue use.

Avoid extravasation during injection. The high pH can result in severe local tissue damage. Complications have occurred from extravasation: Sloughing of skin, superficial phlebitis, SC granuloma and toxic neuritis along the median curve in the antecubital area. Extravasation can cause severe pain in the arm for several hours. When significant extravasation occurs, discontinue injection and use conservative measures to treat damaged tissue and relieve pain.

Pregnancy: (Category C – topical). Avoid parenteral fluorescein angiography in pregnancy, especially in first trimester. There are no reports of fetal complications during pregnancy.

Lactation: Safety for use in the nursing mother has not been established.

Children: Safety and efficacy for use in children have not been established.

Adverse Reactions:

Injection: Nausea, headache, GI distress, vomiting, syncope, hypotension and other symptoms and signs of hypersensitivity; cardiac arrest; basilar artery ischemia; thrombophlebitis at injection site; severe shock; convulsions; death (rare); temporary yellowish skin discoloration. Occasionally, hives, itching, bronchospasm, anaphylaxis, pyrexia, transient dyspnea, urticaria, pruritus, angioneurotic edema and slight dizziness may occur. A strong taste may develop following high dosage. Urine becomes bright yellow. Skin discoloration fades in 6 to 12 hours, urine fluorescence in 24 to 36 hours. Extravasation at injection site causes intense pain at the site and dull aching in the injected arm.

Administration and Dosage:

Topical: To detect foreign bodies and corneal abrasions, instill 1 or 2 drops of 2% solution; allow a few seconds for staining. Wash out excess with sterile irrigating solution.

Strips – Moisten strip with sterile water or irrigating solution. Touch conjunctiva or fornix as required with moistened tip. Have patient blink several times after application.

Injection: To avoid serious allergic reactions, perform intradermal skin test before use. In 9 to 30 sec, luminescence can be seen in retinal and choroidal vessels.

Adults – 500 to 750 mg injected rapidly into the antecubital vein.

Children – 3.5 mg/lb (7.5 mg/kg) injected rapidly into the antecubital vein.

Have epinephrine 1:1000, an antihistamine and oxygen available.

(Products listed on following page)

Refer to the general discussion of these products on page 2253

Diagnostic Products (Cont.)

FLUORESCEIN SODIUM (Cont.)

	Product	Form	Packaging	C.I.
Rx	**AK-Fluor** (Akorn)	**Injection:** 10%	In 5 ml amps.	75
Rx	**Fluorescite** (Alcon)		In 5 ml amps and 5 ml in 10 ml disp. syringe.	131
Rx	**Funduscein-10** (Iolab)		In 5 ml amps.	147
Rx	**I-Rescein** (Americal)		In 5 ml amps.	113
Rx	**AK-Fluor** (Akorn)	**Injection:** 25%	In 2 ml amps and vials.	188
Rx	**Fluorescite** (Alcon)		In 2 ml amps.	391
Rx	**Funduscein-25** (Iolab)		In 3 ml amps.	288
Rx	**I-Rescein** (Americal)		In 2 ml amps.	113
Rx	**Fluorescein** (Various, eg, Alcon, Iolab)	**Solution:** 2%	In 1, 2 and 15 ml.	46+
Rx	**Ful-Glo** (Sola/Barnes-Hind)	**Strips:** 0.6 mg	In 300s.	143
Rx	**Fluorets** (Akorn)	**Strips:** 1 mg	In 100s.	165
Rx	**Fluor-I-Strip-A.T.** (Wyeth-Ayerst)		In 300s.[1]	170
Rx	**Fluor-I-Strip** (Wyeth-Ayerst)	**Strips:** 9 mg	In 300s.[1]	171

FLUOREXON

Indications: A large molecule of fluorescein for use as a diagnostic and fitting aid for patients with hydrogel (soft) contact lenses. Use in eye, with or without lens in place, when fluorescein is contraindicated, to avoid staining lenses.

Warnings: When used with lenses with > 55% hydration, some color may remain on lens. Remove by washing lens repeatedly; rinse with saline or water.

With highly hydrated lenses, the amount of coloring picked up will vary with exposure. Avoid unnecessary delays in examination procedure.

Precautions: Do not use hydrogen peroxide solutions to clean or sterilize lenses until all traces of fluorexon are removed because fluorexon molecules may bind to the lens.

Administration and Dosage:

Place 1 drop on the concave surface of the lens and place the lens immediately on the eye. Alternately place 1 or 2 drops in the lower cul-de-sac and have the patient blink several times. Additional drops may be necessary during a prolonged examination. Rinse both the eye and the lens with saline following examination.

	Product	Form	Packaging	C.I.*
Rx	**Fluoresoft** (Holles[2])	**Solution:** 0.35%	In 0.5 ml Pipettes (12s).	181

ROSE BENGAL

Actions: Stains dead or degenerated epithelial cells of the cornea and conjunctiva including the nuclei and cell walls. It will also stain the mucus of the precorneal tear film.

Indications: A diagnostic agent for routine ocular examinations or when superficial corneal or conjunctival tissue change is suspected. Effective aid for diagnosis of keratitis, keratoconjunctivitis sicca, corrosions or abrasions, and for the detection of foreign bodies.

Contraindications: Hypersensitivity to rose bengal.

Precautions: The solution may be irritating. Prior to instillation, anesthetize the eye.

Administration and Dosage:

Solution: Instill 1 or 2 drops into the conjunctival sac before examination.

Strips: Thoroughly saturate tip of strip with sterile irrigating solution; remove excess before application. Touch conjunctiva or lower fornix with moistened strip. The patient should blink several times after application.

	Product	Form	Packaging	C.I.*
Rx	**Rose Bengal 1%** (Akorn)	**Solution:** 1% w/povidone, sodium borate, PEG p-isooctylphenol 10, 0.01% thimerosal	In 5 ml dropper bottle.	150
Rx	**Rose Bengal** (Americal)		In 5 ml dropper bottle.	74
Rx	**Rose Bengal** (Sola/Barnes-Hind)	**Strips:** 1.3 mg per strip	In 100s.	253
Rx	**Rosets** (Smith & Nephew)		In 100s.	N/A

* Cost Index based on cost per ml or 20 strips.
[1] With boric acid, polysorbate 80, 0.5% chlorobutanol.
[2] Holles Labs., Inc., Cohasset, MA 02025, 617/383-0741.

Miscellaneous Preparations

SODIUM HYALURONATE

Actions: Sodium hyaluronate is widely distributed in extracellular matrix of connective tissues. It is found in synovial fluid, skin, umbilical cord and vitreous and aqueous humor of the eye.

This preparation is a specific fraction of sodium hyaluronate developed for use in anterior segment and vitreous procedures as a viscoelastic agent. It has high molecular weight, is nonantigenic, does not cause inflammatory or foreign body reactions and has a high viscosity. The 1% solution is transparent and remains in the anterior chamber for $<$ 6 days. It protects corneal endothelial cells and other ocular structures. It does not interfere with epithelialization and normal wound healing.

In surgical procedures in the anterior segment of the eye, instillation maintains a deep anterior chamber during surgery, allowing for more efficient manipulation with less trauma to the corneal endothelium and surrounding tissues. Its viscoelasticity helps push back the vitreous face and prevent formation of a postoperative flat chamber.

Indications: As a surgical aid in various anterior segment procedures, ie, intracapsular and extracapsular cataract surgery, intraocular lens (IOL) implantation, corneal transplant and glaucoma surgery; vitreous replacement after retinal attachment surgery.

In posterior segment surgery, the drug serves as a surgical aid to gently separate, maneuver and hold tissues. It also creates a clear field of vision, thereby facilitating photocoagulation and intra- and postoperative inspection of the retina.

Unlabeled Use: Has been used in the treatment of refractory dry eye syndrome.

Precautions: *Postoperative intraocular pressure* (IOP) may be elevated as a result of preexisting glaucoma and by operative procedures and sequelae, including enzymatic zonulysis, absence of an iridectomy, trauma to filtration structures and by blood and lenticular remnants in the anterior chamber. Since the exact role of these factors is difficult to predict in any individual case, the following precautions are recommended:

Do not overfill the anterior chamber; remove some of the preparation by irrigation or aspiration at the close of surgery (except in glaucoma surgery).

Carefully monitor IOP, especially during the immediate postoperative period. Treat significant increases appropriately. Avoid trapping air bubbles behind the drug.

In posterior segment surgery, IOP rises have been reported, especially in aphakic diabetics, after injection of large amounts of the drug.

Hypersensitivity: Because this preparation is extracted from avian tissues and contains minute amounts of protein, potential risks of hypersensitivity may exist.

Adverse Reactions:

Although well tolerated, a transient postoperative increase of IOP has been reported.

Causal relationship not established: Postoperative inflammatory reactions (iritis, hypopyon); corneal edema; corneal decompensation.

Administration and Dosage:

Cataract surgery - IOL implantation: Slowly introduce a sufficient amount (using cannula or needle) into anterior chamber. Inject either before or after delivery of lens. Injection before lens delivery protects corneal endothelium from possible damage from removal of the cataractous lens. May use to coat surgical instruments and the IOL prior to insertion. May inject additional amounts during surgery to replace any of the drug lost.

Glaucoma filtration surgery: In conjunction with the performance of the trabeculectomy, inject slowly and carefully through a corneal paracentesis to reconstitute the anterior chamber. Further injection can be continued to allow it to extrude into the subconjunctival filtration site through and around the sutured outer scleral flap.

Corneal transplant surgery: After removal of the corneal button, fill the anterior chamber with the drug. Then, suture the donor graft in place. An additional amount may be injected to replace the lost amount as a result of surgical manipulation.

Sodium hyaluronate has also been used in the anterior chamber of the donor eye prior to trepanation to protect the corneal endothelial cells of the graft.

Retinal attachment surgery: Slowly introduce into the vitreous cavity. May direct the injection to separate membranes from retina for safe excision and release of traction. Also serves to maneuver tissues into desired position, eg, to gently push back a detached retina or unroll a retinal flap; aids in holding retina against the sclera for reattachment.

Storage: Store at 2° to 8°C. Do not freeze. Use the drug at room temperature.

Rx	**Amvisc** (Iolab)	**Injection:** 10 mg per ml	In 0.25, 0.5, 0.8 or 4 ml disp. syringe.
Rx	**Healon** (Pharmacia)		In 0.4, 0.75 or 2 ml disp. syringe.
Rx	**Amvisc Plus** (Iolab)	**Injection:** 16 mg per ml	In 0.25, 0.5 or 8 ml disp. syringe.
Rx	**Vitrax** (Edward Weck)	**Injection:** 30 mg per ml	In 0.5 or 0.8 ml disp. syringe with cannula.

Miscellaneous Preparations (Cont.)

ZINC SULFATE SOLUTION

Indications:
A mild astringent for temporary relief of minor eye irritation.

Warnings:
If irritation persists or increases, discontinue use and consult physician.

Administration and Dosage:
Instill 2 drops into eye(s) 2 or 3 times daily.

				C.I.*
otc	**Eye-Sed Ophthalmic** (Scherer)	**Solution:** 0.217%	With 2.17% boric acid and 0.01% benzalkonium chloride. In 15 ml.	17

ROSE PETAL AQUEOUS INFUSION

Indications:
Provides relief from minor eye irritation.

Warnings:
If irritation persists or increases, discontinue use and consult physician.

Administration and Dosage:
Mild irritations: Instill 1 drop into each eye as needed.

				C.I.*
otc	**Estivin Ophthalmic** (Alcon)	**Solution:** Aqueous infusion of rose petals	With 0.01% thimerosal. In 7.5 ml w/ dropper.	71

BORIC ACID

Indications:
For the treatment of irritated and inflamed eyelids.

Warnings:
If irritation persists or increases, discontinue use and consult physician.

Administration and Dosage:
Apply a small quantity to the inner surface of the lower eyelid 1 or 2 times daily, or as directed.

				C.I.*
otc	**Boric Acid Ophthalmic** (Various, eg, Balan, Lilly, Major, Moore, Pharmaderm, Pharmafair, Raway, Rugby, Schein)	**Ointment:** 5%	In 3.5, 3.75, 30, 60 and 480 g.	26+
otc	**Boric Acid Ophthalmic** (Various, eg, Ambix, Dixon-Shane, Lilly, Moore, URL)	**Ointment:** 10%	In 3.5, 3.75, 30, 60 and 480 g.	60+

CHONDROITIN SULFATE and SODIUM HYALURONATE

Indications:
A surgical aid in anterior segment procedures including cataract extraction and intraocular lens implantation.

Administration and Dosage:
Carefully introduce (using a needle or cannula) into the anterior chamber after thoroughly cleaning the chamber with a balanced salt solution. May inject prior to or following delivery of the crystalline lens. Instillation prior to lens delivery provides additional protection to corneal endothelium, protecting it from possible damage arising from surgical instrumentation. May also be used to coat intraocular lens and tips of surgical instruments prior to implantation surgery. May inject additional solution during anterior segment surgery to fully maintain the chamber or to replace solution lost during surgery. At the end of surgery, remove solution by thoroughly irrigating with a balanced salt solution containing sodium citrate.

Rx	**Viscoat** (Alcon Surgical)	**Solution:** 40 mg sodium chondroitin, 30 mg sodium hyaluronate, 0.45 mg sodium dihydrogen phosphate hydrate, 2.65 mg disodium hydrogen phosphate, 4.3 mg sodium chloride.	In 0.25 or 0.5 ml.

* Cost Index based on cost per g or ml.

HYDROXYPROPYL METHYLCELLULOSE

Indications:

2% Solution: An ophthalmic surgical aid in anterior segment surgical procedures including cataract extraction and intraocular lens implantation.

2.5% Solution: For professional use in gonioscopic examinations.

Administration and Dosage:

Anterior segment surgery: Carefully introduce into the anterior chamber using a 20 gauge or larger cannula. The 2% solution may be injected into the chamber prior to or following delivery of the crystalline lens. Injection of 2% solution prior to lens delivery will provide additional protection to the corneal endothelium and other ocular tissues.

The 2% solution may also be used to coat an intraocular lens and tips of surgical instruments prior to implantation surgery. May inject during anterior segment surgery to fully maintain the chamber, or to replace fluid lost during the surgical procedure. Remove solution from the anterior chamber at the end of surgery.

Gonioscopic examinations: Fill gonioscopic prism with solution, as necessary.

	Product	Formulation	Package	C.I.*
Rx	**Occucoat** (Storz)	**Solution:** 2%	In 1 ml syringe with cannula.	N/A
otc	**Gonak** (Akorn)	**Solution:** 2.5%	In 15 ml.[1]	42
otc	**Goniosol** (Iolab)		In 15 ml.[2]	57
otc	**Enuclene** (Alcon) **Solution:** 0.25% tyloxapol and 0.02% benzalkonium chloride *Use:* Cleaning, wetting and lubricating agent for artificial eyes. *Dose:* 1 to 2 drops onto artificial eye, 3 or 4 times daily.		In 15 ml.	35
otc	**Gonioscopic Prism Solution** (Alcon) **Solution:** Hydroxyethylcellulose, 0.004% thimerosal, 0.1% EDTA *Use:* For bonding gonioscopic prisms to the eye.		In 15 ml.	54
otc	**I-Scrub** (Spectra) **Solution:** PEG-200 glyceryl monotallawate, disodium laureth sulfosuccinate, cocoamido propyl amine oxide, PEG-78 glyceryl monococoate, benzyl alcohol and EDTA. *Use:* Hygienic management of blepharitis; general eyelid cleaning. *Dose:* Apply with cleansing pad as directed.		In 15 and 240 ml.	3
otc	**SIS** (Spectra) **Sterile Solution:** PEG-200 glyceryl monotallawate, disodium laureth sulfosuccinate, cocoamido propyl amine oxide, PEG-78 glyceryl monococoate, benzyl alcohol and EDTA *Use:* For cleansing the surgical site before application of a germicide and to cleanse structures around the eye prior to noninvasive procedures. To cleanse hands. *Dose:* Wet gauze pad with SIS, lather, wipe area. Apply germicide.		In 15 ml.	11
otc	**Stye** (Commerce) **Ointment:** Boric acid, 1% yellow mercuric oxide, zinc sulfate, light mineral oil, white petrolatum, cod liver oil, anhydrous lanolin *Use:* For relief of discomfort of styes and for the treatment of irritation and minor infection of the eyelids. *Dose:* Apply morning and night directly to the affected lid.		In 3.75 g.	97
Rx	**Succus Cineraria Maritima** (Walker Pharm.) **Solution:** An aqueous and glycerin solution of senecio compositae, hamamelis water and boric acid *Use:* The manufacturer claims usefulness for the treatment of "optic opacity caused by cataract". Not intended for use in glaucoma. *Dose:* Instill 2 drops, morning and night into affected eye.		In 7 ml.	71
Rx	**Sno strips** (Akorn) **Strip:** Sterile tear flow test strips. *Use:* Apply to lower temporal lid margin of eye. Distance between notch and shoulder of strip is 10 mm which should be wetted in ≈ 3 minutes. Repeat if in excess of 5 minutes; > 10 minutes indicates reduced tear secretion.		100 strips per box	N/A

* Cost Index based on cost per g or ml.

[1] With 0.01% benzalkonium chloride, EDTA, boric acid and sodium borate.

[2] With 0.01% benzalkonium chloride.

BOTULINUM TOXIN TYPE A

Actions:

Pharmacology: Botulinum toxin is a sterile, lyophilized form of purified botulinum toxin type A, produced from a culture of the Hall strain of *Clostridium botulinum* grown in a medium containing N-Z amine and yeast extract. Botulinum toxin type A blocks neuromuscular conduction by binding to receptor sites on motor nerve terminals, entering the nerve terminals, and inhibiting the release of acetylcholine. When injected IM at therapeutic doses, botulinum toxin type A produces a localized chemical denervation muscle paralysis. When the muscle is chemically denervated, it atrophies and may develop extrajunctional acetylcholine receptors. There is evidence that the nerve can sprout and reinnervate the muscle, with the weakness thus being reversible.

The paralytic effect on muscles injected with botulinum toxin type A is useful in reducing the excessive, abnormal contractions associated with blepharospasm. When used for the treatment of strabismus, the administration of botulinum toxin type A may affect muscle pairs by inducing an atrophic lengthening of the injected muscle and a corresponding shortening of the muscle's antagonist. Following peri-ocular injection of botulinum toxin type A, distant muscles show electrophysiologic changes, but no clinical weakness or other clinical change for a period of several weeks or months, parallel to the duration of local clinical paralysis.

Clinical trials: In one study, botulinum toxin was evaluated in 27 patients with essential blepharospasm; 26 had previously undergone drug treatment utilizing benztropine mesylate, clonazepam or baclofen without adequate clinical results. Three of these patients then underwent muscle stripping surgery still without an adequate outcome. Upon using botulinum toxin, 25 of the 27 patients reported improvement within 48 hours. One of the other patients was later controlled with a higher dosage. The remaining patient reported only mild improvement but remained functionally impaired.

In another study, 12 patients with blepharospasm were evaluated in a double-blind, placebo controlled study. All patients receiving botulinum toxin (n = 8) were improved compared with no improvements in the placebo group (n = 4). The mean dystonia score improved by 72%, the self-assessment score rating improved by 61%, and a videotape evaluation rating improved by 39%. The effects of the treatment lasted a mean of 12.5 weeks.

Patients with blepharospasm (n = 1684) evaluated in an open trial showed clinical improvement lasting an average of 12.5 weeks prior to the need for retreatment.

Patients with strabismus (n = 677) treated with one or more injections of botulinum toxin type A were evaluated in an open trial; 55% were improved to an alignment of ≤ 10 prism diopters when evaluated ≥ 6 months following injection. These results are consistent with results from additional open label trials.

Indications:

Treatment of strabismus and blepharospasm associated with dystonia, including benign essential blepharospasm or VII nerve disorders in patients ≥ 12 years of age.

The efficacy of botulinum toxin type A in deviations > 50 prism diopters, in restrictive strabismus, in Duane's syndrome with lateral rectus weakness, and in secondary strabismus caused by prior surgical over-recession of the antagonist is doubtful, or multiple injections over time may be required. Botulinum toxin type A is ineffective in chronic paralytic strabismus except to reduce antagonist contracture in conjunction with surgical repair.

Contraindications:

Hypersensitivity to any ingredient in the formulation.

Warnings:

Do not exceed the recommended dosages and frequencies of administration. There have been no reported instances of systemic toxicity resulting from accidental injection or oral ingestion of botulinum toxin type A. Should accidental injection or oral ingestion occur, medically supervise the person for several days on an office or outpatient basis for signs or symptoms of systemic weakness or muscle paralysis. The entire contents of a vial is below the estimated dose for systemic toxicity in humans weighing ≥ 6 kg.

Hypersensitivity: As with all biologic products, epinephrine and other precautions as necessary should be available should an anaphylactic reaction occur. Refer to General Management of Acute Hypersensitivity Reactions.

Pregnancy: Category C. It is not known whether botulinum toxin type A can cause fetal harm when administered to a pregnant woman or can affect reproduction capacity. Administer to pregnant women only if clearly needed.

Lactation: It is not known whether this drug is excreted in breast milk. Exercise caution when botulinum toxin type A is administered to a nursing woman.

Children: Safety and efficacy in children < 12 years of age have not been established.

(Continued on following page)

BOTULINUM TOXIN TYPE A (Cont.)

Precautions:

Safe and effective use of botulinum toxin type A depends upon proper storage of the product, selection of the correct dose and proper reconstitution and administration techniques. Physicians administering botulinum toxin type A must understand the relevant neuromuscular and orbital anatomy and any alterations to the anatomy due to prior surgical procedures, and standard electromyographic techniques.

Retrobulbar hemorrhages: During the administration of botulinum toxin type A for the treatment of strabismus, retrobulbar hemorrhages sufficient to compromise retinal circulation have occurred from needle penetrations into the orbit. Have appropriate instruments to decompress the orbit accessible. Ocular (globe) penetrations by needles have also occurred. An ophthalmoscope to diagnose this condition should be available.

Reduced blinking from botulinum toxin type A injection of the orbicularis muscle can lead to corneal exposure, persistent epithelial defect and corneal ulceration, especially in patients with VII nerve disorders. One case of corneal perforation in an aphakic eye requiring corneal grafting has occurred because of this effect. Carefully test corneal sensation in eyes previously operated upon, avoid injection into the lower lid area to avoid ectropion and vigorously treat any epithelial defect. This may require protective drops, ointment, therapeutic soft contact lenses, or closure of the eye by patching or other means.

Presence of antibodies to botulinum toxin type A may reduce the effectiveness of therapy. In clinical studies, reduction in effectiveness due to antibody production has occurred in one patient with blepharospasm receiving 3 doses over a 6 week period totaling 92 U and in several patients with torticollis who received multiple doses experimentally, totaling over 300 U in 1 month. For this reason, keep the dose of botulinum toxin type A for strabismus and blepharospasm as low as possible in any case < 200 U in a 1 month period.

Drug Interactions:

Aminoglycosides: The effect of botulinum toxin may be potentiated by aminoglycoside antibiotics or any other drug that interferes with neuromuscular transmission. Exercise caution when botulinum toxin type A is used in patients taking any of these drugs.

Adverse Reactions:

Local: Diffuse skin rash (n = 7) and local swelling of the eyelid skin (n = 2) lasting for several days following eyelid injection have occurred.

Strabismus: Inducing paralysis in one or more extraocular muscles may produce spatial disorientation, double vision or past-pointing. Covering the affected eye may alleviate these symptoms. Extraocular muscles adjacent to the injection site are often affected, causing ptosis or vertical deviation, especially with higher doses. Side effects in 2058 adults who received 3650 injections for horizontal strabismus: Ptosis (15.7%); vertical deviation (16.9%). The incidence of ptosis was much less after inferior rectus injection (0.9%) and much greater after superior rectus injection (37.7%).

Side effects persisting for > 6 months in an enlarged series of 5587, injections of horizontal muscles in 3104 patients: Ptosis lasting over 180 days (0.3%); Vertical deviation > 2 prism diopters lasting over 180 days (2.1%).

In these patients, the injection procedure itself caused 9 scleral perforations. A vitreous hemorrhage occurred and later cleared in one case. No retinal detachment or visual loss occurred in any case; 16 retrobulbar hemorrhages occurred. Decompression of the orbit after 5 minutes was done to restore retinal circulation in one case. No eye lost vision from retrobulbar hemorrhage. Five eyes had pupillary change consistent with ciliary ganglion damage (Andies pupil).

(Adverse Reactions continued on following page)

BOTULINUM TOXIN TYPE A (Cont.)

Adverse Reactions (Cont.):

Blepharospasm: In 1684 patients who received 4258 treatments (involving multiple injections) for blepharospasm, the incidence rates of adverse reactions per treated eye were: Ptosis (11%); irritation/tearing, includes dry eye, lagophthalmos, and photophobia (10%); ectropion, keratitis, diplopia and entropion occurred rarely (< 1%).

Ecchymosis occurs easily in the soft eyelid tissues. This can be prevented by applying pressure at the injection site immediately after the injection. In two cases of VII nerve disorder (one case of an aphakic eye), reduced blinking from botulinum toxin type A injection of the orbicularis muscle led to serious corneal exposure, persistent epithelial defect and corneal ulceration. Perforation requiring corneal grafting occurred in one case, an aphakic eye. Avoidance of injection into the lower lid area to avoid ectropion may reduce this hazard. Vigorously treat any corneal epithelial defect. This may require protective drops, ointment, therapeutic soft contact lenses, or closure of the eye by patching or other means.

Two patients previously incapacitated by blepharospasm experienced cardiac collapse attributed to over-exertion within 3 weeks following botulinum toxin type A therapy. Caution sedentary patients to resume activity slowly and carefully following the administration of botulinum toxin type A.

Overdosage:

In the event of overdosage or injection into the wrong muscle, additional information may be obtained by contacting Allergan Pharmaceuticals at (800) 347-5063 from 8 am to 4 pm Pacific Time, or at (714) 724-5954 for a recorded message at other times.

Patient Information:

Patients with blepharospasm may have been extremely sedentary for a long time. Caution sedentary patients to resume activity slowly and carefully following administration.

Administration and Dosage:

Strabismus: Botulinum toxin type A is intended for injection into extraocular muscles utilizing the electrical activity recorded from the tip of the injection needle as a guide to placement within the target muscle. Injection without surgical exposure or electromyographic guidance should not be attempted. Physicians should be familiar with electromyographic technique.

An injection of botulinum toxin type A is prepared by drawing into a sterile 1 ml tuberculin syringe an amount of the properly diluted toxin (see Dilution Table) slightly greater than the intended dose. Air bubbles in the syringe barrel are expelled and the syringe is attached to the electromyographic injection needle, preferably a 1-½ inch, 27 gauge needle. Injection volume in excess of the intended dose is expelled through the needle into an appropriate waste container to assure patency of the needle and to confirm that there is no syringe-needle leakage. Use a new, sterile needle and syringe to enter the vial on each occasion for dilution or removal of botulinum toxin type A.

To prepare the eye for botulinum toxin type A injection, give several drops of a local anesthetic and an ocular decongestant several minutes prior to injection.

Note: The volume of botulinum toxin type A injected for treatment of strabismus should be between 0.05 to 0.15 ml per muscle.

The initial listed doses of the diluted botulinum toxin type A (see Dilution Table) typically create paralysis of injected muscles beginning 1 to 2 days after injection and increasing in intensity during the first week. The paralysis lasts for 2 to 6 weeks and gradually resolves over a similar time period. Overcorrections lasting > 6 months have been rare. About one half of patients will require subsequent doses because of inadequate paralytic response of the muscle to the initial dose, or because of mechanical factors such as large deviations or restrictions, or because of the lack of binocular motor fusion to stabilize the alignment.

I. Initial doses in units (U). Use the lower listed doses for treatment of small deviations. Use the larger doses only for large deviations.
   A. For vertical muscles, and for horizontal strabismus of < 20 prism diopters: 1.25 to 2.5 U in any one muscle.
   B. For horizontal strabismus of 20 prism diopters to 50 prism diopters: 2.5 to 5 U in any one muscle.
   C. For persistent VI nerve palsy of ≥ 1 month duration: 1.25 to 2.5 U in the medial rectus muscle.

(Administration and Dosage continued on following page)

BOTULINUM TOXIN TYPE A (Cont.)

Administration and Dosage (Cont.):

II. Subsequent doses for residual or recurrent strabismus.

A. Re-examine patients 7 to 14 days after each injection to assess the effect of that dose.

B. Patients experiencing adequate paralysis of the target muscle that require subsequent injections should receive a dose comparable to the initial dose.

C. Subsequent doses for patients experiencing incomplete paralysis of the target muscle may be increased up to twice the size of the previously administered dose.

D. Subsequent injections should not be administered until the effects of the previous dose have dissipated as evidenced by substantial function in the injected and adjacent muscles.

E. The maximum recommended dose as a single injection for any one muscle is 25 U.

Blepharospasm: Diluted botulinum toxin type A (see Dilution Table) is injected using a sterile, 27 to 30 gauge needle without electromyographic guidance. 1.25 to 2.5 U (0.05 to 0.1 ml volume at each site) injected into the medial and lateral pre-tarsal orbicularis oculi of the upper lid and into the lateral pre-tarsal orbicularis oculi of the lower lid is the initial recommended dose. In general, the initial effect of the injections is seen within 3 days and reaches a peak at 1 to 2 weeks post-treatment. Each treatment lasts approximately 3 months, following which the procedure can be repeated indefinitely. At repeat treatment sessions, the dose may be increased up to two-fold if the response from the initial treatment is considered insufficient (usually defined as an effect that does not last longer than 2 months). However, there appears to be little benefit obtainable from injecting more than 5 U per site. Some tolerance may be found when botulinum toxin type A is used in treating blepharospasm if treatments are given any more frequently than every 3 months, and it is rare to have the effect be permanent.

The cumulative dose of botulinum toxin type A in a 30 day period should not exceed 200 U.

Dilution Technique: To reconstitute lyophilized botulinum toxin type A, use sterile normal saline without a preservative; 0.9% Sodium Chloride Injection is the recommended diluent. Draw up the proper amount of diluent in the appropriate size syringe. Since botulinum toxin type A is denatured by bubbling or similar violent agitation, inject the diluent into the vial gently. Discard the vial if a vacuum does not pull the diluent into the vial. Record the date and time of reconstitution on the space on the label. Administer within 4 hours after reconstitution.

During this time period, store reconstituted botulinum toxin type A in a refrigerator (2° to 8°C; 36° to 46°F). Reconstituted botulinum toxin type A should be clear, colorless and free of particulate matter. The use of one vial for more than one patient is not recommended because the product and diluent do not contain a preservative.

Dilution of Botulinum Toxin Type A	
Diluent Added (0.9% Sodium Chloride Injection)	Resulting dose
1 ml	10 U
2 ml	5 U
4 ml	2.5 U
8 ml	1.25 U

Note: These dilutions are calculated for an injection volume of 0.1 ml. A decrease or increase in the botulinum toxin type A dose is also possible by administering a smaller or larger injection volume – from 0.05 ml (50% decrease in dose) to 0.15 ml (50% increase in dose).

Storage: Store the lyophilized product in a freezer at or below -5°C (23°F). Administer within 4 hours after the vial is removed from the freezer and reconstituted. During these 4 hours, store reconstituted botulinum toxin type A in a refrigerator (2° to 8°C; 36° to 46°F). Reconstituted botulinum toxin type A should be clear, colorless and free of particulate matter.

Rx	**Oculinum** (Allergan)	**Powder for Injection (lyophilized):** 100 units of lyophilized *Clostridium botulinum* Toxin type A[1]	In vials with 0.05 mg albumin (human) and 0.9 mg sodium chloride. Preservative free.

[1] One unit corresponds to the calculated median lethal intraperitoneal dose (LD/50) in mice of the reconstituted drug injected.

The Ear Preparations on the following pages are divided into groups as follows:
- Antibiotics
- Steroid and Antibiotic Combinations
- Miscellaneous Preparations

Patient Information:

Notify physician if burning or itching occurs or if condition persists.

Proper use of ear drops:

- Wash hands thoroughly.
- Avoid touching the dropper to the ear or any other surface. For accuracy and to avoid contamination, another person should insert the ear drops when possible.
- Hold container in the hand for a few minutes to warm to near body temperature.
- If the drops are in a suspension form, shake well for 10 seconds before using.
- Lie on your side or tilt the affected ear up for ease of administration.
- To allow the drops to run in:
  Adults - Hold the earlobe up and back.
  Children - Hold the earlobe down and back.
- Instill the prescribed number of drops in the ear.
- Do not insert the dropper into the ear.
- Maintain the ear tilted for about 2 minutes, or insert a soft cotton plug, whichever is recommended.

Antibiotics

CHLORAMPHENICOL

Actions:

Chloramphenicol is a broad-spectrum antibiotic originally isolated from *Streptomyces venezuelae.* It is primarily bacteriostatic and acts by inhibition of protein synthesis by interfering with the transfer of activated amino acids from soluble RNA to ribosomes. Development of resistance to chloramphenicol can be regarded as minimal for staphylococci and many other species of bacteria.

Indications:

For treating superficial infections involving the external auditory canal. For inner ear infections, use systemic antibiotic therapy.

Do not use when less potentially dangerous agents would be expected to provide effective treatment.

Contraindications:

Hypersensitivity to any component.

Warnings:

Bone marrow hypoplasia, including aplastic anemia and death, has been reported following local application of chloramphenicol.

Precautions:

Superinfection: Use of antibiotics (especially prolonged or repeated therapy) may result in bacterial or fungal overgrowth of nonsusceptible organisms. Such overgrowth may lead to secondary infection. Take appropriate measures if superinfection occurs.

Except in superficial infections, therapy should include systemic medication.

Adverse Reactions:

Signs of local irritation (itching or burning, angioneurotic edema, urticaria, vesicular and maculopapular dermatitis) have occurred in patients sensitive to chloramphenicol. Blood dyscrasias have occurred with systemic absorption of topical chloramphenicol. Similar sensitivity reactions to other materials in topical preparations may also occur.

Administration and Dosage:

Instill 2 or 3 drops into the ear 3 times daily.

				C.I.*
Rx	**Chloromycetin Otic** (Parke-Davis)	**Solution:** 0.5% in propylene glycol	In 15 ml w/dropper.	131

* Cost Index based on cost per ml.

Refer also to Patient Information on page 2262 for instructions on the use of these products.

Steroid and Antibiotic Combinations

In these combinations:

HYDROCORTISONE is used for its antiallergic, antipruritic and anti-inflammatory effects.

ANTIBIOTICS are used for their antibacterial actions.

Indications: Treatment of superficial bacterial infections of the external auditory canal. The *suspension* is also used to treat infections of mastoidectomy and fenestration cavities.

Contraindications:

Hypersensitivity to any component; prolonged treatment may result in overgrowth of non-susceptible organisms and fungi (ie, herpes simplex, vaccinia and varicella).

Dosage: The usual adult dose is 4 drops instilled 3 or 4 times daily.

	Product	Formulation	Supplied	C.I.*
Rx	**AK-Spore H.C. Otic** (Akorn)	**Solution:** 1% hydrocortisone, 5 mg neomycin sulfate and 10,000 units polymyxin B sulfate per ml	In 10 ml w/dropper.[1]	47
Rx	**Cortatrigen Modified Ear Drops** (Goldline)		In 10 ml.[1]	41
Rx	**Cortisporin Otic** (Burroughs Wellcome)		In 10 ml.[2]	94
Rx	**Drotic** (Ascher)		In 10 ml w/dropper.[1]	94
Rx	**LazerSporin-C** (Pedinol)		In 10 ml w/dropper.	53
Rx	**My Cort Otic #1-20** (Scrip)		In 10 ml.[1]	53
Rx	**Ortega Otic M** (Ortega)		In 10 ml w/dropper.[1]	43
Rx	**Otic-Care** (Parmed)		In 10 ml.[3]	NA
Rx	**Otocort** (Lemmon)		In 10 ml w/dropper.	41
Rx	**Otomycin-Hpn Otic** (Misemer)		In 10 ml w/dropper.[1]	66
Rx	**Otoreid-HC** (Solvay)		In 10 ml w/dropper.[1]	93
Rx	**Otobiotic Otic** (Schering)	**Solution:** 0.5% hydrocortisone and 10,000 units polymyxin B sulfate per ml	In 15 ml w/dropper.[4]	61
Rx	**Pyocidin-Otic** (Forest Pharm.)		In 10 ml w/dropper.[5]	98
Rx	**AK-Spore H.C. Otic** (Akorn)	**Suspension:** 1% hydrocortisone, 5 mg neomycin sulfate and 10,000 units polymyxin B sulfate per ml	In 10 ml w/dropper.[6]	56
Rx	**Cortatrigen Modified Otic** (Goldline)		In 10 ml.[7]	51
Rx	**Cortisporin Otic** (Burroughs Wellcome)		In 10 ml w/dropper.[6]	94
Rx	**Mayotic** (Mayrand)		In 10 ml w/dropper.[8]	NA
Rx	**Otocort** (Lemmon)		In 10 ml w/dropper.[6]	47
Rx	**Pediotic** (Burroughs W)		In 7.5 ml w/dropper.[9]	125
Rx	**UAD Otic** (UAD)		In 10 ml w/dropper.[8]	NA
Rx	**Coly-Mycin S Otic** (Parke-Davis)	**Suspension:** 1% hydrocortisone acetate, 3.3 mg neomycin (as sulfate), 3 mg colistin (as sulfate) and 0.05% thonzonium Br/ml	In 5 and 10 ml w/dropper.[10]	96

* Cost Index based on cost per ml.

[1] With propylene glycol, glycerin and potassium metabisulfite.

[2] With cupric sulfate, propylene glycol, glycerin and potassium metabisulfite.

[3] With glycerin, hydrochloric acid, propylene glycol and potassium metabisulfite.

[4] With propylene glycol, glycerin, EDTA, sodium bisulfite and anhydrous sodium sulfite.

[5] With propylene glycol.

[6] With cetyl alcohol, propylene glycol, polysorbate 80 and thimerosal.

[7] With cetyl alcohol, polyoxyl 40 stearate, polysorbate 80, propylene glycol and benzalkonium Cl.

[8] With 0.01% thimerosal, cetyl alcohol, propylene glycol and polysorbate 80.

[9] With 0.001% thimerosal, cetyl alcohol, glyceryl monostearate, mineral oil, polyoxyl 40 stearate and propylene glycol.

[10] With polysorbate 80, acetic acid, sodium acetate and thimerosal.

Refer also to Patient Information on page 2262 for instructions on the use of these products.

Miscellaneous Preparations

In these combinations:

HYDROCORTISONE and *DESONIDE* are steroids used for their anti-inflammatory, antipruritic and vasoconstrictive effects.

PHENYLEPHRINE is a vasoconstrictor which may be a decongestant.

CHLOROXYLENOL, PARACHLOROMETAXYLENOL, BORIC ACID, BENZALKONIUM CHLORIDE, BENZETHONIUM CHLORIDE and *ALUMINUM ACETATE* provide antibacterial or antifungal action.

ACETIC ACID and *M-CRESYL ACETATE* provide an acid medium and have antibacterial and antifungal actions.

CARBAMIDE PEROXIDE and *TRIETHANOLAMINE* emulsify and disperse ear wax.

GLYCERIN is a solvent and vehicle; it has emollient, hygroscopic and humectant properties.

PRAMOXINE and *BENZOCAINE* are local anesthetics.

ANTIPYRINE is an analgesic.

	Product	Description	Package	C.I.*
Rx	**VōSol HC Otic** (Wallace)	**Solution:** 1% hydrocortisone and 2% acetic acid. With 3% propylene glycol diacetate and 0.02% benzethonium chloride. In 10 ml dropper bottle. *Dose:* Insert saturated wick; keep moist 24 hours. Remove wick and instill 5 drops 3 or 4 times daily.		114
Rx	**Ear-Eze** (Hyrex)	**Solution:** 1% hydrocortisone, 1% pramoxine and 0.1% chloroxylenol. With propylene glycol, acetic acid and benzalkonium chloride. *Dose:* Insert saturated wick; keep moist 24 hours. Remove wick and instill 5 drops 3 or 4 times daily.	In 15 ml dropper bottle.	46
Rx	**Otic-HC Ear Drops** (Hauck)		In 10 ml dropper bottle.	74
Rx	**Tega-Otic** (Ortega)		In 10 ml dropper bottle.	49
Rx	**Otic Tridesilon** (Miles Pharm.)	**Solution:** 0.05% desonide and 2% acetic acid. In propylene glycol. In 10 ml w/dropper. *Dose:* 3 to 4 drops 3 or 4 times daily.		122
Rx	**Otic-Plain** (Hauck)	**Solution:** 1% pramoxine HCl and 2% acetic acid. With 0.1% parachlorometaxylenol and 0.02% benzalkonium chloride in propylene glycol. In 10 ml dropper bottle. *Dose:* Insert saturated wick; keep moist 24 hours. Remove wick and instill 5 drops 3 or 4 times daily.		63

* Cost Index based on cost per ml.

(Continued on following page)

Refer to the general discussion of these products on page 2264
Refer also to Patient Information on page 2262 for instructions on the use of these products.

Miscellaneous Preparations (Cont.)

	Product (Manufacturer)	Composition / Dose	How Supplied	C.I.*
Rx	**Allergen Ear Drops** (Goldline)	**Solution:** 1.4% benzocaine, 5.4% antipyrine, glycerin and oxyquinoline sulfate. *Dose:* Fill ear canal; insert saturated cotton pledget. Repeat 3 or 4 times daily, or up to once every 1 to 2 hours.	In 15 ml w/dropper.	9
Rx	**Auralgan Otic** (Ayerst)		In 15 ml w/dropper.	34
Rx	**Auromid** (Vangard)		In 15 ml w/dropper.	12
Rx	**Auroto Otic** (Barre)		In 15 ml w/dropper.	15
Rx	**Earocol Ear Drops** (Mallard)		In 15 ml w/dropper.	20
Rx	**Oto Ear Drops** (Vortech)		In 15 ml.	22
Rx	**Tympagesic** (Adria)	**Solution:** 5% benzocaine, 5% antipyrine and 0.25% phenylephrine HCl in propylene glycol. In 13 ml dropper bottle. *Dose:* Fill ear canal; plug with saturated cotton. Repeat every 2 to 4 hours.		35
Rx	**Americaine-Otic** (American Critical Care)	**Solution:** 20% benzocaine, with 0.1% benzethonium chloride in 1% glycerin and polyethylene glycol. *Dose:* Instill 4 or 5 drops. Insert cotton pledget. Repeat every 1 to 2 hours.	In 15 ml.	26
Rx	**Otocain** (Holloway)		In 15 ml dropper bottle.	21
Rx	**Cresylate** (Recsei)	**Solution:** 25% m-Cresyl acetate, 25% isopropanol, 1% chlorobutanol, 1% benzyl alcohol and 5% castor oil in propylene glycol. In 15 ml dropper bottles and pt. *Dose:* 2 to 4 drops as required.		21
Rx	**Acetic Acid Otic** (Various)	**Solution:** 2% acetic acid with 3% propylene glycol diacetate, 0.02% benzethonium chloride and 0.015% sodium acetate. *Dose:* Insert saturated wick; keep moist 24 hours. Remove wick and instill 5 drops 3 or 4 times daily.	In 15, 30 and 60 ml.	20+
Rx	**VōSoL Otic** (Wallace)		In 15 and 30 ml.	60
Rx	**Borofair Otic** (Pharmafair)	**Solution:** 2% acetic acid. In aluminum acetate solution. *Dose:* Instill 4 to 6 drops every 2 to 3 hours.	In 60 ml.	6
Rx	**BurOtic** (Parnell)		In 60 ml.	10
Rx	**Otic Domeboro** (Miles Pharm.)		In 60 ml dropper bottle.	19
Rx	**Cerumenex Drops** (Purdue Frederick)	**Solution:** 10% triethanolamine polypeptide oleate-condensate. With 0.5% chlorobutanol in propylene glycol. In 6 and 12 ml w/dropper. *Dose:* Fill ear canal. Insert cotton plug, allow to remain 15 to 30 minutes. Flush ear.		111
otc	**Aurocaine 2** (Republic)	**Solution:** 2.75% boric acid in isopropyl alcohol. *Dose:* Instill 3 to 6 drops in each ear.	In 30 ml.	11
otc	**Auro-Dri** (Commerce)		In 30 ml dropper bottle.	6
otc	**Dri/Ear** (Pfeiffer)		In 30 ml dropper bottle.	5
otc	**Ear-Dry** (Scherer)		In 30 ml dropper bottle.	7
otc	**Swim Ear** (Fougera)		In 30 ml.	6

* Cost Index based on cost per ml.

(Continued on following page)

Refer to the general discussion of these products on page 2264
Refer also to Patient Information on page 2262 for instructions on the use of these products.

Miscellaneous Preparations (Cont.)

	Product	Composition / Dose	How Supplied	C.I.*
otc	**Aurinol Ear Drops** (Various)	**Solution:** Chloroxylenol and acetic acid. With benzalkonium chloride and glycerin. *Dose:* Instill warm drops in affected ear 3 times daily.	In 15 ml.	11+
otc	**Benzodyne Drops** (Kay Pharm.)		In 15 ml.	16
otc	**Halogen Ear Drops** (Halsey)		In 15 ml w/dropper.	11
otc	**Star-Otic** (Stellar)	**Solution:** Nonaqueous acetic acid, Burow's solution and boric acid in propylene glycol. In 15 ml dropper bottles. *Dose:* Instill 2 to 3 drops before and after swimming or showering.		NA
otc	**Debrox Drops** (Marion Merrell Dow)	**Solution:** 6.5% carbamide peroxide. In glycerin and propylene glycol. In 15 and 30 ml dropper bottle. *Dose:* Instill 5 to 10 drops twice daily up to 4 days.		30
otc	**Murine Ear Drops** (Abbott)	**Solution:** 6.5% carbamide peroxide. In anhydrous glycerin. In 15 ml with or without 30 ml ear syringe. *Dose:* Instill 5 to 10 drops twice daily up to 4 days.		29
otc	**Auro Ear Drops** (Commerce)	**Solution:** 6.5% carbamide peroxide. In 15 ml. *Dose:* Instill 5 to 10 drops twice daily for 3 to 4 days.		22
otc	**Aurocaine Ear Drops** (Republic)	**Solution:** Carbamide, glycerin and propylene glycol. With 0.5% chlorobutanol. In 15 ml. *Dose:* Instill 5 to 10 drops twice daily for 3 to 4 days.		16
otc	**Kerid Ear Drops** (Blair)	**Solution:** Urea and glycerin in propylene glycol. In 8 ml w/dropper. *Dose:* Fill ear canal. Insert cotton plug, allow to remain 30 to 60 minutes. Flush with warm water.		49
otc	**E•R•O Ear Drops** (Scherer)	**Solution:** Glycerin and propylene glycol. In 15 ml. *Dose:* Instill 3 to 5 warm drops with saturated cotton. Swab or flush with warm water.		14
otc	**Mollifene Ear Drops** (Pfeiffer)	**Solution:** Glycerin, camphor, cajuput oil, eucalyptus oil and thyme oil. In 24 ml dropper bottle. *Dose:* Instill 3 to 5 drops in affected ear. Swab or flush with a warm water and baking soda solution.		8
otc	**Swim-Ear** (Fougera)	**Liquid:** 95% isopropyl alcohol, 5% anhydrous glycerin. In 30 ml. *Dose:* Instill 4 or 5 drops in affected ear.		NA

* Cost Index based on cost per ml.

NYSTATIN

Actions:

Nystatin, an antifungal antibiotic, is both fungistatic and fungicidal in vitro against a wide variety of yeasts and yeast-like fungi. It is a polyene antibiotic of undetermined structural formula that is obtained from *Streptomyces noursei.* It binds to sterols in the cell membrane of the fungus with a resultant change in membrane permeability.

Following oral administration, nystatin is sparingly absorbed with no detectable blood levels. Most of the orally administered drug is passed unchanged in the stool.

Indications:

Treatment of oral candidiasis.

Contraindications:

Hypersensitivity to nystatin.

Warnings:

Usage in Pregnancy: Category C. Safety for use during pregnancy has not been established. Use only if clearly needed and when the potential benefits outweigh the potential hazards to the fetus.

Adverse Reactions:

GI: Nausea, vomiting, GI distress and diarrhea occur occasionally with large doses.

Patient Information:

Retain the drug in the mouth as long as possible.

Continue use at least 2 days after symptoms have subsided.

Administration and Dosage:

Oral suspension: Adults and children – 400,000 to 600,000 units 4 times daily (½ of dose in each side of mouth, retaining the drug as long as possible before swallowing).

Infants – 200,000 units 4 times daily (100,000 units in each side of mouth).

Premature and low birth weight infants – Limited clinical studies indicate that 100,000 units 4 times daily is effective.

Pastilles: Adults and children – 200,000 to 400,000 units 4 or 5 times daily, for as long as 14 days, if necessary. Do not chew or swallow.

Powder for extemporaneous compounding: Adults & children – Add ⅛ tsp (approx. 500,000 units) to ≈ ½ to 1 cup (120 to 240 ml, or 4 to 8 oz) of water and stir well. Administer 4 times daily. Use immediately after mixing; do not store.

Continue local treatment at least 48 hours after perioral signs and symptoms have disappeared and cultures have returned to normal.

Nystatin vaginal tablets (p. 528) can be given orally for treatment of oral candidiasis.

To improve oral retention of the drug, nystatin (250,000 units) has been administered for oral candidiasis in the form of flavored frozen popsicles.

				C.I.*
Rx	**Nystatin** (Various)	**Oral Suspension:** 100,000 units per ml	In 5, 60 and 480 ml.	10+
Rx	**Mycostatin** (Apothecon)		< 1% alcohol, saccharin and 50% sucrose. In 60 ml w/dropper.	34
Rx	**Nilstat** (Lederle)		Cherry flavor. In 60 ml w/dropper and pt.	31
Rx	**Nystex** (Savage)		< 1% alcohol and 50% sucrose. In 60 ml.	13
Rx	**Mycostatin Pastilles** (Squibb)	**Troches:** 200,000 units	Light to dark gold. Licorice flavor. In 30s.	66
Rx	**Nystatin** (Paddock)	**Powder for Extemporaneous Preparation of Oral Suspension:** 50,000,000 units		
Rx	**Nilstat** (Lederle)	**Powder for Extemporaneous Preparation of Oral Suspension:** 150,000,000 units		
Rx	**Nystatin** (Paddock)			
Rx	**Nystatin** (Paddock)	**Powder for Extemporaneous Preparation of Oral Suspension:** 500,000,000 units		
Rx	**Nilstat** (Lederle)	**Powder for Extemporaneous Preparation of Oral Suspension:** 1,000,000,000 units		
Rx	**Nilstat** (Lederle)	**Powder for Extemporaneous Preparation of Oral Suspension:** 2,000,000,000 units		
Rx	**Nystatin** (Paddock)	**Powder for Extemporaneous Preparation of Oral Suspension:** 5,000,000,000 units		

* Cost Index based on cost per ml or troche.

CLOTRIMAZOLE

Actions:

A broad spectrum antifungal agent that inhibits yeast growth by altering cell membrane permeability. It is fungicidal in vitro against *Candida albicans* and other *Candida* sp.

Following oral administration, long-term concentration in saliva appears related to the slow release of drug from the oral mucosa to which clotrimazole is apparently bound. Dosing every 3 hours maintains effective salivary levels for most strains of *Candida*.

Indications:

Treatment of oropharyngeal candidiasis.

Contraindications:

Hypersensitivity to clotrimazole.

Warnings:

Clotrimazole is not indicated for the treatment of systemic mycoses.

Usage in Pregnancy: Category C. There are no adequate and well controlled studies in pregnant women. Use only when clearly needed and when the potential benefits outweigh the potential hazards to the fetus.

Usage in Children: Safety and efficacy for use in children less than 3 years of age have not been established; therefore, use in these patients is not recommended.

Precautions:

Abnormal liver function tests; SGOT levels were minimally elevated in ≈ 15% of patients in clinical trials. It was often impossible to distinguish effects of clotrimazole from other therapy and the underlying disease (malignancy in most cases). Assess hepatic function periodically, particularly in patients with preexisting hepatic impairment.

Adverse Reactions:

Abnormal liver function tests; elevated SGOT levels were reported in about 15% of patients in clinical trials (see Precautions).

Nausea and vomiting occurred in about 5% of patients.

Patient Information:

To achieve maximum effect, allow troche to dissolve slowly in the mouth.

Administration and Dosage:

Dissolve troche slowly in mouth.

Administer 1 troche 5 times a day for 14 consecutive days. Only limited data are available on safety and efficacy after prolonged administration.

				C.I.*
Rx	**Mycelex** (Miles Pharm.)	**Troches:** 10 mg	(#Miles 095). White. In 70s and 140s.	56

TANNIC ACID

Actions:

Forms a thin pliable film over sores or blisters within 60 seconds of application. This protective film, if used in the mouth, normally withstands eating and drinking.

Indications:

For temporary relief of pain, burning and itching caused by cold sores, fever blisters and canker sores.

Precautions:

Do not use in or around eyes. If contact occurs, flush immediately and continuously with clear water for 10 minutes. Consult physician immediately if pain or irritation persists.

A slight, temporary burning sensation may occur when the drug is applied to an open sore or blister.

If infection persists beyond 10 days, discontinue use and consult a physician.

Administration and Dosage:

At first symptoms, apply 4 times daily for a minimum of 2 days. Wipe affected areas dry before applying.

				C.I.*
otc	**Zilactol Medicated** (Zila Pharm.)	**Liquid:** 7% in 80.8% SD alcohol 37	In 7.5 ml.	NA
otc	**Zilactin Medicated** (Zila Pharm.)	**Gel:** 7% suspended in 80.8% SD alcohol 37	In 7.5 g.	75

* Cost Index based on cost per troche or g.

Product identification code.

CHLORHEXIDINE GLUCONATE

Actions:

Pharmacology: Chlorhexidine provides microbicidal activity during oral rinsing. The clinical significance is not clear. Microbiological sampling of plaque has shown a reduction of aerobic and anaerobic bacteria, ranging from 54% to 97% through 6 months' use.

In a 6 month clinical study, there were no significant changes in bacterial resistance, overgrowth of potentially opportunistic organisms or other adverse changes in the oral microbial ecosystem. Three months after use was discontinued, the number and resistance of bacteria in plaque had returned to baseline levels.

Pharmacokinetics: Approximately 30% of chlorhexidine is retained in the oral cavity following rinsing and is slowly released into the oral fluids. Chlorhexidine is poorly absorbed from the GI tract. The mean peak plasma level of 0.206 mcg/g was reached 30 minutes after ingestion of 300 mg. Detectable levels were not present in the plasma 12 hours after administration. Excretion occurred primarily through the feces (≈ 90%); < 1% was excreted in the urine.

Indications:

For the treatment of gingivitis as characterized by gingival redness and swelling, including bleeding upon probing. It has not been tested in acute necrotizing ulcerative gingivitis.

Contraindications: Hypersensitivity to chlorhexidine gluconate.

Warnings:

An increase in supragingival calculus was noted in clinical testing in chlorhexidine users. It is not known if use results in an increase in subgingival calculus. Remove calculus deposits by dental prophylaxis at 6 month intervals.

Hypersensitivity and generalized *allergic reactions* have been reported rarely. Have epinephrine 1:1000 immediately available. Refer to Management of Acute Hypersensitivity Reactions on p. viii.

Usage in Pregnancy: Category B. Weigh the benefits of the drug against possible risk to the fetus.

Usage in Lactation: It is not known whether this drug is excreted in breast milk. Exercise caution when administering to a nursing mother.

Usage in Children: Efficacy has not been established in children < 18 years of age.

Precautions:

Gingivitis and periodontitis: The presence or absence of gingival inflammation following treatment should not be used as a major indicator of underlying periodontitis.

Staining of oral surfaces, such as tooth surfaces, restorations and the dorsum of the tongue may occur. In clinical testing, 56% of users exhibited a measurable increase in facial anterior stain, compared to 35% of control users after 6 months. Stain will be more pronounced in patients who have heavier accumulations of unremoved plaque.

Stain resulting from use does not adversely affect health of the gingivae or other oral tissues. Stain can be removed from most tooth surfaces by conventional professional prophylactic techniques. Use discretion when prescribing to patients with anterior facial restorations with rough surfaces or margins. If natural stain cannot be removed from these surfaces by dental prophylaxis, exclude patients from treatment if permanent discoloration is unacceptable. Stain in these areas may be difficult to remove and may rarely necessitate replacement of restorations.

Taste perception alteration may occur while undergoing treatment. Most patients accommodate with continued use. Permanent taste alteration has not been reported.

Adverse Reactions:

Most common: Increase in staining of teeth and other oral surfaces, increase in calculus formation and altered taste perception. (See Warnings and Precautions.)

Local: Minor irritation and superficial desquamation of the oral mucosa, particularly among children. Transient parotitis.

Overdosage:

Ingestion of 30 to 60 ml by a small child (≈ 10 kg body weight) might result in gastric distress, including nausea, or signs of alcohol intoxication. Seek medical attention if a small child ingests 120 ml or if signs of alcohol intoxication develop.

Administration and Dosage:

Initiate therapy directly following dental prophylaxis. Reevaluate and give a thorough prophylaxis every 6 months.

Use twice daily as an oral rinse for 30 seconds, morning and evening after toothbrushing. Usual dosage is 15 ml (marked in cap) of undiluted drug. Not intended for ingestion; expectorate after rinsing.

				C.I.*
Rx	**Peridex** (Procter & Gamble)	**Oral Rinse:** 0.12%	Saccharin and 11.6% alcohol. Mint flavor. In 480 ml.[1]	18

* Cost Index based on cost per ml.

[1] Do not freeze.

CARBAMIDE PEROXIDE (Urea Peroxide)

Actions:

Releases oxygen on contact with mouth tissues to provide cleansing effects. Helps reduce inflammation, relieve pain and inhibit odor-forming bacteria.

Indications:

For relief of minor inflammation of gums and other oral mucosal surfaces and lips. Also helpful against discomfort of canker and denture irritation, postdental procedure irritation, and irritation related to inflamed gums. Used to aid oral hygiene when normal cleansing measures are inadequate or when patient wears orthodontic or dental appliances. Useful for debridement and cleansing of accessible oral lesions.

Warnings:

Discontinue use and consult physician or dentist promptly if irritation persists or worsens or if inflammation develops.

Patient Information:

Severe or persistent oral inflammation or denture irritation may be serious. If these or unexpected effects occur, consult physician or dentist promptly.

Discontinue use if condition persists or worsens.

Do not use for more than 7 days or in children less than 3 years of age, unless directed by physician or dentist.

Administration and Dosage:

Solution: Apply undiluted, 4 times daily after meals and at bedtime, or as directed. Place several drops on affected area (expectorate after 2 to 3 minutes; or place 10 drops on tongue, mix with saliva, swish for several minutes and expectorate).

Gel: Do not dilute. Use 4 times a day, or as directed. Gently massage medication on affected area. Do not drink or rinse mouth for 5 minutes after use.

	Product (Manufacturer)	Formulation	How supplied	C.I.*
otc	**Cankaid** (Becton Dickinson)	**Solution:** 10% in anhydrous glycerol	In 22.5 ml.	16
otc	**Gly-Oxide Liquid** (Marion Merrell Dow)		In 15 and 60 ml w/applicator.	30
otc *sf*	**Orajel Brace-aid Rinse** (Commerce)		In 30 ml.	7
otc	**Proxigel** (Reed & Carnrick)	**Gel:** 11% in a water free gel base	In 36 g w/applicator.	15

SALIVA SUBSTITUTES

These products contain electrolytes in a carboxymethylcellulose base. They are used as a saliva substitute for relief of dry mouth and throat in xerostomia.

	Product (Manufacturer)	Formulation	How supplied	C.I.*
otc	**Saliva Substitute** (Roxane)	**Solution:** Sorbitol, sodium carboxymethylcellulose and methylparaben	Dye free. In 120 ml.	3
otc	**Orex** (Young Dental)	**Solution:** Monobasic and dibasic potassium phosphates, magnesium, potassium, calcium and sodium chlorides, sodium fluoride, sorbitol solution, sodium carboxymethylcellulose and methylparaben	In 180 ml.	3
otc *sf*	**Xero-Lube** (Scherer)		In 180 ml w/pump spray.	3
otc *sf*	**Moi-Stir** (Kingswood Lab)	**Solution:** Dibasic sodium phosphate, magnesium, calcium, sodium and potassium chlorides, sorbitol, sodium carboxymethylcellulose and methyl and propyl parabens	Mint flavor. In 120 ml w/pump spray.	3
otc *sf*	**Moi-Stir Swabsticks** (Kingswood Lab)		In 300s.	16
otc *sf*	**Moi-Stir 10** (Kingswood Lab)	**Solution:** Sodium carboxymethylcellulose, potassium chloride, dibasic sodium phosphate and methyl and propyl parabens	In 60 ml pump spray.	5
otc *sf*	**Salivart** (Westport Pharm.)	**Solution:** Sodium carboxymethylcellulose, sorbitol, sodium, potassium, calcium and magnesium chlorides, dibasic potassium phosphate and nitrogen (as propellant)	In 75 ml spray cans.	8
otc *sf*	**Mouthkote** (Parnell)	**Solution:** Xylitol, sorbitol, mucoprotective factor (MPF), yerba santa, saccharin	Alcohol free. Citrus flavor. In 60 and 240 ml and UD 5 ml.	NA

* Cost Index based on cost per g, ml or swabstick.

sf – Sugar free.

Lozenges and Troches

These products are indicated in minor sore throat and in minor irritation of the throat or mouth. Severe and persistent sore throat or sore throat accompanied by high fever, headache, nausea and vomiting may be serious. Consult physician promptly. Do not use more than 2 days or in children less than 3 years of age, unless directed by physician.

In these combinations:

BENZOCAINE is a local anesthetic.

CETYLPYRIDINIUM CHLORIDE, EUCALYPTUS OIL, THYMOL, SODIUM and *HEXYLRESORCINOL* have antiseptic activity.

TERPIN HYDRATE is an expectorant.

MENTHOL, CAMPHOR, DYCLONINE and *PHENOL* are used for their antipruritic, mild local anesthetic and counterirritant activities.

ANTIPYRINE is an analgesic.

	Product	Composition	Description	C.I.*
otc	**Soretts** (Lannett)	**Lozenges:** 32 mg benzocaine, 8 mg licorice extract and 0.5 mg menthol	In 500s and 1000s.	1
otc sf	**Cylex Sugar Free** (Pharmakon)	**Lozenges:** 15 mg benzocaine, 5 mg cetylpyridinium chloride and sorbitol	Cherry flavor. In 12s.	NA
otc	**Cylex Throat** (Pharmakon)		Cherry flavor. In 12s.	NA
otc sf	**Mycinettes** (Pfeiffer)	**Lozenges:** 15 mg benzocaine, cetylpyridinium chloride, terpin hydrate, sodium citrate and sorbitol in a demulcent base	In 12s.	17
otc sf	**Medamint** (Dal Med)	**Lozenges:** 10 mg benzocaine	Cherry mint flavor. In 12s and 24s.	NA
otc	**Spec-T** (Apothecon)		(848). In 10s.	17
otc	**Tyrobenz** (Mallard)		In 500s.	4
otc	**Colrex** (Solvay Pharm.)	**Troches:** 10 mg benzocaine and 2.5 mg cetylpyridinium chloride	Red. In 20s.	16
otc	**Medikets** (Halsey)		In 10s and 18s.	17
otc	**Oradex-C** (Commerce)		In 10s.	17
otc	**Protac** (Republic)		In 10s.	27
otc	**Trocaine** (Vortech)	**Lozenges:** 10 mg benzocaine, 2.5 mg cetylpyridinium chloride and 15 mg terpin hydrate	In 1000s.	4
otc	**Cēpacol Anesthetic** (Lakeside Pharm.)	**Troches:** 10 mg benzocaine and 0.07% cetylpyridinium chloride	Tartrazine. In 18s and 324s.	15
otc sf	**Oracin** (Vicks Health Care)	**Lozenges:** 6.25 mg benzocaine and 0.1% menthol in a sorbitol base	Tartrazine. In 18s.	14
otc sf	**Oracin (Cherry)** (Vicks Health Care)	**Lozenges:** 6.25 mg benzocaine and 0.08% menthol	Sorbitol. Cherry flavor. In 18s.	14
otc	**Children's Chloraseptic** (Vicks Health Care)	**Lozenges:** 5 mg benzocaine	Grape flavor. In 18s.	11
otc	**T-Caine** (Schein)		In 1000s.	1
otc	**Lanazets Improved** (Lannett)	**Lozenges:** 5 mg benzocaine and 1 mg cetylpyridinium chloride	In 500s and 1000s.	1
otc	**Tymatro** (Bowman)	**Troches:** 5 mg benzocaine and 1.5 mg cetylpyridinium chloride	Mint flavor. In 1000s.	2
otc	**Vicks Throat** (Vicks Health Care)	**Lozenges:** 5 mg benzocaine, 1.66 mg cetylpyridinium Cl, menthol, camphor and eucalyptus oil	In 12s.	13
otc	**Conex** (Forest)	**Lozenges:** 5 mg benzocaine, 0.5 mg cetylpyridinium chloride	In 1000s.	2
otc	**Semets** (Beecham Labs)	**Troches:** 3 mg benzocaine and 1:1500 cetylpyridinium chloride	(BMP 135). Red. Cherry flavor. In 450s.	9
otc	**Sucrets Children's Formula** (SK Beecham)	**Lozenges:** 1.2 mg dyclonine HCl, corn syrup and sucrose	Cherry flavor. In 24s.	NA

* Cost Index based on cost per lozenge or troche. *sf* – Sugar free.

(Continued on following page)

Lozenges and Troches (Cont.)

	Product	Composition	Supplied	C.I.*
otc	**Cēpacol Throat** (Lakeside Pharm.)	**Lozenges:** 0.07% cetylpyridinium chloride and 0.3% benzyl alcohol	Tartrazine. In 27s and 400s.	8
otc	**Vapor Lemon Sucrets** (SK-Beecham)	**Lozenges:** 2 mg dyclonine HCl, sucrose	In 24s.	NA
otc	**Sucrets Maximum Strength** (Beecham Products)	**Lozenges:** 3 mg dyclonine HCl	In 24s, 48s and 55s.	9
otc	**Listerine Maximum Strength Throat** (Warner-Lambert)	**Lozenges:** 4 mg hexylresorcinol	In 24s.	8
otc	**Listerine Antiseptic** (Warner-Lambert)	**Lozenges:** 2.4 mg hexylresorcinol	Regular, cherry and lemon-mint flavors. In 24s.	8
otc	**Sucrets Sore Throat** (Beecham Products)		In regular and mentholated flavors. In 24s.	10
otc	**Cēpastat** (Lakeside Pharm.)	**Lozenges:** 1.45% phenol, 0.12% menthol, eucalyptus oil	Saccharin, sorbitol. In 18s.	14
otc	**Cēpastat Cherry** (Lakeside Pharm.)	**Lozenges:** 0.72% phenol and 0.12% menthol	Cherry flavor. Saccharin, sorbitol. In 18s.	14
otc	**Chloraseptic** (Vicks Health Care)	**Lozenges:** 32.5 mg phenol (as phenol and sodium phenolate)	Menthol and cherry flavors. In 18s and 36s.	11
otc	**Hall's Mentho-Lyptus** (Warner-Lambert)	**Lozenges:** Menthol and eucalyptus oil	Regular, sugar free regular, herbal, honey-lemon, cherry and ice blue flavors. In 9s and 30s.	3
otc	**Victors Vapor Cough** (Vicks Health Care)		In 10s.	4
otc	**Robitussin Cough Drops** (Robins Consumer)	**Lozenges:** 7.4 mg menthol (cherry and menthol eucalyptus flavors) or 10 mg menthol (honey-lemon) eucalyptus oil, sucrose, corn syrup	In 9s and 25s.	NA
otc	**Extra Strength Vicks Cough Drops** (Richardson-Vicks)	**Lozenges:** 8.4 mg menthol (menthol flavor) or 10 mg menthol (cherry and honey-lemon flavors), corn syrup and sucrose	In 9s and 30s.	NA
otc *sf*	**N'ice** (Beecham Products)	**Lozenges:** Menthol in a sorbitol base	Cherry, citrus, menthol eucalyptus and menthol mint flavors. In 8s and 16s.	14
otc	**Vicks Ice Blue Throat** (Vicks Health Care)	**Lozenges:** Menthol	Peppermint. In 14s and 40s.	3
otc	**Vicks Throat (Cherry)** (Vicks Health Care)		Cherry flavor. In 14s and 40s.	3
otc	**Vicks Throat (Lemon)** (Vicks Health Care)		Tartrazine. Lemon flavor. In 14s and 40s.	3
otc	**Vicks Throat** (Vicks Health Care)	**Lozenges:** Menthol, thymol, eucalyptus oil, camphor, tolu balsam and benzyl alcohol	Menthol flavor. In 14s and 40s.	3
otc	**Vicks Victors Dual Action Cough Drops** (Richardson-Vicks)	**Lozenges:** Menthol, eucalyptus oil, corn syrup, sucrose	Cherry flavor. In 30s.	NA
otc	**Throat Discs** (Marion)	**Lozenges:** Capsicum, peppermint, anise, cubeb, licorice and linseed	In 60s.	3

* Cost Index based on cost per lozenge.
sf –Sugar free.

Mouthwashes and Sprays

	Product	Composition	Supplied	C.I.*
otc	**Cēpacol** (Lakeside Pharm.)	**Mouthwash:** 0.05% cetylpyridinium chloride with 14% alcohol	Tartrazine, saccharin. In 360, 540, 720, 960 ml.	4
otc	**Scope** (Procter & Gamble)	**Mouthwash:** 0.45% cetylpyridinium chloride, 0.005% domiphen bromide and 18.5% SD alcohol 38F	Tartrazine, saccharin. Wintergreen flavor. In 180, 360, 540, 720, 960 and 1200 ml.	5
otc	**Listerine** (Warner-Lambert)	**Mouthwash:** Thymol, eucalyptol, methyl salicylate, menthol and 26.9% alcohol	In 90, 180, 360, 540, 720 and 960 ml.	56
otc	**Dobell's** (Purepac)	**Mouthwash/gargle:** 0.3% phenol glycerin, sodium borate and sodium bicarbonate	In 480 ml.	2
otc *sf*	**Chloraseptic** (Vicks Health Care)	**Mouthwash/gargle:** 1.4% phenol (as phenol and sodium phenolate)	In menthol and cherry flavors. Saccharin. In 180 and 360 ml.	10
		Throat Spray: 1.4% phenol (as phenol and sodium phenolate)	In menthol and cherry flavors. Saccharin. In 45, 240 and 360 ml.	30
otc	**Phenaseptic** (Barre)	**Mouthwash/gargle:** 1.4% phenol (as phenol and sodium phenolate), sodium borate, glycerin, menthol and thymol	In 240 ml.	5
otc *sf*	**Sucrets Maximum Strength** (Beecham)	**Mouthwash/gargle:** 0.1% dyclonine HCl and 10% alcohol	Sorbitol. Mint flavor. In 180 and 360 ml.	6
otc *sf*	**Sucrets Wintergreen** (Beecham Products)	**Throat Spray:** 0.1% dyclonine HCl and 10% alcohol	Sorbitol. In 90 ml.	NA
otc *sf*	**Larylgan** (Ayerst)	**Throat Spray:** 0.3% antipyrine, 0.05% pyrilamine maleate and 0.5% sodium caprylate. With menthol, gentian violet, methyl salicylate, benzyl alcohol, ethyl alcohol, glycerin, castor oil, parabens and other aromatics	Saccharin. In 28.2 ml.	51
otc	**Orasept** (Pharmakon)	**Throat Spray:** 10.16 mg benzocaine and 10.57 mg methylbenzethonium Cl per ml. With 67.36% ethanol, 70% sorbitol solution, glycerin and menthol	Saccharin and peppermint. In 45 ml.	NA
otc *sf*	**Ora Fresh** (AVP)	**Mouthwash:** Propylene glycol, sodium benzoate, methylparaben and zinc chloride	Saccharin. Alcohol free. Cinnamon flavor. In 30, 120 and 480 ml.	3
otc *sf*	**Ora Fresh** (AVP)	**Mouthwash:** Propylene glycol, glycerin, phenol and sodium phenate	Saccharin. Alcohol free. Peppermint flavor. In 480 ml.	3

MISCELLANEOUS PREPARATIONS C.I.*

These products contain:
STEROIDS (see p. 495), ANESTHETICS (see p. 280b), ANTISEPTICS (see p. 634).

	Product	Composition	Supplied	C.I.*
otc	**Numzident** (Purepac)	**Gel:** Benzocaine, oil of cloves, peppermint oil For alleviating the discomfort of denture irritation, toothache, sore gums, irritation from braces, fever blisters and cold sores.	In 14.1 g.	91
otc	**Maximum Strength Orajel** (Commerce)	**Gel:** 20% benzocaine For temporary relief of toothache.	In 5.3 and 9.45 g.	183
otc	**Maximum Strength Anbesol** (Whitehall)	**Liquid:** 20% benzocaine and 60% alcohol	In 9 ml.	NA
		Gel: 20% benzocaine and 60% alcohol To relieve minor irritations of teeth, mouth and lips.	In 7.2 g.	NA

* Cost Index based on cost per 5 ml or 5 g. *sf* – Sugar free.

(Continued on following page)

Miscellaneous Preparations (Cont.)

	Product	Description	Packaging	C.I.*
otc	**Orabase-O** (Colgate-Hoyt)	**Gel:** 20% benzocaine in polyethylene, mineral oil For temporary relief of pain caused by orthodontic appliances and sores of the mouth and gums.	In 15 g.	19
otc *sf*	**Orajel Brace-aid** (Commerce)	**Gel:** 20% benzocaine and allantoin For temporary relief of pain, soreness and irritation caused by orthodontic appliances.	Saccharin. In 14.1 g.	92
otc	**Benzodent** (Vicks Personal Care)	**Ointment:** 20% benzocaine, 0.1% hydroxyquinoline sulfate and 0.4% eugenol For relief of denture pain and discomfort.	In 7.5 and 30 g.	80
otc *sf*	**Orajel Mouth-Aid** (Commerce)	**Gel:** 20% benzocaine, 0.12% benzalkonium chloride, 0.1% zinc chloride and allantoin For minor mouth irritations.	Saccharin. In 9.45 g.	241
otc	**Orajel Mouth-Aid** (Commerce)	**Liquid:** 20% benzocaine, 0.1% cetylpyridinium chloride, 70% ethyl alcohol, ethyl cellulose, monoammonium glycyrrhizinate and povidone.	Tartrazine, saccharin. In 13.3 ml.	NA
otc *sf*	**Rid-A-Pain** (Pfeiffer)	**Gel:** 10% benzocaine and 7.5% alcohol For the temporary relief of pain from new or poorly fitting dentures and braces.	Dye free. In 10 g.	123
otc	**Oratect** (MGI)	**Gel:** 15% benzocaine in 65.8% SD alcohol	In 10.5 g.	NA
otc	**Orajel** (Commerce)	**Gel:** 10% benzocaine For temporary relief from toothache pain.	Saccharin. In 5.3 & 9.45 g.	146
otc	**Baby Anbesol** (Whitehall)	**Gel:** 7.5% benzocaine For the relief of teething pain.	Saccharin. In 7.2 g	NA
otc *sf*	**Baby Orajel** (Commerce)		In 9.45 g.	140
otc	**Orabase Baby** (Colgate-Hoyt)		Saccharin. In 7.2 g.	NA
otc *sf*	**Anbesol** (Whitehall)	**Liquid:** 6.3% benzocaine, 0.5% phenol, 70% alcohol, menthol, camphor and povidone-iodine **Gel:** 6.3% benzocaine, 0.5% phenol, 70% alcohol For relief of denture irritation, toothache, teething, sore gums, cold sores and fever blisters.	In 9 and 22 ml. In 7.2 g.	126 218
otc *sf*	**Orajel/d** (Commerce)	**Gel:** 10% benzocaine and eugenol To relieve pain and discomfort from dentures.	Saccharin. In 9.45 g.	127
otc	**Poloris Dental Poultice** (Block)	**Poultice:** 7.5 mg benzocaine and 4.6 mg capsicum To relieve minor irritations of teeth and gums.	In 5s and 12s.	28
otc	**Kank-a** (Blistex)	**Liquid:** 5% benzocaine, 0.5% cetylpyridinium chloride, castor oil and benzoin compound For mouth pain, canker and denture sores.	In 3.75 ml.	290
otc	**Jiffy Toothache Drops** (Block)	**Liquid:** 5% benzocaine, 9% eugenol, 2% menthol and 76% SD alcohol 38-B For relief of toothache due to cavity only.	In 3.75 ml.	190
otc	**Orasept** (Pharmakon Labs)	**Liquid:** 114.9 mg tannic acid, 14.4 mg methylbenzethonium HCl, 14.4 mg benzocaine and 61% ethyl alcohol per ml. With camphor, menthol, benzyl alcohol, spearmint oil and oil of Cassia. For mouth and gum irritations.	In 15 ml.	NA
otc	**Medadyne** (Dal Med)	**Liquid:** Methylbenzethonium chloride, benzocaine, tannic acid, camphor, chlorothymol, menthol, benzyl alcohol. With 61% alcohol. For the treatment of various oral conditions.	In 15 and 30 ml.	NA
otc	**Banadyne-3** (Norstar)	**Solution:** 4% lidocaine, 1% menthol, 45% alcohol	In 3 ml.	NA
otc *sf*	**Babee Teething Lotion** (Pfeiffer)	**Solution:** 2.5% benzocaine, 0.02% cetalkonium chloride, 20% alcohol, hamamelis water, propylene glycol, sodium benzoate, urea, menthol and camphor For teething discomfort or denture irritation.	Dye free. In 15 ml.	69
otc *sf*	**Rid-A-Pain Drops** (Pfeiffer)		In 15 ml.	69

* Cost Index based on cost per 5 ml, 5 g or poultice. *sf* – Sugar free.

(Continued on following page)

Miscellaneous Preparations (Cont.)

	Product (Manufacturer)	Composition / Use		C.I.*
otc	**Num-zit jel** (Purepac)	**Gel:** Benzocaine and menthol. For temporary relief of pain due to teething.	In 10 g.	129
otc	**Probax** (T/I Pharm)	**Gel:** 2% propolis, petrolatum, mineral oil and lanolin. For relief of cold sores and fever blisters.	In 3.5 g.	60
otc	**Num-zit** (Purepac)	**Lotion:** Benzocaine, menthol, glycerin, methylparaben and 12% alcohol. For relief of teething pain.	In 22.5 ml.	61
otc	**Pfeiffer's Cold Sore** (Pfeiffer)	**Lotion:** 7% gum benzoin, camphor, menthol, thymol, eucalyptol and 85% alcohol. For cold sores, fever blisters and cracked lips.	In 15 ml.	65
otc *sf*	**Tanac** (Commerce)	**Liquid:** 10% benzocaine, 0.12% benzalkonium chloride and 6% tannic acid. For mouth sores, canker sores, cold sores and fever blisters.	Saccharin. In 9 and 15 ml.	99
otc *sf*	**Tanac** (Commerce)	**Stick:** 7.5% benzocaine, 6% tannic acid, 0.75% octyl dimethyl PABA, 0.2% allantoin and 0.12% benzalkonium chloride. To relieve pain and discomfort of chapped or sun or wind burned lips, cold sores and fever blisters.	Saccharin. In 2.84 g stick.	44
otc *sf*	**Tanac Roll-On** (Commerce)	**Liquid:** 5% benzocaine, 6% tannic acid and 0.12% benzalkonium chloride. To relieve pain and promote healing of cold sores and fever blisters, and to soothe chapped or sun or wind burned lips.	Saccharin. In 10 ml.	138
otc	**Orabase Lip Healer** (Colgate-Hoyt)	**Cream:** 5% benzocaine, 1% allantoin, 0.5% menthol, petrolatum, lanolin, camphor, phenol	In 10 g.	NA
otc	**Orabase w/Benzocaine** (Colgate-Hoyt)	**Paste:** 20% benzocaine, gelatin, pectin and sodium carboxymethylcellulose in a polyethylene and mineral oil gel base. For relief from canker and denture sores and minor irritations of mouth and gums.	In 5 and 15 g.	150
Rx	**Kenalog in Orabase** (Apothecon)	**Paste:** 0.1% triamcinolone acetonide, gelatin, pectin and sodium carboxymethylcellulose in a polyethylene and mineral oil gel base. For adjunctive treatment and for the temporary relief of symptoms associated with oral inflammatory lesions and ulcerative lesions.	In 5 g.	788
Rx	**Oralone Dental** (Thames)		In 5 g.	500
Rx	**Orabase HCA** (Colgate-Hoyt)	**Paste:** 0.5% hydrocortisone acetate, gelatin, pectin and sodium carboxymethylcellulose in 5% polyethylene in mineral oil. For adjunctive treatment and for the temporary relief of symptoms associated with oral inflammatory lesions and ulcerative lesions.	Vanilla flavor. In 5 g.	500
otc	**HVS 1 + 2** (Chemi-Tech)	**Solution:** Benzalkonium chloride. For cold sores, fever blisters and herpes virus.	In 15 ml.	NA
otc	**Blistex Lip** (Blistex)	**Ointment:** 0.5% camphor, 0.5% phenol and 1% allantoin in a lanolin and mineral oil base. For dry, chapped lips, cold sores, fever blisters and sunburned or blistered lips.	In 4.2 and 10.5 g.	86
otc	**Herpecin-L** (Campbell Labs)	**Lip Balm:** Pyridoxine HCl, allantoin, padimate O and titanium dioxide in a balanced, acidic lipid system. For relief of dry and chapped lips, recurrent cold sores, and sun and fever blisters.	In 2.5 g.	60
otc	**Orabase Plain** (Colgate-Hoyt)	**Paste:** Gelatin, pectin & sodium carboxymethylcellulose in polyethylene and mineral oil gel. For temporary relief from minor irritations of the mouth and gums and denture discomfort.	In 5 and 15 g.	119

* Cost Index based on cost per 5 g or 5 ml. *sf* – Sugar free

(Continued on following page)

		Miscellaneous Preparations (Cont.)		C.I.*
otc	**Amosan** (Oral-B)	**Powder:** Sodium peroxyborate monohydrate derived from sodium perborate For adjunctive treatment of oral infections.	Saccharin. Peppermint, menthol and vanilla flavors. In 1.7 g UD packets (20s and 40s).	11
otc	**Peroxyl Mouthrinse** (Colgate-Hoyt)	**Solution:** 1.5% hydrogen peroxide and 6% alcohol For canker sores and minor dental inflammation.	Mint flavor. In 240 ml.	2
otc	**Perimed** (Olin)	**Rinse:** 1.5% hydrogen peroxide and 5% povidone-iodine For relief from minor gum inflammation and mouth and gum wounds.	Saccharin. In 20 ml pouches.	NA
otc	**Peroxyl** (Colgate-Hoyt)	**Gel:** 1.5% hydrogen peroxide For canker sores and cleaning minor wounds or gum inflammation.	Mint flavor. In 15 g.	25
otc	**Banadyne-3** (Inter-Hermes)	**Solution:** 4% lidocaine. For relief of cold sores, sun and fever blisters.	In 3 g.	NA
otc	**Medadyne** (Dal Med)	**Throat Spray:** Lidocaine, cetyl dimethyl ammonium chloride and ethyl alcohol. For relief of sore throat pain.	Spearmint flavor. In 30 ml.	NA
otc	**MG Cold Sore Formula** (Outdoor Recreations)	**Solution:** 1% menthol and lidocaine in a propylene glycol/alcohol base For the temporary relief of discomfort due to cold sores and fever blisters.	In 7.5 ml.	25
otc	**Lenate** (International Pharm.)	**Solution:** Menthol, guaifenesin, strong iodine tincture, phenol, glycerin and 2.5% alcohol For relief of cough, minor sore throat and minor skin irritations.	In 30, 120, 240 and 480 ml.	7
otc	**Butyn** (Abbott)	**Ointment:** 4% butacaine, 1% benzyl alcohol and eugenol For temporary relief of denture pain.	In 7.5 g.	45
otc	**Lip Medex** (Blistex)	**Ointment:** Petrolatum, 1% camphor, 0.54% phenol, cocoa butter, dimethyl oxazolidine and lanolin For treatment of fever blisters and sore, dry and cracked lips.	In 210 g.	4
otc	**ORA5** (McHenry)	**Liquid:** Copper sulfate, iodine, potassium iodide and 1.5% alcohol For relief of soreness and inflammation due to irritation.	In 3.75 and 30 ml.	87
otc	**Phylorinol** (Schaffer)	**Liquid:** 0.6% phenol, boric acid, strong iodine solution, sorbitol 70% solution, sodium copper chlorophyll For oral wounds and infections.	In 240 ml.	NA

PREPARATIONS FOR SENSITIVE TEETH

These toothpastes are specially formulated to replace regular toothpaste for persons with sensitive teeth. Use daily as in regular dental care.

				C.I.*
otc	**Denquel Sensitive Teeth** (Procter & G)	**Toothpaste:** 5% potassium nitrate	Mint flavor. In 48, 90 and 135 g.	3
otc	**Mint Sensodyne** (Block)		Saccharin, sorbitol. Mint flavor. In 28.3 g.	NA
otc	**Promise with Fluoride** (Block)	**Toothpaste:** 5% potassium nitrate and 0.76% sodium monofluorophosphate	Saccharin, sorbitol. In 48 and 90 g.	3
otc	**Sensodyne-F** (Block)		Saccharin, sorbitol. In 72 and 138 g.	3
otc	**Original Sensodyne** (Block)	**Toothpaste:** 10% strontium Cl hexahydrate	Saccharin, sorbitol. In 59.5 g.	NA

* Cost Index based on cost per g, ml or packet.

Antifungal Agents

Treatment of vaginal candidiasis (moniliasis) is complicated by a high recurrence rate due to the ubiquitous nature of *Candida albicans.* Predisposing factors include diabetes, antibiotics, pregnancy, corticosteroids, oral contraceptives and decreased host immunity.

Agents approved for local treatment of vulvovaginal candidiasis include nystatin (the polyene antibiotic), the imidazoles (butoconazole, clotrimazole, miconazole, tioconazole), terconazole (a triazole derivative) and gentian violet (a rosaniline dye). All these agents are fungicidal against *Candida.* Nystatin and gentian violet are fungistatic and fungicidal.

Confirm the diagnosis of vulvovaginal candidiasis prior to therapy by KOH smears or cultures. Terconazole is effective only for vulvovaginitis caused by the genus *Candida.* Tioconazole also exhibits fungicidal activity in vitro against *Torulopsis glabrata.* Other pathogens commonly associated with vulvovaginitis *(Trichomonas* and *Hemophilus vaginalis)* do not respond to these antifungal agents.

Actions:

Nystatin binds to sterols in the cell membrane of the fungus with a resultant change in membrane permeability allowing leakage of intracellular components. The primary action of imidazoles appears to be alteration of the permeability of the fungus cell membrane which allows leakage of essential intracellular components. The mechanism of action of **gentian violet** is unknown.

Terconazole's exact pharmacologic mode of action is uncertain. It may exert antifungal activity by disruption of normal fungal cell membrane permeability.

Pharmacokinetics: Approximately 5.5% of butoconazole is absorbed after vaginal administration; plasma half-life is 21 to 24 hours.

Terconazole – Following intravaginal administration, absorption ranged from 5% to 8% in three hysterectomized subjects and 12% to 16% in two non-hysterectomized subjects with tubal ligations.

Tioconazole – Systemic absorption in nonpregnant patients is negligible.

Indications:

Local treatment of vulvovaginal candidiasis (moniliasis).

Contraindications:

Hypersensitivity to specific drug or component of the product.

Warnings:

Pregnancy: Category A – Nystatin; Category B – Clotrimazole; Category C – Butoconazole, terconazole, tioconazole: No adverse effects or complications are reported in infants born to women treated with these agents. During pregnancy, use of a vaginal applicator may be contraindicated; manual insertion of tablets may be preferred. Use only on advice of physician.

Since small amounts of these drugs may be absorbed from the vagina, use during the first trimester only when essential. Use **butoconazole** only during the second and third trimesters. Possible exposure of the fetus through direct transfer of **terconazole** from an irritated vagina to the fetus by diffusion across amniotic membranes may occur.

Lactation: It is not known whether these drugs are excreted in breast milk. Safety for use during lactation has not been established. Temporarily discontinue nursing during administration.

Terconazole – Because of the potential for adverse reaction in nursing infants from terconazole, decide whether to discontinue nursing or to discontinue the drug, taking into account the importance of the drug to the mother.

Children: Terconazole, tioconazole – Safety and efficacy have not been established.

Precautions:

If irritation or sensitization occurs, discontinue use.

Intractable candidiasis may be a symptom of unrecognized diabetes mellitus. Perform urine and blood glucose studies on patients who do not respond to treatment. A persistently resistant infection may actually be due to reinfection; evaluate sources of reinfection.

Laboratory Tests: If there is lack of response, repeat microbiological studies to confirm diagnosis and rule out other pathogens before reinstituting antimycotic therapy.

Adverse Reactions:

Irritation, sensitization or vulvovaginal burning are generally rare.

Clotrimazole: Skin rash, lower abdominal cramps, bloating, slight urinary frequency; burning or irritation in the sexual partner occurs rarely. Intercurrent cystitis was reported in one vaginal cream user. Vaginal soreness with coitus, vaginal irritation, itching, burning and dyspareunia have also been reported.

Miconazole: Vulvovaginal symptoms (6.6%); pelvic cramps, hives, skin rash and headache were reported in $< 0.2\%$ of patients.

(Adverse Reactions continued on following page)

Refer to the general discussion of these products on page 2277

Antifungal Agents (Cont.)

Adverse Reactions (Cont.):

Butoconazole: Vulvar/vaginal burning (2.3%); patients discontinuing therapy (1.6%); vulvar itching (0.9%); discharge, soreness, swelling, itchy fingers (0.2%).

Terconazole: Headache (26%), body pain (2.1%). Vulvovaginal burning (5.2%), itching (2.3%) or irritation (3.1%) occurred less frequently with terconazole 0.4% vaginal cream than with the vehicle placebo. Rate of patients discontinuing therapy was 1.9%. Most frequent reason for discontinuing was vulvovaginal itching (0.6%), which was lower than the incidence for placebo (0.9%).

Photosensitivity reactions may occur following repeated dermal application of terconazole 2% and 0.8% creams under conditions of filtered artificial ultraviolet light.

Tioconazole: Burning (6%); itching (5%); irritation, discharge, vulvar edema and swelling, vaginal pain, dysuria, nocturia, dyspareunia, dryness of vaginal secretions, desquamation (< 1%).

Gentian violet: Staining of the skin.

Patient Information:

Patient instructions are enclosed with product.

Open applicator just prior to administration to prevent contamination *(tioconazole).*

Insert high into the vagina.

Complete full course of therapy. Use continuously, even during menstrual period.

Notify physician if burning or irritation occurs.

Refrain from sexual intercourse or advise partner to use condom to avoid reinfection.

Use sanitary napkin to prevent staining of clothing.

NYSTATIN

Administration and Dosage:

For oral use of nystatin, refer to page 2267 .

The usual dosage is 1 tablet (100,000 units) intravaginally daily for 2 weeks.

Symptomatic relief may occur in a few days; continue full course of treatment. **C.I.***

	Product	Form	Supplied	C.I.*
Rx	**Nystatin** (Various, eg, Balan, Bioline, Geneva, Goldline, Harber, Major, Moore, Purepac, Rugby, Schein)	**Vaginal Tablets:** 100,000 units	In 15s and 30s.	24+
Rx	**Mycostatin**[1] (Squibb)		(#Squibb 457). In 15s, 30s and UD 50s w/applicator.	93
Rx	**Nilstat** (Lederle)		(#LL N6). Yellow. In 15s and 30s w/applicator.	75
Rx	**O-V Statin**[1] (Squibb)	**Oral/Vaginal Therapy Pack:** 42 oral tablets (500,000 units nystatin) and 14 vaginal tablets (100,000 units nystatin) with applicator.		181

BUTOCONAZOLE NITRATE

Administration and Dosage:

Pregnant patients: (2nd and 3rd trimesters only): 1 applicatorful (≈ 5 g) intravaginally at bedtime for 6 days (see Warnings).

Nonpregnant patients: 1 applicatorful (≈ 5 g) intravaginally at bedtime for 3 days. May be extended to 6 days, if necessary. **C.I.***

	Product	Form	Supplied	C.I.*
Rx	**Femstat**[2] (Syntex)	**Vaginal Cream:** 2%	In 28 g with applicators.	277

TIOCONAZOLE

Administration and Dosage:

As a single dose; insert 1 applicatorful (≈ 4.6 g) intravaginally just prior to bedtime. **C.I.***

	Product	Form	Supplied	C.I.*
Rx	**Vagistat**[6] (Fujisawa SmithKline)	**Vaginal Ointment:** 6.5%	In 4.6 g prefilled applicator.	NA

* Cost Index based on cost per minimum daily dose.
\# Product identification code.
[1] Refrigerate below 15°C (59°F).
[2] Do not store above 40°C (104°F).
[3] Store between 2° and 30°C (36° & 86°F).
[4] Do not store above 35°C (95°F).
[5] Store below 30°C (86°F).
[6] Store between 15° and 30°C (59° & 86°F).

Refer to the general discussion of these products on page 2277

Antifungal Agents (Cont.)

CLOTRIMAZOLE

Administration and Dosage:

Tablets: Insert one 100 mg tablet intravaginally at bedtime for 7 nights or two 100 mg tablets intravaginally at bedtime for 3 nights.

Insert one 500 mg tablet intravaginally, one time only, preferably at bedtime.

Cream: One applicatorful (5 g) a day, preferably at bedtime, for 7 to 14 consecutive days. Patients treated for 14 days had a significantly higher cure rate. **C.I.***

	Product	Form/Strength	Description/Package	C.I.
otc	**Gyne-Lotrimin**[1] (Schering)	**Vaginal Tablets:** 100 mg	(Gyne-Lotrimin or Schering 734). White. In 6s or 7s with applicator.	248
Rx	**Mycelex-G**[2] (Miles Pharm.)		(Miles 093). White. In 7s with applicator.	213
Rx	**Gyne-Lotrimin**[3] (Schering)	**Vaginal Tablets:** 500 mg	(Schering 396). White. In 1s with applicator.	1244
Rx	**Mycelex-G**[3] (Miles Pharm.)		(Miles 097). White. In 1s with applicator.	1244
otc	**Mycelex-7** (Miles)	**Vaginal Tablets:** 100 mg with lactose	In 7s with applicator.	NA
		Vaginal Cream: 1%	In 45 g (7 day therapy) with applicator.	NA
Rx	**Mycelex Twin Pack** (Miles Pharm.)	**Cream:** 1%	In 7 g tube.	NA
		Tablets: 500 mg	(Miles 097). White. In twin packs.	1414
otc	**Gyne-Lotrimin**[1] (Schering)	**Vaginal Cream:** 1%	In 45 g (7 day) and 45 g twin-packs (14 day) w/applicator.	203
Rx	**Mycelex-G**[1] (Miles Pharm.)		In 45 g (7 day) and 90 g (14 day) with applicator.	203

MICONAZOLE NITRATE

Administration and Dosage:

Monistat 3: Insert 1 suppository intravaginally once daily at bedtime for 3 days.

Monistat 7: One applicatorful cream or 1 suppository intravaginally daily at bedtime for 7 days. Repeat course, if necessary, after ruling out other pathogens. **C.I.***

	Product	Form/Strength	Description/Package	C.I.
Rx	**Monistat 3** (Ortho Pharm.)	**Vaginal Suppositories:**[4] 200 mg	In 3s with applicator.	569
otc	**Monistat 7** (Ortho)	**Vaginal Cream:** 2%	45 g (7 doses) w/applicator.	244
		Vaginal Suppositories:[4] 100 mg	In 7s with applicator.	273
Rx	**Monistat Dual-Pak** (Ortho)	**Lotion:** 2%	In 30 and 60 ml.	NA
		Suppositories:[4] 200 mg	In 3s.	NA
		Cream: 2%	In 7s.	NA

TERCONAZOLE

Administration and Dosage:

Administer one full applicator (5 g) intravaginally once daily at bedtime for seven consecutive days. Before prescribing another course of therapy, reconfirm diagnosis by smears or cultures and rule out other pathogens commonly associated with vulvovaginitis. The therapeutic effect of terconazole is not affected by menstruation. **C.I.***

	Product	Form/Strength	Description/Package	C.I.
Rx	**Terazol 7** (Ortho)	**Vaginal Cream:**[5] 0.4%	In 45 g tube with applicator.	NA
Rx	**Terazol 3** (Ortho)	**Cream:** 0.8%	In 20 g tube with applicator.	NA
		Vaginal Suppositories:[5] 80 mg	In 3s w/applicator.	666

GENTIAN VIOLET

Administration and Dosage:

Insert one tampon intravaginally for 3 to 4 hours. Use once or twice daily for 12 days, or until vulvitis has disappeared. In resistant cases, use an additional tampon overnight. If infection persists, a second course of treatment may be required. **C.I.***

	Product	Form/Strength	Description/Package	C.I.
Rx	**Genapax** (Key Pharm.)	**Tampons:**[4] 5 mg	In 12s.	189

* Cost Index based on cost per minimum daily dose.
[1] Store at 2° to 30°C (36° to 86°F).
[2] Do not store above 35°C (95°F).
[3] Store below 30°C (86°F).
[4] Refrigerate below 15°C (59°F).
[5] Store at 13° to 30°C (59° to 86°F).

Miscellaneous Anti-infectives

SULFONAMIDES

Actions:

Sulfonamides exert a bacteriostatic action by competitive antagonism of para-aminobenzoic acid (PABA), an essential component of folic acid synthesis. Refer to page 1900 for additional information on sulfonamides.

Indications:

Triple Sulfa: Treatment of *Hemophilus vaginalis* vaginitis.

Sulfanilamide: For the treatment of *Candida albicans* vulvovaginitis only. Not effective against *Trichomonas vaginalis* or *Hemophilus vaginalis* vaginitis.

Contraindications:

Hypersensitivity to any component; kidney disease.

Warnings:

If local irritation develops or if systemic toxicity is evident, discontinue treatment.

Adverse Reactions:

Local irritations and, rarely, allergic reactions, pruritus and urticaria.

Patient Information:

Patient instructions are included with product.

Insert high into vagina (with applicator provided).

Complete full course of therapy.

Notify physician if burning, irritation or signs of a systemic allergic reaction occur.

	TRIPLE SULFA			C.I.*
Rx	**Sultrin Triple Sulfa** (Ortho)	**Vaginal Tablets:** 172.5 mg sulfathiazole, 143.75 mg sulfacetamide, 184 mg sulfabenzamide and urea *Dose:* 1 tablet intravaginally am and pm for 10 days; repeat if necessary.	In 20s with applicator.	118
Rx	**Triple Sulfa** (Various)	**Vaginal Cream:** 3.42% sulfathiazole, 2.86% sulfacetamide, 3.7% sulfabenzamide and 0.64% urea *Dose:* 1 applicatorful intravaginally twice daily for 4 to 6 days; treatment may then be reduced one half to one quarter.	In 78, 80, 82.5, 90 and 120 g.	5+
Rx	**Dayto Sulf** (Dayton)		In 78 g with applicator.	
Rx	**Femguard** (Reid-Rowell)		In 78 g with applicator.	24
Rx	**Gyne-Sulf** (G & W)		In 82.5 g with applicator	6
Rx	**Sulfa-Gyn** (Mayrand)		In 85 g with applicator.	11
Rx	**Sulfa-Trip** (Major)		In 82.5 g with applicator.	7
Rx	**Sultrin Triple Sulfa** (Ortho)		In 78 g with applicator.	28
Rx	**Trysul** (Savage)		In 78 g with applicator.	14
Rx	**V.V.S.** (Econo Med)		In 90 g with applicator.	13
	SULFANILAMIDE			
Rx	**Vagitrol** (Lemmon)	**Vaginal Cream:** 15% sulfanilamide *Dose:* 1 applicatorful intravaginally once or twice daily continued through one complete menstrual cycle.	In 120 g with applicator.	9
Rx	**AVC** (Merrell Dow)		In 120 g with applicator	114
Rx	**AVC** (Merrell Dow)	**Vaginal Suppositories:** 1.05 g sulfanilamide *Dose:* One suppository intravaginally once or twice daily; continue for 30 days.	In 16s.	114

* Cost Index based on cost per g, tablet or suppository.

In these combinations:

ANTIBIOTICS are used for infections due to susceptible organisms. Consult monographs on individual agents for spectrum of antimicrobial action.

SULFONAMIDES are used for infections due to susceptible organisms (see p. 2280).

ESTROGENS aid in a return to normal of the vaginal mucosa (see p 350).

COPPER SULFATE has mild antifungal activity.

OXYQUINOLINE BENZOATE and *AMINACRINE* are antiseptics.

ALLANTOIN may aid in debriding necrotic tissue and in tissue regeneration.

POLYOXYETHYLENE NONYL PHENOL, ALKYL ARYL SULFONATE, SODIUM LAURYL SULFATE and *DOCUSATE SODIUM* are wetting agents.

	Product	Formulation	Packaging	C.I.*
Rx	**Terramycin w/Polymyxin B Sulfate** (Roerig)	**Vaginal Tablets:** 100 mg oxytetracycline (as HCl) and 100,000 units polymyxin B sulfate *Dose:* 1 tablet twice daily, usually for 2 to 4 days.	In 10s.	70
Rx	**Par-Vag** (Parmed)	**Vaginal Suppositories:** 1.05 g sulfanilamide, 0.014 g aminacrine HCl and 0.14 g allantoin *Dose:* 1 twice daily. Continue through 1 complete menstrual cycle.	In 16s with applicator.	49
Rx	**Vagisec Plus** (Schmid)	**Vaginal Suppositories:** 6 mg aminacrine HCl, 5.25 mg polyoxyethylene nonyl phenol, 0.66 mg EDTA and 0.07 mg docusate sodium *Dose:* 1 twice daily. Continue through 2 menstrual cycles.	In 28s with applicator.	39
Rx	**Cantri** (Hauck)	**Vaginal Cream:** 10% sulfisoxazole, 0.2% aminacrine HCl and 2% allantoin. *Dose:* 1 applicatorful once or twice daily. Continue through 1 complete menstrual cycle.	In 90 g with applicator.	16
Rx	**Vagilia** (Lemmon)		In 90 g with applicator.	15
Rx	**Nil** (Century Pharm.)	**Vaginal Cream:** 15% sulfanilamide, 0.2% aminacrine HCl and 1.5% allantoin *Dose:* 1 applicatorful twice daily. Continue through 1 complete menstrual cycle.	In 120 g with applicator.	4
Rx	**Alasulf** (Major)	**Vaginal Cream:** 15% sulfanilamide, 0.2% aminacrine HCl and 2% allantoin *Dose:* 1 applicatorful once or twice daily. Continue through 1 complete menstrual cycle.	In 120 g.	4
Rx	**Benegyn** (Vortech)		In 96 g.	7
Rx	**Deltavac** (Trimen)		In 113.4 g with applicator.	10
Rx	**D.I.T.I-2** (Dunhall)		In 142 g.	9
Rx	**Par** (Parmed)		In 120 g with applicator.	7
Rx	**Vag** (Parmed)		In 113 g with applicator.	3

* Cost Index based on cost per tablet, suppository or g.

Vaginal douches are for general cleansing of the vaginal and perineal areas; for deodorizing; for relief of itching, burning and edema; for removing vaginal secretions or discharge; or for altering vaginal acidity.

BORIC ACID, POVIDONE-IODINE, CETYLPYRIDINIUM CHLORIDE, EUCALYPTOL, MENTHOL, OXYQUINOLINE, PHENOL, SODIUM PERBORATE and *THYMOL* may have antiseptic or germicidal activity.

Povidine-iodine also relieves minor irritation. It may be absorbed from the vagina; advise patients with thyroid disorders and pregnant patients to avoid iodine-containing douches.

EUCALYPTOL, MENTHOL, PHENOL, METHYL SALICYLATE and *THYMOL* are counterirritants used for their anesthetic or antipruritic effects.

AMMONIUM and *POTASSIUM ALUM, MICRONIZED ALUMINUM* and *ZINC SULFATE* are astringents that reduce local edema and inflammation; high concentrations can be irritating.

DOCUSATE SODIUM, OCTOXYNOL 9, ALKYL ARYL SULFONATE, SODIUM LAURYL SULFATE and *BENZALKONIUM CHLORIDE* are surfactants that facilitate douche spread over vaginal mucosa.

SODIUM PERBORATE, SODIUM BICARBONATE, LACTIC ACID, SODIUM ACETATE and *CITRIC ACID* affect pH.

Patient Information:

Consult manufacturers' recommendations for proper dilution and use of these products.

Vaginal douches are not contraceptive agents.

Douche no sooner than 6 hours after use of a vaginal spermicide.

If irritation occurs, discontinue use.

If infection or disease is suspected, consult physician.

	Product	Content	How Supplied
otc	**Triva Douche** (Boyle)	**Powder:** 2% oxyquinoline sulfate, 35% alkyl aryl sulfonate, 0.33% EDTA, 53% sodium sulfate and 9.67% lactose	In 3 g packets (24s).
otc	**Massengill Douche** (Beecham Products)	**Powder:** Ammonium alum, phenol, methyl salicylate, eucalyptus oil, menthol, thymol and sodium chloride	In 120, 240, 480 and 660 g and UD packets (10s and 12s).
otc	**Trichotine Douche** (Reed & Carnrick)	**Powder:** Sodium lauryl sulfate, sodium perborate and sodium chloride	In 150 and 360 g.
otc	**Inner Rinse Concentrate Douche** (Block Drug)	**Powder:** Sodium edetate, sodium lauryl sulfate, sodium borate and citric acid	In 60 and 120 g.
Rx	**Vagisec Douche** (Schmid)	**Solution:** Polyoxyethylene nonyl phenol, sodium edetate and docusate sodium	In 120 ml.
otc	**Trichotine Douche** (Reed & Carnrick)	**Solution:** Sodium lauryl sulfate, sodium borate and 8% alcohol	In 120 and 240 ml.
otc	**Zonite Douche** (Norcliff Thayer)	**Solution Concentrate:** 0.1% benzalkonium chloride, EDTA, sodium acetate, propylene glycol, menthol and thymol	In 240 and 360 ml.
otc	**Massengill Douche** (Beecham Products)	**Solution Concentrate:** Lactic acid, sodium lactate, sodium bicarbonate, SD alcohol 40 and octoxynol 9	In 120 and 240 ml.
otc	**Feminique Disposable Douche** (Schmid)	**Solution:** Sodium benzoate, sorbic acid, lactic acid and octoxynol 9	Baby powder or wildflower scents. In 150 ml twin-packs.
otc	**Massengill Baking Soda Freshness** (Beecham Products)	**Solution:** Sanitized water and sodium bicarbonate	In 180 ml.
otc	**Massengill Unscented** (Beecham Products)	**Solution:** Water, SD alcohol 40, lactic acid, sodium lactate, octoxynol-9, cetylpyridinium chloride, propylene glycol, diazolidinyl urea, parabens and EDTA	In 180 ml.

(Continued on following page)

	Product	Content	How Supplied
otc	**Acu-dyne Douche** (Acme United)	**Solution:** Povidone-iodine	In 195 ml packets.
otc	**Femidine Douche** (AVP)		In 240 ml.
otc	**Operand Douche** (Redi Products)		In 60, 240 and UD 15 ml.
otc	**Massengill Medicated Douche w/Cepticin** (Beecham Products)	**Liquid concentrate:** 12% povidone-iodine	In 120 and 240 ml.
otc	**Betadine Medicated Douche** (Purdue Frederick)	**Solution:** 10% povidone-iodine (0.3% when diluted)	In 15 and 240 ml packets.
otc	**Betadine Medicated Disposable Douche** (Purdue Frederick)	**Solution:** 0.3% povidone-iodine	In 6 ml vials with 180 ml bottle sanitized water.
otc	**Betadine Medicated Premixed Disposable Douche** (Purdue Frederick)		In 180 ml bottle.
otc	**Massengill Medicated Disposable Douche w/Cepticin** (Beecham Products)		In 180 ml bottle of sanitized water with 5 ml vial povidone-iodine.
otc	**Summer's Eve Medicated Disposable Douche** (Fleet)	**Solution:** 0.23% povidone-iodine when reconstituted	In 135 ml and 135 ml twin-packs.
otc	**Massengill Disposable Douche** (Beecham Products)	**Solution:** Alcohol, lactic acid, sodium lactate, octoxynol 9, propylene glycol and cetylpyridinium chloride[1]	In Belle-Mai, country flowers and mountain herbs scents. In 180 ml.
otc	**Summer's Eve Disposable Douche** (Fleet)	**Solution, regular:** Sodium citrate, citric acid and sodium benzoate **Solution, scented:** Sodium citrate, citric acid, octoxynol 9 and sodium benzoate	In 135 ml and 135 ml twin-packs. In herbal, musk[1] and white flowers scents. In 135 ml and 135 ml twin-packs.
otc	**Summer's Eve Post-Menstrual Disposable Douche** (Fleet)	**Solution:** Sodium lauryl sulfate, monosodium and disodium phosphates, sodium chloride and EDTA	In 135 ml and 135 ml twin-packs.
otc	**Feminique Disposable Douche** (Schmid)	**Solution:** Vinegar and water	In 150 ml twin-packs.
otc	**Massengill Disposable Douche** (Beecham Products)		In 180 ml.
otc	**Massengill Vinegar & Water Extra Mild** (Beecham Products)		Preservative free. In 180 ml.
otc	**Summer's Eve Disposable Douche** (Fleet)		In 135 ml and 135 ml twin-packs.
otc	**Massengill Vinegar & Water Extra Cleansing with Puraclean** (Beecham Products)	**Solution:** Vinegar, water, cetylpyridinium chloride, diazolidinyl urea and EDTA	In 180 ml.
otc	**New Freshness Douche** (Fleet)	**Solution:** Vinegar, water, octoxynol 9 and sorbic acid	**Concentrate:** In 120 and 240 ml. **Disposable:** In 135 ml and 135 ml twin-packs.

[1] With diazolidinyl urea.

Topical contraceptive agents provide spermicidal action which is generally reliable when properly used, either in conjunction with a vaginal diaphragm or as the sole method of contraception. These agents are generally less effective than oral contraceptives. To minimize the potential for conception, follow directions for use carefully.

Condom use and STD: The CDC advises the use of condoms to prevent sexually transmitted diseases (STD). If used properly, condoms help prevent infection by *Chlamydia trachomatis, Ureaplasma urealyticum, Trichomonas vaginalis, Candida albicans,* herpes simplex 1 and 2 (when lesions are on penis or female genital area), human papilloma virus, *Treponema pallidum, Hemophilus ducreyi* and human T-cell lymphotropic virus type III/lymphadenopathy-associated virus (AIDS).

Contraceptive vaginal sponge and nonoxynol 9 have been shown to protect against chlamydia and, to a lesser degree, gonorrhea; they have shown an increased risk of candida.

The following table gives ranges of pregnancy rates reported for various means of contraception. *The efficacy of these means of contraception (except IUD) depends upon the degree of adherence to the method.*

Method of Contraception	Pregnancies per 100 Woman-Years[1]
Oral Contraceptives	
35 mcg or more ethinyl estradiol	<1
50 mcg or more mestranol	<1
35 mcg or less ethinyl estradiol	>1
Progestin only	3
Mechanical/Chemical	
IUD	<1 to 3
Vaginal Sponge	9 to 16
Diaphragm (with cream or gel)	2 to 20
Condoms	3 to 20
Aerosol Foams	2 to 25
Gels and Creams	4 to 36
Rhythm (all types)	<1 to 47
Temperature method (intercourse only in postovulatory phase)	<1 to 7
Temperature method	1 to 20
Mucus method	1 to 25
Calendar method	14 to 47
Withdrawal	9 to 25
No contraception	60 to 80

[1] Number of pregnancies occurring per 100 women-years' exposure or number of pregnancies occurring in 100 sexually active women in 1 year.

Patient Information:

Consult manufacturers' recommendations for proper use of these products. The following general principles should be noted:

Use product prior to intercourse, but not more than 1 hour in advance.

Allow suppositories adequate time to disperse.

Reapply each time intercourse takes place.

Douching is not necessary; however, if a douche is desired for cleansing purposes, wait at least 6 hours following sexual intercourse.

Warnings:

Burning or irritation of the vagina or penis has been reported. In such cases, discontinue use and consult physician.

Controversy surrounds the relationship between the use of vaginal spermicides and congenital malformations. One study has suggested an association between vaginal spermicides and congenital anomalies (eg, limb-reduction deformities, neoplasms and chromosomal abnormalities). However, several other studies do not support these findings. The FDA concurs with the Advisory Committee on Fertility and Maternal Health Drugs that there is currently no need for a labeling revision of spermicidal products.

Toxic shock syndrome has been reported among a few women using the contraceptive sponge. Users who experience difficulty removing a sponge or sponge fragmentation should consult a physician.

(Products listed on following page)

Complete prescribing information for these products begins on page 2284				C.I.*
otc	**Delfen Contraceptive** (Ortho)	**Vaginal Foam:** 12.5% nonoxynol 9	In 20 g w/applicator and 20 & 50 g refills.	47
otc	**Koromex** (Schmid)		In 40 g.	14
otc	**Because** (Schering)	**Vaginal Foam:** 8% nonoxynol 9	In 10 g (6 dose contraceptor unit).	58
otc	**Emko** (Schering)		In 40 g w/applicator and 40 & 90 g refills.	24
otc	**Emko Pre-Fil** (Schering)		In 30 g w/applicator and 60 g refills.	35
otc	**Ramses** (Schmid)	**Vaginal Jelly:** 5% nonoxynol 9	In 150 g.	4
otc	**Koromex** (Schmid)	**Vaginal Jelly:** 3% nonoxynol 9	In 126 g.	5
otc	**Shur-Seal Gel** (Milex)	**Vaginal Jelly:** 2% nonoxynol 9	In 24 UD gel paks.	32
otc	**Conceptrol Disposable Contraceptive** (Ortho)	**Vaginal Gel:** 100 mg nonoxynol 9 per dose	In 2.5 g (6s and 10s).	43
otc	**Conceptrol Birth Control** (Ortho)	**Vaginal Cream:** 5% nonoxynol 9	In 70 g w/applicator and 70 g refills.	17
otc	**Intercept Contraceptive Inserts** (Ortho)	**Vaginal Suppositories:** 100 mg nonoxynol 9	In 12s with applicator and 12 refills.	54
otc	**Encare** (Thompson Medical)	**Vaginal Suppositories:** 2.27% nonoxynol 9	In 12s and 24s.	49
otc	**Semicid** (Whitehall)	**Vaginal Suppositories:** 100 mg nonoxynol 9	In 10s and 20s.	65
otc	**VCF** (Apothecus)	**Vaginal Film:** 28% nonoxynol 9	In 3, 6s and 12s.	

The following products are for use in conjunction with a vaginal diaphragm:

otc	**Ortho-Gynol Contraceptive** (Ortho)	**Vaginal Jelly:** 1% octoxynol 9	In 75 g w/applicator and 75 and 114 g refills.	13
otc	**Gynol II Contraceptive** (Ortho)	**Vaginal Jelly:** 2% nonoxynol 9	In 75 g w/applicator and 75 and 114 g refills.	14
otc	**Koromex Crystal Clear** (Schmid)	**Vaginal Gel:** 2% nonoxynol 9	In 126 g and 126 g w/applicator.	6
otc	**Ortho-Creme Contraceptive** (Ortho)	**Vaginal Cream:** 2% nonoxynol 9	In 64.5 g and 103.5 g.	12
otc	**Koromex** (Schmid)	**Vaginal Cream:** 3% octoxynol	In 115 g w/applicator.	6

A disposable vaginal contraceptive sponge permeated with the spermicide nonoxynol 9. The sponge provides barrier protection by blocking the cervix. Semen is absorbed by the sponge and spermicide is released even during multiple acts of intercourse. Effective for up to 24 hours, the sponge must remain in place for at least 6 hours after intercourse.

otc	**Today** (VLI)	**Sponge:** 1 g nonoxynol 9	In 3s, 6s and 12s.	111

A latex condom with a lubricant containing the spermicide nonoxynol 9. The combination of barrier protection combined with the spermicide improves contraceptive effectiveness over traditional condoms.

otc	**Excita Extra** (Schmid)	**Condom:** 5.6% nonoxynol 9	Ribbed. In 12s.	83
otc	**Koromex** (Schmid)		In 12s.	90
otc	**Ramses Extra** (Schmid)		In 12s.	80
otc	**Sheik Elite** (Schmid)		In 12s.	68

* Cost Index based on cost per g or suppository.

	Product	Supplied	C.I.*
otc	**Betadine** (Purdue Frederick) **Gel:** 10% povidone iodine **Suppositories:** 10% povidone-iodine **Indications:** Relief of irritation, itching & soreness. **Dosage:** 1 applicator of gel or 1 supp. at night for 7 days.	In 0.006, 18 and 120 g w/applicator. In 7s w/applicator.	27 105
otc	**Lubrin** (Upsher-Smith) **Inserts:** Caprylic/capric triglyceride, glycerin and laureth-23 **Indications:** Prolonged lubrication for sexual intercourse. **Dosage:** 1 intravaginally 5 to 30 minutes before intercourse. Allow 5 to 10 minutes for insert to dissolve.	In 5s.	54
otc	**Vaginex** (Schmid) **Cream:** Tripelennamine HCl **Indications:** Temporary relief of external vaginal irritation. **Dosage:** Apply externally 3 or 4 times a day.	In 30 g.	7
Rx	**Aci-Jel** (Ortho) **Jelly:** 0.92% acetic acid, 0.025% oxyquinoline sulfate, 0.7% ricinoleic acid and 5% glycerin **Indications:** Restoration and maintenance of vaginal acidity. **Dosage:** 1 applicatorful intravaginally morning and evening.	In 85 g w/ applicator.	22
otc	**Replens** (Warner Labs.) **Gel:** Glycerin, mineral oil, polycarbophil, carbomer 934P, hydrogenated palm oil glyceride, methylparaben, sorbic acid **Indications:** Replenishes vaginal moisture. **Dosage:** Apply internally.	In 12 pre-filled applicators.	NA
otc	**Astroglide** (Astro-Lube) **Gel:** Glycerin, propylene glycol, polyquaternium #5, methyl and propyl parabens. **Indications:** Vaginal lubricant. **Dosage:** Apply externally or internally.	In 70.5 ml bottle and 3 ml travel packets.	NA
otc	**K-Y** (Johnson & Johnson) **Jelly:** Glucono delta lactate, sodium hydroxide, glycerin, chlorhexidine gluconate and hydroxyethylcellulose **Indications:** As a sexual lubricant and aid for easy insertion of rectal thermometers and tampons. **Dosage:** Apply to area and repeat if necessary.	In 2.7 and 5 g single-use and 5 and 60 g tubes.	3
otc	**Maxilube Personal Lubricant** (Mission) **Jelly:** Water, silicone oil, glycerin, carbomer 934, triethanolamine, sodium lauryl sulfate, parabens. **Indications:** Vaginal lubricant.	In 90 g.	NA
otc	**Personal Lubricant** (Ortho) **Gel:** Glycerin, propylene glycol and sodium carboxymethylcellulose, sodium alginate, sorbic acid **Indications:** Lubricant for sexual intercourse and easy insertion of rectal thermometers, tampons, douches, enemas. **Dosage:** Apply externally or internally.	In 60 and 120 g tubes.	4
otc	**Surgel** (Ulmer) **Gel:** Sodium carboxymethylcellulose, propylene glycol, glycerin and phenylmercuric nitrate **Indications:** Vaginal lubricant.	In 120, 240 and pt and gal.	NA
otc	**Gyne-Moistrin** (Schering-Plough) **Gel:** Polyglyceryl methacrylate, propylene glycerol, parabens	In 45 g.	NA
otc	**Trimo-San** (Milex) **Jelly:** 0.025% oxyquinoline sulfate, 1% boric acid, 0.7% sodium borate, sodium lauryl sulfate & glycerin **Indications:** Controls odor-causing bacteria. **Dosage:** ⅕ to 1 full applicator no more than twice a week.	In 120 g w/ applicator.	9
Rx	**Amino-Cerv pH 5.5 Creme** (Milex) **Cream:** 8.34% urea, 0.5% sodium propionate, 0.83% methionine, 0.35% cystine, 0.83% inositol, benzalkonium chloride **Indications:** Mild cervicitis, postpartum cervicitis/cervical tears, postcauterization, postcryosurgery & postconization. **Dosage:** See manufacturer's information for complete administration and dosage.	Water miscible base. In 82.5 g w/applicator and 82.5 g refill.	14

* Cost Index based on cost per g, suppository or insert.

The anorectal preparations are used primarily for the symptomatic relief of the discomfort associated with hemorrhoids and perianal itching or irritation. In addition to the products specifically listed in this section, many of the Topical Local Anesthetics and Topical Corticosteroids may also be used locally in anorectal therapy.

Ingredients:

The various components of these products are briefly discussed below. For complete information on specific indications, contraindications, precautions and adverse effects of ingredients, refer to the appropriate monographs as indicated.

HYDROCORTISONE (see page 2370) reduces inflammation, itching and swelling. Steroids are contraindicated in fungal and most viral lesions of the skin, including herpes, vaccinia and varicella.

LOCAL ANESTHETICS (benzocaine, dibucaine, diperodon, pramoxine) temporarily relieve pain, itching and irritation. The most frequent adverse effect of topical local anesthetic use are allergic reactions (ie, burning and itching). Their safety and efficacy when used intrarectally require further evaluation. (See page 2387).

VASOCONSTRICTORS (ephedrine, epinephrine or phenylephrine) reduce swelling and congestion of anorectal tissues. They relieve local itching by a slight anesthetic effect. These agents are not effective in stopping bleeding from venous tissues.

ASTRINGENTS (witch hazel, zinc oxide) coagulate the protein in skin cells, protecting the underlying tissue and decreasing the cell volume. They lessen mucus and other secretions, and relieve anorectal irritation and inflammation.

ANTISEPTICS (benzalkonium chloride, boric acid, cetalkonium, cetylpyridinium Cl, hydroxyquinoline, phenol, phenylmercuric nitrate) are not of therapeutic value when applied to the anorectal area. There is no convincing evidence that they prevent infection in the anorectal area. Many are present as preservatives.

EMOLLIENTS/PROTECTANTS (cod liver oil, glycerin, lanolin, mineral oil, petrolatum, zinc oxide, cocoa butter, shark liver oil, bismuth salts) form a physical barrier on the skin and lubricate tissues, preventing irritation of the anorectal area and water loss from the stratum corneum. Many of these substances are used as bases and carriers of pharmacologically active compounds.

COUNTERIRRITANTS (menthol, camphor) evoke a feeling of comfort, cooling, tingling or warmth and distract the perception of pain and itching.

KERATOLYTICS (alcloxa, allantoin, resorcinol) cause desquamation and sloughing of epidermal surface cells and may help to expose underlying tissue to therapeutic agents.

WOUND-HEALING AGENTS (balsam Peru; skin respiratory factor or SRF; yeast cell derivative) are claimed to promote wound healing or tissue repair. Effectiveness of these compounds has not been conclusively demonstrated.

ANTICHOLINERGIC AGENTS (belladonna extract, pyrilamine) inhibit the action of acetylcholine. Since these agents produce their action systemically, they are not effective in ameliorating local symptoms of anorectal disease.

MISCELLANEOUS – *Laxatives* may be added to ease constipation. *Escherichia coli* vaccines have not been proven safe and effective for anorectal disorders.

Patient Information:

Maintain normal bowel function by proper diet, adequate fluid intake and regular exercise.

Avoid excessive laxative use.

Stool softeners or bulk laxatives may be useful adjunctive therapy.

If anorectal symptoms do not improve in 7 days, or if bleeding, protrusion or seepage occurs, consult a physician.

(Products listed on following pages)

Refer to the general discussion of these products on page 538.

		Steroid-Containing Products		C.I.*
Rx	**Proctocort** (Solvay Pharm.)	**Cream:** 1% hydrocortisone	In 30 g with applicator.	27
Rx	**Analpram-HC** (Ferndale)	**Cream:** 1% hydrocortisone acetate and 1% pramoxine HCl	In 30 g with applicators.	36
Rx	**ProctoCream-HC** (Reed & Carnrick)		In 30 g.	56
Rx	**Proctofoam-HC** (Reed & Carnrick)	**Aerosol Foam:** 1% hydrocortisone acetate and 1% pramoxine HCl in a hydrophilic foam base	In 10 g with applicator.	153
Rx	**Anucort-HC** (G & W Labs)	**Suppositories:** 25 mg hydrocortisone acetate	In 12, 24s and 100s.	NA
Rx	**Anuprep HC** (Great Southern)		In 12s.	77
Rx	**Anusol-HC** (Parke-Davis)		In 12s and 24s.	157
Rx	**Cort-Dome High Potency** (Miles Pharm.)		In 12s.	284
Rx	**Hemril-HC Uniserts** (Upsher-Smith)		In 12s.	NA
Rx	**Anumed HC** (Major)	**Suppositories:** 10 mg hydrocortisone acetate, 2.25% bismuth subgallate, 1.75% bismuth resorcin compound, 1.2% benzyl benzoate, 1.8% balsam Peru and 11% zinc oxide	In 12s.	63
Rx	**Hemorrhoidal HC** (Various)		In 12s, 50s, 100s & UD 12s.	40+
Rx	**Rectacort** (Century)		In 12s.	46

* Cost Index based on cost per g or suppository.

Refer to the general discussion of these products on page 2287

Local Anesthetic-Containing Products

	Product	Composition	Supplied	C.I.*
otc	**Rectagene Medicated Rectal Balm** (Pfeiffer)	**Ointment:** 3% benzocaine, 0.2% phenylephrine HCl, 1% bismuth subgallate, 1.5% zinc oxide, pyrilamine maleate and cetalkonium Cl in a polyethylene glycol base	In 30 g.	9
otc	**Medicone Rectal** (Medicone)	**Ointment:** 2% benzocaine, 0.5% hydroxyquinoline sulfate, 10% zinc oxide, 0.4% menthol, 1.26% castor oil and 1.26% balsam Peru in 83.6% petrolatum-lanolin	In 45 g with applicator.	10
otc	**Pazo Hemorrhoid** (Bristol-Myers)	**Ointment:** 0.8% benzocaine, 0.2% ephedrine sulfate, 2.18% camphor, 4% zinc oxide, lanolin and petrolatum	In 30 and 60 g with applicator.	12
otc	**Primaderm-B** (Arrow Medical)	**Ointment:** Benzocaine, zinc oxide, cod liver oil in a petrolatum-lanolin base	In 30 and 60 g.	14
otc	**Americaine** (Fisons)	**Ointment:** 20% benzocaine and 0.1% benzethonium chloride in a water-soluble base	In 30 g.	11
otc	**Fleet Relief Anesthetic Hemorrhoidal** (Fleet)	**Ointment:** 1% pramoxine HCl in a greaseless, water-soluble base	In 30 g with applicator and 6s prefilled.	11
otc	**Anusol** (Parke-Davis)	**Ointment:** 1% pramoxine HCl, 1.2% benzyl benzoate, 1.8% balsam Peru and 11% zinc oxide with mineral oil and polyethylene wax	In 30 and 60 g with applicator.	11
otc	**A-Caine Rectal** (A.V.P.)	**Ointment:** 0.25% diperodon HCl, 0.1% pyrilamine maleate, 0.25% phenylephrine HCl, 0.2% bismuth subcarbonate and 5% zinc oxide in a cod liver oil and petrolatum base	In 45 g.	9
otc	**Hemocaine** (Mallard)		In 37.5 g.	8
otc	**Hemet Rectal** (Halsey)		In 37.5 g.	7
otc	**Tronolane** (Ross)	**Cream:** 1% pramoxine HCl in a nongreasy zinc oxide base	In 30 and 60 g.	13
otc	**Rectal Medicone** (Medicone)	**Suppositories:** 130 mg benzocaine, 16 mg hydroxyquinoline sulfate, 195 mg zinc oxide, 9 mg menthol and 65 mg balsam Peru in a vegetable and petroleum oil base	Green. In 12s and 24s.	36
otc	**Pazo Hemorrhoid** (Bristol-Myers USP)	**Suppositories:** 15.4 mg benzocaine, 3.8 mg ephedrine sulfate, 42 mg camphor and 77.2 mg zinc oxide in a vegetable oil base	In 12s and 24s.	37
otc	**Hem-Prep** (G & W)	**Suppositories:** Shark liver oil, 1:10,000 phenylmercuric nitrate, bismuth subgallate, zinc oxide and benzocaine	In 12s and 24s.	16
otc	**Medicone** (Dickinson)	**Suppositories:** Live yeast cell extract, 3% shark liver oil in cocoa butter base	In 12s.	NA
otc	**Anocaine Hemorrhoidal** (Mallard)	**Suppositories:** Benzocaine, zinc oxide, bismuth subgallate and balsam Peru in a vegetable oil base	In 12s.	30
otc	**Hemet Hemorrhoidal** (Halsey)		In 12s.	19
otc	**Tronolane** (Ross)	**Suppositories:** 1% pramoxine and pramoxine HCl in a zinc oxide base	In 10s and 20s.	42
otc	**Perifoam** (Reid-Rowell)	**Aerosol Foam:** 1% pramoxine HCl, 0.1% benzalkonium chloride, 0.3% allantoin, solubilized lanolin and 35% witch hazel with methyl and propyl parabens	In 45 g.	13
otc	**ProctoFoam** (Reed & Carnrick)	**Aerosol Foam:** 1% pramoxine HCl in an anesthetic mucoadhesive foam base	In 15 g with applicator.	61

* Cost Index based on cost per g or suppository.

Refer to the general discussion of these products on page 2287

Miscellaneous Combinations

	Product	Composition	How Supplied	C.I.*
otc	**Preparation H** (Whitehall)	**Ointment:** Live yeast cell derivative supplying 2000 units skin respiratory factor per 30 g with 3% shark liver oil, petrolatum, cellulose gum, citric acid, EDTA, glycerin, glyceryl stearate, lanolin, parabens, propylene glycol, simethicone, sodium lauryl sulfate, glyceryl oleate	In 27 and 54 g.	14
otc	**Rectagene Medicated Balm** (Pfeiffer)	**Ointment:** Live yeast cell derivative supplying 2000 units Skin Respiratory Factor per 30 g, 3% refined shark liver oil, white petrolatum, lanolin, thyme oil, 1:10,000 phenyl mercuric nitrate	In 56.7 g.	NA
otc	**Preparation H** (Whitehall)	**Suppositories:** Live yeast cell derivative supplying 2000 units Skin Respiratory Factor per ounce of suppository base, 3% shark liver oil, 1:10,000 phenylmercuric nitrate and PEG 600 dilaurate	In 12s, 24s, 36s and 48s.	43
otc	**Calmol 4** (Mentholatum)	**Suppositories:** 80% cocoa butter, 10% zinc oxide and bismuth subgallate	In 12s and 24s.	36
otc	**Nupercainal** (Ciba Consumer)	**Suppositories:** 2.4 g cocoa butter, 0.25 g zinc oxide and bismuth subgallate	In 12s and 24s.	39
otc	**Wyanoids** (Wyeth)	**Suppositories:** 3 mg ephedrine sulfate and 15 mg extract belladonna with boric acid, zinc oxide, bismuth oxyiodide, bismuth subcarbonate and balsam Peru	In 12s.	39
otc	**Anumed** (Major)	**Suppositories:** 2.25% bismuth subgallate, 1.75% bismuth resorcin compound, 1.2% benzyl benzoate, 11% zinc oxide and 1.8% balsam Peru in a hydrogenated vegetable oil base	In 12s.	21
otc	**Anuprep Hemorrhoidal** (Great Southern)		In 12s and 24s.	NA
otc	**Anusol** (Parke-Davis)		In 12s, 24s, 48s.	37
otc	**CPI** (Century Pharm.)		In 12s.	14
otc	**Hemril Uniserts** (Up-S)		In 12s and 50s.	NA
otc	**Rectagene II** (Pfeiffer)	**Suppositories:** 2.25% bismuth subgallate, 1.75% bismuth resorcin compound, 1.2% benzyl benzoate, 1.8% balsam Peru, 11% zinc oxide, bismuth subiodide and calcium phosphate	In 12s.	NA

Perianal Hygiene Products

	Product	Composition	How Supplied	C.I.*
otc	**Gentz** (Roxane)	**Wipes:** 1% pramoxine HCl, 0.2% alcloxa, 50% witch hazel, 10% propylene glycol	In 120s and UD 100s.	25
otc	**Tucks** (Parke-Davis)	**Pads:** 50% witch hazel and 10% glycerin with 0.003% benzalkonium Cl, citric acid	In 40s & 100s.	10
otc	**Tucks Take-Alongs** (P-D)		In 12s.	18
otc	**Mediconet** (Medicone)	**Wipes:** 50% witch hazel, 10% glycerin, 0.02% benzalkonium Cl, 0.5% ethoxylated lanolin with 0.15% methylparaben	In 20s.	23
otc	**Preparation H Cleansing** (Whitehall)	**Pads:** 50% witch hazel, 7.4% alcohol, glycerin, octoxynol 9 and methylparaben	In 40s and 100s.	9
otc	**Balneol Perianal Cleansing** (Solvay)	**Lotion:** Mineral oil, propylene glycol, glyceryl stearate, PEG-100 stearate, PEG-40 stearate, laureth-4, PEG-4 dilaurate, lanolin oil, sodium acetate, carbomer 934, triethanolamine, methylparaben, docusate sodium and acetic acid	In 120 ml.	4
otc	**Aloe Vesta Perineal** (Vestal Labs)	**Solution:** Sodium C_{14-16} olefin sulfonate, amphoteric 2, propylene glycol, aloe vera gel, TEA-coco hydrolyzed protein with sorbitol and DMDM hydantoin	In 120 and 240 ml and gal.	1
otc	**Preparation H Cleansing Tissues** (Whitehall)	**Tissues:** Propylene glycol, phenoxyethanol, parabens, citric acid	In travel pack and 40s.	NA

* Cost Index based on cost per g, suppository, ml or wipe.

TRETINOIN (*trans*-Retinoic Acid, Vitamin A Acid)

Actions:

Although the exact mode of action of tretinoin is unknown, current evidence suggests that topical tretinoin decreases cohesiveness of follicular epithelial cells with decreased microcomedone formation. Additionally, tretinoin stimulates mitotic activity and increased turnover of follicular epithelial cells, causing extrusion of the comedones. It does not alter bacterial skin counts.

Indications:

Topical treatment of acne vulgaris.

Unlabeled Use: Tretinoin has been used to treat several different forms of skin cancer, lamellar ichthyosis and Darier's disease.

Contraindications:

Hypersensitivity to any component.

Warnings:

Photosensitivity: Studies in mice suggest that tretinoin may accelerate the tumorigenic potential of ultraviolet radiation. Although the significance to man is not clear, avoid or minimize exposure to sun.

It is advisable to "rest" a patient's skin until effects of keratolytic agents subside before beginning tretinoin. Minimize exposure to sunlight and sunlamps and advise patients with sunburn not to use tretinoin until fully recovered because of heightened susceptibility to sunlight as a result of use. Patients who undergo considerable sun exposure due to occupation and those with inherent sun sensitivity should exercise particular caution. Use sunscreen products and protective clothing over treated areas. Other weather extremes, such as wind and cold, also may be irritating.

Keep tretinoin away from the eyes, mouth, angles of the nose and mucous membranes.

Tretinoin may induce severe local erythema and peeling at the application site. If the degree of local irritation warrants, use medication less frequently, discontinue use temporarily or completely. Tretinoin may cause severe irritation to eczematous skin; use with caution in patients with this condition.

Usage in Pregnancy: Category B. Reproduction studies performed in rats and rabbits at dermal doses up to 50 times the human dose (assuming the human dose to be 500 mg of gel per day) have revealed no evidence of impaired fertility or fetal harm. There was, however, a slightly higher incidence of irregularly contoured or partially ossified skull bones in some fetuses. There are no adequate and well controlled studies in pregnant women. Use this drug during pregnancy only if clearly needed.

Usage in Lactation: It is not known whether this drug is excreted in breast milk. Exercise caution when tretinoin is administered to a nursing mother.

Precautions:

Redness, peeling or discomfort may occur if medication is applied excessively, and results will not be improved.

Drug Interactions:

Sulfur, resorcinol, benzoyl peroxide or **salicylic acid:** Cautiously use concomitant topical keratolytic medications because of possible interactions with tretinoin. Significant skin irritation may result.

Use medicated or abrasive soaps and cleansers, soaps and cosmetics that have a strong drying effect and products with high concentrations of alcohol, astringents, spices or lime cautiously because of possible interaction with tretinoin.

Adverse Reactions:

Sensitive skin may become excessively red, edematous, blistered or crusted. If these effects occur, discontinue medication until skin integrity is restored or adjust to a tolerable level. True contact allergy is rare.

Temporary hyperpigmentation or hypopigmentation has been reported with repeated application. Some individuals have a heightened susceptibility to sunlight while under treatment.

All adverse effects have been reversible upon discontinuation.

(Continued on following page)

TRETINOIN (*trans*-Retinoic Acid, Vitamin A Acid) (Cont.)

Patient Information:

Patient instructions available with product.

Keep away from eyes, mouth, angles of nose and mucous membranes.

Avoid excessive exposure to sunlight and sunlamps.

Application may cause transitory feeling of warmth and slight stinging. Redness and peeling may occur; if excessive redness or discomfort occurs, decrease or discontinue use temporarily.

Normal use of cosmetics is permissible.

Administration and Dosage:

Apply once a day, before retiring. Cover the entire affected area lightly. Thoroughly wash hands immediately after applying tretinoin.

Liquid: Apply with fingertip, gauze pad or cotton swab. Do not oversaturate gauze or cotton to the extent that liquid will run into unaffected areas.

Gel: Excessive application results in "pilling" of the gel, which minimizes the likelihood of overapplication by the patient.

Some patients require less frequent applications or the lower strength dosage forms; others may respond better to more frequent applications. Closely monitor alterations of vehicle, drug concentration or dose frequency. During the early weeks of therapy, an exacerbation of inflammatory lesions may occur due to the action of the medication on deep, previously undetected lesions; this is not a reason to discontinue therapy.

Therapeutic results should be seen after 2 to 3 weeks, but may not be optimal until after 6 weeks. Once lesions have responded satisfactorily, maintain therapy with less frequent applications or other dosage forms.

Patients may use cosmetics, but thoroughly cleanse area to be treated before applying medication.

				C.I.*
Rx	**Retin-A** (Ortho)	**Cream:** 0.025% in a hydrophilic vehicle	In 20 and 45 g.	650
		0.05% in a hydrophilic vehicle	In 20 and 45 g.	742
		0.1% in a hydrophilic vehicle	In 20 g.	927
		Gel: 0.025% with 90% alcohol	In 15 and 45 g.	870
		0.01% with 90% alcohol	In 15 and 45 g.	870
		Liquid: 0.05% with PEG-400, butylated hydroxytoluene and 55% alcohol	In 28 ml.	908

* Cost Index based on cost per g or ml.

ISOTRETINOIN (13-*cis*-Retinoic Acid)

Warnings:

Women who are pregnant or who may become pregnant must not use isotretinoin. There is an extremely high risk that a deformed infant will result if pregnancy occurs while taking this drug in any amount even for short periods. Potentially all exposed fetuses can be affected.

Contraindicated in women of childbearing potential unless the **patient meets all of the following conditions:**

- has severe disfiguring cystic acne that is recalcitrant to standard therapies
- is reliable in understanding and carrying out instructions
- is capable of complying with the mandatory contraceptive measures
- has received both oral and written warnings of the hazards of taking isotretinoin during pregnancy and the risk of possible contraception failure and has acknowledged her understanding of these warnings in writing
- has had a negative **serum** pregnancy test within 2 weeks prior to beginning therapy. (It is also recommended that pregnancy testing and contraception counseling be repeated on a monthly basis.)
- will begin therapy only on the second or third day of the next normal menstrual period

Major human fetal abnormalities related to use of the drug have included hydrocephalus, microcephalus, external ear abnormalities (micropinna, small or absent external auditory canals), microphthalmia, facial dysmorphia, cleft palate, cardiovascular abnormalities, thymus gland abnormalities, parathyroid hormone deficiency and cerebellar malformation. There is also an increased risk of spontaneous abortion.

Effective contraception must be used for at least 1 month before beginning therapy, during therapy and for 1 month following discontinuation of therapy. It is recommended that two reliable forms of contraception be used simultaneously unless abstinence is the chosen method.

In 47 patients treated chronically with **etretinate** *(Tegison),* another retinoid, five had detectable serum drug levels 2.1 to 2.9 years after therapy was discontinued.

Counsel women fully on the serious risk to the fetus if they become pregnant during treatment. If pregnancy occurs, discuss continuing the pregnancy.

Actions:

Isotretinoin is an isomer of retinoic acid, a metabolite of retinol (vitamin A).

Pharmacology: The exact mechanism of action is unknown. Clinical improvement in cystic acne patients is associated with reduction in sebum secretion. This temporary decrease is related to dose and treatment duration; it reflects a reduction in sebaceous gland size and inhibition of sebaceous gland differentiation. Isotretinoin and other retinoids may also prevent abnormal keratinization.

Sebum lipid composition is altered during isotretinoin therapy, but returns to pretreatment composition upon discontinuation, even though sebum production may not return to pretreatment levels.

Pharmacokinetics: Absorption/Distribution – Oral bioavailability from oil-filled capsules is ≈ 23% to 25%. Plasma levels may be better maintained if the drug is taken with meals. After oral administration of 80 mg, peak plasma concentrations of 98 to 535 ng/ml (mean 256 to 262 ng/ml) were measured at 2.9 to 3.2 hours. The minimum steady-state blood concentration of isotretinoin averaged 160 ± 19 ng/ml with 40 mg twice daily administration. The drug is 99.9% bound to plasma albumin. Maximum concentrations of 4-*oxo*-isotretinoin, the major metabolite, were 87 to 399 ng/ml, and were reached in 6 to 20 hours.

Metabolism/Excretion – The major metabolite in blood, 4-*oxo*-isotretinoin (activity unknown), generally exceeds the concentration of isotretinoin after 6 hours. Terminal elimination half-life of isotretinoin is 10 to 20 hours. Elimination half-life of 4-*oxo*-isotretinoin ranges from 11 to 50 hours (average 24.5 hours).

In adults with normal renal and hepatic function, 65% to 85% of an 80 mg dose is excreted in the urine and feces in approximately equal proportions; enterohepatic circulation probably occurs.

(Continued on following page)

ISOTRETINOIN (13-*cis*-Retinoic Acid) (Cont.)

Indications:

Severe recalcitrant cystic acne. Adverse effects are significant; reserve treatment for patients unresponsive to conventional therapy, including systemic antibiotics. A single course has resulted in complete, prolonged remission in many patients. Patients may continue to improve while not receiving the drug.

Unlabeled Uses: Isotretinoin has been used in the treatment of keratinization disorders such as keratosis follicularis (Darier-White disease), pityriasis rubra pilaris, lamellar ichthyosis, congenital ichthyosiform erythroderma, hyperkeratosis palmaris et plantaris and other ichthyotic conditions. Response is variable and doses higher than usual are required. Success has also been reported in the treatment of cutaneous T-cell lymphoma (mycosis fungoides) and leukoplakia. High dose isotretinoin (2 mg/kg/day) has been used in the prevention of skin cancers in patients with xeroderma pigmentosum.

Contraindications:

Pregnancy: Category X. See boxed Warning.

Do not give to patients sensitive to parabens used as preservatives in the formulation.

Warnings:

Pseudotumor cerebri (benign intracranial hypertension) has occurred with isotretinoin. Early signs and symptoms include papilledema, headache, nausea, vomiting and visual disturbances. Screen patients with these symptoms for papilledema; if present, discontinue drug immediately and consult a neurologist. **Minocycline** and **tetracycline** have been associated with pseudotumor cerebri or papilledema in isotretinoin patients.

Corneal opacities have appeared in patients receiving isotretinoin for acne and in patients on higher dosages for keratinization disorders. If visual difficulties occur, discontinue the drug and perform an ophthalmological examination. Corneal opacities have either completely resolved or were resolving at follow-up 6 to 7 weeks after discontinuation.

Decreased night vision has occurred during therapy. Because the onset in some patients was sudden, advise patients of this potential problem and warn them to be cautious when driving or operating any vehicle at night. Carefully monitor visual problems.

Inflammatory bowel disease (including regional ileitis) has been temporally associated with isotretinoin in patients with no history of intestinal disorders. Discontinue treatment immediately if abdominal pain, rectal bleeding or severe diarrhea occurs.

Hypertriglyceridemia occurs in ≈ 25% of patients; 15% develop a *decrease* in high density lipoproteins (HDL) and ≈ 7% show an increase in cholesterol. After alcohol consumption, wait at least 36 hours before making these determinations; alcohol consumption may potentiate serum triglyceride elevations. Obtain baseline values, then perform tests weekly or biweekly until lipid response is established (usually 4 weeks).

These effects are reversible generally within 8 weeks after cessation of therapy. Patients with increased tendency to develop hypertriglyceridemia include those with diabetes mellitus, obesity, increased alcohol intake and a familial history.

Cardiovascular consequences of hypertriglyceridemia are not well understood, but may increase risk status. Serum triglycerides > 800 mg/dl have been associated with acute pancreatitis. Control significant triglyceride elevation. Reduction of weight, dietary fat, alcohol intake and dose may lower serum triglycerides, allowing patients to continue therapy.

An obese male patient with Darier's disease developed elevated triglycerides and subsequent eruptive xanthomas.

Musculoskeletal symptoms (including arthralgia) develop in ≈ 16% of patients. In general, these are mild to moderate and occasionally require discontinuation. They generally clear rapidly after discontinuing isotretinoin, and rarely persist.

In clinical trials of keratinization, a high prevalence of skeletal hyperostosis was noted with a mean dose of 2.24 mg/kg/day . Two children showed x-ray findings suggestive of premature closure of the epiphyses. Additionally, skeletal hyperostosis was noted in six of eight patients in a prospective study of keratinization disorders.

Minimal skeletal hyperostosis has been observed by x-ray in prospective studies of cystic acne patients treated with a single course of therapy at recommended doses.

Hepatotoxicity: Several cases of clinical hepatitis are possibly or probably related to isotretinoin therapy. Additionally, mild to moderate elevations of liver enzymes have been observed in ≈ 15% of patients, some of which normalized with dosage reduction or continued administration of the drug. If normalization does not readily occur, or if hepatitis is suspected, discontinue the drug and further investigate etiology.

Usage in Pregnancy: Category X. See boxed Warning.

Usage in Lactation: It is not known whether this drug is excreted in breast milk. Because of the potential for adverse effects, do not give to a nursing mother.

Usage in Children: Safety and efficacy have not been established. However, two children showed x-ray findings suggestive of premature closure of the epiphyses.

(Continued on following page)

ISOTRETINOIN (13-*cis*-Retinoic Acid) (Cont.)

Precautions:

As may be seen with healing cystic acne lesions, an occasional exaggerated healing response, manifested by exuberant granulation with crusting, has occurred.

Exacerbation of acne (transient) has occurred, generally during initial period of therapy.

Photosensitivity: Photosensitization (photoallergy or phototoxicity) may occur; caution patients to take protective measures (ie, sunscreens, protective clothing) against exposure to ultraviolet light or sunlight until tolerance is determined.

Contact lens tolerance may decrease.

Diabetes: Certain patients have experienced problems in the control of their blood sugar. In addition, new cases of diabetes have been diagnosed during therapy, although no causal relationship has been established.

Blood donation: Due to the teratogenic potential of isotretinoin, patients receiving the drug should not donate blood for transfusion for 30 days after discontinuing therapy.

Topical agents (eg, benzoyl peroxide, sulfur, tretinoin) should be discontinued before beginning isotretinoin therapy. These agents may potentiate the drying effects of isotretinoin.

Drug Interactions:

Vitamin A: To avoid additive toxic effects, do not take concomitantly with isotretinoin.

Adverse Reactions:

Most adverse reactions are reversible upon discontinuation; however, some have persisted after cessation of therapy. Many are similar to those described in patients taking high doses of vitamin A.

The percentages of adverse reactions reflect the total experience in isotretinoin studies, including investigational studies of disorders of keratinization, with the exception of those pertaining to dry skin and mucous membranes. These latter reflect the experience only in patients with cystic acne because reactions relating to dryness are more commonly recognized as adverse reactions in this disease. Included in this category are dry skin, skin fragility, pruritus, epistaxis, dry nose and dry mouth, which may be seen in up to 80% of cystic acne patients.

Most frequent: Cheilitis, usually dose-related (> 90%); conjunctivitis (40%); skin fragility, dry skin, pruritus, epistaxis, dry nose, dry mouth (up to 80% of cystic acne patients).

Dermatologic: Cheilitis (> 90%); dry skin, pruritus; skin fragility (up to 80%); facial skin desquamation, drying of mucous membranes (30%); nail brittleness (10%); rash (including erythema), thinning of hair which has rarely persisted (< 10%); skin infections, photosensitivity, palmoplantar desquamation (5%); erythema nodosum, paronychia, hypo- or hyperpigmentation, urticaria, hirsutism, hair problems other than thinning, nail dystrophy (< 1%); exaggerated healing response manifested by exuberant granulation tissue with crusting; pyogenic granuloma; petechiae (25%); bruising.

GI: Dry mouth (up to 80%); nausea, vomiting, abdominal pain (20%); nonspecific GI symptoms (5%); anorexia (4%); inflammatory bowel disease including regional enteritis (see Warnings), weight loss, bleeding and inflammation of the gums (< 1%).

Ophthalmic: Conjunctivitis (40%); optic neuritis, photophobia, eyelid inflammation (< 1%); corneal opacities (see Warnings); cataracts; visual disturbances. Dry eyes and decrease in night vision have occurred and, in rare instances, have persisted.

CNS: Fatigue, headache (5%); pseudotumor cerebri, including headache, visual disturbances and papilledema (some associated with tetracyclines). Depression has occurred, and has subsided with discontinuation of therapy and recurred upon reinstitution.

GU: White cells in urine (10% to 20%); proteinuria, microscopic or gross hematuria (< 10%), nonspecific urogenital findings (5%); abnormal menses (< 1%).

(Adverse Reactions continued on following page)

ISOTRETINOIN (13-*cis*-Retinoic Acid) (Cont.)

Adverse Reactions (Cont.)

Musculoskeletal: Mild to moderate musculoskeletal symptoms which occasionally required drug discontinuation (16%). They rarely persisted after discontinuation. Skeletal hyperostosis; arthralgia, bone, joint and muscle pain and stiffness (16% to 17%). (See Warnings.)

Other: Epistaxis, dry nose (up to 80%); flushing, anemia, palpitation, tachycardia, lymphadenopathy, disseminated herpes simplex, edema, respiratory infections (< 1%); transient chest pain (rarely persists after discontinuation); vasculitis.

Laboratory abnormalities: Elevated sedimentation rate (40%); reversible dose-related triglyceride elevation (25%; approximately 4% to 11% showed triglyceride elevation above 500 mg/dl); reversible mild to moderate decrease in HDL (16%), changes in serum lipids; decreased red blood cell parameters and white blood cell counts, elevated platelet counts, and increased alkaline phosphatase, SGOT, SGPT, GGTP and LDH (10% to 20%); increased fasting serum glucose, hyperuricemia; elevated CPK levels in patients who undergo vigorous physical activity (< 10%), reversible minimal elevation of cholesterol (7%).

Overdosage:

Overdosage has been associated with transient headache, vomiting, facial flushing, cheilosis, abdominal pain, headache, dizziness and ataxia. All symptoms quickly resolved without apparent residual effects.

Patient Information:

Patient information leaflet available with product.

Patient consent form, included with package insert, should be completed prior to use.

Do not crush. Take with meals. Do not take vitamin supplements containing vitamin A.

Women of childbearing potential should practice contraception during therapy and for 1 month before and after therapy. Notify physician immediately if pregnancy is suspected.

A transient exacerbation of acne may occur during the initial period of therapy.

May cause photosensitivity; avoid prolonged exposure to sunlight.

Minimize or eliminate alcohol consumption, which may potentiate serum triglyceride elevation.

Administration and Dosage:

Individualize dosage. Adjust the dose according to side effects and disease response.

Recommended course of therapy: Initial dose is 0.5 to 1 mg/kg/day (range, 0.5 to 2 mg/kg/day) divided into 2 doses, for 15 to 20 weeks. Patients whose disease is very severe or is primarily manifest on the body may require up to the maximum recommended dose, 2 mg/kg/day. If the total cyst count decreases by more than 70% prior to this time, the drug may be discontinued. After 2 months or more off therapy, and if warranted by persistent or recurring severe cystic acne, a second course of therapy may be initiated.

In studies comparing 0.1, 0.5 and 1 mg/kg/day, all doses provided initial clearing of disease, but there was a greater need for retreatment with the lower doses.

Doses as low as 0.05 mg/kg/day have been effective with minimal toxicity; however, relapses were more frequent.

DOSING ISOTRETINOIN BY BODY WEIGHT

Body Weight		Total mg/day		
kilograms	pounds	0.5 mg/kg	1 mg/kg	2 mg/kg
40	88	20	40	80
50	110	25	50	100
60	132	30	60	120
70	154	35	70	140
80	176	40	80	160
90	198	45	90	180
100	220	50	100	200

				C.I.*
Rx	**Accutane** (Roche)	**Capsules**[1]: 10 mg	(#Accutane 10 Roche). Light pink. In 30s.	1966
		20 mg	(#Accutane 20 Roche). Maroon. In 30s.	1267
		40 mg	(#Accutane 40 Roche). Yellow. In 30s.	769

* Cost Index based on cost per 10 mg. # Product identification code.

[1] Capsule contains suspension of drug in soybean oil; also contains EDTA and glycerin, with parabens.

BENZOYL PEROXIDE

Actions:

Effectiveness of benzoyl peroxide is primarily attributable to its antibacterial activity, especially against *Propionibacterium acnes,* the predominant organism in sebaceous follicles and comedones. This activity is presumably due to the release of active or free-radical oxygen capable of oxidizing bacterial proteins. Resolution of the acne coincides with reduction in the levels of *P acnes* and of free fatty acids on the skin's surface. This is aided by a drying action, removal of excess sebum, mild desquamation and sebostatic effects.

Benzoyl peroxide is absorbed by the skin, where it is metabolized to benzoic acid and then excreted as benzoate in the urine.

Indications:

Treatment of mild to moderate acne.

Contraindications:

Hypersensitivity to benzoyl peroxide.

Warnings:

Usage in Pregnancy: Category C. It is not known whether benzoyl peroxide can cause fetal harm when administered to a pregnant woman or can affect reproductive capacity. Use in pregnant women only if clearly needed.

Usage in Lactation: It is not known whether this drug is excreted in breast milk. Administer with caution to nursing mothers.

Usage in Children: Safety and efficacy in children less than 12 years of age have not been established.

Precautions:

External use only. Avoid contact with eyelids, lips, mucous membranes and highly inflamed or denuded skin.

Benzoyl peroxide is an oxidizing agent; it may bleach hair and colored fabric.

Cross-sensitization with **benzoic acid derivatives** (eg, cinnamon and certain topical anesthetics) may occur.

Concomitant use of **tretinoin** may cause significant skin irritation.

Adverse Reactions:

Excessive drying (manifested by marked peeling, erythema and possible edema); allergic contact sensitization.

Overdosage:

Symptoms: Excessive scaling, erythema or edema.

Treatment: Discontinue use. If reaction is due to excessive use and not allergy, cautiously reinstate at a reduced dosage schedule after signs and symptoms subside. To hasten resolution of adverse effects, use emollients, cool compresses or topical corticosteroids.

Patient Information:

Keep away from eyes, mouth, inside the nose and mucous membranes.

May cause transitory feeling of warmth or slight stinging. Expect dryness and peeling; if excessive redness or discomfort occurs, decrease or discontinue use temporarily.

Avoid other sources of skin irritation (eg, sunlight, sun lamps, other topical acne medications) unless directed by a physician.

Avoid contact with hair or colored fabric.

Normal use of water-based cosmetics is permissible.

Administration and Dosage:

Cleansers: Wash once or twice daily. Wet skin areas to be treated prior to administration. Rinse thoroughly. Control amount of drying or peeling by modifying dose frequency or concentration.

Other doseforms: Apply once daily for the first few days. After cleansing the skin, smooth a small amount over the affected area. If dryness, redness or peeling does not occur in 3 days, increase application to twice daily. If bothersome dryness or peeling occurs, reduce dosage. If excessive stinging or burning occurs after any single application, remove with mild soap and water, resuming application the next day.

(Products listed on following pages)

BENZOYL PEROXIDE, CLEANSERS				C.I.*
Rx	**Benzac W Wash 5** (Owen/Allercreme)	**Liquid:** 5%	Water base. In 120 and 240 ml.	60
Rx	**Desquam-X 5 Wash** (Westwood)		Water base. In 150 ml.	69
Rx	**Benzac W Wash 10** (Owen/Allercreme)	**Liquid:** 10%	Water base. In 240 ml.	46
Rx	**Desquam-X 10 Wash** (Westwood)		Water base. In 150 ml.	77
otc	**Fostex 10% BPO Wash** (Westwood)		Water base. In 150 ml.	33
otc	**Oxy 10 Wash** (SK Beecham)		In 120 ml.	41
otc	**Propa P.H. Liquid Acne Soap** (Commerce)		In 120 ml.	36
Rx	**Theroxide Wash** (Medicis)		In 120 ml.	NA
otc	**PanOxyl 5** (Stiefel)	**Bar:** 5%	In a soap free detergent base. In 120 g.	46
otc	**Fostex 10% BPO Cleansing** (Westwood)	**Bar:** 10%	In 112.5 g.	30
otc	**PanOxyl 10** (Stiefel)		In a soap free detergent base. In 120 g.	50
otc	**Neutrogena Acne Mask** (Neutrogena)	**Mask:** 5%	With glycerin, bentonite, titanium dioxide. In 60 g.	NA
BENZOYL PEROXIDE, LOTIONS				
otc	**Benzoyl Peroxide** (Various)	**Lotion:** 5%	In 30 and 60 ml.	60+
otc	**Ben-Aqua 5** (Syosset)		Greaseless vanishing base. In 60 ml.	NA
otc	**Benoxyl 5** (Stiefel)		Greaseless vanishing base. In 30, 60 ml.	170
otc	**Dry and Clear** (Whitehall)		Greaseless base. In 30 and 60 ml.	130
otc	**Oxy 5** (SK Beecham)		Greaseless vanishing base. In 30 ml.	123
otc	**Oxy 5 Tinted** (SK-Beecham)		With titanium dioxide. In 30 ml.	NA
Rx	**Theroxide** (Medicis)		In 42.5 g.	NA
otc	**Vanoxide** (Dermik)		Vanishing base. In 25 and 50 ml.	293
otc	**Loroxide** (Dermik)	**Lotion:** 5.5%	Tinted. In 25 ml.	353
otc	**Benzoyl Peroxide** (Various)	**Lotion:** 10%	In 30 and 60 ml.	66+
otc	**Acne-10** (Various)		Greaseless vanishing base. In 30 ml.	74+
otc	**Ben-Aqua 10** (Syosset)		Greaseless vanishing base. In 30 ml.	NA
otc	**Benoxyl 10** (Stiefel)		Greaseless vanishing base. In 30 & 60 ml.	170
otc	**Clearasil 10%** (Vicks Personal Care)		Greaseless base. In 30 ml.	174
otc	**Oxy 10** (SK Beeccham)		Greaseless vanishing base. In 30 ml.	164
Rx	**Theroxide** (Medicis)		In 42.5 g.	NA
BENZOYL PEROXIDE, CREAMS				
Rx	**Benzashave** (Medicis)	**Cream:** 5%	In 113.4 g.	NA
otc	**Cuticura Acne** (DEP)		Tinted. In 30 g.	199
otc	**Acne-Aid** (Stiefel)	**Cream:** 10%	In 54 g.	90
otc	**Ambi 10** (Kiwi Brands)		In 28.3 g.	NA
Rx	**Benzashave** (Medicis)		In 113.4 g.	NA
otc	**Clearasil Maximum Strength Acne Treatment** (Vicks Personal Care)		Tinted or vanishing greaseless base. In 19.5 and 30 g.	174
otc	**Fostex 10% BPO Tinted** (Westwood)		In 45 g.	116
otc	**Oxy 10 Cover** (SK Beecham)		Tinted greaseless base. With silica. In 30 g.	164
otc	**pHisoAc BP** (Winthrop)		Greaseless base. In 22.5 and 45 g.	88
otc	**Dry and Clear Double Strength** (Whitehall)		Vanishing base. In 30 g.	179

* Cost Index based on cost per g or ml.

	BENZOYL PEROXIDE, GELS			C.I.*
Rx	**Benzac AC 2.5%** (Owen/Galderma)	**Gel:** 2.5%	Water base. EDTA. In 60 g.	NA
Rx	**Benzac W 2½** (Owen/Galderma)		Water base. In 60 and 90 g.	111
otc	**Clear By Design** (SmithKline)		Greaseless, invisible base. In 45 and 90 g.	147
Rx	**Desquam-E** (Westwood)		In 42.5 g.	202
Rx	**Desquam-X2.5** (Westwood)		Water base vehicle containing 6% laureth-4. In 45 g.	173
Rx	**PanOxyl AQ 2½** (Stiefel)		Aqueous base.[1] In 60 and 120 g.	121
Rx	**Brevoxyl** (Stiefel)	**Gel:** 4%	Simethicone. In 42.5 g.	NA
Rx	**Benzoyl Peroxide** (Various)	**Gel:** 5%	In 45 g.	42+
Rx	**Ben-Aqua-5** (Syosset)		In 45 and 120 g.[1]	35
Rx	**Benzac AC 5%** (Owen/Galderma)		Water base. EDTA. In 60 g.	NA
Rx	**Benzac 5** (Owen/Galderma)		12% alcohol and 6% polyoxyethylene lauryl ether. In 60 g.	143
Rx	**Benzac W 5** (Owen/Galderma)		Water base. In 60 and 90 g.	133
Rx	**5-Benzagel** (Dermik)		14% alcohol. In 45 and 90 g.	137
otc	**Del Aqua-5** (Del-Ray)		Water base.[1] In 45 g.	81
Rx	**Desquam-E** (Westwood)		In 42.5 g.	202
Rx	**Desquam-X5** (Westwood)		Water base vehicle containing 6% laureth-4. In 45 and 90 g.	172
otc	**Fostex 5% BPO** (Westwood)		Laureth-4. In 45 g.	118
Rx	**PanOxyl 5** (Stiefel)		20% alcohol.[1] In 60 and 120 g.	125
Rx	**PanOxyl AQ 5** (Stiefel)		Aqueous base.[1] In 60 and 120 g.	125
Rx	**Persa-Gel** (Ortho Derm)		Acetone base. In 45 and 90 g.	169
Rx	**Persa-Gel W 5%** (Ortho Derm)		Water base gel. Containing laureth-4. In 45 and 90 g.	169
otc	**Xerac BP5** (Person & Covey)		Laureth-4. In 45 and 90 g.	110
Rx	**Zeroxin-5** (Syosset)		Acetone base. In 42.5 and 113 g.	30
Rx	**Benzoyl Peroxide** (Various)	**Gel:** 10%	In 45 and 120 g.	44+
Rx	**Ben-Aqua-10** (Syosset)		In 42.5 and 120 g.[1]	37
Rx	**Benzac AC 10%** (Owen/Galderma)		Water base. EDTA. In 60 g.	NA
Rx	**Benzac 10** (Owen/Galderma)		12% alcohol and 6% polyoxyethylene lauryl ether. In 60 g.	151
Rx	**Benzac W 10** (Owen/Galderma)		Water base. In 60 and 90 g.	143
Rx	**10-Benzagel** (Dermik)		14% alcohol. In 45 and 90 g.	142
otc	**Del Aqua-10** (Del-Ray)		Water base.[1] In 45 g.	91
Rx	**Desquam-E** (Westwood)		In 42.5 g.	202
Rx	**Desquam-X10** (Westwood)		Water base vehicle containing 6% laureth-4. In 42.5 and 90 g.	191
otc	**Fostex 10% BPO** (Westwood)		Laureth-4. In 45 g.	122
Rx	**PanOxyl 10** (Stiefel)		20% alcohol.[1] In 60 and 120 g.	130
Rx	**PanOxyl AQ 10** (Stiefel)		Aqueous base.[1] In 60 and 120 g.	125
Rx	**Persa-Gel** (Ortho Derm)		Acetone base. In 45 and 90 g.	175
Rx	**Persa-Gel W 10%** (Ortho Derm)		Laureth-4. Water base gel. In 45 and 90 g.	175
otc	**Xerac BP10** (Person & C)		Laureth-4. In 45 and 90 g.	110
Rx	**Zeroxin-10** (Syosset)		Acetone base. In 45 and 120 g.	30

* Cost Index based on cost per g or ml.

[1] With polyoxyethylene lauryl ether.

BENZOYL PEROXIDE COMBINATIONS

				C.I.*
Rx	**Sulfoxyl Regular** (Stiefel)	**Lotion:** 5% benzoyl peroxide and 2% sulfur	In 30 ml.	291
Rx	**Sulfoxyl Strong** (Stiefel)	**Lotion:** 10% benzoyl peroxide and 5% sulfur	In 30 ml.	311

SULFUR PREPARATIONS

Actions:

Sulfur provides antibacterial, peeling and drying actions. Although it may help to resolve comedones, it may also promote the development of new ones by increasing horny cell adhesion.

Indications:

An aid in the treatment of mild acne and oily skin.

Precautions:

For external use only. Avoid overuse and contact with eyes. Certain individuals may be sensitive to one or more components. If undue skin irritation develops or becomes excessive, discontinue use and consult physician.

Patient Information:

Keep away from the eyes.

May cause irritation of the skin; discontinue use and notify physician if this occurs.

Administration and Dosage:

Apply a thin film. Use 1 to 3 times daily. For best results, cleanse skin thoroughly with a mild cleanser prior to application.

				C.I.*
otc	**Fostex Medicated Cover-Up** (Westwood)	**Cream:** 2% sulfur	Tinted. Greaseless base. In 30 g.	182
otc	**Transact** (Westwood)	**Gel:** 2% sulfur, 40% alcohol and laureth-4	Greaseless base. In 30 g.	218
otc	**Xerac** (Person & Covey)	**Gel:** 4% microcrystalline sulfur and 44% isopropyl alcohol	In 45 g.	100
otc	**Liquimat** (Owen/Allercreme)	**Lotion:** 5% sulfur and 22% alcohol	Tinted. Oil free base. In 45 ml.	114
otc	**Sulpho-Lac** (Bradley)	**Soap:** 5% sulphur	In a coconut and tallow oil soap base. In 85 g.	31
Rx	**Bensulfoid** (Poythress)	**Powder:** A fusion of highly reactive sulfur (33% by weight) onto colloidal bentonite *Used for extemporaneous prescription compounding. Topical prescriptions should not contain > 40 gr highly reactive sulfur per 30 g of compounded prescription.*	In 30 g.	178
		Tablets: 130 mg (33% sulfur)	In 100s.	66

* Cost Index based on cost per g, ml or tablet.

METRONIDAZOLE

Actions:

Metronidazole is classified therapeutically as an antiprotozoal and antibacterial agent. The mechanisms by which topical metronidazole acts in reducing inflammatory lesions of acne rosacea are unknown, but may include an antibacterial or an anti-inflammatory effect.

Pharmacokinetics: Bioavailability studies on the topical administration of 1 g of topical metronidazole to the face (7.5 mg of metronidazole) of 10 rosacea patients showed a maximum serum concentration of 66 ng/ml in one patient. This concentration is approximately 100 times less than concentrations afforded by a single 250 mg oral tablet. Three of the patients had no detectable serum concentrations of metronidazole at any time point. The mean dose of gel applied during clinical studies was 600 mg which represents 4.5 mg of metronidazole per application. Therefore, under normal usage levels, the formulation affords minimal serum concentrations of metronidazole.

Indications:

Topical application in the treatment of inflammatory papules, pustules and erythema of rosacea.

Contraindications:

History of hypersensitivity to metronidazole, parabens or other ingredients of the formulations.

Warnings:

Usage in Pregnancy: Category B. There has been no experience to date with the use of topical metronidazole in pregnant patients. Metronidazole crosses the placental barrier and enters the fetal circulation rapidly. No fetotoxicity was observed after oral metronidazole in rats or mice. However, since oral metronidazole is a carcinogen in some rodents, use during pregnancy only if clearly needed.

Usage in Lactation: After oral administration, metronidazole is excreted in breast milk in concentrations similar to those found in the plasma. Even though metronidazole blood levels are significantly lower than those achieved after oral metronidazole, decide whether to discontinue nursing or to discontinue the drug, taking into account the importance of the drug to the mother.

Usage in Children: Safety and efficacy in children have not been established.

Precautions:

Because of the minimal absorption of metronidazole and consequently its insignificant plasma concentration after topical administration, the adverse experiences reported with the oral form of the drug have not been reported with topical metronidazole.

Tearing of the eyes has occurred; therefore, avoid contact with the eyes. If a reaction suggesting local irritation occurs, direct patients to use the medication less frequently, discontinue use temporarily, or discontinue use until further instructions. Metronidazole is a nitroimidazole; use with care in patients with evidence of, or history of, blood dyscrasia.

Drug Interactions:

Drug interactions are less likely with topical administration but should be kept in mind when topical metronidazole is prescribed for patients who are receiving anticoagulant treatment. Oral metronidazole may potentiate the anticoagulant effect of warfarin resulting in a prolongation of prothrombin time.

Adverse Reactions:

Watery (tearing) eyes if the gel is applied too closely to this area, transient redness, and mild dryness, burning and skin irritation (2% or less).

Overdosage:

The acute oral toxicity of the topical metronidazole formulation was determined to be greater than 5 g/kg (the highest dose given) in albino rats.

Patient Information:

For external use only. Avoid contact with the eyes.

Administration and Dosage:

Apply and rub in a thin film twice daily, morning and evening, to entire affected areas after washing. Significant therapeutic results should be noticed within 3 weeks. Clinical studies have demonstrated continuing improvement through 9 weeks of therapy.

Areas to be treated should be cleansed before application of topical metronidazole. Patients may use cosmetics after application of topical metronidazole.

				C.I.*
Rx	**MetroGel** (Curatek)	**Gel:** 0.75%	In 30 g tube.	586

* Cost Index based on cost per g.

TETRACYCLINES, TOPICAL

Actions:

These agents deliver the drug to the pilosebaceous apparatus and adjacent tissues. The mechanism of action by which they improve acne is unknown. Systemic tetracycline seems to decrease the amount of free fatty acids present in acne lesions. It appears that these drugs possess a localized effect since they are not absorbed through the skin in sufficient quantities for systemic action.

Indications:

Treatment of acne vulgaris.

Contraindications:

Hypersensitivity to any component or to any of the other tetracyclines.

Warnings:

Usage in impaired hepatic or renal function: Significant percutaneous absorption may result from prolonged use. Therefore, administer with caution to persons with hepatic or renal dysfunction.

Usage in Pregnancy: Category B. Safety for use during pregnancy has not been established. Use only when clearly needed and when the potential benefits outweigh the potential hazards to the fetus.

Oral tetracycline is not recommended for use during pregnancy (see p. 1813).

Usage in Lactation: Safety for use during lactation has not been established.

Usage in Children: Safety and efficacy for use in children less than 11 years of age have not been established.

Precautions:

For external use only. Keep out of eyes, nose and mouth.

Use the meclocycline cream with caution in patients allergic to formaldehyde.

Adverse Reactions:

There is one report each of acute contact dermatitis and severe dermatitis, and isolated reports of skin irritation. Temporary follicular staining may occur with excessive application of the cream. The cream has demonstrated no photosensitivity or contact allergy potential. Treated areas of skin will also fluoresce under an ultraviolet light source.

Topical administration results in low serum levels; it is highly unlikely that systemic side effects will occur.

Tetracycline: About one third of patients may experience a stinging or burning sensation upon application. A slight yellowing of the skin in the areas of application may be noticed. This condition is superficial, and the color can be eliminated by washing.

Patient Information:

Apply generously until skin is thoroughly wet. Avoid the eyes, nose and mouth.

Stinging or burning may occur, but will subside in a few minutes.

A slight yellowing of the skin may occur; this is not harmful and may be removed by washing (tetracycline).

Normal use of cosmetics is permissible.

Administration and Dosage:

Apply to affected areas twice daily, morning and evening. Less frequent application may be used depending upon patient response. Apply generously until the skin is thoroughly wet. Excessive use of the cream may cause staining of some fabrics.

TETRACYCLINE HCl				C.I.*
Rx	**Topicycline** (Procter & Gamble Pharm.)	**Topical Solution:** 2.2 mg per ml	In 70 ml. Each carton contains 1 vial of powder for reconstitution[1] and diluent[2] to make 70 ml solution.	242
MECLOCYCLINE SULFOSALICYLATE				
Rx	**Meclan** (Ortho Derm)	**Cream:** 1%. In a vehicle of glyceryl stearate, propylene glycol stearate and polysorbate 40	In 20 and 45 g.	764

* Cost Index based on cost per g or ml.

[1] With 4-epitetracycline HCl and sodium bisulfite.

[2] With 40% ethanol, citric acid and n-decyl methyl sulfoxide.

ERYTHROMYCIN, TOPICAL

Actions:

Although the mechanism by which topical erythromycin acts in reducing inflammatory lesions of acne vulgaris is unknown, it is presumably due to its antibiotic action.

Indications:

Topical control of acne vulgaris.

Contraindications:

Hypersensitivity to erythromycin or to any component of these products.

Warnings:

Usage in Pregnancy (Category B: T-Stat 2%, Staticin, Erythromycin for compounding). *(Category C: A/T/S, Erymax, Benzamycin).* Safety for use during pregnancy has not been established. Use only when clearly needed and when the potential benefits outweigh unknown hazards to the fetus.

Usage in Lactation: Erythromycin is excreted in breast milk. Exercise caution when administering to a nursing mother.

Usage in Children: Safety and efficacy for use in children less than 12 years of age have not been established.

Precautions:

For external use only. Keep away from the eyes, nose, mouth and other mucous membranes.

Superinfection: Use of antibiotics (especially prolonged or repeated therapy) may result in bacterial or fungal overgrowth of nonsusceptible organisms. Such overgrowth may lead to a secondary infection. Take appropriate measures if superinfection occurs.

Drug Interactions:

Peeling, desquamating or **abrasive agents:** Use concomitant topical acne therapy with caution because a cumulative irritant effect may occur.

Acids inactivate erythromycin by hydrolysis.

Sodium alginate, pectin, bentonite, calamine, silica and **polysorbate 80** all reduce erythromycin's activity.

Alkaline media: Erythromycin is unstable in alkaline media having a pH $>$ 10.5.

Clindamycin: Antagonism has occurred between clindamycin and erythromycin.

Adverse Reactions:

Erythema, desquamation, burning sensation, eye irritation, tenderness, dryness, pruritus and oily skin.

One case has been reported of a generalized urticarial reaction, possibly related to the drug, which required the use of systemic steroids.

Overdosage:

Ingestion may cause nausea and vomiting; small children may experience inebriation or sedation.

Based on amount ingested and time elapsed since ingestion, treatment methods include induced emesis, gastric lavage, demulcent liquids and general supportive measures. Refer to General Management of Acute Overdosage on p. 2895

Patient Information:

Wash, rinse and dry affected areas before application.

Keep away from the eyes, nose and mouth.

Administration and Dosage:

Apply morning and evening to affected areas. Before applying, wash, rinse well and pat dry all areas to be treated. Apply with fingertips or applicator. Wash hands after use.

Preparation of gel – The topical gel is supplied in a package containing 20 g benzoyl peroxide gel and a plastic vial containing 0.8 g erythromycin powder. Prior to dispensing, add 3 ml of ethyl alcohol (to the mark) to vial and shake well to dissolve erythromycin. Add this solution to gel and stir until homogenous in appearance (1-1½ minutes). Refrigerate. Expiration date is 3 months.

Prior to reconstitution, store at room temperature. *After* reconstitution, store in a cold place, preferably refrigerated.

(Products listed on following page)

ERYTHROMYCIN, TOPICAL (Cont.)

	Product	Form	Package	C.I.*
Rx	**Erythromycin** (Various)	**Topical Solution:** 2%	In 60 ml.	66+
Rx	**Akne-mycin** (Hermal)		In 60 ml.[1]	171
Rx	**A/T/S** (Hoechst-Roussel)		In 60 ml.[1]	242
Rx	**C-Solve 2** (Syosset)		In 60 ml.[2]	NA
Rx	**Erycette** (Ortho)		In 60 swabs.[1]	236
Rx	**Eryderm 2%** (Abbott)		In 60 ml.[3]	258
Rx	**Erymax** (Herbert)		In 60 and 120 ml.[1]	243
Rx	**E-Solve 2** (Syosset)		In 60 ml.[4]	83
Rx	**ETS-2%** (Paddock)		In 60 ml.[1]	86
Rx	**Theramycin Z** (Medicis)		In 60 ml.[5]	NA
Rx	**T-Stat 2%** (Westwood)		In 60 ml.[5]	246
Rx	**Erythromycin** (Various)	**Topical Solution:** 1.5%	In 60 ml.	69+
Rx	**Staticin** (Westwood)		In 60 ml.[6]	285
Rx	**Erythromycin** (Paddock)	**Powder:** For extemporaneous compounding of topical solutions	In 10, 25 and 100 g bottles.	800
Rx	**A/T/S** (Hoechst-Roussel)	**Gel:** 2%	In 30 g.	NA

ERYTHROMYCIN TOPICAL COMBINATIONS

	Product	Form	Package	C.I.*
Rx	**Benzamycin** (Dermik)	**Gel:** 30 mg erythromycin and 50 mg benzoyl peroxide per g	In 23.3 g after reconstitution.[7]	773

* Cost Index based on cost per g, ml or swab.
[1] With 66% alcohol, propylene glycol and citric acid.
[2] With 81% alcohol, propylene glycol, lauramide DEA, zinc acetate and hydroxypropyl cellulose.
[3] With 77% alcohol, polyethylene glycol and acetone.
[4] With 80% alcohol, propylene glycol, lauramide DEA, zinc acetate, hydroxypropyl cellulose and iron oxides.
[5] With 86% alcohol, hydroxypropyl cellulose, zinc acetate, propylene glycol and lauramide DEA.
[6] With 71% alcohol, propylene glycol and citric acid.
[7] With 55% alcohol, propylene glycol and laureth-4.
[8] With 22% alcohol, carbomer 940 and docusate sodium.

CLINDAMYCIN, TOPICAL

Actions:

Clindamycin demonstrates in vitro activity against isolates of *Propionibacterium acnes* which may account for its usefulness in acne. Free fatty acids on the skin surface decrease from approximately 14% to 2% following application.

Following multiple topical applications at a concentration equivalent to 10 mg/ml, very low levels (0 to 3 ng/ml) are present in the serum and less than 0.2% of the dose is recovered in urine as clindamycin. The mean concentration of activity in comedonal extracts from acne patients was 597 mcg/g (range 0 to 1490 mcg/g). Clindamycin in vitro inhibits all *P acnes* cultures tested.

Indications:

Treatment of acne vulgaris.

Unlabeled Use: Clindamycin lotion has been used in the treatment of rosacea.

Contraindications:

Hypersensitivity to clindamycin or lincomycin, a history of regional enteritis or ulcerative colitis or a history of antibiotic-associated colitis.

Warnings:

Colitis: Diarrhea, bloody diarrhea and colitis (including pseudomembranous colitis) have been reported with the use of topical and systemic clindamycin. Symptoms can occur after a few days, weeks or months following initiation of therapy, but have also begun up to several weeks after cessation of therapy. Toxin(s) produced by *Clostridium difficile* is one primary cause of antibiotic-associated colitis, which is usually characterized by severe persistent diarrhea, severe abdominal cramps and the passage of blood and mucus. When significant diarrhea occurs, discontinue the drug. Consider large bowel endoscopy in cases of severe diarrhea.

Treatment – Mild cases of colitis may respond to drug discontinuation. Manage moderate to severe cases promptly with fluid, electrolyte and protein supplementation as indicated. Vancomycin is effective in the treatment of antibiotic-associated pseudomembranous colitis produced by *C difficile* (See page 1842).

Cholestyramine and colestipol resins bind the toxin in vitro. Systemic steroids and steroid retention enemas may help relieve colitis. Antiperistaltic agents such as opiates and diphenoxylate with atropine may prolong or worsen the condition.

Usage in Pregnancy: Category B. Animal studies have revealed no evidence of impaired fertility or fetal harm. Safety for use during pregnancy has not been established. Use only when clearly needed and when the potential benefits outweigh the unknown potential hazards to the fetus.

Usage in Lactation: Safety for use during lactation has not been established. It is not known whether topical clindamycin is excreted in breast milk, although oral and parenteral clindamycin have been reported to appear in breast milk.

Precautions:

Clindamycin topical solution has an alcohol base which will cause burning and irritation of the eye. In case of accidental contact with eyes, abraded skin or mucous membranes, bathe with copious amounts of cool tap water. Use caution when applying medication around the mouth.

Prescribe with caution in atopic individuals.

Drug Interactions:

Erythromycin: Antagonism has been demonstrated with clindamycin.

Adverse Reactions:

GI: Diarrhea, bloody diarrhea, abdominal pains and colitis (including pseudomembranous colitis); GI disturbance.

Other: Skin dryness is the most common adverse reaction seen with the solution. Contact dermatitis; gram-negative folliculitis; irritation; oily skin; sensitization; stinging of eyes.

Patient Information:

Notify physician if abdominal pain or diarrhea occurs.

Avoid contact with eyes, abraded skin or mucous membranes; clindamycin may cause burning and irritation.

Administration and Dosage: Apply a thin film to affected area twice daily.

				C.I.*
Rx	**Cleocin T** (Upjohn)	**Gel:** 10 mg (as phosphate) per ml[1]	In 7.5 and 30 g.	691
		Lotion: 10 mg (as phosphate) per ml[3]	In 60 ml.	550
		Topical Solution: 10 mg (as phosphate) per ml[2]	In 30 and 60 ml & pt.	298

* Cost Index based on cost per g or ml.

[1] With allantoin, carbomer 934P, methylparaben, polyethylene glycol 400 and propylene glycol.

[2] With 50% isopropyl alcohol and propylene glycol.

[3] With cetostearyl alcohol, glycerin, glyceryl stearate SE, isostearyl alcohol, methylparaben, sodium lauryl sarcosinate and stearic acid.

Creams, Lotions and Gels

The following products contain keratolytics and astringents to aid in removing keratin and to dry the skin. Many products also have hydroalcoholic or organic solvent bases to aid in removal of sebum. Individual components include:

ANTIMICROBIAL: Benzalkonium Cl, parachlorometaxylenol (p. 2336), sodium thiosulfate and sodium sulfacetamide (p.2337).

ANTIPRURITIC: Sodium borate.

ANTISEPTIC: Oxyquinoline, methylbenzethonium Cl, ethanol, isopropyl alcohol, phenol, triclosan, thymol, sulfur (p. 2301) and acetone.

ASTRINGENTS: Zinc oxide (p. 2441), zinc sulfate, alcohol and calamine.

COUNTERIRRITANT (local anesthetic): Methylsalicylate.

KERATOLYTICS: Salicylic acid (p 2416), resorcinol and urea (carbamide).

PROTECTIVES and *ADSORBANTS:* Titanium dioxide and zinc oxide.

Hydrocortisone-containing acne products are listed under Topical Corticosteroid Combinations, page 597.

		Sulfur	Salicylic Acid	Resorcinol	Other Content	How Supplied	C.I.*
otc	**Cuticura Ointment** (DEP Corp.)	0.5%[1]			0.1% phenol, 0.05% oxyquinoline	In 52.5 g.	96
otc	**Fostril Lotion** (Westwood)	2%			Laureth-4, bentonite, zinc oxide	In 30 ml.	220
otc	**Finac Lotion** (C & M Pharm.)	2%			Methylbenzethonium chloride, 8% isopropyl alcohol	Tinted. In 60 ml.	60
Rx	**Sulfacet-R Lotion** (Dermik)	5%			10% sodium sulfacetamide, zinc oxide, titanium dioxide	Tinted. In 25 ml.	374
otc	**Acnederm Lotion** (Lannett)	5%			1% zinc sulfate, 10% zinc oxide, 21% isopropyl alcohol	Greaseless water washable base. Tinted. In 60 ml.	47
otc	**Acnophill Ointment** (Torch)	5%[1]			10% zinc oxide, 5% potassium & zinc sulfides-polysulfides	Water washable base. Plain or tinted. In 60 g and 1 lb.	60
otc	**Seale's Lotion Modified** (C & M Pharm.)	6.4%			Zinc oxide, bentonite, sodium borate, acetone	In pt.	27
otc	**Acno Lotion** (Baker/Cummins)	3%	2%			Greaseless base. In 120 ml.	104
otc	**Therac Lotion** (C & M Pharm.)	4%[2]	2.35%			Aqueous base. In 60 ml.	60
otc	**Acnotex Lotion** (C & M Pharm.)	8%	2.25%		Methylbenzethonium chloride, 22% isopropyl alcohol, acetone	In 60 ml.	75
otc	**Sulforcin Lotion** (Owen)	5%		2%	11.65% alcohol	In 120 ml.	45
otc	**Rezamid Lotion** (Summers)	5%		2%	SD-40 alcohol, zinc oxide, talc, propylene glycol, sodium bisulfate, EDTA, parabens	Tinted. In 56.7 g.	135

* Cost Index based on cost per g or ml.

[1] As precipitated sulfur.

[2] As colloidal sulfur.

(Continued on following page)

Creams, Lotions and Gels (Cont.)

		Sulfur	Salicylic Acid	Resorcinol	Other Content	How Supplied	C.I.*
otc	**Clearasil Adult Care Medicated Blemish Stick** (Vicks Personal)	8%		1%	4% bentonite, laureth-4, titanium dioxide	Tinted. In 3.75 g.	438
otc	**Acnomel Cream** (SmithKline)	8%		2%	11% alcohol, bentonite, titanium dioxide	Greaseless base. In 28 g.	206
otc	**Bensulfoid Cream** (Poythress)	8%		2%	10% alcohol	In 15 g.	85
otc	**Sebasorb Liquid** (Summers)	2%[2]	2%		10% attapulgite, polysorbate 80	In 60 ml.	50
otc	**Zinc Sulfide Compound Lotion, Improved** (Paddock)				27 mg zinc and 48 mg sulfur/ml with sodium borate, boric acid and Al hydroxide	In 120 ml.	22
otc	**Saligel Acne Gel** (Stiefel)		5%		14% alcohol	In 60 g.	91
otc	**Buf-Puf Medicated Maximum Strength Pads** (3M Pharm.)		2%		Alcohols benzoate, EDTA, triethanolamine, vitamin E acetate	In 30s.	NA
otc	**Clearasil Double Clear Maximum Strength Pads** (Richardson-Vicks)		2%		40% alcohol, witch hazel distillate, quaternium-22, aloe vera gel, menthol	In 32s.	NA
otc	**Komed Lotion** (Barnes-Hind)		2%		8% sodium thiosulfate, 25% isopropyl alcohol	Thixotropic gel base. In 52.5 ml.	180
otc	**Propa P.H. Medicated Acne Cream w/Aloe** (Commerce)		2%			Greaseless vanishing base. In 30 g.	217
otc	**Propa P.H. Medicated Acne Stick w/Aloe** (Commerce)		2%		Aloe extract, bentonite	Greaseless. In 0.75 g.	2529
otc	**Clearasil Double Clear Regular Strength Pads** (Richardson-Vicks)		1.25%		40% alcohol, witch hazel distillate, quaternium-22, aloe vera gel, menthol	In 32s.	NA
otc	**Oxy Night Watch Lotion** (SK-Beecham)		1%		Cetyl alcohol, silica, propylene glycol, stearyl alcohol, sodium lauryl sulfate, parabens and EDTA	In 60 ml.	NA
otc	**Buf-Puf Medicated Regular Strength Pads** (3M Pharm.)		0.5%		Alcohols benzoate, EDTA, triethanolamine, vitamin E acetate	In 30s.	NA
otc	**Propa P.H. Medicated Cleansing Pads w/Aloe** (Commerce)		0.5%		25% SD alcohol 40, aloe	In 45s.	602
otc	**RA Lotion** (Medco Labs)			3%	Calamine, starch, 43% alcohol, sodium borate, bentonite	In 120, 240 and 480 ml.	23

* Cost Index based on cost per g, ml, stick or pad. [1] From 33% colloidal sulfur. [2] Colloidal sulfur.

Medicated Bar Cleansers

	Product	Composition	Size	C.I.*
otc	**Clearasil Antibacterial Soap** (Vicks Personal Care)	**Bar:** 0.75% triclosan, glycerin, bentonite and titanium dioxide	In 97.5 g.	20
otc	**Oxy Medicated Soap** (SmithKline Beecham)	**Bar:** 1% triclosan, bentonite, cocoamphodipropionate, iron oxides, glycerin, magnesium silicate, sodium borohydride, sodium cocoate, sodium tallowate, talc, EDTA and titanium dioxide	In 97.5 g.	NA
otc	**Acne-Aid Cleansing Bar** (Stiefel)	**Bar:** 6.3% surfactant blend	In 112 and 174 g.	24
otc	**Oxy Clean Soap** (Norcliff Thayer)	**Bar:** 3.5% salicylic acid and sodium borate	In 97.5 g.	19
otc	**Salicylic Acid Soap** (Stiefel)	**Bar:** 3.5% salicylic acid	In 120 g.	26
otc	**Sulfur Soap** (Stiefel)	**Bar:** 10% precipitated sulfur	In 123 g.	25
otc	**Buf-Bar** (3M Personal Care)	**Bar:** 3% sulfur and titanium dioxide	In 105 g.	21
otc	**Fostex Medicated Cleansing Bar** (Westwood)	**Bar:** 2% sulfur, 2% salicylic acid, boric acid, docusate sodium and urea	In 112.5 g.	30
otc	**Salicylic Acid and Sulfur Soap** (Stiefel)	**Bar:** 10% precipitated sulfur and 3% salicylic acid	In 123 g.	26
otc	**Sastid Soap** (Stiefel)		In 123 g.	26
otc	**Aveeno Cleansing Bar** (Rydelle)	**Bar:** 2% sulfur, 2% salicylic acid, 50% colloidal oatmeal and mild surfactant. Soap free.	In 105 g.	21

Abrasive Cleansers

	Product	Composition	Size	C.I.*
otc	**Sastid (AL) Scrub** (Stiefel)	**Cleanser:** 1.6% sulfur and 1.6% salicylic acid with 20% aluminum oxide scrub particles in soapless surfactants	In 87 g.	54
otc	**Pernox Scrub** (Westwood)	**Cleanser:** 2% sulfur and 1.5% salicylic acid with polyethylene and docusate sodium	Lemon or regular scent. In 60 and 120 ml.	110
otc	**Pernox Lathering Lotion** (Westwood)	**Cleanser:** 2% sulfur, 2% salicylic acid, docusate sodium and polyethylene	In 150 ml.	58
otc	**Brasivol** (Stiefel)	**Cleanser, Fine:** Aluminum oxide particles in a surfactant cleansing base with sodium lauryl sulfate	In 153 g.	40
		Cleanser, Medium: Aluminum oxide particles in a surfactant cleansing base with sodium lauryl sulfate	In 180 g.	34
		Cleanser, Rough: Aluminum oxide particles in a surfactant cleansing base with sodium lauryl sulfate	In 195 g.	31
otc	**Ionax** (Owen)	**Scrub:** Polyethylene granules, benzalkonium chloride, 10% alcohol and polyoxyethylene ethers	In 60 and 120 g.	96
otc	**Komex** (Barnes-Hind)	**Scrub:** Sodium tetraborate decahydrate dissolving particles in a base of surfactant cleaning agents. Soap free.	In 75 g.	107
otc	**Oxy Clean Lathering Facial** (Norcliff Thayer)		In 79.5 g.	58
otc	**Seba-Nil Cleansing Mask** (Owen)	**Suspension:** Astringent face mask containing bentonite, polyethylene, SD alcohol-40, sulfated castor oil, titanium dioxide, kaolin, chromium oxide and methylparaben	In 105 g.	62

* Cost Index based on cost per g or ml.

Liquid Cleansers

	Product	Composition	How Supplied	C.I.*
otc	**Sulpho-Lac Acne Medication** (Bradley)	5% sulfur and 27% zinc sulfate in 53% Vleminickx's solution base	In 28.35 g.	NA
otc	**Sastid Plain Therapeutic Shampoo and Acne Wash** (Stiefel)	1.6% sulfur and 1.6% salicylic acid in a surfactant base	In 75 ml.	55
otc	**SalAc Cleanser** (GenDerm)	2% salicylic acid in a surfactant blend	In 177 ml.	17
otc	**Sebacide Cleanser** (Paddock)	Coconut oil, pine oil, alrosol, tri-potassium EDTA, DSS, castor oil, alromine RA, sodium lauryl sarcosinate, lecithin, tetrasodium pyrophosphate, potassium carbonate and 0.35% parachlorometaxylenol	In 120 ml, pt and gal.	14
otc	**Clearasil Medicated Astringent** (Vicks Personal Care)	0.5% salicylic acid and 43% alcohol	In 120 ml.	22
otc	**Stri-Dex Pads** (Glenbrook)	**Regular Strength:** 0.5% salicylic acid, 28% SD alcohol and citric acid **Maximum Strength:** 2% salicylic acid, 44% SD alcohol and citric acid	In 42s and 75s. In 42s.	65 74
otc	**Oxy Clean Medicated Cleanser and Pads** (Norcliff Thayer)	**Cleanser and regular strength pads:** 0.5% salicylic acid, 40% SD alcohol 40B, citric acid, menthol and sodium lauryl sulfate **Maximum strength pads:** 2% salicylic acid, 50% SD alcohol 40B, citric acid, menthol and sodium lauryl sulfate	**Cleanser:** In 120 ml. **Pads (regular):** In 50s. **Pads (maximum):** In 50s.	22 57 57
otc	**Ionax Astringent Skin Cleanser** (Owen)	Salicylic acid, allantoin, acetone, polyoxyethylene ethers and 48% isopropyl alcohol	In 240 ml.	27
otc	**Listerex Scrub** (Warner-Lambert)	**Lotion:** 2% salicylic acid	Herbal or Golden. In 120 and 240 ml.	22
otc	**Drytex Lotion** (C & M Pharm.)	Salicylic acid, 10% acetone, 40% isopropyl alcohol, polysorbate 20 and methylbenzethonium chloride	Tartrazine. In 240 ml.	21
otc	**Seba-Nil Liquid Cleanser** (Owen)	49.7% alcohol, acetone and polysorbate 20	In 240 ml and pt.	23
otc	**Tyrosum Cleanser** (Summers)	50% isopropanol, 10% acetone and 2% polysorbate 80	**Liquid:** In 120 ml and pt. **Packets:** In 24s and 50s.	19 113
otc	**Acno Cleanser** (Baker/Cummins)	60% isopropyl alcohol, laureth-23 and tetrasodium EDTA	In 240 ml.	35
otc	**Brasivol Base** (Stiefel)	A surfactant cleansing base with neutral soaps and polyoxyethylene lauryl ether	In 116 g.	49
otc	**Oxy Clean Medicated Pads for Sensitive Skin** (SK-Beecham)	**Pads:** 0.5% salicylic acid, 16% SD alcohol 40B	In 50s.	NA
Rx	**Xerac AC** (Person & Covey)	6.25% aluminum chloride hexahydrate in 96% anhydrous ethyl alcohol	In 35 and 60 ml.	186
otc	**Ionax Foam** (Owen)	0.2% benzalkonium chloride and polyoxyethylene ethers in a soapless surfactant	In 75 and 150 g aerosol.	74

* Cost Index based on cost per ml, g or pad.

These products are recommended for patients with sensitive, dry or irritated skin, who may react adversely to common soap products. Therapeutic cleansers include "soap free" cleansers, which are less irritating to sensitive skin, and "modified" soap products, which may contain emollient components or may be adjusted to a neutral or slightly acidic pH.

Soap Free Cleansers

				C.I.*
otc	**Aveeno Cleansing Bar** (Rydelle)	**Normal to Oily Skin Formula:** Soap free. 50% colloidal oatmeal, lanolin derivative and a mild surfactant	In 96 and 132 g.	25
otc	**Aveeno Cleansing Bar** (Rydelle)	**Dry Skin Formula:** Soap free, emollient. 30% colloidal oatmeal, vegetable oils, lanolin derivative and 29% glycerin in a mild surfactant base	In 90 g.	25
otc	**Lowila Cake** (Westwood)	**Cleanser:** Soap free, pH adjusted. Dextrin, sodium lauryl sulfoacetate, boric acid, urea, sorbitol, mineral oil, PEG-14 M, lactic acid, cellulose gum and DSS	In 112.5 g.	26
otc	**Cetaphil Cream and Lotion** (Owen)	Lipid free. Cetyl alcohol, stearyl alcohol, sodium lauryl sulfate, propylene glycol and parabens	**Cream:** In 480 g. **Lotion:** In 240 and 480 ml.	25 20
otc	**Keri Facial Cleanser** (Westwood)	**Liquid:** Soap free. Glycerin, squalane, propylene glycol, glyceryl stearate, PEG-100 stearate, stearic acid, steareth-20, lanolin alcohol, magnesium aluminum silicate, cetyl alcohol, beeswax, PEG-20-sorbitan beeswax, methyl and propyl parabens and quaternium-15	In 120 ml.	64
otc	**pHisoDerm** (Winthrop Pharm.)	**Liquid:** Soap free, pH adjusted, octoxynol 3, petrolatum, lanolin alcohol, sodium benzoate, mineral oil, sodium octoxynol 2 ethane sulfonate solution, oleyl alcohol, cocamide MEA, imidazolidinyl urea, tetrasodium EDTA and methylcellulose	**Regular:** In 150 ml, pt and gal. **Dry Skin Formula:** In 150 and 480 ml. **Oily Skin Formula:** In 150 and 480 ml.	27 20 20
otc	**Spectro-Jel** (Recsei)	**Liquid:** Soap free. Methylcellulose, carboxypolymethylene, cetyl alcohol, sorbitan monooleate, fumed silica, triethanolamine stearate, glycol polysiloxane, propylene glycol, glycerin and 5% isopropyl alcohol	In 127.5 ml, pt and gal.	17
otc	**Lobana Body Shampoo** (Ulmer)	**Liquid:** Emollient. Chloroxylenol in a mild sudsing base. pH adjusted	In 240 ml and gal.	18
otc	**Sulfoil** (C & M Pharm.)	**Liquid:** Soap free. Sulfonated castor oil	In pt and gal.	15
otc	**Liquid Lather** (Ulmer)	**Body wash:** Sodium laureth sulfate, sodium lauroyl sarcosinate, lauramide DEA, linoleamide DEA, actyl hydroxystearate, polyquarternium 7, tetrasodium EDTA and quaternium 15	In 240 ml and gal.	NA
otc	**Eucerin Cleansing** (Beiersdorf)	**Lotion:** Sodium laureth sulfate, cocoamphocarboxyglycinate, cocamidopropyl betaine, cocamide MEA, PEG-7 glyceryl cocoate, PEG-5 lanolate, PEG-120 methyl glucose dioleate, lanolin alcohol, imidazolidinyl urea	Soap free. In 240 ml.	NA

* Cost Index based on cost per g or ml.

Refer to the general discussion of these products on page 2310

	Modified Bar Soaps			C.I.*
otc	**Basis, Superfatted Soap** (Beiersdorf)	**Bar:** Sodium tallowate, sodium cocoate, petrolatum, glycerin, zinc oxide, NaCl, titanium dioxide, lanolin alcohol, beeswax, BHT and EDTA	Emollient, superfatted. In 99 and 225 g.	17
otc	**Phisoderm Gentle Cleansing Bar** (Winthrop Consumer)	**Bar:** Sodium tallowate, sodium cocoate, petrolatum, glycerin, lanolin, sodium chloride, BHT, trisodium EDTA and titanium dioxide	Nondetergent, moisturizing. Scented or unscented. In 99 g.	19
otc	**Oilatum Soap** (Stiefel)	**Bar:** 7.5% polyunsaturated vegetable oil	Scented or unscented. In 112 g.	23
otc	**Neutrogena Baby Cleansing Formula Soap** (Neutrogena Corp.)	**Bar:** Triethanolamine, glycerin, stearic acid, tallow, coconut oil, castor oil, sodium hydroxide, oleic acid, laneth-10 acetate, cocamide DEA, nonoxynol 14 and PEG-4 octoate	Transparent, emollient, pH adjusted, moisturizing. In 105 g.	21
otc	**Neutrogena Dry Skin Soap** (Neutrogena Corp.)	**Bar:** Triethanolamine, stearic acid, tallow, glycerin, coconut oil, castor oil, sodium hydroxide, oleic acid, laneth-10 acetate, cocamide DEA, nonoxynol 14, PEG-4 octoate, BHT and O-tolyl biguanide	Transparent, emollient, pH adjusted, moisturizing. Scented or unscented. In 105 and 165 g.	21
otc	**Neutrogena Soap** (Neutrogena Corp.)	**Bar:** Triethanolamine, glycerin, stearic acid, tallow, coconut oil, castor oil, sodium hydroxide, oleic acid and cocamide DEA	Transparent, nondetergent, nonmedicated, pH adjusted. Scented or unscented. In 105 and 165 g.	21
otc	**Neutrogena Acne Cleansing Soap** (Neutrogena Corp.)	**Bar:** Triethanolamine, glycerin, stearic acid, tallow, coconut oil, castor oil, sodium hydroxide, oleic acid, acetylated lanolin alcohol, cocamide DEA, alcohol and TEA lauryl sulfate	Transparent, nonmedicated. In 105 g.	23
otc	**Ambi 10** (Kiwi Brands)	**Bar:** Triclosan, sodium tallowate, PEG-20, titanium dioxide	In 99 g.	NA
otc	**Basis, Glycerin Soap** (Beiersdorf)	**Bar:** Tallow, coconut oil and glycerin	Transparent. **Sensitive:** In 90 and 150 g. **Normal to dry:** In 90 and 150 g.	21 21
otc	**Alpha Keri Moisturizing Soap** (Westwood)	**Bar:** Sodium tallowate, sodium cocoate, mineral oil, lanolin oil, PEG-75, glycerin, titanium dioxide, sodium chloride, BHT and trisodium HEDTA	Nondetergent, emollient. In 120 g.	21
otc	**Purpose Soap** (Ortho Derm.)	**Bar:** Sodium salts of fatty acids and glycerin	Nondetergent, nonmedicated. In 108 and 180 g.	23
otc	**Shepard's Moisturizing Soap** (Dermik)	**Bar:** Soap (sodium tallowate and cocoate types), glycerin, coconut acid, sodium chloride, lanolin, BHT, trisodium HEDTA and titanium dioxide	Nondetergent, moisturizing. In 120 g.	35
otc	**Nivea Creme Soap** (Beiersdorf)	**Bar:** Saponified fatty acids, petrolatum, titanium dioxide, sodium thiosulfate, wool wax alcohol and beeswax	In 90 and 150 g.	13
otc	**Cuticura Medicated Soap** (DEP Corp.)	**Bar:** 1% triclocarban, sodium tallowate, sodium cocoate, glycerin, mineral oil, petrolatum, sodium chloride, tetrasodium EDTA, sodium bicarbonate, magnesium silicate and iron oxides	Phosphorus free. Emollient. Mildly antibacterial. In 97.5 and 142 g.	22

* Cost Index based on cost per g.

In addition to the products described here, other products for treatment of psoriasis include: *COAL TAR*, see pages 2335, 2410 and 2408 *CORTICOSTEROIDS* (Systemic, page 465; Topical, page 2370). *SALICYLIC ACID*, see page 2416.

ANTHRALIN (Dithranol)

Actions:

Anthralin reduces the mitotic rate and proliferation of epidermal cells in psoriasis by inhibiting synthesis of nucleic protein. In vitro evidence suggests that anthralin's antimitotic effect results from inhibition of DNA synthesis.

Indications: Psoriasis.

Contraindications: Acute psoriasis; hypersensitivity to anthralin or any of the components.

Warnings:

Absorption in man has not been finally determined.

Renal and Hepatic Impairment: Although no renal, hepatic or hematologic abnormalities have occurred with topical application, use caution in patients with renal disease and in those having extensive and prolonged applications. Perform periodic urine tests for albuminuria. Discontinue use if sensitivity reactions occur.

Use only on quiescent or chronic patches; not in acute eruptions or where inflammation is present.

Usage in Pregnancy: Category C. Safety for use has not been established. It is not known whether anthralin can cause fetal harm when administered to a pregnant woman. Administer only if clearly needed.

Usage in Lactation: It is not known whether this drug is excreted in breast milk. Because of the potential for tumorigenicity in animal studies, discontinue nursing or the drug.

Usage in Children: Safety and efficacy have not been established.

Precautions:

When redness is observed, reduce frequency of dosage, or discontinue application. Higher concentrations may produce excessive irritation.

Keep away from eyes; if accidentally applied, severe conjunctivitis may result. Do not apply to the face, genitalia or intertriginous skin. If sensitivity reactions occur, especially on the normal skin surrounding the plaque site, discontinue use. Wash hands thoroughly after using. May stain fabrics or skin and may temporarily discolor gray or white hair.

Carcinogenesis, mutagenesis or impairment of fertility: In long-term studies with mice, anthralin demonstrated carcinogenic and tumorigenic activity.

Adverse Reactions:

Excessive irritation; sensitivity reaction. May temporarily discolor fingernails or gray or white hair; may stain fabrics.

Patient Information:

Patient instructions are available with products.

Administration and Dosage:

Apply a thin layer to affected areas, as directed, and a protective film of petrolatum to the areas surrounding the plaque. Initiate therapy with the 0.1% strength. The strength may be gradually increased, depending on patient tolerance. Use plastic gloves and wear a plastic cap over treated scalp at bedtime to prevent staining.

Skin: Apply at bedtime to plaque sites. In the morning, wash off remaining drug.

Scalp: Massage into affected areas. Shampoo scalp in the morning.

	Product	Form/Strength	Package	C.I.*
Rx	**Anthra-Derm** (Dermik)	**Ointment:** 0.1%	In 42.5 g	268
		0.25%	In 42.5 g.	268
		0.5%	In 42.5 g.	284
		1%	In 42.5 g.	284
Rx	**Lasan** (Stiefel)	**Ointment:** 0.4%	In 60 g.	203
Rx	**Lasan** (Stiefel)	**Cream:** 0.1%	In 65 g.	182
		0.2%	In 65 g.	189
		0.4%	In 65 g.	209
Rx	**Dritho-Scalp** (American Dermal)	**Cream:** 0.25%	In 50 g w/applicator.	308
		0.5%	In 50 g w/applicator.	340
Rx	**Drithocreme** (American Dermal)	**Cream:** 0.1%	In 50 g.	277
		0.25%	In 50 g.	298
		0.5%	In 50 g.	333
Rx	**Lasan HP-1** (Stiefel)	**Cream:** 1%	In 65 g.	218
Rx	**Drithocreme HP 1%** (American Dermal)	**Cream:** 1%	In 50 g.	417

* Cost Index based on cost per g.

AMMONIATED MERCURY

Indications:

Psoriasis, seborrheic dermatitis, impetigo contagiosa, dermatomycoses, superficial pyodermas and pediculosis pubis.

Since more effective and less toxic therapies are available, the use of ammoniated mercury is not recommended.

Combination with salicyclic acid in the management of seborrheic dermatitis and psoriasis.

Contraindications:

Hypersensitivity to ammoniated mercury.

Warnings:

May cause skin irritation. Frequent or prolonged application to large areas may cause mercury poisoning.

Usage in Children: Avoid use of ammoniated mercury in infants and young children, it may cause acrodynia (pink disease).

Precautions:

For external use only. Do not apply to highly inflamed skin, sunburn or open wounds. Consult physician in case of deep or puncture wounds or serious burns. If redness, swelling or pain persists or increases, or if infection, rash or irritation occurs, discontinue use and consult physician.

Drug Interactions:

Sulfur or **iodine-containing** preparations: Do not use in conjunction with ammoniated mercury.

Adverse Reactions:

Ammoniated mercury is a potential sensitizer, capable of evoking allergic reactions following topical application.

Patient Information:

Avoid concomitant use of topical iodine or sulfur-containing products.

Administration and Dosage:

Apply 1 or 2 times daily.

Storage: Protect from light. Store in a well-closed, tight container.

				C.I.*
otc	**Ammoniated Mercury** (Various)	**Ointment:** 5%	In 30 g and 1 lb.	114+
otc	**Ammoniated Mercury** (Lilly)		In 30 g.	122
Rx	**Ammoniated Mercury** (Truxton)	**Ointment:** 10%	In 1 lb.	18
Rx	**Emersal** (Medco Lab)	**Lotion:** 5% with 2.5% salicylic acid	In 120 ml.	54

TAR DERIVATIVES, TOPICAL

Indications:

To help control psoriasis affecting the nails.

Precautions:

Exercise caution when used in conjunction with phototherapy. Excessive exposure to sunlight after use should be avoided.

Adverse Reactions:

May stain fabrics.

Administration and Dosage:

Apply a small amount twice daily to edges, surface and base of affected nails. Do not wash nails for several minutes after application. Use for at least 8 weeks.

otc	**PsoriNail** (Summers)	**Liquid:** 2.5% coal tar solution, isopropyl alcohol, 1,3-butylene glycol and acetyl mandelic acid	In 30 ml.	NA

* Cost Index based on cost per g or ml.

This is an abbreviated monograph. For complete prescribing information and use of methotrexate as an antineoplastic agent, see page 2511.

METHOTREXATE (Amethopterin; MTX)

Warnings:

Due to the possibility of fatal or severe toxic reactions, inform patient of risks involved; keep under constant supervision. Deaths have occurred. Restrict use to severe, recalcitrant, disabling psoriasis not adequately responsive to other therapy when diagnosis is established by biopsy or after dermatologic consultation.

May produce marked depression of bone marrow, anemia, leukopenia, thrombocytopenia and bleeding.

May be hepatotoxic, particularly at high dosage or with prolonged therapy. Liver atrophy, necrosis, cirrhosis, fatty changes and periportal fibrosis may occur. Since changes may occur without previous signs of GI or hematologic toxicity, determine hepatic function prior to initiation of treatment; monitor regularly. Use caution in presence of preexisting liver damage or impaired hepatic function. Avoid concomitant use of other drugs with hepatotoxic potential (including alcohol).

Methotrexate may cause fetal death or congenital anomalies; do not use in women of childbearing potential unless benefits outweigh risks. Contraindicated in pregnancy.

Impaired renal function is usually a contraindication.

Diarrhea and ulcerative stomatitis are frequent and require interruption of therapy; otherwise, hemorrhagic enteritis and death from intestinal perforation may occur.

Actions:

Pharmacology: Actively proliferating tissues are generally more sensitive to the effect of methotrexate. In psoriasis, the rate of production of epithelial cells in the skin is greatly increased over normal skin. This differential in reproductive rates is the basis for the use of this drug to control the psoriatic process.

Indications:

For the symptomatic control of severe, recalcitrant, disabling psoriasis which is not adequately responsive to other therapy. Use only when the diagnosis has been established by biopsy or after dermatologic consultation.

Methotrexate is also used as an antineoplastic agent (see p.2511).

Unlabeled Uses: Methotrexate has shown potential value in the treatment of rheumatoid arthritis, psoriatic arthritis and Reiter's disease.

Administration and Dosage:

Severe, recalcitrant, disabling psoriasis: Individualize dosage. Schedules below pertain to a 70 kg adult. Perform test dose (5 to 10 mg parenterally) 1 week prior to therapy.

Weekly single oral, IM or IV dosage schedule – 10 to 25 mg/week until adequate response is achieved. Do not exceed 50 mg per week.

Divided oral dose schedule – 2.5 mg at 12 hour intervals for 3 doses or at 8 hour intervals for 4 doses each week. Do not exceed 30 mg per week.

Daily oral dose schedule – 2.5 mg daily for 5 days followed by at least a 2 day rest period. Do not exceed 6.25 mg per day. This schedule may carry an increased risk of serious liver pathology.

Once optimal clinical response is achieved, reduce to lowest possible amount of drug with the longest possible rest period. Methotrexate may permit return to conventional topical therapy, which should be encouraged.

Rx	**Methotrexate** (Lederle)	**Powder for Injection:** 1 g (as sodium) per vial	Preservative free. In single use vials.[2]
Rx	**Methotrexate** (Lederle)	**Tablets:** 2.5 mg	(LL M1). Yellow, scored. In 100s.
Rx	**Methotrexate** (Various)	**Injection:** 2.5 mg (as sodium) per ml	In 2 ml vials.
		25 mg (as sodium) per ml	In 2, 4 & 8 ml vials.
		Preservative Free Injection: 25 mg (as sodium) per ml[1]	In 2, 4 and 8 ml vials.
		Powder for Injection: 20, 50, 100 and 250 mg (as sodium) per vial for reconstitution	In 20 ml vials.
Rx	**Abitrexate** (Americal)	**Injection:** 25 mg (as sodium) per ml	In 2, 4 and 8 ml vials.
Rx	**Folex** (Adria)	**Powder for Injection:** 25, 50, 100 and 250 mg (as sodium) per vial for reconstitution[1]	In single-use vials.
Rx	**Folex PFS** (Adria)	**Injection:** 25 mg (as sodium) per ml[1]	In 2, 4 and 8 ml vials.

[1] Contains no preservative. For single use only.

[2] Contains ≈ 7 mcg sodium per vial.

ETRETINATE

Warnings:

Etretinate must not be used by females who are pregnant, who intend to become pregnant or who may not use reliable contraception while undergoing treatment. The period of time during which pregnancy must be avoided after treatment has not been determined. Blood levels of 0.5 to 12 ng/ml have been reported in 5 of 47 patients 2.1 to 2.9 years after treatment was concluded.

Major human fetal abnormalities related to administration have been reported, including meningomyelocoele, meningoencephalocoele, multiple synostoses, facial dysmorphia, syndactylies, absence of terminal phalanges, malformations of hip, ankle and forearm, low set ears, high palate, decreased cranial volume and alterations of the skull and cervical vertebrae on x-ray.

Women of childbearing potential must not be given etretinate until pregnancy is excluded. Perform a pregnancy test within 2 weeks prior to initiating therapy. Start therapy on the second or third day of the next normal menstrual period. An effective form of contraception must be used for at least one month before therapy, during therapy and following discontinuation of therapy for an indefinite period of time.

Counsel women on the serious risks to the fetus should they become pregnant while undergoing treatment or after discontinuation of therapy. If pregnancy does occur, the physician and patient should discuss the desirability of continuing the pregnancy.

Actions:

Etretinate is related to retinoic acid and retinol (vitamin A). The mechanism of action is unknown. Improvement in psoriatic patients occurs in association with a decrease in scale, erythema and thickness of lesions, as well as histological evidence of normalization of epidermal differentiation, decreased stratum corneum thickness and decreased inflammation in the epidermis and dermis.

Clinical Pharmacology: Etretinate resulted in clinical improvement in most patients treated. Complete clearing of the disease was observed after 4 to 9 months of therapy in 13% of all patients treated for severe psoriasis. This included complete clearing in 16% of patients with erythrodermic psoriasis and 37% of patients with generalized pustular psoriasis. After discontinuation, most patients experienced some degree of relapse by the end of 2 months. After relapse, subsequent 4 to 9 month courses of therapy resulted in a similar clinical response as experienced during initial therapy.

Pharmacokinetics: The pharmacokinetic profile is linear. The absorption of etretinate was increased by whole milk or a high-lipid diet. Etretinate is extensively metabolized following oral dosing, with significant first-pass metabolism to the acid form, which is pharmacologically active. Subsequent metabolism results in conjugates that are ultimately excreted in the bile and urine.

C_{max} values range from 102 to 389 ng/ml and occur at T_{max} values of 2 to 6 hours. In another study of 47 patients treated chronically with etretinate, 5 had detectable serum drug levels (0.5 to 12 ng/ml) 2.1 to 2.9 years after therapy was discontinued. In one study, the apparent terminal half-life after 6 months of therapy was approximately 120 days. The long half-life appears to be due to storage of etretinate in adipose tissue.

Etretinate is $>$ 99% bound to plasma proteins, predominantly lipoproteins; its active metabolite is predominantly bound to albumin. Concentrations of etretinate in blister fluid after 6 weeks of dosing were approximately one-tenth those observed in plasma. Concentrations of etretinate and its metabolite in epidermal specimens obtained after 1 to 36 months were a function of location; subcutis $>>$ serum $>$ epidermis $>$ dermis. Similarly, liver concentrations of etretinate in patients receiving therapy for 6 months were generally higher than concomitant plasma concentrations.

Indications:

Treatment of severe recalcitrant psoriasis, including the erythrodermic and generalized pustular types.

Because of its significant adverse effects, etretinate should be prescribed only by physicians knowledgeable in the systemic use of retinoids and reserved for patients with severe recalcitrant psoriasis who are unresponsive to or intolerant of standard therapies: Topical tar plus UVB light; psoralens plus UVA light; systemic corticosteroids; and methotrexate.

Contraindications:

Pregnancy (see boxed Warnings).

(Continued on following page)

ETRETINATE (Cont.)

Warnings:

Pseudotumor cerebri: Retinoids have been associated with pseudotumor cerebri (benign intracranial hypertension). Early signs and symptoms include papilledema, headache, nausea, vomiting and visual disturbances. If present, discontinue the drug immediately and refer the patient for neurologic diagnosis and care.

Hepatotoxicity: Of 652 patients treated in US clinical trials, 10 had clinical or histologic hepatitis possibly related to etretinate treatment. Liver function tests returned to normal in 8 patients after the drug was discontinued; one patient had histologic changes resembling chronic active hepatitis 6 months off therapy, and one patient had no follow-up available. There have been four reports of hepatitis-related deaths worldwide.

Elevations of AST (SGOT), ALT (SGPT) or LDH have occurred in 18%, 23% and 15%, respectively, of individuals treated. If hepatotoxicity is suspected during treatment, discontinue the drug and investigate the etiology. These tests should be performed prior to initiation of therapy, at 1 to 2 week intervals for the first 1 to 2 months of therapy, and thereafter at intervals of 1 to 3 months, depending on the response to etretinate.

Ophthalmic effects: Corneal erosion, abrasion, irregularity and punctate staining have occurred, although these effects were absent or improved after therapy was stopped in those patients who had follow-up examinations. Corneal opacities have occurred in patients receiving isotretinoin; they had either completely resolved or were resolving at follow-up 6 to 7 weeks after discontinuation of the drug. Other ophthalmic effects that have occurred include decreased visual acuity and blurring of vision, night vision decrease, minimal posterior subcapsular cataract, iritis, blot retinal hemorrhage, scotoma and photophobia. Any patient experiencing visual difficulties should discontinue the drug and have an ophthalmological examination.

Hyperostosis: In clinical trials, 45 patients with a mean age of 40 years were retrospectively evaluated. They received a mean dose of 0.8 mg/kg for a mean duration of 33 months at time of x-ray. Eleven patients had psoriasis, while 34 patients had a disorder of keratinization. Of 38 patients who continued to receive etretinate for an average of 60 months, 32 (84%) had radiographic evidence of extraspinal tendon and ligament calcification. The most common sites of involvement were the ankles (76%), pelvis (53%) and knees (42%); spinal changes were uncommon. Involvement tended to be bilateral and multifocal. There were no bone or joint symptoms in 47% of the affected patients.

Lipids: Perform blood lipid determinations before etretinate is administered and then at intervals of 1 or 2 weeks until the lipid response is established; this usually occurs within 4 to 8 weeks. Approximately 45% of patients experienced an elevation of plasma triglycerides, 37% developed a decrease in high density lipoproteins (HDL) and about 16% showed an increase in cholesterol levels. They were reversible after discontinuation of therapy.

Patients with a tendency to develop hypertriglyceridemia include those with diabetes mellitus, obesity, increased alcohol intake or a familial history of these conditions.

Cardiovascular effects: Two cases of myocardial infarction have been reported. One possibly related to etretinate therapy and one for which a relationship was not specified.

Usage in Pregnancy: Category X. See Warning Box.

Usage in Lactation: Etretinate is excreted in the milk of lactating rats; however, it is not known whether this drug is excreted in breast milk. Because of the potential for adverse effects, nursing mothers should not receive etretinate.

Usage in Children: Ossification of interosseous ligaments and tendons of the extremities has been reported. Two children showed x-ray changes suggestive of premature epiphyseal closure during treatment. Skeletal hyperostosis has also been reported after treatment with isotretinoin. It is not known if any of these effects occur more commonly in children, but concern is greater because of the growth process. Pretreatment x-rays for bone age including x-rays of the knees, followed by yearly monitoring, are advised. Evaluate pain or limitation of motion with appropriate radiological examination. Because of the lack of data and the possibility of children being more sensitive to effects of the drug, use only when all alternative therapies have been exhausted.

Drug Interactions:

Milk consumption increases the absorption of etretinate.

Adverse Reactions:

Adverse events generally resemble those of the hypervitaminosis A syndrome.

Mucocutaneous: Dry nose, chapped lips (> 75%); thirst, sore mouth (50% to 75%); nosebleed (25% to 50%); cheilitis, sore tongue (10% to 25%); dry eyes, mucous membrane abnormalities, dry mouth, gingival bleeding/inflammation (1% to 10%); decreased mucus secretion, rhinorrhea (< 1%).

(Adverse Reactions continued on following page)

ETRETINATE (Cont.)

Adverse Reactions (Cont.):

Dermatologic: Hair loss, palm/sole/fingertip peeling (> 75%); dry skin, itching, rash, red scaly face, skin fragility (50% to 75%); bruising, sunburn (25% to 50%); nail disorder, skin peeling (10% to 25%); hair abnormalities, bullous eruption, cold/clammy skin, onycholysis, paronychia, pyogenic granuloma, changes in perspiration (1% to 10%); abnormal skin odor, granulation tissue, healing impairment, herpes simplex, hirsutism, increased pore size, sensory skin changes, skin atrophy, fissures, infection, nodules and ulceration, urticaria (< 1%).

Musculoskeletal: Hyperostosis (> 75%); bone/joint pain (50% to 75%); muscle cramps (25% to 50%); myalgia (1% to 10%); gout, hyperkinesia, hypertonia (< 1%).

CNS: Fatigue (50% to 75%); headache (25% to 50%); fever (10% to 25%); dizziness, lethargy, sensation change, pain, rigors (1% to 10%); abnormal thinking, amnesia, anxiety, depression, pseudotumor cerebri (see Warnings), emotional lability (< 1%).

Special senses: Eye irritation (50% to 75%); eyeball pain, eyelid abnormalities (25% to 50%); abnormalities of conjunctiva, cornea, lens and retina; decreased visual acuity, double vision (10% to 25%); abnormalities of lacrimation, vision, extraocular musculature, ocular tension, pupil and vitreous; earache, otitis externa (1% to 10%); equilibrium change, ear drainage or infection, hearing change, decreased night vision, photophobia, visual change, scotoma (< 1%).

GI: Abdominal pain, appetite change (25% to 50%); nausea (10% to 25%); hepatitis (see Warnings) (1% to 10%); constipation, diarrhea, melena, flatulence, weight loss, oral ulcers, taste perversion, tooth caries (< 1%).

Cardiovascular: Cardiovascular, thrombotic or obstructive events, edema (1% to 10%); atrial fibrillation, chest pain, coagulation disorder, phlebitis, postural hypotension, syncope (< 1%).

Respiratory: Dyspnea (1% to 10%); coughing, increased sputum, dysphonia, pharyngitis (< 1%).

Hematologic: Increased MCHC (60%); increased MCH, reticulocytes, PTT, ESR (25% to 50%). Decreased hemoglobin/HCT, RBC and MCV; increased platelets; increased or decreased WBC and components or prothrombin time (10% to 25%). Decreased platelets, MCH, MCHC and PTT; increased hemoglobin/HCT and RBC (1% to 10%).

Urinary: WBC in urine (10% to 25%), proteinuria, glycosuria, microscopic hematuria, casts, acetonuria, hemoglobinuria (1% to 10%); dysuria, polyuria, urinary retention (< 1%).

Hepatic: Increased triglycerides (25% to 50%); increased AST (SGOT), ALT (SGPT), alkaline phosphatase, GGTP, globulin, cholesterol (10% to 25%); increased bilirubin, increased or decreased total protein albumin (1% to 10%).

Renal: Increased BUN and creatinine (1% to 10%); kidney stones (< 1%).

Electrolytes: Increased or decreased potassium, calcium, phosphorus (25% to 50%); increased or decreased venous CO_2, sodium, chloride (10% to 25%).

Miscellaneous: Increased or decreased FBS (10% to 25%); increased CPK and malignant neoplasms (1% to 10%). Abnormal menses, atrophic vaginitis.

Overdosage:

There has been no experience with acute overdosage in humans.

Patient Information:

Advise women of childbearing potential that they must not be pregnant when therapy is initiated; they should use effective contraception for 1 month prior to therapy, while taking etretinate and after it has been discontinued. Etretinate has been found in the blood of some patients 2 to 3 years after its discontinuation. See Warning box.

Patients should not take vitamin A supplements because of possible additive toxic effects.

Transient exacerbation of psoriasis is common during the initial period of therapy.

Patients may experience decreased tolerance to contact lenses during and after therapy.

Administer with food.

Administration and Dosage:

Individualize dosage. Initiate at 0.75 to 1 mg/kg/day in divided doses; maximum dose, 1.5 mg/kg/day. Erythrodermic psoriasis may respond to lower initial doses of 0.25 mg/kg/day increased weekly by 0.25 mg/kg/day until optimal initial response.

Maintenance doses of 0.5 to 0.75 mg/kg/day generally begin after 8 to 16 weeks of therapy. Therapy is usually terminated in patients whose lesions have sufficiently resolved. Relapses may be treated as outlined for initial therapy.

Rx	**Tegison** (Roche)	**Capsules:** 10 mg	(#Tegison 10 Roche). Brown and green. In 30s.
		25 mg	(#Tegison 25 Roche). Brown and caramel. In 30s.

Product identification code.

NITROFURAZONE

Actions:

Nitrofurazone, a synthetic nitrofuran with a broad antibacterial spectrum, is bactericidal against most bacteria commonly causing surface infections, including *Staphylococcus aureus, Streptococcus, Escherichia coli, Clostridium perfringens, Aerobacter aerogenes* and *Proteus* sp.

Indications:

Adjunctive therapy of patients with second and third degree burns when bacterial resistance to other agents is a real or potential problem; skin grafting where bacterial contamination may cause graft rejection or donor site infection, particularly in hospitals with historical resistant bacteria epidemics.

Contraindications:

Known sensitization to nitrofurazone.

Warnings:

There is no evidence of effectiveness in treatment of minor burns or surface bacterial infections involving wounds, cutaneous ulcers or the various pyodermas.

Renal impairment: Use the soluble burn dressing with caution in patients with known or suspected renal impairment. The polyethylene glycol present in the base can be absorbed through denuded skin and may not be excreted normally by a compromised kidney, leading to symptoms of progressive renal impairment including increased BUN, anion gap and metabolic acidosis.

Usage in Pregnancy: Category C. Safety for use during pregnancy has not been established. Use only when clearly needed and when the potential benefits outweigh the unknown potential hazards to the fetus.

Usage in Lactation: It is not known whether this drug is excreted in breast milk. Safety for use in the nursing mother has not been established.

Usage in Children: Safety and efficacy for use in children have not been established.

Precautions:

Superinfection: Use may result in bacterial or fungal overgrowth of nonsusceptible organisms, including fungi and *Pseudomonas.* Such overgrowth may lead to a secondary infection. If this occurs, or if irritation, sensitization or superinfection develops, discontinue treatment and institute appropriate therapy.

G-6-PD Deficiency: Use with caution in individuals with glucose-6-phosphate dehydrogenase deficiency.

Drug Interactions:

Sutilains enzyme activity may be impaired by nitrofurazone.

Adverse Reactions:

In studies, symptoms appeared as varying degrees of contact dermatitis such as rash, pruritus and local edema. Treat allergic reactions symptomatically.

Patient Information:

Notify physician if condition worsens or if irritation occurs.

Administration and Dosage:

For the treatment of burns, apply directly to the lesion or place on gauze. Reapply once daily or every few days, depending on dressing technique.

Storage: Avoid exposure at all times to direct sunlight, excessive heat, strong fluorescent lighting and alkaline materials.

				C.I.*
Rx	**Nitrofurazone** (Various)	**Topical Solution:** 0.2%	In pt and gal.	10+
Rx	**Nitrofurazone** (Various)	**Ointment (soluble dressing):** 0.2%	In 480 g.	12+
Rx	**Furacin** (Procter & Gamble Pharm.)		In a polyethylene glycol base. In 28, 56 and 454 g.	144
Rx	**Furacin** (Procter & Gamble Pharm.)	**Cream:** 0.2%	In a water miscible base. In 28 g.	251

* Cost Index based on cost per ml or g.

MAFENIDE

Actions:

Mafenide, a sulfonamide, is bacteriostatic against many gram-negative and gram-positive organisms, including *Pseudomonas aeruginosa* and certain strains of anaerobes. It is active in the presence of pus and serum; its activity is not altered by changes in the acidity of the environment.

Mafenide reduces the bacterial population present in the avascular tissues of second and third degree burns. This permits spontaneous healing of deep partial-thickness burns and prevents conversion of burn wounds from partial thickness to full thickness. However, delayed eschar separation has occurred in some cases.

Pharmacokinetics: Applied topically, mafenide diffuses through devascularized areas and is absorbed and rapidly metabolized to p-carboxybenzenesulfonamide which is cleared through the kidneys. The metabolite has no antibacterial activity but retains the ability to inhibit carbonic anhydrase.

Indications:

Adjunctive therapy of second and third degree burns.

Contraindications:

In patients who are hypersensitive to the drug. It is a not known whether there is cross-sensitivity to other sulfonamides.

Warnings:

Superinfection: Use may result in bacterial or fungal overgrowth of nonsusceptible organisms. Such overgrowth may lead to a secondary infection. Appropriate measures should be taken if superinfection occurs.

Fungal colonization in and below the eschar may occur concomitantly with reduction of bacterial growth in the burn wound. However, fungal dissemination through the infected burn wound is rare.

Usage in Pregnancy: Category C. Animal reproduction studies have not been conducted. It is not known whether mafenide can cause fetal harm when administered to a pregnant woman or can affect reproduction capacity. Not recommended for the treatment of women of childbearing potential unless the burned area covers more than 20% of the total body surface or benefit is greater than the possible risk to the fetus.

Usage in Lactation: It is not known whether mafenide is excreted in breast milk. Because of the potential for serious adverse reactions in nursing infants, a decision should be made to discontinue nursing or discontinue the drug, taking into account the importance of the drug to the mother.

Precautions:

Metabolic acidosis: Mafenide and its metabolite inhibit carbonic anhydrase, which may result in metabolic acidosis, usually compensated by hyperventilation. High blood levels of mafenide and its metabolite may exaggerate the carbonic anhydrase inhibition. Therefore, close monitoring of acid-base balance is necessary, particularly in patients with extensive second degree or partial thickness burns and in those with pulmonary and renal dysfunction. Some burn patients treated with mafenide have also manifested an unexplained syndrome of marked hyperventilation with resulting respiratory alkalosis (slightly alkaline blood pH, low arterial pCO_2 and decreased total CO_2); change in arterial pO_2 is variable. The etiology and significance of these findings are unknown.

If acidosis occurs and becomes difficult to control, particularly in patients with pulmonary dysfunction, discontinuing therapy for 24 to 48 hours while continuing fluid therapy may aid in restoring acid-base balance.

Acute renal failure: Use with caution in patients with acute renal failure.

Sulfite sensitivity: This product contains sulfites, which may cause allergic-type reactions (eg, hives, itching, wheezing, anaphylaxis) in certain susceptible persons. Although the overall prevalence of sulfite sensitivity in the general population is probably low, it is seen more frequently in asthmatics or in atopic nonasthmatic persons.

(Continued on following page)

MAFENIDE (Cont.)

Adverse Reactions:

It is difficult to distinguish a reaction to mafenide from the effect of a severe burn.

Dermatologic: The most frequently reported reaction was pain on application or a burning sensation. Rare – Excoriation of new skin; bleeding of skin.

Allergic: Rash, itching, facial edema, swelling, hives, blisters, erythema and eosinophilia.

Respiratory: Tachypnea or hyperventilation, decrease in arterial pCO_2.

Metabolic: Acidosis, increase in serum chloride.

Other: One case of bone marrow depression and one case of an acute attack of porphyria have been reported. Fatal hemolytic anemia with disseminated intravascular coagulation, presumably related to a glucose-6-phosphate dehydrogenase deficiency, has been reported. Accidental ingestion has resulted in diarrhea.

Patient Information:

Notify physician if condition worsens or if irritation occurs.

Notify physician if marked hyperventilation occurs.

Administration and Dosage:

Application: Apply to the clean and debrided wound with a sterile gloved hand, once or twice daily, to a thickness of approximately 1⁄16 inch; thicker application is not recommended. Cover the burned areas with mafenide at all times. Reapply to any areas from which it has been removed (eg, by patient activity). Dressings are usually not required, but if necessary, use only a thin layer of dressing.

Bathing: When feasible, bathe the patient daily to aid in debridement. A whirlpool bath is particularly helpful, but the patient may be bathed in bed or in a shower.

Duration of therapy: Continue treatment until healing is progressing well or until the site is ready for grafting. Do not withdraw mafenide while infection is still possible. However, if allergic manifestations occur, discontinue treatment.

				C.I.*
Rx	**Sulfamylon** (Winthrop Pharm.)	**Cream:** 85 mg (as acetate) per g[1]	In 60, 120 and 435 g.	200

* Cost Index based on cost per g.

[1] Contains EDTA, parabens and metabisulfite.

SILVER SULFADIAZINE

Actions:

Pharmacology: Silver sulfadiazine acts only on the cell membrane and cell wall to produce its bactericidal effect. Silver is slowly released from the preparation in concentrations that are selectively toxic to bacteria. Both components in the complex are active. It is not a carbonic anhydrase inhibitor. Acidosis has not been reported; therefore, it may be of particular value in treating pediatric burn patients. While less than 1% of the silver content is absorbed, up to 10% of the sulfadiazine may be absorbed. Serum concentrations of 10 to 20 mcg/ml have been reported when extensive areas were involved.

Microbiology: Silver sulfadiazine is bactericidal for many gram-negative and gram-positive bacteria and is effective against yeast. Silver sulfadiazine will inhibit bacteria resistant to other antimicrobial agents and is superior to sulfadiazine.

Silver sulfadiazine has been shown to be effective against the following organisms:

Pseudomonas species
Pseudomonas aeruginosa
Pseudomonas cepacia
Pseudomonas maltophilia
Enterobacter species
Enterobacter aerogenes
Enterobacter agglomerans
Enterobacter cloacae
Herellea species
Mima species
Klebsiella species
Klebsiella pneumoniae
Escherichia coli
Serratia species
Serratia liquifaciens
Serratia marcescens
Serratia rubidae
Proteus mirabilis
Proteus morganii
Proteus rettgeri
Proteus vulgaris
Providencia species
Citrobacter diversus
Shigella species
Acinetobacter anitratum
Aeromonas hydrophilia
Arizona hinshawii
Alcaligenes faecalis
Staphylococcus aureus
Staphylococcus epidermidis
β-hemolytic *staphylococcus*
Streptococcus Group D (including *Enterococcus*)
Bacillus species
Candida species
Candida albicans
Corynebacterium diphtheriae
Clostridium perfringens

Indications:

Prevention and treatment of sepsis in second and third degree burns.

Contraindications:

Because sulfonamides may increase the possibility of kernicterus, do not use in pregnant women at or near term, in premature infants or in infants less than 2 months old.

Warnings:

Hypersensitivity: Administer with great caution to patients with a history of hypersensitivity to silver sulfadiazine. It is not known whether there is cross-sensitivity to other sulfonamides. If allergic reactions occur, consider discontinuation. Refer to Management of Acute Hypersensitivity Reactions on p. viii.

Use in glucose-6-phosphate dehydrogenase deficient individuals may be hazardous, as hemolysis may occur.

Fungal colonization in and below the eschar may occur concomitantly with reduction of bacterial growth; however, fungal dissemination is rare.

Serum sulfonamide concentrations: In the treatment of burn wounds involving extensive areas of the body, the serum sulfa concentration may approach adult therapeutic levels (8 to 12 mg%). Therefore, in these patients, monitor serum sulfa concentrations. Monitor renal function carefully and check the urine for sulfa crystals.

Usage in Pregnancy: Category C. Safety for use during pregnancy has not been established. Not recommended in women of childbearing potential, unless the burned area covers more than 20% of the total body surface area or the benefit is greater than the possible risk to the fetus.

Usage in Lactation: It is not known whether silver sulfadiazine cream is excreted in breast milk. However, since all sulfonamide derivatives increase the possibility of kernicterus, exercise caution when administering to a nursing mother.

(Continued on following page)

SILVER SULFADIAZINE (Cont.)

Precautions:

If hepatic or renal functions become impaired and drug elimination decreases, accumulation may occur. Weigh discontinuation against the therapeutic benefit being achieved.

Reduction in bacterial colonization has caused delayed separation, in some cases necessitating escharotomy to prevent contracture.

Drug Interactions:

Topical proteolytic enzymes: Silver may inactivate such enzymes if these agents are used in conjunction with silver sulfadiazine.

Adverse Reactions:

It is difficult to distinguish an adverse reaction due to silver sulfadiazine from one due to concomitant use of other therapeutic agents. In 2,297 treated patients, there were 59 drug-related reactions (2.5%). These included burning (51), rash (5), itching (2) and interstitial nephritis (1). Therapy was discontinued in only 0.9% of the patient population.

Leukopenia (< 5000 WBC/mm³) has been reported which reverted to normal upon drug discontinuation or recovered spontaneously.

Since significant quantities of sulfadiazine are absorbed, it is possible that any of the adverse reactions attributable to sulfonamides may occur (p.1903).

Administration and Dosage:

Application: Apply with a sterile gloved hand once or twice daily to a thickness of approximately 1/16 inch to the clean and debrided wound. Cover the burn areas with silver sulfadiazine at all times. Whenever necessary, reapply the cream to any areas from which it has been removed by patient activity. Dressings are not required, but may be used if individual patient requirements make them necessary.

Bathing: When feasible, bathe patient daily to aid in debridement. A whirlpool bath is particularly helpful, but the patient may be bathed in bed or in a shower.

Duration of therapy: Continue treatment until satisfactory healing occurs or until the site is ready for grafting. Do not withdraw the drug while the possibility of infection remains, unless a significant adverse reaction occurs.

	Product	Form	Package	C.I.*
Rx	**SSD Cream** (Boots)	**Cream:** 10 mg per g in a water miscible base[1]	In 50, 400 and 1000 g.	71
Rx	**Silvadene** (Marion Merrell Dow)		In 20, 50, 400 and 1000 g.	85
Rx	**Thermazene** (Sherwood)		In 50, 400 and 1000 g.	NA
Rx	**SSD AF** (Boots)	**Cream:** 1%[1]	In 50, 400 and 1000 g.	NA

* Cost Index based on cost per g.

[1] Cream base contains white petrolatum, stearyl alcohol, isopropyl myristate, sorbitan monooleate, polyoxyl 40 stearate, propylene glycol and methylparaben.

Actions:

Sunscreens provide either a chemical or a physical barrier to sunlight. These agents help to prevent sunburn, actinic keratosis, premature aging and photosensitivity reactions, and to reduce incidences of skin cancer. Chemical sunscreens act by absorbing ultraviolet (UV) rays in the medium wavelength range of 290 to 320 nm (UV-B range). This is the spectrum of UV light primarily responsible for sunburning and suntanning. Long wavelength UV light in the 320 to 400 nm (UV-A range) can cause tanning and is responsible for most photosensitivity reactions which occur with many drugs and cosmetics; it is also a major risk factor for serious skin damage. UV-A irradiation can exceed that of UV-B by 10 to 1000-fold. UV-A deeply penetrates into the dermis; UV-B is primarily absorbed in the epidermis. Physical sunscreens reflect or scatter light in both the visible and UV spectrum (290 to 700 nm), preventing penetration of the skin.

Sunscreen effectiveness is dependent on UV absorption spectrum, concentration, vehicle and ability to withstand swimming or sweating.

The following ingredients are used as sunscreening agents in the concentrations indicated:

Sunscreen Ingredients

	Sunscreens	UV Spectrum (nm)	Concentrations (%)
Chemical	*Benzophenones*	UV-A and UV-B	
	Oxybenzone	270-350	2-6
	Dioxybenzone	250-390	3
	PABA and PABA esters	UV-B	
	p-aminobenzoic acid	260-313	5-15
	Ethyl dihydroxy propyl PABA	280-330	1-5
	Padimate O (octyl dimethyl PABA)	290-315	1.4-8
	Glyceryl PABA	264-315	2-3
	Cinnamates	UV-B	
	Cinoxate	280-320	1-3
	Ethylhexyl p-methoxycinnamate	290-380	2-7.5
	Octocrylene	250-360	—
	Octyl methoxycinnamate	290-320	—
	Salicylates	UV-B[1]	
	Ethylhexyl salicylate	280-320	3-5
	Homosalate	295-315	4-15
	Octyl salicylate	280-320	3-5
	Miscellaneous	UV-B	
	Methyl anthranilate	260-320	3.5-5
	Digalloyl trioleate	270-320	2-5
	Butyl-methoxydibenzoylmethane (Parsol 1789)	UV-A 320-400	3
Physical	Titanium dioxide	290-700	2-25
	Red petrolatum	290-365[2]	30-100
	Zinc oxide	290-700	—

[1] Primarily UV-B, but has about ⅓ the absorbency of PABA.
[2] At 334nm, 16% UV radiation is transmitted; at 365nm, 58% is transmitted.

Indications:

To prevent sunburn. Overexposure to the sun may cause premature skin aging and skin cancer. The liberal and regular use of these products may help reduce the occurrence of these harmful effects.

For persons with conditions such as systemic lupus erythematosus, solar urticaria, erythropoietic protoporphyria or those taking photosensitizing drugs. A brief list of drugs that may cause photosensitivity include:

- Tricyclic antidepressants (eg, amitriptyline)
- Antihistamines (eg, cyproheptadine, diphenhydramine)
- Anti-infectives (eg, tetracyclines, nalidixic acid, sulfonamides)
- Antineoplastic agents (eg, fluorouracil, methotrexate, procarbazine)
- Antipsychotic agents (eg, phenothiazines, haloperidol)
- Diuretics (eg, thiazides, acetazolamide, amiloride)
- Hypoglycemic agents (eg, sulfonylureas)
- Nonsteroidal anti-inflammatory drugs (eg, phenylbutazone, ketoprofen, naproxen)
- Sunscreens (see Precautions)
- Miscellaneous (eg, bergamot oils, etc, used in cosmetics; coal tar; psoralens; amiodarone; oral contraceptives; quinidine; disopyramide; gold salts; isotretinoin; captopril; carbamazepine)

(Continued on following page)

Precautions:

Avoid prolonged exposure to sun and to tanning lamps. Sun sensitive persons particularly should exercise caution. If irritation or sensitization occur, discontinue use.

Do not use sunscreens containing PABA or its derivatives if sensitive to benzocaine, procaine, sulfonamides, thiazides, aniline dyes, PABA or PABA esters.

Avoid contact with eyes.

Do not use sunscreens in highly alcoholic vehicles on eczematous or inflamed skin.

Para-aminobenzoic acid (PABA) may cause a permanent yellow stain on clothing.

Vitamin D deficiency may occur in elderly patients; sunscreens that block UV-B may block cutaneous vitamin D synthesis.

The amount of UV exposure is influenced by many factors (eg, time of day, season, latitude, altitude, atmospheric conditions). UV-B radiation is strongest between 10 am and 2 pm; UV-A is relatively constant. Each 1000 foot increase in altitude adds 4% to UV light intensity. Reflectance from water depends on the angle of exposure, with almost 100% when the sun is directly overhead. Fresh snow reflects approximately 85% of UV light, and sand reflects 20% to 25%.

Adverse Reactions:

Contact dermatitis may develop with PABA or its esters (especially glyceryl PABA), benzophenones and cinnamates. Sunscreens are occlusive; miliaria or folliculitis may occur.

Patient Information:

Follow directions on product container concerning frequency of application; reapply after swimming or sweating. Reapplication does not extend the protection period.

For external use only; do not swallow.

Avoid contact with the eyes.

Discontinue use if signs of irritation or rash appear.

PABA may permanently stain clothing yellow.

Wear protective eye coverings or sunglasses; UV light can cause corneal damage.

Directions for Use:

Apply liberally to all exposed areas (2 mg/cm² is recommended) at least 30 minutes prior to sun exposure (up to 2 hours for aminobenzoic acid and its esters) to allow for penetration and binding to the skin. Reapply after swimming or excessive sweating.

Children: Do not use sunscreens on infants < 6 months old. Do not use sunscreen products with SPF 2 or 3 on children < 2 years old.

Sun protection factor (SPF): Most sunscreen products now include SPF ratings. This factor indicates the amount of increased resistance to sunburning the product provides, relative to unprotected skin. (Example: Using a product with an SPF value of 6 would permit 6 times as much sun exposure.) Base product selection on the patient's history of response to sun exposure.

Suggested SPF Based on Patient Characteristics

Skin Type	Patient Characteristics[1]	Suggested Product SPF
I	Always burns easily; never tans (sensitive)	≥ 15
II	Always burns easily; tans minimally (sensitive)	≥ 15
III	Burns moderately; tans gradually (light brown; normal)	10-15
IV	Burns minimally; always tans well (moderate brown; normal)	6-10
V	Rarely burns; tans profusely (dark brown; insensitive)	4-6
VI	Never burns; deeply pigmented (insensitive)	None indicated

[1] Based on first 45 to 60 minutes sun exposure after winter season or no sun exposure.

Waterproof formulas maintain sunburn protection after being in the water up to 80 minutes.

Water resistant formulas maintain sunburn protection after being in the water up to 40 minutes.

SPFs over 15 are not recommended by the 1978 FDA advisory panel on sunscreens. The agency has not yet issued a tentative final monograph on this product class. It has told the industry that it is reevaluating the SPF numbering system. (*F-D-C Reports* 1986;[Oct 13]:T&G11). An SPF of at least 15 for most individuals is recommended by the Skin Cancer Foundation.

In addition to the products listed on the following pages, there are other sunscreens available from various cosmetic manufacturers.

(Products listed on following pages)

Refer to the general discussion of these products beginning on page 2323

		SPF			C.I.*
otc	**Solbar PF** (Person & Covey)	50	**Cream:** Oxybenzone, octyl methoxycinnamate, octocrylene. PABA free	Waterproof. In 120 g.	65
otc	**Water Babies Sunblock** (Plough)	45	**Lotion:** Ethylhexyl p-methoxycinnamate, 2-ethylhexyl salicylate, octocrylene, oxybenzone, benzyl alcohol.	PABA free. Waterproof. In 120 ml.	62
otc	**Shade Sunblock** (Plough)	45	**Lotion:** Ethylhexyl p-methoxycinnamate, octocrylene, oxybenzone, 2-ethylhexyl salicylate, benzyl alcohol. PABA free	Waterproof. In 120 ml.	62
otc	**PreSun 39 Creamy Sunscreen** (Westwood)	39	**Cream:** Padimate O, oxybenzone, cetyl alcohol	Waterproof. In 120 ml.	NA
otc	**Bullfrog** (Chattem)	36	**Gel:** Benzophenone-3, octocrylene, octyl methoxycinnamate, isostearyl alcohol	Waterproof. In 30 g.	NA
otc	**Sundown Sunblock Ultra** (Johnson & Johnson)	30	**Lotion:** Octyl methoxycinnamate, octyl salicylate, oxybenzone, titanium dioxide, cetyl alcohol. PABA free	Waterproof. In 120 ml.	NA
otc	**Johnson's Baby Sunblock** (Johnson & Johnson)	30	**Lotion:** Benzophenone-3, octyl methoxycinnamate, octyl salicylate, titanium dioxide. PABA free.	Waterproof. In 120 ml.	NA
otc	**Shade Sunblock** (Plough)	30	**Stick:** Ethylhexyl p-methoxycinnamate, oxybenzone, 2-ethylhexyl salicylate, homosalate. PABA free	Waterproof. In 18 g.	224
otc	**Shade Sunblock** (Plough)	30	**Lotion:** Ethylhexyl p-methoxycinnamate, 2-ethylhexyl salicylate, homosalate, oxybenzone, benzyl alcohol, phenethyl alcohol. PABA free	Waterproof. In 120 ml.	62
otc	**Water Babies Sunblock** (Plough)	30	**Lotion:** Ethylhexyl p-methoxycinnamate, 2-ethylhexyl salicylate, homosalate, oxybenzone, benzyl alcohol.	PABA free. Waterproof. In 120 ml.	62
otc	**Bain de Soleil Protecteur Gentil Under Eye Protecteur** (Richardson-Vicks)	30	**Stick:** Ethylhexyl p-methoxycinnamate, oxybenzone, 2-ethylhexyl salicylate	In 1.5 g.	3143
otc	**SolBar PF** (Person & Covey)	30	**Liquid:** Octocrylene, octyl methoxycinnamate, oxybenzone, SD alcohol 40. PABA free	In 114 ml.	NA
otc	**PreSun 29 Sensitive Skin Sunscreen** (Westwood)	29	**Cream:** Octyl methoxycinnamate, oxybenzone, octyl salicylate, cetyl alcohol. PABA free	Waterproof. In 120 ml.	NA
otc	**PreSun for Kids** (Westwood)	29	**Cream:** Octyl methoxycinnamate, oxybenzone, octyl salicylate, cetyl alcohol. PABA free	Waterproof. In 120 ml.	NA
otc	**Water Babies Sunblock** (Plough)	25	**Cream:** Ethylhexyl p-methoxycinnamate, 2-ethylhexyl salicylate, homosalate, oxybenzone, benzyl alcohol. PABA free	Waterproof. In 90 g.	76
otc	**Coppertone Moisturizing Sunblock** (Plough)	25	**Lotion:** Ethylhexyl p-methoxycinnamate, 2-ethylhexyl salicylate, homosalate, oxybenzone, benzyl alcohol, vitamin E, aloe. PABA free	Waterproof. In 118 ml.	NA
otc	**Shade Sunblock** (Plough)	25	**Gel:** Ethylhexyl p-methoxycinnamate, octyl salicylate, homosalate, oxybenzone, SD alcohol 40. PABA free	In 120 g.	NA
otc	**Bain de Soleil Protecteur Gentil Body Silkening Crème** (Richardson Vicks)	25	**Cream:** Padimate O, ethylhexyl p-methoxycinnamate, oxybenzone, benzyl alcohol	Waterproof. In 94 g.	78

* Cost Index based on cost per g or ml.

(Continued on following page)

Refer to the general discussion of these products beginning on page 2323

		SPF			C.I.*
otc	**Bain de Soleil Protecteur Gentil Face Crème** (Richardson Vicks)	25	**Cream:** Padimate O, ethylhexyl p-methoxycinnamate, oxybenzone	Waterproof. In 60 g.	96
otc	**Bain de Soleil Protecteur Gentil Body Silkening** (Richardson Vicks)	25	**Stick:** Padimate O, ethylhexyl p-methoxycinnamate, oxybenzone, dioxybenzone	In 53 g.	137
otc	**Hawaiian Tropic Baby Faces Sunblock** (Tanning R)	25	**Lotion:** 2-ethylhexyl p-methoxycinnamate, oxybenzone, octyl salicylate, methyl anthranilate, PABA free	Waterproof. In 120 ml.	77
otc	**Sundown Sunscreen Ultra** (Johnson & Johnson)	25	**Lotion:** Octyl methoxycinnamate, oxybenzone, octyl salicylate, titanium dioxide, cetyl alcohol	In 120 ml.	NA
otc	**Sundown Sunblock Ultra** (J & J)	24	**Cream:** Padimate O, oxybenzone	Waterproof. In 105 g.	NA
otc	**PreSun 23** (Westwood)	23	**Spray Mist:** Padimate O, octyl methoxycinnamate, oxybenzone, octyl salicylate, 19% SD alcohol 40	Waterproof. In 105 ml.	NA
otc	**PreSun for Kids** (Westwood)			Waterproof. In 105 ml.	NA
otc	**Sundown Sunblock Ultra** (Johnson & Johnson)	20	**Lotion:** Octyl methoxycinnamate, octyl salicylate, oxybenzone, titanium dioxide, cetyl alcohol, PABA free	Waterproof. In 120 ml.	68
otc	**Bain de Soleil Protecteur Gentil Body Silkening Spray** (Richardson Vicks)	20	**Lotion:** Padimate O, oxybenzone, ethylhexyl p-methoxycinnamate	Waterproof. In 240 ml.	34
otc	**Bullfrog** (Chattem)	18	**Gel:** Octocrylene, benzophenone-3, octyl methoxycinnamate, isostearyl alcohol	Waterproof. 120, 30 g.	NA
			Stick: Benzophenone-3, octyl methoxycinnamate, isostearyl alcohol	Waterproof. In 16.5 g.	NA
otc	**Bullfrog for Kids** (Chattem)	18	**Gel:** Octocrylene, octyl methoxycinnamate, octyl salicylate	Waterproof. In 60 g.	NA
otc	**Filteray Broad Spectrum Sunscreen** (Burroughs-W)	15	**Lotion:** 3% avobenzone, 7% padimate O, benzyl alcohol	In 120 ml.	NA
otc	**Noskote Sunblock Creme** (Plough)	15	**Cream:** Ethylhexyl p-methoxycinnamate, 2-ethylhexyl salicylate, oxybenzone, benzyl alcohol, PABA free	Waterproof. In 34 g.	NA
otc	**Aquaderm** (Baker Cummins)	15	**Cream:** 7.5% octyl methoxycinnamate, 6% oxybenzone, 2% titanium dioxide	In 105 g.	NA
otc	**Solbar PF Sunscreen** (Person & Covey)	15	**Liquid:** 7.5% octyl methoxycinnamate, 6% oxybenzone, 76% SD alcohol 40	PABA free. In 120 ml.	NA
otc	**Shade Sunblock** (Plough)	15	**Gel:** Ethylhexyl p-methoxycinnamate, octyl salicylate, oxybenzone, SD alcohol 40, PABA free	Waterproof. In 120 g.	57
			Lotion: Ethylhexyl p-methoxycinnamate, oxybenzone, benzyl alcohol, phenethyl alcohol, PABA free	Waterproof. In 120 ml.	57
otc	**Sundown Sunblock Ultra** (Johnson & Johnson)	15	**Cream:** Octyl methoxycinnamate, octyl salicylate, oxybenzone, titanium dioxide, stearyl alcohol, cetyl alcohol	PABA free. Waterproof. In 60 g.	NA
otc	**Photoplex Broad Spectrum Sunscreen** (Herbert Labs)	15	**Lotion:** 7% padimate O, 3% butyl methoxydibenzoylmethane, benzyl alcohol	Water resistant. In 120 ml.	97
otc	**PreSun Facial** (Westwood)	15	**Cream:** 8% padimate O, 3% oxybenzone, benzyl alcohol, cetyl alcohol	In 60 g.	111

* Cost Index based on cost per g or ml.

(Continued on following page)

Refer to the general discussion of these products beginning on page 2323

		SPF			C.I.*
otc	**PreSun 15 Creamy** (Westwood)	15	**Cream:** Padimate O, oxybenzone and cetyl alcohol	Waterproof. In 120 g.	67
otc	**Coppertone Moisturizing Sunblock** (Plough)	15	**Lotion:** Ethylhexyl p-methoxycinnamate, oxybenzone, benzyl alcohol, vitamin E, aloe. PABA free	Waterproof. In 236 ml.	29
otc	**Hawaiian Tropic 15 Plus Sunblock** (Tanning Research)	15	**Lotion:** 2-ethylhexyl p-methoxycinnamate, oxybenzone, methyl anthranilate. PABA free	Waterproof. In 120 ml.	81
otc	**Block Out by Sea & Ski** (Carter)	15	**Cream:** Padimate O, octyl methoxycinnamate, oxybenzone	Waterproof. In 120 g.	56
otc	**Sundown Sunblock Ultra** (Johnson & Johnson)	15	**Lotion:** Padimate O, octyl methoxycinnamate, oxybenzone, benzyl alcohol, stearyl alcohol	Waterproof. In 120 ml.	57
otc	**Ray Block** (Del Ray)	15	**Lotion:** 5% padimate O, 3% benzophenone-3, SD alcohol	In 118.3 ml.	49
otc	**PreSun 15 Sensitive Skin Sunscreen** (Westwood)	15	**Cream:** Octyl methoxycinnamate, oxybenzone, octyl salicylate, cetyl alcohol. PABA free	Waterproof. In 120 ml.	NA
otc	**PreSun 15 Facial** (Westwood)	15	**Stick:** 8% Padimate O, 3% oxybenzone, petrolatum	In 12.6 g.	NA
otc	**Johnson's Baby Sunblock** (Johnson & Johnson)	15	**Cream and Lotion:** Octyl methoxycinnamate, octyl salicylate, oxybenzone, titanium dioxide, benzyl alcohol, cetyl alcohol. PABA free	Waterproof. In 60 g.	NA
				Waterproof. In 120 ml.	NA
otc	**Total Eclipse Oily and Acne Prone Skin Sunscreen** (Eclipse)	15	**Lotion:** Padimate O, oxybenzone, glyceryl PABA, 77% alcohol	In 120 ml.	50
otc	**Total Eclipse Moisturizing** (Eclipse)	15	**Lotion:** Padimate O, oxybenzone, octyl salicylate. Moisturizing base	In 120 ml.	50
otc	**Block Out Clear by Sea & Ski** (Carter)	15	**Lotion:** Padimate O, octyl methoxycinnamate, octyl salicylate	Waterproof. In 120 ml.	56
otc	**Solbar Plus 15** (Person & Covey)	15	**Cream:** 6% Padimate O, 4% oxybenzone, 2% dioxybenzone	In 30 and 113 g.	57
otc	**Solbar PF** (Person & Covey)	15	**Cream:** 7.5% octyl methoxycinnamate and 5% oxybenzone. PABA free	In 75 g.	50
otc	**Water Babies Sunblock by Coppertone** (Plough)	15	**Lotion:** Ethylhexyl p-methoxycinnamate, oxybenzone, benzyl alcohol. PABA free	Waterproof. In 120 ml.	57
otc	**Solar Shield** (Akorn)	15	**Lotion:** 7.5% ethylhexyl-p-methoxycinnamate, 5% oxybenzone. PABA free	Waterproof. In 120 ml.	NA
otc	**TI•Screen** (T/I Pharmaceuticals)	15	**Lotion:** 7.5% ethylhexyl-p-methoxycinnamate, 5% oxybenzone. PABA free	Water resistant. In 120 ml.	62
otc	**DML Facial Moisturizer** (Person & Covey)	15	**Moisturizer:** 8% octyl methoxycinnamate, 4% oxybenzone, propylene glycol dioctanoate, glycerin, benzyl alcohol	In 45 g.	NA
otc	**Hawaiian Tropic Sunscreen** (Tan. Res.)	10	**Lotion:** Padimate O and oxybenzone	Waterproof. In 120 ml.	69
otc	**Original Eclipse Sunscreen** (Eclipse)	10	**Lotion:** Padimate O and glyceryl PABA	In 120 ml.	48
otc	**Snootie by Sea & Ski** (Carter)	10	**Lotion:** Padimate O	In 30 ml.	119

* Cost Index based on cost per g or ml.

(Continued on following page)

Refer to the general discussion of these products beginning on page 2323

		SPF			C.I.*
otc	**Bullfrog** (Chattem)	9	**Gel:** Benzophenone-3, octyl methoxycinnamate, isostearyl alcohol	Waterproof. In 120 g.	NA
otc	**PreSun 8 Creamy** (Westwood)	8	**Cream:** Padimate O, oxybenzone, cetyl alcohol	Waterproof. In 120 g.	67
otc	**Hawaiian Tropic Aloe PABA Sunscreen** (Tanning Research)	8	**Cream:** Padimate O, oxybenzone, aloe	Waterproof. In 120 g.	69
otc	**TI•Screen** (T/I Pharmaceuticals)	8	**Lotion:** 6% ethylhexyl p-methoxycinnamate and 2% oxybenzone. PABA free	Water resistant. In 120 ml.	55
otc	**Coppertone Moisturizing Sunscreen** (Plough)	8	**Lotion:** Ethylhexl p-methoxycinnamate, oxybenzone, benzyl alcohol, vitamin E, aloe. PABA free	Waterproof. In 118 ml.	29
otc	**Sundown Maximal** (J & J)	8	**Lotion:** Padimate O, oxybenzone, benzyl alcohol, stearyl alcohol	Waterproof. In 120 ml.	55
otc	**Hawaiian Tropic Protective Tanning** (Tanning Research)	6	**Lotion:** Padimate O and oxybenzone	Waterproof. In 120 ml.	43
otc	**Coppertone Moisturizing Sunscreen** (Plough)	6	**Lotion:** Ethylhexl p-methoxycinnamate, oxybenzone, benzyl alcohol, vitamin E, aloe. PABA free	Waterproof. In 118 ml.	NA
otc	**Sundown Extra** (J & J)	6	**Lotion:** Padimate O, oxybenzone, benzyl alcohol, stearyl alcohol	Waterproof. In 120 ml.	49
otc	**Sea & Ski Golden Tan** (Carter)	4	**Lotion:** Padimate O	Waterproof. In 120 ml.	57
otc	**Sundown Moderate** (J & J)	4	**Lotion:** Padimate O, oxybenzone, benzyl alcohol, stearyl alcohol	Waterproof. In 120 ml.	60
otc	**Hawaiian Tropic Dark Tanning with Sunscreen** (Tanning Research)	4	**Lotion:** 2-Ethylhexyl p-methoxycinnamate and methyl anthranilate. PABA free	Waterproof. In 240 ml.	29
otc	**Coppertone Lite Tanning** (Plough)	4	**Lotion:** Ethylhexyl p-methoxycinnamate. PABA free	Waterproof. In 118 ml.	240
otc	**Coppertone Moisturizing Suntan** (Plough)	4	**Lotion:** Ethylhexyl p-methoxycinnamate, oxybenzone, benzyl alcohol, vitamin E, aloe. PABA free	Waterproof. In 236 ml.	NA
otc	**Coppertone Moisturizing Suntan** (Plough)	2	**Oil:** Homosalate, vitamin E, aloe. PABA free	Waterproof. In 236 ml.	NA
otc	**Coppertone Lite Tanning** (Plough)	2	**Oil:** 2-ethylhexyl salicylate. PABA free	In 118 ml.	34
otc	**Sea & Ski Baby Lotion Formula** (Carter)	2	**Lotion:** Padimate O	In 120 ml.	33
otc	**Coppertone Dark Tanning Spray** (Plough)	2	**Oil:** Ethylhexyl p-methoxycinnamate, vitamin E, aloe. PABA free	Waterproof. In 236 ml.	30
otc	**Maxafil** (GenDerm)	‡	**Cream:** 4% cinoxate and 5% methyl anthranilate	In 30 g.	134
otc	**A-Fil** (GenDerm)	‡	**Cream:** 5% methyl anthranilate and 5% titanium dioxide. Dark or neutral tint	In 45 g.	113
otc	**Ray-Nox** (Torch)	‡	**Cream:** PABA, stearyl alcohol, cetyl alcohol	In 60 g and lb.	51
otc	**RVPaque** (ICN Pharm)	‡	**Cream:** Red petrolatum, zinc oxide & cinoxate in a water resistant base	In 15 and 35 g.	328

* Cost Index based on cost per g or ml.

‡ SPF data not provided by distributor.

Refer to the general discussion of these products beginning on page 2323

		SPF	Lip Protectants		C.I.*
otc	**Water Babies Little Licks by Coppertone** (Plough)	30	**Lip balm:** Ethylhexyl p-methoxycinnamate, oxybenzone, 2-ethylhexyl salicylate	Cherry flavor. In 4.8 g.	NA
otc	**Bain de Soleil Lip Protecteur** (Richardson-Vicks)	30	**Lip balm:** Ethylhexyl p-methoxycinnamate, oxybenzone, 2-ethylhexyl salicylate, oleyl alcohol, petrolatum. PABA free	In 3 g.	157
otc	**PreSun 15 Lip Protector** (Westwood)	15	**Lipstick:** 8% padimate O, 3% oxybenzone, petrolatum	In 4.5 g.	997
otc	**Chapstick Sunblock 15** (Robins Consumer)	15	**Lip balm:** 7% padimate O, 3% oxybenzone, 0.5% cetyl alcohol, tartrazine	In 4.25 g.	145
otc	**Eclipse Lip and Face Protectant** (Eclipse)	15	**Stick:** Padimate O and oxybenzone	In 4.5 g.	492
otc	**Hawaiian Tropic 15 Plus Sunblock Lip Balm** (Tanning Research)			Waterproof. In 4.2 g.	321
otc	**Lipkote by Coppertone** (Plough)	15	**Lip balm:** Ethylhexyl p-methoxycinnamate, oxybenzone, vitamin E, aloe. PABA free	In 4.8 g.	486
otc	**Daily Conditioning Treatment for Lips** (Blistex)	15	**Lip balm:** 7.5% padimate O, 3.5% oxybenzone, petrolatum, cetyl alcohol	In 11.4 g.	126
otc	**Blistik** (Blistex)	10	**Lip balm:** 6.6% padimate O, 2.5% oxybenzone, 2% dimethicone, cetyl alcohol. Regular, mint or berry flavors	In 4.5 g.	171
otc	**RVPaba** (ICN Pharm)	‡	**Lipstick:** 5% PABA	In 4.28 g.	667

* Cost Index based on cost per g or ml. ‡ SPF data not provided by distributor.

METHIONINE

Actions and Indications: Treatment of diaper rash in infants and for control of odor, dermatitis and ulceration caused by ammoniacal urine in incontinent adults. The acid-producing effect of methionine on urine pH creates an ammonia-free urine.

Contraindications: Do not administer to patients with a history of liver disease; large doses of methionine may exaggerate the toxemia of the disease.

Precautions: Excessive methionine added alone to the diet over extended periods may result in a less than normal weight gain when protein intake is insufficient. Maintain adequate protein intake during therapy and do not exceed the recommended dosage.

Patient Information: Take with food, milk or other liquid.

Administration and Dosage: *Diaper rash caused by ammoniacal urine:* 75 mg in formula or other liquid, 3 or 4 times daily for 3 to 5 days.

Control of odor in incontinent adults: 200 to 400 mg, 3 or 4 times daily after meals.

	Product	Form	Packaging	C.I.*
Rx	**Pedameth** (Forest)	**Capsules:** 200 mg	In 50s and 500s.	259
Rx	**M-Caps** (Pal-Pak)		Green and white. In 1000s.	NA
Rx	**Uracid** (Wesley)		In 100s and 1000s.	86
otc	**Uranap** (Vortech)		In 100s.	99
otc	**Uranap 500** (Vortech)	**Capsules:** 500 mg	In 1000s.	NA
Rx	**Methionine** (Various, eg, Lannett, Schein, Tyson & Assoc.)	**Tablets:** 500 mg	In 30s, 100s, 500s and 1000s.	20+
Rx	**Pedameth** (Forest)	**Liquid:** 75 mg per 5 ml	Fruit flavor. In pt.	598

Topical Diaper Rash Products

These products are intended for use in diaper rash or ammonia dermatitis.

The principal active components of these formulations include:

ANTIMICROBIAL AGENTS (methylbenzethonium Cl, triclosan and eucalyptol) to minimize bacterial proliferation.

ASTRINGENTS (zinc oxide and calamine) for drying.

CAMPHOR is a local anesthetic.

BALSAM PERU is claimed to promote wound healing or tissue repair, but effectiveness has not been conclusively demonstrated.

CALCIUM CARBONATE and *KAOLIN* are used for their moisture absorbing abilities.

PROTECTANTS and LUBRICANTS to minimize chafing and irritation.

	Product	Composition	Packaging	C.I.*
otc	**Desitin** (Leeming)	**Ointment:** 40% zinc oxide, cod liver oil, talc in a petrolatum/lanolin base	In 30, 60, 120, 240 g and lb.	29
otc	**Dyprotex** (Blistex)	**Pads:** 40% micronized zinc oxide, 37.6% petrolatum, 2.5% dimethicone, cod liver oil, aloe extract, zinc stearate	In 3 pads (9 applications).	NA
otc	**Diaparene Medicated** (Lehn & Fink)	**Cream:** 0.1% methylbenzethonium Cl with white petrolatum, glycerin, mineral oil, stearyl alcohol	In 30, 60 and 120 g.	30
otc	**Flanders Buttocks** (Flanders Inc.)	**Ointment:** Zinc oxide, castor oil, peruvian balsam, boric acid in emollient base	In 60 g.	22
otc	**Taloin** (Adria)	**Ointment:** Methylbenzethonium Cl, zinc oxide, calamine and eucalyptol in a water repellant base with white petrolatum	In 60 g.	133
otc	**Diaparene Peri-Anal Medicated** (Lehn & Fink)	**Ointment:** 0.1% methylbenzethonium Cl, zinc oxide, cod liver oil, mineral oil, white petrolatum, starch, lanolin, calcium caseinate	In 30, 60 and 120 g.	34
otc	**Balmex Baby** (Macsil)	**Powder:** Balsam peru, zinc oxide, corn starch and calcium carbonate	In 240 g.	13
otc	**Diaparene** (Lehn & Fink)	**Powder:** 0.055% methylbenzethonium Cl, corn starch and magnesium carbonate	In 120, 270 and 420 g.	8
otc	**Mexsana Medicated** (Plough)	**Powder:** Triclosan, zinc oxide, kaolin, eucalyptus oil, camphor, corn starch, almonol and lemon oil	In 90, 187.5 and 330 g.	18
otc	**ZBT Baby** (Glenwood)	**Powder:** Talc, mineral oil, magnesium stearate, propylene glycol and BHT	In 420 g.	46

* Cost Index based on cost per 200 mg methionine or g combination product.

For other products used for relief of symptoms associated with contact dermatoses, see also: Antihistamine-Containing Products, Topical; Local Anesthetics, Topical; Corticosteroids, Topical.

Uses: Relief of itching, pain and discomfort of ivy, oak and sumac poisoning. Some products are also recommended for insect bites and other minor skin irritations.

Precautions:

For external use only. Do not use in the eyes. If the condition for which these preparations are used persists or recurs, or if rash, irritation or sensitivity develops, discontinue use and consult physician.

The principal active components of these products include:

ANTIMICROBIAL: Phenylcarbinol (benzyl alcohol).

ANTISEPTIC: Phenol, isopropyl alcohol, benzalkonium chloride, camphor, menthol.

ASTRINGENTS: Calamine, zinc oxide.

COUNTERIRRITANTS: Camphor, methyl salicylate.

LOCAL ANESTHETICS: Benzocaine, pramoxine, phenol, menthol, phenylcarbinol (benzyl alcohol).

ANTIPRURITICS: Phenylcarbinol (benzyl alcohol), camphor, phenol, menthol.

MISCELLANEOUS: Polyvinylpyrrolidone (povidone).

Administration and Dosage:

Apply to affected area 3 to 4 times daily.

	Product	Composition	Supplied	C.I.*
otc	**Rhuli Cream** (Rydelle)	**Cream:** 5% benzocaine, 3% calamine and 0.3% camphor in a base of glycerin, distearyldimonium chloride, petrolatum, isopropyl palmitate, cetyl alcohol, dimethicone	In 60 g.	NA
otc	**Ivarest** (Blistex)	**Cream & Lotion:** 14% calamine and 5% benzocaine	**Cream:** In 3.75 & 60 g.	4.5
			Lotion: In 120 ml.	2.9
otc	**Calamine** (Various, eg, Barre, Goldline, Major, Moore, Paddock, Purepac, Rugby)	**Lotion:** 8% calamine, 8% zinc oxide, 2% glycerin and bentonite magma in calcium hydroxide solution	In 120, 240 and 480 ml.	1+
otc	**Phenolated Calamine** (Humco)	**Lotion:** 8% calamine, 8% zinc oxide, 2% glycerin, bentonite magma and 1% phenol in calcium hydroxide solution	In 120 and 240 ml.	NA
otc	**Resinol** (Mentholatum)	**Ointment:** 6% calamine, 12% zinc oxide, 2% resorcinol, lanolin, petrolatum, starch	In 35.4 g.	NA
otc	**Calamox** (Hauck)	**Ointment:** Each 100 g contains 17 g prepared calamine	In 60 g and lb.	5.1
otc	**Calamatum** (Blair)	**Spray:** Calamine, zinc oxide, menthol, camphor, 1% benzocaine and isopropyl alcohol	In 85 g aerosol.	4.4
otc	**Rhuli Spray** (Rydelle)	**Spray:** 13.8% calamine, 0.7% camphor, and 5% benzocaine in a base of benzyl alcohol, hydrated silica, isobutane, 70% isopropyl alcohol, oleyl alcohol, sorbitan trioleate	In 120 ml.	4.3

* Cost Index based on cost per g or ml.

(Product listings continued on following page)

				C.I.*
otc	**Aveeno Anti-Itch** (Rydelle)	**Cream & Lotion:** 3% calamine, 1% pramoxine HCl, 0.3% camphor in a base of glycerin, distearyldimonium chloride, petrolatum, oatmeal flour, isopropyl palmitate, cetyl alcohol, dimethicone	**Cream:** In 30 g. **Lotion:** In 120 ml.	NA NA
otc	**Rhuli Gel** (Rydelle)	**Gel:** 2% benzyl alcohol, 0.3% menthol, 0.3% camphor and 31% SD alcohol 23A in a base of propylene glycol, carbomer 940, triethanolamine, benzophenone-4, EDTA	In 60 g.	8.3
otc	**Ivy-Chex** (JMI)	**Spray:** Polyvinylpyrrolidone vinylacetate copolymers, methyl salicylate, benzalkonium chloride and 89.5% SD alcohol 40	In 120 g.	3.8
otc	**Ivy-Rid** (Hauck)	**Spray:** Polyvinylpyrrolidone vinylacetate copolymers, isobutane, methyl chloride, benzalkonium chloride, SDA alcohol and isopropyl myristate	In 82.5 ml aerosol.	3.9

* Cost Index based on cost per g or ml.

TOPICAL POISON IVY PREVENTATIVES

Indications:
Protection from effects of poisonous foliage, plants and grasses.

Administration and Dosage:
Apply to skin before exposure.

otc	**Stoko Gard** (Stockhausen[1])	**Cream:** PPG-3 diamine dilinoleate, mineral oil, petroleum wax, PEG-7 hydrogenated castor oil, glycerin, petrolatum, aluminum distearate	In 100 g.

[1] Stockhausen Inc., Greensboro, NC 27406, 1-800-328-2935.

Uses:

These products, which contain the active toxic principle, urushiol, extracted from leaves of poison ivy, poison oak or poison sumac, are recommended for the prevention of Rhus dermatitis. Hyposensitization is temporary; prophylaxis is neither complete nor permanent. Prophylaxis may result in milder and shorter reactions.

Contraindications:

History of kidney damage. Not recommended for treatment of active Rhus dermatitis.

Warnings:

Hypersensitivity: Use extreme caution in treating hypersensitive individuals. Take precautions to prevent extract from coming in contact with the skin. If contact does occur, wash the area promptly with alcohol.

Pregnancy: Category C. It is not known whether systemic poison ivy treatments can cause fetal harm when administered to a pregnant woman or can affect reproduction capacity. Give to a pregnant woman only if clearly needed.

Pregnancy is occasionally associated with kidney disease, as are Rhus dermatitis and hyposensitization. Exposure to Rhus hyposensitization or dermatitis-producing plants may exacerbate kidney disease in susceptible pregnant patients. Avoid hyposensitization and all contact with dermatitis-producing plants during pregnancy.

Precautions:

Renal effects: Renal complications may follow extensive dermatitis of various types; with severe Rhus dermatitis, there may be an aggravation of symptoms following administration of these extracts.

Adverse Reactions:

Local: Transient burning sensation at injection site. Urticaria and other skin eruptions are rarely observed if the dose is not increased too rapidly. These eruptions are never serious and usually disappear within a few days after temporary cessation of treatment. If such symptoms occur, stop treatment until skin is free of eruptions. Then begin treatment at the same or reduced dosage. Rash and soreness of the lips and mouth have also occurred.

Systemic: Pruritus ani; abdominal discomfort or cramps; loose bowel movements.

Administration and Dosage:

Dosage recommendations vary. Refer to package insert for information.

Rx	**Poison Ivy/Oak Extract** (Hollister-Stier)	**Capsules:** Oleoresin in corn oil	In 3 graduated dilutions with sufficient gelatin capsules for oral desensitization.
Rx	**Poison Ivy Extract** (Parke-Davis)	**Injection:** 1 ml poison ivy extract from Rhus toxicodendron dissolved in almond oil	In 2 ml vials.

SELENIUM SULFIDE

Actions:

Selenium sulfide appears to have a cytostatic effect on cells of the epidermis and follicular epithelium, thus reducing corneocyte production.

Indications:

Treatment of dandruff, seborrheic dermatitis of the scalp and tinea versicolor.

Contraindications:

Allergy to any component of the product.

Warnings:

Pregnancy: Category C (tinea versicolor). It is not known whether selenium sulfide can cause fetal harm when administered to a pregnant woman or can affect reproduction capacity. Give to a pregnant woman only if clearly needed. Under ordinary circumstances, do not use for the treatment of tinea versicolor in pregnant women.

Children: Safety and efficacy in infants have not been established.

Precautions:

Hypersensitivity: If sensitivity reactions occur, discontinue use.

Treatment of tinea versicolor: Selenium sulfide may irritate the skin, especially in the genital area and in skin folds. Rinse these areas thoroughly after application.

For external use only. Avoid contact with the eyes.

Acute inflammation/exudation: Do not use when present; absorption may be increased.

Adverse Reactions:

Skin irritation; greater than normal hair loss; hair discoloration (avoid or minimize by thorough rinsing after treatment); oiliness or dryness of hair and scalp.

Overdosage:

Accidental oral ingestion: Symptoms – Selenium sulfide shampoos have generally low toxicity if ingested. Nausea, vomiting and diarrhea usually occur after oral ingestion. There may also be a burning sensation in the mouth and a garlic-like taste/smell to the breath. The detergents found in selenium sulfide shampoos may act as emetics, thereby preventing significant GI absorption of selenium.

Treatment includes usual supportive measures. Refer to General Management of Acute Overdosage.

Patient Information:

For external use only. Avoid contact with the eyes. Do not use on acutely inflamed skin.

If irritation occurs, discontinue use. Thoroughly rinse after application.

If using before or after bleaching, tinting or permanent waving, rinse hair for at least 5 minutes in cool running water.

May damage jewelry; remove before using.

Administration and Dosage:

Massage 5 to 10 ml of the medicated shampoo into wet scalp. Allow to remain on the scalp for 2 to 3 minutes. Rinse thoroughly. Repeat application and rinse thoroughly. Wash hands well after treatment.

Usually, 2 applications each week for 2 weeks will afford control. After this, it may be used at less frequent intervals – weekly, every 2 weeks or even every 3 or 4 weeks in some cases. Do not apply more frequently than required to maintain control.

Tinea versicolor: Apply to affected areas and lather with a small amount of water. Allow to remain on skin for 10 min; rinse body thoroughly. Repeat once a day for 7 days.

				C.I.*
otc	**Selenium Sulfide** (Various, eg, Barre-National, Moore, Rugby)	**Lotion/Shampoo:** 1%	In 120, 210 and 240 ml.	1+
otc	**Head & Shoulders Intensive Treatment Dandruff Shampoo** (Procter & Gamble)		In regular and conditioning formulas. In 120, 210 and 330 ml.	NA
otc	**Selsun Blue** (Ross)		In dry, normal, oily, extra conditioning and extra medicated formulas. In 120, 210 and 330 ml.	2.2
Rx	**Selenium Sulfide** (Various, eg, Dixon-Shane, Geneva Marsam, IDE, Lannett, PBI, Rugby, Schein)	**Lotion/Shampoo:** 2.5%	In 120 ml.	1.6+
Rx	**Exsel** (Herbert)		In 120 ml.	6.6
Rx	**Selsun** (Abbott)		In 120 ml.	6.7

* Cost Index based on cost per ml.

TAR DERIVATIVES, SHAMPOOS

Actions:

Tar derivatives help correct abnormalities of keratinization by decreasing epidermal proliferation and dermal infiltration; they are also antipruritic and antibacterial.

Indications:

For treatment of scalp psoriasis, eczema, seborrheic dermatitis, dandruff, cradle-cap and other oily, itchy conditions of the body and scalp.

Contraindications:

Acute inflammation; open or infected lesions.

Warnings:

Children: Use on children < 2 years of age only as directed by a physician.

Precautions:

For external use only. Avoid contact with eyes.

Irritation: Discontinue if irritation develops.

If condition worsens or does not improve after regular use as directed, or if excessive dryness or any undesirable effect occurs, discontinue use and contact your physician.

Adverse Reactions:

Minor dermatologic side effects include rash or burning sensation. Photosensitivity may occur. May discolor skin.

Patient Information:

For external use only. Avoid contact with the eyes.

Use caution in the sunlight after applying; it may increase the tendency to sunburn up to 24 hours after application.

Do not use for prolonged periods of time (> 6 months) without consulting a physician.

Administration:

Refer to specific product labeling. Rub shampoo liberally into wet hair and scalp. Rinse thoroughly. Repeat; leave on 5 minutes. Rinse thoroughly. Depending on specific product, use from once daily to at least twice a week. For severe scalp problems, use daily.

				C.I.*
otc	**DHS Tar** (Person & Covey)	**Shampoo:** 0.5% coal tar	**Liquid:** In 120, 240 & 480 ml.	3.5
			Gel: In 240 ml.	2.8
otc	**Doctar** (Savage)	**Shampoo:** 0.5% coal tar with conditioner	In 100 ml.	3.1
otc	**Theraplex T** (Medicis)	**Shampoo:** 1% coal tar, benzyl alcohol	In 240 ml.	2.2
otc	**Zetar** (Dermik)	**Shampoo:** 1% whole coal tar	In 180 ml.	2.9
otc	**Ionil•T Plus** (Owen/Galderma)	**Shampoo:** 2% coal tar	In 120 and 240 ml.	3.5
otc	**Neutrogena T/Gel** (Neutrogena Corp.)	**Shampoo:** 2% coal tar extract	In 132, 255 and 480 ml.	2.7
		Conditioner: 1.5% coal tar extract in a conditioner base	In 132 ml.	2.7
otc	**Pentrax** (GenDerm)	**Shampoo:** 4.3% coal tar with a conditioning agent	In 118 and 237 ml.	4.4
otc	**Tegrin Medicated** (Block)	**Shampoo:** 5% coal tar solution, 4.6% alcohol	**Gel:** In 71 g.	3.1
			Lotion: Regular or herbal. In 110 and 198 ml.	1.9
otc	**Tegrin Medicated Extra Conditioning** (Block)	**Shampoo:** 7% coal tar solution, 6.4% alcohol	In 110 and 198 ml.	1.9
otc	**Denorex** (Whitehall)	**Shampoo:** 9% coal tar solution, 1.5% menthol and 7.5% alcohol	Regular, herbal or w/conditioner. In 120, 240 & 360 ml.	2.4
otc	**Extra Strength Denorex** (Whitehall)	**Shampoo:** 12.5% coal tar solution, 1.5% menthol, 10.4% alcohol	In regular and w/ conditioner. In 120, 240, 360 ml.	NA
otc	**MG 217 Medicated** (Triton)	**Shampoo:** 5% coal tar solution, 2% salicyclic acid, 1.5% colloidal sulfur	In 120 and 240 ml.	NA
		Conditioner: 2% coal tar solution	In 120 ml.	NA

* Cost Index based on cost per ml or g.

(Continued on following page)

TAR DERIVATIVES, SHAMPOOS (Cont.)

	Product	Form	Packaging	C.I.*
otc	**Duplex T** (C & M Pharm.)	**Shampoo:** 10% coal tar soln., 15% sodium lauryl sulfate, 8.3% alcohol	In pt and gal.	2.1
otc	**Iocon** (Owen/Galderma)	**Shampoo, gel:** Coal tar solution and 2.1% alcohol	In 105 g.	4.8
otc	**Polytar** (Stiefel)	**Shampoo:** 2.5% polytar (coal tar solution, solubilized crude coal tar equivalent to 0.5% coal tar)	In 180 and 360 ml.	2.3
otc	**Packer's Pine Tar** (Rydelle)	**Shampoo:** Pine tar	In 180 ml.	2.7

PYRITHIONE ZINC

Actions:

Pyrithione zinc, a cytostatic agent, reduces cell turnover rate. Its action is thought to be due to a nonspecific toxicity for epidermal cells. The compound strongly binds to both hair and external skin layers.

Indications:

Helps control dandruff and seborrheic dermatitis of the body *(ZNP Bar Soap)* and of the scalp, and for effective control of dry scalp and dry scalp symptoms.

Precautions:

For external use only. Keep out of eyes; if contact occurs, rinse thoroughly with water.

Overdosage:

Oral: Refer to General Management of Acute Overdosage.

Administration:

Apply shampoo; lather, rinse and repeat. Use once or twice weekly.

	Product	Form	Packaging	C.I.*
otc	**Danex** (Herbert)	**Shampoo:** 1%	In 120 ml.	3.4
otc	**Zincon** (Lederle)		In 118 and 240 ml.	2
otc	**Head & Shoulders** (Procter & Gamble)		**Cream:** In "normal to oily" and "normal to dry" formulas. In 165 g.	1.8
			Lotion: In "normal to oily" and "normal to dry" formulas. In 120, 210, 330 and 450 ml.	1.2
otc	**Head & Shoulders Dry Scalp** (Procter & Gamble)		In regular and conditioning formulas. In 210, 330 and 450 ml.	NA
otc	**DHS Zinc** (Person & Covey)	**Shampoo:** 2%	In 180 and 360 ml.	2.9
otc	**Sebulon** (Westwood Squibb)		In 120 and 240 ml.	3.7
otc	**Theraplex Z** (Medicis)	**Shampoo:** 2%	In 240 ml.	2.1
otc	**ZNP Bar** (Stiefel)	**Soap:** 2%	In 119 g.	2.4

POVIDONE-IODINE SHAMPOO

Actions:

A broad spectrum antimicrobial agent. Liberates free iodine.

Indications:

Temporary relief of scaling and itching due to dandruff.

Precautions:

For external use only. Avoid contact with eyes.

Irritation/Inflammation: Discontinue if signs of irritation or inflammation develop.

Administration and Dosage:

Apply 2 tsp to hair and scalp; use warm water to lather. Rinse. Repeat application. Massage gently into scalp. Allow to remain on scalp for at least 5 minutes. Work up lather to a golden color, using warm water. Rinse scalp thoroughly. Repeat twice weekly until improvement is noted. Thereafter, shampoo weekly.

	Product	Form	Packaging	C.I.*
otc	**Betadine** (Purdue Frederick)	**Shampoo:** 7.5%	In 118 ml.	4.6

* Cost Index based on cost per g or ml.

SULFACETAMIDE SODIUM

For complete information on the sulfonamides, refer to the group monograph in the Anti-Infectives Section.

Actions:

Exerts a bacteriostatic effect against gram-positive and gram-negative microorganisms commonly isolated from secondary cutaneous pyogenic infections.

Indications:

Topical application in the following scaling dermatoses: Seborrheic dermatitis; seborrhea sicca (dandruff). Also indicated in secondary bacterial infections of the skin.

Contraindications:

Hypersensitivity to sulfonamides or to any of the components of the product.

Warnings:

Stevens-Johnson syndrome has occurred with topical sulfacetamide sodium use.

Drug-induced systemic lupus erythematosus from topical sulfacetamide has occurred; one case was fatal.

Pregnancy: Category C. Safety for use during pregnancy has not been established. Use only when clearly needed and when the potential benefits outweigh the potential hazards to the fetus.

Lactation: It is not known whether this drug is excreted in breast milk. Exercise caution when administering to a nursing woman.

Children: Safety and efficacy in children < 12 years of age are not established.

Precautions:

For external use only.

Systemic absorption of topical sulfonamides is greater following application to large, infected, abraded, denuded or severely burned areas.

Superinfection: Use of antibiotics (especially prolonged or repeated therapy) may result in bacterial or fungal overgrowth of nonsusceptible organisms. Such overgrowth may lead to secondary infection. Take appropriate measures if superinfection occurs.

Hypersensitivity reactions may recur when a sulfonamide is readministered, regardless of the route of administration; cross hypersensitivity between sulfonamides may occur. If signs of hypersensitivity or other untoward reactions occur, discontinue use. Refer to Management of Acute Hypersensitivity Reactions.

Overdosage:

Oral ingestion: Symptoms – Nausea; vomiting. Large doses may cause hematuria, crystalluria and renal shutdown due to precipitation of sulfa crystals in renal tubules and urinary tract.

Treatment – Refer to General Management of Acute Overdosage. Observe kidney function for up to 1 week; have the patient ingest copious amounts of fluid. Mannitol infusions may be helpful at the first sign of oliguria. Alkalinization of urine by bicarbonate ingestion may prevent crystallization of sulfa drug in the kidney.

Patient Information:

For external use only. If irritation occurs or continues, or if rash develops, discontinue use and notify physician. Discontinue promptly if arthritis, fever or mouth sores develop.

Administration and Dosage:

Seborrheic dermatitis: In mild cases involving the scalp and adjacent skin areas, including noninflammatory types with scaling (dandruff), apply at bedtime and allow to remain overnight. Precede application by a shampoo if the hair and scalp are oily or greasy or if there is considerable debris. In severe cases with crusting, heavy scaling and inflammation involving the scalp, apply twice daily. Initially, and as frequently as necessary thereafter, cleanse the hair and scalp with a nonirritating shampoo to ensure complete contact of the medication with the affected skin.

The plastic tube is convenient for applying the lotion, especially for patients with thick hair. Part the hair a section at a time and squeeze a small amount on the scalp from the inverted tube. Completely moisten scalp and gently rub in with fingertips. Brush hair thoroughly for 2 to 3 minutes. The following morning wash the hair and scalp if desired. Wash hair at least once a week. (Rinsing with plain water or thorough brushing will remove any excess medication.) Repeat application at bedtime, as described, for 8 to 10 nights. As eruption subsides, lengthen the interval between applications. Applications once or twice weekly or every other week may prevent recurrence. Should the eruption recur after stopping therapy, reinitiate as at the beginning of treatment.

Secondary cutaneous bacterial infections: Apply 2 to 4 times daily until infection clears.

Sulfacetamide sodium is incompatible with silver preparations.

				C.I.*
Rx	**Sebizon** (Schering)	**Lotion:** 10%	In 85 g.	12

* Cost Index based on cost per g.

CHLOROXINE

Actions:

A synthetic antibacterial compound; also has antifungal activity. Chloroxine reduces excess scaling in patients with scaling or seborrheic dermatitis.

Indications:

Treatment of dandruff and mild to moderately severe seborrheic dermatitis of the scalp.

Contraindications:

Hypersensitivity to any of the ingredients. Do not use on acutely inflamed lesions.

Warnings:

Pregnancy: Category C. Safety for use during pregnancy has not been established. Use only when clearly needed and when the potential benefits outweigh the potential hazards to the fetus.

Lactation: It is not known whether the drug is excreted in breast milk. Exercise caution when administering to a nursing woman.

Children: Safety and efficacy for use in children have not been established.

Precautions:

For external use only. Avoid contact with eyes; if contact occurs, flush with cool water.

Adverse Reactions:

Irritation and burning of the scalp and adjacent areas have occurred. Discoloration of light colored hair has occurred.

Patient Information:

For external use only. Avoid contact with eyes.

If irritation, burning or rash occurs, discontinue use.

May discolor blond, gray or bleached hair.

Administration:

Massage thoroughly into wet scalp. Allow lather to remain on scalp for 3 minutes; rinse. Repeat application and rinse. Two treatments per week are usually sufficient.

				C.I.*
Rx	**Capitrol** (Westwood Squibb)	**Shampoo:** 2%	In 120 ml.	8.8

ANTISEBORRHEIC COMBINATIONS

Precautions:

For external use only. Avoid contact with eyes; in case of contact, flush with water.

If undue skin irritation develops or increases, discontinue use and consult physician. Preparations containing tar may temporarily discolor blond, bleached or tinted hair. Slight staining of clothing may also occur.

In these combinations:

SALICYLIC ACID and *SULFUR* (see individual monographs) are used for antiseborrheic and keratolytic/keratoplastic actions.

TAR PREPARATIONS, PYRITHIONE ZINC (see individual monographs) and *MYRISTYLTRIMETHYLAMMONIUM BROMIDE* are used for their antipruritic, antibacterial or antiseborrheic actions.

MENTHOL is used as an antipruritic.

BENZALKONIUM CHLORIDE, ISOPROPYL ALCOHOL, PHENOL and *MENTHOL* are used as antiseptics.

IODOQUINOL, METHYLBENZETHONIUM CHLORIDE and *BENZYL ALCOHOL* are antimicrobial agents.

	Shampoos			C.I.*
otc	**Maximum Strength Meted** (GenDerm)	**Shampoo:** 5% sulfur and 3% salicylic acid	In 118 ml.	4.1
otc	**MG400** (Triton)	**Shampoo:** 3% salicylic acid, 5% colloidal sulfur in Guy-Base II.	In 240 ml and pt.	1.8
otc	**Fostex Medicated Cleansing** (Westwood Squibb)	**Shampoo:** 2% sulfur and 2% salicylic acid	In 120 g.	4.8
otc	**Sebex** (Rugby)		In 118 ml.	NA
otc	**Sebulex** (Westwood Squibb)		Regular and with conditioners. In 120 and 240 ml.	3.2

* Cost Index based on cost per g or ml.

(Continued on following page)

Refer to the general discussion of these products on page2338.

Antiseborrheic Shampoos (Cont.)

	Product	Composition	How Supplied	C.I.*
otc	**Vanseb Dandruff** (Herbert)	**Shampoo:** 2% sulfur and 1% salicylic acid	**Cream:** In 90 g. **Lotion:** In 120 ml.	4.3 3.4
otc	**Ionil Plus** (Owen/Galderma)	**Shampoo:** 2% salicylic acid	In 120 and 240 ml.	3.5
otc	**P & S** (Baker Cummins)		In 120 ml.	3.8
otc	**Sulfoam** (Bradley)		In 118, 236 and 465 ml.	1.8
otc	**Neutrogena T/Sal** (Triton)	**Shampoo:** 2% salicyclic acid, 2% solubilized coal tar extract	In 135 ml.	NA
otc	**Ionil** (Owen/Galderma)	**Shampoo:** Salicylic acid, benzalkonium chloride, EDTA	In 120 and 240 ml, pt and qt.	3.5
otc	**X•Seb** (Baker Cummins)	**Shampoo:** 4% salicylic acid	In 120 ml.	3.9
otc	**Tarsum** (Summers)	**Shampoo/Gel:** 10% crude coal tar and 5% salicylic acid	In 120 and 240 ml.	NA
otc	**X•Seb T** (Baker Cummins)	**Shampoo:** 10% coal tar solution, 4% salicylic acid	In 120 ml.	4.7
otc	**X•Seb T Plus** (Baker Cummins)	**Shampoo:** 10% coal tar solution, 3% salicylic acid and 1% menthol	In 120 ml.	NA
otc	**Sebutone** (Westwood Squibb)	**Shampoo:** 0.5% coal tar, 2% sulfur, 2% salicylic acid	**Cream:** In 120 g. **Liquid:** In 120 and 240 ml.	5.1 4.1
otc	**Vanseb-T** (Herbert)	**Shampoo:** 5% coal tar solution 2% sulfur, 1% salicylic acid	**Cream:** In 90 g. **Lotion:** In 120 ml.	5.1 4
otc	**Sebex-T** (Rugby)	**Shampoo:** 5% coal tar solution, 2% colloidal sulfur and 2% salicylic acid	Soapless. In 118 ml.	1.6
otc	**Ionil T** (Owen/Galderma)	**Shampoo:** Coal tar solution, salicylic acid, benzalkonium chloride	In 120 and 240 ml, pt and qt.	3.6
otc	**Sebaquin** (Summers)	**Shampoo:** 3% iodoquinol, lanolin	In 120 ml.	NA
otc	**X•Seb Plus** (Baker Cummins)	**Shampoo:** 1% pyrithione zinc and 2% salicylic acid	In 120 ml.	NA

Medicated Hair Dressings

	Product	Composition	How Supplied	C.I.*
Rx	**Sal-Oil-T** (Syosset)	**Solution:** 10% crude coal tar, 6% salicylic acid, vegetable oil	In 59.14 ml.	5.8
otc	**SLT Lotion** (C & M Pharm.)	**Lotion:** 2% coal tar solution, 3% salicylic acid, 5% lactic acid, 65% isopropyl alcohol, 1.6% benzyl alcohol and benzalkonium chloride	In 129 ml.	4.2
otc	**Tarlene** (Medco Lab)	**Lotion:** 2% refined coal tar, 2.5% salicylic acid	In 60 ml.	3.1
otc	**Sebucare** (Westwood Squibb)	**Lotion:** 1.8% salicylic acid with 61% alcohol	In 120 ml.	6.2
otc	**Scadan** (Miles Inc.)	**Lotion:** 1% myristyltrimethylammonium bromide and 0.1% stearyl dimethyl benzyl ammonium chloride	In 120 ml.	8.9
otc	**P & S** (Baker Cummins)	**Liquid:** Phenol, mineral oil and glycerin	In 120 and 240 ml.	4.4
otc	**Diaparene Cradol** (Lehn & Fink)	**Liquid:** 0.07% methylbenzethonium chloride, lanolin, mineral oil, parabens	In 90 ml.	2.6

* Cost Index based on cost per g or ml.

Actions:

Topical antihistamines have some local anesthetic activity and are used to relieve itching. Although some transdermal absorption may occur, they are not absorbed in sufficient quantities to produce systemic side effects. They may cause local irritation and sensitization, especially with prolonged use. Refer to the Antihistamine monograph in the Respiratory Drugs section for further information on systemic antihistamines.

Indications:

Temporary relief of itching due to minor skin disorders, ivy, sumac and oak poisoning, sunburn, insect bites (nonpoisonous) and stings.

Warnings:

Do not apply to blistered, raw or oozing areas of the skin, or around the eyes or other mucous membranes (eg, nose, mouth).

Precautions:

For external use only. Avoid contact with the eyes.

If the condition persists, recurs after a few days or irritation develops, discontinue use.

Avoid prolonged use (> 7 days) or use on extensive skin areas.

Other ingredients used with the antihistamines include:

BENZOCAINE as a local anesthetic.
CHLOROXYLENOL, BENZALKONIUM CHLORIDE, EUCALYPTOL as bacteriostatic agents.
BENZYL ALCOHOL, CAMPHOR, MENTHOL and PHENOL for antipruritic effects.
CALAMINE and ZINC OXIDE as astringents.
DIMETHYL POLYSILOXANE as a skin protectant.
CHLOROPHYLLIN SODIUM promotes healing.
ISOPROPYL ALCOHOL as an antiseptic.
CHLOROBUTANOL for antipruritic and antiseptic effects.

	Product	Preparation	Size	C.I.*
otc	**Maximum Strength Benadryl 2%** (Parke-Davis)	**Cream:** 2% diphenhydramine HCl and parabens in a greaseless base	In 15 g.	19
		Spray, non-aerosol: 2% diphenhydramine HCl, 85% alcohol	In 60 ml.	6.4
otc	**Ziradryl** (Parke-Davis)	**Lotion:** 1% diphenhydramine HCl, 2% zinc oxide, 2% alcohol, camphor, parabens	In 180 ml.	2
otc	**Caladryl Clear** (Warner-Lambert)	**Lotion:** 1% diphenhydramine HCl, 2% zinc oxide, 2% alcohol, camphor, chlorophyllin sodium, parabens	In 180 ml.	3
otc	**Benadryl** (Parke-Davis)	**Cream:** 1% diphenhydramine HCl, parabens in a greaseless base	In 15 g.	16
		Spray, non-aerosol: 1% diphenhydramine HCl, 85% alcohol	In 60 ml.	5.9
otc	**Caladryl** (Parke-Davis)	**Cream:** 1% diphenhydramine HCl, 8% calamine, parabens, camphor	In 45 g.	16
		Lotion: 1% diphenhydramine HCl, 8% calamine, camphor, 2% alcohol	In 75 and 180 ml.	2
		Spray: 1% diphenhydramine, 8% calamine, 10% alcohol, camphor	In 120 ml.	3
otc	**Di-Delamine** (Commerce)	**Gel and Spray, non-aerosol:** 1% diphenhydramine HCl, 0.5% tripelennamine HCl, 0.12% benzalkonium Cl, menthol, EDTA	**Gel:** In 37.5 g.	9
			Spray: In 120 ml.	3
otc	**Cala-gen** (Goldline)	**Lotion:** 1% diphenhydramine HCl, camphor, 2% alcohol	In 178 ml.	1.3
otc	**Sting-Eze** (Wisconsin Pharm.)	**Concentrate:** Diphenhydramine HCl, camphor, phenol, benzocaine and eucalyptol	In 15 ml.	NA
otc	**Medacote** (Dal-Med)	**Lotion:** 1% pyrilamine maleate, dimethyl polysiloxane, zinc oxide, menthol and camphor in a greaseless base	In 120 ml.	3.1
otc	**Derma-Pax** (Recsei Labs)	**Lotion:** 0.44% pyrilamine maleate, 0.06% chlorpheniramine, 1% benzyl alcohol, 35% isopropanol, chlorobutanol	In 120 ml and pt.	1
otc	**Calamycin** (Pfeiffer)	**Lotion:** Zinc oxide and 10% calamine, benzocaine, chloroxylenol, pyrilamine maleate, 2% isopropyl alcohol	In 120 ml.	2

* Cost Index based on cost per g or ml.

For information on systemic acyclovir, refer to the individual monograph in the Anti-infectives section.

Antiviral Agent

ACYCLOVIR (Acycloguanosine)

Actions:

Acyclovir, a synthetic acyclic purine nucleoside analog, has in vitro inhibitory activity against herpes simplex types 1 and 2 (HSV-1 and HSV-2), varicella-zoster, Epstein-Barr and cytomegalovirus. Acyclovir is activated by herpesvirus thymidine kinase which results in phosphorylation to produce acyclovir triphosphate. Acyclovir triphosphate interferes with herpes simplex virus DNA polymerase and inhibits viral DNA replication. It also inhibits cellular alpha-DNA polymerase, but to a lesser degree. In vitro, acyclovir triphosphate can be incorporated into growing chains of DNA by viral DNA polymerase. When incorporation occurs, the DNA chain is terminated. Acyclovir is preferentially taken up and selectively converted to the active triphosphate form by herpesvirus infected cells. Thus, acyclovir is much less toxic in vitro for normal uninfected cells. The relationship between in vitro susceptibility of herpes simplex virus to antiviral drugs and clinical response has not been established.

Systemic absorption of acyclovir after topical application is minimal.

Clinical pharmacology: In clinical trials of initial herpes genitalis, acyclovir decreased healing time and, in some cases, decreased duration of viral shedding and pain. Studies in immunocompromised patients with mainly herpes labialis showed a decrease in duration of viral shedding and a slight decrease in duration of pain. In contrast, studies of recurrent herpes genitalis and herpes labialis in nonimmunocompromised patients showed no clinical benefit; there was some decrease in duration of viral shedding.

Indications:

Management of initial episodes of herpes genitalis and in limited non-life-threatening mucocutaneous herpes simplex virus infections in immunocompromised patients.

Contraindications:

Hypersensitivity or chemical intolerance to the components of the formulation.

Warnings:

For cutaneous use only. Do not use in eyes.

Pregnancy: Category C. There are no adequate and well controlled studies in pregnant women. Use during pregnancy only if the potential benefits outweigh the potential hazards to the fetus.

Lactation: It is not known whether this drug is excreted in breast milk. Exercise caution when applying on a nursing mother.

Precautions:

Do not exceed the recommended administration and dosage. No data demonstrate that acyclovir will either prevent transmission of infection to other persons or prevent recurrent infections when applied in the absence of signs and symptoms. Do not use to prevent recurrent HSV infections. Although clinically significant viral resistance associated with acyclovir use has not been observed, this possibility exists.

Adverse Reactions:

Mild pain with transient burning/stinging (28.3%); pruritus (4%); rash (0.3%); vulvitis (0.3%).

In all studies, there was no significant difference between the drug and placebo groups in the rate or type of reported adverse reactions.

Patient Information:

For external use only.

Apply ointment every 3 hours 6 times daily for 1 week.

Ointment must thoroughly cover all lesions. Use a finger cot or rubber glove to apply ointment to prevent spread of infection.

May cause transient burning, stinging, itching and rash; notify physician if these become pronounced or persist.

Acyclovir ointment is not a cure for herpes simplex infections and it is of little benefit in treating recurrent attacks.

Administration and Dosage:

Initiate therapy as early as possible following onset of signs and symptoms.

Apply sufficient quantity to adequately cover all lesions every 3 hours 6 times daily for 7 days. The dose size per application will vary depending upon the total lesion area; a 0.5 inch ribbon of ointment covers approximately 4 square inches of surface area. Use a finger cot or rubber glove when applying acyclovir to prevent autoinoculation of other body sites and transmission of infection to other persons.

Rx	**Zovirax** (Burroughs Wellcome)	**Ointment:** 5% (50 mg per g)	In a polyethylene glycol base. In 3 and 15 g.

Antibiotics

MUPIROCIN (Pseudomonic Acid A)

Actions:

Pharmacology: Mupirocin, a topical antibacterial structurally unrelated to other agents, is produced by fermentation of the organism *Pseudomonas fluorescens.* Mupirocin inhibits bacterial protein synthesis by reversibly and specifically binding to bacterial isoleucyl transfer-RNA synthetase. Therefore, mupirocin shows no cross resistance with chloramphenicol, erythromycin, gentamicin, lincomycin, methicillin, neomycin, novobiocin, penicillin, streptomycin and tetracycline.

Pharmacokinetics: Application of ^{14}C-labeled mupirocin ointment to the lower arm of healthy males followed by occlusion for 24 hours showed no measurable systemic absorption ($<$ 1.1 ng/ml of whole blood). However, measurable radioactivity was present in the stratum corneum of these subjects 72 hours after application.

Microbiology: The following bacteria are susceptible to the action of mupirocin in vitro: The aerobic isolates of *Staphylococcus aureus* (including methicillin-resistant and β-lactamase producing strains), *S epidermidis, S saprophyticus* and *Streptococcus pyogenes*.

Indications:

For the topical treatment of impetigo due to: *Staphylococcus aureus*, beta-hemolytic *Streptococcus* and *S pyogenes*.

Contraindications:

Hypersensitivity reactions to any components of the product.

Warnings:

For external use only. Avoid contact with the eyes.

Pregnancy: Category B. There are no adequate and well controlled studies in pregnant women. Use during pregnancy only if clearly needed.

Lactation: It is not known whether mupirocin is present in breast milk. Temporarily discontinue nursing while using mupirocin.

Precautions:

Sensitivity reaction: If a reaction suggesting sensitivity or chemical irritation occurs, discontinue treatment and institute appropriate alternative therapy.

Superinfection: Use of antibiotics (especially prolonged or repeated therapy) may result in bacterial or fungal overgrowth of nonsusceptible organisms. Such overgrowth may lead to a secondary infection. Take appropriate measures if superinfection occurs.

Adverse Reactions:

Local: Burning, stinging or pain (1.5%); itching (1%); rash, nausea, erythema, dry skin, tenderness, swelling, contact dermatitis and increased exudate ($<$ 1%).

Patient Information:

For external use only. Avoid contact with eyes.

If a skin reaction develops, stop therapy, wash affected area and call a physician.

Apply 3 times daily. If improvement is not seen in 3 to 5 days, contact a physician.

Administration and Dosage:

Apply a small amount to the affected area 3 times daily. The area treated may be covered with a gauze dressing if desired. Reevaluate patients not showing a clinical response within 3 to 5 days.

				C.I.*
Rx	**Bactroban** (SK-Beecham)	**Ointment:** 2% (20 mg per g) in a polyethylene glycol base	In 15 g.	36

* Cost Index based on cost per g.

Antibiotics

Indications:

These antibiotic preparations are used for infection prophylaxis in minor cuts, wounds, burns and skin abrasions, as an aid to healing and for the treatment of superficial infections of the skin due to susceptible organisms amenable to local treatment. **Erythromycin** is also indicated for control of acne vulgaris.

Contraindications:

Prior sensitization to any of the ingredients.

Do not use in eyes.

Warnings:

For topical use only. Do not use in or near the eyes.

Systemic therapy: Deeper cutaneous infections may require systemic antibiotic therapy in addition to local treatment.

Neomycin toxicity: Due to the potential nephrotoxicity and ototoxicity of **neomycin**, use with care in treating extensive burns, trophic ulceration or other extensive conditions where absorption is possible. Do not apply more than once daily in burn cases where $>$ 20% of body surface is affected, especially if the patient has impaired renal function or is receiving other aminoglycoside antibiotics concurrently.

Blood dyscrasias with **chloramphenicol** have occurred (see Adverse Reactions).

Precautions:

Superinfection: Prolonged use of antibiotics may result in overgrowth of nonsusceptible organisms, particularly fungi. Such overgrowth may lead to a secondary infection. Discontinue the drug and take appropriate measures if superinfection occurs.

Neomycin hypersensitivity: Chronic application of **neomycin sulfate** to inflamed skin of individuals with allergic contact dermatitis and chronic dermatoses (eg, chronic otitis externa or stasis dermatitis) increases the possibility of sensitization. Low grade reddening with swelling, dry scaling and itching or a failure to heal are usually manifestations of this hypersensitivity. During long-term use of neomycin-containing products, perform periodic examinations and discontinue use if symptoms appear. These symptoms regress upon withdrawal of medication, but avoid neomycin-containing products thereafter.

Tetracycline: Discontinue **tetracycline** if redness, irritation, swelling or pain persists or increases or if infection occurs.

Deep or puncture wounds/serious burns: Consult physician.

Adverse Reactions:

Gentamicin: Possible photosensitization has been reported.

Chloramphenicol: Bone marrow hypoplasia, including aplastic anemia and death, has occurred following local application.

Itching or burning, angioneurotic edema, urticaria, vesicular and maculopapular dermatitis have occurred in patients sensitive to chloramphenicol, and are causes for discontinuing medication.

Bacitracin ointment: Allergic contact dermatitis has occurred.

Neomycin: Ototoxicity and nephrotoxicity have occurred (see Warnings).

Erythromycin: Isolated cases of skin irritation such as erythema and peeling have occurred.

Patient Information:

For external use only. Cleanse affected area of skin prior to application (unless directed otherwise).

Notify physician if condition worsens or if rash or irritation develops.

Tetracycline and **chlortetracycline** may stain clothing.

Administration:

Apply 1 to 4 times daily to infected area. Cover with sterile bandage if needed.

(Products listed on following page)

Antibiotics (Cont.)

	Product	Form/Strength	Description/Packaging	C.I.*
TETRACYCLINE HCl				
otc	**Achromycin** (Lederle)	**Ointment:** 3%	In 14.2 and 30 g.	6.9
CHLORTETRACYCLINE HCl				
otc	**Aureomycin** (Lederle)	**Ointment:** 3%	In 14.2 and 30 g.	6.2
CHLORAMPHENICOL				
Rx	**Chloromycetin** (Parke-Davis)	**Cream:** 1%	Water miscible ointment base with liquid petrolatum and propylparaben. In 30 g.	6.2
ERYTHROMYCIN				
Rx	**Akne-mycin** (Hermal)	**Ointment:** 2%	Petrolatum, mineral oil. In 25 g.	7
Rx	**Emgel** (Glaxo)		In 27 g.	NA
Rx	**Erygel** (Herbert)	**Gel:** 2%	92% alcohol. In 30 and 60 g w/5 g travel size included.	9.2
GENTAMICIN				
Rx	**Gentamicin** (Various, eg, Dixon-Shane, Geneva Marsam, Major, NMC, Schein)	**Ointment:** 0.1% (as 1.7 mg sulfate per g) in a bland, unctuous petrolatum base	In 15 g.	3.5+
Rx	**Garamycin** (Schering)		Parabens. In 15 g.	16
Rx	**Gentamicin** (Various, eg, Dixon-Shane, Geneva Marsam, Major, NMC, Rugby, Schein)	**Cream:** 0.1% (as 1.7 mg sulfate per g) in a bland emulsion-type base	In 15 g.	3.5+
Rx	**Garamycin** (Schering)		Parabens. In 15 g.	16
Rx	**G-myticin** (Pedinol)	**Ointment:** Gentamicin sulfate equivalent to 1 mg base	In 15 g.	4.8
		Cream: Gentamicin sulfate equivalent to 1 mg base	In 15 g.	4.8
BACITRACIN				
otc	**Bacitracin** (Various, eg, Geneva Marsam, NMC, Parmed, Rugby, Schein, URL)	**Ointment:** 500 units per g	In 0.94, 15 and 30 g and 1 lb.	1.6+
otc	**Baciguent** (Upjohn)		Anhydrous lanolin, mineral oil, white petrolatum. In 15 and 30 g.	2.9
NEOMYCIN SULFATE				
otc	**Neomycin** (Various, eg, Rugby, Schein)	**Ointment:** 3.5 mg neomycin (as sulfate) per g	In 15 and 30 g.	1+
otc	**Myciguent** (Upjohn)		Lanolin, mineral oil, white petrolatum. In 15 and 30 g.	3.1
otc	**Myciguent** (Upjohn)	**Cream:** 3.5 mg neomycin (as sulfate) per g	Methylparaben. In 15 g.	3.1

* Cost Index based on cost per g.

Refer to the general discussion of these products on page 2343

Antibiotics, Multiple

COMBINATION ANTI-INFECTIVE PRODUCTS

	Product and Distributor	Polymyxin B Sulfate (units/g or ml)	Neomycin (mg/g or ml)[1]	Bacitracin (units/g or ml)	Other (g or ml)	How Supplied	C.I.*
otc	**Polysporin Ointment** (Burroughs Wellcome)	10,000		500		White petrolatum base. in 15, 30 and UD 0.94 g (144s).	4
otc	**Polysporin Powder** (Burroughs Wellcome)					Lactose base. in 10 g.	15
otc	**Neosporin Cream** (Burroughs Wellcome)	10,000	3.5			0.25% parabens, mineral oil, white petrolatum. Non-greasy base. In 15 g and UD 0.94 g (144s).	4.4
otc	**Maximum Strength Neosporin Ointment** (Burroughs Wellcome)	10,000	3.5	500		White petrolatum. In 15 g.	4.2
otc	**Lanabiotic Ointment** (Combe)				40 mg lidocaine	Lanolin, mineral oil and petrolatum. In 15 and 30 g.	2.4
otc	**Triple Antibiotic Ointment** (Various, eg, Dixon-Shane, Geneva Marsam, Goldline, Parmed, Rugby, Schein)	5000	3.5	400		In 2.4, 9.6, 15 and 30 g.	2.2+
otc	**Medi-Quick Ointment** (Mentholatum)					Mineral oil and petrolatum. In 14.2 g.	3.6
otc	**N-B-P Ointment** (Forest)					In 14.2 g.	3.6
otc	**Neomixin Ointment** (Hauck)					Petrolatum base. In 15 g and 1 g (144s).	3.1
otc	**Neosporin Ointment** (Burroughs Wellcome)					White petrolatum. In 15 & 30 g and UD 0.94 g (144s).	4.4
otc	**Septa Ointment** (Circle)					In 28.3 g.	1.5
otc	**Spectrocin Plus Ointment** (Numark Labs)				5 mg lidocaine	Mineral oil and white petrolatum. In 15 and 30 g.	4.1
otc	**Bactine First Aid Antibiotic Plus Anesthetic Ointment** (Miles)				10 mg diperodon HCl	Mineral oil and white petrolatum. In 15 g.	NA
otc	**Maximum Strength Mycitracin Triple Antibiotic Ointment** (Upjohn)	5000	3.5	500		Parabens, mineral oil, white petrolatum. In 15 and 30 g and UD 0.94 g (144s).	3
otc	**Campho-Phenique Antibiotic Plus Pain Reliever Ointment** (Winthrop)				40 mg lidocaine	White petrolatum. In 15 g.	NA
otc	**Mycitracin Plus Ointment** (Upjohn)					Mineral oil, parabens and white petrolatum. In 14.2 and 30 g.	4.2
otc	**Polysporin Spray** (Burroughs Wellcome)	2222		111		In 90 g.	1

* Cost Index based on cost per g.

[1] As base; equivalent to 5 mg neomycin sulfate.

Antifungal Agents

UNDECYLENIC ACID AND DERIVATIVES

Indications:

Antifungal and antibacterial agents for tinea pedis (athlete's foot), exclusive of the nails and hairy areas. Also recommended for the relief and prevention of diaper rash, itching, burning and chafing, prickly heat, tinea cruris (jock itch), excessive perspiration and irritation in the groin area and bromhidrosis.

Warnings:

For external use only. Avoid inhaling and contact with the eyes or other mucous membranes. Patients with impaired circulation, including diabetics, should consult a physician before using. Do not use in children < 2 years old except on advice of physician.

Administration:

Cleanse and dry area well; smooth or spray on. Apply as needed or as directed.

The choice of vehicle is important for these products. Ointments, creams and liquids are used as primary therapy. In general, powders are used as adjunctive therapy, but they may be acceptable as primary therapy in very mild conditions.

	Product	Composition	Vehicle/Package	C.I.*
otc	**Protectol Medicated** (Daniels)	**Powder:** 15% calcium undecylenate	Starch. In 56.7 g.	1.5
otc	**Caldesene** (Fisons)	**Powder:** 10% calcium undecylenate	In 60 and 120 g.	1.5
otc	**Cruex** (Fisons)		Talc. In 45 g.	4.3
otc	**Cruex Aerosol** (Fisons)	**Powder:** 19% total undecylenate as undecylenic acid and zinc undecylenate	Menthol, talc. In 54, 105 and 165 g.	3
otc	**Desenex** (Fisons)		Talc. In 45 and 90 g.	3.5
otc	**Desenex Aerosol** (Fisons)		Menthol, talc. In 81 and 165 g.	2.1
otc	**Phicon F** (T.E. Williams)	**Cream:** 8% undecylenic acid, 0.05% pramoxine HCl	In 60 g.	5.8
otc	**Breezee Mist Aerosol** (Pedinol)	**Powder:** Undecylenic acid, menthol and aluminum chlorhydrate	Talc. In 113 g.	NA
Rx	**Pedi-Dri** (Pedinol)	**Powder:** Zinc undecylenate, aluminum chlorhydroxide, menthol and formaldehyde	Cornstarch. In 60 g.	4
otc	**Pedi-Pro** (Pedinol)	**Powder:** Zinc undecylenate, aluminum chlorhydroxide, menthol, chloroxylenol	Starch. In 60 g.	3.4
otc	**Desenex** (Fisons)	**Ointment:** 22% total undecylenate as undecylenic acid and zinc undecylenate	Lanolin, parabens, white petrolatum. In 15 and 30 g.	14
otc	**Desenex Maximum Strength** (Fisons)	**Ointment:** 25% total undecylenate as undecylenic acid and zinc undecylenate	Lanolin, parabens, white petrolatum. In 15 g.	NA
otc	**Decylenes** (Rugby)	**Ointment:** Undecylenic acid and zinc undecylenate	In 30 g and 1 lb.	3
otc	**Cruex** (Fisons)	**Cream:** 20% total undecylenate as undecylenic acid and zinc undecylenate	Lanolin, parabens, white petrolatum. In 15 g.	15
otc	**Desenex** (Fisons)	**Cream:** 25% total undecylenate as undecylenic acid and zinc undecylenate	Lanolin, parabens, white petrolatum. In 15 g.	13
otc	**Desenex** (Fisons)	**Foam:** 10% undecylenic acid with 35.2% isopropyl alcohol	In 42.5 g.	5
otc	**Desenex** (Fisons)	**Soap:** Undecylenic acid	In 97.5 g.	1

* Cost Index based on cost per g or ml.

Antifungal Agents (Cont.)

CLIOQUINOL (Iodochlorhydroxyquin)

Actions:

Has antibacterial and antifungal properties.

Indications:

Inflamed conditions of the skin such as eczema, athlete's foot and other fungal infections.

Precautions:

For external use only. Avoid contact with the eyes.

Sensitivity: In rare cases, may irritate sensitized skin. If itching, redness, irritation, stinging or swelling persists or increases, discontinue use.

May stain fabric, skin or hair.

Administration:

Apply to affected areas 2 or 3 times daily. Not for use > 1 week.

				C.I.*
otc	**Vioform** (Ciba)	**Cream:** 3%	Water washable base. In 30 g.	NA
		Ointment: 3%	Petrolatum base. In 30 g.	NA

MICONAZOLE NITRATE

For information on systemic and vaginal miconazole, refer to individual monographs.

Actions:

Miconazole alters cellular membrane permeability and interferes with mitochondrial and peroxisomal enzymes, resulting in intracellular necrosis. It inhibits growth of the common dermatophytes, *Trichophyton rubrum, T mentagrophytes, Epidermophyton floccosum, Candida albicans* and the active organism in tinea versicolor, *Malassezia furfur*.

Indications:

Rx and otc: Tinea pedis (athlete's foot), tinea cruris (jock itch) and tinea corporis (ringworm) caused by *T rubrum, T mentagrophytes* and *E floccosum*.

Rx only: Cutaneous candidiasis (moniliasis); tinea versicolor.

Warnings:

For external use only. Avoid contact with the eyes.

Sensitivity: If a reaction occurs suggesting sensitivity or chemical irritation, discontinue use.

Adverse Reactions:

Isolated reports of irritation, burning, maceration and allergic contact dermatitis.

Patient Information:

For external use only.

If condition persists or worsens, or if irritation (burning, itching, stinging, redness) occurs, discontinue use and notify physician.

Use for full treatment time, even if symptoms improve. Notify physician if there is no improvement after 2 weeks (*Candida* infections, tinea cruris and corporis) or 4 weeks (tinea pedis).

Administration and Dosage:

Cream and lotion: Cover affected areas twice daily, morning and evening (once daily in patients with tinea versicolor). Lotion is preferred in intertriginous areas; if cream is used, apply sparingly to avoid maceration effects.

Powder: Spray or sprinkle powder liberally over affected area in the morning and evening.

Early relief of symptoms (2 to 3 days) occurs in most patients; clinical improvement may be seen fairly soon after treatment. However, treat candida, tinea cruris and tinea corporis for 2 weeks, and tinea pedis for 1 month, to reduce possible recurrence. If a patient shows no clinical improvement after 1 month, reevaluate diagnosis. Patients with tinea versicolor usually exhibit clinical and mycological clearing in 2 weeks.

				C.I.*
otc	**Miconazole Nitrate** (Taro)	**Cream:** 2%	Benzoic acid, mineral oil, apricot kernal oil. In 15 and 30 g.	NA
otc	**Micatin** (Ortho)		Mineral oil. In 15 and 30 g.	16
Rx	**Monistat-Derm** (Ortho)		Water miscible, mineral oil base. In 15, 30 and 90 g.	25
otc	**Micatin** (Ortho)	**Powder:** 2%	**Powder:** In 90 g bottle.	5.5
			Aerosol powder: Alcohol. Available with and without deodorant. In 90 g.	2.5
otc	**Micatin Liquid** (Ortho)	**Spray:** 2%	Alcohol. In 105 ml.	2

* Cost Index based on cost per g or ml.

ECONAZOLE NITRATE

Actions:

Microbiology: In vitro studies revealed econazole nitrate's broad spectrum antifungal activity against the dermatophytes, *Trichophyton rubrum, T mentagrophytes, T tonsurans, Microsporum canis, M audouini, M gypseum* and *Epidermophyton floccosum,* the yeasts, *Candida albicans* and *Malassezia furfur* (the organism responsible for tinea versicolor) and certain gram-positive bacteria.

Pharmacokinetics: After topical application to the skin, systemic absorption is extremely low. Although most of the applied drug remains on the skin surface, drug concentrations were found in the stratum corneum which exceeded, by far, the minimum inhibitory concentration for dermatophytes. Inhibitory concentrations were achieved in the epidermis and as deep as the middle region of the dermis. Less than 1% of the applied dose was recovered in the urine and feces.

Indications:

Treatment of tinea pedis (athlete's foot), tinea cruris (jock itch) and tinea corporis (ringworm) caused by *T rubrum, T mentagrophytes, T tonsurans, M canis, M audouini, M gypseum* and *E floccosum;* cutaneous candidiasis; tinea versicolor.

Contraindications:

Hypersensitivity to econazole nitrate or any ingredients of the product.

Warnings:

Pregnancy: Category C. Fetotoxic or embryotoxic effects were observed in animal studies with oral doses 10 to 40 times the human dermal dose.

Do not use in the first trimester of pregnancy, unless essential to the patient's welfare. Use during the second and third trimesters only if clearly needed.

Lactation: It is not known whether econazole is excreted in breast milk. Following oral administration to lactating rats, econazole or its metabolites were excreted in milk. Exercise caution when applying on a nursing mother.

Precautions:

Sensitivity: If sensitivity or chemical irritation occurs, discontinue use.

For external use only. Avoid contact with the eyes.

Adverse Reactions:

Local: Burning, itching, stinging, erythema (3%); pruritic rash (one case).

Patient Information:

For external use only. Avoid contact with the eyes.

Cleanse skin with soap and water and dry thoroughly.

For athlete's foot, wear well-fitting and ventilated shoes and change shoes and socks at least once a day.

If condition persists or worsens, or if irritation (burning, itching, stinging, redness) occurs, discontinue use and notify physician.

Use medication for the full treatment time, even though symptoms may have improved. Notify physician if there is no improvement after 2 weeks (tinea cruris and corporis) or 4 weeks (tinea pedis).

Apply after cleansing affected area (unless directed otherwise).

Administration and Dosage:

Tinea pedis, tinea cruris, tinea corporis and tinea versicolor: Apply sufficient quantity to cover affected areas once daily.

Cutaneous candidiasis: Apply twice daily (morning and evening).

Early relief of symptoms is experienced by most patients, and clinical improvement may be seen fairly soon after treatment is begun. However, treat candidal infections and tinea cruris and corporis for 2 weeks and tinea pedis for 1 month, to reduce the possibility of recurrence. If no clinical improvement occurs after the treatment period, reevaluate diagnosis. Patients with tinea versicolor usually exhibit clinical and mycological clearing after 2 weeks of treatment.

				C.I.*
Rx	**Spectazole** (Ortho)	**Cream:** 1%	Water miscible base. Mineral oil. In 15, 30 and 85 g.	25

* Cost Index based on cost per g.

CICLOPIROX OLAMINE

Actions:

Pharmacology: A broad spectrum, antifungal agent. The primary site of action is the cell membrane. At concentrations < 20 mg/L, ciclopirox blocks transmembrane transport of amino acids into the fungal cell. At higher concentrations, the fungal cell membrane integrity is altered, allowing leakage of intracellular material.

Microbiology: Ciclopirox inhibits the growth of pathogenic dermatophytes, yeasts and *Malassezia furfur.* It exhibits fungicidal activity in vitro against isolates of *Trichophyton rubrum, T mentagrophytes, Epidermophyton floccosum, Microsporum canis* and *Candida albicans.*

Pharmacokinetics: An average of 1.3% was absorbed when applied topically, followed by occlusion for 6 hours. The half-life was 1.7 hours and excretion occurred via the kidney. Fecal excretion was negligible.

Studies in human cadaverous skin from the back with ciclopirox cream 1% showed 0.8% to 1.6% of the dose in stratum corneum 1.5 to 6 hours after application. Levels in the dermis were still 10 to 15 times above the minimum inhibitory concentrations.

Ciclopirox penetrates into the hair and through the epidermis and hair follicles into the sebaceous glands and dermis, while a portion of the drug remains in the stratum corneum.

Indications:

Tinea pedis (athlete's foot), tinea cruris (jock itch) and tinea corporis (ringworm) due to *T rubrum, T mentagrophytes, E floccosum* and *M canis;* candidiasis (moniliasis) due to *C albicans;* tinea (pityriasis) versicolor due to *M furfur.*

Contraindications:

Hypersensitivity to ciclopirox olamine or any of its components.

Warnings:

Pregnancy: Category B. There are no adequate or well controlled studies in pregnant women. Use during pregnancy only if clearly needed.

Lactation: It is not known whether this drug is excreted in breast milk. Exercise caution when applying on a nursing woman.

Children: Safety and efficacy in children < 10 years old have not been established.

Precautions:

For external use only. Avoid contact with the eyes.

Sensitivity: If sensitivity or chemical irritation occurs, discontinue treatment.

Adverse Reactions:

Local reactions consist of irritation, pruritus at applicaiton site, redness, pain, burning, worsening of clinical signs and symptoms.

Patient Information:

For external use only. Avoid contact with the eyes.

Cleanse skin with soap and water and dry thoroughly.

For athlete's foot, wear well-fitting, ventilated shoes and change shoes and socks at least once a day.

Use the medication for the full treatment time, even though symptoms may have improved. Notify the physician if no improvement occurs after 4 weeks.

Inform physician if the area of application shows signs of increased irritation (eg, redness, itching, burning, blistering, swelling, oozing) indicative of possible sensitization.

Avoid the use of occlusive wrappings or dressings.

Administration and Dosage:

Gently massage cream into the affected and surrounding skin areas twice daily, morning and evening. Clinical improvement usually occurs within the first week of treatment. If no improvement occurs after 4 weeks of treatment, reevaluate the diagnosis. Patients with tinea versicolor usually exhibit clinical and mycological clearing after 2 weeks of treatment.

				C.I.*
Rx	**Loprox** (Hoechst-Roussel)	**Cream:** 1%	Water miscible base. 1% benzyl alcohol, mineral oil. In 15, 30 and 90 g.	27
		Lotion: 1%	Water miscible base. 1% benzyl alcohol, mineral oil. In 30 ml.	28

* Cost Index based on cost per g.

For information on oral and vaginal clotrimazole, refer to individual monographs.

Antifungal Agents (Cont.)

CLOTRIMAZOLE

Actions:

Microbiology: Clotrimazole is a broad spectrum antifungal agent that inhibits the growth of pathogenic dermatophytes, yeasts and *Malassezia furfur.* Clotrimazole exhibits fungistatic and fungicidal activity in vitro against isolates of *Trichophyton rubrum, T mentagrophytes, Epidermophyton floccosum, Microsporum canis* and *Candida* species, including *Candida albicans.* No single step or multiple step resistance to clotrimazole has developed during successive passages of *C albicans* and *T mentagrophytes.*

Indications:

Otc products: Topical treatment of tinea pedis (athlete's foot), tinea cruris (jock itch) and tinea corporis (ringworm) due to *T rubrum, T mentagrophytes, E floccosum* and *M canis.*

Mycelex (Rx): Same as *otc* products plus candidiasis due to *C albicans* and tinea versicolor due to *M furfur.*

Lotrimin (Rx): Candidiasis due to *C albicans* and tinea versicolor due to *M furfur.*

Contraindications:

Hypersensitivity to clotrimazole or any product component.

Warnings:

Pregnancy: Category B. In clinical trials, use of vaginally applied clotrimazole in pregnant women in their second and third trimesters has not been associated with ill effects.

There are, however, no adequate and well controlled studies in pregnant women during the first trimester of pregnancy. Use only if clearly indicated during the first trimester.

Lactation: It is not known whether this drug is excreted in breast milk. Exercise caution when applying on a nursing mother.

Precautions:

For external use only. Avoid contact with the eyes.

If irritation or sensitivity develops, discontinue treatment and institute appropriate therapy.

Adverse Reactions:

Erythema; stinging; blistering; peeling; edema; pruritus; urticaria; burning; general skin irritation.

Patient Information:

For external use only. Avoid contact with the eyes.

Apply after cleansing affected area (unless directed otherwise).

If condition persists or worsens, or if irritation occurs, discontinue use and notify physician.

Use the medication for the full treatment time even though the symptoms may have improved. Notify the physician if there is no improvement after 4 weeks of treatment.

Inform the physician if the area of application shows signs of increased irritation (eg, redness, itching, burning, blistering, swelling, oozing) indicative of possible sensitization.

Administration and Dosage:

Gently massage into affected and surrounding skin areas twice daily, morning and evening. Clinical improvement, with relief of pruritus, usually occurs within the first week of treatment. If patient shows no clinical improvement after 4 weeks, reevaluate the diagnosis.

	Product	Form		C.I.*
Rx	**Lotrimin** (Schering)	**Cream:** 1%	In 15, 30, 45 and 90 g.	24
otc	**Lotrimin AF** (Schering-Plough)		In 12 g.	19
Rx	**Mycelex** (Miles)		In 15, 30 and 45 g.	28
otc	**Mycelex OTC** (Miles)		1% benzyl alcohol. In 15 g.	18
Rx	**Lotrimin** (Schering)	**Solution:** 1%	With polyethylene glycol 400. In 10 and 30 ml.	23
otc	**Lotrimin AF** (Schering-Plough)		With polyethylene glycol. In 10 ml.	20
Rx	**Mycelex** (Miles)		In 10 and 30 ml.	37
otc	**Mycelex OTC** (Miles)		With polyethylene glycol 400. In 10 ml.	19
Rx	**Lotrimin** (Schering)	**Lotion:** 1%	In 30 ml.	23

* Cost Index based on cost per g or ml.

Antifungal Agents (Cont.)

TRIACETIN (Glyceryl Triacetate)

Actions:

Pharmacology: Triacetin is a broad spectrum antifungal and antimicrobial agent that inhibits the growth of fungus, yeast and bacterial infections of the skin, intertriginous areas and topical mycoses. Triacetin is effective against the following organisms:

Microbiology: Fungus, yeasts – *Aureobasidium mansonii (Cladosporium werneckii and mansonii); Alternaria solani; Aspergillus niger; Candida albicans; Epidermophyton floccosum; Microsporum audouinii, canis* and *gypseum; Penicillium chrysogenum; Piedraia hortae; Rhizopus (nigricans) arrhizus; Saccharomyces (pastorianus) bayanus; Torula roseus (Candida* sp); *Trichophyton mentagrophytes, rubrum, schoenleinii, tonsurans* and *violaceum; Trichosporon beigelii.*

Gram positive – *Bacillus ammoniagenes (Brevibacterium ammoniagenes), cereus* (subsp. *mycoides*) and *subtilis; Staphylococcus aureus; Streptococcus faecalis.*

Gram negative – *Enterobacter aerogenes; Escherichia coli; Pseudomonas aeruginosa; Proteus vulgaris.*

When used for onychomycosis, it facilitates removal of hyperkeratotic or mycotic tissue before debriding nail groove due to its apparent softening effect.

Indications:

Treatment of onychomycosis (nail fungus), tinea pedis (athlete's foot), tinea cruris (jock itch), tinea corporis (ringworm), monilial impetigo and dermatitis.

Spray and tincture: Only for treatment of onychomycosis.

Contraindications:

Sensitivity to any components of the products.

Precautions:

Irritation or sensitivity: Discontinue treatment and notify physician.

For external use only. Not for ophthalmic use.

Diabetics or patients with impaired blood circulation: Use spray with caution.

Patient Information:

For external use only. Avoid contact with the eyes.

Apply after cleansing affected area (unless directed otherwise).

Notify the physician if there is no improvement after 4 weeks of treatment (except when treating nail fungus, which may take several months).

Inform the physician if the area of application shows signs of increased irritation indicative of possible sensitization.

Administration:

Cream, solution: Cleanse and dry affected areas. Gently massage sufficient amount into affected and surrounding skin areas 3 times daily. Clinical improvement usually occurs within the first week of therapy. If no clinical improvement occurs after 4 weeks of treatment, review the diagnosis.

Tincture: Cleanse and dry affected areas. Use brush to apply twice daily to affected areas of nail surface, beds, edges and under surface of the nail. Continued use may be necessary for several months before results are seen.

Spray: Shake well. Dry affected areas. Spray onto affected nails, holding actuator down 1 to 2 seconds.

				C.I.*
Rx	**Fungoid Tincture** (Pedinol)	**Solution:** Triacetin, cetylpyridinium chloride, chloroxylenol, benzyl alcohol, acetone, benzalkonium chloride	In 30 ml and pt.	13
Rx	**Fungoid** (Pedinol)	**Solution:** Triacetin, PEG-8, cetylpyridinium chloride, chloroxylenol and benzalkonium chloride	In 15 ml.	22
Rx	**Fungoid Creme** (Pedinol)	**Cream:** Triacetin, cetylpyridinium chloride, chloroxylenol, mineral oil, lanolin, propylene glycol, parabens in a vanishing cream base	In 30 g.	13
Rx	**Ony-Clear Nail** (Pedinol)	**Spray, Aerosol:** Triacetin, cetylpyridinium chloride, chloroxylenol, benzalkonium chloride, alcohol	In 45 and 60 ml.	11

* Cost Index based on cost per g or ml.

TOLNAFTATE

Actions:

Effective in the treatment of superficial fungus infections of the skin.

Indications:

Treatment of tinea pedis (athlete's foot), cruris (jock itch) or corporis (ringworm) due to infection with *Trichophyton rubrum, T mentagrophytes, T tonsurans, Microsporum canis, M audouini and Epidermophyton floccosum* and for tinea versicolor due to *Malassezia furfur*.

In onychomycosis, in chronic scalp infections in which fungi are numerous and widely distributed in skin and hair follicles, where kerion has formed and in fungus infections of palms and soles, use tolnaftate concurrently for adjunctive local benefit in these lesions.

Powder and powder aerosol: Also effective prophylactically against athlete's foot.

Warnings:

Sensitization or irritation: Discontinue treatment.

Nail and scalp infections: Not recommended for these infections except as adjunctive therapy to systemic treatment.

If symptoms do not improve after 10 days of use as recommended by the labeling, discontinue use unless otherwise directed.

Precautions:

For external use only. Keep out of eyes.

Reevaluate patient if no improvement occurs after 4 weeks.

Adverse Reactions:

A few cases of sensitization have been confirmed; mild irritation has occurred.

Patient Information:

For external use only. Avoid contact with the eyes.

Cleanse skin with soap and water and dry thoroughly before applying product.

For athlete's foot, wear well-fitting, ventilated shoes; change shoes and socks at least once a day.

Administration and Dosage:

Only small quantities are required. Treatment twice a day for 2 or 3 weeks is usually adequate, although 4 to 6 weeks may be required if the skin has thickened. Continue treatment to maintain remission.

The choice of vehicle is important for these products. Ointments, creams and liquids are used as primary therapy. In general, powders are used as adjunctive therapy, but they may be acceptable as primary therapy in very mild conditions.

	Product	Form	Description	C.I.*
otc	**Absorbine Antifungal** (W.F. Young)	**Cream:** 1%	Glyceryl monostearate, propylene glycol, diazolidinyl urea, parabens. In 21.3 g.	NA
otc	**Tolnaftate** (Various, eg, Dixon-Shane, Fougera, Goldline, IDE, Major, Moore, Parmed, NMC, Rugby, UDL)		In 15 g.	5.5+
otc	**Genaspor** (Goldline)		In 15 g.	7.5
otc	**NP • 27** (Thompson Medical)		In 15 and 30 g.	12
otc	**Tinactin** (Schering-Plough)		In 15 and 30 g.	14
otc	**Tinactin for Jock Itch** (Schering-Plough)		Petrolatum, mineral oil. In 15 g.	14
otc	**Ting** (Fisons)		In 15 g.	7.5
otc	**Tolnaftate** (Various, eg, Copley, Fougera, Goldline, IDE, Major, Moore, NMC, Parmed, Rugby)	**Solution:** 1%	In 10 ml.	8.2+
otc	**NP • 27** (Thompson Medical)		In 15 ml.	12
otc	**Tinactin** (Schering-Plough)		In 10 ml.	18
otc	**Aftate for Athlete's Foot** (Schering-Plough)	**Gel:** 1%	In 15 g.	13
otc	**Aftate for Jock Itch** (Schering-Plough)		In 15 g.	13

(Continued on following page)

Antifungal Agents (Cont.)

TOLNAFTATE (Cont.)

	Product	Form	Description	C.I.
otc	**Tolnaftate** (Various)	**Powder:** 1%	In 45 g.	3+
otc	**Absorbine Antifungal** (W.F. Young)		Corn starch, parabens, zinc stearate. In 56.7 g.	NA
otc	**Absorbine Jock Itch** (W.F. Young)		Corn starch, parabens, zinc stearate. In 56.7 g.	NA
otc	**Aftate for Athlete's Foot** (Schering-Plough)		Starch, talc. In 67.5 g.	2
otc	**Aftate for Jock Itch** (Schering-Plough)		Starch, talc. In 45 g.	3.5
otc	**NP • 27** (Thompson Medical)		Cornstarch, talc. In 45 g.	3.2
otc	**Quinsana Plus** (Mennen)		Cornstarch, talc.	1.8
otc	**Tinactin** (Schering-Plough)		Cornstarch, talc. In 45 and 90 g.	4
otc	**Ting** (Fisons)		Cornstarch, talc. In 45 g.	2.5
otc	**Zeasorb-AF** (Stiefel)		Talc. In 70.9 g.	2
otc	**Tolnaftate** (Various)	**Spray Powder:** 1%	In 105 g.	1.5+
otc	**Aftate for Athlete's Foot** (Schering-Plough)		14% alcohol and talc. In 105 g.	1.6
otc	**Aftate for Jock Itch** (Schering-Plough)		36% alcohol. In 105 g.	1.6
otc	**NP • 27** (Thompson Medical)		14.9% alcohol and talc. In 105 g.	1.8
otc	**Tinactin** (Schering-Plough)		14% alcohol and talc. **Deoderant:** In 100 g. **Regular:** In 150 g.	2
otc	**Tinactin for Jock Itch** (Schering-Plough)		14% alcohol and talc. In 100 g.	1.8
otc	**Ting** (Fisons)		14% alcohol and talc. In 90 g.	1.3
otc	**Absorbine Jr. Antifungal** (W.F. Young)	**Spray Liquid:** 1%	Acetone, chloroxylenol, menthol, wormwood oil. In 59.2 and 118.3 ml.	NA
otc	**Aftate for Athlete's Foot** (Schering-Plough)		36% alcohol. In 120 ml.	3.4
otc	**Desenex** (Fisons)		With PEG 400 and 41% SD alcohol 40-B. In 90 ml.	NA
otc	**Tinactin** (Schering-Plough)		36% alcohol. In 120 ml.	1.5
otc	**Ting** (Fisons)		41% alcohol. In 90 ml.	1.3

GENTIAN VIOLET (Methylrosaniline chloride; Crystal Violet)

Actions:

An antibacterial and antifungal dye. It is bactericidal to gram-positive organisms in very high dilutions. It inhibits the growth of *Monilia, Torula, Epidermophyton* and *Trichophyton.* Because of its cosmetic effects and staining of clothing, gentian violet has generally been replaced in practice by other topical agents.

Indications: Topical anti-infective.

Precautions: *For external use only.* Avoid contact with the eyes.

Patient Information:

For external use only. Avoid contact with the eyes.

Gentian violet will stain skin and clothing.

Do not apply to an ulcerative lesion; may result in "tattooing" of the skin.

Administration and Dosage: Apply locally 2 times daily or as directed.

	Product	Form	Description	C.I.*
otc	**Gentian Violet** (Various)	**Solution:** 1%	In 30 ml.	2.5+
		2%	In 30 ml.	3+

* Cost Index based on cost per g or ml.

OXICONAZOLE NITRATE

Actions:

Pharmacology: Oxiconazole nitrate is a broad spectrum antifungal for topical dermatologic use. The fungicidal activity of oxiconazole results primarily from the inhibition of ergosterol synthesis, which is needed for cytoplasmic membrane integrity. It has in vitro activity against a wide range of organisms. Five hours after application of 2.5 mg/cm² of oxiconazole nitrate cream, the concentration of oxiconazole nitrate in the epidermis, upper corium and deeper corium was 16.2, 3.64 and 1.29 mcmols, respectively. Systemic absorption of oxiconazole nitrate appears to be low. Less than 0.3% of the applied dose was recovered in the urine of subjects up to 5 days after application.

Microbiology: In vitro, oxiconazole is active against many strains of clinical isolates of the following dermatophytic organisms: *Trichophyton rubrum* and *T mentagrophytes.*

Oxiconazole is active against the following microorganisms in vitro; however, clinical efficacy has not been established: *Trichophyton tonsurans, T violaceum, Microsporum canis, M audouini, M gypseum, Epidermophyton floccosum, Candida albicans* and *Malassezia furfur.*

Indications:

Topical treatment of the following dermal infections: Tinea pedis (athlete's foot), tinea cruris (jock itch) and tinea corporis (ringworm) due to *T rubrum* and *T mentagrophytes.*

Contraindications:

Hypersensitivity to oxiconazole or any of the components of the product.

Warnings:

Fertility impairment: At doses > 3 mg/kg/day in female rats and 15 mg/kg/day in male rats, the following effects were observed: Reduction in the fertility parameters; reduction in the number of sperm in vaginal smears; extended estrus cycle; decrease in mating frequency.

Pregnancy: Category B. There are no adequate and well controlled studies in pregnant women. Use during pregnancy only if clearly needed.

Lactation: Since oxiconazole is excreted in breast milk, exercise caution when the drug is applied on a nursing woman. Although human data relating concentrations of oxiconazole in milk were not obtained, after SC administration of 5 mg/kg to female rats, the milk:plasma ratio at 1.5 to 12 hours was in the range of 3 to 8.

Precautions:

Sensitivity: If a reaction suggesting sensitivity or chemical irritation should occur with the use of oxiconazole nitrate, discontinue treatment and institute appropriate therapy.

For external use only. Avoid contact with the eyes.

Adverse Reactions:

Itching (1.6%); burning (1.4%); irritation (0.4%); erythema (0.2%); maceration (0.1%); fissuring (0.1%).

Patient Information:

For external use only. Avoid contact with the eyes.

Administration and Dosage:

Apply to cover affected areas once daily (in the evening) in patients with tinea pedis, tinea corporis and tinea cruris. Treat tinea corporis and tinea cruris for 2 weeks and tinea pedis for 1 month to reduce the possibility of recurrence. If a patient shows no clinical improvement after the treatment period, review the diagnosis.

Rx	**Oxistat** (Glaxo)	**Cream:** 1%	White petrolatum. In 15 and 30 g tubes.	39

SULCONAZOLE NITRATE

Actions:

Sulconazole nitrate, a broad spectrum antifungal agent intended for topical application, is an imidazole derivative with antifungal and antiyeast activity. It inhibits the growth of the common pathogenic dermatophytes including *Trichophyton rubrum* (cream only), *T mentagrophytes, Epidermophyton floccosum* and *Microsporum canis.* It also inhibits the organism responsible for tinea versicolor, *(Malassezia furfur), Candida albicans* (cream only) and certain gram-positive bacteria.

A maximization test showed no evidence of irritation or contact sensitization. A modified Draize test showed no allergic contact dermatitis and a phototoxicity study showed no phototoxic or photoallergic reaction to sulconazole nitrate cream.

Indications:

Treatment of tinea pedis (athlete's foot; *cream only),* tinea cruris (jock itch) and tinea corporis (ringworm) caused by *T rubrum, T mentagrophytes, E floccosum* and *M canis;* tinea versicolor.

Solution: Efficacy has not been proven in tinea pedis (athlete's foot).

Contraindications:

Hypersensitivity to any of the components of the product.

Warnings:

Pregnancy: Category C. There are no adequate and well controlled studies in pregnant women. Use during pregnancy only if clearly needed. Sulconazole is embryotoxic in rats when given in doses 125 times the adult human dose. Sulconazole given orally to rats at a dose 125 times the human dose resulted in prolonged gestation and dystocia. Several females died during the perinatal period, most likely due to labor complications.

Lactation: Use with caution in nursing mothers since it is not known if sulconazole appears in breast milk.

Children: Safety and efficacy for use in children have not been established.

Precautions:

For external use only. Avoid contact with the eyes.

If irritation develops, discontinue the solution and institute appropriate therapy.

Adverse Reactions:

Local: Itching, burning, stinging (3%); redness (1%).

Patient Information:

Use only as directed.

For external use only. Avoid contact with the eyes.

Dosage and Administration:

Gently massage a small amount into the affected and surrounding skin areas once or twice daily, except in tinea pedis, where administration should be twice daily.

Early relief of symptoms is experienced by the majority of patients and clinical improvement may be seen fairly soon after treatment is begun. To reduce the possibility of recurrence, treat tinea cruris, tinea corporis and tinea versicolor for 3 weeks and tinea pedis for 4 weeks.

If significant clinical improvement is not seen after 4 to 6 weeks of treatment, consider an alternate diagnosis.

Rx	**Exelderm** (Westwood Squibb)	**Cream:** 1%	In 15, 30 and 60 g tubes.	28
		Solution: 1%	In 30 ml.	29

For information on the vaginal use of nystatin, refer to the individual monograph.

Antifungal Agents (Cont.)

NYSTATIN

Actions:

Pharmacology: An antifungal antibiotic which is both fungistatic and fungicidal in vitro against a wide variety of yeasts and yeast-like fungi. It probably acts by binding to sterols in the cell membrane of the fungus with a resultant change in membrane permeability allowing leakage of intracellular components. It provides specific therapy for all localized forms of candidiasis, and cure is effected both clinically and mycologically in most localized cases. Symptomatic relief is rapid, often occurring within 24 to 72 hours after initiation of treatment.

Indications:

Treatment of cutaneous or mucocutaneous mycotic infections caused by *Candida (Monilia) albicans* and other *Candida* species.

Contraindications:

Hypersensitivity to any component; not for ophthalmic use.

Precautions:

For external use only. Avoid contact with the eyes.

Hypersensitivity: Should a hypersensitivity reaction occur, withdraw drug and take appropriate measures.

Adverse Reactions:

Virtually nontoxic and nonsensitizing; well tolerated by all age groups including debilitated infants, even on prolonged administration. If irritation occurs, discontinue use.

Patient Information:

For external use only. Avoid contact with the eyes.

Apply after cleansing affected area (unless directed otherwise).

If irritation occurs, discontinue use and notify physician.

Administration and Dosage:

Apply to affected areas 2 to 3 times daily, or as indicated, until healing is complete. For fungal infection of the feet caused by *Candida,* dust the powder freely on the feet as well as in shoes and socks. The cream is usually preferred in candidiasis involving intertriginous areas; very moist lesions, however, are best treated with powder.

	Product	Form	Description	C.I.*
Rx	**Nystatin** (Various, eg, Geneva Marsam, Major, NMC, Parmed, Rugby)	**Cream:** 100,000 units per g	In 15 and 30 g.	7+
Rx	**Mycostatin** (Westwood Squibb)		Aqueous vanishing cream base. In 15 and 30 g.	32
Rx	**Nilstat** (Lederle)		Aqueous vanishing cream base. In 15 and 240 g.	22
Rx	**Nystex** (Savage)		Aqueous vanishing cream base. White petrolatum, parabens. In 15 & 30 g.	15
Rx	**Nystatin** (Various, eg, Dixon-Shane, Genetco, Goldline, Major, Moore, NMC, Rugby, Schein, URL)	**Ointment:** 100,000 units per g	In 15 and 30 g.	5+
Rx	**Mycostatin** (Westwood Squibb)		Polyethylene and mineral oil gel base. In 15 and 30 g.	32
Rx	**Nilstat** (Lederle)		Light mineral oil and plastibase 50W. In 15 g.	22
Rx	**Nystex** (Savage)		Polyethylene and mineral oil base. In 15 g.	15
Rx	**Mycostatin** (Westwood Squibb)	**Powder:** 100,000 units per g	Dispersed in talc. In 15 g.	56

* Cost Index based on cost per g.

For information of the systemic use of amphotericin B, refer to the individual monograph in the Anti-infectives section.

Antifungal Agents (Cont.)

AMPHOTERICIN B

Actions:

An antibiotic with antifungal activity produced by a strain of *Streptomyces nodosus*. It exhibits greater in vitro activity than nystatin against *Candida (Monilia) albicans.* Topical amphotericin B was comparable to nystatin in similar formulations.

Although amphotericin B exhibits some in vitro activity against the superficial dermatophytes (ringworm organisms), it has not demonstrated an effectiveness in vivo on topical application.

Indications:

Treatment of cutaneous and mucocutaneous mycotic infections caused by *Candida* sp.

Contraindications:

Hypersensitivity to any of the components.

Precautions:

For external use only. Avoid contact with the eyes.

Hypersensitivity: If a hypersensitivity reaction occurs, discontinue use; initiate appropriate measures.

Adverse Reactions:

These preparations have only a slight sensitizing potential.

Cream: May have a "drying" effect on some skin. Local irritation (erythema, pruritus or a burning sensation) may occur, particularly in intertriginous areas.

Lotion: Rare local intolerance has included increased pruritus with or without other evidence of local irritation or exacerbation of preexisting candidal lesions. Allergic contact dermatitis is rare.

Ointment: May occasionally irritate when applied to moist, intertriginous areas.

Patient Information:

For external use only. Avoid contact with the eyes.

Cleanse affected area(s) of skin prior to application (unless directed otherwise).

Apply liberally to lesions and rub in gently.

The cream may cause drying and slight discoloration of the skin. The lotion and ointment may cause staining of nail lesions, but not skin, if thoroughly rubbed in. Redness, itching or burning may also occur, particularly in skin folds; notify physician if these effects become bothersome, if skin rash develops or if the condition being treated worsens.

Any discoloration of fabrics from the cream or lotion may be removed by hand washing the fabric with soap and warm water. Any fabric discoloration from the ointment may be removed by applying a standard cleaning fluid.

Administration and Dosage:

Apply liberally to candidal lesions 2 to 4 times daily. Therapy duration depends on patient response. Intertriginous lesions usually respond in a few days; treatment may be complete in 1 to 3 weeks. Similarly, candidiasis of the diaper area, perleche and glabrous skin lesions usually clear in 1 to 2 weeks. Interdigital lesions may require 2 to 4 weeks intensive therapy; paronychias also require relatively prolonged therapy, and onychomycoses that respond may require several months or more of treatment. Relapses are frequent in the last 3 conditions.

				C.I.*
Rx	**Fungizone** (Bristol-Myers Squibb)	**Cream:** 3%	In an aqueous vehicle. In 20 g.	44
		Lotion: 3%	In an aqueous vehicle. In 30 ml.	40
		Ointment: 3%	In a polyethylene and mineral oil gel base with titanium dioxide. In 20 g.	44

* Cost Index based on cost per g or ml.

For information on the systemic use of ketoconazole, refer to the individual monograph in the Anti-infectives section.

Antifungal Agents (Cont.)

KETOCONAZOLE

Actions:

Pharmacology: Ketoconazole is a broad spectrum antifungal agent. In vitro studies suggest it impairs ergosterol synthesis, which is a vital component of fungal cell membranes. The therapeutic effect in seborrheic dermatitis and dandruff may be due to reduction of *Pityrosporum ovale (Malassezia ovale).*

Pharmacokinetics: In animal and human studies, there were no detectable plasma levels following the use of the shampoo.

Clinical trials (shampoo): In a 4 week, double-blind, placebo controlled trial, the decrease in *P ovale* on the scalp was significantly greater with ketoconazole shampoo than with placebo and was comparable to selenium sulfide. Ketoconazole and selenium sulfide reduced the severity of adherent dandruff significantly more than placebo.

Microbiology: Ketoconazole inhibits the growth of the following common dermatophytes and yeasts by altering the permeability of the cell membrane. Dermatophytes: *Trichophyton rubrum, T mentagrophytes, T tonsurans, Microsporum canis, M audouini, M gypseum* and *Epidermophyton floccosum.* Yeasts: *Candida albicans, C tropicalis, P ovale (M ovale);* and *P orbiculare (M furfur,* the organism responsible for tinea versicolor). Development of resistance to the drug has not been reported.

Indications:

Cream: Tinea corporis (ringworm) and tinea cruris (jock itch) caused by *Trichophyton rubrum, T mentagrophytes** and *E floccosum*; tinea (pityriasis) versicolor caused by *P orbiculare (M furfur);* cutaneous candidiasis caused by *Candida* sp; seborrheic dermatitis.

Shampoo: Reduction of scaling due to dandruff.

Contraindications:

Hypersensitivity to any component of the product.

Warnings:

Pregnancy: Category C. There are no adequate and well controlled studies in pregnant women. Use during pregnancy only if the potential benefits outweigh the potential hazards to the fetus.

Lactation: Safety for use in the nursing mother has not been established; however, exercise caution when applying on a nursing woman.

Children: Safety and efficacy in children have not been established.

Precautions:

For external use only. Avoid contact with the eyes.

Sensitivity: Discontinue if sensitivity or chemical irritation occurs.

Sulfite sensitivity: The cream contains sulfites that may cause allergic-type reactions including anaphylactic symptoms and life-threatening or less severe asthmatic episodes in certain susceptible persons. The overall prevalence of sulfite sensitivity in the general population is unknown and probably low. It is seen more frequently in asthmatic or atopic nonasthmatic persons.

Adverse Reactions:

Cream: Severe irritation, pruritus, stinging ($\approx$ 5%); painful allergic reaction (one patient).

Shampoo: Increase in normal hair loss, irritation ($<$ 1%); abnormal hair texture; scalp pustules; mild dryness of skin; itching; oiliness/dryness of hair and scalp.

Overdosage:

Shampoo: In the event of ingestion, employ supportive measures, including gastric lavage with sodium bicarbonate. Refer to General Management of Acute Overdosage.

Patient Information:

For external use only. Avoid contact with the eyes.

Shampoo: Removal of the curl from permanently waved hair may occur.

* Efficacy for this organism in this organ system was studied in fewer than ten infections.

(Continued on following page)

KETOCONAZOLE (Cont.)

Administration and Dosage:

Cream:

Cutaneous candidiasis, tinea corporis, tinea cruris and *tinea (pityriasis) versicolor* – Apply once daily to cover the affected and immediate surrounding area. Clinical improvement may be seen fairly soon after treatment is begun; however, treat candidal infections and tinea cruris and corporis for 2 weeks in order to reduce the possibility of recurrence. Patients with tinea versicolor usually require 2 weeks of treatment.

Seborrheic dermatitis – Apply to the affected area twice daily for 4 weeks or until clinical clearing.

If a patient shows no clinical improvement after the treatment period, redetermine the diagnosis.

Shampoo: Dandruff – Moisten hair and scalp thoroughly with water. Apply sufficient shampoo to produce enough lather to wash scalp and hair and gently massage it over the entire scalp area for ≈ 1 minute. Rinse hair thoroughly with warm water. Repeat, leaving shampoo on scalp for an additional 3 minutes. After the second thorough rinse, dry hair with towel or warm air flow.

Shampoo twice a week for 4 weeks with at least 3 days between each shampooing, and then intermittently as needed to maintain control.

Storage: Do not store above room temperature (25°C; 77°F); protect from light.

				C.I.*
Rx	**Nizoral** (Janssen)	**Cream:** 2% in an aqueous vehicle[1]	In 15, 30 and 60 g.	37
		Shampoo: 2% in an aqueous suspension	In 120 ml.	6

HALOPROGIN

Actions:

A synthetic antifungal agent for treatment of superficial fungal infections of the skin.

Indications:

Treatment of tinea pedis (athlete's foot), tinea cruris (jock itch), tinea corporis (ringworm) and tinea manuum due to *Trichophyton rubrum, T tonsurans, T mentagrophytes, Microsporum canis* and *Epidermophyton floccosum.* Also useful in the topical treatment of tinea versicolor due to *Malassezia furfur*.

Contraindications:

Hypersensitivity to any of the components.

Warnings:

Pregnancy: Category B. There are no adequate and well controlled studies in pregnant women. Use only when clearly needed.

Lactation: It is not known whether this drug is excreted in breast milk. Exercise caution when applying on a nursing woman.

Children: Safety and efficacy for use in children have not been established.

Precautions:

Sensitization or irritation: Discontinue treatment and institute appropriate therapy.

Reevaluate the diagnosis if no improvement occurs after 4 weeks of treatment. In mixed infections where bacteria or nonsusceptible fungi are present, supplementary systemic anti-infective therapy may be indicated.

For external use only. Keep out of eyes.

Adverse Reactions:

Local irritation; burning sensation; vesicle formation; erythema; scaling; itching; folliculitis; pruritus.

Patient Information:

For external use only. Avoid contact with eyes.

If condition worsens, or if irritation, redness, swelling, stinging or burning persists, discontinue use and notify physician.

Complete full course of therapy.

Administration and Dosage:

Apply liberally to the affected area twice daily for 2 to 3 weeks. Intertriginous lesions may require up to 4 weeks of therapy.

				C.I.*
Rx	**Halotex** (Westwood Squibb)	**Cream:** 1% in a water dispersible base	In 15 and 30 g.	33
		Solution: 1% with 75% alcohol	In 10 and 30 ml.	46

* Cost Index based on cost per ml or g.

[1] With sodium sulfite.

NAFTIFINE HCl

Actions:

Pharmacology: Naftifine, a broad spectrum antifungal agent, is a synthetic allylamine derivative. Although the exact mechanism of action against fungi is not known, naftifine appears to interfere with sterol biosynthesis by inhibiting the enzyme squalene 2,3-epoxidase. This inhibition of enzyme activity results in decreased amounts of sterols, especially ergosterol, and a corresponding accumulation of squalene in the cells.

Microbiology: Naftifine exhibits fungicidal activity in vitro against a broad spectrum of organisms including *Trichophyton rubrum, T mentagrophytes, T tonsurans, Epidermophyton floccosum, Microsporum canis, M audouini* and *M gypseum,* and fungistatic activity against *Candida* sp, including *C albicans.*

Pharmacokinetics: Naftifine penetrates the stratum corneum to inhibit the growth of dermatophytes. Following a single topical application of 1% naftifine to the skin of healthy subjects, systemic absorption was ≈ 6% (cream) and ≤ 4.2% (gel). Naftifine or its metabolites are excreted via the urine and feces with a half-life of ≈ 2 to 3 days.

Indications:

Topical treatment of tinea pedis (athlete's foot), tinea cruris (jock itch) and tinea corporis (ringworm) caused by the organisms *T rubrum, T mentagrophytes, T tonsurans*† and *E floccosum*.

Contraindications:

Hypersensitivity to naftifine or any component of the product.

Warnings:

Pregnancy: Category B. There are no adequate studies in pregnant women. Use only when clearly needed and when potential benefits outweigh potential hazards to the fetus.

Lactation: It is not known whether naftifine is excreted in breast milk. Exercise caution when applying on a nursing woman.

Children: Safety and efficacy for use in children have not been established.

Precautions:

For external use only. Avoid contact with the eyes.

If irritation or sensitivity develops, discontinue treatment and institute appropriate therapy.

Adverse Reactions:

Local: Cream – Burning/stinging (6%); dryness (3%); erythema, itching, local irritation (2%).
Gel – Burning/stinging (5%); itching (1%); erythema, rash, tenderness (0.5%).

Patient Information:

Avoid the use of occlusive dressings or wrappings unless otherwise directed by the physician.

For external use only. Keep away from the eyes, nose, mouth and other mucous membranes.

Administration and Dosage:

Gently massage a sufficient quantity into the affected area and surrounding skin once a day with the cream, twice a day (morning and evening) with the gel. Wash hands after application.

If no clinical improvement is seen after 4 weeks of treatment, re-evaluate the patient.

				C.I.*
Rx	**Naftin** (Herbert)	**Cream:** 1%	In 15, 30 and 60 g.	28
		Gel: 1%	In 20, 40 and 60 g.	32

* Cost Index based on cost per g.
† Gel; efficacy studied in < 10 infections.

Antifungal Combinations

The principal active components of these formulations include:

Antifungal agents:

UNDECYLENIC ACID (see individual monograph), *SODIUM PROPIONATE, BENZOIC ACID, SODIUM THIOSULFATE.*

Other components include:

SALICYLIC ACID for its topical keratolytic action (see individual monograph).

BORIC ACID as an astringent and antiseptic.

CHLOROXYLENOL as an antiseptic.

BENZOCAINE as an anesthetic (see individual monograph.)

MENTHOL and *PHENOL* for their antipruritic, anesthetic and antiseptic effects.

RESORCINOL as an antipruritic and antiseptic.

CHLOROPHYLL DERIVATIVES to promote healing, although there is no evidence to support this effect. These agents do have a deodorant action.

BASIC FUCHSIN for its antifungal and antibacterial activity.

Note: The choice of vehicle is important for these products. Ointments, creams and liquids are used as primary therapy. In general, powders are used as adjunctive therapy, but they may be acceptable as primary therapy in very mild conditions.

				C.I.*
otc	**Prophyllin** (Rystan)	**Ointment:** 5% sodium propionate and 0.0125% chlorophyllin derivatives	In 30 g.	4.9
otc	**Dermasept Antifungal** (Pharmakon)	**Liquid:** 6.098% tannic acid, 5.081% zinc Cl, 2.032% benzocaine, 3.049% methylbenzethonium HCl, 1.017% tolnaftate, 5.081% undecylenic acid, 58.539% ethanol 38B, phenol, benzyl alcohol, benzoic acid, coal tar, camphor, menthol	In 30 ml bottle w/spray dispenser.	3.6
otc	**Prophyllin** (Rystan)	**Powder:** Packet or tsp bulk powder in 240 ml water makes a solution containing 1% sodium propionate and 0.0025% water soluble chlorophyllin	In 120 g and 2.3 g packets (12s).	68
Rx	**Gordochom** (Gordon)	**Solution:** 25% undecylenic acid, 3% chloroxylenol in an oil base	In 6 ml, 30 ml bottles w/applicator and pints.	8.2
otc	**Steri Nail** (Dr. Nordyke's Labs)	**Solution:** Undecylenic acid tolnaftate, propylene glycol, acetone, acetic acid, pripionic acid, benzyl alcohol, eucalyptol and benzyl acetate	In 3 step kit with SteriScrub and SteriBrush.	NA
otc	**Blis-To-Sol** (Chattem)	**Liquid:** Undecylenic acid, salicylic acid	In 30 and 55.5 ml.	2.6
otc	**Antinea** (American Dermal)	**Cream:** 6% benzoic acid, 3% salicylic acid	In 28.35 g.	6.3

* Cost Index based on cost per g or ml.

(Continued on following page)

Antifungal Combinations (Cont.)

	Product	Contents	Availability	C.I.*
otc	**Whitfield's** (Various, eg, Dixon-Shane, Fougera, Goldline, Lannett, Lilly, Moore, NMC, Rugby, Schein, URL)	**Ointment:** 6% benzoic acid and 3% salicylic acid	In 30 g and 1 lb.	1.8+
otc	**Blis-To-Sol** (Chattem)	**Powder:** Benzoic acid, salicylic acid	In 60 g.	1.6
Rx	**Tinver** (Sola/Barnes-Hind)	**Lotion:** 25% sodium thiosulfate, 1% salicylic acid, 10% isopropyl alcohol, menthol, propylene glycol, EDTA and colloidal alumina	In 120 and 180 ml.	6
Rx	**Castellani Paint** (Pedinol)	**Liquid:** Basic fuchsin, phenol, resorcinol and acetone.	In 30 and 480 ml.	6.7
		Also available as a colorless solution with alcohol and without basic fuchsin.	In 30 and 480 ml.	6.7
otc	**Castel Minus** (Syosset)	**Liquid:** Resorcinol, acetone, 0.0001% basic fuchsin, hydroxyethylcelluose and 11.5% alcohol	In 29.57 ml.	5.9
otc	**Castel Plus** (Syosset)	**Liquid:** Resorcinol, acetone, 0.3% basic fuchsin, hydroxyethylcellulose and 11.5% alcohol	In 29.57 ml.	5.9
otc	**Fungi-Nail** (Kramer)	**Liquid:** 1% resorcinol, 2% salicylic acid, 2% chloroxylenol, 0.5% benzocaine, 50% isopropyl alcohol	In 30 ml.	17
otc	**Castaderm** (Lannett)	**Liquid:** Resorcinol, boric acid, acetone, basic fuchsin, phenol and 9% alcohol	In 30, 120 and 480 ml.	1.8
otc	**Neo-Castaderm** (Lannett)	**Liquid:** Resorcinol, boric acid, acetone, sodium bisulfite, phenol and alcohol	In 30, 120 and 480 ml.	1.5

* Cost Index based on cost per g or ml.

The following section discusses the various agents used as scabicides and pediculicides. Malathion is used only as a pediculicide; crotamiton is used only as a scabicide; permethrin and lindane are both scabicides and pediculicides. Pyrethrins, available only in combination with piperonyl butoxide, are used only as a pediculicide; piperonyl butoxide is used as a synergist for the pyrethrins.

Malathion acts via cholinesterase inhibition. In contrast, lindane and pyrethrins are nervous system stimulants and permethrin disrupts neuronal repolarization and causes paralysis.

These agents differ in kill time, ovicidal and residual activity. This information is summarized in the table below. Crotamiton is not included since it is not a pediculicide.

Activity of Various Pediculicides

Pediculicide	Kill time (min)	Ovicidal activity	Residual activity	Application time
Lindane	190	45% to 70%	none	4 minutes
Malathion	4.4	95%	up to 4 weeks	8 to 12 hours
Permethrin	10 to 15	70% to 80%	up to 10 days	10 minutes
Pyrethrins and piperonyl butoxide[1]	10.5 to 18.6	≈ 75%	none	10 minutes

[1] Products used for data included *A-200 Pyrinate* and *R & C*.

LINDANE (Gamma Benzene Hexachloride)

Actions:

An ectoparasiticide and ovicide.

Indications:

Treatment of *Pediculus capitis* (head lice) and *Pediculus pubis* (crab lice) and their ova. The cream and lotion forms are also indicated for *Sarcoptes scabiei* (scabies).

Contraindications:

Premature neonates, because their skin may be more permeable than that of full-term infants and their liver enzymes may not be sufficiently developed; patients with known seizure disorders; hypersensitivity to lindane or any component of the products.

Warnings:

Absorption: Simultaneous application of creams, ointments or oils may enhance absorption.

Carcinogenesis: In mice, 600 ppm of lindane was associated with a significant increase in the incidence of hepatomas. Although other derivatives of hexachlorocyclohexane have demonstrated carcinogenicity, lindane has not.

Pregnancy: Category B. There are no adequate and well controlled studies in pregnant women. Do not exceed the recommended dosage; treat no more than twice during a pregnancy.

Lactation: Lindane is secreted in breast milk in low concentrations. The levels of lindane found in blood after topical application make it unlikely that amounts of lindane sufficient to cause serious adverse reactions will be excreted in the milk of nursing mothers. If there is any concern, use an alternate method of feeding for 2 days.

Children: Lindane penetrates human skin and has the potential for CNS toxicity. Studies indicate that potential toxic effects of topically applied lindane are greater in the young. Seizures have occurred after excessive use or ingestion of lindane. No residual effects have been demonstrated; do not use prophylactically.

Precautions:

For external use only. Avoid contact with eyes; if this occurs, immediately flush eyes with water.

Irritation or sensitization: Consult physician.

Oils may enhance absorption. If an oil-based hair dressing is used, shampoo, rinse and dry hair before applying lindane shampoo.

Adverse Reactions:

Adverse reactions occur in $< 0.001\%$ of patients.

CNS: Stimulation ranging from dizziness to convulsions. Cases of convulsions have been reported, although these incidents were almost always associated with accidental oral ingestion or misuse of the product.

Dermatologic: Eczematous eruptions due to irritation.

(Continued on following page)

LINDANE (Gamma Benzene Hexachloride) (Cont.)

Overdosage:

Symptoms: Overdosage or oral ingestion can cause CNS excitation and, if taken in sufficient quantities, seizures may occur. A blood level of 290 ng/ml was associated with convulsions following the accidental ingestion of a lindane-containing product. Analysis of blood taken from subjects before and after the lindane shampoo showed a mean peak blood level of only 3 ng/ml at 6 hours which disappeared 2 hours later.

Treatment: If accidental ingestion occurs, institute prompt gastric emptying. However, since oils favor absorption, give saline cathartics for intestinal evacuation rather than oil laxatives. If CNS manifestations occur, administer pentobarbital, phenobarbital or diazepam. Refer to General Management of Acute Overdosage.

Patient Information:

Patient instructions and information are available with product. Do not exceed prescribed dosage.

For external use only (oral ingestion can lead to serious CNS toxicity). Do not apply to face. Avoid getting in eyes; if there is contact, flush well with water for several minutes. Avoid unnecessary skin contact or contact with mucous membrnes (eg, nose, mouth). Wear rubber gloves, particularly when applying lindane to more than one person.

Notify physician if condition worsens or if itching, redness, swelling, burning or skin rash occurs.

Avoid use on open cuts and extensive excoriations.

Treat sexual contacts simultaneously.

Administration and Dosage:

Cream and lotion: Scabies – Apply a thin layer to dry skin and rub in thoroughly. If crusted lesions are present, a tepid bath preceding the medication is helpful. Allow the skin to dry before application. Usually 2 oz are sufficient for an adult. Make total body application from the neck down. Scabies rarely affects the head of children or adults, but may occur in infants. Leave on 8 to 12 hours; remove by thorough washing. One application is usually curative. Many patients exhibit persistent pruritus after treatment; this does not indicate reapplication unless living mites can be demonstrated.

Lotion: Pediculosis pubis – Apply a sufficient quantity only to thinly cover the hair and skin of the pubic area and, if infested, the thighs, trunk and axillary regions. Rub into the skin and hair, leave in place for 12 hours, then wash thoroughly. Reapplication is usually unnecessary unless there are demonstrable living lice after 7 days. Treat sexual contacts concurrently.

Pediculosis capitis – Apply a sufficient quantity to cover only the affected and adjacent hairy areas. Rub into scalp and hair and leave in place for 12 hours; follow by thorough washing. Reapplication is usually not necessary unless there are demonstrable living lice after 7 days.

Shampoo: Pediculosis capitis and pubis – Apply a sufficient quantity to dry hair (1 oz for short, 1½ oz for medium and 2 oz for long hair). Work thoroughly into the hair and allow to remain in place 4 minutes. Add small quantities of water until a good lather forms. Rinse hair thoroughly and towel briskly. Comb with a fine toothed comb or use tweezers to remove any remaining nits or nit shells.

Pediculosis pubis – Reapplication is usually not necessary. Reapply if there are demonstrable living lice after 7 days. Treat sexual contacts concurrently.

Do not use as a routine shampoo.

				C.I.*
Rx	**Kwell** (Reed & Carnrick)	**Cream:** 1%	In 60 g.	3.3
Rx	**Lindane** (Various, eg, Barre-National, Dixon-Shane, Geneva Marsam, Major, Moore, Parmed, PBI, Rugby, Schein, URL)	**Lotion:** 1%	In 30 and 60 ml, pt and gal.	1+
Rx	**G-well** (Goldline)		In 60 and 480 ml.	1.3
Rx	**Kwell** (Reed & Carnrick)		In 59 and 473 ml and 3.8 L.	3
Rx	**Scabene** (Stiefel)		In 59 and 480 ml.	1.3
Rx	**Lindane** (Various, eg, Barre-National, Dixon-Shane, Geneva Marsam, Major, Moore, Parmed, PBI, Rugby, Schein, URL)	**Shampoo:** 1%	In 30 and 60 ml, pt and gal.	1+
Rx	**G-well** (Goldline)		In 60 ml, pt and gal.	1.3
Rx	**Kwell** (Reed & Carnrick)		In 59 and 473 ml and 3.8 L.	2.8
Rx	**Scabene** (Stiefel)		In 59 and 480 ml.	1.3

* Cost Index based on cost per g or ml.

PERMETHRIN

Actions:

Pharmacology: Permethrin is a synthetic pyrethroid, active against lice, ticks, mites and fleas. It acts on the parasites' nerve cell membranes to disrupt the sodium channel current, resulting in delayed repolarization and paralysis of the pests.

In vitro data indicate permethrin has pediculicidal and ovicidal activity against *Pediculus humanus* var. *capitis.* The high cure rate (97% to 99%) in patients with head lice demonstrated at 14 days following a single application is attributable to a combination of its pediculicidal and ovicidal activities and its residual persistence on the hair which may also prevent reinfestation.

Pharmacokinetics: Permethrin is rapidly metabolized by ester hydrolysis to inactive metabolites which are excreted primarily in the urine. Although the amount of permethrin absorbed after a single application of the 5% cream has not been determined precisely, preliminary data suggest it is < 2% of the amount applied. Residual persistence is detectable on the hair for at least 10 days following a single application.

Indications:

Cream: For the single-application treatment of *Sarcoptes scabiei* (scabies).

Liquid: For the single-application treatment of infestation with *Pediculus humanus* var. *capitis* (the head louse) and its nits (eggs). Treatment for recurrences is required in < 1% of patients since the ovicidal activity may be supplemented by residual persistence in the hair. If live lice are observed ≥ 7 days following the initial application, give a second application.

Contraindications:

Hypersensitivity to any synthetic pyrethroid or pyrethrin, to chrysanthemums or to any component of the product. If hypersensitivity develops, discontinue use.

Warnings:

Carcinogenesis: Species-specific increases in pulmonary adenomas, a common benign tumor of mice, were seen in the mouse studies. In one study, incidence of pulmonary alveolar-cell carcinomas and benign liver adenomas increased only in female mice when permethrin was given in their food at a concentration of 5000 ppm.

Pregnancy: Category B. There are no adequate and well controlled studies in pregnant women. Use during pregnancy only if clearly needed.

Lactation: It is not known whether this drug is excreted in breast milk. Because of the evidence for tumorigenic potential of permethrin in animal studies, consider discontinuing nursing temporarily or withholding the drug while the mother is nursing.

Children: Safety and efficacy for use in children < 2 months of age or < 2 years (liquid) have not been established.

Precautions:

For external use only.

Pruritus, erythema and edema often accompany scabies and head lice infestation. Treatment with permethrin may temporarily exacerbate these conditions.

Adverse Reactions:

The most frequent adverse reaction is pruritus. Usually a consequence of scabies or head lice infestation itself, it may be temporarily aggravated following treatment.

Cream: Mild transient burning/stinging (10%); mild temporary itching (7%); tingling, numbness, mild transient erythema, edema or rash (≤ 2%).

Liquid: Mild temporary itching (5.9%); mild transient burning/stinging, tingling, numbness, discomfort (3.4%); mild transient erythema, edema or rash (2.1%).

Overdosage:

If ingested, perform gastric lavage and employ general supportive measures.

Patient Information:

For external use only. Avoid contact with the mucous membranes (eg, nose, mouth).

Itching, redness or swelling of the scalp may occur; notify physician if irritation persists.

Elimite: May be very mildly irritating to the eyes. Avoid contact with the eyes; flush with water immediately if eye contact with the drug occurs.

Patient instructions and information are available with the product. Do not exceed the prescribed dosage.

(Continued on following page)

PERMETHRIN (Cont.)

Administration and Dosage:

Sarcoptes scabiei – Thoroughly massage into the skin from the head to the soles of the feet. Treat infants on the hairline, neck, scalp, temple and forehead. Remove the cream by washing after 8 to 14 hours. Usually 30 g is sufficient for the average adult. One application is curative.

Pediculus capitis – Use after the hair has been washed with shampoo, rinsed with water and towel dried. Apply a sufficient volume to saturate the hair and scalp. Allow to remain on the hair for 10 minutes before rinsing off with water.

A single treatment eliminates head lice infestation. Combing of nits is not required for therapeutic efficacy, but may be done for cosmetic reasons.

				C.I.*
Rx	**Elimite** (Herbert)	**Cream:** 5%	In 60 g tubes.	5.5
otc	**Nix** (Burroughs Wellcome)	**Liquid (creme rinse):** 1%[1]	In 60 ml with comb.	2.8

[1] With 20% isopropyl alcohol, 0.2% imidazolidinyl urea, parabens.

CROTAMITON

Actions:

Scabicidal and antipruritic; the mechanisms of action are not known.

Indications:

Eradication of scabies *(Sarcoptes scabiei)* and symptomatic treatment of pruritic skin.

Contraindications:

Do not administer to patients who develop a sensitivity to or are allergic to crotamiton or who manifest a primary irritation response.

Warnings:

For external use only. Do not apply to acutely inflamed skin, raw weeping surfaces, eyes or mouth. Defer use until acute inflammation has subsided.

Irritation/sensitization: If severe irritation or sensitization develops, discontinue use.

Pregnancy: Category C. It is not known whether crotamiton can cause fetal harm when applied topically to a pregnant woman or if it can affect reproduction capacity. Use on a pregnant woman only if clearly needed.

Children: Safety and efficacy for use in children have not been established.

Adverse Reactions:

Allergic sensitivity or primary irritation reactions may occur.

Patient Information:

Patient instructions available with product.

Shake well before using.

Patients with scabies should take a routine bath or shower.

Change clothing and bed linen the next day. Contaminated clothing and bed linen may be dry cleaned or washed in the hot cycle of the washing machine.

For external use only. Keep away from the eyes and mucous membranes (eg, nose, mouth); do not apply to inflamed skin.

Discontinue use and notify physician if irritation or sensitization occurs.

Overdosage:

Signs and symptoms of ingestion include burning sensation in mouth, irritation of the buccal, esophageal and gastric mucosa, nausea, vomiting and abdominal pain.

Treatment: There is no specific antidote. General measures to eliminate the drug and reduce its absorption, combined with symptomatic treatment, are recommended. Refer to General Management of Acute Overdosage.

Administration and Dosage:

Scabies: Thoroughly massage into the skin of the whole body from the chin down, paying particular attention to all folds and creases. A second application is advisable 24 hours later. Change clothing and bed linen the next morning. Take a cleansing bath 48 hours after the last application.

Pruritus: Massage gently into affected areas until medication is completely absorbed. Repeat as necessary.

				C.I.*
Rx	**Eurax** (Westwood Squibb)	**Cream:** 10% in a vanishing base	In 60 g.	3
		Lotion: 10% in an emollient base	In 60 and 454 ml.	3.3

* Cost Index based on cost per g.

MALATHION

Actions:

Pharmacology: Malathion is an organophosphate pediculicide liquid for topical application to the hair and scalp. Malathion acts via cholinesterase inhibition and exerts both lousicidal and ovicidal actions in vitro. This activity is selective to insects because malathion is rapidly hydrolyzed and detoxified in mammals.

When in contact with the hair, malathion slowly bonds to the hair shaft via bonding between its own sulfur atoms and the sulfur in structural amino cids of the hair. This can give a residual protective effect against reinfestation. This chemical reaction is slow. No useful protection is sufficiently developed before about 6 hours of continuous exposure and the effect takes about 12 hours to maximize.

Pharmacokinetics: Malathion in an acetone vehicle is absorbed through human skin only to the extent of 8% of the applied dose. However, percutaneous absorption from the *Ovide* lotion formulation has not been studied and the parameters of distribution and excretion after absorption are not known.

Indications:

Treatment of head lice and their ova.

Contraindications:

Sensitivity to malathion or any components of the product.

Warnings:

Pregnancy: Category B. Use during pregnancy only if clearly needed.

Lactation: It is not known whether malathion is excreted in breast milk. However, because malathion is systemically absorbed, exercise caution when using on a nursing mother.

Children: The majority of the subjects participating in clinical trials with malathion lotions ranged from 2 to 11 years of age; no pediatric-related problems have been documented to date. Safety and efficacy in children < 2 years of age have not been established.

Precautions:

Contains flammable alcohol. The lotion and wet hair should not be exposed to open flame or electric heat, including hair dryers. Do not smoke while applying lotion, or while hair is wet. Allow hair to dry naturally and uncovered after application.

For external use only. Avoid contact with the eyes; if accidentally placed in the eye, flush immediately with water.

Systemic toxicity: Although topical malathion used in recommended dosage has not been reported to cause systemic toxicity, the remote possibility exists. Daily application of 10% malathion dust to adult human skin for 3 weeks produces little or no inhibition of blood cholinesterase.

Carbamate or organophosphate-type insecticides or pesticides: Exposure of patients using malathion to these preparations may increase the possibility of systemic effects due to absorption of the insecticide or pesticide through the respiratory tract or skin; advise patients to protect themselves from contact with such insecticides or pesticides during therapy with malathion.

Drug Interactions:

No drug interactions have been reported with the use of malathion lotion. However, since malathion inhibits cholinesterase, interaction with the following medications could theoretically occur if percutaneous absorption of malathion was unexpectedly large.

Aminoglycosides, parenteral: Additive respiratory depression because of the neuromuscular blocking action of the parenteral aminoglycosides may occur.

Anesthetics, local (ester-derivative): Inhibition of the metabolism of ester-derivative local anesthetics, including those topically applied and absorbed in significant amounts, leading to increased risk of systemic toxicity.

Antimyasthenics or cholinesterase inhibitors (including ophthalmic agents): Additive toxicity may result.

Edrophonium: Caution is recommended in administering edrophonium to patients with myasthenic weakness who are also using topical malathion, since symptoms of cholinergic crisis (overdosage) may be similar to symptoms occurring with myasthenic crisis (underdosage) and the patient's condition may be worsened by use of edrophonium.

Succinylcholine: Plasma concentrations or activity of pseudocholinesterase, the enzyme that metabolizes succinylcholine, may be decreased, thereby enhancing the neuromuscular blockade of succinylcholine.

Adverse Reactions:

Irritation of the scalp has occurred.

(Continued on following page)

MALATHION (Cont.)

Overdosage:

Oral:

Symptoms – Malathion, although a weaker cholinesterase inhibitor and therefore safer than other organophosphates, may be expected to exhibit the same symptoms of cholinesterase depletion after accidental ingestion orally. The symptoms of systemic toxicity may be delayed for up to 12 hours and can include: Abdominal cramps; anxiety; unsteadiness; confusion; diarrhea; labored breathing; dizziness; drowsiness; increased sweating; watery eyes; muscle twitching; pinpoint pupils; seizures; slow heartbeat.

Treatment – Induce vomiting promptly or lavage the stomach with 5% sodium bicarbonate solution.

Severe respiratory distress is the major and most serious symptom of organophosphate poisoning requiring artificial respiration and large doses of IM or IV atropine. The usual starting dose of atropine is 1 to 4 mg with supplementation hourly as needed to counteract the symptoms of cholinesterase depletion. Repeat analyses of serum and RBC cholinesterase assist in establishing the diagnosis and formulating a long-range prognosis.

IV pralidoxime chloride may be used to reverse muscle paralysis. It appears to be most effective if administered within a few hours after poisoning occurs; it is usually not effective if initially administered after 48 hours have elapsed.

A short-acting barbiturate may be given to control seizures.

Give consideration, as a part of the treatment program, to the high concentration of isopropyl alcohol in the vehicle.

Observe the patient for signs of deterioration due to delayed absorption.

Patient Information:

For external use only (serious toxicity may occur if ingested). Avoid contact with the eyes.

Administration and Dosage:

1) Sprinkle lotion on *dry* hair and rub gently until the scalp is thoroughly moistened. Pay special attention to the back of the head and neck.
2) Allow to dry naturally; use no heat and leave uncovered.
3) After 8 to 12 hours, wash the hair with a nonmedicated shampoo.
4) Rinse and use a fine toothed comb to remove dead lice and eggs.
5) If required, repeat with second application in 7 to 9 days.

Further treatment is generally not necessary. Evaluate other family members to determine if infested; if so, treat.

Rx	**Ovide** (GenDerm)	**Lotion:** 0.5%[1]	In 59 ml.

[1] In a vehicle of 78% isopropyl alcohol, terpineol, dipentene and pine needle oil.

NIT REMOVAL SYSTEM

Actions:

Appears to loosen the bond which continues to hold both live and dead lice eggs to the hair shaft after pediculicide treatment. Surviving nits can cause reinfestation if not removed. Does not kill head lice or lice eggs.

Indications:

For use following a pediculicide to aid in cleansing lice eggs from the hair shaft.

Patient Information:

For external use only. Avoid contact with the eyes, eyelashes and eyebrows.

Administration:

Shake well before using. Protect eyes with a dry towel. Apply to wet hair after rinsing out the pediculicide. Apply enough to saturate each hair shaft and cover the entire scalp, making sure to cover the area around the ears and back of the neck. Do not apply to eyelashes or eyebrows.

Allow to remain on the hair for approximately 10 minutes. Rinse with lukewarm water and dry with a hair dryer. Avoid contact with eyes.

otc	**Step 2** (GenDerm)	**Creme rinse:** Benzyl alcohol, cetyl alcohol, 8% formic acid, glyceryl stearate, PEG-100 stearate, polyquaternium-10	In 60 ml.

Indications:
Treatment of infestations of head lice, body lice and pubic (crab) lice and their eggs.

Contraindications: Hypersensitivity to ingredients; ragweed sensitized persons.

Precautions:
For external use only; harmful if swallowed or inhaled. May be irritating to the eyes and mucous membranes. In case of contact with eyes, flush with water. Discontinue use and notify physician if irritation or infection occurs.

To prevent reinfestation, sterilize or treat all clothing and bedding concurrently.

Administration and Dosage:
Apply undiluted to infested areas. Allow application to remain no longer than 10 minutes; then wash thoroughly with warm water and soap or shampoo. Dead lice and eggs may be removed with a fine comb. Do not exceed two consecutive applications within 24 hours.

Dosage varies. Refer to individual package inserts for information.

	Product	Formulation	Package	C.I.*
Rx	**Ovide** (GenDerm)	**Lotion:** 0.5% malathion in a vehicle of 78% isopropyl alcohol, terpineol, dipentene, pine needle oil	In 59 ml.	NA
otc	**A-200 Pyrinate** (Beecham)	**Gel:** 0.33% pyrethrins, 4% piperonyl butoxide technical, petroleum distillate	In 30 g.	6.1
otc	**Blue** (Various, eg, Balan, Moore)	**Gel:** 0.3% pyrethrins, 3% piperonyl butoxide technical, 1.2% petroleum distillate	In 30 and 480 g.	2+
otc	**Tisit Blue** (Pfeiffer)		In 30 g.	4.8
otc	**Pyrinyl** (Various, eg, Balan, Veratex)	**Liquid:** 0.2% pyrethrins, 2% piperonyl butoxide technical and 0.8% deodorized kerosene	In 60 and 120 ml.	1.1+
otc	**Barc** (Commerce Drug)	**Liquid:** 0.18% pyrethrins, 2.2% piperonyl butoxide technical, 5.52% petroleum distillate	In 60 ml.	2.7
otc	**Licetrol 400** (Republic)	**Liquid:** 0.2% pyrethrins, 2% piperonyl butoxide technical, 0.8% petroleum distillate	In 60 and 120 ml.	1
otc	**RID** (Leeming)	**Liquid:** 0.3% pyrethrins, 3% piperonyl butoxide technical, 1.2% petroleum distillate, 2.4% benzyl alcohol	In 60, 120 & 240 ml.	3.1
otc	**Triple X Kit** (Carter Products)		W/shampoo and comb.	NA
otc	**End Lice** (Thompson)	**Liquid:** 0.3% pyrethrins, 2% piperonyl butoxide technical	With 2 nit combs. In 177 ml.	NA
otc	**Tisit** (Pfeiffer)		In 60 and 118 ml.	1.7
otc	**Pyrinol II** (Barre)	**Liquid:** 0.3% pyrethrins, 2% piperonyl butoxide technical	In 60 and 120 ml with comb.	NA
otc	**Pyrinex Pediculicide** (Ambix)	**Shampoo:** 0.2% pyrethrins, 2% piperonyl butoxide technical and 0.8% deodorized kerosene	In 118 ml.	NA
otc	**A-200** (Beecham)	**Shampoo:** 0.33% pyrethrins, 4% piperonyl butoxide technical	In 60 and 120 ml.	2.9
otc	**Pronto Concentrate** (Commerce Drug)	**Shampoo:** 0.33% pyrethrins, 4% piperonyl butoxide technical	In 59 and 118 ml.	2.9
otc	**Tisit** (Pfeiffer)	**Shampoo:** 0.3% pyrethrins, 3% piperonyl butoxide technical, 1.2% petroleum distillate, 2.4% benzyl alcohol	In 118 ml.	1.3
otc	**R & C** (Reed & Carnrick)	**Shampoo:** 0.3% pyrethrins, 3% piperonyl butoxide technical, 1.2% petroleum distillate	In 60 and 118 ml.	3
otc	**Lice-Enz** (Copely)	**Shampoo Kit:** 0.3% pyrethrins, 3% piperonyl butoxide	In 60 g w/ nit comb.	NA
otc	**Step 2** (GenDerm)	**Creme rinse:** Formic acid, benzyl alcohol, cetyl alcohol, glyceryl stearate, PEG-100 stearate, polyquaternium-10, sodium hydroxide	In 60 ml with metal nit comb.	NA

* Cost Index based on cost per g or ml.

Actions:

Topical corticosteroids have anti-inflammatory, antipruritic, vasoconstrictive and antiproliferative actions. Clinical efficacy depends on the extent of percutaneous absorption or penetration of the active drug through the stratum corneum and epidermis of the skin. Factors influencing absorption include: Agent used; drug concentration; vehicle used; anatomical application site; use of occlusive dressing; integrity of the epidermal barrier. Occlusive vehicles or transparent plastic wrap enhances absorption ≈ 10-fold or greater. Increased absorption can cause adverse systemic steroid effects in patients with altered skin, as in atopic dermatitis. Once absorbed through the skin, topical corticosteroids are handled through pharmacokinetic pathways similar to systemically administered corticosteroids.

When applied to intact noninflamed forearm skin, ≈ 1% is absorbed. Inflamed or damaged skin may absorb ≥ 33%. Eyelids and genital skin, particularly the scrotum, absorb 25%. Absorption is also higher when used on the jaw, forehead, axilla and scalp. Palms and soles, because of their thick stratum corneum, usually absorb < 1%.

Vehicles: Greasy ointment bases, generally more occlusive, are preferred for dry scaly lesions. Greasy creams may be equally effective and are preferred by patients. Gels are less occlusive. Use aerosols, lotions and solutions on hairy areas. Urea enhances hydration; therefore, it may enhance absorption of the steroid. Steroid impregnated tapes are useful for occlusive therapy of small areas.

Relative potency: Fluorinated derivatives (eg, fluocinonide, betamethasone, triamcinolone) are more potent and less likely to cause sodium retention. Hydrocortisone is less potent, but is effective in less severe dermatoses or those requiring long-term topical therapy.

The relative potency of topical corticosteroid preparations depends on several factors including the characteristics and concentration of the drug and the vehicle used. The estimated relative potency of selected commercial preparations is given in the table below. Group I is the most potent; potency decreases with each group to Group VII, the least potent. There is no significant difference among agents within groups II through VII. In group I, clobetasol ointment is more potent than betamethasone or diflorasone ointments.

Relative Potency of Selected Topical Steroid Products[1]

Drug	*Dosage Form*	*Strength*
I. Augmented betamethasone dipropionate	cream, ointment	0.05%
Clobetasol propionate	cream, ointment	0.05%
Diflorasone diacetate	ointment	0.05%
II. Amcinonide	ointment	0.1%
Betamethasone dipropionate	ointment	0.05%
Desoximetasone	cream, ointment	0.25%
	gel	0.05%
Diflorasone diacetate	ointment (emollient base)	0.05%
Fluocinonide	cream, gel, ointment	0.05%
Halcinonide	cream	0.1%
III. Betamethasone dipropionate	cream	0.05%
Betamethasone valerate	ointment	0.1%
Diflorasone diacetate	cream	0.05%
Triamcinolone acetonide	ointment	0.1%
IV. Desoximetasone	cream	0.05%
Fluocinolone acetonide	ointment	0.025%
Flurandrenolide	ointment	0.05%
Hydrocortisone valerate	ointment	0.2%
Triamcinolone acetonide	cream	0.1%
V. Betamethasone dipropionate	lotion	0.02%
Betamethasone valerate	cream	0.1%
Fluocinolone acetonide	cream	0.025%
Flurandrenolide	cream	0.05%
Hydrocortisone butyrate	cream	0.1%
Hydrocortisone valerate	cream	0.2%
Triamcinolone acetonide	lotion	0.1%
VI. Betamethasone valerate	lotion	0.05%
Desonide	cream	0.05%
Fluocinolone acetonide	solution	0.01%
VII. Dexamethasone	Methylprednisolone	
Hydrocortisone	Prednisolone	

[1] Adapted from: Stoughton RB, Cornell RC. Review of super-potent topical corticosteroids. *Semin Dermatol* 1987;6:72-76.

(Continued on following page)

Indications:

Relief of inflammatory and pruritic manifestations of corticosteroid-responsive dermatoses. This may include, but is not limited to: Contact dermatitis; atopic dermatitis; psoriasis; lichen planus associated with severe pruritis; seborrheic dermatitis; discoid lupus erythematosus; alopecia areata; granulomatous disorders (eg, sarcoidosis, necrobiosis lipoidica, granuloma annulare); mycosis fungoides (early stages); lymphocytic infiltration of the skin; pustulosis; palmoplantaris. In children, the conditions may include, but are not limited to: Atopic eczema; contact dermatitis; infantile seborrheic eczema; discoid or nummular eczema; pompholyx; pityriasis alba; perioral eczema; juvenile plantar dermatosis; diaper dermatitis; psoriasis. The agent to be used in each condition depends on the individual, the location of the condition and the length of therapy.

Nonprescription hydrocortisone products: Temporary relief of minor skin irritations, itching and rashes due to eczema, dermatitis, insect bites, poison ivy, poison oak or sumac, soaps, detergents, cosmetics, jewelry; also for itchy genital and anal areas.

Contraindications:

Hypersensitivity to any component; primary bacterial infections (eg, impetigo, furuncles, carbuncles, cellulitis); *Candida* and dermatophytes; herpes simplex and zoster.

Ophthalmic use: When applied to the eyelids or skin near the eyes, the drug may enter the eyes. Prolonged ocular exposure may cause steroid-induced glaucoma and cataracts.

Warnings:

Pregnancy: Category C. Systemic corticosteroids are teratogenic in animals when administered at relatively low dosages. The more potent corticosteroids are teratogenic after dermal application in animals. There are no adequate and well controlled studies in pregnant women. Therefore, use during pregnancy only if the potential benefits outweigh the potential hazards to the fetus. In pregnant patients, do not use extensively; do not use in large amounts or for prolonged periods of time.

Lactation: It is not known whether topical corticosteroids could result in sufficient systemic absorption to produce detectable quantities in breast milk. Systemic corticosteroids are secreted into breast milk in quantities not likely to have a deleterious effect on the infant. Nevertheless, exercise caution when administering topical corticosteroids to a nursing mother.

Children: Children may be more susceptible to topical corticosteroid-induced hypothalamic-pituitary-adrenal (HPA) axis suppression and Cushing's syndrome than adults because of a larger skin surface area to body weight ratio.

HPA axis suppression, Cushing's syndrome and intracranial hypertension have occurred in children receiving topical corticosteroids. Manifestations of adrenal suppression include linear growth retardation, delayed weight gain, low plasma cortisol levels and absence of response to ACTH stimulation. Manifestations of intracranial hypertension include bulging fontanelles, headaches and bilateral papilledema.

Limit administration to the least amount compatible with effective therapy. Chronic corticosteroid therapy may interfere with the growth and development of children.

Safety and efficacy of **desoximetasone** in children < 10 years old have not been established. **Clobetasol** is not recommended for children < 12 years old.

Precautions:

Systemic effects: Systemic absorption of topical corticosteroids has produced reversible HPA axis suppression, Cushing's syndrome, hyperglycemia and glycosuria. Conditions that augment systemic absorption include the application of the more potent steroids, use over large surface areas, prolonged use and the addition of occlusive dressings.

Periodically evaluate patients for evidence of HPA axis suppression by using the urinary free cortisol and ACTH stimulation tests. If HPA axis suppression is noted, attempt to withdraw the drug, reduce the frequency of application, substitute a less potent steroid or use a sequential approach with the occlusive technique. Also test for impairment of thermal homeostasis.

Recovery of HPA axis function and thermal homeostasis are generally prompt and complete upon discontinuation of the drug. Infrequently, signs and symptoms of steroid withdrawal may occur, requiring supplemental systemic corticosteroids.

Clobetasol suppresses the HPA axis at doses as low as 2 g per day.

Children may absorb proportionally larger amounts of topical corticosteroids and may be more susceptible to systemic toxicity (see Warnings).

As a general rule, little effect on the HPA axis will occur with use of a potent topical corticosteroid in amounts of 50 g weekly for an adult and 15 g weekly for a child, without occlusion. To cover the adult body one time requires 12 to 26 g.

For information regarding systemic corticosteroids, refer to the Adrenal Cortical Steroids, Glucocorticoids group monograph in chapter 3.

(Precautions continued on following page)

Precautions (Cont.):

Local irritation: Discontinue use and institute appropriate therapy. Medications containing alcohol may produce dry skin or burning sensations/irritation in open lesions.

Skin atrophy is common and may be clinically significant in 3 to 4 weeks with potent preparations. Atrophy occurs most readily at sites where percutaneous absorption is high.

Take care when using periorbitally or in the genital area. Avoid use of high potency topical corticosteroids on the face and in intertriginous areas because of resulting striae.

Psoriasis: Do not use topical corticosteroids as sole therapy in widespread plaque psoriasis.

In rare instances, treatment (or withdrawal of treatment) of psoriasis with corticosteroids is thought to have provoked the pustular form of the disease.

Atrophic changes: Certain areas of the body, such as the face, groin and axillae, are more prone to atrophic changes than other areas of the body following treatment with corticosteroids. Frequent observation of the patient is important if these areas are to be treated.

Infections: In the presence of an infection, institute therapy with an antifungal or antibacterial agent. If a favorable response does not occur promptly, discontinue the corticosteroid until the infection has been controlled. Treating skin infections with topical corticosteroids can extensively worsen the infection.

Do not use these agents for the treatment of rosacea, perioral dermatitis or acne.

Avoid inhalation of aerosols, ingestion or contact with eyes.

Vehicles: Many topical corticosteroids are in specially formulated bases designed to maximize their release and potency. Mixing with other bases or vehicles may affect potency far beyond that normally expected from the dilution. Exercise caution before mixing; if necessary, contact the manufacturer to determine if there may be an incompatibility.

Occlusive therapy: Discontinue the use of occlusive dressings if infection develops, and institute appropriate antimicrobial therapy.

Occasionally, a patient may develop a sensitivity reaction to a particular occlusive dressing material or adhesive; a substitute material may be necessary.

Do not use occlusive dressings in **clobetasol, mometasone, augmented betamethasone dipropionate** and **betamethasone dipropionate** treatment regimens.

Adverse Reactions:

Local: Burning; itching; irritation; erythema; dryness; folliculitis; hypertrichosis; acneiform eruptions; hypopigmentation; perioral dermatitis; allergic contact dermatitis; numbness of fingers; stinging and cracking of skin; maceration of the skin; secondary infection; skin atrophy; striae; miliaria. These may occur more frequently with occlusive dressings.

Sensitivity to a particular dressing material or adhesive may occur occasionally.

Systemic absorption of topical corticosteroids has produced reversible HPA axis suppression, manifestations of Cushing's syndrome, hyperglycemia and glycosuria (see Precautions). This is more likely to occur with occlusive dressings and with the more potent steroids. Patients with liver failure or children (see Warnings) may be at at higher risk.

Following prolonged application around the eyes, cataracts and glaucoma may develop. In diffusely atrophied skin, blood vessels may become visible on the skin surface; telangiectasia and purpura may occur at the site of trauma.

The risk of adverse reactions may be minimized by changing to a less potent agent, reducing the dosage or using intermittent therapy.

Overdosage:

Topical corticosteroids can be absorbed in sufficient amounts to produce systemic effects (see Precautions).

Patient Information:

Apply sparingly in a light film; rub in lightly. Washing or soaking the area before application may increase drug penetration.

Notify physician if condition being treated persists or worsens, if burning or irritation occurs or if infection develops.

Advise parents of pediatric patients not to use tight-fitting diapers or plastic pants on a child treated in the diaper area; these garments may constitute occlusive dressings.

Avoid prolonged use, especially near eyes, in genital and rectal areas, on the face and in skin creases. Avoid contact with the eyes.

Administration and Dosage:

Generally, apply sparingly 2 to 4 times daily. Applying the agent 1 to 2 times daily may be as effective as 3 to 6 times daily. Intermittent therapy using high potency agents (eg, every other day, 3 to 4 consecutive days per week, 1 day per week) may be more effective with less severe side effects than continuous use of lower potency agents.

Treatment with clobetasol and alclometasone beyond 2 consecutive weeks is not recommended, and the total dosage should not exceed 50 g per week because of the potential for the drug to suppress the HPA axis.

(Products listed on following page)

Complete prescribing information for these products begins on page 2370

ALCLOMETASONE DIPROPIONATE

Administration: Apply a thin film to affected area 2 or 3 times daily; gently massage until medication disappears. Occlusive dressings may be used for the management of refractory lesions of psoriasis and other deep-seated dermatoses (eg, localized neurodermatitis [lichen simplex chronicus]).

	Product	Form	Description	C.I.*
Rx	**Aclovate** (Glaxo)	**Ointment:** 0.05%	White petrolatum. In 15 and 45 g.	10.8
		Cream: 0.05%	Hydrophilic, emollient base. White petrolatum. In 15 and 45 g.	10.8

AMCINONIDE

	Product	Form	Description	C.I.*
Rx	**Cyclocort** (Lederle)	**Ointment:** 0.1%	White petrolatum base. 2% benzyl alcohol. In 15, 30 and 60 g.	21.5
		Cream: 0.1%	Emulsified hydrophilic base. 2% benzyl alcohol, glycerin. In 15, 30 and 60 g.	21.5
		Lotion: 0.1%	Emulsified hydrophilic base. 1% benzyl alcohol, glycerin. In 20 and 60 ml.	18.2

AUGMENTED BETAMETHASONE DIPROPIONATE

	Product	Form	Description	C.I.*
Rx	**Diprolene** (Schering)	**Ointment:** 0.05% betamethasone	In an optimized vehicle. White petrolatum. In 15 and 45 g.	27.1
Rx	**Diprolene AF** (Schering)	**Cream:** 0.05% betamethasone	White petrolatum, emollient base. In 15 and 45 g.	25.1
Rx	**Diprolene** (Schering)	**Gel:** 0.05% betamethasone (0.064% betamethasone dipropionate)	Propylene glycol, carbomer 940. In 15 and 45 g.	26.5
Rx	**Diprolene** (Schering)	**Lotion:** 0.05% betamethasone	Isopropyl alcohol. In 30 and 60 ml.	13.2

BETAMETHASONE BENZOATE

	Product	Form	Description	C.I.*
Rx	**Uticort** (Parke-Davis)	**Cream:** 0.025%	Water washable, mineral oil, emollient base. In 60 g.	9.2
		Lotion: 0.025%	Water miscible vehicle w/methylparaben. In 15 & 60 ml.	7.7
		Gel: 0.025%	13.8% alcohol, EDTA, greaseless. In 15 and 60 g.	9.2

BETAMETHASONE DIPROPIONATE

	Product	Form	Description	C.I.*
Rx	**Betamethasone Dipropionate** (Various)	**Ointment:** 0.05% betamethasone	In 15 and 45 g.	6.1+
Rx	**Alphatrex** (Savage)		Mineral oil, white petrolatum. In 15 and 45 g.	14.1
Rx	**Diprosone** (Schering)		Mineral oil and white petrolatum base. In 15 and 45 g.	24.6
Rx	**Maxivate** (Westwood)		Mineral oil and white petrolatum base. In 15 and 45 g.	16.9
Rx	**Betamethasone Dipropionate** (Various)	**Cream:** 0.05% betamethasone	In 15 and 45 g.	6.1+
Rx	**Alphatrex** (Savage)		Hydrophilic base. Mineral oil, white petrolatum. In 15 and 45 g.	15.1
Rx	**Diprosone** (Schering)		Hydrophilic emollient base. Mineral oil, white petrolatum. In 15 and 45 g.	24.6
Rx	**Maxivate** (Westwood)		Hydrophilic base. Mineral oil, white petrolatum. In 15 and 45 g.	16.7
Rx	**Teladar** (Dermol)		Mineral oil and white petrolatum. In 15 and 45 g.	NA

* Cost Index based on cost per g or ml.

(Continued on following page)

Complete prescribing information for these products begins on page 2370

BETAMETHASONE DIPROPIONATE (Cont)

	Product	Form	Description	C.I.*
Rx	**Betamethasone Dipropionate** (Various, eg, Balan, Bioline, Geneva, Goldline, Lemmon, Major, Moore, Pharmaderm, Rugby, Schein)	**Lotion:** 0.05% betamethasone	In 20 and 60 ml.	3.4+
Rx	**Alphatrex** (Savage)		30% isopropyl alcohol. In 60 ml.	9.1
Rx	**Diprosone** (Schering)		46.8% isopropyl alcohol. In 20 and 60 ml.	22.8
Rx	**Maxivate** (Westwood)		Isopropyl alcohol. In 60 ml.	11
Rx	**Diprosone** (Schering)	**Aerosol:** 0.1% betamethasone	10% isopropyl alcohol, mineral oil. In 85 g.	4.3

BETAMETHASONE VALERATE

	Product	Form	Description	C.I.*
Rx	**Betamethasone Valerate** (Various, eg, Bioline, Fougera, Goldline, Major, Moore, Pharmafair, Rugby, Schein, URL)	**Ointment:** 0.1% betamethasone	In 15 and 45 g.	3.6+
Rx	**Betatrex** (Savage)		Mineral oil and white petrolatum base. In 15 and 45 g.	13.2
Rx	**Beta-Val** (Lemmon)		Mineral oil, white petrolatum and lanolin base. In 15 and 45 g.	4.3
Rx	**Valisone** (Schering)		Mineral oil, white petrolatum and lanolin base. In 15 and 45 g.	19.4
Rx	**Valisone Reduced Strength** (Schering)	**Cream:** 0.01% betamethasone	Hydrophilic emollient base. Mineral oil, white petrolatum. In 15 and 60 g.	12.6
Rx	**Betamethasone Valerate** (Various, eg, Bioline, Geneva, Goldline, Major, Moore, Parmed, Pharmafair, Rugby, Schein, URL)	**Cream:** 0.1% betamethasone	In 15 and 45 g.	3.6+
Rx	**Betatrex** (Savage)		Hydrophilic base. Mineral oil, white petrolatum. In 15 and 45 g.	13.2
Rx	**Beta-Val** (Lemmon)		Vanishing base. Mineral oil, white petrolatum. In 15 g.	7
Rx	**Dermabet** (Taro)		Vanishing mineral oil and white petrolatum base. In 15 and 45 g.	2.9
Rx	**Valisone** (Schering)		Hydrophilic emollient base. Mineral oil, white petrolatum. In 15, 45, 110 and 430 g.	14.1
Rx	**Betamethasone Valerate** (Various, eg, Barre-National, Bioline, Fougera, Goldline, Major, Moore, Pharmafair, Rugby, Schein, URL)	**Lotion:** 0.1% betamethasone	In 60 ml.	2.4+
Rx	**Betatrex** (Savage)		Isopropyl alcohol. In 60 ml.	7.5
Rx	**Beta-Val** (Lemmon)		47.5% isopropyl alcohol. In 60 ml.	4.3
Rx	**Valisone** (Schering)		47.5% alcohol base. In 20 & 60 ml.	12.2
Rx	**Betamethasone Valerate** (Paddock)	**Powder for Compounding**	In micronized 5 and 10 g.	485.2

* Cost Index based on cost per g or ml.

Complete prescribing information for these products begins on page 2370

	Product	Form	Description	C.I.*
CLOBETASOL PROPIONATE				**C.I.***
Rx	**Temovate** (Glaxo)	**Ointment:** 0.05%	White petro base. In 15, 30 & 45 g.	20
		Cream: 0.05%	In 15, 30 and 45 g.	20
		Scalp application: 0.05%	39.3% isopropyl alcohol and carbomer 934 P. In 25 and 50 ml.	NA
CLOCORTOLONE PIVALATE				
Rx	**Cloderm** (Hermal)	**Cream:** 0.1%	Water washable base. White petrolatum, mineral oil, EDTA, parabens. In 15 and 45 g.	13
DESONIDE				
Rx	**DesOwen** (Owen/Galderma)	**Ointment:** 0.05%	In 15 and 60 g.	15
Rx	**Tridesilon** (Miles Inc.)		White petrolatum. In 15 and 60 g.	16
Rx	**DesOwen** (Owen/Galderma)	**Cream:** 0.05%	In 15 and 60 g.	15
Rx	**Tridesilon** (Miles Inc.)		White petrolatum, glycerin, mineral oil, methylparaben. In 15 & 60 g.	16
DESOXIMETASONE				**C.I.***
Rx	**Topicort** (Hoechst-Roussel)	**Ointment:** 0.25%	White petrolatum base. In 15 and 60 g.	21
Rx	**Desoximetasone** (Taro)	**Cream:** 0.05%	Emollient base. White petrolatum, lanolin alcohols, mineral oil, EDTA. In 15 and 60 g.	8.3
Rx	**Topicort LP** (Hoechst-Roussel)		Emollient base. White petro, mineral oil, lanolin alcohols. In 15 & 60 g.	16
Rx	**Desoximetasone** (Taro)	**Cream:** 0.25%	Emollient base. White petro, lanolin alcohols, mineral oil. In 15 & 60 g.	11
Rx	**Topicort** (Hoechst-Roussel)		Emollient base. White petrolatum, mineral oil, lanolin alcohols. In 15, 60 and 120 g.	21
Rx	**Topicort** (Hoechst-Roussel)	**Gel:** 0.05%	20% alcohol 40, EDTA, DSS. In 15 and 60 g.	18
DEXAMETHASONE				
Rx	**Decaderm** (MSD)	**Gel:** 0.1%	Emollient vehicle. Lanolin alcohol. In 30 g.	16
Rx	**Aeroseb-Dex** (Herbert)	**Aerosol:** 0.01%	59% alcohol. In 58 g.	4.3
Rx	**Decaspray** (MSD)	**Aerosol:** 0.04%	In 25 g.	13
DEXAMETHASONE SODIUM PHOSPHATE				
Rx	**Decadron Phosphate** (MSD)	**Cream:** 0.1% dexamethasone phosphate equivalent	Greaseless base. Mineral oil, EDTA, 0.15% methylparabens. In 15 and 30 g.	17
DIFLORASONE DIACETATE				
Rx	**Florone** (Dermik)	**Ointment:** 0.05%	Emollient occlusive base. Lanolin alcohol, white petrolatum. In 15, 30 and 60 g.	22
Rx	**Maxiflor** (Herbert)		Emollient occlusive base. Lanolin alcohol, white petrolatum. In 15, 30 and 60 g.	23
Rx	**Psorcon** (Dermik)		White petrolatum. In 15, 30, 60 g.	28
Rx	**Florone** (Dermik)	**Cream:** 0.05%	Emulsified hydrophilic base. In 15, 30 and 60 g.	22
Rx	**Florone E** (Dermik)		Emollient hydrophilic base. Mineral oil. In 15, 30 and 60 g.	30
Rx	**Maxiflor** (Herbert)		Emulsified hydrophilic base. In 15, 30 and 60 g.	23

* Cost Index based on cost per g or ml.

Complete prescribing information for these products begins on page 2370

FLUOCINOLONE ACETONIDE				C.I.*
Rx	**Fluocinolone** (Various, eg, Fougera, Major)	**Ointment:** 0.025%	In 15, 30, 60 and 425 g.	4.9+
Rx	**Flurosyn** (Rugby)		White petrolatum base. In 15 & 60 g.	7.5
Rx	**Synalar** (Syntex)		White petrolatum vehicle. In 15, 30, 60 and 425 g.	19
Rx	**Fluocinolone** (Various, eg, Fougera, Geneva, Goldline, Major, Moore)	**Cream:** 0.01%	In 15, 30, 60 and 425 g.	2.2+
Rx	**Flurosyn** (Rugby)		In 15, 60 and 425 g.	2.5
Rx	**Synalar** (Syntex)		Water washable, aqueous base. Mineral oil, EDTA, parabens. In 15, 30, 60 and 425 g.	13
Rx	**Fluocinolone** (Various, eg, American Drug Co., Fougera, Geneva, Goldline, Major, Moore)	**Cream:** 0.025%	In 15, 30, 60 and 425 g.	3.2+
Rx	**Flurosyn** (Rugby)		In 15, 60 and 425 g.	3.2
Rx	**Synalar** (Syntex)		Water washable, aqueous base. Mineral oil, EDTA, parabens. In 15, 30, 60 and 425 g.	19
Rx	**Synemol** (Syntex)		Water washable, aqueous, emollient base. Mineral oil. In 15, 30 and 60 g.	20
Rx	**Synalar-HP** (Syntex)	**Cream:** 0.2%	Water washable, aqueous base. Mineral oil, parabens. In 12 g.	45
Rx	**Fluocinolone** (Various, eg, Geneva, Goldline, Major, Moore)	**Solution:** 0.01%	In 20 and 60 ml.	6.3+
Rx	**Fluonid** (Herbert)		In 20 and 60 ml.	12
Rx	**Synalar** (Syntex)		Water washable base. In 20 & 60 ml.	18
Rx	**Fluocinolone Acetonide** (Torch Labs)	**Powder for compounding**	In 5 g.	6.8

FLUOCINONIDE				
Rx	**Fluocinomide** (Lemmon)	**Ointment:** 0.05%	White petrolatum and castor oil. In 15, 30 and 60 g.	NA
Rx	**Lidex** (Syntex)		Occlusive, white petrolatum base. In 15, 30, 60 and 120 g.	24
Rx	**Fluocinonide** (Various, eg, Geneva, Goldline, Lemmon, Major, Rugby, Schein)	**Cream:** 0.05%	In 15, 30, 60 and 120 g.	9+
Rx	**Fluonex** (ICN)		Ethoxylate alcohol (Behenth-20) base, polyethylene glycol 8000, sorbitol monostearate, propylene glycol, citric acid and anhydrous. In 15 and 30 g.	NA
Rx	**Lidex** (Syntex)		Water miscible, anhydrous greaseless vehicle. In 15, 30, 60 and 120 g.	24
Rx	**Lidex-E** (Syntex)		Water washable, aqueous emollient mineral oil base. In 15, 30, 60, 120 g.	24
Rx	**Vasoderm** (Taro)		Water washable, anhydrous glycerin base. In 15, 30 and 60 g.	6.7
Rx	**Vasoderm-E** (Taro)		Water washable, aqueous, emollient mineral oil and white petrolatum base. In 15, 30, 60 and 120 g.	13

* Cost Index based on cost per g or ml.

(Continued on following page)

Complete prescribing information for these products begins on page 2370

	Product	Form	Description	C.I.*
FLUOCINONIDE (Cont.)				
Rx	**Fluocinonide** (Various, eg, Barre-National, Bioline, Geneva, Lemmon, Major, Moore, Parmed, Rugby, URL)	**Solution:** 0.05%	In 20 and 60 ml.	8.2+
Rx	**Lidex** (Syntex)		35% alcohol. In 20 and 60 ml.	21
Rx	**Fluocinonide** (Various, eg, Lemmon, Moore)	**Gel:** 0.05%	In 60 g.	9.7+
Rx	**Lidex** (Syntex)		Water miscible, greaseless base. EDTA. In 15, 30, 60 and 120 g.	24
FLURANDRENOLIDE				
Rx	**Cordran** (Dista)	**Ointment:** 0.025%	White petrolatum base. In 30, 60 and 225 g.	9.8
Rx	**Cordran** (Dista)	**Ointment:** 0.05%	White petrolatum base. In 15, 30, 60 and 225 g.	13
Rx	**Cordran SP** (Dista)	**Cream:** 0.025%	Emulsified mineral oil base. In 30, 60 and 225 g.	9.8
Rx	**Cordran SP** (Dista)	**Cream:** 0.05%	Emulsified mineral oil base. In 15, 30, 60 and 225 g.	13
Rx	**Flurandrenolide** (Barre-National)	**Lotion:** 0.05%	In 15 and 60 ml.	3
Rx	**Cordran** (Dista)		Oil-in-water mineral oil, glycerin, benzyl alcohol emulsion base. In 15 and 60 ml.	12
Rx	**Cordran** (Dista)	**Tape:** 4 mcg per square cm	In 24" x 3" and 80" x 3" rolls.	
FLUTICASONE PROPIONATE				
Rx	**Cutivate** (Glaxo Dermatology)	**Cream:** 0.05%	Propylene glycol and mineral oil base. In 15, 30 and 60 g.	NA
Rx	**Cutivate** (Glaxo Dermatology)	**Ointment:** 0.005%	Propylene glycol, sorbitan sesquioleate, microcrystalline wax and liquid paraffin base. In 15, 30 and 60 g.	NA
HALCINONIDE				
Rx	**Halog** (Westwood Squibb)	**Ointment:** 0.1%	Polyethylene and mineral oil gel base. In 15, 30, 60 and 240 g.	23
Rx	**Halog** (Westwood Squibb)	**Cream:** 0.025%	In 15, 60 g and 240 g.	21
Rx	**Halog** (Westwood Squibb)	**Cream:** 0.1%	In 15, 30, 60 and 240 g.	23
Rx	**Halog-E** (Westwood Squibb)		Water washable, greaseless hydrophilic vanishing white petrolatum base. In 15, 30 and 60 g.	23
Rx	**Halog** (Westwood Squibb)	**Solution:** 0.1%	EDTA. In 20 and 60 ml.	18
HALOBETASOL PROPIONATE				
Rx	**Ultravate** (Westwood Squibb)	**Ointment:** 0.05%	Aluminum stearate, pentaerythritol cocoate, petrolatum, sorbitan sesquioleate, stearyl citrate. In 15 and 45 g.	NA
		Cream: 0.05%	Glycerin, isopropyl isostearate, isopropyl palmitate, steareth-21, diazolidinyl urea, methylchloroisothiazolinone, methylisothiazolinone. In 15 and 45 g.	NA

* Cost Index based on cost per g or ml.

Complete prescribing information for these products begins on page 2370

HYDROCORTISONE

	Product	Form	Description	C.I.*
Rx[1]	**Hydrocortisone** (Various, eg, Bioline, Fougera, Geneva, Goldline, Major, Moore, Parmed, Rugby, URL)	**Ointment:** 0.5%	In 15 and 30 g and lb.	1.3+
otc	**Cortizone-5** (Thompson Med.)		White petrolatum. In 30 g.	1.7
Rx	**Hydrocortisone** (Various, eg, Bioline, Goldline, Major, Moore, Parmed, PBI, Rugby, Schein, URL)	**Ointment:** 1%	In 20, 30 and 120 g and lb.	2.7+
otc	**Anusol-HC** (Parke-Davis)		In 21 g.	NA
otc	**Cortizone 10** (Thompson)		White petrolatum. In 30 g.	NA
Rx	**Cortril** (Pfizer)		White petrolatum and mineral oil base. Parabens. In 15 g.	9.2
Rx	**Hycort** (Everett)		White petrolatum and mineral oil base. In 30 g.	1.4
Rx	**HydroTex** (Syosset)		In 30 g.	3.5
Rx	**Hytone** (Dermik)		Emollient, mineral oil, white petrolatum base. In 30 g.	5.5
otc	**Maximum Strength Cortaid** (Upjohn)		White petrolatum and mineral oil base. Parabens. In 15 and 30 g.	NA
otc	**Tegrin-HC** (Block)		Mineral oil and white petrolatum. In 28 g.	NA
Rx	**1% HC** (C & M Pharm.)		Water immiscible. Petrolatum base. In 15, 20, 30, 60, 120 and 240 g and lb.	4.6
Rx	**Hydrocortisone** (Various, eg, Bioline, Major, Moore, PBI, Rugby, Schein, URL)	**Ointment:** 2.5%	In 20 g and lb.	2.9+
Rx	**Hytone** (Dermik)		Emollient mineral oil, white petrolatum base. In 30 g.	7.9
Rx	**Cort-Dome** (Miles Inc.)	**Cream:** 0.25%	In 30 and 120 g.	6
Rx[1]	**Hydrocortisone** (Various)	**Cream:** 0.5%	In 15, 30 and 120 g and lb.	1.3+
otc	**Bactine Hydrocortisone** (Miles Inc.)		Glycerin, lanolin alcohol, mineral oil, EDTA, parabens. In 15 g.	3.8
Rx	**Cort-Dome** (Miles Inc.)		Glycerin, white petrolatum, mineral oil. In 30 g.	9.8
otc	**Cortef Feminine Itch** (Upjohn)		Vanishing base. Aloe, parabens. In 15 g.	4.3
otc	**Cortizone-5** (Thompson Med.)		Glycerin, mineral oil, white petrolatum, parabens. In 30 and 45 g.	2.2
otc	**Delcort** (Hauck)		Paraben base. In 1 g packets (144s).	2
otc	**DermiCort** (Republic Drug)		Greaseless base. In 30 g.	2.9
otc	**Dermolate Anti-Itch** (Schering)		Greaseless, vanishing base. Mineral oil and petrolatum. In 15 and 30 g.	4.6
otc	**Dermtex HC with Aloe** (Pfeiffer)		Greaseless, vanishing base. Glycerin, white and light petrolatum, methylparaben. In 30 g.	2.7
otc	**HydroTex** (Syosset)		Mineral oil, lanolin alcohol, sodium bisulfite. In 30 and 60 g.	2.7
Rx	**S-T Cort** (Scot-Tussin)		Water washable base. Parabens. In 120 g.	1.2

* Cost Index based on cost per g or ml.

[1] Products are available *otc* or *Rx* depending on product labeling.

(Continued on following page)

Complete prescribing information for these products begins on page 2370

HYDROCORTISONE (Cont.)

				C.I.*
Rx	**Hydrocortisone** (Various, eg, Balan, Bioline, Goldline, Lemmon, Major, Moore, Parmed, Rugby, Schein, URL)	**Cream:** 1%	In 15, 20, 30 and 120 g and lb.	1.9+
Rx	**Ala-Cort** (Del-Ray)		Glycerin base. In 30 and 90 g.	3.6
Rx	**Alphaderm** (Lemmon)		White petrolatum, 10% urea. In 30 and 100 g.	7.8
Rx	**Cort-Dome** (Miles Inc.)		Glycerin, white petrolatum, mineral oil. In 30 g.	16.2
Rx	**Delcort** (Hauck)		In 20 g and lb.	2.9
Rx	**Dermacort** (Solvay Pharm.)		Benzyl alcohol. In lb.	1.7
Rx	**Hi-Cor 1.0** (C & M Pharm.)		Petrolatum and glycerin base. In 30 and 60 g and lb.	3.9
Rx	**Hycort** (Everett)		Mineral oil and paraben base. In 30 g.	1.4
Rx	**HydroTex** (Syosset)		Mineral oil and lanolin alcohol base. Sodium bisulfite. In 28.4, 113.4 and 454 g.	3.5
Rx	**Hytone** (Dermik)		Water washable base. In 30 and 120 g.	4.7
otc	**Maximum Strength Cortaid** (Upjohn)		Parabens, glycerin, white petrolatum, cetyl and stearyl alcohols. In 15 and 30 g.	NA
Rx	**Nutracort** (Owen/Galderma)		In 30, 60 and 120 g.	4.8
Rx	**Synacort** (Syntex)		Mineral oil base. In 15, 30 and 60 g.	5.1
Rx	**Hydrocortisone** (Various, eg, Balan, Bioline, Goldline, Major, Moore, PBI, Rugby, Schein, URL)	**Cream:** 2.5%	In 20 and 30 g and lb.	2.8+
Rx	**Anusol-HC 2.5%** (Parke-Davis)		Water washable. With benzyl alcohol and petrolatum. In 30 g.	NA
Rx	**Hi-Cor 2.5** (C & M Pharm.)		Petrolatum and glycerin base. In 30 and 60 g and lb.	6.8
Rx	**HydroTex** (Syosset)		In 30 and 60 g.	3.5
Rx	**Hytone** (Dermik)		Water washable base. In 30 and 60 g.	7.3
Rx	**Penecort** (Herbert)		Petrolatum, EDTA. In 30 g.	5.8
Rx	**Synacort** (Syntex)		Mineral oil base. In 30 g.	8.2
Rx	**Cetacort** (Owen/Galderma)	**Lotion:** 0.25%	Parabens. In 120 ml.	2.3
Rx	**Cort-Dome** (Miles Inc.)		Glycerin, parabens. In 30 and 120 ml.	3.7
Rx[1]	**Hydrocortisone** (Various, eg, Balan, Bioline, Goldline, Major, Moore, Rugby, Schein, URL)	**Lotion:** 0.5%	In 30, 60 and 120 ml.	1.3+
Rx	**Cetacort** (Owen/Galderma)		Parabens. In 60 ml.	4.6
otc	**Delacort** (Mericon)		Water washable base. In 60 and 120 ml.	1.3
otc	**DermiCort** (Republic Drug)		Greaseless base. In 60 ml.	1.2
Rx	**S-T Cort** (Scot-Tussin)		Water washable base. With parabens. In 120 ml.	1.2
Rx	**Tega-Cort** (Ortega)		Water washable, lanolin alcohol, mineral oil base. In 60 & 120 ml.	2.2

* Cost Index based on cost per g or ml.

[1] Products are available *otc* or *Rx* depending on product labeling.

(Continued on following page)

Complete prescribing information for these products begins on page 2370

	HYDROCORTISONE (Cont.)			C.I.*
Rx	**Hydrocortisone** (Various)	**Lotion:** 1%	In 120 ml.	1.2+
Rx	**Acticort 100** (Baker Cummins)		EDTA. In 60 ml.	5
Rx	**Ala-Cort** (Del-Ray)		Mineral oil, glycerin base. In 120 ml.	2.2
Rx	**Cetacort** (Owen/Galderma)		Parabens. In 60 ml.	5.3
Rx	**Cort-Dome** (Miles Inc.)		In 30 ml.	20.4
Rx	**Dermacort** (Solvay Pharm.)		Benzyl alcohol. In 120 ml.	1.7
Rx	**Hytone** (Dermik)		In 120 ml.	2.9
Rx	**LactiCare-HC** (Stiefel)		Mineral oil. In 120 ml.	2.3
Rx	**Nutracort** (Owen/Galderma)		Mineral oil, parabens, EDTA. In 60 and 120 ml.	4.8
Rx	**Tega-Cort Forte** (Ortega)		Water washable, lanolin alcohol, mineral oil base. 60 & 120 ml.	4.3
Rx	**Ala-Scalp** (Del-Ray)	**Lotion:** 2%	Isopropyl alcohol base. In 30 ml.	4.5
Rx	**Hytone** (Dermik)	**Lotion:** 2.5%	In 60 ml.	5.8
Rx	**LactiCare-HC** (Stiefel)		Mineral oil. In 60 ml.	6.1
Rx	**Nutracort** (Owen/Galderma)		Mineral oil, parabens, EDTA base. In 60 and 120 ml.	4.5
otc	**CortaGel** (Norstar)	**Gel:** 1%	In 15 and 30 g.	NA
Rx	**Texacort** (GenDerm)	**Solution:** 1%	Lipid free. 33% alcohol. In 30 ml.	5.6
Rx	**Aeroseb-HC** (Herbert)	**Aerosol/Pump Spray:** 0.5%	58% alcohol. In 58 g aerosol.	4.3
otc	**CaldeCort Anti-Itch** (Fisons)		89.5% alcohol. In 45 g aerosol.	1.9
otc	**Cortaid** (Upjohn)		46% alcohol. Glycerin, methylparaben. In 45 ml pump spray.	1.8
	HYDROCORTISONE ACETATE			
otc	**Cortaid with Aloe** (Upjohn)	**Ointment:** 0.5% hydrocortisone equivalent	Aloe, mineral oil, white petrolatum, parabens. In 15 and 30 g.	4.2
otc	**Lanacort 5** (Combe)	**Ointment:** 0.5%	Lanolin alcohols, aloe, petrolatum. In 15 g.	3.1
otc	**Corticaine** (Whitby)	**Cream:** 0.5%	Washable. Glycerin, EDTA base. Parabens. In 30 g.	6.4
otc	**FoilleCort** (Blistex)		In 3.75 g.	1.1
otc	**Gynecort** (Combe)		Parabens. In 15 g.	4.8
otc	**Lanacort 5** (Combe)		Aloe, parabens. In 15 and 30 g.	3.1
otc	**Lanacort 10** (Combe)	**Ointment:** 1%	In 15 g.	NA
Rx	**Anusol-HC** (Parke-Davis)	**Cream:** 1%	Water washable. Glyceryl stearate, mineral oil, parabens and white petrolatum. In 30 g.	7.6
otc	**Extra Strength Gynecort 10** (Combe)		Parabens and zinc pyrithione. In 15 g.	NA
otc	**Lanacort 10** (Combe)		In 15 and 30 g.	NA
Rx	**U-Cort** (Thames)		Water washable. EDTA, sodium bisulfite. In 30 and 120 g.	6.2
otc	**CaldeCort** (Fisons)	**Cream:** 0.5% hydrocortisone equivalent	Lanolin alcohol, white petrolatum, mineral oil. In 15 and 30 g.	3.1
otc	**CaldeCort Light with Aloe** (Fisons)		Aloe, parabens. In 15 g.	3.1
otc	**Cortaid with Aloe** (Upjohn)		In 15 and 30 g.	4.2
otc	**Cortaid** (Upjohn)	**Lotion:** 0.5% hydrocortisone equivalent	Vanishing, greaseless base. Parabens. In 30 ml.	2.9
otc	**CortaGel** (Inter-Hermes)	**Gel:** 0.5%	In 15 and 30 g.	5.7

* Cost Index based on cost per g or ml.

Complete prescribing information for these products begins on page 2370

	Product	Form/Strength	Description	C.I.*
HYDROCORTISONE BUTYRATE				
Rx	**Locoid** (Owen/Galderma)	**Ointment:** 0.1%	Mineral oil. In 15 and 45 g.	10.1
Rx	**Locoid** (Owen/Galderma)	**Cream:** 0.1%	Hydrophilic base. White petrolatum, methylparaben, mineral oil. In 15, 45 and 60 g.	10.1
HYDROCORTISONE VALERATE				
Rx	**Westcort** (Westwood)	**Ointment:** 0.2%	Hydrophilic base. White petrolatum, mineral oil. In 15, 45 and 60 g.	10.2
Rx	**Westcort** (Westwood)	**Cream:** 0.2%	Hydrophilic base. White petrolatum. In 15, 45, 60 and 120 g.	10.2
METHYLPREDNISOLONE ACETATE				
Rx	**Medrol Acetate Topical** (Upjohn)	**Ointment:** 0.25%	0.4% methylparaben, 0.3% butyl paraben. In 30 g.	10.5
Rx	**Medrol Acetate Topical** (Upjohn)	**Ointment:** 1%	0.4% methylparaben, 0.3% butyl paraben. In 30 g.	20.9
MOMETASONE FUROATE				
Administration: Apply a thin film to affected areas once daily. Do not use occlusive dressings.				
Rx	**Elocon** (Schering)	**Ointment:** 0.1%	White petrolatum. In 15 and 45 g.	19
Rx	**Elocon** (Schering)	**Cream:** 0.1%	White petrolatum. In 15 and 45 g.	19
Rx	**Elocon** (Schering)	**Lotion:** 0.1%	40% isopropyl alcohol. In 30 and 60 ml.	NA
TRIAMCINOLONE ACETONIDE				
Rx	**Triamcinolone Acetonide** (Various, eg, Balan, Fougera, Goldline, Major, Moore, Rugby, Schein)	**Ointment:** 0.025%	In 15, 80 and 454 g.	2.1+
Rx	**Flutex** (Syosset)		White petrolatum and mineral oil base. In 30, 60 and 120 g.	3.5
Rx	**Kenalog** (Squibb)		Mineral oil gel base. In 15, 80 and 240 g.	4.6
Rx	**Triamcinolone Acetonide** (Various, eg, Balan, Bioline, Fougera, Geneva, Goldline, Major, Moore, Rugby, Schein, URL)	**Ointment:** 0.1%	In 15 and 80 g and lb.	2.4+
Rx	**Aristocort** (Fujisawa)		White petrolatum base. In 15, 60 and 240 g.	7.2
Rx	**Aristocort A** (Fujisawa)		White petrolatum base. In 15 and 60 g.	11.3
Rx	**Flutex** (Syosset)		White petrolatum and mineral oil base. In 30, 60 and 120 g.	5.3
Rx	**Kenalog** (Squibb)		Mineral oil gel base. In 15, 60, 80 and 240 g.	6.3
Rx	**Triamcinolone Acetonide** (Rugby)	**Ointment:** 0.5%	In 15 g.	6.4+
Rx	**Aristocort** (Fujisawa)		White petrolatum base. In 15 and 240 g.	38.8
Rx	**Flutex** (Syosset)		White petrolatum and mineral oil base. In 30 g.	6.7
Rx	**Kenalog** (Squibb)		Mineral oil gel base. In 20 g.	37

* Cost Index based on cost per g.
[1] Contains methyl and butyl parabens.

(Continued on following page)

Complete prescribing information for these products begins on page 2370

TRIAMCINOLONE ACETONIDE (Cont.)			C.I.*
Rx **Triamcinolone Acetonide** (Various, eg, Balan, Bioline, Geneva, Goldline, Major, Moore, Parmed, Rugby, Schein, URL)	**Cream:** 0.025%	In 15, 80 and 454 g.	1+
Rx **Aristocort** (Fujisawa)		In 15 and 60 g.	5.5
Rx **Aristocort A** (Fujisawa)		Water washable. Glycerin, 2% benzyl alcohol. In 15 and 60 g.	8.6
Rx **Flutex** (Syosset)		Mineral oil, lanolin alcohol, sodium bisulfite. In 60 g.	1.9
Rx **Kenalog** (Squibb)		Vanishing, white petrolatum base. In 15, 80 and 240 g.	7.6
Rx **Triamcinolone Acetonide** (Various, eg, Balan, Bioline, Geneva, Goldline, Major, Moore, Parmed, Rugby, Schein, URL)	**Cream:** 0.1%	In 15, 30, 80 and 454 g.	1.3+
Rx **Aristocort** (Fujisawa)		In 15, 60 and 240 g.	8.7
Rx **Aristocort A** (Fujisawa)		Hydrophilic, water washable base. Glycerin. In 15, 60 and 240 g.	11.3
Rx **Flutex** (Syosset)		Mineral oil, lanolin alcohol, sodium bisulfite. In 30, 60 and 120 g.	3.6
Rx **Kenalog** (Squibb)		Vanishing, white petrolatum base. In 15, 60, 80 and 240 g.	10.9
Rx **Kenalog-H** (Squibb)		Hydrophilic vanishing base. White petrolatum. In 15 and 60 g.	8.1
Rx **Triacet** (Lemmon)		Vanishing base. In 15 and 80 g.	1.4
Rx **Triderm** (Del-Rey)		Mineral oil. In 30 and 90 g.	2
Rx **Triamcinolone Acetonide** (Various, eg, Balan, Bioline, Geneva, Goldline, Major, Moore, Parmed, Rugby, Schein, URL)	**Cream:** 0.5%	In 15 g.	5.6+
Rx **Aristocort** (Fujisawa)		In 15 and 240 g.	38.6
Rx **Aristocort A** (Fujisawa)		Hydrophilic base. Glycerin, 2% benzyl alcohol. In 15 g.	48.5
Rx **Flutex** (Syosset)		Mineral oil, lanolin alcohols, sodium bisulfite. In 30 and 240 g.	2.9
Rx **Kenalog** (Squibb)		Vanishing, white petrolatum base. In 20 g.	26.1
Rx **Triamcinolone Acetonide** (Various, eg, Balan, Barre-National, Major, PBI, Rugby, Schein)	**Lotion:** 0.025%	In 60 ml.	3.5+
Rx **Kenalog** (Squibb)		In 60 ml.	8.9
Rx **Triamcinolone Acetonide** (Various, eg, Balan, Barre-National, Geneva, Goldline, Major, PBI, Rugby, Schein)	**Lotion:** 0.1%	In 15 and 60 ml.	3.7+
Rx **Kenalog** (Squibb)		In 15 and 60 ml.	20
Rx **Kenalog** (Squibb)	**Aerosol:** 2 seconds of spray delivers ≈ 0.2 mg	10.3% alcohol with isopropyl palmitate. In 23 and 63 g.	10.7

* Cost Index based on cost per g or ml.

The following products contain corticosteroids in combination with various other components. They are indicated for a variety of specific and nonspecific dermatoses. For further information see individual monographs. Components of these formulations include:

HYDROCORTISONE, used for its anti-inflammatory, antipruritic and vasoconstrictive effects.

IODOCHLORHYDROXYQUIN, IODOQUINOL and *OXYQUINOLINE* are used for their antifungal, antibacterial and anti-eczematous effects.

LIDOCAINE, DIPERODON, PRAMOXINE HCl and *BENZOCAINE* are used as local anesthetics.

ZINC OXIDE is used as a mild astringent.

MENTHOL is a counterirritant, anesthetic and mild antiseptic.

UREA is a mild keratolytic and hydrates dry skin.

PYRILAMINE, CHLORPHENIRAMINE and *CHLORCYCLIZINE* are antihistamines.

EPHEDRINE is a vasoconstrictor.

BENZOYL PEROXIDE is used for its peeling and drying effects.

	Product & Distributor	Hydrocortisone (%)	Iodochlor-hydroxyquin (%)	Pramoxine (%)	Other Content and How Supplied	C.I.*
Rx	**UAD Lotion** (UAD)	0.25	0.75	†	Cetyl alcohol, glyceryl stearate, lanolin, parabens, mineral oil, propylene glycol. In 120 ml.	NA
Rx	**Hydrocortisone with Iodochlorhydroxyquin Cream** (Various, eg, Moore, Rugby)	0.5	3		In 30 g.	13.3+
Rx	**Ala-Quin Cream** (Del-Ray)				Glycerin. In 30 g	32.8
Rx	**Racet Cream** (Lemmon)				Petrolatum base. With parabens. In 15 & 30 g.	41.8
Rx	**Vioform-Hydrocortisone Mild Cream** (Ciba)				Water washable base. Petrolatum, glycerin. In 15 and 30 g.	99.8
Rx	**Hydrocortisone with Iodochlorhydroxyquin Cream** (Various, eg, Goldline, Moore, Schein, URL)	1	3		In 20, 30 and 480 g.	20.7+
Rx	**Corque Cream** (Geneva)				Mineral oil base. With parabens. In 20 g.	132
Rx	**Cortin Cream** (C & M)				Glycerin and petrolatum base. In 20 g.	104.2
Rx	**Hysone Cream** (Hauck)				Water washable. Mineral oil, lanolin alcohol base. With parabens. In 20 g.	333
Rx	**Lanvisone Cream** (Lannett)				Greaseless. In 20 g.	25
Rx	**Pedi-Cort V Cream** (Pedinol)				In 20 g.	65.5
Rx	**Vioform-Hydrocortisone Cream** (Ciba)				Water washable base. Petrolatum, glycerin. In 20 g.	150.5
Rx	**Hydrocortisone with Iodochlorhydroxyquin Ointment** (Various, eg, Moore, Rugby)	1	3		In 20 and 480 g.	121+
Rx	**Vioform-Hydrocortisone Ointment** (Ciba)				Petrolatum base. In 20 g.	150.5
Rx	**Dermarex Cream** (Hyrex)	1	3	†	Parabens, mineral oil. In 15 g.	93.7
Rx	**UAD Cream** (UAD)				Ceresin, glyceryl oleate, propylene glycol, parabens, mineral oil. In 15 g.	NA
Rx	**1 + 1-F Creme** (Dunhall)	1	3	1	Mineral oil, lanolin alcohol, parabens. In 30 g.	55.5

* Cost Index based on cost per g. † Amount not supplied by manufacturer.

(Continued on following page)

	Product & Distributor	Hydrocortisone (%)	Pramoxine (%)	Other Content	How Supplied	C.I.*
Rx	**Pramosone Cream** (Ferndale)	0.5[1]	1	Hydrophilic base	In 30 g.	36.8
Rx	**Pramosone Lotion** (Ferndale)	0.5[1]	1	Hydrophilic base, glycerin	In 60, 120 and 240 ml.	54.8
Rx	**Analpram-HC Cream** (Ferndale Labs)	1[1]	1		In 30 g.	54.8
Rx	**Pramosone Cream** (Ferndale)			Hydrophilic base	In 30 and 120 g.	43.7
Rx	**ProctoCream-HC Cream** (Reed & Carnrick)			Hydrophilic base	In 30 g.	8
Rx	**Pramosone Ointment** (Ferndale)	1[1]	1	Emollient white petrolatum base	In 30 and 120 g.	77.3
Rx	**Pramosone Lotion** (Ferndale)	1[1]	1	Hydrophilic base, glycerin	In 60, 120 and 240 ml.	34.5
Rx	**Epifoam Aerosol Foam** (Reed & Carnrick)	1[1]	1	With parabens	In 10 g.	199.5
Rx	**ProctoFoam-HC Aerosol Foam** (Reed & Carnrick)			Hydrophilic base with parabens	In 10 g.	20.4
Rx	**Analpram-HC Cream** (Ferndale Labs)	2.5[1]	1		In 30 g.	NA
Rx	**Pramosone Cream** (Ferndale)			Hydrophilic base	In 30 and 120 g.	71.8
Rx	**Pramosone Ointment** (Ferndale)			Emollient white petrolatum base	In 30 and 120 g.	77.3
Rx	**Pramosone Lotion** (Ferndale)			Hydrophilic base, glycerin	In 60 and 120 ml.	56.5
Rx	**Allersone Ointment** (Hauck)	0.5		0.5% diperodon HCl, 5% zinc oxide, white petrolatum	Water washable. In 15 g and lb.	43.6
Rx	**Lida-Mantle-HC Cream** (Miles Inc.)	0.5[1]		3% lidocaine, glycerin, parabens	In 30 g.	230
otc	**HC Derma-Pax Liquid** (Recsei)	0.5		0.44% pyrilamine maleate, 0.06% chlorpheniramine maleate	In 60, 128 and 480 ml.	1
Rx	**Vanoxide-HC Lotion** (Dermik)	0.5		5% benzoyl peroxide, mineral oil	Water washable. In 25 ml.	102
Rx	**Mantadil Cream** (Burroughs Wellcome)	0.5[1]		2% chlorcyclizine HCl, 0.25% methylparaben, white petrolatum	Vanishing base. In 15 g.	183.7
Rx	**Fungoid-HC** (Pedinol)	0.5		Cetyl pyridinium chloride, triacetin chloroxylenol	Vanishing base. In 30 g.	NA
Rx	**Carmol HC Cream** (Syntex)	1[1]		10% urea	Vanishing base. In 30 and 120 g.	69
Rx	**Medicone Derma-HC Ointment** (Medicone)	1[1]		2% benzocaine, 1% oxyquinoline sulfate, 0.1% ephedrine, 0.5% menthol, 1% ichthammol, 13.6% zinc oxide, petrolatum, lanolin	In 7 and 20 g.	88.2
Rx	**Vytone Cream** (Dermik)	1		1% iodoquinol	Greaseless base. In 30 g.	92.8

* Cost Index based on cost per g or ml.

[1] Hydrocortisone acetate.

Consider the information for Topical Corticosteroids, Antibiotics and for Antifungals when using these products (see individual monographs).

		Dosage form	Corticosteroid	Neomycin Sulfate	Other	Base/ How Supplied	C.I.*
Rx	**Neo-Cortef** (Upjohn)	Cream	1% hydrocortisone	0.5%		Water soluble, non-greasy vanishing base. With 0.1% methyl and 0.4% butyl parabens. In 20 g.	8.2
Rx	**Neo-Synalar** (Syntex)		0.025% fluocinolone acetonide	0.5%		Water washable base. Mineral oil, EDTA. With methyl and propyl parabens. In 15, 30 and 60 g.	6.9
Rx	**Cordran-N** (Dista)		0.05% flurandrenolide	0.5%		Mineral oil, glycerin. With parabens. In 15, 30 and 60 g.	6.4
Rx	**Neodecadron** (MSD)		0.1% dexamethasone phosphate	0.5%		Greaseless base. Mineral oil, 0.15% methylparaben, 0.18% sodium bisulfite, EDTA. In 15 and 30 g.	4.6
Rx	**Cortisporin** (Burroughs Wellcome)		0.5% hydrocortisone acetate	0.5%	10,000 units polymyxin B sulfate per g	Petrolatum, 0.25% methylparaben. In 7.5 g.	14.8
Rx	**Myco-Biotic II** (Moore)		0.1% triamcinolone acetonide		100,000 units nystatin per g	Aqueous vanishing base. White petrolatum. In 15, 30, 60 g and lb.	1
Rx	**Neo-Medrol Acetate** (Upjohn)	Lipid Base	0.25% methylprednisolone acetate	0.5%		Methyl and butyl parabens. In 30 g.	1
Rx	**Neo-Medrol Acetate** (Upjohn)		1% methylprednisolone acetate	0.5%		Methyl and butyl parabens. In 30 g.	2
Rx	**Neo-Cortef** (Upjohn)	Ointment	0.5% hydrocortisone acetate	0.5%		White petrolatum, mineral oil, parabens. In 20 g.	4.6
Rx	**Hydrocortisone-Neomycin** (Various, eg, Balan, Rugby)		1% hydrocortisone	0.5%		In 20 g.	1+
Rx	**Neo-Cortef** (Upjohn)		1% hydrocortisone acetate	0.5%		White petrolatum, mineral oil, parabens. In 20 g.	7.9
Rx	**Cordran-N** (Dista)		0.05% flurandrenolide	0.5%		White petrolatum base. In 15, 30 and 60 g.	5.6
Rx	**Cortisporin** (Burroughs Wellcome)		1% hydrocortisone	0.5%	400 units bacitracin zinc and 5000 units polymyxin B sulfate per g	White petrolatum base. In 15 g.	5.2

* Cost Index based on cost per g.

Consider the information given for Corticosteroids, Topical and for Antifungals, Topical when using these products.

		Dosage form	Corticosteroid	Antifungal	Base/How Supplied	C.I.*
Rx	**Fungoid-HC** (Pedinol)	Cream	0.5% hydrocortisone	triacetin, cetyl pyridinium Cl[1], chloroxylenol[1,2]	Vanishing base. In 30 g.	NA
Rx	**Lotrisone** (Schering)		0.05% betamethasone (as dipropionate)	1% clotrimazole	Hydrophilic, emollient base. Mineral oil, white petrolatum and benzyl alcohol. In 15 and 45 g.	9.7
Rx	**Nystatin-Triamcinolone Acetonide** (Various, eg, NMC Labs, Pharmaderm, Pharmafair)		0.1% triamcinolone acetonide	100,000 units nystatin per g	In 15, 30, 60 and 120 g.	1+
Rx	**Derma Comb** (Taro)				Aqueous, vanishing base. White petrolatum, alcohol ether. With parabens. In 15, 30 and 60 g.	1.6
Rx	**Mycogen** II (Goldline)				Aqueous vanishing base with white petrolatum. In 15, 30, 60 and 120 g and lb.	2.3
Rx	**Mycolog**-II (Squibb)				Aqueous, vanishing base. White petrolatum. In 15, 30, 60 and 120 g.	8.8
Rx	**Myco-Triacet** II (Lemmon)				Aqueous, vanishing base. White petrolatum and parabens. In 15, 30 and 60 g.	2.5
Rx	**Mytrex** (Savage)				White petrolatum, benzyl alcohol and alcohol ether. In 15, 30 and 60 g.	4.7
Rx	**N.G.T.** (Geneva)				Aqueous vanishing base. White petrolatum. In 15, 30 and 60 g.	2.2
Rx	**Tri-Statin** II (Rugby)				White petrolatum, parabens. In 15, 30, 60, 120 and 480 g.	27
Rx	**Nystatin-Triamcinolone Acetonide** (Various, eg, Fougera, NMC Labs, Pharmaderm, Pharmafair)	Ointment	0.1% triamcinolone acetonide	100,000 units nystatin per g	In 15, 30, 60 and 120 g.	1+
Rx	**Mycogen** II (Goldline)				Mineral oil and white petrolatum base. In 15, 30 and 60 g.	2.3
Rx	**Mycolog**-II (Squibb)				Mineral oil base. In 15, 30, 60 and 120 g.	8.8
Rx	**Myco-Triacet** II (Lemmon)				White petrolatum and mineral oil. In 15 and 30 g.	2.3
Rx	**Mytrex** (Savage)				Mineral oil base. In 15, 30 and 60 g.	4.7

* Cost Index based on cost per g. [1]Anti-infective agent. [2]Antibacterial, antiseptic.

Since topical anesthetics are available in various forms, products are grouped according to their intended site of application: Topical Anesthetics for Skin Disorders and Topical Anesthetics for Mucous Membranes.

In addition to the single entity products listed in this section, other products containing topical local anesthetics are listed in other sections, based on their specific uses. These include: Anorectal Preparations and Ophthalmic Local Anesthetics (see individual monographs).

Because of the diversity of uses of these products, the following is a general discussion. For information on specific applications of individual products, consult the manufacturer's package literature.

Actions:

Local anesthetics inhibit conduction of nerve impulses from sensory nerves. This action results from an alteration of the cell membrane permeability to ions. Although poorly absorbed through the intact epidermis, these agents are readily absorbed from mucous membranes. When skin permeability has been increased by abrasions or ulcers, the absorption and, subsequently, the efficacy of local anesthetics improves; however, the incidence of side effects also increases.

Topical Local Anesthetics: Indications, Dose, Strength, Peak Effect and Duration

Local anesthetics, topical	Indications		Maximum adult dose (mg)	Available or recommended strengths (%)	Peak[1] effect (minutes)	Duration[1] of effect (minutes)
	Skin	Mucous membrane				
Amides						
Dibucaine	✓		25	0.5-1	< 15	180-240
Lidocaine	✓	✓	750	2-5	2-5	30-60
Esters						
Benzocaine	✓	✓	5000	0.5-20	1	30-60
Butamben picrate	✓			1		
Cocaine		✓	50	4-10	2-5	30-120
Tetracaine	✓	✓	50	0.5-2	3-8	30-60
Miscellaneous						
Dyclonine		✓	100	0.5-1	< 10	< 60
Pramoxine	✓		200	1	3-5	

[1] Based primarily on application to mucous membranes.

Indications:

Skin disorders: For topical anesthesia in local skin disorders, including: Pruritus and pain due to minor burns, fungus infections, skin manifestations of systemic disease (eg, chickenpox), prickly heat, diaper rash, abrasions, sunburn, plant poisoning, insect bites, eczema.

Mucous membranes: For local anesthesia of accessible mucous membranes, including: Oral, nasal and laryngeal mucous membranes; respiratory or urinary tracts. Also for the treatment of pruritus ani, pruritus vulvae and hemorrhoids.

Contraindications:

Hypersensitivity to any component of these products; ophthalmic use.

Warnings:

Systemic effects: Use the lowest dose effective for anesthesia to avoid high plasma levels and serious adverse effects. Repeated doses of **lidocaine** and **dyclonine** may cause significant increases in blood levels with each repeated dose because of slow accumulation of the drug or its metabolites. Have resuscitative equipment available for immediate use.

Pregnancy: Category B (lidocaine). Safety for use during pregnancy has not been established. Use in women of childbearing potential, and particularly in early pregnancy, only when the potential benefits outweigh the potential hazards to the fetus.

Precautions:

Minimal effective dose: Reactions and complications are best averted by using the minimal effective dose. Give debilitated or elderly patients, acutely ill patients and children dosages commensurate with their age, size and physical condition.

Severe shock/heartblock: Use **lidocaine** and **dyclonine** with caution.

Use cautiously in persons with known drug sensitivities or in patients with severely traumatized mucosa and sepsis in the region of the application. If irritation or rash occurs, discontinue treatment and institute appropriate therapy.

(Precautions continued on following page)

Precautions (Cont.):

Oral use: Topical anesthetic agents may impair swallowing and enhance the danger of aspiration. Do not ingest food for 1 hour following use of anesthetics in the mouth or throat. This is particularly important in children because of their frequency of eating.

Tartrazine sensitivity: Some of these products contain tartrazine, which may cause allergic-type reactions (including bronchial asthma) in susceptible individuals. Although the incidence of tartrazine sensitivity in the general population is low, it is frequently seen in patients who also have aspirin hypersensitivity. Specific products containing tartrazine are identified in the product listings.

Sulfite sensitivity: Some of these products contain sulfites which may cause allergic-type reactions including anaphylactic symptoms and life-threatening or less severe asthmatic episodes in certain susceptible persons. The overall prevalence of sulfite sensitivity in the general population is unknown and probably low. Sulfite sensitivity is seen more frequently in asthmatic or atopic non-asthmatic persons. Specific products containing sulfites are identified in the product listings.

Adverse Reactions:

Adverse reactions are, in general, dose-related and may result from high plasma levels due to excessive dosage or rapid absorption, hypersensitivity, idiosyncrasy or diminished tolerance. (See Overdosage.)

Allergic: Cutaneous lesions; urticaria; edema; contact dermatitis; anaphylactoid reactions. The detection of sensitivity by skin testing is of doubtful value.

Local: Burning; stinging; tenderness; sloughing.

Miscellaneous: Urethritis with and without bleeding. Methemoglobinemia characterized by cyanosis has followed topical application of **benzocaine** or **lidocaine** for teething discomfort and as a laryngeal anesthetic spray. Seizures in children have occurred from overuse of **oral lidocaine**.

Overdosage:

Symptoms: Reactions due to overdosage (high plasma levels) are systemic and involve the CNS (convulsions) or the cardiovascular system (hypotension).

CNS – Reactions are excitatory or depressant, and may be characterized by: Nervousness; apprehension; euphoria; confusion; dizziness; lightheadedness; tinnitus; blurred vision; vomiting; sensations of heat, cold or numbness; twitching; tremors; drowsiness; convulsions; unconsciousness; respiratory depression or arrest. The excitatory reactions may be very brief or may not occur at all; in this case, the first manifestation of toxicity may be drowsiness, merging into unconsciousness and respiratory arrest.

Cardiovascular – Reactions are depressant, and may be characterized by: Hypotension; myocardial depression; bradycardia; cardiac arrest; cardiovascular collapse.

Treatment: Maintain an airway and support ventilation. Supportive treatment of the cardiovascular system consists of vasopressors, preferably those that stimulate the myocardium, IV fluids and perhaps blood transfusions. Convulsions may be controlled by the slow IV administration of 0.1 mg/kg diazepam or 10 to 50 mg succinylcholine, with continued oxygen administration. Refer to General Management of Acute Overdosage.

Methemoglobinemia may be treated with methylene blue 1%, 0.1 ml/kg IV over 10 minutes (refer to individual monograph).

Patient Information:

Do not ingest food for 1 hour following use of oral topical anesthetic preparations in the mouth or throat. Topical anesthesia may impair swallowing, thus enhancing the danger of aspiration.

Numbness of the tongue or buccal mucosa may increase the danger of biting trauma. Do not eat or chew gum while the mouth or throat area is anesthetized.

Administration and Dosage:

Topical: Apply to the affected area as needed. Ointments and creams can be applied to gauze or to a bandage prior to applying to the skin.

Mucous membranes: Dosage varies and depends upon the area to be anesthetized, vascularity of tissues, individual tolerance and technique of anesthesia. Administer the lowest dose possible that still provides adequate anesthesia. Apply to affected areas using the proper technique (see individual manufacturer inserts).

In debilitated, elderly patients or children, administer lower concentrations.

A combination of tetracaine 0.5%, epinephrine 1:2000 and cocaine 11.8% (also known as TAC) in a liquid topical formulation has been used for minor skin lacerations, especially of the face and scalp. Use results in decreased level of pain on application, allowing for better compliance and tolerance of repair procedure. This may be beneficial in patients who cannot tolerate injection anesthesia or those who are difficult to control (eg, children).

(Products listed on following pages)

Refer to the general discussion of these products beginning on page 2387

Topical Anesthetics for Skin Disorders

BENZOCAINE (Ethyl Aminobenzoate)				C.I.*
otc	**Americaine Anesthetic** (Fisons)	**Spray:** 20%	In 20, 60 and 120 g aerosol.	13
otc	**Dermoplast** (Whitehall)	**Aerosol:** 20% with 0.5% menthol, m-paraben, aloe, lanolin	In 82.5 ml.	5
otc	**Lanacane** (Combe)	**Spray:** 20% with 0.1% benzethonium Cl, 30% ethanol, aloe extract	In 120 ml.	2.8
otc	**Dermoplast** (Whitehall)	**Lotion:** 8% with 0.5% menthol, parabens, lanolin	In 90 ml.	41
otc	**Solarcaine** (Schering-Plough)	**Aerosol:** 20% with 0.13% triclosan, 35% SD alcohol 40	In 90 and 150 ml.	3.9
otc	**Bicozene** (Sandoz)	**Cream:** 6% with 1.67% resorcinol	In 28.4 g.	8.4
otc	**Foille Plus** (Blistex)	**Aerosol:** 5% with 0.6% chloroxylenol, 57.33% alcohol	In 105 g.	2.4
otc	**Foille** (Blistex)	**Spray:** 5% with 0.63% chloroxylenol	In 97.5 ml.	13
otc	**Benzocaine** (Various, eg, IDE, Schein)	**Cream:** 5%	In 30 g and 1 lb.	4.9+
otc	**Benzocol** (Hauck)	**Cream:** 5% in a greaseless cream base	In 30 g and lb.	7.2
otc	**Foille Medicated First Aid** (Blistex)	**Ointment:** 5% with 0.1% chloroxylenol, benzyl alcohol, EDTA in a corn oil base	In 3.5 and 28 g.	5.9
		Aerosol: 5% with 0.6% chloroxylenol, benzyl alcohol in corn oil base	In 92 ml.	2.6
otc	**Unguentine** (Mentholatum)	**Aerosol:** 0.99 g/oz, alcohol, isobutane, menthol	In 90 ml.	3.4
otc	**Chigger-Tox** (Scherer)	**Liquid:** Benzocaine with benzyl benzoate and soft soap in an isopropanol base	In 30 ml.	8
otc	**Solarcaine** (Schering-Plough)	**Lotion:** Benzocaine with triclosan, mineral oil, menthol, camphor, benzyl alcohol, parabens, EDTA	In 120 ml.	3.1
otc	**Lanacane Creme** (Combe)	**Cream:** Benzocaine, benzethonium Cl, parabens	In 30 and 60 g.	7.6

* Cost Index based on cost per g or ml.

Refer to the general discussion of these products beginning on page 2387

Topical Anesthetics for Skin Disorders (Cont.)

	Product	Form	Description	C.I.*
DIBUCAINE				
otc	**Dibucaine** (Various, eg, Fougera, IDE, Lannett, Major, Moore, NMC, Rugby, URL)	**Ointment:** 1%	In 30 g and lb.	5+
otc	**Nupercainal** (Ciba)		Acetone sodium bisulfites, lanolin, mineral oil, white petrolatum. In 30 and 60 g.	124
otc	**Nupercainal** (Ciba)	**Cream:** 0.5%	Acetone sodium bisulfite. In 45 g.	2.7
LIDOCAINE				
Rx	**Lidocaine HCl** (Moore)	**Ointment:** 5%	In 50 g.	4.4
otc	**Xylocaine** (Astra)	**Ointment:** 2.5%	In water soluble carbowaxes. In 37.5 g.	22
otc	**Solarcaine** (Schering-Plough)	**Cream:** 0.5%	Lanolin, camphor, parabens, EDTA, menthol. In 120 g.	2.2
BUTAMBEN PICRATE				
otc	**Butesin Picrate** (Abbott)	**Ointment:** 1%	Lanolin, parabens, mineral oil. In 28.4 g.	19
TETRACAINE				
otc	**Pontocaine** (Winthrop)	**Ointment:** 0.5% tetracaine base	White petrolatum, light mineral oil. In 30 g.	19
		Cream: 1% (as HCl)	Water miscible base with light mineral oil, paraben, sodium metabisulfite. In 28.35 g.	21
PRAMOXINE HCl				
otc	**Tronothane HCl** (Abbott)	**Cream:** 1%	Water miscible base with parabens. In 28.4 g.	19
otc	**PrameGel** (GenDerm)	**Liquid:** 1%	Emollient base with 0.5% menthol, benzyl alcohol, SD alcohol 40. In 118 ml.	5.1
otc	**Prax** (Ferndale)	**Lotion:** 1%	Hydrophilic base with mineral oil, lanolin, 0.1% potassium sorbate, 0.1% sorbic acid. In 15, 120 and 240 ml.	4.4
		Cream: 1%	Hydrophilic base with white petrolatum. In 30 and 113.4 g and 1 lb.	2.4
otc	**Itch-X** (Ascher & Co.)	**Gel:** 1%	10% benzyl alcohol. In 37.5 g	10
otc	**Phicon** (T.E. Williams)	**Cream:** 0.5%	7500 IU vitamin A and 2000 IU vitamin E/30 g. In 60 g.	13

* Cost Index based on cost per g or ml.

Refer to the general discussion of these products beginning on page 2387

Topical Anesthetics for Skin Disorders (Cont.)

MISCELLANEOUS TOPICAL ANESTHETICS

	Product	Description	How supplied	C.I.*
Rx	**Ethyl Chloride** (Gebauer)	**Spray**: Chloroethane **Indications:** Topical vapo-coolant to control pain associated with minor surgical procedures (eg, lancing boils, incision and drainage of small abscesses), athletic injuries, injections and for treatment of myofascial pain, restricted motion and muscle spasm	In 100 g metal tubes, 105 ml bottles with atomizer, 120 ml bottles (fine, medium, coarse & spray pak nozzles).	5
Rx	**Fluro-Ethyl** (Gebauer)	**Aerosol spray**: 25% ethyl chloride and 75% dichlorotetrafluoroethane **Indications:** Topical refrigerant anesthetic to control pain associated with minor surgical procedures, dermabrasion, injections, contusions and minor strains	In 270 ml.	3.4
Rx	**Fluori-Methane** (Gebauer)	**Spray**: 15% dichlorodifluoromethane and 85% trichloromonofluoro methane. **Indications:** Vapo-coolant for topical application in management of myofascial pain, restricted motion and muscle spasm, and for control of pain associated with injections	In 120 ml glass bottles (fine or medium spray).	7.7

* Cost Index based on cost per g or ml.

Refer to the general discussion of these products beginning on page 2387

Topical Anesthetics for Mucous Membranes

LIDOCAINE HCl				C.I.*
Rx	**Xylocaine 10% Oral** (Astra)	**Spray:** 10% *For* topical anesthesia of the mucous membranes of the mouth and oropharynx.	Saccharin, absolute alcohol. In 26.8 ml aerosol.	64
Rx	**Xylocaine** (Astra)	**Ointment:** 5% *For* anesthesia of accessible mucous membranes of the oropharynx; anesthetic lubricant for intubation; for temporary relief of pain of minor burns, skin abrasions and insect bites.	Saccharin (flavored only). Flavored and unflavored. In 3.5 and 35 g.	22
Rx	**Lidocaine HCl Topical**[1] (Various, eg, Moore, Roxane)	**Solution:** 4% *For* topical anesthesia of accessible mucous membranes of the oral and nasal cavities and proximal portions of the digestive tract.	In 50 ml.	13+
Rx	**Xylocaine** (Astra)		Parabens. In 50 ml.	19
Rx	**Lidocaine 2% Viscous**[2] (Various, eg, Moore, Roxane)	**Solution:** 2% *For* topical anesthesia of irritated or inflamed mucous membranes of the mouth and pharynx. Also used to reduce gagging during the taking of x-rays or dental impressions.	In 50 and 100 ml and UD 20 ml.	3.4+
Rx	**Xylocaine Viscous** (Astra)		Sodium carboxymethylcellulose, parabens, saccharin. In 100 and 450 ml & UD 20 ml (25s).	9.4
Rx	**Xylocaine** (Astra)	**Jelly:** 2% *For* prevention and control of pain in procedures involving the male and female urethra, for topical treatment of painful urethritis and as an anesthetic lubricant for endotracheal intubation.	Hydroxypropylmethylcellulose base, parabens. In 30 ml.	29
Rx	**Anestacon** (Webcon)	**Solution:** 2% *For* prevention and control of pain in procedures involving the male and female urethra and for topical treatment of painful urethritis.	1% hydroxypropylmethylcellulose, 0.01% benzalkonium chloride. In 15 and 240 ml disposable units.	12

* Cost Index based on cost per g or ml.

[1] May contain parabens.

[2] May contain sodium carboxymethylcellulose.

Refer to the general discussion of these products beginning on page 2387

Topical Anesthetics for Mucous Membranes

BENZOCAINE (Ethyl Aminobenzoate)				C.I.*
otc	**Maximum Strength Anbesol** (Whitehall)	**Liquid**: 20%	60% alcohol, saccharin. In 9 ml.	NA
		Gel: 20%	60% alcohol, saccharin. In 7.5 g.	NA
otc	**Hurricaine** (Beutlich)	**Liquid or Gel**: 20%	Cherry or pina colada flavor. In 3.75 and 30 ml (liquid), 3.75 and 30 g (gel).	216
		Spray: 20% *For* oral and mucosal anesthesia to control pain and suppress the gag reflex.	Cherry flavor. In 60 ml.	220
Rx	**Americaine Anesthetic Lubricant** (Fisons)	**Gel**: 20% *For* use as a lubricant and anesthetic on intratracheal catheters and pharyngeal and nasal airways; on nasogastric and endoscopic tubes; urinary catheters; laryngoscopes; proctoscopes; sigmoidoscopes; vaginal specula.	0.1% benzethonium chloride. In 2.5 and 30 g.	35
otc	**Orajel Mouth-Aid** (Commerce)	**Liquid**: 20%	0.1% cetylpyridinium chloride, 70% ethyl alcohol, tartrazine, saccharin. In 13.3 ml.	NA
otc	**ZilaDent** (Zila)	**Gel**: 6%	74.9% alcohol. In 7.5 g tube and single packets.	67
TETRACAINE HCl				
Rx	**Pontocaine HCl** (Winthrop)	**Solution**: 2% *For* anesthesia of nose and throat; also when the laryngeal and esophageal reflexes are to be abolished prior to performing bronchoscopy, bronchography and esophagoscopy.	0.4% chlorobutanol. In 30 and 118 ml.	34
DYCLONINE HCl				
Rx	**Dyclone** (Astra)	**Solution**: 0.5%	Chlorobutanol. In 30 ml.	58
		1% *For* anesthetizing mucous membranes (eg, the mouth, pharynx, larynx, trachea, esophagus and urethra) prior to endoscopic procedures. The 0.5% solution may be used to block the gag reflex and relieve pain associated with oral or anogenital lesions.	Chlorobutanol. In 30 ml.	78

* Cost Index based on cost per g or ml.

COCAINE

Actions:

Pharmacology: Cocaine is an alkaloid derived from the plant *Erythroxylon coca;* chemically, it is benzoylmethylecgonine. Following local application, cocaine blocks the initiation or conduction of the nerve impulse and causes intense vasoconstriction. It not only lessens sensibility to pain and touch but, when applied to the nose or mouth, diminishes the acuity of taste and smell. Its most striking systemic effect is general CNS stimulation, manifested in descending order of frequency as euphoria, stimulation, reduced fatigue, loquacity, sexual stimulation, increased mental ability, alertness and increased sociality. As the dose is increased, tremors and tonic-clonic convulsions may occur. In addition, vomiting centers may also be stimulated. Central stimulation is soon followed by depression. The medullary centers are eventually depressed; death results from respiratory failure.

Small doses of cocaine may slow the heart as a result of central sympathetic stimulation, but after moderate doses, the heart rate increases. Although blood pressure may finally fall, there is at first a prominent rise in blood pressure due to sympathetically mediated tachycardia and vasoconstriction.

Cocaine is markedly pyrogenic. It increases muscular activity which augments heat production; vasoconstriction decreases heat loss. Cocaine may also have a direct action on central heat regulating centers.

Cocaine interferes with the uptake of norepinephrine and dopamine by the presynaptic adrenergic nerve terminals; therefore, it may produce sensitization to catecholamines, causing vasoconstriction and mydriasis.

Pharmacokinetics: Absorption/Distribution – Cocaine is rapidly absorbed from all sites of application and absorption is enhanced in the presence of inflammation. When it is applied to mucous membranes, maximum local anesthesia occurs within 5 minutes. A 10% cocaine solution (1.5 mg/kg) applied to nasal mucosa yielded peak plasma levels in 15 to 60 minutes that declined over 3 to 5 hours. Peak effects occur in 2 to 5 minutes, persisting for 30 minutes. Absorption from mucous membranes may exceed the rate of metabolism and excretion.

Metabolism/Elimination – Cocaine is degraded in the liver to its principal metabolite, benzoylecgonine, which is then excreted in the urine. Cocaine is also metabolized by plasma cholinesterase. At therapeutic doses, $<$ 20% is excreted unchanged in the urine. Half-life is approximately 1 to 2.5 hours.

For comparative data of cocaine with other local anesthetics, refer to the Topical Local Anesthetics group monograph.

Indications:

Topical anesthesia for mucous membranes.

Contraindications:

Systemic use; hypersensitivity to cocaine; ophthalmologic anesthesia (see Warnings).

Warnings:

Dependence: Although cocaine does not produce true physical dependence with definite withdrawal symptoms, continual exposure creates an excessively strong psychological dependence, and sometimes depression, as an indirect effect. Chronic use may cause progression from euphoria to paranoid psychosis; included may be perceptual changes (halo lights) and intense pruritus ("cocaine bugs"). This drug produces the highest degree of psychic dependence seen among recreationally abused drugs; thus, cocaine does produce an addictive syndrome.

"Crack" is a form of cocaine that is prepared with ammonia to alkalinize the solution and precipitate alkaloidal cocaine, thereby making it suitable for smoking. This form of cocaine is widely abused, highly addictive and potentially lethal.

Treatment of dependence: In addition to behavior modification and supportive psychotherapy, several agents may help decrease withdrawal symptoms associated with cocaine abuse or dependence, including: Amantadine; bromocriptine; desipramine; mazindol; carbamazepine.

Systemic effects: Concentrations $>$ 4% are not advisable because of the potential for increasing the incidence and severity of systemic toxic reactions.

Ophthalmic use: Cocaine causes sloughing of the corneal epithelium, causing clouding, pitting and occasionally, ulceration of the cornea. Ophthalmic use is contraindicated.

Elderly: Because elderly patients with vascular disease may be sensitive to the vasoconstrictive effects of the drug and may have slowed cocaine metabolism, a lower dosage is recommended.

(Warnings continued on following page)

COCAINE (Cont.)

Warnings (Cont.):

Pregnancy: Category C. Cocaine is not known to have direct adverse effects on the fetus. However, the anorexigenic effects may increase the risk of ketosis during pregnancy. Cocaine causes placental vasoconstriction, decreasing blood flow to the fetus. An increase in uterine contractility has occurred. A study compared 23 women who used cocaine only (n = 12) or cocaine plus narcotics (n = 11) during pregnancy with a group of women who were on methadone (n = 15) and a control group (n = 15). There was a higher rate of spontaneous abortion in the cocaine group. In addition, infants exposed to cocaine had depression of interactive behavior and a poor organizational response to environmental stimuli. In one retrospective trial, pregnant women who used "crack" delivered infants who were more likely to have a birth weight and head circumference under the tenth percentile for their gestational age. Abnormal mild neurobehavioral signs (eg, irritability, muscular rigidity, tremulousness) were also more prevalent after birth.

Women who use cocaine during pregnancy are at significant risk for shorter gestations, premature delivery, spontaneous abortions, abruptio placentae and death. Use only when clearly needed.

Lactation: Safety for use in the nursing mother has not been established. Cocaine is excreted in breast milk for up to 36 hours after the mother's last dose.

Because of the potential for serious adverse reactions in nursing infants from cocaine, it is recommended that nursing be discontinued for 2 days after drug use. Several case reports indicate that cocaine passes into breast milk, and that infants exposed via breastfeeding developed symptoms of cocaine toxicity within 3 hours (eg, tachycardia, tachypnea, hypertension, irritability, tremulousness). Strongly discourage cocaine use during breastfeeding.

Children: Safety and efficacy for use in children have not been established.

Convulsions have occurred in infants, who may be especially susceptible to cocaine-induced toxicity.

Precautions:

Limit administration to office and surgical procedures. Prolonged use of cocaine causes ischemic damage to nasal mucosa.

Use with caution in patients with severely traumatized mucosa and sepsis in the region of the proposed application. Use with caution in persons with known drug sensitivities.

Drug Interactions:

Epinephrine: Do not use with cocaine. The addition of epinephrine is not only unnecessary, but may increase the likelihood of arrhythmias, ventricular fibrillation and hypertensive episodes.

Adverse Reactions:

CNS reactions are excitatory or depressant. Nervousness, restlessness, euphoria, excitement, tremors and tonic-clonic convulsions may result. Central stimulation is followed by depression, with death resulting from respiratory failure.

Cardiovascular: Small doses of cocaine slow the heart rate; after moderate doses, the rate is increased due to central sympathetic stimulation. Hypertension, tachycardia, tachypnea and myocardial ischemia may occur.

(Continued on the following page)

Topical Anesthetics for Mucous Membranes (Cont.)

COCAINE (Cont.)

Overdosage:

Symptoms: Toxicity may occur following ingestion, parenteral administration, inhalation or absorption from topical administration to mucous membranes. Initial symptoms of acute poisoning are anxiety, restlessness, excitability, hallucinations, tachycardia, dilated pupils, chills or fever, abdominal pain, nausea, vomiting, muscle fasciculation, hyperreflexia, euphoria, mydriasis, hypertension, hyperthermia, cardiac arrhythmias, supraventricular and ventricular tachycardias, premature ventricular contractions; bigeminy, ventricular fibrillation, delirium, psychosis, seizures, strokes, numbness and muscular spasm, followed by irregular respirations, convulsions, coma and circulatory failure. Hypotension, bradycardia and respiratory failure have also occurred with cocaine toxicity. If acute poisoning ends in death, it occurs quickly, from minutes to a maximum of 3 hours.

Chronic poisoning may be similar, but long-term changes involve mental deterioration, weight loss, change of character and perhaps, perforated nasal septum from chronic sniffing of cocaine.

Fatal dose: 500 mg to 1.2 g orally. Severe toxic effects have occurred with doses as low as 20 mg.

Treatment: Maintain airway and respiration. If drug was ingested, attempt delay of absorption with activated charcoal, gastric lavage or emesis. Limit absorption from an injection site by tourniquet or ice pack. Control convulsions with diazepam (0.1 mg/kg orally or slow IV) or 2.5% thiopental sodium slowly IV; in severe cases, use pancuronium bromide or succinylcholine with mechanical ventilation. The drug of choice for tachycardia and other arrhythmias is propranolol (1 mg slowly IV, every 5 minutes, up to a dose of 5 to 8 mg) or lidocaine 1 mg/minute IV.

Maintain blood pressure with fluids (vasopressors are hazardous). For hypertensive reactions, give phentolamine, 5 mg slowly IV. Treat hyperthermia if it occurs.

Refer to General Management of Acute Overdosage. If the patient survives the first 3 hours after acute poisoning, recovery is likely.

Administration and Dosage:

Reduce dosages for children and for elderly and debilitated patients. Cocaine solution can be given by means of cotton applicators or packs, instilled into a cavity or as a spray.

For topical application (ear, nose, throat, bronchoscopy), concentrations of 1% to 4% are used. As a general guide, the maximum single dose should be 1 mg/kg. Concentrations > 4% are not advisable because of the potential for increased incidence and severity of systemic toxic reactions.

Preparation of a 4% solution: Dissolve 135 mg in 3.4 ml distilled water.

c-II	**Cocaine HCl Solvets** (Lilly)	**Soluble Tablets:** 135 mg	Lactose. In 100s.
c-II	**Cocaine HCl** (Roxane)	**Topical Solution:** 40 mg per ml 100 mg per ml	In 10 ml and UD 4 ml. In 10 ml and UD 4 ml.
c-II	**Cocaine Viscous** (Roxane)	**Topical Solution:** 4% per ml 10% per ml	In 10 ml multidose and UD 4 ml.
c-II	**Cocaine HCl** (Mallinckrodt)	**Powder:**	In 5 and 25 g.

Refer to the general discussion of these products beginning on page 2387

	Product	Composition	How supplied	C.I.*
otc	**Americaine First Aid** (Fisons)	**Ointment:** 20% benzocaine with benzethonium chloride	In 22.5 g.	9.4
otc	**Sting-Kill** (Kiwi)	**Swabs:** 18.9% benzocaine, 0.9% menthol	In 0.5 & 14 ml.	NA
Rx	**Cetacaine** (Cetylite)	14% benzocaine, 2% tetracaine HCl, 2% butamben and 0.5% benzalkonium chloride with 0.005% cetyl dimethyl ethyl ammonium bromide in a bland water soluble base	**Gel:** In 29 g. **Liquid:** In 56 ml. **Ointment:** In 37 g. **Aerosol:** In 56 g.	28 18 26 54
otc	**Aerocaine** (Aeroceuticals)	**Aerosol:** 13.6% benzocaine with 0.5% benzethonium Cl	In 15 and 75 ml.	2.4
otc	**Aerotherm** (Aeroceuticals)		In 150 ml.	2.4
otc	**Anbesol** (Whitehall)	**Liquid:** 6.3% benzocaine with 0.5% phenol, povidone-iodine, 70% alcohol, camphor, menthol	In 9.3 & 22.2 ml.	38
		Gel: 6.3% benzocaine, 0.5% phenol, 70% alcohol	In 7.5 g.	NA
otc	**Medicone Derma** (Medicone)	**Ointment:** 2% benzocaine, 13.73% zinc oxide, 1.05% 8-hydroxyquinoline sulfate, 1% ichthammol and 0.48% menthol in a 79.87% petrolatum-lanolin base	In 42.5 g.	9.4
otc	**Medicone Dressing** (Medicone)	**Cream:** 0.5% benzocaine, 0.05% 8-hydroxyquinoline sulfate, 12.5% cod liver oil, 12.5% zinc oxide and 0.18% menthol with 2.99% talcum, 1.66% paraffin in a 65.53% petrolatum-lanolin base	In 42.5 g.	9.4
otc	**Vagisil** (Combe)	**Cream:** Benzocaine and resorcin with lanolin alcohol, parabens, trisodium HEDTA, mineral oil and sodium sulfite	In 30 and 60 g.	6.7
otc	**Chiggerex** (Scherer)	**Ointment:** Benzocaine with camphor, menthol	In 50 g.	3.8
otc	**Dermacoat** (Century)	**Aerosol:** Benzocaine with p-chloro-m-xylenol, menthol, 20% isopropyl alcohol	In 210 g.	1.3
otc	**Skeeter Stik** (Triton)	**Liquid:** 4% lidocaine with 2% phenol in an isopropyl alcohol base	In 14 ml.	12
otc	**Bactine Antiseptic Anesthetic** (Miles)	2.5% lidocaine HCl, 0.13% benzalkonium chloride, EDTA, 3.17% alcohol	**Aerosol:** In 90 g. **Liquid:** In pt. **Spray:** In 60, 120 and 480 ml.	3.8 1 2.6
otc	**Unguentine Plus** (Mentholatum)	**Cream:** 2% lidocaine HCl with 2% chloroxylenol and 0.5% phenol, parabens, mineral oil	In 30 g.	6.8
otc	**Medi-Quik** (Mentholatum)	**Aerosol:** Lidocaine HCl and benzalkonium chloride	In 90 ml.	3.3
		Spray: 2% lidocaine, 0.13% benzalkonium chloride, 0.2% camphor, benzyl alcohol	In 85 ml.	2.4

* Cost Index based on cost per g, ml or swab.

DEXPANTHENOL

Indications:

Relieves itching and aids healing of skin in mild eczemas and dermatoses; itching skin, minor wounds, stings, bites, poison ivy, poison oak (dry stage) and minor skin irritations. Also used in infants and children for diaper rash, chafing and mild skin irritations.

Administration:

For external use only. Avoid contact with the eyes.

Apply to affected areas once or twice daily.

				C.I.*
otc	**Panthoderm** (Jones Medical)	**Cream:** 2% in a water miscible base	In 30 and 60 g.	286

UREA (Carbamide)

Indications:

To promote hydration and remove excess keratin in dry skin and hyperkeratotic conditions.

40% urea: Treatment of nail destruction and dissolution. It removes dystrophic and potentially disabling nails without local anesthesia and surgery.

Administration:

For external use only. Avoid contact with the eyes.

Apply 2 to 4 times daily to affected area or as directed by physician. Rub in completely.

40% urea: Cover surrounding surfaces. Generously apply directly to the diseased nail surface and cover with plastic film, wrap and anchor with adhesive tape. Cover with a "finger" cut from plastic or vinyl glove and anchor with more tape. Keep completely dry. Remove treated nails in either 3, 7 or 14 days. Nail bed usually hardens in 12 to 36 hours when left open to the air.

				C.I.*
otc	**Aquacare** (Menley & James)	**Cream:** 10%	Petrolatum, glycerin, lanolin oil, mineral oil, lanolin alcohol, benzyl alcohol. In 75 g.	86
otc	**Nutraplus** (Owen/Galderma)		Mineral oil, parabens. In lb.	86
otc	**Carmol 20** (Syntex)	**Cream:** 20%	Nonlipid vanishing cream base. In 90 g and lb.	71
otc	**Gormel Creme** (Gordon)		Mineral oil and parabens. In 75 and 120 g and lb.	71
otc	**Lanaphilic** (Medco)		Petrolatum, lanolin oil, PPG, lactic acid, parabens. In lb.	NA
otc	**Ureacin-20** (Pedinol)		Lactic acid, glycerin, mineral oil, parabens, EDTA. In 75 g.	100
Rx	**Gordon's Urea 40%** (Gordon)	**Cream:** 40%	Petrolatum base. In 30 g.	600
Rx	**Ureacin-40** (Pedinol)		Glycerin, parabens. In 30 g.	43
otc	**Aquacare** (Menley & James)	**Lotion:** 10%	Mineral oil, petrolatum, parabens. In 240 ml.	29
otc	**Nutraplus** (Owen/Galderma)		Lanolin alcohol, petrolatum, parabens. In 240 and 480 ml.	36
otc	**Carmol 10** (Syntex)		In 180 ml.	29
otc	**Ureacin-10** (Pedinol)		EDTA, parabens, lactic acid. In 240 ml.	29
otc	**Ultra Mide 25** (Baker Cummins)	**Lotion:** 25%	Mineral oil, glycerin, lanolin, EDTA. In 240 ml.	57

* Cost Index based on cost per g or ml.

VITAMINS A, D and E, TOPICAL

Indications:

For temporary relief of discomfort due to minor burns, sunburn, windburn, abrasions, chapped or chafed skin and other minor non-infected skin irritations including diaper rash and irritations associated with ileostomy and colostomy skin drainage.

Warnings:

For external use only. Avoid contact with the eyes.

Worsened condition: If the condition for which these preparations is used worsens or does not improve within 7 days, consult a physician.

Administration:

Apply locally to affected skin with gentle massage.

(Continued on following page)

VITAMINS A, D and E, TOPICAL (Cont.)

	Product	Form and contents	Packaging	C.I.*
otc	**Vitamin A & D** (Various, eg, Goldline, Rugby)	**Ointment**	In 60 g and lb.	29+
otc	**A and D** (Schering-Plough)	**Ointment:** Fish liver oil, cholecalciferol, lanolin, petrolatum, mineral oil	In 45, 120 and 480 g and 75 g pump dispenser.	29
otc	**Caldesene** (Fisons)	**Ointment:** Cod liver oil (vitamins A and D), 15% zinc oxide, lanolin oil, 54% petrolatum, parabens, talc	In 37.5 g.	71
otc	**Comfortine** (Dermik)	**Ointment:** Vitamins A and D, lanolin, zinc oxide, chloroxylenol, iron oxides, lanolin alcohol, mineral oil, triethanolamine, vegetable oil	In 45 and 120 g.	186
otc	**Desitin** (Pfizer)	**Ointment:** Cod liver oil (vitamins A and D), 40% zinc oxide, talc in a petrolatum-lanolin base	In 30, 60, 120, 240 and 270 g.	57
otc	**Lobana Peri-Garde** (Ulmer)	**Ointment:** Vitamins A, D and E and chloroxylenol in an emollient base	In 240 g.	71
otc	**Clocream** (Roberts)	**Cream:** Cod liver oil (vitamins A and D), cholecalciferol, vitamin A palmitate, cottonseed oil, glycerin, parabens, mineral oil	In a vanishing base. In 30 g.	114
otc	**Lazer Creme** (Pedinol)	**Cream:** Vitamins A (3333.3 units/g) and E (116.67 units/g)	In 60 g.	100
otc	**Lobana Derm-Ade** (Ulmer)	**Cream:** Vitamins A, D and E, moisturizers, emollients, silicone	In a vanishing base. In 270 g.	71
otc	**Retinol** (Nature's Bounty)	**Cream:** 100,000 IU vitamin A, glycol stearate, mineral oil, propylene glycol, lanolin oil, propylene glycol stearate SE, lanolin alcohol, retinol, parabens, EDTA	In 60 g.	NA
otc	**Aloe Grande** (Gordon)	**Lotion:** Vitamins A (3333.3 units/g) and E (50 units/g), petrolatum, mineral oil, sodium lauryl sulfate, oleic acid, parabens, triethanolamine, aloe	In 240 ml.	29

VITAMIN E

Indications:

Temporary relief of minor skin disorders such as diaper rash, burns, sunburn and chapped or dry skin.

Administration:

For external use only. Avoid contact with the eyes.

Apply a thin layer over affected area.

	Product	Form and contents	Packaging	C.I.*
otc	**E-Vitamin** (Forest)	**Ointment:** 30 mg d-alpha tocopheryl acetate per g, petrolatum, lanolin, rose oil	In 45 and 60 g.	257
otc	**Vitamin E** (Various, eg, Nature's Bounty)	**Cream**	In 60 g.	44+
otc	**Vitec** (Pharmaceutical Specialities)	**Cream:** dl-alpha tocopheryl acetate in a vanishing cream base, cetearyl alcohol, sorbitol, propylene glycol, simethicone, glyceryl monostearate, PEG monostearate	In 120 g.	86
otc	**Vite E Creme** (Gordon)	**Cream:** 50 mg dl-alpha tocopheryl acetate per g	In lb.	329
otc	**Vitamin E** (Various, eg, Nature's Bounty)	**Lotion**	In 120 ml.	NA
otc	**Vitamin E** (Various, eg, Mission, Nature's Bounty)	**Oil**	In 30 and 60 ml.[1]	271+

* Cost Index based on cost per g.

[1] May or may not contain aloe.

These preparations lubricate and moisturize the skin, counteracting dryness and itching.				C.I.*
otc	**Balmex** (Macsil)	**Ointment:** Bismuth subnitrate, zinc oxide, Balsam Peru, benzoic acid, beeswax, mineral oil, silicone, synthetic white wax	In 30, 60, 120 and 480 g.	52
otc	**Allercreme Ultra Emollient** (Carme[1])	**Cream:** Mineral oil, petrolatum, lanolin, lanolin alcohol, lanolin oil, glycerin, glyceryl stearate, PEG-100 stearate, squalane, parabens	Unscented. In 60 g.	185
otc	**Aveeno Moisturizing** (Rydelle)	**Cream:** 1% colloidal oatmeal, glycerin, petrolatum, dimethicone, phenylcarbinol	In 120 g.	50
otc	**Catrix Correction** (Donell DerMedex)	**Cream:** Dipentaerythrityl, hexacaprylate/hexacaprate, sesame oil, *Catrix* (bovine derived complex mucopolysaccharide), ceteareth-20, glycerin, caprylic/capric triglyceride, glycereth-7, dimethicone, xanthan gum, tocopheryl linoleate, alanine, glycine, urea, EDTA, imidazolidinyl urea, parabens, phenoxyethanol, orange oil, cardamon oil, titanium dioxide	In 36.9 g.	NA
otc	**Complex 15 Face** (Schering-Plough)	**Cream:** Caprylic/capric triglyceride, squalane, glycerin, glyceryl stearate, lecithin, PEG-50 stearate, propylene glycol, dimethicone, diazolidinyl urea, carbomer-934P, EDTA	In 75 g.	71
otc	**Complex 15 Hand & Body** (Schering-Plough)	**Cream:** Mineral oil, glycerin, squalane, caprylic/capric triglyceride, glycol stearate, PEG-50, carboxylic acid sterol ester, glyceryl stearate, lecithin, dimethicone, diazolidinyl urea, carbomer-934, EDTA	In 120 g.	110
otc	**Curel Moisturizing** (Rydelle)	**Cream:** Glycerin, petrolatum, dimethicone, parabens	In 90 g.	26
otc	**Cūtemol** (Summers)	**Cream:** Allantoin, mineral oil, acetylated lanolin, lanolin alcohols extract, mineral wax, beeswax, sorbitan sesquioleate, parabens	In 60 and 240 g.	94
otc	**DML Forte** (Person & Covey)	**Cream:** Petrolatum, PPG-2 myristyl ether propionate, glyceryl stearate, glycerin, simethicone, benzyl alcohol, silica, EDTA, sodium carbomer 1342	In 113 g.	51
otc	**Hydrisinol** (Pedinol)	**Cream:** Sulfonated hydrogenated castor oil, hydrogenated vegetable oil	In 120 g and lb.	64
otc	**Keri Creme** (Westwood)	**Cream:** Mineral oil, lanolin alcohol, talc, sorbitol, ceresin, propylene glycol, magnesium stearate, glyceryl oleate, parabens	In 75 g.	90
otc	**Lanolor** (Squibb)	**Cream:** Lanolin oil, glyceryl stearates, propylene glycol, sodium lauryl sulfate, simethicone, polyoxyl 40 stearate, cetyl esters wax, methylparaben	In 60 and 240 g.	73
otc	**Lubriderm** (Warner-Lambert)	**Cream:** Mineral oil, petrolatum, lanolin, lanolin alcohol, lanolin oil, glycerin, glyceryl stearate, PEG-100 stearate, sorbitan laurate, parabens	Scented and unscented. In 81 g.	NA
otc	**Massé Breast** (Advanced Care)	**Cream:** Glyceryl stearate, glycerin, peanut oil, sorbitan stearate, sodium benzoate, parabens. For care of the nipples of pregnant and nursing women	In 60 g.	119

* Cost Index based on cost per g or ml. [1] Carme, Inc., 84 Galli, Novato, CA, 94949, (800) 447-6758.

(Continued on following page)

				C.I.*
otc	**Nephro-Derm** (R&D Labs)	**Cream:** Camphor, menthol, *Eucerin,* glyceryl stearate, petrolatum, paraffin wax, mineral oil, vitamin B_{12}, polysorbate, parabens	In 113.6 g.	126
otc	**Neutrogena Norwegian Formula Hand** (Neutrogena)	**Cream:** Glycerin, sodium cetearyl sulfate, sodium sulfate, parabens	Scented and unscented. In 56.7 g.	NA
otc	**Nivea Ultra Moisturizing Creme** (Beiersdorf)	**Cream:** Mineral oil, petrolatum, glycerin, isohexadecane, microcrystalline wax, citric acid, paraffin, lanolin alcohol, magnesium sulfate, decyl oleate, octyldodecanol	In 60 and 120 g.	54
otc	**Nutraderm** (Owen/Galderma)	**Cream:** Mineral oil, sorbitan stearate, stearyl alcohol, sorbitol, citric acid, cetyl esters wax, sodium lauryl sulfate, dimethicone, parabens, diazolidinyl urea	In 90, 240 and 480 g.	61
otc	**Pedi-Vit-A Creme** (Pedinol)	**Cream:** 100,000 units vitamin A per 30 g	In 60 g.	114
otc	**Pen•Kera** (B.F. Ascher)	**Cream:** Glycerin, mineral oil, sorbitan stearate, urea, wheat germ glycerides, carbomer 940, triethanolamine, DMDM hydantoin, diazolidinyl urea	Dye and fragrance free. In 237 ml.	54
otc	**Phicon** (T.E. Williams)	**Cream:** 250 IU vitamin A and 66.7 IU E per g, aloe vera, 5% pramoxine HCl	In 60 g.	165
otc	**Polysorb Hydrate** (Fougera)	**Cream:** Sorbitan sesquioleate in a wax and petrolatum base	In 56.7 g and lb.	94
otc	**Purpose Dry Skin** (J&J-Merck)	**Cream:** Mineral oil, white petrolatum, sweet almond oil, propylene glycol, glyceryl stearate, xanthan gum, steareth-2, steareth-20, sodium lactate, sodium lactate, cetyl esters wax, lactic acid	In 85 g.	83
otc	**Shepard's Skin** (Dermik)	**Cream:** Glycerin, glyceryl stearate, ethoxydiglycol, propylene glycol, urea, lecithin, parabens	Unscented. In 113.4 g.	108
otc	**Allercreme Skin** (Carme[1])	**Lotion:** Mineral oil, sorbitol, triethanolamine, parabens	In 240 ml.	73
otc	**Aquanil** (Person & Covey)	**Lotion:** Glycerin, benzyl alcohol, sodium laureth sulfate, stearyl alcohol, xanthan gum	In 240 and 480 ml.	24
otc	**Aveeno** (Rydelle)	**Lotion:** 1% colloidal oatmeal, 0.5% allantoin, glycerin, distearyldimonium Cl, petrolatum, dimethicone, benzyl alcohol	In 240 ml.	NA
otc	**Balmex Emollient** (Macsil)	**Lotion:** Lanolin oil, silicone, Balsam Peru, glycerol monostearate	In 180 ml.	11
otc	**Complex 15 Hand & Body** (Schering-Plough)	**Lotion:** Caprylic/capric triglyceride, PEG-50 stearate, squalane, carboxylic acid sterol ester, diazolidinyl urea, glycerin, glyceryl stearate, lecithin, dimethicone, glycol stearate, carbomer-934P, EDTA	Unscented. In 30 ml.	38
otc	**Corn Huskers** (Warner-Lambert)	**Lotion:** 6.7% glycerin, 5.7% SD alcohol 40, algin, guar gum, methylparaben	In 120 and 210 ml.	16
otc	**Curel Moisturizing** (Rydelle)	**Lotion:** Glycerin, petrolatum, dimethicone, parabens	Regular and fragrance free. In 180, 300 and 390 ml.	22
otc	**Derma Viva** (Rugby)	**Lotion:** Mineral oil, glyceryl stearate, laureth-4, lanolin oil, PEG-100 stearate, PEG-40 stearate, PEG-4 dilaurate, trolamine, dioctyl sodium sulfosuccinate, parabens	In 237 ml.	13

* Cost Index based on cost per g or ml. [1] Carme, Inc. 84 Galli, Novato, CA, 94949, (800) 447-6758.

(Continued on following page)

				C.I.*
otc	**DML** (Person & Covey)	**Lotion:** Petrolatum, glycerin, dimethicone, benzyl alcohol, volatile silicone, glyceryl stearate, palmitic acid, carbomer 941, xanthan gum	Unscented. In 240 and 480 ml.	37
otc	**Emollia** (Gordon Labs)	**Lotion:** Mineral oil, propylene glycol, white wax, sodium lauryl sulfate, oleic acid, parabens	In 120 and 240 ml and gal.	36
otc	**Epilyt** (Stiefel)	**Lotion concentrate:** Propylene glycol, glycerin, oleic acid, lactic acid	In 118 ml.	NA
otc	**Esotérica Dry Skin Treatment** (SK-Beecham)	**Lotion:** Propylene glycol, dicaprylate/dicaprate, mineral oil, glyceryl stearate, cetyl esters wax, hydrolyzed animal protein, dimethicone, TEA-carbomer-941, parabens	In 37.5 ml.	NA
otc	**Eucerin Moisturizing** (Beiersdorf)	**Lotion:** Mineral oil, PEG-40 sorbitan peroleate, lanolin acid glycerin ester, sorbitol, propylene glycol, cetyl palmitate, lanolin alcohol	Unscented. In 52.5, 120 and 240 ml, pt and gal.	38
otc	**Hydrisea** (Pedinol)	**Lotion:** 8% Dead Sea salts concentrate, NaCl, MgCl, KCl, CaCl, mineral oil, propylene glycol, sorbitan stearate, glyceryl stearate, PEG-75 lanolin, EDTA, imidazolidinyl urea, tartrazine, parabens	In 120 ml.	57
otc	**Hydrisinol** (Pedinol)	**Lotion:** Sulfonated castor oil, hydrogenated vegetable oil, propylene glycol stearate SE, mineral oil, lanolin, lanolin alcohol, sesame oil, sunflower oil, aloe, triethanolamine, sorbitan stearate, parabens, hydroxyethyl cellulose	In 240 ml.	32
otc	**Keri** (Westwood)	**Lotion:** Mineral oil, lanolin oil, propylene glycol, glyceryl stearate, PEG-100 stearate, PEG-40 stearate, PEG-4 dilaurate, laureth-4, carbomer-934, triethanolamine, docusate sodium, parabens	Scented and unscented. In 195, 390 and 600 ml.	30
otc	**Keri Light** (Westwood)	**Lotion:** Glycerin, stearyl alcohol, ceteareth-20, cetearyl octanoate, stearyl heptanoate, squalane, parabens, carbomer-934	In 195 and 390 ml.	NA
Rx	**Lac-Hydrin** (Westwood)	**Lotion:** 12% lactic acid, mineral oil, glyceryl stearate, PEG-100 stearate, propylene glycol, polyoxyl 40 stearate, glycerin, laureth-4, parabens, methylcellulose	In 150 ml.	90
otc	**Lac-Hydrin Five** (Westwood)	**Lotion:** Lactic acid, glycerin, petrolatum, squalane, steareth-2, PCE-21-stearyl ether, propylene glycol dioctanoate, dimethicone, cetyl palmitate, diazolidinyl urea	Unscented. In 120 and 240 ml.	NA
otc	**LactiCare** (Stiefel)	**Lotion:** Lactic acid, mineral oil, sodium hydroxide, glyceryl stearate, PEG-100 stearate, carbomer-940, DMDM hydantoin	In 222 and 345 ml.	29
otc	**Lobana Body** (Ulmer)	**Lotion:** Mineral oil, triethanolamine stearate, lanolin, propylene glycol and parabens	In 120 and 240 ml and gal.	25
otc	**Lubriderm** (Warner-Lambert)	**Lotion:** Mineral oil, petrolatum, sorbitol, lanolin, lanolin alcohol, triethanolamine and parabens	Scented and unscented. In 75, 120, 240, 360, 480 ml.	NA
otc	**Moisturel** (Westwood)	**Lotion:** 3% dimethicone, petrolatum, glycerin, steareth-2, benzyl alcohol, laureth-23, carbomer-934	In 360 and 480 ml.	34

* Cost Index based on cost per g or ml.

(Continued on following page)

				C.I.*
otc	**Neutrogena Body** (Neutrogena)	**Lotion:** Glyceryl stearate, PEG-100 stearate, imidazolidinyl urea, carbomer-954, parabens, sodium lauryl sulfate, triethanolamine	Scented and unscented. In 240 ml.	25
otc	**Nivea After Tan** (Beiersdorf)	**Lotion:** SD alcohol 40B, mineral oil, PEG-40 castor oil, sodium cetearyl sulfate, glyceryl stearate, parabens, aloe extract, lanolin alcohol, imidazolidinyl urea, phenoxyethanol, triethanolamine, chamomile extract, carbomer, simethicone, citric acid	In 120 ml.	NA
otc	**Nivea Moisturizing** (Beiersdorf)	**Lotion:** Mineral oil, glycerin, lanolin alcohol, glyceryl stearate, simethicone	In 120, 240 and 360 ml.	27
otc	**Nivea Moisturizing Extra Enriched** (Beiersdorf)	**Lotion:** Mineral oil, PEG-40 sorbitan peroleate, glycerin, polyglyceryl-3 diisostearate, petrolatum, glyceryl lanolate, lanolin alcohol, phenoxyethanol	In 120, 240 and 360 ml.	29
otc	**Nutraderm** (Owen/Galderma)	**Lotion:** Mineral oil, sorbitan stearate, stearyl alcohol, sodium lauryl sulfate, carbomer 940, diazolidinyl urea, parabens, triethanolamine	In 240 and 480 ml.	21
otc	**Pro-Cute** (Ferndale)	**Lotion:** Glycerin, silicone, triethanolamine, P.V.P., menthol	In 240 ml.	31
otc	**Shepard's Cream** (Dermik)	**Lotion:** Glycerin, sesame oil, vegetable oil, SD alcohol 40-B, propylene glycol, ethoxydiglycol, triethanolamine, glyceryl stearate, simethicone, monoglyceride citrate, citric acid, parabens	Unscented. In 240 and 480 ml.	43
otc	**Sofenol 5** (C & M Pharm.)	**Lotion:** Glycerin, petrolatum, allantoin, dimethicone, soluble collagen, PEG-40-stearate, sunflower seed oil, carbomer 940, kaolin	Unscented. In 240 ml.	33
otc	**Therapeutic Bath** (Goldline)	**Lotion:** Mineral oil, glyceryl stearate, PEG-100 stearate, propylene glycol, PEG-40 stearate, laureth-4, PEG-4 dilaurate, lanolin oil, parabens, carbomer 934, trolamine, dioctyl sodium sulfosuccinate	In 236 ml.	NA
otc	**Ultra Derm** (Baker Cummins)	**Lotion:** Mineral oil, petrolatum, lanolin oil, glycerin, propylene glycol, glyceryl stearate, PEG-50 stearate, propylene glycol stearate SE, sorbitan laurate, potassium sorbate, phosphoric acid, EDTA	In 240 ml.	31
otc	**Wibi** (Owen/Galderma)	**Lotion:** Glycerin, SD alcohol 40, PEG-4, PEG-6-32 stearate, PEG-6-32, carbomer-940, PEG-75, parabens, triethanolamine, menthol	In 240 and 480 ml.	29
otc	**Wondra** (Richardson-Vicks)	**Lotion:** Petrolatum, lanolin acid, glycerin, EDTA, hydrogenated vegetable glycerides phosphate, carbomer, dimethicone, imidazolidinyl urea, EDTA, titanium dioxide, parabens	Scented and unscented. In 300 ml.	11
otc	**Neutrogena Body** (Neutrogena)	**Oil:** Sesame oil, PEG-40 sorbitan peroleate	Scented and unscented. In 240 ml.	48
otc	**Nivea Moisturizing** (Beiersdorf)	**Oil:** Mineral oil, PEG-40 sorbitan peroleate, lanolin acid glycerin ester, sorbitol, propylene glycol, lanolin alcohol	In 120 ml.	NA
otc	**Nivea Skin** (Beiersdorf)	**Oil:** Mineral oil, lanolin, petrolatum, glyceryl lanolate, lanolin alcohol	In 240 ml.	23

* Cost Index based on cost per g or ml.

Uses:
To protect skin against contact irritants.

Contraindications:
Do not use silicone on wet, exudative lesions or inflamed or abraded skin.

				C.I.*
otc	**Hydropel** (C&M Pharm.)	**Ointment:** 30% silicone, 10% hydrophobic starch derivative, petrolatum	In 60 g and lb.	NA
otc	**Silicone No. 2** (C&M Pharm)	**Ointment:** 10% silicone in petrolatum, hydrophobic starch derivative, methylparaben	In 30 and 480 g.	94
otc	**White Cloverine Salve** (Medtech)	**Ointment:** 97% white petrolatum, rectified turpentine oil, white wax	In 30 g.	NA
otc	**Kerodex** (Whitehall)	**Cream:** #51-Bentonite, calcium carbonate, cellulose gum, chloroxylenol, glycerin, iron oxides, isopropyl alcohol, kaolin, parabens, petrolatum, sodium lauryl sulfate, spermaceti. Nongreasy invisible barrier for dry or oily work	In 113 g.	35
		Cream: #71-Calcium carbonate, cetrimonium bromide, iron oxide, isopropyl alcohol, kaolin, parabens, mineral oil, paraffin, petrolatum, sodium hexametaphosphate, sodium lauryl sulfate, zinc oxide. Nongreasy invisible water repellent barrier for wet work	In 113 g.	35
otc	**BlisterGard** (Medtech)	**Liquid:** 6.7% alcohol, pyroxylin solution, oil of cloves, 8-hydroxyquinoline	In 30 ml.	NA
otc	**New-Skin** (Medtech)		In 10 and 30 ml bottle and 3.5 ml tube.	126
otc	**New-Skin Antiseptic** (Medtech)	**Spray Liquid:** Pyroxylin solution, acetone ACS, oil of cloves, 8-hydroxyquinoline, 4.2% alcohol	In 28.5 g.	NA
otc	**Aerozoin** (Graham Field)	**Spray:** 30% tincture of benzoin compound, 44.8% isopropyl alcohol	In 105 ml.	83
otc	**Benzoin** (Various, eg, Humco, Lannett)	**Tincture**	In 60 and 120 ml, pt and gal.	NA
otc	**Benzoin Compound** (Various, eg, Century, Humco, Lannett, Paddock, Purepac)	**Tincture:** Benzoin, aloe, storax, tolu balsam, 74% to 80% alcohol	In 30, 60 and 120 ml, pt and gal.	NA
otc	**TinBen** (Ferndale)	**Tincture:** Benzoin, 75% to 83% alcohol	In 120 ml.	39
otc	**TinCoBen** (Ferndale)	**Tincture:** Benzoin, aloe, tolu balsam, storax, 77% alcohol	In 120 ml.	39

* Cost Index based on cost per g or ml.

Uses:

These products are used as bases for incorporation of various active ingredients in extemporaneously compounded dermatological prescriptions.

				C.I.*
otc	**Lanaphilic** (Medco Labs)	**Ointment:** Stearyl alcohol, white petrolatum, isopropyl palmitate, lanolin oil, propylene glycol, sorbitol, sodium lauryl sulfate, parabens	In lb.	16
otc	**Lanaphilic w/Urea 10%** (Medco Labs)	**Ointment:** Urea, stearyl alcohol, white petrolatum, isopropyl palmitate, lanolin oil, sorbitol, propylene glycol, sodium lauryl sulfate, lactic acid, parabens	In lb.	19
otc	**Petrolatum** (Carolina Medical)	**Ointment:** Petrolatum, mineral oil, ceresin wax, woolwax alcohol	In 430 g.	NA
otc	**Absorbase** (Carolina Medical)	**Ointment:** Petrolatum, mineral oil, ceresin wax, woolwax alcohol, potassium sorbate	Unscented. In 114 and 454 g.	NA
otc	**Hydrophilic** (Rugby)	**Ointment:** White petrolatum, stearyl alcohol, propylene glycol, sodium lauryl sulfate, parabens	In 454 g.	NA
otc	**Aquabase** (Paddock)	**Ointment:** Petrolatum, mineral oil, mineral wax, woolwax alcohol, sorbitan sesquioleate	Unscented. Dye free. In 454 g.	NA
otc	**Aquaphilic** (Medco Labs)	**Ointment:** Stearyl alcohol, white petrolatum, isopropyl palmitate, sorbitol, propylene glycol, sodium lauryl sulfate, parabens	In lb.	16
otc	**Aquaphilic w/Carbamide 10% and 20%** (Medco Labs)	**Ointment:** Urea, stearyl alcohol, white petrolatum, isopropyl palmitate, propylene glycol, sorbitol, sodium lauryl sulfate, lactic acid, parabens	In lb.	19
otc	**Aquaphor Natural Healing** (Beiersdorf)	**Ointment:** Petrolatum, mineral oil, mineral wax, woolwax alcohol, panthenol, glycerin, chamomile essence	In 52.5 g.	111
otc	**Polyethylene Glycol** (Medco)	**Ointment:** Water soluble greaseless base with PEG-8 and PEG-75	In lb.	NA
otc	**Solumol** (C&M Pharm.)	**Ointment:** Petrolatum, mineral oil, cetearyl alcohol, sodium lauryl sulfate, glycerin, propylene glycol	In lb.	NA
otc	**Unibase** (Warner Chilcott)	**Ointment:** Nongreasy, water removable base with white petrolatum, glycerin, sodium lauryl sulfate, propylparaben. Will absorb 30% of its weight in water	In lb.	27
otc	**Acid Mantle** (Sandoz)	**Cream:** Aluminum sulfate, calcium acetate, cetearyl alcohol, glycerin, light mineral oil, methylparaben, sodium lauryl sulfate, synthetic beeswax, white petrolatum, ammonium hydroxide, citric acid	In 120 g.	67
otc	**Velvachol** (Owen/Galderma)	**Cream:** Water miscible vehicle containing petrolatum, mineral oil, stearyl alcohol, sodium lauryl sulfate, cholesterol, parabens	In lb.	30
otc	**Dermabase** (Paddock)	**Cream:** Mineral oil, petrolatum, cetostearyl alcohol, propylene glycol, sodium lauryl sulfate, isopropyl palmitate, imidazolidinyl urea, parabens	In 454 g.	NA
otc	**Dermovan** (Owen/Galderma)	**Cream:** Nonionic, water miscible vanishing cream vehicle containing glyceryl stearate, stearamidoethyl diethylamine, glycerin, mineral oil, cetyl esters, parabens	In lb.	37

* Cost Index based on cost per g or ml.

(Continued on following page)

				C.I.*
otc	**Heb Cream Base** (Sola Barnes/Hind)	**Cream:** Self-emulsifying base containing mineral oil, white petrolatum, stearyl alcohol, sodium lauryl sulfate, parabens	In 454 g.	61
otc	**Hydrocream Base** (Paddock)	**Cream:** Petrolatum, mineral oil, mineral wax, woolwax alcohol, cholesterol, imidazolidinyl urea, parabens	In 454 g.	NA
otc	**Eucerin** (Beiersdorf)	**Cream:** Petrolatum, mineral oil, mineral wax, woolwax alcohol	In 60, 120, 240 and 480 g.	33
otc	**Vanicream** (Pharmaceutical Specialties)	**Cream:** White petrolatum, cetearyl alcohol, ceteareth-20, sorbitol solution, propylene glycol, simethicone, glyceryl monostearate, polyethylene glycol monostearate	In 120 g and lb.	21
otc	**Nutraderm** (Owen/Galderma)	**Lotion:** Mineral oil, sorbitan stearate, stearyl alcohol, sodium lauryl sulfate, cetyl alcohol, carbomer-940, parabens, triethanolamine	In 240 and 480 ml.	26
otc	**E-Solve** (Syosset)	**Lotion:** 85% absolute alcohol, propylene glycol, lauramide-DEA, hydroxypropyl cellulose, titanium dioxide, polysorbate 20, polyvinylpyrrolidone, polysorbate 80, talc, iron oxides	In 50 ml.	113
otc	**C-Solve** (Syosset)	**Lotion:** SD alcohol 40B, glycerin, polysorbate 20 and 80, hydroxyethyl cellulose, polyvinylpyrrolidone, hydrolyzed animal protein, collagen, imidazolidinyl urea	In 50 ml with applicator.	113
otc	**Vehicle/N** (Neutrogena)	**Solution:** 45% SD alcohol 40, laureth-4, propylene glycol, 4% isopropyl alcohol	In 50 ml with applicator.	114
otc	**Vehicle/N Mild** (Neutrogena)	**Solution:** 37.5% SD alcohol 40, laureth-4, 5% isopropyl alcohol	In 50 ml with applicator.	114
otc	**Solvent-G** (Syosset)	**Liquid:** 55% SD alcohol 40B, laureth-4, isopropyl alcohol, propylene glycol	In 50 ml.	100

* Cost Index based on cost per g or ml.

Emollient Preparations

Uses: These products contain colloidal solids and various oils which act as emollients. They are recommended for relief of minor skin irritations and pruritus associated with common dermatoses and dry skin conditions.

Precautions:

For external use only. Avoid contact with the eyes; if this occurs, flush with clear water.

Use caution when using bath oils to avoid slipping in tub.

Do not use on acutely inflamed areas.

				C.I.*
otc	**Aveeno Regular Bath** (Rydelle)	100% natural colloidal oatmeal	In 30 g packets (8).	43
otc	**Aveeno Oilated Bath** (Rydelle)	43% colloidal oatmeal, mineral oil	In 30 g packets (8).	43
otc	**Nutra•Soothe** (Pertussin)	Colloidal oatmeal, light mineral oil	In individual oil (9) & oatmeal powder packets (9).	NA
otc	**Pedi-Bath Salts** (Pedinol)	Colloidal sulfur, potassium iodide, Balsam Peru, sodium hyposulfate, sodium bicarbonate, pine needle oil	In 170 g.	20
otc	**Nutraderm Bath Oil** (Owen/Galderma)	Mineral oil, lanolin oil, PEG-4 dilaurate, benzophenone-3, butylparaben	In 240 ml.	36
otc	**Ultra Derm Bath Oil** (Baker Cummins)	Mineral oil, lanolin oil, octoxynol-3	In 240 ml.	54
otc	**Alpha Keri Therapeutic Bath Oil** (Westwood)	Mineral oil, lanolin oil, PEG-4 dilaurate, benzophenone-3	In 120 and 240 ml and pt.	27
otc	**Therapeutic Bath Oil** (Goldline)		In 473 ml.	11
otc	**LubraSol Bath Oil** (Pharmaceutical Specialties)	Mineral oil, lanolin oil, PEG-200 dilaurate, oxybenzone	In 240 ml.	24
otc	**Domol Bath & Shower Oil** (Miles)	Di-isopropyl sebacate, mineral oil	In 240 ml.	64
otc	**Alpha Keri Spray** (Westwood)	Mineral oil, lanolin oil, 28% SD alcohol 40, PPG-15 stearyl ether, C12-15 alcohols benzoate, PEG-4 dilaurate, polysorbate 85	In 150 g.	65
otc	**Lubriderm Bath Oil** (Warner-Lambert)	Mineral oil, PPG-15, stearyl ether oleth-2, nonoxynol-5	In 480 ml.	24
otc	**Surfol Post-Immersion Bath Oil** (Stiefel)	Mineral oil, isostearic acid, PEG-40 sorbitan peroleate, drometrizole	In 237 ml.	23
otc	**Cameo Oil** (Medco)	Mineral oil, PEG-8 dioleate, lanolin oil	Unscented. In 240, 480 and 960 ml.	
otc	**RoBathol Bath Oil** (Pharmaceutical Specialties)	Cottonseed oil and alkyl aryl polyether alcohol	Lanolin free. Dye free. In 240 ml, pt and gal.	24
otc	**Esoterica Soap** (Medicis)	Sodium tallowate, sodium cocoate, mineral oil, acacia, sodium cocoyl isethionate, lauramide DEA, potassium oleate, titanium dioxide, pentasodium pentetate, tetra sodium etidronate	In 85 g.	NA

* Cost Index based on cost per g, ml or packet.

Tar-Containing Products

Uses:

These products contain tar derivatives which have keratoplastic, antieczematous, emollient and antipruritic effects. They are used as adjuncts in a wide range of pruritic dermatoses including: Psoriasis, seborrheic dermatitis, atopic dermatitis and eczematoid dermatitis.

Contraindications:

Open or infected lesions; when acute inflammation is present.

Warnings:

Pregnancy: Category C. It is not known whether coal tar can cause fetal harm when administered to a pregnant woman or can affect reproduction capacity. Use on a pregnant woman only if clearly needed.

Lactation: It is not known whether this drug is excreted in breast milk. Therefore, decide whether to discontinue nursing or discontinue the drug, taking into account the importance of coal tar to the mother.

Precautions:

For external use only. Avoid contact with the eyes.

Photosensitivity: Coal tar is photosensitizing; for 72 hours after use, avoid exposure to direct sunlight or sunlamps.

Use caution to avoid slipping in the bathtub.

Staining of plastic or fiberglass tubs may occur.

Irritation: If irritation persists, discontinue use. In rare cases, coal tar may cause allergic irritation.

Adverse Reactions:

Dermatitis; allergic sensitization; folliculitis; photosensitization (see Precautions).

Directions:

Add to bath water. Soak 10 to 20 minutes and then pat dry.

				C.I.*
otc	**Balnetar** (Westwood)	**Liquid:** 2.5% coal tar in mineral oil, laureth-4, lanolin oil, PEG-4 dilaurate, docusate sodium	In 225 ml.	63
otc	**Cūtar Bath Oil Emulsion** (Summers)	**Liquid:** 7.5% coal tar in mineral oil, isopropyl myristate, polysorbate 80, sorbitan sesquioleate, lanolin alcohols extract, parabens, xanthan gum, carbomer	In 180 ml and gal.	36
otc	**Polytar Bath** (Stiefel)	**Liquid:** 25% polytar (juniper tar, pine tar, coal tar solution, vegetable oil and solubilized crude coal tar) in a water miscible base	In 240 ml.	43
Rx	**Zetar Emulsion** (Dermik)	**Liquid:** 30% whole coal tar in polysorbates	In 177 ml.	94

* Cost Index based on cost per ml.

For other tar-containing preparations, refer to the Antiseborrheic and Bath Dermotologicals sections.

COAL TAR (or derivatives) is used for its antipruritic, anti-eczematous and keratoplastic actions. Used in psoriasis and other chronic skin disorders.

PRECIPITATED SULFUR is a keratolytic, antifungal and antiparasitic agent. See monograph in Acne Products section.

BENZOCAINE is an anesthetic. See Local Anesthetics, Topical monograph.

SALICYLIC ACID is a keratolytic agent. See individual monograph.

ZINC OXIDE is an astringent, antiseptic and protective agent. See individual monograph.

Contraindications:

Do not use on patients sensitive to any component.

Warnings:

Children: Do not use in children < 2 years of age.

Precautions:

For external use only. Avoid contact with the eyes.

Photosensitivity: Avoid exposure to sunlight for up to 24 hours. Do not use on patients who have a disease characterized by photosensitivity (eg, lupus erythematosus, sunlight allergy).

Do not apply to acutely inflamed or broken skin or to the genital or rectal areas. If the condition covers a large area of the body, consult a physician before using.

Discoloration/Staining: Light-colored, bleached or tinted hair may become temporarily discolored. Slight staining of clothes may also occur; standard laundry procedures will remove most stains.

Psoriasis: Do not use with other forms of psoriasis therapy (eg, ultraviolet radiation, drug therapy) unless directed to do so.

				C.I.*
otc	**Medotar** (Medco Lab.)	**Ointment:** 1% coal tar, 0.5% polysorbate 80, octoxynol-5, zinc oxide, white petrolatum	In 480 g.	21
otc	**Taraphilic** (Medco)	**Ointment:** 1% coal tar, 0.5% polysorbate 20, stearyl alcohol, white petrolatum, sorbitol, propylene glycol, sodium lauryl sulfate, parabens	In lb.	NA
otc	**MG217 Medicated** (Triton)	**Ointment:** 2% coal tar solution, 1.1% colloidal sulfur, 1.5% salicylic acid	In 108 and 480 g.	NA
otc	**Fototar** (ICN Pharm)	**Cream:** 2% coal tar in an emollient moisturizing base	In 85 and 454 g.	162
otc	**Tegrin for Psoriasis** (Reedco)	**Cream:** 5% coal tar solution, acetylated lanolin alcohol, 4.6% alcohol, carbomer 934P, glyceryl tribehenate, mineral oil, potassium hydroxide, lanolin alcohol, petrolatum, titanium dioxide, stearyl alcohol	In 60 and 124 g.	174
otc	**MG217 Dual Treatment** (Triton)	**Lotion:** 5% coal tar solution in a light greaseless moisturizing base with jojoba	In 120 ml.	NA
otc	**Tegrin for Psoriasis** (Reedco)	**Lotion:** 5% coal tar solution, 4.6% alcohol, carbomer-940, parabens, PEG-40 stearate, polysorbate-60, propylene glycol, squalane, propylene glycol dipelargonate, titanium dioxide, triethanolamine	In 177 ml.	70
otc	**Oxipor VHC** (Whitehall)	**Lotion:** 48.5% coal tar solution, 1% salicylic acid, 2% benzocaine, 81% alcohol	In 57 and 118 ml.	214
otc	**Coal Tar or Carbonis Detergens** (Various, eg, Lannett)	**Solution:** 20% coal tar	In 120 ml, pt and gal.	NA

* Cost Index based on cost per g or ml.

(Continued on following page)

				C.I.*
otc	**AquaTar** (Allergan Herbert)	**Gel:** 2.5% coal tar extract, glycerin, imidurea, parabens, mineral oil, poloxamer 407, polysorbate 80	In 90 g.	152
otc	**Estar** (Westwood)	**Gel:** Coal tar extract equivalent to 5% coal tar, benzyl alcohol, carbomer 940, glycereth-7 coconate, laureth-4, polysorbate 80, 15.6% SD alcohol 40, simethicone, sorbitol	In 90 g.	158
otc	**P & S Plus** (Baker Cummins)	**Gel:** 8% coal tar solution (1.6% crude coal tar, 6.4% ethyl alcohol), 2% salicylic acid	In 105 g.	116
otc	**PsoriGel** (Owen/Galderma)	**Gel:** 7.5% coal tar solution, 33% alcohol	In 120 g.	101
otc	**Packer's Pine Tar** (GenDerm)	**Soap:** Soap base. Pine tar, pine oil, iron oxide, PEG-75	In 99 g.	30
otc	**Polytar** (Stiefel)	**Soap:** 1% polytar (juniper tar, pine tar, coal tar solution, solubilized crude coal tar, octoxynol-9, povidone, sodium borohydride, sodium cocoate, sodium tallowate, trisodium HEDTA)	In 99 g.	30
otc	**Tegrin Medicated for Psoriasis** (Reedco)	**Soap:** 5% coal tar solution, chromium hydroxide green, glycerin, titanium dioxide	In 127 g.	36
otc	**Neutrogena T/Derm** (Neutrogena)	**Oil:** 5% solubilized coal tar extract in an oil base	In 120 ml.	100

WET DRESSINGS AND SOAKS

ALUMINUM ACETATE SOLUTION (Burow's or Modified Burow's Solution)

Indications:

An astringent wet dressing for relief of inflammatory conditions of the skin, such as insect bites, poison ivy, swelling, allergy, bruises and athlete's foot.

Precautions:

Discontinue use if intolerance, irritation or extension of inflammatory condition being treated occurs. If symptoms persist > 7 days, discontinue use and consult physician.

Do not use plastic or other impervious material to prevent evaporation.

For external use only. Avoid contact with the eyes.

Drug Interactions:

Collegenase: The enzyme activity of topical collagenase may be inhibited by aluminum acetate solution because of the metal ion and low pH. Cleanse the site of the solution with repeated washings of normal saline before applying the enzyme ointment.

				C.I.*
otc	**Burow's Solution** (Various, eg, Paddock)	Aluminum acetate solution	In 480 ml.	NA
otc	**Bluboro Powder** (Allergan Herbert)	Aluminum sulfate and calcium acetate. One packet or tablet in a pint of water produces a modified 1:40 Burow's solution. Apply every 15 to 30 minutes for 4 to 8 hours.	**Powder packets:** 1.8 g. In 12s and 100s.	635
otc	**Boropak Powder** (Glenwood)		**Powder packets:** 2.4 g. In 12s and 100s.	NA
otc	**Domeboro Powder and Tablets** (Miles)		**Effervescent tablets:** In 12s and 100s.	646
			Powder packets: In 12s and 100s.	646
otc	**Pedi-Boro Soak Paks** (Pedinol)		**Powder packets:** 2.7 g. In 12s and 100s.	643

* Cost Index based on cost per g, ml, packet or tablet.

Indications:

These products are used for relief of pain of muscular aches, neuralgia, rheumatism, arthritis, sprains and like conditions, when skin is intact.

Individual components include:

COUNTERIRRITANTS: Cajuput oil, camphor, capsicum preparations (capsicum oleoresin, capsaicin), eucalyptus oil, menthol, methyl nicotinate, methyl salicylate, mustard oil, wormwood oil.

ANTISEPTICS: Chloroxylenol, thymol.

LOCAL ANESTHETIC: Benzocaine (see Local Anesthetics, Topical).

ANALGESICS: Trolamine salicylate.

Contraindications:

Allergy to components of any formulation or to salicylates.

Warnings:

For external use only. Avoid contact with eyes and mucous membranes.

Precautions:

Apply to affected parts only. Do not apply to irritated skin; if excessive irritation develops, discontinue use. If pain persists for more than 7 to 10 days, or if redness is present, or in conditions affecting children $<$ 10 years of age, consult a physician.

Heat therapy: Do not use an external source of heat (eg, heating pad) with these agents since irritation or burning of the skin may occur.

Protective covering: Applying a tight bandage or wrap over these agents is not recommended since increased absorption may occur.

Drug Interactions:

Anticoagulants: An enhanced anticoagulant effect (eg, increased prothrombin time) occurred in several patients receiving an anticoagulant and using topical methylsalicylate concurrently.

Adverse Reactions:

If applied to large skin areas, salicylate side effects may occur, such as tinnitus, nausea or vomiting. Toxic if ingested.

Counterirritants may cause local irritation, especially in patients with sensitive skin.

		Gels, Creams and Ointments		C.I.*
otc	**Analgesia Creme** (Rugby)	10% trolamine salicylate	In 85 g.	27
otc	**Aspercreme Cream** (Thompson)		In 37.5, 90 and 150 g.	64
otc	**Exocaine Odor Free Creme** (Commerce Drug)		In 90 g.	50
otc	**Mobisyl Creme** (Ascher)		In 35.4, 100 and 227 g.	54
otc	**Myoflex Creme** (Fisons)		In 60, 120 and 240 g and lb.	49
otc	**Sportscreme** (Thompson)		In 37.5 and 90 g.	51
otc	**infraRUB Cream** (Whitehall)	35% methyl salicylate and 10% menthol	In 37.5 and 90 g.	106
otc	**Panalgesic Cream** (E.C. Robins/Poythress)	35% methyl salicylate and 4% menthol	In 120 g.	NA
otc	**Icy Hot Cream** (Chattem)	30% methyl salicylate, 10% menthol, carbomer, cetyl esters wax, emulsifying wax, trolamine	In 37.5 and 90 g.	30
otc	**ArthriCare Triple-Medicated Gel** (Commerce)	30% methyl salicylate, 1.25% menthol, 0.7% methyl nicotinate, isopropyl alcohol, propylene glycol, hydroxypropylmethylcellulose and dioctyl sodium sulfosuccinate	In 90 g.	NA
otc	**Musterole Deep Strength Rub** (Schering-Plough)	30% methyl salicylate, 0.5% methyl nicotinate and 3% menthol	In 37 and 90 g.	103

* Cost Index based on cost per g.

(Continued on following page)

Refer to the general discussion of these products on page 2411

	Gels, Creams and Ointments (Cont.)			C.I.*
otc	**Ben-Gay Ultra Strength Cream** (Pfizer)	30% methyl salicylate, 10% menthol, 4% camphor, EDTA, glyceryl stearate SE, anhydrous lanolin, polysorbate 80, potassium carbomer and stearate, triethanolamine carbomer and stearate	In 35 g.	NA
otc	**Ben-Gay Extra Strength Cream** (Pfizer)	30% methyl salicylate, 8% menthol, glyceryl stearate SE, anhydrous lanolin, polysorbate 85, potassium stearate, sorbitan tristearate, xanthan gum	In 35 g.	NA
otc	**Exocaine Plus Rub** (Commerce Drug)	30% methyl salicylate	In 39 and 120 g.	83
otc	**Icy Hot Stick** (Chattem)	30% methyl salicylate, 10% menthol, ceresin, cyclomethicone, hydrogenated castor oil, microcrystalline wax, paraffin, PEG-150 distearate, propylene glycol	In 52.5 g.	NA
otc	**Icy Hot Balm** (Chattem)	29% methyl salicylate, 7.6% menthol, paraffin, white petrolatum	In 105 g.	50
otc	**Exocaine Medicated Rub** (Commerce)	25% methyl salicylate	In 39 and 120 g.	70
otc	**Improved Analgesic Ointment** (Rugby)	18.3% methyl salicylate, 16% menthol	In 36, 85 and 454 g.	50
otc	**Ben-Gay Original Ointment** (Pfizer)	18.3% methyl salicylate, 16% menthol, anhydrous lanolin, microcrystalline wax, synthetic bees wax	In 35 and 90 g.	NA
otc	**Arthritis Hot Creme** (Thompson)	15% methyl salicylate, 10% menthol, glyceryl stearate, carbomer 934, lanolin, PEG-100 stearate, propylene glycol, trolamine, parabens	In 90 g.	NA
otc	**Ben-Gay Regular Strength Cream** (Pfizer)	15% methyl salicylate, 10% menthol, glyceryl stearate SE, anhydrous lanolin, polysorbate 85, sorbitan tristearate, triethanolamine stearate	In 35, 85 and 142 g.	NA
otc	**Muscle Rub Ointment** (Schein)	15% methyl salicylate, 10% menthol, glyceryl stearate, lanolin, parabens, propylene glycol, trolamine	In 85 g.	31
otc	**Deep-Down Rub** (SK-Beecham)	15% methyl salicylate, 5% menthol, 0.5% camphor, 40.5% SD alcohol	In 37.5 and 90 g.	78
otc	**Minit-Rub** (Bristol-Myers)	15% methyl salicylate, 3.5% menthol, 2.3% camphor, anhydrous lanolin	In 45 and 90 g.	62
otc	**Thera-gesic Cream** (Mission)	15% methyl salicylate, menthol, dimethylpolysiloxane, glycerin, carbopol, triethanolamine, sodium lauryl sulfate, parabens	In 90 and 150 g.	57
otc	**Gordogesic Creme** (Gordon)	10% methyl salicylate, propylene glycol, mineral oil, white wax, triethanolamine, sodium lauryl sulfate, parabens	In 75 g and lb.	57
otc	**Methagual** (Gordon)	8% methyl salicylate, 2% guaiacol, petrolatum, white wax, parabens	In 60 g and lb.	71
otc	**Wonder Ice Gel** (Pedinol)	5.25% menthol	In 113 and 473 g.	NA

* Cost Index based on cost per g or ml.

(Continued on following page)

Refer to the general discussion of these products on page 2411

	Gels, Creams and Ointments (Cont.)			C.I.*
otc	**Double Ice Arthri-Care Gel** (Commerce)	4% menthol, 3.1% camphor, aloe vera gel, carbomer 940, dioctylsodium sulfosuccinate, isopropyl alcohol, propylene glycol, triethanolamine	In 90 g.	NA
otc	**Odor Free ArthriCare Rub** (Commerce)	1.25% menthol, 0.25% methyl nicotinate, 0.025% capsaicin, aloe vera gel, carbomer 940, DMDM hydantoin, emulsifying wax, glyceryl stearate SE, isopropyl alcohol, myristyl propionate, propylparaben, triethanolamine	In 90 g.	NA
otc	**Iodex w/Methyl Salicylate** (Medtech)	4.7% iodine with oleic acid and 4.8% oil of wintergreen in a petrolatum base	In 30 and 480 g.	125
otc	**Soltice Quick-Rub** (Chattem)	Methyl salicylate, camphor, menthol, eucalyptus oil, glycerin, oleic acid	In 40 and 112 g.	58
otc	**Dermal-Rub Balm** (Hauck)	Methyl salicylate, camphor, racemic menthol, cajuput oil	In 30 g and lb.	148
otc	**Analgesic Balm** (Various, eg, Goldline, Major, Schein, URL)	Methyl salicylate, menthol	In 30 and 454 g.	42+
otc	**Argesic Cream** (Econo Med)	Methyl salicylate, triethanolamine	Vanishing base. In 60 g.	93
otc	**Musterole Extra Strength** (Schering-Plough)	5% camphor, 3% menthol, methyl salicylate, lanolin, oil of mustard, petrolatum	In 27, 30 and 67.5 g.	129
otc	**Vicks VapoRub** (Richardson-Vicks)	4.7% camphor, 2.6% menthol, 1.2% eucalyptus oil, cedarleaf oil, 4.5% mineral oil, nutmeg oil, petrolatum, thymol, spirits of turpentine	In 45, 60, 90 and 180 g.	63
otc	**Methalgen Cream** (Alra)	Camphor, menthol, methyl salicylate, oil of mustard	In 60 and 480 g.	25
otc	**Therapeutic Mineral Ice Exercise Formula Gel** (Bristol-Myers)	4% menthol, ammonium hydroxide, carbomer 934P or 934, cupric sulfate, isopropyl alcohol, thymol	In 90 g.	NA
otc	**Ben-Gay Vanishing Scent Gel** (Pfizer)	3% menthol, benzophenone-4, camphor, diazolidinyl urea, EDTA, isopropyl alcohol, potassium carbomer 940	In 35 g.	NA
otc	**Sportscreme Ice Gel** (Thompson)	2% menthol, carbomer 934, styrene/acrylate copolymer, triethanolamine, 38% SD alcohol 40	In 227 g.	51
otc	**Therapeutic Mineral Ice Gel** (Bristol-Myers)	2% menthol, ammonium hydroxide, carbomer 934, cupric sulfate, isopropyl alcohol, thymol	In 105, 240 and 480 g.	NA
otc	**Flex-all 454 Gel** (Chattem)	Menthol in an aloe vera gel, methyl salicylate, alcohol, allantoin, boric acid, carbomer 940, diazolidinyl urea, iodine, polysorbate 60, propylene glycol, potassium iodide, triethanolamine, eucalyptus oil, glycerin, parabens	In 60, 120 and 240 g.	71
otc	**MenthoRub Ointment** (Schein)	2.6% menthol, 4.73% camphor, eucalyptus oil, rectified oil of turpentine, cedarleaf oil, nutmeg oil, petrolatum, thymol	In 100 g.	32
		Liquids		
otc	**Extra Strength Absorbine Jr. Liquid** (W.F. Young)	4% menthol	In 59 and 118 ml.	100

* Cost Index based on cost per g or ml.

(Continued on following page)

Refer to the general discussion of these products on page 2411

		Sprays		C.I.*
otc	**Extra Strength Sports Spray** (Mentholatum)	3.5% methyl salicylate, 10% menthol, 5% camphor, 58% alcohol	In 90 g.	NA
otc	**Heet Spray** (Whitehall)	25% methyl salicylate, 3% camphor, 3% menthol, 1% methyl nicotinate, isopropyl alcohol	In 147 g.	54
		Lotions and Liniments		
otc	**Aspercreme Rub Lotion** (Thompson)	10% trolamine salicylate, glyceryl stearate, lanolin, parabens, potassium phosphate, propylene glycol, sodium lauryl sulfate	In 180 ml.	31
otc	**Panalgesic Liniment** (E.C. Robins/ Poythress)	55% methyl salicylate, 3.1% camphor, 1.25% menthol, 18.6% emollient oils, 22% alcohol	In 120 and 480 ml.	61
otc	**Gordobalm** (Gordon)	Menthol, camphor, methyl salicylate, 16% isopropyl alcohol, tragacanth, thymol, acetone, eucalyptus oil, tartrazine	In gal.	NA
otc	**Heet Liniment** (Whitehall)	15% methyl salicylate, 3.6% camphor, capsicum oleoresin (as 0.025% capsaicin), acetone, 70% alcohol	In 68.5 and 150 ml.	77
otc	**Banalg Hospital Strength Lotion** (Forest)	14% methyl salicylate, 3% menthol	In 60 ml.	79
otc	**Absorbine Arthritic Pain Lotion** (W.F. Young)	10% methyl salicylate, 3.25% camphor, 1.25% menthol, 1% cetyl alcohol, glyceryl tribehenate, parabens, polysorbate 60, sorbitan mono-oleate, 1% methyl nicotinate	In 59 and 118 ml.	71
otc	**Analbalm Emulsion** (Central)	10% methyl salicylate, 3% camphor, 1.25% menthol, DMDM hydantoin, paraben esters, sodium alginate	In gal.	54
otc	**Banalg Lotion** (Forest)	4.9% methyl salicylate, 2% camphor, 1% menthol	In 60 and 480 ml.	66
otc	**Extra Strength Absorbine Jr. Liniment** (W.F. Young)	4% natural menthol, plant extracts of calendula, echinacea and wormwood, acetone, chloroxylenol, iodine, potassium iodide, thymol, wormwood oil	In 59 and 118 ml.	NA
otc	**Absorbine Jr. Liniment** (W.F. Young)	1.27% menthol, plant extracts of calendula, echinacea and artemesia absinthium, iodine, potassium iodide, thymol, oil of artemesia, acetone, chloroxylenol	In 13, 30, 59, 118 and 480 ml.	71
otc	**Avalgesic Lotion** (Various)	Methyl salicylate, menthol, camphor, methyl nicotinate, dipropylene glycol salicylate, oil of cassia, capsicum oleoresins, ginger	In 120 ml, pt and gal.	NA
otc	**Bangesic Liniment** (Various, eg, Schein)	Methyl salicylate, camphor, menthol, eucalyptus oil	In 60 ml and gal.	50+
otc	**Betuline Lotion** (Ferndale)	Methyl salicylate, camphor, menthol, peppermint oil in a water soluble base	In 30, 60 and 480 ml.	54
otc	**Dermolin Liniment** (Hauck)	Methyl salicylate, camphor, racemic menthol, mustard oil, 8% isopropyl alcohol	In 45 and 120 ml, pt and gal.	300
otc	**Epiderm Balm** (Pedinol)	Methyl salicylate, menthol, propylene glycol, isopropyl alcohol	In gal.	NA

* Cost Index based on cost per g or ml.

SALICYLIC ACID

Actions:

Pharmacology: Salicylic acid produces desquamation of the horny layer of skin, while not affecting the structure of the viable epidermis, by dissolving intercellular cement substance. The keratolytic action causes the cornified epithelium to swell, soften, macerate and then desquamate.

Salicylic acid is keratolytic at concentrations of 2% to 6%. Concentrations of 10% to 17% in collodion are safe and effective for the removal of common and plantar warts; up to 50% salicylic acid in plasters are used to remove warts and corns.

Salicylic acid preparations, alone or in combination, have also been used to treat dandruff, seborrheic dermatitis, acne, tinea infections, psoriasis and calluses.

Pharmacokinetics: In a study of the percutaneous absorption of salicylic acid in four patients with extensive active psoriasis, peak serum salicylate levels never exceeded 5 mg/dl even though > 60% of the applied salicylic acid was absorbed. Systemic toxic reactions are usually associated with much higher serum levels (30 to 40 mg/dl). Peak serum levels occurred within 5 hours of the topical application under occlusion.

Salicylate is 50% to 80% bound to albumin. Salicylates compete with the binding of several drugs and can modify the action of these drugs; by similar competitive mechanisms, other drugs can influence the serum levels of salicylate.

The major urinary metabolites identified after topical administration differ from those after oral salicylate administration; those derived from percutaneous absorption contain more salicylate glucuronides (42%) and less salicyluric (52%) and salicylic acid (6%). Almost 95% of a single dose of salicylate is excreted within 24 hours.

Indications:

Dermatologic use: A topical aid in the removal of excessive keratin in hyperkeratotic skin disorders, including verrucae and the various ichthyoses (vulgaris, sex-linked and lamellar), keratosis palmaris and plantaris, keratosis pilaris, pityriasis rubra pilaris and psoriasis (including body, scalp, palms and soles).

Podiatric use: A topical aid in the removal of excessive keratin on dorsal and plantar hyperkeratotic lesions. In adjunctive therapy for verrucae plantaris (plantar warts).

Contraindications:

Sensitivity to salicylic acid; children < 2 years of age; diabetics or patients with impaired circulation; use on moles, birthmarks or unusual warts with hair growing from them, genital or facial warts or warts on mucous membranes.

Warnings:

Salicylate toxicity: Prolonged use over large areas, especially in children and those patients with significant renal or hepatic impairment, could result in salicylism. Limit the area to be treated and monitor for signs of salicylate toxicity (eg, nausea, vomiting, dizziness, loss of hearing, tinnitus, lethargy, hyperpnea, diarrhea, psychic disturbances). Avoid concomitant use of other drugs which may contribute to elevated serum salicylate levels. In the event of salicylic acid toxicity, discontinue use.

Refer to the Salicylate monograph for additional information on the systemic effects of salicylates.

Pregnancy: Category C. Salicylic acid is teratogenic in rats and monkeys. There are no adequate and well controlled studies in pregnant women. Use during pregnancy only if the potential benefit justifies the potential risk to the fetus.

Lactation: Because of the potential for serious adverse reactions in nursing infants, decide whether to discontinue nursing or to discontinue the drug, taking into account the importance of the drug to the mother.

Precautions:

For external use only: Avoid contact with eyes and mucous membranes. If contact with eyes or mucous membranes occurs, immediately flush with water for 15 minutes.

Drug Interactions:

Interactions have been reported with both topical and oral salicylates. Refer to the Salicylate monograph for a complete listing.

(Continued on following page)

SALICYLIC ACID (Cont.)

Adverse Reactions:

Excessive erythema and scaling could result from use on open skin lesions.

Local irritation may occur from contact with normal skin surrounding the affected area. If irritation occurs, temporarily discontinue use and take care to apply only to wart site when treatment is resumed.

Patient Information:

For external use only. Avoid contact with eyes, face, genitals and mucous membranes.

Medication may cause reddening or scaling of skin when used on open skin lesions.

Contact with clothing, fabrics, plastics, wood, metal or other materials may cause damage; avoid contact.

Administration and Dosage:

Apply to affected area and place under occlusion at night. Hydrate skin for at least 5 minutes prior to use to enhance the effect. Remove any loose tissue with brush, wash cloth or emery board and dry thoroughly. Wash off in the morning. If excessive drying or irritation occurs, apply a bland cream or lotion. Once clearing is apparent, occasional use will usually maintain the remission. In those areas where occlusion is difficult or impossible, application may be more frequent. Unless hands are being treated, rinse hands thoroughly after application.

				C.I.*
Rx	**Salacid 60%** (Gordon)	**Ointment:** 60% in a petroleum base	In 60 g and lb.	164
Rx	**Salacid 25%** (Gordon)	**Ointment:** 25% in a petroleum base	In 60 g and lb.	143
otc	**Panscol** (Baker Cummins)	**Ointment:** 3%	In 90 g.	151
otc	**Calicylic Creme** (Gordon)	**Cream:** 10% with mineral oil, propylene glycol, white wax, sodium lauryl sulfate, oleic acid, parabens, triethanolamine	In 60 g.	88
Rx	**Salicylic Acid Creme 60%** (Pedinol)	**Cream:** 60% with primex, soybean oil, propylene glycol, polysorbate 20, 40, 80 and 85	In 56.7 g.	NA
otc	**Panscol** (Baker Cummins)	**Lotion:** 3%	In 120 ml.	129
Rx	**Paplex Ultra** (Medicis)	**Solution:** 26% in flexible collodion	In 15 ml with brush applicator.	857
Rx	**Verukan-HP** (Syosset)	**Solution:** 26% in flexible collodion	In 15 ml with applicator.	NA
Rx	**Paplex** (Medicis)	**Solution:** 17% with 17% lactic acid in flexible collodion	In 15 ml with brush applicator.	714
Rx	**Verukan** (Syosset)	**Solution:** 17% in flexible collodion with 17% lactic acid	In 15 ml with applicator.	NA
otc	**Freezone** (Whitehall)	**Solution:** 13.6% in a collodion vehicle with 20.5% alcohol, 64.8% ether and balsam oregon, castor oil, hypophosphorous acid, zinc chloride	In 9.3 ml.	389
Rx	**Occlusal-HP** (GenDerm)	**Liquid:** 26% in a polyacrylic vehicle with acrylates copolymer, butyl acetate, dibutyl phthalate, isopropyl alcohol, polyvinyl butyral	In 10 ml with brush applicator.	1490
Rx	**Lactisol-Forte** (Palisades)	**Liquid:** 20% with 20% lactic acid in a collodion base	In 15 ml with brush applicator.	954
otc	**Compound W** (Whitehall)	**Liquid:** 17% with acetone collodion, 1.83% alcohol, camphor, castor oil, menthol, polysorbate 80, 63.5% ether	In 9.3 ml.	665
otc	**DuoFilm** (Schering-Plough)	**Liquid:** 17% in flexible collodion with 15.8% alcohol, castor oil, 42.6% ether, ethyl lactate, polybutene	In 15 ml with brush applicator.	639

* Cost Index based on cost per g, ml or unit.

(Continued on following page)

SALICYLIC ACID (Cont.)

	Product	Description	Package	C.I.*
Rx	**Occlusal** (GenDerm)	**Liquid:** 17% in a polyacrylic vehicle with isopropyl alcohol, butyl acetate, polyvinyl butaryl, dibutyl phthalate, acrylates copolymer	In 15 ml with applicator.	803
otc	**Off-Ezy Wart Remover** (Commerce Drug)	**Liquid:** 17% in flexible collodion with 21% alcohol and 65% ether	In 13.5 ml.	423
otc	**Maximum Strength Wart-Off** (Pfizer)	**Liquid:** 17% in flexible collodion with 26.35% alcohol in propylene glycol dipelargonate	In 15 ml with applicator.	389
Rx	**Lactisol** (Palisades)	**Liquid:** 16.7% with 16.7% lactic acid in a collodion base	In 15 ml with brush applicator.	704
Rx	**Gordofilm** (Gordon)	**Liquid:** 16.7% with 16.7% lactic acid in flexible collodion	In 15 ml with brush applicator.	390
Rx	**Salactic Film** (Pedinol)	**Liquid:** 16.7% with 16.7% lactic acid in flexible collodion	In 15 ml with brush applicator.	NA
otc	**Mosco** (Medtech)	**Liquid:** 12% salicylic acid in a flexible collodion base with 23% alcohol and 65.5% ether	In 10 ml.	NA
otc	**Wart Remover** (Rugby)	**Liquid:** Salicylic acid, isopropanol in a flexible collodion	In 14.8 ml.	140
Rx	**Sal-Plant** (Pedinol)	**Gel:** 27% in collodion with lactic acid, hydroxypropyl cellulose, alcohol	In 14 g.	857
Rx	**Viranol Gel Ultra** (American Dermal)	**Gel:** 26% in a collodion-like gel vehicle of camphor, pyroxylin, povidone, 2% ethyl alcohol, acetone	In 8 g with applicator.	NA
otc	**Compound W** (Whitehall)	**Gel:** 17% with 67.5% alcohol, camphor, castor oil, collodion, colloidal silicon dioxide, hydroxypropyl cellulose, hypophosphorous acid, polysorbate 80	In 7.5 g.	825
otc	**DuoPlant for Feet** (Schering-Plough)	**Gel:** 17% in a flexible collodion with 57.6% alcohol, 16.42% ether, ethyl lactate, hydroxypropyl cellulose, polybutane	In 15 g.	639
otc	**Vergogel** (Daywell)	**Gel:** 17% with 67.5% alcohol, collodion, castor oil, camphor, colloidal silicon dioxide, polysorbate 80, hydroxypropyl cellulose, hypophosphorous acid	In 15 g.	376
otc	**Viranol** (American Dermal)	**Gel:** 12% with lactic acid, camphor, pyroxylin, 31% ethyl alcohol, ethyl acetate	In 8 g with applicator.	695
Rx	**Hydrisalic** (Pedinol)	**Gel:** 6% with hydroxyethylcellulose, propylene glycol, SD alcohol 40B	In 28.35 g.	272
Rx	**Keralyt** (Westwood)	**Gel:** 6% in a base containing propylene glycol, 19.4% alcohol, hydroxypropylcellulose	In 28.4 g.	581

* Cost Index based on cost per g, ml or unit.

(Continued on following page)

SALICYLIC ACID (Cont.)

				C.I.*
otc	**DuoFilm** (Schering-Plough)	**Transdermal Patch**: 40% in a rubber-based vehicle	In 18s (containing 3 sizes).	533
otc	**Trans-Plantar** (Tsumura Medical)	**Transdermal Patch**: 21% with karaya, PEG-300, propylene glycol	20 mm patches in 25s with securing tapes and one cleaning file.	1173
otc	**PediaPatch** (Tsumura Medical)	**Transdermal Patch**: 15% in karaya gum base	In 6 mm (20s) with bandage tapes.	427
otc	**Trans-Ver-Sal** (Tsumura Medical)	**Transdermal Patch**: 15% with karaya, PEG-300, propylene glycol	6 or 12 mm patches in 40s with securing tapes and emery file.	750
Rx	**Sal-Acid** (Pedinol)	**Plaster**: 50%	In 8s.	580
otc	**Mediplast** (Beiersdorf)	**Plaster**: 40%	2″ x 3″ patches in 25s.	1342
otc	**Clear Away Plantar** (Schering-Plough)	**Disc**: 40% in a rubber-based vehicle	In 24s (for feet) with comfort cushions.	NA
otc	**Clear Away** (Schering-Plough)		In 18s.	NA

* Cost Index based on cost per g, ml or unit.

PODOPHYLLUM RESIN (Podophyllin)

Actions:

Pharmacology: Podophyllum resin is the powdered mixture of resins removed from the May apple or Mandrake *(Podophyllum peltatum Linne')*, a perennial plant of northern and middle US.

Podophyllum is a cytotoxic agent that has been used topically in the treatment of genital warts. It arrests mitosis in metaphase, an effect it shares with other cytotoxic agents such as the vinca alkaloids. The active agent is podophyllotoxin, whose concentration varies with the type of podophyllum resin used; American podophyllum typically has a reduced level of podophyllotoxin and normally contains one-fourth the amount of the Indian source.

Indications:

For the removal of soft genital (venereal) warts (condyloma acuminata) and other papillomas. Also used for multiple superficial epitheliomatosis and keratoses.

The CDC recommends podophyllum resin as an alternative regimen to cryotherapy for the treatment of external genital/perianal warts, vaginal warts and urethral meatus warts.[1]

Contraindications:

Diabetics; patients using steroids or with poor blood circulation; use on bleeding warts, moles, birthmarks or unusual warts with hair growing from them; pregnancy, lactation (see Warnings).

Warnings:

For external use only: Podophyllum is a powerful caustic and severe irritant. Keep away from the eyes; if eye contact occurs, flush with copious amounts of warm water and consult physician or poison control center immediately for advice.

Physician use (application) only: Podophyllum resin is to be applied only by a physician. It is not to be dispensed to the patient.

Pregnancy: There have been reports of complications associated with the topical use of podophyllum on condylomas of pregnant patients including birth defects, fetal death and stillbirth. Do not use on pregnant patients or patients who plan to become pregnant.

Lactation: It is not known whether podophyllum is excreted in breast milk following topical application. Do not use on nursing patients.

Precautions:

Inflamed/Irritated tissue: Do not use if wart or surrounding tissue is inflamed or irritated. Do not use on bleeding warts, moles, birthmarks or unusual warts with hair growing from them.

Adverse Reactions:

Paresthesia; polyneuritis; paralytic ileus; pyrexia; leukopenia; thrombocytopenia; nausea; vomiting; diarrhea; abdominal pain; confusion; dizziness; stupor; convulsions; coma; death.

Significant neuropathy and death are generally related to large amounts used for multiple and widespread lesions. Onset of neuropathy may occur within hours of application and the duration may range from months to years with some neurologic deficit.

Patient information:

To be applied only by a physician.

For external use only. Avoid contact with eyes and healthy tissue.

Administration and Dosage:

Podophyllum is to be applied only by a physician. It is not to be dispensed to the patient. Thoroughly cleanse affected area. Use applicator to apply sparingly to lesion. Avoid contact with healthy tissue. Allow to dry thoroughly. Treat only intact (no bleeding) lesions. As podophyllum is a powerful caustic and severe irritant, it is recommended the first application be left in contact for only a short time (30 to 40 minutes) to determine patient's sensitivity. To avoid systemic absorption, use the minimum time of contact necessary to produce the desired result (1 to 4 hours, depending on condition of lesion and of patient), with the physician developing their own experience and technique. Do not treat large areas or numerous warts at once. After treatment time has elapsed, remove dried podophyllum resin thoroughly with alcohol or soap and water.

				C.I.*
Rx	**Pod-Ben-25** (Palisades)	**Liquid:** 25% podophyllum resin in tincture of benzoin	In 30 ml.	786
Rx	**Podocon-25** (Paddock)		In 15 ml.	NA
Rx	**Podofin** (Syosset)		In 15 ml.	2857

* Cost Index based on cost per ml.

[1] CDC 1989 Sexually Transmitted Diseases Treatment Guidelines. *Morbidity and Mortality Weekly Report* 1989 Sept 1;38(No.S-8):20-21.

PODOFILOX

Actions:

Pharmacology: Podofilox is a topical antimitotic drug which can be chemically synthesized or purified from the plant families *Coniferae* and *Berberidaceae* (eg, species of *Juniperus* and *Podophyllum*). Treatment of genital warts with podofilox results in necrosis of visible wart tissue. The exact mechanism of action is unknown.

Pharmacokinetics: In systemic absorption studies in 52 patients, topical application of 0.05 ml of 0.5% podofilox solution to external genitalia did not result in detectable serum levels. Applications of 0.1 to 1.5 ml resulted in peak serum levels of 1 to 17 ng/ml 1 to 2 hours after application. The elimination half-life ranged from 1 to 4.5 hours. The drug was not found to accumulate after multiple treatments.

Clinical studies: In double-blind clinical studies, patients were treated for 2 to 4 weeks, and reevaluated at a 2 week follow-up examination. Although the number of patients and warts evaluated at each time period varied, the results among investigators were relatively consistent. The following table represents the responses noted in terms of frequency of response by lesions treated and the overall response by patients. Data are presented for only those patients evaluated at the 2 week follow-up.

Patient Response to Podofilox Treatment[1]

	Initially Cleared	Recurred after clearing	Cleared at 2 week follow-up
Warts (n = 524)	79%	35%	60%
Patients (n = 70)	50%	60%	25%

[1] Cleared and clearing mean no visible wart tissue remained at the treated sites.

Indications:

Topical treatment of external genital warts *(Condyloma acuminatum).* This product is *not* indicated in the treatment of perianal or mucous membrane warts (see Precautions).

Contraindications:

Hypersensitivity or intolerance to any component of the formulation.

Warnings:

Diagnosis: Correct diagnosis of the lesions to be treated is essential. Although genital warts have a characteristic appearance, obtain histopathologic confirmation if there is any doubt of the diagnosis. Differentiating warts from squamous cell carcinoma (so-called "Bowenoid papulosis") is of particular concern. Squamous cell carcinoma may also be associated with human papillomavirus but should not be treated with podofilox.

External use only: Podofilox solution is intended for cutaneous use only. Avoid contact with the eyes. If eye contact occurs, immediately flush the eye with copious quantities of water and seek medical advice.

Carcinogenesis/Mutagenesis: In mouse studies, crude podophyllin resin (containing podofilox) applied topically to the cervix produced changes resembling carcinoma in situ. These changes were reversible at 5 weeks after treatment cessation. In one report, epidermal carcinoma of the vagina and cervix was found in 1 of 18 mice after 120 applications of podophyllin (applied twice weekly over 15 months).

Results from the mouse micronucleus in vivo assay using podofilox 0.5% solution in concentrations up to 25 mg/kg indicate that podofilox should be considered a potential clastogen (a chemical that induces disruption and breakage of chromosomes).

Pregnancy: Category C. Podofilox is embryotoxic in rats when administered systemically in a dose approximately 250 times the recommended maximum human dose. There are no adequate and well controlled studies in pregnant women. Use in pregnancy only if the potential benefit justifies the potential risk to the fetus.

Lactation: It is not known whether this drug is excreted in breast milk. Decide whether to discontinue nursing or to discontinue the drug, taking into account the importance of the drug to the mother.

Children: Safety and efficacy in children have not been established.

Precautions:

Perianal/Mucous membrane warts: Data are not available on the safe and effective use of this product for treatment of warts occurring in the perianal area or on mucous membranes of the genital area (including the urethra, rectum and vagina). Do not exceed the recommended method of application, frequency of application, and duration of usage (see Administration and Dosage).

(Continued on following page)

PODOFILOX (Cont.)

Adverse Reactions:

In clinical trials, the following local adverse reactions occurred at some point during treatment. Reports of burning and pain were more frequent and of greater severity in women than in men.

Podofilox Adverse Reactions		
Adverse Reaction	Males	Females
Burning	64%	78%
Pain	50%	72%
Inflammation	71%	63%
Erosion	67%	67%
Itching	50%	65%

Other (< 5%): Pain with intercourse; insomnia; tingling; bleeding; tenderness; chafing; malodor; dizziness; scarring; vesicle formation; crusting edema; dryness/peeling; foreskin irretraction; hematuria; vomiting; ulceration.

Overdosage:

Symptoms: Topically applied podofilox may be absorbed systemically. Toxicity reported following systemic administration of podofilox in investigational use for cancer treatment included: Nausea; vomiting; fever; diarrhea; bone marrow depression; oral ulcers. Following 5 to 10 daily IV doses of 0.5 to 1 mg/kg/day, significant hematological toxicity occurred but was reversible. Other toxicities occurred at lower doses.

Toxicity reported following systemic administration of podophyllum resin included: Nausea; vomiting; fever; diarrhea; peripheral neuropathy; altered mental status; lethargy; coma; tachypnea; respiratory failure; leukocytosis; pancytosis; hematuria; renal failure; seizures.

Treatment of topical overdosage should include washing the skin free of any remaining drug and symptomatic and supportive therapy. Refer to General Management of Acute Overdosage.

Patient Information:

Provide the patient with a Patient Information leaflet when a podofilox prescription is filled.

Administration and Dosage:

Apply twice daily morning and evening (every 12 hours) for 3 consecutive days, then withhold use for 4 consecutive days. This 1 week cycle of treatment may be repeated up to 4 times until there is no visible wart tissue. If there is incomplete response after 4 treatment weeks, consider alternative treatment. Safety and efficacy of > 4 treatment weeks have not been established.

Podofilox is applied to the warts with a cotton-tipped applicator supplied with the drug. Touch the drug-dampened applicator to the wart to be treated, applying the minimum amount of solution necessary to cover the lesion. Limit treatment to < 10 cm^2 of wart tissue and to ≤ 0.5 ml of the solution per day. There is no evidence to suggest that more frequent application will increase efficacy, but additional applications would be expected to increase the rate of local adverse reactions and systemic absorption.

Take care to allow the solution to dry before allowing the return of opposing skin surfaces to their normal positions. Carefully dispose of the used applicator after each treatment and wash hands.

Storage: Avoid excessive heat. Do not freeze.

Rx	**Condylox** (Oclassen)	**Topical Solution:** 0.5% podofilox	95% alcohol. In 3.5 ml amber glass bottles.

CANTHARIDIN

Actions:

Pharmacology: Effectiveness against warts is presumed to result from the "exfoliation" of the tumor as a consequence of its acantholytic action. The lytic action of cantharidin does not go beyond the epidermal cells, the basal layer remains intact and there is minimal effect on the corium; as a result, there is no scarring from topical application.

Indications:

A vesicant for removal of benign epithelial growths: Warts (including ordinary, periungual, subungual and plantar) and molluscum contagiosum.

Contraindications:

Diabetics or persons with impaired peripheral circulation; use on eyes, mucous membranes, ano-genital or intertriginous areas, moles, birthmarks or unusual warts with hair growing from them, or if lesion is being treated with other agents; if growth or surrounding tissue is inflamed or irritated.

Warnings:

Vesicant properties: Cantharidin is a strong vesicant. Use sparingly. Do not use in ano-genital area. Keep away from eyes and mucosal tissue. Avoid use in intertriginous sites due to problems with spreading and body occlusion which often lead to more intense, painful reactions.

Cantharidin may produce blisters on normal skin or mucous membranes. If spilled on skin, wipe off at once, using acetone, alcohol or tape remover; wash with warm soapy water and rinse well. If spilled on mucous membranes or in eyes, flush with water, remove precipitated collodion; flush with water for an additional 15 minutes.

Physician use (application) only: Cantharidin is a potent vesicant and should be applied only by a physician. It is not to be dispensed to the patient.

Sensitivity: Patients vary in sensitivity to cantharidin; tingling, burning or extreme tenderness may develop rarely. In these cases, remove tape and soak the area in cool water for 10 to 15 minutes; repeat as required for relief. If soreness persists, puncture blister aseptically, apply antiseptic and cover with bandage. Treat only one or two lesions on the first visit, until the sensitivity of the patient is known. Expect a more intense reaction in patients with fair skin and blue eyes. Do not reapply to the same lesion more than once per week. Defer second treatment if inflammation is intense.

Palpebral warts: Use great care if treating palpebral warts. Make certain film is thoroughly dry; warn patient not to touch the eyelid.

Pigmentation: Although rare, use care in the selection of site application since residual pigmentation changes may occur.

Pregnancy: There have been no adequate and well controlled studies in pregnant women; therefore, the use of cantharidin during pregnancy is not recommended.

Lactation: Use in nursing mothers is not recommended.

Adverse Reactions:

Annular warts have occurred in some patients. These are superficial and present little problem, although they may alarm patients. Reassure patient and treat again.

There have been several reports of chemical lymphangitis following use of cantharidin, one in combination with salicylic acid plaster. A case of extreme, painful blistering occurred after treatment of multiple axillary lesions.

Patient Information:

May cause tingling, itching or burning within a few hours after application; site may be extremely tender for 2 to 6 days.

If spilled on skin, wipe off at once with acetone, alcohol or tape remover and wash with soap and water.

For external use only. If spilled in the eyes, flush with water and contact physician.

(Continued on following page)

CANTHARIDIN (Cont.)

Administration and Dosage:

Ordinary and periungual warts: No cutting or prior treatment is required. Apply directly to the lesion and cover the growth completely, extending beyond by about 1 mm. Allow a few minutes for a thin membrane to form. Cover completely with nonporous tape. Remove tape in 24 hours and replace with a loose bandage. On next visit (1 to 2 weeks), remove necrotic tissue and reapply to any remaining growth. Defer second treatment if inflammation is intense. A single treatment frequently suffices.

Plantar warts: Pare away keratin covering the wart; avoid cutting viable tissue. Apply to wart and 1 to 3 mm around the wart. Allow to dry, secure with nonporous tape; application of a protective cut-out cushion over the tape may be helpful. After 24 hours, the patient may bathe and replace dressing. Debride 1 to 2 weeks after treatment. If any viable wart tissue remains, reapply as above; ≥ 3 treatments may be required for large lesions. For large mosaic warts, treat a portion of the wart at a time. Applying cantharidin to open tissue will result in stinging from the solvent. Avoid by paring carefully and scheduling treatments 2 weeks apart.

Molluscum contagiosum: Apply a very small amount of solution to only the top of each lesion. Let dry completely. No occlusive tape or dressing is needed. Alert patient that blistering is the desired result and that temporary hypopigmentation may occur. The patient may bathe after 4 to 6 hours; sooner if discomfort occurs. Blisters are usually formed by about 24 hours and crust up in about 4 days. Mild discomfort or itching can usually be controlled with bathing and night sedation. In 1 week, treat new or remaining lesions the same way and re-treat any resistant lesions. This time, cover with a small piece of occlusive tape. Remove tape in 4 to 6 hours, sooner if discomfort occurs.

Note: Use of a mild antibacterial is recommended until the tissue re-epithelializes.

				C.I.*
Rx	**Cantharone** (Seres)	**Liquid:** 0.7% cantharidin in a film-forming vehicle containing acetone, pyroxylin, castor oil, camphor	In 7.5 ml.	3000
Rx	**Verr-Canth** (Palisades)	**Liquid:** 0.7% cantharidin in an adherent film-forming base of ethylcellulose, cellosolve, castor oil, penederm (octylphenylpolyethylene glycol), acetone	In 7.5 ml.	2952

KERATOLYTIC COMBINATIONS

Rx	**Verrex** (Palisades)	**Liquid:** 30% salicylic acid and 10% podophyllum in an adherent film-forming vehicle of penederm (octylphenylpolyethylene glycol), ethylcellulose, cellosolve, collodion, castor oil, acetone	In 7.5 ml with applicator.	1086
Rx	**Cantharone Plus** (Seres)	**Liquid:** 30% salicylic acid, 2% podophyllum and 1% cantharidin in a film-forming vehicle containing 0.5% penederm (octylphenylpolyethylene glycol), cellosolve, ethocel, pyroxylin, castor oil, acetone	In 7.5 ml.	4629
Rx	**Verrusol** (Palisades)	**Liquid:** 30% salicylic acid, 5% podophyllum and 1% cantharidin in an adherent film-forming vehicle of penederm (octylphenylpolyethylene glycol), ethylcellulose, cellosolve, collodion, castor oil, acetone	In 7.5 ml.	4943
otc	**Gets-It** (Oakhurst)	**Liquid:** Salicylic acid, zinc chloride and collodion in ≈35% ether and ≈28% alcohol	In 12 ml.	150

* Cost Index based on cost per g or ml.

CHLOROACETIC ACIDS

Actions:

Rapidly penetrates and cauterizes skin, keratin and other tissues. Monochloroacetic acid is more deeply destructive than trichloroacetic acid.

Indications:

Dichloroacetic acid: Verrucae (warts); calluses; hard and soft corns; xanthoma palpebrarum; seborrheic keratoses; ingrown nails; cysts and benign erosion of the cervix; endocervicitis; epistaxis.

Monochloroacetic and trichloroacetic acid: Removal of verrucae.

The CDC recommends trichloroacetic acid as an alternative regimen to cryotherapy for the treatment of external genital/perianal warts and vaginal and anal warts.

Contraindications:

Treatment of malignant or premalignant lesions; hypersensitivity to any component.

Warnings:

Cauterant properties: These acids are powerful keratolytics and cauterants. Restrict use to areas where these effects are desired. May cause severe burning, inflammation or tenderness of skin.

Cervical lesions: A careful diagnosis and possibly a biopsy is required to rule out malignancy; treatment is contraindicated in the event of positive findings.

Normal tissue: Apply only to the lesion being treated. To prevent acid from spreading onto normal skin, apply petrolatum around the area to be treated. If any acid is spilled on normal tissue or if too much acid is applied, remove immediately and wash with water. Sodium bicarbonate may be applied as a local antidote.

MONOCHLOROACETIC ACID

Administration and Dosage:

Remove callus tissue. Apply to verruca. Apply bandage and allow to remain in place for 5 to 6 days. Remove verruca tissue and reapply as needed. If crystallization of liquid occurs, place capped bottle in hot water to redissolve.

				C.I.*
Rx	**Monocete** (Pedinol)	**Liquid:** 80%	In 15 ml.	714
Rx	**Mono-Chlor** (Gordon)		In 15 ml.	429

DICHLOROACETIC ACID

Administration and Dosage:

Amount applied varies with the nature of the lesion. Dense horny lesions (corns, warts, calluses, plantar warts) require repeated intensive treatment. Lesions of light density (pedunculated warts, xanthoma palpebrarum, soft corns, seborrheic keratoses, condyloma acuminata) receive lighter applications.

Technique for application depends on the type of lesion. Dense growths are treated by rubbing the acid into the lesion with a pointed wooden applicator or a cotton tipped applicator; 3 or 4 treatments may be necessary. Lesions of light density should receive a lighter application at each visit. Usually 1 or 2 such treatments are sufficient.

Apply thin layer of petrolatum to normal tissue surrounding the lesion. Use microdropper to transfer some acid to small-stemmed acid receptacle. The acid should not contact the microdropper's neoprene bulb. Use the microdropper upright, filling no more than halfway. Moisten a sharpened applicator stick in acid and draw over flared lip to remove excess. There should never be a large excess drop on applicator.

When applying very small amounts, hold applicator level or with the point up so that a tiny fraction of one drop can be transferred to small lesions. Cauterization progress is followed by observing change in color of treated area to gray-white, using a magnifying lens if necessary. It is sometimes advantageous to apply the acid by rolling the applicator over the surface of the lesion, using the point only at the edges. To avoid contamination, do not return any remaining acid from the receptacle to the bottle. Keep the bottle tightly capped except when removing acid. Discard applicators after use.

See manufacturer's package insert for treatment of specific lesions.

				C.I.*
Rx	**Bichloracetic Acid** (Glenwood)	**Liquid:** 10 ml dichloroacetic acid.	In treatment kit with 16 g petrolatum, applicators, acid receptacles, microdropper and holder.	2457

TRICHLOROACETIC ACID

Administration and Dosage:

Debride callus tissue. Apply to verruca. Cover with bandage for 5 to 6 days. Remove verruca. Reapply as needed. If crystallization of liquid occurs, place capped bottle in hot water to redissolve.

				C.I.*
Rx	**Tri-Chlor** (Gordon)	**Liquid:** 80%	In 15 ml.	452

* Cost Index based on cost per ml.

[1] CDC 1989 Sexually Transmitted Diseases Treatment Guidelines. *Morbidity and Mortality Weekly Report* 1989 Sept 1;38(No.S-8):20-21.

SILVER NITRATE

For use in the prevention of gonorrheal ophthalmia neonatorum, see monograph in the Ophthalmic section.

Actions:

Pharmacology: Silver nitrate is a strong caustic and escharotic providing antiseptic, astringent, germicidal, local (epithelial) stimulant or caustic action externally.

The attachment of silver to a reactive group of a protein sharply decreases the protein's solubility; the protein's conformation may also be altered and denaturation may occur. Precipitation of the protein generally results. At low concentrations of silver, precipitation is confined to proteins in the interstices and an astringent action occurs. At high concentrations, membrane and intracellular structures are damaged and there is a caustic or corrosive effect.

Because silver ions attach so readily to the various groups of proteins, the silver ions are captured before they diffuse far into the tissues. Precipitation of silver as silver chloride also limits the extent of movement of the ions. Thus, local effects of silver are self-limiting and spread of damage occurs only when the dose of silver overwhelms the capacity of tissues to fix the ion at the site of application. The antiseptic effects of silver may derive in part from the reaction with bacterial and viral proteins.

Indications:

To treat indolent wounds, destroy exuberant granulations, freshen the edges of ulcers and fissures, touch the bases of vesicular, bullous or aphthous lesions and provide styptic action.

10% Ointment: Podiatry – To treat neurovascular helomas; to cauterize and destroy small nerve endings and blood vessels. It forms a protective covering after the removal of corns and calluses.

10% Solution: Impetigo vulgaris. *Podiatry* – Helomas.

25% Solution: Pruritus. *Podiatry* – Plantar warts.

50% Solution: Podiatry – Plantar warts; granulation tissue; papillomatous growths; granuloma pyogenicum.

Unlabeled uses: Concentrations of 0.1% to 0.5% are used as wet dressings in burns and on lesions.

Contraindications:

Application on wounds, cuts or broken skin.

Warnings:

Skin discoloration: Prolonged or frequent use may result in permanent discoloration of the skin due to deposition of reduced silver. However, topical silver nitrate for localized application to suppress granulation tissue apparently does not produce argyria.

Staining of clothes: Will stain clothing and linens.

Electrolyte abnormalities: If wet dressings are used over extensive areas or prolonged periods, electrolyte abnormalities can result. Sodium and chloride leach into the dressing and hyponatremia or hypochloremia can occur. Absorbed nitrate can cause methemoglobinemia.

Precautions:

Irritation: Discontinue use if redness or irritation occurs.

For external use only: Avoid contact with the eyes.

Overdosage:

Symptoms: The fatal dose of silver nitrate may be as low as 2 g. The oral intake of silver nitrate causes a local corrosive effect including pain and burning of the mouth, salivation, vomiting, diarrhea progressing to anuria, shock, coma, convulsions and death. Blackening of the skin and mucous membranes occurs (sometimes permanent).

Treatment: Administer sodium chloride in water, 10 g/L; this causes precipitation of silver chloride. Follow with catharsis, including sodium chloride solution. Also attend to shock and methemoglobinemia if present.

If splashed in the eyes, wash with copious amounts of water and see a physician.

Administration and Dosage:

Ointment: Apply in an apertured pad on affected area or lesion for approximately 5 days, as needed.

Solution: Apply a cotton applicator dipped in solution on the affected area or lesion 2 or 3 times a week for 2 or 3 weeks, as needed.

Rx	**Silver Nitrate** (Gordon Labs)	**Ointment:** 10%	Petrolatum base. In 30 g.
		Solution: 10%	In 30 ml.
		25%	In 30 ml.
		50%	In 30 ml.
Rx	**Silver Nitrate** (Graham-Field)	**Applicators:** 75% with 25% potassium nitrate	In 100s.

SUTILAINS

Actions:

Pharmacology: Selectively digests necrotic soft tissues by proteolytic action. It dissolves and facilitates removal of necrotic tissues and purulent exudates that otherwise impair formation of granulation tissue and delay wound healing.

Indications:

As an adjunct to wound care for biochemical debridement of the following lesions: Second and third degree burns; decubitus ulcers; incisional, traumatic and pyogenic wounds; ulcers secondary to peripheral vascular disease.

Contraindications:

Wounds communicating with major body cavities; wounds containing exposed major nerves or nerve tissue; fungating neoplastic ulcers.

Warnings:

For external use only: Do not permit ointment to come into contact with the eyes. If this inadvertently occurs, rinse immediately with copious amounts of sterile water.

Pregnancy: Category B. There are no adequate or well controlled studies in pregnant women. Use during pregnancy only if no adequate alternatives are available.

Children: Safety and efficacy for use in children have not been established.

Precautions:

A moist environment is essential for optimal enzyme activity.

Systemic therapy: In cases where there is existent or threatening invasive infection, institute systemic antibiotic therapy.

Antibody response: Although there have been no reports of systemic allergic reactions in humans, there may be an antibody response to absorbed enzyme material.

Impairment of enzyme activity: Enzyme activity may be impaired by certain agents. In vitro, several detergents and antiseptics (**benzalkonium chloride, hexachlorophene, iodine** and **nitrofurazone**) render the substrate indifferent to the action of the enzyme. Compounds such as **thimerosal**, which contain metallic ions, interfere directly with enzyme activity to a slight degree, whereas, **neomycin, mafenide, streptomycin** and **penicillin** do not affect enzyme activity. If adjunctive topical therapy has been used and no dissolution of slough occurs after treatment for 24 to 48 hours, further application, because of interference by adjunctive agents, is unlikely to be successful.

Adverse Reactions:

Local: Mild, transient pain; paresthesias; bleeding; transient dermatitis. If bleeding or dermatitis occurs, discontinue therapy. Pain can usually be controlled with mild analgesics. Side effects severe enough to warrant discontinuation of therapy have occurred.

Systemic toxicity has not been observed as a result of topical application.

Administration and Dosage:

Thoroughly cleanse and irrigate wound area with sodium chloride or water solutions. Wound *must* be cleansed of antiseptics or heavy-metal antibacterials which may denature enzyme or alter substrate characteristics (see Precautions).

Thoroughly moisten wound area through bathing, showering or wet soaks (eg, sodium chloride or water solutions).

Apply ointment in a thin layer (⅛ inch), assuring intimate contact with necrotic tissue and complete wound coverage extending ¼ to ½ inch beyond the area to be debrided.

Apply moist dressings.

Repeat entire procedure 3 to 4 times per day for best results.

Storage: Ointment must be refrigerated at 2° to 8°C (36° to 46°F).

				C.I.*
Rx	**Travase** (Boots)	**Ointment:** 82,000 casein units per g in a hydrophobic base of 95% mineral oil and 5% polyethylene	In 14.2 g.	117

* Cost Index based on cost per g.

COLLAGENASE

Actions:

Pharmacology: Since collagen accounts for 75% of the dry weight of skin tissue, the ability of collagenase to digest collagen in the physiological pH range and temperature makes it effective in the removal of tissue debris. Complete debridement occurs in 10 to 14 days. Collagenase thus contributes to the formation of granulation tissues and subsequent epithelialization of dermal ulcers and severely burned areas. Collagen in healthy tissue or in newly formed granulation tissue is not attacked.

Indications:

For debriding chronic dermal ulcers and severely burned areas.

Contraindications:

Local or systemic hypersensitivity to collagenase.

Precautions:

For external use only. Avoid contact with the eyes.

Optimal pH range of the enzyme is 6 to 8.

Systemic bacterial infections: Monitor debilitated patients for systemic bacterial infections because debriding enzymes may increase the risk of bacteremia.

Slight transient erythema has been noted occasionally in surrounding tissue, particularly when the ointment was not confined to the lesion. Therefore, apply carefully within the area of the lesion. Irritation may be prevented by applying a protectant (eg, zinc oxide paste) to the surrounding tissue.

Inhibition of enzymatic activity: Enzymatic activity is inhibited by **detergents, benzalkonium chloride, hexachlorophene, nitrofurazone, tincture of iodine** and **heavy metal ions** such as **mercury** and **silver** which are used in some antiseptics. When such materials have been used, carefully cleanse the site by repeated washings with normal saline before ointment is applied. Avoid soaks containing metal ions or acidic solutions such as **Burow's solution** because of the metal ion and low pH. Cleansing materials such as hydrogen peroxide, Dakin's solution or normal saline do not interfere with enzyme activity.

Adverse Reactions:

No allergic sensitivity or toxic reactions have been noted in clinical investigations. However, one case of systemic manifestations of hypersensitivity to collagenase in a patient treated for > 1 year with a combination of collagenase and cortisone has been reported.

Overdosage:

Action of the enzyme may be stopped by the application of Burow's solution (pH 3.6 to 4.4) to the lesion.

Administration and Dosage:

Apply once daily (more frequently if the dressing becomes soiled).

Prior to application, cleanse the lesion of debris and digested material by gently rubbing with a gauze pad saturated with hydrogen peroxide or Dakin's solution, followed by sterile normal saline.

When infection is present, use an appropriate topical antibacterial agent. Neomycin-bacitracin-polymyxin B is compatible with collagenase ointment; apply to the lesion prior to the application of collagenase ointment. Should the infection not respond, discontinue therapy until remission of the infection occurs.

Apply ointment (using a wooden tongue depressor or spatula) directly to deep wounds; with shallow wounds, use a sterile gauze pad, apply to wound and secure properly.

Crosshatching thick eschar with a #10 blade allows collagenase more surface contact with necrotic debris. Remove as much loosened tissue debris as possible with forceps and scissors.

Remove all excess ointment each time dressing is changed.

Terminate use of the ointment when debridement of necrotic tissue is complete and granulation tissue is well established.

				C.I.*
Rx	**Santyl** (Knoll)	**Ointment:** 250 units collagenase enzyme per g. In white petrolatum.	In 15 and 30 g.	2459

* Cost Index based on cost per g.

FIBRINOLYSIN AND DESOXYRIBONUCLEASE

Actions:

Pharmacology: Combination of these enzymes is based on the observation that prurulent exudates consist largely of fibrinous material and nucleoprotein. Desoxyribonuclease attacks the deoxyribonucleic acid (DNA) and fibrinolysin attacks principally fibrin of blood clots and fibrinous exudates.

The activity of desoxyribonuclease is limited principally to the production of large polynucleotides, which are less likely to be absorbed than the more diffusible protein fractions liberated by enzyme preparations obtained from bacteria. Fibrinolytic action is directed mainly against denatured proteins, such as those found in devitalized tissue, while protein elements of living cells remain relatively unaffected.

Indications:

Topical: Debriding agent in general surgical wounds; ulcerative lesions (trophic, decubitus, stasis, arteriosclerotic); second- and third-degree burns; circumcision; episiotomy.

In infected lesions such as burns, ulcers and wounds where a topical antibiotic is desired, the product containing the enzymes plus chloramphenicol is indicated. Except in very superficial infections, systemic medication is also indicated.

Intravaginal: Cervicitis (benign, postpartum and postconization) and vaginitis.

Irrigating agent: Infected wounds (abscesses, fistulae and sinus tracts); otorhinolaryngologic wounds; superficial hematomas (except when the hematoma is adjacent to or within adipose tissue).

Contraindications:

Hypersensitivity reactions to any component; parenteral use (bovine fibrinolysin may be antigenic).

Warnings:

Bone marrow hypoplasia, aplastic anemia and death have been reported following the local application of chloramphenicol (present in *Elase-Chloromycetin*).

Precautions:

Hypersensitivity: Observe precautions against allergic reactions, particularly in persons with a history of sensitivity to bovine material. Have epinephrine 1:1000 immediately available. Refer to Management of Acute Hypersensitivity Reactions.

Superinfection: Chloramphenicol – Use of antibiotics (especially prolonged or repeated therapy) may result in bacterial or fungal overgrowth of nonsusceptible organisms and may lead to a secondary infection. Take appropriate measures if superinfection occurs.

Adverse Reactions:

Side effects have not been a problem for the indications and dose recommended. With higher concentrations, local hyperemia may occur.

Administration and Dosage:

After application, these products become rapidly and progressively less active; only insignificant activity remains after 24 hours.

Individualize dosage. Successful use of enzymatic debridement depends on several factors: (1) Remove any dense, dry eschar surgically before enzymatic debridement is attempted; (2) the enzyme must be in constant contact with the substrate; (3) periodically remove accumulated necrotic debris; (4) replenish the enzyme at least once daily; and (5) employ secondary closure or skin grafting as soon as possible after optimal debridement. Administer appropriate systemic antibiotics if indicated.

General topical uses:

Repeat local application for as long as enzyme action is desired.

Procedure – Clean wound with water, peroxide or normal saline and dry area gently. Surgically remove dense, dry eschar before applying ointment. Apply a thin layer of ointment and cover with petrolatum gauze or other nonadhering dressing.

Change dressing at least once a day, preferably 2 or 3 times daily. Frequency of application is more important than amount of ointment used. Flush away the necrotic debris and fibrinous exudates with saline, peroxide or warm water so that newly applied ointment is in direct contact with the substrate.

The solution may be applied topically as a liquid, wet dressing or spray by using a conventional atomizer.

Wet dressing: Mix 1 vial of powder with 10 to 50 ml saline and saturate strips of fine-mesh gauze or unfolded sterile gauze sponge with solution. Pack ulcerated area with gauze so that it remains in contact with the necrotic substrate. Allow gauze to dry in contact with ulcerated lesion (approximately 6 to 8 hours). Remove dried gauze; this mechanically debrides the area. Repeat wet-to-dry procedure 3 or 4 times daily since frequent dressing changes enhance results. After 2 to 4 days, the area will be clean and will begin to fill in with granulation tissue.

(Administration and Dosage continued on following page)

FIBRINOLYSIN AND DESOXYRIBONUCLEASE (Cont.)

Administration and Dosage (Cont.):

Intravaginal use: In mild to moderate vaginitis and cervicitis, apply 5 g of ointment deep into the vagina at bedtime for approximately 5 applications. In more severe cases, instill 10 ml of solution intravaginally, wait 1 or 2 minutes for enzyme to disperse, then insert a cotton tampon in the vaginal canal. Remove tampon the next day. Continue therapy with the ointment.

Abscesses, empyema cavities, fistulae, sinus tracts or SC hematomas: Despite contraindications against parenteral use, the solution has been used to irrigate these conditions. Drain and replace solution at intervals of 6 to 10 hours to reduce amount of by-product accumulation and minimize loss of enzyme activity. Traces of blood in discharge usually indicate active filling in of the cavity.

Preparation of solution: Reconstitute contents of each vial with 10 ml isotonic sodium chloride solution. Higher or lower concentrations can be prepared by varying the amount of diluent.

To be maximally effective, solutions must be freshly prepared before use. The loss in activity is reduced by refrigeration; however, do not use solution ≥ 24 hours after reconstitution, even when refrigerated.

				C.I.*
Rx	**Elase** (Fujisawa)	**Powder, lyophilized:** 25 units (Loomis) fibrinolysin and 15,000 units (modified Christensen method) desoxyribonuclease[1] per vial	In 30 ml vials.	888
		Ointment: 1 unit fibrinolysin and 666.6 units desoxyribonuclease[1] per g in a liquid petrolatum and polyethylene base	In 10 and 30 g tubes.	1717
Rx	**Elase-Chloromycetin** (Fujisawa)	**Ointment:** 10 mg chloramphenicol, 1 unit fibrinolysin & 666.6 units desoxyribonuclease[1] per g in a liquid petrolatum and polyethylene base	In 10 and 30 g tubes.	1876

TOPICAL ENZYME COMBINATIONS

TRYPSIN and *PAPAIN* are used for the enzymatic debridement and promotion of normal healing, especially where healing is retarded by eschar, necrotic tissue and debris.

BALSAM PERU is an effective capillary bed stimulant intended to improve circulation to the wound site. It may have a mildly antiseptic action.

CASTOR OIL (also refer to the Laxative monograph) is used to improve epithelialization by reducing premature epithelial desiccation and cornification, and as a protective covering.

UREA (see monograph in Emollients section) is an emollient and keratolytic.

CHLOROPHYLL DERIVATIVES (see individual monograph) aid wound healing and control wound odor.

Warnings:

Arterial clots: Do not spray trypsin products on fresh arterial clots.

For external use only. Avoid contact with the eyes.

Transient burning may be associated with initial application.

Administration and Dosage:

Apply medication once or twice daily.

Clean wound prior to application (hydrogen peroxide solution may inactivate papain) and at each redressing.

				C.I.*
Rx	**Dermuspray** (Warner Chilcott)	**Aerosol:** 0.1 mg trypsin, 72.5 mg Balsam Peru and 650 mg castor oil per 0.82 ml	In 120 g.	165
Rx	**Granulderm** (Copley)		In 113.4 g.	NA
Rx	**Granulex** (Hickam)		In 60 and 120 g.	209
Rx	**GranuMed** (Rugby)		In 113 g.	127
Rx	**Panafil** (Rystan)	**Ointment:** 10% papain, 10% urea and 0.5% chlorophyllin copper complex in a hydrophilic base with white petrolatum, propylene glycol, sorbitan monostearate, polyoxy-40 stearate, boric acid, sodium borate, chlorobutanol	In 30 g and lb.	414
Rx	**Panafil White** (Rystan)	**Ointment:** 10% papain and 10% urea in a hydrophilic base with white petrolatum, propylene glycol, sorbitan monostearate, polyoxy-40 stearate, boric acid, sodium borate, chlorobutanol	In 30 g.	403

* Cost Index based on cost per g or ml.

[1] From bovine pancreas.

For information on the systemic use of fluorouracil, refer to the monograph in the Antineoplastic chapter.

FLUOROURACIL

Actions:

Pharmacology: Fluorouracil appears to inhibit the synthesis of deoxyribonucleic acid (DNA); to a lesser extent, ribonucleic acid (RNA) is inhibited. These effects are most marked on rapidly growing cells which take up fluorouracil at a rapid pace.

When applied to a lesion, response occurs as follows:

1. Early inflammation – Minimal reaction, erythema for several days.
2. Severe inflammation – Burning, stinging, vesiculation.
3. Disintegration – Erosion, ulceration, necrosis, pain, crusting, reepithelialization.
4. Healing – Complete, with residual erythema and occasional, temporary hyperpigmentation, over 1 to 2 weeks.

Pharmacokinetics: Fluorouracil is not significantly absorbed ($\approx$ 6%).

Indications:

Multiple actinic or solar keratoses.

Superficial basal cell carcinomas: The 5% strength is useful when conventional methods are impractical (ie, multiple lesions, difficult treatment sites). Establish diagnosis prior to treatment.

Unlabeled use: A 1% solution of fluorouracil in 70% ethanol and the 5% cream have been used in the treatment of condylomata acuminata.

Contraindications:

Hypersensitivity to any component; pregnancy (see Warnings).

Warnings:

Occlusive dressings may increase the incidence of inflammatory reactions in the adjacent normal skin. A porous gauze dressing may be applied for cosmetic reasons without increase in reaction.

Inflammation: There is a possibility of increased absorption through ulcerated or inflamed skin.

Photosensitivity: Avoid prolonged exposure to ultraviolet rays while under treatment with fluorouracil because the intensity of the reaction may be increased.

Hypersensitivity: The potential for a delayed hypersensitivity reaction to fluorouracil exists. Patch testing to prove hypersensitivity may be inconclusive.

Pregnancy: Category X. Fluorouracil may cause fetal harm when administered to a pregnant woman. In animal studies, fluorouracil is both teratogenic and embryolethal. The drug is contraindicated in women who are or who may become pregnant. If fluorouracil is used during pregnancy, or if the patient becomes pregnant while taking this drug, apprise her of the potential hazard to the fetus.

Lactation: It is not known whether this drug is excreted in breast milk. Because there is some systemic absorption of the drug after topical administration, mothers should not breast feed while receiving this drug.

Children: Safety and efficacy have not been established.

Precautions:

Biopsies: To rule out the presence of a frank neoplasm, biopsy those areas failing to respond to treatment or recurring after treatment. Perform follow-up biopsies as indicated in the management of superficial basal cell carcinoma.

Adverse Reactions:

Local reactions include: Pain; pruritus; hyperpigmentation; irritation; inflammation; burning at site of application; allergic contact dermatitis; scarring; soreness; tenderness; suppuration; scaling; swelling.

Other reactions include: Alopecia; insomnia; irritability; stomatitis; medicinal taste; photosensitivity (see Warnings); lacrimation; telangiectasia; urticaria; toxic granulation.

Lab test abnormalities: Leukocytosis; thrombocytopenia; eosinophilia.

(Continued on following page)

FLUOROURACIL (Cont.)

Overdosage:

Ordinarily overdosage will not cause acute problems. If fluorouracil accidently comes in contact with the eye, flush the eye with water or normal saline. If fluorouracil is accidentally ingested, induce emesis and gastric lavage. Administer symptomatic and supportive care as needed.

Patient Information:

Avoid prolonged exposure to ultraviolet rays or other forms of ultraviolet irradiation while under treatment; intensity of reaction may be increased.

If applied with fingers, wash hands immediately afterward. Apply with care near the eyes, nose and mouth.

Reaction in the treated areas may be unsightly during therapy and, in some cases, for several weeks following cessation of therapy.

Administration and Dosage:

Actinic or solar keratoses: Apply twice daily to cover lesions. Continue until inflammatory response reaches erosion, necrosis and ulceration stage, then discontinue use. Usual duration of therapy is from 2 to 6 weeks. Complete healing may not be evident for 1 to 2 months following cessation. Increasing the frequency of application and a longer period of administration may be required on areas other than the head and neck.

Superficial basal cell carcinomas: Only the 5% strength is recommended. Apply twice daily in an amount sufficient to cover the lesions. Continue treatment for at least 3 to 6 weeks. Therapy may be required for as long as 10 to 12 weeks.

				C.I.*
Rx	**Efudex** (Roche)	**Cream:** 5%	In a white petrolatum base. In 25 g.	1425
Rx	**Fluoroplex** (Allergan Herbert)	**Cream:** 1%	In a base of benzyl alcohol, emulsifying wax and mineral oil. In 30 g.	966
Rx	**Efudex** (Roche)	**Solution:** 2%	With propylene glycol, EDTA and parabens. In 10 ml with dropper.	2213
		5%	With propylene glycol, EDTA and parabens. In 10 ml with dropper.	3141
Rx	**Fluoroplex** (Allergan Herbert)	**Solution:** 1%	With propylene glycol. In 30 ml.	966

* Cost Index based on cost per g or ml.

MINOXIDIL

Actions:

Pharmacology: Minoxidil topical solution stimulates vertex hair growth in individuals with alopecia androgenetica, expressed in males as baldness of the vertex of the scalp and in females as diffuse hair loss or thinning of the frontoparietal areas. There is no effect in patients with predominantly frontal hair loss. The mechanism is not known, but like minoxidil, some other arterial dilating drugs also stimulate hair growth when given systemically.

In placebo controlled trials involving > 3500 male patients given topical minoxidil for 4 months (longer treatment was given after the placebo group was discontinued), and in > 300 female patients given topical minoxidil for 8 months, typical systemic effects of oral minoxidil (weight gain, edema, tachycardia, fall in blood pressure and their more serious consequences) did not occur more frequently in patients given topical minoxidil than in those given topical placebo.

To study the potential for systemic effects of topical minoxidil, three concentrations (1%, 2% and 5%) applied twice daily were compared to low oral doses (2.5 and 5 mg given once daily) and placebo in hypertensive patients in a double-blind controlled trial. The 5 mg oral dose had readily detectable effects, including a fall in diastolic pressure of about 5 mm Hg and an increase in heart rate of 7 bpm. No other group had a clear effect, although there was some evidence of a weak and inconsistent effect in the 2.5 mg oral, and possibly the 5% topical, treatments.

Pharmacokinetics: Topical minoxidil has poor absorption, averaging ≈ 1.4% (range 0.3% to 4.5%) from normal intact scalp, and about 2% in the hypertensive patients, whose scalps were shaved.

In a comparison of topical and oral absorption, peak serum levels of unchanged drug after 1 ml twice a day of 2% solution (the maximum recommended dose) averaged 5.8% (range, 1.4% to 12.7%) of the level observed after 2.5 mg orally twice a day. Similarly, in the hypertension study where patients had shaved scalps, mean concentrations after 1 ml twice a day of 2% topical solution (1.7 ng/ml) were 1/20 the concentrations seen after daily oral doses of 2.5 mg (32.8 ng/ml) or 5 mg (59.2 ng/ml). Blood levels obtained in the large controlled hair growth trials averaged < 2 ng/ml for the 2% solution (range, up to 30 ng/ml). If more than the recommended dose is applied to inflamed skin in an individual with relatively high absorption, blood levels with systemic effects might rarely be obtained.

Serum levels resulting from topical administration are governed by the drug's percutaneous absorption rate. Following cessation of topical dosing, ≈ 95% of systemically absorbed minoxidil is eliminated within 4 days.

Clinical trials: Males – Three main parameters of efficacy were used: Hair counts in a 1 inch diameter circle on the vertex of the scalp; investigator evaluation of terminal hair regrowth; and patient evaluation of hair regrowth. At the end of 4 month placebo controlled portions of 12 month clinical studies (ie, baseline to month 4), topical minoxidil (20 mg/ml) demonstrated the following efficacy:

Hair counts: Topical minoxidil was significantly more effective than placebo in producing hair regrowth as assessed by hair counts. Patients using topical minoxidil had a mean increase from baseline of 72 nonvellus hairs in the 1 inch diameter circle compared with a mean increase of 39 nonvellus hairs in patients on placebo.

Investigator evaluation: Of patients on topical minoxidil, 8% demonstrated moderate to dense terminal hair regrowth compared with 4% on placebo. During the initial 4 months of treatment, however, very little regrowth of terminal hair can be expected. Although most patients did not demonstrate cosmetically significant hair regrowth, 26% of the patients showed minimal terminal hair regrowth using topical minoxidil compared with 16% of those using placebo.

Patient evaluation: 26% using topical minoxidil demonstrated moderate to dense hair regrowth compared with 11% using placebo.

Patients who continued on topical minoxidil during the remaining 8 months of the 12 month clinical studies (ie, the non-placebo controlled portion of the studies) continued to sustain a regrowth response. At the end of the 8 months, the following results were obtained:

Hair counts: Patients using topical minoxidil had a mean increase of 112 nonvellus hairs in the same 1 inch diameter circle as compared to month 4.

Investigator evaluation: 39% of the patients achieved moderate to dense terminal hair regrowth by month 12.

Patient evaluation: 48% felt they had achieved moderate to dense hair regrowth at month 12.

Trends in the data suggest that those patients who are older, who have been balding for a longer period of time, or who have a larger area of baldness, may do less well.

(Actions continued on following page)

MINOXIDIL (Cont.)

Actions (Cont.):

Females (18 to 45 years of age; 90% Caucasian) – In females with Ludwig grade I and II diffuse frontoparietal hair thinning, the main parameters of efficacy were: Non-vellus hair counts in a designated 1 cm^2 site on the frontoparietal areas of the scalp; investigator evaluation of hair regrowth; and patient evaluation of hair regrowth. Data demonstrate that 44% to 63% of women with androgenetic alopecia will have discernible growth of nonvellus hair when treated with minoxidil for 32 weeks vs 29% to 39% for vehicle control treated women.

Two 8 month placebo controlled studies produced the following results:

Hair counts: Minoxidil was significantly more effective than placebo in producing hair regrowth as assessed by hair counts in both studies. Patients using minoxidil had a mean increase from baseline of 22.7 and 33.2 nonvellus hairs, respectively, in the same 1 cm^2 site compared with a mean increase of 11 and 19.1 nonvellus hairs, respectively, in patients using placebo.

Investigator evaluation: Based on the investigators' evaluation, 63% (13% moderate and 50% minimal) and 44% (12% moderate and 32% minimal), respectively, of the patients using minoxidil in the two studies achieved hair regrowth at week 32, compared with 39% (6% moderate and 33% minimal) and 29% (5% moderate and 24% minimal), respectively, of those using placebo.

Patient evaluation: Based on the patients' self evaluation, 59% (19% moderate and 40% minimal) and 55% (1% dense, 24% moderate and 30% minimal), respectively, of the patients using minoxidil reported hair regrowth at week 32, compared with 40% (7% moderate and 33% minimal) and 41% (12% moderate and 29% minimal), respectively, of those using placebo.

Hair growth was defined as follows:

Investigator evaluation of growth – No visible new hair growth; minimal growth (definite growth but no substantial covering of thinning areas); moderate growth (new growth partially covering thinning areas, less dense than non-thinning areas; readily discernible); dense growth (full covering of thinning areas; hair density similar to non-thinning areas).

Patient evaluation of growth: No visible hair growth; minimal hair growth (barely discernible); moderate new hair growth (readily discernible); dense new hair growth.

Indications:

Treatment of androgenetic alopecia, expressed in males as baldness of the vertex of the scalp and in females as diffuse hair loss or thinning of the frontoparietal areas. At least 4 months of twice daily applications are generally required before evidence of hair growth can be expected.

Unlabeled use: Although further study is needed, topical minoxidil may be useful in the treatment of alopecia areata (a systemic disease in which patches of hair fall out over a period of a few days; any part of the body may be involved).

Contraindications:

Hypersensitivity to any component of the preparation.

Warnings:

Cardiac lesions: Minoxidil produces several cardiac lesions in animals. The significance of these lesions for humans is not clear, as they have not been recognized in patients treated with oral minoxidil at systemically active doses (see the systemic Minoxidil monograph in the Antihypertensive Vasodilators section).

Need for normal scalp: The majority of clinical studies included only healthy patients with normal scalps and no cardiovascular disease. Before starting a patient on topical minoxidil, ascertain that the patient has a healthy, normal scalp. Local abrasion or dermatitis may increase absorption and, hence, increase the risk of side effects.

Systemic effects: Although extensive use has not revealed evidence that enough topical drug is absorbed to cause systemic effects, greater absorption because of misuse, individual variability or unusual sensitivity could lead to a systemic effect.

As is the case with other topically applied drugs, decreased integrity of the epidermal barrier caused by inflammation or disease processes in the skin (eg, excoriations of the scalp, scalp psoriasis, severe sunburn) may increase percutaneous absorption. Also, do not use in conjunction with other topical agents (eg, corticosteroids, retinoids, petrolatum) or agents that are known to enhance cutaneous drug absorption.

(Warnings continued on following page)

MINOXIDIL (Cont.)

Warnings (Cont.):

Heart disease: Adverse effects might be especially serious in patients with a history of underlying heart disease. Be alert for tachycardia and fluid retention and watch for increased heart rate, weight gain or other systemic effects.

Pregnancy: Category C. Adequate and well controlled studies have not been conducted in pregnant women. Do not administer to a pregnant woman.

Lactation: Because of the potential for adverse effects in nursing infants from minoxidil absorption, do not apply on a nursing woman.

Children: Safety and efficacy in patients < 18 years of age have not been established.

Precautions:

Monitoring: Patients being considered for topical minoxidil should have a history and physical examination. Advise of the potential risk; the patient and physician should decide that the benefits outweigh the risks.

Monitor patients at least 1 month after starting topical minoxidil and at least every 6 months thereafter. If systemic effects occur, discontinue use.

Alcohol base: This product contains an alcohol base which will cause burning and irritation of eyes. In the event of accidental contact with sensitive surfaces (eg, eyes, abraded skin, mucous membranes), bathe the area with large amounts of cool tap water.

Avoid inhalation of the spray mist.

For topical use only. Accidental ingestion could lead to adverse systemic effects.

Adverse Reactions:

Respiratory: Bronchitis, upper respiratory infection, sinusitis (7.2%; placebo 8.6%).

Dermatological: Irritant dermatitis, allergic contact dermatitis (7.4%; placebo 5.4%); eczema; hypertrichosis; local erythema; pruritus; dry skin/scalp flaking; exacerbation of hair loss; alopecia.

GI: Diarrhea, nausea, vomiting (4.3%; placebo 6.6%).

CNS: Headache, dizziness, faintness, lightheadedness (3.4%; placebo 3.5%).

Musculoskeletal: Fractures, back pain, tendinitis, aches and pains (2.6%; placebo 2.2%).

Cardiovascular: Edema, chest pain, blood pressure increases/decreases, palpitations, pulse rate increases/decreases (1.5%; placebo 1.6%).

Allergy: Non-specific allergic reactions, hives, allergic rhinitis, facial swelling, sensitivity (1.3%; placebo 1%).

Special senses: Conjunctivitis, ear infections, vertigo (1.2%; placebo 1.2%); visual disturbances including decreased visual acuity.

Metabolic: Edema, weight gain (1.2%; placebo 1.3%).

GU: Urinary tract infections, renal calculi, urethritis, prostatitis, epididymitis, vaginitis, vulvitis, vaginal discharge, itching (0.9%; placebo 0.8% to 1.1%); sexual dysfunction.

Psychiatric: Anxiety, depression, fatigue (0.4%; placebo 1%).

Hematologic: Lymphadenopathy, thrombocytopenia, anemia (0.3%; placebo 0.6%).

Endocrine: Menstrual changes, breast symptoms (0.5%; placebo 0.5%).

Overdosage:

Topical: Increased systemic absorption of minoxidil may potentially occur if more frequent or larger doses than directed are used or if the drug is applied to large surface areas of the body or areas other than the scalp. There are no known cases of minoxidil overdosage resulting from topical administration.

In a 14 day controlled clinical trial, 1 ml of 3% minoxidil solution was applied 8 times daily (6 times the recommended dose) to the scalp of 11 healthy male volunteers and to the chest of 11 other volunteers. No significant systemic effects were observed in these subjects when compared with a similar number of placebo-treated subjects.

Systemic: Because of the high concentration of minoxidil in the topical solution, accidental ingestion has the potential of producing systemic effects related to the pharmacologic action of the drug (5 ml contains 100 mg minoxidil, the maximum adult dose for oral minoxidil administration when used to treat hypertension).

Symptoms – Signs and symptoms of minoxidil overdosage would most likely be cardiovascular effects associated with fluid retention and tachycardia.

Treatment – Manage fluid retention with appropriate diuretic therapy. Control clinically significant tachycardia by administration of a β-adrenergic blocking agent. If encountered, control hypotension by IV administration of normal saline. Avoid sympathomimetic drugs, such as norepinephrine and epinephrine, because of their excessive cardiac-stimulating activity.

(Continued on following page)

MINOXIDIL (Cont.)

Patient Information:

Evidence of hair growth usually will take ≥ 4 months.

First hair growth may be soft, downy, colorless hair that is barely visible. After further treatment, the new hair should be the same color and thickness as the other hair on the scalp.

If there is no response to treatment after a reasonable period of time (≥ 4 months), consult physician as to whether to discontinue use.

If treatment is stopped, new hair will probably be shed within a few months.

If one or two daily applications are missed, restart twice-daily application and return to the usual schedule. Do not attempt to make up for missed applications.

More frequent applications or use of larger doses (> 1 ml twice a day) will not speed up the process of hair growth and may increase the possibility of side effects.

Minoxidil topical solution contains alcohol, which could cause burning or irritation of the eyes, mucous membranes or sensitive skin areas. If accidental contact occurs, bathe the area with large amounts of cool tap water. Consult physician if irritation persists.

Because absorption of minoxidil may be increased and the risk of side effects may become greater, apply only to the scalp; do not use on other parts of the body. Do not use if scalp becomes irritated or is sunburned; do not use along with other topical medication on scalp.

Administration and Dosage:

Dry the hair and scalp prior to application. Apply 1 ml to the total affected areas of the scalp twice daily, once in the morning and at night. The total daily dosage should not exceed 2 ml. If finger tips are used to facilitate drug application, wash hands afterwards. Twice daily application for ≥ 4 months may be required before evidence of hair regrowth is observed. Onset and degree of hair regrowth may be variable among patients. If hair regrowth is realized, twice daily applications are necessary for additional and continued hair regrowth. Some anecdotal patient reports indicate that regrown hair and the balding process return to their untreated state 3 to 4 months following cessation of the drug.

Other topical agents: Do not use in conjunction with other topical agents including topical corticosteroids, retinoids and petrolatum or agents that are known to enhance cutaneous drug absorption.

Rx	**Rogaine** (Upjohn)	**Solution:** 20 mg/ml	In 60 ml bottle with multiple applicators.

DEXTRANOMER

Actions:

Pharmacology: Dextranomer's ability to remove exudates rapidly and continuously from the surface of the wound results in a reduction of inflammation and edema. In vitro evidence suggests that the suction forces created by the drug may remove bacteria and inflammatory exudates from the surface of the wound.

Dextranomer is a hydrophilic dextran polymer in the form of tiny beads or paste. The hydrophilic beads absorb approximately 4 ml of fluid per 1 g of beads. The beads swell to approximately 4 times their original size. This swelling causes significant suction forces and capillary action in the spaces between the beads. This action continues as long as unsaturated beads or paste are in proximity to the wound.

When applied to the surface of wet ulcers or wounds, dextranomer removes various exudates and particles that impede tissue repair. Low molecular weight components of wound exudates are drawn up within the beads or paste, while higher molecular weight components (plasma proteins and fibrinogen) are found between the swollen beads. Removal of these latter components (particularly fibrin and fibrinogen) retards eschar formation.

Indications:

For use in cleaning wet ulcers and wounds such as venous stasis ulcers, decubitus ulcers, infected traumatic and surgical wounds and infected burns.

Precautions:

For external use only. Avoid contact with the eyes.

Wound packing: When treating cratered decubitus ulcers, do not pack wound tightly. Allow for expansion of beads. Maceration of surrounding skin may result if occlusive dressings are used.

Removal of dextranomer: Do not use dextranomer in deep fistulas, sinus tracts or any body cavity where complete removal is not assured.

Remove the beads or paste once they are saturated. This avoids encrustation which makes removal more difficult. All dextranomer must be removed before any surgical procedures to close the wound (ie, graft or flap).

Edema reduction: Wounds may appear larger during the first few days of treatment due to reduction of edema.

Dry wounds: Not effective in cleansing dry wounds.

Complete healing: Not all wounds require treatment with dextranomer to complete healing. When the wound is no longer wet and a healthy granulation base is established, discontinue dextranomer.

Treatment of the underlying condition (eg, venous or arterial flow, pressure) should proceed concurrently with the use of dextranomer.

Adverse Reactions:

Upon application or removal of beads, transitory pain, bleeding, blistering and erythema have occurred. Severe infections have been associated with administration in both diabetic and immunosuppressed patients.

Patient Information:

For external use only. Avoid contact with the eyes.

Administration and Dosage:

Application: Debride and clean the wound (dextranomer is not an enzyme and will not debride). Leave cleansed area moist. Apply to at least a thickness of ¼ inch to achieve desired suction effects. Cover area with a dry dressing and close on all sides.

Removal: When saturated, dextranomer changes colors and should be removed. Removal should be as complete as possible and is best achieved by irrigation. Vigorous irrigation (ie, soaking or whirlpool) may be necessary to remove patches that adhere to the wound surface.

Paste may be needed for hard to reach areas or irregular body surfaces.

Mix beads with glycerin either on the dry dressing or in a receptacle or use premixed paste. Do not mix with any substance but glycerin. (See package insert for complete procedure.) Dress wound in the usual manner. Mix a fresh paste for each application. Do not reuse.

Reapply dextranomer beads or paste every 12 hours or more frequently if necessary. Reduce the number of applications as the exudate diminishes. Discontinue applications when the area is free of exudate and edema, or when a healthy granulation base is present. Consult physician if condition worsens or persists beyond 14 to 21 days.

otc	**Debrisan** (Johnson & Johnson)	**Beads**	In 25, 60 and 120 g containers and 4 g packets (in 7s and 14s).
		Paste	Premixed and sterile. In 10 g packets (6s).

FLEXIBLE HYDROACTIVE DRESSINGS AND GRANULES

Actions:

Pharmacology: The dressings interact with wound exudate producing a soft moist gel at the wound surface enabling removal of the dressing with little or no damage to newly formed tissues. They are designed to remain in place from 1 to 7 days.

Indications:

Dressings: For the local management of: Dermal ulcers; pressure ulcers; leg ulcers; superficial wounds (eg, minor abrasions, donor sites, second-degree burns); protective dressings; postoperative wounds.

Granules: For use in the local management of exudating dermal ulcers in association with the dressings.

Paste: For use in association with *DuoDerm* dressings for local management of exudating dermal ulcers.

Contraindications:

Dermal ulcers involving muscle, tendon or bone; ulcers resulting from infection, such as tuberculosis, syphilis and deep fungal infections; lesions in patients with active vasculitis, such as periarteritis nodosa, systemic lupus erythematosus and cryoglobulinemia; third-degree burns; clinically infected wounds.

Precautions:

Excess exudate: In the presence of excess exudate, the ability of the dressings to remain in place with less frequent leakage may be improved by applying the granules directly into the wound site. Used in this way, with the dressings, the granules may reduce the frequency of dressing change.

Odor: Wounds often have a characteristic disagreeable odor. The odor usually disappears following wound cleansing.

Wound deterioration: When using any occlusive dressing, the wound will increase in size and depth during the initial phase of management as the necrotic debris is cleaned away.

Infection: If clinical infection develops, discontinue *DuoDerm* and institute appropriate treatment. Restart *DuoDerm* when the infection has been eradicated.

Administration and Dosage:

Clean and prepare the wound site before application.

See package labeling for wound management and application/removal instructions for the dressing and granules. Dressings are designed to remain in place from 1 to 7 days.

otc	**IntraSite** (Smith & Nephew)	**Gel:** 2% graft T starch copolymer, 78% water, 20% propylene glycol. Sterile amorphous hydrogel dressing	In UD 25 g (10s).
otc	**Shur-Clens** (Calgon Vestal)	**Solution:** 20% poloxamer 188	In UD 100 and 200 ml.
otc	**DuoDerm** (ConvaTec)	**Dressings, sterile:** 4″ × 4″, 6″ × 8″, 8″ × 8″ and 8″ × 12″	In 3s (8″ x 12″ only), 5s and 20s
		Dressing, adhesive border: 4″ x 4″ 8″ x 8″	In 5s. In 3s.
		Granules, sterile: 5 g per tube	In 5s.
		Paste, sterile	In 30 g tube.
otc	**DuoDerm CGF** (ConvaTec)	**Control gel formula dressing, sterile:** 4″ × 4″, 6″ × 6″, 8″ × 8″	In 5s.
		Control gel formula border dressing, sterile: 2.5″ × 2.5″, 4″ × 4″, 6″ × 6″, 4″ × 5″, 6″ × 7″ with adhesive borders	In 5s.
otc	**DuoDerm Extra Thin** (ConvaTec)	**Control gel formula dressing, extra thin, sterile:** 4″ × 4″, 6″ × 6″	In 10s.
otc	**Sorbsan** (Dow B. Hickam)	**Pads, sterile:** Calcium alginate fiber 2″ × 2″, 3″ × 3″, 4″ × 4″ and 4″ × 8″	In 1s.
		Wound packing fibers, sterile: Calcium alginate fiber. 12″ (2 g)	In 1s.

HYDROQUINONE

Actions:

Pharmacology: Hydroquinone depigments hyperpigmented skin by inhibiting the enzymatic oxidation of tyrosine and suppressing other melanocyte metabolic processes, thereby inhibiting melanin formation. Hydroquinone may also act on the essential subcellular metabolic processes of melanocytes with resultant cytolysis (ie, nonenzyme-mediated depigmentation). Skin color diminution usually occurs after 3 or 4 weeks of treatment. Because the rate of depigmentation varies among individuals, a positive response may require 3 weeks to 6 months.

Exposure to sunlight or ultraviolet light will cause repigmentation, which may be prevented by sunblocking agents. In addition to hydroquinone, some products contain sunscreens (eg, octyl dimethyl PABA, ethyl dihydroxypropyl PABA, dioxybenzone, oxybenzone).

Indications:

Temporary bleaching of hyperpigmented skin conditions (eg, freckles, senile lentigines, chloasma and melasma, and other forms of melanin hyperpigmentation).

Contraindications:

Hypersensitivity to hydroquinone or any of the other ingredients of the products.

Warnings:

Sunscreen use is an essential aspect of hydroquinone therapy because minimal sun exposure sustains melanocytic activity. Therefore, avoid sun exposure by using a sunscreen, a sun block or protective clothing to prevent repigmentation.

Sensitivity testing: Test for skin sensitivity before using. Apply a small amount to an unbroken patch of skin and check in 24 hours. If vesicle formation, itching or excessive inflammation occurs, further treatment is not advised. Minor redness is not a contraindication.

Discontinue use if no bleaching or lightening effect is noted after 2 months of treatment.

Pregnancy: Category C. Safety for use during pregnancy has not been established. It is not known whether hydroquinone can cause fetal harm when used topically on a pregnant woman or affect reproductive capacity. It is also not known to what degree, if any, topical hydroquinone is absorbed systemically. Use only if clearly needed.

Lactation: It is not known whether topical hydroquinone is absorbed or excreted in breast milk. Caution is advised when topical hydroquinone is used by a nursing mother.

Children: Safety and efficacy in children ≤ 12 years of age have not been established.

Precautions:

Lips: A bitter taste and anesthetic effect may occur if applied to lips.

For external use only. If rash or irritation develops, discontinue treatment. Do not use near eyes. Use in paranasal and infraorbital areas increases the chance of irritation.

Peroxide: Concurrent use of peroxide may result in transient dark staining of skin areas due to oxidation of hydroquinone. Staining can be removed by discontinuing concurrent use and by normal soap cleansing.

Sulfite sensitivity: Some of these products contain sulfites which may cause allergic-type reactions (eg, hives, itching, wheezing, anaphylaxis) in certain susceptible persons. Although the overall prevalence of sulfite sensitivity in the general population is probably low, it is seen more frequently in asthmatics or in atopic nonasthmatic persons.

Adverse Reactions:

Dryness and fissuring of paranasal and infraorbital areas; erythema; stinging; irritation; sensitization and contact dermatitis in susceptible individuals.

Overdosage:

There have been no systemic reactions from the use of topical hydroquinone. However, limit treatment to relatively small areas of the body at one time, since some patients experience a transient skin reddening and a mild burning sensation which does not preclude treatment.

Patient Information:

For external use only. Avoid contact with the eyes.

Protection from the sun (eg, sunscreens, clothing) is an essential aspect of therapy.

Do not use on irritated, denuded or damaged skin.

Discontinue use and consult physician if rash or irritation develops.

Administration and Dosage:

Hydroquinone bleaching is faster, more dependable and easier if the treated area is protected from ultraviolet light. Therefore, preparations with a sunscreen may be preferred for use during the day.

Apply to affected skin twice daily.

Not recommended for children ≤ 12 years of age.

(Products listed on following page)

HYDROQUINONE (Cont.)

	Product	Form/Strength	Description	C.I.*
otc	**Esoterica Sensitive Skin Formula** (Medicis)	**Cream:** 1.5%	With mineral oil, sodium bisulfite, parabens, EDTA. In 85 g.	101
otc	**Eldopaque** (ICN)	**Cream:** 2%	With sunblock. In 14.2 and 28.4 g.	749
otc	**Eldoquin** (ICN)		In 14.2 and 28.4 g.	749
otc	**Esoterica Facial** (Medicis)		With 3.3% padimate O, 2.5% oxybenzone, sodium bisulfites, parabens, EDTA. In 85 g.	101
otc	**Esoterica Regular** (Medicis)		With parabens, sodium bisulfite, EDTA. In 85 g.	90
otc	**Esoterica Sunscreen** (Medicis)		With 3.3% padimate O, 2.5% oxybenzone, mineral oil, parabens, sodium bisulfite, EDTA. In 85 g.	101
otc	**Porcelana** (DEP)		In 60 and 120 g.	117
otc	**Porcelana with Sunscreen** (DEP)		With 2.5% padimate O. In 120 g.	77
otc	**Solaquin** (ICN)		With sunscreens. In 28.4 g.	669
Rx	**Eldopaque-Forte** (ICN)	**Cream:** 4%	In a sunblock base. With talc, iron oxides, mineral oil, EDTA, sodium metabisulfite. In 14.2 and 28.4 g.	479
Rx	**Eldoquin-Forte Sunbleaching** (ICN)		In a vanishing cream base. With mineral oil, propylparaben, sodium metabisulfite. In 14.2 and 28.4 g.	479
Rx	**Solaquin Forte** (ICN)		With 5% ethyl dihydroxypropyl PABA, 3% dioxybenzone, 2% oxybenzone, EDTA, sodium metabisulfite. In 14.2 and 28.4 g.	NA
otc	**Ambi Skin Tone** (Kiwi Brands)	**Cream**	Dry, oily and normal skin formulas. With padimate O, sodium metabisulfite, parabens, EDTA, vitamin E. In 57 and 114 g.	66
otc	**Eldoquin** (ICN)	**Lotion:** 2%	In 15 ml.	1137
Rx	**Melanex** (Neutrogena)	**Solution:** 3%	With 45% SD alcohol 40, propylene glycol. In 30 ml.	400
Rx	**Solaquin Forte** (ICN)	**Gel:** 4%	With 5% ethyl dihydroxypropyl PABA, 3% dioxybenzone, EDTA, sodium metabisulfite. Hydroalcoholic base. In 14.2 and 28.4 g.	NA

FORMALDEHYDE

Indications:

Antiperspirant for treatment of hyperhidrosis and bromidrosis. Drying agent for pre- and post-surgical removal of warts or nonsurgical laser treatment of warts.

Contraindications: Hypersensitivity to any ingredients of the product.

Precautions:

For external use only. Avoid contact with eyes or mucous membranes.

Irritation/Sensitivity: May be irritating and sensitizing to the skin of some patients; check skin for sensitivity prior to application. If redness or irritation persists, consult physician.

Administration: Apply once a day to affected areas as directed.

	Product	Form/Strength	Description	C.I.*
Rx	**Formalyde-10** (Pedinol)	**Spray:** 10%	In 60 ml.	5
Rx	**Lazer Formalyde** (Pedinol)	**Solution:** 10%	In 90 ml.	4.4

* Cost Index based on cost per g or ml.

CAPSAICIN

Actions:

Pharmacology: Capsaicin is a natural chemical derived from plants of the solanaceae family. Although the precise mechanism of action is not fully understood, evidence suggests that the drug renders skin and joints insensitive to pain by depleting and preventing reaccumulation of substance P in peripheral sensory neurons. Substance P is thought to be the principle chemomediator of pain impulses from the periphery to the central nervous system.

Indications:

Temporary relief of pain from rheumatoid arthritis, osteoarthritis and relief of neuralgias such as the pain following shingles (herpes zoster) or painful diabetic neuropathy.

Unlabeled uses: Capsaicin is being investigated for use in other disorders including psoriasis, vitiligo and intractable pruritus, as well as postmastectomy and postamputation neuroma (phantom limb syndrome), vulvar vestibulitis, apocrine chromhidrosis and reflex sympathetic dystrophy.

Warnings:

For external use only. Avoid getting in eyes or on broken or irritated skin. Use care when handling contact lenses following application of capsaicin; irritation and burning may occur following lens insertion. Washing hands or using gloves or an applicator may alleviate this problem.

Bandage use: Do not bandage tightly.

Worsened condition: If condition worsens or if symptoms persist 14 to 28 days, discontinue use and consult physician.

Adverse Reactions:

Burning (≥ 30%; usually diminishes with repeated use); stinging; erythema; cough; respiratory irritation

Patient Information:

For external use only. Avoid contact with the eyes. Use caution when handling contact lens following application; washing hands or using gloves or an applicator is recommended.

Do not bandage tightly.

If condition worsens or symptoms persist 14 to 28 days, contact a physician.

Administration and Dosage:

Adults and children ≥ 2 years of age: Apply to affected area not more than 3 or 4 times daily. May cause transient burning on application. This is observed more frequently when application schedules of < 3 or 4 times daily are used. If applied with the fingers, wash hands immediately after application.

				C.I.*
otc	**Zostrix** (GenDerm)	**Cream:** 0.025% in an emollient base	In 45 and 90 g.	850
otc	**Zostrix-HP** (GenDerm)	**Cream:** 0.075% in an emollient base	In 30 and 60 g.	531

ALUMINUM CHLORIDE HEXAHYDRATE

Indications:

An astringent used as an aid in the management of hyperhidrosis.

Warnings:

For external use only. Avoid contact with the eyes.

Discontinue use if irritation or sensitization occurs.

Metals/fabrics: Aluminum chloride hexahydrate may be harmful to certain metals and fabrics.

Precautions:

Burning or prickling sensation may occur. Do not apply to broken, irritated or recently shaved skin.

Administration:

Apply to the affected area once a day, only at bedtime. To help prevent irritation, completely dry area prior to application.

For maximum effect cover the treated area with plastic wrap, held in place by a snug fitting "T" or body shirt, mitten or sock. (Never hold plastic wrap in place with tape.) Wash the treated area the following morning. Excessive sweating may stop after ≥ 2 treatments. Thereafter, apply once or twice weekly or as needed.

				C.I.*
Rx	**Drysol** (Person & Covey)	**Solution:** 20% in 93% SD alcohol 40	In 37.5 ml or 35 ml with Dab-O-Matic applicator.	15

* Cost Index based on cost per g or ml.

MONOBENZONE

Indications:

Final depigmentation in extensive vitiligo.

Contraindications:

Freckling; hyperpigmentation due to photosensitization following use of certain perfumes or following inflammation of the skin; melasma (chloasma) of pregnancy; cafe-au-lait spots; pigmented nevi; malignant melanoma; pigment resulting from pigments other than melanin, including bile, silver and artificial pigments; hypersensitivity to monobenzone or any ingredients of the product.

Warnings:

Extensive vitiligo: Monobenzone is a potent depigmenting agent, not a mild cosmetic bleach; do not use except for final depigmentation in extensive vitiligo.

Pregnancy: Category C. It is not known whether the drug can cause fetal harm when used topically on a pregnant woman. Use only when clearly needed.

Lactation: It is not known whether monobenzone is absorbed or excreted in breast milk. Use with caution in nursing mothers.

Children: Safety and efficacy in children $\leq$ 12 years of age have not been established.

Adverse Reactions:

Irritation; burning sensation; dermatitis.

Administration:

For external use only. Avoid contact with the eyes.

Apply and rub into the pigmented areas to be treated, 2 or 3 times daily. Depigmentation is usually observed after 1 to 4 months of therapy. If satisfactory results have not been obtained within 4 months, discontinue treatment.

				C.I.*
Rx	**Benoquin** (ICN)	**Cream:** 20%. In a water washable base	In 35.4 g.	49

HAMAMELIS WATER (Witch Hazel)

Actions:

Pharmacology: Hamamelis water is a mild astringent prepared from twigs of *Hamamelis virginiana;* the distillate is then adjusted with an appropriate amount of alcohol.

Indications:

Temporary relief of anal or vaginal irritation and itching, hemorrhoids, postepisiotomy discomfort and hemorrhoidectomy discomfort.

Warnings:

Worsened condition: If condition worsens or does not improve within 7 days consult a physician.

Bleeding: In case of bleeding, consult physician promptly.

Precautions:

For external use only. Avoid contact with the eyes.

Administration:

Apply locally up to 6 times daily or after each bowel movement.

				C.I.*
otc	**Witch Hazel** (Various, eg, Humco, Lannett, Purepac)	**Liquid**	In 120 and 240 ml, pt and gal.	2+
otc	**Tucks Hemorrhoidal** (Parke-Davis)	**Cream:** 50%. White petrolatum, 7% alcohol, lanolin	In 42 g.	9
otc	**A•E•R** (Birchwood)	**Pads:** 50%. 12.5% glycerin, methylparaben, benzalkonium chloride	In 40s.	NA

ARNICA

Indications:

Relief of pain from sprains and bruises; of doubtful value.

Precautions:

For external use only. Avoid getting into eyes or mucous membranes.

Irritation: Do not apply to irritated skin or if excessive irritation develops.

Adverse Reactions:

Arnica is an irritant to mucous membranes; when ingested, it has produced severe gastroenteritis, nervous disturbances, tachycardia, bradycardia and collapse.

Arnica may cause dermatitis in sensitive persons.

Administration:

Apply locally with massage 2 or 3 times daily.

				C.I.*
otc	**Arnica** (Various, eg, Humco)	**Tincture:** 20%	In 30, 60 and 120 ml, pt and gal.	2.3+

* Cost Index based on cost per g or ml.

ZINC OXIDE

Indications:

Minor skin irritations, burns, abrasions, chafed skin and diaper rash.

Administration:

For external use only. Avoid contact with the eyes.

Apply to affected areas as required.

				C.I.*
otc	**Zinc Oxide** (Various, eg, Major, Moore, Paddock, Qualitest, Rugby, Schein)	**Ointment:** 20%	In 30 and 60 g and lb.	2.8+

DIHYDROXYACETONE

Indications:

For vitiligo and hypopigmented skin.

Precautions:

For external use only. Do not apply to hair, eyelids and around eyes.

Sun exposure: Does not protect skin from sunlight; use a sunblock on affected areas.

Administration:

Use applicator top to apply evenly to areas of skin to be darkened. Allow to remain on the skin at least 30 minutes before washing. The first effects appear a few hours after initial application. To avoid overapplication, use once at bedtime and allow color to develop overnight. If more color is desired, apply once an hour until proper shade is obtained. The coloration will last 3 to 6 days with gradual and even fading. Any initial overuse will be remedied by natural fading acelerated by gently scrubbing the affected area. Maintenance applications of once a day or less should be sufficient.

otc	**Chromelin Complexion Blender** (Summers)	5% in isopropanol	In 30 ml.

CHLOROPHYLL DERIVATIVES

Actions:

Pharmacology: Aids wound healing by helping to produce a clean, granulating wound base for epithelialization or skin grafting. It also soothes inflamed, painful tissues and controls wound odor, even in malignant lesions. This is a true deodorizing, not a masking, action.

Indications:

Arteriosclerotic, diabetic and varicose ulcers; trophic decubitus ulcers and chronic ulcers of nonspecific origin; malignant lesions (where deodorization is desired); traumatic injuries; skin grafting and skin defects; thermal, chemical and irradiation injuries; a wide variety of dermatoses.

Adverse Reactions:

Sensitivity reactions (rare); itching; irritation.

Administration:

Ointment: Apply generously and cover with gauze, linen or other appropriate dressing. For best results, do not change dressings more often than every 48 to 72 hours.

Solution: Apply full strength as continuous wet dressing, or instill directly into sinus tracts, fistulae, deep ulcers or cavities.

				C.I.*
otc	**Chloresium** (Rystan)	**Ointment:** 0.5% chlorophyllin copper complex in a hydrophilic base	In 30 and 120 g and lb.	12
		Solution: 0.2% chlorophyllin copper complex in isotonic saline	In 240 and 960 ml.	3.2

BORIC ACID OINTMENT

Indications:

A soothing application for chafed skin, abrasions, burns and other skin irritations.

Administration:

For external use only. Avoid contact with the eyes.

Apply directly to affected area once or twice daily.

				C.I.*
otc	**Borofax** (Burroughs Wellcome)	**Ointment:** 5%. Lanolin, glycerin, mineral oil, sodium borate	In 52.5 g.	9.7
otc	**Boric Acid** (Various, eg, Ambix, Clay-Park, Fougera, IDE, Major, Moore, NMC, Rugby, URL)	**Ointment:** 10%	In 30 and 60 g and lb.	2.6+

* Cost Index based on cost per g or ml.

Principal active ingredients of these formulations include:

BORIC ACID, OXYQUINOLINE and *BENZALKONIUM CI* are used as antiseptics.

ZINC OXIDE, CALAMINE, ALUMINUM and *ALUMINUM ACETATE* provide astringent and topical protectant actions.

CAMPHOR, EUCALYPTOL, MENTHOL and *PHENOL* are used as antipruritics, mild local anesthetics and counterirritants.

BENZOCAINE and *LIDOCAINE* are local anesthetics.

PYRILAMINE MALEATE is an antihistamine.

CASTOR OIL (RICINUS OIL), GLYCERIN and *MINERAL OIL* are used as emollients.

BENZYL ALCOHOL is used as an antipruritic.

BISMUTH SUBNITRATE is used as a skin protectant.

BALSAM PERU is used to stimulate tissue growth.

BIEBRICH SCARLET RED is used to promote wound healing.

ICHTHAMMOL is used as an anti-infective.

JUNIPER TAR is used as an antieczematic.

SULFUR provides antibacterial, peeling and drying action.

	Product	Formulation	Supplied	C.I.*
otc	**Boil-Ease** (Commerce)	**Salve:** 5% benzocaine, 0.44% sulfur, 1.86% ichthammol, camphor, anhydrous lanolin, eucalyptus oil, juniper tar, liquified phenol, menthol, paraffin, petrolatum, rosin, sexadecyl alcohol, thymol, yellow wax, zinc oxide Drawing salve for boils.	In 30 g.	13
otc	**Boyol Salve** (Pfeiffer)	**Salve:** 10% ichthammol, benzocaine, lanolin, petrolatum	In 30 g.	6.5
otc	**Dr. Dermi-Heal** (Quality)	**Ointment:** 1% allantoin, zinc oxide, Balsam Peru, castor oil, petrolatum For relief of diaper rash, chafing, minor burns, bed sores, external vaginal itching and irritation, ostomy irritation and heat rash.	In 75 g.	65
otc	**Ichthammol** (NMC)	**Ointment:** 10% or 20% ichthammol, lanolin-petrolatum base For relief of minor skin irritations.	In 28.4 g.	NA
otc	**Mammol** (Abbott)	**Ointment:** 40% bismuth subnitrate, 30% castor oil, 22% anhydrous lanolin, 7% ceresin wax and 1% Balsam Peru For prevention of sore, cracked nipples during lactation.	In 25 g.	22
otc	**Saratoga** (Blair)	**Ointment:** Zinc oxide, boric acid, eucalyptol, acetylated lanolin alcohols, white petrolatum, white beeswax For temporary relief of itching and minor skin irritations, chapped and chafed skin, diaper rash, bed sores, mild burns.	In 28 and 60 g.	12
otc	**Unguentine** (Mentholatum)	**Ointment:** 1% phenol, petrolatum, oleostearine, zinc oxide, eucalyptus oil, thyme oil For pain relief in minor burns.	In 30 g.	2.7
otc	**Ostiderm** (Pedinol)	**Lotion:** 14.5 mg aluminum sulfate, 10 mg phenol per g. Glycerin, zinc oxide, bentonite, silica, propylene glycol alginate, camphor, iron oxides For relief of bromhidrosis, hyperhydrosis, dermatitis, itching and poison ivy.	In 45 ml.	12
otc	**Sarna Anti-Itch** (Stiefel)	**Lotion:** 0.5% camphor, 0.5% menthol, carbomer 940, DMDM hydantoin, glyceryl stearate, PEG-8 stearate, PEG-100 stearate, petrolatum For relief of dry, itching skin, sunburn, poison ivy and poison oak.	In 222 ml.	2.4
otc	**Schamberg** (Paddock)	**Lotion:** 8.25% zinc oxide, 0.25% menthol, 1.5% phenol, 30% cottonseed oil, 15% olive oil and lime water For pruritic eczema.	In 480 ml.	1.2

* Cost Index based on cost per g or ml.

(Continued on following page)

				C.I.*
otc	**Schamberg's** (C & M)	**Lotion:** Zinc oxide, 0.15% menthol, 1% phenol, peanut oil and lime water For the temporary relief of itching.	In 480 ml.	2.8
otc	**Soothaderm** (Pharmakon)	**Lotion:** 2.07 mg pyrilamine maleate, 2.08 mg benzocaine and 41.35 mg zinc oxide per ml with simethicone, parabens, propylene glycol, wysteria oil, apple blossom oil, camphor, menthol For relief of itching due to chicken pox, diaper rash, insect bites, poison ivy/oak, prickly heat and sunburn.	In 118 ml.	2.2
otc	**Outgro** (Whitehall)	**Solution:** 25% tannic acid, 5% chlorobutanol, 83% isopropyl alcohol For temporary pain relief of ingrown toenails.	In 9.3 ml.	41
otc	**Stypto-Caine** (Pedinol)	**Solution:** 250 mg aluminum chloride, 2.5 mg tetracaine HCl, 1 mg oxyquinoline sulfate per g with glycerin To stop bleeding in minor cuts.	In 59 ml.	NA
otc	**Campho-Phenique** (Sterling Health)	**Liquid:** 10.8% camphor, 4.7% phenol, eucalyptus oil, light mineral oil For relief of pain and to combat infections.	In 22.5, 45 and 120 ml.	9
otc	**Oxyzal Wet Dressing** (Gordon)	**Liquid:** Oxyquinoline sulfate, benzalkonium Cl 1:2000 For minor infections.	In 30, 120 and 480 ml.	8.7
otc	**Campho-Phenique** (Sterling Health)	**Gel:** 4.7% phenol, 10.8% camphor, colloidal silicon dioxide, eucalyptus oil, glycerin, light mineral oil Pain relief in cold sores, fever blisters, cuts, scrapes, burns and insect bites.	In 6.9 and 15 g.	34
otc	**Topic** (Syntex)	**Gel:** 5% benzyl alcohol, camphor, menthol, 30% isopropyl alcohol For temporary relief of itching from poison oak/ivy, insect bites, eczema, minor skin allergies and heat rash.	In 60 g.	4.4
otc	**Aluminum Paste** (Paddock)	**Ointment:** 10% metallic aluminum An occlusive skin protectant.	White petrolatum base. In lb.	3.5
otc	**Sarna Anti-Itch** (Stiefel)	**Foam:** 0.5% camphor, 0.5% menthol, carbomer 940, DMDM hydantoin, glyceryl stearate, PEG-8 and PEG-100 stearate, petrolatum For relief of dry, itching skin in sunburn and poison ivy.	In 99 g.	5.3
otc	**ProTech First-Aid Stik** (Triton)	**Liquid:** 10% povidone iodine, 2.5% lidocaine HCl For cleaning and pain relief of cuts, scrapes and burns.	In 14 ml.	NA
otc	**Proderm Topical** (Dow B. Hickam)	**Dressing:** 650 mg castor oil and 72.5 mg Balsam Peru per 0.82 ml For prevention and management of decubitus ulcers.	In 113.4 g.	NA
otc	**Dome-Paste** (Miles)	**Wound dressing:** Zinc oxide, calamine, gelatin For conditions of the extremities (eg, varicose ulcers) requiring protection and support.	3″ by 10 yd or 4″ by 10 yd bandages.	NA
Rx	**Scarlet Red Ointment Dressings** (Sherwood Medical)	**Wound dressings:** 5% scarlet red, lanolin, olive oil and petrolatum in fine mesh absorbent gauze For epithelialization of donor sites, burns and wounds.	In 5″ x 9″ strips.	NA

* Cost Index based on cost per g or ml.

Iodine Compounds

IODINE

Uses:

Iodine preparations are used externally for their broad microbicidal spectrum against bacteria, fungi, viruses, spores, protozoa and yeasts. Iodine may be used to disinfect intact skin preoperatively. Potassium iodide is added to increase the solubility of the iodine. Sodium iodide is present to stabilize the tincture and make it miscible with water in all proportions.

Contraindications:

Hypersensitivity to iodine.

Warnings:

For external use only: Avoid contact with the eyes and mucous membranes.

Highly toxic if ingested. Sodium thiosulfate is the most effective chemical antidote.

Staining: Iodine preparations stain skin and clothing.

Occlusive dressings: Do not use.

				C.I.*
otc	**Iodine Topical** (Various, eg, AA-Spectrum)	**Solution:** 2% iodine and 2.4% sodium iodide in purified water	In 500 and 4000 ml.	5.5+
otc[1]	**Strong Iodine (Lugol's Solution)** (Various, eg, Lannett)	**Solution:** 5% iodine and 10% potassium iodide in water	In pt and gal.	1.1+
otc	**Iodine Tincture** (Various, eg, Century, Lannett, Purepac)	**Solution:** 2% iodine and 2.4% sodium iodide in 47% alcohol, purified water	In pt and gal.	1+
otc	**Strong Iodine Tincture** (Various, eg, A-A Spectrum)	**Solution:** 7% iodine and 5% potassium iodide in 83% alcohol	In 500 and 4000 ml.	5+

POVIDONE-IODINE

Actions:

Water soluble complex of iodine with povidone. Povidone-iodine contains 9% to 12% available iodine. It retains the bactericidal activity of iodine but is less potent, therefore causes less irritation to skin and mucous membranes. In vitro, HIV appears to be completely inactivated by povidone-iodine preparations; further study is needed.

Warnings:

Hypothyroidism: A 6-week-old infant developed low serum total thyroxine concentration and high thyroid stimulating hormone concentration following maternal use of topical povidone-iodine during pregnancy and lactation. In one study, the use of povidone-iodine solution on very-low birthweight infants resulted in neonatal hypothyroidism. In contrast, women who used povidone-iodine douche daily for 14 days did not develop overt hypothyroidism; however, there was a significant increase in serum total iodine concentration and urine iodine excretion. Use with caution during pregnancy and lactation and in infants.

Open wounds: Avoid solutions containing a detergent if treating open wounds with povidone-iodine. The value of povidone-iodine on open wounds has not been established.

Administration and Dosage:

Unlike iodine tincture, treated areas may be bandaged.

				C.I.*
otc	**Povidone-Iodine** (Various, eg, Humco, IDE, Major, NMC, Qualitest, Schein, URL)	**Ointment:** 10%	In 30 g and lb.	7.4+
		Solution: 10%	In pt and gal.	1+
		Liquid	In pt.	1.8+
otc	**ACU-dyne** (Acme United)	**Ointment**	In 1, 1.2 & 2.7 g packets (100s.)	9.2
		Perineal wash concentrate: 1% available iodine	In 240 ml.	3.5
		Prep solution	In 240 ml, pt, qt, gal & 30 & 60 ml packets.	2.1

* Cost Index based on cost per g, ml or unit applicator.

[1] Some of these products may be available *Rx,* depending on distributor discretion.

(Continued on following page)

Iodine Compounds (Cont.)

POVIDONE-IODINE (Cont.)

	Product	Form / Contents	Packaging	C.I.*
otc	**ACU-dyne** (Acme United)	**Skin cleanser**	In 60 and 240 ml, pt, qt and gal.	2.3
		Solution, prep swabs: 1% available iodine	In 100s.	11
		Solution, swabsticks	1 or 3/packet in 25s.	38
otc	**Aerodine** (Graham-Field)	**Aerosol**	In 90 ml.	11
otc	**Betadine** (Purdue-Frederick)	**Aerosol**: 5%. Glycerin, dibasic sodium phosphate	In 88.7 ml.	11
		Antiseptic gauze pads (viscous formula): 10%. Emulsifying wax, poloxamer, polyethylene glycol, propylene glycol, white petrolatum	In 12s (3" x 9").	123
		Antiseptic gauze pads: 10%. Citric acid, dibasic sodium phosphate, glycerin, polyethylene glycols	In 12s (3" x 9").	120
		Antiseptic lubricating gel: 5%. Citric acid, dibasic sodium phosphate, glycerin, hydroxypropyl methylcellulose, propylene glycol	In 5 g.	11
		Cream: 5%. Glycerin, mineral oil, polyoxyethylene stearate, polysorbate, sorbitan monostearate, white petrolatum	In 14 g.	39
		Gel (vaginal): 10%. Polyethylene glycols	In 18 and 90 g w/vaginal applicator.	25
		Mouthwash/Gargle: 0.5%. 8% alcohol, glycerin, saccharin	In 177 ml.	5.9
		Ointment: 10%. Polyethylene glycols	In 28 g tube, lb jar and 0.94 and 3.8 g packets.	28
		Perineal wash concentrate: 10%. Citric acid, dibasic sodium phosphate	In 236 ml with empty dispenser bottle.	3.4
		Skin cleanser: 7.5%. Ammonium nonoxynol-4-sulfate, lauramide DEA	In 30 and 118 ml.	7.8
		Skin cleanser, foam: 7.5%. Ammonium nonoxynol-4-sulfate, lauramide DEA	In 170 g.	7.2
		Solution: 10%. Citric acid, dibasic sodium phosphate, glycerin	In 15, 120 and 237 ml, pt, qt, gal and 30 ml packets.	3.9
		Solution, swab aid: 10%. Citric acid, dibasic sodium phosphate, glycerin	In 100s.	12
		Solution, swabsticks: 10%. Citric acid, dibasic sodium phosphate, glycerin	In packets of 1 (200s) or 3 (50s).	40
		Surgical scrub: 7.5%. Ammonium nonoxynol-4-sulfate, lauramide DEA	In pt with or without pump, qt, gal and 15 ml packets.	3.1
		Surgi-Prep sponge brush: 7.5%. Nonoxynol-4-sulfate, lauramide DEA	In 1s with nail pick.	115
		Vaginal suppositories: 10%. Polyethylene glycol.	In 7s w/applicator.	207

* Cost Index based on cost per g, ml or unit applicator.

(Continued on following page)

Iodine Compounds (Cont.)

POVIDONE-IODINE (Cont.)

				C.I.*
otc	**Betagen** (Goldline)	**Ointment:** 1% available iodine. PEG-8 and PEG-75	In 28.35 g and lb.	NA
		Solution: 10%	In pt and gal.	1.9
		Surgical scrub: 7.5%	In pt.	1.9
otc	**Biodine Topical 1%** (Major)	**Solution:** 1% iodine	In pt and gal.	2.4
otc	**Efodine** (Fougera)	**Ointment:** 1% available iodine	In 30 g, lb and 0.94 g (144s).	6.4
otc	**Iodex** (Medtech)	**Ointment:** 4.7% iodine with oleic acid, petrolatum	In 30 g and lb.	17
otc	**Iodex-p** (Medtech)	**Ointment:** 10%	In 30 g.	18
otc	**Mallisol** (Hauck)	**Ointment**	In 1 g packets.	NA
otc	**Minidyne** (Pedinol)	**Solution:** 10%. Citric acid and sodium phosphate dibasic	In 15 ml.	13
otc	**Operand** (Redi-Products)	**Aerosol:** 0.5% iodine	In 90 ml.	NA
		Iofoam skin cleanser: 1% iodine	In 90 ml.	NA
		Ointment: 1% iodine	In 30 g, 1 lb and 1.2 and 2.7 g packets.	NA
		Perineal wash concentrate: 1% iodine	In 240 ml.	NA
		Prep solution: 1% iodine	In 60, 120 and 240 ml, pt and qt.	NA
		Solution, prep pads	In 100s.	NA
		Solution, swab sticks	In 25s.	NA
		Surgical scrub: 7.5%	In 60, 120 and 240 ml, pt, qt, gal and 22.5 ml packets.	NA
otc	**Polydine** (Century)	**Ointment**	In 30 and 120 g & lb.	6.5
		Scrub	In 30, 120 and 240 ml, pt and gal.	2.5
		Solution	In 30, 120 and 240 ml, pt and gal.	2.4
otc	**Povidine** (Various, eg, Barre-National, Moore, Rugby)	**Ointment: 10%**	In 28.4 g and lb.	NA
		Solution: 10%	In pt and gal.	NA
		Surgical scrub: 5%	In pt and gal.	NA

* Cost Index based on cost per g, ml or unit applicator.

Mercury Compounds

THIMEROSAL (49% mercury)

Actions:

Pharmacology: An organomercurial antiseptic with sustained bacteriostatic and fungistatic activity against common pathogens.

Indications:

Tincture/Solution: For antisepsis of the skin prior to surgery and for first aid treatment.

Spray: For cuts, scratches, wounds, lacerations and abrasions; as a pre- and post-operative antiseptic.

Contraindications:

Hypersensitivity to thimerosal.

Precautions:

For external use only. Avoid contact with the eyes.

Prolonged repeated applications: Frequent or prolonged use or application to large areas may cause serious mercury poisoning.

Incompatibilities: Thimerosal is incompatible with strong acids, salts of heavy metals, potassium permanganate and iodine; do not use in combination with or immediately following their application.

Discontinue and consult physician if redness, swelling, pain, infection, rash or irritation persists or increases.

Adverse Reactions:

Some individuals are hypersensitive to the thio or mercuri radicals in thimerosal. Symptoms include erythematous, papular and vesicular eruptions over the application area.

Overdosage:

For ingestion of the tincture, consider alcohol and acetone content.

Treatment: Supportive therapy. Refer to General Management of Acute Overdosage.

Administration and Dosage:

Apply locally 1 to 3 times a day.

	Product	Form	Description	C.I.*
otc	**Thimerosal** (Lannett)	**Solution:** 1:1000	Stainless. In pt and gal.	1+
otc	**Mersol** (Century Pharm.)		Colorless. In 120 ml, pt and gal.	NA
otc	**Mersol** (Century Pharm.)	**Tincture:** 1:1000 with 50% alcohol	In 120 ml, pt and gal.	3
otc	**Aeroaid** (Graham-Field)	**Antiseptic spray:** 1:1000 with 72% alcohol	In 90 ml.	31

TRICLOSAN (Irgasan)

Actions:

Pharmacology: Triclosan, a bis-phenol disinfectant, is a bacteriostatic agent with activity against a wide range of gram-positive and gram-negative bacteria.

Indications:

Septi-Soft: Skin cleanser. May be used as a hand and body wash, shampoo and bed or towel bath.

Septisol: Healthcare personnel handwash and skin degermer.

Contraindications:

Use on burned or denuded skin or mucous membranes; routine prophylactic total body bathing.

Septi-Soft: Not a surgical scrub; do not use in preparation for surgery.

Precautions:

For external use only. Avoid contact with the eyes.

Administration and Dosage:

Dispense a small amount (5 ml) on hands, rub thoroughly for 30 seconds, rinse thoroughly, dry.

Septi-Soft may also be used as a hand and body wash, shampoo and bed or towel bath.

	Product	Form	Description
otc	**Septi-Soft** (Calgon Vestal)	**Solution:** 0.25%. With glycerin, emollients	In 240 ml, qt and gal.
otc	**Septisol** (Calgon Vestal)		In 240 ml, qt and gal.

* Cost Index based on cost per ml.

HEXACHLOROPHENE

Actions:

Pharmacology: Hexachlorophene is a bacteriostatic agent with activity against staphylococci and other gram-positive bacteria. Cumulative antibacterial action develops with repeated use.

Indications:

Surgical scrub and bacteriostatic skin cleanser; control of an outbreak of gram-positive infection when other procedures are unsuccessful.

Contraindications:

Use on burned or denuded skin; as an occlusive dressing, wet pack or lotion; routine prophylactic total body bathing; as a vaginal pack or tampon or on any mucous membrane; sensitivity to any component; primary light sensitivity to halogenated phenol derivatives because of the possibility of cross sensitivity to hexachlorophene.

Warnings:

Rinse thoroughly after use, especially from sensitive areas (eg, scrotum, perineum).

Rapid absorption of hexachlorophene may occur with resultant toxic blood levels when applied to skin lesions such as ichthyosis congenita, the dermatitis of Letterer-Siwe's syndrome, or other generalized dermatological conditions. Application to burns has produced neurotoxicity and death.

Cerebral irritability: Discontinue promptly if signs and symptoms of cerebral irritability occur.

Fertility impairment: Topical exposure of neonatal rats to 3% hexachlorophene solution caused reduced fertility in 7-month-old males, due to inability to ejaculate.

Pregnancy: Category C. Placental transfer occurs in rats. There are no adequate and well controlled studies in pregnant women. Use during pregnancy only if the potential benefit justifies the risk to the fetus. Hexachlorophene is not recommended as an antiseptic lubricant for vaginal exams during labor because appreciable amounts have been detected in maternal and cord serum.

Lactation: It is not known whether this drug is excreted in breast milk. Decide whether to discontinue nursing or discontinue the drug, taking into account the importance of the drug to the mother.

Children: Infants, especially those who weigh < 1200 g and those with a gestational age of < 35 weeks, or those with dermatoses, are particularly susceptible to hexachlorophene absorption. Systemic toxicity may manifest as CNS stimulation (irritation), sometimes with convulsions.

Infants have developed dermatitis, irritability, generalized clonic muscular contractions and decerebrate rigidity following application of 6% hexachlorophene powder. Examination of brain stems revealed vacuolization. Moreover, histologic sections of premature infants who died of unrelated causes have shown a correlation between hexachlorophene baths and white matter brain lesions.

Precautions:

For external use only. Avoid contact with the eyes. If contact occurs, rinse out promptly and thoroughly with water.

Adverse Reactions:

Dermatitis; photosensitivity. Sensitivity to hexachlorophene is rare; however, persons who have developed photoallergy to similar compounds may also become sensitive to hexachlorophene.

Persons with highly sensitive skin may develop a reaction characterized by redness or mild scaling or dryness, especially when combined with mechanical factors such as excessive rubbing or exposure to heat or cold.

Overdosage:

Symptoms: Ingestion of 30 to 120 ml has caused anorexia, vomiting, abdominal cramps, diarrhea, dehydration, convulsions, hypotension, shock and fatalities.

Treatment: If patients are seen early, evacuate the stomach by emesis or gastric lavage. Administer olive oil or vegetable oil (60 ml) to delay absorption of hexachlorophene, followed by a saline cathartic to hasten removal. Treatment is symptomatic and supportive; IV fluids (5% dextrose in physiologic saline solution) may be given for dehydration. Correct electrolyte imbalance. If marked hypotension occurs, vasopressor therapy is indicated. Consider use of opiates if GI symptoms (eg, cramping, diarrhea) are severe.

(Continued on following page)

HEXACHLOROPHENE (Cont.)

Patient Information:

For external use only.

Avoid getting suds in the eyes; if this occurs, rinse out promptly and thoroughly with water.

Rinse skin thoroughly after washing.

Do not use on burns or mucous membranes.

Administration and Dosage:

Surgical wash or scrub: As indicated.

Bacteriostatic cleansing: Wet hand with water and squeeze ≈ 5 ml into palm; add water; work up a lather; apply to area to be cleansed. Rinse thoroughly after each washing.

Infant care: Do not use routinely for bathing infants (see Warnings). Use of baby skin products containing alcohol may decrease the antibacterial action.

Storage: Prolonged direct exposure to strong light may cause brownish surface discoloration, but this does not affect its action. Shaking disperses the color.

				C.I.*
Rx	**pHisoHex** (Winthrop Pharm.)	**Liquid:** 3%. With petrolatum, lanolin, PEG	In 150 ml, pt and gal and UD 8 ml (50s).	72
Rx	**Septisol** (Calgon Vestal)	**Foam:** 0.23%. With 56% alcohol	In 180 and 600 ml.	42

CHLORHEXIDINE GLUCONATE

Actions:

Pharmacology: Provides a persistent antimicrobial effect against a wide range of microorganisms, including gram-positive and gram-negative bacteria such as *Pseudomonas aeruginosa*.

Indications:

Surgical scrub; skin cleanser; preoperative skin preparation; skin wound cleanser; preoperative showering and bathing *(Hibiclens liquid)*.

Hand rinse: Healthcare personnel germicidal hand rinse; when hands are physically clean, but need degerming, and when routine handwashing is inconvenient or undesirable.

Chlorhexidine gluconate 0.12% is also indicated for the treatment of gingivitis. See monograph in the Mouth and Throat Products section.

Unlabeled use: Chlorhexidine gluconate 4% skin cleanser twice daily appears effective in the treatment of acne vulgaris (significant reduction of papules plus pustules count).

Contraindications:

Hypersensitivity to chlorhexidine gluconate or any component of the product.

Warnings:

Hypersensitivity: There have been several case reports of anaphylaxis following disinfection with 0.05% to 1% chlorhexidine. Symptoms included generalized urticaria, bronchospasm, cough, dyspnea, wheezing and malaise. Symptoms resolved following therapy with various agents including oxygen, aminophylline, epinephrine, corticosteroids or antihistamines. Refer to Management of Acute Hypersensitivity Reactions.

Lactation: In one case report, a mother sprayed chlorhexidine gluconate on her breasts to prevent mastitis. Her 2-day-old infant developed bradycardia episodes after breastfeeding; symptoms resolved when the chlorhexidine was discontinued.

Precautions:

For external use only. Keep out of eyes, ears and mouth; if this accidentally occurs, rinse out promptly and thoroughly with water. Do not use as a preoperative skin preparation of the face or head (except *Hibiclens liquid*). Serious and permanent eye injury has occurred when it enters and remains in the eye during surgery (see Adverse Reactions).

Meninges: Avoid contact with meninges (see Adverse Reactions).

Excessive heat: Avoid exposing the drug to excessive heat (> 40° C; 104°F).

Do not use routinely on wounds involving more than the superficial layers of skin, or for repeated general skin cleansing of large body areas except in those patients whose underlying condition makes it necessary to reduce the bacterial population of the skin.

Deafness: May cause deafness when instilled in the middle ear. Take particular care in the presence of a perforated eardrum to prevent exposure of inner ear tissues.

Adverse Reactions:

Irritation; dermatitis; photosensitivity (rare); deafness (see Precautions). Sensitization and generalized allergic reactions have occurred, especially in the genital areas. If adverse reactions occur, discontinue use immediately. If severe, contact physician.

(Continued on following page)

CHLORHEXIDINE GLUCONATE (Cont.)

Administration and Dosage:

Cleanser: Surgical scrub – Wet hands and forearms with warm water. Apply about 5 ml and scrub 3 minutes using a wet brush, paying particular attention to the nails, cuticles and interdigital spaces. Rinse thoroughly. Wash for an additional 3 minutes with 5 ml and rinse under running water. Dry thoroughly.

Preoperative skin preparation – Apply liberally to surgical site and swab for ≥ 2 minutes. Dry with sterile towel. Repeat for an additional 2 minutes and dry with sterile towel.

Preoperative showering and whole-body bathing (Hibiclens liquid): Instruct patient to wash the entire body, including the scalp, on two consecutive occasions immediately prior to surgery. Each procedure should consist of two consecutive thorough applications followed by thorough rinsing. If the patient's condition allows, showering is recommended for whole-body bathing. The recommended procedure is: Wet the body, including hair. Wash the hair using 25 ml and the body with another 25 ml. Rinse. Repeat. Rinse thoroughly after second application.

Hand wash – Wet hands with water. Apply about 5 ml into cupped hands and wash vigorously for 15 seconds. Rinse and dry thoroughly.

Skin wound and general skin cleanser – Thoroughly rinse affected area with water. Apply a sufficient amount to cover skin or wound area and wash gently. Rinse again thoroughly.

Hand rinse/wipe: Dispense about 5 ml into cupped hand or use one towelette and rub vigorously until dry (about 15 seconds), paying particular attention to nails and interdigital spaces. Rinse dries rapidly; no water or toweling are necessary.

Sponge/Brush for surgical hand scrub: Wet hands. Use nail cleaner under fingernails and to clean cuticles. Wet hands and forearms to the elbow with warm water. Wet sponge side of sponge/brush. Squeeze and pump immediately to work up adequate lather. Apply lather to hands and forearms using sponge side of the product. *Start 3 minute scrub* by using the brush side of the product to scrub *only* nails, cuticles and interdigital areas. Use sponge side for scrubbing hands and forearms (avoid using brush on these more sensitive areas). Rinse thoroughly with warm water. Scrub for an additional 3 minutes *using sponge side* only. To produce additional lather, add a small amount of water and pump the sponge. (While scrubbing, do not use excessive pressure to produce lather – a small amount of lather is all that is required to adequately cleanse skin.) Rinse and dry thoroughly, blotting hands and forearms with a soft sterile towel.

	Product	Form	Supplied	C.I.*
otc	**BactoShield 2** (Amsco)	**Solution:** 2% with 4% isopropyl alcohol	In 960 ml.	NA
otc	**Exidine-2 Scrub** (Baxter)		In 120 ml.	NA
otc	**Bactoshield** (AMSCO)	**Solution:** 4% with 4% isopropyl alcohol	In 960 ml.	NA
otc	**Exidine-4 Scrub Care** (Baxter)		In 120, 240, 480 and 887 ml and gal.	NA
otc	**Dyna-Hex 2 Skin Cleanser** (Western Medical)	**Liquid:** 2% with 4% isopropyl alcohol	In 120, 240, 480 and 960 ml and gal.	NA
otc	**Dyna-Hex Skin Cleanser** (Western Medical)	**Liquid:** 4% with 4% isopropyl alcohol	In 120, 240 and 480 ml and gal.	NA
otc	**Exidine Skin Cleanser** (Baxter Health Care)		In 120 and 240 ml, qt and gal.	NA
otc	**Hibiclens Antiseptic/Antimicrobial Skin Cleanser** (Stuart)		In 120 and 240 ml, pt, ½ gal and gal and UD 15ml.	49
otc	**Hibistat Germicidal Hand Rinse** (Stuart)	**Rinse:** 0.5% with 70% isopropanol and emollients	In 120 and 240 ml.	28
otc	**Hibistat Towelettes** (Stuart)	**Wipes:** 0.5% with 70% isopropanol	In 50s.	314
otc	**Hibiclens** (Stuart)	**Sponge/Brush:** 4% with 4% isopropyl alcohol	In unit-of-use 22 ml.	1171
otc	**Bactoshield** (AMSCO)	**Foam:** 4% with 4% isopropyl alcohol	In 180 ml aerosol.	NA

* Cost Index based on cost per ml or disposable unit.

BENZALKONIUM CHLORIDE (BAC)

Actions:

Pharmacology: Benzalkonium chloride (BAC), a cationic surface-active agent, is also a rapidly acting anti-infective agent with a moderately long duration of action. It is active against bacteria and some viruses, fungi and protozoa. Bacterial spores are resistant. Solutions are bacteriostatic or bactericidal according to their concentration. The exact mechanism of bactericidal action is unknown, but may be due to enzyme inactivation. Solutions also have deodorant, wetting, detergent, keratolytic and emulsifying activity.

Indications:

Aqueous solutions in appropriate dilutions: Antisepsis of skin, mucous membranes and wounds; preoperative preparation of the skin; surgeons' hand and arm soaks; treatment of wounds; preservation of ophthalmic solutions; irrigations of the eye, body cavities, bladder and urethra; vaginal douching.

Tinctures and sprays: Preoperative preparation of the skin and treatment of minor skin wounds and abrasions.

Sterile storage of instruments and hospital utensils.

Contraindications:

Use in occlusive dressings, casts and anal or vaginal packs because irritation or chemical burns may result.

Warnings:

Diluents: Use Sterile Water for Injection as a diluent for aqueous solutions intended for deep wounds or for irrigation of body cavities. Otherwise, use freshly distilled water. Tap water containing metallic ions and organic matter may reduce antibacterial potency. Do not use resin deionized water since it may contain pathogenic bacteria.

Storage: Organic, inorganic and synthetic materials and surfaces may adsorb sufficient quantities to significantly reduce the antibacterial potency in solutions, resulting in serious contamination of solutions with viable pathogenic bacteria. Do not use corks to stopper bottles containing BAC solution. Do not store cotton, wool, rayon or other materials in solutions. Use sterile gauze sponges and fiber pledgets to apply solutions to the skin, and store in separate containers; immerse in BAC solutions immediately prior to application.

Soaps: BAC solutions are inactivated by soaps and anionic detergents; therefore, rinse thoroughly if these agents are employed prior to BAC use.

Sterilization: Do not rely upon antiseptic solutions to achieve complete sterilization; they do not destroy bacterial spores and certain viruses, including the etiologic agent of infectious hepatitis, and may not destroy *Mycobacterium tuberculosis* and other bacteria. In addition, when applied to the skin, BAC may form a film under which bacteria remain viable.

Flammable solvents: The tinted tincture and spray contain flammable organic solvents; do not use near an open flame or cautery.

Eyes/Mucous membranes: If solutions stronger than 1:3000 enter the eyes, irrigate immediately and repeatedly with water; obtain medical attention promptly. Do not use concentrations > 1:5000 on mucous membranes, except the vaginal mucosa (see recommended dilutions). Keep the tinted tincture and spray, which contain irritating organic solvents, away from the eyes or other mucous membranes.

Precautions:

Prolonged contact: In preoperative antisepsis, do not prolong solution contact with the patient's skin. Avoid pooling of the solution on the operating table.

Inflamed/Irritated tissues: Solutions used must be more dilute than those used on normal tissues (see recommended dilutions).

Corrosion of instruments: To prevent corrosion of metal instruments, sodium nitrite (Anti-Rust Tablets) is added to the BAC solution. See Administration and Dosage.

Adverse Reactions:

Solutions in concentrations normally used have low systemic and local toxicity and are generally well tolerated, although a rare individual may exhibit hypersensitivity.

(Continued on following page)

BENZALKONIUM CHLORIDE (BAC) (Cont.)

Overdosage:

Symptoms: Marked local GI tract irritation (eg, nausea, vomiting) may occur after ingestion. Signs of systemic toxicity include restlessness, apprehension, weakness, confusion, dyspnea, cyanosis, collapse, convulsions and coma. Death occurs as a result of respiratory muscle paralysis.

Treatment: Immediately administer several glasses of mild soap solution, milk or egg whites beaten in water. This may be followed by gastric lavage with a mild soap solution. Avoid alcohol as it promotes absorption.

To support respiration, clear airway and administer oxygen; employ artificial respiration if necessary. If convulsions occur, a short-acting parenteral barbiturate may be given with caution.

Administration and Dosage:

Thoroughly rinse anionic detergents and soaps from the skin or other areas prior to use of solutions because they reduce the antibacterial activity of BAC.

Incompatibilities: The following substances are incompatible with BAC solutions: Iodine; silver nitrate; fluorescein; nitrates; peroxide; lanolin; potassium permanganate; aluminum; caramel; kaolin; pine oil; zinc sulfate; zinc oxide; yellow oxide of mercury.

Recommended dilutions for specific applications of BAC solutions:

Bladder retention lavage: 1:20,000 to 1:40,000 aqueous solution.
Bladder and urethral irrigation: 1:5000 to 1:20,000 aqueous solution.
Breast/nipple hygiene: 1:1000 to 1:2000 aqueous solution.
Catheters and other adsorbent articles: 1:500 aqueous solution (replenish frequently).
Deep infected wounds: 1:3000 to 1:20,000 aqueous solution.
Denuded skin and mucous membranes: 1:5000 to 1:10,000 aqueous solution.
Eye irrigation: 1:5000 to 1:10,000 aqueous solution.
Hospital disinfection: 1:750 aqueous solution.
Metallic instruments, ampuls and thermometers: 1:750 aqueous solution (replenish frequently).
Minor wounds/lacerations: 1:750 tincture or spray.
Oozing and open infections: 1:2000 to 1:5000 aqueous solution.
Postepisiotomy care: 1:5000 to 1:10,000 aqueous solution.
Preoperative disinfection of skin: 1:750 tincture, aqueous solution or spray.
Preservation of ophthalmic solutions: 1:5000 to 1:7500 aqueous solution.
Surgeons' hand and arm soaks: 1:750 aqueous solution.
Vaginal douche/irrigation: 1:2000 to 1:5000 aqueous solution.
Wet dressings: 1:5000 or less aqueous solution.

Preoperative prep: Perform preoperative periorbital skin or head prep only before the patient or eye is anesthetized.

Prevention of rust: To protect metal instruments stored in BAC solution, add crushed Anti-Rust Tablets (eg, Sanofi Winthrop, Lannett). Add 4 tablets/quart to the antiseptic solution. Change solution at least once a week. Not for storage of aluminum or zinc instruments, instruments with lenses fastened by cement (such as cystoscopes or optical instruments), lacquered catheters or some synthetic rubber goods.

				C.I.*
otc	**Benzalkonium Chloride** (Various, eg, A-A Spectrum)	**Concentrate:** 17%	In 500 ml and 4 L.	2.4+
otc	**Benza** (Century)	**Solution:** 1:750	In 60 and 120 ml.	1
otc	**Zephiran** (Sanofi Winthrop)	**Solution, aqueous:** 1:750	In 240 ml and gal.	3
		Disinfectant concentrate: 17%	In 120 ml and gal.	9.9
		Tincture: 1:750	In gal.	2
		Tincture spray: 1:750	In 30 and 180 g and gal.	16
		Tissue: 1:750. With chlorothymol, isopropyl alcohol and alcohol (20%)	In individual single use packets.	NA

* Cost Index based on cost per ml.

GLUTARALDEHYDE

Actions:

Pharmacology: Glutaraldehyde (pH 3 to 4) is a mildly acidic dialdehyde. Following alkalinization to a pH of 7.5 to 8.5 with sodium bicarbonate or aqueous potassium salt, it becomes a highly effective antimicrobial agent with potent bactericidal, tuberculocidal, fungicidal, sporicidal and virucidal activity. A high degree of effectiveness is retained even in the presence of organic material (eg, blood, tissue, mucus).

Indications:

Germicidal agent for disinfection and sterilization of rigid and flexible fiberoptic endoscopes, plastic and rubber respiratory and anesthesia equipment, surgical and dental instruments and thermometers.

Precautions:

Avoid contact with eyes, skin and mucous membranes. If contact with skin or mucous membranes occurs, wash promptly with water. Should accidental contact with the eye occur, promptly irrigate with water and report to a physician.

Fumes from the solution may be irritating to the respiratory tract, therefore keep solutions covered and use only in a well ventilated area.

Directions:

To remove debris from equipment thoroughly brush clean with a mild detergent solution that does not contain an emollient; rinse and rough dry equipment prior to placement in the solution.

Place clean, dry instruments or equipment in perforated pail or tray and immerse in container of alkalinized glutaraldehyde solution. Cover container to minimize odor and prevent evaporation.

Disinfection: Follow specific label directions for immersion to destroy vegetative pathogens on inanimate surfaces. Rinse equipment thoroughly before use.

Sterilization: Immerse completely for a minimum of 10 hours to destroy resistant pathogenic spores. Use sterile technique to remove instruments from solution. Rinse thoroughly with sterile water. Carefully flush all lumens and cannulas. Dry prior to use.

Preparation of solution: Add activator to the solution. The activator contains a rust inhibitor; do not add any other such agent. Upon mixing, the colorless solution changes to a nonstaining green.

	Product	Form	Package
otc	**Cidex**[1] (J & J Medical)	**Solution:** 2%	In qt, gal and 2.5 gal.[3]
otc	**Cidex-7**[2] (J & J Medical)		In qt, gal and 5 gal.[4]
otc	**Cidex Plus 28**[2] (J & J Medical)	**Solution:** 3.2%	In qt, gal and 2.5 gal.[5]

SODIUM HYPOCHLORITE

Actions:

Pharmacology: Sodium hypochlorite has germicidal, deodorizing and bleaching properties. It is effective against vegetative bacteria and viruses, and also, to some degree, against spores and fungi.

Indications:

Used to disinfect utensils and equipment.

Precautions:

Wound application: Not suitable for application to wounds.

Chemical burns may be produced; avoid skin or eye contact with this solution.

	Product	Form	Package
otc	**Sodium Hypochlorite** (Century Pharm.)	**Solution:** 5%	In gal.
otc	**Dakin's** (Century Pharm.)	**Solution:** 0.25%	In pt.
		0.5%	In pt and gal.

[1] Activated dialdehyde is stable for 14 days after activation.
[2] Long-life activated dialdehyde is stable for 28 days after activation.
[3] Vial of activator contains solid sodium salts as buffer to adjust pH to 8.2 to 8.9.
[4] Vial of activator contains aqueous potassium salts as buffer to adjust pH to 7.5 to 8.1.
[5] Vial of activator contains aqueous potassium salts as buffer to adjust pH to 7.2 to 7.8.

OXYCHLOROSENE SODIUM

Actions:

Pharmacology: Oxychlorosene sodium is a complex of the sodium salt of dodecylbenzenesulfonic acid and hypochlorous acid. Its action is markedly cidal, rapid and complete against both gram-negative and gram-positive bacteria, fungi, yeast, mold, viruses and spores.

Indications:

Used for treating localized infections, particularly when resistant organisms are present; to remove necrotic debris in massive infections or from radiation necrosis; to counteract odorous discharges; as a preoperative and postoperative irrigant and for the cleansing and disinfection of fistulae, sinus tract, empyemas and wounds.

Contraindications:

Where the site of infection is not exposed to direct contact with the solution; systemic use.

Precautions:

Bladder/Eye instillation: Instillation of 0.2% solution, particularly into the bladder or into the eye, may cause severe discomfort. Pretreat the eye with a topical anesthetic. In the bladder, use a 0.1% concentration for the first treatment, instilling the solution to the capacity of the bladder without over-distention.

Administration:

Apply by irrigation, instillation, spray, soaks or wet compresses, preferably thoroughly cleansing with gravity flow irrigation or syringe to provide copious quantities of fresh solution to remove organic wastes and debris. Also for preoperative skin preparation and postoperative protection. Apply topically as the 0.4% solution in water or isotonic saline. Use dilutions of 0.1% to 0.2% in urology and ophthalmology.

				C.I.*
otc	**Clorpactin XCB** (Guardian)	**Powder for Solution:** 5 g oxychlorosene	In 5 g bottles (4s).	1
otc	**Clorpactin WCS-90** (Guardian)	**Powder for Solution:** 2 g sodium oxychlorosene	In 2 g bottles (5s).	3

Silver Compounds

SILVER PROTEIN, MILD

Indications:

For use on mucous membranes, especially the eye, nose and throat.

Precautions:

Prolonged or frequent use of silver products may produce argyria.

				C.I.*
otc	**Argyrol S.S. 10%** (Iolab)	**Solution:** 10% stabilized solution of mild silver protein (20 mg/ml of silver) with 10 mg EDTA	In 15 and 30 ml.	400

Miscellaneous Antiseptics

otc	**S.T. 37** (Menley & James)	**Solution:** 0.1% hexylresorcinol, 28% glycerin	In 165 and 360 ml.	8.7
otc	**Mercurochrome** (Purepac)	**Solution:** 2% merbromin	In 30 ml.	1
otc	**Tincture of Green Soap** (Paddock)	**Liquid:** With 28% to 32% alcohol	In gal.	NA
otc	**B.F.I. Antiseptic** (Menley & James)	**Powder:** 16% bismuth-formic-iodide, zinc phenol sulfonate, potassium alum, bismuth subgallate, boric acid, menthol, eucalyptol, thymol	In 7.5, 37.5 and 240 g.	78
otc	**Alcare** (Calgon Vestal)	**Foam:** 62% ethyl alcohol	In 210, 330 and 600 ml.	NA

* Cost Index based on cost per g or ml.

PHYSIOLOGICAL IRRIGATING SOLUTION

Indications:

For general irrigation, washing and rinsing purposes which permit use of a sterile, nonpyrogenic electrolyte solution.

Contraindications:

Irrigation during electrosurgical procedures.

Warnings:

For irrigation only, not for injection.

Absorption: Irrigating fluids enter the systemic circulation in relatively large volumes and must be regarded as a systemic drug. Absorption of large amounts can cause fluid or solute overloading resulting in dilution of serum electrolyte concentrations, overhydration, congested states or pulmonary edema.

Dilutional states: The risk of dilutional states is inversely proportional to the electrolyte concentrations of administered parenteral solutions. The risk of solute overload causing congested states with peripheral and pulmonary edema is directly proportional to the electrolyte concentrations of such solutions.

Do not heat to > 66° C (> 150° F).

Precautions:

Continuous irrigation: Observe caution when solution is used for continuous irrigation or allowed to "dwell" inside body cavities because of possible absorption into the blood stream and circulatory overload.

Aseptic technique is essential for irrigation of body cavities, wounds and urethral catheters or for wetting dressings that come in contact with body tissues.

Accidental contamination from careless technique may transmit infection.

Containers: When used as a "pour" irrigation, do not allow any part of the contents to contact the surface below the outer protected thread area of the semi-rigid wide mouth container. When used via irrigation equipment, attach the administration set promptly. Discard unused portions and use a fresh container for the start-up of each cycle or repeat procedure. For repeated irrigations of urethral catheters, use a separate container for each patient.

Displaced catheters/drainage tubes can lead to irrigation or infiltration of unintended structures or cavities.

Additives may be incompatible. When introducing additives, use aseptic technique, mix thoroughly and do not store.

Tissue distention/disruption: Excessive volume or pressure during irrigation of closed cavities may cause undue distention or disruption of tissues.

Pregnancy: Category C. It is not known whether these solutions can cause fetal harm when administered to a pregnant woman or can affect reproduction capacity. Give to a pregnant woman only if clearly needed.

Adverse Reactions:

Should any adverse reaction occur, discontinue the irrigant, evaluate the patient, institute appropriate countermeasures and save the remainder of the fluid for examination.

Overdosage:

In overhydration or solute overload, reevaluate and institute corrective measures.

Administration and Dosage:

The dose depends on the capacity or surface area of the structure to be irrigated and the nature of the procedure. When used as a vehicle for other drugs, follow manufacturer's recommendations.

Storage/Stability: Avoid excessive heat. Do not freeze. Store at 25°C (77°F); however, brief exposure to 40°C (104°F) does not cause adverse effects.

(Products listed on following page)

PHYSIOLOGICAL IRRIGATING SOLUTION (Cont.)

Rx	**0.45% Sodium Chloride Irrigation** (Abbott)	**Solution:** 450 mg sodium chloride per 100 ml	In 250 and 500 ml and 1, 1.5, 2 and 3 L.
Rx	**0.9% Sodium Chloride Irrigation** (Abbott)	**Solution:** 900 mg sodium chloride per 100 ml	In 100, 250 and 500 ml and 1, 1.5, 2 and 3 L.
Rx	**Tis-U-Sol** (Baxter)	**Solution:** 800 mg NaCl, 40 mg KCl, 20 mg magnesium sulfate, 8.75 mg dibasic sodium phosphate heptahydrate and 6.25 mg monobasic potassium phosphate per 100 ml	In 1 L.
Rx	**Lactated Ringer's Irrigation** (Abbott)	**Solution:** 600 mg sodium chloride, 310 mg sodium lactate, anhydrous, 30 mg potassium chloride, 20 mg calcium chloride, dihydration per 100 ml.	In 300 ml.
Rx	**Physiolyte** (American McGaw)	**Solution:** 530 mg NaCl, 370 mg sodium acetate, 500 mg sodium gluconate, 37 mg KCl and 30 mg magnesium Cl per 100 ml	In 1 L.
Rx	**PhysioSol** (Abbott)	**Solution:** 526 mg NaCl, 222 mg sodium acetate, 502 mg sodium gluconate, 37 mg KCl and 30 mg magnesium chloride hexahydrate per 100 ml	In 250 and 500 ml and 1 L.

chapter 11

antineoplastic agents

The chemotherapeutic agents include a wide range of compounds which work by various mechanisms. Although development has been directed toward agents capable of selective actions on neoplastic tissues, those presently available manifest significant toxicity on normal tissues as a major complication of therapy. Thoroughly consider the risks versus benefits of therapy when using these agents.

Because of the complexities and dangers in cancer chemotherapy, use should be restricted to, or under the direct supervision of, physicians experienced in their use. In addition to drug therapy, surgical excision and radiation therapy are also employed when appropriate.

Handling of Cytotoxic Agents – Most antineoplastics are toxic compounds known to be carcinogenic, mutagenic or teratogenic. Direct contact may cause irritation of the skin, eyes and mucous membranes. Safe and aseptic handling of parenteral chemotherapeutic drugs by medical personnel involved in preparation and administration of these agents is mandatory. Potential risks from repeated contact with parenteral antineoplastics can be controlled by a combination of specific containment equipment and proper work techniques. The NIH Division of Safety brochure outlines recommendations for safe handling of these agents.

Mechanisms of Action:

The mechanism of action by which these agents suppress proliferation of neoplasms is not fully understood. Generally, they affect one or more stages of cell growth or replication. Those more active at one specific phase of cellular growth are referred to as *cell cycle specific* agents; those that are active on both proliferating and resting cells are *cell cycle nonspecific* agents. The selectivity of cytotoxic agents inversely follows cell cycle specificity. Major adverse effects on other rapidly dividing normal tissues include bone marrow, blood components, hair follicles and mucous membranes of the GI tract.

Alkylating agents form highly reactive carbonium ions which react with essential cellular components, thereby altering normal biological function. Alkylating agents replace hydrogen atoms with an alkyl radical causing cross-linking and abnormal base pairing in deoxyribonucleic acid (DNA) molecules. They also react with sulfhydryl, phosphate and amine groups resulting in multiple lesions in both dividing and nondividing cells. The resultant defective DNA molecules are unable to carry out normal cellular reproductive functions.

Antimetabolites include a diverse group of compounds which interfere with various metabolic processes, thereby disrupting normal cellular functions. These agents may act by two general mechanisms: By incorporating the drug, rather than a normal cellular constituent, into an essential chemical compound; or by inhibiting a key enzyme from functioning normally. Their primary benefit is the ability to disrupt nucleic acid synthesis. These agents work only on dividing cells during the S phase of nucleic acid synthesis and are most effective on rapidly proliferating neoplasms.

Hormones have been used to treat several types of neoplasms. Hormonal therapy interferes at the cellular membrane level with growth stimulatory receptor proteins. The mechanism of action, however, is still unclear. Adrenocortical steroids are used primarily for their suppressant effect on lymphocytes in leukemias and lymphomas and as a component in many combination regimens. The counterbalancing effect of androgens, estrogens and progestins has been used to advantage in the therapy of malignancies of tissues dependent upon these sex-related hormones (ie, tumors of the breast, endometrium and prostate). These agents have the advantage of greater specificity for tissues responsive to their effects, thus inhibiting proliferation without a direct cytotoxic action. **Tamoxifen** is a specific antagonist of estrogens. **Leuprolide acetate** is a synthetic analog of the gonadotropin releasing hormone.

Antibiotic type agents, unlike their anti-infective relatives, are capable of disrupting cellular functions of host (mammalian) tissues. Their primary mechanisms of action are to inhibit DNA-dependent RNA synthesis and to delay or inhibit mitosis. The antibiotics are cell cycle nonspecific.

Mitotic inhibitors act as mitotic spindle poisons, causing metaphase arrest. These agents are plant alkaloids derived from the periwinkle plant (vincristine, vinblastine, vindesine) or the May-apple plant (etoposide). They are M-phase cell cycle specific agents but may also have some activity in G_2 and S phase.

Radioactive molecules exert a direct toxic effect on exposed tissue via radiation emission. Use is restricted to physicians licensed by the Nuclear Regulatory Commission.

Miscellaneous: It is believed that direct antiproliferative action against tumor cells and modulation of the host immune response play important roles in the antitumor activity of **interferon, alfa-2a, recombinant** and **interferon, alfa-2b, recombinant. Hydroxyurea** inhibits ribonucleotide reductase, thus interfering with RNA synthesis; it may also directly affect DNA. **Procarbazine** produces toxic metabolites which induce chromosomal breakage. The exact mechanism of action of **dacarbazine** is unknown. **Mitotane** has a selective cytotoxic action on the adrenal glands; it may also modify peripheral steroid metabolism. **L-asparaginase** is an enzyme that inhibits protein synthesis of malignant cells by inhibiting asparagine which is required for protein synthesis.

(Continued on following page)

Extravasation occurs when IV fluid and medication leak into interstitial tissue. Damage resulting from extravasation of certain antineoplastic agents can range from painful erythematous swelling to full thickness injury with deep necrotic lesions, requiring surgical debridement and skin grafting.

Prevention of extravasation injury is based on careful and accurate administration of IV drugs. Avoid areas of previous irradiation and extremities with poor venous circulation for IV cannula placement. Dilute drugs properly and administer at an appropriate rate.

Treatment of extravasation includes immediate discontinuation of infusion and appropriate antidote administration. Goals of treatment are palliation and prevention of severe tissue damage. For further information regarding the instillation of a specific antidote, refer to individual product monographs. Consider surgical evaluation if an open wound occurs. Some practitioners recommend leaving the IV cannula in place to aspirate some of the chemotherapeutic agent and administering an antidote to the injured site. Others recommend immediate removal of the cannula and administration of the antidote by intradermal or SC injections. Immediate removal of the cannula followed by application of ice has also been recommended for all agents except etoposide, vinblastine and vincristine (warm compresses are recommended for these agents). Apply the ice every 15 to 20 minutes every 4 to 6 hours for the first 72 hours. Elevate the affected area.

Hydrocortisone sodium succinate or dexamethasone sodium phosphate have been administered to the extravasated site for their anti-inflammatory activity. However, the use of these agents as well as other drugs such as sodium bicarbonate and DMSO is unproven for antidote use. Specific antidotes that are recommended include sodium thiosulfate for mechlorethamine and hyaluronidase for vincristine and vinblastine.

The following drugs are associated with severe local necrosis (vesicants):

Carmustine	Mitomycin
Dacarbazine	Plicamycin
Dactinomycin	Streptozocin
Daunorubicin	Vinblastine
Doxorubicin	Vincristine
Mechlorethamine	

Nausea and vomiting may be the most prominent adverse reactions of cancer chemotherapy from the patient's perspective, with 30% or more of patients experiencing some degree of emesis. Therefore, effective management of these effects is an important aspect of therapy.

The antineoplastic agents with the highest emetic potential are:

Cisplatin	Mechlorethamine
Dacarbazine	Streptozocin
Dactinomycin	

The agents with moderate emetic potential are:

Asparaginase	Fluorouracil
Carmustine	Lomustine
Cyclophosphamide	Methotrexate
Dactinomycin	Mitomycin
Daunorubicin	Plicamycin
Doxorubicin	Procarbazine

However, the incidence of emesis with these and other agents varies greatly among individuals. Dose, schedule, concomitant therapy, other medical complications and psychologic parameters may affect the incidence as well.

Treatment of nausea and vomiting should include measures such as dietary adjustment, restriction of activity and positive support. However, if pharmacologic management is necessary, several agents or groups of agents may prove useful. Some drugs that have been used with varying degrees of success, either alone or in combination, include phenothiazines, butyrophenones, cannabinoids, corticosteroids, antihistamines, benzodiazepines, metoclopramide, ACTH and scopolamine. Since only 30% to 40% of patients are effectively treated with a single agent, studies using combination therapy have increased.

Combinations of antineoplastic agents are superior to single drug therapy in the management of many diseases, leading to higher response rates and increased duration of remissions. Improved response may be due to the use of agents which work by differing mechanisms. Neoplastic cells that acquire rapid resistance to a single agent by random mutation develop resistance less rapidly when treated with a combination of agents.

Selection of agents for combination chemotherapeutic regimens is based on: Mechanism of drug action; cell-cycle specificity of action; responsiveness to dosage schedules; and drug toxicity. Increased responsiveness to combination therapy may permit dosage reductions and, therefore, decrease toxicity.

A number of commonly used combination chemotherapeutic regimens are listed below:

ABDIC

Use: Hodgkin's disease (resistant to MOPP)

Regimen:
Doxorubicin 45 mg/m² IV, day 1
Bleomycin 5 mg/m² IV, days 1 and 5
Dacarbazine 200 mg/m²/day IV, days 1 through 5
CCNU 50 mg/m² PO, day 1
Prednisone 40 mg/m²/day PO, days 1 through 5
Repeat at 4 week intervals

Reference: *J Clin Oncol* 1983;1:432-439.

ABVD

Use: Hodgkin's disease, induction (resistant to MOPP)

Regimen:
Doxorubicin 25 mg/m²/day IV, days 1 and 14
Bleomycin 10 units/m²/day IV, days 1 and 14
Vinblastine 6 mg/m²/day IV, days 1 and 14
Dacarbazine 375 mg/m²/day IV, days 1 and 14
Repeat twice monthly until remission; continue for two additional cycles (medium 8 cycles)

References:
Cancer 1975;36:252-259.
Ann Intern Med 1984;101:440-446.

ACE

Use: Small cell carcinoma of the lung

Regimen:
Doxorubicin 45 mg/m² IV, day 1
Cyclophosphamide 1 mg/m² IV, day 1
Etoposide 50 mg/m²/day IV, days 1 through 5
Repeat every 21 days

Reference: *Cancer Chemother Pharmacol* 1982;7:187-193.

ACe

Use: Breast cancer, metastatic or recurrent disease

Regimen:
Cyclophosphamide 200 mg/m²/day PO, days 3 through 6
Doxorubicin 40 mg/m² IV, day 1
Repeat every 21 or 28 days

Reference: *Cancer* 1975;36:90-97.

A-COPP

Use: Hodgkin's disease, induction (children only)

Regimen:
Doxorubicin 60 mg/m² IV, day 1
Cyclophosphamide 300 mg/m²/day IV, days 14 and 20
Vincristine 1.5 mg/m²/day IV, days 14 and 20 (maximum dose 2 mg)
Procarbazine 100 mg/m²/day PO, days 14 through 28
Prednisone 40 mg/m²/day PO, days 1 through 27 (1st and 4th cycles only)
Prednisone 40 mg/m²/day PO, days 14 through 27 (2nd, 3rd, 5th and 6th cycles)
Repeat every 42 days for 6 cycles

Reference: Sullivan MP, et al. Hodgkin's disease in children. In: Sutow W. Clinical Pediatric Oncology, 2nd ed. St. Louis: C.V. Mosby Co., 1977:408-443.

Adria + BCNU

Use: Multiple myeloma, multiple myeloma in relapse (alkylator resistant)

Regimen:
Doxorubicin 30 mg/m² IV, day 1
Carmustine 30 mg/m² IV, day 1
Repeat every 21 or 28 days

Reference: *Lancet* 1976;1:926-928.

Ara-C + ADR

Use: Acute myelocytic leukemia, induction

Regimen: Cytarabine 100 mg/m²/day, continuous 24 hour IV infusion for 7 to 10 days
Doxorubicin 30 mg/m²/day IV for 3 days

References: *Cancer Treat Rep* 1977;61:89-92.
Proc Am Soc Clin Onc 1979;20:297.

Ara-C + DNR + PRED + MP

Use: Acute myelocytic leukemia (children only)

Induction: Daunorubicin 25 mg/m² IV for 1 day
Cytarabine 80 mg/m²/day IV for 3 days
Prednisolone 40 mg/m² PO, daily
Mercaptopurine 100 mg/m² PO, daily
Repeat weekly until remission

Maintenance: Repeat every month or 28 days

Reference: *Cancer* 1975;36:1547-1551.

Ara-C + 6-TG

Use: Acute myelocytic leukemia

Induction: Cytarabine 100 mg/m²/every 12 hours IV for 10 days
Thioguanine 100 mg/m²/every 12 hours PO for 10 days
Repeat both drugs every 30 days until remission marrow is obtained.

Reference: *Med Pediat Onc* 1975;1:149-158.

Maintenance: Cytarabine 100 mg/m²/every 12 hours IV for 5 days
Thioguanine 100 mg/m²/every 12 hours PO for 5 days
Repeat every month.

Reference: *Cancer Treat Rep* 1976;60:585-589.

B-CAVe

Use: Hodgkin's disease, advanced (resistant to MOPP)

Regimen: Bleomycin 5 mg/m² IV, days 1, 28 and 35
CCNU 100 mg/m² PO, day 1
Doxorubicin 60 mg/m² IV, day 1
Vinblastine 5 mg/m² IV, day 1
Continue until patient receives maximum tolerated dose of doxorubicin

Reference: *Cancer* 1978;41:1670-1675.

BCVPP

Use: Hodgkin's disease, induction

Regimen: Carmustine 100 mg/m² IV, day 1
Cyclophosphamide 600 mg/m² IV, day 1
Vinblastine 5 mg/m² IV, day 1
Procarbazine 50 mg/m²/day PO, day 1
Procarbazine 100 mg/m²/day PO, days 2 through 10
Prednisone 60 mg/m²/day PO, days 1 through 10
Repeat every 28 days for 6 cycles

References: *Proc Am Soc Clin Onc* 1979;20:392.
Ann Intern Med 1984;101:447-456.

CAF

Use: Breast cancer, metastatic disease

Regimen: Cyclophosphamide 100 mg/m²/day PO, days 1 through 14
Doxorubicin 30 mg/m²/day IV, days 1 and 8
Fluorouracil 500 mg/m²/day IV, days 1 and 8
Repeat every 4 weeks until a total cumulative dose of 450 mg/m² of doxorubicin is given, then discontinue doxorubicin and substitute methotrexate 40 mg/m² IV, and increase fluorouracil to 600 mg/m² IV

Reference: *Cancer* 1978;41:1649-1657.

CAMP

Use: Lung cancer, non-oat cell carcinomas

Regimen: Cyclophosphamide 300 mg/m²/day IV, days 1 and 8
Doxorubicin 20 mg/m²/day IV, days 1 and 8
Methotrexate 15 mg/m²/day IV, days 1 and 8
Procarbazine 100 mg/m²/day PO, days 1 through 10
Repeat every 28 days

Reference: *Proc Am Soc Clin Onc* 1979;20:356.

CAP

Use: Non-small cell carcinoma of the lung

Regimen: Cyclophosphamide 400 mg/m² IV, day 1
Doxorubicin 40 mg/m² IV, day 1
Cisplatin 40 mg/m² IV, day 1
Repeat every 4 weeks

Reference: *Cancer Treat Rep* 1977;61:1339-45.
Cancer Treat Rep 1981;65:941-945.

CAV

Use: Small cell lung cancer, induction

Regimen: Cyclophosphamide 750 mg/m² IV every 3 weeks
Doxorubicin 50 mg/m² IV every 3 weeks
Vincristine 2 mg IV every 3 weeks

Reference: *Cancer Chemother Update* 1984;2:1-4.

CAVe

Use: Hodgkin's disease, induction (resistant to MOPP)

Regimen: Lomustine 100 mg/m² PO, day 1
Doxorubicin 60 mg/m² IV, day 1
Vinblastine 5 mg/m² IV, day 1
Repeat every 6 weeks for 9 cycles

Reference: *Cancer* 1975;36:796-803.

CHL + PRED

Use: Chronic lymphocytic leukemia

Regimen: Chlorambucil 0.4 mg/kg/day PO for 1 day every other week
Prednisone 100 mg/day PO for 2 days every other week
Adjust dosage according to blood counts every 2 weeks prior to therapy. Increase initial dose of 0.4 mg/kg by 0.1 mg/kg every 2 weeks until toxicity or disease control is achieved

References: *Cancer* 1973;31:502-508.
Cancer 1974;33:555-562.

CHOP

Use: Non-Hodgkin's lymphoma, lymphomas with unfavorable histology

Regimen: Cyclophosphamide 750 mg/m² IV, day 1
Doxorubicin 50 mg/m² IV, day 1
Vincristine 1.4 mg/m² IV, day 1 (maximum dose 2 mg)
Prednisone 60 mg/day PO, days 1 through 5
Repeat every 21 to 28 days for 6 cycles

Reference: *Cancer* 1976;38:1484-1493.

CHOR

Use: Lung cancer, small cell carcinoma

Regimen: Cyclophosphamide 750 mg/m²/day IV, days 1 and 22
Doxorubicin 50 mg/m²/day IV, days 1 and 22
Vincristine 1 mg IV, days 1, 8, 15, and 22
Radiation total dose 3000 rad, 10 daily fractions over a 2 week period beginning with day 36

Reference: *Ann Intern Med* 1978;88:194-199.

CISCA

Use: Urinary tract, metastatic disease

Regimen: Cyclophosphamide 650 mg/m² IV, day 1
Doxorubicin 50 mg/m² IV, day 1
Cisplatin 100 mg/m² IV infusion over 2 hours, day 2
Repeat every 21 days. Discontinue doxorubicin when it reaches a total cumulative dose of 450 mg/m², then increase cyclophosphamide to 1000 mg/m² IV

Reference: *JAMA* 1977;238:2282-2287.

CISCA$_{II}$/VB$_{IV}$

Use: Germ cell tumors, advanced

Regimen: Cyclophosphamide 1 g/m² IV, days 1 and 2
Doxorubicin 80-90 mg/m² IV, days 1 and 2
Cisplatin 100-120 mg/m² IV, day 3
alternating with
Vinblastine 3 mg/m² IV as continuous infusion for 5 days
Bleomycin 30 mg/day IV continuous infusion for 5 days

Reference: *Am J Med* 1986;81:219-228.

CMC-High dose

Use: Lung cancer, small cell carcinoma

Regimen: Cyclophosphamide 1000 mg/m²/day IV, days 1 and 29
Methotrexate 15 mg/m²/day IV, twice weekly for 6 weeks
Lomustine 100 mg/m² PO, day 1
If disease responds, proceed to maintenance therapy

Reference: *Cancer Treat Rep* 1977;61:349-354.

CMF

Use: Breast cancer, metastatic or recurrent disease and adjuvant therapy (various regimens)

Regimen: Cyclophosphamide 100 mg/m²/day PO, days 1 through 14
Methotrexate 40-60 mg/m²/day IV, days 1 and 8
Fluorouracil 600 mg/m²/day IV, days 1 and 8
Repeat every 28 days

References: *Cancer* 1976;38:1882-1886.
N Engl J Med 1980;302:78-90.

CMFP

Use: Breast cancer, metastatic disease

Regimen: Cyclophosphamide 100 mg/m²/day PO, days 1 through 14
Methotrexate 60 mg/m²/day IV, days 1 and 8
Fluorouracil 700 mg/m²/day IV, days 1 and 8
Prednisone 40 mg/m²/day PO, days 1 through 14
Repeat every 28 days

Reference: *Ann Intern Med* 1976;84:389-392.

CMFVP (Cooper's Regimen)

Use: Breast cancer, metastatic or recurrent disease

Regimen: Cyclophosphamide 2 mg/kg PO, daily
Methotrexate 0.75 mg/kg IV, weekly
Fluorouracil 12 mg/kg IV, weekly
Vincristine 0.025 mg/kg IV, weekly (maximum dose 2 mg)
Prednisone 0.75 mg/kg PO, days 1 through 21, then taper

References: *Cancer Treat Rev* 1976;3:141-174.
Proc Am Assoc Cancer Res 1969;10:15 (Abstr).

COMLA

Use: Non-Hodgkin's lymphoma

Regimen: Cyclophosphamide 1.5 g/m² IV, day 1
Vincristine 1.4 mg/m² IV, days 1, 8 and 15
Cytarabine 300 mg/m² IV, days 22, 29, 36, 43, 50, 57, 64 and 71
Methotrexate 120 mg/m² IV, days 22, 29, 36, 43, 50, 57, 64 and 71
Leucovorin 25 mg/m² PO every 6 hours x 4, beginning 24 hours after the methotrexate

Reference: *J Clin Oncol* 1985;3:1596-1604.

COP

Use: Non-Hodgkin's lymphoma, lymphomas with favorable histology

Regimen: Cyclophosphamide 800 to 1000 mg/m² IV, day 1
Vincristine 1.4 mg/m² IV, day 1 (maximum dose 2 mg)
Prednisone 60 mg/m²/day PO, days 1 through 5
Repeat every 21 days for 6 cycles

References: *Cancer* 1971;28:306-317.
Cancer 1974;34:1023-1029.

COP-BLAM

Use: Non-Hodgkin's lymphoma, advanced histiocytic (stage III or IV)

Regimen: Cyclophosphamide 400 mg/m² IV, day 1
Vincristine 1 mg/m² IV, day 1
Prednisone 40 mg/m² PO, days 1 through 10
Bleomycin 15 mg IV, day 14
Doxorubicin 40 mg/m² IV, day 1
Procarbazine 100 mg/m² PO, days 1 through 10

Reference: *Ann Intern Med* 1982;97:190-195.

COPP or "C" MOPP

Use: Non-Hodgkin's lymphoma, lymphomas with unfavorable histology or Hodgkin's disease

Regimen: Cyclophosphamide 650 mg/m²/day IV, days 1 and 8
Vincristine 1.4 mg/m²/day IV, days 1 and 8 (maximum dose 2 mg)
Procarbazine 100 mg/m²/day PO, days 1 through 14
Prednisone 40 mg/m²/day PO, days 1 through 14
Repeat every 28 days for 6 cycles

References: *Blood* 1974;43:181-189.
Br J Cancer 1975;31 (Suppl. II):465-473.
Cancer 1971;28:886-893.

CVP

Use: Non-Hodgkin's lymphoma, lymphomas with favorable histology

Regimen: Cyclophosphamide 400 mg/m²/day PO, days 2 through 6
Vincristine 1.4 mg/m² IV, day 1 (maximum dose 2 mg)
Prednisone 100 mg/m²/day PO, days 2 through 6
Repeat every 21 days for 6 cycles

References: *Ann Intern Med* 1972;76:227-234.
Cancer Res 1974;34:1857-1861.
Proc AACR 1973;Abstract 458:115.

CY-VA-DIC

Use: Soft tissue sarcomas, adult sarcomas

Regimen: Cyclophosphamide 500 mg/m² IV, day 1
Vincristine 1.4 mg/m²/day IV, days 1 and 5 (maximum dose 2 mg)
Doxorubicin 50 mg/m² IV, day 1
Dacarbazine 250 mg/m²/day IV, days 1 through 5
Repeat every 21 days

Reference: *Cancer* 1975;36:765-769.

FAC

Use: Breast cancer, metastatic disease

Regimen: Fluorouracil 500 mg/m²/day IV, days 1 and 8
Doxorubicin 50 mg/m² IV, day 1
Cyclophosphamide 500 mg/m² IV, day 1
Repeat every 3 weeks

Reference: *Ann Intern Med* 1979;91:847-852.

FAM

Use: Lung cancer, non-oat cell carcinomas

Regimen: Fluorouracil 600 mg/m²/day IV, days 1, 8, 28 and 36
Doxorubicin 30 mg/m²/day IV, days 1 and 28
Mitomycin 10 mg/m² IV, day 1
Repeat every 8 weeks

Reference: *Cancer* 1979;43:1183-1188.

Use: Gastric carcinoma, advanced disease

Regimen: Fluorouracil 600 mg/m²/day IV, days 1, 8, 29 and 36
Doxorubicin 30 mg/m²/day IV, days 1 and 29
Mitomycin 10 mg/m² IV, day 1
Repeat every 8 weeks

Reference: *Cancer* 1979;44:42-47.

Use: Pancreatic carcinoma, advanced disease

Regimen: Fluorouracil 600 mg/m²/week IV, weeks 1, 2, 5, 6 and 9
Doxorubicin 30 mg/m²/week IV, weeks 1, 5 and 9
Mitomycin 10 mg/m²/week IV, weeks 1 and 9

Reference: *Proc Am Soc Clin Onc* 1979;20:415.

FOMi

Use: Non-small cell carcinoma of the lung

Regimen: 5FU 300 mg/m²/day IV, days 1 through 4
Vincristine 2 mg IV, day 1
Mitomycin C 10 mg/m² IV, day 1
Repeat at 3 week intervals for three courses; thereafter, every 6 weeks

Reference: *Cancer Treat Rep* 1980;64:1241-1245.

M-2 Protocol

Use: Multiple myeloma

Regimen: Vincristine 0.03 mg/kg IV, day 1 (maximum dose 2 mg)
Carmustine 0.5 mg/kg IV, day 1
Cyclophosphamide 10 mg/kg IV, day 1
Melphalan 0.25 mg/kg/day PO, days 1 through 4
Prednisone 1.0 mg/kg/day PO, days 1 through 7 then taper to day 21
Continue treatment cycle throughout remission period, until disease progresses.

Reference: *Am J Med* 1977;63:897-903.

MAC

Use: Ovarian carcinoma, advanced

Regimen: Mitomycin C 7 mg/m² IV
Doxorubicin 45 mg/m² IV
Cyclophosphamide 450 mg/m² IV
Repeat at 3 week intervals

Reference: *Am J Clin Oncol* 1983;6:565-570.

MACC

Use: Lung cancer, non-oat cell carcinoma

Regimen: Methotrexate 40 mg/m² IV, day 1
Doxorubicin 40 mg/m² IV, day 1
Cyclophosphamide 400 mg/m² IV, day 1
Lomustine 30 mg/m² PO, day 1
Repeat every 21 days

Reference: *JAMA* 1977;237:2392-2396.

MOPP

Use: Hodgkin's disease, induction

Regimen: Mechlorethamine 6 mg/m²/day IV, days 1 and 8
Vincristine 2 mg/m²/day IV, days 1 and 8 (maximum dose 2 mg)
Procarbazine 50 mg/m²/day PO, day 1
Procarbazine 100 mg/m²/day PO, days 2 through 14
Prednisone 40 mg/m²/day PO, days 1 through 14
Repeat every 28 days for 6 cycles

References: *Ann Intern Med* 1970;73:881-895.
Cancer 1970;25:1018-1025.
Cancer 1976;37:2436-2447.
Ann Intern Med 1984;101:447-456.

MOPP/ABVD

Use: Hodgkin's disease, advanced

Regimen: Mechlorethamine 6 mg/m² IV, days 1 and 8
Vincristine 1.4 mg/m² IV, days 1 and 8
Procarbazine 100 mg/m² PO, days 1 through 14
Prednisone 40 mg/m² PO, days 1 through 14
alternating every other month with
Doxorubicin 25 mg/m² IV, days 1 and 15
Bleomycin 10 mg/m² IV, days 1 and 15
Vinblastine 6 mg/m² IV, days 1 and 15
Dacarbazine 375 mg/m² IV, days 1 and 15

Reference: *N Engl J Med* 1982;306:770-775.

MOPP-LO BLEO

Use: Hodgkin's disease, induction

Regimen: Mechlorethamine 6 mg/m²/day IV, days 1 and 8
Vincristine 1.5 mg/m²/day IV, days 1 and 8 (maximum dose 2 mg)
Procarbazine 100 mg/m²/day PO, days 2 through 7, and 9 through 12
Prednisone 40 mg/m²/day PO, in divided doses days 2 through 7, and 9 through 12
Bleomycin 2 units/m²/day IV, days 1 and 8
Repeat monthly for 6 cycles

Reference: Coltman CA. Bleomycin in malignant lymphoma combinations. In: Soper WT, et al. National Cancer Institute. New Drug Seminar on Bleomycin. Silver Spring, MD: Automation Industries, Inc.; 1977:97-107.

MPL + PRED(MP)

Use: Multiple myeloma

Regimen: Melphalan 8 mg/m²/day PO, days 1 through 14
Prednisone 75 mg/m²/day PO, days 1 through 7
Repeat every 28 days for 6 cycles

Reference: *JAMA* 1969;208:1680-1685.

MTX + MP

Use: Acute lymphocytic leukemia, maintenance therapy

Regimen: Methotrexate 20 mg/m²/week IV
Mercaptopurine 50 mg/m²/day PO
Continue both drugs until relapse of disease or after 3 years of remission

References: *Cancer* 1972;29:381-391.
Semin Hematol 1974;11:25-39.

MTX + MP + CTX

Use: Acute lymphocytic leukemia, maintenance therapy

Regimen: Methotrexate 20 mg/m²/week IV
Mercaptopurine 50 mg/m²/day PO
Cyclophosphamide 200 mg/m²/week IV
Continue all 3 drugs until relapse of disease or after 3 years of remission

Reference: *Cancer* 1975;35:25-35.

M-VAC

Use: Transitional cell carcinoma of the bladder

Regimen: Methotrexate 30 mg/m² IV, day 1
Vinblastine 3 mg/m² IV, days 2, 15 and 22
Doxorubicin 30 mg/m² IV, days 2, 15 and 22
Cisplatin 70 mg/m² IV, day 2

Reference: *J Urol* 1985;133:403-407.

POCC

Use: Lung cancer, small cell carcinoma

Regimen: Procarbazine 100 mg/m²/day PO, days 1 through 14
Vincristine 2 mg/day IV, days 1 and 8 (maximum dose 2 mg)
Cyclophosphamide 600 mg/m²/day IV, days 1 and 8
Lomustine 60 mg/m² PO, day 1
Repeat every 28 days

Reference: *Cancer Treat Rep* 1977;61:1-6.

PVB

Use: Testicular carcinoma

Regimen: Cisplatin 20 mg/m²/day IV, days 1 through 5 every 3 weeks for 4 courses
Vinblastine 0.2-0.4 mg/kg IV, day 1 every 3 weeks for 4 courses
Bleomycin 30u IV, day 1 weekly for 12 consecutive weeks

Reference: *J Urol* 1981;126:493-495.

T-2 Protocol

Use: Ewing's sarcoma

Regimen: *Cycle #1*
- Month one
  - Dactinomycin 0.45 mg/m²/day IV, days 1 through 5
  - Doxorubicin 20 mg/m²/day IV, days 20 through 22
  - Radiation days 1 through 21, then 2 weeks rest period
- Month two
  - Doxorubicin 20 mg/m²/day IV, days 8 through 10
  - Vincristine 1.5-2 mg/m² IV, day 24 (maximum dose 2 mg)
  - Cyclophosphamide 1200 mg/m² IV, day 24
  - Radiation days 8 through 28
- Month three
  - Vincristine 1.5-2 mg/m²/day IV, days 3, 9 and 15 (maximum dose 2 mg)
  - Cyclophosphamide 1200 mg/m² IV, day 9

Cycle #2
- Repeat Cycle #1 without radiation

Cycle #3
- Month one
  - Dactinomycin 0.45 mg/m²/day IV, days 1 through 5
  - Doxorubicin 20 mg/m²/day IV, days 20 through 22
- Month two
  - Vincristine 1.5-2 mg/m²/day IV, days 8, 15, 22 and 28 (maximum dose 2 mg/m²)
  - Cyclophosphamide 1200 mg/m²/day IV, days 8 and 22
- Month three - No drugs for 28 days

Cycle #4
- Repeat Cycle #3

References: *Cancer* 1974;33:384-393.
Cancer 1978;41:888-899.
Pediatr Ann 1978;7:30-51.

VAB-6

Use: Testicular carcinoma

Regimen: *Induction (given every 3 to 4 weeks for 2 courses):*
- Cyclophosphamide 600 mg/m² IV, day 1
- Dactinomycin 1 mg/m² IV, day 1
- Vinblastine 4 mg/m² IV, day 1
- Bleomycin 30 mg IV, day 1
- Bleomycin 20 mg/m²/day by continuous 24 hour infusion, days 1 through 3
- Cisplatin 120 mg/m² IV, day 4

Maintenance (given every 3 weeks for 12 months):
- Vinblastine 6 mg/m² IV
- Dactinomycin 1 mg/m² IV

Reference: *Cancer* 1983;51:5-8.

VAC Pulse

Use: Soft tissue sarcomas, rhabdomyosarcoma (pediatric)

Regimen:
- Vincristine 2 mg/m²/week IV, weeks 1 through 12 (maximum dose 2 mg)
- Dactinomycin 0.015 mg/kg/day IV for 5 days, weeks 1 and 13. Continue 5 day courses every 3 months for 5 to 6 courses (maximum dose 0.5 mg/day)
- Cyclophosphamide 10 mg/kg/day IV or PO for 7 days. Continue every 6 weeks for 2 years

Reference: *Cancer* 1975;36:765-769.

VAC Standard

Use: Soft tissue sarcomas, rhabdomyosarcoma and undifferentiated sarcoma

Regimen:
- Vincristine 2 mg/m²/week IV, weeks 1 through 12 (maximum dose 2 mg)
- Dactinomycin 0.015 mg/kg/day IV for 5 days, every 3 months for 5 to 6 courses (maximum dose 0.5 mg/day)
- Cyclophosphamide 2.5 mg/kg/day PO. Continue daily for 2 years

Reference: *Cancer* 1975;36:765.

(Continued on following page)

VAD

Use: Refractory multiple myeloma

Regimen: Vincristine 0.4 mg/day IV by continuous infusion, days 1 through 4
Doxorubicin 9 mg/m²/day IV by continuous infusion, days 1 through 4
Dexamethasone 40 mg PO every morning for 4 days

Reference: *Ann Intern Med* 1986;105:8-11.

VBP

Use: Disseminated testicular cancer

Regimen: Vinblastine 0.2 mg/kg/day IV, days 1 and 2 (every 3 weeks for 5 courses)
Cisplatin 20 mg/m²/day IV infusion over 15 minutes, 6 hours after vinblastine, days 1 through 5. Repeat every 3 weeks for 3 courses
Bleomycin 30 units/week, IV, 6 hours after vinblastine on the second day of each week for 12 weeks to a total cumulative dose of 360 units

References: *Ann Intern Med* 1977;87:293-298.
Ann Intern Med 1979;90:373-385.

VP

Use: Acute lymphocytic leukemia, induction

Regimen: Vincristine 2 mg/m²/week IV for 4 to 6 weeks (maximum dose 2 mg)
Prednisone 60 mg/m²/day PO, in divided doses for 4 weeks. Taper weeks 5-7

Reference: *Cancer Treat Rev* 1976;3:1741.

VP-L-Asparaginase

Use: Acute lymphocytic leukemia, induction

Regimen: Vincristine 2 mg/m²/week IV for 4 to 6 weeks (maximum dose 2 mg)
Prednisone 60 mg/m²/day PO for 4 to 6 weeks then taper
L-asparaginase 10,000 units/m²/day IV for 14 days

References: *Cancer* 1971;28:819-824.
Cancer Res 1977;37:535.

Nitrogen Mustards

MECHLORETHAMINE HCl (Nitrogen Mustard; HN_2)

Actions:

An alkylating agent with cytotoxic, mutagenic and radiomimetic actions which inhibit rapidly proliferating cells. In either water or body fluids, mechlorethamine rapidly undergoes chemical transformation and reacts with various cellular compounds so the active drug is no longer present within a few minutes. Less than 0.01% of the active drug is recovered in the urine. However, > 50% of inactive metabolites are excreted in the urine in the first 24 hours.

Indications:

IV: Palliative treatment of Hodgkin's disease (Stages III and IV); lymphosarcoma; chronic myelocytic or chronic lymphocytic leukemia; polycythemia vera; mycosis fungoides; bronchogenic carcinoma.

Intrapleurally, intraperitoneally or intrapericardially: Palliative treatment of metastatic carcinoma resulting in effusion.

Unlabeled uses: A topical mechlorethamine solution or ointment has been used to treat patients with cutaneous mycosis fungoides.

Contraindications:

Patients with infectious disease; previous anaphylactic reactions to the drug.

Warnings:

> *Extravasation* of the drug into subcutaneous tissues results in painful inflammation and induration; sloughing may occur. If leakage of drug is obvious, promptly infiltrate the area with sterile isotonic sodium thiosulfate (⅙ molar) and apply an ice compress for 6 to 12 hours.

Inoperable neoplasms or terminal stage: Balance the potential risk and discomfort from use in patients with inoperable neoplasms or in the terminal stage of the disease against the limited gain obtainable. Routine use in cases of widely disseminated neoplasms is discouraged.

Hematologic: In patients with leukopenia, thrombocytopenia and anemia due to bone marrow invasion, a good response to treatment with disappearance of the tumor from the bone marrow may be associated with improvement of bone marrow function. However, in the absence of a positive response or in patients who have previously received chemotherapy, hematopoiesis may be further compromised and leukopenia, thrombocytopenia and anemia may become severe, leading to death.

Chronic lymphatic leukemia: Drug toxicity, especially sensitivity to bone marrow failure, appears to be more common in chronic lymphatic leukemia than in other conditions; administer in this condition with great caution, if at all.

Tumors of bone and nervous tissue respond poorly to therapy. Results are unpredictable in disseminated and malignant tumors of different types.

Amyloidosis: Nitrogen mustard therapy may contribute to extensive and rapid development of amyloidosis; use only if foci of acute and chronic suppurative inflammation are absent.

Hypersensitivity reactions, including anaphylaxis, have occurred. Refer to Management of Acute Hypersensitivity Reactions.

Pregnancy: Category D. Mechlorethamine can cause fetal harm when administered to a pregnant woman. Nitrogen mustards produce fetal malformations in the rat and ferret when given as single SC injections of 1 mg/kg (2 to 3 times the maximum recommended human dose). There are no adequate and well controlled studies in pregnant women. If this drug is used during pregnancy, or if the patient becomes pregnant while taking this drug, apprise her of the potential hazard to the fetus. Advise women of childbearing potential to avoid becoming pregnant.

Lactation: It is not known whether this drug is excreted in breast milk. Because of the potential for serious adverse reactions in nursing infants from nitrogen mustards, decide whether to discontinue nursing or to discontinue the drug, taking into account the importance of the drug to the mother.

Children: Safety and efficacy in children have not been established by well controlled studies. Use in children has been quite limited. Nitrogen mustards have been used in Hodgkin's disease (stages III and IV) in combination with other oncolytic agents (MOPP schedule). The MOPP chemotherapy combination includes mechlorethamine, vincristine, procarbazine and prednisone or prednisolone.

(Continued on following page)

MECHLORETHAMINE HCl (Nitrogen Mustard; HN_2) (Cont.)

Precautions:

Local toxicity: This drug is highly toxic and is a powerful vesicant; both powder and solution must be handled and administered with care. Avoid inhalation of dust or vapors and contact with skin or mucous membranes, especially the eyes. Should accidental eye contact occur, institute copious irrigation with water, normal saline or balanced salt ophthalmic irrigating solution immediately, and follow by prompt ophthalmologic consultation. Should accidental skin contact occur, immediately irrigate the affected part with copious amounts of water for at least 15 minutes, and follow by application of 2% sodium thiosulfate solution.

Concomitant therapy: Hematopoietic function is characteristically depressed by x-ray therapy or other chemotherapy in alternating courses. Neither mechlorethamine following x-ray nor x-ray subsequent to the drug should be given until bone marrow function has recovered. In particular, irradiation of such areas as sternum, ribs and vertebrae shortly after a course of nitrogen mustard may lead to hematologic complications.

Therapy with nitrogen mustard may be associated with an increased incidence of a second malignant tumor, especially when it is combined with other antineoplastic agents or radiation therapy.

Immunosuppression: Immunosuppressive activity has occurred with nitrogen mustard. Use may predispose the patient to bacterial, viral or fungal infection.

Hyperuricemia: Urate precipitation may develop during therapy, particularly in the treatment of lymphomas; institute adequate methods for control of hyperuricemia and maintain adequate fluid intake before treatment.

Monitoring: Many abnormalities of renal, hepatic and bone marrow function occur in patients with neoplastic disease who receive mechlorethamine. Check renal, hepatic and bone marrow functions frequently.

Adverse Reactions:

Clinical use of mechlorethamine is usually accompanied by toxic manifestations.

Local toxicity: Thrombosis and thrombophlebitis. Avoid high concentration and prolonged contact with the drug, especially in cases of elevated pressure in the antebrachial vein (eg, in mediastinal tumor compression from severe vena cava syndrome). Extravasation may progress to tissue necrosis (see Warnings).

Systemic toxicity: Nausea, vomiting and depression of formed elements in the circulating blood are dose-limiting side effects that usually occur with full doses. Hypersensitivity reactions, including anaphylaxis, have occurred (see Warnings).

GI: Onset of nausea and vomiting is usually 1 to 3 hours after use. Vomiting may persist for the first 8 hours, nausea for 24 hours. Vomiting may be so severe as to precipitate vascular accidents in patients with a hemorrhagic tendency. Premedication with antiemetics and sedatives may be beneficial. Diarrhea may also occur. Jaundice occurs infrequently.

Hematologic: The usual course of treatment (total dose, 0.4 mg/kg) produces lymphocytopenia within 24 hours after the first injection; significant granulocytopenia occurs within 6 to 8 days and lasts for 10 days to 3 weeks. Agranulocytosis is infrequent and recovery from leukopenia is usually complete within 2 weeks. Thrombocytopenia is variable, but the time course of appearance and recovery generally parallels the sequence of granulocyte levels. Severe thrombocytopenia may lead to bleeding from the gums and GI tract, petechiae and small subcutaneous hemorrhages; these symptoms appear transient and, in most cases, disappear with return to a normal platelet count. However, a severe and uncontrollable hematopoietic depression occasionally may follow the usual dose, particularly in patients with widespread disease and debility and in patients previously treated with other antineoplastic agents or radiation. Persistent pancytopenia has occurred. In rare instances, hemorrhagic complications may be due to hyperheparinemia. Erythrocyte and hemoglobin levels may decline during the first 2 weeks after therapy, but rarely significantly. Depression of the hematopoietic system may occur up to 50 days or more after starting therapy. Rarely, hemolytic anemia associated with such diseases as the lymphomas and chronic lymphocytic leukemia is precipitated.

(Adverse Reactions continued on following page)

MECHLORETHAMINE HCl (Nitrogen Mustard; HN_2) (Cont.)

Adverse Reactions (Cont.)

Hematologic (Cont.):

Use extreme caution when exceeding the average recommended dose. With total doses exceeding 0.4 mg/kg for a single course, severe leukopenia, anemia, thrombocytopenia and hemorrhagic diathesis with subsequent delayed bleeding may develop. Death may follow. The only treatment for excessive dosage appears to be repeated blood product transfusions, antibiotic treatment of complicating infections and general supportive measures.

Dermatologic: Occasionally, a maculopapular skin eruption occurs; this will not necessarily recur with subsequent courses. Alopecia occurs infrequently. Erythema multiforme has been observed. Herpes zoster, common with lymphomas, may first appear after therapy is instituted and may be precipitated by treatment. Discontinue further treatment during the acute phase of this illness to avoid progression to generalized herpes zoster.

Reproductive: Delayed menses; oligomenorrhea; temporary or permanent amenorrhea. Impaired spermatogenesis, azoospermia and total germinal aplasia have occurred in male patients, especially those receiving combination therapy. Spermatogenesis may return in patients in remission, but this may occur several years after chemotherapy has been discontinued. Warn patients of the potential risks to their reproductive capacity.

Miscellaneous: Anorexia; weakness; vertigo, tinnitus, diminished hearing (infrequent); chromosomal abnormalities.

Intercavitary: Pain occurs rarely with intrapleural use; it is common with intraperitoneal injection and is often associated with nausea, vomiting, and diarrhea of 2 to 3 days duration. Transient cardiac irregularities may occur with intrapericardial injection. Death, possibly accelerated by nitrogen mustard, has occurred following intracavitary use. Although absorption by the intracavitary route is probably not complete because of its rapid deactivation by body fluids, the systemic effect is unpredictable. The acute side effects such as nausea and vomiting are usually mild. Bone marrow depression is generally milder than when the drug is given IV. Avoid use by the intracavitary route when other agents which may suppress bone barrow function are being used systemically.

Administration and Dosage:

IV: Individualize dosage. Give a total dose of 0.4 mg/kg for each course either as a single dose or in 2 to 4 divided doses of 0.1 to 0.2 mg/kg/day. Base dosage on ideal dry body weight. Administration at night is preferred, in case sedation for side effects is required.

Do not give subsequent courses until the patient has recovered hematologically from the previous course; determine by studies of the peripheral blood elements, awaiting their return to normal levels. This is mandatory as a guide to subsequent therapy. It is often possible to give repeated courses of mechlorethamine as early as 3 weeks after treatment.

The margin of safety is narrow; exercise considerable care with dosage.

It is preferable to inject into the rubber or plastic tubing of a flowing IV infusion set. This reduces the possibility of extravasation or high drug concentration; it also minimizes a chemical reaction between the drug and the solution. The rate of injection apparently is not critical provided it is completed within a few minutes.

Intracavitary administration has been used with varying success for the control of pleural, peritoneal and pericardial effusions caused by malignant cells.

Consult product labeling for details of intracavitary administration. The technique and dose used by any of these routes varies. The usual dose is 0.4 mg/kg, although 0.2 mg/kg (or 10 to 20 mg) has been used intrapericardially.

Preparation of solution: Each vial contains 10 mg of mechlorethamine HCl triturated with 100 mg sodium chloride. In neutral or alkaline aqueous solution, it undergoes rapid chemical transformation and is highly unstable. Prepare solutions immediately before each injection, since they will decompose on standing.

Reconstitute with 10 ml of Sterile Water for Injection or Sodium Chloride Injection. The resultant solution contains 1 mg/ml mechlorethamine HCl.

Decontamination: To clean rubber gloves, tubing, glassware, etc, after administration, soak them in an aqueous solution containing equal volumes of sodium thiosulfate (5%) and sodium bicarbonate (5%) for 45 minutes. Excess reagents and reaction products are washed away easily with water. Neutralize any unused injection solution by mixing with an equal volume of sodium thiosulfate/sodium bicarbonate solution. Allow the mixture to stand for 45 minutes. Treat contaminated vials in the same way with thiosulfate/bicarbonate solution before disposal.

Rx	**Mustargen** (MSD)	**Powder for Injection:** 10 mg	In vials.

CHLORAMBUCIL

Warning:
Chlorambucil: Can severely suppress bone marrow function; is carcinogenic in humans; is probably mutagenic and teratogenic in humans; affects human fertility.

Actions:

Chlorambucil is a bifunctional alkylating agent of the nitrogen mustard type. It appears to be relatively free from GI effects or other evidence of toxicity apart from its bone marrow depressant action. A cell cycle nonspecific drug, chlorambucil interacts with cellular DNA to produce a cytotoxic cross-linkage.

Pharmacokinetics: Chlorambucil is rapidly and completely absorbed from the GI tract following oral administration. Peak plasma chlorambucil levels are reached in 1 hour; extensive metabolic degradation occurs with 1% unchanged drug recovered in the urine over 24 hours. The plasma half-life is approximately 60 minutes.

Chlorambucil and its metabolites are extensively bound to plasma and tissue proteins. In vitro, it is 99% bound to plasma proteins, specifically albumin.

Chlorambucil is extensively metabolized in the liver, primarily to phenylacetic acid mustard which has antineoplastic activity. Chlorambucil and its major metabolite spontaneously degrade in vivo, forming monohydroxy and dihydroxy derivatives.

Indications:

Palliation for chronic lymphocytic leukemia, malignant lymphomas including lymphosarcoma, giant follicular lymphoma and Hodgkin's disease. It is not a curative in any of these disorders, but it may produce clinically useful palliation.

Unlabeled uses: Chlorambucil (0.1 mg/kg/day) has been used in the treatment of uveitis and meningoencephalitis associated with Behcet's disease. A chlorambucil dosage of 0.1 to 0.2 mg/kg/day every other month alternating with a corticosteroid for 6 months duration has been successful in the treatment of idiopathic membranous nephropathy. Chlorambucil 0.1 to 0.3 mg/kg/day has been used for rheumatoid arthritis with mixed results. Toxicity is a limiting factor although it may be useful at a lower dosage when combined with other antirheumatic agents.

Contraindications:

Resistance to the agent; hypersensitivity.

There may be cross-hypersensitivity (skin rash) between chlorambucil and other alkylating agents.

Warnings:

Carcinogenesis and leukemogenesis: Because of its carcinogenic properties, do not give to patients with conditions other than chronic lymphatic leukemia or malignant lymphomas. Convulsions, infertility, leukemia and secondary malignancies are observed when chlorambucil is used in the therapy of malignant and non-malignant diseases.

There are many additional reports of acute leukemia arising in patients with both malignant and nonmalignant diseases following chlorambucil treatment. Patients often received additional chemotherapeutic agents or radiation therapy. Leukemogenesis apparently increases with both chronicity of treatment and with large cumulative doses. However, it is impossible to define a cumulative dose below which there is no risk of inducing secondary malignancy. Weigh the potential benefits of therapy against the risk of inducing a secondary malignancy.

Fertility impairment: Chlorambucil has caused chromatid or chromosome damage in man. Both reversible and permanent sterility have occurred in both sexes.

A high incidence of sterility occurs when chlorambucil is administered to prepubertal and pubertal males. Prolonged or permanent azoospermia has also occurred in adult males. While most reports of gonadal dysfunction secondary to chlorambucil are related to males, the induction of amenorrhea in females with alkylating agents is well documented, and chlorambucil can produce amenorrhea. Autopsy studies of the ovaries from women with malignant lymphoma treated with combination chemotherapy including chlorambucil show varying degrees of fibrosis, vasculitis and depletion of primordial follicles.

(Warnings continued on following page)

CHLORAMBUCIL (Cont.)

Warnings (Cont.):

Pregnancy: Category D. Chlorambucil can cause fetal harm when administered to a pregnant woman. Unilateral renal agenesis has been observed in two offspring whose mothers received chlorambucil during the first trimester. Urogenital malformations including absence of a kidney were found in fetuses of rats given chlorambucil. There are no adequate and well controlled studies in pregnant women. If this drug is used during pregnancy, or if the patient becomes pregnant while taking this drug, apprise her of the potential hazard to the fetus. Advise women of childbearing potential to avoid becoming pregnant.

Lactation: It is not known whether this drug is excreted in breast milk. Because of the potential for serious adverse reactions in nursing infants, decide whether to discontinue nursing or to discontinue the drug, taking into account the importance of the drug to the mother.

Children: Safety and efficacy in children have not been established.

Precautions:

Radiation and chemotherapy: Do not give at full dosage before 4 weeks after a full course of radiation therapy or chemotherapy because of the vulnerability of the bone marrow to damage under these conditions. If the pretherapy leukocyte or platelet counts are depressed from bone marrow disease process prior to institution of therapy, institute treatment at a reduced dosage.

Bone marrow damage: Follow patients carefully to avoid life-threatening damage to the bone marrow. Determine weekly hemoglobin levels, total and differential leukocyte counts and quantitative platelet counts. Also, during the first 3 to 6 weeks of therapy, perform white blood cell (WBC) counts 3 to 4 days after each of the weekly complete blood counts. It is dangerous to allow a patient to go more than 2 weeks without hematological and clinical examination.

A slowly progressive lymphopenia may develop during treatment. The lymphocyte count usually returns rapidly to normal levels upon completion of drug therapy. Most patients have some neutropenia after the third week of treatment which may continue for up to 10 days after the last dose. Subsequently, the neutrophil count usually rapidly returns to normal. Severe neutropenia appears to be dose-related and usually occurs only in patients who have received a total dose of ≥ 6.5 mg/kg in one course. About one fourth of all patients receiving this dosage, and one third of those receiving this dosage in ≤ 8 weeks, develop severe neutropenia.

It is not necessary to discontinue chlorambucil at the first evidence of a fall in neutrophil count. Decreases may continue for 10 days after the last dose is given. As the total dose approaches 6.5 mg/kg, irreversible bone marrow damage may occur. Most patients who receive benefit from chlorambucil require a smaller dosage than this amount. Decrease dosage if leukocyte or platelet counts fall below normal values; discontinue if more severe depression occurs. Persistently low neutrophil and platelet counts or peripheral lymphocytosis suggest bone marrow infiltration. If confirmed by bone marrow examination, do not exceed a daily dosage of 0.1 mg/kg.

Adverse Reactions:

Bone marrow depression (see Precautions) is the major adverse effect. Although bone marrow suppression frequently occurs, it is usually reversible if chlorambucil is withdrawn early enough. However, irreversible bone marrow failure has occurred.

GI: Nausea; vomiting; diarrhea; oral ulceration (infrequent).

Hepatic: Hepatotoxicity with jaundice.

Pulmonary: Syndrome of bronchopulmonary dysplasia; pulmonary fibrosis.

Reproductive: A high incidence of sterility occurs when chlorambucil is administered to prepubertal and pubertal males. Prolonged or permanent azoospermia has been observed in adult males. Chlorambucil can produce amenorrhea in females. See Warnings.

CNS: Tremors, muscular twitching, confusion, agitation, ataxia, flaccid paresis, hallucinations (rare). Rare, focal or generalized seizures have occurred in adults and children at therapeutic daily doses, pulse dosing regimens and in acute overdosage.

Children with nephrotic syndrome and patients receiving high pulse doses of the drug may have an increased risk of seizures. Exercise caution when administering chlorambucil to patients with a history of seizure disorders, head trauma or to patients receiving other potentially epileptogenic drugs.

Miscellaneous: Drug fever; skin hypersensitivity; peripheral neuropathy; interstitial pneumonia; sterile cystitis; keratitis.

(Continued on following page)

CHLORAMBUCIL (Cont.)

Overdosage:

Reversible pancytopenia was the main finding. Neurological toxicity ranging from agitated behavior and ataxia to multiple grand mal seizures has also occurred. As there is no known antidote, closely monitor the blood picture and institute general supportive measures, together with appropriate blood transfusions if necessary. Chlorambucil is not dialyzable. Refer to General Management of Acute Overdosage.

Patient Information:

Inform patients that the major toxicities of chlorambucil are related to hypersensitivity, drug fever, myelosuppression, hepatotoxicity, infertility, seizures, GI toxicity and secondary malignancies.

Notify physician of unusual bleeding or bruising, fever, nausea, vomiting, skin rash, chills, sore throat, cough, shortness of breath, seizures, amenorrhea, unusual lumps or masses, flank or stomach pain, joint pain, sores in the mouth or on the lips or yellow discoloration of the skin or eyes.

Contraceptive measures are recommended during therapy.

Administration and Dosage:

Initial and short courses of therapy: Usual dose is 0.1 to 0.2 mg/kg/day for 3 to 6 weeks as required (average, 4 to 10 mg/day). The entire daily dose may be given at one time. Adjust carefully to response of the patient and reduce immediately if there is an abrupt fall in the WBC count. Patients with Hodgkin's disease usually require 0.2 mg/kg/day; patients with other lymphomas or chronic lymphocytic leukemia usually require only 0.1 mg/kg/day. When lymphocytic infiltration of bone marrow is present, or bone marrow is hypoplastic, do not exceed 0.1 mg/kg/day (average, 6 mg/day).

An alternate schedule for the treatment of chronic lymphocytic leukemia using intermittent, bi-weekly or monthly pulse doses of chlorambucil consists of an initial single dose of 0.4 mg/kg. Doses are increased by 0.1 mg/kg until control of lymphocytosis or toxicity is observed. Subsequent doses are modified to produce mild hematologic toxicity. The response rate of chronic lymphocytic leukemia to biweekly or monthly administration is similar to or better than that reported with daily administration, and hematologic toxicity was less than or equal to that encountered using daily chlorambucil.

Radiation and cytotoxic drugs render the bone marrow more vulnerable to damage. Therefore, use chlorambucil with particular caution within 4 weeks of a full course of radiation therapy or chemotherapy. However, small doses of palliative radiation over isolated foci remote from the bone marrow will not usually depress neutrophil and platelet count; chlorambucil may be given in the customary dosage.

Short courses of treatment are safer than continuous maintenance therapy, although both methods have been effective. It must be recognized that continuous therapy may give the appearance of "maintenance" in patients who are actually in remission and have no immediate need for further drug. It may be desirable to withdraw drug after maximal control has been achieved, since intermittent therapy reinstituted at time of relapse may be as effective as continuous treatment.

Maintenance therapy: Do not exceed 0.1 mg/kg/day; may be as low as 0.03 mg/kg/day (usually 2 to 4 mg/day or less depending on blood counts).

Rx	**Leukeran** (Burroughs Wellcome)	**Tablets:** 2 mg	White, sugar coated. In 50s.

MELPHALAN (L-PAM; L-Phenylalanine Mustard; L-Sarcolysin)

Warning:
Melphalan is leukemogenic in humans. It produces chromosomal aberrations in vitro and in vivo; therefore, it is potentially mutagenic in humans.
Melphalan produces amenorrhea.

Actions:
Melphalan, a phenylalanine derivative of nitrogen mustard, is a bifunctional alkylating agent.

Pharmacokinetics: Plasma melphalan levels vary after oral dosing with respect both to the rate of absorption and to the peak concentrations achieved. Whether this results from incomplete absorption or first-pass hepatic metabolism is unknown.

Five patients on both oral and IV single bolus doses of 0.6 mg/kg had areas under plasma concentration-time curves after oral use of 61% ± 26% (range, 25% to 89%) of those after IV use. Plasma half-life is approximately 90 min; approximately 10% is excreted unchanged in urine after 24 hours, suggesting renal clearance is not a major route of elimination of the parent drug.

Indications:
Palliative treatment of multiple myeloma and non-resectable epithelial ovarian carcinoma.

Contraindications:
Hypersensitivity to melphalan; demonstrated prior resistance to the drug.

Warnings:
Bone marrow depression: As with other nitrogen mustard drugs, excessive dosage will produce marked bone marrow depression. Frequent blood counts are essential to determine optimal dosage and to avoid toxicity. Discontinue the drug or decrease the dosage upon evidence of bone marrow depression.

If leukocyte count falls below 3000/mm³ or platelet count below 100,000/mm³, discontinue the drug until peripheral blood cell counts have recovered.

Carcinogenesis/Mutagenesis/Impairment of fertility: Many patients with multiple myeloma have developed acute, non-lymphocytic leukemia or myeloproliferative syndrome following therapy with alkylating agents (including melphalan). According to one study, melphalan is 2 to 3 times more likely to induce leukemia than cyclophosphamide. Reports strongly suggest that melphalan is leukemogenic. Risk of leukemogenesis increases with both chronicity of treatment and with large cumulative doses. However, it is unknown if there is a cumulative dose below which there is no risk of the induction of secondary malignancy. Evaluate the potential benefits and the potential risk of carcinogenesis.

Melphalan causes chromatid or chromosome damage in man and suppression of ovarian function in pre-menopausal women, resulting in amenorrhea in many patients.

Pregnancy: Category D. May cause fetal harm when administered to a pregnant woman. There are no adequate and well controlled studies in pregnant women. If this drug is used during pregnancy, or if the patient becomes pregnant while taking it, apprise her of the potential hazard to the fetus. Advise women of childbearing potential to avoid becoming pregnant.

Lactation: It is not known whether this drug is excreted in breast milk. Because of the potential for serious adverse reactions in nursing infants, decide whether to discontinue nursing or to discontinue the drug, taking into account the importance of the drug to the mother.

Children: Safety and efficacy in children have not been established.

Precautions:
Radiation and chemotherapy: Use with extreme caution in patients whose bone marrow reserve may have been compromised by prior irradiation or chemotherapy or whose marrow function is recovering from previous cytotoxic therapy.

Renal function impairment: Whether routine dosage reductions are needed in patients with impaired creatinine clearance is unknown; only a small amount of the administered dose appears as parent drug in urine of patients with normal renal function. Closely observe patients with azotemia in order to make dosage reductions, if required, at the earliest possible time.

Examine the blood weekly to determine hemoglobin levels, total and differential leukocyte counts and platelet enumeration. Patients may develop symptoms of anemia if hemoglobin falls below 9 to 10 g/dl; they are at risk of severe infection if absolute neutrophil count is < 1000/mm³, and may bleed if platelet count is < 50,000/mm³.

(Continued on following page)

MELPHALAN (L-PAM; L-Phenylalanine Mustard; L-Sarcolysin) (Cont.)

Adverse Reactions:

GI: Nausea; vomiting; diarrhea; oral ulceration (infrequent).

Hematologic: Bone marrow suppression is most common. It is usually reversible if melphalan is withdrawn early enough. However, irreversible bone marrow failure has occurred.

Dermatologic: Skin hypersensitivity; alopecia.

Pulmonary: Pulmonary fibrosis.

Miscellaneous: Interstitial pneumonitis; vasculitis; hemolytic anemia; allergic reaction.

Overdosage:

Immediate effects are likely to be vomiting, mouth ulceration, diarrhea and GI tract hemorrhage. The main toxic effect is on bone marrow, and there is no known antidote. Monitor blood picture for 3 to 6 weeks. Institute general supportive measures, together with appropriate blood transfusions and antibiotics, if necessary. Hemodialysis is ineffective. Refer to General Management of Acute Overdosage.

Patient Information:

Inform patients that the major toxicities of melphalan are related to myelosuppression, hypersensitivity, GI toxicity, pulmonary toxicity, infertility, non-lymphocytic leukemia and myeloproliferative syndrome.

Patients should never take the drug without close medical supervision.

Notify physician of unusual bleeding or bruising, fever, chills, sore throat, shortness of breath, yellow discoloration of skin or eyes, persistent cough, flank or stomach pain, joint pain, mouth sores, black tarry stools, skin rash, vasculitis, amenorrhea, nausea, vomiting, weight loss or unusual lumps or masses.

Contraceptive measures are recommended during therapy.

Administration and Dosage:

Multiple myeloma: The usual oral dose is 6 mg/day. The entire daily dose may be given at one time. Adjust, as required, on the basis of weekly blood counts. After 2 to 3 weeks of treatment, discontinue the drug for up to 4 weeks, and carefully monitor the blood count. When the white blood cell (WBC) and platelet counts are rising, institute a maintenance dose of 2 mg/day. Because of patient-to-patient variations in melphalan plasma levels following oral use, some recommend that dosage be cautiously increased until myelosuppression is observed, to assure that therapeutic drug levels have been reached.

Alternative regimens: Initial course of 10 mg/day for 7 to 10 days. Maximal suppression of the leukocyte and platelet counts occurs within 3 to 5 weeks and recovery within 4 to 8 weeks. Institute maintenance therapy with 2 mg/day when the WBC count is $> 4{,}000/mm^3$ and the platelet count is $> 100{,}000/mm^3$. Adjust dosage to between 1 and 3 mg/day depending on hematological response. Maintain a significant degree of bone marrow depression to keep the leukocyte count in the range of 3,000 to 3,500 cells/mm^3.

Other investigators start treatment with 0.15 mg/kg/day for 7 days, followed by a rest period of at least 2 weeks (up to 5 to 6 weeks). Begin maintenance therapy at ≤ 0.05 mg/kg/day when the WBC and platelet counts are rising; adjust according to the blood count. About ⅓ to ½ of patients with multiple myeloma show a favorable response to oral administration of the drug. One study has shown that melphalan in combination with prednisone significantly improves the percentage of patients with multiple myeloma who achieve palliation. One regimen has been to administer melphalan at 0.25 mg/kg/day for 4 consecutive days (or 0.2 mg/kg/day for 5 consecutive days) for a total dose of 1 mg/kg/course. These 4 to 5 day courses are then repeated every 4 to 6 weeks if the granulocyte and platelet counts have returned to normal.

Response may be very gradual over many months; it is important to give repeated courses or continuous therapy, since improvement may continue over many months and the maximum benefit may be missed if treatment is abandoned too soon.

In patients with moderate to severe renal impairment, current pharmacokinetic data does not justify an absolute recommendation on dosage reduction, but it may be prudent to use a reduced dose initially.

Epithelial ovarian cancer: 0.2 mg/kg/day for 5 days as a single course. Repeat courses every 4 to 5 weeks depending upon hematologic tolerance.

Storage: Protect from light. Dispense in glass.

Rx	**Alkeran** (Burroughs Wellcome)	**Tablets:** 2 mg	(Alkeran A2A). White, scored. In 50s.

IFOSFAMIDE

Warning:

Administer ifosfamide under the supervision of a qualified physician experienced in the use of cancer chemotherapeutic agents.

Urotoxic side effects, especially hemorrhagic cystitis, as well as CNS toxicities such as confusion and coma have been associated with the use of ifosfamide. When they occur, they may require cessation of ifosfamide therapy.

Severe myelosuppression has occurred (see Warnings).

Actions:

Pharmacology: Ifosfamide is a chemotherapeutic agent chemically related to the nitrogen mustards and a synthetic analog of cyclophosphamide. Ifosfamide requires metabolic activation by microsomal liver enzymes to produce biologically active metabolites. Activation occurs by hydroxylation to form the unstable intermediate 4-hydroxyifosfamide. This metabolite rapidly degrades to the stable urinary metabolite 4-ketoifosfamide. Formation of the stable urinary metabolite, 4-carboxyifosfamide also occurs. These urinary metabolites are not cytotoxic. Ifosphoramide and acrolein are also found. Enzymatic oxidation of the chloroethyl side chains and subsequent dealkylation produces the major urinary metabolites, dechloroethyl ifosfamide and dechloroethyl cyclophosphamide. The alkylated metabolites of ifosfamide interact with DNA.

Pharmacokinetics: Ifosfamide exhibits dose-dependent pharmacokinetics. At single doses of 3.8 to 5 g/m^2, the plasma concentrations decay biphasically, and the mean terminal elimination half-life is about 15 hours. At doses of 1.6 to 2.4 g/m^2/day, the plasma decay is monoexponential, and the terminal elimination half-life is about 7 hours. Ifosfamide is extensively metabolized, and the metabolic pathways appear to be saturated at high doses.

After administration of doses of 5 g/m^2 of ^{14}C-labeled ifosfamide, from 70% to 86% of the dosed radioactivity was recovered in the urine, with about 61% of the dose excreted as parent compound. At doses of 1.6 to 2.4 g/m^2, only 12% to 18% of the dose was excreted in the urine as unchanged drug within 72 hours.

Thiodiacetic acid, 4-carboxyifosfamide, cysteine conjugates of chloroacetic acid and two different dechloroethylated derivatives of ifosfamide are the major urinary metabolites of ifosfamide, and only small amounts of 4-hydroxyifosfamide and acrolein are present. Small quantities (nmole/ml) of ifosfamide mustard and 4-hydroxyifosfamide are detectable in plasma. Metabolism of ifosfamide is required for the generation of the biologically active species and while metabolism is extensive, it is also quite variable among patients.

Clinical trials: In one study, 50 fully evaluable patients with germ cell testicular cancer were treated with ifosfamide in combination with cisplatin and either vinblastine or etoposide after failing (47 of 50) at least two prior chemotherapy regimens consisting of cisplatin/vinblastine/bleomycin (PVB), cisplatin/vinblastine/actinomycin D/bleomycin/cyclophosphamide (VAB6), or the combination of cisplatin and etoposide. Patients were selected for remaining cisplatin sensitivity because they had previously responded to a cisplatin-containing regimen and had not progressed while on the regimen or within 3 weeks of stopping it. Patients served as their own control based on the premise that long-term complete responses could not be achieved by retreatment with a regimen to which they had previously responded and subsequently relapsed.

Ten of 50 patients were still alive 2 to 5 years after treatment. Four of the 10 long-term survivors were rendered free of cancer by surgical resection after treatment with the ifosfamide regimen; median survival for the entire group of 50 patients was 53 weeks.

Indications:

In combination with certain other approved antineoplastic agents for third-line chemotherapy of germ cell testicular cancer. It should ordinarily be used in combination with a prophylactic agent for hemorrhagic cystitis, such as mesna (see individual monograph).

Unlabeled uses: Ifosfamide has shown activity in the following conditions: Lung, breast, ovarian, pancreatic and gastric cancer, sarcomas, acute leukemias (except AML) and malignant lymphomas. Further studies are needed with ifosfamide alone as well as in combination with other agents.

Contraindications:

Continued use in patients with severely depressed bone marrow function (see Warnings and Precautions); hypersensitivity to ifosfamide.

(Continued on following page)

IFOSFAMIDE (Cont.)

Warnings:

Urotoxic side effects, especially hemorrhagic cystitis, have been frequently associated with the use of ifosfamide. Obtain a urinalysis prior to each dose. If microscopic hematuria (> 10 RBCs per high power field) is present, then withhold subsequent administration until complete resolution. Use ifosfamide with a protector, such as mesna to prevent hemorrhagic cystitis. In one study, bladder irrigation with acetylcysteine (2000 ml/day) completely prevented the development of hematuria.

Use vigorous oral or parenteral hydration with further administration of ifosfamide.

Myelosuppression: When ifosfamide is given in combination with other chemotherapeutic agents, severe myelosuppression is frequent. In studies, myelosuppression was dose-related and dose-limiting. It consisted mainly of leukopenia and, to a lesser extent, thrombocytopenia. A WBC count < $3000/mm^3$ is expected in 50% of the patients treated with ifosfamide single agent at doses of 1.2 g/m^2/day for 5 consecutive days. At this dose level, thrombocytopenia (platelets < $100,000/mm^3$) occurred in about 20% of the patients. At higher dosages, leukopenia was almost universal, and at total dosages of 10 to 12 g/m^2/cycle, one-half of the patients had a WBC count < $1000/mm^3$ and 8% of patients had platelet counts < $50,000/mm^3$. Myelosuppression was usually reversible and treatment can be given every 3 to 4 weeks. When ifosfamide is used in combination with other myelosuppressive agents, adjustments in dosing may be necessary. Patients who experience severe myelosuppression are potentially at increased risk for infection.

Close hematologic monitoring is recommended. Obtain WBC count, platelet count and hemoglobin prior to each administration and at appropriate intervals. Unless clinically essential, do not administer to patients with a WBC count < $2000/mm^3$ or a platelet count < $50,000/mm^3$.

Neurologic manifestations consisting of somnolence, confusion, hallucinations and in some instances, coma, have occurred. The occurrence of these symptoms requires discontinuing ifosfamide therapy. The symptoms have usually been reversible; maintain supportive therapy until their complete resolution.

Renal function impairment: Use with caution.

Carcinogenesis/Mutagenesis: Ifosfamide is carcinogenic in rats, with female rats showing a significant incidence of leiomyosarcomas and mammary fibroadenomas. The mutagenic potential is documented in bacterial systems in vitro and mammalian cells in vivo. In vivo, ifosfamide has induced mutagenic effects in mice and *Drosophila melanogaster* germ cells, and has induced a significant increase in dominant lethal mutations in male mice as well recessive sex-linked lethal mutations in Drosophila.

Ifosfamide has caused resorptions, fetal anomalies, embryolethality and embryotoxicity in various rodent species in doses ranging from 18 to 88 mg/m^2.

Pregnancy: Category D. Animal studies indicate that the drug is capable of causing gene mutations and chromosomal damage in vivo. Embryotoxic and teratogenic effects have been observed in mice, rats and rabbits at doses 0.05 to 0.075 times the human dose. Ifosfamide can cause fetal damage when administered to a pregnant woman. If ifosfamide is used during pregnancy, or if the patient becomes pregnant while taking this drug, apprise the patient of the potential hazard to the fetus.

Lactation: Ifosfamide is excreted in breast milk. Because of the potential for serious adverse events and the tumorigenicity shown for ifosfamide in animal studies, decide whether to discontinue nursing or to discontinue the drug, taking into account the importance of the drug to the mother.

Children: Safety and efficacy in children have not been established.

Precautions:

Compromised bone marrow reserve: Administer cautiously to patients with compromised bone marrow reserve, as indicated by: Leukopenia; granulocytopenia; extensive bone marrow metastases; prior therapy with radiation or other cytotoxic agents.

Wound healing: Ifosfamide may interfere with normal wound healing.

Monitoring: During treatment, monitor the patient's hematologic profile (particularly neutrophils and platelets) regularly to determine the degree of hematopoietic suppression. Examine regularly for red cells which may precede hemorrhagic cystitis.

Adverse Reactions:

Dose-limiting toxicities are myelosuppression and urotoxicity. Dose fractionation, vigorous hydration and a protector (eg, mesna) can significantly reduce hematuria incidence, especially gross hematuria, associated with hemorrhagic cystitis. At a dose of 1.2 g/m^2/day for 5 consecutive days, leukopenia, when it occurs, is usually mild to moderate.

Other significant side effects: Alopecia (83%); nausea, vomiting (58%); central nervous system toxicities (12%).

(Adverse Reactions continued on following page)

IFOSFAMIDE (Cont.)

Adverse Reactions (Cont.):

GI: Nausea and vomiting (58%); anorexia, diarrhea, constipation ($< 1\%$).

GU: Hematuria (6% to 92%): At doses of 1.2 g/m²/day for 5 consecutive days without a protector, microscopic hematuria is expected in ≈ 50% of the patients and gross hematuria in ≈ 8% of patients. Renal toxicity (6%): Clinical signs (eg, elevation in BUN or serum creatinine or decrease in creatinine clearance) were usually transient and most likely related to tubular damage. Hemorrhagic cystitis; dysuria; urinary frequency; renal tubular acidosis that progressed into chronic renal failure (one episode); proteinuria and acidosis (rare). Metabolic acidosis occurred in 31% of patients in one study with doses of 2 to 2.5 g/m²/day for 4 days.

CNS toxicity (12%): Somnolence; confusion; depressive psychosis; hallucinations. Less frequent: Dizziness; disorientation; cranial nerve dysfunction; seizures; coma. CNS toxicity incidence may be higher with altered renal function.

Miscellaneous: Alopecia (≈ 83%) with ifosfamide as a single agent. In combination, this incidence may be as high as 100%, depending on the other agents. Infection (8%); liver dysfunction (3%); phlebitis (2%); fever of unknown origin (1%); allergic reactions, cardiotoxicity, coagulopathy, dermatitis, fatigue, hypertension, hypotension, malaise, polyneuropathy, pulmonary symptoms, salivation, stomatitis ($< 1\%$).

Laboratory test abnormalities: Increases in liver enzymes or bilirubin (3%).

Overdosage:

Management includes general supportive measures to sustain patient through any toxicity that might occur. Refer to General Management of Acute Overdosage.

Patient Information:

Notify physician of unusual bleeding/bruising, fever, chills, sore throat, cough, shortness of breath, seizures, lack of menstrual flow, unusual lumps or masses, flank, stomach or joint pain, sores in mouth or on lips, yellow discoloration of skin or eyes.

Contraceptive measures are recommended during therapy for both men and women.

Administration and Dosage:

Administer IV at a dose of 1.2 g/m²/day for 5 consecutive days. Treatment is repeated every 3 weeks or after recovery from hematologic toxicity (platelets ≥ 100,000/mm³, WBC ≥ 4,000/mm³). In order to prevent bladder toxicity, give ifosfamide with extensive hydration consisting of at least 2 L of oral or IV fluid per day. Use a protector, such as mesna, to prevent hemorrhagic cystitis. Administer ifosfamide as a slow IV infusion lasting a minimum of 30 minutes. Although ifosfamide has been administered to a small number of patients with compromised hepatic or renal function, studies to establish optimal dose schedules of ifosfamide in such patients have not been conducted.

Preparation: Add Sterile Water for Injection or Bacteriostatic Water for Injection (benzyl alcohol or parabens preserved) to the vial and shake to dissolve. Use the quantity of diluent shown below to reconstitute the product:

Reconstitution of Ifosfamide		
Dosage strength	Quantity of diluent	Final concentration
1 g	20 ml	50 mg/ml
3 g	60 ml	50 mg/ml

Storage/Stability: Reconstituted solutions are chemically and physically stable for 1 week at 30°C (86°F) or 3 weeks at 5°C (41°F).

Solutions of ifosfamide may be diluted further to achieve concentrations of 0.6 to 20 mg/ml in the following fluids: 5% Dextrose Injection; 0.9% Sodium Chloride Injection; Lactated Ringer's Injection; Sterile Water for Injection. Such admixtures, when stored in large volume parenteral glass bottles, Viaflex bags, or *PAB* bags, are physically and chemically stable for at least 1 week at 30°C (86°F) or 6 weeks at 5°C (41°F).

Because essentially identical stability results were obtained for Sterile Water admixtures as for the other admixtures, the use of large volume parenteral glass bottles, Viaflex bags or *PAB* bags that contain intermediate concentrations or mixtures of excipients (eg, 2.5% Dextrose Injection, 0.45% Sodium Chloride Injection, or 5% Dextrose and 0.9% Sodium Chloride Injection) is also acceptable.

Refrigerate dilutions of ifosfamide not prepared by constitution with Bacteriostatic Water for Injection (benzyl alcohol or parabens preserved), and use within 6 hours.

May store dry powder at room temperature. Avoid storage > 40°C (104°F).

Rx	**Ifex** (Mead Johnson Oncology)	**Powder for Injection:** 1 g	In single dose vials.[1]
		3 g	In single dose vials.[2]

[1] Includes 200 mg amps *Mesnex* (mesna). [2] Includes 400 mg amps *Mesnex* (mesna).

CYCLOPHOSPHAMIDE

Actions:

Pharmacology: Cyclophosphamide is a synthetic antineoplastic agent chemically related to the nitrogen mustards. Although generally classified as an alkylating agent, cyclophosphamide itself is not; it interferes with the growth of malignant cells and, to some extent, certain normal tissues. The major alkylating activity is accomplished through a metabolite, phosphoramide mustard.

Cyclophosphamide is first hydroxylated by hepatic mixed function oxidases to the intermediate metabolites 4-hydroxycyclophosphamide and aldophosphamide. These are oxidized to inactive metabolites and to the active antineoplastic alkylating compounds nor-nitrogen mustard and phosphoramide mustard. Acrolein is also formed. The mechanism of action of the active metabolites is alkylation, and is thought to involve cross-linking of tumor cell DNA, which interferes with growth of susceptible neoplasms and to some extent, normal tissues. Acrolein, which is cytotoxic, has been implicated in causing irritation of the bladder mucosa. However, it has not been demonstrated that any single metabolite is responsible for either the therapeutic or toxic effects of cyclophosphamide.

Cyclophosphamide also has immunosuppressive activity that may be partly explained by a marked sensitivity of presuppressor cells for B-cell function to low concentrations of drug metabolites.

Pharmacokinetics: Absorption/Distribution – Cyclophosphamide is well absorbed after oral administration with a bioavailability > 75%. Several cytotoxic and noncytotoxic metabolites have been identified in urine and in plasma. Concentrations of metabolites reach a maximum in plasma 2 to 3 hours after an IV dose. Plasma protein binding of unchanged drug is low, but some metabolites are > 60% bound.

Metabolism/Excretion – The drug is activated/inactivated to alkylating/nonalkylating metabolites in the liver. It is eliminated primarily in the form of metabolites; 5% to 25% of a dose is excreted as unchanged cyclophosphamide which has an elimination half-life of 3 to 12 hours. Although elevated levels of metabolites have occurred in patients with renal failure, increased clinical toxicity has not been demonstrated.

Indications:

Frequently used concurrently or sequentially with other antineoplastics. The following malignancies are often susceptible to cyclophosphamide treatment:

Malignant disease: Malignant lymphomas (Stages III and IV, Ann Arbor Staging System): Hodgkin's disease; lymphocytic lymphoma (nodular or diffuse); mixed-cell type lymphoma; histiocytic lymphoma; Burkitt's lymphoma.

Multiple myeloma.

Leukemias: Chronic lymphocytic leukemia; chronic granulocytic leukemia (ineffective in acute blastic crisis); acute myelogenous and monocytic leukemia; acute lymphoblastic (stem-cell) leukemia in children (given during remission, cyclophosphamide is effective in prolonging remission duration).

Mycosis fungoides (advanced disease); neuroblastoma (disseminated disease); adenocarcinoma of the ovary; retinoblastoma; carcinoma of the breast.

Nonmalignant disease: Biopsy proven "minimal change" nephrotic syndrome in children – Cyclophosphamide is useful in carefully selected cases but should not be used as primary therapy. In children whose disease fails to respond adequately to appropriate corticosteroid therapy or in whom the corticosteroid therapy produces or threatens to produce intolerable side effects, cyclophosphamide may induce a remission. Cyclophosphamide is not indicated for the nephrotic syndrome in adults or for any other renal disease.

Unlabeled uses: Variety of severe rheumatologic conditions: Wegener's granulomatosis, other steroid-resistant vasculidites and in some cases of severe progressive rheumatoid arthritis and systemic lupus erythematosus. Toxicity is limiting.

Cyclophosphamide (total dose 1 to 12 g) has been used to halt the progression of multiple sclerosis or decrease the frequency and duration of episodes. It has also been used in the treatment of polyarteritis nodosa using an initial dose of 2 mg/kg/day orally or 4 mg/kg/day IV. Cyclophosphamide (500 mg over 1 hour every 1 to 3 weeks), alone or in combination with corticosteroids, may be useful in the treatment of polymyositis.

Contraindications:

Previous hypersensitivity to the drug; continued use in severely depressed bone marrow function.

(Continued on following page)

CYCLOPHOSPHAMIDE (Cont.)

Warnings:

Cardiac toxicity: Although a few instances of cardiac dysfunction have occurred following use of recommended doses of cyclophosphamide, no causal relationship has been established. Cardiotoxicity has been observed in some patients receiving high doses of cyclophosphamide ranging from 120 to 270 mg/kg administered over a period of a few days, usually as a portion of an intensive antineoplastic multidrug regimen or in conjunction with transplantation procedures. In a few instances with high doses of cyclophosphamide, severe, and sometimes fatal, congestive heart failure has occurred within a few days after the first cyclophosphamide dose. Histopathologic examination has primarily shown hemorrhagic myocarditis.

No residual cardiac abnormalities as evidenced by electrocardiogram or echocardiogram appear to be present in the patients surviving episodes of apparent cardiac toxicity associated with high doses of cyclophosphamide.

Adrenalectomy patients: Adjustment of the doses of both replacement steroids and cyclophosphamide may be necessary for the adrenalectomized patient.

Wound healing: Cyclophosphamide may interfere with normal wound healing.

GU: Acute hemorrhagic cystitis occurs in 7% to 12% of patients, although some report an occurrence of up to 40%. Hemorrhagic cystitis can be severe, even fatal, and is probably due to urinary metabolites. Nonhemorrhagic cystitis and bladder fibrosis have also been reported. Ample fluid intake and frequent voiding help to prevent cystitis, but when it occurs, it is usually necessary to interrupt therapy. Hematuria usually resolves spontaneously within a few days after therapy is discontinued, but may persist. In protracted cases, medical or surgical supportive treatment may be required.

A formalin (37% formaldehyde solution diluted to a 1% solution) bladder instillation has successfully controlled the cystitis. Complications may occur with the 10% solution; there appears to be no additional value in using > 4% solutions. The use of mesna has reduced the incidence of cyclophosphamide-induced cystitis (see individual monograph).

Hypersensitivity reactions (type I) have occurred, mediated through increased B-cell activity and production of IgE. Refer to Management of Acute Hypersensitivity Reactions.

Rare instances of anaphylactic reaction including one death have occurred. One instance of possible cross sensitivity with other alkylating agents has occurred.

Renal or hepatic function impairment: Use cautiously. Patients with compromised renal function may show some measurable changes in pharmacokinetic parameters of cyclophosphamide metabolism, but there is no evidence indicating a need for modified dosage in these patients.

Carcinogenesis: Secondary neoplasia has developed with cyclophosphamide alone or with other antineoplastic drugs or radiation therapy. These most frequently have been urinary bladder, myeloproliferative and lymphoproliferative malignancies. Secondary malignancies have developed most frequently in patients with primary myeloproliferative and lymphoproliferative malignancies and nonmalignant diseases in which immune processes are pathologically involved. In some cases, the secondary malignancy was detected several years after drug discontinuance. Secondary urinary bladder malignancies generally have occurred in patients who previously developed hemorrhagic cystitis. One case of carcinoma of the renal pelvis occurred with long-term therapy for cerebral vasculitits. Consider the possibility of secondary malignancy in any benefit-to-risk assessment for use of the drug.

(Warnings continued on following page)

CYCLOPHOSPHAMIDE (Cont.)

Warnings (Cont.):

Fertility impairment: Cyclophosphamide interferes with oogenesis and spermatogenesis. It may cause sterility in both sexes. Development of sterility appears to depend on the dose, duration of therapy, and the state of gonadal function at the time of treatment. Cyclophosphamide-induced sterility may be irreversible in some patients.

Amenorrhea associated with decreased estrogen and increased gonadotropin secretion develops in a significant proportion of women treated with cyclophosphamide. Affected patients generally resume regular menses within a few months after cessation of therapy. Girls treated during prepubescence generally develop secondary sexual characteristics normally and have regular menses. Ovarian fibrosis with apparently complete loss of germ cells after prolonged cyclophosphamide treatment in late prepubescence has occurred. Girls treated with cyclophosphamide during prepubescence subsequently have conceived.

Men treated with cyclophosphamide may develop oligospermia or azoospermia associated with increased gonadotropin but normal testosterone secretion. Sexual potency and libido are unimpaired in these patients. Boys treated during prepubescence develop secondary sexual characteristics normally, but may have oligospermia or azoospermia and increased gonadotropin secretion. Some degree of testicular atrophy may occur. Cyclophosphamide-induced azoospermia is reversible in some patients, though the reversibility may not occur for several years after cessation of therapy. Men temporarily rendered sterile by cyclophosphamide have subsequently fathered normal children.

Pregnancy: Category D. Both normal and malformed newborns have been reported following the use of cyclophosphamide in pregnancy. Malformations have included limb abnormalities (missing fingers and toes), cardiac anomalies and hernias. In addition, 40% of infants exposed to anticancer drugs (timing of exposure not considered) were of low birth weight. However, use of cyclophosphamide in the second and third trimesters does not seem to place the infant at risk for congenital defects; this does not include the possibility of physical and mental growth abnormalities.

Also, *paternal* use of combination chemotherapy, including cyclophosphamide prior to conception, has been associated with cardiac and limb abnormalities in an infant.

Occupational exposure – A significant association between fetal loss and occupational exposure (nurses) to cyclophosphamide and other antineoplastics has been reported.

If this drug is used during pregnancy, or if the patient becomes pregnant while taking this drug, apprise the patient of the potential hazard to the fetus. Advise women of childbearing potential to avoid becoming pregnant.

Lactation: Cyclophosphamide is excreted in breast milk. Because of the potential for serious adverse reactions and the potential for tumorigenicity decide whether to discontinue nursing or to discontinue the drug, taking into account the importance of the drug to the mother.

Precautions:

Give cautiously to patients with: Leukopenia; thrombocytopenia; tumor cell infiltration of bone marrow; previous radiation therapy; previous cytotoxic therapy.

Immunosuppression: Treatment with cyclophosphamide may cause significant suppression of immune responses. Serious, sometimes fatal, infections may develop in severely immunosuppressed patients. Treatment may not be indicated or should be interrupted or the dose reduced in patients who have or who develop viral, bacterial, fungal, protozoan or helminthic infections.

Renal effects: A syndrome of inappropriate antidiuretic hormone (SIADH) has occurred with IV doses > 50 mg/kg. It is both a limitation to and consequence of fluid loading. Hemorrhagic ureteritis and renal tubular necrosis have occurred. Such lesions usually resolve following cessation of therapy.

Monitoring: During treatment, monitor the patient's hematologic profile (particularly neutrophils and platelets) regularly to determine the degree of hematopoietic suppression. Examine urine regularly for red cells which may precede hemorrhagic cystitis.

(Continued on following page)

CYCLOPHOSPHAMIDE (Cont.)

Drug Interactions:

Cyclophosphamide Drug Interactions			
Precipitant Drug	Object Drug*		Description
Chloramphenicol	Cyclophosphamide	↓	Cyclophosphamide half-life may increase and metabolite concentrations may be decreased
Thiazide diuretics	Cyclosphosphamide[1]	↑	Antineoplastic-induced leukopenia may be prolonged
Cyclophosphamide	Anticoagulants	↑	Anticoagulant effect is increased
Cyclophosphamide[1]	Digoxin	↓	Digoxin serum levels may be reduced
Cyclophosphamide	Doxorubicin	↑	Doxorubicin-induced cardiotoxicity is potentiated
Cyclophosphamide	Succinylcholine	↑	Neuromuscular blockade may be prolonged

* ↑ = Object drug increased. ↓ = Object drug decreased.

[1] Cyclophosphamide used in combination with other antineoplastics.

Adverse Reactions:

Secondary neoplasia has developed with cyclophosphamide alone or with other neoplastic drugs or radiation therapy. See Warnings.

GU: Acute hemorrhagic cystitis occurs in 7% to 12% of patients and may occur in up to 40%. See Warnings.

Hematopoietic: Leukopenia is an expected effect and is used as a guide to dosage. Leukopenia of < 2000 cells/mm³ develops commonly in patients treated with an initial loading dose of the drug, and less frequently in patients maintained on smaller doses. The degree of neutropenia is particularly important because it correlates with a reduction in resistance to infections. Thrombocytopenia or anemia develop occasionally. These effects are usually reversible when therapy is interrupted. Recovery from leukopenia usually begins in 7 to 10 days after cessation of therapy.

GI: Anorexia; nausea; vomiting; diarrhea; stomatitis; abdominal discomfort or pain. There are isolated reports of hemorrhagic colitis, oral mucosal ulceration and jaundice.

Integumentary: Alopecia is frequent; regrowth of hair can be expected, although it may be of a different color or texture. Skin rash occurs occasionally in patients receiving the drug. Pigmentation of the skin and changes in nails can occur.

Pulmonary: Interstitial pulmonary fibrosis with prolonged high dosage has occurred, although dose, duration or schedule dependency is not established.

Cardiotoxicity (hemorrhagic cardiac necrosis, transmural hemorrhages, coronary artery vasculitis) has occurred with massive doses (120 to 240 mg/kg). See Warnings.

Overdosage:

No specific antidote for cyclophosphamide is known. Use general supportive measures. Refer to General Management of Acute Overdosage. Cyclophosphamide and its metabolites are dialyzable.

Patient Information:

Take tablets preferably on an empty stomach. If GI upset is severe, take with food.

Notify your doctor of unusual bleeding or bruising, fever, chills, sore throat, cough, shortness of breath, seizures, lack of menstrual flow, unusual lumps or masses, flank or stomach pain, joint pain, sores in the mouth or on the lips, or yellow discoloration of the skin or eyes.

Contraceptive measures are recommended during therapy for both men and women.

(Continued on following page)

CYCLOPHOSPHAMIDE (Cont.)

Administration and Dosage:

Malignant diseases (adults and children):

IV – When used as the only oncolytic drug therapy, the initial IV dose for patients with no hematologic deficiency is 40 to 50 mg/kg, usually given in divided doses over 2 to 5 days. Other IV regimens include 10 to 15 mg/kg every 7 to 10 days or 3 to 5 mg/kg twice weekly.

Oral – Usually in the range of 1 to 5 mg/kg/day for both initial and maintenance dosing.

When cyclophosphamide is included in combined cytotoxic regimens, it may be necessary to reduce the dose of cyclophosphamide as well as that of the other drugs.

Nonmalignant diseases: Biopsy proven "minimal change" nephrotic syndrome in children – An oral dose of 2.5 to 3 mg/kg daily for a period of 60 to 90 days is recommended. In males, the incidence of oligospermia and azoospermia increases if the duration of treatment exceeds 60 days. Treatment beyond 90 days increases the probability of sterility. Corticosteroid therapy may be tapered and discontinued during the course of cyclophosphamide therapy. See Precautions section concerning hematologic monitoring.

Preparation of parenteral solution: Add Sterile Water for Injection or Bacteriostatic Water for Injection (paraben preserved only) to the vial and shake to dissolve. Use the quantity of diluent shown in the following table to reconstitute the product.

Reconstitution of Cyclophosphamide

Vial strength	Quantity of diluent (ml)	
	Powder for injection	Lyophilized powder for injection
100 mg	5	5
200 mg	10	10
500 mg	25	20-25
1 g	50	50
2 g	100	80-100

Prepared solutions may be injected IV, IM, intraperitoneally or intrapleurally, or they may be infused IV in 5% Dextrose Injection or 5% Dextrose and 0.9% Sodium Chloride Injection, 5% Dextrose and Ringer's Injection, Lactated Ringer's Injection, 0.45% Sodium Chloride Injection or ⅙ molar Sodium Lactate Injection.

Storage: Use solutions prepared with Bacteriostatic Water for Injection, USP (paraben preserved) within 24 hours if stored at room temperature or within 6 days if stored under refrigeration. If cyclophosphamide is not prepared with Bacteriostatic Water for Injection, USP, use the solution promptly (preferably within 6 hours). Cyclophosphamide does not contain an antimicrobial agent; take care to ensure the sterility of prepared solutions.

Preparation of oral solution: Dissolve injectable cyclophosphamide in Aromatic Elixir; store under refrigeration and use within 14 days.

Rx	**Cytoxan** (Bristol-Myers Oncology)	**Tablets:** 25 mg	White with blue flecks. In 100s.
		50 mg	White with blue flecks. In 100s, 1000s & UD 100s.
		Powder for Injection	In 100, 200 and 500 mg and 1 and 2 g vials.
Rx	**Cytoxan Lyophilized** (Bristol-Myers Oncology)	**Powder for Injection**[1]	In 100, 200 and 500 mg and 1 and 2 g vials, and Compliance Packs.
Rx	**Neosar** (Adria)	**Powder for Injection**	In 100, 200 and 500 mg and 1 and 2 g vials.

[1] With 75 mg mannitol per 100 mg.

URACIL MUSTARD

Actions:

A polyfunctional alkylating agent. It is not a vesicant.

Indications:

Palliative treatment in symptomatic chronic lymphocytic leukemia; non-Hodgkin's lymphomas of the histiocytic or lymphocytic type and chronic myelogenous leukemia. It is not effective in acute blastic crisis or in patients with acute leukemia.

Palliation of early stages of polycythemia vera before the development of leukemia or myelofibrosis; also as palliative therapy in mycosis fungoides.

Contraindications:

Severe leukopenia or thrombocytopenia.

Warnings:

Hematologic effects: Monitor patients to avoid irreversible damage to the bone marrow. Uracil mustard has a cumulative toxic effect against the hematopoietic system. Perform blood counts, including platelet counts, once or twice weekly. If severe bone marrow depression occurs, discontinue therapy.

While therapy need not be discontinued following initial depression of blood counts, maximum depression of bone marrow function may not occur until 2 to 4 weeks after discontinuing the drug. As the total accumulated doses approach 1 mg/kg, there is significant danger of producing irreversible bone marrow damage.

While there is no specific therapy for severe bone marrow depression, frequent blood and blood component transfusions in addition to antibiotics to treat secondary infections may sustain the patient until recovery has occurred.

Carcinogenesis: Alkylating agents are carcinogenic in animals and are suspected carcinogens in humans.

Fertility impairment: Consider the possible effect on fertility; amenorrhea and impaired spermatogenesis have occurred following therapy with alkylating agents.

Pregnancy: Drugs of the nitrogen mustard group produce fetal abnormalities in animals when given during pregnancy. Do not use uracil mustard during pregnancy unless potential benefits outweigh the possible hazards.

Precautions:

Tartrazine sensitivity: This product contains tartrazine, which may cause allergic-type reactions (including bronchial asthma) in certain susceptible individuals. Although the incidence of sensitivity in the general population is low, it is frequently seen in patients who also have aspirin hypersensitivity.

Adverse Reactions:

Hematopoietic: Dose-related bone marrow depression; leukopenia; thrombocytopenia; anemia (see Warnings).

GI: Nausea, vomiting or diarrhea of varying severity. These are dose-related; the greater the dose, the more severe the symptoms.

Dermatologic: Pruritus, dermatitis, hair loss (may or may not be drug-related). No reports of frank alopecia have been cited.

CNS: Nervousness, irritability, depression (may or may not be drug-related).

Other: Hepatotoxicity (rare); amenorrhea; azoospermia.

Patient Information:

May cause nausea, vomiting or diarrhea; notify physician if these effects persist.

Notify your doctor of unusual bleeding or bruising, fever, chills, sore throat, cough, shortness of breath, seizures, lack of menstrual flow, unusual lumps or masses, flank, joint or stomach pain, sores in the mouth or on lips, or yellow discoloration of skin/eyes.

Contraceptive measures are recommended during therapy for both men and women.

Administration and Dosage:

Do not administer until 2 or 3 weeks after the maximum effect of any previous x-ray or cytotoxic drug therapy of the bone marrow has been obtained. This is best determined by an increasing white blood cell count. Some investigators prefer to wait until the blood count has returned to normal before beginning a new course of therapy.

Do not administer in the presence of pronounced leukopenia, thrombocytopenia or aplastic anemia. In the presence of bone marrow infiltrated with malignant cells, hematopoietic toxicity may be increased; use care during administration.

Suggested dosage schedules: Individualize dosage.

Adults – A single weekly dose of 0.15 mg/kg for 4 weeks.

Children – A single weekly dose of 0.3 mg/kg for 4 weeks.

If response occurs, continue the same weekly dose until relapse.

Rx	**Uracil Mustard** (Upjohn)	**Capsules:** 1 mg	Tartrazine. Yellow and blue. In 50s.

LOMUSTINE (CCNU)

Warning:

Bone marrow suppression, notably thrombocytopenia and leukopenia, which may contribute to bleeding and overwhelming infections in an already compromised patient, is the most common and severe of the toxic effects of lomustine.

Since the major toxicity is delayed bone marrow suppression, monitor blood counts weekly for at least 6 weeks after a dose. At the recommended dosage, do not give courses of lomustine more frequently than every 6 weeks.

The bone marrow toxicity is cumulative. Therefore, consider dosage adjustments on the basis of nadir blood counts from prior dosage (see Administration and Dosage).

Actions:

Pharmacology: Lomustine acts as an alkylating agent but, like other nitrosoureas, it may also inhibit several key enzymatic processes.

Pharmacokinetics: Absorption – The lipid soluble nitrosoureas are rapidly and completely absorbed when given orally; appearance in plasma occurs about 10 minutes postadministration, and peak levels of metabolites appear in about 3 hours.

Distribution – The lipid solubility of lomustine results in extensive tissue distribution. Blood-brain penetration is good; cerebrospinal fluid levels of 15% to 50% of those in plasma have been noted.

Metabolism – Lomustine is rapidly degraded, apparently in the liver, to several cytotoxic metabolites. The range of half-lives is broad, partly depending on assay method, and varies between 16 to 72 hours.

Elimination – Metabolites are excreted through the kidneys, 60% in 48 hours (50% within 12 hours). Small amounts are excreted via the feces and lungs.

Indications:

As a single agent in addition to other treatment modalities, or in established combination therapy with other agents in the following:

Brain tumors: Both primary and metastatic, in patients who have already received appropriate surgical or radiotherapeutic procedures.

Hodgkin's disease: Secondary therapy in combination with other drugs in patients who relapse while on primary therapy, or who fail to respond to primary therapy.

Contraindications:

Hypersensitivity to lomustine.

Warnings:

Carcinogenic in rats and mice in approximately clinical doses. Acute leukemia and bone marrow dysplasias have occurred after long term nitrosourea therapy.

Pregnancy: Category D. Lomustine is embryotoxic and teratogenic in animals at dose levels equivalent to the human dose. It can cause fetal harm when administered to a pregnant woman. There are no adequate and well controlled studies in pregnant women. Advise patient of the potential hazard to the fetus if patient becomes pregnant while taking lomustine. Advise women of childbearing potential to avoid becoming pregnant while on lomustine.

Lactation: It is not known whether lomustine is excreted in breast milk. Because of the potential for serious adverse reactions, decide whether to discontinue nursing or to discontinue the drug, taking into account the importance of the drug to the mother.

Precautions:

Monitoring: Major toxicity is delayed bone marrow suppression; monitor blood counts weekly for 6 weeks after a dose. Monitor liver and renal function periodically.

Also conduct baseline pulmonary function studies during treatment. Patients with a baseline below 70% of the predicted Forced Vital Capacity (FVC) or Carbon Monoxide Diffusing Capacity (DL_{CO}) are particularly at risk.

Adverse Reactions:

Most adverse reactions are reversible if detected early. When adverse reactions occur, reduce dosage or discontinue drug and take appropriate corrective measures.

GI: Nausea and vomiting may occur 3 to 6 hours after an oral dose and usually last $<$ 24 hours. Use of antiemetics prior to dosing may be effective in diminishing and sometimes preventing these side effects. Nausea and vomiting may also be reduced by administration to fasting patients.

(Adverse Reactions continued on following page)

Nitrosoureas (Cont.)

LOMUSTINE (CCNU) (Cont.)

Adverse Reactions (Cont.):

Hepatotoxicity: A reversible type of hepatic toxicity, manifested by increased transaminase, alkaline phosphatase and bilirubin levels, has occurred in a small percentage of patients.

Hematologic: The most frequent and most serious toxicity is delayed myelosuppression. It usually occurs 4 to 6 weeks after drug administration and is dose-related. Thrombocytopenia occurs about 4 weeks after a dose and persists for 1 to 2 weeks. Leukopenia occurs about 5 to 6 weeks after a dose and persists for 1 to 2 weeks. About 65% of patients develop white blood cell (WBC) counts < 5000/mm³ and 36% develop WBC counts < 3000/mm³. Thrombocytopenia is generally more severe than leukopenia; however, both may be dose-limiting toxicities. Anemia also occurs, but is less frequent and less severe than thrombocytopenia or leukopenia. Cumulative myelosuppression may occur (usually after 4 to 6 weeks), manifested by more depressed indices or longer duration of suppression after repeated doses.

Renal abnormalities: Decrease in kidney size, progressive azotemia and renal failure have occurred in patients who received large cumulative doses after prolonged therapy. Kidney damage has occurred occasionally in patients receiving lower total doses.

Pulmonary toxicity: Pulmonary toxicity characterized by pulmonary infiltrates or fibrosis occurs rarely and appears to be dose-related. Onset of toxicity has occurred after an interval of ≥ 6 months from start of therapy with cumulative doses usually > 1100 mg/m². There is one report of pulmonary toxicity at a cumulative dose of only 600 mg.

Secondary malignancies: Long-term use of nitrosoureas may be associated with development of secondary malignancies (see Warnings).

Other toxicities: Alopecia and stomatitis are infrequent. Disorientation, lethargy, ataxia and dysarthria have been noted; however, the relationship to medication is unclear.

Overdosage:

There are no proven antidotes for lomustine overdosage. Treatment includes usual supportive measures. Refer to General Management of Acute Overdosage.

Patient Information:

Notify physician if fever, chills, sore throat, unusual bleeding or bruising, shortness of breath, dry cough, swelling of feet or lower legs, yellowing of eyes and skin, confusion, sores on the mouth or lips, or unusual tiredness occurs.

Medication may cause loss of appetite, nausea and vomiting and, less frequently, hair loss, skin rash or itching; notify physician if these reactions become pronounced.

Take on an empty stomach to reduce nausea.

Contraceptive measures are recommended during therapy.

Administration and Dosage:

Adults and children: 130 mg/m² as a single oral dose every 6 weeks. In compromised bone marrow function, reduce dose to 100 mg/m² every 6 weeks. Do not give a repeat course until circulating blood elements have returned to acceptable levels (platelets > 100,000/mm³; leukocytes > 4,000/mm³). Monitor blood counts weekly and do not give repeat courses before 6 weeks; hematologic toxicity is delayed and cumulative.

Adjust doses subsequent to the initial dose according to the hematologic response of the patient to the preceding dose as follows:

Suggested Lomustine Dose Following Initial Dose

Nadir after prior dose		Percentage of prior dose to be given
Leukocytes/mm³	Platelets/mm³	
> 4000	> 100,000	100%
3000-3999	75,000-99,999	100%
2000-2999	25,000-74,999	70%
< 2000	< 25,000	50%

Concomitant therapy: With other myelosuppressive drugs, adjust dosage accordingly.

Storage: Avoid excessive heat (over 40°C; 104°F).

Rx	**CeeNu** (Bristol-Myers Oncology)	**Capsules:** 10 mg	Two-tone white. In 20s.
		40 mg	White/green. In 20s.
		100 mg	Two-tone green. In 20s.
		Dose Pack: Two 100 mg capsules, two 40 mg capsules and two 10 mg capsules.	

CARMUSTINE (BCNU)

> **Warning:**
> Since delayed *bone marrow toxicity* is the major toxic effect, monitor complete blood counts weekly for at least 6 weeks after a dose. Do not give repeat doses more frequently than every 6 weeks. Bone marrow toxicity is cumulative; therefore, adjust dosage on the basis of nadir blood counts from prior dose (see dosage adjustment table under Administration and Dosage).
>
> *Bone marrow suppression,* notably thrombocytopenia and leukopenia, which may contribute to bleeding and overwhelming infections in an already compromised patient, is the most common and severe of the toxic effects of carmustine.
>
> *Pulmonary toxicity* from carmustine appears to be dose-related. Patients receiving > 1400 mg/m² cumulative dose are at significantly higher risk than those receiving less.

Actions:

Pharmacology: Carmustine alkylates deoxyribonucleic acid (DNA) and ribonucleic acid (RNA) and also inhibits several enzymes by carbamoylation of amino acids in proteins. Carmustine is not cross resistant with other alkylators. Antineoplastic and toxic activities may be due to metabolites.

Pharmacokinetics: Because of the high lipid solubility and the lack of ionization at physiological pH, carmustine crosses the blood-brain barrier effectively. Levels of radioactivity in the cerebrospinal fluid (CSF) are $\geq$ 50% of those in plasma.

Following IV administration, it is rapidly degraded with a biological half-life of 15 to 30 minutes; the plasma half-life of radiolabeled metabolites is 67 hours. Approximately 60% to 70% of a total dose is excreted in the urine in 96 hours and about 10% is excreted as respiratory CO_2. The fate of the remainder is undetermined.

Indications:

Palliative therapy as a single agent or combined with other chemotherapeutic agents in the following:

Brain tumors: Glioblastoma, brainstem glioma, medulloblastoma, astrocytoma, ependymoma and metastatic brain tumors.

Multiple myeloma: In combination with prednisone.

Hodgkin's disease and non-Hodgkin's lymphomas: As secondary therapy in combination with other drugs in patients who relapse with, or who fail to respond to, primary therapy.

Contraindications:

Hypersensitivity to carmustine.

Warnings:

Monitoring: Monitor liver and renal function tests periodically.

Ocular toxicity: Carmustine administration through an intra-arterial intracarotid route is investigational and has been associated with ocular toxicity.

Carcinogenicity: Nitrosourea therapy has carcinogenic potential. Acute leukemia and bone marrow dysplasias have occurred following long-term nitrosourea therapy.

Fertility impairment: Carmustine affects fertility in male rats at doses somewhat higher than the human dose.

Pregnancy: Category D. Carmustine is embryotoxic and teratogenic in rats and embryotoxic in rabbits at dose levels equivalent to the human dose. Carmustine may cause fetal harm when administered to a pregnant woman. There are no adequate and well controlled studies in pregnant women. If this drug is used during pregnancy, or if the patient becomes pregnant while taking this drug, advise her of the potential hazard to the fetus. Advise women of childbearing potential to avoid becoming pregnant.

Lactation: It is not known whether this drug is excreted in breast milk. Because of the potential for serious adverse reactions in nursing infants from carmustine, decide whether to discontinue nursing or to discontinue the drug, taking into account the importance of the drug to the mother.

Children: Safety and efficacy for use in children have not been established.

(Continued on following page)

CARMUSTINE (BCNU) (Cont.)

Precautions:

Myelosuppression: Carmustine may produce cumulative myelosuppression, manifested by more depressed indices or longer duration of suppression after repeated doses.

Monitoring: Due to delayed bone marrow suppression, monitor blood counts weekly for at least 6 weeks after a dose.

Conduct baseline pulmonary function studies and frequent pulmonary function tests during treatment. Patients with a baseline below 70% of predicted Forced Vital Capacity (FVC) or Carbon Monoxide Diffusing Capacity (DL_{CO}) are at particular risk.

Monitor liver and renal function tests.

Drug Interactions:

Cimetidine may enhance the myelosuppressive effects of carmustine, possibly to the point of toxicity.

Digoxin serum levels may be reduced and its actions may be decreased by a combination chemotherapy regimen including carmustine.

Phenytoin serum concentrations may be decreased by a combination chemotherapy regimen including carmustine.

Adverse Reactions:

Most adverse reactions are reversible if detected early. When toxic effects or adverse reactions occur, reduce dosage or discontinue carmustine and take appropriate corrective measures. Reinstitute carmustine therapy with caution.

Hematopoietic: The most frequent and serious toxic effect is delayed myelosuppression which usually occurs 4 to 6 weeks after administration and is dose-related. Thrombocytopenia occurs at about 4 weeks post-administration and persists for 1 to 2 weeks. Leukopenia occurs at 5 to 6 weeks after a dose and persists for 1 to 2 weeks. Thrombocytopenia is generally more severe than leukopenia; however, both may be dose-limiting toxicities. Anemia is generally less severe.

GI: Nausea and vomiting after IV administration. This dose-related toxicity appears within 2 hours of dosing and lasts 4 to 6 hours. Prior administration of antiemetics is effective in diminishing or preventing these side effects.

Renal: Decrease in kidney size, progressive azotemia and renal failure have occurred in patients who received large cumulative doses after prolonged therapy; occasionally reported in patients receiving lower total doses.

Hepatic: Reversible hepatic toxicity, manifested by increased transaminase, alkaline phosphatase and bilirubin levels, has occurred in a small percentage of patients.

Local: Burning at the injection site may occur; thrombosis is rare.

Accidental contact of reconstituted carmustine with the skin has caused burning and hyperpigmentation of the affected areas.

Pulmonary infiltrates or fibrosis have occurred, mostly in patients on prolonged total doses $>$ 1400 mg/m². However, there have been reports of pulmonary fibrosis in patients receiving lower total doses. Other risk factors include history of lung disease and duration of treatment. Cases of fatal pulmonary toxicity have occurred.

Ocular toxicity manifested as nerve fiber-layer infarcts and retinal hemorrhages has been associated with high dose therapy. Neuroretinitis has also occurred.

Other: Rapid IV infusion may produce intensive flushing of the skin and suffusion of the conjunctiva within 2 hours, lasting about 4 hours.

(Continued on following page)

CARMUSTINE (BCNU) (Cont.)

Overdosage:

No proven antidotes have been established for carmustine overdosage.

Patient Information:

Contraceptive measures are recommended during therapy.

Administration and Dosage:

Administration precautions: Exercise caution in handling the powder and preparing the solution. Accidental contact of reconstituted carmustine with the skin may cause transient hyperpigmentation of the affected areas. Use gloves. If the powder or solution contacts the skin or mucosa, immediately wash the skin or mucosa thoroughly with soap and water.

Single agent in previously untreated patients: 150 to 200 mg/m² IV every 6 weeks. Give as a single dose or divided daily injections (ie, 75 to 100 mg/m² on 2 successive days).

When used in combination with other myelosuppressive drugs or in patients in whom bone marrow reserve is depleted, adjust doses accordingly.

Do not give a repeat course until circulating blood elements have returned to acceptable levels (platelets > 100,000/mm³; leukocytes > 4,000/mm³). Adequate number of neutrophils should be present on a peripheral blood smear. Monitor blood counts weekly; do not give repeat courses before 6 weeks because of delayed and cumulative toxicity.

The following schedule is suggested as a guide to dosage adjustment based on the patient's hematologic response to the previous dose:

Suggested Carmustine Dose Following Initial Dose

Nadir after prior dose		Percentage of prior dose to be given
Leukocytes/mm³	Platelets/mm³	
> 4000	> 100,000	100%
3000-3999	75,000-99,999	100%
2000-2999	25,000-74,999	70%
< 2000	< 25,000	50%

Preparation/Handling of solutions: Dissolve with 3 ml of the supplied sterile diluent, then add 27 ml of Sterile Water for Injection to the alcohol solution. The resulting solution contains 3.3 mg/ml of carmustine in 10% ethanol; pH is 5.6 to 6.

Reconstitution as recommended results in a clear colorless to yellowish solution which may be further diluted with 0.9% Sodium Chloride for Injection or 5% Dextrose for Injection.

Administer the reconstituted solution by IV drip over 1 to 2 hours. Shorter infusion times may produce intense pain and burning at the injection site.

The lyophilized dosage formulation contains no preservatives and is not intended as a multiple dose vial.

Stability: Store unopened vials of the dry powder in a refrigerator (2° to 8°C; 36° to 46°F). The recommended storage of unopened vials provides a stable product for 2 years. After reconstitution as recommended, carmustine is stable for 8 hours at room temperature (25°C; 77°F) or 24 hours under refrigeration (4°C; 39°F).

Vials reconstituted as directed and further diluted to a concentration of 0.2 mg/ml in 5% Dextrose Injection or 0.9% Sodium Chloride Injection are stable for 48 hours under refrigeration (4°C; 39°F) and an additional 8 hours at room temperature (25°C; 77°F) under normal room fluorescent light.

Glass containers were used for the stability data provided. Only use glass containers.

Carmustine has a low melting point (≈ 30.5° to 32°C; ≈ 87° to 90°F). Exposure of the drug to this temperature or above will cause it to liquefy and appear as an oil film on the bottom of the vials. This is a sign of decomposition; discard the vial. If there is a question of adequate refrigeration upon receipt of this product, immediately inspect the larger vial in each individual carton. Hold the vial to a bright light for inspection. The carmustine will appear as a very small amount of dry flakes or dry congealed mass. If this is evident, the carmustine is suitable for use; refrigerate immediately.

Rx	**BiCNU** (Bristol-Myers Oncology)	**Powder for Injection**: 100 mg	In vials with 3 ml sterile diluent.

STREPTOZOCIN

Warning:

A patient need not be hospitalized but should have access to a facility with laboratory and supportive resources sufficient to monitor drug tolerance and to protect and maintain a patient compromised by drug toxicity. Renal toxicity is dose-related and cumulative and may be severe or fatal. Other major toxicities are nausea and vomiting which may be severe and, at times, treatment limiting. In addition, liver dysfunction, diarrhea and hematological changes have been observed.

Judge the possible benefit against the known toxic effects of this drug.

Actions:

Pharmacology: Streptozocin inhibits DNA synthesis in bacterial and mammalian cells. The biochemical mechanism leading to mammalian cell death has not been established but is at least partially due to DNA alkylation causing intrastrand crosslinks; streptozocin inhibits cell proliferation at a considerably lower level than that needed to inhibit precursor incorporation into DNA or to inhibit several of the enzymes involved in DNA synthesis. The drug is cell cycle nonspecific.

In animals, streptozocin induces a diabetes that resembles human hyperglycemic nonketotic diabetes mellitus. This phenomenon appears to be mediated through a histopathologic alteration of pancreatic islet beta cells. Irreversible damage to the pancreatic beta cell with degranulation and loss of insulin secretion occurs.

Pharmacokinetics: After rapid IV injection, unchanged drug is rapidly cleared from the plasma (half-life, 35 minutes). Two hours after administration, metabolites are detected in spinal fluid in equivalent concentration to plasma. Metabolites persist in plasma over 24 hours and concentrate in the liver and kidney. Approximately 60% to 72% of an administered dose can be detected in the urine within 4 hours; 10% to 20% as parent drug. Most excretion is completed in 24 hours.

Indications:

Metastatic islet cell carcinoma of the pancreas (functional and nonfunctional carcinomas). Because of its inherent renal toxicity, limit therapy with this drug to patients with symptomatic or progressive metastatic disease.

Warnings:

Renal toxicity occurs in up to ⅔ of all patients treated with streptozocin, as evidenced by azotemia, anuria, hypophosphatemia, glycosuria and renal tubular acidosis. *Such toxicity is dose-related and cumulative and may be severe or fatal.* Monitor renal function before and after each course of therapy. Obtain serial urinalysis, BUN, plasma creatinine, serum electrolytes and creatinine clearance prior to, at least weekly during, and for 4 weeks after drug administration. Serial urinalysis is particularly important for the early detection of proteinuria; quantitate with a 24 hour collection when proteinuria is detected. Mild proteinuria is one of the first signs of renal toxicity and may herald further deterioration of renal function. Reduce the dose or discontinue treatment in the presence of significant renal toxicity. In patients with preexisting renal disease, judge potential benefit of streptozocin against known risk of serious renal damage.

Do not use in combination or concomitantly with other potential nephrotoxins.

Carcinogenesis, mutagenesis, impairment of fertility: When administered parenterally, streptozocin induces renal tumors in rats, and liver and other tumors in hamsters. Stomach and pancreatic tumors were observed in rats treated orally with streptozocin. Streptozocin is mutagenic in mammalian cells. It has also been carcinogenic in mice and has adversely affected fertility in rats.

Pregnancy: Category C. Streptozocin is teratogenic in the rat and has abortifacient effects in rabbits. There are no studies in pregnant women. Use during pregnancy only if the potential benefit outweighs the potential risks.

Lactation: It is not known whether streptozocin is excreted in breast milk. Because of the potential for serious adverse reactions in nursing infants, discontinue nursing in patients receiving streptozocin.

(Continued on following page)

STREPTOZOCIN (Cont.)

Precautions:

Monitoring: Closely monitor for evidence of renal, hepatic and hematopoietic toxicity. Perform complete blood counts and liver function tests at least weekly. Dosage adjustments or discontinuance of the drug may be indicated, depending upon the degree of toxicity.

Topical exposure: When exposed dermally, some rats developed benign tumors at the site of application. Consequently, streptozocin may pose a carcinogenic hazard following topical exposure if not properly handled.

Adverse Reactions:

Renal: See Warnings.

GI: Nausea and vomiting occur in > 90% of patients, beginning 1 to 4 hours after administration and lasting about 24 hours; occasionally it requires discontinuation of drug therapy. Diarrhea has also occurred.

Hepatic: Chemical liver dysfunction occurs in approximately 25% of patients. Hepatic toxicity characterized by elevated liver enzymes (AST and LDH), and hypoalbuminemia have also occurred.

Hematological toxicity has been rare, most often involving mild decreases in hematocrit. However, *fatal hematological toxicity* with substantial reductions in leukocyte and platelet counts has been observed.

Metabolic: Mild to moderate abnormalities of glucose tolerance have generally been reversible, but insulin shock with hypoglycemia has occurred.

GU: Two cases of nephrogenic diabetes insipidus have been reported. One had spontaneous recovery; the second responded to indomethacin.

CNS: Confusion, lethargy and depression have occurred with a 5 day continuous infusion regimen which may have facilitated these effects.

Overdosage:

No specific antidote for streptozocin is known.

Administration and Dosage:

Administer IV. Intra-arterial administration is not recommended because of the possibility that adverse renal effects may be evoked more rapidly.

The following two different dosage schedules have been used successfully:

Daily schedule – 500 mg/m² of body surface area (BSA) for 5 consecutive days every 6 weeks until maximum benefit or until treatment limiting toxicity is observed. Dosage increases are not recommended.

Weekly schedule – Initial dose is 1000 mg/m² BSA at weekly intervals for the first 2 courses (weeks). In subsequent courses, increase drug doses in patients who have not achieved a therapeutic response and who have not experienced significant toxicity with the previous course of treatment. However, *do not exceed a single dose of 1500 mg/m² BSA,* as a greater dose may cause azotemia. On this schedule, the median time to onset of response is about 17 days and the median time to maximum response is about 35 days. The median *total* dose to onset of response is about 2000 mg/m² BSA and the median *total* dose to maximum response is about 4000 mg/m² BSA.

The ideal duration of maintenance therapy has not been established for either schedule.

For patients with functional tumors, serial monitoring of fasting insulin levels allows a determination of biochemical response to therapy. For patients with either functional or nonfunctional tumors, response to therapy can be determined by measurable reductions of tumor size (reduction of organomegaly, masses or lymph nodes).

Preparation and storage: Reconstitute with 9.5 ml of Dextrose Injection or 0.9% Sodium Chloride Injection. The resulting pale gold solution contains 100 mg/ml streptozocin. Where more dilute infusion solutions are desirable, further dilution in the above vehicles is recommended. The total storage time for reconstituted streptozocin is 12 hours. This product contains no preservatives and is not intended as a multiple dose vial. Refrigerate unopened vials at 2° to 8°C (35° to 46° F) and protect from light.

Exercise caution in the handling and preparation of the powder and solution; use gloves. If powder or solution contacts the skin or mucosa, immediately wash the affected area with soap and water.

Rx	**Zanosar** (Upjohn)	**Powder for Injection:** 1 g (100 mg per ml when reconstituted)	In vials.

THIOTEPA (Triethylenethiophosphoramide; TSPA; TESPA)

Actions:

A cell cycle nonspecific alkylating agent related to nitrogen mustard. It is not a vesicant, which makes it suitable for administration by all parenteral routes and directly into tumors.

Pharmacology: Its radiomimetic action is believed to occur through the release of ethylenimine radicals which disrupt the bonds of deoxyribonucleic acid (DNA). The drug has no apparent differential affinity for neoplasms.

Pharmacokinetics: Thiotepa is rapidly cleared from the plasma following IV administration. It is partially metabolized to triethylene phosphoramide (TEPA); about 85% of the drug is excreted unchanged in the urine.

Indications:

Adenocarcinoma of the breast; adenocarcinoma of the ovary; controlling intracavitary effusions secondary to diffuse or localized neoplastic disease of various serosal cavities; treatment of superficial papillary carcinoma of the urinary bladder.

While now largely superseded by other treatments, this drug has been effective against lymphomas, such as lymphosarcoma and Hodgkin's disease.

Unlabeled uses: Thiotepa has prevented pterygium recurrences after surgery.

Contraindications:

Existing hepatic, renal or bone marrow damage. If the benefits outweigh the potential risks, use in low doses and monitor hepatic, renal and hematopoietic functions.

Hypersensitivity to thiotepa.

Warnings:

Hematopoietic toxicity: This drug is highly toxic to the hematopoietic system. A rapidly falling white blood cell (WBC) or platelet count indicates a need to discontinue or reduce dosage. Perform weekly blood and platelet counts during therapy and for at least 3 weeks after therapy discontinuation.

The most serious complication of excessive therapy or sensitivity is bone marrow depression, causing leukopenia, thrombocytopenia and anemia. Death from septicemia and hemorrhage has occurred as a result of hematopoietic depression.

The most reliable guide to toxicity is the WBC count; if this falls to $\leq 3000/mm^3$, discontinue use. If the platelet count falls to $150,000/mm^3$, discontinue therapy. Red blood cell (RBC) count is a less accurate indicator of toxicity.

Deaths have occurred after intravesical administration. This was caused by bone marrow depression from systemically absorbed drug.

Carcinogenesis: Like all alkylating agents, this drug is carcinogenic.

Mutagenesis: Thiotepa is mutagenic. In vitro, it causes chromatid-type chromosomal aberrations. The frequency of induced aberrations increases with the patient's age.

Pregnancy: This drug is not recommended unless potential benefits outweigh risk of teratogenicity.

Precautions:

Concomitant therapy: Do not combine therapeutic modalities having the same mechanism of action. Thiotepa combined with other alkylating agents, such as nitrogen mustard or cyclophosphamide, or with irradiation, would intensify toxicity rather than enhance therapeutic response. If these agents must follow each other, it is important that recovery from the first, as indicated by WBC count, be complete before therapy with the second agent is instituted.

Drug Interactions:

Neuromuscular blocking agents: A patient who received thiotepa and other anticancer agents experienced prolonged apnea after **succinylcholine** was administered prior to surgery. It was theorized that this was caused by a decrease of pseudocholinesterase activity caused by the anticancer drugs. In another patient, coadministration of thiotepa and **pancuronium** resulted in prolonged muscular paralysis and respiratory depression.

Adverse Reactions:

GI: Nausea; vomiting; anorexia.

GU: Amenorrhea; interference with spermatogenesis.

There have been rare reports of chemical cystitis or hemorrhagic cystitis following intravesical, but not parenteral, administration.

CNS: Dizziness; headache.

Dermatologic/Local: Allergic reactions are rare, but hives and skin rash occur occasionally. One case of alopecia was reported. Pain at injection site has occurred.

Other: Febrile reactions and weeping from a subcutaneous lesion may occur due to breakdown of tumor.

(Continued on following page)

THIOTEPA (Triethylenethiophosphoramide; TSPA; TESPA) (Cont.)

Overdosage:

There is no known antidote for thiotepa overdosage. Transfusions of whole blood, platelets or leukocytes have proven beneficial for hematopoietic toxicity.

Administration and Dosage:

Parenteral administration is most reliable since GI absorption is variable. IV doses may be given directly and rapidly without need for slow drip or large volumes of diluent. Some prefer to give the drug directly into the tumor mass. This may be effected transrectally, transvaginally or intracerebrally. For the control of malignant effusions, instill directly into the cavity involved.

Individualize dosage. A slow response may be deceptive and may lead to unwarranted frequency of administration with subsequent toxicity. After maximum benefit is obtained by initial therapy, continue with maintenance therapy (1 to 4 week intervals). In order to sustain optimal effect, do not give maintenance doses more frequently than weekly, to preserve correlation between dose and blood counts.

Initial and maintenance doses: Usually, the higher dose in the given range is administered initially. Adjust the maintenance dose weekly, based on pretreatment control blood counts and subsequent blood counts.

IV administration: 0.3 to 0.4 mg/kg at 1 to 4 week intervals by rapid administration.

For conversion of mg/kg to mg/m² or the reverse, a ratio of 1:30 is used as a guideline. The conversion factor varies between 1:20 and 1:40, depending on age and body build.

Intratumor administration: Initial doses of 0.6 to 0.8 mg/kg injected directly into a tumor. Inject a small amount of local anesthetic first; then remove the syringe and inject the drug through the same needle. The drug is diluted in Sterile Water for Injection to 10 mg/ml. Maintenance doses at 1 to 4 week intervals range from 0.07 mg/kg to 0.8 mg/kg, depending on the condition of the patient.

Intracavitary administration: Administer 0.6 to 0.8 mg/kg through the same tubing used to remove fluid from the cavity.

Intravesical administration: Dehydrate patients with papillary carcinoma of the bladder for 8 to 12 hours prior to treatment. Then instill 60 mg in 30 to 60 ml of Sterile Water for Injection into the bladder by catheter. For maximum effect, retain the solution for 2 hours. If the patient finds it impossible to retain 60 ml for 2 hours, give the dose in a volume of 30 ml. If desired, the patient may be repositioned every 15 minutes for maximum area contact. The usual course of treatment is once a week for 4 weeks. Repeat if necessary, but give second and third courses with caution, since bone marrow depression may be increased.

Preparation of solution: Reconstitute with Sterile Water for Injection. The amount of diluent most often used is 1.5 ml, resulting in a drug concentration of 5 mg/0.5 ml of solution. Larger volumes are usually employed for intracavitary use, IV drip or perfusion therapy. The reconstituted preparation may be added to larger volumes of other diluents: Sodium Chloride Injection, Dextrose Injection, Dextrose and Sodium Chloride Injection, Ringer's Injection, or Lactated Ringer's Injection. Reconstituted solutions should be clear to slightly opaque; do not use grossly opaque or precipitated solutions.

Addition of Sterile Water for Injection produces an isotonic solution; other diluents may result in hypertonic solutions, which may cause mild to moderate discomfort on injection.

For local use into single or multiple sites, thiotepa may be mixed with 2% procaine HCl, 1:1000 epinephrine HCl or both.

Storage: Store the original powder and reconstituted solution in the refrigerator at 2° to 8°C (35° to 46°F). Reconstituted solutions are stable for 5 days when refrigerated.

Rx	**Thiotepa** (Lederle)	**Powder for Injection:** 15 mg	In vials.

BUSULFAN

Warning:

Busulfan can induce severe bone marrow hypoplasia. Reduce or discontinue dosage immediately at the first sign of any unusual depression of bone marrow function as reflected by an abnormal decrease in any of the formed elements of the blood. Perform a bone marrow examination if bone marrow status is uncertain.

Actions:

Pharmacology: An alkylsulfonate, busulfan's predominant effect is against cells of the granulocytic series. Although a polyfunctional alkylating agent, it appears to interact with cellular thiol groups. Little crosslinking of nucleoproteins is observed. The drug is cell cycle-phase nonspecific.

The biochemical basis for acquired resistance to busulfan is speculative; altered transport of busulfan into the cell and increased intracellular inactivation before it reaches DNA are possibilities. Resistance to these compounds may reflect an acquired ability of the cell to repair alkylation damage more effectively.

Pharmacokinetics: Busulfan is well absorbed following oral administration. There is a lag period of 0.5 to 2 hours prior to detection in blood. A rapid initial plasma clearance occurs with a subsequent low level plateau. The drug appears to be extensively metabolized with little unchanged drug found in the urine.

Indications:

Palliative treatment of chronic myelogenous leukemia (myeloid, myelocytic, granulocytic): Approximately 90% of adults with previously untreated chronic myelogenous leukemia will obtain hematologic remission with regression or stabilization of organomegaly following busulfan. It is superior to splenic irradiation with respect to survival times and maintenance of hemoglobin levels, and equivalent to irradiation at controlling splenomegaly.

Busulfan is less effective in patients with chronic myelogenous leukemia who lack the Philadelphia (Ph^1) chromosome. Juvenile chronic myelogenous leukemia, associated with the absence of a Philadelphia chromosome, responds poorly to busulfan. The drug is of no benefit in patients whose disease has entered a "blastic" phase.

Contraindications:

Patients whose disease has demonstrated prior resistance to this drug.

Busulfan is of no value in chronic lymphocytic leukemia, acute leukemia or in the "blastic crisis" of chronic myelogenous leukemia.

Warnings:

Hematopoietic toxicity: The most frequent and serious side effect is bone marrow failure (which may or may not be anatomically hypoplastic), resulting in severe pancytopenia that may be more prolonged than that induced with other alkylating agents. The usual cause is the failure to stop administration of the drug soon enough; individual idiosyncrasy appears unimportant. Use with extreme caution in patients whose bone marrow reserve or function may be compromised by or recovering from prior irradiation or chemotherapy. Although recovery from busulfan-induced pancytopenia may take from 1 month to 2 years, it is potentially reversible; vigorously support the patient through any period of severe pancytopenia.

The most consistent dose-related toxicity is bone marrow suppression. This may be manifested by anemia, leukopenia, thrombocytopenia, or any combination of these. Instruct patients to report promptly the development of fever, sore throat, signs of local infection, bleeding from any site, or symptoms suggestive of anemia. Any one of these findings may indicate busulfan toxicity or transformation of the disease to an acute "blastic" form. Since busulfan may have a delayed effect, it is important to withdraw the medication temporarily at the first sign of an abnormally large or exceptionally rapid fall in any of the formed elements of the blood.

Evaluate the hemoglobin or hematocrit, white blood cell (WBC) count, differential count and platelet count weekly. If the cause of fluctuation in the formed element of the peripheral blood is obscure, bone marrow examination may be useful. Individualize therapy based not only on the absolute hematologic values, but also on the rapidity with which changes are occurring. The dosage of busulfan may need to be reduced if the agent is combined with other myelosuppressive drugs. Occasionally, patients may be unusually sensitive to busulfan administered at standard dosage and suffer neutropenia or thrombocytopenia after relatively short exposure to the drug. Do not use busulfan where facilities for complete blood counts, including quantitative platelet counts, are not available at weekly (or more frequent) intervals. Never allow patients to take the drug without supervision.

(Warnings continued on following page)

BUSULFAN (Cont.)

Warnings (Cont.):

Pulmonary: A rare, but important complication of busulfan therapy is the development of bronchopulmonary dysplasia with pulmonary fibrosis. Symptoms have occurred within 8 months to 10 years after initiation of therapy (the average duration of therapy being 4 years). Histologic findings associated with "busulfan lung" mimic those seen following pulmonary irradiation. Clinically, patients report the insidious onset of cough, dyspnea and low-grade fever. Pulmonary function studies reveal diminished diffusion capacity and decreased pulmonary compliance. Exclude more common conditions (such as opportunistic infections or leukemic infiltration of the lungs). If sputum cultures, virologic studies and exfoliative cytology fail to establish an etiology for the pulmonary infiltrates, lung biopsy may be necessary to establish the diagnosis.

Treatment is unsatisfactory; most patients have died within 6 months after diagnosis. There is no specific therapy other than the immediate discontinuation of busulfan. Corticosteroid administration has been suggested, but the results have not been impressive or uniformly successful.

Cellular dysplasia: Busulfan may cause cellular dysplasia in many organs in addition to the lung. Giant, hyperchromatic nuclei have been reported in lymph nodes, pancreas, thyroid, adrenal glands, bone marrow and liver. This cytologic dysplasia may be severe enough to cause difficulty in interpretation of exfoliative cytologic examinations from the lung, bladder, breast and the uterine cervix.

Carcinogenesis, mutagenesis: Malignant tumors have occurred in patients on busulfan therapy; this drug may be a human carcinogen. Four cases of acute leukemia occurred among 243 patients treated with busulfan for 5 to 8 years as adjuvant chemotherapy following surgical resection of bronchogenic carcinoma. Busulfan is mutagenic in mice and, possibly, in humans. Chromosome aberrations have been reported in cells from patients receiving busulfan.

Fertility impairment: Ovarian suppression and amenorrhea with menopausal symptoms commonly occur during busulfan therapy in premenopausal patients. There have been clinical reports of sterility, azoospermia and testicular atrophy in male patients.

Pregnancy: Category D. Busulfan may cause fetal harm when administered to a pregnant woman. Although normal children have been born after busulfan treatment during pregnancy, one malformed baby was delivered by a mother treated with busulfan. During this pregnancy, the mother received x-ray therapy early in the first trimester, mercaptopurine until the third month, then busulfan until delivery. In pregnant rats, busulfan produces sterility in both male and female offspring due to the absence of germinal cells in testes and ovaries. Germinal cell aplasia or sterility in offspring of mothers receiving busulfan during pregnancy has not been reported in humans.

There are reports of small infants being born after the mothers received busulfan during pregnancy; in particular, administration occurred during the third trimester. In one case, an infant had mild anemia and neutropenia at birth after busulfan was administered to the mother from the eighth week of pregnancy to term.

There are no adequate and well controlled studies in pregnant women. If this drug is used during pregnancy or if the patient becomes pregnant while taking this drug, apprise her of the potential hazard to the fetus. Advise women of childbearing potential to avoid becoming pregnant.

Lactation: It is not known whether this drug is excreted in breast milk. Because of the potential for tumorigenicity, decide whether to discontinue nursing or to discontinue the drug, taking into account the importance of the drug to the mother.

Drug Interactions:

Thioguanine: In one study, 12 of approximately 330 patients receiving continued busulfan and thioguanine therapy for treatment of chronic myelogenous leukemia were found to have esophageal varices associated with abnormal liver function tests. Subsequent liver biopsies were performed in four of these patients, all of which showed evidence of nodular regenerative hyperplasia. Duration of combination therapy prior to the appearance of esophageal varices ranged from 6 to 45 months. Use with caution in long-term continuous therapy with thioguanine and busulfan.

Busulfan may cause additive myelosuppression when used with other myelosuppresive drugs.

Adverse Reactions:

Hematological: See Warnings.

Pulmonary: Interstitial pulmonary fibrosis. See Warnings.

Cardiac: One case of endocardial fibrosis occurred in a 79-year-old woman who received a total dose of 7200 mg of busulfan over 9 years. At autopsy, endocardial fibrosis of the left ventricle and interstitial pulmonary fibrosis were found.

(Adverse Reactions continued on following page)

BUSULFAN (Cont.)

Adverse Reactions (Cont.):

Ocular: Busulfan may induce cataracts; in the few cases reported, they occurred only after prolonged administration of the drug.

Dermatologic: Hyperpigmentation (5% to 10%) particularly in those with a dark complexion. Also reported are urticaria, erythema multiforme, erythema nodosum, alopecia, porphyria cutanea tarda, excessive dryness and fragility of the skin with anhidrosis, dryness of the oral mucous membranes and cheilosis.

Metabolic: A clinical syndrome closely resembling adrenal insufficiency and characterized by weakness, severe fatigue, anorexia, weight loss, nausea, vomiting and melanoderma has developed after prolonged therapy. The symptoms have sometimes been reversible when busulfan was withdrawn. Adrenal responsiveness to exogenously administered ACTH is usually normal. However, pituitary function testing with metyrapone revealed a blunted urinary 17-hydroxycorticosteroid excretion in two patients. Following the discontinuation of busulfan (which was associated with clinical improvement), rechallenge with metyrapone revealed normal pituitary-adrenal function.

Hyperuricemia and hyperuricosuria may occur in patients with chronic myelogenous leukemia. Additional rapid destruction of granulocytes may accompany chemotherapy and increase the urate pool. Minimize adverse effects by increased hydration, urine alkalinization and the prophylactic administration of allopurinol.

Miscellaneous: Gynecomastia; cholestatic jaundice; myasthenia gravis. A clear cause-and-effect relationship has not been demonstrated.

Patient Information:

Notify physician if unusual bleeding or bruising, fever, cough, shortness of breath, flank, stomach or joint pain occurs.

Medication may cause darkening of skin, diarrhea, dizziness, fatigue, loss of appetite, mental confusion, nausea and vomiting; notify physician if these become pronounced.

Take medication at the same time each day.

Extra fluid intake may be recommended.

Contraceptive measures are recommended during therapy.

If nausea or vomiting occurs, it may help to take the drug on an empty stomach.

Overdosage:

Symptoms: In animals, two distinct types of toxic responses are seen at median lethal doses given intraperitoneally. Within hours, there are signs of stimulation of the CNS with convulsions and death on the first day. With doses at the LD_{50}, there is also delayed death due to bone marrow damage.

Treatment: The principal toxic effect is on the bone marrow. Survival after a single 140 mg dose has been reported in an 18 kg, 4-year-old child, but hematologic toxicity is likely to be more profound with chronic overdosage. Closely monitor hematologic status and institute vigorous supportive measures if necessary. Induce vomiting or gastric lavage, and follow by administration of charcoal if ingestion is recent. It is not known if busulfan is dialyzable. Refer to General Management of Acute Overdosage.

Administration and Dosage:

Remission induction: 4 to 8 mg/day total dose. Since the rate at which the leukocyte count falls is dose-related, reserve daily doses exceeding 4 mg/day for patients with the most compelling symptoms; the greater the total daily dose, the greater the possibility of inducing bone marrow aplasia.

A decrease in the leukocyte count is not usually seen during the first 10 to 15 days of treatment; the leukocyte count may actually increase during this period and should not be interpreted as drug resistance, nor should the dose be increased. Since the leukocyte count may continue to fall for > 1 month after discontinuing the drug, discontinue busulfan before the total leukocyte count falls into the normal range. When the total leukocyte count has declined to ≈ 15,000/mm³, withdraw the drug.

With a constant dose of busulfan, the total leukocyte count declines exponentially; a weekly plot of the leukocyte count on semilogarithmic graph paper aids in predicting the time when therapy should be discontinued. With the recommended dose of busulfan, a normal leukocyte count is usually achieved in 12 to 20 weeks.

Maintenance therapy: During remission, examine the patient at monthly intervals and resume treatment with the induction dosage when total leukocyte count reaches approximately 50,000/mm³. When remission is < 3 months, maintenance therapy of 1 to 3 mg/day may keep the hematological status under control and prevent rapid relapse.

Rx	**Myleran** (Burroughs Wellcome)	**Tablets**: 2 mg	(Myleran K2A). White, scored. In 25s.

PIPOBROMAN

Actions:

Pipobroman is classed as an alkylating agent, but exact mechanism of action is unknown. It is readily absorbed after oral use. Metabolic fate and excretion route are unknown.

Indications:

Polycythemia vera; chronic granulocytic leukemia in patients refractory to busulfan.

Contraindications:

Patients with bone marrow depression from x-ray or cytotoxic chemotherapy.

Warnings:

Hematologic: Bone marrow depression may not occur for $\geq$ 4 weeks after treatment is initiated. The most reliable guide to bone marrow activity is leukocyte count, but platelet count is also a good index. If leukocyte count falls to $\leq$ 3,000/mm^3, or if platelet count is reduced to $\leq$ 150,000/mm^3, temporarily discontinue drug. Cautiously reinstate therapy when the leukocyte or platelet count has risen.

Dose-dependent anemia frequently develops, but usually responds to blood transfusions and dosage reduction. A rapid drop in hemoglobin, increased bilirubin levels and reticulocytosis suggest a hemolytic process, and the drug should be discontinued.

Pregnancy: Category D. Alkylating agents may cause fetal harm when given to pregnant women. Pipobroman has been teratogenic in mice and rats during the organogenetic period. There are no adequate and well controlled studies in pregnant women. If used during pregnancy, or if patient becomes pregnant while on this drug, apprise her of the potential hazards. Advise women of childbearing potential to avoid becoming pregnant.

Lactation: It is not known if this drug is excreted in breast milk. Because of the potential for serious adverse reactions in nursing infants, decide whether to discontinue nursing or discontinue the drug, taking into account the importance of the drug to the mother.

Children: Safety and efficacy in children $<$ 15 years old are not established.

Precautions:

Monitoring: Initiate therapy in the hospital where patients can be closely observed. Perform bone marrow studies prior to treatment and again at the time of maximal hematologic response. Perform complete blood counts once or twice weekly, and leukocyte counts every other day, until the desired response is obtained or until significant toxic effects intervene.

Perform ancillary laboratory determinations, including liver and kidney function tests, prior to therapy and periodically thereafter.

Adverse Reactions:

In decreasing order of severity: Bone marrow depression resulting in leukopenia, thrombocytopenia, anemia (see Warnings); vomiting; diarrhea; nausea; abdominal cramps; skin rash.

Overdosage:

The principal toxic effect is on the bone marrow. Hematologic toxicity will likely be more profound with chronic overdosage. Closely monitor hematologic status; institute vigorous supportive measures as needed. Refer to General Management of Acute Overdosage.

Patient Information:

Notify physician if nausea, vomiting, abdominal cramps, diarrhea and skin rash become pronounced.

Promptly report fever, sore throat, signs of local infection, easy bruising, bleeding from any site, or symptoms suggestive of anemia.

Contraceptive measures are recommended during therapy.

Administration and Dosage:

Administer in divided daily doses. Individualize maintenance doses. Continue as long as needed to maintain satisfactory clinical response.

Polycythemia vera: Initially, 1 mg/kg/day. Larger doses (1.5 to 3 mg/kg/day) may be required in patients refractory to other treatment, but do not use such doses until a dose of 1 mg/kg/day has been given for at least 30 days without improvement. Initiate maintenance therapy when hematocrit is reduced to 50% to 55%. Maintenance dosage ranges from 0.1 to 0.2 mg/kg/day.

Chronic granulocytic leukemia: Initially, 1.5 to 2.5 mg/kg/day. Generally, continue until a maximal clinical or hematologic response is attained. If leukocyte count falls too rapidly, discontinue until rate of decrease levels off. Initiate maintenance therapy as leukocyte count approaches 10,000/mm^3. If relapse is rapid (doubling of leukocyte count in 70 days), use continuous treatment. Intermittent therapy is adequate if $>$ 70 days are required to double leukocyte count. Maintenance dose range: 7 mg/day (50 mg/week) to 175 mg/day.

Rx	**Vercyte** (Abbott)	**Tablets:** 25 mg	Scored. In 100s.

CISPLATIN (CDDP)

> **Warning:**
> *Cumulative renal toxicity* associated with cisplatin is severe.
> Other major dose-related toxicities are myelosuppression, nausea and vomiting.
> *Ototoxicity,* which may be more pronounced in children, is manifested by tinnitus or loss of high frequency hearing and, occasionally, deafness.
> *Anaphylactic-like reactions* have occurred.

Actions:

Pharmacology: Cisplatin is an inorganic heavy metal coordination complex that has biochemical properties similar to those of bifunctional alkylating agents producing interstrand and intrastrand crosslinks in DNA. It is cell cycle nonspecific.

Pharmacokinetics: Following a single IV dose, the drug concentrates in liver, kidneys and large and small intestines. Although levels in normal brain tissue are low, significant levels can be detected in intracerebral tumors. Protein binding is > 90%. Plasma levels of cisplatin decay in a biphasic manner after an IV bolus. The initial plasma half-life is 25 to 49 minutes, and the post-distribution half-life is 58 to 73 hours. Cisplatin is excreted primarily in urine. The extensive protein and tissue binding results in a prolonged or incomplete excretory phase with cumulative urinary excretion of 27% to 43% of a dose within the first 5 days. There are insufficient data to determine whether biliary or intestinal excretion occurs.

Indications:

For palliative therapy in:

Metastatic testicular tumors: In combination therapy in patients who have received appropriate surgical or radiotherapeutic procedures. Combination therapy consists of cisplatin, bleomycin sulfate and vinblastine sulfate.

Metastatic ovarian tumors: In combination therapy with doxorubicin in patients who have received surgical or radiotherapeutic procedures. Cisplatin, as a single agent, is indicated as secondary therapy in patients refractory to standard chemotherapy who have not previously received cisplatin.

Advanced bladder cancer: As a single agent for patients with transitional cell bladder cancer no longer amenable to surgery or radiotherapy.

Contraindications:

Preexisting renal impairment; myelosuppression; hearing impairment; history of allergic reactions to platinum-containing compounds.

Warnings:

Nephrotoxicity: Dose-related and cumulative renal insufficiency is the major dose-limiting toxicity. Renal toxicity has been noted in 28% to 36% of patients treated with a single dose of 50 mg/m². At higher doses (> 100 mg/m²), the nephrotoxicity may be irreversible. First noted during the second week after a dose, it is manifested by elevations in BUN and creatinine, serum uric acid and a decrease in creatinine clearance. Renal toxicity becomes more prolonged and severe with repeated courses of the drug. Renal function must return to normal before another dose can be given.

Impairment of renal function is associated with renal tubular damage. The administration of cisplatin using a 6 to 8 hour infusion with IV hydration and mannitol has been used to reduce nephrotoxicity. However, renal toxicity can still occur.

Measure the serum creatinine, BUN, creatinine clearance and magnesium, calcium and potassium levels prior to initiating therapy, and prior to each subsequent course. Do not give more frequently than once every 3 to 4 weeks.

Neuropathies: Severe neuropathies have occurred in patients receiving higher doses of cisplatin or greater dose frequencies than those recommended or after prolonged therapy (4 to 7 months). These neuropathies may be irreversible and are seen as paresthesias in a stocking-glove distribution, areflexia and loss of proprioception and vibratory sensation. Loss of motor function has also occurred. Discontinue therapy when symptoms are first observed.

Ototoxicity has occurred in up to 31% of patients given a single 50 mg/m² dose. It is manifested by tinnitus or hearing loss in the high frequency range (4000 to 8000 Hz); decreased ability to hear normal conversational tones occurs occasionally. Ototoxic effects may be more severe in children, especially in those < 12 years of age. Hearing loss can be unilateral or bilateral and is more frequent and severe with repeated doses. It is unclear whether ototoxicity is reversible. Since ototoxicity of cisplatin is cumulative, perform audiometry before starting therapy and prior to subsequent doses. Vestibular toxicity has occurred.

(Warnings continued on following page)

CISPLATIN (CDDP) (Cont.)

Warnings (Cont.)

Hypersensitivity: Anaphylactic-like reactions have occurred. Facial edema, wheezing, bronchoconstriction, tachycardia and hypotension may occur within minutes of use in patients with prior drug exposure. They are alleviated by use of epinephrine, corticosteroids and antihistamines. Refer to Management of Acute Hypersensitivity Reactions.

Pregnancy: Safety for use during pregnancy has not been established. In mice, cisplatin is teratogenic and embryotoxic.

Mutagenesis: The drug is mutagenic in bacteria and produces chromosome aberrations in animal cell tissue cultures.

Precautions:

Monitoring: Monitor peripheral blood counts weekly and liver function periodically. Perform neurologic, renal and auditory examinations regularly.

Drug Interactions:

Aminoglycosides: Cisplatin produces cumulative nephrotoxicity which is potentiated by aminoglycosides (see Warnings).

Loop diuretics and cisplatin coadministration may have an additive ototoxic effect.

Phenytoin: Combination chemotherapy (including cisplatin) may reduce phenytoin plasma levels, requiring an increased dosage to maintain therapeutic plasma levels.

Adverse Reactions:

Nephrotoxicity: Renal insufficiency, renal tubular damage (see Warnings).

Ototoxicity: Tinnitus, high frequency hearing loss, vestibular toxicity (see Warnings).

Hematologic: Myelosuppression (25% to 30%). The nadirs in circulating platelets and leukocytes occur between days 18 and 23 (range 7.5 to 45); most patients recover by day 39 (range 13 to 62). Leukopenia and thrombocytopenia are more pronounced at doses > 50 mg/m². Anemia (decrease of 2 g hemoglobin/dl) occurs at the same frequency and with the same timing as leukopenia and thrombocytopenia.

In addition to anemia secondary to myelosuppression, a Coombs' positive hemolytic anemia has been reported. In the presence of cisplatin hemolytic anemia, increased hemolysis may accompany a further course of treatment. Weigh this risk.

GI: Marked nausea and vomiting occur in almost all patients, and are occasionally so severe that the drug must be discontinued. Nausea and vomiting usually begin 1 to 4 hours after treatment and last up to 24 hours; nausea and anorexia may persist for up to 1 week after treatment. Metoclopramide in high doses has been used in the prophylaxis of vomiting associated with cisplatin therapy.

Vascular toxicities coincident with use of cisplatin in combination with other antineoplastic agents have occurred rarely. The events are clinically heterogeneous and may include myocardial infarction, cerebrovascular accident, thrombotic microangiopathy or cerebral arteritis. Various mechanisms have been proposed for these vascular complications. There are also reports of Raynaud's phenomenon occurring in patients treated with the combination of bleomycin and vinblastine with or without cisplatin. Hypomagnesemia developing coincident with use of cisplatin may be an added, although not essential, factor associated with this event. However, it is currently unknown if the cause of Raynaud's phenomenon in these cases is the disease, underlying vascular compromise, bleomycin, vinblastine, hypomagnesemia, or a combination of any of these factors.

Electrolyte disturbances: Hypomagnesemia, hypocalcemia, hyponatremia, hypokalemia, and hypophosphatemia have occurred and are probably related to renal tubular damage. Tetany has occasionally occurred in those patients with hypocalcemia and hypomagnesemia. Generally, normal serum electrolyte levels are restored by administering supplemental electrolytes and discontinuing cisplatin.

Increased plasma iron levels and inappropriate antidiuretic hormone syndrome have also been reported.

Hyperuricemia occurs at approximately the same frequency as increases in BUN and serum creatinine. It is more pronounced after doses > 50 mg/m², and peak uric acid levels generally occur 3 to 5 days after the dose. Allopurinol is effective.

Neurotoxicity: Peripheral neuropathies; seizures; loss of taste; Lhermitte's sign; autonomic neuropathy (see Warnings).

(Adverse Reactions continued on following page)

CISPLATIN (CDDP) (Cont.)

Adverse Reactions (Cont.):

Ocular toxicity: Optic neuritis, papilledema and cerebral blindness have occurred infrequently in patients receiving standard recommended cisplatin doses. Improvement or total recovery usually occurs after drug discontinuation. Steroids with or without mannitol have been used; however, efficacy has not been established.

Blurred vision and altered color perception have occurred after the use of regimens with higher doses or greater dose frequencies than those recommended. The altered color perception manifests as a loss of color discrimination, particularly in the blue-yellow axis. The only finding on funduscopic exam is irregular retinal pigmentation of the macular area.

Anaphylactic-like reactions have occasionally in patients previously exposed to cisplatin (see Warnings).

Other: Infrequent – Cardiac abnormalities; anorexia; rash; elevated ALT.

Administration and Dosage:

For IV use only.

Metastatic testicular tumors: Remission induction –

Cisplatin: 20 mg/m²/day IV for 5 days (days 1 to 5) every 3 weeks for 3 courses.

Bleomycin: 30 units IV weekly (day 2 of each week) for 12 consecutive doses.

Vinblastine: 0.15 to 0.2 mg/kg IV twice weekly (days 1 and 2) every 3 weeks for 4 courses (a total of 8 doses).

Maintenance therapy for patients who respond to the above regimen consists of vinblastine 0.3 mg/kg IV every 4 weeks for a total of 2 years.

Metastatic ovarian tumors:

Cisplatin – 50 mg/m² IV once every 3 weeks (day 1).

Doxorubicin – 50 mg/m² IV once every 3 weeks (day 1).

In combination therapy, administer cisplatin and doxorubicin sequentially.

As a single agent, administer 100 mg/m² cisplatin IV every 4 weeks.

Advanced bladder cancer: Administer as a single agent. Give 50 to 70 mg/m² IV once every 3 to 4 weeks, depending on prior radiation therapy or chemotherapy. For heavily pretreated patients, give an initial dose of 50 mg/m² repeated every 4 weeks.

Repeat courses: Do not give a repeat course until the serum creatinine is $<$ 1.5 mg/dl, or the BUN is $<$ 25 mg/dl or until circulating blood elements are at an acceptable level (platelets $\geq$ 100,000/mm³, WBC $\geq$ 4,000/mm³). Do not give subsequent doses until an audiometric analysis indicates that auditory acuity is within normal limits.

Note: Do not use needles or IV sets containing aluminum parts for preparation. Aluminum reacts with cisplatin, causing precipitate formation and a loss of potency.

Exercise caution in handling the powder and preparing the solution. Skin reactions associated with accidental exposure may occur. Use gloves. If powder or solution contacts skin or mucosa, wash immediately with soap and water.

Hydration: Perform pretreatment hydration with 1 to 2 L fluid infused for 8 to 12 hours prior to dose. Then dilute the drug in 2 L of 5% Dextrose in ½ or ⅓ Normal Saline containing 37.5 g mannitol, and infuse over 6 to 8 hours. Maintain adequate hydration and urinary output during the following 24 hours.

Preparation of solution: Dissolve contents of the 10 and 50 mg vials with 10 or 50 ml of Sterile Water for Injection, respectively. Resulting solutions contain 1 mg/ml.

Stability: Do not refrigerate the reconstituted solution as a precipitate will form. The reconstituted solution is stable for 20 hours at room temperature (27°C; 81°F).

Rx	**Platinol** (Bristol-Myers Oncology)	**Powder for Injection:** 10 mg	In vials.
		50 mg	In vials.
Rx	**Platinol-AQ** (Bristol-Myers Oncology)	**Injection:** 1 mg/ml	In 50 and 100 mg vials.

CARBOPLATIN

Warning:

Administer carboplatin under the supervision of a qualified physician experienced in the use of cancer chemotherapeutic agents.

Bone marrow suppression is dose-related and may be severe, resulting in infection or bleeding. Anemia may be cumulative and may require transfusion support.

Vomiting is a frequent drug-related side effect.

Anaphylactic-like reactions may occur within minutes of administration. Epinephrine, corticosteroids and antihistamines may alleviate symptoms.

Actions:

Pharmacology: Carboplatin is a platinum coordination compound that is used as a cancer chemotherapeutic agent. Carboplatin, like cisplatin, produces predominantly interstrand DNA cross-links rather than DNA-protein cross-links. This effect is apparently cell-cycle nonspecific. The aquation of carboplatin, which is thought to produce the active species, occurs at a slower rate than cisplatin. Despite this difference, both carboplatin and cisplatin induce equal numbers of drug-DNA cross-links, causing equivalent lesions and biological effects. The differences in potencies for carboplatin and cisplatin appear to be directly related to the difference in aquation rates.

Pharmacokinetics: In patients with creatinine clearances (Ccr) of ≥ 60 ml/min, plasma levels of intact carboplatin decay in a biphasic manner after a 30 minute IV infusion of 300 to 500 mg/m². The initial plasma half-life (alpha) is 1.1 to 2 hours, and the postdistribution plasma half-life (beta) is 2.6 to 5.9 hours. The total body clearance, apparent volume of distribution, and mean residence time for carboplatin are 4.4 L/hour, 16 L and 3.5 hours, respectively.

Carboplatin is not bound to plasma proteins. No significant quantities of protein-free, ultrafilterable platinum-containing species other than carboplatin are present in plasma. However, platinum from carboplatin becomes irreversibly bound to plasma proteins and is slowly eliminated with a minimum half-life of 5 days.

The major route of elimination is renal excretion. Patients with Ccr of ≥ 60 ml/min excrete 65% of the dose in urine within 12 hours and 71% within 24 hours. All of the platinum in the 24 hour urine is present as carboplatin. Only 3% to 5% of the administered platinum is excreted in the urine between 24 and 96 hours.

In patients with Ccr < 60 ml/min, total body and renal clearances of carboplatin decrease as Ccr decreases. Reduce dosages in these patients (see Administration and Dosage).

Clinical trials: Initial treatment – Two randomized controlled studies conducted by the National Cancer Institute of Canada, Clinical Trials Group (NCIC) and the Southwest Oncology Group (SWOG) with carboplatin vs cisplatin, both in combination with cyclophosphamide every 28 days for six courses before surgical re-evaluation, demonstrated equivalent overall survival between the two groups.

Secondary treatment – In two prospective randomized controlled studies in patients with advanced ovarian cancer previously treated with chemotherapy, carboplatin achieved six clinical complete responses in 47 patients. Response duration ranged from 45 to ≥ 71 weeks.

Within the group of patients previously treated with cisplatin, those who have developed progressive disease while receiving cisplatin therapy may have a decreased response rate.

Indications:

Ovarian carcinoma:

Initial treatment of advanced ovarian carcinoma in established combination with other approved chemotherapeutic agents. One established combination regimen consists of carboplatin and cyclophosphamide.

Secondary treatment – Palliative treatment of patients with ovarian carcinoma recurrent after prior chemotherapy, including patients who have been previously treated with cisplatin.

Unlabeled uses: Carboplatin has shown activity as a single agent in previously treated and untreated patients with small cell lung cancer, but is most effective when combined with other agents (eg, etoposide). It is useful either alone or in combination (usually with fluorouracil) in the treatment of advanced or recurrent squamous cell carcinoma of the head and neck. Activity has also been demonstrated in advanced endometrial cancer, in relapsed and refractory acute leukemia and for seminoma of testicular cancer, but further studies are needed.

Contraindications:

History of severe allergic reactions to cisplatin or other platinum compounds or mannitol; severe bone marrow depression (see Warnings); significant bleeding.

(Continued on following page)

CARBOPLATIN (Cont.)

Warnings:

Bone marrow suppression (leukopenia, neutropenia and thrombocytopenia) is dose-dependent and is also the dose-limiting toxicity. Frequently monitor peripheral blood counts during carboplatin treatment and, when appropriate, until recovery. Median nadir occurs at day 21 in patients receiving single-agent carboplatin. By day 28, 90% of patients have platelet counts > 100,000/mm³; 74% have neutrophil counts > 2,000 per mm³; 67% have leukocyte counts < 4,000/mm³. In general, do not repeat single intermittent courses until leukocyte, neutrophil and platelet counts recover.

Since anemia is cumulative, transfusions may be needed during treatment with carboplatin, particularly in patients receiving prolonged therapy.

Bone marrow suppression is increased in patients who have received prior therapy, especially regimens including cisplatin. Marrow suppression is also increased in impaired kidney function. Patients with poor performance status have also had a higher incidence of severe leukopenia and thrombocytopenia. Bone marrow depression may be more severe when carboplatin is combined with other bone marrow suppressing drugs or with radiotherapy. Appropriately reduce initial carboplatin dosages in these patients (see Administration and Dosage) and carefully monitor blood counts between courses. If used in combination with other bone marrow suppressing therapies, carefully manage with respect to dosage and timing to minimize additive effects.

Nephrotoxic potential is limited, but concomitant treatment with aminoglycosides has resulted in increased renal or audiologic toxicity. Exercise caution when a patient receives both drugs. Development of abnormal renal function test results is uncommon, despite the fact that carboplatin, unlike cisplatin, has usually been administered without high-volume fluid hydration or forced diuresis. Most of the reported abnormalities have been mild, and about 50% of them were reversible.

Creatinine clearance has been the most sensitive measure of kidney function in carboplatin patients, and it appears to be the most useful test for correlating drug clearance and bone marrow suppression. Of the patients who had a baseline value of ≥ 60 ml/min, 27% demonstrated a reduction below this value during therapy.

Emesis can be induced which can be more severe in patients previously receiving emetogenic therapy. Carboplatin is significantly less emetogenic than cisplatin. Both nausea and vomiting usually cease within 24 hours of treatment, and the incidence and intensity of emesis have been reduced by using premedication with antiemetics. Although no conclusive efficacy data exist with the following schedules of carboplatin, lengthening the duration of single IV administration to 24 hours or dividing the total dose over five consecutive daily pulse doses has reduced emesis.

Peripheral neurotoxicity is infrequent; however, its incidence is increased in patients > 65 years old and in patients previously treated with cisplatin. Carboplatin produces significantly fewer and less severe neurologic side effects than cisplatin. Preexisting cisplatin-induced neurotoxicity does not worsen in about 70% of the patients receiving carboplatin as secondary treatment. Although the overall incidence of peripheral neurologic side effects induced by carboplatin is low, prolonged treatment, particularly in cisplatin-pretreated patients, may result in cumulative neurotoxicity.

Allergic reactions to carboplatin have occurred and may occur within minutes of administration; manage with appropriate supportive therapy. Refer to Management of Acute Hypersensitivity Reactions.

Carcinogenesis/Mutagenesis: The carcinogenic potential has not been studied, but compounds with similar mechanisms of action and mutagenicity profiles have been carcinogenic. Carboplatin is mutagenic both in vitro and in vivo. It is also embryotoxic and teratogenic in rats receiving the drug during organogenesis.

Pregnancy: Category D. Carboplatin may cause fetal harm when administered to a pregnant woman. Carboplatin is embryotoxic and teratogenic in rats. There are no adequate and well controlled studies in pregnant women. If used during pregnancy, or if the patient becomes pregnant while receiving this drug, apprise the patient of the potential hazard to the fetus. Advise women of childbearing potential to avoid pregnancy.

Lactation: It is not known whether carboplatin is excreted in breast milk. Because there is a possibility of toxicity in nursing infants secondary to carboplatin treatment of the mother, discontinue breastfeeding if the mother is treated with carboplatin.

Precautions:

Aluminum can react with carboplatin, causing precipitate formation and loss of potency. Do not use needles or IV administration sets containing aluminum parts that may come in contact with carboplatin for the preparation or administration of the drug.

(Precautions continued on following page)

CARBOPLATIN (Cont.)

Precautions (Cont.):

Laboratory test abnormalities: High dosages of carboplatin (more than four times the recommended dose) have resulted in severe abnormalities of liver function tests, which have generally been mild and reversible in about 50% of the cases; however, the role of metastatic tumor in the liver may complicate the assessment in many patients. In a limited series of patients receiving very high doses of carboplatin and autologous bone marrow transplantation, severe abnormalities of liver function tests occurred.

Adverse Reactions:

Carboplatin Adverse Reactions in Patients with Ovarian Cancer (%)		
Adverse reaction	First line combination therapy[1] (n = 393)	Second line single agent therapy (n = 553)
Bone marrow		
Thrombocytopenia		
< 100,000/mm³	66	62
< 50,000/mm³	33	35
Neutropenia		
< 2000 cells/mm³	96	67
< 1000 cells/mm³	82	21
Leukopenia		
< 4000 cells/mm³	97	85
< 2000 cells/mm³	71	26
Anemia		
< 11 g/dl	90	90
< 8 g/dl	14	21
Transfusions	35	44
Infections	16	5
Bleeding	8	5
GI		
Nausea and vomiting	93	92
Vomiting	83	81
Other GI side effects	46	21
Neurologic		
Central neurotoxicity	26	5
Peripheral neuropathies	15	6
Ototoxicity	12	1
Other sensory side effects	5	1
Renal/Hepatic		
Alkaline phosphatase elevations	29	37
AST elevations	20	19
Blood urea elevations	17	22
Serum creatinine elevations	6	10
Bilirubin elevations	5	5
Electrolyte loss		
Magnesium	61	43
Calcium	16	31
Potassium	16	28
Sodium	10	47
Other		
Alopecia	49	2
Pain	44	23
Asthenia	41	11
Cardiovascular	19	6
Allergic	11	2
Respiratory	10	6
GU	10	2
Mucositis	8	1

[1] Combination therapy with cyclophosphamide in NCIC and SWOG studies. Combination therapy as well as treatment duration may be responsible for the differences noted with single agent therapy

The following incidences of adverse events are based on data from 1,893 patients with various types of tumors who received carboplatin as single-agent therapy.

GI: Vomiting (65%), severe in about one third of these patients (see Warnings); nausea alone (additional 10% to 15%); pain (17%); diarrhea, constipation (6%).

(Adverse Reactions continued on following page)

CARBOPLATIN (Cont.)

Adverse Reactions (Cont.)

Hematologic: Bone marrow suppression is the dose-limiting toxicity of carboplatin: Thrombocytopenia, platelet count < 50,000/mm³ (25%); neutropenia, granulocyte count < 1,000/mm³ (16%); leukopenia, WBC count < 2,000/mm³ (15%). See Warnings. The hematologic effects, although usually reversible, have resulted in infectious or hemorrhagic complications (5%), and drug-related death (< 1%).

Anemia (hemoglobin < 11 g/dl) occurred in 71% of patients who started therapy with a baseline above that value. Anemia incidence increases with increasing carboplatin exposure. Transfusions have been given to carboplatin-treated patients (26%).

Neurologic: Peripheral neuropathies (4%) with mild paresthesias occurring most frequently (see Warnings). Clinical ototoxicity and other sensory abnormalities such as visual disturbances and change in taste (1%). Central nervous system symptoms (5%) appear to be most often related to the use of antiemetics.

Nephrotoxicity (see Warnings): Abnormal renal function tests – Blood urea nitrogen (14%); serum creatinine (6%).

Electrolyte changes: Abnormally decreased serum electrolyte values (rarely associated with symptoms): Sodium (29%); magnesium (29%); calcium (22%); potassium (20%).

Allergic reactions: Hypersensitivity (2%), including rash, urticaria, erythema, pruritus, and rarely bronchospasm and hypotension (see Warnings).

Other: Pain; asthenia; alopecia (3%); cardiovascular, respiratory, genitourinary and mucosal side effects (≤ 6%). Cardiovascular events (cardiac failure, embolism, cerebrovascular accidents) were fatal in < 1%, and did not appear to be related to chemotherapy. Cancer-associated hemolytic uremic syndrome has occurred rarely.

Laboratory test abnormalities: Alkaline phosphatase (24%); AST (15%); total bilirubin (5%). See Precautions.

Comparative toxicity, carboplatin vs cisplatin: In the NCIC and SWOG studies, when cisplatin and carboplatin were used in combination with cyclophosphamide, the pattern of toxicity exerted by the carboplatin-containing regimen was significantly different from that of the cisplatin-containing combinations. The carboplatin regimens induced significantly more thrombocytopenia and, in one study, significantly more leukopenia and more need for transfusional support. In one study, of the cisplatin regimen produced significantly more anemia, and non-hematologic toxicities (eg, emesis, neurotoxicity, ototoxicity, renal toxicity, hypomagnesemia, alopecia) were significantly more frequent in both studies.

Overdosage:

There is no known antidote for carboplatin overdosage. The anticipated complications of overdosage would be secondary to bone marrow suppression or hepatic toxicity.

Administration and Dosage:

Note: Aluminum reacts with carboplatin, causing precipitate formation and loss of potency; therefore, needles or IV sets containing aluminum parts that may come in contact with the drug must not be used for the preparation or administration of carboplatin.

Carboplatin as a single agent: 360 mg/m² IV on day 1 every 4 weeks. In general, however, do not repeat single intermittent courses of carboplatin until the neutrophil count is at least 2,000/mm³ and the platelet count is at least 100,000/mm³.

Combination therapy with cyclophosphamide: Carboplatin 300 mg/m² IV plus cyclophosphamide 600 mg/m² IV, both on day 1 every 4 weeks for six cycles. Do not repeat intermittent courses of the combination until the neutrophil count is at least 2000/mm³ and the platelet count is at least 100,000/mm³.

Dose adjustment: The dose adjustments in the table for single agent or combination therapy are modified from controlled trials in previously treated and untreated patients with ovarian carcinoma. Blood counts were done weekly; recommendations are based on the lowest post-treatment platelet or neutrophil value.

Carboplatin Dose Adjustments

Platelets/mm³	Neutrophils/mm³	Adjusted dose[1] from prior course
> 100,000	> 2,000	125%
50,000-100,000	500-2,000	No adjustment
< 50,000	< 500	75%

[1] Percentages apply to carboplatin as a single agent or to both carboplatin and cyclophosphamide in combination.

Doses > 125% of the starting dose are not recommended.

Carboplatin is usually administered by an infusion lasting ≥ 15 minutes. No pretreatment or post-treatment hydration or forced diuresis is required.

(Administration and Dosage continued on following page)

CARBOPLATIN (Cont.)

Administration and Dosage (Cont.):

Renal function impairment: Patients with impaired kidney function (Ccr < 60 ml/min) are at increased risk of severe bone marrow suppression. In renally impaired patients who received single-agent carboplatin therapy, the incidence of severe leukopenia, neutropenia or thrombocytopenia was about 25% when the dosage modifications below were used. These dosing recommendations apply to the initial course of treatment. Adjust subsequent dosages according to the patient's tolerance based on degree of bone marrow suppression.

Carboplatin Dosage in Renal Insufficiency

Baseline Ccr (ml/min)	Recommended dose on day 1
41 to 59	250 mg/m²
16 to 40	200 mg/m²
≤ 15	†

† Data too limited to permit a recommendation for treatment.

Preparation of IV solutions – Immediately before use, the content of each vial must be reconstituted with either Sterile Water for Injection, 5% Dextrose in Water or Sodium Chloride Injection, according to the following schedule:

Preparation of Carboplatin Solutions

Vial strength (mg)	Diluent volume (ml)	Concentration (mg/ml)
50	5	10
150	15	10
450	45	10

Carboplatin can be further diluted to concentrations as low as 0.5 mg/ml with 5% Dextrose in Water or Sodium Chloride Injection.

Storage/Stability: Store the unopened vials at controlled room temperature (15° to 30°C; 59° to 86°F). Protect from light. When prepared as directed, solutions are stable for 8 hours at room temperature (25°C; 77°F). Since no antibacterial preservative is contained in the formulations, discard solutions 8 hours after dilution.

Rx	**Paraplatin** (Bristol-Myers Oncology)	**Powder for Injection, lyophilized**: 50 mg[1]	In vials.
		150 mg[1]	In vials.
		450 mg[1]	In vials.

[1] With mannitol.

METHOTREXATE (Amethopterin; MTX)

Warning:

Use of high dose regimens recommended for osteosarcoma requires meticulous care.

Deaths have occurred with the use of methotrexate (MTX) in malignancy, psoriasis and rheumatoid arthritis.

Marked bone marrow depression may occur with resultant anemia, leukopenia or thrombocytopenia.

Unexpectedly severe (sometimes fatal) marrow suppression and GI toxicity have occurred with coadministration of MTX (usually in high dosage) along with some NSAIDs (see Precautions, Drug Interactions).

Periodic monitoring for toxicity, including CBC with differential and platelet counts, and liver and renal function tests is mandatory. Periodic liver biopsies may be indicated in some situations. Monitor patients at increased risk for impaired MTX elimination (eg, renal dysfunction, pleural effusions, ascites) more frequently (see Precautions).

Liver: MTX causes hepatotoxicity, fibrosis and cirrhosis, but generally only after prolonged use. Acutely, liver enzyme elevations are frequent, usually transient and asymptomatic, and also do not appear predictive of subsequent hepatic disease. Liver biopsy after sustained use often shows histologic changes, and fibrosis and cirrhosis have occurred; these latter lesions often are not preceded by symptoms or abnormal liver function tests (see Precautions).

MTX-induced lung disease is a potentially dangerous lesion that may occur acutely at any time during therapy and has occurred at doses as low as 7.5 mg/week. It is not always fully reversible. Pulmonary symptoms (especially a dry, nonproductive cough) may require interruption of treatment and careful investigation.

Pregnancy: Fetal death or congenital anomalies have occurred; do not use in women of childbearing potential unless benefits outweigh possible risks.

Renal use: Use MTX in patients with impaired renal function with extreme caution, and at reduced dosages, because renal dysfunction will prolong elimination.

GI: Diarrhea and ulcerative stomatitis require interruption of therapy; hemorrhagic enteritis and death from intestinal perforation may occur.

MTX has been administered in very high dosage followed by leucovorin rescue for certain neoplastic diseases. This procedure is investigational.

Do not use MTX formulations and diluents containing preservatives for intrathecal or experimental high dose MTX therapy.

Severe reactions: Because of the possibility of severe toxic reactions, fully inform patient of the risks involved and assure constant supervision.

Actions:

Pharmacology: Methotrexate (MTX) competitively inhibits dihydrofolic acid reductase. Dihydrofolates must be reduced to tetrahydrofolic acid by this enzyme in the process of deoxyribonucleic acid (DNA) synthesis and cellular replication.

Actively proliferating tissues such as malignant cells, bone marrow, fetal cells, buccal and intestinal mucosa, and cells of the urinary bladder are generally more sensitive to this effect of MTX. Cellular proliferation in malignant tissue is greater than in most normal tissue; thus, MTX may impair malignant growth without irreversibly damaging normal tissues.

The original rationale for high dose MTX therapy was based on the concept of selective rescue of normal tissues by leucovorin. More recent evidence suggests that high-dose MTX may also overcome MTX resistance caused by impaired active transport, decreased affinity of dihydrofolic acid reductase for MTX, increased levels of dihydrofolic acid reductase resulting from gene amplification, or decreased polyglutamation of MTX. The actual mechanism of action is unknown.

Pharmacokinetics: Absorption/Distribution – In adults, oral absorption appears to be dose-dependent. After oral doses $\leq$ 30 mg/m², MTX is generally well absorbed with a mean bioavailability of about 60%. The absorption of doses $>$ 80 mg/m² is significantly less, possibly due to a saturation effect. Peak serum levels are usually reached in 1 to 2 hours. In leukemic children, oral absorption reportedly varies widely (23% to 95%). A 20-fold difference between highest and lowest peak levels was reported. Significant interindividual variability was also noted in time-to-peak concentration and fraction of dose absorbed. Food delayed absorption and reduced peak concentration.

(Actions continued on following page)

METHOTREXATE (Amethopterin; MTX) (Cont.)

Actions (Cont.):

Pharmacokinetics (Cont.):

After injection, the drug is generally completely absorbed, and peak serum levels are seen in 30 to 60 minutes. After IV administration, the initial volume of distribution is ≈ 0.18 L/kg (18% of body weight) and steady-state volume of distribution is ≈ 0.4 to 0.8 L/kg (40% to 80% of body weight). MTX competes with reduced folates for active transport across cell membranes by means of a single carrier-mediated active transport process. At serum concentrations > 100 micromolar, passive diffusion becomes a major pathway by which effective intracellular concentrations can be achieved. Approximately 50% of the absorbed drug is bound to serum protein. MTX does not penetrate the blood-cerebrospinal fluid barrier in therapeutic amounts. High CSF concentrations of the drug may be attained by direct intrathecal administration.

Metabolism/Excretion – After absorption, MTX undergoes hepatic and intracellular metabolism to polyglutamated forms which can be converted back to MTX by hydrolase enzymes. These polyglutamates act as inhibitors of dihydrofolate reductase and thymidylate synthetase. Small amounts of MTX polyglutamates may remain in tissues for extended periods. The retention and prolonged drug action of these active metabolite(s) vary among different cells, tissues and tumors. A small amount of metabolism to 7-hydroxymethotrexate may occur at doses commonly prescribed. Accumulation of this metabolite may become significant at the high doses used in osteogenic sarcoma. The aqueous solubility of 7-hydroxymethotrexate is threefold to fivefold lower than the parent compound. MTX is partially metabolized by intestinal flora after oral administration.

The terminal half-life is approximately 3 to 10 hours for patients receving low-dose antineoplastic therapy (< 30 mg/m²). For patients on high doses, the terminal half-life is 8 to 15 hours.

Renal excretion is the primary route of elimination and is dependent upon dosage and route of administration. With IV administration, 80% to 90% of the administered dose is excreted unchanged in the urine within 24 hours. There is limited biliary excretion of ≤ 10%. Enterohepatic recirculation of MTX has been proposed. Renal excretion occurs by glomerular filtration and active tubular secretion. Impaired renal function, as well as concurrent use of drugs such as weak organic acids that also undergo tubular secretion, can markedly increase serum levels. Excellent correlation has been reported between MTX clearance and endogenous creatinine clearance.

Clearance rates vary widely and are generally decreased at higher doses. Delayed drug clearance is one of the major factors responsible for toxicity because the toxicity for normal tissues appears more dependent upon the duration of exposure to the drug rather than the peak level achieved. When a patient has delayed drug elimination due to compromised renal function or other causes, MTX serum concentrations may remain elevated for prolonged periods.

The potential for toxicity from high-dose regimens or delayed excretion is reduced by leucovorin calcium during the final phase of MTX plasma elimination. Guidelines for monitoring serum MTX levels, and for adjustment of leucovorin dosing to reduce the risk of toxicity, are provided in Administration and Dosage.

Indications:

Antineoplastic chemotherapy: Treatment of gestational choriocarcinoma, chorioadenoma destruens and hydatidiform mole.

Acute lymphocytic leukemia – Treatment and prophylaxis of meningeal leukemia and maintenance therapy in combination with other chemotherapeutic agents.

MTX alone or in combination with other anticancer agents for treatment of breast cancer, epidermoid cancers of the head and neck, advanced mycosis fungoides and lung cancer, particularly squamous cell and small cell types; in combination therapy in the treatment of advanced-stage non-Hodgkin's lymphomas.

MTX in high doses followed by leucovorin rescue in combination with other chemotherapeutic agents for prolonging relapse-free survival in patients with non-metastatic osteosarcoma who have undergone surgical resection or amputation for the primary tumor.

Psoriasis: Symptomatic control of severe, recalcitrant, disabling psoriasis (see specific monograph).

Rheumatoid arthritis: Management of severe, active, classical or definite rheumatoid arthritis (see specific monograph).

Unlabeled uses: High-dose regimen followed by leucovorin rescue for adjuvant therapy of non-metastatic osteosarcoma (orphan drug designation granted in 1985); to reduce corticosteroid requirements in patients with severe corticosteroid-dependent asthma.

Contraindications:

Hypersensitivity to the drug; nursing mothers.

(Continued on following page)

METHOTREXATE (Amethopterin; MTX) (Cont.)

Warnings:

Renal function impairment: MTX is excreted principally by the kidneys. Its use in impaired renal function may result in accumulation of toxic amounts or additional renal damage. Determine the patient's renal status prior to and during therapy. Exercise caution should significant renal impairment occur. Reduce or discontinue drug dosage until renal function improves or is restored.

Toxic effects, potentially serious, may be related in frequency and severity to dose or frequency of administration, but have been seen at all doses. These effects can occur at any time during therapy; follow patients closely. Most adverse reactions are reversible if detected early. When reactions occur, reduce dosage or discontinue drug and take appropriate corrective measures; this could include use of leucovorin calcium. Use caution if therapy is reinstituted. Consider further need for the drug and possibility of recurrence of toxicity. Pharmacists should dispense no more than a 7 day supply of the drug at one time. Refill of such prescriptions should be by direct order (written or oral) of the physician only.

Mutagenesis and impairment of fertility: Although there is evidence that the drug causes chromosomal damage to animal somatic cells and human bone marrow cells, the clinical significance remains uncertain. Weigh benefit against this potential risk before using MTX alone or in combination with other drugs, especially in children or young adults.

The drug causes embryotoxicity, abortion and fetal defects in humans. It has also caused impairment of fertility, oligospermia and menstrual dysfunction during and for a short period after cessation of therapy.

Elderly: Clinical pharmacology has not been well studied in these patients. Due to diminished hepatic and renal function and increased folate stores in this population, consider relatively low doses. Closely monitor for early signs of toxicity.

Pregnancy: Category D. MTX has caused fetal death and congenital anomalies. Do not use unless benefits outweigh risks. Women of childbearing potential should not receive MTX until pregnancy is excluded and they should be fully counseled on the serious risk to the fetus should they become pregnant while undergoing treatment. Avoid pregnancy if either partner is receiving MTX, during and for a minimum of 3 months after therapy for males, and during and for at least one ovulatory cycle after therapy for females.

Category X. Do not administer to pregnant psoriatic or rheumatoid arthritis patients.

Lactation: Contraindicated in nursing mothers. MTX is excreted in breast milk in low concentrations with a milk:plasma ratio of 0.08. The significance of this small amount is unknown. Since the drug may accumulate in neonatal tissues, breast-feeding is not recommended. Decide whether to discontinue nursing, or to discontinue the drug, taking into account the importance of the drug to the mother.

Children: Safety and efficacy in children have not been established, other than in cancer chemotherapy.

Precautions:

Monitoring: Complete blood count with differential and platelet counts; hepatic enzymes; renal function tests; chest x-ray. During initial or changing doses, or during periods of increased risk of elevated MTX blood levels (eg, dehydration), more frequent monitoring may be indicated.

A relationship between abnormal liver function tests and fibrosis or cirrhosis of the liver has not been established. Transient liver function test abnormalities are observed frequently after MTX administration and are usually not cause for modification of MTX therapy. Persistent liver function test abnormalities just prior to dosing, or depression of serum albumin, may indicate serious liver toxicity; they require evaluation.

Pulmonary function tests may be useful if MTX-induced lung disease is suspected, especially if baseline measurements are available.

Intrathecal therapy: Large doses may cause convulsions. Untoward side effects may occur with any intrathecal injection and are commonly neurological. Intrathecal MTX appears significantly in systemic circulation and may cause systemic toxicity; therefore, adjust systemic antileukemic therapy appropriately. Focal leukemic involvement of the CNS may not respond to intrathecal chemotherapy and is best treated with radiotherapy.

(Precautions continued on following page)

METHOTREXATE (Amethopterin; MTX) (Cont.)

Precautions (Cont.):

Organ system toxicity:

GI – If vomiting, diarrhea or stomatitis occur, which may result in dehydration, discontinue MTX until recovery occurs. Use with extreme caution in the presence of peptic ulcer disease or ulcerative colitis.

Hematologic – MTX can suppress hematopoiesis and cause anemia, leukopenia or thrombocytopenia. Use with caution, if at all, in patients with malignancy and preexisting hematopoietic impairment. Continue MTX only if the potential benefit warrants the risk of severe myelosuppression. Evaluate patients with profound granulocytopenia and fever immediately; they usually require parenteral broad-spectrum antibiotic therapy. In severe bone marrow depression, blood or platelet transfusions may be necessary.

Hepatic – MTX has the potential for acute (elevated transaminases) and chronic (fibrosis and cirrhosis) hepatotoxicity. Chronic toxicity is potentially fatal; it generally occurs after prolonged use (generally $\geq$ 2 years) and after a total dose of at least 1.5 g. An accurate incidence rate is undetermined; the rate of progression and reversibility of lesions is not known. Special caution is indicated in the presence of preexisting liver damage or impaired hepatic function.

Periodically perform liver function tests, including serum albumin, prior to dosing. They are often normal in the face of developing fibrosis or cirrhosis. These lesions may be detectable only by biopsy.

Infection or immunologic states – Use with extreme caution in the presence of active infection; usually contraindicated in patients with overt or laboratory evidence of immunodeficiency syndromes. Immunization may be ineffective when given during MTX therapy. Immunization with live virus vaccines is generally not recommended. Disseminated vaccinia infections after smallpox immunization have occurred in patients receiving MTX. Hypogammaglobulinemia occurs rarely.

Neurologic – There have been reports of leukoencephalopathy following IV administration of MTX to patients who have had craniospinal irradiation. Chronic leukoencephalopathy has also occurred in patients with osteosarcoma who received repeated doses of high-dose MTX with leucovorin rescue even without cranial irradiation. Discontinuation of MTX does not always result in complete recovery.

A transient acute neurologic syndrome has been observed in patients treated with high dosage regimens. Manifestations may include behavioral abnormalities, focal sensorimotor signs and abnormal reflexes. The exact cause is unknown.

After intrathecal use of MTX, the CNS toxicity that may occur can be classified as follows: Chemical arachnoiditis manifested by headache, back pain, nuchal rigidity and fever; paresis, usually transient, manifested by paraplegia associated with involvement with one or more spinal nerve roots; leukoencephalopathy manifested by confusion, irritability, somnolence, ataxia, dementia and convulsions.

Pulmonary symptoms (especially a dry, nonproductive cough) or a non-specific pneumonitis occurring during therapy indicate a potentially dangerous lesion and require interruption of treatment and careful investigation. The typical patient presents with fever, cough, dyspnea, hypoxemia and an infiltrate on chest x-ray; infection needs to be excluded. This lesion can occur at all dosages.

Renal – High doses used in the treatment of osteosarcoma may cause renal damage leading to acute renal failure. Nephrotoxicity is due primarily to the precipitation of MTX and 7-hydroxymethotrexate in the renal tubules. Close attention to renal function including adequate hydration, urine alkalinization and measurement of serum MTX and creatinine levels are essential for safe administration.

Other precautions – Use with extreme caution in the presence of debility.

MTX exits slowly from third space compartments (eg, pleural effusions or ascites). This results in a prolonged terminal plasma half-life and unexpected toxicity. In patients with significant third space accumulations, evacuate the fluid before treatment and monitor plasma MTX levels.

Lesions of psoriasis may be aggravated by concomitant exposure to ultraviolet radiation. Radiation dermatitis and sunburn may be "recalled" by the use of MTX.

Drug Interactions:

Aminoglycosides, oral may decrease the absorption and AUC of concurrent oral MTX, although the effect is unpredictable. Consider parenteral MTX.

Charcoal lowers the plasma levels of both oral and IV MTX and may be particularly significant with high dose therapies. Depending on the clinical situation, this will reduce the effectiveness or toxicity of MTX.

Etretinate: Hepatotoxicity occurred in two patients receiving etretinate and MTX for psoriasis, and MTX plasma levels increased in another patient.

(Drug Interactions continued on following page)

METHOTREXATE (Amethopterin; MTX) (Cont.)

Drug Interactions (Cont.):

Folic acid or its derivatives contained in some vitamins may decrease response to MTX.

Nonsteroidal anti-inflammatory drugs: Concurrent MTX caused fatal interactions in four patients (three with **ketoprofen,** one with **naproxen**). **Indomethacin** and **phenylbutazone** increased MTX plasma levels. The mechanism of action is not known, but may involve inhibition of renal prostaglandin synthesis or competitive renal secretion. Excessive MTX levels did not result when **ketoprofen** was given at least 12 hours after completion of therapy. The possibility of a similar interaction exists with the other NSAIDs. Administer concomitantly with extreme caution, if at all.

Phenytoin serum concentrations may be decreased by a combination chemotherapy regimen including MTX.

Probenecid, salicylates and **sulfonamides** (including **TMP-SMZ**): The therapeutic as well as toxic effects of MTX may be increased by these agents. Inhibition of renal tubular secretion, competition for a common elimination pathway or protein displacement may be the mechanisms involved. However, if protein displacement is the mechanism, it may involve displacement of the highly bound metabolic 7-hydroxymethotrexate since the parent drug is only 50% bound.

Procarbazine may increase the nephrotoxicity of MTX.

Thiopurines: MTX coadministration may increase the AUC and plasma levels of thiopurines.

Drug/Food interaction: Food may delay the absorption and reduce the peak concentration of MTX.

Adverse Reactions:

The incidence and severity of acute side effects are generally related to dose and frequency of administration. See also Precautions section under "Organ System Toxicity."

Most common: Ulcerative stomatitis; leukopenia; nausea; abdominal distress; malaise; fatigue; chills; fever; dizziness; decreased resistance to infection.

Skin: Erythematous rashes; pruritus; urticaria; photosensitivity; pigmentary changes; alopecia; ecchymosis; telangiectasia; acne; furunculosis. Lesions of psoriasis may be aggravated by concomitant exposure to ultraviolet radiation.

Hematologic: Bone marrow depression; leukopenia; thrombocytopenia; anemia; hypogammaglobulinemia; hemorrhage; septicemia.

GI: Gingivitis; stomatitis; pharyngitis; anorexia; nausea; vomiting; diarrhea; hematemesis; melena; GI ulceration and bleeding; enteritis.

GU: Renal failure; azotemia; cystitis; hematuria; severe nephropathy; defective oogenesis or spermatogenesis; transient oligospermia; menstrual dysfunction and vaginal discharge; infertility; abortion; fetal defects.

Pulmonary: Deaths from interstitial pneumonitis; chronic interstitial obstructive pulmonary disease.

CNS: Headaches; drowsiness; blurred vision; aphasia; hemiparesis; paresis; convulsions. Leukoencephalopathy following IV use in patients who have had craniospinal irradiation.

After intrathecal use, the CNS toxicity that may occur can be classified as follows:
(1) Chemical arachnoiditis (headache, back pain, nuchal rigidity, fever);
(2) transient paresis (paraplegia with involvement of spinal nerve roots);
(3) leukoencephalopathy (confusion, irritability, somnolence, ataxia, dementia, occasionally major convulsions).

Other: Rarer reactions related to the use of MTX include arthralgia/myalgia, diabetes, osteoporosis and sudden death. A few cases of anaphylactoid reactions have occurred.

Overdosage:

Leucovorin (citrovorum factor) is used to neutralize toxic effects. Administer leucovorin as promptly as possible. As the time interval between administration and leucovorin rescue increases, leucovorin's effectiveness in counteracting hematologic toxicity diminishes. Leucovorin may be administered as follows: 10 mg/m² orally or parenterally initially, followed by 10 mg/m² orally every 6 hours for 72 hours. Leucovorin rescue is usually begun within 24 hours of antifolate administration. If, after 24 hours following MTX administration, the serum creatinine is 50% or greater than the pre-methotrexate serum creatinine, immediately increase the leucovorin dose to 100 mg/m² every 3 hours until the serum MTX level is $< 5 \times 10^{-8}$ M.

Charcoal hemoperfusion can lower serum MTX levels, and ventriculolumbar perfusion was used in one patient who received an overdose of intrathecal MTX.

In cases of massive overdosage, hydration and urinary alkalinization may be necessary to prevent the precipitation of MTX and its metabolites in the renal tubules. Neither hemodialysis nor peritoneal dialysis improves MTX elimination.

(Continued on following page)

METHOTREXATE (Amethopterin; MTX) (Cont.)

Patient Information:

Avoid alcohol, salicylates and prolonged exposure to sunlight or sunlamps (particularly patients with psoriasis).

May cause nausea, vomiting, loss of appetite, hair loss, skin rash, boils or acne. Notify physician if these effects persist.

Use contraceptive measures during and for at least 3 months (males) or 1 ovulatory cycle (females) after cessation of therapy.

Notify physician if any of the following occurs: Diarrhea; abdominal pain; black tarry stools; fever and chills; sore throat; unusual bleeding or bruising; sores in or around the mouth; cough or shortness of breath; yellow discoloration of the skin or eyes; darkened urine; bloody urine; swelling of the feet or legs; joint pain.

Administration and Dosage:

Oral administration is often preferred. Preservative free MTX preparations may be given IM, IV, intra-arterially or intrathecally. If desired, the solution may be further diluted immediately prior to use with an appropriate sterile preservative free medium such as 5% Dextrose Solution or Sodium Chloride Injection. The preserved formulation contains benzyl alcohol and must not be used for intrathecal or high dose therapy.

Intrathecal use – Reconstitute immediately prior to use. Use preservative free medium such as 0.9% Sodium Chloride Injection. Concentration should be 1 mg/ml.

Powder for injection – Reconstitute 20 and 50 mg vials with an appropriate sterile preservative free medium such as 5% Dextrose Solution or Sodium Chloride Injection to a concentration no greater than 25 mg/ml. Reconstitute the 1 g vial with 19.4 ml to a concentration of 50 mg/ml.

Choriocarcinoma and similar trophoblastic diseases: 15 to 30 mg orally or IM daily for a 5 day course. Repeat courses 3 to 5 times, as required, with rest periods of ≥ 1 weeks between courses, until any toxic symptoms subside. Evaluate the effectiveness of therapy by 24 hour quantitative analysis of urinary chorionic gonadotropin hormone (hCG), which should return to normal or < 50 IU/24 hr usually after the third or fourth course and is usually followed by a complete resolution of measurable lesions in 4 to 6 weeks. One to two courses of MTX after normalization of hCG is usually recommended. Careful clinical assessment is essential before each course of the drug. Cyclic combination therapy with other antitumor drugs may be useful.

Since hydatidiform mole may precede choriocarcinoma, prophylaxis with MTX has been recommended. Chorioadenoma destruens is an invasive form of hydatidiform mole. Administer MTX in doses similar to those for choriocarcinoma.

Leukemia: Acute lymphatic (lymphoblastic) leukemia in children and young adolescents is most responsive. In young adults and older patients, clinical remission is more difficult to obtain and early relapse is more common.

When used for induction, MTX in doses of 3.3 mg/m² in combination with prednisone 60 mg/m² given daily, produced remission in 50% of patients, usually within 4 to 6 weeks. MTX in combination with other agents is the drug of choice for maintenance of remissions. When remission is achieved and supportive care has produced general clinical improvement, initiate maintenance therapy as follows: Give MTX orally or IM 2 times weekly in total weekly doses of 30 mg/m²; or 2.5 mg/kg IV every 14 days. If relapse occurs, repeat initial induction regimen.

Meningeal leukemia: Administer 12 mg/m² intrathecally or an empirical dose of 15 mg. Dilute preservative-free MTX to a concentration of 1 mg/ml with a sterile, preservative-free medium such as 0.9% Sodium Chloride Injection. Administer at intervals of 2 to 5 days, and repeat until the cell count of the CSF returns to normal, then give one additional dose. Administration at intervals of < 1 week may result in increased subacute toxicity. For prophylaxis against meningeal leukemia, the dosage is the same as for treatment, except for the intervals of administration.

The CSF volume is dependent on age and not on body surface area (BSA). The CSF is at 40% of the adult volume at birth and reaches the adult volume in several years.

Intrathecal MTX 12 mg/m² (maximum, 15 mg) has resulted in low CSF MTX concentrations and reduced efficacy in children and high concentrations and neurotoxicity in adults. The following dosage regimen is based on age instead of BSA and appears to result in more consistent CSF MTX concentrations and less neurotoxicity:

Intrathecal MTX Dose Based on Age

Age (years)	Dose (mg)
< 1	6
1	8
2	10
≥ 3	12

(Administration and Dosage continued on following page)

METHOTREXATE (Amethopterin; MTX) (Cont.)

Administration and Dosage (Cont.):

Meningeal leukemia (Cont.):

Because the CSF volume and turnover may decrease with age, a dose reduction may be indicated in elderly patients.

Lymphomas: Burkitt's Tumor, Stages I and II – 10 to 25 mg/day orally for 4 to 8 days. In Stage III, give MTX concomitantly with other antitumor agents. Treatment in all stages generally consists of several courses with 7 to 10 day rest periods. Lymphosarcomas in Stage III may respond to combined drug therapy with MTX 0.625 to 2.5 mg/kg/day.

Mycosis fungoides: MTX therapy produces clinical remissions in 50% of cases. Dosage – 2.5 to 10 mg daily orally for weeks or months. Dose levels of drug are guided by patient response and hematologic monitoring. MTX has also been given IM in doses of 50 mg once weekly or 25 mg twice weekly.

Osteosarcoma: Effective therapy requires several cytotoxic chemotherapeutic agents. In addition to high-dose MTX with leucovorin rescue, these agents may include doxorubicin, cisplatin and the combination of bleomycin, cyclophosphamide and dactinomycin (BCD) in the doses and schedule shown in the table below. The starting dose for high dose MTX treatment is 12 g/m². If this dose is not sufficient to produce a peak serum concentration of 1000 micromolar (10^{-3} mol/L) at the end of the MTX infusion, the dose may be increased to 15 g/m² in subsequent treatments. If the patient is vomiting or is unable to tolerate oral medication, give leucovorin IV or IM at the same dose and schedule.

Chemotherapy Regimens for Osteosarcoma		
Drug*	Dose*	Treatment week after surgery
Methotrexate	12 g/m² IV as 4 hour infusion (starting dose)	4, 5, 6, 7, 11, 12, 15, 16, 29, 30, 44, 45
Leucovorin	15 mg orally every 6 hours for 10 doses starting at 24 hours after start of MTX infusion	
Doxorubicin† as a single drug	30 mg/m²/day IV x 3 days	8, 17
Doxorubicin† Cisplatin†	50 mg/m² IV 100 mg/m² IV	20, 23, 33, 36 20, 23, 33, 36
Bleomycin† Cyclophosphamide† Dactinomycin†	15 units/m² IV x 2 days 600 mg/m² IV x 2 days 0.6 mg/m² IV x 2 days	2, 13, 26, 39, 42 2, 13, 26, 39, 42 2, 13, 26, 39, 42

* Link MP, Goorin AM, Miser AW, et al. The effect of adjuvant chemotherapy on relapse-free survival in patients with osteosarcoma of the extremity. *N Engl J Med* 1986;314(25):1600-6.

† See each respective monograph for more complete information. Dosage modifications may be necessary because of drug-induced toxicity.

When administering high doses of MTX, closely observe the following guidelines.

Guidelines for methotrexate therapy with leucovorin rescue:

Delay MTX administration until recovery if:

- the WBC count is < 1500/mm³
- the neutrophil count is < 200/mm³
- the platelet count is < 75,000/mm³
- the serum bilirubin level is > 1.2 mg/dl
- the ALT level is > 450 U
- mucositis is present, until there is evidence of healing
- persistent pleural effusion is present; drain dry prior to infusion.

Adequate renal function must be documented – Serum creatinine must be normal, and creatinine clearance must be > 60 ml/min, before initiation of therapy.

Serum creatinine must be measured prior to each subsequent course of therapy. If serum creatinine has increased by ≥ 50% compared to a prior value, the creatinine clearance must be measured and documented to be > 60 ml/min (even if serum creatinine is still within the normal range).

Patients must be well hydrated, and must be treated with sodium bicarbonate for urinary alkalinization.

Administer 1 L/m² of IV fluid over 6 hours prior to initiation of the MTX infusion. Continue hydration at 125 ml/m²/hr (3 L/m²/day) during MTX infusion, and for 2 days after the infusion has been completed.

Alkalinize urine to maintain pH above 7 during MTX infusion and leucovorin calcium therapy by giving sodium bicarbonate orally or by incorporation into a separate IV solution.

(Administration and Dosage continued on following page)

METHOTREXATE (Amethopterin; MTX) (Cont.)

Administration and Dosage (Cont.):

Guidelines for methotrexate therapy with leucovorin rescue (Cont.):

Repeat serum creatinine and serum MTX 24 hours after starting MTX and at least once daily until the level is $< 5 \times 10^{-8}$ mol/L (0.05 micromolar).

Guidelines for leucovorin calcium dosage based upon serum MTX levels:

Leucovorin Rescue Schedules Following Treatment With Higher Doses of Methotrexate		
Clinical situation	Laboratory findings	Leucovorin dosage and duration
Normal MTX elimination	Serum MTX level ≈ 10 micromolar at 24 hours after administration, 1 micromolar at 48 hours, and < 0.2 micromolar at 72 hours	15 mg po, IM or IV q 6 hours for 60 hours (10 doses starting at 24 hours after start of MTX infusion)
Delayed late MTX elimination	Serum MTX level remaining > 0.2 micromolar at 72 hours, and > 0.05 micromolar at 96 hours after administration	Continue 15 mg po, IM or IV q 6 hours, until MTX level is < 0.05 micromolar
Delayed early MTX elimination or evidence of acute renal injury	Serum MTX level of ≥ 50 micromolar at 24 hours, or ≥ 5 micromolar at 48 hours after administration, or; a ≥ 100% increase in serum creatinine level at 24 hours after MTX administration (eg, an increase from 0.5 mg/dl to a level of ≥ 1 mg/dl)	150 mg IV q 3 hours, until MTX level is < 1 micromolar; then 15 mg IV q 3 hours until MTX level is < 0.05 micromolar

Patients who experience delayed early MTX elimination are likely to develop nonreversible oliguric renal failure. In addition to appropriate leucovorin therapy, these patients require continuing hydration and urinary alkalinization, and close monitoring of fluid and electrolyte status, until serum MTX level has fallen to < 0.05 micromolar and the renal failure has resolved.

Some patients will have abnormalities in MTX elimination, or abnormalities in renal function following MTX administration, which are significant but less severe than those described in the table; they may or may not be associated with significant clinical toxicity. If significant clinical toxicity is observed, extend leucovorin rescue for an additional 24 hours (total 14 doses over 84 hours) in subsequent courses of therapy. Consider the possibility that the patient is taking other medications which interact with MTX when laboratory abnormalities or clinical toxicities are observed.

Hepatic function impairment: If the bilirubin is between 3 and 5, or AST > 180, reduce dose by 25%. If bilirubin is > 5, omit the dose.

Consider procedures for proper handling and disposal of anticancer drugs.

Rx	**Methotrexate** (Lederle)	**Tablets:** 2.5 mg (as sodium)	(LL M1). Yellow, scored. In 100s.
Rx	**Rheumatrex Dose Pack** (Lederle)		(LLM1). Yellow, scored. 4 cards, each w/2, 3, 4, 5 or 6 tablets.
Rx	**Methotrexate** (Lyphomed[1])	**Injection:** 2.5 mg (as sodium) per ml	In 2 ml vials.
Rx	**Methotrexate** (Various, eg, Americal, Astra, Cetus, Dupont[1], Lederle[2], Lyphomed[1], Quad[2], VHA Supply)	**Injection:** 25 mg (as sodium) per ml	In 2, 4, 8 and 10 ml vials.
Rx	**Methotrexate** (Various, eg, Lederle[1], Quad, VHA Supply)	**Powder for Injection:**	In 20, 50, 100 mg and 1 g (as sodium) per vial for reconstitution.
Rx	**Folex** (Adria)		In 25, 50, 100 or 250 mg (as sodium) per vial for reconstitution.[1]
Rx	**Methotrexate LPF** (Lederle)	**Preservative Free Injection:** 25 mg (as sodium) per ml	In 2, 4, 8 and 10 ml vials.[1]
Rx	**Folex PFS** (Adria)		In 2, 4, 8 and 10 ml vials.[1]

[1] Contains no preservative. For single use only.

[2] Contains benzyl alcohol.

FLUOROURACIL AND FLOXURIDINE

Actions:

Pharmacology: There is evidence that the metabolism of fluorouracil in the anabolic pathway blocks the methylation reaction of deoxyuridylic acid to thymidylic acid. In this manner, fluorouracil interferes with the synthesis of deoxyribonucleic acid (DNA) and to a lesser extent inhibits the formation of ribonucleic acid (RNA). Since DNA and RNA are essential for cell division and growth, the effect of fluorouracil may be to create a thymine deficiency provoking unbalanced growth and death of the cell. DNA and RNA deprivation most effect those cells that grow rapidly and take up fluorouracil at a more rapid pace.

Pharmacokinetics: Following IV injection, fluorouracil distributes into tumors, intestinal mucosa, bone marrow, liver and other body tissues. In spite of its limited lipid solubility, fluorouracil diffuses readily across the blood-brain barrier and distributes into CSF and brain tissue.

The parent drug is excreted unchanged (7% to 20%) in the urine in 6 hours; of this, > 90% is excreted in the first hour. The remaining percentage is metabolized, primarily in the liver. The catabolic metabolism of fluorouracil results in inactive degradation products (eg, CO_2, urea, α-fluoro-β-alanine). The inactive metabolites are excreted in the urine over the next 3 to 4 hours. Approximately 90% is excreted in expired CO_2. Following IV use, 90% of the dose is accounted for during the first 24 hours; the mean half-life of elimination from plasma is ≈ 16 minutes (range, 8 to 20 minutes) and is dose-dependent. No intact drug can be detected in the plasma 3 hours after an IV injection.

Floxuridine is rapidly catabolized to 5-fluorouracil. Thus, the same toxic and antimetabolic effects as 5-fluorouracil occur.

Indications:

See individual product listings.

Contraindications:

Poor nutritional status; depressed bone marrow function; potentially serious infections; hypersensitivity to fluorouracil.

Warnings:

Hospitalize patients during initial course of therapy due to possible severe toxic reactions.

Use with extreme caution in poor-risk patients who have had high-dose pelvic irradiation or previous use of alkylating agents, or who have widespread involvement of bone marrow by metastatic tumors or impaired hepatic or renal function. These drugs are not intended as adjuvants to surgery.

Combination therapy: Any form of therapy which adds to the stress of the patient, interferes with nutrition or depresses bone marrow function will increase toxicity.

Mutagenesis: A positive effect was observed in the micronucleus test on bone marrow cells of the mouse, and fluorouracil at very high concentrations produced chromosomal breaks in hamster fibroblasts in vitro.

Fertility impairment: Intraperitoneal doses of 125 or 250 mg/kg induce chromosomal aberrations and changes in chromosomal organization of spermatogonia in rats. Spermatogonial differentiation was also inhibited by fluorouracil, resulting in transient infertility. In female rats, intraperitoneal fluorouracil 25 or 50 mg/kg/week for 3 weeks during the pre-ovulatory phase of oogenesis, significantly reduced the incidence of fertile matings, delayed pre- and postimplantation embryo development, increased preimplantation lethality incidence and induced chromosomal anomalies in these embryos.

Pregnancy: Category D (fluorouracil) – Fluorouracil crosses the placenta and enters into fetal circulation in the rat, resulting in increased resorptions and embryolethality. In monkeys, maternal doses > 40 mg/kg resulted in abortion of all embryos exposed to fluorouracil. Compounds which inhibit DNA, RNA and protein synthesis might be expected to have adverse effects on peri- and postnatal development.

Fluorouracil may cause fetal harm when administered to a pregnant woman; it is teratogenic and mutagenic in laboratory animals. Malformations included cleft palates, skeletal defects and deformed appendages, paws and tails. Teratogenic dosages in animals are 1 to 3 times the maximum recommended human therapeutic dose. There are no adequate and well controlled studies in pregnant women. Advise women of childbearing potential to avoid becoming pregnant. If the drug is used during pregnancy, or if the patient becomes pregnant while taking the drug, tell the patient of the potential hazard to the fetus. Do not use during pregnancy (particularly in the first trimester) unless the potential benefit justifies the potential risk to the fetus.

(Continued on following page)

FLUOROURACIL AND FLOXURIDINE (Cont.)

Warnings (Cont.):

Lactation: It is not known whether fluorouracil is excreted in breast milk. Because fluorouracil inhibits DNA, RNA and protein synthesis, do not nurse while using this drug.

Children: Safety and efficacy of fluorouracil in children have not been established.

Precautions:

Discontinue if signs of toxicity occur: Stomatitis or esophagopharyngitis (at first visible sign); rapidly falling WBC count; leukopenia (WBC $< 3500/mm^3$); intractable vomiting; diarrhea or frequent bowel movements; GI ulceration and bleeding; thrombocytopenia (platelets $< 100{,}000/mm^3$); hemorrhage.

These are highly toxic drugs with a narrow margin of safety. Therapeutic response is unlikely to occur without some toxicity. Inform patients of toxic effects, particularly oral manifestations. Measure WBC count with differential before each dose. Severe hematological toxicity, GI hemorrhage and death may result, despite meticulous patient selection and dosage adjustment. Although severe toxicity and fatalities are more likely in poor-risk patients, these effects may occur in patients in relatively good condition.

Angina: Coronary vasospasm with episodes of angina may occur in patients receiving fluorouracil. The angina appears to occur $\approx$ 6 hours (range, minutes to 7 days) after the third dose (range, 1 to 13 doses). Patients with preexisting coronary artery disease may be at increased risk. Nitrates or morphine appear effective in relieving the pain; pretreatment with a calcium channel blocker may also be successful.

Drug Interactions:

Leucovorin calcium may enhance the toxicity of fluorouracil.

Drug/Lab test interactions: Elevations in **alkaline phosphatase, serum transaminase, serum bilirubin** and **lactic dehydrogenase** may occur.

Adverse Reactions:

Cardiovascular: Myocardial ischemia; angina (see Precautions).

GI: Stomatitis and esophagopharyngitis (which may lead to sloughing and ulceration), diarrhea, anorexia, nausea, vomiting, enteritis (common); cramps; duodenal ulcer; watery stools; duodenitis; gastritis; glossitis; pharyngitis; possible intra- and extrahepatic biliary sclerosis; acalculus cholecystitis; GI ulceration; bleeding.

Blood: Leukopenia; thrombocytopenia; pancytopenia; agranulocytosis; anemia; thrombophlebitis. Low WBC counts are usually observed between days 9 and 14 after the first course of treatment. The count usually normalizes by day 30.

Dermatologic: Alopecia; dermatitis, often as a pruritic maculopapular rash on the extremities or trunk (usually reversible and responsive to symptomatic treatment); nonspecific skin toxicity; photosensitivity as manifested by erythema or increased skin pigmentation; nail changes including loss of nails; dry skin; fissuring; vein pigmentation.

CNS: Lethargy, malaise, weakness, acute cerebellar syndrome (may persist following discontinuation of treatment); headache.

Allergic: Anaphylaxis; generalized allergic reactions.

Psychiatric: Disorientation; confusion; euphoria.

Lab abnormalities: BSP; prothrombin; total proteins; sedimentation rate; thrombocytopenia.

Ocular: Photophobia; lacrimation; decreased vision; nystagmus; diplopia; lacrimal duct stenosis; visual changes.

Other: Fever; epistaxis.

Regional arterial infusion complications: Arterial aneurysm; arterial ischemia; arterial thrombosis; bleeding at catheter site; catheter blocked, displaced or leaking; embolism; fibromyositis; abscesses; infection at catheter site; thrombophlebitis.

Overdosage:

The possibility of overdosage with fluorouracil is unlikely in view of the mode of administration. Nevertheless, the anticipated manifestations would be nausea, vomiting, diarrhea, GI ulceration and bleeding, bone marrow depression (including thrombocytopenia, leukopenia and agranulocytosis). No specific antidotal therapy exists. Patients who have been exposed to an overdose of fluorouracil should be monitored hematologically for at least 4 weeks. Should abnormalities appear, utilize appropriate therapy.

Patient Information:

Transient alopecia may occur with fluorouracil therapy; alert the patient to this possibility.

Contraceptive measures are recommended for men and women during therapy.

Notify doctor if chills, nausea, vomiting, unusual bleeding or bruising, yellowing of skin or eyes, abdominal pain, flank or joint pain, or swelling of feet or legs occurs.

May cause diarrhea, fever and weakness. Notify doctor if these become pronounced.

Drink plenty of liquids while taking this drug.

(Continued on following page)

Complete prescribing information for these products begins on page 2519

FLUOROURACIL (5-Fluorouracil; 5-FU)

Indications:

Palliative management of carcinoma of the colon, rectum, breast, stomach and pancreas.

Fluorouracil is also used in combination with levamisole (see individual monograph) after surgical resection in patients with Dukes' stage C colon cancer.

In patients with metastatic colorectal carcinoma, the administration of IV leucovorin 200 mg/m²/day for 5 days followed by fluorouracil 370 mg/m²/day for 5 days and repeated every 28 days significantly increased the response rate, decreased time to disease progression and prolonged overall survival compared to fluorouracil alone.

Administration and Dosage:

Individualize dosage. Administer IV; avoid extravasation. No dilution is required. Base dosages on actual weight. Use lean body weight (dry weight) if patient is obese or if there has been spurious weight gain due to edema, ascites or other abnormal fluid retention.

Although not FDA approved, fluorouracil has been administered orally in a small number (< 5%) of patients when more acceptable methods are not possible. Absorption is erratic and plasma concentrations are variable. If given orally, do not dilute the dose in orange or grape juice; mix with water only.

Initial dosage: 12 mg/kg IV once daily for 4 days. Do not exceed 800 mg/day. If no toxicity is observed, give 6 mg/kg on days 6, 8, 10 and 12. No therapy is given on days 5, 7, 9 or 11. Discontinue at end of day 12, even with no apparent toxicity.

Poor-risk patients or those not in an adequate nutritional state receive 6 mg/kg/day for 3 days. If no toxicity is observed, give 3 mg/kg on days 5, 7 and 9. Give no therapy on days 4, 6 or 8. Do not exceed 400 mg/day.

A sequence of injections on either schedule constitutes a "course of therapy" Discontinue therapy promptly when any signs of toxicity appear.

Maintenance therapy: Where toxicity has not been a problem, continue therapy using either of the following schedules: (1) Repeat dosage of first course every 30 days after last day of previous course of treatment; (2) when toxic signs from the initial course of therapy have subsided, administer a maintenance dosage of 10 to 15 mg/kg/week as a single dose. Do not exceed 1 g/week. Use reduced doses for poor risk patients. Consider the patient's reaction to the previous course and adjust dosage accordingly. Some patients have received from 9 to 45 courses of treatment over 12 to 60 months.

Storage: Solution may discolor during storage; potency and safety are not adversely affected. Store at room temperature, 15° to 30°C (59° to 86°F) and protect from light. If precipitate forms due to exposure to low temperatures, heat to 60°C (140°F) with vigorous shaking; cool to body temperature before using.

Rx	**Fluorouracil** (Various, eg, Americal, Cetus, Lyphomed, Quad, VHA Supply)	**Injection:** 50 mg/ml	In 10, 20 and 100 ml vials and 10 ml amps.
Rx	**Fluorouracil** (Roche)		In 10 ml vials.
Rx	**Fluorouracil** (Solopak)		In 10 ml amps, 10 and 50 ml vials and 100 ml bulk vials.
Rx	**Adrucil** (Adria)		In 10 ml amps.

FLOXURIDINE

Indications:

Palliative management of GI adenocarcinoma metastatic to the liver, given by continuous regional intra-arterial infusion in selected patients considered incurable by surgery or other means. Patients with disease extending beyond an area capable of infusion via a single artery should, except in unusual circumstances, be considered for systemic therapy with other agents.

Administration and Dosage:

For intra-arterial infusion only: Continuous arterial infusion of 0.1 to 0.6 mg/kg/day. The higher dose ranges (0.4 to 0.6 mg) are usually employed for hepatic artery infusion because the liver metabolizes the drug, thus reducing the potential for systemic toxicity. Administer until adverse reactions appear. When side effects have subsided, resume therapy. Maintain therapy as long as response continues. Use an infusion pump to overcome pressure in large arteries and to ensure a uniform infusion rate.

Reconstitution/Storage: Powder for injection – Reconstitute with 5 ml sterile water. Refrigerate reconstituted vials at 2° to 8°C (36° to 46°F) for not more than 2 weeks.

Rx	**Floxuridine** (Quad)	**Preservative-Free Injection:** 100 mg/ml	In 5 ml single dose vials.
Rx	**Floxuridine** (Quad)	**Powder for Injection:**	500 mg for reconstitution per 10 ml vial.
Rx	**FUDR** (Roche)		500 mg for reconstitution per 5 ml vial.

CYTARABINE (Cytosine Arabinoside; ARA-C)

Warning:

For induction therapy, treat patients in a facility with laboratory and supportive resources sufficient to monitor drug tolerance and protect and maintain a patient compromised by drug toxicity.

The main toxic effect is bone marrow suppression with leukopenia, thrombocytopenia and anemia. Less serious toxicity includes nausea, vomiting, diarrhea, abdominal pain, oral ulceration and hepatic dysfunction.

Actions:

Pharmacology: Cytarabine exhibits cell phase specificity, primarily killing cells undergoing deoxyribonucleic acid (DNA) synthesis (S-phase) and under certain conditions blocking the progression of cells from the G_1 phase to the S-phase. Although the mechanism of action is not completely understood, it appears that cytarabine inhibits DNA polymerase. Incorporation of cytarabine into both DNA and ribonucleic acid (RNA) has also been reported. Chromosomal damage has been produced in rodent cell cultures. Deoxycytidine prevents or delays (but does not reverse) the cytotoxic activity.

Cell culture studies have shown that cytarabine has an antiviral effect. However, efficacy against herpes zoster or smallpox could not be demonstrated in clinical trials.

Cellular resistance and sensitivity: Cytarabine is metabolized by deoxycytidine kinase and other nucleotide kinases to the nucleotide triphosphate, an effective inhibitor of DNA polymerase; it is inactivated by a pyrimidine nucleoside deaminase, which converts it to the nontoxic uracil derivative. It appears that the balance of kinase and deaminase levels may be an important factor in determining sensitivity or resistance of the cell to cytarabine.

Pharmacokinetics: When given orally, cytarabine is rapidly metabolized by the GI mucosa and liver, resulting in $< 20\%$ systemic availability. After SC or IM use, peak plasma levels are achieved in 20 to 60 minutes and are considerably lower than after IV use.

Following rapid IV injection, the disappearance from plasma is biphasic; the distributive phase half-life is about 10 minutes, and the elimination phase half-life is about 1 to 3 hours. Cytarabine is eliminated by enzymatic deamination to nontoxic uracil arabinoside (ara-U). Within 24 hours, about 80% of a dose is recovered in the urine, approximately 90% of which is ara-U.

Relatively constant plasma levels can be achieved by continuous IV infusion.

Cerebrospinal fluid (CSF) levels of cytarabine are lower than plasma levels after single IV injection. However, in one patient in whom CSF levels were examined after 2 hours of constant IV infusion, levels approached 40% of the steady-state plasma level. With intrathecal administration, CSF levels declined with a first order half-life of about 2 hours. Because CSF levels of deaminase are low, little conversion to ara-U was observed.

Immunosuppressive action: Cytarabine may obliterate immune responses with little or no accompanying toxicity. Suppression of antibody responses to E-coli-VI antigen and tetanus toxoid have been demonstrated. This suppression was obtained during both primary and secondary antibody responses. Following 5 days of therapy, the immune response is suppressed as indicated by the following parameters: Macrophage ingress into skin windows; circulating antibody response following primary antigenic stimulation; lymphocyte blastogenesis with phytohemagglutinin. A few days after termination of therapy there was a rapid return to normal.

Cytarabine also suppresses cell-mediated immune responses such as delayed hypersensitivity skin reaction to dinitrochlorobenzene. However, it had no effect on already established delayed hypersensitivity reactions.

(Continued on following page)

CYTARABINE (Cytosine Arabinoside; ARA-C) (Cont.)

Indications:

Induction and maintenance of remission in acute myelocytic leukemia (AML) of both adults and children. It has also been useful in the treatment of other leukemias, such as acute lymphocytic leukemia (ALL) and chronic myelocytic leukemia (blast phase).

Acute myelocytic leukemia (AML): Response rates are higher in children than in adults with similar treatment schedules. With induction and initial drug responsiveness, childhood AML appears to be more similar to childhood acute lymphocytic leukemia (ALL) than to its adult variant.

Acute lymphocytic leukemia (adults and children): Has been effective singly or in combination in patients relapsed on other therapy. When used with other antineoplastic agents as part of a total therapy program, results were equal to or better than those reported with such programs which did not include cytarabine.

Intrathecal use in meningeal leukemia: Cytarabine has been used intrathecally in acute leukemia. Dosage schedule is usually governed by type and severity of CNS manifestations and response to previous therapy. Focal leukemic involvement of the CNS may not respond to intrathecal cytarabine and may be better treated with radiotherapy. Prophylactic triple therapy following the successful treatment of the acute meningeal episode may be useful.

Unlabeled uses: Cytarabine has been used experimentally in a variety of neoplastic diseases. In general, few patients with solid tumors have benefited.

Contraindications:

Hypersensitivity to cytarabine.

Warnings:

Myelosuppression: Cytarabine is a potent bone marrow suppressant. Start therapy cautiously in patients with preexisting drug-induced bone marrow suppression. Keep patients under close medical supervision and, during induction therapy, perform leukocyte and platelet counts daily. Perform bone marrow examinations frequently after blasts have disappeared from the peripheral blood. Have facilities available for management of bone marrow complications, possibly fatal (infection resulting from granulocytopenia and other impaired body defenses, and hemorrhage secondary to thrombocytopenia).

Hypersensitivity: Cases of anaphylaxis have occurred resulting in acute cardiopulmonary arrest which required resuscitation. Refer to Management of Acute Hypersensitivity Reactions.

Experimental doses: Severe and sometimes fatal CNS, GI and pulmonary toxicity (different from that seen with conventional cytarabine regimens) have occurred. These reactions include reversible corneal toxicity and hemorrhagic conjunctivitis, which may be prevented or diminished by prophylaxis with local corticosteroid eye drops; cerebral and cerebellar dysfunction, usually reversible, including personality changes, dysarthria, ataxia, confusion, somnolence and coma; severe GI ulceration, including pneumatosis cystoides intestinalis leading to peritonitis; sepsis and liver abscess; pulmonary edema; liver damage with increased hyperbilirubinemia; bowel necrosis; and necrotizing colitis. Rarely, severe skin rash leading to desquamation may occur. Complete alopecia is more common with experimental high-dose therapy than with standard cytarabine treatment programs. If experimental high-dose therapy is used, do not use a diluent containing benzyl alcohol. In one report, the CNS toxicity occurred only in those patients greater than 55 years of age.

An increase in cardiomyopathy with subsequent death has occurred following experimental high-dose therapy with cytarabine in combination with cyclophosphamide when used for bone marrow transplant preparation.

A syndrome of sudden respiratory distress, rapidly progressing to pulmonary edema and radiographically pronounced cardiomegaly, has been reported following experimental high-dose therapy with cytarabine used for the treatment of relapsed leukemia from one institution in 16 of 72 patients. The outcome of this syndrome can be fatal.

Ten patients treated with experimental intermediate doses of cytarabine (1 g/m^2) with and without other chemotherapeutic agents (meta-AMSA, daunorubicin, etoposide) at various dose regimens developed a diffuse interstitial pneumonitis without clear cause that it may be related to cytarabine.

(Warnings continued on following page)

CYTARABINE (Cytosine Arabinoside; ARA-C) (Cont.)

Warnings (Cont.):

Benzyl alcohol is contained in the diluent for this product. Benzyl alcohol has been reported to be associated with a fatal "Gasping Syndrome" in premature infants.

Pregnancy: Category D. Cytarabine can cause fetal harm when administered to a pregnant woman. There are no adequate and well controlled studies in pregnant women. If cytarabine is used during pregnancy, or if the patient becomes pregnant while taking cytarabine, apprise the patient of the potential hazard to the fetus. Advise women of childbearing potential to avoid becoming pregnant.

The potential for abnormalities exists, particularly during the first trimester. Inform patient of potential risk to the fetus and advisability of pregnancy continuation. There is a lesser risk if therapy is initiated during the second or third trimester. Normal infants have been delivered to patients treated in all three trimesters of pregnancy; however, follow-up of such infants is advisable.

In 32 reported cases where cytarabine was given during pregnancy, either alone or in combination with other cytotoxic agents; 18 normal infants were delivered. Four infants had first trimester exposure, and five were premature or of low birth weight. Twelve of the 18 normal infants were followed up at ages ranging from 6 weeks to 7 years, and showed no abnormalities. One apparently normal infant died of gastroenteritis at 90 days. Two cases of congenital abnormalities have been reported, one with upper and lower distal limb defects, and the other with extremity and ear deformities. Both of these cases had first trimester exposure.

There were seven infants with various problems in the neonatal period, which included: Pancytopenia; transient depression of WBC, hematocrit or platelets; electrolyte abnormalities; transient eosinophilia; increased IgM levels and hyperpyrexia possibly due to sepsis (one case). Six of the seven infants were also premature. The child with pancytopenia died of sepsis at 21 days.

Therapeutic abortions were done in five cases. Four fetuses were grossly normal, but one had an enlarged spleen and another showed Trisomy C chromosomal abnormality in the chorionic tissue.

Lactation: It is not known whether this drug is excreted in breast milk. Because of the potential for serious adverse reactions in nursing infants from cytarabine, decide whether to discontinue nursing or discontinue the drug, taking into account the importance of the drug to the mother.

Precautions:

Monitoring: Monitor patients closely. Frequent platelet and leukocyte counts and bone marrow examinations are mandatory. Suspend or modify therapy when drug-induced marrow depression results in a platelet count $< 50,000/mm^3$ or a polymorphonuclear granulocyte count $< 1000/mm^3$. Counts of formed elements in the peripheral blood may continue to fall after the drug is stopped and reach lowest values after drug free intervals of 12 to 24 days. Restart therapy when definite signs of marrow recovery appear (on successive bone marrow studies). Patients whose drug is withheld until "normal" peripheral blood values are attained may escape from control.

Perform periodic checks of liver and kidney functions.

Rapid administration: When large IV doses are given rapidly, patients are frequently nauseated and may vomit for several hours. This tends to be less severe when the drug is infused slowly.

Hepatic function impairment: The liver detoxifies much of an administered dose. Use the drug with caution and at reduced doses in patients with poor liver function.

Hyperuricemia may be induced due to lysis of neoplastic cells. Monitor patient's blood uric acid level; use supportive and pharmacologic measures as necessary.

Acute pancreatitis has occurred in patients being treated with cytarabine who have had prior treatment with L-asparaginase.

Two other cases of pancreatitis have occurred following experimental doses of cytarabine and numerous other drugs. Cytarabine could have been the causative agent.

Peripheral motor and sensory neuropathies have occurred in two patients with adult acute non-lymphocytic leukemia after consolidation with high dose cytarabine, daunorubicin and asparaginase. Observe patients on high dose cytarabine for neuropathy since dose schedule alterations may be needed to avoid irreversible neurologic disorders.

(Precautions continued on following page)

CYTARABINE (Cytosine Arabinoside; ARA-C) (Cont.)

Precautions (cont.)

Intrathecal cytarabine may cause systemic toxicity; carefully monitor the hematopoietic system. Modification of other antileukemia therapy may be necessary. Major toxicity is rare. The most frequent reactions after intrathecal administration are nausea, vomiting and fever; these reactions are mild and self-limiting. Paraplegia and neurotoxicity have occurred. Necrotizing leukoencephalopathy occurred in five children who had also been treated with intrathecal methotrexate and hydrocortisone and CNS radiation. Blindness occurred in 2 patients in remission whose treatment had consisted of combination systemic chemotherapy, prophylactic CNS radiation and intrathecal cytarabine. Focal leukemic involvement of the CNS may not respond to intrathecal cytarabine and may be better treated with radiotherapy.

If used intrathecally, do not use a diluent with benzyl alcohol. Two patients with childhood acute myelogenous leukemia who received intrathecal and IV cytarabine at conventional doses (in addition to a number of other coadministered drugs) developed delayed progressive ascending paralysis resulting in death in one patient.

Drug Interactions:

Digoxin: Combination chemotherapy (including cytarabine) may decrease digoxin absorption even several days after stopping chemotherapy. **Digoxin capsules** and **digitoxin** do not appear to be affected.

Adverse Reactions:

Blood: Because cytarabine is a bone marrow suppressant, anemia, leukopenia, thrombocytopenia, megaloblastosis and reduced reticulocytes can be expected. The severity of these reactions is dose and schedule dependent. Expect cellular changes in the morphology of bone marrow and peripheral smears.

Following a 5 day constant infusion or acute injections of 50 to 600 mg/m^2, white cell depression follows a biphasic course. Regardless of initial count, dosage level or schedule, there is an initial fall starting the first 24 hours with a nadir at days 7 to 9. A brief rise follows which peaks around day 12. A second and deeper fall reaches nadir at days 15 to 24, then there is rapid rise to above baseline in the next 10 days. Platelet depression is noticeable at 5 days with a peak depression occurring between days 12 to 15. A rapid rise to above baseline occurs in the next 10 days.

Infection: Viral, bacterial, fungal, parasitic or saprophytic infections in any location in the body may be associated with the use of cytarabrine alone or in combination with other immunosuppressive agents following immunosuppressant doses that affect cellular or humoral immunity. These infections may be mild, but can be severe and sometimes fatal.

A cytarabine syndrome characterized by fever, myalgia, bone pain, occasional chest pain, maculopapular rash, conjunctivitis and malaise has been described. It usually occurs 6 to 12 hours following drug administration. Corticosteroids have been beneficial in treating or preventing this syndrome. If the symptoms are treatable, consider use of corticosteroids as well as continuation of cytarabine therapy.

Most frequent: Anorexia; nausea and vomiting (following rapid IV injection); diarrhea; oral and anal inflammation or ulceration; hepatic dysfunction; fever; rash; thrombophlebitis; bleeding (all sites).

Less frequent: Sepsis; pneumonia; cellulitis at injection site; skin ulceration; urinary retention; renal dysfunction; neuritis or neural toxicity; sore throat; esophageal ulceration; esophagitis; chest pain; bowel necrosis; abdominal pain; freckling; jaundice; conjunctivitis (may occur with rash); dizziness; alopecia; anaphylaxis (see Warnings); allergic edema; pruritus; shortness of breath; urticaria; headache.

Experimental doses: Severe and sometimes fatal CNS, GI and pulmonary toxicity (different from that seen with conventional therapy regimens of cytarabine) have occurred. Cardiomyopathy and a syndrome of sudden respiratory distress are other possibly fatal reactions to experimental doses of cytarabine (see Warnings).

Overdosage:

There is no antidote for cytarabine overdosage. Doses of 4.5 g/m^2 by IV infusion over 1 hour every 12 hours for 12 doses has caused an unacceptable increase in irreversible CNS toxicity and death.

Single doses as high as 3 g/m^2 have been administered by rapid IV infusion without apparent toxicity.

(Continued on following page)

CYTARABINE (Cytosine Arabinoside; ARA-C) (Cont.)

Administration and Dosage:

Cytarabine is not active orally; give SC or intrathecally or by IV infusion or injection. Thrombophlebitis has occurred at the injection or infusion site and, rarely, pain and inflammation occur at SC injection sites. The drug is generally well tolerated.

Patients can tolerate higher total doses when the drug is given by rapid IV injection as compared with slow infusion, due to the drug's rapid inactivation and brief exposure of susceptible normal and neoplastic cells to significant levels after rapid injection. There is no distinct clinical advantage demonstrated for either.

Acute non-lymphocytic leukemia: In combination with other anti-cancer drugs, give 100 mg/m²/day by continuous IV infusion (days 1 to 7) or 100 mg/m² IV every 12 hours (days 1 to 7).

Acute lymphocytic leukemia: Consult the literature for current recommendations.

Refractory acute leukemia: High-dose cytarabine 3 g/m² IV every 12 hours for 4 to 12 doses (repeated at 2 to 3 week intervals) has been used. Remission rates in one study were similar for patients with AML and ALL. Therapies using 4 to 6 doses every 2 weeks or 9 doses every 3 weeks appear equally effective and less toxic.

Intrathecal use in meningeal leukemia: Doses range from 5 to 75 mg/m² once daily for 4 days or once every 4 days. The most common dose is 30 mg/m² every 4 days until CSF findings are normal, followed by one additional treatment.

Preparation of solutions:

Preparation of Cytarabine Solutions		
Vial size	Amount of Bacteriostatic Water 0.9% to add	Resultant solution
100 mg	5 ml	20 mg/ml
500 mg	10 ml	50 mg/ml
1 g	10 ml	100 mg/ml
2 g	20 ml	100 mg/ml

If used intrathecally, do not use a diluent containing benzyl alcohol. Reconstitute with preservative free 0.9% Sodium Chloride for Injection; use immediately.

Many investigators prefer to use a special diluent for intrathecal use which is physiologically similar to spinal fluid (Elliott's B Solution).

Storage: Store solutions at controlled room temperature 15° to 30°C (59° to 86°F) for 48 hours. Discard if a slight haze develops. When repackaged in glass or plastic, maximum stability appears to be provided by glass stored at 5°C (41°F); however, storage of cytarabine in plastic disposable syringes stored at 5°C is an acceptable alternative.

Chemical stability in infusion solutions: When the reconstituted cytarabine was added to Water for Injection, 5% Dextrose in Water or Sodium Chloride Injection, 94% to 96% of the cytarabine was present after 192 hours storage at room temperature.

Rx	**Tarabine PFS** (Adria)	**Injection:** 20 mg/ml	Preservative free. In 5 ml single vials and 50 ml bulk package vials.
Rx	**Cytarabine** (Various, eg, Cetus, Quad, Schein)	**Powder for Injection**[1]: 100 mg	In vials.
Rx	**Cytosar-U** (Upjohn)		In vials.
Rx	**Cytarabine** (Various, eg, Cetus, Quad, Schein)	**Powder for Injection**[1]: 500 mg	In vials.
Rx	**Cytosar-U** (Upjohn)		In vials.
Rx	**Cytarabine** (Quad)	**Powder for Injection**[1]: 1 g	In 30 ml vials.
Rx	**Cytosar-U** (Upjohn)		In vials.
Rx	**Cytosar-U** (Upjohn)	**Powder for Injection**[1]: 2 g	In vials.

[1] Supplied with ampul of Bacteriostatic Water for Injection with benzyl alcohol.

MERCAPTOPURINE (6-Mercaptopurine; 6-MP)

Actions:

Pharmacology: Mercaptopurine (6-MP) competes with hypoxanthine and guanine for the enzyme hypoxanthine-guanine phosphoribosyltransferase and is converted to thioinosinic acid (TIMP). This intracellular nucleotide inhibits several reactions involving inosinic acid (IMP). In addition, 6-methylthioinosinate (MTIMP) is formed by the methylation of TIMP. Both TIMP and MTIMP inhibit *de novo* purine ribonucleotide synthesis. Radiolabeled 6-MP may be recovered from deoxyribonucleic acid (DNA) in the form of deoxythioguanosine. Some mercaptopurine is converted to nucleotide derivatives of 6-thioguanine.

Animal tumors resistant to mercaptopurine often have lost the ability to convert mercaptopurine to TIMP. Resistance may be acquired by other means as well, particularly in human leukemias. It is not known which of the biochemical effects of mercaptopurine and its metabolites are directly or predominantly responsible for cell death.

Pharmacokinetics: Absorption/Distribution – The absorption of oral mercaptopurine is incomplete and variable, averaging 50%. Recent reports using a more sensitive assay indicate bioavailability may be less (range from 5% to 37%). There is negligible entry of mercaptopurine into cerebrospinal fluid. Plasma protein binding averages 19% over the concentration range 10 to 50 mcg/ml.

Metabolism/Excretion – There are two major pathways for hepatic drug metabolism: Methylation of the sulfhydryl group and oxidation by the enzyme xanthine oxidase. Allopurinol inhibits xanthine oxidase and retards the catabolism of mercaptopurine and its active metabolites. Plasma half-life averages 21 and 47 minutes in children and in adults, respectively. Metabolites of mercaptopurine appear in urine within 2 hours after administration. After 24 hours, > 50% of a dose can be recovered in the urine as intact drug and metabolites.

Indications:

For remission induction and maintenance therapy of acute lymphatic leukemia. Response to mercaptopurine depends upon the subclassification of acute lymphatic leukemia and age of patient (child or adult).

Acute lymphatic (lymphocytic, lymphoblastic) leukemia: Given as a single agent, mercaptopurine induces complete remission in ≈ 25% of children and 10% of adults. Reliance upon mercaptopurine alone is not justified for initial remission induction of acute lymphatic leukemia since combination chemotherapy with vincristine, prednisone and L-asparaginase results in more frequent complete remission induction than with mercaptopurine alone or in combination. The duration of complete remission induced in acute lymphatic leukemia is so brief without the use of maintenance therapy that some form of drug therapy is considered essential. Mercaptopurine, as a single agent, is capable of significantly prolonging complete remission duration; however, combination therapy has produced remission duration longer than that achieved with mercaptopurine alone.

Acute myelogenous (and acute myelomonocytic) leukemia: As a single agent, mercaptopurine will induce complete remission in approximately 10% of children and adults. These results are inferior to those achieved with combination chemotherapy.

Contraindications:

Prior resistance to this drug. There is usually complete cross-resistance between mercaptopurine and thioguanine.

Mercaptopurine is not effective for prophylaxis or treatment of CNS leukemia, chronic lymphatic leukemia, the lymphomas (including Hodgkin's disease) or solid tumors.

Warnings:

Bone marrow toxicity: The most consistent dose-related toxicity is bone marrow suppression. It may be manifested by anemia, leukopenia or thrombocytopenia. This may also indicate progression of the underlying disease. Patients should report any fever, sore throat, signs of local infection, bleeding from any site or symptoms suggestive of anemia. Since mercaptopurine may have a delayed effect, withdraw medication temporarily at the first sign of an abnormally large fall in any formed blood elements. Toxic effects are often unavoidable during the induction phase of adult acute leukemia if remission induction is to be successful. Whether these effects demand modifying or ceasing dosage depends upon both the response of the underlying disease and availability of supportive facilities. Life-threatening infections and bleeding have occurred as a result of granulocytopenia and thrombocytopenia. Supportive therapy with platelet transfusions for bleeding, and antibiotics and granulocyte transfusions for sepsis, may be required.

The induction of complete remission of acute lymphatic leukemia frequently is associated with marrow hypoplasia. Maintenance of remission generally involves multiple drug regimens whose component agents cause myelosuppression. Anemia, leukopenia and thrombocytopenia are frequently observed. Dosages and schedules are adjusted to prevent life-threatening cytopenias.

(Warnings continued on following page)

MERCAPTOPURINE (6-Mercaptopurine; 6-MP) (Cont.)

Warnings (Cont.):

Bone marrow toxicity (Cont.):

If it is not the intent to induce bone marrow hypoplasia, discontinue the drug temporarily at the first evidence of any abnormally large fall in white blood cell (WBC) count, platelet count or hemoglobin concentration. With severe depression of the formed elements of the blood due to mercaptopurine, the bone marrow may appear hypoplastic or normocellular on aspiration or biopsy.

Evaluate hemoglobin or hematocrit, total WBC, differential counts and platelet counts weekly during therapy. Where the cause of fluctuation in the formed elements in the peripheral blood is obscure, bone marrow examination may help evaluate marrow status. Base the decision to continue mercaptopurine on the absolute hematologic values and the rate at which changes occur in these values, particularly during the induction phase of acute leukemia. Perform complete blood counts more frequently than once a week to evaluate therapeutic effect. Dosage may need to be reduced when combined with other drugs whose primary or secondary toxicity is myelosuppression.

Hepatotoxicity occurs with greatest frequency when doses of 2.5 mg/kg/day are exceeded. Deaths have occurred from hepatic necrosis. The histologic pattern includes both intrahepatic cholestasis and parenchymal cell necrosis, either of which may predominate. It is not clear how much hepatic damage is due to direct toxicity from the drug and how much may be due to a hypersensitivity reaction.

Published reports cite widely varying incidences of overt hepatotoxicity. In patients with various neoplastic diseases, mercaptopurine was given orally in doses ranging from 2.5 to 5 mg/kg without any hepatotoxicity. No definite clinical evidence of liver damage could be ascribed to the drug, although an occasional case of serum hepatitis occurred in patients receiving 6-MP who previously had transfusions. In smaller cohorts of adult and pediatric leukemic patients, the incidence of hepatotoxicity ranged from 0% to 6%. In one report, jaundice occurred more frequently (40%), especially when doses exceeded 2.5 mg/kg.

Usually, clinically detectable jaundice appears early in treatment (1 to 2 months), but has occurred from 1 week to 8 years after the start of treatment. In some patients, jaundice cleared following withdrawal of the drug and reappeared with reintroduction.

Monitoring of serum transaminase, alkaline phosphatase and bilirubin levels may allow early detection of hepatotoxicity. Monitor at weekly intervals when beginning therapy and at monthly intervals thereafter. More frequent liver function tests may be advisable in patients receiving other hepatotoxic drugs or with known preexisting liver disease. Approach all combination therapy involving mercaptopurine with caution. The combination of mercaptopurine with doxorubicin was hepatotoxic in 19 of 20 patients undergoing remission induction therapy for leukemia resistant to previous therapy.

Hepatotoxicity has been associated with anorexia, jaundice, diarrhea and ascites. Hepatic encephalopathy has occurred. The onset of clinical jaundice, hepatomegaly or anorexia with tenderness in the right hypochondrium are immediate indications for withholding mercaptopurine until the exact etiology can be identified. Likewise, any evidence of deterioration in liver function, toxic hepatitis or biliary stasis should prompt discontinuation and a search for an etiology of hepatotoxicity.

Immunosuppression may be manifested by decreased cellular hypersensitivities and impaired allograft rejection. Immunity to infectious agents or vaccines will be subnormal. The degree of immunosuppression depends on antigen dose and temporal relationship to drug. Carefully consider with regard to intercurrent infections and risk of subsequent neoplasia.

Renal function impairment: Start with smaller doses due to the possibility of slower drug elimination and a greater cumulative effect.

Mutagenesis/Carcinogenesis: Mercaptopurine causes chromosomal aberrations in humans. Carcinogenic potential exists in humans, but risk is unknown.

Pregnancy: Category D. Mercaptopurine can cause fetal harm when administered to a pregnant woman. Women receiving the drug in the first trimester of pregnancy have an increased incidence of abortion; the risk of malformation in offspring surviving first trimester exposure is not known. In a series of 28 women receiving mercaptopurine after the first trimester, three mothers died undelivered, one delivered a stillborn child and one aborted; there were no cases of macroscopically abnormal fetuses. Use during pregnancy, especially the first trimester, only if the benefit justifies the risk to the fetus. The drug's effect on fertility is unknown. There are no adequate and well controlled studies in pregnant women. Inform patient of potential hazard to the fetus. Advise women of childbearing potential to avoid becoming pregnant.

Lactation: It is not known whether mercaptopurine is excreted in breast milk. Because of potential for serious adverse reactions in nursing infants, decide whether to discontinue nursing or the drug, taking into account the importance of the drug to the mother.

(Continued on following page)

MERCAPTOPURINE (6-Mercaptopurine; 6-MP) (Cont.)

Precautions:

Pancreatitis: An increased risk of pancreatitis may be associated with the investigational use of mercaptopurine in inflammatory bowel disease.

Drug Interactions:

Allopurinol: When administered concomitantly with mercaptopurine, reduce mercaptopurine to ⅓ to ¼ the usual dose. Failure to observe this dosage reduction will result in a delayed catabolism of mercaptopurine and the likelihood of severe toxicity.

Trimethoprim-sulfamethoxazole: When coadministered with mercaptopurine, enhanced marrow suppression has occurred.

Adverse Reactions:

Bone marrow toxicity and hepatotoxicity: See Warnings.

Oral lesions are rare and resemble thrush rather than antifolic ulcerations.

GI ulceration has occurred. Nausea, vomiting and anorexia are uncommon during initial administration. Mild diarrhea and sprue-like symptoms have been noted, but it is difficult to attribute these to the medication.

Hyperuricemia occurs as a consequence of rapid cell lysis accompanying the antineoplastic effect. Minimize adverse effects by increasing hydration, urine alkalinization and the prophylactic administration of allopurinol (see Drug Interactions).

Dermatologic reactions can occur as a consequence of disease; however, mercaptopurine may cause skin rashes and hyperpigmentation.

Drug fever has occurred rarely with mercaptopurine. Exclude the more common causes of pyrexia, such as sepsis, in patients with acute leukemia.

Overdosage:

Discontinue the drug immediately when toxicity develops. If a patient is seen immediately following overdosage of the drug, induced emesis may be useful.

Signs and symptoms of overdosage may be immediate (anorexia, nausea, vomiting, diarrhea) or delayed (myelosuppression, liver dysfunction and gastroenteritis). Dialysis cannot be expected to clear mercaptopurine. Hemodialysis is of marginal use due to the rapid intracellular incorporation of mercaptopurine into active metabolites with long persistence. There is no known pharmacologic antagonist of mercaptopurine.

Patient Information:

Contraceptive measures are recommended during therapy for men and women.

Notify physician if fever, sore throat, chills, nausea, vomiting, unusual bleeding or bruising, yellow discoloration of the skin or eyes, abdominal pain, flank or joint pain, swelling of the feet or legs, or symptoms suggestive of anemia occurs.

May cause diarrhea, fever and weakness; notify physician if these become pronounced.

Maintain adequate fluid intake.

Administration and Dosage:

Induction therapy: Individualize dosage.

Usual initial dose is 2.5 mg/kg/day (100 to 200 mg in the average adult and 50 mg in an average 5-year-old). Children with acute leukemia tolerate this dose without difficulty in most cases. Continue daily for several weeks or more. If, after 4 weeks on this dosage there is no clinical improvement and no definite evidence of leukocyte or platelet depression, increase dosage up to 5 mg/kg/day.

A dosage of 2.5 mg/kg/day may result in a rapid fall in leukocyte count within 1 to 2 weeks in some adults with acute lymphatic leukemia and high total leukocyte counts.

Daily dosage may be given at one time. Calculate to the closest multiple of 25 mg.

Monitor the leukocyte count closely; because the drug may have a delayed action, discontinue treatment at the first sign of an abnormally large or rapid fall in leukocyte count or platelet count. If the leukocyte count or platelet count subsequently remains constant for 2 or 3 days, or rises, resume treatment.

Maintenance therapy: If complete hematologic remission is obtained with mercaptopurine alone or in combination with other agents, maintenance therapy is essential. Maintenance doses vary from patient to patient. Usual daily dose – 1.5 to 2.5 mg/kg/day as a single dose. In children with acute lymphatic leukemia in remission, superior results have been obtained when mercaptopurine has been combined with other agents (most frequently with methotrexate) for remission maintenance. Mercaptopurine should rarely be relied upon as a single agent for maintenance of remissions induced in acute leukemia.

Rx	**Purinethol** (Burroughs Wellcome)	**Tablets:** 50 mg	(Purinethol O4A). Off-white, scored. In 25s and 250s.

THIOGUANINE (TG; 6-Thioguanine)

Actions:

Thioguanine, an analog of the nucleic acid constituent guanine, is closely related structurally and functionally to 6-mercaptopurine.

Pharmacology: Thioguanine competes with hypoxanthine and guanine for the enzyme hypoxanthine-guanine phosphoribosyltransferase (HGPRTase) and is converted to 6-thioguanylic acid (TGMP). TGMP interferes at several points with the synthesis of guanine nucleotides. It inhibits *de novo* purine biosynthesis by inhibiting glutamine-5-phosphoribosylpyrophosphate amidotransferase. Thioguanine nucleotides are incorporated into both RNA and DNA by phosphodiester linkages and incorporation of such fraudulent bases may contribute to the cytotoxicity of thioguanine.

Thioguanine has multiple metabolic effects. Its tumor inhibitory properties may be due to one or more of its effects on feedback inhibition of *de novo* purine synthesis; inhibition of purine nucleotide interconversions; incorporation into DNA and RNA. The net consequence of its actions is a sequential blockade of the synthesis and utilization of the purine nucleotides.

Resistance may result from the loss of HGPRTase activity (inability to convert thioguanine to TGMP) or increased catabolism of TGMP by a nonspecific phosphatase. Although variable, cross-resistance with mercaptopurine usually occurs.

Pharmacokinetics: Oral absorption averages 30% (14% to 46%). Following oral administration of ^{35}S-6-thioguanine, total plasma radioactivity reached a maximum at 8 hours and declined slowly thereafter.

Intravenous administration of ^{35}S-6-thioguanine disclosed a median plasma half-life of 80 minutes (25 to 240 minutes) when the compound was given in single doses of 65 to 300 mg/m^2. There was no correlation between the plasma half-life and the dose. Thioguanine does not appear to reach therapeutic concentrations in the CSF.

The catabolism of thioguanine and its metabolites is complex. Only trace quantities of parent drug are excreted in the urine. However, a methylated metabolite unaffected by allopurinol, MTG, appeared very early, rose to a maximum 6 to 8 hours after drug administration, and was still being excreted after 12 to 22 hours. Radiolabeled sulfate appeared somewhat later than MTG, but was the principal metabolite after 8 hours. Thiouric acid and some unidentified products were found in the urine in small amounts.

Indications:

Acute nonlymphocytic leukemias: Remission induction, consolidation and maintenance therapy of acute nonlymphocytic leukemias. Response depends upon the age of the patient (younger patients faring better than older) and previous treatment. Reliance upon thioguanine alone is seldom justified for initial remission induction of acute nonlymphocytic leukemias because combination chemotherapy including thioguanine results in more frequent remission induction and longer duration of remission than thioguanine alone.

Other neoplasms: Thioguanine is not effective in chronic lymphocytic leukemia, Hodgkin's lymphoma, multiple myeloma or solid tumors. Although thioguanine is one of several agents with activity in the treatment of the chronic phase of chronic myelogenous leukemia, more objective responses are observed with **busulfan;** therefore busulfan is usually regarded as the preferred drug.

Contraindications:

Prior resistance to this drug. There is usually complete cross-resistance between mercaptopurine and thioguanine.

(Continued on following page)

THIOGUANINE (TG; 6-Thioguanine) (Cont.)

Warnings:

Bone marrow suppression may be manifested by anemia, leukopenia or thrombocytopenia. Any of these may also reflect progression of the underlying disease. Instruct patients to report promptly any fever, sore throat, jaundice, nausea, vomiting, signs of local infection, bleeding from any site or symptoms suggestive of anemia. Since thioguanine may have a delayed effect, withdraw the medication temporarily at the first sign of an abnormally large fall in any of the formed elements of the blood.

Evaluate hemoglobin concentration or hematocrit, total white blood cell (WBC) and differential counts and quantitative platelet count frequently during therapy. Where the cause of fluctuation in the formed elements in the peripheral blood is obscure, bone marrow examination may help evaluate marrow status. Base the decision to change thioguanine dosage on the absolute and rate of change of hematologic values. During the induction phase of acute leukemia, perform CBCs more frequently to evaluate therapeutic effect. The thioguanine dosage may need to be reduced when combined with other myelosuppressive drugs.

Myelosuppression is often unavoidable during the induction phase of adult acute leukemia if remission response is to be successful. Whether this demands modification or cessation of dosage depends upon both the response of the underlying disease and availability of supportive facilities. Life-threatening infections and bleeding have occurred as a result of thioguanine-induced granulocytopenia and thrombocytopenia.

Carcinogenesis and mutagenesis: Thioguanine is potentially mutagenic and carcinogenic; consider risk of carcinogenesis when administering thioguanine.

Pregnancy: Category D. Drugs such as thioguanine are potential mutagens and teratogens. Thioguanine may cause fetal harm when administered to a pregnant woman. Thioguanine is teratogenic in rats at doses 5 times the human dose. When given to the rat on the 4th and 5th days of gestation, 13% of surviving placentas did not contain fetuses; 19% of offspring were malformed or stunted. Malformations included generalized edema, cranial defects and general skeletal hypoplasia, hydrocephalus, ventral hernia, situs inversus and incomplete limb development. There are no adequate and well controlled studies in pregnant women. Inform patient of the potential hazard to the fetus. Advise women of childbearing potential to avoid becoming pregnant.

Lactation: It is not known whether this drug is excreted in breast milk. Because of the potential for tumorigenicity, decide whether to discontinue nursing or to discontinue the drug, taking into account the importance of the drug to the mother.

Precautions:

Although the primary toxicity of thioguanine is myelosuppresion, other toxicities occasionally occur, particularly when thioguanine is used in combination with other cancer chemotherapeutic agents.

Hepatotoxicity: Jaundice has occurred. Among these were two adult males and four children with acute myelogenous leukemia, and an adult male with acute lymphocytic leukemia who developed veno-occlusive hepatic disease while receiving chemotherapy. Six patients had received cytarabine prior to treatment with thioguanine, and some were receiving other chemotherapy in addition to thioguanine when they became symptomatic. Withhold thioguanine if there is evidence of toxic hepatitis, biliary stasis, clinical jaundice, hepatomegaly or anorexia with tenderness in the right hypochondrium. Initiate appropriate clinical and laboratory investigations to establish the etiology of the hepatic dysfunction.

Monitor liver function tests (serum transaminases, alkaline phosphatase, bilirubin) at weekly intervals when first beginning therapy and at monthly intervals thereafter. More frequent liver function tests may be advisable in patients with preexisting liver disease or who are receiving other hepatotoxic drugs. Instruct patients to discontinue thioguanine immediately if clinical jaundice is detected. If deterioration in liver function studies during thioguanine therapy occurs promptly discontinue treatment and search for an explanation of the hepatotoxicity.

(Continued on following page)

THIOGUANINE (TG; 6-Thioguanine) (Cont.)

Adverse Reactions:

Bone marrow toxicity and hepatotoxicity: See Warnings and Precautions.

Myelosuppression is the most frequent adverse reaction to thioguanine. Induction of complete remission of acute myelogenous leukemia usually requires combination chemotherapy in dosages which produce marrow hypoplasia. Since consolidation and maintenance of remission are also affected by multiple drug regimens whose component agents cause myelosuppression, pancytopenia is observed in nearly all patients.

GI: Nausea, vomiting, anorexia and stomatitis may occur. Intestinal necrosis and perforation have also occurred in patients who received multiple drug chemotherapy including thioguanine.

Hyperuricemia frequently occurs as a consequence of rapid cell lysis accompanying the antineoplastic effect. Minimize adverse effects by increasing hydration, urine alkalinization and the prophylactic administration of allopurinol. Unlike mercaptopurine and azathioprine, continue thioguanine in the usual dosage when allopurinol is used concurrently to inhibit uric acid formation.

Overdosage:

Discontinue immediately if unintended toxicity occurs during treatment. Severe hematologic toxicity may require supportive therapy with platelet transfusions for bleeding, and granulocyte transfusions and antibiotics if sepsis is documented.

If a patient is seen immediately following an acute overdosage, induced emesis may be useful. Signs and symptoms of overdosage may be immediate (nausea, vomiting, malaise, hypertension, diaphoresis) or delayed (myelosuppression and azotemia). Hemodialysis is of marginal use due to the rapid intracellular incorporation of active thioguanine metabolites with long persistence. Symptoms of overdosage may occur after a single dose of as little as 2 to 3 mg/kg thioguanine. As much as 35 mg/kg has been given in a single oral dose with reversible myelosuppression observed. There is no known pharmacologic antagonist of thioguanine.

Patient Information:

Notify physician if fever, chills, nausea, vomiting, sore throat, unusual bleeding or bruising, yellow discoloration of the skin or eyes, swelling of the feet or legs, or abdominal pain or joint or flank pain occurs.

May cause diarrhea, fever and weakness. Notify physician if these become pronounced.

Drink plenty of liquids while taking this drug.

Contraceptive measures are recommended during therapy for men and women.

Administration and Dosage:

Individualize dosage.

Initial dosage for children and adults: 2 mg/kg/day orally. If after 4 weeks, there is no clinical improvement and no leukocyte or platelet depression, the dosage may be cautiously increased to 3 mg/kg/day. The total daily dose may be given at one time.

Combination therapy: Of 163 children with previously untreated acute nonlymphocytic leukemia, 96 (59%) obtained complete remission with a multiple-drug protocol including thioguanine, prednisone, cytarabine, cyclophosphamide and vincristine. Remission was maintained with daily thioguanine, 4 day pulses of cytarabine and cyclophosphamide, and a single dose of vincristine every 28 days. The median duration of remission was 11.5 months. Of previously untreated adults with acute nonlymphocytic leukemias, 53% attained remission following use of the combination of thioguanine and cytarabine. A median duration of remission of 8.8 months was achieved with the multiple-drug maintenance regimen which included thioguanine.

Concomitant therapy: In contrast to mercaptopurine or azathioprine, the dosage of thioguanine does not need to be reduced during coadministration of allopurinol. See Adverse Reactions.

Rx	**Thioguanine** (Burroughs Wellcome)	**Tablets:** 40 mg	(Wellcome U3B). Greenish-yellow, scored. In 25s.

FLUDARABINE PHOSPHATE

Warning:

Administer fludarabine under the supervision of a qualified physician experienced in the use of antineoplastic therapy. Fludarabine can severely suppress bone marrow function. When used at high doses in dose-ranging studies in patients with acute leukemia, fludarabine was associated with severe neurologic effects, including blindness, coma and death. This severe CNS toxicity occurred in 36% of patients treated with doses approximately four times greater (96 mg/m²/day for 5 to 7 days) than the recommended dose. Similar severe CNS toxicity has rarely occurred (≤ 0.2%) in patients treated at doses in the range of the dose recommended for chronic lymphocytic leukemia.

Actions:

Fludarabine was approved by the FDA in April 1991.

Pharmacology: Fludarabine is a fluorinated nucleotide analog of the antiviral agent vidarabine that is relatively resistant to deamination by adenosine deaminase. Fludarabine is rapidly dephosphorylated to 2-fluoro-ara-A and then phosphorylated intracellularly by deoxycytidine kinase to the active triphosphate, 2-fluoro-ara-ATP. This metabolite appears to act by inhibiting DNA polymerase alpha, ribonucleotide reductase and DNA primase, thus inhibiting DNA synthesis. The mechanism of action of this antimetabolite is not completely characterized and may be multi-faceted.

Pharmacokinetics: Fludarabine is rapidly converted to the active metabolite, 2-fluoro-ara-A, within minutes after IV infusion. Consequently, clinical pharmacology studies have focused on 2-fluoro-ara-A pharmacokinetics. In a study with 4 patients treated with 25 mg/m²/day for 5 days, the half-life of 2-fluoro-ara-A was ≈ 10 hours. The mean total plasma clearance was 8.9 L/hr/m² and the mean volume of distribution was 98 L/m². Approximately 23% of the dose was excreted in the urine as unchanged 2-fluoro-ara-A. The mean maximum concentration after the day 1 dose was 0.57 mcg/ml and after the day 5 dose was 0.54 mcg/ml. Total body clearance of 2-fluoro-ara-A is inversely correlated with serum creatinine, suggesting renal elimination of the compound. A correlation was noted between the degree of absolute granulocyte count nadir and increased area under the concentration-time curve (AUC).

Clinical trials: Two single-arm open-label studies have been conducted in patients with chronic lymphocytic leukemia (CLL) refractory to at least one prior standard alkylating agent-containing regimen.

Fludarabine Efficacy in Refractory CLL Patients

Parameter	Studies	
	MDAH[1] (n = 48)	SWOG[2] (n = 31)
Overall objective response	48%	32%
Complete response	13%	13%
Partial response	35%	19%
Median time to response	7 weeks (range, 1 to 68)	21 weeks (range, 1 to 53)
Median duration of disease control	91 weeks	65 weeks
Median survival	43 weeks	52 weeks

[1] M.D. Anderson Cancer Center. Dosage: 22 to 40 mg/m²/day for 5 days every 28 days.

[2] Southwest Oncology Group. Dosage: 15 to 25 mg/m²/day for 5 days every 28 days.

The ability of fludarabine to induce a significant rate of response in refractory patients suggests minimal cross-resistance with commonly used anti-CLL agents.

Rai stage improved to Stage II or better in 7 of 12 MDAH responders (58%) and in 5 of 7 SWOG responders (71%) who were Stage III or IV at baseline. In the combined studies, mean hemoglobin concentration improved from 9 g/dl at baseline to 11.8 g/dl at the time of response in a subgroup of anemic patients. Similarly, average platelet count improved from 63,500/mm³ to 103,300/mm³ at the time of response in a subgroup of patients who were thrombocytopenic at baseline.

(Continued on following page)

FLUDARABINE PHOSPHATE (Cont.)

Indications:

Chronic lymphocytic leukemia (CLL): Treatment of patients with B-cell CLL who have not reponded to or have progressed during treatment with at least one standard alkylating agent-containing regimen.

The safety and efficacy in previously untreated or non-refractory patients with CLL have not been established.

Unlabeled uses: Fludarabine may also be useful in the treatment of non-Hodgkin's lymphoma, macroglobulinemic lymphoma, prolymphocytic leukemia or prolymphocytoid variant of CLL, mycosis fungoides, hairy-cell leukemia and Hodgkin's disease. Further study is needed to determine efficacy and dosage.

Contraindications:

Hypersensitivity to this drug or its components.

Warnings:

Dose-dependent toxicity (see boxed Warning): There are clear dose-dependent toxic effects seen with fludarabine. Dose levels ≈ 4 times greater (96 mg/m²/day for 5 to 7 days) than those recommended for CLL (25 mg/m²/day for 5 days) were associated with a syndrome characterized by delayed blindness, coma and death. Symptoms appeared from 21 to 60 days following the last dose. Thirteen of 36 patients (36%) who received high doses (96 mg/m²/day for 5 to 7 days) developed this severe neurotoxicity. This syndrome has been reported rarely in patients treated with doses in the range of the recommended CLL dose of 25 mg/m²/day for 5 days every 28 days. The effect of chronic administration on the CNS is unknown; however, patients have received the recommended dose for up to 15 courses of therapy.

Severe bone marrow suppression, notably anemia, thrombocytopenia and neutropenia, has occurred in patients treated with fludarabine. In solid tumor patients, the median time to nadir counts was 13 days (range, 3 to 25 days) for granulocytes and 16 days (range, 2 to 32) for platelets. Most patients had hematologic impairment at baseline either as a result of disease or as a result of prior myelosuppressive therapy. Cumulative myelosuppression may be seen. While chemotherapy-induced myelosuppression is often reversible, administration of fludarabine requires careful hematologic monitoring.

Renal insufficiency: Administer cautiously. The total body clearance of 2-fluoro-ara-A is inversely correlated with serum creatinine, suggesting renal elimination of the compound.

Mutagenesis: Chromosomal aberrations were observed in an in vitro assay. In addition, fludarabine was determined to cause increased sister chromatid exchanges in vitro.

Fertility impairment: Studies in mice, rats and dogs have demonstrated dose-related adverse effects on the male reproductive system. Observations consisted of a decrease in mean testicular weights in mice and rats with a trend toward decreased testicular weights in dogs and degeneration and necrosis of spermatogenic epithelium of the testes in mice, rats and dogs.

Pregnancy: Category D. Fludarabine may cause fetal harm when administered to a pregnant woman. Fludarabine was teratogenic in rats and rabbits. At 10 and 30 mg/kg/day in rats, there was an increased incidence of various skeletal malformations; dose-related teratogenic effects manifested by external deformities and skeletal malformations were observed in rabbits at 5 and 8 mg/kg/day. There are no adequate and well controlled studies in pregnant women. If fludarabine is used during pregnancy, or if the patient becomes pregnant while taking this drug, apprise her of the potential hazard to the fetus. Advise women of childbearing potential to avoid becoming pregnant.

Lactation: It is not known whether this drug is excreted in breast milk. Decide whether to discontinue nursing or to discontinue the drug, taking into account the importance of the drug to the mother.

Children: Safety and efficacy have not been established.

(Continued on following page)

FLUDARABINE PHOSPHATE (Cont.)

Precautions:

Hematologic toxicity: Fludarabine is a potent antineoplastic agent with potentially significant toxic side effects. Closely observe patients for signs of hematologic and nonhematologic toxicity. Periodic assessment of peripheral blood counts is recommended to detect the development of anemia, neutropenia and thrombocytopenia.

Tumor lysis syndrome associated with fludarabine treatment has occured in CLL patients with large tumor burdens. Since fludarabine can induce a response as early as the first week of treatment, take precautions in patients at risk of developing this complication.

Monitoring: During treatment, monitor the patient's hematologic profile (particularly neutrophils and platelets) regularly to determine the degree of hematopoietic suppression.

Adverse Reactions:

The most common adverse events include myelosuppression (neutropenia, thrombocytopenia and anemia), fever and chills, infection, and nausea and vomiting. Other commonly reported events include malaise, fatigue, anorexia and weakness. Serious opportunistic infections have occurred in CLL patients treated with fludarabine. The most frequently reported adverse events and those reactions which are more clearly related to the drug are arranged below according to body system.

Hematopoietic: Hematologic events (neutropenia, thrombocytopenia or anemia) were reported in the majority of CLL patients (see Warnings). During treatment of 133 patients with CLL, the absolute neutrophil count decreased to $< 500/mm^3$ in 59% of patients, hemoglobin decreased from pretreatment values by at least 2 g% in 60%, and platelet count decreased from pretreatment values by at least 50% in 55% of patients. Myelosuppression may be severe and cumulative. Bone marrow fibrosis occurred in one CLL patient.

Metabolic: Tumor lysis syndrome, which may include hyperuricemia, hyperphosphatemia, hypocalcemia, metabolic acidosis, hyperkalemia, hematuria, urate crystalluria and renal failure. The onset of this syndrome may be heralded by flank pain and hematuria. See Precautions.

CNS (see Warnings): Objective weakness, agitation, confusion, visual disturbances, coma (at the recommended dose); peripheral neuropathy; wrist-drop (one case).

Pulmonary: Pneumonia (16% to 22%; a frequent manifestation of infection in CLL patients); pulmonary hypersensitivity reactions characterized by dyspnea, cough and interstitial pulmonary infiltrate.

GI: Nausea; vomiting; anorexia; diarrhea; stomatitis; GI bleeding.

Cardiovascular: Edema (frequent); pericardial effusion (one patient).

Dermatologic: Skin toxicity, consisting primarily of skin rashes.

(Adverse Reactions continued on following page)

FLUDARABINE PHOSPHATE (Cont.)

Adverse Reactions (Cont.):

Fludarabine Adverse Reactions in the MDAH and SWOG Studies (%)

Adverse reaction	MDAH (n = 101)	SWOG (n = 32)
Any adverse reaction	88	91
Body as a whole	72	84
Fever	60	69
Chills	11	19
Fatigue	10	38
Infection	33	44
Pain	20	22
Malaise	8	6
Diaphoresis	1	13
Alopecia	0	3
Anaphylaxis	1	0
Hemorrhage	1	0
Hyperglycemia	1	6
Dehydration	1	0
Neurological	21	69
Weakness	9	65
Paresthesia	4	12
Headache	3	0
Visual disturbance	3	15
Hearing loss	2	6
Sleep disorder	1	3
Depression	1	0
Cerebellar syndrome	1	0
Impaired mentation	1	0
Pulmonary	35	69
Cough	10	44
Pneumonia	16	22
Dyspnea	9	22
Sinusitis	5	0
Pharyngitis	0	9
Upper respiratory infection	2	16
Allergic pneumonitis	0	6
Epistaxis	1	0
Hemoptysis	1	6
Bronchitis	1	0
Hypoxia	1	0
GI	46	63
Nausea/Vomiting	36	31
Diarrhea	15	13
Anorexia	7	34
Stomatitis	9	0
GI bleeding	3	13
Esophagitis	3	0
GI (Cont.)		
Mucositis	2	0
Liver failure	1	0
Abnormal liver function test	1	3
Cholelithiasis	0	3
Constipation	1	3
Dysphagia	1	0
Cutaneous	17	18
Rash	15	15
Pruritus	1	3
Seborrhea	1	0
GU	12	22
Dysuria	4	3
Urinary infection	2	15
Hematuria	2	3
Renal failure	1	0
Abnormal renal function test	1	0
Proteinuria	1	0
Hesitancy	0	3
Cardiovascular	12	38
Edema	8	19
Angina	0	6
Congestive heart failure	0	3
Arrhythmia	0	3
Supraventricular tachycardia	0	3
Myocardial infarction	0	3
Deep venous thrombosis	1	3
Phlebitis	1	3
Transient ischemic attack	1	0
Aneurysm	1	0
Cerebrovascular accident	0	3
Musculoskeletal	7	16
Myalgia	4	16
Osteoporosis	2	0
Arthralgia	1	0
Tumor lysis syndrome	1	0

(Continued on following page)

FLUDARABINE PHOSPHATE (Cont.)

Overdosage:

High doses are associated with an irreversible CNS toxicity characterized by delayed blindness, coma and death (see Warnings). High doses are also associated with severe thrombocytopenia and neutropenia due to bone marrow suppression. There is no known specific antidote for fludarabine overdosage. Treatment consists of drug discontinuation and supportive therapy. Refer to General Management of Acute Overdosage.

Administration and Dosage:

Usual dose: 25 mg/m² administered IV over a period of ≈ 30 minutes daily for 5 consecutive days. Commence each 5 day course of treatment every 28 days. Dosage may be decreased or delayed based on evidence of hematologic or nonhematologic toxicity. Physicians should consider delaying or discontinuing the drug if neurotoxicity occurs.

A number of clinical settings may predispose to increased toxicity including advanced age, renal insufficiency and bone marrow impairment. Monitor such patients closely for excessive toxicity and modify the dose accordingly.

Duration: The optimal duration of treatment has not been clearly established. It is recommended that three additional cycles be administered following the achievement of a maximal response and then discontinue the drug.

Preparation of solution: When reconstituted with 2 ml of Sterile Water for Injection, USP, the solid cake should fully dissolve in ≤ 15 seconds; each ml of the resulting solution will contain 25 mg fludarabine phosphate, 25 mg mannitol and sodium hydroxide to adjust the pH to 7.7. The pH range for the final product is 7.2 to 8.2. In clinical studies, the product has been diluted in 100 or 125 ml of 5% Dextrose Injection, USP or 0.9% Sodium Chloride, USP. Reconstituted fludarabine contains no antimicrobial preservative; use within 8 hours of reconstitution.

Handling and disposal: Consider procedures for proper handling and disposal according to guidelines issued for cytotoxic drugs. If the solution contacts the skin or mucous membranes, wash thoroughly with soap and water; rinse eyes thoroughly with plain water. Avoid exposure by inhalation or by direct contact of the skin or mucous membranes.

Storage: Store under refrigeration, between 2° to 8°C (36° to 46°F).

Rx	**Fludara** (Berlex)	**Powder for reconstitution (lyophilized):** 50 mg[1]	In single dose vial (6 ml capacity).

[1] With 50 mg mannitol and sodium hydroxide.

This is an abbreviated monograph. For complete information on Androgens, see the group monograph in the Hormones chapter.

Androgens

TESTOLACTONE

Actions:

The precise mechanism by which testolactone produces a clinical antineoplastic effect is unknown. Testolactone's principal action appears to be inhibition of steroid aromatase activity and consequent reduction in estrone synthesis from adrenal androstenedione, the major source of estrogen in postmenopausal women. Based on in vitro studies, the aromatase inhibition may be noncompetitive and irreversible. This phenomenon may account for the persistence of testolactone's effect on estrogen synthesis after drug withdrawal.

Pharmacology: Testolactone is effective in 15% of patients with advanced or disseminated mammary cancer.

Testolactone is well absorbed from the GI tract. It is metabolized to several derivatives in the liver, all of which preserve the lactone D-ring. These metabolites, as well as some unmetabolized drug, are excreted in the urine. Additional pharmacokinetic data in humans are unavailable.

Indications:

Adjunctive therapy in the palliative treatment of advanced disseminated breast carcinoma in postmenopausal women when hormonal therapy is indicated.

Premenopausal women with disseminated breast carcinoma in whom ovarian function has been subsequently terminated.

Contraindications:

Carcinoma of the male breast; hypersensitivity to the drug.

Warnings:

Pregnancy: Category C. Testolactone is intended for use in postmenopausal women and is not indicated for use during pregnancy.

Lactation: It is not known whether this drug is excreted in breast milk. Decide whether to discontinue nursing or to discontinue the drug, taking into account the importance of the drug to the mother.

Children: Safety and efficacy have not been established.

Precautions:

The usual precautions pertaining to use of androgens apply (see Androgen group monograph).

Consult the physician regarding missed doses.

Monitoring: Routinely monitor plasma calcium levels in any patient receiving therapy for mammary cancer, particularly during periods of active remission of bony metastases. If hypercalcemia occurs, institute appropriate measures.

Drug Interactions:

Anticoagulants, oral: Pharmacologic effects may be increased by testolactone; monitor and adjust the anticoagulant dose accordingly.

Drug/Lab test interactions: Physiologic effects of testolactone may result in decreased estradiol concentrations with radioimmunoassays for estradiol, increased plasma calcium concentrations and increased 24 hour urinary excretion of creatine and 17-ketosteroids.

Adverse Reactions:

GI: Glossitis; anorexia; nausea; vomiting.

CNS: Paresthesia.

Miscellaneous: Maculopapular erythema; aches and edema of the extremities; alopecia; nail growth disturbances (rare); increase in blood pressure.

Patient Information:

Notify physician if numbness or tingling of fingers, toes or face occurs.

Contraceptive measures are recommended during treatment.

Medication may cause diarrhea, loss of appetite, nausea, vomiting, loss of hair, swelling or redness of the tongue; notify physician if these become pronounced.

Administration and Dosage:

Administer 250 mg 4 times daily. To evaluate response, continue therapy for a minimum of 3 months, unless there is active disease progression.

Rx	**Teslac** (Squibb)	**Tablets:** 50 mg	(690). White. In 100s.

Antiandrogen

FLUTAMIDE

Actions:

Pharmacology: Flutamide, a nonsteroidal agent, demonstrates potent antiandrogenic effects in animal studies. It exerts its antiandrogenic action by inhibiting androgen uptake or by inhibiting nuclear binding of androgen in target tissues. Prostatic carcinoma is androgen-sensitive and responds to treatment that counteracts the effect of androgen or removes the source of androgen (eg, castration).

Pharmacokinetics: Analysis of plasma, urine and feces following a single oral 200 mg dose of tritium-labeled flutamide to human volunteers showed that the drug is rapidly and completely absorbed. It is excreted mainly in the urine with only 4.2% of the dose excreted in the feces over 72 hours. Flutamide is rapidly and extensively metabolized, with flutamide comprising only 2.5% of plasma radioactivity 1 hour after administration. At least six metabolites have been identified in plasma. The major plasma metabolite is a biologically active alpha-hydroxylated derivative that accounts for 23% of the plasma tritium 1 hour after drug administration.

Following a single 250 mg oral dose to healthy adult volunteers, low plasma levels of varying amounts of flutamide were detected. The biologically active alpha-hydroxylated metabolite reaches maximum plasma levels in about 2 hours, indicating that it is rapidly formed from flutamide. The plasma half-life for this metabolite is about 6 hours.

Following multiple oral dosing of 250 mg 3 times a day in healthy geriatric volunteers, flutamide and its active metabolite approached steady-state plasma levels (based on pharmacokinetic simulations) after the fourth flutamide dose. The half-life of the active metabolite in geriatric volunteers after a single flutamide dose is about 8 hours and at steady state is 9.6 hours.

Flutamide is 94% to 96% bound to plasma proteins at steady-state plasma concentrations of 24 to 78 ng/ml. The active metabolite of flutamide at steady-state plasma concentrations of 1556 to 2284 ng/ml is 92% to 94% bound to plasma proteins.

In male rats, neither flutamide nor any of its metabolites are preferentially accumulated in any tissue except the prostate after an oral 5 mg/kg dose. Total drug levels were highest 6 hours after drug administration in all tissues. Levels declined at roughly similar rates to low levels at 18 hours. The major metabolite was present at higher concentrations than flutamide in all tissues studied.

Elevations of plasma testosterone and estradiol levels have been noted following flutamide administration.

Clinical studies: Flutamide interferes with testosterone at the cellular level. This can complement medical castration achieved with leuprolide, which suppresses testicular androgen production by inhibiting luteinizing hormone secretion.

To study the effects of combination therapy, 617 patients (311 leuprolide + flutamide; 306 leuprolide + placebo) with previously untreated advanced prostatic carcinoma were enrolled in a large multicenter, controlled clinical trial.

Median survival had been reached 3.5 years after the study was initiated. The median actuarial survival time is 34.9 months for patients treated with leuprolide and flutamide versus 27.9 months for patients treated with leuprolide alone (a 25% improvement in overall survival with the flutamide therapy). Analysis of progression-free survival showed a 2.6 month improvement in patients who received leuprolide plus flutamide (a 19% increment over leuprolide and placebo).

Indications:

In combination with LHRH agonistic analogs (such as leuprolide acetate) for the treatment of metastatic prostatic carcinoma (stage D_2). To achieve the benefit of the adjunctive therapy, treatment must be started simultaneously using both drugs.

Contraindications:

Hypersensitivity to flutamide or any component of the preparation.

(Continued on following page)

FLUTAMIDE (Cont.)

Warnings:

Carcinogenesis, mutagenesis, impairment of fertility: Daily administration of flutamide to rats for 52 weeks at doses of 30, 90 or 180 mg/kg/day (approximately 3, 8 or 17 times the human dose) produced testicular interstitial cell adenomas at all doses.

Reduced sperm counts were observed during a 6 week study of flutamide monotherapy in healthy volunteers. Male rats treated with 150 mg/kg/day (30 times the minimum effective antiandrogenic dose) failed to mate; mating behavior returned to normal after dosing was stopped. Conception rates were decreased in all dosing groups. Suppression of spermatogenesis was observed in animals dosed for 52 to 78 weeks at 1.4 to 17 times the human dose.

Pregnancy: Category D. Flutamide may cause fetal harm when administered to a pregnant woman. There was decreased 24 hour survival in the offspring of rats treated with flutamide at doses of 30, 100 or 200 mg/kg/day (approximately 3, 9 and 19 times the human dose) during pregnancy. A slight increase in minor variations in the development of the sternebra and vertebra was seen in the fetuses of rats at the two higher doses. Feminization of the males also occurred at the two higher dose levels. There was a decreased survival rate in the offspring of rabbits receiving the highest dose (15 mg/kg/day; equal to 1.4 times the human dose).

Precautions:

Inform patients that flutamide and the drug used for medical castration should be administered concomitantly, and that they should not interrupt their dosing or stop taking these medications without consulting their physician.

Laboratory test monitoring: Consider periodic liver function tests in patients on long-term treatment with flutamide since transient abnormalities of transaminases have occurred; however, < 1% of the patients treated with the combination had transaminases greater than 5 to 10 times the normal values.

Adverse Reactions:

The following adverse experiences occurred during treatment with flutamide in combination with LHRH-agonists: Hot flashes (61%); loss of libido (36%); impotence (33%); diarrhea (12%); nausea/vomiting (11%); gynecomastia (9%); other GI disturbances (6%).

The most frequently occurring adverse experiences (hot flashes, impotence, loss of libido) were those associated with low serum androgen levels and that occur with LHRH-agonists alone. The only notable difference was the higher incidence of diarrhea in the flutamide plus LHRH-agonist group (12%), which was severe in 5% as opposed to the placebo plus LHRH agonist (4%), which was severe in < 1%.

Other (drug relationship not established):

CNS: Drowsiness, confusion, depression, anxiety, nervousness (1%).

GI: Diarrhea (12%); nausea/vomiting (11%); other GI reactions (6%).

Hematopoietic: Anemia (6%); leukopenia (3%); thrombocytopenia (1%); hemolytic and macrocytic anemia.

Hepatic: Hepatitis, jaundice (< 1%); cholestatic jaundice; hepatic encephalopathy; hepatic necrosis. These conditions were usually reversible after discontinuing therapy.

Dermatologic: Injection site irritation, rash (3%); photosensitivity (five patients).

Other: Gynecomastia (9%); edema, anorexia (4%); neuromuscular, GU symptoms (2%); hypertension (1%); pulmonary symptoms (< 1%).

Abnormal laboratory values: Elevated AST, ALT and bilirubin values (7 patients); elevated creatinine values (11 patients); elevated alpha-glutamyl transferase values.

Overdosage:

Symptoms: In animal studies with flutamide alone, signs of overdose included: Hypoactivity; piloerection; slow respiration; ataxia; lacrimation; anorexia; tranquilization; emesis.

Clinical trials have been conducted with flutamide in doses up to 1500 mg/day for periods up to 36 weeks with no serious adverse effects reported. Those adverse reactions reported included gynecomastia, breast tenderness and some increases in AST. The single dose of flutamide ordinarily associated with symptoms of overdose or considered to be life-threatening has not been established.

Treatment: Since flutamide is highly protein bound, dialysis may not be of any use. Induce vomiting if it does not occur spontaneously if the patient is alert. General supportive care, including frequent monitoring of the vital signs and close observation of the patient, is indicated. Refer to General Management of Acute Overdosage.

Administration and Dosage:

Two capsules 3 times a day at 8 hour intervals for a total daily dosage of 750 mg.

Rx	**Eulexin** (Schering)	**Capsules:** 125 mg	(Schering 525). Brown. In 100s, 500s and UD 100s.

Progestins

This is an abbreviated monograph. For complete information on progestins, see page 363

MEGESTROL ACETATE

> **Warning:**
> The use of megestrol is not recommended during the first 4 months of pregnancy.

Actions:

Pharmacology: The exact mechanism by which megestrol acetate produces its antineoplastic effects is unknown. An antiluteinizing effect mediated via the pituitary has been postulated. Evidence also suggests a local effect as a result of the marked changes from direct instillation of progestational agents into the endometrial cavity.

Indications:

Palliative treatment of advanced carcinoma of the breast or endometrium (ie, recurrent, inoperable or metastatic disease). Do not use instead of surgery, radiation or chemotherapy.

Unlabeled use: Megestrol is currently being studied for and appears effective as an appetite stimulant in HIV-related cachexia. The dosage used has been 80 mg 4 times daily; average weight gain was 0.5 kg/week.

Contraindications:

As a diagnostic test for pregnancy.

Warnings:

The use of megestrol acetate in other types of neoplastic disease is not recommended.

Pregnancy: The use of progestational agents during the first 4 months of pregnancy is not recommended. Reports suggest an association between intrauterine exposure to female sex hormones and congenital anomalies. The risk of hypospadias, 5 to 8 per 1,000 male births in the general population, may be approximately doubled with exposure to these drugs. There are insufficient data to quantify the risk to exposed female fetuses, but because some of these drugs induce mild virilization of external genitalia of the female fetus, and because of the increased association of hypospadias in the male fetus, it is prudent to avoid the use of these drugs during the first trimester.

If the patient is exposed to megestrol during the first 4 months of pregnancy or becomes pregnant while taking this drug, apprise her of potential risks to the fetus.

Precautions:

Use with caution in patients with a history of thrombophlebitis.

Adverse Reactions:

Weight gain is a frequent side effect of megestrol acetate. This effect has been associated with increased appetite, not necessarily with fluid retention.

Thromboembolic phenomena, including thrombophlebitis and pulmonary embolism have occurred rarely.

Other: Nausea/vomiting; edema; breakthrough bleeding; dyspnea; tumor flare (with or without hypercalcemia); hyperglycemia; alopecia; carpal tunnel syndrome; rash.

Patient Information:

Medication may cause back or abdominal pain, headache, nausea, vomiting or breast tenderness; notify physician if these effects become pronounced.

Contraceptive measures are recommended during therapy.

Administration and Dosage:

Breast cancer: 160 mg/day (40 mg 4 times daily).

Endometrial carcinoma: 40 to 320 mg/day in divided doses.

At least 2 months of continuous treatment is adequate for determining efficacy.

No serious side effects have resulted from studies involving megestrol acetate administered in dosages as high as 800 mg/day.

Rx	**Megestrol Acetate** (Various, eg, Balan, Bioline, Geneva, Goldline, Major, Moore, Parmed, PBI, Rugby, Schein)	**Tablets:** 20 mg	In 100s and UD 100s.
Rx	**Megace** (Mead Johnson Oncology)		Blue, scored. In 100s.
Rx	**Megestrol Acetate** (Various, eg, Balan, Bioline, Geneva, Goldline, Major, Moore, Parmed, Rugby, Schein, URL)	**Tablets:** 40 mg	In 100s, 250s, 500s and UD 100s.
Rx	**Megace** (Mead Johnson Oncology)		Blue, scored. In 100s, 250s and 500s.

This is an abbreviated monograph. For complete information on progestins, see page 363

MEDROXYPROGESTERONE ACETATE

Warning:
The use of medroxyprogesterone is not recommended during the first 4 months of pregnancy.

Actions:

Pharmacology: Administered parenterally in the recommended doses to women with adequate endogenous estrogen, it transforms proliferative endometrium into secretory endometrium. Medroxyprogesterone inhibits (in the usual dose range) the secretion of pituitary gonadotropin which, in turn, prevents follicular maturation and ovulation.

Indications:

Adjunctive therapy and palliative treatment of inoperable, recurrent and metastatic endometrial carcinoma or renal carcinoma.

Unlabeled uses: Depot medroxyprogesterone acetate has been used as a long-acting contraceptive (150 mg IM every 3 months or 450 mg every 6 months) and in the treatment of advanced breast cancer.

Contraindications:

Thrombophlebitis, thromboembolic disorders, stroke or patients with past history of these conditions; carcinoma of the breast; undiagnosed vaginal bleeding; missed abortion; known sensitivity to medroxyprogesterone acetate; as a diagnostic test for pregnancy.

Warnings:

Hepatic function impairment: Upon earliest manifestations of impaired liver function, discontinue the drug and re-evaluate the patient's status.

Pregnancy: The use of progestational agents during the first 4 months of pregnancy is not recommended. Several reports suggest an association between intrauterine exposure to female sex hormones and congenital anomalies. The risk of hypospadias, 5 to 8 per 1,000 male births in the general population, may be approximately doubled with exposure to progestational agents. There are insufficient data to quantify the risk to exposed female fetuses, but because some of these drugs induce mild virilization of the external genitalia of the female fetus, and because of the increased association of hypospadias in the male fetus, it is prudent to avoid the use of these drugs during the first trimester of pregnancy.

If the patient is exposed to medroxyprogesterone acetate during the first 4 months of pregnancy or if she becomes pregnant while taking this drug, she should be apprised of the potential risks to the fetus.

Lactation: Medroxyprogesterone does not adversely affect lactation; if breastfeeding is desired, it may be used safely. Milk production and duration of lactation may be increased if given in the puerperium.

Adverse Reactions:

Following repeated injections, amenorrhea and infertility may persist for up to 18 months and occasionally longer.

In a few instances there have been undesirable sequelae at the site of injection, such as residual lump, change in color of skin or sterile abscess.

Thromboembolic phenomena: Thrombophlebitis; pulmonary embolism.

CNS: Nervousness; insomnia; somnolence; fatigue; dizziness; headache (rare).

Skin and mucous membranes: Angioneurotic edema; pruritus; urticaria; generalized rash; acne; alopecia; hirsutism.

GI: Nausea (rare); jaundice, including neonatal jaundice.

Miscellaneous: Hyperpyrexia (rare); anaphylaxis.

Administration and Dosage:

For IM administration only.

Endometrial or renal carcinoma: Initially, 400 to 1000 mg IM per week. If improvement occurs within a few weeks or months and the disease appears stabilized, it may be possible to maintain improvement with as little as 400 mg/month.

Rx	**Depo-Provera** (Upjohn)	**Injection:** 100 mg per ml[1]	In 5 ml vials.
		400 mg per ml[2]	In 2.5 and 10 ml vials and 1 ml U-ject.

[1] With polyethylene glycol 3350, polysorbate 80 and parabens.
[2] With polyethylene glycol 3350, sodium sulfate anhydrous and myristyl-gamma-picolinium chloride.

Estrogens

In addition to the Estrogens discussed in the monograph beginning on page 350 diethylstilbestrol diphosphate and polyestradiol phosphate are specifically indicated in the palliative therapy of advanced prostatic carcinoma. For a complete discussion of the effects and uses of estrogens, refer to the general estrogen monograph beginning on page 350

Actions:

These agents are synthetic estrogens.

Pharmacology: Putative receptor proteins for estrogens have been detected in estrogen-responsive tissues. Estrogens are first bound to a cytoplasmic receptor protein. Following modification, the estrogen-protein complex is translocated to the nucleus where ultimate binding of the estrogen-containing complex occurs. As a result of such binding characteristic metabolic alterations ensue. In the male patient with androgenic hormone dependent conditions such as metastatic carcinoma of the prostate gland, estrogens counter the androgenic influence by competing for receptor sites. Metastatic bone lesions may also show improvement.

Pharmacokinetics: Metabolism and inactivation occur primarily in the liver. Some estrogens are excreted into the bile; however, they are reabsorbed from the intestine and returned to the liver through the portal venous system. Water soluble estrogen conjugates are strongly acidic and are ionized in body fluids, which favor excretion through the kidneys since tubular reabsorption is minimal.

Indications:

Inoperable, progressing prostatic cancer.

Diethylstilbestrol diphosphate is not indicated in the treatment of any disorder in women.

Estrogens should not be used in men with any of the following conditions:

Known or suspected cancer of the breast except in appropriately selected patients being treated for metastatic disease.

Known or suspected estrogen-dependent neoplasia.

Active thrombophlebitis or thromboembolic disorders.

Adverse Reactions:

Estrogen use has been associated with thrombophlebitis, pulmonary embolism, cerebral thrombosis and possibly coronary thrombosis.

Diethylstilbestrol has been associated with hepatic cutaneous porphyria, erythema nodosum and erythema multiforme.

Patient Information:

Medication may cause nausea, vomiting, headache, abdominal pain, painful swelling of breasts; notify physician if these become pronounced.

Diethylstilbestrol diphosphate should not be used by women.

Promptly report the following side effects: Bloating, loss of appetite, skin rash, mood changes, depression, nervousness, dizziness, chest pain, shortness of breath, numbness or tingling about the nose or mouth, fluid accumulation, disturbance in vision, frequent or painful urination, painful swelling of extremities.

Consult a physician regularly for evaluation of blood pressure and heart rate.

Diabetic patients should monitor urine very carefully. Test of blood sugar may be necessary as well.

DIETHYLSTILBESTROL DIPHOSPHATE

Administration and Dosage:

Oral: Initially, 50 mg 3 times daily; increase to ≥ 200 mg 3 times daily, depending on patient tolerance. Maximum daily dose not to exceed 1 g. If relief is not obtained with high oral doses, administer IV.

Parenteral: On the first day, give 0.5 g IV, dissolved in 250 ml of saline or 5% dextrose. On subsequent days give 1 g dissolved in ≈ 250 to 500 ml of saline or dextrose. Administer slowly (20 to 30 drops per minute) during the first 10 to 15 minutes and then adjust the flow rate so that the entire amount is given in 1 hour. Follow this procedure for ≥ 5 days, depending upon patient response. Following this first intensive course of therapy, administer 0.25 to 0.5 g in a similar manner once or twice weekly, or obtain maintenance with oral administration.

Stability of solution: After reconstitution, keep the solution at room temperature and away from direct light. Under these conditions the solution is stable for about 5 days, as long as cloudiness or evidence of a precipitate has not occurred.

Rx	**Stilphostrol** (Miles Inc.)	**Tablets:** 50 mg	(Miles 132). White to off-white with gray/tan mottling, scored. In 50s.
		Injection: 0.25 g (as sodium salt)	In 5 ml amps.

POLYESTRADIOL PHOSPHATE

Biologically active estradiol units are gradually split off from the large parent molecule to provide a continuous level of active estrogen over a prolonged period. The liberated estradiol is metabolized by the body in the same manner as the endogenous hormone.

There is no depot effect at the site of injection; 90% of the injected dose leaves the bloodstream within 24 hours. Passive storage occurs in the reticuloendothelial system. As circulating levels of estradiol drop, more returns to the bloodstream from the storage site for an even, continuous therapeutic effect. Increasing the dose acts to prolong the duration of pharmacologic action rather than increase blood levels.

Administration and Dosage:

Administer by deep IM injection only. Initially, some patients may experience a burning sensation at the injection site. This is transitory; it may not recur with subsequent injections, or it may be obviated by concomitant administration of a local anesthetic.

Inoperable progressing prostatic cancer: 40 mg IM every 2 to 4 weeks or less frequently, depending on patient response. If the response is not satisfactory, administer up to 80 mg. Increasing the dose prolongs the duration of action, but the amount of estrogen available at any one time is not significantly increased. Individualize dosage.

Response should occur within 3 months of beginning therapy. If response occurs, continue the hormone until the disease is again progressive. Then discontinue the hormone, and the patient may obtain another period of improvement known as "rebound regression." This occurs in 30% of the patients who show objective improvement on estrogens.

Preparation of solution: Introduce sterile diluent into the vial, preferably with a 20 gauge needle affixed to a 5 ml syringe. Swirl gently until a solution is effected. Do not agitate violently.

Stability and storage: After reconstitution, store solution at room temperature and away from direct light. The solution is stable for about 10 days, as long as cloudiness or evidence of a precipitate has not occurred.

Rx	**Estradurin** (Wyeth-Ayerst)	**Powder for Injection:** 40 mg per secule[1] with 2 ml ampul of sterile diluent.

[1] With 0.022 mg phenylmercuric nitrate, 25 mg niacinamide and 4 mg propylene glycol.

ESTRAMUSTINE PHOSPHATE SODIUM

Actions:

Estramustine phosphate combines estradiol and nornitrogen mustard by a carbamate link. The molecule is phosphorylated to make it water soluble.

Pharmacology: Mechanism of action – Estramustine appears to act as a relatively weak alkylating agent and imparts a weak estrogenic activity. The estrogenic portion of the molecule acts as a carrier to facilitate selective uptake of the drug into estrogen receptor-positive cells. Due to the selective steroidal uptake, the alkylating effect of the nitrogen mustard is enhanced in these cells.

Pharmacokinetics: Absorption/Distribution – Estramustine phosphate is readily dephosphorylated during absorption, and the major metabolites in plasma are estromustine, the estrone analog, estradiol and estrone.

Prolonged treatment produces elevated total plasma concentrations of estradiol that are within ranges similar to the elevated estradiol levels found in prostatic cancer patients given conventional estradiol therapy. Estrogenic effects, as demonstrated by changes in circulating levels of steroids and pituitary hormones, are similar in patients treated with either estramustine phosphate or conventional estradiol.

Metabolism/Excretion – Estromustine (17-keto analog) is the major metabolite. Estrone and estradiol are also present, as a result of cleavage of the nitrogen mustard from the steroid. Terminal half-life of estramustine phosphate is approximately 20 hours.

The metabolic urinary patterns of estradiol and the estradiol moiety of estramustine phosphate are very similar, although the metabolites derived from estramustine phosphate are excreted at a slower rate. The majority of the drug is excreted in the stool.

Indications:

Palliative treatment of metastatic or progressive carcinoma of the prostate.

Contraindications:

Hypersensitivity to estradiol or nitrogen mustard.

Active thrombophlebitis or thromboembolic disorders, except where the actual tumor mass is the cause of the thromboembolic phenomenon and the benefits of therapy outweigh the risks.

Warnings:

Thrombosis: The risk of thrombosis, including nonfatal myocardial infarction, increases in men receiving estrogens for prostatic cancer. Use with caution in patients with a history of thrombophlebitis, thrombosis or thromboembolic disorders, especially if they were associated with estrogen therapy. Use with caution in patients with cerebral vascular or coronary artery disease.

Glucose tolerance may be decreased; observe diabetic patients receiving this drug.

Elevated blood pressure may occur; monitor blood pressure periodically during therapy.

Hepatic function impairment: Estramustine may be poorly metabolized in patients with impaired liver function. Administer with caution.

Carcinogenesis, mutagenesis, impairment of fertility: Long-term continuous administration of estrogens in certain animal species increases frequency of carcinomas of the breast and liver. Compounds structurally similar to estramustine are carcinogenic in mice.

Although testing by the Ames method failed to demonstrate mutagenicity for estramustine, both estradiol and nitrogen mustard are mutagenic. For this reason, and because some patients who had been impotent while on estrogen therapy have regained potency while taking the drug, advise use of contraceptive measures.

Precautions:

Fluid retention: Exacerbation of preexisting or incipient peripheral edema or congestive heart disease may occur in some patients. Other conditions potentially influenced by fluid retention, such as epilepsy, migraine or renal dysfunction, require careful observation.

Calcium/Phosphorus metabolism may be influenced by estramustine; use with caution in patients with metabolic bone diseases associated with hypercalcemia or in patients with renal insufficiency.

Laboratory test abnormalities: Abnormalities of hepatic enzymes and of bilirubin have occurred, but have seldom required cessation of therapy. Perform such tests at appropriate intervals during therapy and repeat after the drug has been withdrawn for 2 months.

Drug Interactions:

Drug/Food interactions: Milk, milk products and calcium-rich foods or drugs may impair the absorption of estramustine phosphate sodium.

(Continued on following page)

ESTRAMUSTINE PHOSPHATE SODIUM (Cont.)

Adverse Reactions:

Cardiovascular/Respiratory: Cerebrovascular accident; myocardial infarction; thrombophlebitis; pulmonary emboli; congestive heart failure; edema; dyspnea; leg cramps; upper respiratory discharge; hoarseness.

GI: Nausea; vomiting; diarrhea; anorexia; flatulence; GI bleeding; burning throat; thirst; minor GI upset.

Dermatologic: Rash; pruritus; dry skin; peeling skin of fingertips; easy bruising; flushing; thinning hair.

Miscellaneous: Lethargy; emotional lability; insomnia; headache; anxiety; chest pain; tearing of eyes; breast tenderness; mild to moderate breast enlargement.

Laboratory abnormalities in hematologic tests for leukopenia and thrombocytopenia. Also abnormalities of bilirubin, LDH and AST.

Overdosage:

Although there has been no experience with overdosage, it may produce pronounced manifestations of the adverse reactions. In the event of overdosage, evacuate gastric contents by gastric lavage and initiate symptomatic therapy. Monitor hematologic and hepatic parameters for at least 6 weeks after overdosage.

Patient Information:

Because of the possibility of mutagenic effects, use contraceptive measures.

Take with water at least 1 hour before or 2 hours after meals.

Milk, milk products and calcium-rich foods or drugs (such as calcium-containing antacids) must not be taken simultaneously with estramustine phosphate sodium.

Administration and Dosage:

Recommended daily dosage: 14 mg/kg/day (ie, one 140 mg capsule for each 10 kg or 22 lb) in 3 or 4 divided doses (dosage range, 10 to 16 mg/kg/day).

Treat for 30 to 90 days before assessing the possible benefits of continued therapy. Continue therapy as long as response is favorable. Some patients have been maintained on therapy for > 3 years at doses ranging from 10 to 16 mg/kg/day.

Storage: Refrigerate at 2° to 8°C (36° to 46°F). Capsules may be left out of the refrigerator for 24 to 48 hours without affecting potency.

Rx	**Emcyt** (Pharmacia)	**Capsules:** Estramustine phosphate sodium equivalent to 140 mg estramustine phosphate (12.5 mg sodium/capsule)	(Emcyt Pharmacia 132). White. In 100s.

Antiestrogen

TAMOXIFEN CITRATE

Actions:

Pharmacology: A nonsteroidal agent with potent antiestrogenic properties due to its ability to compete with estrogen for binding sites in target tissues such as the breast. Tumor hormone receptors may help predict which patients will benefit from the adjuvant therapy, but not all breast cancer adjuvant tamoxifen studies have shown a clear relationship between hormone receptor status and treatment effect. Tamoxifen competes with estradiol for estrogen receptor protein.

Pharmacokinetics: Blood levels following single oral doses of 0.3 mg/kg reached peak values of 0.06 to 0.14 mcg/ml 4 to 7 hours after dosing, with 20% to 30% of the drug present as tamoxifen. There is an initial half-life of 7 to 14 hours with secondary plateau peaks ≥ 4 days later. Prolongation of blood levels and fecal excretion may be due to enterohepatic circulation, probably of drug metabolites. A primary metabolite, desmethyl tamoxifen, has antitumor potency equivalent to the parent drug. Significant accumulation of this metabolite may occur. Most of the drug is slowly excreted in the feces; only small amounts appear in the urine. Excreted mainly as conjugates, unchanged drug and hydroxylated metabolites account for 30% of the total.

Indications:

Effective in the treatment of metastatic breast cancer in women. In premenopausal women with metastatic breast cancer, tamoxifen is an alternative to oophorectomy or ovarian irradiation. Evidence indicates that patients whose tumors are estrogen receptor positive are more likely to benefit from tamoxifen therapy.

Effective in delaying recurrence following total mastectomy and axillary dissection or segmental mastectomy, axillary dissection and breast irradiation in women with axillary node-negative breast cancer. Data are insufficient to predict which women are most likely to benefit and to determine if tamoxifen provides any benefit in women with tumors < 1 cm. The incidence of second primary breast tumors was reduced in all studies.

Unlabeled uses: Tamoxifen has been used in the treatment of mastalgia (10 mg/day for 4 months) and for decreasing the size and pain of gynecomastia. Studies are currently being considered for use of tamoxifen as chemosuppressive (preventive) therapy in women at high risk for primary breast cancer. Tamoxifen may also be useful in the treatment of male patients with breast cancer and in pancreatic carcinoma.

Contraindications:

Hypersensitivity to the drug.

Warnings:

Ophthalmologic effects occurred in a few patients treated > 1 year at doses at least 4 times the highest recommended daily dose and consisted of retinopathy, corneal changes and decreased visual acuity. A few cases of ocular changes (eg, visual disturbance, cataracts, corneal changes, retinopathy) have occurred in patients treated at recommended doses. It is uncertain whether these effects are due to tamoxifen.

Hypercalcemia has occurred in some breast cancer patients with bone metastases within a few weeks of starting therapy with tamoxifen. If hypercalcemia occurs, institute appropriate measures and, if severe, discontinue use.

Carcinogenicity/Impairment of fertility: A study in rats revealed hepatocellular carcinomas at doses 35 mg/kg/day (206.5 mg/m^2) within 31 to 37 weeks and cataracts at doses of 20 and 35 mg/kg/day within 6 months. In addition, preliminary data from two independent reports revealed liver tumors that one study classified as malignant. Granulosa cell ovarian tumors and interstitial cell testicular tumors were found in mice.

In one study, an increased frequency of endometrial cancer occurred in postmenopausal patients receiving tamoxifen (13 of 931); the risk was highest in patients who continued the drug for > 2 years. However, in a review of > 12,000 patients entered into twelve other large ongoing adjuvant studies in which patients have received tamoxifen 20 to 40 mg/day for 1 to 5 plus years vs control, no increased incidence of uterine cancer was seen.

Endometrial hyperplasia and endometrial polyps have occurred in a small number of cases in association with tamoxifen treatment. A definitive relationship has not been established.

Fertility in female rats decreased following 0.04 mg/kg for 2 weeks prior to mating through day 7 of pregnancy. There was a decreased number of implantations, and all fetuses were found dead.

(Warnings continued on following page)

TAMOXIFEN CITRATE (Cont.)

Warnings (Cont.):

Pregnancy: Category D. Tamoxifen may cause fetal harm when administered to a pregnant woman. Individuals should not become pregnant while taking tamoxifen. Effects on reproductive functions are expected from the antiestrogenic properties of the drug. In reproductive studies in rats at dose levels equal to or below the human dose, nonteratogenic developmental skeletal changes were seen and were found to be reversible. In fertility and teratology studies in rats and rabbits using doses at or below those in humans, a lower incidence of embryo implantation and a higher incidence of fetal death or retarded in utero growth were observed, with slower learning behavior in some rat pups. The impairment of learning behavior did not achieve statistical significance.

There are no adequate and well controlled studies in pregnant women. There have been reports of spontaneous abortions, birth defects, fetal deaths and vaginal bleeding. If this drug is used during pregnancy or if the patient becomes pregnant while taking this drug, apprise her of the potential hazard to the fetus.

Lactation: It is not known whether this drug is excreted in breast milk. Because there is potential for serious adverse reactions in nursing infants, decide whether to discontinue nursing or discontinue the drug.

Precautions:

Leukopenia or thrombocytopenia: Use cautiously. Transient decreases in platelet counts (usually to 50,000 to 100,000/mm³) have occurred. No hemorrhagic tendency has been recorded; platelet counts returned to normal although treatment continued. Perform periodic complete blood counts, including platelet counts.

Hyperlipidemias have occurred infrequently. Periodic monitoring of plasma triglycerides and cholesterol may be indicated in patients with pre-existing hyperlipidemias.

Drug Interactions:

Anticoagulants, oral: The hypoprothrombinemic effect may be increased by concurrent tamoxifen.

Drug/Lab test interactions: Tamoxifen may produce a transient increase in **serum calcium.** T_4 elevations occurred in a few postmenopausal patients but were not accompanied by clinical hyperthyroidism. An increase in thyroid-binding globulin in postmenopausal women on tamoxifen may explain T_4 elevations during treatment.

Variations in the karyopyknotic index on vaginal smears and various degrees of estrogen effect on Pap smears have been infrequently seen in postmenopausal patients.

Adverse Reactions:

Adverse reactions to tamoxifen are relatively mild and rarely require discontinuation of therapy. If adverse reactions are severe, it is sometimes possible to control severe adverse reactions by dosage reduction without losing control of the disease.

Most frequent: Hot flashes, nausea and vomiting (up to 25% of patients), rarely severe.

Less frequent: Vaginal bleeding; vaginal discharge; menstrual irregularities; skin rash. Usually not severe enough to require dosage reduction or discontinuation.

Infrequent: Hypercalcemia; peripheral edema; food distaste; pruritus vulvae; depression; dizziness; lightheadedness; headache; corneal opacity; decreased visual acuity; retinopathy; thrombocytopenia; leukopenia. Thromboembolic events have occurred infrequently during tamoxifen therapy; a causal relationship remains conjectural. An increased incidence has occurred when cytotoxins are combined with tamoxifen.

Ovarian cysts have been observed in a small number of premenopausal patients with advanced breast cancer who have been treated with tamoxifen.

Increased bone and tumor pain and local disease flare are sometimes associated with a good tumor response shortly after starting tamoxifen, and generally subside rapidly. Lesion size may increase suddenly in soft tissue disease, sometimes with new lesions or with erythema in or around the lesion.

Overdosage:

In animals, respiratory difficulties and convulsions occurred at high doses. Treatment includes usual supportive measures. Refer to General Management of Acute Overdosage.

Patient Information:

Contraceptive measures are recommended during treatment.

Notify physician if marked weakness, sleepiness, mental confusion, pain/swelling of legs, shortness of breath, blurred vision, bone pain, hot flashes, nausea, vomiting, weight gain, menstrual irregularities, dizziness, headache or loss of appetite occurs.

Administration and Dosage:

10 or 20 mg twice daily (morning and evening).

Rx	**Nolvadex** (ICI Pharma)	**Tablets:** 10 mg (as citrate)	(Nolvadex 600). White. In 60s and 250s.

Gonadotropin-Releasing Hormone Analog

LEUPROLIDE ACETATE

Actions:

Pharmacology: Leuprolide acetate, an LH-RH agonist, is a synthetic nonapeptide analog of naturally occurring gonadotropin-releasing hormone (GnRH or LH-RH) that has greater potency than the natural hormone. It occupies pituitary GnRH receptors and desensitizes them; thus, it inhibits gonadotropin secretion when given continuously and in therapeutic doses. Following an initial stimulation, chronic leuprolide results in suppression of ovarian and testicular steroidogenesis. This effect is reversible upon drug discontinuation.

Leuprolide injection has a plasma half-life of approximately 3 hours. Following a single depot injection, mean peak leuprolide plasma concentration was almost 20 ng/ml at 4 hours and 0.36 ng/ml at 4 weeks. Nondetectable leuprolide acetate plasma concentrations have been seen during chronic use, but testosterone levels appear to be maintained at castrate levels.

Clinical pharmacology: Advanced prostatic cancer – In humans, administration of leuprolide results in an initial increase in circulating levels of luteinizing hormone (LH) and follicle stimulating hormone (FSH), leading to a transient increase in levels of the gonadal steroids (testosterone and dihydrotestosterone in males, and estrone and estradiol in premenopausal females). However, continuous daily administration of leuprolide results in decreased levels of LH and FSH in all patients. In males, testosterone is reduced to castrate levels. In premenopausal females, estrogens are reduced to postmenopausal levels. These decreases occur within 2 to 4 weeks after initiation of treatment, and castrate levels of testosterone in prostatic cancer patients have been demonstrated for 3 to 5 years.

In a controlled study comparing leuprolide 1 mg/day SC to diethylstilbestrol (DES) 3 mg/day, the survival rate for the two groups was comparable after 2 years of treatment. The objective response to treatment was also similar for the two groups. In clinical trials, the safety and efficacy of leuprolide depot did not differ from that of the SC injection.

Endometriosis – Leuprolide depot 3.75 mg monthly for 6 months was comparable to danazol 800 mg/day in relieving clinical symptoms (eg, pelvic pain, dysmenorrhea, dyspareunia, pelvic tenderness, induration) and in reducing the size of endometrial implants.

Indications:

Advanced prostatic cancer: Palliative treatment as an alternative when orchiectomy or estrogen administration are either not indicated or are unacceptable to the patient.

Leuprolide is also used in combination with flutamide (see individual monograph) for the treatment of metastatic prostatic carcinoma. One study reported that the use of this combination is superior to leuprolide alone.

Endometriosis (leuprolide depot 3.75 mg): Management of endometriosis, including pain relief and reduction of endometriotic lesions. Experience is limited to women ≥ 18 years of age treated for 6 months.

Unlabeled uses: Leuprolide may be useful in the treatment of: Breast, ovarian and endometrial cancer; leiomyoma uteri; precocious puberty; infertility; prostatic hypertrophy.

Contraindications:

Leuprolide depot: Pregnancy and lactation (see Warnings); hypersensitivity to GnRH, GnRH agonist analogs of any excipients in the product; undiagnosed abnormal vaginal bleeding.

Warnings:

Worsening of signs and symptoms may occur during the first few weeks of treatment and are usually manifested by an increase in bone pain. Temporary weakness and paresthesia of the lower limbs have occurred. In a report with another LH-RH analog, such worsening may have contributed to a rapid fatal outcome in two cases.

Closely observe patients with metastatic vertebral lesions or urinary tract obstruction during the first few weeks of therapy. In a few cases, a temporary worsening of existing hematuria and urinary tract obstruction occurred during the first week.

Carcinogenesis/Impairment of fertility: In rats, a dose-related increase in benign pituitary hyperplasia and benign pituitary adenomas was noted after 2 years when high daily doses were administered.

Studies with analogs similar to leuprolide have shown full reversibility of fertility suppression when the drug is discontinued after continuous administration for up to 24 weeks.

(Warnings continued on following page)

LEUPROLIDE ACETATE (Cont.)

Warnings (Cont.):

Pregnancy: Category X (leuprolide depot). The depot injection is contraindicated in women who are or may become pregnant while receiving the drug. When given on day 6 of pregnancy at test dosages of 0.00024, 0.0024 and 0.024 mg/kg (1/600 to 1/6 the human dose) to rabbits, the depot injection produced a dose-related increase in major fetal abnormalities. There was increased fetal mortality and decreased fetal weights with the two higher doses in rabbits and with the highest dose in rats. The effects on fetal mortality are logical consequences of the alterations in hormonal levels brought about by this drug. Therefore, the possibility exists that spontaneous abortion may occur if the drug is given during pregnancy.

Before starting therapy, pregnancy must be excluded. When used monthly at the recommended dose, leuprolide depot usually inhibits ovulation and stops menstruation; however, contraception is not insured. Therefore, patients should use nonhormonal methods of contraception. Advise patients to see their physician if they believe they may be pregnant. If the patient becomes pregnant during treatment, discontinue the drug and apprise the patient of the potential risk to the fetus.

Lactation: It is not known whether leuprolide depot is excreted in breast milk. Do not use during nursing.

Children: Safety and efficacy have not been established.

Precautions:

Bone density changes: After 6 months of leuprolide depot treatment, vertebral trabecular bone density decreased by an average of 13.5% compared to pretreatment levels. There was partial to complete recovery of bone density in the post-treatment period in a small number of patients who were retested. Use of leuprolide depot for > 6 months or in the presence of other known risk factors for decreased bone mineral content may cause additional bone loss.

Monitor response by measuring serum levels of testosterone and acid phosphatase. In the majority of patients, testosterone levels increased above baseline during the first week, declining thereafter to baseline levels or below by the end of the second week. Castrate levels were reached within 2 to 4 weeks and were maintained for as long as drug administration continued. Occasional transient increases in acid phosphatase levels occurred. By the fourth week, the elevated levels usually decreased to values at or near baseline.

Hypersensitivity: Patients with known allergies to benzyl alcohol, an ingredient in the vehicle of leuprolide injection, may present symptoms of hypersensitivity, usually local, in the form of erythema and induration at the injection site. Leuprolide depot contains no preservatives.

Drug Interactions:

Drug/Lab test interactions: Diagnostic tests of pituitary gonadotropic and gonadal functions conducted during treatment and up to 4 to 8 weeks after discontinuing leuprolide depot therapy may be misleading.

(Continued on following page)

Gonadotropin-Releasing Hormone Analog (Cont.)

LEUPROLIDE ACETATE (Cont.)

Adverse Reactions:

Prostatic cancer: In a comparative trial of leuprolide injection vs DES, the adverse reactions in the table below occurred in ≥ 5% of patients. Leuprolide depot 7.5 mg was not compared to DES; however, similar adverse reactions are listed in this table.

Endometriosis: In controlled studies comparing leuprolide depot 3.75 mg and danazol, the adverse reactions in the table below were the most frequently reported.

Leuprolide Acetate Adverse Reactions (%)

	Prostatic cancer			Endometriosis[1]	
Adverse Reaction	Leuprolide Injection (n = 98)	DES (n = 101)	Leuprolide Depot 7.5 mg (n = 56)	Leuprolide Depot 3.75 mg (n = 166)	Danazol (n = 136)
Cardiovascular					
ECG changes/ischemia	19.4	21.7			
High blood pressure	8.2	5			
Murmur	3.1	7.9			
Congestive heart failure	1	5			
Thrombosis/phlebitis	2	9.9			
Edema (peripheral)	12.2	29.7	12.5	6	14
CNS					
Depression/emotional lability	†			21	16
Insomnia/sleep disorders	7.1	5	†	2	3
Pain	13.2	12.9	7.1	19	16
Headache	7.1	4		31	21
Dizziness/lightheadedness	5.1	6.9		11	4
Nervousness	†			6	8
Paresthesias	†		†	7	8
Endocrine					
Androgen-like effects				14	32
Decreased testicular size	7.1	10.9	5.4		
Impotence/decreased libido	4.1	11.9	5.4	11	5
Gynecomastia/breast tenderness	7.1	62.4	†	6	8
Hot flashes/sweats	56.1	11.9	58.9	80	57
GI					
GI disturbances				8	6
Anorexia	6.1	5	†		
Constipation	7.1	8.9			
Nausea/vomiting	5.1	16.8	5.4	13	13
Musculoskeletal					
Joint disorder				8	8
Myalgia	3	8.9	†	2	6
Bone pain	5.1	2	†		
Neuromuscular disorders				7	12
GU					
Vaginitis				28	16
Urinary frequency/urgency	6.1	7.9	†		
Hematuria	6.1	4	†		
Urinary tract infection	3.1	6.9			
Respiratory					
Dyspnea	2	7.9	5.4		
Sinus congestion	5.1	5.9			
Miscellaneous					
Weight gain/loss			†	12	26
Anemia	5.1	5			
Dermatitis/skin reactions	5.1	7.9	†	9	15
Asthenia	10.2	9.9	5.4	4	8

[1] Percentages approximate.

† < 5% of patients

(Adverse Reactions continued on following page)

LEUPROLIDE ACETATE (Cont.)

Adverse Reactions (Cont.):

The following adverse reactions occurred in $<$ 5% of patients:

Leuprolide injection and depot:

Cardiovascular – Angina; cardiac arrhythmias.

GI/GU – Diarrhea; dysuria; testicular pain.

Respiratory – Hemoptysis.

Miscellaneous – Diabetes; fever; chills; increased calcium.

Leuprolide depot:

Dermatologic – Hair growth.

Miscellaneous – Hard nodule in throat; increased uric acid; changes in bone density (see Precautions).

Laboratory test abnormalities – Increased AST, LDH, alkaline phosphatase, cholesterol, LDL and triglycerides; decreased WBC counts and HDL.

Leuprolide injection:

Cardiovascular – Myocardial infarction; pulmonary emboli; hypotension; transient ischemic attack/stroke.

GI – Dysphagia; GI bleeding; GI disturbance; peptic ulcer; rectal polyps; hepatic dysfunction.

Musculoskeletal – Joint pain; ankylosing spondylosis; pelvic fibrosis.

CNS – Anxiety; blurred vision; lethargy; memory disorder; mood swings; numbness; hearing disorder; peripheral neuropathy; spinal fracture/paralysis; syncope/blackouts; taste disorders.

Respiratory – Cough; pleural rub; pneumonia; pulmonary fibrosis; pulmonary infiltrate.

Dermatologic – Carcinoma of skin/ear; dry skin; ecchymosis; hair loss; itching; pigmentation; skin lesions.

GU – Bladder spasms; incontinence; urinary obstruction; penile swelling; prostate pain.

Miscellaneous – Fatigue; hypoglycemia; increased BUN; increased creatinine; infection/inflammation; ophthalmologic disorders; swelling (temporal bone); libido increase; decreased WBC; hypoproteinemia; thyroid enlargement.

Overdosage:

In rats, SC administration of 250 to 500 times the recommended human dose, expressed on a per body weight basis, resulted in dyspnea, decreased activity and local irritation at the injection site.

Patient Information:

Patient package insert is available with each injection kit. Patient information is available from the manufacturer (1-800-622-2011).

Do not discontinue medication except on advice of physician.

May cause increased bone pain and increased difficulty in urinating during the first few weeks of treatment. May cause hot flashes, injection site irritation (eg, burning, itching, swelling) and may cause or aggravate nerve symptoms; notify physician if these become pronounced.

Administration and Dosage:

Advanced prostate cancer: Injection – 1 mg SC daily. Use the syringes included in the kit or low-dose insulin syringes.

Depot – 7.5 mg IM monthly (every 28 to 33 days). Do not use needles smaller than 22 gauge. Reconstitute only with the diluent provided.

Endometriosis (depot only): 3.75 mg as a single monthly IM injection. Use a syringe with a 22 gauge neeedle. Reconstitute with 1 ml of diluent provided.

Recommended duration is 6 months. Retreatment cannot be recommended since safety data are not available.

Storage: Injection – Refrigerate until dispensed. Patients may store at room temperature ≤ 30°C (86°F). Avoid freezing. Protect from light; store vial in carton until use.

Depot – May be stored at room temperature. The suspension is stable for 24 hours following reconstitution; however, since the product does not contain a preservative, discard if not used immediately.

Rx	**Lupron** (TAP Pharm.)	**Injection:** 5 mg/ml	In 2.8 ml[1] multiple dose vials supplied with 14 (2 week kit) or 28 (4 week kit) syringes, or 6-pack vials only.
		Depot suspension: 3.75 mg/ml	Single dose vial with diluent.
		7.5 mg/ml	Single dose vial with diluent and syringe.

[1] With benzyl alcohol.

GOSERELIN ACETATE

Actions:

Pharmacology: Goserelin acetate is a synthetic decapeptide analog of luteinizing hormone-releasing hormone (LHRH or GnRH). It acts as a potent inhibitor of pituitary gonadotropin secretion when administered in the biodegradable formulation. Following initial administration, the drug causes an initial increase in serum luteinizing hormone (LH) and follicle stimulating hormone (FSH) values with subsequent increases in serum levels of testosterone. Chronic administration leads to sustained suppression of pituitary gonadotropins; serum levels of testosterone consequently fall into the range normally seen in surgically castrated men approximately 2 to 4 weeks after initiation of therapy. This leads to accessory sex organ regression. In animal and in in vitro studies, administration of goserelin resulted in the regression or inhibition of growth of the hormonally sensitive dimethylbenzanthracene-induced rat mammary tumor and Dunning R3327 prostate tumor. In clinical trials with follow-up of > 2 years, suppression of serum testosterone to castrate levels has been maintained for the duration of therapy.

Clinical studies: In controlled studies of patients with advanced prostatic cancer comparing goserelin to orchiectomy, the long-term endocrine responses and objective responses were similar between the two treatments. Additionally, duration of survival was similar between the two treatments in a major comparative trial.

Pharmacokinetics: Peak serum concentrations are achieved 12 to 15 days after SC administration; mean peak serum concentrations are ≈ 2.5 ng/ml.

Goserelin is absorbed at a much slower rate initially for the first 8 days, and then there is more rapid and continuous absorption for the remainder of the 28 day dosing period. Despite the change in the absorption rate of goserelin, administration every 28 days resulted in testosterone levels that were suppressed to and maintained in the range normally seen in surgically castrated men. There is no significant evidence of drug accumulation in patients with normal renal and hepatic function. In patients treated for ≤ 3 years, no antibodies to the drug have been detected.

In clinical trials with the solution formulation of goserelin, subjects with impaired renal function (creatinine clearance < 20 ml/min) had a serum elimination half-life of 12.1 hours compared to 4.2 hours for subjects with normal renal function (creatinine clearance > 70 ml/min). However, in clinical trials with the monthly formulation of goserelin, the incidence of adverse events was not increased in patients with impaired renal function.

Indications:

Palliative treatment of advanced carcinoma of the prostate. Goserelin offers an alternative treatment of prostatic cancer when orchiectomy or estrogen administration are either not indicated or unacceptable to the patient.

Contraindications:

Pregnancy (see Warnings).

Warnings:

Prostatic cancer worsening: Initially, goserelin, like other LHRH agonists, transiently increases serum levels of testosterone. Transient worsening of symptoms, or the occurrence of additional signs and symptoms of prostatic cancer, may occasionally develop during the first few weeks of treatment. A small number of patients may experience a temporary increase in bone pain, which can be managed symptomatically.

As with other LHRH agonists, isolated cases of exacerbation of disease symptoms, either ureteral obstruction or spinal cord compression, have been observed. Closely monitor patients during the first month of therapy. If spinal cord compression or renal impairment due to ureteral obstruction develops, institute standard treatment of these complications; in extreme cases, consider an immediate orchiectomy.

Carcinogenesis: After SC implant injections once every 4 weeks for 1 year at two dose levels to male and female rats equivalent to 31.5 and 62.4 times and 21.5 and 42.4 times the recommended monthly dose for a 70 kg human, respectively, an increased incidence of benign pituitary macroadenomas was found. No increase in pituitary adenomas was seen in mice receiving injections of goserelin every 3 weeks for 2 years at doses up to 2400 mcg/kg/day (1200 times the recommended human dose). An increased incidence of histiocytic sarcomas of the bone marrow in vertebral column and femur were observed at both doses in mice. No evidence of pituitary adenomas was seen in a 1 year study in dogs at doses up to 100 times the human dose or in a 6 month study in monkeys at doses up to 200 times the human dose.

(Warnings continued on following page)

GOSERELIN ACETATE (Cont.)

Warnings (Cont.):

Impairment of fertility: Administration of goserelin led to gonadal suppression in both male and female rats as a result of its endocrine action. In male rats treated at 30 to 60 times the recommended monthly dose for a 70 kg human, a decrease in weight and atrophic histological changes were observed in the testes, epididymis, seminal vesicle, and prostate gland with complete suppression of spermatogenesis. In female rats treated with 20 to 40 times the recommended monthly dose for a 70 kg human, suppression of ovarian function led to decreased size and weight of ovaries and secondary sex organs, follicular development was arrested at the antral stage and the corpora lutea were reduced in size and number. Except for the testes, almost complete histologic reversal of these effects in males and females was observed several weeks after dosing was stopped; however, fertility and general reproductive performance were reduced in those that became pregnant after the drug was discontinued. Fertile matings occurred within 2 weeks after cessation of dosing, even though total recovery of reproductive function may not have occurred before mating took place; ovulation rate, corresponding implantation rate, and number of live fetuses were reduced.

In male and female dogs, the suppression of fertility was fully reversible when drug treatment was stopped after continuous administration for 1 year at 100 times the recommended monthly dose.

Pregnancy: Category X. Studies in both rats and rabbits at doses up to 25 times and 500 times the maximum recommended dose to a 70 kg human have confirmed that this drug will increase pregnancy loss in a dose-related manner. Goserelin increased preimplantation loss, resorptions and abortions. In rats and dogs, the drug suppressed ovarian function, decreased ovarian weight and size and led to atrophic changes in secondary sex organs. These effects are an expected consequence of the hormonal alterations produced by goserelin in humans.

In rats and rabbits, there was no evidence that goserelin was teratogenic.

Do not use in women who are or who may become pregnant while receiving the drug. If goserelin is used during pregnancy or if pregnancy occurs while taking this drug, apprise the patient of the potential hazard to the fetus.

Lactation: It is not known if goserelin is excreted in breast milk. Because of the potential for serious adverse reactions in nursing infants from goserelin, decide whether to discontinue nursing or delay use of the drug, taking into account the importance of the drug to the mother.

Children: Safety and efficacy in patients < 18 years old have not been established.

Adverse Reactions:

Goserelin Adverse Reactions (%)

Adverse Reaction	Goserelin (n = 242)	Orchiectomy (n = 254)
Hot flashes	62	53
Sexual dysfunction	21	15
Decreased erections	18	16
Lower urinary tract symptoms	13	8
Lethargy	8	4
Pain (worsened in the first 30 days)	8	3
Edema	7	8
Upper respiratory infection	7	2
Rash	6	1
Sweating	6	4
Anorexia	5	2
Chronic obstructive pulmonary disease	5	3
Congestive heart failure	5	1
Dizziness	5	4
Insomnia	5	1
Nausea	5	2
Complications of surgery	0	18[1]

[1] Complications related to surgery were reported in 18% of the orchiectomy patients, while only 3% of goserelin patients reported adverse reactions at the injection site. The surgical complications included: Scrotal infection (5.9%); groin pain (4.7%); wound seepage (3.1%); scrotal hematoma (2.8%); incisional discomfort (1.6%); skin necrosis (1.2%).

(Adverse Reactions continued on following page)

GOSERELIN ACETATE (Cont.)

Adverse Reactions (Cont.):

Goserelin is generally well tolerated; withdrawal from treatment was rare. As seen with other hormonal therapies, the most commonly observed adverse events were due to the expected physiological effects from decreased testosterone levels, including hot flashes, sexual dysfunction and decreased erections.

Adverse reactions (1% to < 5%):

Cardiovascular – Arrhythmia; cerebrovascular accident; hypertension; myocardial infarction; peripheral vascular disorder; chest pain.

CNS – Anxiety; depression; headache.

GI – Constipation; diarrhea; ulcer; vomiting.

GU – Renal insufficiency; urinary obstruction; urinary tract infection.

Metabolic/Nutritional – Gout; hyperglycemia; weight increase.

Miscellaneous – Anemia; chills; fever; breast swelling and tenderness.

Overdosage:

There is no experience of overdosage from clinical trials. Animal studies indicate that no increased pharmacologic effect occurred at higher doses or more frequent administration. SC doses as high as 1 mg/kg/day in rats and dogs did not produce any nonendocrine-related sequelae; this dose is > 400 times that proposed for human use. If overdosage occurs, manage symptomatically. Refer to General Management of Acute Overdosage.

Administration and Dosage:

Administer a 3.6 mg dose SC every 28 days into the upper abdominal wall using sterile technique under the supervision of a physician. Local anesthesia may be used prior to injection.

While a delay of a few days is permissible, attempt to adhere to the 28 day schedule.

Administration technique: 1) If package is damaged, do not use syringe. Do not remove the sterile syringe until immediately before use. Examine syringe for damage and make sure the drug is visible in the translucent chamber. 2) After cleaning with an alcohol swab, a local anesthetic may be used on an area of skin on the upper abdominal wall. 3) Stretch the patient's skin with one hand, and grip the needle with fingers around the barrel of the syringe. Insert the hypodermic needle into the SC fat. Do not aspirate. If the hypodermic needle penetrates a large vessel, blood will be seen instantly in the syringe chamber. If a vessel is penetrated, withdraw the needle and inject with a new syringe elsewhere. 4) Change the direction of the needle so it parallels the abdominal wall. Push the needle in until the barrel hub touches the patient's skin. Withdraw the needle 1 cm to create a space to discharge the drug; fully depress the plunger to discharge. 5) Withdraw needle and bandage the site. Confirm discharge by ensuring tip of the plunger is visible within the tip of the needle.

In the unlikely event of the need to surgically remove goserelin, it can be localized by ultrasound.

Storage: Store at room temperature; do not exceed 25°C (77°F).

Rx	**Zoladex** (ICI Pharma)	**Implant:** 3.6 mg	In preloaded syringes.

BLEOMYCIN SULFATE (BLM)

Warning:

Pulmonary fibrosis is the most severe toxicity. It is most frequently seen as pneumonitis, which occasionally progresses to pulmonary fibrosis. Its occurrence is higher in elderly patients and in those receiving > 400 units total dose, but pulmonary toxicity has been observed in young patients and those treated with low doses.

A severe idiosyncratic reaction consisting of hypotension, mental confusion, fever, chills and wheezing has occurred in approximately 1% of lymphoma patients.

Actions:

Pharmacology: Bleomycin sulfate is a mixture of cytotoxic glycopeptide antibiotics isolated from a strain of *Streptomyces verticillus.* The exact mechanism of action is unknown; however, the main mode of action appears to be inhibition of deoxyribonucleic acid (DNA) synthesis with lesser inhibition of ribonucleic acid (RNA) and protein synthesis. Bleomycin is cell cycle phase specific, with major effects in G_2 and M phases.

Pharmacokinetics:

Absorption/Distribution – Following IV administration, bleomycin has a rapid initial distribution half-life of 10 to 20 minutes. IM injection produces peak blood levels in 30 to 60 minutes that are approximately ⅓ of those produced IV.

Metabolism/Excretion – 60% to 70% of an administered dose is recovered in the urine as active bleomycin. Only 20% to 40% of this amount is active drug. In patients with a creatinine clearance of >35 ml/min, the plasma terminal elimination half-life is approximately 2 hours. At creatinine clearances of < 35 ml/min, the plasma terminal elimination half-life increases exponentially as the creatinine clearance decreases.

Indications:

Palliative treatment in the following neoplasms as either a single agent or in combination with other chemotherapeutic agents:

Squamous cell carcinoma: Head and neck including mouth, tongue, tonsil, nasopharynx, oropharynx, sinus, palate, lip, buccal mucosa, gingiva, epiglottis, skin and larynx. Response is poorer in patients with head and neck cancer previously irradiated. Bleomycin is also indicated in carcinoma of the skin, penis, cervix and vulva.

Lymphomas: Hodgkin's, reticulum cell sarcoma and lymphosarcoma.

Testicular carcinoma: Embryonal cell, choriocarcinoma and teratocarcinoma.

Contraindications: Hypersensitivity or idiosyncrasy to bleomycin sulfate.

Warnings:

Idiosyncratic reactions similar to anaphylaxis occur in approximately 1% of lymphoma patients. These reactions (hypotension, confusion, fever, chills and wheezing) may be immediate or delayed for several hours, and usually occur after the first or second dose; careful monitoring is essential. Symptomatic treatment includes volume expansion, pressor agents, antihistamines and steroids. Refer to Management of Acute Hypersensitivity Reactions.

Renal or hepatic toxicity, beginning as a deterioration in renal or liver function tests, has occurred infrequently. These toxicities may occur at any time.

Pulmonary toxicities, the most serious side effect, occur in 10% of treated patients. In approximately 1%, the drug-induced nonspecific pneumonitis progresses to pulmonary fibrosis and death. Although this is age- and dose-related, it is unpredictable. It is more common in patients > 70 years of age and in those receiving > 400 units total dose. However, pulmonary toxicity has been seen in young patients receiving low doses. Concomitant use of radiation therapy may also increase the incidence of pulmonary toxicity. Conversely, one study suggests that administration by continuous infusion over several days may decrease the risk.

Identifying patients with pulmonary toxicity is extremely difficult because of lack of specificity of the clinical syndrome. The earliest symptom is dyspnea, and the earliest sign is fine rales.

Radiographically, the pneumonitis produces nonspecific patchy opacities, usually of the lower lung field. Pulmonary function tests demonstrate a decrease in total lung volume and vital capacity. However, these changes are not predictive of fibrosis development.

The nonspecific microscopic tissue changes include bronchiolar squamous metaplasia, reactive macrophages, atypical alveolar epithelial cells, fibrinous edema and interstitial fibrosis. The acute stage may involve capillary changes and subsequent fibrinous exudation into alveoli, producing a change similar to hyaline membrane formation and progressing to a diffuse interstitial fibrosis resembling the Hamman-Rich syndrome.

(Warnings continued on following page)

BLEOMYCIN SULFATE (BLM) (Cont.)

Warnings (Cont.):

Pulmonary toxicities (Cont.): Take chest x-rays every 1 to 2 weeks to monitor the onset of pulmonary toxicity. If changes are noted, discontinue treatment until it is determined if they are drug-related. Sequential measurements of the pulmonary diffusion capacity for carbon monoxide (DL_{CO}) may indicate subclinical pulmonary toxicity. Monitor the DL_{CO} monthly; discontinue the drug when the DL_{CO} falls below 30% to 35% of the pretreatment value. Because of bleomycin's sensitization of lung tissue, patients are at greater risk of developing pulmonary toxicity when oxygen is given in surgery. Long exposure to very high oxygen concentrations is a known cause of lung damage; however, after bleomycin administration, lung damage can occur at concentrations usually considered safe. Suggested preventive measures are to maintain FI O_2 at concentrations approximating that of room air (25%) during surgery and the postoperative period and to carefully monitor fluid replacement, focusing more on colloid administration rather than crystalloid.

Pregnancy: Safety for use during pregnancy has not been established.

Drug Interactions:

Digoxin serum levels may be decreased by combination chemotherapy (including bleomycin). Digitoxin and digoxin capsules do not appear to be affected.

Phenytoin serum concentrations may be decreased by combination chemotherapy.

Adverse Reactions:

Pulmonary: Pneumonitis, pulmonary fibrosis (see Warnings).

Idiosyncratic: (See Warnings).

Integument and mucous membranes (50%): Erythema; rash; striae; vesiculation; hyperpigmentation; skin tenderness; hyperkeratosis; nail changes; alopecia; pruritus; stomatitis. Drug therapy was discontinued in 2% of treated patients because of these toxicities.

Skin toxicity, a relatively late manifestation, appears to be related to the cumulative dose; it usually develops in the second and third week of treatment after administration of 150 to 200 units of drug.

Other: Fever, chills, vomiting (frequent); anorexia, weight loss (common, may persist long after termination of the drug); pain at tumor site, phlebitis (infrequent).

Combination therapy: Vascular toxicities coincident with the use of bleomycin in combination with other antineoplastic agents have occurred rarely. The events are clinically heterogeneous and may include myocardial infarction, cerebrovascular accident, thrombotic microangiopathy or cerebral arteritis. There are also reports of Raynaud's phenomenon occurring with bleomycin alone or with vinblastine with or without cisplatin.

Sudden onset of an acute chest pain syndrome suggestive of pleuropericarditis has occurred rarely during bleomycin sulfate infusions. Although each patient must be individually evaluated, further courses of bleomycin do not appear to be contraindicated.

Administration and Dosage:

May administer IM, IV or SC.

Because of the possibility of anaphylactoid reaction, treat lymphoma patients with ≤ 2 units for the first 2 doses. If no acute reaction occurs, follow the regular dosage schedule. The following schedule is recommended:

Squamous cell carcinoma, lymphosarcoma, reticulum cell sarcoma, testicular carcinoma: 0.25 to 0.5 units/kg (10 to 20 units/m^2) given IV, IM or SC once or twice weekly.

Hodgkin's disease: 0.25 to 0.5 units/kg (10 to 20 units/m^2) IV, IM or SC once or twice weekly. After a 50% response, administer a maintenance dose of 1 unit daily or 5 units weekly IV or IM. Improvement of Hodgkin's disease and testicular tumors is prompt (≤ 2 weeks). If no improvement is seen by this time, it is unlikely to occur. Squamous cell cancers respond more slowly, sometimes requiring 3 weeks before improvement is noted.

Pulmonary toxicity of bleomycin appears to be dose-related with a striking increase when the total dose is > 400 units. Give total doses > 400 units with great caution.

When bleomycin is used in combination with other antineoplastic agents, pulmonary toxicities may occur at lower doses.

Preparation of solutions: IM or SC – Dissolve vial contents with 1 to 5 ml Sterile Water for Injection, NaCl for Injection, 5% Dextrose Injection or Bacteriostatic Water for Injection.

IV solution: Dissolve contents of vial with ≥ 5 ml of physiologic saline or glucose; administer slowly over 10 minutes.

Stability: Bleomycin is stable for 24 hours at room temperature in NaCl, 5% Dextrose solution and 5% Dextrose containing heparin 100 or 1000 units/ml. The powder is stable under refrigeration (2° to 8°C; 36 to 46°F).

Rx	**Blenoxane** (Bristol-Myers Oncology)	**Powder for Injection:** 15 units	In vials.

PENTOSTATIN (2′-deoxycoformycin; DCF)

Warning:

Administer under the supervision of a physician qualified and experienced in the use of cancer chemotherapeutic agents. The use of higher doses than those specified is not recommended. Dose-limiting severe renal, liver, pulmonary and CNS toxicities occurred in Phase I studies that used pentostatin at higher doses than recommended (20 to 50 mg/m² in divided doses over 5 days).

In a clinical investigation in patients with refractory chronic lymphocytic leukemia using pentostatin at the recommended dose in combination with fludarabine phosphate, four of six patients had severe or fatal pulmonary toxicity. The use of pentostatin in combination with fludarabine phosphate is not recommended.

Actions:

Pentostatin was approved by the FDA in October 1991.

Pharmacology: Pentostatin is a potent transition state inhibitor of the enzyme adenosine deaminase (ADA) and is isolated from fermentation cultures of *Streptomyces antibioticus.* The greatest activity of ADA is found in cells of the lymphoid system with T-cells having higher activity than B-cells and T-cell malignancies having higher ADA activity than B-cell malignancies. Pentostatin inhibition of ADA, particularly in the presence of adenosine or deoxyadenosine, leads to cytotoxicity due to elevated intracellular levels of dATP which can block DNA synthesis through inhibition of ribonucleotide reductase. Pentostatin can also inhibit RNA synthesis as well as cause increased DNA damage. In addition to elevated dATP, these mechanisms may contribute to the overall cytotoxic effect of pentostatin. However, the precise mechanism of pentostatin's antitumor effect in hairy cell leukemia is not known.

Pharmacokinetics: In rats pentostatin concentrations were highest in the kidneys with very little CNS penetration.

In man, following a single dose of 4 mg/m² pentostatin infused over 5 minutes, the distribution half-life was 11 minutes, the mean terminal half-life was 5.7 hours, the mean plasma clearance was 68 ml/min/m², and ≈ 90% of the dose was excreted in the urine as unchanged pentostatin or metabolites as measured by adenosine deaminase inhibitory activity. The plasma protein binding of pentostatin is low, ≈ 4%.

A positive correlation was observed between pentostatin clearance and creatinine clearance (Ccr) in patients with Ccr values ranging from 60 to 130 ml/min. Pentostatin half-life in patients with renal impairment (Ccr < 50 ml/min) was 18 hours, which was much longer than that observed in patients with normal renal function (Ccr > 60 ml/min), which was about 6 hours.

Clinical trials: Patients with hairy cell leukemia (n = 133) previously treated with alpha-interferon were treated with pentostatin in five clinical studies. Forty-four of these patients were refractory to alpha-interferon and were evaluable for response to pentostatin. Pentostatin was administered at a dose of 4 mg/m² every other week for 3 months; responding patients received 3 additional months (M.D. Anderson Hospital study). Another group of patients received 4 mg/m² pentostatin every other week for 3 months; responding patients were treated monthly for up to 9 additional months (Cancer and Leukemia Group B study; CALGB). A complete response required clearing of the peripheral blood and bone marrow of hairy cells, normalization of organomegaly and lymphadenopathy, and recovery of the hemoglobin to at least 12 g/dl, platelet count to at least 100,000/mm³ and granulocyte count to at least 1500/mm³. A partial response required that the percentage of hairy cells in the blood and bone marrow decrease by > 50%, enlarged organs and lymph nodes had to decrease by > 50%, and hematologic parameters had to meet the same criteria as for a complete response. For those patients who were clearly refractory to alpha-interferon, the complete response rate was 58% and the partial response rate was 28% giving a total response rate (complete plus partial responses) of 86%. Median time to achieve a response was 4.7 months (range, 2.9 to 24.1 months). Duration of response ranged from 1.4 to 35.1+ months in the CALGB study (median > 7.7 months) and from 1.3+ to 31.2+ months for the M.D. Anderson study (median > 15.2 months). Median duration of follow-up ranged from 3.9 months in the CALGB study to 19.3 months in the M.D. Anderson study. Only 4 of 20 and 2 of 13 responding patients had relapsed, respectively.

Responding patients with abnormal peripheral blood counts at the start of therapy showed increases in their hemoglobin, granulocyte count and platelet count in response to treatment with pentostatin.

Indications:

Single agent for adult patients with alpha-interferon-refractory hairy cell leukemia, defined as progressive disease after a minimum of 3 months of alpha-interferon treatment or no response after a minimum of 6 months of alpha-interferon treatment.

(Continued on following page)

PENTOSTATIN (2′-deoxycoformycin; DCF) (Cont.)

Contraindications:

Hypersensitivity to pentostatin.

Warnings:

Myelosuppression: Patients with hairy cell leukemia may experience myelosuppression, primarily during the first few courses of treatment. Patients with infections prior to pentostatin treatment have in some cases developed worsening of their condition leading to death, whereas others have achieved complete response. Treat patients with infection only when the potential benefit justifies the potential risk to the patient. Attempt to control the infection before treatment is initiated or resumed.

In patients with progressive hairy cell leukemia, the initial courses of pentostatin treatment were associated with worsening of neutropenia. Therefore, frequent monitoring of complete blood counts during this time is necessary. If severe neutropenia continues beyond the initial cycles, evaluate patients for disease status, including a bone marrow examination.

Renal toxicity was observed at higher doses in early studies; however, in patients treated at the recommended dose, elevations in serum creatinine were usually minor and reversible. There were some patients who began treatment with normal renal function who had evidence of mild to moderate toxicity at a final assessment.

Rashes, occasionally severe, were commonly reported and may worsen with continued treatment. Withholding of treatment may be required.

Mutagenesis: Pentostatin was nonmutagenic when tested with various *Salmonella typhimurium* strains; however, when tested with strain TA-100, a repeatable statistically significant response trend was observed with and without metabolic activation. Formulated pentostatin was clastogenic in the in vivo mouse bone marrow micronucleus assay at 20, 120 and 240 mg/kg.

Fertility impairment: In a 5 day IV toxicity study in dogs, mild seminiferous tubular degeneration was observed with doses of 1 and 4 mg/kg. The possible adverse effects on fertility in humans have not been determined.

Pregnancy: Category D. Pentostatin can cause fetal harm when administered to a pregnant woman. Pentostatin was administered IV to pregnant rats on days 6 through 15 of gestation; drug-related maternal toxicity occurred at doses of 0.1 and 0.75 mg/kg/day (0.6 and 4.5 mg/m^2). Teratogenic effects were observed at 0.75 mg/kg/day manifested by increased incidence of various skeletal malformations. In another study, fetal malformations that occurred were an omphalocele at 0.05 mg/kg (0.3 mg/m^2), gastroschisis at 0.75 and 1 mg/kg/day (4.5 and 6 mg/m^2), and a flexure defect of the hind limbs at 0.75 mg/kg/day (4.5 mg/m^2). Pentostatin was also teratogenic in mice when administered as a single 2 mg/kg (6 mg/m^2) intraperitoneal injection on day 7 of gestation. Pentostatin was not teratogenic in rabbits when administered IV on days 6 through 18 of gestation; however, maternal toxicity, abortions, early deliveries and deaths occurred in all drug-treated groups. There are no adequate and well controlled studies in pregnant women. If pentostatin is used during pregnancy, or if the patient becomes pregnant while taking this drug, apprise her of the potential hazard to the fetus. Advise women of childbearing potential to avoid becoming pregnant while taking this drug.

Lactation: It is not known whether pentostatin is excreted in breast milk. Decide whether to discontinue nursing or discontinue the drug, taking into account the importance of the drug to the mother.

Children: Safety and efficacy in children or adolescents have not been established.

Precautions:

Monitoring: Therapy with pentostatin requires regular patient observation and monitoring of hematologic parameters and blood chemistry values. If severe adverse reactions occur, withhold the drug and take appropriate corrective measures.

Prior to initiating therapy, assess renal function with a serum creatinine or a Ccr assay. Perform complete blood counts and serum creatinine before each dose and at other appropriate periods during therapy. Severe neutropenia has been observed following the early courses of treatment; therefore, frequent monitoring of complete blood counts is recommended during this time. If hematologic parameters do not improve with subsequent courses, evaluate patients for disease status, including a bone marrow examination. Perform periodic monitoring of the peripheral blood for hairy cells to assess the response to treatment.

In addition, bone marrow aspirates and biopsies may be required at 2 to 3 month intervals to assess the response to treatment.

CNS toxicity: Withhold or discontinue therapy in patients with evidence of CNS toxicity.

(Continued on following page)

PENTOSTATIN (2′-deoxycoformycin; DCF) (Cont.)

Drug Interactions:

Allopurinol and pentostatin are both associated with skin rashes. Based on clinical studies in 25 refractory patients, combined use did not appear to produce a higher incidence of skin rashes than observed with pentostatin alone. One patient received both drugs and experienced a hypersensitivity vasculitis that resulted in death. It was unclear whether this adverse event and subsequent death resulted from the drug combination.

Fludarabine: Concurrent use with pentostatin is not recommended because it may be associated with an increased risk of fatal pulmonary toxicity (see Warning box).

Vidarabine: Pentostatin enhances the effects of vidarabine. The combined use may result in an increase in adverse reactions associated with each drug. The therapeutic benefit of the drug combination has not been established.

Adverse Reactions:

Pentostatin Adverse Reactions (%)			
Adverse reaction	Incidence	Adverse reaction	Incidence
Hematologic/Lymphatic		*Hepatic*	
Leukopenia	60	Hepatic disorder/elevated liver function tests	19
Anemia	35	*Respiratory*	
Thrombocytopenia	32	Cough	17
Ecchymosis	3-10	Upper respiratory infection	16
Lymphadenopathy	3-10	Lung disorder	12
Petechia	3-10	Bronchitis	3-10
GI		Dyspnea	3-10
Nausea/Vomiting	22-53	Epistaxis	3-10
Anorexia	16	Lung edema	3-10
Diarrhea	15	Pneumonia	3-10
Constipation	3-10	Pharyngitis	3-10
Flatulence	3-10	Rhinitis	3-10
Stomatitis	3-10	Sinusitis	3-10
Dermatologic		*GU*	
Rash	26	Genitourinary disorder	15
Skin disorder	17	Hematuria	3-10
Eczema	3-10	Dysuria	3-10
Dry skin	3-10	Increased BUN	3-10
Herpes simplex/zoster	3-10	Increased creatinine	3-10
Maculopapular rash	3-10	*CNS*	
Vesiculobullous rash	3-10	Headache	13
Pruritus	3-10	Neurologic, CNS	11
Seborrhea	3-10	Anxiety	3-10
Skin discoloration	3-10	Confusion	3-10
Sweating	3-10	Depression	3-10
Body as a whole		Dizziness	3-10
Fever	42	Insomnia	3-10
Infection	36	Nervousness	3-10
Fatigue	29	Paresthesia	3-10
Pain	20	Somnolence	3-10
Allergic reaction	11	Abnormal thinking	3-10
Chills	11	*Musculoskeletal*	
Death	3-10	Myalgia	11
Sepsis	3-10	Arthralgia	3-10
Chest pain	3-10	*Cardiovascular*	
Abdominal pain	3-10	Arrhythmia	3-10
Back pain	3-10	Abnormal ECG	3-10
Flu syndrome	3-10	Thrombophlebitis	3-10
Asthenia	3-10	Hemorrhage	3-10
Malaise	3-10	*Special senses*	
Neoplasm	3-10	Abnormal vision	3-10
Metabolic/Nutritional		Conjunctivitis	3-10
Weight loss	3-10	Ear pain	3-10
Peripheral edema	3-10	Eye pain	3-10
Increased LDH	3-10		

(Adverse Reactions continued on following page)

PENTOSTATIN (2′-deoxycoformycin; DCF) (Cont.)

Adverse Reactions:

The adverse events listed in the preceding table were reported during clinical studies with pentostatin in patients with hairy cell leukemia who were refractory to alpha-interferon therapy. Most patients experienced an adverse event. The drug association is uncertain since the adverse reactions may be associated with the disease itself (eg, fever, infection, anemia), but other events, such as the GI symptoms, hematologic suppression, rashes and abnormal liver function tests, can in many cases be attributed to the drug. Most adverse events that were assessed for severity were either mild (52%) or moderate (26%) and diminished in frequency with continued therapy; 11% of patients withdrew from treatment due to an adverse event.

The remaining adverse events occurred in < 3% of patients; their relationship to pentostatin is uncertain:

Body as a whole: Abscess; enlarged abdomen; ascites; cellulitis; cyst; face edema; fibrosis; granuloma; hernia; injection-site hemorrhage or inflammation; moniliasis; neck rigidity; pelvic pain; photosensitivity reaction; anaphylactoid reaction; immune system disorder; mucous membrane disorder; neck pain.

Cardiovascular: Aortic stenosis; arterial anomaly; cardiomegaly; congestive heart failure; cardiac arrest; flushing; hypertension; myocardial infarct; palpitation; shock; varicose vein.

GI: Colitis; dysphagia; eructation; gastritis; GI hemorrhage; gum hemorrhage; hepatitis; hepatomegaly; intestinal obstruction; jaundice; leukoplakia; melena; periodontal abscess; proctitis; abnormal stools; dyspepsia; esophagitis; gingivitis; hepatic failure; mouth disorder.

Hemic/Lymphatic: Abnormal erythrocytes; leukocytosis; pancytopenia; purpura; splenomegaly; eosinophilia; hematologic disorder; hemolysis; lymphoma-like reaction; thrombocythemia.

Metabolic/Nutritional: Acidosis; increased creatine phosphokinase; dehydration; diabetes mellitus; increased gamma globulins; gout; abnormal healing; hypocholesterolemia; weight gain; hyponatremia.

Musculoskeletal: Arthritis; bone pain; osteomyelitis; pathological fracture.

CNS: Agitation; amnesia; apathy; ataxia; CNS depression; coma; convulsions; abnormal dreams; depersonalization; emotional lability; facial paralysis; abnormal gait; hyperesthesia; hypesthesia; hypertonia; incoordination; decreased libido; neuropathy; postural dizziness; decreased reflexes; stupor; tremor; vertigo.

Respiratory: Asthma; atelectasis; hemoptysis; hyperventilation; hypoventilation; laryngitis; larynx edema; lung fibrosis; pleural effusion; pneumothorax; pulmonary embolus; increased sputum.

Skin and appendages: Acne; alopecia; contact dermatitis; exfoliative dermatitis; fungal dermatitis; psoriasis; benign skin neoplasm; subcutaneous nodule; skin hypertrophy; urticaria.

Special senses: Blepharitis; cataract; deafness; diplopia; exophthalmos; lacrimation disorder; optic neuritis; otitis media; parosmia; retinal detachment; taste perversion; tinnitus. One patient developed unilateral uveitis with vision loss.

GU: Albuminuria; fibrocystic breast; glycosuria; gynecomastia; hydronephrosis; kidney failure; oliguria; polyuria; pyuria; toxic nephropathy; urinary frequency/retention/urgency; urinary tract infection; impaired urination; urolithiasis; vaginitis.

Lab test abnormalities: Liver function test elevations occurred during treatment and were generally reversible.

Overdosage:

Symptoms: Pentostatin administered at higher doses than recommended (20 to 50 mg/m^2 in divided doses over 5 days) was associated with deaths due to severe renal, hepatic, pulmonary and CNS toxicity.

Treatment: Management would include general supportive measures through any period of toxicity that occurs. Refer to General Management of Acute Overdosage.

(Continued on following page)

PENTOSTATIN (2′-deoxycoformycin; DCF) (Cont.)

Administration and Dosage:

Hydrate with 500 to 1000 ml of 5% Dextrose in 0.5 Normal Saline or equivalent before pentostatin administration. Administer an additional 500 ml of 5% Dextrose or equivalent after pentostatin is given.

Alpha-interferon-refractory hairy cell leukemia: 4 mg/m² every other week. Pentostatin may be administered IV by bolus injection or diluted in a larger volume and given over 20 to 30 minutes. (See Preparation of IV Solution.)

Higher doses are not recommended.

No extravasation injuries were reported in clinical studies.

Duration/Response: The optimal duration of treatment has not been determined. In the absence of major toxicity and with observed continuing improvement, treat the patient until a complete response has been achieved. Although not established, the administration of two additional doses has been recommended following the achievement of a complete response.

Assess all patients receiving pentostatin at 6 months for response to treatment. If the patient has not achieved a complete or partial response, discontinue treatment.

If the patient has achieved a partial response, continue treatment in an effort to achieve a complete response. At any time that a complete response is achieved thereafter, two additional doses of pentostatin are recommended; then stop treatment. If the best response to treatment at the end of 12 months is a partial response, stop treatment with pentostatin.

Therapy/Dose discontinuation: Withholding or discontinuing individual doses may be needed when severe adverse reactions occur. Withhold drug treatment in patients with severe rash, and withhold or discontinue in patients showing evidence of CNS toxicity.

Withhold treatment in patients with active infection occurring during the treatment; may resume treatment when the infection is controlled.

Patients who have elevated serum creatinine should have their dose withheld and a Ccr determined. There are insufficient data to recommend a starting or a subsequent dose for patients with impaired renal function (Ccr < 60 ml/min).

Renal function impairment: Treat patients only when potential benefit justifies potential risk. Two patients with impaired renal function (Ccr 50 to 60 ml/min) achieved complete response without unusual adverse events when treated with 2 mg/m².

Hematologic effects: No dosage reduction is recommended at the start of therapy in patients with anemia, neutropenia or thrombocytopenia. In addition, dosage reductions are not recommended during treatment in patients with anemia and thrombocytopenia if patients can be otherwise supported hematologically. Temporarily withhold pentostatin if the absolute neutrophil count falls below 200 cells/mm³ during treatment in a patient who had an initial neutrophil count > 500 cells/mm³; treatment may be resumed when the count returns to predose levels.

Preparation of IV solution:

1. Follow procedures for proper handling and disposal of anticancer drugs. Treat spills and wastes with 5% sodium hypochlorite solution prior to disposal.
2. Protective clothing including polyethylene gloves must be worn.
3. Transfer 5 ml Sterile Water for Injection, USP to the vial containing pentostatin and mix thoroughly to obtain complete dissolution of a solution yielding 2 mg/ml.
4. Pentostatin may be given IV by bolus injection or diluted in a larger volume (25 to 50 ml) with 5% Dextrose Injection, USP or 0.9% Sodium Chloride Injection, USP. Dilution of the entire contents of a reconstituted vial with 25 or 50 ml provides a pentostatin concentration of 0.33 or 0.18 mg/ml, respectively, for the diluted solutions.
5. Pentostatin solution, when diluted for infusion with 5% Dextrose Injection, USP or 0.9% Sodium Chloride Injection, USP does not interact with PVC infusion containers or administration sets at concentrations of 0.18 to 0.33 mg/ml.

Storage/Stability: Pentostatin vials are stable when stored at refrigerated temperatures (2° to 8°C; 36° to 46°F) for the period stated on the package. Vials reconstituted or reconstituted and further diluted as directed may be stored at room temperature and ambient light; however, use within 8 hours because pentostatin contains no preservatives.

Rx	**Nipent** (Parke-Davis)	**Powder for Injection:** 10 mg/vial[1]	In single dose vials.

[1] With 50 mg mannitol per vial.

Anthracyclines

IDARUBICIN HCl

Warnings:

Give idarubicin slowly into a freely flowing IV infusion. It must *never* be given IM or SC. Severe local tissue necrosis can occur if there is extravasation during administration.

Idarubicin can cause myocardial toxicity leading to congestive heart failure. Cardiac toxicity is more common in patients who have received prior anthracyclines or who have pre-existing cardiac disease.

Severe myelosuppression occurs when idarubicin is used at therapeutic doses.

The physician and institution must be capable of responding rapidly and completely to severe hemorrhagic conditions or overwhelming infection.

Reduce dosage in patients with impaired hepatic or renal function. (See Administration and Dosage.)

Actions:

Pharmacology: Idarubicin HCl is a synthetic antineoplastic anthracycline for IV use; it is a DNA-intercalating analog of daunorubicin which has an inhibitory effect on nucleic acid synthesis and interacts with the enzyme topoisomerase II. The compound has a high lipophilicity which results in an increased rate of cellular uptake compared with other anthracyclines.

Pharmacokinetics: Following IV administration of 10 to 12 mg/m² daily for 3 to 4 days (as a single agent or combined with cytarabine) to adult leukemia patients with normal renal and hepatic function, there is a rapid distributive phase with a very high volume of distribution presumably reflecting extensive tissue binding. The plasma clearance is twice the expected hepatic plasma flow indicating extensive extrahepatic metabolism. The drug is eliminated predominantly by biliary and to a lesser extent by renal excretion, mostly in the form of the primary metabolite, 13-dihydroidarubicin (idarubicinol).

The estimated mean terminal half-life is 22 hours (range, 4 to 46 hours) when used as a single agent and 20 hours (range, 7 to 38 hours) when used in combination with cytarabine. The elimination of idarubicinol is considerably slower with an estimated mean terminal half-life that exceeds 45 hours; hence, its plasma levels are sustained for a period > 8 days. As idarubicinol has cytotoxic activity, it presumably contributes to the effects of idarubicin.

The extent of drug and metabolite accumulation predicted in leukemia patients for days 2 and 3 of dosing is 1.7- and 2.3-fold, respectively, and suggests no change in kinetics following a 3 times daily regimen.

In patients with moderate or severe hepatic dysfunction, the metabolism of idarubicin may be impaired and lead to higher systemic drug levels. See Warnings.

Peak cellular idarubicin concentrations are reached a few minutes after injection. Idarubicin and idarubicinol concentrations in nucleated blood and bone marrow cells are > 100 times the plasma concentrations. Idarubicin disappearance rates in plasma and cells were comparable with a terminal half-life of about 15 hours. The terminal half-life of idarubicinol in cells was about 72 hours.

The percentages of idarubicin and idarubicinol bound to human plasma proteins averaged 97% and 94%, respectively. The binding is concentration-independent.

Idarubicin studies in pediatric leukemia patients, at doses of 4.2 to 13.3 mg/m²/day for 3 days, suggest dose-independent kinetics. There is no difference between the half-lives of the drug following 3 times daily or 3 times weekly administration.

Cerebrospinal fluid (CSF) levels of idarubicin and idarubicinol were measured in pediatric leukemia patients. Idarubicin was detected in 2 of 21 CSF samples (0.14 and 1.56 ng/ml), while idarubicinol was detected in 20 of these 21 CSF samples obtained 18 to 30 hours after dosing (mean, ≈ 0.51 ng/ml, range, 0.22 to 1.05 ng/ml). The clinical relevance of these findings is currently being evaluated.

(Actions continued on following page)

IDARUBICIN HCl (Cont.)

Actions (Cont.):

Clinical studies: Four prospective randomized studies have been conducted to compare the safety and efficacy of idarubicin (IDR) to that of daunorubicin (DNR), each in combination with cytarabine (Ara-C) as induction therapy in previously untreated adult patients with acute myeloid leukemia (AML). These data are summarized in the following table and demonstrate significantly greater complete remission rates and significantly longer overall survival for the IDR regimen in two of the studies.

Efficacy of Idarubicin vs Daunorubicin in AML

Studies	Induction[1] regimen dose in mg/m² daily x 3 days		Complete remission rate		Median survival (days)	
	IDR	DNR	IDR	DNR	IDR	DNR
1. Age ≤ 60 years	12[2]	50[2]	51/65[4] (78%)	38/65 (58%)	508[4]	435
2. Age ≥ 15 years	12[3]	45[3]	76/111[4] (69%)	65/119 (55%)	328	277
3. Age ≥ 18 years	13[3]	45[3]	68/101 (67%)	66/113 (58%)	393[4]	281
4. Age ≥ 55 years	12[3]	45[3]	49/124 (40%)	49/125 (39%)	87	169

[1] Patients who had persistent leukemia after the first induction course received a second course
[2] Ara-C 25 mg/m² bolus IV followed by 200 mg/m² daily x 5 days by continuous infusion
[3] Ara-C 100 mg/m² daily x 7 days by continuous infusion
[4] Overall $p < 0.05$, unadjusted for prognostic factors or multiple endpoints

The following consolidation regimens were used in US controlled trials: Patients received the same anthracycline for consolidation as was used for induction.

Studies 1 and 3 utilized 2 courses of consolidation therapy consisting of IDR 12 or 13 mg/m² daily for 2 days, respectively (or DNR 50 or 45 mg/m² daily for 2 days), and Ara-C, either 25 mg/m² daily by IV bolus followed by 200 mg/m² daily by continuous infusion for 4 days (Study 1), or 100 mg/m² daily for 5 days by continuous infusion (Study 3). A rest period of 4 to 6 weeks is recommended prior to initiation of consolidation and between the courses; hematologic recovery is mandatory prior to initiation of each consolidation course.

Study 2 utilized 3 consolidation courses, administered at intervals of 21 days or upon hematologic recovery. Each course consisted of IDR 15 mg/m² IV for 1 dose (or DNR 50 mg/m² IV for 1 dose), Ara-C 100 mg/m² every 12 hours for 10 doses and 6-thioguanine 100 mg/m² for 10 doses. If severe myelosuppression occurred, subsequent courses were given with 25% reduction in the doses of all drugs. In addition, this study included 4 courses of maintenance therapy (2 days of the same anthracycline as was used in induction and 5 days of Ara-C).

Toxicities and duration of aplasia were similar during induction except for an increase in mucositis on the IDR arm in one study. During consolidation, duration of aplasia on the IDR arm was longer in all three studies and mucositis was more frequent in two studies. During consolidation, transfusion requirements were higher on the IDR arm in the two studies in which they were tabulated, and patients on the IDR arm in Study 3 spent more days on IV antibiotics (Study 3 used a higher dose of IDR).

The benefit of consolidation and maintenance therapy in prolonging the duration of remission and survival is not proven.

Intensive maintenance with IDR is not recommended in view of the considerable toxicity (including deaths in remission) experienced by patients during the maintenance phase of Study 2.

Indications:

In combination with other approved antileukemic drugs for the treatment of AML in adults. This includes French-American-British (FAB) classifications M1 through M7.

(Continued on following page)

IDARUBICIN HCl (Cont.)

Warnings:

Bone marrow suppression: Idarubicin is a potent bone marrow suppressant. Do not give to patients with pre-existing bone marrow suppression induced by previous drug therapy or radiotherapy unless the benefit warrants the risk.

Severe myelosuppression will occur in all patients given a therapeutic dose of this agent for induction, consolidation or maintenance. Careful hematologic monitoring is required. Deaths due to infection or bleeding have occurred during the period of severe myelosuppression. Facilities with laboratory and supportive resources adequate to monitor drug tolerability and protect and maintain a patient compromised by drug toxicity should be available. It must be possible to treat rapidly and completely a severe hemorrhagic condition or a severe infection.

Cardiotoxicity: Pre-existing heart disease and previous therapy with anthracyclines at high cumulative doses or other potentially cardiotoxic agents are co-factors for increased risk of idarubicin-induced cardiac toxicity; weigh the benefit-to-risk ratio of idarubicin therapy in such patients before starting treatment.

Myocardial toxicity, as manifested by potentially fatal congestive heart failure, acute life-threatening arrhythmias or other cardiomyopathies, may occur following therapy with idarubicin. Appropriate therapeutic measures for the management of congestive heart failure or arrhythmias are indicated.

Carefully monitor cardiac function during treatment in order to minimize the risk of cardiac toxicity of the type described for other anthracycline compounds. The risk of such myocardial toxicity may be higher following concomitant or previous radiation to the mediastinal-pericardial area or in patients with anemia, bone marrow depression, infections, leukemic pericarditis or myocarditis. While there are no reliable means for predicting congestive heart failure, cardiomyopathy induced by anthracyclines is usually associated with a decrease of the left ventricular ejection fraction (LVEF) from pretreatment baseline values.

Hepatic and renal function impairment can affect the disposition of idarubicin. Evaluate liver and kidney function with conventional clinical laboratory tests (using serum bilirubin and serum creatinine as indicators) prior to and during treatment. Consider dose reduction if the bilirubin or creatinine levels are above the normal range. (See Administration and Dosage.)

Carcinogenesis, mutagenesis, impairment of fertility: Idarubicin and related compounds have mutagenic and carcinogenic properties when tested in experimental models (including bacterial systems, mammalian cells in culture and female Sprague-Dawley rats).

In male dogs given $\geq$ 1.8 mg/m²/day idarubicin (3 times per week for 13 weeks), testicular atrophy was observed with inhibition of spermiogenesis and sperm maturation, and few or no mature sperm. Effects were not readily reversible after an 8 week recovery period.

Pregnancy: Category D. Idarubicin was embryotoxic and teratogenic in the rat at a dose of 1.2 mg/m²/day or one-tenth the human dose, which was nontoxic to dams. Idarubicin was embryotoxic but not teratogenic in the rabbit. Even at a dose of 2.4 mg/m²/day or two-tenths the human dose, which was toxic to dams. There is no conclusive information about idarubicin adversely affecting human fertility or causing teratogenesis. There are no adequate and well controlled studies in pregnant women. If idarubicin is to be used during pregnancy, or if the patient becomes pregnant during therapy, apprise the patient of the potential hazard to the fetus. Advise women of childbearing potential to avoid pregnancy.

Lactation: It is not known whether this drug is excreted in breast milk. Because of the potential for serious adverse reactions in nursing infants from idarubicin, mothers should discontinue nursing prior to taking this drug.

Children: Safety and efficacy in children have not been established.

Precautions:

Monitoring: Therapy with idarubicin requires close observation of the patient and careful laboratory monitoring. Frequent complete blood counts and monitoring of hepatic and renal function tests are recommended.

Hyperuricemia secondary to rapid lysis of leukemic cells may be induced. Take appropriate measures to prevent hyperuricemia and to control any systemic infection before beginning therapy.

Administer slowly (over 10 to 15 minutes) into the tubing of a freely running IV infusion of 0.9% Sodium Chloride Injection, USP or 5% Dextrose Injection, USP. Attach the tubing to a Butterfly needle or other suitable device and insert preferably into a large vein.

(Precautions continued on following page)

IDARUBICIN HCl (Cont.)

Precautions (Cont.):

Extravasation of idarubicin can cause severe local tissue necrosis. Extravasation may occur with or without an accompanying stinging or burning sensation even if blood returns well on aspiration of the infusion needle. If signs or symptoms of extravasation occur, terminate the injection or infusion immediately and restart in another vein.

Care in the administration of idarubicin will reduce the chance of perivenous infiltration. It may also decrease the chance of local reactions such as urticaria and erythematous streaking. If it is known or suspected that SC extravasation has occurred, it is recommended that intermittent ice packs (½ hour immediately, then ½ hour 4 times per day for 3 days) be placed over the area of extravasation and that the affected extremity be elevated. Because of the progressive nature of extravasation reactions, frequently examine the area of injection and obtain plastic surgery consultation early if there is any sign of a local reaction such as pain, erythema, edema or vesication. If ulceration begins or there is severe persistent pain at the site of extravasation, consider early wide excision of the involved area.

Adverse Reactions:

The table below lists the adverse experiences reported in one US study and is representative of the experiences in other studies.

Adverse Reactions: Idarubicin vs Daunorubicin		
Adverse Reactions	IDR (n = 110)	DNR (n = 118)
Infection	95%	97%
Nausea and vomiting	82%	80%
Hair loss	77%	72%
Abdominal cramps/Diarrhea	73%	68%
Hemorrhage	63%	65%
Mucositis	50%	55%
Dermatologic	46%	40%
Mental status	41%	34%
Pulmonary-clinical	39%	39%
Fever	26%	28%
Headache	20%	24%
Cardiac-clinical	16%	24%
Neurologic-peripheral nerves	7%	9%
Seizure	4%	5%
Cerebellar	4%	5%
Pulmonary allergy	2%	4%

The duration of aplasia and incidence of mucositis were greater on the IDR arm than the DNR arm, especially during consolidation in some US controlled trials (see Clinical studies).

The following information reflects experience based on US controlled clinical trials.

Myelosuppression: Severe myelosuppression is the major toxicity associated with idarubicin therapy, but this effect of the drug is required in order to eradicate the leukemic clone. During the period of myelosuppression, patients are at risk of developing infection and bleeding which may be life-threatening or fatal. (See Warnings.)

GI: Nausea or vomiting, mucositis, abdominal pain and diarrhea occurred frequently, but were severe in $< 5\%$ of patients. Severe enterocolitis with perforation has occurred rarely. The risk of perforation may be increased by instrumental intervention. Consider the possibility of perforation in patients who develop severe abdominal pain and take appropriate steps for diagnosis and management.

Dermatologic: Alopecia occurred frequently and dermatologic reactions including generalized rash, urticaria and a bullous erythrodermatous rash of the palms and soles have occurred. The dermatologic reactions were usually attributed to concomitant antibiotic therapy. Local reactions including hives at the injection site have occurred.

Hepatic and renal: Changes in hepatic and renal function tests have been observed. These changes were usually transient and occurred in the setting of sepsis and while patients were receiving potentially hepatotoxic and nephrotoxic antibiotics and antifungal agents. Severe changes in renal function occurred in no more than 1% of patients, while severe changes in hepatic function occurred in $< 5\%$ of patients.

(Adverse Reactions continued on following page)

IDARUBICIN HCl (Cont.)

Adverse Reactions (Cont.):

Cardiac: Congestive heart failure (frequently attributed to fluid overload), serious arrhythmias including atrial fibrillation, chest pain, myocardial infarction and asymptomatic declines in LVEF have occurred in patients undergoing induction therapy for AML. Myocardial insufficiency and arrhythmias were usually reversible and occurred in the setting of sepsis, anemia and aggressive IV fluid administration. The events were reported more frequently in patients > 60 years old and in those with pre-existing cardiac disease. (See Warnings.)

Overdosage:

Two cases of fatal overdosage in patients receiving therapy for AML have been reported. The doses were 135 mg/m² over 3 days and 45 mg/m² of idarubicin and 90 mg/m² of daunorubicin over a 3 day period.

It is anticipated that overdosage with idarubicin will result in severe and prolonged myelosuppression and possibly in increased severity of GI toxicity. Adequate supportive care including platelet transfusions, antibiotics and symptomatic treatment of mucositis is required. The effect of acute overdose on cardiac function is not fully known, but severe arrhythmia occurred in one of the two patients exposed. It is anticipated that very high doses of idarubicin may cause acute cardiac toxicity and may be associated with a higher incidence of delayed cardiac failure.

The profound multicompartment behavior, extensive extravascular distribution and tissue binding, coupled with the low unbound fraction available in the plasma pool make it unlikely that therapeutic efficacy or toxicity would be altered by conventional peritoneal or hemodialysis.

Administration and Dosage:

Induction therapy in adult patients with AML: 12 mg/m² daily for 3 days by slow (10 to 15 min) IV injection in combination with Ara-C, 100 mg/m² daily given by continuous infusion for 7 days or as a 25 mg/m² IV bolus followed by 200 mg/m² daily for 5 days by continuous infusion. In patients with unequivocal evidence of leukemia after the first induction course, a second course may be administered. Delay administration of the second course in patients who experience severe mucositis until recovery from this toxicity has occurred; a dose reduction of 25% is recommended. In patients with hepatic or renal impairment, consider a dose reduction of idarubicin. Do not administer if the bilirubin level is > 5 mg/dl. (See Warnings.)

Preparation of solution: Caution in handling of the powder and in preparation of the solution must be exercised as skin reactions associated with idarubicin may occur. If skin is accidently exposed to idarubicin, thoroughly wash with soap and water; if the eyes are involved, use standard irrigation techniques immediately. The use of goggles, gloves and protective gowns is recommended during preparation and administration of the drug.

Reconstitute 5 and 10 mg vials with 5 and 10 ml, respectively, of 0.9% Sodium Chloride Injection, USP to give a final concentration of 1 mg/ml. Bacteriostatic diluents are not recommended.

The vial contents are under a negative pressure to minimize aerosol formation during reconstitution; therefore, take particular care when the needle is inserted. Avoid inhalation of any aerosol produced during reconstitution.

IV incompatibility: Unless specific compatability data are available, idarubicin should not be mixed with other drugs. Precipitation occurs with heparin. Prolonged contact with any solution of any alkaline pH will result in degradation of the drug.

Storage/Stability: Reconstituted solutions are physicially and chemically stable for at least 168 hours (7 days) under refrigeration (2° to 8° C; 36° to 46°F) and 72 hours (3 days) at controlled room temperature (15° to 30°C; 59° to 86°F). Discard unused solutions in an appropriate manner.

Rx	**Idamycin** (Adria)	**Powder for Injection (lyophilized):** 5 mg	In single-dose vials with 50 mg lactose.
		10 mg	In single-dose vials with 100 mg lactose.

DOXORUBICIN HCl (ADR)

Warning:

Severe local tissue necrosis will result if extravasation occurs. Do not give IM or SC.

Serious irreversible myocardial toxicity with delayed congestive failure often unresponsive to supportive therapy may occur as total dosage approaches 550 mg/m².

Reduce dosage in patients with impaired hepatic function.

Severe myelosuppression may occur.

Actions:

Pharmacology: Doxorubicin is a cytotoxic anthracycline antibiotic isolated from cultures of *Streptomyces peucetius* var. *caesius.* The drug's mechanism of action is related to its ability to bind to DNA and inhibit nucleic acid synthesis. Cell culture studies have demonstrated rapid cell penetration and perinucleolar chromatin binding, rapid inhibition of mitotic activity and nucleic acid synthesis, mutagenesis and chromosomal aberrations.

Pharmacokinetics: Absorption/Distribution – Following IV administration, doxorubicin undergoes rapid and extensive binding to tissue and plasma proteins. It does not cross the blood-brain barrier.

Metabolism/Excretion – Plasma disappearance of doxorubicin follows a triphasic pattern with mean half-lives of 12 minutes, 3.3 hours and 29.6 hours. Doxorubicin is metabolized by carbonyl reduction to the active alcohol, doxorubicinol and inactive aglycones. Other inactive metabolites have been identified in urine and bile.

Impairment of liver function, as reflected by elevated serum bilirubin, results in slower excretion and increased retention and accumulation of doxorubicin and its metabolites in plasma and tissues. Other liver function abnormalities are not predictive. Urinary excretion accounts for approximately 4% to 5% of the administered dose in 5 days. Biliary excretion represents the major excretion route; 40% to 50% of the administered dose is recovered in the bile or feces in 7 days.

Indications:

To produce regression in the following: Acute lymphoblastic leukemia, acute myeloblastic leukemia, Wilms' tumor, neuroblastoma, soft tissue and bone sarcomas, breast carcinoma, ovarian carcinoma, transitional cell bladder carcinoma, thyroid carcinoma, Hodgkin's and non-Hodgkin's lymphomas, bronchogenic carcinoma (the small cell histologic type is the most responsive) and gastric carcinoma.

Contraindications:

Malignant melanoma, kidney carcinoma, large bowel carcinoma, brain tumors and metastases to the CNS are *not* significantly responsive to doxorubicin therapy.

Do not initiate therapy in patients with marked myelosuppression induced by previous treatment with other antitumor agents or by radiotherapy.

Conclusive data are not available on preexisting heart disease as a cofactor of increased risk of drug-induced cardiac toxicity. In such cases cardiac toxicity may occur at doses lower than the recommended cumulative limit. Do not start doxorubicin in such cases.

Patients who received previous treatment with complete cumulative doses of doxorubicin or daunorubicin.

Warnings:

Myelosuppression (60% to 84% of patients), primarily of leukocytes, requires careful monitoring. With the recommended dosage schedule, leukopenia is usually transient, reaching its nadir 10 to 14 days after treatment, with recovery usually by the 21st day. Expect white blood cell counts as low as 1000/mm³ during treatment. Monitor red blood cell and platelet levels, since they may also be depressed. Hematologic toxicity may require dose reduction, suspension or delay of therapy. Persistent, severe myelosuppression may result in superinfection or hemorrhage.

Necrotizing colitis manifested by typhlitis (cecal inflammation), bloody stools and severe and sometimes fatal infections have been associated with a combination of doxorubicin given by IV push daily for 3 days and cytarabine given by continuous infusion daily for $\geq$ 7 days.

Cardiac toxicity must be given special attention. Although uncommon, acute left ventricular failure has occurred, particularly in patients who have received total dosage exceeding the recommended limit of 550 mg/m². Dose-related incidences range from $<$ 2% at total doses of $\leq$ 400 mg/m² to $>$ 20% at total doses of $>$ 700 mg/m². This limit appears to be lower (400 mg/m²) in patients who received radiotherapy to the mediastinal area. The total dose of the drug should also take into account any previous or concomitant therapy with other potentially cardiotoxic agents such as cyclophosphamide or daunorubicin. Cardiomyopathy or CHF may occur several weeks after discontinuation of the drug and is often unresponsive to medical or physical therapy.

(Warnings continued on following page)

DOXORUBICIN HCl (ADR) (Cont.)

Warnings (Cont.):

Cardiac toxicity (Cont.): Early diagnosis of drug-induced heart failure is essential for successful treatment with digitalis, diuretics, low salt diet and bed rest. Severe cardiac toxicity may occur precipitously without antecedent ECG changes. Perform a baseline ECG and prior to each dose or after 300 mg/m² cumulative dose. Transient ECG changes (eg, T wave flattening, ST depression, arrhythmias) lasting up to 2 weeks after a dose are not indications for therapy suspension. Doxorubicin cardiomyopathy is associated with persistent reduction in voltage of the QRS wave, prolongation of the systolic time interval and reduction of ejection fraction. None of these tests have consistently identified patients approaching their maximally tolerated cumulative dose. If test results indicate cardiac function change, carefully evaluate benefit of continued therapy against risk of producing irreversible cardiac damage. Some clinicians recommend discontinuing therapy if ejection fraction is < 0.45 with a drop of 0.15 from baseline. Acute life-threatening arrhythmias occurred during or within a few hours of use. Preliminary evidence suggests cardiotoxicity may be reduced and total dosage safely increased by giving the drug on a weekly schedule or as a prolonged (48 to 96 hrs) continuous infusion.

Hepatic function impairment: Since doxorubicin is excreted primarily via the bile, toxicity is enhanced by hepatic impairment; therefore, prior to dosing, evaluate hepatic function using clinical laboratory tests such as AST, ALT, alkaline phosphatase and bilirubin.

Extravasation at injection site with or without a stinging or burning sensation may occur, even if blood returns well on aspiration of the infusion needle. If any signs of extravasation occur, terminate the infusion immediately and restart in another vein. For management, see the Antineoplastic Introduction.

Carcinogenesis/Mutagenesis: Doxorubicin and related compounds have mutagenic and carcinogenic properties in experimental models.

Pregnancy: Safety for use during pregnancy not established. Use only when the potential benefits outweigh the potential hazards to the fetus. Doxorubicin is embryotoxic and teratogenic in rats and embryotoxic and abortifacient in rabbits. Doxorubicin has been given during pregnancy without adverse fetal effect and has been detected in fetal tissue; however, its effect on the human fetus is unknown.

Precautions:

Monitoring: Initial treatment requires close patient observation and extensive laboratory monitoring. Hospitalize patients at least during the first phase of treatment.

Hyperuricemia may be induced by doxorubicin secondary to rapid lysis of neoplastic cells. Monitor patient's blood uric acid level.

Urine discoloration: Doxorubicin imparts a red color to the urine for 1 to 2 days after administration; advise patients to expect this during active therapy.

Drug Interactions:

Antineoplastic agents: Doxorubicin may potentiate the toxicity of other antineoplastics. Exacerbation of **cyclophosphamide**-induced hemorrhagic cystitis and enhancement of the hepatotoxicity of **6-mercaptopurine** have occurred.

Barbiturates may increase the total plasma clearance of doxorubicin.

Digoxin: Serum levels may be decreased by combination chemotherapy (including doxorubicin). Digitoxin and digoxin capsules do not appear to be affected.

Radiation-induced toxicity to the myocardium, mucosa, skin and liver have been increased by doxorubicin administration.

Adverse Reactions:

Dose-limiting toxicities are *myelosuppression* and *cardiotoxicity* (see Warnings).

GI: Acute nausea and vomiting (21% to 55%) may be severe. This may be alleviated by antiemetic therapy. Mucositis (stomatitis and esophagitis) may occur 5 to 10 days after administration, leading to ulceration, and may represent a site of origin for severe infections. The incidence and severity of mucositis is greater with the 3 successive daily dosage regimen. Ulceration and necrosis of the colon, especially the cecum, may occur leading to bleeding or severe infections which can be fatal. This reaction has occurred in patients with acute non-lymphocytic leukemia treated with a 3 day course of doxorubicin plus cytarabine. Occasionally, anorexia and diarrhea occur.

Cutaneous: Reversible complete alopecia (85% to 100%); hyperpigmentation of nailbeds and dermal creases (primarily in children); onycholysis; recall of skin reaction due to prior radiotherapy. If powder or solution contacts the skin or mucosa, wash thoroughly with soap and water.

Vascular: Phlebosclerosis, especially when small veins are used or a single vein is used for repeated administration. Facial flushing may occur if injection is given too rapidly.

(Adverse Reactions continued on following page)

Anthracyclines (Cont.)

DOXORUBICIN HCl (ADR) (Cont.)

Adverse Reactions (Cont):

Local: Severe cellulitis, vesication and tissue necrosis will occur if doxorubicin is extravasated. Erythematous streaking along the vein next to the injection site has occurred.

Hypersensitivity: Fever; chills; urticaria; anaphylaxis; lincomycin cross-sensitivity.

Ocular: Conjunctivitis and lacrimation occur rarely.

Overdosage:

Acute overdosage enhances the toxic effects of mucositis, leukopenia and thrombocytopenia. Treat the severely myelosuppressed patient by hospitalization, antibiotics, platelet and granulocyte transfusions and give symptomatic treatment of mucositis.

Chronic overdosage with cumulative doses exceeding 550 mg/m² increases the risk of cardiomyopathy and resultant CHF. Treatment consists of vigorous management of CHF with digitalis preparations and diuretics. Use of peripheral vasodilators is recommended.

Administration and Dosage:

For IV use only.

Recommended dosage schedule: 60 to 75 mg/m², as a single IV injection administered at 21 day intervals. Give the lower dose to patients with inadequate marrow reserves due to old age, prior therapy or neoplastic marrow infiltration.

Alternative dose schedules: 30 mg/m² on each of 3 successive days, repeated every 4 weeks. Another alternative dose schedule is weekly doses of 20 mg/m² which may produce a lower incidence of CHF.

Dosage in patients with elevated bilirubin: Serum bilirubin 1.2 to 3 mg/dl, give 50% of normal dose; >3 mg/dl, give 25% of normal dose.

IV infusion: Administer doxorubicin slowly into the tubing of a freely running IV infusion of Sodium Chloride Injection or 5% Dextrose Injection. Attach the tubing to a Butterfly needle inserted into a large vein. Avoid veins over joints or in extremities with compromised venous or lymphatic drainage. Rate depends on the size of the vein and the dosage; however, do not administer in less than 3 to 5 minutes. Local erythematous streaking along the vein as well as facial flushing may indicate too rapid administration.

Extravasation – A burning or stinging sensation may indicate perivenous infiltration; perivenous infiltration may occur painlessly. See Warnings.

Preparation and storage of solution: Dilute the 10 mg vial with 5 ml, the 20 mg vial with 10 ml, the 50 mg vial with 25 ml, the 100 mg vial with 50 ml, and the 150 mg vial with 75 ml of 0.9% Sodium Chloride to give a final concentration of 2 mg/ml. Bacteriostatic diluents are not recommended. Reconstituted solution is stable for 24 hours at room temperature and 48 hours at 2° to 8°C (36° to 46°F). Protect from sunlight; discard unused solution.

IV incompatibilities: Incompatible with **heparin, cephalothin** and **dexamethasone sodium phosphate;** a precipitate will form. A color change in doxorubicin from red to blue-purple which denotes decomposition occurs with **aminophylline** and **5-fluorouracil**. Until specific data are available, do not mix doxorubicin with other drugs. One study reported that a solution of doxorubicin and vinblastine in 0.9% Sodium Chloride is compatible and relatively stable for at least 5 days.

Rx	**Doxorubicin HCl** (Cetus)	**Powder for Injection (lyophilized)**: 10 mg	With 50 mg lactose. In vials.
Rx	**Rubex** (Bristol-Myers Oncology)		With 50 mg lactose. In vials.
Rx	**Doxorubicin HCl** (Cetus)	**Powder for Injection (lyophilized)**: 20 mg	With 100 mg lactose. In vials.
Rx	**Doxorubicin HCl** (Cetus)	**Powder for Injection (lyophilized)**: 50 mg	With 250 mg lactose. In vials.
Rx	**Rubex** (Bristol-Myers Oncology)		With 250 mg lactose. In vials.
Rx	**Rubex** (Bristol-Myers Oncology)	**Powder for Injection (lyophilized)**: 100 mg	With 500 mg lactose. In vials.
Rx	**Adriamycin RDF** (Adria)	**Powder for Injection (lyophilized)**: 10, 20, 50 and 150[1] mg	In vials.[2] *Rapid dissolution formula.*
Rx	**Doxorubicin HCl** (Cetus)	**Injection, aqueous**: 2 mg/ml	With 0.9% sodium chloride. In 5, 10 and 25 ml vials.
Rx	**Adriamycin PFS** (Adria Labs)	**Preservative Free Injection:** 2 mg/ml	In 5, 10, 25 and 100 ml vials.

[1] Multiple-dose vial.
[2] With methylparaben and 50, 100, 250 and 750 mg lactose, respectively.

DAUNORUBICIN HCl (DNR)

Warning:

Give daunorubicin into a rapidly flowing IV infusion. *Never* administer IM or SC. Severe local tissue necrosis will result if extravasation occurs.

Myocardial toxicity, in its most severe form, potentially fatal congestive heart failure (CHF), may occur when total cumulative dosage exceeds 550 mg/m² in adults, 300 mg/m² in children > 2 years old, or 10 mg/kg in children < 2 years old. This may occur during therapy or several months after therapy. Treatment includes digitalis, diuretics, sodium restriction and bed rest.

The physician and institution must be capable of responding rapidly and completely to severe hemorrhagic conditions or overwhelming infection.

Severe myelosuppression occurs when used in therapeutic doses.

Reduce dosage in patients with impaired hepatic or renal function.

Actions:

An anthracycline cytotoxic antibiotic produced by *Streptomyces coeruleorubidus*.

Pharmacology: Inhibits nucleic acid synthesis by insertion into the DNA double helix. Other binding or free radical reactions may occur. The drug has antimitotic, cytotoxic and immunosuppressive activity, but the precise mode of action is unknown.

Pharmacokinetics: Absorption/Distribution - Following IV injection, daunorubicin undergoes rapid tissue uptake and concentration. It does not cross the blood-brain barrier. Plasma and tissue protein binding is rapid and extensive; 25% concentrates in the liver.

Metabolism/Excretion - Daunorubicin is metabolized by carbonyl reduction to the active alcohol daunorubicinol, the predominant plasma compound. Further metabolism by reduction and conjugation occurs. Terminal half-lives for daunorubicin and daunorubicinol are 18.5 and 26.7 hours, respectively. About 25% is eliminated in active form by urinary excretion and 40% by biliary excretion.

Indications:

For remission induction in acute nonlymphocytic leukemia (myelogenous, monocytic, erythroid) of adults and for remission induction in acute lymphocytic leukemia of children and adults. In the treatment of adult acute nonlymphocytic leukemia, daunorubicin used as a single agent produces complete remission rates of 40% to 50%; in combination with cytarabine, it produces complete remission rates of 53% to 65%.

In children receiving identical CNS prophylaxis and maintenance therapy for childhood acute lymphocytic leukemia (without consolidation) after induction, there is a prolongation of complete remission duration induced with the three drug (daunorubicin-vincristine-prednisone) regimen, as compared to two drugs (vincristine-prednisone). There is no evidence that daunorubicin has any impact on the duration of complete remission when a consolidation (intensification) phase is used as part of a total treatment program.

In adult acute lymphocytic leukemia, in contrast to childhood acute lymphocytic leukemia, daunorubicin during induction significantly increases the rate of complete remission, but not remission duration, compared to that obtained with vincristine, prednisone and L-asparaginase alone. Daunorubicin combined with vincristine, prednisone and L-asparaginase produces complete remission rates of 83% in contrast to a 47% remission in patients not receiving daunorubicin.

Warnings:

Bone marrow suppression will occur in all patients given a therapeutic dose of this drug. Do not start therapy in patients with preexisting drug-induced bone marrow suppression unless the benefit from such treatment warrants the risk.

Cardiac toxicity: Preexisting heart disease or previous doxorubicin therapy are co-factors of increased risk of cardiac toxicity; weigh benefit-to-risk ratio before starting therapy. Give attention to the drug's potential cardiac toxicity, particularly in infants and children.

In adults, at total cumulative doses < 550 mg/m², acute CHF is seldom encountered. However, rare instances of pericarditis-myocarditis, not dose-related, have occurred. At cumulative doses > 550 mg/m², there is an increased incidence of CHF. This limit appears lower (400 mg/m²) in patients receiving radiation therapy that encompassed the heart. In infants and children, there is a greater susceptibility to anthracycline-induced cardiotoxicity compared to that in adults, which is more clearly dose-related. However, there is very little risk for children > 2 years old below a cumulative dose of 300 mg/m², or in children < 2 years old (or < 0.5 m² body surface area) below a cumulative dose of 10 mg/kg. Furthermore, the total dose given to both children and adults should take into account any previous or concomitant therapy with other potentially cardiotoxic agents or related compounds such as doxorubicin.

(Warnings continued on following page)

DAUNORUBICIN HCl (DNR) (Cont.)

Warnings (Cont.):

Cardiac toxicity (Cont.): There is no reliable method for predicting patients who will develop acute CHF; certain ECG changes and a decrease in the systolic ejection fraction from pretreatment baseline may aid in recognizing those patients at greatest risk. A decrease of $\geq$ 30% in limb lead QRS voltage has been associated with significant risk of drug-induced cardiomyopathy. Perform an ECG or determine systolic ejection fraction before each course. If one or the other of these predictive parameters should occur, weigh the benefit of continued therapy against the risk of producing cardiac damage.

Early clinical diagnosis of drug-induced CHF is essential for successful treatment with digitalis, diuretics, sodium restriction and bed rest.

Hepatic and renal function impairment can enhance toxicity; therefore, prior to administration, evaluate hepatic and renal function using conventional clinical laboratory tests.

Extravasation at injection site can cause severe local tissue necrosis. Stop the injection immediately. For management see the Antineoplastic Introduction.

Carcinogenesis, mutagenesis, impairment of fertility: Daunorubicin injected SC into mice causes fibrosarcomas to develop at the injection site.

In male dogs, at a daily dose of 0.25 mg/kg administered IV, testicular atrophy was noted at autopsy. Histologic examination revealed total aplasia of the spermatocyte series in the seminiferous tubules with complete aspermatogenesis.

Pregnancy: Category D. Due to its teratogenic potential, daunorubicin can cause fetal harm if administered to a pregnant woman. An increased incidence of fetal abnormalities (parieto-occipital cranioschisis, umbilical hernias or rachischisis) and abortions occurred in rabbits. Decreases in fetal birth weight and postdelivery growth rate were observed in mice. If used during pregnancy, or if the patient becomes pregnant while taking this drug, inform her of the potential hazard. There are no adequate and well controlled studies in pregnant women. Advise women of childbearing potential to avoid becoming pregnant.

Precautions:

Observe patient closely and monitor chemical and laboratory tests extensively. Evaluate cardiac, renal and hepatic function prior to each course of treatment.

Hyperuricemia may be induced secondary to rapid lysis of leukemic cells. As a precaution, administer allopurinol prior to initiating antileukemic therapy. Monitor serum uric acid levels; initiate therapy if hyperuricemia develops.

Urine discoloration (red) may occur transiently; advise patient appropriately.

Control any systemic infection before beginning therapy.

Adverse Reactions:

Dose-limiting toxicity includes myelosuppression and cardiotoxicity (see Warnings).

Cutaneous: Reversible alopecia.

GI: Acute nausea and vomiting (usually mild). Antiemetic therapy may help. Mucositis may occur 3 to 7 days after administration. Diarrhea occurs occasionally.

Local: If extravasation occurs, tissue necrosis can result at the site.

Acute reactions: Fever, chills and skin rash occur rarely.

(Continued on following page)

Anthracyclines (Cont.)

DAUNORUBICIN HCl (DNR) (Cont.)

Administration and Dosage:

For IV use only.

To eradicate the leukemic cells and induce a complete remission, a profound suppression of bone marrow is usually required. Evaluation of both the peripheral blood and bone marrow are mandatory in the formulation of treatment plans.

Representative dose schedules and combination for the approved indication of remission induction in adult acute nonlymphocytic leukemia: Patients < 60 yrs – Daunorubicin 45 $mg/m^2/day$ IV on days 1, 2 and 3 of the first course and on days 1 and 2 of subsequent courses and cytosine arabinoside 100 $mg/m^2/day$ IV infusion daily for 7 days for the first course and for 5 days for subsequent courses.

Patients ≥ 60 yrs – Daunorubicin 30 $mg/m^2/day$ IV on days 1, 2 and 3 of the first course and on days 1 and 2 of subsequent courses and cytosine arabinoside 100 $mg/m^2/day$ IV infusion daily for 7 days for the first course and for 5 days for subsequent courses. This daunorubicin dose reduction is based on a single study and may not be appropriate if optimal supportive care is available.

Attaining a normal appearing bone marrow may require up to 3 courses of induction therapy. Evaluate bone marrow following recovery from the previous induction course to determine the need for a further course of induction treatment.

Representative dose schedule and combination for the approved indication of remission induction in pediatric acute lymphocytic leukemia: Daunorubicin 25 mg/m^2 IV on day 1 every week, vincristine 1.5 mg/m^2 IV on day 1 every week, oral prednisone 40 $mg/m^2/day$. Generally, complete remission will be obtained with four such courses of therapy; however, if after four courses the patient is in partial remission, an additional one or, if necessary, two courses may be given in an effort to obtain a complete remission.

In children < 2 years of age or < 0.5 m^2, calculate dosage on the basis of weight (mg/kg) instead of body surface area.

Representative dose schedules and combination for the approved indication of remission induction in adult acute lymphocytic leukemia: Daunorubicin 45 $mg/m^2/day$ IV on days 1, 2 and 3 and vincristine 2 mg IV on days 1, 8 and 15; prednisone 40 $mg/m^2/day$ orally on days 1 through 22, then tapered between days 22 to 29; L-asparaginase 500 IU/kg/day × 10 days IV on days 22 through 32.

Hepatic or renal function impairment: Reduce dosage.

Daunorubicin Dosage in Hepatic or Renal Function Impairment		
Serum bilirubin	Serum creatinine	Recommended dose
1.2 to 3 mg/dl		¾ normal dose
> 3 mg mg/dl	> 3 mg/dl	½ normal dose

Preparation and storage: Reconstitute vial contents with 4 ml Sterile Water for Injection to prepare a solution of 5 mg of daunorubicin activity per ml. Withdraw the desired dose into a syringe containing 10 to 15 ml of normal saline; inject into the tubing or sidearm of a rapidly flowing IV infusion of 5% glucose or normal saline solution. The reconstituted solution is stable for 24 hours at room temperature and 48 hours under refrigeration. Protect from exposure to sunlight. Do not mix with other drugs or heparin.

Rx	**Cerubidine** (Wyeth-Ayerst)	**Lyophilized Powder for Injection:** 20 mg (as HCl)	In vials.[1]

[1] With 100 mg mannitol.

MITOXANTRONE HCl

Actions:

Mitoxantrone is a synthetic antineoplastic anthracenedione for IV use.

Pharmacology: Although its mechanism of action is not fully elucidated, mitoxantrone is a DNA-reactive agent. It has a cytocidal effect on both proliferating and nonproliferating cultured human cells, suggesting lack of cell cycle phase specificity.

Pharmacokinetics: Absorption/Distribution – Pharmacokinetic studies in adults following a single IV administration have demonstrated multi-exponential plasma clearance. Distribution to tissues is rapid and extensive. Multiple IV doses in dogs daily for 5 days resulted in a fourfold accumulation in plasma and tissue. The apparent steady-state volume of distribution exceeds 1000 L/m^2. Elimination is slow with an apparent mean terminal plasma half-life of 5.8 days (range, 2.3 to 13). The half-life in tissues may be longer. Mitoxantrone is 78% bound to plasma proteins in the concentration range of 26 to 455 ng/ml.

Metabolism/Excretion – Excretion is via the renal and hepatobiliary systems. Renal excretion is limited; only 6% to 11% of the dose is recovered in the urine within 5 days after administration. Of the material recovered in the urine, 65% is unchanged drug; the remaining 35% is comprised of two inactive metabolites and their glucuronide conjugates (mono- and dicarboxylic acid derivatives). Hepatobiliary elimination of drug appears to be of greater significance; 25% of the dose is recovered in the feces within 5 days of IV dosing. No significant difference in pharmacokinetics was observed in seven patients with moderately impaired liver function (serum bilirubin 1.3 to 3.4 mg/dl) as compared with 16 patients without hepatic dysfunction. Results of pharmacokinetic studies on four patients with severe hepatic dysfunction (bilirubin $>$ 3.4 mg/dl) suggest that these patients have a lower total body clearance and a larger area under curve than other patients at a comparable dose.

Clinical pharmacology: The benefit of consolidation therapy in acute nonlymphocytic leukemia (ANLL) patients who achieve a complete remission remains controversial. However, in the only well controlled prospective, randomized multicenter trials with mitoxantrone in ANLL, consolidation therapy was given to all patients who achieved a complete remission. During consolidation in the US study, two myelosuppression-related deaths occurred in mitoxantrone patients and one in daunorubicin patients. However, in the foreign study, there were eight deaths in mitoxantrone patients during consolidation that were related to the myelosuppression, and none in daunorubicin patients where less myelosuppression occurred.

Indications:

In combination with other approved drug(s) in the initial therapy of ANLL in adults. This includes myelogenous, promyelocytic, monocytic and erythroid acute leukemias.

Unlabeled uses: Mitoxantrone may be beneficial, alone or in combination with other agents, in the treatment of breast cancer and refractory lymphomas. Response rates for breast cancer have been as high as 40% when used as a single agent. For non-Hodgkin's lymphoma, a high-dose intermittent dosage schedule appears to be more effective than a lower-dose weekly schedule.

Contraindications:

Hypersensitivity to mitoxantrone.

Warnings:

When used in doses indicated for the treatment of leukemia, severe myelosuppression will occur. Therefore, it is recommended that the drug be administered only by physicians experienced in the chemotherapy of this disease. Laboratory and supportive services must be available for hematologic and chemistry monitoring and adjunctive therapies, including antibiotics. Blood and blood products must be available to support patients during the expected period of medullary hypoplasia and severe myelosuppression. Give particular care to assuring full hematologic recovery before undertaking consolidation therapy (if this treatment is used); monitor patients closely during this phase.

Myelosuppression: Patients with preexisting myelosuppression as the result of prior drug therapy should not receive mitoxantrone unless it is felt that the possible benefit from such treatment warrants the risk of further medullary suppression.

(Warnings continued on following page.)

MITOXANTRONE HCl (Cont.)

Warnings (Cont.)

Cardiac: Functional cardiac changes including congestive heart failure (CHF) and decreases in left ventricular ejection fraction (LVEF) occur. Cardiac toxicity may be more common in patients with prior treatment with anthracyclines, prior mediastinal radiotherapy, or with preexisting cardiovascular disease. Such patients should have regular cardiac monitoring of LVEF from the initiation of therapy. In investigational trials of intermittent single doses in other tumor types, patients who received up to the cumulative dose of 140 mg/m^2 had a cumulative 2.6% probability of clinical CHF. The overall cumulative probability rate of moderate or serious decreases in LVEF at this dose was 13% in comparative trials.

Acute CHF may occasionally occur in patients treated for ANLL. In first-line comparative trials of mitoxantrone plus cytosine arabinoside in adult patients with previously untreated ANLL, therapy was associated with CHF in 6.5% of patients. A causal relationship between drug therapy and cardiac effects is difficult to establish in this setting since myocardial function is frequently depressed by the anemia, fever, infection and hemorrhage which often accompany the underlying disease.

Carcinogenesis/Mutagenesis: Mitoxantrone can result in chromosomal aberrations in animals and it is mutagenic in bacterial systems. Mitoxantrone caused DNA damage and sister chromatid exchanges in vitro.

Pregnancy: Category D. May cause fetal harm when administered to a pregnant woman. In treated rats, low fetal birth weight and retarded development of the fetal kidney were seen in greater frequency. In rabbits, an increased incidence of premature delivery was observed. Mitoxantrone was not teratogenic in rabbits. There are no adequate and well controlled studies in pregnant women. If this drug is used during pregnancy, or if the patient becomes pregnant while taking this drug, apprise her of the potential hazard to the fetus. Advise women of childbearing potential to avoid becoming pregnant.

Lactation: It is not known whether this drug is excreted in breast milk. Because of the potential for serious adverse reactions in infants, discontinue breastfeeding before starting treatment.

Children: Safety and efficacy for use in children have not been established.

Precautions:

For IV use only: Safety for use by routes other than IV administration has not been established. Do not use intrathecally.

Monitoring: Accompany therapy by close and frequent monitoring of hematologic and chemical laboratory parameters, as well as frequent patient observation. Serial complete blood counts and liver function tests are necessary for appropriate dose adjustments.

Hyperuricemia may occur as a result of rapid lysis of tumor cells. Monitor serum uric acid levels and institute hypouricemic therapy prior to initiation of antileukemic therapy.

Systemic infections: Treat concomitantly with or just before starting mitoxantrone.

Hepatotoxicity: Patients have developed transient elevations of AST and ALT following mitoxantrone administration (4 to 24 days after treatment).

Adverse Reactions:

Mitoxantrone has been studied in approximately 600 patients with ANLL. The following table summarizes adverse reactions occurring in patients treated with mitoxantrone plus cytosine arabinoside for therapy of ANLL in a large multicenter randomized prospective US trial. Adverse reactions are presented as major categories and selected examples of clinically significant subcategories. Experience in the large foreign study was similar. A much wider experience in a variety of other tumor types revealed no additional important reactions other than cardiomyopathy. Note that the listed adverse reaction categories include overlapping clinical symptoms related to the same condition (eg, dyspnea, cough, pneumonia). In addition, the listed adverse reactions cannot all necessarily be attributed to chemotherapy as it is often impossible to distinguish effects of the drug from effects of the underlying disease. It is clear, however, that the combination of mitoxantrone plus cytosine arabinoside was responsible for nausea and vomiting, alopecia, mucositis/stomatitis and myelosuppression.

(Adverse Reactions continued on following page.)

MITOXANTRONE HCl (Cont.)

Adverse Reactions (Cont.):

Mitoxantrone Adverse Reactions		
	Induction (%)	Consolidation (%)
Cardiovascular	26	11
CHF	5	0
Arrhythmias	3	4
Bleeding	37	20
GI bleeding	16	2
Petechiae/Ecchymosis	7	11
GI	88	58
Nausea/Vomiting	72	31
Diarrhea	47	18
Abdominal pain	15	9
Mucositis/Stomatitis	29	18
Hepatic	10	14
Jaundice	3	7
Infections	66	60
UTI	7	7
Pneumonia	9	9
Sepsis	34	31
Fungal infections	15	9
Pulmonary	43	24
Cough	13	9
Dyspnea	18	6
CNS	30	34
Seizures	4	2
Headache	10	13
Eye	7	2
Conjunctivitis	5	0
Other		
Renal failure	8	0
Fever	78	24
Alopecia	37	22

Other adverse reactions include: Chest pain; asymptomatic decreases in LVEF; tachycardia; ECG changes; myelosuppression; hypotension, urticaria, dyspnea, rashes (occasionally); phlebitis at infusion site (infrequent); tissue necrosis following extravasation (rare).

Overdosage:

There is no known specific antidote. Accidental overdoses have occurred. Four patients receiving 140 to 180 mg/m² as a single bolus injection died as a result of severe leukopenia with infection. Hematologic support and antimicrobial therapy may be required during prolonged periods of medullary hypoplasia.

Although patients with severe renal failure have not been studied, mitoxantrone is extensively tissue bound and it is unlikely that the therapeutic effect or toxicity would be mitigated by peritoneal or hemodialysis.

(Continued on following page)

MITOXANTRONE HCl (Cont.)

Patient Information:

Mitoxantrone may impart a blue-green color to the urine for 24 hours after administration; advise patients to expect this during therapy. Bluish discoloration of the sclera may also occur. Advise patients of the signs and symptoms of myelosuppression.

Administration and Dosage:

Mitoxantrone solution must be diluted prior to use.

Combination initial therapy for ANLL in adults: For induction, 12 mg/m²/day on days 1 to 3 given as an IV infusion, and 100 mg/m² of cytosine arabinoside for 7 days given as a continuous 24 hour infusion on days 1 to 7.

Most complete remissions will occur following the initial course of induction therapy. In the event of an incomplete antileukemic response, a second induction course may be given. Give mitoxantrone for 2 days and cytosine arabinoside for 5 days using the same daily dosage levels.

If severe or life-threatening nonhematologic toxicity is observed during the first induction course, withhold the second induction course until toxicity clears.

Consolidation therapy used in two large randomized multicenter trials consisted of mitoxantrone 12 mg/m² given by IV infusion daily for days 1 and 2, and cytosine arabinoside 100 mg/m² for 5 days given as a continuous 24 hour infusion on days 1 to 5. The first course was given ≈ 6 weeks after the final induction course, the second was generally administered 4 weeks after the first. Severe myelosuppression occurred.

Preparation of solution: Dilute solution to at least 50 ml with either 0.9% Sodium Chloride Injection or 5% Dextrose Injection. Introduce this solution slowly into the tubing as a freely running IV infusion of 0.9% Sodium Chloride Injection or 5% Dextrose Injection over a period of not less than 3 minutes. Discard unused infusion solutions in an appropriate fashion. If extravasation occurs, stop administration immediately and restart in another vein. The nonvesicant properties of mitoxantrone minimize the possibility of severe local reactions following extravasation. However, take care to avoid extravasation at the infusion site and to avoid contact with the skin, mucous membranes or eyes.

Mitoxantrone may be further diluted into Dextrose 5% in Water, Normal Saline or Dextrose 5% with Normal Saline and used immediately.

If skin is accidentally exposed to mitoxantrone, rinse copiously with warm water; if the eyes are involved, use standard irrigation techniques immediately. The use of goggles, gloves and protective gowns is recommended during preparation and administration of the drug. Spills on equipment and environmental surfaces may be cleaned using an aqueous solution of calcium hypochlorite (5.5 parts calcium hypochlorite in 13 parts by weight of water for each 1 part of mitoxantrone). Absorb the solution with gauze or towels and dispose of these in a safe manner. Wear appropriate safety equipment such as goggles and gloves while working with calcium hypochlorite.

IV incompatibility: Do not mix in the same infusion as heparin; a precipitate may form. Because specific compatibility data are not available, it is recommended that mitoxantrone not be mixed in the same infusion with other drugs.

Storage: Do not freeze.

Rx	**Novantrone** (Lederle)	**Injection:** 2 mg mitoxantrone base per ml	In 10, 12.5 and 15 ml vials.

MITOMYCIN (Mitomycin-C; MTC)

Warning:

Bone marrow suppression, notably thrombocytopenia and leukopenia, which may contribute to overwhelming infection in an already compromised patient, is the most common and severe toxic effect of mitomycin (see Warnings and Adverse Reactions).

Hemolytic uremic syndrome, a serious syndrome of microangiopathic hemolytic anemia, thrombocytopenia and irreversible renal failure has occurred (see Warnings).

Actions:

Pharmacology: Mitomycin is an antibiotic with antitumor activity isolated from *Streptomyces caespitosus*. It selectively inhibits the synthesis of deoxyribonucleic acid (DNA). The guanine and cytosine content correlates with the degree of mitomycin-induced cross-linking. At high concentrations, cellular ribonucleic acid (RNA) and protein synthesis are also suppressed.

Pharmacokinetics: Absorption/Distribution – IV mitomycin is rapidly cleared from the serum. Maximal serum concentrations were 2.4 mcg/ml after IV injection of 30 mg; 1.7 mcg/ml after a 20 mg dose, and 0.52 mcg/ml after 10 mg. Serum half-life after a 30 mg bolus injection is 17 minutes.

Metabolism/Excretion - Clearance is effected primarily by hepatic metabolism, but metabolism occurs in other tissues as well. The rate of clearance is inversely proportional to the maximal serum concentration due to saturation of degradative pathways. Approximately 10% of a dose is excreted unchanged in urine. Because of saturable metabolic pathways, the percent excreted in urine increases with increasing dose.

Indications:

Therapy of disseminated adenocarcinoma of stomach or pancreas combined with other chemotherapeutic agents, and as palliative treatment when other modalities fail.

Unlabeled uses: Mitomycin has been given by the intravesical route for the management of superficial bladder cancer. Mitomycin as an ophthalmic solution appears beneficial as an adjunct to surgical excision in the treatment of primary or recurrent pterygia.

Contraindications:

Primary therapy as a single agent; to replace surgery or radiotherapy; hypersensitivity or idiosyncratic reaction to mitomycin; patients with thrombocytopenia, coagulation disorder or an increase in bleeding tendency due to other causes.

Warnings:

Bone marrow suppression, particularly thrombocytopenia and leukopenia, occurring in 64% of patients, is the most serious toxicity and is cumulative. Thrombocytopenia or leukopenia may occur any time within 8 weeks (average 4 weeks) of therapy; recovery after therapy is within 10 weeks. About 25% of the patients did not recover.

Perform the following during and for at least 8 weeks following therapy: Platelet count, WBC, differential and hemoglobin. A platelet count $< 100{,}000/mm^3$ or a WBC $< 4{,}000/mm^3$, or a progressive decline in either, is an indication to interrupt therapy. Observe patients frequently during and after therapy. Advise patients of potential toxicity, particularly bone marrow suppression. Deaths have occurred due to septicemia as a result of leukopenia.

Renal function: Observe patients for evidence of renal toxicity. Do not give to patients with a serum creatinine > 1.7 mg/dl.

Carcinogenesis: At doses approximating the recommended clinical dose in man, mitomycin produces a 50% to 100% increase in tumor incidence in rats and mice.

Pregnancy: Safety for use during pregnancy has not been established. Teratological changes have been noted in animal studies.

Precautions:

Adult respiratory distress syndrome: A few cases have occurred in patients receiving mitomycin in combination with other chemotherapy and maintained at FIO_2 concentrations $> 50\%$ perioperatively. Exercise caution to use only enough oxygen to provide adequate arterial saturation since oxygen itself is toxic to the lungs. Pay careful attention to fluid balance; avoid overhydration.

Drug Interactions:

Vinca alkaloids: Acute shortness of breath and severe bronchospasm have occurred following use of vinca alkaloids in patients who had previously or simultaneously received mitomycin. Onset of this acute respiratory distress occurs within minutes to hours after the vinca alkaloid injection. Total number of doses for each drug varies considerably. Bronchodilators, steroids or oxygen produce symptomatic relief.

(Continued on following page)

MITOMYCIN (Mitomycin-C; MTC) (Cont.)

Adverse Reactions:

Bone marrow toxicity (64%): Thrombocytopenia and leukopenia (see Warnings).

Integument and mucous membrane (4%): Cellulitis at injection site is occasionally severe; stomatitis; alopecia. Rashes occur rarely.

Extravasation – The most important dermatological problem with this drug is necrosis and consequent tissue sloughing if the drug is extravasated during injection, which may occur with or without stinging or burning and even if there is adequate blood return when the needle is aspirated. Delayed erythema or ulceration may occur either at or distant from injection site, weeks to months after use, even when no evidence of extravasation was seen during use. For management, see Antineoplastics Introduction.

Renal: 2% of 1281 patients had a significant rise in serum creatinine. There was no correlation between total dose or duration of therapy and degree of renal impairment.

Pulmonary toxicity: Occurs infrequently, but can be severe or life-threatening. Dyspnea with nonproductive cough and radiographic evidence of pulmonary infiltrates may indicate pulmonary toxicity. If other etiologies are eliminated, discontinue therapy. Steroids have been employed as treatment of this toxicity, but therapeutic value has not been determined. Adult respiratory distress syndrome may also occur (see Precautions).

Hemolytic uremic syndrome (HUS): This serious complication of chemotherapy, consisting primarily of microangiopathic hemolytic anemia (hematocrit ≤ 25%), thrombocytopenia (≤ 100,000/mm³) and irreversible renal failure (serum creatinine ≥ 1.6 mg/dl) has occurred in patients receiving mitomycin. Microangiopathic hemolysis with fragmented red blood cells on peripheral blood smears has occurred in 98% of patients with the syndrome. Other less frequent complications may include: Pulmonary edema (65%); neurologic abnormalities (16%); hypertension. Exacerbation of the symptoms associated with HUS has occurred in some patients receiving blood product transfusions. A high mortality rate (52%) has been associated with this syndrome.

The syndrome may occur at any time during therapy with mitomycin as a single agent or in combination with other cytotoxic drugs. Closely monitor patients receiving ≥ 60 mg for unexplained anemia with fragmented cells on peripheral blood smear, thrombocytopenia and decreased renal function.

Acute side effects (14%): Fever; anorexia; nausea; vomiting.

Other: Headache; blurred vision; confusion; drowsiness; syncope; fatigue; edema; thrombophlebitis; hematemesis; diarrhea; pain. These did not appear to be dose-related and were not unequivocally drug-related.

Administration and Dosage:

Give IV only. If extravasation occurs, cellulitis, ulceration and sloughing may result.

After hematological recovery (see dosage adjustment guide) from previous chemotherapy use 20 mg/m² IV as a single dose at 6 to 8 week intervals.

Because of cumulative myelosuppression, reevaluate patients after each course of therapy; reduce dose if patient experiences any toxicity. Doses > 20 mg/m² are not more effective, and are more toxic than lower doses. Do not repeat dosage until leukocyte count has returned to 4000/mm³ and platelet count to 100,000/mm³. If disease continues to progress after two courses, discontinue; chances of response are minimal. When used with other myelosuppressive agents, adjust dosage appropriately.

Dosage Adjustment for Mitomycin

Nadir after prior dose per mm³		% of prior dose to be given
Leukocytes	Platelets	
>4000	>100,000	100
3000-3999	75,000-99,999	100
2000-2999	25,000-74,999	70
<2000	<25,000	50

Preparation of solution: Reconstitute 5, 20 or 40 mg vial with 10, 40 or 80 ml Sterile Water for Injection, respectively. If product does not dissolve immediately, allow to stand at room temperature until solution is obtained.

Stability: Avoid excessive heat (> 40°C). Reconstituted with Sterile Water for Injection to 0.5 mg/ml, solution is stable for 14 days under refrigeration, 7 days at room temp.

Diluted in various IV fluids at room temperature to a concentration of 20 to 40 mcg/ml, stability is as follows: 5% Dextrose Injection, 3 hours; 0.9% NaCl Injection, 12 hours; Sodium Lactate Injection, 24 hours.

The combination of mitomycin (5 to 15 mg) and heparin (1,000 to 10,000 units) in 30 ml of 0.9% Sodium Chloride Injection is stable for 48 hours at room temperature.

Rx	**Mutamycin** (Bristol-Myers Oncology)	**Powder for Injection:** 5, 20 and 40 mg	In vials. With 10, 40 and 80 mg mannitol, respectively.

DACTINOMYCIN (Actinomycin D; ACT)

Warning:
Dactinomycin is extremely corrosive to soft tissue. If extravasation occurs during IV use, severe damage to soft tissues will occur. In at least one instance, this has led to contracture of the arms.

Actions:

Pharmacology: Dactinomycin is the principal component of the mixture of actinomycins produced by *Streptomyces parvullus.* Dactinomycin exerts an inhibitory effect on gram-positive and gram-negative bacteria and on some fungi. However, its toxic properties preclude its use as an antibiotic in treating infectious diseases.

Dactinomycin anchors into a purine-pyrimidine (DNA) base pair by intercalation, inhibiting messenger RNA synthesis. Although maximal cell-kill is noted in G_1 phase, the cytotoxic action is primarily cell cycle nonspecific. Actively proliferating cells are more sensitive.

Pharmacokinetics: Very little active drug can be detected in circulating blood 2 minutes after IV injection. It concentrates in nucleated cells and does not cross the blood-brain barrier. Dactinomycin is minimally metabolized. Plasma half-life is ≈ 36 hours.

Indications:

Wilms' tumor: Combinations with vincristine, radiotherapy and surgery.

Rhabdomyosarcoma: Combinations with vincristine, cyclophosphamide and doxorubicin.

Metastatic and nonmetastatic choriocarcinoma: Combination with methotrexate.

Nonseminomatous testicular carcinoma.

Ewing's sarcoma: Palliative treatment alone, with other antineoplastics or x-ray.
Nonmetastatic Ewing's – Cyclosphosphamide and radiotherapy.

Sarcoma botryoides: Palliative treatment alone, with other antineoplastics or radiotherapy.

Radiation therapy effects may be potentiated by dactinomycin; the converse also appears likely. Dactinomycin may be tried in radiosensitive tumors not responding to x-ray therapy. Objective improvement in tumor size and activity may be observed when lower, better tolerated doses of both types of therapy are employed.

Perfusion technique: Dactinomycin alone or with other antineoplastics has been given by the isolation-perfusion technique, either as palliative treatment or as an adjunct to tumor resection; some tumors resistant to chemotherapy and radiation therapy may respond. Neoplasms in which dactinomycin has been tried using this technique include various types of sarcoma, carcinoma and adenocarcinoma. This technique offers advantages, provided drug leakage into the general circulation is minimal. By this technique the drug is in continuous contact with the tumor for the duration of treatment. The dose may be increased well over that used by the systemic route, usually without added toxicity.

Contraindications:

If given at or about the time of infection with chicken pox or herpes zoster, a severe generalized disease may occur, which could result in death.

Warnings:

Radiation: With combined dactinomycin-radiation therapy, the normal skin, as well as the buccal and pharyngeal mucosa, show early erythema. A smaller than usual x-ray dose, when given with dactinomycin, causes erythema and vesiculation which progress more rapidly through the tanning and desquamation stages. Healing may occur in 4 to 6 weeks rather than 2 to 3 months. Erythema from previous x-ray therapy may be reactivated by dactinomycin alone, even when irradiation occurred many months earlier, and especially when the interval between the two forms of therapy is brief. When the nasopharynx is irradiated, the combination may produce severe oropharyngeal mucositis. Severe reactions may appear if high doses are used or if the patient is particularly sensitive to such combined therapy.

Increased incidence of GI toxicity and marrow suppression has occurred when dactinomycin was given with x-ray therapy. Use particular caution in the first 2 months after irradiation for the treatment of right-sided Wilms' tumor, since hepatomegaly and elevated AST levels have been noted.

Reports indicate an increased incidence of second primary tumors following treatment with radiation and dactinomycin.

(Warnings continued on following page)

DACTINOMYCIN (Actinomycin D; ACT)(Cont.)

Warnings (Cont.):

Carcinogenesis/Mutagenesis: The International Agency on Research on Cancer has judged that dactinomycin is a positive carcinogen in animals. Local sarcomas were produced in mice and rats after repeated SC or intraperitoneal injection. Mesenchymal tumors occurred in male rats given intraperitoneal injections of 0.05 mg/kg, 2 to 5 times per week for 18 weeks. The first tumor appeared at 23 weeks.

Dactinomycin has been mutagenic in a number of test systems in vitro and in vivo including human fibroblasts and leukocytes, and HELA cells. DNA damage and cytogenetic effects have been demonstrated in the mouse and the rat.

Pregnancy: Category C. The drug has caused malformations and embryotoxicity in the rat, rabbit and hamster in doses 3 to 7 times the maximum recommended human dose. There are no adequate and well controlled studies in pregnant women. Safety for use during pregnancy has not been established. Use only when clearly needed and when potential benefits outweigh potential hazards to the fetus.

Lactation: It is not known whether this drug is excreted in breast milk. Because of the potential for serious adverse reactions in nursing infants decide whether to discontinue nursing or to discontinue the drug, taking into account the importance of the drug to the mother.

Infants: Do not give to infants < 6 to 12 months of age because of greater frequency of toxic effects.

Precautions:

Reactions may involve any body tissue; anaphylactoid reactions may occur.

Nausea and vomiting due to dactinomycin necessitates intermittent administration. Observe the patient daily for toxic side effects when multiple chemotherapy is used; a full course of therapy occasionally is not tolerated. If stomatitis, diarrhea or severe hematopoietic depression appear, discontinue use until the patient has recovered.

Renal, hepatic and bone marrow function: Many abnormalities have occurred.

This drug is highly toxic. Handle and administer both powder and solution with care. Avoid inhalation of dust or vapors and contact with skin or mucous membranes, especially those of the eyes. Should accidental eye contact occur, immediately institute copious irrigation with water, followed by prompt ophthalmologic consultation. Should accidental skin contact occur, immediately irrigate the affected part with copious amounts of water for at least 15 minutes.

Extravasation: Dactinomycin is extremely corrosive. Extravasation during IV administration causes severe damage to soft tissues. This has led to contracture of the arms in at least one instance. If extravasation occurs, immediately discontinue the infusion. Apply cold compresses to the area. Local infiltration with an injectable corticosteroid may lessen the local reaction. Dilute the drug by infusing saline injection through the line into the infiltrated area.

Drug Interactions:

Drug/Lab test interactions: Dactinomycin may interfere with bioassay procedures for the determination of antibacterial drug levels.

Adverse Reactions:

Toxic effects usually do not become apparent until 2 to 4 days after a course of therapy and may not be maximal before 1 to 2 weeks. Adverse reactions are usually reversible with discontinuation of therapy.

Oral: Cheilitis; dysphagia; esophagitis; ulcerative stomatitis; pharyngitis.

GI: Anorexia; abdominal pain; diarrhea; GI ulceration; proctitis; liver toxicity (including ascites, hepatomegaly, hepatitis and liver function test abnormalities). Alleviate nausea and vomiting occurring during the first few hours after use by giving antiemetics.

Hematologic: Anemia (including aplastic anemia); agranulocytosis; leukopenia; thrombocytopenia; pancytopenia; reticulopenia. Perform platelet and white cell counts daily. If either count markedly decreases, withhold drug until marrow recovery occurs; this often takes up to 3 weeks.

Dermatologic: Alopecia; skin eruptions; acne; flare-up of erythema; increased pigmentation of previously irradiated skin.

Miscellaneous: Malaise; fatigue; lethargy; fever; myalgia; hypocalcemia; death.

Perfusion technique complications may consist of hematopoietic depression, absorption of toxic products from massive destruction of neoplastic tissue, increased susceptibility to infection, impaired wound healing and superficial ulceration of the gastric mucosa. Other side effects may include edema of the extremity involved, damage to soft tissues of the perfused area and (potentially) venous thrombosis.

(Continued on following page)

DACTINOMYCIN (Actinomycin D; ACT) (Cont.)

Administration and Dosage:

Toxic reactions are frequent and may limit the amount of drug that may be given. Severity of toxicity varies and is only partly dependent on dose. Administer the drug in short courses.

IV: Individualize dosage. Do not exceed 15 mcg/kg or 400 to 600 mcg/m² daily IV for 5 days. Calculate the dosage for obese or edematous patients on the basis of surface area in an effort to relate dosage to lean body mass.

Adults: 0.5 mg/day IV for a maximum of 5 days.

Children: 0.015 mg/kg/day IV for 5 days. Alternative schedule is a total dosage of 2.5 mg/m² IV over 1 week.

In both adults and children, administer a second course after at least 3 weeks, provided all signs of toxicity have disappeared.

Isolation-perfusion technique: 0.05 mg/kg for lower extremity or pelvis; 0.035 mg/kg for upper extremity. Use lower doses in obese patients, or when previous therapy has been employed. Complications are related to amount of drug that escapes into systemic circulation.

Use "two-needle technique" if given directly into the vein without use of an infusion. Reconstitute and withdraw dose from vial with one sterile needle. Use another needle for direct injection into vein.

Preparation of solution: Reconstitute by adding 1.1 ml Sterile Water for Injection (without preservative). The resulting solution contains approximately 0.5 mg/ml. Add directly to infusion solutions of 5% Dextrose or Sodium Chloride Injection or to the tubing of a running IV infusion. Although chemically stable after reconstitution, the product does not contain a preservative; discard any unused portion. Use of water that contains preservatives (benzyl alcohol or parabens) to reconstitute the drug for injection results in precipitate formation.

Partial removal of dactinomycin from IV solutions by cellulose ester membrane filters used in some IV in-line filters has been reported.

Storage: Protect from light.

Rx	**Cosmegen** (MSD)	**Lyophilized Powder for Injection:** 0.5 mg	In vials.[1]

[1] With 20 mg mannitol.

PLICAMYCIN (Mithramycin)

Warning:
Severe thrombocytopenia, hemorrhagic tendency and even death may result from use. Although severe toxicity is more apt to occur in patients with advanced disease or patients otherwise considered poor risks for therapy, serious toxicity may also occasionally occur in patients who are in relatively good condition.

Actions:

Pharmacology: Plicamycin is a compound produced by the organism *Streptomyces plicatus.* The exact mechanism of tumor inhibition is unknown; the drug forms a complex with deoxyribonucleic acid (DNA) and inhibits cellular ribonucleic acid (RNA) and enzymatic RNA synthesis. The binding to DNA in the presence of Mg^{++} (or other divalent cations) is responsible for the inhibition of DNA-dependent or DNA-directed RNA synthesis. This action presumably accounts for plicamycin's biological properties.

Plicamycin demonstrates a consistent calcium-lowering effect not related to its tumoricidal activity. It may block the hypercalcemic action of pharmacologic doses of vitamin D. It also acts on osteoclasts and blocks the action of parathyroid hormone. Plicamycin's inhibition of DNA-dependent RNA synthesis appears to render osteoclasts unable to fully respond to parathyroid hormone with the biosynthesis necessary for osteolysis. Decreases in serum phosphate levels and urinary calcium excretion accompany the lowering of serum calcium concentrations.

Pharmacokinetics: Plicamycin is rapidly cleared from the blood within the first 2 hours and excretion is also rapid. Of measured excretion, 67% occurs within 4 hours, 75% within 8 hours, and 90% in the first 24 hours after injection. Plicamycin crosses the blood-brain barrier; the concentration found in brain tissue is low, but it persists longer than in other tissues.

Clinical pharmacology: Inoperable testicular tumors – In a combined series of 305 patients with inoperable testicular tumors treated with plicamycin, 33 patients (11%) showed a complete disappearance of tumor masses; 80 (26%) responded with significant partial regression. The longest duration of a continuing complete response is > 8.5 years.

Plicamycin may be useful in testicular tumors resistant to other chemotherapeutic agents. Prior radiation or chemotherapy did not alter response rate, suggesting no significant cross-resistance between plicamycin and other antineoplastics.

Hypercalcemia/Hypercalciuria – A limited number of patients with hypercalcemia (range: 12 to 25.8 mg/dl) and hypercalciuria (range: 215 to 492 mg/day) associated with malignant disease and treated with plicamycin had reversal of these abnormal levels. In some patients, the primary malignancy was of nontesticular origin.

Indications:

Malignant testicular tumors when surgery or radiation is impossible.

Hypercalcemia and hypercalciuria in symptomatic patients (NOT responsive to conventional treatment) associated with advanced neoplasms.

Contraindications:

Thrombocytopenia, thrombocytopathy, coagulation disorders or increased susceptibility to bleeding due to other causes; impairment of bone marrow function; pregnancy (see Warnings).

Warnings:

Hemorrhagic syndrome, the most important form of toxicity, usually begins with epistaxis. It may only consist of a single or several episodes of epistaxis and progress no further. It can start with hematemesis which may progress to more widespread GI hemorrhage or to a more generalized bleeding tendency. It is most likely due to abnormalities in multiple clotting factors and is dose-related. With doses of ≤ 30 mcg/kg/day for ≤ 10 doses, the incidence of bleeding episodes has been 5.4% with a mortality rate of 1.6%. With doses > 30 mcg/kg/day for ≥ 10 doses, bleeding episodes increased to 11.9% with a mortality rate of 5.7%.

Renal or hepatic function impairment: Use extreme caution. Monitor renal function carefully before, during and after treatment.

Mutagenesis: Histologic evidence of inhibition of spermatogenesis occurs in some male rats receiving doses of ≥ 0.6 mg/kg/day.

Pregnancy: Category X. Use only when clearly needed and when the benefits outweigh the potential toxicity to the embryo or fetus. Plicamycin may cause fetal harm when given to a pregnant woman, and is contraindicated in women who are or may become pregnant. If used during pregnancy or if patient becomes pregnant while taking this drug, inform her of the potential hazard to the fetus.

Lactation: It is not known whether plicamycin is excreted in breast milk. Because of the potential for serious adverse reactions in nursing infants, decide whether to discontinue nursing or the drug, taking into account the importance of the drug to the mother.

(Continued on following page)

PLICAMYCIN (Mithramycin) (Cont.)

Precautions:

Electrolyte imbalance (especially hypocalcemia, hypokalemia and hypophosphatemia): Correct with appropriate therapy prior to treatment.

Monitoring: Obtain platelet count, prothrombin and bleeding times frequently during therapy and for several days following the last dose. Discontinue therapy if thrombocytopenia or a significant prolongation of prothrombin or bleeding times occurs.

Adverse Reactions:

Most common: GI symptoms (anorexia, nausea, vomiting, diarrhea and stomatitis).

Less frequent: Fever; drowsiness; weakness; lethargy; malaise; headache; depression; phlebitis; facial flushing; skin rash; hepatotoxicity (mild, reversible).

Laboratory abnormalities: Generally reversible following cessation of treatment.

Hematologic – Depression of platelet count, white count, hemoglobin and prothrombin; elevation of clotting time and bleeding time; abnormal clot retraction. Thrombocytopenia may be rapid in onset and may occur at any time during therapy or within several days following the last dose. The infusion of platelet concentrates of platelet-rich plasma may help elevate the platelet count. Leukopenia is relatively uncommon (≈ 6%).

Abnormalities in clotting time or clot retraction are not commonly demonstrated prior to the onset of an overt bleeding episode. Perform these tests periodically; abnormalities may serve as a warning of impending serious toxicity.

Liver function – Increased AST, ALT, lactic dehydrogenase, alkaline phosphatase, serum bilirubin, ornithine carbamyl transferase, isocitric dehydrogenase and bromsulphalein retention.

Renal function – Increased BUN and serum creatinine; proteinuria.

Electrolyte abnormalities – Depression of serum calcium, phosphorus and potassium.

Overdosage:

Expect exaggeration of usual adverse effects. Closely monitor hematologic picture including factors involved in clotting mechanism, hepatic and renal functions and serum electrolytes. No specific antidote is known. Management includes general supportive measures.

Patient Information:

Notify physician of any of the following: Fever; sore throat; rashes; chills; unusual bleeding or bruising; bloody nose; black tarry stools; dark urine; yellowing of skin/eyes.

Most common side effects: Nausea, vomiting; stomach upset. Avoid sweet, fried or fatty foods. Eat smaller light meals several times a day. Dry foods (eg, toast, crackers) and liquids (eg, soups, unsweetened apple juice) may be more easily digested. Do not lie down after eating. If this does not help, antinausea drugs may be prescribed.

Contraceptive measures are recommended during treatment.

Calcium supplements are sometimes needed during plicamycin therapy.

Administration and Dosage:

Base daily dose on body weight. Use ideal weight if patient has abnormal fluid retention.

Testicular tumors: 25 to 30 mcg/kg/day for 8 to 10 days unless significant side effects or toxicity occurs. Do not use > 10 daily doses. Do not exceed 30 mcg/kg/day.

In responsive tumors, some degree of regression is usually evident within 3 or 4 weeks following the initial course of therapy. If tumor masses remain unchanged, additional courses at monthly intervals are warranted.

When significant tumor regression is obtained, give additional courses of therapy at monthly intervals until complete regression is obtained or until definite tumor progression or new tumor masses occur, in spite of continued therapy.

Hypercalcemia and hypercalciuria (associated with advanced malignancy): 25 mcg/kg/day for 3 or 4 days. If desired degree of reversal is not achieved with initial course of therapy, repeat at intervals of ≥ 1 week to achieve desired result or to maintain serum and urinary calcium excretion at normal levels. It may be possible to maintain normal calcium balance with single, weekly doses or with 2 or 3 doses per week.

Administer IV only. Dilute daily dose in 1 L of 5% Dextrose Injection or Sodium Chloride Injection, and administer by slow IV infusion over 4 to 6 hours. Avoid rapid direct IV injection because it may be associated with a higher incidence and greater severity of GI side effects. Extravasation of solutions may cause local irritation and cellulitis at injection sites. Should thrombophlebitis or perivascular cellulitis occur, terminate infusion and reinstitute at another site. The application of moderate heat to the extravasation site may help disperse the compound and minimize discomfort and local tissue irritation. Antiemetic compounds may help relieve nausea and vomiting.

Preparation of solution: Reconstitute with 4.9 ml of Sterile Water for Injection to make 500 mcg plicamycin per ml. Discard unused solution. Prepare fresh solutions daily.

Storage: Refrigerate unreconstituted vials at 2° to 8°C (36° to 46°F).

Rx	**Mithracin** (Miles Inc.)	**Powder for Injection:** 2500 mcg per vial with 100 mg mannitol.

Podophyllotoxin Derivatives

Warning:

Severe myelosuppression with resulting infection or bleeding may occur.

Hypersensitivity reactions, including anaphylaxis-like symptoms, may occur with initial dosing or at repeated exposure to teniposide. Epinephrine, with or without corticosteroids and antihistamines, has been used to alleviate symptoms.

Actions:

Pharmacology: Etoposide and teniposide are semisynthetic derivatives of podophyllotoxin.

Etoposide – Its main effect appears to be at the G_2 portion of the cell cycle. Two dose-dependent responses occur: At high concentrations (≥ 10 mcg/ml), lysis of cells entering mitosis is seen; at low concentrations (0.3 to 10 mcg/ml), cells are inhibited from entering prophase. The predominant macromolecular effect appears to be DNA synthesis inhibition.

Teniposide is a phase-specific cytotoxic drug, acting in the late S or early G_2 phase of the cell cycle, thus preventing cells from entering mitosis. Teniposide causes dose-dependent single- and double-stranded breaks in DNA and DNA:protein cross-links. The mechanism of action appears to be related to the inhibition of type II topoisomerase activity since teniposide does not intercalate into DNA or bind strongly to DNA. The cytotoxic effects of teniposide are related to the relative number of double-stranded DNA breaks produced in cells, which are a reflection of the stabilization of a topoisomerase II-DNA intermediate. Teniposide has a broad spectrum of in vivo antitumor activity against murine tumors, including hematologic malignancies and various solid tumors. Notably, it is active against sublines of certain murine leukemias with acquired resistance to cisplatin, doxorubicin, amsacrine, daunorubicin, mitoxantrone or vincristine.

Pharmacokinetics: The pharmacokinetic characteristics of teniposide differ from those of etoposide. Teniposide is more extensively bound to plasma proteins and its cellular uptake is greater. Teniposide also has a lower systemic clearance, a longer elimination half-life and is excreted in the urine as parent drug to a lesser extent than etoposide.

Various Pharmacokinetic Parameters for Etoposide and Teniposide

Parameter	Etoposide	Teniposide
Total body clearance (ml/min)	33-48	10.3
Terminal half-life (hrs)	4-11	5
Volume of distribution (L)	18-29	3-11 (children) 8-44 (adults)
Protein binding (%)	97	> 99
Elimination	Renal (35%) and nonrenal (ie, mostly metabolism, ≤ 6% bile)	Renal (44%) and fecal (≤ 10%)
Excreted unchanged in urine (%)	< 50	4-12

Etoposide – Absorption/Distribution: The mean oral bioavailability is approximately 50% (range, 25% to 75%). There is no evidence of a first-pass effect for etoposide. On IV administration, the disposition of etoposide is a biphasic process with a distribution half-life of about 1.5 hours. The areas under the plasma concentration-time curves (AUC) and maximum plasma concentration (C_{max}) values increase linearly with dose. Etoposide does not accumulate in the plasma following daily administration of 100 mg/m² for 4 to 5 days. After either IV infusion or oral administration, C_{max} and AUC values exhibit marked intra- and intersubject variability. These values for oral etoposide consistently fall in the same range as the C_{max} and AUC values for an IV dose of half the size of the oral dose.

Although detectable in CSF and intracerebral tumors, the concentrations are lower than in extracerebral tumors and plasma. Concentrations are higher in normal lung than in lung metastases and are similar in primary tumors and normal tissues of the myometrium. An inverse relationship between plasma albumin levels and renal clearance is found in children.

Metabolism/Excretion – The major urinary metabolite is the hydroxy acid. Glucuronide or sulfate conjugates of etoposide are excreted in human urine and represent 5% to 22% of the dose.

In adults, the total body clearance of etoposide is correlated with creatinine clearance, serum albumin concentration and nonrenal clearance. In children, elevated serum ALT levels are associated with reduced drug total body clearance. Prior use of cisplatin may also result in a decrease of etoposide total body clearance in children.

(Actions continued on following page)

Actions (Cont.):

Pharmacokinetics (Cont.):

Teniposide – Plasma drug levels decline biexponentially following IV infusion in children. In adults, plasma levels increase linearly with dose. Drug accumulation did not occur after daily administration for 3 days. In children, C_{max} after infusions of 137 to 203 mg/m² over a period of 1 to 2 hours exceeded 40 mcg/ml; by 20 to 24 hours after infusion plasma levels were generally < 2 mcg/ml.

The blood-brain barrier appears to limit diffusion of teniposide into the brain, although in a study in patients with brain tumors, CSF levels were higher than in patients without brain tumors.

Clinical trials: Teniposide – Nine children with acute lymphocytic leukemia (ALL) failing induction therapy with a cytarabine-containing regimen were treated with teniposide plus cytarabine. Three of these patients were induced into complete remission with durations of remission of 30 weeks, 59 weeks and 13 years. In another study, 16 children with ALL refractory to vincristine/prednisone-containing regimens were treated with teniposide plus vincristine and prednisone. Three patients were induced into complete remission with durations of remission of 5.5, 37 and 73 weeks.

Indications:

Etoposide: Refractory testicular tumors in combination with other chemotherapeutic agents in patients who have received surgery, chemotherapy and radiotherapy. Adequate data on the use of oral etoposide are not available.

Small cell lung cancer in combination with other agents as first line treatment.

Teniposide: In combination with other approved anticancer agents for induction therapy in patients with refractory childhood acute lymphoblastic leukemia (ALL). Teniposide has been available under a Treatment IND since 1988 for treatment of relapsed or refractory ALL.

Unlabeled uses: Etoposide has also been used alone or in combination in the treatment of acute nonlymphocytic leukemias (monocytic), Hodgkin's disease, non-Hodgkin's lymphomas, Kaposi's sarcoma and neuroblastoma. Other tumors with a response rate of 5% to 20% to etoposide as a single agent include: Choriocarcinoma; rhabdomyosarcoma; hepatocellular carcinoma; epithelial ovarian, non-small and small cell lung, testicular, gastric, endometrial and breast cancers; acute lymphocytic leukemia; soft tissue sarcoma.

Contraindications:

Hypersensitivity to etoposide, teniposide or *Cremophor EL* (polyoxyethylated castor oil, present in the teniposide preparation).

Warnings:

Myelosuppression: Observe patients for myelosuppression during and after therapy. Dose-limiting bone marrow suppression is the most significant toxicity.

Laboratory studies – Perform at the start of therapy and prior to each subsequent dose: Platelet count, hemoglobin, white blood cell count and differential. A platelet count < 50,000/mm³ or an absolute neutrophil count < 500/mm³ is an indication to withhold further therapy until the blood counts have sufficiently recovered.

Anaphylaxis manifested by chills, fever, tachycardia, bronchospasm, dyspnea, facial flushing, hypertension or hypotension may occur (etoposide, 0.7% to 2%; teniposide, ≈ 5%). The reactions usually respond to cessation of infusion and institution of appropriate therapy. Refer to Management of Acute Hypersensitivity Reactions.

This reaction may occur with the first dose of teniposide and may be life threatening if not treated promptly with antihistamines, corticosteroids, epinephrine, IV fluids and other supportive measures as clinically indicated. The exact cause of these reactions is unknown; they may be due to the polyoxyethylated castor oil component of the vehicle or to teniposide itself. The incidence appears to be increased in patients with brain tumors and neuroblastoma. Patients who have experienced prior hypersensitivity reactions to teniposide are at risk for recurrence of symptoms and should only be retreated if the antileukemic benefit already demonstrated clearly outweighs the risk of a probable hypersensitivity reaction for that patient. When a decision is made to retreat a patient, pretreat with corticosteroids and antihistamines and carefully observe during and after the infusion. To date, there is no evidence to suggest cross-sensitization between teniposide and etoposide.

Monitoring: In addition to hematologic tests, carefully monitor renal and hepatic function tests prior to and during therapy.

Hypotension: Administer by slow IV infusion (30 to 60 minutes or longer) since hypotension may occur with rapid IV injection. With teniposide, it may also be due to a direct effect of the polyoxyethylated castor oil component. If hypotension occurs, stop infusion and give fluids or other supportive therapy, as appropriate. When restarting infusion, use a slower rate.

(Warnings continued on following page)

Podophyllotoxin Derivatives (Cont.)

Warnings (Cont.):

Benzyl alcohol: Teniposide contains benzyl alcohol, which has been associated with a fatal "gasping" syndrome in premature infants.

CNS depression: Acute CNS depression and hypotension have occurred in patients receiving investigational infusions of high-dose teniposide who were pretreated with antiemetic drugs. The depressant effects of the antiemetic agents and the alcohol content of the teniposide formulation may place patients receiving higher than recommended doses at risk for CNS depression.

Down's syndrome patients: Patients with both Down's syndrome and leukemia may be especially sensitive to myelosuppressive chemotherapy; therefore, reduce initial dosing with teniposide in these patients. It is suggested that the first course be given at half the usual dose. Subsequent courses may be administered at higher dosages depending on the degree of myelosuppression and mucositis encountered in earlier courses in an individual patient.

Hepatic function impairment: There appears to be some association between an increase in serum alkaline phosphatase or gamma glutamyl-transpeptidase and a decrease in plasma clearance of teniposide. Therefore, exercise caution if teniposide is administered to patients with hepatic dysfunction. In children, elevated serum ALT levels are associated with reduced drug total body clearance of etoposide.

Carcinogenesis/Mutagenesis: These agents are possible carcinogens. Mutagenic and genotoxic potential has been established in mammalian cells.

Children with ALL in remission who received maintenance therapy with teniposide at weekly or twice weekly doses (plus other chemotherapeutic agents) had a relative risk of developing secondary acute nonlymphocytic leukemia (ANLL) approximately 12 times that of patients treated according to other less intensive schedules. A short course of teniposide for remission-induction or consolidation therapy was not associated with an increased risk of secondary ANLL, but the number of patients assessed was small. The potential benefit must be weighed on a case by case basis against the potential risk of the induction of a secondary leukemia.

Pregnancy: Category D. Etoposide and teniposide may cause fetal harm. They are teratogenic and embryotoxic in animals. There are no adequate and well controlled studies in pregnant women. If used during pregnancy, or if the patient becomes pregnant while receiving this drug, apprise her of the potential hazard to the fetus. Avoid becoming pregnant.

Lactation: It is not known whether this drug is excreted in breast milk. Because of the potential for serious adverse reactions in nursing infants, decide whether to discontinue nursing or the drug, accounting for the importance of the drug to the mother.

Children: Safety and efficacy for use of etoposide in children have not been established. Teniposide is indicated for use in children.

Drug Interactions:

Etoposide/Teniposide Drug Interactions			
Precipitant drug	Object drug *		Description
Etoposide	Warfarin	↑	Prolongation of the prothrombin time may occur.
Teniposide	Methotrexate	↑	Plasma clearance of methotrexate may be slightly increased. In vitro, increased intracellular levels were observed.
Sodium salicylate Sulfamethizole Tolbutamide	Teniposide	↑	Teniposide was displaced from protein-binding sites by these agents to a small but significant extent. Because of the extremely high binding of teniposide to plasma proteins, these small decreases in binding could cause substantial increases in free drug levels, resulting in potentiation of toxicity.

* ↑ = Object drug increased

(Continued on following page)

Adverse Reactions:

Most adverse reactions are reversible if detected early. If severe reactions occur, reduce or discontinue dosage and institute corrective measures. Reinstitute therapy with caution, consider further need for the drug and be alert to recurrence of toxicity.

Etoposide/Teniposide Adverse Reactions (%)		
Adverse reaction	Etoposide	Teniposide
Hematologic		
Myelosuppression, nonspecified	✓	75
Leukopenia (WBC/mm³)		
< 4000	60-91	—
< 3000	—	89
< 1000	3-17	—
Neutropenia (ANC/mm³)		
< 2000	—	95
Thrombocytopenia (platelets/mm³)		
< 100,000	22-41	85
< 50,000	1-20	—
Anemia	≤ 33	88
GI		
Mucositis	—	76
Nausea/Vomiting	31-43	29
Anorexia	10-13	—
Diarrhea	1-13	33
Abdominal pain	≤ 2	—
Stomatitis	1-6	—
Hepatic dysfunction/toxicity	≤ 3	< 1
Dysphagia	✓	—
Constipation	✓	—
Dermatologic		
Alopecia (reversible)[1]	≤ 66	9
Rash	✓	3
Pigmentation	✓	—
Pruritus	✓	—
Radiation recall dermatitis	one report	—
Cardiovascular		
Hypotension[2]	1-2	2
Hypertension	✓	—
Miscellaneous		
Hypersensitivity/Anaphylactic reactions[2]	0.7-2 (< 1 oral)	≈ 5
Peripheral neurotoxicity	1-2	< 1
Aftertaste	✓	—
Fever	✓	3
Transient cortical blindness	✓	—
Infection	—	12
Bleeding	—	5
Renal dysfunction	—	< 1
Metabolic abnormalities	—	< 1

[1] Sometimes progressing to total baldness
[2] See Warnings
✓ = Adverse reaction observed, incidence not reported
— = Not reported

Overdosage:

Symptoms: The anticipated complications of overdosage are secondary to bone marrow suppression.

Treatment: There is no known antidote for overdosage. Treatment should consist of supportive care including blood products and antibiotics as indicated.

Patient Information:

Contraceptive measures are recommended during treatment.

Notify physician of any of the following: Fever; chills; rapid heartbeat; difficult breathing.

(Products listed on following pages)

Podophyllotoxin Derivatives (Cont.)

ETOPOSIDE (VP-16-213)

Administration and Dosage:

Approved by the FDA in 1983.

Modify the dosage, by either route, to account for the myelosuppressive effects of other drugs in combination, the effects of prior x-ray therapy or chemotherapy which may have compromised bone marrow reserve.

Administer solution over 30 to 60 minutes or longer. Do not give by rapid IV injection.

Testicular cancer: Parenteral – Usual dose is 50 to 100 mg/m²/day on days 1 to 5 to 100 mg/m²/day on days 1, 3 and 5.

Small cell lung cancer: Parenteral – 35 mg/m²/day for 4 days to 50 mg/m²/day for 5 days. Courses are repeated at 3 to 4 week intervals after recovery from toxicity.

Oral – 2 times the IV dose rounded to the nearest 50 mg.

Preparation for IV administration: Dilute with either 5% Dextrose Injection or 0.9% Sodium Chloride Injection to give a final concentration of 0.2 or 0.4 mg/ml.

Plastic devices made of acrylic or ABS have cracked and leaked when used with undiluted etoposide. This has not been reported with diluted solutions.

Handling: Skin reactions may occur with accidental exposure. Use gloves. If solution contacts the skin or mucosa, immediately wash the area thoroughly with soap and water.

Storage/Stability: Unopened vials are stable for 2 years at room temperature (25°C; 77°F). Diluted solutions (concentration of 0.2 or 0.4 mg/ml) are stable for 96 and 48 hours, respectively, at room temperature under normal room fluorescent light in both glass and plastic containers. Capsules must be stored at 2° to 8°C (36° to 46°F). Stable for 2 years under refrigeration, 3 months at room temperature. Do not freeze.

Rx	**VePesid** (Bristol-Myers Oncology)	**Capsules:** 50 mg	Sorbitol. (Bristol 3091). Pink. In blisterpack 20s.
		Injection: 20 mg/ml[1]	In 5 ml vials.

[1] With 30 mg benzyl alcohol, 80 mg polysorbate 80, 650 mg polyethylene glycol 300, 30.5% alcohol.

TENIPOSIDE (VM-26)

Administration and Dosage:

Approved by the FDA on July 14, 1992.

Teniposide must be administered as an IV infusion. Take care to ensure that the IV catheter or needle is in the proper position and functional prior to infusion. Improper administration may result in extravasation causing local tissue necrosis or thrombophlebitis. In some instances, occlusion of central venous access devices has occurred during 24-hour infusion at a concentration of 0.1 to 0.2 mg/ml. Frequent observation during these infusions is necessary to minimize this risk.

Administer over 30 to 60 minutes or longer. Do not give by rapid IV injection. Hypotension has been reported following rapid IV administration.

In one study, childhood ALL patients failing induction therapy with a cytarabine-containing regimen were treated with the combination of teniposide 165 mg/m² and cytarabine 300 mg/m² IV twice weekly for 8 to 9 doses. In another study, patients with childhood ALL refractory to vincristine/prednisone-containing regimens were treated with the combinationn of teniposide 250 mg/m² and vincristine 1.5 mg/m² IV weekly for 4 to 8 weeks and prednisone 40 mg/m² orally for 28 days.

Hepatic/Renal function impairment: Adequate data in patients with hepatic or renal insufficiency are lacking, but dose adjustments may be necessary for patients with significant renal or hepatic impairment.

Down's syndrome patients: Reduce initial dosing; give the first course at half the usual dose (see Warnings).

Preparation for IV administration: Teniposide must be diluted with either 5% Dextrose Injection, USP, or 0.9% Sodium Chloride Injection, USP, to give final teniposide concentrations of 0.1, 0.2, 0.4 or 1 mg/ml.

Contact of undiluted teniposide with plastic equipment or devices used to prepare solutions for infusion may result in softening or cracking and possible drug product leakage. This effect has not been reported with diluted solutions.

In order to prevent extraction of the plasticizer DEHP, prepare and administer solutions in non-DEHP-containing LVP containers such as glass or polyolefin plastic bags or containers. The use of PVC containers is not recommended.

Lipid administration sets or low DEHP containing nitroglycerin sets will keep patients' exposure to DEHP at low levels and are suitable for use. The diluted solutions are chemically and physically compatible with the recommended IV administration sets and LVP containers for up to 24 hours at ambient room temperature and lighting conditions.

(Administration and Dosage continued on following page)

TENIPOSIDE (VM-26) (Cont.)

Administration and Dosage (Cont.):

Teniposide is a cytotoxic anticancer drug; use caution in handling and preparing the solution. Skin reactions associated with accidental exposure may occur. The use of gloves is recommended. If teniposide solution contacts the skin, immediately wash the skin thoroughly with soap and water. If the drug contacts mucous membranes, flush thoroughly with water.

Admixture incompatibilities: Heparin solution can cause precipitation of teniposide, therefore, flush the administration apparatus thoroughly with 5% Dextrose Injection or 0.9% Sodium Chloride Injection, USP before and after administration of teniposide. Because of the potential for precipitation, compatibility with other drugs, infusion materials or IV pumps cannot be assured.

Storage/Stability: Unopened amps are stable until the date indicated on the package when stored under refrigeration (2° to 8°C; 36° to 46°F) in the original package (to protect from light). Freezing does not adversely affect the product. Reconstituted solutions are stable at room temperature for up to 24 hours after preparation. Administer 1 mg/ml solutions within 4 hours of preparation to reduce the potential for precipitation. Refrigeration of solutions is not recommended. Stability and use times are identical in glass and plastic containers.

Although solutions are chemically stable under the conditions indicated, precipitation of teniposide may occur at the recommended concentrations, especially if the diluted solution is subjected to more agitation than is recommended to prepare the drug solution for parenteral administration. In addition, minimize storage time prior to administration and take care to avoid contact of the diluted solution with other drugs or fluids. Precipitation has been reported during 24-hour infusions of teniposide concentrations of 0.1 to 0.2 mg/ml, resulting in occlusion of central venous access catheters in several patients.

Rx	**Vumon** (Bristol-Myers Oncology)	**Injection**[1]: 50 mg (10 mg/ml)	In 5 ml amps.[2]

[1] Must be diluted prior to administration.

[2] With 30 mg benzyl alcohol and 500 mg *Cremophor EL* (polyoxyethylated castor oil) per ml, with 42.7% dehydrated alcohol.

VINCRISTINE SULFATE (VCR; LCR)

> **Warnings:**
> It is extremely important that the IV needle or catheter be properly positioned before any vincristine is injected. Leakage into surrounding tissue during IV administration may cause considerable irritation.
> This preparation is for IV use only. Intrathecal use usually results in death.

Actions:

Pharmacology: Vincristine sulfate is an alkaloid obtained from the periwinkle (*Vinca rosea* Linn). The mode of action of vincristine is unknown. In vitro, it arrests mitotic division at the stage of metaphase. The antineoplastic effects of vinca alkaloids are related to interference with intracellular tubulin function. It reversibly binds to microtubule and spindle proteins in the S phase.

Pharmacokinetics: Absorption/Distribution – Within 15 to 30 minutes following IV administration, > 90% of the drug is distributed from blood into tissue where it remains tightly, but not irreversibly, bound. Penetration across the blood-brain barrier is poor.

Metabolism/Excretion – Pharmacokinetic studies in cancer patients show a triphasic serum decay pattern following rapid IV injection. The initial, middle and terminal half-lives are 5 minutes, 2.3 hours and 85 hours, respectively; however, the range of the terminal half-life is from 19 to 155 hours. The liver is the major excretory organ; about 80% of an injected dose appears in the feces and 10% to 20% in the urine. Hepatic dysfunction may alter the elimination kinetics and augment toxicity.

Combination cancer chemotherapy involves simultaneous use of several agents. Generally, each agent has a unique toxicity and mechanism of action so that therapeutic enhancement occurs without additive toxicity. It is rarely possible to achieve equally good results with single agent methods of treatment. Thus, vincristine is often chosen as part of polychemotherapy because of lack of significant bone marrow suppression (at recommended doses) and of unique clinical toxicity (neuropathy). See Administration and Dosage for possible increased toxicity when used in combination therapy.

Indications:

Acute leukemia.

Combination therapy in Hodgkin's disease, non-Hodgkin's malignant lymphomas (lymphocytic, mixed-cell, histiocytic, undifferentiated, nodular and diffuse types), rhabdomyosarcoma, neuroblastoma and Wilms' tumor.

Unlabeled use: Vincristine has been used in the treatment of idiopathic thrombocytopenic purpura, Kaposi's sarcoma, breast cancer and bladder cancer.

Contraindications:

Do not give to patients with demyelinating form of Charcot-Marie-Tooth syndrome.

Warnings:

Administer IV only; intrathecal administration is uniformly fatal.

Hypersensitivity, temporally related to vincristine therapy, has occurred. Refer to Management of Acute Hypersensitivity Reactions. See Adverse Reactions.

Carcinogenesis, mutagenesis, impairment of fertility: Patients who received vincristine with anticancer drugs known to be carcinogenic have developed secondary malignancies. Vincristine's contributing role in this development has not been determined.

Laboratory tests have failed to demonstrate conclusively that this drug is mutagenic. Clinical reports of both male and female patients who received multiple agent chemotherapy that included vincristine indicate that azoospermia and amenorrhea can occur in postpubertal patients. Recovery occurred many months after completion of chemotherapy in some patients. It is much less likely to cause permanent azoospermia and amenorrhea in prepubertal patients.

Pregnancy: Category D. Vincristine can cause fetal harm when administered to a pregnant woman. In several animal species, the drug can induce teratogenic effects and embryolethality with doses that are nontoxic to the mother. There are no adequate and well controlled studies in pregnant women. If this drug is used during pregnancy or if the patient becomes pregnant while receiving it, apprise her of the potential hazard to the fetus. Advise women of childbearing potential to avoid becoming pregnant.

Lactation: It is not known whether this drug is excreted in breast milk. Because of the potential for serious adverse reactions in nursing infants, decide whether to discontinue nursing or the drug, taking into account importance of the drug to the mother.

Precautions:

Acute uric acid nephropathy has occurred.

CNS leukemia has occurred in patients undergoing otherwise successful therapy with vincristine. If CNS leukemia is diagnosed, additional agents may be required, since this drug does not adequately cross the blood-brain barrier.

(Precautions continued on following page)

VINCRISTINE SULFATE (VCR; LCR) (Cont.)

Precautions (Cont.):

Leukopenia or complicating infection: In the presence of these conditions, administration of the next dose warrants careful consideration.

Neuromuscular disease: Pay particular attention to dosage and neurological side effects if administered to patients with preexisting neuromuscular disease or when other neurotoxic drugs are used.

Eye contamination should be avoided with concentrations used clinically. If accidental contamination occurs, severe irritation (or, if the drug was delivered under pressure, even corneal ulceration) may result. Wash the eyes immediately and thoroughly.

Pulmonary reactions: Acute shortness of breath and severe bronchospasm have followed administration of vinca alkaloids, most frequently when the vinca alkaloid was used in combination with mitomycin-C. The onset may be within minutes or several hours after the vinca is injected and may occur up to 2 weeks following the dose of mitomycin.

Concomitant radiation therapy: Do not give to patients receiving radiation therapy through ports that include the liver.

Monitoring: Since dose-limiting clinical toxicity is manifested as neurotoxicity, clinical evaluation (history, physical examination) is necessary to detect the need for dosage modification. Following vincristine administration, some individuals may have a fall in the WBC count or platelet count, particularly when previous therapy or the disease itself has reduced bone marrow function. Therefore, perform a complete blood count before each dose. Acute elevation of serum uric acid may also occur during induction of remission in acute leukemia; thus determine such levels frequently during the first 3 to 4 weeks of treatment or take appropriate measures to prevent uric acid nephropathy.

Drug Interactions:

Digoxin: Combination chemotherapy (including vincristine) may decrease digoxin plasma levels and renal excretion.

L-asparaginase: Administering L-asparaginase first may reduce the hepatic clearance of vincristine. Give vincristine 12 to 24 hours before L-asparaginase administration to minimize toxicity.

Mitomycin-C: Acute pulmonary reactions may occur (see Precautions).

Phenytoin: Combination chemotherapy (including vincristine) may reduce phenytoin plasma levels, requiring an increased dosage to maintain therapeutic plasma levels.

Adverse Reactions:

Adverse reactions are generally reversible and dose-related. With single weekly doses, leukopenia, neuritic pain and constipation may occur and are usually of short duration (ie, < 7 days). When dosage is reduced, reactions may lessen or disappear. They seem to increase when the drug is given in divided doses. Other adverse reactions, such as hair loss, sensory loss, paresthesia, difficulty in walking, slapping gait, loss of deep tendon reflexes and muscle wasting, may persist for at least as long as therapy is continued. Generalized sensorimotor dysfunction may become progressively more severe with continued treatment. Neuromuscular difficulties usually disappear by the sixth week after treatment is discontinued, but they may persist for prolonged periods in some patients. Hair regrowth may occur while maintenance therapy continues.

Neurologic: Loss of deep-tendon reflexes, ataxia, footdrop and paralysis have been seen with continued use. Cranial nerve manifestations, including isolated paresis or paralysis of muscles may occur; extraocular and laryngeal muscles are most commonly involved. Severe pain may occur in the jaw, pharynx, parotid gland, bones, back and limbs. Myalgias have occurred. Reduced intestinal motility results in constipation. Convulsions, often with hypertension, have occurred in a few patients. Convulsions followed by coma have been seen in children. Frequently, there is a sequence in the development of neuropathy: Initially, sensory impairment and paresthesias, then neuritic pain may appear and later, motor difficulties. Neurotoxicity is dose-related and cumulative to where therapy must be stopped after a cumulative dose of 30 to 50 mg. It is reversible upon discontinuation, but recovery takes several months.

In one study, the administration of glutamic acid (500 mg 3 times daily) decreased the neurotoxicity induced by vincristine.

GI: Oral ulceration; abdominal cramps; nausea; vomiting; diarrhea; anorexia; intestinal necrosis or perforation.

Constipation may take the form of upper colon impaction, and, on examination, the rectum may be empty. Colicky abdominal pain may accompany an empty rectum. A flat film of the abdomen demonstrates this condition. Cases respond to high enemas and laxatives. Use routine prophylaxis for constipation.

Paralytic ileus which mimics the "surgical abdomen" may occur, particularly in young children. The ileus will reverse itself upon temporary discontinuation of vincristine and with symptomatic care.

(Adverse Reactions continued on following page)

VINCRISTINE SULFATE (VCR; LCR) (Cont.)

Adverse Reactions (Cont.):

SIADH: The syndrome of inappropriate antidiuretic hormone secretion (SIADH), including high urinary sodium excretion in the presence of hyponatremia, has occurred rarely. Renal or adrenal disease, hypotension, dehydration, azotemia and clinical edema are absent. With fluid deprivation, the hyponatremia and renal sodium loss improve.

Hematologic: Serious bone marrow depression (usually not dose-limiting); anemia; leukopenia; thrombocytopenia. Thrombocytopenia, if present when therapy is begun, may improve before the appearance of marrow remission.

Hypersensitivity: Rare cases of allergic type reactions, such as anaphylaxis, rash and edema, that are temporally related to vincristine therapy have occurred in patients receiving vincristine as a part of multi-drug chemotherapy regimens. See Warnings.

GU: Polyuria; dysuria; urinary retention due to bladder atony. Discontinue other drugs known to cause urinary retention (particularly in the elderly), if possible, for the first few days following administration.

Ophthalmic: Optic atrophy with blindness; transient cortical blindness; ptosis; diplopia; photophobia.

Pulmonary: Acute shortness of breath, severe bronchospasm (see Precautions).

Other: Hypertension; hypotension; weight loss; fever; alopecia; rash; headache.

Overdosage:

Symptoms: Side effects are dose-related. After an overdose, expect exaggerated side effects. In children < 13 years of age, death has occurred after doses 10 times those recommended; severe symptoms may occur with 3 to 4 mg/m^2. Adults may experience severe symptoms after single doses ≥ 3 mg/m^2.

Treatment: Supportive care should include prevention of side effects resulting from SIADH (ie, restriction of fluid intake and perhaps the administration of a diuretic affecting the function of Henle's loop and the distal tubule); phenobarbital (anticonvulsant); enemas or cathartics to prevent ileus (in some instances, decompression of the GI tract may be necessary); monitor the cardiovascular system; determine daily blood counts for guidance in transfusion requirements.

Folinic acid, 100 mg IV every 3 hours for 24 hours and then every 6 hours for at least 48 hours, may be helpful in treating a vincristine overdose. Treatment with folinic acid does not eliminate the need for supportive measures.

Most of an IV dose is excreted into the bile after rapid tissue binding. Hemodialysis is not likely to be helpful. Patients with liver disease sufficient to decrease biliary excretion may experience increased severity of side effects.

Administration and Dosage:

Cautiously calculate and administer dose; overdosage may be serious or fatal.

Administer IV only, at weekly intervals. Inject solution either directly into a vein or into the tubing of a running IV infusion. Injection may be completed in about 1 minute.

Adults: 1.4 mg/m^2. *Children:* 2 mg/m^2. For children weighing ≤ 10 kg or having a body surface area < 1 m^2, give 0.05 mg/kg once a week.

Hepatic function impairment – A 50% reduction in the dose is recommended for patients having a direct serum bilirubin value > 3 mg/dl.

Extravasation: Properly position the needle in the vein before injecting vincristine. Leakage into surrounding tissue during IV administration may cause considerable irritation. Discontinue injection immediately; introduce any remaining portion of the dose into another vein. Locally inject hyaluronidase and apply moderate heat to the area to disperse the drug and minimize discomfort and the possibility of cellulitis.

Compatibility: Do not dilute in solutions that raise or lower the pH outside the range of 3.5 to 5.5. Do not mix with anything other than normal saline or glucose in water.

Consider procedures for proper handling and disposal of anticancer drugs.

Rx	**Vincristine Sulfate** (Various, eg, Americal, Balan, Lyphomed, Moore, Quad, VHA Supply)	**Injection:** 1 mg/ml	In 1, 2 and 5 ml vials.
Rx	**Oncovin** (Lilly)		In 1, 2 and 5 ml vials and 1 and 2 ml Hyporets.[1]
Rx	**Vincasar PFS** (Adria)		In 1, 2 and 5 ml flip-top vials.[2]

[1] With 100 mg mannitol, 1.3 mg methylparaben and 0.2 mg propylparaben per ml. Refrigerate.
[2] With 100 mg mannitol. Refrigerate.

VINBLASTINE SULFATE (VLB)

Actions:

Pharmacology: Vinblastine sulfate, an alkaloid extracted from *Vinca rosea* Linn, interferes with metabolic pathways of amino acids leading from glutamic acid to the citric acid cycle and urea. Studies have demonstrated an antimitotic effect and various atypical mitotic figures. However, therapeutic responses are not fully explained by the cytologic changes, since these changes are sometimes observed clinically and experimentally in the absence of any oncolytic effects.

Vinblastine has an effect on cell energy production required for mitosis and interferes with nucleic acid synthesis. In vitro, the drug arrests growing cells in metaphase.

Reversal of the antitumor effect by glutamic acid or tryptophan has occurred.

Pharmacokinetics:

Absorption/Distribution – Similar to vincristine, vinblastine undergoes rapid distribution and extensive tissue binding following IV injection. Approximately 75% is bound to serum proteins. Vinblastine also localizes in platelets and leukocyte fractions of whole blood.

Metabolism/Excretion – Vinblastine is partially metabolized to deacetyl vinblastine which is more active than the parent drug. Plasma decline follows a triphasic pattern. The initial, middle and terminal half-lives are 3.7 minutes, 1.6 hours and 24.8 hours, respectively. Toxicity may be increased if liver disease is present.

Vinblastine is metabolized in the liver and the major route of excretion may be through the biliary system.

Indications:

Palliative treatment of the following:

Frequently responsive malignancies: Generalized Hodgkin's disease (stages III and IV, Ann Arbor modification of Rye staging system), lymphocytic lymphoma (nodular and diffuse, poorly and well differentiated); histiocytic lymphoma; mycosis fungoides (advanced stages); advanced testicular carcinoma; Kaposi's sarcoma and Letterer-Siwe disease (histiocytosis X).

Less frequently responsive malignancies: Choriocarcinoma resistant to other chemotherapy; breast cancer unresponsive to surgery and hormonal therapy.

Multiple drug protocols: Vinblastine, effective as a single agent, is usually administered with other antineoplastics. Combination therapy enhances therapeutic effect without additive toxicity when agents with different dose-limiting toxicities and mechanisms of action are selected.

Hodgkin's disease: Vinblastine used as a single agent; advanced Hodgkin's disease has also been successfully treated with multiple-drug regimens that included vinblastine.

Advanced testicular germinal-cell cancers (embryonal carcinoma, teratocarcinoma and choriocarcinoma) are sensitive to vinblastine alone, but better clinical results are achieved with combination therapy. Vinblastine enhances the effect of bleomycin if given 6 to 8 hours prior to bleomycin administration; this schedule permits more cells to be arrested during metaphase, the stage in which bleomycin is active.

Contraindications:

Leukopenia.

Presence of bacterial infection; infections must be under control prior to initiating therapy.

Significant granulocytopenia unless it is a result of the disease being treated.

(Continued on following page)

VINBLASTINE SULFATE (VLB) (Cont.)

Warnings:

Hematologic effects: Leukopenia is expected; leukocyte count is an important guide to therapy. In general, the larger the dose, the more profound and longer lasting the leukopenia will be. If the WBC count returns to normal after drug-induced leukopenia, the white cell-producing mechanism is not permanently depressed. Usually, WBC count has completely returned to normal after virtual disappearance of white cells from peripheral blood. The nadir in WBC count occurs 5 to 10 days after the last dose of drug is given. Recovery of the WBC count is usually complete within 7 to 14 days. With smaller doses employed for maintenance therapy, leukopenia may not occur.

Although the thrombocyte count ordinarily is not significantly lowered by therapy, recently impaired bone marrow by prior therapy with radiation or with other oncolytic drugs may show thrombocytopenia (< 200,000 platelets/cu mm). When other chemotherapy or radiation has not been previously employed, thrombocytopenia is rare, even when vinblastine may be causing significant leukopenia. Rapid recovery (within a few days) from thrombocytopenia is the rule.

The effect on red blood cell count and hemoglobin is usually insignificant in the absence of other therapy; however, patients with malignant disease may exhibit anemia in the absence of any therapy.

If leukopenia (< 2000 WBC/cu mm) occurs following a dose of this drug, carefully watch the patient for evidence of infection until a safe WBC count has returned.

When cachexia or ulcerated skin surface occur, a more profound leukopenic response may occur; avoid use in older persons suffering from these conditions.

In patients with malignant cell infiltration of bone marrow, leukocyte and platelet counts have sometimes fallen precipitously after moderate doses, making further use of the drug inadvisable.

Leukopenia (granulocytopenia) may reach dangerously low levels following use of the higher recommended doses. Follow recommended dosage technique. Stomatitis and neurologic toxicity, although not common or permanent, can be disabling.

Impairment of Fertility: Aspermia has been reported. Amenorrhea has occurred in some patients treated with a combination of an alkylating agent, procarbazine, prednisone and vinblastine. Its occurrence was related to the total dose of these agents. Recovery of menses was frequent. The same combination of drugs given to male patients produced azoospermia; if spermatogenesis did return, it was not likely to do so with less than 2 years of unmaintained remission.

Usage in Pregnancy: Category D. Information is very limited. Animal studies suggest teratogenicity may occur. Animals given the drug early in pregnancy suffer resorption of the conceptus; surviving fetuses demonstrate gross deformities. There are no adequate and well controlled studies in pregnant women, but the drug can cause fatal harm. If the drug is used during pregnancy, or if the patient becomes pregnant while receiving this drug, apprise her of the potential hazard to the fetus. Advise women of childbearing potential to avoid becoming pregnant.

Usage in Lactation: It is not known whether this drug is excreted in breast milk. Because of the potential for serious adverse reactions in nursing infants, decide whether to discontinue nursing or to discontinue the drug, taking into account the importance of the drug to the mother.

Precautions:

Toxicity may be enhanced in the presence of hepatic insufficiency.

Using small amounts of drug daily for long periods is not advised, even though the resulting total weekly dose may be similar to that recommended. Strict adherence to the recommended dosage schedule is very important. When amounts equal to several times the recommended weekly dosage were given in 7 daily installments for long periods, convulsions, severe and permanent CNS damage and death occurred.

Avoid eye contamination; severe irritation or corneal ulceration (if the drug was delivered under pressure) may result. Thoroughly wash the eye with water immediately.

Pulmonary reactions: Acute shortness of breath and severe bronchospasm have occurred following use of vinca alkaloids. These reactions occur most frequently when the vinca alkaloid is used with mitomycin-C. Onset may be within minutes or several hours after the vinca is injected and may occur up to 2 weeks after the dose of mitomycin.

Drug Interactions:

Mitomycin-C: Acute shortness of breath and severe bronchospasm have occurred following use of vinca alkaloids in patients who had previously or simultaneously received mitomycin. Onset may be within minutes or several hours after the vinca alkaloid is injected and may occur up to 2 weeks after the dose of mitomycin.

Phenytoin: Combination chemotherapy (including vinblastine) may reduce phenytoin plasma levels, requiring increased dosage to maintain therapeutic plasma levels.

(Continued on following page)

VINBLASTINE SULFATE (VLB) (Cont.)

Adverse Reactions:

Incidence of adverse reactions is dose-related. Except for epilation, leukopenia and neurologic side effects, adverse reactions have not usually persisted for longer than 24 hours. Neurologic side effects are not common; when they occur, they often last for more than 24 hours. Leukopenia, the most common adverse reaction, is usually the dose-limiting factor.

Hematologic: Leukopenia (granulocytopenia), anemia, thrombocytopenia (myelosuppression). See Warnings.

Cardiovascular: Hypertension. Cases of unexpected myocardial infarction and cerebrovascular accidents have occurred in patients undergoing combination chemotherapy with vinblastine, bleomycin and cisplatin.

GI: Nausea and vomiting (may be controlled by antiemetics); pharyngitis; vesiculation of the mouth; ileus; diarrhea; constipation; anorexia; abdominal pain; rectal bleeding; hemorrhagic enterocolitis; bleeding from an old peptic ulcer.

Neurologic: Numbness of digits; paresthesias; peripheral neuritis; mental depression; loss of deep tendon reflexes; headache; convulsions.

Dermatologic: Total epilation infrequently develops. In some cases, hair regrows during maintenance therapy. Vesiculation of the skin may occur. A single case of light sensitivity has been associated with this drug.

Miscellaneous: Malaise; weakness; dizziness; pain in tumor site; bone and jaw pain. The syndrome of inappropriate secretion of antidiuretic hormone has occurred with higher than recommended doses.

Extravasation during IV injection may lead to cellulitis and phlebitis; sloughing may occur.

There are isolated reports of Raynaud's phenomenon occurring in patients with testicular carcinoma treated with bleomycin, cisplatin and vinblastine sulfate. It is unknown whether the cause was the disease, the drugs or a combination of these.

Overdose:

Symptoms: Side effects are dose-related. After an overdose, expected exaggerated effects. In addition, neurotoxicity similar to that with vincristine may occur.

Treatment: Supportive care should include prevention of side effects that result from the syndrome of inappropriate secretion of antidiuretic hormone (ie, restriction of the volume of daily fluid intake to that of the urine output plus insensible loss and perhaps use of a diuretic affecting the function of the loop of Henle and the distal tubule); administration of an anticonvulsant; prevention of ileus; monitoring the cardiovascular system; and determining daily blood counts for guidance in transfusion requirements and assessing the risk of infection. The major effect of excessive doses will be myelosuppression, which may be life-threatening. There is no information regarding the effectiveness of dialysis nor of cholestyramine for the treatment of overdosage.

In the dry state, the drug is irregularly and unpredictably absorbed from the GI tract following oral administration. Absorption of the solution has not been studied. If vinblastine is swallowed, oral activated charcoal in a water slurry may be given along with a cathartic. The use of cholestyramine in this situation has not been reported.

Patient Information:

Immediately report sore throat, fever, chills or sore mouth to the physician.

The following may occur: Alopecia, jaw pain, pain in the organs containing tumor tissue, nausea and vomiting. Scalp hair will regrow to its pretreatment extent, even with continued treatment. Report any other serious medical event to the physician.

Avoid constipation.

(Continued on following page)

VINBLASTINE SULFATE (VLB) (Cont.)

Administration and Dosage:

For IV use only. It is anticipated that intrathecal use would be fatal, as with vincristine.

Leukopenic responses vary following therapy. For this reason, do not administer drug more than once weekly. Initiate therapy for adults with a single IV dose of 3.7 mg/m^2 of body surface. Thereafter, measure WBC counts to determine patient's sensitivity. A 50% dose reduction is recommended for patients having a direct serum bilirubin value > 3 mg/dl. Since metabolism and excretion are primarily hepatic, no modification is recommended for patients with impaired renal function.

A simplified and conservative incremental dosage at *weekly intervals* is as follows:

	Adult Dose (mg/m^2)	Pediatric Dose (mg/m^2)
First dose	3.7	2.5
Second dose	5.5	3.75
Third dose	7.4	5.0
Fourth dose	9.25	6.25
Fifth dose	11.1	7.5

Use the same increments until a max. dose not exceeding 18.5 mg/m^2 for adults and 12.5 mg/m^2 for children is reached. Do not increase dose after WBC count is reduced to $\approx$ 3000 cells/cu mm. For most adults the weekly dosage range is 5.5 to 7.4 mg/m^2.

Maintenance therapy: When the dose produces the above degree of leukopenia, administer a dose one increment smaller at weekly intervals for maintenance. Even though 7 days have elapsed, do not give the next dose until the WBC count has returned to at least 4000/cu mm. In some cases, oncolytic activity may be encountered before leukopenic effect but do not increase the size of subsequent doses.

Duration of maintenance therapy varies according to the disease and the combination of antineoplastics used. Prolonged chemotherapy for maintaining remission involves several risks: Life-threatening infections, sterility, secondary cancers through suppression of immune surveillance. In some disorders, survival following complete remission may not be as prolonged as that achieved with shorter periods of maintenance therapy. Conversely, failure to provide maintenance therapy may lead to unnecessary relapse; complete remission in patients with testicular cancer, unless maintained for at least 2 years, often results in early relapse.

IV: Inject into either the tubing of a running IV infusion or directly into a vein over 1 minute. Secure the needle within the vein so that no solution extravasates, to prevent cellulitis or phlebitis. To further minimize extravasation, rinse syringe and needle with venous blood before withdrawal of needle. Do not dilute the dose in large volumes of diluent (ie, 100 to 250 ml) or give IV for prolonged periods (30 to 60 min. or more), since this often results in vein irritation and increases the chance of extravasation.

Because of the enhanced possibility of thrombosis, do not inject solution into an extremity in which circulation is impaired or potentially impaired by conditions such as compressing or invading neoplasm, phlebitis or varicosity.

Extravasation may cause considerable irritation. Discontinue the injection immediately; introduce any remaining portion of the dose into another vein. Locally inject hyaluronidase and apply moderate heat to the area of leakage to disperse the drug and minimize discomfort and the possibility of cellulitis.

Preparation of solution: Add 10 ml of Sodium Chloride Injection (preserved with phenol or benzyl alcohol) to the vial for a concentration of 1 mg/ml. The drug dissolves instantly to give a clear solution. A preservative-containing solvent is unnecessary if unused portions are discarded immediately.

Compatability: Do not dilute with solvents that raise or lower the pH of the resulting solution from between 3.5 and 5. Solutions should be made with either normal saline or 5% glucose in water (each with or without preservative) and should not be combined in the same container with any other chemical.

Storage: After reconstitution and if a portion is removed from the vial, refrigerate the remainder for 30 days without loss of potency. Refrigerate unopened vials at 2° to 8°C (36° to 46°F) to ensure stability. Consider procedures for proper handling and disposal.

	Product	Form	Packaging
Rx	**Vinblastine Sulfate** (Various)	**Powder for Injection:** 10 mg per vial	
Rx	**Velban** (Lilly)		
Rx	**Velsar** (Adria)		
Rx	**Vinblastine Sulfate** (LyphoMed)	**Injection:** 1 mg/ml	In 10 ml vials[1]
Rx	**Alkaban-AQ** (Quad)		In 10 ml vials[1].

[1]With 0.9% benzyl alcohol.

SODIUM IODIDE I 131

Actions:

After rapid GI absorption, iodine 131 is primarily distributed within extracellular fluid. It is trapped and rapidly converted to protein-bound iodine by the thyroid; it is concentrated, but not protein bound, by the stomach and salivary glands. It is promptly excreted by kidneys.

About 90% of the local irradiation is caused by beta radiation and 10% is caused by gamma radiation. Iodine 131 has a physical half-life of 8.06 days.

Indications:

Selected cases of thyroid carcinoma. Palliative effects may occur in patients with papillary or follicular thyroid carcinoma. Stimulation of radioiodide uptake may be achieved by giving thyrotropin. (Radioiodide will not be taken up by giant cell and spindle cell carcinoma of the thyroid or by amyloid solid carcinomas.)

Treatment of *hyperthyroidism* (see page 535).

Contraindications:

Preexisting vomiting and diarrhea; women who are or may become pregnant.

Warnings:

Use of radiopharmaceuticals should be restricted to physicians qualified in the safe use and handling of radionuclides and whose experience and training have been approved by the appropriate government agency.

Usage in Pregnancy: Category X. Do not administer to pregnant women (see Contraindications). Do not use in women who are or may become pregnant. Iodine 131 may cause fetal harm when administered to a pregnant woman. Permanent damage to the fetal thyroid may occur. If this drug is used during pregnancy or if patient becomes pregnant while taking this drug, inform patient of the potential hazard to the fetus.

Usage in Lactation: Iodine 131 is excreted in breast milk; discontinue nursing during therapy. Do not resume nursing until all radiation is absent from breast milk.

Usage in Children: Safety and efficacy in children have not been established.

Precautions:

Ensure minimum radiation exposure to patients and occupational workers consistent with proper patient management.

Drug Interactions:

Uptake of iodine 131 will be affected by recent intake of **stable iodine** in any form, or by use of **thyroid, antithyroid** and certain other drugs. Question the patient regarding previous medication and procedures involving radiographic contrast media.

Adverse Reactions:

Following large doses used to treat thyroid carcinoma, adverse reactions may be severe and present special problems.

Hematologic: Depression of hematopoietic system with large doses; bone marrow depression; acute leukemia; anemia; blood dyscrasia; leukopenia; thrombocytopenia; death.

Endocrine: Severe sialoadenitis; acute thyroid crises.

Miscellaneous: Radiation sickness (nausea and vomiting); increased clinical symptoms; chest pain, tachycardia, rash, hives, chromosomal abnormalities; tenderness and swelling of the neck, pain on swallowing, sore throat and cough may occur around the third day after treatment (usually amenable to analgesics); temporary hair thinning (may occur 2 to 3 months after treatment).

Allergic reactions occur infrequently.

Administration and Dosage:

Measure dose by a suitable radioactivity calibration system immediately prior to use.

Carcinoma of the thyroid: Individualize dosage. *Usual dose for ablation of normal thyroid tissue:* 50 mCi, with subsequent therapeutic doses usually 100 to 150 mCi.

Preparation of oral solution: To prepare a stock solution use Purified Water with 0.2% sodium thiosulfate as a reducing agent. Acidic diluents may cause pH to drop below 7.5 and stimulate volatilization of iodine 131-hydriodic acid. Equipment used to prepare the stock solution must be thoroughly rinsed and free of acidic cleaning agents.

Physical characteristics: Consult product literature for specific calibration and dosimetry.

Rx	**Iodotope** (Squibb)	**Capsules**	Radioactivity ranging from 1 to 50 mCi per capsule at time of calibration. Blue/buff.
		Oral Solution	Radioactivity concentration of 7.05 mCi/ml at time of calibration. In vials[1] containing approximately 7, 14, 28, 70 or 106 mCi at time of calibration.
Rx	**Sodium Iodide I 131** (Mallinckrodt)	**Capsules**	Radioactivity ranging from 0.8 to 100 mCi per capsule.
		Oral Solution	Radioactivity ranging from 3.5 to 150 mCi per vial.[2]

[1] With 1 mg EDTA per ml.

[2] With 0.1% sodium bisulfite and 0.2% EDTA.

SODIUM PHOSPHATE P 32

Actions:

Phosphorus is necessary to the metabolic and proliferative activity of cells. Radioactive phosphorus concentrates to a very high degree in rapidly proliferating tissue.

Sodium phosphate P 32 decays by beta emission with a physical half-life of 14.3 days. The mean energy of the P 32 beta particle is 695 keV.

Indications:

Treatment of polycythemia vera, chronic myelocytic leukemia and chronic lymphocytic leukemia.

Palliative treatment of selected patients with multiple areas of skeletal metastases.

Contraindications:

Sequential therapy: Do not use as part of sequential treatment with a chemotherapeutic agent.

Polycythemia vera: Do not administer when the leukocyte count is < 5,000/cu mm or platelet count is < 150,000/cu mm.

Chronic myelocytic leukemia: Do not administer when the leukocyte count is < 20,000/cu mm.

Treatment of bone metastases: Usually not administered when the leukocyte count is < 5,000/cu mm and the platelet count is < 100,000/cu mm.

Warnings:

Do not administer as an intracavitary injection.

Use of radiopharmaceuticals should be restricted to physicians who are qualified in the safe use and handling of radionuclides and whose experience and training have been approved by the appropriate government agency.

Perform examinations using radiopharmaceuticals (especially elective examinations) to women of childbearing capacity during the first 10 days following the onset of menses.

Usage in Pregnancy: Category C. Safey for use during pregnancy has not been established. Use only when clearly needed and when the potential benefits outweigh the potential hazards to the fetus.

Usage in Lactation: It is not known whether sodium phosphate is excreted in breast milk. Discontinue nursing during therapy.

Usage in Children: Safety and efficacy in children have not been established.

Precautions:

Ensure minimum radiation exposure to patients and occupational workers consistent with proper patient management.

Sodium phosphate P 32 does not usually localize in retinoblastomas.

Adverse Reactions:

None known.

Overdosage:

May produce serious effects on the hematopoietic system. Monitor blood and bone marrow at regular intervals.

Administration and Dosage:

Administer IV only.

Measure dose by a suitable radioactivity calibration system immediately before use.

Polycythemia vera: 1 to 8 mCi IV are given, depending upon the stage of disease and size of the patient. Individualize repeat doses.

Chronic leukemia: 6 to 15 mCi usually with concomitant hormone manipulation.

Storage: Store at room temperature, 30°C (< 86°F).

Physical characteristics: Consult product literature for specific calibration and dosimetry information.

Rx	**Sodium Phosphate P 32** (Mallinckrodt)	**Injection:** 0.67 mCi/ml	In 10 ml vials containing 5 mCi radioactivity.

CHROMIC PHOSPHATE P 32

Actions:

Local irradiation by beta emission.

P 32 decays by beta emission with a physical half-life of 14.3 days. The mean energy of the beta particle is 695 keV.

Indications:

Intracavitary instillation: Treatment of peritoneal or pleural effusions caused by metastatic disease.

Interstitial injection: Treatment of cancer.

Contraindications:

Presence of ulcerative tumors; administration in exposed cavities or where there is evidence of loculation unless its extent is determined.

Warnings:

Not for intravascular use.

Radiopharmaceuticals: Restrict use to physicians qualified in the safe use and handling of radionuclides produced by nuclear reactor or particle accelerator and whose experience and training have been approved by the appropriate government agency.

Pregnancy and lactation: Use only when clearly needed and when the potential benefits outweigh the potential hazards to the fetus or nursing infant.

Precautions:

Radioactive material: Ensure minimum radiation exposure to the patient and occupational workers consistent with proper patient management.

Intracavitary use: Careful intracavitary instillation is required to avoid placing the dose of chromic phosphate P 32 into intrapleural or intraperitoneal loculations, bowel lumen or the body wall. Intestinal fibrosis or necrosis and chronic fibrosis of the body wall have resulted from unrecognized misplacement of the therapeutic agent.

Large tumor masses indicate the need for other forms of treatment; however, when other forms of treatment fail to control the effusion, chromic phosphate P 32 may be useful. In bloody effusion, treatment may be less effective.

Adverse Reactions:

Transitory radiation sickness, bone marrow depression, pleuritis, peritonitis, nausea and abdominal cramping.

Radiation damage may occur if injected interstitially or into a loculation.

Administration and Dosage:

For interstitial or intracavitary use only.

Measure dose by suitable radioactivity calibration system immediately prior to use.

The suggested dose range in the average patient (70 kg) is:

Intraperitoneal instillation: 10 to 20 mCi.
Intrapleural instillation: 6 to 12 mCi.
Interstitial use: 0.1 to 0.5 mCi/g of estimated weight of tumor.

Physical characteristics: Consult product literature for specific calibration and dosimetry information.

Rx	**Phosphocol P 32** (Mallinckrodt)	**Suspension:** 10 or 15 mCi with a concentration of up to 5 mCi/ml and specific activity of up to 5 mCi/mg at time of standardization.	In 10 ml vials.[1]

[1] With 2% benzyl alcohol.

INTERFERON ALFA-2a (rIFN-A; IFLrA)

Actions:

Pharmacology: Interferon alfa-2a is a sterile protein product manufactured by recombinant DNA technology that employs a genetically engineered *Escherichia coli* bacterium. Interferon alfa-2a is a highly purified protein containing 165 amino acids.

The mechanism by which interferons exert antitumor activity is not clearly understood. However, direct antiproliferative action against tumor cells and modulation of the host immune response may play important roles.

Using human cells in culture, interferon alfa-2a has antiproliferative and immunomodulatory activities that are very similar to those of the mixture of interferon alfa subtypes produced by human leukocytes. In vivo, interferon alfa-2a inhibits the growth of several human tumors growing in immunocompromised (nude) mice.

Pharmacokinetics: Absorption/Distribution – In healthy people, interferon alfa-2a exhibited an elimination half-life of 3.7 to 8.5 hours (mean, 5.1 hours), volume of distribution at steady state of 0.223 to 0.748 L/kg (mean, 0.4 L/kg) and a total body clearance of 2.14 to 3.62 ml/min/kg (mean, 2.79 ml/min/kg) after a 36 million IU (2.2 x 10^8 pg) IV infusion. After IM and SC administrations of 36 million IU, peak serum concentrations ranged from 1500 to 2580 pg/ml (mean, 2020 pg/ml) at a mean time to peak of 3.8 hours and from 1250 to 2320 pg/ml (mean, 1730 pg/ml) at a mean time to peak of 7.3 hours, respectively. The serum concentrations of interferon alfa-2a reflected a large intersubject variation. Dose proportional increases in serum concentrations were observed after single doses up to 198 million IU. There were no changes in the distribution or elimination of interferon alfa-2a during twice daily (0.5 to 36 million IU), once daily (1 to 54 million IU) or 3 times weekly (1 to 136 million IU) dosing regimens up to 28 days of dosing. Multiple IM doses resulted in accumulation of 2 to 4 times the single dose serum concentrations. The apparent fraction of the dose absorbed after IM injection was greater than 80%.

Metabolism/Excretion – Alpha interferons are filtered through the glomeruli and undergo rapid proteolytic degradation during tubular reabsorption, rendering a negligible reappearance of intact alpha interferon in the systemic circulation, suggesting near complete reabsorption of interferon alfa-2a catabolites. Liver metabolism and subsequent biliary excretion are minor pathways of elimination.

Clinical pharmacology: Hairy cell leukemia – During the first 1 to 2 months of treatment, significant depression of hematopoiesis was likely to occur. Subsequently, there was improvement in circulating blood cell counts.

Of the 75 patients evaluated for at least 16 weeks of therapy, 46 (61%) achieved complete or partial response. Twenty-one patients (28%) had a minor remission, eight (11%) remained stable and none had worsening of disease. All patients who achieved either a complete or partial response had complete or partial normalization of all peripheral blood elements with a concomitant decrease in peripheral blood and bone marrow hairy cells. Responding patients also exhibited a marked reduction in red blood cell and platelet transfusion requirements, a decrease in infectious episodes, and improvement in performance status. The probability of survival for 2 years in patients receiving interferon alfa-2a (94%) was statistically increased compared to a historical control group (75%).

AIDS-related Kaposi's sarcoma: Doses of 3 to 54 million IU daily were evaluated in more than 350 patients. An additional 91 patients received interferon alfa-2a in combination with vinblastine. The best response rate associated with acceptable toxicity was observed when interferon alfa-2a was administered as a single agent at a dose of 36 million IU daily. The escalating regimen of 3 to 36 million IU provided equivalent therapeutic benefit with some amelioration of acute toxicity in some patients. Lower doses were less effective in inducing tumor regression and doses higher than 36 million IU daily were associated with unacceptable toxicity.

The likelihood of response to interferon alfa-2a varies with the clinical manifestations of human immunodeficiency virus (HIV) infection but not to extent of tumor involvement. Patients with prior opportunistic infection or B symptoms (eg, night sweats, weight loss > 10% of body weight or 15 lbs, fever > 100°F without identifiable source of infection) are unlikely to respond to treatment.

Patients who were otherwise asymptomatic, with no prior opportunistic infection and near-normal levels of CD_4 lymphocytes, experienced higher response rates. Responding patients with a baseline CD_4 lymphocyte count > 200 cells/mm³ had a distinct survival advantage over both responding patients with a baseline CD_4 lymphocyte count of ≤ 200 cells/mm³ and nonresponding patients regardless of their baseline CD_4 lymphocyte count.

The median time to response was 2.7 months. The median duration of response for patients achieving a partial or complete response was 6.3 and 20.7 months, respectively. Complete and partial responses lasting in excess of 3 years have been observed.

(Continued on following page)

INTERFERON ALFA-2a (rIFN-A; IFLrA) (Cont.)

Indications:

Hairy cell leukemia: In select patients 18 years of age and older.

AIDS-related Kaposi's sarcoma: In select patients 18 years of age and older.

Unlabeled uses: Alpha interferons have been used for a variety of conditions. Clinical trials are in progress to further determine clinical efficacy, optimal dosage and length of treatment.

Interferon Alfa Unlabeled Uses		
Neoplastic Diseases		
Significant activity	*Limited activity*	*No activity*
Bladder tumors (local use for superficial tumors) Carcinoid tumor Chronic myelogenous leukemia Cutaneous T-cell lymphoma Essential thrombocythemia Non-Hodgkin's lymphoma (low-grade)	Acute leukemias Cervical carcinoma Chronic lymphocytic leukemia Hodgkin's disease Malignant gliomas Melanoma Multiple myeloma Mycosis fungoides/Sézary syndrome Nasopharyngeal carcinoma Osteosarcoma Ovarian carcinoma Renal carcinoma	Breast cancer Colorectal carcinoma Gastric carcinoma Lung carcinoma Pancreatic carcinoma Prostatic carcinoma Soft tissue carcinoma
Viral Infections		**Miscellaneous**
Chronic non-A, non-B hepatitis Condyloma acuminatum Cutaneous warts Cytomegaloviruses Herpes keratoconjunctivitis	Herpes simplex Papillomaviruses Rhinoviruses Vaccinia virus Varicella zoster Viral hepatitis B[1]	Hemangiomas of infancy (life-threatening) Multiple sclerosis

[1] May be more effective following prednisone withdrawal (immunologic priming).

Contraindications:

Hypersensitivity to alpha interferon or any component of the product.

Warnings:

Laboratory tests: Prior to initiation of therapy, perform tests to quantitate peripheral blood hemoglobin, platelets, granulocytes and hairy cells and bone marrow hairy cells. Monitor periodically (eg, monthly) during treatment to determine response to treatment. If a patient does not respond within 6 months, discontinue treatment. If a response occurs, continue treatment until no further improvement is observed and these laboratory parameters have been stable for about 3 months. It is not known whether continued treatment after that time is beneficial.

Exercise caution in the following: In patients with severe renal or hepatic disease, seizure disorders or compromised CNS function.

Administer with caution to patients with cardiac disease or with any history of cardiac illness. No direct cardiotoxic effect has been demonstrated, but it is likely that acute, self-limited toxicities (ie, fever, chills) frequently associated with interferon alfa administration may exacerbate preexisting cardiac conditions. Rarely, myocardial infarction has occurred.

Exercise caution when administering to patients with myelosuppression.

CNS reactions have occurred in a number of patients and included decreased mental status, exaggerated CNS function and dizziness. More severe obtundation and coma have been rarely observed. Most of these were mild and reversible within a few days to 3 weeks upon dose reduction or drug discontinuation. Careful periodic neuropsychiatric monitoring of all patients is recommended.

Leukopenia and elevation of hepatic enzymes occurred frequently but were rarely dose-limiting. Thrombocytopenia occurred less frequently. Proteinuria and increased cells in urinary sediment were also seen infrequently. Rarely, significant hepatic, renal and myelosuppressive toxicities were noted.

(Warnings continued on following page)

INTERFERON ALFA-2a (rIFN-A; IFLrA)(Cont.)

Warnings (Cont.):

Fertility impairment: Nonpregnant rhesus female monkeys treated with interferon alfa-2a at doses of 5 and 25 million IU/kg/day have shown menstrual cycle irregularities, and were considered to be anovulatory. The monkeys returned to normal menstrual rhythm following drug discontinuation.

Pregnancy: Category C. Safety in pregnancy has not been established. Use during pregnancy only if the potential benefit justifies the potential risk to the fetus. Information from primate studies showed dose-related menstrual irregularities and an increased incidence of spontaneous abortions. Fertile women should not receive interferon alfa-2a unless they are using effective contraception during therapy.

Lactation: It is not known whether this drug is excreted in breast milk. Because of the potential for serious adverse reactions in nursing infants, decide whether to discontinue nursing or to discontinue the drug, taking into account the importance of the drug to the mother.

Children: Safety and efficacy in children < 18 years of age have not been established.

Precautions:

Monitoring: Perform periodic complete blood counts and liver function tests during the course of treatment. Perform prior to therapy and at appropriate periods during therapy. Since responses of hairy cell leukemia are not generally observed for 1 to 3 months after initiation of treatment, very careful monitoring for severe depression of blood cell counts is warranted during the initial phase of treatment.

Those patients who have preexisting cardiac abnormalities or who are in advanced stages of cancer should have ECGs taken prior to and during the course of treatment.

Drug Interactions:

Aminophylline: In one study, a single IM injection of interferon alfa-2a significantly reduced the clearance of aminophylline 33% to 81% in 8 of 9 subjects, probably due to inhibition of the cytochrome P-450 enzyme system.

Adverse Reactions:

Most adverse reactions are reversible if detected early. If severe reactions occur, reduce dosage or discontinue the drug; take appropriate corrective measures according to physician's clinical judgment. Reinstitute therapy with caution; consider further need for the drug, and be alert to possible recurrence of toxicity.

The following data are based on the SC or IM administration of interferon alfa as a single agent. Interferon alfa was also evaluated for treatment of many other types of cancer. These studies generally used higher doses (12 to 50 million IU/m²). Incidence of most adverse reactions was similar, but tended to be more severe with higher doses.

Flu-like syndromes consisting of fever (74% to 98%), fatigue (89% to 95%), myalgias (69% to 73%), headache (66% to 71%), chills (41% to 64%) and arthralgia (5% to 24%) occurred in the majority of patients and tended to diminish with continuing therapy.

GI: Anorexia (46% to 65%); nausea (32% to 51%); diarrhea (29% to 42%), emesis (10% to 17%); abdominal pain (15%); flatulence and constipation (< 3%); abdominal fullness, hypermotility, gastric distress, hepatitis (< 1%).

CNS: Dizziness (21% to 41%); decreased mental status (17%); depression (16%); confusion (8% to 10%); diaphoresis (7% to 8%); paresthesias (6% to 8%); numbness (3% to 6%); lethargy (3%); visual disturbances, sleep disturbances (5%); nervousness, vertigo, anxiety and forgetfulness (< 3%); gait disturbance, poor coordination, hallucinations, seizures, encephalopathy, psychomotor retardation, stroke, coma, aphasia, aphonia, ataxia, dysarthria, dysphasia, amnesia, sedation, apathy, anxiety, emotional lability, irritability, hyperactivity, weakness, involuntary movements, claustrophobia, loss of libido, neuropathy, tremor (< 1%).

Cardiovascular and pulmonary: Coughing (27%); dyspnea (11%); hypotension (4% to 6%); edema (3% to 9%); chest pain (4%); hypertension, arrhythmias, chest congestion and palpitations (< 3%); syncope, stroke, transient ischemic attacks, congestive heart failure, pulmonary edema, myocardial infarction, Raynaud's phenomenon, hot flashes (< 1%).

Dermatologic: Partial alopecia (8% to 22%); rash (11% to 18%); dryness or inflammation of the oropharynx (14% to 16%); dry skin or pruritus (5% to 13%); urticaria (< 3%); flushing of the skin (< 1%).

Other: Weight loss (14% to 25%); change in taste (13% to 25%); reactivation of herpes labialis (8%); transient impotence (6%); night sweats (8%); rhinorrhea (4%); sinusitis (< 3%); conjunctivitis, injection site inflammation (rare); muscle contractions, bronchospasm, tachypnea, excessive salivation, cyanosis, earache, eye irritation, rhinitis (< 1%).

Rare reactions (possibly related to underlying disease): Epistaxis; bleeding gums; ecchymoses; petechiae.

(Adverse Reactions continued on following page)

INTERFERON ALFA-2a (rIFN-A; IFLrA) (Cont.)

Adverse Reactions (Cont.):

Abnormal laboratory test values:

Hematologic – Leukopenia (49%); neutropenia (52%); thrombocytopenia (35%); decreased hemoglobin (27%).

Hepatic – AST (42% to 46%); alkaline phosphatase (8% to 11%); LDH (10% to 13%); bilirubin (≤ 2%).

Renal/urinary – Proteinuria (< 1%); uric acid (< 5%); serum creatinine (≤ 2%); BUN (4%).

Other – Hypocalcemia; elevated fasting serum glucose and elevated serum phosphorus (< 5%).

Neutralizing antibodies were detected in approximately 27% of all patients (3.4% for patients with hairy cell leukemia). No clinical sequelae have been documented. Antibodies to human leukocyte interferon may occur spontaneously in certain clinical conditions (cancer, systemic lupus erythematosus, herpes zoster) in patients who have never received exogenous interferon.

Patient Information:

Patient package insert available with product.

Warn patients not to change brands of interferon; changes in dosage may result.

Instruct patients on proper home technique.

Patients should be well hydrated, especially during initial treatment.

Administration and Dosage:

Approved by the FDA in 1986.

Give SC or IM. Subcutaneous administration is suggested for, but not limited to, patients who are thrombocytopenic (platelet count < 50,000/mm³) or who are at risk for bleeding.

Hairy cell leukemia: Induction dose – 3 million IU daily for 16 to 24 weeks, SC or IM.

Maintenance dose – 3 million IU 3 times per week. Dosage reduction by one-half or withholding of individual doses may be needed when severe adverse reactions occur.

The use of doses higher than 3 million IU is not recommended.

Treat patients for approximately 6 months before determining whether to continue therapy. Patients with hairy cell leukemia have been treated for up to 20 consecutive months. The optimal duration of treatment for this disease has not been determined.

AIDS-related Kaposi's sarcoma: Induction dose – 36 million IU daily for 10 to 12 weeks, administered IM or SC.

Maintenance dose – 36 million IU, 3 times per week. Dose reductions by one-half or withholding of individual doses may be required when severe adverse reactions occur. An escalating schedule of 3, 9 and 18 million IU daily for 3 days followed by 36 million IU daily for the remainder of the 10 to 12 week induction period has also produced equivalent therapeutic benefit with some amelioration of the acute toxicity in some patients.

When disease stabilization or a response to treatment occurs, treatment should continue until there is no further evidence of tumor or until discontinuation is required because of a severe opportunistic infection or adverse effects. The optimal duration of treatment for this disease has not been determined.

If severe reactions occur, modify dosage (50% reduction) or temporarily discontinue therapy until the adverse reactions abate. The need for dosage reduction should take into account the effects of prior x-ray therapy or chemotherapy that may have compromised bone marrow reserve. Minimum effective doses have not been established.

Storage: Refrigerate 2° to 8°C (36° to 46°F). Do not freeze; do not shake. Once the powder is reconstituted, use within 30 days.

Rx	**Roferon-A** (Roche)	**Injection Solution:** 3 million IU/ml	In 1 ml vials (3 million IU per vial).[1]
		6 million IU/ml	In 3 ml vials (18 million IU per vial).[1]
		36 million IU/ml[2]	In 1 ml vials (36 million IU per vial).[1]
		Powder for Injection: 6 million IU/ml when reconstituted	In 18 million IU per vial with diluent.[1]

[1] With human serum albumin and phenol.

[2] Do not use this dosage form for the treatment of hairy cell leukemia.

INTERFERON ALFA-2b (IFN-alpha 2; rIFN-α2; α-2-interferon)

Actions:

Pharmacology: Interferon alfa is a protein produced by recombinant DNA techniques. It is obtained from a strain of *Escherichia coli* bearing a genetically engineered plasmid containing an interferon alfa-2b gene from human leukocytes.

The content is expressed in terms of International Units (IU). International Units are determined by comparison of the antiviral activity of the interferon alfa-2b, recombinant, with the activity of the international reference preparation of human leukocyte interferon established by the World Health Organization (WHO).

The interferons are naturally occurring small protein molecules. They are produced and secreted by cells in response to viral infections or synthetic and biological inducers. Three major classes of interferons have been identified: Alpha, beta and gamma. These classes are not homogenous; each may contain several different molecular species. At least 14 genetically distinct human alpha interferons have been identified thus far.

Interferons exert their cellular activities by binding to specific membrane receptors on the cell surface. Once bound to the cell membrane, interferon initiates a complex sequence of intracellular events that includes the induction of certain enzymes. This process, at least in part, may be responsible for the various cellular responses to interferon, including inhibition of virus replication in virus-infected cells, suppression of cell proliferation and such immunomodulating activities as enhancement of the phagocytic activity of macrophages and augmentation of the specific cytotoxicity of lymphocytes for target cells.

Pharmacokinetics: Twelve healthy male volunteers were studied following single doses of 5 million IU/m^2 administered IM, SC and as a 30 minute IV infusion in a crossover design. Interferon concentrations were determined by using a radioimmunoassay (RIA) with a detection limit equal to 10 IU/ml.

Mean serum concentrations following IM and SC injections were comparable. Maximum serum concentrations obtained were $\approx$ 18 to 116 IU/ml and occurred 3 to 12 hours after administration. Elimination half-lives were approximately 2 to 3 hours. Serum concentrations were below the detection limit by 16 hours after the injections.

After IV administration, serum concentrations peaked (135 to 273 IU/ml) by the end of the infusion, then declined at a slightly more rapid rate than after IM or SC drug administration, becoming undetectable 4 hours after the infusion. Elimination half-life was approximately 2 hours.

Interferon could not be detected in urine; the kidney may be the main site of interferon catabolism.

Clinical pharmacology: Hairy cell leukemia – In clinical trials, there was depression of circulating red blood cells, white blood cells and platelets during the first 1 to 2 months of treatment. Subsequently, both splenectomized and nonsplenectomized patients achieved substantial and sustained improvements in granulocytes, platelets and hemoglobin levels in 75% of treated patients, and at least some improvement (minor responses) occurred in 90%. For the entire study group, median platelet counts were within the normal range after 2 months, median hemoglobin levels were in the normal range after 4 months and median granulocyte counts were in the normal range after 5 months of treatment.

Treatment resulted in a decrease in bone marrow hypercellularity and hairy cell infiltrates. The hairy cell index was $\geq$ 50% at the beginning of the study in 87% of patients. The percentage of patients with such an index decreased to 25% after 6 months and to 14% after 1 year. Prolonged treatment may be required to obtain maximal reduction in tumor cell infiltrates in the bone marrow.

The percentage of patients with hairy cell leukemia who required red blood cell or platelet transfusions decreased significantly during treatment. Additionally, the percentage of patients with confirmed and serious infections declined during treatment as granulocyte counts improved.

Reduced risk of major complications of hairy cell leukemia (serious infections, bleeding diatheses, transfusion requirements) was apparent within 3 months of initiation of treatment. No deaths occurred in interferon alfa-2b patients during the next 9 months of treatment and follow-up, while the mortality rate in the control group was 20%. During the initial 3 months of treatment, interferon-mediated suppression of hematopoiesis may occur.

(Actions continued on following page)

INTERFERON ALFA-2b (IFN-alpha 2; rIFN-α2; α-2-interferon) (Cont.)

Actions (Cont.):

Clinical pharmacology (Cont.):

Condylomata acuminata – A total of 192 patients were injected intralesionally with 1 million IU interferon alfa-2b per lesion. Up to five lesions per patient were treated 3 times a week for 3 weeks, and the patients were then observed for up to 16 weeks after the full treatment course. Interferon alfa-2b was significantly more effective than placebo in the treatment of condylomata, as measured by disappearance of lesions, decreases in lesion size and by an overall change in disease status. In the 192 patients evaluated, 42% experienced clearing of all treated lesions, while 24% experienced marked and 18% experienced moderate reduction in lesion size, and 10% of patients had a slight reduction in lesion size.

In one study, overall percentage of patients who had all their treated lesions clear after two courses of treatment ranged from 57% to 85%. Treated lesions showed improvement within 2 to 4 weeks after the start of treatment, and the maximal response was noted 4 to 8 weeks after initiation of treatment.

AIDS-related Kaposi's sarcoma – A total of 144 patients were treated in three clinical trials with various dosage regimens. Significantly greater activity occurred in asymptomatic (afebrile and without weight loss) patients than systemic symptom patients (57% vs 23%) in one study. In another study, a 44% response rate occurred in asymptomatic patients vs 7% in symptomatic patients. Median time to response was ≈ 2 months and median duration of response ≈ 3 months for asymptomatic patients. For symptomatic patients, median time to response and median duration of response were both 1 month. In a third study, median time to response was 2 months and median duration of response 5 months in asymptomatic patients. In all studies, response likelihood was greatest in those with relatively intact immune systems as assessed by baseline T4 counts (interchangeable with CD4) or T4/T8 ratios. Results at doses of 30 million IU/m^2 3 times/week and 35 million IU/day SC were similar.

Chronic hepatitis non-A, non-B/C (NANB/C) – A total of 332 patients were given interferon alfa-2b SC at doses of 1, 2 or 3 million IU 3 times a week for 6 months in four controlled studies. Interferon alfa-2b produced a statistically significant improvement in serum alanine aminotransferase (ALT) levels in all studies. Of the 54% of responding patients at a dose of 3 million IU, 70% achieved reductions in ALT levels to normal, 18% achieved reductions to near normal levels and 12% achieved partial response. Combined analysis for three studies showed a statistically significant histological improvement, due primarily to decreases in severity of necrosis and degeneration in the lobular and periportal regions, in 65% of patients vs 46% of controls. The ALT response was maintained in 51% of responding patients 6 months after the end of therapy. Of patients who relapsed during follow-up and were retreated, 83% responded to retreatment.

Serum anti-interferon neutralizing antibodies were detected in 15% of patients who received 3 million IU 3 times a week for 6 months. The titers were low and the significance is not known.

Chronic hepatitis B – A total of 86 patients received either 5 million IU every day (n = 38) or 10 million IU 3 times a week (n = 48) for 16 weeks. Compared to untreated controls, a significantly greater proportion of interferon alfa-2b-treated patients exhibited a virologic response (7% vs 39% to 48%). No patient responding to therapy relapsed during a follow-up period of 2 to 6 months. Loss of serum HBeAg and HBV-DNA (indicators of HBV replication) was maintained in 100% of 19 responding patients for 3.5 to 36 months of follow-up. In a pilot study, 100% of 12 patients responding to treatment remained serum HBeAg negative for 3.8 to 6.6 years after treatment. Normalization of serum ALT also occurred in a significantly greater proportion of treated patients vs controls. Virologic response was associated with a reduction of serum ALT to normal or near normal (≤ 1.5 times upper limit of normal) in 87% of patients responding to 5 million IU/day and 100% of patients responding to 10 million IU 3 times per week.

Indications:

Hairy cell leukemia: In select patients ≥ 18 years of age, both previously splenectomized and nonsplenectomized.

Condylomata acuminata: Intralesional treatment of genital or venereal warts in patients who do not respond to other treatment modalities or whose lesions are more readily treatable by interferon alfa-2b.

AIDS-related Kaposi's sarcoma: In select patients ≥ 18 years of age.

Chronic hepatitis non-A, non-B/C: In patients ≥ 18 years of age with compensated liver disease and a history of blood or blood product exposure or are HCV antibody positive.

Chronic hepatitis B: In patients ≥ 18 years of age with compensated liver disease and HBV replication. Patients must be serum HBsAg positive for at least 6 months and have HBV replication (serum HBeAg positive) with elevated serum ALT.

(Indications continued on following page)

INTERFERON ALFA-2b (IFN-alpha 2; rIFN-α2; α-2-interferon) (Cont.)

Indications (Cont.):

Unlabeled uses: Alpha interferons have been used for a variety of conditions, a list of which follows. Clinical trials are currently in progress to further determine clinical efficacy, optimal dosage and length of treatment.

Interferon Alfa Unlabeled Uses		
Neoplastic Diseases		
Significant activity	*Limited activity*	*No activity*
Bladder tumors (local use for superficial tumors) Carcinoid tumor Chronic myelogenous leukemia Cutaneous T-cell lymphoma Essential thrombocythemia Non-Hodgkin's lymphoma (low-grade)	Acute leukemias Cervical carcinoma Chronic lymphocytic leukemia Hodgkin's disease Malignant gliomas Melanoma Multiple myeloma Nasopharyngeal carcinoma Osteosarcoma Ovarian carcinoma Renal carcinoma	Breast cancer Colorectal carcinoma Gastric carcinoma Lung carcinoma Pancreatic carcinoma Prostatic carcinoma Soft tissue carcinoma
Viral Infections		**Miscellaneous**
Cutaneous warts Cytomegaloviruses Herpes keratoconjunctivitis Herpes simplex	Papillomaviruses Rhinoviruses Vaccinia virus Varicella zoster	Multiple sclerosis

Contraindications:

Hypersensitivity to interferon alfa-2b or any components of the product.

Warnings:

Hairy cell leukemia:

Monitoring – Prior to initiation of therapy, perform tests to quantitate peripheral blood hemoglobin, platelets, granulocytes and hairy cells and bone marrow hairy cells. Monitor periodically to determine response. If a patient does not respond within 6 months, discontinue treatment. If a response does occur, continue treatment until no further improvement is observed and these laboratory parameters have been stable for about 3 months. It is not known if continued treatment after that point is beneficial.

Do not give IM to patients with platelet counts $< 50,000/mm^3$. Instead, give SC.

Cardiovascular adverse experiences such as significant hypotension, arrhythmia or tachycardia ($\geq$ 150 beats/min), were observed in $\approx$ 3% of patients studied who had various malignancies and were treated at doses higher than those for hairy cell leukemia. Incidence of these complications in patients with preexisting heart disease is unknown. Hypotension may occur during administration, or for up to 2 days post-therapy, and may require supportive therapy, including fluid replacement, to maintain intravascular volume. Supraventricular arrhythmias occurred rarely and appeared to be correlated with preexisting conditions and prior therapy with cardiotoxic agents. These adverse experiences were controlled by modifying dose or discontinuing treatment, but they may require specific additional therapy. Closely monitor patients with a recent history of myocardial infarction or previous or current arrhythmic disorder.

CNS effects (eg, depression, confusion, other alterations of mental status) were observed in about 2% of hairy cell leukemia patients. The overall incidence in a larger patient population with other malignancies treated with higher doses was 10%. More significant obtundation and coma may occur in some patients, usually elderly, treated at higher doses for other malignant diseases. These effects are usually rapidly reversible. In a few severe episodes, full resolution of symptoms takes up to 3 weeks. Closely monitor patients until these effects resolve. Discontinuation of therapy may be required. Narcotics, hypnotics or sedatives may be used concurrently with caution.

Condylomata acuminata:

Do not use the 3, 5 and 25 million IU strengths intralesionally since the dilution would result in a hypertonic solution. The 50 million IU strength is not to be used for condylomata.

AIDS-related Kaposi's sarcoma:

Monitoring – Perform lesion measurements and blood counts prior to initiation of therapy; monitor periodically during treatment.

Rapidly progressive visceral disease – Do not use.

(Warnings continued on following page)

INTERFERON ALFA-2b (IFN-alpha 2; rIFN-α2; α-2-interferon) (Cont.)

Warnings (Cont.):

Chronic hepatitis – NANB/C:

Monitoring – Perform a liver biopsy to establish diagnosis. Test for presence of antibody to HCV. Exclude patients with other causes of chronic hepatitis, including autoimmune hepatitis. Establish that the patient has compensated liver disease. Before treatment, establish and consider the following criteria: Bilirubin ≤ 2 mg/dl; albumin stable and within normal limits; prothrombin time (PT) < 3 seconds prolonged; WBC ≥ 3000/mm³; platelets > 70,000/mm³; serum creatinine normal or near normal. Evaluate CBC and platelet counts, then repeat at weeks 1 and 2 following therapy initiation, monthly thereafter. Evaluate ALT levels after 2, 16 and 24 weeks.

Preexisting psychiatric condition/history of severe psychiatric disorder – Do not treat; discontinue therapy in any patient developing severe depression.

Preexisting thyroid abnormalities – Patients whose thyroid function cannot be maintained in the normal range by medication should not be treated. Discontinue therapy in patients developing thyroid abnormalities during treatment.

Chronic hepatitis B:

Monitoring – Perform a liver biopsy to establish presence of chronic hepatitis and extent of liver damage. Establish that the patient has compensated liver disease. Before treatment, establish and consider the following criteria: Bilirubin normal; albumin stable and within normal limits; PT < 3 seconds prolonged; WBC ≥ 4000/mm³; platelets ≥ 100,000/mm³. Evaluate CBC and platelet counts, then repeat at weeks 1, 2, 4, 8, 12 and 16. Evaluate liver function tests, including serum ALT, albumin and bilirubin at treatment weeks 1, 2, 4, 8, 12 and 16. Evaluate HBeAg, HBsAg and ALT at the end of therapy and 3 and 6 months post-therapy.

ALT increase – A transient increase in ALT ≥ 2 times baseline (flare) can occur, generally 8 to 12 weeks after therapy initiation, and is more frequent in responders. Continue therapy unless signs and symptoms of hepatic failure occur. During the ALT flare, monitor clinical symptomatology and liver function tests (including ALT, PT, alkaline phosphatase, albumin and bilirubin) at ≈ 2 week intervals.

Chronic hepatitis B patients with evidence of decreasing hepatic synthetic functions (eg, decreasing albumin levels, prolongation of PT) may be at increased risk of clinical decompensation in association with a flare of aminotransferases. Evaluate the potential risks vs potential benefits of treatment.

Chronic hepatitis NANB/C and B: Do not treat patients with decompensated liver disease, autoimmune hepatitis or a history of autoimmune disease, or patients who are immunosuppressed transplant recipients. In these patients, worsening liver disease, including jaundice, hepatic encephalopathy, hepatic failure and death have occurred following therapy. Discontinue therapy for any patient developing signs and symptoms of liver failure.

Moderate to severe adverse experiences may require modification of the patient's dosage regimen, or in some cases, termination of therapy.

Fever/"flu-like" symptoms: Because of fever and other "flu-like" symptoms associated with this drug, use cautiously in debilitating medical conditions, such as those with a history of cardiovascular disease (eg, unstable angina, uncontrolled CHF), pulmonary disease (eg, chronic obstructive pulmonary disease) or diabetes mellitus prone to ketoacidosis. Observe caution in coagulation disorders (eg, thrombophlebitis, pulmonary embolism) or severe myelosuppression.

Hypersensitivity reactions (eg, urticaria, angioedema, bronchoconstriction, anaphylaxis) have not been observed in patients receiving interferon alfa-2b; however, if such an acute reaction develops, discontinue the drug immediately and institute appropriate medical therapy. Have epinephrine 1:1000 immediately available. Refer to Management of Acute Hypersensitivity Reactions. Transient cutaneous rashes have occurred following injection, but have not necessitated treatment interruption.

Fertility impairment: Interferon may impair fertility. In non-human primates, abnormalities of the menstrual cycle have been observed. Decreases in serum estradiol and progesterone concentrations have occurred in women treated with human leukocyte interferon. Fertile women should not receive interferon alfa-2b unless they are using effective contraception. Use with caution in fertile men.

Pregnancy: Category C. Another interferon alfa preparation has abortifacient effects in rhesus monkeys when given at 20 to 500 times the human dose. Therefore, use during pregnancy only if the potential benefit justifies the potential risk to the fetus.

Lactation: It is not known if this drug is excreted in breast milk. Because of the potential for serious reactions in nursing infants, decide whether to stop nursing or to stop the drug, taking into account the importance of the drug to the mother.

Children: Safety and efficacy in children < 18 years of age have not been established.

(Continued on following page)

INTERFERON ALFA-2b (IFN-alpha 2; rIFN-α2; α-2-interferon) (Cont.)

Precautions:

Monitoring: In addition to tests normally required for monitoring patients, the following are recommended for all patients on interferon therapy, prior to beginning treatment and periodically thereafter: Standard hematologic tests with complete blood counts and differential, platelet counts, blood chemistries, electrolytes and liver function tests. Patients with preexisting cardiac abnormalities, or in advanced stages of cancer, should have ECGs taken before and during treatment. Refer also to the monitoring sections under Warnings for each indication.

Photosensitivity may occur; therefore, caution patients to take protective measures (ie, sunscreens, protective clothing) against exposure to ultraviolet light or sunlight until tolerance is determined.

Drug Interactions:

Interferon Alfa-2b Drug Interactions			
Precipitant drug	Object drug*		Description
Interferon alfa-2b	Aminophylline	⬆	In one study, a single IM injection of interferon alfa-2a significantly reduced the clearance of aminophylline by 33% to 81% in 8 of 9 subjects, probably due to inhibition of the cytochrome P-450 enzyme system.
Interferon alfa-2b	Zidovudine	⬆	There may be synergistic adverse effects between interferon alfa-2b and zidovudine. Patients have had a higher incidence of neutropenia than that expected with zidovudine alone. Carefully monitor WBC count.

* ⬆ = Object drug increased

Adverse Reactions:

Adverse reactions are dose-related. Most reactions are mild to moderate in severity. Some are transient and most diminish with continued therapy. The most frequently reported reactions are flu-like symptoms, particularly fever, headache, chills, myalgia and fatigue.

Interferon Alfa-2b Adverse Reactions Based on Indication (%)						
	Adverse reaction	Hairy cell leukemia (n = 145)	Condylomata acuminata (n = 352)	AIDS-related Kaposi's sarcoma[1] (n = 103)	Chronic hepatitis non-A non-B/C (n = 159)	Chronic hepatitis B[1] (n = 179)
Flu-like symptoms	Fever	68	56	47-55	43	66-86
	Fatigue	61	18	48-84	19	69-75
	Chills	46	45	—	—	—
	Headache	39	47	21-36	43	44-61
	Myalgia	39	44	28-34	42	40-59
Central & peripheral nervous systems	Dizziness	12	9	7-24	9	10-13
	Paresthesia	6	1	3-21	1	3-6
	Depression	6	3	9-28	8	6-17
	Anxiety	5	< 1	1-3	1	2
	Confusion	< 5	4	10-12	1	—
	Hypoesthesia	< 5	1	10	—	—
	Amnesia	< 5	—	14	—	—
	Impaired concentration	—	< 1	3-14	4	5-8
	Nervousness	—	1	3	—	3
	Irritability	—	—	—	4	12-16
	Somnolence	< 5	3	3	1	9-14
	Decreased libido	< 5	—	—	1	1-5
GI	Nausea	21	17	21-28	23	33-50
	Diarrhea	18	2	18-45	13	8-19
	Vomiting	6	2	11-14	3	7-10
	Anorexia	19	1	38-41	13	43-53
	Dyspepsia	—	2	4	3	3-8
	Constipation	< 1	—	1-10	< 1	5
	Loose stools	—	<1	10	3	2
	Abdominal pain	< 5	1	5-21	6	4-5

[1] Incidence related to dosage. — = Not reported.

(Adverse Reactions continued on following page)

INTERFERON ALFA-2b (IFN-alpha 2; rIFN-α2; α-2-interferon) (Cont.)

Adverse Reactions (Cont.):

Interferon Alfa-2b Adverse Reactions Based on Indication (%) (Cont.)

	Adverse reaction	Hairy cell leukemia (n = 145)	Condylomata acuminata (n = 352)	AIDS-related Kaposi's sarcoma[1] (n = 103)	Chronic hepatitis non-A non-B/C (n = 159)	Chronic hepatitis B[1] (n = 179)
Respiratory	Pharyngitis	<5	1	1-31	1	1-7
	Nasal congestion	—	1	10	—	4
	Dyspnea	<1	—	1-34	<1	5
	Coughing	<1	—	14-31	<1	1-4
	Sinusitis	—	—	21	—	—
	Dry mouth/thirst	19	<5	22-28	<5	5-6
Bone, joint, muscle	Arthralgia	8	9	3	19	8-19
	Asthenia	7	—	11	24	5-15
	Rigors	—	—	14-30	27	38-42
	Back pain	19	6	1-3	3	—
	Muscle pain/weakness	<5	<5	<5	<5	≤9
Dermatologic	Rash	25	—	9-10	6	1-8
	Pruritus	11	1	7	6	4-6
	Dry skin	9	—	9-10	<1	3
	Dermatitis	8	—	—	—	1
	Alopecia	8	—	12-31	17	26-38
	Moniliasis	—	<1	17	—	—
	Edema/facial edema	—	<1	10	1	1-3
	Injection site reaction (eg, inflammation, burning, pain, bleeding)	20	<5	<5	7	3-<5
Miscellaneous	Pain	18	3	3	—	—
	Chest pain	<1	<1	1-28	1	4
	Increased sweating	8	2	4-21	3	1
	Malaise	—	14	5	3	6-9
	Taste alteration	13	<1	5-7	1	10
	Insomnia	—	<1	3	4	6-11
	Weight loss	<1	<1	3-5	<1	2-5
	Herpes simplex	—	1	3	—	5
	Gingivitis	—	—	14	—	1
Lab test abnormalities	Hemoglobin	na	—	1-15	15	23-32
	WBC count	na	17	10-22	18	34-68
	Platelet count	na	—	8	9	5-12
	Serum creatinine	0	—	—	2	3
	Alkaline phosphatase	4	—	—	3	4-8
	Serum urea nitrogen	0	—	—	1	—
	AST	4	12	11-41	—	—
	ALT	13	—	10-15	—	—
	Granulocyte count					
	Total	na	—	31-39	37	61-71
	1000-<1500/mm³	—	—	—	—	31-32
	750-<1000/mm³	—	—	—	—	18-23
	500-<750/mm³	—	—	—	—	9-15
	<500/mm³	—	—	—	—	2

[1] Incidence related to dosage. — = Not reported. na = Not applicable.

Additional reactions reported for all indications and occurring at an incidence of < 5% are as follows:

Hematologic: Anemia; granulocytopenia; hemolytic anemia; leukopenia; thrombocytopenia.

Cardiovascular: Arrhythmia; atrial fibrillation; bradycardia; cardiac failure; cardiomyopathy; extrasystoles; hypertension; hypotension; palpitations; postural hypotension; tachycardia.

Endocrine: Aggravation of diabetes mellitus; gynecomastia; thyroid disorder; virilism.

Respiratory: Bronchospasm; cyanosis; epistaxis; pleural pain; pneumonia; rhinitis; rhinorrhea; sneezing; wheezing.

(Adverse Reactions continued on following page)

INTERFERON ALFA-2b (IFN-alpha 2; rIFN-α2; α-2-interferon) (Cont.)

Adverse Reactions (Cont):

GI: Abdominal distention; dysphagia; eructation; esophagitis; flatulence; gastric ulcer; GI hemorrhage; GI mucosal discoloration; gingival bleeding; gum hyperplasia; increased appetite; increased saliva; melena; oral leukoplakia; rectal bleeding after stool; rectal hemorrhage; stomatitis; ulcerative stomatitis.

Hepatic/Biliary: Abnormal hepatic function tests; bilirubinemia; increased transaminases; jaundice; right upper quadrant pain; hepatic encephalopathy; hepatic failure.

Musculoskeletal: Arthritis; arthrosis; bone pain; leg cramps.

CNS: Abnormal coordination, dreaming, gait and thinking; aggravated depression; aggressive reaction; agitation; apathy; aphasia; ataxia; CNS dysfunction; coma; convulsions; dysphonia; emotional lability; extrapyramidal disorder; feeling of ebriety; flushing; hot flashes; hyperesthesia; hyperkinesia; hypertonia; hypokinesia; impaired consciousness; migraine; neuropathy; neurosis; paresis; paroniria; parosmia; personality disorder; polyneuropathy; suicide attempt; syncope; tremor.

GU: Amenorrhea; impotence; increased BUN; hematuria; leukorrhea; menorrhagia; micturition disorder/frequency; nocturia; polyuria; uterine bleeding.

Dermatologic: Abnormal hair texture; acne; cyanosis of the hand; cold/clammy skin; dermatitis lichenoides; epidermal necrolysis; erythema; furunculosis; increased hair growth; melanosis; nail disorders; nonherpetic cold sores; peripheral ischemia; photosensitivity (see Precautions); purpura; skin depigmentation; skin discoloration; urticaria; vitiligo.

Special senses: Abnormal/Blurred vision; conjunctivitis; diplopia; dry eyes; earache; eye pain; hearing disorder; lacrimal gland disorder; periorbital edema; photophobia; speech disorder; taste loss; tinnitus; vertigo.

Miscellaneous: Abscess; cachexia; dehydration; hypercalcemia; lymphadenopathy; peripheral edema; sepsis; stye; substernal chest pain; weakness.

Patient Information:

Patient package insert available with product.

Do not change brands of interferon; changes in dosage may result.

The most common adverse effects are "flu-like" symptoms, such as fever, headache, fatigue, anorexia, nausea and vomiting. These appear to decrease in severity as treatment continues. Some of these "flu-like" symptoms may be minimized by bedtime doses. Use acetaminophen to prevent or partially alleviate fever and headache.

Patients should be well hydrated, especially during the initial stages of treatment.

Administration and Dosage:

Hairy cell leukemia: 2 million IU/m², IM or SC 3 times per week. The normalization of one or more hematologic variables usually begins within 2 months of initiation of therapy. Improvement in all 3 hematologic variables may require $\geq$ 6 months of therapy.

Maintain this dosage regimen unless the disease progresses rapidly, or severe intolerance occurs. If severe adverse reactions develop, modify dosage (50% reduction) or discontinue therapy until reactions abate. Discontinue if intolerance persists or recurs following adequate dosage adjustment, or if disease progresses.

At the physician's discretion, the patient may self-administer the dose; it may be administered at bedtime. Use sterilized glass or disposable syringes.

Condylomata acuminata: 1 million IU/lesion 3 times/wk for 3 weeks intralesionally. Use only 10 million IU vial since dilution of other strengths required for intralesional use results in a hypertonic solution. Do not reconstitute 10 million IU vial with $>$ 1 ml diluent. Use tuberculin or similar syringe and 25 to 30 gauge needle. Do not go beneath lesion too deeply or inject too superficially. As many as 5 lesions can be treated at one time. To alleviate side effects, give in evening with acetaminophen.

Maximum response usually occurs 4 to 8 weeks after initiation of therapy. If results are not satisfactory after 12 to 16 weeks, a second course may be instituted. Patients with six to ten condylomata may receive a second sequential course of treatment. Patients with greater than ten condylomata may receive additional sequences.

AIDS-related Kaposi's sarcoma: 30 million IU/m² 3 times a week administered SC or IM. Use only 50 million IU vial. Maintain the selected dosage regimen unless the disease progresses rapidly or severe intolerance occurs. If severe adverse reactions develop, modify dosage (50% reduction) or temporarily discontinue therapy until adverse reactions abate. When patients initiate therapy at 30 million IU/m² 3 times a week, average dose tolerated at end of 12 weeks therapy is 110 million IU/week and 75 million IU/week at end of 24 weeks therapy.

When disease stabilization or response to treatment occurs, continue treatment until there is no further evidence of tumor or until discontinuation is required by evidence of a severe opportunistic infection or adverse effect.

(Administration and Dosage continued on following page)

INTERFERON ALFA-2b (IFN-alpha 2; rIFN-α2; α-2-interferon) (Cont.)

Administration and Dosage (Cont.):

Chronic hepatitis non-A, non-B/C: 3 million IU 3 times/week SC or IM. Normalization of ALT levels may occur in some patients as early as 2 weeks after treatment initiation; however, current experience suggests completing a 6 month course of therapy in responding patients. Consider discontinuing therapy in nonresponders after 16 weeks. If severe adverse reactions develop, modify the dose (50% reduction) or temporarily discontinue therapy until reactions abate. Patients who relapse may be retreated with the same dosage regimen to which they had previously responded. At the physician's discretion, the patient may self-administer the medication.

Chronic hepatitis B: 30 to 35 million IU per week SC or IM, either as 5 million IU daily or 10 million IU 3 times a week for 16 weeks. If serious adverse reactions or lab abnormalities develop during therapy, decrease the dose by 50% or discontinue if appropriate until adverse reactions abate. If intolerance persists after dose adjustment, discontinue the drug.

Decreased granulocyte or platelet counts – Use the following guidelines:

Interferon Alfa-2b Dose with Decreased Granulocyte or Platelet Counts		
Granulocyte count	Platelet count	Interferon alfa-2b dose
$< 750/mm^3$	$< 50,000/mm^3$	Reduce by 50%
$< 500/mm^3$	$< 30,000/mm^3$	Interrupt

When platelet or granulocyte counts return to normal or baseline values, reinstitute therapy at up to 100% of initial dose.

Preparation of solution: Inject diluent (Bacteriostatic Water for Injection) amount stated in chart below into vial. Agitate gently, withdraw with sterile syringe, inject IM or SC.

Preparation of Interferon Alfa-2b Solution Based on Indication		
Vial strength	Amount of diluent	Final concentration
Hairy cell leukemia		
3 million IU	1 ml	3 million IU/ml
5 million IU	1 ml	5 million IU/ml
10 million IU	2 ml	5 million IU/ml
18 million IU[1]	3.8 ml	6 million IU/ml
25 million IU	5 ml	5 million IU/ml
Condylomata acuminata		
10 million IU	1 ml	10 million IU/ml
AIDS-related Kaposi's sarcoma		
50 million IU	1 ml	50 million IU/ml
Chronic hepatitis – NANB/C		
3 million IU	1 ml	3 million IU/ml
18 million IU[1]	3.8 ml	6 million IU/ml
Chronic hepatitis B		
5 million IU	1 ml	5 million IU/ml
10 million IU	1 ml	10 million IU/ml

[1] Multi-dose vial.

Stability and storage: After reconstitution, solution is stable for 1 month at 2° to 8°C (36° to 46°F). Store solution before and after reconstitution between 2° and 8°C.

Rx	**Intron A** (Schering)	**Powder for Injection, lyophilized:**[2]	
		3 million IU per vial	In vials with 1 ml diluent[3] vial or syringe.
		5 million IU per vial	In vials with 1 ml diluent[3] vial or syringe.
		10 million IU per vial	In vials with 2 ml diluent[3] vial or 1 ml diluent[3] syringe.
		18 million IU per vial	In multi-dose vial with 3.8 ml diluent[3] vial.
		25 million IU per vial	In vials with 5 ml diluent[3] vial.
		50 million IU per vial[4]	In vials with 1 ml diluent[3] vial.

[2] Refer to table above for amount of diluent to use to achieve the desired final concentration.
[3] Bacteriostatic Water for Injection. Formulation includes human albumin.
[4] To be used *only* for treatment of AIDS-related Kaposi's sarcoma.

INTERFERON ALFA-n3

Actions:

Pharmacology: Interferon alfa-n3 (Human Leukocyte Derived) is a sterile aqueous formulation of purified, natural, human interferon alpha proteins for use by injection comprising approximately 166 amino acids. It is manufactured from pooled units of human leukocytes induced by incomplete infection with an avian virus (Sendai virus) to produce interferon alfa-n3.

Since interferon alfa-n3 is manufactured using human leukocytes, donors are screened to minimize the risk that the leukocytes could contain infectious agents including hepatitis B surface antigen (HBsAg) and antibodies to human immunodeficiency virus (HIV-1) and human T lymphotropic virus-I (HTLV-I). In addition, the manufacturing process contains steps which inactivate viruses, and there has been no evidence of infection transmission to recipients in clinical trials.

Clinical Pharmacology: Interferons are naturally occurring proteins with both antiviral and antiproliferative properties. They are produced and secreted in response to viral infections and to a variety of other synthetic and biological inducers. Three major families of interferons have been identified: alpha, beta, and gamma. The interferon alpha family contains at least 15 different molecular species.

Interferons bind to specific membrane receptors on cell surfaces. Interferon alfa-n3 binds to the same receptors as interferon alfa-2b with high species specificity.

Binding of interferon to membrane receptors initiates a series of events including induction of protein synthesis. These actions are followed by a variety of cellular responses, including inhibition of virus replication and suppression of cell proliferation. Immunomodulation, including enhancement of phagocytosis by macrophages, augmentation of the cytotoxicity of lymphocytes and enhancement of human leukocyte antigen expression occurs in response to exposure to interferons.

Pharmacokinetics: In a study of intralesional use of interferon alfa-n3 injection for the treatment of condylomata acuminata, plasma concentrations of interferon were below the detection limit of the assay (≤ 3 IU/ml). Minor systemic effects (eg, myalgias, fever, headaches) were noted, indicating that some of the injected interferon entered the systemic circulation (see Adverse Reactions).

Clinical trials: Condylomata acuminata (venereal or genital warts) are associated with infections of human papilloma virus (HPV), especially HPV type-6 and possibly type-11.

In a multicenter randomized double-blind, placebo controlled clinical trial, intralesional administration of interferon alfa-n3 was an effective treatment for condylomata acuminata. Patients (n = 81) had a mean of five warts (range: 2 to 14) and were injected intralesionally with a mean of 225,000 IU per wart 2 times a week for up to 8 weeks.

Overall, 80% of patients treated had a complete or partial resolution of warts compared with 44% (n = 75) of placebo-treated patients. Interferon alfa-n3 was significantly more effective than placebo in producing a complete resolution of warts, as shown by the following table:

Degree of Wart Resolution with Interferon Alfa-n3				
	Complete Resolution	Partial (≥ 50%) Resolution	Minor (< 50%) Resolution	Progression/ No Change
Interferon alfa-n3 (n = 81)	54%	26%	15%	5%
Placebo (n = 75)	20%	24%	13%	43%

Of the patients who had a complete resolution of warts, approximately 50% of patients had complete resolution by the end of treatment, and 50% had complete resolution during the 3 months after treatment cessation. Patients with complete resolution were followed for a median of 48 weeks. Overall, 76% of interferon alfa-n3-treated patients remained clear of all treated lesions during follow-up.

A total of 762 evaluable warts were injected in this trial. Of the 407 interferon alfa-n3-treated warts, 73% completely resolved, as compared to 35% of the placebo-treated warts. Interferon alfa-n3 was effective in treating lesions of all sizes, and there was no difference in resolution for perianal, penile or vulvar lesions. Among patients with recalcitrant warts, 82% of patients had complete or partial resolution of warts due to intralesional administration of interferon alfa-n3 compared to 43% of placebo patients.

In an open clinical trial using a once-a-week treatment schedule for up to 16 weeks, 28 patients were evaluable for efficacy; 89% had a complete or partial resolution of warts following treatment with interferon alfa-n3. The condylomata acuminata resolved completely in 46% of the patients. Of the 154 warts treated, 77% resolved completely.

(Actions continued on following page)

INTERFERON ALFA-n3 (Cont.)

Actions (Cont.):

Antigenicity: To date, no antibodies to interferon alfa-n3 have been detected in tested patients. No hypersensitivity reactions to the components of interferon alfa-n3 have been observed. Interferon alfa-n3 uses a murine monoclonal antibody in one of the purification procedures. A possibility exists that patients treated with interferon alfa-n3 may develop hypersensitivity to the mouse proteins. However, none of the patients developed antibodies or hypersensitivity to mouse proteins (see Contraindications).

Although no egg protein (ovalbumin) has been detected in the initial stage of interferon manufacture, a possibility exists that patients treated with interferon alfa-n3 may develop hypersensitivity to egg protein (see Contraindications).

The leukocyte nutrient medium contains the antibiotic neomycin sulfate at a concentration of 35 mg/L; however, neomycin sulfate is not detectable in the final product.

Indications:

Condylomata acuminata: For the intralesional treatment of refractory or recurring external condylomata acuminata in patients ≥ 18 years of age.

Select patients for treatment after consideration of a number of factors: Locations and sizes of the lesions, past treatment and response, and the patient's ability to comply with the treatment regimen. Interferon alfa-n3 is particularly useful for patients who have not responded satisfactorily to other treatment modalities (eg, podophyllin resin, surgery, laser or cryotherapy).

Unlabeled Uses: Alpha interferons have been used for a variety of conditions, a list of which follows. Clinical trials are currently in progress to further determine clinical efficacy, optimal dosage and length of treatment.

Interferon Alpha Unlabeled Uses		
Neoplastic Diseases		
Significant Activity	*Limited Activity*	*No Activity*
Bladder tumors (local use for superficial tumors)	Acute leukemias	Breast cancer
Carcinoid tumor	Cervical carcinoma	Colorectal carcinoma
Chronic myelogenous leukemia	Chronic lymphocytic leukemia	Gastric carcinoma
Cutaneous T-cell lymphoma	Hodgkin's disease	Lung carcinoma
Essential thrombocythemia	Malignant gliomas	Pancreatic carcinoma
Hairy cell leukemia†	Melanoma	Prostatic carcinoma
Non-Hodgkin's lymphoma (low-grade)	Multiple myeloma	Soft tissue carcinoma
	Nasopharyngeal sarcoma	
	Osteosarcoma	
	Ovarian carcinoma	
	Renal carcinoma	
Viral Infections		
AIDS-related Kaposi's sarcoma†		
Chronic non-A, non-B hepatitis		
Cutaneous warts		
Cytomegaloviruses		
Herpes keratoconjunctivitis		
Herpes simplex		
Papillomaviruses		
Rhinoviruses		
Vaccinia virus		
Varicella zoster		
Viral hepatitis B		

† Interferon alfa-2a and -2b indicated for this use.

Contraindications:

Hypersensitivity to human interferon alpha or any component of the product; patients who have anaphylactic sensitivity to mouse immunoglobulin (IgG), egg protein or neomycin (see Actions).

Warnings:

Debilitating medical conditions: Because of the fever and other "flu-like" symptoms associated with interferon alfa-n3, use cautiously in patients with debilitating medical conditions such as cardiovascular disease (eg, unstable angina and uncontrolled congestive heart failure), severe pulmonary disease (eg, chronic obstructive pulmonary disease), diabetes mellitus with ketoacidosis, coagulation disorders (eg, thrombophlebitis, pulmonary embolism and hemophilia), severe myelosuppression or seizure disorders.

(Warnings continued on following page)

INTERFERON ALFA-n3 (Cont.)

Warnings (Cont.):

Hypersensitivity: Acute, serious hypersensitivity reactions (eg, urticaria, angioedema, bronchoconstriction, anaphylaxis) have not been observed in patients receiving interferon alfa-n3. However, if such reactions develop, discontinue administration immediately and institute appropriate medical therapy. Refer to Management of Acute Hypersensitivity Reactions on page 2897

Impairment of fertility: In studies with adult females, interferon alpha affects the menstrual cycle and decreases serum estradiol and progesterone levels. Caution fertile women to use effective contraception while being treated with interferon alfa-n3. Use caution in fertile men.

Changes in the menstrual cycle and abortions have occurred in primates given extremely high doses of recombinant interferon alpha. When given at daily IM doses 326 times the average intralesional dose (120 times the maximum recommended dose), this recombinant interferon formulation produced menstrual cycle changes in monkeys. In human clinical trials of 51 women, there was no significant difference between interferon alfa-n3 and placebo treatment groups with regard to menstrual cycle changes.

Pregnancy: Category C. It is not known whether interferon alfa-n3 can cause fetal harm when administered to a pregnant woman or can affect reproductive capacity. Use in pregnant women only if clearly needed.

Changes in the menstrual cycle and abortions occurred in primates given extremely high doses of recombinant interferon alpha. Abortifacient effects were noted when the recombinant interferon alpha was given daily during early to mid-gestation at IM doses of 978 times the average intralesional dose of interferon alfa-n3 (360 times the maximum recommended dose).

Lactation: It is not known whether interferon alfa-n3 is excreted in breast milk. Studies in mice have shown that mouse interferons are excreted in milk. Because of the potential for serious adverse reactions in nursing infants, decide whether to discontinue nursing or to not initiate drug treatment, taking into account the importance of the drug to the mother and the potential risks to the infant.

Children: Safety and effectiveness have not been established in patients < 18 years of age.

Precautions:

Product interchange: Because the manufacturing process, strength, and type of interferon (eg, natural, human leukocyte interferon vs single-subspecies recombinant interferon) may vary for different interferon formulations, changing brands may require a change in dosage. Therefore, physicians are cautioned not to change from one interferon product to another without considering these factors.

Adverse Reactions:

In the double-blind efficacy trial for the treatment of condylomata acuminata, 104 patients were treated with doses of interferon alfa-n3 of 0.05 to 2.5 million IU per treatment session (average dose = 0.92 million IU/treatment session) by intralesional injection. In open trials, an additional 98 patients received a dose range of 0.05 to 4.6 million IU of interferon alfa-n3/treatment session (average dose = 1.12 million IU/treatment session). Patients with cancer were given doses of interferon alfa-n3 injection of 3, 9, or 15 million IU/day for 10 days by IM injection.

In a total of 104 patients with condylomata acuminata, adverse reactions consisted primarily of "flu-like" symptoms (myalgias, fever or headache) which were in most cases mild or moderate and transient, and did not interfere with treatment.

The "flu-like" adverse reactions, consisting of fever, myalgias, or headache, occurred primarily after the first treatment session and were reported by 30% of the patients. The frequency of "flu-like" adverse reactions abated with repeated dosing so that the incidences due to interferon alfa-n3 and placebo were similar after 3 to 4 weeks of treatment (after six to eight treatment sessions). "Flu-like" symptoms were relieved by acetaminophen.

(Adverse Reactions continued on following page)

INTERFERON ALFA-n3 (Cont.)

Adverse Reactions (Cont.):

Adverse Reactions of Interferon Alfa-n3			
	Condylomata acuminata		Cancer
Adverse Reactions	Interferon alfa-n3 (n = 104)	Placebo (n = 85)	Interferon alfa-n3 (n = 31)
Autonomic Nervous System			
Sweating	2%	1%	0.3%
Vasovagal reaction	2%	0%	
Body as a Whole			
Fever	40%	19%	81%
Chills	14%	2%	87%
Fatigue	14%	6%	6%
Malaise	9%	9%	65%
Central & Peripheral Nervous System			
Dizziness/Lightheadedness	9%	4%	0.3%
Insomnia	2%	1%	
Sleepiness			10%
GI System			
Nausea	4%	7%	48%
Vomiting	3%	0%	29%
Dyspepsia/Heartburn	3%	1%	0.3%
Diarrhea	2%	2%	6%
Constipation			0.3%
Anorexia			68%
Sore mouth/Stomatitis Dry mouth/Mucositis			0.3-6%
Musculoskeletal System			
Myalgias	45%	15%	16%
Headache	31%	15%	10%
Arthralgia	5%	1%	10%
Back pain	4%	1%	0.3%
Miscellaneous			
Depression	2%	1%	0.3%
Nose/Sinus drainage	2%	2%	
Generalized pruritis	2%	0%	
Sore injection site			10%
Blurred vision/Ocular rotation pain			0.3-6%
Chest pains			10%
Low blood pressure			6%

Most of the systemic adverse reactions were mild or moderate. Severe systemic adverse reactions were reported by 18% of interferon alfa-n3-treated patients and 13% of placebo-treated patients. Most of the severe systemic adverse reactions reported were "flu-like". Other severe systemic adverse reactions included back pain, insomnia and sensitivity to allergens.

Adverse reactions reported by 1% of patients treated with interferon alfa-n3 in the double-blind and open clinical trials included: Left groin lymph node swelling; tongue hyperesthesia; thirst; tingling of legs/feet; hot sensation on bottom of feet; strange taste in mouth; increased salivation; heat intolerance; visual disturbances; pharyngitis; sensitivity to allergens; muscle cramps; nose bleed; throat tightness and papular rash on neck; herpes labialis; hot flashes; nervousness; decrease in concentration; dysuria; photosensitivity; swollen lymph nodes.

Laboratory test abnormality: Decreased WBC (11%).

(Adverse Reactions continued on following page)

INTERFERON ALFA-n3 (Cont.)

Adverse Reactions (Cont.)

Adverse reactions in patients with cancer: Thirty-one patients with cancer were treated with a maximum of 10 IM injections of interferon alfa-n3 in doses of 3, 9, or 15 million IU/treatment session. The occurrence of adverse reactions was judged to be unrelated to the dose of interferon alfa-n3. See table for major adverse reactions. Those adverse reactions which were each reported by only one patient treated with interferon alfa-n3 included: Face flushed; edema; coughing; numbness; numbness in hands or fingers; ringing in ears; cramps; confusion.

Abnormal Laboratory Test Values with Interferon Alfa-n3

Laboratory Test	Cancer Patients (n = 31)
Hemoglobin Level	2 (7%)
WBC Count	1 (3%)
Platelet Count	1 (3%)
GGT	1 (6%)
AST	1 (3%)
Alkaline Phosphatase	2 (8%)
Total Bilirubin	1 (4%)

Patient Information:

Inform patients of the early signs of hypersensitivity reactions including hives, generalized urticaria, tightness of the chest, wheezing, hypotension and anaphylaxis, and advise them to contact their physician if these symptoms occur.

Inform patients of benefits and risks associated with treatment.

Caution patients not to change brands of interferon without medical consultation, as a change in dosage may occur.

Administration and Dosage:

Condylomata acuminata: 0.05 ml (250,000 IU) per wart. Administer twice weekly for up to 8 weeks. The maximum recommended dose/treatment session is 0.5 ml (2.5 million IU). Inject into the base of each wart, preferably using a 30 gauge needle. For large warts, interferon alfa-n3 may be injected at several points around the periphery of the wart, using a total dose of 0.05 ml per wart.

The minimum effective dose for the treatment of condylomata acuminata has not been established. Moderate to severe adverse experiences may require modification of the dosage regimen or, in some cases, termination of therapy.

Genital warts usually begin to disappear after several weeks of treatment. Continue treatment for a maximum of 8 weeks. In clinical trials, many patients who had partial resolution of warts during treatment experienced further resolution of their warts after treatment cessation. Of the patients who had complete resolution of warts due to treatment, half the patients had complete resolution by the end of the treatment and half had complete resolution during the 3 months after cessation of treatment. Thus, it is recommended that no further therapy (interferon alfa-n3 or conventional therapy) be administered for 3 months after the initial 8 week course of treatment unless the warts enlarge or new warts appear. Studies to determine the safety and efficacy of a second course of treatment with interferon alfa-n3 have not been conducted.

Storage: Store at 2° to 8°C (36° to 46°F). Do not freeze. Do not shake.

Rx	**Alferon N** (Purdue Frederick)	**Injection:** 5 mIU/vial	In 1 ml vials.[1]

[1] With 3.3 mg phenol and 1 mg albumin.

LEVAMISOLE HCl

Actions:

Pharmacology: Levamisole is an immunomodulator. The mechanism of action of levamisole in combination with fluorouracil is unknown. The effects of levamisole on the immune system are complex. The drug appears to restore depressed immune function rather than to stimulate response to above normal levels. Levamisole can stimulate formation of antibodies to various antigens, enhance T-cell responses by stimulating T-cell activation and proliferation, potentiate monocyte and macrophage functions including phagocytosis and chemotaxis, and increase neutrophil mobility adherence and chemotaxis. Other drugs have similar short-term effects, and the clinical relevance is unclear.

Besides its immunomodulatory function, levamisole also inhibits alkaline phosphatase and has cholinergic activity.

Pharmacokinetics: The pharmacokinetics of levamisole have not been studied in the dosage regimen recommended with fluorouracil nor in patients with hepatic insufficiency. It appears that levamisole is rapidly absorbed from the GI tract. Mean peak plasma concentrations of 0.13 mcg/ml are attained within 1.5 to 2 hours. The plasma elimination half-life is between 3 to 4 hours. Levamisole 150 mg is extensively metabolized by the liver, and the metabolites are excreted mainly by the kidneys (70% over 3 days). The elimination half-life of metabolite excretion is 16 hours. Approximately 5% is excreted in the feces; $< 5\%$ is excreted unchanged in the urine and $< 0.2\%$ in the feces. Approximately 12% is recovered in urine as the glucuronide of p-hydroxy-levamisole.

Clinical trials: Two clinical trials having essentially the same design have demonstrated an increase in survival and a reduction in recurrence rate in patients with resected Dukes' C colon cancer treated with levamisole plus fluorouracil. After surgery patients were randomized to no further therapy, levamisole alone, or levamisole plus fluorouracil.

In one clinical trial, 262 Dukes' C colorectal cancer patients were evaluated for a minimum follow-up of 5 years. The estimated reduction in death rate was 27% for levamisole plus fluorouracil and 28% for levamisole alone. The estimated reduction in recurrence rate was 36% for levamisole plus fluorouracil and 28% for levamisole alone. In another clinical trial designed to confirm these results, 929 Dukes' C colon cancer patients were evaluated for a minimum follow-up of 2 years. The estimated reduction in death rate and recurrence rate was 33% and 41%, respectively for levamisole plus fluorouracil. The group on levamisole alone did not show advantage over the group receiving no treatment on improving recurrence or survival rates. There are presently insufficient data to evaluate the effect of the combination of levamisole plus fluorouracil in Dukes' B patients. There are also insufficient data to evaluate the effect of levamisole plus fluorouracil in patients with rectal cancer.

Indications:

Only as adjuvant treatment in combination with fluorouracil after surgical resection in patients with Dukes' stage C colon cancer.

Contraindications:

Hypersensitivity to the drug or its components.

Warnings:

Agranulocytosis: Levamisole has been associated with agranulocytosis, sometimes fatal. The onset of agranulocytosis is frequently accompanied by a flu-like syndrome (eg, fever, chills); however, in a small number of patients, it is asymptomatic. A flu-like syndrome may also occur in the absence of agranulocytosis. It is essential that appropriate hematological monitoring be done routinely during therapy with levamisole and fluorouracil. Neutropenia is usually reversible following discontinuation of therapy. Instruct patients to report immediately any flu-like symptoms.

Higher than recommended doses of levamisole may be associated with an increased incidence of agranulocytosis, so do not exceed the recommended dose.

The combination of levamisole and fluorouracil has been associated with frequent neutropenia, anemia and thrombocytopenia.

Fertility impairment: In rats given 20, 60 and 180 mg/kg, copulation period was increased, duration of pregnancy was slightly increased, and fertility, pup viability and weight, lactation index and number of fetuses were decreased at 60 mg/kg.

Pregnancy: Category C. In rats, embryotoxicity was present at 160 mg/kg; in rabbits, at 180 mg/kg. There are no adequate and well controlled studies in pregnant women. Do not be administer levamsiole unless the potential benefits outweigh the risks. Advise women taking the combination of levamisole and fluorouracil not to become pregnant.

(Warnings continued on following page)

LEVAMISOLE HCl (Cont.)

Warnings (Cont.):

Lactation: It is not known whether levamisole is excreted in breast milk; it is excreted in cows' milk. Because of the potential for serious adverse reactions in nursing infants from levamisole, decide whether to discontinue nursing or discontinue the drug, taking into account the importance of the drug to the mother.

Children: Safety and efficacy of levamisole in children have not been established.

Precautions:

Monitoring: On the first day of therapy with levamisole and fluorouracil, patients should have a CBC with differential and platelets, electrolytes and liver function tests performed. Thereafter, perform a CBC with differential and platelets weekly prior to each treatment with fluorouracil; perform electrolyte and liver function tests every 3 months for a total of 1 year. Institute dosage modifications (see Administration and Dosage).

Drug Interactions:

Alcohol: Levamisole may produce disulfiram-like effects with alcohol coadministration.

Phenytoin: Coadministration with levamisole and fluorouracil has led to increased phenytoin plasma levels. Monitor phenytoin plasma levels and decrease the dose if necessary.

Adverse Reactions:

Levamisole and Levamisole/Fluorouracil Adverse Reactions (%)		
Adverse Reaction	Levamisole (n = 440)	Levamisole plus fluorouracil (n = 599)
Hematological		
Leukopenia		
< 2,000/mm^3	< 1	1
≥ 2,000 to < 4,000/mm^3	4	19
≥ 4,000/mm^3	2	33
unscored category	0	< 1
Thrombocytopenia		
< 50,000/mm^3	0	0
≥ 50,000 to < 130,000/mm^3	1	8
≥ 130,000/mm^3	1	10
Anemia	0	6
Granulocytopenia	< 1	2
Epistaxis	0	1
Skin and appendages		
Dermatitis	8	23
Alopecia	3	22
Pruritus	1	2
Skin discoloration	0	2
Urticaria	< 1	0
Body as a whole		
Fatigue	6	11
Fever	3	5
Rigors	3	5
Chest pain	< 1	1
Edema	1	1
GI		
Nausea	22	65
Diarrhea	13	52
Stomatitis	3	39
Vomiting	6	20
GI (Cont.)		
Anorexia	2	6
Abdominal pain	2	5
Constipation	2	3
Flatulence	< 1	2
Dyspepsia	< 1	1
Special senses		
Taste perversion	8	8
Altered sense of smell	1	1
Musculoskeletal system		
Arthralgia	5	4
Myalgia	3	2
Central and peripheral nervous system		
Dizziness	3	4
Headache	3	4
Paresthesia	2	3
Ataxia	0	2
Psychiatric		
Somnolence	3	2
Depression	1	2
Nervousness	1	2
Insomnia	1	1
Anxiety	1	1
Forgetfulness	0	1
Vision		
Abnormal tearing	0	4
Blurred vision	1	2
Conjunctivitis	< 1	2
Other		
Infection	5	12
Hyperbilirubinemia	< 1	1

Less frequent adverse experiences included: Exfoliative dermatitis; periorbital edema; vaginal bleeding; anaphylaxis; confusion; convulsions; hallucinations; impaired concentration; renal failure; elevated serum creatinine; increased alkaline phosphatase. An encephalopathy-like syndrome has occurred.

(Adverse Reactions continued on following page)

LEVAMISOLE HCl (Cont.)

Adverse Reactions (Cont.):

Almost all patients receiving levamisole and fluorouracil reported adverse experiences. In a clinical trial, 66 of 463 patients (14%) discontinued the combination of levamisole plus fluorouracil because of adverse reactions; 43 (9%) developed isolated or a combination of GI toxicities (eg, nausea, vomiting, diarrhea, stomatitis, anorexia). Ten patients developed rash or pruritus. Five patients discontinued therapy because of flu-like symptoms or fever with chills; 10 patients developed CNS symptoms such as dizziness, ataxia, depression, confusion, memory loss, weakness, inability to concentrate and headache. Two patients developed reversible neutropenia and sepsis: One because of thrombocytopenia, one because of hyperbilirubinemia. One patient in the levamisole plus fluorouracil group developed agranulocytosis and sepsis, and died.

In the levamisole alone arm of the trial, 15 of 310 patients (4.8%) discontinued therapy because of adverse experiences. Six of these (2%) discontinued because of rash, six because of arthralgia/myalgia, and one each for fever and neutropenia, urinary infection and cough.

Overdosage:

Fatalities have occurred in a 3-year-old child who ingested 15 mg/kg and in an adult who ingested 32 mg/kg. No further clinical information is available. In cases of overdosage, gastric lavage is recommended together with symptomatic and supportive measures. Refer to General Management of Acute Overdosage.

Patient Information:

Immediately notify the physician if flu-like symptoms or malaise occurs.

Administration and Dosage:

Adjuvant use of levamisole and fluorouracil is limited to the following schedule:

Initial therapy:

Levamisole – 50 mg orally every 8 hours for 3 days (starting 7 to 30 days post-surgery).

Fluorouracil – 450 mg/m²/day IV for 5 days concomitant with a 3 day course of levamisole (starting 21 to 34 days post-surgery).

Maintenance:

Levamisole – 50 mg orally every 8 hours for 3 days every 2 weeks.

Fluorouracil – 450 mg/m²/day IV once a week beginning 28 days after the initiation of the 5 day course.

Treatment: Initiate levamisole no earlier than 7 and no later than 30 days post-surgery at a dose of 50 mg every 8 hours for 3 days repeated every 14 days for 1 year. Initiate fluorouracil therapy no earlier than 21 days and no later than 35 days after surgery providing the patient is out of the hospital, ambulatory, maintaining normal oral nutrition, has well healed wounds and is fully recovered from any postoperative complications. If levamisole has been initiated from 7 to 20 days after surgery, initiate fluorouracil therapy coincident with the second course of levamisole, ie, at 21 to 34 days. If levamisole is initiated from 21 to 30 days after surgery, initiate fluorouracil simultaneously with the first course of levamisole.

Administer fluorouracil by rapid IV push at a dosage of 450 mg/m²/day for 5 consecutive days. Dosage is based on actual weight (estimated dry weight). If the patient develops any stomatitis or diarrhea (≥ 5 loose stools), discontinue this course before the full 5 doses are administered. Twenty-eight days after initiation of this course, institute weekly fluorouracil at 450 mg/m²/week and continue for a total treatment time of 1 year. If stomatitis or diarrhea develop during weekly therapy, defer the next dose of fluorouracil until these side effects have subsided. If these side effects are moderate to severe, reduce the fluorouracil dose 20% when it is resumed.

Institute dosage medications as follows: If WBC is 2500 to 3500/mm³ defer the fluorouracil dose until WBC is > 3500/mm³. If WBC is < 2500/mm³, defer the fluorouracil dose until WBC is > 3500/mm³, then resume the fluorouracil dose reduced by 20%. If WBC remains < 2500/mm³ for > 10 days despite deferring fluorouracil, discontinue administration of levamisole. Defer both drugs unless platelets are adequate (≥ 100,000/mm³).

Levamisole should not be used at doses exceeding the recommended dose or frequency. Clinical studies suggest a relationship between levamisole adverse experiences and increasing dose, and some of these (eg, agranulocytosis) may be life-threatening (see Warnings).

Before beginning this combination adjuvant treatment, the physician should become familiar with the labeling for fluorouracil.

Rx	**Ergamisol** (Janssen)	**Tablets:** 50 mg levamisole base	(Janssen L 50). White. In blister pack 36s.

ALTRETAMINE (Hexamethylmelamine)

Warning:

Administer only under the supervision of a physician experienced in the use of antineoplastic agents.

Monitor peripheral blood counts at least monthly, prior to the initiation of each course of altretamine therapy and as clinically indicated (see Adverse Reactions).

Because of the possibility of altretamine-related neurotoxicity, perform neurologic examination regularly during administration (see Adverse Reactions).

Actions:

Pharmacology: Altretamine, formerly known as hexamethylmelamine, is a synthetic cytotoxic antineoplastic s-triazine derivative. The precise mechanism by which altretamine exerts its cytotoxic effect is unknown, although a number of theoretical possibilities have been studied. Structurally, altretamine resembles the alkylating agent triethylenemelamine, yet in vitro tests for alkylating activity of altretamine and its metabolites have been negative. Altretamine is efficacious for certain ovarian tumors resistant to classical alkylating agents. Metabolism of altretamine is a requirement for cytotoxicity. Synthetic monohydroxymethylmelamines and products of altretamine metabolism in vitro and in vivo can form covalent adducts with tissue macromolecules including DNA, but the relevance of these reactions to antitumor activity is unknown.

Pharmacokinetics: Altretamine is well absorbed following oral administration, but undergoes rapid and extensive demethylation in the liver, producing variations in altretamine plasma levels. The principal metabolites are pentamethylmelamine and tetramethylmelamine. After oral administration to 11 patients with advanced ovarian cancer in doses of 120 to 300 mg/m², peak plasma levels were reached between 0.5 and 3 hours, varying from 0.2 to 20.8 mg/L. Half-life of the β-phase of elimination ranged from 4.7 to 10.2 hours. Altretamine and metabolites show binding to plasma proteins. The free fractions of altretamine, pentamethylmelamine and tetramethylmelamine are 6%, 25% and 50%, respectively.

Following oral administration of 4 mg/kg, urinary recovery was 61% at 24 hours and 90% at 72 hours. Human urinary metabolites were N-demethylated homologues of altretamine with $<$ 1% unmetabolized altretamine excreted at 24 hours. After intraperitoneal administration to mice, tissue distribution was rapid in all organs, reaching a maximum at 30 minutes. The excretory organs (liver and kidney) and the small intestine showed high concentrations, whereas relatively low concentrations were found in other organs, including the brain.

Clinical trials: In two studies in patients with persistent or recurrent ovarian cancer following first-line treatment with cisplatin or alkylating agent-based combinations, altretamine was administered as a single agent for 14 or 21 days of a 28 day cycle. In the 51 patients with measurable or evaluable disease, there were 6 clinical complete responses, 1 pathologic complete response, and 2 partial responses for an overall response rate of 18%. The duration of these responses ranged from 2 months in a patient with a palpable pelvic mass to 36 months in a patient who achieved a pathologic complete response. In some patients, tumor regression was associated with improvement in symptoms and performance status.

Indications:

For use as a single agent in the palliative treatment of patients with persistent or recurrent ovarian cancer following first-line therapy with a cisplatin- or alkylating agent-based combination.

Contraindications:

Hypersensitivity to altretamine.

Pre-existing severe bone marrow depression or severe neurologic toxicity; however, altretamine has been administered safely to patients heavily pretreated with cisplatin or alkylating agents including patients with pre-existing cisplatin neuropathies. Careful monitoring of neurologic function in these patients is essential.

Warnings:

Neurotoxicity: Altretamine causes mild to moderate neurotoxicity. Peripheral neuropathy and CNS symptoms (eg, mood disorders, disorders of consciousness, ataxia, dizziness, vertigo) have occurred. They are more likely to occur in patients receiving continuous high-dose daily altretamine than moderate-dose altretamine administered on an intermittent schedule. Neurologic toxicity appears to be reversible when therapy is discontinued. It has been suggested that the incidence and severity of neurotoxicity may be decreased by concomitant administration of pyridoxine, but this remains unproven. Perform a neurologic examination prior to the initiation of each course of therapy.

(Warnings continued on following page)

ALTRETAMINE (Hexamethylmelamine) (Cont.)

Warnings (Cont.):

Hematologic: Altretamine causes mild to moderate dose-related myelosuppression. Leukopenia $<$ 3000 WBC/mm^3 occurred in $<$ 15% of patients on a variety of intermittent or continuous dose regimens; $<$ 1% had leukopenia $<$ 1000 WBC/mm^3. Thrombocytopenia $<$ 50,000 platelets/mm^3 was seen in $<$ 10% of patients. When given in doses of 8 to 12 mg/kg/day over a 21 day course, nadirs of leukocyte and platelet counts were reached by 3 to 4 weeks, and normal counts were regained by 6 weeks. With continuous administration at doses of 6 to 8 mg/kg/day, nadirs are reached in 6 to 8 weeks (median). Monitor peripheral blood counts prior to the initiation of each course of therapy, monthly, and as clinically indicated. Adjust the dose as necessary (see Administration and Dosage).

Carcinogenesis, mutagenesis and impairment of fertility: Drugs with similar mechanisms of action are carcinogenic. Altretamine was weakly mutagenic when tested in strain TA100 of *Salmonella typhimurium*. Altretamine administered to female rats 14 days prior to breeding through the gestation period had no adverse effect on fertility but decreased postnatal survival at 120 mg/m^2/day and was embryocidal at 240 mg/m^2/day. Administration of 120 mg/m^2/day to male rats for 60 days prior to mating resulted in testicular atrophy, reduced fertility and a possible dominant lethal mutagenic effect. Male rats treated with 450 mg/m^2/day for 10 days had decreased spermatogenesis and atrophy of testes, seminal vesicles and ventral prostate.

Pregnancy: Category D. Altretamine is embryotoxic and teratogenic in rats and rabbits when given at doses 2 and 10 times the human dose, and it may cause fetal damage when administered to a pregnant woman. If altretamine is used during pregnancy, or if the patient becomes pregnant while taking the drug, apprise the patient of the potential hazard to the fetus. Advise women to avoid becoming pregnant.

Lactation: It is not known whether altretamine is excreted in breast milk. Because there is a possibility of toxicity in nursing infants secondary to altretamine treatment of the mother, it is recommended that breastfeeding be discontinued if the mother is treated with altretamine.

Children: Safety and efficacy in children have not been established.

Precautions:

Nausea and vomiting: With continuous high-dose daily altretamine, nausea and vomiting of gradual onset occur frequently. In most instances, these symptoms are controllable with antiemetics; at times, however, the severity requires dose reduction or, rarely, discontinuation of therapy. In some instances, a tolerance of these symptoms develops after several weeks of therapy. The incidence and severity of nausea and vomiting are reduced with moderate-dose administration of altretamine. In two clinical studies of single-agent altretamine utilizing a moderate, intermittent dose and schedule, only 1 patient (1%) discontinued altretamine due to severe nausea and vomiting.

Drug Interactions:

Cimetidine, an inhibitor of microsomal drug metabolism, increased altretamine's half-life and toxicity in a rat model.

Monoamine oxidase inhibitors and concurrent altretamine may cause severe orthostatic hypotension. Four patients, all $>$ 60 years of age, experienced symptomatic hypotension after 4 to 7 days of concomitant therapy.

(Continued on following page)

ALTRETAMINE (Hexamethylmelamine) (Cont.)

Adverse Reactions:

The most common adverse reactions are: Nausea and vomiting (see Precautions); peripheral neuropathy, CNS symptoms and myelosuppression (see Warnings).

Data in the following table are based on the experience of 76 patients with ovarian cancer previously treated with a cisplatin-based combination regimen who received single-agent altretamine. In one study, altretamine 260 mg/m²/day was administered for 14 days of a 28 day cycle. In another study, altretamine 6 to 8 mg/kg/day was administered for 21 days of a 28 day cycle.

Altretamine Adverse Reactions in Previously Treated Ovarian Cancer Patients (n = 76)	
Adverse reaction	Incidence (%)
GI	
Nausea and vomiting	
Mild to moderate	32
Severe	1
Increased alkaline phosphatase	9
Neurologic	
Peripheral sensory neuropathy	
Mild	22
Moderate to severe	9
Anorexia and fatigue	1
Seizures	1
Hematologic	
Leukopenia	
WBC 2000 to 2999/mm³	4
WBC < 2000/mm³	1
Thrombocytopenia	
Platelets 75,000 to 99,000/mm³	6
Platelets < 75,000/mm³	3
Anemia	
Mild	20
Moderate to severe	13
Renal	
Serum creatinine 1.6 to 3.75 mg/dl	7
BUN	
25-40 mg/dl	5
41-60 mg/dl	3
> 60 mg/dl	1

Additional adverse reaction information is available from 13 single-agent altretamine studies (total of 1014 patients). The treated patients had a variety of tumors and many were heavily pretreated with other chemotherapies; most of these trials utilized high, continuous daily doses of altretamine (6 to 12 mg/kg/day). In general, adverse reaction experiences were similar in the two trials described above. Additional toxicities not reported in the above table included hepatic toxicity, skin rash, pruritus and alopecia, each occurring in < 1% of patients.

Administration and Dosage:

Altretamine is administered orally. Calculate doses on the basis of body surface area.

Altretamine may be administered either for 14 or 21 consecutive days in a 28 day cycle at a dose of 260 mg/m²/day. Give the total daily dose as 4 divided oral doses after meals and at bedtime.

Temporarily discontinue altretamine (for ≥ 14 days) and subsequently restart at 200 mg/m²/day for any of the following situations: GI intolerance unresponsive to symptomatic measures; WBC < 2000/mm³ or granulocyte count < 1000/mm³; platelet count < 75,000/mm³; progressive neurotoxicity.

If neurologic symptoms fail to stabilize on the reduced dose schedule, discontinue altretamine indefinitely.

Rx	**Hexalen** (US Bioscience)	**Capsules:** 50 mg	Lactose. (USB001 Hexalen 50 mg). Clear. In 100s.

HYDROXYUREA

Actions:

Pharmacology: The precise mechanism of cytotoxic action is unknown. Hydroxyurea causes an immediate inhibition of deoxyribonucleic acid (DNA) synthesis without interfering with the synthesis of ribonucleic acid (RNA) or protein. It may also inhibit the incorporation of thymidine into DNA.

Three mechanisms have been postulated for the effectiveness of hydroxyurea with irradiation on squamous cell (epidermoid) carcinomas of the head and neck. In vitro, hydroxyurea is lethal to normally radioresistant S-stage cells, and holds other cells in the G-1 or pre-DNA synthesis stage where they are most susceptible to the irradiation effects. Also, hydroxyurea, by inhibiting DNA synthesis, hinders the normal repair process of cells damaged but not killed by irradiation, decreasing their survival rate; RNA and protein synthesis have shown no alteration.

Pharmacokinetics: Absorption/Distribution - Hydroxyurea is readily absorbed from the GI tract, reaching peak serum concentrations within 2 hours; by 24 hours the serum concentration is essentially zero. Hydroxyurea readily crosses the blood-brain barrier with peak CSF levels at 3 hours.

Metabolism/Excretion - About 50% of an oral dose is degraded in the liver and excreted into the urine as urea and as respiratory carbon dioxide; the remainder is excreted intact in the urine. Approximately 80% may be recovered in the urine within 12 hours.

Indications:

Melanoma; resistant chronic myelocytic leukemia; recurrent, metastatic or inoperable carcinoma of the ovary.

Concomitant administration with irradiation therapy in the local control of primary squamous cell (epidermoid) carcinomas of the head and neck, excluding the lip.

Contraindications:

Marked bone marrow depression, ie, leukopenia ($<$ 2500/cu mm WBC) or thrombocytopenia ($<$ 100,000/cu mm platelets), or severe anemia.

Warnings:

Patients who have received prior irradiation therapy may have an exacerbation of post-irradiation erythema.

Bone marrow suppression may occur, and leukopenia is generally the first and most common manifestation. Thrombocytopenia and anemia occur less often, seldom without a preceding leukopenia. Recovery from myelosuppression is rapid when therapy is interrupted. Bone marrow depression is more likely in patients who have previously received radiotherapy or cytotoxic antineoplastics. Correct severe anemia with whole blood replacement before initiating hydroxyurea therapy.

Erythrocytic abnormalities: Self-limiting megaloblastic erythropoiesis is often seen early in hydroxyurea therapy. The morphologic changes resemble pernicious anemia but are not related to vitamin B-12 or folic acid deficiency. Hydroxyurea may delay plasma iron clearance and reduce the rate of iron utilization by erythrocytes, but it does not alter the RBC survival time.

Use in impaired renal function: Hydroxyurea is excreted by the kidneys; therefore, use with caution in patients with marked renal dysfunction.

Elderly patients may be more sensitive to the effects of hydroxyurea and may require a lower dosage regimen.

Usage in Pregnancy: Drugs which affect DNA synthesis may be mutagenic. Hydroxyurea is a known teratogen in animals. Do not use in women who are or who may become pregnant, unless the potential benefits outweigh the possible hazards.

Usage in Children: Dosage regimens for children have not been established.

Precautions:

Therapy requires close supervision. Determine the complete status of the blood, including bone marrow examination if indicated, as well as renal and liver function prior to and during treatment.

Hematology: Monitor hemoglobin, total leukocyte counts and platelet counts at least once a week throughout therapy. If WBC decreases to less than 2500/cu mm or the platelet count to less than 100,000/cu mm, interrupt therapy until values rise significantly toward normal. Treat anemia with whole blood replacement; do not interrupt therapy.

Drug Interactions:

Drug/Lab Tests: **Serum uric acid, BUN** and **creatinine** levels may be increased by hydroxyurea.

(Continued on following page)

HYDROXYUREA (Cont.)

Adverse Reactions:

Most frequent: Primarily bone marrow depression (leukopenia, anemia and occasionally thrombocytopenia).

Less frequent:

GI – Stomatitis, anorexia, nausea, vomiting, diarrhea, and constipation.

Dermatologic – Maculopapular rash and facial erythema. Alopecia occurs very rarely.

Neurological: Headache, dizziness, disorientation, hallucinations and convulsions are extremely rare. Large doses may produce moderate drowsiness.

Renal impairment: May temporarily impair renal tubular function accompanied by elevated serum uric acid, BUN and creatinine levels.

Other: Fever, chills, malaise and elevation of hepatic enzymes have been reported. Abnormal BSP retention has been reported. Dysuria occurs rarely.

Combination therapy: Adverse reactions observed with combined hydroxyurea and irradiation therapy are similar to those reported using either one alone, primarily bone marrow depression (anemia and leukopenia) and gastric irritation. Combined therapy may cause an increase in the incidence and severity of these side effects. Almost all patients receiving an adequate course of combined therapy will demonstrate concurrent leukopenia. Platelet depression ($<$ 100,000 cells/cu mm) has occurred rarely and only in the presence of marked leukopenia.

Mucositis at the site is attributed to irradiation, although more severe cases may be due to combination therapy. Control pain or discomfort with topical anesthetics and oral analgesics. If the reaction is severe, temporarily interrupt hydroxyurea therapy; if it is extremely severe, irradiation dosage may be temporarily postponed. This is rarely necessary.

Control severe gastric distress by temporary interruption of hydroxyurea administration; interruption of irradiation is rarely necessary.

Patient Information:

Notify physician if fever, chills, sore throat, nausea, vomiting, loss of appetite, diarrhea, sores in the mouth and on the lips, unusual bleeding or bruising occur.

Medication may cause drowsiness, constipation, redness of the face, skin rash, itching, and loss of hair; notify physician if these become pronounced.

Extra fluid intake is recommended.

Contraceptive measures are recommended during therapy.

Administration and Dosage:

Base dosage on the patient's actual or ideal weight, whichever is less. If the patient prefers, or is unable to swallow capsules, empty the contents of the capsules into a glass of water and take immediately. Some inert material may not dissolve.

An adequate trial period to determine effectiveness is 6 weeks. When there is regression in tumor size or arrest in tumor growth, continue therapy indefinitely. Interrupt therapy if the WBC drops below 2500/cu mm or the platelet count below 100,000/cu mm. In these cases, recheck counts after 3 days, and resume therapy when the counts rise significantly toward normal. Since the hematopoietic rebound is prompt, it is usually necessary to omit only a few doses. If prompt rebound has not occurred during combined hydroxyurea and irradiation therapy, irradiation may also be interrupted. However, this is rare. Correct anemia with whole blood replacement; do not interrupt hydroxyurea therapy.

Because hematopoiesis may be compromised, administer cautiously to patients who have recently received extensive radiation therapy or cytotoxic chemotherapy.

Solid tumors: Patients on intermittent therapy rarely require complete discontinuation of therapy because of toxicity.

Intermittent therapy – 80 mg/kg as a single dose every third day.

Continuous therapy – 20 to 30 mg/kg as a single daily dose.

Concomitant therapy with irradiation (carcinoma of the head and neck): 80 mg/kg as a single dose every third day. Begin hydroxyurea at least 7 days before initiation of irradiation and continue during radiotherapy and indefinitely afterwards, provided the patient is adequately observed and exhibits no unusual or severe reactions. Administer irradiation at the maximum dose appropriate for the therapeutic situation; adjustment of irradiation dosage is not usually necessary with concomitant hydroxyurea.

Resistant chronic myelocytic leukemia: Continuous therapy (20 to 30 mg/kg as a single daily dose) is recommended.

Usage in Children: Dosage regimens have not been established.

Storage: Avoid excessive heat.

Rx	**Hydrea** (Squibb)	**Capsules:** 500 mg. (#Squibb 830). In 100s.

Product identification code.

BCG, INTRAVESICAL

Actions:

BCG is a freeze-dried suspension of an attenuated strain of *Mycobacterium bovis* (Bacillus Calmette and Guérin) used in the non-specific active therapy of carcinoma in situ of the urinary bladder. BCG live *(TheraCys)* is used only for carcinoma in situ of the urinary bladder; BCG Vaccine *(TICE BCG)* is also used for immunization against tuberculosis (see individual monograph in Biologicals section).

Pharmacology: BCG promotes a local inflammatory reaction with histiocytic and leukocytic infiltration in the urinary bladder. The local inflammatory effects are associated with an apparent elimination or reduction of superficial cancerous lesions of the urinary bladder. The exact mechanism is unknown.

Clinical trials: TheraCys – In a randomized, actively controlled multicenter study, *TheraCys* was compared to doxorubicin HCl in the treatment of carcinoma in situ of the urinary bladder. The response of 114 patients is given in the following table. Among the 54 patients receiving *TheraCys*, 74% had a complete response. The estimated median time to treatment failure (recurrence, progression or death) was 48.2 months.

Response of Patients with Carcinoma In Situ to Treatment with *TheraCys* (n = 54) or Doxorubicin (n = 60)

Response	*TheraCys*	Doxorubicin
Complete response[1]	74%	42%
No response[2]	11%	10%
Progressive disease[3]	13%	42%
No evaluation	2%	7%
Number of failures	27	46
Median time to treatment failure (TTF)	48.2 months	5.9 months

[1] Confirmed by cytology and cystoscopic examination.
[2] Less than a CR or stable disease. [3] Increase of stage or grade.

The effect of chemotherapy (other than *TheraCys* or doxorubicin) prior to entry into the controlled study was analyzed.

Prior vs No Prior Treatment for Carcinoma In Situ of the Urinary Bladder

Prior treatment	Study arm	Response rate	Median TTF (# events/n)
Yes	BCG live	81%	Not reached (11/26)
Yes	Doxorubicin	53%	7 months (22/30)
No	BCG live	68%	32.8 months (16/28)
No	Doxorubicin	30%	3.7 months (24/30)

No survival advantage for *TheraCys* therapy over that for doxorubicin was demonstrated after a 40 to 72 month follow-up. The median time to death for each group was 23 and 21 months for *TheraCys* and doxorubicin, respectively.

The clinical trials carried out with *TheraCys* included percutaneous administration of 0.5 ml, which was reconstituted in the diluent provided and further diluted in 50 ml sterile preservative-free saline with each intravesical dose. Some studies have suggested that this may not be necessary. If severe reactions (eg, ulceration) occurred, the percutaneous treatment was discontinued.

TICE BCG – In 119 evaluable patients, 54 (45.4%) had a complete histological response and 36 (30.2%) had a complete clinical response without cytology. Of the 54 patients classified as complete histological response, 30 remained without evidence of disease after a median follow-up of 47 months. Of the 90 (75.6%) overall responders, 36.7% relapsed; 13.3% died of other diseases, and 50% remained in complete response. In addition, two patients who relapsed were reinduced in complete response by a second course of *TICE BCG*. Among the 119 evaluable patients there was no significant difference in response rates between patients with or without prior intravesical chemotherapy. The median duration of response is estimated at $\geq$ 4 years.

Indications:

Intravesical use in the treatment of primary and relapsed carcinoma in situ of the urinary bladder to eliminate residual tumor cells and to reduce the frequency of tumor recurrence (*TheraCys*); primary or secondary treatment in absence of invasive cancer for patients with medical contraindications to radical surgery *(TICE BCG)*.

Treatment of carcinoma in situ with or without associated papillary tumors. Not indicated for the treatment of papillary tumors occurring alone.

Therapy for patients with carcinoma in situ of the bladder following failure to respond to other treatment regimens.

BCG vaccines for tuberculosis prevention are discussed in the Biologicals section.

(Continued on following page)

BCG, INTRAVESICAL (Cont.)

Contraindications:

Patients on immunosuppressive or corticosteroid therapy, with compromised immune systems, or asymptomatic carriers with a positive HIV serology due to the risk of overwhelming systemic mycobacterial sepsis.

Fever, unless the cause of the fever is determined and evaluated. If the fever is due to an infection, withhold therapy until the patient is afebrile and off all therapy.

Urinary tract infection because administration may result in the risk of disseminated BCG infection or in an increased severity of bladder irritation.

Not a vaccine for the prevention of cancer.

TheraCys: As an immunizing agent for the prevention of tuberculosis.

TICE BCG: Positive Mantoux test, only if there is evidence of an active TB infection.

Warnings:

Tuberculosis prevention: TheraCys should not be administered as an immunizing agent for the prevention of TB. These agents may cause TB sensitivity. Since this is a valuable aid in TB diagnosis, it may be useful to determine tuberculin reactivity by PPD skin testing before treatment.

Cancer prevention: These agents are not vaccines for cancer prevention.

Urinary status monitoring: Since administration of intravesical BCG causes an inflammatory response in the bladder and has been associated with hematuria, urinary frequency, dysuria and bacterial urinary tract infection, careful monitoring of urinary status is required. If there is an increase in the patient's existing symptoms, if symptoms persist, or if any of these symptoms develop, evaluate and manage the patient for urinary tract infection or BCG toxicity.

BCG infection, systemic: Since death has occurred due to systemic BCG infection, closely monitor patients for symptoms of such an infection. Withhold BCG therapy upon any suspicion of systemic infection (eg, granulomatous hepatitis). If systemic BCG infection is suspected (ie, fever > 39°C [103°F], persistent fever > 38°C [101°F] over 2 days or severe malaise), consult an infectious disease specialist and initiate fast-acting antituberculosis therapy. BCG systemic infections are rarely evidenced by positive cultures.

Antimicrobial therapy: Evaluate patients undergoing antimicrobial therapy for other infections to assess whether the therapy will obviate the effects of BCG actions.

Small bladder capacity: Consider increased risk of severity of local irritation when deciding to treat with these agents.

Hypersensitivity: Consider the possibility of allergic reactions in individuals sensitive to the components of the product. Refer to Management of Acute Hypersensitivity Reactions.

Pregnancy: Category C. It is not known whether BCG can cause fetal harm when administered to a pregnant woman. Give to a pregnant woman only if clearly needed. Advise women not to become pregnant while on therapy.

Lactation: It is not known whether BCG is excreted in breast milk. Exercise caution when BCG is administered to a nursing woman.

Children: Safety and efficacy for use in children have not been established.

Precautions:

Contains viable attenuated mycobacteria. Handle as infectious. Use aseptic technique.

Instillation equipment disposal: After usage, immediately place all equipment and materials (eg, syringes, catheters and containers that may have come into contact with BCG) used for instillation of the product into the bladder into plastic bags labeled "Infectious Waste" and dispose of accordingly as biohazardous waste.

Aseptic technique must be used during administration so as not to introduce contaminants into the urinary tract or to unduly traumatize the urinary mucosa.

Urine disinfection: Disinfect urine voided for 6 hours after instillation with an equal volume of 5% hypochlorite solution (undiluted household bleach) and allow to stand for 15 minutes before flushing.

Transurethral resection: It is recommended that intravesical BCG not be administered any sooner than 1 to 2 weeks following transurethral resection because fatalities due to disseminated BCG infection have occurred with BCG use after traumatic catheterization.

If the physician believes that the bladder catheterization has been traumatic (eg, associated with bleeding or possible false passage), then BCG should not be administered, and there must be a treatment delay of at least 1 to 2 weeks. Resume subsequent treatment as if no interruption in the schedule had occurred. That is, administer all doses even after a temporary halt in administration.

Drug Interactions:

Bone marrow depressants, immunosuppressants or **radiation** may impair the response to BCG or increase the risk of osteomyelitis or disseminated BCG infection.

(Continued on following page)

BCG, INTRAVESICAL (Cont.)

Adverse Reactions:

BCG therapy can affect several organs (or parts) of the body in addition to the cancer cells. Most local adverse reactions occur following the third intravesical instillation. Symptoms usually begin 2 to 4 hours after instillation and persist for 24 to 72 hours. Systemic reactions usually last for 1 to 3 days after each intravesical instillation.

BCG Adverse Reactions (≥ 1% of patients)[1]

Local			Systemic		
Adverse Reaction	Total (%)	Severe[2] %	Adverse Reaction	Total (%)	Severe[2] %
Dysuria	51.8-59.5	3.6-10.7	Malaise/Fatigue	7.4-40.2	2
Urinary frequency	≈ 40.4	1.8-7.4	Fever (> 38°C)	19.9-38.4	2.6-7.6
Hematuria	26-39.3	7.4-17	Chills	3.3-33.9	1-2.6
Cystitis	5.9-29.5	0-1.9	Anemia	1.3-20.5	0-0.4
Urinary urgency	5.8-17.9	0-1.3	Nausea/Vomiting	3-16.1	0-0.3
Urinary tract infection	1.5-17.9	0.9-1	Anorexia	2.2-10.7	0-0.1
Urinary incontinence	2.4-6.3	0	Renal toxicity	0-9.8	0-2
Cramps/Pain	4-6.3	0-0.9	Genital pain	0-9.8	0
Decreased bladder capacity	0-5.4	0	Myalgia/Arthralgia/Arthritis	2.7-7.1	0.4-1
Nocturia	0-4.5	0-0.6	Diarrhea	1.2-6.3	0-0.1
Urinary debris	0.9-2.2	0-0.4	Leukopenia	0.3-5.4	0
Genital inflammation/Abscess	0-1.8	0-0.4	Mild liver involvement/Hepatitis/Hepatic granuloma	0.2-2.7	0-0.4
Urethritis	0-1.2	0	Mild abdominal pain	1.5-2.7	0-0.6
			Systemic infection[3]	0.4-2.7	0.4-2
			Pulmonary infection[3]	0-2.7	0
			Cardiac	1.9-2.7	0-1.3
			Coagulopathy	0.3-2.7	0-0.3
			Headache/Dizziness	2.4-2.7	0
			Allergic	1.8-2.1	0-0.4
			Respiratory	0-1.6	0-0.2
			Pneumonitis	0-1.2	0-0.6

[1] Pooled data from two products: *TheraCys* (n = 112); *TICE BCG* (n = 674).
[2] Severe is defined as grade 3 (severe) or grade 4 (life-threatening).
[3] Includes both BCG and other infections.

Irritative bladder symptoms associated with BCG administration can be managed symptomatically with phenazopyridine HCl, propantheline bromide or oxybutynin and acetaminophen or ibuprofen.

Systemic side effects (such as malaise, fever and chills) may represent hypersensitivity reactions and can be treated with antihistamines. Systemic infection as a result of the spread of BCG organisms has occasionally occurred with intravesical BCG administration (see Warnings). At least two deaths occurred as a result of systemic BCG infection and sepsis. There have been two cases of nephrogenic adenoma, a benign lesion of bladder epithelium, associated wtih intravesical BCG therapy.

Overdosage:

Overdosage occurs if more than one amp of TICE BCG is administered per instillation. Closely monitor the patient for signs of systemic BCG infection and treat with antituberculous medication.

Patient Information:

Advise patients to check with their doctor as soon as possible if there is an increase in their existing symptoms, or if their symptoms persist even after receiving a number of treatments, or if any of the following symptoms develop:

Patient Information for BCG: Notify Physician if Listed Symptoms Occur

More Common	Rare
Blood in urine	Cough
Fever and chills	Skin rash
Frequent urge to urinate	
Increased frequency of urination	
Joint pain	
Nausea and vomiting	
Painful urination	

(Continued on following page)

BCG, INTRAVESICAL (Cont.)

Patient Information (Cont.)

A cough that develops after administration of BCG could indicate a BCG systemic infection that is life-threatening. Notify the physician immediately.

All patients should sit while voiding following instillation of solution.

Disinfect urine voided for 6 hours after instillation with an equal volume of 5% hypochlorite solution (undiluted household bleach) and allowed to stand for 15 minutes before flushing.

Administration and Dosage:

Intravesical treatment and prophylaxis for carcinoma in situ of the urinary bladder:

TheraCys – Begin between 7 to 14 days after biopsy or transurethral resection. Give a dose of 3 vials intravesically under aseptic conditions once weekly for 6 weeks (induction therapy). Each dose (3 reconstituted vials) is further diluted in an additional 50 ml sterile, preservative free saline for a total of 53 ml. Follow the induction therapy by one treatment given 3, 6, 12, 18 and 24 months following the initial treatment.

TICE BCG – Allow 7 to 14 days to elapse after bladder biopsy or transurethral resection before administration. Patients should not drink fluids for 4 hours before treatment and should empty their bladder prior to administration. The dose consists of one amp suspended in 50 ml preservative free saline. A standard treatment schedule consists of one instillation per week for 6 weeks. This may be repeated once if tumor remission has not been achieved and if the clinical circumstances warrant. Thereafter, continue at approximately monthly intervals for at least 6 to 12 months.

TheraCys and TICE BCG – A urethral catheter is inserted into the bladder under aseptic conditions, the bladder is drained, and then the suspension is instilled slowly by gravity, following which the catheter is withdrawn.

During the first hour following instillation, the patient should lie for 15 minutes each in the prone and supine positions and also on each side. The patient is then allowed to be up but should retain the suspension for another 60 minutes for a total of 2 hours. All patients may not be able to retain the suspension for the 2 hours and should be instructed to void in less time if necessary. At the end of 2 hours, all patients should void in a seated position for safety reasons. Maintain adequate hydration.

If the bladder catheterization has been traumatic (eg, associated with bleeding or possible false passage), BCG should not be administered, and there must be a treatment delay of at least 1 week. Resume subsequent treatment as if no interruption in the schedule had occurred (ie, administer all doses even after a temporary halt in administration).

Preparation of TheraCys solution: Do not remove the rubber stopper from the vial.

Reconstitute and dilute immediately prior to use.

Persons handling product should be masked and gloved.

TheraCys should not be handled by persons with a known immunologic deficiency.

TheraCys should be handled as infectious material.

Reconstitute only with the diluent provided to ensure proper dispersion of the organisms.

The reconstituted material from three vials (1 dose) is further diluted in an additional 50 ml sterile, preservative free saline to a final volume of 53 ml for intravesical instillation (and percutaneous injection if it is given).

Preparation of TICE BCG solution: Draw 1 ml of sterile, preservative free saline into a small (eg, 3 ml) syringe and add to one amp of *TICE BCG*. Draw the mixture into the syringe and gently expel back into the amp three times to ensure thorough mixing and minimize clumping of the mycobacteria. Dispense the cloudy BCG suspension into the top end of a catheter-tip syringe which contains 49 ml saline diluent bringing the total volume to 50 ml. Gently rotate the syringe. Do not filter the contents. Perform all mixing operations in sterile glass or thermosetting plastic containers and syringes.

Stability/Storage: Keep BCG and any accompanying diluent in a refrigerator at a temperature between 2° and 8°C (36° and 46°F). It should not be used after the expiration date marked on the vial, otherwise it may be inactive. Use immediately after reconstitution. Do not use after 2 hours. Any reconstituted product which exhibits flocculation or clumping that cannot be dispersed with gentle shaking should not be used. At no time should the freeze-dried or reconstituted BCG be exposed to sunlight, direct or indirect. Exposure to artificial light should be kept to a minimum.

Rx	**TICE BCG** (Organon)	**Freeze-dried suspension for reconstitution:** 1 to 8 x 10^8 CFU (equivalent to approximately 50 mg)	In 2 ml amps.
Rx	**TheraCys** (Connaught)	**Freeze-dried suspension for reconstitution:** 27 mg (3.4 ± 3 x 10^8 CFU)/vial	In 3 vials with 3 vials diluent (1 ml/vial).

ALDESLEUKIN (Interleukin-2; IL-2)

Warning:

Administer aldesleukin only in a hospital setting under the supervision of a qualified physician experienced in the use of anti-cancer agents. An intensive care facility and specialists skilled in cardiopulmonary or intensive care medicine must be available.

Aldesleukin administration has been associated with capillary leak syndrome (CLS). CLS results in hypotension and reduced organ perfusion which may be severe and can result in death (see Warnings).

Restrict therapy to patients with normal cardiac and pulmonary functions as defined by thallium stress testing and formal pulmonary function testing. Use extreme caution in patients with normal thallium stress tests and pulmonary function tests who have a history of prior cardiac or pulmonary disease.

Hold aldesleukin administration in patients developing moderate to severe lethargy or somnolence; continued administration may result in coma.

Actions:

Pharmacology: Aldesleukin, a human recombinant interleukin-2 product, is a highly purified protein (lymphokine) produced by recombinant DNA technology using a genetically engineered *Eschericia coli* strain containing an analog of the human interleukin-2 gene. The human IL-2 gene is modified, and the resulting expression clone encodes a modified human interleukin-2. This recombinant form differs from native interleukin-2 in the following ways: 1) Aldesleukin is not glycosylated; 2) the molecule has no N-terminal alanine; 3) the molecule has serine substituted for cysteine at amino acid position 125; and 4) the aggregation state of aldesleukin is likely to be different from that of native interleukin-2. Aldesleukin exists as biologically active, non-covalently bound microaggregates with an average size of 27 recombinant IL-2 molecules.

Aldesleukin possesses the biological activity of human native interleukin-2. In vitro, the immunoregulatory properties of aldesleukin include: 1) Enhancement of lymphocyte mitogenesis and stimulation of long-term growth of human interleukin-2 dependent cell lines; 2) enhancement of lymphocyte cytotoxicity; 3) induction of killer cell (lymphokine-activated [LAK] and natural [NK]) activity; and 4) induction of interferon-gamma production.

Administration produces multiple immunological effects in a dose-dependent manner. These effects include activation of cellular immunity with profound lymphocytosis, eosinophilia and thrombocytopenia, the production of cytokines (including tumor necrosis factor, IL-1 and gamma interferon) and inhibition of tumor growth. The exact mechanism by which aldesleukin mediates its antitumor activity is unknown.

Pharmacokinetics: The solubilizing agent, sodium dodecyl sulfate, may affect the kinetic properties of this product. The pharmacokinetic profile of aldesleukin is characterized by high plasma concentrations following a short IV infusion, rapid distribution to extravascular, extracellular space and elimination from the body by metabolism in the kidneys with little or no bioactive protein excreted in the urine. Approximately 30% of the dose initially distributes to the plasma. This is consistent with studies in rats that demonstrate a rapid ($<$ 1 minute) and preferential uptake of approximately 70% of an administered dose into the liver, kidney and lung.

The serum distribution and elimination half-lives in 52 cancer patients following a 5 minute IV infusion were 13 and 85 minutes, respectively.

The relatively rapid clearance rate of aldesleukin has led to dosage schedules characterized by frequent, short infusions. Observed serum levels are proportional to the dose.

Following the initial rapid organ distribution, the primary route of clearance of circulating aldesleukin is the kidney; it is cleared from the circulation by both glomerular filtration and peritubular extraction. This may account for the preservation of clearance in patients with rising serum creatinine values. Greater than 80% of the amount distributed to plasma, cleared from the circulation and presented to the kidney is metabolized to amino acids in the cells lining the proximal convoluted tubules. The mean clearance rate in cancer patients is 268 ml/min.

Immunogenicity: Of 76 renal cancer patients, 58 (76%) treated with the every 8 hour regimen developed low titers of non-neutralizing anti-interleukin-2 antibodies. Neutralizing antibodies were not detected in this group of patients, but have been detected in $<$ 1% treated with IV aldesleukin using a wide variety of schedules and doses. The clinical significance of anti-interleukin-2 antibodies is unknown.

(Actions continued on following page)

ALDESLEUKIN (Interleukin-2; IL-2) (Cont.)

Actions (Cont.):

Clinical trials: Patients with metastatic renal cell cancer (n = 255) were treated with single agent aldesleukin. Patients were required to have bidimensionally measurable disease, Eastern Cooperative Oncology Group (ECOG) Performance Status (PS) of 0 or 1 (see table), and normal organ function; 218 (85%) patients had undergone nephrectomy prior to treatment. All patients were treated with 28 doses or until dose-limiting toxicity occurred requiring ICU-level support. Patients received a median of 20 of 28 scheduled doses.

Objective response was seen in 37 patients (15%) with 9 (4%) complete and 28 (11%) partial responders. Onset of tumor regression has been observed as early as 4 weeks after completion of the first course of treatment and tumor regression may continue for up to 12 months after the start of treatment. Median duration of objective (partial or complete) response was 23.2 months (1 to 50 months); the median duration of objective partial response was 18.2 months. The proportion of responding patients who will have response durations of ≥ 12 months is projected to be 85% for all responders and 79% for patients with partial responses. Response was observed in both lung and non-lung sites (eg, liver, lymph node, renal bed recurrences, soft tissue). Patients with individual bulky lesions as well as large cumulative tumor burden achieved durable responses.

An analysis of prognostic factors showed that performance status as defined by the ECOG (see table) was a significant predictor of response. In addition, the frequency of toxicity was related to the performance status. As a group, PS 0 patients, when compared with PS 1 patients, had lower rates of adverse events with fewer on-study deaths (4% vs 6%), less frequent intubations (8% vs 25%), gangrene (0% vs 6%), coma (1% vs 6%), GI bleeding (4% vs 8%) and sepsis (6% vs 18%).

Eastern Cooperative Oncology Group (ECOG) Performance Status (PS) Scale

Performance status equivalent		Performance status definitions
ECOG	Karnofsky	
0	100	Asymptomatic
1	80-90	Symptomatic; fully ambulatory
2	60-70	Symptomatic; in bed < 50% of day
3	40-50	Symptomatic; in bed > 50% of day
4	20-30	Bedridden

Aldesleukin Response Analyzed by ECOG Performance Status

Pretreatment ECOG PS	Patients treated (n = 255)	Response		Patients responding (%)	On-study death rate
		Complete	Partial		
0	166	9	21	18	4%
1	80	0	7	9	6%
≥ 2	9	0	0	0	0%

Indications:

Metastatic renal cell carcinoma in adults (≥ 18 years of age).

Careful patient selection is mandatory prior to administration. Patients with more favorable ECOG performance status (ECOG PS 0) at treatment initiation respond better to aldesleukin with a higher response rate and lower toxicity. Experience in patients with PS > 1 is extremely limited.

Unlabeled uses: Aldesleukin is being investigated in the treatment of Kaposi's sarcoma in combination with zidovudine. Aldesleukin may be beneficial for metastatic melanoma; 20% to 30% response rates have been reported in combination with low-dose cyclophosphamide. Aldesleukin has been used with some success in the treatment of colorectal cancer and non-Hodgkin's lymphoma, often in combination with lymphokine activated killer (LAK) cells.

(Continued on following page)

ALDESLEUKIN (Interleukin-2; IL-2) (Cont.)

Contraindications:

Hypersensitivity to interleukin-2 or any component of the formulation; abnormal thallium stress test or pulmonary function tests; organ allografts.

Retreatment is contraindicated in patients who experienced the following toxicities while receiving an earlier course of therapy: Sustained ventricular tachycardia (≥ 5 beats); cardiac rhythm disturbances uncontrolled or unresponsive; recurrent chest pain with ECG changes, consistent with angina or myocardial infarction (MI); intubation required > 72 hours; pericardial tamponade; renal dysfunction requiring dialysis > 72 hours; coma or toxic psychosis lasting > 48 hours; repetitive or difficult to control seizures; bowel ischemia/perforation; GI bleeding requiring surgery.

Warnings:

Capillary leak syndrome (CLS): Aldesleukin has been associated with CLS which begins immediately after treatment starts and results from extravasation of plasma proteins and fluid into the extravascular space and loss of vascular tone. This usually results in a concomitant drop in mean arterial blood pressure within 2 to 12 hours after the start of treatment and reduced organ perfusion which may be severe and can result in death. With continued therapy, clinically significant hypotension (systolic blood pressure < 90 mm Hg or a 20 mm Hg drop from baseline systolic pressure) and hypoperfusion will occur. In addition, extravasation will lead to edema and effusions. The CLS may be associated with cardiac arrhythmias (supraventricular and ventricular), angina, MI, respiratory insufficiency requiring intubation, GI bleeding or infarction, renal insufficiency and mental status changes.

Medical management of CLS begins with careful monitoring of the patient's fluid and organ perfusion status. Frequently determine blood pressure and pulse, and monitor organ function, including assessment of mental status and urine output. Assess hypovolemia by catheterization and central pressure monitoring.

Flexibility in fluid and pressor management is essential for maintaining organ perfusion and blood pressure. Consequently, use extreme caution in treating patients with fixed requirements for large volumes of fluid (eg, patients with hypercalcemia).

Patients with hypovolemia are managed by administering IV fluids, either colloids or crystalloids. IV fluids are usually given when the central venous pressure (CVP) is < 3 to 4 mm H_2O. Correction of hypovolemia may require large volumes of IV fluids but use caution because unrestrained fluid administration may exacerbate problems associated with edema or effusions.

With extravascular fluid accumulation, edema is common and some patients may develop ascites or pleural effusions. Carefully balance the effects of fluid shifts so that neither the consequences of hypovolemia (eg, impaired organ perfusion) nor the consequences of fluid accumulations (eg, pulmonary edema) exceeds the patient's tolerance.

Early administration of dopamine (1 to 5 mcg/kg/min) to patients manifesting CLS, before the onset of hypotension, can help maintain organ perfusion particularly to the kidney and thus preserve urine output. Carefully monitor weight and urine output. If organ perfusion and blood pressure are not sustained by dopamine therapy, the dose of dopamine may be increased to 6 to 10 mcg/kg/min or phenylephrine HCl (1 to 5 mcg/kg/min) may be added to low-dose dopamine. Prolonged use of pressors, either in combination or as individual agents at relatively high doses, may be associated with cardiac rhythm disturbances.

Failure to maintain organ perfusion, demonstrated by altered mental status, reduced urine output, a fall in the systolic blood pressure < 90 mm Hg or onset of cardiac arrhythmias, should lead to holding the subsequent doses until recovery of organ perfusion and a return of systolic blood pressure > 90 mm Hg are observed.

Recovery from CLS begins soon after cessation of therapy, within a few hours. If there has been excessive weight gain or edema formation, particularly if associated with shortness of breath from pulmonary congestion, use of diuretics, once blood pressure has normalized, hastens recovery. Oxygen is given if pulmonary function monitoring confirms that P_aO_2 is decreased.

(Warnings continued on following page)

ALDESLEUKIN (Interleukin-2; IL-2) (Cont.)

Warnings (Cont.):

Clinical evaluation: Because of the severe adverse events which generally accompany therapy at the recommended dosages, perform thorough clinical evaluation to exclude from treatment patients with significant cardiac, pulmonary, renal, hepatic or CNS impairment. Patients who have had a nephrectomy are still eligible for treatment if they have serum creatinine levels ≤ 1.5 mg/dl.

CNS metastases: Aldesleukin may exacerbate disease symptoms in patients with clinically unrecognized or untreated CNS metastases. Thoroughly evaluate all patients and treat CNS metastases prior to therapy. Patients should be neurologically stable with a negative CT scan. In addition, exercise extreme caution in treating patients with a history of seizure disorder because aldesleukin may cause seizures.

Bacterial infections: Intensive treatment is associated with impaired neutrophil function (reduced chemotaxis) and with an increased risk of disseminated infection, including sepsis and bacterial endocarditis. Consequently, adequately treat preexisting bacterial infections prior to initiation of therapy. Additionally, give all patients with indwelling central lines antibiotic prophylaxis effective against *Staphylococcus aureus*. Antibiotic prophylaxis which has been associated with a reduced incidence of staphylococcal infections in aldesleukin studies includes the use of oxacillin, nafcillin, ciprofloxacin or vancomycin. Disseminated infections acquired in the course of treatment are a major contributor to treatment morbidity; use of antibiotic prophylaxis and aggressive treatment of suspected and documented infections may reduce the morbidity.

Renal/Hepatic function impairment occurs during treatment. Use of concomitant medications known to be nephrotoxic or hepatotoxic may further increase toxicity to the kidney or liver. In addition, reduced kidney and liver function secondary to treatment may delay elimination of concomitant medications and increase their risk of adverse events.

Fertility impairment: It is recommended that this drug not be administered to fertile persons of either sex not practicing effective contraception.

Pregnancy: Category C. It is not known whether aldesleukin can cause fetal harm when administered to a pregnant woman or can affect reproduction capacity. In view of the known adverse effects of aldesleukin, only give to a pregnant woman with extreme caution, weighing the potential benefit with the risks associated with therapy.

Lactation: It is not known whether this drug is excreted in breast milk. Because of the potential for serious adverse reactions in nursing infants, decide whether to discontinue nursing or to discontinue the drug, taking into the account the importance of the drug to the mother.

Children: Safety and efficacy in children < 18 years of age have not been established.

Precautions:

Anemia/Thrombocytopenia may occur. Packed red blood cell transfusions have been given both for relief of anemia and to ensure maximal oxygen carrying capacity. Platelet transfusions have been given to resolve absolute thrombocytopenia and to reduce the risk of GI bleeding. In addition, leukopenia and neutropenia have been observed.

Mental status changes including irritability, confusion or depression may occur and may be indicators of bacteremia or early bacterial sepsis. Mental status changes due solely to aldesleukin are generally reversible when drug administration is discontinued. However, alterations in mental status may progress for several days before recovery begins.

Thyroid function impairment has occurred following treatment. Some patients went on to require thyroid replacement therapy. This impairment of thyroid function may be a manifestation of autoimmunity; consequently, exercise extra caution when treating patients with known autoimmune disease.

Allograft rejection: Aldesleukin enhancement of cellular immune function may increase the risk of allograft rejection in transplant patients.

(Precautions continued on following page)

ALDESLEUKIN (Interleukin-2; IL-2) (Cont.)

Precautions (Cont.):

Monitoring: The following clinical evaluations are recommended for all patients prior to beginning treatment and then daily during drug administration: Standard hematologic tests, including CBC, differential and platelet counts; blood chemistries, including electrolytes, renal and hepatic function tests; chest x-rays.

All patients should have baseline pulmonary function tests with arterial blood gases. Document adequate pulmonary function ($FEV_1 > 2$ L or $\geq 75\%$ of predicted for height and age) prior to initiating therapy. Screen all patients with a stress thallium study. Document normal ejection fraction and unimpaired wall motion. If a thallium stress test suggests minor wall motion abnormalities of questionable significance, a stress echocardiogram to document normal wall motion may be useful to exclude significant coronary artery disease.

Daily monitoring during therapy should include vital signs (temperature, pulse, blood pressure and respiration rate) and weight. In a patient with a decreased blood pressure, especially $<$ 90 mm Hg, conduct constant cardiac monitoring for rhythm. If an abnormal complex or rhythm is seen, perform an ECG. Take vital signs in these hypotensive patients hourly and check CVP.

During treatment monitor pulmonary function on a regular basis by clinical examination, assessment of vital signs and pulse oximetry. Further assess patients with dyspnea or clinical signs of respiratory impairment (tachypnea or rales) with arterial blood gas determination. Repeat these tests as often as clincally indicated.

Cardiac function is assessed daily by clinical examination and assessment of vital signs. Further assess patients with signs or symptoms of chest pain, murmurs, gallops, irregular rhythm or palpitations with an ECG examination and CPK evaluation. If there is evidence of cardiac ischemia or CHF, perform a repeat thallium study.

Drug Interactions:

Aldesleukin Drug Interactions

Precipitant drug	Object drug*		Description
Antihypertensives	Aldesleukin	↑	Antihypertensives may potentiate the hypotension seen with aldesleukin.
Corticosteroids	Aldesleukin	↓	Although glucocorticoids reduce the side effects of aldesleukin including fever, renal insufficiency, hyperbilirubinemia and dyspnea, concomitant use may reduce the antitumor effectiveness of aldesleukin; avoid concurrent use.
Cardiotoxic agents (eg, doxorubicin) Hepatotoxic agents (eg, methotrexate, asparaginase) Myelotoxic agents (eg, cytotoxic chemotherapy) Nephrotoxic agents (eg, aminoglycosides, indomethacin)	Aldesleukin	↑	Increased toxicity in these organ systems may occur during concomitant administration.
Aldesleukin	Psychotropic agents	↔	Aldesleukin may affect CNS function. Therefore, interactions could occur following concurrent use of these agents.

* ↑ = Object drug increased ↓ = Object drug decreased ↔ = Undetermined effect

Adverse Reactions:

Adverse events are frequent, often serious and sometimes fatal. Administration results in fever, chills, rigors, pruritus and GI side effects in most patients treated at recommended doses. The rate of drug-related deaths in the 255 metastatic renal cell carcinoma patients who received single-agent aldesleukin was 4% (11/255). Frequency and severity of adverse reactions have generally been dose-related and schedule-dependent. Most adverse reactions are self-limiting and are usually, but not invariably, reversible within 2 or 3 days of discontinuation of therapy. The incidence of these events has been higher in PS 1 patients than in PS 0 patients. Examples of adverse reactions with permanent sequelae include MI, bowel perforation/infarction and gangrene. Should adverse events occur which require dose modification, withhold rather than reduce dosage.

(Adverse Reactions continued on following page)

ALDESLEUKIN (Interleukin-2; IL-2) (Cont.)

Adverse Reactions (Cont.):

Aldesleukin Adverse Reactions (n = 373[1])	
Adverse reaction	Incidence (%)
Cardiovascular	
Hypotension	85
(requiring pressors)	71
Sinus tachycardia	70
Arrhythmias	22
Atrial	8
Supraventricular	5
Ventricular	3
Junctional	1
Bradycardia	7
PVCs	5
Premature atrial contractions	4
Myocardial ischemia	3
Myocardial infarction	2
Cardiac arrest	2
Congestive heart failure	1
Myocarditis/Endocarditis	1
Stroke	1
Gangrene	1
Pericardial effusion	1
Thrombosis	1
Pulmonary	
Pulmonary congestion	54
Dyspnea	52
Pulmonary edema	10
Respiratory failure	9
Tachypnea	8
Pleural effusion	7
Wheezing	6
Apnea	1
Pneumothorax	1
Hemoptysis	1
Hepatic	
Jaundice	11
Ascites	4
Hepatomegaly	1
Hematologic	
Anemia	77
Thrombocytopenia	64
Leukopenia	34
Coagulation disorders	10
Leukocytosis	9
Eosinophilia	6
Laboratory test abnormalities	
Elevated bilirubin	64
BUN ↑	63
Serum creatinine ↑	61
Transaminase ↑	56
Alkaline phosphatase ↑	56
Hypomagnesemia	16
Acidosis	16
Hypocalcemia	15
Hypophosphatemia	11
Hypokalemia	9
Hyperuricemia	9
Hypoalbuminemia	8
Hypoproteinemia	7
Hyponatremia	4
Hyperkalemia	4
Alkalosis	4
Hypo/Hyperglycemia	2
Hypocholesterolemia	1
Hypercalcemia	1
Hypernatremia	1
Hyperphosphatemia	1
GI	
Nausea and vomiting	87
Diarrhea	76
Stomatitis	32
Anorexia	27
GI bleeding	13
(requiring surgery)	2
Dyspepsia	7
Constipation	5
Intestinal perforation/ileus	2
Pancreatitis	< 1
CNS	
Mental status changes	73
Dizziness	17
Sensory dysfunction	10
Special sensory disorders (vision, speech, taste)	7
Syncope	3
Motor dysfunction	2
Coma	1
Seizure (grand mal)	1
Renal	
Oliguria/Anuria	76
Proteinuria	12
Hematuria	9
Dysuria	3
Renal impairment requiring dialysis	2
Urinary retention	1
Urinary frequency	1
Dermatologic	
Pruritus	48
Erythema	41
Rash	26
Dry skin	15
Exfoliative dermatitis	14
Purpura/Petechiae	4
Urticaria	2
Alopecia	1
Musculoskeletal	
Arthralgia	6
Myalgia	6
Arthritis	1
Muscle spasm	1
Miscellaneous	
Fever/Chills	89
Pain (all sites)	54
Abdominal	15
Chest	12
Back	9
Fatigue/Weakness/Malaise	53
Edema	47
Infection (including urinary tract, injection site, catheter tip, phlebitis, sepsis)	23
Weight gain (≥ 10%)	23
Headache	12
Weight loss (≥ 10%)	5
Conjunctivitis	4
Injection site reactions	3
Allergic reactions	1
Hypothyroidism	< 1

[1] 255 patients with renal cell cancer, 118 with other tumors receiving the recommended every 8 hour, 15 minute infusion dosing regimen.

(Adverse Reactions continued on following page)

ALDESLEUKIN (Interleukin-2; IL-2) (Cont.)

Adverse Reactions (Cont.):

Other serious adverse events were derived from trials involving > 1800 patients treated with aldesleukin-based regimens. These events each occurred with a frequency of < 1% and included: Liver or renal failure resulting in death; duodenal ulceration; fatal intestinal perforation; bowel necrosis; fatal cardiac arrest, myocarditis and supraventricular tachycardia; permanent or transient blindness secondary to optic neuritis; fatal malignant hyperthermia; pulmonary edema resulting in death; respiratory arrest; fatal respiratory failure; fatal stroke; transient ischemic attack; meningitis; cerebral edema; pericarditis; allergic interstitial nephritis; tracheo-esophageal fistula; fatal pulmonary emboli; severe depression leading to suicide.

Overdosage:

Symptoms: Side effects following the use of aldesleukin are dose-related. Administration of more than the recommended dose has been associated with a more rapid onset of expected dose-limiting toxicities.

Treatment: Adverse reactions generally will reverse when the drug is stopped, particularly because its serum half-life is short. Treat any continuing symptoms supportively. Refer to General Management of Acute Overdosage. Life-threatening toxicities have been ameliorated by the IV administration of dexamethasone, which may result in loss of therapeutic effect of aldesleukin.

Administration and Dosage:

Approved by the FDA on May 5, 1992.

Administer by a 15 minute IV infusion every 8 hours. Before initiating treatment, carefully review the prescribing information, particularly regarding patient selection, possible serious adverse events, patient monitoring and withholding dosage.

Metastatic renal cell carcinoma in adults: Each course of treatment consists of two 5 day treatment cycles separated by a rest period:

1) 600,000 IU/kg (0.037 mg/kg) administered every 8 hours by a 15 minute IV infusion for a total of 14 doses. Following 9 days of rest, repeat the schedule for another 14 doses, for a maximum of 28 doses per course.
2) Patients treated with this schedule received a median of 20 of the 28 doses during the first course of therapy due to toxicity.

Retreatment: Evaluate patients for response approximately 4 weeks after completion of a course of therapy and again immediately prior to the scheduled start of the next treatment course. Additional courses of treatment may be given to patients only if there is some tumor shrinkage following the last course and retreatment is not contraindicated (see Contraindications). Separate each treatment course by a rest period of at least 7 weeks from the date of hospital discharge. Tumors have continued to regress up to 12 months following the initiation of therapy.

Dose modification: Accomplish dose modification for toxicity by holding or interrupting a dose rather than reducing the dose to be given. Decisions to stop, hold or restart therapy must be made after a global assessment of the patient with use the following guidelines:

Guidelines for Discontinuation of Aldesleukin Therapy	
Organ system	Permanently discontinue treatment for the following toxicities:
Cardiovascular	Sustained ventricular tachycardia (≥ 5 beats) Cardiac rhythm disturbances not controlled or unresponsive Recurrent chest pain with ECG changes, documented angina or MI Pericardial tamponade
Pulmonary	Intubation required > 72 hours
Renal	Renal dysfunction requiring dialysis > 72 hours
CNS	Coma or toxic psychosis lasting > 48 hours Repetitive or difficult to control seizures
GI	Bowel ischemia/perforation/GI bleeding requiring surgery

(Administration and Dosage continued on following page)

ALDESLEUKIN (Interleukin-2; IL-2) (Cont.)

Administration and Dosage (Cont.):

Guidelines for Held Doses and Subsequent Doses of Aldesleukin		
Organ system	Hold dose for:	Subsequent doses may be given if:
Cardiovascular	Atrial fibrillation, supraventricular tachycardia or bradycardia that requires treatment or is recurrent or persistent.	Patient is asymptomatic with full recovery to normal sinus rhythm.
	Systolic bp $<$ 90 mm Hg with increasing needs for pressors.	Systolic bp $\geq$ 90 mm Hg and stable or improving needs for pressors.
	Any ECG change consistent with MI or ischemia with/without chest pain; suspicion of cardiac ischemia.	Patient is asymptomatic. MI has been ruled out, clinical suspicion of angina is low.
Pulmonary	O_2 saturation $<$ 94% on room air or $<$ 90% w/2 L O_2 by nasal prongs.	O_2 saturation $\geq$ 94% on room air or $\geq$ 90% w/2 L O_2 by nasal prongs.
CNS	Mental status changes, including moderate confusion or agitation.	Mental status changes completely resolved.
Systemic	Sepsis syndrome, patient is clinically unstable.	Sepsis syndrome has resolved, patient is clinically stable, infection is under treatment.
Renal	Serum creatinine $\geq$ 4.5 mg/dl or a serum creatinine of 4 mg/dl in the presence of severe volume overload, acidosis or hyperkalemia.	Serum creatinine $<$ 4 mg/dl and fluid and electrolyte status is stable.
	Persistent oliguria, urine output of $\leq$ 10 ml/hr for 16 to 24 hours with rising serum creatinine.	Urine output $>$ 10 ml/hour with a decrease of serum creatinine $\geq$ 1.5 mg/dl or normalization of serum creatinine.
Hepatic	Signs of hepatic failure including encephalopathy, increasing ascites, pain, hypoglycemia.	All signs of hepatic failure have resolved[1].
GI	Stool guaiac repeatedly 3 to 4+.	Stool guaiac negative.
Skin	Bullous dermatitis or marked worsening of preexisting skin condition (avoid topical steroid therapy).	Resolution of all signs of bullous dermatitis.

[1] Discontinue all further treatment for that course. Consider starting a new course of treatment at least 7 weeks after cessation of adverse event and hospital discharge.

Reconstitution and dilutions: Reconstitute and dilute only as recommended since the delivery or pharmacology of aldesleukin may be altered.

1) Each vial contains 22 million IU (1.3 mg) aldesleukin; reconstitute aseptically with 1.2 ml Sterile Water for Injection, USP. When reconstituted as directed, each ml contains 18 million IU (1.1 mg). The resulting solution should be a clear, colorless to slightly yellow liquid. The vial is for single-use only; discard unused portion.

2) During reconstitution, direct the Sterile Water for Injection, USP at the side of the vial and swirl the contents gently to avoid excess foaming. Do not shake.

3) Dilute the dose of aldesleukin reconstituted in Sterile Water for Injection, USP (without preservative) in 50 ml of 5% Dextrose Injection, USP and infuse over 15 minutes. Although glass bottles and plastic (polyvinyl chloride) bags have been used in clinical trials with comparable results, use plastic bags as the dilution container since experimental studies suggest that use of plastic containers results in more consistent drug delivery. Do not use in-line filters when administering aldesleukin.

4) Avoid reconstitution or dilution with Bacteriostatic Water for Injection, USP or 0.9% Sodium Chloride Injection, USP because of increased aggregation. Dilution with albumin can alter the pharmacology of aldesleukin. Do not mix with other drugs.

Storage/Stability: Before and after reconstitution and dilution, store vials in a refrigerator at 2° to 8°C (36° to 46°F). Do not freeze. Administer within 48 hours of reconstitution. Bring the solution to room temperature prior to infusion in the patient. This product contains no preservative; discard unused portion.

Rx	**Proleukin** (Cetus Oncology)	**Powder for Injection, lyophilized:** 22 x 10^6 IU per vial (18 million IU [1.1 mg] per ml when reconstituted).	In single-use vials (10s).[1]

[1] Preservative free. With 50 mg mannitol, 0.18 mg sodium dodecyl sulfate and 0.17 mg monobasic and 0.89 mg dibasic sodium phosphate.

PROCARBAZINE HCl (N-Methylhydrazine; MIH)

Actions:

Pharmacology: The mode of cytotoxic action is not clear; procarbazine may inhibit protein, ribonucleic acid (RNA) and deoxyribonucleic acid (DNA) synthesis. Procarbazine may inhibit transmethylation of methyl groups of methionine into t-RNA. The absence of functional t-RNA could cause the cessation of protein synthesis and consequently DNA and RNA synthesis. In addition, procarbazine may directly damage DNA. Hydrogen peroxide, formed during the auto-oxidation of the drug, may attack protein sulfhydryl groups contained in residual protein which is tightly bound to DNA. Procarbazine is metabolized primarily in the liver and kidneys. No cross-resistance with other agents, radiotherapy or steroids has been demonstrated.

Pharmacokinetics: Absorption/Distribution – Procarbazine is rapidly and completely absorbed from the GI tract and quickly equilibrates between plasma and cerebrospinal fluid (CSF). Peak CSF levels occur in 30 to 90 minutes. Following oral administration, maximum peak plasma concentrations occur within 60 minutes.

Metabolism/Excretion – The drug is metabolized in the liver to cytotoxic products. The major portion of drug is excreted in the urine as N-isopropylterephthalamic acid (≈ 70% within 24 hours following oral and IV administration). Less than 5% is excreted in urine unchanged.

After IV injection, the plasma half-life is ≈ 10 minutes. Procarbazine crosses the blood-brain barrier.

Indications:

In combination with other antineoplastics for treatment of Stage III and IV Hodgkin's disease. Use procarbazine as part of the MOPP (nitrogen mustard, vincristine, procarbazine, prednisone) regimen.

Contraindications:

Hypersensitivity to procarbazine. Inadequate marrow reserve demonstrated by bone marrow aspiration; consider in any patient with leukopenia, thrombocytopenia or anemia.

Warnings:

Give procarbazine only under supervision of a physician experienced in the use of potent antineoplastic drugs. Have adequate clinical and laboratory facilities available for proper monitoring.

Because procarbazine exhibits some monoamine oxidase inhibitory activity, avoid sympathomimetics, antihistamines, tricyclic antidepressants (eg, amitriptyline HCl, imipramine HCl) and other drugs and foods with known high tyramine content, such as wine, yogurt, ripe cheese and bananas.

Do not use prescription drugs without consent of physician.

Toxicity common to many hydrazine derivatives is hemolysis and the appearance of Heinz-Ehrlich inclusion bodies in erythrocytes.

Usage in Pregnancy: Category D. Procarbazine can cause fetal harm when administered to a pregnant woman. There are no adequate and well controlled studies in pregnant women. If this drug is used during pregnancy, inform patient of the potential hazard to the fetus. Advise women of childbearing potential to avoid becoming pregnant.

Administration in first trimester of pregnancy has been described in five patients; congenital malformations were observed in four. The other pregnancy was electively terminated. When combined with other antineoplastics, procarbazine may produce gonadal dysfunction in males and females. Use only when clearly needed and when the potential benefits outweigh the potential hazards.

Procarbazine is teratogenic in the rat when given at doses approximately 4 to 13 times the maximum recommended human therapeutic dose of 6 mg/kg/day.

Usage in Lactation: It is not known whether procarbazine is excreted in human milk. Because of the potential for tumorigenicity shown in animal studies, mothers should not nurse while receiving this drug.

(Continued on following page)

PROCARBAZINE HCl (N-Methylhydrazine; MIH) (Cont.)

Precautions:

Use in impaired renal and hepatic function: Undue toxicity may occur if used in patients with known impairment of renal or hepatic function. Consider hospitalization for the initial treatment course.

Use following radiation or other chemotherapy is known to have marrow depressant activity. Wait 1 month or longer before starting procarbazine. Interval length may also be determined by evidence of bone marrow recovery based on successive bone marrow studies.

Carcinogenesis, mutagenesis and impairment of fertility: Carcinogenesis in mice, rats and monkeys has been reported including: Instances of a second non-lymphoid malignancy, including acute myelocytic leukemia, (in patients with Hodgkin's disease treated with procarbazine in combination with other chemotherapy or radiation). The International Agency for Research on Cancer (IARC) considers that there is "sufficient evidence" for the human carcinogenicity of procarbazine HCl when it is given in intensive regimens which include other antineoplastic agents but there is inadequate evidence of carcinogenicity in humans given procarbazine HCl alone.

Procarbazine is mutagenic in a variety of bacterial and mammalian test systems.

Azoospermia and antifertility effects associated with procarbazine coadministered with other antineoplastics for treating Hodgkin's disease have been reported in human clinical studies. Since these patients received multicombination therapy, it is difficult to determine to what extent procarbazine alone was involved in the male germ-cell damage. Compounds which inhibit DNA, RNA or protein synthesis might be expected to have adverse effects on gametogenesis. Unscheduled DNA synthesis in the testis of rabbits and decreased fertility in male mice treated with procarbazine HCl have been reported.

Drug Interactions:

Digitalis glycosides: Combination chemotherapy (including procarbazine) may result in a decrease in **digoxin** plasma levels, even several days after stopping chemotherapy.

Procarbazine, which possesses weak monoamine oxidase (MAO) inhibitor activity, may interact with the following agents in a manner similar to the MAO inhibitors:

Levodopa – Coadministration may result in flushing and a significant rise in blood pressure within 1 hour of levodopa administration.

Narcotics – Concomitant use may result in depressant effects on the CNS leading to deep coma and death.

Sympathomimetics (indirect acting) and ingestion of **foods with high tyramine content** (see p. 1312) may cause an abrupt increase in blood pressure, resulting in a potentially fatal hypertensive crisis.

Tricyclic antidepressants – Severe toxic and fatal reactions including excitability, fluctuations in blood pressure, convulsions and coma may occur. However, some studies report uneventful concurrent use with MAO inhibitors.

Adverse Reactions:

Frequent: Leukopenia, anemia, thrombocytopenia, nausea and vomiting.

GI: Anorexia, stomatitis, dry mouth, dysphagia, abdominal pain, diarrhea and constipation.

Hematologic: Pancytopenia, eosinophilia, hemolytic anemia, bleeding tendencies such as petechiae, purpura, epistaxis, hemoptysis, hematemesis and melena.

Cardiovascular: Hypotension, tachycardia, syncope.

GU: Hematuria, urinary frequency, nocturia.

Endocrine: Gynecomastia in prepubertal and early pubertal boys.

Dermatologic: Dermatitis, pruritus, rash, urticaria, herpes, hyperpigmentation, flushing, alopecia and jaundice.

CNS: Paresthesias and neuropathies, headache, dizziness, depression, apprehension, nervousness, insomnia, nightmares, hallucinations, falling, weakness, fatigue, lethargy, drowsiness, unsteadiness, ataxia, foot drop, decreased reflexes, tremors, coma, confusion and convulsions.

Miscellaneous: Pain, including myalgia and arthralgia, hepatic dysfunction, pyrexia, diaphoresis, chills, intercurrent infections, pleural effusion, edema, cough, pneumonitis, hoarseness, photosensitivity, fainting, generalized allergic reactions, hearing loss, slurred speech.

Ocular: Retinal hemorrhage; nystagmus; photophobia; diplopia; inability to focus; papilledema.

Second nonlymphoid malignancies, including acute myelocytic leukemia and malignant myelosclerosis and azoospermia have been reported in patients with Hodgkin's disease treated with procarbazine in combination with other chemotherapy or radiation.

(Continued on following page)

PROCARBAZINE HCl (N-Methylhydrazine; MIH) (Cont.)

Overdosage:

The major manifestations of overdosage with procarbazine would be anticipated to be nausea, vomiting, enteritis, diarrhea, hypotension, tremors, convulsions and coma. Treatment consists of either the administration of an emetic or gastric lavage. Use general supportive measures such as IV fluids. Since the major toxicity of procarbazine is hematologic and hepatic, perform frequent complete blood counts and liver function tests throughout recovery period and for a minimum of 2 weeks thereafter. Should abnormalities appear in any of these determinations, immediately undertake appropriate measures for correction and stabilization.

Patient Information:

May produce drowsiness and dizziness; patients should observe caution while driving or performing other tasks requiring alertness.

Avoid ingestion of the following: Tyramine-containing foods (see page 1312), certain cold, hay fever or weight-reducing preparations (containing sympathomimetics).

Notify physician if cough, shortness of breath, thickened bronchial secretions, fever, chills, sore throat, unusual bleeding or bruising, vomiting of blood, or black tarry stools occurs.

Medication may cause muscle or joint pain, nausea, vomiting, sweating, tiredness, weakness, constipation, headache, difficulty swallowing, loss of appetite, loss of hair, and mental depression; notify physician if these become pronounced.

Avoid prolonged exposure to sunlight; photosensitivity may occur.

Contraceptive measures are recommended during therapy for both men and women.

Administration and Dosage:

Base dosages on the patient's actual weight. Use estimated lean body mass (dry weight) if patient is obese or if there has been a spurious weight gain due to edema, ascites or other forms of abnormal fluid retention.

The following doses are for administration of procarbazine as a single agent. When used in combination with other anticancer drugs, appropriately reduce procarbazine dosage eg, in the MOPP regimen, the procarbazine dose is 100 mg/m^2 daily for 14 days.

Adults: To minimize nausea and vomiting, give single or divided doses of 2 to 4 mg/kg/day for the first week. Maintain daily dosage at 4 to 6 mg/kg/day until the WBC falls below 4,000/cu mm or the platelets fall below 100,000/cu mm, or until maximum response is obtained. Upon evidence of hematologic toxicity, discontinue the drug until there has been satisfactory recovery. Resume treatment at 1 to 2 mg/kg/day. When maximum response is obtained, maintain the dose at 1 to 2 mg/kg/day.

Children: Close clinical monitoring is mandatory. Toxicity, evidenced by tremors, coma and convulsions, has occurred. Individualize dosage. This dosage schedule is a guideline only: 50 mg/m^2 daily for the first week. Maintain daily dosage at 100 mg/m^2 until leukopenia or thrombocytopenia occurs or maximum response is obtained. Upon evidence of hematologic toxicity, discontinue drug until there has been satisfactory response. When maximum response is attained, maintain the dose at 50 mg/m^2/day.

Monitoring Therapy: Obtain baseline laboratory data prior to initiation of therapy. Monitor hemoglobin, hematocrit, WBC, differential, reticulocytes and platelets at least every 3 or 4 days. Bone marrow depression often occurs 2 to 8 weeks after the start of treatment. If leukopenia occurs, hospitalization may be needed to prevent systemic infection.

Evaluate hepatic and renal function prior to initiation of therapy.

Repeat urinalysis, transaminase, alkaline phosphatase and BUN at least weekly.

Promptly cease therapy if any of the following occurs: CNS signs or symptoms; leukopenia (WBC $<$ 4000/cu mm); thrombocytopenia (platelets $<$ 100,000/cu mm); hypersensitivity reaction; stomatitis (the first small ulceration or persistent spot soreness); diarrhea; hemorrhage or bleeding tendencies.

Resume therapy after side effects clear; adjust to a lower dosage schedule.

Rx	**Matulane** (Roche)	**Capsules:** 50 mg	(#Roche Matulane). Ivory. In 100s.

Product identification code.

DACARBAZINE (DTIC; Imidazole Carboxamide)

Warning:

Hemopoietic depression is the most common toxicity (see Warnings).

Hepatic necrosis has been reported (see Warnings).

Administer under the supervision of a qualified physician experienced in the use of antineoplastic agents.

Actions:

Pharmacology: The exact mechanism of action is unknown. There is some evidence for activity via three mechanisms: Alkylation through an activated carbonium ion; inhibition of DNA synthesis by acting as a purine analog; and interaction with sulfhydryl groups in proteins. Both deoxyribonucleic acid (DNA) and ribonucleic acid (RNA) synthesis are inhibited. Although dacarbazine appears to be more active on cells in late G_2 phase, it is considered cell cycle phase nonspecific.

Pharmacokinetics: Absorption/Distribution - After IV administration of dacarbazine, the volume of distribution exceeds total body water content suggesting tissue localization, probably in the liver. There is relatively little distribution into the cerebrospinal fluid (CSF). At therapeutic concentrations, the drug is not appreciably bound to plasma protein.

Metabolism/Excretion - Plasma disappearance is biphasic with an initial half-life of 19 minutes and a terminal half-life of 5 hours. In renal and hepatic dysfunction, half-lives increase to 55 minutes and 7.2 hours.

An average of 40% of dacarbazine is excreted unchanged in the urine in 6 hours. Dacarbazine is subject to renal tubular secretion rather than glomerular filtration. Besides unchanged dacarbazine, 5-aminoimidazole-4 carboxamide (AIC) is a major metabolite in the urine.

Indications:

Metastatic malignant melanoma.

Second-line therapy in Hodgkin's disease in combination with other agents.

Contraindications:

Hypersensitivity to dacarbazine.

Warnings:

Hemopoietic depression is the most common toxicity and involves primarily the leukocytes and platelets, although anemia sometimes occurs. Leukopenia and thrombocytopenia may be severe enough to cause death. Possible bone marrow depression requires careful monitoring of WBC, RBC and platelet levels. Hemopoietic toxicity may warrant temporary suspension or cessation of therapy.

Hepatotoxicity, accompanied by hepatic vein thrombosis and hepatocellular necrosis resulting in death, has been reported in approximately 0.01% of patients treated. This toxicity has been observed mostly when dacarbazine was coadministered with other antineoplastics, but it has also been reported with dacarbazine alone.

Anaphylaxis can occur following the administration of dacarbazine.

Usage in Pregnancy: Category C. Teratogenicity has been demonstrated in animals given 7 to 20 times the human dose. There are no adequate and well controlled studies in pregnant women. Use during pregnancy only if the potential benefit justifies the potential risk to the fetus.

Usage in Lactation: It is not known if this drug is excreted in breast milk. Because of the potential for tumorigenicity, decide whether to discontinue nursing or to discontinue the drug, taking into account the importance of the drug to the mother.

Precautions:

Hospitalization is not always necessary, but adequate laboratory facilities must be available.

Extravasation of the drug may result in tissue damage and severe pain. Locally applied hot packs may relieve pain, burning sensation and irritation at the injection site.

Carcinogenicity: Angiosarcomas of the spleen and proliferative endocardial lesions, including fibrosarcomas and sarcomas, were induced in small animals after administration.

Photosensitivity: Photosensitization (photoallergy or phototoxicity) may occur; therefore, caution patients to take protective measures (ie, sunscreens, protective clothing) against exposure to ultraviolet light or sunlight until tolerance is determined.

(Continued on following page)

DACARBAZINE (DTIC, Imidazole Carboxamide) (Cont.)

Adverse Reactions:

GI: Anorexia, nausea and vomiting occur in over 90% of patients with the initial few doses. The vomiting lasts 1 to 12 hours and is incompletely and unpredictably palliated with phenobarbital or prochlorperazine. Rarely, intractable nausea and vomiting have necessitated discontinuation of therapy. Diarrhea occurs rarely. Restricting the patient's oral intake of fluids and food for 4 to 6 hours prior to treatment may be beneficial. Rapid tolerance to these symptoms suggests that a CNS mechanism may be involved; symptoms usually subside after the first 1 or 2 days.

A flu-like syndrome of fever to 39°C, myalgia and malaise has been reported. Symptoms usually occur after large single doses, may last for several days and may occur with successive treatments.

Laboratory findings of significant liver or renal function test abnormalities have been few.

Dermatologic: Erythematous and urticarial rashes (infrequent) and alopecia. Photosensitivity reactions may occur rarely (see Precautions).

Miscellaneous: Facial flushing and facial paresthesia.

Overdosage:

Give supportive treatment and monitor blood cell counts.

Administration and Dosage:

Administer IV only. Extravasation of the drug subcutaneously during IV administration may result in tissue damage and severe pain.

Malignant melanoma: 2 to 4.5 mg/kg/day IV for 10 days. Repeat at 4 week intervals.

Alternatively, administer 250 mg/m²/day IV for 5 days. Repeat every 3 weeks.

Hodgkin's disease: 150 mg/m²/day for 5 days, in combination with other effective drugs. Repeat every 4 weeks.

Alternatively, administer 375 mg/m² on day 1, in combination with other effective drugs; repeat every 15 days.

Preparation of the solution: Reconstitute the 100 mg vials with 9.9 ml and the 200 mg vials with 19.7 ml of Sterile Water for Injection. The resulting solution contains 10 mg/ml of dacarbazine with a pH of 3 to 4. The reconstituted solution may be further diluted with 5% Dextrose Injection or Sodium Chloride Injection, and administered as an IV infusion.

Storage/Stability: After reconstitution, store the solution in the vial at 4°C up to 72 hours or at normal room conditions (temperature and light) up to 8 hours. If the reconstituted solution is further diluted in 5% Dextrose Injection or Sodium Chloride Injection, store the resulting solution at 4°C up to 24 hours or at normal room conditions up to 8 hours. A white flocculent precipitate was observed when IV tubing containing dacarbazine (25 mg/ml) in 0.9% Sodium Chloride was flushed with heparin sodium. However, no precipitate was observed when 10 mg/ml of dacarbazine was used.

Rx	**Dacarbazine** (Various)	**Injection:** 100 mg per 10 ml vial 100 mg per 20 ml vial 200 mg per 20 ml vial 200 mg per 30 ml vial 500 mg per 50 ml vial
Rx	**DTIC-Dome** (Miles Pharm.)	**Injection:** 100 mg per 10 ml vial[1] 200 mg per 20 ml vial[1]

[1] With mannitol.

MITOTANE (o, p'-DDD)

Warning:
Discontinue temporarily following shock or severe trauma since the prime action of mitotane is adrenal suppression. Administer exogenous steroids in such circumstances, since the depressed adrenal may not immediately start to function.

Actions:

Pharmacology: Mitotane is an adrenal cytotoxic agent, although it can cause adrenal inhibition without cellular destruction. The primary action is upon the adrenal cortex. The production of adrenal steroids is reduced. The biochemical mechanism of action is unknown. Data suggest that the drug modifies the peripheral metabolism of steroids and directly suppresses the adrenal cortex.

Use of mitotane alters the peripheral metabolism of cortisol, leading to a reduction in measurable 17-hydroxycorticosteroids, even though plasma levels of corticosteroids do not fall. The drug causes increased formation of 6-β-hydroxycortisol.

Pharmacokinetics: Absorption/Distribution – Approximately 40% of oral mitotane is absorbed; it can be found in all body tissues but is primarily stored in fat. Blood levels detectable for up to 10 weeks after discontinuation of therapy may be related to a slow persistent release of drug from lipid storage sites. Blood levels do not appear to correlate with therapeutic or toxic effects.

Metabolism/Excretion – The primary metabolites of mitotane are oxidation products; several polar metabolites are also produced. Approximately 10% to 25% of the drug is excreted in the urine as an unidentified water soluble metabolite. A variable amount of metabolite (1% to 17%) is excreted in the bile and the balance is apparently stored in tissues. Up to 60% is excreted unchanged in the stool. Following discontinuation of the drug, plasma terminal half-life has ranged from 18 to 159 days.

No unchanged mitotane has been found in the urine or bile.

Clinical Pharmacology: A number of patients have been treated intermittently, restarting treatment when severe symptoms reappeared. Patients often do not respond after the third or fourth such course. Continuous treatment with the maximum possible dosage may be the best approach.

A substantial percentage of patients show signs of adrenal insufficiency. Watch for this condition and institute steroid therapy if necessary. The metabolism of exogenous steroids is modified with mitotane; somewhat higher doses than just replacement therapy may be required.

Clinical effectiveness can be shown by reductions in tumor mass, pain, weakness or anorexia and steroid symptoms.

Indications:
Treatment of inoperable adrenal cortical carcinoma (functional and nonfunctional).

Contraindications:
Hypersensitivity to mitotane.

Warnings:
Temporarily discontinue mitotane immediately following shock or severe trauma, since adrenal suppression is its prime action. Use exogenous steroids in such circumstances, since the depressed adrenal may not immediately start to secrete steroids.

Usage in impaired hepatic function: Administer with care to patients with liver disease other than metastatic lesions of the adrenal cortex. Interference with mitotane metabolism may occur, causing drug accumulation.

Surgically remove all possible tumor tissue from large metastatic masses before administration to minimize the possibility of infarction and hemorrhage in the tumor due to a rapid, cytotoxic effect of the drug.

Long-term therapy: Continuous administration of high doses may lead to brain damage and impairment of function. Conduct behavioral and neurological assessments at regular intervals when continuous treatment exceeds 2 years.

Carcinogenesis, Mutagenesis, Impairment of Fertility: The carcinogenic and mutagenic potential is unknown. However, the mechanism of action suggests that the drug probably has less carcinogenic potential than other cytotoxic chemotherapeutic drugs.

Usage in Pregnancy: Category C. Safety for use during pregnancy has not been established. Use only when clearly needed and when the potential benefits outweigh the potential hazards to the fetus.

Usage in Lactation: It is not known whether this drug is excreted in breast milk. Because of the potential for adverse reactions in nursing infants, decide whether to discontinue nursing or discontinue the drug.

(Continued on following page)

MITOTANE (o, p′-DDD) (Cont.)

Precautions:

Adrenal insufficiency may develop; consider adrenal steroid replacement in these patients.

Potentially hazardous tasks: May produce sedation, lethargy, vertigo or other CNS side effects; observe caution while driving or performing other tasks requiring alertness.

Drug Interactions:

Corticosteroid metabolism may be altered by mitotane; higher dosages may be required.

Warfarin: The metabolism of warfarin may be accelerated by the mechanism of hepatic microsomal enzyme induction, leading to an increase in dosage requirements for warfarin. Monitor patients for a change in anticoagulant dosage requirements when administering mitotane to patients on coumarin-type anticoagulants.

Give with caution to patients receiving other drugs susceptible to the influence of hepatic enzyme reduction.

Drug/Lab Tests: **Protein-bound iodine** (PBI) levels and **urinary 17-hydroxycorticosteroids** may be decreased by mitotane.

Adverse Reactions:

GI: Anorexia, nausea or vomiting and diarrhea (80%).

CNS (40%): Primarily depression as manifested by lethargy and somnolence (25%), and dizziness or vertigo (15%).

Dermatologic (15%): Primarily transient skin rashes. In some instances, this side effect subsided while patients were maintained on the drug.

Infrequent:

Ophthalmic - Visual blurring, diplopia, lens opacity and toxic retinopathy.
GU - Hematuria, hemorrhagic cystitis and proteinuria.
Cardiovascular - Hypertension, orthostatic hypotension and flushing.
Miscellaneous - Generalized aching, hyperpyrexia and lowered PBI.

Patient Information:

Notify physician if nausea, vomiting, loss of appetite, diarrhea, mental depression, skin rash or darkening of the skin occurs.

Medication may cause aching muscles, fever, flushing or muscle twitching; notify physician if these become pronounced.

May produce drowsiness, dizziness and tiredness; patients should observe caution when driving or performing other tasks requiring alertness.

Contraceptive measures are recommended during therapy.

Administration and Dosage:

Start at 2 to 6 g/day in divided doses, 3 or 4 times daily. Increase dose incrementally to 9 to 10 g per day. If severe side effects appear, reduce to the maximum tolerated dose. If the patient can tolerate higher doses, and if improved clinical response appears possible, increase the dose until adverse reactions interfere. Maximum tolerated dose varies from 2 to 16 g/day (usually 9 to 10 g). The highest doses used in studies were 18 to 19 g/day.

Institute treatment in the hospital until dosage regimen is stable.

Continue treatment as long as clinical benefits are observed (ie, maintenance of clinical status or slowing of growth of metastatic lesions). If no clinical benefits are observed after 3 months at the maximum tolerated dose, consider the case a clinical failure. However, 10% of the patients who showed a measurable response required more than 3 months at the maximum tolerated dose. Early diagnosis and prompt institution of treatment improve the probability of a positive clinical response.

Rx	**Lysodren** (Bristol-Myers Oncology)	**Tablets:** 500 mg	Scored. In 100s.

ASPARAGINASE

Warning:

Because of possible severe reactions, including anaphylaxis and sudden death, administer only in a hospital setting under the supervision of a physician qualified by training and experience in antineoplastic agents. Be prepared to treat anaphylaxis at each administration.

Actions:

Asparaginase contains the enzyme L-asparagine amidohydrolase, type EC-2, derived from *Escherichia coli*.

Pharmacology: In a significant number of patients with acute (particularly lymphocytic) leukemia, the malignant cells depend on exogenous asparagine for survival. Normal cells are able to synthesize asparagine and thus are affected less by the rapid depletion produced by treatment. Administration of asparaginase hydrolyzes serum asparagine to nonfunctional asparatic acid and ammonia, depriving tumor cells of a required amino acid. Tumor cell proliferation is blocked due to interruption of asparagine-dependent protein synthesis. The inhibitory activity is maximal in the postmitotic (G_1) phase of the cell cycle.

Pharmacokinetics:

Absorption/Distribution – Initial plasma levels of L-asparaginase following IV administration are correlated to dose. Daily administration results in a cumulative increase in plasma levels. Asparaginase serum levels following IM use are approximately one-half those achieved with IV administration. Apparent volume of distribution is approximately 70% to 80% of estimated plasma volume. There is some slow movement from vascular to extravascular, extracellular space. L-asparaginase is detected in the lymph. Cerebrospinal fluid levels usually are less than 1% of concurrent plasma levels.

Metabolism/Excretion – Plasma half-life varied from 8 to 30 hours. Half-life is not influenced by dosage and cannot be correlated with age, sex, surface area, renal or hepatic function, diagnosis or extent of disease. Only minimal urinary and biliary excretion occurs.

Indications:

Acute lymphocytic leukemia primarily in combination with other chemotherapeutic agents in the induction of remissions of disease in children. Do not use as the sole induction agent unless combination therapy is deemed inappropriate.

Not recommended for maintenance therapy.

Contraindications:

Anaphylactic reactions to asparaginase; pancreatitis or a history of pancreatitis.

Warnings:

Because of the unpredictability of adverse reactions, use only in a hospital.

Hypersensitivity reactions are frequent and may occur during the primary course of therapy. They are not completely predictable based on the intradermal skin test. Anaphylaxis and death have occurred.

Once a patient has received asparaginase, there is an increased risk of hypersensitivity reactions with retreatment. In patients found to be hypersensitive by skin testing, and in any patient previously under therapy with asparaginase, administer the drug only after successful desensitization. Even then, the possible benefit should be judged as greater than the increased risk since desensitization may also be hazardous (see Administration and Dosage).

Alternatively, asparaginase derived from a source other than *E coli* may be appropriate. Erwinia asparaginase is available from the National Cancer Institute for selected cases (see page 2647).

Hepatotoxicity occurs in the majority of patients. Therapy may increase preexisting liver impairment caused by prior therapy or underlying disease; asparaginase may increase the toxicity of other medications.

Usage in Pregnancy: Category C. Asparaginase has been shown to retard the weight gain of mothers and fetuses, has caused resorptions, and has resulted in dose-dependent embryotoxicity and gross abnormalities in various rodent species when given in doses ranging from 0.05 to 1 times the human dose. There are no adequate and well controlled studies in pregnant women. Use during pregnancy only if the potential benefit justifies the potential risk to the fetus.

Usage in Lactation: It is not known whether this drug is excreted in breast milk. Because of potential serious adverse reactions in nursing infants, discontinue nursing or discontinue the drug, considering the importance of the drug to the mother.

(Continued on following page)

ASPARAGINASE (Cont.)

Precautions:

Monitoring: The fall in circulating lymphoblasts is often quite marked; normal or below normal leukocyte counts are noted frequently several days after initiating therapy and may be accompanied by a marked rise in serum uric acid. Uric acid nephropathy may develop; take appropriate preventive measures (eg, allopurinol, increased fluid intake, alkalinization of urine). Monitor peripheral blood count and bone marrow frequently.

Obtain frequent serum amylase determinations to detect early evidence of pancreatitis. If pancreatitis occurs, discontinue therapy.

Monitor blood sugar during therapy since hyperglycemia may occur.

Asparaginase has immunosuppressive activity in animals; consider the possibility of predisposition to infection.

This drug may be a contact irritant. Handle and administer with care. Avoid inhalation of dust or vapors and contact with skin or mucous membranes, especially the eyes. If contact occurs, wash with copious amounts of water for at least 15 minutes.

Drug Interactions:

Vincristine and **prednisone**: IV administration of asparaginase concurrently with or immediately before a course of these drugs may be associated with increased toxicity.

Methotrexate: Asparaginase may diminish or abolish methotrexate's effect on malignant cells; this effect persists as long as plasma asparagine levels are suppressed. Do not use methotrexate with, or following asparaginase, while asparagine levels are below normal.

Drug/Lab Test Interactions: L-asparaginase may interfere with the interpretation of **thyroid function tests** by producing a rapid and marked reduction in serum concentrations of thyroxine-binding globulin within 2 days after the first dose. Serum concentrations of thyroxine-binding globulin returned to pretreatment values within 4 weeks of the last dose of L-asparaginase.

Adverse Reactions:

Asparaginase toxicity is reported to be greater in adults than in children.

Hypersensitivity reactions include skin rashes, urticaria, arthralgia, respiratory distress, and acute anaphylaxis. Acute reactions have occurred in the absence of a positive skin test and during maintenance of therapeutic serum levels of the drug.

In children with advanced leukemia, a lower incidence of anaphylaxis has occurred with IM use, although there was a higher incidence of milder hypersensitivity reactions than with IV use (see Warnings).

Hyperglycemia with glucosuria and polyuria has been reported in low incidence. Serum and urine acetone are usually absent or negligible; this syndrome thus resembles hyperosmolar, nonketotic hyperglycemia. It usually responds to drug discontinuation and judicious use of IV fluid and insulin, but it may be fatal.

Bone marrow depression: Rarely, transient bone marrow depression has been seen as evidenced by a delay in return of hemoglobin or hematocrit levels to normal in patients undergoing hematologic remission of leukemia. Marked leukopenia has been reported.

Bleeding: In addition to hypofibrinogenemia, other clotting factors may be depressed. Most marked has been a decrease in factors V and VIII with a variable decrease in factors VII and IX. A decrease in circulating platelets has occurred in low incidence which, with the increased levels of fibrin degradation products in the serum, may indicate consumption coagulopathy. Bleeding has been a problem in only a few patients; however, intracranial hemorrhage and fatal bleeding associated with low fibrinogen levels have been reported. Increased compensatory fibrinolytic activity has also occurred.

CNS: Depression, somnolence, fatigue, coma, confusion, agitation and hallucinations varying from mild to severe. Rarely, a Parkinson-like syndrome has occurred, with tremor and a progressive increase in muscular tone. These effects usually reversed spontaneously after stopping treatment. No clear correlation exists between elevated blood ammonia levels and CNS changes. Headache and irritability (usually mild) have occurred.

(Adverse Reactions continued on following page)

ASPARAGINASE (Cont.)

Adverse Reactions (Cont.):

Renal: Azotemia, usually prerenal, occurs frequently. Acute renal shut-down and fatal renal insufficiency have been reported. Proteinuria has occurred infrequently.

Hepatic: Elevations of serum glutamic-oxaloacetic transaminase (SGOT), serum glutamic-pyruvic transaminase (SGPT), alkaline phosphatase, bilirubin (direct and indirect), and depression of serum albumin, cholesterol (total and esters) and plasma fibrinogen. Increases and decreases of total lipids; marked hypoalbuminemia associated with peripheral edema. These abnormalities usually are reversible on discontinuation of therapy and some reversal may occur during the course of therapy. Fatty changes in the liver (documented by biopsy) and malabsorption syndrome have been reported.

Hematologic: Rarely, transient bone marrow depression, evidenced by a delayed return of hemoglobin or hematocrit levels to normal. Marked leukopenia has been reported.

GI: Nausea, vomiting, anorexia, abdominal cramps (usually mild). Pancreatitis, sometimes fulminant, and acute hemorrhagic pancreatitis have occurred; both may be fatal.

Miscellaneous: Chills, fever, weight loss (usually mild). Fatal hyperthermia has occurred.

Administration and Dosage:

As a component of multiple agent induction regimens, administer the drug IV or IM.

IV: Give over not less than 30 minutes through the side arm of an already running infusion of Sodium Chloride Injection or 5% Dextrose Injection. The drug has little tendency to cause phlebitis when given IV.

IM: Limit the volume at a single injection site to 2 ml. For a volume greater than 2 ml, use 2 injection sites.

Induction regimens: One of the following combination regimens is recommended for acute lymphocytic leukemia in *children*. (Day 1 is considered the first day of therapy.)

Regimen I –

Prednisone 40 mg/m²/day orally in 3 divided doses for 15 days, followed by tapering of the dosage as follows: 20 mg/m² for 2 days, 10 mg/m² for 2 days, 5 mg/m² for 2 days, 2.5 mg/m² for 2 days and then discontinue.

Vincristine sulfate 2 mg/m² IV once weekly on days 1, 8 and 15. The maximum single dose should not exceed 2 mg.

Asparaginase 1,000 IU/kg/day IV for 10 successive days beginning on day 22.

Regimen II –

Prednisone 40 mg/m²/day orally in 3 divided doses for 28 days (the total daily dose to the nearest 2.5 mg), then gradual discontinuation over 14 days.

Vincristine sulfate 1.5 mg/m² IV weekly for 4 doses, on days 1, 8, 15 and 22. The maximum single dose should not exceed 2 mg.

Asparaginase 6,000 IU/m² IM on days 4, 7, 10, 13, 16, 19, 22, 25 and 28.

When remission is obtained with either of the above regimens, institute appropriate maintenance therapy. Do not use asparaginase as part of a maintenance regimen.

The above regimens do not preclude the need for special therapy to prevent CNS leukemia.

Asparaginase has been used in other combination regimens. Administering the drug IV concurrently with or immediately before a course of vincristine and prednisone may be associated with increased toxicity.

Single agent induction therapy: Use asparaginase as the sole induction agent only when a combined regimen is inappropriate because of toxicity or other specific patient-related factors, or in cases refractory to other therapy.

Children or adults – 200 IU/kg/day IV for 28 days. Complete remissions are of short duration, 1 to 3 months. Asparaginase has been used as the sole induction agent in other regimens.

Dosage adjustments: Carefully monitor patients undergoing induction therapy; individualize dosage. Adjustments always involve decreasing dosages of one or more agents or discontinuation. Patients who have received a course of therapy, if treated again, have an increased risk of hypersensitivity reactions. Therefore, repeat treatment only when the benefit of such therapy is weighed against the increased risk.

(Administration and Dosage continued on following page)

ASPARAGINASE (Cont.)

Administration and Dosage (Cont.):

Intradermal skin test: Perform an intradermal skin test prior to initial administration of asparaginase and when it is given after a week or more has elapsed between doses.

Prepare the skin test solution as follows: Reconstitute a 10,000 IU vial with 5 ml of diluent. From this solution (2,000 IU/ml), withdraw 0.1 ml and inject it into another vial containing 9.9 ml of diluent, yielding a skin test solution of approximately 20 IU/ml. Use 0.1 ml of this solution (about 2 IU) for the intradermal skin test. Observe the skin test site for at least 1 hour for a wheal or erythema that indicates a positive reaction. An allergic reaction even to the skin test dose may occur rarely. A negative skin test reaction does not preclude possible development of an allergic reaction.

Desensitization: Perform desensitization before giving the first treatment dose of asparaginase in positive reactors, and on retreatment of any patient. Attempt rapid desensitization of the patient by progressively increasing amounts of the drug IV. Take adequate precautions to treat an acute allergic reaction. One schedule begins with 1 IU given IV and doubles the dose every 10 minutes if no reaction has occurred, until the accumulated total amount given equals the planned doses for that day. For convenience, the following table is included to calculate the number of doses necessary to reach the patient's total dose for that day:

Injection Number	Dose (IU)	Accumulated Total Dose (IU)
1	1	1
2	2	3
3	4	7
4	8	15
5	16	31
6	32	63
7	64	127
8	128	255
9	256	511
10	512	1,023
11	1,024	2,047
12	2,048	4,095
13	4,096	8,191
14	8,192	16,383
15	16,384	32,767
16	32,768	65,535
17	65,536	131,071
18	131,072	262,143

Preparation of solutions: Solution should be clear and colorless. If it becomes cloudy, discard.

IV – Reconstitute the 10,000 unit vial with 5 ml Sterile Water for Injection or with Sodium Chloride Injection. Ordinary shaking during reconstitution does not inactivate the enzyme. This solution may be used for direct IV administration within 8 hours following reconstitution. For administration by infusion, dilute solutions with Sodium Chloride Injection or 5% Dextrose Injection. Infuse within 8 hours and only if clear.

Occasionally, gelatinous fiber-like particles may develop on standing. Filtration through a 5 micron filter during administration will remove the particles with no loss of potency. Some loss of potency has been observed with the use of a 0.2 micron filter.

IM – Reconstitute by adding 2 ml Sodium Chloride Injection to the 10,000 unit vial. Use the resulting solution within 8 hours and only if clear.

Storage: Store at 2° to 8°C (36 ° to 46°F). Because it does not contain a preservative, store reconstituted solution at 2° to 8°C (36° to 46°F); discard after 8 hours or sooner if cloudy.

Rx	**Elspar** (MSD)	**Powder for Injection:** 10,000 IU	In 10 ml vials.[1]

[1] With 80 mg mannitol.

The National Cancer Institute (NCI), Division of Cancer Treatment (DCT) is involved in the development and research of antineoplastic drugs. Agents under investigation are categorized and distributed as follows:

Group A: Used in Phase I and II clinical studies. Distribution is limited to intramural investigators, members of the Phase I Working Group, Cancer Therapy Evaluation Program contractors and cooperative groups who have been given permission to do Phase I and II studies with these agents.

Group B: Agents tested in Phase II studies and considered worthy of further clinical studies by the New Drug Liaison Meetings and the Cancer Therapy Evaluation Program staff. They are distributed to cooperative groups, NCI contractors and cancer center directors through the New Drug Studies mechanism.

Group C: Agents found effective in the treatment of a specific neoplasm through multiple studies that have changed the approach to therapy. They can be distributed to any properly trained physician for use without specialized supportive care facilities.

Use of Group C Agents:

Physicians desiring to use Group C investigational agents must: (1) register as an investigator with NCI by submitting FD-form 1573; (2) submit a request for the drugs, indicating the disease to be treated; (3) follow NCI established protocol; (4) report all adverse reactions to the NCI Investigational Drug Branch. For further information contact: Investigational Drug Branch, National Cancer Institute, Executive Plaza North, Room 715, Bethesda, Maryland 20892, (301) 496-1196.

The following Group C agents are available from NCI for the conditions indicated:

Amsacrine

Other Names: NSC-249992, m-AMSA, Acridinyl Anisidide

Use: Refractory adult acute myelogenous leukemia

Azacitidine

Other Names: NSC-102816, 5-Azacytidine, AZA-CR, 5-AZC, Ladakamycin

Use: Refractory acute myelogenous leukemia (AML)

Erwinia Asparaginase

Other Names: NSC-106977, Porton Asparaginase

Use: Acute lymphocytic leukemia (ALL) in patients sensitive to *E Coli* L-asparaginase

chapter 12

miscellaneous products

This information on local anesthetics is not intended to be comprehensive. Consult standard textbooks for further discussion of techniques and applications.

Actions:

Pharmacology: Local anesthetics prevent the generation and conduction of nerve impulses by reducing sodium permeability, increasing the electrical excitation threshold, slowing the nerve impulse propagation and reducing the rate of rise of the action potential; the exact mechanism is unknown. The progression of anesthesia is related to the diameter, myelination and conduction velocity of affected nerve fibers. The order of loss of nerve function is as follows: Pain, temperature, touch, proprioception and skeletal muscle tone.

Systemic absorption of local anesthetics affects the cardiovascular system and CNS. At blood concentrations achieved with normal therapeutic doses, changes in cardiac conduction, excitability, refractoriness, contractility and peripheral vascular resistance are minimal. However, toxic blood concentrations depress cardiac conduction and excitability, which may lead to atrioventricular block and ultimately to cardiac arrest. In addition, with toxic blood concentrations, myocardial contractility may be depressed and peripheral vasodilation may occur, leading to decreased cardiac output and arterial blood pressure.

Following systemic absorption, toxic blood concentrations of local anesthetics can produce CNS stimulation, depression or both. Apparent central stimulation may be manifested as restlessness, tremors and shivering, which may progress to convulsions. Depression and coma may occur, possibly progressing ultimately to respiratory arrest. The local anesthetics have a primary depressant effect on the medulla and on higher centers. The depressed stage may occur without a prior stage of central nervous system stimulation.

The use of *vasoconstrictors* (eg, epinephrine, norepinephrine or levonordefrin) in conjunction with local anesthetics promotes local hemostasis, decreases systemic absorption and prolongs the duration of action. Levonordefrin is similar to epinephrine; it is less potent than epinephrine in raising blood pressure and as a vasoconstrictor, but is more stable.

Pharmacokinetics: Various pharmacokinetic parameters of the local anesthetics can be significantly altered by the presence of hepatic or renal disease, addition of epinephrine, factors affecting urinary pH, renal blood flow, the route of administration, and age of patient. Pharmacokinetic parameters for injectable local anesthetics are summarized below:

Anesthetic	Onset (minutes)	Duration (hours)	Equivalent Anesthetic Concentration (%)	pKa	Partition[3] Coefficient	Systemic Protein Binding (%)
ESTERS						
Procaine[1]	2-5	0.25-0.5	2	8.9	0.02	5
(w/Epinephrine)	nd	0.5-1.5				
(Epidural)[2]	15-25	0.5-1.5				
Chloroprocaine[1]	6-12	0.25-0.5	2	8.7	0.14	nd
(w/Epinephrine)	nd	0.5-1.5				
(Epidural)[2]	5-15	0.5-1.5				
Tetracaine[1]	up to 15	2-3	0.25	8.5	4.1	85
(Epidural)[2]	20-30	3-5				
(Spinal)	nd	1.25-2.5				
AMIDES						
Lidocaine[1]	0.5-1	0.5-1	1	7.9	2.9	55-65
(w/Epinephrine)	nd	2-6				
(Epidural)[2]	5-15	1-3				
(Spinal)	nd	0.5-1.5				
Prilocaine[1]	1-2	0.5-1.5	1	7.9	0.9	55
(w/Epinephrine)	nd	2-6				
(Epidural)[2]	5-15	1-3				
Mepivacaine[1]	3-5	0.75-1.5	1	7.6	0.8	65-77
(w/Epinephrine)	nd	2-6				
(Epidural)[2]	5-15	1-3				
(Spinal)	nd	0.5-1.5				
Bupivacaine[1]	5	2-4	0.25	8.1	27.5	84-95
(w/Epinephrine)	nd	3-7				
(Epidural)[2]	10-20	3-5				
(Spinal)	nd	1.25-2.5				
Etidocaine[1]	3-5	2-3	0.5	7.7	141	94
(w/Epinephrine)	nd	3-7				
(Epidural)[2]	5-15	3-5				

[1] Values in this line represent those for infiltrative anesthesia. nd – No data.
[2] With epinephrine 1:200,000.
[3] n-Heptane/Buffer, pH 7.4.

(Actions continued on following page)

Actions (Cont.):

Pharmacokinetics (Cont.): Rate of systemic absorption depends on total dose and concentration of drug, vascularity of administration site and presence of vasoconstrictors. Depending on route, local anesthetics are distributed to some extent to all body tissues. High concentrations are found in highly perfused organs (eg, liver, lungs, heart, brain). The rate and extent of placental diffusion is determined by plasma protein binding, ionization and lipid solubility. It is the nonionized form of the drug which crosses cellular membranes to the site of action. Fetal/maternal ratios are inversely related to degree of protein binding. Only the free, unbound drug is available for placental transfer. Drugs with the highest protein binding capacity may have the lowest fetal/maternal ratios. Lipid soluble, nonionized drugs readily enter the fetal blood from the maternal circulation.

Onset of local anesthesia is dependent on the dissociation constant (pKa), lipid solubility, pH of the solution, protein binding and molecular size. In general, local anesthetics with high lipid solubility or low pKa have a faster onset.

Local anesthetics are divided into two groups: *Esters* which are derivatives of para-aminobenzoic acid and *amides* which are derivatives of aniline. The "ester" local anesthetics are metabolized by hydrolysis of the ester linkage by plasma esterase, probably plasma cholinesterase. The "amide" local anesthetics are metabolized primarily in the liver, then excreted primarily in the urine as metabolites, with a small fraction of unchanged drug. Biliary excretion may contribute to the disposition of lidocaine, mepivacaine and tetracaine. Hypersensitivity reactions may occur with local anesthetics of the ester type (see Precautions).

Indications:

Refer to individual product listings.

Contraindications:

Hypersensitivity to local anesthetics, para-aminobenzoic acid or parabens.

Do not use large doses of local anesthetics in patients with heart block.

Do not use **prilocaine** in patients with methemoglobinemia.

Bupivacaine is contraindicated in obstetrical paracervical block anesthesia; use in this technique has resulted in fetal bradycardia and death. Bupivacaine is not recommended for IV regional anesthesia (Bier block); cardiac arrest and death have occurred. See Warnings.

Spinal anesthesia is contraindicated in septicemia.

Do not use **chloroprocaine HCl** for subarachnoid administration.

Warnings:

The 0.75% concentration of **bupivacaine** is not recommended for obstetrical anesthesia. Cardiac arrest with difficult resuscitation or death has occurred during use for epidural anesthesia in obstetrical patients. Resuscitation has been difficult or impossible despite adequate preparation and appropriate management. Cardiac arrest has occurred after convulsions resulting from systemic toxicity, presumably following unintentional intravascular injection. Reserve the 0.75% concentration for surgical procedures where a high degree of muscle relaxation and prolonged effect are necessary.

Have resuscitative equipment and drugs immediately available when any local anesthetic is used.

Do NOT use preparations containing preservatives for spinal or epidural anesthesia. When using preparations without preservatives, discard any unused drug remaining in vial.

Usage in Pregnancy: Category B (etidocaine, lidocaine, prilocaine). *Category C* (bupivacaine, chloroprocaine, mepivacaine, tetracaine). Safety for use in pregnant women, other than those in labor, has not been established. Local anesthetics rapidly cross the placenta. When used for epidural, caudal or pudendal block, they can cause varying degrees of maternal, fetal and neonatal toxicity involving alterations of the CNS, peripheral vascular tone and cardiac function. The incidence and degree of toxicity depend upon the procedure, type and amount of drug used and technique of administration.

(Warnings continued on following page)

Warnings: (Cont.):

Usage in Labor, Delivery and Abortion: Fetal bradycardia may occur in 20% to 30% of patients receiving amide-type anesthetics for paracervical block and may be associated with fetal acidosis. Always monitor fetal heart rate during paracervical anesthesia. Added risk appears to be present in prematurity, toxemia of pregnancy and fetal distress. Weigh the possible advantages against dangers when considering paracervical block in these conditions. The use of some local anesthetics during labor and delivery may be followed by diminished muscle strength and tone for the infant's first day or two of life.

Careful adherence to recommended dosage is extremely important. Failure to achieve adequate analgesia via intended paracervical or pudendal block or both with these doses may indicate intravascular or fetal intracranial injection. Babies so affected present with unexplained neonatal depression at birth and usually manifest seizures within 6 hours. Prompt use of supportive measures and forced urinary excretion of the local anesthetic have been used successfully.

Maternal hypotension has resulted from regional anesthesia. Local anesthetics produce vasodilation by blocking sympathetic nerves. Elevating the patient's legs and positioning her on her left side will help prevent decreases in blood pressure. Continuously monitor fetal heart rate; electronic monitoring is advisable. It is extremely important to avoid aorto-caval compression by the gravid uterus during administration of regional block.

Epidural, caudal or pudendal anesthesia may alter the forces of parturition through changes in uterine contractility or maternal expulsive efforts. Epidural anesthesia has been reported to prolong the second stage of labor by removing the parturient's reflex urge to bear down or by interfering with motor function. The use of obstetrical anesthesia may increase the need for forceps assistance.

Maternal convulsions and cardiovascular collapse following use of **mepivacaine** for paracervical block in early pregnancy (as anesthesia for elective abortion) suggest that systemic absorption may be rapid. Therefore, do not exceed the recommended maximum dose of 100 mg per side. Inject slowly, with frequent aspirations. Allow a 5 minute interval between sides.

Head and Neck Area: Small doses of local anesthetics injected into the head and neck area, including retrobulbar, dental and stellate ganglion blocks, may produce adverse reactions similar to systemic toxicity seen with unintentional intravascular injections of larger doses. Fatalities have occurred. The injection procedures require the utmost care. Confusion, convulsions, respiratory depression or arrest, and cardiovascular stimulation or depression have been reported. These reactions may be due to intra-arterial injection of the local anesthetic with retrograde flow to cerebral circulation. They may also be due to puncture of the dural sheath of the optic nerve during retrobulbar block with diffusion of any local anesthetic along the subdural space to the midbrain. Observe patient carefully. Monitor respiration and circulation. Do not exceed dosage recommendations.

When local anesthetic solutions are used for retrobulbar block, complete corneal anesthesia usually precedes onset of clinically acceptable external ocular muscle akinesia. Therefore, presence of akinesia rather than anesthesia alone should determine readiness of the patient for surgery.

Dentistry: Because of the long duration of anesthesia of **bupivacaine with epinephrine**, caution patients about the possibility of inadvertent trauma to tongue, lips and buccal mucosa and advise against chewing solid foods or testing anesthetized area by biting or probing.

Cardiovascular reactions are depressant. They may be the result of direct drug effect, or, more commonly in dental practice, the result of vasovagal reaction, particularly if the patient is in the sitting position. Failure to recognize premonitory signs such as sweating, feeling of faintness, changes in pulse or sensorium may result in progressive cerebral hypoxia and seizure, or serious cardiovascular catastrophe. Place patient in recumbent position and administer oxygen. Vasoactive drugs such as ephedrine or methoxamine may be administered IV.

Usage in Lactation: Safety for use in the nursing mother has not been established. It is not known whether local anesthetic drugs are excreted in breast milk.

Usage in Children: Due to lack of clinical experience, the administration of **bupivacaine** to children under 12 is not recommended.

(Continued on following page)

Precautions:

Use with inflammation or sepsis: Use local anesthetic procedures with caution when there is inflammation or sepsis in the region of proposed injection.

Monitor cardiovascular and respiratory vital signs and state of consciousness after each injection. Restlessness, anxiety, incoherent speech, lightheadedness, numbness and tingling of the mouth and lips, metallic taste, tinnitus, dizziness, blurred vision, tremors, twitching, depression or drowsiness may be early signs of CNS toxicity.

Debilitated or elderly patients, acutely ill patients, children, obstetric delivery patients, and patients with increased intra-abdominal pressure: Repeated doses may cause accumulation of the drug or its metabolites or slow metabolic degradation. Give reduced doses. Use anesthetics with caution in patients with severe shock or heart block.

Malignant hyperthermia: Many drugs used during anesthesia are considered potential triggering agents for familial malignant hyperthermia. It is not known whether amide-type local anesthetics may trigger this reaction and the need for supplemental general anesthesia cannot be predicted in advance; therefore, have a standard protocol for management available.

Epidural and caudal anesthesia: Use with extreme caution in pediatric patients and in persons with existing neurological disease, spinal deformities, septicemia and severe hypertension.

Vasoconstrictors: Use solutions containing a vasoconstrictor with caution and in carefully circumscribed quantities in areas of the body supplied by end arteries or having otherwise compromised blood supply. Use with extreme caution in patients whose medical history and physical evaluation suggest the existence of hypertension, peripheral vascular disease, arteriosclerotic heart disease, cerebral vascular insufficiency, heart block, thyrotoxicosis or diabetes. These individuals may exhibit exaggerated vasoconstrictor response.

Intravenous regional anesthesia: Proper tourniquet technique is essential. Do NOT use solutions containing epinephrine or other vasoconstrictors for this technique.

Cardiac arrest and death are reported with the use of **bupivacaine** for IV regional anesthesia (Bier block). Bupivacaine is not recommended for this technique.

Hypersensitivity reactions including anaphylaxis may occur in a small segment of the population allergic to para-aminobenzoic acid derivatives (procaine, tetracaine, benzocaine, etc). The amide-type local anesthetics have not shown cross-sensitivity with the esters. Hypersensitivity reactions and anaphylaxis have occurred rarely with lidocaine. See also Management of Acute Hypersensitivity Reactions on p. 2897

Administer ester-type local anesthetics cautiously to patients with abnormal or reduced levels of plasma esterases.

Sulfite hypersensitivity: Some of these products contain sulfites. Sulfites may cause allergic-type reactions (eg, hives, itching, wheezing, anaphylaxis) in certain susceptible persons. Although the overall prevalence of sulfite sensitivity in the general population is probably low, it is seen more frequently in asthmatics or in atopic nonasthmatic persons.

Usage in impaired hepatic function: Because amide-type local anesthetics are metabolized primarily in the liver, patients with hepatic disease, especially severe hepatic disease, may be more susceptible to potential toxicity. Use cautiously in such patients.

Usage in renal disease: Use **mepivacaine** with caution in patients with renal disease.

(Continued on following page)

Drug Interactions:

Intercurrent use: Mixtures of local anesthetics are sometimes employed to compensate for the slower onset of one drug and the shorter duration of action of the second drug. Toxicity is probably additive with mixtures of local anesthetics, but some experiments suggest synergisms. Exercise caution regarding toxic equivalence when mixtures of local anesthetics are employed.

Prior use of **chloroprocaine** may interfere with subsequent use of **bupivacaine**. Because of this, and because safety of intercurrent use of bupivacaine and chloroprocaine has not been established, such use is not recommended.

Vasopressors (for the treatment of hypotension related to obstetric blocks) and **ergot-type oxytocics:** Concurrent administration may cause severe, persistent hypertension or cerebrovascular accidents.

MAO inhibitors, tricyclic antidepressants, phenothiazines: Use solutions containing a vasoconstrictor with extreme caution in patients receiving drugs that produce blood pressure alterations; severe and sustained hypotension or hypertension may occur.

Inhalation anesthetics: Serious dose-related cardiac arrhythmias may occur if preparations containing a vasoconstrictor such as epinephrine are employed in patients during or following the administration of potent inhalation anesthetics. Consider the combined action of both agents upon the myocardium, the concentration and volume of vasoconstrictor used and the time since injection.

Sulfonamides: The para-aminobenzoic acid metabolite of procaine, chloroprocaine and tetracaine inhibits the action of sulfonamides. Despite adequate sulfonamide therapy, local infections have occurred in areas infiltrated with procaine prior to diagnostic punctures and drainage procedures. Therefore, do not use procaine, chloroprocaine or tetracaine in any condition in which a sulfonamide drug is employed.

Sedatives: If employed to reduce patient apprehension during dental procedures, use reduced doses, since local anesthetics used in combination with CNS depressants may have additive effects. Give young children minimal doses of each agent.

Metals react with local anesthetics and cause the release of the metals' respective ions which, if injected, may cause severe local irritation. Do not use disinfecting agents containing heavy metals for skin or mucous membrane disinfection.

Adverse Reactions:

The most common acute adverse reactions are related to the CNS and cardiovascular systems. These are generally dose-related and may result from rapid absorption from the injection site, from diminished tolerance or from unintentional intravascular injection.

CNS: Restlessness, anxiety, dizziness, tinnitus, transient loss of hearing acuity, blurred vision, nausea, vomiting, chills, pupil constriction or tremors may occur, possibly proceeding to convulsions (≈ 0.1% of local anesthetic epidural administrations). Excitement may be transient or absent, with depression being the first manifestation. This may quickly be followed by drowsiness merging into unconsciousness and respiratory arrest.

Postspinal headache, meningismus, arachnoiditis, palsies and spinal nerve paralysis (spinal anesthesia) have also occurred.

Cardiovascular: Peripheral vasodilation, myocardial depression, hypotension (with spinal anesthesia due to vasomotor paralysis and pooling of blood in the venous bed) or hypertension, decreased cardiac output, heart block, bradycardia, ventricular arrhythmias (including tachycardia and fibrillation), cardiac arrest and fetal bradycardia (see Warnings).

Allergic: Cutaneous lesions of delayed onset, urticaria, pruritis, erythema, angioneurotic edema (including laryngeal edema), sneezing, syncope, excessive sweating, elevated temperature and anaphylactoid symptoms (including severe hypotension). Sensitivity reactions to methylparaben or sulfites may occur. Skin testing is of limited value. Fatal reactions have occurred rarely.

Respiratory: Respiratory impairment or paralysis due to level of anesthesia (spinal) extending to upper thoracic and cervical segments. Respiratory arrest (following retrobulbar block injection). See Warnings.

Lumbar, epidural or caudal anesthesia: Occasional unintentional penetration of the subarachnoid space by the catheter may occur. Subsequent adverse effects may depend partially on amount of drug administered subdurally. These may include: High or total spinal block; hypotension secondary to spinal block; urinary retention; fecal or urinary incontinence; loss of perineal sensation and sexual function; persistent analgesia/anesthesia; paresthesia, weakness and paralysis of the lower extremities and loss of sphincter control; headache and backache; septic meningitis; meningismus; slowing of labor and increased incidence of forceps delivery; cranial nerve palsies due to traction on nerves from loss of cerebrospinal fluid; arachnoiditis; persistent motor, sensory or autonomic deficit of some lower spinal segments with slow (several months) or incomplete recovery.

(Adverse Reactions continued on following page)

Adverse Reactions (Cont.):

Prilocaine HCl may produce dose-dependent methemoglobinemia due to the metabolite o-toluidine. Administration of prilocaine in doses exceeding 400 mg has been associated with methemoglobinemia in adult patients and with proportionately lower doses in children. While methemoglobin values of less than 20% do not generally produce any clinical symptoms, evalute the appearance of cyanosis at 2 to 4 hours following administration in terms of the patient's status.

Treat methemoglobinemia with 1 to 2 mg/kg of methylene blue administered IV over 5 minutes (see page 2697).

Overdosage:

Acute emergencies from local anesthetics are generally related to high plasma levels encountered during therapeutic use or to unintended subarachnoid injection.

Management: The first consideration is prevention.

Convulsions, as well as underventilation or apnea, are due to unintentional subarachnoid injection; maintain patent airway and assist or control ventilation with oxygen and a delivery system capable of permitting immediate positive airway pressure by mask. Evaluate circulation. If convulsions persist despite respiratory support, and if the status of the circulation permits, give small increments of an ultra short-acting barbiturate (ie, thiopental or thiamylal) or a benzodiazepine (ie, diazepam) IV. Circulatory depression may require administration of IV fluids and a vasopressor.

If not treated immediately, convulsions and cardiovascular depression can result in hypoxia, acidosis, bradycardia, arrhythmias and cardiac arrest. Underventilation or apnea may produce these same signs and also lead to cardiac arrest if ventilatory support is not instituted. If cardiac arrest occurs, institute standard cardiopulmonary resuscitative measures.

Endotracheal intubation may be indicated.

Patient Information:

When appropriate, inform patients in advance that they may experience temporary loss of sensation and motor activity, usually in the lower half of the body, following proper administration of caudal or epidural anesthesia.

Administration and Dosage:

The dose of local anesthetic administered varies with the procedure, vascularity of the tissues, depth of anesthesia, degree of required muscle relaxation, duration of anesthesia desired, and the physical condition of the patient. Reduce dosages for children, elderly and debilitated patients and patients with cardiac or liver disease.

Infiltration or regional block anesthesia: Always inject slowly, with frequent aspirations.

Prevent intravascular injection. Inject slowly with frequent aspirations to avoid systemic reactions.

(Products listed on following pages)

Complete prescribing information for these products begins on page 2654.

PROCAINE HCl, INJECTABLE

Indications:

Infiltration anesthesia: 0.25% to 0.5% solution.

Peripheral nerve block: 0.5% to 2% solution.

Spinal anesthesia: 10% solution.

Dilution instructions: To prepare 60 ml of a 0.5% solution (5 mg/ml), dilute 30 ml of the 1% solution with 30 ml sterile distilled water. To prepare 60 ml of a 0.25% solution (2.5 mg/ml), dilute 15 ml of the 1% solution with 45 ml sterile distilled water. Add 0.5 to 1 ml of epinephrine 1:1000 per 100 ml anesthetic solution for vasoconstrictive effect (1:200,000 to 1:100,000).

	Product	Form	Package	C.I.*
Rx	**Procaine HCl** (Various)	**Injection:** 1%	In 2 ml amps and 30 and 100 ml vials.	2+
Rx	**Novocain** (Winthrop Pharm.)		In 2 and 6 ml amps and 30 ml vials.	4
Rx	**Procaine HCl** (Various)	**Injection:** 2%	In 30 and 100 ml vials.	2+
Rx	**Novocain** (Winthrop Pharm.)		In 30 ml vials.	28
Rx	**Novocain** (Winthrop Pharm.)	**Injection:** 10%	In 2 ml amps.[1]	208

CHLOROPROCAINE HCl

Indications:

Infiltration and peripheral nerve block: 1% to 2% solution.

Mandibular - 2% solution.
Infraorbital - 2% solution.
Brachial Plexus - 2% solution.
Digital (without epinephrine) - 1% solution.
Pudendal block - 2% solution.
Paracervical block - 1% solution.

Infiltration, peripheral and central nerve block, including caudal and epidural block: 2% or 3% solution (without preservatives).

	Product	Form	Package	C.I.*
Rx	**Nesacaine** (Astra)	**Injection:**[2] 1%	In 30 ml vials.	35
		2% (Not for epidural or caudal block.)	In 30 ml vials.	36
Rx	**Nesacaine-MPF** (Astra)	**Injection:**[3,4] 2%	In 30 ml vials.	39
		3%	In 30 ml vials.	41

TETRACAINE HCl

Indications:

Spinal anesthesia (high, median, low and saddle blocks): 0.2% to 0.3% solution.

Spinal anesthesia, prolonged (2 to 3 hours): 1% solution.

Store under refrigeration.

	Product	Form	Package	C.I.*
Rx	**Pontocaine HCl** (Winthrop Pharm.)	**Injection:** 1%	In 2 ml amps.[1]	158
		0.2% with 6% dextrose	In 2 ml amps.	155
		0.3% with 6% dextrose	In 5 ml amps.	79
		Powder for reconstitution	In 20 mg Niphanoid (instantly soluble) amps.	32

* Cost Index based on cost per ml.
[1] With acetone sodium bisulfite.
[2] With methylparaben and EDTA.
[3] Preservative free.
[4] With EDTA.

Complete prescribing information for these products begins on page 2654.

PROPOXYCAINE HCl and PROCAINE HCl

Indications:

For local anesthesia by nerve block or infiltration in dental procedures.

			C.I.*
Rx	**Ravocaine and Novocain with Levophed** (Cook-Waite)	**Injection:** 7.2 mg propoxycaine HCl, 36 mg procaine with norepinephrine 0.12 mg per 1.8 ml dental cartridge.[1]	†
Rx	**Ravocaine and Novocain with Neo-Cobefrin** (Cook-Waite)	**Injection:** 7.2 mg propoxycaine HCl, 36 mg procaine with levonordefrin 0.09 mg per 1.8 ml dental cartridge.[1]	†

LIDOCAINE HCl

Indications:

Infiltration:
- *Percutaneous* - 0.5% or 1% solution.
- *IV regional* - 0.5% solution.

Peripheral nerve block:
- *Brachial* - 1.5% solution.
- *Dental* - 2% solution.
- *Intercostal or paravertebral* - 1% solution.
- *Pudendal or paracervical obstetrical (each side)* - 1% solution.

Sympathetic nerve blocks:
- *Cervical (stellate ganglion) or lumbar* - 1% solution.

Central neural blocks:
- *Epidural* -
  - *Thoracic:* 1% solution.
  - *Lumbar:*
    - *Analgesia* - 1% solution.
    - *Anesthesia* - 1.5% or 2% solution.

Caudal:
- *Obstetrical analgesia* - 1% solution.
- *Surgical anesthesia* - 1.5% solution.

Spinal anesthesia - 5% solution with glucose.

Low spinal or "saddle block" anesthesia: 1.5% solution with dextrose.

Retrobulbar or transtracheal injection: 4% solution.

				C.I.*
Rx	**Xylocaine HCl** (Astra)	**Injection:** 0.5%	In 50 ml single and multiple[2] dose vials.	7
Rx	**Lidocaine HCl** (Various)	**Injection:** 1%	In 2 and 5 ml amps, 2, 30 and 50 ml vials, and 5, 10, 20 and 30 ml syringes.	2+
Rx	**Caine-1** (Parnell)		In 50 ml vials.	5
Rx	**Dilocaine** (Hauck)		In 50 ml vials.	6
Rx	**L-Caine** (Century)		In 50 ml vials.	4
Rx	**Lidoject-1** (Mayrand)		In 50 ml vials.	10
Rx	**Nervocaine 1%** (Keene)		In 50 ml vials.	6
Rx	**Nulicaine** (Kay)		In 50 ml vials.[2]	4
Rx	**Xylocaine HCl** (Astra)		In 2, 5 and 30 ml amps, 20 & 50 ml multiple dose vials[2] and 30 ml single dose vials.	4
Rx	**Lidocaine HCl** (Various)	**Injection:** 1.5%	In 20 ml amps.	27+
Rx	**Xylocaine HCl** (Astra)		In 20 ml single dose amps & 20 ml single dose vials.	36

* Cost Index based on cost per ml.
† Price not available from distributor.
[1] With acetone sodium bisulfite.
[2] With methylparaben.

(Continued on following page)

Complete prescribing information for these products begins on page 2654.

LIDOCAINE HCl (Cont.)

	Product	Strength	How supplied	C.I.*
Rx	**Lidocaine HCl** (Various)	**Injection:** 2%	In 2 and 10 ml amps, 2, 5, 30 and 50 ml vials, and 5 and 10 ml syringes.	2+
Rx	**Caine-2** (Parnell)		In 50 ml vials.	5
Rx	**Dalcaine** (Forest)		In 5 ml vials.[1]	52
Rx	**Dilocaine** (Hauck)		In 50 ml vials.[2]	6
Rx	**Lidoject-2** (Mayrand)		In 50 ml vials.	10
Rx	**Nervocaine 2%** (Keene)		In 50 ml vials.	6
Rx	**Nulicaine** (Kay)		In 50 ml vials.[2]	4
Rx	**Xylocaine HCl** (Astra)		In 2, 5 and 10 ml amps, 20[2] and 50[2] ml vials, 5 ml syringes and 1.8 ml dental cartridge.	7
Rx	**Xylocaine HCl** (Astra)	**Injection:** 4%	In 5 ml amps.	93
Rx	**Duo-Trach Kit** (Astra)		In 5 ml disp. syringe with laryngotracheal cannula.	151
Rx	**Lidocaine HCl** (Various)	**Injection:** 10%	In 10 ml vials.	86+
Rx	**Lidocaine HCl** (Various)	**Injection:** 20%	In 10 and 20 ml vials and 5 ml syringes.	108+
Rx	**Xylocaine HCl** (Astra)	**Injection:** 0.5% with 1:200,000 epinephrine	In 50 ml vials.[3]	7
Rx	**Xylocaine HCl** (Astra)	**Injection:** 1% with 1:100,000 epinephrine	In 20 and 50 ml vials.[3]	10
Rx	**Xylocaine HCl** (Astra)	**Injection:** 1% with 1:200,000 epinephrine	In 30 ml amps[4] and 30 ml vials.[4]	25
Rx	**Lidocaine HCl** (Abbott)	**Injection:** 1.5% with 1:200,000 epinephrine	In 5 ml amps.	69
Rx	**Xylocaine HCl** (Astra)		In 30 ml amps[4] and 10 and 30 ml single dose vials.[4]	26
Rx	**Octocaine HCl** (Novocol)	**Injection:** 2% with 1:50,000 epinephrine	In 1.8 ml dental cartridge.[5]	†
Rx	**Xylocaine HCl** (Astra)		In 1.8 ml dental cartridge.	134
Rx	**Octocaine HCl** (Novocol)	**Injection:** 2% with 1:100,000 epinephrine	In 1.8 ml dental cartridge.[5]	†
Rx	**Xylocaine HCl** (Astra)		In 20 and 50 ml vials[3] and 1.8 ml dental cartridge.	11
Rx	**Xylocaine HCl** (Astra)	**Injection:** 2% with 1:200,000 epinephrine	In 20 ml amps[4] and 20 ml single dose vials.[4]	43
Rx	**Xylocaine HCl** (Astra)	**Injection:** 1.5% with 7.5% dextrose	In 2 ml amps.	357
Rx	**Xylocaine HCl** (Astra)	**Injection:** 5% with 7.5% glucose	In 2 ml amps.	321

* Cost Index based on cost per ml.
† Price not available from distributor.
[1] Preservative free.
[2] With methylparaben.
[3] With methylparaben and sodium metabisulfite.
[4] With sodium metabisulfite.
[5] With sodium bisulfite.

Complete prescribing information for these products begins on page 2654

PRILOCAINE HCl

Indications:

For local anesthesia by nerve block or infiltration in dental procedures: 4% solution.

				C.I.*
Rx	**Citanest HCl** (Astra)	**Injection, Plain:** 4%	In 1.8 ml dental cartridge.	17
		Injection, Forte: 4% with 1:200,000 epinephrine	In 1.8 ml dental cartridge.[1]	17

MEPIVACAINE HCl

Indications:

Nerve block (eg, cervical, brachial, intercostal, pudendal): 1% or 2% solution.
Transvaginal block (paracervical plus pudendal): 1% solution.
Paracervical block in obstetrics: 1% solution.
Caudal and epidural block: 1%, 1.5% or 2% solution.
Infiltration: 1% solution.
Therapeutic block: 1% or 2% solution.
Dental procedures (infiltration or nerve block): 3% solution or 2% solution with levonordefrin.

				C.I.*
Rx	**Carbocaine** (Winthrop Pharm.)	**Injection:** 1%	In 30 ml vials and 50 ml[2] vials.	21
Rx	**Mepivacaine HCl** (Goldline)		In 50 ml[2] multiple dose vials.	NA
Rx	**Polocaine** (Astra)		In 30 and 50 ml vials.	20
Rx	**Carbocaine** (Winthrop Pharm.)	**Injection:** 1.5%	In 30 ml vials.	28
Rx	**Polocaine** (Astra)		In 30 ml vials.	26
Rx	**Carbocaine** (Winthrop Pharm.)	**Injection:** 2%	In 20 ml vials and 50 ml[2] vials.	35
Rx	**Polocaine** (Astra)		In 30 and 50 ml vials.	30
Rx	**Carbocaine** (Cook-Waite)	**Injection:** 3%	In 1.8 ml dental cartridge.	†
Rx	**Isocaine HCl** (Novocol)		In 1.8 ml dental cartridge.	†
Rx	**Polocaine** (Astra)		In 1.8 ml dental cartridge.	18
Rx	**Carbocaine with Neo-Cobefrin** (Cook-Waite)	**Injection:** 2% with 1:20,000 levonordefrin	In 1.8 ml dental cartridge.[3]	†
Rx	**Isocaine HCl** (Novocol)		In 1.8 ml dental cartridge.[4]	†

* Cost Index based on cost per ml.
† Price not available from distributor.
[1] With sodium metabisulfite.
[2] With methylparaben.
[3] With acetone sodium bisulfite.
[4] With sodium bisulfite.

Complete prescribing information for these products begins on page2654

BUPIVACAINE HCl

Indications:

Local infiltration: 0.25% solution.
Lumbar epidural: 0.25%, 0.5% and 0.75% solutions (0.75% nonobstetrical).
Subarachnoid block: 0.75% solution.
Caudal block: 0.25% and 0.5% solutions.
Peripheral nerve block: 0.25% and 0.5% solutions.
Retrobulbar block: 0.75% solution.
Sympathetic block: 0.25% solution.
Dental block: 0.5% solution with epinephrine.

				C.I.*
Rx	**Bupivacaine HCl** (Abbott)	**Injection:** 0.25%	In 20 ml amps and 50 ml syringes.	45
Rx	**Marcaine HCl** (Winthrop Pharm.)		In 50 ml amps and 10, 30 and 50[1] ml vials.	21
Rx	**Sensorcaine** (Astra)		In 30 ml amps and 30 and 50[1] ml vials.	19
Rx	**Bupivacaine HCl** (Abbott)	**Injection:** 0.5%	In 20 ml amps and 30 ml syringes.	48
Rx	**Marcaine HCl** (Winthrop Pharm.)		In 30 ml amps and 10, 30 and 50[1] ml vials.	29
Rx	**Sensorcaine** (Astra)		In 30 ml amps and 10, 30 and 50[1] ml vials.	19
Rx	**Bupivacaine HCl** (Abbott)	**Injection:** 0.75%	In 20 ml amps and 20 ml syringes.	41
Rx	**Marcaine HCl** (Winthrop Pharm.)		In 30 ml amps and 10 and 30 ml vials.	34
Rx	**Marcaine Spinal** (Winthrop Pharm.)		In 2 ml single dose amps.[2]	192
Rx	**Sensorcaine** (Astra)		In 30 ml amps.	22
Rx	**Marcaine HCl** (Winthrop Pharm.)	**Injection:** 0.25% with 1:200,000 epinephrine	In 50 ml amps[3] and 10,[3] 30[3] and 50[4] ml vials.	21
		0.5% with 1:200,000 epinephrine	In 3 and 30 ml amps[3] and 10,[3] 30[3] and 50[4] ml vials.	29
		0.75% with 1:200,000 epinephrine	In 30 ml amps.[3]	30
Rx	**Marcaine with Epinephrine** (Cook-Waite)	**Injection:** 0.5% with 1:200,000 epinephrine	In 1.8 ml dental cartridges.[3]	†
Rx	**Sensorcaine** (Astra)	**Injection:** 0.5% with 1:200,000 epinephrine	In 5 and 30 ml amps[4] and 30 ml vials.[5]	22
		0.75% with 1:200,000 epinephrine	In 30 ml amps[4] and 30 ml vials.[5]	21

ETIDOCAINE HCl

Indications:

Peripheral nerve block, central nerve block or lumbar peridural: 1% solution.
Intra-abdominal or pelvic surgery, lower limb surgery or caesarean section: 1% or 1.5% solution.
Caudal: 1% solution.
Maxillary infiltration or inferior alveolar nerve block: 1.5% solution.

				C.I.*
Rx	**Duranest HCl** (Astra)	**Injection:** 1%	In 30 ml single dose vials.	48
		1% with 1:200,000 epinephrine	In 30 ml single dose vials.[5]	52
		1.5% with 1:200,000 epinephrine	In 20 ml amps.[5]	82

* Cost Index based on cost per ml.
† Price not available from distributor.
[1] With methylparaben.
[2] With 8.25% dextrose.
[3] With sodium metabisulfite and EDTA.
[4] With sodium metabisulfite, EDTA and methylparaben.
[5] With sodium metabisulfite.

ADENOSINE PHOSPHATE (A_5MP)

Actions:

Adenosine monophosphate (A_5MP) is converted to adenosine which is associated with many normal biochemical processes. The mechanism of action is not understood. Clinical benefit may result from correction of underlying biochemical imbalances or deficiencies at the cellular level. Beneficial therapeutic effects may be due in part to the drug's vasodilating action. The drug may also be a neurotransmitter.

Indications:

Symptomatic relief of varicose vein complications with stasis dermatitis.

Unlabeled Uses: Adenosine monophosphate has been used in the treatment of herpes infections.

Adenosine is currently being investigated for use in supraventricular tachycardia and in increasing blood flow to brain tumors.

Contraindications:

History of myocardial infarction; cerebral hemorrhage.

Warnings:

Anaphylactoid reactions: If a patient complains of dyspnea and chest tightness following an injection, do not administer further injections. Immediately institute treatment for allergic reactions.

Toxic effects: AMP is converted to adenosine which may inhibit immune system function. Use with caution.

Usage in Pregnancy: Safe use has not been established with respect to adverse effects upon fetal development. Do not use in women of childbearing potential and particularly during early pregnancy unless the benefits outweigh the potential hazards.

Usage in Children: Not recommended for use in children. Clinical experience has been insufficient to establish safety or a suitable dosage regimen.

Adverse Reactions:

Flushing, dizziness and palpitations. Hypotension, dyspnea, epigastric discomfort, nausea, occasional local rash and diuresis, increase in symptoms of bursitis and tendinitis.

Administration and Dosage:

Not for IV use. Administer IM only.

Initial: Administer 25 to 50 mg once or twice daily until symptoms subside.

Maintenance: 25 mg 2 or 3 times weekly.

				C.I.*
Rx	**Adenosine Phosphate** (Various)	**Injection:** 25 mg per ml in an aqueous solution	In 10 and 30 ml vials.	25+
Rx	**Cobalasine** (Keene)		In 10 ml vials.	103
Rx	**Kaysine** (Kay Pharm)		In 10 ml vials.	40

* Cost Index based on cost per 25 mg.

LIVER DERIVATIVE COMPLEX

Actions: Claimed to enhance the resolution of inflammation and edema.

Indications: Management of acne vulgaris, herpes zoster, "poison ivy" dermatitis, pityriasis rosea, seborrheic dermatitis, urticaria and eczema, severe sunburn, rosacea.

Contraindications: Hypersensitivity or intolerance to liver.

Warnings: Use with caution in patients suspected of being hypersensitive to liver or with other allergic diatheses.

Adverse Reactions: No serious side effects have been reported.

Administration and Dosage: The usual dose is 2 ml SC or IM daily or as indicated.

Rx	**Kutapressin** (Kremers-Urban)	**Injection:** Liver derivative complex composed of peptides and amino acids	In 20 ml vials.[1]

SYSTEMIC DEODORIZERS

CHLOROPHYLL DERIVATIVES (Chlorophyllin)

Indications:

Oral: To control fecal and urinary odors in colostomy, ileostomy or incontinence; also for certain breath and body odors.

Topical: To promote normal healing, relieve pain and inflammation and reduce malodors in wounds, burns, surface ulcers, cuts, abrasions and skin irritations.

Adverse Reactions:

Oral: No toxic effects have been reported. A temporary mild laxative effect may occur; the stool is commonly stained dark green.

Topical: Sensitivity reactions are extremely rare; only a few instances of slight itching or irritation have been reported.

Administration and Dosage:

Topical: Ointment – Apply generously and cover with gauze, linen or other appropriate dressing. Change no more often than every 48 to 72 hours.

Solution – Apply full strength as continuous wet dressing, or instill directly into sinus tracts, fistulae, deep ulcers or cavities. As a mouthwash, use half strength.

Oral: Adults & Children (> 12) – 1 to 2 tabs/day. *Children (< 12)* – Consult physician.

Ostomies: In ostomies, take tablets orally or place in the appliance.

otc	**Chlorophyll** (Freeda)	**Tablets:** 20 mg chlorophyll	Sugar free. In 100s, 250s and 500s.
otc	**Derifil** (Rystan)	**Tablets:** 100 mg water-soluble chlorophyll derivatives	In 30s, 100s and 1000s.
otc	**PALS** (Palisades)	**Tablets:** 100 mg chlorophyllin copper complex	Coated. In 30s, 100s, 1000s and UD 30s.
otc	**Nullo** (Chattem Consumer)	**Tablets:** 33.3 mg water-soluble chlorophyllin copper complex	In 30s, 60s and 135s.
otc	**Chloresium** (Rystan)	**Tablets:** 14 mg chlorophyllin copper complex	In 100s and 1000s.
otc	**Chloresium** (Rystan)	**Solution:** 0.2% chlorophyllin copper complex in an isotonic saline solution	In 240 ml and qt.
otc	**Chloresium** (Rystan)	**Ointment:** 0.5% water-soluble chlorophyllin copper complex in a hydrophilic base	In 30 and 120 g and lb.

AMMONIA INHALANTS

AROMATIC AMMONIA SPIRIT

Ammonia vapor is a respiratory and circulatory stimulant; it is used as "smelling salts" to treat or prevent fainting.

				C.I.*
otc	**Aromatic Ammonia** (Various)	**Inhalants:** 0.33 ml	In 10s, 12s and 100s.	170+
otc	**Aromatic Ammonia Vaporole** (B-W)		36% alcohol. In 12s.	220
otc	**Aromatic Ammonia Aspirols** (Lilly)	**Inhalants:** 0.4 ml	36% alcohol. In 12s.	208
otc	**Aromatic Ammonia Spirit** (Various)	**Solution**	In 30, 60 and 120 ml, pt and gal.	37+

* Cost Index based on cost per ammonia inhaler or ml solution.

[1] Contains 0.5% phenol.

PERITONEAL DIALYSIS SOLUTIONS

Indications: Acute or chronic renal failure; acute poisoning by dialyzable toxins; intractable edema; hyperkalemia, hypercalcemia, azotemia and uremia; hepatic coma. Refer to manufacturer's package literature for specific prescribing information.

	Product and Distributor	Dextrose (g/liter)	Electrolyte content given in mEq/liter							Osmolarity (mOsm/liter)	How Supplied
			Na^+	K^+	Ca^{++}	Mg^{++}	Cl^-	Lactate	Acetate		
Rx	**Dianeal w/1.5% Dextrose** (Travenol)	15	141		3.5	1.5	101	45		364	In 1000 and 2000 ml.
Rx	**Inpersol-LM w/1.5% Dextrose** (Abbott)	15	132		3.5	0.5	96	40		346	In 1000 and 2000 ml.
Rx	**Dianeal 137 w/1.5% Dextrose** (Travenol)	15	132		3.5	1.5	102	35		347	In 2000 ml.
Rx	**Inpersol w/1.5% Dextrose** (Abbott)	15	132		3.5	1.5	102	35		347	In 1000 and 2000 ml.
Rx	**Dialyte Pattern LM w/1.5% Dextrose** (Gambro)	15	131		3.5	0.5	94	40		345	In 1000 and 2000 ml.
Rx	**Dialyte Pattern LM w/2.5% Dextrose** (Gambro)	25	131.5		3.5	0.5	94	40		395	In 2000 ml.
Rx	**Inpersol w/2.5% Dextrose** (Abbott)	25	132		3.5	1.5	102	35		398	In 1000 and 2000 ml.
Rx	**Inpersol-LM w/2.5% Dextrose** (Abbott)	25	132		3.5	0.5	96	40		396	In 1000 and 2000 ml.
Rx	**Inpersol-LM w/4.25% Dextrose** (Abbott)	42.5	132		3.5	0.5	96	40		485	In 2000 ml.
Rx	**Dianeal w/4.25% Dextrose** (Travenol)	42.5	141		3.5	1.5	101	45		503	In 2000 ml.
Rx	**Dianeal 137 w/4.25% Dextrose** (Travenol)	42.5	132		3.5	1.5	102	35		486	In 2000 ml.
Rx	**Inpersol w/4.25% Dextrose** (Abbott)	42.5	132		3.5	1.5	102	35		486	In 2000 ml.
Rx	**Dialyte Pattern LM w/4.25% Dextrose** (Gambro)	42.5	131.5		3.5	0.5	94	40		485	In 2000 ml.

[1] Concentration of formulation after dilution with 19 parts water.

Rx **Cyanide Antidote Package** (Lilly)
For the treatment of cyanide poisoning.
Package includes:
Sodium nitrite, 300 mg in 10 ml (2 amps).
Sodium thiosulfate, 12.5 g in 50 ml (2 amps).
Amyl nitrite inhalant, 0.3 ml (12 aspirols).
Also disposable syringes, stomach tube, tourniquet and instructions.

Rx **Cyanide Antidote** (Quad)
For the treatment of cyanide poisoning.
Package includes:
Sodium nitrite, 300 mg in 10 ml (2 amps).
Sodium thiosulfate, 12.5 g in 50 ml (2 amps).
Amyl nitrate inhalant, 0.3 ml (12 amps).
Also 10 ml disposable syringe with needle, stomach tube, 60 ml disposable syringe, disposable needle, 60 ml syringe tourniquet and an instruction book.

Rx **AtroPen Auto-Injector** (Survival Technology)
For toxic exposure to organophosphorus or carbamate insecticides.
Atropine sulfate with phenol, 2 mg. In prefilled automatic injection device.

Rx **LidoPen Auto-Injector** (Survival Technology)
For cardiac arrhythmias.
Lidocaine HCl, 10% solution. In 3 ml (300 mg) disposable, prefilled automatic injection device for self-administration.

Rx **EpiPen Auto-Injector** (Center Labs.[1])
For insect sting emergencies in adults.
Delivers 0.3 mg IM dose of epinephrine 1:1000 with sodium metabisulfite. In 2 ml disposable injectors.

Rx **EpiPen Jr. Auto-Injector** (Center Labs.[1])
For insect sting emergencies in children.
Delivers 0.15 mg IM dose of epinephrine 1:2000 with sodium metabisulfite.
In 2 ml disposable injectors.

Rx **Ana-Guard Epinephrine** (Hollister Stier/Miles)
Injection: 1:1000 epinephrine, < 5 mg chorobutanol and 1.5 mg sodium bisulfite per ml. In 1 ml syringes designed to deliver 2 doses of 0.3 ml each.

Rx **Ana-Kit** (Hollister Stier/Miles)
Emergency insect sting treatment.
Package includes:
Epinephrine 1:1000 in 1 ml (1 sterile syringe)
Chlorpheniramine maleate, 2 mg (4 chewable tablets)
Sterile alcohol pads (2 each)
Tourniquet (1 each)

Rx **Emergent-Ez Kit** (Healthfirst Corp.)
Adrenalin (2 amps)
Aminophylline (1 amp)
Ammonia Inhalants (3 each)
Amyl Nitrite Inhalants (2 each)
Atropine (2 amps)
Benadryl (2 amps)
Nitroglycerin (1 bottle)
Solu-cortef (1 Mix-o-vial)
Talwin (1 amp)
Tigan (1 amp)
Valium (2 amps)
Wyamine (2 amps)
Plastic Airway (1 each)
Disposable Syringes
Tracheotomy Needle (1 each)
Tourniquet (1 each)

Rx **Glucagon Emergency Kit** (Lilly)
For treatment of severe insulin reactions (low blood glucose).
1 mg glycagon and 49 mg lactose with diluent. In 1 ml Hyporets for injection.

---

otc **Poison Antidote Kit** (Bowman)
Emergency poison treatment.
Package includes:
Syrup of Ipecac in 30 ml (1 bottle)
Charcoal suspension in 60 ml (4 bottles)

---

otc **Potable Aqua** (Wisconsin)
For emergency disinfection of drinking water.
Tablets for solution: 16.7% tetraglycine hydroperiodide (6.68% titrable iodine). In 50s.

---

[1] Center Labs., 35 Channel Dr., Port Washington, NY 11050-0110.

Drug	Trade Name (Distributor)	Toxic/Overdosed Substance	Page #
Dimercaprol (BAL)	*BAL In Oil* (H, W & D)	Arsenic, gold, mercury, lead	2670
Deferoxamine Mesylate	*Desferal Mesylate* (Ciba)	Iron	2671
Edetate Calcium Disodium	*Calcium Disodium Versenate* (Riker)	Lead	2672
Sodium Thiosulfate		Arsenic, cyanide	2673
Narcotic Antagonists		Opioids	2674
Naloxone	*Narcan* (DuPont)		2674
Physostigmine Salicylate	*Antilirium* (Forest Pharm.)	Anticholinergics (including tricyclic antidepressants) Diazepam, Morphine (CNS depression)	2686
Pralidoxime Cl	*Protopam* (Ayerst)	Organophosphates; Anticholinesterases	2687
Digoxin Immune Fab	*Digibind* (Burroughs Wellcome)	Digoxin	2690
Methylene Blue	(Various)	Cyanide	2698
Other agents used additionally as antidotes			
Leucovorin Calcium	*Wellcovorin* (Burroughs-Wellcome) *Leucovorin Calcium* (Lederle)	Folic acid antagonists (eg, methotrexate)	231
Hydroxocobalamin	(Various)	Cyanide poisoning from nitroprusside	240
Vitamin K	(Various)	Oral anticoagulants	241
Protamine Sulfate	(Various)	Heparin	286
Glucagon	(Lilly)	Insulin-induced hypoglycemia	509
Edetate Disodium	(Various)	Hypercalcemia Digitalis toxicity	862
Acetylcysteine	*Mucomyst* (Bristol-Myers) *Mucosol* (Dey Labs)	Acetaminophen	930
Atropine	(Various)	Cholinergic agents: Organophosphates, carbamates, pilocarpine, physostigmine or isofluorophate	1586
Amyl nitrite, Sodium Nitrite, Sodium Thiosulfate	*Cyanide antidote kit* (Lilly)	Cyanide	2668
Anticholinesterases		Anticholinergics, Nondepolarizing muscle relaxants	2712
Pyridostigmine Br	*Mestinon* (Roche) *Regonol* (Organon)		2714
Neostigmine	*Prostigmin* (Roche)		2716
Edrophonium Cl	*Tensilon* (Roche)		2717
Nonspecific therapy of overdoses include:			
Osmotic diuretics		Nonspecific, supportive therapies of overdoses. See also page vi for general management guidelines	584
Cathartics			1642
Peritoneal Dialysis Solutions			2667
Emetics			
Apomorphine	(Lilly)		2694
Syrup of Ipecac	(Various)		2695
Activated Charcoal	(Various)		2696
Urinary Alkalinizers			2721
Urinary Acidifiers			2722

DIMERCAPROL

Actions:

Pharmacology: Dimercaprol promotes excretion of arsenic, gold and mercury by chelation. The chelate complexes form between dimercaprol sulfhydryl groups and the metals. Formation of the chelate increases urinary and fecal elimination of the metals. Dimercaprol will be most effective in preventing sulfhydryl enzyme inhibition in the body if it is administered 1 to 2 hours after exposure. To a lesser degree, dimercaprol may reactivate affected enzymes. Dimercaprol is also used in combination with calcium edetate disodium to promote the excretion of lead.

Pharmacokinetics: After IM administration, peak concentrations are attained in 30 to 60 minutes. It has a short half-life; metabolism and excretion are complete within 4 hours.

Indications:

Treatment of arsenic, gold and mercury poisoning.

Acute lead poisoning when used with calcium edetate disodium.

Acute mercury poisoning if therapy is begun within 1 or 2 hours; not effective for chronic mercury poisoning.

Dimercaprol injection is of questionable value in poisoning caused by other heavy metals such as antimony and bismuth.

Contraindications:

Hepatic insufficiency, except postarsenical jaundice. Discontinue or use only with extreme caution if acute renal insufficiency develops during therapy.

Do not use in iron, cadmium or selenium poisoning; the resulting dimercaprol-metal complexes are more toxic than the metal alone, especially to the kidneys.

Warnings:

There may be local pain at the site of injection.

Usage in Pregnancy: Do not use unless necessary in the treatment of life-threatening acute poisoning.

Usage in Children: Fever, a reaction apparently peculiar to children, may persist during therapy. It occurs in approximately 30% of children. A transient reduction of the percentage of polymorphonuclear leukocytes may also be observed.

Precautions:

Urinary alkalinization is recommended because the dimercaprol-metal complex breaks down easily in an acid medium. Alkaline urine protects the kidney during therapy.

G-6-PD deficiency: Use with caution in these patients, especially in the presence of infection or other stressful situations; hemolysis may occur.

Drug Interactions:

Iron: Do not administer to patients under therapy with dimercaprol.

Adverse Reactions:

One of the most consistent responses to dimercaprol is a rise in blood pressure accompanied by tachycardia, roughly proportional to the dose. Larger than recommended doses may cause other transitory signs and symptoms in approximate order of frequency as follows: Nausea and vomiting; headache; a burning sensation in the lips, mouth and throat; a feeling of constriction, even pain, in the throat, chest or hands; conjunctivitis, lacrimation, blepharal spasm, rhinorrhea and salivation; tingling of the hands; a burning sensation in the penis; sweating of the forehead, hands and other areas; abdominal pain; and occasional appearance of painful sterile abscesses. Many of the above symptoms are accompanied by anxiety, weakness and unrest and often are relieved by administration of an antihistamine.

Administration and Dosage:

Give by deep IM injection only. Begin therapy as early as possible along with other supportive measures.

Mild arsenic or gold poisoning: 2.5 mg/kg 4 times daily for 2 days, then 2 times on the third day, and once daily thereafter for 10 days.

Severe arsenic or gold poisoning: 3 mg/kg every 4 hours for 2 days, then 4 times on the third day, then twice daily thereafter for 10 days.

Mercury poisoning: 5 mg/kg initially, followed by 2.5 mg/kg 1 or 2 times daily for 10 days.

Acute lead encephalopathy: 4 mg/kg alone in the first dose and thereafter at 4 hour intervals in combination with calcium edetate disodium administered at a separate site. For less severe poisoning, the dose can be reduced to 3 mg/kg after the first dose. Maintain treatment for 2 to 7 days, depending on clinical response.

Rx	**BAL In Oil** (H, W & D)	**Injection:** 100 mg per ml	In 3 ml ampuls.[1]

[1] In peanut oil with benzyl benzoate.

DEFEROXAMINE MESYLATE

Actions:

Pharmacology: Deferoxamine chelates iron and prevents it from entering into chemical reactions. It binds free serum iron, iron of ferritin and hemosiderin, but it minimally affects iron of transferrin. The iron of cytochromes and hemoglobin is inaccessible. Theoretically, 100 parts by weight can bind 8.5 parts of ferric iron. It does not demonstrably increase the excretion of electrolytes and trace metals.

Pharmacokinetics: Parenteral use is required for systemic activity. It is rapidly metabolized by plasma enzymes and excreted in urine. The iron chelate is excreted renally, giving urine a reddish color. Some is also excreted in feces via the bile. Half-life after IV use is 1 hour.

Indications:

Acute iron intoxication: An adjunct to standard treatment measures.

Chronic iron overload: Can promote iron excretion in patients who have secondary iron overload from multiple transfusions. Deferoxamine slows accumulation of hepatic iron and retards or eliminates progression of hepatic fibrosis.

Unlabeled Uses: Management of aluminum accumulation in bone in renal failure patients, and in aluminum-induced dialysis encephalopathy.

Contraindications: Severe renal disease or anuria; primary hemochromatosis.

Warnings:

Cataracts occur rarely in patients treated for prolonged periods. Perform periodic slit-lamp exams on patients treated for chronic iron overload. Other ocular disturbances (rare) include: Decreased visual acuity; impaired peripheral, color and night vision; retinal pigmentary abnormalities. Disturbances were usually reversible on treatment cessation.

Auditory disturbances: Neurotoxicity-related auditory abnormalities have been reported including high-frequency sensorineural hearing loss.

Usage in Pregnancy: Skeletal anomalies were seen in animal fetuses at doses just above those recommended for humans. A case of infant iron deficiency followed deferoxamine in a mother hours before delivery. Do not use unless clearly needed.

Usage in Children: Iron mobilization by deferoxamine is relatively poor in patients under 3 years old with relatively small degrees of iron overload; withhold the drug in such patients unless significant iron mobilization (eg, $\geq$ 1 mg of iron/day) is demonstrated.

Precautions: Flushing of the skin, urticaria, hypotension and shock have occurred with rapid IV injection. Give IM, or by slow SC or IV infusion.

Adverse Reactions:

Occasional pain and induration at injection site. *Acute iron intoxication:* Generalized erythema, urticaria and hypotension (with rapid IV injection). *Long-term therapy:* Allergic-type reactions (cutaneous wheal formation, generalized itching, rash, anaphylactic reaction), blurred vision, dysuria, abdominal discomfort, diarrhea, leg cramps, tachycardia, fever. *SC therapy:* Localized pain, pruritus, erythema, skin irritation and swelling, which might also occur in a patient treated for acute intoxication.

Administration and Dosage:

May administer IM, by continuous SC mini-infusion or by slow IV infusion. Net iron excretion with SC use is greater than with equal IM doses because the labile (chelatable) intracellular iron pool is constantly exposed to the drug.

Acute iron intoxication:

IM – Preferred route; use for all patients not in shock. Initially, 1 g; then 0.5 g every 4 hrs for 2 doses. Subsequently, give 0.5 g every 4 to 12 hrs based on clinical response. Do not exceed 6 g/day.

IV – Use only for patients in cardiovascular collapse and then only by slow infusion. Dosage is the same as with IM use; do not exceed 15 mg/kg/hr. As soon as possible, discontinue IV and give IM. Some authorities prefer IV use in most cases, assuring the slow infusion rate.

Oral use is controversial and unlabeled (binding iron in the GI tract) but appears to be generally discouraged.

Chronic iron overload: Individualize dosage.

IM – 0.5 to 1 g daily. Give 2 g IV with, but separate from, each unit of blood. The rate of IV infusion must not exceed 15 mg/kg/hour.

SC – 1 to 2 g/day (20 to 40 mg/kg/day) over 8 to 24 hrs with continuous mini-infusion pump. Individualize infusion duration. In some patients, iron excretion will be as great after a short infusion (8 to 12 hrs) as if the same dose is given over 24 hrs.

Children: 50 mg/kg/dose IM or IV every 6 hours or up to 15 mg/kg/hr by continuous IV infusion, to a maximum of 6 g/24 hr or 2 g/dose.

Preparation and storage: Add 2 ml Sterile Water for Injection to each vial. For IV use, add to saline, glucose in water or Ringer's Lactate solution. Do not store solutions reconstituted with sterile water longer than 1 week. Protect from light.

Rx	**Desferal Mesylate** (Ciba)	**Powder for Injection:** 500 mg	In vials.

EDETATE CALCIUM DISODIUM (Calcium EDTA)

Actions:

The calcium in edetate calcium disodium is readily displaced by heavy metals, such as lead, to form stable complexes which are excreted in the urine. The elimination half-life is 20 to 60 minutes. About 50% is excreted in the urine in 1 hour; 95% in 24 hours.

Edetate calcium disodium is poorly absorbed (< 5%) from the GI tract.

Indications:

Acute and chronic lead poisoning and lead encephalopathy.

Contraindications:

Anuria.

Warnings:

Do not exceed recommended dosage. EDTA can produce toxic and potentially fatal effects. In lead encephalopathy, avoid rapid infusion; the IM route is preferred.

Usage in Pregnancy: Safety for use during pregnancy has not been established; do not use during pregnancy unless potential benefits outweigh potential hazards to the fetus.

Precautions:

Renal damage: Severe acute lead poisoning may cause proteinuria and microscopic hematuria. EDTA may produce the same signs of renal damage. Perform urinalysis daily during therapy to monitor for progression of renal tubular damage. The presence of large renal epithelial cells, increasing numbers of red blood cells in the urinary sediment or greater proteinuria call for immediate discontinuation. Perform periodic BUN determinations before and during each course of therapy.

Hydration: Avoid excess fluids in patients with lead encephalopathy and increased intracranial pressure. In such cases, mix a 20% solution with procaine to give a final concentration of 0.5% procaine and administer IM.

Acutely ill individuals may be dehydrated from vomiting. Since EDTA is excreted in the urine, establish urine flow by IV infusion before administering the first dose. Once urine flow is established, restrict further IV fluid to basal water and electrolyte requirements. Stop EDTA when urine flow ceases.

Adverse Reactions:

The principal toxic effect is renal tubular necrosis.

Administration and Dosage:

Effective IV, SC or IM; however, because of convenience and greater safety in treating symptomatic children, the IM route is preferred and is recommended in patients with overt or incipient lead encephalopathy. Rapid IV infusion may be lethal by suddenly increasing intracranial pressure in this group of patients with cerebral edema.

Do not administer larger than recommended doses.

IV: Dilute the 5 ml ampul with 250 to 500 ml of Normal Saline or 5% dextrose solution. In asymptomatic adults, administer this dilution over at least 1 hour twice daily for up to 5 days. Interrupt therapy for 2 days; follow with another 5 days of treatment, if indicated.

In mildly affected or asymptomatic individuals, do not exceed 50 mg/kg/day. In symptomatic adults, keep fluids to basal levels and increase administration time to 2 hours. Give second daily infusion 6 or more hours after the first.

IM: Do not exceed 35 mg/kg (0.5 g/30 lbs) twice a day; total, ≈ 75 mg/kg/day (1 g/30 lbs/day). In mild cases, do not exceed 50 mg/kg/day. For young children, give total daily dose in divided doses every 8 or 12 hours for 3 to 5 days; give a second course after a rest period of 4 or more days. Add procaine to produce a concentration of 0.5% to minimize pain at injection site.

Lead encephalopathy is relatively rare in adults, but is common in children and has a high mortality rate. Though some investigators have employed a combination of EDTA and dimercaprol, EDTA alone has been used over a longer period of time. When administered concurrently, inject dimercaprol and EDTA at separate deep IM sites.

Rx	**Calcium Disodium Versenate** (Riker)	**Injection:** 200 mg per ml	In 5 ml amps.

SODIUM THIOSULFATE

Actions:

Pharmacology: The primary mechanism of cyanide detoxification involves conversion of cyanide to the relatively nontoxic thiocyanate ion. This reaction involves the enzyme rhodanese (thiosulfate cyanide sulfurtransferase) found in many body tissues, but with major activity in the liver. The body has the capability to detoxify cyanide; however, the rhodanese enzyme system responds slowly to large amounts of cyanide. The rhodanese enzyme reaction can be accelerated by supplying an exogenous source of sulfur, accomplished by administering sodium thiosulfate.

Following IV injection, sodium thiosulfate is distributed throughout the extracellular fluid and excreted unchanged in the urine. The biological half-life is 0.65 hours.

Indications:

Used alone or as adjunctive therapy with sodium nitrite or amyl nitrite in cyanide toxicity.

Warnings:

Usage in Pregnancy: Category C. Safety for use during pregnancy has not been established. Use only when clearly needed and when the potential benefits outweigh the potential hazards to the fetus.

Administration and Dosage:

Sodium thiosulfate injection is meant for slow IV use only.

Arsenic poisoning: Initially, 1 ml, then 2 ml, 3 ml and 4 ml on successive days. Thereafter, 5 ml on alternate days or as needed.

Cyanide poisoning: Following administration of 300 mg IV sodium nitrite, inject 12.5 g sodium thiosulfate IV (over ≈ 10 minutes). If needed, injection of both sodium nitrite and sodium thiosulfate may be repeated, but each in one-half the original dose.

Rx	**Sodium Thiosulfate** (Various)	**Injection:** 1 g/10 ml	In 10 ml amps and 10 ml vials.
Rx	**Sodium Thiosulfate** (Quad)		In 10 ml vials.
Rx	**Sodium Thiosulfate** (Various)	**Injection:** 2.5 g/10 ml	In 50 ml vials.
Rx	**Sodium Thiosulfate** (Quad)		In 50 ml vials.

Narcotic Antagonists

NALOXONE HCl

Actions:

The narcotic antagonist naloxone is clinically useful in the reversal of narcotic-induced respiratory depression. Naloxone, a pure narcotic antagonist, will precipitate abstinence syndrome in the presence of narcotic addiction. Since it is devoid of undesirable agonist properties, naloxone is the preferred agent in the reversal of narcotic-induced respiratory depression. Naloxone prevents or reverses the effects of opioids including respiratory depression, sedation and hypotension; it can reverse the psychotomimetic and dysphoric effects of agonist-antagonists such as pentazocine.

Pharmacology: Mechanism – The mechanism of action is not fully understood; evidence suggests that it antagonizes the opioid effects by competing for the same receptor sites. Naloxone is an essentially pure narcotic antagonist, ie, it does not possess "agonistic" or morphine-like properties.

Effects – Naloxone does not produce respiratory depression, psychotomimetic effects or pupillary constriction. In the absence of narcotics or agonistic effects of other narcotic antagonists, naloxone exhibits essentially no pharmacologic activity; doses up to 24 mg cause only slight drowsiness. Naloxone has not produced tolerance or caused physical or psychological dependence.

Pharmacokinetics:

Distribution/Metabolism – After parenteral use, naloxone is rapidly distributed in the body. It is metabolized in the liver, primarily by glucuronide conjugation.

Excretion – Naloxone is excreted in the urine. The serum half-life in adults ranged from 30 to 81 minutes (mean 64 ± 12 minutes); in neonates, 3.1 ± 0.5 hours.

Onset, peak and duration – The onset of action of IV naloxone is generally apparent within 2 minutes; it is only slightly less rapid when it is administered SC or IM. Naloxone has a duration of action of 1 to 4 hours dependent upon dose and route. Administration IM produces a more prolonged effect than IV use. The requirement for repeat doses will also depend upon amount, type and route of the narcotic being antagonized.

Indications:

For the complete or partial reversal of narcotic depression, including respiratory depression, induced by opioids including natural and synthetic narcotics, propoxyphene, methadone, nalbuphine, butorphanol and pentazocine. Also indicated for the diagnosis of suspected acute opioid overdosage.

Unlabeled Uses: Naloxone has been used to improve circulation in refractory shock. It appears to antagonize the effect of β-endorphin and allows prostaglandins and catecholamines to reestablish control of circulation. Naloxone has also been used for the reversal of alcoholic coma, dementia of the Alzheimer type and schizophrenia.

Contraindications:

Hypersensitivity to these agents.

Warnings:

Drug dependence: Administer cautiously to persons who are known or suspected to be physically dependent on opioids, including newborns of mothers with narcotic dependence. Reversal of narcotic effects will precipitate an acute abstinence syndrome.

Repeat administration: The patient who has satisfactorily responded should be kept under continued surveillance. Administer repeated doses as necessary, since the duration of action of some narcotics may exceed that of the narcotic antagonist.

Respiratory depression: Not effective against respiratory depression due to nonopioid drugs.

Usage in Pregnancy: Category B. Reproductive studies in mice and rats at doses up to 1000 times the human dose revealed no evidence of impaired fertility or fetal harm. There are, however, no adequate and well controlled studies in pregnant women. Use during pregnancy only when clearly needed.

Usage in Lactation: It is not known whether the drug is excreted in breast milk. Use caution when administering to a nursing woman.

Precautions:

Other supportive therapy: Maintain a free airway and provide artificial ventilation, cardiac massage and vasopressor agents; employ when necessary to counteract acute narcotic overdosage.

Cardiovascular effects: Several instances of hypotension, hypertension, pulmonary edema and ventricular tachycardia and fibrillation have been reported in postoperative patients, most of whom had preexisting cardiovascular disorders or who received other drugs which may have similar adverse cardiovascular effects. A direct cause and effect relationship has not been established; use caution in patients with preexisting cardiac disease or patients who have received potentially cardiotoxic drugs.

(Continued on following page)

NALOXONE HCl (Cont.)

Adverse Reactions:

Abrupt reversal of narcotic depression may result in nausea, vomiting, sweating, tachycardia, increased blood pressure and tremulousness.

In postoperative patients, excessive dosage may result in excitement and significant reversal of analgesia, hypotension, hypertension, pulmonary edema and ventricular tachycardia and fibrillation. Seizures have been reported infrequently after administration, however, a causal relationship has not been established.

Administration and Dosage:

Give IV, IM or SC. The most rapid onset of action is achieved with IV use which is recommended in emergency situations. Duration of action of some narcotics may exceed that of naloxone. Keep patient under continued surveillance and give repeat doses as necessary.

Adults:

Narcotic overdose (known or suspected) – Initial dose is 0.4 to 2 mg IV; may repeat IV at 2 to 3 minute intervals. If no response is observed after 10 mg has been administered, question the diagnosis of narcotic-induced or partial narcotic-induced toxicity. IM or SC administration may be necessary if the IV route is not available.

Postoperative narcotic depression (partial reversal) – Smaller doses are usually sufficient. Titrate dose according to the patient's response. Excessive dosage may result in significant reversal of analgesia and increase in blood pressure. Similarly, too rapid reversal may induce nausea, vomiting, sweating or circulatory stress.

Initial dose: Inject in increments of 0.1 to 0.2 mg IV at 2 to 3 minute intervals to the desired degree of reversal (ie, adequate ventilation and alertness without significant pain or discomfort).

Repeat dose: Repeat doses may be required within 1 or 2 hour intervals depending upon the amount, type (ie, short- or long-acting) and time interval since last administration of narcotic. Supplemental IM doses have produced a longer lasting effect.

Children:

Narcotic overdose (known or suspected) – Initial dose is 0.01 mg/kg IV; give a subsequent dose of 0.1 mg/kg if needed. If an IV route is not available, naloxone may be given IM or SC in divided doses. If necessary, dilute with Sterile Water for Injection.

Postoperative narcotic depression – Follow the recommendations and cautions under adult administration guidelines. For initial reversal of respiratory depression, inject in increments of 0.005 to 0.01 mg IV at 2 to 3 minute intervals to desired degree of reversal.

Neonates:

Narcotic-induced depression – Initial dose is 0.01 mg/kg IV, IM or SC; may be repeated in accordance with adult administration guidelines.

Intravenous infusion: Dilute in normal saline or 5% dextrose solutions. The addition of 2 mg in 500 ml of either solution provides a concentration of 0.004 mg/ml. Titrate the administration rate in accordance with the patient's response.

Incompatibilities – Do not mix naloxone with preparations containing bisulfite, metabisulfite, long-chain or high molecular weight anions, or any solution having an alkaline pH. Do not add any drug or chemical agent unless its effect on the chemical and physical stability of the solution has first been established.

Stability – Use mixtures within 24 hours. After 24 hours, discard unused solution.

				C.I.*
Rx	**Naloxone HCl** (Various)	**Injection:** 0.4 mg/ml	In 1 ml amps, 1 ml disp. syringes and 1, 2 and 10 ml vials.	2175+
Rx	**Narcan** (DuPont Pharm.)		In 1 ml amps, 1 ml disp. syringes and 10 ml vials.[1]	4810
Rx	**Naloxone HCl** (Elkins-Sinn)	**Injection:** 1 mg/ml	In 2 ml vials.	1540
Rx	**Narcan** (DuPont Pharm.)		In 2 ml amps and 10 ml vials.[2]	1709
Rx	**Naloxone HCl** (Various)	**Neonatal Injection:** 0.02 mg per ml	In 2 ml amps, disp. syringes and vials.	19,750+
Rx	**Narcan** (DuPont Pharm.)		In 2 ml amps.[1]	27,200

* Cost Index based on cost per 0.4 mg.

[1] Available with or without methyl and propylparabens.

[2] With methyl and propyl parabens.

See also page 2674 for naloxone, indicated for acute reversal of narcotic depression. Naltrexone is discussed separately because of its unique pharmacokinetics and indications.

NALTREXONE HCl

Actions:

Pharmacology: Naltrexone, a pure opioid antagonist, partially or completely, reversibly blocks the subjective effects of IV opioids including analgesics possessing agonist and antagonist activity (eg, butorphanol, nalbuphine and pentazocine). When coadministered with morphine on a chronic basis, it blocks the physical dependence to morphine and presumably other opioids. It has few other, if any, intrinsic actions.

Naltrexone 50 mg will block the pharmacologic effects of 25 mg IV heroin for as long as 24 hours. Data suggest that doubling the dose of naltrexone provides blockade for 48 hours and tripling the dose provides blockade for about 72 hours.

While the mechanism of action is not fully understood, naltrexone appears to block the effects of opioids by competitive binding at opioid receptors. This makes the blockade produced potentially surmountable.

Pharmacokinetics:

Absorption/Distribution – Following the administration of 50 mg tablets to 24 healthy adult male volunteers, peak levels of naltrexone and 6-β-naltrexol were 8.6 ng/ml and 99.3 ng/ml, respectively; time to peak was 1 hour. The maximum concentration, area under the curve (AUC) and the amount excreted in the urine increased proportionally as the amount of naltrexone administered increased from 50 mg to 200 mg. Plasma protein binding was 21%.

Metabolism/Excretion – Naltrexone undergoes extensive "first-pass" hepatic metabolism; approximately 95% of the absorbed drug is converted to several metabolites. The major metabolite is 6-β-naltrexol; like naltrexone, it is believed to be a pure antagonist and may contribute to the opioid receptor blockade. Minor metabolites are also conjugated to form additional metabolic products. Mean elimination half-lives for naltrexone and 6-β-naltrexol are 3.9 hours and 12.9 hours, respectively; pharmacologic effects range from 24 to 72 hours and are independent of dose. The drug does not accumulate during chronic dosing. As predicted by its longer half-life, plasma levels of 6-β-naltrexol increase by 40% during chronic dosing. Naltrexone and its metabolites are excreted primarily by the kidney; fecal excretion is a minor elimination pathway. The urinary excretion of unchanged drug is less than 1% of an oral dose; urinary excretion of unchanged and conjugated 6-β-naltrexol accounts for approximately 38% of a dose. Naltrexone and its metabolites appear to undergo enterohepatic recycling.

Total body clearance is 1.5 L/min which approximates the liver blood flow and suggests naltrexone is a highly extracted compound. It is cleared by glomerular filtration. However, 6-β-naltrexol may have an additional renal tubular secretory mechanism.

Indications:

Adjunct to the maintenance of the opioid-free state in detoxified, formerly opioid-dependent individuals.

Unlabeled Uses: Naltrexone has been used in the treatment of postconcussional syndrome unresponsive to other treatments, and in eating disorders. To increase patient compliance, an SC implant is being studied.

Contraindications:

Patients receiving opioid analgesics; opioid-dependent patients; patients in acute opioid withdrawal. Also contraindicated in any individual who: Fails a naloxone challenge; has a positive urine screen for opioids; has a history of sensitivity to naltrexone (it is not known if there is any cross-sensitivity with naloxone or other phenanthrene-containing opioids); has acute hepatitis or liver failure.

Warnings:

Hepatotoxicity: Naltrexone can cause dose-related hepatocellular injury. Prior to treatment, perform baseline liver function studies. Carefully consider its use in patients with liver disease or a history of recent liver disease. The margin of separation between the apparently safe and the hepatotoxic doses appears only fivefold or less. Monitor liver function tests monthly during the first 6 months and at appropriate intervals thereafter.

Evidence of its hepatotoxic potential is derived primarily from a placebo controlled study in which naltrexone was administered to obese subjects at a dose approximately fivefold that recommended (300 mg per day). Five of 26 naltrexone recipients developed elevations of serum transaminases 3 to 19 times their baseline values after 3 to 8 weeks of treatment. The patients involved were generally clinically asymptomatic and the transaminase levels of all patients on whom follow-up was obtained returned to (or toward) baseline values in a matter of weeks. The lack of any transaminase elevations of similar magnitude in any of the 24 placebo patients indicates that naltrexone is a direct hepatotoxin.

(Warnings continued on following page)

NALTREXONE HCl (Cont.)

Warnings (Cont.):

Unintended precipitation of abstinence or exacerbation of a preexisting subclinical abstinence syndrome may occur; therefore, patients should remain opioid-free for a minimum of 7 to 10 days before starting naltrexone. The absence of opioid in urine is not sufficient proof that a patient is opioid-free. Perform a naloxone challenge to exclude the possibility of precipitating a withdrawal reaction. See Administration and Dosage.

Severe opioid withdrawal syndromes precipitated by the accidental ingestion of naltrexone have been reported in opioid-dependent individuals. Withdrawal symptoms usually appear within 5 minutes of ingestion and have lasted for up to 48 hours. Mental status changes, including confusion, somnolence and visual hallucinations have occurred. Significant fluid losses from vomiting and diarrhea have required IV fluids.

Surmountable blockade: While naltrexone is a potent antagonist with a prolonged pharmacologic effect (24 to 72 hours), the blockade produced by naltrexone is surmountable. This poses a potential risk to individuals who attempt to overcome the blockade by self-administering large amounts of opioids. Any attempt by a patient to overcome the antagonism by taking opioids is very dangerous and may lead to fatal overdose. Also, lesser amounts of exogenous opioids are dangerous if they are taken in a manner (ie, relatively long after the last dose of naltrexone) and in an amount that persists in the body longer than effective concentrations of naltrexone and its metabolites.

In an emergency situation requiring analgesia which can only be achieved with opioids, amount of opioid required may be greater than usual and resulting respiratory depression may be deeper and more prolonged. A rapidly acting analgesic which minimizes respiratory depression is preferred. Individualize dosage and monitor closely.

Additionally, nonreceptor-mediated actions may occur (eg, facial swelling, itching, generalized erythema presumably due to histamine release).

Use with narcotics: Patients taking naltrexone may not benefit from opioid-containing medicines, such as cough and cold preparations, antidiarrheal preparations and opioid analgesics. Use a nonopioid-containing alternative, if available.

Usage in Pregnancy: Category C. Naltrexone is embryocidal in rats and rabbits when given in doses approximately 140 times the human therapeutic dose. There are no adequate and well controlled studies in pregnant women. Use naltrexone in pregnancy only when the potential benefit justifies the potential risk to the fetus.

Usage in Lactation: Whether naltrexone is excreted in human milk is unknown. Exercise caution when naltrexone is administered to a nursing mother.

Usage in Children: Safety for use in children under 18 years has not been established.

Adverse Reactions:

CNS: Difficulty sleeping, anxiety, nervousness, headache, low energy (> 10%); increased energy, irritability, dizziness (< 10%); depression, paranoia, fatigue, drowsiness, restlessness, confusion, disorientation, hallucinations, nightmares, bad dreams (< 1%).

Cardiovascular: Phlebitis, edema, increased blood pressure, nonspecific ECG changes, palpitations, tachycardia (< 1%).

GI: Abdominal cramps/pain, nausea, vomiting (> 10%); loss of appetite, diarrhea, constipation (< 10%); excess gas, hemorrhoids, ulcer, dry mouth (< 1%); hepatotoxicity (see Warnings).

Respiratory: Nasal congestion, rhinorrhea, sneezing, sore throat, excess mucus or phlegm, sinus trouble, heavy breathing, hoarseness, cough, shortness of breath (< 1%).

Musculoskeletal: Joint and muscle pain (> 10%); painful shoulders, legs or knees, tremors, twitching (< 1%).

GU: Delayed ejaculation, decreased potency (< 10%); increased frequency/discomfort during urination, increased or decreased sexual interest (< 1%).

Dermatologic: Skin rash (< 10%); itching, oily skin, pruritus, acne, athlete's foot, cold sores, alopecia (< 1%).

Special senses: Blurred vision, burning, light-sensitive, swollen, aching or strained eyes, "clogged" or aching ears, tinnitus (< 1%).

Other: Chills, increased thirst (< 10%); increased appetite, weight loss or gain, yawning, nose bleeds, fever, inguinal pain, swollen glands, "side" pains, head "pounding", cold feet, hot spells (< 1%). Idiopathic thrombocytopenic purpura was reported in one patient but cleared without sequelae after discontinuation of naltrexone and corticosteroid treatment.

Laboratory Tests: Liver test abnormalities, lymphocytosis.

(Continued on following page)

NALTREXONE HCl (Cont.)

Overdosage:

Symptoms: In one study, subjects who received 800 mg/day for up to 1 week showed no evidence of toxicity. In acute toxicity studies in animals, death was due to clonic-tonic convulsions or respiratory failure.

Treatment: Treat symptomatically. See also General Management of Acute Overdosage on p. vi.

Patient Information:

Patients should wear identification indicating naltrexone use.

If patients attempt self-administration of heroin or any other opiate in small doses, they will perceive no effect. However, self-administration of large doses of heroin or other narcotics can overcome the blockade and may cause death, serious injury or coma.

Administration and Dosage:

Do not attempt treatment until naloxone challenge is negative. Initiate treatment using the following guidelines:

1. Do not attempt treatment until the patient has remained opioid-free for 7 to 10 days. Verify by analyzing urine for opioids. The patient should not be manifesting withdrawal signs or reporting withdrawal symptoms.
2. Administer a naloxone challenge test (see below). If signs of opioid withdrawal are still observed following challenge, do not treat with naltrexone. The naloxone challenge can be repeated in 24 hours.
3. Initiate treatment carefully, slowly increasing the dose. Administer 25 mg initially; observe patient for 1 hour. If no withdrawal signs occur, give the rest of the daily dose.

Naloxone challenge test: Do not perform in a patient showing clinical signs of opioid withdrawal or in a patient whose urine contains opioids. Administer the challe' ge test either IV or SC.

IV challenge – Draw 2 ampuls of naloxone, 2 ml (0.8 mg) into a syringe. Inject 0.5 ml (0.2 mg); while the needle is still in the patient's vein, observe for 30 seconds for withdrawal signs or symptoms. If there is no evidence of withdrawal, inject the remaining 1.5 ml (0.6 mg) and observe for an additional 20 minutes for signs and symptoms of withdrawal.

SC challenge – Administer 2 ml (0.8 mg) SC, and observe the patient for signs and symptoms of withdrawal for 45 minutes.

Monitor the patient's vital signs and watch for signs and symptoms of opioid withdrawal. Question the patient carefully. The signs and symptoms of opioid withdrawal include, but are not limited to, the following: Stuffiness or runny nose, tearing, yawning, sweating, tremor, vomiting or piloerection, feeling of temperature change, joint or bone and muscle pain, abdominal cramps, skin crawling, etc.

Interpretation of the challenge – The elicitation of the enumerated signs or symptoms indicates a potential risk for the subject, and naltrexone should not be administered. If there are no signs or symptoms of withdrawal, naltrexone may be administered. If there is any doubt in the observer's mind that the patient is not opioid-free, or is in continuing withdrawal, readminister naloxone as follows:

Confirmatory rechallenge – Inject 4 ml (1.6 mg) of naloxone IV and observe the patient again for signs and symptoms of withdrawal. If none are present, naltrexone may be administered. If signs and symptoms of withdrawal are present, delay naltrexone until repeated naloxone challenge indicates the patient is no longer at risk.

Maintenance treatment: Once the patient has been started on naltrexone, 50 mg every 24 hours will produce adequate clinical blockade of the actions of parenterally administered opioids (ie, this dose will block the effects of a 25 mg IV heroin challenge). A flexible dosing regimen may be employed. Thus, patients may receive 50 mg every weekday with a 100 mg dose on Saturday, 100 mg every other day, or 150 mg every third day. While the degree of opioid blockade may be somewhat reduced by using higher doses at longer dosing intervals, improved patient compliance may result from dosing every 48 to 72 hours. Several studies have employed the following dosing regimen with success: 100 mg Monday, 100 mg Wednesday and 150 mg Friday.

				C.I.*
Rx	**Trexan** (DuPont)	**Tablets:** 50 mg	(#DuPont Trexan). Scored. In 50s.	1008

* Cost Index based on cost per 50 mg.

Product identification code.

FLUMAZENIL

Actions:

Flumazenil was approved by the FDA in December 1991.

Pharmacology: Flumazenil is a benzodiazepine receptor antagonist available for IV administration. Flumazenil, an imidazobenzodiazepine derivative, antagonizes the actions of benzodiazepines on the CNS and competitively inhibits the activity at the benzodiazepine recognition site on the GABA/benzodiazepine receptor complex. It is a weak partial agonist in some animal models of activity, but has little or no agonist activity in man. The drug does not antagonize the CNS effects of drugs affecting the GABA-ergic neurons by means other than the benzodiazepine receptor (including ethanol, barbiturates or general anesthetics) and does not reverse the effects of opioids.

Flumazenil antagonizes sedation, impairment of recall and psychomotor impairment produced by benzodiazepines in healthy volunteers. The duration and degree of reversal of benzodiazepine effects are related to the dose and plasma concentrations of flumazenil. Generally, doses of approximately 0.1 to 0.2 mg (corresponding to peak plasma levels of 3 to 6 ng/ml) produce partial antagonism, whereas higher doses of 0.4 to 1 mg (peak plasma levels of 12 to 28 ng/ml) usually produce complete antagonism in patients who have received the usual sedating doses of benzodiazepines. The onset of reversal is usually evident within 1 to 2 minutes after the injection is completed. Within 3 minutes, 80% response will be reached, with the peak effect occurring at 6 to 10 minutes. The duration and degree of reversal are related to the plasma concentration of the sedating benzodiazepine as well as the dose of flumazenil given.

In healthy volunteers, flumazenil did not alter intraocular pressure when given alone or reverse the decrease in intraocular pressure seen after midazolam administration.

Pharmacokinetics: After IV administration, plasma concentrations of flumazenil follow a two compartment open pharmacokinetic model with an initial distribution half-life of 7 to 15 minutes and a terminal half-life of 41 to 79 minutes. Peak concentrations of flumazenil are proportional to dose, with an apparent initial volume of distribution of 0.5 L/kg. After redistribution the apparent volume of distribution ranges from 0.77 to 1.6 L/kg. Protein binding is approximately 50% and the drug shows no preferential partitioning into red blood cells.

Flumazenil is a highly extracted drug. Clearance of flumazenil occurs primarily by hepatic metabolism and is dependent on hepatic blood flow. In healthy volunteers, total clearance ranges from 0.7 to 1.3 L/hr/kg, with < 1% of the administered dose eliminated unchanged in the urine. The major metabolites of flumazenil identified in urine are in the deethylated free acid and its glucuronide conjugate. In preclinical studies there was no evidence of pharmacologic activity exhibited by the deethylated free acid. Elimination of drug is essentially complete within 72 hours, with 90% to 95% appearing in urine and 5% to 10% in the feces.

Pharmacokinetic Parameters of Flumazenil Following a 5 min 1 mg Infusion	
Parameter	Mean (Range)
Maximum concentration	24 ng/ml (11-43)
AUC	15 ng • hr/ml (10-22)
Apparent volume of distribution	1 L/kg (0.8-1.6)
Clearance	1 L/hr/kg (0.7-1.4)
Half-life	54 min (41-79)

The pharmacokinetics of flumazenil are not significantly affected by gender, age, renal failure (creatinine clearance < 10 ml/min) or hemodialysis beginning 1 hour after drug administration. Mean total clearance is decreased to 40% to 60% of normal in patients with moderate liver dysfunction and to 25% of normal in patients with severe liver dysfunction compared with age-matched healthy subjects. This results in a prolongation of the half-life from 0.8 hours in healthy subjects to 1.3 hours in patients with moderate hepatic impairment and 2.4 hours in severely impaired patients. Ingestion of food during an IV infusion results in a 50% increase in clearance, most likely due to the increased hepatic blood flow that accompanies a meal. The pharmacokinetic profile of flumazenil is unaltered in the presence of benzodiazepine agonists and the kinetic profiles of those benzodiazepines are unaltered by flumazenil.

(Actions continued on following page)

FLUMAZENIL (Cont.)

Actions (Cont.):

Clinical trials: Flumazenil has been administered to reverse the effects of benzodiazepines in conscious sedation, general anesthesia and the management of suspected benzodiazepine overdose.

Conscious sedation – In four trials in 970 patients who received an average of 30 mg diazepam or 10 mg midazolam for sedation (with or without a narcotic) in conjunction with both inpatient and outpatient diagnostic or surgical procedures, flumazenil was effective in reversing the sedating and psychomotor effects of the benzodiazepine; however, amnesia was less completely and less consistently reversed. In these studies, flumazenil was administered as an initial dose of 0.4 mg IV (two doses of 0.2 mg) with additional 0.2 mg doses as needed to achieve complete awakening, up to a maximum total dose of 1 mg.

Of patients receiving flumazenil, 78% responded by becoming completely alert. Of those patients, approximately half responded to doses of 0.4 to 0.6 mg, while the other half responded to doses of 0.8 to 1 mg. Adverse effects were infrequent in patients who received ≤ 1 mg, although injection site pain, agitation and anxiety did occur. Reversal of sedation was not associated with any increase in the frequency of inadequate analgesia or increase in narcotic demand in these studies. While most patients remained alert throughout the 3 hour post-procedure observation period, resedation was observed to occur in 3% to 9% of the patients, and was most common in patients who had received high doses of benzodiazepine (see Precautions).

General anesthesia – In four trials, 644 patients received midazolam as an induction or maintenance agent in both balanced and inhalational anesthesia. Midazolam was generally administered in doses ranging from 5 to 80 mg, alone or in conjunction with muscle relaxants, nitrous oxide, regional or local anesthetics, narcotics or inhalational anesthetics. Flumazenil was given as an initial dose of 0.2 mg IV, with additional 0.2 mg doses as needed to reach a complete response, up to a maximum total dose of 1 mg. These doses were effective in reversing sedation and restoring psychomotor function, but did not completely restore memory as tested by picture recall. Flumazenil was not as effective in the reversal of sedation in patients who had received multiple anesthetic agents in addition to benzodiazepines.

Of patients sedated with midazolam, 81% responded to flumazenil by becoming completely alert or just slightly drowsy. Of those patients, 36% responded to doses of 0.4 to 0.6 mg, while 64% responded to doses of 0.8 to 1 mg.

Resedation in patients who responded to flumazenil occurred in 10% to 15% of patients studied and was more common with larger doses of midazolam (> 20 mg), long procedures (> 60 minutes) and use of neuromuscular blocking agents (see Precautions).

Management of suspected benzodiazepine overdose – In two trials, 497 patients were presumed to have taken an overdose of a benzodiazepine, either alone or in combination with a variety of other agents. In these trials, 299 patients were proven to have taken a benzodiazepine as part of the overdose, and 80% of the 148 who received flumazenil responded by an improvement in level of consciousness. Of the patients who responded to flumazenil, 75% responded to a total dose of 1 to 3 mg.

Reversal of sedation was associated with an increased frequency of symptoms of CNS excitation. Of the patients treated with flumazenil, 1% to 3% were treated for agitation or anxiety. Serious side effects were uncommon, but six seizures were observed in 446 patients treated with flumazenil. Four of these six patients had ingested a large dose of cyclic antidepressants, which increased the risk of seizures (see Warnings).

Indications:

For the complete or partial reversal of the sedative effects of benzodiazepines in cases where general anesthesia has been induced or maintained with benzodiazepines, where sedation has been produced with benzodiazepines for diagnostic and therapeutic procedures, and for the management of benzodiazepine overdose.

Contraindications:

Hypersensitivity to flumazenil or to benzodiazepines; in patients who have been given a benzodiazepine for control of a potentially life-threatening condition (eg, control of intracranial pressure or status epilepticus); in patients who are showing signs of serious cyclic antidepressant overdose (see Warnings).

Warnings:

The use of flumazenil has been associated with the occurrence of seizures. These are most frequent in patients who have been on benzodiazepines for long-term sedation or in overdose cases where patients are showing signs of serious cyclic antidepressant overdose. Individualize the dosage of flumazenil and be prepared to manage seizures.

(Warnings continued on following page)

FLUMAZENIL (Cont.)

Warnings (Cont.):

Seizure risk: The reversal of benzodiazepine effects may be associated with the onset of seizures in certain high-risk populations. Possible risk factors for seizures include: Concurrent major sedative-hypnotic drug withdrawal; recent therapy with repeated doses of parenteral benzodiazepines; myoclonic jerking or seizure activity prior to flumazenil administration in overdose cases; concurrent cyclic antidepressant poisoning.

Flumazenil is not recommended in cases of serious cyclic antidepressant poisoning, as manifested by motor abnormalities (twitching, rigidity, focal seizure), dysrhythmia (wide QRS, ventricular dysrhythmia, heart block), anticholinergic signs (mydriasis, dry mucosa, hypoperistalsis) and cardiovascular collapse at presentation. In such cases withhold flumazenil and allow the patient to remain sedated (with ventilatory and circulatory support as needed) until the signs of antidepressant toxicity have subsided. Treatment with flumazenil has no known benefit to the seriously ill mixed-overdose patient other than reversing sedation and should not be used in cases where seizures (from any cause) are likely.

Most convulsions associated with flumazenil administration require treatment and have been successfully managed with benzodiazepines, phenytoin or barbiturates. Because of the presence of flumazenil, higher than usual doses of benzodiazepines may be required.

Hypoventilation: Monitor patients who have received flumazenil for the reversal of benzodiazepine effects (after conscious sedation or general anesthesia) for resedation, respiratory depression or other residual benzodiazepine effects for an appropriate period (up to 120 minutes) based on the dose and duration of effect of the benzodiazepine employed, because flumazenil has not been established as an effective treatment for hypoventilation due to benzodiazepine administration. The availability of flumazenil does not diminish the need for prompt detection of hypoventilation and the ability to effectively intervene by establishing an airway and assisting ventilation.

Flumazenil may not fully reverse postoperative airway problems or ventilatory insufficiency induced by benzodiazepines. In addition, even if flumazenil is initially effective, such problems may recur because the effects of flumazenil wear off before the effects of many benzodiazepines. Always monitor overdose cases for resedation until the patients are stable and resedation is unlikely.

Hepatic function impairment: The clearance of flumazenil is reduced to 40% to 60% of normal in patients with mild to moderate hepatic disease and to 25% of normal in patients with severe hepatic dysfunction (see Pharmacokinetics). While the dose of flumazenil used for initial reversal of benzodiazepine effects is not affected, reduce the size and frequency of repeat doses of the drug in liver disease.

Elderly: The pharmacokinetics of flumazenil have been studied in the elderly and are not significantly different from younger patients. Several studies in patients > 65 years of age and one study in patients > 80 years of age suggest that while the doses of benzodiazepines used to induce sedation should be reduced, ordinary doses of flumazenil may be used for reversal.

Pregnancy: Category C. In rabbits, embryocidal effects (as evidenced by increased pre- and post-implantation losses) were observed at 50 mg/kg or 200 times the human exposure from a maximum recommended IV dose of 5 mg. In rats at oral dosages of 5, 25 and 125 mg/kg/day of flumazenil, pup survival was decreased during the lactating period, pup liver weight at weaning was increased for the high-dose group (125 mg/kg/day) and incisor eruption and ear opening in the offspring were delayed; the delay in ear opening was associated with a delay in the appearance of the auditory startle response. There are no adequate and well controlled studies in pregnant women. Use during pregnancy only if the potential benefit justifies the potential risk to the fetus.

Labor and delivery: The use of flumazenil to reverse the effects of benzodiazepines used during labor and delivery is not recommended because the effects of the drug in the newborn are unknown.

Lactation: Exercise caution when deciding to administer flumazenil to a nursing woman because it is not known whether flumazenil is excreted in breast milk.

Children: Flumazenil is not recommended for use in children (either for reversal of sedation, management of overdose or resuscitation of the newborn), as no clinical studies have been performed to determine the risks, benefits and dosage to be used.

(Continued on following page)

FLUMAZENIL (Cont.)

Precautions:

Return of sedation: Flumazenil may be expected to improve the alertness of patients recovering from a procedure involving sedation or anesthesia with benzodiazepines, but should not be substituted for an adequate period of post-procedure monitoring. The availability of flumazenil does not reduce the risks associated with the use of large doses of benzodiazepine for sedation. Monitor patients for resedation, respiratory depression (see Warnings) or other persistent or recurrent agonist effects for an adequate period of time after administration of flumazenil.

Resedation is least likely in cases where flumazenil is adminstered to reverse a low dose of a short-acting benzodiazepine (< 10 mg midazolam). It is most likely in cases where a large single or cumulative dose of a benzodiazepine has been given in the course of a long procedure along with neuromuscular blocking agents and multiple anesthetic agents.

Profound resedation was observed in 1% to 3% of patients in the clinical studies. In clinical situations where resedation must be prevented, physicians may wish to repeat the initial dose (up to 1 mg given at 0.2 mg/min) at 30 minutes and possibly again at 60 minutes. This dosage schedule, although not studied in clinical trials, was effective in preventing resedation in a pharmacologic study in healthy volunteers.

Intensive Care Unit (ICU): Use with caution in the ICU because of the increased risk of unrecognized benzodiazepine dependence in such settings. Flumazenil may produce convulsions in patients physically dependent on benzodiazepines (see Administration and Dosage and Warnings).

The use of flumazenil to diagnose benzodiazepine-induced sedation in the ICU is not recommended due to the risk of adverse events as described above. In addition, the prognostic significance of a patient's failure to respond to flumazenil in cases confounded by metabolic disorder, traumatic injury, drugs other than benzodiazepines or any other reasons not associated with benzodiazepine receptor occupancy is not known.

Overdose situations: Flumazenil is intended as an adjunct to, not as a substitute for, proper management of airway, assisted breathing, circulatory access and support, internal decontamination by lavage and charcoal, and adequate clinical evaluation. Institute necessary measures to secure airway, ventilation and IV access prior to administering flumazenil. Upon arousal patients may attempt to withdraw endotracheal tubes or IV lines as the result of confusion and agitation following awakening.

Head injury: Use with caution in patients with head injury as flumazenil may be capable of precipitating convulsions or altering cerebral blood flow in patients receiving benzodiazepines. It should be used only by practitioners prepared to manage such complications should they occur.

Neuromuscular blocking agents: Do not use flumazenil until the effects of neuromuscular blockade have been fully reversed.

Psychiatric patients: Flumazenil may provoke panic attacks in patients with a history of panic disorder.

Drug and alcohol dependent patients: Use with caution in patients with alcoholism and other drug dependencies due to the increased frequency of benzodiazepine tolerance and dependence observed in these patient populations. Flumazenil is not recommended either as a treatment for benzodiazepine dependence or for the management of protracted benzodiazepine abstinence syndromes, as such use has not been studied.

The administration of flumazenil can precipitate benzodiazepine withdrawal in animals and man. This has been seen in healthy volunteers treated with therapeutic doses of oral lorazepam for up to 2 weeks who exhibited effects such as hot flushes, agitation and tremor when treated with cumulative doses of up to 3 mg flumazenil.

Similar adverse experiences suggestive of flumazenil precipitation of benzodiazepine withdrawal have occurred in some patients in clinical trials. Such patients had a short-lived syndrome characterized by dizziness, mild confusion, emotional lability, agitation (with signs and symptoms of anxiety) and mild sensory distortions. This response was dose-related, most common at doses > 1 mg, rarely required treatment other than reassurance and was usually short-lived. When required (5 to 10 cases), these patients were successfully treated with usual doses of a barbiturate, a benzodiazepine or other sedative drug.

Assume that flumazenil administration may trigger dose-dependent withdrawal syndromes in patients with established physical dependence on benzodiazepines and may complicate the management of withdrawal syndrome for alcohol, barbiturates and cross-tolerant sedatives.

(Precautions continued on following page)

FLUMAZENIL (Cont.)

Precautions (Cont.):

Tolerance to benzodiazepines: Flumazenil may cause benzodiazepine withdrawal symptoms in individuals who have been taking benzodiazepines long enough to have some degree of tolerance. Patients who had been taking benzodiazepines prior to entry into the flumazenil trials who were given flumazenil in doses > 1 mg experienced withdrawal-like events 2 to 5 times more frequently than patients who received < 1 mg.

In patients who may have tolerance to benzodiazepines, as indicated by clinical history or by the need for larger than usual doses of benzodiazepines, slower titration rates of 0.1 mg/min and lower total doses may help reduce the frequency of emergent confusion and agitation. In such cases, take special care to monitor the patients for resedation because of the lower doses of flumazenil used.

Physical dependence on benzodiazepines: Flumazenil is known to precipitate withdrawal seizures in patients who are physically dependent on benzodiazepines, even if such dependence was established in a relatively few days of high-dose sedation in ICU environments. The risk of either seizures or resedation in such cases is high and patients have experienced seizures before regaining consciousness. Use flumazenil in such settings with extreme caution, since the use of flumazenil in this situation has not been studied and no information as to dose and rate of titration is available. Use in such patients only if potential benefits of using the drug outweigh the risks of precipitated seizures.

Pain on injection: To minimize the likelihood of pain or inflammation at the injection site, administer flumazenil through a freely flowing IV infusion into a large vein. Local irritation may occur following extravasation into perivascular tissues.

Respiratory disease: Appropriate ventilatory support is the primary treatment of patients with serious lung disease who experience serious respiratory depression due to benzodiazepines rather than the administration of flumazenil. Flumazenil is capable of partially reversing benzodiazepine-induced alterations in ventilatory drive in healthy volunteers, but is not clinically effective.

Cardiovascular disease: Flumazenil did not increase the work of the heart when used to reverse benzodiazepines in cardiac patients when given at a rate of 0.1 mg/min in total doses of < 0.5 mg. Flumazenil alone had no significant effects on cardiovascular parameters when administered to patients with stable ischemic heart disease.

Ambulatory patients: The effects of flumazenil may wear off before a long-acting benzodiazepine is completely cleared from the body. In general, if a patient shows no signs of sedation within 2 hours after a 1 mg dose of flumazenil, serious resedation at a later time is unlikely. Provide an adequate period of observation for any patient in whom either long-acting benzodiazepines (eg, diazepam) or large doses of short-acting benzodiazepines (eg, > 10 mg midazolam) have been used (see Administration and Dosage).

Because of the increased risk of adverse reactions in patients who have been taking benzodiazepines on a regular basis, it is particularly important that physicians query carefully about benzodiazepine, alcohol and sedative use as part of the history prior to any procedure in which the use of flumazenil is planned (see Drug and Alcohol Dependent Patients).

Drug abuse and dependence: Flumazenil acts as a benzodiazepine antagonist, blocks the effects of benzodiazepines in animals and man, antagonizes benzodiazepine reinforcement in animal models, produces dysphoria in normal subjects and has had no reported abuse in foreign marketing. Flumazenil has a benzodiazepine-like structure, but it does not act as a benzodiazepine agonist in man and is not a controlled substance.

Monitoring: No specific laboratory tests are recommended to follow the patient's response or to identify possible adverse reactions.

Drug Interactions:

CNS depressants: Interaction with CNS depressants other than benzodiazepines has not been specifically studied; however, no deleterious interactions were seen when flumazenil was administered after narcotics, inhalational anesthetics, muscle relaxants and muscle relaxant antagonists administered in conjunction with sedation or anesthesia.

Mixed drug overdosage: Particular caution is necessary when using flumazenil in cases of mixed drug overdosage since the toxic effects (eg, convulsions, cardiac dysrhythmias) of other drugs taken in overdose (especially cyclic antidepressants) may emerge with the reversal of the benzodiazepine effect by flumazenil (see Warnings).

Benzodiazepine pharmacokinetics are unaltered in the presence of flumazenil.

Drug/Food interaction: Ingestion of food during an IV infusion of flumazenil results in a 50% increase in flumazenil clearance, most likely due to the increased hepatic blood flow that accompanies a meal.

(Continued on following page)

FLUMAZENIL (Cont.)

Adverse Reactions:

Serious adverse reactions: Deaths have occurred in patients who received flumazenil in a variety of clinical settings. The majority of deaths occurred in patients with serious underlying disease or in patients who had ingested large amounts of non-benzodiazepine drugs (usually cyclic antidepressants) as part of an overdose.

Serious adverse events have occurred in all clinical settings, and convulsions are the most common serious adverse event reported. Flumazenil administration has been associated with the onset of convulsions in patients who are relying on benzodiazepine effects to control seizures, are physically dependent on benzodiazepines, or who have ingested large doses of other drugs (see Warnings).

Two of the 446 patients who received flumazenil in controlled clinical trials for the management of a benzodiazepine overdosage had cardiac dysrhythmias (one ventricular tachycardia, one junctional tachycardia).

Body as a whole: Headache, injection site pain, increased sweating (3% to 9%); injection site reaction (thrombophlebitis, skin abnormality, rash), fatigue (asthenia, malaise) (1% to 3%); rigors, shivering (< 1%).

Cardiovascular: Cutaneous vasodilation (sweating, flushing, hot flushes) (1% to 3%); arrhythmia (atrial, nodal, ventricular extrasystoles), bradycardia, tachycardia, hypertension, chest pain (< 1%).

GI: Nausea, vomiting (11%); hiccups (< 1%).

CNS: Dizziness (vertigo, ataxia) (10%); agitation (anxiety, nervousness, dry mouth, tremor, palpitations, insomnia, dyspnea, hyperventilation) (3% to 9%); emotional lability (abnormal crying, depersonalization, euphoria, increased tears, depression, dysphoria, paranoia) (1% to 3%); confusion (difficulty concentrating, delirium), convulsions (see Warnings), somnolence (stupor), speech disorder (dysphonia, thick tongue) (< 1%).

Special senses: Abnormal vision (visual field defect, diplopia), blurred vision (3% to 9%); paresthesia (sensation abnormal, hypoesthesia) (1% to 3%); abnormal hearing (transient hearing impairment, hyperacusis, tinnitus) (< 1%).

Overdosage:

Large IV doses of flumazenil, when administered to healthy volunteers in the absence of a benzodiazepine agonist, produced no serious adverse reactions, severe signs or symptoms, or clinically significant laboratory test abnormalities. In clinical studies, most adverse reactions to flumazenil were an extension of the pharmacologic effects of the drug in reversing benzodiazepine effects.

Reversal with an excessively high dose of flumazenil may produce anxiety, agitation, increased muscle tone, hyperesthesia and possibly convulsions. Convulsions have been treated with barbiturates, benzodiazepines and phenytoin, generally with prompt resolution of the seizures (see Warnings).

Patient Information:

Flumazenil does not consistently reverse amnesia. Patients cannot be expected to remember information told to them in the post-procedure period; reinforce instructions given to patients in writing or give to a responsible family member. Discuss with patients, both before surgery and at discharge, that although they may feel alert at the time of discharge, the effects of the benzodiazepine may recur. As a result, instruct the patient, preferably in writing, that their memory and judgment may be impaired and specifically advise patients:

1. Not to engage in any activities requiring complete alertness, and not to operate hazardous machinery or a motor vehicle until at least 18 to 24 hours after discharge, and it is certain no residual sedative effects of the benzodiazepine remain.
2. Not to take any alcohol or non-prescription drugs for 18 to 24 hours after flumazenil administration or if the effects of the benzodiazepine persist.

Administration and Dosage:

For IV use only. To minimize the likelihood of pain at the injection site, administer flumazenil through a freely running IV infusion into a large vein.

Individualization of dosage: The serious adverse effects of flumazenil are related to the reversal of benzodiazepine effects. Using more than the minimally effective dose of flumazenil is tolerated by most patients but may complicate the management of patients who are physically dependent on benzodiazepines or patients who are depending on benzodiazepines for therapeutic effect (such as suppression of seizures in cyclic antidepressant overdose).

In high-risk patients, it is important to administer the smallest amount of flumazenil that is effective. The 1 minute wait between individual doses in the dose-titration recommended for general clinical populations may be too short for high-risk patients because it takes 6 to 10 minutes for any single dose of flumazenil to reach full effects. Slow the rate of administration of flumazenil administered to high-risk patients.

(Administration and Dosage continued on following page)

FLUMAZENIL (Cont.)

Administration and Dosage (Cont.):

Reversal of conscious sedation or in general anesthesia: For the reversal of the sedative effects of benzodiazepines administered for conscious sedation or general anesthesia, the recommended initial dose is 0.2 mg (2 ml) administered IV over 15 seconds. If the desired level of consciousness is not obtained after waiting an additional 45 seconds, a further dose of 0.2 mg (2 ml) can be injected and repeated at 60 second intervals where necessary (up to a maximum of 4 additional times) to a maximum total dose of 1 mg (10 ml). Individualize the dose based on the patient's response, with most patients responding to doses of 0.6 to 1 mg.

The major risk will be resedation because the duration of effect of a long-acting (or large dose of a short-acting) benzodiazepine may exceed that of flumazenil. In the event of resedation, repeated doses may be administered at 20 minute intervals as needed. For repeat treatment, administer no more than 1 mg (given as 0.2 mg/min) at any one time, and give no more than 3 mg in any one hour.

It is recommended that flumazenil be administered as the series of small injections described (not as a single bolus injection) to allow the practitioner to control the reversal of sedation to the approximate endpoint desired and to minimize the possibility of adverse effects.

Management of suspected benzodiazepine overdose: For initial management of a known or suspected benzodiazepine overdose, the recommended initial dose is 0.2 mg (2 ml) administered IV over 30 seconds. If the desired level of consciousness is not obtained after waiting 30 seconds, a further dose of 0.3 mg (3 ml) can be administered over another 30 seconds. Further doses of 0.5 mg (5 ml) can be administered over 30 seconds at 1 minute intervals up to a cumulative dose of 3 mg.

The risk of confusion, agitation, emotional lability and perceptual distortion with the doses recommended in patients with benzodiazepine overdose (3 to 5 mg administered as 0.5 mg/min) may be greater than that expected with lower doses and slower administration. The recommended doses represent a compromise between a desirable slow awakening and the need for prompt response and a persistent effect in the overdose situation. If circumstances permit, the physician may elect to use the 0.2 mg/min titration rate to slowly awaken the patient over 5 to 10 minutes, which may help to reduce signs and symptoms on emergence.

Do not rush the administration of flumazenil. Patients should have a secure airway and IV access before administration of the drug and be awakened gradually (see Precautions).

Most patients with benzodiazepine overdose will respond to a cumulative dose of 1 to 3 mg, and doses beyond 3 mg do not reliably produce additional effects. On rare occasions, patients with a partial response at 3 mg may require additional titration up to a total dose of 5 mg (administered slowly in the same manner).

If a patient has not responded 5 minutes after receiving a cumulative dose of 5 mg, the major cause of sedation is likely not to be due to benzodiazepines, and additional flumazenil is likely to have no effect.

In the event of resedation, repeated doses may be given at 20 minute intervals if needed. For repeat treatment, give no more than 1 mg (given as 0.5 mg/min) at any one time and give no more than 3 mg in any 1 hour.

IV compatibility: Flumazenil is compatible with 5% Dextrose in Water, Lactated Ringer's and normal saline solutions. If flumazenil is drawn into a syringe or mixed with any of these solutions, it should be discarded after 24 hours. For optimum sterility, flumazenil should remain in the vial until just before use.

Rx	**Mazicon** (Hoffman-La Roche)	**Injection:** 0.1 mg/ml	In 5 and 10 ml vials[1].

[1] With parabens and EDTA.

Refer to the general discussion of these products on page 2671.

PHYSOSTIGMINE SALICYLATE

Actions:

Pharmacology: The action of acetylcholine is transient because of hydrolysis by acetylcholinesterase. Physostigmine, a reversible anticholinesterase drug, increases the concentration of acetylcholine at the sites of cholinergic transmission and prolongs and exaggerates the effect of acetylcholine.

Physostigmine reverses the following central and peripheral anticholinergic effects:

Central toxic effects – Anxiety, delirium, disorientation, hallucinations, hyperactivity and seizures. Severe poisoning due to anticholinergics may produce coma, medullary paralysis and death.

Peripheral toxic effects – Tachycardia, hyperpyrexia, mydriasis, vasodilatation, urinary retention, decreased GI motility, decreased secretion in salivary and sweat glands, loss of secretions in the pharynx, bronchi and nasal passages.

Dramatic reversal of the effects of anticholinergic symptoms occurs minutes after IV administration if the patient has not suffered anoxia or other trauma.

Pharmacokinetics: Physostigmine, a tertiary amine, is readily absorbed and freely crosses the blood-brain barrier following IM or IV administration. Peak effects are seen within 5 minutes and persist for 45 to 60 minutes following IV administration. Physostigmine is rapidly hydrolyzed by cholinesterase, the enzyme which it inhibits. Plasma half-life is approximately 1 to 2 hours. Renal impairment does NOT require dosage alteration.

Indications:

To reverse toxic CNS effects caused by anticholinergic drugs (including tricyclic antidepressants).

May antagonize the CNS depressant effects of diazepam.

Unlabeled Uses: Physostigmine has been used in the treatment of delirium tremens and Alzheimer's disease.

Contraindications:

Asthma; gangrene; diabetes; cardiovascular disease; intestinal or urogenital tract obstruction; any vagotonic state; patients receiving choline esters or depolarizing neuromuscular blocking agents (decamethonium, succinylcholine).

Warnings:

Discontinue drug if symptoms of excessive salivation or emesis, frequent urination or diarrhea occur. If excessive sweating or nausea occurs, reduce dosage.

Administer IV slowly, at a controlled rate, no more than 1 mg/minute. Rapid administration can cause bradycardia, hypersalivation leading to respiratory difficulties and seizures.

Usage in Pregnancy: There have been no reports linking physostigmine with congenital defects. Transient muscular weakness has been noted in neonates whose mothers had been treated with other cholinesterase inhibitors for myasthenia gravis. Use only when clearly needed and when the potential benefits outweigh the potential hazards to the fetus.

Usage in Lactation: Safety for use has not been established.

Precautions:

Because of the possibility of hypersensitivity, atropine sulfate should be available as an antagonist and antidote for physostigmine.

Adverse Reactions:

Nausea, vomiting, salivation; bradycardia and convulsions (if IV administration is too rapid).

Overdosage:

Can cause cholinergic crisis. Atropine sulfate is an appropriate antidote.

Administration and Dosage:

Post-Anesthesia: 0.5 to 1 mg IM or IV. Administer IV slowly, no more than 1 mg/min. Repeat at 10 to 30 minute intervals if desired response is not obtained.

Overdosage of anticholinergic drugs: 2 mg IM or IV; give IV slowly, no more than 1 mg/min. Repeat if life-threatening signs such as arrhythmia, convulsions or coma occur.

Pediatric: Reserve for life-threatening situations only. Recommended dosage is 0.02 mg/kg IM or by slow IV injection, no more than 0.5 mg per minute. If necessary, repeat at 5 to 10 minute intervals until a therapeutic effect or a maximum dose of 2 mg is attained.

Rx	**Antilirium** (Forest Pharm.)	**Injection:** 1 mg per ml	In 2 ml amps[1] and 1 ml syringes.[1]

[1] With 2% benzyl alcohol and 0.1% sodium bisulfite.

Refer to the general discussion of these products on page2671.

PRALIDOXIME CHLORIDE (2-PAM)

Actions:

Pharmacology: Pralidoxime reactivates cholinesterase (mainly outside the CNS) inactivated by phosphorylation due to an organophosphate pesticide or related compound. Destruction of accumulated acetylcholine can then proceed, allowing neuromuscular junctions to function normally. It also slows the "aging" of phosphorylated cholinesterase to a nonreactive form, and detoxifies certain organophosphates by direct chemical reaction. The drug's most critical effect is relieving respiratory muscle paralysis. Because pralidoxime is less effective in relieving depression of the respiratory center, concomitant atropine is required to block the effect of accumulated acetylcholine at this site. Pralidoxime relieves muscarinic signs and symptoms (salivation, bronchospasm), but this is relatively unimportant since atropine is adequate for this purpose.

Pralidoxime does not antagonize the effects on the neuromuscular junction of the carbamate anticholinesterases, neostigmine, pyridostigmine and ambenonium, used in the treatment of myasthenia gravis. It has been used in carbamate poisoning, however, it is not as effective an antidote to these drugs as it is to the organophosphates.

Pharmacokinetics: Pralidoxime is slowly absorbed from the GI tract; blood concentrations are more rapidly achieved with IM or IV administration. Pralidoxime is distributed throughout the extracellular water; it is not bound to plasma protein and does not readily pass into the CNS. The drug is rapidly excreted in the urine, partly unchanged and partly as a metabolite produced by the liver. Average half-life is around 1.7 hours. It is relatively short-acting and repeated doses may be needed, especially when poison absorption continues. Renal dysfunction will increase drug blood levels.

Indications:

Antidote in poisoning due to organophosphate pesticides and chemicals with anticholinesterase activity (eg, dichlorvos, dioxathion, echothiophate iodide, endothion, fenthion, formothion, isoflurophate, malathion, methyl parathion, parathion, TEPP, diazinon).

Control of overdosage by anticholinesterase drugs used to treat myasthenia gravis.

Pralidoxime chloride auto-injector: Specifically for IM use as an adjunct to atropine, in poisoning by nerve agents having anticholinesterase activity.

Contraindications:

Hypersensitivity to any component.

Warnings:

Until further information is available, no recommendation is made for use in intoxication by pesticides of the carbamate class.

Usage in Pregnancy: Category C. It is not known whether pralidoxime can cause fetal harm when administered to a pregnant woman or can affect reproduction capacity. Give pralidoxime to a pregnant woman only if clearly needed.

Usage in Lactation: It is not known whether this drug is excreted in human milk. Exercise caution when pralidoxime is administered to a nursing woman.

Usage in Children: Safety and efficacy in children have not been established.

Precautions:

Institute treatment of organophosphate poisoning without waiting for laboratory test results. Red blood cell, plasma cholinesterase and urinary paranitrophenol measurements (in the case of parathion exposure) may help confirm diagnosis and follow course of the illness. A reduction in red blood cell cholinesterase concentration to below 50% of normal has been seen only with organophosphate ester poisoning.

Generally well tolerated; however, the desperate condition of the organophosphate-poisoned patient will mask the minor signs and symptoms noted in normal subjects.

Administer slowly by IV infusion, since tachycardia, laryngospasm and muscle rigidity have occurred with a too rapid rate of injection. (See Administration and Dosage.)

Usage in impaired renal function: A decrease in renal function will result in increased drug blood levels; reduce dosage in the presence of renal insufficiency.

Auto-injector users must understand the indications and use. Review symptoms of poisoning and operation instructions of the mechanism.

Myasthenia gravis: Use with caution in treating organophosphate overdosage in cases of myasthenia gravis, since it may precipitate a myasthenic crisis.

Drug Interactions:

Barbiturates are potentiated by the anticholinesterases; therefore, use with caution in the treatment of convulsions.

Morphine, theophylline, aminophylline, succinylcholine, reserpine and **phenothiazines:** Avoid in patients with organophosphate poisoning.

(Continued on following page)

PRALIDOXIME CHLORIDE (2-PAM) (Cont.)

Adverse Reactions:

Mild to moderate pain at the injection site 40 to 60 minutes after IM injection.

SGOT and SGPT elevations which return to normal in 2 weeks. Transient elevations in CPK have also been observed.

Dizziness, blurred vision, diplopia and impaired accommodation, headache, drowsiness, nausea, tachycardia, hyperventilation and muscular weakness.

When atropine and pralidoxime are used together, atropinization may occur earlier than expected, especially if the total dose of atropine has been large and the administration of pralidoxime has been delayed. Excitement and manic behavior immediately following recovery of consciousness have been reported. However, similar behavior has occurred in cases of organophosphate poisoning that were not treated with pralidoxime.

Overdosage:

Symptoms: Dizziness, headache, blurred vision, diplopia, impaired accommodation, nausea, slight tachycardia. In therapy, it has been difficult to differentiate side effects due to the drug from those due to the poison.

Treatment: Administer artificial respiration and other supportive therapy as needed.

Administration and Dosage:

Organophosphate poisoning: Initial measures include removal of secretions, maintenance of a patent airway and artificial ventilation. In the absence of cyanosis, give atropine 2 to 4 mg IV; when cyanosis is present, give 2 to 4 mg atropine IM while improving ventilation. Repeat every 5 to 10 minutes until signs of atropine toxicity appear. Maintain atropinization for at least 48 hours. Begin pralidoxime concomitantly with atropine.

Adults – Initial dose of 1 to 2 g IV, preferably as a 15 to 30 minute infusion in 100 ml of saline. If this is not practicable or if pulmonary edema is present, give slowly IV as a 5% solution in water over not less than 5 minutes. After about an hour, give a second dose of 1 to 2 g if muscle weakness is not relieved. Give additional doses cautiously if muscle weakness persists. If IV administration is not feasible, give IM or SC.

Children – 20 to 40 mg/kg/dose, given as above.

Treatment is most effective if begun within a few hours after poisoning. Usually, the drug is ineffective if first administered more than 36 to 48 hours after exposure. However, it is indicated in severe poisoning since patients may still respond. In severe cases, especially after ingestion of the poison, monitor the effect of therapy by ECG because of possible heart block due to the anticholinesterase. Where the poison has been ingested, consider the likelihood of continuing absorption from the lower bowel; additional doses of pralidoxime may be needed every 3 to 8 hours or continued for several days.

Oral: 1 to 3 g every 5 hours in the absence of severe GI symptoms resulting from the anticholinesterase intoxication. Observe patient closely for at least 24 to 72 hours.

If dermal exposure has occurred, remove clothing and thoroughly wash hair and skin with sodium bicarbonate or alcohol as soon as possible.

If convulsions interfere with respiration, carefully give 2.5% IV sodium thiopental or diazepam.

Anticholinesterase overdosage (eg, neostigmine, pyridostigmine and ambenonium used in the treatment of myasthenia gravis): 1 to 2 g IV followed by increments of 250 mg every 5 minutes.

Exposure to nerve agents: Administer atropine and pralidoxime as soon as possible after exposure. Depending on the severity of symptoms, immediately administer one atropine-containing auto-injector, followed by one pralidoxime-containing auto-injector. Atropine must be given first until its effects become apparent; then administer pralidoxime. If nerve agent symptoms are present after 15 minutes, repeat injections. If symptoms exist after an additional 15 minutes, repeat injections. If symptoms remain after the third set of injections, seek medical help.

Rx	**Protopam Chloride** (Ayerst)	**Emergency Kit:** One 20 ml vial containing 1 g each pralidoxime chloride with one 20 ml amp diluent, disposable syringe, needle and alcohol swab. **Hospital Package:** Six 20 ml vials containing 1 g each pralidoxime chloride without diluent or syringe. **Tablets:** 500 mg. In 100s.
Rx	**Pralidoxime Chloride** (Survival Technology)	**Injection:** One auto-injector containing 600 mg pralidoxime chloride in 2 ml.[1]

[1] Contains benzyl alcohol and aminoacetic acid.

DIGOXIN IMMUNE FAB (Ovine)

Actions:

Digoxin immune fab (ovine) are antigen binding fragments (fab) derived from specific anti-digoxin antibodies produced in sheep. Production involves conjugation of digoxin as a hapten to human albumin. Sheep are immunized with this material to produce antibodies specific for the digoxin molecule. The antibody is then papain digested, and digoxin-specific fab fragments are isolated and purified.

Pharmacokinetics: After IV injection in humans with normal renal function, the half-life appears to be 15 to 20 hours. Studies in animals indicate that these antibody fragments have a large volume of distribution in the extracellular space. Ordinarily, improvement in signs and symptoms of intoxication begins in less than half an hour.

Fab fragments bind molecules of digoxin, making them unavailable for binding at their site of action. The fab fragment-digoxin complex accumulates in the blood and is excreted by the kidneys.

Indications:

Treatment of potentially life-threatening digoxin intoxication. It has also been used successfully to treat life-threatening digitoxin overdose.

Manifestations of life-threatening toxicity include severe arrhythmias, ie, ventricular tachycardia or ventricular fibrillation, or progressive bradyarrhythmias such as severe sinus bradycardia or second or third degree heart block not responsive to atropine.

Ingestion of more than 10 mg digoxin by healthy adults or 4 mg digoxin by healthy children, or steady-state serum concentrations > 10 ng/ml, often results in cardiac arrest. Digitalis-induced progressive elevation of serum potassium concentration also suggests imminent cardiac arrest. If the potassium concentration exceeds 5 mEq/L in the setting of digitalis intoxication, digoxin fab therapy is indicated.

Contraindications:

None known.

Warnings:

Suicidal ingestion often involves more than one drug; consider toxicity from other drugs.

Allergic reactions have not yet occurred, but consider the possibility of anaphylactic, hypersensitivity or febrile reactions. If an anaphylactoid reaction occurs, discontinue the drug infusion and initiate appropriate therapy. Have epinephrine 1:1000 immediately available. Refer to Management of Acute Hypersensitivity Reactions on p. viii.

Patients allergic to ovine proteins are particularly at risk, as are individuals who have previously received antibodies or fab fragments raised in sheep.

Skin testing for allergy was performed during the clinical investigation of this agent. Only one patient developed erythema at the site of skin testing. The patient had no adverse reaction to systemic treatment. Allergy testing is not routinely required before treatment of life-threatening digitalis toxicity.

Skin testing may be appropriate for high risk individuals, especially patients with known allergy to sheep proteins or those previously treated with digoxin immune fab. The intradermal skin test can be performed by: 1) Diluting 0.1 ml of reconstituted drug (10 mg/ml) in 10 ml sterile isotonic saline (1:100 dilution, 100 mcg/ml); 2) Injecting 0.1 ml of the 1:100 dilution (10 mcg) intradermally and observing for an urticarial wheal surrounded by a zone of erythema. Read the test at 20 minutes.

The scratch test procedure is performed by placing one drop of a 1:100 dilution on the skin and then making a ¼-inch scratch through the drop with a sterile needle. The scratch site is inspected at 20 minutes for an urticarial wheal surrounded by erythema.

If skin testing causes a systemic reaction, apply a tourniquet above the site of testing and treat anaphylaxis. Avoid further administration of the drug unless its use is absolutely essential; in this case, pretreat the patient with corticosteroids and diphenhydramine, and make preparations for treating anaphylaxis.

Usage in Pregnancy: Category C. It is not known whether this agent can cause fetal harm or affect reproduction capacity. Use only if clearly needed and if the potential benefits outweigh the potential hazards to the fetus.

Usage in Lactation: It is not known whether this drug is excreted in breast milk. Exercise caution when administering to a nursing mother.

Usage in Children: This agent has been used successfully in infants with no apparent adverse sequelae. Use in infants only if the potential benefits outweigh the hazards.

(Continued on following page)

DIGOXIN IMMUNE FAB (Ovine) (Cont.):

Precautions:

For standard therapy of digitalis intoxication see page 596 .

Impaired cardiac function: Patients may deteriorate from withdrawal of digoxin. Additional support can be provided by use of IV inotropes (ie, dopamine or dobutamine) or vasodilators. With catecholamines, take care not to aggravate digitalis toxic rhythm disturbances. Do not use other types of digitalis glycosides or redigitalize until the fab fragments have been eliminated from the body; this may require several days. Patients with impaired renal function may require a week or longer.

Impaired renal function: The elimination half-life in renal failure has not been clearly defined. Several patients with mild to moderate renal dysfunction have been successfully treated. There is no evidence to suggest any difference between these patients and patients with normal renal function, but excretion of the fab fragment-digoxin complex from the body is probably delayed. In patients who are functionally anephric, anticipate failure to clear the fab fragment-digoxin complex from the blood by glomerular filtration and renal excretion; the reticuloendothelial system might eliminate the complex. Whether this would lead to detoxification or to reintoxication by release of newly unbound digoxin into the blood is not known.

Laboratory Tests: Obtain serum concentrations before administration. These measurements may be difficult to interpret if drawn soon after the last digitalis dose, since at least 6 to 8 hours are required for equilibration of digoxin between serum and tissue. Closely monitor the patient's temperature, blood pressure, ECG and potassium concentration during and after drug administration. The total serum digoxin concentration may rise precipitously following administration of the drug, but this will be almost entirely bound to the fab fragment. Fab fragments will interfere with digitalis immunoassay measurements. The standard serum digoxin concentration measurement can be clinically misleading until the fab fragment is eliminated from the body, which may require several days. Patients with impaired renal function may require a week or longer before the standard serum digoxin concentration assay will give reliable results.

Severe digitalis intoxication can cause life-threatening elevation in serum potassium concentration by shifting potassium from inside to outside the cell. This can lead to increased renal excretion of potassium. These patients may have hyperkalemia with a total body deficit of potassium. When the effect of digitalis is reversed, potassium shifts back inside the cell with a resulting decline in serum potassium concentration. Hypokalemia may develop rapidly. Monitor serum potassium concentration repeatedly, especially over the first several hours after the drug is given, and cautiously treat when necessary.

Adverse Reactions:

In a few instances, low cardiac output states and congestive heart failure could have been exacerbated by withdrawal of the inotropic effects of digitalis. Hypokalemia may occur from reactivation of ATPase (sodium, potassium). Patients with atrial fibrillation may develop a rapid ventricular response from withdrawal of the effects of digitalis on the AV node.

Administration and Dosage:

Digoxin immune fab is administered IV over 30 minutes and infused through a 0.22 μm membrane filter. If cardiac arrest is imminent, give as a bolus injection.

Dosage varies according to the amount of digoxin to be neutralized. Dosing guidelines are given on the following page. If, after several hours, toxicity has not reversed or appears to recur, readministration may be required. If a patient presents with digitalis toxicity from an acute ingestion, and neither a serum digitalis concentration nor an estimated ingestion amount is available, administer 20 vials (800 mg). This will be adequate to treat most life-threatening ingestions in adults and children. However, in small children, it is important to monitor for volume overload.

Dosage estimates: The dose need not be exactly equimolar. In general, a large dose has a faster onset but enhances the possibility of an allergic or febrile reaction. The tables on the following page give approximate doses.

(Administration and Dosage continued on following page)

DIGOXIN IMMUNE FAB (Ovine) (Cont.):

Administration and Dosage (Cont.):

TABLE 1: Approximate Dose for Reversal of a Single Ingestion Digoxin Overdose

Number of Digoxin Tablets or Capsules Ingested*	Dose	
	mg	# of Vials
25	340	8.5
50	680	17
75	1000	25
100	1360	34
150	2000	50
200	2680	67

* 0.25 mg tablets with 80% bioavailability or 0.2 mg *Lanoxicaps* Capsules

Since infants can have much smaller dosage requirements, reconstitute the 40 mg vial as directed and administer with a tuberculin syringe. For very small doses, dilute a reconstituted vial with 36 ml sterile isotonic saline to achieve a 1 mg/ml concentration.

Table 2: Estimates of Fab Fragments From Serum Digoxin Concentration

Patient	Weight (kg)	Serum Digoxin Concentration (ng/ml)						
		1	2	4	8	12	16	20
Infants/ Children (dose given in mg)	1	0.5 mg†	1 mg†	1.5 mg†	3 mg	5 mg	6 mg	8 mg
	3	1 mg†	2 mg†	5 mg	9 mg	13 mg	18 mg	22 mg
	5	2 mg†	4 mg	8 mg	15 mg	22 mg	30 mg	40 mg
	10	4 mg	8 mg	15 mg	30 mg	40 mg	60 mg	80 mg
	20	8 mg	15 mg	30 mg	60 mg	80 mg	120 mg	160 mg
Adults (dose given in vials [v])	40	0.5 v	1 v	2 v	3 v	5 v	6 v	8 v
	60	0.5 v	1 v	2 v	5 v	7 v	9 v	11 v
	70	1 v	2 v	3 v	5 v	8 v	11 v	13 v
	80	1 v	2 v	3 v	6 v	9 v	12 v	15 v
	100	1 v	2 v	4 v	8 v	11 v	15 v	19 v

† Dilution of reconstituted vial to 1 mg/ml may be desirable. v = vials.

Exact dosage calculation: The equimolar dose required is calculated from the total amount of digoxin (or digitoxin) in the patient's body. An estimate of total body load is based either on the known acutely ingested dose or is estimated by using a steady-state serum concentration. For toxicity from an acute ingestion, the total body load of digoxin (mg) will be approximately equal to the dose ingested (mg); multiply by 0.8 to correct for incomplete absorption of tablets. Total body load of digitoxin (mg) is equal to the dose ingested (mg). To estimate total load from the steady-state serum concentration, the patient's serum digoxin concentration (SDC) in ng/ml is multiplied by the mean volume of distribution of digoxin (5.6 L/kg times patient weight in kg) to give total body load in mcg. Divide by 1000 to obtain the estimated mg amount of digoxin in the body.

Digoxin: Body load in mg = (SDC) (5.6) (weight in kg) ÷ 1000.

For patients toxic from digitoxin, estimate total body load by using the value 0.56 L/kg volume of distribution in place of the 5.6 L/kg for digoxin.

Digitoxin: Body load in mg = (SDC) (0.56) (weight in kg) ÷ 1000.

Each vial contains 40 mg purified digoxin-specific fab fragments which will bind approximately 0.6 mg digoxin (or digitoxin). Calculate the total number of vials required by dividing the total body load in mg by 0.6 mg/vial.

$$\text{Dose (in \# of vials)} = \frac{\text{Body load (mg)}}{\text{0.6 (mg/vial)}}$$

If the calculation based on ingested dose differs substantially from the calculation based on serum digoxin or digitoxin concentration, it may be preferable to administer an amount based on the higher calculation. Inaccurate serum digoxin concentration measurements are a source of error, especially for very high values.

Reconstitution: Dissolve the contents in each vial with 4 ml of Sterile Water for Injection. Mix gently to give an approximately isosmotic solution with a protein concentration of 10 mg/ml. Use reconstituted product promptly. If it is not used immediately, store at 2° to 8°C (36° to 46°F) for up to 4 hours. The reconstituted product may be diluted with sterile isotonic saline to a convenient volume.

Rx	**Digibind**[1] (Burroughs Wellcome)	**Injection, lyophilized:** 40 mg per vial with 75 mg sorbitol. Each vial will bind ≈ 0.6 mg digoxin or digitoxin.

[1] This is an orphan drug; therefore, availability is limited. For further information, contact Burroughs Wellcome, 3030 Cornwallis Road, Research Triangle Park, North Carolina 27709 (919) 248-3000.

MESNA

Actions:

Pharmacology: Mesna injection is a detoxifying agent used to inhibit the hemorrhagic cystitis induced by ifosfamide (see ifosfamide monograph). In the kidney, the mesna disulfide is reduced to the free thiol compound, mesna, which reacts chemically with the urotoxic ifosfamide metabolites (acrolein and 4-hydroxy-ifosfamide) resulting in their detoxification. The first step in the detoxification process is the binding of mesna to 4-hydroxy-ifosfamide forming a non-urotoxic 4-sulfoethylthioifosfamide. Mesna also binds to the double bonds of acrolein and other urotoxic metabolites.

Pharmacokinetics: Analogous to the physiological cysteine-cystine system, following IV administration mesna is rapidly oxidized to its only metabolite, mesna disulfide (dimesna). Mesna disulfide remains in the intravascular compartment and is rapidly eliminated by the kidneys.

After administration of an 800 mg dose, the half-lives of mesna and dimesna in the blood are 0.36 and 1.17 hours, respectively. Approximately 32% and 33% of the administered dose is eliminated in the urine in 24 hours as mesna and dimesna, respectively. The majority of the dose recovered is eliminated within 4 hours. Mesna has a volume of distribution of 0.652 L/kg and a plasma clearance of 1.23 L/kg/hour.

Ifosfamide has dose-dependent pharmacokinetics. At doses of 2 to 4 g, its terminal elimination half-life is about 7 hours. As a result, in order to maintain adequate levels of mesna in the urinary bladder during the course of elimination of the urotoxic ifosfamide metabolites, repeated doses of mesna are required.

Clinical Pharmacology: Mesna was given as bolus doses prior to ifosfamide and at 4 and 8 hours after ifosfamide administration. The hemorrhagic cystitis produced by ifosfamide is dose dependent. At a dose of 1.2 g/m² ifosfamide administered daily for 5 days, 16% to 26% of the patients who received conventional uroprophylaxis (high fluid intake, alkalinization of the urine and the administration of diuretics) developed hematuria (> 50 rbc/hpf or macrohematuria). In contrast, none of the patients who received mesna together with this dose of ifosfamide developed hematuria. Higher doses of ifosfamide from 2 to 4 g/m² administered for 3 to 5 days produced hematuria in 31% to 100% of the patients. When mesna was administered together with these doses of ifosfamide, the incidence of hematuria was < 7%.

Indications:

Prophylactic agent to reduce the incidence of ifosfamide-induced hemorrhagic cystitis.

Unlabeled Use: Mesna may be useful in reducing the incidence of cyclophosphamide-induced hemorrhagic cystitis.

Contraindications:

Hypersensitivity to mesna or other thiol compounds.

Warnings:

Mesna prevents ifosfamide-induced hemorrhagic cystitis. It will not prevent or alleviate other adverse reactions or toxicities associated with ifosfamide therapy.

Mesna does not prevent hemorrhagic cystitis in all patients. Up to 6% of patients treated with mesna have developed hematuria (> 50 rbc/hpf or WHO grade 2 and above). As a result, examine a morning specimen of urine for hematuria (red blood cells) each day prior to ifosfamide therapy. If hematuria develops when mesna is given with ifosfamide according to the dosage schedule, depending on the severity of the hematuria, dosage reductions or discontinuation of ifosfamide therapy may be initiated.

Mesna must be administered with each dose of ifosfamide (see Administration and Dosage). Mesna is not effective in preventing hematuria due to other pathological conditions such as thrombocytopenia.

Usage in Pregnancy: Category B. Reproduction studies in rats and rabbits with oral doses up to 1000 mg/kg have revealed no harm to the fetus. It is not known whether mesna can cause fetal harm when administered to a pregnant woman or can effect reproductive capacity. Mesna should be given to a pregnant woman only if the benefits clearly outweigh any possible risks.

Usage in Lactation: It is not known whether mesna or dimesna is excreted in breast milk. Because of the potential for adverse reactions in nursing infants, decide whether to discontinue nursing or to discontinue the drug, taking into account the importance of the drug to the mother.

(Continued on following page)

MESNA (Cont.)

Drug Interactions:

Drug/Lab Test Interaction: A false positive test for urinary ketones may arise in patients treated with mesna. In this test, a red-violet color develops which, with the addition of glacial acetic acid, will return to violet.

Adverse Reactions:

Because mesna is used in combination with ifosfamide and other chemotherapeutic agents with documented toxicities, it is difficult to distinguish the adverse reactions which may be due to mesna. As a result, the adverse reaction profile of mesna was determined in three Phase I studies (16 subjects) with IV and oral use and two controlled studies in which ifosfamide and mesna were compared to ifosfamide and standard prophylaxis.

In Phase I studies in which IV bolus doses of 0.8 to 1.6 g/m^2 mesna were administered as single or three repeated doses to a total of 10 patients, a bad taste in the mouth (100%) and soft stools (70%) were reported. At IV and oral bolus doses of 2.4 g/m^2 which are approximately 10 times the recommended clinical doses (0.24 g/m^2), diarrhea (83%), limb pain (50%), headache (50%), fatigue (33%), nausea (33%), hypotension (17%) and allergy (17%) occurred in 6 patients.

In controlled clinical studies, adverse reactions were vomiting, diarrhea and nausea.

Overdosage:

There is no known antidote for mesna.

Administration and Dosage:

For the prophylaxis of ifosfamide-induced hemorrhagic cystitis, mesna is given as IV bolus injections in a dosage equal to 20% of the ifosfamide dosage (w/w) at the time of ifosfamide administration and 4 and 8 hours after each dose of ifosfamide. The total daily dose of mesna is 60% of the ifosfamide dose.

Dosing Schedule for Mesna			
	0 Hours	4 Hours	8 Hours
Ifosfamide	1.2 g/m^2	—	—
Mesna	240 mg/m^2	240 mg/m^2	240 mg/m^2

To maintain adequate protection, repeat this dosing schedule on each day that ifosfamide is administered. When the dosage of ifosfamide is adjusted (either increased or decreased), modify the dose of mesna accordingly.

Preparations of IV Solutions: For IV administration, the drug can be diluted by adding the contents of a mesna amp to any of the following fluids obtaining final concentrations of 20 mg mesna/ml fluid: 5% Dextrose Injection, 5% Dextrose and Sodium Chloride Injection, 0.9% Sodium Chloride Injection or Lactated Ringer's Injection.

For example: One 200 mg/2 ml amp may be added to 8 ml, or one 400 mg/4 ml amp may be added to 16 ml, of any of the solutions listed above to create a final concentration of 20 mg mesna/ml fluid.

Storage/stability: Diluted solutions – Chemically and physically stable for 24 hours at 25°C (77°F). Refrigerate and use within 6 hours. *Ampule* – Store at room temperature.

When exposed to oxygen, mesna is oxidized to the disulfide, dimesna. As a result, any unused drug remaining in the amps after dosing should be discarded and a new amp used for each administration.

Admixture incompatibility: Mesna is not compatible with cisplatin.

Rx	**Mesnex** (Mead Johnson Oncology)	**Injection:** 100 mg/ml[1]	In 2, 4 and 10 ml ampules.

[1] With 0.25 mg/ml EDTA.

Emetics

APOMORPHINE HCl

Actions:

Apomorphine, a dopaminergic agonist, causes vomiting by directly stimulating the chemoreceptor trigger zone. Results are usually obtained within 5 to 10 minutes after parenteral administration.

Indications:

A centrally acting emetic.

Contraindications:

Do not use in impending shock; in corrosive poisoning; in narcosis due to opiates, barbiturates, alcohol or other CNS depressants; in patients too inebriated to stand unaided; in patients sensitive to morphine derivatives.

Warnings:

Usage in Pregnancy: Category C. It is not known whether the drug can cause fetal harm when administered to a pregnant woman or can affect reproduction capacity. Give apomorphine to a pregnant woman only if clearly needed.

Usage in Labor and Delivery: Apomorphine with scopolamine produces analgesia and amnesia during labor. Doses of 0.6 to 1.2 mg SC apomorphine appear to potentiate scopolamine analgesia, and the combination decreases the need for inhalation anesthesia. No untoward effects have been observed.

Usage in Lactation: It is not known whether this drug is excreted in human milk. Exercise caution when apomorphine is administered to a nursing woman.

Precautions:

Use with caution in children, debilitated individuals, those with cardiac decompensation, or persons predisposed to nausea and vomiting.

In narcotic poisoning, apomorphine is often ineffective because the vomiting center has been depressed. If vomiting does not result from the first dose, do not repeat.

Adverse Reactions:

Therapeutic doses may cause CNS depression, euphoria, tachypnea, restlessness and tremors. Peripheral vascular collapse has been reported. Dangerous depression (even death) may occur when the drug is used in patients who are in shock (from corrosive poisons) or in those narcotized from overdoses of opiates, barbiturates, alcohol or other CNS depressants.

Overdosage:

Symptoms: Violent vomiting, retching, cardiac depression, acute circulatory failure and death.

Treatment: CNS depression can usually be reversed by a narcotic antagonist (eg, naloxone). A narcotic antagonist is usually unnecessary; however, it is used to terminate vomiting and to alleviate drowsiness.

Administration and Dosage:

Adults: 5 mg SC (range 2 to 10 mg). *Do not repeat.*

Infants and Children: 0.1 mg/kg SC. *Do not repeat.*

Storage: Protect from light and keep in tightly closed bottles. This preparation changes with age; discoloration may occur. Do not use the solution if it has turned green or brown.

Rx	**Apomorphine HCl** (Lilly)	**Tablets, soluble:** 6 mg with lactose	In 100s.

Emetics

IPECAC SYRUP

Actions:

Ipecac produces vomiting by a local irritant effect on the GI mucosa and a central medullary effect (stimulation of the chemoreceptor trigger zone). The central effect is caused by emetine and cephaeline, the two alkaloids in ipecac. An adequate dose causes vomiting within 30 minutes in > 90% of patients (average time is < 20 minutes).

Indications:

Treatment of drug overdose and in certain poisonings.

Contraindications:

Do not use in semiconscious or unconscious patients, or in pregnant or lactating women. Do not use if strychnine, corrosives such as alkalies and strong acids, or petroleum distillates have been ingested.

Warnings:

Syrup/fluid extract: Do not confuse ipecac syrup with ipecac fluid extract, which is 14 times stronger and has caused some deaths.

Call an emergency room, Poison Control Center or physician before using; if vomiting does not occur within 30 minutes after the second dose, perform gastric lavage.

Ipecac syrup abuse: Ipecac syrup may be abused by bulimic and anorexic patients. It has been implicated as the causative factor of severe cardiomyopathies, and even death, in several persons with eating disorders who used it regularly to induce vomiting.

Usage in Pregnancy: Category C. It is not known whether the drug can cause harm when administered to a pregnant woman or can affect reproductive capacity. Minimal systemic absorption is expected when used as directed (see Administration and Dosage).

Usage in Lactation: It is not known whether ipecac alkaloids are excreted in human milk. Exercise caution if ipecac syrup is used for treatment of a nursing woman.

Precautions:

May not be effective in those cases in which the ingested substance is an antiemetic. Ipecac syrup can be cardiotoxic if not vomited and allowed to be absorbed.

Drug Interactions:

Activated charcoal will adsorb ipecac syrup. If both are to be used, give the activated charcoal only after vomiting has been produced by the ipecac syrup.

Milk or **carbonated beverages:** Do not administer with ipecac syrup.

Adverse Reactions:

When ipecac syrup does not cause emesis, absorption of the alkaloid emetine may occur and may cause heart conduction disturbances, atrial fibrillation or fatal myocarditis.

After therapeutic doses, diarrhea and mild CNS depression are common; GI upset may last several hours after emesis. An anorexia nervosa patient developed fatal cardiomyopathy due to chronic ingestion (60 to 90 ml ipecac syrup/day for 21 days). Autopsy revealed myopathic and degenerative changes in heart and skeletal muscles. See Warnings.

Overdosage:

Symptoms: Ipecac is cardiotoxic if absorbed and may cause cardiac conduction disturbances, bradycardia, atrial fibrillation, hypotension or fatal myocarditis.

Treatment: Activated charcoal may be given to adsorb ipecac syrup; perform gastric lavage. Support cardiovascular system by symptomatic treatment.

Patient Information:

Always consult a physician or poison control center in cases of accidental ingestion.

Give with adequate amounts of water. Do not exceed recommended dosage.

Administration and Dosage:

Ipecac syrup may not work on an empty stomach. Have patient sit upright with head forward before administering dose.

Children (< 1 year): 5 to 10 ml followed by one-half to one glass of water. Syrup of ipecac should *probably* be administered only with medical supervision. There is controversy as to whether or not ipecac should be given to children less than 6 months of age.

Children (> 1 year to 12 years): 15 ml followed by 1 to 2 glasses of water.

Adults: 15 to 30 ml followed by 3 to 4 glasses of water.

Repeat the dosage (15 ml) once if vomiting does not occur within 20 minutes. If vomiting does not occur within 30 minutes after the second dose, perform gastric lavage.

otc[1]	**Ipecac** (Various)	**Syrup:** 1.5% alcohol	In 15 and 30 ml and UD 15 ml (40s, 50s and 100s) and UD 30 ml (50s and 100s).
Rx	**Ipecac** (Various)	**Syrup:** 2% alcohol	In 30 ml, pt & gal & UD 15 & 30 ml (25s).

[1] Product may be *otc* or *Rx*, depending on manufacturer's discretion.

CHARCOAL, ACTIVATED

Actions:

Activated charcoal is a carbon residue derived from organic material by exposing it to an oxidizing gas compound of steam, oxygen and acids at high temperatures resulting in the production of increased surface area through the creation of external and internal pores. Activation (to make a fine network of pores) of the charcoal surface increases adsorptive properties. The total surface area of a good quality activated charcoal is about 1000 m^2/g, and a pore volume of about 1 ml/g. The maximum amount of drug adsorbed by such charcoal is approximately 100 to 1000 mg/g charcoal. Activated charcoal is insoluble in water.

Sorbitol may be added to some activated charcoal products because it improves the taste, and it does not have a gritty oral residue. Sorbitol also reduces intestinal transit time from 25 hours to ≈ 1 hour.

Pharmacology: Activated charcoal adsorbs toxic substances by forming an effective barrier between any remaining particulate material and the GI mucosa, thus inhibiting GI adsorption. The adsorptive properties of the activated charcoal in a liquid base are slightly decreased during its shelf life but are still capable of adsorbing at least 99% of the substances tested.

Indications:

For use as an emergency treatment in poisoning by most drugs and chemicals.

Contraindications:

Ineffective for poisoning or overdosage of cyanide, mineral acids and alkalies.

Although not necessarily contraindicated, activated charcoal is not particularly effective in poisonings of ethanol, methanol and iron salts.

Warnings:

Induce emesis before giving activated charcoal. Administer to conscious persons only.

Drug Interactions:

Syrup of Ipecac: Do not administer concomitantly. Activated charcoal will adsorb and inactivate this agent.

The effectiveness of other medication may be decreased when used concurrently because of adsorption by the activated charcoal.

Drug/food interactions: Do not mix charcoal with **milk, ice cream** or **sherbet** since it will decrease the adsorptive capacity of the activated charcoal.

Adverse Reactions:

GI: Rapid ingestion of high doses may cause vomiting. Constipation or diarrhea may occur. Stools will be black.

Sorbitol may cause loose stools and vomiting.

Administration and Dosage:

Acute intoxication: Adult initial dose – 30 to 100 g (or 1 g/kg or approximately 5 to 10 times the amount of poison ingested) as a suspension (6 to 8 ounces water). For maximum effect, administer activated charcoal solution within 30 minutes after ingestion of poison. When large doses of drugs are ingested, remove as much of the ingested poison as possible by gastric lavage. After ipecac-induced vomiting, the patient may be intolerant of activated charcoal for 1 to 2 hours.

Gastrointestinal dialysis: Multiple administration (eg, 20 to 40 g every 6 hours for 1 to 2 days) may be used in severe poisonings to prevent desorption from the charcoal; also promoted to increase GI clearance and rate of elimination of drugs that undergo an enteral recirculation pattern.

Five to six tablespoonsful is approximately equal to one ounce of activated charcoal.

Storage: Activated charcoal adsorbs gases from the air; therefore, store in closed containers. Sealed aqueous suspensions can be stored for at least 1 year without loss of activity.

(Products listed on following page)

CHARCOAL, ACTIVATED (Cont.)

otc	**Charcoal, Activated** (Various)	**Powder:**	In 15, 30, 40, 120 and 240 g and UD 30 g.
otc	**Superchar** (Gulf Bio-Systems)	**Powder:**	In 30 g.
otc	**Activated Charcoal** (Various)	**Liquid:**	12.5 g with propylene glycol. In 60 ml bottle. 25 g with propylene glycol. In 120 ml bottle.
otc	**Actidose-Aqua** (Paddock)	**Liquid:**	25 g in 120 ml suspension. 50 g in 240 ml suspension.
otc	**Actidose with Sorbitol** (Paddock)	**Liquid:**	25 g in 120 ml suspension with sorbitol. 50 g in 240 ml suspension with sorbitol.
otc	**Charcoaid** (Requa)	**Liquid:**	30 g in 150 ml suspension with sorbitol.
otc	**Liqui-Char** (Jones Medical)	**Liquid:**	12.5 g in 60 ml bottle, 15 g in 75 ml bottle, 25 g in 120 ml squeeze container, 50 g in 240 ml squeeze container, 30 g in 120 ml squeeze container.
otc	**Superchar** (Gulf Bio-System)	**Liquid:**	30 g in 240 ml suspension. 30 g in 240 ml suspension with sorbitol.

UNIVERSAL ANTIDOTE

Actions:

The universal antidote has been used as an alternative to activated charcoal to bind unabsorbed poisons in the GI tract. It consists of a mixture of two parts activated charcoal, one part antacid (usually magnesium oxide) and one part tannic acid. Tannic acid and magnesium oxide interfere with or inactivate the absorptive capacity of activated charcoal. Tannic acid precipitates organic and inorganic compounds including metals, alkaloids and some glucosides (aluminum, apomorphine, lead, silver salts, strychnine, veratrine); however, it may produce hepatotoxicity and should only be used when specifically indicated.

Activated charcoal alone is the preferred mode of therapy for general detoxification and adsorption of poisons.

Administration and Dosage:

Empty ½ of contents into full glass of warm water. Stir 20 seconds and drink. Repeat dosage in 5 or 10 minutes.

otc	**Res-Q** (Boyle)	**Powder:** 50% activated charcoal, 25% magnesium hydroxide and tannic acid	In 15 g packets.

METHYLENE BLUE

Actions:

This compound has an oxidation/reduction action and a tissue-staining property. It has opposite actions on hemoglobin depending on concentration. In high concentrations, it converts the ferrous iron of reduced hemoglobin to the ferric form, and, as a result, methemoglobin is produced. This action is the basis for the antidotal action of methylene blue in cyanide poisoning. In contrast, low concentrations of methylene blue are capable of hastening the conversion of methemoglobin to hemoglobin.

Methylene blue is a dye that is a weak germicide and is used as a mild GU antiseptic.

Indications:

In the treatment of cyanide poisoning and drug-induced methemoglobinemia.

Oral: Mild GU antiseptic for cystitis and urethritis.

Unlabeled Uses: Delineation of body structures and fistulas through its dye effect; diagnosis/confirmation of rupture of amniotic membranes.

Contraindications:

Patients allergic to methylene blue; renal insufficiency; intraspinal injection.

Precautions:

Methylene blue may induce hemolysis in glucose-6-phosphate dehydrogenase deficient patients.

Continued administration may cause a marked anemia due to accelerated destruction of erythrocytes; check the hemoglobin frequently.

Cyanosis and cardiovascular abnormalities have accompanied treatment.

Inject IV over a period of several minutes to prevent local high concentration from producing additional methemoglobin. Do not exceed recommended dosage.

Adverse Reactions:

Discolors the urine, and sometimes the stool, blue-green. May cause bladder irritation, nausea, vomiting and diarrhea. Large doses produce abdominal and precordial pain, dizziness, headache, profuse sweating, fever, mental confusion and methemoglobin.

When injected subcutaneously, it has caused necrotic abscesses. When injected intrathecally, neural damage, including paraplegia, has resulted. Intraamniotic injection has resulted in fetal tachycardia and neonatal hemolytic anemia, hyperbilirubinemia, methemoglobinemia and blue skin.

Methylene blue stains skin blue. The staining may be removed by hypochlorite solution.

Patient Information:

Take oral form after meals with a glass of water.

May discolor the urine, and sometimes the stool, blue-green.

Administration and Dosage:

Oral: 65 to 130 mg 3 times daily after meals with a full glass of water.

Parenteral: 1 to 2 mg/kg (0.1 to 0.2 ml/kg). Inject IV over several minutes.

				C.I.*
Rx	**Methylene Blue** (Kenneth Manne)	**Tablets:** 65 mg	In 100s and 1000s.	2
Rx	**Urolene Blue** (Star)		Blue. In 100s and 1000s.	5
Rx	**Methylene Blue** (Various)	**Injection:** 10 mg per ml	In 1 and 10 ml amps.	20+

* Cost Index based on cost per 10 mg.

TRIENTINE HCl

Actions:

Pharmacology: Wilson's disease (hepatolenticular degeneration) is a metabolic defect resulting in excess copper accumulation, possibly because the liver lacks the mechanism to excrete free copper into the bile. Hepatocytes store excess copper, but when their capacity is exceeded copper is released into the blood and is taken up into extrahepatic sites. Treat this condition with a low copper diet and with chelating agents that bind copper to facilitate its excretion from the body. Trientine HCl is a chelating compound for removal of excess copper from the body.

Clinical Pharmacology: Forty-one patients (aged 6 to 54) with Wilson's disease who were intolerant of penicillamine were treated in two separate studies with trientine. The average dosage required to achieve an optimal clinical response varied between 1000 and 2000 mg per day (range, 450 to 2400 mg). The mean duration of therapy was 48.7 months (range, 2 to 164 months). Thirty-four patients improved, four had no change in clinical global response, two were lost to follow-up and one showed deterioration in clinical condition. One of the patients who improved while on trientine experienced a recurrence of the systemic lupus erythematosus symptoms which had appeared originally during penicillamine therapy; trientine was discontinued. No other adverse reactions, except iron deficiency, were noted among any of these 41 patients.

One investigator treated 13 patients with trientine following their development of intolerance to penicillamine. Retrospectively, he compared these patients to an additional group of 12 patients with Wilson's disease who were both tolerant of, and controlled with, penicillamine therapy, but who failed to continue copper chelation therapy. Various laboratory parameters showed changes in favor of the trientine patients. In the 13 patients treated with trientine, previous symptoms and signs relating to penicillamine intolerance disappeared in eight patients, improved in four patients and remained unchanged in one. The neurological status in the trientine group was unchanged or improved over baseline, whereas in the untreated group, six patients remained unchanged and six worsened. Kayser-Fleischer rings improved significantly during trientine treatment. Of the 13 patients on therapy with trientine (mean duration, 4.1 years; range, 1 to 13 years), all were alive at the data cutoff date, and in the non-treated group (mean years with no therapy, 2.7 years; range, 3 months to 9 years), 9 of the 12 died of hepatic disease.

Studies: Renal clearance studies were carried out with penicillamine and trientine on separate occasions in selected patients treated with penicillamine for at least 1 year. Six hour excretion rates of copper were determined off treatment, and after a single dose of 500 mg of penicillamine or 1.2 g of trientine. Results demonstrated that trientine is effective as a cupriuretic agent in patients with Wilson's disease, although on a molar basis, the drug appears to be less potent or less effective than penicillamine.

Indications:

Treatment of patients with Wilson's disease who are intolerant of penicillamine.

Contraindications:

Hypersensitivity to trientine.

Not recommended for use in cystinuria, rheumatoid arthritis or biliary cirrhosis.

Warnings:

Patient experience with trientine is limited. Patients should remain under regular medical supervision throughout the period of drug administration.

Iron deficiency anemia: Closely monitor patients (especially women) for evidence of iron deficiency anemia.

Usage in Pregnancy: Category C. Trientine was teratogenic in rats at doses similar to the human dose. The frequencies of both resorptions and fetal abnormalities, including hemorrhage and edema, increased while fetal copper levels decreased. There are no adequate and well controlled studies in pregnant women. Use during pregnancy only when the potential benefits outweigh the potential hazards to the fetus.

Usage in Lactation: It is not known whether this drug is excreted in breast milk. Exercise caution when administering to a nursing woman.

Usage in Children: Safety and efficacy for use in children have not been established. Trientine has been used clinically in children as young as 6 years of age with no reported adverse effects.

(Continued on following page)

TRIENTINE HCl (Cont.)

Precautions:

Hypersensitivity: There are no reports of hypersensitivity in patients given trientine for Wilson's disease. However, there have been reports of asthma, bronchitis and dermatitis occurring after prolonged environmental exposure in workers who use trientine HCl as a hardener of epoxy resins. Observe patients closely for signs of possible hypersensitivity. Refer to Management of Hypersensitivity Reactions.

Monitoring: The most reliable index for monitoring treatment is the determination of free copper in the serum, which equals the difference between quantitatively determined total copper and ceruloplasmin-copper. Adequately treated patients will usually have less than 10 mcg free copper/dl of serum.

Therapy may be monitored with a 24 hour urinary copper analysis periodically (ie, every 6 to 12 months). Urine must be collected in copper free glassware. Since a low copper diet should keep copper absorption down to less than 1 mg/day, the patient probably will be in the desired state of negative copper balance if 0.5 to 1 mg of copper is present in a 24 hour collection of urine.

Drug Interactions:

Iron: In general, do not give mineral supplements; they may block the absorption of trientine. However, iron deficiency may develop, especially in children and menstruating or pregnant women, or as a result of the low copper diet recommended for Wilson's disease. If necessary, iron may be given in short courses, but since iron and trientine each inhibit absorption of the other, allow 2 hours to elapse between administration of trientine and iron.

Adverse Reactions:

Iron deficiency and systemic lupus erythematosus have occurred in patients with Wilson's disease who were on therapy with trientine.

Trientine is not indicated for treatment of biliary cirrhosis, but in one study of four patients treated with trientine for primary biliary cirrhosis, the following adverse reactions were reported: Heartburn; epigastric pain and tenderness; thickening, fissuring and flaking of the skin; hypochromic microcytic anemia; acute gastritis; aphthoid ulcers; abdominal pain; melena; anorexia; malaise; cramps; muscle pain; weakness; rhabdomyolysis. A causal relationship to drug therapy could not be rejected or established.

Overdosage:

There is a report of an adult woman who ingested 30 g trientine without apparent ill effects.

Patient Information:

Take on an empty stomach, at least 1 hour before meals or 2 hours after meals and at least 1 hour apart from any other drug, food or milk.

Swallow capsules whole with water. Do not open or chew.

Because of the potential for contact dermatitis, any site of exposure to the capsule contents should be promptly washed with water.

Take temperature nightly, and report any symptoms such as fever or skin eruption for the first month of treatment.

Administration and Dosage:

Adults: Initially, 750 mg to 1.25 g/day, in divided doses, 2, 3 or 4 times daily. May increase to a maximum of 2 g/day.

Children ≤ 12 years: Initially, 500 to 750 mg/day, in divided doses, 2, 3 or 4 times daily. May increase to a maximum of 1.5 g/day.

Increase the daily dose only when the clinical response is not adequate or the concentration of free serum copper is persistently above 20 mcg/dl. Determine optimal long-term maintenance dosage at 6 to 12 month intervals.

Storage: Store at 2° to 8°C (36° to 46°F).

Rx	**Syprine** (MSD)	**Capsules:** 250 mg.	(MSD 661). Light brown. In 100s.

SUCCIMER

Actions:

Succimer was approved by the FDA in February 1991.

Pharmacology: Succimer is an orally active, heavy metal chelating agent; it forms water soluble chelates and, consequently, increases the urinary excretion of lead.

Toxicology: In oral toxicity studies up to 28 days, doses of succimer up to 200 mg/kg/day did not produce any significant overt toxicity in rats and dogs. However, in 6 and 28 day oral toxicity studies, doses of ≥ 300 mg/kg/day were toxic and lethal to some dogs. The kidney and the GI tract were the major target organs for succimer toxicity. Toxicity was manifested by anorexia, emesis, mucoid or bloody diarrhea, increased blood urea nitrogen concentration, increased AST, ALT and alkaline phosphatase levels, renal tubular necrosis, purulent nephritis and severe GI bleeding and ulceration. Deaths were due to renal failure.

Pharmacokinetics: In a study in healthy adult volunteers, after a single dose of 16, 32 or 48 mg/kg, absorption was rapid but variable, with peak blood levels between 1 and 2 hours. Approximately 49% of the dose was excreted: 39% in the feces, 9% in the urine and 1% as carbon dioxide from the lungs. Since fecal excretion probably represented non-absorbed drug, most of the absorbed drug was excreted by the kidneys. The apparent elimination half-life was about 2 days.

In other studies of healthy adult volunteers receiving a single oral dose of 10 mg/kg, succimer was rapidly and extensively metabolized. Approximately 25% of the dose was excreted in the urine with the peak blood level and urinary excretion occurring between 2 and 4 hours. Of the total amount of drug eliminated in the urine, approximately 90% was eliminated in altered form as mixed succimer-cysteine disulfides; the remaining 10% was eliminated unchanged.

Clinical trials: Studies were performed in 18 men with blood lead levels of 44 to 96 mcg/dl. Three groups of 6 patients received either 10, 6.7 or 3.3 mg/kg every 8 hours for 5 days. After 5 days the mean blood levels of the three groups decreased 72.5%, 58.3% and 35.5%, respectively. The mean urinary lead excretions in the initial 24 hours were 28.6, 18.6 and 12.3 times the pretreatment 24 hour urinary lead excretion. As the chelatable pool was reduced during therapy, urinary lead output decreased. A mean of 19 mg lead was excreted during a 5 day course of 30 mg/kg/day. Clinical symptoms, such as headache and colic, and biochemical indices of lead toxicity also improved. Decrease in urinary excretion of d-aminolevulinic acid (ALA) and coproporphyrin paralleled the improvement in erythrocyte ALA dehydratase. Three control patients with lead poisoning of similar severity received edetate calcium disodium (EDTA) IV at a dose of 50 mg/kg/day for 5 days. The mean blood lead level decreased 47.4% and the mean urinary lead excretion was 21 mg in the control patients.

Effect on essential minerals – In the above studies, succimer had no significant effect on the urinary elimination of iron, calcium or magnesium. Zinc excretion doubled during treatment. The effect of succimer on the excretion of essential minerals was small compared to that of EDTA, which can induce more than a tenfold increase in urinary excretion of zinc and doubling of copper and iron excretion.

Succimer vs EDTA – A study was performed in 15 children ages 2 to 7 years with blood lead levels of 30 to 49 mcg/dl and positive EDTA lead mobilization tests. Each group of five patients received 350, 233 or 116 mg/m² succimer every 8 hours for 5 days. These doses corresponded to 10, 6.7 and 3.3 mg/kg. Six control patients received 1000 mg/m²/day EDTA IV for 5 days. Following therapy, the mean blood lead levels decreased 78%, 63% and 42%, respectively, in the three groups treated with succimer. The response of the 350 mg/m² every 8 hours (10 mg/kg every 8 hrs) group was significantly better than that of the other succimer-treated groups as well as that of the control group, whose mean blood lead level fell 48%. No adverse reactions or changes in essential mineral excretion were reported in the succimer-treated groups. In the EDTA-treated group, the cumulative amount of urinary lead excreted was slightly but significantly greater than in the succimer group. After EDTA, the urinary excretion of copper, zinc, iron and calcium were significantly increased.

As with other chelators, both adults and children experienced a rebound in blood lead levels after discontinuing succimer. In these studies, after treatment with 350 mg/m² (10 mg/kg) every 8 hours for 5 days, the mean lead level rebounded and plateaued at 80% to 85% of pretreatment levels 2 weeks after therapy. The rebound plateau was somewhat higher with lower doses of succimer and with IV EDTA.

(Actions continued on following page)

SUCCIMER (Cont.)

Actions (Cont.):

Clinical trials (Cont.):

In an attempt to control rebound of blood lead levels, 19 children, ages 1 to 7 years, with blood lead levels of 42 to 67 mcg/dl were treated with 350 mg/m² every 8 hours for 5 days and then divided into three groups. One group was followed for 2 weeks with no further therapy, the second group was treated for 2 weeks with 350 mg/m² daily, and the third with 350 mg/m² every 12 hours. After the initial 5 days of therapy, the mean blood lead level in all subjects declined 61%, while the untreated group and the group treated with 350 mg/m² daily experienced rebound during the ensuing 2 weeks, the group who received the 350 mg/m² every 12 hours experienced no such rebound during the treatment period and less rebound following cessation of therapy.

In another study, ten children, ages 21 to 72 months old, with blood lead levels of 30 to 57 mcg/dl, were treated with succimer 350 mg/m² every 8 hours for 5 days, followed by an additional 19 to 22 days of therapy at a dose of 350 mg/m² every 12 hours. The mean blood lead levels decreased and remained stable at under 15 mcg/dl during the extended dosing period.

In addition to the controlled studies, approximately 250 patients with lead poisoning have been treated with succimer either orally or parenterally in open US and foreign studies with similar results reported. Succimer has been used for the treatment of lead poisoning in one patient with sickle cell anemia and in five patients with glucose-6-phosphodehydrogenase (G-6-PD) deficiency without adverse reactions.

Lead encephalopathy – Three adults with lead encephalopathy have improved with succimer therapy. However, data are not available for the use of succimer for treatment of this rare and sometimes fatal complication of lead poisoning in children.

Other heavy metal poisoning – A limited number of patients have received succimer for mercury or arsenic poisoning. These patients showed increased urinary excretion of the heavy metal and varying degrees of symptomatic improvement.

Indications:

Treatment of lead poisoning in children with blood lead levels > 45 mcg/dl. Not indicated for prophylaxis of lead poisoning in a lead-containing environment; always accompany the use of succimer with identification and removal of the source of the lead exposure.

Unlabeled uses: Succimer may be beneficial in the treatment of other heavy metal poisonings (eg, mercury, arsenic); further study is needed.

Contraindications:

History of allergy to the drug.

Warnings:

Keep out of reach of children.

Not a substitute for effective abatement of lead exposure.

Pregnancy: Category C. Succimer is teratogenic and fetotoxic in pregnant mice when given SC in a dose range of 410 to 1640 mg/kg/day during the period of organogenesis. There are no adequate and well controlled studies in pregnant women. Use during pregnancy only if the potential benefit justifies the potential risk to the fetus.

Lactation: It is not known whether this drug is excreted in breast milk. Discourage mothers requiring therapy from nursing their infants.

Children: Refer to the Indications and Administration and Dosage sections. There is no therapeutic experience with succimer in children < 1 year of age.

Precautions:

Carefully observe patients during treatment due to limited clinical experience with succimer.

Elevated blood lead levels and associated symptoms may return rapidly after discontinuation of succimer because of redistribution of lead from bone stores to soft tissues and blood. After therapy, monitor patients for rebound of blood lead levels by measuring the levels at least once weekly until stable. However, use the severity of lead intoxication (as measured by the initial blood lead level and the rate and degree of rebound of blood lead) as a guide for more frequent blood lead monitoring.

Renal function: Adequately hydrate all patients undergoing treatment. Exercise caution in using succimer therapy in patients with compromised renal function. Limited data suggest that succimer is dialyzable, but that the lead chelates are not.

Hepatic function: Transient mild elevations of serum transaminases have been observed in 6% to 10% of patients during the course of therapy. Monitor serum transaminases before the start of therapy and at least weekly during therapy. Closely monitor patients with a history of liver disease. No data are available regarding the metabolism of succimer in patients with liver disease.

(Precautions continued on following page)

SUCCIMER (Cont.)

Precautions (Cont.):

Repeated courses: Clinical experience is limited. The safety of uninterrupted dosing > 3 weeks has not been established and is not recommended.

Allergic reactions: The possibility of allergic or other mucocutaneous reactions to the drug must be borne in mind on readministration (as well as during initial courses). Monitor patients requiring repeated courses during each treatment course. One patient experienced recurrent mucocutaneous vesicular eruptions of increasing severity affecting the oral mucosa, the external urethral meatus and the perianal area on the third, fourth and fifth courses of the drug. The reaction resolved between courses and on discontinuation of therapy.

Drug Interactions:

Chelation therapy (eg, EDTA): Coadministration of succimer with other chelation therapy is not recommended.

Drug/lab test interactions: Succimer may interfere with serum and urinary laboratory tests. In vitro, succimer caused false-positive results for ketones in urine using nitroprusside reagents such as *Ketostix* and falsely decreased measurements of serum uric acid and CPK.

Adverse Reactions:

The most common events attributable to succimer (ie, GI symptoms or increases in serum transaminases) have been observed in about 10% of patients (see Precautions). Rashes, some necessitating discontinuation of therapy, have occurred in about 4% of patients. If rash occurs, consider other causes (eg, measles) before ascribing the reaction to succimer. Rechallenge with succimer may be considered if lead levels are high enough to warrant retreatment. One allergic mucocutaneous reaction has occurred on repeated administration of the drug (see Precautions). The following table presents adverse events reported with the administration of succimer for the treatment of lead and other heavy metal intoxication.

Succimer Adverse Reactions (%)[1]

Body system/adverse reaction	Children (n = 191)	Adults (n = 134)
Digestive:		
Nausea; vomiting; diarrhea; appetite loss; hemorrhoidal symptoms; loose stools; metallic taste in mouth	12	20.9
Body as a whole:		
Back, stomach, head, rib, flank pain; abdominal cramps; chills; fever; flu-like symptoms; heavy head/tired; head cold; headache; moniliasis	5.2	15.7
Metabolic:		
Elevated AST, ALT, alkaline phosphatase, serum cholesterol	4.2	10.4
CNS:		
Drowsiness; dizziness; sensorimotor neuropathy; sleepiness; paresthesia	1	12.7
Skin and appendages:		
Papular rash; herpetic rash; rash; mucocutaneous eruptions; pruritus	2.6	11.2
Special senses:		
Cloudy film in eye; ears plugged; otitis media; watery eyes	1	3.7
Respiratory:		
Sore throat; rhinorrhea; nasal congestion; cough	3.7	0.7
GU:		
Decreased urination; voiding difficulty; proteinuria increased	0	3.7
Other:		
Arrhythmia	0	1.8
Increased platelet count; intermittent eosinophilia	0.5	1.5
Kneecap pain; leg pains	0	3

[1] Incidence regardless of attribution or dosage.

(Continued on following page)

SUCCIMER (Cont.)

Overdosage:

Doses of 2300 to 2400 mg/kg in the rat and mouse produced ataxia, convulsions, labored respiration and frequently death. Induction of vomiting or gastric lavage followed by administration of an activated charcoal slurry and appropriate supportive therapy are recommended. Refer to General Management of Acute Overdosage.

Limited data indicate that succimer is dialyzable.

Patient Information:

Instruct patients to maintain adequate fluid intake. If rash occurs, patients should consult their physician.

In young children unable to swallow capsules, the contents of the capsule can be administered in a small amount of food (see Administration and Dosage).

Administration and Dosage:

Start dosage at 10 mg/kg or 350 mg/m^2 every 8 hours for 5 days; initiation of therapy at higher doses is not recommended (see table). Reduce frequency of administration to 10 mg/kg or 350 mg/m^2 every 12 hours (two-thirds of initial daily dosage) for an additional 2 weeks of therapy. A course of treatment lasts 19 days. Repeated courses may be necessary if indicated by weekly monitoring of blood lead concentration. A minimum of 2 weeks between courses is recommended unless blood lead levels indicate the need for more prompt treatment.

Succimer Pediatric Dosing Chart

Weight		Dose (mg)[1]	Number of capsules[1]
lbs	kg		
18-35	8-15	100	1
36-55	16-23	200	2
56-75	24-34	300	3
76-100	35-44	400	4
> 100	> 45	500	5

[1]To be administered every 8 hours for 5 days, followed by dosing every 12 hours for 14 days.

In young children who cannot swallow capsules, succimer can be administered by separating the capsule and sprinkling the medicated beads on a small amount of soft food or putting them in a spoon and following with a fruit drink.

Identification of the lead source in the child's environment and its abatement are critical to successful therapy. Chelation therapy is not a substitute for preventing further exposure to lead and should not be used to permit continued exposure to lead.

Patients who have received EDTA with or without BAL may use succimer for subsequent treatment after an interval of 4 weeks. Data on the concomitant use of succimer with EDTA with or without BAL are not available, and such use is not recommended.

Rx	**Chemet** (McNeil-CPC)	**Capsules:** 100 mg	Sucrose. (Chemet 100.) White. In 100s.

PENICILLAMINE

Actions:

Rheumatoid arthritis: The mechanism of action of penicillamine in rheumatoid arthritis is unknown. Penicillamine markedly lowers IgM rheumatoid factor, but produces no significant depression in absolute levels of serum immunoglobulins; it dissociates macroglobulins (rheumatoid factor). The drug may decrease cell-mediated immune response by selectively inhibiting T-lymphocyte function. Penicillamine may also act as an anti-inflammatory agent by inhibiting release of lysosomal enzymes and oxygen radicals protecting lymphocytes from the harmful effects of hydrogen peroxide formed at inflammatory sites.

The onset of therapeutic response may not be seen for 2 or 3 months in those patients who respond. The optimum duration of therapy has not been determined. If remissions occur, they may last from months to years, but usually require continued treatment (see Administration and Dosage).

Wilson's disease: Penicillamine is a chelating agent that removes excess copper in patients with Wilson's disease. From in vitro studies which indicate that one atom of copper combines with two molecules of penicillamine, it would appear that 1 g penicillamine should be followed by the excretion of about 200 mg of copper; however, the actual amount excreted is about 1% of this. Noticeable improvement may not occur for 1 to 3 months. Occasionally, neurologic symptoms become worse during initiation of therapy.

Poisoning: Penicillamine also forms soluble complexes with iron, mercury, lead and arsenic which are readily excreted by the kidneys. The drug may be used to treat poisoning by these metals.

Cystinuria: Penicillamine reduces excess cystine excretion in cystinuria. Penicillamine with conventional therapy decreases crystalluria and stone formation and may decrease the size of or dissolve existing stones. This is done, at least in part, by disulfide interchange between penicillamine and cystine, resulting in a substance more soluble than cystine and readily excreted.

Pharmacokinetics: It is well absorbed from the GI tract after oral administration (40% to 70%); peak plasma levels occur in 1 to 3 hours. Most (80%) of the plasma penicillamine is protein bound, primarily to albumin. Penicillamine is rapidly excreted in the urine (42.1 ± 6.2% in 24 hours); 50% is excreted in the feces. Metabolites may be detected in the urine for up to 3 months after stopping the drug. Half-life ranges are 1.7 to 3.2 hours (average 2.1 hours).

Indications:

Rheumatoid arthritis: Because penicillamine can cause severe adverse reactions, restrict its use in rheumatoid arthritis to patients who have severe, active disease and who have failed to respond to an adequate trial of conventional therapy. Carefully consider the benefit-to-risk ratio. Use other measures, such as rest, physiotherapy, salicylates and corticosteroids, when indicated in conjunction with the drug.

Wilson's disease (hepatolenticular degeneration) is an abnormality in copper metabolism. As a result, copper is deposited in several organs and produces pathologic effects most prominently seen in brain, liver, kidneys and eyes. Penicillamine is a copper chelating agent intended to promote excretion of copper deposited in tissues.

Cystinuria: Cystinuria is characterized by excessive urinary excretion of amino acids, including cystine. Stone formation is the only known pathology in cystinuria.

Penicillamine may be used as additional therapy, when conventional measures (ie, dilution and alkalinization of the urine, methionine restricted diet) are inadequate to control recurrent stone formation.

Unlabeled uses: The benefits of penicillamine's copper chelating and immunological effects have been investigated for use in the treatment of primary biliary cirrhosis. Doses of 600 to 900 mg/day have been used with both success and failure. Some data suggest that penicillamine may be beneficial in scleroderma.

Contraindications:

History of penicillamine-related aplastic anemia or agranulocytosis; rheumatoid arthritis patients with a history or other evidence of renal insufficiency (due to potential for causing renal damage); pregnancy; breastfeeding.

(Continued on following page)

PENICILLAMINE (Cont.)

Warnings:

Penicillamine has been associated with fatalities due to aplastic anemia, agranulocytosis, thrombocytopenia, Goodpasture's syndrome and myasthenia gravis.

Monitoring: When indicated, monitor drug toxicity or efficacy through urinalysis. In rheumatoid arthritis patients, discontinue the drug if unexplained gross hematuria or persistent microscopic hematuria develops. Perform liver function tests and an annual x-ray for renal stones.

Because of the potential for serious adverse hematological reactions, monitor white and differential blood cell count, hemoglobin determination, and direct platelet count every 2 weeks for the first 6 months of penicillamine therapy and monthly thereafter. Instruct patients to report promptly signs and symptoms of granulocytopenia or thrombocytopenia such as fever, sore throat, chills, bruising or bleeding.

Hematologic: Leukopenia (2%) and thrombocytopenia (4%) have occurred. A reduction in WBC below 3500, neutrophils $< 2000/mm^3$, or monocytes $> 500/mm^3$ mandate permanent withdrawal of therapy. Thrombocytopenia may be idiosyncratic, with decreased or absent megakaryocytes in marrow, when it is part of an aplastic anemia. In other cases, thrombocytopenia is presumably on an immune basis since the number of megakaryocytes in the marrow has been normal or sometimes increased. Platelet count below 100,000, even in the absence of clinical bleeding, or a progressive fall in either platelet count or WBC in three successive determinations, even though values are still in the normal range, requires at least temporary cessation of therapy.

Renal: Proteinuria or hematuria may develop and may be a warning sign of membranous glomerulopathy which can progress to a nephrotic syndrome. In some patients, proteinuria disappears with continued therapy; in others, penicillamine must be discontinued. When proteinuria or hematuria develops, ascertain whether it is a sign of drug-induced glomerulopathy or is unrelated to penicillamine. History of proteinuria secondary to gold therapy may be a risk factor for penicillamine proteinuria.

Cautiously continue penicillamine in rheumatoid arthritis patients developing moderate degrees of proteinuria; obtain quantitative 24 hour urinary protein determinations at 1 to 2 week intervals. Do not increase dosage. If proteinuria exceeds 1 g/24 hours, or progressively increases, discontinue drug or reduce dosage. Proteinuria has cleared after dosage reduction. One year or more may be required for any urinary abnormalities to disappear after penicillamine has been discontinued.

Autoimmune syndromes which may be caused by penicillamine include *polymyositis, diffuse alveolitis* and *dermatomyositis* and the following:

Goodpasture's syndrome is rare. Development of abnormal urinary findings associated with hemoptysis and pulmonary infiltrates on x-ray requires immediate drug cessation.

Obliterative bronchiolitis has been reported rarely. Caution the patient to report immediately pulmonary symptoms such as exertional dyspnea or unexplained cough or wheezing. Consider pulmonary function studies at this time.

Myasthenic syndrome sometimes progressing to myasthenia gravis has been reported. In most cases, symptoms have receded after withdrawal of the drug.

Pemphigoid-type reactions characterized by bullous lesions have required discontinuation of penicillamine and treatment with corticosteroids.

Lupus erythematosus: Certain patients will develop a positive antinuclear antibody (ANA) test and some may show a lupus erythematosus-like syndrome similar to other drug-induced lupus, but it is not associated with hypocomplementemia and may be present without nephropathy. A positive ANA test does not mandate drug discontinuance; however, a lupus erythematosus-like syndrome may develop later.

Sensitivity reactions: Once instituted for Wilson's disease or cystinuria, continue treatment with penicillamine on a daily basis. Interruptions for even a few days have been followed by sensitivity reactions after reinstitution of therapy.

Usage in Pregnancy: In 89 known pregnancies, penicillamine was given throughout and three infants had birth defects deemed attributable to the drug. All infants exhibited cutis laxia; one had hypotonia, hyperflexion of hips and shoulders, pyloric stenosis, vein fragility and varicosities; another showed growth retardation, hernia, perforated bowel and simian crease. The latter two died.

Use only when clearly needed and when the potential benefits outweigh the potential hazards to the fetus. Inform women of childbearing potential or who are pregnant of the possible hazards of penicillamine to the developing fetus and advise them to report promptly any missed menstrual periods or other indications of possible pregnancy.

Usage in Lactation: Safety has not been established. See Contraindications.

Usage in Children: The efficacy of penicillamine in juvenile rheumatoid arthritis has not been established.

(Continued on following page)

PENICILLAMINE (Cont.)

Precautions:

Drug fever may appear in some patients, usually in the second to third week of therapy; it is sometimes accompanied by a macular cutaneous eruption.

In patients with Wilson's disease or cystinuria, because no alternative treatment is available, temporarily discontinue penicillamine until the reaction subsides. Reinstitute therapy with a small dose and gradually increase until the desired dosage is attained. Systemic steroid therapy may be necessary, and is usually helpful, in patients who develop toxic reactions a second or third time.

In rheumatoid arthritis patients, discontinue penicillamine and try another therapeutic alternative since the febrile reaction will recur in a high percentage of patients upon readministration.

Dermatologic: Skin rashes (44% to 50%) are the most frequent adverse reactions. *Early rash* occurs during the first few months of treatment and is more common. It is usually a generalized pruritic, erythematous, maculopapular or morbilliform rash and resembles the allergic rash seen with other drugs. It usually disappears within days after stopping penicillamine and seldom recurs when the drug is restarted at a lower dosage. Pruritus and early rash are often controlled by antihistamine coadministration.

A late rash is less commonly seen, usually after 6 months or more of treatment, and requires drug discontinuation. It usually appears on the trunk, is accompanied by intense pruritus, and is usually unresponsive to topical corticosteroids. It may take weeks to disappear after penicillamine is stopped and usually recurs if the drug is restarted.

Pemphigoid rash, the most serious dermatologic adverse reaction occurs most often after 6 to 9 months of penicillamine. From 1 to 2 months may be required for resolution. Do not rechallenge patient.

The appearance of a drug eruption accompanied by fever, arthralgia, lymphadenopathy, or other allergic manifestations usually requires drug discontinuation.

Oral ulcerations may develop which may have the appearance of aphthous stomatitis; it usually recurs on rechallenge but often clears on a lower dosage. Although rare, cheilosis, glossitis and gingivostomatitis have been reported. They are frequently dose-related and may preclude further increase in dosage or require drug discontinuation.

Hypogeusia occurs in 25% to 33% of patients, except for a lesser incidence in Wilson's disease (4%). Most cases are established within 6 weeks, but most commonly resolve in 2 to 6 months despite continued treatment. Total loss of taste has occurred.

Hypoglycemia has been reported in 4 patients receiving penicillamine therapy for rheumatoid arthritis. The mechanism of hypoglycemia is unknown. Two insulin dependent diabetic patients experienced nighttime hypoglycemia after the addition of penicillamine. Both patients required a reduction in their insulin dosage.

Two nondiabetic patients who had never received insulin or oral hypoglycemics developed anti-insulin antibodies. In these patients, penicillamine was suspected to be responsible for the antibody formation because it has been known to induce autoimmune complexes (see Warnings).

Cross-sensitivity may theoretically appear in patients allergic to penicillin. Reactions from contamination of penicillamine by trace amounts of penicillin have been eliminated now that penicillamine is produced synthetically rather than as a degradation product of penicillin.

Dietary supplementation: Because of their dietary restriction, give patients with Wilson's disease, cystinuria and rheumatoid arthritis whose nutrition is impaired 25 mg/day of pyridoxine during therapy, since penicillamine increases the requirement for this vitamin. In Wilson's disease, multivitamin preparations must be copper free. Do not give mineral supplements, since they may block the response to penicillamine.

Iron deficiency may develop, especially in children and in menstruating women. If necessary, give iron in short courses. A period of 2 hours should elapse between administration of penicillamine and iron, since orally administered iron reduces the effects of penicillamine.

Effects of penicillamine on collagen and elastin make it advisable to consider a reduction in dosage to 250 mg/day when surgery is contemplated. Delay full therapy until wound healing is complete.

Penicillamine causes an increase in the amount of soluble collagen. This may cause increased skin friability at sites subject to pressure or trauma, such as shoulders, elbows, knees, toes and buttocks. Extravasations of blood may occur and may appear as purpuric areas, with external bleeding if the skin is broken, or as vesicles containing dark blood. Neither type is progressive. Therapy with penicillamine may be continued in the presence of the lesions. They may not recur if dosage is reduced. Other related effects are excessive wrinkling of the skin and development of small, white papules at venipuncture and surgical sites.

(Continued on following page)

PENICILLAMINE (Cont.)

Drug Interactions:

Gold therapy, antimalarial or **cytotoxic drugs, oxyphenbutazone** or **phenylbutazone** should not be used in patients who are concurrently receiving penicillamine. These drugs are associated with similar serious hematologic and renal reactions.

Patients who have had **gold salt** therapy discontinued due to a major toxic reaction may be at greater risk of serious adverse reactions with penicillamine, but not necessarily of the same type. However, this is controversial.

Iron salts (ferrous sulfate 35%), **antacids** (aluminum hydroxide, magnesium hydroxide, simethicone mixture; 66%) and **food** (52% to 63%): The absorption of penicillamine is significantly decreased by these drugs. Avoid concomitant administration.

Digoxin serum levels may be reduced, possibly decreasing its pharmacological effects. The digoxin dose may need to be increased.

Adverse Reactions:

Penicillamine has a high incidence (over 50%) of untoward reactions, some of which are potentially fatal. Medical supervision throughout administration is mandatory.

Allergic/immunologic: Generalized pruritus, early and late rashes (5% to 50%); lupus erythematosus-like syndrome (2%), similar to other drug-induced lupus; pemphigoid-type reactions; drug eruptions (may be accompanied by fever, arthralgia or lymphadenopathy); urticaria and exfoliative dermatitis; thyroiditis and hypoglycemia (extremely rare); migratory polyarthralgia, often with objective synovitis; polymyositis (some fatal); Goodpasture's syndrome (a severe and ultimately fatal glomerular nephritis associated with intra-alveolar hemorrhage); allergic alveolitis; obliterative bronchiolitis. See Warnings.

GI: Anorexia, epigastric pain, nausea, vomiting or occasional diarrhea (17%); altered taste perception (4% to 33%); blunting, diminution or total loss of taste perception (12%); stomatitis (10%); reactivated peptic ulcer; hepatic dysfunction; pancreatitis; intrahepatic cholestasis and toxic hepatitis (rare); increased serum alkaline phosphatase and LDH and positive cephalin flocculation and thymol turbidity tests; oral ulcerations; cheilosis, glossitis and gingivostomatitis (rare); colitis.

Hematologic: Bone marrow depression. Leukopenia (2%); thrombocytopenia (4%). Fatalities have resulted from thrombocytopenia, agranulocytosis and aplastic anemia.

Thrombotic thrombocytopenic purpura, hemolytic anemia, red cell aplasia, monocytosis, leukocytosis, eosinophilia and thrombocytosis have also been reported.

There have been reports associating penicillamine with leukemia; cause and effect relationship has not been established.

Renal: Proteinuria (6%) or hematuria which may progress to the nephrotic syndrome as a result of an immune complex membranous glomerulopathy.

CNS: Tinnitus. Reversible optic neuritis with racemic penicillamine (may be related to pyridoxine deficiency). Pyridoxine-responsive motor neuropathy with D-penicillamine.

Other (rare): Thrombophlebitis; hyperpyrexia; falling hair or alopecia; lichen planus; myasthenia gravis; dermatomyositis; mammary hyperplasia; elastosis perforans serpiginosa; toxic epidermal necrolysis; anetoderma (cutaneous macular atrophy); fatal renal vasculitis; interstitial pneumonitis and pulmonary fibrosis; bronchial asthma; hot flashes (2.5%).

Increased skin friability, excessive wrinkling of skin and development of small white papules at venipuncture and surgical sites have been reported. Penicillamine toxicity may be twice as common in elderly patients. The chelating action of the drug may cause increased excretion of other heavy metals such as zinc, mercury and lead.

Patient Information:

Take on an empty stomach, 1 hour before or 2 hours after meals and at least 1 hour apart from any other drug, food or milk.

Patients with *cystinuria* should drink copious amounts of water.

Notify physician if skin rash, unusual bruising or bleeding, sore throat, exertional dyspnea, unexplained coughing or wheezing, fever, chills, or any other unusual effects occur.

Administration and Dosage:

Wilson's disease: Initial dosage is 1 g/day for children or adults. This may be increased, as indicated by the urinary copper analyses, but it is seldom necessary to exceed 2 g/day. In patients who cannot tolerate 1 g/day initially, initiating dosage with 250 mg/day and increasing gradually allows closer control of the drug. Give on an empty stomach in 4 divided doses, 30 minutes to 1 hour before meals and at bedtime (at least 2 hours after the evening meal).

Determine optimal dosage by measurement of urinary copper excretion. Quantitatively analyze for copper before and soon after initiation of therapy. Monitor therapy with a 24 hour urinary copper analysis every 3 months for the duration of therapy. The patient probably will be in negative copper balance of 0.5 to 1 mg of copper present in a 24 hour collection of urine.

(Administration and Dosage continued on following page)

PENICILLAMINE (Cont.)

Administration and Dosage (Cont.):

Cystinuria:

Adult dosage – 2 g/day (range 1 to 4 g/day) in 4 divided doses. *Pediatric dosage* – 30 mg/kg/day in 4 divided doses. Divide the total daily amount into 4 doses. If 4 equal doses are not feasible, give the larger portion at bedtime. If adverse reactions necessitate a reduction in dosage, it is important to retain the bedtime dose. Initiating dosage with 250 mg/day, and increasing gradually, allows closer control of the drug and may reduce the incidence of adverse reactions.

Patients should drink about a pint of fluid at bedtime and another pint once during the night when urine is more concentrated and more acid than during the day. The greater the fluid intake, the lower the dosage of penicillamine required.

Individualize dosage to limit cystine excretion to 100 to 200 mg/day in those with no history of stones, and below 100 mg/day in those who have had stone formation or pain. Consider the inherent tubular defect and the patient's size, age and rate of growth, as well as diet and water intake.

Rheumatoid arthritis: 2 or 3 months may be required before a clinical response is noted.

Administer on an empty stomach at least 1 hour before meals and at least 1 hour apart from any other drug, food or milk.

When treatment has been interrupted because of adverse reactions or other reasons, cautiously reintroduce the drug at a lower dosage and increase slowly.

Initial therapy – A single daily dose of 125 or 250 mg. Thereafter, increase dose at 1 to 3 month intervals by 125 or 250 mg/day as patient response and tolerance indicate. If satisfactory remission is achieved, continue the dose. If there is no improvement and if there are no signs of potentially serious toxicity after 2 to 3 months with doses of 500 to 750 mg/day, continue increases of 250 mg/day at 2 to 3 month intervals until satisfactory remission occurs or toxicity develops. If there is no discernible improvement after 3 to 4 months of treatment with 1 to 1.5 g/day, assume the patient will not respond and discontinue the drug.

Maintenance therapy – Individualize dosage. Many patients respond to 500 to 750 mg/day or less. Changes in dosage level may not be reflected clinically or in the erythrocyte sedimentation rate for 2 to 3 months after each adjustment. Some patients will subsequently require an increase in dosage to achieve maximal disease suppression. In patients who respond but who evidence incomplete disease suppression after the first 6 to 9 months of treatment, increase daily dosage by 125 or 250 mg/day at 3 month intervals. Dosage above 1 g/day is unusual, but up to 1.5 g/day has been required.

Management of exacerbations – Following an initial good response, some patients may experience a self-limited exacerbation of disease activity which can subside within 12 weeks. They are usually controlled by adding nonsteroidal anti-inflammatory drugs. Consider an increase in maintenance dose only if the patient has demonstrated a true "escape" phenomenon (as evidenced by failure of the flare to subside within this time period).

Migratory polyarthralgia due to penicillamine is extremely difficult to differentiate from an exacerbation of the rheumatoid arthritis. Discontinuation or substantial reduction in dosage for several weeks will usually determine which of these processes is responsible for the arthralgia.

Duration of therapy has not been determined. If the patient has been in remission for 6 months or more, attempt a gradual, stepwise dosage reduction in decrements of 125 or 250 mg/day at approximately 3 month intervals.

Concomitant drug therapy – See Drug Interactions. Salicylates, other nonsteroidal anti-inflammatory drugs or systemic corticosteroids may be continued when penicillamine is initiated. After improvement begins, analgesic and anti-inflammatory drugs may be discontinued slowly as symptoms permit. Months of penicillamine treatment may be required before steroids can be completely eliminated.

				C.I.*
Rx	**Cuprimine** (MSD)	**Capsules:** 125 mg	(#MSD 672). Yellow and gray. In 100s.	407
		250 mg	(#MSD 602). Ivory. In 100s.	290
Rx	**Depen** (Wallace)	**Tablets:** 250 mg	(#37-4401). White, scored. In 100s.	249

* Cost Index based on cost per 250 mg.
# Product identification code.

TIOPRONIN

Actions:

Tiopronin is an active reducing and complexing thiol compound for the prevention of cystine (kidney) stone formation. It undergoes thiol-disulfide exchange with cystine to form a mixed disulfide of tiopronin-cysteine; a water-soluble mixed disulfide is formed and the amount of sparingly soluble cystine is reduced.

Pharmacokinetics: Up to 48% of a dose appears in urine during the first 4 hours and up to 78% by 72 hours. Thus, in patients with cystinuria, a sufficient amount of tiopronin or its active metabolites could appear in urine to react with cystine, lowering cystine excretion.

The decrement in urinary cystine produced by tiopronin is generally proportional to the dose. A reduction in urinary cystine of 250 to 300 and 500 mg/day at a dosage of 1 and 2 g/day, respectively, might be expected. Tiopronin causes a sustained reduction in cystine excretion without loss of effectiveness. It has a rapid onset and offset of action, showing a fall in cystine excretion on the first day of administration and a rise on the first day of drug withdrawal.

Clinical Pharmacology: Cystine stones typically occur in approximately 10,000 persons in the U.S. who are homozygous for cystinuria. These persons excrete abnormal amounts of cystine in urine, as well as excessive amounts of other dibasic amino acids (lysine, arginine and ornithine). They also show varying intestinal transport defects for these same amino acids. The stone formation is the result of poor aqueous solubility of cystine. Stone formation is determined primarily by the urinary supersaturation of cystine. Thus, cystine stones, theoretically, form whenever urinary cystine concentration exceeds the solubility limit. Cystine solubility in urine is pH-dependent, and ranges from 170 to 300 mg/L at pH 5 to 220 to 500 mg/L at pH 7.5.

The goal of therapy is to reduce urinary cystine concentration below its solubility limit. It may be accomplished by dietary means to reduce cystine synthesis and by a high fluid intake to increase urine volume and thereby lower cystine concentration. These conservative measures alone may be ineffective. In such patients, d-penicillamine has been used as an additional therapy. However, d-penicillamine treatment is frequently accompanied by adverse reactions.

Indications:

Prevention of cystine (kidney) stone formation in patients with severe homozygous cystinuria with urinary cystine greater than 500 mg/day, who are resistant to treatment with conservative measures of high fluid intake, alkali and diet modification, or who have adverse reactions to d-penicillamine.

Contraindications:

History of agranulocytosis, aplastic anemia or thrombocytopenia on this medication.

Warnings:

A fatal outcome from tiopronin is possible (but not reported), as has been reported with d-penicillamine from such complications as aplastic anemia, agranulocytosis, thrombocytopenia, Goodpasture's syndrome or myasthenia gravis.

Hematologic: Leukopenia of the granulocytic series may develop without eosinophilia. Thrombocytopenia may be immunologic in origin or idiosyncratic. The reduction in peripheral blood white count to less than 3500/cu mm or in platelet count to below 100,000/cu mm mandates cessation of therapy. Instruct patients to report promptly any symptom or sign of these hematological abnormalities, such as fever, sore throat, chills, bleeding or easy bruisability.

Proteinuria, sometimes sufficiently severe to cause nephrotic syndrome, may develop from membranous glomerulopathy. Close observation of patients is mandatory.

Complications (rare) have occurred during d-penicillamine therapy and could occur during tiopronin treatment. Stop therapy if the following occurs: Abnormal urinary findings with hemoptysis and pulmonary infiltrates suggestive of Goodpasture's syndrome; appearance of myasthenic syndrome or myasthenia gravis; development of pemphigus-type reactions.

Usage in Pregnancy. Category C. Skeletal defects and cleft palates occur in the fetus when d-penicillamine is given to pregnant rats at 10 times the dose recommended for humans. A similar teratogenicity might be expected for tiopronin. There are no adequate and well controlled studies in pregnant women. Use during pregnancy only if the potential benefit justifies potential risk to the fetus.

(Warnings continued on following page)

TIOPRONIN (Cont.)

Warnings (Cont.):

Usage in Lactation: Because tiopronin may be excreted in breast milk, and because of potential serious adverse reactions of nursing infants, advise mothers taking tiopronin not to nurse their infants.

Usage in Children: Safety and effectiveness in children < 9 have not been established.

Precautions:

Monitoring tests are recommended, including: Peripheral blood counts, direct platelet count, hemoglobin, serum albumin, liver function tests, 24 hour urinary protein and routine urinalysis at 3 to 6 month intervals during treatment. In order to assess effect on stone disease, monitor urinary cystine frequently during the first 6 months when the optimum dose schedule is being determined, and at 6 month intervals thereafter. Abdominal roentgenogram (KUB) is advised yearly to monitor the size and appearance of stone(s).

Adverse Reactions:

Drug fever may develop, usually during the first month of therapy; discontinue until the fever subsides. It may be reinstated at a small dose, with a gradual increase in dosage until the desired level is achieved.

Generalized rash (erythematous, maculopapular or morbilliform) accompanied by pruritis may develop during the first few months of treatment. It may be controlled by antihistamine therapy, typically recedes when tiopronin is discontinued and seldom recurs when tiopronin is restarted at a lower dosage. Less commonly, rash may appear late in treatment (after more than 6 months). Located usually on the trunk, the late rash is associated with intense pruritis, recedes slowly after discontinuing treatment, and usually recurs upon resumption of treatment.

Lupus erythematous-like reaction, manifested by fever, arthralgia and lymphadenopathy may develop. It may be associated with a positive antinuclear antibody test, but not necessarily with nephropathy. It may require discontinuance of tiopronin treatment.

Wrinkling and friability of skin usually occurs after long-term treatment, and results from the effect of tiopronin on collagen.

Hypogeusia, often self-limiting may develop, the result of trace metal chelation by tiopronin.

Vitamin B_6 deficiency is uncommonly associated with tiopronin treatment, unlike during d-penicillamine therapy.

Versus penicillamine: A multiclinic trial involving 66 cystinuric patients indicated that tiopronin is associated with fewer or less severe adverse reactions than d-penicillamine. Among those stopping d-penicillamine due to toxicity, 64.7% could take tiopronin. In those without a history of d-penicillamine treatment, only 5.9% developed reactions of sufficient severity to require tiopronin withdrawal.

Administration and Dosage:

Attempt a conservative treatment program first. Provide at least 3 L of fluid, including two glasses with each meal and at bedtime. Advise the patient to awake at night to urinate, and to drink two more glasses of fluids before returning to bed. Additional fluids should be consumed if there is excessive sweating or intestinal fluid loss. Seek a minimum urine output of 2 L/day on a consistent basis. Provide a modest amount of alkali in order to maintain urinary pH at a high normal range (6.5 to 7).

Excessive alkali therapy is not advisable. When urinary pH increases above 7 with alkali therapy, calcium phosphate nephrolithiasis may ensue because of the enhanced urinary supersaturation of hydroxyapatite in an alkaline environment. Potassium alkali are advantageous over sodium alkali, because they do not cause hypercalciuria and are less likely to cause the complication of calcium stones.

In patients who continue to form cystine stones on the above conservative program, tiopronin may be added. Tiopronin may also be substituted for d-penicillamine in patients who have developed toxicity to the latter drug. In both situations, continue the conservative treatment program.

Base tiopronin dosage on that amount required to reduce urinary cystine concentration to below its solubility limit (generally < 250 mg/L). The extent of the decline in cystine excretion is generally dosage dependent.

Initial adult dosage – 800 mg/day in adults with cystine stones; average dose is 1000 mg/day. However, some patients require less. *Children* – Initial dosage may be based on 15 mg/kg/day. Measure urinary cystine 1 month after treatment, and every 3 months thereafter. Readjust dosage depending on urinary cystine value. Whenever possible, give in divided doses 3 times/day at least 1 hour before or 2 hours after meals. In patients with severe toxicity to d-penicillamine, initiate tiopronin at a lower dosage.

Rx	**Thiola** (Mission)	**Tablets:** 100 mg	White, sugar coated. In 100s.

Anticholinesterase Muscle Stimulants

Actions:

These drugs facilitate transmission of impulses across the myoneural junction by inhibiting the destruction of acetylcholine by cholinesterase. They differ in duration of action and in adverse effects. Equivalent doses, onset and duration of action are summarized below:

Drug	Route	Equivalent Dosage (mg)	Onset (min)	Duration (hours)	Indications
Pyridostigmine	PO	60	20-30	3-6	Myasthenia gravis
	IM	2	< 15	2-4	Myasthenia gravis
	IV	2	2-5	2-4	Myasthenia gravis; Nondepolarizing muscle relaxant antagonist
Ambenonium	PO	5-10	20-30	3-8	Myasthenia gravis
Neostigmine	PO	15	45-75	2-4	Myasthenia gravis
	IM	1.5	20-30	2-4	Myasthenia gravis
	IV	0.5	4-8	2-4	Diagnosis myasthenia gravis; Nondepolarizing muscle relaxant antagonist
Edrophonium	IM	10	2-10	0.17-0.67	Diagnosis myasthenia gravis
	IV	10	< 1	0.08-0.33	Diagnosis myasthenia gravis;[1] Nondepolarizing muscle relaxant antagonist

[1] Also used to evaluate treatment requirements in myasthenia gravis.

Indications:

Diagnosis of myasthenia gravis: Parenteral administration will rapidly improve muscle strength in myasthenia patients. Because of its rapid and brief duration of action, edrophonium is usually preferred.

Small parenteral doses are also used to evaluate the adequacy of therapy in patients on maintenance therapy and to differentiate myasthenic from cholinergic states.

Maintenance therapy in myasthenia: Pyridostigmine is most widely used for its prolonged duration of action. Ambenonium is particularly useful in patients sensitive to bromides.

Reversal of nondepolarizing muscle relaxants.

Contraindications:

Hypersensitivity to anticholinesterases; mechanical intestinal and urinary obstructions.

Neostigmine is contraindicated in patients with peritonitis.

Neostigmine bromide or **pyridostigmine bromide** are contraindicated in patients with a history of reaction to bromides.

Because **ambenonium** has a more prolonged action than other antimyasthenic drugs, simultaneous use with other cholinergics is contraindicated except under strict supervision. Therefore, when a patient is to be given the drug, suspend use of all other cholinergics until the patient has been stabilized. In most instances, the myasthenic symptoms are effectively controlled by ambenonium alone.

Warnings:

Use with caution in patients with bronchial asthma, epilepsy, bradycardia, recent coronary occlusion, vagotonia, hyperthyroidism, cardiac arrhythmias or peptic ulcer. Treat transient bradycardia with atropine sulfate. Isolated instances of cardiac and respiratory arrest believed to be vagotonic effects have occurred. When large doses are given, prior or simultaneous injection of atropine sulfate may be advisable. Use separate syringes.

Hypersensitivity: Because of possible hypersensitivity in an occasional patient, have atropine and epinephrine readily available when using parenteral therapy.

Cholinergic/Myasthenic crisis: Overdosage may result in *cholinergic crisis*, characterized by increasing muscle weakness which, through involvement of the respiratory muscles, may lead to death. *Myasthenic crisis* due to an increase in disease severity is also accompanied by extreme muscle weakness and may be difficult to distinguish from cholinergic crisis. Differentiation is extremely important; use edrophonium and clinical judgment.

Treatment of the two conditions differs radically: *Myasthenic crisis* requires more intensive anticholinesterase therapy; *cholinergic crisis* calls for withdrawal of all drugs of this type and immediate use of atropine. Have a syringe containing 1 mg of atropine sulfate immediately available to be given IV to counteract severe cholinergic reactions. Use atropine to abolish or blunt GI side effects or other muscarinic reactions; however, such use may lead to inadvertent induction of cholinergic crisis by masking signs of overdosage.

(Warnings continued on following page)

Warnings (Cont.):

Used as antagonists to nondepolarizing muscle relaxants: Obtain adequate recovery of voluntary respiration and neuromuscular transmission prior to discontinuing respiratory assistance. Observe patient continuously. If there is doubt concerning the adequacy of recovery from the nondepolarizing muscle relaxant, continue artificial ventilation.

Ambenonium chloride: Great care and supervision are required, since the warning of overdosage is minimal and requirements of patients vary tremendously. A narrow margin exists between first appearance of side effects and serious toxic effects.

Usage in Pregnancy: (Category C – neostigmine.) Safety for use during pregnancy has not been established. Although cholinesterase inhibitors are apparently safe for the fetus, they may affect the condition of the neonate. Transient muscular weakness occurred in about 20% of infants born to mothers treated with these drugs during pregnancy. Use only when clearly needed and when the potential benefits outweigh the potential hazards to the fetus.

Anticholinesterase drugs may cause uterine irritability and induce premature labor when given IV to pregnant women near term.

Usage in Lactation: It is not known whether these drugs are excreted in breast milk. Because of the potential for serious adverse reactions in the nursing infant, decide whether to discontinue nursing or to discontinue the drug, taking into account the importance of the drug to the mother.

Usage in Children: Safety and efficacy for use of **neostigmine** in children have not been established.

Precautions:

Anticholinesterase insensitivity may develop for brief or prolonged periods. Carefully monitor the patient; respiratory assistance may be needed. Reduce or withhold dosages until the patient again becomes sensitive.

Drug Interactions:

Aminoglycoside antibiotics (eg, neomycin, streptomycin, kanamycin) have a mild but definite nondepolarizing blocking action which may accentuate neuromuscular block.

Anticholinesterase drugs: Exercise caution in patients with myasthenic symptoms who are receiving other anticholinesterase muscle stimulants. Since symptoms of anticholinesterase overdose (cholinergic crisis) may mimic underdosage (myasthenic weakness), the condition may be worsened.

Routine administration of **atropine** or **belladonna derivatives** with these agents may suppress the parasympathomimetic (muscarinic) symptoms of excessive GI stimulation, leaving only the more serious symptoms of fasciculation and paralysis of voluntary muscles as signs of overdosage.

Corticosteroids may decrease the anticholinesterase effects of these agents. Conversely, anticholinesterase effects may increase after stopping corticosteroids. Provide respiratory support as needed.

Depolarizing muscle relaxants (eg, succinylcholine, decamethonium): Neostigmine may prolong the Phase I block of these drugs. Use these drugs in myasthenic patients only where definitely indicated. Make careful adjustment of the anticholinesterase dosage.

Local and **some general anesthetics, antiarrhythmics** and other drugs that interfere with neuromuscular transmission: Use cautiously, if at all, in patients with myasthenia gravis. The neostigmine dose may have to be increased accordingly.

Magnesium has a direct depressant effect on skeletal muscle, and it may antagonize the beneficial effects of anticholinesterase therapy.

Mecamylamine: Do not administer to patients receiving this ganglionic blocking agent.

Methocarbamol: A single case report indicates this drug may have impaired the effect of pyridostigmine in a patient with myasthenia gravis.

Succinylcholine neuromuscular blocking effects may be increased. Prolonged respiratory depression with extended periods of apnea may occur. Provide respiratory support as needed.

(Continued on following page)

Anticholinesterase Muscle Stimulants (Cont.)

Adverse Reactions:

Observe for severe cholinergic reactions in the hyperreactive individual. Observe the myasthenic patient in crisis for bradycardia or cardiac standstill and cholinergic reactions if an overdose is given. The following reactions may occur:

Ocular: Lacrimation; miosis; spasm of accommodation; diplopia; conjunctival hyperemia; visual changes.

CNS: Convulsions; dysarthria; dysphonia; dizziness; loss of consciousness; drowsiness; headache.

Respiratory: Increased tracheobronchial secretions; laryngospasm; bronchiolar constriction; respiratory muscle paralysis; central respiratory paralysis; dyspnea; respiratory depression; respiratory arrest; bronchospasm.

Cardiac: Arrhythmias (especially bradycardia); fall in cardiac output leading to hypotension; tachycardia; AV block; nodal rhythm; nonspecific ECG changes; cardiac arrest; syncope.

GI: Increased salivary, gastric and intestinal secretions; nausea; vomiting; dysphagia; increased peristalsis; diarrhea; abdominal cramps; flatulence.

Skeletal muscle: Weakness; fasciculations; muscle cramps and spasms; arthralgia.

Allergic: Allergic reactions and anaphylaxis.

Miscellaneous: Urinary frequency and incontinence; urinary urgency; diaphoresis; rash; urticaria; flushing. Alopecia (pyridostigmine).

Pyridostigmine or **neostigmine bromide** may occasionally cause skin rash which may subside upon discontinuation. Thrombophlebitis has been reported after IV use.

Overdosage:

Symptoms: When the drug produces overstimulation, the clinical picture is one of increasing parasympathomimetic action that is more or less characteristic when not masked by the use of atropine. Signs and symptoms of overdosage, including cholinergic crises, vary considerably. They are usually manifested by increasing GI stimulation with epigastric distress, abdominal cramps, diarrhea and vomiting, excessive salivation, pallor, cold sweating, urinary urgency, blurring of vision, and eventually fasciculation and paralysis of voluntary muscles, including those of the tongue (thick tongue and difficulty in swallowing), shoulder, neck and arms. Miosis, increase in blood pressure with or without bradycardia, and finally, subjective sensations of internal trembling, and often severe anxiety and panic may complete the picture. A cholinergic crisis is usually differentiated from the weakness and paralysis of myasthenia gravis insufficiently treated by cholinergic drugs by the fact that myasthenic weakness is not accompanied by any of the above signs and symptoms, except the last two subjective ones (anxiety and panic).

Management: Since the warning of overdosage is minimal, the existence of a narrow margin between the first appearance of side effects and serious toxic effects must be borne in mind constantly. If signs of overdosage occur (excessive GI stimulation, excessive salivation, miosis and more serious fasciculations of voluntary muscles), discontinue temporarily all cholinergic medication and administer from 0.5 mg to 1 mg (1/120 to 1/60 grain) of atropine IV. A total atropine dose of 5 to 10 mg or more may be required. Give other supportive treatment as indicated (artificial respiration, tracheotomy, oxygen, etc).

Patient Information:

Notify physician if nausea, vomiting, diarrhea, sweating, increased salivary secretions, irregular heartbeat, muscle weakness, severe abdominal pain or difficulty in breathing occurs.

(Products listed on following page)

Complete prescribing information for these products begins on page2712.

Anticholinesterase Muscle Stimulants (Cont.)

PYRIDOSTIGMINE BROMIDE

Indications:

Treatment of myasthenia gravis. The injectable form is also used to reverse or antagonize nondepolarizing muscle relaxants such as curariform drugs and gallamine triethiodide.

Administration and Dosage:

Myasthenia Gravis:

Oral – Individualize dosage. *Adults:* 600 mg/day (range 60 to 1500 mg), spaced to provide maximum relief. *Children:* 7 mg/kg/24 hours divided into 5 or 6 doses.

Sustained release tablets: 180 to 540 mg once or twice daily. Individual needs may vary markedly. Use dosage intervals of at least 6 hrs. Do not crush or chew. For optimum control, the more rapidly acting regular tablets or syrup may also be needed.

Parenteral – To supplement oral dosage preoperatively and postoperatively, during labor and postpartum, during myasthenic crisis or when oral therapy is impractical, give approximately 1/30th the oral dose, either IM or very slowly IV. Observe patient closely for cholinergic reactions, particularly if the IV route is used.

Neonates of myasthenic mothers may have transient difficulty in swallowing, sucking and breathing. Injectable pyridostigmine may be indicated (by symptoms and use of the edrophonium test) until syrup can be taken. Dosage requirements range from 0.05 to 0.15 mg/kg IM. It is important to differentiate between cholinergic and myasthenic crises in neonates.

Pyridostigmine, given parenterally 1 hour before second stage labor is complete, enables patients to have adequate strength during labor and provides protection to infants in the immediate postnatal state.

Reversal of Nondepolarizing Muscle Relaxants: Give atropine sulfate (0.6 to 1.2 mg) IV immediately prior to pyridostigmine to minimize side effects. Reversal dosages range from 0.1 to 0.25 mg/kg. Pyridostigmine 10 or 20 mg IV will usually be sufficient. Although full recovery usually occurs within 15 minutes, 30 minutes or more may be required. Satisfactory reversal is evident by adequate voluntary respiration, respiratory measurements and use of a peripheral nerve stimulator device. Keep patient well ventilated and maintain a patent airway until complete recovery of normal respiration.

Once satisfactory reversal has been attained, recurarization has not been reported. Failure of pyridostigmine injection to provide prompt (within 30 minutes) reversal may occur (eg, extreme debilitation, carcinomatosis or with concomitant use of certain broad-spectrum antibiotics or anesthetic agents, notably ether).

				C.I.*
Rx	**Mestinon** (ICN)	**Tablets:** 60 mg	(#Mestinon 60 Roche). In 100s and 500s.	4
		Syrup: 60 mg per 5 ml	5% alcohol. Sorbitol. Raspberry flavor. In 480 ml.	3
		Sustained Release Tablets: 180 mg	(#Roche 34). In 100s.	3
Rx	**Mestinon** (ICN)	**Injection:** 5 mg per ml	In 2 ml amps.[1]	14
Rx	**Regonol** (Organon)		In 2 ml amps[2] and 5 ml vials.[2]	7

AMBENONIUM CHLORIDE

Indications:

Treatment of myasthenia gravis.

Administration and Dosage:

Individualize dosage. The amount of medication necessary to control symptoms may also fluctuate in each patient. Since maximum therapeutic effectiveness (optimal muscle strength and no GI disturbances) is highly critical, close supervision is necessary.

Ambenonium has a longer duration of action than other agents and requires administration only every 3 or 4 hours, depending on clinical response. Medication is usually not required throughout the night.

Moderately severe myasthenia: 5 to 25 mg 3 or 4 times daily (range from 5 mg to 75 mg per dose). Start with 5 mg and increase gradually to determine optimum dose. Adjust dosage at 1 to 2 day intervals to avoid drug accumulation and overdosage.

A few patients require greater doses for adequate control, but increasing dosage above 200 mg daily requires exacting supervision to avoid overdosage.

Edrophonium may be used to evaluate adequacy of maintenance dose. See p.2717.

				C.I.*
Rx	**Mytelase Caplets** (Winthrop Pharm.)	**Tablets:** 10 mg	Scored. In 100s.	8

* Cost Index based on cost per 60 mg oral or 2 mg parenteral pyridostigmine bromide or 10 mg ambenonium chloride.

\# Product identification code.

[1] With 0.2% methyl and propyl parabens.

[2] With 1% benzyl alcohol.

Complete prescribing information for these products begins on page 2712

Anticholinesterase Muscle Stimulants (Cont.)

NEOSTIGMINE

Indications:

Symptomatic control of myasthenia gravis: In acute myasthenic crisis where difficulty in breathing and swallowing is present, use the parenteral form; transfer to oral therapy as soon as it can be tolerated.

Diagnosis of myasthenia gravis: The parenteral form can be used; however, edrophonium is preferred because of its more rapid onset and brief duration of action.

Antidote for nondepolarizing neuromuscular blocking agents (eg, tubocurarine, metocurine, gallamine or pancuronium) after surgery.

For additional indications refer to p. 2730

Administration and Dosage:

Symptomatic control of myasthenia gravis:

Oral – Dosage requirements vary from 15 to 375 mg/day. It may be necessary to exceed these dosages, but consider the possibility of cholinergic crisis. The average dosage is 150 mg given over 24 hours; for children, 2 mg/kg/day divided every 3 to 4 hours. The interval between doses is of paramount importance; it must be individualized. Frequently, therapy is required day and night. Larger portions of the total daily dose may be given at times of greater fatigue (afternoon, mealtimes, etc). Encourage patients to keep a daily record to assist in optimal therapy.

Parenteral – Inject 1 ml of the 1:2000 solution (0.5 mg) SC or IM. Individualize subsequent doses. For children, 0.01 to 0.04 mg/kg/dose IM, IV or SC every 2 to 3 hours as needed.

Diagnosis of myasthenia gravis: Adults – 0.022 mg/kg IM. *Children* – 0.04 mg/kg IM.

Antidote for nondepolarizing neuromuscular blocking agents: When administered IV, also give atropine sulfate (0.6 to 1.2 mg) IV several minutes before the neostigmine rather than concomitantly. Give 0.5 to 2 mg neostigmine by slow IV injection and repeat as required; however, only in exceptional cases should total dose exceed 5 mg.

Children – 0.07 to 0.08 mg/kg/dose IV neostigmine with 0.008 to 0.025 mg/kg/dose atropine sulfate.

Keep the patient well ventilated and maintain a patent airway until complete recovery of normal respiration is assured. The optimum time to administer the drug is when the patient is being hyperventilated and the carbon dioxide level of blood is low.

Never administer in the presence of high concentrations of halothane or cyclopropane. In cardiac cases and severely ill patients, titrate the exact dose of neostigmine required using a peripheral nerve stimulator. In the presence of bradycardia, increase pulse rate to about 80/minute with atropine before administering neostigmine.

	Product	Form	Description	C.I.*
Rx	**Neostigmine Bromide** (Lannett)	**Tablets:** 15 mg	In 100s and 1000s.	1
Rx	**Prostigmin** (ICN)		(#Roche Prostigmin). White, scored. In 100s and 1000s.	4
Rx	**Neostigmine Methylsulfate** (Various)	**Injection:** 1:1000	In 10 ml vials.	5+
Rx	**Prostigmin** (ICN)		In 10 ml vials.[1]	22
Rx	**Neostigmine Methylsulfate** (Various)	**Injection:** 1:2000	In 1 ml amps and 10 ml vials.	3+
Rx	**Prostigmin** (ICN)		In 1 ml amps[2] and 10 ml vials.[1]	26
Rx	**Neostigmine Methylsulfate** (Various)	**Injection:** 1:4000	In 1 ml amps.	15+
Rx	**Prostigmin** (ICN)		In 1 ml amps.[2]	69

* Cost Index based on cost per 15 mg oral or 1 mg parenteral.

Product identification code.

[1] With 0.45% phenol.

[2] With 0.2% methyl and propyl parabens.

Complete prescribing information for these products begins on page 2712

NEOSTIGMINE METHYLSULFATE and ATROPINE SULFATE INJECTION

Indications:

Neostigmine methylsulfate can be used as an antidote to curare principles. When it is administered IV, it is recommended that atropine sulfate also be given IV.

Administration and Dosage:

When neostigmine methylsulfate is administered IV, it is recommended that atropine sulfate (0.6 to 1.2 mg) also be given IV. Some authorities recommend that the atropine be injected several minutes prior to the neostigmine methylsulfate injection, rather than concomitantly. Usual dose is 0.5 to 2 mg neostigmine methylsulfate given by slow IV injection, repeated as required; only in exceptional cases should the total dose of neostigmine methylsulfate exceed 5 mg.

The patient should be well ventilated and a patent airway maintained until complete recovery of normal respiration is assured. The optimum time to administer neostigmine methylsulfate is when the patient is being hyperventilated and the carbon dioxide level of the blood is low.

It should never be administered in the presence of high concentrations of halothane or cyclopropane. In small children, cardiac cases, and severely ill patients, titrate the exact dose of neostigmine methylsulfate required, using a peripheral nerve stimulator. In the presence of a bradycardia, the pulse rate should be increased to about 80/minute with atropine before administering neostigmine.

Preparation of solution: Using the system, transfer the contents of the neostigmine methylsulfate vial into the atropine sulfate vial. The 3.5 ml resultant mixture contains 1.2 mg atropine sulfate and 2.5 mg neostigmine methylsulfate.

Rx	**Neostigmine Methylsulfate Min-I-Mix** (IMS)	**Injection:** Dual chambered vial containing 1.2 mg atropine sulfate and 2.5 mg neostigmine methylsulfate when mixed.

Complete prescribing information for these products begins on page 2712

EDROPHONIUM CHLORIDE

Indications:

Differential diagnosis of myasthenia gravis; adjunct in evaluating treatment requirements in myasthenia gravis; evaluate emergency treatment in myasthenic crises. Because of its brief duration of action, it is not useful in maintenance therapy.

Curare antagonist to reverse neuromuscular block produced by curare, tubocurarine or gallamine; adjunct in treating respiratory depression caused by curare overdosage.

Administration and Dosage:

Differential diagnosis of myasthenia gravis:

Adults, IV – Prepare tuberculin syringe containing 10 mg edrophonium with IV needle. Inject 2 mg IV in 15 to 30 seconds. Leave needle in situ. If no reaction occurs after 45 seconds, inject the remaining 8 mg. If a cholinergic reaction (muscarinic side effects, skeletal muscle fasciculations or increased muscle weakness) occurs after injection of 2 mg, discontinue the test and administer atropine sulfate 0.4 to 0.5 mg IV. After 30 minutes, the test may be repeated.

Adults, IM – In adults with inaccessible veins, inject 10 mg IM. Retest subjects who demonstrate hyperreactivity (cholinergic reaction) after 30 minutes with 2 mg IM to rule out false-negative reactions.

Children, IV – Up to 34 kg (75 lbs), 1 mg; > 34 kg (> 75 lbs), 2 mg. If no response after 45 seconds, may titrate up to 5 mg in children < 34 kg (< 75 lbs), and up to 10 mg in heavier children, given in 1 mg increments every 30 to 45 seconds. In infants, give 0.5 mg. Alternatively, the following schedule is recommended: Total dose is 0.2 mg/kg. Give 0.04 mg/kg initially as a test dose, then in 1 mg increments if no reaction occurs within 1 minute. Maximum dose is 10 mg total.

Children, IM – Up to 34 kg (75 lbs), 2 mg; > 34 kg (> 75 lbs), 5 mg. There is a 2 to 10 minute delay in reaction.

Evaluation of treatment requirements in myasthenia gravis: 1 to 2 mg IV 1 hour after oral intake of the treatment drug. Responses are summarized below:

Response to Edrophonium Test in Myasthenia Gravis

Response to edrophonium test	Myasthenic[1]	Adequate[2]	Cholinergic[3]
Muscle strength (ptosis, diplopia, dysphonia, dysphagia, dysarthria, respiration, limb strength)	Increased	No change	Decreased
Fasciculations (orbicularis oculi, facial muscles, limb muscles)	Absent	Present or absent	Present or absent
Side effects (lacrimation, diaphoresis, salivation, abdominal cramps, nausea, vomiting, diarrhea)	Absent	Minimal	Severe

[1] *Myasthenic response:* Occurs in untreated myasthenics and may establish diagnosis; in patients under treatment, it indicates inadequate therapy.

[2] *Adequate response:* Observed in stabilized patients; a typical response in normal individuals. In addition, forced lid closure is often observed in psychoneurotics.

[3] *Cholinergic response:* Seen in myasthenics overtreated with anticholinesterases.

Edrophonium test in crisis: When a patient is apneic, secure controlled ventilation immediately. Do not test with edrophonium until respiration is adequate. If the patient is *cholinergic,* edrophonium will increase oropharyngeal secretions and further weaken respiratory muscles. If the crisis is *myasthenic,* the test clearly improves respiration and the patient can be treated with a longer acting IV anticholinesterase. Do not have > 2 mg in the syringe. Give 1 mg IV initially; carefully observe patient's cardiac response. If, after 1 minute, this dose does not further impair the patient, inject the remaining 1 mg. If no clear improvement of respiration occurs after 2 mg, discontinue all anticholinesterase therapy and control ventilation by tracheostomy and assisted respiration.

Curare antagonist: Give 10 mg slowly IV over 30 to 45 seconds to detect onset of cholinergic reaction. Repeat when necessary. Maximal dose is 40 mg. Do not give before use of curare, tubocurarine or gallamine triethiodide; use when needed. When given to counteract curare overdosage, carefully observe the effect of each dose on respiration before repeating, and employ assisted ventilation.

				C.I.*
Rx	**Enlon** (Anaquest)	**Injection:** 10 mg per ml	In 15 ml vials.[1]	16
Rx	**Reversol** (Organon)		In 10 ml vials (25s).[1]	20
Rx	**Tensilon** (ICN)		In 1 ml amps[2] & 10 ml vials.[1]	24

* Cost Index based on cost per 10 mg edrophonium.

[1] With 0.45% phenol and 0.2% sodium sulfite.

[2] With 0.2% sodium sulfite.

Complete prescribing information for edrophonium begins on page 2712 Refer also to the atropine prescribing information in the GI Anticholinergic/Antispasmodic section.

Anticholinesterase Muscle Stimulants (Cont.)

EDROPHONIUM CHLORIDE/ATROPINE SULFATE

Actions:

Atropine is added to edrophonium to counteract the unavoidable muscarinic side effects (eg, bradycardia, bronchoconstriction, increased secretions) of edrophonium.

Indications:

As a reversal agent or antagonist of nondepolarizing neuromuscular blocking agents.

Adjunctively in the treatment of respiratory depression caused by curare overdosage.

Not effective against depolarizing neuromuscular blocking agents. Not recommended for use in the differential diagnosis of myasthenia gravis.

Administration and Dosage:

Approved by the FDA on November 6, 1991.

Dosages of edrophonium and atropine injection range from 0.05 to 0.1 ml/kg given slowly over 45 seconds to 1 minute at a point of at least 5% recovery of twitch response to neuromuscular stimulation (95% block). The dosage delivered is 0.5 to 1 mg/kg edrophonium and 0.007 to 0.014 mg/kg atropine. A total dosage of 1 mg/kg edrophonium should rarely be exceeded. Monitor response carefully and secure assisted or controlled ventilation. Satisfactory reversal permits adequate voluntary respiration and neuromuscular transmission (as tested with a peripheral nerve stimulator). Recurarization has not been reported after satisfactory reversal has been attained.

Storage: Store between 15° to 26° C (59° to 78° F).

Rx	**Enlon-Plus** (Anaquest)	**Injection:** 10 mg edrophonium chloride and 0.14 mg atropine sulfate	In 5 ml amps[1] and 15 ml multidose vials.[2]

[1] With 2 mg sodium sulfite.

[2] With 2 mg sodium sulfite and 4.5 mg phenol.

GUANIDINE HCl

Actions:

Guanidine enhances the release of acetylcholine following a nerve impulse. It appears to slow the rates of depolarization and repolarization of muscle cell membranes.

Indications:

For reduction of the symptoms of muscle weakness and easy fatigability associated with the myasthenic syndrome of Eaton-Lambert. Not indicated for myasthenia gravis.

Contraindications:

History of intolerance or allergy to guanidine.

Warnings:

Fatal bone marrow suppression, apparently dose-related, can occur. Follow baseline blood studies by frequent complete blood cell (CBC) count and differential counts. Discontinue use if bone marrow suppression occurs. Do not continue treatment longer than necessary. Avoid concurrent therapy with other drugs that may cause bone marrow suppression.

Pregnancy: Safety for use during pregnancy has not been established. Use only when clearly needed and when the potential benefits outweigh the potential hazards to the fetus.

Lactation: Guanidine is excreted in breast milk; patients taking this drug should discontinue breastfeeding.

Children: Safety for use in children has not been established.

Precautions:

Renal effects: Renal function may be affected in some patients. Perform regular urine examinations and serum creatinine determinations.

Adverse Reactions:

Hematologic: Bone marrow depression with anemia (see Warnings), leukopenia and thrombocytopenia.

CNS/Neurologic: Paresthesia of lips, face, hands and feet; cold sensations in hands and feet; nervousness; lightheadedness; increased irritability; jitteriness; tremor; trembling sensations; ataxia; emotional lability; psychotic state; confusion; mood changes; hallucinations.

GI: Dry mouth; anorexia; gastric irritation; nausea; diarrhea; abdominal cramping. GI side effects may preclude use.

Dermatologic: Rash; flushing or pink complexion; folliculitis; petechiae; purpura; ecchymoses; sweating; skin eruptions; dryness and scaling of the skin.

Renal: Elevation of creatinine; uremia; chronic interstitial nephritis; renal tubular necrosis.

Hepatic: Abnormal liver function tests.

Cardiac: Palpitations; tachycardia; atrial fibrillation; hypotension.

General: Sore throat; fever.

Overdosage:

Symptoms: Mild GI disorders (anorexia, increased peristalsis or diarrhea) are early warnings that tolerance is being exceeded. These symptoms may be relieved by atropine, but consider dosage reduction. Slight numbness or tingling of the lips and fingertips has occurred shortly after taking a guanidine dose; this is not an indication to discontinue treatment or reduce dosage.

Severe intoxication is characterized by nervous hyperirritability, fibrillary tremors and convulsive contractions of muscle, salivation, vomiting, diarrhea, hypoglycemia and circulatory disturbances.

Treatment: Calcium gluconate IV may control the neuromuscular and convulsive symptoms and relieve other toxic manifestations. Atropine relieves the GI symptoms, circulatory disturbances and changes in blood sugar.

Patient Information:

Notify physician if sore throat, fever, skin rash, flushing, GI upset (nausea, vomiting, diarrhea), nervousness or tremor occurs.

Administration and Dosage:

Initial dosage is 10 to 15 mg/kg/day in 3 or 4 divided doses; gradually increase to 35 mg/kg/day or up to the development of side effects. Continue the tolerable dose. Occasionally, removal of the primary neoplastic lesion may result in improvement of symptoms, permitting drug discontinuation.

Rx	**Guanidine HCl** (Key Pharm.)	**Tablets:** 125 mg	In 100s.

Prescribing information on the Urinary Tract Anti-Infectives begins on page 2036

Alkalinizers

Urinary alkalinizing agents are bases or salts of bases which increase the excretion of free base in the urine, thus effectively raising the urinary pH.

These agents are used to correct acidosis in renal tubular disorders, and to minimize uric acid crystallization as adjuvants to uricosuric agents in gout. Urine alkalinization increases the antimicrobial effectiveness of aminoglycosides and the solubility of sulfonamides.

SODIUM BICARBONATE

For information on parenteral sodium bicarbonate, refer to page 145

One gram of sodium bicarbonate provides 11.9 mEq sodium and 11.9 mEq bicarbonate.

Precautions:

Use cautiously in edematous sodium-retaining states, CHF, liver cirrhosis, toxemia of pregnancy or renal impairment. Prolonged therapy may lead to systemic alkalosis.

Dose: 325 mg to 2 g, up to 4 times daily. The maximum daily intake is 17 g (200 mEq) in patients under 60 years old and 8 g (100 mEq) in those over 60.

	Product	Form	Packaging	C.I.*
otc	**Sodium Bicarbonate** (Various)	**Tablets:** 325 mg	In 100s & 1000s.	2+
		650 mg	In 100s, 200s and 1000s.	2+
		Powder:	In 120 & 480 g.	1+

POTASSIUM CITRATE

Administration and Dosage:

Severe hypocitraturia: Initially, 60 mEq/day (20 mEq 3 times per day or 15 mEq 4 times per day with meals or within 30 minutes after meals).

Mild to moderate hypocitraturia: 30 mEq/day (10 mEq 3 times per day with meals). Do not exceed 100 mEq/day.

	Product	Form	Packaging	C.I.*
Rx	**Urocit-K** (Mission)	**Tablets:** 5 mEq	In 100s.	17

POTASSIUM CITRATE COMBINATIONS

For complete prescribing information on citrate and citric acid preparations, see page 54.

Administration and Dosage:

Liquids: 15 to 20 ml 4 times daily usually maintains a urinary pH of 7 to 7.6 throughout 24 hours; 10 to 15 ml 4 times daily usually maintains a urinary pH of 6.5 to 7.4.

Adults – 15 to 30 ml diluted with water, after meals and at bedtime.

Children – 5 to 15 ml diluted with water, after meals and at bedtime.

Neutralizing buffer: 15 ml diluted in 15 ml water, as a single dose.

Tablets: 1 to 4 tablets with a full glass of water, after meals and at bedtime.

	Product	Form	Packaging	C.I.*
Rx	**Citrolith** (Beach Pharm.)	**Tablets:** 50 mg potassium citrate and 950 mg sodium citrate	(Beach 1136). In 100s & 500s.	11
Rx	**Polycitra** (Willen)	**Syrup:** 550 mg potassium citrate, 500 mg sodium citrate and 334 mg citric acid per 5 ml. (1 mEq potassium, 1 mEq sodium per ml; equivalent to 2 mEq bicarbonate)	Alcohol free. In 120 and 480 ml.	4
Rx sf	**Polycitra-LC** (Willen)	**Solution:** 550 mg potassium citrate, 500 mg sodium citrate and 334 mg citric acid per 5 ml. (1 mEq potassium, 1 mEq sodium per ml; equivalent to 2 mEq bicarbonate)	Alcohol free. In 120 and 480 ml.	4
Rx sf	**Polycitra-K** (Willen)	**Solution:** 1100 mg potassium citrate and 334 mg citric acid per 5 ml. (2 mEq potassium/ml; equivalent to 2 mEq bicarbonate)	Alcohol free. In 120 and 480 ml.	4
		Crystals for Reconstitution: 3300 mg potassium citrate and 1002 mg citric acid per UD packet (equivalent to 30 mEq bicarbonate)	Alcohol free. In single dose packets.	NA

SODIUM CITRATE AND CITRIC ACID SOLUTION (Shohl's Solution, Modified)

Administration and Dosage:

Systemic alkalinization:

Adults – 10 to 30 ml diluted in 30 to 90 ml water, after meals and at bedtime.

Neutralizing buffer: 15 ml diluted in 15 ml water, as a single dose.

	Product	Form	Packaging	C.I.*
Rx sf	**Bicitra** (Willen)	**Solution:** 500 mg sodium citrate and 334 mg citric acid per 5 ml. (1 mEq sodium/ml)	Alcohol free. In 120 & UD 15 & 30 ml, pt & gal.	3

* Cost Index based on cost per tablet, g or 5 ml. *sf* – Sugar free.

Acidifiers

AMMONIUM CHLORIDE

For information on parenteral ammonium chloride, refer to page 155

Indications:
Used as a diuretic or systemic and urinary acidifying agent.

Contraindications:
Markedly impaired renal or hepatic function.

Adverse Reactions:
Gastric irritation, nausea, vomiting; acidosis with large doses.

Overdosage:
Symptoms: Nausea, vomiting, thirst, headache, hyperventilation and progressive drowsiness leading to profound acidosis and hypokalemia.

Treatment: Correct acidosis and electrolyte loss by administering IV sodium bicarbonate or sodium lactate. Hypokalemia may be treated by oral potassium salts.

Administration and Dosage:
Usual dose is 1 g 3 times daily for no longer than 6 days.

				C.I.*
otc	**Ammonium Cl** (Various)	**Tablets:** 500 mg	In 100s and 1000s.	2+
		Tablets, enteric coated: 500 mg	In 100s and 1000s.	4+
otc	**Ammonium Cl** (Lilly)	**Tablets, enteric coated:** 500 mg	In 100s.	11

AMMONIUM BIPHOSPHATE, SODIUM BIPHOSPHATE AND SODIUM ACID PYROPHOSPHATE

Indications:
Used to increase solubility of calcium in urine to assist in preventing formation of urinary calculi. Can decrease urinary pH to 5 to 5.5 in conjunction with an acid ash diet.

Precautions:
Administer with caution in cases of severe or extensive renal damage.

Adverse Reactions:
Occasional hyperacidity, particularly when gastritis or ulceration exists; occasional nausea with high dosage. This may be decreased or eliminated by use of enteric coated tablets. Excessive doses may act as a saline cathartic and cause diarrhea. In such cases, decrease dosage until symptoms disappear.

Patient Information:
Take with a full glass of water.

Administration and Dosage:
Usual dose is 1 g, followed by a glass of water 3 times daily. Use in conjunction with an acidifying diet. Occasionally, higher dosage is required.

				C.I.*
Rx	**pHos-pHaid** (Guardian)	**Tablets (enteric coated):** 0.5 g – 190 mg ammonium biphosphate, 200 mg sodium biphosphate and 110 mg sodium acid pyrophosphate. < 65 mg sodium per tablet	In 90s and 500s.	14
		0.25 g – 95 mg ammonium biphosphate, 100 mg sodium biphosphate and 55 mg sodium acid pyrophosphate. < 32 mg sodium per tablet	In 150s.	8

ASCORBIC ACID

While controversy exists regarding the efficacy of ascorbic acid as a urinary acidifier, it is frequently used for this purpose. Refer to the "Actions" section of the ascorbic acid monograph on page 25 for dosage guidelines.

* Cost Index based on cost per tablet.

ACID PHOSPHATES

Indications:

To acidify the urine and lower urinary calcium concentration.

Increases the antibacterial activity of methenamine.

Reduces odor and rash caused by ammoniacal urine.

Contraindications:

Renal insufficiency (less than 30% of normal), infected magnesium ammonium phosphate stones, hyperphosphatemia and hyperkalemia.

Warnings:

Concurrent potassium supplementation: Consider potassium content of these products. Decrease supplemental potassium dosage to avoid hyperkalemia.

Usage in Pregnancy: Category C. Safety for use during pregnancy has not been established. Use only when clearly needed and when the potential benefits outweigh the potential hazards to the fetus.

Usage in Lactation: Safety for use in the nursing mother has not been established. It is not known whether this drug is excreted in breast milk. Exercise caution when administering to a nursing woman.

Precautions:

Use with caution if regulation of potassium is desired. Use sodium acid phosphate cautiously in patients on sodium restriction.

Exercise caution in following conditions: Cardiac disease (particularly digitalized patients), Addison's disease, acute dehydration, severe renal insufficiency or chronic renal disease, extensive tissue breakdown (such as severe burns), myotonia congenita, cardiac failure, cirrhosis of the liver or severe hepatic disease, peripheral and pulmonary edema, hypernatremia, hypertension, toxemia of pregnancy, hypoparathyroidism, osteomalacia, acute pancreatitis and rickets.

Patient Information: Warn patients with kidney stones of possibility of passing old stones when phosphate therapy is started. Advise patients to avoid antacids containing aluminum, calcium or magnesium which may prevent phosphate absorption. To assure against GI injury associated with oral ingestion of concentrated potassium salt preparations, dissolve tablets completely in an appropriate amount of water before taking.

Laboratory Tests: Carefully monitor renal function and serum electrolytes (calcium, phosphorus, potassium) at periodic intervals during phosphate therapy if required. High serum phosphate levels increase incidence of extraskeletal calcification.

Drug Interactions:

Antacids containing magnesium, calcium or aluminum in conjunction with phosphate preparations may bind the phosphate and prevent absorption.

Potassium-containing medications or potassium-sparing diuretics may cause hyperkalemia when used concurrently with potassium phosphates. Perform periodic serum potassium level determinations.

Salicylates: Concurrent use may lead to increased serum salicylate levels since salicylate excretion is reduced in acidified urine. Use of monobasic phosphates in patients stabilized on salicylates may lead to salicylate toxicity. Monitor serum salicylate levels closely.

Antihypertensives, especially diazoxide, guanethidine, hydralazine, methyldopa or rauwolfia alkaloids; or corticosteroids, especially mineralocorticoids or corticotropin: Concurrent use of sodium phosphate may result in hypernatremia.

Adverse Reactions:

Mild laxation may occur; it usually subsides with dosage reduction. If laxation persists, discontinue use. Abdominal discomfort, diarrhea, nausea and vomiting may occur.

Less frequent: Fast or irregular heartbeat, dizziness, headache, mental confusion, seizures, weakness or heaviness of legs, unusual tiredness, muscle cramps, numbness, tingling, pain or weakness in hands or feet, numbness or tingling around lips, shortness of breath or troubled breathing, swelling of feet or legs, unusual weight gain, low urine output, thirst, bone and joint pain.

Patient Information:

Notify physician if abdominal pain, nausea or vomiting occurs.

Warn patients with kidney stones of possibility of passing old stones when phosphate therapy is started. Advise patients to avoid antacids containing aluminum, calcium or magnesium which may prevent phosphate absorption. To assure against GI injury associated with oral ingestion of concentrated potassium salt preparations, instruct patients to dissolve tablets completely in an appropriate amount of water before taking.

(Products listed on following page)

Acidifiers (Cont.)

POTASSIUM ACID PHOSPHATE

Administration and Dosage:

1 g dissolved in 180 to 240 ml water 4 times daily with meals and at bedtime. For best results, soak tablets in water for 2 to 5 minutes. Stir vigorously and swallow. **C.I.***

Rx	**K-Phos Original** (Beach)	**Tablets:** 500 mg (contains 3.7 mEq potassium)	Sodium free. (#Beach 1111). White, scored. In 100s and 500s.	11

POTASSIUM ACID PHOSPHATE AND SODIUM ACID PHOSPHATE

Administration and Dosage:

1 to 2 tablets 4 times daily with a full glass of water. When the urine is difficult to acidify, administer 1 tablet every 2 hours. Do not exceed 8 tablets in 24 hours. **C.I.***

Rx	**K-Phos M.F.** (Beach)	**Tablets:** 155 mg potassium acid phosphate and 350 mg sodium acid phosphate (contains 1.1 mEq potassium and 2.9 mEq sodium)	(#Beach 1135). White, scored. In 100s and 500s.	11
Rx	**K-Phos No. 2** (Beach)	**Tablets:** 305 mg potassium acid phosphate and 700 mg sodium acid phosphate (contains 2.3 mEq potassium and 5.8 mEq sodium)	(#Beach 1134). Brown. In 100s and 500s.	18

* Cost Index based on cost per tablet.

Product identification code.

Antispasmodics

In addition to the GI antispasmodics (refer to the Gastrointestinal chapter), many of which are recommended for urologic conditions, the following agents are indicated specifically for urologic disorders. Urinary antispasmodics in combination with urinary anti-infective agents are listed in the Anti-Infectives chapter. Urinary antispasmodics in combination with urinary analgesics are also available.

FLAVOXATE HCl

Actions:

Counteracts smooth muscle spasm of the urinary tract. Flavoxate relaxes the detrusor and other smooth muscle by cholinergic blockade. It also exerts a direct effect on the muscle. It has anticholinergic, local anesthetic and analgesic properties.

Indications:

For the symptomatic relief of dysuria, urgency, nocturia, suprapubic pain, frequency and incontinence as may occur in cystitis, prostatitis, urethritis, urethrocystitis/urethrotrigonitis.

NOT indicated for definitive treatment, but is compatible with drugs used to treat urinary tract infections.

Contraindications:

Pyloric or duodenal obstruction; obstructive intestinal lesions or ileus; achalasia; GI hemorrhage; obstructive uropathies of the lower urinary tract.

Warnings:

Glaucoma: Give cautiously in patients with suspected glaucoma.

Pregnancy: Category B. There are no well controlled studies in pregnant women. Therefore, use during pregnancy only when clearly needed.

Lactation: It is not known whether this drug is excreted in breast milk. Use caution when flavoxate is administered to a nursing woman.

Children: Safety and efficacy in children $<$ 12 years old have not been established.

Adverse Reactions:

Nausea; vomiting; dry mouth; nervousness; vertigo; headache; drowsiness; mental confusion (especially in the elderly patient); hyperpyrexia; blurred vision; increased ocular tension, disturbance in accommodation; urticaria and other dermatoses; dysuria; tachycardia; palpitations; eosinophilia; leukopenia.

Patient Information:

These agents may cause drowsiness or blurred vision; observe caution while driving or performing other tasks requiring alertness, coordination or physical dexterity.

May cause dry mouth.

Administration and Dosage:

Adults and children $>$ 12 years of age: 100 or 200 mg 3 or 4 times daily. Reduce the dose when symptoms improve.

In one study, investigators used doses up to 1200 mg/day for treatment of urinary urgency following pelvic radiotherapy. The 1200 mg/day dose was superior to the 600 mg/day dose.

				C.I.*
Rx	**Urispas** (SK-Beecham)	**Tablets:** 100 mg	(SKF Urispas). White. Film coated. In 100s and UD 100s.	3.3

* Cost Index based on cost per 300 mg.

OXYBUTYNIN CHLORIDE

Actions:

Pharmacology: Oxybutynin exerts direct antispasmodic effect on smooth muscle and inhibits the muscarinic action of acetylcholine on smooth muscle. It exhibits one-fifth of the anticholinergic activity of atropine, but 4 to 10 times the antispasmodic activity. No blocking effects occur at skeletal neuromuscular junctions or autonomic ganglia (antinicotinic effects).

In patients with conditions characterized by involuntary bladder contractions, oxybutynin increases vesical capacity, diminishes frequency of uninhibited contractions of the detrusor muscle and delays initial desire to void. These effects are more consistently improved in patients with uninhibited neurogenic bladder. Oxybutynin thus decreases urgency and the frequency of both incontinent episodes and voluntary urination.

The drug is well tolerated in patients administered the drug from 30 days to 2 years.

Indications:

For the relief of symptoms of bladder instability associated with voiding in patients with uninhibited and reflex neurogenic bladder (eg, urgency, frequency, urinary leakage, urge incontinence, dysuria).

Contraindications:

Glaucoma (angle closure); GI obstruction; paralytic ileus; intestinal atony of the elderly or debilitated; megacolon; toxic megacolon complicating ulcerative colitis; severe colitis; myasthenia gravis; obstructive uropathy; unstable cardiovascular status in acute hemorrhage; hypersensitivity to the product.

Warnings:

Heat prostration: When administered in the presence of high environmental temperature, heat prostration (fever and heat stroke) may occur due to decreased sweating.

Diarrhea may be an early symptom of incomplete intestinal obstruction, especially in patients with ileostomy or colostomy; discontinue treatment.

Pregnancy: Category B. Safety for use during pregnancy has not been established. Use only when clearly needed and when the potential benefits outweigh the potential hazards to the fetus.

Lactation: It is not known whether this drug is excreted in breast milk. Exercise caution when administering to a nursing woman.

Children: Safety and efficacy in children $<$ 5 years of age have not been established.

Precautions:

Use with caution in the elderly and patients with autonomic neuropathy, hepatic or renal disease. Doses administered to patients with ulcerative colitis may suppress GI motility and produce paralytic ileus and precipitate or aggravate toxic megacolon.

Cardiac effects: Symptoms of hyperthyroidism, coronary heart disease, congestive heart failure, cardiac arrhythmias, tachycardia, hypertension, hiatal hernia and prostatic hypertrophy may be aggravated.

Potentially hazardous tasks: May produce drowsiness or dizziness; patients should observe caution while driving or performing other tasks requiring alertness, coordination or physical dexterity.

Drug Interactions:

Oxybutynin Drug Interactions			
Precipitant Drug	Object Drug*		Description
Oxybutynin	Digoxin	↑	Serum levels of digoxin (administered as slow dissolution tablets) may be increased.
Oxybutynin	Haloperidol	↓	Worsening of schizophrenic symptoms, decreased serum concentration of haloperidol, development of tardive dyskinesia.
Oxybutynin	Phenothiazines	↔	Increased incidence of anticholinergic side effects, and decreased or increased phenothiazine levels may occur.

* ↑ = Object drug increased; ↓ = Object drug decreased; ↔ = Undetermined effect.

Adverse Reactions:

Dry mouth; decreased sweating; rash; urinary hesitancy and retention; decreased lacrimation; mydriasis; amblyopia; cycloplegia; tachycardia; palpitations; vasodilation; drowsiness; hallucinations; insomnia; restlessness; asthenia; dizziness; nausea; vomiting; constipation; decreased GI motility; impotence; suppression of lactation.

(Continued on following page)

OXYBUTYNIN CHLORIDE (Cont.)

Overdosage:

Symptoms include: Signs of CNS excitation (eg, restlessness, tremor, irritability, convulsions, delirium, hallucinations); flushing; fever; nausea; vomiting; tachycardia; hypotension or hypertension; respiratory failure; paralysis; coma.

Treatment should be symptomatic and supportive. Maintain respiration and induce emesis or perform gastric lavage (emesis is contraindicated in precomatose, convulsive or psychotic state). Activated charcoal may be administered as well as a cathartic. Physostigmine may be considered to reverse symptoms of anticholinergic intoxication. Treat hyperpyrexia symptomatically with ice bags or other cold applications and alcohol sponges. Refer to General Management of Acute Overdosage.

Patient Information:

May cause drowsiness, dizziness or blurred vision; alcohol or sedatives may enhance this effect. Observe caution while driving or performing other tasks requiring alertness, coordination or physical dexterity.

May cause dry mouth.

Administration and Dosage:

Adults: 5 mg 2 or 3 times daily. Maximum dose is 5 mg 4 times daily.

Children (> 5 years): 5 mg twice a day. Maximum dose is 5 mg 3 times daily.

				C.I.*
Rx	**Oxybutynin Chloride** (Various, eg, Geneva Marsam, Goldline, Major, Moore, Parmed, Rugby, Schein, URL)	**Tablets:** 5 mg	In 100s, 500s and 1000s and UD 100s.	1+
Rx	**Ditropan** (Marion Merrell Dow)		Lactose. (Marion 1375). Blue, scored. Biconvex. In 100s, 1000s and UD 100s.	2.5
Rx	**Ditropan** (Marion Merrell Dow)	**Syrup:** 5 mg per 5 ml	Sorbitol, sucrose. In 473 ml.	2.8

* Cost Index based on cost per 15 mg.

Cholinergic Stimulants

BETHANECHOL CHLORIDE

Actions:

Pharmacology: Bethanechol is an ester of a choline-like compound. It acts principally by stimulating the parasympathetic nervous system. It increases the tone of the detrusor urinae muscle, usually producing a contraction strong enough to initiate micturition and empty the bladder. It stimulates gastric motility, increases gastric tone and often restores impaired rhythmic peristalsis.

When spontaneous stimulation of the parasympathomimetic system is reduced, acetylcholine can be given, but it is rapidly hydrolyzed by cholinesterase and its effects are transient. Bethanechol is not destroyed by cholinesterase and its effects are more prolonged than those of acetylcholine.

It has predominant muscarinic action and only slight nicotinic action. Doses that stimulate micturition and defecation and increase peristalsis do not ordinarily stimulate ganglia or voluntary muscles. Therapeutic test doses in healthy human subjects have little effect on heart rate, blood pressure or peripheral circulation.

Pharmacokinetics: Effects appear within 30 to 90 minutes after oral administration. Usual duration is 1 hour, although large doses (eg, 300 to 400 mg) may persist for up to 6 hours. Administration SC is usually effective in 5 to 15 minutes.

A clinical study was conducted on the relative efficacy of oral and SC bethanechol on the stretch response of bladder muscle in patients with urinary retention. A 5 mg SC dose stimulated a response that was more rapid in onset and of larger magnitude than an oral dose of 50, 100 or 200 mg. The oral doses, however, had a longer duration of effect than the SC dose. Although the 50 mg oral dose caused little change in intravesical pressure, this dose is effective in the rehabilitation of patients with decompensated bladders.

Indications:

Acute postoperative and postpartum nonobstructive (functional) urinary retention and neurogenic atony of the urinary bladder with retention.

Unlabeled uses: Bethanechol has been used in adults and children for treatment (25 mg 4 times daily) and diagnosis (two 50 mcg/kg SC doses 15 minutes apart) of reflux esophagitis. In infants and children, an oral dosage of 3 mg/m^2/dose 3 times a day has been used for gastroesophageal reflux.

Contraindications:

Hypersensitivity to bethanechol; hyperthyroidism; peptic ulcer; latent or active asthma; pronounced bradycardia; atrio-ventricular conduction defects; vasomotor instability; coronary artery disease; epilepsy; parkinsonism; coronary occlusion; hypotension; hypertension; when the strength or integrity of the GI or bladder wall is in question or in the presence of mechanical obstruction; when increased muscular activity of the GI tract or urinary bladder might prove harmful, as following recent urinary bladder surgery, GI resection and anastomosis, or when there is possible GI obstruction; bladder neck obstruction; spastic GI disturbances; acute inflammatory lesions of the GI tract; peritonitis; marked vagotonia.

Warnings:

Parenteral dosage form: For SC injection only; do not give IM or IV. Violent symptoms of cholinergic overstimulation, such as circulatory collapse, fall in blood pressure, abdominal cramps, bloody diarrhea, shock or sudden cardiac arrest are likely if given IM or IV. These symptoms occur rarely after SC injection and may occur in cases of hypersensitivity or overdosage.

Pregnancy: Category C. It is not known whether bethanechol can cause fetal harm when administered to a pregnant woman or can affect reproduction capacity. Give to a pregnant woman only if clearly needed.

Lactation: It is not known whether this drug is excreted in breast milk. Because of the potential for serious adverse reactions, decide whether to discontinue nursing or discontinue the drug, taking into account the importance of the drug to the mother.

Children: Safety and efficacy have not been established. See Unlabeled uses.

Precautions:

Reflux infection: In urinary retention, if the sphincter fails to relax as bethanechol contracts the bladder, urine may be forced up the ureter into the kidney pelvis. If there is bacteriuria, this may cause reflux infection.

Tartrazine sensitivity: Some of these products contain tartrazine, which may cause allergic-type reactions (including bronchial asthma) in susceptible individuals. Although the incidence of sensitivity is low, it is frequently seen in patients who also have aspirin hypersensitivity. Specific products containing tartrazine are identified in the product listings.

(Continued on following page)

BETHANECHOL CHLORIDE (Cont.)

Drug Interactions:

Quinidine or procainamide may antagonize cholinergic effects of bethanechol.

Cholinergic drugs (particularly cholinesterase inhibitors): Additive effects may occur.

Ganglionic blocking compounds: A critical fall in blood pressure may occur, which is usually preceded by severe abdominal symptoms.

Adverse Reactions:

Adverse reactions are rare following oral administration of bethanechol, but are more common following SC injection. Adverse reactions are more likely to occur when dosage is increased.

GI: Abdominal cramps or discomfort; colicky pain; nausea; belching; diarrhea; borborygmi (rumbling/gurgling of stomach); salivation.

Cardiovascular: Fall in blood pressure with reflex tachycardia; vasomotor response.

Dermatologic: Flushing producing a feeling of warmth; sensation of heat about the face; sweating.

Respiratory: Bronchial constriction; asthmatic attacks.

Special senses: Lacrimation; miosis.

Other: Malaise; urinary urgency; headache.

Overdosage:

Symptoms: Abdominal discomfort, salivation, flushing of the skin ("hot feeling"), sweating, nausea and vomiting are early signs of overdosage.

Treatment: Atropine is a specific antidote. The recommended dose for adults is 0.6 mg. Repeat doses may be given every 2 hours according to clinical response.

The recommended dosage in infants and children up to 12 years of age is 0.01 mg/kg repeated every 2 hours as needed until the desired effect is obtained or adverse effects of atropine preclude further usage. The maximum single dose should not exceed 0.4 mg.

Subcutaneous injection of atropine is preferred except in emergencies when the IV route may be used. When administering bethanechol SC, always have a syringe containing atropine available.

Patient Information:

To avoid nausea and vomiting, take on an empty stomach. If taken soon after eating, nausea and vomiting may occur.

May cause abdominal discomfort, salivation, sweating or flushing; notify physician if these effects are pronounced.

Dizziness, lightheadedness or fainting may occur, especially when getting up from a lying or sitting position.

Administration and Dosage:

Individualize dose and route. Administer preferably when the stomach is empty. If taken soon after eating, nausea and vomiting may occur.

Oral: Adults 10 to 50 mg 3 to 4 times daily. The minimum effective dose is determined by giving 5 or 10 mg initially; repeat the same amount hourly to a maximum of 50 mg until satisfactory response occurs.

SC: Do not give IV or IM (see Warnings). Usual dose is 5 mg; some patients respond to as little as 2.5 mg. The minimum effective dose is determined by injecting 2.5 mg initially and repeating the same amount at 15 to 30 minute intervals to a maximum of 4 doses until satisfactory response is obtained, unless disturbing reactions appear. The minimum effective dose may be repeated 3 or 4 times a day as required.

Rarely, single doses up to 10 mg are required. Such large doses may cause severe reactions; use only after determining that single doses of 2.5 to 5 mg are not sufficient.

If necessary, drug effects can be abolished promptly by atropine.

(Products listed on following page)

Cholinergic Stimulants (Cont.)

BETHANECHOL CHLORIDE (Cont.)

	Product	Form	Description	C.I.*
Rx	**Bethanechol Chloride** (Various, eg, Bolar, Danbury, Genetco, Goldline, Lannett, Sidmak, UDL, Vangard)	**Tablets:** 5 mg	In 100s, 500s, 1000s and UD 100s.	3.9+
Rx	**Urecholine** (MSD)		Lactose. (MSD 403). White, scored. In 100s & UD 100s.	40
Rx	**Bethanechol Chloride** (Various, eg, Geneva, Goldline, Lannett, Major, Moore, Parmed, Rugby, Schein, UDL, URL)	**Tablets:** 10 mg	In 100s, 250s, 500s, 1000s and UD 100s.	2+
Rx	**Duvoid** (Roberts[1])		(Eaton 045). Orange, scored. In 100s and UD 100s.	35
Rx	**Myotonachol** (Glenwood)		Tartrazine. Scored. In 100s.	16
Rx	**Urecholine** (MSD)		Lactose. (MSD 412). Pink, scored. In 100s & UD 100s.	37
Rx	**Bethanechol Chloride** (Various, eg, Dixon-Shane, Geneva Marsam, Goldline, Moore, Parmed, Rugby, Schein, Sidmak, UDL, URL)	**Tablets:** 25 mg	In 100s, 500s, 1000s and UD 100s.	1.1+
Rx	**Duvoid** (Roberts[1])		(Eaton 046). White, scored. In 100s and UD 100s.	21
Rx	**Myotonachol** (Glenwood)		Tartrazine. Scored. In 100s.	14
Rx	**Urecholine** (MSD)		Lactose. (MSD 457). Yellow, scored. In 100s & UD 100s.	23
Rx	**Bethanechol Chloride** (Various, eg, Danbury, Dixon-Shane, Genetco, Moore, Parmed, Rugby, Schein, Sidmak, URL)	**Tablets:** 50 mg	In 100s, 500s, 1000s and UD 100s.	1+
Rx	**Duvoid** (Roberts[1])		(Eaton 047). Tan, scored. In 100s and UD 100s.	16
Rx	**Urecholine** (MSD)		Lactose. (MSD 460). Yellow, scored. In 100s.	16
Rx	**Urecholine** (MSD)	**Injection:** 5 mg per ml	In 1 ml vials.	579

* Cost Index based on cost per 5 mg.

[1] Roberts Pharmaceutical Corp., Meridian Center III, 6 Industrial Way West, Eatontown, NJ 07724 (800) 828-8566.

Neostigmine is also used in the diagnosis and treatment of myasthenia gravis and as an antidote for nondepolarizing neuromuscular blockers; refer to Anticholinesterase Muscle Stimulants.

Cholinergic Stimulants (Cont.)

NEOSTIGMINE METHYLSULFATE

Actions:

Pharmacology: Neostigmine inhibits acetylcholine hydrolysis by competing for attachment to acetylcholinesterase at sites of cholinergic transmission. It enhances cholinergic action by facilitating the transmission of impulses across neuromuscular junctions. It also has a direct cholinomimetic effect on skeletal muscle and possibly on autonomic ganglion cells and neurons of the CNS.

Pharmacokinetics: Absorption/Distribution – Neostigmine is poorly absorbed orally. Following IM administration, the drug is rapidly absorbed and eliminated. Serum albumin binding ranges from 15% to 25%.

Metabolism/Excretion – Neostigmine undergoes hydrolysis by cholinesterase and is metabolized by microsomal enzymes in the liver. Approximately 80% is eliminated in the urine within 24 hours, 50% as the unchanged drug and 30% as metabolites. Following IV administration, plasma half-life is 47 to 60 minutes (mean 53 minutes).

Onset/Duration – Clinical effects usually begin within 20 to 30 minutes after IM injection and last 2.5 to 4 hours.

Indications:

Prevention and treatment of postoperative distention and urinary retention.

Contraindications:

Hypersensitivity to neostigmine; peritonitis; mechanical intestinal or urinary tract obstruction.

Warnings:

Use with caution in patients with epilepsy, bronchial asthma, bradycardia, recent coronary occlusion, vagotonia, hyperthyroidism, cardiac arrhythmias or peptic ulcer.

Concomitant atropine administration: When large doses are administered, the prior or simultaneous injection of atropine sulfate may be advisable. Use separate syringes for neostigmine and atropine.

Hypersensitivity: Have atropine and antishock medication immediately available. Refer to Management of Acute Hypersensitivity Reactions.

Pregnancy: Category C. There are no adequate or well controlled studies. It is not known whether neostigmine can cause fetal harm when administered to a pregnant woman or can affect reproductive capacity. Anticholinesterase drugs may cause uterine irritability and induce premature labor when given IV to pregnant women near term. Give to a pregnant woman only if clearly needed.

Lactation: It is not known whether neostigmine is excreted in breast milk. Because of the potential for serious adverse reactions in nursing infants, decide whether to discontinue nursing or to discontinue the drug, taking into account the importance of the drug to the mother.

Children: Safety and efficacy for use in children have not been established.

Adverse Reactions:

Side effects are generally due to exaggerated pharmacological effects; salivation and fasciculation are the most common.

CNS: Dizziness; convulsions; loss of consciousness; drowsiness; headache; weakness; dysarthria; miosis; visual changes.

Cardiovascular: Cardiac arrhythmias (bradycardia, tachycardia, AV block and nodal rhythm); nonspecific ECG changes; cardiac arrest; syncope; hypotension.

Respiratory: Increased oral, pharyngeal and bronchial secretions; dyspnea; respiratory depression; respiratory arrest; bronchospasm.

Dermatologic: Rash; urticaria.

GI: Nausea; emesis; flatulence; increased peristalsis; bowel cramps; diarrhea.

Musculoskeletal: Muscle cramps and spasms; arthralgia.

Miscellaneous: Diaphoresis; flushing; allergic reactions; anaphylaxis; urinary frequency.

(Continued on following page)

NEOSTIGMINE METHYLSULFATE (Cont.)

Overdosage:

Symptoms: Overdosage may result in cholinergic crisis, characterized by increasing muscle weakness. This, through involvement of respiratory muscles, may lead to death.

Treatment: Cholinergic crisis calls for the prompt withdrawal of all drugs of this type and the immediate use of atropine (see Anticholinergics/Antispasmodics in the Gastrointestinal chapter).

Atropine may also be used to abolish or minimize GI side effects or other muscarinic reactions; such use can lead to inadvertent induction of cholinergic crisis by masking signs of overdosage.

Administration and Dosage:

Prevention of postoperative distention and urinary retention: 1 ml of the 1:4000 solution (0.25 mg) SC or IM as soon as possible after operation; repeat every 4 to 6 hours for 2 or 3 days.

Treatment of postoperative distention: 1 ml of the 1:2000 solution (0.5 mg) SC or IM, as required.

Treatment of urinary retention: 1 ml of the 1:2000 solution (0.5 mg) SC or IM. If urination does not occur within 1 hour, catheterize the patient. After the bladder is emptied, continue 0.5 mg injections every 3 hours for at least 5 injections.

				C.I.*
Rx	**Prostigmin** (ICN)	**Injection:** 1:4000 (0.25 mg/ml) solution	In 1 ml amps.[1]	555
Rx	**Neostigmine Methylsulfate** (Various, eg, Elkins-Sinn, Geneva Marsam, Lyphomed, Schein)	**Injection:** 1:2000 (0.5 mg/ml) solution	In 10 ml vials.	237+
Rx	**Prostigmin** (ICN)		In 1 ml amps[1] and 10 ml vials.[2]	344
Rx	**Neostigmine Methylsulfate** (Various, eg, Elkins-Sinn, Geneva Marsam, Lyphomed, Schein)	**Injection:** 1:1000 (1 mg/ml) solution	In 10 ml vials.	119+
Rx	**Prostigmin** (ICN)		In 10 ml vials.[2]	182

* Cost Index based on cost per mg.

[1] With 0.2% methyl and propyl parabens.

[2] With 0.45% phenol.

Urinary analgesics in combination with urinary anti-infectives are listed in the Anti-Infectives chapter.

Analgesics

PHENAZOPYRIDINE HCl (Phenylazo Diamino Pyridine HCl)

Actions:

Pharmacology: Phenazopyridine, an azo dye, is excreted in the urine where it exerts a topical analgesic effect on urinary tract mucosa; therefore, use only for relief of symptoms. Its mechanism of action is unknown. Phenazopyridine is compatible with antibacterial therapy and can help relieve pain and discomfort before antibacterial therapy controls the infection.

Pharmacokinetics: Phenazopyridine is rapidly excreted by kidneys; 65% is excreted unchanged in urine.

Indications:

Symptomatic relief of pain, burning, urgency, frequency and other discomforts arising from irritation of the lower urinary tract mucosa caused by infection, trauma, surgery, endoscopic procedures or passage of sounds or catheters. Its analgesic action may reduce or eliminate the need for systemic analgesics or narcotics.

Contraindications:

Hypersensitivity to phenazopyridine; renal insufficiency.

Warnings:

Carcinogenesis: Long-term administration of phenazopyridine has induced neoplasia in rats (large intestine) and mice (liver).

Pregnancy: Category B. There are no adequate and well controlled studies in pregnant women. Use during pregnancy only if clearly needed.

Lactation: No information is available on the appearance of this drug or its metabolites in breast milk.

Children: Do not administer to children < 12 years of age unless directed by a physician.

Precautions:

Skin/sclera discoloration: A yellowish tinge of the skin or sclera may indicate accumulation due to impaired renal excretion and the need to discontinue therapy.

Duration of therapy: Treatment of a urinary tract infection (UTI) with phenazopyridine should not exceed 2 days because there is a lack of evidence that the combined administration of phenazopyridine and an antibacterial provides greater benefit than administration of the antibacterial alone after 2 days.

Drug Interactions:

Drug/Lab test interaction: An azo dye, phenazopyridine may interfere with urinalysis based on spectrometry or color reactions.

Adverse Reactions:

Headache; rash; pruritus; occasional GI disturbances; anaphylactoid-like reaction; methemoglobinemia, hemolytic anemia, renal and hepatic toxicity (usually at overdosage levels).

Overdosage:

Symptoms: Exceeding the recommended dose or administering the usual dose to patients with impaired renal function (common in elderly patients), may lead to toxic reactions. Methemoglobinemia generally follows a massive, acute overdose. Oxidative Heinz body hemolytic anemia may occur, and "bite cells" (degmacytes) may be present in chronic overdosage. Red blood cell G-6-PD deficiency may predispose to hemolysis. Renal and hepatic impairment and failure, usually due to hypersensitivity, may also occur.

Treatment: Methylene blue, 1 to 2 mg/kg IV (see individual monograph), or 100 to 200 mg ascorbic acid orally should cause prompt reduction of methemoglobinemia and disappearance of cyanosis. Refer to General Management of Acute Overdosage.

Patient Information:

May cause GI upset; take after meals.

May cause a reddish-orange discoloration of the urine and may stain fabric. This is not abnormal and represents no cause for alarm. Staining of contact lenses has also occurred.

Do not use long-term to treat undiagnosed urinary tract pain. This product treats painful symptoms but not the source or cause of the pain.

(Continued on following page)

Analgesics (Cont.)

PHENAZOPYRIDINE HCl (Phenylazo Diamino Pyridine HCl) (Cont.)

Administration and Dosage:

Do not use chronically to treat undiagnosed pain of the urinary tract. Such use could lead to serious delays in appropriate diagnosis and treatment. This product treats painful symptoms but does not treat the source or cause of the disorder causing the pain.

Adults: 200 mg 3 times a day after meals. Administration should not exceed 2 days when used concomitantly with an antibacterial agent for the treatment of UTI.

Children (6 to 12 years): 12 mg/kg/24 hr divided into three oral doses for 2 days.

	Product	Form	Description	C.I.*
otc	**Azo-Standard** (Alcon)	**Tablets:** 95 mg	(W). In 30s.	25
Rx	**Phenazopyridine HCl** (Various, eg, Dixon-Shane, Geneva Marsam, Moore, Parmed, UDL, URL)	**Tablets:** 100 mg	In 100s, 1000s and UD 100s.	1.7+
otc	**Baridium** (Pfeiffer)		In 32s.	18
Rx	**Eridium** (Hauck)		Red. In 1000s.	1
Rx	**Geridium** (Goldline)		Burgundy. Sugar coated. In 100s and 1000s.	8.5
Rx	**Phenazodine** (Lannett)		Maroon. Sugar coated. In 100s and 1000s.	4
Rx	**Pyridiate** (Rugby)		In 100s.	4.3
Rx	**Pyridium** (Parke-Davis)		Sucrose, lactose. (P-D 180). Maroon. In 100s, 1000s and UD 100s.	43
Rx	**Urodine** (Various, eg, IDE, Schein)		In 100s and 1000s.	8.3+
Rx	**Urogesic** (Edwards)		In 100s.	25
Rx	**Phenazopyridine HCl** (Various, eg, Dixon-Shane, Geneva Marsam, Moore, Parmed, UDL, URL)	**Tablets:** 200 mg	In 100s, 1000s and UD 100s.	1.2+
Rx	**Geridium** (Goldline)		Burgundy. Sugar coated. In 100s.	5.4
Rx	**Phenazodine** (Lannett)		Sugar coated. In 1000s.	2.5
Rx	**Pyridium** (Parke-Davis)		Sucrose, lactose. (P-D 181). Maroon. In 100s, 1000s and UD 100s.	41
Rx	**Urodine** (Schein)		In 100s and 1000s.	5.4

Analgesic Combinations

These products combine phenazopyridine HCl with antispasmodics (belladonna alkaloids; see Anticholinergics/Antispasmodics in the Gastrointestinal chapter) and sedatives (butabarbital; see Sedatives and Hypnotics, Barbiturate monograph).

	Product	Content	Description	C.I.*
Rx	**Pyridium Plus** (Parke-Davis)	**Tablets:** 150 mg phenazopyridine HCl, 0.3 mg hyoscyamine HBr and 15 mg butabarbital *Dose: Adults* – 1 tablet 4 times daily after meals and at bedtime.	Lactose, sucrose. (P-D 182). Maroon. Square. In 100s.	36

Miscellaneous

Indications:

Applied topically following sexual contact; for prophylaxis of syphilis and gonorrhea. Not for application over large areas of the body. Use within 1 hour after exposure.

Warnings:

Discontinue use if rash or irritation develops. Consult physician if a sore appears.

	Product	Content	Description	C.I.*
otc	**Sanitube** (Sanitube Co.)	**Ointment:** 30% calomel, oxyquinoline benzoate and triethanolamine soap in a nonirritating base with lanolin and a phenol derivative	In 5 g.	NA

* Cost Index based on cost per daily adult dose.

DIMETHYL SULFOXIDE (DMSO)

Dimethyl sulfoxide (DMSO) is available in a variety of forms not intended for human use (ie, veterinary and industrial solvents). Discourage human use of such products because of their unknown purity. Because of its cutaneous transport characteristics, impurities and contaminants may be systemically absorbed from topical use.

Actions:

Pharmacology: DMSO is a clear, colorless liquid which is miscible with water and most organic solvents. Its broad range of pharmacological properties include: Anti-inflammatory action, nerve blockade, diuresis, cholinesterase inhibition, vasodilation and muscle relaxation.

Pharmacokinetics: Following topical application, DMSO is absorbed and widely distributed in tissue and body fluids. It is metabolized to dimethyl sulfone and dimethyl sulfide; DMSO and dimethyl sulfone are excreted in the urine and feces. DMSO is eliminated through the breath and skin and is responsible for the characteristic garlic odor. Unchanged DMSO has a half-life of 12 to 15 hours. Dimethyl sulfone can persist in serum $>$ 2 weeks after a single intravesical instillation. No residual accumulation of DMSO has occurred after treatment for protracted periods of time.

Indications:

Symptomatic relief of interstitial cystitis.

Unlabeled uses: DMSO has been used in the topical treatment of a wide variety of musculoskeletal disorders, related collagen diseases and to enhance the percutaneous absorption of other drugs.

Other topical systemic uses include: Scleroderma; arthritis; tendinitis; breast and prostate malignancies; retinitis pigmentosa; herpesvirus infections; head and spinal cord injury; stroke. Some reports claim limited extravasation injury and enhanced antineoplastic activity when DMSO is used with some chemotherapy agents. It has been used in renal amyloidosis.

Warnings:

Urinary tract infections, bacterial: There is no clinical evidence of effectiveness in the treatment of bacterial urinary tract infections.

Hypersensitivity reactions: DMSO can liberate histamine; hypersensitivity reactions may occur. If anaphylactoid symptoms develop, institute appropriate therapy. Refer to Management of Acute Hypersensitivity Reactions.

Pregnancy: Category C. Safety for use during pregnancy has not been established. Use only when clearly needed and when the potential benefits outweigh the potential hazards to the fetus.

High intraperitoneal doses of DMSO caused teratogenesis in small animals, but oral or topical doses did not. Two studies in rabbits using large topical doses produced conflicting reproductive results.

Lactation: It is not known whether this drug is excreted in breast milk. Exercise caution when administering to a nursing woman.

Children: Safety and efficacy for use in children have not been established.

(Continued on following page)

DIMETHYL SULFOXIDE (DMSO) (Cont.)

Precautions:

Ophthalmic effects: Lens opacities and changes in the refractive index have been seen in animals given chronic high doses of DMSO. Perform full eye evaluations, including slit-lamp examinations, prior to and periodically during treatment.

Monitoring: Perform liver and renal function tests and complete blood counts every 6 months.

Intravesical instillation may be harmful to patients with urinary tract malignancy because of DMSO-induced vasodilation.

Drug Interactions:

Sulindac's pharmacologic effects may be decreased by DMSO. DMSO impairs sulindac conversion to its sulfide metabolite by competitive inhibition of sulfide reductase.

Severe peripheral neuropathy characterized by increasing numbness and weakness of the extremities has been associate with concurrent use of sulindac and topical DMSO. These effects may last for several days after discontinuing DMSO.

Adverse Reactions:

Garlic-like taste within a few minutes after instillation. This taste may last several hours; odor on the breath and skin may remain for 72 hours.

Transient chemical cystitis has followed instillation of DMSO. Moderately severe discomfort on administration usually becomes less prominent with repeated use.

Topical administration (80% to 90% DMSO): Garlic-like breath, local dermatitis, sedation, nausea, vomiting, headache, burning or aching eyes.

Overdosage:

In case of accidental oral ingestion, induce emesis. Additional measures which may be considered are gastric lavage, activated charcoal and forced diuresis. Refer to General Management of Acute Overdosage on p. vi.

Patient Information:

A garlic-like taste may be noted within a few minutes of administration; odor on the breath and skin may be present and remain for up to 72 hours.

Administration and Dosage:

Not for IM or IV injection.

Instill 50 ml DMSO solution directly into the bladder by catheter or asepto syringe and allow to remain for 15 minutes. Apply an analgesic lubricant gel, such as lidocaine jelly, to the urethra prior to inserting the catheter to avoid spasm. The medication is expelled by spontaneous voiding. Repeat every 2 weeks until maximum symptomatic relief is obtained. Thereafter, increase time intervals between treatments.

To reduce bladder spasm, administer oral analgesics or suppositories containing belladonna and opium prior to instillation. In patients with severe interstitial cystitis and very sensitive bladders, perform the initial treatment, and possibly the second and third (depending on patient response), under anesthesia (saddle block has been suggested.)

Rx	**Rimso-50** (Research Industries[1])	**Solution:** 50% aqueous solution	In 50 ml.

[1]Research Industries Corp., 1847 West 2300 South, Salt Lake City, Utah 84119, 801/972-5500.

CELLULOSE SODIUM PHOSPHATE

Actions:

Cellulose Sodium Phosphate (CSP), a synthetic compound made by phosphorylation of cellulose, is insoluble in water and is nonabsorbable. CSP has excellent ion exchange properties, the sodium ion exchanging for calcium. When taken orally, CSP binds calcium; the complex of calcium and cellulose phosphate is then excreted in feces.

Pharmacology: CSP alters urinary composition of calcium, magnesium, phosphate and oxalate by affecting their absorption in the intestinal tract. When given orally with meals, CSP binds dietary and secreted calcium and reduces urinary calcium by approximately 50 mg/5 g of CSP. It also binds dietary magnesium and lowers urinary magnesium. Oral magnesium supplementation given separately from CSP partially overcomes this effect.

CSP administration increases urinary phosphorus and oxalate. The usual rise in urinary phosphorus of 150 to 250 mg/15 g CSP largely reflects the hydrolysis of 7% to 30% of CSP in the intestinal tract and absorption of released phosphorus. An increase in urinary oxalate occurs. Since CSP binds divalent cations, the cations are not available to complex oxalate and limit its absorption. The rise in urinary oxalate may be largely prevented by moderate dietary oxalate restriction and a modest dose of CSP (10 to 15 g/day).

The marked reduction in urinary calcium, with only slightly increased urinary phosphorus and oxalate, leads to a reduction in urinary saturation and propensity for spontaneous nucleation of calcium oxalate and calcium phosphate (brushite).

CSP apparently does not alter the serum concentration of copper, zinc or iron.

Indications:

Absorptive hypercalciuria Type I with recurrent calcium oxalate or calcium phosphate nephrolithiasis. Appropriate use of CSP substantially reduces the incidence of new stone formation. Do not expect causes of hypercalciuria other than hyperabsorption to respond to CSP.

Characteristics of absorptive hypercalciuria Type I - Recurrent passage or formation of calcium oxalate or calcium phosphate renal stones; no evidence of bone disease; normal serum calcium and phosphorus; increased intestinal calcium absorption; hypercalciuria; normal urinary calcium during fasting; normal parathyroid function; and lack of renal "leak" or excessive skeletal mobilization of calcium.

Absorptive hypercalciuria Type II is identical, except it can be eliminated by a low calcium diet.

Contraindications:

Primary or secondary hyperparathyroidism, including renal hypercalciuria (renal calcium leak); hypomagnesemic states (serum Mg < 1.5 mg/dl); osteoporosis, osteomalacia, osteitis; hypocalcemic states (eg, hypoparathyroidism, intestinal malabsorption); normal or low intestinal absorption and renal excretion of calcium; enteric hyperoxaluria.

Do not use in patients with high fasting urinary calcium or hypophosphatemia, unless a high skeletal mobilization of calcium can be excluded.

Warnings:

CHF or ascites: The sodium contained in CSP (35 to 48 mEq exchangeable sodium per 15 g CSP) may represent a hazard.

Usage in Pregnancy: Category C. Safety for use during pregnancy has not been established. Because of the increased dietary calcium requirement in pregnant women, use only when clearly needed and when the potential benefits outweigh potential hazards to the fetus.

Usage in Children: Because of the increased requirement for dietary calcium in growing children, the use of CSP in children less than 16 years of age is not recommended.

(Continued on following page)

CELLULOSE SODIUM PHOSPHATE (Cont.)

Precautions:

Parathyroid effects: By inhibiting intestinal calcium absorption, CSP may stimulate parathyroid function, leading to hyperparathyroid bone disease. Monitor parathyroid hormone levels. CSP treatment can maintain parathyroid function within normal limits if it is used only in absorptive hypercalciuria Type I at a dosage just sufficient to restore normal calcium absorption, but not sufficient to cause subnormal absorption.

Complications may potentially develop during long-term use: Hyperoxaluria and hypomagnesiuria, which would negate the beneficial effect of hypocalciuria on new stone formation; magnesium depletion; depletion of trace metals (Cu, Zn, Fe). Minimize effects by restricting the use of CSP to only absorptive hypercalciuria Type I by monitoring serum Ca, Mg, Cu, Zn, Fe, parathyroid hormone and by performing complete blood counts every 3 to 6 months.

Repeat borderline values for parathyroid hormone and calcium promptly. Obtain serum PTH at least once between the first 2 weeks to 3 months; adjust or stop treatment if serum PTH rises above normal. If there is an inadequate hypocalciuric response to CSP treatment (a reduction in urinary calcium of less than 30 mg/5 g of CSP), while patients are maintained on moderate calcium and sodium restriction, discontinue treatment. Consider the cessation of treatment if urinary oxalate exceeds 55 mg/day on moderate dietary oxalate restriction.

Dietary measures: Moderate calcium intake; avoid dairy products. Moderately restrict dietary oxalate by avoiding spinach (and similar dark greens), rhubarb, chocolate and brewed tea. Avoid vitamin C supplementation because of its potential metabolism to oxalate. Discourage a high sodium intake to achieve an intake of $<$ 150 mEq/day. Encourage fluid intake to achieve a minimum urine output of 2 L/day.

Adverse Reactions:

GI: Poor taste of the drug; loose bowel movements; diarrhea; dyspepsia.

Administration and Dosage:

Initial dose of CSP is 15 g/day (5 g with each meal) in patients with urinary calcium $>$ 300 mg/day (on moderate calcium restricted diet). When urinary calcium declines to $<$ 150 mg/day, reduce to 10 g/day (5 g with supper, 2.5 g each with remaining meal). Begin patients with controlled urinary calcium on moderate calcium restricted diet $<$ 300 mg/day (but $>$ 200 mg/day) on 10 g/day.

Suspend each dose of CSP (powder) in a glass of water, soft drink or fruit juice; ingest within 30 minutes of a meal. Do not take with magnesium gluconate. The amount of dietary calcium bound is considerably reduced when CSP is administered more than 1 hour after a meal. Base the initial and maintenance doses of CSP on measurements of 24 hour urinary calcium excretion.

Concomitant magnesium supplements: The dose of oral magnesium supplements, given as magnesium gluconate, depends upon the dose of CSP. Those receiving 15 g of CSP/day should take 1.5 g of magnesium gluconate before breakfast and again at bedtime (separately from CSP). Those taking 10 g of CSP/day should take 1 g of magnesium gluconate twice a day. To avoid binding of magnesium by CSP, give supplemental magnesium at least 1 hour before or after a dose of CSP.

Rx	**Calcibind** (Mission)	**Powder:** 2.5 g packets. Inorganic phosphate content ≈ 34% and sodium content ≈ 11%	In 90 single dose packets and 300 g bulk pak.

ACETOHYDROXAMIC ACID (AHA)

Actions:

Pharmacology: Acetohydroxamic acid (AHA) reversibly inhibits the bacterial enzyme urease, thereby inhibiting the hydrolysis of urea and production of ammonia in urine infected with urea-splitting organisms. The reduced ammonia levels and decreased pH enhance the effectiveness of antimicrobial agents and increase the cure rate of these infections. AHA does not acidify urine directly, nor does it have an antibacterial effect.

In patients with urea-splitting urinary infections (often accompanied by struvite stone disease) that are recalcitrant to other management, AHA reduces the pathologically elevated urinary ammonia and pH levels.

Pharmacokinetics: Absorption/Distribution – AHA is well absorbed from the GI tract after oral administration; peak blood levels occur in 0.25 to 1 hour after a given dose; it is distributed throughout body water. AHA chelates with dietary iron and may interfere with iron absorption. Treat concomitant hypochromic anemia with parenteral iron.

Excretion – From 36% to 65% of the drug is excreted unchanged in the urine and provides the therapeutic effect, but the concentration of AHA in urine that is necessary to inhibit urease is unknown. Concentrations as low as 8 mcg/ml may be beneficial; expect higher concentrations (ie, 30 mcg/ml) to provide more complete urease inhibition. Plasma half-life of AHA is approximately 5 to 10 hours with normal renal function and is prolonged in patients with reduced renal function.

Indications:

Adjunctive therapy in chronic urea-splitting urinary infection; do not use in lieu of curative surgical treatment (for patients with stones) or antimicrobial treatment. Long-term treatment may be warranted to maintain urease inhibition as long as urea-splitting infection is present.

Contraindications:

In patients whose physical state and disease are amenable to surgery or antimicrobial agents, whose urine is infected by nonurease-producing organisms, whose renal function is poor (ie, serum creatinine $>$ 2.5 mg/dl or Ccr $<$ 20 ml/min), in females without a satisfactory method of contraception.

Contraindicated in pregnancy: Category X. May cause fetal harm when administered to a pregnant woman. AHA was teratogenic (retarded or clubbed rear leg at 750 mg/kg and exencephaly and encephalocele at 1500 mg/kg) when given to rats. Do not use in women who are or who may become pregnant. If a patient becomes pregnant while taking this drug, inform her of the potential hazard to the fetus.

Warnings:

Coombs negative hemolytic anemia has occurred. GI upset characterized by nausea, vomiting, anorexia and generalized malaise have accompanied the most severe forms of hemolytic anemia. Approximately 3% of patients developed hemolytic anemia of sufficient magnitude to interrupt treatment. Approximately 15% of patients on AHA have had only laboratory findings of an anemia. However, most patients developed a mild reticulocytosis. The untoward reactions have reverted to normal following treatment cessation. A complete blood count, including reticulocytes, is recommended after 2 weeks of treatment. If reticulocyte count exceeds 6%, reduce dosage. Perform a CBC and reticulocyte count at 3 month intervals for the duration of treatment.

Hematologic effects: Bone marrow depression (leukopenia, anemia and thrombocytopenia) has occurred in animals receiving large doses of AHA, but has not been seen in man. Its bone marrow suppression is probably related to its ability to inhibit DNA synthesis, but anemia could also be related to depletion of iron stores. Hemolysis, with a decrease in the circulating RBCs, hemoglobin and HCT has been noted. Platelet or white blood cell abnormalities have not been noted, but clinical monitoring is recommended.

Usage in Pregnancy: Category X. See Contraindications

Usage in Lactation: It is not known if AHA is secreted in breast milk. Discontinue nursing or the drug, taking into account the importance of the drug to the mother.

Usage in Children: Children with chronic, recalcitrant, urea-splitting urinary infection may benefit from AHA. Dosage has not been established, although 10 mg/kg/day, taken in 2 or 3 divided doses for up to 1 year, have been tolerated. Monitor patients.

Precautions:

Liver function: Abnormalities have not been reported, but close monitoring is recommended because a derivative of AHA has caused significant liver dysfunction.

Renal impairment: Since AHA is eliminated primarily by the kidneys, closely monitor patients and reduce daily dose to avoid excessive drug accumulation.

Carcinogenesis, mutagenesis, impairment of fertility: Acetamide, a metabolite of AHA, caused hepatocellular carcinoma in rats at doses 1500 times the human dose. AHA is cytotoxic and was positive for mutagenicity in the Ames test.

(Continued on following page)

ACETOHYDROXAMIC ACID (AHA) (Cont.)

Drug Interactions:

Alcoholic beverages taken with AHA has resulted in a rash.

Heavy metals: AHA chelates heavy metals, notably iron. The absorption of iron and AHA from the intestinal lumen may be reduced when both drugs are taken concomitantly. When iron is indicated, administer parenterally.

Adverse Reactions:

Of 150 patients treated, most for more than a year, adverse reactions have occurred in up to 30%. Adverse reactions seem more prevalent in patients with preexisting thrombophlebitis, phlebothrombosis or advanced degrees of renal insufficiency. The risk of adverse reactions is highest during the first year of treatment. Chronic treatment does not seem to increase risk or severity of adverse reactions.

CNS: Mild headaches (30%) during the first 48 hours of treatment respond to oral salicylate analgesics and usually disappear spontaneously.

Depression, anxiety, nervousness, malaise and tremulousness (20%). In most patients, the symptoms were mild and transitory; however, in about 6%, symptoms warranted interruption or discontinuation of treatment.

GI: Nausea, vomiting, anorexia (20% to 25%). In most, symptoms were mild, transitory and did not interrupt treatment.

Hematologic: A mild reticulocytosis (5%) without anemia is even more prevalent than anemia. The laboratory findings are occasionally accompanied by malaise, lethargy, fatigue and GI symptoms which improve following cessation of treatment. Hematological abnormalities are more prevalent in patients with advanced renal failure (see Warnings).

Cardiovascular: Superficial phlebitis involving the lower extremities. One patient developed deep vein thrombosis of the lower extremities. All resolved following therapy.

Radiographic evidence of small pulmonary emboli was seen in three patients with phlebitis in their lower legs; this resolved following discontinuation of AHA and implementation of medical therapy. Several patients have resumed AHA treatment without ill effect. Palpitations have also been reported.

Dermatological: Nonpruritic, macular skin rash in the upper extremities and on the face, usually when AHA has been taken long-term and concomitantly with alcohol. The rash commonly appears 30 to 45 minutes after ingestion of alcohol, may be associated with a general sensation of warmth and disappears spontaneously in 30 to 60 minutes. In some patients, the rash may warrant drug discontinuation. Alopecia has been reported.

Overdosage:

Symptoms: Mild overdosages resulting in hemolysis have occurred in reduced renal function after several weeks or months of continuous treatment.

Acute deliberate overdosage has not occurred, but would be expected to induce the following: Anorexia, malaise, lethargy, diminished sense of well being, tremulousness, anxiety, nausea and vomiting. Laboratory findings are likely to include an elevated reticulocyte count and a severe hemolytic reaction requiring hospitalization, symptomatic treatment and possibly, blood transfusions. Anticipate concomitant reduction in platelets or white blood cells.

Treatment: Cessation of treatment, monitoring of hematologic status, symptomatic treatment and blood transfusions as required. The drug is probably dialyzable, but has not been clinically tested. Refer to General Management of Acute Overdosage on p. 2711

Administration and Dosage:

Adults: 250 mg, 3 to 4 times a day for a total dose of 10 to 15 mg/kg/day. The recommended starting dose is 12 mg/kg/day, administered at 6 to 8 hour intervals on an empty stomach. The maximum daily dose is no more than 1.5 g.

Children: Initial dose is 10 mg/kg/day. Monitor clinical condition and hematologic status; dosage titration may be required.

Renal dysfunction: Patients with serum creatinine of > 1.8 mg/dl should take no more than 1 g/day, dosed at 12 hour intervals. Further dosage reductions to prevent accumulation may be desirable. Do not treat patients with advanced (ie, serum creatinine > 2.5 mg/dl) renal insufficiency.

Rx	**Lithostat** (Mission)	**Tablets:** 250 mg	Scored. In unit-of-use 120s.

YOHIMBINE HCl

Yohimbine, an indolalkylamine alkaloid, has chemical similarity to reserpine. It is the principal alkaloid of the bark of the West African *Corynanthe yohimbe* tree and is also found in Rauwolfia Serpentina (L) Benth. It is believed to have properties similar to rauwolfia alkaloids.

Actions:

Yohimbine is primarily an α_2-adrenergic blocker. It blocks presynaptic α_2-adrenoreceptors causing release of norepinephrine.

Pharmacology: Its peripheral autonomic nervous system effect is to increase parasympathetic (cholinergic) and decrease sympathetic (adrenergic) activity. In male sexual performance, erection is linked to cholinergic activity which theoretically results in increased penile blood inflow, decreased penile blood outflow or both, causing erectile stimulation without increasing sexual desire.

Yohimbine exerts a stimulating action on mood and may increase anxiety. Such actions are not adequately studied, although they appear to require high doses. Yohimbine has a mild antidiuretic action, probably via stimulation of hypothalmic centers and release of posterior pituitary hormone. It may also have a local anesthetic effect.

Its action on peripheral blood vessels resembles that of reserpine, though it is weaker and of short duration. The drug reportedly exerts no significant influence on cardiac stimulation and other effects mediated by β-adrenergic receptors. Its effect on blood pressure, if any, would be to lower it; however, no adequate studies quantitate this effect and some reports indicate that it may increase blood pressure.

Indications:

Yohimbine has no FDA sanctioned indications.

Unlabeled Uses: Sympatholytic and mydriatic. It may have activity as an aphrodisiac.

Impotence has been successfully treated with yohimbine in patients with vascular or diabetic origins (18 mg/day), but data are sparse. Urologists have used yohimbine experimentally for the treatment and the diagnostic classification of certain types of male erectile impotence.

Orthostatic hypotension may be favorably affected by yohimbine 12.5 mg/day, but much more research is needed.

Contraindications:

In patients with renal disease; hypersensitivity to any component.

Warnings:

Not for use in geriatric patients, psychiatric patients or cardio-renal patients with a history of gastric or duodenal ulcer. Generally not for use in females.

Usage in Pregnancy: Do not use during pregnancy.

Usage in Children: Do not use in children.

Drug Interactions:

Antidepressants and other mood-modifying drugs: Do not use with yohimbine.

Adverse Reactions:

CNS: Yohimbine readily penetrates the CNS and produces a complex pattern of responses in lower doses than those required to produce peripheral α-adrenergic blockade. These include: Antidiuresis and central excitation including elevated blood pressure and heart rate, increased motor activity, nervousness, irritability and tremor. Dizziness, headache and skin flushing have been reported.

Sweating, nausea and vomiting are common after parenteral administration.

Overdosage:

Daily doses of 20 to 30 mg may produce increases in heart rate and blood pressure, piloerection and rhinorrhea. More severe symptoms may include paresthesias, incoordination, tremulousness and a dissociative state (resembling phencyclidine ingestion) with higher doses. Death occurs via respiratory paralysis.

For treatment, refer to the General Management of Acute Overdosage on p. vi.

Administration and Dosage:

Male erectile impotence: Experimental dosage has been 1 tablet 3 times/day. If side effects occur, reduce to ½ tablet 3 times/day, followed by gradual increases to 1 tablet 3 times a day. Results of therapy for > 10 weeks have not been reported.

	Product	Form	Package	C.I.*
Rx	**Aphrodyne** (Star)	**Tablets:** 5.4 mg	In 100s and 1000s.	24
Rx	**Dayto Himbin** (Dayton)		In 60s.	
Rx	**Yocon** (Palisades)		In 100s and 1000s.	31
Rx	**Yohimex** (Kramer)		Pink. In 100s.	30

* Cost Index based on cost per tablet.

Actions:

Clinical Pharmacology: Sodium benzoate and sodium phenylacetate are metabolically active compounds which decrease elevated blood ammonia concentrations in patients with inborn errors of ureagenesis. The mechanisms for this action are conjugation reactions involving acylation of amino acids which results in decreased ammonia formation. Benzoate and phenylacetate activate conjugation pathways which then substitute for or supplement the defective ureagenic pathway in patients with urea cycle enzymopathies (UCE), preventing the accumulation of ammonia.

The therapeutic regimens of sodium benzoate and sodium phenylacetate, which also included dietary manipulation and amino acid supplementation, were effective in long-term management of UCE patients. Survival rate in patients with complete enzyme deficiencies was ≈ 80% with this combined regimen in what was previously an almost universally fatal disease within the first year of life. The survival rate for each complete enzyme deficiency studied was: Carbamylphosphate synthetase, 75%; ornithine transcarbamylase (males), 59%; argininosuccinate synthetase, 96%. Survival in heterozygous females with partial ornithine transcarbamylase deficiency was 95%; for patients with other partial deficiencies, 86%. Early diagnosis and treatment are important in minimizing developmental disabilities. Reversal of preexisting neurologic impairment is not likely to occur with treatment, and neurologic deterioration may continue in some patients.

Pharmacokinetics: Studies have not been conducted in the primary patient population (neonates, infants and children). Preliminary pharmacokinetic data were obtained from only three normal adult subjects and the overall disposition of sodium benzoate, sodium phenylacetate and their metabolites has not been fully characterized. Peak blood levels of benzoate or phenylacetate occur within 1 hour after a single oral dose of sodium benzoate or sodium phenylacetate, respectively. A majority of the administered compound (approximately 80% to 100%) was excreted by the kidneys within 24 hours as the respective conjugation product, hippurate or phenylacetylglutamine. The major sites for metabolism of benzoate and phenylacetate are the liver and kidneys.

Indications:

Adjunctive therapy for the prevention and treatment of hyperammonemia in the chronic management of patients with UCE involving partial or complete deficiencies of carbamylphosphate synthetase, ornithine transcarbamylase or argininosuccinate synthetase.

Warnings:

Solutions containing sodium ions should be used with great care, if at all, in patients with congestive heart failure, severe renal insufficiency, and in clinical states in which there is sodium retention with edema. In patients with diminished renal function, administration of solutions containing sodium ions may result in sodium retention.

Usage in Pregnancy: Category C. Safety for use during pregnancy has not been established. Use only when clearly needed and when the potential benefits outweigh the potential hazards to the fetus.

Usage in Lactation: It is not known whether this drug is excreted in breast milk. Use caution when administering to a nursing woman.

Precautions:

Not intended as sole therapy for UCE patients. Combine as adjunctive therapy with dietary management (low protein diet) and amino acid supplementation for optimal results.

Use with caution in neonates with hyperbilirubinemia, since in vitro experiments suggest that benzoate competes for bilirubin binding sites on albumin.

The benefits of treating neonatal hyperammonemic coma with this drug have not been established. The treatment of choice in neonatal hyperammonemic coma is hemodialysis. Peritoneal dialysis may be helpful if hemodialysis is not available.

Do not administer to patients with known hypersensitivities to sodium benzoate or sodium phenylacetate. No such cases of hypersensitivities have been reported.

Drug Interactions:

Penicillin may compete with conjugated products of sodium benzoate and sodium phenylacetate for active secretion by renal tubules.

Probenecid inhibits the renal transport of many organic compounds, including amino hippuric acid and may affect renal excretion of the conjugation products of sodium benzoate and sodium phenylacetate.

(Continued on following page)

Adverse Reactions:

Nausea and vomiting.

Side effects associated with salicylates such as exacerbation of peptic ulcers, mild hyperventilation and mild respiratory alkalosis may occur due to structural similarities between benzoate and salicylates.

If an adverse reaction does occur, discontinue administration, evaluate the patient and institute appropriate therapeutic countermeasures.

Overdosage:

Four overdoses of sodium phenylacetate or sodium benzoate in UCE patients have been reported, two cases following the use of an IV infusion. Two patients became irritable and vomited after receiving three-fold overdoses of oral sodium benzoate. Both patients recovered without treatment within 24 hours after the drug was discontinued.

Treatment: Discontinue the drug and institute supportive measures for metabolic acidosis and circulatory collapse. Hemodialysis or peritoneal dialysis may be beneficial.

Administration and Dosage:

For oral use only. Must be diluted before use.

The usual total daily dose for adjunctive therapy of UCE patients is 2.5 ml/kg/day (250 mg sodium benzoate and 250 mg sodium phenylacetate) in 3 to 6 equally divided doses. Total daily dose should not exceed 100 ml (10 g each of sodium benzoate and sodium phenylacetate).

Dilute each dose in 4 to 8 ounces of infant formula or milk and administer with meals. If other beverages are used, particularly acidic beverages, precipitation of the drug may occur depending on pH and the final concentration. Inspect the mixture for compatibility before administration.

Because this is a concentrated solution, exercise care in calculating the dose to avoid the possibility of overdosage.

Not intended as sole therapy for UCE patients. Combine as adjunctive therapy with dietary management (low protein diet) and amino acid supplementation for optimal results.

Because sodium phenylacetate has a lingering odor, exercise care in mixing and administering the drug to minimize contact with skin and clothing.

Storage: Store at room temperature. Avoid excessive heat.

Rx	**Ucephan** (Kendall McGaw)	**Solution:** 10 g sodium benzoate & 10 g sodium phenylacetate per 100 ml	In 100 ml multiple unit bottles.

ALPROSTADIL (Prostaglandin E_1; PGE_1)

Warning:
Apnea occurs in about 10% to 12% of neonates with congenital heart defects treated with alprostadil. Apnea is most often seen in neonates weighing less than 2 kg at birth and usually appears during the first hour of drug infusion. Monitor respiratory status throughout treatment; have ventilatory assistance immediately available.

Actions:

Pharmacology: Alprostadil (prostaglandin E_1) produces vasodilation, inhibits platelet aggregation and stimulates intestinal and uterine smooth muscle; IV doses of 1 to 10 mcg/kg lower the blood pressure in mammals by decreasing peripheral resistance. Reflex increases in cardiac output and rate accompany the reduction in blood pressure.

Smooth muscle of the ductus arteriosus, especially sensitive to alprostadil, relaxes in the presence of the drug. These effects are beneficial in infants who have congenital defects which restrict the pulmonary or systemic blood flow and who depend on a patent ductus arteriosus for adequate blood oxygenation and lower body perfusion.

In infants with restricted pulmonary blood flow, about 50% responded to alprostadil infusion with at least 10 mm Hg increase in blood pO_2 (mean increase about 14 mm Hg and mean increase in oxygen saturation about 23%). In general, patients who responded best had low pretreatment blood pO_2 and were 4 days old or less.

The increase in blood oxygenation is inversely proportional to pretreatment pO_2 values; patients with a low pO_2 respond best, and patients with a $pO_2 \geq 40$ mm Hg usually have little response.

In infants with restricted systemic blood flow, alprostadil often increased pH in those with acidosis. It also increased systemic blood pressure and decreased the ratio of pulmonary artery pressure to aortic pressure.

Pharmacokinetics: Alprostadil is rapidly metabolized. As much as 80% may be metabolized in one pass through the lungs, primarily by oxidation. Metabolites are excreted primarily by the kidneys, and excretion is essentially complete within 24 hours. No unchanged alprostadil has been found in the urine, and there is no evidence of tissue retention.

Indications:

For palliative, not definitive, therapy to temporarily maintain the patency of the ductus arteriosus until corrective or palliative surgery can be performed in neonates who have congenital heart defects and who depend upon the patent ductus for survival. Such defects include pulmonary atresia or stenosis, tricuspid atresia, tetralogy of Fallot, interruption of the aortic arch, coarctation of the aorta or transposition of the great vessels with or without other defects.

Contraindications:

None known.

Warnings:

Administer only by trained personnel in facilities that provide pediatric intensive care.

Precautions:

Skeletal effects: Cortical proliferation of the long bones has been observed in infants during long-term infusions of alprostadil. This regressed after drug withdrawal.

Duration of infusion: Infuse for the shortest time and at the lowest dose that will produce the desired effects. Weigh the risks of long-term infusion against the possible benefits that critically ill infants may derive from its administration.

Hemostatic effects: Because alprostadil inhibits platelet aggregation, use cautiously in neonates with bleeding tendencies.

Respiratory distress syndrome: Do not use alprostadil in respiratory distress syndrome. Make a differential diagnosis between respiratory distress syndrome (hyaline membrane disease) and cyanotic heart disease (restricted pulmonary blood flow). If full diagnostic facilities are not immediately available, cyanosis (pO_2 less than 40 mm Hg) and restricted pulmonary blood flow apparent on an X-ray are appropriate indicators of congenital heart defects.

Monitor arterial pressure intermittently by umbilical artery catheter, auscultation or with a Doppler transducer. If arterial pressure falls significantly, decrease the infusion rate immediately.

In infants with restricted pulmonary blood flow, measure efficacy of alprostadil by monitoring blood oxygenation. To measure efficacy in infants with restricted systemic blood flow, monitor systemic blood pressure and blood pH.

(Continued on following page)

ALPROSTADIL (Prostaglandin E_1; PGE_1) (Cont.)

Adverse Reactions:

CNS: Fever (14%); seizures (4%); cerebral bleeding, hyperextension of the neck, hyperirritability, hypothermia, jitteriness, lethargy and stiffness (< 1%).

Cardiovascular: Flushing (10%, more common after intra-arterial dosing); bradycardia (7%); hypotension (4%); tachycardia (3%); cardiac arrest, edema (1%); congestive heart failure, hyperemia, second degree heart block, shock, spasm of the right ventricle infundibulum, supraventricular tachycardia and ventricular fibrillation (< 1%).

Respiratory: Apnea (12%); bradypnea, bronchial wheezing, hypercapnia, respiratory depression, respiratory distress and tachypnea (< 1%).

GI: Diarrhea (2%); gastric regurgitation and hyperbilirubinemia (< 1%).

Hematologic: Disseminated intravascular coagulation (1%); anemia, bleeding and thrombocytopenia (< 1%).

Renal: Anuria and hematuria (< 1%).

Skeletal: Cortical proliferation of the long bones.

Miscellaneous: Sepsis (2%); hypokalemia (1%); peritonitis, hypoglycemia and hyperkalemia (< 1%).

Overdosage:

Symptoms: Apnea, bradycardia, pyrexia, hypotension and flushing.

Treatment: If apnea or bradycardia occurs, discontinue infusion and provide appropriate medical treatment. Use caution in restarting the infusion. If pyrexia or hypotension occurs, reduce the infusion rate until symptoms subside. Flushing is usually a result of incorrect intra-arterial catheter placement; reposition catheter.

Administration and Dosage:

The preferred administration route is continuous IV infusion into a large vein. Alternatively, the drug may be administered through an umbilical artery catheter placed at the ductal opening. Increases in blood pO_2 have been the same by either route.

Begin infusion with 0.05 to 0.1 mcg/kg/minute. A starting dose of 0.1 mcg/kg/min is recommended; however, adequate clinical response has been reported using a starting dose of 0.05 mcg/kg/min. After a therapeutic response is achieved (increased pO_2 in infants with restricted pulmonary blood flow or increased systemic blood pressure and blood pH in infants with restricted systemic blood flow), reduce the infusion rate to the lowest dosage that maintains the response. This may be accomplished by reducing the dosage from 0.1 to 0.05 to 0.025 to 0.01 mcg/kg/minute. If response to 0.05 mcg/kg/minute is inadequate, dosage can be increased up to 0.4 mcg/kg/minute, although in general, higher infusion rates do not produce greater effects.

Preparation of solution: Dilute 500 mcg alprostadil with Sodium Chloride Injection or Dextrose Injection. Dilute to volumes appropriate for the pump delivery system available. Discard and prepare fresh infusion solutions every 24 hours.

Sample Dilutions and Infusion Rates to Provide a Dosage of 0.1 mcg/kg/min

Add 500 mcg alprostadil to:	Approximate concentration of resulting solution (mcg/ml)	Infusion rate (ml/min/kg)
250 ml	2	0.05
100 ml	5	0.02
50 ml	10	0.01
25 ml	20	0.005

Storage: Refrigerate at 2° to 8°C (35° to 46°F).

Rx	**Prostin VR Pediatric** (Upjohn)	**Injection:** 500 mcg per ml[1]	In 1 ml amps.

[1] In 1 ml dehydrated alcohol.

INDOMETHACIN SODIUM TRIHYDRATE

Actions:

Pharmacology: Indomethacin sodium trihydrate is an injectable formulation of indomethacin used for closure of a patent ductus arteriosus in premature infants. Indomethacin is a potent inhibitor of prostaglandin synthesis, both in vitro and in vivo. The exact mechanism of action through which indomethacin causes closure of a patent ductus arteriosus is unknown, but it is believed to be through inhibition of prostaglandin synthesis.

In double-blind, placebo controlled studies of 460 preterm infants who weighed < 1750 g, those treated with IV indomethacin had a 75% to 80% closure rate, thus avoiding surgery.

Pharmacokinetics: Plasma half-life is variable among premature infants and varies inversely with postnatal age and weight. In a study of 28 infants, the plasma half-life of those less than 7 days old averaged 20 hours; in infants older than 7 days, the mean plasma half-life was 12 hours. The mean plasma half-life was 21 hours in infants weighing < 1000 g and 15 hours in those weighing > 1000 g.

Following IV administration in adults, indomethacin is eliminated via renal excretion, metabolism and biliary excretion, and it undergoes appreciable enterohepatic circulation. The mean plasma half-life of indomethacin is 4.5 hours; in the absence of enterohepatic circulation, it is 90 minutes.

Indications:

For closure of a hemodynamically significant patent ductus arteriosus in premature infants weighing between 500 and 1750 g if, after 48 hours, usual medical management is ineffective. Clinical evidence of a hemodynamically significant patent ductus arteriosus should be present (ie, respiratory distress, a continuous murmur, a hyperactive precordium, cardiomegaly and pulmonary plethora on chest x-ray).

Unlabeled Use: Indomethacin IV has been used prophylactically to reduce the incidence of symptomatic patent ductus arteriosus in premature infants with a high probability of developing this condition; a single dose of 0.2 mg/kg 24 hours after birth has been used. However, no study has shown a significant decrease in neonatal morbidity.

Contraindications:

Proven or suspected untreated infection; bleeding, especially active intracranial hemorrhage or GI bleeding; thrombocytopenia; coagulation defects; necrotizing enterocolitis; significant renal impairment; congenital heart disease patients in whom patency of the ductus arteriosus is necessary for satisfactory pulmonary or systemic blood flow (eg, pulmonary atresia, severe tetralogy of Fallot, severe coarctation of the aorta).

Warnings:

GI effects: Minor GI bleeding (ie, chemical detection of blood in the stool) has been reported.

Hemorrhage: Prematurity per se is associated with an increased incidence of spontaneous intraventricular hemorrhage. Indomethacin may inhibit platelet aggregation and increase the potential for intraventricular bleeding.

Renal effects: Indomethacin may cause significant reduction in urine output (50% or more) with concomitant elevations of BUN and creatinine and reductions in glomerular filtration rate and creatinine clearance. In most infants, these effects are transient and disappear with cessation of therapy. Indomethacin may precipitate renal insufficiency, including acute renal failure, especially in infants with other conditions that may adversely affect renal function during therapy.

When significant suppression of urine volume occurs after a dose, do not give additional doses until the urine output returns to normal levels.

Electrolyte balance: Indomethacin may suppress water excretion to a greater extent than sodium excretion. Perform serum electrolyte determinations and monitor renal function during therapy.

Precautions:

Infection: Indomethacin may mask the usual signs and symptoms of infection. Use with extra care in the presence of existing controlled infection.

Hepatic effects: Severe hepatic reactions have been reported in adults treated chronically with oral indomethacin. If clinical signs and symptoms consistent with liver disease develop in the neonate, or if systemic manifestations occur, discontinue the drug.

Avoid extravascular injection or leakage; the solution may irritate tissue.

(Continued on following page)

INDOMETHACIN SODIUM TRIHYDRATE (Cont.)

Drug Interactions:

Aminoglycosides: In one study of premature infants treated with indomethacin IV and also receiving either gentamicin or amikacin, both peak and trough levels of these aminoglycosides were significantly elevated.

Digitalis: In premature infants, the half-life of digitalis may be further prolonged, due to reduced renal function during therapy with indomethacin.

Frequent ECGs and serum digitalis levels may be required to prevent or detect digitalis toxicity early.

Furosemide: Indomethacin may blunt furosemide's natriuretic effect; this is attributed to inhibition of prostaglandin synthesis. In 19 premature infants with patent ductus arteriosus, infants receiving both agents had significantly higher urinary output, higher levels of sodium and chloride excretion and higher glomerular filtration rates than did those infants receiving indomethacin alone. Data suggest that furosemide helped to maintain renal function in the premature infant when indomethacin was added.

Adverse Reactions:

Coagulation: Decreased platelet aggregation. There was greater incidence of bleeding problems, ie, gross or microscopic bleeding into the GI tract, oozing from skin after needle stick, pulmonary hemorrhage and disseminated intravascular coagulopathy.

Renal: Renal dysfunction in 41% of infants, including one or more of the following: Oliguria; reduced urine sodium, chloride or potassium, urine osmolality, free water clearance or glomerular filtration rate; elevated serum creatinine or BUN; uremia.

Cardiovascular: Pulmonary hypertension.

GI: GI bleeding (3% to 9%); vomiting, abdominal distention, transient ileus, localized perforation of small or large intestines (1% to 3%).

Metabolic: Hyponatremia; elevated serum potassium (3% to 9%); hypoglycemia, fluid retention (1% to 3%).

The following adverse reactions have also been reported in infants treated with indomethacin; however, a causal relationship has not been established:

Cardiovascular - Intracranial bleeding (3% to 9%); bradycardia (< 3%).
Respiratory - Apnea; exacerbation of preexisting pulmonary infection.
Metabolic - Acidosis/alkalosis.
GI - Necrotizing enterocolitis.
Ophthalmic - Retrolental fibroplasia (3% to 9%).

Additional adverse reactions have been reported with oral indomethacin. Relevance to the preterm neonate receiving indomethacin IV is unknown.

Administration and Dosage:

For IV use only.

A course of therapy is defined as 3 IV doses given at 12 to 24 hour intervals.

Renal impairment: If anuria or marked oliguria (urinary output < 0.6 ml/kg/hr) is evident at the scheduled time of the second or third dose, do not give additional doses until laboratory studies indicate that renal function has returned to normal.

Dosage According to Age			
Age at 1st dose	Dose (mg/kg)		
	1st	2nd	3rd
< 48 hours	0.2	0.1	0.1
2-7 days	0.2	0.2	0.2
> 7 days	0.2	0.25	0.25

If the ductus arteriosus closes or is significantly reduced in size after 48 hours or more from completion of the first course, no further doses are necessary. If the ductus arteriosus reopens, a second course of 1 to 3 doses may be given, each dose separated by a 12 to 24 hour interval as described above.

If the infant remains unresponsive to therapy after 2 courses, surgery may be necessary. If severe adverse reactions occur, stop the drug.

Preparation of solution: Prepare with 1 to 2 ml of Sodium Chloride Injection 0.9% or Water for Injection. All diluents should be preservative free (ie, without benzyl alcohol). If 1 ml of diluent is used, the concentration of indomethacin ≈ 0.1 mg/0.1 ml; if 2 ml of diluent are used, the concentration of the solution ≈ 0.05 mg/0.1 ml. Discard any unused portion of the solution. Prepare a fresh solution just prior to each administration. Once reconstituted, inject IV over 5 to 10 seconds.

Further dilution with IV infusion solutions is not recommended.

Rx	**Indocin I.V.** (MSD)	**Powder for injection:** 1 mg (as sodium trihydrate)	In single dose vials.

ETHANOLAMINE OLEATE

Actions:

Pharmacology: Ethanolamine oleate is a mild sclerosing agent. When injected IV, it acts primarily by irritation of the intimal endothelium of the vein and produces a sterile dose-related inflammatory response. This results in fibrosis and occlusion of the vein. Ethanolamine oleate also rapidly diffuses through the venous wall and produces a dose-related extravascular inflammatory reaction.

The oleic acid component of ethanolamine oleate is responsible for the inflammatory response, and may also activate coagulation in vivo by release of tissue factor and activation of Hageman factor. The ethanolamine component, however, may inhibit fibrin clot formation by chelating calcium, so that a procoagulant action of ethanolamine oleate has not been demonstrated.

Pharmacokinetics: Ethanolamine oleate disappears from the injection site within 5 minutes via the portal vein. When volumes larger than 20 ml are injected, some ethanolamine oleate also flows into the azygos vein through the periesophageal vein. Within 4 days after injection, there is neutrophil infiltration of the esophageal wall and hemorrhage within 6 days. Granulation tissue is first seen at 10 days, red thrombi obliterating the varices by 20 days, and sclerosis of the varices by 2½ months. Sclerosis of esophageal varices will be a delayed rather than an immediate effect of the drug.

In dogs, ethanolamine oleate 1 ml/kg injected into the right atrium over 1 minute increases extravascular lung water. The concentration of ethanolamine oleate reaching the lung in human treatment will be less than in the dog studies, but pleural effusions, pulmonary edema, pulmonary infiltration and pneumonitis have occurred. Minimize the total per session dose, especially in those with concomitant cardiopulmonary disease.

Indications:

Treatment of patients with esophageal varices that have recently bled, to prevent rebleeding.

Not indicated for the treatment of patients with esophageal varices that have not bled.

Contraindications:

Hypersensitivity to ethanolamine, oleic acid or ethanolamine oleate.

Warnings:

Sclerotherapy with ethanolamine oleate has no beneficial effect upon portal hypertension, the cause of esophageal varices, so that recanalization and collateralization may occur, necessitating reinjection.

Varicosities of the leg: Use of ethanolamine oleate injection is not supported by adequately controlled clinical trials and is not recommended.

Hypersensitivity: Fatal anaphylactic shock was reported following injection of a larger than normal volume of ethanolamine oleate injection into a male who had a known allergic disposition. There are only three reports of anaphylaxis. Be prepared to treat anaphylaxis appropriately. In emergencies, administer 0.25 ml of a 1:1000 IV solution of epinephrine (0.25 mg); control allergic reactions with antihistamines. Have epinephrine 1:1000 immediately available. Refer to Management of Acute Hypersensitivity Reactions on p. viii.

Usage in Pregnancy: Category C. It is not known whether ethanolamine oleate injection can cause fetal harm when administered to a pregnant woman or can affect reproduction capacity. Give to pregnant women only if clearly needed.

Usage in Lactation: It is not known whether this drug is excreted in breast milk. Exercise caution when ethanolamine oleate is administered to a nursing woman.

Usage in Children: Safety and efficacy in children have not been established. In one study, 21 children with esophageal varices were treated with ethanolamine oleate via an endotracheal tube using 2 to 5 ml injection per varix to a maximum of 20 ml. Variceal obliteration occurred in 18 of the children.

(Continued on following page)

ETHANOLAMINE OLEATE (Cont.):

Precautions:

Acute renal failure with spontaneous recovery followed injections of 15 to 20 ml in two women.

Severe injection necrosis may result from direct injection of sclerosing agents, especially if excessive volumes are used. At least one fatal case of extensive esophageal necrosis and death has occurred. The drug should be administered by physicians who are familiar with an acceptable injection technique.

Child Class C patients are more likely to develop esophageal ulceration than those in Classes A and B. Complications of ulceration, necrosis and delayed esophageal perforation appear to occur more frequently when ethanolamine oleate is injected submucosally. This route is not recommended.

Concomitant cardiorespiratory disease: Careful monitoring and minimization of the total dose per session is recommended.

Fatal aspiration pneumonia has occurred in elderly patients undergoing esophageal variceal sclerotherapy with ethanolamine oleate. It appears to be procedure-related rather than drug-related, but as aspiration of blood or stomach contents is not uncommon in patients with bleeding esophageal varices, take special precautions to prevent its occurrence, especially in the elderly and critically ill subjects.

Adverse Reactions:

The frequency of complications/adverse events per injection session was 13%.

Most common: Pleural effusion/infiltration (2.1%); esophageal ulcer (2.1%); pyrexia (1.8%); retrosternal pain (1.6%); esophageal stricture (1.3%); pneumonia (1.2%).

Local esophageal reactions: Pleural effusion/infiltration (2.1%); esophageal ulcer (2.1%); esophageal stricture (1.3%); esophagitis, tearing of the esophagus, sloughing of the mucosa overlying the injected varix, necrosis, periesophageal abscess and perforation (0.1% to 0.4%) (see Precautions). These complications appear to be dependent upon the dose and the patient's clinical state.

Other: Pyrexia (1.8%); retrosternal pain (1.6%); fatal aspiration pneumonia (see Precautions); pneumonia (1.2%); bacteremia; anaphylactic shock (see Warnings); acute renal failure with spontaneous recovery (see Precautions). Spinal cord paralysis due to occlusion of the anterior spinal artery has been reported in one child 8 hours after ethanolamine oleate sclerotherapy.

Overdosage:

Overdosage of ethanolamine oleate injection can result in severe intramural necrosis of the esophagus; complications have resulted in death. The minimum lethal dose of ethanolamine oleate injection administered IV to rabbits is 130 mg/kg.

Administration and Dosage:

Local ethanolamine oleate injection sclerotherapy of esophageal varices should be performed by physicians who are familiar with an acceptable technique.

Usual IV dose is 1.5 to 5 ml per varix.

Maximum total dose per treatment session should not exceed 20 ml or 0.4 ml/kg for a 50 kg patient. Patients with significant liver dysfunction (Child Class C) or concomitant cardiopulmonary disease should usually receive less than the recommended maximum dose.

Submucosal injections are not recommended as they are reportedly more likely to result in ulceration at the site of injection.

To obliterate the varix, injections may be made at the time of the acute bleeding espisode and then after 1 week, 6 weeks, 3 months and 6 months as indicated.

Storage: Store at controlled room temperature 15°C to 30°C (59°F to 86°F). Protect from light.

Rx	**Ethamolin** (Reed & Carnrick)	**Injection:** 5%	In 2 ml amps.[1]

[1] With 2% benzyl alcohol.

Actions:

These agents are mild sclerosing drugs used in the treatment of varicose veins. They produce their effect by irritation and inflammation of the venous intimal endothelium and formation of a thrombus. This blood clot occludes the injected vein and fibrous tissue develops, resulting in the obliteration of the vein.

Sodium tetradecyl is an anionic surface active agent. Morrhuate sodium is a mixture of the sodium salts of the saturated and unsaturated fatty acids of cod liver oil.

Indications:

Treatment of small, uncomplicated varicose veins of the lower extremities.

Sclerosing agents may be useful as a supplement to venous ligation to obliterate residual varicosed veins or in patients who have conditions which increase the risk of surgery. Ineffective sclerotherapy may decrease the potential success of later surgery.

Morrhuate sodium has been used for the treatment of internal hemorrhoids; there is no substantial evidence for this indication.

Unlabeled uses: Sclerosing agents have been used to treat esophageal varices, introduced via a flexible fiberoptic esophagoscope.

Contraindications:

Hypersensitivity to any component of these drugs; acute superficial thrombophlebitis; underlying arterial disease; varicosities caused by abdominal and pelvic tumors; uncontrolled diabetes mellitus; sepsis; blood dyscrasia; thyrotoxicosis; tuberculosis; neoplasms; asthma; acute respiratory or skin diseases; any condition which causes the patient to be bedridden; extensive injection treatment in patients who are severely debilitated or senile; an unusual local reaction at the injection site or any systemic reaction; persistent occlusion of deep veins.

Delay treatment if there is any acute local or systemic infection, including infected ulcers.

Do not use if there is significant valvular or deep venous incompetence.

Warnings:

Anaphylactoid and allergic reactions have occurred. Anaphylactoid reactions may occur within a few minutes after the injection and are most likely to occur when therapy is reinstituted after several weeks. Refer to Management of Acute Hypersensitivity Reactions on p. viii.

Usage in Pregnancy: (Category C – sodium tetradecyl sulfate). Safety for use during pregnancy has not been established. Use only when clearly needed and when the potential benefits outweigh the potential hazards to the fetus.

Precautions:

Do not undertake sclerotherapy for the treatment of varicosities unless valvular competency and deep vein patency and competency are determined. Perform the Trendelenburg test, Perthes' test and angiography. Because of the danger of extension of thrombosis into the deep veins, perform a thorough preinjection evaluation for valvular competence and slowly inject a small amount (not more than 2 ml) of the preparation into the varicosity. Necrosis may result from direct injection of sclerosing agents.

Initially treat most patients with symptomatic primary varicosed veins with compression stockings. If this treatment is inadequate, surgery may be required.

For IV use only. Inadvertent intra-arterial injection may result in severe ischemic damage.

Adverse Reactions:

Local: Burning; cramping sensations; urticaria; tissue sloughing and necrosis may occur with extravasation (morrhuate).

A permanent discoloration, usually small and barely noticeable, can occur at the injection site with sodium tetradecyl sulfate and may be cosmetically objectionable.

Hypersensitivity (rare): Dizziness; weakness; vascular collapse; asthma; respiratory depression; GI disturbances (ie, nausea and vomiting); urticaria (see Warnings).

Postoperative sloughing can occur.

Pulmonary embolism has occurred. Drowsiness and headache may occur rarely with morrhuate.

(Products listed on following page)

SODIUM TETRADECYL SULFATE

Administration and Dosage:

For IV use only. Do not use if precipitated. The strength of solution required depends on the size and degree of varicosity. In general, the 3% solution will be most useful, with the 1% solution preferred for small varicosities. The dosage should be small, using 0.5 to 2 ml for each injection; do not exceed 10 ml of a 3% solution.

As a precaution against anaphylactic shock, give 0.5 ml; observe patient for several hours before administering a larger injection.

Rx	**Sotradecol** (Elkins-Sinn)	**Injection:** 1%	In 2 ml Dosette amps.[1]
Rx	**Sotradecol** (Elkins-Sinn)	**Injection:** 3%	In 2 ml Dosette amps.[1]

MORRHUATE SODIUM

Administration and Dosage:

For IV use only. Avoid extravasation. Dosage depends on the size and degree of varicosity.

To determine possible sensitivity: 0.25 to 1 ml of 5% injection into a varicosity 24 hours before administration of a large dose.

Usual adult dose for obliteration of small or medium veins: 50 to 100 mg (1 to 2 ml). *For large veins:* 150 to 250 mg (3 to 5 ml). The drug may be given as multiple injections at one time or in single doses. Therapy may be repeated at 5 to 7 day intervals, according to the patient's response.

Following injection, the vein promptly becomes hard and swollen for 2 to 4 inches, depending on the size and response of the vein. After 24 hours, the vein is hard and slightly tender to the touch (with little or no periphlebitis). The skin around the injection becomes light-bronze; this color usually disappears quickly. An aching sensation and feeling of stiffness usually occurs and lasts approximately 48 hours.

When small veins are injected, or the injection solution is cold, or when solid matter has separated in the solution, warm the ampul or vial by immersing in hot water. The solution should become clear on warming; use only a clear solution that contains no solid matter. Because the solution froths easily, use a large bore needle to fill the syringe; however, use a small bore needle for the injection.

Storage: Store below 40°C (104°F); refrigerate preferably between 15°C and 30°C (59° and 86°F).

Rx	**Morrhuate Sodium** (Pasadena Research Labs)	**Injection:** 50 mg/ml	In 30 ml multiple use vials.
Rx	**Scleromate** (Palisades Pharm.)		In 5 ml amps, 10 ml vials and 10 ml fill in 20 ml vials.

[1] With 0.02 ml benzyl alcohol per ml.

CHYMOPAPAIN

Warning:

Use chymopapain only in a hospital setting by physicians experienced and trained in the diagnosis of lumbar disc disease and all acceptable treatment modalities, including surgery and in the management of all potential complications from chymopapain. Anaphylaxis has occurred in about 0.5% of patients (0.4% under local anesthesia versus 0.5% under general anesthesia); it can be fatal.

Paraplegia or paraparesis, central nervous system hemorrhage and other serious neurologic adverse events have been observed within hours or days after chymopapain injection at a rate of about 1 in 2,000. Acute transverse myelitis/acute transverse myelopathy has been observed 2 to 3 weeks following chymopapain injection at a rate of about 1 in 18,000. A cause and effect relationship between these neurologic events and chymopapain when properly injected has not been established.

Chymopapain is extremely toxic when injected intrathecally, as are some radiopaque contrast media used for discography. Therefore, take great care to assure that the dura is not penetrated and that chymopapain, or contrast medium if used, does not enter the subarachnoid space. If there is any question regarding needle tip location within the nucleus of the disc or if contrast medium is used and it extravasates into the subarachnoid space, abandon the procedure and do not inject chymopapain.

Discography at the time of chemonucleolysis is not recommended unless it is determined that the benefits outweigh the risks. Limit chemonucleolysis to the disc producing the patient's signs and symptoms and use supplemented local anesthesia whenever possible.

Actions:

Pharmacology: Chymopapain is a nonpyrogenic proteolytic enzyme derived from the crude latex of *Carica papaya.* Sodium L-cysteinate hydrochloride is added as a reducing agent for this sulphur-containing enzyme to maintain the sulphur in the sulphydryl form. The pH of the reconstituted drug is 5.5 to 6.5.

When injected into the nucleus pulposus of the lumbar intervertebral disc, chymopapain rapidly hydrolyzes the noncollagenous polypeptides or proteins that maintain the tertiary structure of the chondromucoprotein. This degradation lessens the intradiscal osmotic activity, thereby decreasing fluid absorption, reducing intradiscal pressure and relieving compressive symptoms.

Pharmacokinetics: Although the mechanism of action has not been directly established, operative findings in patients undergoing surgery following injection usually revealed the nucleus pulposus to be absent from its former site. A temporary increase in urinary mucopolysaccharide occurs following intradiscal injection of chymopapain, and it appears the inhibitory activity of the alpha$_2$-macroglobulin prevents expression of any significant proteolytic activity outside the disc. Also, due to the inhibitory activity of the plasma alpha$_2$-macroglobulin and the low concentration of chymopapain's reactive fragments (CIP), it is unlikely that any proteolytic activity is expressed outside the disc. Chymopapain and CIP are detectable in plasma at 30 minutes and decline at 24 hours. Small amounts of CIP are also detected in the urine. The liquified nucleus diffuses into the circulation, where the enzyme is inactivated. However, because chymopapain is injected directly into the herniated lumbar intervertebral disc, absorption, distribution and metabolism are not necessary for it to achieve its intended purpose.

Clinical pharmacology: Approximately 75% of patients responded successfully to the drug, compared to approximately 45% for placebo. When the placebo failures were then treated with drug, 90% of them responded with partial or total relief of their symptoms. In open studies success rates ranged from 80% to 89%.

Indications:

For the treatment of documented herniated lumbar intervertebral discs, whose symptoms and signs, particularly sciatica, have not responded to adequate conservative therapy. The drug has not been studied in treatment of herniated discs in areas other than the lumbar spine.

Contraindications:

Known sensitivity to chymopapain, papaya or papaya derivatives (eg, papain-containing contact lens cleaner); severe spondylolisthesis; significant spinal stenosis; severe progressing paralysis, as indicated by rapidly progressing neurologic dysfunction; evidence of spinal cord tumor or other lesions producing spinal motor or sensory dysfunction (eg, a cauda equina lesion); previous injection of chymopapain; any spinal region other than the lumbar area.

(Continued on following page)

CHYMOPAPAIN (Cont.)

Warnings:

Proper selection of patients is mandatory since nerve root compression resulting from conditions other than herniated disc can produce similar signs and symptoms.

Anaphylaxis (severe to mild) occurs in about 0.5% of patients and may be life threatening if not treated promptly and correctly. Females, particularly those with an elevated erythrocyte sedimentation rate, may be prone to develop such a reaction (approximately tenfold more common).

Data obtained from surveillance of over 71,000 patients demonstrate the incidence of anaphylaxis secondary to chymopapain injection varies by gender and type of anesthesia:

Anaphylaxis Incidence with Chymopapain			
	Local	General	Overall
Male	0.3%	0.3%	0.3%
Female	0.6%	0.9%	0.8%
Overall	0.4%	0.5%	0.5%

The anaphylaxis rate is significantly higher for females (0.8% v. 0.3% for males) and for patients who received general anesthesia (0.5% v. 0.4% for local anesthesia). In the population where race has been reported, the incidence is significantly higher in black females.

Preoperative pretreatment regimens to prevent anaphylactic reactions have been used, although there are no clinical studies demonstrating efficacy. Recommended regimens include cimetidine with either diphenhydramine or chlorpheniramine (see Administration and Dosage), diphenhydramine and dexamethasone with prednisone, and doxepin and terbutaline with an optional long-acting corticosteroid. Allergy testing to determine chymopapain-sensitive patients is available; however, the radioallergosorbent test and chymopapain fluorescence assay sensitivity test have excessively high false negative rates, and the skin test may be likely to produce false positives. Also, skin testing itself may sensitize patients.

Symptoms can be immediate or delayed up to 2 hours after injection and can last for minutes to several hours or longer. The patient may have almost immediate hypotension (more common) or bronchospasm and may proceed to laryngeal edema, cardiac arrhythmia, cardiac arrest, coma and death. Instruct patients to anticipate any delayed reactions (rash, urticaria or itching), which may occur for up to 15 days after injection.

Treatment – Clinical judgment, speed of therapy, and choice of agents all enter into treatment. The use of a preoperative screening test for chymopapain-specific IgE antibody should be considered to identify patients at risk for anaphylaxis. Keep at least one open IV line in place to permit rapid management. Epinephrine is indicated for immediate treatment. Beta-blocker therapy may inhibit the action of epinephrine. Reserve other agents such as steroids for cases where epinephrine is not appropriate. Refer to Management of Acute Hypersensitivity Reactions on p. viii.

Fatalities such as those due to anaphylaxis or complications of anaphylaxis (see Warnings), disc space infection, or central nervous system hemorrhage, may be associated with either the drug or the procedure. Others appear to be coincidental. The overall mortality rate following chymopapain injection is approximately 1 in 5,000 patients (0.02%). In comparison, mortality associated with laminectomy ranges from 0.02% to 0.1%.

(Warnings continued on following page)

CHYMOPAPAIN (Cont.)

Warnings (Cont.):

Neurological events: Paraplegia, paraparesis (eg, as are seen in the cauda equina syndrome), other serious neurologic adverse events, subarachnoid and intracerebral hemorrhage, and seizures have been observed soon after (within hours or days) chymopapain injection at a rate of about 1 in 2,000. Causal relationships to the drug when properly injected have not been established. Needle trauma or injection of chymopapain and contrast media into the spinal fluid may be causes in some of these reported cases. Other less severe neurologic reactions have included burning sacral pain, leg pain, hypalgesia, leg weakness, foot drop, cramping in both calves, pain in the opposite leg, paresthesia, tingling in legs and numbness of legs/toes.

Acute transverse myelitis/myelopathy has been associated with chymopapain, injection at a rate of about 1 in 18,000, although cause and effect relationship to the injection of chymopapain itself has not been established. These patients are characterized clinically by the delayed (2 to 3 weeks) onset of paraplegia or paraparesis without prior signs or symptoms.

In nearly all cases of serious neurologic adverse events, discography was performed as part of the procedure. Injection of contrast agent and chymopapain into the spinal fluid may be a cause in some cases. Additionally, several patients experiencing neurologic adverse events who did not have discography performed prior to the procedure experienced only transient problems. Therefore, it is recommended that discography not be performed as part of the chemonucleolysis procedure unless, in the judgment of the surgeon, the benefits outweigh the risks for a particular patient. A water or saline acceptance test may be used as an alternative to discography to indicate that the disc is abnormal and to attempt reproduction of sciatic pain in the patient receiving local anesthesia.

Patients receiving injections at two or more disc spaces appear to be at increased risk of serious neurologic adverse events. Therefore, limit chemonucleolysis to the one disc producing the patient's symptoms unless definitive signs, symptoms, and diagnostic procedures indicate that more than one disc is at fault.

Nearly all patients experiencing a serious neurologic adverse event had the procedure performed under general anesthesia. Local anesthesia provides an awake patient, more likely to experience pain and complain if the needle impinges on the nerve tissue. Also, it is unlikely that a patient under local anesthesia will tolerate an excessive number of attempts to place the needle. Although the final choice of anesthetic rests with the patient's physician, it is recommended that local or supplemented local anesthesia be used for chemonucleolysis whenever possible.

Patients who have had prior surgery of the lumbar spine appear to be at increased risk of experiencing a serious neurologic adverse event. Therefore, it is recommended that such patients be selelcted for chemonucleolysis only after careful consideration of the risk/benefit ratio.

Several patients with a history of hypertension, known or suspected cerebrovascular anomaly, previous cerebrovascular accident or a strong family history of cerebrovascular accident have experienced extensive, severe or fatal central nervous system hemorrhage following chemonucleolysis.

Immunological response: Chymopapain, a foreign protein, has the potential to cause an immunological response. Therefore, do not reinject patients who have already received any form of chymopapain injection.

Toxicity: The drug is extremely toxic when injected intrathecally in animals. Exercise caution to assure that chymopapain is not intrathecally injected into the dural canal; avoid transdural or posterior needle placement.

Certain radiopaque contrast media used for discography are neurotoxic when injected intrathecally. Toxicity may be enhanced by intrathecal bleeding. If chymopapain is inadvertently administered intrathecally, disruption of the capillaries may occur resulting in intrathecal bleeding.

Usage in Pregnancy: Category C. Safety for use during pregnancy has not been established. Use only when clearly needed and when the potential benefits outweigh the potential hazards to the fetus.

Usage in Children: Safety and efficacy for use in children have not been established.

Precautions:

Determine if the patient has multiple allergies, especially papaya, papaya derivatives or iodine. Do not use absorbable iodine during myelography or discography in patients allergic to iodine.

Postinjection pain: Patients may experience pain or involuntary muscle spasm in the lower back for several days. A residual stiffness or soreness may persist for several months.

(Continued on following page)

CHYMOPAPAIN (Cont.)

Adverse Reactions:

Allergic reactions: Erythema; pilomotor erection; rash; pruritic urticaria; conjunctivitis; vasomotor rhinitis; angioedema; various GI disturbances; anaphylaxis (see Warnings).

Frequent: Back pain, stiffness, soreness (≈ 50%); back spasm (≈ 30%).

Less frequent (< 1%): Itching; nausea; paralytic ileus; urinary retention; headache; dizziness; sacral burning; leg pain; hypalgesia; leg weakness; cramping in both calves; pain in the opposite leg; paresthesia; foot drop; tingling and numbness of legs/toes.

Discitis, both bacterial and aseptic.

Causal relationship unknown: Transverse myelitis/myelopathy (see Warning Box and Warnings).

Overdosage:

In animal studies, doses up to 100 times greater than that required to remove the nucleus pulposus were well tolerated when injected IV, intradiscally and epidurally.

Administration and Dosage:

Pretreatment: Prior to injection of chymopapain, pretreat with histamine receptor (H_1 and H_2) antagonists to lessen the severity of an anaphylactic reaction. One widely used regimen is cimetidine 300 mg orally every 6 hours and diphenhydramine 50 mg orally every 6 hours for 24 hours prior to chemonucleolysis.

Because of the abrupt decrease in intravascular volume during anaphylaxis, patients should be well hydrated by oral or IV fluids prior to chemonucleolysis. Always have at least one open IV line in place to permit rapid and adequate management of anaphylaxis.

Note: The unit of chymopapain activity is the nanoKatal (nKat). In general, 1 mg of chymopapain contains at least 0.5 nKat units. Each 2 ml vial of chymopapain contains 4 nKat units of enzyme for reconstitution with 2 ml Sterile Water for Injection, USP. Each 5 ml vial contains 10 nKat units of the enzyme for reconstitution with 5 ml Sterile Water for Injection, USP. The concentration of solution in the reconstituted vial is 2 nKat units of drug per ml.

Dosage is 2 to 4 nKat units per disc, usually 3 nKat units per disc, or a volume injection of 1 to 2 ml, usually 1.5 ml per disc. Maximum dose in a single patient with multiple disc herniation (see Warnings) is 8 nKat units.

Intradiscal administration: Treat each herniated disc with a single injection of chymopapain. Refer to package literature for detailed administration procedure.

Preparation of solution: Use alcohol to cleanse the vial stopper prior to insertion of needles into the vial. However, since alcohol inactivates the enzyme, allow to air dry before continuing the reconstitution process. The manufacturing process results in a residual vacuum in the vial; therefore, do not use automatic filling syringes.

Reconstitution – Reconstitute with 5 ml Sterile Water for Injection, which is supplied with each vial of chymopapain. (Use only 2 ml Sterile Water solution when reconstituting 4 nKat unit vial.) Do not use Bacteriostatic Water for Injection because it may inactivate the enzyme.

Stability and storage: Although it can be shipped unrefrigerated, store chymopapain at 2° to 8°C (36° to 46°F) until reconstitution.

Chymopapain must be used within 2 hours of its reconstitution; promptly discard unused drug.

Rx	**Chymodiactin** (Boots-Flint)	**Powder for Injection:** 4 nKat units and 1.4 mg sodium L-cysteinate HCl per vial w/diluent. (2 nKat units/ml after reconstitution)	In 2 ml vials.
		10 nKat units and 3.6 mg sodium L-cysteinate HCl per vial w/diluent.[1] (2 nKat units/ml after reconstitution)	In 5 ml vials.

[1] Contains no preservatives.

DISULFIRAM

Warning:
Never give to a patient in a state of alcohol intoxication, or without the patient's full knowledge. Instruct the patient's relatives accordingly.

Actions:

Pharmacology: Disulfiram produces an intolerance to alcohol which results in a highly unpleasant reaction when the patient under treatment ingests even small amounts of alcohol. Disulfiram blocks oxidation of alcohol at the acetaldehyde stage by inhibiting aldehyde dehydrogenase. The concentration of acetaldehyde in the blood may be 5 to 10 times higher than that achieved during normal alcohol metabolism. Accumulation of acetaldehyde produces the disulfiram-alcohol reaction (see Warnings). This reaction persists as long as alcohol is being metabolized. Disulfiram does not influence alcohol elimination.

Pharmacokinetics: Disulfiram is rapidly absorbed from the GI tract and eliminated slowly from the body. About 12 hours are required for its full action. Disulfiram is metabolized to diethyldithiocarbamate, which is oxidized to carbon disulfide and diethylamine. Approximately 20% of the drug remains after 1 week. Ingestion of alcohol may produce unpleasant symptoms for 1 to 2 weeks after the last dose of disulfiram. Prolonged administration of disulfiram does not produce tolerance; the longer a patient remains on therapy, the more sensitive he becomes to alcohol.

Indications:

An aid in the management of selected chronic alcoholics who want to remain in a state of enforced sobriety.

Effectiveness in promoting abstinence is limited. Compliance with the disulfiram regimen and regular follow-ups correlate with abstinence.

Contraindications:

Severe myocardial disease or coronary occlusion; psychoses; hypersensitivity to disulfiram or to other thiuram derivatives used in pesticides and rubber vulcanization; patients receiving or who have recently received metronidazole, paraldehyde, alcohol, or alcohol-containing preparations (eg, cough syrups, tonics).

Warnings:

Never administer to an intoxicated patient or without the patient's knowledge (see Warning box).

Disulfiram-alcohol reaction: Disulfiram plus alcohol, even small amounts, produces flushing, throbbing in head and neck, throbbing headaches, respiratory difficulty, nausea, copious vomiting, sweating, thirst, chest pain, palpitations, dyspnea, hyperventilation, tachycardia, hypotension, syncope, marked uneasiness, weakness, vertigo, blurred vision and confusion. In severe reactions there may be respiratory depression, cardiovascular collapse, arrhythmias, myocardial infarction, acute congestive heart failure, unconsciousness, convulsions and death. The intensity of the reaction is proportional to the amounts of disulfiram and alcohol ingested. Mild reactions may occur in the sensitive individual when the blood alcohol concentration is as low as 5 to 10 mg/dl. Symptoms are fully developed at 50 mg/dl, and unconsciousness usually results at 125 to 150 mg/dl. The duration of the reaction varies from 30 to 60 minutes to several hours.

Concomitant conditions: Because of the possibility of an accidental reaction, use with caution in patients with diabetes mellitus, hypothyroidism, epilepsy, cerebral damage, chronic and acute nephritis, hepatic cirrhosis or insufficiency.

Hypersensitivity: Evaluate patients with a history of rubber contact dermatitis for hypersensitivity to thiuram derivatives before administering disulfiram. Refer to General Management of Acute Hypersensitivity Reactions.

Pregnancy: Safety for use during pregnancy has not been established.

Precautions:

Dependence and addiction: Alcoholism may accompany or be followed by dependence on narcotics or sedatives. Barbiturates have been coadministered with disulfiram without untoward effects, but consider the possibility of initiating a new abuse.

Ethylene dibromide: Patients should not be exposed to ethylene dibromide or its vapors. This precaution is based on preliminary results of animal research which suggest a toxic interaction between inhaled ethylene dibromide and ingested disulfiram resulting in higher incidence of tumors and mortality in rats.

Monitoring: Perform baseline and follow-up transaminase tests (10 to 14 days) to detect hepatic dysfunction resulting from therapy. Perform a CBC and SMA-12 test every 6 months.

(Continued on following page)

DISULFIRAM (Cont.)

Drug Interactions:

Alcohol: Disulfiram causes a severe alcohol-intolerance reaction. Avoid alcohol in all forms. See Warnings.

Benzodiazepines: Disulfiram decreases the plasma clearance of benzodiazepines metabolized by oxidation, possibly resulting in increased CNS depressant actions. When benzodiazepine therapy is indicated, use oxazepam, alprazolam or lorazepam since they are metabolized by glucuronidation.

Caffeine: Cardiovascular and CNS stimulation effects of caffeine may be increased by disulfiram.

Hydantoins: Serum hydantoin levels may be increased by disulfiram, resulting in an increase in the pharmacologic and toxic effects. Monitor hydantoin levels and adjust the dosage as needed.

Isoniazid: Observe patients receiving isoniazid and disulfiram for the appearance of unsteady gait or marked changes in behavior; discontinue disulfiram or reduce the dose if such signs appear.

Metronidazole: Patients may exhibit acute toxic psychosis or confusional state when taking metronidazole in combination with disulfiram, requiring discontinuation of one or both of the agents.

Tricyclic antidepressants and disulfiram coadministration may result in acute organic brain syndrome. The bioavailability of the antidepressant may also be increased.

Warfarin: Disulfiram may increase the anticoagulant effect of warfarin. Monitor prothrombin time and adjust the warfarin dosage as necessary.

Adverse Reactions:

CNS: Drowsiness (most common); fatigability; headache; restlessness. Psychotic reactions have been noted, often attributable to high dosage, combined toxicity (metronidazole or isoniazid), or to the unmasking of underlying psychoses.

Neurologic: Peripheral neuropathy (with axonal degeneration); polyneuritis; optic or retrobulbar neuritis (with impaired vision, color perceptions and blindness).

Dermatologic: Occasional skin eruptions are, as a rule, readily controlled by antihistamines; acneiform eruptions; allergic dermatitis.

GI: Metallic or garlic-like aftertaste, usually during the first 2 weeks of therapy.

Hepatotoxicity resembling viral or alcoholic hepatitis; probably due to hypersensitivity, but toxic metabolite formation has also been proposed.

Multiple cases of both cholestatic and fulminant hepatitis have been associated with disulfiram use.

Miscellaneous: Arthropathy; acetonemia; impotence.

Patient Information:

Never use in intoxicated individuals or without an individual's knowledge.

Do not take for at least 12 hours after drinking alcohol. A reaction may occur for up to 2 weeks after disulfiram has been stopped.

Avoid alcohol in all forms. This includes: Alcoholic beverages, vinegars, many liquid medications (including prescription and nonprescription products), some sauces, aftershave lotions, colognes, liniments, etc.

Always read product labels or ask your pharmacist about alcohol content of all liquid medications before choosing one.

Tablets can be crushed or mixed with liquid.

May cause drowsiness. Use caution while driving or performing other tasks requiring alertness.

The alcohol-disulfiram reaction can have serious effects on the heart and respiratory systems.

Always carry identification indicating you are taking disulfiram. Include the phone numbers of your doctor or the medical facility that should be contacted in case of reaction.

Administration and Dosage:

Do NOT administer until the patient has abstained from alcohol for at least 12 hours.

Initial dosage schedule: Administer a maximum of 500 mg daily in a single dose for 1 to 2 weeks. If a sedative effect is experienced, take at bedtime or decrease dosage.

Maintenance regimen: The average maintenance dose is 250 mg daily (range, 125 to 500 mg), not to exceed 500 mg daily. NOTE: Occasional disulfiram patients report that they are able to drink alcoholic beverages with impunity and without any symptomatology. Such patients must be presumed to be disposing of their tablets without actually taking them. Until such patients are observed reliably taking their daily tablets (preferably crushed and well mixed with liquid), do not assume that disulfiram is ineffective.

(Administration and Dosage continued on following page)

DISULFIRAM (Cont.)

Administration and Dosage (Cont.):

Duration of therapy: Continue use until the patient is fully recovered socially and a basis for permanent self-control is established. Maintenance therapy may be required for months or even years.

Trial with alcohol: The test reaction has been largely abandoned. Do not administer a test reaction to a patient > 50 years of age. A clear, detailed and convincing description of the reaction is felt to be sufficient in most cases.

Where a test reaction is deemed necessary, the suggested procedure is: After the first 1 to 2 weeks of therapy with 500 mg daily, a drink of 15 ml of 100 proof whiskey or equivalent is taken slowly. This test dose may be repeated once only so that total dose does not exceed 30 ml (1 g) whiskey. Once a reaction develops, no more alcohol should be consumed. Only perform such tests when the patient is hospitalized and facilities are available.

Management of disulfiram-alcohol reaction: In severe reactions, institute supportive measures to restore blood pressure and treat shock. Other recommendations include: Oxygen or carbogen (95% oxygen and 5% carbon dioxide), vitamin C IV in massive doses (1 g) and ephedrine sulfate. Antihistamines have also been used IV. Monitor potassium levels, particularly in patients on digitalis, since hypokalemia has been reported.

Extemporaneous aqueous suspensions of disulfiram powder or tablets (2.5 g, with 2 g acacia and 100 mg sodium benzoate, with water to make 100 ml) have been reported stable up to 295 days when stored at 24°C (room temperature) in amber-colored bottles under fluorescent light.

	Product	Form	Packaging	**C.I.***
Rx	**Disulfiram** (Various, eg, Danbury, Geneva, Goldline, Major, Moore, Qualitest, Rugby, Schein, Sidmak, URL)	**Tablets:** 250 mg	In 100s and 1000s.	20+
Rx	**Antabuse** (Wyeth-Ayerst)		Scored. In 100s.	176
Rx	**Disulfiram** (Various, eg, Danbury, Geneva, Goldline, Major, Qualitest, Rugby, Schein, Sidmak)	**Tablets:** 500 mg	In 50s, 100s and 500s.	22+
Rx	**Antabuse** (Wyeth-Ayerst)		Scored. In 50s and 1000s.	106

* Cost Index based on cost per 500 mg.

NICOTINE

Actions:

Pharmacology: Nicotine polacrilex contains nicotine bound to an ion exchange resin in a chewing gum base. The nicotine transdermal system is a multilayered unit containing nicotine as the active agent that provides systemic delivery of nicotine for 24 hours following its application to intact skin.

Nicotine, the chief alkaloid in tobacco products, binds stereoselectively to acetylcholine receptors at the autonomic ganglia, in the adrenal medulla, at neuromuscular junctions and in the brain. Two types of CNS effects are believed to be the basis of nicotine's positively reinforcing properties. A stimulating effect, exerted mainly in the cortex via the locus ceruleus, produces increased alertness and cognitive performance. A "reward" effect via the "pleasure system" in the brain is exerted in the limbic system. At low doses the stimulant effects predominate, while at high doses the reward effects predominate. Intermittent IV administration of nicotine activates neurohormonal pathways, releasing acetylcholine, norepinephrine, dopamine, serotonin, vasopressin, beta-endorphin, growth hormone and ACTH.

The cardiovascular effects of nicotine include peripheral vasoconstriction, tachycardia and elevated blood pressure. Acute and chronic tolerance to nicotine develops from smoking tobacco or ingesting nicotine preparations. Acute tolerance (a reduction in reponse for a given dose) develops rapidly (< 1 hour), but at distinct rates for different physiologic effects (skin temperature, heart rate, subjective effects). Withdrawal symptoms, such as cigarette craving, can be reduced in some individuals by plasma nicotine levels lower than those for smoking.

Withdrawal from nicotine in addicted individuals is characterized by craving, nervousness, restlessness, irritability, mood lability, anxiety, drowsiness, sleep disturbances, impaired concentration, increased appetite, minor somatic complaints (headache, myalgia, constipation, fatigue) and weight gain. Nicotine toxicity is characterized by nausea, abdominal pain, vomiting, diarrhea, diaphoresis, flushing, dizziness, disturbed hearing/vision, confusion, weakness, palpitations, altered respiration and hypotension.

Nicotine's effects are generally dose-dependent. In nonsmokers, CNS-mediated symptoms of hiccoughs, nausea and emesis are commonly associated with the use of even small doses of inhaled smoke or nicotine gum. However, in smokers these symptoms occur only with much larger doses. If nicotine gum (2 mg/piece) is used by smokers at a rate not exceeding 1 piece/hour or if transdermal nicotine is used (21 mg/day), the cardiovascular effects produced do not differ from those seen with placebo.

Pharmacokinetics: Nicotine gum – Absorption/Distribution: The nicotine is bound to an ion exchange resin and is released only during chewing; nicotine will not be released in significant amounts if the gum is swallowed. The blood level of nicotine will depend upon the vigor, rapidity and duration of chewing. The trough level of nicotine obtained by smoking one cigarette per hour is approximately twice that of chewing one 2 mg piece of gum per hour.

Metabolism/Excretion – Nicotine is metabolized mainly by the liver, and to a lesser extent, by the kidney and lung. There is no significant skin metabolism of nicotine. More than 20 metabolites of nicotine have been identified, all of which are believed to be less active than the parent compound. The half-life of nicotine ranges from 1 to 2 hours. The primary metabolite of nicotine in plasma, cotinine, has a half-life of 15 to 20 hours and concentrations that exceed nicotine by 10-fold. Plasma protein binding of nicotine is < 5%. The primary urinary metabolites are cotinine (15% of the dose) and trans-3-hydroxycotinine (45% of the dose). About 10% of nicotine is excreted unchanged in the urine. As much as 30% may be excreted in the urine with high urine flow rates and urine acidification below pH5.

Nicotine transdermal system: All systems are labeled by the actual amount of nicotine absorbed by the patient.

Nicoderm – Following application, ≈ 68% of the nicotine released from the system enters the systemic circulation. The remainder of the nicotine released from the system is lost via evaporation from the edge. After application, plasma concentrations rise rapidly, plateau within 2 to 4 hours, and then slowly decline until the system is removed, after which they decline more rapidly. Nicotine in the adhesive layer is absorbed into and then through the skin, causing the initial rapid rise in plasma concentrations. The nicotine from the reservoir is released slowly through the membrane with a release rate constant approximately 20 times smaller than the skin absorption rate constant. Therefore, the slow decline of plasma nicotine concentrations during 4 to 24 hours is determined primarily by the release of nicotine from the system.

Habitrol – Following an initial lag time of 1 to 2 hours, nicotine concentrations increase to a broad peak between 6 and 12 hours and then decrease gradually.

(Actions continued on following page)

NICOTINE (Cont.)

Actions (Cont.):

Pharmacokinetics (Cont.):

Habitrol/Nicoderm: Following the second daily system application (or within 2 days of initiating treatment), steady-state plasma nicotine concentrations are achieved and are on average 25% to 30% higher compared with single-dose applications. Plasma nicotine concentrations are proportional to dose for the three dosages of the transdermal systems. Nicotine kinetics are similar for all sites of application on the upper body and upper outer arm. Plasma nicotine concentrations from the 21 mg/day system are the same as those from simultaneous use of 14 and 7 mg/day systems.

Following removal of the system, plasma nicotine concentrations decline in an exponential fashion with an apparent mean half-life of 3 to 4 hours compared with 1 to 2 hours for IV administration, due to continued absorption from the skin depot. Most nonsmoking patients will have nondetectable nicotine concentrations in 10 to 12 hours.

Half-hourly smoking of cigarettes produces average plasma nicotine concentrations of approximately 44 ng/ml. In comparison, average plasma nicotine concentrations from transdermal nicotine 21 mg/day are about 17 ng/ml.

Obese men using transdermal systems had significantly lower AUC and C_{max} values than normal weight men. Men and women having low body weight are expected to have higher AUC and C_{max} values.

Clinical trials: Nicotine gum – In the varied controlled trials conducted, the success rate of smoking cessation has been approximately doubled using nicotine gum.

Nicoderm – In two trials of transdermal nicotine vs placebo, treatment with 21 mg/day for 6 weeks provided significantly higher quit rates than the 14 mg/day and placebo treatments at 6 weeks (32% to 92%, 30% to 61% and 15% to 46%, respectively). Quit rates were still significantly different after an additional 6 week weaning period (18% to 63%, 15% to 52% and 0% to 38%, respectively) and at follow-up 3 months later (3% to 50%, 0% to 48% and 0% to 35%, respectively).

Habitrol – In two trials in otherwise healthy smokers with concomitant support, transdermal therapy resulted in higher quit rates than placebo after 7 weeks (19% to 54% vs 9% to 30%). Quit rates were still significantly different after an additional 3 week weaning period (8% to 43% vs 8% to 30%). When transdermal nicotine was used without concomitant support, greater variability and decreased quit rates were demonstrated with both treatment and placebo after 7 weeks (4% to 28% vs 0% to 24%) as well as after an additional 3 week weaning period (4% to 20% vs 0% to 22%).

Indications:

As an aid to smoking cessation for the relief of nicotine withdrawal symptoms. Use as part of a comprehensive behavioral smoking-cessation program.

In general, smokers who have a high "physical" type of nicotine dependence are most likely to benefit from the use of nicotine gum or transdermal systems. The following characteristics correlate with a "physical" type of nicotine dependence: (1) Smoke $>$ 15 cigarettes per day, (2) prefer brands of cigarettes with nicotine levels $>$ 0.9 mg, (3) usually inhale the smoke frequently and deeply, (4) smoke the first cigarette within 30 minutes of arising, (5) find the first cigarette in the morning the hardest to give up, (6) smoke most frequently during the morning, (7) find it difficult to refrain from smoking in places where it is forbidden, or (8) smoke even when they are so ill they are confined to bed most of the day.

The benefits of use beyond 3 months have not been demonstrated.

Unlabeled uses: In two children, use of nicotine polacrilex gum and haloperidol resulted in improvement of symptoms (eg, tics) of Tourette's syndrome. Further study is needed.

Contraindications:

Hypersensitivity to nicotine or any components of the transdermal system; nonsmokers; during the immediate postmyocardial infarction period; life-threatening arrhythmias; severe or worsening angina pectoris; active temporomandibular joint disease (nicotine polacrilex); pregnancy (see Warnings).

Warnings:

Cardiovascular: Weigh the benefits against the risks of nicotine in patients with certain cardiovascular diseases. Specifically, screen and evaluate patients with coronary heart disease (history of myocardial infarction or angina pectoris), serious cardiac arrhythmias or vasospastic diseases (Buerger's disease, Prinzmetal variant angina) before nicotine is prescribed. There have been occasional reports of tachyarrhythmias associated with nicotine use; therefore, if an increase in cardiovascular symptoms occurs, discontinue the drug. Generally, do not use during the immediate post-myocardial infarction period, with serious arrhythmias or with severe or worsening angina pectoris.

Cigarette smoking may play a perpetuating role in hypertension. Therefore, use nicotine in patients with systemic hypertension only when the benefits of such a smoking cessation program outweigh the risks.

(Warnings continued on following page)

NICOTINE (Cont.)

Warnings (Cont.):

Endocrine: Because of the action of nicotine on the adrenal medulla (release of catecholamines), use with caution in patients with hyperthyroidism, pheochromocytoma or insulin-dependent diabetes.

Hepatic/Renal function impairment: Since nicotine is extensively metabolized and its total system clearance is dependent on liver blood flow, anticipate some influence of hepatic impairment on drug kinetics (reduced clearance). Only severe renal impairment would be expected to affect the clearance of nicotine or its metabolites from the circulation.

Fertility impairment: A decrease of litter size in rats treated with nicotine during the time of fertilization has occurred. Rare reports of miscarriages have been received. A relationship to drug therapy as a contributing factor cannot be excluded.

Elderly: Transdermal nicotine therapy appeared to be as effective in elderly patients > 60 years of age as in younger smokers. However, asthenia, various body aches and dizziness occurred slightly more often in elderly patients.

Pregnancy: Category X (nicotine polacrilex), *Category D* (transdermal nicotine). Nicotine may cause fetal harm when administered to a pregnant woman. Use of cigarettes or nicotine gum during the last trimester has been associated with a decrease in fetal breathing movements. These effects may be the result of decreased placental perfusion caused by nicotine. Rare reports of miscarriages have been received, and a relationship to drug therapy as a contributing factor cannot be excluded. Nicotine is contraindicated in women who are or may become pregnant; advise patients to use contraceptive measures. If this drug is used during pregnancy, or if the patient becomes pregnant while taking this drug, apprise the patient of the potential hazard to the fetus.

The specific effects of transdermal nicotine on fetal development are unknown. Therefore, encourage pregnant smokers to attempt cessation before using pharmacological approaches. Use during pregnancy only if the likelihood of smoking cessation justifies the potential risk of use of nicotine replacement by the patient who may continue to smoke.

Lactation: Nicotine passes freely into breast milk and has the potential for serious adverse reactions in nursing infants. Nicotine concentrations in milk can be expected to be lower with transdermal nicotine therapy when used as directed than with cigarette smoking, as maternal plasma nicotine concentrations are generally reduced with nicotine replacement. Decide whether to discontinue nursing or to discontinue the drug, weighing the risk of exposure of the infant to nicotine from replacement therapy against the risks associated with the infant's exposure to nicotine from continued smoking by the mother and from nicotine therapy alone or in combination with continued smoking.

Children: Safety and efficacy in children/adolescents who smoke have not been evaluated.

The amounts of nicotine that are tolerated by adult smokers can produce symptoms of poisoning and could prove fatal if the transdermal nicotine system is applied or ingested by children or pets. Used 21 mg/day *Nicoderm* and *Habitrol* systems contain about 73% (83 mg) and 60% (32 mg) of their initial drug content, respectively. Therefore, caution patients to keep both the used and unused systems out of the reach of children and pets.

Precautions:

Oral/GI: Use with caution in patients with oral or pharyngeal inflammation and in patients with a history of esophagitis or peptic ulcer. Since nicotine delays healing in peptic ulcer disease, use in patients with active or inactive peptic ulcer only when the benefits of including nicotine in a smoking cessation program outweigh the risks.

Skin disease: Systems are usually well tolerated by patients with normal skin, but may be irritating for patients with some skin disorders (atopic or eczematous dermatitis).

Allergic reactions: In two studies, 29 of 450 patients exhibited definite erythema at 24 hours after application of the transdermal system. Upon rechallenge, 7 patients exhibited mild to moderate contact allergy. Caution patients with contact sensitization that a serious reaction could occur from exposure to other nicotine-containing products or smoking. Erythema following system removal was typically seen in 14% to 17% of patients, some edema in 3% to 4% and dropouts due to skin reactions in 2% to 6%.

Instruct patients to promptly discontinue the use of nicotine systems and contact their physicians if they experience severe or persistent local skin reactions (eg, severe erythema, pruritus, edema) at the site of application or a generalized skin reaction (eg, urticaria, hives, generalized rash).

Patients using transdermal nicotine concurrently with other transdermal products may exhibit local reactions at both application sites. Reactions were seen in 2 of 7 patients using concomitant estradiol transdermal system. In such patients, use of one or both systems may have to be discontinued.

Dental problems might be exacerbated by chewing nicotine gum.

(Precautions continued on following page)

NICOTINE (Cont.)

Precautions (Cont.):

Drug abuse and dependence: Urge patients to stop smoking completely when initiating therapy. If patients continue to smoke while using nicotine therapy, they may experience adverse effects due to peak nicotine levels higher than those experienced from smoking alone.

The possibility of transference of nicotine dependence exists. The use of transdermal nicotine or nicotine gum beyond 3 months has not been demonstrated to increase the smoking cessation rate. To minimize the risk of dependence, encourage patients to gradually withdraw or stop gum usage at 3 months, transdermal nicotine after 4 to 8 weeks of use (progressively decrease the dose every 2 to 4 weeks). The chronic consumption of nicotine is toxic and addicting. Weigh the relative risks of a possible return to smoking and continued, long-term use of the gum.

Drug Interactions:

Smoking cessation, with or without nicotine substitutes, may alter response to concomitant medication in ex-smokers. Smoking is considered to increase metabolism and lower blood levels of the following drugs through enzyme induction (smoking cessation may reverse these actions).

Acetaminophen	**Oxazepam**	**Propranolol**
Caffeine	**Pentazocine**	**Theophylline**
Imipramine		

Catecholamines and cortisol: Both smoking and nicotine can increase circulating cortisol and catecholamines. Therapy with **adrenergic agonists** or with **adrenergic blockers** may need to be adjusted according to changes in nicotine therapy or smoking status.

Furosemide: Smoking may reduce diuretic effects of furosemide and decrease cardiac output. Smoking cessation may reverse these actions.

Glutethimide absorption may be decreased with smoking cessation.

Insulin: Increase in subcutaneous insulin absorption with smoking cessation may occur.

Propoxyphene: The first-pass metabolism of propoxyphene may be decreased by smoking cessation.

Drug/Food interaction: Effective absorption of nicotine polacrilex relies on a mildly alkaline saliva (produced from the release of buffering agents). Therefore, since coffee, cola and other drinks or food may reduce salivary pH, it may be beneficial for patients to not ingest food or drink during or immediately before the use of nicotine gum.

Adverse Reactions:

Nicotine polacrilex: Local reactions – Mechanical effects of gum chewing include traumatic injury to oral mucosa or teeth, jaw ache and eructation secondary to air swallowing. Minimize by modifying chewing technique. Oral mucosal changes such as stomatitis, glossitis, gingivitis, pharyngitis and aphthous ulcers, in addition to changes in taste perception, can occur during smoking cessation efforts with or without nicotine gum.

Systemic – Although the systemic effects seen in trials were generally similar, the reported frequency of adverse drug effects was highly variable.

Nicotine Polacrilex Adverse Reactions (%)

	US studies		British studies	
	Drug (n = 94)	Placebo (n = 95)	Drug (n = 58)	Placebo (n = 58)
CNS				
Insomnia	1.1	1.1		
Dizziness/Lightheadedness	2.1	2.1	19	13.8
Irritability/Fussiness	1.1	1.1		
Headache	1.1	5.3	24.1	29.3
GI				
Nonspecific GI distress	9.6	6.3		
Eructation	6.4	1.1		
Indigestion			41.4	20.7
Nausea/Vomiting	18.1	4.2	31	15.5
Oropharyngeal				
Mouth or throat soreness	37.2	31.6	56.9	53.4
Jaw muscle ache	18.1	9.5	44.8	44.8
Other				
Anorexia	1.1	1.1		
Excess salivation	2.1	0		
Hiccoughs	14.9	0	22.4	3.4

(Adverse Reactions continued on following page)

NICOTINE (Cont.)

Adverse Reactions (Cont.):

Nicotine polacrilex (Cont.):

Cardiovascular – Edema; flushing; hypertension; palpitations; tachyarrhythmias; tachycardia. One patient displayed what may have been nicotine-induced, but reversible, atrial fibrillation. Cardiac irritability is a well known consequence of cigarette smoking.

Deaths, myocardial infarction, congestive heart failure, cerebrovascular accident and cardiac arrest have occurred (a cause and effect relationship has not been established).

CNS – Confusion; convulsions; depression; euphoria; numbness; paresthesia; syncope; tinnitus; weakness.

Dermatologic – Erythema; itching; rash; urticaria.

GI – Alteration of liver function tests; constipation; diarrhea.

Respiratory – Breathing difficulty; cough; hoarseness; sneezing; wheezing.

Miscellaneous – Dry mouth; systemic nicotine intoxication.

Transdermal nicotine: The most common adverse event associated with topical nicotine is a short-lived erythema, pruritus or burning at the application site, which was seen at least once in 35% to 47% of patients in the clinical trials. Local erythema after system removal was noted at least once in 14% to 17% of patients and local edema in 3% to 4%. Erythema generally resolved within 24 hours. Cutaneous hypersensitivity (contact sensitization) occurred in 2% of patients (see Precautions).

Body as a whole: Asthenia, back pain, pain (3% to 9%); chest pain, allergy (1% to 3%).

GI: Diarrhea, dyspepsia, constipation, nausea (3% to 9%); abdominal pain, vomiting, dry mouth (1% to 3%).

CNS: Headache (17% to 29%); insomnia (3% to 23%); abnormal dreams, nervousness, dizziness (3% to 9%); paresthesia, somnolence, impaired concentration (1% to 3%).

Respiratory: Increased cough, pharyngitis (3% to 9%); sinusitis (1% to 3%).

Skin and appendages: Rash (3% to 9%).

Musculoskeletal: Myalgia, arthralgia (3% to 9%).

Miscellaneous: Taste perversion, dysmenorrhea (3% to 9%); sweating, hypertension (1% to 3%).

Overdosage:

Symptoms: Overdose will probably be minimized by the early nausea and vomiting that occur with excessive nicotine intake. Signs and symptoms of acute nicotine poisoning include: Nausea; salivation; abdominal pain; vomiting; diarrhea; cold sweat; headache; dizziness; disturbed hearing and vision; mental confusion; marked weakness. Faintness and prostration will ensue and hypotension may occur; breathing is difficult; the pulse may be rapid, weak and irregular; respiratory collapse may be followed by terminal convulsions. Death may result within a few minutes from paralysis of respiratory muscles. The oral minimum lethal dose for nicotine in adults is 40 to 60 mg.

Treatment: Nicotine polacrilex – If emesis has not occurred, induce with ipecac syrup in conscious patients. A saline cathartic will speed GI passage of the gum. In unconscious patients with a secure airway, gastric lavage followed by suspension of activated charcoal will aid in nicotine removal. Mechanical ventilation for respiratory paralysis may be necessary. Hypotension or cardiovascular collapse may occur; treat vigorously. Refer to General Management of Acute Overdosage.

Transdermal nicotine – Topical exposure: Remove the transdermal system immediately if the patient shows signs of overdosage and seek immediate medical care. The skin surface may be flushed with water and dried. Do not use soap, since it may increase nicotine absorption. Nicotine will continue to be delivered into the bloodstream for several hours after removal of the system because of a depot of nicotine in the skin.

Ingestion: Refer patients to a health care facility for management. Due to the possibility of nicotine-induced seizures, administer activated charcoal. In unconscious patients with a secure airway, instill activated charcoal via a nasogastric tube. A saline cathartic or sorbitol added to the first dose of activated charcoal may speed GI passage of the system. Administer repeated doses of activated charcoal as long as the system remains in the GI tract since it will continue to release nicotine for many hours.

Other supportive measures include diazepam or barbiturates for seizures, atropine for excessive bronchial secretions or diarrhea, respiratory support for respiratory failure and vigorous fluid support for hypotension and cardiovascular collapse.

(Continued on following page)

NICOTINE TRANSDERMAL SYSTEM

Patient Information:

A patient instruction sheet, included in the package dispensed to the patient, contains important information and instructions on proper use and disposal of the transdermal system. Encourage patients to ask questions of the physician and pharmacist.

Advise patients to keep used and unused systems out of reach of children and pets.

Administration and Dosage:

Approved by the FDA in November 1991.

Patients must desire to stop smoking. Instruct them to *stop smoking immediately* as they begin using therapy, to read the patient instruction sheet and to ask questions. Initiate treatment according to the recommended dosing schedule (see table below).

Once the appropriate dosage is selected, the patient should begin 4 to 12 weeks of therapy at that dosage (refer to specific product guidelines for duration). The patient should stop smoking cigarettes completely during this period. If the patient is unable to stop cigarette smoking within 4 weeks, therapy probably should be stopped, since few additional patients in clinical trials were able to quit after this time. Use beyond 3 months (5 months for *Nicotrol*) has not been studied.

Recommended Dosing Schedule of Transdermal Nicotine for Healthy Patients

	Duration	
Dose	Per strength of patch	Entire course of therapy
Habitrol[1]		
21 mg/day	First 6 weeks	
14 mg/day	Next 2 weeks[2]	8 to 12 weeks
7 mg/day	Last 2 weeks[3]	
Nicoderm[1]		
21 mg/day	First 6 weeks	
14 mg/day	Next 2 weeks[2]	8 to 12 weeks
7 mg/day	Last 2 weeks	
Nicotrol		
15 mg/day	First 12 weeks	
10 mg/day	Next 2 weeks[2]	14 to 20 weeks
5 mg/day	Last 2 weeks	
ProStep[3]		
22 mg/day	4 to 8 weeks	6 to 12 weeks
11 mg/day[4]	2 to 4 weeks	

[1] Start with 14 mg/day for 6 weeks for patients who: Have cardiovascular disease; weigh < 100 lbs; smoke < ½ pack of cigarettes/day. Decrease dose to 7 mg/day for the final 2 to 4 weeks.

[2] Patients who have successfully abstained from smoking should have their dose reduced after each 2 to 4 weeks of treatment until the 7 mg/day dose *(Habitrol; Nicoderm)* or 5 mg/day dose *(Nicotrol)* has been used for 2 to 4 weeks.

[3] Start with 22 mg/day except for patients who weigh < 100 lbs; they may start with 11 mg/day with the dose increased as appropriate.

[4] Optional weaning dose.

Application of system: Apply the system promptly upon its removal from the protective pouch to prevent evaporative loss of nicotine from the system. Use only when the pouch is intact to ensure that the product has not been tampered with. Apply only once a day to a non-hairy, clean, dry skin site on the upper body or upper outer arm.

Habitrol, Nicoderm, ProStep – After 24 hours, remove the used system and apply a new system to an alternate skin site. Skin sites should not be reused for at least a week. Caution patients not to continue to use the same system for > 24 hours.

Nicotrol – Each day apply a new system upon waking and remove at bedtime.

Individualization of dosage: Patients who fail to quit on any attempt may benefit from interventions to improve their chances for success on subsequent attempts. These patients should be counselled to determine why they failed and then probably be given a "therapy holiday" before the next attempt. Encourage a new quit attempt when the factors that contributed to failure can be eliminated or reduced, and conditions are more favorable.

(Administration and Dosage continued on following page)

NICOTINE TRANSDERMAL SYSTEM (Cont.)

Administration and Dosage (Cont.):

Safety/Handling: The transdermal nicotine system can be a dermal irritant and can cause contact sensitization. Instruct patients in the proper use of the systems by using demonstration systems. Although exposure of health care workers to nicotine from the systems should be minimal, take care to avoid unnecessary contact with active systems. If you do handle active systems, wash with water alone, since soap may increase nicotine absorption. Do not touch your eyes.

Disposal: When the used system is removed from the skin, fold it over and place in the protective pouch that contained the new system. Immediately dispose of the used system in such a way to prevent its access by children or pets.

Storage/Stability: Do not store above 30°C (86°F) because the transdermal systems are sensitive to heat. A slight discoloration of the system is not significant. Do not store out of the pouch. Once removed from the protective pouch, apply promptly since nicotine is volatile and the system may lose strength.

	Product/ Distributor	Dose absorbed in 24 hours (mg/day)	Surface area (cm^2)	Total nicotine content (mg)	How supplied
Rx	**Habitrol** (Basel Pharm.)	21[1] 14 7	30 20 10	52.5 35 17.5	30 systems per box.
Rx	**Nicoderm** (Marion Merrell Dow)	21 14 7	22 15 7	114 78 36	14 systems per box.
Rx	**Nicotrol** (Parke-Davis)	15[2] 10[2] 5[2]	30 20 10	24.9 16.6 8.3	14 systems per box.
Rx	**ProStep** (Lederle)	22 11	7 3.5	30 15	7 systems per box.

NICOTINE POLACRILEX (Nicotine resin complex)

Patient Information:

A patient instruction sheet is included in the package dispensed to the patient. See also Administration and Dosage.

Administration and Dosage:

Approved by the FDA in January 1984.

Individualize dosage. A candidate for nicotine therapy must desire to stop smoking and should *stop smoking immediately*. Give the patient an instruction sheet on nicotine gum chewing, and allow patient to read the instruction sheet and ask any questions. Arrange patient follow-up visits at intervals not greater than 1 month. Successful abstainers at 3 months should stop using gum or gradually withdraw from gum usage. Consider patients who chew gum beyond 3 months as possibly using the gum as a substitute source for their nicotine dependence. (See Drug abuse and dependence in Precautions section of the Smoking Deterrents monograph). Most patients who returned to smoking in nicotine-assisted programs did so within 6 months of treatment. Therefore, initiate gradual withdrawal after 3 months of usage and complete by 6 months. The use of nicotine beyond 6 months is not recommended.

At the initial visit, instruct patients to chew one piece of gum whenever they have the urge to smoke. Chew each piece slowly and intermittently for about 30 minutes to promote even, slow, buccal absorption of the nicotine. Chewing quickly can release the nicotine too rapidly, leading to effects similar to oversmoking (eg, nausea, hiccoughs or throat irritation). The patient must learn to self-titrate the nicotine dose to minimize side effects (see Patient Instruction Sheet).

Most patients require approximately 10 to 12 pieces of gum per day during the first month of treatment. Do not exceed 30 pieces of gum per day.

Rx *sf*	**Nicorette** (Marion Merrell Dow)	**Chewing gum:** 2 mg nicotine (as polacrilex) per square	Beige. In 96s (12 × 8s).

sf – Sugar free.

[1] Pouch contains patch labeled 23 mg/24 hr, which delivers 21 mg/day.

[2] Dose absorbed in 16 hours (mg/day).

LOBELINE

Actions:

Lobeline, an alkaloid of *Lobelia inflata,* produces pharmacologic effects similar to, yet weaker than, those produced by nicotine on the peripheral circulation, neuromuscular junctions and the CNS. The majority of controlled studies show that lobeline has only a placebo effect in decreasing the physical craving for cigarettes.

Indications:

A temporary aid to break the cigarette habit. The FDA OTC Advisory Panel has classified it as Category III (ie, safety, but not efficacy, has been established).

Warnings:

Pregnancy: Neither smoking nor lobeline is recommended during pregnancy.

Children: Not intended for use by children.

Precautions:

A single dose of 8 mg can cause epigastric pain, heartburn, belching, nausea, vomiting and faintness. These effects may be lessened by an antacid.

Because of the lack of data, do not use lobeline for longer than 6 weeks.

Adverse Reactions:

GI: Epigastric pain, severe heartburn, nausea and vomiting in higher doses.

Other: Coughing; dizziness.

Overdosage:

Symptoms: Sinus arrhythmia; tachycardia; extrasystoles; partial bundle branch block. Profuse diaphoresis, hypotension, muscular twitching, convulsions, paresis, hypothermia and coma may occur. Death has occurred from paralysis of the respiratory center.

Treatment: Empty the stomach. Employ supportive therapy, including ventilatory support, as required. Refer to General Management of Acute Overdosage.

Patient Information:

Do not exceed recommended dosage. Do not use this product longer than 6 weeks.

Notify physician if any of the following occurs: Nausea, vomiting, palpitations, convulsions.

Administration and Dosage:

One tablet after each meal with a half glass of water. Do not use longer than 6 weeks.

otc	**Bantron** (DEP Corp.)	**Tablets:** 2 mg lobeline sulfate alkaloids, 130 mg tribasic calcium phosphate and 130 mg magnesium carbonate	In 18s and 36s.

AZATHIOPRINE

Warning:
Chronic immunosuppression with azathioprine increases the risk of neoplasia. Physicians using this drug should be familiar with this risk as well as with the mutagenic potential to both men and women and with possible hematologic toxicities.

Actions:
Azathioprine, an imidazolyl derivative of 6-mercaptopurine (6-MP), has many biological effects similar to those of the parent compound.

Pharmacology:

Homograft survival – Although the use of azathioprine for inhibition of renal homograft rejection is well established, the mechanism(s) for this action are somewhat obscure. The drug suppresses cell-mediated hypersensitivities and alters antibody production. Suppression of T-cell effects, including ablation of T-cell suppression, depends on the temporal relationship to antigenic stimulus or engraftment. This agent has little effect on established graft rejections or secondary responses.

Alterations in specific immune responses or immunologic functions in transplant recipients are difficult to relate specifically to immunosuppression by azathioprine. These patients have subnormal responses to vaccines, low numbers of T-cells and abnormal phagocytosis by peripheral blood cells, but their mitogenic responses, serum immunoglobulins and secondary antibody responses are usually normal.

Immunoinflammatory response – The severity of adjuvant arthritis is reduced by azathioprine. The mechanisms whereby it affects autoimmune diseases are not known. Azathioprine is immunosuppressive; delayed hypersensitivity and cellular cytotoxicity tests are suppressed to a greater degree than are antibody responses. In the rat model of adjuvant arthritis, azathioprine inhibits the lymph node hyperplasia that precedes the onset of the signs of the disease. Both the immunosuppressive and therapeutic effects in animal models are dose-related. Azathioprine is a slow-acting drug and effects may persist after the drug has been discontinued.

Pharmacokinetics: Maximum serum radioactivity occurs at 1 to 2 hours after oral radioactive azathioprine and decays with a half-life of 5 hours. This is not an estimate of the half-life of azathioprine itself but is the decay rate for all radioactive metabolites of the drug. Because of extensive metabolism, only a fraction of the radioactivity is present as azathioprine. Usual doses produce blood levels of <1 mcg/ml azathioprine and 6-MP. Blood levels are of little value for therapy since the magnitude and duration of clinical effects correlate with thiopurine nucleotide levels in tissues rather than with plasma drug levels. Azathioprine and 6-MP are 30% bound to serum proteins.

Azathioprine is cleaved in vivo to 6-MP. Both compounds are rapidly eliminated from blood and are oxidized or methylated in erythrocytes and liver; no azathioprine or 6-MP is detectable in urine after 8 hours. Conversion to inactive 6-thiouric acid by xanthine oxidase is an important degradative pathway. Proportions of metabolites are different in individual patients, and this presumably accounts for variable magnitude and duration of drug effects. Renal clearance is probably not important in predicting effectiveness or toxicity, although dose reduction is practiced in patients with poor renal function. Azathioprine and 6-MP are partially dialyzable.

(Continued on following page)

AZATHIOPRINE (Cont.)

Indications:

Renal homotransplantation: As an adjunct for the prevention of rejection in renal homotransplantation. Experience with over 16,000 transplants shows a 5 year patient survival rate of 35% to 55%, but this is dependent on donor and many other variables.

Rheumatoid arthritis: Indicated only in adult patients meeting criteria for classic or definite rheumatoid arthritis as specified by the American Rheumatism Association. Restrict use to patients with severe, active and erosive disease not responsive to conventional management. Continue rest, physiotherapy and salicylates while azathioprine is given, but it may be possible to reduce the dose of corticosteroids.

Unlabeled use: Azathioprine has been used in the treatment of chronic ulcerative colitis; however, serious adverse effects may offset its limited value.

Contraindications:

Hypersensitivity to azathioprine.

Pregnant rheumatoid arthritis patients.

Rheumatoid arthritis patients previously treated with alkylating agents (cyclophosphamide, chlorambucil, melphalan or others) may have a prohibitive risk of neoplasia if treated with azathioprine.

Warnings:

Severe leukopenia or thrombocytopenia, macrocytic anemia and severe bone marrow depression may occur in patients on azathioprine. Hematologic toxicities are dose-related, may occur late in the course of therapy and may be more severe in renal transplant patients whose homograft is undergoing rejection. Perform complete blood counts, including platelet counts, weekly during the first month, twice monthly for the second and third months of treatment, then monthly or more frequently if dosage alterations or other therapy changes are necessary. Delayed hematologic suppression may occur. Prompt reduction in dosage or temporary withdrawal of the drug may be necessary if there is a rapid fall in, or persistently low leukocyte count or other evidence of bone marrow depression. Leukopenia does not correlate with therapeutic effect; do not increase the dose intentionally to lower the white blood cell count.

Serious infections are a constant hazard for patients on chronic immunosuppression, especially for homograft recipients. Fungal, viral, bacterial and protozoal infections may be fatal and should be treated vigorously. Infection may occur as a secondary manifestation of bone marrow suppression or leukopenia. Consider reduction of azathioprine dosage or use of other drugs.

Carcinogenicity: Azathioprine is carcinogenic in animals and may increase the patient's risk of neoplasia. Renal transplant patients have an increased risk of malignancy, predominantly skin cancer and reticulum cell or lymphomatous tumors. The precise risk of neoplasia due to azathioprine has not been defined, but the risk is lower for patients with rheumatoid arthritis than for transplant recipients. However, acute myelogenous leukemia as well as solid tumors have been reported in patients with rheumatoid arthritis who have received azathioprine.

Usage in Pregnancy: Whenever possible, avoid use in pregnant patients. Azathioprine is mutagenic in both male and female animals. Chromosomal abnormalities have also been documented in patients; however, the abnormalities in humans were reversed upon discontinuance of the drug.

Azathioprine is teratogenic in rodents. Transplacental transmission of azathioprine and its metabolites has been reported in humans. Limited immunologic and other abnormalities have occurred in some infants born of renal homograft recipients. Weigh benefit versus risk before use in patients of reproductive potential. Do not use to treat rheumatoid arthritis in pregnant women.

(Continued on following page)

AZATHIOPRINE (Cont.)

Drug Interactions:

Allopurinol decreases the hepatic metabolism of azathioprine by inhibiting xanthine oxidase, thereby increasing the pharmacologic effects of azathioprine. Reduce the dose of azathioprine to approximately ⅓ to ¼ the usual dose.

Azathioprine has been reported to resist or reverse the neuromuscular blockade of **nondepolarizing muscle relaxants** (eg, tubocurarine, pancuronium).

The combined use of azathioprine with **gold, antimalarials** or **penicillamine** has not been evaluated; therefore, their use with azathioprine cannot be recommended.

Adverse Reactions:

The principal and potentially serious toxic effects are hematologic and gastrointestinal. The risks of secondary infection and neoplasia are also important. The frequency and severity of adverse reactions depend on the dose and duration, as well as on the patient's underlying disease or concomitant therapies. The incidence of hematologic toxicities and neoplasia encountered in groups of renal homograft recipients is significantly higher than that in rheumatoid arthritis patients. The relative incidences in clinical studies are summarized below:

Toxicity	Renal Homograft	Rheumatoid Arthritis
Leukopenia		
Any Degree	< 50%	28%
< 2500/mm³	16%	5.3%
Neoplasia		
Lymphoma	0.5%	*
Others	2.8%	

* 18 reported cases; denominator unknown.

Hematologic: Leukopenia or thrombocytopenia; dose reduction or temporary withdrawal allows reversal. The incidence of infection in renal homotransplantation is 30 to 60 times that in rheumatoid arthritis. Macrocytic anemia or bleeding and selective erythrocyte aplasia have also been reported.

GI: Nausea and vomiting may occur within the first few months of therapy (12% of 676 rheumatoid arthritis patients). The frequency of gastric disturbance can be reduced by administration in divided doses or after meals. Vomiting with abdominal pain may occur rarely with a hypersensitivity pancreatitis. Diarrhea and steatorrhea have been reported (< 1%).

Hepatotoxicity with elevated serum alkaline phosphatase and bilirubin may occur. This toxic hepatitis with biliary stasis is known to occur in homograft recipients and has been generally reversible after interruption of azathioprine. Hepatotoxicity has been uncommon in rheumatoid arthritis patients (< 1%).

Other: Skin rashes (≈ 2%); alopecia, fever, arthralgias and negative nitrogen balance (< 1%); hypotension (rare).

(Continued on following page)

AZATHIOPRINE (Cont.)

Patient Information:

If GI upset occurs, administer in divided doses or take with food.

Notify physician if any of the following occurs: Unusual bleeding or bruising, fever, sore throat, mouth sores, signs of infection, abdominal pain, pale stools or darkened urine.

May cause nausea, vomiting, skin rash, fever, arthralgias and diarrhea; notify physician if these persist or become bothersome.

Administration and Dosage:

Renal homotransplantation: The dose required to prevent rejection and minimize toxicity varies. Initial dose is usually 3 to 5 mg/kg/day, given as a single daily dose on the day of transplantation, and in a minority of cases, 1 to 3 days before transplantation. It is often initiated IV, with subsequent use of tablets (at the same dose level) after the post-operative period. Reserve IV administration for patients unable to tolerate oral medications. Maintenance levels are 1 to 3 mg/kg/day. Do not increase the dose to toxic levels because of threatened rejection. Discontinuation may be necessary for severe hematologic or other toxicity, even if homograft rejection may be a consequence.

Rheumatoid arthritis: Usually given daily. Initial dose should be approximately 1 mg/kg (50 to 100 mg) given as a single dose or twice daily. The dose may be increased, beginning at 6 to 8 weeks and thereafter by steps at 4 week intervals, if there are no serious toxicities and if initial response is unsatisfactory. Dose increments should be 0.5 mg/kg/day, up to a maximum dose of 2.5 mg/kg/day.

Therapeutic response occurs after 6 to 8 weeks of treatment; an adequate trial should be a minimum of 12 weeks. Patients not improved after 12 weeks are refractory. Continue the drug in patients with clinical response, but monitor carefully, and attempt gradual dosage reduction to reduce risk of toxicity. Maintenance therapy should be at the lowest effective dose; lower incrementally with changes of 0.5 mg/kg or approximately 25 mg/day every 4 weeks while other therapy is kept constant. Azathioprine can be discontinued abruptly, but delayed effects are possible.

Use in renal dysfunction: Relatively oliguric patients, especially those with tubular necrosis in the immediate postcadaveric transplant period, may have delayed clearance of azathioprine or its metabolites. They may be particularly sensitive to this drug and may require lower doses.

Use with allopurinol: Reduce dose of azathioprine to approximately ⅓ to ¼ the usual dose.

Parenteral administration: For IV use only. Add 10 ml Sterile Water for Injection; use within 24 hours. Further dilution into sterile saline or dextrose is usually made for infusion. The final volume depends on the infusion time, it is usually 30 to 60 minutes, but ranges from 5 minutes to 8 hours for the daily dose.

Rx	**Azathioprine Sodium** (Quad)	**Injection:** 100 mg (as sodium) per vial. In 20 ml vials.
Rx	**Imuran** (Burroughs Wellcome)	**Tablets:** 50 mg. (#Imuran 50). Yellow, scored. In 100s. **Injection:** 100 mg (as sodium) per vial. In 20 ml vials.

Product identification code.

CYCLOSPORINE (Cyclosporin A)

Warning:

Only physicians experienced in immunosuppressive therapy and management of organ transplant patients should prescribe cyclosporine. Manage patients in facilities equipped and staffed with adequate laboratory and supportive medical resources.

Administer cyclosporine with adrenal corticosteroids but not with other immunosuppressive agents. Increased susceptibility to infection and the possible development of lymphoma may result from immunosuppression.

Absorption during chronic use is erratic. Monitor blood levels at repeated intervals in patients taking the oral solution or capsules and make dose adjustments to avoid toxicity (high levels) or possible organ rejection (low absorption). This is of special importance in liver transplants (see Administration and Dosage).

Actions:

Cyclosporine is a cyclic polypeptide immunosuppressant consisting of 11 amino acids. It is produced as a metabolite by the fungus species *Tolypocladium inflatum Gams*. It is a potent immunosuppressive agent which prolongs survival of allogeneic transplants involving skin, heart, kidneys, pancreas, bone marrow, small intestine and lungs in animals. Cyclosporine suppresses some humoral immunity and, to a greater extent, cell-mediated reactions such as allograft rejection, delayed hypersensitivity, experimental allergic encephalomyelitis, Freund's adjuvant arthritis and graft vs host disease in many animal species for a variety of organs.

Pharmacology: Exact mechanism of action is unknown. Experimental evidence suggests that the action is due to specific and reversible inhibition of immunocompetent lymphocytes in the G_0 or G_1-phase of the cell cycle. T-lymphocytes are preferentially inhibited. The T-helper cell is the main target, but the T-suppressor cell may also be suppressed. Cyclosporine also inhibits lymphokine production and release including interleukin-2 or T-cell growth factor (TCGF). Cyclosporine does not cause bone marrow suppression.

Pharmacokinetics: Absorption from the GI tract is incomplete and variable. Peak blood and plasma concentrations are achieved at about 3.5 hours. Peak concentrations and area under the plasma or blood concentration-time curve (AUC) increase with administered dose; for blood, the relationship is curvilinear (parabolic) between 0 and 1400 mg. Peak concentration is ≈ 1 ng/ml/mg of dose for plasma and 2.7 to 1.4 ng/ml/mg of dose for blood (for low to high doses). Absolute bioavailability of oral solution or capsules shows a wide patient variability (4% to 89%). Factors which may affect bioavailability include: 1) Food that may delay and impair absorption, 2) enterohepatic recirculation, 3) radioimmunoassay (RIA) vs high pressure liquid chromatography (HPLC) assay (RIA cross reacts with metabolites), 4) whole blood vs plasma specimen.

Distribution is largely outside the blood volume; ≈ 33% to 47% is in plasma, 4% to 9% in lymphocytes, 5% to 12% in granulocytes and 41% to 58% in erythrocytes. At high concentrations, the uptake by leukocytes and erythrocytes becomes saturated. In plasma, ≈ 90% is bound to proteins, primarily lipoproteins.

Blood level monitoring of cyclosporine may be useful in patient management. While no fixed relationships have been established, 24 hour trough values of 250 to 800 ng/ml (whole blood, RIA) or 50 to 300 ng/ml (plasma, RIA) appear to minimize side effects and rejection events. Blood level monitoring is not a replacement for renal function monitoring with serum creatinines, creatinine clearance or tissue biopsies.

Metabolism – Cyclosporine is metabolized by the cytochrome P-450 hepatic enzyme system. It is extensively metabolized to at least 17 metabolites. Only 0.1% of the dose is excreted unchanged in urine. The disposition from blood is biphasic with a terminal half-life of ≈ 19 hours (range, 10 to 27 hours).

Elimination is primarily biliary. Only 6% of the dose is excreted in urine.

Indications:

Prophylaxis of organ rejection in kidney, liver and heart allogeneic transplants in conjunction with adrenal corticosteroids; treatment of chronic rejection in patients previously treated with other immunosuppressive agents.

Unlabeled uses: Cyclosporine has had limited but successful use in other procedures including pancreas, bone marrow and heart/lung transplantation.

The following conditions have been treated with cyclosporine; oral dosages have ranged from 1 to 10 mg/kg/day: Alopecia areata; aplastic anemia; atopic dermatitis; Behcet's disease; biliary cirrhosis; Crohn's disease; dermatomyositis; Graves' ophthalmopathy; insulin-dependent diabetes mellitus (see Glucose Metabolism in Warnings); lupus nephritis; multiple sclerosis; myasthenia gravis; nephrotic syndrome; pemphigus and pemphigoid; polymyositis; psoriatic arthritis; pulmonary sarcoidosis; pyoderma gangrenosum; rheumatoid arthritis; severe psoriasis; ulcerative colitis; uveitis.

Contraindications:

Hypersensitivity to cyclosporine or polyoxyethylated castor oil.

(Continued on following page)

CYCLOSPORINE (Cyclosporin A) (Cont.)

Warnings:

Nephrotoxicity has been noted in 25%, 38% and 37% of renal, cardiac and liver transplantation cases, respectively. Mild nephrotoxicity was generally noted 2 to 3 months after transplant and consisted of an arrest in the fall of preoperative elevations of BUN and creatinine at a range of 35 to 45 mg/dl and 2 to 2.5 mg/dl, respectively. These elevations were often responsive to dosage reduction. More overt nephrotoxicity was seen early after transplantation and was characterized by a rapidly rising BUN and creatinine. These elevations in renal transplant patients do not necessarily indicate rejection; this form of nephrotoxicity is also usually responsive to dosage reduction. In one study, the use of transdermal clonidine before and after surgery decreased the frequency of nephrotoxicity.

Hepatotoxicity has been noted in 4%, 7% and 4% of renal, cardiac and liver transplantation cases, respectively. This usually occurred during the first month of therapy when high doses of cyclosporine were used and consisted of elevations of hepatic enzymes and bilirubin. The chemistry elevations usually decreased with a reduction in dosage.

Thrombocytopenia and microangiopathic hemolytic anemia syndrome, which may result in graft failure, occasionally develops. Neither pathogenesis nor management of this syndrome is clear.

Significant hyperkalemia and hyperuricemia occasionally occur.

Lymphomas have developed in patients receiving cyclosporine and other forms of immunosuppressive therapy after transplantation, although no causal relationship has been established. With cyclosporine, some patients have developed a lymphoproliferative disorder, which regresses when the drug is discontinued.

Convulsions have occurred in adult and pediatric patients receiving cyclosporine, particularly in combination with high-dose methylprednisolone.

Anaphylactic reactions are rare (≈ 1 in 1000) in patients on cyclosporine IV. Although the exact cause of these reactions is unknown, it is believed to be due to the polyoxyethylated castor oil used as vehicle for IV formulation. Reactions have consisted of flushing of face and upper thorax, acute respiratory distress with dyspnea and wheezing, blood pressure changes and tachycardia. One patient died after respiratory arrest and aspiration pneumonia. In some cases, the reaction subsided after infusion was stopped.

Continuously observe patients on IV cyclosporine for at least the first 30 minutes after start of infusion and frequently thereafter. If anaphylaxis occurs, stop infusion. Have available an aqueous solution of epinephrine 1:1000 and an oxygen source.

Anaphylactic reactions have not been reported with oral doseforms which lack polyoxyethylated castor oil. Patients experiencing anaphylactic reactions were treated subsequently with capsules or with oral solution without incident.

CNS toxicity may include: Headache; flushing; confusion; seizures; ataxia; hallucinations; mania; depression; encephalopathy; sleep problems; blurred vision. Various studies have associated these symptoms with low cholesterol, low magnesium, aluminum overload, high-dose methylprednisolone, nephrotoxicity and hypertension.

Lipids: In one study, cyclosporine significantly increased total cholesterol, LDL and apolipoprotein B levels. It is not known if these changes persist over long periods.

Glucose metabolism: There are conflicting reports of the drug's effects on glucose metabolism. Kidney transplant patients have developed insulin-dependent diabetes mellitus after treatment with cyclosporine and prednisolone. The diabetes caused by β-cell toxicity appears dose-related and reversible. Conversely, cyclosporine preserved β-cell function and produced an insulin-independent state in many newly diagnosed insulin-dependent diabetics.

Renal function impairment at any time requires close monitoring and possibly frequent dosage adjustment. In patients with persistent high elevations of BUN and creatinine who are unresponsive to dosage adjustments, consider switching to other immunosuppressive therapy. In the event of severe and unremitting rejection, it is preferable to allow the kidney transplant to be rejected and removed rather than increase the cyclosporine dosage to a very high level in an attempt to reverse the rejection.

Pregnancy: Category C. Cyclosporine is embryotoxic and fetotoxic in rats and rabbits when given in doses 2 to 5 times the human dose. The drug readily crosses the placenta. Safety for use during pregnancy has not been established; however, based on a relatively small number of cases, cyclosporine use during pregnancy does not pose a major fetal risk, and limited experience indicates that it is unlikely that it is a teratogen in humans. Use only when clearly needed and when the potential benefits outweigh the potential hazards to the fetus.

Lactation: Avoid nursing; cyclosporine is excreted in breast milk.

Children: Safety and efficacy have not been established. Patients as young as 6 months of age have received the drug with no unusual adverse effects.

(Continued on following page)

CYCLOSPORINE (Cyclosporin A) (Cont.)

Precautions:

Malabsorption: Patients with malabsorption may have difficulty achieving therapeutic levels with oral use.

Potassium-sparing diuretics should not be used concomitantly with cyclosporine, given its hyperkalemic effect.

Hypertension is a fairly common side effect. In some patients with cardiac transplants, antihypertensive therapy was required.

Hypertension appears to be most severe in children. It is not consistently associated with dose, concentration, duration or prior history of hypertension. Although no specific antihypertensive treatment has been shown to be more effective, angiotensin converting enzyme inhibitors do not appear to be effective.

Laboratory test monitoring: Repeatedly assess renal and liver functions by measurement of BUN, serum creatinine, serum bilirubin and liver enzymes. Inform patients of the necessity of repeated laboratory tests while receiving the drug.

Drug Interactions:

Pharmacokinetic Interactions with Cyclosporine		
Drug	Effects on cyclosporine	Mechanism
Carbamazepine Phenobarbital Phenytoin Rifampin	Decreased half-life and blood levels; possible rejection of transplanted organ	Increased cyclosporine metabolism; induction of P-450 enzyme system; decreased absorption (phenytoin)
Sulfamethazine/ Trimethoprim IV	Decreased serum levels and possible rejection of transplanted organ	Unknown
Diltiazem Erythromycin Fluconazole Ketoconazole[1] Nicardipine	Increased half-life, blood levels and immunosuppression; possible nephrotoxicity	Inhibition of cyclosporine metabolism; inhibition of biliary excretion and increased absorption (erythromycin); unknown (fluconazole)
Imipenem-cilastatin	Increased blood levels and CNS toxicity	Possible inhibition of cyclosporine metabolism
Methylprednisolone (high-dose) Prednisolone	Increased plasma levels (RIA); decreased blood levels (HPLC)	Inhibition of cyclosporine metabolism (inhibition of P-450 enzyme system)
Metoclopramide	Increased bioavailability and plasma levels	Increased absorption

Pharmacologic Interactions with Cyclosporine		
Drug	Effects	Mechanism
Aminoglycosides Amphotericin B NSAIDs TMP-SMZ	Nephrotoxicity	Interacts at tubular or glomerular level; possible effect on prostaglandins (NSAIDs)
Melphalan Quinolones	Nephrotoxicity	Unknown
Methylprednisolone	Convulsions	Unknown
Azathioprine Corticosteroids Cyclophosphamide	Increased immunosuppression; possible infection; malignancy (see Warning box)	Lymphocytes suppressed
Verapamil	Increased immunosuppression	Lymphocytes suppressed
Digoxin	Elevated digoxin levels with toxicity may occur	Unknown; most likely pharmacokinetic in origin
Nondepolarizing muscle relaxants	Prolonged neuromuscular blockade	Unknown; however, possible inhibition of metabolism by cyclosporine may be involved

[1] Since the effect on cyclosporine levels is consistent and predictable, this interaction has been used beneficially to decrease cyclosporine dosage in some patients.

(Continued on following page)

CYCLOSPORINE (Cyclosporin A) (Cont.)

Adverse Reactions:

Principal reactions: Renal dysfunction; tremor; hirsutism; hypertension; gum hyperplasia.

Cyclosporine Adverse Reactions

Body system/ adverse reaction	Randomized kidney patients: Cyclosporine (n = 227)	Randomized kidney patients: Azathioprine (n = 228)	All cyclosporine patients (n = 892) (kidney, heart, liver transplants)
GU			
Renal dysfunction	32%	6%	25%-38%
Hematuria			Rare
Cardiovascular			
Hypertension	26%	18%	13%-53%
Cramps	4%	< 1%	≤ 2%
Myocardial infarction			Rare
Skin			
Hirsutism	21%	< 1%	21%-45%
Acne	6%	8%	1%-2%
Brittle finger nails			≤ 2%
Hair breaking, pruritus			Rare
CNS			
Tremor	12%	0	21%-55%
Convulsions	3%	1%	1%-5%
Headache	2%	< 1%	2%-15%
Confusion			≤ 2%
Anxiety, depression, lethargy, weakness			Rare
GI			
Gum hyperplasia	4%	0	5%-16%
Diarrhea	3%	< 1%	3%-8%
Nausea/vomiting	2%	< 1%	4%-10%
Hepatotoxicity	< 1%	< 1%	4%-7%
Abdominal discomfort	< 1%	0	≤ 7%
Anorexia, gastritis, peptic ulcer, hiccoughs			≤ 2%
Mouth sores, swallowing difficulty, upper GI bleeding, pancreatitis, constipation			Rare
Autonomic nervous system			
Paresthesia	3%	0	1%-2%
Flushing	< 1%	0	≤ 4%
Night sweats			Rare
Hematopoietic			
Leukopenia	2%	19%	≤ 6%
Lymphoma	< 1%	0	1%-6%
Anemia, thrombocytopenia			≤ 2%
Miscellaneous			
Gynecomastia	< 1%	0	≤ 4%
Sinusitis	< 1%	0	3%-7%
Allergic reactions, conjunctivitis, edema, fever, hearing loss, tinnitus, hyperglycemia, muscle pain			≤ 2%
Chest/joint pain, tingling, visual disturbances, weight loss			Rare

Infectious complications developed in approximately 74% of patients on cyclosporine, compared to 94% receiving standard therapy.

Discontinuation of cyclosporine therapy occurred in 10% to 11.3% of 705 patients, primarily because of renal toxicity, infection, acute tubular necrosis and lack of efficacy.

Polyoxyethylated castor oil is known to cause hyperlipemia and electrophoretic abnormalities of lipoproteins. These effects are reversible upon discontinuation of treatment but are usually not a reason to stop treatment.

Overdosage:

There is minimal experience with overdosage. Because of the slow absorption of oral cyclosporine, forced emesis would be of value up to 2 hours after administration. Transient hepatotoxicity and nephrotoxicity may occur, which should resolve following drug withdrawal. In two children, cyclosporine levels were only moderately increased above therapeutic levels despite a tenfold oral overdose. Follow general supportive measures and symptomatic treatment in all cases of overdosage. Refer to General Management of Acute Overdosage. Cyclosporine is not dialyzable to any great extent, nor is it cleared well by charcoal hemoperfusion.

(Continued on following page)

CYCLOSPORINE (Cyclosporin A) (Cont.)

Patient Information:

To improve the flavor of the oral solution, dilute with milk, chocolate milk or orange juice (preferably at room temperature). Use a glass container when taking this medication. Do not allow it to stand before drinking. Stir oral solution well and drink all at once. Rinse glass and drink again to assure that the entire dose was taken.

See your physician regularly to assure that the drug is working properly and that no serious side effects are developing. Do not stop taking this medication unless advised to do so. Contact your physician if fever, sore throat, tiredness or unusual bleeding or bruising occurs.

Use mechanical contraceptive measures (eg, diaphragm, condom) during cyclosporine treatment. Do not use oral contraceptives.

Administration and Dosage:

Oral: Initially – 15 mg/kg/day 4 to 12 hours prior to transplantation (14 to 18 mg/kg/day were used in most clinical trials). Continue dose postoperatively for 1 to 2 weeks, then taper by 5% per week to a maintenance level of 5 to 10 mg/kg/day. In several studies, pediatric patients tolerated and required higher doses of cyclosporine. Some centers successfully tapered the dose to as low as 3 mg/kg in selected renal transplant patients without an apparent rise in rejection rate.

Solution may be mixed with milk, chocolate milk or orange juice, preferably at room temperature. Stir well and drink at once. Do not allow it to stand before drinking. Use a glass container and rinse with more diluent to ensure that the total dose is taken. After use, dry outside of pipette and replace in cover. Do not rinse with water or other cleaning agents.

In one large controlled study in renal transplantation, a lower initial dose of 10 mg/kg/day was used after a preoperative oral dose of 20 mg/kg. Dosage was adjusted to achieve specific plasma levels as determined by RIA. During the first few weeks after transplant, trough plasma levels of 150 to 250 ng/ml were sought. By 3 months post-transplant, trough plasma levels of 50 to 150 ng/ml were sought. These values correspond to trough whole blood levels of 450 to 750 ng/ml and 150 to 450 ng/ml. Overt nephrotoxicity was uncommon in that trial (although BUN and creatinine were somewhat increased on the average), perhaps because of the lower dose. However, do not consider such a dose unless cyclosporine level monitoring can be obtained.

Parenteral: Patients unable to take the oral solution or capsules preoperatively or postoperatively may be given the IV concentrate. Use the IV form at ⅓ the oral dose.

Initial dose – 5 to 6 mg/kg/day given 4 to 12 hours prior to transplantation as a single IV dose. Give each dose as dilute solution (50 mg per 20 to 100 ml) and administer as a slow infusion over 2 to 6 hours. Continue this daily single dose postoperatively until the patient can tolerate the oral doseforms. Switch patients to oral therapy as soon as possible after surgery.

Dilution – Immediately before use, dilute 1 ml concentrate in 20 to 100 ml of 0.9% Sodium Chloride Injection or 5% Dextrose Injection; give in a slow IV infusion over approximately 2 to 6 hours. The polyoxyethylated castor oil contained in the concentrate for IV infusion can cause phthalate stripping from PVC.

Children: The same dose and dosing regimen may be used although higher doses may be required.

Adjunctive steroid therapy. Studies used prednisone in different tapering schedules with seemingly similar results. One center started with 2 mg/kg/day for days 0 to 4, tapered to 1 mg/kg/day by 1 week, 0.6 mg/kg/day by 2 weeks, 0.3 mg/kg/day by 1 month and reached a maintenance dose of 0.15 mg/kg/day by 2 months.

Another center started with a 200 mg dose initially, tapered by 40 mg/day until reaching 20 mg/day, and continued at this level for 60 days. A further reduction to 10 mg/day was made during the following months. Adjustments in dosage were made according to the clinical situation (see also Drug Interactions).

In one study, the coadministration of misoprostol in patients receiving cyclosporine and steroids improved renal function and reduced the incidence of acute rejection in renal transplant patients.

Storage: Store at < 30°C (86°F). Protect *IV solution* from light. Do not store *oral solution* in the refrigerator and use contents within 2 months once opened. Do not freeze.

Rx	**Sandimmune** (Sandoz)	**Capsules, soft gelatin:** 25 mg	(78/240). Pink. Oblong. In UD 30s.
		100 mg	(78/241). Rose. Oblong. In UD 30s.
		Oral Solution: 100 mg/ml[1]	In 50 ml bottles with graduated pipette.
		IV Solution: 50 mg/ml[2]	In 5 ml amps.

[1] With 12.5% alcohol. [2] With 650 mg polyoxyethylated castor oil and 32.9% alcohol.

MUROMONAB-CD3

Warnings:

Only physicians experienced in immunosuppressive therapy and management of renal transplant patients should use muromonab-CD3.

Patients receiving muromonab-CD3 should be managed in facilities equipped and staffed for cardiopulmonary resuscitation. Severe pulmonary edema has occurred in patients with fluid overload prior to treatment.

Actions:

Muromonab-CD3 is a murine monoclonal antibody to the T3 (CD3) antigen of human T cells which functions as an immunosuppressant. Muromonab-CD3 is for IV use only. The antibody is a biochemically purified IgG_{2a} immunoglobulin.

Pharmacology: Muromonab-CD3 reverses graft rejection, probably by blocking the T cell function, which plays a major role in acute renal rejection. It reacts with, and blocks the function of, a molecule (CD3) in the membrane of human T cells that is associated with the antigen recognition structure of T cells and is essential for signal transduction. Muromonab-CD3 blocks all known T cell functions, and it reacts with most peripheral T cells in blood and in body tissues.

A rapid concomitant decrease in the number of circulating CD3, CD4 and CD8 positive T cells was observed within minutes after administration. Between days 2 and 7, increasing numbers of circulating CD4 and CD8 positive cells have been observed, although CD3 positive cells are not detectable. CD3 positive cells reappear rapidly and reach pretreatment levels within a week after therapy termination. Increasing numbers of CD3 positive cells have been observed in patients during week 2 of therapy, possibly due to the development of neutralizing antibodies.

Antibodies have occurred (incidence of 21% for IgM, 86% for IgG and 29% for IgE). Mean time of appearance of IgG antibodies was 20 ± 2 days. Early IgG antibodies occur towards the end of the second week of treatment in 3% (n = 86) of patients.

Pharmacokinetics: Serum levels are measured with an enzyme-linked immunosorbent assay (ELISA). During treatment with 5 mg/day for 14 days, mean serum trough levels rose over the first 3 days and then averaged 0.9 mcg/ml on days 3 to 14.

Indications:

Treatment of acute allograft rejection in renal transplant patients.

Contraindications:

Hypersensitivity to this or any product of murine origin; patients in fluid overload, as evidenced by chest x-ray or $>$ 3% weight gain within the week prior to treatment.

Warnings:

Lymphomas: Immunosuppressive therapy can lead to increased susceptibility to infection. Further, lymphomas may follow immunosuppressive therapy, and data suggest that their occurrence is related to the intensity and duration of immunosuppression rather than the use of specific agents.

First dose: Significant fever, chills, dyspnea and malaise may occur 30 minutes to 6 hours after the first dose. Therefore, begin treatment in a facility where the patient can be monitored and which is equipped for cardiopulmonary resuscitation. The most serious first-dose reaction, potentially fatal severe pulmonary edema, has occurred infrequently (4.7% of the initial 107 patients and 0% in the subsequent 311 patients treated with first-dose restrictions). In each case, fluid overload was present before treatment. Therefore, evaluate patients for fluid overload by chest x-ray or weight gain of $>$ 3%. Weight should be $\leq$ 3% above minimum weight the week before treatment begins.

First-dose reactions may be minimized by using the recommended regimen:

Suggested Prevention/Treatment of Muromonab-CD3 First-Dose Effects		
Adverse reaction	Effective prevention or palliation	Supportive treatment
Severe pulmonary edema	• Clear chest x-ray within 24 hrs preinjection • Weight restriction to $\leq$ 3% gain over 7 days preinjection	• Prompt intubation and oxygenation • 24 hr close observation
Fever, chills	• 1 mg/kg methylprednisolone sodium succinate preinjection • Fever reduction below 37.8°C (100°F) preinjection	• Cooling blanket • Acetaminophen prn
Respiratory effects	• 100 mg hydrocortisone sodium succinate 30 min postinjection	• Additional 100 mg hydrocortisone sodium succinate prn

(Warnings continued on following page)

MUROMONAB-CD3 (Cont.)

Warnings (Cont.):

Usage in Pregnancy: Category C. It is not known whether the drug can cause fetal harm when administered to a pregnant woman or can affect reproduction capacity. Use during pregnancy only if potential benefits outweigh potential hazards to the fetus.

Usage in Children: Safety and efficacy for use in children have not been established. Patients as young as 2 years of age have had no unexpected adverse effects.

Precautions:

Bone marrow: This product contains polysorbate 80; do not use for the in vitro treatment of bone marrow.

Fever: If the patient temperature exceeds 37.8°C (100°F), lower with antipyretics before muromonab-CD3 administration.

Antibodies: The drug is a heterologous protein and induces antibodies in most patients. Presence of antibodies could limit its efficacy upon readministration and may cause serious reactions. Use caution if a second course is given.

Monitoring: Chest x-ray taken within 24 hours before initiating treatment must be clear of fluid; monitor WBCs and differentials at intervals during treatment. Monitor the drug's effect on circulating T cells expressing the CD3 antigen by in vitro assay.

Adverse Reactions:

Determinations of adverse reactions with muromonab have been primarily documented in clinical trials of renal rejection following cadaveric transplantation. These patients simultaneously received low-dose immunosuppressive therapy, primarily azathioprine and corticosteroids.

Compared to conventional treatment, patients treated with muromonab-CD3 experienced increased adverse reactions during the first 2 days. The majority (73%) of patients experienced pyrexia; of these, 2% had fevers of 40°C (104°F) or above. Other reactions included chills (57%); dyspnea (21%); chest pain (14%); vomiting (13%); wheezing (11%); nausea (11%); diarrhea (10%); tremor (10%); severe pulmonary edema ($<$ 2%). See Warnings.

Infections commonly observed in the first 45 days of therapy were due to cytomegalovirus (19%) and herpes simplex (27%). Other severe and life-threatening infections were *Staphylococcus epidermidis* (4.8%), *Pneumocystis carinii* (3.1%), *Legionella, Cryptococcus, Serratia* and gram-negative bacteria (1.6%). The incidence was not statistically different with muromonab-CD3 than with high dose steroids.

Causal relationship unclear: Anaphylaxis (one patient); serum sickness (two patients); lymphoma (two patients).

A monoclonal B-lymphoproliferative disorder, similar to Epstein-Barr virus (EBV), occurred in 1 of 22 bone marrow transplant patients. One patient with acute renal rejection developed generalized lymphoma 3 weeks after receiving 3 days of muromonab-CD3.

Patient Information:

Inform patients of expected first dose effects, which are markedly reduced on successive days of treatment.

Administration and Dosage:

Administer as an IV bolus in $<$ 1 minute. Do not give by IV infusion or in conjunction with other drug solutions.

Acute renal allograft rejection: 5 mg/day for 10 to 14 days. Begin treatment once acute renal rejection is diagnosed.

Monitor patients closely for 48 hours after the first dose. Methylprednisolone sodium succinate 1 mg/kg IV given prior to muromonab-CD3 administration, and IV hydrocortisone sodium succinate 100 mg given 30 minutes after administration, are strongly recommended to decrease the incidence of reactions to the first dose. Acetaminophen and antihistamines, given concomitantly, may reduce early reactions. Patient temperature should not exceed 37.8°C (100°F) at time of first administration (see Warnings).

Reduce concomitant immunosuppressive therapy during muromonab-CD3 administration to a daily dose of prednisone 0.5 mg/kg and azathioprine 25 mg. Reduce or discontinue cyclosporine. Resume maintenance immunosuppression $\approx$ 3 days prior to cessation of muromonab-CD3.

Preparation of solution: Draw solution into a syringe through a low protein-binding 0.2 or 0.22 micrometer (μm) filter. Discard filter and attach needle for IV bolus injection.

Because this drug is a protein solution, it may develop a few fine translucent particles which do not affect its potency.

Storage and stability: Refrigerate at 2° to 8°C (36° to 46°F). Do not freeze or shake.

Rx	**Orthoclone OKT3** (Ortho)	**Injection:** 5 mg per 5 ml	In 5 ml amps.[1]

[1]With 1 mg polysorbate 80.

Bromocriptine is also used for Parkinson's disease; refer to page 1553 for information.

BROMOCRIPTINE MESYLATE

Actions:

Pharmacology: Bromocriptine mesylate is a semisynthetic ergot alkaloid derivative which inhibits prolactin secretion with little or no effect on other pituitary hormones, except in acromegaly, where it lowers elevated blood levels of growth hormone.

It is a dopamine receptor agonist that activates postsynaptic dopamine receptors. The dopaminergic neurons in the tuberoinfundibular process modulate the secretion of prolactin from the anterior pituitary by secreting a prolactin inhibitory factor (thought to be dopamine) in the corpus striatum; the dopaminergic neurons are involved in the control of motor function. Bromocriptine significantly reduces plasma levels of prolactin in patients with hyperprolactinemia.

Clinical Pharmacology: Amenorrhea/galactorrhea/female infertility – In about 75% of cases of galactorrhea associated with amenorrhea, bromocriptine suppresses the galactorrhea and reinitiates normal ovulatory menstrual cycles, usually in 6 to 8 weeks. However, some patients respond within a few days. Others may take up to 8 months. Menses are usually reinitiated prior to complete suppression of galactorrhea.

Galactorrhea may take longer to control, depending on the degree of stimulation of the mammary tissue prior to therapy. At least a 75% reduction in secretion is usually observed after 8 to 12 weeks. Some patients fail to respond, even after 12 months.

Prevention of physiological lactation - Bromocriptine, because it inhibits prolactin secretion, prevents physiological lactation when therapy is started after delivery and is continued for 2 to 3 weeks. The drug does not act on mammary tissue to prevent lactation, as do estrogen-containing preparations.

Acromegaly - Bromocriptine produces a prompt and sustained reduction in circulating levels of serum growth hormone. Since the effects of external pituitary radiation may not become maximal for several years, adjunctive therapy with bromocriptine offers potential benefit before the effects of irradiation are manifested (see Precautions).

Pharmacokinetics: Absorption/Distribution - Peak levels are reached in 1 to 3 hours; 28% of an oral dose is absorbed from the GI tract. Blood levels following a 2.5 mg dose range from 2 to 3 ng equivalents/ml. Plasma levels range from 4 to 6 ng equivalents/ml. The drug undergoes first-pass metabolism and only 6% of the absorbed dose reaches the systemic circulation unchanged. Plasma half-life is ≈ 3 hours. Bromocriptine is 90% to 96% bound to serum albumin. Serum prolactin levels remain suppressed up to 14 hours after a single dose.

Metabolism/Excretion - Bromocriptine is completely metabolized prior to excretion; 85% to 98% of the dose is excreted in the feces. Only 2.5% to 5.5% is excreted in the urine. The major route of excretion of absorbed drug is via the bile.

Indications:

Hyperprolactinemia-associated dysfunctions: Amenorrhea with or without galactorrhea, infertility or hypogonadism. Indicated in patients with prolactin-secreting adenomas, which may be the basic underlying endocrinopathy contributing to above clinical presentations. Reduction in tumor size has been demonstrated in both male and female patients with macroadenomas. In cases where adenectomy is elected, a course of bromocriptine therapy may be used to reduce tumor mass prior to surgery.

Female infertility associated with hyperprolactinemia.

Prevention of physiological lactation (secretion, congestion and engorgement) occurring after parturition when the mother does not breast-feed, or after stillbirth or abortion.

The incidence of painful engorgement is low and usually responds to supportive therapy. Once therapy is stopped, 18% to 40% of patients experience rebound of breast secretion, congestion or engorgement (usually mild to moderate in severity).

Acromegaly: Bromocriptine, alone or as adjunctive therapy with pituitary irradiation or surgery, reduces serum growth hormone by 50% or more in approximately one-half of patients treated, although not usually to normal levels.

Parkinson's disease: See page 1553

Unlabeled Uses: Bromocriptine has been used to treat hyperprolactinemia associated with pituitary adenomas; it has caused elevated prolactin levels to normalize, causing shrinkage of macroprolactinomas. Maintenance doses of 0.625 to 10 mg/day have been used for 6 to 52 months.

Bromocriptine has also been used to treat neuroleptic malignant syndrome and cocaine addiction.

(Continued on following page)

BROMOCRIPTINE MESYLATE (Cont.)

Contraindications:

Sensitivity to ergot alkaloids; severe ischemic heart disease or peripheral vascular disease; pregnancy (see Warnings).

Warnings:

Pituitary tumors: Since hyperprolactinemia with amenorrhea/galactorrhea and infertility has been found in patients with pituitary tumors, perform evaluation of pituitary before treatment.

Symptomatic hypotension: In postpartum studies, hypotension (decrease in supine systolic and diastolic pressures of > 20 and 10 mm Hg, respectively) was observed in almost 30% of patients. On occasion, the drop in supine systolic pressure was as great as 50 to 59 mm Hg. Since decreases in blood pressure are frequently noted during the puerperium independent of drug therapy, it is likely that hypotension was not drug-induced. However, since bromocriptine causes hypotension and, rarely, hypertension, do not initiate therapy until the vital signs are stabilized and no sooner than 4 hours after delivery.

Give particular attention to patients with preeclampsia and to those who have received within the preceding 24 hours other ergot alkaloids or drugs which can alter blood pressure. Monitor blood pressure, particularly during the first few days of therapy. Exercise care when bromocriptine is administered concomitantly with other medications known to lower blood pressure.

Pregnancy: Since pregnancy is often the therapeutic objective in many hyperprolactinemic patients presenting with amenorrhea/galactorrhea and infertility, assess pituitary to detect the presence of a prolactin secreting adenoma. Advise patients not seeking pregnancy, or those harboring large adenomas, to use contraceptive measures other than oral contraceptives during treatment. Since pregnancy may occur prior to reinitiation of menses, perform a pregnancy test at least every 4 weeks during the amenorrheic period, and, once menses are reinitiated, every time a patient misses a menstrual period. Use barrier contraceptive methods during therapy since estrogen-containing oral contraceptives may increase the risk of stimulating prolactin-secreting cells. Discontinuation of bromocriptine treatment in patients with known macroadenomas has been associated with rapid regrowth of tumor and increase in serum prolactin in most cases.

Safe use of bromocriptine has not been demonstrated in pregnancy and use in pregnancy is contraindicated. If pregnancy occurs, discontinue treatment immediately and carefully observe these patients throughout pregnancy for signs and symptoms which may develop if a previously undetected prolactin-secreting tumor enlarges.

Compression of optic or other cranial nerves may occur and emergency pituitary surgery may be necessary. In most cases, compression resolves before delivery. Reinitiation of bromocriptine has produced improvement in visual fields of patients in whom nerve compression has occurred during pregnancy. The relative efficacy of bromocriptine vs surgery in preserving visual fields is not known. Evaluate patients with rapidly progressive visual field loss to decide on the most appropriate therapy.

Of 1276 reported pregnancies in women who took bromocriptine during early pregnancy, there were 1109 live born infants and 4 stillborn infants. Several patients received the drug for up to 3 months, and five were treated for the entire period of gestation. Bromocriptine has been used during the final week of pregnancy to reduce plasma levels of prolactin in cases where possible pituitary tumor expansion has occurred. Among the 1113 infants, 37 cases of congenital anomalies have been reported (9 major malformations which included 3 limb reduction defects and 28 minor malformations).

The total incidence of malformations (3.3%) and spontaneous abortions (11%) does not exceed that of the population at large. There were three hydatidiform moles, two in the same patient.

Lactation: Since bromocriptine prevents lactation, do not administer to mothers who will breastfeed.

Children: Safety and efficacy in children < 15 years of age have not been established.

(Continued on following page)

BROMOCRIPTINE MESYLATE (Cont.)

Precautions:

Acromegaly: Cold sensitive digital vasospasm has occurred in some acromegalic patients treated with bromocriptine. The response can be reversed by reducing the dosage and may be prevented by keeping the fingers warm. Cases of severe GI bleeding from peptic ulcers have been reported, some fatal. Although there is no evidence that bromocriptine increases the incidence of peptic ulcers in acromegalic patients, thoroughly investigate symptoms suggestive of peptic ulcer and treat appropriately.

Possible tumor expansion during therapy has occurred. The natural history of growth hormone secreting tumors is unknown; monitor patients. If evidence of tumor expansion develops, discontinue treatment and consider alternative procedures.

Parkinson's disease: Safety for use for > 2 years at the doses required for parkinsonism has not been established. Periodically evaluate hepatic, hematopoietic, cardiovascular and renal functions. Symptomatic hypotension can occur; therefore, use caution when treating patients receiving antihypertensive drugs (see Warnings).

High doses of bromocriptine may be associated with confusion and mental disturbances. Since parkinsonian patients may manifest mild degrees of dementia, use caution when treating such patients.

Bromocriptine, given alone or with levodopa, may cause hallucinations (auditory or visual) which usually resolve with dosage reduction; discontinuation may be required. Rarely, these have persisted for several weeks after discontinuing high dose therapy.

As with levodopa, exercise caution when administering to patients with a history of myocardial infarction who have a residual atrial, nodal or ventricular arrhythmia.

Pulmonary effects: Long-term treatment (6 to 36 months) in doses of 20 to 100 mg/day is associated with pulmonary infiltrates, pleural effusion and pleural thickening. When treatment was terminated, the changes slowly reverted towards normal.

Drug Interactions:

Antihypertensives: Exercise care when administering bromocriptine concomitantly with other medications which lower blood pressure. See Warnings.

Dopamine antagonists: Lack of or decrease in efficacy may occur in patients receiving bromocriptine concurrently with phenothiazines, butyrophenones, etc. This may be a problem particularly for patients treated with bromocriptine for macroadenomas.

Adverse Reactions:

Hyperprolactinemic indications: The incidence of adverse effects is high (69%), but they are generally mild to moderate. Therapy was discontinued in approximately 5% of patients. Adverse reactions include: Nausea (49%); headache (19%); dizziness (17%); fatigue (7%); lightheadedness, vomiting (5%); abdominal cramps (4%); nasal congestion, constipation, diarrhea, drowsiness (3%); psychosis. Occurrence of these effects may be lessened by temporarily reducing dosage to ½ tablet 2 to 3 times daily.

A slight hypotensive effect may accompany bromocriptine treatment.

A few cases of cerebrospinal fluid rhinorrhea occurred in patients receiving bromocriptine for treatment of large prolactinomas. This has occurred rarely, usually only in patients who have received previous transsphenoidal surgery, pituitary radiation, or both, and who were receiving bromocriptine for tumor recurrence. It may also occur in previously untreated patients whose tumor extends into the sphenoid sinus.

Physiological lactation: Of patients treated, 23% had at least one side effect, generally mild to moderate; therapy was discontinued in approximately 3%. Most frequent: Headache (10%); dizziness (8%); nausea (7%); vomiting (3%); fatigue (1%); syncope (0.7%); diarrhea, cramps (0.4%). Usually transient decreases in blood pressure (≥ 20 mm Hg systolic and ≥ 10 mm Hg diastolic) occurred in 28% of patients at least once during the first 3 postpartum days. Two reports of fainting during the puerperium may be related.

Six cases of isolated hypertension, three cases of hypertension and stroke (including one fatal cerebral hemorrhage), three cases of hypertension and seizures and three cases of isolated seizures have occurred. Some of these patients had toxemia (including postpartum eclampsia), and some received concomitant ergot alkaloids or other drugs which can raise the blood pressure, so that the relationship between the adverse reactions and bromocriptine is not certain.

(Adverse Reactions continued on following page)

BROMOCRIPTINE MESYLATE (Cont.)

Adverse Reactions (Cont.):

Acromegaly: Most frequent – Nausea (18%), constipation (14%), postural/orthostatic hypotension (6%), anorexia (4%), dry mouth/nasal stuffiness and indigestion/dyspepsia (4%), digital vasospasm and drowsiness/tiredness (3%) and vomiting (2%).

Less frequent (< 2%) – GI bleeding, dizziness, exacerbation of Raynaud's syndrome, headache and syncope.

Rarely (< 1%) – Hair loss, alcohol potentiation, faintness, lightheadedness, arrhythmias, ventricular tachycardia, decreased sleep requirement, visual hallucinations, lassitude, shortness of breath, bradycardia, vertigo, paresthesia, sluggishness, vasovagal attack, delusional psychosis, paranoia, insomnia, heavy headedness, reduced tolerance to cold, tingling of ears, facial pallor and muscle cramps.

Parkinson's disease: Most common – Nausea, abnormal involuntary movements, hallucinations, confusion, "on-off" phenomenon, dizziness, drowsiness, fainting, vomiting, asthenia, abdominal discomfort, visual disturbance, ataxia, insomnia, depression, hypotension, shortness of breath, constipation, vertigo.

Less common – Anorexia, anxiety, blepharospasm, dry mouth, dysphagia, edema of the feet and ankles, erythromelalgia, epileptiform seizure, fatigue, headache, lethargy, skin mottling, nasal stuffiness, nervousness, nightmares, paresthesia, skin rash, urinary frequency, urinary incontinence, urinary retention, and rarely, signs and symptoms of ergotism such as tingling of fingers, cold feet, numbness, muscle cramps of feet and legs or exacerbation of Raynaud's syndrome.

Laboratory test abnormalities: Elevations in BUN, SGOT, SGPT, GGPT, CPK, alkaline phosphatase and uric acid are usually transient and not clinically significant.

Patient Information:

Take with meals or food.

Dizziness or fainting may occur, particularly following the first dose; take the first dose while lying down. Avoid sudden changes in posture, such as rising from a sitting position. Observe caution while driving or performing other tasks requiring alertness.

Advise patients receiving bromocriptine for hyperprolactinemic states associated with macroadenoma or those who have had previous transsphenoidal surgery to report any persistent watery nasal discharge to their physician. Advise patients receiving bromocriptine for treatment of a macroadenoma that discontinuation of drug may be associated with rapid regrowth of the tumor and recurrence of original symptoms.

Use contraceptive measures (other than oral contraceptives) during treatment.

Administration and Dosage:

Hyperprolactinemic indications: Initial – 1.25 to 2.5 mg daily with meals; 2.5 mg may be added as tolerated every 3 to 7 days until optimal therapeutic response is achieved. Therapeutic dosage usually is 5 to 7.5 mg (range 2.5 to 15 mg/day).

Use a mechanical contraceptive in conjunction with therapy until normal ovulatory menstrual cycles have been restored. Contraception should then be discontinued. If menstruation does not occur within 3 days of the expected date, discontinue therapy and perform a pregnancy test.

Prevention of physiological lactation: Start therapy only after vital signs have been stabilized and no sooner than 4 hours after delivery. Dosage is 2.5 mg twice daily with meals; usual range is 2.5 mg daily to 2.5 mg, 3 times daily with meals. Continue therapy for 14 days, up to 21 days, if necessary.

Acromegaly: Virtually all patients receiving therapeutic benefit show reductions in circulating levels of growth hormone. Periodically assess growth hormone levels. If no significant reduction in hormone levels has occurred after a brief trial, adjust dosage or discontinue the drug.

Initial – 1.25 to 2.5 mg for 3 days (with food) on retiring. Add an additional 1.25 to 2.5 mg as tolerated every 3 to 7 days until the patient obtains optimal therapeutic benefit. Reevaluate patients monthly and adjust the dosage based on reductions of growth hormone. The usual optimal therapeutic dosage range varies from 20 to 30 mg per day. Maximal dosage should not exceed 100 mg per day.

Withdraw patients treated with pituitary irradiation from bromocriptine therapy on a yearly basis to assess both the clinical effects of radiation on the disease process as well as the effects of bromocriptine. Usually, a 4 to 8 week withdrawal period is adequate. Recurrence of symptoms or growth hormone increases indicates the disease process is still active. Consider further courses of bromocriptine.

Rx	**Parlodel** (Sandoz)	**Capsules:** 5 mg (as mesylate)	(#Parlodel 5 mg 78 102). Caramel and white. In 30s and 100s.
		Tablets: 2.5 mg (as mesylate)	(#Parlodel 2½ 78 17). White, scored. In 30s.

Product identification code.

HYALURONIDASE

Actions:

Hyaluronidase, a protein enzyme, is a preparation of highly purified bovine testicular hyaluronidase. The exact chemical structure of this enzyme is unknown. Hyaluronidase is available in two dosage forms.

Pharmacology: Hyaluronidase is a spreading or diffusing substance which modifies the permeability of connective tissue through the hydrolysis of hyaluronic acid, a polysaccharide found in the intracellular ground substance of connective tissue, and of certain specialized tissues. This temporarily decreases the viscosity of the cellular cement and promotes diffusion of injected fluids or of localized transudates or exudates, thus facilitating their absorption.

The rate of diffusion is proportionate to the amount of enzyme, and the extent is proportionate to the volume of solution.

Studies have demonstrated that hyaluronidase is antigenic; repeated injections of relatively large amounts of this enzyme may result in the formation of neutralizing antibodies. The reconstitution of the dermal barrier removed by intradermal injection of hyaluronidase (20, 2, 0.2, 0.02 and 0.002 U/ml) to adult humans indicated that at 24 hours the restoration of the barrier is incomplete and inversely related to the dosage of enzyme; at 48 hours, the barrier is completely restored in all treated areas.

Indications:

Adjuvant to increase the absorption and dispersion of other injected drugs.

Hypodermoclysis.

Adjunct in SC urography for improving resorption of radiopaque agents. When IV administration cannot be successfully accomplished, particularly in infants and small children.

Contraindications:

Hypersensitivity to hyaluronidase. Conduct a preliminary test for sensitivity.

Because of the danger of spreading a localized infection, do not inject into or around an infected or acutely inflamed area; do not inject into an area that is known or suspected to be cancerous.

Warnings:

When considering the administration of any other drug with hyaluronidase, consult appropriate references to determine the usual precautions for the use of the other drug; eg, when epinephrine is injected along with hyaluronidase, observe the precautions for the use of epinephrine in cardiovascular disease, thyroid disease, diabetes, digital nerve block, ischemia of the fingers and toes, etc.

Laboratory Tests: A preliminary skin test for sensitivity to hyaluronidase should be performed with an intradermal injection of approximately 0.02 ml of the solution. A positive reaction consists of a wheal with pseudopods appearing within 5 minutes, persisting for 20 to 30 minutes and accompanied by localized itching. Transient vasodilation at the site of the test, ie, erythema, is not a positive reaction.

Usage in Pregnancy: Category C. It is not known whether hyaluronidase can cause fetal harm when administered to a pregnant woman. Give hyaluronidase to a pregnant woman only if clearly needed.

Human studies on the effect of intravaginal hyaluronidase in sterility due to oligospermia indicated that hyaluronidase may aid conception. Thus, it appears that hyaluronidase may not adversely affect fertility in females.

Usage in Labor and Delivery: Administration of hyaluronidase during labor has caused no complications. No increase in blood loss or differences in cervical trauma were seen.

Usage in Lactation: It is not known whether hyaluronidase is excreted in breast milk. Exercise caution when hyaluronidase is administered to a nursing woman.

Usage in Children: Hyaluronidase may be added to small volumes of solution (up to 200 ml), such as a small clysis for infants or solutions of drugs for SC injection. Remember the potential for chemical or physical incompatibilities.

Drug Interactions:

When hyaluronidase is added to a local anesthetic agent, it hastens the onset of analgesia and tends to reduce the swelling caused by local infiltration, but the wider spread of the local anesthetic solution increases its absorption; this shortens its duration of action and tends to increase the incidence of systemic reaction.

(Continued on following page)

HYALURONIDASE (Cont.)

Adverse Reactions:

The SC administration of hyaluronidase has been associated with very few adverse reactions. Allergic reactions (urticaria) are rare. Anaphylactic-like reactions following retrobulbar block or IV injections have occurred in isolated cases. Cardiac fibrillation has been encountered once.

Overdosage:

Symptoms: Local edema or urticaria, erythema, chills, nausea, vomiting, dizziness, tachycardia and hypotension.

Treatment: Discontinue enzyme and initiate supportive measures immediately. Agents such as epinephrine, corticosteroids and antihistamines should always be available for emergency treatment. Refer to General Management of Acute Overdosage on p. vi.

Administration and Dosage:

Lyophilized powder for injection: Add 1 ml of 0.9% sodium chloride to a vial containing 150 U of hyaluronidase, and 10 ml of 0.9% sodium chloride to a vial containing 1,500 U of hyaluronidase, respectively, to provide a solution containing approximately 150 U/ml.

Absorption and dispersion of injected drugs: Add 150 U hyaluronidase to the injection solution. To prepare a solution containing epinephrine, add 0.5 ml epinephrine HCl injection (1:1000) to the above solution. Before adding hyaluronidase to a solution containing another drug, consult appropriate references regarding physical or chemical incompatibilities.

Hypodermoclysis: Insert needle with tip lying free and movable between skin and muscle; begin clysis. Fluid should start in readily without pain or lump. Then inject hyaluronidase solution into rubber tubing close to needle. An alternate method is to inject the solution under skin prior to clysis. 150 U will facilitate absorption of 1,000 ml or more of solution. Observe same precautions for restoring fluid and electrolyte balance as in IV injections. Individualize dosage, administration, and type of solution (saline, glucose, Ringer's, etc). When solutions devoid of inorganic electrolytes are given by hypodermoclysis, hypovolemia may occur. This may be prevented by using solutions containing adequate amounts of inorganic electrolytes or controlling the volume and speed of administration.

Hyaluronidase may be added to small volumes of solution (up to 200 ml), such as small clysis for infants or solutions of drugs for SC injection.

For children less than 3 years old. Limit the volume of a single clysis to 200 ml.

Premature infants or during the neonatal period. Do not exceed 25 ml/kg/day. The rate of administration should not be greater than 2 ml/minute.

Older patients – Do not exceed the rate and volume of administration employed for IV infusion.

Subcutaneous urography: With the patient prone, 75 U of hyaluronidase is injected SC over each scapula, followed by injection of the contrast medium at the same sites.

Not recommended for IV use.

Storage and Stability: Keep lyophilized hyaluronidase in a dry place. Sterile reconstituted solution may be stored below 30°C (86°F) for 2 weeks without significant loss of potency. Hyaluronidase solution must be refrigerated.

Rx	**Wydase** (Wyeth-Ayerst)	Purified bovine testicular hyaluronidase.	
		Injection, lyophilized powder:	
		150 units per vial	In 1 ml vials.[1]
		1500 units per vial	In 10 ml vials.[1]
		Injection, stabilized solution:	
		150 units per ml	In 1 and 10 ml vials.[2]

[1] With lactose and thimerosal.
[2] With sodium chloride, EDTA and thimerosal.

Warning:

Methoxsalen with ultraviolet (UV) radiation should be used only by physicians with competence in diagnosis and treatment of psoriasis and vitiligo, and with special training and experience in photochemotherapy. Constantly supervise psoralen and UV radiation therapy. For psoriasis, restrict photochemotherapy to patients with severe, recalcitrant, disabling psoriasis not adequately responsive to other forms of therapy, and only when diagnosis is supported by biopsy. Because of possible ocular damage, skin aging and skin cancer (including melanoma), inform patient of risks.

Never dispense methoxsalen lotion to a patient.

These are potent drugs, capable of producing severe burns if improperly used. Read entire monograph before prescribing or dispensing these medications.

CAUTION: *Oxsoralen-Ultra* should not be used interchangeably with regular *Oxsoralen.* This new dosage form of methoxsalen exhibits significantly greater bioavailability and earlier photosensitization onset time than previous methoxsalen dosage forms. Treat patients in accordance with the dosimetry specifically recommended for this product. Determine the minimum phototoxic dose (MPD) and phototoxic peak time after drug administration prior to onset of photochemotherapy with this dosage form.

Actions:

Pharmacology: Normal skin pigmentation is due to melanin formed by the oxidation of tyrosine to dopa (dihydroxyphenylalanine). Melanin must be activated by radiant energy in the form of UV light, preferably between 290 and 380 nm. The combination treatment regimen of psoralen (P) and UV radiation of 320 to 400 nm wavelength (UVA) is known by the acronym PUVA. Skin reactivity to UVA radiation is markedly enhanced by the ingestion of methoxsalen.

Orally administered methoxsalen reaches the skin via the blood and UVA penetrates well into the skin. If sufficient cell injury occurs in the skin, an inflammatory reaction occurs. The most obvious manifestation of this reaction is delayed erythema, which may not begin for several hours and peaks at 48 to 72 hours. The inflammation is followed over several days to weeks by repair which is manifested by increased melanization of the epidermis and thickening of the stratum corneum.

The exact mechanism of action of psoralens in the process of melanogenesis is not known. The action of these drugs depends upon the presence of functional melanocytes and their proliferation (mitotic activation) by the photoactivated psoralen. One belief is that exposure of methoxsalen-treated patients to UV light thickens the stratum corneum, induces an inflammatory reaction and increases the amount of melanin in exposed areas. The exact mechanism of action of methoxsalen with the epidermal melanocytes and keratinocytes is not known.

Methoxsalen acts as a photosensitizer; subsequent exposure to UVA can lead to cell injury. In the treatment of psoriasis, the mechanism is assumed to be DNA photodamage and resulting decrease in cell proliferation, but other vascular, leukocyte or cell regulatory mechanisms may also be involved. The best known biochemical reaction of methoxsalen is with DNA. Methoxsalen, upon photoactivation, conjugates and forms covalent bonds with DNA which leads to the formation of both monofunctional (addition to a single strand of DNA) and bifunctional (crosslinking of psoralen to both strands of DNA) adducts. Reactions with proteins have also been described.

Pharmacokinetics: Oral psoralen is more than 95% absorbed from the GI tract. Concomitant administration with food increases peak serum concentrations.

Oxsoralen-Ultra Capsules reach peak drug levels in 0.5 to 1 hour (mean = 1.8 hours) as compared to 1.5 to 6 hours (mean = 3 hours) for regular *Osxoralen* when administered with 8 ounces of milk. The maximum bioavailability of *8-MOP* is reached in 1.5 to 3 hours (mean 2 hours). Peak drug levels were twofold to threefold greater when the overall extent of drug absorption was approximately twofold greater for *Oxsoralen-Ultra Capsules* as compared to *Oxsoralen Capsules.* Detectable methoxsalen levels were observed up to 12 hours post-dose. The half-life is ≈ 2 hours. Photosensitivity studies demonstrate a shorter time of peak photosensitivity of 1.5 to 2.1 hours vs 3.9 to 4.25 hours for *Oxsoralen.* In addition, the mean minimal erythema dose for *Oxsoralen-Ultra* is substantially less than that required for *Oxsoralen.*

Methoxsalen is reversibly bound to serum albumin and is preferentially taken up by epidermal cells. Methoxsalen is rapidly metabolized. Accumulation does not occur during continuous administration; metabolism occurs in hepatic microsomal enzymes. Approximately 95% is excreted in the urine within 24 hours; 4% to 10% is excreted in the feces.

Trioxsalen possesses greater activity than methoxsalen, yet its median lethal dose is 6 times that of methoxsalen.

(Continued on following page)

Indications:

Oxsoralen, Oxsoralen-Ultra, 8-MOP: Symptomatic control of severe recalcitrant disabling psoriasis not responsive to other therapy when the diagnosis has been supported by biopsy. Administer only in conjunction with a schedule of controlled doses of long wave UV radiation.

Oxsoralen (oral and topical), 8-MOP, trioxsalen: With long wave UV radiation for repigmentation of idiopathic vitiligo.

8-MOP: With long wave UV radiation of white blood cells (photopheresis) and the UVAR System in the palliative treatment of the skin manifestations of cutaneous T-cell lymphoma (CTCL) in persons who have not been responsive to other forms of treatment. Refer to the UVAR System Operator's Manual for specific warnings, cautions, indications and instructions related to photopheresis.

Trioxsalen: For increasing tolerance to sunlight and for enhancing pigmentation.

Contraindications:

Idiosyncratic reactions to psoralen compounds; melanoma or a history of melanoma; invasive squamous cell carcinomas; aphakia (increased risk of retinal damage due to the absence of lenses). Diseases associated with photosensitivity, such as porphyria, acute lupus erythematosus, porphyria cutanea tarda, erythropoietic protoporphyria, variegate porphyria, xeroderma pigmentosum, leukoderma of infectious origin and in albinism.

Do not use with any preparation having internal or external photosensitizing capacity.

Oral trioxsalen and methoxsalen lotion are contraindicated in children $\leq$ 12 years of age.

Warnings:

Skin burning: Serious burns from either UVA or sunlight (even through window glass) can result if the recommended dosage of the drug or exposure schedules are not maintained.

Carcinoma: A 5 year prospective study of 1380 patients revealed an $\approx$ ninefold increase in risks of squamous cell carcinoma among PUVA patients. This appears greatest among patients who are fair skinned or who had pre-PUVA exposure to prolonged tar and UVB treatment, ionizing radiation or arsenic. An $\approx$ twofold increase in risk of basal cell carcinoma was also noted. Two patients developed malignant melanoma, and more than 1/5 developed macular pigmented lesions on buttocks. Observe patients with a history of previous grenz or x-ray therapy, basal cell carcinoma and arsenic therapy for signs of carcinoma.

A study in 690 patients for up to 4 years showed no increase in risk of non-melanoma skin cancer. However, patients had significantly less PUVA exposure. There is no evidence of an increased risk of melanoma in PUVA patients, but there is a need for continued evaluation of melanoma risk in these patients.

In a study in Indian patients treated for 4 years for vitiligo, 12% developed keratoses, but not cancer, in the depigmented, vitiliginous areas.

Cataracts: The concentration of methoxsalen in the lens is proportional to the serum level. If the lens is exposed to UVA during the presence of methoxsalen in the lens, photochemical action may lead to irreversible binding of methoxsalen to proteins and the DNA components of the lens. However, if the lens is shielded from UVA, the methoxsalen will diffuse out of the lens in a 24 hour period. Emphatically instruct patients to wear UVA-absorbing, wrap-around sunglasses for the 24 hours following ingestion of methoxsalen, whether exposed to direct or indirect sunlight in the open, or through window glass.

Among patients using proper eye protection, there is no evidence for a significantly increased risk of cataracts in association with PUVA therapy. Of 1380 patients, 35 have developed cataracts in the 5 years since their first PUVA treatment, an incidence comparable to that expected in a population of this size and age distribution. No relationship between PUVA dose and cataract risk has been noted.

Actinic degeneration: Exposure to sunlight or UV radiation may prematurely age the skin.

Hepatic diseases: Since hepatic biotransformation is necessary for drug urinary excretion, treat patients with hepatic insufficiency with caution.

Cardiac diseases: Do not treat patients with cardiac disease or those who may be unable to tolerate prolonged standing or exposure to heat stress in a vertical UVA chamber.

Total cumulative safe UVA dosage over long periods of time is not established.

Do not increase the dosage of **trioxsalen** and exposure time. To prevent harmful effects, instruct the patient to adhere to the prescribed dosage schedule and procedure.

Usage in Pregnancy: Category C. It is not known whether psoralens can cause fetal harm when administered to a pregnant woman or can affect reproduction capacity. Use only if clearly needed.

Usage in Lactation: It is not known whether these agents are excreted in breast milk. Exercise caution when administering to a nursing woman.

Usage in Children: Safety of methoxsalen use has not been established. Potential hazards include possible carcinogenicity and cataractogenicity, and probable actinic degeneration. Oral trioxsalen and methoxsalen lotion are contraindicated in children $\leq$ 12 years of age.

(Continued on following page)

Precautions:

Vitiligo therapy: Do not increase the dosage of methoxsalen above 0.6 mg/kg; overdosage may result in serious burning of the skin. Provide eye and skin sun protection.

Laboratory monitoring: Perform the following before therapy, retest in 6 to 12 months and conduct additional tests at more extended time periods as indicated: CBC (hemoglobin or hematocrit; WBC, if abnormal, a differential count), antinuclear antibodies, liver and renal function tests and ophthalmologic examination.

Furocoumarin-containing foods: No clinical reports or tests verify that more severe reactions may result from concomitant ingestion, but warn the patient that eating limes, figs, parsley, parsnips, mustard, carrots and celery might be dangerous.

Tartrazine sensitivity: Some of these products contain tartrazine, which may cause allergic-type reactions (including bronchial asthma) in susceptible individuals. Although the incidence of tartrazine sensitivity in the general population is low, it is frequently seen in patients who also have aspirin hypersensitivity. Specific products containing tartrazine are identified in the product listings.

Photosensitizing agents: Exercise special care in treating patients who are receiving concomitant therapy (either topically or systemically) with known photosensitizing agents such as **anthralin, coal tar** or **coal tar derivatives, griseofulvin, phenothiazines, nalidixic acid, halogenated salicylanilides** (bacteriostatic soaps), **sulfonamides, tetracyclines, thiazides** and certain organic staining dyes such as **methylene blue, toluidine blue, rose bengal** and **methyl orange**.

Adverse Reactions:

Severe burns can result from excessive sunlight or sunlamp UV exposure.

Basal cell epitheliomas have been removed from exposed and unexposed areas.

Nausea is common (10%).

Other effects of **methoxsalen** include nervousness; insomnia; psychological depression; edema; dizziness; headache; malaise; hypopigmentation; vesiculation and bullae formation; nonspecific rash; herpes simplex; miliaria; urticaria; folliculitis; GI disturbances; cutaneous tenderness; leg cramps; hypotension; extension of psoriasis and depression.

Combined methoxsalen/UVA therapy:

Pruritus (approximately 10%) - Alleviate with frequent application of bland emollients or other topical agents; severe pruritus may require systemic treatment. If pruritus is unresponsive, shield pruritic areas from further UVA exposure until the condition resolves. If intractable pruritus is generalized, discontinue UVA treatment until pruritus disappears.

Erythema - Mild, transient erythema 24 to 48 hours after PUVA therapy is expected; it indicates a therapeutic interaction between methoxsalen and UVA. Shield any area showing moderate erythema during subsequent UVA exposures until the erythema has resolved. Erythema greater than Grade 2 which appears within 24 hours after UVA treatment may signal a potentially severe burn. Erythema may worsen progressively over the next 24 hours since peak erythemal reaction characteristically occurs 48 hours or later after methoxsalen ingestion. Protect the patient from further UVA exposures and sunlight; monitor closely.

Overdosage:

Induce emesis within the first 2 to 3 hours after ingestion of **methoxsalen,** since maximum blood levels are reached by this time. Follow accepted procedures for treatment of severe burns. Keep the individual in a darkened room for 8 to 24 or more hours or until cutaneous reactions subside.

Patient Information:

Use **topical methoxsalen** only on small, well defined lesions which can be protected by clothing from subsequent exposure to radiant energy. If used to treat vitiligo of face or hands, keep the treated area protected from light by use of protective clothing or sunscreens. The area of application may be highly photosensitive for several days and may result in severe burns if exposed to additional UV or sunlight.

Before methoxsalen ingestion: Do not sunbathe during the 24 hours prior to methoxsalen ingestion and UV exposure. Sunburn may prevent an accurate evaluation of the patient's response to photochemotherapy.

(Patient Information continued on following page)

Patient Information (Cont.):

After methoxsalen ingestion: Wear UVA-absorbing wrap-around sunglasses during daylight for 24 hours to prevent cataracts (see Warnings). The protective eyewear must prevent entry of stray radiation to the eyes, including that which may enter from the sides of the eyewear. Visual discrimination should be permitted by the eyewear for patient well-being and comfort.

Avoid sun exposure, even through window glass or cloud cover, for at least 8 hours after methoxsalen ingestion. If sun exposure cannot be avoided, wear protective devices such as a hat and gloves, or apply sunscreens that filter out UVA radiation (eg, sunscreens with SPF $\geq$ 15). Apply sunscreens to all areas that might be exposed to the sun (including lips). Do not apply sunscreens to areas affected by psoriasis until after treatment in the UVA chamber.

During PUVA therapy, wear total UVA-absorbing/blocking goggles mechanically designed to give maximal ocular protection. Failure to do so may increase the risk of cataract formation. A radiometer can verify elimination of UVA transmission through the goggles.

Protect abdominal skin, breasts, genitalia and other sensitive areas for approximately one-third of the initial exposure time until tanning occurs. Unless affected by disease, shield male genitalia.

After combined methoxsalen/UVA therapy: Wear UVA-absorbing wrap-around sunglasses during the daylight for 24 hours after therapy. Do not sunbathe for 48 hours after therapy. Erythema or burning due to photochemotherapy and sunburn are additive.

Minimize or avoid nausea by taking the drug with milk or food, or by dividing into two doses, taken ½ hour apart.

Do not exceed prescribed dosage or exposure time.

Avoid furocoumarin-containing foods (eg, limes, figs, parsley, parsnips, mustard, carrots, celery).

METHOXSALEN (8-Methoxypsoralen, 8-MOP), ORAL

Indications:

Oxsoralen, Oxsoralen-Ultra, 8-MOP: Symptomatic control of severe, recalcitrant disabling psoriasis not responsive to other therapy when the diagnosis has been supported by biopsy. Administer only in conjunction with a schedule of controlled doses of long wave UV radiation.

Oxsoralen, 8-MOP: With long wave UV radiation for repigmentation of idiopathic vitiligo.

8-MOP: With long wave UV radiation of white blood cells (photopheresis) and the UVAR System in the palliative treatment of the skin manifestations of cutaneous T-cell lymphoma (CTCL) in persons who have not been responsive to other forms of treatment. Refer to the UVAR System Operator's Manual for specific warnings, cautions, indications and instructions related to photopheresis.

Administration and Dosage:

> **Caution:** *Oxsoralen-Ultra* represents a new methoxsalen dose form. It exhibits significantly greater bioavailability and earlier photosensitization onset time than previous forms. Evaluate patients by determining minimum phototoxic dose (MPD) and phototoxic peak time after administration prior to onset of photochemotherapy with this dosage form. Human bioavailability studies indicate the following dosage and administration directions are to be used as a guideline only.

Vitiligo (Oxsoralen, 8-MOP): 20 mg daily in one dose with milk or food, taken 2 to 4 hours before UV exposure. Therapy should be on alternate days, and never on consecutive days.

Limit exposure time to sunlight according to the following table:

SUGGESTED SUN EXPOSURE GUIDE			
	Basic Skin Color		
Exposure	Light	Medium	Dark
Initial Exposure	15 min	20 min	25 min
Second Exposure	20 min	25 min	30 min
Third Exposure	25 min	30 min	35 min
Fourth Exposure	30 min	35 min	40 min
Subsequent Exposure	Gradually increase exposure based on erythema and tenderness of amelanotic skin.		

(Administration and Dosage continued on following page)

Complete prescribing information for these products begins on page 2784

METHOXSALEN (8-Methoxypsoralen, 8-MOP), ORAL (Cont.)

Administration and Dosage (Cont.):

Psoriasis: Initial therapy – Take dose 2 hours before UVA exposure (*Oxsoralen-Ultra* – 1½ to 2 hours with low fat food or milk), according to the following table:

METHOXSALEN DOSING								
	Patient Weight							
	kg lb	< 30 < 65	30-50 65-100	51-65 101-145	66-80 146-175	81-90 176-200	91-115 201-250	> 115 > 250
Oxsoralen, 8-MOP: mg		10	20	30	40	50	60	70
Oxsoralen-Ultra Low dose: mg mg/kg		10 0.33	10 0.33	20 0.39	20 0.30	30 0.37	30 0.33	40 0.35
High-dose: mg mg/kg		10 0.33	20 0.67	30 0.59	40 0.61	50 0.62	60 0.66	70 0.61

Weight change: If the patient's weight changes during treatment and falls into an adjacent weight range/dose category, no dose change is usually required. If a weight change is sufficiently great to modify dose, adjust UVA exposure.

Doses/week: Determine the number of doses per week of methoxsalen capsules by the patient's schedule of UVA exposures. Never give treatments more often than once every other day (*Oxsoralen-Ultra* – once every day), because the full extent of phototoxic reactions may not be evident until 48 hours after each exposure.

Dosage increase: If there is no response, or only minimal response, after 15 treatments, increase dosage by 10 mg (a one-time increase). Continue this increased dosage for the remainder of the course of treatment, but do not exceed it.

Cutaneous T-cell lymphoma: Two hours after 8-MOP administration, a pint of blood is withdrawn from the patient and infused into the UVAR system. The red cells and plasma are immediately returned to the patient; before the leukocyte fraction is returned to the patient, it is exposed to UV radiation, which activates the methoxsalen. The methoxsalen becomes an alkylating agent that deactivates when no longer exposed to light. The treated white cells (unable to reproduce) are then returned to the patient. Refer to the UVAR Photopheresis System (by Therakos) for further details.

For UVA source specifications and PUVA protocols, see manufacturer information.

Rx	**Oxsoralen** (ICN Pharm)	**Capsules:** 10 mg (hard capsules)	Tartrazine. (#Elder 600). In 30s and 100s.
Rx	**Oxsoralen-Ultra**[1] (ICN Pharm)	**Capsules:** 10 mg (soft capsules)	In 50s and 100s.
Rx	**8-MOP** (ICN Pharm)	**Capsules:** 10 mg	Tartrazine. In 8s.

METHOXSALEN (8-Methoxypsoralen, 8-MOP), TOPICAL

Note: *Never dispense this product to the patient.*

Indications:

Repigmenting agent in vitiligo, used in conjunction with controlled doses of UVA (320 to 400 nm) or sunlight.

Patient Information:

Protect treated areas from light by use of a bandage, gloves or a sunscreen (particularly when treating vitiligo of the face or hands).

Administration and Dosage:

Apply lotion to a small, well defined, vitiliginous lesion, then expose this area to UVA light. Initial exposure time must not exceed one-half the minimal erythema dose.

Regulate treatment intervals by erythema response (once a week or less, depending on the results).

Pigmentation may begin after a few weeks; significant repigmentation may take up to 6 to 9 months. Periodic treatment may be needed to retain the new pigment.

Essentially, idiopathic vitiligo is reversible, but not equally in every patient. Repigmentation varies in completeness, time of onset and duration; it occurs more rapidly on fleshy regions such as the face, abdomen and buttocks, and less rapidly over bony areas such as the dorsum of the hands and feet.

Rx	**Oxsoralen** (ICN Pharm)	**Lotion:** 1%	In 30 ml.

[1] Not interchangeable with *Oxsoralen*. Refer to manufacturer's literature for complete information.

Complete prescribing information for these products begins on page 2784

TRIOXSALEN, ORAL

Indications:

Taken 2 hours before measured periods of exposure to UV light, trioxsalen facilitates:

Repigmentation of idiopathic vitiligo, not equally reversible in every patient, will vary in completeness, time of onset and duration. Repigmentation occurs more rapidly on fleshy regions (face, abdomen and buttocks), and less rapidly over bony areas (dorsum of the hands and feet). Repigmentation may begin after a few weeks; however, significant results may take 6 to 9 months, and repigmentation at the optimum level may require maintenance dosage. If follicular repigmentation is not apparent after 3 months of daily treatment, discontinue treatment.

Increasing tolerance to sunlight: In blond persons and those with fair complexions who suffer painful reactions when exposed to sunlight, trioxsalen aids in increasing resistance to solar damage. Persons who are allergic to sunlight or who exhibit sun sensitivity may benefit from the protective action. In albinism, trioxsalen will increase tolerance to sunlight, although no pigment is formed. This protective action seems to be related to the thickening of the horny layer and retention of melanin which produces a thickened melanized stratum corneum and formation of a stratum lucidum.

Enhancing pigmentation: Use of trioxsalen accelerates pigmentation only when followed by exposure to sunlight or UV irradiation. The increase in pigmentation occurs gradually within a few days of repeated exposure and may become equivalent in degree to that achieved by a full summer of sun exposure. Since sufficient pigment will have been formed within 2 weeks of continuous therapy, discontinue use beyond this period. Maintain pigmentation by periodic exposure to sunlight.

Administration and Dosage:

Wear sunglasses during exposure and protect lips with a light-screening lipstick. May be taken with food or milk.

Adults and children over 12 years of age:

Vitiligo – 10 mg daily, 2 to 4 hours before measured periods of exposure.

To increase tolerance to sunlight or to enhance pigmentation – 10 mg daily, 2 hours before measured periods of exposure to sun or UV irradiation; do not continue for longer than 14 days. Do NOT increase the dosage, as severe burning may occur.

Limit exposure time according to the following:

SUGGESTED SUN EXPOSURE GUIDE		
Exposure	**Basic Skin Color**	
	Light	Medium
Initial Exposure	15 min	20 min
Second Exposure	20 min	25 min
Third Exposure	25 min	30 min
Fourth Exposure	30 min	35 min
Subsequent Exposure	Gradually increase exposure based on erythema and tenderness.	

Rx	**Trisoralen** (ICN Pharm)	**Tablets:** 5 mg	Tartrazine. In 28s and 100s.

BETA-CAROTENE

Actions:

Beta-carotene, a vitamin A precursor, is a carotenoid pigment occurring naturally in green and yellow vegetables. In terms of vitamin activity, 0.6 mcg of dietary beta-carotene is equivalent to 0.3 mcg of vitamin A (retinol). Bioavailability of beta-carotene depends on fat in the diet to act as a carrier, and on bile in the intestinal tract for its absorption. Beta-carotene is metabolized, primarily in the intestine, to vitamin A at a rate of approximately 50% to 60% of normal dietary intake. The rate falls off rapidly as intake goes up. In humans, an appreciable amount of unchanged beta-carotene is absorbed and stored in various tissues, especially the depot fat. Small amounts may be converted to vitamin A in the liver. The vitamin A derived from beta-carotene follows the same metabolic pathway as that from dietary sources. The major route of elimination is fecal excretion.

Indications:

To reduce severity of photosensitivity reactions in patients with erythropoietic protoporphyria.

Contraindications:

Hypersensitivity to beta-carotene.

Warnings:

Beta-carotene has not been proven effective as a sunscreen.

Usage in Pregnancy: Category C. Beta-carotene caused an increase in resorption rate but was not teratogenic when given to rats at higher than recommended human doses. There are no adequate and well controlled studies in pregnant women. Use only when clearly needed and when potential benefits outweigh potential hazards to the fetus.

Usage in Lactation: It is not known whether this drug is excreted in breast milk. Exercise caution when beta-carotene is administered to a nursing mother.

Precautions:

Usage in impaired renal or hepatic function: Give with caution to patients with impaired renal or hepatic function, because safety in these conditions has not been established.

Beta-carotene fulfills normal vitamin A requirements; do not prescribe additional vitamin A.

Adverse Reactions:

Some patients may have occasional loose stools; this is sporadic and may not require drug discontinuation. Ecchymoses and arthralgia (rare) have also been reported.

Patient Information:

Take with meals.

The skin may appear slightly yellow while receiving beta-carotene therapy.

Do not increase exposure to sunlight until carotenemic (first seen as yellowness of palms and soles), usually after 2 to 6 weeks of therapy. Then increase sun exposure gradually. The protective effect is not total; patients must establish their own limits of exposure. Continue sun protection.

Administration and Dosage:

Adjust dosage depending on severity of the symptoms and patient response. Several weeks of therapy are necessary to accumulate enough beta-carotene in the skin to exert its effect. Administer either as a single daily dose or in divided doses, preferably with meals.

Adults: 30 to 300 mg/day.

Children (under 14 years of age): 30 to 150 mg/day. Capsules may be opened and contents mixed in orange or tomato juice to aid administration.

otc	**Max-Caro** (Marlyn)	**Capsules:** 15 mg	Lecithin. In 250s.
otc	**Provatene** (Solgar)	**Soft Gel Perles:** 15 mg	In 60s and 180s.
Rx	**Solatene** (Roche)	**Capsules:** 30 mg	(#Solatene/Roche). Blue and green. In 100s.

Product identification code.

The following is a list of available diagnostic aids used in office practice or by the patient at home. Those tests requiring special equipment and used primarily by commercial laboratories are not included. For complete information on specific uses, directions and characteristics of these products, consult the manufacturers' package literature.

IN VITRO DIAGNOSTIC AIDS

ACETONE (Ketone) TESTS

To detect the presence of ketones in the urine or serum.

Product	Description	Supplied
Acetest Reagent (Ames)	Tablets for urine or blood test	In 100s.
Chemstrip K (Boehringer Mannheim)	Reagent papers for urine test	In 25s and 100s.
Ketostix Strips (Ames)	Reagent strips for urine test	In 50s, 100s and UD 20s.

ALBUMIN TESTS

Screening tests to detect protein in the urine.

Product	Description	Supplied
Albustix Strips (Ames)	Reagent strips for urine test	In 100s.
Chemstrip Micral (Boehringer Mannheim)	Reagent strips for urine test	In 5s and 30s.

BACTERIURIA TESTS

Product	Description	Supplied
Microstix-3 Strips (Ames)	Test for nitrite in urine and for bacterial growth	In 25s.
Uricult (Medical Technology)	Urine culture test to detect bacteriuria and identify uropathogens	In 10s.
Isocult for Bacteriuria (SmithKline Diagnostics)	Culture test for bacteriuria	In 4s.

BILIRUBIN TEST

Product	Description	Supplied
Ictotest Tablets (Ames)	Reagent for urine test	In 100s.

BLOOD UREA NITROGEN TEST

To estimate the amount of urea nitrogen in whole blood.

Product	Description	Supplied
Azostix Strips (Ames)	Reagent strips for blood test	In 25s.

CANDIDA TEST

Product	Description	Supplied
Isocult for Candida (SmithKline Diagnostics)	Culture test for vagina.	In 4s.

CHLAMYDIA TRACHOMATIS TEST

To detect and identify *Chlamydia trachomatis* in patient specimens.

Product	Description	Supplied
Chlamydiazyme (Abbott)	Solid phase enzyme immunoassay	In 100s and 500s.
MicroTrak *Chlamydia trachomatis* Direct Specimen Test (Syva)	Slide test	In 60s.
Sure Cell Chlamydia Test (Kodak)	Antibody-based enzyme-linked immunosorbent assay	In 10s, 25s and 100s.

COLOR ALLERGY SCREENING TEST – For Professional Office Use.

For determination of Immunoglobulin E in serum.

Product	Description	Supplied
CAST (Biomerica)	Reagent test for immunoglobulin E in serum	In kit for 25 assay tubes.

GASTROINTESTINAL TESTS

Diagnostic tool for recovery of upper GI fluid without gastric intubation or chemical analysis.

Product	Description	Supplied
Entero-Test Capsules (HDC Corp.)	To identify duodenal parasites; to diagnose and locate upper GI bleeding, pH disorders, achlorhydria and esophageal reflux	In 10s and 25s.
Entero-Test Pediatric Capsules (HDC Corp.)		In 10s and 25s.
Gastro-Test (HDC Corp.)	For determining stomach pH and to diagnose and locate gastric bleeding	In 25s.

Refer to the general statement concerning these products on page 745.

GLUCOSE, BLOOD TESTS – Home Test Kits

Chemstrip bG Strips (Boehringer Mannheim)	To measure glucose in blood	In 25s and 50s.
Dextrostix Reagent Strips (Ames)		In 25s, 100s and UD 10s.
Diascan-S Reagent Strips (Home Diagnostics, Inc.)		In 50s.
Glucostix Strips (Ames)		In 50s, 100s and UD 25s.
Tracer bG Reagent Strips (Boehringer Mannheim)		In 25s and 50s.
Visidex II Reagent Strips (Ames)		In 25s.

GLUCOSE, URINE TESTS – Home Test Kits

To detect glucose in the urine to monitor diabetes mellitus.

Clinitest Tablets (Ames)	Copper sulfate reduction method	In 36s, 100s and UD 100s.
Chemstrip uG Strips (Boehringer Mannheim)	Glucose oxidase method	In 100s.
Clinistix Strips (Ames)		In 50s.
Diastix Strips (Ames)		In 50s and 100s.
Tes-Tape (Lilly)		In 100 test tape dispenser.

GONORRHEA TESTS

Used as a presumptive test for *Neisseria gonorrhoeae.*

Product	Test	Supplied
Biocult-GC (Medical Technology)	Swab test for endocervical, urethral, rectal and pharyngeal cultures	1 test per kit.
Gonodecten Test Kit (United States Packaging)[1]	Tube test for urethral discharge from males	In 10s and 25s.
Gonozyme Diagnostic Kit (Abbott)	Enzyme immunoassay for urogenital swab specimens	In 100 test kits.
Isocult for *Neisseria gonorrhoeae* (SmithKline Diagnostics)	Culture test for endocervix, rectum, urethra and pharynx	In 4s.
MicroTrak *Neisseria gonorrhoeae* Culture Test (Syva)	Slide test for endocervical, urethral, rectal, conjunctival and pharyngeal cultures	In 85 test kits.

LUNG CELL TESTS – Home Test Kit

For early detection of precancerous lung cells.

Product	Test	Supplied
Lung Check (Nix-O-Tine)	Sputum cytology test	In 3 day test kits.

MONONUCLEOSIS TESTS – For Professional Office Use

For qualitative and quantitative identification of heterophilic antibodies for the diagnosis of infectious mononucleosis.

Mono-Diff Test (Wampole)	In 20 test kits.
Mono-Latex (Wampole)	In 20, 50 and 1000 test kits.
Mono-Lisa (Medical Technology)	In 20 test kits.
Mono-Plus (Wampole)	In 24 test kits.
Monospot (Ortho Diagnostics)	In 20 test kits.
Monosticon (Organon Teknika)	In 30 and 150 test kits.
Monosticon Dri-Dot (Organon Teknika)	In 25 and 100 test kits.
Mono-Sure Test (Wampole)	In 20 test kits.
Mono-Test (Wampole)	In 40 test kits.
Mono-Test (FTB) (Wampole)	In 10 test kits.

[1] United States Packaging Corporation, 506 Clay St., LaPorte, IN 46350, (219) 362-9782.

Refer to the general statement concerning these products on page 2791

OCCULT BLOOD SCREENING TESTS

Used to detect occult blood in urine, feces or gastric contents.

Product	Use	Supplied
ColoCare (Helena Labs)	For in-home fecal testing	3 test per kit
CS-T (Helena Labs)		In 12, 25, 50, 100 test kits.
Early Detector (Warner-Lambert)		1 test per kit.
EZ Detect (Biomerica)		5 tests per kit.
Hemoccult II (SmithKline Diagnostics)	For in-home fecal sample sent to lab for assessment	In 40s, 100s and 102s.
Gastroccult (SmithKline Diagnostics)	For gastric content testing	In 40s.
Hema-Chek Slides (Ames)	For fecal testing	In 100s, 300s and 1000s.
Hematest Tablets (Ames)		In 100s.
HemeSelect (SmithKline Diagnostics)		In 40 test kits.
Hemoccult Slides (SmithKline Diagnostics)		In 100s and 1000s.
Hemoccult SENSA (SmithKline Diagnostics)		In 40 test kits.
Hemastix Strips (Ames)	For urine testing	In 50s.
EZ Detect (Biomerica)		In 50s.

OVULATION TESTS

Tests to predict time of ovulation.

Product	Use	Supplied
Answer Ovulation (Carter)	Home test	In 6 day test kits.
Clearplan Easy (Whitehall)		In 5 day test kits.
OvuGen (BioGenex)		In 6 and 10 day test kits.
OvuQUICK Self-Test (Monoclonal Antibodies)[1]		In 9 day test kits.
Color Ovulation Test (Biomerica)	Monoclonal antibody-based enzyme immunoassay test for hLH in urine	In 9 day test kits.
First Response Ovulation Predictor Test Kit (Carter Products)		1 test per kit.
Fortel Home Ovulation Test (Biomerica)		In 9 day test kits.
OvuKIT Self-Test (Monoclonal Antibodies)[1]		In 6 and 9 day test kits.

PREGNANCY TESTS – Home Test Kits

Product	Use	Supplied
Advance (Advanced Care)	Reagent in-home kit for urine testing	1 test per kit.
Answer (Carter)		1 test per kit.
Answer 2 (Carter)		2 tests per kit.
Answer Plus (Carter)		1 test per kit.
Answer Plus 2 (Carter)		2 tests per kit.
Answer Quick & Simple (Carter)		1 test per kit.
Clearblue (Whitehall)		2 tests per kit.
Clearblue Easy (Whitehall)		1 or 2 tests per kit.
Daisy 2 (Advanced Care Products)		2 tests per kit.
e.p.t. Stick Test (Warner-L)		1 test per kit.
Fact Plus (Advanced Care Products)		1 and 2 tests per kit.
First Response (Carter)		1 test per kit.

[1] Monoclonal Antibodies, 995 Benicia Avenue, Sunnyvale, CA 94086, (408) 739-2700.

Refer to the general statement concerning these products on page 2791

PREGNANCY TESTS – For Professional Office Use

Rapid screening tests for pregnancy based on presence of chorionic gonadotropin in urine.

Product	Description	How supplied
Pregnosis (Roche Labs)	Latex agglutination inhibition slide test	In 50s and 200s.
UCG-Slide Test (Wampole)		In 30s, 100s and 300s.
Abbott TestPack Plus hCG-Urine (Abbott)	Monoclonal antibody-based enzyme immunoassay	In 20s.
HCG-nostick (Organon Teknika)		In 30s.
Nimbus[1] (Biomerica)		In 25s, 50s and 100s.
Nimbus II[1] (Biomerica)		In 25s.
RAMP Urine hCG Assay (Monoclonal Antibodies)[2]		In 50s.
Wampole One-Step hCG (Wampole)	In vitro detection of human chorionic gonadotropin in serum and urine	In 3s, 24s, 96s and 500s test kits.

PSEUDOMONAS TEST

Product	Description	How supplied
Isocult for *Pseudomonas aeruginosa* (SmithKline Diagnostics)	Culture test for exudate or urine	In 4s.

RHEUMATOID FACTOR TEST

For detection of rheumatoid factor in the blood.

Product	Description	How supplied
Rheumanosticon Dri-Dot (Organon Teknika)	One-minute latex agglutination slide test	In 25s and 100s.
Rheumatex (Wampole)		In 100 test kits.
Immunex CRP (Wampole)	Two-minute latex slide test for C-reactive protein in serum	In 100 test kits.
Rheumaton (Wampole)	In vitro 2-minute hemagglutination slide test	In 20s, 50s and 150s test kits.

SICKLE CELL TEST – For Professional Office Use

A qualitative tube test for detecting hemoglobin S.

Product	Description	How supplied
Sickledex Test (Ortho Diag.)		In 12s and 100s.

STAPHYLOCOCCUS TEST

Product	Description	How supplied
Isocult for *Staphylococcus aureus* (SmithKline Diagnostics)	Culture test for exudate	In 4s.

STREPTOCOCCI TESTS – For Professional Office Use

Product	Description	How supplied
Abbott TestPack Strep A (Abbott)	Enzyme immunoassay for group A streptococci from throat	In 20s and 40s.
Sure Cell Strep A Test (Kodak)		In 10s, 25s and 100s.
Culturette 10 Minute Group A Strep ID (BD)	Latex slide agglutination test for group A streptococcal antigen on throat swabs	Kits contain materials for 55 or 200 determinations.
RapidTest Strep (SmithKline Diagnostics)		In 25s and 100s.
EZ Detect Strep-A Test (Biomerica)	Coated stick test for detection of group A streptococci from throat swab	In 3s.
Isocult Throat Streptococci (SmithKline Diagnostics)	Culture test for group A β-hemolytic streptococci	In 4s.
Respiracult-Strep (Medical Technology)	Culture test for group A β-hemolytic streptococci from throat and nasopharynx	In 10s.
Respiralex (Medical Technology)	Latex agglutination test to detect group A streptococci in throat and pharynx	In 30s and 150s.
Streptonase-B (Wampole)	Tube test for determination of streptococcal infection by serum DNase-B antibodies	1 test per kit.

[1] For serum or urine.

[2] Monoclonal Antibodies, 995 Benicia Avenue, Sunnyvale CA 94086. (408) 739-2700.

Refer to the general statement concerning these products on page 2791

TASTE FUNCTION TEST

Used to measure taste function; also used to measure taste dysfunction which may be associated with a disease condition.

Accusens T (Westport Pharmaceuticals)		Kit of 15 bottles totaling 60 ml of tastant.

TOXOPLASMOSIS TEST

TPM Test (Wampole)	Indirect hemagglutination test for *Toxoplasma gondii* antibodies in serum	In 120s.

TRICHOMONAS TEST

Isocult for *Trichomonas vaginalis* (SmithKline Diagnostics)	Culture test for urethra (or centrifuged urine) or vagina	In 4s.

VIRUS TESTS

Abbott HIVAB HIV-1 EIA (Abbott)	Enzyme immunoassay for the antibody to human immunodeficiency virus type 1 (HIV-1) in serum or plasma	In 100s and 1000s.
Abbott HIVAG-1 (Abbott)	Enzyme immunoassay for the human immunodeficiency virus type 1 (HIV-1) antigens in serum or plasma	In 100s and 1000s.
Abbott HTLV I EIA (Abbott)	To detect antibody to Human T-Lymphotropic Virus Type I in serum or plasma	In 100 test kits.
Abbott HTLV III Confirmatory EIA (Abbott)	Enzyme immunoassay for confirmation of specimens found to be positive to antibody to HTLV III	In 100s.
MicroTrak HSV 1/HSV 2 Culture Identification/Typing Test (Syva)	For identification and typing of herpes simplex virus in tissue culture	1 test per kit.
MicroTrak HSV1/HSV2 Direct Specimen Identification/Typing Test (Syva)	Slide test for identification and typing of herpes simplex virus from external lesions	In 60 test kits.
Sure Cell Herpes Test (HSV)	Monoclonal antibody-based enzyme immunoassay for HSV-1 and 2 antigens from lesions	In 10s and 25s.
Recombigen HIV-1 LA Test (Cambridge BioScience)	Recombinant antigen-latex agglutination test for detection of human antibody to HIV-1	In 100s.
Rotalex Test (Medical Technology)	Latex slide agglutination test for rotavirus in feces	1 kit.
Rubacell II (Abbott)	Passive hemagglutination (PHA) test to detect antibody to rubella virus in serum or recalcified plasma	In 100s and 1000s.
Rubazyme (Abbott)	Enzyme immunoassay for IgG antibody to rubella virus in serum	In 100s and 500s.

(Continued on following page)

Refer to the general statement concerning these products on page 2791

VIRUS TESTS (Cont.)

Product	Description	How Supplied
Virogen Herpes Slide Test (Wampole)	Latex agglutination slide test for the detection of herpes simplex virus antigens directly from lesions or cell culture	In 100s.
Virogen HSV Antibody Test (Wampole)	Latex agglutination slide test for the qualitative and quantitative detection of herpes simplex virus antibody in serum	In 100s.
Virogen Rotatest (Wampole)	Latex agglutination assay for the detection of rotavirus in feces	In 50s.
Virogen Rubella Microlatex Test (Wampole)	Latex agglutination micro latex test for the detection of rubella virus antibody in serum	In 500s.
Virogen Rubella Slide Test (Wampole)	Latex agglutination slide test for the qualitative and quantitative detection of rubella virus antibody in serum	In 100s, 500s, 3000s and 5000s.

COMBINATION TESTS

Product	Description	How Supplied
Bactigen Meningitis Panel (Wampole)	Latex agglutination slide test for the qualitative detection of *Hemophilus influenzae* type b, *Neisseria meningitidis* serogroups A/B/C/Y/W135 and *Streptococcus pneumoniae* antigens in cerebrospinal fluid, serum, urine and blood culture	In 54s.
Bactigen *Salmonella-Shigella* (Wampole)	Latex agglutination slide test for the qualitative detection of *Salmonella* or *Shigella* from cultures	In 96s.
Isocult for *N gonorrhoeae* and Candida (SmithKline Diagnostics)	Culture test for endocervix, rectum, urethra, pharynx and vagina	In 4s.
Isocult for *T vaginalis* and Candida (SmithKline Diagnostics)	Culture test for vagina and urethra (or centrifuged urine)	In 4s.

MISCELLANEOUS URINE TESTS

Product	Description	How Supplied
Nitrazine Paper (Apothecon)	For pH determination of 4.5 to 7.5 range	In rolls.
Phenistix Reagent Strips (Ames)	Test for phenylketonuria	In 50s.

Refer to general statement concerning these products on page 2791

MULTIPLE URINE TEST PRODUCTS

These products are used to make simultaneous determinations of two or more urine tests.

	Glucose	Protein	pH	Blood	Ketones	Bilirubin	Urobilinogen	Nitrite	Leukocytes	How Supplied
Chemstrip 2 GP (Boehringer Mannheim)	X	X								In 100s.
Uristix (Ames)	X	X								In 100s.
Combistix (Ames)	X	X	X							In 100s.
Hema-Combistix (Ames)	X	X	X	X						In 100s.
Uristix 4 (Ames)	X	X						X	X	In 100s.
Chemstrip 4 the OB (Boehringer Mannheim)	X	X		X					X	In 100s.
Chemstrip uGK (Boehringer Mannheim)	X				X					In 100s.
Glucose & Ketone Urine Test (Major)	X				X					In 100s.
Keto-Diastix (Ames)	X				X					In 50s and 100s.
Chemstrip 6 (Boehringer Mannheim)	X	X	X	X	X				X	In 100s.
Labstix (Ames)	X	X	X	X	X					In 100s.
Bili-Labstix (Ames)	X	X	X	X	X	X				In 100s.
Chemstrip 7 (Boehringer Mannheim)	X	X	X	X	X	X			X	In 100s.
Multistix (Ames)	X	X	X	X	X	X	X			In 100s.
Multistix SG[1] (Ames)	X	X	X	X	X	X	X			In 100s.
Multistix 7 (Ames)	X	X	X	X	X			X	X	In 100s.
Multistix 8 SG[1] (Ames)	X	X	X	X	X			X	X	In 100s.
Chemstrip 8 (Boehringer Mannheim)	X	X	X	X	X	X	X		X	In 100s.
N-Multistix (Ames)	X	X	X	X	X	X	X	X		In 100s.
N-Multistix SG[1] (Ames)	X	X	X	X	X	X	X	X		In 100s.
Multistix 9 SG[1] (Ames)	X	X	X	X	X	X		X	X	In 100s.
Multistix 10 SG[1] (Ames)	X	X	X	X	X	X	X	X	X	In 100s.
Chemstrip 10 With SG[1] (Boehringer Mannheim)	X	X	X	X	X	X	X	X	X	In 100s.
Chemstrip 9 (Boehringer Mannheim)	X	X	X	X	X	X	X	X	X	In 100s.
Multistix 9 (Ames)	X	X	X	X	X	X	X	X	X	In 100s.
Chemstrip 2 LN (Boehringer Mannheim)								X	X	In 100s.
Multistix 2 (Ames)								X	X	In 100s.

[1] Also tests specific gravity.

Refer to the general statement concerning these products on page 2791

AMINOHIPPURATE SODIUM (PAH)

For the estimation of renal plasma flow and to measure the functional capacity of the renal tubular secretory mechanism.

	Product	Form	Packaging
Rx	**Aminohippurate Sodium** (MSD)	**Injection:** 20% aqueous solution	In 10 ml vials.

HYSTEROSCOPY FLUID

For use with the hysteroscope as an aid in distending the uterine cavity and in irrigating and visualizing its surfaces.

	Product	Form	Packaging
Rx	**Hyskon** (Pharmacia)	32% w/v dextran 70 in 10% w/v dextrose	In 100 and 250 ml.

INDIGOTINDISULFONATE SODIUM INJECTION

For localizing ureteral orifices during cystoscopy and ureteral catheterization.

	Product	Form	Packaging
Rx	**Indigo Carmine Solution Ampules** (American Regent)	0.8% aqueous solution	In 5 ml amps.

INDOCYANINE GREEN

For determining cardiac output, hepatic function and liver blood flow and for ophthalmic angiography.

	Product	Form	Packaging
Rx	**Cardio-Green** (Becton Dickinson)	**Powder**	In 25 and 50 mg vials w/solvent.

INULIN

For measurement of glomerular filtration rate (GFR).

	Product	Form	Packaging
Rx	**Inulin Injection** (Iso-Tex Diagnostics)	**Injection:** 100 mg per ml	In 50 ml vials.[1]

MANNITOL

For measurement of glomerular filtration rate (GFR). For therapeutic indications, refer to pages 585 and 2054

	Product	Form	Packaging
Rx	**Mannitol IV** (Various, eg, Kendall McGaw)	**Injection:** 10%	In 1000 ml.
Rx	**Mannitol IV** (Various, eg, Abbott, Kendall McGaw)	**Injection:** 15%	In 150 and 500 ml.
Rx	**Mannitol IV** (Various, eg, Abbott, Kendall McGaw)	**Injection:** 20%	In 250 and 500 ml.
Rx	**Mannitol IV** (Various, eg, American Regent, Astra, IMS, Lyphomed, Pasadena, Schein, Steris)	**Injection:** 25%	In 50 ml vials and syringes.

D-XYLOSE

For evaluating intestinal absorption and diagnosing malabsorptive states.

	Product	Form	Packaging
otc	**Xylo-Pfan** (Adria)	**Powder**	In 25 g bottles.

[1] With 0.9% Sodium Chloride in Water for Injection.

Thyroid Function Test

PROTIRELIN

Actions:

Pharmacology: Protirelin, a synthetic tripeptide, is probably structurally identical to the natural thyrotropin-releasing hormone produced by the hypothalamus. Protirelin increases release of thyroid stimulating hormone (TSH) from the anterior pituitary. Prolactin release is also increased. Approximately 65% of acromegalic patients respond with a rise in circulating growth hormone levels; clinical significance of this is unclear.

Pharmacokinetics: Following IV administration, the mean plasma half-life is approximately 5 minutes. TSH levels rise rapidly and reach a peak in 20 to 30 minutes. The decline in TSH levels approaches baseline levels after approximately 3 hours.

Indications:

An adjunct in the diagnostic assessment of thyroid function, and an adjunct to other diagnostic procedures in patients with pituitary or hypothalamic dysfunction.

An adjunct to evaluate the effectiveness of thyrotropin suppression with a particular dose of T_4 in patients with nodular or diffuse goiter. A normal TSH baseline value and a minimal difference between the 30 minute and baseline response to protirelin injection indicates adequate suppression of the pituitary secretion of TSH.

May be used adjunctively for adjustment of thyroid hormone dosage in patients with primary hypothyroidism. A normal or slightly blunted TSH response, 30 minutes following injection, indicates adequate replacement therapy.

Warnings:

Blood pressure: Transient blood pressure changes are common. Measure blood pressure before and at frequent intervals during the first 15 minutes after administration. To minimize incidence or severity of hypotension, the patient should be supine before, during and after administration. If a clinically important change occurs, continue monitoring blood pressure until it returns to baseline. Increased systolic (usually $<$ 30 mm Hg) or diastolic pressures (usually $<$ 20 mm Hg) are observed more often than decreased pressure. These changes do not ordinarily persist $>$ 15 minutes.

More severe degrees of hypertension or hypotension, with or without syncope, have occurred in a few patients. In patients in whom such changes would be hazardous, weigh the benefit/risk ratio carefully.

Pregnancy: Reproduction studies in rabbits at 1.5 and 6 times the human dose revealed an increased number of resorption sites. There are no studies in pregnant women; safety for use has not been established. Use only when clearly needed and when potential benefits outweigh potential hazards to the fetus.

Drug Interactions:

Adrenocortical drugs: Do not withdraw maintenance doses used in the therapy of documented hypopituitarism. Glucocorticoids at physiologic doses have no significant effect on the TSH response to thyrotropin-releasing hormone, but pharmacologic doses of steroids reduce the TSH response.

Aspirin: Therapeutic doses (2 to 3.6 g/day) inhibit the TSH response to protirelin. Aspirin ingestion caused the peak level of TSH to decrease approximately 30%, as compared to values obtained without aspirin administration. In both cases, the TSH peak occurred 30 minutes after protirelin administration.

Levodopa: Chronic administration of levodopa may inhibit TSH response to protirelin.

Thyroid hormones reduce the TSH response to protirelin. Discontinue liothyronine (T_3) $\approx$ 7 days prior to testing and discontinue medications containing levothyroxine (T_4) (eg, desiccated thyroid, thyroglobulin or liotrix) at least 14 days before testing.

Do not discontinue hormone therapy when the test is used to evaluate the effectiveness of thyroid suppression with T_4 in patients with nodular or diffuse goiter, or for adjustment of thyroid dosage in patients with primary hypothyroidism.

Adverse Reactions:

Side effects, reported in about 50% of patients tested, are generally minor, occur promptly and persist for only a few minutes.

Cardiovascular: Blood pressure changes (see Warnings).

Endocrine: Breast enlargement and leakage in lactating women for up to 2 to 3 days.

Other: Most frequent – Nausea; urge to urinate; flushed sensation; lightheadedness; bad taste in mouth; abdominal discomfort; headache; dry mouth.

Less frequent – Anxiety; sweating; tightness in the throat; pressure in the chest; tingling sensation; drowsiness; headaches (sometimes severe); transient amaurosis in patients with pituitary tumors. Rarely, convulsions may occur in patients with predisposing conditions (eg, epilepsy, brain damage).

(Continued on following page)

PROTIRELIN (Cont.)

Administration and Dosage:

Administer IV bolus over 15 to 30 seconds with the patient remaining supine for an additional 15 minutes; during this time, monitor blood pressure.

Draw one blood sample for TSH assay immediately prior to injection, and obtain a second sample 30 minutes after injection.

The TSH response to protirelin is reduced by repetitive administration. If the protirelin test is repeated, an interval of 7 days is recommended.

Elevated serum lipids may interfere with the TSH assay. Thus, fasting (except in patients with hypopituitarism) or a low-fat meal is recommended prior to the test.

Adults: 500 mcg IV (range 200 to 500 mcg); 500 mcg is the optimum dose to give the maximum response. Doses > 500 mcg are unlikely to elicit a greater TSH response.

Children (6 to 16 years old): 7 mcg/kg, up to 500 mcg.

Infants and children (up to 6 years): Experience is limited in this age group; doses of 7 mcg/kg have been administered.

Interpretation of test results: TSH test results vary with the laboratory; therefore, be familiar with the TSH assay method used and the normal range for the laboratory performing the assay.

Characterization of Thyroid Function with Protirelin

Thyroid function	Baseline serum TSH (microU/ml)	Change of serum TSH (microU/ml) at 30 minutes
Euthyroidism (normal thyroid function)	≤ 10 (usually ≤ 6; 20% have < 1.5)	≥ 2 (usually 6 to 30)
Hyperthyroidism	≤ 10 (usually ≤ 4)	< 2
Primary hypothyroidism (thyroidal)	> 10 (usually 15 to 200)	≥ 2 (usually ≥ 20)
Secondary hypothyroidism (pituitary)	≤ 10 (usually ≤ 6)	< 2 (59%) 2 to 50 (41%)
Tertiary hypothyroidism (hypothalamic)	≤ 10 (often < 2)	≥ 2

Primary (thyroidal) hypothyroidism – The diagnosis is frequently supported by the finding of clearly elevated baseline TSH levels; protirelin administration to these patients generally would not be expected to yield additional useful information. Since the same response in 30 minutes is also found in normal subjects, protirelin testing does not differentiate primary hypothyroidism from normal.

Secondary (pituitary) and tertiary (hypothalamic) hypothyroidism – In the presence of evidence of hypothyroidism, a baseline TSH level < 10 microU/ml should suggest secondary or tertiary hypothyroidism. A response > 2 microU/ml is not helpful in differentiating between secondary and tertiary hypothyroidism.

Establishing the diagnosis of secondary or tertiary hypothyroidism requires a careful history and physical examination along with appropriate tests of anterior pituitary or target gland function. Do not use the protirelin test as the only laboratory determinant for establishing these diagnoses.

Rx	**Thypinone** (Abbott)	**Injection:** 500 mcg per ml	In 1 ml amps.[1]
Rx	**Relefact TRH** (Ferring)		In 1 ml amps.

[1] With 0.9 mg sodium chloride.

SODIUM IODIDE I^{123}

Actions:

Pharmacology: Sodium Iodide I^{123} ($Na^{123}I$) is readily absorbed from the upper GI tract. The iodide is distributed primarily within the extracellular fluid of the body. It is trapped and organically bound by the thyroid and concentrated by the stomach, choroid plexus and salivary glands. It is excreted by the kidneys.

The fraction of the administered dose that is accumulated in the thyroid gland may be a measure of thyroid function in the absence of unusually high or low iodine intake or administration of certain drugs which influence iodine accumulation by the thyroid gland. Accordingly, question the patient carefully regarding previous medications or procedures involving radiographic media. Healthy subjects can accumulate approximately 10% to 50% of the administered iodine dose in the thyroid gland; however, the normal and abnormal ranges are established by individual physician's criteria.

Indications:

As a diagnostic procedure in evaluating thyroid function or morphology.

Warnings:

Pregnancy: Category C. It is not known whether Sodium Iodide I^{123} can cause fetal harm when administered to a pregnant woman or can affect reproductive capacity. Give to a pregnant woman only if clearly needed. Females of childbearing age should not be studied unless the benefits anticipated from the test outweigh the possible risk of exposure to the amount of ionizing radiation associated with the test. Ideally, perform examinations using radiopharmaceuticals, especially those elective in nature, during the first few (approximately 10) days following the onset of menses.

Lactation: Since I^{123} is excreted in breast milk, substitute formula feeding for breastfeeding if the agent must be administered to the mother during lactation.

Children: Safety and efficacy in children have not been established. Children under the age of 18 should not be studied unless the benefits anticipated from the test outweigh the possible risk of exposure to the amount of ionizing radiation associated with the test.

Precautions:

The contents of the capsule are radioactive. Adequate shielding of the preparation must be maintained at all times.

Do not use after the expiration time and date stated on the label. Administer the prescribed Sodium Iodide I^{123} dose as soon as practical from the time of receipt of product (ie, as close to calibration time as possible), in order to minimize the fraction of radiation exposure due to the relative increase of radionuclidic contaminants with time.

Handle with care. Use appropriate safety measures to minimize radiation exposure to clinical personnel. Take care to minimize radiation exposure to the patient consistent with proper patient management.

Radiopharmaceuticals should be used only by physicians who are qualified by training and experience in the safe use and handling of radionuclides, and whose experience and training have been approved by the appropriate government agency authorized to license the use of radionuclides.

Adverse Reactions:

Although rare, reactions include, in decreasing order of frequency: Nausea; vomiting; chest pain; tachycardia; itching skin; rash; hives.

Administration and Dosage

The recommended oral dose for the average patient (70 kg) is 3.7 to 14.8 MBq (100 to 400 mcCi). The lower part of the dosage range is recommended for uptake studies alone, and the higher part for thyroid imaging. The determination of I^{123} concentration in the thyroid gland may be initiated at 6 hours after administering the dose; measure in accordance with standardized procedures.

Measure the patient dose by a suitable radioactivity calibration system immediately prior to administration. The capsules can be utilized up to 30 hours after calibration time and date. Thereafter, discard the capsules in accordance with standard safety procedures. The user should wear waterproof gloves at all times when handling the capsules or container.

Storage: The contents of the vial are radioactive and adequate shielding and handling precautions must be maintained. Dispense and preserve capsules in tightly closed containers that are adequately shielded. Control the storage and disposal of Sodium Iodide I^{123} capsules in a manner that is in compliance with the appropriate regulations of the government agency authorized to license the use of this radionuclide.

Rx	**Sodium Iodide I 123** (Mallinckrodt Diagnostic)	**Capsules:** 3.7 MBq sodium iodide I 123	Sucrose. Red and white. In 1s, 3s and 5s.
		7.4 MBq sodium iodide I 123	Sucrose. Green and white. In 1s, 3s and 5s.

THYROTROPIN (Thyroid Stimulating Hormone; TSH)

Actions:

Pharmacology: Thyrotropin or thyroid stimulating hormone (TSH) is a highly purified and lyophilized thyrotropic isolated from bovine anterior pituitary. The potency is designated in International-Thyrotropin units and is free of significant amounts of adrenocorticotropic, gonadotropic, somatotropic, and posterior pituitary hormones. It is a glycoprotein with a molecular weight in the range of 28,000 to 30,000. Thyrotropin produces increased uptake of iodine by the thyroid, increased formation of thyroid hormone, increased release of thyroid hormone, and cellular hyperplasia of the thyroid on prolonged stimulation.

After injection, the effect on the thyroid in normal individuals is evident within 8 hours, reaching a maximum in 24 to 48 hours.

Indications:

As a diagnostic agent to differentiate thyroid failure and to establish a diagnosis of decreased thyroid reserve.

Thyrotropin can be used for PBI or I^{131} uptake determinations.

Contraindications:

Hypersensitivity to thyrotropin; coronary thrombosis; untreated Addison's disease.

Warnings:

Anaphylactic reactions have occurred with repeated administration.

Pregnancy: Category C. It is not known whether thyrotropin can cause fetal harm when administered to a pregnant woman or can affect reproduction capacity. Give to a pregnant woman only when clearly needed.

Lactation: It is not known whether this drug is excreted in breast milk. Exercise caution when administering thyrotropin to a nursing woman.

Children: Safety and efficacy for use in children have not been established.

Precautions:

Thyrotropin can stimulate thyroid secretion; use cautiously in patients with cardiac disease who are unable to tolerate additional stress.

Adverse Reactions:

Most common: Nausea; vomiting; headache; urticaria.

Cardiovascular: Transitory hypotension; tachycardia (probably related to sensitivity reaction).

Other: Anaphylactic reactions with patient collapse; thyroid gland swelling (particularly with doses $>$ 10 IU).

Overdosage:

Symptoms: Headache; irritability; nervousness; sweating; tachycardia; increased bowel motility; menstrual irregularities. Angina pectoris or congestive heart failure may be induced or aggravated. Shock may develop. Excessive doses may result in symptoms resembling thyroid storm. Chronic excessive dosage will produce signs and symptoms of hyperthyroidism.

Treatment: Discontinue thyrotropin. In shock, consider supportive measures and treatment of unrecognized adrenal insufficiency.

Administration and Dosage:

Administer IM or SC.

Usual dose: 10 IU for 1 to 3 days. Follow by a radioiodine study 24 hours after the last injection. No response will occur in thyroid failure, but substantial response will occur in pituitary failure.

Storage: After reconstitution, store between 2° to 8°C (36° to 46°F), for not $>$ 2 weeks.

Rx	**Thytropar** (Armour)	**Powder for Injection (lyophilized):** 10 IU of thyrotropic activity/vial	With vial of diluent.

GONADORELIN HCl

Actions:

Pharmacology: A synthetic luteinizing hormone releasing hormone (LH-RH), also referred to as gonadotropin releasing hormone (GnRH). It is structurally identical to natural LH-RH.

Gonadorelin has gonadotropin releasing effects upon the anterior pituitary. Normal baseline luteinizing hormone (LH) levels are 5 to 25 mIU/ml in postpubertal males and postpubertal and premenopausal females, but levels vary with the assay method.

In menopausal and postmenopausal females, the baseline LH levels are elevated; maximum LH increases are exaggerated when compared to premenopausal levels.

Patients with clinically diagnosed or suspected pituitary or hypothalamic dysfunction often had subnormal or no LH responses following administration.

Indications:

Evaluating functional capacity and response of the gonadotropes of the anterior pituitary; testing suspected gonadotropin deficiency; evaluating residual gonadotropic function of the pituitary following removal of a pituitary tumor by surgery or irradiation.

Unlabeled uses: Ovulation inhibition (contraceptive effect); treatment of precocious puberty. Gonadorelin acetate *(Lutrepulse)* is used for the induction of ovulation in women with primary hypothalamic amenorrhea. See individual monograph in Gonadotropin Releasing Hormones section.

Contraindications:

Hypersensitivity to gonadorelin or any of the components of the product.

Warnings:

Pregnancy: Category B. No adequate and well controlled studies have been conducted in pregnant women. Repetitive, high doses of gonadorelin may cause luteolysis and inhibition of spermatogenesis. Safety for use during pregnancy has not been established; use only when clearly needed.

Precautions:

Hypersensitivity and anaphylactic reactions have occurred following multiple-dose administration. Refer to Management of Acute Hypersensitivity Reactions.

Antibody formation has rarely occurred after chronic administration of large doses.

Drug Interactions:

Androgen, estrogen, glucocorticoid and progestin containing preparations directly affect pituitary secretion of the gonadotropins. Do not conduct tests during administration of these agents.

Digoxin and oral contraceptives may suppress gonadotropin levels.

Levodopa and spironolactone may transiently elevate gonadotropin levels.

Phenothiazines and dopamine antagonists which increase prolactin may blunt the response to gonadorelin.

Adverse Reactions:

Systemic (rare): Headache; nausea; lightheadedness; abdominal discomfort; flushing.

Local: Swelling, with occasional pain, and pruritus at the SC injection site may occur. Local and generalized skin rash have been noted after chronic SC administration. See Warnings.

Rare instances of hypersensitivity reaction (bronchospasm, tachycardia, flushing, urticaria, induration at injection site) and anaphylactic reactions have occurred following multiple-dose administration. See Warnings.

Overdosage:

Administer symptomatic treatment as required. Refer to General Management of Acute Overdosage.

Administration and Dosage:

Adults: 100 mcg SC or IV. In females, perform the test in the early follicular phase (days 1 to 7) of the menstrual cycle.

For specific test methodology and interpretation of test results, refer to manufacturer's full prescribing product information.

Preparation of solution: Reconstitute 100 mcg vial with 1 ml and the 500 mcg vial with 2 ml of accompanying diluent. Prepare immediately before use. After reconstitution, store at room temperature (≈ 25°C; ≈ 77°F); use within 1 day. Discard unused solution and diluent.

Rx	**Factrel** (Wyeth-Ayerst)	**Powder for Injection:** 100 mcg (as HCl) per vial.[1] 500 mcg (as HCl) per vial.[1]	With 2 ml sterile diluent.[2]

[1] With 100 mg lactose.
[2] With 2% benzyl alcohol.

TOLBUTAMIDE SODIUM

Actions:

Patients with functioning insulinomas exhibit hypoglycemic responses to IV tolbutamide, which are distinctive from responses of normal individuals.

Administration of 1 g to healthy subjects results in a rapid fall in blood sugar levels for 30 to 45 minutes, followed by a secondary rise into the normal range in the ensuing 90 to 180 minutes. The initial hypoglycemia results from the rapid release of insulin from the pancreatic beta cells, while the secondary rise is due to activation of counter-regulatory factors. Serum insulin levels rise from a fasting mean value of 19 microU/ml to a peak mean value of ≈ 40 microU/ml (range, 27 to 89), 20 minutes after injection.

In contrast, patients with insulinomas exhibit tolbutamide-induced blood sugar decreases of greater magnitude associated with an excessive, prompt rise in serum insulin (118 to 1055 microU/ml). The magnitude of blood sugar fall in these patients is of greater significance than the persistence of hypoglycemia for 3 hours after administration. Persistent tolbutamide-induced hypoglycemia, rather than degree of blood sugar decrease, is important in the diagnosis of pancreatic islet cell adenomas.

Indications:

As an aid in the diagnosis of pancreatic islet cell adenoma. Accurate differential diagnosis of spontaneous hypoglycemia is essential to avoid subtotal pancreatic resection in patients in whom surgery is not indicated.

Contraindications:

Children (see Warnings); previous allergy to tolbutamide or related sulfonylureas.

Warnings:

False-positive responses occurred in a few patients with liver disease, alcohol hypoglycemia, idiopathic hypoglycemia of infancy, severe undernutrition, azotemia, sarcoma, and other extrapancreatic insulin-producing tumors.

Renal or hepatic function impairment: Use cautiously because severe and prolonged hypoglycemia following oral tolbutamide has occurred.

Hypoglycemia may develop, particularly in patients with fasting hypoglycemic blood sugar levels. If it occurs, terminate the test immediately; inject 12.5 to 25 g glucose IV in a 25% to 50% solution.

Anaphylaxis: Epinephrine and other resuscitative drugs should be available. Refer to Management of Acute Hypersensitivity Reactions.

Pregnancy: Category C. Teratogenic effects – Tolbutamide sodium was teratogenic in rats given doses 25 to 100 times the human dose (increased mortality in offspring and ocular and bony abnormalities). There are no adequate and well controlled studies in pregnant women. Tolbutamide is not recommended for the treatment of pregnant diabetic patients. Consider the possible hazards of the use in women of childbearing potential who might become pregnant while using the drug.

Nonteratogenic effects – Prolonged severe hypoglycemia (4 to 10 days) occurred in neonates born to mothers who were receiving a sulfonylurea drug at the time of delivery. This has occurred more frequently with the use of agents with prolonged half-lives. Use of the drug in pregnant patients is not recommended.

Lactation: Tolbutamide is excreted in small amounts in the breast milk of nursing mothers. Because of the potential for serious adverse reactions in nursing infants, discontinue nursing or discontinue the drug.

Children: Not recommended in children because of the lack of data to establish ideal dosage and the inability to interpret results.

Precautions:

Test dose-induced hypoglycemic symptoms are usually not severe; however, certain nondiabetics may develop moderate to severe symptoms. To avoid this occurrence, terminate the diagnostic test by administering carbohydrates immediately after obtaining the 30 minute blood sample, especially in the testing of persons with atherosclerosis.

Use only a true glucose procedure (Somogyi-Nelson, Modified Folin-Wu, AutoAnalyzer, or glucose oxidase) to eliminate highly variable amounts of nonglucose-reducing substances as a major source of error.

(Continued on following page)

TOLBUTAMIDE SODIUM (Cont.)

Drug Interactions:

Salicylates, sulfonamides, oxyphenbutazone, phenylbutazone, probenecid, and MAOIs may interfere with results of a tolbutamide tolerance test.

Since the tolbutamide diagnostic test involves a single injection, drug interactions that may occur with chronic tolbutamide use may not occur in this situation. However, for further information refer to the Sulfonylureas monograph.

Drug/Laboratory test interaction: On rare occasions, urine containing the tolbutamide metabolite may give a false-positive reaction for **albumin** by the usual test (acidification after boiling). Circumvent this problem by using bromphenol reagent strips.

Adverse Reactions:

Rare: Mild shoulder pain or slight burning sensation along the course of the vein during the IV injection may occur. It lasts no more than 2 to 3 minutes, is attributed to venospasm and may be obviated by administering the solution over 2 to 3 minutes.

Thrombophlebitis with thrombosis of the injected vein occurs in 0.8% to 2.4% of patients. These are usually painless, detectable only by careful palpation and may not appear for 1 or 2 weeks after injection. No sequelae have been noted. The vein gradually shrinks or recanalizes.

Overdosage:

The dose which may cause hypoglycemia is variable; usual therapeutic doses have caused symptomatic hypoglycemia.

Symptoms: Overdose of sulfonylureas, including tolbutamide, will produce symptoms of hypoglycemia. Seizures may occur with marked hypoglycemia.

Mild – Sweating; trembling; weakness; fatigue; nervousness; hunger; nausea.

Severe – Lethargy; confusion; stupor; loss of consciousness; coma.

Treatment: Treat mild symptoms of hypoglycemia without loss of consciousness with oral glucose and adjustment in drug dosage and meal patterns. Continue monitoring until the patient is out of danger. Severe hypoglycemic reactions with coma, seizure or other neurological impairment are rare, but require immediate hospitalization; give a rapid IV injection of 50% dextrose solution. Repeat as needed. Follow by a continuous infusion of 10% dextrose solution to maintain the blood glucose level above 100 mg/dl. Closely monitor patients in hospital for a minimum of 24 to 48 hours, since hypoglycemia may recur after apparent clinical recovery.

Overdosage with sulfonylurea drugs has not responded to peritoneal dialysis or hemodialysis. Experience, however, is quite limited.

Administration and Dosage:

For IV use only.

Fajans test:

1. Eat a high carbohydrate diet of 150 to 300 g/day for at least 3 days prior to test.
2. On the morning of the test, after an overnight fast, obtain a fasting blood specimen.
3. Inject 20 ml tolbutamide solution IV at a constant rate over 2 to 3 minutes.
4. Withdraw blood specimens at the following intervals (in minutes) after the midpoint of the injection: 20, 30, 45, 60, 90, 120, 150, and 180. The determination of serum insulin levels before, and at 10, 20 and 30 minutes after the IV administration, provides a specific and safer test for insulinoma, and permits the performance of the test in the presence of moderate fasting hypoglycemia, since interpretation is not based on the decline of the blood glucose.
5. Blood glucose determinations are made by the true glucose procedures.
6. Terminate the procedure with readily assimilable carbohydrates or breakfast.

Interpretation of results: Healthy subjects – A decrease in blood sugar (38% to 79% of the fasting level) may be expected. At 90 to 120 minutes, 78% to 100% of the initial level may be seen. Similar responses occur in patients with functional hyperinsulinism.

Insulinoma patients – Minimum blood sugar levels of 17% to 50% of fasting values are seen. In 90 to 180 minutes, levels range from 40% to 64%. Patients with liver disease may show the same type of blood glucose response as patients with insulinomas; use appropriate laboratory and clinical tests to distinguish between these conditions.

Inject 1 g IV at a constant rate over 2 to 3 minutes.

For specific test methodology (Fajans test) and interpretation of test results, refer to the manufacturer's full prescribing product information.

Storage: Use within 1 hour after reconstitution, but only if solution is complete and clear.

Rx	**Orinase Diagnostic** (Upjohn)	**Powder for Injection:** 1 g (as sodium) per vial with 20 ml amp of diluent.

METHACHOLINE CHLORIDE

Warnings:

Methacholine is a bronchoconstrictor for diagnostic purposes only. Perform inhalation challenge under the supervision of a physician trained in and thoroughly familiar with all aspects of the technique, all contraindications, warnings and precautions of methacholine challenge and the management of respiratory distress. Have emergency equipment and medication immediately available to treat acute respiratory distress.

Administer only by inhalation; severe bronchoconstriction and reduction in respiratory function can result. Patients with severe hyperreactivity of the airways can experience bronchoconstriction at a dosage as low as 0.025 mg/ml (0.125 cumulative units). If severe bronchoconstriction occurs, reverse immediately by administration of a rapid-acting inhaled bronchodilator (β-agonist). Do not perform methacholine challenge in any patient with clinically apparent asthma, wheezing or very low baseline pulmonary function tests (ie, FEV_1 less than 1 to 1.5 L or less than 70% of the predicted values). Consult standard nomograms for predicted values.

Actions:

Pharmacology: Methacholine Cl is a parasympathomimetic (cholinergic) bronchoconstrictor, the β-methyl homolog of acetylcholine, and differs from the latter primarily in its greater duration and selectivity of action. Bronchial smooth muscle contains significant parasympathetic innervation. Bronchoconstriction occurs when the vagus nerve is stimulated releasing acetylcholine from the nerve endings. Muscle constriction is essentially confined to the local site of release because acetylcholine is rapidly inactivated by acetylcholinesterase. Methacholine is more slowly hydrolyzed by acetylcholinesterase and is almost totally resistant to inactivation by nonspecific cholinesterase or pseudocholinesterase. Asthmatics are markedly more sensitive to inhaled methacholine-induced bronchoconstriction than are healthy subjects. This difference in response is the pharmacologic basis for the methacholine inhalation challenge.

Indications:

For the diagnosis of bronchial airway hyperreactivity in subjects who do not have clinically apparent asthma.

Contraindications:

Hypersensitivity to methacholine or other parasympathomimetics.

Repeated administration other than challenge with increasing doses.

Do not perform inhalation challenge in patients receiving any β-adrenergic blocking agent because, in such patients, responses to methacholine Cl can be exaggerated or prolonged, and may not respond as readily to treatment.

Warnings:

Usage in Pregnancy: Category C. It is not known whether this drug can cause fetal harm when administered to a pregnant patient or can affect reproductive capacity. Give to a pregnant woman only if clearly needed. In females of childbearing potential, perform inhalation challenge either within 10 days following the onset of menses or within 2 weeks of a negative pregnancy test.

Usage in Lactation: It is not known whether methacholine Cl is excreted in breast milk. Do not administer to nursing women.

Usage in Children: Safety and efficacy for use in children less than 5 years of age have not been established.

Precautions:

Do not administer to patients with epilepsy, cardiovascular disease accompanied by bradycardia, vagotonia, peptic ulcer disease, thyroid disease, urinary tract obstruction or other condition that could be adversely affected by a cholinergic agent unless the benefit to the individual outweighs the potential risk.

Adverse Reactions:

Adverse reactions associated with 153 inhaled methacholine Cl challenges include one occurrence each of headache, throat irritation, lightheadedness and itching.

Administered orally or by injection, methacholine Cl is associated with nausea, vomiting, substernal pain or pressure, hypotension, fainting and transient complete heart block.

Overdosage:

When administered orally or by injection, overdosage with methacholine Cl can result in a syncopal reaction with cardiac arrest and loss of consciousness. Treat serious toxic reactions with 0.5 to 1 mg of atropine sulfate, IM or IV.

(Continued on following page)

METHACHOLINE CHLORIDE (Cont.)

Patient Information:

Instruct patients about symptoms that may occur as a result of the test, and explain how to manage such symptoms.

Female patients should inform physician of pregnancy, the date of last onset of menses or the date and result of last pregnancy test.

Administration and Dosage:

Before inhalation challenge is begun, perform baseline pulmonary function tests. The subject to be challenged must have an FEV_1 of at least 70% of the predicted value.

The target level for a positive challenge is a 20% reduction in the FEV_1 compared with the baseline value after inhalation of the control sodium chloride solution. Calculate and record the target value before challenge is started.

Procedure: Perform the challenge by giving a subject ascending serial concentrations of methacholine. At each concentration, five breaths are administered by a nebulizer that permits intermittent delivery time of 0.6 seconds by either a Y-tube or a breath-actuated timing device (dosimeter).

At each of five inhalations of a serial concentration, the subject begins at functional residual capacity (FRC) and slowly and completely inhales the dose delivered. Within 5 minutes, FEV_1 values are determined. The procedure ends either when there is a 20% or greater reduction in the FEV_1 compared with the baseline sodium chloride solution value (ie, a positive response) or if 188.88 total cumulative units have been given (see table below) and FEV_1 has been reduced by $\leq$ 14% (ie, a negative response). If there is a reduction of 15% to 19% in the FEV_1 compared with baseline, either repeat the challenge at that concentration or give a higher concentration as long as the dosage administered does not result in total cumulative units exceeding 188.88.

The following is a suggested schedule for administration of methacholine challenge. Calculate cumulative units by multiplying number of breaths by concentration given. Total cumulative units is the sum of cumulative units for each concentration given.

Vial	Serial Concentration	Number of Breaths	Cumulative Units per Concentration	Total Cumulative Units
E	0.025 mg/ml	5	0.125	0.125
D	0.25 mg/ml	5	1.25	1.375
C	2.5 mg/ml	5	12.5	13.88
B	10 mg/ml	5	50	63.88
A	25 mg/ml	5	125	188.88

An inhaled β-agonist may be administered after methacholine challenge to expedite the return of the FEV_1 to baseline and to relieve the discomfort of the subject. Most patients revert to normal pulmonary function within 5 minutes following bronchodilators or within 30 to 45 minutes without any bronchodilator.

Dilutions: (Do not inhale powder. Do not handle this material if you have asthma or hay fever.) Make all dilutions with 0.9% sodium chloride injection containing 0.4% phenol (pH 7). Use a bacterial-retentive filter (porosity 0.22 μ) when transferring solution from vial to nebulizer. After adding the sodium chloride solution, shake each vial to obtain a clear solution.

Vial A: Add 4 ml of 0.9% sodium chloride injection containing 0.4% phenol (pH 7) to the 5 ml vial containing 100 mg (25 mg/ml).

Vial B: Remove 3 ml from vial A, transfer to another vial and add 4.5 ml of the 0.9% sodium chloride solution (10 mg/ml). An alternative method of preparing vial B is to remove 1 ml from vial A and add 1.5 ml of the 0.9% sodium chloride solution.

Vial C: Remove 1 ml from vial A, transfer to another vial and add 9 ml of the 0.9% sodium chloride solution (2.5 mg/ml). This step depletes contents of vial A if the first dilution method under vial B directions is used.

Vial D: Remove 1 ml from vial C, transfer to another vial and add 9 ml of the 0.9% sodium chloride solution (0.25 mg/ml).

Vial E: Remove 1 ml from vial D, transfer to another vial and add 9 ml of the 0.9% sodium chloride solution (0.025 mg/ml).

Storage: Store dilutions A through D in refrigerator (36° to 46°F) for up to 2 weeks, then discard the vials. Freezing does not affect the stability of dilutions A through D. Vial E must be prepared on the day of the challenge. Store the unreconstituted powder at 59° to 86°F.

Rx	**Provocholine** (Roche)	**Powder for reconstitution of solution for inhalation:** 100 mg per 5 ml	In 5 ml vials.

TERIPARATIDE ACETATE

Actions:

Teriparatide acetate (hPTH 1-34) is a synthetic polypeptide hormone consisting of the 1-34 fragment of human parathyroid hormone, the biologically active N-terminal region of the 84 amino acid native hormone.

Pharmacology: Parathyroid hormone is secreted by the four parathyroid glands found on or embedded in the two lateral lobes of the thyroid gland. Human parathyroid hormone 1-34 acts on bone to mobilize calcium; it also acts on the kidney to reduce calcium clearance, increase phosphate excretion, stimulate the release of cyclic AMP in the urine, and stimulate the conversion of 25-hydroxyvitamin D_3 (25-OH-D_3) to the active form 1, 25-dihydroxyvitamin D_3 [1,25$(OH)_2D_3$].

The initial effect of teriparatide acetate on bone is to promote an increased rate of release of calcium from bone into blood.

The kidney effects, which may be due to a direct action of the hormone on its receptors, include a reduction of calcium clearance and an inhibition of tubular phosphate reabsorption as well as an increased excretion of sodium and potassium. Parathyroid hormone stimulates the conversion of 25-OH-D to 1,25$(OH)_2$D by the kidney.

Intestinal transport of calcium is increased by the PTH indirectly by increasing renal 1,25$(OH)_2$D production.

The primary mode of action is the stimulation of adenylate cyclase in the involved organ.

Indications:

Diagnostic agent to assist in establishing the diagnosis in patients presenting with clinical laboratory evidence of hypocalcemia due to either hypoparathyroidism or pseudohypoparathyroidism. The test will distinguish between hypoparathyroidism and pseudohypoparathyroidism, but not between these conditions and normal. The discriminant power of its effect on urinary cAMP is much greater than that of the effect on urinary phosphate.

Contraindications:

Hypersensitivity to teriparatide or any component of this preparation.

Warnings:

Hypercalcemia may develop with the administration of teriparatide. Teriparatide is not intended for recurrent or chronic use.

Allergic Reactions: Because teriparatide acetate is a peptide, systemic allergic reactions are possible. This product may contain up to 35% extraneous peptides, the chemical structures of which have not been determined. Have epinephrine 1:1000 immediately available. Refer to Management of Acute Hypersensitivity Reactions on p. viii.

Usage in Pregnancy: Category C. It is not known whether teriparatide can cause fetal harm when administered to a pregnant woman or can affect reproductive capacity. Give to a pregnant woman only if clearly needed.

Usage in Lactation: It is not known to what degree teriparatide is excreted in human milk, but the peptide would not be expected to be absorbed in an active form from the infant's GI tract. However, exercise caution when administering to a nursing woman.

Usage in Children: Use in children 3 years of age and older was uneventful and the response to the drug followed expected patterns. Limited data are available.

Adverse Reactions:

Hypertensive crisis occurred in one patient 8 hours after a study. This patient had experienced previous hypertensive episodes not related to teriparatide acetate injection.

Metabolic: Hypocalcemia was not reversed in one patient, and a hypocalcemic convulsion occurred 4½ hours following injection; this was corrected by calcium administration.

GI: Nausea, abdominal cramps, urge to defecate, diarrhea ($< 2\%$).

Other: Tingling of the extremities, metallic taste and pain at the injection site during or shortly following the infusion ($< 2\%$).

Overdosage:

Repeated doses in excess of 500 units may produce hypercalcemia. In those who are borderline hypercalcemic (10.5 mg/dl), a dose of 200 units could produce mild hypercalcemia for a brief period. If hypercalcemia develops, discontinue the drug and ensure adequate hydration.

(Continued on following page)

TERIPARATIDE ACETATE (Cont.)

Administration and Dosage:

Diagnostic use in patients with hypocalcemia:

Adult dose – 200 units. Reconstitute by adding the 10 ml diluent to the 10 ml vial. The 10 ml of solution is infused IV over 10 minutes.

Children (≥ 3 years) – 3 units/kg (maximum of 200 units).

Use reconstituted solution within 4 hours. Discard any unused portion.

Modified Ellsworth Howard Test: Test subjects should be in a fasting state when starting the test period. Initiate and maintain an active urine output by the ingestion of 200 ml of water/hour for 2 hours prior to study and continuing through the study. Make a baseline urine collection in the 60 minute period preceding the infusion. Following the hPTH (1-34) infusion (time 0), collect urine as separate collections in the 0 to 30 minute, 30 to 60 minute and 60 to 120 minute postinfusion time periods. Confidence in the test will be influenced by adequate hydration and urine flow and complete collection of urine specimens.

Interpretation of Test: The measurement of urinary cAMP and phosphate must be corrected for creatinine excretion.

Hypoparathyroidism patients – In the clinical trials, these patients showed a tenfold or greater increase over baseline of urinary cAMP at the 0 to 30 minute postinfusion period, and 92% of these patients showed a threefold or greater urinary phosphate excretion in the 0 to 60 minute collection.

Pseudohypoparathyroid patients with end-organ resistance pseudohypoparathyroidism showed a blunted response of less than sixfold increase of urinary cAMP excretion over baseline in the 0 to 30 minute period, and 88% showed a less than threefold increase in urinary phosphate excretion in the 0 to 60 minute collection period.

Although this test does not discriminate between normal and abnormal in most cases, it does discriminate between hypoparathyroidism and pseudohypoparathyroidism. The change in the urinary cAMP excretion in the 0 to 30 minute period is the most sensitive indicator for separation of hypoparathyroidisms.

Rx	**Parathar** (Rorer)	**Powder for Injection (lyophilized):** 200 units hPTH activity	In 10 ml vials[1] w/10 ml vial of diluent.

[1] With 20 mg gelatin.

PENTAGASTRIN

Actions:

Pentagastrin contains the C-terminal tetrapeptide responsible for the actions of the natural gastrins and, therefore, acts as a physiologic gastric acid secretagogue. The recommended dose of 6 mcg/kg SC produces a peak acid output which is reproducible when used in the same individual. It stimulates gastric acid secretion approximately 10 minutes after SC injection, with peak responses occurring in most cases 20 to 30 minutes after administration. Duration of activity is usually between 60 and 80 minutes.

Indications:

A diagnostic agent to evaluate gastric acid secretory function in:

Anacidity - In suspected pernicious anemia, atrophic gastritis or gastric carcinoma.

Hypersecretion - In suspected duodenal ulcer or postoperative stomal ulcer; Zollinger-Ellison tumor.

It is also useful in determining the adequacy of acid-reducing operations for peptic ulcer.

Contraindications:

Hypersensitivity or idiosyncrasy to pentagastrin.

Warnings:

Effects on gastric acid secretion: In amounts in excess of the recommended dose, pentagastrin may cause inhibition of gastric acid secretion.

Usage in Pregnancy: Safety for use during pregnancy has not been established. Use only when clearly needed and when the potential benefits outweigh the unknown potential hazards to the fetus.

Usage in Children: Safety and efficacy for use in children have not been established.

Precautions:

Use with caution in patients with pancreatic, hepatic or biliary disease. Like gastrin, pentagastrin could, in some cases, have the physiologic effect of stimulating pancreatic enzyme and bicarbonate secretion, as well as biliary flow.

Adverse Reactions:

Causes fewer and less severe cardiovascular and other adverse reactions than histamine. The majority of reactions are related to the GI tract.

GI: Abdominal pain; urge to defecate; nausea; vomiting; borborygmi; blood-tinged mucus.

Cardiovascular: Flushing; tachycardia.

CNS: Dizziness; faintness; lightheadedness; drowsiness; sinking feeling; transient blurring of vision; tiredness; headache.

Allergic and hypersensitivity reactions may occur in some patients.

Miscellaneous: Shortness of breath; heavy sensation in arms and legs; tingling fingers; chills; sweating; generalized burning sensation; warmth; pain at injection site; bile in collected specimens.

Overdosage:

In case of overdosage or idiosyncrasy, administer symptomatic treatment, as required.

Refer to General Management of Acute Overdosage on p. vi.

Administration and Dosage:

Adults: 6 mcg/kg SC.

Rx	**Peptavlon** (Ayerst)	**Injection:** 0.25 mg (250 mcg) per ml. In 2 ml amps.

HISTAMINE PHOSPHATE

Actions:

Histamine acts on the vascular system, smooth muscle and exocrine glands increasing the volume and acidity of the gastric juice and stimulating the smooth muscle of the respiratory and GI tracts. It has little effect on the smooth muscle of the uterus. It stimulates exocrine gland secretion, including secretion of the gastric, duodenal, salivary, pancreatic, bronchial and lacrimal glands. Histamine causes an increase in the secretion of gastric juice of high acidity apparently by a direct action on the gastric parietal cells. Histamine also causes an increase in the secretion of pepsin. The stimulating effect of histamine on gastric secretion is not antagonized by antihistamines; the antagonism exerted by atropine is inconsistent.

Absorption/Distribution: Readily absorbed following parenteral administration. Its action is very transient since the drug rapidly diffuses into body tissues and is metabolized.

Metabolism/Excretion: About half of a dose is metabolized to 1-methylimidazole acetic acid. Most of the remainder is oxidized to imidazole acetic acid and its riboside. Following an intradermal dose, 4% to 8% is excreted in the urine as methylhistamine, 42% to 47% as methylimidazole acetic acid, 9% to 11% as imidazole acetic acid, 16% to 23% as imidazole acetic acid riboside and 2% to 3% as free histamine.

Histamine is the most vigorous stimulant of gastric acid secretion available. The absence of free hydrochloric acid in the gastric juice after an injection of histamine indicates the absence of acid-secreting cells from the stomach. Gastric achlorhydria after administration of histamine is an essential finding in the diagnosis of pernicious anemia. The response to histamine persists after section of the vagus nerve.

Indications:

Gastric histamine test: Used SC to test the gastric mucosa's ability to produce hydrochloric acid.

Pheochromocytoma test: Used IV for the presumptive diagnosis of pheochromocytoma.

Contraindications:

Gastric histamine test: Hypersensitivity to histamine products; hypotension; severe hypertension; vasomotor instability; bronchial asthma (past or present); urticaria (past or present); severe cardiac, pulmonary or renal disease; elderly patients.

Pheochromocytoma test: Contraindicated in elderly or severely hypertensive patients.

Warnings:

Usage in bronchial disease/allergic conditions: May precipitate attacks of severe asthma or other serious allergic conditions. Carefully weigh the possible benefit against the serious untoward reactions that may develop in patients with allergic diseases. Small doses may precipitate asthma in patients with bronchial disease; extreme caution is advised. Patients with an allergic diathesis may react severely.

Gastric test: Avoid accidental introduction into a vein or artery. Pull back on the syringe plunger before the injection is made to be sure the end of the needle is not in a blood vessel. Epinephrine 1:1000 should be immediately available.

Weigh the risk/benefit ratio when considering the use of the gastric histamine test in patients with pheochromocytoma.

Usage in Pregnancy: Category C. Animal reproduction studies have not been conducted. Safety for use during pregnancy has not been established. Use only when clearly needed and when the potential benefits outweigh the unknown potential hazards to the fetus.

Usage in Lactation: It is not known whether this drug is excreted in breast milk. Decide whether to discontinue nursing or to not administer the drug, taking into account the importance of the test to the mother.

Usage in Children: Safety and efficacy have not been established.

Precautions:

Average or large doses may cause alarming, potentially dangerous reactions. (See Adverse Reactions.) Histamine increases the acid of the gastric juice and may cause symptoms of peptic ulcer.

Gastric test: Local reactions at the site of injection may include erythema and edema. Use with caution in patients with any cardiac abnormalities.

(Continued on following page)

HISTAMINE PHOSPHATE (Cont.)

Adverse Reactions:

Average or large doses may produce flushing, dizziness, headache, bronchial constriction, dyspnea, visual disturbances, faintness, syncope, urticaria, asthma, marked hypertension or hypotension, palpitation, tachycardia, nervousness, abdominal cramps, diarrhea, vomiting, metallic taste, local or generalized allergic manifestations, collapse with convulsions, severe occipital headache, blurred vision, anginal pain, a rapid drop in blood pressure and cyanosis of the face.

Frequently check blood pressure and pulse during IV injection. Promptly give an epinephrine injection if a dangerous fall in blood pressure is noted.

Gastric test: Erythema, edema, weakness and nausea.

Overdosage:

Symptoms: May cause severe symptoms, including circulatory or vasomotor collapse, shock and even death.

Treatment: If accidental overdosage is discovered early, temporary application of a tourniquet proximally to the injection site may slow the absorption of the drug. Epinephrine is indicated if hypotension or acute asthma occur. Antidotes to histamine are as follows:

Epinephrine HCl, 0.1 to 0.5 ml of a 1:1000 aqueous solution, given SC in case of emergency due to severe reactions.

An antihistamine preparation given IM to prevent or ameliorate systemic reactions.

Administration and Dosage:

Gastric test: The physician should be thoroughly familiar with the technique of performing the gastric histamine test or the augmented histamine test and with the interpretation of the results from standard reference texts.

Histamine test: After the basal gastric secretion has been collected, give 0.0275 mg of histamine phosphate (or 0.01 mg histamine base) per kg SC. Collect the gastric contents in four 15 minute specimens for 1 hour and analyze for volume, acidity, pH and acid output.

Augmented histamine test: Initially, give a suitable dose of antihistamine IM (eg, 10 mg chlorpheniramine maleate or 50 mg diphenhydramine HCl). After conclusion of the basal secretion study, give 0.04 mg/kg SC.

Pheochromocytoma histamine test: Withhold antihypertensives, sympathomimetics, sedatives and narcotics for at least 24 hours, preferably 72 hours, before performing the histamine test. *Do not withhold food.*

The pheochromocytoma histamine test is a provocative test, indicated only for the occasional patient with paroxysmal signs of excessive catecholamine secretion and normal urinary values for assays of catecholamines and metabolites during asymptomatic periods. It provides information on the symptomatic and physiologic responses and changes in urinary catecholamine levels. Use only in patients with resting blood pressure ≤ 150/110 mm Hg.

Have epinephrine available in case of a severe hypotensive response. Have phentolamine on hand to depress any alarming increase in blood pressure.

The patient should rest in bed while a slow IV infusion of either 5% dextrose or isotonic saline solution is established. Record blood pressure until it is stable, then start a 2 hour urine collection for catecholamine assay. At the end of the period, rapidly administer histamine through the infusion and start another 2 hour urine collection.

The first IV dose of histamine should be 0.01 mg (10 mcg). If no response is observed within 5 minutes, administer a dose of 0.05 mg (50 mcg). Record blood pressure and pulse every 30 seconds for 15 minutes. The expected responses are headache, flushing and a decrease in blood pressure followed within 2 minutes by an increase.

Interpretation of test results:

Positive tests have been defined as:

1. An increase in blood pressure of at least 20/10 mm Hg greater than that obtained with the cold pressor test.

2. An increase in blood pressure of at least 60/40 mm Hg above baseline and greater than that with the cold pressor test.

An increase in urinary catecholamine levels from normal during the pretest control period to abnormally high during the test lessens the possibility of false-positive results.

Rx	**Histamine Phosphate** (Lilly)	**Gastric test:** 0.55 mg (equivalent to 0.2 mg histamine base) per ml	In 5 ml vials.[1]
		2.75 mg (equivalent to 1 mg histamine base) per ml	In 1 ml amps.[1]
		Pheochromocytoma test: 0.275 mg (equivalent to 0.1 mg histamine) per ml	In 1 ml amps.

[1] With glycerin and phenol.

BENTIROMIDE

Actions:

Bentiromide is a peptide which carries the marker para-aminobenzoic acid (PABA); 500 mg of bentiromide contains 170 mg PABA.

Pharmacokinetics: Following oral administration, bentiromide is selectively cleaved by pancreatic chymotrypsin with the liberation of PABA. PABA is readily absorbed through the intestinal mucosa under normal conditions, and is conjugated primarily by the liver and rapidly excreted in the urine. Under conditions of normal exocrine pancreatic function, gastric emptying, and gut and kidney function, over 50% of the PABA contained in bentiromide appears in the urine within 6 hours following administration. It is not known whether bentiromide or PABA crosses the placental barrier or the blood brain barrier.

PABA is detected in the urine using the Smith modification of the Bratton-Marshall test for arylamines, which detects both conjugated and unconjugated arylamines.

Indications:

Screening test for pancreatic exocrine insufficiency; to monitor the adequacy of supplemental pancreatic therapy.

Contraindications:

Hypersensitivity to bentiromide.

Warnings:

Usage in Pregnancy: Category B. Reproduction studies in small animals revealed no evidence of impaired fertility or fetal harm due to bentiromide doses 50 and 100 times the human dose. Safety for use during pregnancy has not been established. Use only when clearly needed and when the potential benefits outweigh the unknown potential hazards to the fetus.

Usage in Lactation: It is not known whether this drug is excreted in breast milk. Safety for use in the nursing mother has not been established.

Usage in Children: Safety and efficacy for use in children below the age of 6 years have not been established.

Precautions:

Proper use of bentiromide requires close attention to the technical details of drug administration and of urine collection, handling and assay for arylamine levels and awareness that "false-positive" and "false-negative" results can occur.

Schedule repeat dosings, if needed, at intervals of 7 days or more to assure complete metabolism and excretion of prior doses of the drug.

Diabetics: Insulin may need adjustment to accommodate the fasting patient.

Usage in impaired hepatic or renal function: May alter test interpretation due to altered handling of PABA.

Gastrointestinal absorption defects may falsely indicate decreased chymotrypsin secretion.

Hypersensitivity: A single case of bentiromide hypersensitivity has been reported (see Adverse Reactions). The frequency of sensitization is unknown. Following administration of bentiromide, patients should remain in a medical setting for observation.

Have epinephrine 1:1000 immediately available. Refer to Management of Acute Hypersensitivity Reactions on p. viii.

Laboratory Tests: It has not been established whether concurrent GI diagnostic testing interferes with the results of this test; conduct GI testing at least 24 hours before or after dosing with bentiromide.

Drug Interactions:

Methotrexate may compete for binding sites with PABA.

Sulfa drugs: PABA interferes with antibacterial action.

Salicylates: Therapeutic and toxic effects may be increased with concurrent administration of PABA.

Assay Interactions: Drugs metabolized to primary arylamines may cause assay interference and falsely elevate test results. These drugs include: **Acetaminophen, benzocaine, chloramphenicol, lidocaine, procaine, procainamide** and **thiazide diuretics. PABA-containing drugs** such as sunscreens or certain multiple vitamins may also falsely elevate test results. Discontinue any of these drugs 3 days prior to bentiromide administration.

In adults, discontinue oral pancreatic enzyme supplements 5 days prior to bentiromide administration. In cystic fibrotic children, reduce the time interval to 1 day.

(Continued on following page)

BENTIROMIDE (Cont.)

Adverse Reactions:

Most frequent: Diarrhea, headache (< 2%).

Rare: Flatulence, nausea, vomiting and weakness (0.6%) are transient and rarely require symptomatic therapy.

Acute respiratory distress and stridor requiring symptomatic therapy has been reported in one patient following a second dose of bentiromide; the patient developed coughing and choking after his first dose.

Causal relationship unknown: Abdominal pain; drowsiness; lightheadedness; heartburn; transient elevations of liver function tests.

Overdosage:

Treatment includes usual supportive measures. Refer to General Management of Acute Overdosage on p. vi.

Patient Information:

Patient package insert available with product.

Fast after midnight before taking bentiromide.

Urinate before taking the drug.

Notify physician if you are taking any drugs that may interfere with the test (see Drug Interactions). Discontinue pancreatic supplements 5 days before the test.

Diarrhea, headache, nausea, vomiting, flatulence and weakness have been reported. If any discomfort or unusual change is experienced, notify physician.

Administration and Dosage:

Administer following an overnight fast. Urinate prior to drug administration. Administer a single 500 mg dose; follow immediately by 250 ml of water. In patients less than 12 years of age, calculate the dose on the basis of 14 mg/kg. Drinking water is encouraged to promote diuresis. Give the patient 250 ml of water at post-dosing hour 2 and up to an additional 500 ml during post-dosing hours 2 through 6. Obtain a total urine collection during 0 to 6 hours post-dosing. Measure the volume of the collection and retain a 10 ml sample for analysis. Break the fast following completion of urine collection. Should re-testing be necessary, separate subsequent administrations by at least 7 day intervals to avoid interference of test results by prior bentiromide dosings.

Analysis of urine: Use the Smith modification of the Bratton-Marshall test for arylamines.

A negative bentiromide test suggesting pancreatic exocrine insufficiency should not lead to termination of the search for a pancreatic etiology of maldigestion or other pancreatic disease. A good response to an oral pancreatic enzyme supplement would be confirmatory of a positive bentiromide test.

For test interpretations, see manufacturer's package insert.

Rx	**Chymex** (Adria)	**Solution:** 500 mg (170 mg PABA) in 40% propylene glycol. In 7.5 ml.

SECRETIN

Actions:

Pharmacology: The main action of secretin is to increase the volume and bicarbonate content of pancreatic juice. In one study of 6 healthy subjects, the elimination half-life was about 4 minutes and the clearance rate was 540 ml/min. Normal ranges and values for pancreatic secretory response to IV secretin in patients with specific pancreatic diseases can vary significantly from one investigator to another, presumably because of differences in technique. However, a constant and reliable response can be obtained. The results of a properly performed test when compared to results obtained in an adequate series of normal subjects will reliably identify pancreatic disease.

A set of typical values (± S.D.) for pancreatic secretory responses to secretin in normal subjects and patients with well documented pancreatitis is given in the table below:

Parameters	Normal Subjects	Pancreatitis
Volume (ml/hr)	235 ± 60	63 ± 42
Bicarbonate (mEq/L)	114 ± 20	71 ± 33
Bicarbonate output (mEq/kg/hr)	0.436 ± 0.141	0.105 ± 0.093

These values are derived from a single study. Use them as guidelines only. When performing secretin testing for diagnosis of pancreatic disease for the first time, begin by assessing normal subjects to develop proficiency in proper technique and to generate normal ranges for the three commonly assessed parameters of pancreatic exocrine response.

Secretin IV stimulates gastrin release in patients with gastrinoma (Zollinger-Ellison syndrome), and either does not affect, or produces small changes in, serum gastrin concentrations in normal subjects. It may produce a small decrease in gastrin in patients with duodenal ulcer disease. This action is the basis for its use as a provocative test in the evaluation of patients in whom gastrinoma is a diagnostic consideration.

Indications:

Diagnosis of pancreatic exocrine disease.

Diagnosis of gastrinoma (Zollinger-Ellison syndrome).

As an adjunct in obtaining desquamated pancreatic cells for cytopathologic examination.

Contraindications:

Do not give to patients with acute pancreatitis until the attack has subsided.

Warnings:

Usage in Pregnancy: It is not known whether secretin can cause fetal harm when administered to pregnant women or can affect reproductive capacity. Since fluoroscopic guidance is usually necessary to position the duodenal lumen of the double-lumen tube used for the pancreatic function test, postpone the test until after delivery in pregnant women.

Usage in Lactation: It is not known whether secretin is excreted in breast milk. Exercise caution when administering to the nursing mother. Normal values for pancreatic secretory and serum gastrin response to secretin have not been established for nursing mothers.

Precautions:

Test dose: Administer an IV test dose of 0.1 to 1 CU secretin, especially to patients with a history of atopic allergy or asthma. One minute later, if there has been no allergic reaction, administer the recommended dose by injection over approximately 1 minute.

Patients who have undergone vagotomy, who are receiving anticholinergics at the time of secretin testing, or who have inflammatory bowel disease may be hyporesponsive to secretin stimulation. This does not indicate pancreatic disease.

A greater than normal volume response to secretin stimulation, which can mask coexisting pancreatic disease, is occasionally encountered in patients with alcoholic or other liver disease.

(Continued on following page)

SECRETIN (Cont.)

Adverse Reactions:

None reported.

Administration and Dosage:

Pancreatic function testing: Pass a Dreiling type, radiopaque, double-lumen tube through the mouth after a 12 to 15 hour fast. Under fluoroscopic guidance, place the proximal lumen of the tube in the gastric antrum and the distal lumen just beyond the papilla of Vater. Confirm the position of the tube and secure the tube in place prior to testing. Apply suction at a negative pressure of 25 to 40 mm Hg to both lumens and maintain throughout the test. Interruption of suction at intervals of about 1 minute improves the reliability of collection. When uncontaminated duodenal contents are obtained (ie, clear, although possibly bile stained, with a pH of 6 or higher), collect a baseline sample of duodenal fluid for 2 consecutive 10 minute periods. Subsequent to the baseline collections, slowly inject secretin in a dose of 1 CU/kg IV over approximately 1 minute. Then, collect duodenal fluid for 60 minutes after administration. The aspirate is fractioned into four collection periods, the first two at 10 minute intervals, and the last two at 20 minute intervals. Clear the duodenal lumen of the tube with an injection of air after collection of each fraction. Wide variations in volume of the aspirate suggest incomplete aspiration or contamination. Place each fraction of duodenal fluid on ice and subsequently analyze for volume and bicarbonate concentration. The duodenal aspirate may also be submitted for cytopathological examination.

Diagnosis of gastrinoma (Zollinger-Ellison syndrome): The patient should fast for 12 hours prior to the test. Prior to injection of secretin, draw 2 blood samples for determination of baseline serum gastrin levels. Subsequently, give 2 CU/kg IV over 1 minute and collect post-injection blood samples at 1, 2, 5, 10 and 30 minutes for determination of serum gastrin concentrations.

Gastrinoma is strongly suggested in patients with elevated fasting serum gastrin concentrations in the 120 to 500 pg/ml range (determined by RIA using an antibody to gastrin similar to that prepared by Rehfeld) and an increase in serum gastrin concentration of more than 110 pg/ml over basal level in response to IV secretin.

Preparation of solution: Prepare immediately prior to use. Dissolve contents of a vial in 7.5 ml Sodium Chloride Injection, to give a concentration of 10 CU/ml. Avoid vigorous shaking.

Storage: Store in freezer at -20°C. Can be stored at 25°C or below for up to 3 weeks.

Rx	**Secretin-Ferring** (Ferring)	**Powder for Injection:** 75 CU per vial (10 CU/ml when reconstituted with 7.5 ml). In 10 ml vials.[1]

[1] With 1 mg l-cysteine HCl and 20 mg mannitol.

SINCALIDE

Actions:

Sincalide IV substantially reduces gallbladder size by causing it to contract. The evacuation of bile that results is similar to the physiological response to endogenous cholecystokinin. Bolus IV administration causes a prompt contraction of the gallbladder that becomes maximal in 5 to 15 minutes. The stimulus of a fatty meal causes a progressive contraction that becomes maximal after approximately 40 minutes. A 40% reduction in radiographic area of the gallbladder is satisfactory.

Like cholecystokinin, sincalide given in conjunction with secretin stimulates pancreatic secretion; concurrent administration increases the volume of pancreatic secretion and the output of bicarbonate and protein (enzymes). This combined effect of secretin and sincalide permits the assessment of specific pancreatic function through measurement and analysis of the duodenal aspirate. The parameters determined are: Volume of the secretion; bicarbonate concentration; and amylase content (which parallels the content of trypsin and total protein).

Indications:

Used to provide a sample of gallbladder bile for analysis of its composition (eg, to determine the degree of cholesterol saturation).

Use in conjunction with secretin (see Administration and Dosage) to stimulate pancreatic secretion for analysis of its composition and examination of cytology (eg, in suspected cancer of the pancreas).

For postevacuation cholecystography, when this procedure is indicated but the physician wishes to avoid the fatty meal.

Contraindications:

Patients sensitive to sincalide.

Warnings:

Usage in Pregnancy: No teratogenic or antifertility effects were seen in animal studies. Data are inadequate to determine safety in human pregnancy. Use in pregnant women only when the benefits outweigh the possible risk to the fetus.

Usage in Children: The safety for use in children has not been established.

Precautions:

Stimulation of gallbladder contraction in patients with small gallbladder stones may lead to the evacuation of the stones, resulting in their lodging in the cystic duct or in the common bile duct. The risk is minimal because sincalide, when given as directed, does not ordinarily cause complete contraction of the gallbladder.

Adverse Reactions:

Gastrointestinal symptoms such as abdominal discomfort or pain and an urge to defecate frequently accompany the injection of sincalide. These phenomena are manifestations of the physiologic actions of the drug including delayed gastric emptying and increased intestinal motility. The reactions do not necessarily indicate a biliary tract abnormality unless there is other clinical or radiologic evidence of disease. Nausea, dizziness and flushing occur occasionally.

Administration and Dosage:

Contraction of the gallbladder: A dose of 0.02 mcg/kg (1.4 mcg/70 kg) is injected IV over 30 to 60 seconds; if satisfactory gallbladder contraction does not occur in 15 minutes, a second dose (0.04 mcg/kg) may be given. In cholecystography, roentgenograms are usually taken at 5 minute intervals after the injection. For visualization of the cystic duct, it may be necessary to take roentgenograms at 1 minute intervals during the first 5 minutes after the injection.

Secretin-Sincalide test of pancreatic function: A dose of 0.25 units/kg of secretin is infused IV over 60 minutes. Thirty minutes after initiating secretin, give a separate IV infusion of sincalide at a total dose of 0.02 mcg/kg over 30 minutes. For example, the total dose for a 70 kg patient is 1.4 mcg sincalide; therefore, dilute 1.4 ml reconstituted sincalide solution to 30 ml with Sodium Chloride Injection and administer at a rate of 1 ml/minute.

Preparation of solution: To reconstitute, add 5 ml Sterile Water for Injection to the vial; the solution may be kept at room temperature. Use within 24 hours after reconstitution; discard any unused portion.

Storage: Store at room temperature prior to reconstitution.

Rx	**Kinevac** (Squibb)	**Powder for Injection:** 5 mcg per vial for reconstitution (1 mcg/ml when reconstituted).

BENZYLPENICILLOYL-POLYLYSINE

Actions:

Benzylpenicilloyl-polylysine is a skin test antigen that reacts specifically with benzylpenicilloyl skin sensitizing antibodies (reagins: IgE class) to produce an immediate wheal and flare reaction at a skin test site. Individuals exhibiting a positive response possess reagins against the benzylpenicilloyl group.

Individuals who have previously received therapeutic penicillin may have positive skin test reactions to benzylpenicilloyl-polylysine and to other non-benzylpenicilloyl haptenes of minor determinants. The major metabolite of penicillin is the penicilloyl group; this "major determinant" is thought to be responsible for accelerated reactions, but not anaphylaxis. Other breakdown products or "minor determinants" are felt to be responsible for anaphylaxis and immediate systemic reactions. Virtually everyone who receives penicillin develops specific antibodies, but skin tests to penicillin and penicillin-derived reagents become positive in less than 10% of patients who have tolerated penicillin in the past; allergic responses are infrequent (< 1%).

Many individuals reacting positively will not develop a systemic allergic reaction on subsequent exposure to therapeutic penicillin; this skin test facilitates assessing the local allergic skin reactivity to benzylpenicilloyl.

Indications:

An adjunct in assessing the risk of administering penicillin (benzylpenicillin or penicillin G) in adults with a history of clinical penicillin hypersensitivity. A negative skin test is associated with an incidence of allergic reactions of < 5% after the administration of penicillin; the incidence may be > 20% in the presence of a positive skin test.

Contraindications:

Systemic or marked local reaction to previous administration. Do not test patients known to be extremely hypersensitive to penicillin.

Warnings:

Systemic allergic reactions rarely follow a skin test. Avoid by making the first application by scratch test. Use the intradermal route only if the scratch test is entirely negative. Do not perform skin testing with penicillin or other penicillin derived reagents simultaneously.

Usage in Pregnancy: Safety for use during pregnancy has not been established. Use only when clearly needed and when potential benefits outweigh unknown potential hazards.

Precautions:

Allergic reactions are predominantly dermatologic. Data are insufficient to document that a decreased incidence of anaphylactic reactions following penicillin administration will occur in patients with a negative skin test. Similarly, data are insufficient to determine the value of this skin test as a means of assessing the risk of administering therapeutic penicillin (when penicillin is the drug of choice) in adult patients with no history of clinical penicillin hypersensitivity or in pediatric patients.

No reagent, test or combination of tests will completely assure a reaction to penicillin therapy will not occur.

Data are insufficient to assess the potential danger of sensitization to penicillin from repeated skin testing.

There are no data to assess the clinical value of benzylpenicilloyl-polylysine skin test where exposure to penicillin is suspected as a cause of a drug reaction and in patients who are undergoing routine allergy evaluation.

There are no data relating the clinical value of skin tests to the risk of administering semi-synthetic penicillins (phenoxymethyl penicillin, ampicillin, carbenicillin, dicloxacillin, methicillin, nafcillin, oxacillin) and cephalosporin-derived antibiotics.

(Precautions continued on following page)

BENZYLPENICILLOYL-POLYLYSINE (Cont.)

Precautions (Cont.):

Consider the following clinical outcomes when the decision to administer or not to administer penicillin is based in part on the skin test: (1) An allergic reaction to penicillin may occur in a patient with a negative skin test. (2) A patient may have an anaphylactic reaction to penicillin in the presence of a negative skin test and a negative history of clinical penicillin hypersensitivity. (3) If penicillin is the absolute drug of choice in a life-threatening situation, successful desensitization with therapeutic penicillin may be possible, despite a positive skin test or a positive history of clinical penicillin hypersensitivity.

Adverse Reactions:

Local: Occasional intense inflammatory response at the skin test site.

Systemic: Generalized erythema, pruritis, urticaria, angioneurotic edema, dyspnea or hypotension. The usual methods of treating a skin test antigen-induced reaction (application of a venous occlusion tourniquet proximal to the skin test site and administration of epinephrine or antihistamine) are recommended and will usually control the reaction. Systemic allergic reactions following skin test procedures usually are of short duration and controllable, but observe the patient for several hours.

Acute Hypersensitivity Reaction: Have epinephrine 1:1000 immediately available. Refer to Management of Acute Hypersensitivity Reactions on p. viii.

Administration and Dosage:

Scratch testing: Perform skin testing on the inner volar aspect of the forearm. **Always** apply the skin test material first by the scratch technique. After preparing the skin surface, use a sterile 20 gauge needle to make a 3 to 5 mm scratch on the epidermis. Very little pressure is required to break the epidermal continuity. If bleeding occurs, prepare a second site and scratch more lightly with the needle, sufficient to produce a nonbleeding scratched surface. Apply a small drop of solution to the scratch and rub gently with an applicator, toothpick or the side of the needle.

Interpretation of test results - Observe for the appearance of a wheal, erythema and itching at the test site during the next 15 minutes, then wipe off the solution over the scratch. A positive reaction consists of development of a pale wheal, usually with pseudopods, surrounding the scratch site within 10 minutes. It varies in diameter from 5 to 15 mm (or more). This wheal may be surrounded by erythema and accompanied by itching. The most sensitive individuals develop itching instantly, and the wheal and erythema promptly appear. As soon as a positive response is clearly evident, wipe off the solution over the scratch. If the scratch test is either negative or equivocally positive (< 5 mm wheal, little or no erythema, no itching), perform an intradermal test.

Intradermal test: Using a tuberculin syringe with a ⅜" to ⅝", 26 to 30 gauge, short bevel needle, withdraw the contents of the ampule. Prepare a sterile skin test area on the upper, outer arm, sufficiently below the deltoid muscle to permit proximal application of a tourniquet, if necessary. Inject an amount of benzylpenicilloyl-polylysine sufficient to raise the smallest possible perceptible bleb. This volume will be 0.01 to 0.02 ml. Using a separate syringe and needle, inject a like amount of saline as a control at least 1½ inches from the test site.

Interpretation of test results - Most skin reactions develop within 5 to 15 minutes.

Negative (−): No increase in size of original bleb or no greater reaction than the control site.

Ambiguous (±): Wheal only slightly larger than initial injection bleb, with or without accompanying erythematous flare and larger than the control site.

Positive (+): Itching and marked increase in size of original bleb. Wheal may exceed 20 mm in diameter and exhibit pseudopods.

The control site should be completely reactionless. If it exhibits a wheal greater than 2 to 3 mm, repeat the test. If the same reaction is observed, consult a physician experienced with allergy skin testing.

Storage: Stable only when kept under refrigeration; discard test materials subjected to ambient temperatures for over a day.

Rx **Pre-Pen** (Kremers-Urban) **Solution:** 0.25 ml per amp.

Dipyridamole oral is used as an antiplatelet and antianginal agent. For further information refer to the individual monographs in the Blood Modifiers and Cardiovascular chapters.

DIPYRIDAMOLE

Actions:

Pharmacology: Dipyridamole for IV injection is a coronary vasodilator used for the evaluation of coronary artery disease. The mechanism of vasodilation has not been fully elucidated, but may result from inhibition of adenosine uptake, an important mediator of coronary vasodilation. How dipyridamole-induced vasodilation leads to abnormalities in thallium distribution ventriculation function is also uncertain, but presumably represents a "steal" phenomenon in which relatively intact vessels dilate, and sustain enhanced flow, leaving reduced pressure and flow across areas of hemodynamically important coronary vascular constriction.

In a study of 10 patients with angiographically normal or minimally stenosed coronary vessels, IV dipyridamole 0.56 mg/kg infused over 4 minutes resulted in an average fivefold increase in coronary blood flow velocity compared to resting coronary flow velocity. The mean time to peak flow velocity was 6.5 minutes from the start of the 4 minute infusion. Cardiovascular responses, when given to patients in the supine position, include a mild but significant increase in heart rate of ≈ 20% and mild, but significant decreases in both systolic and diastolic blood pressure of ≈ 2% to 8%, with vital signs returning to baseline values in ≈ 30 minutes.

Pharmacokinetics: Plasma dipyridamole concentrations decline in a triexponential fashion following IV infusion with half-lives averaging 3 to 12 minutes, 33 to 62 minutes and 11.6 to 15 hours. The mean dipyridamole serum concentration is 4.6 ± 1.3 mcg/ml 2 minutes after a 4 minute 0.568 mg/kg infusion. The average plasma protein binding of dipyridamole is ≈ 99%, primarily to α_1-glycoprotein. Dipyridamole is metabolized in the liver to the glucuronic acid conjugate and excreted with the bile. The average total body clearance is 2.3 to 3.5 ml/min/kg, with an apparent volume of distribution at steady state of 1 to 2.5 L/kg and a central apparent volume of 3 to 5 L.

Clinical trials: In a study of about 1100 patients who underwent coronary arteriography and IV dipyridamole-assisted thallium imaging, the sensitivity of the dipyridamole test (true positive dipyridamole divided by the total number of patients with positive angiography) was about 85%. The specificity (true negative divided by the number of patients with negative angiograms) was about 50%. In a subset of patients who had exercise thallium imaging as well as dipyridamole thallium imaging, sensitivity and specificity of the two tests were almost identical.

Indications:

As an alternative to exercise in thallium myocardial perfusion imaging for the evaluation of coronary artery disease in patients who cannot exercise adequately.

Contraindications:

Hypersensitivity to dipyridamole.

Warnings:

Cardiotoxicity and bronchospasm: Serious adverse reactions have included fatal and non-fatal myocardial infarction, ventricular fibrillation, symptomatic ventricular tachycardia, transient cerebral ischemia and bronchospasm.

In a study of 3911 patients given IV dipyridamole as an adjunct to thallium myocardial perfusion imaging, two types of serious adverse events occurred: Four cases of myocardial infarction (0.1%; two fatal, two non-fatal); and six cases of severe bronchospasm (0.2%). Although the incidence was small (0.3%; 10 of 3911), the potential clinical information to be gained through use of IV dipyridamole thallium imaging must be weighed against the patient risk. Patients with a history of unstable angina may be at a greater risk for severe myocardial ischemia, and patients with a history of asthma may be at a greater risk for bronchospasm.

When thallium myocardial perfusion imaging is performed with IV dipyridamole, parenteral aminophylline should be readily available for relieving adverse events such as bronchospasm or chest pain. Monitor vital signs during, and for 10 to 15 minutes following, the IV infusion of dipyridamole, and obtain an ECG tracing using at least one chest lead. Should severe chest pain or bronchospasm occur, administer parenteral aminophylline by slow IV injection (50 to 100 mg over 30 to 60 seconds) in doses ranging from 50 to 250 mg. In the case of severe hypotension, place the patient in a supine position with the head tilted down, if necessary, before administration of aminophylline. If 250 mg does not relieve chest pain symptoms within a few minutes, SL nitroglycerin may be administered. If chest pain continues despite use of aminophylline and nitroglycerin, consider the possibility of myocardial infarction. If the clinical condition of a patient with an adverse event permits a 1 minute delay in the use of aminophylline, thallium-201 may be injected and allowed to circulate for 1 minute before the injection of aminophylline. This will allow initial thallium perfusion imaging to be performed before reversal of the pharmacologic effects of dipyridamole on the coronary circulation.

(Warnings continued on following page)

DIPYRIDAMOLE (Cont.)

Warnings (Cont.)

Fertility impairment: A significant reduction in number of corpora lutea with consequent reduction in implantations and live fetuses occurred in rats following 1250 mg/day.

Pregnancy: Category B. There are no adequate and well controlled studies in pregnant women. Use during pregnancy only if clearly needed.

Lactation: Dipyridamole is excreted in breast milk.

Children: Safety and efficacy in children have not been established.

Drug Interactions:

Theophylline may abolish the coronary vasodilation induced by IV dipyridamole. This could lead to a false negative thallium imaging result.

Adverse Reactions:

Adverse reaction information is derived from a study of 3911 patients, from spontaneous reports and from the published literature.

IV Dipyridamole Adverse Reactions (> 1%)	
Adverse Reaction	Incidence (%)
Chest pain/angina pectoris	19.7
Headache	12.2
Dizziness	11.8
ECG abnormalities/ST-T changes	7.5
ECG abnormalities/extrasystoles	5.2
Hypotension	4.6
Nausea	4.6
Flushing	3.4
ECG abnormalities/tachycardia	3.2
Dyspnea	2.6
Pain unspecified	2.6
Blood pressure lability	1.6
Hypertension	1.5
Paresthesia	1.3
Fatigue	1.2

Other adverse reactions (≤ 1%):

Cardiovascular: ECG abnormalities unspecified (0.8%); arrhythmia unspecified (0.6%); palpitation (0.3%); ventricular tachycardia (see Warnings), bradycardia (0.2%); myocardial infarction (see Warnings), AV block, syncope, orthostatic hypotension, atrial fibrillation, supraventricular tachycardia (0.1%); ventricular arrhythmia unspecified (see Warnings), heart block unspecified, cardiomyopathy, edema (0.03%).

Central and peripheral nervous system: Hypothesia (0.5%); hypertonia (0.3%); nervousness/anxiety (0.2%); tremor (0.1%); abnormal coordination, somnolence, dysphonia, migraine, vertigo (0.03%).

GI: Dyspepsia (1%); dry mouth (0.8%); abdominal pain (0.7%); flatulence (0.6%); vomiting (0.4%); eructation (0.1%); dysphagia, tenesmus, increased appetite (0.03%).

Respiratory: Pharyngitis (0.3%); bronchospasm (0.2%, see Warnings); hyperventilation, rhinitis (0.1%); coughing, pleural pain (0.03%).

Other: Myalgia (0.9%); back pain (0.6%); injection site reaction unspecified, diaphoresis (0.4%); asthenia, malaise, arthralgia (0.3%); injection site pain, rigor, earache, tinnitus, vision abnormalities unspecified, dysgeusia (0.1%); thirst, depersonalization, eye pain, renal pain, perineal pain, breast pain, intermittent claudication, leg cramping (0.03%).

Overdosage:

It is unlikely that overdosage will occur because of the nature of use (ie, single IV administration in controlled settings).

Administration and Dosage:

Adjust the dose according to the weight of the patient. The recommended dose is 0.142 mg/kg/minute (0.57 mg/kg total) infused over 4 minutes. Although the maximum tolerated dose has not been determined, clinical experience suggests that a total dose beyond 60 mg is not needed for any patient. Prior to IV administration, dilute in at least a 1:2 ratio with 0.5N Sodium Chloride Injection, 1N Sodium Chloride Injection, or 5% Dextrose Injection for a total volume of approximately 20 to 50 ml. Infusion of undiluted dipyridamole may cause local irritation. Inject thallium-201 within 5 minutes following the 4 minute infusion of dipyridamole.

Storage: Avoid freezing. Protect from direct light.

Rx	**Persantine IV** (DuPont-Merck)	**Injection:** 10 mg[1]	In 2 ml amps.

[1] With 100 mg polyethylene glycol 600 and 4 mg tartaric acid.

SERMORELIN ACETATE

Actions:

Pharmacology: Sermorelin is for diagnostic use only. It increases plasma growth hormone (GH) concentrations by direct stimulation of the pituitary gland to release GH. Sermorelin is an acetate salt of a synthetic, 29-amino acid polypeptide that is the amino-terminal segment of the naturally occurring human growth hormone-releasing hormone (GHRH or GRH) consisting of 44 amino acid residues. Sermorelin appears to be equivalent to GRH (1-44) in its ability to stimulate growth hormone secretion in humans. It has also been called GRH (1-29) and GHRH (1-29).

Because baseline GH levels are generally very low (< 4 ng/ml), provocative tests may be useful in determining the functional GH-secreting capability of the pituitary somatotroph. Adults and children with normal responses to standard provocative tests of GH secretion were used to define the range of normal plasma GH-level responses to sermorelin. It was found that the absolute peak GH level following sermorelin infusion and the time elapsed from infusion to that peak are appropriate measures to evaluate the response to GH infusion. Doses used in children and adults in these studies ranged from 0.3 to 6.06 mcg/kg with a majority of patients receiving 1 mcg/kg. Based on these studies and published reports, 1 mcg/kg was chosen as the recommended dose for diagnostic purposes.

Clinical trials: A total of 71 sermorelin injection tests were performed on 47 boys and 24 girls who showed normal responses to standard, indirect provocative tests such as clonidine, L-dopa and arginine. The GH peak plasma response to sermorelin was 28 ± 15 ng/ml and the time to this peak was 30 ± 27 minutes.

Of all children who had GH responses of > 7 ng/ml to standard provocative tests, 96% also had responses to sermorelin of > 7 ng/ml. In 77 patients who failed to respond to standard provocative tests, mean GH peak responses to sermorelin were significantly lower compared to the mean GH peak response of normal control children. However, 53% of the children who failed to respond to standard tests had a GH response to sermorelin of > 7 ng/ml suggesting that clinical GH deficiency is frequently not due to somatotroph failure.

Preliminary studies have demonstrated an age-related decline in GH responsiveness to GRH in persons > 40 years old, but the normal range of GH response to sermorelin in older adults has not been established.

Indications:

As a single IV injection for evaluating the ability of the somatotroph of the pituitary gland to secrete growth hormone.

Contraindications:

Hypersensitivity to sermorelin or any of the excipients.

Warnings:

Hypersensitivity: Although hypersensitivity reactions have been observed with other polypeptide hormones, to date no such reactions have been reported following the administration of a single dose of sermorelin.

Antibody formation has occurred in humans after chronic SC administration of large doses of sermorelin. Approximately one in four patients given repeated doses of one or more of the three forms of GRH (1-29, 1-40 and 1-44) has developed antibodies to GRH. The clinical significance of these antibodies is unknown. One patient who developed antibodies to GRH (1-44) also experienced an allergic reaction described as severe redness, swelling and urticaria at the injection sites. No long-lasting effects from this reaction were reported. No symptomatic allergic reactions to GRH (1-29) have been reported.

GH deficiency: A normal plasma GH response to sermorelin demonstrates that the somatotroph is intact. However, a normal response does not exclude GH deficiency because this deficiency is frequently the result of hypothalamic dysfunction in the presence of an intact somatotroph. The sermorelin stimulation test is most easily interpreted when there is a subnormal response to conventional provocative testing and a normal response to sermorelin. Such findings suggest that hypothalamic dysfunction is the cause for the growth hormone deficiency. When both conventional and sermorelin testing result in subnormal GH responses, the site of dysfunction cannot be determined with certainty because some patients with GH deficiency due to hypothalamic dysfunction require repeated sermorelin administration before demonstrating a normal response.

(Warnings continued on following page)

SERMORELIN ACETATE (Cont.)

Warnings (Cont.):

Acromegaly: The sermorelin test has not been found useful in the diagnosis of acromegaly.

Pregnancy: Category C. Sermorelin produces minor variations in fetuses of rats and rabbits when given in SC doses of 50, 150 and 500 mcg/kg. In the rat teratology study, external malformations (thin tail) were observed in the higher dose groups, and there was an increase in minor skeletal variants at the high dose. Some visceral malformations (hydroureter) were observed in all treatment groups, with the incidence greatest in the high-dose group. In rabbits, minor skeletal anomalies were significantly greater in the treated animals than in the controls. There are no adequate and well controlled studies in pregnant women. Use sermorelin during pregnancy only if the potential benefit justifies the potential risk to the fetus.

Lactation: It is not known whether this drug is excreted in breast milk. Exercise caution when administering to a nursing woman.

Precautions:

Subnormal GH response: Obesity, hyperglycemia and elevated plasma fatty acids generally are associated with subnormal GH responses to sermorelin.

Drug Interactions:

The sermorelin test should not be conducted in the presence of drugs that directly affect the pituitary secretion of somatotropin. These include preparations that contain or release somatostatin, insulin, glucocorticoids, or cyclooxygenase inhibitors such as aspirin or indomethacin. Somatotropin levels may be transiently elevated by clonidine, levodopa and insulin-induced hypoglycemia. Response to sermorelin may be blunted in patients who are receiving muscarinic antagonists (atropine) or who are hypothyroid or being treated with antithyroid medications such as propylthiouracil. Discontinue exogenous growth hormone therapy at least 1 week before administering the test.

Adverse Reactions:

The following adverse reactions, in decreasing order of frequency, have occurred following sermorelin administration: Transient warmth or flushing of the face; injection site pain; redness or swelling at injection site; nausea; headache; vomiting; strange taste in the mouth; paleness; tightness in the chest. Antibody formation has been reported (see Warnings).

Overdosage:

Changes of heart rate and blood pressure have occurred with the various GRH peptides in IV doses exceeding 10 mcg/kg. Cardiovascular collapse is a conceivable, but as of yet, unreported, complication of overdosage with GRH (1-29).

Administration and Dosage:

Approved by the FDA in 1991.

Individualize dosage for each patient according to weight. Administer in a single IV dose of 1 mcg/kg in the morning following an overnight fast.

Children (or subjects < 50 kg):

1) Reconstitute the contents of one 50 mcg amp with a minimum of 0.5 ml of the accompanying sterile diluent.

2) Draw venous blood samples for GH determinations 15 minutes before and immediately prior to administration.

3) Administer a bolus of 1 mcg/kg IV followed by a 3 ml normal saline flush.

4) Draw venous blood samples for GH determinations at 15, 30, 45 and 60 minutes after administration.

Adults (or subjects > 50 kg):

1) Determine the number of amps needed, based on a dose of 1 mcg/kg.

2) Reconstitute the contents of each amp with a minimum of 0.5 ml of the accompanying sterile diluent.

3) Follow steps 2 through 4 in the Children's section.

Storage/Stability: The lyophilized product must be stored under refrigeration (2° to 8°C; 36° to 46°F). Use immediately after reconstitution. Discard unused material.

Rx	**Geref** (Serono Labs)	**Powder for Injection, lyophilized:** 50 mcg (as the acetate)[1]	In amps with 2 ml of 0.9% Sodium Chloride Injection, USP as a diluent in vials.

[1] With 5 mg mannitol, 0.66 mg monobasic sodium phosphate and 0.04 mg dibasic sodium phosphate; may contain up to 1% albumin (Human).

Radiopaque agents, except barium sulfate, include a number of iodinated compounds; these agents are used to visualize various organ systems upon x-ray examination. The radiopacity of these agents is a function of the percentage of iodine in the molecule and the concentration of compound present.

The most important characteristic of contrast media is the iodine content. The relatively high atomic weight of iodine contributes sufficient radiodensity for radiographic contrast with surrounding tissues. The enteral radiopaque agents are substituted, triiodinated, benzoic acid derivatives.

Parenteral radiopaque diagnostic agents are water soluble, triiodinated, benzoic acid salts. Due to organically bound iodine (5.1% to 48.25% by weight), the injectable radiopaque agents can opacify internal structures for x-ray visualization and fluoroscopy.

Nonionic vs ionic agents: Iohexol, iopamidol and metrizamide are nonionic iodine contrast media. The other iodinated contrast media currently available are ionic. The nonionic media have a lower osmolality than the ionic contrast media and are associated with a lower incidence of adverse effects. The nonionic media are also associated with a lower incidence of anaphylactoid reactions.

Anaphylactoid reactions occur in 1% to 2% of patients receiving radiopaque agents. The incidence increases to 17% to 35% when radiocontrast procedures are repeated in patients with a history of anaphylactoid reactions to radiopaque agents. Pretreatment of the high risk patients with a regimen including diphenhydramine, prednisone and ephedrine has reduced the incidence of repeated and possibly more severe reactions to ≈ 3.1%. Use extreme caution. Refer to Management of Acute Hypersensitivity Reactions.

Tartrazine sensitivity: Some of these products contain tartrazine which may cause allergic-type reactions (including bronchial asthma) in certain susceptible individuals. Although the overall incidence of tartrazine sensitivity in the general population is low, it is frequently seen in patients who also have aspirin hypersensitivity. Specific products containing tartrazine are identified in the product listings.

Patient Information:

Oral and rectal iodinated agents:

Take all medication with water following a fat-free dinner on the evening prior to the test. Thereafter, take nothing except water until the test has been completed.

Inform physician of pregnancy or of allergy to iodine, any foods or x-ray materials.

These agents may cause mild and transient abdominal cramping, nausea, vomiting, diarrhea, skin rashes, itching, heartburn, dizziness or headache.

Consult physician if thyroid tests are planned; iodine may interfere with thyroid tests.

Parenteral iodinated agents:

Prior to these procedures, notify physician if any of the following conditions exist: Pregnancy, diabetes, multiple myeloma, pheochromocytoma, homozygous sickle cell disease, thyroid disease, allergy to any drugs or food, reactions to previous injections of dyes used for x-ray procedures. Also notify physician if you are taking any other medications, including *otc* drugs.

These agents should be given only by personnel experienced in their use, and only in facilities with the proper equipment to deal with possible untoward effects of the drug.

The following table summarizes the radiopaque agents and their uses. Due to the specificity of use and the multiplicity of administrations for these agents, this table and the product listings in this section are not intended to provide comprehensive information necessary for the safe and effective use of these agents. Consult the package literature for complete prescribing information.

Indications and Uses of the Radiopaque Agents

Radiopaque Agents	% Iodine (Approx.)	Cholecystography	Cholangiography	Gastrointestinal	Urography	Pyelography	Cystourethrography	Arthrography	Myelography	Angiography	Angiocardiography	Arteriography	Aortography	Ventriculography	Venography	Hysterosalpingography	Splenoportography	Computed Tomography	Lymphography
Oral Cholecystographics																			
Iocetamic acid	62	✓																	
Iopanoic acid	67	✓	✓																
Ipodate calcium	62	✓	✓																
Ipodate sodium	61	✓	✓																
Tyropanoate sodium	57	✓																	

(Indications table continued on following page)

Indications and Uses of the Radiopaque Agents (Cont.)

Radiopaque Agents	% Iodine (Approx.)	Cholecystography	Cholangiography	Gastrointestinal	Urography	Pyelography	Cystourethrography	Arthrography	Myelography	Angiography	Angiocardiography	Arteriography	Aortography	Ventriculography	Venography	Hysterosalpingography	Splenoportography	Computed Tomography	Lymphography
GI Contrast																			
Barium	0			✓														✓	
Diatrizoate sodium 41.66%	25			✓															
Diatrizoate sodium powder	60			✓															
Diatrizoate meglumine 66%/ Diatrizoate sodium 10%	37			✓														✓	
Parenteral																			
Diatrizoate meglumine 30%	14				✓	✓									✓			✓	
Diatrizoate meglumine 60%[1]	28		✓		✓	✓		✓		✓		✓			✓		✓	✓	
Diatrizoate meglumine 76%	36				✓					✓		✓	✓						
Diatrizoate sodium 25%	15				✓													✓	
Diatrizoate sodium 50%	30		✓		✓					✓			✓		✓	✓	✓	✓	
Gadopentetate dimeglumine[2]	0																		
Iodamide meglumine 24%	11				✓	✓												✓	
Iodamide meglumine 65%	30				✓														
Iodipamide meglumine 10.3%	5	✓	✓																
Iodipamide meglumine 52%	26	✓	✓																
Iohexol	46				✓				✓	✓	✓	✓	✓	✓	✓			✓	
Iopamidol 26%	13									✓									
Iopamidol 41%	20				✓					✓	✓	✓	✓	✓	✓			✓	
Iopamidol 61%	30				✓					✓	✓	✓	✓	✓	✓			✓	
Iopamidol 76%	37				✓					✓	✓	✓	✓	✓	✓			✓	
Iothalamate meglumine 30%	14				✓					✓								✓	
Iothalamate meglumine 43%	20				✓	✓	✓			✓					✓			✓	
Iothalamate meglumine 60%[3]	28		✓		✓			✓		✓		✓			✓			✓	
Iothalamate sodium 54.3%	33				✓														
Iothalamate sodium 66.8%	40				✓						✓		✓					✓	
Iothalamate sodium 80%	48										✓		✓						
Metrizamide[4]	48								✓		✓	✓		✓				✓	
Diatrizoate meglumine 28.5%/ Diatrizoate sodium 29.1%[5]	31				✓						✓	✓	✓		✓				
Diatrizoate meglumine 34.3%/ Diatrizoate sodium 35%[5]	37				✓						✓	✓	✓		✓				
Diatrizoate meglumine 50%/ Diatrizoate sodium 25%	39				✓					✓	✓		✓					✓	
Diatrizoate meglumine 52%/ Diatrizoate sodium 8%[1]	29		✓		✓			✓		✓		✓			✓		✓	✓	
Diatrizoate meglumine 60%/ Diatrizoate sodium 30%	46				✓					✓	✓		✓			✓		✓	
Diatrizoate meglumine 66%/ Diatrizoate sodium 10%	37				✓					✓	✓	✓	✓	✓	✓			✓	
Iothalamate meglumine 52%/ Iothalamate sodium 26%	40				✓					✓	✓	✓	✓					✓	
Ioxaglate meglumine 39.3%/ Ioxaglate sodium 19.6%	32				✓			✓		✓	✓	✓	✓	✓	✓	✓		✓	
Ioversol 34%	16									✓									
Ioversol 51%	24									✓					✓				
Ioversol 68%	32				✓					✓		✓	✓	✓				✓	
Miscellaneous																			
Diatrizoate meglumine 18%	9						✓												
Diatrizoate meglumine 30%	14					✓	✓												
Diatrizoate sodium 20%	12					✓													
Iothalamate meglumine 17.2%[6]	8						✓												
Iothalamate meglumine 43%[6]	20					✓	✓												
Diatrizoate meglumine 52.7%/ Iodipamide meglumine 26.8%	38															✓			
Ethiodized oil	37															✓			✓
Propyliodone oil[7]	34																		

[1] Also discography.
[2] With MRI for intracranial, spine and associated tissues.
[3] Also cholangiopancreatography.
[4] Also cisternography.
[5] Also venocavography.
[6] Also cystography.
[7] Also bronchography.

Oral Cholecystographic Agents

IOCETAMIC ACID (62% iodine)

Rx	**Cholebrine** (Mallinckrodt)	**Tablets:** 750 mg	White, scored. In 150s.

IOPANOIC ACID (66.68% iodine)

Rx	**Telepaque** (Winthrop Pharm.)	**Tablets:** 500 mg	Off-white, scored. In 150s.

IPODATE CALCIUM (61.7% iodine)

Rx	**Oragrafin Calcium** (Squibb Diagnostics)	**Granules for Oral Suspension:** 3 g/packet	Sucrose. In 25 g packets.

IPODATE SODIUM (61.4% iodine)

Rx	**Bilivist** (Berlex)	**Capsules:** 500 mg	D-sorbitol, lecithin. (162). In 120s.
Rx	**Oragrafin Sodium** (Squibb Diagnostics)		Tartrazine, lecithin. (455). Yellow. In 100s, 144s and UD 100s.

TYROPANOATE SODIUM (57.4% iodine)

Rx	**Bilopaque** (Winthrop Pharm.)	**Capsules:** 750 mg	Benzyl alcohol. In 100s.

GI Contrast Agents (Iodinated)

DIATRIZOATE SODIUM 41.66% (24.9% iodine)

Rx	**Hypaque Sodium** (Winthrop Pharm.)	**Solution**	In 120 ml.[1]

DIATRIZOATE SODIUM (59.87% iodine)

Rx	**Hypaque Sodium** (Winthrop Pharm.)	**Powder**	In 10 and 250 g.[2]

DIATRIZOATE MEGLUMINE 66% and DIATRIZOATE SODIUM 10% (37% iodine)

Rx	**Gastrografin** (Squibb Diagnostics)	**Solution**	Lemon flavor. In 120 ml.[3]
Rx	**MD-Gastroview** (Mallinckrodt)		Vanilla-lemon flavor. In 120 and 240 ml.[4]

GI Contrast Agents (Miscellaneous)

RADIOPAQUE POLYVINYL CHLORIDE

Rx	**Sitzmarks** (Lafayette Pharm.)	**Capsules:** Contain 20 radiopaque rings (1 mm x 4.5 mm)	In 10s.

SODIUM BICARBONATE

Rx	**Baros** (Lafayette)	**Granules, Effervescent:** 460 mg (126 mg sodium) and 420 mg tartaric acid	Simethicone. In 3 g plastic ampules.

[1] Parabens, polysorbate 80, saccharin, sucrose.
[2] Polysorbate 80.
[3] EDTA, polysorbate 80, saccharin.
[4] EDTA, saccharin.

GI Contrast Agents (Miscellaneous) (Cont.)

BARIUM SULFATE

Rx	**Baro-cat** (Lafayette Pharm.)	**Suspension:** 1.5%	Sorbitol. Pineapple-banana flavor. In 300, 900 and 1900 ml.
Rx	**Prepcat** (Lafayette Pharm.)		Sorbitol. Strawberry flavor. In 450 ml.
Rx	**Enecat** (Lafayette Pharm.)	**Concentrated Suspension:** 5%	Sorbitol. In 110 ml with 480 ml bottle for dilution.
Rx	**Tomocat** (Lafayette Pharm.)		Sorbitol. Strawberry flavor. In 145 ml with 480 ml bottle for dilution and 225 ml with two 1000 ml bottles for dilution.
Rx	**Entrobar** (Lafayette Pharm.)	**Suspension:** 50%	In 500 ml.
Rx	**Liquid Barosperse** (Lafayette Pharm.)	**Suspension:** 60%	Vanilla flavor. In 355 ml.
Rx	**HD 85** (Lafayette Pharm.)	**Suspension:** 85%	Raspberry flavor. In 150, 450 and 1900 ml.
Rx	**Barobag** (Lafayette Pharm.)	**Suspension:** 97%	In 340 and 454 g kits.
Rx	**Liquipake** (Lafayette Pharm.)	**Suspension:** 100%	In 1850 ml.
Rx	**Flo-Coat** (Lafayette Pharm.)		In 1850 ml.
Rx	**Epi-C** (Lafayette Pharm.)	**Concentrated Suspension:** 150%	Spearmint flavor. In 450 ml.
Rx	**Barium Sulfate, USP** (Various, eg, Humco)	**Powder**	In 500 g, 1 lb and 5 lb.
Rx	**Baroflave** (Lannett)	**Powder**	Raspberry flavor. In 5 and 25 lb.
Rx	**Tonopaque** (Lafayette Pharm)	**Powder for Suspension:** 95%	Sorbitol. Strawberry flavor. In 180 and 1200 g.
Rx	**Baricon** (Lafayette Pharm.)	**Powder for Suspension:** 98%	Vanilla-lemon flavor. In UD 340 g.
Rx	**HD 200 Plus** (Lafayette Pharm.)		Strawberry flavor. In 312 g.
Rx	**Barosperse** (Lafayette Pharm.)	**Powder for Suspension:** 95% and suspending agent	Vanilla flavor. In UD 225 and 900 g.
Rx	**Anatrast** (Lafayette Pharm.)	**Paste:** 100%	In 500 g tubes.

Parenteral Agents

DIATRIZOATE MEGLUMINE 30% (14.1% iodine)

	Product	Form	How Supplied
Rx	**Hypaque Meglumine 30%** (Winthrop Pharm.)	Injection	In 100 ml bottles[1] and 300 ml bottles[1] with or without infusion set.
Rx	**Reno-M-Dip** (Squibb Diagnostics)		In 300 ml bottles[1] with or without infusion set.
Rx	**Urovist Meglumine DIU/CT** (Berlex)		In 300 ml bottles[1] with or without infusion set.

DIATRIZOATE MEGLUMINE 60% (28% iodine)

	Product	Form	How Supplied
Rx	**Angiovist 282** (Berlex)	Injection	In 50, 100, 150, 500 and 1000 ml vials.[1]
Rx	**Hypaque Meglumine 60%** (Winthrop Pharm.)		In 20, 30, 50 and 100 ml vials and 150 and 200 ml bottles, and 100 & 150 ml with infusion sets.[1]
Rx	**Reno-M-60** (Squibb Diagnostics)		In 10, 30, 50 and 100 ml vials[1] and 100 and 150 ml bottles[1] with or without infusion sets.

DIATRIZOATE MEGLUMINE 76% (35.8% iodine)

	Product	Form	How Supplied
Rx	**Diatrizoate Meglumine 76%** (Squibb Diagnostics)	Injection	In 50 ml vials.[1]

DIATRIZOATE SODIUM 25% (15% iodine)

	Product	Form	How Supplied
Rx	**Hypaque Sodium 25%** (Winthrop Pharm.)	Injection	In 300 ml bottles with or without infusion set.[1]

DIATRIZOATE SODIUM 50% (30% iodine)

	Product	Form	How Supplied
Rx	**Hypaque Sodium 50%** (Winthrop Pharm.)	Injection	In 20, 30 and 50 ml vials[1] and 150 and 200 ml dilution bottles.[1]
Rx	**Urovist Sodium 300** (Berlex)		In 50 ml vials.[1]

GADOPENTETATE DIMEGLUMINE 46.9%

	Product	Form	How Supplied
Rx	**Magnevist** (Berlex)	Injection	In 20 ml.

IODAMIDE MEGLUMINE 24% (11.1% iodine)

	Product	Form	How Supplied
Rx	**Renovue-Dip** (Squibb Diagnostics)	Injection	In 300 ml bottles.[1]

IODAMIDE MEGLUMINE 65% (30% iodine)

	Product	Form	How Supplied
Rx	**Renovue-65** (Squibb Diagnostics)	Injection	In 50 ml vials.[1]

IODIPAMIDE MEGLUMINE 10.3% (5.1% iodine)

	Product	Form	How Supplied
Rx	**Cholografin Meglumine** (Squibb Diagnostics)	Injection	In 100 ml vials.[1]

IODIPAMIDE MEGLUMINE 52% (25.7% iodine)

	Product	Form	How Supplied
Rx	**Cholografin Meglumine** (Squibb Diagnostics)	Injection	In 20 ml vials.[1]

IOHEXOL (46.36% iodine)

	Product	Form	How Supplied
Rx	**Omnipaque** (Winthrop Pharm.)	**Injection:** 140 mg/ml (intrathecal only)	In 50 ml vials and bottles.[1]
		180 mg/ml	In 10 and 20 ml vials.[1]
		210 mg/ml	In 15 ml.[1]
		240 mg/ml	In 10, 20 and 50 ml vials[1] and 50, 100, 150 and 200 ml bottles.[1]
		300 mg/ml	In 10, 30 and 50 ml vials[1] and 50, 100 and 150 ml bottles.
		350 mg/ml	In 50 ml vials[1] & 50, 75, 100, 125, 150, 175 & 200 ml bottles.

[1] With EDTA.

Parenteral Agents (Cont.)

IOPAMIDOL 26% (12.8% iodine)			
Rx	**Isovue-128** (Squibb Diagnostics)	**Injection**	In 50 ml vials.[1]
IOPAMIDOL 41% (20% iodine)			
Rx	**Isovue-200** (Squibb Diagnostics)	**Injection**	In 50 ml vials[1] and 100 and 200 ml bottles.[1]
Rx	**Isovue-M 200** (Squibb Diagnostics)	**Injection**	In 20 ml vials.[1] *For intrathecal use.*
IOPAMIDOL 61% (30% iodine)			
Rx	**Isovue-300** (Squibb Diagnostics)	**Injection**	In 30, 50, 75, 100 and 150 ml.[2]
Rx	**Isovue-M 300** (Squibb Diagnostics)	**Injection**	In 15 ml vials.[2] *For intrathecal use.*
IOPAMIDOL 76% (37% iodine)			
Rx	**Isovue-370** (Squibb Diagnostics)	**Injection**	In 20, 30, 50, 75, 100, 150, 175 and 200 ml.[2]
IOTHALAMATE MEGLUMINE 30% (14.1% iodine)			
Rx	**Conray 30** (Mallinckrodt)	**Injection**	In 50, 100, 150 and 300 ml.[1]
IOTHALAMATE MEGLUMINE 43% (20.2% iodine)			
Rx	**Conray 43** (Mallinckrodt)	**Injection**	In 50, 100, 150, 200 and 250 ml vials[1] and 50, 95 and 125 ml prefilled syringes.[1]
IOTHALAMATE MEGLUMINE 60% (28.2% iodine)			
Rx	**Conray** (Mallinckrodt)	**Injection**	In 20, 30, 50, 100, 150 and 200 ml vials[1] and 30, 50, 95 and 125 ml prefilled syringes.[1]
IOTHALAMATE SODIUM 54.3% (32.5% iodine)			
Rx	**Conray 325** (Mallinckrodt)	**Injection**	In 30 and 50 ml vials[1] and 50 ml prefilled syringes.[1]
IOTHALAMATE SODIUM 66.8% (40% iodine)			
Rx	**Conray 400** (Mallinckrodt)	**Injection**	In 25 and 50 ml vials[1] and 30 and 50 ml prefilled syringes.[1]
IOTHALAMATE SODIUM 80% (48% iodine)			
Rx	**Angio Conray** (Mallinckrodt)	**Injection**	In 50 ml vials.[1]
IOVERSOL 34% (16% iodine)			
Rx	**Optiray 160** (Mallinckrodt)	**Injection**	In 50 and 100 ml vials.[2]
IOVERSOL 51% (24% iodine)			
Rx	**Optiray 240** (Mallinckrodt)	**Injection**	In 50, 100 and 200 ml.[2]
IOVERSOL 68% (32% iodine)			
Rx	**Optiray 320** (Mallinckrodt)	**Injection**	In 20, 30, 50, 100, 150 and 200 ml.[2]
METRIZAMIDE (48.25% iodine)			
Rx	**Amipaque** (Winthrop Pharm.)	**Powder for Injection, lyophilized:**	
		13.5%	In 50 ml vial[2] w/diluent.
		18.75%	In 20 ml vial[2] w/diluent.

[1] With EDTA.
[2] With EDTA and tromethamine.

Parenteral Agents (Cont.)

DIATRIZOATE MEGLUMINE 28.5% and DIATRIZOATE SODIUM 29.1% (31% iodine)

	Product	Form	How Supplied
Rx	**Renovist II** (Squibb Diagnostics)	**Injection**	In 30 and 60 ml vials.[1]

DIATRIZOATE MEGLUMINE 34.3% and DIATRIZOATE SODIUM 35% (37% iodine)

	Product	Form	How Supplied
Rx	**Renovist** (Squibb Diagnostics)	**Injection**	In 50 ml vials.[1]

DIATRIZOATE MEGLUMINE 50% and DIATRIZOATE SODIUM 25% (38.5% iodine)

	Product	Form	How Supplied
Rx	**Hypaque-M, 75%** (Winthrop Pharm.)	**Injection**	In 20 and 50 ml vials.[1]

DIATRIZOATE MEGLUMINE 52% and DIATRIZOATE SODIUM 8% (29.3% iodine)

	Product	Form	How Supplied
Rx	**Angiovist 292** (Berlex)	**Injection**	In 30, 50 and 100 ml vials.[1]
Rx	**MD-60** (Mallinckrodt)		In 30 and 50 ml vials.[1]
Rx	**Renografin-60** (Squibb Diagnostics)		In 10, 30, 50 and 100 ml vials.[1]

DIATRIZOATE MEGLUMINE 60% and DIATRIZOATE SODIUM 30% (46.2% iodine)

	Product	Form	How Supplied
Rx	**Hypaque-M, 90%** (Winthrop Pharm.)	**Injection**	In 50 ml vials.[1]

DIATRIZOATE MEGLUMINE 66% and DIATRIZOATE SODIUM 10% (37% iodine)

	Product	Form	How Supplied
Rx	**Angiovist 370** (Berlex)	**Injection**	In 50, 100, 150 and 200 ml vials & 500 ml w/infusion set.[1]
Rx	**Hypaque-76** (Winthrop Pharm.)		In 30, 50, 100, 150 and 200 ml.[1]
Rx	**MD-76** (Mallinckrodt)		In 50, 100, 150 and 200 ml vials and 95 and 125 ml syringes.[1]
Rx	**Renografin-76** (Squibb Diagnostics)		In 20, 50, 100 and 200 ml.[1]

IOTHALAMATE MEGLUMINE 52% and IOTHALAMATE SODIUM 26% (40% iodine)

	Product	Form	How Supplied
Rx	**Vascoray** (Mallinckrodt)	**Injection**	In 50 ml vials and 100, 150 and 200 ml bottles.[1]

IOXAGLATE MEGLUMINE 39.3% and IOXAGLATE SODIUM 19.6% (32% iodine)

	Product	Form	How Supplied
Rx	**Hexabrix** (Mallinckrodt)	**Injection**	In 20, 30 and 50 ml vials, 75 ml fill in 150 ml bottles, 100 ml fill in 150 ml, 200 ml fill in 250 ml, 150 ml bottles, 95 and 125 ml prefilled syringes.[1]

[1] With EDTA.

Miscellaneous Agents

The following products are used for instillation into various cavities. They are NOT intended for intravascular administration.

DIATRIZOATE MEGLUMINE 18% (8.5% iodine)

Rx	**Cystografin Dilute** (Squibb Diagnostics)	**Injection**	In 300 and 500 ml[1] with or without administration sets.

DIATRIZOATE MEGLUMINE 30% (14.1% iodine)

Rx	**Cystografin** (Squibb Diagnostics)	**Injection**	In 100 and 300 ml.[1]
Rx	**Hypaque-Cysto** (Winthrop Pharm.)		In 100 ml in a pediatric 300 ml bottle[1] and 250 ml in a 500 ml bottle.[1]
Rx	**Reno-M-30** (Squibb Diagnostics)		In 50 and 100 ml.[2]
Rx	**Urovist Cysto** (Berlex)		In 100 ml in a pediatric 300 ml bottle[1] and 300 ml in a 500 ml bottle.[1]

DIATRIZOATE SODIUM 20% (12% iodine)

Rx	**Hypaque Sodium 20%** (Winthrop Pharm.)	**Injection**	In 100 ml.[1]

IOTHALAMATE MEGLUMINE 17.2% (8.1% iodine)

Rx	**Cysto-Conray II** (Mallinckrodt)	**Injection**	In 250 and 500 ml.[1]

IOTHALAMATE MEGLUMINE 43% (20.2% iodine)

Rx	**Cysto-Conray** (Mallinckrodt)	**Injection**	In 50 and 100 ml vials and 250 ml bottles and 50 ml prefilled syringes.[1]

DIATRIZOATE MEGLUMINE 52.7% & IODIPAMIDE MEGLUMINE 26.8% (38% iodine)

Rx	**Sinografin** (Squibb Diagnostics)	**Injection**	In 10 ml vials.[1]

ETHIODIZED OIL (37% iodine)

Rx	**Ethiodol** (Savage)	**Injection**	In 10 ml amps.

PROPYLIODONE 60% in peanut oil (≈ 34% iodine)

Rx	**Dionosil Oily** (Allen & Hanburys)	**Suspension**	In 20 ml vials. *For intratracheal use.*

ISOSULFAN BLUE

Indications:

Delineates the lymphatic vessels. Adjunct to lymphography for visualization of the lymphatic system draining the region of injection.

Rx	**Lymphazurin 1%** (Hirsch Industries, Inc.)	**Injection:** 1% (10 mg/ml)	In 5 ml vials.

POTASSIUM PERCHLORATE

Indications:

To minimize the accumulation of pertechnetate Tc 99m in the choroid plexus and in the salivary and thyroid glands of patients receiving sodium pertechnetate Tc 99m for brain and blood pool imaging and placenta localization.

Unlabeled use: Treatment of hyperthyroidism.

Rx	**Perchloracap** (Mallinckrodt)	**Capsules:** 200 mg	(19-N025) Opaque gray. In 100s.

[1] With EDTA.

[2] With EDTA and methyl and propyl parabens.

The National Information Center for Orphan Drugs and Rare Diseases (NICODARD) provides information about the treatment of rare diseases, the availability of orphan drugs, grant program materials and an information packet (including general information on NICODARD, an overview of the OPD grants program, etc). The Orphan Drug Act defines an orphan drug as a drug or biological product for the diagnosis, treatment or prevention of a rare disease or condition. A rare disease is one which affects < 200,000 persons in the US or one which affects > 200,000 persons but for which there is no reasonable expectation that the cost of developing the drug and making it available will be recovered from sales of that drug.

Inquiries can be made to:

National Information Center for Orphan Drugs and Rare Diseases (NICODARD)
PO Box 1133
Washington, DC 20013-1133
(800) 456-3505 or (202) 565-4167
(Washington DC metropolitan area)

or

Office of Orphan Products Development
5600 Fishers Lane
Rockville, Maryland 20857
(301) 443-4903

Orphan Drug/Biological Designations

Drug *(Trade Name)*	Proposed Use	Sponsor
Acetylcysteine *(Mucomyst/Mucomyst 10)*	IV for moderate to severe acetaminophen overdose	Bristol-Myers
Aconiazide	Tuberculosis	Lincoln Diagnostics
Adenosine	In conjunction with BCNU in the treatment of brain tumors	Medco Research
Allopurinol riboside	Chagus' disease; cutaneous and visceral leishmaniasis	Burroughs Wellcome
Allopurinol sodium *(Zyloprim)*	Ex vivo preservation of cadaveric kidneys for transplantation	Burroughs Wellcome
Alpha-1-antitrypsin (recombinant DNA origin)	Supplementation therapy for alpha-1-antitrypsin deficiency in the ZZ phenotype population	Cooper Biomedical
Alpha-fetoprotein radioimmunodetection with TC-99M	Detection of alpha-fetoprotein producing germ cell tumors and hepatocellular carcinoma and hepatoblastoma	Immunomedics
Alpha-Galactoside A *(FABRase)*	Fabry's Disease	Robert J. Desnick, MD, PhD
Alpha-1-proteinase inhibitor[1]	Replacement therapy in the alpha-1-proteinase inhibitor congenital deficiency state	Cutter
Amiloride HCl for inhalation	Cystic fibrosis	Glaxo
4-Aminopyridine	Relief of symptoms of multiple sclerosis	Rush-Presby-St. Luke's
4-Aminosalicylic acid *Pamisyl (P-D); Rezipas (Squibb)*	Mild to moderate ulcerative colitis in patients intolerant to sulfasalazine	Warren L. Becker, MD
Amsacrine *(Amsidyl)*	Acute adult leukemia	Warner-Lambert
Anagrelide	Polycythemia vera; essential thrombocythemia; thrombocytosis in chronic myelogenous leukemia	Bristol-Myers
Ancrod *(Arvin)*	Antithrombotic in patients with heparin-induced thrombocytopenia or thrombosis	Knoll
Anti-cytomegalovirus monoclonal antibodies	To treat/prevent cytomegalovirus infection in AIDS, bone marrow and organ transplant patients	Medimorphics
Antiepilepsirine	Drug-resistant generalized tonic-clonic (GTC) epilepsy in children and adults	Children's Hospital, Columbus, OH

[1] Approved for marketing.

(Continued on following page)

Orphan Drug/Biological Designations		
Drug *(Trade Name)*	Proposed Use	Sponsor
Antihemophilic factor XIII	To treat bleeding in hemophilia A; for prophylaxis when surgery is required	Miles
Anti-J5MAB	Patients with gram-negative bacteremia which has progressed to endotoxin shock	Centocor
Antimelanoma antibody XMMME-001-RTA	Stage III melanoma not amenable to surgical resection	Xoma
Anti-MY9-blocked ricin	Myeloid leukemia, including AML, and blast crisis of CML; ex vivo purging of leukemic cells from the bone marrow of acute myelocytic leukemia patients	Immunogen
Antipyrine	Test as an index of hepatic drug-metabolizing capacity	Upsher-Smith
Anti-TAP-72 Immunotoxin *(Xomazyme-791)*	Metastatic colorectal cancer adenocarcinoma treatment	Xoma
Antithrombin III (eg, *Kybernin*)	Prophylaxis/treatment of thromboembolic episodes in genetic-AT-III deficiency	Hoechst-Roussel; Cutter
Antithrombin III human (eg, *Antithrombin*)	Patients with hereditary antithrombin III deficiency in connection with surgical or obstetrical procedures; thromboembolism	Kabi Vitrum; American Red Cross
AS-101	AIDS	Wyeth-Ayerst
5-AZA-2 Deoxycytidine	Acute leukemia	Pharmachemie B.V.
3-Azido-2, 3 Dideoxyuridine	AIDS	Triton Biosciences
Bacitracin *(Altracin)*	Antibiotic-associated pseudomembranous enterocolitis caused by toxins A and B elaborated by *Clostridium difficile*	A.L. Labs
Baclofen (intrathecal) *(Lioresal)*	Intractable spasticity due to spinal cord injury or multiple sclerosis	Medtronic
Benzoate and phenylacetate *(Ucephan[1])*	Adjunctive therapy to prevent/treat hyperammonemia in patients with urea cycle enzymopathy due to certain enzyme deficiencies	Kendall McGaw
Benzylpenicillin, Benzylpenicilloic acid, Benzylpenilloic acid *(Pre-Pen/MDM)*	Assessing risk of using penicillin when it is the preferred drug of choice in adults with a history of clinical penicillin sensitivity	Schwarz Pharma Kremers Urban
Bethanidine sulfate	To treat/prevent primary ventricular fibrillation	Medco Research
Biodegradable polymer implant containing carmustine *(Biodel Implant/BCNU)*	For localized placement in the brain for the treatment of recurrent malignant glioma	Nova Pharmaceutical
Botulinum toxin *(Ortholinum)*	Spasmodic torticollis	Alan B. Scott, MD
Botulinum toxin type A *(Oculinum)*	Blepharospasm; strabismus	Oculinum
Botulism immune globulin	Infant botulism	California Dept. Health Service
Branched chain amino acids	Amyotrophic lateral sclerosis	Mount Sinai Medical Center
Bromhexine	Mild/moderate keratoconjunctivitis sicca in Sjogren's syndrome	Boehringer Ingelheim
BW 12C	Sickle cell disease	Burroughs Wellcome

[1] Approved for marketing.

(Continued on following page)

Orphan Drug/Biological Designations		
Drug *(Trade Name)*	Proposed Use	Sponsor
BW B759U (DHPG)	Human cytomegalovirus infections in specific immunosuppressed patients (eg, bone marrow transplant recipients, AIDS)	Burroughs Wellcome
C1-Inhibitor *(C1-Inhibitor (Human) Vapor Heated)*	To prevent/treat acute attacks of angioedema, including short-term prophylaxis in dental or other surgical procedures	Immuno Clinical Research
Caffeine	Apnea of prematurity	Pediatric Pharms
Calcitonin-Human *(Cibacalcin[1])*	Symptomatic Paget's Disease of bone (osteitis deformans)	Ciba-Geigy
Calcium acetate *(Phos-Lo)*	Hyperphosphatemia in end stage renal failure	Braintree Laboratories; Pharmedic
Carbovir	AIDS; symptomatic HIV infection and CD4 count $< 200/mm^3$	Glaxo
Cascara sagrada fluid extract	For oral drug overdosage to speed lower bowel evacuation	Intramed
CD4 human truncated 369 AA polypeptide *(Soluble T4)*	AIDS	SKF
CD4 (human, recombinant)	Treatment of AIDS in patients infected with HIV virus	Genentech
CD5-T lymphocyte immunotoxin *(Xomazyme-H65)*	Graft vs host disease or rejection in bone marrow transplants; ex vivo treatment to eliminate mature T cells from potential bone marrow grafts	Xoma
Ceramide trihexosidase/alpha-galactosidase A	Fabry's Disease	Genzyme
Cetiedil citrate	Sickle cell crisis	Medical Market Specialties
Chenodiol *(Chenix[1])*	For radiolucent stones in well opacifying gallbladders, where elective surgery would be undertaken except for presence of increased surgical risk	Reid-Rowell
Chlorhexidine gluconate mouth rinse *(Peridex)*	Amelioration of oral mucositis associated with cytoreductive therapy for conditioning patients for bone marrow transplantation	Procter and Gamble
2-Chloro-2-Deoxyadenosine	Acute myeloid leukemia	St. Jude Children's Hospital
Citric acid, glucono-delta-lactone and mag carbonate *(Renacidin Solution[1])*	Renal and bladder calculi of the apatite or struvite variety	United-Guardian
Clindamycin *(Cleocin)*	*Pneumocystis carinii* pneumonia associated with AIDS	Upjohn
Clofazimine *(Lamprene[1])*	Lepromatous leprosy, including dapsone-resistant lepromatous leprosy and lepromatous leprosy complicated by erythema nodosum leprosum	Ciba-Geigy
Clonidine HCl	Epidural use for pain in cancer patients tolerant/unresponsive to intraspinal opiates	Lyphomed
Clostridium botulinum toxin type A *(Dysport)*	Blepharospasm	Parton Products

[1] Approved for marketing.

(Continued on following page)

Orphan Drug/Biological Designations		
Drug *(Trade Name)*	Proposed Use	Sponsor
Coagulation factor IX (human) *(Alphanine)*	Replacement therapy in hemophilia B for prevention of bleeding episodes; during surgery to correct defective hemostasis	Alpha Therapeutic
Colchicine	Arresting progression of neurologic disability due to chronic progressive multiple sclerosis	Pharmacontrol
Colfosceril palmitate, synthetic pulmonary surfactant *(Exosurf[1])*	To prevent hyaline membrane disease (respiratory distress syndrome) in infants born at ≤ 32 weeks gestation; to treat established hyaline membrane disease at all gestational ages	Burroughs Wellcome
Copolymer 1 (COP 1)	Multiple sclerosis	TAG
Cromolyn sodium *(Gastrocrom[1])*; Cromolyn sodium 4% ophthalmic solution *(Opticrom 4% Ophthalmic Solution[1])*	Mastocytosis Vernal keratoconjunctivitis	Fisons
Cyclosporine ophthalmic *(Optimmune)*	Severe keratoconjunctivitis sicca with Sjogren's syndrome	University of Georgia
Cyproterone acetate *(Androcur)*	Severe hirsutism	Berlex Labs
Cysteamine (2-aminoethanethiol)	Nephropathic cystinosis	Jess G. Thoene, MD
Cytomegalovirus immune globulin (human[1])	Prevention or attenuation of primary cytomegalovirus disease in immunosuppressed recipients of organ transplants	Mass. Pub. Health Bio. Labs
D, 1-Sotalol HCl	Treat/prevent life-threatening ventricular arrhythmias	Bristol-Myers
Dantrolene sodium *(Dantrium)*	Neuroleptic malignant syndrome	Procter & Gamble
Defibrotide	Thrombotic thrombocytopenic purpura	Crinos International
Dehydrex	Recurrent corneal erosion	Holles Labs
Deslorelin *(Somagard)*	Central precocious puberty	Roberts Pharmaceuticals
Dextran sulfate sodium	AIDS	Ueno Fine Chemicals
Diaziquone	Primary brain malignancies (Grade III-IV astrocytomas)	Warner-Lambert
2, 3-Dideoxycytidine	AIDS	Hoffman LaRoche; NCI; Bristol-Myers
Diethyldithiocarbamate	AIDS	Merieux Institute
Digoxin immune fab (Ovine) *(Digibind[1])*	Treatment of potentially life-threatening digitalis intoxication	Burroughs Wellcome
Digoxin immune fab (Ovine) *(Digidote)*	Life-threatening acute cardiac glycoside intoxication	Boehringer Mannheim
Dihematoporphyrin ethers *(Photofrin II)*	Photodynamic therapy of transitional cell carcinoma in situ of urinary bladder or primary recurrent obstructing esophageal carcinoma	QLT Phototherapeutics
24, 25 Dihydroxycholecalciferol	Uremic osteodystrophy	Lemmon/TAG
2, 3-Dimercaptosuccinic acid	Lead poisoning in children	Johnson & Johnson
Dimethyl sulfoxide (DMSO) *(Sclerosol)*	Cutaneous manifestations of scleroderma	Research Medical

[1] Approved for marketing.

(Continued on following page)

Orphan Drug/Biological Designations		
Drug *(Trade Name)*	Proposed Use	Sponsor
Dipalmitoylphosphatidylcholine/Phosphatidylglycerol	Prevention and treatment of respiratory distress syndrome in premature newborns	Alec
Disaccharide tripeptide glycerol dipalmitoyl *(Immther)*	Pulmonary and hepatic metastases in colorectal adenocarcinoma	Immuno Therapeutics
Disodium clodronate tetrahydrate *(Bonefos)*	Increased bone resorption due to malignancy	Leiras Pharmaceuticals
Disodium silibinin dihemisuccinate *(Legalon)*	Hepatic intoxication by amanita phalloides (poison mushroom)	Pharmaquest
Dynamine	Lambert Eaton myasthenic syndrome	Mayo Foundation
Eflornithine HCl (DFMO) *(Ornidyl)*	Trypanosoma brucei gambiense sleeping sickness; *Pneumocystis carinii* pneumonia in AIDS	Merrell Dow Research
Enisoprost	With cyclosporine in organ transplant recipients to reduce acute transplant rejection and cyclosporine nephrotoxicity	Searle
Epidermal growth factor (Human)	Acceleration of corneal epithelial regeneration and healing of stromal incisions from corneal transplant surgery and of non-healing corneal defects; promotes cutaneous wound healing in extreme burns	Chiron; Ethicon
Epoetin alfa *(Epogen*[1]*)*	Anemia associated with end stage renal disease	Amgen
Epoprostenol *(Flolan; Cyclo-prostin)*	Primary pulmonary hypertension; replacement of heparin in patients requiring hemodialysis at increased risk of hemorrhage	Burroughs Wellcome; Upjohn
Erwinia L-asparaginase	Acute lymphocytic leukemia	Porton
Erythropoietin (recombinant human) *(Eprex)*	Anemia in AIDS and ARC; anemia associated with end stage renal disease; anemia of premature infants	R.W. Johnson Research
Erythropoietin (recombinant human) (eg, *Marogen*)	Anemia associated with end stage renal disease	McDonnell Douglas Corp; Chugai; Organon
Ethanolamine oleate *(Ethamolin*[1]*)*	Bleeding esophageal varices	Glaxo
Ethinyl estradiol, USP	Turner's syndrome	Gynex
Ethiofos *(Ethyol)*	Chemoprotective agent for cisplatin in metastatic melanoma; for cyclophosphamide/cisplatin in advanced ovarian carcinoma	U.S. Bioscience
Etidronate disodium *(Didronel*[1]*)*	Hypercalcemia of a malignancy	Procter & Gamble
Factor VII-A (recombinant, DNA origin)	Patients with hemophilia A and B with and without antibodies against Factors VIII/IX; Von Willebrand's Disease	Novo
Factor XIII (placenta-derived)	Congenital Factor XIII deficiency	Hoechst-Roussel
Felbamate	Lennox-Gastrant syndrome	Wallace
Fibronectin (human plasma)	Nonhealing corneal ulcers or epithelial defects	New York Blood Center; Chiron Ophthalmics

[1] Approved for marketing.

(Continued on following page)

Orphan Drug/Biological Designations		
Drug *(Trade Name)*	Proposed Use	Sponsor
Fludarabine monophosphate	Non-Hodgkin's lymphoma	Triton Biosciences
Flumecinol *(Zixoryn)*	Hyperbilirubinemia in newborns unresponsive to phototherapy	Farmacon
Flunarizine *(Sibelium)*	Alternating hemiplegia	Janssen
Fluorouracil *(Adrucil)*	With leucovorin for colon/rectum metastatic adenocarcinoma	Lederle
Fluorouracil	In combination with interferon alpha-2a, for esophageal and advanced colorectal carcinoma	Hoffman LaRoche
Gallium nitrate	Hypercalcemia of malignancy	Lyphomed
Ganciclovir sodium *(Cytovene[1])*	Cytomegalovirus retinitis in AIDS patients	Syntex (USA)
Gangliosides as sodium salts *(Cronassial)*	Retinitis pigmentosa	FIDIA Pharmaceutical
Gentamicin liposome injection	Disseminated *mycobacterium avium-intracellulare* infection	Liposome Company
Glucocerebrosidase-beta-glucosidase (placenta-derived)	Replacement therapy in Gaucher's Disease type I	Genzyme
Gonadorelin acetate *(Lutrepulse[1])*	Ovulation induction in women with hypothalamic amenorrhea due to a deficiency or absence in endogenous Gn-RH secretion	R.W. Johnson Research Institute
Granulocyte-colony stimulating factor, recombinant (G-CSF)	Myelodysplastic syndrome	Amgen
Granulocyte macrophage-colony stimulating factor (GM-CSF)	AIDS patients with neutropenia due to the disease, zidovudine or ganciclovir; myelodysplastic syndrome; aplastic anemia; hairy cell leukemia; neutropenia associated with bone marrow transplants; chronic lymphocytic leukemia; severe thermal injuries in patients with > 40% full or partial thickness burns	Schering
Group B streptococcus immune globulin	Disseminated Group B streptococcal infection in neonates	Univax
Guanethidine monosulfate *(Ismelin)*	Moderate/severe reflex sympathetic dystrophy and causalgia	Ciba-Geigy
hCG radioimmunodetection with TC-99M *(Immuraid, HCGTC99M)*	Detection of hCG-producing tumors (eg, germ and trophoblastic cell tumors)	Immunomedics
Heme arginate *(Normosang)*	Symptomatic stage of acute porphyria	Huhtamaki Oy
Hemin *(Panhematin[1])*	Amelioration of recurrent attacks of acute intermittent porphyria temporarily related to menstrual cycle and similar symptoms which occur in other patients with AIP, porphyria variegata and heredita coproporphyria	Abbott
Hexamethylmelamine *(Hexastat)*	Advanced ovarian adenocarcinoma	U.S. Biosciences

[1] Approved for marketing.

(Continued on following page)

Orphan Drug/Biological Designations		
Drug *(Trade Name)*	Proposed Use	Sponsor
Histrelin	Central precocious puberty	Ortho
HPA-23	AIDS	Rhone-Poulenc
Human growth hormone releasing factor (1-44) amide	Long-term treatment of children who have growth failure due to a lack of adequate endogenous growth hormone secretion	Hoffman LaRoche
Human growth hormone, recombinant	Growth retardation associated with chronic renal failure	Genentech
Human IgM monoclonal antibody (C-58) to CMV *(Centovir)*	Treatment and prophylaxis of cytomegalovirus infections in allogenic bone marrow transplant patients	Centocor
Human immunodeficiency virus immune globulin	AIDS	Abbott
Human T-lymphotropic virus type III gp160 antigens *(Vaxsyn HIV-1)*	AIDS	Micro GeneSys
4-Hydroperoxycyclophosphamide (4-HC)	Ex vivo treatment of autologous bone marrow and subsequent reinfusion in patients with acute myelogenous leukemia (acute nonlymphocytic leukemia)	Nova Pharmaceutical
Hydroxocobalamin/sodium thiosulfate	Severe acute cyanide poisoning	Evreka
Idarubicin *(Idamycin[1])*	Acute nonlymphocytic leukemia	Adria
Ifosfamide *(Ifex[1])*	Testicular cancer; bone sarcomas; soft tissue sarcomas	Bristol-Myers
Iloprost	Raynaud's phenomenon secondary to systemic sclerosis; heparin-associated thrombocytopenia	Berlex
Immune globulin, aerosolized, pooled	Respiratory syncytial virus; lower respiratory tract disease	Pediatric Pharmaceuticals
Indium in 111 murine anti-CEA monoclonal antibody type ZCE 025 *(CEAker)*	Detection of tumor foci of recurrent colorectal carcinoma	Hybritech
Indium in 111 antimelanoma antibody XMMME-0001-DTPA	Diagnostic use in imaging systemic and nodal melanoma metastasis	Xoma
Indium in 111 murine monoclonal antibody B72.3 *(Oncoscint OV103)*	Detection of ovarian carcinoma	Cytogen
Indium in 111 murine monoclonal antibody fab to myosin *(Myoscint)*	Aid in diagnosis of myocarditis; detecting early necrosis as indication of rejection of orthotopic cardiac transplants	Centocor
Inosine pranobex *(Isoprinosine)*	Subacute sclerosing panencephalitis	Newport
Interferon alfa-2a *(Roferon A)*	Chronic myelogenous leukemia; with fluorouracil for advanced colorectal cancer; with teceleukin for metastatic malignant melanoma and renal cell carcinoma; AIDS-related Kaposi's sarcoma; renal cell carcinoma	Hoffmann LaRoche

[1] Approved for marketing.

(Continued on following page)

Orphan Drug/Biological Designations		
Drug *(Trade Name)*	Proposed Use	Sponsor
Interferon alfa-2b (recombinant) *(Intron A)*	Chronic myelogenous leukemia; metastatic renal cell carcinoma; AIDS-related Kaposi's sarcoma; ovarian carcinoma; invasive carcinoma of cervix; primary malignant brain tumors; laryngeal (respiratory) papillomatosis; carcinoma in situ of urinary bladder; chronic delta hepatitis; acute hepatitis B	Schering
Interferon alfa-n1 *(Wellferon)*	AIDS-related Kaposi's sarcoma; human papillomavirus in severe resistant/recurrent respiratory (laryngeal) papillomatosis	Burroughs Wellcome
Interferon beta, recombinant human *(Betaseron)*	AIDS; multiple sclerosis	Triton Biosciences
Interferon gamma 1-B	Chronic granulomatous disease	Genentech
Interleukin-2, recombinant *(Proleukin)*	Metastatic renal cell carcinoma; primary immunodeficiency disease associated with T-cell defects	Cetus
Interleukin-2, recombinant, human *(Teceleukin)*	With interferon alfa-2a for metastatic renal cell carcinoma and malignant melanoma; metastatic malignant melanoma	Hoffman LaRoche
Iodine I^{123} murine monoclonal antibody to alpha-fetoprotein	Detection of hepatocellular carcinoma and hepatoblastoma; detection of alpha-fetoprotein producing germ cell tumors	Immunomedics
Iodine I^{131} 6B-iodomethyl-19-norcholesterol	Adrenal cortical imaging	William Beierwaltes, MD
Iodine I^{131} lym-1 monoclonal antibody	B-cell lymphoma	Lederle
Iodine I^{131} meta-iodobenzylguanidine	Diagnostic adjunct in patients with pheochromocytoma	William Beierwaltes, MD
Iodine I^{131} murine monoclonal antibody IgG2A to B cell *(Immurait; LL-2-I-131)*	Radioimmunotherapy of B-cell lymphomas and leukemias	Immunomedics
Iodine I^{131} murine monoclonal antibody to alpha-fetoprotein	Hepatocellular carcinoma and hepatoblastoma; alpha-fetoprotein producing germ cell tumors	Immunomedics
Iodine I^{131} murine monoclonal antibody to hCG	hCG-producing tumors (eg, germ cell/trophoblastic cell tumors)	Immunomedics
L-5-Hydroxytryptophan (L-5HTP)	Postanoxic intention myoclonus	Bolar
L-Alpha-acetyl-methadol	Heroin addicts suitable for maintenance on opiate agonists	Dixon & Williams Pharm.
L-Baclofen	Trigeminal neuralgia	Gerhard H. Fromm, MD
L-Carnitine *(Vitacarn)*	Genetic carnitine deficiency[1]; manifestations of carnitine deficiency in dialysis patients with end stage renal disease (ESRD); prevent/treat secondary carnitine deficiency in valproic acid toxicity	Kendall McGaw
(Carnitor)	Genetic primary/secondary carnitine deficiency; manifestations of carnitine deficiency in dialysis patients with ESRD	Sigma Tau
L-Cycloserine	Gaucher's Disease	City College, NY Med. School

[1] Approved for marketing.

(Continued on following page)

Orphan Drug/Biological Designations		
Drug *(Trade Name)*	Proposed Use	Sponsor
L-Threonine *(Threostat)*	Amyotrophic lateral sclerosis	Tyson and Associates
Leucovorin *(Leucovorin calcium; Wellcovorin)*	With 5-fluorouracil for colon/rectum metastatic adenocarcinoma; after high-dose methotrexate in osteosarcoma	Lederle; Burroughs Wellcome
Leukopoietin *(Leukine)*	Neutropenia assoc. with bone marrow transplant; treatment of graft failure and delay of engraftment; promotion of early engraftment	Immunex
Leuprolide acetate *(Lupron Injection)*	Central precocious puberty	TAP Pharmaceuticals
Levocabastine ophthalmic suspension 0.05%	Vernal keratoconjunctivitis	Iolab
Liothyronine sodium injection	Myxedema coma	SKF
Lysine acetylsalicylate *(Aspegic)*	Pain and fever secondary to sickle cell crisis	Searle
Mafenide acetate solution *(Sulfamylon Solution)*	Prevention of graft loss of meshed autografts on excised burn wounds	Sterling Drug
Mazindol *(Sanorex)*	Duchenne muscular dystrophy	Platon J. Collipp, MD
Mefloquine HCl *(Mephaquin; Lariam)*	Treat/prevent chloroquine-resistant falciparum malaria; acute malaria due to *Plasmodium falciparum* and plasmodium; prophylaxis of resistant *P falciparum* malaria	Mephra AG; Hoffman LaRoche
Megestrol acetate *(Megace)*	Anorexia/cachexia assoc. with positive laboratory findings for HIV or confirmed AIDS diagnosis	Bristol-Myers
Melanoma vaccine *(Melaccine)*	Stage III-IV melanoma	Ribi Immunochem Research
Mesna (eg, *Mesnex*[1])	Prophylactic in reducing incidence of ifosfamide-induced hemorrhagic cystitis; inhibition of the urotoxic effects induced by oxazaphosphamide compounds (eg, cyclophosphamide)	Degussa Corp; Adria
Methotrexate sodium	Osteogenic sarcoma	Lederle
4-Methylpyrazole *(4 MP)*	Methanol or ethylene glycol poisoning	Louisiana State University
Metronidazole (topical) *(Flagyl)*	Grade III and IV, anaerobically infected, decubitus ulcers	Searle
Metronidazole (topical) gel *(Metrogel*[1]*)*	Acne rosacea	Curatek
Midodrine HCl *(Midamine)*	Idiopathic orthostatic hypotension	Roberts
Mitolactol *(Dibromodulcitol)*	Recurrent invasive/metastatic squamous cervix carcinoma	Amswiss
Mitoxantrone HCl *(Novantrone*[1]*)*	Acute myelogenous leukemia (acute nonlymphocytic leukemia)	Lederle
Molecusol-Carbamazepine	Emergency rescue treatment of status epilepticus, grand mal type	Pharmatec
Monoclonal antibodies (murine or human) B-cell lymphoma	B-cell lymphoma	Idec

[1] Approved for marketing.

(Continued on following page)

Orphan Drug/Biological Designations		
Drug *(Trade Name)*	Proposed Use	Sponsor
Monoclonal antibodies PM-81 and AML-2-23	Patients with acute myelogenous leukemia undergoing bone marrow transplant	Medarex
Monoclonal antibody 17-1A *(Panorex)*	Pancreatic cancer	Centocor
Monoclonal antiendotoxin antibody XMMEN-0E5	Gram-negative sepsis which has progressed to shock	Pfizer
Monoclonal factor IX	Replacement treatment and prophylaxis of the hemorrhagic complications of hemophilia B	Armour
Monooctanoin *(Moctanin[1])*	Dissolution of cholesterol gallstones retained in the common bile duct	Ethitek
Morphine sulfate concentrate (preservative-free) *(Duramorph)*	Via microinfusion devices. Epidural: Severe chronic pain unresponsive to systemic analgesics or when preferable to systemic use; Intrathecal: Refractory pain due to malignancy	Elkins-Sinn
Morphine sulfate concentrate (preservative-free) *(Infumorph)*	Via microinfusion devices for intraspinal in intractable chronic pain	Elkins-Sinn
MVI neonatal formula	Establishment/maintenance of total parenteral nutrition in very low birth weight infants	Armour
N-Acetylprocainamide *(NAPA)*	To lower defibrillation energy requirement to allow automatic implantable cardioverter defibrillator therapy	Medco Research
Nafarelin acetate *(Synarel)*	Central precocious puberty	Syntex
Naltrexone HCl *(Trexan[1])*	Blockade of opioid effects as adjunct to maintenance of detoxified, formerly opioid-dependent, individuals	E.I. du Pont de Nemours
NG-29	Diagnostic measure of the capacity of the pituitary gland to release growth hormone	Ferring Labs
OncoRad OV103	Ovarian cancer	Cytogen
Ovine corticotropin releasing hormone	Differentiating pituitary and ectopic production of ACTH in patients with ACTH-dependent Cushings syndrome	Ferring Labs
Oxandrolone	Short stature associated with Turner's syndrome	Gynex
Oxymorphone HCl *(Numorphan H.P.)*	Relief of severe intractable pain in narcotic-tolerant patients	Du Pont
PEG-adenosine deaminase (PEG-ADA) *(Adagen[1])*	Enzyme replacement therapy for ADA deficiency in severe combined immunodeficiency	Enzon
PEG-interleukin-2	Primary immunodeficiencies associated with T-cell defects	Cetus
PEG-L-asparaginase	Acute lymphocytic leukemia	Enzon
Pentamidine isethionate	Pneumonia; PCP	Rhone-Poulenc
Pentamidine isethionate (inhalation) *(Aeropent)*	PCP prevention in high-risk patients	Fisons
Pentamidine isethionate *(Pentam 300[1]; NebuPent)*	Treatment of *Pneumocystis carinii* pneumonia (PCP); PCP prevention in high-risk patients	Lyphomed

[1] Approved for marketing.

(Continued on following page)

Orphan Drug/Biological Designations		
Drug *(Trade Name)*	Proposed Use	Sponsor
Pentastarch *(Pentaspan[1])*	Adjunct in leukapheresis to improve the harvesting and increase the yield of leukocytes by centrifugal means	Du Pont
Pentostatin	Hairy cell leukemia	Warner-Lambert
Phosphocysteamine	Cystinosis	Medea Research
Physostigmine salicylate *(Antilirium)*	Friedreich's and other inherited ataxias	Forest
Piracetam *(Nootropil)*	Myoclonus	U.C.B. Secteur
Piritrexim isethionate	*P carinii, Toxoplasma gondii, Mycobacterium avium-intracellulare* infections	Burroughs Wellcome
Poloxamer 188 *(Rheothrx Copolymer)*	Sickle cell crisis; severe burns requiring hospitalization	Cytrx
Polyribonucleotide *(Ampligen)*	AIDS	Hem Research
Potassium citrate *(Urocit K[1])*	Prevention of uric acid nephrolithiasis; prevention of calcium renal stones in patients with hypocitraturia; avoidance of the complication of calcium stone formation in uric lithiasis	Univ. of Texas Health Sciences
Potassium citrate and citric acid *(Polycitra-K)*	Dissolution/control of urinary tract uric acid/cysteine calculi	Willen Drug
Praziquantel *(Cysticide)*	Neurocysticercosis	Em Labs
Prednimustine *(Sterecyt)*	Malignant non-Hodgkin's lymphomas	Pharmacia
Propamidine isethionate 0.1% ophthalmic soln *(Brolene)*	Acanthamoeba keratitis	Bausch & Lomb
Protirelin (TRH) *(Thymone)*	Amyotrophic lateral sclerosis	Abbott
Pulmonary surfactant replacement	Prevent/treat infant respiratory distress syndrome	California Biotechnology Inc
Redox-Acyclovir	Herpes simplex encephalitis in AIDS patients	Pharmatec
Redox-Penicillin G	AIDS-associated neurosyphilis	Pharmatec
Redox-Phenytoin	Emergency rescue treatment of status epilepticus, grand mal type	Pharmatec
Ricin (blocked) conjugated murine monoclonal antibody	B-cell leukemia and lymphoma	Immunogen
Rifabutin	Disseminated *Mycobacterium avium* complex disease; prevention of disease in patients with AIDS or patients with CD4 counts $< 200/mm^3$	Adria
Rifampin *(Rifadin I.V.[1])*	Antituberculosis treatment when oral doseform is not feasible	Merrell Dow
Rifampin, Isoniazid, Pyrazinamide *(Rifater V)*	Short course treatment of tuberculosis	Merrell Dow
Selegiline HCl *(Deprenyl[1])*	Adjuvant to levodopa/carbidopa in idiopathic Parkinson's Disease (paralysis agitans), postencephalitic parkinsonism and symptomatic parkinsonism	Somerset

[1] Approved for marketing.

(Continued on following page)

Orphan Drug/Biological Designations		
Drug *(Trade Name)*	Proposed Use	Sponsor
Sermorelin acetate *(Geref)*	Idiopathic or organic growth hormone deficiency in children with growth failure; adjunct to gonadotropin in ovulation induction in anovulatory or oligoovulatory infertility after treatment with clomiphene citrate or gonadotropin alone	Serono Labs
Serratia marcescens extract (polyribosomes)	Primary brain malignancies	Cell Technology
Short chain fatty acid solution	Active phase of ulcerative colitis with involvement restricted to the left side of the colon	Richard Breuer, MD
SK&F 110679	Long-term treatment of children who have growth failure due to a lack of adequate endogenous growth hormone secretion	SKF
Sodium oxybate (Gammahydroxybutyrate)	Narcolepsy and the auxiliary symptoms of cataplexy, sleep paralysis, hypnagogic hallucinations and automatic behavior	Sigma Chemical; Biocraft
Sodium pentosan polysulphate *(Elmiron)*	Interstitial cystitis	Medical Market Spec
Sodium tetradecyl sulfate *(Sotradecol)*	Bleeding esophageal varices	Elkins-Sinn
Somatostatin *(Reducin)*	Adjunct to the non-operative management of secreting cutaneous fistulas of the stomach, duodenum, small intestine or pancreas	Ferring
Somatrem *(Protropin)*	Long-term treatment of children who have growth failure due to a lack of adequate endogenous growth hormone secretion[1]; short stature associated with Turner's syndrome	Genentech
Somatropin *(Humatrope[1]; Saizen; Protropin II; Norditropin)*	Long-term treatment of children who have growth failure due to inadequate secretion of normal endogenous growth hormone; treatment of short stature associated with Turner's syndrome; adjunct for ovulation induction in infertility due to hypogonadotropic hypogonadism, bilateral tubal occlusion or unexplained infertility (women undergoing in vivo/in vitro fertilization procedures); enhancement of nitrogen retention with severe burns	Lilly; Serono; Genentech; Nordisk-USA
Spiramycin *(Rovamycine)*	Symptomatic relief and parasitic cure of chronic cryptosporidiosis in immunodeficiency	Rhone-Poulenc
ST1-RTA immunotoxin	B-chronic lymphocytic leukemia; prevention of acute graft vs host disease in allogenic bone marrow transplantation	Sanofi
Sucralfate	Oral complications of chemotherapy in bone marrow transplant	Naska Pharmacal

[1] Approved for marketing.

(Continued on following page)

Orphan Drug/Biological Designations		
Drug *(Trade Name)*	Proposed Use	Sponsor
Superoxide dismutase (recombinant human)	Prevention of reperfusion injury or damage to donor organ tissue	Bristol-Myers; Pharmacia-Chiron
Surface active extract of saline lavage of bovine lungs *(Infasurf)*	To treat/prevent respiratory failure due to pulmonary surfactant deficiency in preterm infants	Ony
Surfactant (human) (amniotic fluid-derived) *(Human Surf)*	To prevent/treat neonatal respiratory distress syndrome	Allan T. Merritt, MD
Surfactant TA (modified bovine lung surfactant extract) *(Survanta)*	To prevent/treat neonatal respiratory distress syndrome	Ross
T4 endonuclease, B liposome encapsulated *(T4N5)*	Prevent cutaneous neoplasms and other skin abnormalities in xeroderma pigmentosum	Applied Genetics
Technetium TC-99M anti-melanoma murine monoclonal antibody	Detecting, by imaging, metastases of malignant melanoma	Neorx
Teleleukin	Metastatic renal cell carcinoma	Hoffman LaRoche
Teniposide	Refractory childhood acute lymphocytic leukemia	Bristol-Myers
Teriparatide *(Parathar[1])*	Diagnostic agent for patients presenting with clinical and laboratory evidence of hypocalcemia due to either hypoparathyroidism or pseudohypoparathyroidism	Rorer
Terlipressin *(Glypressin)*	Bleeding esophageal varices	Ferring AB
Thalidomide	Prevent/treat graft vs host disease in bone marrow transplantation; treatment/maintenance of reactional lepromatous leprosy	Pediatric Pharmaceuticals; Andrulis Research
Thymoxamine HCl	Reversal of phenylephrine-induced mydriasis in patients with narrow anterior angles at risk of developing acute angle-closure glaucoma attack	Iolab
Tiopronin *(Thiola[1])*	Prevention of cystine nephrolithiasis in patients with homozygous cystinuria	Charles Y.C. Pak, MD
Tocophersolan oral solution (Vitamin E-TPGS)	Vitamin E deficiency from malabsorption due to prolonged cholestatic hepatobiliary disease	Eastman
Tranexamic acid *(Cyklokapron)*	Hereditary angioneurotic edema; prostatectomy when there is hemorrhage or risk of hemorrhage as a result of increased fibrinolysis or fibrinogenolysis; patients with congenital coagulopathies undergoing surgical procedures (eg, dental extractions)	Kabi Vitrum
Tretinoin	Squamous metaplasia of ocular surface epithelia (conjunctiva or cornea) with mucous deficiency and keratinization	Spectra

[1] Approved for marketing.

(Continued on following page)

Orphan Drug/Biological Designations		
Drug *(Trade Name)*	Proposed Use	Sponsor
Trientine HCl *(Cuprid[1])*	Patients with Wilson's Disease intolerant or inadequately responsive to penicillamine	Merck Sharp & Dohme
Trimetrexate	Advanced non-small cell carcinoma of the lung; PCP in AIDS patients; metastatic carcinoma of head and neck; metastatic colorectal adenocarcinoma; pancreatic adenocarcinoma	Warner-Lambert
Triptorelin pamoate *(Decapeptyl Injection)*	Palliative treatment of advanced ovarian carcinoma of epithelial origin	Organon
Trisaccharides A and B	Moderate/severe forms of hemolytic disease of the newborn arising from placental transfer of antibodies against blood group substances A and B; ABO-incompatible solid organ transplantation; moderate/very severe forms of transfusion reactions arising from ABO-incompatible transfusion; prevention of ABO medical hemolytic reactions arising from ABO-incompatible bone marrow transplantation	Chembiomed
Troleandomycin	Severe steroid-requiring asthma	Stanley J. Szefler, MD
Urofollitropin *(Metrodin[1])*	Induction of ovulation in patients with polycystic ovarian disease who have an elevated LH/FSH ratio and who have failed to respond to adequate clomiphene citrate therapy	Serono
Viloxazine HCl *(Vivalan)*	Cataplexy; narcolepsy	Stuart
Zidovudine *(Retrovir[1])*	AIDS and AIDS-related complex	Burroughs Wellcome
Zinc acetate	Wilson's Disease	Lemmon

[1] Approved for marketing.

PHENFORMIN – Available under IND exemption.

The biguanide hypoglycemic agent, phenformin, was removed from the US market on October 23, 1977, as a result of concern over the unacceptably high risk of lactic acidosis associated with its use. Phenformin is now available only through an Investigational New Drug (IND) Application which must be filed with the US Food and Drug Administration. Use of phenformin is restricted to specific clearly defined situations and requires registration and reporting to the FDA. Complete information on use of phenformin, physician sponsor applications, patient consent forms and request forms for ordering phenformin tablets or capsules are available from:

Center for Drug Evaluation and Research
Division of Metabolism and Endocrine
Drug Products (HFD-510)
Room 14B03
5600 Fishers Lane
Rockville, Maryland 20857
301-443-3510

Indications: May be used only in adult-onset, nonketotic diabetics who meet *all* of the following criteria: In addition to elevated blood glucose, have symptoms such as polydipsia; symptoms are not controlled with diet and sulfonylureas or cannot take sulfonylureas because of nontolerance or allergy; symptoms are controlled by phenformin; no underlying risk factors which contraindicate the use; (a) occupation is such that the risk of hypoglycemia from insulin would threaten their jobs or be a hazard to them or others, or (b) cannot take insulin because of disability and have no practical way to receive assistance.

Phenformin is also available under a separate IND for a dermatological condition called atrophie blanche or livedo vasculitis.

Contraindications: Although there is no absolute way to predict the population at risk for lactic acidosis, the following are recognized contraindications: Insulin-dependent diabetes; hypersensitivity to phenformin; renal disease with even mild degrees of impaired renal function; liver disease; history of lactic acidosis; alcohol abuse; any acute medical situation such as cardiovascular collapse (shock), congestive heart failure, myocardial infarction, surgery or septicemia; disease states that may be associated with hypoxemia; complications of diabetes such as metabolic acidosis, coma, infection or gangrene; acute gastrointestinal disturbances (vomiting or diarrhea) which are likely to result in dehydration and prerenal azotemia.

Lactic acidosis in patients taking phenformin has been estimated to occur in 0.25 to 4 cases per 1000 phenformin treatment years. Lactic acidosis is characterized by elevated lactate levels, increased lactate-to-pyruvate ratio and decreased blood pH. In many of the reported cases, azotemia ranging from mild to severe was present.

Nausea, vomiting, hyperventilation, malaise or abdominal pain may herald the onset of lactic acidosis. Instruct the patient to discontinue phenformin and notify the physician immediately if any of these symptoms occur.

Warn patients against using alcohol while receiving phenformin, since ethanol and phenformin potentiate the tendency of each to cause an elevation of blood lactate levels.

Conclusions: Although phenformin has been removed from the market because of the potential for adverse effects, a select group of patients may require use of this agent. Careful patient selection is necessary to assure a reasonable risk-benefit ratio. Supplies of phenformin are available to practicing physicians from the FDA under an IND exemption.

KETOTIFEN (*Zaditen* by Sandoz) – An antiasthmatic agent.

Asthma is a chronic respiratory disease characterized by episodes of reversible airway obstruction due to bronchospasms. Although a variety of effective agents are available for the prophylaxis and treatment of asthmatic conditions, both the incidence of side effects and inconvenience of administration by inhalation encourage the search for new modes of therapy. Ketotifen is an orally active agent with significant antihistamine and antianaphylactic properties which may prove useful in asthma prophylaxis.

Pharmacology of asthma: The factors responsible for intrinsic asthma are poorly understood. Extrinsic allergic asthma results from a series of events triggered by an allergen (antigen) which activates the release of chemical mediators of bronchoconstriction (histamine and the slow-reacting substance of anaphylaxis) from sensitized mast cells. Bronchodilators (beta-adrenergic agonists or theophylline) counteract these bronchoconstrictor effects. Antihistamines are somewhat useful in blocking the effects of histamine. The introduction of cromolyn sodium was the advent of a true prophylactic measure for allergic asthma. Although not effective during an acute asthma episode, chronic therapy with cromolyn stabilizes the mast cell membrane and inhibits the release of histamine and slow-reacting substance of anaphylaxis.

Ketotifen appears to act by the same pharmacological mechanism as cromolyn; however, it has the advantage of being active on oral administration. Ketotifen is a benzocycloheptathiophene derivative with antihistaminic and antianaphylactic activity. It is well absorbed orally; effects are sustained for up to 12 hours. As with cromolyn, the onset of its prophylactic activity is slow; 4 to 6 weeks are required to achieve full prophylactic value. Therapeutic serum levels range between 1 and 4 mcg/ml.

Clinical studies: Ketotifen, 1 mg orally, twice daily was found to be equivalent to 20 mg sodium cromolyn 4 times daily (via spinhaler). No statistically significant differences were demonstrated between the two drugs for daily peak respiratory flow rates and spirometry during the 3 months that each drug was administered to 35 skin test positive (allergic) asthmatic adults. Ketotifen prevented histamine-induced bronchoconstriction in 24 patients with mild to moderate extrinsic (allergic) asthma. Histamine challenge was used to evaluate bronchial reactivity following 1 week of treatment with theophylline and salbutamol spray. Ketotifen, 1 mg twice daily, was then added to the regimen. Patients were rechallenged with histamine after 4, 8 and 12 weeks of ketotifen therapy. Decrease in bronchial reactivity to histamine was noted at 4 weeks and maintained for 12 weeks.

In a double-blind study of 50 patients with allergic asthma, ketotifen, 1 or 2 mg twice daily, was added to existing inhalation therapy of salbutamol or corticosteroid. Ketotifen, 2 mg twice daily, slightly decreased the number of puffs per week of salbutamol and improved breathing. No improvement was noted in patients using inhaled corticosteroids. Ketotifen, 1 mg twice daily, failed to provide prophylaxis in adults with intrinsic (nonallergic) asthma; however, there was no deterioration of the condition.

In a double-blind study in 23 children with asthma, 0.5 to 0.94 mg/kg ketotifen failed to provide protection against bronchoconstriction. Ketotifen 1 mg twice daily for 3 days was compared to cromolyn 20 mg administered 15 minutes prior to exercise. Ketotifen was ineffective in preventing exercise-induced bronchospasm, while cromolyn was effective.

Side effects: The most frequently reported side effects, sedation and drowsiness, may require dosage reduction or discontinuation if the severity does not decrease with continued therapy. Alcohol may potentiate these adverse reactions. Weight gain, dry mouth, headache, dizziness and giddiness have also been reported. In addition, symptoms of overdosage have included: Mild abdominal pain, confusion, hyperexcitability, bradycardia, tachycardia, dyspnea, tachypnea, cyanosis, convulsions and unconsciousness.

Summary: Ketotifen appears to be a potential alternative in the prophylaxis of asthma; however, it is unlikely to replace established drugs. Several weeks of administration are required to produce maximum prophylactic effects; additionally, it frequently produces marked drowsiness. Ketotifen is long-acting and offers the convenience of oral administration which may be useful in individuals who develop bronchospasms following inhalation of other products. Ketotifen is available in Britain and Europe; Sandoz filed a New Drug Application (NDA) in November 1982 which is pending, and plans to market the drug under the name *Zaditen*.

DOMPERIDONE (*Motilium* by Janssen Pharmaceutica) – An investigational antiemetic.

Acute nausea and vomiting induced by cytotoxic chemotherapy are frequent and serious toxicities distressful to cancer patients. Symptoms can be so pronounced and refractory that they interfere with therapeutic measures and patient nutrition. Available antiemetics block the chemoreceptor trigger zone (CTZ) (neuroleptics), sedate the vomiting centers (antihistamines), block afferent impulses at the vomiting center (anticholinergics), act peripherally and in the CNS (metoclopramide), or by less defined central mechanisms (cannabinoids). These agents are effective in most patients; however, side effects (eg, drowsiness, dry mouth, hypotension, extrapyramidal effects) are limitations. Domperidone, an investigational antiemetic, appears to act with minimum adverse effects.

Pharmacology: Domperidone is chemically unrelated to the butyrophenones, phenothiazines or metoclopramide; however, it shares pharmacological properties with these agents. In the medulla it produces a direct blocking effect of dopamine receptors in the CTZ. Like metoclopramide and haloperidol, domperidone is a peripheral dopamine antagonist; however, it contrasts in that it does not cross the blood-brain barrier and produce CNS effects. It selectively blocks peripheral dopamine receptors in the gastrointestinal wall, thus enhancing normal synchronized GI peristalsis and motility in the proximal portion of the GI tract; it may also counteract anticholinergic-induced relaxation of the lower esophageal sphincter (LES).

Pharmacokinetics: Peak plasma levels are achieved within 30 minutes following IM or oral administration and between 1 to 4 hours after rectal administration. Approximately 40% of a dose is rapidly distributed into peripheral compartments. It is metabolized in the liver and eliminated in the urine, primarily as conjugates. Less than 1% appears in the urine as unchanged drug. Excretion is almost complete within 4 days. The duration of activity is between 2 and 4 hours following IV administration.

Clinical studies: The effectiveness of domperidone in the treatment of nausea and vomiting associated with cytotoxic chemotherapy has been evaluated. Several double-blind studies were conducted in patients with Hodgkin's disease. Domperidone 16 mg IV was preferred and superior to placebo; it was effective and well tolerated, and decreased the duration of nausea and vomiting by greater than ⅓ when injected 1 hour before the start of cytostatic treatment. Domperidone, 1 to 40 mg IV daily, was administered with chemotherapy infusion in 172 patients. Vomiting induced by agents considered to be moderate emetics (eg, cyclophosphamide, 5-fluorouracil, vinblastine) was reduced; however, patients with emesis induced by doxorubicin or mechlorethamine did not respond as well. The higher dosages of domperidone did not achieve a proportionally augmented response rate. In another study, domperidone 4 mg IV produced excellent or good response in 72% of patients receiving varied chemotherapy; poor responses occurred in patients receiving dacarbazine. When domperidone 12 mg IV was compared to metoclopramide 10 mg IV, both drugs produced a good or excellent response in 70% of patients; however, metoclopramide had a higher incidence of side effects. Domperidone 1 mg/kg IV or metoclopramide 0.5 mg/kg IV was used to prevent chemotherapy-induced nausea and vomiting in children. In the random crossover trial, domperidone decreased nausea and vomiting to a significantly greater extent than metoclopramide.

Other uses: Domperidone has been compared favorably to cimetidine in 20 gastric ulcer patients; it may also have value in treating symptoms of gastroesophageal reflux and postoperative- or bromocriptine-induced nausea and vomiting.

Side effects: Domperidone does not appear to produce significant side effects or toxicities. Doses of 40 mg IV or 100 mg orally have not been reported to produce CNS or cardiovascular side effects, only facial flushing, headache, slight somnolence and dry mouth. Unlike metoclopramide, domperidone does not cross the blood-brain barrier; therefore, the incidence of extrapyramidal or psychotropic effects should be low. Yet there have been isolated reports of idiosyncratic extrapyramidal reactions. Domperidone does not stimulate aldosterone secretion.

Summary: Domperidone selectively blocks peripheral dopamine receptors both in the GI wall and in the CTZ. Its major advantage appears to be the lack of significant side effects; it may be an effective alternative to available antiemetics, including metoclopramide. Domperidone, like other antiemetics, produces variable effects on cytotoxic chemotherapy-induced nausea and vomiting, depending on the agent administered. There is limited or no data available comparing domperidone to more standard antiemetic agents other than metoclopramide. Domperidone was developed in Belgium by Janssen Pharmaceutica; it is available in Europe. Clinical trials are still in progress in the US; a New Drug Application (NDA) was filed in 1985.

Bibliography Available on Request

Brogden RN, Carmine AA, Heel RC, et al. Domperidone: A review of its pharmacological activity, pharmacokinetics and therapeutic efficacy in the symptomatic treatment of chronic dyspepsia and as an antiemetic. *Drugs* 1982;24:360-400.

TWO (MORE) INVESTIGATIONAL BENZODIAZEPINES

Clobazam and nitrazepam are investigational benzodiazepine derivatives. The profile of these agents parallels those of approved benzodiazepines; subtle differences account for individual product distinction.

Clobazam (*Frisium* by Hoechst Roussel) is structurally and pharmacologically related to approved benzodiazepines. Antianxiety and anticonvulsant properties are similar to diazepam; the usual adult dose is 20 to 30 mg daily. Initially, clobazam is effective against all varieties of epilepsy; however, efficacy decreases within a few days to a few weeks in approximately one-third of patients. Success has also been demonstrated in cyclic exacerbations of epilepsy associated with menstruation. Clobazam is a weak hypnotic agent.

The pharmacokinetics are independent of dose and concentration. Oral clobazam is 87% absorbed. Concomitant administration with alcohol increases clobazam's bioavailability by 50%. Food may slow the rate, but does not alter total absorption. Absorption is not influenced by age or sex. Clobazam is 85% bound to human serum protein; peak serum concentrations occur 1 to 4 hours after ingestion. It is metabolized via dealkylation and hydroxylation to a pharmacologically active metabolite, N-desmethylclobazam, and several inactive metabolites. The mean half-life of the unchanged drug is 18 hours, and up to 77 hours for metabolites. Clobazam is 81% to 97% excreted in the urine; accumulation is expected in impaired renal function.

The most frequent (10% to 44%) side effects include: Drowsiness, hangover effects, dizziness, weakness and lightheadedness. Less frequent (5% to 10%) adverse reactions include: Weight gain, orthostatic hypotension, syncope, headache, dry mouth and incoordination.

Nitrazepam (*Mogadon* by Roche) has been widely used for many years in Europe and Canada as a sedative/hypnotic in doses of 2.5 to 10 mg, and in the management of myoclonic seizures of childhood epilepsy. Its structure and clinical effects are also analogous to other benzodiazepines.

Nitrazepam is 80% bioavailable following oral administration. Absorption is rapid: 0.5 to 5 hours to peak concentration; concomitant administration with food decreases peak levels by 30%. Nitrazepam is lipophilic and is widely distributed in the body; 10% to 15% is found in the cerebrospinal fluid; 85% to 90% is plasma protein bound. It crosses the placenta and is found in breast milk (50% and about 50% to 100% of maternal plasma concentration, respectively). Metabolism is extensive and excretion is urinary, primarily as inactive metabolites; only 1% is excreted as the unchanged drug. The elimination half-life is approximately 30 hours.

The frequency of adverse reactions increases with age and dosage, and parallels those of other benzodiazepines. The most common include: Fatigue, dizziness, lightheadedness, drowsiness, lethargy, mental confusion, staggering, ataxia and falling. Nightmares, insomnia, agitation, rash, pruritus, headache and GI disturbances have also been reported. The hangover effect is also common and may be a function of nitrazepam's long half-life.

Summary: Nitrazepam and clobazam appear to be safe and effective agents with antianxiety, anticonvulsant and hypnotic properties. These agents have long elimination half-lives; this enhances the potential for drug accumulation and increases the potential for residual side effects. These agents are unlikely to replace established benzodiazepine derivatives; however, they may provide viable therapeutic alternatives.

Bibliography Available on Request

ISOXICAM (*Maxicam* by Warner-Lambert) – A nonsteroidal anti-inflammatory drug (NSAID).

Isoxicam, like piroxicam *(Feldene),* is a member of the oxicam class of drugs. It is about one-tenth as potent (on a weight basis) as piroxicam and has a long duration of action which permits once-daily dosing. Clinical studies show it to be as effective as or superior to other NSAIDs. Isoxicam is well tolerated; GI disturbance is the most common side effect.

Pharmacology: Rheumatoid arthritis (RA) and degenerative joint disease (DJD) are common chronic rheumatic disorders which cause considerable human suffering and disability. The NSAIDs are first line agents for pain relief in both disorders and for the reduction of inflammation in RA. Salicylates have long been established as analgesic anti-inflammatory drugs and are usually drugs of first choice. However, since therapeutic failure and side effects are frequent, newer agents are steadily being introduced as alternatives.

Isoxicam has potent and prolonged antipyretic, analgesic and anti-inflammatory activity. It inhibits the synthesis of prostaglandins which may contribute to the development of the cardinal signs/symptoms of inflammation. It is also a potent inhibitor of platelet aggregation. This effect likely underlies its potentiation of sodium warfarin's anticoagulant action (see below).

Pharmacokinetics: Isoxicam is well absorbed orally and generally reaches peak plasma concentration 4 to 8 hours after administration. Both its rate and extent of absorption increase when given with meals.

Isoxicam is 95% to 98% protein bound. It is extensively metabolized with only 1% to 2% of the dose appearing in the urine as unchanged drug. This suggests that the drug's dose need not be changed in patients with renal dysfunction. Isoxicam has a half-life of approximately 31 hours (range, 21 to 70 hours) which permits once-daily dosing. Because of its long half-life, steady-state levels occur after 1 to 2 weeks of daily administration. As a result, a continual increase in response is expected until steady state is achieved.

Clinical studies: In a placebo controlled multicenter study, isoxicam was superior to placebo for the treatment of patients with RA or DJD. Morning stiffness was reduced by more than 60% in the isoxicam group, compared to 19% for patients in the placebo group; 52% of patients in the placebo group withdrew from the study because of lack of treatment efficacy, compared to 18% withdrawal in the isoxicam group.

An aspirin (3.6 g/day) and placebo controlled study of isoxicam (200 mg/day) in the treatment of RA found isoxicam superior to aspirin and placebo. Patient withdrawal rates for insufficient efficacy were 17.1%, 31.1% and 58.5% for isoxicam, aspirin and placebo, respectively.

In comparative studies of isoxicam (200 mg/day) vs naproxen (750 mg/day) and ibuprofen (1200 mg/day) in patients with RA, no significant efficacy differences were observed. In similar studies involving patients with DJD, isoxicam (200 mg/day) was as effective as naproxen (750 mg/day) and indomethacin (150 mg/day) in relieving pain and improving articular function. Patients on isoxicam experienced significantly fewer adverse effects than those on indomethacin.

Side effects: Isoxicam has so far been well tolerated and has caused few problems other than gastrointestinal effects. Other less commonly reported adverse effects include headache, dizziness and tinnitus. A higher than anticipated rate of skin reactions has occurred in foreign countries where isoxicam is available.

Drug interactions: The use of aspirin with NSAIDs is not generally recommended because of aspirin-induced reductions of NSAID blood levels and a lack of therapeutic advantage with concomitant use. However, the use of aspirin with isoxicam does not appear to lower plasma isoxicam levels, but the combination increases GI blood loss. It remains to be determined whether an isoxicam-aspirin combination offers any therapeutic advantage. When used with sodium warfarin, isoxicam potentiates warfarin's anticoagulant effect. Monitor the prothrombin time in patients on both agents more frequently and adjust the sodium warfarin dosage if needed. No interaction occurs between cimetidine and isoxicam.

Summary: Isoxicam is a novel NSAID of the oxicam class. It appears to be as effective as or superior to aspirin and nonaspirin agents for the treatment of common rheumatic disorders. The ability to administer isoxicam once a day is an important advantage. Parke-Davis (Warner-Lambert) submitted an NDA for isoxicam in August 1983, to be marketed under the name *Maxicam.* The drug was withdrawn from the European market in October 1985 following reports of adverse skin reactions during which time the NDA was pending in the US. In 1987, Warner-Lambert asked the FDA to reactivate the NDA since the skin reactions were apparently due to a manufacturing byproduct.

Bibliography Available on Request

Talbott JH, ed. Isoxicam: A new nonsteroidal anti-inflammatory agent. *Semin Arthritis Rheum* 1982 Nov;12(Suppl 2):153-83.

L-5-HYDROXYTRYPTOPHAN (L-5HTP)

L-5HTP is available as an "orphan" drug for the treatment of post-anoxic intention myoclonus. Myoclonus is an uncommon neuromuscular movement disorder characterized by involuntary, irregular muscle contraction; it is associated with a variety of brain lesions. There is evidence that at least some of these disorders are related to brain neurotransmitter levels or function, specifically serotonin. L-5HTP is an aromatic amino acid, the immediate precursor of serotonin.

L-5HTP is administered with carbidopa (see page 290d), a peripheral dopa-decarboxylase inhibitor that decreases the conversion of L-5HTP to serotonin in the extracerebral tissues. This permits the administration of lower doses of L-5HTP and reduces the peripheral GI side effects such as diarrhea and nausea.

Pharmacokinetics: When administered orally with carbidopa (which produces a 5 to 15 fold increase in plasma L-5HTP), the systemic availability of L-5HTP is 47% to 84%; peak plasma concentrations of L-5HTP are reached at 1 to 3 hours. The biological half-life of L-5HTP, after pretreatment with carbidopa, is 2 to 7 hours. The major metabolic pathway of L-5HTP is decarboxylation to serotonin by L-aromatic amino acid decarboxylase; the highest activity is in the kidney, liver and small intestine. However, carbidopa-decarboxylase inhibition is incomplete; this may account for the GI side effects.

Indications: L-5HTP in combination with carbidopa is effective in the therapy of post-anoxic intention myoclonus. In 41 patients, 65% experienced a 50% or more improvement. However, patients with intention myoclonus associated with head trauma and methyl bromide toxicity, progressive myoclonus epilepsy, essential myoclonus and palatal myoclonus also show improvement. In addition, L-5HTP has shown some success in treating depression and in migraine prophylaxis.

Contraindications: L-5HTP/carbidopa is contraindicated in patients with renal disease, peptic ulcer, platelet disorders, scleroderma and Parkinson's disease.

Drug Interactions: Do not give **monoamine oxidase inhibitors** or **reserpine** concurrently with L-5HTP/carbidopa. Discontinue these drugs at least 2 weeks prior to initiating treatment with L-5HTP/carbidopa.

Discontinue **tricyclic antidepressants** with a major serotonin reuptake inhibition mechanism (ie, imipramine) prior to L-5HTP/carbidopa therapy. Also, avoid serotonin receptor antagonists like **methysergide** or **cyproheptadine,** which may reduce the therapeutic effects of L-5HTP/carbidopa.

Fenfluramine releases brain serotonin from serotonergic nerve terminals and may potentiate L-5HTP/carbidopa.

Precautions: Use L-5HTP/carbidopa with caution in patients with severe emotional or psychiatric disorders because of occasional mental side effects. Mental depression has improved in some patients.

Adverse Effects: Most common (GI) – Anorexia, nausea, diarrhea and vomiting. These can usually be avoided or minimized by gradual increases of L-5HTP dosage; they rapidly disappear when the dose is reduced or discontinued. The diarrhea will respond to therapy with diphenoxylate; the other GI symptoms respond to treatment with prochlorperazine or trimethobenzamide. These side effects eventually disappear or diminish.

Other adverse effects include mental changes (ie, euphoria) which may progress to hypomania, restlessness, rapid speech, anxiety, insomnia, aggressiveness and agitation; mydriasis, lightheadedness, sleepiness, blurring of vision and bradycardia. Dyspnea, sometimes accompanied by hyperventilation and lightheadedness, is rare. L-5HTP/carbidopa might unmask subclinical scleroderma in patients with an abnormality in kynurenine metabolism.

Overdosage of L-5HTP/carbidopa can produce respiratory difficulties and hypotension.

Administration and Dosage: Begin with 25 mg L-5HTP 4 times daily; increase by 100 mg/day every 3 to 5 days if there are no significant side effects. If significant GI side effects develop, reduce the rate of increase to every 1 to 2 weeks. A reduction in myoclonus is usually first observed at 600 to 1000 mg/day (with carbidopa); the usual optimal dose of L-5HTP is between 1000 and 2000 mg/day in 4 divided doses.

Summary: L-5HTP is available through a treatment IND under the FDA's orphan drug program from Bolar Pharmaceuticals, Inc., 130 Lincoln Street, Copiague, NY 11726; (516) 842-8383. The drug will be beneficial to a small number of patients; further research may elucidate additional uses as we increase our understanding of the brain's complex chemistry. Carbidopa may be obtained for use with L-5HTP by contacting Audrey A. Geist, MD, Professional Information, MSD, West Point, PA 19486; (215) 661-7300.

Bibliography Available on Request

VINDESINE SULFATE (*Eldisine* by Lilly) – An investigational anticancer drug.

Vindesine sulfate (Lilly 99094, NSC-245467, DAVA, desacetyl vinblastine amide sulfate) is a synthetic vinca alkaloid derived from vinblastine sulfate, but more closely resembling the activity of vincristine.

A large number of studies support its utility in a diverse group of cancer types. Major and dose-limiting toxicities include myelosuppression and neurotoxicity.

Pharmacology: The mechanism of vindesine's anticancer action is probably like that of the other vinca alkaloids; it is cell-cycle specific and blocks mitosis with metaphase arrest. Vinca alkaloids bind specifically to cellular microtubules of the mitotic apparatus and disrupt their function. This leads to inability of the dividing cell to correctly segregate chromosomes and ultimately, to cell death.

Pharmacokinetics: Vindesine sulfate appears to have similar pharmacokinetics to vincristine and vinblastine. The triphasic clearance profile of IV vindesine is summarized below:

Phase	Half-life (minutes)	Volume of distribution (liters)
Alpha (α)	3 ± 1	5 ± 2
Beta (β)	99 ± 45	58 ± 51
Gamma (γ)	1213 ± 493	598 ± 294

Elimination in the urine in the first 24 hours accounts for 13.2% of the total dose administered. The remainder is sequestered in the body or eliminated in the bile.

Clinical studies: Overall, vindesine demonstrates good activity in difficult-to-treat and refractory cancer types. Responses to vindesine in patients who have received vincristine or vinblastine therapy suggest a lack of cross-resistance between these agents. Doses have ranged from 3 to 4.5 mg/m² as an IV bolus every 1 to 2 weeks *or* 1 to 2 mg/m²/day for 2 to 10 days every 2 to 3 weeks. The results of clinical studies are summarized below:

Cancer Type	Number of Patients Treated	Response Rate		
		Range (%)	Average (%)	Complete No. of Patients
Lung	234	17-43	30	10
Esophageal	76	17-55	43	0
Colorectal	33	6	6	1
Metastatic Breast	120	0-28	18	0
Lymphoma	61	34-50	41	4
Leukemias	26	15-61	38	4
TOTAL	550	0-61	29	19

Side effects: Major dose-limiting toxicities include myelosuppression and neuropathy. The primary *hematologic* toxicity is leukopenia, which is reversible with dosage reduction or discontinuation. Anemia and thrombocytopenia occur, but are rarely severe. *Neurotoxicity* appears to be a function of cumulative dose. Patients with hepatic dysfunction and those over 60 years old may be at greater risk. Neurotoxic manifestations include peripheral paresthesia, decreased tendon reflexes, muscle weakness and myalgia, headache, parotid and jaw pain, constipation and paralytic ileus.

Other side effects: Nausea; vomiting; stomatitis; hoarseness; transient hepatic dysfunction; inappropriate antidiuretic hormone secretion; fever; skin rash; alopecia; local cellulitis. Vindesine sulfate is a potent vesicant; avoid extravasation into the SC tissues.

Summary: Vindesine sulfate is a vinca alkaloid which demonstrates promise for a wide variety of cancer types; however, its full extent of activity remains to be determined. Its major toxicities are similar to those of its family, myelotoxicity and neurotoxicity. It was recommended for approval by FDA's Oncologic Drugs Advisory Committee in September 1982. A New Drug Application (NDA) is pending.

Bibliography Available on Request

Cersosimo RJ, et al. Pharmacology, clinical efficacy and adverse effects of vindesine sulfate, a new vinca alkaloid. *Pharmacotherapy* 1983;3:259-74.

PIRENZEPINE HCl (*Gastrozepine* by Boehringer Ingelheim) – An investigational antiulcer agent.

Pirenzepine is a tricyclic benzodiazepine antiulcer agent comparable to standard antiulcer agents such as cimetidine and ranitidine. However, its uniqueness and mechanism of action hinge on *selective* antimuscarinic activity for gastric acid secretory cells.

Pharmacology: Pirenzepine selectively suppresses both basal and stimulated acid and pepsin secretion with lesser effects on other muscarinic sites (eg, salivary secretion) compared to atropine and other classic anticholinergic agents. Controlled trials show that 50 mg, 2 to 3 times daily, inhibits acid secretion at least up to 4.5 hours after dosing. Higher doses inhibit esophageal and colonic motility and decrease lower esophageal sphincter pressure. Pirenzepine may also have cytoprotective effects; however, this is of questionable significance since it has little or no effect on gastric mucus and endogenous gastric prostaglandin production.

Pharmacokinetics: Pirenzepine is a hydrophilic molecule which has systemic bioavailability after oral dosing of 20% to 30%. Approximately 10% of the drug is protein bound. Little drug is found in the brain; brain to serum concentration is 1 to 10.

At least 80% is renally excreted unchanged. Most metabolites are of a desmethyl variety. The parent molecule has a half-life of about 10 hours.

These data indicate the potential for few CNS effects and the need to adjust dosage in patients with impaired renal function.

Clinical studies: Numerous short-term (1 to 6 weeks) studies have been conducted comparing pirenzepine to placebo and other antiulcer drugs in ulcer patients. In small doses (50 to 75 mg/day) duodenal ulcer healing percentages with pirenzepine are not superior to placebo. Doses of 100 to 150 mg/day produce healing in 70% to 90% of patients. Statistically significant symptomatic improvement (decreased antacid use and pain) occurs with both dosage levels.

Short-term double-blind studies comparing duodenal ulcer healing rates of pirenzepine (100 to 150 mg/day) and cimetidine (1 g/day) produced similar results (60% to 79% for pirenzepine and 53% to 85% for cimetidine). A single study comparing pirenzepine (100 mg/day) to cimetidine (1 g/day) and ranitidine (300 mg/day) found similar rates of ulcer healing. However, pirenzepine showed a slower effect on symptom disappearance.

Fewer studies have been conducted in patients with gastric ulcer. Double-blind studies comparing pirenzepine to placebo show a need to use adequate doses (100 to 150 mg/day). Pirenzepine and cimetidine have produced similar healing rates (50% *vs* 48%) in patients with gastric ulcer, but more studies are indicated.

Trials were performed comparing maintenance doses of pirenzepine (30 to 50 mg/day) to placebo and cimetidine (400 mg/day) in duodenal ulcer patients for 12 months. Results indicate statistically significant reductions in ulcer recurrences for active treatment groups *vs* placebo (24% recurrence in active treatment group *vs* 80% in placebo-treated patients). No difference was demonstrated in recurrence rates between pirenzepine and cimetidine patients.

Combined use of pirenzepine with ranitidine or cimetidine shows more effective inhibition of gastric acid secretion than with use of a single agent. Such combinations may be useful in peptic ulcer conditions resistant to single drug therapy and in the Zollinger-Ellison syndrome.

Side effects: Pirenzepine is well tolerated with few reported adverse effects. Dry mouth is the most common effect, but nausea, vomiting, diarrhea, constipation, increased appetite, anorexia, tiredness and difficulty of accommodation have all occurred. Daily doses of less than 150 mg seem to significantly reduce the incidence of at least some of these problems.

Summary: In clinical studies, pirenzepine is equally effective as cimetidine in the treatment of peptic ulcer disease. Its low incidence of side effects and selective inhibition of muscarinic gastric acid secretion will make it a valuable addition to existing agents used to treat ulcers. Pirenzepine is currently available in some European countries; expected date of availability in the United States is unknown. A New Drug Application (NDA) is pending.

Bibliography Available on Request

Bianchi Porro G, Petrillo M. Pirenzepine in the treatment of peptic ulcer disease: Review and commentary. *Scand J Gastroenterol* 1982;17 (Suppl 72):229-35.

Berardi RR, Caplan NB. Agents with tricyclic structures for treating peptic ulcer disease. *Clin Pharm* 1983;2:425-31.

MILRINONE (*Primacor* by Sterling Winthrop) – A cardiotonic agent.

Milrinone (Win-47203 by Sterling Winthrop) is a new and potent analog of the positive inotropic cardiac bipyridine, amrinone *(Inocor)*.

Pharmacology: For years, the digitalis glycosides have been the principal drugs in the treatment of cardiac dysfunction. They increase the inotropic activity of the myocardium, resulting in increased oxygen utilization. More recently, application of peripheral vasodilators to reduce ventricular afterload and improve cardiac performance has led to their use in the treatment of heart failure. Experimental and clinical data emphasize the advantages of combining ventricular afterload reduction and positive inotropic stimulation to provide the most efficient pharmacologic enhancement of cardiac pump function.

Milrinone has combined positive inotropic and vasodilatory properties. The mechanism for its effects remains to be fully elucidated. Milrinone is an inhibitor of cardiac adenosine 3', 5' monophosphate (cAMP) phosphodiesterase with resultant increases in cardiac cAMP levels. However, the time course for this increase does not seem to correspond to milrinone's positive inotropic effect. A more likely mechanism may involve the direct or indirect enhancement of calcium ion movement into or storage within the myocardial cell.

Milrinone's vasodilatory effects may be due in part to a reduction in excess baseline sympathetic tone after improvement in myocardial contractility and a direct vasodilating action via relaxation of vascular smooth muscle.

Pharmacokinetics: The drug is well absorbed after oral administration with a bioavailability of 75%. The mean total clearance and volume of distribution of milrinone following IV administration has been reported as 0.15 L/hr/kg and 0.3 L/kg, respectively. The plasma half-life following IV and oral administration was 1.52 hours and 1.2 to 2.1 hours, respectively.

From this data and the clinical observation that cardiac symptoms tend to return prior to the next dose in patients given the drug every 6 hours (duration of effects, 3 to 5 hours), frequent dosing or a sustained release form of the drug will be required to achieve a continuous effect throughout the day.

Clinical studies: Milrinone has nearly 20 times the inotropic potency of amrinone, the parent compound. It has the ability to increase cardiac contractile force and output with minimal increase of heart rate. Other favorable effects include significant reductions in left ventricular end-diastolic pressure, pulmonary wedge pressure, right atrial pressure, systemic vascular resistance, as well as slight reduction of mean arterial pressure.

In one long-term study, 19 of 20 patients receiving oral milrinone (29 ± 2 mg/day) for up to 11 months showed sustained improvement in symptoms of severe heart failure. Another study in seven patients over 2 to 15 weeks achieved results with 10 to 20 mg/day.

In addition, animal studies confirm the drug's ability to counteract the negative inotropic effects of cardiac depressants such as calcium channel blocking agents, propranolol and pentobarbital.

Side effects: In contrast to digitalis glycosides, milrinone has a high toxic-to-therapeutic ratio. It appears to be remarkably free of adverse effects. No side effects have been noted with either short-term or long-term IV infusion; headache and worsening of angina pectoris have occurred with chronic oral use. However, of the patients reporting worsening of their angina, all had severe underlying coronary artery disease.

The lack of milrinone-induced side effects is in contrast to amrinone. Long-term oral amrinone therapy is associated with a 10% to 15% incidence of dose-related, reversible thrombocytopenia and idiosyncratic reactions such as fever. Use of oral amrinone is also associated with a 5% to 10% incidence of GI side effects (vomiting, dyspepsia, cramps and diarrhea) severe enough to require dose reduction or drug withdrawal.

Summary: Milrinone is a safe and effective agent for patients with severe congestive heart failure. It is a unique agent which combines the properties of positive inotropism and vasodilation. It appears to be very well tolerated; however, because of its short half-life, a sustained-release form of the drug would seem clinically and commercially desirable. Milrinone IV (*Primacor,* formerly *I.V. Corotrope*) was approved by the FDA in December 1987, but has yet to be released. An NDA was filed for the oral dosage form on March 19, 1987. The controlled-release form is in Phase II. However, in 1990 the manufacturer decided to discontinue further development of oral milrinone. This decision is based on results of a 2 year survival study that indicate the oral form has a deleterious effect on the survival of patients with advanced CHF.

Bibliography Available on Request

Weintraub M, Standish R. Milrinone shows potential for the long term treatment of congestive heart failure. *Hosp Formul* 1984;19:25, 26, 32.

INOSIPLEX (*Isoprinosine* by Newport) – An immunomodulating agent.

Inosiplex (inosine pranobex, BAN) is a synthetic complex formed from the p-acetamidobenzoic acid salt of N-N dimethylamino-2-propanol and inosine in a 3:1 molar ratio. Early studies examined inosiplex as an antiviral agent. However, recent research has focused on its immunomodulating properties and suggests that its antiviral activity involves enhancement of host defenses rather than direct inhibition of viral replication. Inosiplex may be more appropriately classed with those agents that regulate immunity, eg, levamisole.

Pharmacology: Inosiplex augments immunological events triggered by such agents as mitogens, antigens, phagocyte stimulants or lymphokines. Inosiplex alone does not appear to affect lymphocytes or macrophages. In the presence of triggering agents, it results in an increase in mitogen responses, T-lymphocyte differentiation, total rosette-forming T-cells, lymphotoxin production, virus-induced lymphoproliferative responses, lymphocyte cytotoxicity to viral-infected target cells and skin test responses. This augmentation of responses occurs at inosiplex levels of 0.1 to > 100 mcg/ml with a biphasic profile. Such a profile suggests action on more than one cell population or, more likely, a dual action on a single cell population which is concentration-dependent. Exactly how the drug acts on the lymphocyte to alter the magnitude of triggered responses is unclear. It may involve one or several cell surfaces and nuclear metabolic events linked to RNA metabolism, cyclic nucleotide levels or calcium ion flux. Inosiplex also potentiates interferon activity through mechanisms which remain unclear.

Pharmacokinetics: Inosiplex is rapidly metabolized after both oral and IV administration. The half-life of the inosine portion of the parent complex is 3 minutes after IV administration and 50 minutes after oral administration. In animal models, 90% of the inosine moiety is excreted in the urine as allantoin and uric acid, along with small amounts of hypoxanthine, xanthine and adenine. The p-acetamidobenzoic acid moiety and the N-N-dimethylamino-2-propanol moiety are excreted in the urine after glucuronidation and oxidation, respectively.

Clinical trials examining the use of inosiplex in a variety of viral disorders (eg, herpes zoster, herpes simplex, rhinovirus, influenza A and subacute sclerosing panencephalitis), rheumatoid arthritis and solid tumors have not been able to establish definite efficacy of the drug in any of these disorders. A preliminary study involving four patients with a pre-Acquired Immune Deficiency Syndrome (AIDS) complex (a prodrome of AIDS) and five patients with AIDS given 4 g inosiplex per day for 4 weeks showed enhancement of mitogen-induced lymphocyte proliferative responses in two patients with the pre-AIDS complex. These results agreed with data from an in vitro study of inosiplex's effect on lymphocytes from pre-AIDS patients, patients with AIDS and healthy heterosexual controls which demonstrated that inosiplex could partially restore some of the depressed lymphocyte functions associated with AIDS. The data also suggested, however, that this effect was likely to have clinical significance only in those patients with the milder, pre-AIDS condition. After examination of the combined preliminary results of three studies (unpublished data), Newport Pharmaceuticals reported to FDA officials that there appeared to be a trend toward a delay in the development of fully developed AIDS in pre-AIDS patients treated with inosiplex for 28 days. A multicenter study is in progress to evaluate the use of inosiplex in pre-AIDS patients.

Side effects: In tolerance studies involving healthy volunteers and in clinical trials involving various patient groups, no serious side effects were reported after continuous inosiplex administration for 1 week to 7 years at doses of 1 to 8 g/day. Occasional transient nausea was associated with the ingestion of large numbers of tablets; a transient rise in serum and urinary uric acid, related to the metabolism of the drug, occurred in a small number of patients. Initiate concomitant administration of drugs that increase uric acid levels with caution, since the potential for additive effects has not been studied.

Summary: Inosiplex is a new immunomodulating agent. Preliminary data indicate that the compound may improve the immunologic status of some pre-AIDS patients and may delay progression of pre-AIDS to AIDS. Inosiplex could presumably be used long-term in these patients, since it is administered orally and has not been associated with serious side effects. However, more extensive clinical trials are needed to establish the safety and efficacy of the agent. Newport Pharmaceuticals submitted a New Drug Application (NDA) September 3, 1985, requesting approval of inosiplex *(Isoprinosine)* for immunorestoration in pre-AIDS patients, but it was rejected by the FDA in February 1986. Research continues.

Bibliography Available on Request

Hadden JW, Giner-Sorolla A. Isoprinosine and NPT 15392: Modulators of lymphocyte and macrophage development and function. In: Hersh EM, Chirigos MA, Mastrangelo MJ, eds. Progress in Cancer Research and Therapy. *Augmenting Agents in Cancer Therapy.* Vol. 16. New York: Raven Press, 1981:497-515.

Chang T-W, Heel RC. Ribavirin and inosiplex: A review of their present status in viral diseases. *Drugs* 1981;22:111-28.

FENOTEROL HBr (*Berotec* by Boehringer Ingelheim) -A β_2 agonist.

Fenoterol HBr is a β_2-adrenergic agonist undergoing investigation in the US as a bronchodilating agent. It has been available outside the US since the early 1970s as a metered dose inhaler (MDI), a solution for nebulization, a powder for inhalation and an oral dosage form.

Pharmacology: Stimulation of β_2-adrenoreceptors activates adenyl cyclase which converts adenosine triphosphate into cyclic AMP (cAMP). Increased levels of cAMP inhibit mediator release and produce bronchodilation. Although controversial, an increase in mucociliary transport may also occur. In addition, β_2-adrenoreceptor stimulation causes vasodilatation of peripheral blood vessels. This peripheral vasodilatory effect can result in a baroreceptor-mediated reflex-positive chronotropic response (increase in heart rate) and stimulation of skeletal muscle, leading to tremor. Fenoterol has greater β_2-adrenoreceptor selectivity than metaproterenol, but it is approximately equal in selectivity to albuterol and terbutaline. Bronchoselectivity is enhanced by administering fenoterol by inhalation; this allows for use of a lower dose to achieve a therapeutic effect and reduce dose-related side effects.

Usual therapeutic doses (200 to 400 mcg) of inhaled fenoterol do not significantly affect the cardiovascular system; however, marked cardiovascular effects have been observed after oral, SC, IM or IV administration. Fenoterol prevents immediate antigen-induced bronchospasm but does not prevent delayed allergic reactions. A transient reduction in serum potassium levels (representing the uptake of potassium into the intracellular space), and an increase in serum glucose levels have been observed, but the clinical significance remains unclear.

Pharmacokinetics: Approximately 60% of an oral dose is absorbed, with peak plasma levels reached in 2 hours. After inhalation, fenoterol appears to undergo a two-stage absorption process; the first stage is independent of dose, while the second is similar to that seen after oral administration. This is consistent with the observation that, when a drug is administered by inhalation, as much as 90% of the dose is swallowed. Fenoterol undergoes extensive first-pass metabolism. The half-life of total radioactive-labelled drug is 7 hours; however, this does not represent a true half-life for the parent compound. Although maximum effect of inhaled fenoterol is not achieved for 1 to 2 hours, 60% of the maximal response is seen within the first few minutes. The duration of action of fenoterol is approximately 4 to 6 hours. However, since the lower therapeutic dose produces near maximal bronchodilatation, increasing the dose to near maximal effective concentrations will increase the duration of action without affecting the intensity of the peak response. After oral administration, $<$ 2% of the dose is eliminated unchanged in the urine; the balance is excreted as acid conjugates in the urine and feces (40%).

Clinical studies: Clinical trials have established the efficacy of fenoterol for maintenance therapy in patients with moderate to severe asthma, therapy of chronic obstructive lung disease (COLD), protection against exercise-induced asthma and treatment of acute asthma attacks. It is difficult to evaluate many of the studies because they are single-dose studies, or because they do not compare equipotent doses when evaluated against albuterol and terbutaline. However, at equipotent doses (1 puff fenoterol [200 mcg/puff] = 2 puffs albuterol [100 mcg/puff] = 2 puffs terbutaline [250 mcg/puff]), there appears to be no clinically significant difference in duration of action, bronchoselectivity or therapeutic efficacy among the three agents. The dose of fenoterol used to treat an acute asthma attack is 200 mcg (1 puff) repeated once in 5 minutes for the pediatric patient, and 1 to 3 puffs for adults. Maintenance therapy is 1 to 2 puffs 2 to 4 times daily for adults; give one puff twice daily to the pediatric patient. Increasing an inhaled dose of fenoterol to $>$ 600 mcg (3 puffs) does not appear to increase the therapeutic response but may increase the incidence of side effects. In one study, an 800 mcg dose increased the heart rate 10% with a slow return to baseline over 2 hours. Although inhaled bronchodilators have many advantages, as many as 10% of the patients may not receive maximal therapeutic benefit due to improper use of the MDI.

Side effects: After inhalation of therapeutic doses of fenoterol, side effects are rare. After oral therapy, skeletal muscle tremor, tachycardia, palpitations and nervousness occur occasionally. Fenoterol is not recommended for use in patients with hyperthyroidism, and should be used with caution in patients with cardiovascular disease, diabetes mellitus and hepatic or renal dysfunction until further studies have clarified the possible risks.

Summary: Fenoterol by inhalation appears to be a safe and effective treatment for prophylaxis of exercise-induced bronchospasm, acute attacks of mild to moderate asthma and maintenance therapy for chronic asthma or COLD. However, no apparent advantage of fenoterol over equipotent doses of the currently available β_2-selective agonists, albuterol or terbutaline, has yet been demonstrated. A New Drug Application (NDA) is pending. Fenoterol will be marketed as *Berotec* from Boehringer Ingelheim.

Bibliography Available on Request

Svedmyr N. Fenoterol: A beta₂-adrenergic agonist for use in asthma. *Pharmacotherapy* 1985;5:109-26.

NITRENDIPINE (*Baypress* by Miles): A Type II calcium channel blocking agent.

Pharmacology: Nitrendipine is a 1,4-dihydropyridine derivative calcium entry blocker, structurally similar to nifedipine. It is further classified as a Type II calcium antagonist because, at usual doses and concentrations, it is devoid of electrophysiologic effects, but is a potent peripheral vasodilator. Relaxation of peripheral vascular smooth muscle occurs as a result of inhibition of calcium influx across cellular membranes.

Nitrendipine causes a decrease in both systolic and diastolic blood pressure, primarily due to arteriolar dilatation. Significant peripheral venodilation is unlikely, since postural hypotension is usually not seen. Reflex increases in heart rate, AV nodal conduction and myocardial contractility occur frequently at therapeutic doses and may precipitate myocardial ischemia in patients with coronary artery disease. Plasma renin activity and catecholamine concentrations increase during therapy with nitrendipine; however, the fact that it reduces the pressor response to norepinephrine but affects no change in responses to angiotensin II may explain its greater effectiveness in the treatment of low-renin hypertension. Nitrendipine does not alter glomerular filtration rate (GFR), renal blood flow or plasma aldosterone levels. A short-term, modest diuretic and natriuretic effect has been observed on initiation of therapy.

The dose/response relationship for this effect appears to be flat; a 10 mg dose produces maximum diuresis. It is unlikely that this has any therapeutic implications during long-term therapy. Preliminary data suggest that nitrendipine has no effect on blood glucose, total cholesterol, triglyceride or uric acid levels.

Pharmacokinetics: Available pharmacokinetic data are based on experience with small numbers of patients using assays of varying sensitivity; data vary.

Nitrendipine appears to be well absorbed after oral administration. Peak serum concentrations are seen at 1 to 2 hours; peak effect is seen at approximately 4 hours. The distribution half-life ($t_{1/2}$-α) is approximately 1 hour. Beta elimination half-life ($t_{1/2}$-β) averages 8 to 11 hours. Nitrendipine is metabolized by the liver to an inactive pyridine analog and to several more polar metabolites that are excreted in the urine. Dosage adjustments appear to be necessary in patients with hepatic dysfunction, but specific guidelines are not established. A single-dose study in 16 patients with various degrees of renal dysfunction found no alterations in any kinetic parameters; dosage adjustments appear unnecessary in renal patients.

Clinical studies: Nitrendipine is effective in the treatment of mild to moderate hypertension (diastolic blood pressure 90 to 114 mm Hg). Initial data suggest that the drug is particularly useful in low-renin hypertension, which accounts for 20% to 30% of the hypertensive population. Doses of 10 to 80 mg/day have been used, administered as a single dose or in 2 to 3 divided doses per day. Although a single daily dose will decrease blood pressure for 24 hours, most patients require twice-daily dosing for optimal blood pressure control. Due to reflex increases in heart rate and contractility, concomitant β-blocker therapy may be required in some patients. It has not been determined whether nitrendipine, like verapamil and nifedipine, tends to be more effective in older patients.

Side effects: Nitrendipine has a side effect profile similar to nifedipine. The side effect reported most frequently is headache. Fatigue, peripheral edema, flushing, palpitations, dizziness, polyuria and mild elevations in liver function (in two patients) have also occurred.

Summary: Nitrendipine is a potent vasodilator which effectively reduces blood pressure when given 1 to 3 times daily. The drug appears most useful in low-renin hypertensives. Biochemical abnormalities common to other currently used antihypertensives (eg, hypokalemia, hyperglycemia, increased uric acid and lipids) are not seen with this class of drugs and may represent an advantage over β-blockers and diuretics. Although most patients will require twice-daily dosing, the only other available dihydropyridine (nifedipine) usually requires dosing 3 to 4 times a day.

A New Drug Application (NDA) is pending with the FDA for an antihypertensive indication. Nitrendipine will be co-marketed by Miles and Roche.

Bibliography Available on Request

Pedrinelli R, Fouad FM, Tarazi RC, et al. Nitrendipine, a calcium-entry blocker; renal and humoral effects in human arterial hypertension. *Arch Intern Med* 1986;146:62-65.

Moser M. Nitrendipine in the treatment of mild to moderate hypertension. *J Vasc Dis* 1988;39:73-80.

PINACIDIL (*Pindac* by Lilly) – A new antihypertensive agent.

Pharmacology: Pinacidil is a new vasodilator under investigation for use as an antihypertensive agent. Pinacidil acts at the level of the precapillary, arteriolar (resistance) vessels, causing direct relaxation of vascular smooth muscle. Its vasodilator effect is not altered by blockade of β-adrenergic, cholinergic or histaminic receptors, or by the presence of prostaglandin inhibitors such as indomethacin.

When compared to other vasodilators with similar sites of action (eg, minoxidil [*Loniten*], guancydine, diazoxide [*Hyperstat*]), pinacidil, at comparable levels of blood pressure reduction, produces quantitatively identical increases in heart rate, reflex sympathetic mediated cardiac contractility and cardiac output. However, when compared to hydralazine (another precapillary arteriolar vasodilator), pinacidil, at doses which produce equivalent reductions in total peripheral resistance, is a more potent blood pressure lowering agent. Since blood pressure is a function of the cardiac output multiplied by the total peripheral resistance, this difference may be explained by the fact that hydralazine appears to have a direct (as well as the indirect) cardiostimulatory effect which offsets some of the blood pressure reduction caused by vasodilation. As would be expected from their differing effects on cardiac output, pinacidil produces less of an increase in myocardial oxygen consumption than hydralazine.

Although an active metabolite has been identified, it does not appear to contribute significantly to the overall antihypertensive activity.

There is a linear correlation between pinacidil drug levels and the fall in mean blood pressure and total peripheral resistance; minimal therapeutic levels are reported to be 50 ng/ml.

Pharmacokinetics: Absorption/Distribution – Available pharmacokinetic data are complicated by the fact that at least two different oral formulations have been used in clinical trials. However, in general, bioavailability approaches 100% after oral administration, with both peak serum concentrations and peak effect occurring at 1 hour. Coadministration of food does not alter bioavailability but slightly delays absorption. Approximately 60% of a dose is protein bound.

Metabolism/Excretion – Pinacidil is metabolized by the liver to a number of metabolites, the most significant being the active metabolite, pinacidil N-oxide. Within the first 24 hours, 55% to 60% of an administered dose appears in the urine as pinacidil or the N-oxide, 20% to 30% is excreted in the urine as other metabolites and 3% is recovered in the feces. The elimination half-life (t½) varies between 1.5 to 3 hours. Average clearance values are 42 ± 5 L/hr.

Although exact dosage guidelines have not been established, patients with liver disease should have therapy initiated slowly, at low doses, and with careful blood pressure monitoring. Eight patients with chronic, stable cirrhosis showed a 50% reduction in clearance, prolongation of the half-life and a decrease in the percentage of parent compound converted to the N-oxide metabolite.

Clinical studies: Only a limited number of clinical studies, each involving only a few patients, have been published. This may reflect that pinacidil is not considered to be a first- or second-line drug in the stepped-care approach.

Pinacidil use has generally been confined to patients with moderate to severe hypertension. It is safe and effective, especially when added to a regimen of a diuretic and β-blocker in patients who failed the initial combination regimen.

Pinacidil has been particularly effective in selected patients with renal impairment (both dialysis and non-dialysis patients) with drug-resistant, non-volume dependent hypertension.

Although most studies have used doses of 10 to 100 mg twice daily, some clinicians feel that the drug may require 3 times daily dosing. The most effective dose range appears to be 12.5 or 25 mg twice daily.

Side effects: Pinacidil appears to be well tolerated. Only a few reports of mild side effects (eg, dizziness, headache and facial flushing) have been noted.

Edema has occurred in 23.5% to 45.2% of patients on doses of pinacidil alone of 25 to 50 mg. Concomitant diuretics may be required in most patients.

Two patients have developed positive anti-nuclear antibody (ANA) titers while receiving pinacidil. Neither had clinical manifestations of a lupus-like syndrome, and a direct cause and effect relationship could not be linked to pinacidil. However, further studies are necessary to investigate the potential for pinacidil to cause a drug-induced lupus syndrome.

Summary: Pinacidil appears to be a promising alternative agent for the treatment of moderate to severe hypertension. However, further studies are needed to clarify the drug's optimal dosing schedule, long-term side effects and optimal drug combinations.

The FDA's Cardio-Renal Drugs Advisory Committee recommended approval of pinacidil on May 28, 1987, with the stipulation that it be used concomitantly with diuretics. The drug was approved by the FDA in December 1989; however, Lilly has no plans to market pinacidil at this time.

Bibliography Available on Request

LORATADINE (*Claritin* by Schering) – A new long-acting, nonsedating antihistamine.

Pharmacology: Loratadine is a new, oral, long-acting antihistamine with minimal central nervous sytem and anticholinergic effects. Loratadine is a selective histamine-1 (H_1) receptor antagonist which shows greater affinity for peripheral than central nervous system histamine receptors. This selectivity, along with loratadine's poor penetration into the central nervous system, are thought to account for its lack of sedation. In in vivo experimental models, loratadine's action is similar to terfenadine *(Seldane)*; however, loratadine is approximately four times more potent. In addition to its antihistaminic activity, loratadine may also have some slight inhibitory activity on PAF, a phospholipid released from a variety of cells which is a potent mediator of systemic anaphylactoid reactions, including bronchospasm and acute inflammatory responses.

Pharmacokinetics: Loratadine is rapidly absorbed after oral administration; the rate is directly proportional to the dose administered. A multiple-dose study of loratadine 40 mg once daily has reported the following pharmacokinetic profile: Time to peak serum concentration – 1.5 hours; peak concentration – 26 ng/ml; elimination half-life ($t_{1/2}$) – 14.4 hours.

Loratadine undergoes extensive pre-systemic (first-pass) metabolism. An active metabolite, descarboethoxyloratadine (DCL) has been identified, but is present only in very low concentrations due to further metabolism. The pharmacokinetic profile of DCL after multiple dosing of the parent compound (40 mg once daily) is almost identical to that of loratadine; time to peak serum concentration – 1.8 to 3 hours; peak serum concentration – 26 to 29 ng/ml; elimination half-life ($t_{1/2}$) – 18.7 hours.

This pharmacokinetic profile, as well as clinical observations, supports once-daily dosing of loratadine.

Clinical trials with loratadine suggest that the onset rate of the therapeutic effect, total therapeutic effect, duration of therapeutic effect, and side effects are dose-related. Loratadine 10 mg is reportedly as effective as 12 mg chlorpheniramine maleate (eg, *Chlor-Trimeton*) in suppression of histamine-induced wheal formation. Greater suppression was produced by 20 and 40 mg loratadine. In a multicenter trial, loratadine 10 mg daily was as effective as clemastine *(Tavist)* 1 mg twice daily for treatment of seasonal allergic rhinitis. Using equipotent doses, loratadine has also been as effective as terfenadine for treatment of seasonal rhinitis.

Development of tolerance has not been noted in studies of continuous administration for up to 28 days.

Side effects: The major limiting side effects of drugs in this therapeutic class are sedation and functional impairment. Preliminary studies suggest that 10 to 20 mg/day loratadine does not cause sedation or impairment of performance criteria such as visual-motor coordination and short-term memory. However, 40 mg of loratadine slightly impairs performance criteria, but does not cause sedation. Sedation caused by 10 mg loratadine once daily appears to be about the same as 60 mg terfenadine twice daily. No other significant side effects have been reported. However, more extensive studies are required to accurately assess the side effect profile of loratadine. In addition, published studies have not included geriatric patients who may be more sensitive to this drug's side effects.

Summary: Preliminary data suggest that loratadine is effective for the control of histamine mediated disorders, such as seasonal and allergic rhinitis. Sedation and functional impairment are minimal, especially at doses less than 40 mg per day. Once-daily dosing may be considered an advantage over the currently available twice a day regimen.

Loratadine was recommended for approval by the FDA's Pharmacy-Allergy Drugs Advisory Committee October 23, 1987. It will be marketed as *Claritin* by Schering. Schering also has an NDA pending for a combination of loratidine with pseudoephedrine *(Claritin D)*.

Bibliography Available on Request

Dockhorn RJ, Bergner A, Connell JT, et al. Safety and efficacy of loratadine (SCH-29851): A new non-sedating antihistamine in seasonal allergic rhinitis, *Ann Allergy* 1987;58:407-11.

Bedard PM, Del Carpio J, Gutkowski A, et al. Comparison of efficacy and safety of SCH 29851, terfenadine, and placebo in the treatment of seasonal rhinitis, *Ann Allergy* 1985;55:233.

CARPROFEN (*Rimadyl* by Roche) – A new nonsteroidal anti-inflammatory agent.

Pharmacology: Carprofen [(D,L)-6-chloro-alpha-methylcarbazole-2-acetic acid] is a member of the arylpropionic acid class of nonsteroidal anti-inflammatory drugs (NSAIDs) which includes ibuprofen (eg, *Motrin, Rufen, Advil*), naproxen (*Naprosyn*) and others. The drug also possesses analgesic and antipyretic activity.

Although the site and exact mechanism of action of the NSAIDs has not been fully elucidated, most investigators agree that these drugs owe their analgesic and anti-inflammatory activity, as well as their gastric irritant properties, to their ability to inhibit prostaglandin synthetase. Carprofen is considered to be a less potent inhibitor of prostaglandin biosynthesis than naproxen or ibuprofen, and is only 1% to 4% as potent as indomethacin (eg, *Indocin*).

Considerable evidence suggests that the anti-inflammatory activity of carprofen is due primarily to the D-isomer; the L-isomer is only about one-seventh as potent.

Pharmacokinetics: Absorption/Distribution – Carprofen is rapidly and extensively absorbed after oral administration. Peak concentrations of approximately 6 to 12 mcg/ml are achieved in 1 to 3 hours; absolute bioavailability is approximately 90%. Ingestion of food results in a slight reduction in the rate of absorption as well as the peak plasma concentration. However, the total amount of the drug absorbed is not reduced. Peak plasma concentrations may be higher in the elderly. Carprofen is highly protein bound ($>$ 98%). In patients with osteoarthritis (OA) or rheumatoid arthritis (RA), the drug enters the synovial fluid rapidly, where it may achieve concentrations in excess of plasma concentrations.

Metabolism – Approximately 65% to 70% of an administered dose is metabolized by direct conjugation to an ester glucuronide. The elimination half-life ($t_{1/2}$) is between 13 to 25 hours. Despite the extensive hepatic metabolism, no difference has been observed in pharmacokinetics between cirrhotics and normal volunteers. Thus, dosage adjustments are unnecessary in patients with renal or hepatic insufficiency.

Excretion – Most of an orally administered dose of carprofen (65% to 70%) is eliminated in the urine as the glucuronide metabolite; only 3% to 12% of a dose is excreted unchanged. The remainder of the drug is excreted in the feces after undergoing extensive enterohepatic recycling.

Clinical trials: Carprofen is effective in a variety of clinical settings including treatment of rheumatoid arthritis, osteoarthritis, ankylosing spondylitis, extra-articular inflammatory processes (eg, tendonitis, bursitis), acute pain syndromes (eg, dental and post-traumatic pain) and acute gouty arthritis. Dosages have ranged from 150 to 600 mg/day in two or three divided doses. The few available comparative studies have usually shown carprofen to be equal to, or superior to, aspirin up to 3600 mg/day. Comparisons with indomethacin 75 to 150 mg/day have usually shown the lower doses (up to 300 mg/day) of carprofen to be slightly less effective but better tolerated than indomethacin. Larger doses of carprofen (400 to 600 mg/day) have been used in the treatment of OA; however, the use of larger doses may not produce any additional response over lower doses.

Side effects: Gastrointestinal effects have occurred in approximately 15% of patients. Pain, nausea, heartburn and dyspepsia are most common, while diarrhea is uncommon (approximately 1%). More serious GI side effects such as peptic ulceration are rare. Carprofen has been used along with antacids in patients with active peptic ulcer disease and has been well tolerated.

Renal or urinary adverse reactions including urinary frequency, dysuria, burning, hematuria, nephritis, proteinuria and acute renal failure occurred in 3.4% of 1521 patients in premarketing clinical trials.

Cutaneous reactions such as eczema, skin rash, urticaria and photosensitivity have occurred in 6% to 10% of patients.

Hepatic enzyme elevation occurred in 1.4% of patients in European trials and in as many as 14% of patients in large American trials. These enzyme elevations are usually asymptomatic.

Summary: Carprofen appears to be an effective NSAID which offers convenient twice daily dosing. Despite a low incidence of serious GI side effects, the drug does not appear superior to currently available agents.

Carprofen was approved by the FDA December 31, 1987. However, Roche has made a decision not to market carprofen at this time.

Bibliography Available on Request

Brogden RN. Non-steroidal anti-inflammatory analgesics other than salicylates. *Drugs* 1986;32(suppl 4):27-45.

O'Brien WM, Bagby GF. Carprofen: A new nonsteroidal antiinflammatory drug. *Pharmacotherapy* 1987;7:16-24.

ACECAINIDE HCl (*Napa* by Medco Research/Parke-Davis) – An antiarrhythmic agent.

Pharmacology: Acecainide (also known as N-acetylprocainamide, NAPA and acetylprocainamide) is an antiarrhythmic agent which was first identified as the major active metabolite produced by N-acetylation of procainamide (eg, *Pronestyl, Procan SR*). The drug has distinct electrophysiologic and pharmacologic effects which differ from the parent compound.

Acecainide is classified as a Type III (Vaughn-Williams classification) antiarrhythmic agent, along with amiodarone *(Cordarone)* and bretylium (eg, *Bretylol*), because of its ability to prolong atrial and ventricular action potential durations and refractory periods. This occurs without significant depression of conduction velocity. Sinus cycle length, sinus node recovery time, atrioventricular (AV) node refractory period and conduction intervals (eg, atrio-His, His-ventricular) are also not affected by therapeutic concentrations of the drug. Electrocardiographically, the PR interval and QRS duration show no significant changes during acecainide therapy. However, the rate corrected QT interval (QTc) is significantly increased at concentrations of the drug which produce arrhythmia suppression (12 to 35 mcg/ml).

Blood pressure and heart rate may be reduced, but this effect is not consistently seen. There is no significant effect on cardiac output or pulmonary artery wedge pressure. Several studies have shown that acecainide increases myocardial contractility.

Pharmacokinetics: Acecainide is well absorbed after oral administration, with bioavailability values ranging from 82% to 100% using capsule and tablet dosage formulations. Peak levels occur within 1 to 3 hours after oral administration. Protein binding averages 10% and is independent of plasma concentration.

Metabolism of acecainide is limited. A small amount (2% to 5%) is deacetylated back to the parent compound, procainamide, or converted to desethyl N-acetylprocainamide (< 1%). The majority of the drug (59% to 87%) is excreted unchanged in the urine, and there appears to be a strong correlation between renal clearance and creatinine clearance. Additional metabolic or excretion pathways are presumed to exist since approximately 10% to 15% of an administered dose cannot be accounted for in present studies.

The half-life ranges from 4 to 13 hours in patients with normal renal function to as long as 42 hours in functionally anephric patients. Elderly patients show a reduction in acecainide clearance which may reflect both age-related decrease in renal function and reduced renal tubular secretion of the drug.

Hemodialysis and continuous arteriovenous hemofiltration enhance acecainide clearance.

Clinical trials: The fact that acecainide produces electrophysiologic effects which are distinctly different from procainamide requires that the drug be evaluated separately. A positive response to procainamide is not necessarily predictive of a positive response to acecainide.

Acecainide has been used to suppress premature ventricular complexes (PVCs) and refractory ventricular arrhythmias. About 50% of patients with at least one PVC/minute achieved 50% suppression of arrhythmia; 40% achieved 75% suppression at plasma levels which averaged 22 mcg/ml. In the only published long-term trial of acecainide in drug refractory ventricular arrhythmias, 63% of patients were effectively controlled at 12 months.

Animal studies suggest acecainide may be useful in converting atrial flutter to sinus rhythm.

Side effects: Side effects are common, approximately 45%. Discontinuation of therapy due to side effects, however, is only required in approximately 10% of patients. Gastrointestinal disturbances are the most common (nausea, vomiting), followed by neurologic symptoms such as dizziness, lightheadedness, blurred vision, numbness and tingling.

Acecainide has little tendency to cause a drug-induced lupus-like syndrome which frequently limits the usefulness of procainamide. This reaction appears to be caused by the parent compound; however, a small amount of administered acecainide is converted back to procainamide. Like all antiarrhythmics, acecainide may have a proarrhythmic effect. Although not systematically studied in humans, reports of acecainide-induced torsade de pointes have been recorded.

Summary: Acecainide appears to be a potentially useful antiarrhythmic. The fact that it has little tendency to induce the lupus-like syndrome frequently associated with procainamide is of interest, but other alternatives to procainamide also exist. Additional studies are necessary to compare the efficacy of this drug to currently available agents and further define its place in therapy. An NDA is pending with the FDA for the oral form of acecainide.

Bibliography Available on Request

Singh, BN, ed. Therapeutic applications of a new antiarrhythmic compound; a clinical overview. *Angiology* 1986;37 (12 pt 2):929-81.

Feld GK, Singh BN. N-acetylprocainamide (acecainide HCl): Electrophysiology and antiarrhythmic effects. *Hosp Form* 1987;22:1038-46.

CIFENLINE SUCCINATE (*Cipralan* by Hoffman-LaRoche) – An anriarrhythmic agent.

Pharmacology: Cifenline succinate (formerly cibenzoline) is a new antiarrhythmic agent. It is an imidazoline derivative, structurally unrelated to any other currently available antiarrhythmic.

Cifenline's primary electrophysiologic effects are similar to those produced by quinidine (eg, *Duraquin, Quinidex*). The drug acts predominantly on the fast sodium current, reducing the rate of rise of phase 0 of the action potential and prolonging the effective refractory period. These effects are characteristic of Class IA (Vaughn-Williams classification) agents such as quinidine, procainamide (eg, *Pronestyl, Procan SR*) and disopyramide (eg, *Norpace*).

The drug has also been shown to increase the action potential duration, a property of Class III agents, and may produce blockade of the slow inward calcium channel similar to the Class IV agents. The contribution of these secondary effects to the drug's clinical usefulness has not been clearly delineated.

The drug produces a plasma concentration-dependent prolongation of the QRS duration. Prolongation of the PR interval and the rate-corrected QT interval have not been consistently observed, but these effects are compatible with the drug's known electrophysiologic effects and may be seen at higher doses or in patients with underlying conduction disturbances.

Pharmacokinetics: Cifenline is well absorbed after oral administration. Absolute bioavailability is approximately 85%, with peak plasma concentrations occurring approximately 1.5 hours after administration. Coadministration with food slightly decreases the rate, but not the extent, of absorption. Approximately 55% of the drug is bound to plasma proteins, primarily albumin.

Following multiple doses, the elimination half-life of the drug is approximately 12 hours (range, 8 to 12 hours). As much as 60% of a dose is excreted unchanged in the urine, and total body clearance correlates closely with creatinine clearance. Therefore, in patients with chronic renal failure, dosage should be reduced. Older patients also clear the drug more slowly, probably as a result of age-related reductions in renal function. The plasma concentrations of unchanged drug are apparently responsible for its antiarrhythmic effect. Studies have shown that the antiarrhythmic response following twice daily administration of cifenline is equivalent to a 4 times a day regimen.

Clinical trials: Cifenline is effective in suppressing a variety of ventricular arrhythmias, including complex PVCs and nonsustained ventricular tachycardia. In these applications, the drug has produced response rates similar to or higher than those reported for quinidine, procainamide, disopyramide and tocainide *(Tonocard)*. Data for patients with sustained ventricular tachycardia resistant to conventional therapy is limited; however, response rates of 25% have occurred. Long-term follow-up studies (12 to 24 months) have reported sustained therapeutic efficacy in 36% to 80% of initial responders.

Side effects: Cifenline appears to be well tolerated, especially when compared to the other Class IA antiarrhythmics. Gastrointestinal intolerance is the most common reason cited for discontinuation of therapy due to side effects. Other adverse effects reported include: Lightheadedness, dizziness, nervousness, tremulousness, blurred vision and dry mouth.

Worsening of pre-existing left ventricular dysfunction has occurred. The drug should be used with caution in patients with CHF, especially if baseline ejection fraction is less than 30%. The proarrhythmic effect that may occur (as with all antiarrhythmic agents) has occurred in 10% to 15% of patients receiving cifenline.

No serious hematologic or laboratory abnormalities have been reported.

Summary: Cifenline is a unique antiarrhythmic agent which may offer similar efficacy with a more favorable side effect profile than currently available Class IA agents. The long half-life which permits twice daily dosing may also be considered an advantage. FDA approval for cifenline, which will be co-marketed as *Cipralan* by Roche and Glaxo, is expected in 1990. The NDA has been pending since December 1985. The official generic name was recently changed from cibenzoline to cifenline.

Bibliography Available on Request

Seals AA, et al. Antiarrhythmic efficacy and hemodynamic effects of cibenzoline in patients with nonsustained ventricular tachycardia and left ventricular dysfunction. *Circulation* 1987;75:800-8.

Mohiuddin SM, et al. Long-term antiarrhythmic therapy with cibenzoline. *J Clin Pharmacol* 1987;27:400-6.

RIMANTADINE HYDROCHLORIDE *(Flumadine* by Roche) – An antiviral agent.

Pharmacology: Rimantadine is an antiviral agent structurally related to amantadine *(Symmetrel).* It effectively inhibits the replication of all human subtypes of influenza virus (H1N1, H2N2 and H3N2).

Although the exact mechanism of action of rimantadine is unknown, influenza A virus replication is delayed in the presence of the drug and is restored upon removal of the drug. It has been proposed that this effect is due to interference with viral uncoating.

Although rimantadine is transported more readily than amantadine across cerebral capillaries (blood-brain barrier), there is no evidence to support that it is effective in the treatment of Parkinson's disease, as is amantadine.

Pharmacokinetics: Absorption/Distribution – Rimantadine is well absorbed after oral administration. Absolute bioavailability data are unobtainable due to the lack of an intravenous form of the drug, but it is estimated to be in excess of 90%. Food does not appear to affect the absorption of rimantadine. Peak serum concentrations are achieved in 3 to 6 hours after oral administration, and protein binding is approximately 40%. The drug is concentrated in respiratory secretions (nasal mucus/plasma ratio of 1.73).

Metabolism/Excretion – Rimantadine is almost completely metabolized in the liver, with less than 1% of the parent compound excreted unchanged in the urine. Three metabolites have been identified: The ortho-, para-, and metahydroxylated forms. Whether these metabolites are active has not been established. Despite extensive hepatic metabolism, dosage reductions in patients with less severe forms of liver disease (eg, normal prothrombin time, total bilirubin < 2.7 mg/dl, and albumin > 2.5 g/dl without ascites) do not appear to be necessary.

Rimantadine has a longer elimination half-life than amantadine (33 hours vs 20 hours). The drug follows linear pharmacokinetics. Single-dose studies using small study groups with patients ranging from 5 to 70 years of age have shown no significant age-related differences in rimantadine clearance. However, lower doses may be warranted in the elderly who may be more sensitive to the drug's side effects.

Clinical trials: Rimantadine is highly effective in the prophylaxis of infections caused by influenza A viruses. When compared to placebo, rimantadine 200 mg/day as a single or divided (twice-daily) dose, has been shown to reduce the incidence of influenza-like illnesses in 70% to 90% of treated patients. Preliminary evidence suggests that the combined use of influenza vaccine with rimantadine chemoprophylaxis may provide additive protection.

The drug also appears to be useful for shortening the duration of infectivity (viral shedding) and severity of symptoms when administered within the first 24 to 48 hours of symptoms.

Side effects: The side effect profile of rimantadine is similar to that seen with amantadine. However, the incidence of these adverse effects is much lower with rimantadine.

Dose-related CNS disturbances occur in 10% to 30% of patients receiving amantadine, but are reported in only approximately 3% of rimantadine-treated patients. Nervousness, lightheadedness, difficulty in concentrating, sleep disturbances and fatigue are most commonly reported and occur early in the course of therapy. Nausea, vomiting and diarrhea have occasionally been linked to rimantadine administration. Long-term administration (mean, 80 days) has been studied in a nursing home population, with no evidence of cumulative toxicity.

Summary: Rimantadine appears to be as effective as amantadine in the prophylaxis of infections caused by influenza type A. Side effects, however, are much less common with equally effective doses of rimantadine. An adult dose of 200 mg twice daily and a children's dose of 5 to 7 mg/kg/day for up to 6 weeks duration for prophylaxis and 5 days for treatment has been suggested. The availability of a better tolerated form of chemoprophylaxis may further enhance efforts to control outbreaks of influenza, especially in high-risk populations.

A New Drug Application (NDA) was filed for rimantadine for treatment and prophylaxis of influenza A in November 1986. The FDA's Anti-Infective Drugs Advisory Committee recommended the drug for approval October 27, 1987. Rimantadine will be marketed as *Flumadine* by Roche.

Bibliography Available on Request

Deeter RG, Khanderia U. Recent advances in antiviral therapy. *Clin Pharm* 1986;5:961-76.

Dolin R, Reichman RC, Madore HC, et al. A controlled trial of amantadine and rimantadine in the prophylaxis of Influenza A infection. *N Engl J Med* 1982;307:580-84.

TOLRESTAT (*Alredase* by Wyeth-Ayerst) – An aldose reductase inhibitor.

Pharmacology: Tolrestat, a carboxylic acid, is an aldose reductase inhibitor currently undergoing clinical trials to assess its value in controlling the biochemical abnormalities responsible for the late complications of diabetes (eg, diabetic neuropathy and retinopathy).

Diabetic neuropathy, characterized by postural hypotension, diarrhea, pain and tingling in muscle groups, impotence, etc, occurs in about 10% of diabetic patients with good glycemic control and in up to 70% of patients with poorly controlled diabetes. Diabetic retinopathy occurs in approximately 75% of long-standing (up to 20 years) diabetics. These late complications of insulin-dependent diabetes appear to be related to the accumulation of intracellular sorbitol and galactitol which results in cellular damage. A deficit of myo-inositol may also be involved, especially in the diabetic neuropathies.

Aldose reductase is the first enzyme in the sorbitol (polyol) pathway. This pathway is responsible for the conversion of glucose to sorbitol and the conversion of galactose to galactitol. Under conditions of hyperglycemia, sorbitol accumulation occurs. By inhibiting aldose reductase, tolrestat prevents the accumulation of intracellular sorbitol.

Pharmacokinetics: Tolrestat is almost completely absorbed after oral administration in healthy subjects. Bioavailability is reduced in diabetic patients, but the difference is not statistically significant. Peak plasma concentrations are achieved in 1 to 2 hours. Maximum decreases in red blood cell (RBC) sorbitol levels occur after 3 days of treatment with 100 mg twice daily. The distribution half-life averages 2 to 3 hours, whereas the elimination half-life averages 10 to 13 hours. Protein binding is extensive (99.5%).

Metabolism of tolrestat is minimal. The drug is excreted primarily by the kidneys as unchanged drug. The need for dosage reductions in patients with compromised renal function has not been established.

Clinical trials: The majority of published data on tolrestat involves animal or in vitro studies. However, a study of 23 diabetic patients receiving tolrestat 25 or 100 mg twice daily showed a dose-dependent reduction of RBC sorbitol levels of 21% and 57%, respectively.

In two unpublished clinical efficacy trials, tolrestat was administered to patients with diabetic neuropathy in a randomized, double-blind placebo controlled fashion. The short-term (8 week) trial in 260 patients compared placebo to 200 mg twice daily or 400 mg once daily; the long-term (1 year) trial in 548 patients compared placebo to 50, 100 or 200 mg once daily or 100 mg twice daily. Compared with placebo, 28% of patients in the long-term study receiving tolrestat 200 mg once daily showed improvement of nerve conduction velocity and paresthesias but not pain. Improvement was seen in both trials with a once-daily dose of 200 or 400 mg, but not when the same dose was given twice daily.

Side effects: The most common side effect reported by the manufacturer in unpublished clinical trials was dizziness, which occurred in 11% of patients receiving 200 mg tolrestat daily. Other adverse effects that have occurred include skin rash and liver enzyme elevations. A clear cause and effect relationship between tolrestat therapy and these adverse effects has not been established.

Drug interactions: Studies with warfarin (eg, *Coumadin*) indicated that no drug interaction occurred due to protein binding displacement at therapeutic doses. Salicylates at concentrations of 100 to 200 mcg/ml displace tolrestat (21% and 35%, respectively). Tolbutamide (eg, *Orinase*) also displaces tolrestat (22% displacement at tolbutamide concentrations of 160 mcg/ml).

Summary: Published data, although scant, suggest that tolrestat is safe and well tolerated. The ability of aldose reductase inhibition to decrease RBC sorbitol accumulation has been demonstrated in humans. Despite evidence for a favorable biochemical effect, supporting evidence for a beneficial clinical effect (ie, prevention of late complications of diabetes) has yet to be conclusively established. Furthermore, the groups most likely to benefit from this form of therapy, those with poor glycemic control or long-standing diabetes, present methodologic problems for assessing cause and effect relationships with any form of therapy.

The NDA for tolrestat was filed on April 4, 1986 for diabetic neuropathy. It is in Phase III trials for diabetic retinopathy. Tolrestat will be marketed as *Alredase* by Wyeth-Ayerst.

Bibliography Available on Request

Raskin P, Rosenstock J, Challis P, et al. Effect of tolrestat on red blood cell sorbitol levels in patients with diabetes. *Clin Pharmacol Ther* 1985;38:625-30.

Hicks DR, Kraml M, Cayen MN, et al. Tolrestat kinetics. *Clin Pharmacol Ther* 1984;36:493-99.

DILEVALOL (*Unicard* by Key) – A β-adrenergic blocking agent.

Pharmacology: Dilevalol, a noncardioselective β-adrenergic blocking agent, is the R,R-isomer of labetalol *(Normodyne, Trandate),* one of four optical isomers of the drug. Although dilevalol is virtually devoid of α_1-blocking activity, having only one-fourth to one-third the activity of labetalol, it has ≈ 7 times the vasodilatory effect. However, this effect appears to be mediated via a β_2-agonist effect as opposed to an α_1-blocking effect. Dilevalol also has ≈ 4 times the β-blocking (β_1 and β_2) effect of labetalol. The degree of β_1 receptor blockade appears to be similar to propranolol (eg, *Inderal*).

The β-agonist activity of dilevalol appears to be selective for β_2 receptors. The vasodilatory response is blocked by propranolol, but not metoprolol *(Lopressor)* pretreatment, indicating the vasodilatory actions are mediated by β_2 receptor stimulation. Pindolol *(Visken),* which has significant intrinsic sympathomimetic activity (ISA), differs from dilevalol in that its agonist activity is not β_2 selective.

Dilevalol appears to decrease peripheral vascular resistance with no effect on cardiac output. The reflex increase in heart rate that might be expected with vasodilation is counteracted by the drug's β-blocking activity. In one study of 29 patients, heart rate actually decreased by 8 beats per minute compared to placebo. Dilevalol slightly decreased plasma renin activity in one study. In a study comparing dilevalol and metoprolol on the lipid profile of 309 patients, dilevalol increased HDL cholesterol and slightly decreased LDL cholesterol, a finding that is opposite that seen with other agents in this class besides pindolol and acebutolol *(Sectral).*

Pharmacokinetics: Absorption/Distribution – Dilevalol is rapidly absorbed following oral administration, reaching peak concentrations within 1 hour. Following absorption, it is rapidly distributed in the extravascular system. In one study of 12 volunteers, the mean maximum concentration was 62 ng/ml. Plasma levels appear to increase in a dose-related manner.

Metabolism/Excretion – Dilevalol undergoes extensive first-pass metabolism (85% to 95%), resulting in an absolute bioavailability of 11% to 14%. The half-life is ≈ 8 hours following oral administration, and 12 hours following IV, indicating dilevalol need only be given once daily. The metabolites are conjugated with glucuronides and are excreted in urine. Approximately 3% of the drug was excreted unchanged after an IV dose in 12 volunteers.

Plasma concentrations do not appear altered in severe renal impairment. In a study of six volunteers, only 0.007% (mean, 27 mcg) of a dose was excreted in breast milk over 48 hours.

Clinical trials: Dilevalol, in once-daily doses of 100 to 800 mg, is effective in the treatment of mild to moderate hypertension. Because of its vasodilatory effects, it may be more useful than other agents of this class in hypertensive patients with compromised myocardial function or peripheral vascular insufficiency. Since it does not affect glomerular filtration rate, renal plasma flow, renal blood flow or renal vascular resistance, it may be useful in patients with renal insufficiency. Some studies also indicate a possible benefit in Black patients. It is effective when administered orally and IV. In several studies, dilevalol was equal to or greater than labetalol, metoprolol and atenolol *(Tenormin)* in antihypertensive efficacy, with less side effects. In one study comparing dilevalol with atenolol, patients receiving dilevalol showed a greater and longer-lasting decrease in mean arterial pressure.

Although only reported in two patients, dilevalol may be useful for the treatment of pheochromocytoma. It may also be useful, administered IV, in the management of severe hypertension. Further studies are needed.

Side effects: Dilevalol appears to be very well tolerated. It has a relatively low incidence of CNS side effects, despite its lipid solubility. When compared to placebo, the most common side effects associated with dilevalol were dizziness, somnolence and nausea.

Drug interactions: In one study involving nine healthy subjects, cimetidine *(Tagamet)* slightly increased dilevalol's bioavailability. The clinical significance was not determined.

Summary: Dilevalol, an isomer of labetalol, is a noncardioselective β-adrenergic blocking agent with significant vasodilatory (β_2 agonist) activity; therefore, it may have advantages over other agents in this class in certain hypertensive patients with altered cardiac conduction. Black patients and patients with renal insufficiency may also benefit. It also appears to be well tolerated, with minimal side effects reported. It is usually administered once daily, and can be given orally or IV.

An NDA for the oral form was filed in 1986. In January 1990, the FDA's Cardio-Renal Advisory Committee recommended approval for dilevalol. However, due to an increasing incidence of hepatotoxicity, the manufacturer decided to withdraw the NDA and discontinue the worldwide marketing of the drug.

Bibliography Available on Request

Weintraub M, Standish R. Dilevalol: The R,R-isomer of labetalol. *Hosp Formul* 1988;23:639-45.

Soberman J, Greenberg S, Frishman W. The safety and efficacy of once-daily dilevalol in patients with mild hypertension: A placebo-controlled study. *J Clin Hypertens* 1987;3:271-77.

INDECAINIDE HCl (*Decabid* by Eli Lilly) – An antiarrhythmic agent.

Pharmacology: Indecainide is a class IC antiarrhythmic agent that is structurally similar to the investigational agent aprindine. Other available class IC antiarrhythmics are encainide (*Enkaid*) and flecainide (*Tambocor*). This class of drugs markedly suppresses premature ventricular complexes (PVCs) and depresses intramyocardial conduction. Indecainide prolongs the PR and QRS intervals, significantly increasing intraventricular conduction time without significantly affecting atrial or ventricular refractoriness. There appear to be no significant hemodynamic effects.

Pharmacokinetics: Indecainide is completely absorbed following oral administration. In animals, the half-life is 3 to 5 hours; however, the half-life in patients is considerably longer (9 to 10 hours), suggesting that twice-daily dosing may be effective in some patients. Indecainide is metabolized in the liver to desisopropyl indecainide. This metabolite appears to have a longer half-life than the parent drug, although the plasma levels of the metabolite are only approximately 10% those of indecainide. It is not known if desisopropyl indecainide possesses any antiarrhythmic effects. Approximately 63% of indecainide is recovered in the urine, with < 10% recovered as the metabolite. In one study, there was no correlation between percent suppression of ventricular ectopic depolarizations and plasma levels or half-life of either indecainide or the metabolite.

Clinical trials: Clinical information regarding the efficacy of indecainide is available only through several studies using small patient populations. Antiarrhythmic efficacy appears similar to encainide and flecainide. Efficacy was maintained in some patients for up to 2 years. Indecainide IV or orally markedly suppresses the frequency of PVCs, particularly repetitive forms. In one study, 63% to 82% of patients had suppression of PVCs, 60% to 82% had more than a 95% elimination of couplets, and 56% to 74% had complete elimination of ventricular tachycardia. The average suppression of PVCs with most available antiarrhythmics ranges from 50% to 75%. The degree of suppression was comparable to encainide and flecainide. Other studies have reported a 90% reduction in PVCs in approximately 85% of patients, and elimination of ventricular tachycardia in approximately 86% of patients. In a study involving 231 patients, indecainide reduced PVCs by 93%, while disopyramide reduced PVCs by 80%; suppression of runs of ventricular tachycardia were equivalent for both drugs. In a study of 11 patients, indecainide suppressed ventricular premature beats in 90% of patients, but suppression of ventricular tachycardia was achieved in only 45% of patients.

In data from five clinical trials through the manufacturer involving 792 patients, 70% receiving indecainide responded to ≤ 200 mg/day, and 90% responded to 300 mg/day.

Side effects: In clinical trials, the following side effects were noted: Dizziness (18% with the 200 mg dose, 12% with 150 mg and 9% with 100 mg); proarrhythmias (14.8%); congestive heart failure (3.9%). Each of these effects appeared to be dose-related. Other adverse reactions reported in the smaller patient population studies included headache, blurry vision, impotence, lightheadedness, confusion, thought disorders, nausea and constipation. Most reactions appear mild and may respond to dosage adjustment.

Drug interactions: In five patients receiving concurrent indecainide and digoxin, the digoxin concentration increased (range, 47% to 300%) in three of the five patients. The digoxin concentration decreased significantly when indecainide was discontinued. The clinical significance of this pharmacokinetic interaction was not determined.

Summary: Indecainide is an effective class IC antiarrhythmic agent that may offer an alternative for the patients who cannot tolerate the GI side effects of quinidine or the CNS effects of the other class IC agents. Lilly is recommending a dosage of 100 to 200 mg/day, and they plan to market only the twice-daily formulation (an immediate release form for 4 times daily administration was also tested in clinical trials).

Because of the recent findings of the Cardiac Arrhythmia Suppression Trial (CAST), which reduced the indications for encainide and flecainide to treatment of life-threatening arrhythmias only, Lilly is reviewing the CAST study data to determine if there is any potential relevance to indecainide.

In November, 1988, the FDA's Cardio-Renal Drugs Advisory Committee unanimously recommended approval for indecainide for sustained ventricular tachycardia, ventricular fibrillation, nonsustained ventricular and chronic benign PVCs. Indecainide was approved by the FDA in December, 1989. However, Lilly has made a decision not to market the drug at this time.

Bibliography Available on Request

Salerno DM, Krejci J, Granrud G, et al. Indecainide for treatment of ventricular ectopic depolarizations: Efficacy, pharmacokinetics, hemodynamic effects and safety. *J Am Coll Cardiol* 1988;11:843-50.

Nestico PF, Morganroth J, Horowitz LN, et al. Efficacy of oral and intravenous indecainide in ventricular arrhythmias. *Am J Cardiol* 1987;59:1332-36.

DOTHIEPIN HCl (*Prothiaden* by Boots) – A tricyclic antidepressant.

Pharmacology – Dothiepin, a thio analog of amitriptyline (eg, *Elavil*), is a tricyclic antidepressant (TCA) used for the treatment of depression. It is also structurally related to doxepin (eg, *Sinequan*). The efficacy of dothiepin does not appear to differ significantly from other available TCAs, and it appears comparable in efficacy to other antidepressants including fluoxetine *(Prozac)* and trazodone (eg, *Desyrel*). The anticholinergic effects may be less than with amitriptyline, although the sedative and anxiolytic activity appears to be similar.

Dothiepin and its metabolites inhibit the neuronal uptake of norepinephrine in vitro, thereby facilitating noradrenergic neurotransmission. The drug may also enhance serotonergic neurotransmission by inhibiting serotonin uptake. In vitro, dothiepin is a potent antagonist of histamine H_1-receptors, an effect common with other antidepressants. As with other TCAs, the therapeutic effects may not occur for 2 to 4 weeks following initiation of therapy.

Pharmacokinetics: Absorption/Distribution – Following oral administration, dothiepin is rapidly and completely absorbed. Peak plasma concentrations are achieved in 2 to 4 hours, and reach steady-state concentrations within 12 days (1 or 3 times daily administration).

Metabolism/Elimination – Dothiepin undergoes extensive hepatic metabolism resulting from N-demethylation and S-oxidation. Following the first-pass effect, oral bioavailability of dothiepin is approximately 30%. In one study in healthy volunteers, peak plasma concentrations and AUC of dothiepin-S-oxide were higher than the parent drug; the peak plasma concentrations of the other two metabolites were lower. It is not known if the metabolites contribute to the therapeutic efficacy of the drug. The terminal elimination half-lives of dothiepin and its metabolites are: Dothiepin 14.4 to 23.9 hrs; dothiepin-S-oxide 22.7 to 25.5 hrs; northiaden 34.7 to 45.7 hrs; northiaden-S-oxide 24.2 to 33.5 hrs. In two subjects, within 96 hours of administration, ≈ 56% of a dothiepin dose was recovered in the urine, and 15% in the feces. Unchanged dothiepin accounted for only 0.5% of the dose.

In elderly subjects, the time to peak plasma concentration, elimination half-life and AUC of dothiepin are increased, and the absorption rate constant, volume of distribution and plasma clearance are decreased. Dothiepin also appears in the breast milk in a concentration of ≥ 1 mcg/dl (dose: 75 mg/day).

Clinical trials: In several noncomparative studies using dothiepin doses of 75 to 300 mg per day for 4 to 24 weeks, a marked improvement in the symptoms of depression occurred in a large percentage of patients. However, the results are difficult to assess due to lack of controls and the short duration of therapy in some cases. Although one study showed the efficacy of dothiepin (75 to 225 mg/day) to be greater with a single dose at night vs a 3 times daily regimen, others have reported no statistically significant difference in efficacy.

In randomized double-blind comparative studies of amitriptyline and dothiepin (50 to 300 mg/day) for 4 to 12 weeks, no significant difference in efficacy was noted, although dothiepin may have a faster onset of action. Dothiepin is also comparable in efficacy to doxepin, imipramine (eg, *Tofranil*), maprotiline *(Ludiomil)*, fluoxetine and trazodone. In patients with mixed depression and anxiety symptoms, dothiepin is equally effective as alprazolam *(Xanax)*, and equal or superior to chlordiazepoxide (eg, *Librium*).

Dothiepin also appears to have significant analgesic activity and may be useful in patients with idiopathic fibromyalgia syndrome (eg, generalized musculoskeletal aching, multiple tender points, fatigue, stiffness, sleep disturbances), rheumatoid arthritis or psychogenic facial pain.

Side effects: The adverse effects are similar to those seen with other TCAs. The following occurred in data pooled from 12 double-blind and noncomparative studies involving 5755 patients: Dry mouth (24%); drowsiness (16.8%); GI disorders (10.8%); dizziness (10.3%); tremor (8.5%); sweating, insomnia (5.7%); blurred vision (4.5%); weight gain (3.5%); palpitations (2.8%); hypotension, headache (1.9); cardiac dysrhythmias (0.1%). Approximately 5% of patients withdrew from treatment due to side effects. Dothiepin appears to produce a lower incidence of anticholinergic, cardiac and sedative effects than amitriptyline; tolerability is similar to doxepin and imipramine. Consider drug interactions that may occur with TCAs.

Summary: Dothiepin is a tricyclic antidepressant agent that is effective in the treatment of depression but appears to offer no significant advantage over existing agents. The lower incidence of anticholinergic effects compared to amitriptyline may make it a more useful agent in elderly patients. The initial dosage appears to be 75 mg/day either divided 3 times daily or as a single nighttime dose. Dosage range appears to be 75 to 300 mg/day.

The NDA for dothiepin was originally submitted in 1979 by Boots licensee Marion. In 1982 the drug was recommended for approval by the FDA's Psychopharmacologic Drugs Advisory Committee; however, in 1987 the FDA requested additional safety information for the higher dosage ranges (200 to 300 mg) approximately 6 months after Boots reacquired rights to the drug. A 1992 approval is expected. Dothiepin will be marketed as *Prothiaden*.

Bibliography Available on Request

TACRINE HCl (*Cognex* by Warner-Lambert) – A cholinergic agent for Alzheimer's disease.

Pharmacology – Tacrine, also known as tetrahydroaminoacridine (THA), is a potent centrally acting anticholinesterase being investigated for use in the treatment of memory deficits in patients with Alzheimer's disease. A chemical analog of 4-aminopyridine, tacrine is approximately 100 times more potent in blocking pseudocholinesterase than tissue cholinesterase. Through its reversible inhibition of acetylcholinesterase, it is believed that tacrine may be useful in Alzheimer's disease; this is based on a 1976 discovery of a link between Alzheimer's and a deficit in neural choline acetyltransferase.

Other mechanisms of action may also exist, including: Selective blockade of potassium channels in the CNS; alteration in phosphorylation; presynaptic and postsynaptic blockade of muscarinic and nicotinic receptors.

Lecithin has been used in conjunction with tacrine in several trials since anticholinesterase agents increase the need for free choline; lecithin contains choline and is a precursor of acetylcholine. Lecithin alone has been advocated for presenile dementia.

Pharmacokinetics: The pharmacokinetics of tacrine have not been well defined. Most of the data are from a single study involving eight patients with Alzheimer's disease. Serum concentrations of tacrine and its metabolite were measured after a 25 and 50 mg single oral dose, after 50 mg orally three times daily for 1 month and after a single 50 mg IV dose. Absorption of tacrine was rapid; peak serum concentrations were achieved after 1.5 hours. Half-life was 1.59 and 2.14 hours following the 25 and 50 mg single dose, respectively. Following continuous administration of tacrine, half-life was 2.91 hours. Oral bioavailability was $< 5\%$ and urine recovery was $< 3\%$ of the dose. Half-life of the metabolite was 3.56, 4.11 and 5.07 hours following the 25 and 50 mg single doses and the 50 mg repeated dosing, respectively. It appears that tacrine is rapidly metabolized by the liver. Also, the AUC for the metabolite compared to the parent drug (oral vs IV) indicated that first-pass metabolism occurs.

Clinical trials: In the largest published study to date, tacrine was administered to 17 patients with moderate to severe Alzheimer's disease in a three phase study. In phase I, patients received tacrine at a peak dose of 150 to 200 mg/day; phase II included 14 patients who received the optimal tacrine dose determined in phase I for 3 weeks (patients served as their own control); phase III consisted of 12 patients involved in a long-term study of tacrine administration. All patients were encouraged to take 10 to 15 g of lecithin each day. Patients in all phases receiving tacrine showed significant improvement in the Alzheimer's Deficit Scale and Orientation Test compared to placebo. Although the results were promising, this trial has been criticized for several serious flaws in its design as well as interpretation of the data.

Tacrine has also been used in the treatment of tricyclic antidepressant overdose, myasthenia gravis, tardive dyskinesia, to potentiate narcotic analgesics, to ameliorate opiate withdrawal, to decrease morphine-induced respiratory depression and as a decurarizing agent.

Side effects: The most frequent side effect of tacrine appears to be cholinergic effects including sweating, diarrhea, increased urination, nausea and abdominal discomfort. In the clinical trial, reduction of the dose, administration of glycopyrrolate (eg, *Robinul*), or both, reversed these effects. Tacrine is a monoamine acridine, which may be associated with hepatic, hematologic and neurologic toxicity. Hepatotoxicity, which takes the form of an autoimmune granulomatous hepatitis, has occurred. In one trial 8 of 45 patients had abnormal liver function tests; however, there appeared to be no evidence of hepatotoxicity, and the liver function tests returned to baseline when the dose was decreased.

Summary: Preliminary results suggest that tacrine may be beneficial in the treatment of memory deficits in Alzheimer's disease in some patients. Many more studies are needed, however, to assess the actual benefit in these patients. Tacrine is not a cure for Alzheimer's and will not halt the progression of the disease. It is also possible that any beneficial effects of tacrine may decrease as the disease progresses.

Phase III trials of tacrine are ongoing. Trials were suspended at one time because of the concerns about potential hepatotoxicity. The US National Institute of Aging is a partial sponsor of the trials along with Warner-Lambert. If the drug is approved, Warner-Lambert may get 5 years of exclusivity; the drug, first synthesized in 1908, is not patentable. An NDA for tacrine was filed in June 1990, and has received a 1A rating from the FDA (new molecular entity with important therapeutic gain), indicating a high priority review. In March 1991, the FDA's Peripheral and Central Nervous System Drugs Advisory Committee did not recommend approval for tacrine because of unresolved questions about the drug's efficacy; however, the agency will continue its review. On December 2, 1991, the FDA approved a Treatment IND for tacrine involving up to 15,000 to 20,000 patients in a dose-escalation study (40 mg/day for 6 weeks, 80 mg/day for 6 weeks if no evidence of hepatic toxicity exists, then 120 mg/day for 12 weeks). Another study is underway using doses of 160 mg/day in 500 patients. Tacrine will be available as *Cognex*. For further information call 1-800-45-COGNEX.

Bibliography Available on Request

MIFEPRISTONE (RU 486) – An antiprogesterone.

Pharmacology: Mifepristone is a synthetic progesterone and glucocorticosteroid receptor antagonist.

Mifepristone's antagonist activity at the glucocorticosteroid receptor disrupts the negative pituitary feedback resulting from the normal morning rise in cortisol level.

When used as an abortifacient, mifepristone acts as an antagonist at progesterone receptors in the endometrium and the trophoblast, allowing prostaglandins to stimulate uterine contractions and causing the conceptus to detach from the uterine wall. Various vascular changes are produced which may decrease placental viability as well as decrease glandular secretory activity, accelerate degenerative changes, and increase stromal but not glandular mitotic activity in the endometrium causing sloughing of the endometrium.

Pharmacokinetics: Mifepristone is rapidly absorbed after oral administration. After a single dose of 25 mg and up to 25 mg/kg, peak plasma levels of 3.5 to 7.5 mcmol/L have been reported at 1 to 3 hours after administration. The drug is 94% bound to protein, with the majority (91%) bound to albumin. The volume of distribution is ≈ 1.5 L/kg. Cerebrospinal fluid levels equal to 4% of the plasma concentration have occurred. The half-life is 20 or 54 hours, depending on the method of pharmacokinetic analysis used in the study. Three active metabolites have been identified. Less than 0.5% of the drug is excreted in the urine.

Mifepristone also crosses the placental barrier, achieving levels equal to one-third of the maternal plasma levels in the fetal circulation.

Clinical trials: Clinical trials have demonstrated that mifepristone is an effective abortifacient in early pregnancy (< 56 days of amenorrhea). A variety of dosing regimens have been successful. Dosages from 25 mg twice daily for 4 days to 50 mg 3 times daily for 4 days have resulted in success rates of 61% to 85%. Once-daily administration of 50 to 100 mg for 7 days was successful in 50% to 73% of cases. A single 600 mg dose has a success rate of 72% to 100%. Menses typically begins within 5 days of initiation of therapy and continues for 1 to 2 weeks. Preliminary evidence suggests that the combination of a single dose of mifepristone followed within 48 hours by the administration of gemeprost, an investigational synthetic prostaglandin in vaginal suppository form, may improve the success rate by stimulating myometrial contraction, cervical softening and dilation. Patients are treated as outpatients unless complications occur.

Preliminary data suggest that the antiglucocorticosteroid action of mifepristone 20 mg/kg/day is useful in the treatment of Cushing's syndrome in some patients.

Mifepristone has also been used in patients with tamoxifen *(Nolvadex)* resistant breast cancer who have evidence of progesterone receptors. A dose of 200 mg/day resulted in a response rate of 18% at 3 months in one study.

Other uses under investigation are treatment of open-angle glaucoma, postcoital contraception and induction of labor. Due to the transplacental passage of mifepristone, the latter application requires further clarification of the drug's effect on a viable fetus.

Side effects: The most common side effect of mifepristone used as an abortifacient is heavy bleeding. Dilation and curettage or transfusion may be required to manage this side effect in some cases. The severity of bleeding is directly related to the use of higher doses (> 800 mg) and a longer duration of gestation before therapy.

Other common side effects include abdominal pain (80%), mild to moderate nausea and vomiting (43%), mild to moderate uterine pain (26%), headache (15%) and diarrhea (7.5%). These can usually be controlled with mild analgesics and antiemetic agents.

Summary: Mifepristone appears to be a safe and effective alternative to presently available forms of abortion. Efficacy is increased when used concurrently with a prostaglandin. It also shows promise in several disease states, such as Cushing's syndrome and breast cancer, which may respond to its specific receptor antagonist effects.

Mifepristone is currently marketed in France as *Mifegyne* by Roussel-Uclaf, and it also is approved in China. Hoechst, Roussel's marketing partner, may seek approval of mifepristone in the U.K., Scandinavia and the Netherlands in 1990. There appear to be no plans to test the drug in the US in the near future.

Bibliography Available on Request

Couzinet B, Schaison G. Mifegyne (mifepristone), a new antiprogestagen with potential therapeutic use in human fertility control. *Drugs* 1988;35:187-91.

Grimes DA, Mishell DR, Shoupe D, et al. Early abortion with a single dose of the antiprogestin RU-486. *Am J Obstet Gynecol* 1988;158:1307-12.

Silvestre L, Dubois C, Renault M, et al. Voluntary interruption of pregnancy with mifepristone (RU 486) and a prostaglandin analogue. *N Engl J Med* 1990;322:645-48.

FLUPIRTINE MALEATE (by Carter-Wallace) – A nonnarcotic analgesic.

Pharmacology: Flupirtine maleate, a triaminopyridine derivative, is a nonnarcotic analgesic structurally unrelated to other analgesic agents. Although its exact mechanism of action is not known, flupirtine lacks affinity for any type of opiate receptor and therefore, has a mechanism that differs from the opiates. Flupirtine also appears to lack some of the side effects of the opiates including constipation, respiratory depression, withdrawal phenomena, development of tolerance and abuse potential. It is suggested that flupirtine is a medium to strong analgesic; its duration of action is comparable to codeine, and it is up to three times as potent as codeine and propoxyphene (eg, *Darvon*), up to twice as potent as meperidine (eg, *Demerol*) and approximately ten times as potent as acetaminophen (eg, *Tylenol*).

Pharmacokinetics: The pharmacokinetics of flupirtine have not been well defined. The drug appears to have linear kinetics. A dosage of 100 mg 3 times daily achieves average steady-state blood levels equivalent to the peak for a single 200 mg dose. In one study of 55 patients, the analgesic effect occurred within 45 minutes to 2 hours; the duration of action was 4 to 6 hours. The half-life of flupirtine appears to be 7 to 10 hours.

In 13 elderly patients receiving flupirtine 100 mg 3 times daily for 12 days, the mean elimination half-life was higher than in healthy young subjects (mean, 18.6 hours on day 12 vs 6.5 hours). This was associated with an increased maximum serum concentration and reduced clearance in the elderly subjects.

In 12 patients with renal impairment, the half-life of flupirtine was higher compared to healthy subjects (mean, 9.8 hours vs 6.5 hours) following a single oral 100 mg dose.

Flupirtine peak levels and area under the curve may be higher in patients with primary biliary cirrhosis. In a study of ten patients, flupirtine did not induce hepatic microsomal enzymes.

Clinical trials: Flupirtine is effective in the treatment of pain resulting from various procedures or conditions including episiotomy, cancer, and postoperative and dental pain. Dosages used have ranged from 100 to 600 mg/day; the most common dosages were 100 mg once daily or 100 mg 3 times daily. Capsules were used in most studies although the suppository form was also used. Analgesic efficacy of flupirtine was judged to be as effective as other analgesics used in the studies including acetaminophen, codeine, pentazocine *(Talwin NX)*, oxycodone plus acetaminophen (eg, *Percocet*), naproxen (eg, *Naprosyn*) and diclofenac *(Voltaren)*. Flupirtine appears to have no tolerance or addiction potential. In one study, the average number of capsules taken per month remained constant for 12 months, as did the analgesic effect.

Flupirtine significantly reduced seizure frequency in eight of nine patients with minimal side effects; however, since other derivatives of the drug may have greater activity, no further studies in the treatment of epilepsy are planned at this time.

Side effects: Flupirtine does not appear to share the common side effects of the opiates such as respiratory depression and constipation. The drug is generally well tolerated. In a study of 55 patients, the most common adverse effects were dizziness (11%), drowsiness (9% to 10%), pruritis (9%) and dry mouth (5%). Other side effects that occurred included: Pain in forehead; sensation of excessive fullness in stomach; muscular tremor; nausea; other GI disturbances (eg, vomiting, abdominal discomfort).

Summary: Flupirtine is a nonnarcotic analgesic that compares favorably in efficacy with other available analgesics. At this time, however, it offers no clear advantage over the nonsteroidal anti-inflammatory agents except perhaps in the GI and CNS side effect profile. It does offer an advantage over the opiates in side effect profile, abuse potential, withdrawal phenomena and development of tolerance. The average dose appears to be 100 mg 1 to 3 times daily. It has been used in both a capsule and suppository formulation.

An NDA was filed for flupirtine by Carter-Wallace in April 1986. At one time, a 1989 approval was anticipated; however, there has been no recent projected approval date. The company is also working with a combination product of flupirtine with codeine.

Bibliography Available on Request

McMahon FG, Arndt WF, Newton JJ, et al. Clinical experience with flupirtine in the U.S. *Postgrad Med J* 1987;63:81-85.

Herrmann WM, Kern U, Aigner M. On the adverse reactions and efficacy of long-term treatment with flupirtine: Preliminary results of an ongoing twelve-month study with 200 patients suffering from chronic pain states in arthrosis or arthritis. *Postgrad Med J* 1987;63:87-103.

NEDOCROMIL SODIUM (*Tilade* by Fisons) – A second generation antiasthmatic agent.

Pharmacology: Nedocromil sodium, a cromolyn sodium-like drug (eg, *Intal*), is a new agent for the management of reversible obstructive airway disease (ROAD). The drug, used by inhalation, is for use in adults and children > 12 years of age. Nedocromil is to be used prophylactically, not on an as needed basis (eg, for an acute asthma attack).

In patients with ROAD, there may be chronic inflammatory changes in the airways, which is caused by the release of mediators from different cell types including mast cells, eosinophils, neutrophils, monocytes, platelets and macrophages in the bronchial mucosa and lumen. In vitro, nedocromil inhibits the release and activation of these mediators from these inflammatory cells. Nedocromil also inhibits release of histamine, leukotriene C_4 and prostaglandin D_2 from mucosal mast cells in vitro. The drug also appears to have anti-allergic activity as demonstrated in animals.

Pharmacokinetics: Absorption/Distribution – Following inhalation of nedocromil, approximately 90% of the dose is swallowed; however, the portion reaching the lung is completely absorbed. Bioavailability is 6% to 9%, with GI absorption contributing 2.5% to 3%. The absorption of swallowed drug makes a negligible contribution to the plasma concentration profile. After a 4 mg inhalation dose, mean maximum plasma concentration is 3.3 mcg/L. Peak levels are achieved quickly and decline slowly. The half-life is approximately 1.5 to 2.3 hours.

Metabolism/Excretion – Following IV administration, there is no detectable metabolism of the drug. Elimination is mainly via the kidneys, with 55% and 64% recovered in urine in 2 and 96 hours, respectively, after an 18 mcg/kg IV dose. By 96 hours, 36% of the dose was recovered in the feces.

Clinical trials: There have been many double-blind, placebo controlled and long-term noncomparative studies done with nedocromil. However, it is difficult to conduct and evaluate clinical trials in patients with asthma due to the variability of the disease. Therefore, a statistical analysis of 40 double-blind, placebo controlled studies involving > 1000 asthmatic patients was done. The patients were not homogenous in asthma type, and their condition was moderate to severe. The following variables were evaluated: Clinician's and patient's global assessment of efficacy; assessment of day and night asthma symptoms; lung function as assessed by morning and evening peak expiratory flow rate. A "good effect" of drug treatment was based only on opinions of moderately or very effective results. Clinicians and patients favored nedocromil over placebo in 32 and 31 of 40 studies, respectively. In 26 studies of similar design, nedocromil was reported as being effective in 73% to 76% of patients.

Nedocromil may also allow patients maintained on inhalational corticosteroids to reduce the dosage of the corticosteroid by ≥ 50%, and the resultant therapeutic effect may be additive. Nedocromil cannot, however, completely replace the use of the corticosteroid.

In one study involving 100 patients, nedocromil was compared to cromolyn sodium. There was a clinically insignificant difference between the two drugs when assessing improvement in pulmonary function and symptoms associated with daytime and nighttime asthma.

There has been conflicting data regarding efficacy of nedocromil in children. Some studies report improvement in symptoms, others indicate no difference compared to placebo.

Nedocromil appears effective in patients with ragweed-allergic rhinitis when administered as a 1% nasal spray. In addition, a 2% ophthalmic solution of nedocromil appears effective for the treatment of seasonal allergic conjunctivitis.

Side effects: Nedocromil 2 or 4 mg 2 to 4 times per day has been generally well tolerated in healthy volunteers and patients with ROAD. The most frequent adverse reactions reported include: Unpleasant taste (13.6%; approximately 5% find it intolerable); headache (4.8%); nausea (4%); vomiting (1.8%); dizziness (1% to 2%). In a comparison of 1041 patients or volunteers receiving nedocromil, 3% withdrew due to side effects including nausea or vomiting, sore throat, unpleasant taste, headache and chest tightness.

Summary: Nedocromil is a second generation inhalational antiasthmatic drug with anti-allergic and anti-inflammatory properties that is effective as maintenance therapy in patients with ROAD. It is not intended for the treatment of acute asthma attacks. The use of nedocromil may allow patients to decrease the dosage of concurrent corticosteroid or bronchodilator therapy, although it will not replace the use of these agents. The recommended dosage is 4 mg 2 to 4 times daily in adults and children over 12 years of age.

On June 11, 1990, the FDA's Pulmonary-Allergy Drugs Advisory Committee recommended approval for nedocromil for asthma. A 1992 approval is anticipated. The drug will be marketed as *Tilade* by Fisons.

Bibliography Available on Request

Gonzalez JP, Brogden RN. Nedocromil sodium. A preliminary review of its pharmacodynamic and pharmacokinetic properties, and therapeutic efficacy in the treatment of reversible obstructive airways disease. *Drugs* 1987;34:560-577.

CILAZAPRIL (*Inhibace* by Roche/Glaxo) – A non-sulfhydryl-containing ACE inhibitor.

Pharmacology: Cilazapril is a potent, structurally new, non-sulfhydryl-containing orally active angiotensin-converting enzyme (ACE) inhibitor prodrug currently under investigation for use in patients with hypertension and congestive heart failure. Following oral administration, cilazapril is de-esterified in the liver and other tissues to the active diacid form, cilazaprilat. Cilazaprilat is approximately ten times more potent than captopril *(Capoten)* and five times more potent than enalaprilat, the active form of enalapril *(Vasotec)*, in a variety of test systems.

The ACE inhibitors block the enzymatic conversion of angiotensin I to the potent vasoconstrictor angiotensin II. While this inhibition also results in reduced metabolism of bradykinin, alterations in the prostaglandin system and reductions in plasma aldosterone and antidiuretic hormone (ADH), these responses do not appear to be responsible for the primary therapeutic effects of these agents. Blockade of angiotensin II production reduces supine and standing blood pressure in hypertensive patients. In patients with congestive heart failure (CHF), the vasodilatory response reduces afterload, leading to an increase in cardiac output. These beneficial responses may be facilitated by the responses mentioned above.

After administration of cilazapril, ACE activity, angiotensin II and plasma aldosterone concentrations, total peripheral resistance, blood pressure (systolic, diastolic and mean), and the response to exogenous angiotension I are all reduced, while heart rate, baroreceptor reflex sensitivity, cardiovascular reflexes and glomerular filtration rate are usually unchanged.

Pharmacokinetics: Cilazapril is rapidly absorbed after oral administration, with peak levels of the parent compound achieved at ≈ 1 hour. Conversion to cilazaprilat, the active form, is rapid and extensive, with peak levels attained at ≈ 1.8 hours with 57% absolute bioavailability of the active compound. In contrast to some other ACE inhibitors, the bioavailability of a therapeutic dose of cilazapril is not significantly reduced by food. After single doses of 0.5, 1, 2.5 and 5 mg, peak plasma concentrations of cilazaprilat were 5.4, 12.4, 37.7 and 94.2 ng/ml, respectively, indicating that greater than proportional increases in the active compound are achieved over this dose range. The elimination of cilazaprilat is biphasic, with an initial half-life of 1 to 2 hours controlled by the rate of conversion to this active form, followed by a prolonged terminal elimination half-life of 30 to 50 hours consistent with tight, saturation binding to ACE resulting in non-linear kinetics. The volume of distribution is ≈ 20 L.

Clearance of cilazaprilat is almost exclusively renal. Patients with severe renal or hepatic impairment require smaller or less frequent doses; however, specific guidelines for dose adjustment have not been established. One study suggests that hypertensive patients undergoing hemodialysis can be controlled on 0.5 mg cilazapril post-dialysis. The presence of CHF or advanced age has not been shown to significantly alter pharmacokinetic parameters.

Clinical trials: Clinical trials in > 4500 hypertensive patients have evaluated the efficacy of cilazapril. Single daily doses of 2.5 to 5 mg are as effective as single daily doses of: Hydrochlorothiazide (HCTZ; eg, *Esidrix*) 25 to 50 mg; atenolol *(Tenormin)* 50 to 100 mg; sustained release propranolol (eg, *Inderal LA*) 80 to 160 mg; and enalapril 10 to 20 mg. In patients with mild to moderate hypertension, a 5 mg cilazapril dose produces a maximal effect, which can be enhanced by the addition of 12.5 to 25 mg HCTZ. In patients with severe hypertension, including patients with left ventricular hypertrophy, the mean effective dose was 10 mg in combination with 12.5 to 25 mg of HCTZ daily.

Side effects: Cilazapril appears to be well tolerated. In controlled trials of cilazapril monotherapy in > 3500 patients, the most frequently reported side effects were: Headache (4.5%); dizziness (3.3%); fatigue (1.7%); cough (1.6%); chest pain (0.8%); rash, somnolence (0.6%). In patients ≥ 65 years of age, cough, dizziness, palpitations and somnolence occurred slightly more frequently than in younger patients. The addition of HCTZ in an additional 1000 patients resulted in a slightly higher incidence of dizziness, cough and somnolence, while the incidence of other side effects was comparable to cilazapril monotherapy. Dizziness, fatigue and somnolence are commonly seen in treated hypertensives, regardless of the drug used.

Drug interactions: Indomethacin (eg, *Indocin*) considerably attenuates the antihypertensive activity of cilazapril. This attenuation was most pronounced when cilazapril was added to indomethacin, while the addition of indomethacin to a stable cilazapril regimen resulted in a degree of attenuation of effect which was considered to be clinically insignificant. Thus, the significance of this interaction appears to be dependent on the order of drug administration.

Summary: Cilazapril is a long-acting, potent ACE inhibitor. It appears to be well tolerated, while offering the advantage of once-daily dosing; this property may make it a useful addition to a class of drugs whose efficacy and safety continue to be confirmed in a variety of disease states. An NDA for cilazapril was filed in September 1989 for hypertension. Roche and Glaxo will comarket cilazapril as *Inhibace*. A 1992 approval is expected. A combination of cilazapril/HCTZ *(Inhibace HCTZ)* is in early clinical trials.

Bibliography Available on Request

TERODILINE HCl (*Micturin* by Forest Labs) – An agent for urinary incontinence.

Pharmacology: Terodiline is a secondary amine which has non-selective anticholinergic and calcium blocking effects. Although originally investigated as an anti-anginal agent, terodiline is presently undergoing clinical trials to evaluate its safety and efficacy in the treatment of patients with bladder incontinence. Terodiline provides the advantage of both anticholinergic and calcium blocking effects within the same plasma concentration range, with anticholinergic effects predominating at lower plasma concentrations and calcium entry blocking action predominating at higher plasma concentrations.

The motor nerve supply to the bladder and urethra is from the parasympathetic system; the neurotransmitter active in this system is acetycholine. Therefore, anticholinergic agents have been used to treat incontinence, but side effects often limit their usefulness. In addition to parasympathetic activity, it appears that calcium entry from the extracellular space is important in the contractile activity of urinary tract smooth muscle. Calcium blockers reduce frequency and amplitude of detrusor contractions and improve bladder capacity; however, side effects associated with their use have prevented their use in treating incontinence.

Pharmacokinetics: Terodiline is well absorbed after oral administration with a bioavailability of ≈ 90%. Peak serum concentrations occur 2 to 8 hours (average, 4 hours) after administration. Although therapeutic plasma levels have not been clearly established, a steady-state concentration of 0.6 mg/L is generally well tolerated. Higher concentrations of 0.8 to 1.1 mg/L can be maintained in some patients without serious adverse effects. One probable fatal overdose has occurred at a postmortem terodiline level of 10 mg/L.

The volume of distribution of terodiline is 500 L, ≈ 80% to 85% is bound to serum proteins, and the serum half-life is ≈ 60 hours. Due to the long serum half-life, maximum clinical effects will not be seen until ≈ 10 days after initiation of therapy.

It is uncertain if terodiline undergoes enterohepatic circulation, although it is extensively metabolized in liver. The major metabolite, parahydroxyterodiline, is minimally active compared to the parent. Approximately 15% of the drug can be recovered unchanged in urine.

Major pharmacokinetic changes occurred in patients with an average age of 85 years (eg, prolongation of half-life, decreased unbound drug fraction and body clearance, increased time to reach steady-state plasma concentrations). A 25 mg/day dose achieved similar plasma concentrations as a 37.5 to 50 mg/day dose in younger, healthier patients. This suggests that elderly patients should have therapy initiated at a dose not to exceed 12.5 mg twice daily, and increased doses should not occur prior to 4 weeks post-initiation.

Clinical trials: Terodiline 12.5 to 25 mg twice daily was effective in the treatment of some patients with urge urinary incontinence. Patients treated with terodiline have a decrease in both pre-micturition symptoms such as urgency and in urinary frequency. One study reported a decrease in voluntary micturitions from a mean of 10.8 to 7.9/day after 6 months of treatment. Another group reported a decrease in involuntary micturitions from 2.5 to 1.5/day with greater effects in those patients with higher baseline micturition frequency.

An increase in bladder capacity has been observed in several studies with one group reporting an average increase from 252 to 335 ml after 6 months of therapy. An expanded maximum cystometric capacity without increased residual urine values has also been observed.

A preliminary study suggests that terodiline may be safe and effective in children 6 to 14 years of age involved in a bladder training program to correct urgency or urge incontinence.

Side effects: Up to 50% of patients in some studies reported side effects during the first 3 months of therapy vs 35% in placebo groups. Most side effects were mild, anticholinergic-related and decreased in frequency (34%) between 3 and 6 months of continuous therapy. The most commonly reported effect was dry mouth (27% during first 3 months, 19% between 3 and 6 months). Other side effects reported during the first 3 months include: Blurred vision (15%); tremor (14%); weight gain (11%); tachycardia (4%); ankle edema (2%). The incidence of these effects between 3 and 6 months decreased to 1%, 7%, 4%, 3% and 1%, respectively. One study reported a small, statistically significant increase (2 mm Hg) in resting diastolic blood pressure after 6 months. Other side effects include: Vertigo; headache; nausea; balance disturbances. Polymorphic ventricular tachycardia (PVT) has been reported in other countries.

Summary: Studies to date suggest that terodiline is a safe and effective agent for the treatment of urinary incontinence. Its unique combination of both anticholinergic and calcium blocking activity may provide an advantage over presently available treatments. However, further studies are required to clarify long-term safety and to identify those patients most likely to benefit from terodiline therapy. Forest Labs acquired US licensing rights for the oral tablets from KabiPharmacia in December 1987. Kabi temporarily discontinued the sale of terodiline world wide following reports of an association with PVT. Clinical trials in the US have been put on hold at the request of the FDA. Forest submitted an NDA on August 30, 1989. An anticipated approval date for the drug, which will be marketed as *Micturin,* is now unknown.

Bibliography Available on Request

CELIPROLOL HCl (*Selecor* by Upjohn and Rhone-Poulenc Rorer Pharmaceuticals) – A cardioselective beta-adrenergic blocking agent.

Pharmacology: Celiprolol HCl is a third-generation, cardioselective, hydrophilic beta-adrenoreceptor blocking agent. It possesses weak vasodilating and bronchodilating effects attributed to partial, selective β_2-adrenoreceptor agonist activity and, possibly, direct papaverine-like smooth muscle relaxation. There is evidence for intrinsic sympathomimetic activity (ISA) at the β_2-receptor. The drug is devoid of membrane stabilizing activity (MSA, or quinidine-like effect). Weak alpha$_2$-antagonist properties are also present but are not considered clinically significant at therapeutic doses.

At therapeutic doses, celiprolol reduces heart rate and blood pressure. While the drug dose not generally produce any ECG changes, it can increase the AV nodal functional refractory period. Blood glucose levels and insulin requirements are not significantly altered in Type I diabetics. Celiprolol does not appear to alter pulmonary function, not inhibit bronchodilation induced by agents such as aminophylline (eg, *Phyllocontin*), albuterol (eg, *Proventil*) and ipratropium *(Atrovent)*. Triglycerides, LDL cholesterol and total cholesterol are decreased in some patients while HDL is increased; it appears that total lipid levels are not increased. A reduction in fibrinogen levels has occurred, which may be of some benefit in hypertensive patients with hypercoagulability.

Pharmacokinetics: Absorption/Distribution – Following oral administration, absorption is non-linear and dose-dependent. Bioavailability ranges from 30% to 70% following a single 100 mg dose and averages 74% after a 400 mg dose. Single-dose bioavailability is reduced by chlorthalidone (eg, *Hygroton*), hydrochlorothiazide (eg, *Esidrix*) and theophylline (eg, *Theo-Dur*). Food has also reduced bioavailability in some studies, but data are conflicting. Peak plasma concentrations and pharmacodynamic activity are seen 2 to 4 hours after oral administration; pharmacodynamic activity persists for 24 hours. Protein binding is approximately 25% and the drug follows a hydrophilic pattern of distribution.

Metabolism/Excretion: Celiprolol is largely unmetabolized and is excreted unchanged in urine and feces. It does not undergo first-pass hepatic metabolism and there are no significant active metabolites. Approximately 15% (range, 3% to 22%) of an oral dose and 50% of an IV dose is recovered in the urine within 3 days, the rest being excreted in the feces. Steady-state concentrations are achieved after 2 to 3 days. The predominant mode of excretion of active drug is renal; renal dysfunction may cause a reduction in systemic clearance and the need for dose reduction. Bioavailability is decreased and the extent of renal elimination increased in patients with cirrhosis. The pharmacokinetics are not significantly different in the elderly. The elimination half-life averages 4 to 5 hours. Placental transfer averages 3% at steady state compared to 18% for propranolol (eg, *Inderal*) and 6% for atenolol *(Tenormin)*.

Clinical trials: Celiprolol is a safe and effective drug for treatment of hypertension and angina. In doses of 200 to 500 mg once daily in the morning, celiprolol reduces blood pressure to comparable levels seen with other β-blockers, calcium channel blockers and angiotensin-converting enzyme inhibitors. In comparative trials in patients with mild to moderate hypertension, a 200 to 600 mg celiprolol dose was similar in efficacy to 80 to 160 mg/day propranolol or 100 mg/day atenolol. In patients with angina, celiprolol 300 to 600 mg daily was as effective as propranolol 80 to 160 mg/day or atenolol 50 to 100 mg/day in improving exercise performance, reducing the number of angina attacks and nitroglycerin requirements, and increasing the time to, or reducing the degree of, ST segment depression. The addition of a diuretic to doses of 200 to 400 mg/day may be more effective at controlling blood pressure than the use of celiprolol monotherapy in doses of 300 to 600 mg/day.

Side effects: In a study of > 2300 patients, side effects were mild and similar to placebo. GI symptoms (eg, nausea, abdominal discomfort, diarrhea), the most frequently reported complaints, were responsible for drug discontinuation in 13 patients. Headache, fatigue, dizziness and insomnia occurred in 6%, 4%, 3% and 1% of patients, respectively. Cardiovascular symptoms included development of a modest degree of CHF (n = 2), AV nodal block (n = 3) and bradycardia (n = 1). Other side effects included: Raynaud's phenomenon; orthostatic hypotension; bronchial obstruction; tremor; rash; muscle cramps; impotence.

Summary: Celiprolol appears to be well tolerated and effective for the treatment of hypertension and angina. Its combination of cardioselectivity, β_2-agonist activity, hydrophilicity and long duration of action make it unique among currently available drugs in this class. Whether these properties will be useful in the myriad of other applications for which β-blockers have been used (eg, post-MI prophylaxis, migraine, selected arrhythmias) will require additional experience. Until additional data is available, follow the usual precautions which apply to the use of any β-blocker. The NDA for celiprolol was filed by Rhone-Poulenc Rorer in June 1987 for long-term use in controlling hypertension and angina. The drug will be co-marketed by Upjohn under the name *Selecor*. A late 1992 approval is expected.

Bibliography Available on Request

SUMATRIPTAN (*Imitrex* by Glaxo) – A serotonin agonist for treatment of migraine and cluster headaches.

Pharmacology: Sumatriptan is a selective serotonin (5-HT) receptor agonist being investigated for the treatment of migraine and cluster headaches; both an oral and subcutaneous form are currently in clinical trials.

Serotonin appears to play a large role in the pathophysiology of migraine headaches. During the prodromal phase, serotonin is spontaneously released from platelets, enters the vessel wall and lowers the pain threshold. Also, serotonin enters into the brain by increasing permeability, thereby causing arterial vasoconstriction. Serotonin is then rapidly taken up by the platelets and spleen and excreted by the kidney. Without serotonin, the extracranial arteries are dilated and distended, resulting in headache.

Sumatriptan is chemically related to serotonin, but is highly selective for the 5-HT_1 receptor subtype (possibly 5-HT_{1D}). It is less potent at the 5-HT_{1A} receptor and inactive at other neurotransmitter receptor binding sites including adrenergic, dopaminergic and muscarinic receptors. In vitro, both sumatriptan and dihydroergotamine *(D.H.E. 45)* share a high affinity for 5-HT_{1D} and 5-HT_{1A} receptors. This 5-HT_1 receptor is mainly localized in certain cranial blood vessels; therefore, sumatriptan may have selective cranial vasoconstrictor activity, which is possibly the mechanism involved in its treatment of migraine. In vitro studies show constriction of meningeal circulation; the fact that sumatriptan is effective in alleviating migraine headache is consistent with the suggestion that dilation of blood vessels in the meningeal circulation is involved with migraine headache pathogenesis. In animals, the drug has no analgesic activity, and there was no effect on peripheral arteries in eight healthy volunteers.

Pharmacokinetics: The pharmacokinetic profile of sumatriptan is not well defined; data are obtained from a small number of subjects. Following oral dosing, the drug is rapidly absorbed with a mean absolute bioavailability of 14%, partly due to first-pass metabolism. Sumatriptan has a high plasma clearance, mostly due to non-renal clearance and a large volume of distribution. In 6 healthy subjects, maximum plasma concentration was 37 ng/ml (IV) and 44 ng/ml (oral); time to reach maximum plasma concentration was 0.25 hours (IV) and 2.3 hours (oral); half-life was 1.7 hours (IV) and 2.6 hours (oral); AUC was 25.5 hr • ng/ml (IV) and 180.2 hr • ng/ml (oral). Values listed are means.

In a study of 10 patients with acute migraine, peak sumatriptan plasma levels occurred within 10 to 20 minutes following SC use; relapse in severity of headache did not occur when the plasma concentration declined.

Clinical trials: In clinical trials involving patients with common or classic migraine headache, the administration of IV, SC or oral sumatriptan was effective in reducing pain in up to 96% of patients. Following SC administration (1 to 4 mg), complete relief occurred in 86% to 96% of patients within 20 to 60 minutes; SC doses of 3 to 4 mg appeared to be most effective. IV use (64 mcg/kg) resulted in abolition of all migraine symptoms within 10 to 30 minutes in 90% of cases. In nine patients, oral sumatriptan (140 to 280 mg) resulted in complete relief of all symptoms within 2 hours. In another study, sumatriptan 3 to 6 mg SC aborted migraine attacks in seven of eight patients; however, headache recurred in four patients who received the lower dose (3 mg) within 4 to 12 hours. A decrease in the symptoms associated with migraine (eg, nausea, vomiting, photophobia) and an increased ability to perform daily activities have also occurred following therapy. The response to therapy is seen at any stage that the migraine headache is treated.

Sumatriptan also appears to provide effective treatment for cluster (Horton's) headache.

Side effects: Sumatriptan is well tolerated. Adverse reactions have been mild and transient and included: Pressure in the head; feelings of heaviness, warmth or tingling; vertigo; malaise; fatigue; local irritation at the injection site (patients who injected themselves had a lower incidence). There were no changes in heart rate, blood pressure or ECG.

Summary: Sumatriptan is a selective serotonin agonist that appears to be highly effective in the treatment of migraine and cluster headache. The recommended SC dose is 6 mg as a single dose (maximum, 12 mg/day). The recommended oral dose is 100 mg. The SC form has a quicker onset and peak; however, the oral form may be preferred in patients who can anticipate a migraine attack or who have relatively mild attacks.

Glaxo filed an NDA for the SC formulation on July 3, 1990, and for the oral dose form on December 17, 1990. In October 1991, the FDA's Peripheral and CNS Drugs Advisory Committee unanimously recommended sumatriptan for approval. Glaxo anticipates approval in late 1992 or early 1993. Sumatriptan will be marketed as *Imitrex*.

Bibliography Available on Request

Humphrey PP, Feniuk W, Perren MJ, et al. Serotonin and migraine. *Ann NY Acad Sci* 1990;600:587-600.

FLUVOXAMINE (*Floxyfral* by Solvay/Duphar) – A serotonin reuptake inhibitor for depression.

Pharmacology: Fluvoxamine, a potent and selective inhibitor of presynaptic neuronal reuptake of serotonin, is currently being investigated for the treatment of a number of psychiatric disorders, including major depression and obsessive-compulsive behavior.

Inhibition of serotonin reuptake results in an increase in the concentration of serotonin in the synaptic cleft and a reduction in serotonin turnover mediated through a negative feedback mechanism. This facilitation of serotonergic neurotransmission is hypothesized to be responsible for the antidepressant activity of fluvoxamine. The mechanism of action in obsessive-compulsive disorder may be related to chronic treatment-induced adaptive changes in serotonin receptor function (ie, autoreceptor desensitization), or indirect influences on dopaminergic function. Fluvoxamine does not inhibit monoamine oxidase.

Pharmacokinetics: Fluvoxamine is rapidly and almost completely absorbed after oral administration. Peak plasma concentrations occur in 2 to 8 hours. Time to peak and peak plasma concentrations are unaffected by food. Plasma protein binding averages 77%. The elimination half-life is 15 hours; volume of distribution is > 5 L/kg (data extrapolated from canine studies).

Following an oral dose, 94% is recovered in the urine in the form of at least 11 inactive metabolites; no unchanged drug is recovered. Four major metabolic pathways have been identified. Although a linear relationship between fluvoxamine plasma levels and clinical response has been suggested, therapeutic plasma levels have not been established. Preliminary data suggest that pharmacokinetics are not altered in healthy elderly (> 60 yrs) patients.

Clinical trials: Fluvoxamine was effective in the treatment of depressive disorders in both open and placebo controlled trials. In comparative studies, fluvoxamine 50 to 300 mg/day in single or divided doses was as effective as clomipramine *(Anafranil)*, desipramine (eg, *Norpramin*) or imipramine (eg, *Tofranil*) for the treatment of depression. Therapy was initiated with 50 or 100 mg/day for 1 week, then titrated to clinical response. Maximum response to a given dose usually takes approximately 4 weeks. Maximum benefit and minimum side effects are achieved with single bedtime doses. Although not demonstrated to be superior to tricyclic antidepressants, some patients refractory to traditional therapy may respond to fluvoxamine, and it may be more effective than imipramine in treating the anxiety component of depressed patients.

In open and placebo controlled trials, doses used for the treatment of depression were also effective in the treatment of obsessive-compulsive disorders. The addition of lithium (eg, *Eskalith*) or a neuroleptic agent may result in improvement despite an inadequate initial response to fluvoxamine, especially in patients with the additional diagnosis of tic spectrum disorders (eg, Tourette's syndrome) and schizotypal personality disorders.

Fluvoxamine may be useful in the treatment of panic attacks and to improve episodic memory in patients with alcohol amnestic disorder (eg, Korsakoff's psychosis).

Side effects: The following side effects were reported during clinical trials: Nausea/vomiting (37%); somnolence, dry mouth (26%); headache (22%); constipation (18%); agitation (16%); anorexia, insomnia (15%); dizziness, syncope (14%); tremor (11%); hypokinesia (8%); asthenia (7%). The incidence of side effects was similar in elderly (> 60 yrs) patients. Overall, 12% of patients discontinued therapy due to side effects, usually during the first 8 days of therapy due to nausea, vomiting and insomnia. Abnormal liver function tests have been reported; assess liver function at baseline and weekly during the first month of therapy. Anecdotal data suggest that fluvoxamine therapy may precipitate mania in some bipolar patients.

Drug interactions: The coadministration of fluvoxamine 100 mg/day and propranolol (eg, *Inderal*) resulted in a fivefold increase in propranolol plasma concentrations and a slight (3 bpm) decrease in heart rate; diastolic blood pressure during exercise was reduced but overall blood pressure control was unaffected. Coadministration of atenolol *(Tenormin)* and fluvoxamine 100 mg/day resulted in no change in plasma concentration but a slight potentiation of heart rate reduction and slight antagonism of hypotensive effect. Closely monitor β-blocker and fluvoxamine coadministration. The addition of fluvoxamine to stable warfarin (eg, *Coumadin*) regimens has resulted in a 65% increase in warfarin concentrations and a prolongation of prothrombin time.

Summary: Fluvoxamine provides a safe and effective treatment option for patients who do not respond to or cannot tolerate the side effects of tricyclic antidepressant therapy. It also provides an important therapeutic alternative for patients with obsessive-compulsive disorder. Additional trials are required to establish the safety and efficacy of long-term treatment and in patients with concomitant disease states.

An NDA for fluvoxamine was filed in late 1984 and is currently pending at the FDA. A 1992 approval is expected. Fluvoxamine will be marketed as *Floxyfral* by Solvay (formerly Reid Rowell).

Bibliography Available on Request

SOTALOL (*Betapace* by Berlex) – An antiarrhythmic agent.

Pharmacology: Sotalol is a unique investigational antiarrhythmic agent for the treatment of atrial, AV-nodal and ventricular arrhythmias. The drug exhibits properties of both Class II (Singh-Vaughan Williams classification) antiarrhythmics, characterized by β-adrenergic blockade as is seen with propranolol (eg, *Inderal*), and Class III agents, which produce prolongation of the action potential duration (APD) as is seen with amiodarone *(Cordarone)*.

As a β-blocker, sotalol is a hydrophilic, non-cardioselective compound, devoid of intrinsic sympathomimetic activity (ISA), local anesthetic effects, and membrane stabilizing activity (except at very high doses). The majority of the β-blocking activity resides in the levorotatory form of this racemic compound.

Electrophysiologic studies have established that sotalol prolongs the monophasic APD in the atria and ventricles, increases the effective refractory period in atrial, ventricular, AV nodal and bypass tracts while lengthening the intranodal conduction time. The drug produces a dose- and concentration-dependent prolongation of the QT interval, an effect which is accentuated at slower heart rates. There is minimal change in the QRS duration.

Hemodynamic effects include a significant reduction in resting heart rate and blunting of exercise-induced tachycardia, a modest reduction in systolic blood pressure, an increase in systemic vascular resistance and a reduction in cardiac output. The latter is due primarily to a reduction in heart rate, since stroke volume is unchanged.

Pharmacokinetics: The bioavailability of oral sotalol approaches 100% and peak plasma concentrations are reached in 2 to 3 hours. Administration with food (especially milk and milk products) results in a slight, but clinically unimportant, reduction in absorption. There is no first-pass metabolism and no metabolites have been detected. The drug is not bound to plasma proteins. More than 75% of an IV or oral dose is eliminated unchanged in the urine.

Volume of distribution is 1.6 to 2.4 L/kg; elimination half-life ranges from 7 to 18 hours in patients with normal renal function, prolonging to 24 hours with moderate renal dysfunction and 33 hours with dialysis. A therapeutic range of 1 to 4 mcg/ml has been reported.

In elderly patients, the half-life may be slightly increased; however, no dose adjustments are usually required if renal function is adequate. The drug crosses the placenta (maternal:fetal concentration ratio of 1:18) and is found in breast milk (milk:serum ratio of 2.4 to 5.6).

Clinical trials: In doses of 160 to 320 mg/day, sotalol was effective in suppressing chronic PVCs, especially in patients with complex (multi-focal) or repetitive (couplets, triplets) forms in a variety of settings, including ischemic heart disease, post-MI and cardiomyopathy patients. In comparison studies it is usually superior to procainamide (eg, *Pronestyl*), quinidine (eg, *Cin-Quin*) and conventional β-blockers for these indications. In patients with ventricular tachycardia or fibrillation induced by programmed electrical stimulation, sotalol rendered 46% to 67% of patients non-inducible and it was superior to a wide range of Class I agents in most studies. The drug has been used safely in patients with depressed left ventricular function, but caution is advised with this group.

Intravenous sotalol (0.4 to 1.5 mg/kg) has effectively converted 46% of patients with paroxysmal atrial fibrillation in open label studies. Oral sotalol 160 to 320 mg/day was compared to quinidine (1200 mg/day) for maintenance of sinus rhythm following successful direct current cardioversion; 52% of the sotalol patients and 48% of the quinidine patients remained in sinus rhythm at the end of a 6 month follow-up. Although the drugs were equally effective, sotalol was better tolerated.

Both oral and IV sotalol are effective in preventing induction of sustained, paroxysmal supraventricular tachycardia; oral sotalol is superior to metoprolol *(Lopressor)* and atenolol *(Tenormin)* for this indication.

Side effects: Most side effects can be attributed to sotalol's β-blocking action and include: Dyspnea (19%); bradycardia (8.6%); chest pain (16.8%); CHF (2.1%; worsening or precipitation is most frequent during the first 30 days of therapy); palpitations (15.8%); fatigue (21.2%); dizziness (21.2%); asthenia (11.5%); headache (10%); nausea/vomiting (9.6%); diarrhea (6.7%). Proarrhythmia is the most serious side effect and has been reported in 4.3% to 7% of treated patients. Torsade de pointes was the arrhythmia recorded in 1.9% of the study population. Slight decreases in HDL and increases in VLDL and LDL cholesterol and triglycerides have been reported.

Summary: Sotalol is an effective and well tolerated agent in a variety of supraventricular and ventricular arrhythmias. It has the potential to become a first-line agent, replacing less effective or more toxic agents. Twice daily dosing may also be considered an advantage.

On December 13, 1990, the FDA's Cardio-Renal Advisory Committee recommended conditional approval for the drug, with approval contingent on data obtained from a trial sponsored by the National Heart, Lung and Blood Institute comparing sotalol with other antiarrhythmics. The study, completed in February 1992, showed sotalol significantly reduces the risk of ventricular arrhythmia recurrence. Sotalol, which will be available as *Betapace* from Berlex, was originally developed by Bristol-Myers Squibb. A 1992 approval is expected.

Bibliography Available on Request

AMLODIPINE (*Norvasc* by Pfizer) – Another calcium channel blocker.

Pharmacology: Amlodipine is a calcium channel blocker currently being investigated for the treatment of hypertension and angina. It is a 1,4 dihydropyridine derivative, structurally related to nifedipine (eg, *Procardia*), but containing a basic amino group substitution that appears to confer unique pharmacokinetic and pharmacodynamic properties.

The effects of amlodipine appear to be dose-dependent and are characterized by a gradual onset and a prolonged duration of action. The drug is a potent vasodilator, especially in the peripheral vasculature, although coronary vasodilation accounts, in part, for its usefulness as an antianginal agent.

In hypertensive patients, mean, systolic and diastolic blood pressures and systemic and renovascular resistance are reduced, while renal blood flow and glomerular filtration rate are increased. In patients with ischemic heart disease, coronary vascular resistance and myocardial oxygen consumption are reduced; coronary blood flow and cardiac index are increased.

Reflex tachycardia occurs rarely and has been attributed to the drug's gradual onset of action since it occurs more frequently after IV administration. In limited studies, the drug appears to have no significant effects on cardiac conduction; no significant ECG changes have been noted. At high concentrations, weak negative inotropic effects are observed.

Pharmacokinetics: Following oral administration, amlodipine is slowly absorbed; peak plasma concentrations occur within 6 to 9 hours. Bioavailability is high (65%) relative to other drugs in this class and is not affected by administration with food; protein binding is 97%. Volume of distribution is 21 L/kg.

Presystemic metabolism of amlodipine is limited. The drug is extensively but slowly metabolized in the liver to a number of metabolites which lack significant activity; < 10% of an oral dose is eliminated unchanged. Unchanged drug and metabolites are eliminated primarily in the urine (60%) and feces (25%). The elimination half-life averages 35 hours but is prolonged in the elderly (48 to 65 hours) and in patients with cirrhosis (66 hours), suggesting that reduced dosages should be used in these patients. Renal dysfunction does not appear to significantly influence the pharmacokinetics of amlodipine.

Clinical trials: The majority of clinical trials with amlodipine have involved small numbers of patients (10 to 200) but with consistent results, possibly due to the similarity of study design.

In doses of 2.5 to 10 mg/day, amlodipine is effective monotherapy for the treatment of mild to moderate essential hypertension. Sustained blood pressure reductions of 10% to 20% occurred in both placebo controlled and comparative studies. The drug produces prolonged (24 hour) blood pressure control with single daily dosing that is equal or superior to placebo, atenolol (eg, *Tenormin;* 50 to 100 mg/day), verapamil (eg, *Isoptin;* 160 to 320 mg/day), captopril (eg, *Capoten;* 50 to 100 mg/day) or hydrochlorothiazide (eg, *Esidrix;* 25 to 100 mg/day). Blood pressure reductions tended to be equivalent in both elderly and younger hypertensives, although elderly patients with primarily systolic hypertension showed greater reductions in systolic blood pressure.

Amlodipine, in doses of 2.5 to 10 mg/day, is effective in the treatment of chronic stable, exercise-induced and vasospastic angina when exercise time, time to onset, frequency, nitroglycerin use, ST segment changes, or a combination of these endpoints was used to evaluate efficacy. In patients with chronic stable angina, several small trials showed that the antianginal effect of amlodipine 10 mg/day was similar to nadolol *(Corgard)* 100 mg/day and diltiazem *(Cardizem)* 180 to 360 mg/day.

Side effects: Pooled data from 40 studies involving 4227 subjects (2495 amlodipine, 1213 placebo, 519 active comparisons) indicate that amlodipine is well tolerated with a side effect frequency of 29.8% for the amlodipine-treated group vs 22.1% for the placebo group. Withdrawal due to side effects was reported in 1.1% of amlodipine and 0.7% of placebo treated patients. The most frequently reported side effects in the amlodipine and placebo groups, respectively, included: Edema (9.8% vs 2.3%); headache (8.1% for both groups); dizziness (3% vs 3.4%); fatigue (4.6% vs 2.9%); nausea (2.8% vs 1.9%); flushing (2.4% vs 0.5%).

Summary: Amlodipine appears to be a safe and effective agent for the treatment of hypertension (monotherapy and combination therapy) and various anginal states. Its long half-life, which allows once-daily dosing without the need for modified formulations, lack of active metabolites and tolerability promise to make it a useful addition to a class of drugs which continues to find new applications.

The NDA for amlodipine was filed in December 1987. On June 7, 1991, the FDA's Cardiovascular and Renal Drugs Advisory Committee recommended approval for amlodipine for treatment of angina and hypertension. A late 1992 approval is anticipated for amlodipine, which will be marketed as *Norvasc* by Pfizer.

Bibliography Available on Request

Acquired Immune Deficiency Syndrome (AIDS) is an immunodeficiency state caused by an infection with the human immunodeficiency virus, HIV. This retrovirus has also been referred to as human T-cell lymphotropic virus, type III (HTLV-III), lymphadenopathy-associated virus (LAV) and the AIDS-related virus. There are several drugs being studied for AIDS, AIDS-Related Complex (ARC), AIDS-associated infections (*Pneumocystis carinii, Mycobacterium avium-intracellulare,* cryptosporidiosis, cytomegalovirus) and Kaposi's sarcoma. Listed below are some antiviral, cytokine and immunomodulating drugs currently undergoing clinical trials. To date, only three drugs, zidovudine *(Retrovir),* didanosine *(Videx)* and zalcitabine *(Hivid),* have been approved by the FDA for AIDS.

AIDS Drugs in Development			
Drug	Drug type	FDA status	Treatment sponsor
Acemannan *(Carrisyn)*	antiviral, immunomodulator	Phase I AIDS, ARC	Carrington Laboratories
AL-721	antiviral	Phase I/II AIDS, ARC, HIV positive	Matrix Laboratories
Ampligen	immunomodulator	Phase II/III AIDS	HEM Pharmaceutical
Ansamycin (*Rifabutin,* LM-427)	antiviral	Phase II ARC	Adria Laboratories
AS-101	immunomodulator	Phase I/II ARC, AIDS	Wyeth-Ayerst
Azidouridine (AZDU)	antiviral	Phase I HIV positive symptomatic, ARC, AIDS	Berlex
Bropirimine *(ABPP)*	immunomodulator	Phase II Kaposi's	Upjohn
CD4, soluble human, recombinant	antiviral	Phase II ARC, AIDS	Biogen
CD4-IgG	antiviral	Phase I maternal/fetal HIV transfer	Genentech
sCD4-PE40	antiviral	Phase I AIDS	Upjohn/NIH
d-ala-peptide T (Peptide T)	antiviral	Phase II AIDS-associated neuro-cognitive impairment	Carl Biotech/National Institute of Mental Health
Deoxynojirmycin (Butyl-DNJ)	antiviral	Phase II ARC, AIDS	Searle
Dextran sulfate *(Uendex)*	antiviral	Phase II AIDS, ARC, HIV positive asymptomatic	Ueno Fine Chem. Industry Ltd.
Diethyl-dithiocarbamate *(Imuthiol)*	immunomodulator	Phase II/III AIDS, ARC, HIV, pediatric HIV	Connaught

(Continued on following page)

AIDS Drugs in Development (Cont.)

Drug	Drug type	FDA status	Treatment sponsor
EL10 (DHEA)	antiviral, immunomodulator	IND approved; HIV infection	Elan Corporation
Fiacitabine (FIAC)	antiviral	Phase I/II HIV, ARC, AIDS	Oclassen
Fialuridine (FIAU)	antiviral	Phase I HIV, ARC, AIDS	Oclassen
Filgrastim[1] (granulocyte colony stimulating factor; G-CSF; *Neupogen*)	cytokine	Phase I/II AIDS	Amgen
FK-565	immunomodulator	Phase I HIV	Fujisawa
Fluorothymidine (FLT)	antiviral	Phase I HIV, ARC, AIDS	Lederle
Hypericin *(VIMRxyn)*	antiviral	Phase I AIDS	VIMRx Pharm/NIH
Immune globulin IV[1] (IGIV; eg, *Gamimune-N*)	immunomodulator	Phase II/III Pediatric HIV; with zidovudine for AIDS, ARC	Alpha Therapeutics/ Cutter Biological/Sandoz
Imreg-1 and *Imreg-2*	immunomodulator	Phase II/III AIDS, ARC, Kaposi's	Imreg
Interferon alfa *(Wellferon)*	cytokine	Phase II/III Kaposi's sarcoma	Burroughs Wellcome
Interferon, alfa-2b[1] *(Intron A)*	cytokine	Phase II With zidovudine for AIDS, ARC	Schering-Plough
Interferon, alfa-n3[1] (*Alferon LDO* [low-dose oral])	cytokine	Phase I/II ARC, AIDS	Interferon Sciences
Interferon, beta *(Betaseron)*	cytokine	Phase II/III Kaposi's, AIDS, ARC	Triton Biosciences
Interleukin-2[1] (IL-2; aldesleukin; eg, *Proleukin*)	cytokine	Phase I AIDS, advanced ARC, with zidovudine for HIV	Hoffmann-LaRoche/ Immunex
Interleukin-2 PEG	cytokine	Phase I/II With zidovudine for AIDS	Cetus
Interleukin-3, recombinant human	cytokine	Phase I HIV with cytopenia	Sandoz
Iscador	antiviral	Phase I HIV, ARC, AIDS	Hiscia
Isoprinosine (Inosine pranobex, inosiplex, methisoprinol)	antiviral, immunomodulator	Phase III ARC, HIV seropositive asymptomatic; NDA rejected February 1986	Newport Pharmaceuticals
Lentinan *(Lentinan-Ajinomoto)*	immunomodulator	Phase I/II HIV positive asymptomatic and symptomatic, ARC, AIDS, pediatric AIDS	Lenti-Chemico Pharmaceuticals

[1] Approved for other indications; refer to individual monographs.

(Continued on following page)

AIDS Drugs in Development (Cont.)			
Drug	Drug type	FDA status	Treatment sponsor
Methionine-enkephalin	immunomodulator	Phase I Stimulation of cellular function in immune deficiency states	TNI Pharmaceuticals
Monoclonal antibody (MSL-109; MAb)	antiviral	Phase I AIDS	Sandoz
Muramyl-tripeptide (MTP-PE)	immunomodulator	Phase II Kaposi's	Ciba-Geigy
Nevirapine (BI-RG-587)	antiviral	Phase II HIV	Boehringer-Ingelheim
Novapren	antiviral	Phase I HIV inhibitor	Novaferon Labs
Oxothiazolidine carboxylate *(Procysteine)*	immunomodulator	Phase I Restoration of glutathione depletion in HIV, ARC, AIDS; prevention of inflammation-induced HIV replication	Clintec Nutritional/Ben Venue Labs
Protease inhibitor	antiviral	Phase I ARC, AIDS	Hoffman-LaRoche
Ribavirin[1] *(Virazole)*	antiviral	Phase II/III Asymptomatic HIV positive, ARC; IND denied April 1987	Viratek/ICN
Roquinimex *(Linomide)*	immunomodulator	Phase II HIV	Kabi Pharmacia
Sargramostim[1] (granulocyte macrophage colony stimulating factor; GM-CSF; eg, *Leucomax, Leukine, Prokine*)	cytokine	Phase III ARC, AIDS; with zidovudine for AIDS; with interferon alfa-2a and zidovudine for Kaposi's	Immunex/Hoechst-Roussel/Sandoz/ Genetics Institute/ Schering-Plough
Stavudine (didehydrodideoxythymidine; d4T)	antiviral	Phase I/II HIV, ARC, AIDS	B-M Squibb
T4, soluble human, recombinant	antiviral	Phase I/II HIV	Biogen
Thymic humoral factor	immunomodulator	Phase I HIV positive	Adria
Thymopentin *(Timunox)*	immunomodulator	Phase III HIV	Immunobiology Research Institute
Thymostimuline *(TP-1)*	immunomodulator	Phase III AIDS	Serono Laboratories
Trichosanthin (*GLQ223*; Compound Q)	antiviral	Phase II HIV, ARC, AIDS	Genelabs
Tumor necrosis factor (TNF)	immunomodulator	Phase I With gamma interferon for ARC	Genentech

[1] Approved for other indications; refer to individual monographs.

Bibliography Available on Request

TEICOPLANIN (*Targocid* by Marion-Merrell Dow) – A glycopeptide antibiotic.

Pharmacology: Teicoplanin (teichomycin A2) is a glycopeptide antibiotic complex structurally related to vancomycin (eg, *Vancocin*). It has a similar spectrum of activity but a longer half-life which allows less frequent dosing. It may be administered by IM as well as IV injection and brief (30 minute) infusion. Teicoplanin is a mixture of six closely related glycopeptide components designated as teicoplanin-A2 (1 through 5) and teicoplanin-A3. The components of the A2 complex account for 90% to 95% of teicoplanin. The drug interferes with cell wall synthesis in susceptible organisms by inhibiting peptidoglycan polymerization.

Like vancomycin, teicoplanin is active only against gram-positive organisms. It is bactericidal against most susceptible strains, with the possible exception of some coagulase-negative staphylococci (which may show reduced susceptibility), where it may be bacteriostatic. It has equivalent or superior activity (based on MIC data) to vancomycin against staphylococci, including both methicillin-sensitive and -resistant *S aureus, S epidermidis,* streptococci (including viridans group, and groups B, C, F and G), enterococci, and many anaerobic gram-positive bacteria, including *Clostridium difficile, C perfringens, Listeria monocytogenes* and *Corynebacterium jeikeium.* Vancomycin-resistant enterococci may be resistant to teicoplanin.

Teicoplanin is usually synergistic with aminoglycosides and imipenem, and additive with rifampin (eg, *Rifadin*). A post-antibiotic effect of 2.4 to 4.1 hours has been reported with both methicillin-sensitive and -resistant strains of *S aureus.*

Pharmacokinetics: Absorption/Distribution – Like vancomycin, teicoplanin is minimally absorbed after oral administration; this route is acceptable only for the treatment of pseudomembranous colitis.

Following IM administration of 3 mg/kg, peak levels of 5 to 7 mcg/ml are achieved at 2 to 4 hours; bioavailability is 90%. Peak serum levels after IV administration are dependent on the dose and the method of administration. Following administration of 3 mg/kg, peak levels after a 30 second injection or a 30 minute infusion average 53 and 20 mcg/ml, respectively. Trough (24 hour) levels are not influenced. The drug is widely distributed in most tissues and fluids (with the exception of the CSF), although the rate and extent varies. Volume of distribution (Vd) at steady state averages 0.6 to 0.8 L/kg. Protein binding is 90%.

Metabolism/Excretion – The drug does not appear to undergo metabolism and is excreted in the urine almost entirely by glomerular filtration. Disposition kinetics are linear with relation to dose and are best described by a three compartment model. The terminal elimination half-life averages 45 to 70 hours. In patients with renal dysfunction and the elderly, the elimination half-life is increased but the Vd is unchanged. Current dosing recommendations for renal impairment state that usual doses be given for the first 3 days. Thereafter, either the dose is reduced or the interval prolonged, based on the degree of renal insufficiency according to the following scheme: Creatinine clearance (Ccr) 40 to 60 ml/min, half the dose or twice the interval; Ccr $<$ 40 ml/min, one-third the dose or triple the interval.

Clinical trials: Reported response rates by type of infection are: Skin and soft tissue (90%); septicemia, bone and joint (89%); endocarditis (83%); respiratory tract (77%). Other applications in which the drug has demonstrated efficacy include: Endocarditis prophylaxis in dental surgery; Hickman catheter and other indwelling device-related infections; neurosurgical shunt ventriculitis (intraventricular administration); CAPD-related peritonitis (added to dialysate); surgical prophylaxis; presumed gram-positive infections in immunocompromised patients. The usual loading and maintenance doses of 6 mg/kg followed by 3 mg/kg/24 hours may need to be increased in children and in the treatment of *S aureus* endocarditis and septicemia. A reduction in efficacy has been noted in diabetics, immunocompromised patients (including malignancy) and when foreign bodies are present.

Side effects: The overall incidence of side effects is 10.3%. Most commonly reported effects include: Non-specific complaints (fatigue, headache, diarrhea) (5.1%); injection site intolerance (pain, redness, phlebitis) (3%); hypersensitivity skin reactions (pruritus, urticaria, maculopapular rash) (2.4%); hematologic abnormalities (eosinophilia, reversible neutropenia, increased platelet count) (2.2%); transient elevation of LFTs (1.7%); nephrotoxicity (0.35% to 0.6%); high-frequency hearing loss which may be irreversible (0.28%); bronchospasm (0.2%); anaphylactoid reactions (0.07%). Teicoplanin does not appear to cause the dose or infusion rate-related histamine release associated with the "red man syndrome", as does vancomycin. Concomitant use of an aminoglycoside appears to increase the incidence of nephrotoxicity.

Summary: Teicoplanin appears to be a safe and effective alternative to vancomycin. Potential advantages appear to be the availability of IM administration, reduced infusion times and volume requirements, the lack of infusion-related reactions and once daily dosing.

The NDA for teicoplanin was filed in March 1991. The FDA has given the drug a "1A" priority review rating. Teicoplanin is currently available in 13 countries, including Germany, France, Italy and the U.K. It will be available as *Targocid* by Marion Merrell Dow. A 1993 approval is anticipated.

Bibliography Available on Request

PAROXETINE (*Paxil* by SK-Beecham) – A serotonin reuptake inhibitor for depression.

Pharmacology: Paroxetine, a phenylpiperidine derivative, is a potent and selective inhibitor of serotonin (5-hydroxytryptamine, 5-HT) reuptake, possessing marked antidepressant activity. It inhibits the active membrane transport mechanism responsible for the reuptake of serotonin, causing accumulation of serotonin in the synaptic cleft and prolonging the activity at postsynaptic receptor sites. It is postulated that inhibition of serotonin reuptake leads to a reduction in turnover rate via a negative feedback mechanism.

After long-term therapy, paroxetine may decrease the responsiveness of the terminal serotonin autoreceptors without desensitizing postsynaptic receptors, allowing an increased amount of serotonin to be released for each action potential. Long-term therapy does not result in beta-adrenoreceptor down-regulation as is seen with fluoxetine *(Prozac)*, sertraline *(Zoloft)* and the investigational agent fluvoxamine *(Floxyfral)*. Paroxetine has no effect on norepinephrine reuptake or dopaminergic or cholinergic neurotransmission.

At doses up to 40 mg/day, paroxetine appears to have no significant effect on heart rate, blood pressure or the electrocardiogram. Psychomotor function is unchanged at doses up to 30 mg/day; the effect with higher doses has not been studied. Psychomotor impairment caused by haloperidol (eg, *Haldol*), alcohol or oxazepam (eg, *Serax*) is not potentiated by paroxetine. Paroxetine 15 mg/day reduces total rapid eye movement (REM) sleep, while 30 mg/day also increases the number of awakenings, decreases total sleep time and prolongs stage 1 sleep.

Pharmacokinetics: Paroxetine is well absorbed after oral administration and undergoes 50% first-pass metabolism which is partially saturable. Absorption is not affected by food, fat content of the diet or antacid administration. After a single oral dose, the mean time to peak plasma concentration is 5 hours but considerable interpatient variability exists (range, 0.5 to 11 hours). Steady-state concentrations are achieved in 7 to 14 days; however, no correlation has been established between plasma concentrations and clinical efficacy. Paroxetine is lipophilic and distributes widely into tissues; only 1% remains in the systemic circulation. Concentrations in breast milk are equal to plasma concentrations. Protein binding is 95%.

Approximately 85% of a dose is oxidized to a catechol intermediate which undergoes methylation and conjugation to glucuronide and sulfate metabolites. While active, these metabolites are not considered to contribute to the antidepressant activity. The mean terminal elimination half-life is 24 hours, but significant interpatient variability exists (range, 3 to 65 hours). Approximately 1% to 2% of the drug is eliminated unchanged in the urine; 64% is excreted by the kidneys in the form of metabolites.

Although specific dosage guidelines have not been established, initiate therapy cautiously, and closely monitor elderly patients and patients with hepatic dysfunction and severe renal impairment (creatinine clearance < 30 ml/min) since clearance may be reduced in these populations.

Clinical trials: In open label, placebo controlled and comparative trials, paroxetine appears to be effective in the treatment of major depression. Comparative trials with amitriptyline (eg, *Elavil*) and the investigational drugs dothiepin and mianserin have shown equal efficacy, while comparisons with imipramine (eg, *Tofranil*) and clomipramine *(Anafranil)* have reported variable results. Clinical trials have established a usual starting dose of 20 mg given in the morning with food to minimize sleep and GI disturbances. The dose is increased according to clinical response every 3 to 4 weeks to a maximum of 50 mg/day (40 mg/day in the elderly). No comparative trials to other serotonin reuptake inhibitors (eg, fluoxetine, sertraline) have been published to date.

Side effects: Side effects are generally mild, dose-related, and occur most commonly during the first week of therapy. Tolerance may develop. In short-term studies (< 6 weeks), most commonly reported side effects included: Nausea (12%); somnolence (11%); sweating (9%); tremor (8%); asthenia, dry mouth (7%); insomnia (6%); constipation, dizziness, decreased libido, blurred vision, abnormal ejaculation (< 5%). In long-term studies (> 6 weeks), headache (15%), sweating (12%) and weight gain (9%) were the most commonly reported side effects. No anorectic effect has been reported with paroxetine. In the largest overdose reported, 850 mg paroxetine was not associated with any adverse cardiac effects or seizure activity.

Summary: Paroxetine appears to be a safe and effective agent for the treatment of major depression and can be given once daily. Additional studies in select patient populations and comparative trials to other serotonin reuptake inhibitors are needed to establish its place in therapy.

The NDA for paroxetine was filed in November 1989. The drug is also in Phase II clinical trials for the treatment of anxiety. Paroxetine will be available as *Paxil* by SK-Beecham. It is currently available in the UK as *Seroxat*. A 1992 approval is expected.

Bibliography Available on Request

REMOXIPRIDE (*Roxiam* by MSD) – An antipsychotic agent.

Pharmacology: Remoxipride, a substituted benzamide, is an atypical antipsychotic agent. It is a weak, but selective, dopamine-2 (D_2) receptor antagonist. D_2 receptors are thought to act in an inhibitory manner on adenylate cyclase, while dopamine-1 (D_1) receptors are associated with adenylate cyclase stimulation. The presynaptic dopamine "autoreceptors", which regulate the synthesis and release of dopamine, appear to be of the D_2 subtype. Many investigators have suggested that it is blockade of the D_2 receptor that mediates the clinical effects of most antipsychotic agents.

Remoxipride has a marked affinity for sigma receptors, which mediate opioid effects; clinical significance is unknown. There is a wide range between the dose that blocks apomorphine-induced hyperactivity and the dose that produces catalepsy, suggesting a favorable separation between the dose associated with antipsychotic effects and that producing extrapyramidal symptoms. The administration of remoxipride causes a significant, transient increase in prolactin release; however, prolonged administration (> 15 days) results in a reduction in this response.

Pharmacokinetics: Remoxipride is almost completely absorbed after oral administration with a bioavailability of 96% for both standard and controlled release (CR) formulations. There is no first-pass metabolism. Plasma concentrations peak within 1 to 2 hours after administration of standard formulations and within 2 to 6 hours after administration of CR formulations and are linearly related to dose. Volume of distribution averages 0.5 to 0.7 L/kg. Protein binding, primarily to alpha-1 acid glycoprotein, averages 80%. CSF levels average 6% to 17% of total plasma concentrations. Breast milk concentrations are $\approx$ 30% of those in plasma.

Approximately 70% of an administered dose is metabolized in the liver to six inactive oxidized metabolites. Plasma concentrations of unchanged remoxipride are higher in slow debrisoquine metabolizers. Between 10% and 40% of an oral dose is excreted unchanged in the urine. Plasma elimination half-life averages 4 to 7 hours.

Remoxipride is a weak base (pKa 8.9). Urinary elimination is reduced and plasma half-life is prolonged in alkaline urine (pH 7.2). Conversely, acidification of urine (pH 5.2) results in increased urinary elimination and a reduction in half-life. Mean plasma concentrations are increased and the half-life is prolonged in the elderly, in patients with creatinine clearances < 25 ml/min, and in severe liver disease. Most investigators recommend initiating therapy with one-half the usual dose in the elderly.

Clinical trials: Remoxipride is an effective treatment for chronic schizophrenia and acute exacerbations of chronic schizophrenia. Improvement was documented in both positive (eg, thought disturbances, hostility/suspiciousness, hallucinations, delusions) and negative (eg, emotional withdrawal, motor retardation) symptoms. In doses of 150 to 600 mg/day, remoxipride had similar antipsychotic efficacy to haloperidol (eg, *Haldol*) 5 to 45 mg/day and thioridazine (eg, *Mellaril*) 150 to 750 mg/day. The addition of anticholinergic agents to the treatment regimen was three times as frequent in the haloperidol-treated groups.

In most clinical trials, therapy was initiated with 300 mg/day. Patients responded to total daily doses of 300 to 450 mg/day (maximum dose, 600 mg/day) during initiation of therapy, and were tapered to usual maintenance doses of 150 to 300 mg/day. Dosage adjustments were made no more frequently than every 3 days and were based on patient response. A controlled release formulation has been evaluated, which allows once-daily administration with similar therapeutic efficacy.

Remoxipride may also be effective in the treatment of acute mania.

Side effects: Remoxipride, like other atypical antipsychotic agents (eg, clozapine *[Clozaril]*), causes less frequent extrapyramidal symptoms (EPS) than the classic antipsychotic agents (eg, haloperidol). Long-term, comparative trials reported an EPS incidence of 2% to 15% and 7% to 27% in the remoxipride- and haloperidol-treated groups, respectively. Pooled data from nine comparative trials with haloperidol also showed a lower incidence of insomnia, tiredness/drowsiness, difficulty in concentration and dry mouth in the remoxipride-treated group. Although isolated reports of cardiovascular effects such as postural hypotension are documented, they are not considered to be clinically significant. There are no reports of remoxipride-induced tardive dyskinesia.

Summary: Available data suggests that remoxipride is a safe and effective treatment for schizophrenia. Its favorable side effect profile makes it an important therapeutic option for patients unable to tolerate traditional antipsychotic agents. Additional comparative and long-term studies are necessary to clarify its overall role in the treatment of schizophrenia and evaluate its potential to cause tardive dyskinesia.

An NDA for remoxipride was filed in December, 1988. It is currently in phase III clinical trials for the treatment of acute and chronic schizophrenia. The drug, which will be marketed as *Roxiam* by MSD, is currently available in the UK, Denmark and Luxembourg. A 1992 or 1993 approval is anticipated.

Bibliography Available on Request

TAXOL (by Bristol-Myers Squibb) – An investigational antineoplastic agent.

Pharmacology: Taxol, a dipterene plant product derived from the needles and bark of the western yew evergreen tree, *Taxus brevifolia,* is being investigated for the treatment of various cancers, especially ovarian. The yew has been used in herbal medicine for centuries. Taxol has unique antineoplastic characteristics, combining activity as a mitotic inhibitor, and blocking cells in the G2 and M phases of the cell cycle while also enhancing the rate and yield of microtubular assembly and preventing microtubular depolymerization. In addition to ovarian cancer, preliminary studies suggest taxol may have at least marginal activity in acute leukemia, non-small cell lung cancer, melanoma and some other tumors; however, due to the limited supply, more extensive testing of taxol for these indications is awaiting development of a synthetic source.

Pharmacokinetics: Data on taxol are lacking. Elimination half-life is approximately 4.3 hours. Approximately 8% of the dose is excreted unchanged in the urine within 24 hours.

Clinical trials: In one study, 47 patients with advanced, progressive, and drug-refractory epithelial ovarian cancer were treated with 250 mg/m² taxol as a 24 hour continuous IV infusion for patients who had received only a single previous chemotherapeutic regimen and 200 mg/m² for patients having received two or more previous chemotherapeutic regimens or previous wide-field radiation. In response to unacceptable hematologic toxicity, initial doses were reduced to 200 and 170 mg/m², respectively, with further reduction to 135 and 110 mg/m² in some heavily pretreated patients. Repeat courses were administered every 22 days if there was no evidence of tumor regression and if blood counts had returned to pretreatment levels. A total of 281 courses of therapy were administered, with the majority being in the dose range of 110 to 170 mg/m². Overall, 12 patients had either partial response or complete response with duration of 66 to 462 days (median, 182 days). A clinical response was noted in 24% of patients whose cancer was refractory to cisplatin *(Platinol)* and 40% not showing clear refractoriness to cisplatin. Seven additional patients had a minor response. The number of courses required to obtain a response ranged from one to six. Overall, the response rate was similar to that seen in early trials with cisplatin. Taxol is also being evaluated in advanced as well as previously untreated ovarian cancer.

In a recent study, a $>$ 20% response rate (24% complete, 21% partial) occurred in 24 patients treated with taxol for non-small cell lung cancer. Patients received a 200 mg/m² infusion over 24 hours every 3 weeks.

Side effects: Neutropenia; thrombocytopenia; leukopenia; diarrhea; alopecia; arthralgias; myalgias; fever; headache; fatigue; nausea; vomiting; peripheral neuropathy; mucositis; bradycardia; taste perversion. A number of these reactions are dose-related. Hematologic effects are dose limiting. Neutropenia, although significant, was of relatively short duration (5 to 10 days). Alopecia was complete in all patients in one study. GI toxicity was very mild.

Hypersensitivity reactions occurred at a variety of doses and were characterized most frequently by dyspnea, hypotension, bronchospasm, urticaria and erythematous rashes. In later studies, IV administration time was prolonged and routine premedication was implemented to decrease the incidence of hypersensitivity reaction.

Summary: Taxol appears to be effective in the treatment of drug-refractory ovarian carcinoma. However, efficacy in the treatment of other cancers remains to be established. The dose used in clinical trials for 24 hour taxol IV infusion ranged from 170 mg/m² for heavily pretreated patients to 250 mg/m² for patients with minimal or no previous cytotoxic therapy. Taxol is administered IV over 6 to 24 hours to minimize the incidence of hypersensitivity reaction; the 24 hour infusion is preferred.

Presently, taxol supplies are limited, which is the greatest hindrance in its evaluation and approval. It is currently derived from the bark of the Pacific Yew tree and it takes 25,000 lbs of bark to derive 1 kg of finished taxol; patients require 1200 to 1500 mg over the average course of treatment. Work is currently progressing on a synthetic form of taxol by altering the chemical structure of pinene, a similar compound. Other alternate sources are also being considered such as cultivated yew biomass, semi-synthesis and plant cell cultures. Also, Rhone-Poulenc Rorer is investigating a semi-synthetic taxol analog called taxotere, which is extracted from the needles, rather than the bark, of the yew tree, and Bristol-Myers Squibb signed an agreement with an Italian firm (Indena) in June 1992 to derive taxol from needles and twigs of yew species in Europe and Asia. The natural chemical 10-deacetyl baccatin III, a precursor for taxol, will be processed into the natural chemical taxol via a semi-synthetic process..

Bristol-Myers Squibb plans to file an NDA in mid-1992 for taxol and an NDA in 1993 for the new source of taxol (ie, from the needles). A 1993 approval is anticipated. Taxol has received compassionate use designation from the National Cancer Institute.

Bibliography Available on Request

Brown T, Havlin K, Weiss G, et al. A phase I trial of taxol given by a 6-hour intravenous infusion. *J Clin Oncol* 1991;9:1261-67.

McGuire WP, Rowinsky EK, Rosenshein NB, et al. Taxol: A unique antineoplastic agent with significant activity in advanced ovarian epithelial neoplasms. *Ann Intern Med* 1989;111:273-79.

BISOPROLOL (*Probeta* by Lederle) – Another cardioselective beta blocker.

Pharmacology: Bisoprolol is a relatively selective β_1 adrenoreceptor antagonist. At oral doses up to 10 mg/day, there is no significant blockade of β_2 receptors, while doses up to 40 mg/day show only slight antagonism at the β_2 receptor. This selectivity is greater than that seen with equivalent doses of atenolol (eg, *Tenormin*). It is devoid of membrane depressant activity (eg, propranolol [eg, *Inderal*]), or intrinsic sympathomimetic activity (eg, pindolol [*Visken*]).

Bisoprolol, in oral doses up to 40 mg/day, produces a dose-dependent reduction in exercise-induced increases in heart rate, blood pressure and myocardial oxygen consumption, with most of the effect seen at doses up to 20 mg/day. Effects persist for at least 24 hours following once daily doses.

In studies in asthmatic patients, doses up to 20 mg/day produced only minor effects on airway resistance, forced expiratory volume in 1 second (FEV_1), and forced vital capacity (FVC).

Left ventricular function, assessed by ejection fraction and changes in pulmonary artery wedge pressure, is not significantly depressed by doses up to 20 mg/day. The electrophysiologic effects of IV doses up to 10 mg include depression of sinus rate, prolongation of the sinus cycle length, sinus node recovery time, and the functional and effective refractory periods of the atrioventricular (AV) node.

In acute and long-term studies, bisoprolol has either no effect, or a slight negative effect, on total cholesterol and HDL cholesterol, while triglycerides consistently showed a slight increase.

Pharmacokinetics: Oral absorption is > 90% and is not affected by food. Peak plasma concentrations are achieved between 1.7 and 3 hours and are linearly proportional to dose. The drug is rapidly and widely distributed, with highest concentrations found in lungs, liver and kidneys; V_d is approximately 3 L/kg. Protein binding is low (26% to 33%).

About 50% of the drug is metabolized in the liver by O-dealkylation followed by oxidation to 3 inactive carboxylic acid metabolites. Metabolism is independent of genetic polymorphism; first-pass metabolism is < 10%. The remainder of the drug is excreted unchanged in the urine; thus it is described as having "balanced" elimination.

The elimination half-life averages 9 to 12 hours in healthy individuals, but may be prolonged in patients with end-stage renal or hepatic disease (up to 28 and 21 hours, respectively), necessitating dosage reduction.

Clinical trials: Bisoprolol is both safe and effective in those cardiovascular conditions in which other beta blockers have been successfully employed.

In patients with mild to moderate hypertension, doses of 5 to 20 mg/day are as effective as atenolol 50 to 100 mg/day, metoprolol *(Lopressor, Toprol XL)* 100 mg/day and nifedipine sustained release (*Procardia XL*) 40 to 80 mg/day, and more effective than the combination of hydrochlorothiazide/amiloride (*Moduretic;* 50 and 5 mg, respectively).

In stable angina pectoris, 5 to 10 mg/day is as effective as atenolol 100 mg. Doses of 2.5 to 20 mg/day have similar efficacy to propranolol in the treatment of supraventricular tachycardias and beta blocker responsive patients with premature ventricular contractions.

Side effects: Bisoprolol is generally well tolerated; < 3% of patients discontinued the drug in published clinical trials. Effects are usually dose-related and occur during the first 6 to 8 weeks of therapy.

The side effect profile is similar to other beta blockers and includes: Bradycardia; weakness; edema; vivid dreams; insomnia; cold extremities; abdominal pain; nausea; vomiting; diarrhea; headache; anxiety.

Summary: Bisoprolol appears to be a safe and effective alternative to currently available beta blockers. The long half-life allows once daily administration and may facilitate compliance, although the drug is not unique in this respect. The "balanced" elimination may be useful in selected patients, however, these drugs are usually titrated to clinical effect and the value of this has yet to be demonstrated. Additional studies in selected patient populations will help determine its place among currently available drugs in this class.

On June 6, 1991, the FDA's Cardiovascular and Renal Drugs Advisory Committee unanimously recommended approval for bisoprolol for the treatment of hypertension. The committee also recommended approval for the combination of bisoprolol and low-dose hydrochlorothiazide (eg, *Esidrix*) as first-line treatment for hypertension; they recommended that the labeling forego the standard requirement that each drug in the combination be titrated to individual needs. Bisoprolol will be marketed as *Probeta* by Lederle; the previous trade name being considered was *Monocor.* A 1992 approval is anticipated.

Bibliography Available on Request

Lancaster SG, Sorkin EM. Bisoprolol: A preliminary review of its pharmacodynamic properties, and therapeutic efficacy in hypertension and angina pectoris. *Drugs* 1988;36:256-85.

GEPIRONE HCl (by Bristol-Myers Squibb) – An anxiolytic and antidepressant.

Pharmacology: Gepirone, an azapirone, is chemically related to buspirone *(Buspar)* but unrelated to the benzodiazepines in structure or pharmacology. Gepirone does not directly or indirectly interact with the benzodiazepine-gamma-aminobutyric acid receptor-chloride ion channel complex. Differing from buspirone, gepirone does not interact with dopamine receptors. Its principle effect relates to its action on brain serotonin activity.

The biochemical basis of the psychiatric disorders of anxiety and depression may be viewed as a dynamic serotonergic continuum with anxiety representing a relative serotonin (5-HT) excess disease and depression a relative 5-HT deficit disease. Gepirone acts as a *total* agonist on presynaptic 5-HT_{1A} autoreceptors (these inhibit neuronal firing and decrease 5-HT synthesis) and as a *partial* agonist at postsynaptic 5-HT_{1A} receptors (these are linked to cyclic-AMP and probably modulate signal transfer).

Partial agonists recognize and bind to receptors, but exert less activity than the *full* agonist. In the absence of the endogenous full agonist (serotonin), gepirone would exert its agonist effects. However, when full agonists are also present, partial agonists compete for receptors. When partial agonists (which have less intrinsic activity) displace full agonists from receptor sites, they decrease synaptic neurotransmission relative to what would have been achieved by the full agonist alone, and thus essentially act as functional antagonists. Therefore, the effects that 5-HT partial agonists (eg, buspirone, gepirone) ultimately exert on 5-HT neurotransmission depend on the serotonergic tone of the synapse in which the drug is working.

In the 5-HT excess state of anxiety, gepirone would act as an agonist on presynaptic 5-HT_{1A} receptors to decrease 5-HT synthesis and neuronal firing and on the postsynaptic 5-HT_{1A} receptor as a functional antagonist. The result would be a reduction of hyperserotonergic tone in the brain and an amelioration of anxiety symptomatology. However, the effects of gepirone in the relative serotonin deficit disease of depression would be quite different. Gepirone would bind to presynaptic 5-HT_{1A} receptors and exert its agonist effects to decrease neuron activity. In the 5-HT-deficit state of depression, this action would allow 5-HT depleted neurons to replenish their serotonin stores and thus serve 5-HT homeostasis. Gepirone would also bind to postsynaptic 5-HT_{1A} receptors, but in the 5-HT-deficient state of depression it would express its agonist effects thus causing normosensitization of postsynaptic 5-HT_{1A} receptors and restoration of postsynaptic serotonergic activity. This normalization of hyposerotonergic tone in depression would produce antidepressant effects and improvement of depressive symptoms.

Pharmacokinetics: Gepirone is rapidly absorbed after oral administration, reaching peak levels in about 1 hour. It undergoes extensive first-pass metabolism by the liver and has an oral bioavailability of only 15%. Both it and buspirone are hepatically metabolized to the major active metabolite 1-(2-pyrimidinyl) piperazine (1-PP). The plasma half life of gepirone is 2 to 3 hours. No change in dosing would be anticipated in patients with renal insufficiency or failure.

Clinical trials: Gepirone 30 to 60 mg/day and placebo were compared in a 6 week double-blind trial in 30 outpatients with generalized anxiety disorder. According to the Hamilton Anxiety Scale, the Clinical Global Impressions Severity of Illness scale, and physician and patient Clinical Global Impressions Improvement ratings, gepirone was significantly superior to placebo and produced improvement in both somatic and psychic anxiety. Significant improvement was delayed and occurred after 2 to 3 weeks of treatment. Predictors of clinical improvement included high levels of baseline anxiety and length of time off anxiolytic therapy (ie, the longer the time off benzodiazepines, etc, the more likely a positive response).

Both a single blind study using doses of 25 to 75 mg/day and a double-blind, placebo controlled study using doses ranging from 5 to 90 mg/day found gepirone exerted significant antidepressant effects in patients with major depression.

Side effects: Gepirone is well tolerated with most side effects reported as mild to moderate. The most frequently reported adverse effects were dizziness, nausea, headache, drowsiness and weakness. Gepirone does not impair memory, verbal fluency or psychomotor performance.

Like buspirone, gepirone does not appear to have a potential for causing physical dependence or addiction in humans, and it is expected that gepirone will not interact with alcohol or sedative/hypnotic drugs.

Summary: Gepirone is a nonbenzodiazepine drug similar in structure to buspirone. It lacks the sedative and adverse psychomotor and memory impairment effects of the benzodiazepines and does not appear to have the potential for causing physical dependence or addiction. Gepirone selectively affects the serotonergic system, targeting specifically the serotonin 5-HT_{1A} receptor subtype. Clinical studies indicate that it possesses both antianxiety and antidepressant properties and is well tolerated.

Gepirone is currently in Phase II/III clinical trials and will be available from Bristol-Myers Squibb. An anticipated approval date is unknown.

Bibliography Available on Request

APPENDIX

APPENDIX

Controlled Substances

The Controlled Substances Act of 1970 regulates the manufacturing, distribution and dispensing of drugs which have potential for abuse. The Drug Enforcement Administration (DEA) within the US Department of Justice is the lead federal agency responsible for enforcement of the Act.

DEA Schedules: Drugs under jurisdiction of the Controlled Substances Act are divided into five schedules based on their potential for abuse, physical and psychological dependence. All controlled substances listed in *Drug Facts and Comparisons* are identified by schedule as follows:

Schedule I (*C-I*): High abuse potential and no accepted medical use (heroin, marijuana, LSD).

Schedule II (*C-II*): High abuse potential with severe dependence liability (narcotics, amphetamines and barbiturates).

Schedule III (*C-III*): Less abuse potential than schedule II drugs and moderate dependence liability (nonbarbiturate sedatives, nonamphetamine stimulants, limited amounts of certain narcotics).

Schedule IV (*C-IV*): Less abuse potential than schedule III and limited dependence liability (some sedatives, antianxiety agents and nonnarcotic analgesics).

Schedule V (*C-V*): Limited abuse potential. Primarily small amounts of narcotics (codeine) used as antitussives or antidiarrheals. Under federal law, limited quantities of certain *c-v* drugs may be purchased without a prescription directly from a pharmacist. The purchaser must be at least 18 years of age and must furnish suitable identification. All such transactions must be recorded by the dispensing pharmacist.

Registration: Prescribing physicians and dispensing pharmacies must be registered with the DEA, PO Box 28083, Central Station, Washington DC 20005.

Order Forms: A triplicate order form is necessary for the transfer of controlled substances in schedules I and II. Forms are available at no charge from the DEA.

Inventory: Separate records must be kept of purchases and dispensing of controlled drugs. An inventory of controlled substances must be made every 2 years.

Prescriptions: Prescriptions for controlled substances must be written in ink and include: Date; name and address of the patient; name, address and DEA number of the physician. Oral prescriptions must be promptly committed to writing. Controlled substance prescriptions may not be dispensed or refilled more than 6 months after the date issued or be refilled more than 5 times. A written prescription signed by the physician is required for schedule II drugs. In case of emergency, oral prescriptions for schedule II substances may be filled; however, the physician must provide a signed prescription within 72 hours. Schedule II prescriptions cannot be refilled.

State Laws: In many cases, state laws are more restrictive than federal law and therefore impose additional requirements.

FDA Pregnancy Categories

The rational use of any medication requires a risk versus benefit assessment. Among the myriad of risk factors which complicate this assessment, pregnancy is one of the most perplexing.

The FDA has established five categories to indicate a systemically absorbed drug's potential for causing birth defects. The key differentiation among the categories rests upon the degree (reliability) of documentation and the risk:benefit ratio. Pregnancy Category X is particularly notable in that if any data exists that may implicate a drug as a teratogen and the risk:benefit ratio is clearly negative, the drug is contraindicated during pregnancy.

These categories are summarized below:

Pregnancy Category	*Definition*
A	Adequate studies in pregnant women have not demonstrated a risk to the fetus in the first trimester of pregnancy and there is no evidence of risk in later trimesters.
B	Animal studies have not demonstrated a risk to the fetus but there are no adequate studies in pregnant women . . . or . . . Animal studies have shown an adverse effect, but adequate studies in pregnant women have not demonstrated a risk to the fetus during the first trimester of pregnancy and there is no evidence of risk in later trimesters.
C	Animal studies have shown an adverse effect on the fetus but, there are no adequate studies in humans; the benefits from the use of the drug in pregnant women may be acceptable despite its potential risks . . . or . . . There are no animal reproduction studies and no adequate studies in humans.
D	There is evidence of human fetal risk, but the potential benefits from the use of the drug in pregnant women may be acceptable despite its potential risks.
X	Studies in animals or humans or adverse reaction reports or both have demonstrated fetal abnormalities; the risk of use in a pregnant woman clearly outweighs any possible benefit.

Regardless of the designated Pregnancy Category or presumed safety, no drug should be administered during pregnancy unless it is clearly needed.

Acute Overdosage

Rapid intervention is essential to minimize morbidity and mortality in an acute toxic ingestion. Institute measures to prevent absorption and hasten elimination as soon as possible; however, symptomatic and supportive care takes precedence over other therapy. It is assumed that basic life support measures, ie, cardiopulmonary resuscitation (CPR), have been instituted. Specific antidotes are discussed in the overdosage section of individual drug monographs. The discussion below outlines procedures used in the management of acute overdosage of orally ingested systemic drugs.

Advanced Life Support Measures:

Adequate Airway must be established and maintained, generally via oropharyngeal or endotracheal airways, cricothyrotomy or tracheostomy.

Ventilation may then be performed via mouth-to-mouth insufflation, hand-operated bag (ambu bag) or a mechanical ventilator.

Circulation must be maintained.

- *Hypotension:* If hypotension/hypoperfusion occurs, place the patient in shock position (head lowered, feet elevated); specific therapy may include:

  Establish intravenous (IV) access and initiate IV fluids (eg, normal saline, ½ normal saline; Ringer's lactate; dextrose solutions; etc). A maintenance flow rate is generally 100 to 200 ml/hour; individualize as necessary.

  Plasma, plasma protein fractions, whole blood or plasma expanders may be required.

  Severe hypotension may require judicious use of vasopressors. The most commonly recommended agents are dopamine, dobutamine, norepinephrine and phenylephrine.

- *Arrhythmia* treatment is dictated by the offending drug.

- *Hypertension,* sometimes severe, may occur. (See Agents for Hypertensive Emergencies.)

For specific information on these individual drugs or drug classes, see individual or group monographs.

Seizures: Simple isolated seizures may require only observation and supportive care. Repetitive seizures or status epilepticus require therapy. Diazepam IV is generally the agent of choice; the barbiturates have also been used.

Reduction of Drug Absorption:

Gastric emptying is generally recommended as soon as possible. Syrup of ipecac and gastric lavage are the two most commonly employed methods.

- *Syrup of ipecac* is the method of choice outside the hospital, but administer only on the advice of a qualified health professional.
- *Gastric lavage* is indicated in the comatose patient and for those in whom syrup of ipecac fails to produce emesis. Airway protection via endotracheal intubation is appropriate for the patient without a gag reflex. Position the patient on their left side and use a large bore tube. Instill warm water or saline (37°C), (100 to 300 ml per wash for adults; 10 ml/kg to a maximum of 250 ml for children) until lavage solution returns clear. Instill the fluid over 1 to 2 minutes, leave in place about 1 minute and drain over 3 to 4 minutes.

Adsorption, using activated charcoal after completion of emesis or lavage, is indicated for virtually all significant toxic ingestions. It adsorbs a wide variety of toxins and there are no contraindications. However, it adsorbs many orally administered antidotes as well, so space dosage properly.

Catharsis is often recommended, generally using a saline cathartic (ie, magnesium sulfate, magnesium citrate, etc) to promote passage of the toxin through the gastrointestinal tract.

Elimination of Absorbed Drug:

Interruption of enterohepatic circulation by "gastric dialysis" uses scheduled doses of activated charcoal for 1 to 2 days. Gastric dialysis not only interrupts the enterohepatic cycle of some drugs, but also creates an osmotic gradient, drawing drug from the plasma back into the gastrointestinal lumen where it is bound by the charcoal and excreted in the feces.

Diuresis may be effective as identified in the individual drug monographs.

- *Forced diuresis* is occasionally useful. The most common agents employed are furosemide and osmotic diuretics.
- *Alkaline diuresis* is appropriate for certain compounds (eg, phenobarbital, salicylates) and is usually accomplished by the administration of IV sodium bicarbonate.
- *Acid diuresis* may be indicated (eg, amphetamines, fenfluramine, quinine) but use caution in patients with renal or liver disease. It is usually accomplished with oral or IV ascorbic acid or ammonium chloride.

Dialysis is indicated in a minority of severe overdose cases. Drug factors that alter dialysis effectiveness include volume of distribution, drug compartmentalization, protein binding and lipid/water solubility.

- *Peritoneal dialysis* and *hemodialysis* have been the most common methods used. *Charcoal or resin hemoperfusion* is a relatively new procedure with promising clinical potential (eg, theophylline).

Poison Control Center:

Consultation with a regional poison control center is highly recommended.

Poison Control Center: ______________________________

Management of

Acute Hypersensitivity Reactions

Type I hypersensitivity reactions (immediate hypersensitivity or anaphylaxis) are immunologic responses to a foreign antigen to which a patient has been previously sensitized. Anaphylact*oid* reactions are not immunologically mediated; however, symptoms and treatment are similar.

Signs and Symptoms:

Anaphylactic reactions typically begin within 1 to 30 minutes of exposure to the offending antigen. Tingling sensations and a generalized flush may proceed to a fullness in the throat, chest tightness or a "feeling of impending doom". Generalized urticaria and sweating are common. *Severe* reactions include life-threatening involvement of the airway and cardiovascular system.

Treatment:

Appropriate and immediate treatment is imperative. The following general measures are commonly employed:

Epinephrine 1:1000, 0.2 to 0.5 mg (0.2 to 0.5 ml) SC is the primary treatment. In children, administer 0.01 to 0.03 ml/kg or 0.1 to 0.3 ml. Doses may be repeated every 30 to 60 minutes. Additionally, 0.1 to 0.3 ml may be introduced into an injection site (if it is the administration site of the offending drug). If appropriate, the use of a tourniquet above the site of injection of the causative agent may stop its distribution. However, remove the tourniquet every 10 to 15 minutes.

Epinephrine IV (generally indicated in the presence of hypotension) is often recommended in a 1:10,000 dilution, 3 to 5 ml over 5 minutes; repeat every 15 minutes, if necessary. In children, inject 1 to 2 ml or 0.1 ml/kg/dose over 5 minutes; repeat every 30 minutes.

A conservative IV epinephrine protocol includes 10 ml of a 1:100,000 dilution (0.1 ml of a 1:1000 dilution mixed in 10 ml normal saline) given over 5 to 10 minutes. If an IV infusion is necessary, administer at a rate of 1 to 4 mcg/min. In children, infuse 0.1 to 1.5 (maximum) mcg/kg/min.

Hypotension: The patient should be recumbent with feet elevated. Depending upon the severity, consider the following measures:

- Establish a patent IV catheter in a suitable vein.
- Administer IV fluids (eg, normal saline, lactated Ringer's).
- Administer plasma expanders.
- Administer vasopressors (see group and individual monographs). Commonly recommended agents include dopamine, dobutamine, norepinephrine and phenylephrine.

Airway: Ensure a patent airway via endotracheal intubation or cricothyrotomy and administer oxygen. Severe respiratory difficulty may respond to IV aminophylline or to other bronchodilators.

Adjunctive therapy does not alter acute reactions, but may modify an ongoing or slow-onset process and shorten the course of the reaction.

- *Antihistamines: Diphenhydramine* - 50 to 100 mg IM or IV, continued orally at 5 mg/kg/day or 50 mg every 6 hours for 1 to 2 days. For children, give 5 mg/kg/day, maximum 300 mg per day.
  Chlorpheniramine (adults, 10 to 20 mg; children, 5 to 10 mg) IM or slowly IV.
- *Corticosteroids,* eg, hydrocortisone IV 100 to 1000 mg or equivalent, followed by 7 mg/kg/day IV or oral for 1 to 2 days.
- *Hydroxyzine* 10 to 25 mg orally 3 to 4 times daily.
- *Cimetidine* 25 to 30 mg/kg/day IV in six divided doses.

Calculations

To calculate milliequivalent weight: $mEq = \frac{\text{gram molecular weight/valence}}{1000}$

$$mEq = \frac{mg}{eq\ wt} \qquad \text{equivalent weight or eq wt} = \frac{\text{gram molecular weight}}{\text{valence}}$$

Commonly used mEq weights	
Chloride	35.5 mg = 1 mEq
Sodium	23 mg = 1 mEq
Calcium	20 mg = 1 mEq
Magnesium	12 mg = 1 mEq
Potassium	39 mg = 1 mEq

To convert temperature °C ↔ °F:

$$\frac{°C}{°F - 32} = \frac{5}{9} \quad \text{or} \quad °C = \frac{5}{9}(°F - 32) \qquad °F = 32 + \frac{9}{5}\,°C$$

To calculate creatinine clearance from serum creatinine:

$$\text{Male: Ccr} = \frac{\text{weight (kg)} \times (140\text{-age})}{72 \times \text{serum creatinine (mg/100 ml)}}$$

Female: Ccr = 0.85 × above value

To calculate ideal body weight (kg):

Male = 50 kg + 2.3 kg (each inch over 5 foot)

Female = 45.5 kg + 2.3 kg (each inch over 5 foot)

To approximate surface area (m^2) of children from weight (kg):

WEIGHT RANGE (kg)	APPROXIMATE SURFACE AREA (m^2)
1 to 5	(0.05 × kg) + 0.05
6 to 10	(0.04 × kg) + 0.10
11 to 20	(0.03 × kg) + 0.20
21 to 40	(0.02 × kg) + 0.40

DESIRABLE HEIGHT AND WEIGHT

	Weight (lb)					
	MEN[1]			WOMEN[2]		
Height	Small frame	Medium frame	Large frame	Small frame	Medium frame	Large frame
4′10″				102-111	109-121	118-131
4′11″				103-113	111-123	120-134
5′ 0″				104-115	113-126	122-137
5′ 1″				106-118	115-129	125-140
5′ 2″	128-134	131-141	138-150	108-121	118-132	128-143
5′ 3″	130-136	133-143	140-153	111-124	121-135	131-147
5′ 4″	132-138	135-145	142-156	114-127	124-138	134-151
5′ 5″	134-140	137-148	144-160	117-130	127-141	137-155
5′ 6″	136-142	139-151	146-164	120-133	130-144	140-159
5′ 7″	138-145	142-154	149-168	123-136	133-147	143-163
5′ 8″	140-148	145-157	152-172	126-139	136-150	146-167
5′ 9″	142-151	148-160	155-176	129-142	139-153	149-170
5′10″	144-154	151-163	158-180	132-145	142-156	152-173
5′11″	146-157	154-166	161-184	135-148	145-159	155-176
6′ 0″	149-160	157-170	164-188	138-151	148-162	158-179
6′ 1″	152-164	160-174	168-192			
6′ 2″	155-168	164-178	172-197			
6′ 3″	158-172	167-182	176-202			
6′ 4″	162-176	171-187	181-207			

Based on the Metropolitan Insurance Company *Height and Weight Tables* 1983. Source: 1979 Build Study, Society of Actuaries and Association of Life Insurance Medical Doctors of America, 1980.

[1] Weight in shoes and 5 lbs of indoor clothing.

[2] Weight in shoes and 3 lbs of indoor clothing.

International System of Units

The *Système international d'unités* (International System of Units) or *SI* is a modernized version of the metric system. The primary goal of the conversion to SI units is to revise the present confused measurement system and to improve test-result communications.

The SI has 7 basic units from which other units are derived:

Base Units of SI

Physical Quantity	Base Unit	SI Symbol
length	meter	m
mass	kilogram	kg
time	second	s
amount of substance	mole	mol
thermodynamic temperature	kelvin	K
electric current	ampere	A
luminous intensity	candela	cd

Combinations of these base units can express any property although, for simplicity, special names are given to some of these derived units.

Representative Derived Units

Derived Unit	Name and Symbol	Derivation from Base Units
area	square meter	m^2
volume	cubic meter	m^3
force	newton (N)	$kg{\cdot}m{\cdot}s^{-2}$
pressure	pascal (Pa)	$kg{\cdot}m^{-1}{\cdot}s^{-2}$ (N/m^2)
work, energy	joule (J)	$kg{\cdot}m^2{\cdot}s^{-2}$ ($N{\cdot}m$)
mass density	kilogram per cubic meter	kg/m^3
frequency	hertz (Hz)	s^{-1}
temperature	degree Celsius (°C)	°C = °K -273.15
concentration		
mass	kilogram/liter	kg/L
substance	mole/liter	mol/L
molality	mole/kilogram	mol/kg
density	kilogram/liter	kg/L

Prefixes to the base unit are used in this system to form decimal multiples and submultiples. The preferred multiples and submultiples listed below change the quantity by increments of 10^3 or 10^{-3}. The exceptions to these recommended factors are outlined by the rectangle.

Prefixes and Symbols for Decimal Multiples and Submultiples

Factor	Prefix	Symbol
10^{18}	exa	E
10^{15}	peta	P
10^{12}	tera	T
10^{9}	giga	G
10^{6}	mega	M
10^{3}	kilo	k
10^{2}	hecto	h
10^{1}	deka	da
10^{-1}	deci	d
10^{-2}	centi	c
10^{-3}	milli	m
10^{-6}	micro	μ
10^{-9}	nano	n
10^{-12}	pico	p
10^{-15}	femto	f
10^{-18}	atto	a

Normal Laboratory Values

In the following tables, normal reference values for commonly requested laboratory tests are listed in traditional units and in SI units. The tables are a guideline only. Values are method dependent and "normal values" may vary between laboratories.

BLOOD, PLASMA or SERUM

Determination	Reference Value: Conventional Units	Reference Value: SI Units
Ammonia	10-80 μg/dl	5-50 μmol/L
Amylase	0-130 U/L	0-130 U/L
Antinuclear antibodies	negative at 1:8 dilution of serum	
Bilirubin: direct	≤ 0.2 mg/dl	≤ 4 μmol/L
total	0.1-1 mg/dl	2-18 μmol/L
Calcitonin, male	0-14 pg/ml	0-4.1 pmol/L
female	0-28 pg/ml	0-8.2 pmol/L
medullary carcinoma	> 100 pg/ml	> 29.3 pmol/L
Calcium[1]	8.8-10.3 mg/dl	2.2-2.6 mmol/L
Carbon dioxide content	22-28 mEq/L	22-28 mmol/L
Chloride	95-105 mEq/L	95-105 mmol/L
Coagulation screen:		
Bleeding time	3-9.5 min	180-570 sec
Prothrombin time	< 2 sec from control	< 2 sec from control
Partial thromboplastin time (activated)	25-38 sec	25-38 sec
Copper, total	70-140 μg/dl	11-22 μmol/L
Corticotropin (ACTH)	20-100 pg/ml	4-22 pmol/L
Cortisol: 8 am	5-25 μg/dl	0.14-0.69 μmol/L
8 pm	< 10 μg/dl	< 0.28 μmol/L
4 hr ACTH test	30-45 μg/dl	0.83-1.24 μmol/L
Overnight suppression test	< 5 μg/dl	< 0.14 μmol/L
Creatine phosphokinase, total (CK, CPK)	≤ 130 U/L	≤ 130 U/L
Creatine phosphokinase isoenzymes	CK-MB = ≤ 5% total CK	≤ 0.05
Creatinine	0.6-1.2 mg/dl	50-110 μmol/L
Follicle stimulating hormone (FSH),		
female	2-15 mIU/ml	2-15 IU/L
peak production	20-50 mIU/ml	20-50 IU/L
male	1-10 mIU/ml	1-10 IU/L
Glucose, fasting	70-110 mg/dl	3.9-6.1 mmol/L
Hematologic tests:		
Hematocrit (Hct), female	33%-43%	0.33-0.43
male	39%-49%	0.39-0.49
Hemoglobin (Hb), female	12-15 g/dl	120-150 g/L
male	13.6-17.2 g/dl	136-172 g/L
Leukocyte count (WBC)	3200-9800/mm³	3.2-9.8 x 10⁹/L
Erythrocyte count (RBC), female	3.5-5 million/mm³	3.5-5 x 10¹²/L
male	4.3-5.9 million/mm³	4.3-5.9 x 10¹²/L
Mean Corpuscular Volume (MCV)	76-100 μm³/cell	76-100 fl/cell
Mean Corpuscular Hemoglobin (MCH)	27-33 pg/RBC	27-33 pg/RBC
Mean Corpuscular Hemoglobin Concentration (MCHC)	33-37 g/dl	330-370 g/L

[1] Slightly higher in children.

(Table continued on following page)

BLOOD, PLASMA or SERUM (Cont.)		
	Reference Value	
Determination	Conventional Units	SI Units
Hematologic tests (cont.):		
Erythrocyte sedimentation rate (sedrate, ESR): female	≤ 30 mm/hr	≤ 30 mm/hr
male	≤ 20 mm/hr	≤ 20 mm/hr
Erythrocyte enzymes:		
Glucose-6-phosphate dehydrogenase (G6PD)	5-15 U/g Hb	5-15 U/g Hb
Pyruvate kinase	13-17 U/g Hb	13-17 U/g Hb
Ferritin (serum): Iron deficiency	0-12 ng/ml	0-4.8 nmol/L
Borderline	13-20 ng/ml	5.2-8 nmol/L
Iron excess	> 400 ng/L	> 160 nmol/L
Folic acid: normal	> 3.3 ng/ml	> 7.3 nmol/L
borderline	2.5-3.2 ng/ml	5.75-7.39 nmol/L
Platelet count	150,000-450,000/mm^3	150-450 x 10^9/L
Vitamin B_{12}: normal	205-876 pg/ml	150-674 pmol/L
borderline	140-204 pg/ml	102.6-149 pmol/L
Iron		
female	60-160 μg/dl	11-29 μmol/L
male	80-180 μg/dl	14-32 μmol/L
Iron Binding Capacity	250-460 μg/dl	45-82 μmol/L
Lactic Acid	0.5-2.2 mmol/L	0.5-2.2 mmol/L
Lactic dehydrogenase	50-150 U/L	50-150 U/L
Lead	≤ 50 μg/dl	≤ 2.4 μmol/L
Lipids: Cholesterol		
< 29 yr	< 200 mg/dl	< 5.2 mmol/L
30-39 yr	< 225 mg/dl	< 5.85 mmol/L
40-49 yr	< 245 mg/dl	< 6.35 mmol/L
> 50 yr	< 265 mg/dl	< 6.85 mmol/L
Triglycerides	40-150 mg/dl	0.4-1.5 g/L
LDL	50-190 mg/dl	1.3-4.9 mmol/L
HDL		
female	30-90 mg/dl	0.8-2.35 mmol/L
male	30-70 mg/dl	0.8-1.8 mmol/L
Magnesium	1.8-3 mEq/L	0.8-1.2 mmol/L
Osmolality	280-296 mOsm/kg water	280-296 mmol/kg
Oxygen saturation (arterial)	96%-100%	0.96-1
PCO_2, Arterial	35-45 mm Hg	4.7-6 kPa
pH, Arterial	7.35-7.45	7.35-7.45
PO_2, Arterial: breathing room air[2]	75-100 mm Hg	10-13.3 kPa
on 100% O_2	> 500 mm Hg	
Phosphatase (acid), total:	≤ 3 King-Armstrong units/dl	≤ 5.5 U/L
	≤ 3 Bodansky units/dl	≤ 16.1 U/L
Phosphatase (alkaline)[3]	30-120 U/L	30-120 U/L
Phosphorus, inorganic[4]	3-4.5 mg/dl	1-1.5 mmol/L
Potassium	3.5-5 mEq/L	3.5-5 mmol/L

[1] Higher in males.
[2] Age dependent.
[3] Infants and adolescents up to 104 U/L.
[4] Infants in the first year up to 6 mg/dl.

BLOOD, PLASMA or SERUM (Cont.)		
	Reference Value	
Determination	**Conventional Units**	**SI Units**
Progesterone		
Follicular phase	< 2 ng/ml	< 6 nmol/L
Luteal phase	2-20 ng/ml	6-64 nmol/L
Prolactin	2-15 ng/ml	0.08-6 nmol/L
Protein: Total	6-8 g/dl	60-80 g/L
Albumin	4-6 g/dl	40-60 g/L
Globulin	2.3-3.5 g/dl	23-35 g/L
Rheumatoid factor	< 60 IU/ml	
Sodium	135-147 mEq/L	135-147 mmol/L
Testosterone, female	< 0.6 ng/ml	< 2 nmol/L
male	4-8 ng/ml	14-28 nmol/L
Thyroid Hormone Function Tests:		
Thyroid-stimulating hormone (TSH)	0.5-5 μU/ml	0.5-5 arb unit
Thyroxine-binding globulin capacity	15-25 μg T_4/dl	193-322 nmol/L
Total triiodothyronine (T_3)	75-220 ng/dl	1.2-3.4 nmol/L
Total thyroxine by RIA (T_4)	4-12 μg/dl	52-154 nmol/L
T_3 resin uptake	25%-35%	0.25-0.35
Transaminase, AST (Aspartate aminotransferase, SGOT)	7-27 U/L	117-450 nmol/sec/L
Transaminase, ALT (Alanine aminotransferase, SGPT)	1-21 U/L	17-350 nmol/sec/L
Urea nitrogen (BUN)	8-18 mg/dl	3-6.5 mmol/L
Uric acid	2-7 mg/dl	120-420 μmol/L
Vitamin A	0.15-0.6 μg/ml	0.5-2.1 μmol/L
Zinc	75-120 μg/dl	11.5-18.5 μmol/L

URINE						
		Reference Value				
Determination		**Conventional Units**		**SI Units**		
Catecholamines: Epinephrine		< 20 μg/day		< 109 nmol/day		
Norepinephrine		< 100 μg/day		< 590 nmol/day		
Creatinine		15-25 mg/kg/day		0.13-0.22 mmol/kg/day		
Potassium[1]		25-125 mEq/day		25-125 mmol/day		
Protein, quantitative		< 150 mg/day		< 0.15 g/day		
Sodium[1]		40-220 mEq/day		40-220 mmol/day		
Steroids:		(mg/day)		(μmol/day)		
	Age (yrs)	male	female	male	female	
17-Ketosteroids	10	1-4	1-4	3-14	3-14	
	20	6-21	4-16	21-73	14-56	
	30	8-26	4-14	28-90	14-49	
	50	5-18	3-9	17-62	10-31	
	70	2-10	1-7	7-35	3-24	
17-Hydroxycorticosteroids (as cortisol), female		2-8 mg/day		5-25 μmol/day		
male		3-10 mg/day		10-30 μmol/day		

[1] Varies with intake.

DRUG LEVELS†		
	Reference Value	
Drug Determination	Conventional Units	SI Units
Aminoglycosides (peak levels):		
Amikacin	8-16 μg/ml	nd
Gentamicin	4-8 μg/ml	nd
Kanamycin	8-16 μg/ml	nd
Netilmicin	0.5-10 μg/ml	nd
Streptomycin	25 μg/ml	nd
Tobramycin	4-8 μg/ml	nd
Antiarrhythmics:		
Amiodarone	0.5-2.5 μg/ml	nd
Bretylium	0.5-1.5 μg/ml	nd
Digitoxin	9-25 μg/L	11.8-32.8 nmol/L
Digoxin	0.5-2.2 ng/ml	0.6-2.8 nmol/L
Disopyramide	2-6 μg/ml	6-18 μmol/L
Flecainide	0.2-1 μg/ml	nd
Lidocaine	1-5 μg/ml	4.5-21.5 μmol/L
Mexiletine	0.5-2 μg/ml	nd
Phenytoin	10-20 μg/ml	40-80 μmol/L
Procainamide	4-8 μg/ml	17-34 μmol/L
Propranolol	50-200 ng/ml	190-770 nmol/L
Quinidine	1.5-3 μg/ml	4.6-9.2 μmol/L
Tocainide	4-10 μg/ml	nd
Verapamil	0.08-0.3 μg/ml	nd
Anticonvulsants:		
Carbamazepine	4-12 μg/ml	17-51 μmol/L
Phenobarbital	15-40 μg/ml	65-172 μmol/L
Phenytoin	5-20 μg/ml	40-80 μmol/L
Primidone	6-10 μg/ml	25-46 μmol/L
Valproic acid	50-100 μg/ml	350-7000 μmol/L
Chloramphenicol	10-20 μg/ml	31-62 μmol/L
Ethanol[1]	0 mg/dl	0 mmol/L
Lithium	0.5-1.5 mEq/L	0.5-1.5 mmol/L
Salicylate	100-200 mg/L	724-1448 μmol/L
Sulfonamide	5-15 mg/dl	nd
Theophylline	10-20 μg/ml	55-110 μmol/L

† The values given are generally accepted as desirable for achieving therapeutic effect without toxicity for most patients. However, exceptions are not uncommon.

[1] Toxic: 50-100 mg/dl (10.9-21.7 mmol/L).

nd – No data available.

Standard Abbreviations

ac	before meals
bid	twice daily
°C	Celsius
Ca	calcium
Cal	Calorie (kilocalorie)
Ccr	creatinine clearance
CDC	Centers for Disease Control
ci	curie
Cl	chloride
cu	cubic
Cu	copper
dl	deciliter (100 ml)
DNA	Deoxyribonucleic acid
ECG	electrocardiogram
F	fluoride
°F	Fahrenheit
FA	folic acid
FDA	Food and Drug Administration
Fe	iron
g	gram
G-6-PD	glucose-6-phosphate dehydrogenase
gal	gallon
h	hour
hs	bedtime
I	iodine
IM	intramuscular
IU	international units
IV	intravenous
K	potassium
kg	kilogram
L	liter
lb	pound
m	meter
m^2	square meter
mcg	microgram
mCi	millicurie
mEq	milliequivalent
mg	milligram
Mg	magnesium
MIC	Minimum Inhibitory Concentration
ml	milliliter
mm	millimeter
Mn	manganese
Mo	molybdenum
mOsm	milliosmole
Na	sodium
NF	National Formulary
ng	nanogram
otc	over the counter (nonprescription)
oz	ounce
P	phosphorus
pc	after meals
po	by mouth
ppm	parts per million
prn	as needed
pt	pint
qid	four times daily
qt	quart
RDA	Recommended Dietary Allowance
RNA	Ribonucleic acid
Rx	prescription only
SC	subcutaneous
Se	selenium
t½	half-life
tid	three times daily
tbsp	tablespoon
tsp	teaspoon
U	unit
UD	unit dose package
USP	United States Pharmacopeia
WHO	World Health Organization
Zn	zinc

Distributor Abbreviations

This listing includes only those manufacturers whose names are abbreviated in *Drug Facts and Comparisons*. It is not a complete list of all manufacturers whose products are listed in this book.

ACC	American Critical Care
AOC	American Optical Corporation
Baker-C	Baker/Cummins
B-H	Barnes-Hind
B I	Boehringer Ingelheim
B W	Burroughs Wellcome
CMC	Consolidated Midland Corporation
Hoechst	Hoechst-Roussel
HW&D	Hynson, Westcott & Dunning
IMS	International Medication Systems
J & J	Johnson & Johnson
K-U	Kremers-Urban
Mead J	Mead Johnson
MSD	Merck, Sharp and Dohme
P-D	Parke-Davis
P & G	Procter & Gamble
Purdue F	Purdue Frederick
Reed & C	Reed and Carnrick
SKF	Smith, Kline and French
Upsher-S	Upsher-Smith
USV	USV Pharmaceutical Corporation
Whittaker	Whittaker General Medical

Trademark Glossary

Many companies use trademarks to identify specific dosage forms or unique packaging materials. The following list is provided as a guide to the interpretation of these descriptions.

Abbo-Pac (Abbott)
Unit dose package

Accu-Pak (Ciba)
Unit dose blister pack

Act-O-Vial (Upjohn)
Vial system

ADD-Vantage (Burroughs Wellcome)
Sterile dissolution system for admixture

ADT (Upjohn)
Alternate day therapy

Ambot (Cutter)
Additive syringe

Aspirol (Lilly)
Crushable ampule for inhalation

Back-Pack (MSD)
Unit-of-use package

bidCAP (Bristol Labs)
Double strength capsule

Bitab (Merrell Dow)
Double strength tablet

Bristoject (Bristol Labs)
Unit dose syringe

Caplet
Capsule shaped tablet

Capsulet (Marion)
Capsule shaped tablet

Carpuject (Winthrop Pharm.)
Cartridge needle unit

Chronosule (Schering)
Sustained action capsule

Chronotab (Schering)
Sustained action tablet

Clinipak (Wyeth-Ayerst)
Unit dose package

ControlPak (Sandoz)
Unit dose rolls, tamper resistant

Detecto-Seal (Winthrop Pharm.)
Tamper resistant parenteral package

Dialpak (Ortho)
Compliance package

Dis-Co Pack (Robins)
Unit dose package

Disket (Lilly)
Dispersible tablet

Dispenserpak (Burroughs Wellcome)
Unit-of-use package

Dispertab (Abbott)
Particles in tablet

Dispette (Lederle)
Disposable pipette

Divide-Tab (Abbott)
Scored tablet

Dividose (Mead Johnson)
Tablet, bisected/trisected

D·Lay (Lemmon)
Timed release tablet

Dosette (Elkins-Sinn)
Single dose ampule or vial

Dosepak (Upjohn)
Compliance package

Dospan (Merrell Dow)
Controlled release tablet

Drop Dose (Burroughs Wellcome)
Ophthalmic dropper dispenser

Drop-Tainer (Alcon)
Ophthalmic dropper dispenser

Dulcet (Abbott)
Chewable tablet

Duracap (Glaxo)
Timed release capsule

Dura-Tab (Berlex)
Sustained release tablet

Enduret (Boehringer Ingelheim)
Prolonged action tablet

Enseal (Lilly)
Enteric coated tablet

EN-tabs (Pharmacia)
Enteric coated tablet

Extencap (Robins)
Controlled release capsule

Extentab (Robins)
Continuous release tablet

Filmlok (Squibb)
Veneer coated tablet

Filmseal (Parke-Davis)
Film coated tablet

Filmtab (Abbott)
Film coated tablet

Flo-Pack (Burroughs Wellcome)
Vial for preparation of IV drips

Gelseal (Lilly)
Soft gelatin capsule

Gradumet (Abbott)
Controlled release tablet

Granucap (Reid-Rowell)
Sustained release capsule

Gy-Pak (Geigy)
Unit-of-issue package

Gyrocap (Rorer)
Timed release capsule

Hyporet (Lilly)
Unit dose syringe

Identi-Dose (Lilly)
Unit dose package

Infatab (Parke-Davis)
Chewable pediatric tablet

Inject-all (Bristol Labs)
Prefilled disposable dilution syringe

Inlay-Tabs (Dorsey/Sandoz)
Inlaid tablets

Isoject (Pfizer)
Unit dose syringe

Kapseal (Parke-Davis)
Banded (sealed) capsule

Kronocap (Ferndale)
Sustained release capsule

Lanacap (Lannett)
Timed release capsule

Lederject (Lederle)
Disposable syringe

Linguet (Ciba)
Buccal tablet

Liquitab (Mission)
Chewable tablet

Lontab (Ciba)
Long acting tablet

Memorette (Syntex)
Compliance package

Mix-O-Vial (Upjohn)
Dual compartment vial

Mono-Drop (Winthrop Pharm.)
Ophthalmic plastic dropper

Ocumeter (MSD)
Ophthalmic dropper dispenser

Ovoid (Winthrop Pharm.)
Sugar coated tablet

Perle (Endo)
Soft gelatin capsule

Pilpak (Wyeth-Ayerst)
Compliance pack

Plateau CAP (Marion)
Controlled release capsule

Pulvule (Lilly)
Bullet-shaped capsule

Rap-Add (American Critical Care)
Unit dose additive syringe

Rediject (Organon)
Unit dose syringe

Redipak (Wyeth-Ayerst)
Unit dose or unit-of-issue package

Redi Vial (Lilly)
Dual compartment vial

Repetab (Schering)
Repeat action tablet

Respihaler (MSD)
Aerosol for inhalation

Robicap (Robins)
Capsule

Robitab (Robins)
Tablet

SandoPak (Sandoz)
Unit dose blister package

Sani-Pak (Hauck)
Sanitary dispensing box

Secule (Wyeth-Ayerst)
Single dose vial

Sequels (Lederle)
Sustained release capsule or tablet

SigPak (Sandoz)
Unit-of-use package

Softab (Stuart)
Chewable tablet

Solvet (Lilly)
Soluble tablet

Spansule (SKF)
Sustained release capsule

Stat-Pak (Adria)
Unit dose package

Steri-Dose (Parke-Davis)
Unit dose syringe

Steri-Vial (Parke-Davis)
Ampule

Supprette (Webcon)
Suppository

Supule (Lemmon)
Suppository

Tab-In (Marion)
Delayed release tablet

Tabloid (Burroughs Wellcome)
Branded tablet (with raised lettering)

Tamp-R-Tel (Wyeth-Ayerst)
Tubex, tamper resistant

Tel-E-Amp (Roche)
Single dose amp

Tel-E-Dose (Roche)
Unit dose strip package

Tel-E-Ject (Roche)
Unit dose syringe

Tel-E-Pack (Roche)
Packaging system

Tel-E-Vial (Roche)
Single dose vial

Tembid (Wyeth-Ayerst)
Sustained action capsule

Tempule (Armour)
Timed release capsule or tablet

Ten-Tab (3M Riker)
Controlled release tablet

Thera-Ject (Beecham Labs)
Unit dose syringe

Tiltab (SKF)
Tablet shape

Timecap (Schwarz Pharma Kremers Urban)
Sustained release capsule

Timecelle (Hauck)
Timed release capsule

Timespan (Roche)
Timed release tablet

Titradose (Wyeth-Ayerst)
Scored tablet

Traypak (Lilly)
Multivial carton

Tubex (Wyeth-Ayerst)
Cartridge-needle unit

Turbinaire (MSD)
Aerosol for nasal inhalation

U-Ject (Upjohn)
Unit dose syringe

Uni-Amp (Winthrop Pharm.)
Single dose ampule

Unimatic (Squibb)
Unit dose syringe

Uni-nest (Winthrop Pharm.)
Ampule

Unisert (Upsher-Smith)
Suppository

Vaporole (Burroughs Wellcome)
Crushable ampule for inhalation

Visipak (Upjohn)
Reverse numbered pack

Wyseal (Wyeth-Ayerst)
Film coated tablet

12463
Abana Pharmaceuticals
230 Oxmoor Circle, Suite 1111
Birmingham, AL 35209
205-942-1808

00074
Abbott Diagnostics
Customer Support Cnt.
Dept 94P
Abbott Park, IL 60064
800-323-9100

00074
Abbott Hospital Products
Div. of Abbott Laboratories
1 Abbott Park Rd. D39b AP30
Abbott Park, IL 60064
708-937-6100

00074
Abbott Laboratories
D-305, Bldg AP30 4E
1 Abbott Road
Abbott Park, IL 60064
708-937-6100

Acme United Corporation
75 Kings Highway Cutoff
Fairfield, CT 06430
203-332-7330

53014
Adams Laboratories
14801 Sovereign Road
Ft. Worth, TX 76155-2645
817-545-7791

Adolphs
Div. of Chesebrough-Ponds
Ragu Foods, Inc.
75 Merritt Blvd
Trumbull, CT 06611
203-381-3500

00013
Adria Laboratories
Division of Erbamont Inc.
P.O. Box 16529
Columbus, OH 43216-6529
614-764-8100

Advanced Care Products
Div. of Ortho
Route 202
Raritan, NJ 08869
201-524-0171

10888
Advanced Nutrit. Tech. Inc.
P.O. Box 3225
Elizabeth, NJ 07207
201-354-2740

17478
Akorn, Inc.
100 Akorn Drive
Abita Springs, LA 70420
504-893-9300

00065
Alcon Laboratories, Inc.
6201 South Freeway
Ft. Worth, TX 76134
817-293-0450

00023
Alk America
132 Research Dr.
Milford, CT 06460
203-877-4782

A.L. Labs
One Executive Dr.
P.O. Box 1399
Ft. Lee, NJ 07024
201-947-7774

00173
Allen & Hanburys
Div. of Glaxo
5 Moore Drive
Research Triangle Pk.,
NC 27709
919-248-2500

00299
Allercreme
Div. of Owen Laboratories
P.O. Box 6600
Ft. Worth, TX 76115
817-293-0450

00023
Allergan Pharmaceuticals
2525 DuPont Drive
Irvine, CA 92713-1599
714-752-4500

54569
Allscripts
1033 Butterfield Rd.
Vernon Hills, IL 60061
708-680-3515

49669
Alpha Therapeutic Corp.
5555 Valley Blvd.
Los Angeles, CA 90032
213-225-2221

51641
Alra Laboratories, Inc.
3850 Clearview Court
Gurnee, IL 60031
708-244-9440

Altana
60 Baylis Road
Melville, NY 11747
516-454-7677

00731
Alto Pharmaceuticals, Inc.
P.O. Box 1910
Land O' Lakes, FL 34639-
1910
813-949-7464

Alva Laboratories
6625 Avondale Ave.
Chicago, IL 60631
312-792-0200

17314
Alza Corporation
950 Page Mill Road
Palo Alto, CA 94304
415-494-5000

10038
Ambix Laboratories Inc.
210 Orchard Street
East Rutherford, NJ 07073
201-939-2200

89709
Amcon Laboratories
40 N. Rock Hill Rd.
St. Louis, MO 63119
314-961-5758

53443
Americal Pharmaceutical Inc.
Div. of Akorn
1340 N. Jefferson St.
Anaheim, CA 92807
714-579-7545

51201
American Dermal Corp.
P.O. Box 900
Plumsteadville, PA 18949-
0900
215-766-2110

57506
American Drug Industries
8510-20 S. Perry Ave.
Chicago, IL 60621
312-667-7070

00517
American Regent
Subsidiary, Luitpold Pharm. Inc.
1 Luitpold Dr.
Shirley, NY 11967
516-924-4000

50349
American Therapeutics, Inc.
83 Carlough Rd.
Bohemia, NY 11716
516-563-1830

00539
American Urologicals, Inc.
7881 Hollywood Blvd. Suite 4
Pembroke Pines, FL 33024
305-651-6575

00193
Ames Company
Div. of Miles Labs., Inc.
P.O. Box 70
Elkhart, IN 46515
219-264-8111

05551
Amgen Inc.
1900 Oak Terrace Lane
Thousand Oaks, CA 91320-1789
805-499-5725

52152
Amide Pharmaceuticals, Inc.
101 East Main Street
Little Falls, NJ 07424
201-890-1440

10019
Anaquest
2005 W. Beltline Hwy.
Madison, WI 53173
608-273-0019

Apothecary Products, Inc.
11531 Rupp Drive
Burnsville, MN 55337
612-890-1940

00003
Apothecon
Div. of Bristol-Myers Squibb
P.O. Box 4000
Princeton, NJ 08543-4000
609-987-6800

48723
Apothecus, Inc.
132 South Street
Oyster Bay, NY 11771
516-624-8200

Applied Genetics
205 Buffalo Avenue
Freeport, NY 11520
516-868-9026

00598
Approved Pharmaceuticals
1643 E. Genesee St.
P.O. Box 6669
Syracuse, NY 13217-6669
315-478-6303

00275
Arco Pharmaceuticals, Inc.
90 Orville Drive
Bohemia, NY 11716
516-567-9500

00053
Armour Pharmaceutical
Div. of Rhone-Poulenc Rorer
500 Virginia Drive
Ft. Washington, PA 19034
215-628-6085

48558
Arther, Inc.
P.O. Box 1455
W. Caldwell, NJ 07007
201-263-2050

00225
B. F. Ascher and Company
15501 W. 109th St.
Lenexa, KS 66219
913-888-1880

00186
Astra Pharmaceutical Prod.
50 Otis
Westborough, MA 01581
508-366-1100

Astro Lube Inc.
P.O. Box 965302
Marietta, GA 30066
404-565-6078

10003
A.V.P. Pharmaceuticals, Inc.
9829 Main Street, P.O. Box N
Clarence, NY 14031
716-688-9676

00575
Baker Cummins Pharm., Inc.
Subsidiary of Ivax
8800 N.W. 36th St.
Miami, FL 33178-2404
305-590-2282

10106
J. T. Baker, Inc.
222 Red School Lane
Phillipsburg, NJ 08865
201-859-2151

00304
J.J. Balan, Inc.
5725 Foster Ave.
Brooklyn, NY 11234
718-251-8663

00555
Barr Laboratories, Inc.
2 Quaker Road
Pomona, NY 10970
914-362-1100

00472
Barre-National Inc.
7205 Windsor Blvd.
Baltimore, MD 21207
301-298-1000

Basel Pharmaceuticals
Div. of Ciba-Geigy Corp.
566 Morris Avenue
Summit, NJ 07901
908-277-5000

10119
Bausch and Lomb Consumer
1400 N. Goodman St.
Rochester, NY 14692
716-338-6000

10119
Bausch and Lomb Pharm.
8500 Hidden River Parkway
Tampa, FL 33637
813-975-7700

47679
Baxter Healthcare Corporation
1425 Lake Cook Road
Deerfield, IL 60015
708-940-5000

00944
Baxter Hyland
Div. of Baxter Healthcare
550 North Brand Blvd.
Glendale, CA 91203
818-956-3200

00486
Beach Pharmaceuticals
Div. of Beach Products
P.O. Box 128
Conestee, SC 29636
803-277-7282

31280
Becton Dickinson & Company
One Becton Drive
Franklin Lakes, NJ 07417-1881
201-848-6900

10356
Beiersdorf, Inc.
P.O. Box 5529
S. Norwalk, CT 06856
203-853-8008

38697
Berkeley Biologicals
1831 Second St.
Berkeley, CA 94710
415-843-6846

50419
Berlex Laboratories, Inc.
300 Fairfield Rd.
Wayne, NJ 07470
201-694-4100

58337
Berna Products Corporation
4216 Ponce De Leon Blvd.
Coral Gables, FL 33146
305-443-2900

54274
Best Generics
19589 N.E. 10th Avenue
North Miami Beach,
FL 33179-3501
305-653-2378

00283
Beutlich, Inc.
7149 North Austin Ave.
Niles, IL 60648
708-647-8110

53191
Bio-Tech
P.O. Box 1992
Fayetteville, AR 72702
501-443-9148

00332
Biocraft Laboratories, Inc.
18-01 River Road
Fair Lawn, NJ 07410
800-631-0165

Biogen
14 Cambridge Center
Cambridge, MA 02142
617-864-8900

Bioline Labs, see Goldline

Biomerica, Inc.
1533 Monrovia Avenue
Newport Beach, CA 92663
714-645-2111

52311
Biosearch Medical Products
P.O. Box 1700
Somerville, NJ 00876
201-722-5000

12136
Bird Corporation
3101 E. Alejo Road
Palm Springs, CA 92262
619-778-7200

00165
Blaine Company, Inc.
2700 Dixie Highway
Ft. Mitchell, KY 41017
606-341-9437

00154
Blair Laboratories
100 Connecticut Ave.
Norwalk, CT 06856
203-853-0123

50486
Blairex Labs., Inc.
4810 Tecumseh Ln.
P.O. Box 15190
Evansville, IN 47716-0190
812-476-8077

10157
Blistex, Inc.
1800 Swift Drive
Oak Brook, IL 60521
708-571-2870

10158
Block Drug Company, Inc.
257 Cornelison Ave.
Jersey City, NJ 07302
201-434-3000

00563
Bock Pharmacal Company
P.O. Box 8519
St. Louis, MO 63126-0519
314-343-0994

00597
Boehringer Ingelheim, Inc.
90 East Ridge
Ridgefield, CT 06877
203-798-9988

50924
Boehringer Mannheim Diagnostic
Div. Boehringer Ingelheim
9115 Hague Rd.
Indianapolis, IN 46250-0100
800-428-5074

44437
Bolan Pharmaceutical, Inc.
P.O. Box 230
Hurst, TX 76053
817-268-6110

00725
Bolar Pharmaceutical Co.
33 Ralph Avenue
Copiague, NY 11726-0030
516-842-8383

00822, 00524
Boots
Div. of The Boots Co.(USA) Inc
300 Tri-State Internat. Center
Lincolnshire, IL 60069-4415
708-405-7400

00048
Boots-Flint
Div. of The Boots Co.(USA) Inc
300 Tri-State Internat. Center
Lincolnshire, IL 60069-4415
708-405-7400

00222
Boyle and Company Pharm.
1030 S. Arroyo Parkway
Pasadena, CA 91105
818-441-0284

52268
Braintree Laboratories Inc.
60 Columbian, P.O. Box 361
Braintree, MA 02184
617-843-2202

72363
Brimms Inc.
Div. Pertussin Laboratories
425 Fillmore Ave.
Tonawanda, NY 14150
716-694-7100

19810
Bristol-Myers Oncology Div.
Div. Bristol-Myers Squibb
P.O. Box 4755
Evansville, IN 47721-0001
812-429-5000

19810
Bristol-Myers Products
Div. Bristol-Myers Squibb
1350 Liberty Ave.
Hillside, NJ 07205
908-851-2400

00087
Bristol-Myers U.S. Pharm.
Div. Bristol-Myers Squibb
2404 West Pennsylvania Street
Evansville, IN 47721-0001
812-429-5000

00081
Burroughs Wellcome Co.
3030 Cornwallis Road
Research Triangle Pk.,
NC 27709
919-248-3000

00398
C & M Pharmacal, Inc.
1721 Maple Lane
Hazel Park, MI 48030-2696
313-548-7846

55559
Calgon Vestal Laboratories
Division of Calgon Corporation
P.O. Box 147
St. Louis, MO 63166-0147
314-535-1810

California Biotechnology Inc.
2450 Bayshore Parkway
Mountain View, CA 94043
415-966-1550

00147
Camall Company, Inc.
P.O. Box 307
Romeo, MI 48065-0307
313-752-9683

38083
Campbell Laboratories
P.O. Box 812 FDR Station
New York, NY 10150
212-688-7684

J.R. Carlson Labs, Inc.
15 College Drive
Arlington Heights, IL 60004
708-255-1600

00086
Carnrick Laboratories, Inc.
65 Horse Hill Road
Cedar Knolls, NJ 07927
201-267-2670

46287
Carolina Medical Products
P.O. Box 147
Farmville, NC 27828
919-753-7111

Carrington Labs
1300 E. Rochelle Blvd.
Irving, TX 75062
214-518-1300

00164
Carter Products
Div. Carter-Wallace, Inc.
One-Half Acre Road
Cranbury, NJ 08512
609-655-6000

CDC, see Centers for Disease Control

Cell Technology
1668 Valtec Lane
Boulder, CO 80301
303-443-8155

00556
H.R. Cenci Labs., Inc.
1420 Tuolumne St.
P.O. Box 12524
Fresno, CA 93778-2524
209-268-4401

00268
Center Laboratories
Div. of EM Industries
35 Channel Drive
Port Washington, NY 11050
516-767-1800

Centers for Disease Control
1600 Clifton Rd, Mail Stop
D-09
Atlanta, GA 30333
404-639-3311

Centocor
244 Great Valley Parkway
Malvern, PA 19355
215-296-4488

00131
Central Pharmaceuticals, Inc.
120 East Third Street
P.O. Box 328
Seymour, IN 47274-9985
812-522-3915

00436
Century Pharmaceuticals, Inc.
10377 Hague Road
Indianapolis, IN 46256
317-849-4210

53905
Cetus
1400 53rd Street
Emeryville, CA 94608
415-420-3300

10223
Cetylite Industries, Inc.
9051 River Road
P.O. Box CN6
Pennsauken, NJ 08110
609-665-6111

54429
Chase Laboratories
280 Chestnut Street
Newark, NJ 07105-1598
201-589-8181

49447
Chattem Consumer Products
Div. of Chattem Inc.
1715 W. 38th Street
Chattanooga, TN 37409
615-821-4571

52489
Chemi-Tech Laboratories
74-80 Marine Street
Farmingdale, NY 11735

00521
Chesebrough-Pond's, Inc.
33 Benedict Place
Greenwich, CT 06830
203-661-2000

Chiron Ophthalmics
9342 Geronimo Road
Irvine, CA 92718-1903
714-768-4690

00083
Ciba Consumer Pharmaceuticals
Div. of Ciba-Geigy Corp.
Raritan Plaza III
Edison, NJ 08837
201-225-6000

00083
Ciba Pharmaceutical
Div. of Ciba-Geigy Corp.
556 Morris Avenue
Summit, NJ 07901
908-277-5000

00346
Ciba Vision Care
2910 Amwiler Court
Atlanta, GA 30360
404-448-1200

00659
Circle Pharmaceuticals, Inc.
10377 Hague Road
Indianapolis, IN 46256
317-842-5463

City Chemical Corporation
132 W. 22nd Street
New York, NY 10011
212-929-2723

00338
Clintec Nutrition
Three Parkway North Suite 500
Deerfield, IL 60015
708-940-5000

00126
Colgate-Hoyt
1 Colgate Way
Canton, MA 02021
617-769-6850

Colgate-Palmolive Co.
300 Park Avenue
New York, NY 10022
212-310-2000

00837
Columbia Laboratories, Inc.
4000 Hollywood Blvd., 3rd Fl
So.
Hollywood, FL 33021
800-749-1919

11509
Combe Incorporated
1101 Westchester Ave.
White Plains, NY 10604
914-694-5454

10310
Commerce Drug Company
565 Broad Hollow Road
Farmingdale, NY 11735
516-293-7070

49281
Connaught Laboratories, Inc.
Route 611, P.O. Box 187
Swiftwater, PA 18370-0187
717-839-7187

00223
Consolidated Midland Corp.
195 E. Main St.
Brewster, NY 10509
914-279-6108

00003
ConvaTec Research/ Development
Div. of Bristol-Myers Squibb
P.O. Box 5254
Princeton, NJ 08543-5254
201-359-9200

00961
Cook-Waite Laboratories, Inc.
90 Park Avenue
New York, NY 10016
212-907-2712

CooperBiomedical, Inc.
One Technology Court
Malvern, PA 19355
215-251-2000

CooperVision
3495 Winton Place
Rochester, NY 14623-2807
408-434-7000

38245
Copley Pharmaceutical, Inc.
25 John Road
Canton, MA 02021
617-268-1208

01020
Cumberland Packing Corp.
#2 Cumberland St.
Brooklyn, NY 11205
914-835-4826

55326
Curatek (Ltd. Partnership)
1965 Pratt Boulevard
Elk Grove Village, IL 60004
708-806-7680

00161
Cutter Biological
Div. of Miles Labs, Inc.
400 Morgan Lane
West Haven, CT 06516-4175
203-937-2000

00161
Cutter Medical
Div. of Miles Labs, Inc.
2200 Powell St.
Emeryville, CA 94662
415-420-4000

CytRx
150 Technology Parkway
Norcross, GA 30092
404-368-9500

Cytogen
Princeton Forrestal Center
600 College Road East
Princeton, NJ 08540
609-987-8200

55994
Dakryon Pharmaceuticals
301 Utica Ave
Lubbock, TX 79416
806-797-9941

55425
Dal-Med Pharmaceuticals
5701 North Pine Island Road
Tamarac, FL 33321
800-543-9151

00591
Danbury Pharmacal
Subsidiary of Henry Schein
131 West Street
Danbury, CT 06810
203-744-7200

00689
Daniels Pharmaceuticals, Inc.
2517 25th Avenue North
St. Petersburg, FL 33713
813-323-5151

58869
Dartmouth Pharmaceuticals
19 Whaler's Way
North Dartmouth, MA 02747
508-636-5553

00938
Davis and Geck
Div. of American Cyanamid
One Cyanamid Plaza
Wayne, NJ 07470
201-831-2000

52041
Dayton Laboratories, Inc.
3307 N.W. 74th Ave.
Miami, FL 33122
305-594-0988

00744
Daywell Laboratories Corp.
78 Unquowa Place
Fairfield, CT 06430
203-255-3154

Degussa Corporation
65 Challenger Road
Ridgefield Park, NJ 07660
201-641-6100

48532
Delmont Laboratories, Inc.
Biological Specialties
P.O. Box 269
Swarthmore, PA 19081
215-543-3365

00316
Del-Ray Laboratory, Inc.
27 20th Avenue N.W.
Birmingham, AL 35215
205-853-8247

00295
Denison Laboratories, Inc.
60 Dunnell Lane
Pawtucket, RI 02860
401-723-5500

10486
C. S. Dent & Co. Division
The Grandpa Brands Co.
317 E. Eighth St.
Cincinnati, OH 45202
513-241-1677

11588
DEP Corporation
2101 East Via Arado
Rancho Dominguez,
CA 90220
213-604-0777

00066
Dermik Laboratories, Inc.
920A Harvest Drive Suite 200
Blue Bell, PA 19422
215-540-8300

17271
Deseret Medical, Inc.
9450 South State
Sandy, UT 84070
801-255-6851

49502
Dey Laboratories, Inc.
2751 Napa Valley Corporate Dr.
Napa, CA 94558
707-224-3200

10331
E. E. Dickinson Co.
2 Enterprise Dr.
Shelton, CT 06484
203-929-1197

00777
Dista Products Co.
Div. of Eli Lilly
Bldg. 11/3 Lilly Corp. Center
Indianapolis, IN 46285
317-276-4000

17236
Dixon-Shane Inc.
256 Geiger Road
Philadelphia, PA 19115
215-673-7770

25358
Donell DerMedex
342 Madison Ave. Suite 1422
New York, NY 10173
800-526-3461

00261
Drug Industries Co.
3237 Hilton Road
Ferndale, MI 48220
313-547-3784

00217
Dunhall Pharmaceuticals, Inc.
P.O. Box 100
Gravette, AR 72736
501-787-5232

00094, 00590, 00056
DuPont Critical Care
Barley Mill Plaza
P.O. Box 80027
Wilmington, DE 19880-0027
302-892-1564

00060
DuPont Pharm., Caribe
Barley Mill Plaza
P.O. Box 80027
Wilmington, DE 19880-0027
800-543-8693

51479
Dura Pharmaceuticals
11175 Flintkote
San Diego, CA 92121
800-488-4844

51285
Duramed Pharmaceuticals
5040 Lester Road
Cincinnati, OH 45213
513-731-9900

55516
Dyna Pharm, Inc.
P.O. Box 2141
Del Mar, CA 92014-2141
619-792-9523

Eagle Vision, Inc.
6263 Poplar Avenue Ste. 650
Memphis, TN 38119
901-767-3937

Eastman Kodak
343 State Street
Rochester, NY 14650
800-445-6325

Eastman Pharmaceuticals
90 Park Ave.
New York, NY 10016
212-907-2000

Eaton Medical Corporation
Eye Care Division
2288 Dunn Ave.
Memphis, TN 38114
901-744-8024

19458
Eckerd Drug Company
8333 Bryan Dairy
P.O. Box 4689
Clearwater, FL 34618
813-397-7461

00803
Eclipse
Div. of Triangle Laboratories
100 Robins Road
Lynchburg, VA 24506
804-846-7161

38130
Econo Med Pharmaceuticals
4305 Sartin Rd.
Burlington, NC 27217-7522
919-226-1091

00485
Edwards Pharmaceuticals Inc.
111 Mulberry St.
Ripley, MS 38663
601-837-8182

Elan Corporation
1300 Gould Drive
Gainesville, GA 30501
404-534-8239

00641
Elkins-Sinn, Inc.
2 Esterbrook Lane
Cherry Hill, NJ 08003
609-424-3700

EM Pharmaceuticals
5 Skyline Drive
Hawthorne, NY 10532
914-592-4660

57665
Enzon, Inc.
40 Cragwood Road
South Plainfield, NJ 07080-
2480
908-668-1800

58177
Ethex Corporation
10888 Metro Court
St. Louis, MO 63043-2413
314-567-3307

Ethicon
Route 22 West
Somerville, NJ 08876
201-218-0707

54686
Ethitek Pharmaceuticals
7855 Gross Point Road
Skokie, IL 60077

00642
Everett Laboratories, Inc.
71 Glenwood Place
East Orange, NJ 07017-3004
201-674-8455

Evreka
Telos Associates L.P.
600 Montgomery Street
San Francisco, CA 94111
415-627-2040

Farmacon
P.O. Box 586
Westport, CT 06881

00496
Ferndale Laboratories, Inc.
780 W. Eight Mile Road
Ferndale, MI 48220-1218
313-548-0900

55566
Ferring Laboratories, Inc.
75 Montebello Road
Suffern, NY 10901
914-368-2244

31795
Fibertone Co.
6324 Ferris Sq.
San Diego, CA 92121
619-452-3100

00729
Fidelity Halsom
1330 Farr Drive at Stanley
Dayton, OH 45404
513-224-7636

Fidia Pharmaceutical
1775 K Street, N.W.
Washington, DC 20006
202-466-7066

00421
The Fielding Company
94 Weldon Parkway
Maryland Heights, MO 63043
314-567-5462

Fiske Industries
339 N. Main St.
New York, NY 10956
914-634-5099

00235
Fisons Consumer Health
P.O. Box 1212
Rochester, NY 14603-1212
716-475-9000

00585
Fisons Corp.
P.O. Box 1766
Rochester, NY 14623
716-475-9000

54323
Flanders Incorporated
P.O. Box 39143
Charleston, SC 29047
803-571-6768

00132
C. B. Fleet Co., Inc.
4615 Murray Place
Lynchburg, VA 24506
804-528-4000

00256
Fleming & Co.
1600 Fenpark Drive
Fenton, MO 63026
314-343-8200

00288
Fluoritab Corp.
P.O. Box 507
Temperance, MI 48182-0507
313-847-3985

00456, 00535
Forest Pharmaceutical, Inc.
Subs. of Forest Labs. Inc.
2510 Metro Blvd.
Maryland Heights, MO 63043-9979
314-569-3610

00168
E. Fougera and Co.
60 Baylis Road
Melville, NY 11747
516-454-6996

10432
Freeda Vitamins, Inc.
36 East 41st St.
New York, NY 10017-6203
212-685-4980

57317
Fujisawa SmithKline Corp.
3 Parkway North Center
Deerfield, IL 60015-2548
708-317-0600

00713
G & W Laboratories
111 Coolidge St.
South Plainfield, NJ 07080
201-753-2000

57284
Galen Pharma Inc.
2905 MacArthur Blvd.
Northbrook, IL 60062
708-498-0045

51552
Gallipot Inc.
2401 Pilot Knob Rd.
St. Paul, MN 55120
612-681-9517

Gambro, Inc.
1185 Oak Str.
Lakewood, CO 80215
800-525-2623

00386
Gebauer Chemical Company
9410 St. Catherine Ave.
Cleveland, OH 44104
216-271-5252

00028
Geigy Pharmaceuticals
Div. of Ciba-Geigy Corp.
556 Morris Avenue
Summit, NJ 07901
201-277-5000

35470
Gen-King
Div. of Kinray Inc.
80-25 Cornish Ave.
Elmhurst, NY 11373
718-478-8800

52761
GenDerm Corporation
600 Knightsbridge Parkway
Lincolnshire, IL 60069-3657
708-564-5435

00502, 50242
Genentech, Inc.
460 Point San Bruno Blvd.
South San Francisco, CA 94080
415-266-1000

50272
General Generics, Inc.
P.O. Box 510
Oxford, MS 38655
601-234-0130

52584
General Inj. & Vac., Inc.
U.S. Highway 52/P.O. Box 9
Bastian, VA 24314-0009
703-688-4121

00302
Genetco, Inc.
711 Union Parkway
Ronkonkoma, NY 11779
516-585-1000

00781
Geneva Pharmaceuticals
Div. of Ciba-Geigy
2599 W. Midway Blvd.
P.O. Box 469
Broomfield, CO 80038-0469
800-525-2492

58468
Genzyme Corporation
One Kendall Square
Cambridge, MA 02139
617-252-7500

00249
Geriatric Pharm. Corp.
P.O. Box 99
Butler, WI 53007
414-272-2552

00173
Glaxo, Inc.
Five Moore Dr.
Research Triangle Pk,
NC 27709
919-248-2100

12843
Glenbrook Laboratories
90 Park Avenue, 17th Floor
New York, NY 10016
212-907-2000

00516
Glenwood Inc.
83 N. Summit St.
Tenafly, NJ 07670
201-569-0050

00182
Goldline Laboratories, Inc.
1900 W. Commercial Blvd.
Ft. Lauderdale, FL 33324
305-491-4002

74684
Goody's Manufacturing Corp.
436 Salt Street
Winston-Salem, NC 27108
919-723-1831

10481
Gordon Laboratories
State and Parkview Roads
Upper Darby, PA 19082-1694
215-789-3055

00152
Gray Pharmaceutical Co.
100 Connecticut Ave.
Norwalk, CT 06856
203-853-0123

51301
Great Southern Laboratories
10863 Rockley Road
Houston, TX 77099
713-530-3077

00327
Guardian Laboratories
Div. of United-Guardian, Inc.
P.O. Box 2500
Smithtown, NY 11787-2500
516-273-0900

Gynex Labs
1175 Corporate Woods
Parkway
Vernon Hills, IL 60061
708-948-9300

54765
GynoPharma Laboratories
50 Division Street
Somerville, NJ 08876
201-725-3100

00879
Halsey Drug Company
Blue Cross Product, Inc.
1827 Pacific Street
Brooklyn, NY 11233
718-467-7500

51432
Harber Pharmaceutical Co.
350 Meadowlands Pkwy.
Secaucus, NJ 07094
201-348-3700

43797
W. E. Hauck, Inc.
P.O. Box 1065
Alpharetta, GA 30239-1065
404-475-4758

HDC Corporation
2109 O'Toole Ave.
San Jose, CA 95131
408-954-1909

00534
Health & Medical Techniques
P.O. Box A
Rahway, NJ 07065-1175
201-382-9300

51662
Healthfirst Corporation
P.O. Box 279
Edmonds, WA 98020
206-771-5733

00586
Heather Drug Company Inc.
1 Fellowship Road
Cherry Hill, NJ 08003
609-424-3663

Helena Laboratories
Home Health Care Division
P.O. Box 572
Beaumont, TX 77704-0752
409-842-3714

HEM Research
1617 John F. Kennedy Blvd.
Philadelphia, PA 19103
215-988-0080

00023
Herbert Laboratories
Div. of Allergan
18600 Von Karman Avenue
Irvine, CA 92713-9534
714-955-6200

48017
Hermal Pharmaceutical Labs
163 Delaware Avenue
Delmar, NY 12460
518-475-0175

00514
Dow B. Hickam, Inc.
P.O. Box 2006
Sugarland, TX 77478
713-491-1900

Hirsch Industries, Inc.
4912 West Broad St. Suite 201
Richmond, VA 23230
804-355-4500

Hiscia
Institut Hiscia
CH-4144, Arlesheim Kirshweg
Switzerland
4106172-2323

00039
Hoechst-Roussel Pharm., Inc.
Route 202-206 P.O. Box 2500
Somerville, NJ 08876-1258
201-231-2000

Holles Laboratories
30 Forest Notch
Cohasset, MA 02025-1198
617-383-0741

00118
Hollister-Stier
Div. of Miles Laboratories
P.O. Box 3145
Spokane, WA 99220-3153
509-489-5656

25077
The Hudson Corporation
Div. of Nature's Bounty
90 Orville Dr.
Bohemia, NY 11716
516-567-9500

00395
Humco Laboratory, Inc.
P.O. Box 2550
Texarkana, TX 75503
903-793-3174

Hybritech
11095 Torreyana Rd.
P.O. Box 269006
San Diego, CA 92126-9006
619-455-6700

00011
Hynson, Westcott & Dunning
Div. of Becton Dickinson
250 Schilling Circle
Cockeysville, MD 21030
301-771-0100

00314
Hyrex Pharmaceuticals
P.O. Box 18385
Memphis, TN 38181-0385
901-794-9050

00310
ICI Pharma
ICI Americas, Inc.
Concord Pike and Murphy Road
Wilmington, DE 19897
302-886-2231

00187
ICN Pharmaceuticals, Inc.
3300 Hyland Avenue
Costa Mesa, CA 92626
714-545-0100

51244
I.C.P. Pharmaceuticals
P.O. Box 294
Cudahy, WI 53110
414-521-4647

IDEC Pharmaceuticals
11099 North Torrey Pines Road
La Jolla, CA 92037
619-458-0600

Immunex
51 University Street
Seattle, WA 98101
206-587-0430

Immunobiology Rsch Inst.
Route 22 East, P.O. Box 999
Annandale, NJ 08801-0999
201-730-0999

ImmunoGen
148 Cambridge Street
Cambridge, MA 02139
617-661-9312

Immunomedics
150 Mt. Bethel Road
Warren, NJ 07060
201-647-5400

Immunotherapeutics
3505 Riverview Circle
Morehead, MN 56560
701-232-9575

Immuno U.S., Inc.
1200 Parkdale Rd.
Rochester, MI 48063
212-759-3520

Imreg
144 Elk Place
New Orleans, LA 70112
504-523-2875

00548
I.M.S. Ltd.
1886 Santa Anita Ave.
South El Monte, CA 91733
818-442-6757

Interferon Sciences
783 Jersey Avenue
New Brunswick, NJ 08901
201-249-3250

55077
Inter-Hermes Pharma, Inc.
4 Reuten Drive
Closter, NJ 07624
201-784-1436

11584
International Ethical Labs
Reparto Metropolitano
Rio Piedras, PR 00921
809-765-3510

00665
International Laboratories
Div. of Solvay Pharmaceuticals
901 Sawyer Road
Marietta, GA 30062
404-578-5583

Interpro
P.O. Box 1823
Haverhill, MA 01831
508-373-2438

00814
Interstate Drug Exchange
1500 New Horizons Blvd.
Amityville, NY 11701-1130
516-957-8300

Intramed
102 Tremont Way
Augusta, GA 30907

52189
Invamed Incorporated
12 Dwight Place
Fairfield, NJ 07006
201-575-3303

00258
Inwood Laboratories
300 Prospect Street
Inwood, NY 11696
516-371-1155

00058
Iolab Pharmaceuticals
500 Iolab Drive
Claremont, CA 91711
714-624-2020

11808
ION Laboratories, Inc.
7171 Pebble Drive
Ft. Worth, TX 76118
817-589-7257

50914
Iso Tex Diagnostics, Inc.
P.O. Box 909
Friendswood, TX 77546
713-482-1231

49938
Jacobus Pharmaceutical Co.
37 Cleveland Lane
Princeton, NJ 08540
609-921-7447

50458
Janssen Pharmaceutica, Inc.
40 Kingsbridge Road
Piscataway, NJ 08854
201-524-9100

00252
JMI-Canton Pharmaceuticals
119 Schroyer Ave. S.W.
Canton, OH 44702
216-456-2873

00137
Johnson & Johnson
Consumer Products Inc.
Grandview Rd.
Skillman, NJ 08558-9418
908-874-2670

56091
Johnson & Johnson Medical
P.O. Box 130
Arlington, TX 76004-0130
800-433-5009

S.C. Johnson & Son, Inc.
1525 Howe Street
Racine, WI 53403
414-631-2618

52604
Jones Medical Industries
P.O. Box 46903
St. Louis, MO 63146-6903
314-432-7557

00601
KabiVitrum, Inc.
160 Industrial Drive
Franklin, OH 45005
800-526-5224

00588
Keene Pharmaceuticals Inc.
P.O. Box 7
Keene, TX 76059-0007
817-645-8083

28851
Kendall Company
One Federal Steet
Boston, MA 02110-2003
617-574-7000

00482
Kenwood Laboratories
Div. of Bradley Pharm., Inc.
383 Rt. 46 W.
Fairfield, NJ 07006-2402
201-882-1505

00085
Key Pharmaceuticals
c/o Schering Corporation
Galloping Hill Road
Kenilworth, NJ 07033
201-298-4000

Kingswood Laboratories, Inc.
10375 Hague
Indianapolis, IN 46256
316-849-9513

00098
Kirkman Sales Company
P.O. Box 1009
Wilsonville, OR 97070
503-694-1600

00044
Knoll Pharmaceuticals
30 N. Jefferson Rd.
Whippany, NJ 07981
201-887-8300

00224
Konsyl Pharmaceuticals
4200 South Hulen Street
Ft. Worth, TX 76109
817-763-8011

55505
Kramer Laboratories, Inc.
8778 S.W. 8th Street
Miami, FL 33174-9990
305-223-1287

41383
LactAid Inc.
P.O. Box 111
Pleasantville, NJ 08232
609-653-6100

Lakeside Pharmaceuticals
P.O. Box 429553
Cincinnati, OH 45242-9553
513-948-9110

00527
The Lannett Co., Inc.
9000 State Rd.
Philadelphia, PA 19136
215-333-9000

00277
Laser, Inc.
P.O. Box 905, 2000 N.Main St.
Crown Point, IN 46307
219-663-1165

10651
Lavoptik Co., Inc.
661 Western Ave. N.
St. Paul, MN 55103
612-489-1351

00005
Lederle Laboratories
Div. of American Cyanamid Co.
North Middletown Road
Pearl River, NY 10965-1299
914-732-5000

74300
Leeming/Pacquin
Div. of Pfizer, Inc.
235 East 42nd St.
New York, NY 10017
212-573-3131

25332
Legere Pharmaceuticals, Inc.
7326 E. Evans Rd.
Scottsdale, AZ 85260
602-991-4033

19200
Lehn & Fink
225 Summit Avenue
Montvale, NJ 07645
201-573-5700

P. Leiner Nutritional Products
1845 W. 205th St.
Torrance, CA 90501
213-328-9610

Lemar Laboratories, Inc.
10 Perimeter Way
NW Bldg B-200
Atlanta, GA 30339
404-952-3922

00093
Lemmon Company
P.O. Box 30
Sellersville, PA 18960
215-723-5544

Lenti-Chemico Pharmaceuticals
Glenpointe Centre West
500 Frank W. Burr Blvd.
Teaneck, NJ 07666
201-836-1196

00454
Lexis Laboratories
P.O. Box 202887
Austin, TX 78720
512-474-7724

00737
Life Labs
9380 San Fernando Rd.
Sun Valley, CA 91532
213-875-0330

00002
Eli Lilly and Co.
Bldg. 11/3 Lilly Corp. Center
Indianapolis, IN 46285
317-276-2000

Lincoln Diagnostics
240 East Hickory Point Road
Decatur, IL 62526
217-877-2531

The Liposome Company
Princeton Forrestal Center
One Research Way
Princeton, NJ 08540
609-452-7060

55390
Loch Pharmaceuticals
270 Northfield Rd.
P.O. Box 46568
Bedford, OH 44146
516-742-7040

41470
Loma Linda Foods, Inc.
11503 Pierce St.
Riverside, CA 92505
714-687-7800

00273
Lorvic Corporation
8810 Frost Ave.
St. Louis, MO 63134-1095
314-524-7444

50732
LuChem Pharmaceuticals
8910 Linwood Ave.
P.O. Box 6038
Shreveport, LA 71106
318-688-4800

00374
Lyne Laboratories
260 Tosca Drive
Stoughton, MA 02072
617-344-4676

00469
Lyphomed
3 Pkwy N.
Deerfield, IL 60015-2548
708-317-8800

00466
Macsil, Inc.
1326 Frankford Ave.
Philadelphia, PA 19125-0976
215-739-7300

00904
Major Pharmaceuticals
Michigan Division
3720 Lapeer Road
Auburn Hills, MI 48321
313-370-0680

00019
Mallinckrodt Medical, Inc.
675 McDonnell Blvd.
P.O. Box 5840
St. Louis, MO 63134
314-895-2000

10706
Kenneth A. Manne Co.
1522 Cleveland Ave. N.W.
Canton, OH 44711
216-455-5717

00068
Marion Merrell Dow Inc.
Consumer Products Division
P.O. Box 429553
Cincinnati, OH 45242-9553
513-948-9111

00068
Marion Merrell Dow Inc.
Prescription Products Division
P.O. Box 8480
Kansas City, MO 64114
800-362-7466

Marlin Industries
Div. of J. L. M. Inc.
P.O. Box 560
Grover City, CA 93483-0560
213-393-3644

10712
Marlyn Company Inc.
6324 Ferris Square
San Diego, CA 92121
619-453-5600

52555
Martec Pharmaceutical, Inc.
1800 N. Topping
Kansas City, MO 64120
800-822-6782

11845
Mason Distributors, Inc.
5105 N.W. 159th Street
Hialeah, FL 33014-6370
305-624-5557

12758
Mason Pharmaceuticals, Inc.
4425 Jamboree
Newport Beach, CA 92660
714-851-6860

14362
Mass. Public Health Bio. Lab.
305 South St.
Jamaica Plains, MA 02130
617-522-3700

Matrix Laboratories
1430 O'Brian Drive
Menlo Park, CA 94025
415-326-6100

10719
Maurry Biological Co., Inc.
6109 South Western Ave.
Los Angeles, CA 90047
213-759-1127

00259
Mayrand, Inc.
P.O. Box 8869
Greensboro, NC 27419
919-292-5347

00264
McGaw, Inc.
ASC2 P.O. Box 19791
Irvine, CA 92713-9791
714-660-2000

11089
McGregor Pharmaceuticals
8420 Ulmenton Road #305
Largo, FL 34641
813-530-4361

49072
McGuff Company, Inc.
3617 W. MacArthur Blvd. #507
Santa Ana, CA 92704
800-854-7220

50185
McHenry Laboratories Inc.
118 N. Wells-Lee Bldg.
Edna, TX 77957
512-782-5438

00045
McNeil Consumer Products
Camp Hill Road
Ft. Washington, PA 19034-2292
215-233-7000

00045
McNeil Pharmaceutical
Welsh and McKean Rds.
Spring House, PA 19477-0776
215-628-5000

00087
Mead Johnson
Div. of Bristol-Myers Squibb
2404 Pennsylvania Street
Evansville, IN 47721
812-426-6000

00015
Mead Johnson Oncology
Div. of Bristol-Myers Squibb
2400 West Lloyd Expressway
Evansville, IN 47721-0001
812-429-5000

Medarex
12 Commerce Avenue
West Lebanon, NH 03784
603-298-8456

MedChem
444 Washington St.
Woburn, MA 01801
617-938-9328

11940
Medco Lab, Inc.
P.O. Box 864
Sioux City, IA 51102-0864
712-255-8770

Medco Research
8733 Beverly Blvd.
Los Angeles, CA 90048
213-854-1954

44081
Med-Corp
Div. of Life Medical Sys., Inc.
5001 Spring Valley Road
Dallas, TX 75244-3910
214-385-7214

45565
Med-Derm Pharmaceuticals
P.O. Box 5193
Kingsport, TN 37663
615-477-3991

Medea Research Laboratories
200 Wilson Street
Port Washington, NY 11776
516-331-7718

Medi Aid Corporation
8250 S. Akron Street Suite 205
Englewood, CO 80155
303-790-1655

52891
Medical Market Specialties
P.O. Box 150
Boonton, NJ 07005
201-263-4243

Medical Technology Corp.
71 Veronica Avenue
Somerset, NJ 08875-0218
201-246-3366

99207
Medicis Dermatologicals, Inc.
100 East 42nd St.
New York, NY 10017
212-599-2000

00244
Medicone Company
225 Varick St.
New York, NY 10014
212-924-5166

Medimorphics
245 East 6th Street
St. Paul, MN 55101
612-224-2800

17156
Medi-Physics, Inc.
Div. of Hoffmann-LaRoche
140 East Ridgewood
P.O. Box 289
Paramus, NJ 07653-0289
201-599-8931

00348
Medtech Laboratories, Inc.
3510 N. Lake Creek
P.O. Box 1108
Jackson, WY 83001
307-733-1680

Medtronic
7000 Central Ave., N.E.
Minneapolis, MN 55432
612-574-4000

87900
Menley & James Labs
A Div. of WKW Inc.
100 Tournament Drive
Horsham, PA 19044
215-441-6509

22200
Mennen Company
Hanover Ave. Box 1000
Morristown, NJ 07960
201-631-9000

10742
Mentholatum Co., Inc.
1360 Niagara St.
Buffalo, NJ 14213
716-882-7660

16837
J & J Merck Cons. Pharm.
Camp Hill Road
Ft. Washington, PA 19034
215-233-7000

00006
Merck Sharp and Dohme
Div. of Merck & Co.
WP 38M-2
West Point, PA 19486
215-661-5000

00394
Mericon Industries, Inc.
8819 N. Pioneer Road
Peoria, IL 61615
309-676-0744

50361
Merieux Institute, Inc.
7855 N.W. 12th St. Suite #114
Miami, FL 33126-1818
305-593-9577

58063
MGI Pharma, Inc.
9900 Bren Rd. East Ste 300-E
Minneapolis, MN 55343-9667
612-939-4672

32954
MiLance Laboratories, Inc.
P.O. Box 39
Maplewood, NJ 07040

52836
Milance Laboratories, Inc.
P.O. Box 368
Millington, NJ 07946
201-508-1591

16500, 00192
Miles Inc.
1127 Myrtle Street
P.O. Box 340
Elkhart, IN 46515-0340
219-264-8111

00026
Miles Inc.
Pharmaceutical Division
400 Morgan Lane
West Haven, CT 06516
203-937-2000

00396
Milex Products, Inc.
5915 Northwest Highway
Chicago, IL 60631-1032
312-631-6484

17204
Miller Pharmacal Group Inc.
245 W. Roosevelt Rd.
West Chicago, IL 60186-0279
800-323-2935

53118
Millgood Laboratories, Inc.
250 D Arizona Ave.
P.O. Box 170159
Atlanta, GA 30317
404-377-6538

00276
Misemer Pharmaceuticals
4553 S. Campbell
Springfield, MO 65810-5918
417-881-0660

00178
Mission Pharmacal Company
P.O. Box 1676
San Antonio, TX 78296-1676
512-650-3273

Monoclonal Antibodies, Inc.
2319 Charleston Rd.
Mountain View, CA 94043
408-739-2700

00839
H. L. Moore Drug Exchange
389 John Downey Dr.
New Britain, CT 06050
203-826-3600

Morton Salt
Div. Morton-Thiokol
110 North Wacker Dr.
Chicago, IL 60606
312-621-5200

Murdock Pharmaceuticals Inc.
1400 Mountain Springs Park
Springvale, UT 84663
801-489-3633

00451
Muro Pharmaceutical, Inc.
890 East St.
Tewksbury, MA 01876-9987
508-851-5981

00150
Murray Drug Corporation
415 S. 4th Street
Murray, KY 42071
502-753-6654

53489
Mutual Pharmaceutical Co.
1100 Orthodox Street
Philadelphia, PA 19124
215-288-6500

00378
Mylan Pharmaceuticals
P.O. Box 4310
Morgantown, WV 26505
304-599-2595

Naska Pharmacal
Riverview Road, P.O. Box 898
Lincolnton, NC 28093
704-735-5700

05745
Nastech Pharmaceutical Co.
P.O. Box 13322
Hauppauge, NY 11788
800-962-3442

National Patent Medical
Div. National Patent Develop.
P.O. Box 419
Dayville, CT 06241
800-243-1172

74312
Nature's Bounty, Inc.
105 Orville Drive
Bohemia, NY 11716
516-567-9500

76611
Navaco Laboratories
Pro-Mix Brand Products
512 Ash Avenue
McAllen, TX 78501
512-682-0188

55437
Nelson Pharmaceutical, Inc.
3101 Louisiana Avenue N.
Minneapolis, MN 55424
612-542-3232

00487
Nephron Corporation
P.O. Box 1974
Tacoma, WA 98401-1974
206-475-3452

NeuroGenesis/MATRIX Tech.
1020 Bay Area Boulevard
Houston, TX 77058
800-345-8912

10812
Neutrogena Dermatologic
5760 W. 96th Street
Los Angeles, CA 90045
213-642-1150

Newport Pharmaceuticals
897 West 16th
Newport Beach, CA 92663
714-642-7511

12934
Nion Corporation
11581 Federal Drive
El Monte, CA 91731
213-686-2105

23317
NMC Laboratories
70-36 83rd Street
Glendale, NY 11385
800-431-5014

51801
Nomax, Inc.
40 North Rock Hill Rd.
St. Louis, MO 63119
314-961-2500

00149
Norwich Eaton Pharm.
P.O. Box 191
Norwich, NY 13815
607-335-2111

Novaferon Labs
2658 Patton Road
Roseville, MN 55713

Nova Pharmaceutical
6200 Freeport Centre
Baltimore, MD 21224
301-558-7000

00362
Novocol Chemical Mfr. Co.
485-09 S. Broadway
Hicksville, NY 10801
516-496-7200

00003, 50445
Novo/Nordisk Pharm., Inc.
100 Overlook Dr. Ste. 200
Princeton, NJ 08540
609-987-5827

55953
Novopharm, Inc.
165 E. Commerce
Suite 100/200
Schaumberg, IL 60173-5326
708-882-4200

55499
Numark Laboratories, Inc.
P.O. Box 6321
Edison, NJ 08818
800-338-8079

51081
Nutripharm Laboratories, Inc.
8 Bartles Corner Road Ste. 101
Flemington, NJ 08822
908-806-8954

10797
Oakhurst Company
3000 Hempstead Turnpike
Levittown, NY 11756
516-731-5380

00477
Obetrol Pharmaceuticals
Div. of Rexar Pharm. Corp.
396 Rockway Ave.
P.O. Box 397
Valley Stream, NY 11582
516-561-7662

55515
Oclassen
100 Pelican Way
San Rafael, CA 94901
415-258-4500

O'Connor Pharmaceuticals, see Columbia Laboratories

Ocular Pharmaceuticals, Inc.
712 Ginesi Drive
Morganville NJ 07751
201-972-8585

OHM Laboratories, Inc.
P.O. Box 279
Franklin Park, NJ 08823
908-297-3030

12622
Olin Corporation
120 Long Ridge Road
Stamford, CT 06904-1355
203-356-2000

ONY
1576 Sweet Home Road
Amherst, NY 14221
716-636-9096

Optikem International, Inc.
2172 S. Jason Street
Denver, CO 80223
303-936-1137

50520
Optimox Corporation
2720 Monterey, Suite 406
Torrance, CA 90503
213-618-9370

52238
Optopics Laboratories, Corp.
Main Street, P.O. Box 210
Fairton, NJ 08320-0210
800-223-0865

00041
Oral-B Laboratories, Inc.
170 S. Whisman Road
Mountain View, CA 94041
415-961-8130

00052
Organon, Inc.
375 Mt. Pleasant Ave.
West Orange, NJ 07052
201-325-4500

Organon Teknika Corp.
100 Akzo Avenue
Durham, NC 27704
919-620-2000

00191
Ortega Pharm. Co., Inc.
586 S. Edgewood Ave.
Jacksonville, FL 33205
904-387-0536

00062
Ortho Dermatologic
c/o Ortho Pharmaceutical
Route 202, P.O. Box 300
Raritan, NJ 08869-0602
908-218-6000

00062
Ortho Diagnostic Systems
Route 202, P.O. Box 300
Raritan, NJ 08869
908-218-6000

00062
Ortho Pharmaceutical Corp.
Route 202, P.O. Box 300
Raritan, NJ 08869
908-524-0400

00299
Owen/Galderma Laboratories
P.O. Box 660
Ft. Worth, TX 76115
817-293-0450

00574
Paddock Laboratories
3101 Louisiana Ave. North
Minneapolis, MN 55427
612-546-4676

00377
Pal-Pak, Inc.
1201 Liberty St., P.O. Box 299
Allentown, PA 18105
215-433-7579

53159
Palisades Pharmaceuticals
219 County Road
Tenafly, NJ 07670
201-569-8502

49884
Par Pharmaceuticals
Div. of Pharm. Resources
One Ram Ridge Rd
Spring Valley, NY 10977
914-425-7100

00071
Parke-Davis
Div. of Warner-Lambert Co.
201 Tabor Road
Morris Plains, NJ 07950
201-540-2000

00349
Parmed Pharmaceuticals Inc.
4220 Hyde Park Blvd.
Niagara Falls, NY 14305
716-284-5666

50930
Parnell Pharmaceuticals, Inc.
373-G Vintage Park Drive
Foster City, CA 94404
415-574-1500

The Parthenon Co., Inc.
3311 West 2400 South
Salt Lake City, UT 84119
801-972-5184

00418
Pasadena Research Labs
940 Calle Amancer Suite L
San Clemente, CA 92672
714-492-4030

Pediatric Pharmaceuticals
379 Thornall Street
Edison, NJ 08837
201-906-4615

00884
Pedinol Pharmacal, Inc.
30 Banfi Plaza North
Farmingdale, NY 11735
516-293-9500

10974
Pegasus Medical, Inc.
1 Technology Dr Bldg 1C
Ste. 527
Irvine, CA 92718-2325
714-753-9055

00096
Person and Covey, Inc.
616 Allen Avenue
Glendale, CA 91201
818-240-1030

00927
Pfeiffer Company
P.O. Box 100
Wilkes-Barre, PA 18773
717-826-9000

00995
Pfipharmecs, see Pfizer

00069
Pfizer Laboratories
235 E. 42nd St.
New York, NY 10017-5755
212-573-2323

00121
Pharmaceutical Associates
Div. of Beach Products
P.O. Box 128
Conestee, SC 29636
803-277-7282

00832
Pharmaceutical Basics Inc.
(Liquids Only)
6451 West Main Street
Morton Grove, IL 60053
708-967-5600

00832
Pharmaceutical Basics, Inc.
(Solids Only)
8755 W. Higgins Rd. Suite 810
Chicago, IL 60631
312-380-0080

51655
Pharmaceutical Corporation of America
12348 Hancock
Carmel, IN 46032
317-573-8000

45334
Pharmaceutical Specialties Inc
P.O. Box 729
Rochester, MN 55903-0729
507-288-8500

00016
Pharmacia Inc.
Medical Products Division
800 Centennial Ave.
Piscataway, NJ 08855-1327
201-457-8000

PharmaControl
661 Palisade Ave.
P.O. Box 931
Englewood Cliffs, NJ 07632
201-567-9004

00462
Pharmaderm
Div. of Altana Inc.
60 Baylis Road
Melville, NY 11747
516-454-7677

24208
Pharmafair, Inc.
205C Kelsey Lane
Tampa, FL 33619
813-972-7705

00554
Pharmakon Laboratories, Inc.
6050 Jet Port Industrial Blvd.
Tampa, FL 33634
813-886-3216

Pharmatec
County Rd 2054, P.O. Box 730
Alachua, FL 32615
904-462-1210

39822
Pharma Tek, Inc.
P.O. Box AB
Huntington, NY 11743
516-757-5522

00813
Pharmics Incorporated
1878 South Redwood Rd.
Salt Lake City, UT 84104
801-972-4138

60104
Pioneer Pharmaceuticals Inc.
Subs. of Essex Chemical Corp.
209 40th Street
Irvington, NJ 07111
201-372-6200

41100
Plough, Inc.
Div. of Schering-Plough HealthCare Products
110 Allen Rd
Liberty Bell, NJ 07938
908-604-1995

Polymer Technology
100 Research Drive
Wilmington, MA 01887
800-343-1445

55688
Porton Product Limited
30401 Agoura Rd.
Agoura Hills, CA 91301
818-879-2200

00095
Poythress Laboratories. Inc.
16 N. 22nd St.
Richmond, VA 23261
804-644-8591

53124
Praxis Biologics, Inc.
30 Corporate Woods, Suite 300
Rochester, NY 14623-1493
716-272-7000

Precision-Cosmet
500 Iolab Drive
Claremont, CA 91711
800-423-1871

00684
Primedics Laboratories
Ethical Div., Irenda Corp.,
1852 West 169th Street
Gardenia, CA 90247
213-770-3005

00003
Princeton Pharm. Products
Div. of Bristol-Myers Squibb
P.O. Box 4000
New Brunswick, NJ 08543-4000
609-243-6000

37000
The Procter and Gamble Co.
P.O. Box 599
Cincinnati, OH 45201-0599
513-983-1100

Professional Supplies, Inc.
1153 Main St.
Stevens Point, WI 54481
715-345-0404

00034
Purdue Frederick Co.
100 Connecticut Ave.
Norwalk, CT 06856
203-853-0123

00228
Purepac Pharmaceutical Co.
Div. of Kalipharma, Inc.
200 Elmora Ave.
Elizabeth, NJ 07207
201-527-9100

51309
Quad Pharmaceuticals, Inc.
Div. of Pharm. Resources
6340 LaPas Trail
Indianapolis, IN 46268
317-299-6611

52446
Qualitest Products Inc.
1025 Jordan Road
Huntsville, AL 35811
205-859-4011

12225
Quality Formulations, Inc.
P.O. Box 827
Zachary, LA 70791-0827
504-654-6880

52273
Quantum Pharmics, Ltd.
26 Edison Street
Amityville, NY 11701
516-842-4200

54391
R & D Laboratories, Inc.
4204 Glencoe Avenue
Marina Del Rey, CA 90292-5612
213-305-8053

00196
Rachelle Laboratories, Inc.
P.O. Box 187
Culver, IN 46511
219-842-3305

30103
Randob Laboratories, Ltd.
508 Franklin Ave.
Mt. Vernon, NY 10550
914-699-3131

00686
Raway Pharmacal, Inc.
Lower Granit Road
Accord, NY 12404
914-626-8133

10952
Recsei Laboratories
330 S. Kellogg Bldg. M
Goleta, CA 93117-3875
805-964-2912

53506
Redi-Med, Inc.
801-N N. Blacklawn Rd.
P.O. Box 1407
Conyers, GA 30207
404-929-0961

48028
Redi-Products Labs, Inc.
P.O. Box 126
Prichard, WV 25555
800-624-3413

00021
Reed & Carnrick
One New England Ave.
Piscataway, NJ 08855
201-981-0070

10956
Reese Chemical Co.
10617 Frank Ave.
Cleveland, OH 44106
216-231-6441

00102
Regal Laboratories
1925 Enterprise Parkway
Twinsburg, OH 44087
216-425-9811

10960
Republic Drug Company
P.O. Box 186
Buffalo, NY 14216
716-874-5060

10961
Requa
1 Seneca Place, P.O. Box 4008
Greenwich, CT 06830
203-869-2445

00433
Research Industries Corp.
1847 West 2300 South
Salt Lake City, UT 84119
801-972-5500

00122
Rexall Group
4031 N.E. 12th Terrace
Ft. Lauderdale, FL 33334
800-255-7399

00195, 00067
Rhone-Poulenc Rorer
500 Virginia Dr
Ft. Washington, PA 19034
215-628-6000

Ribi ImmunoChem Research
553 Old Corvallis Rd
P.O. Box 1409
Hamilton, MT 59840
406-363-6214

76660
Richardson-Vicks, Inc.
A Procter & Gamble Company
1 Far Mill Crossing
P.O. Box 854
Shelton, CT 06484-0925
203-925-6000

12071
Richie Pharmacal Co., Inc.
197 State Avenue
P.O. Box 460
Glasgow, KY 42141
800-626-0250

00115
Richlyn Laboratories, Inc.
Castor & Kensington Avenues
Philadelphia, PA 19124
215-289-2220

54807
R.I.D. Inc.
525 Mednik Avenue
Los Angeles, CA 90022
213-268-0635

54092
Roberts Pharmaceutical Corp.
Meridian Center III
6 Industrial Way West
Eatontown, NJ 07724
908-389-1182

00031
A. H. Robins Company, Inc.
P.O. Box 8299
Philadelphia, PA 19101-1245
215-688-4400

00031
A.H. Robins Cons. Prod. Div.
1211 Sherwood Ave.
Richmond, VA 23261-6609
804-257-2735

00004
Roche Dermatologics Prod.
340 Kingsland Street
Nutley, NJ 07110-1199
201-812-2000

00004, 00140
Roche Laboratories
Div. of Hoffman-La Roche
340 Kingsland St.
Nutley, NJ 07110-1199
800-526-6367
201-235-3139

00049
J. B. Roerig Division
235 E. 42nd St.
New York, NY 10017
212-573-2323

00074
Ross Laboratories
625 Cleveland Ave.
Columbus, OH 43215
614-227-3333

00054
Roxane Laboratories, Inc.
P.O. Box 16532
Columbus, OH 43216-6532
614-276-4000

51875
Royce Laboratories, Inc.
16600 N.W. 54 Avenue
Miami, FL 33014
800-537-3593

00536
Rugby Labs., Inc.
898 Orlando Ave.
West Hempstead, NY 11552
516-536-8565

46500
Rydelle Laboratories
1525 Howe Street
Racine, WI 53403-5011
414-631-2000

00263
Rystan Company, Inc.
P.O. Box 214
Little Falls, NJ 07424-0214
201-256-3737

00212
Sandoz Nutrition
5320 W. 23rd Street
Minneapolis, MN 55440
612-925-2100

00043, 00078
Sandoz Pharmaceutical Corp.
59 Route 10
East Hanover, NJ 07936
201-503-7500

51353
The Sanitube Company
19 Concord St.
S. Norwalk, CT 06854
203-853-7856

Sanofi
101 Park Ave.
New York, NY 10178
212-682-8580

00281
Savage Laboratories
Div. of Altana Inc.
60 Baylis Road
Melville, NY 11747-2006
516-454-9071

11012
Schaffer Laboratories
1058 North Allen Ave.
Pasadena, CA 91104
818-798-8644

00364
Schein Pharmaceutical, Inc.
26 Harbor Park Dr.
Port Washington, NY 11050
516-625-9000

00274
Scherer Laboratories, Inc.
315 Gilmer Ferry Road
Ball Ground, GA 30107
800-858-9888

00085
Schering-Plough Corporation
Schering-Plough HealthCare
110 Allen Road
Liberty Corner, NJ 07938
908-604-1995

00085
Schering-Plough Corporation
2000 Galloping Hill Road
Kenilworth, NJ 07033
908-298-4000

00905
Schiapparelli Searle
P.O. Box 5110
Chicago, IL 60680-5110
708-982-7000

00234
Schmid Products Co.
Route 46 West
Little Falls, NJ 07424
201-256-5500

Scholl, Inc.
3030 Jackson, P.O. Box 377
Memphis, TN 38151
901-320-2011

00091
Schwarz Pharma Kremers Urban
5600 W. County Line
Mequon, WI 53092
414-354-4300

42021
Sclavo, Inc.
5 Mansard Court
Wayne, NJ 07470
201-696-8300

00372
Scot-Tussin Pharmacal Co.
50 Clemence St.
P.O. Box 8217
Cranston, RI 02920-0217
401-942-8555

00444
Scrip, Inc.
101 South St.
Peoria, IL 61602-1986
309-674-3488

54977
Scripts America Corp.
5317 N.W. 35 Terrace
Ft. Lauderdale, FL 33309
305-486-7880

00014
Searle & Company
c/o Searle Pharmaceuticals
P.O. Box 5110
Chicago, IL 60680
708-470-9710

00025
Searle Laboratories
c/o Searle Pharmaceuticals, Inc
P.O. Box 5110
Chicago, IL 60680-5110
708-982-7000

00551
The Seatrace Company
P.O. Box 363
Gadsden, AL 35902-0363
205-442-5023

50694
Seres Laboratories
3331 Industrial Dr.
P.O. Box 470
Santa Rosa, CA 95401
707-526-4526

44087
Serono Laboratories, Inc.
100 Longwater Circle
Norwell, MA 02061
617-982-9000

97692
S.G. Labs, Incorporated
500 North Broadway
Jericho, NY 11753
516-822-2900

49731
Sherman Laboratories, Inc.
P.O. Box 368
Abita Springs, LA 70420
504-893-0007

08880, 08881, 08884, 08889
Sherwood Medical
1831 Olive Street
St. Louis, MO 63103
314-621-7788

45809
Shionogi USA
3848 Carson St., #206
Torrance, CA 90503
213-540-1161

50111
Sidmak Laboratories, Inc.
17 West St., P.O. Box 371
East Hanover, NJ 07936
201-386-5566

54482
Sigma-Tau Pharmaceuticals
200 Orchard Ridge Drive
Gaithersburg, MD 20878
301-948-1041

39769
Smith + Nephew SoloPak
Div. of Smith + Nephew
1845 Tonne
Elk Grove Village, IL 60007-5125
708-806-0080

08026
Smith + Nephew United
Div. of Smith + Nephew
11775 Starkey Rd.
P.O. Box 197
Largo, FL 34649
800-876-1261

00766, 00128, 49692
SmithKline Beecham
100 Beecham Drive
Pittsburgh, PA 15205
412-928-1000

00029, 00007
SmithKline Beecham Pharm.
P.O. Box 7929
Philadelphia, PA 19103
215-751-4000

00978
SmithKline Diagnostics
225 Baypoint Parkway
San Jose, CA 95134-1622
800-877-6242

Soft Rinse Corp.
2411 Third Street South
Wisconsin Rapids, WI 54494
800-826-0457

00077
Sola/Barnes-Hind
810 Kifer Road
Sunnyvale, CA 94086-5200
619-277-9873

Solgar Company, Inc.
P.O. Box 330
Lynbrook, NY 11563
516-599-2442

00032
Solvay
901 Sawyer Road
Marietta, GA 30062-2224
404-578-9000

39506
Somerset Pharmaceuticals
400 Morris Avenue, Suite 7S
Denville, NJ 07834
201-586-2310

54027
Spectra Pharm. Service
155 Webster Street
Hanover, MA 02339
617-871-3991

38137
Spectrum Chemical Mfg.
14422 S. San Pedro St.
Gardena, CA 90248-9985
800-772-8786

00537
Spencer Mead, Inc.
5000 Kingshighway
Brooklyn, NY 11234
800-645-3737

Sphinx Pharmaceutical Corp.
Two University Place
P.O. Box 52330
Durham, NC 27717
919-489-9090

00003
Squibb Diagnostic Division
Div. Bristol-Myers Squibb
P.O. Box 4500
Princeton, NJ 08543-4500
609-987-1813

00003
Squibb-Marsam
Div. Bristol-Myers Squibb
P.O. Box 1022
Cherry Hill, NJ 08034
609-424-5600

00003
E. R. Squibb & Sons, Inc.
Div. Bristol-Myers Squibb
P.O. Box 4000
Princeton, NJ 08543-4000
609-921-4000

53385
Standard Drug Company
P.O. Box 710
Riverton, IL 62561
217-629-9884

00076
Star Pharmaceuticals, Inc.
1990 N.W. 44th Street
Pompano Beach, FL 33064-1278
305-971-9704

51318
Stellar Pharmacal Corp.
1990 44th Street
Pompano Beach, FL 33064
800-845-7827

00402
Steris Laboratories Inc.
620 North 51st Avenue
Phoenix, AZ 85043
602-278-1400

00145
Stiefel Laboratories, Inc.
2801 Ponce de Leon Blvd.
Coral Gables, FL 33134
305-443-3807

89223
Stockhausen Inc.
408 Doyle St.
Greensboro, NC 27406
800-334-0242

Storz Ophthalmics
Subs. American Cyanamid
3365 Tree Court Industrial
St. Louis, MO 63122-6694

00038
Stuart Pharmaceuticals
Concord Pike & New Murphy Rd.
Wilmington, DE 19897
302-886-2231

11086
Summers Laboratories, Inc.
Morris Rd. & Wissahickon Creek
Ft. Washington, PA 19034
215-646-1477

57267
Summit Medical Products
1075 Central Park Ave.
Scarsdale, NY 10583
914-472-2737

11704
Survival Technology, Inc.
8101 Glenbrook Rd.
Bethesda, MD 20814
301-656-5600

00033
Syntex Laboratories
3401 Hillview Ave.
Palo Alto, CA 94304
415-855-5050

47854
Syosset Laboratories Co., Inc.
150 Eileen Way
Syosset, NY 11791
516-921-6306

Syva Company
929 Queensbridge
St. Louis, MO 63021
314-391-5374

Tag Pharmaceuticals
P.O. Box 904
Sellersville, PA 18960
215-723-5544

Tambrands Incorporated
1 Marcus Ave.
Lake Success, NY 11042
516-358-8300

Tanning Research Labs. Inc.
1190 U.S. 1 North
Ormond Beach, FL 32174
904-677-9559

00300
Tap Pharmaceuticals
2355 Waukegan Rd
Deerfield, IL 60015
708-317-5700

51672
Taro Pharmaceuticals U.S.A.
Six Skyline Drive
Hawthorne, NY 10532
914-345-9001

49158
Thames Pharmacal Co., Inc.
2100 Fifth Ave.
Ronkonkoma, NY 11779-6906
516-737-1155

11290
Thompson Medical Co.
222 Lakeview Ave.
West Palm Beach, FL 33401
407-820-9900

00089
3M Personal Care Products
3M Center, Bldg. 223-4N-10
St. Paul, MN 55144-1000
612-733-1110

00089
3M Pharmaceutical
Medical Service Dept
225-1N-07 3M Center
St. Paul, MN 55144-1000
612-736-4930

51687
T/I Pharmaceuticals
15231 Barranca Parkway
Irvine, CA 92718
714-727-7466

TNI Pharmaceuticals
5105 North Pearl Street
Schiller Park, IL 60176
708-678-3067

11299
Torch Laboratories, Inc.
P.O. Box 248
Reistertown, MD 21136
301-363-6350

11311
Trimen Laboratories, Inc.
80-26th Street
Pittsburgh, PA 15222
412-261-0339

Triton Bioscience
1501 Harbor Bay Parkway
Alameda, CA 94501
415-769-5200

79511
Triton Consumer Products
Div. M. George Research, Inc.
5105 Tollview Dr., Suite 190
Rolling Meadows, IL 60008
708-228-7650

00463
C. O. Truxton Inc.
P.O. Box 1594
Camden, NJ 08101
609-365-4118

Tsumura Medical
104 Peavey Road
Chaska, MN 55318
612-448-4181

53335
Tyson & Associates, Inc.
12832 Chadron Ave.
Hawthorne, CA 90250-5525
213-675-1080

00785
UAD Laboratories, Inc.
P.O. Box 10587
8839 Hwy 18 W
Jackson, MS 39289-0587
601-372-7773

51079
UDL Laboratories, Inc.
Div. American Cyanamid
P.O. Box 10319
Rockford, IL 61131-3019
815-282-1201

Ueno Fine Chemicals Industry
31, Koraibashi 2-chome
Osaka 541, Japan
06-203-0761

00127
Ulmer Pharmacal
Div. of James Phillips Co.
2440 Fernbrook Lane
Plymouth, MN 55447-9987
612-559-3333

Unimed
35 Columbia Rd
Somerville, NJ 08876
201-526-6894

00677
United Research Laboratories
3600 Meadow Lane
Bensalem, PA 19020-8546
215-638-2626

48663
Unitek Corporation
2724 South Peck Rd.
Monrovia, CA 91016
818-445-7960

Univax Biologics
12111 Parklawn
Rockville, MD 20852
301-770-3099

00009
The Upjohn Company
7000 Portage Rd.
Kalamazoo, MI 49001
616-323-4000

00245
Upsher-Smith Labs., Inc.
14905-23rd Ave. N.
Minneapolis, MN 55447
612-473-4412

58178
US Bioscience
One Tower Bridge
100 Front St. Suite 400
West Conshohocken,
PA 19428
215-832-0570

US Packaging Corp. Medical
506 Clay Street
LaPorte, IN 46350
219-362-9782

52747
US Pharmaceutical Corp.
2500 Park Central Blvd.
Decatur, GA 30035
404-987-4745

51626
US Products, Inc.
16636 N.W. 54th St.
Miami Lakes, FL 33014
305-620-9540

54627
ValMed, Inc.
410 Great Road
Littleton, MA 01460
508-486-8300

00615
Vangard Labs, Inc.
31-E Bypass
Glasgow, KY 42141
502-651-6188

17022
Veratex Corp.
1304 E. Maple Road
P.O. Box 4031
Troy, MI 48084
313-588-2970

53258
VHA Supply Company
320 Deker Dr.
P.O. Box 160909
Irving, TX 75016
214-650-4444

23900
Vicks Health Care Products
Div. Richardson-Vicks, Inc.
One Far Mill Crossing
Shelton, CT 06484
203-925-7701

25866
Vicks Pharmacy Products
Div. Richardson-Vicks, Inc.
One Far Mill Crossing
Shelton, CT 06484
203-929-2500

Viratek
3300 Hyland Avenue
Costa Mesa, CA 92627
714-540-1866

54891
Vision Pharmaceuticals Inc.
P.O. Box 400
Mitchell, SD 57301-0400
605-996-3356

54022
Vitaline Corporation
722 Jefferson Ave.
Ashland, OR 97520
503-482-9231

00185
Vitarine Pharmaceuticals, Inc.
227-15 North Conduit Ave.
Springfield Gardens,
NY 11413-3199
718-276-8600

49727
Vita-Rx Corporation
P.O. Box 8229
Columbus, GA 31908
404-568-1881

Vivan Pharmacol Inc.
1000 Bennett Blvd.
Lakewood, NJ 08701
201-364-9700

00298
Vortech Pharmaceuticals
6851 Chase Rd., P.O. Box 189
Dearborn, MI 48121
313-584-4088

00741
Walker Corp.
P.O. Box 1320
Syracuse, NY 13201
315-463-4511

00619
Walker Pharmacal Company
4200 Laclede Ave.
St. Louis, MO 63108
314-533-9600

00037
Wallace Laboratories
Div. of Carter-Wallace, Inc.
P.O. Box 1
Cranbury, NJ 08512
609-655-6000

00017
Wampole Laboratories
Div. of Carter-Wallace, Inc.
Half Acre Rd., P.O. Box 1001
Cranbury, NJ 08515-0181
609-655-6000

00047
Warner Chilcott Laboratories
Div. of Warner-Lambert Co.
182 Tabor Rd.
Morris Plains, NJ 07950
201-540-2000

11370
Warner-Lambert Cons. Hlth
170 Tabor Road
Morris Plains, NJ 07950
201-540-2000

52544
Watson Laboratories
132-A Business Center Drive
Corona, CA 91720
714-736-8444

00998
Webcon Products
Div. Alcon Laboratories, Inc.
6201 South Freeway T4-4
Ft. Worth, TX 76134-2099
817-293-0450

00917
Wesley Pharmacal Co., Inc.
114 Railroad Dr.
Ivyland, PA 18974
215-953-1680

50893
Westport Pharmaceuticals
1 Turkey Hill Rd South
Westport, CT 06880
203-226-0622

00143
West-Ward, Inc.
465 Industrial Way
Eatontown, NJ 07724
201-542-1191

00072
Westwood Pharmaceuticals
Div. of Westwood-Squibb
100 Forest Avenue
Buffalo, NY 14213
716-887-3400

00003
Westwood-Squibb Pharm.
100 Forest Avenue
Buffalo, NY 14213
716-887-3400

50474
Whitby Pharmaceuticals, Inc.
1211 Sherwood Ave.
Richmond, VA 23261-7426
804-254-4478

00573
Whitehall Laboratories
Div. of American Home Prod.
685 Third Avenue
New York, NY 10017-4076
212-878-5500

00918
Whittaker General Medical
8741 Landmark Rd.
Richmond, VA 23261
804-264-7500

00317
Whorton Pharmaceuticals
4202 Gary Ave.
Fairfield, AL 35064
205-786-2584

11414
Willen Drug Co.
18 North High Street
Baltimore, MD 21202-4785
301-752-1865

51189
T.E. Williams Pharmaceuticals
P.O. Box 312
Divide, CO 80814-0312
719-687-3092

00024
Winthrop
Div. of Sterling Drug
90 Park Avenue
New York, NY 10016
212-907-2000

12120
Wisconsin Pharmacal Co.
2977 Hwy 60
Jackson, WI 53037
414-677-4121

00008
Wyeth-Ayerst Laboratories
P.O. Box 8299
Philadelphia, PA 19101
215-688-4400

50962
Xactdose, Inc.
722 Progressive Lane
South Beloit, IL 61080
815-624-8523

Xoma
2910 Seventh Street
Berkeley, CA 94710
415-644-1170

00116
Xttrium Laboratories, Inc.
415 West Pershing Road
Chicago, IL 60609
312-268-5800

60077
Young Dental
13705 Shoreline Court East
St. Louis, MO 63045
314-344-0010

11444
W. F. Young, Inc.
111 Lyman Street
Springfield, MA 01101
413-737-0201

00172
Zenith Laboratories, Inc.
140 Legrand Avenue
Northvale, NJ 07647
201-767-1700

05128
Zila Pharmaceuticals, Inc.
5227 North 7th St.
Phoenix, AZ 85014-2800
602-266-6700

INDEX

NOTES

NOTES

NOTES

NOTES

NOTES

NOTES

NOTES

NOTES

NOTES

NOTES

NOTES

NOTES

NOTES

NOTES

NOTES

NOTES

ISBN 0-932686-93-1
90000
9 780932 686930